Heat exhaustion and heat stroke | I
High-altitude sickness | I
Hypothermia | I
Lyme disease | I
Malaria | I
Microsporidosis | I
Mushroom poisoning | I
Radiation exposure | I
Rocky Mountain spotted fever | I
Salmonellosis | I
Shigellosis | I
Southern tick-associated rash illness (STARI) | I
Tapeworm infestation | I
Vaccinations for international travel | V
Zika virus | I

GASTROENTEROLOGY

Abdominal compartment syndrome | I
Abdominal pain, chronic lower | II
Abdominal pain, nonsurgical causes | II
Achalasia | I
Acute colonic pseudo-obstruction | I
Acute liver failure | I
Acute lower gastrointestinal bleeding | I
Acute mesenteric ischemia | I
Alcoholic hepatitis | I
Anal abscess and fistula | II
Anorectal fistula | I
Anorectal stricture | I
Anorexia | II
Aphthous ulcers | I
Appendicitis | I
Ascariasis | I
Ascites | I
Autoimmune hepatitis | I
Bacterial overgrowth, small intestine | II
Barrett esophagus | I
Bile duct, dilated | II
Bleeding, gastrointestinal, algorithm | III
Bleeding, rectal | II
Bleeding, variceal | III
Budd-Chiari syndrome | I
Calcifications, liver on x-ray | II
Calcifications, pancreas on x-ray | II
Calcifications, spleen on x-ray | II
Celiac disease | I
Cholangiocarcinoma | I
Cholangitis | I
Cholecystitis | I
Choledocholithiasis | I
Cholelithiasis | I
Chronic pancreatitis | I
Cirrhosis | I
Cirrhosis, primary biliary | I
Cirrhotic cardiomyopathy | I
Colic, acute abdominal | II
Colorectal cancer | I
Colostridium difficile infection | I
Constipation, adult patient | II
Constipation | I, III
Crohn disease | I
Cryptosporidium infection | I
Delayed passage of meconium | II
Diarrhea, acute | III
Diarrhea, acute watery and bloody | II
Diarrhea, chronic | III
Diarrhea, chronic, in patients with HIV infection, algorithm | III
Diarrhea, infectious | II
Diarrhea, non-infectious | II
Diarrhea, persistent | I
Diverticular disease (diverticulosis, diverticulitis) | I
Drug-induced liver injury | I
Dyspepsia | III
Dyspepsia, nonulcerative | I
Dysphagia, oropharyngeal | II
Echinococcosis | I
Eosinophilic esophagitis | I
Epigastric pain | II
Esophageal tumors | I
Esophageal varices | I
Esophagitis | II
Familial adenomatous polyps and Gardner syndrome | I
Fetal alcohol spectrum disorder | I
Food poisoning, bacterial | I
Functional gallbladder disorder | I
Gallbladder carcinoma | I
Gallbladder polyps | I
Gastric cancer | I
Gastric dilatation | II
Gastric emptying, delayed | II
Gastritis | I
Gastroenteritis | I
Gastroesophageal reflux disease | I
Giardiasis | I
Gilbert disease | I
Glossitis | I
Glossodynia | II
Helicobacter pylori infection | I
Hematemesis | II
Hemochromatosis | I
Hemoperitoneum | II

Hemoptysis | I
Hepatic encephalopathy | I
Hepatitis A | I
Hepatitis, acute | I
Hepatitis B | I
Hepatitis B prophylaxis | I
Hepatitis C | I
Hepatitis D | I
Hepatitis E | I
Hepatitis, viral | III
Hepatomegaly, algorithm | III
Hepatomegaly, by shape of liver | II
Hepatopulmonary syndrome | I
Hepatorenal syndrome | I
Hookworm | I
Hypergastrinemia | II
Hypersplenism, associated conditions | II
Hypoglycemia | II
Incontinence, fecal | II
Inguinal hernia | I
Irritable bowel syndrome | I
Ischemia, colon | III
Ischemic colitis | I
Ischemic hepatitis | I
Jaundice and hyperbilirubinemia in the newborn | I
Jaundice, classification | II
Jaundice in the adult patient | I
Jaundice, neonatal | II
Jaundice, neonatal, algorithm | III
Lactose intolerance | I
Large bowel obstruction | I
Large bowel stricture | II
Levator ani syndrome | I
Liver abscess | I
Liver disease, pregnancy | II
Liver lesions, benign | II
Liver transplantation | I
Lynch syndrome | I
Malabsorption | II
Malabsorption algorithm | III
Mallory-Weiss tear | I
Microscopic colitis | I
Nonalcoholic fatty liver disease | I
Non-celiac disease gluten sensitivity | I
Nutrition assessment and intervention in cancer patient | III
Odynophagia | II
Pancreas transplantation | I
Pancreatic calcifications | II
Pancreatic cancer (exocrine) | I
Pancreatitis, drug-induced | II
Peptic ulcer disease | I
Perianal pain | II
Peritonitis, secondary | I
Peutz-Jeghers syndrome and other polyposis syndromes | I
Pinworms | I
Pneumatosis intestinalis in neonate and older child | II
Portal hypertension | I
Portal vein thrombosis | I
Primary sclerosing cholangitis | I
Rectal mass, palpable | II
Retropharyngeal abscess | I
Rumination syndrome | I
Shigellosis | I
Short bowel syndrome | I
Small bowel masses | II
Small bowel obstruction | I
Small bowel intestinal bacterial overgrowth | I
Small intestine ulceration | II
Spontaneous bacterial peritonitis | I
Subphrenic abscess | I
Tapeworm infestation | I
Toxic megacolon | I
Traveler's diarrhea | I
Ulcerative colitis | I
Vitamin deficiency (hypovitaminosis) | I

GYNECOLOGY AND OBSTETRICS

Abruptio placentae | I
Abnormal uterine bleeding | I
Acute fatty liver of pregnancy | I
Acute pelvic pain in women | I
Adnexal masses | I
Amniotic fluid alpha-fetoprotein elevation | II
Anovulatory uterine bleeding | I
Asherman syndrome | I
Bartholin gland abscess | I
Bleeding, early pregnancy | III
Bleeding neonate | III
Bleeding, vaginal | III
Bone mineral density, increased | II
Breast cancer | I
Breastfeeding difficulties | III
Breast, nipple discharge evaluation | III
Breast, radiologic evaluation | III
Breast, routine screen or palpable mass evaluation | III
Cervical cancer | I
Cervical dysplasia | I
Cervicitis | I
Chlamydia genital infections | I
Condyloma acuminatum | I

| | III
| | II
| | I
| | III
| | I
| | I

Endometrial cancer | I
Endometriosis | I
Endometritis | I
Erosions, genitalia | I
Fallopian tube cancer | I
Fertility preservation in women | I
Fibrocystic breast disease | I
Genital lesions or ulcers, algorithm | III
Genitopelvic pain/penetration syndrome | I
Gestational trophoblastic disease | I
Gonococcal urethritis | I
Gonorrhea | I
Groin masses | II
Heart failure, pregnancy | II
Heavy menstrual bleeding | I
Hemorrhagic ovarian cyst | I
Hereditary breast and ovarian cancer syndrome | I
Herpes simplex | I
Hot flashes | I
Hyperemesis gravidarum | I
Hypoactive sexual desire disorder | I
Hypogonadism | III
Immunizations during pregnancy | V
Incontinence (urinary) | I
Infertility | I
Mastitis | I
Mastodynia | I
Meigs syndrome | I
Menopause | I
Molar pregnancy | I
Nipple lesions | II
Nongonococcal urethritis | I
Ovarian cancer | I
Ovarian neoplasm, benign | I
Ovarian torsion | I
Paget's disease of the breast | I
Pelvic abscess | I
Pelvic congestion syndrome | I
Pelvic inflammatory disease | I
Pelvic mass, algorithm | III
Pelvic organ prolapse (uterine prolapse) | I
Pelvic pain, causes in women | II
Pelvic pain, reproductive-age woman | III
Perirectal abscess | I
Placenta previa | I
Polycystic ovary syndrome | I
Postpartum depression | I
Postpartum hemorrhage | I
Preeclampsia | I
Premature rupture of membranes | I
Premenstrual syndrome | I
Preterm labor | I
Primary ovarian insufficiency | I
Pruritus, pregnant patient | III
Pruritus vulvae | I, II
Rh incompatibility | I
Sexual assault | I
Sexual dysfunction | III
Sexual dysfunction in women | I, II
Spontaneous abortion | I
Syphilis | I
Thrombocytopenia, in pregnancy | II
Toxic shock syndrome | I
Urinary tract infection | I
Uterine fibroids | I
Uterine malignancy | I
Vaginal bleeding during pregnancy | I
Vaginal discharge, algorithm | III
Vaginal fistulas | I
Vaginal cancer | I
Vaginal prolapse | III
Vaginitis, estrogen-deficient | I
Vaginitis, fungal | I
Vaginitis, prepubescent | I
Vaginitis, *Trichomonas* | I
Vaginosis, bacterial | I

HEMATOLOGY/ONCOLOGY

Acute lymphoblastic leukemia | I
Acute myeloid leukemia | I
Anal cancer | I
Anemia, algorithm | III
Anemia, aplastic | I, II
Anemia, aplastic due to drugs and chemicals | II
Anemia, autoimmune hemolytic | I
Anemia, hypochromic | II
Anemia, inflammatory | I
Anemia in newborn | III
Anemia, iron deficiency | I
Anemia, macrocytic | III
Anemia, microcytic | III
Anemia, pernicious | I
Anemia with reticulocytosis | III

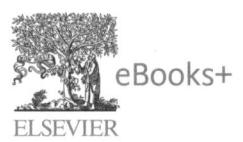
eBooks+

ELSEVIER

Any screen.
Any time.
Anywhere.

Activate the eBook version
of this title at no additional charge.

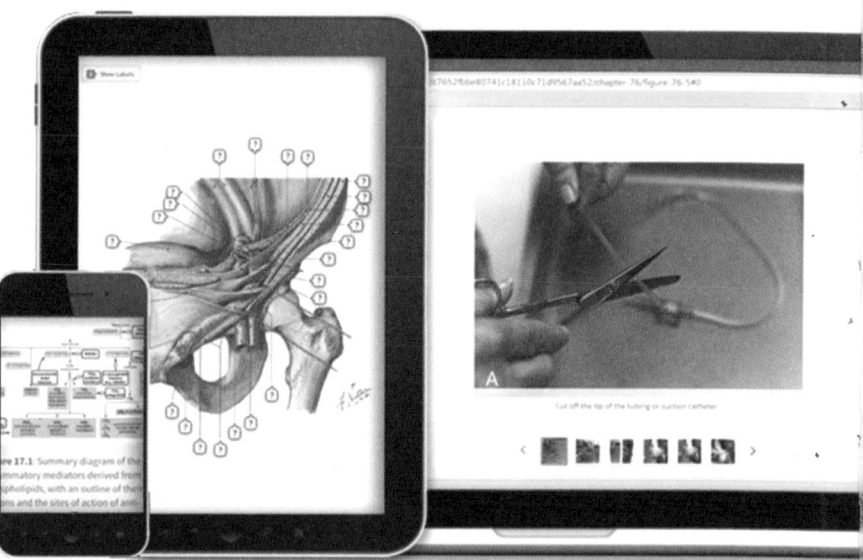

Elsevier eBooks+ gives you the power to browse, search, and customize your content,
make notes and highlights, and have content read aloud.

Unlock your eBook today.

1. Visit **http://ebooks.health.elsevier.com/**
2. Log in or Sign up
3. Scratch box below to reveal your code
4. Type your access code into the "Redeem
   Access Code" box
5. Click "Redeem"

It's that easy!

For technical assistance:
email textbookscom.support@elsevier.com
call 1-800-545-2522 (inside the US)
call +44 1 865 844 640 (outside the US)

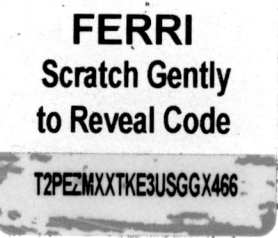

FERRI
**Scratch Gently
to Reveal Code**

T2PEZMXXTKE3USGGX466

2022v1 0

2024

Ferri's
CLINICAL
ADVISOR

FRED F. FERRI, MD, FACP

Clinical Professor
Department of Medicine
Warren Alpert Medical School
Brown University
Providence, Rhode Island

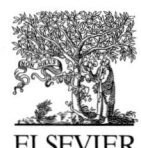

ELSEVIER

Elsevier
1600 John F. Kennedy Blvd.
Ste 1800
Philadelphia, PA 19103-2899

International Standard Book Number: 978-0-323-75576-4

Publisher: Sarah Barth
Senior Content Development Manager: Meghan Andress
Publishing Services Manager: Catherine Jackson
Senior Project Manager: Douglas Turner
Design Direction: Bridget Hoette

Printed in Canada

Last digit is the print number: 9 8 7 6 5 4 3 2 1

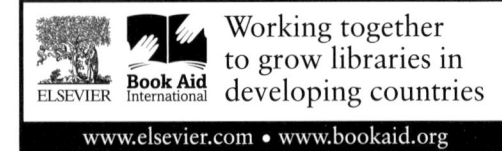

Contributors

Mohamed A. Abdelazeem, MD
Department of Internal Medicine
St. Elizabeth's Medical Center
Boston, MA

Rebecca A. Abelman, MD
Division of Infectious Diseases
University of California San Francisco
San Francisco, CA

Sarah Abu Kar, MD
Department of Nephrology
Vanderbilt University Medical Center
Nashville, TN

Maxwell Eyram Afari, MD
Attending Physician
Advanced Heart Failure and Transplant Cardiology
Maine Medical Center
Portland, ME

Ali Ahmad, MD
Neurocritical Care Fellow
Department of Neurology
Baylor College of Medicine
Houston, TX

Hammood Ahmed, MD
Department of Nephrology
Vanderbilt University Medical Center
Nashville, TN

Benjamin J. Ahn, BS
Warren Alpert Medical School of Brown University
Providence, RI

Rosa Ahn-Horst, MD, MPH
Department of Psychiatry
Massachusetts General Hospital and McLean Hospital
Boston, MA

Shanice Akoto, MD, MPH
Department of Obstetrics & Gynecology
CCHS
Newark, DE

Abrar AlAbdulhadi, MD
Department of Pediatrics
Children's Hospital of Philadelphia
Philadelphia, PA

Yoseph A. Aldras, MD
Department of Internal Medicine
Warren Alpert Medical School of Brown University, Lifespan
Providence, RI

Fahad Ali, MD
Emergency Department
Warren Alpert Medical School of Brown University
Providence, RI

Tanya Ali, MD
Clinical Assistant Professor of Medicine
Department of Medicine
Warren Alpert Medical School of Brown University
Providence, RI

Narges Alipanah-Lechner, MD
Pulmonary and Critical Care Medicine
Division of Pulmonary, Critical Care, Allergy and Sleep Medicine
University of California San Francisco
San Francisco, CA

Erdem Altunel, MD
Division of Hematology-Oncology
University of Massachusetts Medical School
Worcester, MA

Lama Alzoebie, MD
Pediatric Endocrinology
Division of Endocrinology and Diabetes
Children's Hospital of Philadelphia
Philadelphia, PA

Chelsie Anderson, MD, MS
Department of Surgery
University of California San Francisco
San Francisco, CA

Christine B. Andrews, MD, MPH
Pediatric Gastroenterology
Department of Pediatric Gastroenterology, Hepatology and Nutrition
Hasbro Children's Hospital
Providence, RI

Kathryn Taylor Anilowski, MS, PT, CLT-LANA
Physical Therapist
Kinder Touch Lymphedema Center
Saratoga Springs, NY

Anngene Anthony, MD, MPH, FAAFP
Teaching Faculty
HMH Mountainside Family Medicine Residency Program
Assistant Professor of Family Medicine
Associate Clerkship Director/Site Director–Family Medicine Clerkship
Hackensack Meridian School of Medicine
Nutley, NJ

Joseph A. Asaro, DO
Attending Neonatologist
AtlantiCare Regional Medical Center
Children's Hospital of Philadelphia Newborn Care Network
Galloway, NJ

Daniel K. Asiedu, MD, PhD, FACP
Staff Physician
Coastal Medical, Inc.
Lincoln, RI

Contributors

Artem Astsaturov, MD
Cardiac Electrophysiology
St. Elizabeth's Medical Center, A Boston University Teaching Hospital
Boston, MA

Sudeep K. Aulakh, MD, FACP, FRCPC
Director Ambulatory Education, Internal Medicine Residency
Department of Medicine
UMASS Medical School-Baystate
Springfield, MA

Matthew Authement, MD
Pediatric Hospitalist
Department of Pediatrics
Children's Hospital and Medical Center
Omaha, NE

Rupali S. Avasare, MD
Assistant Professor
Department of Internal Medicine
Oregon Health Sciences University
Portland, OR

Tania B. Babar, MD
Cardiologist
Charleston Area Medical Center
Charleston, WV

Emelia Argyropoulos Bachman, MD, FACOG
Delaware Institute for Reproductive Medicine
Department of Obstetrics & Gynecology
ChristianaCare Health System
Newark, DE

Muhammad Baig, MD
Preventive Cardiology
Division of Cardiology
Providence VA Medical Center and Brown University
Providence, RI

Ashika Bains, MD, MS
Attending Physician
Psychiatry Department
Massachusetts General Hospital
Boston, MA

Pedro Balaguera, MD
Assistant Professor of Neurology
University of Texas Health Science Center at Houston
McGovern Medical School
Houston, TX

Javier Balda, MD
Cardiovascular Medicine
St. Elizabeth's Medical Center
Boston, MA

T. Caroline Bank, MD
Department of Obstetrics & Gynecology
ChristianaCare Health System
Newark, DE

Brenda Banwell, MD
Chief of Division of Neurology
Neurology and Pediatrics
Children's Hospital of Philadelphia
Philadelphia, PA

Craig L. Basman, MD, FACC, FSCAI
Structural Interventional Cardiologist
Attending Physician
Department of Cardiology and Cardiothoracic Surgery,
Assistant Professor at Northwell Health
Northwell Health – Lenox Hill Hospital
New York, NY

Crystal T. Bass, MD
Attending Neonatologist
AtlantiCare Regional Medical Center
Children's Hospital of Philadelphia Newborn Care Network
Galloway, NJ

Sarah D. Bayefsky, MD
Divisions of Pediatric & Adult Rheumatology
The Children's Hospital of Philadelphia & Hospital of the University of
  Pennsylvania
Philadelphia, PA

Jasjit Beausang, MD
Female Pelvic Medicine and Reconstructive Surgery
Department of Obstetrics and Gynecology
Cooper University Hospital
Camden, NJ

Ren Belcher, MD
Lecturer in Psychiatry
Harvard Medical School
Clinical Associate
McLean Hospital
Boston, MA

Jennifer Bell, MD
Advanced Heart Failure and Transplant Cardiology
Assistant Professor University of Connecticut School of Medicine
Hartford HealthCare
Hartford, CT

Amy L. Bellinghausen, MD
Assistant Clinical Professor
Pulmonary, Critical Care and Sleep Medicine
University of California San Diego
San Diego, CA

Colleen E. Bennett, MD, MSHP
Assistant Professor
Clinical Pediatrics, Department of Pediatrics
University of Pennsylvania School of Medicine
Philadelphia, PA

John W. Benninger, MD, PhD
Director of Research and Clinical Training
Benson-Henry Institute for Mind Body Medicine
Department of Psychiatry
Massachusetts General Hospital/Harvard Medical School
Boston, MA

Michael A. Bergen, MD
Department of Orthopaedics
Brown/Rhode Island Hospital
Providence, RI

Agatha Berger, MD, MPH
Faculty
Department of Obstetrics & Gynecology
ChristianaCare Health System
Newark, DE

Carol D. Berkowitz, MD
Chief, Division of General Pediatrics
Harbor-UCLA Medical Center
Torrance, CA

Julia Berkowitz, MD
Internal Medicine
Department of Medicine
Warren Alpert Medical School of Brown University
Providence, RI

Omkar Betageri, MD
Department of Cardiology
Maine Medical Center
Portland, ME

Vicky H. Bhagat, MD, MPH
Department of Gastroenterology
Robert Wood Johnson University Hospital
New Brunswick, NJ

Murtaza Bharmal, MD
Division of Cardiology
University of California, Irvine
Orange, CA

Harikrashna B. Bhatt, MD
Assistant Professor, Clinician Educator
Division of Endocrinology
Department of Medicine
Warren Alpert Medical School of Brown University
Providence, RI

Prachi H. Bhuptani, PhD
Post-Doctoral Research Associate
Department of Psychiatry and Human Behavior
Warren Alpert Medical School of Brown University
Department of Adult Psychiatry, Rhode Island Hospital
Providence, RI

Richard O. Bido-Medina, MD, PhD
Department of Psychiatry
Harvard Medical School
Massachusetts General Hospital and McLean Hospital
Boston, MA

Kendall M.H. Bielak, MD
Obstetrics & Gynecology
ChristianaCare Health System
Newark, DE

Courtney Clark Bilodeau, MD, FACP
Assistant Professor
Department of Obstetric Medicine
Warren Alpert Medical School of Brown University
Attending Physician
Internal Medicine
Women's Medicine Collaborative
Miriam Hospital
Providence, RI

Lisa Bird, MD
Resident Physician
Department of Obstetrics & Gynecology
TriHealth
Cincinnati, OH

Erin Bishop, MD
Department of Obstetrics & Gynecology
ChristianaCare Health System
Newark, DE

Ghamar Bitar, MD
Maternal Fetal Medicine
The University of Texas Health Science Center at Houston (UTHealth)
Houston, TX

Craig Blakeney, MD
Emergency Medicine
UTHSC
Memphis, TN

Brian Block, MD
Assistant Professor of Medicine
University of California San Francisco
San Francisco, CA

Risa Bochner, MD
Pediatric Hospitalist, Patient Safety Officer
Department of Pediatrics and Quality Management
New York City Health and Hospitals/Harlem
New York, NY

Christina M. Bortz, MD, FACP
Assistant Professor of Medicine
Warren Alpert Medical School of Brown University
Attending Physician, Internal Medicine
Women's Medicine Collaborative
Providence, RI

Kristopher R. Bosse, MD
Assistant Professor of Pediatrics
Perelman School of Medicine at the University of Pennsylvania
Division of Oncology, The Children's Hospital of Philadelphia
Philadelphia, PA

Tara C. Bouton, MD, MPH
Assistant Professor of Medicine
Section of Infectious Disease
Boston Medical Center
Boston University School of Medicine
Boston, MA

Mary E. Bove, MD
Pediatric Attending
CHOP Care Network Delaware County
Philadelphia, PA

Lynn A. Bowlby, MD, FACP
Center for Primary Care
Warren Alpert Medical School of Brown University
Providence, RI

Mark F. Brady, MD, MPH, MMSc
Assistant Professor
Department of Emergency Medicine
Warren Alpert Medical School of Brown University
Providence, RI

Russell E. Bratman, MD
Assistant Professor, Clinician Educator
Division of Endocrinology
Department of Medicine
Warren Alpert Medical School of Brown University
Providence, RI

Keith Brennan, MD
Department of Geriatric Medicine
Stony Brook University
Stony Brook, NY

Austin K. Brown, MD
Department of Emergency Medicine
University of Tennessee Health Science Center
Memphis, TN

Emily C.B. Brown, MD
Safe Children and Adolescent Network (SCAN)
Department of Pediatrics
Seattle Children's Hospital
University of Washington School of Medicine
Seattle, WA

Eric Bui, MD, PhD
Professor of Psychiatry
Department of Psychiatry
Caen University Hospital
Caen, France

Christine Burke, MD
Obstetrics & Gynecology
ChristianaCare Health System
Newark, DE

William Butler, MD
Massachusetts General Hospital
McLean Hospital
Harvard Medical School
Boston, MA

Katerina L. Byanova, MD, MS
Division of Pulmonary, Critical Care, Allergy and Sleep Medicine
University of California San Francisco
San Francisco, CA

Marcin Byra, DO
Assistant Professor
Department of Emergency Medicine
UTHSC
Memphis, TN

Tucker C. Callanan, MD
Orthopedic Surgery
Brown University
Providence, RI

Taylor Campbell, MD
Department of Emergency Medicine
UTHSC
Memphis, TN

Adriana Cantos, MD
Department of Psychiatry
Massachusetts General Hospital
McLean Hospital
Boston, MA

Ethan Canty, MD, MPH
Department of Pediatrics
Oregon Health & Sciences University
Portland, OR

Katherine W. Canty, MD
Attending Physician
Child Protection Program
Division of General Pediatrics
Boston Children's Hospital
Boston, MA

Andrew Caraganis, MD
Internal Medicine
Boston University School of Medicine
Roger Williams Medical Center
Providence, RI

Randy S. Carpenter, BA
University of Tennessee Health Science Center
Memphis, TN

Eugene Carragee, MD
Department of Anesthesia and Perioperative Care
University of California San Francisco
San Francisco, CA

Meredith Carrel-Lammert, MD
OB/GYN Faculty
TriHealth OB/GYN Residency
Cincinnati, OH

Ashlie Sewdass Carter, MD
Department of Obstetrics & Gynecology
ChristianaCare Health System
Newark, DE

Ernesto Casillas, Jr., MD
Pulmonary & Critical Care Medicine
University of California, San Francisco
San Francisco, CA

Ana Castaneda-Guarderas, MD
Assistant Professor, University of Tennessee Regional One Physicians
Emergency Medicine Department
Memphis, TN

Jorge J. Castillo, MD
Associate Professor
Harvard Medical School
Senior Physician
Dana-Farber Cancer Institute
Boston, MA

Daniel Chait, MD, MEd
Department of Psychiatry
Massachusetts General Hospital
Harvard Medical School
Boston, MA

Philip A. Chan, MD, MS
Associate Professor
Department of Medicine
Brown University
Providence, RI

Kenny Chang, BS
Warren Alpert Medical School of Brown University
Providence, RI

Arlene B. Chapman, MD
Professor of Medicine
Chief, Section of Nephrology
University of Chicago
Chicago, IL

Sudeshna Chatterjee-Paer, MD
Department of Gynecologic & Oncology
Helen Graham Cancer Center
ChristianaCare Health System
Newark, DE

Richard S. Chaudhary, MD
Department of Medicine
Beth Israel Deaconess Medical Center
Harvard Medical School
Boston, MA

Vicky Cheng, MD
Assistant Professor
Division of Endocrinology
Department of Medicine
Warren Alpert Medical School of Brown University
Providence, RI

Daniel Chilcote, MD
Department of Anesthesiology and Critical Care Medicine
The Children's Hospital of Philadelphia
Philadelphia, PA

Dana Ricci Chofay, MD
Assistant Professor of Medicine and Medical Science
Warren Alpert Medical School of Brown University
Providence, RI

Jonathan Chou, MD, MS
Department of Psychiatry
Massachusetts General Hospital/McLean Hospital
Boston, MA

Stella T. Chou, MD
Chief, Division of Transfusion Medicine
Department of Pathology and Laboratory Medicine
Attending Physician, Division of Hematology
Department of Pediatrics
Children's Hospital of Philadelphia
Philadelphia, PA

Natasha Choudhury, MD
Division of Multiple Sclerosis and Neuroimmunology
Department of Neurology
Northwestern University Feinberg School of Medicine
Chicago, IL

Shivali Choxi, MD
Pediatrician and Director of Pediatric Primary Care Innovation
Department of Pediatrics
New York City Health + Hospitals/Jacobi
New York, NY

Winona Chua, MD
Clinical Associate Professor of Pediatrics
Perelman School of Medicine
University of Pennsylvania
Attending Physician
Department of Pediatrics
Children's Hospital of Philadelphia
Philadelphia, PA

Rhiannon E. Chubb, MD
Physician
Rhode Island Hospital
Providence, RI

Michael P. Cinelli, DO
Department of Cardiology
Northwell Health Staten Island University Hospital
Staten Island, NY

David Claman, MD
Professor of Medicine and Medical Director of Sleep Disorders Center
Division of Pulmonary, Critical Care, Allergy and Sleep Medicine
University of California San Francisco
San Francisco, CA

Grace V. Clark, MD, BA
Obstetrics & Gynecology
ChristianaCare Health Services
Newark, DE

Seth Clark, MD, MPH, FASAM
Assistant Professor
Department of Medicine
Department of Psychiatry and Human Behavior
Warren Alpert Medical School of Brown University
Providence, RI

Nathan Clarke, MD
Assistant Professor
Department of Neurology
University of Michigan
Ann Arbor, MI

Karl T. Clebak, MD, MHA, FAAFP
Associate Professor, Program Director
Department of Family and Community Medicine Residency Program
Penn State Health M. S. Hershey Medical Center
Hershey, PA

Derrick Cleland, DO, MPH
Department of Medicine
Loma Linda University Health
Loma Linda, CA

Michael Lawrenz Co, MD, MSc
Division of Cardiology
Thomas Jefferson University Hospital
Philadelphia, PA

Debbie L. Cohen, MD
Professor of Medicine
Renal, Electrolyte and Hypertension Division
Perelman School of Medicine at the University of Pennsylvania
Philadelphia, PA

Lisa Cohen, PharmD
Associate Professor of Pharmacy
University of Rhode Island
Kingston, RI

Morgan Congdon, MD, MPH
Clinical Assistant Professor of Pediatrics
Children's Hospital of Philadelphia
Philadelphia, PA

Maria Constantinou, MD
Clinical Assistant Professor of Medicine
Warren Alpert Medical School of Brown University
Medical Oncologist
Lifespan Cancer
Providence, RI

James Earl Corley, III, MD
Faculty, Department of Emergency Medicine
University of Tennessee Health Science Center
Memphis, TN

Abigail Cosgrove, MD
Assistant Professor
Emergency Medicine
University of Tennessee Health Science Center
Memphis, TN

Rebecca Craine, MSEd, CCC-SLP
Speech Language Pathologist, Rehabilitation
Bradley Hospital
East Providence, RI

Patricia Cristofaro, MD
Assistant Professor
Department of Infectious Diseases
Brown (Warren Alpert) University Medical School
Providence, RI

Aristides I. Cruz, MD
Department of Orthopaedic Surgery
Brown University
Providence, RI

Karlene Cunningham, PhD
Clinical Assistant Professor
Department of Psychiatry and Behavioral Medicine
Brody School of Medicine, East Carolina University
Greenville, NC

Alicia J. Curtin, PhD
Assistant Professor
Division of Geriatrics
Warren Alpert Medical School at Brown University
Providence, RI

Joseph Cusano, MD
Department of Orthopedic Surgery
Rhode Island Hospital/Brown University
Providence, RI

Frank B. D'Alessandro, MD
Endocrinologist
Providence, RI

Lynn Dado, MD
Primary Care Physician, Internal Medicine
Henry Ford Health System
Bloomfield Hills, MI

Deepansh Dalela, MD
Department of Urology/Vattikuti Urology Institute
Henry Ford Hospital
Detroit, MI

Abhijit Das, MD
Child Neurology
Department of Pediatrics
Baylor College of Medicine
Houston, TX

Manuel F. DaSilva, MD
Associate Professor
Department of Orthopedics
Warren Alpert Medical School of Brown University
Providence, RI

Mackenzie Davis, MD
Clinical Fellow in Department of Psychiatry
Harvard Medical School
Massachusetts General Hospital/McLean Hospital Adult Psychiatry
Boston, MA

Carlos De La Garza, MD
Department of Adult Neurology
Baylor College of Medicine
Houston, TX

Alison DeDent, MD
Assistant Professor
Division of Pulmonary and Critical Care Medicine
University of California San Francisco
San Francisco, CA

Maya Deeb, MD
Division of Gastroenterology, Department of Medicine
University of Toronto
Toronto, Ontario
Canada

Tyler DeJong, MD
University of Tennessee Health Sciences Center
Memphis, TN

Colette Desrochers, MD
Primary Care Attending Physician
Children's Hospital of Philadelphia
Associate Professor of Pediatrics
Associated Faculty of the Perelman School of Medicine
Philadelphia, PA

Joseph A. Diaz, MD, MPH
Associate Dean for Diversity and Multicultural Affairs
Associate Professor of Medicine and Medical Science
Warren Alpert Medical School of Brown University
Providence, RI

Jason L. Dickherber, MD, MS
Department of Orthopedic Surgery
Brown University
Providence, RI

Toan Do, MD
Department of Medicine
Oregon Health & Science University
Portland, OR

Kathleen Doo, MD, MHPE
Associate Program Director
Kaiser Permanente Northern California Pulmonary and Critical Care Medicine Fellowship
Department of Pulmonary Medicine
The Permanente Medical Group
Oakland, CA

James H. Dove, MD
Department of Orthopedic Surgery
Brown University
Providence, RI

Alexandre Dubanchet, MD
Department of Psychiatry
Caen University Hospital
Caen, France

Carol Duh-Leong, MD
Clinical Assistant Professor
NYU Grossman School of Medicine
New York, NY

Roop Dutta, MD
Department of Medicine, Division of Cardiology
St. Elizabeth's Medical Center
Boston, MA

Myles Dworkin, MD, MPH
Department of Orthopedics
Brown University
Providence, RI

Timothy G. Dyster, MD
Division of Pulmonary, Critical Care, Allergy, and Sleep Medicine
University of California San Francisco
San Francisco, CA

Eric Ebert, MD
Department of Emergency Medicine
Brown Emergency Medicine
Providence, RI

Joseph Edmund, MD
Division of Hematology/Oncology
Roger Williams Medical Center
Providence, RI

Erica Eggers, MD
Female Pelvic Medicine & Reconstructive Surgery
Department of Obstetrics & Gynecology
Cooper University Hospital
Camden, NJ

Christine Eisenhower, PharmD
Clinical Associate Professor
Pharmacy Practice
University of Rhode Island
Kingston, RI

Pamela Ellsworth, MD
Chief, Division of Urology
Vice Chair, Academics, Department of Surgery
Nemours Children's Health
Orlando, FL

César E. Escamilla-Ocañas, MD
Department of Neurology
Baylor College of Medicine
Houston, TX

Patricio Sebastian Espinosa, MD, MPH, FAAN
Professor of Neurology
Chief and Institute Director
Neurology Department
Espinosa Neuroscience Institute
Boca Raton, FL

Marisol Esqueda, MD
Department of Medicine
OHSU Hillsboro Medical Center
Hillsboro, OR

Eileen Everly, MD
Attending Physician
Department of General Pediatrics
The Children's Hospital of Philadelphia
Philadelphia, PA

Mark D. Faber, MD
Senior Staff
Division of Nephrology and Hypertension
Henry Ford Hospital
Associate Professor, Internal Medicine
Wayne State University School of Medicine
Detroit, MI

Rachel Faber, MD
Department of Orthopaedic Surgery
Warren Alpert Medical School of Brown University
Providence, RI

Evan Facer, DO
Pediatric Infectious Diseases
UPMC Children's Hospital of Pittsburgh
Pittsburgh, PA

Paul D. Fadale, MD
Department of Orthopaedic Surgery
Warren Alpert Medical School of Brown University
Providence, RI

Benyamin Farahvash, MD
Department of Endocrinology
Warren Alpert Medical School of Brown University
Providence, RI

Michael J. Farias, BS
Warren Alpert Medical School of Brown University
Providence, RI

Jon Farkas, MD
Pediatric Hospital Medicine Attending
Pediatrics
NYU School of Medicine
New York, NY

Erica Farrand, MD
Assistant Professor
Division of Pulmonary and Critical Care Medicine
University of California San Francisco
San Francisco, CA

Kevin Fay, MD
Assistant Professor of Clinical Medicine
Renal, Electrolyte and Hypertension Division
Penn Presbyterian Medical Center
Philadelphia, PA

Samantha Fernandez Hernandez, MD
Department of Neurology
Baylor College of Medicine
Houston, TX

Contributors

Carlos Fernandez-Robles, MD, MBA
Chief of Psychiatry
Vice Chair of Brigham and Women's Faulkner Psychiatry
Brigham and Women's Hospital
Boston, MA

Jason D. Ferreira, MD
Clinical Assistant Professor of Medicine at Brown University
Gastroenterology
University Gastroenterology, LLC/Miriam Hospital
Providence, RI

Fred F. Ferri, MD
Clinical Professor
Department of Medicine
Warren Alpert Medical School of Brown University
Providence, RI

Heather Ferri, DO
Department of Medicine
Warren Alpert Medical School at Brown University
Rhode Island Hospital
Providence, RI

Staci A. Fischer, MD
Staff Member
Accreditation Council for Graduate Medical Education
Chicago, IL

Hannah Fiske, MD
Department of Internal Medicine
Brown University
Providence, RI

Maria Camila Velez Florez, MD
Department of Psychiatry
Massachusetts General Hospital
McLean Hospital
Boston, MA

Cristina Font, MD
Department of Internal Medicine
Warren Alpert Medical School of Brown University
Providence, RI

Kellie C. Forbes, MD
Department of Obstetrics & Gynecology
ChristianaCare Health System
Newark, DE

Michelle Forcier, MD, MPH
Professor Pediatrics
Alpert School of Medicine Brown University
Providence, RI

Sydney Ford, MD, MPH
Department of Obstetrics & Gynecology
ChristianaCare Health System
Newark, DE

Frank G. Fort, MD, FACS, RPHS
Medical Director
Capital Region Vein Centre
Schenectady, NY

Glenn G. Fort, MD, MPH
Clinical Associate Professor of Medicine
The Warren Alpert School of Medicine at Brown University
Providence, RI
Chief of Infectious Diseases
Landmark Medical Center
Woonsocket, RI

Nancy Freeman, MD
Chief, Hematology/Oncology
Providence VA Medical Center
Clinical Associate Professor of Medicine
Brown University
Providence, RI

Daniel R. Frisch, MD
Associate Professor
Division of Cardiology
Thomas Jefferson University
Philadelphia, PA

Relindis Azenwi Fru, MD
Department of Hematology and Oncology
Doctors Hospital at Renaissance
Edinburg, TX

Lynn C. Fullenkamp, MD, JD
Assistant Professor
Pediatric Hospital Medicine & Child Advocacy Team
Children's Hospital and Medical Center/University of Nebraska Medical Center
Omaha, NE

Michael Gaffney, MD
Department of Pediatrics
New York University Grossman School of Medicine
New York, NY

Paloma Jolin Garcia, MD
Division of Human Genetics
The Children's Hospital of Philadelphia and Perelman School of Medicine of the University of Pennsylvania
Philadelphia, PA

Connie Ge, BA
University of Massachusetts Chan Medical School
Worcester, MA

Yaron B. Gesthalter, MD
Assistant Professor of Medicine
Co-director of Interventional Pulmonary Medicine
University of California, San Francisco
San Francisco, CA

Anil Ghimire, MD
Associate Clinical Professor
Director, Adult CF Program
PCCSM Division, Dept of Medicine
University of California, San Francisco
Fresno, CA

Christopher Gibson, MD
Pediatric Endocrinology Physician
Division of Endocrinology and Diabetes
Children's Hospital of Philadelphia
Assistant Professor of Clinical Medicine
University of Pennsylvania Perelman School of Medicine
Philadelphia, PA

Nisha H. Gidwani, MD
Associate Professor of Clinical Medicine
Division of Pulmonary, Critical Care, Allergy and Sleep Medicine
University of California, San Francisco
San Francisco, CA

Joseph Gil, MD
Department of Orthopaedic Surgery
Warren Alpert Medical School of Brown University
Providence, RI

Raphaela Gold, MD, MSc
Division of Women's Mental Health
McLean Hospital
Belmont, MA

Alla Goldburt, MD
Assistant Clinical Professor, Family Medicine
Warren Alpert Medical School at Brown University
Providence, RI

Corey Elam Goldsmith, MD, FAAN
Associate Professor of Neurology
Department of Neurology
Baylor College of Medicine
Houston, TX

Maheswara Satya Gangadhara Rao Golla, MD
Interventional Cardiology
Parkersburg Cardiology Associates
Camden Clark Medical Center
Parkersburg, WV

Alexander Gomez, MD
Assistant Clinical Professor
Division of Pulmonary, Critical Care, Allergy, and Sleep Medicine
University of California San Francisco
San Francisco, CA

Helen B. Gomez Slagle, MD
Obstetrics & Gynecology
ChristianaCare Health System
Newark, DE

Morgan Greenfield, MD
Attending Physician
Department of Pediatrics
The Children's Hospital of Philadelphia
Philadelphia, PA

Lindsey Anne Grisham, MD
Clinical Faculty, Emergency Medicine
University of Tennessee Health Science Center
Memphis, TN

Joey Gu, BS
Warren Alpert Medical School of Brown University
Providence, RI

Cara E. Guardino, MD
Division of Cardiology
Warren Alpert Medical School of Brown University and Lifespan
Cardiovascular Institute
Providence, RI

Lindsay Gugerty, MD
Department of Obstetrics & Gynecology
ChristianaCare Health System
Newark, DE

Fahad Gul, MD
Division of Cardiology
University of California, Irvine
Orange, CA

Patan Gultawatvichai, MD
Assistant Professor
Division of Hematology-Oncology
University of Massachusetts Medical School
Worcester, MA

Samantha Gunning, MD
Assistant Professor of Medicine
Department of Nephrology
The University of Chicago Medicine
Chicago, IL

Averill Guo, MD
Fellow
Division of Gastroenterology
Warren Alpert Medical School of Brown University
Providence, RI

David Guo, MD
Affiliate Clinical Assistant Professor
Department of Urology
Stanford Medical School
Kaiser Santa Clara Medical Center
Santa Clara, CA

Simran Gupta, MD
Rhode Island Hospital
Brown University
Providence, RI

Brittany Guttadauria, MD
Pediatric Emergency Medicine
Children's Hospital of Philadelphia
Philadelphia, PA

Herodes Guzman, MD, MPH
General Pediatrics
Children's Hospital of Philadelphia
Philadelphia, PA

Meghan Gwinn, MD
Division of Internal Medicine
Henry Ford Hospital
Detroit, MI

Ryan Hadden, MD
Department of Orthopaedic Surgery
Warren Alpert Medical School of Brown University
Providence, RI

Muhammad Ubaid Hafeez, MD
Department of Neurology
University of Texas Health Science Center
Houston, TX

Hayden Hall, DO
Department of Neurology
Baylor College of Medicine
Houston, TX

Sarah Hall, MD
Generalist Faculty Attending
Department of Obstetrics & Gynecology
ChristianaCare Health System
Newark, DE

Sajeev Handa, MD, SFHM
Chief, Hospital Medicine
Lifespan Physician Group
Rhode Island Hospital/The Miriam Hospital/Newport Hospital
Clinical Assistant Professor of Medicine & Clinical Assistant Professor of Neurology
Warren Alpert Medical School of Brown University
Providence, RI

Stacy N. Handler, MD
Department of Medicine
Brown University/Rhode Island Hospital
Providence, RI

James Hanna, MD
Henry Ford Health Department of Nephrology
Henry Ford Hospital
Detroit, MI

John Hanna, MD
Department of Orthopaedics
Brown/Rhode Island Hospital
Providence, RI

Nikolas Harbord, MD
Division Chief
Nephrology & Hypertension
Mount Sinai Beth Israel
New York, NY

Kyle Hardacker, MD
Orthopedic Surgery
Brown University
Providence, RI

Anna Hardesty, MD
Department of Internal Medicine
Warren Alpert Medical School of Brown University
Providence, RI

Nirav Haribhakti, MD, PharmD
Department of Internal Medicine
Rhode Island Hospital
Warren Alpert Medical School of Brown University
Providence, RI

Daniel J. Harris, MD
Department of Psychiatry
Massachusetts General Hospital
Boston, MA

Davis A. Hartnett, BS
Research Fellow
Department of Orthopaedics
Brown University
Providence, RI

Nathan Hartvigsen, MD
Harvard Medical School Instructor in Psychiatry
Massachusetts General Hospital
Boston, MA

Brian Hawkins, MD
Assistant Professor
Emergency Medicine
University of Tennessee Health Science Center
Memphis, TN

Rachel Wright Heinle, MD, FACOG
Attending Physician
Department of Obstetrics & Gynecology
ChristianaCare Health System
Newark, DE

Leesha A. Helm, MD, MPH
Assistant Professor
Department of Family and Community Medicine
Penn State Medical Center
Hershey, PA

Matthew F. Helm, MD
Assistant Professor
Department of Dermatology
Penn State Medical Center
Hershey, PA

Thomas Herlevich, MD
Department of Emergency Medicine
UTHSC
Memphis, TN

Klodia M. Hermez, DO
Division of Nephrology
Henry Ford Hospital
Detroit, MI

Ross W. Hilliard, MD, FACP
Associate Professor (Clinician)
Department of Medicine
Warren Alpert Medical School of Brown University
Providence, RI

Katherine Hladky, MD
Faculty
Department of Obstetrics & Gynecology
ChristianaCare Health System
Newark, DE

Ashley Hodges, MD
Obstetrics & Gynecology
ChristianaCare Health System
Newark, DE

Ryan Hoffman, MD
Department of Orthopedics
Brown University
Providence, RI

R. Scott Hoffman, MD
Ophthalmologist
Assistant Clinical Professor
University of Louisville School of Medicine
Doctors Eye Institute and U of L Ophthalmology
Louisville, KY

Dawn Hogan, MD
Clinical Assistant Professor of Family Medicine
Warren Alpert Medical School at Brown University
Providence, RI

Jennifer J. Holiman, MSN, APRN, PMHNP-BC
Staff Clinician
Division of Geriatric Psychiatry
McLean Hospital
Belmont, MA

N. Wilson Holland, MD
Associate Professor of Medicine
Division of Geriatrics and Gerontology
Emory University School of Medicine
Acting Designated Learning Officer
Atlanta Veterans Administration Medical Center
Atlanta, GA

Siri M. Holton, MD
Attending Physician
Department of Obstetrics & Gynecology
ChristianaCare Health System
Newark, DE

Benjamin J. Homer, BS
Department of Orthopaedic Surgery
Warren Alpert Medical School of Brown University
Providence, RI

Benjamin E. Hook, MD
Department of Emergency Medicine
UTHSC
Memphis, TN

Cody Howell, MD
Emergency Medicine Department
University of Tennessee Health Science Center
Memphis, TN

Raymond Hsu, MD
Department of Orthopedic Surgery
Brown University
Providence, RI

Laurence Huang, MD, FCCP, ATSF
Professor of Medicine
Chief, HIV/AIDS Chest Clinic, Zuckerberg San Francisco General Hospital and Trauma Center
Division of HIV, Infectious Diseases and Global Medicine
Division of Pulmonary, Critical Care, Allergy and Sleep Medicine
University of California, San Francisco
San Francisco, CA

Mariam Hull, MD
Assistant Professor
Pediatric Movement Disorders Clinic
Section of Child Neurology and Neurodevelopmental Disabilities
Texas Children's Hospital/Baylor College of Medicine
Houston, TX

Anne L. Hume, PharmD
Professor of Pharmacy
Department of Pharmacy Practice
University of Rhode Island
Kingston, RI

Zilla Hussain, MD
Attending Physician
Gastroenterology
Greater Baltimore Medical Center
Baltimore, MD

Donny V. Huynh, MD
Mcleod Oncology and Hematology Associates at Seascoast
Department of Medicine Chair
Mcleod Health
Little River, SC

Sarah Hyder, MD, MBA
Director of Endoscopic Ultrasound
Rhode Island Hospital
Providence, RI

Zainab Ibrahim, MD
Department of Orthopaedic Surgery
Warren Alpert Medical School of Brown University
Providence, RI

Caitlin Ingraham, MD
Gyn Surgery
Department of Obstetrics & Gynecology
ChristianaCare Health System
Newark, DE

Nicholas J. Inman, MD
Clinical Faculty
Emergency Medicine
University of Tennessee Health Science Center
Memphis, TN

Louis F. Insalaco, MD
Department of Otolaryngology
Mass Eye and Ear, Stoneham
Harvard Medical School
Stoneham, MA

Rishubh Jain, BA
Warren Alpert Medical School of Brown University
Providence, RI

Vanita B.D. Jain, MD
Physician
ChristianaCare Health System
Delaware Center for Maternal Fetal Medicine
Newark, DE

Vipul V. Jain, MD, MS
Professor of Clinical Medicine
Division Chief–PCCSM
Executive Vice Chief, Dept of Medicine
UCSF
Fresno, CA

Fariha Jamal, MD
Assistant Professor of Neurology
Baylor College of Medicine
Michael E. DeBakey VA Medical Center
Houston, TX

Kaushal Jani, MD
DM Clinical Research
Clinical Research Coordinator

Robert H. Janigian, Jr., MD
Clinical Associate Professor of Surgery
The Warren Alpert Medical School at Brown University
Providence, RI

Sonia Jasuja, MD
Clinical Instructor
Division of Pulmonary, Critical Care, and Sleep Medicine
University of California Los Angeles
Los Angeles, CA

Noelle Marie Javier, MD
Associate Professor
Department of Geriatrics and Palliative Medicine
Icahn School of Medicine at Mount Sinai
New York, NY

Vybhav Jetty, MD, MHA
Cardiac Clinical Electrophysiology
Division of Electrophysiology
St. Elizabeth's Medical Center
Boston, MA

Jennie E. Johnson, MD
Assistant Professor of Medicine
Warren Alpert Medical School of Brown University
Associate Director
Infectious Diseases & Immunology Center at Miriam Hospital
Providence, RI

Michael P. Johnson, MD
MDVIP-Affiliated Physician
Providence, RI

Steven D. Johnson, MD
Attending Physician
Department of Obstetrics and Gynecology
TriHealth
Cincinnati, OH

Angad Jolly, MD, PhD
Postdoctoral Associate
Baylor College of Medicine
Houston, TX

Amanda Jones, MD
Department of Obstetrics & Gynecology
ChristianaCare Health System
Newark, DE

Shyam Joshi, MD
Assistant Professor of Medicine
Section of Allergy and Immunology
Oregon Health & Science University
Portland, OR

Kareem Joudi, BA
MD Candidate
Warren Alpert School of Medicine
Providence, RI

Joshua Justice, MD
Assistant Professor
Department of Emergency Medicine
University of Tennessee Health Science Center
Memphis, TN

Timothy Kaddis, MD
House Officer, Internal Medicine
Department of Medicine
Oregon Health and Science University
Portland, OR

Markos Kalligeros, MD
Department of Internal Medicine
Warren Alpert Medical School
Providence, RI

Omar Karim, BS
Department of Orthopaedic Surgery
Warren Alpert Medical School of Brown University
Providence, RI

Vanji Karthikeyan, MD
Senior Staff
Division of Nephrology
Henry Ford Hospital
Detroit, MI

Benjamin Kartub, MD
Department of Emergency Medicine
University of Tennessee Health Science Center
Memphis, TN

Vania Kasper, MD
Assistant Professor
Department of Pediatric Gastroenterology
Hepatology and Nutrition
Hasbro Children's Hospital
Providence, RI

Joseph S. Kass, MD, JD, FAAN
Associate Dean of Student Affairs
Professor of Neurology, Psychiatry, and Medical Ethics
Director, Alzheimer's Disease and Memory Disorders Center
Baylor College of Medicine
Chief of Neurology
Director of Comprehensive Stroke Program
Ben Taub General Hospital
Houston, TX

Naomi R. Kass, BA
Baylor College of Medicine
Houston, TX

Viknesh S. Kasthuri, AB
Warren Alpert Medical School of Brown University
Providence, RI

Luca Katz, BA
Warren Alpert Medical School of Brown University
Providence, RI

Bhavika Kaul, MD
Assistant Professor
Division of Pulmonary and Critical Care Medicine
University of California San Francisco
San Francisco, CA

Arpanjeet Kaur, MD
Department of Medicine
Mount Sinai Morningside/West
New York, NY

Jennifer L. Keim, MD, MPH
Clinical Assistant Professor of Pediatrics
General Pediatrics
Children's Hospital of Philadelphia
Philadelphia, PA

Vasken Keleshian, MD
Department of Medicine, Division of Cardiology
University of California, Irvine
Orange, CA

Abigail Keogh, MD
Physician, Child Protection Program
Division of General Pediatrics
Boston Children's Hospital
Boston, MA

Dennis Keselman, MD
Department of Neurology
Children's Hospital of Philadelphia
Philadelphia, PA

Adeeba Khan, DO
Department of Neurology
Baylor College of Medicine
Houston, TX

Sarthak Khare, MD
Department of Cardiovascular Medicine
St. Elizabeth Medical Center
Boston, MA

Hussain R. Khawaja, MD, FACP
Assistant Professor of Medicine, Clinician Educator
Warren Alpert Medical School of Brown University
Division of General Internal Medicine
Department of Medicine
Rhode Island Hospital
Providence, RI

Vishal Khetpal, MD, MSc
Brown University Department of Internal Medicine
Warren Alpert Medical School
Providence, RI

Saranya S. Khurana, MD, MPH
Department of Psychiatry
Massachusetts General Hospital
Boston, MA

Betelhem Kifle, MD
Department of Medicine
University of California San Francisco
San Francisco, CA

Eun Kyung (Ellen) Kim, MD
Psychiatry
Massachusetts General Hospital/McLean Hospital
Boston, MA

Jinseong Kim, MD
Department of Orthopaedic Surgery
Warren Alpert Medical School of Brown University
Providence, RI

Julianne Kleitsch, BA
Department of Dermatology
Autoimmune Skin Disease Unit
University of Pennsylvania
Philadelphia, PA

Tess Knudson-Fitzpatrick, MD
Pulmonary and Critical Care Fellow
Kaiser Permanente Northern California Pulmonary and Critical Care Medicine
Fellowship
Kaiser Hospital Foundation
Oakland, CA

Samuel I. Kohrman, MD
Department of Psychiatry
Massachusetts General Hospital
Boston, MA

Aravind Rao Kokkirala, MD, FACC
Division of Cardiology, Department of Medicine
Warren Alpert Medical School of Brown University
Providence Veterans Affairs Medical Center
Providence, RI

Yuval Konstantino, MD
Cardiac Electrophysiology and Pacing Unit
Department of Cardiology
Soroka University Medical Center
Beer-Sheba, Israel

Nelson Kopyt, DO
Staff Nephrologist
Department of Medicine
Lehigh Valley Hospital
Allentown, PA

Savan Kothadia, MD
Department of Internal Medicine
Rhode Island Hospital
Providence, RI

Ajay Koti, MD
Safe Children and Adolescent Network (SCAN)
Department of Pediatrics
Seattle Children's Hospital
University of Washington School of Medicine
Seattle, WA

Ioannis Koulouridis, MD, MSc
Division of Cardiology
St. Elizabeth's Medical Center
Boston, MA

Timothy R. Kreider, MD, PHD
Assistant Professor
Department of Psychiatry
Donald and Barbara Zucker School of Medicine at Hofstra/Northwell
Hempstead, NY

Van S. Krueger, MD
Department of Orthopedic Surgery
Warren Alpert Medical School of Brown University
Providence, RI

Ilana Krumm, MD
Division of Pulmonary, Critical Care, Allergy and Sleep
University of California San Francisco
San Francisco, CA

Lalathaksha Kumbar, MD
Nephrology Attending
Henry Ford Hospital
Division of Nephrology and Hypertension
Detroit, MI

Eren O. Kuris, MD
Assistant Professor
Department of Orthopaedic Surgery
Warren Alpert Medical School of Brown University
Providence, RI

David I. Kurss, MD, FACOG, NCMP
Attending Physician
Women's Wellness Center of Western New York
Invision Health
Clinical Assistant Professor
School of Medicine
Department of Obstetrics and Gynecology
State University of New York at Buffalo
Buffalo, NY

Nathan L'Etoile, MD
The Children's Hospital of Philadelphia
Philadelphia, PA

Uyen T. Lam, MD
Noninvasive Cardiologist
Division of Cardiology
St. Elizabeth's Medical Center
Boston, MA

William Lam, MD
Associate Professor
Baylor College of Medicine
Departments of Medicine and Pediatrics
Division of Cardiology
Houston, TX

Mary Larijani, MD
Assistant Professor of Pediatrics; Attending Physician
Dermatology Section
Department of Pediatrics
Perelman School of Medicine
Children's Hospital of Philadelphia
Philadelphia, PA

Michael Lawrenz Co, MD, MSc
Electrophysiology
Division of Cardiology
Thomas Jefferson University
Philadelphia, PA

Peter Le, MD
Pulmonary and Critical Care Physician
Kaiser Permanente Oakland Medical Center
Department of Pulmonary Medicine
The Permanente Medical Group
Oakland, CA

Lorriana E. Leard, MD
Professor of Clinical Medicine
Vice Chief, Clinical Operations
Division of Pulmonary, Critical Care, Allergy and Sleep Medicine
University of California San Francisco
San Francisco, CA

David A. Leavitt, MD
Associate Director of Endourology
Director of Laser Surgery
Vattikuti Urology Institute
Henry Ford Hospital Health System
Detroit, MI

Christopher T. Leba, MD, MPH
Pulmonary and Critical Care Medicine Fellow
Division of Pulmonary, Critical Care, Allergy and Sleep Medicine
University of California San Francisco
San Francisco, CA

Kachiu C. Lee, MD, MPH
Assistant Professor
Department of Dermatology
Temple University
Philadelphia, PA

Nicholas J. Lemme, MD
Department of Orthopaedic Surgery
Warren Alpert Medical School of Brown University
Providence, RI

Jian Li, MD, PhD
Clinical Assistant Professor
Wayne State University School of Medicine/Henry Ford Hospital
Division of Nephrology and Hypertension
Detroit, MI

Leora Lieberman, MD
Hospitalist Physician
Department of Anesthesiology and Critical Care Medicine
The Children's Hospital of Philadelphia
Philadelphia, PA

Carol Lim, MD, MPH
Psychiatrist
Massachusetts General Hospital
Instructor of Psychiatry
Harvard Medical School
Boston, MA

Jason Lin, BA
Department of Orthopaedic Surgery
UT Southwestern
Dallas, TX

Jordan Lippincott, MD
Depeartment of Emergency Medicine
University of Tennessee Health Science Center
Memphis, TN

Jonathan Liu, MD
Orthopedic Surgery
Warren Alpert Medical School of Brown University
Providence, RI

Teresa C. Logue, MD, MPH
Obstetrics & Gynecology
ChristianaCare Health System
Newark, DE

Gabriela López, PhD
Brown University, Center for Alcohol and Addiction Studies (CAAS)
Providence, RI

Kito Akin Lord, MD, MBA
Assistant Professor
Department of Emergency Medicine
University of Tennessee Health Science Center
Memphis, TN

Mathew J. Lucas, MD
Department of Pediatrics
The Children's Hospital of Philadelphia
Philadelphia, PA

David J. Lucier, Jr., MD, MBA, MPH, CPPS
Director of Quality and Patient Safety, Hospital Medicine
Division of General Internal Medicine
Massachusetts General Hospital
Boston, MA

Marwan Ma'ayeh, MD, BCh
Maternal-Fetal Medicine
ChristianaCare Health System
Newark, DE

Rachel L. Maclean, MD
Department of Psychiatry
Massachusetts General Hospital
Boston, MA

Maeve G. MacMurdo, MBChB, MPH
Clinical Associate
Respiratory Institute
Cleveland Clinic
Cleveland, OH

Elizabeth N. Madva, MD
Member of the Faculty of Psychiatry
Department of Psychiatry
Massachusetts General Hospital
Harvard Medical School
Boston, MA

Sahar Mahani, MD
Department of Internal Medicine
Northwell Health, Lenox Hill Hospital
New York, NY

Gretchen Makai, MD
Director, Division of Minimally Invasive Gynecologic Surgery
Department of Obstetrics & Gynecology
ChristianaCare Health System
Newark, DE

Luis Malpica, MD
Assistant Professor
The University of Texas
Physician
The University of Texas MD Anderson Cancer Center
Houston, TX

Stephen E. Marcaccio, MD
Department of Orthopaedic Surgery
Warren Alpert Medical School of Brown University
Providence, RI

Ana Paula Marques Pinheiro, MD
Department of Psychiatry MGH/McLean
Boston, MA

Peter J. Mazzaglia, MD
Associate Professor of Surgery
Warren Alpert Medical School of Brown University
Providence, RI

Nadine N. Mbuyi, MD
Assistant Professor of Medicine
Department of Medicine
Washington, DC

Russell J. McCulloh, MD
Professor, Pediatrics
University of Nebraska Medical Center
Omaha, NE

Christopher L. McDonald, MD
Department of Orthopedic Surgery
Warren Alpert Medical School of Brown University
Providence, RI

Donna M. McDonald-McGinn, MS, LCGC
Professor of Clinical Pediatrics
Director, 22q and You Center
Chief, Section of Genetic Counseling
Associate Director, Clinical Genetics Center
Research Scientist
The Children's Hospital of Philadelphia
Perelman School of Medicine of the University of Pennsylvania
Philadelphia, PA

Alexandra McGowen, MD
Department of Emergency Medicine
UTHSC
Memphis, TN

Katherine Elizabeth McGraw, MD
Pediatrician
Children's Hospital & Medical Center
Omaha, NE

Jaclyn McKenna, MD
Primary Care Sports Medicine
University of South Carolina/Prisma Health
Columbia, SC

Kelly McNamara, MD
Obstetrics & Gynecology Attending Generalist Physician
Obstetrics & Gynecology
ChristianaCare Health System
Newark, DE

Kelly C. Mead, MD
Department of Orthopaedic Surgery
Warren Alpert Medical School of Brown University
Providence, RI

Caroline P. Meehan, MD
Hospice & Palliative Medicine
Brown University
Providence, RI

Ozair K. Meghani, BA
Department of Orthopaedics
Warren Alpert Medical School of Brown University
Providence, RI

Kapil S. Meleveedu, MD
Director, Blood and Marrow Transplant and Head of Hematological Malignancies
Department of Hematology-Oncology
University of Connecticut
Farmington, CT

Dianelys Mendez, MD
Department of Clinical Endocrinology
Warren Alpert Medical School of Brown University
Providence, RI

Megan Mendez-Miller, DO
Associate Professor
Department of Family and Community Medicine Residency Program
Penn State Health M.S. Hershey Medical Center
Hershey, PA

Jorge Mercado, MD
Clinical Associate Professor of Medicine
NYU School of Medicine
New York, NY
Director of Pulmonary Section
Director of Bronchoscopy
Associate Director, Pulmonary and Critical Care Section
NYU Langone Brooklyn Hospital
Brooklyn, NY

Osvaldo Mercado, MD
Division of Neonatology
Children's Hospital of Philadelphia
Philadelphia, PA

Scott J. Merrill, MD
Obstetrics & Gynecology
ChristianaCare Health System
Newark, DE

Rory Merritt, MD, MEHP
Assistant Dean of Medicine – PLME Advising
Assistant Professor of Emergency Medicine
Warren Alpert Medical School of Brown University
Providence, RI

Marian G. Michaels, MD, MPH
Professor of Pediatrics and Surgery
Division of Infectious Diseases
Children's Hospital of Pittsburgh of UPMC
Pittsburgh, PA

Jeremy Michel, MD, MHS
Attending Physician
Department of Pediatrics
Children's Hospital of Philadelphia
Philadelphia, PA

Brian D. Mikolasko, MD
Assistant Professor of Medicine
Division of Geriatric and Palliative Medicine
Warren Alpert Medical School of Brown University
Providence, RI

John D. Milner, MD
Department of Orthopaedic Surgery
Warren Alpert Medical School of Brown University
Providence, RI

May Min, MD
Attending Physician
Division of Gastroenterology
Warren Alpert Medical School of Brown University
Providence, RI

Taro Minami, MD
Director, Intensive Care Unit (ICU) at Kent Hospital
Division of Pulmonary, Critical Care, and Sleep Medicine, Care New England
Director of Medical Simulation and Point-of-Care Ultrasound (POCUS)
  Training
Department of Medicine at Kent Hospital and Care New England
Associate Professor of Medicine, Clinician Educator
Associate Professor of Medical Science, Clinician Educator
Warren Alpert Medical School of Brown University
Providence, RI

Rei Mitsuyama, MD
Department of Medicine
Brown University
Providence, RI

Laura Miyares, MD
Department of Pediatrics
Children's Hospital of Philadelphia
Philadelphia, PA

Ankur Mogla, MD
Nephrology and Hypertension
Henry Ford Hospital
Detroit, MI

Javad Najjar Mojarrab, MD, MBA
Fellow in Nephrology/Critical Care
Henry Ford Hospital
Detroit, MI

Philippe Montgrain, MD
Professor of Medicine
Division of Pulmonary, Critical Care and Sleep Medicine
University of California San Diego
La Jolla, CA

Michael Z. Moore, MD
Multiple Sclerosis Clinical Fellow
Maxine Mesinger Multiple Sclerosis Clinic
Baylor College of Medicine
Houston, TX

Shawn D. Moore, MD
Department of Adult Neurology
Baylor College of Medicine
Houston, TX

Leah Morelli, MD
Child & Adolescent Psychiatry
Department of Child Psychiatry
Massachusetts General Hospital
Boston, MA

Patrick J. Morrissey, MD
Orthopaedic Surgery
Brown University
Providence, RI

Aleem I. Mughal, MD, FHRS
Cardiac Electrophysiologist
Department of Electrophysiology
Heart Center of North Texas
Medical Director
Department of Electrophysiology
Baylor All Saints Hospital
Baylor Heart and Vascular Hospital
Fort Worth, TX

Shiva Kumar R. Mukkamalla, MD, MPH
Attending Physician
Hematology/Oncology
Presbyterian Healthcare Services
Rio Rancho, NM
Assistant Professor
Burrell College of Osteopathic Medicine
Las Cruces, NM

Katherine M. Mullersman, MD
Massachusetts General Hospital
McLean Hospital
Harvard Medical School
Boston, MA

Ahmad Mumtaz, MD
Department of Neurology
Baylor College of Medicine
Houston, TX

Fadeke Muraina, MD
Department of Psychiatry
Massachusetts General Hospital/McLean Hospital
Boston, MA

Ahmad Mustafa, MD
Department of Internal Medicine
Northwell Health – Staten Island University Hospital
New York, NY

Ellen Myers, MD
Obstetrician/Gynecologist
ChristianaCare Health System
Newark, DE

Emily Mylhousen, MD
Department of Emergency Medicine
The University of Tennessee Health Sciences Center
Memphis, TN

Akash Nadella, BS
Warren Alpert Medical School of Brown University
Providence, RI

Mohnish Nadella, BS
Warren Alpert Medical of Brown University
Providence, RI

Nikita Nagpal, MD
Assistant Professor of Pediatrics
Department of Pediatrics
NYU Grossman School of Medicine/Bellevue Hospital Center
New York, NY

Minesh Nandi, MD
Department of Hematology/Oncology
University of Massachusetts Medical School
Worcester, MA

Uzma Nasir, MD
Assistant Professor, Clinical Anesthesia and Pain Management
SUNY at Stony Brook University Hospital, VA Hospital
Northport, NY

George H. Nasr, MD
Department of Cardiovascular Disease
UC Irvine Health
Division of Cardiology
Orange, CA

Asim Naveed, MD
Neurohospitalist
Willis-Knighton Healthcare System
Shreveport, LA

Robert Neff, MD
TriHealth Cancer Institute
Division of Gynecologic Oncology
Cincinnati, OH

Adrienne B. Neithardt, MD
Physician
Boston IVF
Waltham, MA & Newburgh, IN

Timothy Nelin, MD
Department of Neonatology
Children's Hospital of Philadelphia
Philadelphia, PA

Christina Nestlerode, DO
Department of OB/GYN
TriHealth
Cincinnati, OH

Samantha Ni, MD
Department of Emergency Medicine
University of Tennessee Health Science Center
Emergency Medicine Residency
Memphis, TN

Azfar K. Niazi, MD
Department of Internal Medicine
Greater Baltimore Medical Center
Baltimore, MD

Jonathan Nichols, DO
Cardiology Fellow
Maine Medical Center
Portland, ME

Natalie Nokoff, MD, MSCS
Assistant Professor
Department of Pediatrics
Section of Endocrinology
University of Colorado Anschutz Medical Campus
Aurora, CO

Ibrahim Z.D. Noorbhai, MD
Department of Neurology
Baylor College of Medicine
Houston, TX

James E. Novak, MD, PhD
Nephrology Program Director
Henry Ford Hospital and Professor of Clinical Medicine
Michigan State University
Detroit, MI

Austin Novarra, MD
MGH/McLean Department of Psychiatry
Mass General Brigham
Boston, MA

Emily E. Nuss, MD
Department of Obstetrics & Gynecology
ChristianaCare Health System
Newark, DE

Rebecca Oliver, DO
Obstetrician/Gynecologist
TriHealth Obstetrics and Gynecology
Cincinnati, OH

Adam J. Olszewski, MD
Associate Professor of Medicine
Warren Alpert Medical School of Brown University
Providence, RI

Henry K. Onyeaka, MD, MPH
MGH/McLean Department of Psychiatry
Mass General Brigham
Boston, MA

Lindsay M. Orchowski, PhD
Associate Professor (Research)
Department of Psychiatry and Human Behavior
Warren Alpert Medical School of Brown University
Rhode Island Hospital
Providence, RI

Jasmine Outlaw, MD
Department of Psychiatry
Massachusetts General Hospital/McLean Hospital
Boston, MA

Brett D. Owens, MD
Orthopedic Sports Medicine Surgeon
Complex Shoulder and Knee Specialist
Warren Alpert Medical School of Brown University
Providence, RI

Ayotomide Oyelakin, MD, MPH
Assistant Professor of Psychiatry
Department of Psychiatry & Behavioral Sciences
McGovern Medical School at UTHealth
Houston, TX

Paolo G. Pace, MASc, MD
Department of Internal Medicine
Roger Williams Medical Center
Providence, RI

Isaac Palma-Zamora, MD
Vattikuti Urology Institute
Henry Ford Health System
Detroit, MI

Rachita Pandya, BA
Department of Dermatology
University of Pennsylvania
Philadelphia, PA

Lisa Pappas-Taffer, MD
Medical Director
Department of Dermatology
University of Pennsylvania
Philadelphia, PA

Sneha Paranandi, MD
Department of Obstetrics & Gynecology
ChristianaCare Health System
Newark, DE

Mihir Parikh, MD
Instructor in Medicine
Division of Thoracic Surgery & Interventional Pulmonology
Beth Israel Deaconess Medical Center
Department of Medicine
Harvard Medical School
Boston, MA

Sara Park, MD
Department of Anesthesiology
Brown University
Providence, RI

Michael T. Partin, MD
Assistant Professor
Department of Family and Community Medicine
Penn State Health M. S. Hershey Medical Center
Hershey, PA

Birju B. Patel, MD
Assistant Professor of Medicine
Department of Medicine
Division of Geriatrics and Gerontology
Emory University School of Medicine
Atlanta Veterans Affairs Medical Center
Atlanta, GA

Melissa D. Patel, MD, MPH
Associate Professor of Clinical Pediatrics
University of Pennsylvania School of Medicine
Section Chief, Pediatric Hospital Medicine
The Children's Hospital of Philadelphia
Philadelphia, PA

Minta Patel, MD
Internal Medicine
Cambridge Memorial Hospital
Cambridge, Ontario
Canada

Nima R. Patel, MD, MS
Minimally Invasive Gynecologic Surgeon & Residency Program Director
Department of Obstetrics and Gynecology
TriHealth
Cincinnati, OH

Pranav M. Patel, MD, FACC, FAHA, FSCAI
Professor of Medicine and Biomedical Engineering
Chief, Division of Cardiology
University of California, Irvine
Orange, CA

Vidhi Patel, MBBS
Clinical Research Coordinator
Department of Cardiovascular Surgery–Lenox Hill Hospital
Northwell Health
New York, NY

Brett Patrick, MD
Residency Curriculum Director
Emergency Medicine
University of Tennessee Health Science Center
Memphis, TN

Shreedhar Paudel, MD, MPH
Psychiatrist
Massachusetts General Hospital
Assistant Professor of Psychiatry
Harvard Medical School
Boston, MA

E. Scott Paxton, MD
Attending Orthopaedic Surgeon
Department of Orthopedics
Brown University
Providence, RI

Celeste Peay, MD, JD
Department of Psychiatry
Harvard Medical School
House Officer in Psychiatry
Massachusetts General Hospital and McLean Hospital
Boston, MA

Mark A. Perazella, MD, FASN, FNKF
Professor of Medicine
Section of Nephrology
Department of Internal Medicine
Yale University School of Medicine
New Haven, CT

David L. Perez, MD, MMSc
Associate Professor of Neurology
Departments of Neurology and Psychiatry
Massachusetts General Hospital
Harvard Medical School
Boston, MA

Jose J. Hermina Perez, MD
Department of Psychiatry
Massachusetts General Hospital/McLean Hospital
Harvard Medical School
Boston, MA

Erin Pete Devon, MD
Assistant Professor of Clinical Pediatrics
Children's Hospital of Philadelphia
Perelman School of Medicine
University of Pennsylvania
Philadelphia, PA

Courtney Pfeuti, MD
Department of Obstetrics & Gynecology
ChristianaCare Health System
Newark, DE

Lily C. Pham, MD
Assistant Professor
Department of Neurology, Division of Neuro-Oncology
University of Maryland School of Medicine
Baltimore, MD

Kendall Phelps-Polirer, MD
Department of Internal Medicine
HCA Florida Blake Medical Center
Bradenton, FL

Katharine A. Phillips, MD
DeWitt Wallace Senior Scholar
Professor of Psychiatry
Department of Psychiatry
Weill Cornell Medical College
Attending Psychiatrist
New York-Presbyterian Hospital
New York, NY

Oliver W. Phillips, MD
Movement Disorders
Center for Neurological Restoration
Cleveland Clinic
Cleveland, OH

Tara M. Phillips, CRNP
Pediatric Nurse Practitioner
Department of Urology
Children's Hospital of Philadelphia
Philadelphia, PA

Lauren E. Piana, MD
Department of Orthopaedic Surgery
Warren Alpert Medical School of Brown University
Providence, RI

Brandon Portnoff, BS
Department of Orthopedics
Brown University
Providence, RI

Mitchell Powell, MD
Department of Neurology
Baylor College of Medicine
Houston, TX

Alexander Powers, MD
Department of Psychiatry
Harvard Medical School
Resident, Adult Psychiatry
Massachusetts General Hospital/McLean Hospital
Boston, MA

Rohini Prashar, MD
Senior Staff
Division of Nephrology
Henry Ford Hospital
Detroit, MI

Ned Premyodhin, MD
Division of Cardiology
University of California, Irvine
Orange, CA

Dana Price, MD
Department of Cardiology
Warren Alpert Medical School of Brown University
Providence, RI

Margaret Priestley, MD
Senior Medical Director, Pediatric Intensive Care Unit
Department of Anesthesiology and Critical Care Medicine
Children's Hospital of Philadelphia
Philadelphia, PA

Christian Provenza, MD
Department of Emergency Medicine
University of Tennessee Health Science Center
Memphis, TN

Christine Pulice, DO
Clinical Professor of Pediatrics
General Pediatrics
The Children's Hospital of Philadelphia
Philadelphia, PA

Diana Punko, MD, MS
Instructor
Department of Psychiatry
Harvard Medical School
Boston, MA

Imran Puthawala, MD
Division of Hematology/Oncology
University of Massachusetts Memorial Medical Center
Worcester, MA

Imrana Qawi, MD
Assistant Professor
Pulmonary and Critical Care Medicine
Tufts Medical Center
Boston, MA

David Qu, MD
Emergency Medicine
University of Tennessee Health Science Center
Memphis, TN

Adrian Quesada, MD
Attending Physician
Department of Obstetrics & Gynecology
ChristianaCare Health System
Newark, DE

Matthew Quinn, MD
Department of Orthopaedics
Brown University/Rhode Island Hospital
Providence, RI

Gregory S. Rachu, MD, MPH
Assistant Professor of Medicine
Division of Geriatrics and Palliative Medicine
Warren Alpert Medical School of Brown University
Providence, RI

Amulya Rajagopal, MD
Physician
Henry Ford Hospital
Detroit, MI

Bharti Rathore, MD
Assistant Professor
Boston University School of Medicine
Program Director, Hematology/Oncology Fellowship
Roger Williams Medical Center
Providence, RI

Ritesh Rathore, MD
Associate Professor
Boston University School of Medicine
Director, Hematology/Oncology
Roger Williams Medical Center
Providence, RI

Neha P. Raukar, MD, MS
Consultant, Emergency Medicine
Mayo Clinic
Rochester, MN

Lakshmi Ravindra, MD
Department of Medicine
Warren Alpert Medical School of Brown University
Providence, RI

John L. Reagan, MD
Hematologist-Oncologist
Division of Hematology/Oncology
Warren Alpert Medical School of Brown University
Providence, RI

P.K. Reardon, MD, DPhil
Department of Psychiatry
Massachusetts General Hospital and McLean Hospital
Clinical Fellow
Harvard Medical School
Boston, MA

Bharathi V. Reddy, MD
Associate Professor of Medicine
Department of Medicine
Section of Nephrology
University of Chicago
Chicago, IL

Snigdha T. Reddy, MD
Division of Nephrology
Henry Ford Hospital
Detroit, MI

Anne Reed-Weston, MD
Resident, Obstetrics and Gynecology
ChristianaCare Health System
Newark, DE

Anthony M. Reginato, PhD, MD
Division of Rheumatology
Interim Director, Division of Rheumatology
Associate Professor of Medicine
Warren Alpert Medical School of Brown University
Director of Rheumatology Research and Musculoskeletal Ultrasound
Rhode Island Hospital
Chief, Division of Rheumatology
Providence Veteran Affairs Medical Center
Providence, RI

James P. Reichart, MD
Department of Medicine
Lehigh Valley Health Network
Allentown, PA

Victor I. Reus, MD
Emeritus Distinguished Professor
Department of Psychiatry and Behavioral Sciences
Weill Institute for Neurosciences
University of California (UCSF)
San Francisco School of Medicine
San Francisco, CA

Harlan G. Rich, MD, FACP, AGAF
Associate Professor of Medicine
Division of Gastroenterology
Brown University
Providence, RI

Lauren Davis Rivera, MD, MSEd
Obstetrics & Gynecology
ChristianaCare Health Services
Newark, DE

Melena J. Robertson, DO
Pediatric Infectious Diseases
Division of Infectious Diseases
Children's Hospital of Pittsburgh of UPMC
Pittsburgh, PA

Lauren Roby, MD
Obstetrics & Gynecology
ChristianaCare Health Services
Newark, DE

Meaghan Roche, MD
Clinical Assistant Professor
Department of Medicine
Michigan State University College of Human Medicine
Senior Staff Physician
Henry Ford Health
Detroit, MI

Alejandra E. Morfin Rodriguez, MD
Massachusetts General Hospital/Mclean Hospital Adult Psychiatry Residency
Harvard Medical School
Boston, MA

Perla M. Romero Gómez, MD
Department of Psychiatry
University of New Mexico
Albuquerque, NM

Hayley A. Ron, MD
Medical Geneticist
The Children's Hospital of Philadelphia
Philadelphia, PA

Blake L. Rosenbaum, MD
Department of Psychiatry
Massachusetts General Hospital
Boston, MA

Michael Rossi, MD
Department of Infectious Disease
Rhode Island Hospital/The Miriam Hospital
Warren Alpert Medical School of Brown University
Providence, RI

Breton Roussel, MD
Department of Gastroenterology
Rhode Island Hospital
Providence, RI

David Rubin, MD
Assistant Professor, Harvard Medical School
Director, Child and Adolescent Psychiatry Residency Training
Massachusetts General Hospital/McLean Hospital
Executive Director, MGH Psychiatry Academy
Boston, MA

Kelly Ruhstaller, MD
Obstetrician/Gynecologist
ChristianaCare Health System
Newark, DE

Beth H. Rutstein, MD, MSCE
Attending Physician
Division of Rheumatology, Department of Pediatrics
The Children's Hospital of Philadelphia
Philadelphia, PA

Noushine Sadeghi, MD
Department of Obstetrics & Gynecology
ChristianaCare Health System
Newark, DE

Ruchi Jalota Sahota, MD
Department of Nephrology
Henry Ford
Detroit, MI

Emily Saks, MD, MSCE
Physician
Female Pelvic Medicine and Reconstructive Surgery
ChristianaCare Health System
Newark, DE

Jeffrey W. Sall, PhD, MD
Professor of Anesthesia and Perioperative Care
University of California San Francisco
San Francisco, CA

Joshua D. Salvi, MD, PhD
Psychiatrist
Department of Psychiatry
Massachusetts General Hospital
Instructor in Psychiatry
Harvard Medical School
Boston, MA

Frank Sanchez, MD, MBA
Physician
Internal Medicine/GME
New York Medical College/Landmark Medical Center
Woonsocket, RI

Martha C. Sanchez, MD
Assistant Professor of Medicine
Division of Infectious Diseases
Warren Alpert Medical School of Brown University
Providence, RI

Pranavi Sanka, MD
Department of Internal Medicine
Warren Alpert Medical School of Brown University
Providence, RI

Lekshmi Santhosh, MD, MAEd
Associate Professor of Clinical Medicine
Division of Pulmonary, Critical Care, Allergy and Sleep Medicine
University of California San Francisco
San Francisco, CA

Linda Herrera Santos, MD, PhD
Psychiatry Department
Massachusetts General Hospital
Boston, MA

Emily Sauck, DO, MBA
Department of Obstetrics & Gynecology
ChristianaCare Health System
Newark, DE

Syeda M. Sayeed, MD
Attending Physician, Department of Rheumatology
South Coast Health
Fall River, MA

Leah Saylor, DO
Department of Obstetrics and Gynecology
TriHealth
Cincinnati, OH

Phillip R. Schmitt, BS
Warren Alpert Medical School of Brown University
Providence, RI

Anthony Sciscione, DO
Professor, Obstetrics and Gynecology
Jefferson Medical College
Philadelphia, PA
Residency Program Director
Director of Maternal-Fetal Medicine
Department of Obstetrics & Gynecology
ChristianaCare Health System
Newark, DE

Bethany K. Sederdahl, MD, MPH
Department of Obstetrics & Gynecology
ChristianaCare Hospital
Newark, DE

Richard E. Seeber, II, MD
Department of Psychiatry
Massachusetts General Hospital and McLean Hospital
Clinical Fellow
Harvard Medical School
Boston, MA

Aritra Sen, MD
Department of Pulmonary/Critical Care
Tufts Medical Center
Boston, MA

Rachel Sewell, MD
Department of Pediatrics
Section of Endocrinology
University of Colorado Anschutz Medical Campus
Aurora, CO

Hesham Shaban, MD, FRCP
Senior Staff
Division of Nephrology and Hypertension
Henry Ford Hospital
Detroit, MI

Ankur Shah, MD
Assistant Professor of Medicine
Division of Kidney Disease and Hypertension
Warren Alpert Medical School of Brown University
Providence, RI

Aaron Ali Shaikh, MD
Department of Cardiology
Maine Medical Center
Portland, ME

Animesh Sharma, MD
Assistant Professor of Pediatrics
Pediatric Endocrinology
Children's Hospital of Colorado
Aurora, CO

Yuvraj Sharma, MD
Senior Staff
Division of Nephrology and Hypertension
Henry Ford Hospital
Detroit, MI

Lydia Sharp, MD
Assistant Professor
Department of Neurology
Baylor College of Medicine
Houston, TX

Wasiq Sheikh, MD, MMSc
Warren Alpert Medical School of Brown University
Providence, RI

Alexander Sherman, MD
Clinical Instructor
Division of Pulmonary, Critical Care, and Sleep Medicine
University of California Los Angeles
Los Angeles, CA

Jessica E. Shill, MD
Senior Staff Physician
Division of Endocrinology, Diabetes and Bone and Mineral Disorders
Henry Ford Health
Detroit, MI
Clinical Associate Professor of Medicine
Wayne State University School of Medicine
Detroit, MI

Alexei Shimanovsky, MD
Clinical Assistant Professor of Medicine
Hematology & Oncology
Brown University/Alpert Medical School
Lifespan Cancer Institute
The Miriam Hospital & Rhode Island Hospital
Providence, RI

Philip A. Shlossman, MD
Managing Partner
Delaware Center for Maternal Fetal Medicine
Newark, DE

Khawja A. Siddiqui, MD
Assistant Professor of Neurology
Baylor College of Medicine
Houston, TX

Alyssa Siegel, MD
Attending Physician
General Pediatrics, Children's Hospital of Philadelphia
Clinical Assistant Professor
Perelman School of Medicine at the University of Pennsylvania
Philadelphia, PA

Mark Sigman, MD
Krishnamurthi Family Professor of Urology
Professor of Surgery (Urology)
Professor of Pathology and Laboratory Medicine
Warren Alpert Medical School of Brown University
Providence, RI

Rebecca Simon, MD
Department of Pediatrics
NYU Langone and Bellevue
New York, NY

Harinder P. Singh, MD
Assistant Professor
Department of Pulmonary and Critical Care Medicine
Carney Hospital, Tufts University
Boston, MA

Brett Slingsby, MD
Assistant Professor of Pediatrics, Clinical Instructor
Warren Alpert Medical School of Brown University
Providence, RI

Amy Sloane, MD
Attending Physician
Holy Redeemer Hospital
Philadelphia, PA

Alexandra H. Smick, MD
Department of Obstetrics & Gynecology
TriHealth
Cincinnati, OH

Devon Smith, DO
Female Pelvic Medicine & Reconstructive Surgery
Department of Obstetrics & Gynecology
Cooper University Hospital
Camden, NJ

Jeanette G. Smith, MD
Assistant Professor
Division of Gastroenterology
Department of Medicine
Warren Alpert Medical School of Brown University
Providence, RI

Matthew J. Smith, MD
Physician
University Orthopedics, Inc.
Providence, RI

Ryann Sohaney, DO, MS
Division of Nephrology
Henry Ford Hospital
Detroit, MI

Vivek Soi, MD
Clinical Associate Professor
Wayne State University
Internal Medicine
Detroit, MI

Rebecca Soinski, MD
Rheumatologist
Women's Medicine Collaborative
Providence, RI

Maria E. Soler, MD, MPH, MBA
Director, Education Division and OB Triage
Department of Obstetrics & Gynecology
ChristianaCare Health System
Newark, DE

Sandeep Soman, MD
Division of Nephrology
Henry Ford Hospital
Detroit, MI

Jeffrey S. Song, MD
Department of Critical Care Nephrology
Henry Ford Health
Detroit, MI

Emily Sorg, MD
Psychiatrist
Massachusetts General Hospital
Boston, MA

C. John Sperati, MD, MHS
Associate Professor of Medicine
Division of Nephrology
Johns Hopkins University School of Medicine
Baltimore, MD

Nathan Stanford, MD
Department of Emergency Medicine
University of Tennessee Health Science Center
Memphis, TN

Seth Daly Stennis, MD
Department of Psychiatry
Massachusetts General Hospital/McLean Hospital
Boston, MA

Michael S. Stephens, MD
Department of Emergency Medicine
Mayo Clinic
Rochester, MN

Ella Stern, MD
Division of Obstetrics & Gynecology
ChristianaCare Health Services
Newark, DE

Philip Stockwell, MD
Associate Professor of Medicine (Clinician Educator)
Warren Alpert Medical School of Brown University
Providence, RI

Edward Suh, MD, MPH
Assistant Professor
Department of Anesthesiology
Brown University
Providence, RI

Jennifer K. Sun, MD, PhD
Internal Medicine-Pediatrics
Children's Hospital of Philadelphia/Hospital of the University of Pennsylvania
Philadelphia, PA

Anjali Sundaramoorthy, DO
Neurologist
Baylor Scott & White Comprehensive Headache Center
Dallas, TX

Varut Supanakorn, MD
Staff Attending of Otolaryngology
Department of Otolaryngology
King Chulalongkorn Memorial Hospital
Bangkok, Thailand

Priyasha Suri, MD
Department of Critical Care
Max Healthcare
Dehradun, Uttarakhand
India

Stephanie Sutter, MD
Department of Anesthesia and Perioperative Care
University of California San Francisco
San Francisco, CA

Hannah Sweeney, MD
Department of Obstetrics & Gynecology
ChristianaCare Health System
Newark, DE

Kaoru Takasaki, MD
Instructor of Hematology
Division of Hematology
Department of Pediatrics
Children's Hospital of Philadelphia
Philadelphia, PA

Ryosuke Takei, MD
Attending Physician
Division of General Pediatrics
Section of Pediatric Hospital Medicine
Children's Hospital of Philadelphia
Philadelphia, PA

Laren Tan, MD, MBA
Associate Professor of Medicine
Chair, Department of Medicine
Division of Pulmonary, Critical Care, Hyperbaric, Allergy and Sleep Medicine
Department of Medicine
Loma Linda University Health
Loma Linda, CA

Alan Taylor, MD
Program Director
Emergency Medicine
University of Tennessee Health Science Center
Memphis, TN

Matthew Taylor, MD
Department of Medicine
Rhode Island Hospital
Providence, RI

S. Trevor Taylor, MD, MPH
Department of Psychiatry
Harvard Medical School
Resident Physician
Massachusetts General Hospital and McLean Hospital
Boston, MA

Tahir Tellioglu, MD
Addiction Psychiatrist
Massachusetts General Hospital
Instructor of Psychiatry
Harvard Medical School
Boston, MA

Edward J. Testa, MD
Department of Orthopedics
Brown University
Providence, RI

Anthony G. Thomas, DO, FACP
Clinical Assistant Professor of Medicine
Hematology & Oncology
Warren Alpert Medical School of Brown University
Lifespan Cancer Institute
The Miriam Hospital & Rhode Island Hospital
Providence, RI

Stefani Thompson, MD
Department of Nephrology and Critical Care
Henry Ford Hospital
Detroit, MI

Alexandra Meyer Tien, MD
Clinical Assistant Professor
Department of Family Medicine
Warren Alpert Medical School of Brown University
Providence, RI

David Robbins Tien, MD
Clinical Associate Professor
Department of Surgery (Ophthalmology)
Warren Alpert Medical School of Brown University
Providence, RI

Anna-Marie Tierney, MD
Attending Physician, Care Network South Philadelphia
Children's Hospital of Philadelphia
Clinical Associate Professor of Pediatrics
University of Pennsylvania School of Medicine
Philadelphia, PA

Patrick Tiffany, MD
Department of Pediatrics
Colorado University School of Medicine
Aurora, CO

Helen Toma, MD, MSPH
Department of Obstetrics & Gynecology
ChristianaCare Health System
Newark, DE

Thomas M. Triplett, MD
Faculty
Emergency Medicine
University of Tennessee Health Science Center
Memphis, TN

Margaret Tryforos, MD
Family Medicine
Care New England Primary Care–Medical Group/Kent Hospital
Pawtucket, RI

Gal Tsaban, MD, MPH
Department of Cardiology
Soroka University Medical Center
Beer-Sheba, Israel

Christine Tschoe, MD
Department of Neurology
Baylor College of Medicine
Houston, TX

Joseph R. Tucci, MD, FACP, FACE
Professor of Medicine
Boston University School of Medicine
Director, Division of Endocrinology
Roger Williams Medical Center/Boston University School of Medicine
Adjunct Professor of Medicine
Warren Alpert Medical School of Brown University
Providence, RI

Julia Turock, MD
Department of Pediatrics
NYU School of Medicine
New York, NY

Junior Uduman, MD, MS
Division of Nephrology & Hypertension
Henry Ford Hospital
Clinical Assistant Professor
Michigan State University
Detroit, MI

Sean H. Uiterwyk, MD
Clinical Assistant Professor, Community and Family Medicine
Geisel School of Medicine at Dartmouth
Hanover, NH
White River Family Practice
White River Junction, VT

Rebecca Ukaegbu, MD
Department of Psychiatry
Massachusetts General Hospital and McLean Hospital
Boston, MA

Kausik Umanath, MD, MS, FASN
Associate Professor of Medicine
Wayne State University
Clinical Associate Professor
Michigan State University
Section Head, Clinical Research
Division of Nephrology and Hypertension
Henry Ford Health
Detroit, MI

Babak Vakili, MD
Faculty
Department of Obstetrics & Gynecology
ChristianaCare Health System
Newark, DE

Emily Van Kirk, MD
Department of Internal Medicine
Roger Williams Medical Center
Providence, RI

Ridhima Vemula, MD
Resident
TriHealth
Cincinnati, OH

Aida Venado, MD, MAS
Assistant Professor of Medicine
Division of Pulmonary, Critical Care, Allergy and Sleep Medicine
University of California, San Francisco
San Francisco, CA

Shilpa Vijayakumar, MD
Division of Cardiology
Department of Medicine
Warren Alpert Medical School of Brown University
Providence, RI

Kathryn G. Vollum, MD
Department of Obstetrics & Gynecology
ChristianaCare Health System
Newark, DE

Ethan Vorel, MD
Department of Pediatric Emergency Medicine
Johns Hopkins Children's Center
Baltimore, MD

Ifeanyi Walson, DO
Department of Psychiatry and Behavioral Medicine
Brody School of Medicine, East Carolina University
Greenville, NC

Angela Wang, MD
Clinical Professor
Pulmonary, Critical Care and Sleep Medicine
University of California San Diego
San Diego, CA

Jarey H. Wang, MD, PhD
Department of Radiation Oncology
Johns Hopkins University
Baltimore, MD

Manuel Shayne Weekley, MD
Clinical Faculty
University of Tennessee Health Sciences Center
Memphis, TN

Marc S. Weinberg, MD, PhD
Staff Psychiatrist, Department of Psychiatry
Staff Clinician, Department of Neurology
Massachusetts General Hospital
Instructor
Harvard Medical School
Boston, MA

Stephen Wendolowski, MD
Department of Orthopaedic Surgery
Warren Alpert Medical School of Brown University
Providence, RI

Roi Westreich, MD, PhD
Department of Cardiology
Soroka University Medical Center and Faculty of Health Sciences
Ben-Gurion University of the Negev
Beer-Sheva, Israel

Colin Whitaker, BA
Warren Alpert Medical School of Brown University
Providence, RI

Morgan Wilhoite, DO
Department of Obstetrics and Gynecology
TriHealth
Cincinnati, OH

Andrew Wilks, MD
Hematology Oncology
University of Massachusetts Medical Center
Worcester, MA

Annise Wilson, MD
Assistant Professor of Neurology and Medicine (Pulmonary, Critical Care and Sleep Medicine)
Baylor College of Medicine
Houston, TX

Jared M. Winikor, MD
Attending Physician
Pediatrics
Children's Hospital of Philadelphia
Philadelphia, PA

Bryce Wininger, MD
Attending Psychiatrist
Department of Psychiatry
Massachusetts General Hospital & Harvard Medical School
Boston, MA

Julia M. Winschel, MPH
Warren Alpert Medical School of Brown University
Providence, RI

Adam J. Wolpaw, MD, PhD
Assistant Professor of Pediatrics
Perelman School of Medicine at the University of Pennsylvania
Division of Oncology
The Children's Hospital of Philadelphia
Philadelphia, PA

Marlene Fishman Wolpert, MPH, CIC, FAPIC
Consultant in Infection Prevention and Control
Long-term Care Infection Preventionist
Infection Control and Epidemiology
Lifespan Health System
Providence, RI

Perry Wu, MD
Department of Medicine
Division of Cardiology
University of California Irvine Medical Center
Orange, CA

John Wylie, MD, FACC
Director, Cardiac Electrophysiology
Steward Health Care System
Associate Professor of Medicine
Tufts University School of Medicine
Adjunct Associate Professor of Medicine
Boston University School of Medicine
Boston, MA

Grace K. Yaguchi, MD
Department of Urology
Henry Ford Hospital
Detroit, MI

Anna Yang, MD
Assistant Professor
Emergency Medicine
University of Tennessee Health Science Center
Memphis, TN

Xuan Yao, MD
Division of Cardiology
St. Elizabeth's Medical Center
Boston, MA

Muhammad Yaseen, MD
Department of Nephrology
Henry Ford Hospital
Detroit, MI

Jerry Yee, MD, MACP, FRCP, FASN, FNKF [†]
Clinical Professor of Medicine
Henry Ford Hospital
Detroit, MI

Gemini Yesodharan, MD
Interventional Cardiology Fellow
Department of Cardiology
St. Elizabeth's Medical Center
Boston, MA

Jennifer Yeung, DO
FPMRS Program Director
TriHealth FPMRS Fellowship
Cincinnati, OH

Chun H. Yin, MD
General Pediatrics
CHOP Primary Care Moorestown
Children's Hospital of Philadelphia
Philadelphia, PA

Agustin G. Yip, MD, PhD
Medical Director
North Belknap 1
Division of Depression and Anxiety Disorders
McLean Hospital
Belmont, MA

Elizabeth An Yu, MD, PhD
Assistant Professor of Medicine
Division of Pulmonary, Critical Care, Allergy and Sleep Medicine
University of California San Francisco
San Francisco, CA

Juliana Zambrano, MD, MPH
Department of Psychiatry
Massachusetts General Hospital/McLean Hospital
Harvard Medical School
Boston, MA

Talia Zenlea, MD
Assistant Professor
Faculty of Medicine
Division of Gastroenterology and Hepatology
University of Toronto
Toronto, Ontario
Canada

B. Shoshana Zha, MD, PhD
Assistant Professor
Division of Pulmonary, Critical Care Allergy and Sleep Medicine
University of California San Francisco
San Francisco, CA

Helen Zhang, BS
Warren Alpert Medical School of Brown University
Providence, RI

Leon Zhao, BS
Orthopedics Research Intern
Warren Alpert Medical School of Brown University
Providence, RI

Diana X. Zhou, MD
Department of Emergency Medicine
University of Tennessee Health Science Center
Memphis, TN

Navid Ziaie, MD
Oregon Health and Science University
Division of Internal Medicine
Portland, OR

Joshua W. Zollman, MD
Department of Psychiatry
Massachusetts General Hospital and McLean Hospital
Boston, MA

Danylo Zorin, MD
Department of Cardiology
St. Elizabeth's Medical Center
Boston, MA

Olivia Zurek, MD
Psychiatrist
Department of Psychiatry
Massachusetts General Hospital and Spaulding Rehabilitation Hospital
Boston, MA

† Deceased.

Section Editors

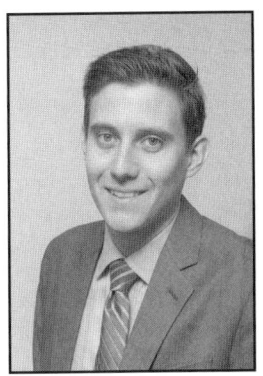

Scott R. Beach, MD, FACLP
Program Director, MGH/McLean Adult
  Psychiatry Residency
Associate Professor of Psychiatry
Harvard Medical School
Boston, Massachusetts

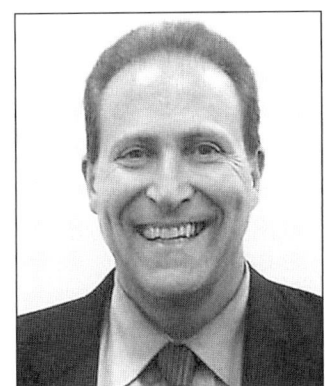

Fred F. Ferri, MD, FACP
Clinical Professor, Department of
  Medicine
Warren Alpert Medical School of
  Brown University
Providence, Rhode Island

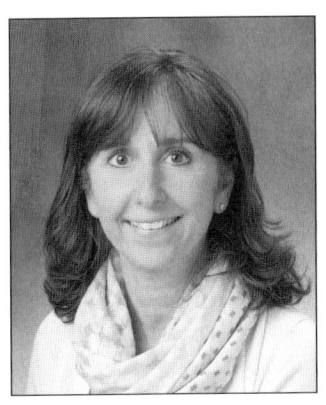

Cindy W. Christian, MD
Anthony A. Latini Chair in Child
  Abuse and Neglect Prevention
Children's Hospital of Philadelphia
Professor of Pediatrics
University of Pennsylvania
Perelman School of Medicine
Philadelphia, Pennsylvania

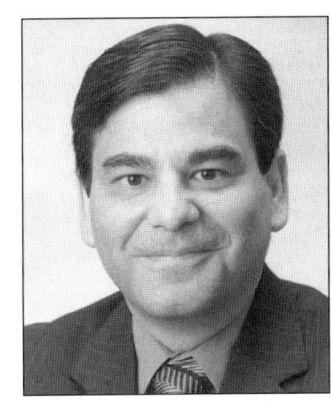

**Glenn G. Fort, MD, MPH,
FACP, FIDSA**
Clinical Associate Professor of
  Medicine
Warren Alpert Medical School of
  Brown University
Chief, Infectious Diseases
Our Lady of Fatima Hospital and
  Landmark Medical Center
Providence, Rhode Island

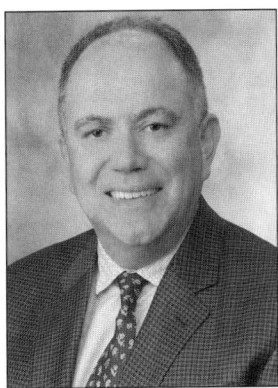

Manuel F. DaSilva, MD
Associate Professor
Director, Medical Student Education
Department of Orthopedic Surgery
Warren Alpert Medical School of Brown
  University
Providence, Rhode Island

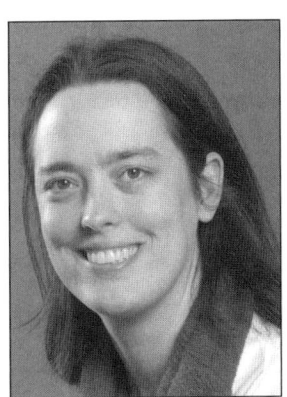

**Corey Elam Goldsmith, MD,
FAAN**
Assistant Professor of Neurology
Neurology Residency Program Director
Baylor College of Medicine
Chief of Neurology Outpatient Clinics
Ben Taub Hospital—Harris Health
  System
Houston, Texas

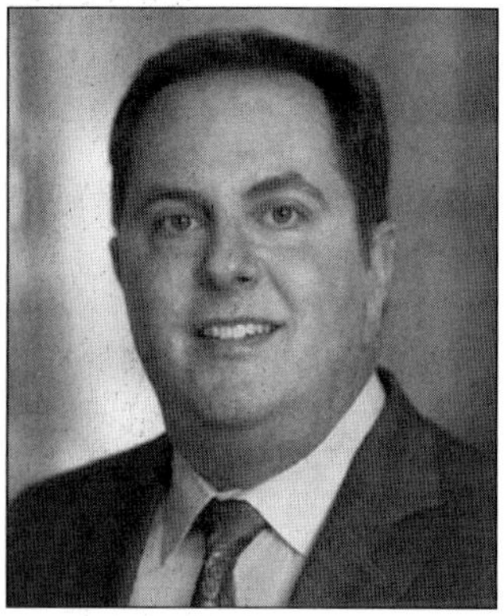

Joseph S. Kass, MD, JD, FAAN
Associate Dean of Student Affairs
Professor of Neurology, Psychiatry, and Medical Ethics
Director, Alzheimer's Disease and Memory Disorders Center
Baylor College of Medicine
Houston, Texas

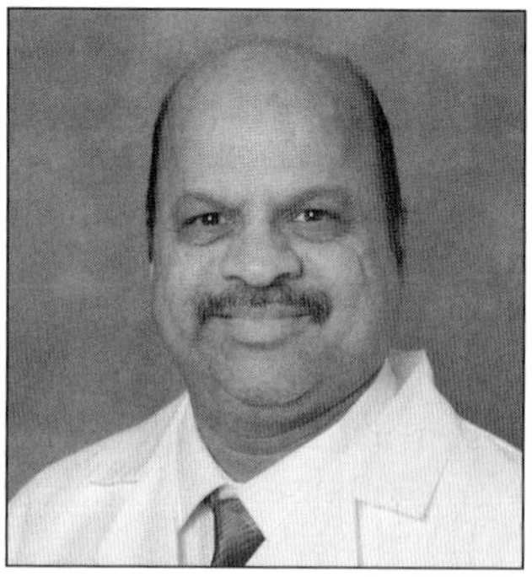

Sandeep S. Soman, MD, FNKF, FAMIA
Physician
Associate Division Head
Division of Nephrology and Hypertension
Henry Ford Hospital
Detroit, Michigan

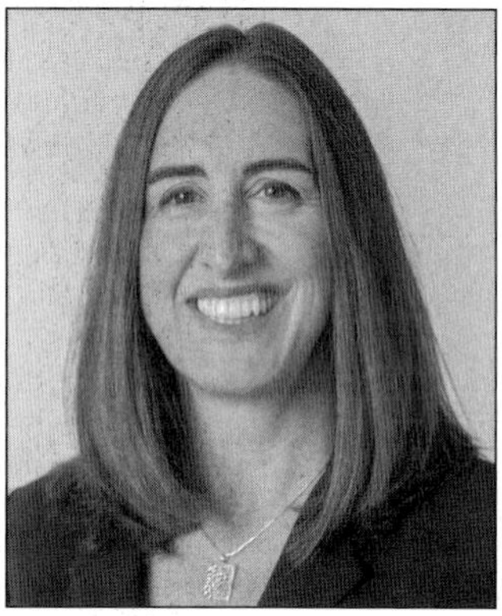

Lorriana E. Leard, MD, FACCP
Professor of Clinical Medicine
Vice Chief, Clinical Operations, Division of Pulmonary, Critical Care, Allergy and Sleep Medicine
University of California San Francisco
San Francisco, California

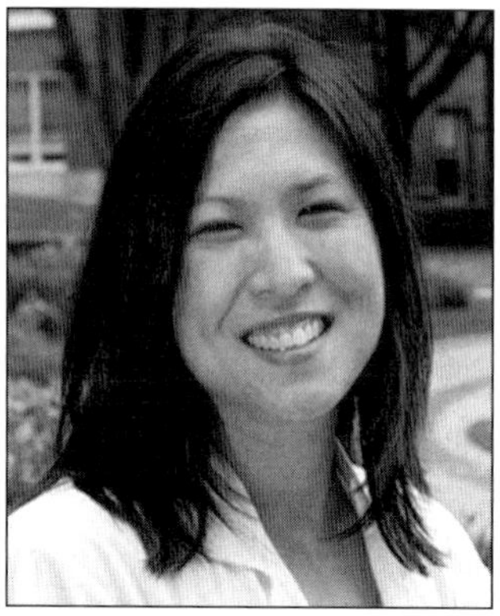

Iris L. Tong, MD
Associate Professor
Department of Medicine
Warren Alpert Medical School of Brown University
Attending Physician
Women's Primary Care
Women's Medicine Collaborative
Providence, Rhode Island

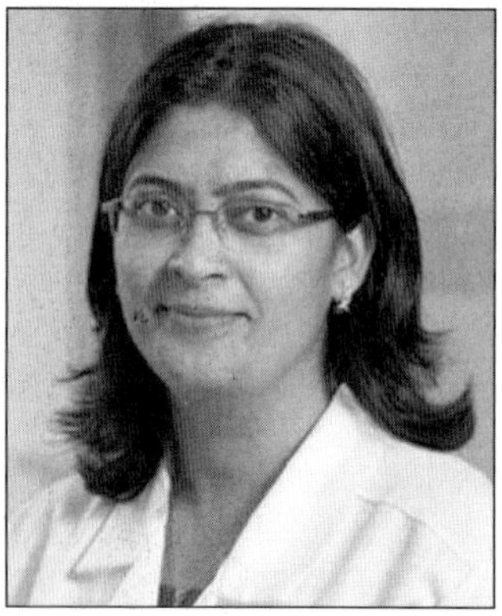

Bharti Rathore, MD
Program Director, Hematology/Oncology Fellowship
Roger Williams Medical Center
Providence, Rhode Island
Assistant Professor of Medicine
Boston University School of Medicine
Boston, Massachusetts

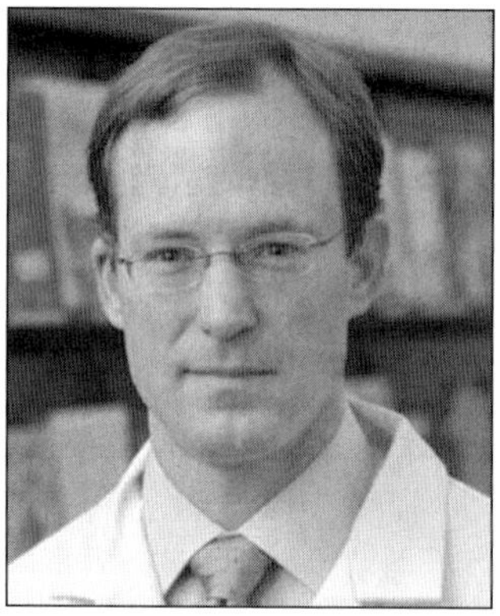

John Wylie, MD, FACC
Director, Cardiac
Electrophysiology
Steward Health Care System
Associate Professor of Medicine
Tufts University School of Medicine
St. Elizabeth's Medical Center
Boston, Massachusetts

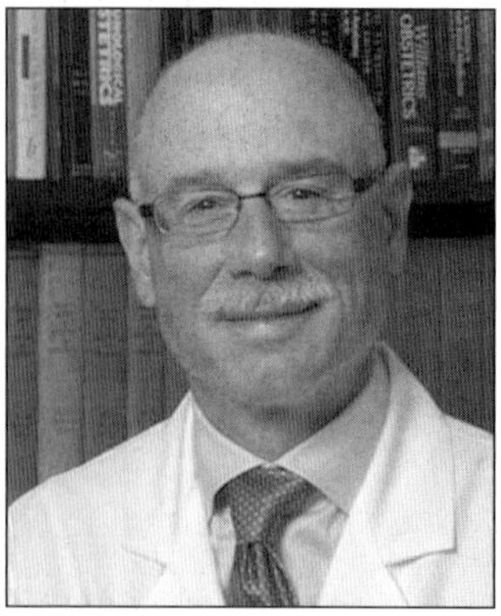

Anthony Sciscione, DO
Professor of Obstetrics and Gynecology
Jefferson Medical College
Philadelphia, Pennsylvania
Residency Program Director
Director of Maternal-Fetal Medicine
Department of Obstetrics and Gynecology
ChristianaCare Health System
Newark, Delaware

To my sons, Dr. Vito F. Ferri and Dr. Christopher A. Ferri, and my daughter-in-law, Dr. Heather A. Ferri, for their help and constant support, and to my wife, Christina, for her patience during manuscript preparation. A special thanks to all the readers who have personally commented on the merits of this book and through their suggestions have helped make this product a bestseller in the medical field.

Fred F. Ferri, MD, FACP
Clinical Professor
Department of Medicine
Warren Alpert Medical School of Brown University
Providence, Rhode Island

Preface

This book is intended to be a clear and concise reference for physicians and allied health professionals. Its user-friendly format is designed to provide a fast and efficient way to identify important clinical information and to offer practical guidance in patient management. The book is divided into five sections and an appendix, each with emphasis on clinical information.

The tremendous success of the previous editions and the enthusiastic comments from numerous colleagues have brought about several positive changes over time. This is the 26th edition of *Ferri's Clinical Advisor*, a bestseller nationally and internationally and now available in multiple languages. Each section has been significantly expanded from prior editions, bringing the total number of medical topics covered in this book to more than 1200. New illustrations, tables, and boxes have been added to this edition to enhance recollection of clinically important facts. The expedited claims submission and reimbursement ICD-10CM codes are included in all topics.

Section I describes in detail over 1000 medical disorders and diseases—including 30 new topics this edition—arranged alphabetically and presented in outline format for ease of retrieval. Topics with an accompanying algorithm are identified with an ALG icon; similarly, those topics with an accompanying online Patient Teaching Guide (PTG) are identified with a PTG symbol. Throughout the text, key quick-access information is consistently highlighted, with clinical photographs to further illustrate selected medical conditions, and relevant ICD-10CM codes listed. Most references focus on current peer-reviewed journal articles rather than outdated textbooks and old review articles.

Topics in **Section I** use the following structured approach:
1. Basic Information (Definition, Synonyms, ICD-10CM Codes, Epidemiology & Demographics, Physical Findings & Clinical Presentation, Etiology)
2. Diagnosis (Differential Diagnosis, Workup, Laboratory Tests, Imaging Studies)
3. Treatment (Nonpharmacologic Therapy, Acute General Rx, Chronic Rx, Disposition, Referral)
4. Pearls & Considerations (Comments, Suggested Readings)

Section II includes the differential diagnosis, etiology, and classification of signs and symptoms. This practical section allows the user investigating a physical complaint or abnormal laboratory value to follow a "workup" leading to a diagnosis. The physician can then easily look up the presumptive diagnosis in Section I for information specific to that illness. Several new signs and symptoms have been added to this section for the 2024 edition.

Section III includes more than 150 clinical algorithms to guide and expedite the patient's workup and therapy. For the 2024 edition, we have continued to update algorithms and colorize online versions for improved readability. Physicians describe this section as particularly valuable in today's managed-care environment.

Section IV includes normal laboratory values and interpretation of results of commonly ordered laboratory tests. By providing interpretation of abnormal results, this section facilitates the diagnosis of medical disorders and further adds to the comprehensive "one-stop" nature of our text. New illustrations and tables have been added for this edition.

Section V focuses on preventive medicine. Information here includes screening recommendations for major diseases and disorders, patient counseling, and immunization and chemoprophylaxis recommendations.

The **Appendix** is divided into nine major sections. Appendix I contains extensive information on complementary and alternative medicine (CAM), including Common Herbs in Integrated Medicine as well as Herbal Activities Against Pain and Chronic Diseases. With this material, we aim to lessen the current scarcity of exposure of allopathic and osteopathic physicians to the diversity of CAM therapies. Appendix II focuses on nutrition, with an emphasis on dietary supplements, vitamins, and minerals. Appendix III deals with diagnosis and treatment of acute poisoning. Appendix IV is a guide on impairment and disability evaluation. Appendix V focuses on the protection of travelers. Appendix VI addresses care of the transgender patient. Appendix VII is a repository of practical patient instruction sheets, organized alphabetically, and covers the majority of topics in this book. These guides can be easily customized and printed and serve as valuable tools for improving physician-patient communication, patient satisfaction, and ultimately quality of care. Appendix VIII and IX offer guidance related to palliative care and preoperative evaluation, respectively.

I believe that we have produced a state-of-the-art information system with significant differences from existing texts. The information offered in all five sections and patient education guides could be sold separately based on their content, yet are available under a single cover, offering the reader tremendous value. I hope that the *Clinical Advisor's* user-friendly approach, numerous unique features, and yearly updates will make this book a valuable medical reference, not only to primary care physicians but also to physicians in other specialties, medical students, and allied health professionals.

Fred F. Ferri, MD, FACP
Clinical Professor
Department of Medicine
Warren Alpert Medical School of Brown University
Providence, Rhode Island

Note: Comments from readers are always appreciated and can be forwarded directly to Dr. Ferri at fred_ferri@brown.edu.

Mouse icon: Indicates content with additional references, figures, or tables available at eBooks.Health.Elsevier.com.

(PTG) PTG icon: Indicates an accompanying Patient Teaching Guide available at eBooks.Health.Elsevier.com. Many additional PTGs are available online that are not connected to topics in Section I.

(ALG) ALG icon: Indicates a topic with an accompanying algorithm.

In Memoriam

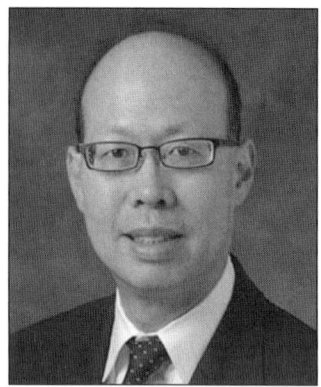

Jerry Yee, MD, MACP, FRCP, FASN, FNKF
August 5, 1959 - June 9, 2022
Clinical Professor of Medicine
Department of Internal Medicine
Wayne State University School of Medicine
Division Head, Nephrology and Hypertension
Henry Ford Hospital
Detroit, Michigan

Contents

Detailed Contents

SECTION I **Diseases and Disorders***

*Italic topics are available online only.

SECTION I **Bonus Content***

SECTION II **Differential Diagnosis**

*Italic topics are available online only.

SECTION III Clinical Algorithms*

*Italic topics are available online only.

Detailed Contents

SECTION IV Laboratory Tests and Interpretation of Results*

*Italic topics are available online only.

SECTION V   Clinical Practice Guidelines*

*Italic topics are available online only.

SECTION I

Diseases and Disorders

Fred F. Ferri, MD

ⓘ BASIC INFORMATION

DEFINITION

An abdominal aortic aneurysm (AAA) is a segmental full-thickness dilation of the abdominal aortic artery to at least 50% greater than the normal vessel diameter. The average diameter of a human infrarenal aorta is approximately 2 cm, thus a threshold of 3 cm is commonly considered aneurysmal.[1]

ICD 10-CM CODES
I71.4 Abdominal aortic aneurysm, without rupture
I71.3 Abdominal aortic aneurysm, ruptured

EPIDEMIOLOGY & DEMOGRAPHICS

- Approximately 13,000 deaths/yr in the U.S. are attributed to AAA.[1]
- AAA is predominantly a disease of older adults and affects men four times more than women.[2]
- The prevalence of AAA ranges 1.2% to 3.3% in men older than 60 yr, which is lower than had been previously reported, likely due to societal reductions in smoking. The prevalence in the U.S. specifically is unclear given that screening is rare in nonsmokers.[3]
- More than half of males with subaneurysmal aorta (2.6 to 2.9 cm) develop an AAA >3.0 cm within 5 yr of their original ultrasound. 28% of male patients with a subaneurysmal aorta will develop a large AAA >5.5 cm within 15 yr.[4]

NATURAL HISTORY

- AAAs tend to develop in the infrarenal aorta and expand at a faster rate the larger the diameter of the AAA, with each 0.5 cm increase in baseline AAA diameter increasing the rate of expansion by 0.59 mm/yr.[5]
- Larger aneurysms are associated with increased rate of expansion, and thus current guidelines recommend more frequent surveillance for larger aneurysms. Frequency of surveillance for aneurysms is as follows: 3.0 to 3.9 cm every 3 yr, 4.0 to 4.9 cm every year, 5.0 to 5.4 every 6 mo.[6] Aneurysmal size is the greatest predictor of rupture.[1]
- Out of hospital AAA rupture is often lethal with mortality ranging from 80% to 90%.[1,3] Female sex, current smoking, and older age are associated with an increased risk of AAA rupture. Current smokers are two times more likely than former smokers to suffer from AAA rupture.[3]
- Annual risk for rupture of the AAA depends on the size of the AAA:[1]
  1. <1% for AAA 5.4 cm or under
  2. 9.4% for AAA between 5.5 cm and 5.9 cm
  3. 10.2% for AAA between 6 cm to 6.9 cm
  4. 32.5% for AAA 7.0 cm or greater

- Heavily calcified AAAs expand at a slower rate than less calcified AAAs.[6a] The presumed mechanism may be stabilization of the aortic wall by calcification.

SCREENING & MONITORING

- The U.S. Preventive Services Task Force (USPSTF) recommends one-time screening for AAA by ultrasonography in men ages 65 to 75 who have a history of smoking, and selectively offer men 65 yr of age or older who have never smoked but have certain risk factors, including family history of AAA in a parent or sibling. These populations have been shown to have a higher prevalence of AAA, and selectively screening this group has been shown to decrease AAA-specific mortality.[3]
- The USPSTF has found little benefit in repeat screening in men with a negative ultrasound and has determined that men over the age of 75 are unlikely to benefit from screening. It was also concluded that the current evidence is insufficient to assess the balance of the harms and benefits of screening for AAA in women ages 65 to 75 who have ever smoked or with family history of AAA.[3]
- The Society for Vascular Surgery recommends one-time ultrasonography screening for AAAs in men and women ages 65 to 75 yr with a history of tobacco use; in men and women 65 to 75 yr with a first-degree relative with an AAA; and in patients 75 yr or older in good health who have either a history of smoking or a first-degree relative with an AAA.[6]
- The Society for Vascular Surgery guidelines recommend monitoring by ultrasound or CT scan should be performed every 6 mo for patients with AAAs measuring 5.0 to 5.4 cm in diameter, every 12 mo for AAAs measuring 4.0 to 4.9 cm in diameter, and every 3 yr for AAAs 3.0 to 3.9 cm in diameter.[6]

PHYSICAL FINDINGS & CLINICAL PRESENTATION

- Most aneurysms are asymptomatic and incidentally discovered on imaging studies.[7,8]
- Physical examination has moderate sensitivity for detection of AAA. Abdominal palpitation may reveal a pulsatile mass and is less than 50% sensitive in detection of AAA. Detection is further limited in individuals with abdominal girth >100 cm. Palpation of the aneurysm does not increase the risk of rupture.[8]
- Symptomatic patients may present with pain of the abdomen, back, flank, or groin or sequelae of the AAA's compression of nearby organs. Early satiety, nausea, and vomiting may be caused by compression of adjacent bowel. Venous thrombosis or insufficiency may occur from iliocaval venous compression. Thromboembolization can cause lower extremity pain and discoloration. Abdominal bruits can be present in case of renal or visceral arterial stenosis. Ureteral obstruction

and hydronephrosis can cause flank and groin pain and lead to obstructive renal failure.[8] Additionally, aneurysmal formation can lead to development of arteriovenous fistulas and aortoenteric fistulas, which may present as heart failure and gastrointestinal blood loss, respectively.[8]
- 50% of patients with AAA rupture will classically present as a triad of abdominal or back pain, hypotension, and a pulsatile abdominal mass. Ruptured aneurysms (Fig. E1) lead to rapid progression to hemorrhagic shock and require emergent surgery within hours to increase chances of survival.[1,7]

ETIOLOGY

- AAA development is characterised by various pathophysiological mechanisms including smooth muscle cell apoptosis and media layer thinning, vascular inflammation from lymphocyte and macrophage infiltration, and extracellular matrix degradation.[1,9] These degenerative processes deplete the normal lamellar elastin matrix leading to vascular remodeling and aneurysmal formation, expansion, and eventual rupture.[9] Matrix metalloproteinases have been implicated in the development of aneurysms as well and have been tested with variable success as a therapeutic target for prevention of AAA.[10]
- Advanced age is significantly associated with AAA. Individuals over the age of 65 (compared to under age 55) are 9.4 times as likely to develop AAA.[2]
- Smoking is considered one of the strongest modifiable risk factors for AAA development. A history of smoking was associated with an odds ratio of 5.07 for formation of AAA over 4 cm. Smoking was considered to be responsible for 75% of the excess prevalence of AAAs ≥4 cm.[11]
- The association of family history of AAA suggests a role of inherited connective tissues diseases such as Marfans and Ehlers-Danlos in the pathogenesis of AAA formation.[2]
- Less impactful risk factors include hyperlipidemia, obesity, prexisting peripheral arterial disease, cerebrovascular disease, coronary artery disease, other aneurysmal vessels, hypertension.[1,2]
- Regular consumption of fruits, vegetables, and nuts along with regular moderate intensity exercise were associated with reduced risk of AAA formation.[2]
- Ethnically, Caucasian race is associated with increased risk of AAA development compared to African American, Hispanic, and Asian origins.[2]

Ⓓⓧ DIAGNOSIS

DIFFERENTIAL DIAGNOSIS

Most patients with AAA are asymptomatic, and the condition is discovered on routine examination or serendipitously when ordering studies for

Abdominal Aortic Aneurysm

other symptoms.[7] Diagnosis of AAA should be considered in the differential with the following symptoms: Abdominal, back, or flank pain and/or a pulsatile abdominal mass. The differential diagnosis of these symptoms can include aortic dissection, ulcerated aortic plaque, renal colic, mesenteric ischemia, pancreatitis, diverticulitis, peptic ulcer disease, biliary tract disease, and others.

LABORATORY TESTS

Not routinely indicated. For suspected infected or inflammatory aneurysms, white blood cell (WBC), erythrocyte sedimentation rate (ESR)/C-reactive protein (CRP), and blood cultures can be considered. An elevated d-dimer may indicate a thrombus within the aneurysm. Fig. 2 describes an algorithm for the diagnosis and treatment of abdominal aortic aneurysms.

IMAGING STUDIES

- Abdominal ultrasound (Fig. 3) is 94% to 100% sensitive and 98% to 100% specific in identifying an aneurysm. Ultrasound is readily available, noninvasive, and accurate. Increasing application in emergency settings has led to a significant reduction in time to diagnosis and treatment of AAA.[3,6]
- Computed tomography (CT) (Fig. 4) scan is recommended for preoperative aneurysm imaging and estimates the size of the AAA to within 0.2 mm.[2] CT scan can identify extension to renal vessels with more precision than ultrasound. It is the imaging modality of choice for symptomatic AAA and can also detect the integrity of the wall (Fig. 5) and exclude rupture.[8]
- Magnetic resonance angiography (MRA) may also be used and is more accurate than CT.[2]
- Plain radiographs may show the outline of an aneurysm in calcified aortas. This is an insensitive test for diagnosing AAA.
- Diagnostic aortography has essentially been replaced by other noninvasive imaging modalities such as CT or MRA. Intraoperative angiography is still used for determining treatment options and postprocedure efficacy (Fig. 6).

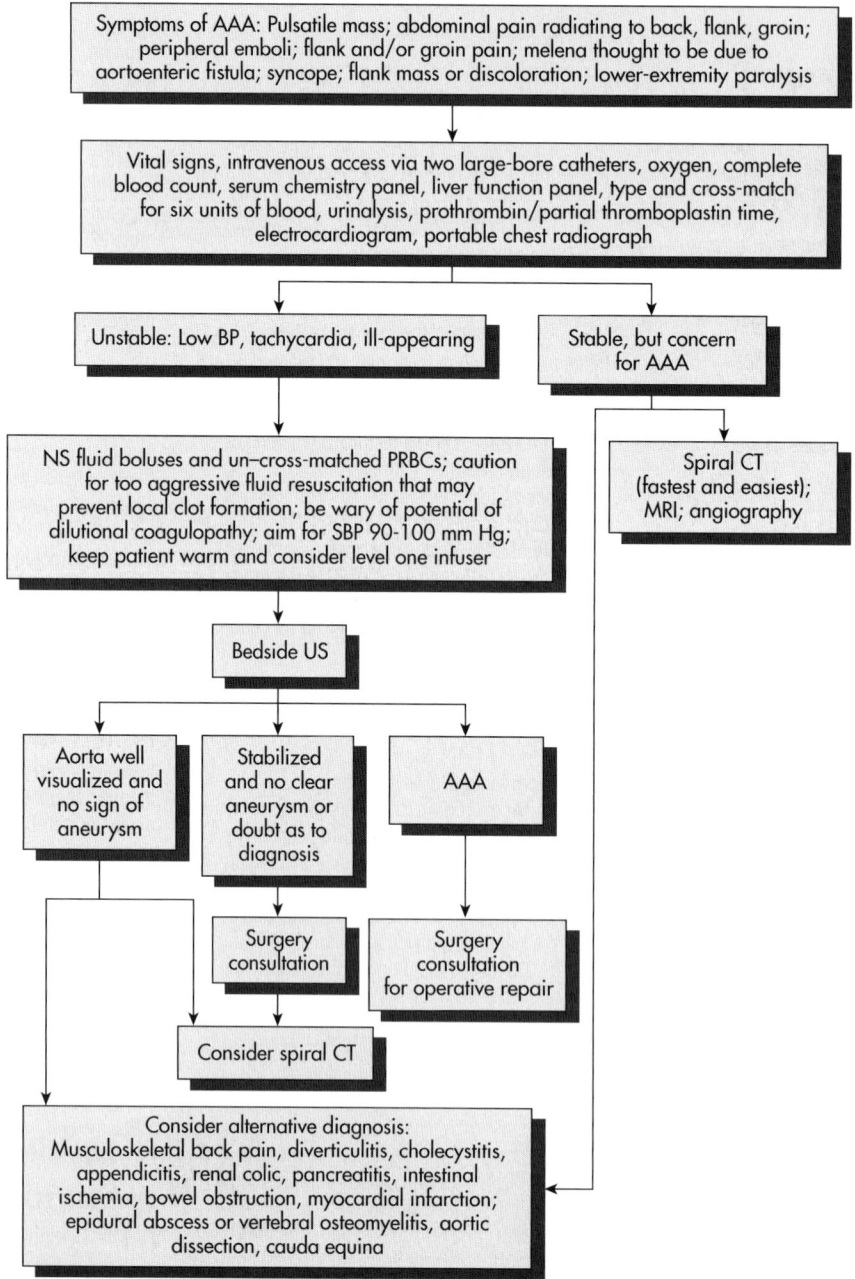

FIG. 2 Algorithm for the diagnosis and treatment of abdominal aortic aneurysms *(AAAs)*. *BP,* Blood pressure; *CT,* computed tomography; *MRI,* magnetic resonance imaging; *NS,* normal saline; *PRBCs,* packed red blood cells; *SBP,* systolic blood pressure; *US,* ultrasonography. (From Adams JG et al: *Emergency medicine, clinical essentials,* ed 2, Philadelphia, 2013, Elsevier.)

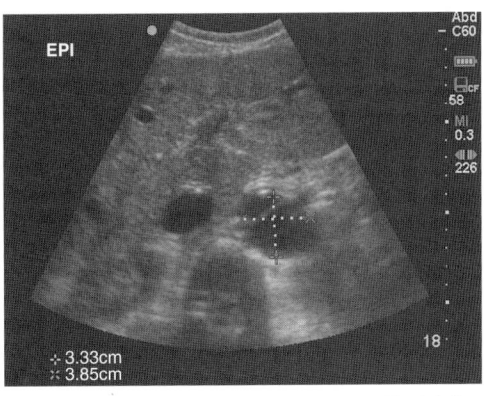

FIG. 3 Transverse image of an abdominal aortic aneurysm. Note the measurements of 3.33 × 3.85 cm. The inferior vena cava is seen to the patient's right of the aorta, and the vertebral body is seen below the two vessels. Note also that there appears to be an echogenic flap within the aorta, possibly representing an aortic dissection. (From Adams JG et al: *Emergency medicine, clinical essentials,* ed 2, Philadelphia, 2013, Elsevier.)

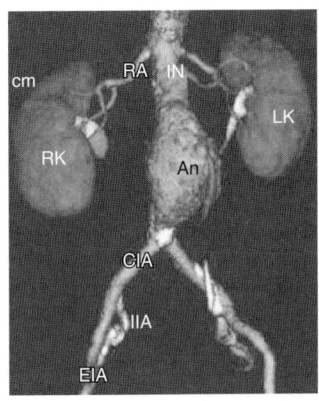

FIG. 4 Three-dimensional computed tomography image illustrates the presence of an infrarenal abdominal aortic aneurysm. *An,* Aneurysm; *CIA,* common iliac artery; *EIA,* external iliac artery; *IIA,* internal iliac artery; *IN,* infrarenal neck; *LK,* left kidney; *RA,* renal artery; *RK,* right kidney. (From Townsend CM et al [eds]: *Sabiston textbook of surgery,* ed 17, Philadelphia, 2004, Saunders.)

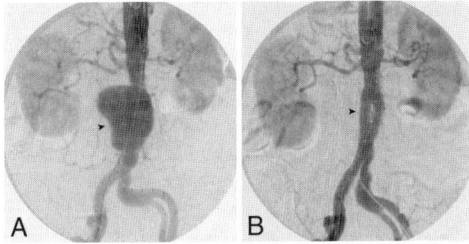

FIG. 6 A, Conventional catheter angiography with bilateral marked catheters in place demonstrates a large, lobulated, infrarenal aortic aneurysm *(arrowhead)* with a 4-cm proximal neck suitable for endovascular repair. **B,** An image after endovascular repair demonstrates complete exclusion of the aneurysm *(arrowhead)* with no endoleak and preservation of the renal and hypogastric arteries. (From Soto JA, Lucey BC: *Emergency radiology, the requisites,* ed 2, Philadelphia, 2017, Elsevier.)

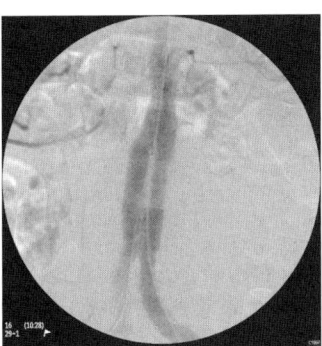

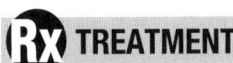

FIG. 7 Digital subtraction angiogram following endovascular aneurysm repair. (From Fillit HM: *Brocklehurst's textbook of geriatric medicine and gerontology,* ed 8, Philadelphia, 2017, Elsevier.)

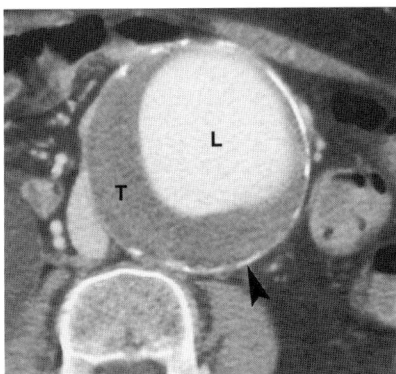

FIG. 5 Aneurysm of the abdominal aorta. A large aortic aneurysm is evident. The aorta exceeds 5 cm in diameter. A large amount of thrombus *(T)* partially surrounds the contrast-enhanced patent lumen *(L).* Note the atherosclerotic calcification *(arrowhead)* in the wall of the aneurysm.

• Endovascular aneurysm repair (EVAR) needs close and lifelong imaging surveillance of the aneurysm site for the timely detection of possible complications, including endoleaks, graft migration, fractures, graft infection, and enlargement of aneurysm sac size with eventual rupture.[6] Contrast-enhanced computed tomography (CTA) is considered the gold standard in EVAR follow-up (Fig. 7); however, routine use is limited given cumulative radiation exposure and risk of contrast-induced renal injury. Guidelines suggest serial ultrasound surveillance if neither endoleak nor AAA enlargement is seen on CTA at 1 yr after EVAR.[6]

🅡🅧 TREATMENT

NONPHARMACOLOGIC THERAPY

• Smoking cessation is critical for treatment of patients with AAAs and can decrease rate of expansion. Patients with known AAA or a family history of aneurysms should be advised to stop smoking and be offered smoking cessation interventions.[11]
• Healthy diet and exercise have been observed to be associated with reduced risk of AAA. Of note, moderate exercise does not increase the rate of aneurysm expansion or the risk of rupture.[2]
• Definitive treatment depends on the size of the aneurysm (see "Chronic Rx").

ACUTE GENERAL RX

• AAA can be treated with open surgical repair (OSR) or EVAR. EVAR is recommended in patients with suitable anatomy given reduced

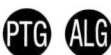
short term morbidity compared to OSR.[6,12,13] Elective, symptomatic, or ruptured AAA repair can be performed via endovascular or open techniques.[6,8] Ruptured AAA requires emergent repair, and symptomatic AAA requires urgent repair.[6]

- Historically, emergent open repair had been the standard of care; however, trials now show no significant difference in 30-day mortality compared to EVAR.[12] There was a higher incidence of reintervention for patients undergoing EVAR, although interventions to deal with procedural complications were generally less invasive and involved catheter-based approaches.[13,14,15]
- The major limitations for EVAR include anatomic issues such as tortuosity or small caliber iliac arteries prohibiting graft deployment, end-organ ischemia from endograft limb occlusion, endoleak from inadequate fixation or sealing of the graft to the vessel wall, and inability to follow up patients to exclude late failure of stent-grafts and development of endoleaks.[6,7,8]

CHRONIC RX

- Blood pressure and fasting lipids should be monitored and controlled as recommended for patients with hypertensive and atherosclerotic disease. AAA formation is recognized as a distinct degenerative process from atherosclerosis, and thus statins and β-blockers are not generally recommended for the sole purpose of reducing the risk of AAA expansion and rupture.[1,6]
- Data are conflicting as to the protective effects of antibiotics such as doxycycline and roxithromycin to limit the expansion of small AAAs.[6,16]
- AAA repair to eliminate the risk for rupture should be performed for patients with infrarenal or juxtarenal AAA of approximately 5.5 cm or larger in diameter. Repair in females can be considered at diameters larger than 5 cm per Society of Vascular Surgery guidelines. Additionally, AAAs with a rate of enlargement greater than 0.5 cm over 6 mo should be considered for repair. All patients who are symptomatic should undergo repair, regardless of size.[6]
- Smoking cessation is recommended for at least 2 wk before surgery.[6] It is reasonable to

delay AAA repair in an effort to optimize comorbid medical conditions. Preoperative nutritional status should be optimized prior to undergoing elective repair. Intravenous antibiotics with a first generation cephalosporin should be administered 30 min to 1 h prior to either OSR or EVAR.[6]

- There is no clear advantage to early repair (open or endovascular) for small asymptomatic AAAs. Meta-analysis has demonstrated no significant difference in all-cause mortality or AAA-related mortality with early treatment (EVAR vs. OSR) compared with surveillance for small AAAs.[17]
- Historically, EVAR was thought to be associated with better short-term outcomes than OSR (lower 30-day mortality and myocardial infarction [MI] rates, shorter hospital stays, and better health-related quality of life up to 12 mo postoperatively) but increased rates of graft-related complications and long-term all-cause mortality. However, there is conflicting evidence about the long-term relative benefits of OSR, with some recent trials demonstrating no significant difference in long-term mortality.[6,8,13,14,15]
- In patients who have undergone EVAR, long-term surveillance is required to assess for an endoleak, stent migration, change in aneurysm size, and need for reintervention.[6] Surveillance for endovascular AAA repair has typically involved use of periodic CT scans, but abdominal ultrasound is gaining widespread adoption for postprocedure monitoring. Surveillance is recommended to occur at least 1 mo and 12 mo postoperatively and then annually thereafter.[6]
- EVAR with proximally fenestrated grafts (FEVAR) is an alternative to open repair in the management of juxtarenal aortic aneurysms and short-neck abdominal aortic aneurysms (the "neck" is the distance from the lowest main renal artery to the beginning of the aneurysm). Contemporary literature shows it is a safe and efficacious treatment, particularly for those deemed surgically high risk.[13]
- For patients with limited life expectancy, elective AAA repair is not recommended.[5]

REFERRAL

- Vascular surgical referral is recommended at the time of diagnosis of AAA.[6]

- It is important to optimize any comorbid conditions along with surgical referral.[6]

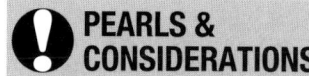

⚠ PEARLS & CONSIDERATIONS

- Smoking is the strongest modifiable risk factor for AAA formation, expansion, and rupture, and cessation should strongly be encouraged through utilization of behavioral support techniques and pharmacological therapy.
- Guidelines suggest elective repair for patients with AAA ≥5.5 cm at low or acceptable surgical risk.
- The results from multiple trials to date demonstrate no advantage to immediate repair for small AAA (4.0 to 5.5 cm).
- 5-yr all-cause mortality remains poor after elective AAA repair despite advances in short-term outcomes.

COMMENTS

- Most AAAs are infrarenal. This is thought to be due in part to decreased lamellar structural proteins in the vascular wall below the renal arteries leading to decreased vascular wall strength.[1,9]
- Surgical risk is increased in patients with coexisting coronary artery disease, pulmonary disease, or chronic renal failure. Evaluation for ischemia and aggressive perioperative hemodynamic monitoring can help identify high-risk patients and decrease postoperative complications.[6]
- AAAs expand at a faster rate the larger the diameter of the AAA, with each 0.5 cm increase in baseline AAA diameter increasing the rate of expansion by 0.59 mm/yr.[5]

REFERENCES
Available at eBooks.Health.Elsevier.com

RELATED CONTENT
Abdominal Aortic Aneurysm (Patient Information)

AUTHORS: **FAHAD GUL, MD,** and
PRANAV M. PATEL, MD, FACC, FAHA, FSCAI

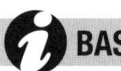

BASIC INFORMATION

DEFINITION

Abnormal uterine bleeding (AUB) describes uterine bleeding that is abnormal in regularity, quantity, frequency, or duration, in the nonpregnant person. Historically, AUB was described as in Table 1. The term *dysfunctional uterine bleeding* was applied when no clear etiology could be identified. These terms have fallen out of favor. In 2011, the FIGO Working Group on Menstrual Disorders released a classification system intended to simplify these definitions. It is known by the acronym PALM-COEIN, which is further described later. This classification system divides the causes of AUB into two groups: structural (PALM) and nonstructural (COEIN). Today, AUB is described according to these criteria.

A normal menstrual cycle is typically described as lasting 21 to 35 days with up to 7 days of bleeding per cycle. Total blood loss for normal menses is thought to be less than 80 mL.

SYNONYMS

Abnormal uterine bleeding (AUB)
Dysfunctional uterine bleeding

ICD-10CM CODES
N91.5   Oligomenorrhea, unspecified
N92.0   Excessive and frequent menstruation with regular cycle
N92.1   Excessive and frequent menstruation with irregular cycle
N92.5   Other specified irregular menstruation
N93.8   Other specified abnormal uterine and vaginal bleeding
N93.9   Abnormal uterine and vaginal bleeding, unspecified

EPIDEMIOLOGY & DEMOGRAPHICS

- One third of outpatient visits to the gynecologist are for AUB.
- Most cases of AUB result from structural (uterine) pathology (the PALM portion of the acronym).
- Up to 20% of women presenting with heavy menstrual bleeding will be found to have a coagulopathy or underlying bleeding disorder.

PHYSICAL FINDINGS & CLINICAL PRESENTATION

- The clinical presentation of AUB is variable. Although many patients complain of the abnormality of their cycles, some will present with symptoms of anemia, with AUB being elicited only with a careful history.
- Physical findings depend on the etiology. For example, an enlarged or irregular uterine contour may suggest fibroids, or a polyp may be seen on the cervix during a speculum examination.
- A thorough physical and pelvic examination should be done in every case.
- Workup should be performed to exclude the other causes of abnormal bleeding such as thyroid or endocrine diseases.

ETIOLOGY

- Table 2 describes many of the various causes of AUB.
- Endocrinopathies, including hyperprolactinemia, hyperthyroidism, and hypothyroidism, may also contribute to heavy or irregular menstrual bleeding.

DIAGNOSIS

DIFFERENTIAL DIAGNOSIS

- PALM–COEIN:
  1. Polyps (AUB-P)
  2. Adenomyosis (AUB-A)
  3. Leiomyoma (AUB-L)
  4. Malignancy/hyperplasia (AUB-M)
  5. Coagulopathy (AUB-C; most commonly von Willebrand disease)
  6. Ovulatory dysfunction (AUB-O; most commonly polycystic ovarian syndrome [PCOS])
  7. Endometrial (AUB-E)
  8. Iatrogenic (AUB-I; e.g., anticoagulants, hormonal contraception, and some herbal remedies)
  9. Not yet classified (AUB-N)

- Anatomic nonuterine causes:
  1. Cervix: Cervical neoplasia, cervicitis
  2. Vagina: Vaginal neoplasia, adhesions, trauma, foreign body, atrophic vaginitis, infections, condyloma
  3. Vulva: Vulvar trauma, infections, neoplasia, condyloma, dystrophy, varices
  4. Urinary tract: Urethral caruncle, diverticulum, hematuria, neoplasia
  5. Gastrointestinal tract: Hemorrhoids, anal fissure, colorectal lesions, or neoplasia
- Systemic diseases/effects:
  1. Exogenous hormone intake: Hormone replacement therapy
  2. Medications
  3. Coagulopathies: Von Willebrand disease, thrombocytopenia, hepatic failure
  4. Endocrinopathies: Thyroid disorder, hyperprolactinemia, diabetes mellitus
  5. Renal diseases: Generally causing acquired coagulopathy
  6. Impaired nutritional status: Anorexia/bulimia, excessive exercise

WORKUP

- Obtain a detailed history, including age of menarche and current and prior menstrual

---

TABLE 1   Definitions of Abnormal Uterine Bleeding

Term	Description
Oligomenorrhea	Bleeding at intervals greater than 35 days
Polymenorrhea	Bleeding at intervals less than 21 days
Hypermenorrhea (menorrhagia)	Excessive flow or bleeding with normal intervals
Metrorrhagia	Bleeding between menses
Menometrorrhagia	Excessive flow or duration with periods and between periods
Withdrawal bleeding	Bleeding after the withdrawal of hormones

From Crum CP et al: *Diagnostic gynecologic and obstetric pathology*, ed 3, Philadelphia, 2018, Elsevier.

TABLE 2   Causes of Abnormal Uterine Bleeding

Age (Years)	Differential Diagnosis
Prepubertal	Precocious puberty (hypothalamic, pituitary, ovarian)
Adolescence	• Immature hypothalamic-pituitary axis (transient)
	• Pregnancy
	• Disorders in folliculogenesis (transient)
	• Sexually transmitted infections
	• Hematologic disorders (von Willebrand disease, hemophilias, factors VII, XI)
Third and fourth decades	• Oral contraceptive pill-related
	• Pregnancy or postpartum
	• Benign organic lesions (polyps, leiomyomata, endometritis)
	• Anovulatory cycle
Fifth decade	• Anovulatory or altered cycle
	• Benign organic lesions (polyps, adenomyosis, leiomyomata, or endometritis)
	• Neoplasia
Sixth decade	• Hormone replacement therapy
	• Benign organic lesions (polyps, adenomyosis, leiomyomata, endometritis)
	• Atrophy
	• Neoplasia

From Crum CP et al: *Diagnostic gynecologic and obstetric pathology*, ed 3, Philadelphia, 2018, Elsevier.

characteristics. The severity of bleeding is important to discern but can be difficult for patients to describe objectively. Asking specifics regarding size of tampon/pads used, frequency of changing menstrual products, use of concomitant tampons and pads, and saturating clothes can be useful to estimate severity. Review of systems should include symptoms of anemia, hyper- or hypothyroidism, and hyperprolactinemia

- Medical and surgical history, which could suggest of other causes/contributors
- Family history of bleeding disorders, gynecologic conditions such as uterine fibroids, endometriosis, or neoplasia
- Thorough physical examination, including a pelvic examination (bimanual and speculum)
  1. Includes thyroid, breast, liver, skin (e.g., presence or absence of ecchymotic lesions)
  2. Patient habitus: Obese and hirsute (e.g., polycystic ovarian disease) or underweight (e.g., anorexia nervosa or excessive exercise)
  3. Presence or absence of vulvar, vaginal, or cervical lesions; uterine (fibroid) or ovarian tumors; urethral caruncles or diverticula; hemorrhoids; anal fissures; colorectal lesions
  4. Complete pelvic exam to identify lesions and the size and shape of the uterus

LABORATORY TESTS (AS INDICATED BY HISTORY AND PHYSICAL)

- Pregnancy test (blood or urine)
- Complete blood count
- Targeted screening for bleeding disorders, when indicated per history or physical exam
  1. Prothrombin/international normalization ratio and partial thromboplastin (or PFA-100 assay) if coagulopathy is suspected
  2. von Willebrand panel, particularly in women with heavy bleeding since menarche if initial testing suggests coagulopathy
- Iron studies
- Thyroid function tests
- Chlamydia trachomatis testing and other sexually transmitted infection testing
- Endometrial biopsy or dilation and curettage. This is a required component of the workup for AUB in patients over 45 yr old. It should also be performed in younger patients with a history of unopposed estrogen exposure (such as in obesity or PCOS) or in patients who have failed medical management and have persistent AUB
- Pap smear if indicated
- Stool testing for occult blood
- Urinalysis for hematuria

IMAGING STUDIES

- Pelvic ultrasound, generally performed transvaginally, including measurement of endometrial thickness in the postmenopausal woman and assessment of myometrial or endometrial defects is considered first line.

- Fluid contrast ultrasound (also called saline sonogram, sonohysterogram, or saline infusion sonogram) may be indicated if the endometrium appears thickened or irregular. It distends the uterine cavity so that "filling defects" of the endometrium can be assessed for possible endometrial polyp, uterine fibroid, or neoplasm.
- Hysteroscopy may be performed to both assess and treat intracavitary fibroids or polyps.
- MRI may help better characterize large fibroids or uterine pathology and can be particularly helpful in diagnosing adenomyosis.

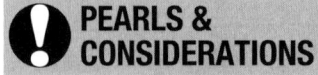

RX TREATMENT

NONPHARMACOLOGIC THERAPY

- Increase dietary iron intake or consider oral iron supplementation for anemia.
- Initiate lifestyle changes, including weight loss, exercise, and low-carb diet, if indicated.

ACUTE THERAPY

- Pharmacologic:
  1. Medroxyprogesterone acetate (oral), up to 20 mg PO tid daily for 7 days
  2. Combined oral contraceptives (containing 35 mcg ethinyl estradiol): One tablet tid for 7 days; patient should then continue on oral contraceptives daily
  3. Tranexamic acid, 1.3 g PO or 10 mg/kg IV (max 600 mg per dose), tid for 5 days
  4. Conjugated equine estrogen 25 mg IV every 4 to 6 h for a maximum of 24 h
  5. NSAIDs
- Nonpharmacologic:
  1. Intrauterine tamponade with 26F foley catheter inflated with 30 cc saline

CHRONIC THERAPY

- Progestins:
  1. Medroxyprogesterone acetate 10 mg daily for 12 days, then either continuously or cyclically to induce monthly withdrawal bleeding. If taken continuously, patients should be counseled about the possibility of irregular breakthrough bleeding.
  2. Norethindrone 2.5 to 10 mg daily for 12 days each month, or can be continued daily, at a dose of 0.35 mg (marketed as the "mini-pill")
  3. Depo-Provera 150 mg IM every 3 mo
  4. Combined hormonal contraceptives, one tablet daily either cyclically or continuously using only active pills (or patch or ring)
  5. Levonorgestrel-releasing intrauterine device (LNG-IUD) – Mirena IUD has an FDA indication for heavy menstrual bleeding and is now approved for use for up to 8 yr.
- Others:
  1. Antiprostaglandins – ibuprofen or naproxen sodium can reduce bleeding by 40%.

2. Danazol – suppresses estrogen and progesterone receptors in the endometrium, leading to endometrial atrophy and reduced menstrual loss but is rarely used due to side-effect profile (androgenism, menopause-like symptoms, weight gain, acne).
3. Gonadotropin-releasing hormone (GnRH) analogues – often used to reduce bleeding and ameliorate anemia in preparation for a surgical procedure.
4. Tranexamic acid – antifibrinolytic agent FDA approved for cyclic heavy menstrual bleeding. Dosage in normal renal function is 3900 mg daily (650 mg tablets, 2 tablets tid) for up to 5 days during menses.
- Surgical treatment:
  1. Dilation and curettage
  2. Operative hysteroscopy
  3. Endometrial ablation
  4. Uterine artery embolization
  5. Hysterectomy for definitive management

DISPOSITION

Can consider cyclical treatment on birth control pills or Provera for several cycles, then discontinue pill and watch patient for onset of regular menses. If the patient does not desire pregnancy, cycle management with a hormonal contraceptive or placement of LNG-IUD are commonly used.

REFERRAL

To gynecologist in case of failure of treatment or for comprehensive workup.

❗ PEARLS & CONSIDERATIONS

- Don't forget a pregnancy test!
- Up to 20% of patients with AUB will have an underlying bleeding disorder.
- Endometrial sampling is a first-line test in patients over age 45 with new AUB.

COMMENTS

Patient education material may be obtained from the American College of Obstetricians and Gynecologists, 409 12th Street SW, Washington, DC, 20024-2188; phone 202-638-5577.

SUGGESTED READINGS
Available at eBooks.Health.Elsevier.com.

RELATED CONTENT
Abnormal Uterine Bleeding (Patient Information)
Endometrial Cancer (Related Key Topic)
Heavy Menstrual Bleeding (Menorrhagia) (Related Key Topic)
Uterine Fibroids (Related Key Topic)

AUTHORS: **SYDNEY FORD, MD, MPH,** and **SIRI M. HOLTON, MD**

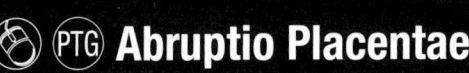

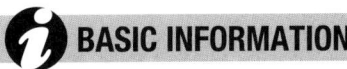 **BASIC INFORMATION**

DEFINITION

Abruptio placentae is the separation of placenta from the uterine wall before delivery of the fetus. The condition occurs in approximately 1% of pregnancies. There are three classes of abruption (Fig. 1) based on maternal and fetal status, including an assessment of uterine contractions, quantity of bleeding, fetal heart rate monitoring, and abnormal coagulation studies (fibrinogen, prothrombin time, partial thromboplastin time).
- Grade I: Mild vaginal bleeding, uterine irritability, stable vital signs, reassuring fetal heart rate, normal coagulation profile (fibrinogen 450 mg/dl). Approximately half of abruptions are grade I.
- Grade II: Moderate vaginal bleeding, hypertonic uterine contractions, orthostatic blood pressure measurements, unfavorable fetal status, fibrinogen 150 to 250 mg. Approximately a quarter of abruptions are grade II.
- Grade III: Severe bleeding (may be concealed), hypertonic uterine contractions, overt signs of hypovolemic shock, fetal death, thrombocytopenia, fibrinogen <150 mg/dl. Approximately a quarter of abruptions are grade III.

SYNONYM

Premature separation of placenta
Placental abruption

ICD-10CM CODES
O45.8X1	Other premature separation of placenta, first trimester
O45.8X2	Other premature separation of placenta, second trimester
O45.8X3	Other premature separation of placenta, third trimester
O45.8X9	Other premature separation of placenta, unspecified trimester
O45.91	Premature separation of placenta, unspecified, first trimester
O45.92	Premature separation of placenta, unspecified, second trimester
O45.93	Premature separation of placenta, unspecified, third trimester

EPIDEMIOLOGY & DEMOGRAPHICS

INCIDENCE (IN U.S.): 9.6/1000 births; 80% occur before the onset of labor.
PREVALENCE: 5% to 17%, some studies showing a 5- to 10-fold increase in risk; with two prior episodes, 25%.

RISK FACTORS: Hypertension (greatest association), trauma, polyhydramnios, multifetal gestation, smoking, use of cocaine, chorioamnionitis, preterm premature rupture of membranes. Table 1 summarizes placental abruption risk factors.

PHYSICAL FINDINGS & CLINICAL PRESENTATION
- Triad of uterine bleeding (concealed or per vagina), hypertonic uterine contractions or signs of preterm labor, and evidence of fetal compromise exists.
- More than 80% of cases have external bleeding; 20% of cases have no bleeding but have indirect evidence of abruption, such as failed tocolysis for preterm labor.
- Tetanic uterine contractions are found in only 17%.

ETIOLOGY
- Primary etiology: Unknown
- Hypertension: Found in 40% to 50% of grade III abruptions
- Rapid decompression of uterine cavity, as can occur in polyhydramnios or multifetal gestation
- Blunt external trauma (motor vehicle accident, spousal abuse)

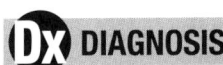 **DIAGNOSIS**

DIFFERENTIAL DIAGNOSIS
- Placenta previa
- Cervical or vaginal trauma
- Labor
- Cervical cancer
- Rupture of membranes
- The differential diagnosis of vaginal bleeding in pregnancy is described in Section III

WORKUP
- Placental abruption is primarily a clinical diagnosis that is supported by laboratory, radiographic (Fig. 2), and pathologic studies.
- Initial assessment should evaluate for the source of bleeding, ruling out placenta previa that may contraindicate any type of vaginal examination (e.g., pelvic speculum examination).
- Continuous fetal heart monitoring is indicated for all viable gestations (60% incidence of fetal distress in labor); may show early signs of

maternal hypovolemia (late decelerations or fetal tachycardia) before overt maternal vital sign changes.
- Actual amount of blood loss is often greater than initially perceived because of the possibility of concealed retroplacental bleeding and apparent "normal" vital signs. The relative hypervolemia of pregnancy initially protects the patient until late in the course of bleeding, when abrupt and sudden cardiovascular collapse can occur.

LABORATORY TESTS
- Baseline serum hemoglobin helps quantify blood loss and establish baseline values for serial comparisons during expectant management.
- Coagulation profile: Platelets, fibrinogen, prothrombin, and partial thromboplastin time. Diffuse intravascular coagulation can develop with severe abruption. If fibrinogen is <150 mg/dl, estimated blood loss is approximately 2000 ml; if fibrinogen is <100 mg/dl, consider fresh frozen plasma to prevent further bleeding.
- Type and antibody screen is important to identify Rh-negative patients who need Rh immune globulin.

IMAGING STUDIES

Ultrasound should include fetal presentation and status, amniotic fluid volume, placental location, as well as any evidence of hematoma (retroplacental, subchorionic, or preplacental) (Fig. 3).

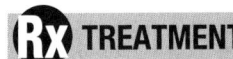 **TREATMENT**

ACUTE GENERAL Rx
- Stabilization of the mother is the first priority.
- Treatment depends on gestational age of the fetus, severity of the abruption, and maternal status.
- Initial assessment for signs of maternal hemodynamic compromise or hemorrhagic shock; large-bore intravenous access, with crystalloid fluid resuscitation using a replacement of 3 ml lactated Ringer solution for every 1 ml estimated blood loss.

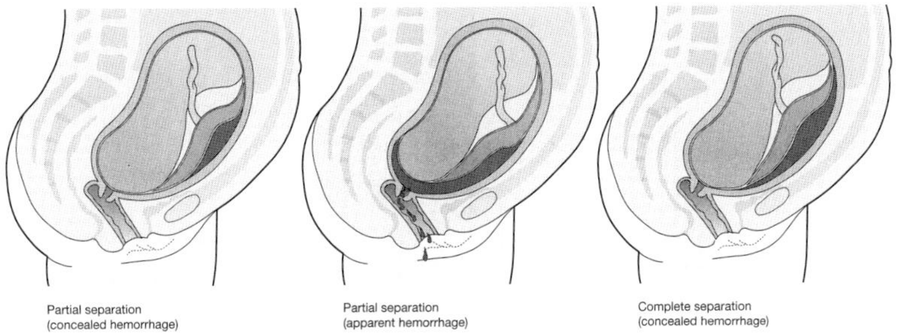

TABLE 1 Placental Abruption Risk Factors

Increasing parity or maternal age
Cigarette smoking
Cocaine abuse
Trauma
Maternal hypertension
Preterm premature rupture of membranes
Rapid uterine decompression associated with multiple gestation and polyhydramnios
Inherited or acquired thrombophilia
Uterine malformations or fibroids
Placental abnormalities or ischemia
Prior abruption

From Gabbe SG: *Obstetrics*, ed 6, Philadelphia, 2012, Saunders.

FIG. 1 Classification of placental abruption. (From Magowan BA: *Clinical obstetrics & gynecology*, ed 4, 2019, Elsevier.)

Partial separation (concealed hemorrhage)   Partial separation (apparent hemorrhage)   Complete separation (concealed hemorrhage)

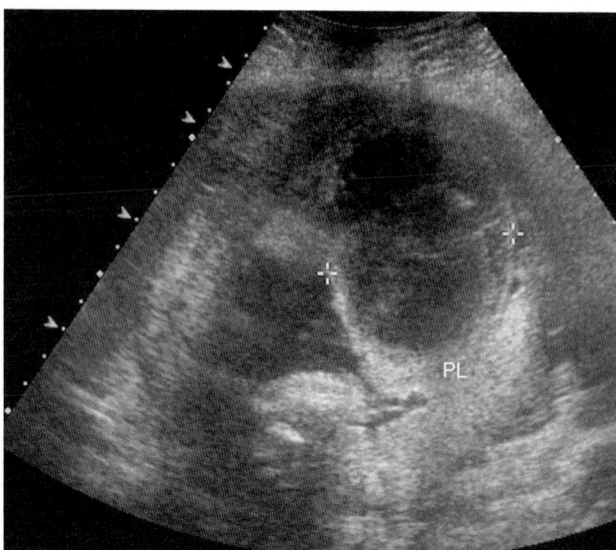

FIG. 2 Placental abruption. Transabdominal sonogram of the placenta *(PL)* with a hematoma *(calipers)* lifting the placenta away from the uterine wall. (From Rumack CM et al [eds]: *Diagnostic ultrasound,* ed 4, Philadelphia, 2011, Mosby.)

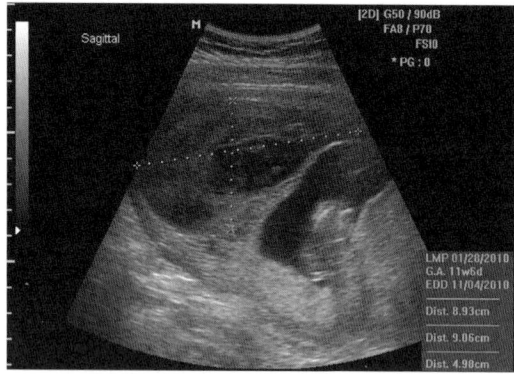

FIG. 3 Ultrasonic image of a subchorionic abruption. (Courtesy K. Francois; from Gabbe SG: *Obstetrics,* ed 6, Philadelphia, 2012, Saunders.)

- Indwelling Foley catheter to monitor urine output and maternal volume status, with a goal of 30 ml/h urine output.

- Assess fetal status and gestational age by sonogram and continuous fetal heart rate monitoring.

- Because of the unpredictable nature of abruptions, cross-matched blood should be made available during the initial resuscitation period.

CHRONIC Rx

- In the term fetus, delivery is indicated.
- In the preterm fetus, consider betamethasone 12.5 mg IM q24h for two doses and then delivery, depending on the severity of the abruption and the likelihood of fetal complications from preterm birth.
- Cesarean delivery should be reserved for cases of fetal distress or for standard obstetric indications. While cesarean delivery may be needed to stabilize the fetal and/or maternal status, the mother's coagulation status may complicate the procedure and availability of blood products may be critical.
- In cases of maternal stability and fetal prematurity, expectant management can occur in the setting of close follow-up, including regular evaluation of fetal growth and reassuring antenatal testing.

DISPOSITION

Because of the unpredictable nature of abruptions, expectant management should occur only under controlled circumstances.

REFERRAL

Abruptio placentae places mother and fetus in a high-risk situation and should be managed by a qualified obstetrician in a facility with capability for neonatal and maternal resuscitation, for supporting a preterm infant if delivery is indicated at an early gestational age, and for performing emergency cesarean deliveries.

RELATED CONTENT

Abruptio Placentae (Patient Information)
Premature Labor (Related Key Topic)
Vaginal Bleeding during Pregnancy (Related Key Topic)

AUTHOR: **KELLY RUHSTALLER, MD**

BASIC INFORMATION

DEFINITION

Absence seizures are a type of generalized seizure characterized by brief episodes of staring with impairment of consciousness (absence). They usually last no more than 20 to 30 sec. The onset and the end of the seizures are sudden. Patients are typically unaware of the seizure and resume the activity they were performing before the seizure. The electroencephalogram signature of absence seizures consists of a generalized 3-Hz spike and slow wave discharges.

SYNONYMS

Childhood absence epilepsy
Seizures, absence

ICD-10CM CODE

G40.309 Generalized idiopathic epilepsy and epileptic syndromes, not intractable, without status epilepticus

EPIDEMIOLOGY & DEMOGRAPHICS

INCIDENCE: 1 to 10 cases per 100,000 population
PREVALENCE: Represents up to 18% of all pediatric epilepsy syndromes
PREDOMINANT SEX AND AGE: More common in girls than in boys, absences typically begin between 4 and 10 yr and remit by age 20[1]
PEAK INCIDENCE: 6 to 7 yr

PHYSICAL FINDINGS & CLINICAL PRESENTATION

- Patients with absence seizures usually have normal physical and neurologic examinations.
- During the seizures, the patients are unresponsive and can have motor phenomena (automatisms, eye blinks, mouth and hand movements).
- Absence seizures are not associated with post-ictal confusion.
- They may be triggered by hyperventilation associated with activity.
- Tonic clonic seizures are not usually a feature of this syndrome. If the patient also experiences tonic clonic seizures, other etiologies should be investigated, such as juvenile absence epilepsy, juvenile myoclonic epilepsy, complex partial seizures, etc.

ETIOLOGY

Genetic

DIAGNOSIS

DIFFERENTIAL DIAGNOSIS

It is important to distinguish between focal onset impaired awareness seizures (previously called complex partial seizures) and absence seizures (Tables E1 and E2).

- Juvenile absence epilepsy
- Juvenile myoclonic epilepsy
- Complex partial seizures
- Focal seizures with altered consciousness
- Nonepileptic spells comprised of staring

WORKUP

- EEG with hyperventilation and photic stimulation is crucial in the diagnosis. (Fig. E1)
- Ambulatory EEG and video EEG are recommended for patients with diagnostic uncertainty.

LABORATORY TESTS

No specific studies needed

IMAGING STUDIES

- MRI of the brain with and without contrast should be performed in all epilepsy patients, especially if the EEG does not show the typical characteristic of absence seizures (3-Hz spike and slow wave discharges).
- Computed tomography scans of the head should be avoided in children due to unnecessary exposure to radiation and low yield of the test except when MRI cannot be obtained.

TREATMENT

The medication of choice based on the best current evidence available is ethosuximide, followed by valproic acid and lamotrigine.[2]

NONPHARMACOLOGIC THERAPY

Not applicable

ACUTE GENERAL Rx

- Ethosuximide: Initial dose: 10 mg/kg/day; then after 7 days, 20 mg/kg
- Divalproex sodium (Depakote): Initial dose: 5 to 10 mg/kg/day (divided bid), maximum dose: 60 mg/kg/day
- Lamotrigine (Lamictal): Dose for patients on no other antiepileptic drugs. Wk 1 and 2: 0.3 mg/kg/day. Wk 3 and 4: 0.6 mg/kg/day. Wk 5 onward: Increase every 1 to 2 wk by 0.6 mg/kg/day. Maintenance: 4.5 to 7.5 mg/kg/day. Warning: Should be used with caution due to the potential for toxicity and Stevens-Johnson syndrome. Patients on other antiepileptic drugs can also have severe adverse reactions (e.g., valproate can cause increased levels of lamotrigine, and lamotrigine must be titrated much more slowly in patients on valproate therapy)

CHRONIC Rx

- Children with recurrent seizures require chronic treatment.
- If children are seizure-free for a period of 1 to 2 yr, a trial on no medications should be considered; children typically outgrow childhood absence seizures.

DISPOSITION

- Response to treatment is excellent.
- Absence seizures tend to remit in teenage yr.
- Epilepsy can be considered as resolved once 10 yr have elapsed since the last event, including 5 yr free from medications.

COMPLEMENTARY & ALTERNATIVE MEDICINE

Not applicable

REFERRAL

Patients with epilepsy should be referred for a consultation by a child neurologist, preferably one specializing in epilepsy.

PEARLS & CONSIDERATIONS

COMMENTS

- Absence seizures can be present in other epilepsy syndromes.
- Valproate should be avoided in girls and women with childbearing potential due to the risk of teratogenicity.
- Carbamazepine and phenytoin should be avoided in the treatment of absence seizures since these medications may worsen seizures and provoke absence status epilepticus.
- All women of childbearing age taking antiepileptic drugs should take folic acid supplementation (1 to 4 mg/day) for the prevention of neural tube defects.

PREVENTION

Sleep deprivation and alcohol consumption should be avoided.

PATIENT & FAMILY EDUCATION

Patients with ongoing seizures are forbidden to drive; check state regulations and laws regarding driving and epilepsy.

REFERENCES

Available at eBooks.Health.Elsevier.com.

RELATED CONTENT

Absence Seizures (Patient Information)

AUTHOR: **JOSEPH S. KASS, MD, JD, FAAN**

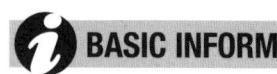
ⓘ BASIC INFORMATION

DEFINITION

Acetaminophen (APAP) poisoning is a disorder caused by excessive intake of APAP and is manifested by jaundice, nausea, vomiting, abdominal discomfort, and potential death from hepatic necrosis if not treated appropriately.

SYNONYM

Paracetamol poisoning

ICD-10CM CODES

T39.1 Poisoning by 4-aminophenol derivatives, accidental

X60 Intentional self-poisoning by 4-aminophenol derivatives

EPIDEMIOLOGY & DEMOGRAPHICS

- APAP is one of the most widely prescribed antipyretics and analgesics in the U.S. Potentially toxic ingestions, both intentional and unintentional, exceed 100,000 cases annually in the U.S.
- APAP is the most commonly potential toxic pharmaceutical reported to U.S. Poison Control Centers.
- APAP is available in more than 100 over-the-counter combination formulations, such as DayQuil/NyQuil Cold and Flu, Excedrin, and Robitussin Cold and Flu.
- APAP toxicity is the number one cause of liver transplant in the U.S. Death rate is approximately 1 in 1000 persons. Nearly 50% of exposures occur in children ≤6 yr.
- Hepatic necrosis is most likely to occur in people who (1) are chronically malnourished, (2) have alcohol use disorder, (3) have chronic liver disease, and (4) use other potentially hepatotoxic medications.
- Combination opioid and acetaminophen medications are an important source of APAP toxicity.

PHYSICAL FINDINGS & CLINICAL PRESENTATION

- The physical examination may vary depending on the amount of time since ingestion.
- Phase I (0-24 hr): Initial symptoms may be mild or absent and may consist of anorexia, diaphoresis, malaise, nausea, vomiting, lethargy, and a subclinical rise in transaminase levels. In a massive APAP ingestion, altered mental status and lactic acidosis can occur in phase I.
- Phase II (24-72 hr): Right upper quadrant pain, vomiting, somnolence, tachycardia, jaundice, hypotension, and continued increase in transaminases.
- Phase III (72-96 hr): Hepatic necrosis with abdominal pain, jaundice, hepatic encephalopathy, coagulopathy, hypoglycemia, renal failure, fatality from multiorgan failure.

- Phase IV (4 days to 2 wk): Complete resolution of symptoms and resolution of organ failure.
- Table E1 summarizes the four phases/stages of acetaminophen poisoning.

ETIOLOGY

- The amount of APAP necessary for hepatic toxicity varies with the patient's body size and hepatic function. APAP hepatotoxicity occurs when its typical metabolism pathway is overwhelmed, resulting in glutathione depletion and accumulation of the toxic metabolite, NAPQI.
- When prescribing APAP, it is recommended that APAP intake should not exceed 3 to 4 g for adults and 90 mg/kg in children within a 24-hr period. A potentially toxic single ingestion of APAP is 7.5 g for adults or 150 mg/kg in a child.
- There is no standard accepted definition, but a massive APAP ingestion is characterized by a single ingestion of >30 g to >50 g or an APAP concentration of greater than 250 mcg/ml or 300 mcg/ml in 4 h.
- A standardized nomogram (Fig. 1) is used to determine potential hepatic toxicity by knowing the APAP plasma level and the number of hr after ingestion. See the APAP ingestion algorithm.

Ⓓⓧ DIAGNOSIS

DIFFERENTIAL DIAGNOSIS

- Liver disease from alcohol use disorder
- Viral hepatitis
- Ingestion of other hepatotoxic substances
- Bacterial/viral gastroenteritis
- Pancreatitis

WORKUP

Initial workup is aimed at confirming APAP overdose with plasma APAP level and assessment of hepatic damage. A careful history should elicit the time of APAP ingestion, amount, preparation (e.g., extended release), and possible coingestants (see "Laboratory Tests").

LABORATORY TESTS

- Initial laboratory evaluation should include an initial plasma APAP level with a second level drawn approximately 4 hr after the initial ingestion. Subsequent levels can be obtained every 2 to 4 hr until the levels stabilize or decline. Levels starting from 4 hr post-ingestion should be plotted on the Rumack-Matthew nomogram (see acetaminophen ingestion algorithm to calculate potential

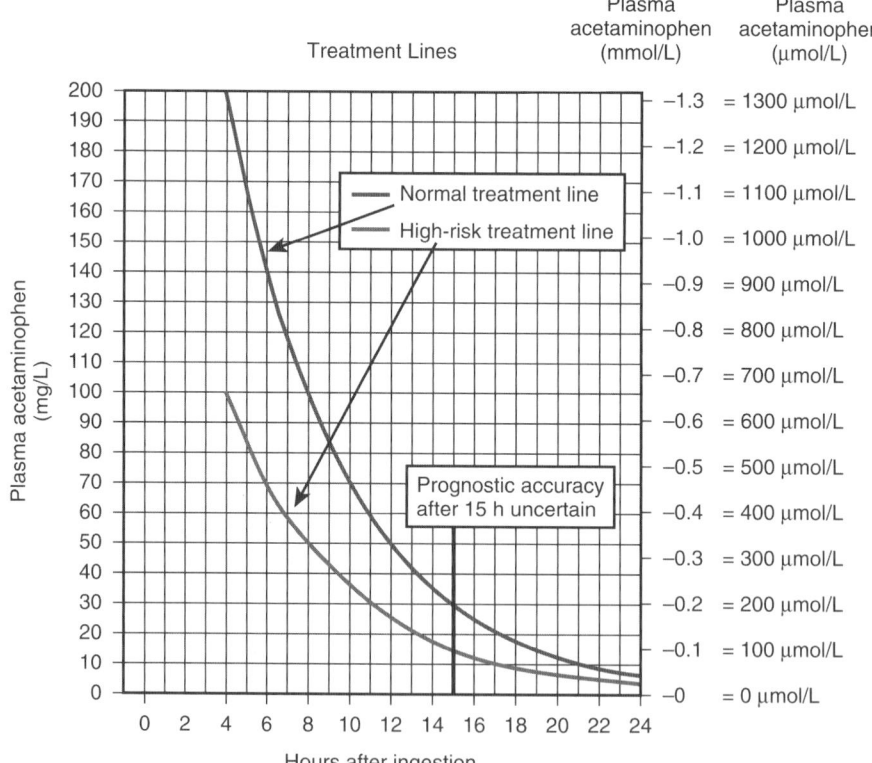

FIG 1 Normal treatment line and high-risk treatment line for the initiation of N-acetylcysteine (NAC) treatment based on serum acetaminophen levels and hours after ingestion. The high-risk line has been adopted as the standard and only treatment line in the United Kingdom. This is done to avoid confusion and to reduce the risk of undertreatment in patients with chronically induced hepatic enzymes, such as those receiving antiepileptic medication, chronic ethanol abusers, or smokers. If there is any doubt about the number of hours since ingestion, or if there is any suggestion of a staggered overdose or chronic overingestion, NAC should be administered. (From Paracetamol overdose: new guidance on treatment with intravenous acetylcysteine, *Drug Safety Update* 6[2]:A1, 2012.)

hepatic toxicity). The nomogram cannot be used with patients who present >24 hr after ingestion, took extended-release preparations, had chronic ingestions, or when the time of ingestion is unknown.

- Transaminases (aminotransferase [AST], alanine aminotransferase [ALT]), serum glucose, bilirubin level, lipase level, prothrombin time (INR), blood urea nitrogen, creatinine, ECG, and urinalysis should be initially obtained on all patients.
- Serum and urine toxicology screens for other potential toxic substances (e.g., salicylate level, ethanol level, urine drugs of abuse screening) are also recommended on admission. Screening for infectious hepatitis should also be considered.
- Urine for β-hCG should be obtained from all women of childbearing age.

Ⓡⓧ TREATMENT

NONPHARMACOLOGIC THERAPY

Consultation with a Poison Control Center (1-800-222-1222 in the United States) is recommended for patients who have ingested a large amount of APAP and/or other toxic substances. In health care encounters where APAP will be prescribed or recommended, it is important for the health care team to educate patients on the potentially toxic effects of APAP if taken in excess.

ACUTE GENERAL RX

- It is important to make the diagnosis and start treatment early, as later initiation of treatment can result in more severe hepatoxicity.
- Hepatotoxicity is defined as any increase in ALT or aspartate AST >1000 IU/L, and hepatic failure manifests as hepatotoxicity with hepatic encephalopathy. For those who cannot be risk stratified using the nomogram, the American College of Emergency Physicians recommends that N-acetylcysteine (NAC) be administered without delay to those >12 yr and >8 hr after ingestion at presentation. This would include anyone with an ingestion of APAP over many days with an APAP level <20 μg/ml (with or without ALT elevation) or anyone with undetectable APAP levels with an elevated ALT and a history of excessive APAP intake.
- Administer activated charcoal 1 g/kg PO if the patient is seen within 4 h of ingestion or the clinician suspects polysubstance ingestion that delays gastric emptying.
- Gastric lavage and whole-bowel irrigation are unnecessary and not helpful in APAP overdose as APAP is rapidly absorbed in the stomach and can delay administration of a very effective antidote if given timely, NAC.
- Determine serum acetaminophen levels 4 h after ingestion; if in the toxic range based on the Rumack-Matthew nomogram, start NAC either IV (Acetadote) or PO (Mucomyst). NAC IV loading dose is 150 mg/kg ×1 diluted in 200 ml D5W over 15 to 60 min. Maintenance dose is 50 mg/kg diluted in 500 ml D5W over 4 h, followed by 100 mg/kg diluted in 1000 ml D5W over 16 h. The dose does not require adjustment for renal or hepatic impairment or for dialysis. Total administration time is 21 h.
- Oral administration is 140 mg/kg PO as a loading dose, followed after 4 h by 70 mg/kg PO q4h for a total of 18 doses. NAC therapy should be started within 24 h of APAP overdose. Total administration time is 72 h.
- Advantages of IV administration include more reliable absorption, fewer doses, and shorter duration of treatment. Disadvantages include cost, lower hepatic concentrations from first-pass flow as compared to oral acetylcysteine, and potential for anaphylactoid reactions. Oral NAC commonly causes nausea, vomiting, diarrhea, or headache in 20% of patients.
- Monitor APAP level; use Rumack-Matthew nomogram to trend hepatic toxicity. Repeat AST/ALT and APAP levels after 12 to 14 h of IV acetylcysteine infusion and continue infusion longer than 16 h if transaminases are elevated, if APAP concentration is still measurable, or if coagulopathy exists (INR >1.5-2.0). Patients with severe, irreversible liver failure may need to continue NAC until liver transplantation is available.
- Provide adequate IV hydration (e.g., D$_{5\frac{1}{2}}$NS at 150 ml/h).
- Patients on IV N-acetylcysteine with liver failure require frequent monitoring of vital signs, oxygen saturation by pulse oximetry, and frequent blood draws. Frequent reassessment for hypoglycemia and infection is also essential.
- If APAP level is nontoxic, N-acetylcysteine therapy may be discontinued.
- Hemodialysis is recommended in APAP poisoning when:
  1. APAP is greater than 1000 and NAC is not administered
  2. Patient has altered mental status, metabolic acidosis, an elevated lactate, and APAP is >900 even if NAC is given
  3. Patient has altered mental status, metabolic acidosis, an elevated lactate, and APAP is >700 and NAC is not administered
- Continue NAC therapy during dialysis at an increased rate.

DISPOSITION

All patients with confirmed APAP poisoning will require admission, usually to an intensive care unit. Most patients (90%) will recover fully without persistent hepatic abnormalities. Hepatic failure is particularly unusual in children <6 yr.

REFERRAL

Psychiatric referral is recommended after intentional ingestions.

SUGGESTED READINGS

Available at eBooks.Health.Elsevier.com.

RELATED CONTENT

Acetaminophen Overdose (Patient Information)

AUTHORS: **Fahad Ali, MD**, and **Rory Merritt, MD, MEHP**

Achalasia 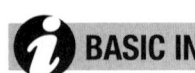 (PTG) (ALG)

BASIC INFORMATION

DEFINITION
Achalasia is a motility disorder of the esophagus classically characterized by incomplete relaxation of the lower esophageal sphincter (LES) and aperistalsis of the esophageal smooth muscle resulting in functional obstruction of the esophagus.

SYNONYMS
Achalasia and cardiospasm
Achalasia (of cardia)
Aperistalsis of esophagus
Megaesophagus
Esophageal achalasia
Esophageal cardiospasm

ICD 10-CM CODES
K22.0 Achalasia of cardia

EPIDEMIOLOGY & DEMOGRAPHICS
- Incidence has increased to approximately to 0.03 to 1.63 in 100,000 persons/yr due to studies using high-resolution esophageal manometry (HRM).[1]
- Prevalence is around 10 per 100,000 persons.
- Although the onset of symptoms may occur at any age, incidence is typically bimodal (between 20 and 40 yr, then after 60 yr) with greater incidence in the elderly.
- Men and women are affected equally.

PHYSICAL FINDINGS & CLINICAL PRESENTATION
Symptoms:
- Dysphagia (most commonly with both solids and liquids) without oropharyngeal transfer difficulties
- Difficulty belching
- Regurgitation or vomiting of undigested food
- Chest pain and/or heartburn
- Globus
- Frequent hiccups
- Symptoms of aspiration such as nocturnal cough; possible dyspnea and pneumonia
- Weight loss
- The Eckardt symptom score (assessing dysphagia, regurgitation, retrosternal pain, and weight loss) is a fairly reliable measure of achalasia severity and may be used to assess response to therapy
- The Brief Esophageal Dysphagia Questionnaire (BEDQ) is more highly sensitive for manometric diagnosis of dysphagia; it is independent of GERD symptoms and has been shown to be a better symptom-generic evaluating tool, while the Eckardt score is a more achalasia-specific metric.[2]
Physical Exam:
- While achalasia patients typically have a benign physical exam, focal lung examination abnormalities and wheezing are possible.

ETIOLOGY
- Etiology is poorly understood.
- Loss of intrinsic inhibitory neurons in the myenteric plexus and smooth muscle portion of the esophagus as well as depletion of networks of interstitial cells of Cajal of the LES result in the loss of inhibitory neurotransmitters nitric oxide and vasoactive intestinal polypeptide and unopposed excitatory cholinergic activity, leading to incomplete relaxation of the lower esophageal sphincter (LES) and loss of esophageal peristalsis.[1,3]
- Loss of myenteric nerve fibers is associated with lymphocytic and eosinophilic infiltrates, capillaritis, plexitis, venulitis, nerve hypertrophy, and fibrosis.
- There is evidence to suggest that esophageal achalasia may be autoimmune mediated, with an increase in immune cells, cytokines, chemokines, and autoimmune antibodies.[4] This disorder may be caused by autoimmune degeneration of the esophageal myenteric plexus in association with several human leucocyte antigen (HLA) class II DQ antigens. An eight amino-acid insertion in the cytoplasmic tail of HLA-DQβ1 has been identified as a strong achalasia risk factor. Antimyenteric plexus and other antineural autoantibodies have also been described. Patients with achalasia are more likely to have other autoimmune diseases.
- Abnormal immune reactions to neurotropic viruses, such as varicella zoster, measles, herpes simplex type 1, and human papilloma virus have been implicated. A host T-cell—mediated response may lead to neuronal injury; this has been suggested as the cause of types I and II achalasia (see "Imaging Studies" section).
- Achalasia is also seen in Allgrove syndrome, a rare autosomal recessive disorder caused by gene mutation on chromosome 12q13 and defined by achalasia, alacrima, autonomic disturbance, and acetylcholine insensitivity. Neurons in this syndrome may be susceptible to oxidative injury.
- Recent studies suggest that type III achalasia (see "Imaging Studies" section) is associated with myenteric inflammation but not neuronal loss; downregulation of nitric oxide synthase expression and increased cholinergic sensitivity are cytokine-mediated.
- A type III achalasia pattern has been described in chronic daily opiate users.

DIAGNOSIS

DIFFERENTIAL DIAGNOSIS
- Primary achalasia:
  1. Idiopathic
- Secondary achalasia:
  1. Chagas disease
  2. Vagal injury
  3. Prior surgery, including fundoplication; achalasia-like esophageal dilation has also been described after laparoscopic gastric banding

- Pseudoachalasia (diseases that may mimic achalasia):
  1. Esophageal cancer
  2. Infiltrating gastric cancer
  3. Oat cell and bronchogenic lung cancer
  4. Lymphoma
  5. Amyloidosis
  6. Paraneoplastic syndrome
- Angina
- Bulimia
- Anorexia nervosa
- Gastric bezoar
- Gastritis
- Peptic ulcer disease
- Postvagotomy dysmotility
- Opioid-induced esophageal dysmotility
- Esophageal disease (Table 1):
  1. Gastroesophageal reflux disease
  2. Sarcoidosis
  3. Amyloidosis
  4. Esophageal stricture
  5. Esophageal webs and rings
  6. Scleroderma
  7. Barrett esophagus
  8. Esophagitis
  9. Diffuse esophageal spasm

WORKUP
- Physical examination and laboratory analyses to rule out other causes (Fig. E1, Table 2) and assess complications
- Imaging studies, manometry, and endoscopy (may be supportive or complementary)

LABORATORY TESTS
- Assessment of nutritional status (evaluate for malnutrition, iron deficiency, vitamin/mineral deficiencies)
- Complete blood count
- ECG and/or stress test as appropriate to exclude cardiac etiologies of substernal chest pain
- Serologic assays for *Trypanosoma cruzi* (Chagas disease) in appropriate individuals

IMAGING STUDIES
Barium swallow with fluoroscopy (particularly a timed barium esophagram (TBE)) may demonstrate:
- Uncoordinated or absent esophageal contractions (loss of peristalsis)
- An acutely tapered contrast column ("bird's beak"; Fig. E2)
- Dilation of the distal esophagus (smooth muscle portion; Fig. E3)
- Esophageal air-fluid level with evidence of poor esophageal emptying
- Late-stage changes include tortuosity, angulation, dilated megaesophagus, retained food, and secretions
Manometry (Fig. E4) is considered the "gold standard" test to confirm the diagnosis. High-resolution manometry (HRM) or high-resolution esophageal pressure topography (HREPT) has defined subsets of patients with achalasia who may have different responses to medical or

TABLE 1 Esophageal Motor Disorders

	Achalasia	Scleroderma	Distal Esophageal Spasm
Symptoms	Dysphagia Regurgitation of nonacidic material	Gastroesophageal reflux disease Dysphagia	Substernal chest pain (angina-like) Dysphagia with pain
Radiographic appearance	Dilated, fluid-filled esophagus Distal *bird-beak* stricture	Aperistaltic esophagus Free reflux Peptic stricture	Simultaneous noncoordinated contractions
Manometric findings	High resting pressure	Low resting pressure	Normal pressure
Lower esophageal sphincter	Incomplete or abnormal relaxation with swallow		
Body	Low-amplitude, simultaneous contractions after swallowing	Low-amplitude peristaltic contractions or no peristalsis	Some peristalsis Diffuse and simultaneous nonperistaltic contractions, occasionally high amplitude

From Andreoli TE et al: *Andreoli and Carpenter's Cecil essentials of medicine*, ed 8, Philadelphia, 2010, Saunders.

TABLE 2 Chicago Classification v4.0 of Esophageal Motility Disorders[5]

Disorder	Diagnostic Criteria
Disorders of EGJ Outflow	
Type I achalasia (classic)	Abnormal median IRP and 100% failed peristalsis
Type II achalasia	Abnormal median IRP, 100% failed peristalsis, and ≥20% of swallows with panesophageal pressurization
Type III achalasia	Abnormal median IRP and ≥20% of swallows with premature/spastic contractions and no evidence of peristalsis
EGJ outflow obstruction	Abnormal median IRP (supine and upright), ≥20% elevated intrabolus pressure (supine), and sufficient evidence of peristalsis such that criteria for achalasia are not met; diagnosis requires clinical symptoms in addition to manometric criteria
Disorders of Peristalsis	
DES	Normal median IRP and ≥20% swallows with premature/spastic contractions with DCI >450 mm Hg•sec•cm; diagnosis requires clinical symptoms in addition to manometric criteria
Hypercontractile (jackhammer) esophagus	Normal median IRP and ≥20% hypercontractile swallows with DCI >8000 mm Hg•sec•cm; diagnosis requires clinical symptoms in addition to manometric criteria
Absent contractility	Normal median IRP and 100% failed peristalsis/absent contractility (DCI <100 mm Hg•sec•cm)
Ineffective esophageal motility (includes the definition of fragmented peristalsis)	>70% ineffective swallows or with DCI <450 mm Hg•sec•cm or ≥50% failed peristalsis

DES, Diffuse esophageal spasm; *DCI*, distal contractile interval; *DL*, distal latency; *EGJ*, esophagogastric junction; *IRP*, integrated relaxation pressure *ULN*, upper limits of normal.

surgical therapies and prognoses. This technique uses the integrated relaxation pressure (IRP) >15 mm Hg to define better the failure of esophagogastric junction relaxation. HRM also utilizes the distal contraction integral (DCI) to define hypercontractile vs. weak swallows vs. failed peristalsis. The distal latency (DL) defines premature contractions.

- In classic (Type I) achalasia, manometric abnormalities include 100% aperistalsis and incomplete or absent LES relaxation (with median IRP ≥15 mm Hg while supine or ≥12 mm Hg while upright) after swallow.
- Type II achalasia shows panesophageal pressurization to greater than 30 mm Hg with ≥20% of test swallows, aperistalsis, and incomplete or absent LES relaxation.
- Type III achalasia shows premature or spastic contractions of the distal esophagus with ≥20% of swallows (reduced DL, normal DCI), aperistalsis, and incomplete or absent LES relaxation.[5]
- HREPT has also defined the achalasia variant esophagogastric junction outflow obstruction (EGJOO), where the IRP is ≥15 mm Hg, but peristalsis is present, excluding the diagnosis of achalasia. Some are associated with secondary causes; a small percentage may progress to achalasia; and, in many, the natural history is unclear, and response to therapy is variable. A clinical diagnosis of EGJOO requires both a manometric diagnosis of EGJOO as well as clinically relevant symptoms (dysphagia and/or noncardiac chest pain) supported by follow-up testing, including pharmacologic provocation, TBE, or functional luminal imaging probe (FLIP) technology.[5] If incidentally found on manometry, asymptomatic EGJOO does not require treatment.

- Multiple rapid swallows and rapid drink challenges are provocative tests done as part of HREPT to distinguish achalasia from other motility disorders.[5]
- Accuracy of manometric classification requires normal foregut anatomy, without prior surgical interventions and without anatomical variants, including hernias, which could alter manometric catheter measurements.[5]
- Direct visualization by endoscopy (Fig. E5), including careful visualization of the esophagogastric junction and cardia, should be performed prior to manometry to exclude other causes of dysphagia, including EGJOO, strictures, secondary causes of achalasia (including infiltrating cancers), and pseudoachalasia. It is important that patients on long-term opioids be weaned off prior to manometric testing to exclude opioid-induced esophageal dysmotility; opioids have been linked to shortened DL, elevated DCI, and elevated IRP.

FLIP is a new technique that can measure compliance and distensibility across the esophagogastric junction and may demonstrate both impaired LES relaxation and response to achalasia therapy.[6]

Rx TREATMENT

NONPHARMACOLOGIC THERAPY

- Achalasia is treatable but incurable. The goals of therapy are to decrease LES pressure to relieve the functional obstruction, improve symptoms, and prevent progression to a dilated esophagus, also referred to as a megaesophagus. Current treatments are unable to improve esophageal peristalsis.
- Pneumatic dilation (PD) uses a fixed-diameter and high-pressure dilating balloon across the LES under fluoroscopic visualization to disrupt the muscle fibers and may benefit 50% to 93% of patients. Most protocols use a graded dilation approach, starting with a 30-mm balloon and repeating if required with a 35-mm or 40-mm balloon. Studies show this may be more effective in females, older patients, and HRM type 2 patients. Esophageal rupture or perforation is a rare complication (2% to 4%). It may be managed conservatively

in stable patients with a small perforation but may require surgery with larger tears or mediastinal contamination. Some patients will experience heartburn after, usually responsive to proton-pump inhibitor therapy.

- Surgical: Laparoscopic, or less commonly open, Heller esophagomyotomy (HM) is effective (90%). Approximately 35% of patients undergoing surgery will develop reflux disease. As a result, some surgeons will perform an anterior Dor or posterior Toupet antireflux repair (fundoplication) as part of the surgical procedure. Studies suggest this may be more effective in men and younger patients. An observational study has suggested that those with prior endoscopic treatment before myotomy may not do as well as those who have a primary myotomy.
- A large European study suggested that patients may expect similar medium-term outcomes from myotomy and balloon dilation. A meta-analysis suggests better long-term durability of myotomy, while balloon dilation may be more cost-effective. About 20% to 30% of patients undergoing either therapy may require retreatment within 5 to 7 yr.
- Endoscopic submucosal myotomy (peroral endoscopic myotomy [POEM]) has a high success rate comparable to laparoscopic HM (particularly in HRM type 3 patients in whom a longer myotomy, tailored to the length of the diseased segment, improves outcome), decreased hospital length of stay, few adverse events (which are similar to those associated with Heller myotomy and include pneumo-mediastinum, pneumothorax, pneumo-peritoneum, pleural effusion, pneumonia, and bleeding), and exceedingly rare mortality. Since no antireflux procedure is performed, there is a modest risk (up to 53%) of developing pathologic reflux. POEM should only be performed at high-volume centers. A randomized multicenter study showed a higher treatment success rate for POEM at 2 yr when compared with pneumatic dilation.[7,8]
- FLIP and TBE may help determine response to therapy.[6]
- Esophagectomy has been performed in patients with end-stage achalasia with a dilated, often sigmoid-shaped or megaesophagus, who have failed myotomy or pneumatic

dilation. Esophagectomy is coupled with either gastric pull-up, colon interposition, or jejunal interposition, where the stomach, colon, or small bowel are used to functionally replace the esophagus.

- Self-expanding metal stents (SEMS) have been studied as a temporary treatment in a few studies with low-quality evidence and are not currently recommended. Patients with SEMS often reported chest pain and regurgitation.
- Transoral incisionless fundoplication (TIF) may be an endoscopic treatment alternative for postprocedural GERD, specifically after POEM.[9]

ACUTE GENERAL RX

- Medications may be useful for short-term symptom relief and in patients with refractory chest pain. They should only be considered in patients unable to receive, or who are scheduled for, more definitive procedures. LES pressure may be lowered temporarily by up to 50% through sublingual use of long-acting nitrates (e.g., isosorbide dinitrate 5 to 20 mg) or calcium channel blockers (e.g., nifedipine 10 to 30 mg). Side effects are common, and duration of relief tends to be short. Sildenafil was shown to be effective in a few small, short-term studies based on manometric results but is generally not recommended given minimal clinical improvement and negative side effect profile. Anticholinergics such as atropine and theophylline are less commonly used.
- Botulinum toxin (BT) injection will benefit up to 85% of patients by inhibiting acetylcholine release from cholinergic nerve endings and blocking the unopposed cholinergic stimulation of the LES, without impacting the myogenic tone. Up to half will require repeat injections by 6 mo. A few studies have suggested that repeated injections may have diminished efficacy and can lead to fibrosis, complicating subsequent attempts at surgical therapy. Studies have identified age >40, type II or III achalasia, and EGJOO to have more favorable response to BT injections. BT is recommended as first-line therapy for patients

who may not be candidates for surgical options.

- Many patients will require proton pump inhibitor therapy for gastroesophageal reflux after effective disruption of the LES.
- For patients with weight loss secondary to achalasia, studies regarding dietary modification as adjunctive treatment are underway to help improve weight after intervention.
- Future therapies, including neural cell transplantation and electrical stimulation, are currently under investigation in animal models, but likely are years away from implementation.

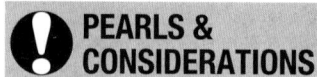

PEARLS & CONSIDERATIONS

COMMENTS

- Medication has a limited role in treatment.
- Botulinum toxin is transiently effective in improving symptoms and should be considered primarily in patients too elderly or ill to be considered for surgery.
- Pneumatic dilation, surgical myotomy, and POEM provide more durable long-term responses and are the treatment of choice for most patients.
- Patients with achalasia may be at long-term risk of squamous cell carcinoma of the esophagus and non–reflux-associated esophagitis. Treated patients may be at long-term risk for reflux esophagitis, Barrett esophagus, and adenocarcinoma. Endoscopic surveillance is not routinely recommended in these patients.

REFERENCES
Available at eBooks.Health.Elsevier.com

RELATED CONTENT
Achalasia (Patient Information)
Dysphagia (Related Key Topic)

AUTHOR: **HANNAH FISKE, MD,** and **HARLAN G. RICH, MD, FACP, AGAF**

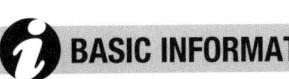

A

I

BASIC INFORMATION

DEFINITION

Acne vulgaris is a chronic disorder of the pilosebaceous apparatus caused by abnormal desquamation of follicular epithelium leading to obstruction of the pilosebaceous canal, resulting in inflammation and subsequent formation of papules, pustules, nodules, comedones, and scarring. Based on their appearance, the acne lesions can be divided into inflammatory (presence of papules, pustules, cysts, and nodules) or noninflammatory (open and closed comedones). For inflammatory acne, lesions can be classified as papulopustular, nodulocystic, or both. There are many classification schemes for categorizing acne severity, but because of variability in these tools, there is no universal grading system for acne.[1,2] In general:

1. Mild acne: Characterized by the presence of comedones (Figs. E1 and E2) (noninflammatory lesions), few papules and pustules (generally <10), but no cysts or nodules.
2. Moderate acne: Presence of several to many papules and pustules (10 to 40) along with comedones (10 to 40). The presence of >40 papules and pustules along with larger, deeper nodulocystic inflamed lesions (Figs. E3 and E4) (up to five) denotes moderately severe acne.
3. Severe acne: Presence of numerous or extensive papules and pustules as well as many nodulocystic lesions (Fig. E5).

In addition, the presence of larger and deep-seated inflammatory lesions distributed along the mandibular and anterolateral neck regions, menstrual flares, and the presence of signs of androgen excess such as hirsutism and menstrual irregularity are suggestive of hormonally-driven acne.

SYNONYM

Acne

ICD-10CM CODES
L70.0 Acne vulgaris
L70.1 Acne conglobata
L70.2 Acne varioliformis
L70.3 Acne tropica
L70.4 Infantile acne; Neonatal acne
L70.5 Acne excoriee
L70.8 Other acne
L70.9 Acne, unspecified
L71.9 Acne rosacea
L73.0 Acne keloidalis nuchae

EPIDEMIOLOGY & DEMOGRAPHICS

- Acne is the most common skin disease in the U.S. Increased incidence of acne mechanica due to prolonged wearing of masks has been seen during the COVID-19 pandemic.
- It is most common in teenagers, with as many as 85% of all teenagers being affected to some degree.[3]
- Highest incidence between ages of 15 and 18 yr in both genders.
- Involution of the disease usually occurs before age 25 yr, but 26% of women and 12% of men will continue to have clinical acne until the mid-40s.

PHYSICAL FINDINGS & CLINICAL PRESENTATION

- Open comedones (blackheads), closed comedones (whiteheads)
- Inflammatory papules, pustules, nodulocystic lesions, and ectatic pores
- Greasiness (oily skin)
- Presence of scars from prior acne cysts (ice pick, crateriform, rolling, keloidal)
- Dyspigmentation (usually hyperpigmentation or erythema)
- Various stages of development and severity may be present concomitantly
- Common distribution of acne: Face, back, and upper chest
- Common distribution of hormonal acne: Mandibular and anterolateral neck regions

ETIOLOGY

- Acne vulgaris is a follicular disease, with the principal abnormality being comedone formation.
- Overactivity of the sebaceous glands and excessive desquamation of the epithelial cells leading to blockage in the ducts. The obstruction leads to the formation of comedones, which can become inflamed because of overgrowth of *Cutibacterium acnes* (formerly known as *P. acnes*).
- Exacerbated by environmental factors (hot, humid, tropical climate), medications (e.g., iodine in cough mixtures, hair greases, anabolic steroids, progestins, lithium), industrial exposure to halogenated hydrocarbons.
- Mechanical or frictional forces can aggravate existing acne (e.g., excessive washing by some patients to help rid them of their blackheads or oiliness, sports gear).
- Stress is also known to exacerbate acne through the Hypothalamic-Pituitary-Adrenal (HPA) axis and increased androgen activation.

DIAGNOSIS

DIFFERENTIAL DIAGNOSIS (TABLE 1)

- Gram-negative folliculitis
- Staphylococcal pyoderma
- Drug eruption
- Sebaceous hyperplasia
- Angiofibromas, basal cell carcinomas, osteoma cutis
- Occupational exposures to oils or grease
- Steroid acne
- Hidradenitis suppurativa
- Perioral dermatitis
- Pseudofolliculitis barbae
- Miliaria
- Seborrheic dermatitis
- Keratosis pilaris

WORKUP

History and physical examination:
- Inquire about previous treatment
- Careful drug history (including all OTC products)
- Family history, history of cyclic menstrual flares
- History of use of cosmetics and cleansers
- Oral contraceptive use
- Use of medications that may worsen acne such as corticosteroids, anabolic steroids, lithium, neuroleptics, cyclosporine
- Consider the possibility of hyperandrogenic state in all women (hirsutism, irregular menses, androgenic alopecia) or children (seborrhea, acanthosis nigricans, onset of acne between ages 1 and 7 yr and no obvious external factors). It is important to consider the timing of puberty, which can occur as early as 6 yr in Black girls.

LABORATORY TESTS

- Laboratory evaluation is generally not helpful. Patients who are candidates for therapy with isotretinoin should have baseline liver enzymes and triglycerides checked because this medication may result in elevation of lipids and liver enzymes.
- A negative serum or urine pregnancy test should also be obtained in females 1 mo before and at the time of initiation of isotretinoin; it is also imperative to maintain effective contraception during and 1 mo after therapy with isotretinoin ends because of its teratogenic effects. Pregnancy status should be rechecked at monthly visits.
- If hyperandrogenism is suspected in female patients, levels of dehydroepiandrosterone sulfate (DHEAS), testosterone (total and free), luteinizing hormone and follicle stimulating hormone levels should be measured. For women with regular menstrual cycles, serum androgen measurements generally are not necessary.

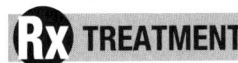 TREATMENT

The cornerstone of acne treatment is combination therapy, which addresses the many pathogenic mechanisms responsible for acne.

NONPHARMACOLOGIC THERAPY

- Blue light (ClearLight therapy system) can be used for treatment of moderate inflammatory acne vulgaris. Light in the violet/blue range can cause bacterial death by a photoreaction in which porphyrins react with oxygen to generate reactive oxygen species, which damage the cell membranes of *P. acnes*. Treatment usually consists of 15-min

TABLE 1 Differential Diagnosis of Acne

ACNE VULGARIS—COMEDONAL

Closed	**Open**
• Milia	• Contact acne (see Closed)
• Osteoma cutis	• Acne exacerbated by systemic corticosteroids‡ or anabolic steroids
• Sebaceous hyperplasia	• Trichostasis spinulosa
• Pseudoacne of the nasal crease	• Favre-Racouchot syndrome
• Syringomas	• Pseudoacne of the nasal crease
• Trichoepitheliomas*	• Nevus comedonicus
• Trichodiscomas, fibrofolliculomas	• Basaloid follicular hamartoma syndrome
• Eruptive vellus hair cysts†, steatocystoma multiplex†	• Familial dyskeratotic comedones
• Colloid milia	• Dowling-Degos disease
• Acne exacerbated by systemic corticosteroids‡ or anabolic steroids	• Radiation-induced comedones
• Contact acne (occupational, pomade, cosmetica, mechanica; chloracne)	• Molluscum-induced comedones
• Follicular mucinosis	• Childhood flexural comedones (often a single double-orifice lesion)
• Follicular mycosis fungoides	• Dilated pore of Winer (single lesion)
	• Trichofolliculoma (usually a single lesion)
	• Follicular spines—in settings such as trichodysplasia spinulosa§, type VI pityriasis rubra pilaris§, multiple myeloma, demodicosis§, follicular mucinosis, and drug-induced (e.g., BRAF inhibitors, cyclosporine§, acitretin)
Acne vulgaris—inflammatory	
• Rosacea	• Keratosis pilaris
• Perioral/periorificial dermatitis	• Trichodysplasia spinulosa (viral-associated trichodysplasia)§
• Demodicosis (adults > children§)	• Lupus miliaris disseminatus faciei
• Folliculitis—culture-negative (normal flora), staphylococcal, gram-negative, eosinophilic§, Pityrosporum	• Psychogenic (neurotic) excoriations, factitial lesions
• Acne/acneiform eruptions due to topical or systemic corticosteroids‡, anabolic steroids, or other medications (e.g., lithium, EGFR inhibitors)	• Follicular mucinosis
	• Follicular mycosis fungoides
• Pseudofolliculitis barbae, acne keloidalis nuchae	• Tinea faciei
• Pseudoacne of the nasal crease	• Molluscum contagiosum (especially inflamed lesions)
• Furuncle/carbuncle	• Angiofibromas
• Idiopathic facial aseptic granuloma (in children)	• Dowling-Degos disease (especially the Haber syndrome variant)
• Neutrophilic dermatoses and neutrophilic eccrine hidradenitis	• Cutaneous Rosai-Dorfman disease
	• Granulomatosis with polyangiitis (Wegener granulomatosis)
	• Syndromes associated with acne, e.g., PAPA, (PA)PASH, SAPHO, Apert syndrome
Neonatal acne (neonatal cephalic pustulosis)	
• Sebaceous hyperplasia	• Candidal infection
• Milia	• Papulopustular eruption of hyper-IgE syndrome
• Miliaria rubra (especially pustular variant)	• Vesiculopustular eruption of transient myeloproliferative disorder
Solid facial edema secondary to acne vulgaris	
• Solid facial edema secondary to rosacea	• Angioedema (lasts <24-72 h), C1 esterase inhibitor deficiency (lasts 2-3 days), blepharochalasis/Ascher syndrome
• Melkersson-Rosenthal syndrome, sarcoidosis (e.g., Heerfordt syndrome), lepromatous leprosy	• Sweet syndrome or cellulitis—more abrupt onset
• Lymphoma (B- or T-cell), leukemia cutis, angiosarcoma	• Superior vena caval obstruction
• Scleromyxedema, myxedema, self-healing (juvenile) cutaneous mucinosis	• Lymphatic malformation
• Autoimmune connective tissue disease (e.g., dermatomyositis, lupus erythematosus, Still disease)	• Pachydermoperiostosis and other genetic disorders with coarse facies
	• Other—trichinosis, primary systemic amyloidosis

EGFR, Epidermal growth factor receptor; *PAPA, pyogenic arthritis, pyoderma gangrenosum, and acne conglobata; (PA)PASH, (pyogenic arthritis), pyoderma gangrenosum, acne, and suppurative hidradenitis; SAPHO, synovitis, acne, pustulosis, hyperostosis, and osteitis.*
*Early or small-sized.
†In the differential diagnosis of cystic lesions of the trunk.
‡Can also lead to rosacea-like picture.
§Often in the setting of HIV infection and/or other immunocompromised states, including trichodysplasia spinulosa in patients receiving cyclosporine.
From Bolognia J: *Dermatology*, ed 4, 2018, Elsevier.

exposures twice weekly for 4 wk. Phototherapy may be effective for short-term treatment of acne, but long-term efficacy and how it compares with conventional acne therapy is unclear.
• Diet: In obese patients, dietary counseling is recommended. A high-glycemic or high-dairy diet as well as low fat or skim milk may worsen acne, although the strength of their influence is controversial.[4]

ACUTE GENERAL Rx

Treatment generally varies with the type of lesions (comedones, papules, pustules, cystic lesions) and the severity of acne. Table 2 summarizes an acne treatment algorithm. First-line treatment for mild acne vulgaris includes benzoyl peroxide, a topical retinoid, or a combination of topical medications, including topical antibiotics. Use of topical treatments for 6 to 8 wk is required to judge their efficacy. Table E3 describes prescription topical therapies for acne.

TABLE 2 Acne Treatment Algorithm

	SEVERITY (LESION TYPE)				
Therapy	Mild (Comedonal)	Mild (Inflammatory/Mixed)	Moderate (Inflammatory/Mixed)	Severe (Inflammatory/Mixed)	Severe (Nodular/Scarring)
Initial therapy options*,†	Topical retinoid BP Salicylic acid cleanser	BP/retinoid combo BP/antibiotic combo Antibiotic/retinoid combo + BP	BP/retinoid combo BP/antibiotic combo ± topical retinoid Antibiotic/retinoid combo + BP ± oral antibiotic	BP/retinoid combo + oral antibiotic BP/antibiotic combo + topical retinoid + oral antibiotic Antibiotic/retinoid combo + BP + oral antibiotic	Isotretinoin
Alternative therapy options*,†,‡	Add BP or retinoid if not already prescribed BP/antibiotic combo BP/retinoid combo Antibiotic/retinoid combo	Substitute another combo product Add missing component (i.e., topical retinoid, BP, topical antibiotic) Change type, strength, or formulation of topical retinoid	Substitute another combo product Add missing component (i.e., topical retinoid, BP, topical antibiotic, oral antibiotic) Change type, strength, or formulation of topical retinoid Consider hormonal therapy for females Consider oral isotretinoin	Consider changing oral antibiotic Consider isotretinoin Consider hormonal therapy for females	Consider hormonal therapy for females
Maintenance therapy	Topical retinoid or BP/retinoid combo	Topical retinoid or BP/retinoid combo	Topical retinoid or BP/retinoid combo	Topical retinoid or BP/retinoid combo	Topical retinoid or BP/retinoid combo

BP, Benzoyl peroxide.

*If combination products not available to patient, consider substitution of individual components as separate prescriptions.

†Topical dapsone may be considered in place of topical antibiotic.

‡If needed as determined by physician assessment and patient satisfaction.

Modified from Zaenglein AL, Thiboutot DM: Expert committee recommendations for acne management, *Pediatrics* 118(3):1188-1199, 2006; Thiboutot D, et al: New insights into the management of acne: an update from the Global Alliance to Improve Outcomes in Acne Group, *J Am Acad Dermatol* 60:S1-S50, 2009; Eichenfield LF, et al: Evidence-based recommendations for the diagnosis and treatment of pediatric acne, *Pediatrics* 131(3):S163-S186, 2013; Thiboutot DM, Gollnick HP: Treatment considerations for inflammatory acne: clinical evidence for adapalene 0.1% in combination therapies, *J Drugs Dermatol* 5(8):785-794, 2006; Gollnick H, et al: Management of acne: a report from a Global Alliance to Improve Outcomes in Acne, *J Am Acad Dermatol* 49(Suppl 1):S1-S37, 2003.

- Comedones (noninflammatory acne) can be treated with retinoids or retinoid analogs. Topical retinoids are comedolytic and work by normalizing follicular keratinization. Commonly available agents are Adapalene (Differin, 0.1% gel or cream, applied once or twice daily), tazarotene (Tazorac 0.1% cream or gel applied once daily), tretinoin (Retin-A 0.1% cream or 0.025 gel applied once daily), tretinoin microsphere (Retin-A Micro, 0.1% gel, applied once daily). Tretinoin and tazarotene are inactivated by ultraviolet light and oxidized by benzoyl peroxide; therefore, it should only be applied at night and not used concomitantly with benzoyl peroxide. Adapalene, rather, is not photolabile and can be used morning or evening.
- Tretinoin is pregnancy category C and tazarotene is pregnancy category X. Salicylic acid preparations (e.g., Neutrogena 2% wash) have keratolytic and antiinflammatory properties, and are also useful in the treatment of comedones. Large, open comedones (blackheads) should be expressed.
- Patients should be reevaluated after 6 to 8 wk.
- Benzoyl peroxide gel (2.5% or 5%) may be added if the comedones become inflamed or form pustules. The most common adverse effects are dryness, erythema, and peeling.
- Topical antibiotics (erythromycin, clindamycin lotions/gels or pads) can also be used in patients with significant inflammation. They reduce *C. acnes* in the pilosebaceous follicle and have some antiinflammatory effects. The combination of 5% benzoyl peroxide and 3% erythromycin (Benzamycin) or 1% clindamycin with 5% benzoyl peroxide (BenzaClin) is highly

effective in patients who have a mixture of comedonal and inflammatory acne lesions.
- Fixed-dose combinations of clindamycin phosphate 1.2% and tretinoin 0.025% are available (Veltin gel, Ziana) and are more effective than either product used alone; however, they are much more expensive than the individual generic components.
- Pustular acne can be treated with tretinoin and benzoyl peroxide gel applied on alternate evenings; drying agents (sulfacetamide-sulfa lotions [Novacet, Sulfacet]) are also effective when used in combination with benzoyl peroxide; oral antibiotics (doxycycline 100 mg qd or bid or erythromycin 1 g qd given in 2 to 3 divided doses) are effective in patients with moderate to severe pustular acne. Patients not responding well to these antibiotics can be switched to minocycline 50 to 100 mg bid. Table E4 summarizes oral antibiotics for acne vulgaris.
- Patients with nodulocystic acne and those with moderate to severe inflammatory acne unresponsive to topical drugs can be treated with systemic agents: Antibiotics (erythromycin, tetracycline, doxycycline, minocycline), isotretinoin (available on a restricted basis), or oral contraceptives. Periodic intralesional triamcinolone (Kenalog) injections by a dermatologist are also effective. The possibility of endocrinopathy should be considered in patients responding poorly to therapy.
- Oral antibiotic use should be limited to 3 to 6 mo to avoid antibiotic resistance and disruption of the microbiome.
- Isotretinoin is the most effective drug available for treatment of severe nodulocystic acne. It is indicated for acne resistant to antibiotic

therapy and severe acne. It inhibits *C. acne's* colonization by reducing sebum production and has antiinflammatory and keratolytic effects. It is available only on a restricted basis. Dosage is 0.5 to 1 mg/kg/day in two divided doses (maximum of 2 mg/kg/day); duration of therapy is generally 24 wk to reach a cumulative dose 120 to 150 mg/kg for severe cystic acne. Before using this medication, patients should undergo baseline laboratory evaluation (see "Laboratory Tests"). This drug is absolutely contraindicated during pregnancy because of its teratogenicity. It should be used with caution in patients with history of depression. Physicians, distributors, pharmacies, and patients must register in the iPLEDGE program (www.ipledgeprogram.com) before using isotretinoin.
- Azelaic acid is a bacteriostatic dicarboxylic acid used to normalize keratinization and reduce inflammation. It can be used in pregnant women.
- Oral contraceptives reduce androgen levels and therefore sebum production. They represent a useful adjunctive therapy for all types of acne in women and adolescent girls. FDA-approved agents for the treatment of hormonal acne include norgestimate/ethinyl estradiol (Ortho Tri-Cyclen), drospirenone/ethinyl estradiol (Yaz), drospirenone/ethinyl estradiol/levomefolate calcium (Beyaz), and norethindrone/ethinyl estradiol/ferrous fumarate (Estrostep Fe).
- In addition to oral contraceptives, topical and oral antiandrogenic agents including clascoterone (Winlevi) 1% cream and spironolactone 25 to 200 mg/day can also be considered as adjuncts for hormonal acne.

TABLE 6 Tips for Topical Acne Therapy

Improve adherence—often compromised due to patients having busy schedules or quitting when the response is not rapid	• Simplify the regimen: Once daily when possible; consider combination products (e.g., benzoyl peroxide + adapalene or clindamycin; tretinoin + clindamycin), especially in less motivated adolescents • Inform patients that it will take 6-8 wk of treatment for substantial improvement • Ask specifically about adherence: "Out of 7 nights, how many times do you apply the medication?"
Educate on proper use	• In general, topical medications (especially retinoids) should be used to the entire acne-prone region rather than as "spot treatment" of individual lesions • Provide instructions on where to apply the medication and how much to use
Minimize irritation—most common in adolescents with atopic dermatitis and adults	• Note that using too much medication or applying it too frequently can increase irritation • Devise a gradual initial approach to improve tolerance in patients with sensitive skin; for example, a single agent may be used for the first 2-3 wk (starting every other day for retinoids), followed by slow introduction of a second medication (e.g., transitioning from alternate days to daily) • Advise to avoid harsh scrubs and other irritating agents (e.g., toners, acne products that are not part of the regimen) • Suggest use of a noncomedogenic sensitive skin moisturizer if dryness occurs
Avoid exacerbation	• Review all skin care products and cosmetics; having patients bring everything that they apply to their face to a visit may help to determine the source of problems • Advise noncomedogenic products (e.g., moisturizers, sunscreens, make-up) and to avoid having oily hair or using pomades that may contribute to acne • Instruct patients not to pick or manipulate lesions
Reinforce the plan—patients often forget what is recommended and are bombarded by advertising and false information about acne	• Provide a written handout with your specific instructions • Recommend additional reliable educational resources about acne and its treatment (e.g., www.aad.org/public/diseases/acne#www.webmd.com/skin-problems-and-treatments/acne/default.htm)

From Bolognia J: *Dermatology,* ed 4, Philadelphia, 2018, Elsevier.

REFERRAL

Referral for intralesional injection, resurfacing lasers, and dermabrasion should be considered in patients with severe acne unresponsive to conventional therapy. Table E5 summarizes alternative treatments for acne vulgaris.

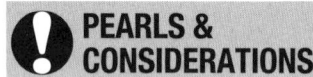

PEARLS & CONSIDERATIONS

• Gram-negative folliculitis should be suspected if inflammatory acne worsens after several months of oral antibiotic therapy.
• Acne may worsen during the first 3 to 4 wk of retinoid therapy before improving.

• Tips for topical acne therapy are summarized in Table 6.

COMMENTS

Indications for systemic therapy of acne are:
• Painful deep papules or nodules
• Extensive lesions
• Active acne with severe scarring, hyperpigmentation, or evidence of acne excoriée
• Patient's morale

Patients should be educated that in most cases acne can be controlled but not cured and that at least 4 to 6 wk of initial therapy should be required before significant improvement is noted.

• The negative psychological effect of acne may be severe and long-lasting.

REFERENCES & SUGGESTED READINGS
Available at eBooks.Health.Elsevier.com

RELATED CONTENT
Acne (Patient Information)

AUTHOR: **MARY LARIJANI, MD**

BASIC INFORMATION

DEFINITION

Acquired immunodeficiency syndrome (AIDS) is a disorder caused by infection with the human immunodeficiency virus (HIV) and marked by progressive deterioration of the cellular immune system, leading to secondary (opportunistic) infections and/or malignancies.

SYNONYM

AIDS

ICD-10CM CODE
B20 Human immunodeficiency virus [HIV] disease

EPIDEMIOLOGY & DEMOGRAPHICS

INCIDENCE (IN U.S.):
- A significant number of persons are diagnosed with AIDS in the U.S. each year.
- There is a disproportionate number of new HIV/AIDS cases among Black/African Americans and Latino/Hispanic Americans compared with white Americans.
- The majority of all new HIV/AIDS diagnoses are among gay, bisexual, or other men who have sex with men (MSM).

PREVALENCE (IN U.S.): Approximately 1.2 million people in the U.S. have HIV. A subset of these have been diagnosed with AIDS.

PREDOMINANT SEX: Men constitute the majority of HIV/AIDS diagnoses in the U.S. with a disproportionate number among MSM.

PREDOMINANT AGE: The predominant age group diagnosed with HIV/AIDS is 25 to 59 yr of age.

PEAK INCIDENCE: Ages 25 to 59 yr

GENETICS:
- Familial disposition: Although there is no proven genetic predisposition, individuals with deletions in the *CCR5* gene are less susceptible to HIV infection with macrophage tropic virus (the predominant virus in sexual transmission) and may progress to AIDS more slowly.
- Congenital infection:
  1. HIV is transmittable from an infected mother to the fetus in utero in as many as 30% of pregnancies if untreated.
  2. No specific congenital malformations associated with infection; low birth weight and spontaneous abortion are possible.

PHYSICAL FINDINGS & CLINICAL PRESENTATION

- Nonspecific findings: Fever, weight loss, anorexia
- Specific syndromes:
  1. Seen in association with specific opportunistic infections and malignancies. These include:
     a. Opportunistic infections:
        (1) Disseminated strongyloidiasis
        (2) Disseminated toxoplasmosis, cryptococcosis, histoplasmosis, cyto-

megalovirus (CMV), herpes simplex virus (HSV), or mycobacterial disease (most common is *Mycobacterium avium* complex)
        (3) *Candida* esophagitis or bronchopulmonary disease
        (4) Chronic cryptosporidiosis diarrhea
        (5) *Pneumocystis jiroveci* pneumonia (PJP)
        (6) Extensive pulmonary and extrapulmonary tuberculosis (TB)
        (7) Recurrent pneumonia or other bacterial infections
        (8) Progressive multifocal leukoencephalopathy (PML)
     b. AIDS-related neoplasms:
        (1) Kaposi sarcoma
        (2) Primary brain lymphoma
        (3) Invasive cervical carcinoma
        (4) High-grade B-cell non-Hodgkin lymphoma, Burkitt lymphoma, undifferentiated non-Hodgkin lymphoma, or immunoblastic lymphoma
  2. Most common:
     a. Respiratory infections (*Pneumocystis jiroveci* [formerly known as *Pneumocystis carinii*] pneumonia, TB, bacterial pneumonia, fungal infection)
     b. CNS infections (toxoplasmosis, TB)
     c. GI (cryptosporidiosis, isosporiasis, CMV); Sections II and III describe organisms associated with diarrhea in patients with AIDS
     d. Eye infections (CMV, toxoplasmosis)
     e. Kaposi sarcoma (cutaneous or visceral) or lymphoma (nodal or extranodal)
- Possibly asymptomatic
- Diagnosis of AIDS if the CD4 cell count is <200 or <14% of total lymphocyte in the presence of proven HIV infection, even in the absence of other infections
- The various manifestations of HIV infection are described in Section II

ETIOLOGY

- Caused by infection with HIV-1 or HIV-2 (less common).
- HIV is transmitted by sexual contact, needle-sharing (during injection drug use), transfusion of contaminated blood or blood products, and from infected mother to fetus or neonate.

DIAGNOSIS

DIFFERENTIAL DIAGNOSIS

- Other wasting illnesses mimicking the nonspecific features of AIDS:
  1. TB
  2. Malignancy
  3. Disseminated fungal infection
  4. Malabsorption syndromes
  5. Depression
- Other disorders associated with dementia or demyelination producing encephalopathy, myelopathy, or neuropathy

WORKUP

Prompt evaluation of respiratory, CNS, and GI complaints. Fig. 1 illustrates a syndromic approach to suspected opportunistic infection in HIV.

LABORATORY TESTS

- HIV antibody testing. See "Human Immunodeficiency Virus" topic for the updated surveillance case definition for HIV infection
- CD4 cell count: Performed to determine the degree of immunodeficiency
- Viral load assay: To plan long-term antiviral therapy and to follow progression and success of treatment (i.e., HIV RNA PCR)
- CSF examination: For meningitis or neurologic disease (if indicated)
- Serologic tests for syphilis, hepatitis A, hepatitis B, hepatitis C, and toxoplasmosis
- Testing for other sexually transmitted infections (STIs) such as syphilis, gonorrhea, and chlamydia
- Genotypic resistance testing: Used to assess for primary resistance in naïve patients and secondary resistance in patients failing a regimen
- Eye exam: To evaluate for CMV retinitis in patients with CD4 counts <50 cells/mm^3
- Cryptococcal antigen: Part of the evaluation in AIDS patients with CD4 counts <100 cells/mm^3 who have fever, diffuse pneumonia, or evidence of meningitis
- Evaluation for infection with mycobacterium (TB or MAI) including a tuberculin skin test (TST) or interferon-gamma release assay (IGRA), sputum cultures, chest radiograph, and blood cultures for acid-fast bacteria, depending on clinical presentation

IMAGING STUDIES

- MRI or CT of head for encephalopathy or focal CNS complications (e.g., toxoplasmosis [Fig. E2], lymphoma)
- Chest radiography or CT to aid in the diagnosis of *Pneumocystis jiroveci* pneumonia (PJP), TB, or bacterial pneumonia

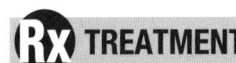 TREATMENT

The most important aspect in management of AIDS due to HIV infection is the timely initiation of antiretroviral therapy. Antiretroviral therapy should be initiated regardless of CD4 cell count.

NONPHARMACOLOGIC THERAPY

- Maintain adequate caloric intake.
- Encourage good oral hygiene and regular dental care.
- Avoid high-risk behaviors that increase the risk of other potential pathogens—use condoms, avoid sharing needles, etc.
- Update vaccines—particularly Tdap (tetanus, diphtheria, and pertussis), pneumococcal, meningococcal, and hepatitis A/B vaccines along with annual influenza vaccines. COVID-19 vaccination is recommended.

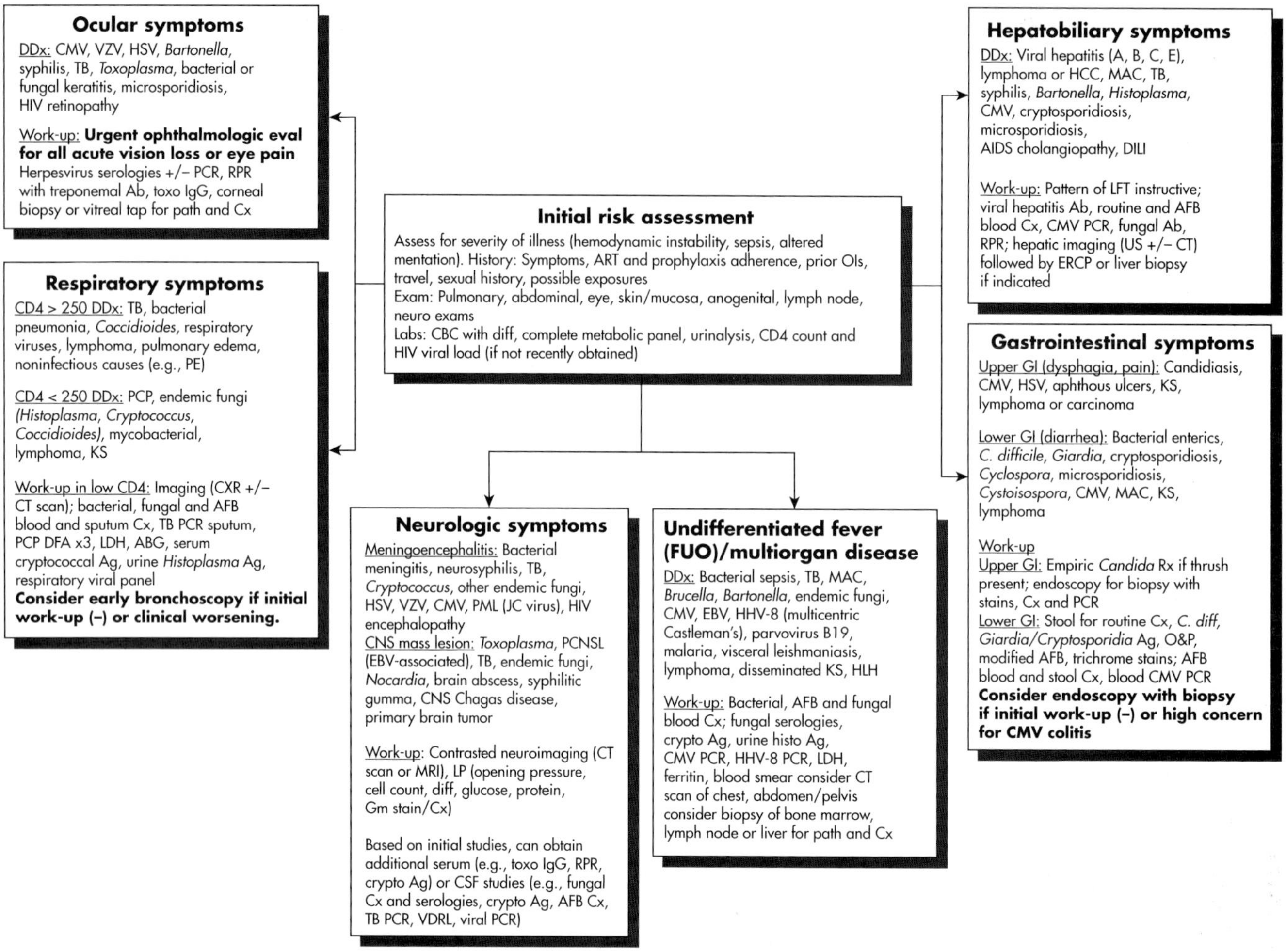

Ocular symptoms
DDx: CMV, VZV, HSV, *Bartonella*, syphilis, TB, *Toxoplasma*, bacterial or fungal keratitis, microsporidiosis, HIV retinopathy

Work-up: **Urgent ophthalmologic eval for all acute vision loss or eye pain**
Herpesvirus serologies +/– PCR, RPR with treponemal Ab, toxo IgG, corneal biopsy or vitreal tap for path and Cx

Respiratory symptoms
CD4 > 250 DDx: TB, bacterial pneumonia, *Coccidioides*, respiratory viruses, lymphoma, pulmonary edema, noninfectious causes (e.g., PE)

CD4 < 250 DDx: PCP, endemic fungi (*Histoplasma, Cryptococcus, Coccidioides*), mycobacterial, lymphoma, KS

Work-up in low CD4: Imaging (CXR +/– CT scan) bacterial, fungal and AFB blood and sputum Cx, TB PCR sputum, PCP DFA x3, LDH, ABG, serum cryptococcal Ag, urine *Histoplasma* Ag, respiratory viral panel
Consider early bronchoscopy if initial work-up (–) or clinical worsening.

Initial risk assessment
Assess for severity of illness (hemodynamic instability, sepsis, altered mentation). History: Symptoms, ART and prophylaxis adherence, prior OIs, travel, sexual history, possible exposures
Exam: Pulmonary, abdominal, eye, skin/mucosa, anogenital, lymph node, neuro exams
Labs: CBC with diff, complete metabolic panel, urinalysis, CD4 count and HIV viral load (if not recently obtained)

Neurologic symptoms
Meningoencephalitis: Bacterial meningitis, neurosyphilis, TB, *Cryptococcus*, other endemic fungi, HSV, VZV, CMV, PML (JC virus), HIV encephalopathy
CNS mass lesion: *Toxoplasma*, PCNSL (EBV-associated), TB, endemic fungi, *Nocardia*, brain abscess, syphilitic gumma, CNS Chagas disease, primary brain tumor

Work-up: Contrasted neuroimaging (CT scan or MRI), LP (opening pressure, cell count, diff, glucose, protein, Gm stain/Cx)

Based on initial studies, can obtain additional serum (e.g., toxo IgG, RPR, crypto Ag) or CSF studies (e.g., fungal Cx and serologies, crypto Ag, AFB Cx, TB PCR, VDRL, viral PCR)

Undifferentiated fever (FUO)/multiorgan disease
DDx: Bacterial sepsis, TB, MAC, *Brucella, Bartonella*, endemic fungi, CMV, EBV, HHV-8 (multicentric Castleman's), parvovirus B19, malaria, visceral leishmaniasis, lymphoma, disseminated KS, HLH

Work-up: Bacterial, AFB and fungal blood Cx; fungal serologies, crypto Ag, urine histo Ag, CMV PCR, HHV-8 PCR, LDH, ferritin, blood smear consider CT scan of chest, abdomen/pelvis consider biopsy of bone marrow, lymph node or liver for path and Cx

Hepatobiliary symptoms
DDx: Viral hepatitis (A, B, C, E), lymphoma or HCC, MAC, TB, syphilis, *Bartonella, Histoplasma*, CMV, cryptosporidiosis, microsporidiosis, AIDS cholangiopathy, DILI

Work-up: Pattern of LFT instructive; viral hepatitis Ab, routine and AFB blood Cx, CMV PCR, fungal Ab, RPR; hepatic imaging (US +/– CT) followed by ERCP or liver biopsy if indicated

Gastrointestinal symptoms
Upper GI (dysphagia, pain): Candidiasis, CMV, HSV, aphthous ulcers, KS, lymphoma or carcinoma

Lower GI (diarrhea): Bacterial enterics, *C. difficile, Giardia*, cryptosporidiosis, *Cyclospora*, microsporidiosis, *Cystoisospora*, CMV, MAC, KS, lymphoma

Work-up
Upper GI: Empiric *Candida* Rx if thrush present; endoscopy for biopsy with stains, Cx and PCR
Lower GI: Stool for routine Cx, *C. diff, Giardia/Cryptosporidia* Ag, O&P, modified AFB, trichrome stains; AFB blood and stool Cx, blood CMV PCR
Consider endoscopy with biopsy if initial work-up (–) or high concern for CMV colitis

FIG. 1 Syndromic approach to suspected opportunistic infection in HIV. *ABG,* Arterial blood gas; *AFB,* acid-fast bacilli; *ART,* antiretroviral therapy; *CBC,* complete blood count; *CMV,* cytomegalovirus; *DFA,* direct fluorescent antibody; *DILI,* drug-induced liver injury; *EBV,* Epstein–Barr virus; *ERCP,* endoscopic retrograde cholangiopancreatography; *FUO,* fever of unknown origin; *HCC,* hepatocellular carcinoma; *HHV-8,* human herpes virus 8; *HLH,* hemophagocytic lymphohistiocytosis; *HSV,* herpes simplex virus; *KS,* Kaposi sarcoma; *LDH,* lactate dehydrogenase; *LP,* lumbar puncture; *MAC, Mycobacterium avium* complex; *O&P,* ova and parasite; *PCNSL,* primary CNS lymphoma; *PCP, Pneumocystis* pneumonia; *PCR,* polymerase chain reaction; *PE,* pulmonary embolism; *PML,* progressive multifocal leukoencephalopathy; *RPR,* rapid plasma reagin; *TB,* tuberculosis; *US,* ultrasound; *VDRL,* Venereal Disease Research Laboratory test; *VZV,* varicella-zoster virus. (From Spec A et al: *Comprehensive review of infectious diseases,* 2020, Elsevier.)

- Avoid administration of any live attenuated vaccines that may be a risk to these immunocompromised patients (e.g., MMR, varicella). (See "Section V" for immunization schedules for HIV-infected children.)
- When feasible, avoid activities that might increase risk of exposure to opportunistic infections (e.g., cleaning out a cat litter box [toxoplasmosis], getting scratched by a cat [*Bartonella* infections], exposure to pet reptiles [salmonellosis], traveling to developing countries [cryptosporidiosis, tuberculosis], eating undercooked foods and drinking from unsafe water supplies, etc.). A description of enteropathogens causing infections in HIV-infected patients is provided in Table 1.

ACUTE GENERAL Rx

Acute management of opportunistic infections is summarized in Table 2 and reviewed elsewhere in this text under specific AIDS-related disorders.

For management of AIDS-related malignancies, please refer to the specific malignancy elsewhere in this text.

CHRONIC Rx

For all HIV-infected patients, particularly those meeting the case definition of AIDS:
- Preventive therapy for *Pneumocystis jiroveci* pneumonia and *Mycobacterium avium* (see specific chapters elsewhere in this text). With appropriate antiretroviral therapy, many patients experience substantial restoration of cellular immune function. Preventive therapy for *Pneumocystis jiroveci* can be safely stopped if the CD4 cell count rises above 200 for at least 3 mo.
- Based on the Department of Health and Human Services (DHHS) Guidelines, active antiretroviral therapy (ART) should be started regardless of CD4 cell count. Individuals with CD4 cell counts <350 and especially CD4 cell

counts <200 should be strongly encouraged to start ART in a timely fashion.
- ART usually includes three-drug combinations of:
  1. Nucleoside reverse transcriptase inhibitors (NRTI): Tenofovir disoproxil fumarate (TDF), tenofovir alafenamide fumarate (TAF), lamivudine (3TC), emtricitabine (FTC), and abacavir (ABC). Older drugs such as zidovudine (AZT), didanosine (ddI), and stavudine (d4T) are generally not recommended.
  2. Protease inhibitors (PI): Darunavir (preferred) or atazanavir.
  3. Nonnucleoside reverse transcriptase inhibitors (NNRTI): Nevirapine, efavirenz (EFV), etravirine, doravirine, and rilpivirine.
  4. Integrase inhibitors: Raltegravir, elvitegravir, bictegravir, dolutegravir, and cabotegravir.
  5. Others: Maraviroc, enfuvirtide, ibalizumab, and fostemsavir.

TABLE 1   Organisms That Cause Gastrointestinal Tract Infections in Patients With HIV/AIDS

	Organisms
Esophagus	*Candida albicans*[a]
	Cytomegalovirus[a]
	Herpes simplex virus[a]
Hepatobiliary	Cytomegalovirus
	Cryptosporidium[a]
	Hepatotropic viruses
	Mycobacterium avium complex[a]
Small intestine	*Campylobacter* species
	Cytomegalovirus[a]
	Cryptosporidium[a]
	Giardia lamblia[a]
	Isospora belli[a]
	Mycobacterium avium complex[a]
	Microsporidia[a] (*Enterocytozoon bieneusi* and *Encephalitozoon intestinalis*)
	Salmonella species[a]
	Enteroaggregative *E. coli*
	Strongyloides stercoralis
Large intestine	*Campylobacter* species
	Clostridium difficile
	Cytomegalovirus[a]
	Entamoeba histolytica
	Herpes simplex virus[a]
	Salmonella species[a]
	Enteroaggregative *E. coli*
	Shigella species

[a]Diseases of the gastrointestinal tract that fulfill the Centers for Disease Control and Prevention surveillance case definition of AIDS.
From Cherry JD et al: *Feigin and Cherry's pediatric infectious diseases,* ed 8, Philadelphia, 2019, Elsevier.

TABLE 2   Treatment of AIDS-Associated Opportunistic Infections

Opportunistic Infection	Preferred Therapy	Alternative Therapy	Other Comments
PJP	• Patients who develop PJP despite TMP-SMX prophylaxis can usually be treated with standard doses of TMP-SMX. • Duration of PJP treatment: 21 days. *For Moderate to Severe PJP:* • TMP-SMX: (TMP 15-20 mg and SMX 75-100 mg/kg/day) IV given q6h or q8h, may switch to PO after clinical improvement. *For Mild to Moderate PJP:* • TMP-SMX: (TMP 15-20 mg and SMX 75-100 mg/kg/day), given PO in 3 divided doses, *or* • TMP-SMX: (160 mg/800 mg or DS) 2 tablets PO tid. *Secondary Prophylaxis, after completion of PJP treatment:* • TMP-SMX DS: 1 tablet PO daily *or* • TMP-SMX (80 mg/400 mg or SS): 1 tablet PO daily.	*For Moderate to Severe PJP:* • Pentamidine 4 mg/kg IV daily infused over ≥60 min; can reduce dose to 3 mg/kg IV daily because of toxicities, *or* • Primaquine 30 mg (base) PO daily + (clindamycin 600 mg q6h IV or 900 mg IV q8h) or (clindamycin 300 mg PO q6h or 450 mg PO q8h). *For Mild to Moderate PJP:* • Dapsone 100 mg PO daily + TMP 5 mg/kg PO tid, *or* • Primaquine 30 mg (base) PO daily + (clindamycin 300 mg PO q6h or 450 mg PO q8h), *or* • Atovaquone 750 mg PO bid with food. *Secondary Prophylaxis, after completion of PJP treatment:* • TMP-SMX DS: 1 tablet PO tiw, *or* • Dapsone 100 mg PO daily, *or* • Dapsone 50 mg PO daily + (pyrimethamine 50 mg + leucovorin 25 mg) PO weekly, *or*	*Indications for Adjunctive Corticosteroids:* • Pao₂ <70 mm Hg at room air, *or* • Alveolar-arterial O₂ gradient >35 mm Hg. *Prednisone Doses (beginning as early as possible and within 72 h of PJP therapy):* • Days 1-5: 40 mg PO bid. • Days 6-10: 40 mg PO daily. • Days 11-21: 20 mg PO daily. • IV methylprednisolone can be administered as 75% of prednisone dose. • Benefit of corticosteroid if started after 72 h of treatment is unknown, but some clinicians will use it for moderate-to-severe PJP. • Whenever possible, patients should be tested for G6PD before use of dapsone or primaquine. Alternative therapy should be used in patients found to have G6PD deficiency. • Patients who are receiving pyrimethamine/sulfadiazine for treatment or suppression of

Continued

TABLE 2 Treatment of AIDS-Associated Opportunistic Infections—cont'd

Opportunistic Infection	Preferred Therapy	Alternative Therapy	Other Comments
		• (Dapsone 200 mg + pyrimethamine 75 mg + leucovorin 25 mg) PO weekly, or • Aerosolized pentamidine 300 mg monthly via Respirgard II nebulizer, or • Atovaquone 1500 mg PO daily, or • (Atovaquone 1500 mg + pyrimethamine 25 mg + leucovorin 10 mg) PO daily.	toxoplasmosis do not require additional PJP prophylaxis. • If TMP-SMX is discontinued because of a mild adverse reaction, reinstitution should be considered after the reaction resolves. The dose can be increased gradually (desensitization) or be reduced, or the frequency can be modified. • TMP-SMX should be permanently discontinued in patients with possible or definite Stevens–Johnson syndrome or toxic epidermal necrosis. • Adjunctive corticosteroids (e.g., dexamethasone) should only be administered when clinically indicated to treat mass effect associated with focal lesions or associated edema; discontinue as soon as clinically feasible. • Anticonvulsants should be administered to patients with a history of seizures and continued through acute treatment but should not be used as seizure prophylaxis. • If clindamycin is used in place of sulfadiazine, additional therapy must be added to prevent PCP.
Toxoplasma gondii encephalitis	*Treatment of Acute Infection:* • Pyrimethamine 200 mg PO 1 time, followed by weight-based therapy: • If <60 kg, pyrimethamine 50 mg PO once daily + sulfadiazine 1000 mg PO q6h + leucovorin 10-25 mg PO once daily. • If ≥60 kg, pyrimethamine 75 mg PO once daily + sulfadiazine 1500 mg PO q6h + leucovorin 10-25 mg PO once daily. • Leucovorin dose can be increased to 50 mg daily or bid. • *Duration for Acute Therapy:* • At least 6 wk; longer duration if clinical or radiologic disease is extensive or response is incomplete at 6 wk. • *Chronic Maintenance Therapy:* • Pyrimethamine 25-50 mg PO daily + sulfadiazine 2000-4000 mg PO daily (in 2-4 divided doses) + leucovorin 10-25 mg PO daily (AI). • *After collecting specimen for culture and molecular diagnostic tests, empiric TB treatment should be started in individuals with clinical and radiographic presentation suggestive of TB.*	*Treatment of Acute Infection:* • Pyrimethamine (leucovorin)* + clindamycin 600 mg IV or PO q6h or • TMP-SMX (TMP 5 mg/kg and SMX 25 mg/kg) IV or PO bid, or • Atovaquone 1500 mg PO bid with food + pyrimethamine (leucovorin), or • Atovaquone 1500 mg PO bid with food + sulfadiazine 1000-1500 mg PO q6h (weight-based dosing, as in preferred therapy) or • Atovaquone 1500 mg PO bid with food, or • Pyrimethamine (leucovorin)* + azithromycin 900-1200 mg PO daily. • *Chronic Maintenance Therapy:* • Clindamycin 600 mg PO q8h + (pyrimethamine 25-50 mg + leucovorin 10-25 mg) PO daily or • TMP-SMX DS 1 tablet bid, or • Atovaquone 750-1500 mg PO bid + (pyrimethamine 25 mg + leucovorin 10 mg) PO daily, or • Atovaquone 750-1500 mg PO bid + sulfadiazine 2000-4000 mg PO daily (in 2-4 divided doses), or • Atovaquone 750-1500 mg PO bid with food.	
Mycobacterium tuberculosis disease (TB)	• *Initial Phase (2 mo, given daily):* • INH + [RIF or RFB] + PZA + EMB. *Continuation Phase:* • INH + (RIF or RFB) daily. • *Total Duration of Therapy (for drug-susceptible TB):* • Pulmonary TB: 6 mo. • Pulmonary TB and culture-positive after 2 mo of TB treatment: 9 mo. • Extrapulmonary TB with CNS infection: 9-12 mo. • Extrapulmonary TB with bone or joint involvement: 6-9 mo. • Extrapulmonary TB in other sites: 6 mo. • Total duration of therapy should be based on number of doses received, not on calendar time.	*Treatment for Drug-Resistant TB* • *Resistant to INH:* • (RIF or RFB) + EMB + PZA + (moxifloxacin or levofloxacin) for 2 mo; followed by (RIF or RFB) + EMB + (moxifloxacin or levofloxacin) for 7 mo. *Treatment for Drug-Resistant TB* • *Resistant to INH:* • (RIF or RFB) + EMB + PZA + (moxifloxacin or levofloxacin) for 2 mo; followed by (RIF or RFB) + EMB + (moxifloxacin or levofloxacin) for 7 mo. • *Resistant to Rifamycins ± Other Drugs:* • Regimen and duration of treatment should be individualized based on resistance pattern, clinical and microbiologic responses, and in close consultation with experienced specialists.	• Adjunctive corticosteroid improves survival for TB meningitis and pericarditis. See text for drug, dose, and duration recommendations. • RIF *is not recommended* for patients receiving HIV PI because of its induction of PI metabolism. • RFB is a less potent CYP3A4 inducer than RIF and is preferred in patients receiving PIs. • Once-weekly rifapentine can result in development of rifamycin resistance in HIV-infected patients and *is not recommended.* • Therapeutic drug monitoring should be considered in patients receiving rifamycin and interacting ART. • Paradoxical IRIS that is not severe can be treated with NSAIDs without a change in TB or HIV therapy. • For severe IRIS reaction, consider prednisone and taper over 4 wk based on clinical symptoms. For example:

TABLE 2   Treatment of AIDS-Associated Opportunistic Infections—cont'd

Opportunistic Infection	Preferred Therapy	Alternative Therapy	Other Comments
			• *If receiving RIF:* Prednisone 1.5 mg/kg/day for 2 wk, then 0.75 mg/kg/day for 2 wk. • *If receiving RFB:* Prednisone 1.0 mg/kg/day for 2 wk, then 0.5 mg/kg/day for 2 wk. • A more gradual tapering schedule over a few mo may be necessary for some patients.
Disseminated MAC disease	*At Least Two Drugs as Initial Therapy With:* Clarithromycin 500 mg PO bid + ethambutol 15 mg/kg PO daily, *or* Azithromycin 500-600 mg + ethambutol 15 mg/kg PO daily if drug interaction or intolerance precludes the use of clarithromycin. *Duration:* At least 12 mo of therapy, can discontinue if no signs and symptoms of MAC disease and sustained (>6 mo) CD4 count >100 cells/μl in response to ART.	• Addition of a third or fourth drug should be considered for patients with advanced immunosuppression (CD4 counts <50 cells/μl), high mycobacterial loads (>2 log CFU/ml of blood), or in the absence of effective ART. *Third or Fourth Drug Options May Include:* • RFB 300 mg PO daily (dosage adjustment may be necessary based on drug interactions), *or* • Amikacin 10-15 mg/kg IV daily, *or* • Streptomycin 1 g IV or IM daily, *or* • Moxifloxacin 400 mg PO daily *or* levofloxacin 500 mg PO daily.	• Testing of susceptibility to clarithromycin and azithromycin is recommended. • NSAIDs can be used for patients who experience moderate to severe symptoms attributed to IRIS. • If IRIS symptoms persist, short-term (4-8 wk) systemic corticosteroids (equivalent to 20-40 mg prednisone) can be used.
Bacterial respiratory diseases (*with focus on pneumonia*)	Empiric antibiotic therapy should be initiated promptly for patients presenting with clinical and radiographic evidence consistent with bacterial pneumonia. The recommendations listed are suggested empiric therapy. The regimen should be modified as needed once microbiologic results are available. *Empiric Outpatient Therapy:* • A PO β-lactam + a PO macrolide (azithromycin or clarithromycin). • *Preferred β-lactams:* Amoxicillin/clavulanate. • *Alternative β-lactams:* Cefpodoxime or cefuroxime, *or* • *For penicillin-allergic patients:* Levofloxacin 750 mg PO once daily, *or* moxifloxacin 400 mg PO once daily. • *Duration:* 7-10 days (a minimum of 5 days). Patients should be afebrile for 48-72 h and clinically stable before stopping antibiotics. • *Empiric Therapy for Non-ICU Hospitalized Patients:* • An IV β-lactam + a macrolide (azithromycin or clarithromycin). • *Preferred β-lactams:* Ceftriaxone, cefotaxime, ceftaroline or ampicillin-sulbactam. • *For penicillin-allergic patients:* • Levofloxacin, 750 mg IV once daily, *or* moxifloxacin, 400 mg IV once daily. • *Empiric Therapy for ICU Patients:* • An IV β-lactam + IV azithromycin, *or* • An IV β-lactam + (levofloxacin 750 mg IV once daily or moxifloxacin 400 mg IV once daily). • *Preferred β-lactams:* Ceftriaxone, cefotaxime, ceftaroline *or* ampicillin-sulbactam. • *Empiric Therapy for Patients at Risk of Pseudomonas Pneumonia:* • An IV antipneumococcal, antipseudomonal β-lactam +	*Empiric Outpatient Therapy:* • A PO β-lactam + PO doxycycline. • Preferred β-lactams: Amoxicillin/clavulanate. • Alternative β-lactams: Cefpodoxime or cefuroxime. • *Empiric Therapy for Non-ICU Hospitalized Patients:* • An IV β-lactam + doxycycline • *Empiric Therapy for ICU Patients:* • *For penicillin-allergic patients:* Aztreonam IV + (levofloxacin 750 mg IV once daily or moxifloxacin 400 mg IV once daily). May add other agents depending on concern for MRSA. *Empiric Therapy for Patients at Risk of Pseudomonas Pneumonia:* • Above β-lactam + an aminoglycoside + (levofloxacin 750 mg IV once daily or moxifloxacin 400 mg IV once daily), *or* • *For penicillin-allergic patients:* Replace the β-lactam with aztreonam. • An IV antipneumococcal, antipseudomonal β-lactam + an aminoglycoside + azithromycin.	• Fluoroquinolones should be used with caution in patients in whom TB is suspected but is not being treated. • Empiric therapy with a macrolide alone should be used with caution in areas with high (>25%)[3] pneumococcal resistance. • Patients receiving a macrolide for MAC prophylaxis should not receive macrolide monotherapy for empiric treatment of bacterial pneumonia. • For patients begun on IV antibiotic therapy, switching to PO should be considered when they are clinically improved and able to tolerate oral medications. • Chemoprophylaxis can be considered for patients with frequent recurrences of serious bacterial pneumonia. • Clinicians should be cautious about using antibiotics to prevent recurrences because of the potential for developing drug resistance and drug toxicities.

Continued

Acquired Immunodeficiency Syndrome 🅟🆃🅖 🅐🅛🅖

TABLE 2 Treatment of AIDS-Associated Opportunistic Infections—cont'd

Opportunistic Infection	Preferred Therapy	Alternative Therapy	Other Comments
	ciprofloxacin 400 mg IV q8-12h or levofloxacin 750 mg IV once daily. • *Preferred β-lactams:* Piperacillin-tazobactam, cefepime, imipenem, or meropenem. • *Empiric Therapy for Patients at Risk for Methicillin-Resistant* Staphylococcus aureus *Pneumonia:* • Add vancomycin IV or linezolid (IV or PO) to the baseline regimen. • Addition of clindamycin to vancomycin (but not to linezolid) can be considered for severe necrotizing pneumonia to minimize bacterial toxin production.		
Bacterial enteric infections	• Diagnostic fecal specimens should be obtained before initiation of empiric antibiotic therapy. • Empiric antibiotic therapy is indicated for patients with advanced HIV (CD4 count <200 cells/μl or concomitant AIDS-defining illnesses), with clinically severe diarrhea (>6 stools/day), and/or accompanying fever or chills. • *Empiric Therapy:* • Ciprofloxacin 500-750 mg PO (or 400 mg IV) q12h. • Therapy should be adjusted based on the results of diagnostic workup. • For patients with chronic diarrhea (>14 days) without severe clinical signs, empiric antibiotic therapy is not necessary; can withhold treatment until a diagnosis is made.	*Empiric Therapy:* Ceftriaxone 1 g IV q24h, *or* Cefotaxime 1 g IV q8h.	• Hospitalization with IV antibiotics should be considered in patients with marked nausea, vomiting, diarrhea, electrolyte abnormalities, acidosis, and blood pressure instability. • Oral or IV rehydration if indicated. • Antimotility agents should be avoided if there is concern about inflammatory diarrhea, including *Clostridium difficile*—associated diarrhea. • If no clinical response after 5-7 days, consider follow-up stool culture with antibiotic susceptibility testing or alternative diagnostic tests (e.g., toxin assays, molecular testing), alternative diagnosis, or antibiotic resistance.
Salmonellosis	All HIV-infected patients with salmonellosis should be treated because of high risk of bacteremia. • Ciprofloxacin 500-750 mg PO (or 400 mg IV) q12h, if susceptible. • *Duration of Therapy:* • *For gastroenteritis without bacteremia:* • If CD4 count ≥200 cells/μl: 7-14 days. • If CD4 count <200 cells/μl: 2-6 wk. *For gastroenteritis with bacteremia:* • If CD4 count ≥200/μl: 14 days; longer duration if bacteremia persists or if the infection is complicated (e.g., if metastatic foci of infection are present). • If CD4 count <200 cells/μl: 2-6 wk. *Secondary Prophylaxis Should Be Considered for:* • Patients with recurrent *Salmonella* gastroenteritis ± bacteremia, *or* • Patients with CD4 <200 cells/μl with severe diarrhea.	• Levofloxacin 750 mg (PO or IV) q24h, *or* • Moxifloxacin 400 mg (PO or IV) q24h, *or* • TMP, 160 mg-SMX 800 mg (PO or IV) q12h, *or* • Ceftriaxone 1 g IV q24h, *or* • Cefotaxime 1 g IV q8h.	• Oral or IV rehydration if indicated. • Antimotility agents should be avoided. • The role of long-term secondary prophylaxis in patients with recurrent *Salmonella* bacteremia is not well established. Must weigh benefit against risks of long-term antibiotic exposure. • Effective ART may reduce the frequency, severity, and recurrence of *Salmonella* infections.
Mucocutaneous candidiasis	*For Oropharyngeal Candidiasis; Initial Episodes (for 7-14 days):* • *Oral Therapy* • Fluconazole 100 mg PO daily, *or* • *Topical Therapy* • Clotrimazole troches, 10 mg PO 5 times daily, *or* • Miconazole mucoadhesive buccal 50-mg tablet—apply to mucosal surface over the canine fossa once daily (do	*For Oropharyngeal Candidiasis; Initial Episodes (for 7-14 days):* • *Oral Therapy* • Itraconazole oral solution 200 mg PO daily, *or* • Posaconazole oral solution 400 mg PO bid for 1 day, then 400 mg daily. • *Topical Therapy* • Nystatin suspension 4-6 ml qid or 1-2 flavored pastilles 4-5 times daily.	• Chronic or prolonged use of azoles may promote development of resistance. • Higher relapse rate for esophageal candidiasis is seen with echinocandins than with fluconazole use. • Suppressive therapy is usually not recommended unless patients have frequent or severe recurrences. *If Decision Is to Use Suppressive Therapy: Oropharyngeal Candidiasis:* • Fluconazole 100 mg PO daily or tiw.

TABLE 2 Treatment of AIDS-Associated Opportunistic Infections—cont'd

Opportunistic Infection	Preferred Therapy	Alternative Therapy	Other Comments
	not swallow, chew, or crush). *For Esophageal Candidiasis (for 14-21 days):* • Fluconazole 100 mg (up to 400 mg) PO or IV daily, *or* • Itraconazole oral solution 200 mg PO daily. *For Uncomplicated Vulvovaginal Candidiasis:* • Oral fluconazole 150 mg for 1 dose, *or* • Topical azoles (clotrimazole, butoconazole, miconazole, tioconazole, or terconazole) for 3-7 days. *For Severe or Recurrent Vulvovaginal Candidiasis:* • Fluconazole 100-200 mg PO daily for ≥7 days, *or* • Topical antifungal ≥7 days.	*For Esophageal Candidiasis (for 14-21 days):* • Voriconazole 200 mg PO or IV bid, *or* • Posaconazole 400 mg PO bid, *or* • Anidulafungin 100 mg IV 1 time, then 50 mg IV daily, *or* • Caspofungin 50 mg IV daily, *or* • Micafungin 150 mg IV daily, *or* • Amphotericin B deoxycholate 0.6 mg/kg IV daily, *or* • Lipid formulation of amphotericin B 3-4 mg/kg IV daily. *For Uncomplicated Vulvovaginal Candidiasis:* • Itraconazole oral solution 200 mg PO daily for 3-7 days.	• Itraconazole oral solution 200 mg PO daily. *Esophageal Candidiasis:* • Fluconazole 100-200 mg PO daily. • Posaconazole 400 mg PO bid. *Vulvovaginal Candidiasis:* • Fluconazole 150 mg PO once weekly.
Cryptococcosis	*Cryptococcal Meningitis* • *Induction Therapy (for at least 2 wk, followed by consolidation therapy):* • Liposomal amphotericin B 3-4 mg/kg IV daily + flucytosine 25 mg/kg PO qid. (NOTE: Flucytosine dose should be adjusted in patients with renal dysfunction.) • *Consolidation Therapy (for at least 8 wk followed by maintenance therapy):* • Fluconazole 800[4] mg PO (or IV) daily. • *Maintenance Therapy:* • Fluconazole 200 mg PO daily for at least 12 mo. *For Non-CNS, Extrapulmonary Cryptococcosis and Diffuse Pulmonary Disease:* • Treatment same as for cryptococcal meningitis. *Non-CNS Cryptococcosis With Mild to Moderate Symptoms and Focal Pulmonary Infiltrates:* • Fluconazole, 400-800 mg PO daily for 12 mo.	*Cryptococcal Meningitis* • *Induction Therapy (for at least 2 wk, followed by consolidation therapy):* • Amphotericin B deoxycholate 0.7 mg/kg IV daily + flucytosine 25 mg/kg PO qid, *or* • Amphotericin B lipid complex 5 mg/kg IV daily + flucytosine 25 mg/kg PO qid, *or* • Liposomal amphotericin B 3-4 mg/kg IV daily + fluconazole 800 mg PO or IV daily, *or* • Amphotericin B deoxycholate 0.7 mg/kg IV daily + fluconazole 800 mg PO or IV daily, *or* • Fluconazole 800-1200 mg[5] PO or IV daily + flucytosine 25 mg/kg PO qid, *or* • Fluconazole 1200 mg PO or IV daily. • *Consolidation Therapy (for at least 8 wk followed by maintenance therapy):* • Itraconazole 200 mg PO bid for 8 wk—less effective than fluconazole. • *Maintenance Therapy:* • No alternative therapy recommendation.	• Addition of flucytosine to amphotericin B has been associated with more rapid sterilization of CSF and decreased risk for subsequent relapse. • Patients receiving flucytosine should have either blood levels monitored (peak level 2 h after dose should be 30-80 μg/ml) or close monitoring of blood counts for development of cytopenia. Dosage should be adjusted in patients with renal insufficiency. • Opening pressure should always be measured when an LP is performed. Repeated LPs or CSF shunting are essential to effectively manage increased intracranial pressure. • Corticosteroids and mannitol are ineffective in reducing intracranial pressure and are not recommended. • Some specialists recommend a brief course of corticosteroid for management of severe IRIS symptoms.
Histoplasmosis	*Moderately Severe to Severe Disseminated Disease Induction Therapy (for at least 2 wk or until clinically improved):* • Liposomal amphotericin B 3 mg/kg IV daily. • *Maintenance Therapy:* • Itraconazole 200 mg PO tid for 3 days, then 200 mg PO bid. *Less Severe Disseminated Disease* • Induction and Maintenance Therapy: • Itraconazole 200 mg PO tid for 3 days, then 200 mg PO bid. • *Duration of Therapy:* • At least 12 mo. *Meningitis*	*Moderately Severe to Severe Disseminated Disease Induction Therapy (for at least 2 wk or until clinically improved):* • Amphotericin B lipid complex 3 mg/kg IV daily, *or* • Amphotericin B cholesteryl sulfate complete 3 mg/kg IV daily. • *Alternatives to Itraconazole for Maintenance Therapy or Treatment of Less Severe Disease:* • Voriconazole 400 mg PO bid for 1 day, then 200 mg bid, *or* • Posaconazole 400 mg PO bid. • Fluconazole 800 mg PO daily. *Meningitis*	• Itraconazole, posaconazole, and voriconazole may have significant interactions with certain ARV agents. These interactions are complex and can be bidirectional. • Therapeutic drug monitoring and dosage adjustment may be necessary to ensure triazole antifungal and ARV efficacy and to reduce concentration-related toxicities. • Random serum concentration of itraconazole + hydroxyitraconazole should be >1 μg/ml. • Clinical experience with voriconazole or posaconazole in the treatment of histoplasmosis is limited. • Acute pulmonary histoplasmosis in HIV-infected patients with CD4 counts >300

Continued

TABLE 2 Treatment of AIDS-Associated Opportunistic Infections—cont'd

Opportunistic Infection	Preferred Therapy	Alternative Therapy	Other Comments
	• *Induction Therapy (4-6 wk):* • Liposomal amphotericin B 5 mg/kg/day. • *Maintenance Therapy:* • Itraconazole 200 mg PO bid to tid for ≥1 yr and until resolution of abnormal CSF findings. • *Long-Term Suppression Therapy:* • For patients with severe disseminated or CNS infection after completion of at least 12 mo of therapy; and those who relapse despite appropriate therapy • Itraconazole 200 mg PO daily.	• No alternative therapy recommendation. • *Long-Term Suppression Therapy:* • Fluconazole 400 mg PO daily.	cells/μl should be managed as nonimmunocompromised host.
Coccidioidomycosis	*Clinically Mild Infections (e.g., focal pneumonia):* • Fluconazole 400 mg PO daily *or* • Itraconazole 200 mg PO bid. *Severe, Nonmeningeal Infection (diffuse pulmonary infection or severely ill patients with extrathoracic, disseminated disease):* • Amphotericin B deoxycholate 0.7-1.0 mg/kg IV daily. • Lipid formulation amphotericin B 4-6 mg/kg IV daily. • Duration of therapy: Continue until clinical improvement, then switch to an azole. *Meningeal Infections:* • Fluconazole 400-800 mg IV or PO daily. *Chronic Suppressive Therapy:* • Fluconazole 400 mg PO daily, *or* • Itraconazole 200 mg PO bid.	*Mild Infections (focal pneumonia) for patients who failed to respond to fluconazole or itraconazole:* • Posaconazole 200 mg PO bid, *or* • Voriconazole 200 mg PO bid. *Severe, Nonmeningeal Infection (diffuse pulmonary infection or severely ill patients with extrathoracic, disseminated disease):* • Some specialists will add a triazole (fluconazole or itraconazole, with itraconazole preferred for bone disease) 400 mg per day to amphotericin B therapy and continue triazole once amphotericin B is stopped. *Meningeal Infections:* • Itraconazole 200 mg PO tid for 3 days, then 200 mg PO bid, *or* • Posaconazole 200 mg PO bid, *or* • Voriconazole 200-400 mg PO bid, *or* • Intrathecal amphotericin B deoxycholate, when triazole antifungals are ineffective. *Chronic Suppressive Therapy:* • Posaconazole 200 mg PO bid, *or* • Voriconazole 200 mg PO bid.	• Some patients with meningitis may develop hydrocephalus and require CSF shunting. • Therapy should be continued indefinitely in patients with diffuse pulmonary or disseminated diseases because relapse can occur in 25%-33% of HIV-negative patients. It can also occur in HIV-infected patients with CD4 counts >250 cells/μL. • Therapy should be lifelong in patients with meningeal infections because relapse occurs in 80% of HIV-infected patients after discontinuation of triazole therapy. • Itraconazole, posaconazole, and voriconazole may have significant interactions with certain ARV agents. These interactions are complex and can be bidirectional. Therapeutic drug monitoring and dosage adjustment may be necessary to ensure triazole antifungal and antiretroviral efficacy and to reduce concentration-related toxicities. • Intrathecal amphotericin B should be given only in consultation with a specialist and should be administered by an individual with experience with the technique.
Aspergillosis, invasive	*Preferred Therapy:* • Voriconazole 6 mg/kg IV q12h for 1 day, then 4 mg/kg IV q12h, followed by voriconazole 200 mg PO q12h after clinical improvement. • *Duration of Therapy:* • Until CD4 cell count >200 cells/μl and the infection appears to be resolved.	*Alternative Therapy:* • Lipid formulation of amphotericin B 5 mg/kg IV daily, *or* • Amphotericin B deoxycholate 1 mg/kg IV daily, *or* • Caspofungin 70 mg IV 1 time, then 50 mg IV daily, *or* • Micafungin 100-150 mg IV daily, *or* • Anidulafungin 200 mg IV 1 time, then 100 mg IV daily, *or* • Posaconazole 200 mg PO qid, then, after condition improved, 400 mg PO bid.	• Potential for significant pharmacokinetic interactions between certain ARV agents and voriconazole; they should be used cautiously in these situations. Consider therapeutic drug monitoring and dosage adjustment if necessary.
CMV disease	*CMV Retinitis Induction Therapy for Immediate Sight-Threatening Lesions (adjacent to the optic nerve or fovea)* • Consult ophthalmologist; ganciclovir implant no longer available: • Ganciclovir 5 mg/kg IV q12h for 14-21 days followed by Valganciclovir 900 mg PO bid. *For Small Peripheral Lesions:*	*CMV Retinitis Induction Therapy:* • Ganciclovir 5 mg/kg IV q12h for 14-21 days, *or* • Foscarnet 90 mg/kg IV q12h or 60 mg q8h for 14-21 days, *or* • Cidofovir 5 mg/kg/wk IV for 2 wk; saline hydration before and after therapy and probenecid, 2 g PO 3 hours before dose, followed by 1 g PO 2 h and 8 h after the dose (total of 4 g). (Note: This regimen should be avoided	• The choice of therapy for CMV retinitis should be individualized, based on location and severity of the lesions, level of immunosuppression, and other factors (e.g., concomitant medications and ability to adhere to treatment). • The choice of chronic maintenance therapy (route of administration and drug choices) should be made in consultation with an ophthalmologist. Considerations should include the anatomic location of

TABLE 2 Treatment of AIDS-Associated Opportunistic Infections—cont'd

Opportunistic Infection	Preferred Therapy	Alternative Therapy	Other Comments
	• Valganciclovir 900 mg PO bid for 14-21 days. • One dose of intravitreal ganciclovir can be administered immediately after diagnosis until steady-state plasma ganciclovir concentration is achieved with oral valganciclovir. • *Chronic Maintenance (secondary prophylaxis):* • Valganciclovir 900 mg PO daily (for small peripheral lesion). *CMV Esophagitis or Colitis:* • Ganciclovir 5 mg/kg IV q12h; may switch to valganciclovir 900 mg PO q12h once patient can tolerate oral therapy. • Duration: 21-42 days or until symptoms have resolved. • Maintenance therapy is usually not necessary but should be considered after relapses. *Well-Documented, Histologically Confirmed CMV Pneumonia:* • Experience for treating CMV pneumonitis in HIV patients is limited. Use of IV ganciclovir or IV foscarnet is reasonable (doses same as for CMV retinitis). • The optimal duration of therapy and the role of oral valganciclovir have not been established. • *CMV Neurologic Disease* • Note: Treatment should be initiated promptly. • Ganciclovir 5 mg/kg IV q12h + (foscarnet 90 mg/kg IV q12h or 60 mg/kg IV q8h) to stabilize disease and maximize response; continue until symptomatic improvement and resolution of neurologic symptoms. • The optimal duration of therapy and the role of oral valganciclovir have not been established.	in patients with sulfa allergy because of cross-hypersensitivity with probenecid.) • *Chronic Maintenance (secondary prophylaxis):* • Ganciclovir 5 mg/kg IV 5-7 times weckly, *or* • Foscarnet 90-120 mg/kg IV once daily, *or* • Cidofovir 5 mg/kg IV every other wk with saline hydration and probenecid as above. *CMV Esophagitis or Colitis:* • Foscarnet 90 mg/kg IV q12h or 60 mg/kg q8h for patients with treatment-limiting toxicities to ganciclovir or with ganciclovir resistance, *or* • Valganciclovir 900 mg PO q12h in milder disease and if able to tolerate PO therapy, *or* • For mild cases, if ART can be initiated without delay, consider withholding CMV therapy. • Duration: 21-42 days or until symptoms have resolved.	the retinal lesion, vision in the contralateral eye, the patients' immunologic and virologic status, and response to ART. • Patients with CMV retinitis who discontinue maintenance therapy should undergo regular eye examinations for early detection of relapse IRU—optimally every 3 mo and then annually after immune reconstitution. • IRU may develop in the setting of immune reconstitution. • *Treatment of IRU:* • Periocular corticosteroid or short courses of systemic steroid. • Initial therapy in patients with CMV retinitis, esophagitis, colitis, and pneumonitis should include initiation or optimization of ART.
HSV disease	*Orolabial Lesions (for 5-10 days):* • Valacyclovir 1 g PO bid *or* • Famciclovir 500 mg PO bid *or* • Acyclovir 400 mg PO tid. *Initial or Recurrent Genital HSV (for 5-14 days):* • Valacyclovir 1 g PO bid, *or* • Famciclovir 500 mg PO bid, *or* • Acyclovir 400 mg PO tid. *Severe Mucocutaneous HSV:* • Initial therapy acyclovir 5 mg/kg IV q8h • After lesions begin to regress, change to PO therapy as previously. Continue until lesions are completely healed. • *Chronic Suppressive Therapy for Patients With Severe Recurrences of Genital Herpes or for Patients Who Want to Minimize Frequency of Recurrences:* • Valacyclovir 500 mg PO bid. • Famciclovir 500 mg PO bid. • Acyclovir 400 mg PO bid.	*For Acyclovir-Resistant HSV* • *Preferred Therapy:* • Foscarnet 80-120 mg/kg/day IV in 2-3 divided doses until clinical response. • *Alternative Therapy* • IV cidofovir (dosage as in CMV retinitis), *or* • Topical trifluridine, *or* • Topical cidofovir, *or* • Topical imiquimod. • *Duration of Therapy:* • 21-28 days or longer.	• Patients with HSV infections can be treated with episodic therapy when symptomatic lesions occur, or with daily suppressive therapy to prevent recurrences. • Topical formulations of trifluridine and cidofovir are not commercially available. • Extemporaneous compounding of topical products can be prepared using trifluridine ophthalmic solution and the IV formulation of cidofovir.

Continued

TABLE 2   Treatment of AIDS-Associated Opportunistic Infections—cont'd

Opportunistic Infection	Preferred Therapy	Alternative Therapy	Other Comments
VZV disease	• Continue indefinitely regardless of CD4 cell count. *Primary Varicella Infection (Chickenpox):* • *Uncomplicated Cases (for 5-7 days):* • Valacyclovir 1 g PO tid *or* • Famciclovir 500 mg PO tid. • *Severe or Complicated Cases:* • Acyclovir 10-15 mg/kg IV q8h for 7-10 days. • May switch to oral valacyclovir, famciclovir, or acyclovir after defervescence if no evidence of visceral involvement. *Herpes Zoster (Shingles) Acute Localized Dermatomal:* • For 7-10 days; consider longer duration if lesions are slow to resolve. • Valacyclovir 1 g PO tid *or* • Famciclovir 500 mg tid. *Extensive Cutaneous Lesion or Visceral Involvement:* • Acyclovir 10-15 mg/kg IV q8h until clinical improvement is evident. • May switch to PO therapy (valacyclovir, famciclovir, or acyclovir) after clinical improvement (i.e., when no new vesicle formation or improvement of signs and symptoms of visceral VZV), to complete a 10- to 14-day course. *Progressive Outer Retinal Necrosis:* • Ganciclovir 5 mg/kg + foscarnet 90 mg/kg IV q12h + ganciclovir 2 mg/0.05 ml ± foscarnet 1.2 mg/0.05 ml intravitreal injection twice weekly *or* • Initiate or optimize ART. *Acute Retinal Necrosis:* • Acyclovir 10 mg/kg IV q8h for 10-14 days, followed by valacyclovir 1 g PO tid for 6 wk.	*Primary Varicella Infection (Chickenpox):* • Uncomplicated Cases (for 5-7 days): • Acyclovir 800 mg PO 5 times/day. *Herpes Zoster (Shingles)* • *Acute Localized Dermatomal:* • For 7-10 days; consider longer duration if lesions are slow to resolve. • Acyclovir 800 mg PO 5 times/day.	• In managing VZV retinitis: Consultation with an ophthalmologist experienced in management of VZV retinitis is strongly recommended. • Duration of therapy for VZV retinitis is not well defined and should be determined based on clinical, virologic, immunologic, and ophthalmologic responses. • Optimization of ART is recommended for serious and difficult-to-treat VZV infections (e.g., retinitis, encephalitis).
Progressive multifocal leukoencephalopathy (JC virus infections)	• There is no specific antiviral therapy for JC virus infection. The main treatment approach is to reverse the immunosuppression caused by HIV. • Initiate ART immediately in ART-naïve patients. • Optimize ART in patients who develop PML in phase of HIV viremia on ART.	None.	• Corticosteroids may be used for PML-IRIS characterized by contrast enhancement, edema, or mass effect and with clinical deterioration.

AIDS, Acquired immunodeficiency syndrome; *ART,* antiretroviral therapy; *ARV,* antiretroviral; *bid,* twice a day; *CD4,* CD4 T lymphocyte cell; *CFU,* colony-forming unit; *CMV,* cytomegalovirus; *CNS,* central nervous system; *CSF,* cerebrospinal fluid; *CYP3A4,* cytochrome P-450 3A4; *DS,* double strength; *EMB,* ethambutol; *G6PD,* glucose-6-phosphate dehydrogenase; *HIV,* human immunodeficiency virus; *HSV,* herpes simplex virus; *ICU,* intensive care unit; *IM,* intramuscular; *INH,* isoniazid; *IRIS,* immune reconstitution inflammatory syndrome; *IRU,* immune recovery uveitis; *IV,* intravenous; *JC,* John Cunningham (virus); *LP,* lumbar puncture; *MAC, Mycobacterium avium* complex; *NSAID,* nonsteroidal antiinflammatory drug; *PCP, Pneumocystis* pneumonia; *PI,* protease inhibitor; *PJP, Pneumocystis jiroveci* pneumonia; *PML,* progressive multifocal leukoencephalopathy; *PO,* oral; *PZA,* pyrazinamide; *qid,* four times a day; *RFB,* rifabutin; *RIF,* rifampin; *SS,* single strength; *TB,* tuberculosis; *tid,* three times daily; *tiw,* three times weekly; *TMP-SMX,* trimethoprim-sulfamethoxazole; *VZV,* varicella zoster virus. *Quality of Evidence for the Recommendation:* I: One or more randomized trials with clinical outcomes and/or validated laboratory endpoints. II: One or more well-designed, nonrandomized trials or observational cohort studies with long-term clinical outcomes. III: Expert opinion.
* Pyrimethamine and leucovorin doses are the same as for preferred therapy.

Diseases and Disorders

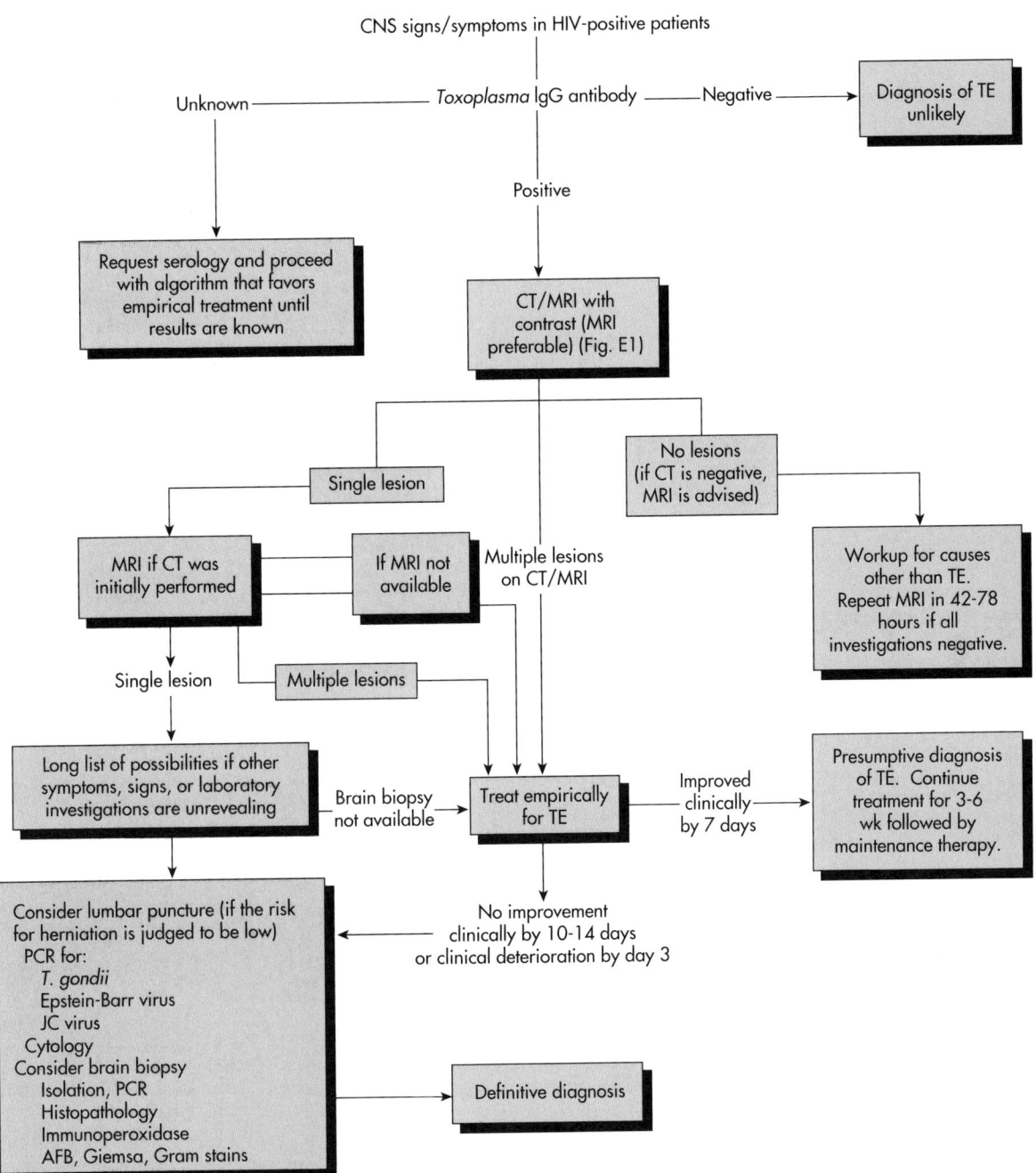

FIG. 3 Diagnostic approach and management algorithm for human immunodeficiency virus *(HIV)*—infected patients with central nervous system *(CNS)* symptoms or signs that might potentially be toxoplasmic encephalitis *(TE)*. *AFB,* Acid-fast bacilli; *CT,* computed tomography; *IgG,* immunoglobulin G; *MRI,* magnetic resonance imaging; *PCR,* polymerase chain reaction. (From Bennett JE et al: *Mandell, Douglas, and Bennett's principles and practice of infectious diseases,* ed 8, Philadelphia, 2015, Saunders.)

The medications ritonavir or cobicistat are usually used in combination with other protease inhibitors or integrase inhibitors to obtain more sustained drug levels. Usual initial dosing regimens include two NRTIs and an NNRTI or PI or integrase inhibitor. Two-drug regimens with dolutegravir and lamivudine can be considered in certain clinical situations. Currently, integrase inhibitors are recommended as first-line drugs because of tolerability. Examples of initial regimens recommended by the guidelines:

1. Bictegravir/tenofovir alafenamide/emtricitabine

2. Dolutegravir/abacavir/lamivudine (in patients who are HLA-B5701 NEGATIVE)*
3. Dolutegravir plus tenofovir/emtricitabine*
4. Dolutegravir and lamivudine (two-drug regimen). This regimen should not be used in individuals with HIV RNA >500,000 copies/ml, HBV coinfection, or in whom ART is to be started before the results of HIV

*Tenofovir-based formulations can include tenofovir disoproxil fumarate (TDF) or tenofovir alafenamide (TAF).

genotypic resistance testing for reverse transcriptase or HBV testing are available.
All these drugs have unique and class-specific side effects and require careful and expert follow-up to achieve optimal antiviral effects, ensure compliance, and maintain efficacy. Antiviral response should be monitored by baseline HIV viral load and CD4 count and repeat measurement at 2 wk and 4 wk into treatment and then periodically (3 to 6 mo) to ensure viral suppression.

1. The approach to a patient with CNS signs and symptoms is described in Fig. 3, and

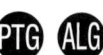
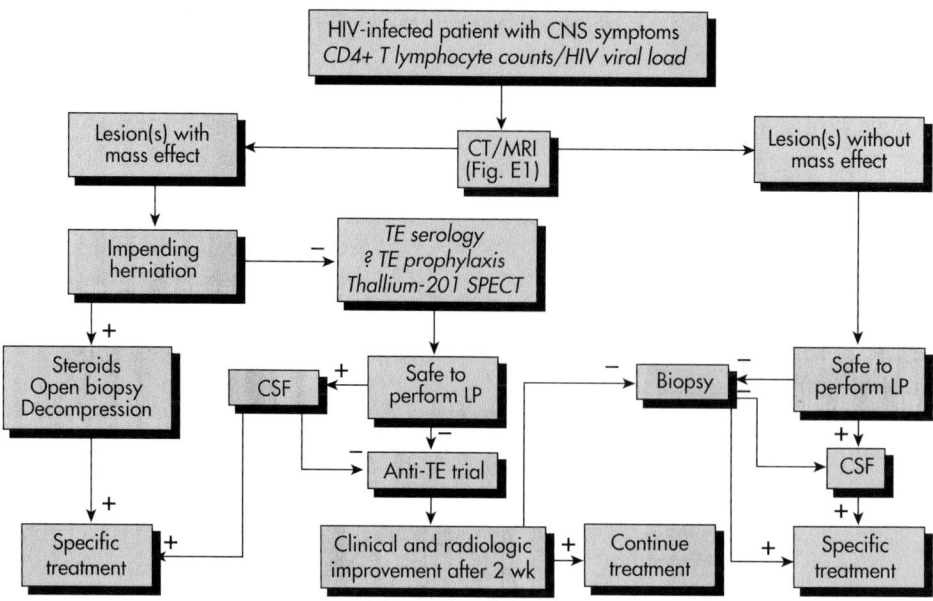

FIG. 4 Management of the human immunodeficiency virus (HIV) type 1–infected patient with central nervous system (CNS) mass lesions. The elements in italics represent data that contribute to the decision-making process (see text for details). *CSF,* Cerebrospinal fluid; *CT,* computed tomography; *LP,* lumbar puncture; *MRI,* magnetic resonance imaging; *SPECT,* single-photon emission computed tomography; *TE, Toxoplasma* encephalitis. (From Bennett JE et al: *Mandell, Douglas, and Bennett's principles and practice of infectious diseases,* ed 8, Philadelphia, 2015, Saunders.)

Fig. 4 describes the management of CNS mass lesions.

2. Genotypic resistance testing is strongly encouraged for all patients initiating treatment and for any patient failing antiretroviral therapy. Poor adherence to therapy, however, often underlies virologic failure.

DISPOSITION

The outlook for HIV has changed radically since the advent of ART from an essentially fatal disease to a chronic medical illness compatible with long-term survival and remarkably good quality of life. Patients should be aggressively treated for severe illnesses as outcomes following ICU admissions remain good. This is accomplished through expert and continuous follow-up, use of ART, and careful detail to compliance to medications and lifestyle modification.

REFERRAL

All patients with HIV should be referred to a physician knowledgeable and experienced in the management of the disease and its complications.

PEARLS & CONSIDERATIONS

- Newer agents effective against HIV have recently been approved:
  1. Ibalizumab-Uiyk (Trogarzo): injectable monoclonal antibody that binds to the surface proteins of CD4 and thus prevents fusion entry of HIV virus into cells
  2. Fostemsavir (Rukobia): is an attachment inhibitor that prevents viral entry into cells used in combination with other agents in patients with multidrug resistant HIV-1.
- Four patients have been cleared of their HIV after stem cell transplant for blood cancer; the most recent case was announced in July 2022: stem cell transplant for AML.

SUGGESTED READINGS
Available at eBooks.Health.Elsevier.com.

RELATED CONTENT
Acquired Immunodeficiency Syndrome (AIDS) (Patient Information)
Candidiasis, Cutaneous (Related Key Topic)
Candidiasis, Invasive (Related Key Topic)
Cryptosporidium Infection (Related Key Topic)
Cytomegalovirus Infection (Related Key Topic)
Herpes Simplex (Related Key Topic)
Histoplasmosis (Related Key Topic)
HIV-Associated Cognitive Dysfunction (Related Key Topic)
Human Immunodeficiency Virus (Related Key Topic)
Kaposi Sarcoma (Related Key Topic)
Pneumonia, *Pneumocystis jiroveci (carinii)* (Related Key Topic)
Progressive Multifocal Leukoencephalopathy (Related Key Topic)
Toxoplasmosis (Related Key Topic)
Tuberculosis, Pulmonary (Related Key Topic)

AUTHOR: **PHILIP A. CHAN, MD, MS**

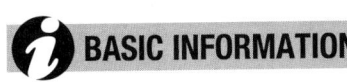
Diseases
and Disorders

I

BASIC INFORMATION

DEFINITION

Acute aortic syndromes are a spectrum of aortic pathologies that include aortic dissection, intramural hematomas (IMHs), and penetrating atherosclerotic ulcers.[1] Aortic dissections are the most common and occur when blood passes through an intimal tear, separating the intima from the medial layers and creating a false lumen.[1] IMH and penetrating aortic ulcer are variants of the classically described aortic dissection. Fig. 1 illustrates acute aortic syndromes.

CLASSIFICATION

Aortic dissection is generally classified according to anatomic location (Fig. 2). Table 1 summarizes classification schemes of acute aortic dissection.
- Stanford (more commonly used classification system): Type A ascending aorta (proximal), type B descending aorta (distal)
- DeBakey: Type I ascending and descending aorta, type II ascending aorta, type III descending aorta

- The Society of Thoracic Surgery and Society of Vascular Surgery have recently proposed a classification system of dissection subtypes to more precisely define the location of disease as extending between two anatomic zones[2]
- Aortic dissection can also be classified by acuity of presentation: Hyperacute (<24 h), acute (2 to 7 days), subacute (8 to 30 days), and chronic (>30 days). The overall survival rate is inversely related to time of presentation, with the highest survival rate in the hyperacute group and the lowest survival rate in the chronic group

SYNONYMS

Aortic dissection
Dissecting aortic aneurysm
AAS

ICD-10CM CODES
I71.00	Dissection of unspecified site of aorta
I71.01	Dissection of thoracic aorta
I71.02	Dissection of abdominal aorta
I71.03	Dissection of thoracoabdominal aorta

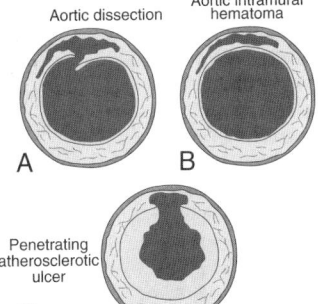

FIG. 1 Acute aortic syndromes. A, Classic aortic dissection. There is a tear in the intima with blood entering the media and a dissecting cleavage plane propagating for variable distances anterograde (and occasionally retrograde) throughout the aortic wall. **B,** Aortic intramural hematoma (IMH). A spontaneous hemorrhage of the vasa vasorum leads to bleeding within the media in the absence of an intimal tear or intimal flap. **C,** Penetrating atherosclerotic aortic ulcer (PAU). An ulcerated aortic plaque ruptures into the media, leading to an outpouching or ulceration in the aortic wall. This may be associated with IMH formation; pseudoaneurysm; or a focal, thick-walled aortic dissection. (From Zipes DP: *Braunwald's heart disease: a textbook of cardiovascular medicine,* ed 11, Philadelphia, 2019, Elsevier.)

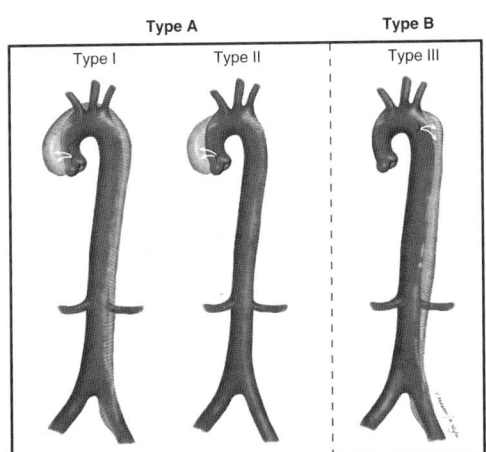

FIG. 2 Classification schemes of acute aortic dissection. (From Mann DL et al: *Braunwald's heart disease,* ed 10, Philadelphia, 2015, Elsevier.)

EPIDEMIOLOGY & DEMOGRAPHICS

INCIDENCE: 2.6 to 3.5 per 100,000 person-yr; more frequent in winter as compared to other seasons, although no clear reason has been identified.[3,4]

PREDOMINANT SEX & AGE: Males (65%) females (35%), ages 60 to 80 yr; mean = 63 yr[1,3,5]

RISK FACTORS: (TABLE 2):
- Hypertension (found in up to 77% of patients with aortic dissection)[3,5]
- Atherosclerosis (found in up to 27% of patients with aortic dissection)[3,5]
- Preexisting aortic aneurysm (found in up to 16% of patients with aortic dissection)[3,5]
- Age (60 to 80 yr)
- Family history of aortic aneurysms/dissection
- History of cardiac surgery, aortic valve replacement, intraaortic catheterization[1,3,5]
- Disorders of collagen (Marfan syndrome, Ehlers-Danlos syndrome)[3,5]
- Vascular inflammation (giant cell arteritis, Takayasu arteritis, rheumatoid arthritis, syphilitic aortitis)
- Aortic coarctation, bicuspid aortic valve
- Turner syndrome
- Cocaine abuse (usually within 12 h of last use of cocaine)[1,3,5]
- Trauma (~20% road accident fatalities found to have ruptured aorta on autopsy)[1]
- Pregnancy and delivery
- Fluoroquinolone use[1]
- Table 3 summarizes genetically triggered conditions associated with aortic dissection

PHYSICAL FINDINGS & CLINICAL PRESENTATION

- Sudden onset of severe sharp, tearing, or ripping chest, back, or abdominal pain.[1,3,5] However, painless dissection occurs in ~6.3% of cases[2]
- Anterior chest pain (79% type A, 63% type B)[3]
- Back pain, abdominal pain (43% type A, 64% type B)[3]
- Syncope (19% type A, 3% type B), generally secondary to cardiac tamponade or stroke[3]
- Congestive heart failure (CHF)[1]
- May present with hypertension (28% for type A, 66% in type B dissection),[5] although 25% present with hypotension (systolic blood pressure <100 mm Hg), which can indicate bleeding, cardiac tamponade, or severe aortic regurgitation.[3] Patients presenting with very high systolic blood pressure (>180 mm Hg for type A, >200 mm Hg for type B dissection), as well as in those with systolic blood pressure ≤100 mm Hg, have significantly higher in-hospital mortality rates
- Pulse and blood pressure differentials (>20 mm Hg between arms) in 19% to 31% of cases caused by partial compression of subclavian arteries[6]
- Aortic regurgitation in 40% to 75% of cases of proximal dissection,[1] often with diastolic decrescendo murmur
- Myocardial ischemia caused by coronary artery occlusion, most commonly involving the right coronary artery

TABLE 1 Classification Schemes of Acute Aortic Dissection

DeBakey Classification

Type I	Originates in the ascending aorta and extends at least to the aortic arch and often to the descending aorta (and beyond)
Type II	Originates in the ascending aorta and confined to this segment
Type III	Originates in the descending aorta, usually just distal to the left subclavian artery, and extends distally

Stanford Classification

Type A	Dissections involving the ascending aorta (with or without extension into the descending aorta)
Type B	Dissections not involving the ascending aorta

From Mann DL et al: *Braunwald's heart disease,* ed 10, Philadelphia, 2015, Elsevier.

TABLE 2 Risk Factors for Aortic Dissection

Hypertension
Heritable or genetic thoracic aortic disease and
   syndromes
   Marfan syndrome
   Loeys-Dietz syndrome
   Familial thoracic aortic aneurysm syndromes
   Vascular Ehlers-Danlos syndrome
   Turner syndrome
Congenital diseases/syndromes
   Bicuspid aortic valve
   Coarctation of the aorta
   Tetralogy of Fallot
Atherosclerosis
   Penetrating atherosclerotic ulcer
Trauma, blunt or iatrogenic
   Catheter/guidewire
   Intra-aortic balloon pump
   Aortic/vascular surgery
   Motor vehicle accident
   Coronary artery bypass grafting/aortic valve
     replacement/TAVR
   Thoracic endovascular aneurysm repair (TEVAR)
Cocaine/methamphetamine use
Inflammatory/infectious diseases
   Giant cell arteritis
   Takayasu arteritis
   Behçet syndrome
   Aortitis
   Syphilis
Pregnancy (with underlying aortopathy)
Weightlifting (with underlying aortopathy)

TAVR, Transcatheter aortic valve replacement.
From Zipes DP: Braunwald's heart disease: a textbook of cardiovascular medicine, ed 11, Philadelphia, 2019, Elsevier.

- Stroke in 5% to 10% of patients (secondary to dissection into or decreased blood flow to the carotids)[1]
- Mesenteric ischemia occurs in 3% to 5% of cases, with external compression, flap prolapse, or involvement of arterial ostia[1]
- Horner syndrome (ptosis, miosis, anhidrosis)
- Vocal cord paralysis or hoarse voice (caused by compression of the left recurrent laryngeal nerve)[1]

ETIOLOGY

Genetics, in addition to other risk factors (Tables 4, 5, 6, and 7), contribute to the development of aortic aneurysms and dissection.

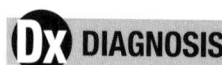 **DIAGNOSIS**

DIFFERENTIAL DIAGNOSIS

- Known as the great imitator: Pulmonary embolism, acute coronary syndrome, aortic stenosis/insufficiency, nondissecting aneurysm, pericarditis, cholecystitis, peptic ulcer disease, pancreatitis, musculoskeletal pain.[3]
- Consider aortic dissection in patients with unexplained stroke, chest pain, syncope, acute-onset CHF, abdominal pain, back pain, and malperfusion of extremities or internal organs.[3] Acute aortic syndromes may be associated with nonspecific signs and symptoms; a high clinical index of suspicion is necessary to detect the disease early in its course as nearly two thirds of patients under medical care are not diagnosed before death. Box E1 summarizes a differential diagnosis of aortic dissection.
- In an emergency situation, a rapid yet comprehensive workup is crucial to reduce diagnostic time delay. This should include clinical assessment, laboratory data (D-dimer and troponin), chest x-ray, ECG, and aortic imaging in the appropriate patient.[1,3,5]
- The Aortic Dissection Detection Risk Score (ADD-RS) can be a useful tool in diagnosing aortic dissection in the emergency room setting.[6] ADD-RS is based on the presence of one or more of the clinical risk markers outlined in Table 8. A high ADD-RS effectively stratifies the risk for acute aortic dissection (score 0 is low risk, score 1 is intermediate risk, and score ≥2 is high risk).[6] Score 0 has 95.6% certainty in ruling out aortic dissection.
- The addition of D-dimer to ADD-RS may further improve diagnostic performance of each of these when used alone for ruling out acute aortic dissection or other acute aortic syndromes.[6] Among low- to intermediate-risk patients (ADD-RS <2), a negative D-dimer (<500 mg/dl) can rule out aortic dissection with 99.7% certainty.[6] Among high-risk patients (ADD-RS ≥2), D-dimer is not discriminatory and requires conclusive imaging.[6]

WORKUP

ECG: Helpful to rule out myocardial infarction, although dissection can lead to coronary ischemia.[1,3,5]

LABORATORY TESTS

- D-Dimer has a high negative predictive value in dissection, but lacks specificity in the setting of acute aortic dissection.[1,3] However, a negative D-dimer does not rule out IMH or penetrating aortic ulcer.[1,3]
- Soluble ST2, a novel biomarker, may have superior diagnostic performance over D-dimer in discriminating acute aortic dissection from other acute chest pain syndromes.[7] At a cutoff level of 34.6 ng/ml, the sensitivity and specificity for acute aortic dissection were 99.1% and 84.9%, respectively.[7]
- Several other biomarkers with different diagnostic windows can be used in the diagnosis of aortic dissection[1,8]:
  1. Smooth muscle myosin heavy chain protein (released from damaged medial smooth muscle) can be used to detect proximal aortic dissections (91% sensitivity and 93% specificity). Myosin heavy chains will peak within 3 h of dissection and clear within 24 h of aortic injury.
  2. CK-BB isoenzyme also peaks within 6 h of dissection.
  3. Calponin, a smooth muscle troponin counterpart, increases in aortic dissection with a wider diagnostic window when compared to smooth muscle myosin heavy chain and CK-BB.
  4. C-reactive protein, fibrinogen and soluble elastin fragments are under investigation.

IMAGING STUDIES

- Multidetector CT (Fig. E3) is considered the gold standard, but its use may be limited in patients with renal failure as it involves the use of intravenous contrast.[1,3,5]
- Transesophageal echocardiography (TEE), multidetector CT, and MRI are all highly sensitive (98% to 100%) and specific (95% to 98%).[9] Test of choice depends on clinical circumstances and hospital availability.
- TEE is study of choice in unstable patients with type A dissection but is operator dependent.[1]
- MRI has high sensitivity and specificity but limited availability; not suitable for unstable patients; contraindicated with noncompatible pacemakers, metal devices; uses gadolinium-based contrast which is less nephrotoxic than iodinated agents in patients without severe renal dysfunction.[1]
- With medium or high pretest probability, a second diagnostic test should be done if the first is negative.
- Coronary computed tomographic angiography (CTA) may be an alternative and useful diagnostic study when evaluating for pulmonary embolism, acute coronary syndrome, and aortic dissection.[1]
- Aortography rarely done, as less sensitive than TEE, CT, or MRI.[1]

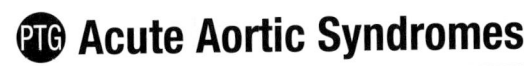
TABLE 3   Genetically Triggered Conditions Associated with Aortic Dissection

Marfan syndrome (MFS)	Autosomal dominant disorder of connective tissue caused by *FBN1* mutation; incidence of 1 in ≈5000 individuals; multisystem manifestations, including ectopia lentis; mitral valve prolapse, aortic root aneurysm, aortic dissection; skeletal features (pectus deformities, scoliosis, arachnodactyly, hyperflexibility, tall stature, elongated fingers and toes); dural ectasia; spontaneous pneumothorax
Loeys-Dietz syndrome (LDS)	Autosomal dominant disorder caused by mutations in *TGFBR1* and *TGFBR2*, associated with aneurysms and dissections involving the aorta and branch vessels, often at relatively small diameters and young age; manifestations include craniofacial features (hypertelorism, craniosynostosis, cleft palate, bifid or broad uvula), bluish sclera, arterial tortuosity, velvety and hyperlucent skin, easily visible veins, clubfeet, skeletal abnormalities; phenotypes may vary, including those with more pronounced craniofacial features and those with more cutaneous features; ectopia lentis has not been described in LDS; mutations in *TGFB2* lead to a syndrome with an overlap in clinical features of LDS and MFS
Familial thoracic aortic aneurysm (FTAA) syndromes	Autosomal dominant disorders with variable expression and penetrance leading to thoracic aortic aneurysms (TAAs) and dissections at variable ages in families; *ACTA2* mutations occur in 10%-15% of cases of FTAA and are associated with bicuspid aortic valve (BAV) disease, cerebral aneurysms, livedo reticularis, iris flocculi, PDA, moyamoya, and premature coronary artery disease; gene mutations causing familial thoracic aortic aneurysm and dissection (TAAD) include *ACTA2, TGFBR1, TGFBR2, FBN1, MYH11, MYLK, TGFB2, SMAD3*
Vascular Ehlers-Danlos syndrome (vEDS)	Autosomal dominant disorder of collagen synthesis caused by a gene mutation in *COL3A1* leading to rupture and dissection of the aorta (usually the descending and abdominal aorta) and branch vessels; manifestations include flexible digits, hyperlucent skin with visible veins, varicose veins, typical facial appearance, and spontaneous rupture of the uterus or bowel
Bicuspid aortic valve (BAV)	Congenital condition affecting ≈1% of the population, familial in ≈9% of cases; often associated with dilation of the ascending aorta and carries increased risk for aortic dissection; gene mutations include *NOTCH1* and loci at 15q, 18q, 5q, and 13q; may be associated with FTAA
Turner syndrome (TS)	Genetic disorder affecting 1 in 2000 live-born girls and caused by complete or partial loss of the second sex chromosome (XO, Xp); women with TS often have BAV and aortic coarctation; associated with ascending aortic dilation for body size and increased risk for aortic dissection, especially when associated with BAV, hypertension, and coarctation
Aneurysms-osteoarthritis syndrome	Autosomal dominant genetic disorder resulting from mutations in the *SMAD3* gene and associated with premature osteoarthritis, osteochondritis dissecans, skeletal features, aortic aneurysms, branch vessel aneurysms, and arterial tortuosity; overlap with LDS phenotype

From Mann DL et al: *Braunwald's heart disease*, ed 10, Philadelphia, 2015, Elsevier.

TABLE 4   Ascending Thoracic Aortic Aneurysms

Degenerative	Associated with Atherosclerosis
Inheritable/connective tissue	Marfan syndrome
	Ehlers-Danlos syndrome
	Loeys-Dietz syndrome
	Turner syndrome
	Osteogenesis imperfecta
	Rheumatoid arthritis
	Bicuspid aortic valve
	Aneurysm of sinus of Valsalva
Arteritis	Giant cell
	Takayasu
	Behçet disease
	Relapsing polychondritis
Infectious	Syphilis
	Mycotic aneurysms

From Soto JA, Lucey BC: *Emergency radiology: the requisites*, ed 2, Philadelphia, 2017, Elsevier.

TABLE 5   Aortic Arch Aneurysms

Degenerative	Resulting from Atherosclerosis
Arteritis	Giant cell
	Takayasu
	Behçet disease
Infectious	Syphilis

From Soto JA, Lucey BC: *Emergency radiology: the requisites*, ed 2, Philadelphia, 2017, Elsevier.

- Chest radiograph may show widened mediastinum (52% in type A dissections and 39% in type B dissections) and displacement of aortic intimal calcium.[4] It is normal in 29% to 36% of patients with aortic dissection.
- Although the diagnostic sensitivity of transthoracic echocardiography is suboptimal (31% to 55%), it is useful in assessing potential high-risk features or complications, such as pericardial effusion and cardiac tamponade, and in making other potential diagnoses. A negative transthoracic echocardiography, however, does not exclude aortic dissection.[1]

Rx TREATMENT

- Urgent surgical consultation should be obtained for all thoracic aortic dissection regardless of anatomic location. Table 9 summarizes size threshold for prophylactic aortic root or ascending aortic aneurysm resection for various conditions.
- Proximal dissections (acute type A) require emergent surgery to prevent rupture or pericardial effusion.[1]
- Distal dissections (Stanford type B) are usually treated medically unless distal organ involvement or impending rupture occurs.
  1. Surgical intervention for distal dissections is reserved for patients who have a complicated course, including occlusion of a major aortic branch, propagation of the dissection, enlarging aneurysm, and evidence of aortic rupture.[1]
  2. Thoracic endovascular aortic repair (TEVAR) is a less invasive option for complicated type B aortic dissections and is associated with lower short-term and midterm

TABLE 6 Descending Thoracic Aortic Aneurysm

Degenerative	Resulting from atherosclerosis
Arteritis	Focal pseudoaneurysm resulting from a penetrating aortic ulcer
	Giant cell
	Takayasu
	Behçet disease
Inherited/connective tissue	Marfan syndrome
	Ductus aneurysm
	Loeys-Dietz syndrome
Infectious	Mycotic aneurysms
Traumatic	Posttraumatic pseudoaneurysms
	Chronic aortic transection

From Soto JA, Lucey BC: *Emergency radiology: the requisites*, ed 2, Philadelphia, 2017, Elsevier.

TABLE 7 Crawford Classification of Thoracoabdominal Aneurysms

I	Descending thoracic aorta to suprarenal aorta
II	Proximal descending thoracic aorta to infrarenal aorta (below the diaphragm)
III	Mid descending thoracic aorta to infrarenal aorta
IV	Supravisceral aorta to infrarenal aorta

From Soto JA, Lucey BC: *Emergency radiology: the requisites*, ed 2, Philadelphia, 2017, Elsevier.

TABLE 8 Aortic Dissection Detection Risk Score (ADD-RS)

Clinical Risk Markers*	Score
High-risk condition such as Marfan syndrome, family history of aortic disease, known aortic valve disease, known thoracic aortic aneurysm, or previous aortic manipulation, including cardiac surgery	1
Pain in the chest, back, or abdomen described as abrupt, of severe intensity, or a ripping/tearing sensation	1
Physical examination findings of perfusion deficit, including pulse deficit, systolic blood pressure difference, or focal neurologic deficit, or with aortic diastolic murmur and hypotension/shock	1

*Presence of ≥1 marker within each of these groups is given a score of 1 with a maximum cumulative score of 3 if all three are present. Modified from Erbel R et al: 2014 ESC guidelines on the diagnosis and treatment of aortic diseases: document covering acute and chronic aortic diseases of the thoracic and abdominal aorta of the adult. The Task Force for the Diagnosis and Treatment of Aortic Diseases of the European Society of Cardiology (ESC), *Eur Heart J* 35:2873-2926, 2014; Hiratzka LF et al: 2010 ACCF/AHA/AATS/ACR/ASA/SCA/SCAI/SIR/STS/SVM guidelines for the diagnosis and management of patients with thoracic aortic disease, *Circulation* 121:e266-369, 2010; and Hiratzka et al: Surgery for aortic dilatation in patients with bicuspid aortic valves: a statement of clarification from the American College of Cardiology/American Heart Association Task Force on Clinical Practice Guidelines, *J Am Coll Cardiol* 67:724-731, 2016.

mortality than medical therapy.[1,3,10] Indications for TEVAR for type B aortic dissection are summarized in Table 10.

3. For acute type B dissections, in-hospital mortality in patients managed surgically has been reported to be 33.9% versus those managed with endovascular treatment at 10.6%.[3]
   a. Independent predictors of complication and mortality in distal dissections include periaortic hematoma and descending aortic diameter >5.5 cm, partial false lumen thrombosis, primary tear >10 mm, one entry tear, and false lumen >22 mm.[1,10,11]
   b. There is ongoing debate about a possible beneficial role of TEVAR for uncomplicated type B dissections. Data suggest that in uncomplicated type B dissections, TEVAR significantly lowers aorta-related mortality and disease progression in 5-yr follow-up.[1]

ACUTE GENERAL Rx
- Admit to ICU for monitoring.
- Target systolic blood pressure 100 to 120 mm Hg; heart rate <60 beats/min to reduce aortic wall stress.[1,8] Treatment with beta-blockers has been associated with improved survival in all patients with acute aortic dissections.
- IV beta-blockers are cornerstones of treatment, but multiple medications may be needed.
  1. Propranolol 1 mg every 3 to 5 min, metoprolol 5 mg IV every 5 min, or labetalol 20 mg IV, then 20 to 80 mg every 10 min, followed by nitroprusside 0.3 to 10 mcg/kg/min.[8]
  2. Vasodilators should not be used without beta-blockade as they can induce reflex sympathetic stimulation and increase aortic shear stress.[8]
  3. IV calcium channel blockers with negative inotropy (i.e., verapamil, diltiazem) may be used if beta-blockers are contraindicated.[8]
- Pain control, often with morphine.[8]

CHRONIC Rx
- Chronic aortic dissection (>2 wk) managed with aggressive blood pressure control; target <130/80 mm Hg in most patients[1,8]
- Statin therapy to reduce low-density lipoprotein <70 mg/dl[8]
- Tobacco cessation[8]
- Minimize strenuous physical activity such as heavy lifting[8]
- Serial imaging of the aorta, with multidetector CT or MRI should be performed at presentation, at 1, 3, 6, and 12 mo given the higher risk of instability early on, followed by yearly clinical and imaging follow-up[8]
- As stated above, endovascular repair should be considered in complicated chronic type B dissections, that is, when the aortic diameter exceeds 5.5 cm, when there is uncontrolled pain or blood pressure, or when there is rapid growth of the dissecting aneurysm (>4 mm per yr)[8]

DISPOSITION
- 90% mortality rate is within 2 wk for an untreated type A dissection.
- Proximal dissection is a surgical emergency. Time is critical; mortality rate is 1% to 3%/h, approaching 70% after 48 h.[1,8]
- Overall, in-hospital mortality rate is 22% with proximal dissections (27% treated surgically and 56% treated medically) and 13% with distal dissections.[3]
- Table 11 summarizes suggested imaging surveillance of asymptomatic thoracic aortic aneurysms.

REFERRAL
For ICU management and surgical intervention

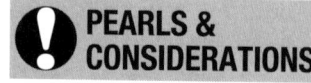
❗ PEARLS & CONSIDERATIONS

- Blood pressure control is essential; beta-blocker is first-line medication.[1,8]
- Proximal dissection is a surgical emergency.[1,3,8]
- Cardiac tamponade is not uncommon in patients with acute type A aortic dissection.[8] Syncope, altered mental status, and a widened mediastinum on chest radiograph on presentation suggest tamponade, which warrants urgent operative therapy.[1,8]

TABLE 9 Size Threshold for Prophylactic Aortic Root or Ascending Aortic Aneurysm Resection for Various Conditions

Condition	Size Threshold*
Degenerative aneurysm	≥5.5 cm
Bicuspid aortic valve	≥5.5 cm
Bicuspid aortic valve with risk factors or low surgical risk[†]	≥5.0 cm
Bicuspid aortic valve requiring aortic valve replacement	>4.5 cm
Marfan syndrome	>5.0 cm
Marfan syndrome with risk factors[‡]	>4.5 cm
Loeys-Dietz syndrome[§]	4.0-4.5 cm
Familial thoracic aortic aneurysm syndromes[¶]	4.5-5.0 cm
Turner syndrome	>2.5 cm/m^2

* Lower thresholds for intervention may be considered according to body surface area in patients of small stature or in the case of rapid growth of the aorta. Age, body size, rapid growth, family history, risk of surgery, and patient and physician wishes may influence aortic size threshold.

[†]Family history of aortic dissection or aortic growth rate of ≥0.5 cm/yr or if the patient is at low surgical risk (<4%) and the surgery is performed by an experienced aortic surgical team in a center with established expertise in these procedures. Other risk factors for aortic dissection include coarctation of the aorta, hypertension, and the root phenotype of bicuspid aortic valve.

[‡]Family history of aortic dissection or rapid aortic growth (>3 mm/yr), or severe aortic or mitral regurgitation. If pregnancy desired, consider prophylactic aortic surgery for aortic diameter of 4.0-4.5 cm.

[§]It is reasonable to consider surgical repair of the aorta in adults with Loeys-Dietz syndrome or a confirmed *TGFBR1* or *TGFBR2* mutation with aortic diameter of 4.2 cm or more by transesophageal echocardiogram or 4.4-4.6 or more by CT or MRI. Aortic surgery at smaller diameters may be recommended when there are severe craniofacial features, rapid growth, or a family history of aortic dissection.

[¶]Surgical thresholds vary depending on the specific gene mutation involved. TAA caused by *ACTA2*, *SMAD3*, and *MYLK* may lead to aortic dissection at relatively small aortic diameters.

From Zipes DP: *Braunwald's heart disease: a textbook of cardiovascular medicine*, ed 11, Philadelphia, 2019, Elsevier.

TABLE 10 Indications for Thoracic Endovascular Aortic Repair for Type B Aortic Dissection*

Rupture
Impending rupture
Malperfusion
Hemorrhagic pleural effusion
Refractory pain
Refractory hypertension
Aneurysmal dilation (>55 mm)
Rapid increase in diameter
Recurrent symptoms

* Or open surgical repair if anatomy is unsuitable for TEVAR.
From Zipes DP: *Braunwald's heart disease: a textbook of cardiovascular medicine*, ed 11, Philadelphia, 2019, Elsevier.

- Surgery for acute type A aortic dissection in patients ≥70 yr old can be performed with acceptable outcomes.[3]

OTHER ACUTE AORTIC SYNDROMES

ACUTE INTRAMURAL HEMATOMA:
- Acute IMH occurs when the vasa vasorum ruptures within the medial wall. It does not involve an intimal tearing unless a dissection develops.

- About 10% to 20% of patients with suspected aortic dissection will be found to have acute IMH.[8]
- The key imaging findings are the absence of intimal tear and absence of blood flow into a false lumen.
- Echocardiography shows crescentic or circumferential thickening of aortic wall without an intimal flap.
- About 8% to 16% of patients with IMH will evolve into aortic dissection.[3]
- Management remains controversial, but in the ascending aorta, IMH is generally treated with urgent surgical repair.
- Similar to aortic dissections, in-hospital mortality is significantly worse among patients with type A IMH compared to type B.[3]

PENETRATING ATHEROSCLEROTIC ULCER:
- Penetrating atherosclerotic ulcers occur in the setting of extensive aortic atherosclerosis and hypertension.[8]
- These are seen mostly in older adults and occurs in descending aorta in over 90% of cases.[8]
- There is an ulceration of atheroma that disrupts the internal elastic lamina and extends into the media and allows hematoma formation.[8]

TABLE 11 Suggested Imaging Surveillance of Asymptomatic Thoracic Aortic Aneurysms*

Initial Discovery of Aneurysm	Repeated Imaging at 6 mo to Document Stability
Degenerative Aneurysm[†]	
3.5-4.4 cm	Annual imaging
4.5-5 cm	Annual to biannual imaging
MFS, BAV with TAA, and Familial TAA	
3.5-4.4 cm	Annual imaging
4.5-5.0 cm	Biannual imaging
LDS[‡]	
<4 cm	At least annual imaging
>4 cm	Biannual imaging

BAV, Bicuspid aortic valve; *LDS*, Loeys-Dietz syndrome; *MFS*, Marfan syndrome; *TAA*, thoracic aortic aneurysm.

*For aneurysms growing rapidly, more frequent imaging is recommended. Management of TAA must take into account the family history, age, body size, sex, rate of aneurysm growth, and underlying disease.

[†]For relatively small degenerative aneurysms found by imaging to be stable from year to year, imaging may be performed every 2-3 yr (Hiratzka et al).

[‡]Some recommend surgery for aortic root dimensions larger than 4 cm in adults with LDS, whereas the American College of Cardiology/American Heart Association guidelines for thoracic aortic disease recommend prophylactic surgery at 4.2 cm by TEE and 4.4-4.6 cm by CT or MRI (Hiratzka et al).

From Hiratzka LF et al: 2010 ACCF/AHA/AATS/ACR/ASA/SCA/SCAI/SIR/STS/SVM guidelines for the diagnosis and management of patients with thoracic aortic disease: a report of the American College of Cardiology Foundation/American Heart Association Task Force on Practice Guidelines, American Association for Thoracic Surgery, American College of Radiology, American Stroke Association, Society of Cardiovascular Anesthesiologists, Society for Cardiovascular Angiography and Interventions, Society of Interventional Radiology, Society of Thoracic Surgeons, and Society for Vascular Medicine, *Circulation* 121:e266, 2010; Mann DL et al: *Braunwald's heart disease*, ed 10, Philadelphia, 2015, Elsevier.

- They should be treated promptly, because there is potential for extensive IMH, pseudoaneurysm or complete rupture of aorta.[8]

The general principles of the treatment of acute IMHs and penetrating atherosclerotic ulcers are similar to acute aortic dissection.[8]

REFERENCES
Available at eBooks.Health.Elsevier.com

RELATED CONTENT
Aortic Dissection (Patient Information)

AUTHORS: **CRISTINA FONT, MD** and **PHILIP STOCKWELL, MD**

Acute Bronchitis

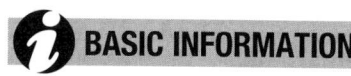

BASIC INFORMATION

DEFINITION
Acute bronchitis is a self-limited inflammation of trachea and bronchi.

SYNONYM
Chest cold

ICD-10CM CODE
J20.9 Acute bronchitis, unspecified

EPIDEMIOLOGY & DEMOGRAPHICS
- Highest incidence in smokers, older adults, and young children and during winter months.
- In the U.S. there are nearly 30 million ambulatory visits annually for cough, leading to more than 12 million diagnoses of "bronchitis."
- Acute lower respiratory tract infection is the most common condition treated in primary care.

PHYSICAL FINDINGS & CLINICAL PRESENTATIONS
- In most cases, acute bronchitis begins with signs and symptoms typical of the common cold syndrome (nasal congestion, sore throat), followed shortly by the onset of cough
- Cough, usually worse in the morning, often productive; mainly caused by transient bronchial hyperresponsiveness
- Low-grade fever
- Substernal discomfort worsened by coughing
- Postnasal drip, pharyngeal injection
- Rhonchi that may clear after cough, occasional wheezing
- Various host factors (age, immune status, smoking, underlying medical conditions) can influence illness severity and clinical presentation
- In mild cases, the illness lasts only 7 to 10 days, whereas in others, cough may persist for up to 3 wk or longer

ETIOLOGY
- Viral infections are the leading cause of bronchitis (rhinovirus, influenza virus, adenovirus, respiratory syncytial virus)
- Atypical organisms (Mycoplasma, Chlamydia pneumoniae)
- Bacterial infections (Bordetella pertussis, Haemophilus influenzae, Moraxella, Streptococcus pneumoniae)
- Table 1 summarizes viral and bacterial causes of acute bronchitis

DIAGNOSIS

DIFFERENTIAL DIAGNOSIS
- Pneumonia
- Asthma
- Sinusitis
- Bronchiolitis
- Aspiration
- Cystic fibrosis
- Pharyngitis
- Cough secondary to medications
- Neoplasm (elderly patients)
- Influenza
- Allergic aspergillosis
- Gastroesophageal reflux disease
- Congestive heart failure (in elderly patients)
- Bronchogenic neoplasm

WORKUP
Seldom necessary (e.g., to rule out pneumonia, neoplasm)

LABORATORY TESTS
Laboratory tests are generally not necessary.

IMAGING STUDIES
Chest x-ray is usually reserved for patients with suspected pneumonia, influenza, or underlying chronic obstructive pulmonary disease (COPD) and no improvement with therapy.

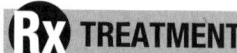

TREATMENT

NONPHARMACOLOGIC THERAPY
- Avoidance of tobacco and other pulmonary irritants
- Increased fluid intake
- Use of vaporizer to increase room humidity

ACUTE GENERAL Rx
- Therapy is generally symptomatic and directed at relief of cough and wheezing.
- Inhaled bronchodilators (e.g., albuterol, metaproterenol) as needed for 1 to 2 wk in patients with wheezing or troublesome cough. Inhaled albuterol has been proven effective in reducing the duration of cough in adults with uncomplicated acute bronchitis.

TABLE 1 Viral and Bacterial Causes of Acute Bronchitis

Pathogen	Seasonality	Comments
Influenza viruses	Winter	Local epidemics last 6-8 wk during which clinical illness of cough and fever has high predictive value; laboratory diagnosis readily available; early neuraminidase inhibitor therapy effective
Rhinoviruses	Fall and spring	Most frequent cause of common cold syndrome; immunity is serotype specific
Coronaviruses	Winter to spring	Cause common cold syndrome; newer strains are difficult to culture and require RT-PCR for diagnosis
Adenoviruses	Year round, winter epidemics	High attack rates in closed populations such as persons living in military barracks or college dormitories; serotype-specific immunity
Respiratory syncytial virus (RSV)	Late fall to early spring	Attack rates approach 75% in neonates, 3%-5% in adults; associated with wheezing in all age groups; rapid antigen test accurate in children but requires culture or RT-PCR to diagnose in adults
Human metapneumovirus (hMPV)	Winter to early spring	Associated with wheezing in adults and in infants; difficult to isolate in tissue culture and often requires RT-PCR
Parainfluenza viruses	Fall to winter	Similar to RSV and hMPV, parainfluenza viruses are primarily pediatric pathogens but can cause severe acute disease in some adults
Measles virus	Year round	Can cause respiratory disease in malnourished children; illness causes transient immune suppression
Mycoplasma pneumoniae	Year round, fall outbreaks	Long incubation period (10-21 days) results in staggered epidemic pattern in families; nonproductive persistent cough typical; diagnosed by IgM serology; treated with macrolide, quinolone, or tetracycline antibiotics
Chlamydia pneumoniae	Year round	Associated with sinusitis; diagnosis by RT-PCR not readily available
Bordetella pertussis	Year round	Severe illness in nonimmunized children; illness milder in partially immune adults; can be associated with prolonged cough; adults are often reservoirs for epidemics; early therapy with antibiotics can reduce spread

IgM, Immunoglobulin M; RT-PCR, reverse-transcriptase polymerase chain reaction. From Bennett JE et al: Mandell, Douglas, and Bennett's principles and practice of infectious diseases, ed 8, Philadelphia, 2015, Saunders.

- Cough suppression with dextromethorphan and guaifenesin is commonly recommended; addition of codeine for cough suppression if cough is severe and is significantly interrupting patient's sleep pattern.
- Use of antibiotics (trimethoprim-sulfamethoxazole, amoxicillin, doxycycline, cefuroxime) for acute bronchitis is generally not indicated; should be considered only in patients with concomitant COPD, increased dyspnea, and purulent sputum or in patients with suspected pertussis. In the few cases of acute bronchitis caused by *B. pertussis* or atypical bacteria such as *C. pneumoniae* or *Mycoplasma pneumoniae*, early use of macrolide antibiotics is reasonable. Clinicians should limit antibiotic treatment duration to 5 days when managing patients with COPD exacerbations and acute uncomplicated bronchitis who have clinical signs of a bacteria infection.
- Antibiotics are overused in patients with acute bronchitis (70% to 90% of office visits for acute bronchitis result in treatment with antibiotics); this practice pattern is contributing to increases in resistant organisms.
- Trials have shown that there are no significant differences in patients receiving antibiotics compared with those receiving placebo in overall clinical improvements or limitations in work or other activities. There was a significant increase in adverse effects in the antibiotic group, particularly GI symptoms.

CHRONIC Rx

Avoidance of tobacco and other pulmonary irritants.

DISPOSITION

- Complete recovery within 7 to 10 days in most patients.
- Patients should be informed to expect to have a cough for 10 to 14 days after the visit.

REFERRAL

For pulmonary function testing only in patients with recurrent bronchitis and suspected underlying pulmonary disease.

⊘ PEARLS & CONSIDERATIONS

COMMENTS

- Patients are more likely to receive prescriptions for antibiotics from mid- or late-career physicians with high patient volumes and from physicians who were trained outside of Canada or the U.S. Intervention studies reveal that patient and physician education are effective in reducing the use of antibiotic therapy. No offer or delayed offer of antibiotics for acute uncomplicated lower respiratory tract infection is acceptable, is associated with little difference in symptom resolution, and is likely to reduce antibiotic use and beliefs in the effectiveness of antibiotics.
- It is helpful to refer to acute bronchitis as a "chest cold." Patients should be informed that antibiotics are probably not going to be beneficial and may result in significant side effects.

SUGGESTED READINGS

Available at eBooks.Health.Elsevier.com

RELATED CONTENT

Acute Bronchitis (Patient Information)

AUTHOR: **FRED F. FERRI, MD**

A

Diseases and Disorders

I

Acute Coronary Syndrome (PTG)

BASIC INFORMATION

Acute coronary syndrome (ACS) represents a spectrum of clinical disorders that results from a sudden and unpredictable decrease of blood flow to the myocardium. ACS is a life-threatening disorder that incurs high, and in some cases immediate, mortality. This syndrome is usually due to interaction of vulnerable atherosclerotic plaque in the coronary arteries with that of activated clotting factors and platelets in the systemic circulation. In the modern era, management of ACS involves highly protocolized and systematic care of both procedural and medical therapies guided toward restoring blood flow to the heart. The spectrum of ACS is predominated by two important subtypes: ST-elevation myocardial infarction (STEMI) and non–ST-elevation myocardial infarction (NSTEMI). The third category of ACS is called unstable angina (UA) and falls within the NSTEMI subtype. The type of ACS dictates the timing of reperfusion, with STEMI being the most severe and always emergent. In this spectrum, UA and NSTEMI are represented by an abnormal ECG without the presence of ST-segment elevation in the appropriate clinical setting (i.e., chest discomfort). NSTEMI is additionally characterized by positive cardiac biomarkers. STEMI is characterized by ST-segment elevation on ECG in the appropriate clinical setting.[1] With the advent and widespread use of the high-sensitivity troponin, the diagnosis of UA has changed to NSTEMI in almost all patients formerly diagnosed with UA. This is in part due to patients previously diagnosed with UA having abnormally elevated high-sensitivity troponin levels.[2] Thus ACS should be thought of as a continuous spectrum as UA will often progress to a myocardial infarction (MI) if left untreated (Table 1). Because of this continuum, the 2014 American College of Cardiology/American Heart Association (ACC/AHA) guidelines have grouped UA and NSTEMI into a single category called non–ST-elevation ACS (NSTE-ACS).[3]

SYNONYMS

ACS
UA
NSTEMI
STEMI
Acute MI

ICD-10CM CODES

I20.0	Unstable angina
I21.0-I21.3	ST elevation (STEMI)
I21.4	Non-ST elevation (NSTEMI) myocardial infarction
I24.9	Acute ischemic heart disease, unspecified

EPIDEMIOLOGY & DEMOGRAPHICS

INCIDENCE: In the U.S., cardiovascular disease accounts for approximately 640,000 deaths each year. The estimated annual incidence of heart attacks in the U.S. is 600,000 new attacks and 200,000 recurrent attacks.[4] Approximately 70% of MIs are listed as NSTEMI, with the remainder being listed as STEMI. Patients presenting with NSTE-ACS have worse long-term prognosis than patients presenting with STEMI. This is due to the higher comorbidity profile of patients presenting with NSTE-ACS (i.e., significantly older population, higher burden of comorbidities, and frequent history of coronary artery disease [CAD]). The underlying etiology, atherosclerotic CAD, remains the number one cause of mortality.[4]

PREDOMINANT SEX AND AGE: In the U.S., the median age at ACS presentation is 68 yr old (interquartile range 56 to 79), and the male:female ratio is approximately 3:2. In a 2005 to 2011 study sponsored by National Heart, Lung, and Blood Institute, the average age-adjusted first MI or fatal coronary heart disease rates per 1000 population in patients age 35 to 84 yr of age were 3.7 for white men, 5.9 for black men, 2.1 for white women, and 4.0 for black women.[4] As noted in this study, heart disease affects African Americans disproportionately. Heart disease is also the leading cause of death in women, surpassing all forms of cancer.[4]

RISK FACTORS: Hypertension, diabetes mellitus, dyslipidemia, tobacco use, and family history of premature CAD (CAD in a male first-degree relative younger than 55 yr or a female younger than 65 yr of age) are all associated risk factors for CAD. There are also female-specific risk factors for CAD, including disorders of pregnancy and early onset of menopause. Refer to the topic "Angina Pectoris" for an extensive list of risk factors. Presence of these risk factors cause damage to the vascular endothelium and progression of atherosclerotic coronary artery plaques.

PHYSICAL FINDINGS & CLINICAL PRESENTATION

- Symptoms often, but not always, include chest discomfort described as a pressure that may radiate to the shoulders, neck, jaw, or back. Typical angina is substernal in location, brought on by emotional or physical stress, and relieved with rest and/or nitroglycerin. The pain and discomfort associated with an ACS event is often diffuse rather than localized and often associated with diaphoresis.
- Women, diabetics, the elderly (>75 yr old), and postoperative patients often have an atypical presentation for ACS.
- UA has three typical presentations:
  1. Rest angina: Angina occurring at rest and usually prolonged for longer than 20 min.
  2. New-onset angina: New-onset angina of at least Canadian Cardiovascular Society (CCS) class III symptoms (Table 2).
  3. Progressive angina: Previously diagnosed angina that has become distinctly more frequent, longer in duration, or lower in threshold (i.e., increased by ≥1 CCS class to at least CCS class III severity).
- "Anginal equivalents" may include dyspnea, nausea, vomiting, and fatigue.
- ECG for NSTE-ACS may reveal transient ST-segment elevation, ST-segment depression, and/or new T-wave inversion. ECG for definition of STEMI will reveal ≥1-mm ST-segment elevation at the J-point in two contiguous leads other than leads V_2-V_3 in which cut-points are ≥2-mm in men ≥40 yr, ≥2.5-mm in men <40 yr, or ≥1.5-mm in women regardless of age.[1]
- Physical examination findings alone are insufficient for the diagnosis of ACS. The physical examination may provide clues as to alternative diagnoses, such as aortic dissection (differences in pulse and blood pressure between the arms, murmur of aortic regurgitation), aortic stenosis, pericarditis (friction rub), cardiac tamponade (pulsus paradoxus), and pneumothorax (absent breath sounds). In ACS, it is important to assess the patient's hemodynamic stability, as signs of heart failure may be present. These signs include elevated jugular venous pressure (JVP), presence of an S3 gallop, rales, and to a lesser extent, peripheral edema. The degree of heart failure with MI can be represented by the Killip classification, with the greater the Killip classification, the greater the mortality noted[5]:
  1. Killip Class 1 is no heart failure.
  2. Killip Class 2 includes individuals with rales, elevated JVP, and S3 on examination.
  3. Killip Class 3 includes individuals with frank pulmonary edema.

TABLE 1 Acute Coronary Syndromes

	SPECTRUM OF ACUTE CORONARY SYNDROME		
	Unstable Angina	**NSTEMI**	**STEMI**
Chest discomfort	1	1	1
Cardiac biomarkers	2	1	1
ECG changes	TWI and/or ST depression	TWI and/or ST depression	ST elevation or presumed new left bundle branch block
Pathophysiology	Partial/transient thrombotic occlusion	Partial/transient thrombotic occlusion	Complete thrombotic occlusion

ECG, Electrocardiogram; *NSTEMI,* non–ST-segment elevation myocardial infarction; *STEMI,* ST-segment myocardial infarction; *TWI,* T-wave inversion.

TABLE 2 Grading of Angina Pectoris According to CCS Classification

Class	Description of Stage
I	"Ordinary physical activity does not cause angina," such as walking or climbing stairs. Angina occurs with strenuous, rapid, or prolonged exertion at work or recreation.
II	"Slight limitation of ordinary activity." Angina occurs on walking or climbing stairs rapidly; walking uphill; walking or stair climbing after meals; in cold, in wind, or under emotional stress; or only during the few hours after awakening. Angina occurs on walking 0.2 blocks on the level and climbing 0.1 flight of ordinary stairs at a normal pace and under normal conditions.
III	"Marked limitations of ordinary physical activity." Angina occurs on walking 1-2 blocks on the level and climbing one flight of stairs under normal conditions and at a normal pace.
IV	"Inability to carry on any physical activity without discomfort—anginal symptoms may be present at rest."

Adapted with permission from Campeau L: Grading of angina pectoris (letter), *Circulation* 54:522-523, 1976. © 1976, American Heart Association, Inc.

From Braunwald E et al: ACC/AHA guidelines for the management of patients with unstable angina and non–ST-segment elevation myocardial infarction: a report of the American College of Cardiology/American Heart Association Task Force on Practice Guidelines (Committee on the Management of Patients With Unstable Angina), *J Am Coll Cardiol* 36:970-1062, 2000.

4. Killip Class 4 describes individuals in cardiogenic shock or hypotension with evidence of vasoconstriction noted.

ETIOLOGY

The hallmark of ACS is vulnerable atherosclerotic plaque, which typically has a thin fibrous cap and a large lipid core. This vulnerable plaque can spontaneously rupture, which leads to platelet activation and aggregation and a systemic inflammatory cascade, leading to thrombus formation. STEMI typically results from complete thrombotic occlusion of a coronary artery, whereas NSTE-ACS often has partial occlusion. Angiographically, it is often the intermediate coronary artery lesions (30% to 50% diameter vessel stenosis) that lead to subtotal or total vessel occlusion in two thirds of STEMI cases.

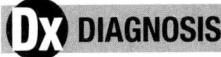 **DIAGNOSIS**

DIFFERENTIAL DIAGNOSIS

Chest pain mimicking ACS may be the result of various underlying disorders, some of which are also accompanied by ECG changes and/or cardiac biomarker release. Examples include acute pulmonary embolism, acute aortic dissection, pericarditis, myocarditis, costochondritis, pneumonia, tension pneumothorax, perforating ulcer, or esophageal perforation (i.e., Boerhaave syndrome). Refer to topics "Angina Pectoris," "Coronary Artery Syndrome," and "Myocardial Infarction" for extensive differential diagnoses of chest pain.

WORKUP

Focused history and physical examination, 12-lead ECG, cardiac biomarkers, and chest radiograph (CXR) are the cornerstone of initial chest pain workup. Initial biomarkers may not be positive early in the disease process. Conventional troponin levels are often drawn every 6 to 8 h for a total of three sets for the purposes of ruling out MI or until peak to determine the severity of an established MI, but with the advent of the high-sensitivity troponin, the time to rule in MI can

be done in as little as 3 h from initial presentation.[1] Echocardiogram may reveal new regional wall motion abnormalities or newly depressed left ventricular (LV) function or aneurysm formation. Fig. 1 summarizes the evaluation of patients for ACS.

LABORATORY TESTS

- Biomarkers and, in particular, the rising and/or falling pattern play an important role in the early detection and diagnosis of ACS. Although troponin is essential to the diagnosis of acute MI, other markers have demonstrated utility in the setting of acute chest pain and ACS. Creatinine kinase-myocardial band (CK-MB) and myoglobin are two traditional markers that are frequently used in combination with troponin and will be elevated in the setting of NSTEMI or STEMI. See Fig. E2, *A*, for timing of release of each biomarker. Troponin is the most sensitive biomarker for cardiac myocyte damage and also predicts 42-day mortality in ACS. Troponin is considered the gold standard biomarker for diagnosis of MI (Fig. E2, *B*). Newer troponin assays, often referred to as high-sensitivity troponin, have the ability to detect troponin levels at thresholds approximately 100 times lower than older assays. These assays allow for improved sensitivity in diagnosis or exclusion of acute MI.[1]
- CK-MB is the cardiac specific isoform of creatinine kinase (CK) and is found in high concentrations in the myocardium. After an acute myocardial injury, CK-MB levels peak within 4 to 6 h. Its shorter half-life leads to normal values within 24 to 48 h after an event. As such, CK-MB is especially useful when assessing a patient for possible reinfarction given troponin levels can remain elevated up to 14 days or more after an acute MI.[1]
- MI is not always the cause of elevated troponin levels. Any form of myocardial injury can cause elevation in troponin. Cardiac conditions that cause supply-demand mismatch without acute coronary obstruction, including arrhythmias, hypotension/hypertension, heart failure, and myocarditis, are a few examples that can lead to elevated levels. Noncardiac

conditions, including renal failure, sepsis, respiratory failure, and neurologic diseases, may similarly lead to elevations in troponin.
- Meanwhile, other biomarkers also have significant prognostic value. Testing for B-type natriuretic peptide (BNP) can help risk-stratify mortality in patients presenting with ACS. Notably, a BNP >80 portends a high risk of death at initial presentation of a STEMI.[1]

RISK MODELS & RISK SCORES

Risk models and scores such as TIMI (see "Risk Assessment" in "Myocardial Infarction" topic), PURSUIT, HEART, and GRACE based on clinical, ECG, risk factors, and laboratory data at presentation help to discriminate patients at high risk versus low risk for short- and intermediate-term adverse outcomes (Fig. E2, *C*).[6] These risk stratification models are helpful in determining the timing and strategy of treatment.

IMAGING STUDIES

- A CXR to assist in evaluating for volume overload and possible widened mediastinum, which could be indicative of an aortic dissection. CXR can be useful in assessing for pneumonia, pneumothorax, intraperitoneal free air, and other noncardiac causes of chest pain.
- In patients for whom ECG and cardiac biomarkers are nondiagnostic but they have high clinical suspicion for ACS, an echocardiogram may be helpful to assess LV function and regional wall motion abnormalities.
- Coronary CT angiography can be performed in patients with suspected ACS but with a normal 12-lead ECG, negative troponin, and no history of coronary artery disease (Class IIa).[7]
- Cardiac stress testing (treadmill ECG, imaging stress studies using echocardiography or nuclear modalities) is helpful in further risk stratification of these patients. (See "Coronary Artery Syndrome" in Section I.)
- Coronary angiogram/cardiac catheterization will reveal coronary artery luminal irregularities/stenotic lesions. In patients with ACS who undergo coronary angiography, approximately 25% will have one-vessel disease, 25% will have two-vessel disease, 25% will have three-vessel disease, 10% will have left main disease, and 15% will have coronary stenosis of <50% or normal coronaries.[4]

Rx TREATMENT

The overall goal for patients with ACS is to relieve myocardial ischemia and to prevent recurrent cardiovascular events. This is achieved by targeting both vulnerable coronary plaque and activated clotting factors and platelets in the blood. Revascularization, whether it is chemical (i.e., thrombolysis) or mechanical (i.e., percutaneous coronary intervention [PCI]), is needed to prevent further events and improve flow within the coronary artery lumen. In the modern era, PCI has improved outcomes for patients presenting with ACS.[8] For patients with STEMI, time from

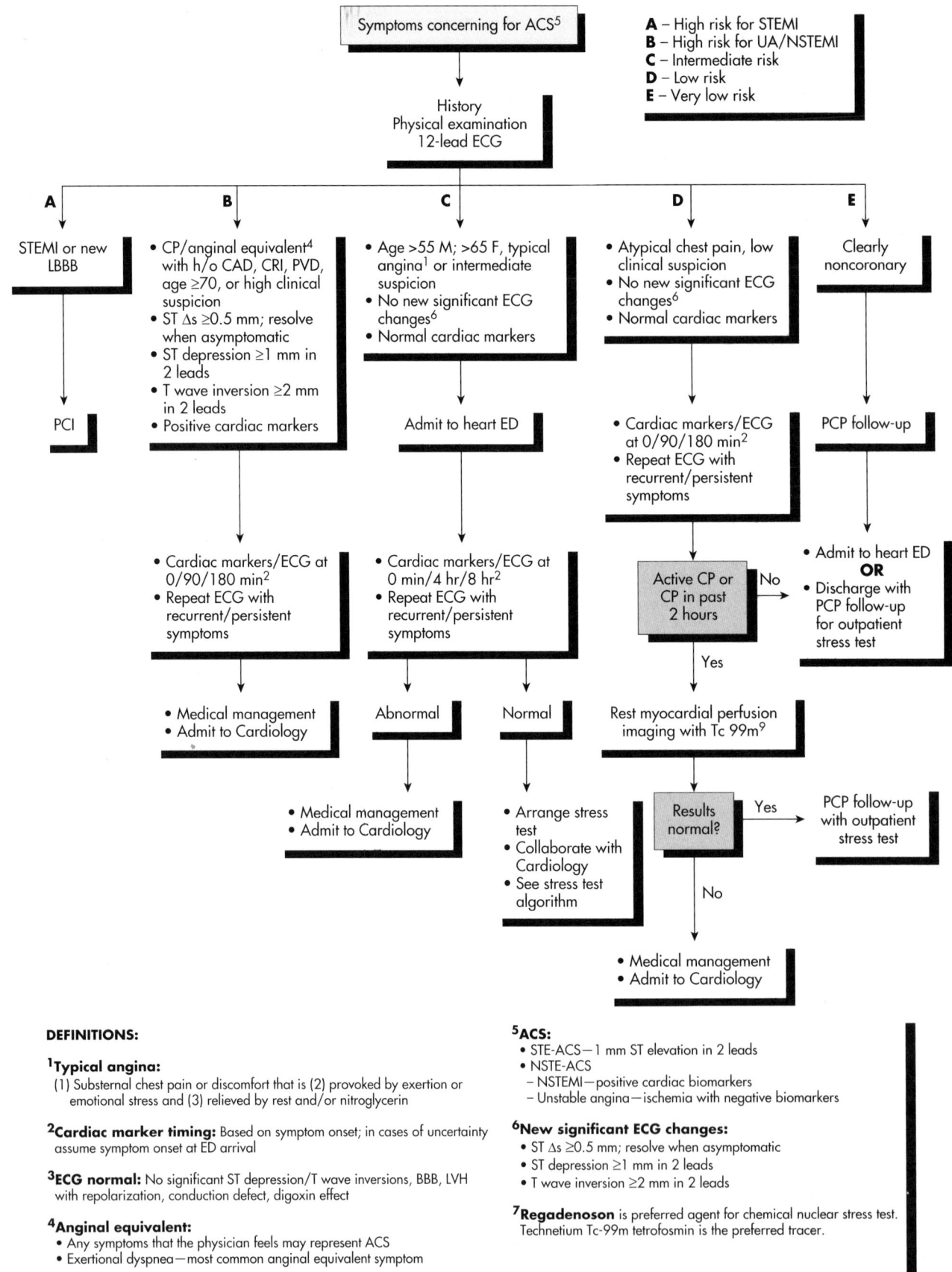

FIG. 1 Evaluation of patients for acute coronary syndrome (ACS). *CAD,* Coronary artery disease; *CP,* chest pain; *CRI,* chronic renal insufficiency; *ECG,* electrocardiogram; *ED,* emergency department; *h/o,* history of; *LBBB,* left bundle branch block; *NSTE,* non–ST-segment elevation; *NSTEMI,* non–ST-segment elevation myocardial infarction; *PCP,* primary care physician; *PVD,* peripheral vascular disease; *STE,* ST-segment elevation; *STEMI,* ST-segment elevation myocardial infarction; *UA,* unstable angina. (From Adams JG et al: *Emergency medicine: clinical essentials,* ed 2, Philadelphia, 2013, Elsevier.)

Text within the figure:

Symptoms concerning for ACS[5]

A – High risk for STEMI
B – High risk for UA/NSTEMI
C – Intermediate risk
D – Low risk
E – Very low risk

History
Physical examination
12-lead ECG

A
STEMI or new LBBB
→ PCI

B
• CP/anginal equivalent[4] with h/o CAD, CRI, PVD, age ≥70, or high clinical suspicion
• ST Δs ≥0.5 mm; resolve when asymptomatic
• ST depression ≥1 mm in 2 leads
• T wave inversion ≥2 mm in 2 leads
• Positive cardiac markers
↓
• Cardiac markers/ECG at 0/90/180 min[2]
• Repeat ECG with recurrent/persistent symptoms
↓
• Medical management
• Admit to Cardiology

C
• Age >55 M; >65 F, typical angina[1] or intermediate suspicion
• No new significant ECG changes[6]
• Normal cardiac markers
↓
Admit to heart ED
↓
• Cardiac markers/ECG at 0 min/4 hr/8 hr[2]
• Repeat ECG with recurrent/persistent symptoms
↓
Abnormal → • Medical management • Admit to Cardiology
Normal → • Arrange stress test • Collaborate with Cardiology • See stress test algorithm

D
• Atypical chest pain, low clinical suspicion
• No new significant ECG changes[6]
• Normal cardiac markers
↓
• Cardiac markers/ECG at 0/90/180 min[2]
• Repeat ECG with recurrent/persistent symptoms
↓
Active CP or CP in past 2 hours — No → • Admit to heart ED **OR** • Discharge with PCP follow-up for outpatient stress test
↓ Yes
Rest myocardial perfusion imaging with Tc 99m[9]
↓
Results normal? — Yes → PCP follow-up with outpatient stress test
↓ No
• Medical management
• Admit to Cardiology

E
Clearly noncoronary
↓
PCP follow-up

DEFINITIONS:

[1]**Typical angina:**
(1) Substernal chest pain or discomfort that is (2) provoked by exertion or emotional stress and (3) relieved by rest and/or nitroglycerin

[2]**Cardiac marker timing:** Based on symptom onset; in cases of uncertainty assume symptom onset at ED arrival

[3]**ECG normal:** No significant ST depression/T wave inversions, BBB, LVH with repolarization, conduction defect, digoxin effect

[4]**Anginal equivalent:**
• Any symptoms that the physician feels may represent ACS
• Exertional dyspnea—most common anginal equivalent symptom

[5]**ACS:**
• STE-ACS—1 mm ST elevation in 2 leads
• NSTE-ACS
  – NSTEMI—positive cardiac biomarkers
  – Unstable angina—ischemia with negative biomarkers

[6]**New significant ECG changes:**
• ST Δs ≥0.5 mm; resolve when asymptomatic
• ST depression ≥1 mm in 2 leads
• T wave inversion ≥2 mm in 2 leads

[7]**Regadenoson** is preferred agent for chemical nuclear stress test. Technetium Tc-99m tetrofosmin is the preferred tracer.

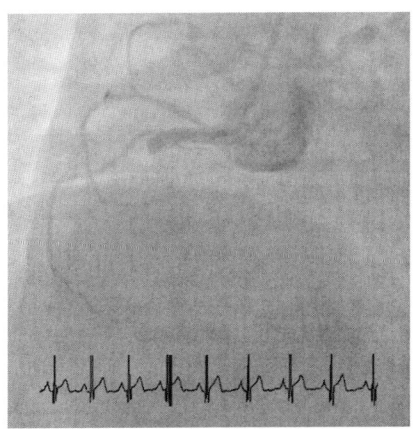

FIG. 3 Right coronary artery totally occluded proximally during ST-elevation myocardial infarction.

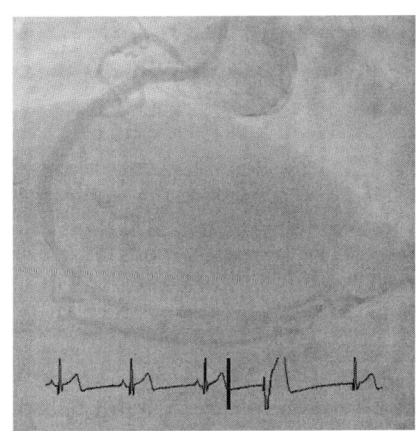

FIG. 4 Right coronary artery after successful percutaneous coronary artery stenting during ST-elevation myocardial infarction.

TABLE 3	Reperfusion Strategies	
Anticipated time from FMC to PCI	>120 min and	<120 min or
Symptom duration?	<12 h and	<24 h or
Thrombolytic eligible?	YES	NO
Reperfusion strategy	Thrombolytics and transfer	Primary PCI

FMC, First medical contact; PCI, percutaneous coronary intervention.

onset of ischemia to revascularization guides the reperfusion strategy. STEMI patients presenting to a hospital with PCI capability should be treated with primary PCI within 90 min of first medical contact (Figs. 3 and 4). At non–PCI-capable hospitals where the first medical contact to PCI is more than 120 min, thrombolytic therapy should be given to eligible patients within the first 12 h after symptom onset; thrombolytics should not be administered 24 h after initial diagnosis of STEMI (Table 3).[8] In patients who receive thrombolytic agents, coronary angiography can be done at a receiving hospital as soon as possible but not within the first 2 to 3 h after administration of a fibrinolytic agent. Thrombolytic agents come in two forms, fibrin specific (alteplase, reteplase, tenecteplase, staphylokinase) and nonfibrin specific (streptokinase, anistreplase, urokinase). Absolute contraindications to thrombolytic therapy include the following: History of intracranial hemorrhage, known structural cerebral vascular lesion, known intracranial neoplasm, ischemic stroke within 3 mo, suspected aortic dissection, active bleeding, head trauma within 3 mo, or intracranial surgery within 2 mo. Relative contraindications include ischemic stroke more than 3 mo prior, dementia, major surgery within 3 wk, current oral anticoagulant therapy, and traumatic or prolonged CPR.[9] Antithrombotic therapy is needed to reduce thrombus burden, prevent further thrombosis, and improve coronary artery flow.

NONPHARMACOLOGIC THERAPY

- STEMI is a medical emergency and requires immediate reperfusion therapy; the best outcomes are seen with cardiac catheterization and primary PCI. Guidelines call for a goal door-to-balloon time of ≤90 min.[9]
- Patients with NSTE-ACS should be risk stratified in conjunction with the cardiology consult service. Risk scores such as the TIMI and GRACE scores can be used to decide between an early invasive strategy and an ischemia-guided strategy. Overall, an early invasive strategy is associated with better outcomes in patients with higher risk (i.e., TIMI score >3 or GRACE >140) and involves cardiac catheterization followed by revascularization with PCI or coronary artery bypass grafting (CABG) within 4 to 24 h of presentation. An ischemia-guided strategy involves aggressive medical management and revascularization only if ischemia recurs or is documented on noninvasive testing.[3] This should be reserved only for selected patients with low-risk scores (TIMI score 0 to 2). The early invasive strategy can be further stratified by timing:
  1. Immediate (within 2 h): Patients with refractory or recurrent angina despite optimal initial treatment, signs or symptoms of heart failure, new or worsening mitral regurgitation, hemodynamic instability, sustained ventricular tachycardia or ventricular fibrillation

  2. Early (within 24 h): No characteristics from the immediate category but new ST-segment depression, a GRACE risk score >140 or temporal change in troponin
  3. Delayed invasive (25 to 72 h): None of the immediate or early characteristics but renal insufficiency, LV ejection fraction (EF) of <40%, early post-infarct angina, history of PCI within the past 6 mo, prior CABG, GRACE risk score of 109 to 140, or TIMI score of ≥2
- Continuous ECG monitoring is recommended for all ACS patients. Supplemental oxygen should be administered to patients with arterial oxygen saturation of <90%, respiratory distress, or other high-risk features of hypoxemia. Finger pulse oximetry should be used to assess arterial oxygen saturation.[8]

ACUTE GENERAL TREATMENT

- Table 4 is a summary of recommendations for standard medical therapy in the early hospital care phase of management of patients with NSTE-ACS.[3]
- Antithrombotic therapy (Table 5) is critical in treating the underlying pathophysiology of ACS. This consists of administering antiplatelet and anticoagulant agents (Table 6).
- Antiplatelet agents (Table 7) inhibit platelet activation and aggregation. Aspirin is an irreversible cyclooxygenase inhibitor that blocks platelet aggregation and should be administered to all ACS patients without contraindications.
- All patients with ACS should receive full-dose nonenteric-coated chewable aspirin of 162 to 325 mg to establish a high blood level for its antiplatelet effects to occur. Thereafter, daily dose of 81 mg should be continued indefinitely.[3]
- Clopidogrel is a thienopyridine agent that inhibits platelet activation and aggregation. It should be administered in all ACS patients, with the timing dependent on the clinical scenario and management strategy. It requires a loading dose of 300 to 600 mg followed by 75 mg/day. It should be discontinued at least 5 days before CABG to avoid excessive bleeding related to surgery. If a patient is unable to take aspirin in the setting of hypersensitivity or major gastrointestinal intolerance, a loading dose of clopidogrel followed by daily maintenance should be started.[3]
- Other antiplatelet agents that can be substituted instead of clopidogrel include prasugrel and ticagrelor. Ticagrelor has a half-life of 12 h with a more rapid onset and more consistent onset of action. In the PLATO trial, there was a reduction in death from vascular causes, MI, and stroke in patients with NSTE-ACS with ticagrelor over clopidogrel without an increase in the rate of overall major bleeding.[10] This benefit is limited to patients taking aspirin 75 to 100 mg/day. Prasugrel is not recommended as the initial antiplatelet agent in patients with NSTE-ACS. Multiple studies have demonstrated an increase in bleeding in patients taking prasugrel; in particular, those who are >75 yr old, with low body weight

TABLE 4 Summary of Recommendations for Standard Medical Therapy in the Early Hospital Care Phase of Management of Patients With Non–ST-Elevation Acute Coronary Syndrome (NSTE-ACS)

Recommendations	COR	LOE
Oxygen		
Administer supplemental oxygen only with oxygen saturation <90%, respiratory distress, or other high-risk features for hypoxemia.	I	C
Nitrates		
Administer sublingual NTG every 5 min ×3 for continuing ischemic pain and then assess need for IV NTG.	I	C
Administer IV NTG for persistent ischemia, HF, or hypertension.	I	B
Nitrates are contraindicated with recent use of a phosphodiesterase inhibitor.	III: Harm	B
Analgesic Therapy		
IV morphine sulfate may be reasonable for continued ischemic chest pain despite maximally tolerated antiischemic medications.	IIb	B
NSAIDs (except aspirin) should not be initiated and should be discontinued during hospitalization for NSTE-ACS because of the increased risk of MACE associated with their use.	III: Harm	B
Beta-Adrenergic Blockers		
Initiate oral beta blockers within the first 24 h in the absence of HF, low-output state, risk for cardiogenic shock, or other contraindications to beta blockade.	I	A
Use of sustained-release metoprolol succinate, carvedilol, or bisoprolol is recommended for beta-blocker therapy with concomitant NSTE-ACS, *stabilized* HF, and reduced systolic function.	I	C
Reevaluate to determine subsequent eligibility in patients with initial contraindications to beta blockers.	I	C
It is reasonable to continue beta-blocker therapy in patients with normal LV function with NSTE-ACS.	IIa	C
IV beta blockers are potentially harmful when risk factors for shock are present.	III: Harm	B
Calcium Channel Blockers (CCBs)		
Administer initial therapy with nondihydropyridine CCBs with recurrent ischemia and contraindications to beta blockers in the absence of LV dysfunction, increased risk for cardiogenic shock, PR interval >0.24 sec, or second- or third-degree atrioventricular block without a cardiac pacemaker.	I	B
Administer oral nondihydropyridine calcium antagonists with recurrent ischemia after use of beta blocker and nitrates in the absence of contraindications.	I	C
CCBs are recommended for ischemic symptoms when beta blockers are not successful, are contraindicated, or cause unacceptable side effects.*	I	C
Long-acting CCBs and nitrates are recommended for patients with coronary artery spasm.	I	C
Immediate-release nifedipine is contraindicated in the absence of a beta-blocker.	III: Harm	B
Cholesterol Management		
Initiate or continue high-intensity statin therapy in patients with no contraindications.	I	A
Obtain a fasting lipid profile, preferably within 24 h.	IIa	C

COR, Class of recommendation; *HF*, heart failure; *IV*, intravenous; *LOE*, level of evidence; *LV*, left ventricular; *MACE*, major adverse cardiovascular events; *N/A*, not available; *NSAIDs*, nonsteroidal anti-inflammatory drugs; *NTG*, nitroglycerin.

*Short-acting dihydropyridine calcium channel antagonists should be avoided.

From Amsterdam EA et al: 2014 AHA/ACC guideline for the management of patients with non–ST-elevation acute coronary syndromes: a report of the American College of Cardiology/American Heart Association task force on practice guidelines, *J Am Coll Cardiol* 64:e139-228, 2014 in Zipes DP: *Braunwald's heart disease: a textbook of cardiovascular medicine*, ed 11, Philadelphia, 2019, Elsevier.

(<60 kg), or with a history of cerebrovascular events.[11] Cangrelor is an IV ADP-P2Y12 receptor antagonist that may be used initially as a load in the emergency department before an invasive strategy, given its initial action and quick platelet recovery time. As a rule, all ACS patients should have two antiplatelet agents initiated and should be continued up to 12 mo regardless of treatment strategy.[3]

- GP IIb/IIIa inhibitors (Table 8) may be considered as an intravenous antiplatelet therapy in addition to aspirin for medium- or high-risk patients with NSTE-ACS in whom an invasive strategy is planned (Class IIb). Eptifibatide and tirofiban are preferred agents over abciximab for NSTE-ACS patients; however, for STEMI patients undergoing primary PCI, IV abciximab has the same Class IIa indication as tirofiban and ptifibatide.[9]

- Anticoagulant agents should be administered to all ACS patients, irrespective of initial treatment strategy. Options include either unfractionated heparin (UFH), or low-molecular-weight heparin (LMWH; enoxaparin), or factor Xa inhibitors such as fondaparinux, or direct thrombin inhibitors such as bivalirudin (Table 9).[9]

- For STEMI, fondaparinux can be used for anticoagulation. It has been shown to decrease bleeding complications as compared with either UFH or LMWH. However, it should not be used as the sole anticoagulant in PCI because of the risk of catheter thrombosis.[9]

- Bivalirudin is a reversible direct thrombin inhibitor and may be considered as an alternative to UFH and GP IIb/IIIa inhibitors in patients with STEMI who are undergoing primary PCI. When bivalirudin was compared to UFH plus a glycoprotein IIb/IIIa inhibitor in patients with STEMI and PCI, less bleeding and a short- and long-term reduction in cardiac events and overall mortality was observed. With bivalirudin, there is no risk of heparin-induced thrombocytopenia, less bleeding is observed, and the anticoagulant effect can be monitored during intervention by the activated clotting time. Similar results were reported in the use of bivalirudin alone in patients with UA/NSTEMI in the ACUITY trial

when compared to enoxaparin/UFH with GP IIb/IIIa arms.[12]

- Beta-blocker therapy reduces ischemia by decreasing myocardial oxygen demand and has a proven long-term mortality benefit. Oral therapy should be initiated within 24 hours of onset of ACS unless signs or symptoms of heart failure and shock are present or bradycardia precludes its use. Oral administration, titrated to a heart rate of 50 to 60 beats/min, is preferred.[9] Intravenous beta-blockers can be administered to STEMI patients who are hypertensive or have ongoing ischemia; they should be avoided if the patients have any of the following:

  1. Signs of heart failure
  2. Evidence of a low output state
  3. Increased risk for cardiogenic shock
  4. Other relative contraindications to beta-blockade (PR interval >0.24 sec, second- or third-degree heart block, active asthma, or reactive airway disease)

- Nitroglycerin is a vasodilator that should be administered to relieve chest discomfort in all

TABLE 5 Summary of Recommendations for Antithrombotic Therapy

Recommendations	Dosing, Special Considerations	COR	LOE
Aspirin			
Nonenteric-coated aspirin to all patients promptly after presentation	162-325 mg	I	A
Aspirin maintenance dose continued indefinitely	81-325 mg/day*	I	A
P2Y12 Inhibitors			
Clopidogrel loading dose followed by daily maintenance dose in patients unable to take aspirin	75 mg	I	B
P2Y12 inhibitor, in addition to aspirin, for up to 12 mo for patients treated initially with either an early invasive or initial ischemia-guided strategy:		I	B
• Clopidogrel	300- or 600-mg loading dose, then 75 mg/day		
• Ticagrelor	180-mg loading dose, then 90 mg twice daily		
P2Y12 inhibitor therapy (clopidogrel, prasugrel, or ticagrelor) continued for at least 12 mo in post-PCI patients treated with coronary stents	N/A	I	B
Ticagrelor in preference to clopidogrel for patients treated with an early invasive or ischemia-guided strategy	N/A	IIa	B
Glycoprotein (GP) IIb/IIIa Inhibitors			
GP IIb/IIIa inhibitor in patients treated with an early invasive strategy and DAPT with intermediate/high-risk features (e.g., positive troponin)	Preferred options are eptifibatide or tirofiban	IIb	B
Parenteral Anticoagulant and Fibrinolytic Therapy			
SC enoxaparin for duration of hospitalization or until PCI is performed	1 mg/kg SC every 12 h (reduce dose to 1 mg/kg/day SC in patients with CrCl <30 ml/min) Initial 30-mg IV loading dose in select patients	I	A
Bivalirudin until diagnostic angiography or PCI is performed in patients with early invasive strategy only	Loading dose 0.10 mg/kg, followed by 0.25 mg/kg/h Only provisional use of GP IIb/IIIa inhibitor in patients also treated with DAPT	I	B
SC fondaparinux for the duration of hospitalization or until PCI is performed	2.5 mg/day SC	I	B
Administer additional anticoagulant with antiIIa activity if PCI is performed while patient is on fondaparinux	N/A	I	B
IV UFH for 48 hr or until PCI is performed	Initial loading dose 60 IU/kg (max 4000 IU) with initial infusion 12 IU/kg/h (max 1000 IU/h) Adjusted to therapeutic APTT range	I	B
IV fibrinolytic treatment not recommended in patients with NSTE-ACS	N/A	III: Harm	A

APTT, Activated partial thromboplastin time; *COR*, class of recommendation; *CrCl*, creatinine clearance; *DAPT*, dual antiplatelet therapy; *IV*, intravenous; *LOE*, level of evidence; *max*, maximum; *N/A*, not available; *NSTE-ACS*, non–ST-elevation acute coronary syndromes; *PCI*, percutaneous coronary intervention; *SC*, subcutaneous; *UFH*, unfractionated heparin.

*The recommended maintenance dose of aspirin to be used with ticagrelor is 81 mg/day.

Modified from Amsterdam EA et al: 2014 AHA/ACC guideline for the management of patients with non–ST-elevation acute coronary syndromes: a report of the American College of Cardiology/American Heart Association task force on practice guidelines, *J Am Coll Cardiol* 64:e139-228, 2014, in Zipes DP: *Braunwald's heart disease: a textbook of cardiovascular medicine*, ed 11, Philadelphia, 2019, Elsevier.

ACS patients. It can be administered sublingually at first, up to 3 doses, followed by intravenous administration if symptoms persist. In the setting of an inferior STEMI, it is necessary to rule out a right ventricular (RV) infarct with a right-sided ECG before the administration of nitroglycerin.[9] This is because RV infarcts are preload dependent and nitroglycerin decreases preload through venodilation, which leads to hypotension in this setting. This can be corrected by discontinuing nitroglycerin and starting bolus intravenous fluids. Nitrates should not be administered in patients who recently received a phosphodiesterase inhibitor. Of note, nitroglycerin provides no mortality benefit in ACS patients.

• Oxygen should be administered to patients with signs of acute heart failure, cardiogenic shock, or an arterial oxyhemoglobin saturation of <90%. The 2014 ACC/AHA guidelines report no demonstrated benefit for routine use of supplemental oxygen in normoxic patients

with NSTE-ACS; rather, emerging data suggest that routine use of oxygen can lead to adverse effects such as increased coronary vascular resistance, reduced coronary blood flow, and increased mortality rate.[3]

• Morphine can be used intravenously in patients with NSTE-ACS if there is continued ischemic chest pain despite treatment with maximally tolerated antiischemic medications (Class IIb).[7]

• Calcium channel blockers (nondihydropyridine) may be used in patients with persisting or recurrent symptoms, despite treatment with beta-blockers and nitroglycerin. They work by having negative inotropic and chronotropic effects and causing coronary vasodilation. They are especially useful when beta-blockers are contraindicated and in patients with coronary artery spasm. Calcium channel blockers should not be used in cases of severe LV dysfunction, pulmonary edema, increased risk for cardiogenic shock or advanced heart blocks.[9]

• Patients routinely taking NSAIDs (except for aspirin), both nonselective as well as COX-2–selective agents, before ACS should discontinue those agents at the time of presentation because of the increased risks of mortality, reinfarction, hypertension, heart failure, myocardial rupture, along with overall cardiovascular and bleeding events. However, there is evolving evidence for the role of colchicine to reduce recurrent event risk in the acute post-MI period, with the COLCOT trial showing a reduction in death from cardiovascular causes, resuscitated cardiac arrest, recurrent MI, stroke or urgent hospitalization for angina leading to coronary revascularization.[13] No guidelines have been published that reflect the results of this trial.

• ACE inhibitors may be added and should be used within 24 h of onset of ACS in all patients with depressed LV function (EF <40%) and those with a history of hypertension, diabetes mellitus, or stable chronic kidney disease. Angiotensin receptor blockers (ARBs) should

TABLE 6 2014 Guideline Recommendations for Antithrombotic Agents in Patients With Non–ST-Elevation Acute Coronary Syndrome

Antiplatelet Therapy

Nonenteric-coated, chewable aspirin (162-325 mg) should be given to all patients without contraindications on presentation, and a maintenance dose of aspirin (81-325 mg/day) continued indefinitely.

In patients who are unable to take aspirin because of hypersensitivity or major gastrointestinal intolerance, a loading dose of clopidogrel (300 or 600 mg) followed by a daily maintenance dose of 75 mg should be substituted.

Either clopidogrel or ticagrelor can be used initially with either an early invasive or ischemic guided strategy (COR I, LOE: B).

Ticagrelor may be preferred over clopidogrel as the initial treatment (COR IIa, LOE: B).

In patients treated with ticagrelor, the preferred aspirin maintenance dose is 81 mg/day.

Use prasugrel only in patients receiving coronary stents (COR I, LOE: B).

The use of glycoprotein IIb/IIIa receptor inhibitors is reserved mainly to the time of PCI in high-risk patients who were not adequately pretreated with P2Y12 inhibitors (COR I, LOE: A) or in those patients who were adequately pretreated with P2Y12 inhibitors but have a high-risk profile (COR IIa, LOE: B).

Clopidogrel and ticagrelor should be discontinued at least 5 days (COR I, LOE: B) and prasugrel at least 7 days (COR I, LOE: C) before major surgery.

Anticoagulant Therapy

Enoxaparin is recommended at presentation (COR I, LOE: A); other options include unfractionated heparin (UFH) (COR I, B) and fondaparinux (COR I, LOE: B). If an early invasive strategy is planned, bivalirudin (COR I, LOE: B) is also an option.

If fondaparinux is used initially, add UFH or bivalirudin just before or during PCI to prevent catheter-related thrombosis (COR I, LOE: B).

Bivalirudin is preferred over UFH plus GP IIb/IIIa inhibitor in patients undergoing PCI who are at high risk of bleeding (COR IIa, LOE: B).

It is reasonable to use enoxaparin during PCI if it was used as the initial anticoagulant (COR IIb, LOE: B).

COR, Class of recommendation; *LOE,* level of evidence; *PCI,* percutaneous coronary intervention.

Modified from Eisen A, Giugliano RP: Antiplatelet and anticoagulation treatment in patients with non–ST-segment elevation acute coronary syndrome: comparison of the updated North American and European guidelines, *Cardiol Rev* 24:170-176, 2016; and Amsterdam EA et al: 2014 AHA/ACC guideline for the management of patients with non–ST-elevation acute coronary syndromes: a report of the American College of Cardiology/American Heart Association Task Force on Practice Guidelines, *J Am Coll Cardiol* 64: e139-228, 2014, in Zipes DP: *Braunwald's heart disease: a textbook of cardiovascular medicine,* ed 11, Philadelphia, 2019, Elsevier.

TABLE 7 Pharmacologic Characteristics of Oral Antiplatelet Drugs Commonly Used in the Management of Acute Coronary Syndrome

Characteristic	Aspirin	ADP RECEPTOR ANTAGONISTS		
		Clopidogrel	Prasugrel	Ticagrelor
Class	COX inhibitor	Thienopyridine (second generation)	Thienopyridine (third generation)	Cyclopentyl triazolopyrimidine
Target	COX-1	P2Y12	P2Y12	P2Y12
Dose	162- to 325-mg loading dose; 75-325 mg/day maintenance dose	300- to 600-mg loading dose; 75 mg/day maintenance dose	60-mg loading dose; 10 mg/day maintenance dose	180-mg loading dose; 90 mg bid maintenance dose
Prodrug	No	Yes	Yes	No
Time to effect[a]	<1 h	4-6 h[b]	<1 h	<1 h
Drug half-life	20 min	Min	Min	12 hr
Reversible	No	No	No	Yes

ADP, Adenosine diphosphate; *bid,* twice daily; *COX,* cyclooxygenase.

[a]After loading dose.

[b]Increased antithrombotic benefit was seen after the first hour in patients enrolled in the COMMIT trial who did not receive a loading dose, but maximum effect is not seen until after 4-6 h.

From Hoffman R et al: *Hematology: basic principles and practice,* ed 7, Philadelphia, 2018, Elsevier.

be used in patients who are ACE inhibitor intolerant.[3]

- Table 10 summarizes indications and cautions for adjunctive medical therapies for patients with STEMI.
- Refer to topic "Cocaine Overdose" for treatment of cocaine-related ACS.

CHRONIC Rx

- Post-ACS medical therapy involves aspirin, statin, beta-blocker, and a second antiplatelet agent such as clopidogrel, ticagrelor, or prasugrel.
- In patients already on an oral anticoagulant for another diagnosis such as atrial fibrillation, the duration of triple therapy should be minimized. Strategies aimed at minimizing the risk of bleeding in patients treated with triple therapy (dual antiplatelet therapy and an oral anticoagulant) are summarized in Table 11. The WOEST trial showed that using clopidogrel along with an oral anticoagulant but without aspirin resulted in a significant reduction in bleeding complications compared with those patients on a triple therapy of oral anticoagulant, aspirin, and clopidogrel.[14] It is a class IIB recommendation in those patients with atrial fibrillation and a CHADS-VASC score of ≥2 after coronary revascularization to consider using clopidogrel concurrently with oral anticoagulant (Table 12) but without aspirin. Similarly, the AUGUSTUS trial in 2019 demonstrated that triple therapy (aspirin, P2Y12 inhibitor, direct oral anticoagulants [DOAC], or warfarin) was associated with substantial increases in bleeding without improved thrombotic protection compared with P2Y12 inhibitor and oral anticoagulation alone.[15]

- Lipid lowering with high-intensity statins has been shown to reduce death, MI, and cardiac events at 16 wk when administered early (within 24 to 96 h after ACS). Additional data demonstrated the benefit of early high-intensity statin therapy with low density lipoprotein (LDL) targets <70 mg/dl in ACS.[3]
- ACE inhibitors may be added to treat hypertension and should be used in all patients with depressed LV function (EF <40%) or pulmonary vascular congestion. ARBs should be used in patients who are ACE inhibitor intolerant.[3]

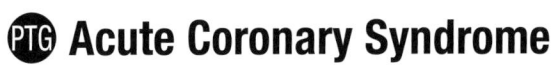

TABLE 8 Pharmacologic Characteristics of Intravenous Antiplatelet Drugs Used in the Management of Acute Coronary Syndrome

	GP IIB/IIIA INHIBITORS			ADP RECEPTOR ANTAGONISTS
Characteristic	Abciximab	Eptifibatide	Tirofiban	Cangrelor
Class	Fab fragment	Nonpeptide	Cyclic heptapeptide	Nonthienopyridine
Onset	Rapid	Rapid	Rapid	Rapid
Drug half-life	10-30 min	2 h	2.5 h	3-6 min
Reversibility of platelet inhibition	Slow	Rapid	Rapid	Rapid
Excretion	Unknown	40%-70% renal	50% renal	Dephosphorylation

ADP, Adenosine diphosphate; *GP,* glycoprotein.
From Hoffman R et al: *Hematology: basic principles and practice,* ed 7, Philadelphia, 2018, Elsevier.

TABLE 9 Pharmacologic Characteristics of Parenteral Anticoagulants Commonly Used in the Management of Patients With Acute Coronary Syndrome

	Unfractionated Heparin	Enoxaparin	Bivalirudin	Fondaparinux
Route of administration	IV	SC (first dose IV[a])	IV	SC (first dose IV[a])
Frequency of dosing	Continuous IV infusion	Twice daily; once daily if CrCl <30 ml/min	Continuous IV infusion	Once-daily injection
Clearance	Primarily nonrenal	Renal	Renal, proteolytic cleavage	Renal
Use in ACS patients with moderate renal impairment	Yes	Yes (dose reduction)	Yes (dose reduction)	Yes[b]
Use in ACS patients undergoing dialysis	Yes	No experience	Yes (dose reduction)	No experience[c]
Routine laboratory monitoring	Yes	No	No[d]	No
Dose	Adjust dose according to the results of the aPTT	Fixed weight adjusted	Fixed weight adjusted	Fixed
Accumulation in renal failure	No	Yes	Yes	Yes
Nonanticoagulant side effects	Allergy, HIT	HIT (rare)	—	—
Nonbleeding contraindications	Allergy, immune HIT	Allergy, immune HIT	Allergy	Allergy
Antidote	Protamine sulfate	Protamine sulfate partially reverses	No	No

ACS, Acute coronary syndromes; *aPTT,* activated partial thromboplastin time; *CrCl,* creatinine clearance; *HIT,* heparin-induced thrombocytopenia; *IV,* intravenous; *SC,* subcutaneous.
[a]The first dose of enoxaparin was given by the intravenous route in the TIMI-11B (Thrombolysis In Myocardial Infarction 11B) and EXTRACT-TIMI 25 (Enoxaparin and Thrombolysis Reperfusion for Acute Myocardial Infarction Treatment, Thrombolysis in Myocardial Infarction 25) studies. The first dose of fondaparinux was given by the intravenous route in the OASIS-6 (Optimal Antiplatelet Strategy for Interventions 6) trial.
[b]Acute coronary syndrome patients with creatinine up to 265 μmol/L were eligible for inclusion in the OASIS-5 and -6 trials (equivalent to an estimated creatinine clearance of 15-20 ml/min in a 70-kg patient who is 70 yr of age).
[c]Fondaparinux is contraindicated in patients with venous thromboembolism who have severe renal impairment.
[d]Monitoring and dose adjustment required in patients with creatinine clearance below 30 ml/min.
From Hoffman R et al: *Hematology: basic principles and practice,* ed 7, Philadelphia, 2018, Elsevier.

TABLE 10   Indications and Cautions for Adjunctive Medical Therapies for Patients With ST-Elevation Myocardial Infarction

Therapy	Indications	Cautions
Beta-adrenergic receptor–blocking agents	Oral: All patients without contraindication IV: Patients with refractory hypertension or ongoing ischemia without contraindication	Signs of congestive heart failure Low-output state Increased risk for cardiogenic shock Prolonged first-degree or high-grade atrioventricular block Reactive airways disease
Angiotensin-converting enzyme (ACE) inhibitors	Anterior myocardial infarction and LVEF $\leq$0.40 or congestive heart failure All patients without contraindication	Hypotension Renal failure Hyperkalemia
Angiotensin receptor–blocking agents (ARBs)	Intolerant of ACE inhibitors	Hypotension Renal failure Hyperkalemia
Statins	All patients without contraindications	With drugs metabolized via CYP3A4, fibrates Monitor for myopathy, hepatotoxicity Adjust dose for lipid targets
Nitroglycerin	Ongoing chest pain Hypertension and congestive heart failure	Suspected right ventricular infarction SBP <90 (or 30 mm Hg below baseline) Recent use of a type 5 PDE inhibitor
Oxygen	Clinically significant hypoxemia (Spo_2 <90) Congestive heart failure Dyspnea	Chronic obstructive pulmonary disease and CO_2 retention
Morphine	Pain Anxiety Pulmonary edema	Lethargic or moribund patient Hypotension Bradycardia Known hypersensitivity

IV, Intravenous; *LVEF,* left ventricular ejection fraction; *PDE,* phosphodiesterase; *SBP,* systolic blood pressure.
From Zipes DP: *Braunwald's heart disease: a textbook of cardiovascular medicine,* ed 11, Philadelphia, 2019, Elsevier.

TABLE 11   Strategies Aimed at Minimizing the Risk of Bleeding in Patients Treated With Triple Therapy (Dual Antiplatelet Therapy and an Oral Anticoagulant)

Proposed Approach	Rationale
Aspirin maintenance dose $\leq$100 mg/day	Higher aspirin maintenance doses increase bleeding, and there is no evidence that they improve efficacy.
PPI with a preference for agents that interfere less with CYP 2C19 (e.g., pantoprazole)	Much of the excess bleeding is from the GI tract. The use of acid-suppressive agents that interfere less with CYP 2C19 minimizes the potential for a negative interaction with clopidogrel.
Preference for a nonvitamin K antagonist oral anticoagulant	Dabigatran 110 mg twice daily and apixaban 2.5 or 5.0 mg twice daily are associated with lower rates of bleeding than warfarin.
For warfarin, use a target INR of 2-2.5	Some evidence that a restricted target INR range reduces the risk of bleeding.
Manage warfarin in a specialized anticoagulation clinic	Compared with usual care, specialist clinics achieve a higher TTR of the INR.
Minimize duration of triple therapy	The risk of bleeding is highest during the first 30 days but remains elevated with long-term treatment.
Avoid NSAIDs	NSAIDs are a common cause of upper GI bleeding.
Avoid prasugrel and ticagrelor	Prasugrel and ticagrelor cannot be recommended because they are more potent than clopidogrel and cause more bleeding.

CYP, Cytochrome P-450; *GI,* gastrointestinal; *INR,* international normalized ratio; *NSAID,* nonsteroidal antiinflammatory drug; *PPI,* proton pump inhibitor; *TTR,* time in therapeutic range.
From Hoffman R et al: *Hematology: basic principles and practice,* ed 7, Philadelphia, 2018, Elsevier.

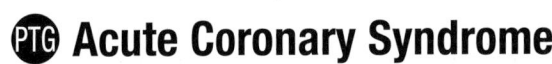

A

I

TABLE 12 Pharmacologic Characteristics of Warfarin and New Oral Anticoagulants Evaluated in Phase III Trials for the Long-Term Management of Acute Coronary Syndrome

Characteristic	Warfarin	Rivaroxaban	Apixaban
Target	VKORC1	Factor Xa	Factor Xa
Prodrug	No	No	No
Bioavailability (%)	100	80	60
Dosing	Variable, once daily	Fixed, 2.5 or 5 mg twice daily[a]	Fixed, 5 mg twice daily (2.5 mg twice daily in selected patients)
Half-life	Mean: 40 h (range: 20-60 h)	7-11 h	12 h
Renal clearance (%)	Nil	66[b]	25
Routine coagulation monitoring	Yes (INR)	No	No
Drug interactions	Multiple	Potent inhibitors of CYP3A4 and P-gp[c]	Potent inhibitors of CYP3A4 and P-gp[c]
Antidote	Yes (vitamin K, PCC, FFP)	Yes (Andexanet alfa)	Yes (Andexanet alfa)
Approved for ACS management	Yes	Yes, in Europe	No

ACS, Acute coronary syndromes; CYP3A4, cytochrome P-450 3A4; FFP, fresh frozen plasma; fXa, activated factor X; INR, international normalized ratio; PCC, prothrombin complex concentrates; P-gp, P-glycoprotein; VKORC1, C1 subunit of vitamin K epoxide reductase.
Strategies Aimed at Minimizing the Risk of Bleeding in Patients Treated With Triple Therapy (Dual Antiplatelet Therapy and an Oral Anticoagulant).
[a]A once-daily regimen was tested in atrial fibrillation.
[b]Half of renally cleared rivaroxaban is cleared as unchanged drug and half as inactive metabolites.
[c]Potent inhibitors of both CYP3A4 and P-glycoprotein include azole antifungals (e.g., ketoconazole, itraconazole, voriconazole, posaconazole) and protease inhibitors, such as ritonavir. Potent inhibitors of CYP3A4 include azole antifungals, macrolide antibiotics (e.g., clarithromycin), and protease inhibitors (e.g., atazanavir).
From Hoffman R et al: Hematology: basic principles and practice, ed 7, Philadelphia, 2018, Elsevier.

- An aldosterone blocker should be used in post-MI patients without significant renal dysfunction (creatinine >2.5 mg/dl in men or creatinine >2.0 mg/dl in women) or hyperkalemia (K >5.0 mEq/L) who have an EF of <40% and are already on therapeutic doses of an ACE inhibitor and a beta-blocker.[3]
- Cardiac rehabilitation and a monitored exercise program should be recommended at the time of discharge.[3]
- Aggressive risk factor management, including smoking cessation, weight loss, diet and exercise, diabetes control, and so on, for secondary prevention of future events is crucial.[3]

REFERRAL

- All ACS patients should be cared for in conjunction with the cardiology consult service.
- When appropriate, referral to a cardiac surgeon may be necessary for CABG and comprehensive heart team approach.

- At the time of discharge, patients should be referred for cardiac rehabilitation.

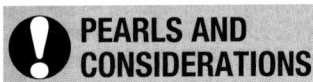

PEARLS AND CONSIDERATIONS

COMMENTS

- ACS is common life-threatening disorder and a leading cause of mortality in the U.S.
- The diagnosis hinges on the basics—history and physical, ECG, biomarkers, and CXR.
- Remember the potentially fatal non-ACS causes of chest discomfort, which include acute pulmonary embolism, acute ascending aortic dissection, pneumothorax, and esophageal rupture (Boerhaave syndrome).
- STEMI patients presenting to a hospital with PCI capability should be treated with primary PCI within 90 min of first medical contact.
- STEMI patients presenting to a hospital without PCI capability and who cannot be transferred to a PCI center and undergo PCI

within 120 min of first medical contact should be treated with fibrinolytic therapy within 30 min of hospital presentation unless fibrinolytic therapy is contraindicated.
- Refer to topics "Angina Pectoris" and "Myocardial Infarction" for additional discussion of this subject matter.

REFERENCES

Available at eBooks.Health.Elsevier.com

RELATED CONTENT

Acute Coronary Syndrome (Patient Information)
Angina Pectoris (Related Key Topic)
Coronary Artery Disease (Related Key Topic)
Myocardial Infarction (Related Key Topic)
Hypertension (Related Key Topic)

AUTHORS: **GEORGE H. NASR, MD**
PRANAV M. PATEL, MD, FACC, FAHA, FSCAI

Acute Glomerulonephritis (PTG)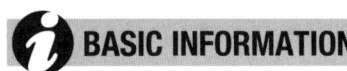

BASIC INFORMATION

DEFINITION

Acute glomerulonephritis (GN) is inflammation of the kidney glomerulus, an intricate mesh of blood vessels, usually caused by an autoimmune reaction resulting in deposition of immunoreactants and recruitment of inflammatory cells. Clinically, patients present with blood and protein in the urine and high blood pressure. If untreated, chronic glomerular inflammation leads to progressive chronic kidney disease.

SYNONYMS

Acute nephritic syndrome
Glomerulonephritis, acute GN

ICD-10CM CODES

N00.0 Acute nephritic syndrome with minor glomerular abnormality
N00.1 Acute nephritic syndrome with focal and segmental glomerular lesions
N00.2 Acute nephritic syndrome with diffuse membranous glomerulonephritis
N00.3 Acute nephritic syndrome with diffuse mesangial proliferative glomerulonephritis
N00.4 Acute nephritic syndrome with diffuse endocapillary proliferative glomerulonephritis
N00.5 Acute nephritic syndrome with diffuse mesangiocapillary glomerulonephritis
N00.6 Acute nephritic syndrome with dense deposit disease
N00.7 Acute nephritic syndrome with diffuse crescentic glomerulonephritis
N00.8 Acute nephritic syndrome with other morphologic changes
N00.9 Acute nephritic syndrome with unspecified morphologic changes

EPIDEMIOLOGY & DEMOGRAPHICS

- Incidence of primary GN varies between 0.2/100,000 (membranoproliferative GN) and 2.5/100,000 (immunoglobulin A [IgA] nephropathy) cases per patient-yr.[1]
- Immunoglobulin A (IgA) nephropathy is the most common form of GN worldwide.
- GN accounts for 23% of end-stage kidney disease cases worldwide.
- GN affects adults and children.

PHYSICAL FINDINGS & CLINICAL PRESENTATION

- Acute onset of hypertension.
- Dark, "tea-colored" urine.
- Edema (peripheral, periorbital, or pulmonary).
- Fatigue.
- Concurrent pulmonary hemorrhage and rapidly progressive decline in kidney function is often associated with "crescentic GN," such as that seen with antineutrophil cytoplasmic antibody (ANCA) vasculitis or antiglomerular basement membrane (anti-GBM) disease.[2]

- Joint pains, oral ulcers, and malar rash are frequently seen with systemic lupus erythematosus (SLE).[3]
- Palpable purpura may be seen in patients with systemic vasculitides, such as IgA vasculitis (formerly Henoch-Schönlein purpura), ANCA-associated vasculitis, SLE, or cryoglobulinemia.[2]
- A recent history of endocarditis, cellulitis, or pharyngitis preceding urinary abnormalities may indicate infection-related GN.
- Hepatitis C virus infection may cause membranoproliferative GN (MPGN) with or without cryoglobulinemia.[4]
- Concurrent upper respiratory tract infection (synpharyngitic infection) and gross hematuria may indicate IgA nephropathy.
- Table 1 summarizes the clinical and laboratory features of the different causes of rapidly progressive GN.

ETIOLOGY

- Acute GN may occur as a renal-limited disease or part of a systemic disorder. A description of target antigens is included in Table E2.
- In the past decade, the knowledge of the pathogenesis of several acute GNs has greatly expanded.
- IgA nephropathy is considered a multi-hit process that involves insufficiently O-galactosylated IgA1, development of O-glycan-specific antibodies, and deposition of IgA1-containing immune complexes in the kidney.[5]
- Hepatitis C causes chronic immune stimulation and production of cryoglobulins that deposit in the kidney.[5]
- Poststreptococcal GN is now part of the broader category termed infection-related GN that includes IgA-dominant *Staphylococcus*-associated GN.
- ANCA-associated vasculitis is associated with antibodies to myeloperoxidase and proteinase 3, although not all studies have supported direct disease causation.[6]
- Paraproteins, which are immunoglobulin components or whole immunoglobulins, may deposit in the kidney and cause a variety of glomerular lesions. When these paraproteins are not associated with a hematologic malignant condition, the kidney condition is termed monoclonal gammopathy of renal significance.[7]
- C3 glomerulopathy, composed of C3 GN and dense deposit disease, is caused by dysregulation of the alternative complement pathway. The alternative complement pathway is now implicated in several different GNs, including IgA nephropathy and ANCA-associated vasculitis. Identification of complement activation in these disorders portends future treatment implications.[8]
- Thrombotic microangiopathy in the native kidney is caused by endothelial damage that can be triggered by drugs, autoimmune

diseases (e.g., atypical hemolytic uremic syndrome, antiphospholipid antibody disease, lupus), infection, and primary genetic disorders.[9]
- Pathologic features of immune glomerular diseases are summarized in Table E3.

DIAGNOSIS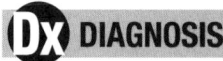

DIFFERENTIAL DIAGNOSIS FOR HEMATURIA AND/OR PROTEINURIA IN ADDITION TO ACUTE GN

- Urinary tract infection
- Nephrolithiasis
- Urothelial malignancy
- Polycystic kidney disease
- Acute interstitial nephritis
- Acute tubular necrosis
- Nephrotic syndrome
- Hereditary nephritis (Alport syndrome and thin basement membrane nephropathy)
- Diabetic nephropathy

WORKUP

Initial evaluation of suspected GN consists of laboratory testing.

LABORATORY TESTS[10]

- Urinalysis with albuminuria (majority of proteinuria in GN is albuminuria) and hematuria (dysmorphic erythrocytes and red cell casts).
- Blood urea nitrogen and serum creatinine.
- 24-h urine collection for total protein excretion (includes albumin plus tubular proteins) and creatinine clearance to document degree of renal dysfunction and accuracy of urine collection. Random urine (spot) specimen for evaluation of the protein-to-creatinine ratio instead of a 24-h collection is also acceptable. Proteinuria in acute GN typically ranges from 500 mg/day to 3 g/day, but nephrotic-range proteinuria (>3.5 g/day) may be present.
- Streptococcal tests (Streptozyme) and anti-streptolysin O (ASO) quantitative titer (highest in 3 to 5 wk). The ASO titer is not related to severity of kidney disease, duration, or prognosis.
- Additional serologic testing, including antinuclear antibody (ANA), antibody directed against double-stranded DNA (anti-dsDNA), C3, C4, hepatitis B and C viral serologies, HIV, ANCA (myeloperoxidase and proteinase-3 antigens), anti-GBM antibodies, cryoglobulins, rheumatoid factor, serum and urine protein electrophoresis with immunofixation, and serum free light chain analysis.
- Hematocrit and platelet count are decreased in thrombotic microangiopathies, although these parameters may be normal in renal-limited thrombotic microangiopathy.
- Blood cultures are obtained from any febrile patient.

TABLE 1 Clinical and Laboratory Features in the Different Causes of Rapidly Progressive Glomerulonephritis

Disease	Typical Clinical Features	Serologic Findings	Complement Levels	Immune Deposits in Glomerulus on Renal Biopsy
Vasculitis				Few/pauci-immune
Granulomatosis with polyangiitis (formerly, Wegener granulomatosis)	Prodrome of nasal stuffiness, blocked ears, arthralgia; then onset of hemoptysis, purpura, peripheral neuropathy	C-ANCA	Normal or increased	
Microscopic polyangiitis	Similar to granulomatosis with polyangiitis (Wegener granulomatosis) or affecting the kidneys only (renal-limited) or overlap with polyarteritis nodosa	P-ANCA	Normal or increased	
Anti-GBM disease	Macroscopic hematuria and hemoptysis	Anti-GBM antibodies	Normal or increased	Linear staining for IgG and C3
SLE (diffuse proliferative, WHO Class IV)	Previous history of SLE, marked hematuria and proteinuria, hypertension "telescoping" urinary sediment	ANA, anti-dsDNA antibodies	Low C3, low C4	Granular immune deposits
IgA disease	Persistent microscopic hematuria with episodes of synpharyngitic macroscopic hematuria, with proteinuria, hypertension	IgA (increased in about half of cases)	Normal or increased	
Poststreptococcal glomerulonephritis	At 1-3 wk after streptococcal pharyngitis or impetigo, macroscopic hematuria, edema, hypertension, oliguria	ASO, anti-DNase B antibodies	Low C3, normal C4	

ANA, Antinuclear antibody; *anti-DNase B*, anti-deoxyribonuclease B antibody; *anti-dsDNA*, anti—double-stranded DNA antibody; *anti-GBM*, glomerular basement membrane antibody; *ASO*, antistreptolysin O antibody; *C-ANCA*, cytoplasmic antineutrophil cytoplasmic antibody; *IgA*, immunoglobulin A; *IgG*, immunoglobin G; *P-ANCA*, perinuclear antineutrophil cytoplasmic antibody; *SLE*, systemic lupus erythematosus; *WHO*, World Health Organization. From Ronco C et al: *Critical care nephrology*, ed 3, Philadelphia, 2019, Elsevier.

IMAGING STUDIES

- Chest radiograph: If opacities are present, consider diffuse alveolar hemorrhage as occurs with ANCA-associated vasculitis and anti-GBM disease (Goodpasture disease).
- Renal ultrasound to exclude structural causes of hematuria and proteinuria. A kidney size of <9 cm in sagittal length may indicate extensive scarring and a low likelihood of reversibility.
- Echocardiogram in patients with new cardiac murmurs or positive blood cultures to rule out endocarditis and pericardial effusion.
- Kidney biopsy with light, electron, and immunofluorescence microscopy.
- Biopsy of other affected organs if systemic vasculitis is suspected.

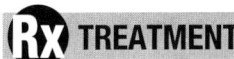 **TREATMENT**

NONPHARMALOGIC THERAPY

- Low-sodium (i.e., 2 g sodium) diet if edema or hypertension is present
- Avoidance of high-potassium foods if patient is hyperkalemic

ACUTE GENERAL Rx

- Acute management is specific to the type of GN and requires urgent nephrology consultation. The Kidney Disease Improving Global Outcome (KDIGO) guidelines for GN management provides evidence-based diagnostic and treatment strategies.
- Diuretics if edema or hypertension is present.
- Correction of electrolyte abnormalities (hypocalcemia, hyperkalemia) and metabolic acidosis.
- Hemodialysis in patients with diuretic-resistant volume overload, refractory hyperkalemia, uremic symptoms, and severe metabolic acidosis. Plasma exchange therapy for antibody removal in cases of diffuse alveolar hemorrhage

or rapidly progressive GN is no longer a standard evidence-based treatment but may be considered in select situations.

CHRONIC RX[11]

- Some types of GN have a relapsing and remitting course. Periodic monitoring of blood pressure, urinalysis, serum creatinine and blood urea nitrogen, serum albumin, and random urine protein-to-creatinine ratio are important to detect relapsing disease.
- ACE inhibitors or angiotensin II type 1 receptor blockers (ARBs) to reduce proteinuria.
- Lipid management with statins and fibrates as indicated.
- Monitor for side effects related to immunosuppression such as infection, leukopenia and anemia, osteoporosis or osteopenia, GI ulcers, high blood pressure, and tumors.
- Routine health maintenance with CDC recommended vaccinations for immunocompromised patients and/or patients with chronic kidney disease, and age-appropriate malignancy screening. Live vaccines are contraindicated in patients actively receiving immunosuppressant therapy.

DISPOSITIION

- Prognosis is generally correlated to initial serum creatinine and degree of fibrosis on kidney biopsy.
- In general, prognosis is worse in patients with heavy albuminuria/proteinuria, low glomerular filtration rate at presentation, severe hypertension, and kidney biopsy-proven crescentic GN with high degree of crescents.

REFERRAL

Nephrology consultation for all patients with suspected GN. Urgent consultation is recommended if hyperkalemia, acidosis, or azotemia is present.

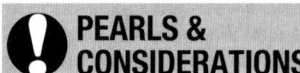 **PEARLS & CONSIDERATIONS**

COMMENTS

- Diagnosis of acute GN is established by kidney biopsy if the biopsy results influence the treatment plan, especially with systemic illnesses, significant proteinuria (>500 mg to 1000 mg/day), or increasing serum creatinine. Exploration for systemic illness, including infections, autoimmune disease, and malignancy is required along with careful history, physical examination, and serologic tests. Some patients with suspected GN may not require a kidney biopsy because of the success of supportive therapies (e.g., infection-related GN).
- Nephrology consultation should be obtained before initiating immunosuppressive therapy. ACE inhibitor or ARB therapy is essential for proteinuria reduction, unless contraindicated. Spironolactone has been added to ACE inhibitor treatment for greater proteinuria reduction.
- Periodic monitoring for side effects of immunosuppressive drugs and complications of corticosteroids is necessary.
- Monitor lipids and treat persistent hyperlipidemia.

REFERENCES & SUGGESTED READINGS
Available at eBooks.Health.Elsevier.com

RELATED CONTENT
Glomerulonephritis (Patient Information)
Acute Kidney Injury (Related Key Topic)

AUTHOR: **RUPALI AVASARE, MD**

Acute Kidney Injury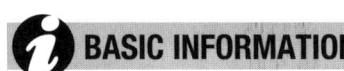

BASIC INFORMATION

DEFINITION

Acute kidney injury (AKI) is defined as a rapid impairment in kidney function that results in oliguria and retention of nitrogenous products in the blood normally excreted by the kidneys, that is, azotemia. The decline in kidney function can result in volume overload and dysregulation of acid-base status and electrolytes. Current consensus criteria for diagnosis of AKI requires an increase in serum creatinine of 0.3 mg/dl within 48 h or 1.5 times baseline serum creatinine over 7 days, and/or a decline in urine in output to <0.5 ml/kg/h for 6 to 12 h. AKI is further graded by severity as described in Table 1.[1]

SYNONYMS

AKI
Acute renal failure (ARF)
Acute kidney failure

ICD—10 CM CODES

N17.0	Acute kidney failure with tubular necrosis
N17.1	Acute kidney failure with acute cortical necrosis
N17.2	Acute kidney failure with medullary necrosis
N17.8	Other acute kidney failure
N17.9	Acute kidney failure, unspecified
N99.0	Postprocedural (acute) (chronic) kidney failure
O90.4	Postpartum acute kidney failure

EPIDEMIOLOGY & DEMOGRAPHICS[2]

- An estimated 20% of hospitalized patients and 60% of intensive care unit patients develop AKI.
- AKI occurs in 20% of patients with moderate sepsis and in >50% of patients with septic shock and positive blood cultures.
- More than 40% of hospital-associated AKI is iatrogenic.
- AKI in hospitalized patients is associated with increased hospital length-of-stay and cost.
- Most common cause of AKI in hospitalized patients is from intrinsic kidney failure due to acute tubular necrosis (ATN).
- Key risk factors for AKI include older age, preexisting chronic kidney disease, diabetes mellitus, and/or preexisting proteinuria.

PHYSICAL FINDINGS & CLINICAL PRESENTATION[3]

- The clinical presentation of AKI depends on the presence of any preexisting conditions, the precipitating conditions, the precipitating event(s) that caused the AKI and the severity of AKI (Fig E1).
- Early or mild AKI is frequently asymptomatic.
- Frequent presenting symptoms include weakness, anorexia, generalized malaise, and nausea.
- Patients may develop oliguric or nonoliguric kidney injury.
- Oliguria is defined as <400 to 500 ml of urine per 24 h. Anuria is frequently seen in ATN or bilateral obstructive uropathy.
- Physical examination should focus on evaluation of volume status, eliciting systemic signs of AKI, and findings supportive of kidney injury etiology.
- Clinical signs and symptoms are numerous; some key findings are highlighted:
  1. Peripheral edema from volume overload, heart failure, liver failure, or nephrotic syndrome.
  2. Pulmonary edema.
  3. Cardiac dysrhythmias.
  4. Neurologic findings include altered mental status, delirium, lethargy, myoclonus, seizures, and asterixis.
  5. Pruritus, uremic odor.
  6. Flank pain.
  7. Painless hematuria may be seen with glomerulonephritis (GN), whereas painful hematuria is more consistent with obstructive uropathy.
  8. Pericardial effusion and/or pericardial rub.
  9. Fever, skin rash, and arthralgia can be seen with systemic vasculitis.
  10. Classic triad of fever, rash, and eosinophilia in the setting of AKI strongly implicates allergic interstitial nephritis (AIN). However, the simultaneous appearance of all three manifestations occurs in only 30% of cases. When AIN is considered the cause of AKI, a careful review of medications is required.

ETIOLOGY[3,4-6]

- **Prerenal:** Inadequate renal perfusion caused by hypovolemia, congestive heart failure (impaired cardiac output), cirrhosis (fluid third-spacing), sepsis (vasodilation), abdominal compartment syndrome, or other. Sixty percent of community-acquired cases of AKI are due to prerenal conditions.
- **Postrenal:** Bladder outlet obstruction (prostatic enlargement, urethral fibrosis), ureteral obstruction (stones, bladder masses, retroperitoneal fibrosis, ureteral fibrosis), or renal vein occlusion. With two functioning kidneys, bilateral obstruction is usually required to produce significant AKI. Postrenal causes of AKI account for 5% to 15% of community-acquired AKI.
- **Intrinsic renal:** ATN, AIN, and GN. Common causes of ATN include ischemia (e.g., hypotension or shock, postcardiac bypass, or aorta surgery), rhabdomyolysis, sepsis, drug toxicity (e.g., aminoglycosides, amphotericin, cisplatin), and iodinated radiocontrast-induced nephropathy. Contrast-induced nephropathy is the third most common cause of new-onset AKI in hospitalized patients. However, most of these cases have multiple confounding factors and are better characterized as contrast-associated nephropathy. AIN can develop after exposure to medications, most commonly NSAIDs, antibiotics, and proton pump inhibitors. Microvascular diseases that cause AKI include thrombotic microangiopathies (e.g., thrombotic

---

TABLE 1 Consensus Acute Kidney Injury Definitions and Classification Systems

Serum Creatinine		Urine Output
RIFLE Criteria		
Risk	Increase in SCr to ≥1.5 times baseline *or* decrease in GFR by >25% within 7 days	<0.5 ml/kg/h for >6 h
Injury	Increase in SCr to >2 times baseline *or* decrease in GFR by >50% within 7 days	<0.5 ml/kg/h for >12 h
Failure	Increase in SCr to >3 times baseline *or* decrease in GFR by >75% within 7 days *or* increase in SCr to ≥4 mg/dl with an acute rise of 0.5 mg/dl	<0.3 ml/kg/h for >24 h *or* anuria for 12 h
Loss	Complete loss of kidney function requiring dialysis for >4 wk	
ESRD	Complete loss of kidney function requiring dialysis for >3 mo	
AKIN Criteria		
Stage 1	Increase in SCr by ≥0.3 mg/dl *or* increase in SCr to ≥1.5 times baseline within 48 h	<0.5 ml/kg/h for ≥6 h
Stage 2	Increase in SCr to >2 times baseline within 48 h	<0.5 ml/kg/h for ≥12 h
Stage 3	Increase in SCr to >3 times baseline within 48 h *or* increase in SCr to ≥4 mg/dl with a rise of 0.5 mg/dl within 24 h *or* initiation of dialysis	<0.3 ml/kg/h for ≥24 h *or* anuria for ≥12 h
KDIGO Criteria		
Stage 1	Increase in SCr by ≥0.3 mg/dl within 48 h *or* increase in SCr to ≥1.5 times baseline within 7 days	<0.5 ml/kg/h for ≥6 h
Stage 2	Increase in SCr to >2 times baseline within 7 days	<0.5 ml/kg/h for ≥12 h
Stage 3	Increase in SCr to >3 times baseline within 7 days *or* increase in SCr to ≥4 mg/dl *or* initiation of dialysis	<0.3 ml/kg/h for ≥24 h *or* anuria for ≥12 h

AKIN, Acute kidney injury network; *ESRD,* end-stage renal disease; *GFR,* glomerular filtration rate; *KDIGO,* kidney disease improving global outcomes; *RIFLE,* risk, injury, failure, loss, end-stage kidney disease; *SCr,* serum creatinine.
From Newman M et al: *Perioperative medicine,* ed 2, Philadelphia, 2022, Elsevier.

thrombocytopenic purpura, classic and atypical hemolytic-uremic syndrome, and preeclampsia) and cholesterol emboli.
- Causes of AKI are listed in Table 2.
- Nearly one third of AKI cases may be prevented or mitigated.

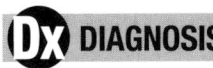 **DIAGNOSIS**

Table 3 summarizes useful clinical features, urinary findings, and confirmatory tests in the differential diagnosis of AKI.

DIFFERENTIAL DIAGNOSIS

Refer to "Etiology." Diagnostic tests to distinguish prerenal and renal AKI are described in Table 4. A diagnostic approach to patients with suspected AKI is shown in Fig. 2.

LABORATORY TESTS[1,3-5]

- Elevated serum creatinine.
- Standard estimating equations for glomerular filtration rate (GFR) require steady-state creatinine levels and are not recommended to estimate GFR during AKI.

- Elevated blood urea nitrogen (BUN): BUN-to-creatinine ratio is commonly >20:1 in prerenal azotemia, postrenal azotemia, and acute GN.
- BUN-to-creatinine ratio is <20:1 in acute interstitial nephritis and ATN.
- Hyperkalemia, hyperphosphatemia, and metabolic acidosis are common.
- Hypocalcemia with hyponatremia or hypernatremia may occur, depending on etiology.
- Urinalysis is the initial diagnostic evaluation. Prerenal and postrenal AKI are typically characterized by a normal urinalysis. Conversely, abnormal findings should prompt further workup for specific intrinsic causes of AKI that may require intervention. Hematuria and proteinuria imply GN; heavy (>3+) proteinuria is associated with leukocyturia and may signify AIN. Microscopic examination of urine sediment may facilitate diagnosis: Granular casts in ATN, dysmorphic red blood cells or red blood cell casts in acute GN, and white blood cell casts in AIN.
- In oliguric patients, obtain urine sodium and creatinine concentrations for determination of fractional excretion of sodium: $FE_{Na} = 100\% \times (U_{Na} \times P_{Cr})/(P_{Na} \times U_{Cr})$. $FE_{Na} < 1\%$ occurs in

prerenal AKI and >1% occurs in intrinsic AKI. FE_{Na} may be falsely elevated in patients taking diuretics or falsely low in several intrinsic renal conditions, including acute GN, contrast-induced nephropathy, and rhabdomyolysis. (U_{Na}, urinary sodium; U_{Cr}, urinary creatinine; P_{Cr}, plasma creatinine; P_{Na}, plasma sodium).
- Fractional excretion of urea (FE_{Urea}) can be used to assess renal dysfunction in AKI. FE_{Urea} is more useful than FE_{Na} during diuretic therapy. FE_{Urea} is calculated as follows: $FE_{Urea} = 100\% \times (U_{Urea} \times P_{Cr})/(P_{Urea} \times U_{Cr})$. If $FE_{Urea} < 35\%$ prerenal AKI is likely, and if $FE_{Urea} > 50\%$ intrinsic AKI is likely. (U_{Urea}, urinary urea; P_{Urea}, plasma urea).
- Urinary osmolality range of 250 mOsm/kg H_2O to 300 mOsm/kg H_2O in ATN (isosthenuria), <400 mOsm/kg H_2O in postrenal azotemia, and >500 mOsm/kg H_2O in prerenal azotemia and acute GN.
- In suspected GN (e.g., hematuria plus proteinuria), additional serologic testing may be warranted. Abnormal liver function tests and elevated inflammatory markers are nonspecific. Immune complex deposition disorders (e.g., infectious GN, lupus nephritis,

TABLE 2	Etiologies of Acute Kidney Injury	
Prerenal Causes (Decreased Renal Blood Flow)	**Intrinsic Renal Causes**	**Postrenal Causes**
Hypovolemia	**Vascular: Large and Small Vessels**	**Ureteral Obstruction**
Renal losses (diuretics, osmotic agents, polyuria)	Trauma	Calculus
Gastrointestinal losses (vomiting, diarrhea)	Renal vein obstruction (thrombosis, ventilation with	Tumor (intrinsic or extrinsic)
Cutaneous losses (burns, exfoliative syndromes)	high-level PEEP, abdominal compartment syndrome)	Fibrosis
Hemorrhage	Microangiopathy (thrombotic thrombocytopenic purpura,	Ligation during pelvic surgery
Pancreatitis	hemolytic-uremic syndrome, disseminated	**Bladder Neck Obstruction**
Decreased Cardiac Output	intravascular coagulation, preeclampsia)	Benign prostatic hypertrophy
Congestive heart failure	Malignant hypertension	Prostate cancer
Pulmonary embolism	Scleroderma renal crisis	Neurogenic bladder
Acute myocardial infarction	Transplant rejection	Tricyclic antidepressants
Severe valvular heart disease	Atheroembolic disease	Ganglionic blockers
Abdominal compartment syndrome	**Glomerular**	Bladder tumor
Renal artery obstruction (stenosis, embolism,	Antiglomerular basement membrane disease (Goodpasture	Calculus
thrombosis, dissection)	syndrome)	Hemorrhage/clot
Systemic Vasodilation	Antineutrophil cytoplasmic antibody-associated	**Urethral Obstruction**
Sepsis	glomerulonephritis (Wegener granulomatosis)	Strictures
Anaphylaxis	Immune complex glomerulonephritis, systemic lupus	Tumor
Anesthetics	erythematosus, postinfectious cryoglobulinemia,	Phimosis
Drug overdose	primary membranoproliferative glomerulonephritis	Renal calcinosis
Afferent Arteriolar Vasoconstriction	**Tubular**	Obstructed urinary catheter, ureteral stent, or ileal conduit
Hypercalcemia	Ischemic	Pelvic trauma, retroperitoneal hematoma
Drugs (NSAIDs, amphotericin B, calcineurin inhibitors,	Cytotoxic	
norepinephrine, radiocontrast agents, aminoglycosides)	Heme pigment (rhabdomyolysis, intravascular hemolysis)	
Hepatorenal syndrome	Crystals (tumor lysis syndrome, seizures, ethylene glycol	
Efferent arteriolar vasodilation (angiotensin converting	poisoning, vitamin C megadose, acyclovir, indinavir,	
enzyme inhibitors, aldosterone receptor blockers)	methotrexate)	
	Drugs (aminoglycosides, lithium, amphotericin B,	
	pentamidine, cisplatin, ifosfamide, radiocontrast	
	agents), synthetic cannabinoid use	
	Interstitial	
	Drugs (penicillins, cephalosporins, NSAIDs, proton pump	
	inhibitors, allopurinol, rifampin, indinavir, mesalamine,	
	sulfonamides, trimethoprim)	
	Infection (pyelonephritis, viral infection)	
	Systemic Disease	
	Sjögren syndrome, sarcoidosis, systemic lupus	
	erythematosus, lymphoma, leukemia, interstitial	
	nephritis, uveitis	

NSAIDs, Nonsteroidal antiinflammatory drugs; *PEEP,* positive end-expiratory pressure.
Modified from Cameron JL, Cameron AM: *Current surgical therapy,* ed 10, Philadelphia, 2011, Saunders.

TABLE 3 Useful Clinical Features, Urinary Findings, and Confirmatory Tests in the Differential Diagnosis of Acute Kidney Injury

Cause of Acute Kidney Injury	Some Suggestive Clinical Features	Typical Urinalysis Results	Some Confirmatory Tests
Prerenal azotemia	Evidence of true volume depletion (thirst, postural or absolute hypotension and tachycardia, low jugular venous pressure, dry mucous membranes and axillas, weight loss, fluid output greater than input) or decreased effective circulatory volume (e.g., heart failure, liver failure), treatment with NSAID, diuretic, or ACE inhibitor/ARB	Hyaline casts $FE_{Na} <1\%$ $U_{Na} <10$ mmol/L SG >1.018	Occasionally requires invasive hemodynamic monitoring; rapid resolution of AKI with restoration of renal perfusion
Diseases Involving Large Renal Vessels			
Renal artery thrombosis	History of atrial fibrillation or recent myocardial infarction, nausea, vomiting, flank or abdominal pain	Mild proteinuria Occasionally RBCs	Elevated LDH level with normal transaminase levels, renal arteriogram, MAG3 renal scan, MRA*
Atheroembolism	Usually age >50 yr, recent manipulation of aorta, retinal plaques, subcutaneous nodules, palpable purpura, livedo reticularis	Often normal Eosinophiluria Rarely casts	Eosinophilia, hypocomplementemia, skin biopsy, renal biopsy
Renal vein thrombosis	Evidence of nephrotic syndrome or pulmonary embolism, flank pain	Proteinuria, hematuria	Inferior venacavogram, Doppler flow studies, MRV*
Diseases of Small Renal Vessels and Glomeruli			
Glomerulonephritis or vasculitis	Compatible clinical history (e.g., recent infection), sinusitis, lung hemorrhage, rash or skin ulcers, arthralgias, hypertension, edema	RBC or granular casts, RBCs, white blood cells, proteinuria	Low complement levels; positive antineutrophil cytoplasmic antibodies, antiglomerular basement membrane antibodies, antistreptolysin O antibodies, anti-DNase, cryoglobulins; renal biopsy
HUS/TTP	Compatible clinical history (e.g., recent gastrointestinal infection, cyclosporine, anovulants), pallor, ecchymoses, neurologic findings	May be normal, RBCs, mild proteinuria, rarely RBC or granular casts	Anemia, thrombocytopenia, schistocytes on peripheral blood smear, low haptoglobin level, increased LDH, renal biopsy
Malignant hypertension	Severe hypertension with headaches, cardiac failure, retinopathy, neurologic dysfunction, papilledema	May be normal, RBCs, mild proteinuria, rarely RBC casts	LVH by echocardiography or ECG, resolution of AKI with BP control
Ischemic or Nephrotoxic Acute Tubular Necrosis			
Ischemia	Recent hemorrhage, hypotension, surgery often in combination with vasoactive medication (e.g., ACE inhibitor, NSAID)	Muddy-brown granular or tubular epithelial cell casts, $FE_{Na} >1\%$, $U_{Na} >20$ mmol/L SG ≈ 1.010	Clinical assessment and urinalysis usually inform diagnosis
Exogenous toxin	Recent contrast medium-enhanced procedure; nephrotoxic medications; certain chemotherapeutic agents often with coexistent volume depletion, sepsis, or chronic kidney disease	Muddy-brown granular or tubular epithelial cell casts $FE_{Na} >1\%$, $U_{Na} >20$ mmol/L SG ≈ 1.010	Clinical assessment and urinalysis usually inform diagnosis
Endogenous toxin	History suggestive of rhabdomyolysis (coma, seizures, drug abuse, trauma)	Urine supernatant tests positive for heme in absence of RBCs	Hyperkalemia, hyperphosphatemia, hypocalcemia, increased CK, myoglobin
	History suggestive of hemolysis (recent blood transfusion)	Urine supernatant pink and tests positive for heme in absence of RBCs	Hyperkalemia, hyperphosphatemia, hypocalcemia, hyperuricemia, and free circulating hemoglobin
	History suggestive of tumor lysis (recent chemotherapy), myeloma (bone pain), or ethylene glycol ingestion	Urate crystals, dipstick-negative proteinuria, oxalate crystals, respectively	Hyperuricemia, hyperkalemia, hyperphosphatemia (for tumor lysis); circulating or urinary monoclonal protein (for myeloma); toxicology screen, acidosis, osmolal gap (for ethylene glycol)
Diseases of the Tubulointerstitium			
Allergic interstitial nephritis	Recent ingestion of drug and fever, rash, loin pain, or arthralgias	White blood cell casts, white blood cells (frequently eosinophiluria), RBCs, rarely RBC casts, proteinuria (occasionally nephritic)	Systemic eosinophilia, renal biopsy
Acute bilateral pyelonephritis	Fever, flank pain and tenderness, toxic state	Leukocytes, occasionally white blood cell casts, RBCs, bacteria	Urine and blood cultures
Postrenal AKI	Abdominal and flank pain, palpable bladder	Frequently normal, hematuria if stones, prostatic hypertrophy	Plain abdominal radiography, renal ultrasonography, postvoid residual bladder volume, computed tomography, retrograde or antegrade pyelography

ACE, Angiotensin-converting enzyme; *AKI,* acute kidney injury; *ARB,* angiotensin receptor blocker; *BP,* blood pressure; *CK,* creatine kinase; *DNase,* deoxyribonuclease; *ECG,* electrocardiography; FE_{Na}, fractional excretion of sodium; *HUS,* hemolytic uremic syndrome; *LDH,* lactate dehydrogenase; *LVH,* left ventricular hypertrophy; *MAG3,* mercaptoacetyltriglycine; *MRA,* magnetic resonance angiography; *MRV,* magnetic resonance venography; *NSAID,* nonsteroidal antiinflammatory drug; *RBC,* red blood cell; *SG,* specific gravity; *TTP,* thrombotic thrombocytopenic purpura; U_{Na}, urinary sodium concentration.
*Contrast-enhanced MRA and MRV should be used with extreme caution in patients with AKI.
From Skorecki K et al: *Brenner & Rector's the kidney,* ed 10, Philadelphia, 2016, Elsevier.

TABLE 4 Diagnostic Tests to Distinguish Between Prerenal and Renal Acute Kidney Injury

Index	Prerenal Causes	Renal Causes
FE_{Na}	<1%	>2%
Urine sodium	<10 mmol/L	>40 mmol/L
Urine/plasma osmolality	>1.5	1-1.5
Renal failure index	<1	>2
BUN-to-serum creatinine ratio	>20	<10

BUN, Blood urea nitrogen; FE_{Na}, fractional excretion of sodium. Calculation of FE_{Na}: (Urine sodium × Plasma creatinine)/(Plasma sodium × Serum creatinine) ×100. Renal failure index: (Urine sodium × Urine creatinine)/Plasma creatinine. From Cameron JL, Cameron AM: *Current surgical therapy,* ed 10, Philadelphia, 2011, Saunders.

cryoglobulinemic vasculitis) are characterized by decreased complement levels (C3, C4). Specific testing includes antinuclear antibodies (lupus), antineutrophil cytoplasmic antibodies (ANCA-associated vasculitis), antiglomerular basement membrane antibodies (Goodpasture disease), and cryoglobulins. Kidney biopsy is frequently required for diagnostic confirmation.

- Creatinine phosphokinase level is indicated if rhabdomyolysis is suspected; positive blood reaction on a urine dipstick with typically few or no red blood cells by microscopy may indicate myoglobinuria from rhabdomyolysis.
- Serum free light chain analysis, serum and urine protein electrophoresis, and serum and urine immunofixation electrophoresis for suspected multiple myeloma or other plasma cell dyscrasias. Myeloma can cause AKI via a variety of mechanisms, including tubular precipitation of filtered light chains (cast nephropathy), hypercalcemia, and amyloidosis, among others.
- Kidney biopsy may be indicated in patients with intrinsic kidney failure when considering specific therapy. The major indications for kidney biopsy include the following: Differential diagnosis of nephrotic syndrome, distinguishing lupus vasculitis from other vasculitides, distinguishing lupus membranous nephropathy from idiopathic membranous nephropathy, confirmation of hereditary nephropathies based on ultrastructure, diagnosis of rapidly progressive GN, distinguishing AIN from ATN, and separation of primary glomerulonephritides. In addition to establishing a diagnosis, biopsy may determine renal prognosis and guide direction of management. Severe interstitial fibrosis is associated with poor renal outcomes.
- Biomarkers of kidney injury have been explored for earlier diagnosis of AKI and to separate intrinsic from prerenal causes. Candidate markers include neutrophil gelatinase-associated lipocalin (NGAL), kidney-injury molecule 1 (KIM-1), and the product of tissue inhibitor of metalloproteinase-2 and insulin-like growth-factor binding protein-7 (TIMP2*IGFBP7).
- TIMP2*IGFBP7 is U.S. FDA approved for risk prediction of AKI. However, there remains little published experience with this test, and the clinical role remains undefined.

IMAGING STUDIES[1,5]

- ECG for arrhythmia detection, especially in hyperkalemia: Peaked T waves in precordial leads, widening QRS interval, and/or bradycardia with AV node blockade.
- Chest radiograph to detect signs of congestive heart failure and pulmonary renal syndromes that frequently present with alveolar hemorrhage (antiglomerular basement membrane or ANCA-associated vasculitis).
- Bladder scan to assess post-void residual urine when urinary obstruction is suspected.
- Kidney ultrasonography to determine kidney sizes (distinguishes acute from chronic kidney disease), presence of obstruction, and renal vascular status (Doppler study).

Rx TREATMENT

Management of AKI depends on the underlying etiology. Some conditions (e.g., GN) require specific therapy. The general focus of treatment for established AKI is supportive care and limiting additional injury. Fig. 3 illustrates an algorithm for management of AKI.

NONPHARMACOLOGIC THERAPY

- Withdraw nephrotoxic medications.
- Evaluate volume status and correct hypovolemia. Goal of therapy is to increase cardiac output and improve tissue perfusion.
- Avoid excessive fluid administration in patients who are nonvolume responsive.[1,5,6]
- Dietary modification: (1) Energy prescription (29 to 36 Kcal/kg/day), (2) potassium restriction (60 mmol/day), (3) sodium restriction (90 mmol/day), (4) phosphorus restriction (<800 mg/day), and (5) high biologic value protein (1.2 g/kg/day) depending on requirement for dialysis.[7]
- Daily weight to monitor for fluid retention, in addition to intake and output measurement.
- Modification of drug dosages or schedules of renally excreted medications. Dosing should consider the trajectory of renal function, during evolving and recovering AKI, and may require additional adjustments in patients who require dialysis.[8]

ACUTE GENERAL Rx

- Correct electrolyte abnormalities and metabolic acidosis.
- Administer loop diuretics for volume overload.

- Administer vasopressors for circulatory shock or vasodilators, when appropriate, to optimize cardiac output in congestive heart failure. Specific treatment is variable and depends on cause of AKI.[8-12]
- Prerenal: Intravenous (IV) volume expansion with isotonic solutions in hypovolemic patients or those with shock. Balanced crystalloid solutions are preferable.
- Intrinsic kidney failure: Discontinue all potential nephrotoxins and treat condition(s) causing kidney failure. In severe AIN cases, consider a trial of corticosteroids. For acute noninfectious GN, high-dose pulse corticosteroids are first-line therapy, typically in conjunction with other immunomodulatory therapy and/or plasma exchange, depending on the clinical scenario.
- Postrenal: Eliminate cause of obstruction. Immediate bladder catheter insertion for suspected bladder outlet obstruction. This maneuver should precede the kidney ultrasonogram during the diagnostic workup. Percutaneous nephrostomy tubes or ureteral stents may be required for upper urinary tract obstruction.
- Hyperkalemia-related ECG changes: IV calcium if electrocardiographic changes are present; IV insulin and/or glucose to shift potassium into cells; and IV bicarbonate therapy when metabolic acidosis is present to shift potassium into cells. These three treatments are temporary, and definitive therapy requires potassium removal via the GI tract by cation exchangers or via the urinary tract by diuretics or dialytic therapy.

Dialysis in AKI:

- General indications for initiation of dialysis during AKI:
  1. Uremic symptoms (e.g., encephalopathy, pericarditis, seizures).
  2. Extracellular fluid volume overload refractory to medical management.
  3. Severe acid-base derangement(s) refractory to medical management.
  4. Significant electrolyte derangement(s) (e.g., hyperkalemia, hyponatremia) refractory to medical management.
- Among critically ill patients, kidney replacement therapy may be required despite an absence of other indications. Optimal timing of initiation of dialysis remains controversial and is not solely dependent on previous metabolic parameters. Multiple recent clinical trials have not shown that early dialysis in AKI is beneficial.
- Intermittent hemodialysis and continuous renal replacement therapy (CRRT) have similar outcomes for patients with AKI. However, CRRT is associated with greater hemodynamic stability and fluid removal compared to conventional intermittent hemodialysis. CRRT is employed in critically ill patients with hemodynamic instability.

ADJUNCTIVE Rx

- Monitoring of renal function parameters and electrolytes.

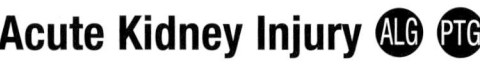
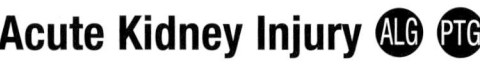

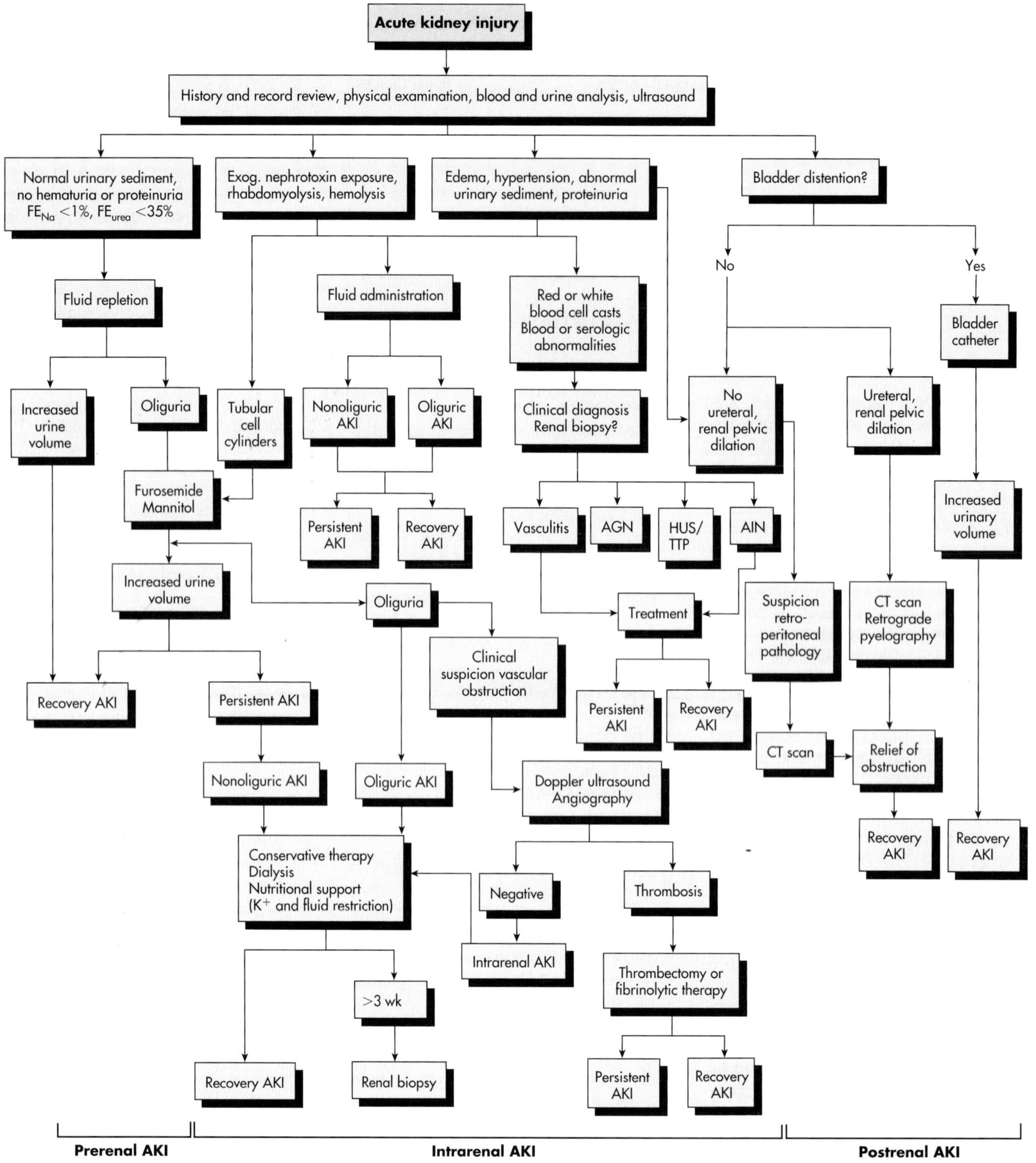

FIG. 2 Diagnostic approach to patients with suspected acute kidney injury (AKI). *AGN,* Acute glomerulonephritis; *AIN,* acute interstitial nephritis; *CT,* computed tomography; *Exog,* exogenous; *HUS/TTP,* hemolytic-uremic syndrome/thrombotic thrombocytopenic purpura. (From Floege J et al: *Comprehensive clinical nephrology,* ed 4, Philadelphia, 2010, Saunders.)

- Renally excreted drugs are adjusted according to creatinine clearance or GFR to prevent further kidney damage or other medication-related toxicities.
- Prevent further renal insult with appropriate volume expansion, particularly before contrast administration, and avoid nephrotoxic agents. Volume expansion with isotonic solutions is more effective than hydration with hypotonic solutions. Isotonic saline or bicarbonate-containing solutions are effective.
- Renal function recovery (ability to discontinue dialysis) varies from 50% to 75% in AKI survivors. Preexisting chronic kidney disease, longer duration of dialysis dependence, congestive heart failure, and older age are negative prognostic factors for renal function recovery.
- Overall mortality rate in AKI is nearly 25% and approaches 50% to 60% in patients who require acute dialysis.
- The combination of AKI and sepsis is associated with a mortality rate as high as 70%.

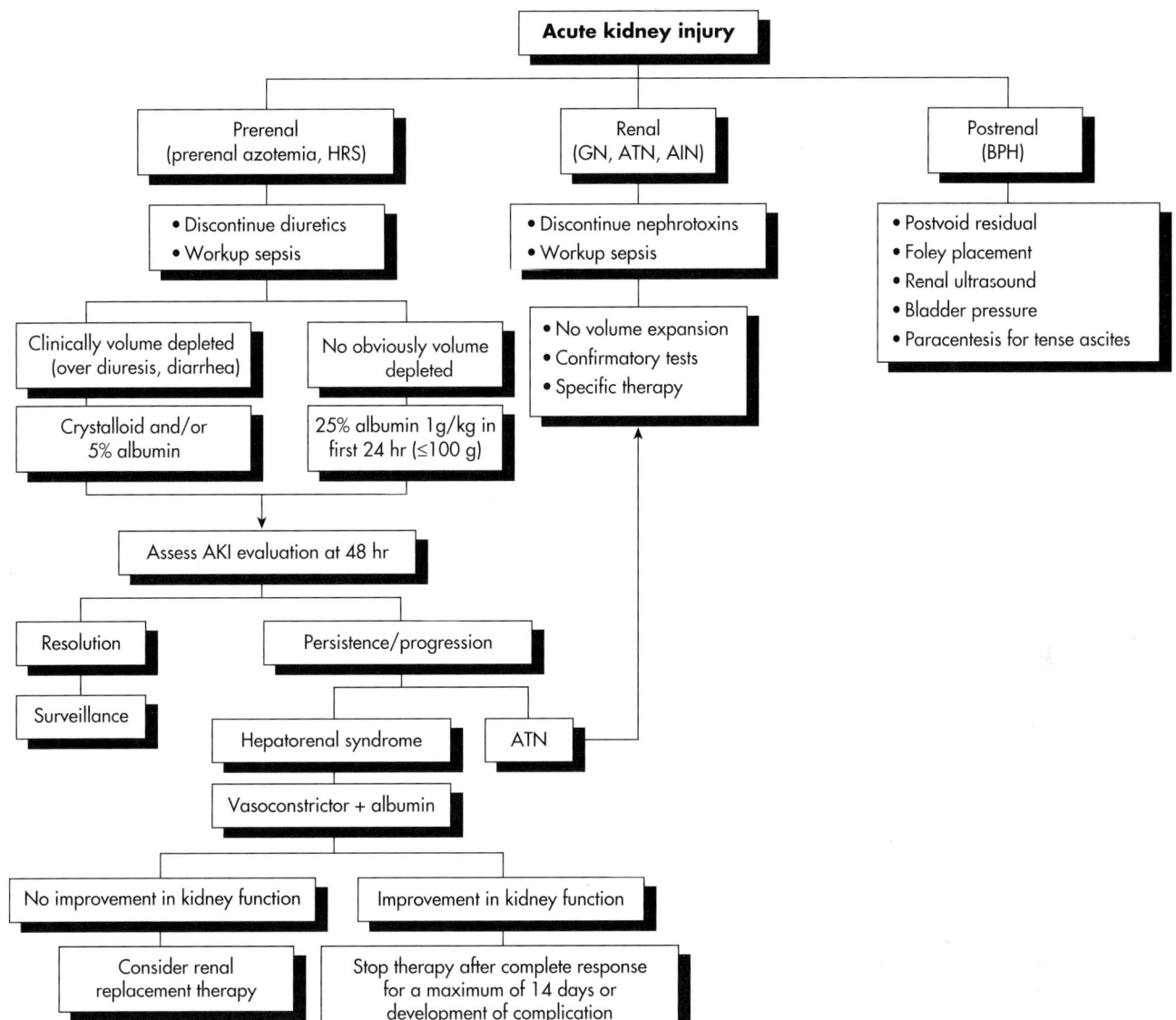

FIG. 3 Algorithm for management of acute kidney injury (AKI). *AIN,* Acute interstitial nephritis; *ATN,* acute tubular necrosis; *BPH,* benign prostatic hypertrophy; *GN,* glomerulonephritis; *HRS,* hepatorenal syndrome. (From Ronco C et al: *Critical care nephrology,* ed 3, Philadelphia, 2019, Elsevier.)

PEARLS & CONSIDERATIONS

- Patients with AKI are susceptible to infections and sepsis.
- In patients with community-acquired AKI, it is important to obtain a thorough medication history, including nonprescription medications and supplements.
- AKI survivors are at risk for development of chronic kidney disease, and follow-up with monitoring of kidney function annually for at least 3 yr is recommended, even with apparent renal recovery. An initial visit within 3 mo after discharge from hospitalization for AKI is recommended.

REFERENCES & SUGGESTED READINGS
Available at eBooks.Health.Elsevier.com.

RELATED CONTENT
Acute Renal Failure (Patient Information)
Chronic Kidney Disease (Related Key Topic)

AUTHOR: **JUNIOR UDUMAN, MD, MS**

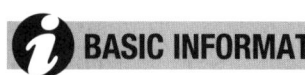

BASIC INFORMATION

DEFINITION

Acute liver failure (ALF) is defined as the rapid progression of liver dysfunction resulting in coagulopathy and altered mentation in patients without previously known liver disease. Practically, it is described as the constellation of acute severe hepatic injury (<26 wk); synthetic liver dysfunction, specifically coagulopathy (international normalized ratio [INR] >1.5); and any degree of mental alteration (encephalopathy) in a patient without preexisting cirrhosis and in the absence of acute alcoholic hepatitis. ALF can also be diagnosed in patients with preexisting liver disease, such as Wilson disease, vertically acquired hepatitis B, and autoimmune hepatitis (despite the possibility of cirrhosis in these patients), provided that diagnosis of these conditions was made within the preceding 26 wk.[1] Box 1 summarizes classifications of ALF. ALF must be distinguished from acute-on-chronic liver failure and acutely decompensated cirrhosis, two syndromes that pertain to acute deterioration in patients with preexisting chronic liver disease.[2] *Acutely decompensated cirrhosis* refers to the development of ascites, encephalopathy, gastrointestinal hemorrhage, or any combination of these disorders in patients with cirrhosis.[1] Acute-on-chronic liver failure is a syndrome where acute and severe hepatic derangements occur secondary to various insults in patients with chronic liver disease, including both cirrhotic and non-cirrhotic. It occurs in the context of intense systemic inflammation (e.g., infections or alcoholic hepatitis) and can be associated with single or multiorgan failure.[2,3]

SYNONYMS

Fulminant hepatic failure
Fulminant hepatitis
Fulminant hepatic necrosis
Acute hepatic necrosis
Acute and subacute necrosis of liver
ALF

ICD-10CM CODES

K72	Hepatic failure, not elsewhere classified
K72.0	Acute and subacute hepatic failure
K72.00	Acute and subacute hepatic failure without coma
K72.01	Acute and subacute hepatic failure with coma

EPIDEMIOLOGY & DEMOGRAPHICS

INCIDENCE: Affects approximately 2000 people/yr in U.S. and 1 to 8 people per million population in the U.K.[1]

PREDOMINANT SEX & AGE: Seen more often in women (90% of cases), often affects younger people

RISK FACTORS[1]:
- Intentional or inadvertent drug overdose
- Risk factors for viral hepatitis:
  1. Intravenous drug use
  2. Occupational exposure to blood or body fluids
  3. Blood transfusions
  4. Hemodialysis
  5. Intranasal cocaine use
  6. Imprisonment
  7. Travel to endemic hepatitis areas
- Previous alcohol use
- Hepatotoxic medications
- Critical illness

PHYSICAL FINDINGS & CLINICAL PRESENTATION[4]

- **Clinical Presentation** Initial symptoms of ALF are mostly nonspecific and depend on the etiology of liver injury. They include fatigue, lethargy, anorexia, and nausea/vomiting. Pruritus, jaundice, and right upper quadrant abdominal pain and distention may be present. Symptoms may also be more serious and consist of severe hypotension, sepsis, and hepatic encephalopathy.
- **Physical Examination** Findings include, by definition, abnormal neurologic findings of encephalopathy (see Table 1). Other findings may include jaundice, asterixis, hepatomegaly, decreased hepatic mass on percussion, and ascites. Multisystem organ failure can ensue. In rare cases, as the hepatic encephalopathy progresses, cerebral edema and increased intracranial pressure can occur, with abnormal pupillary exam findings, hypertension, bradycardia, respiratory depression (Cushing triad), and loss of brain stem reflexes. Seizures secondary to increased intracranial pressure and hypoxia can occur. Vesicular skin lesions are suggestive of HSV.
- Family history of unexplained liver disease/cirrhosis should prompt slit lamp ocular examination for the identification of Kayser-Fleischer rings (copper rings around the iris seen in Wilson disease).

ETIOLOGY[4]

- Common causes in the Western world:
  1. Acetaminophen toxicity (46%)
  2. Indeterminate (14%)
  3. Idiosyncratic drug reaction (12%)
  4. Viral hepatitis (A, B) (10%)

Other, more rare causes include alcoholic hepatitis, autoimmune hepatitis, Wilson disease, ischemic hepatopathy, Budd-Chiari syndrome, acute fatty liver of pregnancy, venoocclusive disease, toxin ingestion (e.g., mushroom poisoning *[Amanita phalloides]*), sepsis, infiltrative malignancy (breast cancer, lymphoma, myeloma, melanoma, small cell lung cancer), and other viruses (adenovirus, hepatitis E, herpes simplex virus [HSV]). Box 2 summarizes possible etiologies of liver failure.

LABORATORY FINDINGS[4]

- Coagulopathy is characteristic of patients with ALF, given decreased synthesis of clotting factors II, V, VII, IX, and X by the liver. Patients with ALF typically have a prolonged prothrombin time (INR >1.5), elevated transaminases, and elevated bilirubin, and may have a low platelet count (<150,000).
- Other possible laboratory findings can include an elevated blood urea nitrogen (BUN)/creatinine (studies show 30% to 50% also have acute kidney injury) and hypoglycemia (impairment of gluconeogenesis). Electrolyte disturbances, hyponatremia, hypophosphatemia, hypomagnesemia, hypokalemia, metabolic acidosis or respiratory alkalosis, elevated lactate dehydrogenase, and elevated ammonia.

BOX 1   Classifications of Acute Liver Failure

Trey and Davidson
Fulminant hepatic failure: Development of HE within 8 wk of onset of symptoms

British Classification
Acute liver failure (includes only patients with encephalopathy)

Subclassification Depending on the Interval between the Onset of Jaundice and HE
- Hyperacute liver failure: 0-7 days
- Acute liver failure: 8-28 days
- Subacute liver failure: 29-72 days
- Late-onset acute liver failure: 56-182 days

French Classification
Acute hepatic failure: A rapidly developing impairment of liver function
  Severe acute hepatic failure: Prothrombin time or factor V concentration below 50% of normal with or without HE

Subclassification
- Fulminant hepatic failure: HE within 2 wk of onset of jaundice
- Subfulminant hepatic failure: HE between 3 and 12 wk of onset of jaundice

International Association for the Study of Acute Liver Failure
Acute liver failure (occurrence of HE within 4 wk after onset of symptoms)

Subclassification
- Acute liver failure—hyperacute: Within 10 days
- Acute liver failure—fulminant: 10-30 days
- Acute liver failure—not otherwise specified
- Subacute liver failure (development of ascites and/or HE from 5-24 wk after onset of symptoms)

HE, Hepatic encephalopathy.
From Vincent JL et al: *Textbook of critical care*, ed 7, Philadelphia, 2017, Elsevier.

BOX 2 Etiologic Classification of Acute Liver Failure

Acetaminophen Toxicity
Idiosyncratic Drug Injury
Infrequent Agents
Isoniazid
Valproate
Halothane
Phenytoin
Sulfonamide
Propylthiouracil
Amiodarone
Disulfiram
Dapsone
Bromfenac
Troglitazone
Zidovudine
Lamivudine
Lamotrigine
Gatifloxacin
Methotrexate
Miscellaneous Agents
Ecstasy
Cocaine
Phencyclidine
Rare Agents
Carbamazepine
Ofloxacin
Ketoconazole
Lisinopril
Nicotinic acid
Labetalol
Etoposide
Imipramine
Interferon alfa
Flutamide
Tolcapone
Nefazodone
Oral contraceptives

Combination Agents with Enhanced Hepatotoxicity
Alcohol-acetaminophen
Trimethoprim-sulfamethoxazole
Rifampicin-isoniazid
Amoxicillin-clavulanic acid
Viral Hepatitides
Hepatitis A, B, C, D, E, G
Human herpesvirus
Cytomegalovirus
Epstein-Barr virus
Herpes simplex virus
Varicella zoster virus
Paramyxovirus
Parvovirus B19
Adenovirus
Togavirus
Parvovirus
SEN virus
TT virus
Yellow fever virus
Toxins
CCl_4
Amanita phalloides
Yellow phosphorus
Herbal products
Vascular
Ischemic
Venooclusive disease
Budd-Chiari syndrome
Malignant infiltration
Non-Hodgkin lymphoma
Miscellaneous
Wilson disease
Autoimmune hepatitis
Acute fatty liver of pregnancy
Reye syndrome

From Vincent JL et al: *Textbook of critical care,* ed 7, Philadelphia, 2017, Elsevier.

BOX 3 Investigations in Fulminant Hepatic Failure

Baseline essential investigations
Biochemistry
- Bilirubin, transaminases
- Alkaline phosphatase
- Albumin
- Urea and electrolytes
- Creatinine
- Calcium, phosphate
- Ammonia
- Acid-base, lactate
- Glucose
Hematology
- Full blood count, platelets
- PT, PTT
- Factors V or VII
- Blood group cross-match
Septic screen
Omitting lumbar puncture
- Radiology
- Chest radiograph
- Abdominal ultrasound
- Head CT scan or MRI
Neurophysiology
- Electroencephalogram
Diagnostic investigations
Serum
- Acetaminophen levels
- Cu, ceruloplasmin (>3 yr)
- Autoantibodies
- Immunoglobulins
- Amino acids
- Lactate
- Pyruvate
- Hepatitis A, B, C, E
- EBV, CMV, HSV viral loads
- Other viruses
Urine
- Toxic metabolites
- Amino acids, succinylacetone
- Organic acids
- Reducing sugars

PT, *Prothrombin time;* PTT, *partial thromboplastin time;* EBV, *Epstein-Barr virus;* CMV, *cytomegalovirus;* HSV, *herpes simplex virus.*
From Fuhrman BP, Zimmerman JJ: *Fuhrman and Zimmerman's pediatric critical care,* ed 4, Philadelphia, 2011, Mosby.

DX DIAGNOSIS

DIFFERENTIAL DIAGNOSIS

- Severe acute hepatitis, also known as acute liver injury (including alcoholic hepatitis): Jaundice and coagulopathy without encephalopathy
- Acute-on-chronic liver failure (in patients with liver disease duration >26 wk)
- Cirrhosis (includes decompensated cirrhosis)
- Hepatocellular carcinoma
- Table 1 describes features distinguishing ALF from chronic hepatic encephalopathy or portal systemic encephalopathy

WORKUP (BOX 3)[1,4-7]

- Fig. 1 describes an algorithm for evaluation of ALF.
- Clinical history is critical, but in the case of patients with severe encephalopathy, the

TABLE 1 Features Distinguishing Acute Liver Failure from Chronic Hepatic Encephalopathy or Portal Systemic Encephalopathy

Feature	Acute Liver Failure	Portal Systemic Encephalopathy
History		
Onset	Usually acute	Varies; may be insidious or subacute
Mental state	Mania may evolve to deep coma	Blunted consciousness
Precipitating factor	Viral infection or hepatotoxin	Gastrointestinal hemorrhage, exogenous protein, drugs, uremia, infection
History of liver disease	No	Usually yes
Symptoms		
Nausea, vomiting	Common	Unusual
Abdominal pain	Common	Unusual
Signs		
Liver	Small, soft, tender	Usually large, firm, no pain
Nutritional state	Normal	Cachectic
Collateral circulation	Absent	May be present
Ascites	Absent	May be present
Laboratory Test		
Transaminases	Very high	Normal or slightly high
Coagulopathy	Present	Often present

From Jankovic J et al: *Bradley and Daroff's neurology in clinical practice,* ed 8, Philadelphia, 2022, Elsevier.

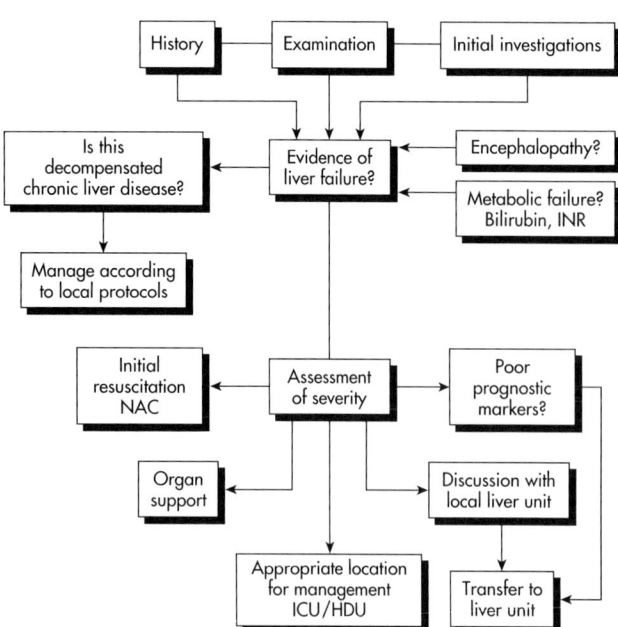

FIG. 1 Initial management of a patient presenting with liver failure. *HDU,* High-dependency unit; *ICU,* intensive care unit; *INR,* international normalized ratio; *NAC,* N-acetylcysteine. (From Parrillo JE, Dellinger RP: *Critical care medicine, principles of diagnosis and management in the adult,* ed 5, Philadelphia, 2019, Elsevier.)

TABLE 2 Grades of Encephalopathy

Grade	Description
I	Changes in behavior with minimal change in level of consciousness (mild confusion, slurred speech, disordered sleep)
II	Gross disorientation, drowsiness, possibly asterixis, inappropriate behavior
III	Marked confusion (stupor), incoherent speech, sleeping most of the time but rousable to vocal stimuli
IV	Comatose, unresponsiveness to pain, decorticate or decerebrate posturing

history may be limited, and efforts should be made to obtain information from the patient's family. Important history components include medication use (6-mo history of prescriptions, over-the-counter medications, herbal supplements), alcohol use, recreational drug use, prior symptoms of jaundice, onset of symptoms, history of depression and prior suicide attempts, recent travel to endemic areas of viral hepatitis, sexual exposures, previous blood transfusions, family history of liver failure/disease, history of malignancy, or hypercoagulable state.

- Physical examination should include assessing for stigmata of chronic liver disease, as their presence has different diagnostic and management implications, and mental status. Grading of hepatic encephalopathy should be performed (Table 2). Perform an asterixis maneuver, consider psychometric tests (i.e., number connection test) to detect subtle degree of encephalopathy.

- Laboratory evaluation should be targeted to assess the severity of ALF, as well as its etiology. Early testing includes CBC, liver function tests (LFTs) including prothrombin time and INR, bilirubin, chemistry panel (sodium, potassium, chloride, bicarbonate, BUN, creatinine, glucose, magnesium, phosphate, calcium), arterial blood gas, arterial lactate, blood type and screen, acetaminophen level, ethanol level, toxicology screen, viral hepatitis serologies (hepatitis A immunoglobulin M [IgM], hepatitis B surface antigen, anti-hepatitis B core IgM, anti-hepatitis C antibody [IgM and IgG]), hepatitis C viral load (HCV RNA), anti-hepatitis E IgM and IgG, HSV-1 IgM and HSV polymerase chain reaction (PCR), Epstein-Barr virus DNA PCR, cytomegalovirus DNA PCR, anti-hepatitis D IgM and IgG, hepatitis D viral load (HDV RNA), ceruloplasmin level (as well as serum copper and 24-h urine copper if high suspicion), pregnancy test, arterial ammonia level, autoimmune markers (antinuclear antibody, anti-smooth muscle antibody, anti-liver kidney microsomal antibody type 1, total IgG levels), HIV-1, HIV-2, amylase, and lipase.

- Imaging studies include abdominal ultrasound with Doppler to evaluate for Budd-Chiari syndrome, portal hypertension, hepatic congestion, and hepatic steatosis. Cirrhosis cannot be diagnosed in the setting of ALF, as the liver may appear nodular in ALF due to massive necrosis. Consider cross-sectional imaging of the liver (triphasic CT, magnetic resonance cholangiopancreatography, or MRI with gadolinium), especially in patients with a history of malignancy, to rule out malignant infiltration. CT or MRI of the head should be considered to ensure no other causes for altered mental status.

- Prompt liver biopsy (via transjugular approach to decrease risk of bleeding) should be performed in cases in which:
  1. The etiology is unknown after the initial workup; *or*
  2. Etiology is thought to be secondary to autoimmune hepatitis, malignancy, or HSV.

COMPLICATIONS

Complications or progression of liver failure may result in cerebral edema due to increased intracranial pressure (in up to 40% of patients). Hypoglycemia and lactic acidosis are common complications of ALF, as well as acute kidney injury and pancreatitis (particularly in acetaminophen-induced ALF). Upper gastrointestinal hemorrhage is uncommon (in 1.5% of patients). Infections can occur due to impaired leukocyte function (in nearly 80% patients). High-output cardiac failure and acute respiratory distress syndrome can also occur. Hypotension occurs due to decreased oral intake as well as extravasation of fluid into extravascular space.

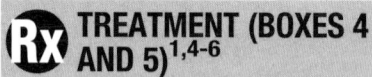

Rx TREATMENT (BOXES 4 AND 5)[1,4-6]

Broadly, the treatment of ALF should include:
- Identification of the etiology of liver injury, if possible, and specific treatment
- Symptomatic and supportive management and transfer to an intensive care unit (ICU) if necessary
- Early involvement of a liver specialist and transfer to a transplant center when required

NONPHARMACOLOGIC THERAPY[1,4-6]

- Initial treatment should focus on the patient's mental status and managing encephalopathy.
  1. Grade I encephalopathy may be managed on a medical ward (neuro vital signs q4h).
  2. Grade II, III, and IV encephalopathy should be managed in an ICU (with elevated head of the bed to 30 degrees). Grade III and IV encephalopathy require intubation and mechanical ventilation.
  3. Decreased stimulation is important (avoiding sedatives; dimly lit, quiet room; no audible monitor alarms).

- A liver specialist should be notified urgently, and arrangements should be made for imminent transfer to a transplant center. Early transport is important, as the patient transport risks increase or even preclude transfer in later stages of encephalopathy.

- Nutritional support should be initiated early. A daily intake goal of 60 g of protein (or amino acids 0.8 to 1.2 g/kg/day) is recommended to prevent catabolism of protein stores. Enteral feeding should be initiated in patients with grade III or IV encephalopathy.

- Fluid support should be initiated if patient is not tolerating oral intake, or signs of hypoperfusion are present. Crystalloid solutions (normal saline in hypotensive patients, ½ normal saline + 75 mEq/L NaCO$_3$ in acidotic

BOX 4 Management of Fulminant Hepatic Failure

No sedation except for procedures
Minimal handling
Enteric precautions until infection ruled out
Monitor:
- Heart and respiratory rate
- Arterial BP, CVP
- Core/toe temperature
- Neurologic observations
- Gastric pH (>5.0)
- Blood glucose (>4 mmol/L)
- Acid-base
- Electrolytes
- PT, PTT
Fluid balance
- 75% maintenance
- Dextrose 10%-50% (provide 6-10 mg/kg/min)
- Sodium (0.5-1 mmol/L)
- Potassium (2-4 mmol/L)
  Maintain circulating volume with colloid/FFP
Coagulation support only if required
Drugs:
- Vitamin K
- H_2 antagonist
- Antacids
- Lactulose
- N-acetylcysteine for acetaminophen toxicity
- Broad-spectrum antibiotics
- Antifungals
Nutrition
- Enteral feeding (1-2 g protein/kg/day)
- PN if ventilated

BP, *Blood pressure;* CVP, *central venous pressure;* PT, *prothrombin time;* PTT, *partial thromboplastin time;* FFP, *fresh frozen plasma;* PN, *parenteral nutrition.* From Fuhrman BP, Zimmerman JJ: *Fuhrman and Zimmerman's pediatric critical care,* ed 4, Philadelphia, 2011, Mosby.

patients, normal saline + dextrose in hypoglycemic patients) can be used.

PHARMACOLOGIC TREATMENT[1,4-6]

- If encephalopathy progresses and cerebral edema develops leading to increased ICP, intravenous mannitol is recommended to reduce cerebral edema transiently. Prophylactic hyperventilation is not recommended in patients with ALF. Serum sodium should be maintained between 140 to 150 mmol/L. In patients with the highest risk of cerebral edema, hypertonic saline is recommended.
- Phenytoin can be used to manage seizures. In patients not responding to phenytoin, short-acting benzodiazepines may be used.
- Sedative medications should be avoided, as they are not cleared well and may mask signs of worsening encephalopathy or cerebral edema.
- Lactulose and rifaximin are not routinely recommended for encephalopathy treatment; neomycin should be avoided due to concerns of nephrotoxicity.

BOX 5 Hepatic Replacement Therapeutic Options Available to Patients with Fulminant Hepatic Failure

Liver Transplantation
- Cadaveric transplantation
- Whole liver
- Reduced-size liver
- Split liver
- Auxiliary partial liver
- Orthotopic position
- Heterotopic position
- Auxiliary whole liver
- Living-related transplantation
- Left lateral segment
- Left lobe
- Extended left lobe
- Right lobe

Artificial Liver Assist Devices
- Non–cell-based systems
- Charcoal hemoperfusion
- High-volume plasmapheresis
- Continuous high-frequency hemodiafiltration
- Molecular adsorbent recirculating system (MARS)
- Cell-based systems (bioartificial liver assist devices)
- Primary porcine hepatocytes
- Human hepatoblastoma cells
- Extracorporeal liver assist device (ELAD)

Hepatocyte Transplantation

From Vincent JL et al: *Textbook of critical care,* ed 6, Philadelphia, 2011, Saunders.

- Broad-spectrum antibiotics should be started immediately if infection is suspected. Sources usually include respiratory, urinary, and blood; there is no evidence for empiric antibiotic treatment. Antifungals should be initiated if no initial improvement with antibiotics occurs.
- In the case of persistent hypotension, norepinephrine is the initial vasopressor of choice; vasopressin can be added as a second pressor to maintain mean arterial pressure (MAP) >75 mm Hg. Persistent hypotension despite fluid resuscitation and pressor support should prompt concern for adrenal insufficiency.
- If dialysis is required for renal support, continuous mode is recommended over intermittent hemodialysis.
- Patients should receive stress ulcer prophylaxis, given the risk of gastrointestinal bleeding.
- Routine correction of thrombocytopenia or INR correction are not recommended in the absence of bleeding. However, in the setting of clinical bleeding or the need for a procedure with a high bleeding risk, plasma or clotting factors are recommended. Vitamin K should be given routinely since in patients with ALF vitamin K deficiency is common.
- Part of the pharmacologic treatment will be specific to the suspected etiology of ALF.

- If acetaminophen is the known or suspected cause, an IV acetylcysteine protocol should be initiated. N-acetylcysteine is not harmful and dramatically alters the course in acetaminophen toxicity, so there should be a low threshold to start, particularly in young patients or those with no known cause of ALF.
- The 20-h protocol is:
  1. Initial loading dose of 150 mg/kg IV given over 60 min followed by
  2. 12.5 mg/kg IV/h over 4 h followed by
  3. 6.25 mg/kg IV/h for 16 h.
- A repeat acetaminophen level and alanine transaminase (ALT) should be checked at hour 18 of NAC treatment. If either the acetaminophen level or the ALT is elevated, the 16-h portion of treatment (6.25 mg/kg) should be extended and another ALT, INR, or acetaminophen level should be checked every 12 h. The acetylcysteine can be stopped once the acetaminophen level is undetectable, INR <2, or ALT is shown to be either normal or decreasing. Additional information on acetaminophen overdose is available in the topic "Acetaminophen Poisoning."
- N-acetylcysteine therapy outside of acetaminophen poisoning has been investigated, but evidence for the benefit is inconclusive. Its routine use is not currently recommended by practice guidelines and is center specific.[8]
- Liver support systems:
  1. Liver support systems have been trialed either to support the patient until the liver recovers or as a bridge to liver transplantation.
  2. High-volume plasma exchange can improve hepatic encephalopathy and transplant-free survival in a patient ineligible for liver transplantation, but no survival benefit has been shown for a patient undergoing liver transplantation with plasma exchange compared with supportive therapy alone.[9]
  3. The molecular absorbents recirculating system (MARS) is an artificial extracorporeal hepatic support system that allows albumin-bound toxins to be removed. MARS has been shown to improve hemodynamics and biochemical variables, and there is emerging evidence that MARS therapy is associated with higher transplant-free survival. However, the routine use of MARS is not currently recommended by practice guidelines.[10]
  4. Bioartificial support systems in the form of hepatocytes (human or other mammalian origin) have also been used in cartridges as part of extracorporeal systems. These have not shown any benefit, with or without transplantation.

MONITORING[1,5]

- In patients with high-grade hepatic encephalopathy (HE) awaiting transplant, intracranial pressure (ICP) monitoring is recommended in centers with expertise in ICP monitoring.

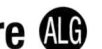

TABLE 3 King's College Hospital Criteria for Liver Transplantation in Acute Liver Failure

Acetaminophen-Induced Acute Liver Failure	Non—Acetaminophen-Induced Acute Liver Failure
Arterial pH <7.3 (irrespective of grade of encephalopathy) *OR* Grade III or IV encephalopathy *and* Prothrombin time >100 sec *and* Serum creatinine >3.4 mg/dL	Prothrombin time >100 sec (irrespective of grade of encephalopathy) *OR* Any of three of the following variables (irrespective of grade of encephalopathy): 1. Age <10 yr or >40 yr 2. Etiology: Non-A hepatitis, non-B hepatitis, halothane hepatitis, idiosyncratic drug reactions 3. Duration of jaundice before onset of encephalopathy >7 days 4. Prothrombin time >50 sec 5. Serum bilirubin >18 mg/dL

Sec, Seconds.

- Neurologic examination every 1 to 4 h is recommended in the absence of ICP monitoring.
- Patients with suspected acetaminophen toxicity should have LFTs monitored every 12 h. Otherwise, LFTs can be monitored daily.
- Chemistry panels and prothrombin time/INR should be monitored every 8 to 12 h. Correction of coagulopathy should be avoided because it can interfere with assessment of liver function. In the setting of life-threatening bleeding, fresh frozen plasma (FFP) and recombinant factor VIIa can be considered.
- Point-of-care glucose should be checked every 4 h initially to evaluate for hypoglycemia. If hypoglycemia is detected, dextrose should be added to crystalloid solution.
- Because of the increased risk of infection, daily urine, sputum, and blood cultures, as well as chest x-ray examinations, should be checked even in the absence of signs or symptoms of infection.

PROGNOSIS[1,4,5]

- Overall mortality from ALF is 30% to 40% and has improved significantly over the last 20 yr.
- Transplant-free survival in ALF in the setting of acetaminophen, hepatitis A, shock liver, and pregnancy-related disease is >50%; for all other causes of ALF, transplant-free survival is <25%.

- Higher-grade hepatic encephalopathy and renal dysfunction in non-acetaminophen ALF predict worse survival.
- Multiple models have been developed to predict spontaneous recovery in ALF patients (King's College criteria, Clichy criteria, MELD score, APACHE II score).
- The King's College criteria form the basis of the model most commonly used for prognostication (Table 3).
- Transplantation:
  1. Patients with ALF are given the highest priority for liver transplantation. ALF accounts for only 10% of the U.S. liver transplants.
  2. Contraindications to listing include medical history of irreversible brain injury, psychiatric illness severe enough to affect patients' survival or likelihood of compliance with medications, active sepsis, severe medical comorbidities including malignancy, increasing dependence on ventilator/inotropic support, acute substance abuse, previous episodes of self-harm (>5 episodes), refractory mental illness, and inadequate family support.
  3. For patients with alcoholic liver disease, many centers require a 6-mo abstinence period, but several transplant centers in North America and Europe have transplanted selected patients with alcoholic hepatitis who were unlikely to survive 6 mo.[11]
  4. Mortality on the waiting list is 25%; 1-yr and 5-yr survival after transplantation are 73% and 67%, respectively.
  5. Various prognostic criteria used for liver transplantation in patients with fulminant hepatic failure are summarized in Box E6.

⚠ PEARLS & CONSIDERATIONS

- ALF is defined as severe hepatic injury (as evidenced by elevated liver enzymes) with INR >1.5 and hepatic encephalopathy occurring <26 wk before presentation in a patient with no prior history of liver disease.
- Close to half of ALF is caused by drug ingestion, usually acetaminophen.
- Given the potential rapidity of deterioration, referral must be made as soon as possible to a liver transplant center.
- There should be a low threshold to start *N*-acetylcysteine.
- Coagulopathy should not be corrected unless life-threatening bleeding occurs or it is recommended by the liver transplant hepatologist.

REFERENCES

Available at eBooks.Health.Elsevier.com

RELATED CONTENT

Acetaminophen Poisoning (Related Key Topic)
Ascites (Related Key Topic)
Encephalopathy (Related Key Topic)
Hepatopulmonary Syndrome (Related Key Topic)
Hepatorenal Syndrome (Related Key Topic)

AUTHORS: **MAYA DEEB, MD,** and **TALIA ZENLEA, MD**

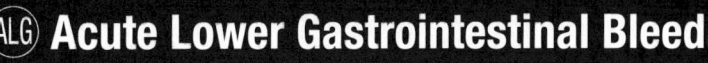
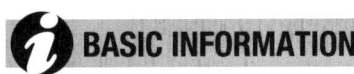 **BASIC INFORMATION**

DEFINITION

Acute lower GI bleeding is classically defined as sudden loss of blood distal to the ligament of Treitz. This has more recently been redefined as bleeding originating from either the colon or the rectum.[1]

SYNONYMS

Acute colonic bleeding
Gastrointestinal hemorrhage
Melena
Hematochezia

ICD-10CM CODES	
K62.5	Hemorrhage of rectum and anus
K92.1	Melena
K92.2	Gastrointestinal hemorrhage, unspecified

EPIDEMIOLOGY & DEMOGRAPHICS

INCIDENCE:
- Annual incidence of hospitalization is 33 to 87/100,000 (about half of that for upper GI bleeding) in the U.S.[2,3]
- Mortality rates of 2.5% to 3.9% during hospitalization.[2,3] Rebleeding rates of 13% to 19% at 1 yr and 46% at 5 yr.[2,4]

PREDOMINANT SEX & AGE: 24.2/100,000 in males vs. 17.2/100,000 in females.[3]

PEAK INCIDENCE: The rate of lower GI bleeding, including that necessitating hospitalization, is higher in the elderly. The risk of lower GI bleed increases 200-fold by the 9th decade of life. Age >65 yr is associated with increased in-hospital mortality.[3-5]

RISK FACTORS: Risk factors include use of antithrombotic agents, NSAID use, aspirin use, alcohol abuse, GI malignancy, atrial fibrillation, coagulopathies, prior GI bleed, cirrhosis, constipation, congenital malformations, radiation exposure, recent infectious illness, recent travel, abdominal aortic aneurysm (AAA) repair, and inflammatory bowel disease.[2,4,5]

PHYSICAL FINDINGS & CLINICAL PRESENTATION

- Attention should be paid in the history to details suggesting the location and etiology of the bleed.[1] For instance, weight loss and abdominal pain suggest inflammatory bowel disease; recent AAA repair, especially with history of a sentinel bleed, raises suspicion for aortoenteric fistula; a history of cirrhosis suggests bleeding from portal hypertension, such as varices. Bright red blood per rectum is typically from a brisk upper GI bleed, distal colon, or anorectal disease. Melena arises from the upper GI tract, small bowel, or proximal colon. Take a detailed medication history, noting NSAIDs or other drugs that may cause or mimic GI bleeding as well as beta blockers that may mask tachycardia in the setting of significant blood loss.
- The clinician should first and foremost check vital signs, including orthostatics, if stable. Check for pallor and signs of volume depletion, such as delayed capillary refill and skin tenting. Observe

for stigmata of liver disease, such as telangiectasias and jaundice. Auscultate for bowel sounds. Absence of bowel sounds may indicate perforation. Palpate the abdomen for pain, masses, and hepatosplenomegaly. Rectal examination should be performed, noting the presence of blood, rate of bleeding, masses, fissures, hemorrhoids, tenderness, and skin changes. If no gross bleed is seen, perform hemoccult testing. Ensure that the bleeding is, in fact, gastrointestinal, excluding hematuria, vaginal bleeding, and wounds.

ETIOLOGY

Diverticulosis is the most common cause of lower GI bleeding at 30%. Internal hemorrhoids are the second most common cause. Colitis (ischemia, infection, inflammatory bowel disease), angioectasia, and rectal ulcers are less common causes. 15% of lower GI bleeds are due to upper GI bleeding.[1,2,5]

DX DIAGNOSIS

DIFFERENTIAL DIAGNOSIS (TABLE 1)

- Upper GI bleed
- Diverticulosis
- Diverticulitis
- Ischemic colitis
- Postpolypectomy bleeding
- Vascular ectasias (angiodysplasia, arteriovenous malformation)
- Anal fissure
- Rectal ulcer
- Colonic polyps
- Advanced neoplasms
- Hemorrhoids
- Intussusception
- Coagulopathies
- Infectious colitis (*E. coli, Shigella, Salmonella, Giardia*)
- Autoimmune (hemolytic uremic syndrome)
- Radiation colitis or proctitis
- Aortoenteric fistula
- Vasculitis
- Inflammatory (ulcerative colitis, Crohn disease)
- Colonic varices
- Drugs (iron, NSAIDs)
- Foreign body

WORKUP

Assess vital signs and ABCs. Establish large-bore intravenous access. If the patient has significant hematochezia without hematemesis, consider performing nasogastric lavage to evaluate for upper GI bleeding. An algorithm for the management of severe hematochezia is illustrated in Fig. 1.[1-3,5,6]

LABORATORY TESTS

- CBC may reveal anemia and/or thrombocytopenia. The hematocrit and hemoglobin should generally be trended every 4 to 6 hr to document the progression of blood loss.
- Order a comprehensive metabolic panel to evaluate the following: Elevated blood urea nitrogen, which may indicate reabsorption of red blood cells; elevated creatinine, which indicates poor renal perfusion; liver function tests, which could reveal liver disease that is exacerbating bleeding.
- International normalized ratio (INR), especially if patient is taking warfarin.
- Partial thromboplastin time, especially if the patient is on heparin.
- Type and screen/cross in anticipation of the need for blood products.
- Stool studies, including white blood cell count, Gram stain, culture, and pathogen-specific testing to identify infectious etiologies.
- Inflammatory markers including procalcitonin, erythrocyte sedimentation rate, and C-reactive protein.

IMAGING STUDIES

- Computed tomography (CT) angiography (sensitivity 85.2%, specificity 92.1%) can potentially identify the location of the bleed as well as abnormal vasculature.[2]
- Perform a tagged red blood cell scan if source is not identified on CT angiography.
- CT scan of the abdomen and pelvis may identify malignancy as the source of bleeding.
- If free air is suspected from perforation, an abdominal or chest plain film should be ordered immediately. An abdominal plain film can also identify radiopaque foreign bodies.
- Abdominal ultrasound if intussusception is suspected.
- Meckel (technetium-99) scan if Meckel diverticulum is suspected.

TABLE 1 Differential Diagnosis of Lower Gastrointestinal Hemorrhage

Colonic bleeding	95%	Small bowel bleeding	5%
Diverticular disease	30%-40%	Angiodysplasias	
Anorectal disease	5%-15%	Erosions or ulcers (potassium, nonsteroidal antiinflammatory drugs)	
Ischemia	5%-10%	Crohn disease	
Neoplasia	5%-10%	Radiation	
Infectious colitis	3%-8%	Meckel diverticulum	
Postpolypectomy	3%-7%	Neoplasia	
Inflammatory bowel disease	3%-4%	Aortoenteric fistula	
Angiodysplasia	3%		
Radiation colitis or proctitis	1%-3%		
Other	1%-5%		
Unknown	10%-25%		

From Townsend CM et al: *Sabiston textbook of surgery*, ed 21, St Louis, 2022, Elsevier.

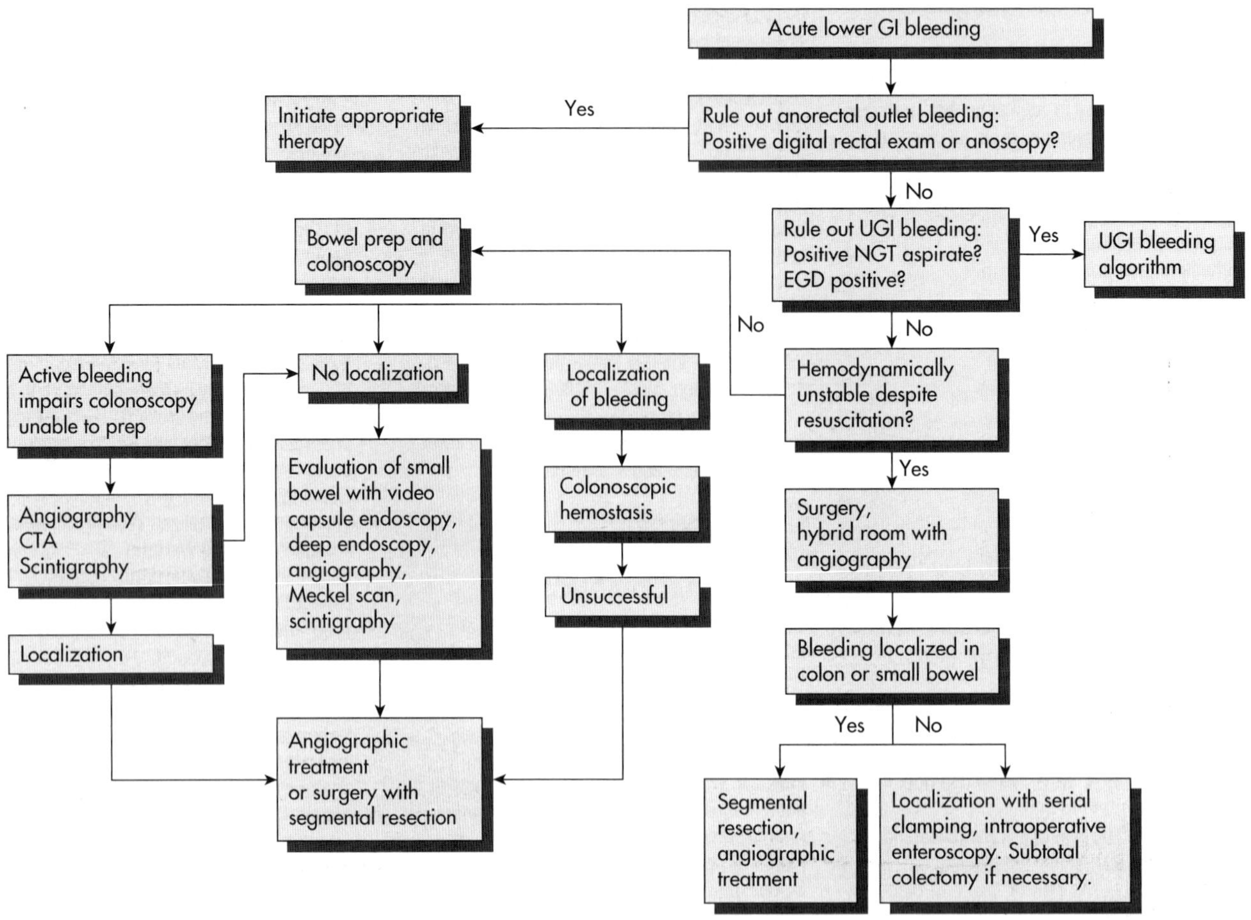

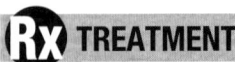

FIG. 1 Algorithm for diagnosis and management of lower GI hemorrhage. *CTA*, Computed tomography angiogram; *EGD*, esophagogastroduodenoscopy; *GI*, gastrointestinal; *NGT*, nasogastric tube; *UGI*, upper GI. (From Townsend CM et al: *Sabiston textbook of surgery*, ed 21, St Louis, 2022, Elsevier.)

Rx TREATMENT

Begin crystalloid bolus to maintain a systolic blood pressure of at least 100 mm Hg. Transfuse for hemoglobin and hematocrit of 7 and 21, respectively, or less. If the patient has coronary artery disease or multiple medical comorbidities and is older than 65 yr, the goal hemoglobin and hematocrit are 8 and 24, respectively. Platelets should be maintained above 50,000 and INR 1.5 or less. If possible, discontinue any antithrombotic agents and NSAIDs after consultation with the appropriate physician who initiated therapy.[1,2]

NONPHARMACOLOGIC THERAPY
- Colonoscopy defines the colonic anatomy, can identify the source of bleeding, and allows for potential therapy.
- Endoscopy can be performed if the source of the bleed is suspected to be proximal to the ligament of Treitz.
- Anoscopy can be performed for bleeding internal hemorrhoids or other anorectal disorders.
- Balloon tamponade of esophageal or anorectal bleeds.
- Perform surgery if the source of the bleed cannot be otherwise identified, for aortoenteric fistula, or if air enema for intussusception is unsuccessful.

- Interventional radiology for embolization.
- Ablation.

ACUTE GENERAL RX
Proton pump inhibitor, histamine-2 blocker if suspecting upper GI blood with rapid transit

CHRONIC RX
Avoid NSAIDs and alcohol. Treat the underlying cause of the bleed, such as coagulopathy, portal hypertension, etc. Most patients are prescribed daily proton pump inhibitors. Fiber, stool softeners, and analgesic creams may alleviate development and/or symptoms of hemorrhoids.

DISPOSITION
Lower GI bleeding will resolve spontaneously in most patients. Therefore if the patient is hemodynamically stable without symptomatic anemia or brisk bleeding, he or she may follow up with his or her primary care physician or a gastroenterologist. However, patients with shock or other hemodynamic compromise, severe bleeding, or significant comorbidities should be admitted to the intensive care unit. These patients are at high risk for acute decompensation and as such require close monitoring and aggressive resuscitation; furthermore, they will require urgent diagnosis and intervention to stop the bleeding.[1]

Clinical factors predictive of severe colonic bleeding include aspirin use, at least two comorbid illnesses, pulse >100 beats/min, and systolic blood pressure <115 mm Hg. The overall mortality rate from colonic bleeding is 2.4% to 3.9%. Independent predictors of in-hospital mortality are age >65 yr, intestinal ischemia, and two or more comorbidities. Inform patients that the risk of rebleeding is fairly high (13% to 19% within 1 yr), and they should continue to closely monitor their symptoms and stool for any signs of recurrence.

REFERRAL
Patients should be referred to gastroenterology for follow-up.[1]

REFERENCES
Available at eBooks.Health.Elsevier.com.

RELATED CONTENT
Bleeding, Gastrointestinal (Algorithm)
Colorectal Cancer (Related Key Topic)
Diverticular Disease (Related Key Topic)
Meckel Diverticulum (Related Key Topic)

AUTHORS: **BENJAMIN KARTUB, MD,** and **JOSHUA JUSTICE, MD**

A

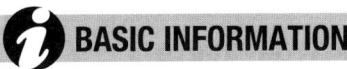 **BASIC INFORMATION**

DEFINITION

Acute lymphoblastic leukemia (ALL) is a malignancy of precursor B or T lymphocytes (lymphoblasts) characterized by uncontrolled proliferation of malignant lymphocytic cells with replacement of normal bone marrow elements and bone marrow failure. Lymphoblastic lymphoma (LBL) is diagnosed when the disease presents in extramedullary sites (most commonly as mediastinal mass in T-cell disease) *and* <20% of the bone marrow is involved.

SYNONYMS

Acute lymphocytic leukemia
Acute lymphoblastic leukemia
ALL

ICD-10CM CODES
C91.00	Acute lymphoblastic leukemia not having achieved remission
C91.01	Acute lymphoblastic leukemia, in remission
C91.02	Acute lymphoblastic leukemia, in relapse

EPIDEMIOLOGY & DEMOGRAPHICS

- ALL is primarily a disease of children, adolescents, and young adults.
- Overall incidence is 1.8/100,000 persons per year; 65% are <34 yr. It is most commonly diagnosed among people aged <20 (SEER database 2015-2019).
- Incidence varies according to race and ethnic group, being more common in Hispanics and whites than blacks.
- Male:female ratio is 55:45.

PHYSICAL FINDINGS & CLINICAL PRESENTATION

- Findings consistent with bone marrow failure and peripheral cytopenias—pallor, bruising, petechiae
- Lymphadenopathy or hepatosplenomegaly
- Fever (disease related or infectious), bone pain, weakness, weight loss, mental status changes, and neurologic findings associated with central nervous system (CNS) involvement (if present)
- T-cell LBL is usually associated with a mediastinal mass
- Table 1 summarizes the clinical presentation of acute LBL

ETIOLOGY

- Most cases are sporadic without established risk factors.
- Ionizing radiation exposure appears to be a risk factor.
- Down syndrome (trisomy 21) is associated with an approximately 3% risk of developing leukemia by age 30, predominantly ALL. ALL may be seen with other hereditary premalignancy syndromes (e.g., ataxia-telangiectasia)

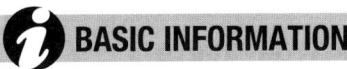 **DIAGNOSIS**

DIFFERENTIAL DIAGNOSIS

Disorders associated with lymphocytosis (lymphocytes >5000/mcl):
- Adults: Chronic lymphocytic leukemia, mantle cell lymphoma, marginal zone lymphoma, hairy cell leukemia
- Adolescents/young adults: Infectious mononucleosis syndromes due to Epstein-Barr virus or cytomegalovirus, among others, may present with lymphocyte abnormalities with appearance suggestive of leukemic blasts
- Disorders associated with circulating blasts or blast-like cells such as acute myeloid leukemia, prolymphocytic leukemia, blastoid mantle cell lymphoma, and Burkitt lymphoma (mature B-cell leukemia/lymphoma)
- LBL
- Aplastic anemia; ALL may present without circulating leukemia cells and with only manifestations of bone marrow failure

WORKUP

- Identification of circulating abnormal cell population by flow cytometry. CD19, cytoplasmic CD22, and/or cCD79a identifies most B lineage cells. Immature leukemic blasts should have *absence* of surface immunoglobulin (sIg) and will usually express CD 10, CD34, and stain positive for terminal deoxynucleotidyltransferase (TdT). A strong expression of CD20, expression of sIg, and negativity of TdT should prompt a workup for a mature B cell neoplasms such as Burkitt ALL because this distinction is critical. Cytoplasmic CD3 and CD7 establish immature T-cell lineage in most cases. Aberrant myeloid markers (CD13, CD33) can be seen. Early T-cell precursor (ETP-ALL) has a unique immunologic signature, as well as different prognosis and treatment approaches.
- Cytochemical stains are sometimes easier to perform and may be available sooner but are less specific. ALL blasts should be negative for myeloperoxidase and esterase stains.
- Bone marrow examination (Fig. E1).
- Genetic studies define important treatment categories, of which the most important is Philadelphia chromosome positive (Ph+) vs. Philadelphia chromosome negative (Ph−) disease, because these are treated differently. Although rare in children (incidence 2% to 5%) Ph+ ALL represents the most common genetic subgroup in ALL in adults with an overall incidence of 20% to 25%. The incidence increases with age and accounts for more than 50% of cases of ALL in patients who are older than 60 years of age.[1] Ph status can be determined rapidly by polymerase chain reaction (PCR) or fluorescence in situ hybridization (FISH) and should be available within 24 to 48 h of diagnosis. The WHO classification recognizes genetic variants of ALL as distinct syndromes (Table 2), and the clinical significance of common abnormalities is outlined in Table 3.
- Genetic profiling for "Ph-like" ALL (genetic profile similar to Ph+ disease, but no BCR/ABL abnormality) or IKZF1 (IKAROS) mutations may provide additional prognostic information but may not be uniformly available. Ph-like ALL may respond to tyrosine kinase inhibitor therapy and may behave more like Ph+ ALL; however, Ph-like ALL cases contain a number of genetic alterations that activate kinase and cytokine receptor signaling. Alterations can be grouped into two major subclasses that include ABL-class fusions involving ABL1, ABL2, SDF1R, and PDGFRB that phenocopy BCR-ABL1, and alteration of CRLF2, JAK2, and EPOR that activate JAK/STAT signaling.
- Other alterations in the Ph-like genomic landscape activate other kinases, including BLNK, DGKH, FGFR1, OL2RB, LYN, NTRK3, PDGFRA, PTK2B, TYK2, and the RAS signaling pathway.
- Lumbar puncture is usually done at diagnosis, if practical, to assess for CNS involvement and to initiate CNS prophylactic therapy.

TABLE 1 Clinical Presentation of Acute Lymphoblastic Leukemia

Symptoms/Signs	Etiology	Management
Fever	Disease or infection	Always conduct fever workup and provide broad antimicrobial coverage until infectious etiology is ruled out
Fatigue, pallor	Anemia (ALL infiltrating bone marrow)	Packed red blood cell transfusion (slow if anemia is severe, avoid in hyperleukocytosis)
Petechiae, bruising, bleeding	Thrombocytopenia (ALL infiltrating bone marrow)	Transfuse with platelets
Pain	Leukemia infiltrating bones/joints, or expanding marrow cavity	Establish diagnosis and start chemotherapy
Respiratory distress/superior vena cava syndrome	Mediastinal mass	Avoid sedation in presence of tracheal compression. Establish diagnosis as soon as possible and start chemotherapy

ALL, Acute lymphoblastic leukemia.
From Hoffman R et al: *Hematology: basic principles and practice,* ed 7, Philadelphia, 2018, Elsevier.

TABLE 2   WHO Classification of Precursor Lymphoid Neoplasms

B-lymphoblastic leukemia/lymphoma, not otherwise specified
B-lymphoblastic leukemia/lymphoma with recurrent cytogenetic abnormalities:
    B-lymphoblastic leukemia/lymphoma with t(9;22)(q34;q11.2); *BCR-ABL1*
    B-lymphoblastic leukemia/lymphoma with t(v;11q23) *KMT2A* rearranged.
    B-lymphoblastic leukemia/lymphoma with t(12;21)(p13;q22); *ETV6-RUNX1*
    B-lymphoblastic leukemia/lymphoma with hyperdiploidy
    B-lymphoblastic leukemia/lymphoma with hypodiploidy
    B-lymphoblastic leukemia/lymphoma with t(5;14)(q32;q32); IL3-IGH
    B-lymphoblastic leukemia/lymphoma with t(1;19)(q23;p13.3); EZA-PBX1 (TCF3-PBX-1)
    B lymphoblastic leukemia/lymphoma with iAMP21
T-lymphoblastic leukemia/lymphoma
NK-lymphoblastic leukemia/lymphoma
Provisional entities:
    B-lymphoblastic leukemia/lymphoma BCR/ABL1-like

NK, Natural killer; *WHO*, World Health Organization.

TABLE 3   More Common Recurrent Cytogenetic Abnormalities in Acute Lymphoblastic Leukemia/Lymphoma

Abnormality	Clinical Relevance
B cell ALL	
t(9;22)(q34;q11.2); *BCR-ABL1*	Incidence approximately 3% in children, 25% in adults, rising with age; requires therapy with ABL1 tyrosine kinase inhibitors.
t(v*;11q23) *MLL* rearranged	Most common variant is t(4;11); often presents with very high WBC; confers worse prognosis; rare in adults; common in infant leukemia. HSCT is often required.
t(12;21)(p13;q22); *TEL-AML1*	Common in children (20%-30%); rare in adults; confers improved prognosis with intensive asparaginase
Hyperdiploidy (>50 chromosomes)	Seen in about 25% of children, less in adults; confers favorable prognosis.
Hypodiploidy (<44 chromosomes)	Uncommon; confers worse prognosis.
t(1;19)(q23;p13.3); *TCF3-PBX1*	Incidence approximately 5%; intermediate/favorable in children, intermediate/poor in adults. Benefits from high dose methotrexate.
BCR-ABL1-like	Adverse prognosis. Might benefit from tyrosine kinase inhibitors and/or JAK2 inhibitors
T cell ALL NOTCH1 mutation	More common in adults 60%-70%.

v*, Variable gene partners.
Many of these disorders also have distinct immunophenotypes by flow cytometry. Additional molecular abnormalities of recently defined relevance include mutations of *IKZF1*, which encodes a lymphoid transcription factor IKAROS, is associated with high relapse rates and gene expression profile similar to *BCR-ABL1* translocated disease. Gene expression profiling has identified a subgroup of "Philadelphia chromosome–like" acute lymphoblastic leukemia (ALL) with a gene expression similar to *BCR-ABL1* translocation associated disease, which confers worse prognosis, but which may identify new opportunities for targeted therapies.

TABLE 4   Tumor Lysis Syndrome

Laboratory Tumor Lysis Syndrome[a]
Uric acid: $\geq$8 mg/dl or 476 μmol/L
Potassium: $\geq$6.0 mmol/L
Phosphorus: $\geq$4.5 mg/dl or 1.5 mmol/L (adults), $\geq$6.5 mg/dl or 2.1 mmol (children)
1. Calcium: Corrected[b] Ca^{++} <7.0 mg/dl or 1.75 mmol/L or ionized Ca^{++} <1.12 mg/dl or 0.3 mmol/L, or 25% increase from baseline uric acid, potassium, phosphorus; 25% decrease for calcium
Clinical Tumor Lysis Syndrome
Acute kidney injury
1. Rise in serum creatinine $\geq$0.3 mg/dl (26.5 μmol/L).
2. Any creatinine >1.5 age-appropriate upper limit normal if no baseline available
3. Oliguria defined as urine output <0.5 ml/kg/h for 6 h
Cardiac arrhythmia
Seizure
Symptomatic hypocalcemia (e.g., neuromuscular irritability such as tetany)

[a]Laboratory tumor lysis syndrome present if two or more abnormalities are present within 3 days before or 7 days after therapy.
[b]Corrected calcium is measured calcium (mg/dl) + 0.8 × (4 − measured albumin g/dl).
From Arber DA et al: The 2016 revision to the World Health Organization classification of myeloid neoplasms and acute leukemia, *Blood* 127:2391-2405, 2016.

LABORATORY TESTS

- CBC reveals normochromic, normocytic anemia, thrombocytopenia.
- Peripheral smear will usually reveal lymphoblasts, but in some cases only the marrow is involved.
- Initial blood work should also include assessment for basic organ function (creatinine, bilirubin), blood glucose (glucocorticoids are part of therapy), and spontaneous tumor lysis syndrome (K^+, Ca^{++}, $PO4^{++}$, uric acid).
- Coagulation studies (full disseminated intravascular coagulation [DIC] screen) before lumbar puncture.
- Studies appropriate to identifying and risk-stratifying leukemia as outlined previously.

IMAGING STUDIES

- Chest x-ray to evaluate fever and for the presence of mediastinal mass.
- CT for symptomatic complaints. Be cautious about contrast dye exposure in patients with evidence of spontaneous tumor lysis syndrome to avoid further renal injury.

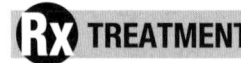 **TREATMENT**

ACUTE GENERAL Rx

- Survival of children with ALL has improved from 10% to 90% in the last 40 yr and is a major success story of modern medical science and research. Adults have fared less well, but cure rates have also improved to about 60% to 70% in standard-risk patients in recent trials. Adults in particular have benefited from tyrosine kinase inhibitor therapy for Ph+ ALL, because this disease is more common in adults and may represent 50% or more of disease in patients over 50.
- **Hyperleukocytic leukemia** (WBC >100,000/mcl) is uncommon in ALL and lymphocyte counts of 100,000 may be well tolerated. Prednisone and vincristine usually offer rapid cytoreduction, and leukapheresis is rarely (but sometimes) required.
- **Tumor lysis syndrome** is common in ALL and was seen in 23% of patients in one large series. It is sometimes spontaneous—that is, present before therapy is given—and is a potential cause of early death. Tumor lysis syndrome is caused by release of intracellular potassium, phosphate, and nucleic acids. The nucleic acids adenosine and guanosine are eventually metabolized to uric acid. Elevated potassium may cause cardiac dysrhythmia and death. Elevated uric acid may cause renal failure through renal urate crystal deposition and possibly other mechanisms. Elevated phosphates cause renal calcium phosphate deposition and kidney injury while also lowering serum calcium, which can cause cardiac dysrhythmia and spasms. Therapy is directed mainly at maintaining renal function through vigorous hydration (3 L normal saline per day if practical, alkalinization not recommended); "forced diuresis" if necessary to

maintain urine output at 2 ml/kg/h; and dialysis if necessary to control K^+, phosphates, or fluid balance. Allopurinol, up to 800 mg/day for adults, 300 to 450 mg/m^2/day for children, is given routinely. Rasburicase is a recombinant urate oxidase that rapidly lowers uric acid levels. The dose is 0.2 mg/kg, and one dose is usually enough. Rasburicase should be avoided in patients with G6PD deficiency. Phosphate binders are of uncertain value but are usually given. Asymptomatic hypocalcemia is not treated to avoid increasing calcium phosphate deposition. Definitions of laboratory and clinical tumor lysis and defined risk categories are outlined in Table 4.

- Numerous protocols have been used for Ph-ALL, and the specific protocol is likely to be determined by institution/physician familiarity and access to clinical trials, among other factors.
- In the 1990s and early 2000s, it was noted that adolescents and young adult (AYA) patients had better outcomes on pediatric trials than on adult trials. Consequently, this group (currently defined as ages 15 to 39) is now often (especially younger AYAs) treated on pediatric protocols by pediatric services or on adult "pediatric inspired" protocols.
- Therapy for Ph-negative ALL generally has four components:
  1. Induction therapy, typically with corticosteroids, cyclophosphamide (some regimens), vincristine, an anthracycline (doxorubicin or daunorubicin usually), and asparaginase. The CD20 directed antibody rituximab has shown benefit in patients with >20% CD20 expression on their blast cells.
  2. Consolidation therapy is high-dose chemotherapy aimed at preventing relapse after remission and commonly consists of cytarabine and methotrexate in combination with other agents.
  3. Maintenance therapy is low-intensity outpatient therapy that is continued for 2 to 3 yr after completion of consolidation. Prednisone, monthly vincristine,

TABLE 5 Risk Factors for Treatment Failure in Recent ALL Trials

t(v*;11q23) *MLL* rearranged

Hypodiploidy

Minimal residual disease after remission or consolidation*

Philadelphia chromosome-like genomic signature (in Ph-ALL)[†]

Early precursor T (ETP) ALL (absent CD1a, CD8, weak CD5, myeloid or stem cell antigen expression)

---

*Measured variously after induction or consolidation therapy.
[†]Standardized testing for this is still in development, but it may have important treatment implications. Note also that many historic risk factors (e.g., T-cell vs B-cell disease) have not been independent risk factors in current trials.
ALL, Acute lymphoblastic leukemia.
From Roberts KG et al: Targetable kinase-activating lesions in Ph-like acute lymphoblastic leukemia, *N Engl J Med* 371(11):1005-1015, 2014.

TABLE 6 Prognostic Factors in Acute Lymphoblastic Leukemia

Factor	Prognosis	Clinical Application
Age		
<1 yr	MLL$^+$ (70%-80% infants) poor outcome; MLL−same outcome as older children	MLL−do well on standard ALL therapy. Potential role for FLT3 inhibitors, proteasome inhibitors, histone deacetylase inhibitors, and hypomethylating agents for MLL$^+$
1-9 yr	Lower (standard) risk	ALL biology may change risk
>9 yr	Higher risk	ALL biology may change risk
WBC		
<50 × 10^9/L in pediatric < 30 x 10^9/L in adults	Lower (standard) risk	ALL biology may change risk
≥50 × 10^9/L in pediatric >30 in B cell ALL or > 100 in T cell ALL	Higher risk	ALL biology may change risk
CNS		
CNS3	Higher risk of CNS and bone marrow relapse	Therapy intensification
CNS2 Traumatic lumbar puncture with blasts	Higher risk of CNS relapse	CNS directed therapy intensification
Testicular	Higher risk	Therapy intensification
Immunophenotype		
T cell	Higher risk	Poor outcome abolished with current therapy
pre-B (cIgM+)	Standard risk	Poor outcome abolished with current therapy
Early pre-B	Standard risk	Genetics may change risk
Early T-cell precursor	Adverse prognosis	Ongoing studies exploring targeted therapies
Ploidy		
>50 (DI >1.16)	Low risk	Good response to antimetabolites
<44	Higher risk	Therapy intensification
Genetic Alterations		
t(9;22)/*BCR-ABL1*	Higher risk	ABL TKI
t(4;11)/*MLL-AF4*	Higher risk	Potential role for FLT3 inhibitors, proteasome inhibitors, histone deacetylase inhibitors, and hypomethylating agents
t(1;19)/*E2A-PBX1*	Higher risk of CNS relapse	Improved outcome with current therapy
t(12;21)/*ETV6-RUNX1*	Low risk	
IKZF1	Poor prognosis. Present in 80% Ph+ and also in Ph-like ALL	Potential role for tyrosine kinase, JAK inhibitors
NUP214-ABL1	High risk	Potential benefits from TKI
CRLF2	In half of Ph-like cases, associated with Hispanic/Latino, poor outcome	Potential role for JAK inhibitors
CREBBP	Associated with drug resistance and relapse	Potential benefit from histone deacetylase inhibitors
MRD		
End of induction <0.01% or negative	Excellent outcome	No benefit from 2nd delayed intensification
Slow early responders	Higher MRD = higher risk of relapse	Benefit from augmented delayed intensification
End of induction ≥0.01%	Poor prognosis	Consider transplantation in first CR
Persistent MRD after end of first consolidation (weeks 12 and 16)	Dismal outcome	Transplantation in first CR

ALL, Acute lymphoblastic leukemia; *CNS*, central nervous system; *CR*, complete remission; *DI*, deoxyribonucleic acid index; *JAK*, Janus kinase; *MLL*, mixed-lineage leukemia; *MRD*, minimal residual disease; *TKI*, tyrosine kinase inhibitor; *WBC*, white blood cell.
From Hoffman R et al: *Hematology: basic principles and practice*, ed 7, Philadelphia, 2018, Elsevier.

TABLE 7 Markers for Poor Prognosis in Adult Acute Lymphoblastic Leukemia

ESTABLISHED RISK FACTORS	
Age	**>60 yr**
Presenting WBC count	>30,000/μL (B-cell ALL); >100,000/μL (T-cell ALL)
Immunophenotype	Pro-B cell; early T cell[a]
Cytogenetics	t(4;11)(q21;q23) and other *MLL* rearrangements
	t(9;22)(q34;q11.2) – Philadelphia chromosome
	Hypodiploidy (<44 chromosomes)
	Complex (>5 abnormalities)
Therapy response	Time to complete remission >4 wk
MRD	≥0.01% at 3-6 mo after initiation of therapy[b]
Emerging Risk Factors	
Immunophenotype	CD20
Molecular	BAALC
	FUS
	ERG
	IKZF1[c]
	Ph-like ALL

[a]Initial report characterizing ETP ALL showed a poor outcome. However, subsequent studies have shown variable association with response to therapy.
[b]Different studies have used different time points for MRD assessment.
[c]Focal deletions in IKZF1 are present in up to 70% of Ph-like ALL. However, IKZF1 deletions are associated with adverse outcome irrespective of association with Ph-like phenotype.
ALL, Acute lymphoblastic leukemia; *ETP,* early T-cell precursor; *MRD,* minimal residual disease; *Ph,* Philadelphia chromosome; *WBC,* white blood cell.
From Hoffman R et al: *Hematolog: basic principles and practice,* ed 7, Philadelphia, 2018, Elsevier.

methotrexate, and oral 6-mercaptopurine (POMP regimen) are commonly used.

4. CNS prophylaxis is universal and is usually done with intrathecal therapy (methotrexate alone or in combination with cytarabine and hydrocortisone) administered by lumbar puncture or an Ommaya reservoir. Due to increased toxicity, cranial radiotherapy is reserved for patients with high-risk features, such as active CNS disease at diagnosis.

- Allogeneic bone marrow transplant in first remission of ALL is controversial because of improving results with current nontransplant therapies. It is usually recommended for patients in whom the likelihood of cure is considered less than 50% to 60% with chemotherapy alone, depending on age and donor availability. Autologous bone marrow transplant is rarely used in Ph-ALL. In 2008, the final results of the MRC/UKALL XII/ECOG E2993 study were published. This study evaluated the relative safety and efficacy of chemotherapy, and autologous and allogeneic transplant after first complete remission (CR) in Ph− patients. This was a randomized trial of 1826 patients with newly diagnosed ALL. Patients who had a matched related donor were offered an allogeneic transplant. Patients without a donor were further randomized to an autologous transplant or chemotherapy and maintenance. The key conclusions of this study were:
  1. Allogeneic transplant in first CR is associated with lower relapse rates versus autologous transplant or chemotherapy/

maintenance therapy alone in Ph− patients.
  2. Allogeneic transplant in first CR improved overall survival in standard risk patients. There was a lower risk of relapse in both standard and high-risk patients. There was high treatment-related mortality in high-risk older patients. The increased mortality offsets the benefit of lower relapse risk for the patient group.

- The findings did not support autologous transplant as replacement therapy in any ALL group.
- Risk factors for treatment failure in recent protocols are outlined in Table 5. Prognostic factors in ALL are summarized in Tables 6 and 7.
- Therapy of Ph+ ALL consists of a tyrosine kinase inhibitor—imatinib, dasatinib, nilotinib, ponatinib have been used—with chemotherapy.
  1. 2-yr survival rates are reported at 50% to 65%, with various regimens.
  2. Low-intensity induction chemotherapy with dasatinib and prednisone or imatinib, vincristine, and prednisone have resulted in remission rates of 100% and 98% and may allow for less toxicity and hospitalization at diagnosis.
  3. Allogeneic bone marrow transplant is commonly used as consolidative therapy if available but has become more controversial. Maintenance therapy with tyrosine kinase inhibitor is usually given after BMT or non-BMT therapy.
- Therapy of relapsed disease:

1. Allogeneic bone marrow transplant is offered for relapsed disease, but relapse after BMT is common, and long-term cure rates have been low at about 20%.
2. In 2017, the FDA approved three new therapies for relapsed ALL: Chimeric antigen receptor T-cell (CAR-T) therapy, a form of targeted immunotherapy, yielded a remission rate of 90% in pediatric and young adult (<26 yr) patients with relapsed B-cell ALL. Chimeric antigen T-cells are created by harvesting the patient's T cells, then transfecting them with lentivirus vector that inserts DNA expressing an anti-CD19 domain (the target antigen on B cells) coupled to a T-cell receptor. The T cells expressing the chimeric anti-CD19/T-cell receptor specifically target CD19-expressing B cells. The CAR-T cell population is then expanded ex vivo and reinfused to the patient. About 70% of remissions were durable at 6 mo. The main side effect is cytokine release syndrome (CRS) associated with "vascular leak," hypotension, respiratory and renal insufficiency, and coagulopathy. CRS is treated with tocilizumab and anti-IL6 receptor blocking antibody. CAR-T cells for ALL have been given the generic designation tisagenlecleucel (trade name Kymriah). It currently costs $475,000 and is available at centers certified for its use.
3. In October 2021, the FDA granted approval for another CD-19 directed CART brexucabtagene autoleucel (trade name Tecartus) for treatment of adult patients (≥18 yr) with relapsed or refractory B- cell ALL. This was based on a single arm multicenter trial (ZUMA-3) where out of 54 patients who were evaluated for efficacy, 28 achieved CR within 3 months. The duration of complete response was estimated to exceed 12 mo for more than half of the patients. CRS occurred in 92% of patients and neurotoxicity in 87%.
4. Blinatumomab is a bispecific antibody that binds CD19 and CD3, redirecting T cells to leukemia cells. It was FDA-approved for relapsed ALL, including Ph+ ALL, in adults and children. Blinatumomab is administered as a continuous infusion for 4 wk (9 μg/day wk 1, 28 μg/day thereafter), with maintenance therapy for 4 wk every 12 wk. In a large phase III trial, the remission rate was 44% (vs. 25% with chemotherapy), a small number durable. In a smaller phase II trial for Ph+ ALL, the remission rate was 36%. A small number of blinatumomab responses have been durable. Blinatumomab can also be associated with cytokine release syndrome.

- Inotuzumab ozogamicin (IO) is an antibody drug conjugate in which chemotherapeutic agent calicheamicin is bound to an anti-CD22 antibody. In a large phase III trial, the remission rate was 81% vs. 33% for standard chemotherapy, with a median duration of 4.6 mo. Approximately 40% of IO patients were successfully bridged to transplant vs. 10% with chemotherapy. A small number of responses were durable.

- Survivorship:
  1. Survivors of childhood and adult ALL are increasingly being seen in primary care practices; as of 2006 there were estimated >50,000 survivors, likely increasing by about 2000+/yr.
  2. Long-term complications of ALL therapy include secondary malignancy from chemotherapy (usually in first 5 to 10 yr) or from radiation: If given, no plateau in risk, congestive heart failure from anthracycline therapy (often manifesting 20 to 30 yr after treatment), osteopenia and avascular necrosis from glucocorticoid therapy, obesity, and neurocognitive defects. Key recommendations include the following:
     a. Echocardiography every 3 to 5 yr for asymptomatic congestive heart failure, more often if anthracycline exposure was >250 to 300 mg/m^2, because asymptomatic congestive heart failure may warrant therapy. This may show up decades after therapy.
     b. Screening for malignancy and endocrinopathies in pertinent radiation fields.
     c. Attention to the increased risk of obesity and metabolic derangement in survivors.
     d. Recent reviews (see references) summarizing current recommendations and guidelines are accessible online (http://www.survivorshipguidelines.org/pdf/LTFUGuidelines_40.pdf).

REFERENCE & SUGGESTED READINGS

Available at eBooks.Health.Elsevier.com.

RELATED CONTENT

Acute Lymphocytic Leukemia (ALL) (Patient Information)
Tumor Lysis Syndrome (Related Key Topic)

AUTHOR: **KAPIL S. MELEVEEDU, MD**

A

Diseases and Disorders

I

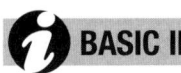

BASIC INFORMATION

DEFINITION

Acute mesenteric ischemia (AMI) is the sudden onset of intestinal hypoperfusion to all or part of the small bowel caused by emboli, arterial or venous thrombosis, vasoconstriction from low-flow states, or arterial vasospasm that ultimately leads to ischemia and secondary inflammatory changes.

SYNONYMS

AMI
Mesenteric ischemia, acute

ICD-10CM CODE
K55.0 Acute vascular disorders of intestine

EPIDEMIOLOGY & DEMOGRAPHICS

INCIDENCE:
- Accounts for 0.09% to 0.2% of all acute admissions to emergency departments.[1]
- Mortality ranges between 50% and 80%.[1]
- The incidence appears to be increasing. Factors for this include increased awareness among clinicians, improved diagnostic modalities, the aging of the population, and improved intensive care leading to longer survival of sicker patients.

PREDOMINANT SEX & AGE:
- AMI caused by arterial embolism or thrombosis occurs more frequently in the elderly.
- AMI due to mesenteric venous thrombosis often presents in younger age groups.

RISK FACTORS:
- Advanced age, atherosclerosis, low cardiac output (especially atrial fibrillation), severe cardiac valvular disease, intraabdominal malignancy.
- In the subgroup of cases caused by venous thrombosis, risk factors include hypercoagulable states, portal hypertension, abdominal infection, blunt trauma, pancreatitis, and portal malignancy.
- Additional risk factors for AMI caused by nonocclusive mesenteric ischemia include recent cardiac or aortic surgery, dialysis, hypovolemia, and vasoconstrictive medications (including illicit drugs such as cocaine).
- Table 1 summarizes risk factors for ischemic bowel disease.
- AMI may also occur rarely in patients with no identifiable risk factors.

GENETICS: No specific genetic predisposition but may be related to underlying factors such as cardiac disease, atherosclerosis, and hypercoagulable states.

PHYSICAL FINDINGS & CLINICAL PRESENTATION

- The classic presentation is rapid onset of severe periumbilical pain "out of proportion to physical examination findings," often followed by nausea/vomiting, diarrhea, and/or blood per rectum.[2]
- Approximately one third of patients present with the triad of abdominal pain, fever, and hemoccult-positive stools. Nausea and vomiting are commonly associated.

- Generally, patients with mesenteric venous thrombosis tend to present with less abrupt onset of abdominal pain than those with acute arterial occlusion.
- Initial abdominal examination may be normal, with no rebound or guarding, or may include minimal distention or stool positive for occult blood. An epigastric bruit may be present in some patients.
- Later in the disease course the patient may present with septic shock, gross abdominal distention, absence of bowel sounds, and peritoneal signs. In the elderly, mental status changes may occur.

- If the physical examination demonstrates signs of peritonitis, there is likely irreversible intestinal ischemia with bowel necrosis.

ETIOLOGY

Conventionally, AMI is stratified into four groups by etiology: Arterial embolism, arterial thrombosis, venous thrombosis, and nonocclusive mesenteric ischemia (NOMI). The pathophysiology behind these different etiologies is summarized in Table 2. Causes and approximate frequencies of AMI are summarized in Table 3. The pathophysiologic mechanisms that cause AMI include:

TABLE 1 Risk Factors for Ischemic Bowel Diseases*

Risk Factor	Arterial Thrombosis	Embolus	Mesenteric Vein Thrombosis	Nonobstructive Mesenteric Ischemia
Advanced age	+	+	+	+
Atherosclerosis	+			
Aortic dissection	+			
Low cardiac output	+	+		+
Congestive heart failure				+
Shock				+
Severe dehydration	+		+	
Cardiac arrhythmias, especially atrial fibrillation		+		+
Severe cardiac valvular disease		+		
Recent myocardial infarction	+			+
Intraabdominal malignancy			+	
Abdominal trauma			+	
Intraabdominal infection			+	
Intraabdominal inflammatory conditions			+	
Parasitic infection (ascariasis)			+	
Hypercoagulable states (venous thrombosis)			+	
Sickle cell anemia			+	
Recent cardiac surgery	+	+		+
Recent abdominal surgery			+	
Vascular aortic prosthetic grafts proximal to the superior mesenteric artery		+		
Hemodialysis				+
Vasculitis	+		+	
Pregnancy			+	
Decompression sickness			+	
Blast lung caused by systemic air embolism		+		
Drugs that cause constriction:				
• Digitalis				+
• Cocaine				+
• Amphetamines				+
• Pseudoephedrine				+
• Vasopressin			+[†]	+
Estrogen therapy			+	

*A plus sign (+) indicates that the factor is a risk for the disease subtype.
[†]Especially after sclerotherapy.
From Adams JG et al: *Emergency medicine: clinical essentials,* ed 2, Philadelphia, 2013, Elsevier.

TABLE 2 Pathophysiology of the Four Different Causes of Acute Mesenteric Ischemia (AMI)

Cause	Pathophysiology
Embolism	• Often in patients with atrial fibrillation • Emboli lodge 3-10 cm distal to origin of SMA, often past branching of middle colic artery • Proximal mid-jejunum is spared
Thrombosis	• Typically these patients have a history of symptomatic stenosis of mesenteric arteries • Any clinical scenario that leads to low flow or hypotension can result in acute-on-chronic arterial thrombosis • Affects the orifice of the SMA • Flush occlusion of the SMA and the entire middle gut is involved during the initial presentation
Nonocclusive	• Low flow state resulting from any type of shock or the use of vasoconstrictors • The entire bowel may be involved
Mesenteric venous thrombosis	• Thrombosis of the veins draining the intestines; SMV, IMV, splenic and portal veins among hypercoagulable patients with cancer or hypercoagulable state • Decreased venous outflow, bowel edema, distention, and decreased mesenteric perfusion

IMV, Inferior mesenteric vein; *SMA,* superior mesenteric artery; *SMV,* superior mesenteric vein.
Modified from Cameron JL, Cameron AM: *Current surgical therapy,* ed 12, Philadelphia, 2017, Elsevier.

TABLE 3 Causes and Approximate Frequencies of Acute Mesenteric Ischemia

Cause	Frequency (%)
SMA thrombosis	54-68
SMA embolus	26-32
Nonocclusive mesenteric ischemia	10
Mesenteric venous thrombosis	5
Focal segmental ischemia of the small intestine	5

SMA, Superior mesenteric artery.
From Feldman M et al: *Sleisenger and Fordtran's gastrointestinal and liver disease,* ed 10, Philadelphia, 2016, Elsevier.

- Mesenteric arterial embolism (40% to 50% of cases of AMI) typically arises from a cardiac source: Left atrium associated with cardiac dysrhythmias such as atrial fibrillation, left ventricle with global myocardial dysfunction associated with poor ejection fraction, or cardiac valves due to endocarditis. The superior mesenteric artery (SMA) is most commonly affected because of its relatively large diameter and low takeoff angle from the aorta.[2]
- Mesenteric arterial thrombosis (20% to 35% of cases of AMI) is often seen in patients with prior progressive atherosclerotic stenosis, with superimposed abdominal trauma or infection. Many of these patients have a history consistent with chronic mesenteric ischemia, including postprandial pain, weight loss, or "food fear."[2]
- Nonocclusive mesenteric ischemia (20% of cases of AMI) is usually a consequence of SMA vasoconstriction associated with low splanchnic blood flow as seen with hypotension, hypovolemia, vasoconstricting drugs, and hemodialysis. Interestingly, NOMI is the most common mechanism of ischemia seen in COVID-19—related AMI.[3]
- Mesenteric venous thrombosis (<10% of cases of AMI) may occur in the setting of hypercoagulable states (acquired or inherited), blunt trauma, abdominal infection, portal hypertension, pancreatitis, and portal malignancy. Other risk factors include intraabdominal sepsis, smoking, oral contraceptives, and liver cirrhosis. In these situations, the consequences of bowel edema and increased vascular resistance secondary to venous thrombosis result in reduced arterial blood flow, leading to bowel ischemia.
- Dissection or inflammation of the mesenteric artery accounts for less than 5% of cases of AMI.

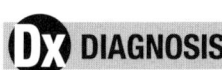 **DIAGNOSIS**

DIFFERENTIAL DIAGNOSIS

Initially include other causes of acute-onset abdominal pain, including perforated peptic ulcer, acute pancreatitis, and early appendicitis, as well as the varied causes of peritonitis.

WORKUP

- Early diagnosis is key, and the key to early diagnosis is a high level of clinical suspicion.
- Treatment success is related to the duration of symptoms before diagnosis. Consider early laparotomy for diagnosis in cases with a high index of suspicion when imaging is not readily available.

LABORATORY TESTS

- Classically, patients with AMI have leukocytosis, metabolic acidosis, elevated D-dimer, and elevated serum lactate[2]; however, these laboratory test results are nonspecific, especially early in the course. Elevated lactic acid, leukocytosis, and elevated hematocrit from hemoconcentration can occur later in the course, often after progression to bowel necrosis has occurred, hence are not useful for early diagnosis.
- D-Dimer has been reported to be an independent risk factor of intestinal ischemia, reflecting ongoing clot formation and endogenous degradation via fibrinolysis. Normal D-dimer testing may help rule out AMI while elevated levels are nonspecific.
- Serum lactate >2 mmol/L is correlated with irreversible transmural intestinal necrosis.[4]
- When a hypercoagulable state is suspected, workup may include proteins C and S, antithrombin III, and factor V Leiden. This will likely not affect the diagnosis of AMI but may help guide long-term therapy.
- Amylase levels may be elevated in up to 50% of individuals with intestinal ischemia; phosphate levels may be elevated in up to 80% of affected individuals.

IMAGING STUDIES

- Contrast-enhanced computed tomography (CT) has replaced conventional angiography as the gold standard imaging modality in AMI.[5] It is more readily available and has similar sensitivity to angiography, the prior gold standard test. Computed tomographic angiography (CTA) has 95% to 100% accuracy for the diagnosis of visceral ischemic syndromes and is also useful in detecting potential sources of emboli and other pathologic processes.
- Plain CT findings are nonspecific and more often found late in the course. Portal venous gas or intramural gas may be seen after the development of gangrene (Fig. E1). In many cases, CT findings remain nonspecific even at advanced stages.
- Gadolinium-enhanced MRI can be used to detect proximal obstruction of the SMA and celiac axis, but it has less value in the evaluation of distal arterial occlusions and other intestinal findings in AMI. Magnetic resonance angiography (MRA) may be more useful in cases of mesenteric vein thrombosis causing AMI. It has also been found useful in monitoring the progress of patients with superior mesenteric venous thrombosis who are treated nonsurgically. MRA, however, takes longer than CTA to perform and can overestimate the degree of stenosis.
- Plain x-rays are not useful in AMI; plain films are normal 25% of the time in early stages. Suggestive findings may include ileus (Fig. E2), bowel wall thickening, or intramural gas. Gas in the portal veins is a sign of extensive intestinal pneumatosis and implies that bowel necrosis has developed. Free air under the diaphragm may support early surgical intervention before further radiologic evaluation.
- Ultrasound is not recommended in AMI if CT is available. Doppler ultrasound evaluation of intestinal blood flow is time consuming and is often limited by the presence of air-filled loops of bowel, body habitus, or recent intraabdominal surgery.
- Angiography may be considered if the diagnosis remains unclear after CT or MRI.

TREATMENT

- The goal of treatment is to restore blood flow to ischemic bowel as rapidly as possible (Fig. E3) before the occurrence of infarction.
- Treatment varies depending on specific etiology.

Acute Mesenteric Ischemia

NONPHARMACOLOGIC THERAPY

- Specific management will depend on patient status and most likely etiology of the ischemia. Signs of peritonitis mandate early laparotomy and resection of infarcted bowel.
- When workup is positive for major SMA embolus, embolectomy is considered standard treatment in the absence of peritoneal signs. Depending on the location and degree of occlusion of the embolus, surgical revascularization, intraarterial infusion of thrombolytics or vasodilators, or systemic anticoagulation may be considered.
- In cases of SMA thrombosis, emergency surgical revascularization is the treatment of choice. Stent placement may be a viable alternative.
- Management of NOMI is based on treatment of the underlying precipitating cause. Fluid resuscitation, optimization of cardiac output, and elimination of vasopressors remain important primary measures. Additional treatment may include systemic anticoagulation and the use of catheter-directed infusion of vasodilatory and antispasmodic agents, most commonly papaverine hydrochloride.
- Two-dimensional perfusion angiography is a new modality that can assess blood flow and tissue perfusion after use of selective intraarterial vasodilator therapy (such as prostaglandin E1 or papaverine) in the treatment of NOMI.[6]
- In patients with mesenteric vein thrombosis, treatment depends on the presence or absence of peritoneal signs. Laparotomy and resection of infarcted bowel is indicated in more advanced cases. If there are no peritoneal signs, immediate anticoagulant therapy with heparin, and ultimately warfarin, may be adequate treatment.
- In general, percutaneous treatment with lytic therapy, balloon angioplasty, or stenting may be limited by the frequent presence of nonviable bowel, which would require laparotomy despite success with percutaneous treatment.

- A "second look" procedure is indicated in most patients, 24 to 48 hours after initial revascularization.

ACUTE GENERAL Rx

- Initial management should include hemodynamic monitoring and support, including fluid resuscitation with crystalloid and blood products, correction of acidosis, pain control (using parenteral opioids), administration of broad-spectrum antibiotics to cover gram-negative and anaerobic organisms, and gastric decompression by nasogastric tube.[1,2]
- Vasopressors should be used with caution and only to avoid fluid overload and abdominal compartment syndrome. Dobutamine, low-dose dopamine, and milrinone to improve cardiac function have been shown to have less impact on mesenteric blood flow.
- In the absence of active bleeding, the use of systemic anticoagulation is usually indicated. The optimal timing of initiation is unclear.

CHRONIC Rx

Patients should be followed up in an outpatient clinical setting at regular intervals.
- Patients who receive endovascular treatment should be managed with 3 to 6 mo of clopidogrel; additionally, periodic surveillance for restenosis with duplex ultrasound or CTA is indicated.
- In the subgroup of patients with mesenteric venous thrombosis, prevention of further thrombosis is indicated. The optimal duration of anticoagulation is unclear.

DISPOSITION

- Prognosis is best in AMI due to mesenteric venous thrombosis and after surgical treatment for acute arterial embolism. It remains poor in cases of arterial thrombosis and non-occlusive ischemia.
- With delayed diagnosis, intestinal infarction—resulting in perforation or gangrenous bowel, sepsis, shock, and death—is typical.

REFERRAL

- Early surgical consultation should be considered. There should be no delay in patients with peritoneal signs.
- Surgery may also be warranted for diagnostic purposes.

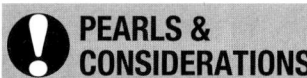 **PEARLS & CONSIDERATIONS**

COMMENTS

- The diagnosis of AMI should be considered in any patient with acute onset of abdominal pain out of proportion to physical findings, particularly in at-risk patients.
- Early diagnosis, before intestinal infarction occurs, is critical and correlates with improved survival rates.
- The use of endovascular procedures for AMI is becoming more common and may be most appropriate for patients with ischemia that is not severe, and for those who have severe coexisting conditions that place them at high risk for complications and death associated with open surgery.

PREVENTION

Prevention of underlying factors, most notably atherosclerotic disease (smoking cessation, management of hypertension, and use of statins) is indicated for primary prevention as well as prevention of recurrence.

REFERENCES & SUGGESTED READINGS

Available at eBooks.Health.Elsevier.com.

RELATED CONTENT

Mesenteric Venous Thrombosis (Related Key Topic)

AUTHORS: **SIMRAN GUPTA, MD,** and **SARAH HYDER, MD, MBA**

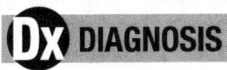

A

BASIC INFORMATION

DEFINITION

Acute myeloid leukemia (AML) is a malignancy of hematopoietic progenitor cells that would normally give rise to mature granulocytes. Strictly speaking, AML is a subset of acute non-lymphocytic leukemia (ANLL), a designation that broadly distinguishes these diseases from the biologically distinct leukemias of lymphocytic origin. ANLL includes leukemias involving the spectrum of myeloid stem cells, including precursors of granulocytes, monocytes, erythrocytes, and megakaryocytes. Acute promyelocytic leukemia is a distinct leukemia syndrome that is part of the ANLL spectrum, but that has very different treatment implications. ANLL is characterized by maturation failure of myeloid progenitors, excessive numbers of immature progenitors ("blasts"), and various degrees of bone marrow failure (neutropenia, thrombocytopenia, anemia).

SYNONYMS

Acute nonlymphocytic leukemia (ANLL)
Acute myelogenous leukemia
AML

ICD-10CM CODES
C92.60	Acute myeloid leukemia with 11q23-abnormality not having achieved remission
C92.61	Acute myeloid leukemia with 11q23-abnormality in remission
C92.62	Acute myeloid leukemia with 11q23-abnormality in relapse
C92.90	Myeloid leukemia, unspecified, not having achieved remission
C92.91	Myeloid leukemia, unspecified in remission
C92.92	Myeloid leukemia, unspecified in relapse
C92.A0	Acute myeloid leukemia with multilineage dysplasia, not having achieved remission
C92.A1	Acute myeloid leukemia with multilineage dysplasia, in remission
C92.A2	Acute myeloid leukemia with multilineage dysplasia, in relapse
C92.Z0	Other myeloid leukemia not having achieved remission
C92.Z1	Other myeloid leukemia, in remission
C92.Z2	Other myeloid leukemia, in relapse
C92.00	Acute myeloblastic leukemia, not having achieved remission
C92.01	Acute myeloblastic leukemia, in remission
C92.02	Acute myeloblastic leukemia, in relapse

EPIDEMIOLOGY & DEMOGRAPHICS

- AML incidence rises with age:
  1. Incidence 20 to 55 yr old: 1 to 3/100,000 persons/yr
  2. Incidence 65 to 80 yr old: 11 to 20/100,000 persons/yr, a 10-fold increase.
  3. Median age at diagnosis is 68 yr (Surveillance, Epidemiology, and End Results [SEER] 2015 to 2019)
- Annual incidence is 4 cases/100,000 persons/yr
- Males slightly > females; European ancestry slightly > African ancestry

PHYSICAL FINDINGS & CLINICAL PRESENTATION

Symptoms/examination findings:
- Complications of bone marrow failure:
  1. Thrombocytopenia-associated bleeding
  2. Fatigue and shortness of breath associated with anemia
  3. Infection(s) associated with neutropenia
- Complications of leukocytosis (hyperleukocytic leukemia, white blood count [WBC] >100,000/mcl):
  1. Retinal hemorrhage with visual symptoms (blurred vision, diplopia)
  2. Intracranial bleeding (headache, somnolence, confusion, delirium, paralysis)
  3. Respiratory symptoms (dyspnea, tachypnea, hypoxia) from pulmonary involvement
  4. Organ ischemia causing cerebral vascular accident, myocardial infarction, priapism
- Systemic symptoms: Fatigue, fever (usually infectious, rarely tumor), bone pain (more common in ALL).
- Hemorrhagic complications of disseminated intravascular coagulation (DIC), especially with acute promyelocytic leukemia (APML).
- Physical examination will reflect consequences of cytopenias (bruising from thrombocytopenia, pallor from anemia) or hyperleukocytosis (papilledema). Enlarged lymph nodes and enlarged liver and spleen are rare. Examination is often normal.
- Rarely disease will present as "extramedullary" with skin lesions (leukemia cutis, blastic plasmacytoid dendritic cell neoplasm [BPDCN]) or soft tissue lesions (granulocytic sarcoma).
- Gum hypertrophy and organ/skin involvement is more common in monocytic leukemia.

ETIOLOGY

- Environmental/exposure related: Benzene (best documented), organic solvents (including gasoline), cigarette smoking (≥20 pack-yr 1.34 relative risk), obesity, best documented in women
- Hereditary disorders: Numerous, including bone marrow failure syndromes (Fanconi anemia, Bloom syndrome, Shwachman Diamond syndrome, Diamond Blackfan anemia), genetic disorders (e.g., Down syndrome), familial AML (e.g., DDX41, RUNX1, GATA2 gene mutations) among others
- Therapy related: This is the most common cause accounting for 10% to 20% of cases
  1. Alkylator (e.g., melphalan, busulfan, cisplatin) related: Typical latency 5 to 7 yr, associated with chromosome 5 and 7 abnormalities and/or mutation in TP53
  2. Topoisomerase II inhibitor (e.g., etoposide, doxorubicin): Typical latency 1 to 3 yr, associated with 11q23 (mixed lineage leukemia [MLL] gene) rearrangements
- Radiation exposures (therapeutic—generally low risk), occupational
- Antecedent hematologic disorders: Myelodysplasia, myeloproliferative disorders, aplastic anemia
- Another increasingly recognized condition is clonal hematopoiesis of indeterminate potential (CHIP), which can predispose to the development of AML many years later

DIAGNOSIS

DIFFERENTIAL DIAGNOSIS

- Disorders that can present with circulating blasts or cells with blast-like appearance:
  1. Acute myeloid leukemia/acute lymphocytic leukemia
  2. Myelodysplasia (up to 20% circulating blasts, if ≥20% = AML)
  3. Primary myelofibrosis
  4. Chronic myeloid leukemia
  5. Blastoid variant of mantle cell lymphoma
  6. Prolymphocytic leukemia
  7. Blastic plasmacytoid dendritic cell neoplasm/BPDCN
  8. Atypical lymphocytes of Epstein-Barr and cytomegalovirus infection may have blast-like appearance

WORKUP

The diagnostic workup consists of a morphologic assessment, immunophenotyping by flow cytometry, assessment of karyotype, and a panel of gene mutations (Fig. 1).

LABORATORY TESTS

- CBC and blood smear evaluation. Note that morphologic evaluation of blasts may suggest myeloid or lymphoid origin, but flow cytometry or cytochemistries (often faster) are needed to confirm. Auer rods are seen in blasts of myeloid origin.
- Lactate dehydrogenase (LDH) is commonly elevated. Other biochemistries to assess organ function (creatinine, liver enzymes) and spontaneous tumor lysis syndrome (TLS) (uric acid, potassium, phosphate, calcium).
- Vitamin B_{12} and folate levels oftentimes are low due to rapid cell turnover and require replacements.
- Coagulation studies (prothrombin time, activated partial thromboplastin time, fibrinogen) to assess DIC. DIC is always present in APML but can be present in all forms of acute leukemia, especially acute monocytic leukemia.
- Human leukocyte antigen (HLA) typing for possible bone marrow transplant and platelet support.
- Cytochemical stains:
  1. Myeloperoxidase can be performed in minutes, + in myeloid origin leukemia.
  2. Alpha naphthyl acetate esterase ("nonspecific esterase") stains mainly monocytic cells.
- Flow cytometry on blood and/or bone marrow (see Table 1).
- Cytogenetic studies, ideally on bone marrow, but can be done on peripheral blood. Fluorescence in situ hybridization (FISH) is often used as an adjunct to conventional chromosome analysis.
- Next-generation sequencing (NGS) by polymerase chain reaction (PCR) to detect specific prognostic gene mutations.
- Molecular studies to further stratify risk and prognosis, which may affect treatment choices

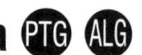
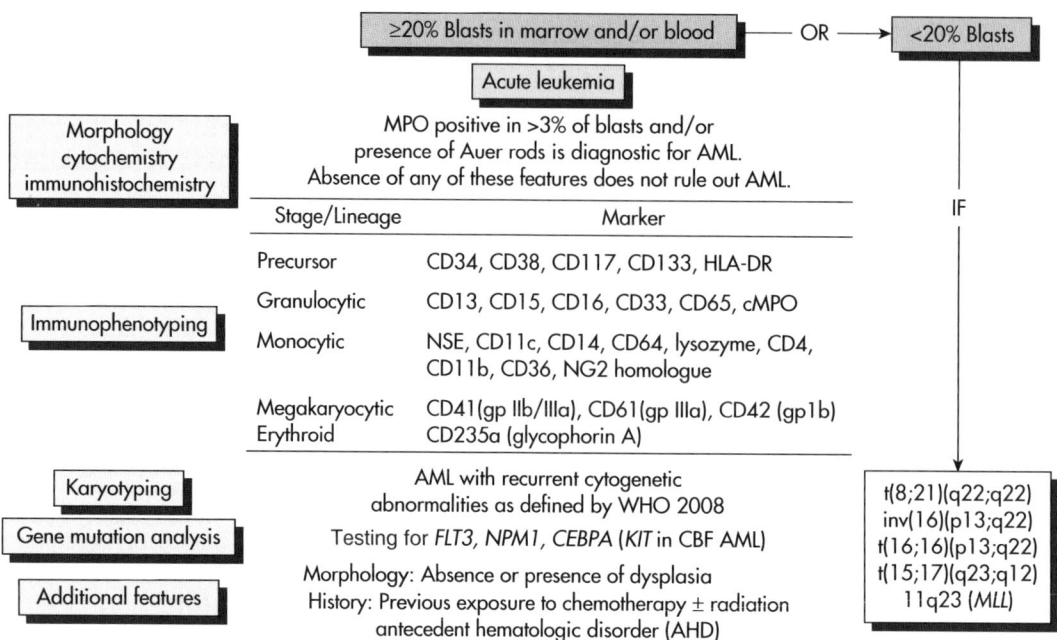

FIG. 1 Workup of acute myeloid leukemia. The diagnostic workup consists of a morphologic assessment, immunophenotyping by flow cytometry, assessment of the karyotype, and a panel of gene mutations. Whereas morphologic assessment by itself is often not sufficient to render a diagnosis, flow cytometry will confirm the lineage assignment (myeloid vs. lymphoid) and stage of differentiation in more than 95% of cases. In the remainder, either no lineage-specific antigens are expressed (acute undifferentiated leukemia) or antigens of more than one lineage are present (mixed-phenotype acute leukemia). In the latter scenario, antigens of several lineages can be found on one (biphenotypic) or separate populations of blasts (bilineal). Karyotyping and gene mutation analysis may add diagnostic information in morphologically ambiguous situations but is otherwise of more interest in determining prognosis. Additional information (exposure to previous chemotherapy and/or radiation therapy, history of an antecedent hematologic disorder, dysplasia) forms the basis for the 2008 revision of the WHO classification of AML. *AML,* acute myeloid leukemia; *ANLL,* acute nonlymphocytic leukemia; *CBF,* core-binding factor; *HLA-DR,* human leukocyte antigen-DR isotope; *MPO,* myeloperoxidase; *NSE,* nonspecific esterase; *WHO,* World Health Organization. (From Hoffman R et al: *Hematology: basic principles and practice,* ed 7, Philadelphia, 2018, Elsevier.)

TABLE 1 Flow Cytometry Markers Used for Diagnosis of ANLL

Precursor stage	CD34, CD117, CD13, CD133, HLA-DR
Granulocytic (myeloid) markers	CD65, cytoplasmic myeloperoxidase
Monocytic markers	CD14, CD36, CD64
Megakaryocytic markers	CD41 (glycoprotein IIb/IIIa), CD61 (glycoprotein IIIa)
Erythroid markers	CD235 (glycophorin A), CD36

ANLL, Acute nonlymphocytic leukemia.
Adapted from Doehner H et al: Diagnosis and management of acute myeloid leukemia in adults, recommendations from an international expert panel, on behalf of the European Leukemia Net, *Blood* 129(4):424-447, 2017.

TABLE 2 Significance of Molecular Abnormalities in Cytogenetically Normal Patients With AML

Molecular Profile	Patients	4-yr Overall Survival
Mutant *CEBPA*	67	62%
Mutant *NPM,* without *FLT-3 ITD*	150	60%
FLT-3 ITD present	164	24%
FLT-3 ITD absent, wild type *NPM,* wild type *CEBPA* (triple negative leukemia)	69	33%

AML, Acute myeloid leukemia; *CEBPA,* CCAAT/enhancer binding protein α gene; *FLT-3 ITD,* FMS-related tyrosine kinase gene internal tandem duplication; *NPM,* nucleophosmin gene. Improved prognosis in patients with *CEBPA* mutations is limited to patients who lack FLT-3 ITD and have biallelic mutations. *CEBPA* mutations are seen in approximately 6%-10% of AML cases, *NPM* mutations in 25%-35% (more common in cytogenetically normal cases) and FLT-3 ITD in approximately 20%-30% of cases.
The updated 2018 NCCN guidelines for AML risk stratification contain favorable, intermediate, and poor risk categories. Molecular abnormalities now included in this updated version in addition to *NPM1, FLT3-ITD,* and biallelic *CEBPA* mutation include TP53 mutation, mutated RUNX1, and mutated ASXL1. Molecular abnormalities validation and prognostication is a rapidly evolving field, and risk stratification should be modified on the continuous evaluation of research data. See the NCCN Guidelines Version 3.2018 AML Risk stratification for specific details.
Data from Schlenk RF et al: Mutations and treatment outcome in cytogenetically normal acute myeloid leukemia, *N Engl J Med* 358:1909-1918, 2008; and Green CL et al: Prognostic significance of *CEBPA* mutations in a large cohort of younger adult patients with acute myeloid leukemia: impact of double *CEBPA* mutations and the interaction with *FLT3* and *NPM1* mutations, *J Clin Oncol* 28:2739-2747, 2010.

(see Tables 2, 3, and 4). Directing this workup should be done with combined hematology and laboratory expertise and typically will consist of studies for fms-related tyrosine kinase gene *(FLT3)* mutations, nucleophosmin gene *(NPM)* mutations, isocitrate dehydrogenase *(IDH 1* and *2)* mutations and CCAAT/enhancer binding protein α gene *(CEBPA)* mutations. Wider molecular panels are increasingly common because of the increasing numbers of potential markers and the potential availability of targeted therapies for *FLT3* mutated disease and those with *IDH* mutations, among others. Table E5 summarizes common recurrent mutations in adult acute myeloid leukemia.

- Formal diagnosis of acute nonlymphocytic leukemia is established if the marrow or peripheral blood blast percentage is ≥20%, unless t (8;21), inv(16), t(16;16) or t(15;17) are present, in which case AML can be diagnosed regardless of the percentage of blasts. Newer WHO classification has additional, albeit rare AML defining recurrent cytogenetics.
  1. Myeloperoxidase (MPO) staining of 3% of blasts establishes myeloid lineage, but MPO may be negative in some AML cases diagnosed by flow cytometry.
  2. Specific criteria exist for diagnosing other forms of ANLL, mainly to distinguish it from myelodysplasia. The WHO AML classification is outlined in Table 6.
  3. Bone marrow findings are described in Fig. E2.

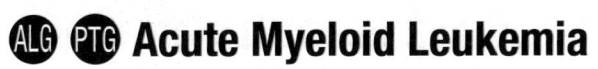

TABLE 3 European LeukemiaNet AML Risk Classification

Genetic Group	Subsets
Favorable	t(8;21)(q22;q22); *RUNX1-RUNX1T1*
	inv(16)(p13.1q22) or t(16;16)(p13.1;q22); *CBFB-MYH11*
	Mutated *NPM1* without *FLT3*-ITD (normal karyotype)
	Mutated *CEBPA* (normal karyotype)
Intermediate-[a] Intermediate	Mutated *NPM1* and *FLT3*-ITD (normal karyotype)
	Wild-type *NPM1* and *FLT3*-ITD (normal karyotype)
	Wild-type *NPM1* without *FLT3*-ITD (normal karyotype)
	t(9;11)(p22;q23); *MLLT3-MLL*
	Cytogenetic abnormalities not classified as favorable or adverse[b]
Adverse	inv(3)(q21q26.2) or t(3;3)(q21;q26.2); *RPN1-EVI1*
	t(6;9)(p23;q34); *DEK-NUP214*
	t(v;11)(v;q23); *MLL* rearranged
	t(9;22)(q34.1;q11.2); *BCR-ABL1*
	Mutated RUNX1, ASXL1 or TP53
	−5 or del(5q); −7; abnl(17p); complex karyotype[c]

[a]Includes all AMLs with normal karyotype except for those included in the favorable subgroup; most of these cases are associated with poor prognosis.
[b]For most abnormalities, adequate numbers have not been studied to draw firm conclusions regarding their prognostic significance.
[c]Three or more chromosome abnormalities in the absence of one of the WHO designated recurring translocations or inversions, that is, t(15;17), t(8;21), inv(16) or t(16;16), t(9;11), t(v;11)(v;q23), t(6;9), inv(3), or t(3;3).
AML, Acute myeloid leukemia
From Hoffman R et al: *Hematology: basic principles and practice*, ed 7, Philadelphia, 2018, Elsevier.

IMAGING STUDIES

- Imaging studies are typically directed to evaluating specific complaints.
- Echocardiogram or multigated acquisition scan is usually performed to verify that cardiac function is adequate to tolerate anthracycline (usually daunorubicin) therapy, with left ventricular ejection fraction (LVEF) of >50% typically considered acceptable.

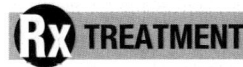 **TREATMENT**

ACUTE GENERAL Rx

- The general approach to AML is summarized in Fig. 3. Therapy of AML typically has three components:
  1. Immediate therapy to correct metabolic, infectious, or hyperleukocytic emergencies (if needed). Therapy for AML is always urgent but not always an emergency. However, treatment for APML should be considered a medical emergency to prevent catastrophic bleeding.
  2. Induction therapy, which is therapy of active disease intended to obtain remission and restore normal bone marrow

TABLE 4 Allogeneic Transplantation Guidelines for Adult Acute Myeloid Leukemia Based on Commonly Assessed Cytogenetic and Molecular Markers

AML Category	Prognostic Impact	Allogeneic Transplantation	Notes
AML-CR1: Younger Adults			
Good-risk disease			
APL	Favorable	No	APL is treatable by chemotherapy.
CBF-AML *without mKIT*	Favorable	No	t(8;21) AML with high WBC count at diagnosis may have worse prognosis.
CBF-AML *with mKIT*	Intermediate	Possible: MRD, MUD Uncertain: MMUD, UCB, haplo	
Intermediate-Risk Disease			
CN-AML *with CEBPA*	Favorable	No	Benefit likely restricted to *DM-CEBPA*.
CN-AML *with mutant NPM1 but not FLT-3-ITD*	Favorable	Possible: MRD	Emerging data suggests allogeneic HSCT benefit for this category, with reduced relapse and improved DFS in patients >40 yr.
CN-AML *with FLT-3-ITD*	Unfavorable[a]	Yes: MRD, MUD Possible: Haplo > MMUD, UCB	Unfavorable risk may be restricted to AML *with FLT-3-ITD allelic ratio >0.51*.
Other intermediate-risk disease	Intermediate or Unfavorable	Yes: MRD Likely acceptable[a]: MUD Possible[b]: Haplo > MMUD, UCB	Likely considerable underlying clinical heterogeneity. Molecular risk profiling may further delineate risk in this category.
Poor-Risk Disease			
Monosomal karyotype *absent*	Unfavorable	Yes: MRD, MUD Likely acceptable[b]: Haplo >MMUD, UCB	
Monosomal karyotype *present*	Very unfavorable	Yes: MRD, MUD Acceptable[b]: Haplo >MMUD, UCB	
Abnormal 17(p)	Very unfavorable	Yes: MRD, MUD Acceptable[b]: Haplo >MMUD, UCB	
AML-CR1: Older adults	Unfavorable	Yes: MRD, MUD Likely acceptable[b]: Haplo >MMUD, UCB	
AML-CR1: t-AML, AML/MDS	Unfavorable	Yes: MRD, MUD Acceptable[b]: Haplo >MMUD, UCB	Molecular risk profiling may supersede clinical classification of secondary AML, especially in older patients.
AML-CR2	Very unfavorable	Yes: MRD, MUD Acceptable[b]: Haplo >MMUD, UCB	
AML not in remission	Very unfavorable	Yes: MRD, MUD Uncertain: MMUD, UCB, haplo	For selected patients: Good performance status, little comorbidity, lower leukemic burden; CIBMTR risk score may be useful.

[a]If no sibling donor available.
[b]If no timely matched donor available.
AML, Acute myeloid leukemia; *APL*, acute promyelocytic leukemia; *CBF*, core binding factor; *CIBMTR*, Center for International Blood and Marrow Transplant Research; *CN*, cytogenetically normal; *CR1*, first complete remission; *CR2*, second complete remission; *haplo*, haploidentical; *MDS*, myelodysplastic syndrome; *MMUD*, mismatched unrelated donor; *MRD*, matched related donor; *MUD*, matched unrelated donor; *t-AML*, therapy-related AML; *UCB*, umbilical cord blood; *WBC*, white blood cell.
From Hoffman R et al: *Hematology: basic principles and practice*, ed 7, Philadelphia, 2018, Elsevier.

A

Diseases and Disorders

I

TABLE 6 Classification of Acute Myeloid Leukemia According to the Revised World Health Organization Classification (2016)

Category	Subtype/Definition*
AML with recurrent cytogenetic abnormalities	t(8;21)(q22;q22); RUNX1-RUNX1T1[†]inv(16)(p13.1q22); CBFB-MYH11[†]
	t(16;16)(p13.1q22); CBFB-MYH11[†]
	t(15;17)(q22;q12); PML-RARA[†] (= acute promyelocytic leukemia)
	t(9;11)(p22;q23); MLLT3-KMT2A
	t(6;9)(p23;q34); DEK-NUP214
	inv(3)(q21q26.2); GATA2, MECOM
	t(3;3)(q21;q26.2); RPN1-EVI1
	t(1;22)(p13q13); RBM15-MKL1 (megakaryoblastic)
	with mutated NPM1
	with biallelic mutations of *CEBPA*
AML with MDS-related changes	Morphologic features of MDS, or prior history of MDS or MDS/MPN, or MDS-related karyotype, and none of the recurrent genetic abnormalities above
Therapy-related myeloid neoplasms	Late complications of cytotoxic chemotherapy (alkylating agents, topoisomerase II inhibitors) and/or ionizing radiation therapy[†]
AML, not otherwise specified	AML with minimal differentiation
	AML without maturation
	AML with maturation
	Acute myelomonocytic leukemia
	Acute monoblastic/monocytic leukemia
	Pure erythroid leukemia
	Acute megakaryoblastic leukemia
	Acute basophilic leukemia
	Acute panmyelosis with myelofibrosis
Myeloid Sarcoma	
Myeloid proliferations related to Down syndrome	Transient abnormal myelopoiesis
	Myeloid leukemia associated with Down syndrome
Blastic Plasmacytoid Dendritic Cell Neoplasm	
Acute leukemia of ambiguous lineage	Acute undifferentiated leukemia
	Mixed-phenotype acute leukemia with: t(9;22)(q34;q11.2); BCR-ABL1
	t(v;11q23); KMT2A rearranged
	Mixed-phenotype acute leukemia, B/myeloid, NOS
	Mixed-phenotype acute leukemia, T/myeloid, NOS
Provisional entities	AML with mutated *NPM1*
	AML with mutated *CEBPA*
	NK-cell lymphoblastic leukemia/lymphoma

*Diagnosis of AML regardless of percentage of blasts.
[†]Excluded are patients with AML who have transformed from MPN.
AML, Acute myeloid leukemia; *MDS*, myelodysplastic syndrome; *MPN*, myeloproliferative neoplasm; *NK*, natural killer; *NOS*, not otherwise specified. For AML with recurrent genetic abnormalities, specific genes rearranged follow the chromosome rearrangement. In 2016, the *MLL* gene has been renamed *KMT2A*.

function. Remission is defined as blasts <5% in the bone marrow, absolute neutrophils (ANC) of >1000/mcl, platelets >100,000/mcl, and transfusion independence. Complete remission with incomplete marrow recovery (CRi) indicates absence of leukemic blasts in the marrow but persistent cytopenias. Cytogenetic remissions and molecular remissions indicate absence of previously detectable cytogenetic mutations/translocations and molecular mutations. Measurable residual disease or MRD is rapidly evolving as a desirable goal for deep remissions.

3. Consolidation therapy, typically some form of intensive chemotherapy or stem cell transplant therapy intended to prevent relapse.

4. Hyperleukocytic symptoms are typically seen with WBC >100,000/ml.

Leukapheresis requires catheter placement and pheresis but spares tumor lysis. Rapid cytoreduction with chemotherapy (hydroxyurea 3 to 6 g orally or cytarabine) is often adequate and easier but risks tumor lysis. Optimal management is therefore individualized.

5. TLS is associated with a rise in uric acid, potassium, and serum phosphate, the last causing a reciprocal fall in calcium. The metabolic changes may result in renal failure, cardiac dysrhythmias, muscle spasms (due to low calcium), seizures, and death (a more detailed discussion is in the section on acute lymphocytic leukemia).

6. The mainstays of therapy for AML are medications dating from the 1970s—daunorubicin and cytarabine—but since 2017, the U.S. FDA has approved

nine new agents for treatment of AML. The role of these agents and their relation to standard therapy is outlined below.

7. Induction chemotherapy typically consists of daunorubicin 60 or 90 mg/m^2 intravenous for 3 days and cytarabine (Ara-C) 100 or 200 mg/m^2/day as continuous infusion for 7 days ("7+3"). Success rates are 60% to 80% and have been better in recent trials. Other agents that are used include etoposide, idarubicin, fludarabine, and cladribine. Bone marrow examination is usually performed at day 14 of therapy to assess the response.

8. Gemtuzumab ozogamicin (GO, Mylotarg) is an antibody-drug conjugate binding an anti-CD33 antibody to the chemotherapeutic agent calicheamicin that was approved in 2017 for therapy of newly diagnosed CD33+ AML. In newly diagnosed AML, the use of low-dose GO when added (3 mg/m^2 given on Day 1 or 2 or 3 or 4) to standard 7+3 induction had a success rate of 81%, with 2-yr relapse-free survival improving from 22.7% to 50.3% compared with standard therapy alone. The benefit was seen only in favorable and intermediate-risk patients and not in adverse risk AML.

9. Midostaurin was also approved in 2017 for treatment of newly diagnosed AML with mutations in the fms-related tyrosine kinase 3 *(FLT3)* gene in combination with standard induction therapy. Four-year overall survival was 51.4% in *FLT3*-positive patients receiving midostaurin (50 mg orally every 12 h on days 8 to 21) vs. 44.3% in the placebo arm, with improved durability of remissions in patients achieving remission. The optimal use of these therapies requires rapid access to genetic data at the time of diagnosis.

10. Also approved in 2017 was CPX-351, a liposomal formulation of cytarabine and daunorubicin encapsulated in a 5:1 ratio, for patients with AML related to previous therapy (t-AML) or with AML with myelodysplasia-related change (AML-MRC). In a trial of t-AML and AML evolving from myelodysplasia or with WHO-defined myelodysplasia-related cytogenetic changes in patients ages 60 to 75 yr, CPX-351 (given on days 1, 3, and 5) improved survival to 9.56 mo vs. 5.95 mo with standard 7+3 induction.

11. Mutations in genes isocitrate dehydrogenase 1 *(IDH1)* and *IDH2* are found in nearly 10% to 20% of AML cases. Two oral *IDH* inhibitors, enasidenib *(IDH2* inhibitor) and ivosidenib *(IDH1* inhibitor), were approved in 2017 and 2018, respectively, for AML harboring these mutations. Enasidenib at a dose of 100 mg showed a response rate of 40.3%, with 19.3% achieving remission, some durable. In the case of ivosidenib, a Ph 1 trial showed remission (complete remission and complete remission with

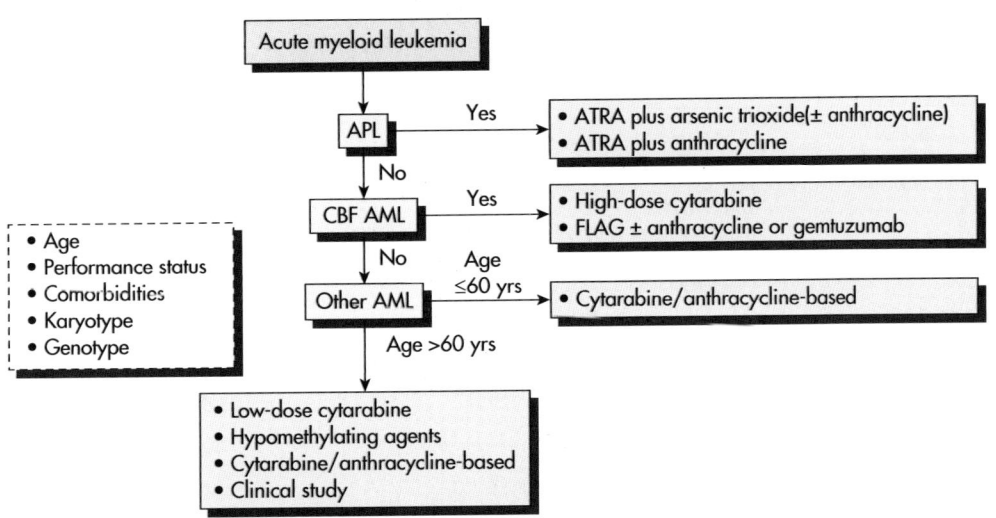

FIG. 3 General approach to acute myeloid leukemia therapy. *AML,* Acute myeloid leukemia; *APL,* acute promyelocytic leukemia; *ATRA,* all-trans retinoic acid; *CBF,* core binding factor; *FLAG,* fludarabine, cytarabine (Ara-C), and granulocyte colony-stimulating factor. (From Hoffman R et al: *Hematology: basic principles and practice,* ed 7, Philadelphia, 2018, Elsevier.)

partial hematologic improvement) of 32.8%, the median duration of remission being 8.2 mo. These agents have a distinctive side effect of differentiation syndrome, characterized by fever, dyspnea, hypotension, weight gain, and pulmonary infiltrates, which can be life-threatening; early detection with supportive care is of paramount importance.

12. Gilteritinib was FDA approved in 2018 for treatment of adult patients who have relapsed or refractory acute myeloid leukemia with a *FLT3* mutation. Approval was based on an interim analysis of a trial, which included 138 adult patients with relapsed or refractory AML having an *FLT3* ITD, D835, or I836 mutation. Gilteritinib was given orally at a dose of 120 mg/day until unacceptable toxicity or lack of clinical benefit. After a median follow-up of 4.6 mo, 21% of patients achieved complete remission (CR) or CR with partial hematologic recovery (CRh).

13. Glasdegib, an oral inhibitor of hedgehog signaling pathway, was approved in combination with low-dose cytarabine in 2018 for older/unfit AML patients Approval was based upon a multicenter, open-label, randomized study that randomized eligible patients 2:1 to receive glasdegib, 100 mg/day, with LDAC 20 mg subcutaneously twice daily on days 1 to 10 of a 28-day cycle or LDAC alone in 28-day cycles until disease progression or unacceptable toxicity. Efficacy was established based on an improvement in overall survival, 8.3 mo for LDAC + glasdegib versus 4.3 mo for LDAC alone. HR of 0.46 (95% confidence interval: 0.30, 0.71; $p = 0.0002$). However, it has not been widely adopted in clinical practice relative to venetoclax-based treatments.

14. In 2018, the FDA granted accelerated approval to venetoclax, an oral BCL-2

inhibitor, in combination with azacitidine or decitabine or low-dose cytarabine for the treatment of newly diagnosed acute myeloid leukemia in adults who are age 75 yr or older, or who have comorbidities that preclude the use of intensive induction chemotherapy. In a major breakthrough phase 3 trial (VIALE-A), compared to hypomethylating agents alone, the combination increased the CR rate (66.4% vs 28.3%; $p <0.001$) and OS (14.7 mo vs. 9.6 mo; $p <0.001$) setting a new standard of care for these patients. The ease of administration and tolerability has resulted in a quick uptake in clinical practice as well. The unprecedented results have stirred tremendous interest on venetoclax with ongoing trials evaluating its use in younger patients, as a partner combination in all kinds of therapeutic strategies in AML including "7+3" as well as a bridge to allogeneic transplant.

15. In September 2020, CC-486 an oral formulation of azacitidine was approved as maintenance therapy in AML in patients who receives intensive chemotherapy but cannot proceed or are considered ineligible for an allogeneic stem cell transplantation. In the pivotal randomized phase 3 trial (QUAZAR AML-001) that randomized 472 patients who were 55 yr or older, oral azacitidine improved OS compared to placebo (median OS, 24.7 vs. 14.8 mo) in patients who achieved CR after intensive chemotherapy. This agent is not considered as a bioequivalent to standard injectable azacitidine and such use is currently discouraged.

• Consolidation therapy is controversial. For patients managed with chemotherapy, cytarabine 3 g/m² for six doses is commonly used (day 1, 3, 5), but intermediate doses (1000 to 1500 mg/m²) for six doses appear equally

effective and less toxic. Doses above 1000 mg/m² are poorly tolerated in patients over 60 yr because of cerebellar toxicity. Renal insufficiency also increases the risk of cerebellar toxicity from Ara-C, which can be severe.

1. For favorable risk disease, consolidation with chemotherapy alone with two to four cycles of intermediate/high-dose cytarabine is typically given, with long-term survival of 60% to 70%.

2. For intermediate-risk and unfavorable-risk disease, first-remission allogeneic stem cell marrow transplant is often recommended if a donor is available. If not, chemotherapy consolidation chemotherapy is offered, although the optimal therapy and schedule, especially for unfavorable disease, is uncertain.

3. In the trial of GO as initial therapy, GO was also used in consolidation with high-dose cytarabine and daunorubicin.

4. The role of autologous bone marrow transplant is controversial, with some evidence of decreased relapse rates after chemotherapy but no clear benefit in overall survival.

5. Allogeneic bone marrow transplant is offered to patients with relapsed disease if a second remission can be obtained in good-risk patients. It is offered to high-risk and intermediate-risk patients in first remission if a donor is available. In 2023, most patients will be able to find a donor from either a matched related donor, matched unrelated donor, mismatched unrelated donor, haploidentical donor, or cord blood donor. The Center for International Blood and Marrow Transplant Research (CIBMTR) has published data for 12,309 patients receiving an HLA-matched sibling transplant and 15,632 patients receiving a matched unrelated donor for AML between 2002 and 2012. Their disease status at the time of transplant and the donor type were

Acute Myeloid Leukemia ⓅⓉⒼ ⒶⓁⒼ

TABLE 7 Prognostic Models in Older Patients With Acute Myeloid Leukemia

Study	Outcome	Unfavorable Characteristics
Study Alliance Leukemia	Survival Disease-free survival	CD34 expression >10% WBC >20 × 10^9/L Age >65 yr LDH >700 U/L *NPM1* status wild-type[a]
UK Medical Research Council	Survival	Adverse cytogenetic group Elevated WBC[b] Poor performance status[b] Older age[b] Secondary AML
Acute Leukemia French Association	Survival	High-risk cytogenetics ± Age ≥75 yr Performance status ≥2 WBC ≥50 × 10^9/L
MD Anderson Cancer Center	Remission rate Induction mortality Survival	Age ≥75 yr Secondary AML[c] AHD duration ≥6[c] (12) mo Treatment outside LAFR Unfavorable cytogenetics WBC ≥25 × 10^9/L[c] Hemoglobin ≤8 g/dl[c] Creatinine >1.3 mg/dl Performance status >2 LDH >600 U/L[d]
Hematopoietic Cell Transplantation Comorbidity Index	Early mortality Survival	Dyspnea Coronary artery disease, CHF, MI, or EF <50% Chronic hepatitis, elevation of bilirubin and/or transaminases Cirrhosis Elevations of creatinine, dialysis, renal transplant Secondary AML Depression/anxiety requiring therapy Continued use of antimicrobial therapy after day 0 BMI >35 kg/m²

AHD, Antecedent hematologic disorder; *AML*, acute myeloid leukemia; *BMI*, body mass index; *CEBPA*, CCAAT/enhancer binding protein α gene; *CHF*, congestive heart failure; *EF*, ejection fraction; *LAFR*, laminar air flow room (isolation floor); *LDH*, lactate dehydrogenase; *MI*, myocardial infarction; *WBC*, white blood cell count.

[a]Favorable and high-risk groups were defined solely by cytogenetic aberrations. Above factors served to further divide the intermediate-risk group into good intermediate versus adverse intermediate.

[b]As continuous variables.

[c]Only significant for prediction of remission.

[d]Only significant for prediction of survival.

From Hoffman R et al: *Hematology: basic principles and practice*, ed 7, Philadelphia, 2018, Elsevier.

found to be the best predictors of post-transplant survival. The 3-yr probabilities of survival after HLA-matched sibling transplant in this cohort was 58% ± 1%, 50% ± 1%, and 24% ± 1% for patients with early, intermediate, and advanced disease, respectively. The probabilities of survival after an unrelated donor transplant were 49% ± 1%, 47% ± 1%, and 22% ± 1% for patients with early, intermediate, and advanced disease, respectively.

6. Relapses after bone marrow transplant can sometimes be managed with donor lymphocyte infusions, adjustment of immune suppression, and chemotherapy (often low intensity). In general, outcomes are poor with posttransplant relapses.

- Treatment of older patients (>60 yr) is problematic, with cure rates of 10% to 15%. Older patients do worse because they are more likely to have high-risk features and less likely to tolerate therapy. Several models have been devised to identify variables that predict which patients may do well with conventional therapy versus those who will not (Table 7). Options for these patients include:

1. Standard induction therapy is reasonable for patients likely to tolerate it. Even in the absence of cure, quality of life is often excellent in remission. More recent studies suggest that the early death rate (within 30 days of diagnosis) was lower for patients in their 70s and 80s receiving standard induction. There is no standardized approach to evaluating fitness for therapy.

2. Hypomethylating agents—decitabine and azacytidine—may be considered in patients unlikely to tolerate induction therapy. Azacytidine (75 mg/m²/day for 7 days every 28 days) and decitabine (20 mg/m² for 5 days every 28 days) are considered in older patients who are not considered appropriate for induction chemotherapy. Both are outpatient regimens, and decitabine especially is very well tolerated. Recent data with azacytidine suggest benefit in about 20% to 30%

lasting 14 to 16 mo in responders, with equivalent results in low blast count (20% to 30% in the bone marrow) vs. higher blast count disease.

3. Single-agent gemtuzumab ozogamicin is an option for treatment of CD33+ AML in patients considered unfit for induction. The benefit compared to best supportive care (BSC) was mainly seen in patients with CD33 expression of greater than 80% and favorable/intermediate cytogenetics (1 yr survival 22% and 37% respectively, BSC <10%), with no benefit in patients with high-risk cytogenetics.

4. Low-dose cytarabine 20 mg/m² twice daily or 40 mg/m²/day for 10 days subcutaneously) has shown survival benefit over hydroxyurea in low-/intermediate-risk patients.

5. Venetoclax (a bcl-2 protein inhibitor) in combination with azacitidine or decitabine or low-dose cytarabine is the new standard of care for treatment of newly diagnosed acute myeloid leukemia in adults who are age 75 yr or older, or who have comorbidities that preclude use of intensive induction chemotherapy. The recommended venetoclax dose depends upon the combination regimen and is described in prescribing information of venetoclax.

6. In patients who harbor *IDH* 1 or 2 mutations and ineligible for any intensive treatments due severe comorbidities or poor performance status, Ivosidenib 500 mg PO (*IDH1* mutated AML) or Enasidenib (*IDH2* mutated AML) can be used alone or in combination with hypomethylating agents.

7. Glasdegib (a small molecule inhibitor of Sonic hedgehog pathway) in combination with low-dose cytarabine (LDAC) is another option for newly diagnosed acute myeloid leukemia in patients who are ≥75 yr or who have comorbidities that preclude intensive induction chemotherapy.

8. Oral hydroxyurea dosed to counts and cytopenias.

9. Best supportive care.

10. Reduced-intensity allogeneic stem cell transplant is an option for patients in remission after standard therapy. A meta-analysis of studies including 749 patients over 60 receiving radioimmunotherapy (RIT) identified a 3-yr relapse-free survival of 35%. A recent prospective AML trial (AML16) of patients aged 60 to 70 yr undergoing RIC transplant versus chemotherapy survival was significantly improved (37% vs. 20%, HR 0.67 [0.53 to 0.84] p <0.001).

- **Acute Promyelocytic Leukemia (APML):** APML is a distinct leukemia syndrome with very different treatment implications. Cure rates greater than 95% have been seen in current protocols in the absence of high-risk features. It is associated with t(15;17), which translocates the PML gene to retinoic acid receptor α (PML-RARa). Uncommon variants are t(11;17) and t(5;17). Risk groups for relapse were defined in studies using retinoic acid and chemotherapy. Patients with presenting WBC >10,000/mcl were considered high risk, patients with WBC <10,000 and platelets >40,000 were considered low risk, and all others were considered intermediate risk. In current protocols, high-risk patients receive some form of intensified therapy.

- APML is a medical emergency because of the high risk of bleeding complications.
  1. All patients with APML have DIC, caused by overexpression of annexin II (which increases generation of plasmin, degrading fibrin), elastases (which degrade fibrinogen and fibrinolytic inhibitors), and increased endothelial tissue plasminogen activator release.
  2. Occurs more often in younger population (median age at diagnosis 44 yr) than other AML subtypes.
  3. Early death due to hemorrhage is seen in 5% to 17% of newly diagnosed APML patients, usually intracranial or pulmonary. Risk factors include elevated WBC, increased age, and elevated creatinine.
  4. Retinoic acid rapidly stabilizes the coagulopathy of APML; consideration should be given to starting this immediately for suspected cases.
  5. Cryoprecipitate (usual dose 10 bags) to raise the fibrinogen level to 150 mg/dl and platelet transfusion to raise the count to >50,000 mcl should be given as needed.
  6. Unfractionated heparin may paradoxically stop bleeding in APML by inhibiting DIC but is rarely used in the retinoic acid treatment era.
- Diagnosis of APML.
  1. Rapid diagnosis is essential due to treatment implications.

2. Diagnosis by classic APML blast morphology and clinical syndrome (especially DIC with low fibrinogen) is sufficient to justify starting treatment with retinoic acid pending confirmation with molecular studies. Immediate therapy with retinoic acid will rapidly stabilize the coagulopathy and help prevent catastrophic bleeding.
3. Polymerase chain reaction for PML/RARa.
4. FISH or cytogenetics for t(15;17) or variants.
5. Flow cytometry is typically distinct with lack of HLA-DR and CD34; CD13, CD33, and CD64 are usually positive.
- Therapy of APML.
  1. Emergency measures to stabilize coagulopathy as outlined previously.
  2. Patients with WBC ≤10,000 (low/intermediate risk) are treated with retinoic acid and arsenic trioxide ("differentiation therapy").
  3. Therapy of high-risk patients is less well standardized but has included intensification with cytarabine, anthracyclines, and gemtuzumab ozogamicin. A recent trial using arsenic and retinoic acid with GO demonstrated 100% 4-yr survival in high-risk patients after 30 days, emphasizing the importance of preventing early deaths in APML.
  4. Maintenance therapy for 2 yr is given in some APML protocols.
  5. Patients with high-risk disease receive central nervous system prophylaxis with intrathecal chemotherapy.
  6. Treatment of relapsed disease typically consists of autologous bone marrow transplant after obtaining second remission.
- Differentiation syndrome (DS) is a potentially fatal complication of therapy with retinoic acid and arsenic trioxide. It is associated with fever, interstitial pulmonary infiltrates, peripheral

edema, pleural and pericardial effusions, and renal failure; it is commonly associated with rising WBC seen in patients on differentiation therapy.
1. Therapy for suspected differentiation syndrome is dexamethasone 10 mg/m^2 every 12 h. Cytoreductive therapy (hydroxyurea, idarubicin) and stopping retinoic acid and arsenic are appropriate for inadequate response to dexamethasone.
2. Prophylaxis for differentiation syndrome with dexamethasone 2.5 mg/m^2 every 12 h has been suggested for WBC >5000 or creatinine >1.4 mg/dl. Hydroxyurea is used to keep the WBC below 10,000/mcl in some protocols.

! PEARLS & CONSIDERATIONS

- The diagnosis of acute myeloid leukemia or variants is often, but not always, a medical emergency requiring rapid clinical and laboratory assessment by appropriate expertise.
- APML is a distinct clinical entity that has a high cure rate with current protocols, but which requires intensive supportive care at the time of diagnosis.

SUGGESTED READINGS
Available at eBooks.Health.Elsevier.com.

RELATED CONTENT
Acute Myelogenous Leukemia (Patient Information)

AUTHOR: **KAPIL S. MELEVEEDU, MD**

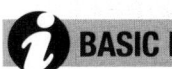
BASIC INFORMATION

DEFINITION

Acute respiratory distress syndrome (ARDS) is a form of noncardiogenic pulmonary edema that results from acute damage to the alveoli. It is characterized by diffuse infiltrative lung lesions with resulting interstitial and alveolar edema, severe hypoxemia, and respiratory failure.[1-3] The cardinal feature of ARDS, refractory hypoxemia, is caused by formation of protein-rich alveolar edema after damage to the integrity of the lung's alveolar-capillary barrier.

The initial definition of ARDS was based on the American–European Consensus Conference (AECC) from 1994 and included the following components:

- The syndrome must present acutely.
- A ratio of Pao_2 to Fio_2 ≤ 200 regardless of the level of positive end-expiratory pressure (PEEP).
- The detection of bilateral pulmonary infiltrates on frontal chest x-ray examination
- Absence of congestive heart failure (pulmonary artery wedge pressure [PAWP] ≤ 18 mm Hg or no clinical evidence of elevated left atrial pressure on the basis of chest x-ray examination or other clinical data)

The 2012 Berlin definition of ARDS (Table 1) addresses some of the limitations of the AECC definition and establishes the criteria for ARDS:

- Timing: Within 1 week of a known clinical insult or new or worsening respiratory symptoms

- Chest imaging (chest x-ray examination or computed tomography [CT] scan): Bilateral opacities, not fully explained by effusions, lobar/lung collapse, or nodules
- Origin of edema: Respiratory failure not fully explained by cardiac failure or fluid overload. Need objective assessment (e.g., echocardiography) to exclude hydrostatic edema if no risk factors are present
- Oxygenation (if altitude is higher than 1000 m, the correction factor should be calculated as follows: [$Pao_2/Fio_2 \times$ {barometric pressure/ 760}]
- Mild: 200 mm Hg $< Pao_2/Fio_2 \leq 300$ mm Hg with PEEP or continuous positive airway pressure (CPAP) ≥ 5 cm H_2O (this may be delivered noninvasively in the mild ARDS group)
- Moderate: 100 mm Hg $< Pao_2/Fio_2 \leq 200$ mm Hg with PEEP or CPAP ≥ 5 cm H_2O
- Severe: $Pao_2/Fio_2 \leq 100$ mm Hg with PEEP or CPAP ≥ 5 cm H_2O

SYNONYMS

ARDS
Adult respiratory distress syndrome
Acute lung injury

ICD-10CM CODE
J80   Acute respiratory distress syndrome

EPIDEMIOLOGY & DEMOGRAPHICS

- More than 150,000 ARDS cases per year in the U.S.

- 7.1% of all patients admitted to an intensive care unit (ICU) and 16.1% of all patients on mechanical ventilation develop ARDS.
- An international study in 50 countries revealed that 10% of patients admitted to an ICU fulfilled criteria for ARDS, and 93% developed it within 48 h of admission. The study reinforced that ARDS is underrecognized.[4]
- Black, Hispanic, and other patients belonging to racial minority groups in the U.S. were observed to exhibit significantly higher in-hospital sepsis-related respiratory failure and associated mortality.[5]

PHYSICAL FINDINGS & CLINICAL PRESENTATION[6]

- Signs and symptoms:
  1. Dyspnea
  2. Chest discomfort
  3. Cough
  4. Anxiety
- Physical examination:
  1. Tachypnea
  2. Tachycardia
  3. Hypertension
  4. Paradoxic breathing and use of accessory muscles
  5. Coarse crepitations or crackles of both lungs
  6. Fever may be present if infection is the underlying etiology

ETIOLOGY (TABLE 2)

- Sepsis (>40% of cases)
- Aspiration: Near-drowning, aspiration of gastric contents (>30% of cases)
- Trauma (>20% of cases)
- Pneumonia
- Multiple transfusions, blood products
- Drugs (e.g., overdose of morphine, methadone, heroin; reaction to nitrofurantoin)
- Noxious inhalation (e.g., chlorine gas, high O_2 concentration)
- Postresuscitation
- Cardiopulmonary bypass
- Burns
- Pancreatitis
- Table 3 describes risk factors associated with development of ARDS
- History of chronic alcohol abuse significantly increases the risk of developing ARDS in critically ill patients

TABLE 1   2012 Berlin Definition of Acute Respiratory Distress Syndrome (All Components Must Be Present)

Timing	Within 1 wk of a known clinical insult or new/worsening respiratory symptoms		
Chest imaging	Bilateral opacities: Not fully explained by effusions, lobar/lung collapse, or nodules		
Origin of edema	Respiratory failure not fully explained by cardiac failure or fluid overload; need objective assessment (e.g., echocardiography) to exclude hydrostatic edema if no risk factor for ARDS is present		
Oxygenation	*Mild ARDS*	*Moderate ARDS*	*Severe ARDS*
	$200 < Pao_2/Fio_2 \leq 300$ with PEEP or CPAP ≥ 5 cm H_2O	$100 < Pao_2/Fio_2 \leq 200$ with PEEP ≥ 5 cm H_2O	$Pao_2/Fio_2 \leq 100$ with PEEP ≥ 5 cm H_2O

ARDS, Acute respiratory distress syndrome; *CPAP,* continuous positive airway pressure; *PEEP,* positive end-expiratory pressure.
From Weinberger SE: *Principles of pulmonary medicine,* ed 7, Philadelphia, 2019, Elsevier.

TABLE 2   Conditions Associated with Acute Respiratory Distress Syndrome by Possible Mechanisms of Injury

Direct Injury (Pulmonary)	Indirect Injury (Nonpulmonary)
Pneumonia (bacterial, viral [e.g., influenza, COVID-19])	Sepsis
	Major trauma
Aspiration	Multiple blood transfusions
Pulmonary contusion	Pancreatitis
Toxic inhalation	Cardiopulmonary bypass
Near-drowning	Drug overdose
Reperfusion injury (e.g., post–lung transplant)	Adverse effects of medication

COVID-19, Coronavirus disease 2019.
From Broaddus VC et al: *Murray & Nadel's textbook of respiratory medicine,* ed 7, Philadelphia 2022, Elsevier.

DIAGNOSIS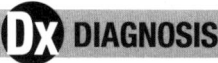

DIFFERENTIAL DIAGNOSIS

- Cardiogenic pulmonary edema
- Interstitial lung disease (acute interstitial pneumonia, nonspecific interstitial pneumonia, cryptogenic organizing pneumonia, acute eosinophilic pneumonia, hypersensitivity pneumonia, pulmonary alveolar proteinosis)
- Connective tissue diseases, such as polymyositis
- Diffuse alveolar hemorrhage
- Lymphangitic carcinomatosis from T-cell or B-cell lymphomas

- Drug-induced lung diseases (amiodarone, bleomycin)

WORKUP

The search for an underlying cause should focus on treatable causes (e.g., infections such as sepsis or pneumonia).
- Arterial blood gases (ABGs)
- Hemodynamic monitoring
- Bronchoalveolar lavage (selected patients)
- Transthoracic echocardiogram

LABORATORY TESTS

- ABGs:
  1. Initially: Varying degrees of hypoxemia, generally resistant to supplemental oxygen
  2. Respiratory alkalosis, decreased P_{CO_2}
  3. Widened alveolar-arterial gradient
  4. Hypercapnia as the disease progresses
- Bronchoalveolar lavage:
  1. The most prominent finding is an increased number of polymorphonucleocytes.
  2. The presence of eosinophilia has therapeutic implications because these patients respond to corticosteroids.
- Blood and urine cultures
- Blood work:
  1. Increased or reduced white blood cell count with left shift if concomitant infectious process
  2. Normal or mildly elevated B-type natriuretic peptide level

3. Increased lactate level if concomitant sepsis or septic shock

IMAGING STUDIES

Chest x-ray examination (Fig. 1).
- The initial chest x-ray examination might be normal in the initial hours after the precipitating event.
- Bilateral interstitial infiltrates are usually seen within 24 to 72 h; they often are more prominent in the bases and periphery.
- CT scan of chest: Bilateral diffuse, dense consolidations with air bronchograms.

Rx TREATMENT

NONPHARMACOLOGIC THERAPY

Treatment of ARDS is supportive. There is no specific pharmacotherapy for ARDS. Management principles are summarized in Table 4.
Hemodynamic monitoring:
- Can be used for the initial evaluation of ARDS (in ruling out cardiogenic pulmonary edema) and its subsequent management. However, a pulmonary catheter is not indicated in the routine management of ARDS. Trials have shown that clinical management involving the early use of pulmonary artery catheters in patients with ARDS did not significantly affect mortality and morbidity rates and may result in more complications as compared with a central venous catheter.

- Although no dynamic profile is diagnostic of ARDS, the presence of pulmonary edema, a high cardiac output, and a low pulmonary capillary wedge pressure (PCWP) is characteristic of ARDS.
- It is important to remember that partially treated intravascular volume overload and flash pulmonary edema can have the hemodynamic features of ARDS; filling pressures can also be elevated by increased intrathoracic pressures or with fluid administration; cardiac function can be depressed by acidosis, hypoxemia, or other factors associated with sepsis.
Ventilatory support:
- Noninvasive positive-pressure ventilation (NIPPV) (i.e., BiPAP) should only be used in selected cases in patients with hypoxic respiratory failure.
- A randomized multicenter, open-label trial showed that high-flow oxygen by nasal cannula increased ventilator-free days and reduced 90-day mortality compared with NIPPV in patients with hypoxemic respiratory failure without hypercapnia. Either modality should not delay intubation and mechanical ventilation initiation in patients with rapidly progressing clinical deterioration.
- Mechanical ventilation is generally necessary to maintain adequate gas exchange. Ventilatory strategy for patients with ARDS as proposed by the ARDS Network is summarized in Fig. 2. A low tidal volume and low plateau pressure ventilator strategy are recommended to avoid ventilator-induced injury. Assist-control is generally preferred initially with the following ventilator settings:
  1. F_{IO_2} 1.0 (until a lower value can be used to achieve adequate oxygenation). When possible, minimize oxygen toxicity by maintaining F_{IO_2} at <60%.
  2. Tidal volume: Set initial tidal volume at 6 ml/kg of predicted body weight (PBW). Tidal volumes are reduced from 6 mL/kg of PBW to a minimum of 4 mL/kg if plateau airway pressures exceed 30 cm of water. The concept of using PBW is based on the fact that lung size depends most strongly on height and sex; PBW normalizes the tidal

TABLE 3 Risk Factors Associated with Development of Acute Lung Injury and Acute Respiratory Distress Syndrome	
Direct Lung Injury	**Indirect Lung Injury**
Pneumonia	Sepsis
Aspiration of gastric contents	Multiple trauma
Pulmonary contusion	Cardiopulmonary bypass
Fat, amniotic fluid, or air emboli	Drug overdose
Near-drowning	Acute pancreatitis
Inhalational injury	Transfusion of blood products
Reperfusion pulmonary edema	

From Vincent JL et al: *Textbook of critical care*, ed 6, Philadelphia, 2011, Saunders.

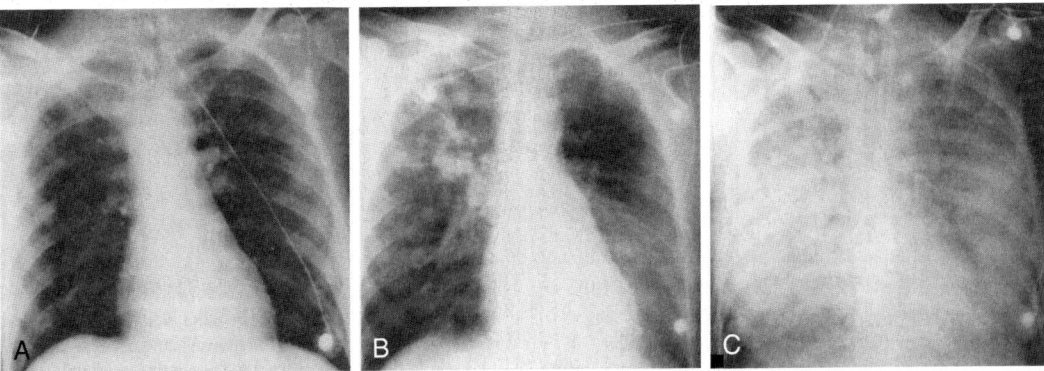

FIG. 1 Acute respiratory distress syndrome. X-ray of a young man who had sustained severe trauma and blood loss in a road traffic accident; the lungs cover a period of 5 days from a relatively normal x-ray **(A),** to bilateral infiltrates **(B),** to bilateral "whiteout" **(C),** accompanied by severe hypoxemia. A Swan-Ganz catheter for measurement of pulmonary artery "wedge" pressure (as a reflection of left atrial pressure) can be seen in situ on the x-ray film in **C.** The patient died shortly after the last film.

TABLE 4 ARDS Management Principles

Supportive Care

Supplemental oxygen to ensure adequate oxygenation

Lung-protective ventilation
- Volume and pressure limited
- Ensure ventilator synchrony
- Prone position if Pao_2/Fio_2 <150 despite protective ventilation

Reduce oxygen consumption if hypoxia is critical

Support adequate perfusion for other organs; focus on both cardiac output and blood pressure

Find and Treat Underlying Cause

Consider infections, mimics

Minimize Further Edema Accumulation

Seek lowest pulmonary microvascular pressure that maintains adequate perfusion

Diurese/reduce vascular volume while maintaining adequate perfusion

Avoid Harm

Volume- and pressure-limited ventilation strategy

Avoid both hypotension and volume overload

Goal-directed sedation with frequent reassessment

Avoid hyperoxia

Consider early physical rehabilitation

Seek and treat neuromuscular, cognitive, and psychological impairments during recovery

ARDS, Acute respiratory distress syndrome; *Fio₂*, fractional concentration of oxygen in inspired gas; *Pao₂*, partial pressure of arterial oxygen.
From Broaddus VC et al: *Murray & Nadel's textbook of respiratory medicine*, ed 7, Philadelphia 2022, Elsevier.

volume to lung size. Aim to maintain plateau pressure (P_{plat}) at <30 mm Hg PEEP 5 cm H_2O or greater (to increase lung volume and keep alveoli open).

3. PEEP should be increased in small increments of 3 to 5 cm H_2O to achieve acceptable arterial saturation (>0.9) with nontoxic Fio_2 values (<0.6) and acceptable airway plateau pressures (<30 to 35 cm H_2O). It is important to remember that an increase in PEEP may lower cardiac output and, despite improvement in Pao_2, may actually have a negative effect on tissue oxygenation (the major determinants of tissue oxygenation are hemoglobin, percent saturation, and cardiac output). The optimal level of PEEP remains unestablished.[7] Although higher levels of PEEP may help prevent life-threatening hypoxemia and be associated with lower hospital mortality in patients meeting criteria for ARDS, such benefit is unlikely in patients with less severe lung injury (Pao_2/Fio_2 >200) and a strategy of treating such patients with high PEEP levels may be harmful. A study published in 2017 demonstrated that the open lung approach increases mortality in patients with moderate to severe ARDS.[8]

Ventilatory Strategy for Patients With ARDS*

Goal 1: Low Vt /P_{plat}

Initiation:
Calculate PBW
—Male:
  50 + 2. 3 (height [inches] – 60)
—Female:
  45.5 + 2.3 (height [inches] – 60)
Initiate volume assist control
—start with 8 mL/kg, and ↓ to
  6 mL/kg over a few hours

Keep P_{plat} (based on 0.5-sec pause)
< 35 cm H_2O
If P_{plat} > 30 cm H_2O, ↓ Vt by
  1 mL/kg to 5 or 4 mL/kg
If P_{plat} < 25 AND Vt < 6 mL/kg,
  ↑ Vt by 1 mL/kg until P_{plat} >
  25 cm H_2O OR Vt = 6 mL/kg
If patient severely distressed
  and/or breath stacking, consider
  ↑ Vt to 7 or 8 mL/kg, as long as
  P_{plat} ≤ 30 cm H_2O †

Goal 2: Adequate Oxygenation

Specific goal:
Pao_2 55-80 mm Hg
or
Spo_2 88-95%
Use only Fio_2 /PEEP combinations shown below to achieve this target
- if oxygenation is low, choose Fio_2 /PEEP combination (from Fio_2 /PEEP table) to the right
- if oxygenation is high, choose Fio_2 /PEEP combination to the left

Goal 3: Arterial pH

Goal:
pH: 7.30–7.45
Acidosis algorithm
If pH 7.15–7.30
- ↑ set rate until pH > 7.30 or $Paco_2$ < 25 mm Hg (max RR = 35)
- if RR = 35 & pH < 7.30 $NaHCO_3$ may be given
If pH < 7.15
- ↑ set RR to 35
- if set RR = 35 & pH < 7.15, Vt may be ↑ in 1 mL/kg steps until pH > 7.15
(P_{plat} target may be exceeded)
Alkalosis algorithm
If pH > 7.45
- ↓ set RR until patient RR > set RR
(minimum set RR = 6/min)

Fio_2/PEEP Table

Fio_2	0.3	0.4	0.4	0.5	0.5	0.6	0.7	0.7	0.7	0.8	0.9	0.9	0.9	1.0
PEEP	5	5	8	8	10	10	10	12	14	14	14	16	18	18–24

*Based on ARDS Network Algorithm
†If compliance of the chest wall is markedly decreased (e.g., massive ascites), it may be reasonable or necessary (if the patient is very hypoxemic) to allow a P_{plat} >30 cm H_2O.

FIG. 2 Ventilatory strategy for patients with the acute respiratory distress syndrome (ARDS) as proposed by the ARDS Network. Several caveats should be considered in using the low tidal volume strategy. (1) Tidal volume (VT) is based on predicted body weight (PBW), not actual body weight; PBW tends to be about 20% lower than actual body weight. (2) The protocol mandates decreases in the VT lower than 6 mL/kg of PBW if the plateau pressure (P_{plat}) is greater than 30 cm H_2O and allows small increases in VT if the patient is severely distressed or if there is breath stacking, as long as P_{plat} remains at 30 cm H_2O or lower. (3) Because arterial carbon dioxide (CO_2) levels will rise, pH will fall; acidosis is treated with increasingly aggressive strategies dependent on the arterial pH. (4) The protocol has no specific provisions for the patient with a stiff chest wall, which in this context refers to the rib cage and abdomen; in such patients, it seems reasonable to allow P_{plat} to increase to more than 30 cm H_2O, even though it is not mandated by the protocol; in such cases, the limit on P_{plat} may be modified on the basis of analysis of abdominal pressure, which can be estimated by measuring bladder pressure. *Fio₂*, Fraction of inspired oxygen; *Paco₂*, arterial partial pressure of carbon dioxide; *Pao₂*, arterial partial pressure of oxygen; *PBW*, predicted body weight; *P_{plat}*, plateau pressure; *PEEP*, positive end-expiratory pressure; *RR*, respiratory rate; *Spo₂*, oxygen saturation based on pulse oximeter; *VT*, tidal volume. (From Goldman L, Shafer AI: *Goldman-Cecil medicine*, ed 26, Elsevier, 2020.)

4. Inspiratory flow: 60 L/min.
5. Ventilatory rate: High ventilatory rates of up to 35 breaths/min are often necessary in patients with ARDS to achieve the desired minute ventilation because of their increased physiologic dead space and smaller lung volumes. Patients must be monitored for excessive intrathoracic gas trapping (auto-PEEP or intrinsic PEEP) that can depress cardiac output.
- Permissive hypercapnia: To maintain a low plateau pressure, a low tidal volume is frequently required, leading to a reduced minute ventilation and hypoventilation with consequently a respiratory acidosis (elevated P_{CO_2} and reduced pH). Most patients (excluding patients with cerebral edema, acute coronary syndrome, seizures, cardiac arrhythmias, and so on) can tolerate a low pH without major consequences. Bicarbonate replacement is suggested when the pH falls to below 7.20.
- Sedation: Gamma-aminobutyric acid (GABA) receptor agonists (including propofol and benzodiazepines) have traditionally been the most commonly administered sedative drugs for ICU patients. Recent trials indicate that the alpha-2 agonist dexmedetomidine (Precedex) may have

distinct advantages. At comparable sedation levels, dexmedetomidine-treated patients spent less time on ventilator, experienced less delirium, and developed less tachycardia and hypertension. The most notable adverse effect of dexmedetomidine was bradycardia.
- Neuromuscular blockade: The benefits of early continuous neuromuscular blockade in patients with ARDS who are receiving mechanical ventilation remains unclear. In a trial among patients with moderate-to-severe ARDS who were treated with a strategy involving a high PEEP, there was no significant difference in mortality at 90 days between patients who received an early and continuous infusion of the neuromuscular blocking agent cisatracurium and those who were treated with a usual-care approach with lighter sedation targets.[9,10]
- Discontinuing ventilation/extubation: Fig. 3 is an algorithm for assessing whether a patient is ready to be liberated from mechanical ventilation and extubated.

ACUTE GENERAL Rx

Identify and treat precipitating conditions:
- Blood and urine cultures and trial of antibiotics in presumed sepsis (routine administration of

antibiotics in all cases of ARDS is not recommended).
- Prompt repair of bone fractures in patients with major trauma.
- Crystalloid resuscitation in pancreatitis.
- Fluid management: In most patients with ARDS, fluid restriction is associated with better outcomes than a liberal fluid policy. Optimal fluid and hemodynamic management of patients with ARDS should be patient specific; in general, administration of crystalloids is recommended if a downward trend in PCWP is associated with diminished cardiac index, resulting in prerenal azotemia, oliguria, and relative tachycardia.[11]
- Positioning the patient: Changes in position can improve oxygenation by improving the distribution of perfusion to ventilated lung regions; repositioning (lateral decubitus positioning) should be attempted in patients with hypoxemia that is not responsive to other medical interventions. Placing patients with moderate and severe hypoxemia in a prone position may improve their oxygenation. A meta-analysis that included the recent trials by Guerin et al[12] have shown that in patients with severe ARDS, early application of prolonged (over 16 h/day) prone-positioning sessions

Approach to Discontinuing Ventilation/Extubation

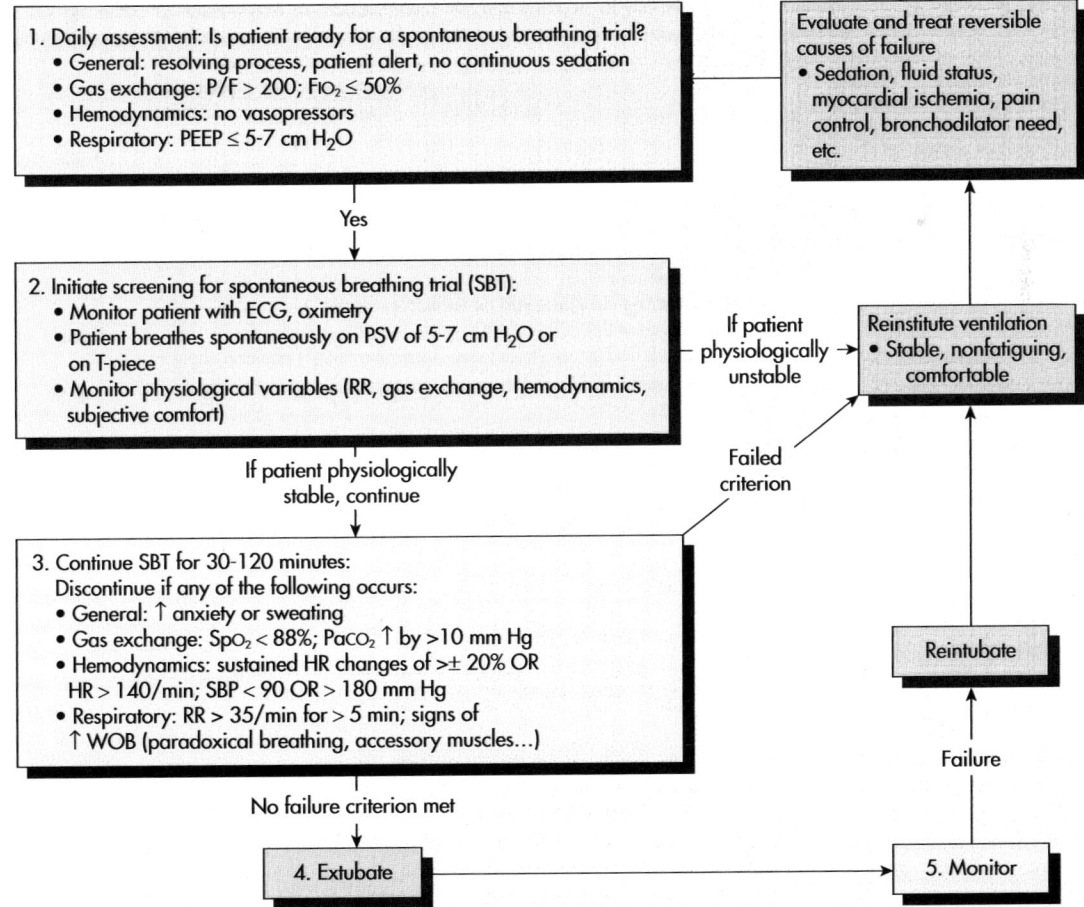

FIG. 3 Algorithm for assessing whether a patient is ready to be liberated from mechanical ventilation and extubated. *ECG,* Electrocardiogram; *HR,* heart rate; *Paco₂,* arterial partial pressure of carbon dioxide; *PEEP,* positive end-expiratory pressure; *P/F,* Pao₂/Fio₂; *PSV,* pressure support ventilation; *RR,* respiratory rate; *SBP,* systolic blood pressure; *Spo₂,* oxygen saturation based on pulse oximeter; *WOB,* work of breathing. (From Goldman L, Shafer AI: *Goldman-Cecil medicine,* ed 26, Elsevier, 2020.)

significantly decreases 28-day and 90-day mortality.

- Corticosteroids: Routine use of corticosteroids in ARDS is not recommended; corticosteroids may be beneficial in patients with many eosinophils in the bronchoalveolar lavage fluid or in patients with severe pneumonia. Systemic infections should be ruled out or adequately treated before administration of corticosteroids. Use of methylprednisolone has not been

shown to increase the rate of infectious complications but is associated with a higher rate of neuromuscular weakness. In addition, starting methylprednisolone therapy more than 2 wk after the onset of ARDS may increase the risk of death.

- Nutritional support: Nutritional support, preferably administered by the enteral route, is necessary to maintain adequate colloid oncotic pressure and intravascular volume. The use of

antioxidants and dietary oil supplements is still equivocal and cannot be recommended at this time.

- Tracheostomy: Tracheostomy is warranted in patients requiring >2 wk of mechanical ventilation; discussion regarding tracheostomy should begin with patient (if alert and oriented) and/or family members/legal guardian after 5 to 7 days of ventilatory support. Early tracheostomy (within 4 days of

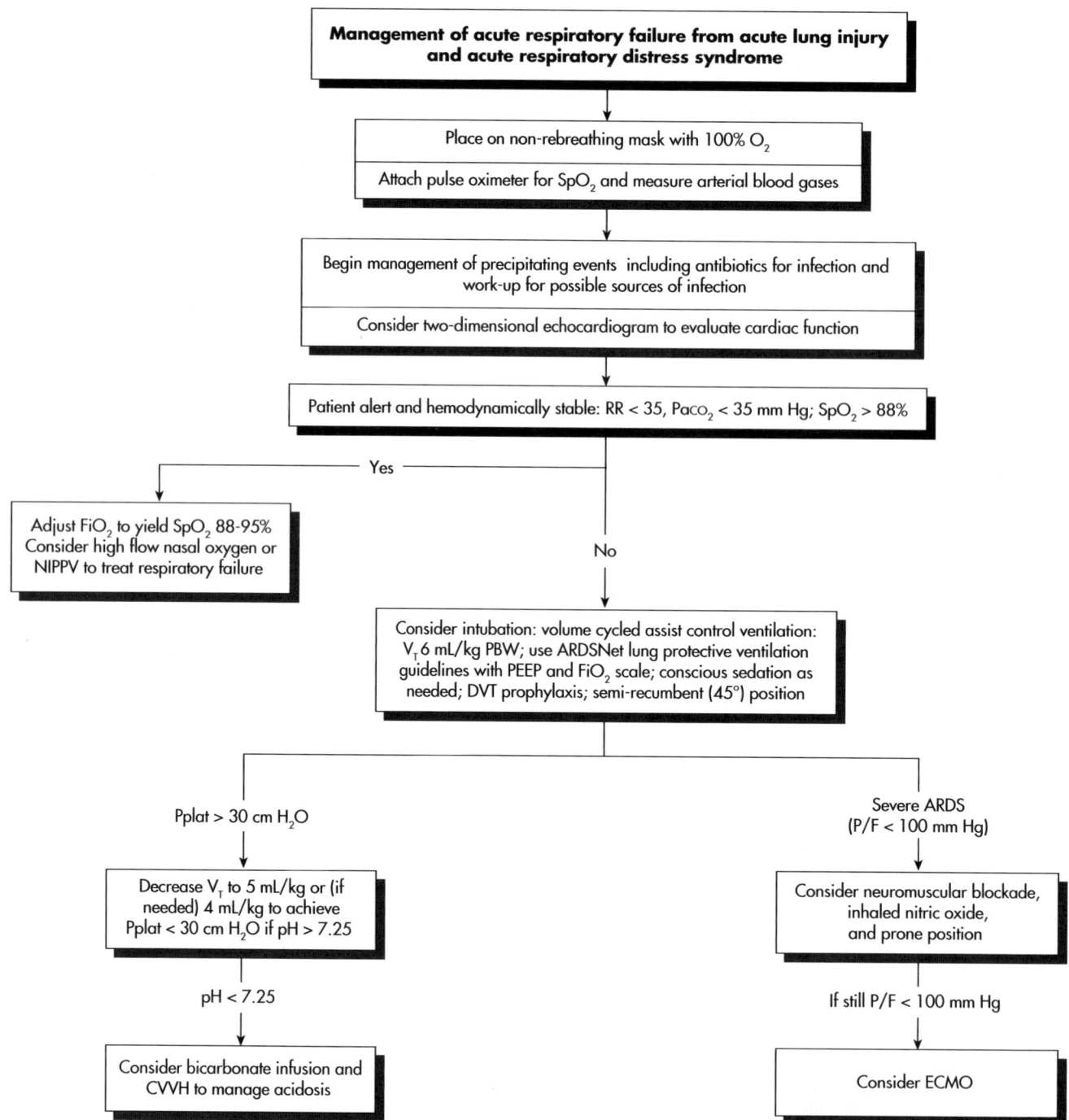

FIG. 4 Management of acute respiratory failure from acute lung injury and acute respiratory distress syndrome. *CVVH,* Continuous venovenous hemofiltration; *DVT,* deep venous thrombosis; *ECMO,* extracorporeal membrane oxygenation; *NIPPV,* noninvasive positive pressure ventilation; *PBW,* predicted body weight; *PEEP,* positive end-expiration pressure; *P/F,* Pao_2/Fio_2; P_{plat}, plateau airway pressure; *RR,* respiratory rate; Spo_2, arterial oxygen saturation; *VT,* tidal volume. (From Goldman L, Shafer AI: *Goldman-Cecil medicine,* ed 26, Elsevier, 2020.)

admission to critical care) does not limit mortality and results in many unneeded procedures.[12]
- Some form of deep vein thrombosis prophylaxis is indicated in all patients with ARDS.
- Stress ulcer prophylaxis with sucralfate suspension (by nasogastric tube), or proton pump inhibitors (PO or IV) or histamine-2 blockers (PO or IV). Should be reserved for seriously ill patients who are at high risk for this complication.[13]
- The use of surfactant remains controversial. Patients who receive surfactant have a greater improvement in gas exchange in the initial 24-h period than patients who receive standard therapy alone; however, the use of exogenous surfactant does not improve survival.
- Fig. 4 illustrates the management of acute respiratory failure from acute lung injury and ARDS.
- The SARS-CoV-2 virus first identified in 2019 can lead to severe ARDS. There was debate on whether ARDS caused by the virus merited special management. There is now consensus and sufficient evidence that it should not be treated differently than other ARDS resulting from other etiologies. (See chapter on viral pneumonia.)[14,15]

DISPOSITION
- Patients who survive ARDS are at risk of diminished functional capacity, mental illness, and decreased quality of life. Prognosis for ARDS varies with the underlying cause. Prognosis is worse in patients with chronic liver disease, nonpulmonary organ dysfunction, sepsis, and advanced age. ARDS survivors are at high risk for incident joblessness and substantial loss of wages, and 58% of those returning to work received disability.
- Elevated values of dead space fraction ([$Paco_2$ >2 $Peco_2$]/$Paco_2$; normal is <0.3) is associated with an increased risk of death.
- In ARDS, the percentage of potentially recruitable lung is variable and associated with the response to PEEP.
- Overall mortality rate varies between 32% and 45%. Most deaths are attributable to sepsis or multiorgan dysfunction rather than primary respiratory causes.
- Trials have shown that as compared with the current standard of care, a ventilator strategy using esophageal measures to estimate the transpulmonary pressure significantly improves oxygenation and compliance. Further trials will determine if this approach should be widely adopted.
- Other strategies for treatment of life-threatening refractory hypoxemia (inhaled nitric acid, extracorporeal membrane oxygenation [ECMO], high-frequency oscillatory ventilation, recruitment maneuvers) may improve oxygenation, but their impact on mortality remains unproven. Use of ECMO in combination with lung-protective ventilation was found to be beneficial as a treatment strategy early in the course of ARDS related to H1N1 infection. Extracorporeal gas exchange may allow the use of low tidal volumes and lower levels of inspired oxygen and use of higher PEEP if desired. ECMO is costly and labor-intensive. The role and proper use of ECMO for patients with ARDS have not been clearly defined.[16,17]

- General indications for ECMO in severe cases of ARDS are:
  1. Severe hypoxemia (e.g., ratio of Pao_2 to Fio_2 <80 despite the application of high levels of PEEP [typically 15 to 20 cm H_2O]) for at least 6 h in patients with potentially reversible respiratory failure
  2. Uncompensated hypercapnia with acidemia (pH <7.15) despite the best accepted standard of care for management with a ventilator
  3. Excessively high-end inspiratory plateau pressure (>35 to 45 cm H_2O, according to the patient's body size) despite the best accepted standard of care for management with a ventilator

REFERRAL
Surgical referral for tracheostomy (see "Acute General Rx").
Referral to ECMO team or center in severe cases when indicated.

REFERENCES & SUGGESTED READINGS
Available at eBooks.Health.Elsevier.com.

RELATED CONTENT
Acute Respiratory Distress Syndrome (ARDS) (Patient Information)
Pneumonia, Viral (Related Key Topic)

AUTHOR: **JORGE MERCADO, MD**

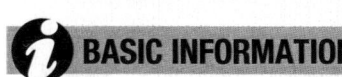
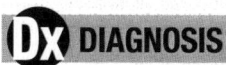 BASIC INFORMATION

DEFINITION

Respiratory failure is a condition in which the respiratory system fails in one or both of its gas exchanging functions (oxygenation and carbon dioxide elimination). There are two major types of acute respiratory failure (ARF): type I (hypoxemic) and type II (hypercapnic). In addition, type III (associated with atelectasis) and type IV (hypoperfusion of respiratory muscles in patients with shock) have also been described. Table 1 summarizes the classification of ARF.

Hypoxemic respiratory failure is characterized by a low arterial partial pressure of oxygen, usually <60 mm Hg while breathing room air. A major cause of hypoxemic respiratory failure is Acute Respiratory Distress Syndrome (see "ARDS" chapter), but other etiologies include heart failure and pneumonia. See Table 2 for list of potential etiologies for acute hypoxemic respiratory failure.

Hypercapnic respiratory failure is defined as an elevation in arterial partial pressure of carbon dioxide to >45 mm Hg. This is directly proportional to the rate of CO_2 production and inversely proportional to the rate of CO_2 elimination by the lungs. Both hypoxemia and hypercapnia can occur at the same time, depending on the location of the underlying disorder and mechanism. Table 3 summarizes etiologies for acute hypercapnic respiratory failure.

Respiratory failure can be acute or chronic. The acute presentation occurs within minutes to hours, whereas the chronic form develops over days or longer.[1] Hypoxemia is dangerous because it can lead to tissue hypoxia. Oxygen concentration is one factor that contributes to delivery of oxygen to tissues but is not the only one. Oxygen capacity of the blood, hemoglobin capacity, cardiac output, and blood flow also contribute to oxygenation of the tissues.

SYNONYMS

Respiratory insufficiency
Hypercarbic respiratory failure
Hypoxemic respiratory failure
ARF

ICD-10CM CODES
J96.00	Acute respiratory failure
J96.01	Acute respiratory failure with hypoxia
J96.02	Acute respiratory failure with hypercapnia
J96.90	Respiratory failure, unspecified
J96.91	Respiratory failure, unspecified with hypoxia
J96.92	Respiratory failure, unspecified with hypercapnia

EPIDEMIOLOGY & DEMOGRAPHICS

- An estimated 1.9 million patients discharged from acute care hospitals nationwide meet criteria for ARF.
- The peak incidence of ARF is in the winter months, when upper and lower respiratory tract infections are more prevalent.
- Comorbid conditions, including chronic disorders of the cardiac, pulmonary, neurologic, renal, hepatic systems, and the patient's advanced age, increase the risk of mortality.

PHYSICAL FINDINGS & CLINICAL PRESENTATION

- Hypoperfusion to brain occurs within seconds
- Decreased myocardial contractility, tachycardia early, bradycardia in late presentation
- Decreased diaphragmatic function
- Shift of the oxyhemoglobin dissociation curve to the right
- Physical symptoms:
  1. Dyspnea
  2. Somnolence
  3. Headaches
  4. Confusion
  5. Asterixis
  6. Coma

ETIOLOGY
See Tables 2 and 3.

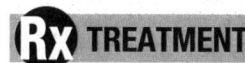 DIAGNOSIS

Diagnosis is made clinically according to physical examination findings and is confirmed by arterial blood gas. Table 4 summarizes common clues obtained from the history and physical examination.

DIFFERENTIAL DIAGNOSIS
See Tables 2 and 3.

WORKUP

After supportive therapy is initiated, a careful search for the underlying cause of the respiratory failure is critical, as this may have important implications on ultimate therapy.

LABORATORY TESTS
- Arterial blood gas (Fig. 1)
- Basal metabolic panel
- CBC

IMAGING STUDIES
- Chest imaging studies include:
  1. Chest x-ray examination
  2. Computed tomography scan of the chest (with angiography when suspecting pulmonary embolism)
  3. Chest ultrasound
  4. Ventilation perfusion scan

RX TREATMENT

The treatment of respiratory failure is initially supportive, aiming to determine first the acuity and/or severity of the presentation. Correction of the hypoxemia, hypercapnia, and management of the underlying etiology of the condition are essential to its treatment.[1] Potential indications for mechanical ventilation are summarized in Table 5.[2] The

---

TABLE 1 Classification of Acute Respiratory Failure

	Type I	Type II	Type III	Type IV
Mechanism of hypoxemia	Low Fio$_2$ ventilation/perfusion (V/Q) mismatch Shunting Reduced diffusing capacity	Hypoventilation	Shunting Hypoventilation V/Q mismatch	Hypoperfusion or inadequate oxygenation of peripheral tissues
Location of pathologic process	Inhaled air composition Alveolar-capillary unit Oxygen-carrying capacity of blood	Airway Central nervous system (CNS) Neuromuscular system Chest wall	Alveolar-capillary unit collapse with regional hypoventilation	Cardiovascular system Peripheral tissues
Clinical syndromes	Cardiogenic pulmonary edema Acute respiratory distress syndrome Pneumonia Interstitial lung disease Pulmonary embolism Pulmonary hypertension Atelectasis Alveolar hemorrhage Carbon monoxide poisoning Anatomic shunts	Chronic obstructive pulmonary disease Asthma CNS depression (intoxication) CNS trauma or injury Neuromuscular disorders Skeletal disorders Obesity-hypoventilation syndrome	Thoracic or upper abdominal surgery or trauma Inadequate postoperative analgesia Pleural tumor or inflammation Trapped lung Subdiaphragmatic tumor or inflammation Obesity	Septic (distributive) shock Hypovolemic shock Cardiogenic shock Compromised cellular oxidation Hypermetabolic states

Fio$_2$, Fraction of inspired oxygen.
Modified from Jean-Louis V: *Intensive care medicine: annual update 2008*, Berlin Heidelberg, 2008, Springer-Verlag.

TABLE 2   Pathophysiologic Mechanisms of Acute Hypoxemic Respiratory Failure

Extrapulmonary processes, including chest wall and skeletal abnormalities (hypoxic hypoxia)	Deficiency of oxygen in inspired air (high altitude, suffocation) Hypoactive hypoventilation (central nervous system trauma, drug toxicities, and neuromuscular and skeletal disorders) Upper airway obstruction leading to hypoventilation (trauma and angioedema)
Pulmonary etiologies (hypoxic hypoxia)	Hypoventilation caused by increased airway resistance (chronic obstructive pulmonary disease and asthma) Abnormal alveolar ventilation-perfusion ratio (pulmonary embolism, pneumonia, aspiration, and emphysema) Diminished diffusing capacity via the alveolar-capillary membrane (interstitial lung disease and pulmonary vascular disease) Pulmonary shunting (atelectasis, pneumonia, hepatopulmonary syndrome, and arteriovenous malformations)
Cardiac right-to-left shunts; e.g., atrial septal defect (hypoxic hypoxia)	—
Inadequate capacity of blood to transport oxygen (anemic hypoxia)	Anemia Hemoglobinopathies (methemoglobinemia and carbon monoxide poisoning)
Inadequate oxygen transport due to a circulatory defect (static hypoxia)	General circulatory deficiency or collapse (shock or cardiac failure) Localized circulatory deficiency (peripheral, cerebral, and coronary vessels)
Abnormal tissue capability for using oxygen (histotoxic hypoxia)	Late-stage irreversible shock Poisoning of cellular oxidation enzymes (cyanide or arsenic toxicity and heavy ethanol intoxication) Diminished cellular metabolic capacity for using oxygen (severe vitamin deficiencies; e.g., beri-beri)

From Vincent JL et al: *Textbook of critical care,* ed 7, Philadelphia, 2017, Elsevier.

TABLE 3   Potential Causes of Acute Hypercapnic Respiratory Failure

Central Nervous System	Spinal Cord, Nerves, Muscle	Chest Wall, Thoracic Cage	Increased Dead Space
Medications (anesthetics and/or opioids) Alveolar hypoventilation Trauma Meningoencephalitis Localized tumors or vascular abnormalities of the medulla Strokes affecting medullary control centers Severe alkalosis	Medications Trauma Myasthenia gravis Guillain-Barré syndrome Electrolyte abnormalities	Trauma Kyphoscoliosis Flail chest Pleural disease Scleroderma Morbid obesity Ascites Severe ileus	Obstructive airways disorders Upper: Acute epiglottitis, foreign body aspiration, tracheal tumor Lower: COPD, asthma, cystic fibrosis

COPD, Chronic obstructive pulmonary disease.

TABLE 4   Common Clues Obtained from the History, Symptoms, and Clinical Examination Findings That Can Help in the Initial Diagnostic Workup and Management of Acute Respiratory Failure

History and Symptoms	Signs on Physical Examination	Diagnosis
Cough, sputum, secretions	Rales or wheezing	Pneumonia, chronic obstructive pulmonary disease (COPD) exacerbation, bronchiectasis
Sudden onset of shortness of breath	Normal auscultation and percussion, possible signs of leg swelling to suggest deep vein thrombosis	Pulmonary embolism
History of heavy smoking	Wheezing, rhonchi	Emphysema, chronic bronchitis
Orthopnea, chest pain, paroxysmal nocturnal dyspnea	Arrhythmia, peripheral edema, jugular venous distention, peripheral hypoperfusion	Congestive heart failure or acute coronary syndrome
Trauma, aspiration, blood transfusions	Diffuse crackles	Acute respiratory distress syndrome
History of allergies, wheezing, or airway disease	Wheezing	Asthma, COPD
Exposure to heavy metals, handling of animals, dust or other significant environmental exposures	"Velcro" rales, clubbing	Chronic interstitial lung disease
Choking, aspiration, vomiting, dental procedures	Inspiratory stridor, poor air entry	Foreign body
Drug abuse	Constricted or dilated pupils, altered mental status, skin marks, perforated nasal septum, hypersalivation, decreased respiratory frequency	Central nervous system depression, intoxication
Exposure to a new drug/chemical or foods known to be allergenic	Swollen oral mucosa and tongue; stridor or wheezing	Angioedema, anaphylaxis
Progressive muscle weakness or immobility	Sensory abnormalities	Neuromuscular disorders
Trauma, procedures, inhalational injury	Absent breath sounds unilaterally, hypertympanic, tracheal deviation	Pneumothorax
Trauma, procedures	Absent breath sounds, dull on percussion, tracheal deviation	Hemothorax

From Vincent JL et al: *Textbook of critical care,* ed 7, Philadelphia, 2017, Elsevier.

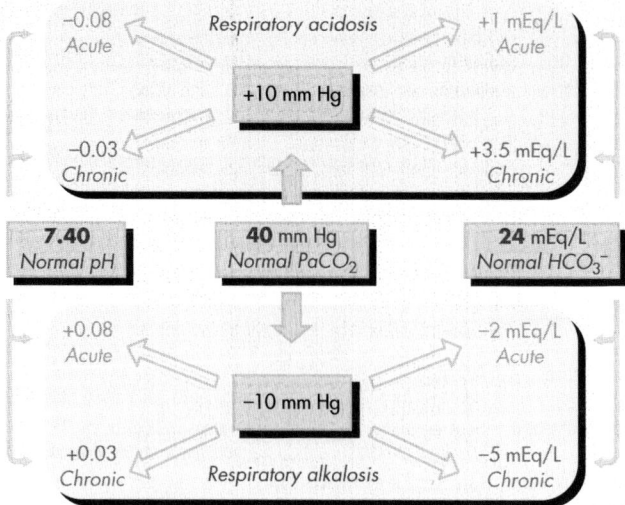

FIG. 1 Interpretation of an arterial blood gas in the setting of respiratory failure. $PaCO_2$, Partial pressure of carbon dioxide; HCO_3, bicarbonate; *Hg,* mercury. (From Vincent JL et al: *Textbook of critical care,* ed 7, Philadelphia, 2017, Elsevier.)

TABLE 5 Potential Indications for Mechanical Ventilation

Physiologic Mechanism	Clinical Assessment	Normal Range	Value(s)/Finding(s) Supporting Need for Mechanical Ventilation
Hypoxemia	$P(A-a)O_2$ gradient (mm Hg)	25-65	>350
	PaO_2/FiO_2 ratio	425-475	<300
	SaO_2	98%	<90% despite supplemental oxygen
Hypercarbia/inadequate alveolar ventilation	$PaCO_2$	35-45 mm Hg	Acute increase from patient's baseline pH <7.20 Mental status decline
Oxygen delivery/oxygen consumption imbalance	Elevated lactate	≤2.2 mg/dL	≥4 mg/dL despite adequate resuscitation
	Decreased mixed venous oxygen saturation	70%	<70% despite adequate acute resuscitation
Increased work of breathing	Minute ventilation	5-10 L/min	>15-20 L/min
	Dead space	0.15-0.30	≥0.5 (acute)
Inspiratory muscle weakness	NIP	80-100 cm H_2O	<20-30
	VC	60-75 mL/kg	<15-20
Acute decompensated heart failure	Jugular venous distention Pulmonary edema Decreased EF		Clinical judgment combined with the listed factors
Inadequate lung expansion	V_T (mL/kg)	5-8	<4-5
	VC (mL/kg)	60-75	<10-15
	Respiratory rate (breaths/min)	12-20	≥35

EF, Ejection fraction; *FiO_2,* fraction of inspired oxygen; *NIP,* negative inspiratory pressure; *$P(A-a)O_2$,* alveolar-arterial oxygen pressure difference; *PaO_2,* partial pressure of oxygen; *$PaCO_2$,* partial pressure of carbon dioxide; *SaO_2,* arterial oxygen saturation; *VC,* vital capacity; *V_T,* tidal volume.
From Parrillo JE, Dellinger RP: *Critical care medicine: principles of diagnosis and management in the adult,* ed 5, Philadelphia, 2019, Elsevier.

decision windows for noninvasive ventilation (NIV) or endotracheal intubation are illustrated in Fig. 2.

NONPHARMACOLOGIC THERAPY
- Hypoxemia may require treatment with supplemental oxygen, positive pressure support in the form of NIV, or mechanical ventilation.[3,4]
- Hypercapnia may require treatment with ventilatory support, NIV, or mechanical ventilation. The decision for either can be difficult and is primarily based on clinical presentation, severity of symptoms, comorbidities, and level of acid base derangement, as well as mental status.
- Contraindications to NIV include respiratory arrest, hemodynamic or cardiac instability, or inability to protect the airway.

- Monitoring carbon dioxide levels has not been standardized, but a change in symptoms and/or worsening in mental status can prompt a repeat in blood gas analysis.
- Worsening blood gas levels can be remediated with changes in the pressures on the noninvasive ventilator or by switching to a mechanical ventilator.

ACUTE GENERAL Rx
- Ventilatory support, either invasive (mechanical ventilation) or noninvasive, is often required. Early clinical identification of failure is important to circumvent delayed intubation, and therefore careful monitoring is required.[5] Table 6 provides an overview of features of selected modes of mechanical

ventilation. Potential advantages and disadvantages of each mode are summarized in Table 7.
- Compared with NIV, high-flow nasal oxygen (HFNO) as initial ARF management may improve several clinical outcomes. Compared with conventional oxygenation therapy, HFNO as postextubation management may reduce reintubation and improve patient comfort.[6,7]

REFERRAL
Pulmonologist

REFERENCES
Available at eBooks.Health.Elsevier.com

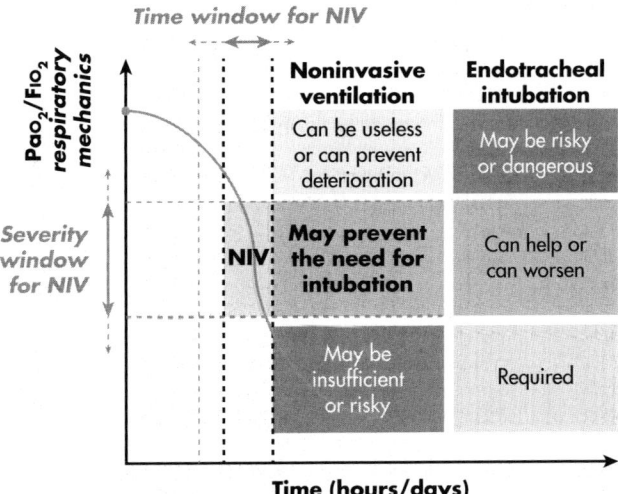

FIG. 2 The decision windows for noninvasive ventilation (NIV) or endotracheal intubation. There is an optimal window of time and severity of injury in which to consider NIV. As a patient worsens over time (see curve of patient course), one must consider whether the severity is appropriate for NIV or intubation and invasive mechanical ventilation. For the right level of severity, NIV can be valuable in offering needed support and perhaps preventing the need for intubation. If the severity worsens further, NIV may be insufficient or risky, and intubation may then be required. If the condition is mild, neither NIV nor invasive mechanical ventilation would be warranted. Unfortunately, there are no strictly objective criteria that delineate the windows of severity or of time for determining exactly when NIV should be used. *FIO₂*, Fraction of inspired oxygen; *PaO₂*, partial pressure of oxygen. (From Broaddus VC et al: *Murray & Nadel's textbook of respiratory medicine,* ed 7, Philadelphia 2022, Elsevier.)

TABLE 6 Overview of Features of Selected Modes of Mechanical Ventilation

Ventilator Mode	Trigger	Control	Cycling	Inspiratory Flow
Continuous mandatory ventilation	Time	Flow or pressure	Volume or time	Selected or decelerating
Volume control/assist control (VC/AC)	Patient or time	Flow	Volume	Square, decelerating, or sinusoidal
Pressure control/assist control (PC/AC)	Patient or time	Pressure	Time	Decelerating
Synchronized intermittent mandatory ventilation	Patient or time	Pressure for patient breaths	Flow for spontaneous breaths	Decelerating for spontaneous breath
		Flow (VC) or pressure (PC) for ventilator breaths	Volume or time for ventilator breaths	Square (VC), decelerating (VC or PC), sinusoidal for spontaneous breaths
Stand-alone pressure-support ventilation	Patient	None	Flow	Decelerating

From Parrillo JE, Dellinger RP: *Critical care medicine: principles of diagnosis and management in the adult,* ed 5, Philadelphia, 2019, Elsevier.

TABLE 7 Potential Advantages and Disadvantages of Selected Modes of Mechanical Ventilation

Mode	Advantage(s)	Disadvantage(s)
Controlled mechanical ventilation	Rests muscles of respiration	Requires use of heavy sedation/neuromuscular blockade
Assist volume control	Reduced work of breathing Guarantees delivery of set tidal volume (unless peak pressure limit alarm is exceeded)	Potential adverse hemodynamic effects May lead to inappropriate hyperventilation and excessive inspiration pressures
Assist pressure control	Allows limitation of peak inspiratory pressures	Same as for assist volume control Potential hyperventilation or hypoventilation with lung resistance/compliance changes
Synchronized intermittent mandatory ventilation	Less interference with normal cardiovascular function	Increased work of breathing compared with assist control Patient may find it difficult to adjust to two different types of ventilator breaths
Stand-alone pressure-support ventilation	Patient comfort Improved patient-ventilator interaction Decreased work of breathing	Apnea alarm is only backup Variable patient tolerance

From Parrillo JE, Dellinger RP: *Critical care medicine: principles of diagnosis and management in the adult,* ed 5, Philadelphia, 2019, Elsevier.

RELATED CONTENT

Acute Respiratory Distress Syndrome (Related Key Topic)
Asthma (Related Key Topic)
Carbon Monoxide Poisoning (Related Key Topic)

Chronic Obstructive Pulmonary Disease (Related Key Topic)
Interstitial Lung Disease (Related Key Topic)
Pneumonia, Bacterial (Related Key Topic)
Pneumonia, Mycoplasma (Related Key Topic)
Pneumonia, Pneumocystis jiroveci (Related Key Topic)

Pneumonia, Viral (Related Key Topic)
Pulmonary Embolism (Related Key Topic)
Pulmonary Edema (Related Key Topic)

AUTHOR: **JORGE MERCADO, MD**

BASIC INFORMATION

DEFINITION

An acute inability to urinate when the bladder is full. Acute urinary retention (AUR) is often, but not always, painful. The distended bladder may be palpable and percussible. AUR is distinct from chronic urinary retention, a condition in which patients can still void but chronically retain a significant volume of urine in the bladder after voiding.[1] Chronic urinary retention is not painful.

SYNONYMS

AUR
Urinary retention
Retaining urine

ICD-10CM CODES	
R33	Retention of urine
R33.8	Other retention of urine
R33.9	Retention of urine, unspecified

EPIDEMIOLOGY & DEMOGRAPHICS

INCIDENCE:
- One of the most common urologic emergencies.
- Typically occurs in aging men, especially those older than 60 yr. However, it may occur in any age group and in either sex.[1-3]
- Over a 5 yr period, AUR will occur in 10% of men older than 70 yr and in one third of men older than 80 yr. There is a near-linear increase in age-specific incidence for men ages 40 to 80 yr.[1,2]

PREVALENCE: Estimates are 40/100,000 men and 3/100,000 women. Prevalence increases as average lifespan increases.[1,2]

GENETICS: None known.

PHYSICAL FINDINGS & CLINICAL PRESENTATION

- Acute inability to pass urine or the tendency to pass only small amounts of urine.
- Pain and/or pressure in the lower abdomen and suprapubic region is typical. Low back pain may also occur. Pain may be absent, especially in older adults, patients with underlying neurologic disorders, and during chronic urinary retention.[1,2]
- Palpable and/or percussible bladder may be detected during abdominal examination in the suprapubic region.
- Suprapubic or bladder tenderness with deep palpation may be elicited.
- Increased urge to urinate with palpation of bladder (pressure applied to suprapubic region).
- Rarely, flank pain and costovertebral angle tenderness are present when high bladder pressures are transmitted to the ureters and kidney.
- Increased severity of lower urinary tract symptoms (LUTS) is associated with increased AUR risk. Patients may complain of worsening LUTS prior to episode, including increased urinary urgency, incontinence, nocturia, stranguria, hesitancy, and intermittency. These symptoms usually develop between 1 day and a few wk prior to AUR.[1]
- Patients with cognitive deficits or inability to communicate may present with restlessness, discomfort, confusion, and/or delirium.
- Acute kidney injury, electrolyte abnormalities, nausea, and lower extremity edema may be present with delayed presentation.[1,3-5]

ETIOLOGY

- AUR may be spontaneous or precipitated by a triggering event. Spontaneous AUR may arise from the natural progression of bladder outlet obstruction, more commonly from benign prostatic hyperplasia (BPH) and less commonly from pelvic masses and urethral stricture disease. Conversely, precipitated AUR episodes have an identifiable triggering event, such as acute trauma, surgical procedures (e.g., spinal, orthopedic, and urologic), medications (e.g., over-the-counter antihistamines and sympathomimetic agents commonly found in cough medications, anticholinergic drugs, and opioids), excessive fluid intake (e.g., alcohol), urinary tract infection, central nervous system insults (e.g., strokes, hemorrhage, spinal cord injuries), and severe constipation. There is overlap between spontaneous and precipitated AUR, particularly when triggering events are superimposed on underlying obstructive risk factors.[1,2]
- Urinary retention generally results from one of three categories: (1) Increased bladder outflow obstruction, as seen in BPH, urethral stricture disease, extrinsic compression from malignancy, constipation, and in gross hematuria where large clots can obstruct the urethra or bladder neck; (2) disruption of detrusor muscle innervation in association with diabetic neuropathy, spinal cord injury, progressive neurologic pathologies, and bladder contractile dysfunction and decompensation secondary to prolonged outlet obstruction; and (3) bladder overdistension that leads to impaired contractility and may result from general anesthesia, epidural anesthesia, or anticholinergic use.[1,2]
- Acute retention is often multifactorial in older patients, with an underlying obstructive risk factor and an acute precipitant.
- In women, obstructive factors can include benign tumors (especially fibroid tumors); malignant tumors of pelvic, urethral, or vaginal origin; urethral strictures and urethral meatal stenosis; postpartum vulvar edema; and labial fusion. Pelvic organ prolapse, including cystocele, rectocele, and uterine prolapse, can also lead to urinary retention.[1,6]
- Infection including prostatitis, urethritis, cystitis, genital herpes, and herpes zoster may also produce AUR.
- AUR is common in the postoperative period when patients are less mobile, are constipated, or have received opioid medications.[1,2]

DIAGNOSIS

DIFFERENTIAL DIAGNOSIS

- AUR is typically self-evident to the cognitively intact patient and the treating physician.
- Chronic urinary retention.
- Pelvic masses, fluid collections, uterine fibroids, pregnancies, or ascites may be confused for a full bladder, particularly when using bedside ultrasonic bladder capacity-measuring instruments.

WORKUP

- History is focused on urologic symptoms: Dysuria, hematuria, baseline voiding symptoms (caliber and force of stream, nocturia, sensation of incomplete emptying, double-voiding, incontinence, hesitancy), past episodes of retention, surgical history (urologic and other surgical procedures, particularly recent ones), pelvic/perineal trauma, and urologic cancer.
- History should include a complete list of prescribed and over-the-counter medications and recent medication changes.
- Review of symptoms should include presence of fever, back pain, neurologic symptoms, and rash.
- Rectal examination for masses, fecal impaction, perineal and perianal sensation, prostate size, and sphincter tone.
- Genitourinary examination in men, with special attention for meatal stenosis and phimosis or paraphimosis.
- Pelvic examination in women to assess for evidence of pelvic organ prolapse(s).
- Neurologic examination, with particular evaluation for "saddle" anesthesia (i.e., cauda equina syndrome) and pelvic sensory or motor deficits to rule out an underlying neurologic cause.

LABORATORY TESTS

- Electrolytes, blood urea nitrogen (BUN), and serum creatinine.
- Urinalysis and culture obtained via bladder or suprapubic catheterization.
- Prostate-specific antigen (PSA) testing is not helpful in AUR and may be falsely elevated after catheter placement. This test should not be routinely checked in the acute setting.[1]

IMAGING STUDIES

- Bladder ultrasound or a bedside postvoid residual urine scan (bladder scan) can be diagnostic. Ascites, pelvic fluid collections, body habitus, and presence of surgical implants (e.g., reservoirs for inflatable penile prostheses or artificial urinary sphincters) may confound accurate volume measurement with these devices.[1,3]
- Abdominal ultrasound or computed tomography (CT) may be helpful if there is suspicion of a pelvic mass.
- CT (Fig. 1) can be helpful when high volumes are measured by a bedside bladder scan, but low volumes are returned upon bladder catheterization.
- Magnetic resonance imaging (MRI) should be obtained when a spinal cord problem is suspected.
- Renal ultrasound or abdominopelvic CT may be obtained when there is kidney functional impairment and/or hydronephrosis is suspected.

Acute Urinary Retention (AUR)

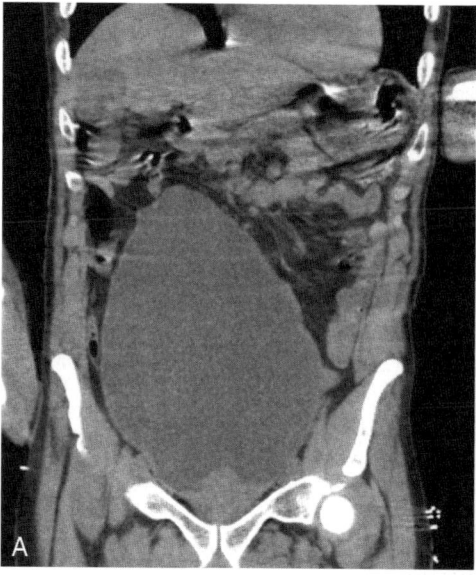
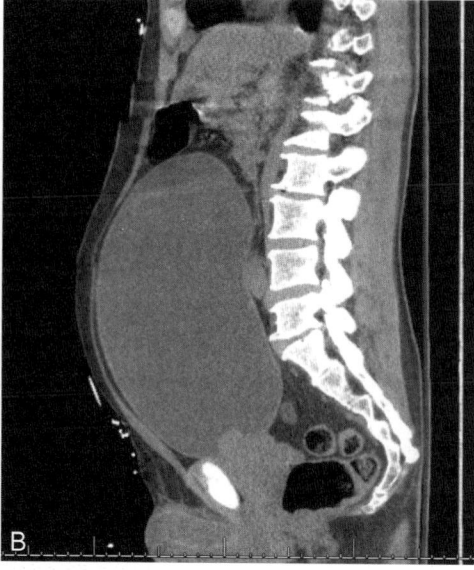

FIG. 1 Large volume urinary retention. Computed tomography images of coronal view **(A)** and sagittal view **(B)** of greatly distended bladder. The bladder extends into the midabdomen and above the pubic symphysis. More than 2 liters of urine were drained on bladder catheterization.

- Evaluation of bladder function by urodynamic testing may be conducted after initial management, particularly in women with no evidence of anatomic obstruction or in patients with longstanding obstruction and/or other neurologic conditions that affect bladder contractility.
- X-rays are of limited utility in evaluating AUR, but may show underlying constipation.

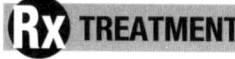 **TREATMENT**

ACUTE GENERAL Rx

- Prompt bladder decompression and drainage is the initial management of AUR, generally by indwelling urethral catheterization. Coude-tip (angled-tip) catheters can facilitate catheter placement in men with large prostates.[1,3,4] Clean intermittent catheterization is an option for patients with sufficient dexterity, vision, and motivation.
- Urologic consultation is advised after recent genitourinary surgery or a history of urethral stricture disease or difficult urethral catheterizations.
- When urethral catheterization is not possible or is contraindicated, suprapubic catheter placement is required.[1,3,5]
- Postdecompression hematuria may develop shortly after bladder drainage from small vessel injury of the overstretched bladder wall. This complication is usually self-limiting.[1,4]
- Monitor for postobstructive diuresis that results from a mixed osmotic and saline diuresis from salt and urea accumulation during the period of obstruction.[1,4]
- Avoid and/or discontinue medications that precipitate AUR (e.g., narcotics, anticholinergics, antihistamines).

CHRONIC Rx

- A voiding trial is reasonable 5 to 7 days after relief of obstruction in most patients.
- α-Blockers are effective for treatment of BPH symptoms in men. These agents increase the success rate of early catheter removal and should be initiated, unless contraindicated. There is limited evidence to suggest benefit in women.[1]
- If feasible, discontinue medications that increase the risk of AUR.
- Correct constipation and increase patient mobility.
- Inability to void after 5 to 7 days of catheterization mandates urologic consultation with more intensive evaluation of AUR, including possible cystoscopic evaluation and/or urodynamic studies.
- For patients who are unable to void after a voiding trial, either initiate clean intermittent catheterization, often two to three times a day, or have the urinary bladder catheter replaced.[1]

DISPOSITION

- Patients can be discharged home when close follow-up is feasible and progressive kidney injury and postobstructive diuresis are absent.[1,3-5]
- Hospital admission if patients have the following: Sepsis; complicated urinary tract infection; acute kidney injury; severe postobstructive diuresis; hyperkalemia; acidemia or azotemia; or if AUR is from malignancy, hematuria, or spinal cord compression.[1,3-5]

REFERRAL

- Urologist, if initial bladder catheterization is unsuccessful, or in surgical scenarios of radical prostatectomy, transurethral resection of prostate, urethral stricture surgery, and other bladder/prostate surgeries

- Urologic referral for recurrent AUR in men
- Gynecologic referral is mandatory if a pelvic mass is identified as etiology of AUR in women.

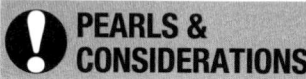 **PEARLS & CONSIDERATIONS**

- AUR is often painful.
- Rapid bladder drainage is of paramount importance.
- Monitor for postobstructive diuresis and correct electrolyte abnormalities.
- Request urologic advice or referral for AUR after urologic surgery.

PREVENTION

- Avoid and/or treat constipation.
- Avoid and/or discontinue medications that precipitate AUR (e.g., narcotics, anticholinergics, antihistamines).
- Patients with BPH should be cautious regarding medications that may precipitate AUR, including antihistamines, sympathomimetics, sedatives, and anticholinergics. On a chronic basis, 5-α reductase inhibitors (e.g., finasteride, dutasteride) may reduce the risk of AUR in men with BPH and large prostates.

REFERENCES
Available at eBooks.Health.Elsevier.com.

RELATED CONTENT
Benign Prostatic Hyperplasia (Related Key Topic)

AUTHORS: **GRACE K. YAGUCHI, MD,** and **DAVID A. LEAVITT, MD**

ℹ️ BASIC INFORMATION

DEFINITION

Adrenal insufficiency is characterized by inadequate secretion of corticosteroids resulting from partial or complete destruction of the adrenal glands (primary adrenal failure). Inadequate secretion of cortisol from the adrenals due to critical illness and pituitary insufficiency is known as secondary cortisol deficiency.

SYNONYMS

Primary adrenocortical insufficiency
Addison disease

ICD-10CM CODES
E23.3	Hypopituitarism
E27.1	Primary adrenocortical insufficiency
E27.2	Addisonian crisis
E27.3	Drug-induced adrenocortical insufficiency
E27.40	Unspecified adrenocortical insufficiency
E27.49	Other adrenocortical insufficiency

EPIDEMIOLOGY & DEMOGRAPHICS

PREVALENCE: 10 to 15 per 100,000 persons
PREDOMINANT SEX: Female:male ratio of 2:1

PHYSICAL FINDINGS & CLINICAL PRESENTATION

- Adrenal insufficiency may present insidiously with nonspecific symptoms. A high index of suspicion is required for diagnosis. About half of patients may present acutely with adrenal crises. Table 1 summarizes the clinical features of primary adrenal insufficiency
- Hyperpigmentation of skin (Figs. E1 and E2) and mucous membranes is a cardinal sign of adrenal insufficiency: More prominent in palmar creases, buccal mucosa, pressure points (elbows, knees, knuckles), perianal mucosa, and around areolas of nipples
- Hypotension, postural dizziness
- Generalized weakness, chronic fatigue, malaise, anorexia
- Amenorrhea and loss of axillary hair in females

ETIOLOGY

- Autoimmune destruction of the adrenal glands (80% of cases)
- Tuberculosis (TB) (7% to 20% of cases)
- Carcinomatous destruction of the adrenal glands, lymphoma
- Adrenal hemorrhage (anticoagulants, trauma, coagulopathies, pregnancy, sepsis)
- Adrenal infarction (antiphospholipid syndrome, arteritis, thrombosis)
- AIDS (adrenal insufficiency develops in 30% of patients with AIDS, often cytomegalovirus [CMV] adrenalitis)
- Genetic causes: Autoimmune polyglandular syndromes (APS) types 1 and 2, X-linked adrenoleukodystrophy, congenital adrenal hyperplasia
- Other: Sarcoidosis, amyloidosis, hemochromatosis, Wegener granulomatosis, postoperative, fungal infections (candidiasis, histoplasmosis)

🅳🆇 DIAGNOSIS

DIFFERENTIAL DIAGNOSIS

Sepsis, hypovolemic shock, acute abdomen, apathetic hyperthyroidism in the elderly, myopathies, gastrointestinal malignancy, major depression, anorexia nervosa, hemochromatosis, salt-losing nephritis, chronic infection

WORKUP (FIG. 3)

- An early morning (8 A.M.) serum cortisol <3 mcg/dl (82.8 mmol/L) is consistent with cortisol deficiency.
- If the cortisol level is 3 to 15 mcg/dl, the diagnosis can be confirmed with the rapid adrenocorticotropic hormone (ACTH) test:
  1. Give 250 mcg ACTH (Synacthen, tetracosactrin) by IV push and measure cortisol levels at 0, 30, and 60 min.
  2. An increase in serum cortisol level to peak concentration >500 nmol/L (18 mcg/dl) indicates a normal response. Cortisol level ≤18 mcg/dl at 30 or 60 min is suggestive of adrenal insufficiency.
  3. Measure plasma ACTH. A high ACTH level (>200 pg/ml [44 pmol/L]) confirms primary adrenal insufficiency.

Critical illness-related corticosteroid insufficiency (e.g., in sepsis) is best established with the 1-mcg ACTH stimulation test in which cortisol levels are measured at baseline and 30 min after administration of ACTH. A level <25 mcg/dl (690 nmol/L) or an increment over baseline of <9 mcg (250 nmol/L) represents an inadequate adrenal response.

- Secondary adrenocortical insufficiency (caused by pituitary dysfunction) can be distinguished from primary adrenal insufficiency by the following:
  1. Normal or low plasma ACTH level after rapid ACTH.
  2. Absence of hyperpigmentation.
  3. No significant impairment of aldosterone secretion (because aldosterone secretion is under control of the renin-angiotensin system).
  4. Additional evidence of hypopituitarism (e.g., hypogonadism, hypothyroidism).

LABORATORY TESTS

- Hyponatremia, hyperkalemia
- Decreased glucose
- Increased blood urea nitrogen/creatinine ratio (prerenal azotemia)

TABLE 1 Clinical Features of Primary Adrenal Insufficiency

Feature	Frequency (%)
Symptoms	
Weakness, tiredness, fatigue	100
Anorexia	100
Gastrointestinal symptoms	92
Nausea	86
Vomiting	75
Constipation	33
Abdominal pain	31
Diarrhea	16
Salt craving	16
Postural dizziness	12
Muscle or joint pains	13
Signs	
Weight loss	100
Hyperpigmentation	94
Hypotension (<110 mm Hg systolic)	88-94
Vitiligo	10-20
Auricular calcification	5
Laboratory Findings	
Electrolyte disturbances	92
Hyponatremia	88
Hyperkalemia	64
Hypercalcemia	6
Azotemia	55
Anemia	40
Eosinophilia	17

From Melmed SZ et al: *Williams textbook of endocrinology,* ed 14, Philadelphia, 2019, Saunders.

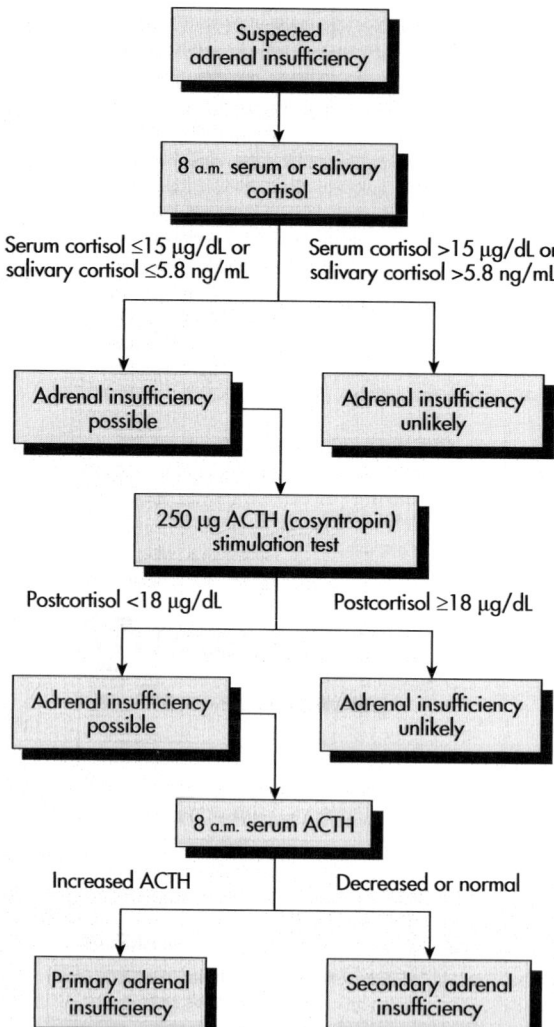

FIG. 3 Algorithm for the diagnosis of adrenal insufficiency. The adequacy of cortisol production is initially assessed with morning cortisol level measurement. Patients with low or borderline values undergo provocative adrenocorticotropic hormone (ACTH) stimulation testing, with serum cortisol levels measured before and 30 to 60 min after the administration of ACTH. Failure to mount an adequate response to ACTH usually establishes the diagnosis of adrenal insufficiency. The cause of adrenal insufficiency is then investigated with a morning ACTH level measurement. (From Townsend CM et al: *Sabiston textbook of surgery,* ed 21, St Louis, 2022, Elsevier.)

Mild normocytic, normochromic anemia, neutropenia, lymphocytosis, eosinophilia (significant dehydration may mask hyponatremia and anemia), hypercalcemia, metabolic acidosis

- A morning cortisol level >500 mmol/L (18 mcg/dl) generally excludes the diagnosis, whereas a level <165 mmol/L (6 mcg/dl) is suggestive of Addison disease and a level <3 mcg/dl requires further evaluation (see "Workup")
- Additional evaluation may include 21-hydroxylase antibodies present in 90% of autoimmune adrenalitis cases. If negative, obtain computed tomographic (CT) scan of adrenal glands
- PPD or QuantiFERON Gold test to rule out TB

IMAGING STUDIES
- Imaging is not necessary for diagnosis but may help identify potential causes.

- Abdominal CT scan (Fig. E4): Small adrenal glands generally indicate either idiopathic atrophy or longstanding TB, whereas enlarged glands are suggestive of early TB or potentially treatable diseases.
- Chest x-ray may reveal a small heart (Fig. E5).
- Abdominal x-ray: Adrenal calcifications may be noted if the adrenocortical insufficiency is secondary to TB or fungal infection.

℞ TREATMENT

NONPHARMACOLOGIC THERAPY
- Perform periodic monitoring of serum electrolytes, vital signs, and body weight; liberal sodium intake is suggested.
- Periodic measurement of bone density may be helpful in identifying patients at risk for the development of osteoporosis.

- Patients should carry a MedicAlert bracelet and an emergency pack containing hydrocortisone 100-mg ampule, syringe, and needle.
- Patients and partners should be educated on how to give IM injection in case of vomiting or coma.

ACUTE GENERAL Rx
- Adrenal crisis is an acute complication of adrenal insufficiency characterized by circulatory collapse, dehydration, nausea, vomiting, hypoglycemia, and hyperkalemia. Table 2 summarizes the treatment of acute adrenal insufficiency (adrenal crisis) in adults.
  1. Draw plasma cortisol level; do not delay therapy while waiting for confirming laboratory results.
  2. Administer hydrocortisone 100 mg IV immediately and every 6 h; if patient shows good

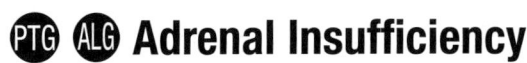

TABLE 2 Treatment of Acute Adrenal Insufficiency (Adrenal Crisis) in Adults

Emergency Measures

1. Establish intravenous access with a large-gauge needle.
2. Draw blood for immediate serum electrolytes and glucose and routine measurement of plasma cortisol and ACTH. Do not wait for laboratory results.
3. Infuse 2-3 L of 154 mmol/L NaCl (0.9% saline) solution, or 50 g/L (5%) dextrose in 154 mmol/L NaCl (0.9% saline) solution, as quickly as possible. Monitor for signs of fluid overload by measuring central or peripheral venous pressure and listening for pulmonary rales. Reduce infusion rate if indicated.
4. Inject intravenous hydrocortisone (100 mg immediately and every 6 h).
5. Use supportive measures as needed.

Subacute Measures after Stabilization of the Patient

1. Continue intravenous 154 mmol/L NaCl (0.9% saline) solution at a slower rate for next 24-48 h.
2. Search for and treat possible infectious precipitating causes of the adrenal crisis.
3. Perform a short ACTH stimulation test to confirm the diagnosis of adrenal insufficiency (if patient does not have known adrenal insufficiency).
4. Determine the type of adrenal insufficiency and its cause, if not already known.
5. Taper glucocorticoids to maintenance dosage over 1-3 days, if precipitating or complicating illness permits.
6. Begin mineralocorticoid replacement with fludrocortisone (0.1 mg by mouth daily) when saline infusion is stopped.

ACTH, Adrenocorticotropic hormone.
From Melmed S et al: *Williams textbook of endocrinology,* ed 14, 2019, Elsevier.

TABLE 3 Treatment of Chronic Primary Adrenal Insufficiency in Adults

Maintenance Therapy

Glucocorticoid Replacement

- Hydrocortisone 15-20 mg on awakening and 5-10 mg in early afternoon.
- Monitor clinical symptoms and morning plasma ACTH.

Mineralocorticoid Replacement

- Fludrocortisone 0.1 (0.05-0.4) mg orally.
- Liberal salt intake.
- Monitor lying and standing blood pressure and pulse, edema, serum potassium, and plasma renin activity.
- Educate patient about the disease, how to manage minor illnesses and major stresses, and how to inject steroid intramuscularly.
- Obtain MedicAlert bracelet/necklace, Emergency Medical Information card.

Treatment of Minor Febrile Illness or Stress

- Increase glucocorticoid dose twofold to threefold for the few days of illness; do not change mineralocorticoid dose.
- Contact physician if illness worsens or persists for more than 3 days or if vomiting develops.
- No extra supplementation is needed for most uncomplicated, outpatient dental procedures with local anesthesia. General anesthesia or intravenous sedation should not be used in the office.

Emergency Treatment of Severe Stress or Trauma

- Inject contents of prefilled dexamethasone (4-mg) syringe or contents of hydrocortisone hemisuccinate rapid reconstitution vial (100-mg) intramuscularly.
- Get to physician as quickly as possible.

Steroid Coverage for Illness or Surgery in Hospital

- For moderate illness, give hydrocortisone 50 mg bid PO or IV. Taper rapidly to maintenance dose as patient recovers.
- For severe illness, give hydrocortisone 100 mg IV q8h. Taper to maintenance level by decreasing by half every day. Adjust dose according to course of illness.
- For minor procedures under local anesthesia and most radiologic studies, no extra supplementation is needed.
- For moderately stressful procedures such as barium enema, endoscopy, or arteriography, give a single 100-mg IV dose of hydrocortisone just before the procedure.
- For major surgery, give hydrocortisone 100 mg IV just before induction of anesthesia and continue q8h for first 24 h. Taper dose rapidly, decreasing by half per day, to maintenance level.

ACTH, Adrenocorticotropic hormone; *bid,* twice a day; *IV,* intravenous; *PO,* orally; *q,* every.
From Melmed S et al: *Williams textbook of endocrinology,* ed 14, 2019, Elsevier.

TABLE 4 Suggested Plan for Steroid Replacement in Patients Withdrawing From Chronic Corticosteroid Therapy

Pred Dose (mg/day)	DURATION OF GLUCOCORTICOID TREATMENT			
	≤3 wk[a]			>3 wk
≥7.5	Can stop	↓ rapidly (e.g., 2.5 mg q3-4d) THEN		
5-7.5	Can stop	↓ 1 mg q2-4wk THEN	OR	Convert 5 mg pred to 20 mg HC, then ↓ 2.5 mg/wk to 10 mg/day THEN
<5	Can stop	↓ 1 mg q2-4wk		After 2-3 mo HC 10 mg/day, administer SST/ITT: Pass → Withdraw Fail → Continue

HC, Hydrocortisone; *ITT*, insulin tolerance test; *pred*, prednisolone; *SST*, short Synacthen test. Basal 0900h ACTH can be used to monitor for recovery of HPA axis and levels may be above the normal range ahead of a "pass" on an SST.

[a]Beware of frequent steroid courses (e.g., in asthma).

From Melmed S et al: *Williams textbook of endocrinology*, ed 14, 2019, Elsevier.

clinical response, gradually taper dosage over 1 to 3 days and change to oral maintenance dose (usually prednisone 7.5 mg/day).

3. Provide adequate volume replacement with D_5NS solution until hypotension, dehydration, and hypoglycemia are completely corrected. Large volumes (2 to 3 L) under continuous cardiac monitoring may be necessary in the first 2 to 3 h to correct the volume deficit and hypoglycemia and to avoid further hyponatremia.

- Identify and correct any precipitating factor (e.g., sepsis, hemorrhage).

CHRONIC Rx

- Table 3 summarizes the treatment of chronic primary adrenal insufficiency in adults.
- Give hydrocortisone 15 to 20 mg PO every morning and 5 to 10 mg in late afternoon or prednisone 5 mg in morning and 2.5 mg hs.
- Give oral fludrocortisone 0.05 mg/day to 0.4 mg/day. This mineralocorticoid is necessary if the patient has primary adrenocortical insufficiency. The dose is adjusted based on the serum sodium level and the presence of postural hypotension or marked orthostasis.
- Instruct patients to increase glucocorticoid replacement in times of stress and to receive parenteral glucocorticoids if diarrhea or vomiting occurs. Typical supplementation varies from 25 mg PO qd of hydrocortisone for minor medical and surgical stress to 50 to 100 mg IV hydrocortisone q8h for sepsis-induced hypotension or shock.
- The administration of dehydroepiandrosterone (DHEA) is controversial due to lack of robust data. It is not indicated in men but may be considered in women with primary adrenal failure. A dose of 50 mg PO qd may improve well-being and sexuality in women with adrenal insufficiency.
- Patients with concomitant hypothyroidism should be treated with glucocorticoids first before correcting hypothyroidism because correction of thyroid hormone deficiency will accelerate cortisol clearance and can precipitate adrenal crisis.
- A plan for steroid replacement in patients withdrawing from chronic corticosteroid therapy is outlined in Table 4.

SUGGESTED READINGS
Available at eBooks.Health.Elsevier.com

RELATED CONTENT
Addison Disease (Patient Information)

AUTHOR: **FRED F. FERRI, MD**

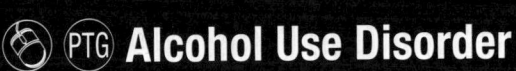

A

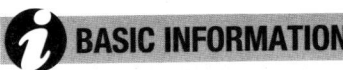 **BASIC INFORMATION**

DEFINITION

- "Moderate drinking": Moderate drinking has been defined as two standard drinks (e.g., 12 oz of beer) per day for men and one drink per day for women and persons older than 65 yr.
- "Hazardous" or "at-risk drinking": For men, at-risk drinking or *harmful alcohol use* is defined as more than 14 drinks/wk or more than four drinks/occasion. For women, at-risk drinking is defined as four or more drinks on one occasion or eight or more drinks per week.
- "Alcohol withdrawal": The American Psychiatric Association defines diagnostic criteria for *alcohol withdrawal* as follows:
  1. Cessation of (or reduction in) alcohol use that has been heavy and prolonged
  2. Two (or more) of the following, developing within several hours to a few days:
     a. Autonomic hyperactivity (e.g., sweating or pulse rate >100 beats/min)
     b. Increased hand tremor
     c. Insomnia
     d. Nausea and vomiting
     e. Transient visual, tactile, or auditory hallucinations or illusions
     f. Psychomotor agitation
     g. Anxiety
     h. Grand mal seizures
  3. The symptoms cause clinically significant distress or impairment in social, occupational, or other important areas of functioning
- The symptoms are not attributable to a general medical condition and are not better accounted for by another mental disorder.

SYNONYMS

Alcohol dependence syndrome
Substance abuse
Alcohol withdrawal syndrome
Alcoholism

ICD-10CM CODES
F10	Mental and behavioral disorders due to use of alcohol
F10.1	Mental and behavioral disorders due to use of alcohol: Harmful use
F10.2	Mental and behavioral disorders due to use of alcohol: Dependence syndrome
F10.3	Mental and behavioral disorders due to use of alcohol: Withdrawal state
F10.4	Mental and behavioral disorders due to use of alcohol: Withdrawal state with delirium
F10.5	Mental and behavioral disorders due to use of alcohol: Psychotic disorder
F10.6	Mental and behavioral disorders due to use of alcohol: Amnesic syndrome

EPIDEMIOLOGY & DEMOGRAPHICS

INCIDENCE (IN U.S.):
- The clinical history suggests alcohol problems in 15% to 20% of patients in primary care and hospitalized patients. In the U.S., alcohol use disorder generates nearly $223 billion in annual economic costs. An estimated 14% of adults in the U.S. have alcohol dependence. Alcohol accounts for 6.8% of age-standardized deaths in men and 2.2% in women.
- Data from the 2020 National Survey on Drug Use and Health indicate that 7% of adults reported heavy alcohol use in the previous month, and only 4.2% of adults with alcohol use disorder received treatment.[1a]
- Alcohol-associated liver disease (ALD) is among the most common liver diseases, and more than 2 million people in the U.S. in 2017 had alcohol-associated cirrhosis.[1]
- 20% achieve abstinence without help; 70% achieve sobriety for 1 yr.

PREVALENCE (IN U.S.): 7% of population ≥18 yr
PREDOMINANT SEX:
- Lifetime risk for males 8% to 10%
- Lifetime risk for females 3% to 5%

PEAK INCIDENCE: 20 to 40 yr. The most common age range for initial treatment of alcohol dependence is 35 to 45 yr. However, the peak period for meeting alcohol dependence criteria is ≥10 yr earlier.

GENETICS: More common with a family history of alcoholism and in patients of Irish, Scandinavian, and Native American descent

PHYSICAL FINDINGS & CLINICAL PRESENTATION

- Recurring minor trauma
- Gastrointestinal bleeding from gastritis and/or varices
- Pancreatitis (acute and chronic)
- Liver disease
- Odor of alcohol on breath
- Tremulousness
- Tachycardia
- Peripheral neuropathy
- Recent memory loss

ETIOLOGY

- Social and genetic factors important
- Risk factors:
  1. Broken homes
  2. Unemployment
  3. Divorce
  4. Recurrent depression
  5. Addiction to another substance, including tobacco
  6. Working long hours (≥55 hours/wk)

Dx DIAGNOSIS

WORKUP

- The United States Preventive Services Task Force (USPSTF) recommends that clinicians screen adults 18 yr and older for alcohol misuse and provide persons engaged in risky or hazardous drinking with brief behavioral counseling interventions to reduce alcohol misuse. Several screening tests (CAGE [Table 1], TWEAK, CRAFFT, Alcohol Use Disorders Identification Test-Concise [AUDIT-C; Table 2]) are available. The four-item CAGE (feeling need to Cut down, Annoyed by criticism, Guilty about drinking, and need for an Eye-opener in the morning) is the most popular screening test in primary care. A positive response should lead to further questioning. The sensitivity of the CAGE ranges from 43% to 94% and its specificity ranges from 70% to 97%. The five-item TWEAK scale (Tolerance, Worry, Eye-openers, Amnesia, [K] cut down) and the TACE questionnaire (Tolerance, Annoyance, Cut down, Eye-opener) are designed to screen pregnant women for alcohol misuse. They detect lower levels of alcohol consumption that may pose risks during pregnancy. The CRAFFT questionnaire (riding in Car with someone who was drinking, using alcohol to Relax, using alcohol while Alone, Forgetfulness, criticism from Friends and Family, Trouble) is useful as a screening tool for adolescents. Its sensitivity is 92% and specificity 64% for alcohol use disorder. Single-question screening about alcohol consumption in a day ("When was the last time you had more than X drinks in a day?" [where X is five for men and four for women]) with the threshold set at "in the past 3 mo" is 85% sensitive and 70% specific in men and 82% and 70% in women for unhealthy alcohol use. The three-question AUDIT-C is a shorter form of the 10-item AUDIT, and the questions center on the quantity and frequency of alcohol use. It asks how often someone has had a drink containing alcohol, how many standard drinks containing alcohol one consumes on a typical day when one is drinking, and how often one

TABLE 1 CAGE Questionnaire for Alcohol Problems Screening

C	Have you felt the need to Cut down on your drinking?
A	Have people Annoyed you by criticizing your drinking?
G	Have you ever felt bad or Guilty about your drinking?
E	Have you had a drink first thing in the morning to steady your nerves or to get rid of a hangover (i.e., an "Eye opener")?

From Stern TA et al: *Massachusetts General Hospital handbook of general hospital psychiatry*, ed 7, Philadelphia, 2018, Elsevier.

TABLE 2 AUDIT-C Questionnaire for Alcohol Problems Screening[a]

Question	Score
How often did you have a drink containing alcohol in the past year?	Never (0 points) Monthly or less (1 point) 2-4 times per month (2 points) 2-3 times per week (3 points) >4 times per week (4 points)

AUDIT-C, Alcohol Use Disorders Identification Test-Concise.
[a]AUDIT-C is scored 0-12, with score >4 (men) and >3 (women) considered positive for problematic drinking.
From Stern TA et al: *Massachusetts General Hospital handbook of general hospital psychiatry*, ed 7, Philadelphia, 2018, Elsevier.

has six or more drinks on one occasion. Scoring ranges from 0 to 4 on each question with a total score range of 0 to 12. A total score of 3 or higher for women and 4 or higher for men indicates alcohol use disorder and need for further assessment. Its sensitivity ranges from 85% in Hispanic women to 95% in white men.
- Laboratory evaluation (see below).

LABORATORY TESTS

Lab tests alone do not accurately detect alcohol problems but can help identify medical complications related to alcohol use, such as pancreatitis or cirrhosis.
- Gamma-glutamyltransferase (GGTP), generally elevated
- Liver transaminases (alanine aminotransferase [ALT], aspartate aminotransferase [AST]), often elevated, may be normal or low in advanced liver disease
- Low albumin level, hypophosphatemia, hypomagnesemia from malnutrition
- Complete blood count (CBC) reveals elevated mean corpuscular volume from toxic effect of alcohol on erythrocyte development in nutritional deficiencies
- Stool for occult blood may be positive as a result of gastritis or variceal bleeding
- Red blood cell (RBC) folate, vitamin B_{12} level, vitamin B_6, vitamin B_1 level

IMAGING STUDIES

Indicated only with a history of trauma. CT or ultrasound of abdomen may reveal fatty liver or cirrhosis in advanced stages.

(Rx) TREATMENT

NONPHARMACOLOGIC THERAPY

- Twelve-step facilitation, cognitive behavioral therapy, and motivational enhancement therapy improve the chances of recovery in patients with alcohol use disorder and dependence.
- Depression, if present, should be treated at same time alcohol is withdrawn.

ACUTE GENERAL Rx

Alcohol withdrawal syndrome (AWS) occurs when a person stops ingesting alcohol after prolonged consumption. It can result in four possible clinical patterns depending on the severity of the patient's alcohol use and the time from the patient's previous alcohol ingestion. Blood ethanol level decreases by ~20 mg/dl/h in a normal person. Although discussed separately, these withdrawal states blend together in real life. Table 3 summarizes medications for the treatment of alcohol dependence. The cornerstone of treatment for alcohol withdrawal syndrome is the use of benzodiazepines.
- **Tremulous state** (early alcohol withdrawal, "impending delirium tremens [DTs]," "shakes," "jitters")
  1. Time interval: Usually occurs 6 to 8 h after the last drink or 12 to 48 h after reduction of alcohol intake; becomes most pronounced at 24 to 36 h
  2. Manifestation: Tremors, mild agitation, insomnia, tachycardia; symptoms are relieved by alcohol

3. Detoxification can be in the outpatient (ambulatory) or inpatient setting. Candidates for outpatient detoxification should have a reasonable support system (e.g., reliable contact person) who can monitor progress and lack of any significant comorbid conditions (e.g., suicide risk, seizure disorder, coexisting benzodiazepine dependence, prior unsuccessful outpatient detoxification, pregnancy, cirrhosis) or risk factors for severe withdrawal (age >40 yr, drinking >100 g of ethanol daily [e.g., 1 pint of liquor or eight 12-oz cans of beer, random blood alcohol concentration >200 mg/dl])
4. Inpatient treatment:
   a. The management of alcohol withdrawal is facilitated by the use of ethanol withdrawal charts. An example of such a chart is shown in Fig. 1
   b. Admit to medical floor (private room); monitor vital signs q4h; institute seizure precautions; maintain adequate sedation
   c. Administer lorazepam as follows:
      (1) Day 1: 2 mg PO q4h while awake and not lethargic
      (2) Day 2: 1 mg PO q4h while awake and not lethargic
      (3) Day 3: 0.5 mg PO q4h while awake and not lethargic
      (4) NOTE: Hold sedation for lethargy or abnormal vital or neurologic signs. The preceding doses are only guidelines; it is best to titrate the dose case by case

---

TABLE 3 Medications for the Treatment of Alcohol Dependence*

Medication	Dose and Route	Frequency	Effects	Major Common Adverse Effects
Alcohol Withdrawal				
		Benzodiazepines[†]		
Chlordiazepoxide*	25-100 mg, PO/IV/IM[†]	Every 4-6 h	Decreased severity of withdrawal; stabilization of vital signs; prevention of seizures and delirium tremens	Confusion, oversedation, respiratory depression
Diazepam[‡]	5-10 mg, PO/IV/IM[†]	Every 6-8 h		
Oxazepam[‡]	15-30 mg, PO[†]	Every 6-8 h		
Lorazepam[‡]	1-4 mg, PO/IV/IM[†]	Every 4-8 h		
		β-Blockers		
Atenolol	25-50 mg, PO	Once a day	Improvement in vital signs	Bradycardia, hypotension
Propranolol	10-40 mg, PO	Every 6-8 h	Reduction in craving	
		α-Agonists		
Clonidine	0.1-0.2 mg, PO	Every 6 h	Decreased withdrawal symptoms	Hypotension, fatigue
		Antiepileptics		
Carbamazepine	200 mg, PO	Every 6-8 h	Decreased severity of withdrawal; prevention of seizures	Dizziness, fatigue, red blood cell abnormalities
		Prevention of Relapse		
Disulfiram[‡]	125-500 mg, PO	Daily	Decreased alcohol use among those who relapse	Disulfiram-alcohol reaction, rash, drowsiness, peripheral neuropathy
Naltrexone[‡]	50 mg, PO	Daily	Increased abstinence, decreased drinking days	Nausea, abdominal pain, myalgias-arthralgias
	380 mg, IM	Every 4 wk		
Acamprosate[‡]	666 mg, PO	Three times a day	Increased abstinence	Diarrhea

IM, intramuscular; *IV*, intravenous; *PO*, by mouth.
*Most commonly used medications listed.
[†]Currently approved by U.S. Food and Drug Administration for the indication noted.
[‡]Dose and routes given for standard fixed-dose regimens, which include dose tapers over time.
From Goldman L, Schafer AI: *Goldman's Cecil medicine,* ed 24, Philadelphia, 2012, Saunders.

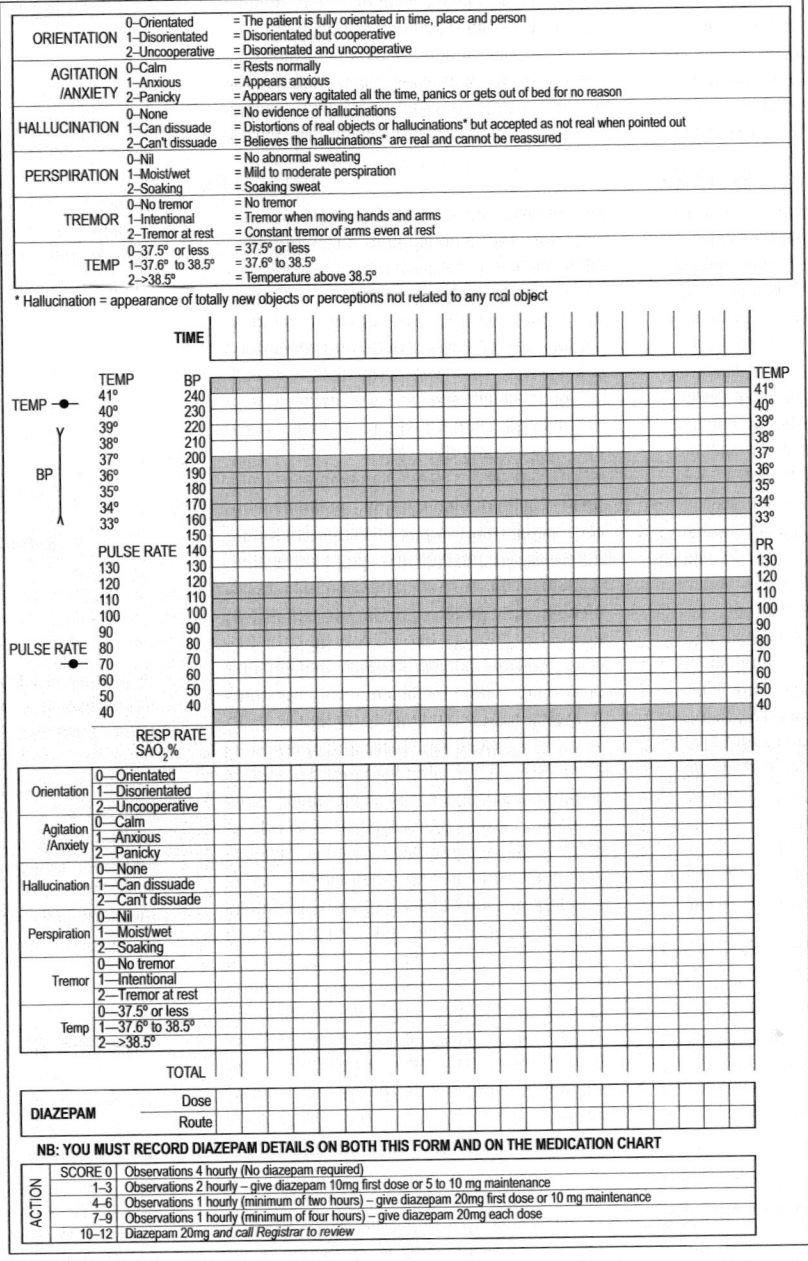

ORIENTATION	0–Orientated	= The patient is fully orientated in time, place and person
	1–Disorientated	= Disorientated but cooperative
	2–Uncooperative	= Disorientated and uncooperative
AGITATION /ANXIETY	0–Calm	= Rests normally
	1–Anxious	= Appears anxious
	2–Panicky	= Appears very agitated all the time, panics or gets out of bed for no reason
HALLUCINATION	0–None	= No evidence of hallucinations
	1–Can dissuade	= Distortions of real objects or hallucinations* but accepted as not real when pointed out
	2–Can't dissuade	= Believes the hallucinations* are real and cannot be reassured
PERSPIRATION	0–Nil	= No abnormal sweating
	1–Moist/wet	= Mild to moderate perspiration
	2–Soaking	= Soaking sweat
TREMOR	0–No tremor	= No tremor
	1–Intentional	= Tremor when moving hands and arms
	2–Tremor at rest	= Constant tremor of arms even at rest
TEMP	0–37.5° or less	= 37.5° or less
	1–37.6° to 38.5°	= 37.6° to 38.5°
	2–>38.5°	= Temperature above 38.5°

* Hallucination = appearance of totally new objects or perceptions not related to any real object

ACTION	SCORE 0	Observations 4 hourly (No diazepam required)
	1–3	Observations 2 hourly – give diazepam 10mg first dose or 5 to 10 mg maintenance
	4–6	Observations 1 hourly (minimum of two hours) – give diazepam 20mg first dose or 10 mg maintenance
	7–9	Observations 1 hourly (minimum of four hours) – give diazepam 20mg each dose
	10–12	Diazepam 20mg *and call Registrar to review*

NB: YOU MUST RECORD DIAZEPAM DETAILS ON BOTH THIS FORM AND ON THE MEDICATION CHART

FIG. 1 An example of an alcohol withdrawal chart. (From Cameron P et al: *Textbook of adult emergency medicine,* ed 5, 2020, Elsevier.)

d. In patients with mild to moderate withdrawal and without history of seizures, individualized benzodiazepine administration (rather than a fixed-dose regimen) results in lower benzodiazepine administration and avoids unnecessary sedation. The Clinical Institute Withdrawal Assessment Scale for Alcohol, Revised (CIWA-Ar) scale (Box 1) can be used to measure the severity of alcohol withdrawal. It consists of 10 items: Nausea; tremor; autonomic hyperactivity; anxiety; agitation; tactile, visual, and auditory disturbances; headache; and disorientation. Each item is assigned a score from 0 to 7. For example, in the "agitation" category 0 indicates normal activity, and 7 indicates that the patient constantly thrashes about. For the category of "tremor," 0 indicates that tremor is not present and 7 that tremor is severe, even with arms not extended. The maximum total score is 67. Patients with mild AWS symptoms (CIWA-Ar score <8) can be monitored on an outpatient basis. Benzodiazepines are beneficial for most patients with a CIWA-AR score ≥8 and are strongly recommended in patients with substantial withdrawal symptoms (CIWA-Ar score >12). Patients with CIWA-Ar score of ≥15 should be admitted to detox unit. In-patient treatment is also recommended for patients with history of withdrawal seizures and for those with suicidal ideation and significant comorbidities

e. Beta-adrenergic blockers: Beta-blockers are useful for controlling blood pressure and tachyarrhythmias. However, they do not prevent progression to more serious symptoms of withdrawal and, if used, should not be administered alone but in conjunction with benzodiazepines. Beta-blockers should be avoided in patients with contraindications to their use (e.g., bronchospasm, bradycardia, or severe congestive heart failure). Centrally acting alpha-adrenergic agonists such as clonidine ameliorate symptoms in patients with mild to moderate withdrawal but do not reduce delirium or seizures

f. Vitamin replacement: Thiamine 100 mg IV or IM for at least 5 days plus oral multivitamins. The IV administration of glucose can precipitate Wernicke encephalopathy in alcoholics with thiamine deficiency; therefore thiamine administration should precede IV dextrose

g. Hydration PO or IV (high-caloric solution): If IV, glucose with Na^+, K^+, Mg^{2+}, and phosphate replacement prn

h. Laboratory studies:
   (1) CBC, platelet count, international normalized ratio (INR)
   (2) Electrolytes, glucose, blood urea nitrogen, creatinine
   (3) GGTP, ALT, AST
   (4) Phosphorus and magnesium
   (5) Serum vitamin B_{12} and folic acid (if megaloblastic features in blood smear)

i. Diagnostic imaging: Generally not necessary; if subdural hematoma is suspected (evidence of trauma, persistent lethargy), a CT scan should be ordered

j. Social rehabilitation: Group therapy such as Alcoholics Anonymous; identification and treatment of social and family problems should be initiated during the patient's hospital stay

- **Alcoholic hallucinosis:**
  1. Manifestations: Hallucinations usually are auditory, but hallucinations occasionally are visual, tactile, or olfactory; usually there is no clouding of sensorium as in delirium (clinical presentation may be mistaken for an acute schizophrenic episode). Disordered perceptions become most pronounced after 24 to 36 h of abstinence.
  2. Treatment: Same as for DTs (see "Withdrawal seizures").

- **Withdrawal seizures ("rum fits"):**
  1. Time interval: Usually occurs 7 to 30 h after cessation of drinking, with a peak incidence between 13 and 24 h
  2. Manifestations: Generalized convulsions with loss of consciousness; focal signs are usually absent; consider further investigation with CT scan of head and electroencephalography if clearly indicated (e.g., presence of focal neurologic deficits, prolonged postictal confusion state). In addition, in a febrile patient who is having a seizure or altered mental state, a lumbar puncture is necessary.
  3. Treatment:
     a. Diazepam 2.5 mg/min IV until seizure is controlled (check for respiratory depression or hypotension) may be beneficial for prolonged seizure activity; IV lorazepam 1 to 2 mg q2h can be used in place of diazepam. Withdrawal seizures generally are self-limited and treatment is not required; the use of phenytoin or other anticonvulsants for short-term treatment of alcohol withdrawal seizures is not recommended
     b. Thiamine 100 mg IV, followed by IV dextrose, should also be administered.
     c. Electrolyte imbalances (increased Mg^{2+}, decreased K^+, increased or decreased Na^+, decreased PO_4^{3-}) that may exacerbate seizures should be corrected.

BOX 1 Alcohol Withdrawal Assessment Scoring Guidelines (Revised Clinical Institute Withdrawal Assessment for Alcohol Scale)

Nausea and Vomiting (0-7)
0, none; 1, mild nausea with no vomiting; 4, intermittent nausea; 7, constant nausea, frequent dry heaves and vomiting

Tremor (0-7)
0, no tremor; 1, not visible, but can be felt fingertip to fingertip; 4, moderate, with patient's arms extended; 7, severe, even with arms not extended

Paroxysmal Sweats (0-7)
0, no sweats; 1, barely perceptible sweating, palms moist; 4, beads of sweat obvious on forehead; 7, drenching sweats

Anxiety (0-7)
0, no anxiety, patient at ease; 1, mildly anxious; 4, moderately anxious or guarded, so anxiety is inferred; 7, equivalent to acute panic states seen in severe delirium or acute schizophrenic reactions

Agitation (0-7)
0, normal activity; 1, somewhat more than normal activity; 4, moderately fidgety and restless; 7, pacing back and forth during, or constantly thrashing about

Tactile Disturbances (0-7)
Ask, "Have you experienced any itching, pins and needles sensation, burning or numbness, or a feeling of bugs crawling on or under your skin?"
0, none; 1, very mild itching, pins and needles, burning, or numbness; 2, mild itching, pins and needles, burning, or numbness; 3, moderate itching, pins and needles, burning, or numbness; 4, moderately severe tactile hallucinations; 5, severe hallucinations; 6, extremely severe hallucinations; 7, continuous hallucinations

Auditory Disturbances (0-7)
Ask, "Are you more aware of sounds around you? Are they harsh? Do they startle you? Do you hear anything that disturbs you or that you know isn't there?"
0, not present; 1, very mild harshness or ability to startle; 2, mild harshness or ability to startle; 3, moderate harshness or ability to startle; 4, moderate hallucinations; 5, severe hallucinations; 6, extremely severe hallucinations; 7, continuous hallucinations

Visual Disturbances (0-7)
Ask, "Does the light appear to be too bright? Is its color different than normal? Does it hurt your eyes? Are you seeing anything that disturbs you?"
0, not present; 1, very mild sensitivity to light; 2, mild sensitivity; 3, moderate sensitivity; 4, moderate hallucinations; 5, severe hallucinations; 6, extremely severe hallucinations; 7, continuous hallucinations

Headache (0-7)
0, not present; 1, very mild; 2, mild; 3, moderate; 4, moderately severe; 5, severe; 6, very severe; 7, extremely severe

Orientation and Clouding of Sensorium (0-4)
Ask, "What day is this? Where are you? Who am I?"
0, oriented; 1, cannot do serial additions or is uncertain about date; 2, disoriented to date by no more than 2 calendar days; 3, disoriented to date by more than 2 calendar days; 4, disoriented to place and/or person

Total Score
0-9: Absent or minimal withdrawal
10-19: Mild to moderate withdrawal
More than 20: Severe withdrawal

From Sullivan JT et al: Assessment of alcohol withdrawal: the revised Clinical Institute Withdrawal Assessment for Alcohol Scale (CIWA-Ar), *Br J Addict* 84:1353-1357, 1989.

- **DTs:**
  1. Time interval: Variable; usually occurs within 1 wk after reduction or cessation of heavy alcohol intake and persists for 1 to 3 days. Peak incidence is 72 h and 96 h after the cessation of alcohol consumption.
  2. Manifestations: Profound confusion, tremors, vivid visual and tactile hallucinations, autonomic hyperactivity; this is the most serious clinical presentation of alcohol withdrawal (mortality rate is approximately 15% in untreated patients).
  3. Treatment:
     a. Admission to a detoxification unit where patient can be observed closely
     b. Vital signs q30min (neurologic signs, if necessary)
     c. Use of lateral decubitus or prone position if restraints are necessary
     d. NPO: Nasogastric tube for abdominal distention may be necessary but should not be routinely used
     e. Laboratory studies: Same as for early alcohol withdrawal
     f. Vigorous hydration (4 to 6 L/day): IV with glucose (Na^+, K^+, PO_4^{3-} and Mg^{2+} replacement [if patient has hypophosphatemia or hypomagnesemia])
     g. Vitamins: Thiamine 100 mg IV qd. The initial dose of thiamine should precede the administration of IV dextrose; multivitamins (may be added to the hydrating solution)
     h. Sedation: Control of agitation should be achieved with rapid-acting sedative-hypnotic agents in adequate doses to maintain light somnolence for the duration of delirium
        (1) Initially: Lorazepam 2 to 5 mg IM/IV repeated prn
        (2) Maintenance (individualized dosage): Chlordiazepoxide, 50 to 100 mg PO q4 to 6h, lorazepam 2 mg PO q4h, or diazepam 5 to 10 mg PO tid; withhold doses or decrease subsequent doses if signs of oversedation are apparent
        (3) Midazolam is also effective for managing DTs. Its rapid onset (sedation within 2 to 4 min of IV injection) and short duration of action (approximately 30 min) make it an ideal agent for titration in continuous infusion
     i. Treatment of seizures (as previously described)
     j. Diagnosis and treatment of concomitant medical, surgical, or psychiatric conditions

CHRONIC Rx

- See "Referral."
- Pharmacotherapies for alcoholism include:
  1. Acamprosate is a synthetic compound with a chemical structure similar to the neurotransmitter gamma-aminobutyric acid and the amino acid neuromodulator taurine. Its mechanism of action is not completely understood. It is indicated for the maintenance of abstinence from alcohol in patients with alcohol dependence who are abstinent at treatment initiation. It should be used only as part of a comprehensive psychosocial treatment program. It does not cause a disulfiram-like reaction as a result of ethanol ingestion. Dose is two 333-mg tablets tid. Treatment should be initiated as soon as possible after the period of alcohol withdrawal, when the patient has achieved abstinence, and should be maintained if the patient relapses. Avoid acamprosate if severe renal impairment is present.
  2. The long-acting opiate antagonist naltrexone inhibits the rewarding effects of alcohol. The starting dose is 25 mg/day, increased to 50 mg PO qd after 1 wk. An extended-release, once-monthly injection of naltrexone is also available and can be used along with psychosocial support to maintain alcohol abstinence. In patients with opioid dependence, naltrexone can precipitate acute withdrawal syndrome and should not be used at least 7 days from last opioid use. There are no established guidelines on the appropriate length of naltrexone treatment for alcohol dependence. One study recommends at least 3 mo of treatment. Avoid naltrexone if acute hepatitis, hepatic failure, or ongoing opioid use is present.
  3. Disulfiram (Antabuse): Dosage is 500 mg max qd for 1 to 2 wk, then 125 to 500 mg qd. It interferes with the metabolism of alcohol by inhibiting aldehyde dehydrogenase, causing an accumulation of acetaldehyde. It produces unpleasant symptoms (nausea, flushing, elevated blood pressure, headache, weakness) when alcohol is ingested. It is an older drug that is now rarely used.
  4. Topiramate, baclofen, or gabapentin can be offered as second line drugs; to patients with moderate to severe alcohol use disorder topiramate might be preferable.
  5. Avoid pharmacological treatments in pregnant or breastfeeding women.

DISPOSITION

See "Referral."

REFERRAL

- To Alcoholics Anonymous or Adult Children of Alcoholics
- Family members to Al-Anon or Al-A-Teen
- Many cities have Salvation Army Adult Rehabilitation centers; all patients accepted, regardless of ability to pay

PEARLS & CONSIDERATIONS

COMMENTS

- Relative indications for inpatient alcohol detoxification are as follows: History of DTs or withdrawal seizures, severe withdrawal symptoms, concomitant psychiatric or medical illness, pregnancy, multiple previous detoxifications, recent high levels of alcohol consumption, and lack of reliable support network.
- Detoxification is not a stand-alone treatment but should serve as a bridge to a formal treatment program for alcohol dependence.
- The cure rate for alcoholism is highly disappointing, regardless of the modality. Only those who want to be helped will be helped. An effective strategy for the primary care physician is a prominently displayed sign in the office that states, "If you think you consume too many alcoholic beverages, please discuss it with me." Those who do open up the discussion can be given the facts in a nonjudgmental way and often can be helped. All too often problem drinkers lie on the questionnaire until they face a life-threatening health issue—and even then denial often reigns supreme.
- Alcohol-associated liver disease is among the most common liver diseases, and more than 2 million people in the U.S. in 2017 had alcohol-associated cirrhosis.[1]

REFERENCES & SUGGESTED READINGS

Available at eBooks.Health.Elsevier.com

RELATED CONTENT

Alcohol Use Disorder (Patient Information)
Drug Use Disorder (Related Key Topic)
Alcoholic Hepatitis (Related Key Topic)
Substance Use Disorder (Related Key Topic)
Wernicke Syndrome (Related Key Topic)

AUTHOR: **FRED F. FERRI, MD**

Alcoholic Hepatitis 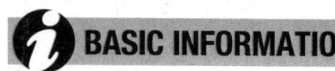 ⒜⒧⒢ ⒫⒯⒢ ⊘

ⓘ BASIC INFORMATION

DEFINITION

Alcoholic hepatitis (AH) is a severe, progressive, inflammatory, and cholestatic liver disease occurring in patients with long-term heavy alcohol use (60 to 80 g/day in men and 20 to 40 g/day in women). Main characteristics include rapid onset of jaundice, hepatomegaly, generalized malaise, and subtle systemic inflammatory response features.

SYNONYM

AH

ICD-10CM CODES	
K70.10	Alcoholic hepatitis without ascites
K70.9	Alcoholic liver disease, unspecified

EPIDEMIOLOGY & DEMOGRAPHICS

- Approximately 2 million people in the U.S. (about 1% of the population) are affected by alcoholic liver disease.
- Alcoholic hepatitis accounts for 0.08% to 0.09% of admissions in the U.S.
- Typical presentation age: 40 to 50 yr. Majority occurs before age 60.
- Patients with alcoholic hepatitis typically drink more than 100 g of alcohol daily for two or more decades.
- Excessive alcohol intake is the third leading preventable cause of death in the U.S.

PREVALENCE: Approximately 25% to 30%
PREDOMINANT SEX & AGE: The majority of patients are males. Males are two times as likely as women to abuse alcohol. However, women develop alcoholic hepatitis after a shorter time and smaller amount of alcoholic exposure than men.
RISK FACTORS: Drinking multiple alcohol types, drinking alcohol between meal times, poor nutrition, female gender, obesity, Hispanic ethnicity, long-term ingestion of >10 to 20 g/day of alcohol in women and >20 to 40 g/day in men
GENETICS: No genetic predilection for any one race. In the U.S., however, there is increased incidence in minority groups.

PHYSICAL FINDINGS & CLINICAL PRESENTATION

Common presenting symptoms include:
- Rapid onset of jaundice within 60 days of heavy alcohol consumption (>50 g/day) for at least 6 mo
- Jaundice with duration <3 mo
- Right upper quadrant abdominal/epigastric pain
- Nausea/vomiting
- Malaise
- Low-grade fever
- Anorexia
- Abdominal distention/pain (due to ascites)
- Weight loss or malnourishment

- Proximal muscle wasting and weakness
- Complications of liver impairment (GI bleed; confusion, lethargy, ascites)

Findings on physical examination include:
- Jaundice and ascites
- Hepatomegaly, with tender liver on palpation
- Fever (first exclude other causes of fever, such as spontaneous bacterial peritonitis, urinary tract infection [UTI], pneumonia)
- Asterixis (a flapping tremor)
- Splenomegaly
- Tachycardia/tachypnea
- Hypotension
- Peripheral edema
- Abdominal distention with shifting dullness (ascites)
- Hepatic bruit (may occur in >50% of patients)
- With coexistent cirrhosis, look for:
  1. Gynecomastia
  2. Proximal muscles wasting
  3. Spider angiomata
  4. Altered hair distribution

⒟⒳ DIAGNOSIS

DIFFERENTIAL DIAGNOSIS

- Hepatitis B
- Hepatitis C
- Nonalcoholic steatohepatitis (NASH)
- Chronic pancreatitis
- Drug-induced liver injury
- Hemochromatosis
- Cholangitis

WORKUP

- Diagnosis of AH is clinically supported by laboratory findings.
- The standard screening test for alcohol abuse is the Alcohol Use Disorders Identification Test (AUDIT).
- A thorough and detailed history is needed.
- Relevant questions may include:
  1. When patient started drinking
  2. Number of times patient drinks per day
  3. How many years of regular/daily drinking
  4. Types of alcohol
  5. Home or bar drinking
  6. Rehabilitation for drinking
  7. Social problems (e.g., arrest for public intoxication or driving under the influence, marital discord due to alcoholism)
  8. A typical patient may have a long history of excessive alcohol intake (>100 g of alcohol per day for at least 20 yr)
- Abdominal imaging with ultrasound (the imaging of choice) to rule out gallstones, biliary, and other liver diseases such as liver abscess or hepatocellular carcinoma.

LABORATORY TESTS

The best biomarkers of harmful ethanol use are gamma glutamyltransferase (GGT), aspartate aminotransferase (AST), ethyl glucuronide (ETG), and phosphatidyl ethanol.

- Elevated transaminase (aspartate aminotransferase [AST] >45 U/L but <500 U/L; however, some patients may not have elevations in ALT, AST in early phases)
- AST: Alanine aminotransferase [ALT] ratio ≥2:1
- S-bilirubin >5 mg/dl
- Increased prothrombin time [PT]/international normalized ratio [INR]
- Elevated gamma glutamyltransferase (GGT)
- Carbohydrate-deficient transferrin (CDT) is a reliable marker for chronic alcoholism
- Elevated C-Reactive Protein [CRP is a good marker of alcoholic hepatitis]
- Electrolyte disorder (hypokalemia, hypomagnesemia, low zinc, hypophosphatemia)
- Hypoalbuminemia
- Hyperferritinemia
- CBC (may reveal leukocytosis with bandemia or anemia or thrombocytopenia); mean corpuscular volume (MCV) may be elevated
- Screening tests to rule out other conditions include checking:
  1. Hepatitis B surface antigen (HBsAg), hepatitis B core antibody (HB_cAb) (IgM), hepatitis A antibody (IgM)
  2. Antihepatitis C antibody, hepatitis C ribonucleic acid (RNA)
  3. Ferritin-transferrin saturation
  4. Alpha-fetoprotein
  5. Alkaline phosphatase
- Laboratory criteria of severe alcoholic hepatitis are defined as
  1. Maddrey Discriminant Function (MDF) score >32, which is calculated as follows: MDF = 4.6 × prothrombin time−control-prothrombin time + total bilirubin (mg/dl)
     OR
  2. Model for End-Stage Liver Disease (MELD) >21
     AND/OR
  3. Hepatic encephalopathy. There are other models for determining severity such as the Alcohol Hepatitis Histologic Score (AHHS) or for prognostication such as the MELD + Lille combination models.

IMAGING STUDIES

Ultrasonography is the preferred imaging study. The earliest histologic change in alcoholic liver disease is macrovesicular steatosis.

LIVER BIOPSY

- Liver biopsy is rarely needed
- Useful to:
  1. Confirm the diagnosis
  2. Evaluate the effect of coexisting disease
  3. Rule out cirrhosis
  4. Exclude other diagnoses (especially other causes of liver diseases, biliary obstruction, Budd-Chiari syndrome)

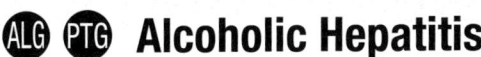

- Typical histologic findings include:
  1. Micro- or macrovesicular steatosis
  2. Hepatocyte injury (ballooning degeneration and focal hepatocyte necrosis)
  3. Mallory-Denk bodies (characteristic of alcoholic hepatitis)
  4. Perivenular fibrosis
  5. Portal and lobular inflammation with neutrophils or lymphocyte infiltration

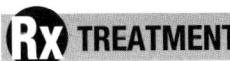 **TREATMENT**

An algorithm for the management of patients with alcoholic hepatitis is described in Fig. E1. Treatment can be divided into three main components:
1. Determining the severity of the disease using Maddrey Discriminant Function (DF) and Model for End Stage Liver Disease (MELD)
2. Supportive care which includes lifestyle modifications and nutritional support
3. Pharmacologic therapy

LIFESTYLE MODIFICATIONS

- Abstinence, together with adequate nutritional support, is the cornerstone of management.
- Abstinence from alcohol (this improves both short- and long-term survival). Fig. E2 describes the effect of subsequent alcohol intake on 5-yr survival in patients with alcoholic hepatitis.
- Nonpharmacologic methods to promote abstinence include cognitive-behavioral therapy (CBT), Alcoholics Anonymous (AA) attendance, and motivational interviewing.
- Pharmacologic aids include using naltrexone, acamprosate, or baclofen.
- Monitor abstinence with breath test or urine drug screen (for use in past 3 days) or hair sample analysis for ethyl glucuronide (test alcohol intake within the last few months).
- Smoking cessation (to decrease oxidative stress).
- Treatment of substance abuse.

NUTRITIONAL SUPPORT:

- Good nutrition is an essential part of treatment because many patients with alcoholic hepatitis have severe protein-calorie malnutrition as well as deficiencies of trace minerals and several vitamins.
- Nutritional support includes:
  1. Liberal vitamin supplementation (especially thiamine, folic acid, vitamin K)
  2. Mineral supplementation **(but not iron)**
  3. Calorie counting is essential. A high calorie intake (1.2 to 1.4 times the normal resting intake) may be required

4. Protein intake of 1.2 to 1.5 g/kg of ideal body weight per day will provide adequate support. **Exception: In patients with severe encephalopathy, protein restriction may be required.**
5. Fluid management

PHARMACOLOGIC THERAPY

Severe alcoholic hepatitis may require treatment. Severity can be assessed by calculating the MELD score or MDF score or the Glasgow score.
- An MDF score ≥ 32 indicates significant or severe alcoholic hepatitis (30-day mortality of 50%).
- MELD score can easily be calculated (visit https://optn.transplant.hrsa.gov/resources/allocation-calculators/meld-calculator/). This score predicts short-term survival in patients with cirrhosis. A score >20 predicts increased short-term mortality.
- Glasgow score: Contains four variables (BUN, PT, WBC count, and bilirubin). A score ≥ 9 indicates increased mortality.

Indications for hospitalization include:
1. MDF ≥ 32
2. MELD >20
3. Glasgow score >8
4. Hepatic encephalopathy

Patients with severe alcoholic hepatitis may be treated with glucocorticosteroids (prednisolone 40 mg/day for 28 days with a 2-wk taper). Glucocorticosteroids reduce hepatic injury, suppress inflammation, and promote liver regeneration. However, not all studies have demonstrated consistent therapeutic benefits for steroids, even in high-risk patients.[1] Prednisolone should be discontinued if bilirubin does not decrease by day 17. An alternative agent for patients with contraindications to corticosteroids is pentoxifylline. Pentoxifylline is not effective in patients who do not respond to prednisone, and data supporting its use is weak.

LIVER TRANSPLANTATION

- Liver transplantation could be considered for patients with MELD >26 and unresponsive to steroids.
- Usually reserved for patients with end-stage liver disease. Patients whose hepatitis is not responding to medical therapy have a 6-mo survival rate of approximately 30%. Since most hepatitis deaths occur within 2 mo, early liver transplantation is attractive and associated with higher than 80% survival at 3 yr.
- Patients with alcoholic hepatitis must be sober for at least 6 mo before they can be eligible for

consideration for liver transplantation. However, transplantation candidates should not be based solely on 6 mo abstinence, and other factors, such as social support and need for rehabilitation, should be considered.

REFERRAL

Severe acute alcoholic hepatitis may require intensive care unit (ICU) care and referral to different subspecialists:
- GI/hepatology (for patients with evidence of GI hemorrhage)
- Nutritional services
- Nephrology (for acute renal failure, hepatorenal syndrome)
- Neurology (for change in mental status, seizures)
- Infectious disease (for fever/leukocytosis)

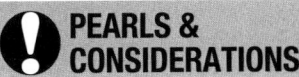 **PEARLS & CONSIDERATIONS**

COMMENTS

- Referral to substance abuse treatment programs may be helpful.
  1. Stress to patients that there are limited long-term drug treatments for alcoholic hepatitis.
  2. Maintaining good general nutrition is important.
  3. Advise patient about the risk of taking certain medications, especially acetaminophen.
- Periodic follow-up to monitor patient's response to check basic metabolic panel (BMP) and liver function tests (LFTs).
- Encourage alcohol abstinence. Abstinence improves long-term survival.
- If patient develops liver cirrhosis, check serum alpha-fetoprotein every 6 mo and liver ultrasound annually to rule out hepatocellular carcinoma.
- Vaccinate patient against hepatitis A and B viruses, pneumococci, influenza A virus, and routine adult vaccinations, if appropriate.

REFERENCE AND SUGGESTED READINGS
Available at eBooks.Health.Elsevier.com.

RELATED CONTENT
Alcoholic Hepatitis (Patient Information)

AUTHOR: **DANIEL K. ASIEDU, MD, PHD, FACP**

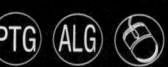
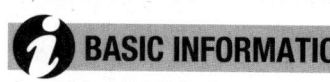 **BASIC INFORMATION**

DEFINITION

Primary aldosteronism is a group of disorders distinguished by inappropriate, autonomous, and excessive aldosterone production that results in renal sodium retention, plasma renin suppression, and secondary hypertension, which is classically characterized by hypokalemia and metabolic alkalosis.

SYNONYMS

Hyperaldosteronism
Conn syndrome

ICD-10CM CODES
E26.0	Primary hyperaldosteronism
E26.01	Conn syndrome
E26.02	Glucocorticoid-remediable aldosteronism
E26.1	Secondary hyperaldosteronism
E26.9	Hyperaldosteronism, unspecified

EPIDEMIOLOGY & DEMOGRAPHICS

PREVALENCE: Recent studies show that primary aldosteronism in hypertensive patients is much more common than previously recognized. Primary aldosteronism is increasingly prevalent with worsening severity of hypertension and, while estimates vary widely across observational studies, is likely present in 17.2% to 26.8% of patients with resistant hypertension.[1]
GENETICS: Familial hyperaldosteronism is a subset of hyperaldosteronism with five known heritable forms. It should be suspected in patients with any of the following:
- Onset of hypertension before age 21 yr and a family history of hypertension
- Family history of primary aldosteronism
- Family history of stroke before age 40 yr

ETIOLOGY (TABLE E1)
- Bilateral idiopathic adrenal hyperplasia (60% to 70%)
- Unilateral adenoma or Conn syndrome (30% to 40%)
- Unilateral adrenal hyperplasia (2%)
- Familial hyperaldosteronism (<1%)
- Carcinoma (<0.1%)
- Ectopic production (<0.1%)

PHYSICAL FINDINGS & CLINICAL PRESENTATION
- Generally asymptomatic
- Hypertension that is often resistant
- Spontaneous hypokalemia
- Family history of early-onset hypertension or stroke at age <40 yr

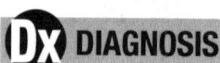 **DIAGNOSIS**

DIFFERENTIAL DIAGNOSIS
- Hypokalemia from diuretic use
- Hypokalemia from vomiting and/or diarrhea
- Renovascular hypertension

- Other endocrine neoplasm (pheochromocytoma, deoxycorticosterone-producing tumor, renin-secreting tumor)

WORKUP

Primary aldosteronism is characterized by suppressed plasma renin activity (PRA) and an elevated serum aldosterone level, usually exceeding 15 ng/dL. Box 1 provides guidance on when to consider testing for primary aldosteronism. Fig. 1 describes a diagnostic approach to patients with suspected primary aldosteronism. Computed tomography (CT), magnetic resonance imaging (MRI), and adrenal vein sampling (AVS) are used to distinguish unilateral from bilateral increased aldosterone secretion. This distinction affects treatment options. Unilateral secretion ideally is treated surgically if the patient is a surgical candidate, and bilateral secretion is treated medically.[2]

LABORATORY TESTS
- A 24-h urinary aldosterone excretion under aldosterone-suppressing conditions should be used when aldosterone and renin testing remains nondiagnostic. The sensitivity of plasma aldosterone/plasma renin activity ratio (ARR) to exclude primary aldosteronism is only 32%.
- Routine laboratory tests may suggest primary aldosteronism but are not diagnostic. Common abnormalities include the following:
  1. Spontaneous hypokalemia (9% to 37%) or severe hypokalemia while receiving conventional doses of diuretics
  2. Possible metabolic alkalosis and/or mild hypernatremia

IMAGING STUDIES
- Adrenal CT scan (Fig. E2) is the preferred imaging technique because adrenal adenomas have a high lipid content and are better visualized on CT scan.
- MRI may be used as an alternative.

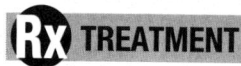 **TREATMENT**

NONPHARMACOLOGIC THERAPY
Regular blood pressure monitoring, low-sodium diet, tobacco avoidance, maintenance of ideal body weight, and regular exercise

---

BOX 1 Indications for Testing for Primary Aldosteronism

- Resistant hypertension
- Onset of hypertension at a young age (<20 yr)
- Hypertension with one of the following:
  1. Spontaneous or diuretic-induced hypokalemia
  2. Adrenal incidentaloma
  3. Sleep apnea
- Hypertension with a family history of:
  1. Primary aldosteronism
  2. Stroke before age 40 yr

ACUTE GENERAL RX
- Control of blood pressure and hypokalemia with spironolactone, eplerenone, or amiloride
- Surgery (unilateral adrenalectomy) for aldosterone-producing adenoma or unilateral adrenal hyperplasia

CHRONIC RX

A mineralocorticoid receptor antagonist, spironolactone (starting dose 25 mg daily), or eplerenone (starting dose, 25 mg twice daily) is titrated upward until a mid- to high-normal serum potassium concentration is achieved without potassium supplementation. The dose is increased at 2-wk intervals. Eplerenone causes less gynecomastia in men and less menstrual irregularities in women because of greater mineralocorticoid receptor selectivity. Amiloride (starting dose, 5 mg twice daily) may be used for patients intolerant of spironolactone and eplerenone.

DISPOSITION

Treatment of primary aldosteronism with mineralocorticoid receptor antagonism or unilateral adrenalectomy resolves hypokalemia, reduces blood pressure, and improves impaired cardiac and renal function.

Hypertension persists in 40% to 65% of patients after unilateral adrenalectomy. Patients who are more likely to experience complete resolution of hypertension are younger, take two or fewer antihypertensive agents preoperatively, have short duration of hypertension, have no family history of hypertension, and/or have a higher ARR.[3]

REFERRAL

Referral to an experienced interventional radiologist for adrenal vein sampling. If lateralization occurs, surgical referral for unilateral adrenalectomy should proceed after confirmation of a unilateral aldosterone-producing adenoma, unilateral adrenal hyperplasia, or carcinoma.

PEARLS & CONSIDERATIONS

- Primary aldosteronism is more common than previously thought and should be considered in all patients with apparent treatment-resistant hypertension.
- There is a more rapid decline in estimated glomerular filtration rate (eGFR) and increased occurrence of left ventricular mass, as well as increased relative risk of stroke, myocardial infarction, and atrial fibrillation in patients with primary aldosteronism than in patients with essential hypertension matched for age, gender, and blood pressure. Increased risk is attenuated but persists when treated with a mineralocorticoid antagonist. Adrenalectomy decreases these risks to below that of a matched patient with essential hypertension.[4]

A

I

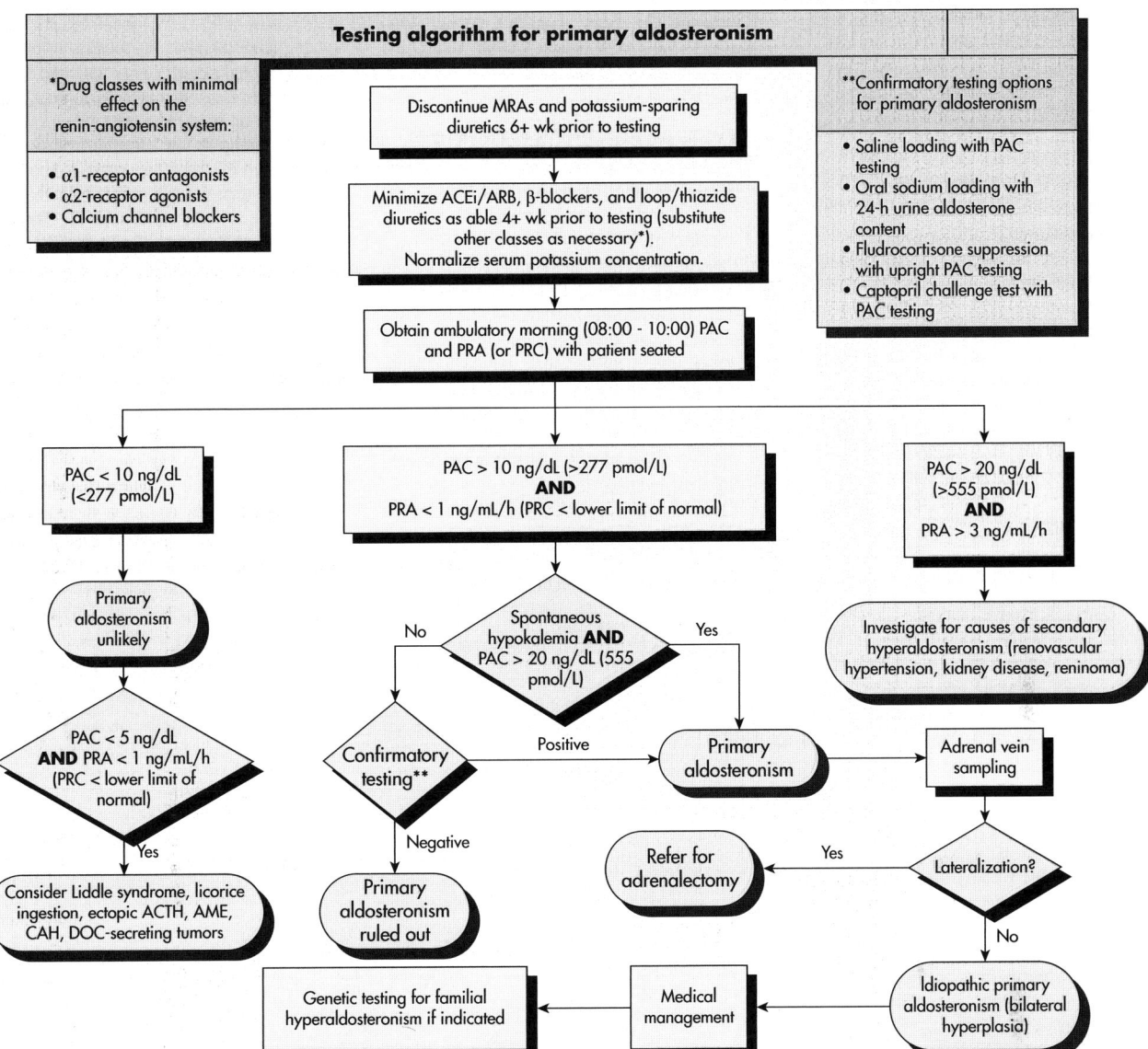

FIG. 1 Diagnostic approach to patients with suspected primary aldosteronism. The authors' preferred confirmatory test for primary aldosteronism is oral sodium loading with 300 mmol/day of sodium and 75 mmol/day of potassium for 3 days prior to a 24-h urine collection with measurement of urine sodium, potassium, creatinine, and aldosterone secretion. Excessive urine aldosterone excretion (>12 μg/day [33 nmol/day]) in this setting is consistent with primary aldosteronism. Adrenal vein sampling shows lateralization if the lateralization index (aldosterone-to-cortisol ratio measured in an adrenal vein divided by the aldosterone-to-cortisol ratio of the contralateral adrenal vein) is >4. A lateralization index <3 indicates bilateral adrenal hyperplasia. *ACEi,* Angiotensin-converting-enzyme inhibitor; *ACTH,* adrenocorticotropic hormone; *ARB,* angiotensin II receptor blocker; *AME,* Apparent mineralocorticoid excess; *CAH,* congenital adrenal hyperplasia; *DOC,* deoxycorticosterone; *MRA,* mineralocorticoid receptor antagonist; *PAC,* plasma aldosterone concentration; *PRA,* plasma renin activity; *PRC,* plasma renin concentration.

- Frequent monitoring of blood pressure and electrolytes after adrenalectomy is required because normalization of blood pressure after unilateral adrenalectomy may take up to 4 mo.
- Caution must be taken during interpretation of direct renin concentration (DRC) and PRA testing results because of different units used for each assay. The aldosterone-to-DRC ratio is yet to be as widely validated as the ARR.

REFERENCES
Available at eBooks.Health.Elsevier.com.

RELATED CONTENT
Aldosteronism (Hyperaldosteronism, Primary) (Patient Information)
Hypertension (Related Key Topic)

AUTHORS: **KEVIN S. FAY, MD** and **DEBBIE L. COHEN, MD**

Alzheimer Disease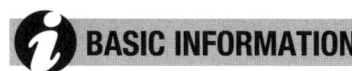

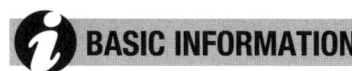

BASIC INFORMATION

DEFINITION

Dementia is a syndrome characterized by progressive loss of previously acquired cognitive skills, including memory, language, insight, and judgment. Alzheimer disease (AD) is thought to account for the majority of all cases of dementia.

ICD-10CM CODES
G30.0   Alzheimer disease with early onset
G30.1   Alzheimer disease with late onset
G30.8   Other Alzheimer disease
G30.9   Alzheimer disease, unspecified

EPIDEMIOLOGY & DEMOGRAPHICS

INCIDENCE: Risk doubles every 5 yr after the age of 65. The Chicago Health and Aging Population study found that the average annual incidence in people ages 65 and above was 2.3%, with Blacks having a significantly increased risk compared to Whites.[1]

PREVALENCE: Approximately 1/9 people (10.7%) ages ≥65 has Alzheimer dementia. Currently an estimated 6.5 million Americans have AD; 5% of the population between the ages of 65 and 74, 13.1% between 75 and 84, and 33.2% at ≥85 yr. Between 12% and 18% of Americans over age 60 are thought to have mild cognitive impairment (MCI).[2]

PREDOMINANT SEX: Females greater than males. In the U.S. 4 million women versus 2.5 million men are affected (12% of women, 9% of men ≥65).[2]

PHYSICAL FINDINGS & CLINICAL PRESENTATION

- Spouse or other family member, usually not the patient, notes insidious memory impairment.
- Patients have difficulties learning and retaining new information and handling complex tasks (e.g., balancing the checkbook) and have impairments in reasoning, judgment, spatial ability, and orientation (e.g., difficulty driving, getting lost away from home).
- Behavioral changes, such as mood changes and apathy, may accompany memory impairment. In later stages, patients may develop agitation and psychosis.
- Rare variants: Atypical presentations include early and severe behavioral changes, focal findings on examination, parkinsonism, hallucinations, falls, or onset of symptoms ≤65 yr.

DIAGNOSIS

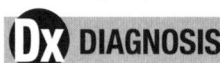

Diagnosis of AD has evolved with the development of biomarkers that indicate AD pathology in vivo such as brain amyloidosis and pathologic tau accumulation. The National Institute on Aging (NIA) and the Alzheimer Association (AA) recommended new diagnostic criteria and guidelines for AD in 2011, and these criteria were further revised in 2018 (Table 1). The NIA-AA criteria differed from prior DSM or NINDCS-ADRDA criteria in the following ways: (1) They recommend AD be considered a disease well before the onset of symptoms by incorporating biomarkers in diagnosis, and (2) they define three distinct stages of AD: (1) *Preclinical* AD, in which there is measurable biologic evidence of AD pathology but no symptoms; (2) MCI due to AD, in which the patient experiences mild memory loss but experiences no functional impairment at home or work but demonstrates biomarker evidence of AD; and (3) *dementia* due to AD, in which the patient experiences cognitive decline causing functional impairment and demonstrates biomarker evidence of AD. The 2018 NIA-AA criteria define AD not as three clinical syndromes but as a biologic process defined by biomarkers indicating the presence of beta amyloid (A+), pathologic tau (T+), and neurodegeneration or neuronal injury (N+). Using the ATN system and clinical status together allows an entire study population to be characterized (Fig. 1).

Although not yet commonly used in the clinic but invariably used in AD clinical trials, biomarkers transform the diagnosis of AD into one that can be established definitively while the

TABLE 1   New Diagnostic Criteria

Criteria for Probable Alzheimer Disease	RESEARCH CRITERIA		
	DSM-5 2013	NINCDS—ADRDA 2007	NIA-AA 2018
Insidious onset	X	X	X
Onset over months to years		X	X
Progressive decline	X	X	X
Deficits are not explained by delirium or other medical or psychiatric conditions	X	X	X
Social/occupational impairment	X		X
Presence of episodic memory deficit	X	X	
Cognitive deficits in at least two domains	X		X
Neuropsychologic testing required for diagnosis?	Preferably	X	Only if routine history and mental status testing are inconclusive
Abnormal PET or MRI scan		Supportive feature*	Required if needed to show biomarker evidence of amyloidosis, tauopathy, neurodegeneration as part of the biomarker-based AT(N) diagnostic schema
Genetic markers?	X	Supportive feature*	For research purposes
	Required only if there is evidence of multiple causes and no clear evidence of progression and decline in memory and another cognitive domain		
Abnormal cerebrospinal fluid marker required?		Supportive feature*	Required if needed to show biomarker evidence of amyloidosis, tauopathy, neurodegeneration as part of the biomarker-based AT(N) diagnostic schema

DSM-5, Diagnostic and Statistical Manual of Mental Disorders, fifth edition; *MRI*, magnetic resonance imaging; *NIA-AA*, National Institute on Aging—Alzheimer's Association; *NINCDS-ADRDA*, National Institute of Neurological and Communicative Disorders and Stroke—Alzheimer's Disease and Related Disorders Association; *PET*, positron emission tomography.
*At least one supportive feature is required for diagnosis of probable AD.
Modified from Fillit HM: *Brocklehurst's textbook of geriatric medicine and gerontology*, ed 8, Philadelphia, 2017, Elsevier.

	Biomarker Profile	Cognitive Stage		
		Cognitively Unimpaired	**Mild Cognitive Impairment**	**Dementia**
Biomarker Profile	**A⁻ T⁻ (N)⁻**	normal AD biomarkers, cognitively unimpaired	normal AD biomarkers with MCI	normal AD biomarkers with dementia
	A⁺ T⁻ (N)⁻	Preclinical Alzheimer pathologic change	Alzheimer pathologic change with MCI	Alzheimer pathologic change with dementia
	A⁺ T⁺ (N)⁻ / **A⁺ T⁺ (N)⁺**	Preclinical Alzheimer disease	Alzheimer disease with MCI (Prodromal AD)	Alzheimer disease with dementia
	A⁺ T⁻ (N)⁺	Alzheimer and concomitant suspected non-Alzheimer pathologic change, cognitively unimpaired	Alzheimer and concomitant suspected non-Alzheimer pathologic change with MCI	Alzheimer and concomitant suspected non-Alzheimer pathologic change with dementia
	A⁻ T⁺ (N)⁻ / **A⁻ T⁻ (N)⁺** / **A⁻ T⁺ (N)⁺**	non-Alzheimer pathologic change, cognitively unimpaired	non-Alzheimer pathologic change with MCI	non-Alzheimer pathologic change with dementia

FIG. 1 Descriptive nomenclature: Syndromal cognitive staging combined with biomarkers. *AD,* Alzheimer disease; *MCI,* mild cognitive impairment.
NOTE: Formatting denotes three general biomarker "categories" based on biomarker profiles: Those with normal AD biomarkers *(no color),* those with non-AD pathologic change *(dark gray),* and those who are in the Alzheimer continuum *(light gray).* (From Clifford RJ Jr et al: NIA-AA research framework: toward a biological definition of Alzheimer's disease, *Alzheimer Dement* 14:535-562, 2018.)

BOX 1   Red Flags for an Alzheimer Disease Diagnosis

- Age <65yr
- Fluctuating level of consciousness (consider toxic-metabolic encephalopathy, dementia with Lewy bodies)
- Behavioral, emotional, or personality disturbances overshadowing cognitive impairment (consider frontotemporal dementia, HIV dementia)
- Rapidly (6-12 mo) progressive development (consider Creutzfeldt–Jakob disease, paraneoplastic limbic encephalitis, autoimmune encephalitis, HIV dementia, frontotemporal dementia)
- Presence of physical abnormalities:
  1. Gait impairment (consider vascular dementia, HIV dementia, NPH, chronic subdural hematomas, Parkinson disease and atypical Parkinsonian disorders)
  2. Lateralized signs, e.g., hemiparesis, spasticity, other corticospinal tract signs (consider vascular dementia)
  3. Movement disorders
  4. Myoclonus (consider Creutzfeldt–Jakob disease, paraneoplastic encephalitis)
  5. Rigidity, bradykinesia (parkinsonism) (consider dementia with Lewy bodies and Parkinson disease)

Modified from Kaufman DM, et al: *Kaufman's clinical neurology for psychiatrists,* ed 8, Philadelphia, 2017, Elsevier.

---

patient is still alive. In clinical practice, the diagnosis is commonly made based on clinical history, a thorough physical and neurologic examination, and use of reliable and valid diagnostic criteria (i.e., DSM or NINDCS-ADRDA) such as the following:

- Loss of memory and one or more additional cognitive abilities (aphasia, apraxia, agnosia, or other disturbance in executive functioning)
- Impairment in social or occupational functioning that represents a decline from a previous level of functioning and results in significant disability
- Deficits that do not occur exclusively during the course of delirium
- Insidious onset and gradual progression of symptoms

- Cognitive loss documented by neuropsychologic tests
- No physical signs, neuroimaging, or laboratory evidence of other diseases that can cause dementia (i.e., metabolic abnormalities, medication or toxin effects, infection, stroke, Parkinson disease, subdural hematoma, or tumors)

Red flags for an AD diagnosis are summarized in Box 1.

DIFFERENTIAL DIAGNOSIS (TABLE 2)

- Other neurodegenerative dementia (Table 3):
  1. Primary age-related tauopathy
  2. Limbic predominant age-related TDP-43 encephalopathy (LATE)

  3. Argyrophilic grain disease
  4. Frontotemporal lobar degeneration
  5. Dementia with Lewy bodies
  6. Parkinson disease dementia
  7. Corticobasal syndrome
  8. Progressive supranuclear palsy
- Vascular cognitive impairment disorder (vascular dementia due to multiple strokes, severe small vessel changes, chronic vasculitis, or chronic subdural hematoma)
- Subjective memory loss
- Depression (pseudodementia) (Table 4)
- Neoplasm (benign or malignant brain tumor, leptomeningeal disease)
- Infection (HIV-associated dementia, neurosyphilis, progressive multifocal leukoencephalopathy [PML])

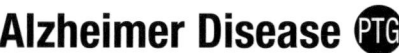

TABLE 2 Cognitive Disorders in Older Adults

Diagnosis (% of Dementias Attributable)	History	Physical Examination Findings	Imaging Findings	Comment
Normal aging changes (n/a)	Delayed retrieval (forgetting names, dates), slower processing (takes longer to learn new things). No functional limitations	None	Mild generalized cortical atrophy, mild ventricular enlargement. No focal findings	Patients may have white matter disease and/or prior lacunar infarcts related to HTN, DM, and cardiovascular disease, etc., but unrelated to memory complaints
Mild cognitive impairment (n/a)	Cognitive deficits beyond what is expected for age across one or more domains	None	Variable depending on etiology. Atrophy of medial temporal lobe and/or hippocampus (pre-Alzheimer disease)	• Clinical course highly dependent on etiology. Amnestic MCI most likely to progress to dementia (50%) • Neuropsychologic testing may help to clarify diagnosis
Alzheimer disease (67%)	Progressive memory loss and other cognitive deficits	• Essentially normal in early stages • Moderate: Patients may develop apraxia, aphasia	Medial temporal, parietal lobe, and/or hippocampal atrophy on MRI. Positivity on amyloid PET scan	• Patients will occasionally present with unusual variants based on atypical neuroanatomic pathology; for example, fixed delusions or behavioral manifestations (dysexecutive variant) or prominent visual symptoms (posterior cortical atrophy)
Vascular dementia (20%, includes mixed dementia)	Prominent vascular risk factors, possible history of stroke/TIA, possible stepwise disease progression. Executive dysfunction may be prominent early symptom	Variable depending on distribution of disease	Cortical and subcortical infarcts and white matter disease	Commonly present in conjunction with Alzheimer disease—known as mixed dementia
Lewy body dementia and Parkinson dementia (15%)	Fluctuating cognition, well-formed visual hallucinations, REM sleep disorder, falls, sensitivity to neuroleptics	Orthostatic hypotension, postural instability, hyposmia, bradykinesia, resting tremor, rigidity	No specific findings on MRI. Positivity on dopamine transporter PET scan	Parkinson dementia occurs in patients with preexisting Parkinson disease of at least 1-yr duration, followed by onset of cognitive deficits
Frontotemporal dementia (<5%)	Two variants: • Behavioral variant (50%) presents with progressive personality and behavioral changes • Primary progressive aphasia presents with progressive language impairment	Frontal release signs	Frontal and temporal lobe atrophy	Executive function and episodic memory generally preserved in early stages of disease
Chronic traumatic encephalopathy (CTE, unknown)	History of multiple concussions and/or traumatic brain injury, most commonly in former athletes or military personnel. Concurrent behavioral changes and psychiatric disease common	None	Nonspecific white matter changes	Tauopathy in cortical and perivascular regions of the brain. CTE can only definitely be diagnosed by autopsy; there is currently no definitive clinical criteria for diagnosis
Rapidly progressive dementia (<1%)	Memory symptoms progressive over weeks to months	• Variable depending on etiology • Myoclonus/startle reflex suggestive of prion disease	Variable depending on etiology	• Rapidly progressive dementias are rare and merit urgent referral to a neurologist • Specialized testing should be based on patient-specific risk factors
Delirium (n/a)	Identifiable toxic, metabolic, or infectious etiology and/or precipitants (e.g., acute hospital admission). Rapid onset	Inattention, disorganized thinking, and/or altered level of consciousness. Fluctuating course	No specific findings	• EEG will demonstrate acute slowing • Generally reversible with correction of precipitant(s)

DM, Diabetes mellitus; *EEG,* electroencephalogram; *HTN,* hypertension; *MCI,* mild cognitive impairment; *MRI,* magnetic resonance imaging; *PET,* positron emission tomography; *REM,* rapid eye movement; *TIA,* transient ischemic attack.
From Warshaw G et al: *Ham's primary care geriatrics,* ed 7, Philadelphia, 2022, Elsevier.

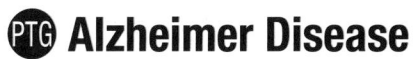

TABLE 3 Features Distinguishing Alzheimer Disease and Frontotemporal Dementia

Feature	Alzheimer Disease	Frontotemporal Dementia
Age at onset (yr)	>65	53 (mean)
Memory impairments	Early, pronounced	Subtle, at least initially, with preserved visuospatial ability
Behavior abnormalities	None until middle or late stage	Early and prominent perseverative and compulsive behavior; hyperorality; impaired executive ability
Language impairment	Except for anomia, none until late stage	Paraphasias, anomia, decreased fluency
CT/MRI appearance	General atrophy, but especially parietal and temporal lobes	Frontal and temporal lobe atrophy
Histologic marker	Aβ accumulation	Tau accumulation

CT, Computed tomography; *MRI,* magnetic resonance imaging.
From Kaufman DM et al: *Kaufman's clinical neurology for psychiatrists,* ed 8, Philadelphia, 2017, Elsevier.

TABLE 4 Clinical Features of Delirium, Depression, and Alzheimer's Disease

	DELIRIUM	DEPRESSION	ALZHEIMER'S DISEASE
Onset of initial symptoms	Abrupt	Relatively discrete	Insidious
	Difficulty with attention and disturbed consciousness	Dysphoric mood or lack of pleasure	Memory deficits—verbal and/or spatial
Course	Fluctuating—over days to weeks	Persistent—usually lasting months if untreated	Gradually progressive, over years
Family history	Not contributory	May be positive for depression	May be positive for AD
Memory	Poor registration	Patchy/inconsistent	Recent > remote
Memory complaints	Absent	Present	Variable—usually absent
Language deficits	Dysgraphia	Increased speech latency	Confrontation naming difficulties
Affect	Labile	Depressed/irritable	Variable—may be neutral

From Stern TA: *Massachusetts General Hospital handbook of general hospital psychiatry,* ed 7. Philadelphia, 2018, Elsevier.

- Toxic/metabolic (EtOH, myxedema coma, subacute combined degeneration, pellagra, mercury exposure, drug effects)
- Organ failure (hepatic encephalopathy)

WORKUP
HISTORY & GENERAL PHYSICAL EXAMINATION:
- Medication lists should always be reviewed for drugs or home remedies that may cause mental status changes, especially anticholinergic medications, benzodiazepines, opiates, barbiturates, and neuroleptics.
- Patients should be screened for depression, because it can sometimes mimic dementia but often occurs as a coexisting condition and should be treated.
- On examination, look for signs of metabolic disturbance, presence of psychiatric features, or focal neurologic deficits.
- Symptoms and preserved abilities of Alzheimer dementia by disease stage are summarized in Table 5.

MENTAL STATUS TESTING: Brief mental status testing can be done easily and quickly in the office. Formal neuropsychologic testing offers more nuanced data about a patient's current cognitive and emotional function but is not required for straightforward cases. Formal neuropsychologic testing is indicated when patients present with atypical symptoms, have significant psychiatric comorbidities, and when patients' or families'

report of cognitive dysfunction differs from findings on a bedside cognitive assessment. Also, neuropsychologic testing may be beneficial if there are concerns that in the future, the patient's testamentary capacity will be challenged.

Commonly used cognitive tests to detect dementia include the Folstein Mini-Mental State Examination (MMSE), the Mini-Cog test, and the Montreal Cognitive Assessment. A newer self-administered gerocognitive examination (SAGE) which patients complete by themselves, usually in 15 minutes is now available and consists of a validated 11-item instrument that compares favorably with MMSE and has the advantage of self-administration at home.[3] A meta-analysis examining the performance of commonly used screening tests for dementia identified 11 commonly used tests, with the MMSE having the most data. The combined sensitivity and specificity for detecting dementia were 0.81 and 0.89, respectively, for the MMSE and 0.91 and 0.86, respectively, for the Mini-Cog. Subgroup analysis revealed that only the Montreal Cognitive Assessment had comparable performance to the MMSE for detecting MCI with 0.89 sensitivity and 0.75 specificity.

The Mini-Cog (https://mini-cog.com/) is a 3-min instrument consisting of a 3-item recall test for memory and a simply scored clock drawing test. The Montreal Cognitive Assessment (MoCA, www.mocatest.org/) is a 30-point test that takes approximately 10 min to administer and includes

tests of visuospatial function, attention, verbal recall, language, abstraction, and orientation. A score of 25 points or less (26 points if the patient has <12 yr of education) indicates cognitive impairment. The test is available in >35 languages, and multiple forms in English allow for repeated assessments over time. A summary of commonly used tests may be found in Table E6.

Mental status testing should include tests that assess the following cognitive functions:
- Orientation: Ask the patient to give the day, date, month, year, and place and to name the current president.
- Attention: Ask the patient to recite the months of the year forward and in reverse.
- Verbal recall: Ask the patient to remember three items; test for recall after a 1- and 5-min delay.
- Language: Ask the patient to write and then read a sentence; have the patient name both common and less common objects.
- Visuospatial: Ask the patient to draw a clock and to set the hands of the clock at 11:10.

Patients with AD typically have trouble with verbal recall in addition to experiencing visuospatial or language deficits. Attention is usually preserved until the later stages of AD, so consider alternative diagnoses in patients who perform poorly on tests of attention early in their disease. A summary of the pattern of cognitive deficits associated with different dementias and depression may be found in Table 7.

TABLE 5 Symptoms and Preserved Abilities of Alzheimer Dementia by Disease Stage Symptoms and Preserved Abilities by Cognitive Domain Across Various Stages of Alzheimer Dementia

	Mild	Moderate	Severe
Memory			
Symptoms	• Loss of short-term memory; may recall some aspects of important events • May lose enjoyment in reading because of difficulty following a story line	• Forgets entire events have occurred, some long-term memories remain • Repetitive questioning may become troublesome for caregivers	• Complete loss of short-term memory • May not recognize familiar individuals • Long-term memories fade
Preserved abilities	• May benefit from simple reminders, routines, and habits • May still derive enjoyment from reminiscing	• May still enjoy reminiscing with the assistance of visual or verbal stimulation	• Implicit memory may still be preserved • Familiar environments and persons may be comforting
Executive Function			
Symptoms	• Difficulty acting on desired goals, resulting in irritation • Judgment may be poor • Social graces may suffer • May demonstrate anhedonia or apathy	• Problem-solving ability very limited • Angry outbursts • Impulsive • Difficulty in new situations • Requires reminders or physical support to complete ADLs	• Requires assistance with all ADLs • Cannot independently set goals or act upon them • Gradual loss of motor abilities, including dysphagia
Preserved abilities	• Decision-making capacity is likely to be intact • Comprehension may increase if information presentation is adapted	• Capacity for simple, every-day decision making may be preserved, even if capacity for complex decision making is lost	
Language and Communication			
Symptoms	• Some word-finding difficulties	• More pronounced difficulty understanding written or spoken language • Difficulty making needs known	• Gradual loss of speech
Preserved abilities	• Can engage in conversations, but may require environmental supports, such as those recommended by speech and language pathologists		• Ability to communicate needs nonverbally through emotional expression or other cues (e.g., grimacing to indicate pain)
Sensory/Perceptual			
Symptoms	• Difficulty with interpreting complex visual figures or displays	• May develop hallucinations or delusions	• May react poorly to noxious stimulation from the environment
Preserved abilities	• Ability to follow and enjoy simplified visual displays		• May enjoy individually enhanced sensory environments • Tactile stimulation may be preferable to auditory or visual
	• May respond positively to interventions, such as personalized music		

ADLs, Activities of daily living.
From Warshaw G et al: *Ham's primary care geriatrics,* ed 7, Philadelphia, 2022, Elsevier.

In addition to the common amnestic presentation, AD rarely presents as one of three rare nonamnestic syndromes that affect memory later in the course of the disease. These three rare presentations should also raise suspicion of another dementia type. A primary language variant presents as either logopenic expressive aphasia or progressive nonfluent aphasia and may be either a form of AD or of frontotemporal lobar degeneration. A primary visuospatial variant called posterior cortical atrophy presents with disturbances in complex visual processing and may be a form of either AD or dementia with Lewy bodies. An executive/behavioral variant presents with impaired executive function and/or behavior derangement and may represent either a frontal variant of AD or behavioral variant frontotemporal dementia.

LABORATORY TESTS (TABLE 8)
• CBC
• Serum electrolytes
• Glucose

• BUN/creatinine
• Liver and thyroid function tests
• Serum vitamin B_{12}
• Syphilis serology (rapid plasma reagin [RPR]), if supported by clinical history
• HIV screening as appropriate
• Lumbar puncture if history or signs of cancer, infectious process, or unusual clinical presentation (e.g., rapid progression of symptoms)
• EEG if there is history of seizures, episodic confusion, rapid clinical decline, or suspicion of Creutzfeldt-Jakob disease
• Apolipoprotein E genotyping, measurement of CSF tau, and amyloid and functional imaging including positron emission tomography (PET [Fig E2]), single-photon emission computed tomography (SPECT), amyloid PET imaging, and tau PET imaging are not yet routinely used outside of clinical trials because insurers generally do not pay for these tests.
• Brain biopsy is usually reserved for diagnoses such as prion disease and cerebral vasculitis.

Generally performed postmortem

IMAGING STUDIES
• MRI (Fig. E3) to rule out hydrocephalus, cerebrovascular disease, and mass lesions, including subdural hematoma and to look for typical patterns of neurodegeneration (i.e., regional brain atrophy) such as hippocampal atrophy. CT can be used if MRI is contraindicated.
• Amyloid PET: The FDA has approved several agents for beta-amyloid PET imaging, including florbetapir, flutemetamol, and florbetaben. As with these other imaging agents, a positive amyloid scan does not establish a diagnosis of AD or any other cognitive disorder, but a negative scan indicating sparse to no amyloid plaques is inconsistent with a neuropathologic diagnosis of AD. A positive amyloid scan indicates the presence of moderate to frequent amyloid neuritic plaques; neuropathologic examination has shown this amount of amyloid plaque is present in AD patients but may also be present in

TABLE 7   Patterns of Cognitive Impairment by Domain and Dementia

Episodic Memory	Attention	Language	Executive	Visuospatial		BEHAVIORAL SYMPTOMS
Alzheimer disease	(I)	Simple (P) Divided (I)	Phonemic (P) Semantic (I) Naming (I)	(I)	Simple (P) Complex (I)	Early apathy, late psychotic symptoms
Mild cognitive impairment—amnestic	Immediate and Delayed recall (I) Recognition (I)	Simple (P) Divided (P)	(P)	(P)	(P)	(P)
Vascular dementia	Immediate and Delayed recall (V) Recognition (P)	Simple (P) Divided (I)	(I)	(I)	(P)	Depression
Behavioral variant FTLD	(V)	Simple (P) Divided (I)	(I)	(I)	(P)	Disinhibition, apathy, hyperorality, inappropriate social interaction
Semantic variant PPA	(P)	(P)	(I) Comprehension (I) Fluency	(P)	(P)(I) Visual agnosia	(P)
Nonfluent variant PPA	(P)	(P)	(I) Fluency (P) Comprehension, (I) Expressive speech	(P)	(P)	(P)
Parkinson disease dementia	(V) Immediate and Delayed recall (P) Recognition	(I)	(P)	(I)	(I)	Depression, possible hallucinations, psychomotor slowing
Dementia with Lewy bodies	(V) Immediate and Delayed recall (P) Recognition	(V)	(V)	(I)	(I)	Hallucinations, delusions
Depression	(V) Immediate and Delayed recall (P) Recognition	(V)	(V) Fluency (P) Naming	I/V	(P)	Psychomotor slowing, apathy

FTLD, Frontotemporal lobar degeneration; *I,* impaired; *P,* preserved; *PPA,* primary progressive aphasia; *V,* variable.
From Fillit HM: *Brocklehurst's textbook of geriatric medicine and gerontology,* ed 8, Philadelphia, 2017, Elsevier.

TABLE 8   Laboratory Evaluation of Patients with Dementia

Type of Study	Examples
Basic studies, excluding reversible with specific indication from history for causes of dementia or examination	• Complete blood count (CBC) • Chemistry or metabolic panel (SM-17) • Thyroid function tests (thyroid-stimulating hormone [TSH]) • Vitamin B_{12}, folate levels • Computed tomography (CT) or magnetic resonance imaging (MRI) • HIV testing • Sedimentation rate • Hemoglobin A1C (HbA1C) • Urinalysis • Chest x-ray • Urine or plasma for drugs or heavy metals
Adjuvant studies to Aid Diagnosis	
Other tests as indicated by history or physical or neurologic examination	• Single-photon emission computed tomography (SPECT) • Positron emission tomography (PET) • Lumbar puncture with cerebrospinal fluid for β-amyloid

From Fillit HM: *Brocklehurst's textbook of geriatric medicine and gerontology,* ed 8, Philadelphia, 2017, Elsevier.

individuals with other types of neurologic conditions as well as in cognitively normal older adults.

• Tau PET: The FDA has approved one agent for tau imaging: Flortaucipir. Flortaucipir is used to estimate the density and distribution of aggregated tau neurofibrillary tangles in adult patients with cognitive impairment under evaluation for AD. It is not indicated for use in patients undergoing evaluation for chronic traumatic encephalopathy, which is also a tauopathy.

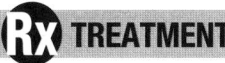 **TREATMENT**

NONPHARMACOLOGIC THERAPY

• Patient safety, including risks associated with impaired driving, wandering behavior, leaving stoves unattended, and accidents, must be addressed with the patient and family early and appropriate measures implemented.
• Wandering, hoarding, or hiding objects, repetitive questioning, withdrawal, and social inappropriateness often respond to behavioral therapies.
• Cognitive stimulation programs are beneficial for maintenance of cognitive function and improved self-reported quality of life in patients with mild to moderate AD.
• Person-centered care approach applied to care of people living with dementia is summarized in Table 9.

ACUTE GENERAL Rx
None

CHRONIC Rx
• Symptomatic treatment of memory disturbance (Table 10):
  1. Cholinesterase inhibitors (ChEls [Table 11]): Donepezil (Aricept), galantamine (Razadyne), and rivastigmine (Exelon)
     a. FDA approved for the treatment of mild to moderate AD with the exception of

TABLE 9 Person-Centered Care Approach Applied to Care of People Living with Dementia

Key Component	Early Stage	Middle Stage	Late Stage
Develop a personalized, goal-oriented care plan, based on a thorough medical, functional, and social assessment	• Conduct a functional assessment, including sensory status, language abilities • Establish stage-appropriate, personally meaningful goals • Encourage advance care planning, including naming a surrogate decision maker		• Engage with family members and surrogate decision makers to interpret patient's nonverbal communication • If on ChE-I, consider discontinuation
	• Discuss advantages and disadvantages of pharmacotherapy to help with cognitive or behavioral symptoms and monitor regularly for side effects		
Periodically review the person's goals and care plan to assess ongoing effectiveness and to address evolving goals	• Refer to community resources to promote the person's ongoing connection with and engagement in personally meaningful activities • Assess and address caregiver stress • Consider referral to senior centers or adult day programs to promote social engagement • In-home care services may be helpful		• Personalized music programs may be helpful • Hospice consultation may be indicated
Engage an interprofessional team that adapts its composition in response to the needs of the person living with dementia	• Care managers to refer to resources in community • SLP referral to teach caregivers supported communication approaches • PT/OT: In-home safety evaluation and customization of activities	• Care managers: Assist with symptom management, respite services • SLP consultation for assistance with supported communication approaches and feeding techniques • OT consultation to maximize functional independence	• Care managers: Assistance managing symptoms, referral for respite services • Palliative care or hospice consultation for symptom management and end-of-life care • OT sensory stimulation approaches to promote wellbeing
	• Pharmacy to assist with deprescribing and simplification of medication regimen • Specialty referrals (psychiatry, dementia care clinics) for management of BPSD		
A specified team leader to facilitate information transfer, care coordination, and continuity	• Primary care provider or specialty-trained care manager, such as nurse specialist or social worker	• Primary care provider or specialty-trained care manager	• Primary care provider or hospice team

BPSD, Behavioral and psychologic symptoms of dementia; *CHe-I*, acetylcholinesterase inhibitors; *OT*, occupational therapy; *PT*, physical therapy; *SLP*, speech language pathology.
From Warshaw G et al: *Ham's primary care geriatrics*, ed 7, Philadelphia, 2022, Elsevier.

TABLE 10 Symptomatic Treatment of Memory Disturbance

	Initial Dose	Target Dose
Donepezil	5 mg qd for 4-6 wk	10 mg qd
Rivastigmine	1.5 mg bid with food, increase by 1.5 mg bid weekly	3-6 mg bid
Galantamine	4 mg bid with food, increase by 4 mg bid every 4 wk	8-12 mg bid
Memantine	5 mg qd, increase by 5 mg weekly	10 mg bid

TABLE 11 Acetylcholinesterase Inhibitor Dosing

Drug	Initial Dose	Recommended Dose	Minimum Therapeutic Dose	Formulations
Donepezil	5 mg daily	10 mg daily	5 mg daily	5, 10, 23 mg
Galantamine IR	4 mg bid	12 mg bid	8 mg bid	4, 8, 12 mg
Galantamine ER	8 mg daily	24 mg daily	16 mg daily	8, 12, 24 mg
Rivastigmine	1.5 mg bid	6 mg bid	3 mg bid	1.5, 3, 4.5, 6 mg
Rivastigmine patch	4.6 mg daily	9.5 mg daily	9.5 mg daily	4.6, 9.5, 13.3 mg

bid, Twice daily.
Acetylcholinesterase inhibitor dosing and suggested titration intervals. From US Department of Veterans Affairs. *Pharmacy Benefits Management Services*. 2018 [cited October 15, 2019]. Available at: http://www.pbm.va.gov/. Note that medication doses can be increased every 4 wk as patient tolerates.
From Warshaw G et al: *Ham's primary care geriatrics*, ed 7, Philadelphia, 2022, Elsevier.

donepezil, which is approved for mild, moderate, and severe dementia. Common side effects include vivid dreams, bradycardia, and GI side effects (nausea, diarrhea, and anorexia). GI side effects may be bothersome enough to require either a slower escalation of dosage or switching to another agent. The rivastigmine patch has lower rates of GI side effects than the oral agents. Table 12 summarizes some instruments used to monitor clinical response of AD to pharmacologic therapy.

2. NMDA receptor antagonist: Memantine (Namenda).
   a. FDA approved for the treatment of moderate to severe AD. Common side effects include constipation, dizziness, or headache. Memantine is contraindicated in patients with renal insufficiency or history of seizures.

3. Antiamyloid monoclonal antibodies: Aducanumab (Aduhelm): Aducanumab is a human immunoglobulin G1 (IgG1) monoclonal antibody that targets aggravated forms of amyloid beta protein that accumulate in the brain of patients with AD. Several trails with other

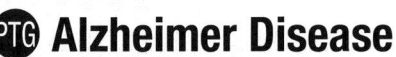
TABLE 12 Instruments Used to Monitor Clinical Response of Alzheimer Disease (AD) to Pharmacologic Therapy

Mini-Mental State Examination
- Global measure of cognition widely used by physicians and third-party caregivers
- Assesses orientation, registration, recall, language, and attention
- Uses a 30-point scale
- Requires ≈5-10 min to complete
- Sensitivity, 80%-90%; specificity, 80%
- Administered by psychometricians, nurses, and physicians
- AD typically advances by 3 points/yr

Clock Drawing
- Global measure of cognition widely used by physicians
- Multiple scoring systems with proven validity; sensitivity, 59%; specificity, 90%
- Assesses multiple cognitive domains in a single test
- 1-2 min to complete
- Minimal training to administer

Geriatric Depression Scale
- Evaluates depressive symptoms in patients
- Requires 5 min to complete
- Very useful in assessing depression in new patients and in follow-up
- Minimal training to administer
- Ease of administration has led to rapid spread in its use

From Fillit HM: *Brocklehurst's textbook of geriatric medicine and gerontology,* ed 8, Philadelphia, 2017, Elsevier.

TABLE 13 Treatment of Behavioral and Neuropsychiatric Symptoms

	Initial Dose	Maximum Dose
Atypical Antipsychotics		
Olanzapine	2.5 mg qd to bid, may increase by 2.5 mg as needed	7.5 mg bid
Quetiapine	25 mg bid, may increase by 25 mg every 2 days	250 mg tid
Antidepressants		
Sertraline	25-50 mg qd, may increase by 25 mg every week	200 mg qd
Escitalopram	10 mg qd, may increase after 1 wk to 20 mg qd	10 mg qd

agents have failed to demonstrate that reducing amyloid beta plaques in the brain of patients with AD produces meaningful clinical benefit.[1,2]

a. In June 2021, the FDA granted Aduhelm accelerated approval for all AD patients. This approval was controversial because, of the two studies used to support the drug's approval, one showed that cognitive and functional decline occurred at a lower rate in treated patients and the other trial did not demonstrate this effect. Furthermore, the drug was studied in patients with MCI and mild AD, but the initial approval did not limit use to these two groups. In July 2021, the FDA revised the approval, limiting it to patients with MCI and mild AD. However, the trial did not include patients with poorly controlled vascular risk factors, those with evidence of ischemic white matter changes, and individuals taking anticoagulants.

b. Aducanumab, like most other anti-amyloid monoclonal antibodies in clinical trials, can result in a potentially serious side effect called amyloid related imaging abnormalities (ARIA). ARIA can take two forms, ARIA-E (edema) and ARIA-H (hemosiderin deposition). ARIA-E is diagnosed when the MRI demonstrates focal cerebral vasogenic edema or sulcal effusions, and ARIA-H is diagnosed with the development of microhemorrhage and/or superficial siderosis. ARIA may be mild, moderate, or severe, and even severe ARIA may be asymptomatic. ARIA of any time and severity is common with aducanumab. Taking the two clinical trials together, 41% of treated patients were found to have ARIA and 24% of patients had symptomatic ARIA.

c. Prescribing aducanumab requires demonstrating the presence of amyloidosis using either CFS or amyloid PET. A baseline MRI is also required. ARIA usually occurs early in administration, so the drug label recommends an MRI monitoring protocol when using this medication. Given the complexity of this medication and the restrictions surrounding Medicare reimbursement for this medication, patients should be referred to special centers with established protocols for the safe administration and monitoring of this medication.

- Lecanemab, a humanized IgG1 monoclonal antibody that binds to A β souluble protofibrils was recently FAD approved for persons with early Alzheimer disease. Trials have shown that Lecanemab reduces markers of amyloid in early Alzheimer disease and results in moderately less decline on measures of cognition and function than placebo but it is associated with adverse events[4] Symptomatic treatment of neuropsychiatric and behavioral disturbances (Table 13).
- Depression, agitation, delusions, or hallucinations may respond to medications.
- A recent review and meta-analysis of cholinesterase inhibitors, memantine, and supplements determined that cholinesterase inhibitors and memantine slightly reduced short-term cognitive decline, and cholinesterase inhibitors slightly reduced reported functional decline, but differences versus placebo were of uncertain clinical importance. Evidence was mostly insufficient on drug treatment of behavioral and psychologic symptoms of dementia and on supplements for all outcomes.

DISPOSITION & REFERRAL
- Patients with complex or atypical presentations or challenging management issues should be referred to a neurologist, geriatric psychiatrist, or geriatrician with expertise in dementia.
- Approximately one in eight hospitalized patients with AD who develop delirium will have at least one adverse outcome (e.g., institutionalization, cognitive decline, death) associated with delirium.
- Family education and support may help reduce need for skilled nursing facility and reduce caregiver stress, depression, and burnout.

⚠ PEARLS & CONSIDERATIONS

The physician should make a thorough search for the treatable causes of dementia. Current American Academy of Neurology practice parameters recommend:
- Treat cognitive symptoms of AD with ChEIs.
- Treat depression.
- Treat agitation and psychosis using non-pharmacologic interventions first and use pharmacologic interventions at the lowest possible dose if other interventions have failed.
- Encourage caregivers to participate in educational programs and support groups.

TABLE 14 Strategies for Prevention of Dementia

Recommendation	Quality of Evidence
Engage in physical activity	Moderate
In adults with **mild cognitive impairment,** engage in physical activity to slow cognitive decline	Low
Tobacco cessation	Low
Do not exceed maximum daily recommended amount of alcohol intake	Moderate[a]
Follow a healthy diet based on WHO recommendations[b]	Moderate[c]
Follow a Mediterranean diet	Moderate
Maintain a healthy weight	Low
Participate in cognitively stimulating activities or cognitive training	Low
Treatment of hypertension	High
Treatment of *diabetes mellitus*	Moderate
Treatment of dyslipidemia	Low

Strategies for Prevention of Dementia, as based on World Health Organization (WHO) 2019 Guidelines for Risk Reduction of Cognitive Impairment and Dementia.
[a]4 units of alcohol per week for men, 7 units of alcohol per week for women.
[b]Components include: 5 daily servings of nonstarchy vegetables, <10% dietary intake of free sugars, <30% dietary intake of fats (preferentially unsaturated fats), <5 g daily of salt.
[c]Strength of evidence is variable based on individual dietary components.
From Warshaw G et al: *Ham's primary care geriatrics,* ed 7, Philadelphia, 2022, Elsevier.

TABLE 15 Genes Implicated in the Development of Alzheimer Disease

Gene	Comment
APP	>30 known mutations associated with EOAD; located on chromosome 21; associated with elevated risk of AD in Down syndrome
PSEN1	>150 known mutations associated with EOAD
PSEN2	<20 known mutations associated with EOAD
APOE	Three known alleles: • ε2 — protective of LOAD • ε3 — Neutral risk of LOAD • ε4 — Increased risk of LOAD

AD, Alzheimer disease; *EOAD,* early-onset Alzheimer disease; *LOAD,* late-onset Alzheimer disease.
From Warshaw G et al: *Ham's primary care geriatrics,* ed 7, Philadelphia, 2022, Elsevier.

COMMENTS

- Ginkgo biloba is marketed widely as effective in delaying cognitive impairment; however, trials have shown that it is not effective in reducing the incidence of Alzheimer dementia or dementia overall.
- Higher midlife fitness levels seem to be associated with lower hazards of developing all-cause dementia later in life independent of cerebrovascular disease. Exercise also may slow the rate of functional deterioration in mild AD.
- Even moderate adherence to the MIND (the Mediterranean-DASH Intervention for Neurodegenerative Delay) diet, a hybrid of the Mediterranean and DASH diets specifically designed to optimize brain health, has been shown to reduce the incidence of AD.
- Strategies for prevention of dementia are summarized in Table 14.

- Antipsychotics should be used with extreme caution in treating dementia-related psychosis. All antipsychotics carry a warning from the FDA stating that the medication is not approved for dementia-related psychosis because elderly patients on either conventional or atypical antipsychotics experience an increased risk of death due to cardiovascular or infectious causes.
- Apolipoprotein E (APOE) is the main cholesterol-carrying molecule in the brain, and it exists in three allelic variants: E2, E3, and E4. The E3 allele is most common and has a neutral influence on developing AD, whereas the E2 allele, the rarest allele, may be protective against AD. The E4 allele increases the risk of developing AD and advances the age of first symptoms in those who experience the disease. However, neither E4 heterozygosity or homozygosity is required or sufficient to cause AD. Among Caucasians, E4 heterozygosity increases the risk of developing AD approximately threefold, whereas E4 homozygosity increases AD risk by approximately 15 times compared to the E3/E3 baseline. The APOE E4 allele is also associated with an earlier age of onset of AD. Because the benefits of genetic testing are often modest, and the tests themselves are often imprecise in identifying risk, the test is generally discouraged. Genes implicated in the development of AD are summarized in Table 15. Recent trials, however, reveal that the disclosure of *APOE* genotyping results to adult children of patients with AD did not result in significant short-term psychologic risks. Test-related distress was reduced among those who learned that they were *APOE4* negative. Persons with high levels of emotional distress before undergoing genetic testing are more likely to have emotional difficulties after disclosure.

For additional information for patients, families, and clinicians, contact the following organizations:
- Alzheimer's Association (http://www.alz.org/; 800-272-3900)
- Alzheimer's Disease Education and Referral Center (www.nia.nih.gov/Alzheimers; 800-438-4380)

REFERENCES & SUGGESTED READINGS

Available at eBooks.Health.Elsevier.com

AUTHOR: **JOSEPH S. KASS, MD, JD, FAAN**

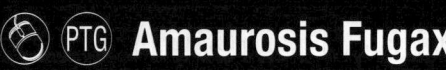
A

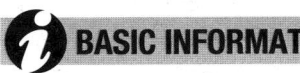 **BASIC INFORMATION**

DEFINITION

Amaurosis fugax is a temporary loss of monocular vision caused by transient retinal ischemia due to reversible occlusion within the ophthalmic artery or its branches. The ophthalmic artery is a branch of the internal carotid artery, and the central retinal artery is a branch of the ophthalmic artery.[1]

ICD-10CM CODE
G45.3 Amaurosis fugax

EPIDEMIOLOGY & DEMOGRAPHICS

INCIDENCE (IN U.S.): An uncommon but important presentation of carotid artery disease
PEAK INCIDENCE: Approximately 55 yr

PHYSICAL FINDINGS & CLINICAL PRESENTATION

- Onset is sudden, typically lasting seconds to minutes, and often accompanied by scotomas such as a shade or curtain being pulled over the front of the eye (usually downward).
- Vision loss can be complete, hemianopic, or quadratic.
- Acute stage: Cholesterol emboli may be seen in retinal artery (Hollenhorst plaque).

ETIOLOGY

- Usually embolic from either the internal carotid artery or the heart
- Cardiac embolus most commonly due to atrial fibrillation
- Internal carotid artery embolus will be apparent as carotid stenosis on carotid imaging such as CT angiography, MR angiography, or carotid ultrasound
- Giant cell arteritis (GCA) causing inflammation of retinal arteries
- Hyperviscosity syndromes, such as sickle cell disease, which causes ischemia in the vascular territory of the ophthalmic artery
- Hypercoagulable states
- Reversible cerebral vasoconstriction syndrome

DIAGNOSIS

DIFFERENTIAL DIAGNOSIS

- Retinal migraine: In contrast to amaurosis, the onset of visual loss develops more slowly, usually over 15 to 20 min.
- Transient visual obscurations occur in the setting of papilledema due to elevated intracranial pressure; intermittent rises in intracranial pressure briefly compromise optic disc perfusion and cause transient visual loss lasting 1 to 2 seconds. The episodes may be binocular. If the visual loss persists at the time of evaluation (i.e., vision has not yet recovered), then the differential diagnosis should be broadened to include:
  1. Anterior ischemic optic neuropathy: Arteritic (classically GCA) or nonarteritic
  2. Central retinal artery occlusion
  3. Branch retinal artery occlusion

WORKUP

- Workup should focus on embolic sources, but GCA should always be considered.
- Careful examination of retina; embolus may be visible and confirm the diagnosis (Fig. 1).
- Auscultation of arteries for carotid bruits.
- Examination of all pulses and for temporal artery tenderness.
- Inquire about symptoms of GCA (scalp tenderness, headache, fever, jaw claudication).
- Examine for signs of hemispheric stroke resulting from intracranial atherosclerosis (contralateral limb and facial weakness or sensory loss, aphasia, etc.).

LABORATORY TESTS

- CBC with erythrocyte sedimentation rate and C-reactive protein.
- Serum chemistries, including lipid profile and hemoglobin A1C.
- Cardiac enzymes and ECG.
- Hypercoagulable workup is discretionary based on younger age and history.

IMAGING STUDIES

- CT or MR angiography of head and neck preferred to examine carotid and intracranial vasculature. Carotid ultrasound if contraindication to MR or CT angiography
- MRI of the brain with diffusion-weighted imaging to look for infarcts, especially those presenting with focal neurologic disturbances
- Transthoracic echocardiography is indicated to screen for sources of emboli in patients with evidence of heart disease and in patients without an evident source for transient neurologic deficit. Transesophageal echocardiography is more sensitive for detecting cardiac sources of emboli (ventricular mural thrombus, atrial appendage, patent foramen ovale, aortic arch)
- Extended monitoring for atrial fibrillation if neither carotid stenosis nor GCA is found to be the etiology

TREATMENT

NONPHARMACOLOGIC THERAPY

- Diet (decrease saturated fatty acids and high-cholesterol foods)

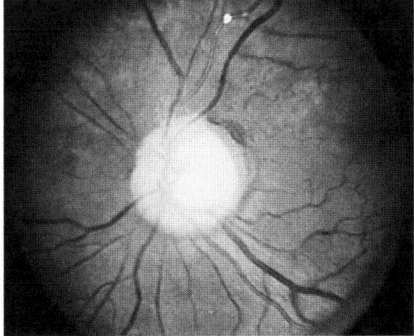

FIG. 1 A cholesterol crystal embolus lodged at an arterial bifurcation. (From Stein JH [ed]: *Internal medicine*, ed 5, St Louis, 1998, Mosby.)

- Exercise
- Cessation of tobacco use and illicit drug use

ACUTE GENERAL Rx

- Investigate as an emergency.
- Aspirin.
- If GCA is suspected, start prednisone and refer for temporal artery biopsy within 48 h (see "Giant Cell Arteritis" in Section I).

CHRONIC Rx

- Reduce risks by carotid endarterectomy if stenosis >50%. Carotid stenting may be performed in high-risk surgical candidates.
- Manage vascular risk factors such as hypertension, hyperlipidemia (statin therapy), diabetes, smoking cessation, etc.
- Antiplatelet therapy due to arterial atherosclerosis and postcarotid intervention; anticoagulation if etiology is atrial fibrillation.

DISPOSITION

Among patients with >50% carotid stenosis who do not undergo carotid endarterectomy, those who present with transient monocular blindness have an approximate 10% risk of stroke within 3 yr compared with an approximate 20% risk in patients who present with a hemispheric transient ischemic attack (TIA).

REFERRAL

- As with any TIA, emergent inpatient workup in a hospital that is a certified stroke center, if possible.
- If significant carotid stenosis, consider either carotid endarterectomy or carotid stenting for the following:
  1. Ipsilateral high-grade (≥70%) stenosis, but consider for ipsilateral stenosis of 50% to 69%
  2. Multiple TIAs despite medical therapy in the setting of high-grade or ulcerative disease

PEARLS & CONSIDERATIONS

- Cholesterol emboli in retinal arteries on fundoscopy confirm the diagnosis.
- Recognize that transient visual loss has multiple other causes.
- Refer to emergent evaluation like any other TIA.

REFERENCE
Available at eBooks.Health.Elsevier.com.

RELATED CONTENT
Amaurosis Fugax (Patient Information)
Carotid Artery Stenosis (Related Key Topic)
Giant Cell Arteritis (Related Key Topic)
Transient Ischemic Attack (Related Key Topic)

AUTHOR: **JOSEPH S. KASS, MD, JD, FAAN**

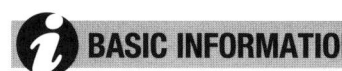

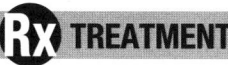 BASIC INFORMATION

DEFINITION

Anaphylaxis is a severe allergic reaction that is rapid in onset and life-threatening. In anaphylaxis, immunoglobulin E (IgE)– and non–IgE-mediated systemic degranulation of mast cells causes respiratory, cardiovascular, GI, and/or mucocutaneous signs and symptoms.

SYNONYM

Anaphylactic reaction

ICD-10CM CODES
T78.2	Anaphylactic shock, unspecified, initial encounter
T78.00XA	Anaphylactic reaction due to unspecified food, initial encounter
T80.52XA	Anaphylactic reaction due to vaccination, initial encounter
T63.94XA	Toxic effect of contact with unspecified venomous animal, undetermined, initial encounter

EPIDEMIOLOGY & DEMOGRAPHICS

INCIDENCE: The incidence of anaphylaxis in the U.S. is 50 to 2000 episodes/100,000 persons with a lifetime prevalence of 1.6% to 5.1%. Incidence is on the rise with emergency department visits for anaphylaxis increasing by 101% between 2005 and 2014. Despite this increase, anaphylaxis-related fatalities remain stable at 0.7 per million adults/yr. Medications and insect stings are leading triggers in adults, whereas foods and insect stings are the leading triggers in children and adolescents.

RISK FACTORS: Atopy is a risk factor for anaphylaxis triggered by food, exercise, and latex. Risk factors for severe anaphylaxis include cardiovascular disease, asthma, older age, mast cell disorder, beta-blocker use, and ACE inhibitor use.

PHYSICAL FINDINGS & CLINICAL PRESENTATION

- Mucocutaneous: Urticaria, pruritus, skin flushing, angioedema (Table 1)
- Respiratory: Dyspnea, cough, wheezing, hypoxia, stridor, rhinitis
- Cardiovascular: Hypotension, tachycardia, weakness, dizziness, syncope, malaise, vascular collapse (Table 2)
- Gastrointestinal: Nausea, vomiting, diarrhea, dysphagia, abdominal pain

ETIOLOGY (BOX 1)

Anaphylaxis results from a sudden systematic release of histamine and other inflammatory mediators from basophils and mast cells due to both IgE and non–IgE-mediated mechanisms. Virtually any substance may induce anaphylaxis. In an acute setting, the cause of anaphylaxis is often unidentifiable (30% to 60% of cases):

- Foods and food additives: Peanuts, tree nuts, eggs, shellfish, fish, cow's milk, fruits, soy

1. Alpha-1,3-galactose (alpha-gal): Lone star tick bite causes IgE sensitization to alpha-gal (carbohydrate moiety found in red meat) causing delayed anaphylaxis when consuming mammalian products
- Medications: Antibiotics (especially penicillins and sulfa-based agents), insulin, allergen extracts, opiates, vaccines, NSAIDs, contrast media, streptokinase, immunomodulators, IV iron
- Environmental exposures: Bee or wasp sting, snake venom, fire ant venom
- Blood products: Plasma, immunoglobulin, cryoprecipitate, whole blood
- Latex
- Exercise

Box 2 summarizes agents frequently associated with immune and nonimmune types of anaphylaxis.

DX DIAGNOSIS

DIFFERENTIAL DIAGNOSIS

- Allergic reaction
- Other causes of shock such as sepsis or pulmonary embolism
- Endocrine disorders (carcinoid, adrenal crisis, paradoxical pheochromocytoma)
- Systemic mastocytosis
- Serum sickness
- Severe asthma (the key clinical difference is the abrupt onset of symptoms in anaphylaxis versus a history of progressive worsening of symptoms)
- Scombroid poisoning
- Localized angioedema
- Acute urticaria
- Presyncopal syndromes including vasovagal reactions
- Airway foreign body, vocal cord dysfunction
- Globus hystericus, anxiety disorder

WORKUP

Workup is aimed at ruling out other conditions that may mimic anaphylaxis. Given the potentially life-threatening nature of anaphylaxis, treatment should not be delayed. Clinical criteria for diagnosing anaphylaxis are summarized in Box 3.

LABORATORY TESTS

Laboratory evaluation is generally not helpful because anaphylaxis is a clinical diagnosis. Elevated serum and urine histamine levels and serum tryptase levels (measured 30 min to 2 h after symptom onset compared to baseline) can be useful for diagnosis of anaphylaxis, but these tests are not commonly available in the emergency setting and normal levels do not preclude the diagnosis.

IMAGING STUDIES

Are generally not helpful. Chest radiography for evaluation of foreign body aspiration or pulmonary pathology is indicated in patients with acute respiratory compromise. Consider ECG in all patients with sudden loss of consciousness or reports of chest pain or dyspnea and in any elderly

patient. ECG in anaphylaxis usually reveals sinus tachycardia.

RX TREATMENT

NONPHARMACOLOGIC THERAPY

- Remove the trigger. Establish and protect airway. Provide supplemental O_2 if indicated.
- Rapidly establish intravenous (IV) access and administer IV fluids (i.e., normal saline).
- Cardiac monitoring is recommended.

ACUTE GENERAL RX

- 0.3 to 0.5 mg intramuscular (IM) epinephrine (1:1000 concentration) should be rapidly administered for adults and children >30 kg in the anterolateral thigh. Any patient weighing over 50 kg should receive 0.5 mg IM. 0.01 mg/kg IM epinephrine (1:1000 concentration) should be administered for children <30 kg. IM administration is preferred because it provides more reliable and quicker rise to effective plasma levels. The dose may be repeated within minutes if symptoms do not improve.
- Adjunct therapies include histamine-1 H_1 and H_2 receptor antagonists such as diphenhydramine and famotidine. Although useful to improve cutaneous erythema and pruritus, H_1 antagonists are not effective in reversing upper airway obstruction, respiratory compromise, or hypotension and their onset of action is delayed 1 to 2 h.
- Corticosteroids are not useful in the acute episode because of their slow onset of action and have not been shown to decrease the risk of or prevent prolonged or biphasic anaphylaxis (recurrent anaphylaxis after complete improvement). Despite this they are commonly used in clinical practice and are considered secondary treatment.
- Vasopressor therapy with IV epinephrine (1:10,000 concentration) is indicated in patients with refractory hypotension/cardiovascular collapse despite crystalloid resuscitation and IM epinephrine. Small IV boluses of epinephrine can also be used in the periarrest state.
- Aerosolized β-agonists are useful to control bronchospasm.
- Patients taking beta-blocking medications may be refractory to initial treatment; consider administration of IV glucagon.
- Table 3 summarizes drugs and other agents used in anaphylaxis therapy.
- Fig. E1 illustrates an algorithm for the management of a patient with severe anaphylaxis.

DISPOSITION

- Patients with mild episodes should be observed for 1 h after resolution of symptoms. Patients with severe symptoms (cyanosis, pulse oxygen <92%, systolic BP <90 mm Hg, confusion, loss of consciousness, incontinence), >1 dose of epinephrine, wide pulse pressure, unknown trigger, cutaneous signs or symptoms, and medication trigger in children should be observed for at least 6 h to monitor for biphasic anaphylaxis.

TABLE 1 Dynamics of Cardiovascular Abnormalities in Anaphylactic Shock

	At Onset of Reaction	Early Stage (Minutes) With No Treatment	Prolonged Shock
Blood pressure	↓	↓↓	↓↓↓
Pulse	↑	↑	↑↑
Cardiac output	↑	↓	↓↓
PVR	↓	→ ↓*	→ ↑↓*
Intravascular volume	→ ↓	↓	↓↓↓

*Peripheral vascular resistance (PVR) can vary, likely depending on internal compensation response.
From LoVerde D et al: Anaphylaxis, *Chest* 153(2):528-543, 2018. https://doi.org/10.1016/j.chest.2017.07.033.

TABLE 2 Signs and Symptoms of Anaphylaxis: Frequency of Occurrence[2]

Sign or Symptom	Percentage of Cases (%)
Cutaneous	>90
Urticaria and angioedema	85-90
Flush	45-55
Pruritus without rash	2-5
Respiratory	40-60
Dyspnea, wheeze	45-50
Upper airway angioedema	50-60
Rhinitis	15-20
Dizziness, syncope, hypotension	30-35
Abdominal	
Nausea, vomiting, diarrhea, cramping pain	25-30
Miscellaneous	
Headache	5-8
Substernal pain	4-6
Seizure	1-2

BOX 1 Causes of Anaphylaxis

IgE-dependent mechanisms
Drugs, chemicals, and biologic agents
Penicillins, cephalosporins, sulfonamides, muscle relaxants, vaccines, insulin, thiamine, protamine, gamma globulin, cis-carboplatin and doxorubicin, monoclonal antibodies cetuximab/rituximab, antivenoms, formaldehyde, ethylene oxide, chlorhexidine, semen
Foods
Peanuts, tree nuts, shellfish, fin fish, milk, egg, fruits, vegetables, sesame, flour
Hymenoptera sting venom, insect saliva, other venoms
Bees, wasps, ants, hornets, ticks, triatomine "kissing bugs," snakes, scorpions, jellyfish
Natural rubber latex
Environmental
Pollen, horse dander, hydatid cyst rupture
Non–IgE-dependent mechanisms
Physical factors
Exercise, cold, heat, sunlight
Medications and biologic agents
Opiates, aspirin and NSAIDs, ACE inhibitors, vancomycin, radiocontrast media, N-acetylcysteine, fluorescein
Food additives
Metabisulphite, tartrazine
Idiopathic
Exclusion of all known causes including mastocytosis

Several mechanisms may coexist, such as exercise-induced following food.
Non–IgE-dependent mechanisms include complement activation, kinin production, or potentiation and direct mediator release.
ACE inhibitor use is an important cause of unexplained angioedema, occurring in up to 1:200 patients on these drugs; it may develop at any interval after starting (most commonly early on).
NOTE: Cross-reactivity is seen; both IgE-dependent and non–IgE-dependent reactions may occur with the same agent.
ACE, Angiotensin-converting enzyme inhibitors; *NSAIDs,* nonsteroidal, antiinflammatory drugs.
From Cameron P et al: *Textbook of adult emergency medicine,* 5th ed, Elsevier, 2019, Sydney, Australia.

CHRONIC RX
- Patients appropriate for discharge after remaining asymptomatic should have two epinephrine autoinjectors prescribed. Include instructions on when and how to use.

REFERRAL
- Referral to an allergist can be help determine a cause if unclear in the emergent setting.

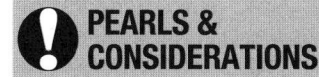
PEARLS & CONSIDERATIONS

COMMENTS
- Patient education regarding the nature of the illness and preventive measures is recommended. A documented history of previous anaphylactic episodes or known triggers is the most reliable method of identifying individuals at risk.
- Prescription for a prefilled epinephrine syringe (EpiPen or EpiPen Jr.) should be given, and the patient should be instructed on the use of this emergency kit, and to carry it with them at all times. School-aged children should keep an additional EpiPen at school with the appropriate staff.
- Patients should also be advised to carry or wear a MedicAlert ID describing substances that have caused anaphylaxis.
- Avoidance of radiologic contrast is also recommended in those who have had a prior reaction. However, pretreatment regimens with methylprednisolone or diphenhydramine, exist for those who have had contrast reactions in the past.
- Venom immunotherapy immediately after a sting is effective and recommended for up to 5 yr after the anaphylactic incident.

SUGGESTED READINGS
Available at eBooks.Health.Elsevier.com.

AUTHORS: **RORY MERRITT, MD, MEHP** and **ERIC EBERT, MD**

BOX 2   Agents Frequently Associated With Immune and Nonimmune Types of Anaphylaxis

Immunologic Mechanisms
Immunoglobulin E (IgE)-mediated:
    Food (nuts, shellfish, fruits, etc.)
    Venoms (stinging insects)
    Medications (β-lactam antibiotics, NSAIDs, neuromuscular blocking agents, etc.)
    Natural rubber latex
    Seminal fluid
    Radiocontrast media (in some cases)

IgE-independent
Radiocontrast media (in most cases)
    Dextrans
    Monoclonal antibodies (rituximab)
    Medications (β-lactam antibiotics, NSAIDs, etc.)
    Natural rubber latex
    Seminal fluid

Nonimmunologic Mechanisms
Medications (opioids, protamine, etc.)

NSAIDs, Nonsteroidal antiinflammatory drugs.
From Parrillo JE, Dellinger RP: Critical care medicine: principles of diagnosis and management in the adult, ed 5, Philadelphia, 2019, Elsevier.

BOX 3   Clinical Criteria for Diagnosing Anaphylaxis

Anaphylaxis is highly likely when any one of the following three criteria is fulfilled:
1. Acute onset of an illness (minutes to several hours) with involvement of the skin, mucosal tissue, or both (e.g., generalized urticaria, itching or flushing, swollen lips/tongue/uvula) and at least one of the following:
    a. Respiratory compromise (e.g., dyspnea, wheeze/bronchospasm, stridor, reduced PEF, hypoxemia)
    a. Reduced blood pressure or associated symptoms of end-organ dysfunction (e.g., hypotonia collapse, syncope, incontinence)
    OR
2. Two or more of the following that occur rapidly after exposure to a likely allergen for that patient (minutes to several hours):
    a. Involvement of the skin-mucosal tissue (e.g., generalized urticaria, itch/flush, swollen lips/tongue/uvula)
    b. Respiratory compromise (e.g., dyspnea, wheeze/bronchospasm, stridor, reduced PEF, hypoxemia)
    c. Reduced blood pressure or associated symptoms (e.g., hypotonia collapse, syncope, incontinence)
    5. Persistent gastrointestinal symptoms (e.g., crampy abdominal pain, vomiting)
    OR
3. Reduced blood pressure after exposure to known allergen for that patient (minutes to several hours)
    a. Infants and children: Low systolic blood pressure (age-specific) or >30% decrease in systolic blood pressure
    b. Adults: Systolic blood pressure of <90 mm Hg or >30% decrease from that person's baseline

PEF, Peak expiratory flow.
From Sampson HA et al: Second symposium on the definition and management of anaphylaxis: summary report—Second National Institute of Allergy and Infectious Disease/Food Allergy and Anaphylaxis Network symposium, J Allergy Clin Immunol 117(2):391-397, 2006. https://doi.org/10.1016/j.jaci.2005.12.1303.

TABLE 3	Management of a Patient With Anaphylaxis		
Treatment	**Mechanism(s) of Effect**	**Dosage(s)**	**Comments; Adverse Reactions**
Patient Emergency Management (Dependent on Severity of Symptoms)			
Epinephrine (adrenaline)	α_1-, β_1-, β_2-Adrenergic effects	0.01 mg/kg, up to 0.5 mg IM in lateral thigh Adrenaclick, Auvi-Q, EpiPen Jr./EpiPen: 0.15 mg IM for 8-25 kg 0.3 mg IM for 25 kg or more Epinephrine autoinjector: 0.1 mg for 7.5-15 kg 0.15 mg for 15-25 kg 0.3 mg for 25 kg or more	Tachycardia, hypertension, nervousness, headache, nausea, irritability, tremor
Cetirizine (liquid)	Antihistamine (competitive of H_1 receptor)	Cetirizine liquid: 5 mg/5 ml, 0.25 mg/kg, up to 10 mg PO	Hypotension, tachycardia, somnolence
Alternative: Diphenhydramine	Antihistamine (competitive of H_1 receptor)	1.25 mg/kg up to 50 mg PO or IM	Hypotension, tachycardia, somnolence, paradoxical excitement
Transport to an Emergency Facility			
Emergency Personnel Management (Dependent on Severity of Symptoms)			
Epinephrine (adrenaline)	α_1-, β_1-, β_2-Adrenergic effects	0.01 mg/kg, up to 0.5 mg IM in lateral thigh Epinephrine autoinjector: 0.1 mg for 7.5-15 kg 0.15 mg for 15-25 kg 0.3 mg for 25 kg or more 0.01 ml/kg/dose of 1:1,000 (vial) solution, up to 0.5 ml IM May repeat every 10-15 min For severe hypotension: 0.01 ml/kg/dose of 1:10,000 slow IV push	Tachycardia, hypertension, nervousness, headache, nausea, irritability, tremor
Supplemental Oxygen and Airway Management			
Volume Expanders			
Crystalloids (normal saline or Ringer lactate)		30 ml/kg in 1st hr	Rate titrated against BP response If tolerated, place patient supine with legs raised
Colloids (hydroxyethyl starch)		10 ml/kg rapidly followed by slow infusion	Rate titrated against BP response If tolerated, place patient supine with legs raised
Antihistamines			
Cetirizine (liquid)	Antihistamine (competitive of H_1 receptor)	Cetirizine liquid: 5 mg/5 ml 0.25 mg/kg, up to 10 mg PO	Hypotension, tachycardia, somnolence
Alternative: Diphenhydramine	Antihistamine (competitive of H_1 receptor)	1.25 mg/kg, up to 50 mg PO, IM, or IV	Hypotension, tachycardia, somnolence, paradoxic excitement
Ranitidine	Antihistamine (competitive of H_2 receptor)	1 mg/kg, up to 50 mg IV Should be administered slowly	Headache, mental confusion
Alternative: Cimetidine	Antihistamine (competitive of H_2 receptor)	4 mg/kg, up to 200 mg IV Should be administered slowly	Headache, mental confusion
Corticosteroids			
Methylprednisolone	Antiinflammatory	Solu-Medrol (IV): 1-2 mg/kg, up to 125 mg IV Depo-Medrol (IM): 1 mg/kg, up to 80 mg IM	Hypertension, edema, nervousness, agitation
Prednisone	Antiinflammatory	1 mg/kg up, to 75 mg PO	Hypertension, edema, nervousness, agitation
Nebulized albuterol	β-Agonist	0.83 mg/ml (3 ml) via mask with O_2	Palpitations, nervousness, CNS stimulation, tachycardia; use to supplement epinephrine when bronchospasm appears unresponsive; may repeat
Postemergency Management			
Antihistamine		Cetirizine (5-10 mg qd) or loratadine (5-10 mg qd) for 3 days	
Corticosteroids		*Optional:* Oral prednisone (1 mg/kg up to 75 mg) daily for 3 days	

Preventive Treatment
Prescription for epinephrine autoinjector and antihistamine
Provide written plan outlining patient emergency management (may download form from http://www.aap.org or http://www.foodallergy.org)
Follow-up evaluation to determine/confirm etiology
Immunotherapy for insect sting allergy

Patient Education
Instruction on avoidance of causative agent
Information on recognizing early signs of anaphylaxis
Stress early treatment of allergic symptoms to avoid systemic anaphylaxis
Encourage wearing medical identification jewelry

BP, Blood pressure; *CNS,* central nervous system; *IM,* intramuscularly; *IV,* intravenously; *PO,* orally; *qd,* every day.
From Kliegman RM, Geme JS: *Nelson textbook of pediatrics,* Philadelphia, 2019, Elsevier.

BASIC INFORMATION

DEFINITION

Anti-neutrophil cytoplasmic antibody (ANCA)—associated vasculitis (AAV) describes a family of small to medium vessel systemic vasculitides that shares many overlapping features, including clinical manifestations and therapies but also has distinct differences among each condition (granulomatosis with polyangiitis [GPA], microscopic polyangiitis [MPA], and eosinophilic granulomatosis with polyangiitis [EGPA]). These vasculitides are characterized by necrotizing, pauci-immune small vessel vasculitis with GPA and without MPA granulomatous inflammation. Most patients present with both renal and pulmonary involvement, but the skin, nervous system, and gastrointestinal tract can also be affected. In a limited form of GPA, disease is generally confined to the upper respiratory tract and can be managed less aggressively.

SYNONYMS

Anti-neutrophil cytoplasm antibody—associated vasculitis
Anti-neutrophil cytoplasmic antibody—positive vasculitis
Granulomatosis with polyangiitis
GPA
Wegener granulomatosis (WG)
MPA
Microscopic polyangiitis
Eosinophilic granulomatosis with polyangiitis
EGPA

ICD-10CM CODES
I77.6   Arteritis, unspecified
M31.3   Granulomatosis with polyangiitis
M31.7   Microscopic polyangiitis
M30.1   EGPA

EPIDEMIOLOGY & DEMOGRAPHICS

INCIDENCE: 6 to 12 cases per million per year in Western Europe and Japan, but statistics vary globally[1]
PREVALENCE: Varies between 94 and 160 per million[1]
PREDOMINANT SEX & AGE: Slightly higher incidence in males, peak 60 to 70 yr[1]
PEAK INCIDENCE: Increases with age, peak 60 to 70 yr of age[1]
RISK FACTORS: Infections (e.g., *Staphylococcus aureus*), silica exposure, hydrocarbon exposure, cigarette smoking, pesticides, medications (e.g., hydralazine, minocycline, propylthiouracil, levamisole-cocaine, allopurinol)
GENETICS: Familial forms have been described but are rare; GPA associated with single nucleotide polymorphisms (SNP) in HLA-DP, PRTN3, SERPINA1; MPA associated with HLA-DQ polymorphisms.

PHYSICAL FINDINGS & CLINICAL PRESENTATION (TABLES 1 AND 2)

• Constitutional symptoms: Fever, fatigue, weight loss, myalgia, arthralgia.

• Upper respiratory tract (URT): Chronic sinusitis, chronic otitis media, mastoiditis, nasal crusting, obstruction and epistaxis, nasal septal perforation, nasal lacrimal duct stenosis, saddle nose deformities (Fig. 1), tracheal and subglottic stenosis. Up to 90% of patients with GPA have one or more URT manifestations.
• Eyes: Conjunctivitis, ulcerative keratosis, episcleritis or scleritis, optic neuropathy, nasolacrimal duct obstruction, retinal vasculitis, uveitis, proptosis.
• Ears: Sensorineural and conductive hearing loss, otorrhea, and polychondritis.
• Mouth: Chronic ulcerative lesions of the oral mucosa, "mulberry" gingivitis, can be seen in GPA.
• Pulmonary: Dyspnea, hemoptysis, pleuritic chest pain. Imaging may show nodules, infiltrates, cavitary lesions, effusion, or alveolar hemorrhage.
• Gastrointestinal: Ischemic abdominal pain, peritonitis, bloody diarrhea, bowel ulceration or perforation, most commonly in MPA.
• Renal: Most affected organ in GPA and MPA. Elevated blood pressure, edema, decreased urine output. Rapidly progressive glomerulonephritis (38% to 70%), microscopic hematuria with or without red cell casts, and proteinuria.
• Nervous system: Mononeuritis multiplex and peripheral neuropathies (15% to 50% in both), meningeal inflammation (pachymeningitis), headaches, and rarely central nervous system (CNS) involvement with seizures or strokes.
• Skin: Cutaneous nodules over extensor surfaces of joints, necrotizing skin lesions (Fig. E2), palpable purpura (30% to 46%), urticaria, livedo reticularis, and digital gangrene.

ETIOLOGY

The etiology of this complex immune-mediated disorder remains unclear and is likely multifactorial in nature. ANCAs play a major role in the pathogenesis. When PR3 and MPO are expressed on cell surfaces of neutrophils, they can cause endothelial damage as well as local tissue necrosis if activated in extravascular tissue. Other risk factors including genetic, environmental exposure to silica or certain strains of *S. aureus* have been proposed.

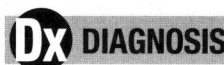 **DIAGNOSIS**

DIFFERENTIAL DIAGNOSIS

• Other granulomatous lung diseases for GPA (e.g., sarcoidosis, lymphomatoid granulomatosis, EGPA, necrotizing bronchocentric granulomatosis). The differential diagnosis of granulomatous lung disease is described in Section II. Table 3 describes differential diagnostic features of ANCA-associated vasculitis.
• Other ANCA-associated vasculitides and systemic vasculitis.
• Goodpasture disease, other causes of glomerulonephritis (e.g., poststreptococcal nephritis).
• Neoplasms (especially lymphoproliferative disease).
• Bacterial or fungal sinusitis for GPA.
• Viral infections.
• Cocaine-induced midline destructive lesions and levamisole-induced vasculitis.

WORKUP (TABLE 4)

• Thorough medical history and physical examination. Suspect GPA/MPA if patient has pulmonary and renal symptoms and is

---

TABLE 1 Preliminary Criteria for the Classification of Catastrophic Antiphospholipid Syndrome (APS)

• Evidence of involvement of three or more organs, systems, or tissues[a]
• Development of manifestations simultaneously or in <1 wk
• Confirmation by histopathology of small vessel occlusion in at least one organ or tissue[b]
• Laboratory confirmation of the presence of antiphospholipid antibody (lupus anticoagulant or anticardiolipin or anti—β_2-glycoprotein I antibodies)[c]

Definite Catastrophic APS

All four criteria

Probable Catastrophic APS

Criteria 2 through 4 and two organs, systems, or tissues involved

Criteria 1 through 3, except no confirmation 6 wk apart owing to early death of patient not tested before catastrophic episode

Criteria 1, 2, and 4

Criteria 1, 3, and 4 and development of a third event more than 1 wk but less than 1 mo after the first, despite anticoagulation

---

[a]Usually, clinical evidence of vessel occlusions, confirmed by imaging techniques when appropriate. Renal involvement is defined by a 50% rise in serum creatinine, severe systemic hypertension, proteinuria, or some combination of these.

[b]For histopathologic confirmation, significant evidence of thrombosis must be present, although vasculitis may coexist occasionally.

[c]If the patient has not been diagnosed previously with APS, laboratory confirmation requires that the presence of antiphospholipid antibody be detected on two or more occasions at least 6 wk apart (not necessarily at the time of the event), according to proposed preliminary criteria for the classification of APS.

From Asherson RA et al: Catastrophic antiphospholipid syndrome: international consensus statement on classification criteria and treatment guidelines, *Lupus* 12:530-534, 2003.

TABLE 2 Clinical Findings in the ANCA-Associated Vasculitides[9-36]

	GPA	EGPA	MPA
Constitutional	Common. Includes fatigue, malaise, fevers, and weight loss.	Common. Weight loss, fatigue, fevers, myalgias and arthralgias.	Very common. Generally precedes renal disease by months.
Pulmonary	70%-95% of patients with respiratory symptoms or chest imaging abnormalities. Tracheobronchial and endobronchial disease in 10%-50%.	Asthma essentially universal. Patchy, heterogenous radiographic infiltrates in >70%.	10%-30% with diffuse alveolar hemorrhage.
Renal	50%-90% of patients.	20%-50% of patients.	RPGN almost universal.
Upper airway	70%-95% of patients. Destructive or ulcerating lesions are suggestive.	Sinusitis, polyposis, and/or rhinitis in ≥70% of patients. Generally not destructive.	5%-30%, with sinus disease most common.
Musculoskeletal	Arthralgias, synovitis, and myalgias in up to 80%.	Arthralgias and myalgias in up to 50%.	Arthralgias and myalgias in at least 50% of patients.
Eyes	25%-60% of patients. Vision-threatening disease including uveitis, ocular ulcers.	<5%.	0%-30% of patients. May be clinically silent.
Cardiac	5%-25% of patients. Conduction delays or other ECG abnormality, systolic or diastolic dysfunction, pericarditis, or coronary artery vasculitis.	30%-50% of patients and a major cause of mortality. Conduction delays or other ECG abnormality, systolic or diastolic dysfunction, pericarditis, or coronary artery vasculitis.	10%-20%. CHF and pericarditis have been described.
Gastrointestinal	<10%	30%-50% of patients and a major cause of morbidity and mortality. Hemorrhage, abdominal pain, infarct or perforated viscus.	35%-55% of patients. Findings similar to PAN. Pain, bleeding, and ischemia. Rare visceral aneurysms.
Dermatologic	Up to 60%. Palpable purpura, ulcers, nodules or vesicles.	50%-70% purpura, nodules, papules, leukocytoclastic vasculitis with or without eosinophils.	35%-60% of patients with purpura common.
Neurologic	Both central and peripheral nervous system involvement.	Mononeuritis multiplex in 50%-75%. CNS in 5%-40%.	Mononeuritis multiplex in 10%-50%.
Chest imaging	Abnormal in >80%. Alveolar, interstitial or mixed infiltrates, often with nodular and/or cavitary disease.	Infiltrates in >70%. Airways disease common (airway wall thickening, hyperinflation).	Infiltrates in 10%-30%. Pleural effusions in 5%-20%.
ANCA	ANCA positive >90% (PR3-ANCA 75%, MPO-ANCA 20%).	ANCA positive in 50% (PR3-ANCA 5%, MPO-ANCA 45%).	ANCA positive in 90% (PR3-ANCA 30%, MPO-ANCA 60%).

ANCA, Antineutrophil cytoplasmic antibodies; *CHF,* congestive heart failure; *CNS,* central nervous system; *ECG,* electrocardiography; *EGPA,* eosinophilic granulomatosis with polyangiitis; *GPA,* granulomatosis with polyangiitis; *MPA,* microscopic polyangiitis; *MPO,* myeloperoxidase; *PAN,* polyarteritis nodosa; *PR3,* proteinase 3; *RPGN,* rapidly progressive glomerulonephritis.
From Broaddus VC et al: *Murray & Nadel's textbook of respiratory medicine,* ed 7, Philadelphia 2022, Elsevier.

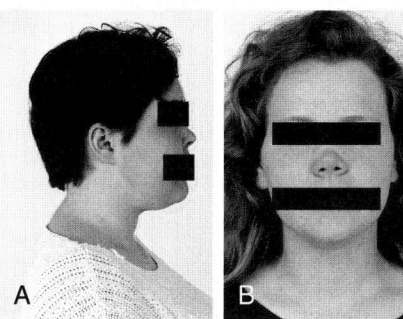

FIG. 1 Saddle-nose deformity in a patient with Wegener granulomatosis. (From *Kelley's textbook of rheumatology,* ed 8, Philadelphia, 2009, Elsevier.)

TABLE 3 Differential Diagnostic Features of the Anti-Neutrophil Cytoplasm Antibody–Associated Vasculitides

Feature	Microscopic Polyangiitis (MPA)	GPA (Wegener Granulomatosis)	EGPA (Churg-Strauss Syndrome)	Comments
Glomerulonephritis	+++	+++	+	Progressive renal failure uncommon in EGPA
Pulmonary infiltrates or nodules	++	+++	+++	Asthma and eosinophilia in EGPA
Alveolar hemorrhage	++	++	+	
Upper airway disease	+	+++	++	Ear, nose, and throat disease usually favors GPA
Skin, purpura	+++	+	++	
Peripheral nerve involvement	+	++	+++	Often a prominent feature of EGPA
Central nervous system involvement	+	+	+	

+++, Very commonly seen; ++, seen often; +, uncommon finding; *EGPA,* eosinophilic granulomatosis with polyangiitis; *GPA,* granulomatosis with polyangiitis.
From Firestein GS et al: *Kelly's textbook of rheumatology,* ed 9, Philadelphia, 2013, Saunders.

refractory to conventional treatment. Suspect GPA if sinus disease.

- Chest x-ray, laboratory evaluation, pulmonary function tests, and tissue (lung or kidney) biopsy for granulomatous lesions in GPA (Fig. E3) or non-granulomatous vasculitis in MPA.

LABORATORY TESTS

- ANCA serology (see Table 4): Most patients with GPA have a cytoplasmic pattern of ANCA (c-ANCA), which are predominantly directed against proteinase 3 (PR3). Whereas in MPA, the majority of patients have a perinuclear pattern (p-ANCA) directed against myeloperoxidase (MPO). Up to 15% of GPA patients have p-ANCA/MPO and about 25% of MPA patients have c-ANCA/PR3. Approximately 10% to 15% of AAV patients are ANCA negative
- CBC: Anemia, leukocytosis, thrombocytosis (>400,000/μL)
- Chemistry: Elevated serum creatinine, decreased creatinine clearance
- Urinalysis: May reveal hematuria, red blood cell (RBC) casts, and proteinuria
- Inflammatory markers: Increased erythrocyte sedimentation rate (ESR), positive rheumatoid factor, and elevated C-reactive protein may be found
- Liver function, hepatitis serologies, cryoglobulins, HIV screens, ANA, C3, C4, anti—glomerular basement membrane, and cultures to exclude other processes with similar constitutional symptoms

IMAGING STUDIES

- Chest x-ray: Pulmonary infiltrates, nodules, pleural effusions, and cavitary lesions (Fig. 4)
- CT of sinuses (Fig. 5), CT of chest, mesenteric angiography (if renal function permits), MRI of brain depending on symptoms
- Fiber optic bronchoscopy with bronchoalveolar lavage (BAL) and endoscopic ear, nose, and throat (ENT) examination: Nasal crusting ("golden crusts") are typical on evaluation
- Electromyography/nerve conduction study: Sensorimotor peripheral neuropathy
- Biopsy of one or more affected organs should be attempted, including the lung, skin, nasopharynx, or kidneys

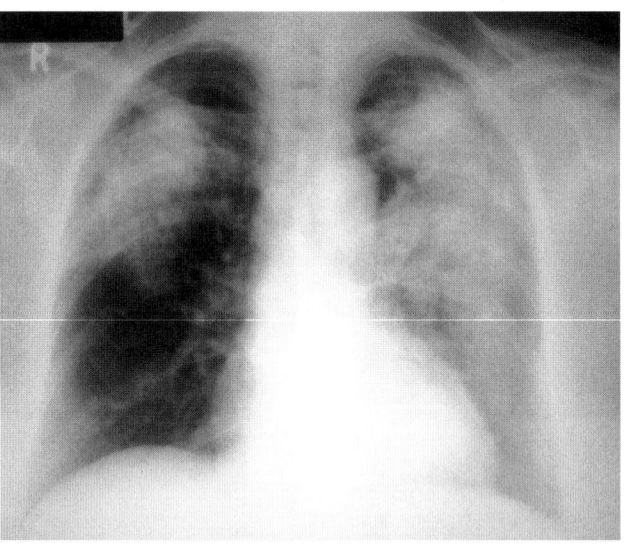

FIG. 4 Pulmonary hemorrhage in microscopic polyangiitis. (From Hochberg MC et al: *Rheumatology*, ed 5, St Louis, 2011, Mosby.)

TABLE 4 Clinical Settings in Which It Is Appropriate to Check ANCA and in Which Positive Testing for Antiproteinase 3 or Antimyeloperoxidase Antibodies Could Be Considered Diagnostic of GPA or MPA[a]

Disease	Manifestation	Examination Technique	Laboratory and Other Testing	Imaging	Problems With Biopsy
GPA > MPA	Scleritis	Ophthalmologic examination			
GPA	Orbital pseudotumor	Routine inspection, or with measurement tool		CT or MRI	
GPA > MPA	Sensorineural hearing loss		Audiography		Impossible
GPA	Sinonasal inflammation	Otoscope or fiberoptic examination		CT of sinuses	All three characteristic features[b] seen in only 10% of GPA
GPA	Subglottic inflammation	Laryngoscopy		CT of neck	Correlates poorly with examination or outcome
GPA	Pulmonary nodule(s)			CT of chest	1. Transbronchial: All three diagnostic features[b] are seldom seen. 2. Surgical biopsy: Invasive
GPA/MPA	Alveolar hemorrhage	Inspection (witnessed hemoptysis) or bronchoscopy with BAL		CT of chest	Invasive, and patient is often critically ill
GPA/MPA	Digit ischemia	Routine inspection		Angiography	Impossible
GPA/MPA	Peripheral neuropathy	Neurologic examination: Sensory and motor	Nerve conduction studies/electromyography		Likely to result in an area of permanent sensory deficit; small chance of chronic pain
GPA/MPA	Nephritis		Urine sediment: RBC casts		

BAL, Bronchoalveolar lavage; *EGPA*, eosinophilic granulomatosis with polyangiitis; *GPA*, granulomatosis with polyangiitis (Wegener's); *MPA*, microscopic polyangiitis.

[a]If accompanied by marked peripheral eosinophilia, then EGPA would be the most probable diagnosis. Biopsy is often unnecessary to diagnose scleritis or alveolar hemorrhage, is often nonspecific or nondiagnostic for GPA in sinonasal or subglottic or orbital disease, and is impossible in digit ischemia or sensorineural hearing loss. The value of biopsy of a pulmonary nodule or peripheral nerve depends on how typical or atypical the overall presentation is for anti-neutrophil cytoplasmic antibodies—associated vasculitides. Some experts recommend a kidney biopsy for all patients with suspected nephritis. Skin disease is not included in the table because the appearances of cutaneous vasculitis are nonspecific; skin biopsy is therefore particularly valuable for diagnosing vasculitis, although differentiation from other causes of cutaneous vasculitis is often impossible.

[b]Granulomatous inflammation, necrosis, and small vessel vasculitis.

From Firestein GS et al: *Firestein & Kelley's textbook of rheumatology*, ed 11, Philadelphia 2021, Elsevier.

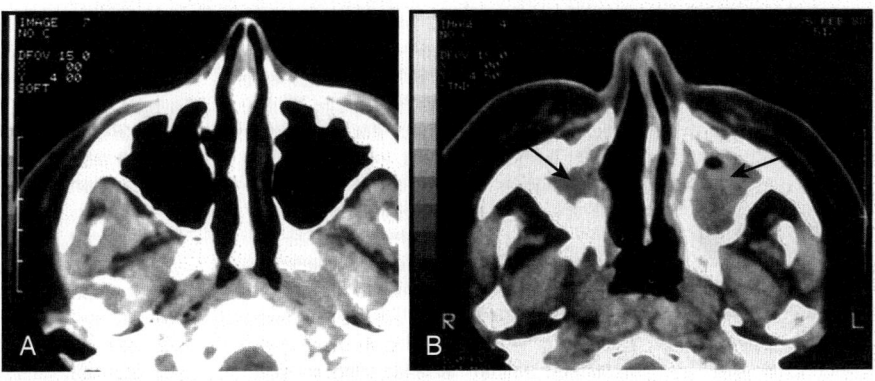

FIG. 5 CT scans of the sinuses. A, Normal maxillary sinuses in a patient recently diagnosed with granulomatosis with polyangiitis. **B,** Sinus CT scan of a patient with long-standing Wegener granulomatosis. Nasal septal deviation to the left, destruction of the medial walls of the right maxillary sinus, opacification of both sinuses with soft tissue densities *(arrows)*, and neo-ossification of all maxillary bony structures due to chronic inflammation. (From Hochberg MC et al: *Rheumatology,* ed 5, St Louis, 2011, Mosby.)

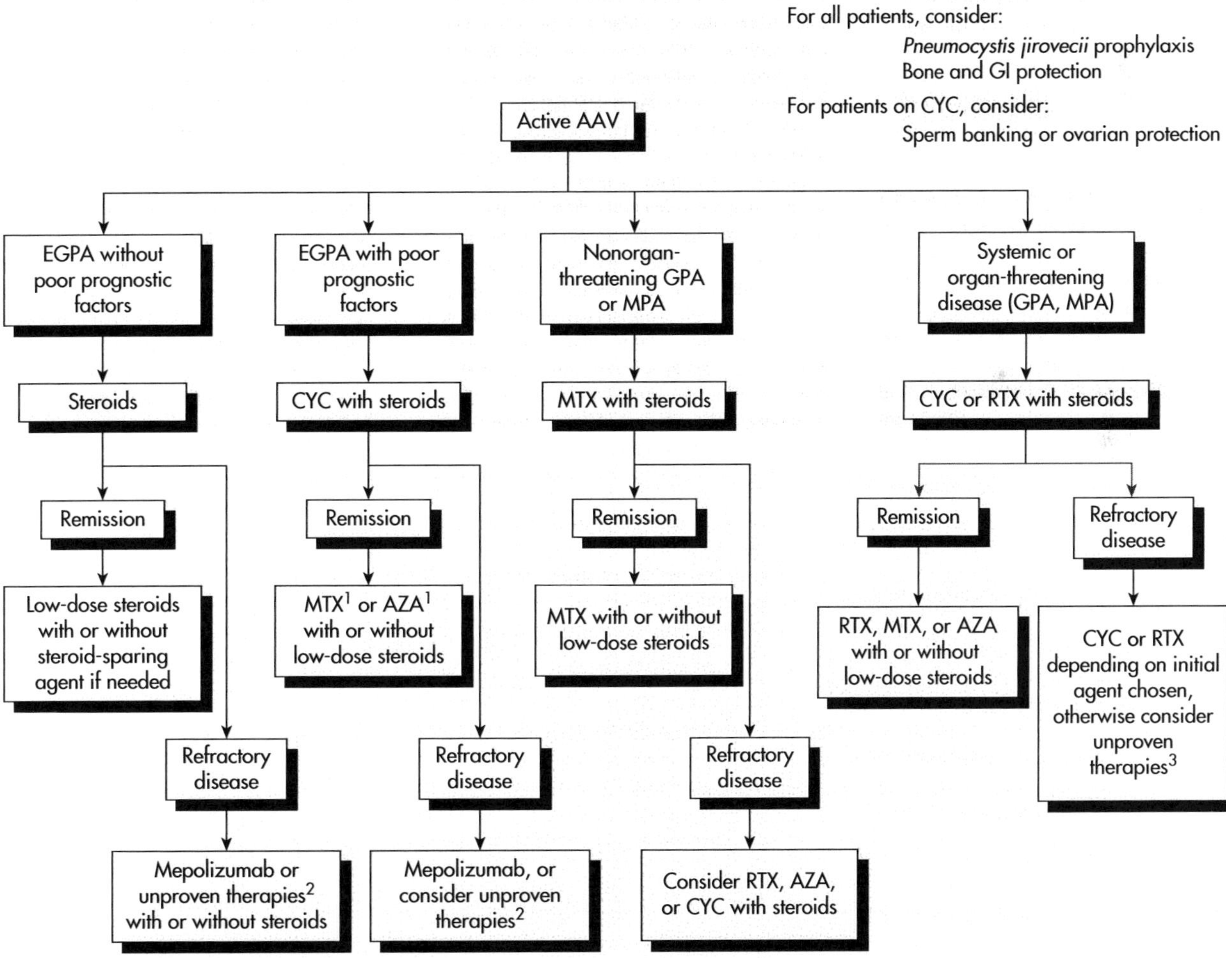

For all patients, consider:
> *Pneumocystis jirovecii* prophylaxis
> Bone and GI protection

For patients on CYC, consider:
> Sperm banking or ovarian protection

Active AAV

- **EGPA without poor prognostic factors**
  - Steroids
    - Remission
      - Low-dose steroids with or without steroid-sparing agent if needed
        - Refractory disease
          - Mepolizumab or unproven therapies[2] with or without steroids

- **EGPA with poor prognostic factors**
  - CYC with steroids
    - Remission
      - MTX[1] or AZA[1] with or without low-dose steroids
        - Refractory disease
          - Mepolizumab, or consider unproven therapies[2]

- **Nonorgan-threatening GPA or MPA**
  - MTX with steroids
    - Remission
      - MTX with or without low-dose steroids
        - Refractory disease
          - Consider RTX, AZA, or CYC with steroids

- **Systemic or organ-threatening disease (GPA, MPA)**
  - CYC or RTX with steroids
    - Remission
      - RTX, MTX, or AZA with or without low-dose steroids
    - Refractory disease
      - CYC or RTX depending on initial agent chosen, otherwise consider unproven therapies[3]

[1]Widely used but without strong evidence of efficacy
[2]Includes RTX, hydroxurea, MTX, AZA, and MMF
[3]Includes infliximab, MMF, intravenous immunoglobulin, and 15-deoxyspergualin

FIG. 7 Treatment algorithm for the anti-neutrophil cytoplasmic antibody (ANCA)-associated vasculitides (AAV). *AZA,* Azathioprine; *Cr,* serum creatinine; *CYC,* cyclophosphamide; *EGPA,* eosinophilic granulomatosis with polyangiitis; *GI,* gastrointestinal; *GPA,* granulomatosis with polyangiitis; *MPA,* microscopic polyangiitis; *MTX,* methotrexate; *PEX,* plasma exchange; *RTX,* rituximab. (From Firestein GS et al: *Firestein & Kelley's textbook of rheumatology,* ed 11, Philadelphia 2021, Elsevier.)

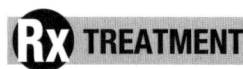 **TREATMENT**

NONPHARMACOLOGIC THERAPY
- Ensure proper airway drainage
- Give nutritional counseling

ACUTE GENERAL Rx (Fig. 7)
- Immunosuppressive therapy should be considered in all patients with GPA.
- Induction therapy consists of glucocorticoid with either cyclophosphamide or rituximab. Selected patients with severe disease, including alveolar hemorrhage or rapidly progressive glomerulonephritis, may benefit from the addition of plasma exchange to this regimen.
- The gold standard for treatment is pulse methylprednisolone followed by prednisone 60 to 80 mg/day. Based on the PEXIVAS trial, a reduced dose glucocorticoid regimen demonstrated equal efficacy as compared to the standard dose glucocorticoid regimen.
- Based on the RAVE trial, rituximab (375 mg/m/wk × 4 wk) appears to be more effective than traditional therapy in treating GPA/MPA that presents with disease flares and is at least as effective as traditional therapy for the induction of remission.[2] The RITUXVAS trial concluded that a combined cyclophosphamide-rituximab regimen was not inferior to pulse cyclophosphamide alone. Both studies used concurrent methylprednisolone followed by prednisone. If cyclophosphamide is used, MESNA can be given to prevent cyclophosphamide-induced hemorrhagic cystitis.[3]
- Methotrexate and glucocorticoids alone may be used with mild extrarenal disease or little to no renal involvement, or with limited sinus and upper airway involvement.
- The initial MEPEX trial demonstrated that plasma exchange in addition to cyclophosphamide and glucocorticoids may enhance renal function recovery. However, the more recent PEXIVAS trials showed no additional benefit in reducing mortality or progression to end-stage renal disease with plasma exchange.[4]
- Ongoing ADVOCATE trial of investigating the oral C5a receptor blocker, avacopan, as a

steroid sparing agent, in addition to rituximab or cyclophosphamide shows promising preliminary results of comparable remission rate and serious adverse events.[5]

CHRONIC Rx
- Potentially useful agents for maintenance therapy include rituximab, methotrexate, azathioprine, and mycophenolate mofetil. The MAINRITSAN trial showed that rituximab may be preferable for maintenance therapy. MAINRITSAN2 further demonstrated that patients who received tailored rituximab injections that corresponded with elevated CD19+ B lymphocyte or ANCA counts, rather than fixed-scheduled administrations, demonstrated similar relapse presentation rates, even with the former receiving much lower doses of rituximab.[6] A recent trial demonstrated that extended therapy with biannual rituximab infusions over 18 mo is associated with a lower incidence of AAV.[6]
- The CYCAZAREM (for azathioprine) and LEM (for leflunomide) trials showed that these agents can also be used. The WEGENT study showed oral methotrexate and azathioprine were noninferior for maintenance than intravenous cyclophosphamide.[7]
- Maintenance therapy should generally be continued for at least 18 to 24 mo, and ultimate duration of immunosuppression is decided on a case-by-case basis.
- Mepolizumab, an anti−interleukin-5 (IL-5) monoclonal antibody, is approved for the treatment of EGPA and is used in patients who are not controlled with oral steroids alone.[8]
- Treatment with TMP-SMX (160 mg/800 mg bid) may reduce the incidence of relapses in patients with GPA in remission. It is also useful in preventing *Pneumocystis jiroveci* pneumonia (PJP), which occurs in 10% of patients receiving induction therapy. Dose of trimethoprim-sulfamethoxazole (TMP-SMX) (160 mg/800 mg) for prophylaxis is 1 tablet three times/wk. If the patient is unable to tolerate TMP-SMX, PJP prophylaxis can also be achieved with dapsone, atovaquone, or inhaled pentamidine.[1]

DISPOSITION
- 5-yr survival with prompt initiation and aggressive treatment is approximately 80%; without treatment 2-yr survival is 20%.
- Renal failure and pulmonary involvement are major causes of morbidity and mortality. Age over 50 yr and lack of ENT changes at diagnosis are also associated with worse outcomes and increased mortality in GPA.
- Remission rate can be achieved in the majority of patients, but relapse is frequent.

REFERRAL
- Rheumatology referral for continued treatment.
- Multidisciplinary consultation including nephrology, ENT, pulmonary, and dermatology may be required depending on other organ involvement.

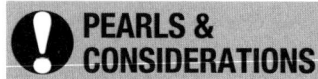 **PEARLS & CONSIDERATIONS**

COMMENTS
The goal with treatment of AAV is to achieve rapid, long-standing remission, based on induction therapy and then maintenance regimens. Without treatment there is a very high rate of mortality, and treatment is complicated by serious infections and renal disease.

PATIENT & FAMILY EDUCATION
Support can be found with the Vasculitis Foundation.

REFERENCES & SUGGESTED READINGS
Available at eBooks.Health.Elsevier.com.

RELATED CONTENT
Systemic Vasculitis (Related Key Topic)

AUTHORS: **OMAR KARIM, BS,** and **MANUEL F DASILVA, MD**

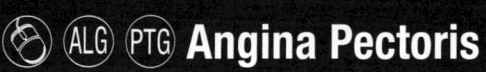

A

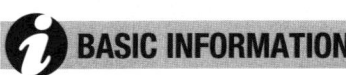 **BASIC INFORMATION**

DEFINITION

Angina pectoris is a term used to describe a clinical syndrome, typically characterized by chest, jaw, shoulder, back, or arm discomfort that is caused by myocardial ischemia. This is most commonly related to atheromatous plaque in one or more than one large epicardial coronary artery; however, myocardial ischemia may occur in the absence of obstructive coronary artery disease (CAD), such as uncontrolled hypertension, microvascular disease, valvular heart disease, hypertrophic cardiomyopathy, coronary spasm, or endothelial dysfunction. Any situation that causes an imbalance in myocardial oxygen supply and demand can cause an angina syndrome. Angina can be classified as follows:

- Chronic stable angina, stable ischemic heart disease (SIHD), or chronic CAD:
  1. Predictable. Usually follows a precipitating event (e.g., climbing stairs, sexual intercourse, a heavy meal, emotional stress, cold weather)
  2. Generally, has the same severity as previous attacks; relieved by rest or by the customary dose of sublingual nitroglycerin
  3. Caused by a fixed coronary artery obstruction secondary to atherosclerosis. The presence of one or more obstructions in major coronary arteries is likely; the severity of stenosis is usually >70%
- Unstable (rest, recent onset, crescendo angina; will be reviewed under "Acute Coronary Syndrome"):
  1. Rest angina: Angina occurring at rest and usually prolonged >20 min, occurring within 1 wk of presentation
  2. Recent onset: Angina of at least CCS Class III severity occurring less than 2 mo after the onset of the symptoms
  3. Crescendo angina: Previously diagnosed angina that is distinctly more frequent, longer in duration, or lower in threshold (i.e., increased by >1 CCS class within 2 mo of initial presentation to at least CCS Class III severity)
- Prinzmetal variant:
  1. Occurs at rest, common after cold exposure
  2. Cyclical in nature
  3. ECG finding of episodic ST-segment elevations
  4. Caused by coronary artery spasm with or without superimposed CAD
  5. Patients are more likely to develop ventricular arrhythmias
- Microvascular angina (syndrome X):
  1. Refers to patients with angina symptoms, positive exercise test, normal coronary angiograms, and no coronary spasm. Defective endothelium-dependent dilation in the coronary microcirculation contributes to the altered regulation of myocardial perfusion and the ischemic manifestations in these patients.
  2. Patients with chest pain and normal or nonobstructive coronary angiograms are predominantly women, and many have a

prognosis that is not as benign as commonly thought (2% risk of death or myocardial infarction [MI] at 30 days of follow-up).
- Refractory angina:
  1. Refers to patients who, despite optimal medical therapy with at least maximal doses, or as tolerated of two antianginal medications, in addition to aspirin, aggressive risk factor modification, such as smoking cessation, adequate control of hypertension, diabetes, and hyperlipidemia, still have both angina and objective evidence of ischemia
- Other:
  1. Angina due to aortic stenosis and idiopathic hypertrophic subaortic stenosis, cocaine-induced coronary vasoconstriction

FUNCTIONAL CLASSIFICATION:

Stable angina should be classified using a grading system. The most commonly adopted is that of the Canadian Cardiovascular Society (CCS):

- Class I: Ordinary physical activity, such as walking or climbing stairs, does not cause angina. Angina occurs with strenuous, rapid, or prolonged exertion at work or recreation.
- Class II: Slight limitation of ordinary activity. Angina occurs on walking or climbing stairs rapidly; walking uphill; walking or stair climbing after meals, in cold, in wind, or under emotional stress; or only during the few hours after awakening. Angina occurs on walking more than two level blocks and climbing more than one flight of ordinary stairs at a normal pace and in normal conditions.
- Class III: Marked limitations of ordinary physical activity. Angina occurs on walking one to two level blocks and climbing one flight of stairs in normal conditions and at a normal pace.
- Class IV: Inability to carry on any physical activity without discomfort; anginal symptoms may be present at rest.

ICD-10CM CODES
I20.1	Angina pectoris with documented spasm
I20.8	Other forms of angina pectoris
I20.9	Angina pectoris, unspecified
I25.110	Atherosclerotic heart disease of native coronary artery with unstable angina pectoris
I25.111	Atherosclerotic heart disease of native coronary artery with angina pectoris with documented spasm
I25.118	Atherosclerotic heart disease of native coronary artery with other forms of angina pectoris
I25.119	Atherosclerotic heart disease of native coronary artery with unspecified angina pectoris
I25.700	Atherosclerosis of coronary artery bypass graft(s), unspecified, with unstable angina pectoris
I25.790	Atherosclerosis of other coronary artery bypass graft(s) with unstable angina pectoris
I25.791	Atherosclerosis of other coronary artery bypass graft(s) with angina pectoris with documented spasm
I25.798	Atherosclerosis of other coronary artery bypass graft(s) with other forms of angina pectoris
I25.799	Atherosclerosis of other coronary artery bypass graft(s) with unspecified angina pectoris

EPIDEMIOLOGY & DEMOGRAPHICS

- It is estimated that one in three adults in the U.S. (about 81 million) has some form of cardiovascular disease. Based on the NHANES survey 2007 to 2010, an estimated 15.4 million have coronary heart disease (CHD) of which 7.8 million have angina.
- Angina is most common in middle-aged and elderly men. Among persons 60 to 79 yr of age, approximately 25% of men and 16% of women have CHD, and these figures rise to 37% and 23% among men and women >80 yr of age, respectively.
- The incidence of CHD and angina in women after menopause is similar to that of men.
- Although the survival rate has steadily improved over time, SIHD remains the number one cause of death in men and women (27% of deaths).
- The initial manifestation of ischemic heart disease is angina pectoris in 50%, and about 50% of patients presenting to the hospital with acute coronary syndrome have preceding angina.
- Two older population-based studies from Olmstead County, MN, and Framingham, MA, showed annual rate of MI in patients with symptomatic angina of 3% to 3.5%/yr.
- Within 12 mo of initial diagnosis, 10% to 20% of patients with diagnosis of stable angina progress to MI or unstable angina.

PHYSICAL FINDINGS & CLINICAL PRESENTATION

- The assessment of chest pain should include quality, location, severity, and duration of pain; radiation; associated symptoms; provocative factors; and alleviating factors. Anginal pain can be described as "squeezing," "griplike," "suffocating," and "heavy," but it is rarely sharp or stabbing and typically does not vary with position or respiration. The classic Levine sign is placing a clenched fist over the precordium to describe the pain. Many patients do not, however, describe angina as frank pain but as tightness, pressure, or discomfort. Other patients, in particular women and older adults, can present with atypical symptoms such as nausea, vomiting, midepigastric discomfort, sharp (atypical) chest pain, dizziness, or syncope.
- Ischemic pain of more than 20 minutes' duration should raise concern for possible acute coronary syndrome.
- Women are more likely than men to report atypical chest pain or discomfort (65%

reported on Women's Ischemic Syndrome Evaluation [WISE] study).
- Elderly and diabetics may report symptoms other than chest pain, such as dyspnea, fatigue, or diaphoresis.

ETIOLOGY
RISK FACTORS:
- Advanced age.
- Male sex.
- Genetic predisposition, family history of premature CAD in first-degree relatives (men <55 yr of age, and women <65 yr of age).
- Smoking (risk of first MI is increased by near threefold).
- Hypertension.
- Hyperlipidemia.
- Impaired glucose tolerance or diabetes mellitus.
- History of stroke or peripheral arterial disease.
- Chronic kidney disease (CKD).
- Metabolic syndrome.
- Physical inactivity.
- Obesity (body mass index [BMI] >30% over ideal). A higher BMI during childhood is also associated with an increased risk of CHD in adulthood.
- Entities that cause increased oxygen demand include hyperthermia (particularly if accompanied by volume contraction), hyperthyroidism, and cocaine or methamphetamine abuse.
- Cocaine is used by >5 million Americans regularly and is responsible for >64,000 emergency department (ED) evaluations yearly to rule out myocardial ischemia. Cocaine causes sympathomimetic toxicity and not only increases myocardial oxygen demand but also induces coronary vasospasm and can cause infarction in young patients. Long-term cocaine use can cause premature development of SIHD.
- Severe uncontrolled hypertension causes increased myocardial oxygen demand and decreased subendocardial perfusion that increases left ventricular (LV) wall tension. Hypertrophic cardiomyopathy and aortic stenosis can induce even more severe LV hypertrophy and resultant wall tension.
- Other causes of increased myocardial oxygen demand are ventricular or supraventricular tachycardias. Ambulatory monitoring may be required to diagnose these.
- Entities that limit myocardial oxygen supply such as anemia may cause angina when the hemoglobin drops to <9 g/dl, and ST-T-wave changes (depression or inversion) can occur at levels <7 g/dl.
- Hypoxemia resulting from pulmonary disease (e.g., pneumonia, asthma, chronic obstructive pulmonary disease, pulmonary hypertension, interstitial fibrosis, or obstructive sleep apnea) can also precipitate angina.
- Polycythemia, leukemia, thrombocytosis, and hypergammaglobulinemia.
- Oral contraceptive and hormone replacement therapy use.
- Coronary artery calcium is associated with an increased risk of MI.

- Long-term use of NSAIDs.
- Exposure to air pollution from traffic (dilute diesel exhaust) promotes myocardial ischemia and is associated with adverse cardiovascular events.
- Low serum folate levels required for conversion of homocysteine to methionine are associated with an increased risk of fatal CHD. Hyperhomocysteinemia has a toxic effect on vascular endothelium and interferes with proliferation of arterial wall smooth muscle cells. Elevated plasma homocysteine level is a strong and independent risk factor for CHD events, especially in patients with type 2 diabetes mellitus.
- Elevated levels of highly sensitive C-reactive protein (hs-CRP, cardio CRP). Diseases associated with systemic inflammation can lead to accelerated atherosclerosis.
- Depression.
- Vasculitis.
- Elevated levels of lipoprotein-associated phospholipase A_2.
- Elevated fibrinogen levels.
- Low level of red blood cell glutathione peroxidase-1 activity.
- Radiation therapy.

🅓🅧 DIAGNOSIS

DIFFERENTIAL DIAGNOSIS
- Nonischemic cardiovascular: Aortic dissection, pericarditis
- Pulmonary: Pulmonary embolism, pneumothorax, pneumonia, pleuritis
- Gastrointestinal: Esophageal, esophagitis, spasm, reflux, biliary colic, cholecystitis, choledocholithiasis, cholangitis, peptic ulcer, pancreatitis
- Chest wall: Costochondritis, fibrositis, rib fracture, sternoclavicular arthritis, herpes zoster (before the rash)
- Psychiatric: Anxiety disorders, hyperventilation, panic disorder, primary anxiety, affective disorders (i.e., depression), somatoform disorders, thought disorders (i.e., fixed delusions)

WORKUP
- In patients with chest pain, the probability of CAD should be estimated on the basis of patient age, sex, cardiovascular risk factors, and pain characteristics.
- The most important diagnostic element is the history. Chest pain or left arm pain or discomfort occurring with exertion and relieved by rest in a patient with cardiovascular risk factors is consistent with a high likelihood of CAD.
- In assessing the likelihood of underlying SIHD it is helpful to classify the chest pain as typical angina, atypical angina, and/or noncardiac chest pain.
- Typical angina, (definite) will have the following three features: (1) Substernal chest discomfort with a characteristic quality and duration, (2) provoked by exertion or emotional stress, and (3) relieved by rest and/or sublingual nitroglycerin.

- Atypical angina, (probable) will have two of the above listed three features.
- Noncardiac chest pain will have one or none of the previously listed features.
- Physical examination may be completely normal in many patients; however, certain findings may be helpful in the assessment of the patient with suspected SIHD. Some findings may identify consequences of ischemia or possible causes of the anginal syndrome other than CAD. The presence of hypertension, arcus senilis, xanthelasma, carotid or peripheral bruits, and a prominent S4 are all physical signs that could raise concern for the presence of CAD. A murmur of mitral regurgitation may be a marker of an ischemic cardiomyopathy or transient ischemia. A murmur suggestive of hypertrophic cardiomyopathy or aortic stenosis may suggest a cause of angina other than CAD.
- The ultimate goal for an SIHD patient's evaluation is to identify high-risk CAD patients with minimal use of resources. In general, four common steps would help a clinician to assess high feature of SIHD. Those are (1) CAD risk assessment based on various classic risk factors, (2) functional capacity and stress test result, (3) LV and right ventricular (RV) function, and (4) coronary anatomy. Every patient does not need each of the modalities. One should classify stable angina without history of CAD patients to low, intermediate, and high pretest probability or likelihood for CAD after assessment of comorbidities and atherosclerotic vascular disease risk factors. Consider functional capacity and stress test (ETT [exercise tolerance test], ETT-MIBI [ETT-myocardial perfusion imaging (multiplex ion beam imaging with dipyridamole/technetium sestamibi)] or stress echo) for low and intermediate pretest probability patients. Exercise testing (Fig. 1) is preferred to pharmacologic stress tests when possible. Functional capacity and stress test results categorize SIHD patients based on their risk of annual mortality. Patients with an estimated annual mortality of <1% classify as low risk, 1% to 3% are considered as intermediate risk, and >3% annual mortality belongs to high-risk patient population (please see "Coronary Artery Disease" chapter).[1,2]

LABORATORY TESTS
- Screen for hypertension, diabetes, and hyperlipidemia per routine guidelines.
- Electrocardiogram should be obtained during pain and when the patient is free of any discomfort. A normal resting electrocardiogram is not unusual in patients with SIHD; in patients who present with chest pain, 1% to 6% who have an acute MI will have a normal or nondiagnostic electrocardiogram.
- Chest x-ray PA and lateral if symptoms suggestive of heart failure, pericardial disease, aortic aneurysm/dissection.
- Cardio-CRP (hs-CRP): Its elevation is a relatively moderate predictor of CHD, and it adds prognostic information to that conveyed by the Framingham risk score.

EXERCISE TESTING AND IMAGING STUDIES (SEE "CORONARY ARTERY DISEASE" CHAPTER, FIG. 1):

- Exercise testing is used for diagnosis as well as prognosis of SIHD. If the patient is physically capable to perform at least moderate physical exercise, exercise stress testing see (see Fig. 1) is useful because of the important prognostic information obtained from exercise performance and the hemodynamic response. Risk stratification based on noninvasive testing is summarized in Table 1. Patients who have an intermediate likelihood of CAD, as patients in a low-risk or high-likelihood category are more likely to have a false-positive or false-negative result, respectively. Risk assessment is also indicated in patients with SIHD who are being considered for revascularization of known coronary stenosis of unclear physiologic significance. The exercise treadmill test is contraindicated in patients with presence of ST depression >0.5 mm or Wolff-Parkinson-White syndrome, left bundle branch block, or pacemaker rhythm in baseline ECG.
- Stress echocardiography or stress testing with myocardial perfusion imaging may be employed when baseline electrocardiographic abnormalities are present that render the electrocardiographic response to exercise uninterpretable. Stress echocardiography has the advantage of higher specificity and a lower cost. Stress radionuclide perfusion imaging has a higher sensitivity, particularly for single-vessel coronary disease, and has a higher technical success rate. When the patient is unable to exercise adequately, pharmacologic stress testing (i.e., dobutamine, adenosine, regadenoson) may be used with these imaging modalities.

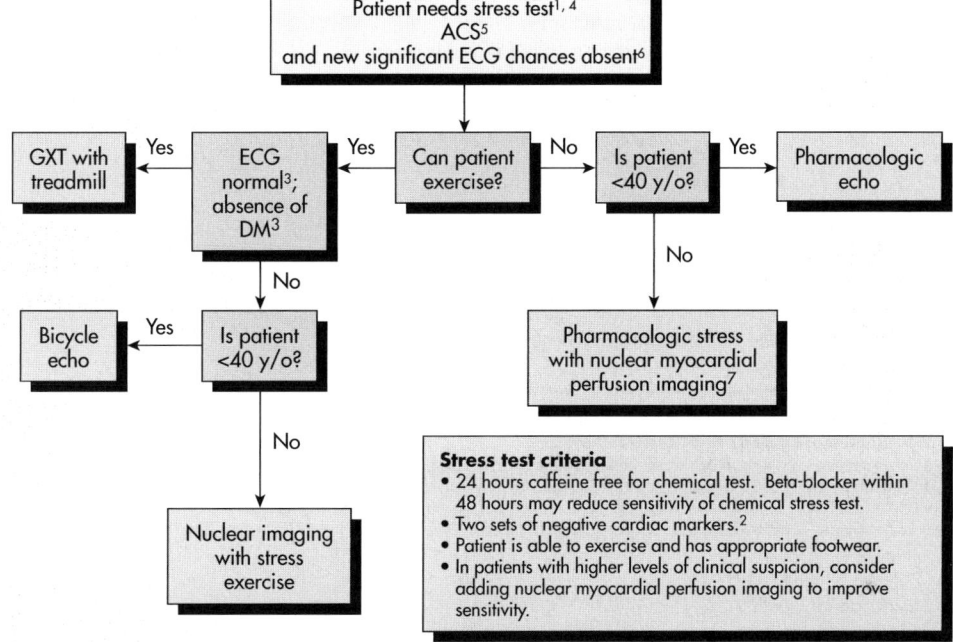

DEFINITIONS:

[1]Typical angina:
(1) Substernal chest pain or discomfort that is (2) provoked by exertion or emotional stress and (3) relieved by rest and/or nitroglycerin

[2]Cardiac marker timing: Based on symptom onset; in cases of uncertainty assume symptom onset at ED arrival

[3]ECG normal: No significant ST depression/T wave inversions, BBB, LVH with repolarization, conduction defect, digoxin effect

[4]Anginal equivalent:
- Any symptoms that the physician feels may represent ACS
- Exertional dyspnea—most common anginal equivalent symptom

[5]ACS:
- STE-ACS—1 mm ST elevation in 2 leads
- NSTE-ACS
  - NSTEMI—positive cardiac biomarkers
  - Unstable angina—ischemia with negative biomarkers

[6]New significant ECG changes:
- ST Δs $\geq$ 0.5 mm; resolve when asymptomatic
- ST depression $\geq$1 mm in 2 leads
- T wave inversion $\geq$2 mm in 2 leads

[7]Regadenoson is preferred agent for chemical nuclear stress test. Technetium Tc 99m tetrofosmin is the preferred tracer.

FIG. 1 Stress test algorithm. *ACS,* Acute coronary syndrome; *BBB,* bundle branch block; *DM,* diabetes mellitus; *ECG,* electrocardiogram; *echo,* echocardiography; *ED,* emergency department; *GTX,* graded exercise test; *LVH,* left ventricular hypertrophy; *NSTE,* non—ST-segment elevation; *NSTEMI,* NSTE myocardial infarction; *STE,* ST-segment elevation; *y/o,* years old. (From Adams JG et al: *Emergency medicine: clinical essentials,* ed 2, Philadelphia, 2013, Saunders.)

TABLE 1   Risk Stratification Based on Noninvasive Testing

High Risk (>3% Annual Risk for Death or Myocardial Infarction)

1. Severe resting left ventricular dysfunction (LVEF <35%) not readily explained by noncoronary causes
2. Resting perfusion abnormalities involving ≥10% of the myocardium without previous known MI
3. High-risk stress findings on the ECG, including:
   - ≥2-mm ST-segment depression at low workload or persisting into recovery
   - Exercise-induced ST-segment elevation
   - Exercise-induced VT/VF
4. Severe stress-induced LV dysfunction (peak exercise LVEF <45% or drop in LVEF with stress ≥10%)
5. Stress-induced perfusion abnormalities encumbering ≥10% of the myocardium or stress segmental scores indicating multiple vascular territories with abnormalities
6. Stress-induced LV dilation
7. Inducible wall motion abnormality (involving >2 segments or 2 coronary beds)
8. Wall motion abnormality developing at a low dose of dobutamine (≤10 mg/kg/min) or at a low heart rate (<120 beats/min)
9. Multivessel obstructive CAD (≥70% stenosis) or left main stenosis (≥50% stenosis) on CCTA

Intermediate Risk (1%-3% Annual Risk for Death or Myocardial Infarction)

1. Mild to moderate resting LV dysfunction (LVEF of 35%-49%) not readily explained by noncoronary causes
2. Resting perfusion abnormalities involving 5%-9.9% of the myocardium in patients without a history or previous evidence of MI
3. ≥1-mm ST-segment depression occurring with exertional symptoms
4. Stress-induced perfusion abnormalities encumbering 5%-9.9% of the myocardium or stress segmental scores indicating 1 vascular territory with abnormalities but without LV dilation
5. Small wall motion abnormality involving 1-2 segments and only 1 coronary bed
6. Single-vessel CAD with ≥70% stenosis or moderate CAD stenosis (50%-69% stenosis) in ≥2 arteries on CCTA

Low Risk (<1% Annual Risk for Death or Myocardial Infarction)

1. Low-risk treadmill score (score ≥5) or no new ST-segment changes or exercise-induced chest pain symptoms when achieving maximal levels of exercise
2. Normal or small myocardial perfusion defect at rest or with stress encumbering <5% of the myocardium*
3. Normal stress or no change in limited resting wall motion abnormalities during stress
4. No coronary stenosis >50% on CCTA

CCTA, Cardiac computed tomography angiography; *LVEF*, left ventricular ejection fraction; *VF*, ventricular fibrillation; *VT*, ventricular tachycardia.
Assessment of coronary artery calcium can also be used to contribute to risk assessment.
*Although the published data are limited, patients with these findings will probably not be at low risk in the presence of either a high-risk treadmill score or severe resting LV dysfunction (LVEF <35%).
Modified from Fihn SD et al: ACCF/AHA/ACP/AATS/PCNA/SCAI/STS guideline for the diagnosis and management of patients with stable ischemic heart disease: a report of the American College of Cardiology Foundation/American Heart Association Task Force on Practice Guidelines, and the American College of Physicians, American Association for Thoracic Surgery, Preventive Cardiovascular Nurses Association, Society for Cardiovascular Angiography and Interventions, and Society of Thoracic Surgeons, *Circulation* 126:e354, 2012; in Zipes DP: *Braunwald's heart disease: a textbook of cardiovascular medicine*, ed 11, Philadelphia, 2019, Elsevier.

- A good predictor of risk for a patient with stable angina is the Duke treadmill score, which incorporates the patient's functional status (METS or time in minutes during the Bruce protocol), ST-segment depression in millimeters, and an angina index (yes or no). Patients with favorable Duke scores (>5) have a 5-yr survival rate of >97%; this is independent of other factors such as coronary anatomy and LV function.
- Echocardiography is indicated in patients with murmurs suggestive of aortic stenosis, hypertrophic cardiomyopathy, mitral regurgitation, mitral valve prolapse, previous MI, pathologic Q waves, complex ventricular arrhythmias, heart failure, hypertension, diabetes, and abnormal ECG.
- Cardiac computed tomography (CCTA; Fig. 2) is useful for the detection of subclinical CAD in asymptomatic patients with an intermediate Framingham 10-yr risk estimate of 10% to 20%. 2021 ACC/AHA/ASE chest pain guidelines recommend cardiac CT angiogram (CCTA) as a front-line imaging modality for stable angina. Trials comparing CCTA to invasive coronary angiography (ICA) in patients with stable angina have shown that an initial strategy of CCTA for anatomic imaging is associated with similar outcomes but fewer procedural complications and invasive angiograms.[3] CCTA detects and quantifies coronary calcium and evaluates the lumen and wall of the coronary artery. CCTA can be useful as a first-line test for risk assessment in patients with SIHD who are unable to exercise to an adequate workload regardless of interpretability of ECG. Also can be used when a functional test has an indeterminate result and to assess bypass graft patency or patency of previous stents >3 mm diameter. CCTA CT cost and radiation exposure are limiting factors to recommending widespread routine use of this marker. CCTA has an excellent negative predictive value to rule out severe CAD in the setting of active chest pain evaluation in the emergency room (ROMICAT-II trial). In 2018 the SCOT-HEART trial showed coronary CTA resulted in a lower risk of nonfatal MI than standard care alone (ETT) in stable angina patients. Myocardial perfusion imaging and noninvasive fractional flow ratio would be possible with cardiac CTA as well.
- Coronary artery calcium score is a strong predictor of incidence of CAD and provides predictive information in patients with low to intermediate pretest probability of CAD beyond that provided by standard risk factors. A score <100 indicates low risk and a score >400 high risk.
- Cardiac magnetic resonance imaging, in addition to its use for diagnosis of arrhythmogenic right ventricular dysplasia, can also be used to assess myocardial perfusion and viability as well as function in patients unable to exercise. Additional studies are needed to determine the cost effectiveness of these studies in patients with ischemic cardiomyopathy.
- Invasive coronary angiography remains the gold standard for the identification of clinically significant CAD. Angiography is performed to define the location and extent of coronary disease; indicated in selected patients who are candidates for coronary revascularization (either coronary artery bypass graft [CABG] surgery or angioplasty).

ⓇⓍ TREATMENT

FIVE FUNDAMENTAL OVERLAPPING STRATEGIES ARE RECOMMENDED

- Patient education: Support active participation of patients in the decision-making process of their treatment.
- Management of comorbid conditions that contribute to or worsen SIHD.

A

Diseases and Disorders

I

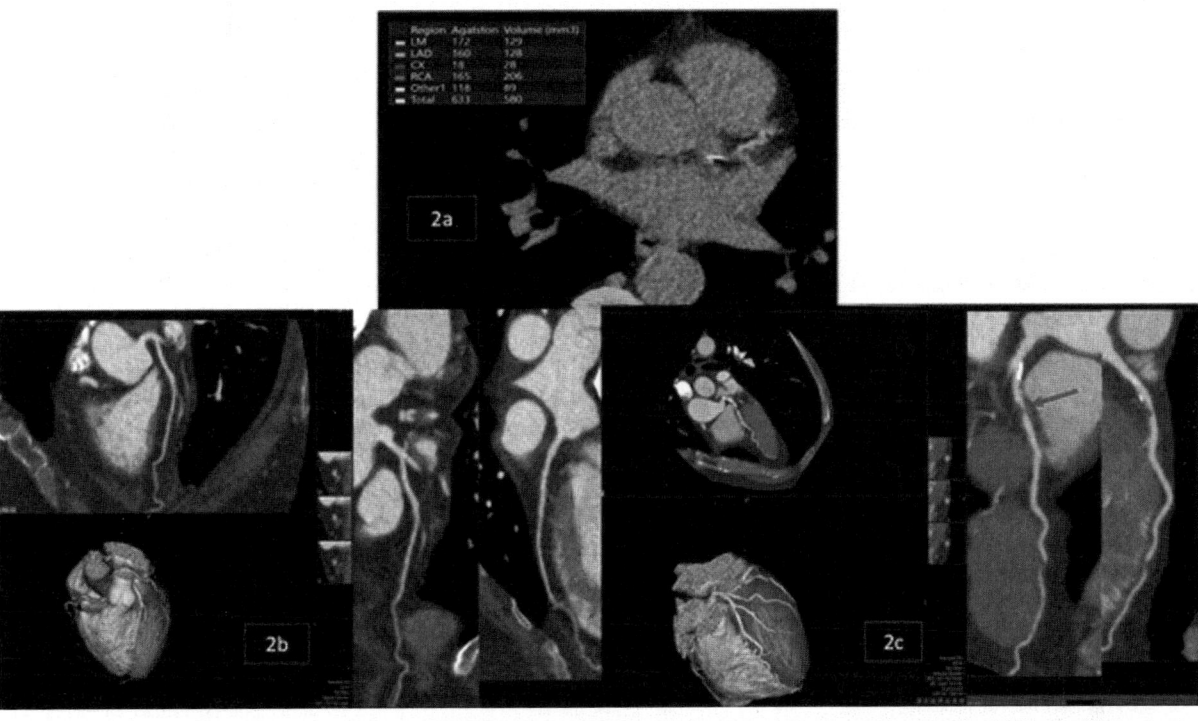

FIG. 2 *2a,* Example of coronary artery calcium scoring in which calcified foci are identified within the left anterior descending *(green)* and left main *(blue)* coronary arteries; table shows individual and total Agatston scores. *2b,* Cardiac CTA showed normal coronary arteries. *2c,* Cardiac CTA showed proximal to mid—left anterior descending artery stenosis (∼80%) *(red arrow).* (Courtesy Maheswara Satya Gangadhara Rao Golla, MD.)

- Aggressive modification of preventable risk factors such as smoking cessation, weight reduction in obese patients, regular aerobic exercise program (at least 30 to 60 min/day for 5 days a week), correction of folate deficiency, reduced intake of saturated fats (to <7% of total calories) and trans-fatty acids (to <1% of total calories), low-sodium diet (<2 g/day), and teaching importance of medication adherence. Whole grains as the main form of carbohydrates, an abundance of fruits and vegetables, and adequate omega-3 fatty acids are optimal for prevention of SIHD.
- Evidence-based pharmacologic management to improve quality of life and survival.
- Use appropriate revascularization procedures to improve survival and long-term outcomes in selected patients.

PHARMACOLOGIC THERAPY (SEE "CORONARY ARTERY DISEASE")

Treatment can be classified based on medications that prevent MI and death.
- Aspirin reduces cardiovascular mortality and morbidity rates by 20% to 25% among patients with CAD. Appropriate dose is 75 to 162 mg/day in the absence of contraindications. It inhibits the enzyme cyclooxygenase and synthesis of thromboxane A2 and reduces the risk of adverse cardiovascular events by 33% in patients with unstable angina. Patients intolerant to aspirin can be treated with clopidogrel or can undergo aspirin desensitization. Clopidogrel irreversibly blocks the P2Y12 adenosine diphosphate receptor on the platelet surface, thereby interrupting platelet activation and aggregation. Clopidogrel can be combined with ASA in high-risk patients with SIHD with low risk for bleeding complications or can be given alone in patients that are aspirin intolerant. Dose is 75 mg/day.
- Ticagrelor, in the PEGASUS-TIMI-54, reduced the risk of death, cardiovascular MI, or stroke in patients after 1 yr of MI. However, it is associated with an increased risk of bleeding when compared to placebo.
- Dipyridamole is not recommended as an antiplatelet therapy for the treatment of patients with SIHD.
- Beta-adrenergic blockers, which prevent MI and death, are first-line therapy in the management of angina pectoris. They achieve their major antianginal effect by decreasing myocardial oxygen demand in reducing heart rate and systolic blood pressure product, atrioventricular nodal conduction, and myocardial contractility, in this manner contributing to a reduction in angina onset, with improvement in the ischemic threshold during exercise and during the usual daily activities. Absent contraindications, they should be regarded as initial therapy for stable angina for all patients. Their dose should generally be adjusted to reduce the resting heart rate to 55 to 60 beats/min. Despite the difference among the available beta-blockers, they all seem to be equally efficacious in SIHD. Beta-blockers recommended for at least 2 to 3 yr after MI, and lifelong for patients with LV ejection fraction of <40% with heart failure or prior MI.
- Nitrates cause venodilation and relaxation of vascular smooth muscle; the decreased venous return from venodilation decreases diastolic ventricular wall tension (preload) and thereby reduces mechanical activity (and myocardial oxygen consumption) during systole. Relaxation of vascular smooth muscle increases coronary blood flow and reduces systemic pressure. Dilation of the arterial wall will not be affected by plaque, but independent of an intact endothelium, leads to reduced resistance across the obstructed lumen. Nitroglycerin contributes to coronary blood flow redistribution by augmenting collateral flow and lowering ventricular diastolic pressure from areas of normal perfusion to ischemic zones. Nitroglycerin also has demonstrated antithrombotic and antiplatelet effects. Sublingual nitroglycerin or nitroglycerin spray should be prescribed to all patients with SIHD for immediate angina relief. Tolerance to nitrates can be minimized by avoiding sustained blood levels with a daily nitrate-free period (e.g., omission of bedtime dose of oral isosorbide dinitrate or 12 h on/12 h off transdermal nitroglycerin therapy). Nitrates are relatively contraindicated in patients with hypertrophic obstructive cardiomyopathy, and should also be avoided in patients with severe aortic stenosis. Nitrates should not be used within 24 h of sildenafil (Viagra) or vardenafil (Levitra) or within 48 h of tadalafil (Cialis) because of the potential for hypotension.
- Calcium channel blockers are antiischemic medications that have no proven mortality benefit in SIHD. They improve myocardial oxygen supply by decreasing coronary vascular resistance and augmenting epicardial conduit vessel and systemic arterial blood flow. Myocardial demand is decreased by a

reduction in myocardial contractility, systemic vascular resistance, and arterial pressure. They are first-line treatment when beta-blockers are contraindicated. They play a major role in preventing and terminating myocardial ischemia induced by coronary artery spasm. They are particularly effective in treating microvascular angina. All classes of calcium channel blockers reduce anginal episodes, increase exercise duration, and reduce use of sublingual nitroglycerin in patients with effort-induced angina. Short-acting calcium channel blockers should be avoided. Calcium channel blockers (particularly nondihydropyridine) should generally also be avoided in patients with CHF secondary to systolic dysfunction due to its negative inotropic effect.

- Ranolazine, which has been tested in four different studies with a total of 1737 patients (MARISA, CARISA, RANO80, and ERICA), inhibits the late inward sodium current, indirectly reducing the sodium-dependent calcium current during ischemic conditions and leading to improvement in ventricular diastolic tension and oxygen consumption. It seems to increase the efficiency of energy production in the heart, maintaining cardiac function. Its anti-anginal and antiischemic effects do not depend on reductions in heart rate or blood pressure. It is indicated for treatment of chronic angina that is inadequately controlled with other antianginals. It represents a new class of drugs known as metabolic modulators and can be useful when prescribed as substitute for beta-blockers or in combination with them for relief of symptoms when initial treatment with beta-blockers is not successful or is contraindicated. Side effects include prolongation of QT interval. Low doses of diltiazem and verapamil should be used with ranolazine. The extended-release preparation reduces the frequency of angina, improves exercise performance, and delays the development of exercise-induced angina and ST-segment depression.
- ACE inhibition through changes in the physiologic balance between angiotensin II and bradykinin could contribute to the reductions in LV and vascular hypertrophy, atherosclerosis progression, plaque rupture, and thrombosis; the favorable changes in cardiac hemodynamics; and the improved myocardial oxygen supply/demand. It has been shown to be effective in reducing cardiovascular death, MI, and stroke in patients who are at risk for or who had vascular disease. They are indicated in patients with hypertension, diabetes, LVEF <40%, and CKD. Angiotensin receptor blockers (ARBs) can be given to patients with SIHD who are intolerant to ACE inhibitors and qualify for them.
- Use of high-intensity statin drugs is recommended in all patients with CAD. In late 2018 the American College of Cardiology (ACC) recommended an low density lipoprotein (LDL) goal of <70 mg/dl for secondary prevention of atherosclerotic cardiovascular disease. There is no LDL goal for primary prevention. The FDA

approved PCSK9 (proprotein convertase subtilisin/kexin type 9) inhibitors (alirocumab and evolocumab) for heterozygous familial hypercholesterolemia in those who maximally tolerated statins. Newer 2018 lipid guidelines suggested starting PCSK9 inhibitor in very-high-risk atherosclerotic cardiovascular disease patients who did not meet the LDL goal on high-intensity statin and ezetimibe. One should always consider adding ezetimibe to high-intensity statin prior to initiation of PCSK9 inhibitor due to cost issues. Inclisiran, evinacumab, and bempedoic acid are reasonable nonstatin therapy alternatives in patients who are unable to tolerate statin and reach target LDL levels.
- Influenza vaccine is recommended for patients with SIHD on annual basis to prevent all-cause mortality, morbidity, and hospitalization caused by the exacerbation of underlying medical conditions produced by influenza.
- The EMPAREG OUTCOME, CANVAS, DECLARE-TIMI 58, and CREDENCE trial showed that SGLT2 inhibitors significantly reduce cardiovascular events in type 2 diabetic patients.

NEW MODALITIES FOR THE TREATMENT OF CHRONIC STABLE ANGINA PECTORIS:

- Although a significant amount of progress has been made in the management of CAD with percutaneous coronary intervention (PCI) and CABG, many patients with the condition require additional therapeutic modalities for relief of symptoms and improvement in quality of life. This group of patients includes those with diffuse CAD who are not suitable for revascularization, patients with previous multiple PCIs or CABG limiting the chances for further revascularization, the lack of vascular conduits for CABG, severe LV systolic dysfunction in patients with previous CABG or PCI, and comorbidities that would render the patients at high risk for revascularization.
- The following pharmacologic agents have been used for the management of stable angina in combination with the standard protocol of nitrates, beta-blockers, calcium channel blockers, and ranolazine: High-dose statin therapy, trimetazidine, perhexiline, nicorandil, allopurinol, ivabradine, fasudil, and testosterone.
- Other, nonpharmacologic modalities that are highly experimental include stem cell therapy, therapeutic angiogenesis, and mechanical therapies such as external counterpulsation, spinal cord stimulation, transmyocardial laser revascularization, and coronary sinus reducing device.
- In TACT (Trial to Assess Chelation Therapy), ethylenediaminetetraacetic acid (EDTA) intravenous infusion resulted in significant decrease in total mortality, recurrent MI, stroke, coronary revascularization, or hospitalization for angina. Thus chelation therapy was upgraded from Class III (not recommended) to Class IIb in the 2014 SIHD guidelines. Allopurinol, a xanthine oxidase inhibitor, was shown to reduce myocardial oxygen

demand per unit of cardiac output in patients with heart failure in a small crossover study of 65 patients given 600 mg of allopurinol daily for 6 wk. Allopurinol increased the median time to ST depression from 232 sec at baseline to 393 sec. Further and larger studies are necessary to recommend allopurinol as an adjunctive therapy for stable angina.
- Testosterone improves endothelial dysfunction and may be an effective antiangina agent. However, given the potential side effects, additional trials are necessary to recommend testosterone as an adjunctive drug for chronic angina.

The value of enhanced external counterpulsation (EECP) was assessed with the MUST-EECP trial, which randomly assigned 139 outpatients with angina, documented CAD, and a positive stress test to 35 h of active EECP. The results indicated the following regarding EECP: (1) Was well tolerated; (2) exercise duration increased in both groups; (3) active EECP patients had a significant increase in time to 1-mm ST-segment depression, whereas there was no change in the inactive group; (4) more patients undergoing active EECP had a decrease in angina episodes, and fewer had an increase in angina symptoms compared with the active group. These data corroborate similar data from multicenter registries. The American Heart Association, American College of Cardiology, Society for Cardiovascular Angiography and Interventions, American Thoracic Society, and Society of Thoracic Surgeons focused update states that EECP may be considered for relief of refractory angina.

The following treatments have NOT been shown to be beneficial in reducing cardiovascular risk or improving clinical outcomes: Estrogen therapy, vitamin C, vitamin E, and beta-carotene supplementation; treatment of elevated homocysteine with folate or vitamins B_6 and B_{12}; chelation therapy; garlic; coenzyme Q10; selenium; and chromium.

REFERRAL

Revascularization:

- Revascularization methods should be formulated taking into consideration improved survival or improved symptoms. Revascularization includes either PCI (balloon angioplasty and stenting) or CABG. However, note that although the role of PCI is unquestionable in the presence of an acute MI, its role is not so clear in stable CAD. The utilization of PCI for stable CAD was reduced by 51.7% from 2007 to 2011, and hospitals with higher volumes of PCI had the largest reduction of these procedures.
- **To improve survival:**
1. Perform CABG for patients with significant (>50% diameter stenosis) left main coronary artery stenosis, more than 70% diameter stenosis in proximal left anterior descending artery (LAD), or more than 70% diameter stenosis in three major epicardial vessels, >70% diameter stenosis in two major coronary arteries with severe or extensive myocardial ischemia, and in

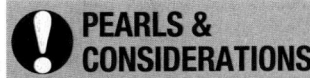

patients with mild to moderate LV systolic dysfunction (EF 35% to 50%) and significant multivessel CAD. Left internal mammary artery (LIMA) graft improves survival when used to bypass a proximal LAD artery stenosis. CABG is recommended in preference to PCI to improve survival in patients with multivessel CAD with Syntax score of >22 and multivessel CAD with diabetes, particularly if a LIMA graft to LAD is used.[2]

2. PCI is reasonable as an alternative to CABG in selected stable patients (low or intermediate SYNTAX score and/or high STS score) with unprotected left main CAD, low risk of PCI procedural complications, and a high likelihood of good long-term outcome *and* clinical characteristics that predict a significantly increased risk of adverse surgical outcomes (e.g., STS-predicted risk of operative mortality >5).

- **To improve symptoms:**

CABG or PCI to improve symptoms is beneficial in patients with one or more significant (>70% diameter) coronary artery stenosis amenable to revascularization and unacceptable angina despite maximal medical treatment, or in whom increasing medical therapy cannot be implemented because of medication contraindications, adverse effects, or patient preferences. In 2017, ORBITA trial showed no significant improvement in angina score after PCI for optimally treated stable angina patients. However, 85% of study patients in placebo group underwent PCI within 6 wk after ORBITA trial completed. In 2020, the Ischemia trial showed no benefit with routine invasive therapy compared to conservative treatment in moderate to severe ischemia patients. However, this study excludes patients with ACS, severe and frequent symptoms, EF <35%, and left main stenosis. Hybrid coronary revascularization: LIMA-to-LAD artery grafting and of

>1 non-LAD coronary artery can be used in patients who have an unfavorable aorta, have poor target vessels for CABG, have unsuitable graft conduits, or have unfavorable LAD for PCI.

- Compared with PCI, CABG is more effective in relieving angina and leads to fewer repeated revascularizations but has a higher risk for procedural stroke. Survival to 10 yr is similar for both procedures.
- Angioplasty and coronary stents (Fig. E3).
- PCI has an established place in treating angina but is not superior to intensive medical therapy to prevent MI and death in symptomatic or asymptomatic patients. Patients selected for PCI should also be candidates for CABG. Approximately 80% of patients show immediate benefit after PCI. The development of coronary stents has increased the number of patients who can be treated in the cardiac laboratory. Cardiac stents (Fig. E4) are currently used in nearly 95% of all patients with PCI lesions. The rate of restenosis is reduced by placing a stent electively in primary atheromatous lesions. The major limitations of stenting are subacute thrombosis, restenosis within the stent, bleeding complications when antiplatelets are used after stenting, and higher cost. The combination of aspirin and P2Y12 antagonists is effective in preventing coronary stent thrombosis and the duration of therapy depends on whether bare metal stents (BMS) or drug-eluting stents (DES) are used. Duration of dual antiplatelet therapy can be as short as 4 wk for BMS, but 6 to 12 mo of therapy is generally required for DES. This difference in duration is due to the lack of endothelium proliferation in DES initially. New drug-eluting stents with thin struts releasing Limus-family analogs from durable polymers have lowered the risk of stent thrombosis compared with early-generation

stents releasing sirolimus or paclitaxel. Current evidence supports the use of drug-eluting stents in most clinical settings without safety concerns (unless there are contraindications to use of dual antiplatelet therapy).[2]

PEARLS & CONSIDERATIONS

COMMENTS

- Although nitrate responsiveness is usually an integral part of a diagnostic strategy for SIHD, recent reports question its value and conclude that in a general population admitted for chest pain, relief of pain after nitroglycerin treatment does not predict active CAD and should not be used to guide diagnosis in the acute care setting.
- CABG is associated with higher long-term survival rates and lower rates of repeat revascularization than PCI and stenting; however, patients often prefer stenting because it is less invasive, involves a shorter hospital stay, and has a lower in-hospital mortality rate.

REFERENCES
Available at eBooks.Health.Elsevier.com

RELATED CONTENT
Angina (Patient Information)
Unstable Angina (Patient Information)
Acute Coronary Syndrome (Related Key Topic)
Coronary Artery Disease (Related Key Topic)
Myocardial Infarction (Related Key Topic)

AUTHOR: **MAHESWARA SATYA GANGADHARA RAO GOLLA, MD**

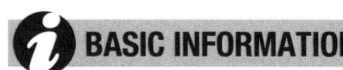

BASIC INFORMATION

DEFINITION

- The mucocutaneous swelling caused by the release of vasoactive mediators is called urticaria and angioedema.[1]
- Urticaria causes edema of the superficial dermis.
- Angioedema is due to a transient increase in vascular permeability of the mucosal/submucosal or dermal/subcutaneous tissues resulting in tissue swelling.[2]

SYNONYMS

Angioneurotic edema
Hereditary angioedema (HAE)

ICD-10CM CODES	
T78.3	Angioedema
D84.1	Angioedema, hereditary

EPIDEMIOLOGY & DEMOGRAPHICS

INCIDENCE: 100 to 3000/100,000 persons for urticaria and angioedema. Approximately 7.4% of the general population will experience angioedema alone.[3]
LIFETIME PREVALENCE: Approximately 25% of the population experiences urticaria and/or angioedema at some time during life. The prevalence of hereditary angioedema is one case/50,000 persons.[1,2,4,5]

DEMOGRAPHICS:

- Race: African Americans have higher rates of ACE inhibitor–induced angioedema.[6]
- Sex: More occurrences in women than men.
- Angioedema commonly occurs after adolescence in the third decade of life.
- Angioedema can occur together with urticaria (40%) or alone (20%); the remaining 40% have urticaria alone.
- The mean age of onset of hereditary angioedema with C1 inhibitor is 8 to 12 yr and rarely occurs before 1 yr of age.

PHYSICAL FINDINGS & CLINICAL PRESENTATION

- Angioedema may be acute or chronic:
  1. Acute angioedema is defined as symptoms lasting 6 wk.
  2. Chronic angioedema is defined as symptoms lasting >6 wk.
- Angioedema is characterized by the following:
  1. Nonpruritic, nonpitting, burning, occasionally painful swelling of deep skin layers or submucosal membranes.
  2. Poorly demarcated.
  3. Commonly involve eyelids, lips (Fig. E1), tongue, and extremities.
  4. Can involve the upper airway, causing respiratory distress.
  5. Can involve the GI tract, leading to cyclic abdominal pain, nausea, vomiting, and diarrhea.
  6. Resolves slowly within hours to a few days.

ETIOLOGY

- Angioedema, with or without urticaria, is classified as histaminergic (mast cell mediated or idiopathic) or bradykinin-mediated (e.g., hereditary).[7]
- Angioedema is primarily caused by immune activation with release of vasoactive mediators (e.g., histamine, serotonin, bradykinins), resulting in postcapillary venule inflammation, vascular leakage, and edema in the deep layers of the dermis and subcutaneous tissue.
- Pathologically, angioedema has both immunologic- and nonimmunologic-mediated mechanisms (Fig. 2).
  1. Immunoglobulin E–mediated angioedema may result from antigen exposure (e.g., foods [milk, eggs, peanuts, shellfish] or drugs [beta-lactam antibiotics, aspirin, NSAIDs, phenytoin, sulfonamide antibiotics, recombinant tissue plasminogen activator]).
  2. Complement-mediated angioedema involving immune complex mechanisms can also lead to mast cell activation that manifests as serum sickness.
  3. Hereditary angioedema is subdivided into three different groups: HAE with deficit

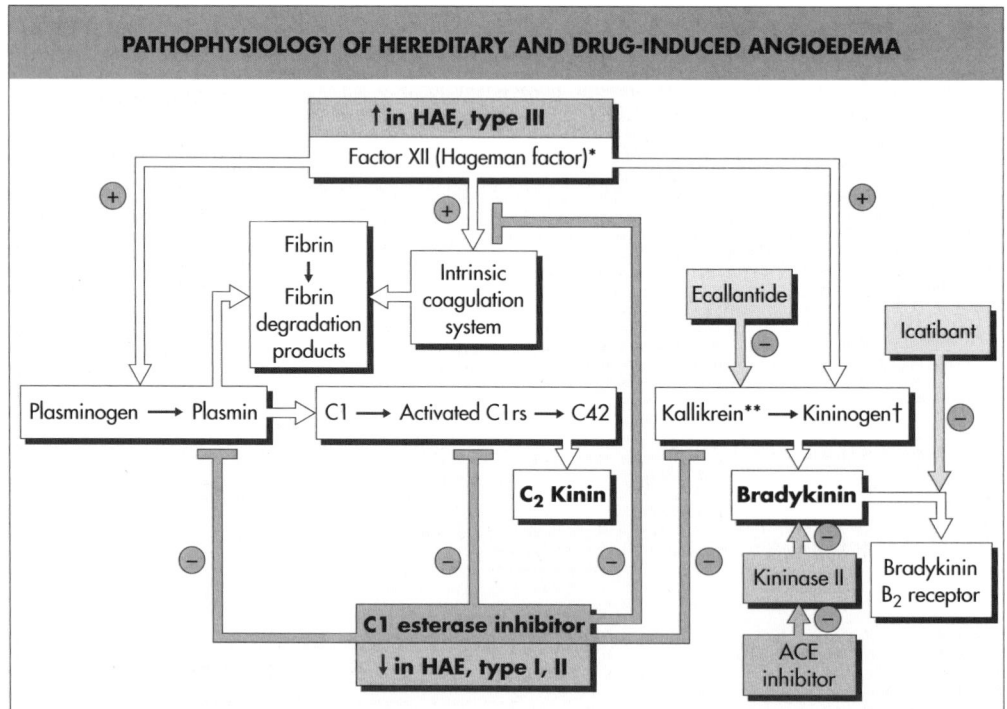

FIG. 2 Pathophysiology of hereditary and drug-induced angioedema. Angiotensin-converting enzyme *(ACE)* inhibitor-induced urticaria is believed to result from the inhibition of endogenous kininase and a subsequent increase in bradykinin. Icatibant and ecallantide have been approved for the emergency treatment of hereditary angioedema *(HAE)* as alternatives to C1 esterase inhibitor (C1-INH) concentrate (derived from human plasma) or recombinant C1-INH (derived from milk of transgenic rabbits). Icatibant, a decapeptide, is a specific bradykinin B2 receptor antagonist. Ecallantide, a 60-amino acid recombinant protein, selectively inhibits kallikrein. Off label, icatibant has been used to treat ACE inhibitor-induced angioedema. Two forms of C1-INH, one of which is administered intravenously and the other subcutaneously, are approved for prevention of attacks. At the time of writing, twice-monthly administration of lanadelumab, a human monoclonal antibody that inhibits plasma kallikrein, is under investigation for prevention of attacks. *The active form of factor XII (Hageman factor) is XIIa. **Kallikrein is formed from prekallikrein. †High-molecular-weight. (From Bolognia J et al: *Dermatology,* ed 4, London, 2018, Elsevier Limited.)

C1-inhibitor (HAE-1), HAE with dysfunctional C1-inhibitor (HAE-2), and HAE with normal C1-inhibitor function (HAE nC1-INH). HAE-1 and HAE-2 result from the autosomal dominant mutation in the *SERPING1* gene, which codes for a serine protease inhibitor called C1 esterase inhibitor (C1-INH). C1-INH serves many functions, one of which is to inhibit plasma kallikrein, a protease that cleaves kininogen and releases bradykinin. Bradykinin is a powerful vasodilator resulting in increased capillary permeability and activation of pain receptors. Deficiency or dysfunctional C1-INH inhibitory activity results in excess bradykinin leading to angioedema. Both types are characterized by low serum C4 levels from activation of the complement cascade, for which C1 inhibitor is a key regulatory protein.[2]

4. Acquired angioedema is usually associated with other diseases, most commonly B-cell lymphoproliferative disorders, but may also result from the formation of autoantibodies directed against C1 inhibitor protein.
5. Other causes of angioedema include infection (e.g., herpes simplex, hepatitis B, Coxsackie A and B, *Streptococcus, Candida, Ascaris*, and *Strongyloides*), insect bites and stings, stress, physical factors (e.g., cold, exercise, pressure, and vibration), connective tissue diseases (e.g., systemic lupus erythematosus, Henoch-Schönlein purpura), and idiopathic causes. ACE inhibitors can increase kinin activity and lead to angioedema. Other medications include antibiotics (beta-lactams and quinolones), opiates, and muscle relaxants (succinylcholine).[8,9]

Dx DIAGNOSIS

A detailed history and physical examination usually establish the diagnosis of angioedema. Extensive laboratory testing is of limited value.

DIFFERENTIAL DIAGNOSIS

- Anaphylaxis
- Contact dermatitis
- Cellulitis
- Lymphedema
- Arthropod bite
- Hypothyroidism
- Atopic dermatitis
- Mastocytosis
- Granulomatous cheilitis
- Bullous pemphigoid
- Urticaria pigmentosa
- Erythema multiforme
- Epiglottitis
- Peritonsillar abscess
- Parasite infection
- Superior vena cava syndrome

WORKUP

- An extensive workup searching for the cause of angioedema is often unrevealing (40%).
- Workup, including diagnostic blood tests and allergy testing, is performed according to results of the history and physical examination. Fig. 3 illustrates an algorithm for the diagnosis of angioedema.

LABORATORY TESTS

- CBC, erythrocyte sedimentation rate, and urinalysis are sometimes helpful as part of the initial evaluation.
- Serum total tryptase helpful in confirming mast cell—mediated anaphylaxis.
- C4 levels are usually reduced in acquired and hereditary angioedema (occurring without

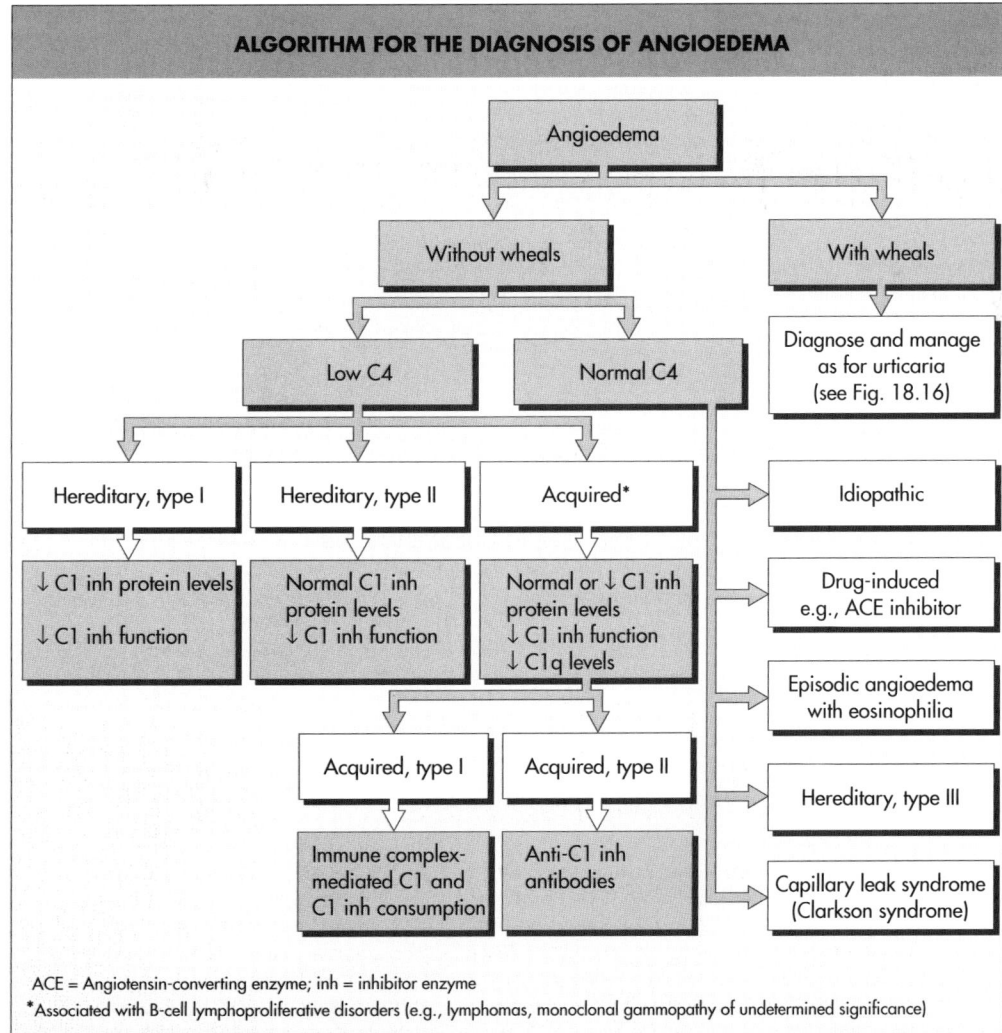

ALGORITHM FOR THE DIAGNOSIS OF ANGIOEDEMA

ACE = Angiotensin-converting enzyme; inh = inhibitor enzyme
*Associated with B-cell lymphoproliferative disorders (e.g., lymphomas, monoclonal gammopathy of undetermined significance)

FIG. 3 Algorithm for the diagnosis of angioedema. Episodic angioedema with hypereosinophilia, along with weight gain and fever, is known as Gleich syndrome. (From Bolognia J et al: *Dermatology*, ed 4, London, 2018, Elsevier Limited.)

urticaria). If C4 levels are low, C1-INH levels and activity should be obtained. There are isolated reports of hereditary angioedema with normal C4 levels but reduced C1-INH levels.
- Skin prick and in vitro sIgE (ImmunoCAP) testing may be done if food allergies are suspected.
- Skin biopsy is usually done in patients with chronic angioedema refractory to corticosteroid treatment.
- Stools for ova and parasites.

Rx TREATMENT

NONPHARMACOLOGIC THERAPY
- Eliminate the offending agent
- Avoid triggering factors (e.g., cold, stress, certain medications, including ACE inhibitor)
- Cold compresses to affected areas

ACUTE GENERAL Rx
- Acute life-threatening angioedema involving the larynx is treated with the following. However, it should be noted that bradykinin-mediated angioedema will have minimal response to these medications.
  1. Epinephrine 0.3 mg in a solution of 1:1000 given SC
  2. Diphenhydramine 25 to 50 mg IV or IM or cetirizine 10 mg IV
  3. Cimetidine 300 mg IV or famotidine 20 mg IV
  4. Methylprednisolone 125 mg IV
- Maintenance therapy in mast cell–mediated, nonhereditary angioedema is H_1 antihistamines:
  1. Cetirizine 10 mg/day (may require up to 4 times the FDA-approved dosing)
  2. Fexofenadine 180 mg/day (may require up to 4 times the FDA-approved dosing)
  3. Hydroxyzine 10 to 25 mg q6h
  4. Diphenhydramine 25 to 50 mg q6h
- H_2 antihistamines can be added to H_1 antihistamines:
  1. Cimetidine 400 mg bid
  2. Famotidine 20 mg bid
- Tricyclic antidepressants:
  1. Doxepin 25 to 50 mg qHS
- Corticosteroids may be used for symptomatic relief of refractory acute angioedema.
- Antihistamines are ineffective in hereditary angioedema.

- Purified plasma-derived C1-INH replacement therapy is effective and safe in treating acute attacks of hereditary angioedema caused by C1 inhibitor deficiency. All of the following therapies are approved as abortive therapies for HAE.[2,10]
  1. Purified C1 inhibitor concentrate (Berinert)
  2. Icatibant (Firazyr), a bradykinin–B2-receptor antagonist
  3. Ecallantide (Kalbitor), a kallikrein inhibitor

CHRONIC Rx
- Chronic histaminergic angioedema is treated as described under "Acute General Rx" with H_1 antihistamines, H_2 antihistamines, and corticosteroids for refractory cases. Prednisone 1 mg/kg/day for 5 days and then tapered over 7 days). Omalizumab is an anti-IgE monoclonal antibody that has shown efficacy in cases refractory to antihistamines alone although is not FDA approved for this indication.
- For HAE, long-term prophylaxis includes androgens (danazol, stanozolol, oxandrolone, methyltestosterone) and antifibrinolytic agents, but these agents are associated with many adverse effects. Intravenous plasma-derived C1 inhibitors (Cinryze, Berinert) are safe and effective and may be used in patients who have frequent or severe attacks. Cost can be a limiting factor. A twice-weekly subcutaneous formulation (Haegarda/CSL830, CSL Behring) is approved by the FDA to treat HAE-1 and HAE-2 hereditary angioedema. Lanadelumab and berotralstat are kallikrein inhibitors that have recently received FDA approval for prophylaxis therapy of HAE.[2,10,11]

In a recent phase 2 trial among patients with hereditary angioedema, selective inhibition of plasma prekallikrein production by antisense oligonucleotide treatment (donidalorsen) resulted in a significantly lower rate of angioedema attacks than placebo.[12]

DISPOSITION
- Antihistamines achieve symptomatic relief in more than 85% of patients with nonhereditary acute angioedema.[13]
- For chronic nonhereditary angioedema, antihistamines remain the mainstay in therapy and systemic steroids should be reserved for severe or refractory cases.

- A small percentage of people will have recurrence of symptoms after completion of treatment.
- Chronic angioedema can last for months to years but possibly longer in the situation of HAE.

REFERRAL
Consultation with dermatologist and/or allergist is recommended in patients with chronic angioedema, hereditary angioedema, and recurring angioedema.

ⓘ PEARLS & CONSIDERATIONS

ACE inhibitors can cause angioedema months or years after initiation.[14] There are multiple case reports and case series of angiotensin receptor blocker (ARB)–induced angioedema, although the risk is substantially less than that of ACE inhibitors. Approximately 10% of patients with recurrent angioedema had ACE inhibitor exposure with median duration of 1 yr prior to symptom onset. Incidence rates per 1000 person-yr are 4.38 cases for ACE inhibitors, 1.66 cases for ARBs. The incidence rate is also very high for the direct renin inhibitor aliskiren (4.67).

COMMENTS
- Identifying a cause for angioedema in patients is often difficult and met with frustration.
- Chronic angioedema, unlike acute angioedema, is rarely caused by an allergic reaction.
- HAE is a life-threatening condition and should be managed by an allergist.

REFERENCES
Available at eBooks.Health.Elsevier.com.

RELATED CONTENT
Angioedema (Patient Information)

AUTHORS: **TOAN DO, MD,** and **SHYAM JOSHI, MD**

BASIC INFORMATION

DEFINITION

Ankylosing spondylitis (AS) is a type of inflammatory arthritis involving the sacroiliac joints and axial skeleton characterized by ankylosis (abnormal stiffening of a joint) and enthesitis (inflammation at tendon insertions). It is part of a family of overlapping syndromes called seronegative spondyloarthropathies (SpA) that includes reactive arthritis (formerly Reiter syndrome), psoriatic spondylitis, and enteropathic arthritis.[1]

SYNONYMS

Marie-Strümpell disease
Bechterew disease

ICD-10CM CODES

M45.9 Ankylosing spondylitis of unspecified sites in spine
M08.1 Juvenile ankylosing spondylitis
M45.0 Ankylosing spondylitis of multiple sites in spine
M45.1 Ankylosing spondylitis of occipito-atlanto-axial region
M45.2 Ankylosing spondylitis of cervical region
M45.3 Ankylosing spondylitis of cervicothoracic region
M45.4 Ankylosing spondylitis of thoracic region
M45.5 Ankylosing spondylitis of thoracolumbar region
M45.6 Ankylosing spondylitis lumbar region
M45.7 Ankylosing spondylitis of lumbosacral region
M45.8 Ankylosing spondylitis sacral and sacrococcygeal region

EPIDEMIOLOGY & DEMOGRAPHICS

PREVALENCE: Between 0.1% and 1% of the population. Varies with prevalence of HLA-B27 and ethnicity. The U.S. prevalence of AS has been reported between 5% and 6% in HLA-B27 populations. Much higher in those with positive family history of spondyloarthropathy.[2]
PREDOMINANT SEX: 70.4% male predominance
PREDOMINANT AGE: 15 to 35 yr, usually symptoms present before age 45

PHYSICAL FINDINGS & CLINICAL PRESENTATION (TABLES E1 AND E2)

- Prolonged morning back stiffness of insidious onset lasting more than 3 mo
- Bilateral sacroiliac joint tenderness (sacroiliitis)
- Inflammatory back pain; often improves with exercise and is worse with rest
- Limited lumbar spine motion
- Tenderness at tendon insertion sites, especially the Achilles tendons and plantar fascia
- Loss of chest expansion reflecting rib cage involvement
- Possible to have peripheral joint arthritis, usually involving lower extremities
- In advanced cases the typical posture consists of compensatory hyperextension of neck, fixed flexion of hips, and compensatory flexion of knees (Fig. 1)

- There is an increased incidence of iritis and uveitis (30% to 40% lifetime prevalence)
- Other extra-skeletal manifestations include effects on the cardiovascular system (aortic insufficiency, cardiovascular disease), cerebrovascular system, and lungs (pulmonary fibrosis). There is also an increased risk for osteoporosis.[3,4]

ETIOLOGY

Although significant progress has been made, the etiology of AS still remains unclear to an extent. To date, it is believed that genetic background, immune reactions, infection, and endocrinal

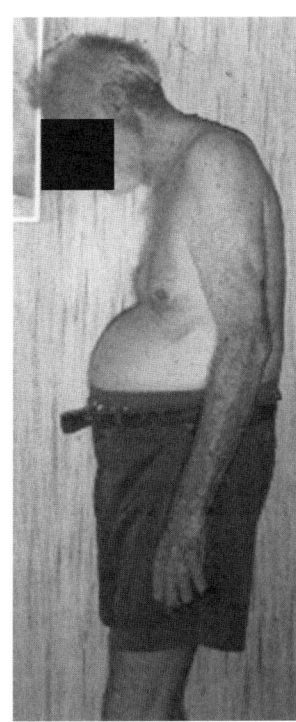

FIG 1 Typical posture of patient with ankylosing spondylitis; note the flexed neck, protuberant abdomen, and loss of lumbar lordosis. (From Talley NJ et al: *Essentials of internal medicine*, ed 4, Chatswood, NSW, 2021, Elsevier Australia.)

abnormities play a role in susceptibility to the spondyloarthropathies. Major histocompatibility complex class I allele HLA-B27 has been described as the predominant genetic predisposing factor. Infections such as *Klebsiella pneumonia*, an opportunistic pathogen that makes up part of the normal gut microflora, may be an exacerbating agent in the autoimmune process of AS. Tumor necrosis factor is important in the inflammatory response.[5]

DIAGNOSIS

DIFFERENTIAL DIAGNOSIS

- Diffuse idiopathic skeletal hyperostosis (Forestier disease)
- Noninflammatory back pain (a clinical algorithm for the evaluation of back pain is described in Section III)
- Table 3 compares ankylosing spondylitis and related disorders

LABORATORY TESTS

- Elevated sedimentation rate, C-reactive protein
- Mild hyperchromic anemia
- Demonstration of inflammatory sacroiliitis by radiography or MRI is diagnostic for most patients, although some patients may meet criteria for "nonradiographic spondyloarthropathy" based on compelling clinical evaluation[6]
- HLA-B27 antigen is not useful in the evaluation of noninflammatory back pain because it is present in up to 10% of the normal population (varies based on ethnicity)

IMAGING STUDIES

- Classic feature is bilateral sacroiliitis on pelvic x-rays (modified NY criteria).
- Vertebral bodies lose anterior concave shape and become square.
- With progression, calcification of the annulus fibrosus and paravertebral ligaments develops, giving rise to the so-called *bamboo spine* (Figs. E2 through Fig. E6).
- Severe diskovertebral erosions and destruction may occur (Andersson lesion, Fig. 7).

TABLE 3 Comparison of Ankylosing Spondylitis and Related Disorders

Feature	Ankylosing Spondylitis	Psoriatic Arthritis	Reactive Arthritis	Enteropathic Arthropathy
Gender (male:female)	2-3:1	1:1	1:1	1:1
Age of onset	<40 yr	35-55 yr	20-40 yr	Any age
Sacroiliitis or spondylitis (%)	100	~20	~40	<20
Symmetry of sacroiliitis	Symmetric	Asymmetric	Asymmetric	Symmetric
Peripheral arthritis (%)	~25	95	90	5-20
Distribution	Axial and lower limbs	Variable	Lower limbs	Variable
HLA-B27 positivity (%)	85-95	25-60*	30-70	7-70†
Uveitis (%)	0-40	~20	~50	<15

*60% when spondylitis is present.
†60% when spondylitis is present.
~, approximately.
From Hochberg MC: *Rheumatology*, ed 7, Philadelphia, 2019, Elsevier.

A

Diseases and Disorders

I

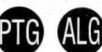
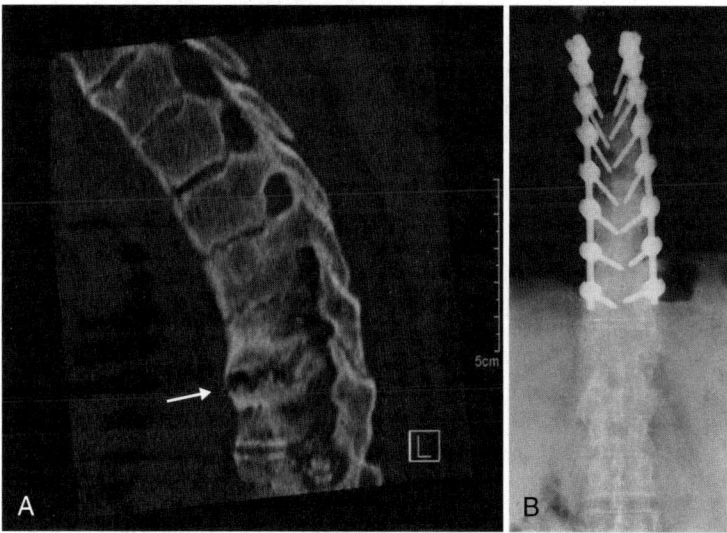

FIG. 7 Severe Andersson lesion (diskovertebral erosions and destruction) (**A**, *arrow*) of the thoracic spine in a patient with ankylosing spondylitis resulting in instability and severe pain, which was treated with a fusion operation (**B**). (From Hochberg MC: *Rheumatology*, ed 7, Philadelphia, 2019, Elsevier.)

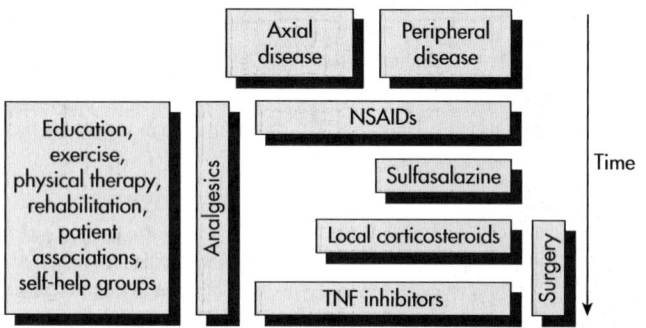

FIG. 10 Recommended management of ankylosing spondylitis (AS), based on clinical expertise and research evidence. The disease progression with time moves vertically from top to bottom. These recommendations were developed before the availability of secukinumab. Secukinumab is approved but was not available at the time of these recommendations. *ASAS/EULAR*, Assessment in Ankylosing Spondylitis/European League against Rheumatism; *NSAIDs*, nonsteroidal antiinflammatory drugs; *TNF*, tumor necrosis factor. (From Firestein GS et al: *Firestein & Kelley's textbook of rheumatology*, ed 11, Philadelphia 2021, Elsevier.)

- MRI (Fig. E8) may be useful in detecting early inflammatory lesions and is especially helpful when the history is suggestive but x-rays are equivocal; can see bone marrow edema, fatty metaplasia, sacroiliitis, erosions, shiny corners.[7]

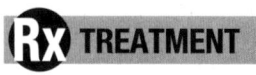 **TREATMENT**

NONPHARMACOLOGIC THERAPY
- Exercises primarily to maintain flexibility and aerobic activity are important (Fig. E9).

- Postural training:
  1. Patients must be instructed on spinal extension exercises to avoid fusion in a flexed position.
  2. Sleeping should be in the supine position on a firm mattress; pillows should not be placed under the head or knees.

PHARMACOLOGIC THERAPY
- NSAIDs: Patients with ankylosing spondylitis should be trialed on full-dose continuous NSAID therapy. There is anecdotal evidence suggesting that indomethacin may be more effective than other NSAIDs, but other NSAIDs are also efficacious and may be better tolerated. One study suggested that continuous NSAID therapy may retard the radiographic progression of ankylosing spondylitis, but data are conflicting.[5]
- Sulfasalazine may be efficacious in patients with peripheral arthritis.[5]
- Numerous controlled trials have shown that tumor necrosis factor (TNF) antagonists such as etanercept, infliximab, and adalimumab are very effective for relieving symptoms of spinal inflammatory arthritis. Anti-TNF therapy should be recommended for patients whose symptoms are not completely controlled with NSAIDs, and it can result in dramatic improvement in symptoms, range of motion of the spine, and quality of life for these patients. There is evidence suggesting that anti-TNF therapy slows the radiographic progression of the disease. Etanercept should generally be avoided if history of uveitis.[5]
- Secukinumab, an antiinterleukin-17A monoclonal antibody, has been approved for treating AS. Ixekizumab, another interleukin-17A antibody, was also approved in 2019.[8]
- Fig. 10 shows American College of Rheumatology (ACR)/The European League Against Rheumatism (EULAR) recommendations for management.

DISPOSITION

Most patients have a normal life span, but many can suffer significant disability from loss of spinal mobility.

REFERRAL

All patients with seronegative spondyloarthropathy should be referred to a rheumatologist for further evaluation and treatment.

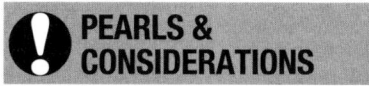 **PEARLS & CONSIDERATIONS**

A family history of seronegative spondyloarthropathy increases the specificity of testing for HLA-B27. Surgical osteotomy may benefit selected patients with severe spinal deformity. Recent data suggest that men with AS have increased risk of vascular mortality.

REFERENCES
Available at eBooks.Health.Elsevier.com.

RELATED CONTENT
Ankylosing Spondylitis (Patient Information)

AUTHORS: **BENJAMIN J. AHN, BS, JOHN D. MILNER, MD**, and **MANUEL F. DASILVA, MD**

A

Diseases and Disorders

I

BASIC INFORMATION

DEFINITION

Antiphospholipid antibody syndrome (APS), the most common acquired thrombophilia, is characterized by clinical features of arterial or venous thrombosis and/or pregnancy morbidity, as well as the persistence of at least one type of antiphospholipid autoantibody (aPL). aPLs are antibodies directed against anionic phospholipids and phospholipid-binding protein cofactors. These autoantibodies lead to stimulation of procoagulant factors and inhibition of the fibrinolytic system. This further triggers downstream pathways, including mTOR upregulation, Toll-like receptor signaling, and activation of vascular endothelium, monocytes, neutrophils, platelets, complement, and proinflammatory cytokines.

Three types of aPLs have been characterized:
- Anticardiolipin antibodies (detected in approximately 2% to 44% of patients)
- Lupus anticoagulants (detected in approximately 34% of patients)
- Anti–β2-glycoprotein-I (anti–β2-GPI) antibodies (detected in approximately 20% of patients)[1]

APS can be a primary condition or secondary to a rheumatic disease, with the most common being systemic lupus erythematosus (SLE). APS can affect all organ systems and includes venous and arterial thrombosis, recurrent fetal losses, and cytopenias, including thrombocytopenia and microangiopathic hemolytic anemia.

SYNONYM

Antiphospholipid syndrome

ICD-10CM CODE
D68.61 Antiphospholipid syndrome

EPIDEMIOLOGY & DEMOGRAPHICS

PREVALENCE:
- Up to 5% of healthy individuals without a history of thrombosis have positive aPLs.
- aPLs are positive in approximately 13% of patients with stroke, 11% with myocardial infarction, 10% of patients with deep vein thrombosis (DVT), and 6% of patients with pregnancy complications.[2]
- Nearly 20% of women under 50 who have a cerebrovascular accident test positive for aPLs.[3]
- 10% to 15% of women with recurrent miscarriages have aPLs.[4]
- aPLs without APS can be seen in patients with certain medications, infections, malignancies, and autoimmune conditions.

PREDOMINANT AGE: Young to middle-aged adults.

RISK FACTORS:
- Underlying SLE and collagen-vascular diseases; other autoimmune disorders, including rheumatoid arthritis, Sjögren syndrome, Behçet syndrome, primary immune thrombocytopenia (also known as idiopathic thrombocytopenic purpura), acquired immunodeficiency syndrome (AIDS).

- However, most individuals are otherwise healthy and have no underlying medical condition.

Thrombotic risk is increased by the presence of other etiologies of systemic hypercoagulability, including genetic thrombophilia, as well as acquired risk factors such as oral contraceptive use, pregnancy, smoking, prolonged immobilization, malignancy, and hyperlipidemia.

PROGNOSIS:
- 91% survival at 10-yr follow-up
- 71% success rate in pregnancy with recommended therapies; prematurity and intrauterine growth restriction are common complications[5]

GENETICS: Some APS-positive families exist, and human leukocyte antigen (HLA) studies have suggested associations with HLA DR7, DR4, and Dqw7+Drw53.

PHYSICAL FINDINGS & CLINICAL PRESENTATION

No pathognomonic findings on examination; Table 1 summarizes other features suggesting the presence of antiphospholipid antibodies, including abnormal findings consistent with ischemia or infarction.

- Thrombosis (Fig. E1): Patients with APS are at risk for both venous and arterial thromboses. Venous thromboses are more common, occurring as the initial manifestation of APS in approximately 30% of APS patients. The most common site for DVT is the calf, but thromboses may also occur in the renal, hepatic, axillary, subclavian, vena cava, and retinal

---

TABLE 1 Other Features Suggesting the Presence of Antiphospholipid Antibodies

Clinical

Livedo reticularis

Thrombocytopenia (usually 50,000-100,000 platelets/mm³)

Autoimmune hemolytic anemia

Cardiac valve disease (vegetations or thickening)

Multiple sclerosis–like syndrome, chorea, or other myelopathy

From Firestein GS et al: *Kelley's textbook of rheumatology,* ed 9, Philadelphia, 2013, Saunders.

---

veins. The most common site of arterial thrombosis are the cerebral vessels, followed by the coronary, renal, mesenteric, and bypass arteries. Recurrent thrombosis is common with APS.

- Commonly involved organ systems include:
  1. Central nervous system: Stroke, transient ischemic attack, migraine, multi-infarct dementia, epilepsy, movement disorders, transverse myelopathy, retinal venous or arterial occlusion
  2. Pulmonary: Pulmonary embolism and infarction, pulmonary hypertension, acute respiratory distress syndrome, diffuse alveolar hemorrhage
  3. Cardiology: Libman-Sacks endocarditis, intracardiac thrombosis, coronary artery disease, myocardial infarction, valvulopathy, left ventricular diastolic dysfunction
  4. Gastrointestinal: Abdominal pain, gastrointestinal bleed secondary to esophageal/mesenteric ischemia, splenic or pancreatic infarction, hepatic vein thrombosis, Budd-Chiari syndrome
  5. Renal: Hypertension, renal infarct, renal artery or vein thrombosis, acute renal failure, glomerular damage including membranous nephropathy, minimal change disease, and pauci-immune glomerulonephritis
  6. Hematology: Thrombocytopenia, hemolytic anemia
  7. Endocrine: Addison disease secondary to adrenal hemorrhage and, less frequently, thrombosis
  8. Cutaneous: Livedo reticularis, cutaneous necrosis, skin ulcerations, phlegmasia cerulea dolens, gangrene of digits (Fig. E2)
  9. Obstetric: Recurrent spontaneous abortion, premature delivery, fetal growth restriction, preeclampsia/eclampsia, abruptio placentae
  10. Vascular: DVT, arterial thrombosis in extremities, superficial thrombophlebitis, amaurosis fugax

- **Catastrophic APS** (CAPS) (Table 2): CAPS is a rapidly progressive multiorgan thrombotic disease. Approximately 1% of APS is CAPS; approximately 45% of patients with CAPS do not present as APS initially. To make the diagnosis of catastrophic APS, four criteria must be satisfied:

TABLE 2 Differential Diagnosis of Catastrophic Antiphospholipid Syndrome (CAPS)

Laboratory Abnormalities	CAPS	TTP	DIC
Microangiopathic hemolytic anemia	−	+	+
Thrombocytopenia	+	+	+
Fibrinogen/FDP	Normal/normal	Normal/increased	Decreased/increased
Anticardiolipin antibody	+	−	−
Lupus anticoagulant	+	−	−

DIC, Disseminated intravascular coagulation; *FDP,* fibrin degradation products; *TTP,* time to progression.

1. Evidence of involvement of three or more organs, systems, and/or tissues. The most common symptoms are abdominal pain, dyspnea, neurologic symptoms, chest pain, and skin rash
2. Development of manifestations simultaneously or in ≤1 wk
3. Confirmation by histopathology of small-vessel occlusion in at least one organ or tissue
4. Laboratory confirmation of the presence of aPL[6,7]

ETIOLOGY/PATHOPHYSIOLOGY

- Endothelial cells are activated by aPLs causing upregulation of adhesion and procoagulant molecules such as tissue factor and von Willebrand factor.
- Table E3 and Box E1 summarize proposed pathogenic mechanisms of antiphospholipid syndrome. Mechanisms of pregnancy loss in antiphospholipid syndrome are summarized in Box E2.
- Monocyte activation by aPLs yields expression of inflammatory cytokines and additional tissue factor, contributing to the procoagulant state.
- Neutrophil activation by aPLs via complement is proposed to cause the release of neutrophil extracellular traps leading to increased thrombin.
- aPL binding to glycoprotein 1b and ApoE receptor 2 causes platelet activation and increased platelet adhesion.
- aPL binding decreases activation of antithrombin and protein C, while also reducing the ability of activated protein C to inactivate coagulation factors V and VIII.
- aPL binding to annexin A2 (tissue plasminogen activator receptor) contributes to the prothrombotic state seen in APS.
- The mammalian target of rapamycin complex (mTORC) has been shown to be involved in endothelial activation and in regulating expression of tissue factor and interleukin 8 in monocytes.
- Toll-like receptors 4 and 7 and triggering of the innate immune system are involved in endothelial activation and the development of the prothrombotic state.
- Autoantibodies against other antigens, such as phosphatidylserine, phosphatidyl ethanolamine, and other complexes have been identified in APS patients, but their clinical significance has yet to be elucidated.[8]

🄳🅧 DIAGNOSIS

DIFFERENTIAL DIAGNOSIS

Other hypercoagulable states (inherited or acquired):
- Inherited: Antithrombin III, protein C and protein S deficiencies, factor V Leiden, prothrombin gene mutation
- Acquired: Malignancy, heparin-induced thrombocytopenia, myeloproliferative syndromes
- Alternative causes of recurrent pregnancy loss should also be considered (e.g., anatomic abnormalities, chromosomal abnormalities, or endocrine disorders such as hypothyroidism)

WORKUP

Diagnostic criteria of APS include at least one clinical criterion and at least one laboratory criterion.
- Clinical (Box 3):
  1. Venous, arterial, or small vessel thrombosis *or*
  2. Morbidity with pregnancy, defined as:
     a. Unexplained fetal death at ≥10 wk gestation *or*
     b. ≥1 premature births before 34 wk gestation secondary to eclampsia, preeclampsia, or severe placental insufficiency *or*
     c. ≥3 unexplained spontaneous abortions before 10 wk gestation.
- Laboratory:
  1. Lupus anticoagulant present in plasma on two or more occasions at least 12 wk apart, *or*
  2. Anticardiolipin antibody, IgG or IgM present in serum or plasma at >40 MP or GPL units (titer), or >99th percentile on two or more occasions at least 12 wk apart, *or*
  3. Anti–β2-GPI antibodies present in serum or plasma at >99th percentile on two or more occasions at least 12 wk apart
- Screening tests:
  1. Partial thromboplastin time (PTT): Elevated. Activated PTT prolongation indicating either the presence of a clotting factor deficiency, or the presence of an inhibitor such as a lupus anticoagulant.
  2. Mixing study: Normal plasma is incubated with the patient's plasma. In cases of clotting factor deficiencies, the PTT will correct. If an inhibitor is present as in the case with APS, the PTT will not correct.
  3. Dilute Russell viper venom time: Elevated. Laboratory clotting requires the addition of phospholipids and calcium to plasma samples. Antiphospholipid antibodies bind the phospholipids in the test tube, thereby preventing clot formation. The addition of Russell viper venom to plasma results in immediate activation of factor X (common pathway). Therefore it will not be prolonged in intrinsic or extrinsic factor deficiencies but will be prolonged in the presence of an antiphospholipid antibody.
  4. The lupus anticoagulant screen is the addition of Russell viper venom to plasma. In the lupus anticoagulant confirmatory testing, massive doses of phospholipids are added to saturate the antiphospholipid antibody, thereby correcting the prolonged PTT.
- Initial testing for presence of aPL:
  1. Anticardiolipin (aCL) enzyme-linked immunosorbent assay (ELISA) antibodies (immunoglobulin G [IgG] or IgM), *or*
  2. Lupus anticoagulant (LA) activity identified, *or*
  3. Anti–β2-GPI ELISA antibodies (IgG or IgM).
- Confirmatory aPL testing: Repeat testing after 12 wk is required to confirm the persistence of a positive aCL, anti–β2-GPI, or LA test because transient aPL elevations can occur.
- Note that patients on anticoagulants may have falsely prolonged aPTT and interfere with the LA screening test. These patients should be tested for aCL and anti–β2-GPI antibodies, as these assays are unaffected by the presence of an anticoagulant.[9]

LABORATORY TESTS

Diagnostic evaluation of aPLs is indicated in:
- Patient with underlying SLE or collagen-vascular disease with thrombosis. (European League Against Rheumatism [EULAR] recommendation)
- Patient with recurrent, familial, or juvenile DVT or thrombosis in an unusual location (mesenteric or cerebral).
- One or more unexplained thrombotic events. Do not test those at low risk, such as elderly patients with other thrombotic risk factors.
- One or more specific pregnancy events such as early fetal death, premature birth due to severe preeclampsia or placental insufficiency, embryonic losses within 10 wk of gestation.
- Thrombotic complications associated with autoimmune diseases.
- Patients with an unexplained elevation in PTT, or less commonly, in prothrombin time/international normalization ratio (PT/INR).[10]

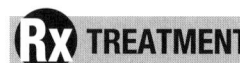 TREATMENT

ACUTE RX

- Initial anticoagulation with heparin or low-molecular-weight heparin (LMWH), before transitioning to a vitamin K antagonist (VKA) such as warfarin, is recommended. Direct oral anticoagulants are not recommended due to recent a study in high-risk APS (positivity for all three antiphospholipid antibodies), which showed an increased risk of recurrent thromboembolism for patients on rivaroxaban compared to warfarin.[11,12]
- Standard intensity (INR 2.0 to 3.0) anticoagulation with warfarin is preferred in venous thrombosis, as prior randomized trials failed to show a decrease in recurrent thromboses with high-intensity anticoagulation (INR 3.0 to 4.0).[10] Task-force reports have not reached a consensus regarding intensity of anticoagulation in secondary thromboprophylaxis of arterial events.
- Unfractionated heparin (UFH) is preferred if quick reversibility is needed.[11]

PRIMARY PREVENTION

- Modifiable risk factors for thrombosis, such as smoking and immobility, should be controlled.
- Cardiovascular risk factors, such as hypertension, obesity, and hyperlipidemia, should also be addressed.
- Aspirin use for primary prevention remains controversial.
- Adding low-dose warfarin to aspirin for primary prevention seems to confer no benefit.

BOX 3   Preliminary Criteria for Classification of Antiphospholipid Syndrome

Clinical criteria

Vascular thrombosis

One or more clinical events of arterial, venous, or small-vessel thrombosis in any tissue or organ. Thrombosis must be confirmed by Doppler ultrasonography, other imaging, or histopathologic analysis, with the exception of superficial venous thrombosis. The histopathologic study does not have to demonstrate significant evidence of inflammation of the blood vessel.

Pregnancy morbidity

- One or more unexplained deaths of morphologically normal fetuses at 10 or more wk of gestation, with a normal fetal morphology confirmed by ultrasound or direct examination of the fetus.
- One or more premature births of a morphologically normal newborn at 34 wk of gestation or before caused by
  - Severe preeclampsia or eclampsia defined according to current standards, or
  - Recognized placental insufficiency
- Three or more consecutive spontaneous abortions without explanation before 10 wk of gestation, excluding those associated with hormonal or anatomic alterations in the mother or chromosomal alterations inherited from either parent.

Laboratory criteria

The presence of at least one of the following test results:

- Lupus anticoagulant in the plasma on two or more separate occasions within a period of 12 wk, detected according to the guidelines of the International Society of Thrombosis and Haemostasis (Scientific Subcommittee on lupus anticoagulant/phospholipid-dependent antibodies).
- IgG or IgM anticardiolipin antibodies in plasma or serum in medium-high titers (more than 40 GPL or MPL units, respectively) on two or more separate occasions within a period of 12 wk, as measured by standardized ELISA.
- IgG or IgM anti–β_2-GPI antibodies in the serum or plasma (in titer above the 99th percentile) on two or more separate occasions within a period of 12 wk, as measured by standardized ELISA according to recommended procedures.

From Hochberg MC: *Rheumatology,* ed 7, Philadelphia, 2019, Elsevier.

- Hydroxychloroquine may be useful in those patients with SLE and aPL; it has been shown to reduce the incidence of thrombotic complications in this population.
- For pregnant women with a positive test for aPL antibodies without a history of DVT or pregnancy morbidity, decision to treat with low-dose subcutaneous UFH or LMWH and/or low-dose aspirin, or to manage with surveillance should be made on an individual basis as there is no clear consensus data.[13]

SECONDARY PREVENTION

- For men and nonpregnant women, long-term anticoagulation with warfarin, or with UFH or LMWH if warfarin is contraindicated, should be used (Table 4).
- Modifiable risk factors for thrombosis should be reduced when possible.
- For pregnant women with previously diagnosed APS:
  1. Warfarin should be discontinued before pregnancy due to its teratogenic effects.
  2. For women with APS without prior thrombosis but with pregnancy morbidities of either unexplained fetal death at $\geq$10 wk gestation or $\geq$3 unexplained spontaneous abortions before 10 wk gestation, aspirin 81 mg in combination with subcutaneous

TABLE 4   Risk Stratification and Treatment of Various Phenotypes of Antiphospholipid Syndrome

Risk	Laboratory Result	Clinical Manifestation	Treatment
High	Triple positive for LA, aCL (IgG or IgM >40 GPL) and anti–β_2-GPI (IgG or IgM >99th percentile)	Venous thrombosis	Long-term vitamin K antagonist, INR 2.0-3.0
		Arterial thrombosis	Stroke: Long-term vitamin K antagonist, INR 2.0-3.0 plus low dose aspirin
			Myocardial infarction: Long-term vitamin K antagonist, INR 2.0-3.0 plus low-dose aspirin or Long-term vitamin K antagonist, INR 3.0-4.0
			Myocardial infarction with percutaneous coronary interventions and stent placement: Long-term vitamin K antagonist, INR 2.0-3.0, low-dose aspirin, and clopidogrel 75 mg per day
		Pregnant women with history of pregnancy complications or thrombotic events	Unfractionated heparin plus low-dose aspirin
		Asymptomatic	Consider anticoagulant prophylaxis for high risk situations, e.g., immobilization, surgery, air travel
			Consider long-term vitamin K antagonist recommended to prevent thromboembolic events
			Consider low-dose aspirin and possible unfractionated heparin for pregnant patients
Medium	Double positive for LA, aCL (IgG or IgM >40 GPL) or anti–β_2-GPI (IgG or IgM >99th percentile) or Single positive for LA	Venous thrombosis	Long-term vitamin K antagonist, INR 2.0-3.0
		Arterial thrombosis	Long-term vitamin K antagonist, INR 2.0-3.0 plus low-dose aspirin
		Pregnant women with history of pregnancy complications or thrombotic events	Unfractionated heparin plus low-dose aspirin
		Asymptomatic	No treatment, consider prophylaxis treatment in situations with increased risk: Surgery or prolonged immobilization
Low	Single positive for aCL (IgG or IgM >40 GPL) or anti–β_2-GPI (IgG or IgM >99th percentile)	Venous thrombosis	Long-term vitamin K antagonist, INR 2.0-3.0
		Arterial thrombosis	Long-term vitamin K antagonist, INR 2.0-3.0
		Pregnant women with history of pregnancy complications or thrombotic events	Early miscarriage (does not meet clinical criteria for obstetric APS): Consider low-dose aspirin
			Late miscarriage: Unfractionated heparin plus low-dose aspirin
		Asymptomatic	No treatment; however, consider prophylaxis treatment in situations with increased risk: Surgery or prolonged immobilization

aCL, Anticardiolipin; *β_2-GPI,* β_2-glycoprotein I; *Ig,* immunoglobulin; *INR,* international normalized ratio; *LA,* lupus anticoagulant.
Adapted from Rand J, Wolgast L: The antiphospholipid syndrome. In *Hematology: basic principles and practice,* ed 7, Philadelphia, 2018, Elsevier.

TABLE 5 Alternative Therapies for Antiphospholipid Syndrome

Treatment	Target Effect (in vitro and/or animal studies)	Results of Human Studies
Hydroxychloroquine	aPL-induced platelet activation Inhibition of aPL-mediated thrombosis in mice Protection of aPL-induced displacement of annexin A5 from phospholipid bilayers	Decreases thrombotic risk in SLE Increases survival in SLE Protective against thrombosis in aPL+ individuals Decreases aPL and/or LAC in SLE patients
Statins	Reversal of aPL-induced endothelial cell activation and TF upregulation Abrogation of enhanced thrombus formation in mice	Decrease proinflammatory and prothrombotic markers in APS Contraindicated in pregnancy
Rituximab	Blocking of B-cell activating factor, which can prevent disease onset in APS mouse model	Effective for aPL-related cytopenias Effective for catastrophic APS Increases response in APS (off-label use) RITAPS trial: Effective for some noncriteria manifestations of APS
Potential immunomodulatory approaches	Anticomplement peptides Inhibition of TF Inhibition of nuclear factor κB Inhibition of p38 MAPK Inhibition of TLR-4 Inhibition of TNF-α, or IL-6 Inhibition of apo ER2 Inhibition of mTORC Peptides mimicking domains of β_2-GPI or β_2-GPI receptor blockers Other biologics (eculizumab belimumab, abatacept)	Experimental studies (MBB2: A single-chain fragment variable recognizing β_2-GP1) Eculizumab (complement-5 inhibitor): Based on case reports/series has been effective in treating CAPS, limited data in pregnancy; currently ongoing clinical trials[1]
Experimental Tx	Autologous hematopoietic stem cell transplantation	Limited data; appears to be effective and safe in APS patients

[1]Dobrowolski C, Erkan D: Treatment of antiphospholipid syndrome beyond anticoagulation, *Clin Immunol* 206:53-62, 2019.
aPL, Antiphospholipid antibody; *APS*, antiphospholipid syndrome; *β_2-GPI*, β_2-glycoprotein I; *IL-6*, interleukin-6; *LAC*, lupus anticoagulant; *MAPK*, mitogen-activated protein kinase; *mTORC*, mammalian target of rapamycin complex; *RITAPS*, rituximab in antiphospholipid syndrome; *SLE*, systemic lupus erythematosus; *TF*, tissue factor; *TLR*, Toll-like receptor; *TNF*, tumor necrosis factor.
Modified from Hochberg MC: *Rheumatology*, ed 7, Philadelphia, 2019, Elsevier.

UFH or LMWH is recommended to improve pregnancy outcomes.

3. For women with APS without prior thrombosis but with pregnancy morbidity of ≥1 premature births before 34 wk gestation secondary to eclampsia, preeclampsia, or severe placental insufficiency, aspirin 81 mg is recommended to improve pregnancy outcomes.

4. For pregnant women with APS and prior thrombosis, aspirin in combination with subcutaneous UFH or LMWH should be used.
5. Pregnant patients taking LMWH should be transitioned to unfractionated heparin before delivery for ease of reversibility.
6. Hypertension, obesity, and hyperlipidemia, if present, should be controlled.[14,15]

FOR CATASTROPHIC ANTIPHOSPHOLIPID ANTIBODY SYNDROME (CAPSS)

- The combination of anticoagulation with heparin products, high-dose corticosteroids, and supportive care, including debriding necrotic tissue and treating underlying infections is the mainstay of therapy.
- Patients may be transitioned to oral anticoagulation with warfarin once clinically stable.
- Plasma exchange with or without intravenous immunoglobulin (IVIG) has been shown to improve mortality; however, the decision to use IVIG should be made on an individual basis (e.g., avoid in patients in whom anticoagulation has been discontinued).
- Eculizumab (monoclonal antibody against complement protein C5) and rituximab

TABLE 6 Treatment Recommendations for Persistently Antiphospholipid Antibody–Positive Individuals

Clinical Circumstance	Recommendation
Asymptomatic	No treatment[a]
Venous thrombosis	Warfarin INR 2.5-3[a]
Arterial thrombosis	Warfarin INR 2.5-3[a]
Recurrent thrombosis	Warfarin INR 3-4 ± low-dose aspirin
Pregnancy:	
First pregnancy	No treatment[b]
Single pregnancy loss at <10 wk	No treatment[b]
≥1 Fetal or ≥3 (pre)-embryonic losses, no thrombosis	Prophylactic heparin[c] + low-dose aspirin throughout pregnancy, discontinue 6-12 wk postpartum
Thrombosis regardless of pregnancy history	Therapeutic heparin[d] or low-dose aspirin throughout pregnancy, warfarin postpartum
Valve nodules or deformity	No known effective treatment; full anticoagulation if emboli or intracardiac thrombi demonstrated
Thrombocytopenia >50,000/mm³	No treatment
Thrombocytopenia <50,000/mm³	Prednisone, IVIG, rituximab
Catastrophic antiphospholipid syndrome	Anticoagulation + corticosteroids + IVIG or plasmapheresis

INR, International normalized ratio; *IVIG*, intravenous immunoglobulin.
[a]Aspirin (81 mg/day) may be considered in high-risk patients with multiple non-aPL cardiovascular risk factors.
[b]Aspirin (81 mg/day) may be considered.
[c]Enoxaparin 0.5 mg/kg subcutaneously once daily.
[d]Enoxaparin 1 mg/kg subcutaneously twice daily or 1.5 mg/kg subcutaneously once daily.
From Firestein GS et al: *Firestein & Kelley's Textbook of Rheumatology*, ed 11, Philadelphia 2021, Elsevier.

(monoclonal antibody against CD20) have been used successfully in refractory cases.
- Immunosuppressant therapy with cyclophosphamide should be considered in patients with CAPS and SLE as it has been demonstrated to decrease mortality in this group.[7]

CHRONIC Rx

- Anticoagulation with VKAs, such as warfarin, remains the standard of care. The potential role of new oral anticoagulants in APS remains uncertain. Meta-analyses of patients with APS treated with direct oral anticoagulants demonstrate higher rates of recurrent thrombosis, which are increased up to fourfold in patients with triple positivity (positive for all three APS antibodies). Trials involving rivaroxaban showed a nonstatistically significant near doubling of the risk for recurrent thrombosis and a trial involving apixaban showed an increase in arterial thrombosis compared to warfarin.[11,12,16]

- Duration of treatment is unknown and should be determined on an individual basis. However, in the absence of any contraindication to anticoagulation, indefinite therapy is recommended, as the lifelong recurrence rate reached nearly 30% in some studies.
- Evidence on length of therapy is unclear in provoked DVTs (prolonged hospitalization, estrogen supplementation) in patients who later test negative for aPL.
- Immunosuppressive agents such as corticosteroids and cyclophosphamide have not been shown to be effective for chronic treatment of APS.
- Limited data suggest that hydroxychloroquine may be effective in patients with APS and SLE, although efficacy in primary APS remains unproven.
- Recurrent thrombosis can occur even in the setting of "therapeutic" anticoagulation, and multiple assays have been studied to monitor the adequacy of anticoagulation in APS.
- In cases of recurrent thrombosis, hydroxychloroquine and statins (antiinflammatory and antithrombotic activity) may be considered as adjuvant therapies.

- Table 5 summarizes alternative therapies for antiphospholipid syndrome.[17]

DISPOSITION

- APS patients have a 20% to 70% risk for recurrent thrombosis. Positivity in more than one aPL assay is associated with increased thrombotic risk. Treatment recommendations for persistently antiphospholipid antibody-positive individuals are summarized in Table 6.
- Initial arterial thrombosis tends to be followed by arterial events, and initial venous thrombosis tends to be followed by venous events.
- Incidence of developing catastrophic APS is approximately 1.0% among APS patients. CAPS is associated with a high mortality rate (35% to 45%, primarily due to cerebral and cardiac involvement).

REFERRAL

Referrals to hematology, rheumatology, and/or obstetric medicine should be placed when diagnosis is made.

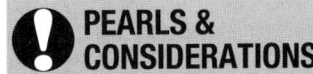

PEARLS & CONSIDERATIONS

COMMENTS

- Observational studies show APS is associated with a 10% mortality over a 10-yr period. Causes of death included arterial and venous thrombotic events (stroke, myocardial infarction), as well as infection and CAPS.[17,18]

Cerebral features of SLE may be more related to thrombosis than inflammation and may respond better to anticoagulants than immunosuppression.

PREVENTION

Prophylaxis for asymptomatic patients with positive aPL tests without previous thrombosis:

- No routine prophylaxis is recommended.
- Questionable whether low-dose aspirin is effective.
- Antithrombotic prophylaxis for major surgery, prolonged immobilization, and pregnancy is appropriate.
- Avoid combination oral contraceptive pills in women with positive aPL tests.

REFERENCES

Available at eBooks.Health.Elsevier.com.

RELATED CONTENT

Antiphospholipid Antibody Syndrome (Patient Information)
Deep Vein Thrombosis (Related Key Topic)
Hypercoagulable State (Related Key Topic)
Pulmonary Embolism (Related Key Topic)

AUTHORS: **PRANAVI SANKA, MD** and **JOHN L. REAGAN, MD**

Aortic Regurgitation (PTG) (ALG)

BASIC INFORMATION

DEFINITION

Aortic regurgitation (AR) is abnormal retrograde blood flow into the left ventricle from the aorta due to an inadequately closing aortic valve (AV). The inadequate closure of the valve can result from either disease of the ascending aorta (ex., dilation) and aortic root or disease of aortic valve leaflets. In addition, it can be acute or chronic in nature.

Stages of chronic aortic regurgitation:
- Stage A = at risk of aortic insufficiency (AI) without even trace AR (e.g., bicuspid AV, AV sclerosis, diseases of the ascending aorta, history of rheumatic heart disease, or infective endocarditis)
- Stage B = progressive AI with mild to moderate AR and preserved left ventricular ejection fraction (LVEF)
- Stage C = asymptomatic severe AR with preserved (stage C1) or reduced (stage C2) LVEF
- Stage D = symptomatic severe AR

SYNONYMS

Aortic insufficiency
AI
AR

ICD-10CM CODES

I35.1	Nonrheumatic aortic (valve) insufficiency
I35.2	Nonrheumatic aortic (valve) stenosis with insufficiency
I06.1	Rheumatic aortic insufficiency
I06.2	Rheumatic aortic stenosis with insufficiency
Q23.1	Congenital insufficiency of aortic valve

EPIDEMIOLOGY & DEMOGRAPHICS

Prevalence varies with severity of AR, age, and gender, as summarized in Table 1.
- Most common cause in the developing world is rheumatic heart disease.
- Most common causes in developed countries are aortic root dilation, congenital bicuspid aortic valve, and calcific valve disease.
- Infectious endocarditis (IE) is the most frequent cause of acute AR.

TABLE 1 Prevalence of Aortic Regurgitation (AR)

Mild AR Prevalence	Males	Females
Age 50-59	3.7 %	1.9%
Age 60-69	12.1%	6%
Age 70-83	12.2%	14.6%
Moderate-Severe AR Prevalence	Males	Females
Age 50-59	0.5%	0.2%
Age 60-69	0.6%	0.8%
Age 70-83	2.2%	2.3%

From Singh JP et al: Prevalence and clinical determinants of mitral, tricuspid, and aortic regurgitation (the Framingham Heart Study), *Am J Cardiol* 83:897, 1999.

PHYSICAL FINDINGS & CLINICAL PRESENTATION

Clinical presentation varies depending on whether AR is acute or chronic. Chronic AR is well tolerated (except when secondary to IE), and patients remain asymptomatic for years. Common manifestations after significant deterioration of LVEF are dyspnea on exertion, syncope, chest pain, and congestive heart failure (CHF). The stages of chronic AR are summarized in Table 2. Acute severe AR manifests primarily with hypotension caused by a sudden fall in cardiac output and resultant cardiogenic shock. A rapid rise in left ventricular diastolic pressure results in a further decrease in coronary blood flow.

Physical findings in chronic AR:
- Widened pulse pressure (markedly increased systolic blood pressure with decreased diastolic blood pressure). Fig. 1 illustrates characteristics of the AR murmur
- Findings associated with widened pulse pressure:
  1. Bounding, "water hammer," or collapsing pulse (***Corrigan*** pulse) can be palpated at the wrist or femoral artery and is caused by the rapid rise and sudden collapse of arterial pressure during late systole
  2. Head "bobbing" with each heart beat (***de Musset*** sign)
  3. "Pistol shot femorals" (***Traube*** sign) describes a loud sound over the femoral artery with systole and diastole
  4. Capillary pulsations (***Quincke*** sign) may occur on the lips or at the base of the nail beds
- A to-and-fro intermittent femoral murmur (***Duroziez*** sign) may be heard with slight compression of the femoral arteries. Popliteal systolic pressure increased >20 mm Hg over the brachial systolic pressure (***Hill*** sign); a 40 to 60 mm difference represents moderate AR and >60 mm difference, severe AR
- Findings more of historical than practical interest, which are neither sensitive nor specific, include:
  1. ***Mueller*** sign—Systolic pulsations of the uvula
  2. ***Becker*** sign—Visible pulsations of the retinal arteries and pupils
  3. ***Mayne*** sign—More than a 15 mm Hg decrease in diastolic blood pressure with arm elevation from the value obtained with the arm in the standard position
  4. ***Rosenbach*** sign—Systolic pulsations of the liver
  5. ***Gerhard*** sign—Systolic pulsations of the spleen
  6. ***Landolfi*** sign—Pupil dilation and constriction with each heartbeat on the ocular exam

Cardiac auscultation reveals:
- Displacement of cardiac impulse downward and to the patient's left
- S_3 heard over the apex
- Decrescendo, blowing diastolic murmur heard along left sternal border
- Low-pitched apical diastolic rumble (***Austin Flint*** murmur)—the precise etiology is uncertain, but it is generally believed to be related to increased velocity of mitral inflow consequent to the AR
- Early systolic ejection sound and systolic ejection murmur

In patients with acute aortic insufficiency, both the wide pulse pressure and the large stroke volume are absent. A short, blowing diastolic murmur may be the only finding on physical examination.

ETIOLOGY

- Leaflet abnormalities:
  1. Infective endocarditis
  2. Rheumatic fibrosis (most common cause in developing countries)
  3. Trauma with valvular rupture
  4. Congenital heart disease (bicuspid aortic valve—most common cause in the U.S., sinus of Valsalva aneurysm)
  5. Myxomatous degeneration
  6. Calcific AV disease
  7. Drug-induced (fenfluramine, dexfenfluramine, pergolide, cabergoline)
  8. Systemic rheumatic disorders (ankylosing spondylitis, rheumatoid arthritis, systemic lupus erythematosus)
  9. Iatrogenic (ex., Aortic balloon valvotomy)
- Aortic root or ascending aorta abnormalities:
  1. Annuloaortic ectasia
  2. Genetic syndromes (Ehlers-Danlos, Marfan)
  3. Trauma
  4. Ankylosing spondylitis
  5. Syphilitic aortitis
  6. Systemic hypertension
  7. Aortic dissection
- Postprocedural AR, usually due to a paravalvular leak, occurs in 10% to 20% of patients undergoing transcatheter aortic valve replacement (TAVR). Patients with more than mild AR after TAVR have worse outcomes than those without AR

DIAGNOSIS

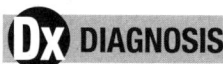

DIFFERENTIAL DIAGNOSIS

- Patent ductus arteriosus, pulmonary regurgitation, and other valvular abnormalities.
- The differential diagnosis of cardiac murmurs is described in Sections II and III.

WORKUP

- Echocardiogram, chest radiograph, electrocardiogram (ECG), cardiac magnetic resonance (CMR) imaging, and cardiac catheterization (selected patients)
- Medical history and physical examination focused on dyspnea on exertion, syncope, chest pain, and CHF

IMAGING STUDIES

- Chest radiography:
  1. Left ventricular hypertrophy (LVH) (chronic AR).
  2. Aortic dilation.
  3. Normal cardiac silhouette with pulmonary edema: Possible in patients with acute AR.

TABLE 2 Stages of Chronic Aortic Regurgitation

Stage	Definition	Valve Anatomy	Valve Hemodynamics	Hemodynamic Consequences	Symptoms
A	At risk of AR	Bicuspid aortic valve (or other congenital valve anomaly)Aortic valve sclerosis Diseases of the aortic sinuses or ascending aorta History of rheumatic fever or known rheumatic heart disease IE	AR severity none or trace	None	None
B	Progressive AR	Mild to moderate calcification of a trileaflet valve bicuspid aortic valve (or other congenital valve anomaly) Dilated aortic sinuses Rheumatic valve changes Previous IE	*Mild AR:* Jet width <25% of LVOT vena contracta <0.3 cm RVol <30 ml/beat RF <30% ERO <0.10 cm^2 Angiography grade 1+ *Moderate AR:* Jet width 25%-64% of LVOT Vena contracta 0.3-0.6 cm RVol 30-59 ml/beat RF 30%-49% ERO 0.10-0.29 cm^2 Angiography grade 2+	Normal LV systolic function Normal LV volume or mild LV dilation	None
C	Asymptomatic severe AR	Calcific aortic valve disease Bicuspid valve (or other congenital abnormality) Dilated aortic sinuses or ascending aorta Rheumatic valve changes IE with abnormal leaflet closure or perforation	*Severe AR:* Jet width ≥65% of LVOT Vena contracta >0.6 cm Holodiastolic flow reversal in the proximal abdominal aorta RVol ≥60 ml/beat RF ≥50% ERO ≥0.3 cm^2 Angiography grade 3+ to 4+ In addition, diagnosis of chronic severe AR requires evidence of LV dilation	C1: Normal LVEF (≥55%) and mild-to-moderate LV dilation (LVESD ≤50 mm) C2: Abnormal LV systolic function with depressed LVEF (<55%) or severe LV dilation (LVESD >50 mm or indexed LVESD >25 mm/m^2)	None; exercise testing is reasonable to confirm symptom status
D	Symptomatic severe AR	Calcific valve disease Bicuspid valve (or other congenital abnormality) Dilated aortic sinuses or ascending aorta Rheumatic valve changes Previous IE with abnormal leaflet closure or perforation	*Severe AR:* Doppler jet width ≥65% of LVOT Vena contracta >0.6 cm Holodiastolic flow reversal in the proximal abdominal aorta RVol ≥60 ml/beat RF ≥50% ERO ≥0.3 cm^2 Angiography grade 3+ to 4+ In addition, diagnosis of chronic severe AR requires evidence of LV dilation	Symptomatic severe AR may occur with normal systolic function (LVEF ≥55%), mild-to-moderate LV dysfunction (LVEF 40%-55%), or severe LV dysfunction (LVEF <40%). Moderate-to-severe LV dilation is present	Exertional dyspnea or angina, or more severe HF symptoms

AR, Aortic regurgitation; *ERO*, effective regurgitant orifice; *HF*, heart failure; *IE*, infective endocarditis; *LV*, left ventricle; *LVEF*, left ventricular ejection fraction; *LVESD*, left ventricular end-systolic dimension; *LVOT*, left ventricular outflow tract; *RF*, regurgitant fraction; *RVol*, regurgitant volume.
From Otto CM et al: 2020 ACC/AHA Guideline for the Management of Patients With Valvular Heart Disease: Executive Summary: A Report of the American College of Cardiology/American Heart Association Joint Committee on Clinical Practice Guidelines [published correction appears in *Circulation* 143(5):e228, 2021] [published correction appears in *Circulation* 143(10):e784, 2021]. *Circulation* 143(5):e35-e71, 2021. https://doi.org/10.1161/CIR.0000000000000932

- ECG is not useful for diagnostic purposes but is commonly used in evaluation of patients with chronic AR to exclude associated arrhythmia. Typical findings on an ECG are LVH as a result of volume overload.
- Echocardiography (Fig. E2) is the main imaging modality to diagnose AR and assess left ventricular size and function. Quantification of the severity of regurgitation can be made either qualitatively by Doppler vena contracta width (severe if >0.6 cm) or quantitatively by effective regurgitant orifice area (severe if >0.30 cm^2), regurgitant

volume (severe if >60 ml per/beat) and/or regurgitant fraction ≥ 50%.[1]
- Echocardiography can also be used for periodic monitoring of asymptomatic patients with normal LV systolic function and chronic AR.
- TTE (Class I) is indicated to assess severity and presence of AR in patients with bicuspid aortic valve or with known dilation of the aortic sinuses or ascending aorta.[1]
- TEE, CMR, or cardiac catheterization is indicated (class 1) in patients with moderate or severe AR and suboptimal echocardiographic

images or discrepancy between TTE and clinical findings in order to assess AR severity, LV systolic function, and aortic size.[1,2]

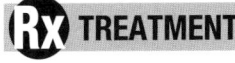 **TREATMENT**

NONPHARMACOLOGIC THERAPY

- Avoidance of competitive sports and heavy weight lifting if severe AR, patient is symptomatic, ejection fraction <50%, AR is associated with aortic root dilation
- Salt restriction

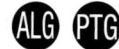

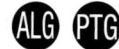

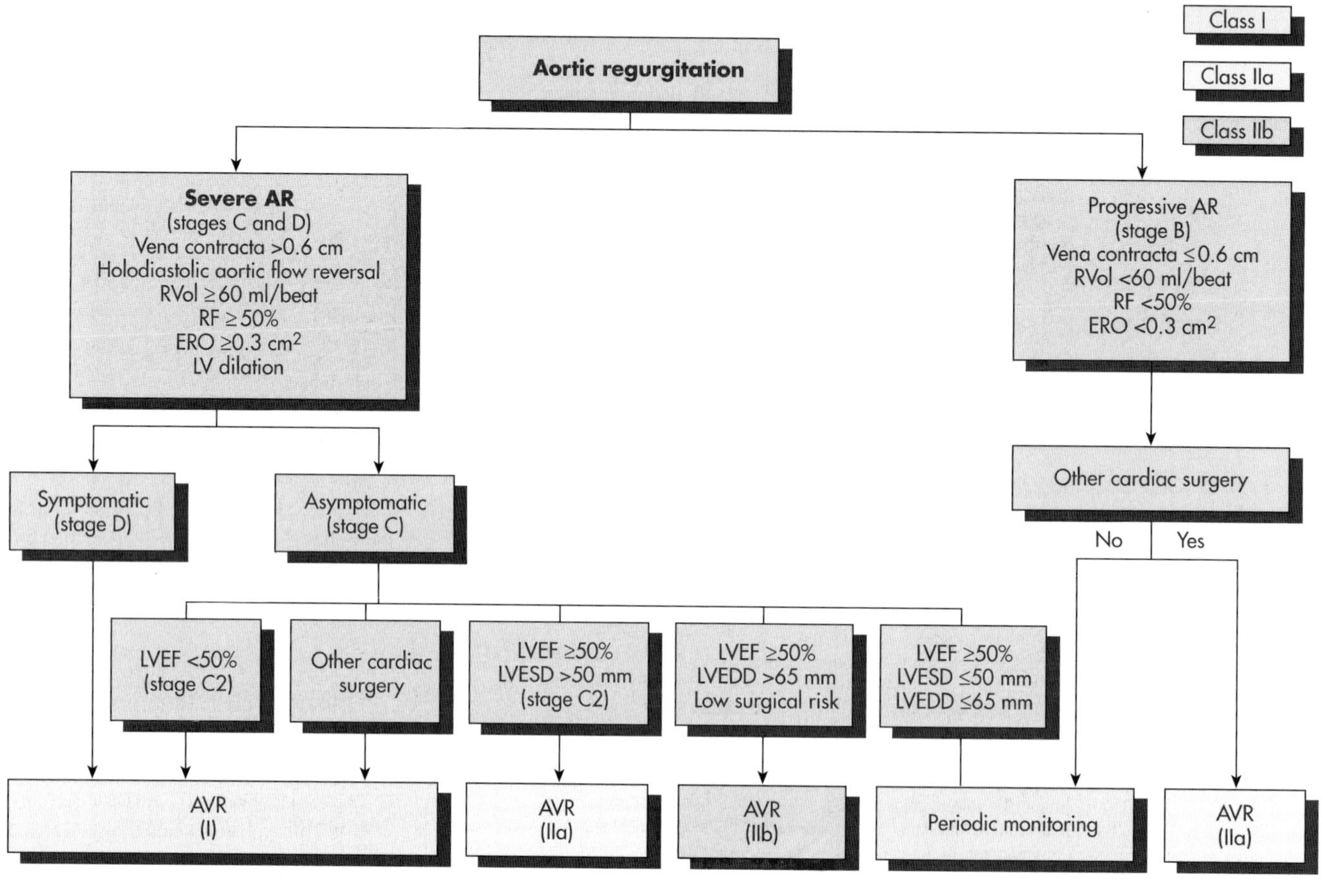

FIG. 1 **Aortic regurgitation as an example of an early diastolic murmur.** (From Epstein O et al: *Pocket guide to clinical examination,* ed 4, St Louis, 2009, Mosby.)

TABLE 3 American College of Cardiology/American Heart Association Guidelines for Aortic Valve Replacement (AVR) for Chronic Aortic Regurgitation (AR)

Class	Indication	LOE
I	AVR for symptomatic patients with severe AR regardless of LV systolic function (stage D).	B
	AVR for asymptomatic patients with chronic severe AR and LV systolic dysfunction (LVEF <55%) (stage C2).	B
	AVR for patients with severe AR (stage C or D) while undergoing cardiac surgery for other indications.	C
IIa	AVR is reasonable for asymptomatic patients with severe AR with normal LV systolic function (LVEF ≥55%), but severe LV dilation (stage C2, LVESD >50 mm).	B
	AVR is reasonable in patients with moderate AR (stage B) who are undergoing other cardiac surgery.	C
IIb	AVR may be considered for asymptomatic patients with severe AR and normal LV systolic function (stage C1, LVEF ≥55%) but severe LV dilation (LVEDD >65 mm) if surgical risk is low.*	C

LOE, Level of evidence; *LV,* left ventricular; *LVEDD,* LV end-diastolic dimension; *LVEF,* LV ejection fraction; *LVESD,* LV end-systolic dimension.

* Particularly in the setting of progressive LV enlargement.

From Zipes DP et al: *Braunwald's heart disease, a textbook of cardiovascular disease,* ed 11, Philadelphia, 2019, Elsevier.

- Endocarditis prophylaxis is not recommended for chronic AR patients with native valves undergoing invasive procedures. However, antibiotic prophylaxis is recommended for patients with a prior history of infective endocarditis or a presence of prosthetic heart valve

ACUTE GENERAL RX:
- Emergent AV replacement (preferred) or repair for acute, severe AR.[3]
- Intraaortic balloon pump is contraindicated
- Afterload reduction: Angiotensin-converting enzyme (ACE) inhibitors and vasodilators (i.e., nitroprusside) in acute AR; diuretics for pulmonary edema
- Avoid beta-blockers that can prolong diastole
- Emergent surgical referral for cardiogenic shock

CHRONIC RX: Management depends on whether patients are symptomatic and candidates for valve surgery. ACC/AHA guidelines for aortic valve replacement for chronic aortic regurgitation are summarized in Table 3.

- Symptomatic patients with severe AR who are candidates for valve surgery should proceed with valve replacement after medical optimization of heart failure.
- A trial comparing the outcomes of transcatheter aortic valve replacement (TAVR) with surgical aortic valve replacement (SAVR) in patients with pure aortic insufficiency (PAI) revealed no significant statistical difference in in-hospital mortality, fewer respiratory complications, acute kidney injuries, septic shock, and mechanical ventilation with TAVR but significantly more cardiopulmonary resuscitation and permanent pacemaker placements. TAVR could be considered for patients with PAI who are not candidates for surgery.[4]
- Patients with severe AR who have LV systolic dysfunction and/or symptomatic but have a high and prohibitive surgical risk, guideline directed medical therapy is recommended including ACE inhibitors, ARBs, and sacubitril/valsartan.

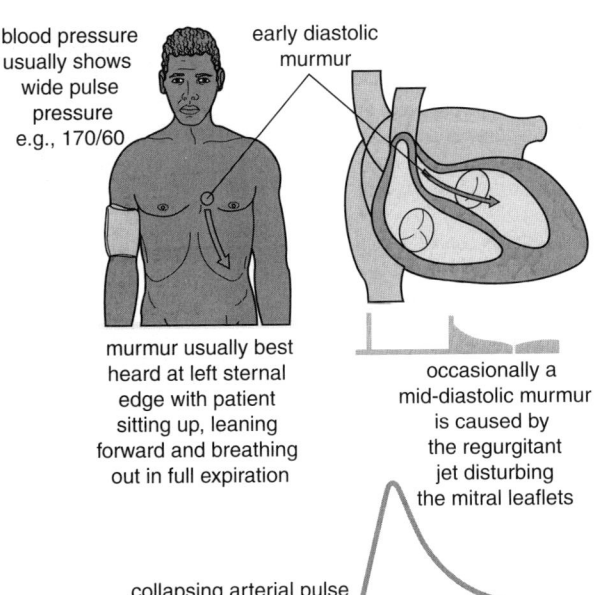

blood pressure usually shows wide pulse pressure e.g., 170/60

early diastolic murmur

murmur usually best heard at left sternal edge with patient sitting up, leaning forward and breathing out in full expiration

occasionally a mid-diastolic murmur is caused by the regurgitant jet disturbing the mitral leaflets

collapsing arterial pulse

FIG. 3 Management strategy for patients with chronic severe aortic regurgitation (AR). *AVR,* Aortic valve replacement (valve repair may be appropriate in selected patients); *ERO,* effective regurgitant orifice; *LV,* left ventricle; *LVEDD,* left ventricular end-diastolic dimension; *LVEF,* left ventricular ejection fraction; *LVESD,* left ventricular end-systolic dimension; *RF,* regurgitant fraction; *RVol,* regurgitant volume. (From Zipes DP et al: *Braunwald's heart disease, a textbook of cardiovascular disease,* ed 11, Philadelphia, 2019, Elsevier.)

- Other medical treatments for AR are based on limited studies. Beta-blocker use is controversial but has been associated with a higher survival rate in severe AR. Vasodilatory therapies (nifedipine and enalapril) have failed to show benefit in reducing the need for or delaying AV replacement in asymptomatic, severe AR with normal systolic function, but ACE/ARB therapy may indeed benefit moderate to severe AR.[5] Long-term vasodilator therapy with ACE inhibitors or nifedipine may be used in patients who have concomitant hypertension. There is no current definitive indication of medical therapy with afterload reduction for aortic regurgitation other than hypertension control specifically a systolic blood pressure >140 mm Hg.[1]

- Beta-blockers in combination with ACE inhibitors are reasonable in patients with symptomatic severe AR or LV dysfunction when surgery cannot be performed because of concomitant comorbidities. In a retrospective cohort study of 756 patients with chronic AR, beta-blocker therapy was associated with decreased mortality. Patients treated with beta-blockers were more likely to be taking ACE inhibitors and dihydropyridine calcium channel blockers as well (53% vs. 40%). In the same study, patients treated with beta-blockers and undergoing AVR were also noted to have a mortality benefit.[6]

- Diuretics and sodium restriction for CHF.
- Fig. 3 describes a management strategy for patients with chronic severe AR.

REFERRAL

Surgical referral is reserved for the following patients:

- Patients with acute severe AR (i.e., infective endocarditis) and cardiogenic shock
- Symptomatic patients with severe AR regardless of LV systolic function (Class I)
- Patients with hemodynamically stable severe AR undergoing CABG or surgery on the aorta or other heart valves
- Evidence of systolic dysfunction with left ventricular ejection fraction of less than 55% and asymptomatic patients with chronic severe AR[7]
- Patients with moderate AR who are undergoing other forms of cardiac surgery
- Asymptomatic patients with severe AR and left ventricular ejection fraction >55% but with left ventricular dilation:
  1. Echocardiographic end-systolic dimension >50 mm (Class IIa level of evidence) *or;*
  2. Echocardiographic end-diastolic dimension >65 mm with low surgical risk (Class IIb)

REFERENCES
Available at eBooks.Health.Elsevier.com

RELATED CONTENT
Aortic Insufficiency (Patient Information)

AUTHOR: **SARTHAK KHARE, MD**

Diseases and Disorders

I

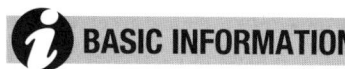
BASIC INFORMATION

DEFINITION

Aortic stenosis (AS) is obstruction of left ventricular systolic outflow due to aortic valve thickening/calcification generating a significant pressure gradient. Symptoms typically appear when the valve orifice decreases to <1 cm^2 (normal orifice is 3 to 4 cm^2). Criteria for severe AS include a valve area <1.0 cm^2, a mean gradient >40 mm Hg, or a peak velocity >4 m/s (correlating with a peak gradient of 64 mm Hg). Doppler aortic jet velocities >5 m/sec is defined as very severe.[1]

SYNONYMS

Aortic valve stenosis
AS

ICD-10CM CODES

I35.0	Nonrheumatic aortic (valve) stenosis
I35.2	Nonrheumatic aortic (valve) stenosis with insufficiency
Q23.0	Congenital stenosis of aortic valve

EPIDEMIOLOGY & DEMOGRAPHICS

- Aortic stenosis is the most common valve lesion in adults in North America and Europe.
- The prevalence demonstrates a strong relationship with age, affecting 0.2% between ages 50 and 59 yr, 1.3% between 60 and 69 yr, 3.9% between 70 and 79 yr, and 9.8% between ages 80 and 89.

PHYSICAL FINDINGS & CLINICAL PRESENTATION

- Harsh midsystolic, crescendo-decrescendo murmur (Fig. 1) best heard at base of heart and radiating into neck vessels; often associated with a thrill or ejection click; may also be heard well at the apex.
- Signs of severe AS include absent or diminished intensity of the second heart sound and/or slow-rising carotid upstroke with delayed amplitude (pulsus parvus et tardus), presence of S4, and a reverse splitting of the second heart sound.
- Early symptoms include decreased exercise tolerance, dyspnea on exertion, exertional dizziness or syncope, and exertional angina.
- Late symptoms include angina (secondary primarily to reduced coronary blood flow and increased total left ventricle [LV] oxygen demand), syncope, and heart failure.
- Table 1 summarizes the stages of valvular aortic stenosis.
- Pathophysiology: Antegrade velocities remain normal until the cross-sectional area of the left ventricular outflow tract (typically 3 to 4 cm^2) is reduced by roughly half. At this point, secondary to the increased resistance, the left ventricle systolic pressure starts to increase, and the LV adapts with concentric hypertrophy. The hypertrophy allows for normalization of the wall stress and preservation of the ejection fraction, cardiac output, and left ventricular

end diastolic pressures despite the LV/peripheral arterial system pressure gradient.
- LV hypertrophy eventually leads to LV diastolic dysfunction, which may herald early symptoms. That said, symptoms generally do not begin until stenosis becomes severe (valve area <1.0 cm^2, a mean gradient >40 mm Hg, or a peak gradient >4 m/s).
- For most patients, after becoming symptomatic, LV systolic function will begin to drop (decreased cardiac output and stroke volume) with development of signs and symptoms of overt heart failure. At this point, if a symptomatic severe AS patient does not undergo valve replacement, their mortality drastically increases.[1,2]
- Acquired von Willebrand disease is seen in approximately 20% of severe AS, which can lead to GI bleeding from angiodysplasia (Heyde syndrome) that resolves after aortic valve replacement.

ETIOLOGY

- Idiopathic calcification of the aortic valve (most common cause in North America and Europe, presents at ages 60 to 80).
- Rheumatic heart disease: Characterized by commissural fusion leaving a small central orifice (most common cause worldwide).
- Progressive stenosis of congenital unicuspid or bicuspid valve (found in 1% to 2% of the population, presents at ages <30 yr for unicuspid and at ages 40 to 60 for bicuspid valves).[3]
- Less common causes include rare metabolic disease (Fabry disease), systemic lupus erythematosus, radiation, end-stage renal

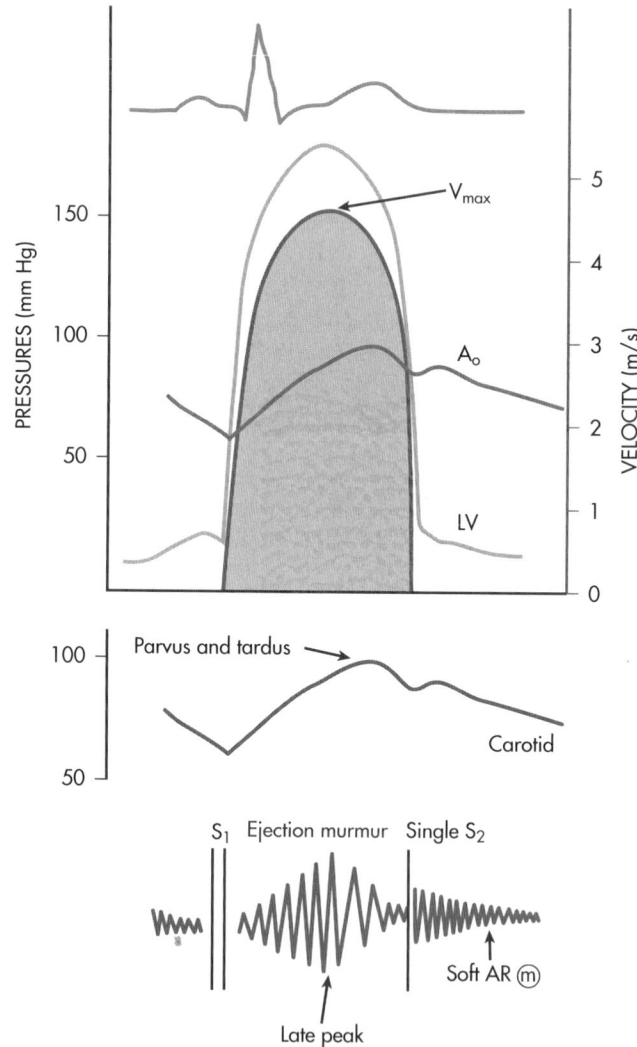

FIG. 1 Relationship between left ventricle (LV) and aortic (Ao) pressures and the Doppler aortic stenosis velocity curve (*in red*). The pressure difference between the LV and aorta in systole is four times the velocity squared (the Bernoulli equation). Thus a maximum velocity (V $_{max}$) of 4.3 m/sec corresponds to a maximum LV to Ao pressure difference of 74 mm Hg and a mean systolic gradient of 44 mm Hg. On physical examination, the slow rate of rise and delayed peak in the carotid pulse (or parvus and tardus) matches the contour of the aortic pressure waveform. The murmur corresponds to the Doppler velocity curve with a harsh crescendo-decrescendo late-peaking systolic murmur, best heard at the aortic region (upper right sternal border). Often, a soft, high-pitched diastolic decrescendo murmur of aortic regurgitation also is appreciated. *AR,* Aortic regurgitation. (From Bonow et al [eds]: *Braunwald's heart disease,* ed 9, Philadelphia, 2012, Saunders.)

TABLE 1 Stages of Valvular Aortic Stenosis

Stage	Definition	Valve Anatomy	Valve Hemodynamics	Hemodynamic Consequences	Symptoms
A	**At risk of AS**	Bicuspid aortic valve (or other congenital valve anomaly) Aortic valve sclerosis	Aortic V_{max} <2 m/sec	None	None
B	**Progressive AS**	Mild to moderate leaflet calcification of a bicuspid or trileaflet valve with some reduction in systolic motion or rheumatic valve changes with commissural fusion	***Mild AS:*** Aortic V_{max} 2.0-2.9 m/sec or mean ΔP <20 mm Hg ***Moderate AS:*** Aortic V_{max} 3.0-3.9 m/sec or mean ΔP 20-39 mm Hg	Early LV diastolic dysfunction may be present Normal LVEF	None
C	**Asymptomatic severe AS**				
C1	Asymptomatic severe AS with preserved LVEF	Severe leaflet calcification or congenital stenosis with severely reduced leaflet opening	***Severe AS:*** Aortic V_{max} ≥4 m/sec or mean ΔP ≥40 mm Hg AVA typically is ≤1 cm^2 (or AVAi ≤0.6 cm^2/m^2) Very severe AS is an aortic V_{max} ≥5 m/sec, or mean ΔP ≥60 mm Hg	LV diastolic dysfunction Mild LV hypertrophy Normal LVEF	None; exercise testing is reasonable to confirm symptom status
C2	Asymptomatic severe AS with LV dysfunction	Severe leaflet calcification or congenital stenosis with severely reduced leaflet opening	Aortic V_{max} ≥4 m/sec or mean ΔP ≥40 mm Hg AVA typically is ≤1 cm^2 (or AVAi ≤0.6 cm^2/m^2)	LVEF <50%	None
D	**Symptomatic severe AS**				
D1	Symptomatic severe high-gradient AS	Severe leaflet calcification or congenital stenosis with severely reduced leaflet opening	***Severe AS:*** Aortic V_{max} ≥4 m/sec, or mean ΔP ≥40 mm Hg AVA typically is ≤1 cm^2 (or AVAi ≤0.6 cm^2/m^2), but may be larger with mixed AS/AR	LV diastolic dysfunction LV hypertrophy Pulmonary hypertension may be present	Exertional dyspnea or decreased exercise tolerance Exertional angina Exertional syncope or presyncope
D2	Symptomatic severe low-flow/low-gradient AS with reduced LVEF	Severe leaflet calcification with severely reduced leaflet motion	AVA ≤1 cm^2 with resting aortic V_{max} <4 m/sec, or mean ΔP <40 mm Hg Dobutamine stress echo shows AVA ≤1 cm^2 with V_{max} ≥4 m/sec at any flow rate	LV diastolic dysfunction LV hypertrophy LVEF <50%	HF, angina, syncope or presyncope
D3	Symptomatic severe low-gradient AS with normal LVEF or paradoxical low-flow severe AS	Severe leaflet calcification with severely reduced leaflet motion	AVA ≤1 cm^2 with aortic V_{max} <4 m/sec, or mean ΔP <40 mm Hg AVAi ≤0.6 cm^2/m^2 Stroke volume index <35 ml/m^2 Measured when the patient is normotensive (systolic BP <140 mm Hg)	Increased LV relative wall thickness Small LV chamber with low-stroke volume. Restrictive diastolic filling LVEF ≥50%	HF, angina, syncope or presyncope

AR, Aortic regurgitation; *AS*, aortic stenosis; *AVA*, aortic valve area; *AVAi*, aortic valve area indexed to body surface area; *BP*, blood pressure; *HF*, heart failure; *LV*, left ventricle; *LVEF*, left ventricular ejection fraction; *ΔP*, pressure gradient; *V_{max}*, maximum aortic velocity.

From Nishimura RA et al: 2014 AHA/ACCF guideline for the management of patients with valvular heart disease: a report of the American College of Cardiology Foundation/American Heart Association Task Force on Practice Guidelines. In Mann DL et al (eds): *Braunwald's heart disease*, ed 10, Philadelphia, 2015, Elsevier.

disease, and obstructive vegetations/endocarditis may all cause early development of AS.
- Genetic variation in the LPA locus, mediated by Lp(2) levels, is associated with aortic valve calcification across multiple ethnic groups and with incidental clinical aortic stenosis.[4]

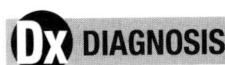 **DIAGNOSIS**

DIFFERENTIAL DIAGNOSIS
- Hypertrophic cardiomyopathy
- Mitral regurgitation
- Ventricular septal defect
- Aortic sclerosis. Aortic stenosis is distinguished from aortic sclerosis by the degree of valve impairment. In aortic sclerosis, the valve leaflets are abnormally thickened but obstruction to outflow is absent or minimal
- Subvalvular membrane or supravalvular AS
- Stages of valvular AS
  1. Stage A = at risk of AS
  2. Stage B = progressive AS (formerly known as mild and moderate AS)
  3. Stage C = asymptomatic severe AS
  4. Stage D = symptomatic severe AS

WORKUP
- Echocardiography: The primary test for diagnosis (see "Imaging Studies")
- ECG: May demonstrate left ventricular hypertrophy and/or left atrial abnormality
- Chest radiograph: May demonstrate cardiomegaly. Poststenotic dilation of the ascending aorta may also be evident
- Cardiac catheterization in selected patients (see "Imaging Studies")
- Dobutamine challenge (for low-flow, low-gradient AS)[5]

IMAGING STUDIES
- Doppler echocardiography: Used to evaluate structure and anatomy of the valve. Hemodynamics can easily be assessed; allows calculation of both aortic valve area and estimation of pressure gradients to determine severity of AS (Fig. 2). Furthermore, allows evaluation of the LV size and function and pulmonary pressures.
- Chest x-ray:
  1. Poststenotic dilation of the ascending aorta
  2. Calcification of aortic cusps
  3. Rounding of left ventricle (LV) apex

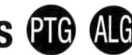
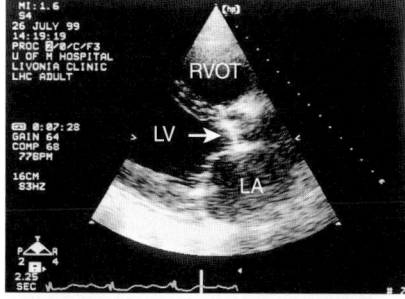

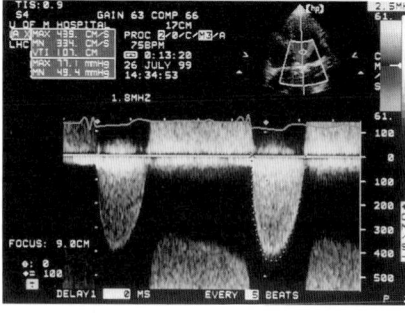

FIG. 2 Echocardiogram recorded in a patient with severe aortic stenosis. The *top panel* is a parasternal long-axis view recorded in systole. Left ventricular function is diminished. The aortic valve is markedly thickened and partially calcified. Its motion is markedly reduced, and in systole it appears that the valve occludes the orifice *(arrow)*. The *lower panel* is a continuous-wave Doppler recorded from the apex of the left ventricle along a line aimed through the stenotic aortic valve. Note the aortic stenosis signal below the zero crossing line. The peak velocity is 430 cm/sec, which corresponds to a maximum gradient of 77 mm Hg and a mean gradient of 49.4 mm Hg. *LA,* Left atrium; *LV,* left ventricle; *RVOT,* right ventricular outflow tract. (From Zipes DP et al [eds]: *Braunwald's heart disease,* ed 7, Philadelphia, 2005, Saunders.)

- ECG:
  1. Left ventricular hypertrophy (found in 80% of patients)
  2. Left atrial enlargement
  3. Atrial fibrillation (in late disease)
- Cardiac catheterization: Indicated in symptomatic patients awaiting aortic valve replacement (AVR) in order to detect coexisting coronary artery stenosis that may need bypass at the same time as aortic valve replacement. Cardiac catheterization can also be used to determine invasive aortic gradients (which may be underestimated on echocardiography).
- A CT with contrast for imaging the aorta may be needed for annular sizing, aortic measurements, and if a transcatheter aortic valve replacement (TAVR) is planned, the CT scan is crucial to planning TAVR approach.[1]
- Exercise testing: Strongly encouraged for any patient with stage C "asymptomatic" severe AS to evaluate exercise tolerance and to look

for a fall in systemic blood pressure while exercising.

Rx TREATMENT

GENERAL Rx
MEDICAL:
- Once symptomatic, the mainstay of treatment is replacement of the valve. AS is a surgical disease. Fig. 3 summarizes a treatment strategy for patients with severe AS.[1,6]
- Optimize loading conditions by keeping a normal volume status (gentle diuresis for volume overload as preload dependent) and controlling hypertension (HTN) but avoid vasodilators (nitrates); maintain sinus rhythm.
- In 2007, the AHA guidelines for prevention of infectious endocarditis were revised, and routine antibiotic prophylaxis to undergo dental or other invasive procedures is no longer recommended, unless the patient has prior endocarditis.[7]

INDICATIONS FOR AORTIC VALVE REPLACEMENT: Valve replacement is the treatment of choice in symptomatic patients because there is a 50% mortality rate at 2 yr with medical therapy alone. If a patient does not have a >1 yr life expectancy, then replacement should not be considered, but rather palliative therapies should be discussed. ACC/AHA guidelines for aortic valve replacement for aortic stenosis are summarized in Table 2.

Percutaneous balloon aortic valvuloplasty (BAV) serves best as palliative therapy in severely symptomatic patients who are not surgical candidates and as a bridge to therapy in patients not ready for TAVR/SAVR or a bridge to decision (for patients with unclear candidacy for TAVR/SAVR). Restenosis occurs in most adult patients within 6 mo, so BAV is not a long-term therapy. The 2020 updated ACC /AHA guidelines for choice of surgical versus transcatheter treatment of aortic stenosis are summarized in Table 3.[1]

Valve replacement is a **Class I indication** for any patients with:
- Stage D1: Symptomatic severe AS
- Stage C2: Asymptomatic severe AS with LV ejection fraction (EF) <50%
- Stage C1 or C2: Asymptomatic severe AS undergoing CABG or surgery on the aorta or other heart valves

Valve replacement is a **Class IIa indication** for patients with:
- Stage D2: Low-flow/low gradient (with low ejection fraction <50%) with a positive low-dose dobutamine stress echo
- Stage D3: Symptomatic patients with low-flow/low gradient severe AS with a **normal LVEF** ≥50%, a valve area ≤1.0 cm², and a stroke volume index <35 ml/m²
- Stage C: Asymptomatic severe AS and abnormal blood pressure response (decrease in systolic blood pressure) or decreased exercise tolerance during exercise

- Stage C: Asymptomatic patients with critical AS (peak velocity >5 m/s or mean pressure gradient >60 mm Hg) with low surgical risk
- Stage B: Patients with moderate AS who are undergoing cardiac surgery for other indications

Valve replacement is a **Class IIb indication** for patients with:
- Stage C: Asymptomatic severe AS in a low-risk patient showing rapid progression of disease (V$_{max}$ >0.3m/s/yr).
- When deciding replacement strategy, surgical aortic valve replacement (SAVR) vs. transcatheter aortic valve replacement (TAVR), in all cases a heart team approach is a Class I indication. TAVR is a catheter-based technology that allows for implantation of a prosthetic valve without open heart surgery, decreasing recovery time and hospital stay.
- Historically, the choice of SAVR versus TAVR strategy had been driven by patient surgical risk. Primarily due to TAVR trial design, patients were classified by their STS-PROM score into four categories: Extreme surgical risk (absolute surgical contraindication), high surgical risk (STS-PROM score >8), intermediate surgical risk (STS-PROM score 4 to 8), and low surgical risk (STS-PROM score <4). As more data have been collected, the two approaches, SAVR versus TAVR, appear to be more and more comparable with regard to valve durability. TAVR is associated with slightly lower mortality, shorter hospital length of stay, less bleeding, lower risk of transient or permanent atrial fibrillation, more rapid return to normal activities, and less pain post-procedure than SAVR.
- SAVR, on the other hand, has less need for permanent pacemaker placement, lower rate of valve reintervention, and is associated with a lower risk of paravalvular leak. As such, deciding between the two approaches now focuses on patient's age, anatomic contraindications for transfemoral TAVR, high risk or prohibitive surgical risk, the life expectancy of the patient, and the patient's values and preferences.

AVR criteria is listed in Table 2.
- For patients who are **>80 yr of age** or for younger patients with a life expectancy <10 yr and no anatomic contraindications to transfemoral TAVR, transfemoral TAVR is recommended in preference to SAVR.
- For patients who are **65 to 80 yr of age** and have no anatomic contraindications to transfemoral TAVR, either SAVR or transfemoral TAVR is recommended after shared decision making about the balance between expected patient longevity and valve durability.

For patients who are **<65 yr of age** or have a life expectancy >20 yr, SAVR is recommended. For patients with a bicuspid valve, a heart team approach, as with all aortic valve replacements, is strongly advised.

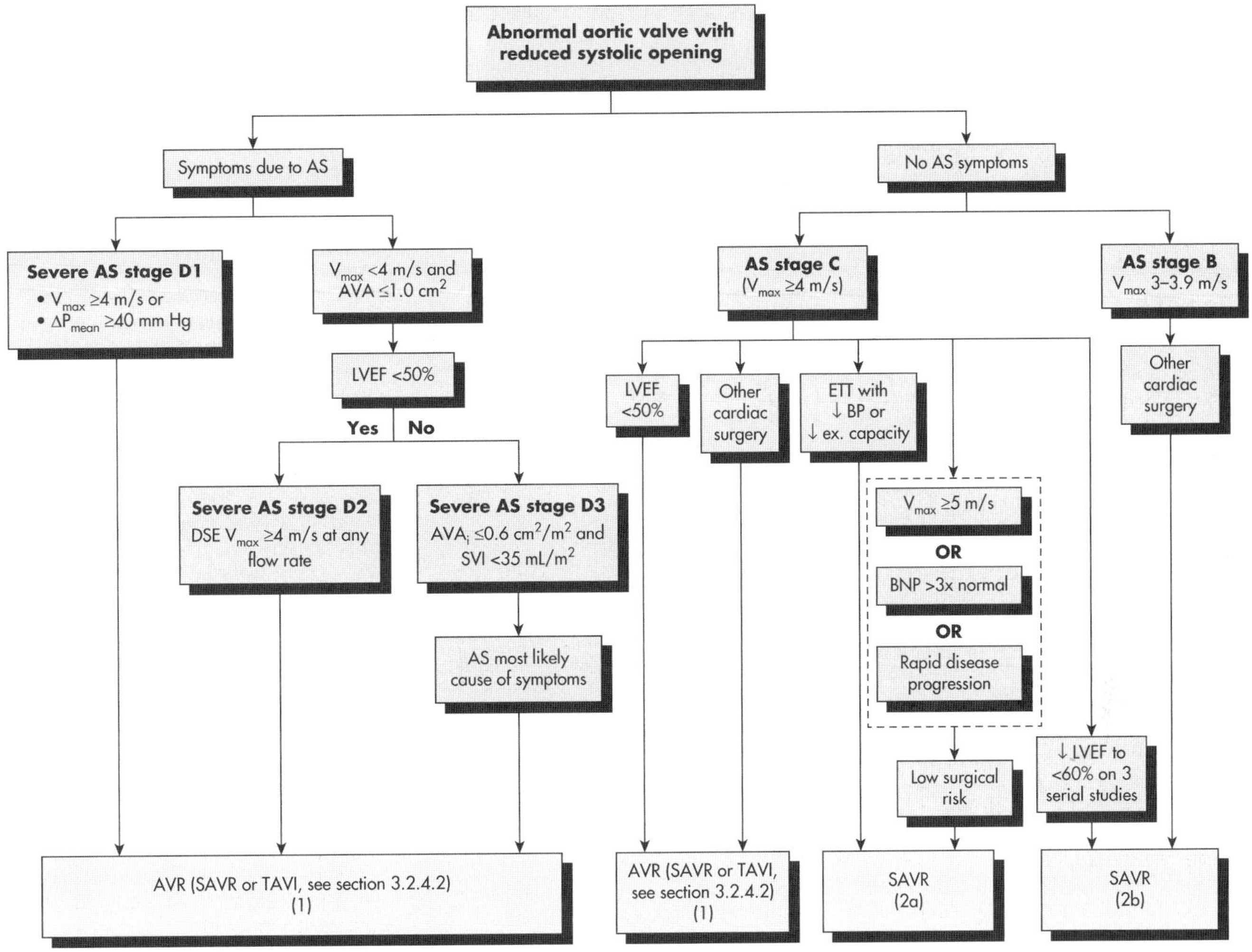

FIG. 3 Management strategy for patients with severe AS. Arrows show the decision pathways that result in a recommendation for AVR. Periodic monitoring is indicated for all patients in whom AVR is not yet indicated, including those with asymptomatic (Stage C) and symptomatic (Stage D) AS and those with low-gradient AS (Stage D2 or D3) who do not meet the criteria for intervention. *AS,* Aortic stenosis; *AVA,* aortic valve area; *AVAi,* aortic valve area index; *AVR,* aortic valve replacement; *BNP,* B-type natriuretic peptide; *BP,* blood pressure; *DPmean,* mean systolic pressure gradient between LV and aorta; *DSE,* dobutamine stress echocardiography; *ETT,* exercise treadmill test; *LVEF,* left ventricular ejection fraction; *SAVR,* surgical aortic valve replacement; *SVI,* stroke volume index; *TAVI,* transcatheter aortic valve implantation; *TAVR,* transcatheter aortic valve replacement; *V$_{max}$,* maximum velocity. (From Otto CM et al: 2020 AHA/ACC Guideline for the management of patients with valvular heart disease: a report of the American College of Cardiology/American Heart Association Task Force on Practice Guidelines, *JACC* 77(4):e25-197, 2021.)

DISPOSITION

- The presence of even mild symptoms is an indicator of poor survival for patients with AS. The average duration of symptoms before death is angina, 5 yr; syncope, 3 yr; CHF, 2 yr.
- Approximately 75% of patients with symptomatic AS will die within 3 yr of symptom onset unless the aortic valve is replaced.

REFERRAL

- A heart team referral for valve replacement in all symptomatic AS patients (Class I indication). There are studies that are examining the presence of moderate or severe valvular calcification, together with a rapid increase in aortic jet velocity and elevated BNP, to identify patients with a very poor prognosis who should be considered for early valve replacement rather than delayed until symptoms develop. Additionally, patients with severe AS who are asymptomatic should be considered for exercise stress test to see if they are truly without symptoms (low exercise tolerance) or if the BP drops with exercise, both which would be indications for a heart team referral.
- In asymptomatic patients, Doppler echocardiography is recommended every 6 to 12 mo for severe aortic stenosis, every 1 to 2 yr for moderate disease, and every 2 to 3 yr for mild disease. Should have a low threshold to repeated echocardiogram for any change in symptoms or exam.
- Referral to cardiology should be considered in any patients with severe AS and in particular those with low-flow, low-gradient (low ejection fraction) symptomatic aortic stenosis for further workup (dobutamine stress echo).
- Balloon valvuloplasty is useful in infants and children or poor surgical candidates who do not have calcified valve apparatus; it can be done as an intermediate procedure to stabilize high-risk patients before surgery.
- Role of palliative care:
  If life expectancy with aortic valve replacement (SAVR or TAVR) is <1 yr **or** the patient's quality of

TABLE 2 ACC/AHA Guidelines for Aortic Valve Replacement (AVR) for Aortic Stenosis (AS)

Class	Indication	LOE
I	AVR with severe high-gradient AS who have symptoms by history or on exercise testing (stage D1).	B
	AVR for asymptomatic patients with severe AS (stage C2) and LVEF less than 50%.	B
	AVR for patients with severe AS (stage C or D) when undergoing other cardiac surgery.	B
IIa	AVR is reasonable for asymptomatic patients with very severe AS (stage C1, aortic velocity ≥5 m/sec) and low surgical risk.	B
	AVR is reasonable in asymptomatic patients (stage C1) with severe AS and decreased exercise tolerance or an exercise fall in blood pressure.	B
	AVR is reasonable in symptomatic patients with low-flow/low-gradient severe AS with reduced LVEF (stage D2) with a low-dose dobutamine stress study that shows an aortic velocity of 4 m/sec or more (or mean pressure gradient ≥40 mm Hg) with a valve area of 1.0 cm^2 or less at any dobutamine dose.	B
	AVR is reasonable in symptomatic patients with low-flow, low-gradient severe AS (stage D3) who are normotensive and have LVEF of 50% or greater, if clinical, hemodynamic, and anatomic data support valve obstruction as the most likely cause of symptoms.	C
	AVR is reasonable for patients with moderate AS (stage B) (aortic velocity, 3.0-3.9 m/sec) who are undergoing other cardiac surgery.	C
IIb	AVR may be considered for asymptomatic patients with severe AS (stage C1) and rapid disease progression and low surgical risk.	C

LOE, Level of evidence; *LVEF,* left ventricular ejection fraction.
From Zipes DP: *Braunwald's heart disease, a textbook of cardiovascular medicine*, ed 11, Philadelphia, 2019, Elsevier.

TABLE 3 Updated 2020 ACC/AHA Guidelines for Choice of Surgical Versus Transcatheter Treatment of Aortic Stenosis (AS)

Class	Indication	LOE
I	For patients in whom TAVR or high-risk surgical AVR is being considered, members of a heart valve team should collaborate to provide optimal patient care.	A
	For symptomatic and asymptomatic patients with severe AS and any indication for AVR who are **<65 yr of age** or have a life expectancy >20 yr, SAVR is recommended. (*Modified 2020*)	A
	For symptomatic patients with severe AS who are **65 to 80 yr of age** and have no anatomic contraindication to transfemoral TAVI, either SAVR or transfemoral TAVI is recommended after shared decision making about the balance between expected patient longevity and valve durability. (*Modified 2020*)	A
	For symptomatic patients with severe AS who are **>80 yr of age** or for younger patients with a life expectancy <10 yr and no anatomic contraindication to transfemoral TAVI, transfemoral TAVI is recommended in preference to SAVR. (*Modified 2020*)	A
I	For patients with an indication for AVR for whom a bioprosthetic valve is preferred but valve or vascular anatomy or other factors are not suitable for transfemoral TAVI, SAVR is recommended. (*Modified 2020*)	A
I	For symptomatic patients of any age with severe AS and a high or prohibitive surgical risk, TAVI is recommended if predicted post-TAVI survival is >12 mo with an acceptable quality of life. (*Modified 2020*)	A
IIb	Percutaneous aortic balloon dilation may be considered as a bridge to surgical or transcatheter AVR in severely symptomatic/critically ill patients with severe AS.	C

ACC, American College of Cardiology; *AHA,* American Heart Association; *AVR,* aortic valve replacement; *LOE,* level of evidence; *TAVR,* transcatheter AVR.
From Otto CM et al: Guideline for the management of valvular heart disease, *JACC* 77(4):e25-197, 2021.

life is unlikely to improve after aortic valve replacement (due to coexisting significant comorbidities), palliative care consultation is extremely valuable as it focuses on shared decision making as well as improving quality of life without interruption of conservative medical therapy.[1]

REFERENCES
Available at eBooks.Health.Elsevier.com.

RELATED CONTENT
Aortic Stenosis (Patient Information)

AUTHORS: **AHMAD MUSTAFA, MD** and **CRAIG L. BASMAN, MD, FACC, FSCAI**

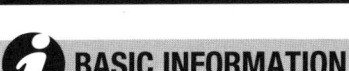

BASIC INFORMATION

DEFINITION

- Aphasia is an acquired disorder of language resulting from brain damage to the dominant (typically left) hemisphere. Brain lesions causing aphasia are illustrated in Fig. E1. The damage may be vascular, traumatic, neuro-degenerative, neoplastic, infectious, or inflammatory. Stroke is by far the most common cause of aphasia.
- Aphasia is not the same as dysarthria (a disorder of the neuromuscular control of speech) dysphonia (a disorder of the voice), apraxia of speech (disorder of programming of articulation of sequences of phonemes, especially consonants), aphemia (muteness with normal reading, writing, and comprehension), or stuttering.
- Language has a specific neuroanatomy, and aphasia manifests differently depending on the part of the language system that is damaged. Fig. E2 depicts most of the major nodes of the language system. Fig. E3 is a schematic of how the brain processes and produces language.

SYNONYMS

- Aphasia conductive
- Aphasia, expressive (difficulty speaking)
- Aphasia, expressive and receptive
- Aphasia, receptive
- Aphasia-angular gyrus syndrome
- Conduction aphasia
- Expressive dysphasia
- Global aphasia
- Psycho-sensory aphasia

ICD-10 CM CODES
R47.01	Aphasia
I69.320	Aphasia following cerebral infarction
I69.020	Aphasia following nontraumatic subarachnoid hemorrhage
I69.120	Aphasia following nontraumatic intracerebral hemorrhage
I69.920	Aphasia following unspecified cerebrovascular disease

EPIDEMIOLOGY & DEMOGRAPHICS

PREVALENCE: The United States has >1 million survivors of stroke-related aphasia. Aphasia is common after acute stroke, with 21% to 38% of stroke patients experiencing aphasia and almost 80% still experiencing aphasia at 12 mo after the stroke.

DIAGNOSIS

- Although aphasia can arise from any acquired damage to the language network, stroke-related aphasia is the most common cause.
- Box 1 summarizes the clinical evaluation of a patient with aphasia. Salient features of nonfluent (Table 1) and fluent (Table 2) are described in Table 3.
- The presence of aphasia may be obvious when listening to a patient's spontaneous speech

BOX 1   Clinical Evaluation for Aphasia

Spontaneous speech: Fluent versus nonfluent
Verbal tests
  Comprehension
    Ability to follow simple requests, e.g., "Please, pick up your hand"
    Ability to follow complex requests, e.g., "Please, show me your left ring finger, and stick out your tongue"
  Naming
    Common objects: Tie, keys, pen
    Uncommon objects: Watchband, belt buckle
  Repetition
    Simple phrases: e.g., "The boy went to the store"
    Complex phrases: e.g., "No if's, and's, or but's"
Reading and writing tests

From Kaufman DM et al: *Kaufman's clinical neurology for psychiatrists,* ed 9, Philadelphia, 2023, Elsevier.

TABLE 1   Nonfluent Aphasias

	Comprehension	Repetition
Broca's	Intact	Lost
Transcortical motor	Intact	Intact
Mixed transcortical	Lost (isolation)	Intact
Global	Lost	Lost

From Kaufman DM et al: *Kaufman's clinical neurology for psychiatrists,* ed 9, Philadelphia, 2023, Elsevier.

TABLE 2   Fluent Aphasias

	Comprehension	Repetition
Wernicke's	Lost	Lost
Transcortical sensory	Lost	Intact
Conduction	Intact	Lost
Anomic	Intact	Intact

From Kaufman DM et al: *Kaufman's clinical neurology for psychiatrists,* ed 9, Philadelphia, 2023, Elsevier.

TABLE 3   Salient Features of the Nonfluent and Fluent Aphasias

Feature	Nonfluent	Fluent
Other terms	Expressive Motor Brocass	Receptive Sensory Wernickeee
Spontaneous speech		
Content	Paucity of words, mostly nouns and verbs	Complete sentences with normal syntax
Articulation	Dysarthric, slow, stuttering	Good
Errors	Telegraphic speech	Paraphasic errors, circumlocutions, tangentialities, clang associations
Associated deficits	Right hemiparesis (arm, face, leg)	Hemianopsia, hemisensory loss
Localization of lesion	Frontal lobe	Temporal or parietal lobe Occasionally diffuse

From Kaufman DM et al: *Kaufman's clinical neurology for psychiatrists,* ed 9, Philadelphia, 2023, Elsevier.

but can be mistaken for or coexist with encephalopathy or delirium, making the diagnosis more difficult in the acute setting.
- Stroke-related aphasia will arise suddenly and will have associated neurologic signs and symptoms referable to the affected vascular

territory, typically the territory of the left middle cerebral artery or its branches or even more severely, the left internal carotid artery.
- When an acute cerebrovascular event is suspected, the history, physical examination, evaluation, and treatment are all geared to

determining the underlying cause of the acute change and implementing appropriate therapies in a timely manner.

- Once a patient with acute onset of aphasia is stabilized, evaluated, and treated with time-sensitive interventions, a more thorough examination of the patient's language deficit may be undertaken. This same approach to the bedside evaluation of aphasia applies to patients presenting with subacute and chronic language complaints. This evaluation allows for localization of the aphasia and the generation of an appropriate differential diagnosis (Table 4).
- The history should include questions about the time of onset (acute vs. insidious), the duration and tempo of symptom progression (acute change, rapid deterioration, or slowly progressive), accompanying constitutional, autonomic (e.g., orthostasis, bowel or bladder incontinence), neurologic (e.g., focal weakness or numbness, falls, Parkinsonism, seizures), and neuropsychiatric (e.g., apathy, disinhibition, lack of empathy, aggression,

depression, visual or auditory hallucinations, delusions, changes in sleep, acting out of dreams) symptoms.

- In addition to performing a neurologic examination, the patient presenting with a language complaint should undergo a thorough assessment of language function as well as cognitive screening. Language assessment begins with an analysis of a patient's fluency and speech content, most easily achieved by listening to a patient's spontaneous speech during the interview or by asking open-ended questions. Other critical elements of the bedside language examination include assessing comprehension (asking the patient to follow increasingly complex commands or to interpret the meaning of sentences with complex syntax), naming (of both common and uncommon objects), reading (regular and irregular words aloud as well as assessing reading comprehension), writing (spontaneously, to dictation, and copying), and repetition (of both simple and grammatically complex phrases).

DIFFERENTIAL DIAGNOSIS
NEURODEGENERATIVE CAUSES OF APHASIA:

- Language function is among the cognitive domains affected by Alzheimer disease (AD) even in early clinical stages. Patients develop difficulty understanding others, will sometimes use the incorrect word, and will have trouble getting words out and finding the correct word.
- Primary progressive aphasias (PPAs) are a group of neurodegenerative disorders in which an aspect of the language network is the primary target of degeneration. The PPAs include nonfluent/agrammatic variant of PPA (nfvPPA) and the semantic variant of PPA (svPPA), both classified under the umbrella of frontotemporal lobar degeneration (FTLD), as well as logopenic progressive aphasia (lvPPA), an atypical variant of AD pathology. Table 5 outlines the clinical features and localization.
- In nfvPPA, patients present with nonfluent, agrammatic speech, with some also experiencing apraxia of speech. Degeneration of

TABLE 4 Principal Aphasia Syndromes Due to Stroke

Type	Lesion Site	Fluency	Comprehension	Repetition	Naming	Other Signs
Broca (expressive)	Inferior frontal lobe	↓	Good	↓	↓	Contralateral weakness
Wernicke (receptive)	Posterior superior temporal lobe	Good	↓	↓	↓	Homonymous hemianopia
Transcortical motor	Inferior frontal gyrus	↓	Good	Good	May be normal	May be contralateral weakness
Transcortical sensory	Middle temporal gyrus, thalamus	Good	↓	Good	Usually normal	May be normal
Conduction	Supramarginal gyrus	Good	Good	↓	↓	None
Global	Frontal lobe (large)	↓	↓	↓	↓	Hemiplegia

↓, Reduced.
From Wing EJ, Schiffman FJ: *Cecil essentials of medicine*, ed 10, Philadelphia, 2022, Elsevier.

TABLE 5 Clinical Characteristics of Primary Progressive Aphasia

	Clinical Features*	Cortical Atrophy	Pathologic Changes†	Alternative Nomenclature
Nonfluent/agrammatic PPA	Grammatical simplification and errors in language production Effortful, halting speech with speech sound errors Two or more of the following: Impaired syntactic comprehension, spared content word comprehension, or spared object knowledge	Left inferior frontal and insula	FTLD-tau (52%), AD (25%), FTLD-TDP (19%), and other (4%)	Progressive nonfluent aphasia (PNFA) Agrammatic PPA (PPA-G)
Semantic variant PPA	Poor confrontation naming Impaired single-word comprehension Three or more of the following: Poor object or person knowledge or both; surface dyslexia; spared repetition; or spared motor speech	Anterior and ventral temporal lobe	FTLD-TDP (69%), AD (25%), and FTLD-tau (6%)	Semantic dementia (SD) Semantic PPA (PPA-S)
Logopenic variant PPA	Impaired single-word retrieval Impaired repetition of phrases and sentences Three or more of the following: Speech sound errors, spared motor speech, spared single-word comprehension and object knowledge, or absence of agrammatism	Left posterior superior temporal and inferior parietal	AD (50%), FTLD-TDP (38%), and FTLD-tau (12%)	Logopenic progressive aphasia (LPA) Logopenic PPA (PPA-L) Progressive mixed aphasia (PMA)

AD, Alzheimer disease; *FTLD-tau*, frontotemporal lobar degeneration with tau-positive pathology; *FTLD-TDP*, frontotemporal lobar degeneration with ubiquitin-positive and TDP-43-positive pathology; *PPA*, primary progressive aphasia.
*Based on expert consensus.
†From a literature review of confirmed pathologic changes in patients with PPA recruited without a-priori bias.
Reprinted with permission from Elsevier. From Grossman M: The non-fluent/agrammatic variant of primary progressive aphasia, *Lancet Neurol* 11(6):545-555, 2012. https://doi.org/10.1016/s1474-4422(12)70099-6.

TABLE 6   Supportive Communication Strategies for Aphasia

Verbal Strategies	Environmental Strategies	Visual Strategies
• Speak slowly but with a natural tone and rhythm • Use short, simple sentences • Gently give two or three options when providing choices • Ask yes or no questions • Use writing, gestures, or drawing in addition to speaking • Give the person more time to speak • Repeat your question or instructions if the person asks or seems unsure • Repeat what the person says to make sure you understood correctly • Ignore simple mistakes that do not change the meaning of the message (do not correct the person)	• Remove distractions (e.g., turn off the TV, close the door) • Adjust lighting so the person can see you easily • Sit or stand facing the person when speaking or listening to the person; make eye contact • Keep communication tools nearby (e.g., pen/paper, communication book, picture) • Limit group conversations to only a few people	• Use direct eye contact • Use gestures to enhance your message (e.g., thumbs up/down) • Write important words you are saying to help the person understand • Write notes when communication breakdown occurs and return to them later • Point to objects/pictures as you talk to give the person a visual of what you are saying • If written information is being provided, leave extra white space on the paper, use short sentences, and use simple language

From Armour M et al: Supportive communication for individuals with aphasia, *Arch Phys Med Rehabil* 102(7);1437-1439, 2021. https://doi.org/10.1016/j.apmr.2021.03.008.

BOX 2   Stimulation-Facilitation Approaches for Aphasia Therapy

- Gestural expression and pointing
- Word-to-picture matching
- Yes/no response reliability
- Oral-motor imitation
- Phoneme, then word repetition
- Verbal cueing for words and sentence completion
- Contextual cueing
- Phonemic and semantic word-retrieval strategies
- Priming for responses
- Auditory processing at phrase level and then sentence level
- Word-, phrase-, then sentence-level reading
- Melodic stimulation
- Graphic tasks: Tracing, copying, word completions
- Calculations
- Pragmatic linguistic and nonlinguistic conversational skills
- Psychosocial supports

From Jankovic J et al: *Bradley and Daroff's neurology in clinical practice,* ed 8, Philadelphia, 2022, Elsevier.

the left posterior frontoinsular association cortex is the cause of this language-based dementia.

- In svPPA, patients develop difficulty naming, loss of object knowledge, and surface dyslexia (the inability to read irregular words properly) typically to the result of left anterior temporal lobe degeneration. However, this variant can begin in the right anterior temporal lobe, causing difficulty recognizing faces and meaning of facial expressions, before spreading to the left anterior temporal lobe and causing semantic language dysfunction.
- In lvPPA, patients have impaired naming and sentence repetition, develop long pauses in their speech, and experience phonologic errors in their speech. This variant arises from left posterior perisylvian or parietal association cortex degeneration.

WORKUP

- Targeted to the underlying etiology of the aphasia but will always include neuroimaging, preferably MRI of the brain.
- In nonstroke aphasia and in patients without significant kidney disease, MRI should be done with and without contrast.
- In stroke-related aphasia, acute neuroimaging will include a brain computed tomography (CT) and CT angiogram of the head and neck. An MRI can be performed after acute interventions have been performed.
- Advanced neuroimaging techniques such as fluorodeoxyglucose (FDG)-PET may be appropriate for neurodegenerative aphasias.

LABORATORY TESTS

Targeted to the underlying etiology of the aphasia. In stroke-related aphasia, the laboratory workup will include an assessment of vascular risk factors. In a neurodegenerative aphasia, the assessment will be similar to that for AD.

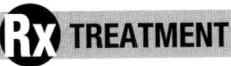 TREATMENT

NONPHARMACOLOGIC THERAPY

Speech language therapy. Commonly used techniques include script training, response elaboration training, constraint-induced aphasia therapy, speech entrainment, and melodic intonation therapy.

ACUTE GENERAL Rx

Target the underlying cause of the aphasia

CHRONIC Rx

Target the underlying cause of aphasia and include speech language therapy.

REFERRAL

- Neurology
- Speech language pathology
- Neuropsychology
- Physical medicine and rehabilitation
- Psychiatry

❗ PEARLS & CONSIDERATIONS

COMMENTS

- Recovery from poststroke aphasia is very difficult to predict. The most important factors correlating with recovery are the lesion location and size, aphasia type and severity, and to some extent the nature of early hemodynamic response to acute interventions such as thrombolysis, and treatment received.
- Most studies attest that recovery is inversely related to the size of lesion, with a preserved left superior temporal gyrus as one of the most important factors for satisfactory recovery and intact basal ganglia also contributing significantly to better recovery.
- Broca and conduction aphasia enjoy better recovery than global and anomic aphasia.

PREVENTION

Prevention of stroke-related aphasia involves modification of vascular risk factors.

PATIENT/FAMILY EDUCATION

Teach families of aphasia patients about supportive communication strategies (Table 6)

SUGGESTED READINGS

Available at eBooks.Health.Elsevier.com.

RELATED CONTENT

Stroke, Ischemic (Related key Topic)
Alzheimer Disease (Related key Topic)
Frontotemporal Dementia (Related key Topic)

AUTHOR: **JOSEPH S. KASS, MD, JD, FAAN**

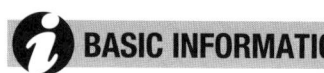
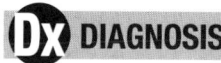

BASIC INFORMATION

DEFINITION

Appendicitis is the acute inflammation of the vermiform appendix.

ICD-10CM CODES

K35.2	Acute appendicitis with generalized peritonitis
K35.3	Acute appendicitis with localized peritonitis
K35.80	Unspecified acute appendicitis
K35.89	Other acute appendicitis
K36	Other appendicitis
K37	Unspecified appendicitis

EPIDEMIOLOGY & DEMOGRAPHICS

- Appendicitis occurs in 10% of the population, most commonly between the ages of 10 and 30 yr. Median age is 22 yr. Lifetime risk is 7% to 8%.[1]
- Approximately 300,000 appendectomies are performed in the U.S. each yr.
- It is the most common abdominal surgical emergency.
- Incidence of appendicitis has declined over the past 30 yr.
- Male:female ratio is 3:2 until mid-20s; it equalizes after age 30 yr.

PHYSICAL FINDINGS & CLINICAL PRESENTATION

- In children with abdominal pain, fever is the single most useful sign associated with appendicitis. Vomiting, rectal tenderness, and rebound tenderness along with fever are more indicative of appendicitis in children than in adults.
- Abdominal pain: Initially the pain may be epigastric or periumbilical in nearly 50% of patients; it subsequently localizes to the right lower quadrant within 12 to 18 h. Pain can be found in back or right flank if appendix is retrocecal or in other abdominal locations if there is malrotation of the appendix.
- Pain with right thigh extension *(psoas sign)*, low-grade fever: Temperature may be >38° C (100.4° F) if there is appendiceal perforation.
- Pain with internal rotation of the flexed right thigh *(obturator sign)* is present.
- Right lower quadrant (RLQ) pain on palpation of the left lower quadrant (LLQ) *(Rovsing sign):* Physical examination may reveal right-sided tenderness in patients with pelvic appendix.
- Point of maximum tenderness is in the RLQ *(McBurney point)*.
- Nausea, vomiting, tachycardia, cutaneous hyperesthesias at the level of T12 can be present.

ETIOLOGY

Obstruction of the appendiceal lumen with subsequent vascular congestion, inflammation, and edema; common causes of obstruction are:

- Fecaliths: 30% to 35% of cases (most common in adults)
- Foreign body: 4% (fruit seeds, pinworms, tapeworms, roundworms, calculi)
- Inflammation: 50% to 60% of cases (submucosal lymphoid hyperplasia [most common etiology in children, teens])
- Neoplasms: 1% (carcinoids, metastatic disease, carcinoma)

DIAGNOSIS

DIFFERENTIAL DIAGNOSIS

- Intestinal: Regional cecal enteritis, incarcerated hernia, cecal diverticulitis, intestinal obstruction, perforated ulcer, perforated cecum, Meckel diverticulitis
- Reproductive: Ectopic pregnancy, ovarian cyst, torsion of ovarian cyst, salpingitis, tuboovarian abscess, mittelschmerz, endometriosis, seminal vesiculitis
- Renal: Renal and ureteral calculi, neoplasms, pyelonephritis
- Vascular: Leaking aortic aneurysm
- Psoas abscess
- Trauma
- Cholecystitis
- Mesenteric adenitis
- Table 1 summarizes the differential diagnosis of appendicitis

WORKUP (FIG. 1)

Patients with RLQ pain, nausea, vomiting, anorexia, and RLQ rebound tenderness should undergo prompt clinical and laboratory evaluation. Imaging studies are generally not necessary in typical appendicitis and generally reserved for patients with an equivocal likelihood of

---

TABLE 1   Differential Diagnosis of Appendicitis

Diagnosis	Findings That Help Differentiate Entity From Appendicitis
Bacterial or viral enteritis	Nausea, vomiting, and diarrhea are severe; pain usually develops after vomiting.
Epiploic appendagitis	Focal abdominal pain and tenderness without migration or progression of the pain; patients have a paucity of other GI symptoms such as anorexia or nausea. Laboratory findings are usually normal.
Mesenteric adenitis	Duration of symptoms is longer; fever is uncommon; RLQ physical findings are less marked; WBC count is usually normal.
Pyelonephritis	Pain is more likely to be felt in the right flank; high fever and rigors are common; marked pyuria or bacteriuria and urinary symptoms are present; abdominal rigidity is less marked.
Renal colic	Pain radiates to the right groin; significant hematuria; character of the pain is clearly colicky.
Acute pancreatitis	Pain and vomiting are more severe; tenderness is less well localized; serum amylase and lipase levels are elevated.
Crohn disease	History of recurrent similar attacks; diarrhea is more common; palpable mass is more common; extraintestinal manifestations may have occurred or be present.
Cholecystitis	History of prior attacks is common; pain and tenderness are greater; radiation of pain is to the right shoulder; nausea is more marked; liver biochemical tests are more likely to be abnormal.
Meckel diverticulitis	Nearly impossible to distinguish preoperatively from appendicitis.
Cecal diverticulitis	Difficult to distinguish preoperatively from appendicitis; symptoms are milder and of longer duration; CT is helpful; patients are usually older.
Sigmoid diverticulitis	Usually occurs in older patients; changes in bowel habits are more common; radiation of the pain is to the suprapubic area, not RLQ; fever and WBC count are higher.
Small bowel obstruction	History of abdominal surgery; pain is colicky; vomiting and distention are more marked; RLQ localization is uncommon.
Ectopic pregnancy	History of menstrual irregularities; characteristic progression of symptoms is absent; syncope; positive pregnancy test.
Ruptured ovarian cyst	Occurs in the middle of the menstrual cycle; pain is of sudden onset; nausea and vomiting are less common; WBC count is normal.
Ovarian torsion	Vomiting is more marked and occurs at the same time as the pain; progression of symptoms is absent; abdominal or pelvic mass often is palpable.
Acute salpingitis or tuboovarian abscess	Longer duration of symptoms; pain begins in the lower abdomen; often there is a history of STDs; vaginal discharge and marked cervical tenderness often are present.

CT, Computed tomography; *GI,* gastrointestinal; *IV,* intravenous; *RLQ,* right lower quadrant; *STD,* sexually transmitted disease; *WBC,* white blood cell.
From Feldman M et al: *Sleisenger and Fordtran's gastrointestinal and liver disease,* ed 10, Philadelphia, 2016, Elsevier.

General approach to the patient with suspected appendicitis

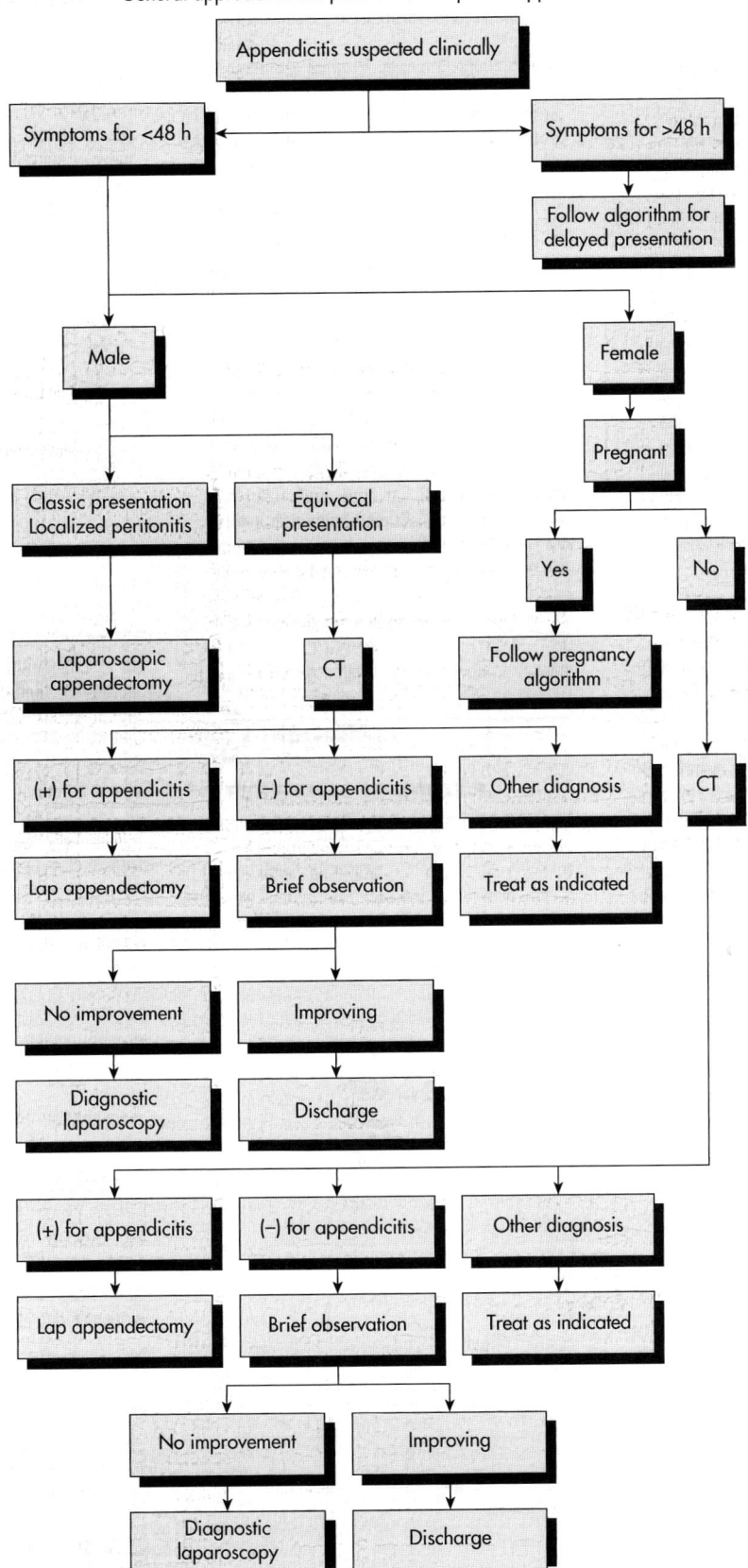

FIG. 1 Suggested algorithm for the approach to the patient with possible appendicitis. *CT,* Computed tomography; *Lap,* laparoscopic. (From Townsend CM et al: *Sabiston textbook of surgery,* ed 21, St Louis, 2022, Elsevier.)

appendicitis. They are useful when the diagnosis is uncertain. Several clinical decision tools such as the Alvarado score (also known as the MANTRELS criteria) are available to assist in the diagnosis of appendicitis (Table 2). Laparoscopy may be useful as both a diagnostic and a therapeutic modality.

LABORATORY TESTS

- Complete blood count with differential reveals leukocytosis with a left shift in 90% of patients with appendicitis. Total white blood cell (WBC) count is generally lower than 20,000/mm^3. Higher counts may be indicative of perforation. Less than 4% have a normal WBC and differential. A WBC count <10,000/mm^3 decreases the likelihood of appendicitis. Low hemoglobin and hematocrit levels in an older patient should raise suspicion for gastrointestinal tract carcinoma.
- Microscopic hematuria and pyuria may occur in <20% of patients.
- Human chorionic gonadotropin to rule out pregnancy in females of reproductive age.

IMAGING STUDIES

- Multidetector computed tomography (CT; Fig. 2) is a useful test for routine evaluation of suspected appendicitis in adults. CT of the abdomen/pelvis without contrast has a sensitivity of >90% and an accuracy >94% for acute appendicitis. A distended appendix, periappendiceal inflammation, and a thickened appendiceal wall are indicative of appendicitis. Table 3 describes CT findings of appendicitis. In children and young adults, exposure to CT radiation is of particular concern. Trials with low-dose CT (116 mGy cm) have shown that low-dose CT is not inferior to standard-dose CT (521 mGy cm)

with respect to negative (unnecessary) appendectomy rates in young adults with suspected appendicitis.
- Ultrasonography (Fig. E3) has a sensitivity of 75% to 90% for the diagnosis of acute appendicitis, although it is highly operator dependent and difficult in patients with large body habitus. Ultrasound is useful, especially in pregnancy and in younger women when

diagnosis is unclear. Normal ultrasonographic findings should not deter surgery if the history and physical examination are indicative of appendicitis.
- MRI of the abdomen and pelvis can also be used to accurately diagnose acute appendicitis in pregnant patients (100% sensitivity, 93.6% specificity) without exposure to ionizing radiation.

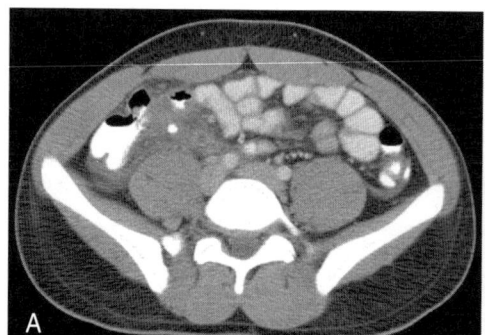
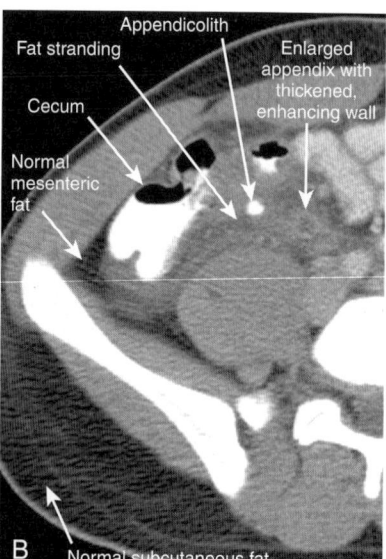

FIG. 2 Appendicitis, computed tomography (CT) with intravenous (IV) and oral contrast. This CT demonstrates classic findings of appendicitis in an 18-yr-old male with right lower quadrant pain, as seen with CT with IV and oral contrast. Studies suggest that CT without contrast has similar sensitivity and specificity. An enlarged appendix is seen near the cecum as a right lower quadrant tubular structure in short-axis cross section, giving it a circular appearance. The surrounding fat shows stranding, a smoky appearance indicating inflammation (compare with normal mesenteric and subcutaneous fat, which is nearly black). The appendiceal wall shows enhancement, a brightening after administration of IV contrast. This slice also shows an appendicolith, an occasional finding of appendicitis. It does not appear to be within the appendix in this slice, because the appendix bends in and out of the plane of this slice. An appendicolith usually appears as a calcified (white) rounded structure, visible without any contrast. **A**, Axial CT image. **B**, Close-up. (From Broder JS: *Diagnostic imaging for the emergency physician*, Philadelphia, 2011, Saunders.)

TABLE 2 Alvarado Score (MANTRELS Criteria)

Criterion		Point(s)
Symptoms		
M	Migration of pain to RLQ	1
A	Anorexia	1
N	Nausea and vomiting	1
Signs		
T	Tenderness in RLQ	2
R	Rebound pain	1
E	Elevated temperature	1
Laboratory Findings		
L	Leukocytosis	2
S	Shift of WBCs to left	1
Total Score		10
Interpretation		
1-4	Appendicitis unlikely	
5-6	Appendicitis possible	
7-8	Probable appendicitis	
9-10	Surgery indicated	

RLQ, Right lower quadrant; *WBCs*, white blood cells.
From Cameron P et al: *Textbook of adult emergency medicine*, ed 5, Philadelphia, 2019, Elsevier.

TABLE 3 Computed Tomography Findings of Appendicitis: SCALPEL Mnemonic

Term	Description
Stranding	Fat stranding suggests regional inflammation, possibly because of appendicitis.
Cecum	The appendix originates from the cecum, which should be identified first to help localize the appendix. The cecum may show wall thickening, suggesting appendicitis.
Air	Air outside of the lumen of the appendix is pathologic and suggests perforation. Air within the appendiceal wall is also abnormal.
Large	The normal appendix is <6 mm; an enlarged appendix >6 mm suggests appendicitis. Wall thickening >1 mm also suggests appendicitis.
Phlegmon	Inflammatory changes surrounding the appendix suggest a perforated appendix. A heterogeneous collection called a phlegmon may be seen. If the appendix has ruptured, a pericecal phlegmon may be the only remaining evidence, because the appendix itself may not be seen.
Enhancement	The wall of an abnormal appendix enhances with IV contrast and appears brighter than the normal bowel or the normal psoas muscle.
Lith	An appendicolith is a calcified stone sometimes found in the lumen of an inflamed appendix.

IV, Intravenous.
From Broder JS: *Diagnostic imaging for the emergency physician*, Philadelphia, 2011, Saunders.

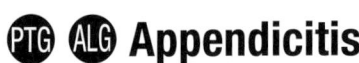
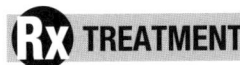 **TREATMENT**

NONPHARMACOLOGIC THERAPY

- Nothing by mouth
- Do not administer analgesics until the diagnosis is made

ACUTE GENERAL Rx

- Urgent appendectomy (laparoscopic [Fig. E4] or open), correction of fluid and electrolyte imbalance with vigorous intravenous (IV) hydration, and electrolyte replacement.
- IV antibiotic prophylaxis to cover gram-negative bacilli and anaerobes (ampicillin/sulbactam 3 g IV q6h or piperacillin/tazobactam 4.5 g IV q8h in adults). For patients who undergo appendectomy, antibiotics should be discontinued postoperatively.[1]
- If nonoperative treatment is anticipated, then the administration of a long active parenteral antibiotic (ertapenem or ceftriaxone). Along with high dose, once daily metronidazole can facilitate early discharge. Parenteral antibiotics are followed by oral regimen of metronidazole plus advanced generation cephalosporin or fluoroquinolones for 7 to 10 days.[1]
  Management of Complicated Appendicitis:
- Fig. E5 is an algorithm for managing the patient with delayed presentation of appendicitis and possible diffuse peritonitis
- The management of the pregnant patient with possible appendicitis is illustrated in Fig. E6

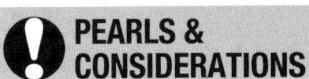 **PEARLS & CONSIDERATIONS**

COMMENTS

- Perforation is common (20% in adult patients). Indicators of perforation are pain lasting >24 h, leukocytosis >20,000/mm^3, temperature >102° F (38.9° C), palpable abdominal mass, and peritoneal findings (Fig. E7).

- In general, prognosis is excellent. Mortality rate is <1% in young adults without complications; however, it exceeds 10% in elderly patients with ruptured appendix.
- In approximately 20% of patients who undergo exploratory laparotomy because of suspected appendicitis, the appendix is normal.
- An increasing amount of evidence[2,3] supports the use of antibiotics instead of surgery for treating patients with uncomplicated appendicitis.[4] Fig. E8 illustrates an algorithm for the nonoperative management of appendicitis. A trial assessing the feasibility of nonoperative management for uncomplicated acute appendicitis in children using either IV piperacillin-tazobactam or ciprofloxacin metronidazole therapy for at least 24 h followed by oral antibiotics for 10 days revealed that 90% of children managed nonoperatively had no progression within 30 days. Another trial among patients with CT-proven, uncomplicated appendicitis revealed that antibiotic treatment did not meet the prescribed criterion for noninferiority compared with appendectomy. Most patients randomized to antibiotic treatment for uncomplicated appendicitis did not require appendectomy during the 1-yr follow-up period, and those who required appendectomy did not experience significant complications. A 5-yr follow-up of antibiotic therapy for uncomplicated acute appendicitis in the APPAC randomized clinical trial revealed that among patients who were initially treated with antibiotics for uncomplicated acute appendicitis, the likelihood of late recurrence within 5 yr was 39.1%. A more recent trial also confirmed that antibiotics are not inferior to appendectomy on the basis of a health status questionnaire; however, in the antibiotics group nearly 3 in 10 participants had unresolved appendectomy by 90 days and those with an appendicolith had a higher risk for appendectomy and for complications. It remains to be determined whether the benefits of potentially avoiding an operation with antibiotics-first approach are outweighed by the burden to the patient related to future appendicitis episodes, more days of antibiotic therapy, lingering symptoms, and uncertainty that may affect quality of life. Factors associated with primary nonresponsiveness to antibiotics in adults with uncomplicated are the presence of an appendicolith, appendiceal diameter of ≥15 mm on imaging, and fever >38° C.[5]

REFERENCES & SUGGESTED READINGS

Available at eBooks.Health.Elsevier.com.

RELATED CONTENT

Appendicitis (Patient Information)

AUTHOR: **FRED F. FERRI, MD**

A

Diseases and Disorders

I

Arrhythmogenic Right Ventricular Dysplasia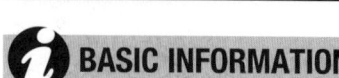

BASIC INFORMATION

DEFINITION

Arrhythmogenic right ventricular dysplasia (ARVD) is a cardiomyopathy characterized by replacement of the normal myocardium with fibrous or fibrofatty tissue, mainly of the right ventricle but also occasionally with involvement of the lateral or posterior left ventricle. Historically, these macroscropic pathologic changes appeared in the "triangle" of dysplasia, which involves the right ventricular inflow tract, outflow tract, and apex. It is defined clinically by palpitations, syncope, and potentially life-threatening right-sided ventricular arrhythmias and, at later stages, heart failure.[1]

SYNONYMS

Arrhythmogenic right ventricular cardiomyopathy
ARVC

ICD-10CM CODE
I42.8 Arrhythmogenic ventricular dysplasia

EPIDEMIOLOGY & DEMOGRAPHICS

PREVALENCE: The current prevalence of ARVD in adults is 1:2000 to 5000 persons. It is one of the leading causes of arrhythmic cardiac arrest in young people and athletes.
PREDOMINANT SEX & AGE: Mean age, 31 yr (range, 12 to 50 yr), predominantly male
RISK FACTORS: Family history of ARVD (present in nearly 50% of affected patients)

GENETICS:
- Autosomal dominant (most common) with variable penetrance and polymorphic phenotypic expression
- Autosomal recessive (rarely, e.g., Naxos disease)
- Several different gene mutations in desmosomal proteins
- Gene mutations can be identified in 50% of affected individuals

PHYSICAL FINDINGS & CLINICAL PRESENTATION
- ARVD can present with a wide range of clinical symptoms and severity from palpitations, syncope, and chest discomfort to ventricular tachycardia, sudden cardiac arrest, and signs of right ventricular failure such as dyspnea, edema, and fatigue. Patients may be clinically asymptomatic for many years.
- Cardiac arrest after exertion or at rest may be the initial presentation.
- Physical examination will be normal in most patients. Widely split S2 is an important diagnostic clue.

ETIOLOGY

ARVD is characterized by progressive replacement of mainly the right ventricular myocardium with fatty or fibrofatty tissue after apoptotic myocardial cell death caused by mutations of desmosomal proteins with isolated residual cardiac cells. Historically, these macroscropic pathologic changes appeared in the "triangle" of dysplasia, which involves the right ventricular inflow tract, outflow tract, and apex. However, it is now recognized that there is sparing of the right ventricular apex early in disease. There can be involvement of the posterolateral LV with sparing of the LV septum.[2]

DIAGNOSIS

A major criterion equals 2 points; a minor criterion equals 1 point. The diagnosis of ARVD is considered definite if the patient has 4 points and probable with 3 points. See Table 1 for diagnostic criteria.

DIFFERENTIAL DIAGNOSIS
- Cardiomyopathy with involvement of the right ventricle
- Uhl anomaly: Rare anomaly that presents mainly in childhood with signs and symptoms of right heart failure and characterized by a "paper-thin" right ventricle resulting from death of the myocytes throughout the right ventricle
- Idiopathic RV tachycardia
- Sarcoidosis
- Right ventricular infarction

WORKUP
- Initial workup includes history with focus on sudden death in the family, resting ECG, 24-Holter ECG, signal-averaged ECG, and imaging studies with echocardiography and cardiac MRI.
- ECG will have diagnostic findings in 50% to 90% of patients with ARVD, including T-wave inversions in anterior precordial leads V_1 to V_6, epsilon waves, and a QRS duration longer than 110 ms in V1 or >40 ms longer in V1 than V6 (Fig. 1).
- Ventricular tachycardia (VT) with a characteristic left bundle branch block pattern and frequent PVC's (>500 in 24 hr) might be detected by 24-hr Holter monitoring.
- An abnormal signal-averaged ECG is a minor diagnostic criteria.
- Echocardiography will show right ventricular dilation with regional wall motion abnormalities, increased diameter of the right ventricular outflow tract, aneurysms, and depressed RV function that varies with the severity of the disease.
- MRI (Fig. 2) is a noninvasive method to detect structural abnormalities (fibrofatty changes) and regional dysfunction. Cardiac MRI (CMR) is the most sensitive method to detect ARVD, but it has high false-positive rates. Cardiac CT angiogram (Fig. E3) will reveal thinning and aneurysmal dilation of the RV anterior wall and outflow tract.
- If the routine tests are not conclusive, endomyocardial biopsy and electrophysiologic testing can be considered. However, biopsies and radionuclide ventriculography are rarely performed in the U.S.

TREATMENT

There is no curative treatment available. The treatment goals are focused on preventing sudden cardiac death, symptomatic treatment of right heart failure, and pharmacologic and invasive treatment of arrhythmias. Therapy with cardio-selective beta-blockers, such as metoprolol succinate, is recommended in both those with a history of ventricular arrythmias and those with a history of ventricular arrythmias for prophylaxis. Family members with a negative phenotype (either healthy gene carriers or those with an unknown genotype) do not need any specific treatment other than sports restriction; however, lifelong clinical assessment with the use of noninvasive tests at least every 2 yr is warranted.

NONPHARMACOLOGIC THERAPY
- Avoidance of activity, especially moderate and high instensity exercise, that may trigger ventricular tachycardia and may lead to disease progression.
- For those with a definitive diagnosis of ARVD, implantable cardiodefibrillator (ICD) implantation needs to be considered if they are survivors of sudden cardiac arrest, have symptomatic ventricular tachycardia or ventricular fibrillation, have documented asymptomatic ventricular tachycardia or fibrillation, or have a left ventricular ejection fraction of 35% or less. Patients with unexplained syncope, advanced disease, documented ventricular arrhythmias, or a family history of sudden cardiac death or who have been resuscitated from cardiac arrest are at high risk. A subcutaneous ICD might be an alternative option instead of transvenous implantation.[3,4]
- Radiofrequency catheter ablation is used in cases of refractory VT or frequent tachycardia after defibrillator placement.
- Cardiac transplantation.
- Fig. 4 describes a management algorithm for ARVD.

PHARMACOLOGIC TREATMENT

Antiarrhythmic therapy with sotalol (first-line treatment) or amiodarone, often in combination with beta-blockers, is used for tachycardia suppression.

REFERRAL
- Early cardiology and electrophysiology referral
- Consider referring for genetic counseling

PEARLS & CONSIDERATIONS

PREVENTION

All first-degree relatives should be tested if ARVD is confirmed. Sports activity increases the risk of sudden cardiac death among adolescents and young adults with ARVC. The estimated overall mortality ranges from 0.08% to 3.6% per year.

REFERENCES
Available at eBooks.Health.Elsevier.com.

AUTHOR: **ROOP DUTTA, MD**

TABLE 1 Global or Regional Dysfunction and Structural Alterations

Major

2D echo criteria

Regional RV akinesia, dyskinesia, or aneurysm and one of the following measured at end diastole:

    PLAX RVOT $\geq$32 mm or

    PSAX RVOT $\geq$36

    Fractional area change $\leq$33%

    MRI criteria

Regional RV akinesia or dyskinesia or dyssynchronous RV contraction and one of the following:

    Ratio of RV end-diastolic volume to BSA >100, <110 ml/m^2 (male) or >100 ml/m^2

    RV ejection fraction >40% $\leq$45%

    RV angiography criteria

    Regional RV akinesia, dyskinesia, or aneurysm

Minor

2D echo criteria

Regional RV akinesia or dyskinesia or dyssynchronous RV contraction and one of the following measured at end diastole:

    PLAX RVOT $\geq$29 <32 mm or

    PSAX RVOT $\geq$32 <36

    Fractional area change >33% $\leq$40%

    MRI criteria

Regional RV akinesia or dyskinesia or dyssynchronous RV contraction and one of the following:

    Ratio of RV end-diastolic volume to BSA $\geq$110 ml/m^2 (male) or $\geq$100 ml/m^2

    RV ejection fraction $\leq$40%

Tissue characterization of wall

Major

Residual myocytes <60% by morphometric analysis (or <50% if estimated) with fibrous replacement of the RV free wall myocardium in >1 sample, with or without fatty replacement of tissue on endomyocardial biopsy

Minor

Residual myocytes 60%-75% by morphometric analysis (or 50%-65% if estimated), with fibrous replacement of the RV free wall myocardium in >1 sample with or without fatty replacement of tissue on endomyocardial biopsy

Repolarization abnormalities

Major

Inverted T waves in right precordial leads (V1, V2, and V3) or beyond in individuals >14 yr of age (in the absence of complete RBBB QRS $\geq$120 ms)

Minor

Inverted T waves in V1 and V2 in individuals >14 yr of age (in the absence of complete RBBB) or in V4, V5, and V6

Inverted T waves in leads V1, V2, V3, and V4 in individuals >14 yr of age in the presence of a complete RBBB

Depolarization or conduction abnormalities

Major

Epsilon wave (reproducible low-amplitude signals between end of QRS complex to onset of T wave) in the right precordial leads (V1-V3)

Minor

Late potentials by SAECG in $\geq$1 of 3 parameters in the absence of a QRSd of $\geq$110 ms on standard ECG

Filtered QRS $\geq$114 ms

Duration of terminal QRS <40 mV $\geq$38 ms

Root-mean-square voltage of terminal 40 ms $\leq$20 μV

Terminal activation duration $\geq$55 ms measured from the nadir of the end of the QRS, including R', in V1, V2, or V3 in absence of complete RBBB

Arrhythmias

Major

Nonsustained or sustained VT of LBBB morph with superior axis

Minor

Nonsustained or sustained VT of RVOT configuration, LBBB morph with inferior axis or of unknown axis

>500 PVCs per 24 hr (Holter)

Family history

Major

ARVD/C in first-degree relative who meets Task Force criteria

ARVD/C confirmed pathologically at autopsy or surgery in first-degree relative

Identification of pathogenic mutation categorized as associated or probably associated with ARVD/C in the patient under evaluation

Minor

History of ARVD/C in first-degree relative in whom it is not possible to determine whether the family member meets Task Force criteria

Premature sudden death (<35 yr of age) caused by suspected ARVD/C in a first-degree relative

ARVD/C confirmed pathologically or by current Task Force criteria in second-degree relative

A major criterion equals 2 points, a minor criterion 1 point. The diagnosis of arrhythmogenic right ventricular dysplasia (ARVD) is considered definite if the patient has 4 points and probable with 3 points. *BSA,* Body surface area; *ECG,* electrocardiogram; *MRI,* magnetic resonance imaging; *PLAX,* parasternal long axis; *PSAX,* parasternal short axis; *PVCs,* premature ventricular contractions; *RBBB,* right bundle branch block; *RV,* right ventricle; *RVOT,* right ventricular outflow tract; *SAECG,* signal-averaged electrocardiogram; *2D,* two dimensional; *VT,* ventricular tachycardia.

From Marcus IM: Diagnosis of arrhythmogenic right ventricular cardiomyopathy/dysplasia proposed modification of the Task Force criteria, *Circulation* 121:1533-1541, 2010.

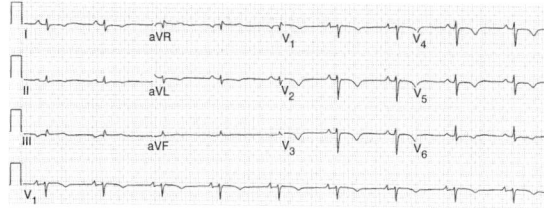

FIG. 1 Arrhythmogenic right ventricular cardiomyopathy—Epsilon wave. This 12-lead electrocardiogram tracing with lead Vfn[11] rhythm strip shows sinus rhythm with T-wave inversion over the right precordial leads. In addition, there is an epsilon wave (small deflection at the end of the QRS complex), evident in lead V[1], which is characteristic of arrhythmogenic right ventricular cardiomyopathy. (From Olshansky B et al: *Arrhythmia essentials,* ed 2, Philadelphia, 2017, Elsevier.)

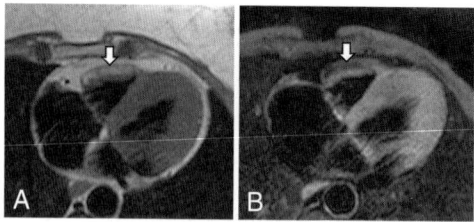

FIG. 2 Arrhythmogenic right ventricular cardiomyopathy. Spin-echo cardiovascular magnetic resonance without **(A)** and with **(B),** a fat-suppression prepulse. There is bright signal in the free wall of the right ventricle that suppresses with fat suppression *(arrows).* (From Selke FW et al: *Sabiston & Spencer surgery of the chest,* ed 9, Philadelphia, 2016, Elsevier.)

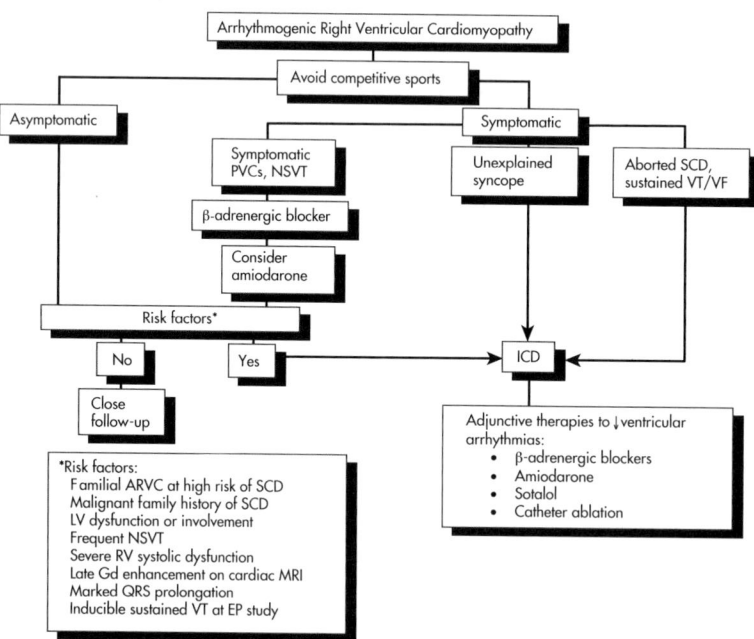

FIG. 4 Arrhythmogenic right ventricular cardiomyopathy. *ARVC,* Arrhythmogenic right ventricular cardiomyopathy; *EP,* electrophysiology; *Gd,* gadolinium; *ICD,* implantable cardiodefibrillator; *NSVT,* nonsustained ventricular tachycardia; *PVCs,* premature ventricular contractions; *SCD,* sequential compression device; *VF,* ventricular fibrillation; *VT,* ventricular tachycardia. (From Olshansky B et al: *Arrhythmia essentials,* ed 2, Philadelphia, 2017, Elsevier.)

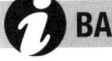
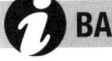 BASIC INFORMATION

DEFINITION

Asbestosis is a slow, progressive diffuse interstitial fibrosis as a consequence of dose-related inhalation exposure to fibers of asbestos in miners, millers, workers of asbestos textiles, and insulators. Clinically, the lung involvement is characterized by bilateral diffuse interstitial fibrosis, more pronounced in the lower lobes, and pleural thickening, leading to shortness of breath and dry cough.

Asbestos exposure can lead to the spectrum of pulmonary pathology, including pulmonary fibrosis; asbestos-related pleural plaque disease (ARPD), both focal and diffuse; and malignancies (lung cancer or mesothelioma).

ICD-10CM CODE
J61 Pneumoconiosis due to asbestos and other mineral fibers

EPIDEMIOLOGY & DEMOGRAPHICS

- 5 to 10 new cases per 100,000 persons per year in the U.S.
- Prolonged interval (20 to 30 years) between exposures to inhaled fibers and clinical manifestations of disease.
- Most common in workers over age 40 years involved in the primary extraction of asbestos from rock deposits and in those involved in the fabrication and installation of products containing asbestos (e.g., naval shipyards in World War II; installation of floor tiles, ceiling tiles, acoustic ceiling coverings, wall insulation, and pipe coverings in public buildings).
- Smokers and heavy drinkers have the greatest risk of developing this disease.

PHYSICAL FINDINGS & CLINICAL PRESENTATION

- Insidious onset of shortness of breath and dry cough with exertion is usually the first sign of asbestosis.
- Dyspnea becomes more severe as the disease advances; with time, progressively less exertion is tolerated.
- Cough is frequent and usually paroxysmal, dry, and nonproductive. Hemoptysis is rare but reported. Scant mucoid sputum may accompany the cough in the later stages of the disease.
- Fine end-respiratory crackles (rales, crepitations) are heard more predominantly in the lung bases.
- Digital clubbing, edema, and jugular venous distention may be present.
- Advanced cases may have signs of right heart failure.

ETIOLOGY/PATHOGENESIS

Inhalation of asbestos fibers. The pathogenesis of pulmonary interstitial inflammation and fibrosis is related to immune mechanisms. Asbestosis is known to be associated with positive serum antinuclear antibody (ANA) and rheumatoid factor (RF). An important role of interleukin-1beta (IL-1beta) in the pathogenesis of asbestosis and its systemic autoimmune manifestations has been reported.

Asbestos-Related Pulmonary Manifestations[1]:
- *Pleural Plaques:* Pleural plaques are the most common manifestation of prior asbestos exposure. They are usually a radiographic finding, and they do not cause any pulmonary symptoms. Usual presentation 20-30 yr after exposure.
- *Diffuse Pleural Thickening (DPT):* It is usually due to involvement of the visceral pleura. Occurs few years after exposure. It is thought to be due to fibrosis from chronic pleural irritation from asbestos. It is a radiographic finding and usually does not cause symptoms.
- *Rounded Atelectasis:* Always adjacent to the pleura, and vessels and bronchi entering the area of collapse appear bent, forming a "comet tail," which is typical for rounded atelectasis. Usually is asymptomatic, but if presenting with pleural effusion should be investigated further to rule out malignancy or infection.
- *Benign Asbestos Pleural Effusion:* Usually unilateral, though Bilateral presentation can occur. These effusions often spontaneously resolve in a few months, but some may persist or recur for several years. Effusion usually exudative, with eosinophil predominance.
- *Asbestos-Related Interstitial Lung Disease:* Can be mild or can progress to diffuse pulmonary fibrosis. Needs to be differentiated from usual interstitial pneumonia (UIP) and other interstitial lung disease (ILD).
- *Asbestos-Associated Cancer:* Asbestos exposure is linked to increased risk of lung cancer and mesothelioma. Risk increases in smokers. Mesothelioma is associated with asbestos exposure, but the most common cancer associated with asbestos exposure is bronchogenic carcinoma.

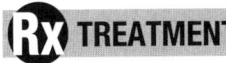 DIAGNOSIS

DIFFERENTIAL DIAGNOSIS

- Silicosis
- Siderosis, other pneumonoconioses
- Interstitial lung disease
- Lung cancer

WORKUP

Documentation of exposure history
Pulmonary function testing
Diagnostic imaging studies

LABORATORY TESTS

- Generally not helpful
- Arterial blood gases: May show hypoxemia and/or hypercarbia in advanced stages
Pulmonary function testing:
- Most often shows decreased vital capacity (VC), decreased total lung capacity (TLC), and decreased carbon monoxide gas transfer (DLco)
- FEV1 might be reduced in concomitant smokers
Bronchoscopy with bronchoalveolar lavage:
- Clinical utility of bronchoscopy is limited. It can be helpful in ruling out infection, or hypersensitivity pneumonitis. Asbestos bodies are found in sputum and bronchoalveolar lavage (BAL) fluid of asbestos workers but utility in diagnosis of asbestos-related lung disease and progression is limited.

IMAGING STUDIES

- Chest x-ray (Figs. 1): Imaging findings associated with asbestos exposure may vary from benign pleural disease (including discrete plaques, pleural calcification, diffuse pleural thickening with blunting of costophrenic angles, and thickening of the interlobar fissure) to asbestosis (diffuse interstitial pulmonary fibrosis).
- CT scan of chest (Fig. 2): Typical findings of asbestosis on high-resolution CT of the chest include increased interstitial markings found mainly at the bases (Fig. 3). As the disease progresses, honeycombing is noted.

(Rx) TREATMENT

NONPHARMACOLOGIC THERAPY

- Smoking cessation
- Exercise program to maximize available lung function. Pulmonary rehabilitation can be considered in advanced cases for improved cardiopulmonary capacity
- Supplemental oxygen on a PRN basis
- Removal of patient from further asbestos fiber exposure

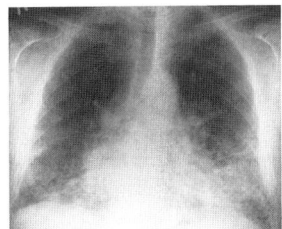

FIG. 1 Asbestosis. Posteroanterior radiograph shows coarse linear opacities at both lung bases obscuring the cardiac borders. (From McLoud TC: *Thoracic radiology: the requisites,* St Louis, 1998, Mosby.)

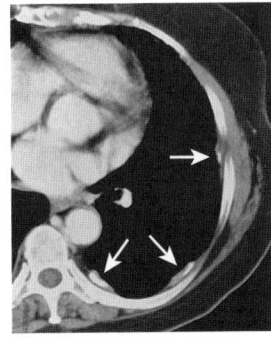

FIG. 2 Asbestos-related pleural plaques. Typical calcified pleural plaques *(arrows)* are visible. They are often internal to the ribs. (From Webb WR et al: *Fundamentals of body CT,* ed 4, Philadelphia, 2014, Saunders.)

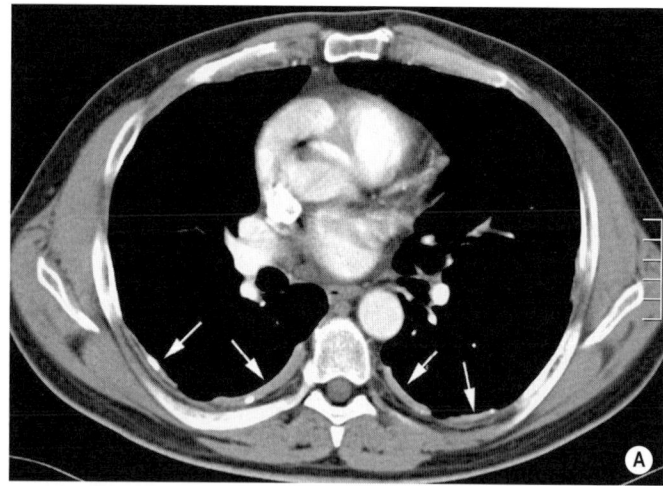 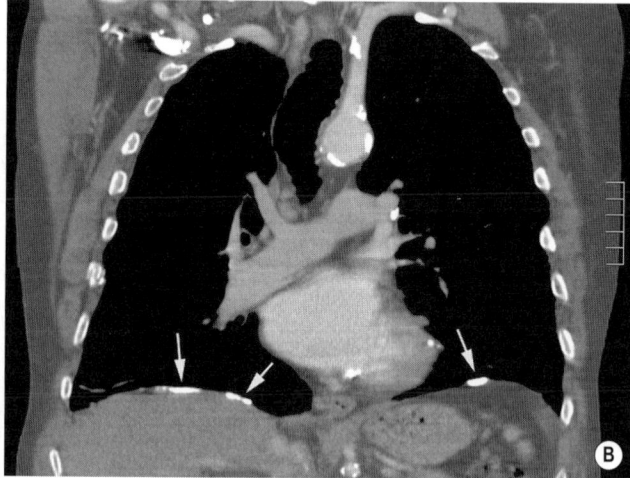

FIG. 3 Pleural plaques caused by asbestos exposure. (A) Axial and **(B)** coronal computed tomography. Pleural plaques are most commonly found along the lower thorax and on the diaphragmatic pleura *(arrows)*. They can partially or completely calcify or ossify. (From Adam A et al: *Grainger & Allison's diagnostic radiology,* ed 5, 2007, Churchill Livingstone: In Grant LA: *Grainger & Allison's diagnostic radiology essentials,* ed 2, 2019, Elsevier.)

- Prompt identification and treatment of respiratory infections
- Pneumococcal vaccination and annual influenza vaccination

PHARMACOLOGIC THERAPY
- There is no specific pharmacologic treatment for asbestosis
- Some new data are coming out targeting IL-1beta therapy on the progression of lung fibrosis that suggest a new perspective for the treatment of systemic autoimmune features of asbestosis and, possibly, of lung involvement.[2]

DISPOSITION
- Death is usually from respiratory failure from cor pulmonale.
- Survival in patients after development of mesothelioma is 4 to 6 yr.

- Benign asbestos pleural effusions (BAPEs) are usually small and unilateral and occur years before the onset of interstitial disease.
- Diffuse pleural thickening and asbestosis are associated with increased risks of malignant peritoneal mesothelioma beyond the risk calculated to be associated with the degree of asbestos exposure.[3]
- None of the benign pleural diseases or ARPD was associated with an increased risk of malignant pleural mesothelioma.
- Asbestos increases the risk for development of lung cancer regardless of smoking status. The joint effect of asbestos and smoking is additive and depends in part on the presence of asbestosis. Patients with a history of tobacco smoking who have diffuse parenchymal disease secondary to asbestos, have a 40-fold increased risk of lung cancer compared to never-smokers. Asbestos workers who stop smoking experience a dramatic decline in lung cancer risk, which approaches that of non-smokers after 30 yr.
- Low-dose chest CT scanning offers an excellent opportunity to detect early-stage lung cancers in asbestos-exposed workers.
- Computed tomography is more sensitive than radiography, computed tomography without contrast generally suffices for evaluation, and PET scan (fluorodeoxyglucose-positron emission tomography) may have utility in patients with mesothelioma.

REFERENCES
Available at eBooks.Health.Elsevier.com.

RELATED CONTENT
Asbestosis (Patient Information)

AUTHOR: **IMRANA QAWI, MD**

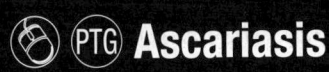
BASIC INFORMATION

DEFINITION

Ascariasis is a parasitic infection caused by the nematode *Ascaris lumbricoides*. The majority of those infected are asymptomatic; however, clinical disease may arise from pulmonary hypersensitivity, intestinal obstruction, or nutrient depletion and other secondary complications.

SYNONYMS

Round worms
Worms

ICD-10CM CODES
B77.0 Ascariasis with intestinal complications
B77.81 Ascariasis pneumonia
B77.89 Ascariasis with other complications
B77.9 Ascariasis, unspecified

EPIDEMIOLOGY & DEMOGRAPHICS

INCIDENCE (IN U.S.):
- Unknown. Worldwide, *A. lumbricoides* is the most common helminthic infection of humans, infecting as many as 1 billion or more persons. 71% of persons at risk for infection live in Asia and the Western Pacific.
- Three times the infection rates found in blacks as in whites.

PREVALENCE (IN U.S.): Estimated at 4 million, the majority of which live in the rural southeastern part of the country; ascariasis is associated with poor sanitation.

PREDOMINANT SEX: Both sexes probably equally affected, with a possible slight female preponderance.

PREDOMINANT AGE: Most common in children from ages 2 to 10 yr old and decreases after age 15; infections tend to cluster in families.

PEAK INCIDENCE: Unknown

NEONATAL INFECTION: Probable transmission, though not specifically studied

PHYSICAL FINDINGS & CLINICAL PRESENTATION

- Most people infected with *Ascaris* are asymptomatic
- Occurs approximately 9 to 12 days after ingestion of eggs (corresponding to the larval migration through the lungs)
- Nonproductive cough
- Substernal chest discomfort
- Fever
- In patients with large worm burdens, especially children, intestinal obstruction associated with perforation, volvulus, and intussusception
- Migration of worms into the biliary tree giving clinical appearance of biliary colic and pancreatitis as well as acute appendicitis with movement into that appendage

- Rarely, infection with *A. lumbricoides* producing interstitial nephritis and acute renal failure
- In endemic areas in Asia and Africa, malabsorption of dietary proteins and vitamins as a consequence of chronic worm intestinal carriage; 1 billion people worldwide are infected with this nematode

ETIOLOGY

- Transmission is usually hand to mouth, but eggs may be ingested via transported vegetables grown in contaminated soil.
- Eggs are hatched in the small intestine, with larvae penetrating intestinal mucosa and migrating via the circulation to the lungs.
- Larval forms proceed through the alveoli, ascend the bronchial tree, and return to the intestines after swallowing, where they mature into adult worms.
- Estimated time until the female adult worm begins producing eggs is 2 to 3 mo.
- Eggs are passed out of the intestines with feces and can survive for years in warm, moist, shaded soil.
- Within human host, adult worm life span is 1 to 2 yr.
- Fig. 1 illustrates the life cycle of *A. lumbricoides*.

DIAGNOSIS

DIFFERENTIAL DIAGNOSIS

- Radiologic manifestations and eosinophilia to be distinguished from drug hypersensitivity and Löffler syndrome.
- Table 1 compares features of major intestinal nematodes.

LABORATORY TESTS

- Examination of the stool for *Ascaris* ova (Fig. E2).
- The World Health Organization (WHO) recommends the Kato-Katz thick smear kit for soil-transmitted helminths.
- Expectoration or fecal passage of adult worm.
- Adult male worms: 10 to 30 cm long; adult female worms: Larger than male, up to 40 cm.
- Eosinophilia: Most prominent early in the infection and subsides as the adult worm infestation established in the intestines; usually in 5% to 12% range but can be up to 50%.
- Serology: Patients develop immunoglobulin G (IgG) antibodies, but they cross react with antigens from other helminths and are not protective; thus, serology is used more for epidemiologic purposes than for individual diagnosis.
- Polymerase chain reaction (PCR) on stool samples; multiplex PCR can differentiate multiple different parasite species (*A. lumbricoides*, *T. trichiura*, and *N. americanus*).

IMAGING STUDIES

- Chest x-ray to reveal bilateral oval or round infiltrates of varying size (Löffler syndrome); NOTE: Infiltrates are transient and eventually resolve.
- Plain films of the abdomen and contrast studies to reveal worm masses in loops of bowel.
- Ultrasonography and endoscopic retrograde cholangiopancreatography (ERCP) to identify worms in the pancreaticobiliary tract.
- CT scan with oral contrast can also assist in the detection of GI foreign bodies such as parasites.

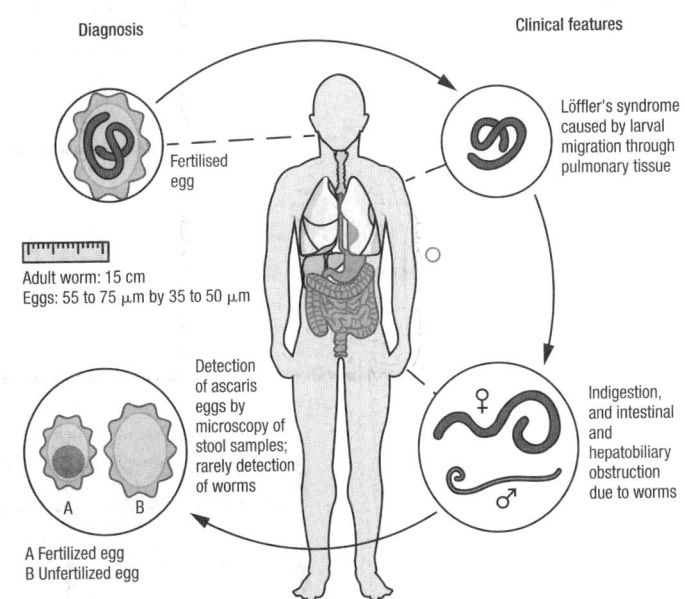

FIG 1 Life cycle of Ascaris lumbricoides. (Reprinted with permission from Jourdan PM et al. Soil-transmitted helminth infections, Elsevier (The Lancet 2018;391:252–265).)

TABLE 1 Features of Major Intestinal Nematodes

Nematode	Transmission	Direct Person-to-Person Transmission	Geographic Distribution	Duration of Infection	Location of Adult Worm(s)	Treatment*
Ascaris lumbricoides	Ingestion of infective eggs	No	Warm, humid areas; temperate zones in warmer months	1-2 yr	Free in lumen of small bowel, primarily jejunum	Albendazole Mebendazole Pyrantel Ivermectin Levamisole Piperazine
Trichuris trichiura (whipworm)	Ingestion of infective eggs	No	Warm, humid areas; temperate zones in warmer months	1-3 yr	Anchored in superficial mucosa of cecum and colon	Albendazole Mebendazole
Necator americanus, Ancylostoma duodenale (hookworm)	Penetration of skin by filariform larvae	No	Warm, humid areas; temperate zones in warmer months	3-5 yr *(Necator)*; 1 yr *(Ancylostoma)*	Attached to mucosa of mid to upper portion of small bowel	Albendazole Mebendazole Levamisole Pyrantel
Strongyloides stercoralis	Penetration of skin or bowel mucosa by filariform larvae	Yes	Primarily warm, humid areas but can be worldwide	Lifetime of host	Embedded in mucosa of duodenum, jejunum	Ivermectin† Albendazole Thiabendazole
Enterobius vermicularis (pinworm)	Ingestion of infective eggs	Yes	Worldwide	1 mo	Free in lumen of cecum, appendix, adjacent colon	Albendazole Mebendazole Pyrantel Ivermectin Levamisole Piperazine

*Nitazoxanide has been shown to be effective in the treatment of ascariasis, trichuriasis, and enterobiasis in several trials in Mexico. Tribendimidine, which is licensed in China, was shown to be efficacious against *Ascaris* spp. and had moderate efficacy against *Strongyloides* spp. in a randomized trial.
†Drug of choice.
From Bennett et al: *Mandell, Douglas, and Bennett's principles and practice of infectious diseases*, ed 8, Philadelphia, 2015, Saunders.

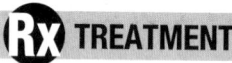

TREATMENT

NONPHARMACOLOGIC THERAPY
Aggressive IV hydration, especially in children with fever, severe vomiting, and resultant dehydration

ACUTE GENERAL Rx
- All infected patients, including asymptomatic ones, should be treated.
  1. Albendazole: 400 mg PO × 1 dose is the first-line agent.
  2. Mebendazole 100 mg PO bid × 3 days for persons >1 yr of age or mebendazole 500 mg PO × 1 dose for persons >1 yr of age (not available as 500 mg in the U.S.).
- Cure rate with these agents is 95% to 100%, but they are considered FDA pregnancy risk Class C. The WHO allows use of albendazole in second and third trimesters.
- Side effects: GI discomfort, headache, and rarely leukopenia.
- Alternative agent or for use in pregnancy: Pyrantel pamoate (Antiminth):
  1. Given at a dose of 11 mg/kg PO (maximum dose of 1 g/day).
  2. Considered safe for use in pregnant women.
- Other alternative agents:
  1. Ivermectin: 150 to 200 mcg/kg orally once.
  2. Nitazoxanide: Ages 2 to 3 yr: 100 mg/5 ml bid × 3 days, and ages 4 to 11 yr: 200 mg/10 ml bid × 3 days. Cure rates in heavy worm burden are only 50% to 80%.
  3. Piperazine citrate: No longer first-line agent due to toxicity but still used in cases of intestinal or biliary obstruction, as drug paralyzes the worm, helping its expulsion. Dose: 50 to 75 mg/kg once daily up to maximum of 3.5 g for 2 days.
  4. Levamisole: 2.5 mg/kg once orally is recommended by the WHO as alternative therapy, but not available in the U.S.
- Complete obstruction should be managed surgically.

DISPOSITION
Overall prognosis is good. Patients should be reevaluated in 2 to 3 mo. Reinfection is common.

REFERRAL
- To gastroenterologist in cases of visualized pancreaticobiliary tract or appendiceal obstruction
- To surgeon in cases of complete obstruction or suspected secondary complication (e.g., perforation or volvulus)

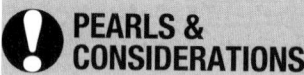

PEARLS & CONSIDERATIONS

COMMENTS
- Hepatic abscess, containing both viable and dead worms, complicating *Ascaris*-induced biliary duct disease has been documented.
- Given the known transmission of the parasite, routine hand washing with soap and proper disposal of human waste would significantly decrease the prevalence of this disease.
- Other protective measures to avoid ingestion of worm eggs:
  1. Peel or cook food.
  2. Boil drinking water.
  3. Do not place small children directly on soil.

SUGGESTED READINGS
Available at eBooks.Health.Elsevier.com.

RELATED CONTENT
Ascariasis (Patient Information)

AUTHOR: **GLENN G. FORT, MD, MPH**

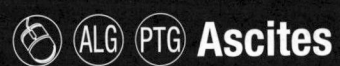

A

I

BASIC INFORMATION

DEFINITIONS

Ascites is a pathologic accumulation of fluid in the peritoneal cavity, most commonly due to portal hypertension caused by cirrhosis.

- **Diuretic-resistant ascites:** Ascites that cannot be mobilized or the early occurrence of ascites that cannot be prevented because of a lack of response to dietary sodium restriction and intensive diuretic treatment
- **Diuretic-intractable ascites:** Ascites that cannot be mobilized or the early recurrence of ascites that cannot be prevented because of the development of diuretic-induced complications that preclude the use of effective doses of diuretics
- Ascites may be graded according to the amount of fluid in the peritoneal cavity[1,2]:
  1. Grade 1 (mild ascites): Ascites only detectable by ultrasound
  2. Grade 2 (moderate ascites): Ascites with moderate symmetric abdominal distention
  3. Grade 3 (large ascites): Ascites with marked abdominal distention

SYNONYMS

Peritoneal cavity fluid
Hydroperitoneum
Hydroperitonia
Hydrops abdominis

ICD-10CM CODES
R18	Ascites
K70.11	Alcoholic hepatitis with ascites
K70.31	Alcoholic cirrhosis of liver with ascites
K71.51	Toxic liver disease with chronic active hepatitis with ascites
R18.8	Other ascites

EPIDEMIOLOGY & DEMOGRAPHICS

Ascites is the most common decompensation-defining complication of cirrhosis and is associated with worse prognosis. Ascites occurs at a rate of 7% to 10% annually in cirrhotic patients and occurs in ~60% of individuals with cirrhosis within 10 yr of diagnosis.[3] Cirrhosis is the cause of more than 80% of cases of ascites.[4]

CLINICAL PRESENTATION & PHYSICAL FINDINGS

- Important information to elicit within history:
  1. History of viral hepatitis
  2. Ongoing or previous heavy alcohol use
  3. Current or previous intravenous drug use and/or intranasal cocaine use
  4. Sexual history (e.g., unprotected sex with multiple partners, men who have sex with men)
  5. History of transfusions, tattoos, piercings, or incarceration
  6. Travel history and time spent in endemic regions for hepatitis
  7. Symptoms suggestive of peritoneal malignancy (e.g., weight loss, pain, palpable masses, rectal/vaginal bleeding)
  8. Other liver disease symptoms (e.g., increasing abdominal girth, jaundice, pruritus, confusion, pedal edema)
  9. Cardiac symptoms (e.g., pedal edema, shortness of breath, orthopnea, chest pain)
  10. Hypothyroid disease (fatigue, weight gain, constipation)
  11. History of ascites, prior treatment, large volume paracentesis (LVP) requirements and frequency
- Important physical exam findings:
  1. Protuberant abdomen (Fig. E1)
  2. Bulging flanks (can be present in obesity)
  3. Flank dullness to percussion (requires ~1500 mL of fluid)
  4. Fluid wave on abdominal exam
  5. Lower extremity edema
  6. Shifting dullness on abdominal exam
  7. Physical signs associated with liver cirrhosis: Spider angiomas, jaundice, loss of body hair, skeletal muscle wasting (sarcopenia), Dupuytren contracture, bruising, palmar erythema, gynecomastia, testicular atrophy, rectal varices, and caput medusa

ETIOLOGY

Pathophysiology of ascites (Fig. E2): Increased hepatic resistance to portal flow leads to portal hypertension. A portal pressure >12 mm Hg appears to be required for fluid retention.[5] The splanchnic vessels respond by increased secretion of nitric oxide, causing splanchnic artery vasodilation. Vasodilation appears also to be mediated by the translocation of enteric bacteria and bacterial products. Early in the disease, increased plasma volume and increased cardiac output compensate for this vasodilation. However, as the disease progresses, the effective arterial blood volume decreases, causing sodium and fluid retention through activation of the renin-angiotensin system. Over time, activation of the sympathetic system causes renal vascular perfusion to decrease and may lead to hepatorenal syndrome. The change in capillary pressure causes increased permeability and retention of fluid in the abdomen.[5] Principal causes of ascites formation categorized by underlying pathophysiology are summarized in Box E1.

DIAGNOSIS

DIFFERENTIAL DIAGNOSIS

- Chronic parenchymal liver disease, leading to portal hypertension
- Acute liver failure
- Noncirrhotic portal hypertension (e.g., portal vein clot)
- Peritoneal carcinomatosis
- Cardiac disease (e.g., heart failure, constrictive pericarditis)
- Hepatic venous outflow obstruction (e.g., Budd-Chiari syndrome, IVC webs)
- Protein losing enteropathy
- Peritoneal tuberculosis
- Nephrotic syndrome
- Pancreatitis

LABORATORY TESTS

- Initial evaluation should always include:
  1. Diagnostic paracentesis. Initial laboratory tests on ascitic fluid should include a cell count and differential, albumin, total protein, culture, and Gram stain. A serum-ascites albumin gradient (SAAG) should be calculated in all patients. The SAAG is measured by subtracting the level of albumin in the ascitic fluid from a concurrent serum albumin measurement: SAAG = serum albumin−ascites albumin.
     a. If the SAAG is greater than 1.1 g/dL, the cause of ascites can be attributed to portal hypertension (e.g., cirrhosis, or post-sinusoidal elevated pressures as in Budd-Chiari syndrome or heart failure). A total ascitic protein level >2.5 g/dL may be indicative of cardiac ascites.[4]
     b. If SAAG is less than 1.1 g/dL, the cause of ascites is not portal hypertension (e.g., peritoneal carcinomatosis, tuberculous ascites, nephrotic syndrome). Optional tests on ascitis fluid that may aid in diagnosis include amylase, lactic dehydrogenase, acid-fast bacilli, and glucose levels.
     c. Cell count and differential: Ascitic fluid with greater than 250 neutrophils per cubic mm is diagnostic of spontaneous bacterial peritonitis (SBP).[4]
     d. Total ascitic fluid protein: Patients with protein concentration <1.5 g/dL have an increased risk of SBP.[1]
     e. Cytology: Obtain in patients with a high index of suspicion for associated malignancy.[2]
  2. Aspartate aminotransferase, alanine transaminase, total and direct bilirubin, albumin, alkaline phosphatase, gamma-glutamyl transpeptidase.
  3. CBC, coagulation studies (prothrombin time/INR).
  4. Electrolytes, blood urea nitrogen (BUN), creatinine.
- Causes of ascites in the normal or diseased peritoneum by SAAG are summarized in Table 1.
- Fig. 3 illustrates an algorithm for the approach to the differential diagnosis of ascites.

IMAGING STUDIES

- Abdominal ultrasound (Fig. E4) is the most sensitive measure for detecting ascitic fluid; a computed tomography or MRI scan is a viable alternative. Doppler studies of portal and hepatic veins should be added to rule out vascular etiology of ascites.
- Endoscopy of the upper GI tract to evaluate for esophageal and gastric varices if ascites is secondary to portal hypertension.

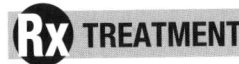 TREATMENT

NONPHARMACOLOGIC THERAPY

- Sodium-restricted diet (88 mmol/day or <2 g/day) is recommended for all patients with grade 2 ascites.

TABLE 1   Diagnosis of Ascites

CLASSIFICATION OF ASCITES BY SERUM ASCITES—ALBUMIN GRADIENT (SAAG)

SAAG High (≥1.1 g/dL)	SAAG Low (<1.1 g/dL)
Cirrhosis	Peritoneal carcinomatosis
Alcoholic hepatitis	Tuberculous peritonitis
Cardiac ascites	Pancreatic ascites
Massive liver metastases	Bile leak
Fulminant hepatic failure	Inflammation e.g. systemic lupus erythematosus
Cirrhosis plus another cause	Nephrotic syndrome

CHARACTERISTICS OF PARACENTESIS FLUID

Etiology	Color	Saag (g/L)	RBCs	WBCs (Cells/Microl)	Cytology	Other
Cirrhosis	Straw	≥11	Few	<250		Protein <25 g/L
Infected ascites	Straw	≥11	Few	≥250 polymorphs or >500 cells		Positive culture
Neoplastic	Straw/ hemorrhagic/ mucinous	<11	Variable	Variable	Malignant cells	Protein >25 g/L
Tuberculosis	Clear/turbid/ hemorrhagic	<11	High	>1000, 70% lymphocytes		Acid-fast bacilli + culture Protein >25 g/L
Cardiac failure	Straw	≥11	0	<250		Protein >25 g/L
Pancreatic	Turbid/ hemorrhagic	<11	Variable	Variable		Amylase increased
Lymphatic obstruction or disruption	White	<11	0	0		Fat globules on staining

RBC, Red blood cell; *WBC*, white blood cell.
From Talley NJ et al: *Essentials of internal medicine*, ed 4, Chatswood NSW, 2021, Elsevier Australia.

- Fluid restriction is only indicated in patients with hyponatremia (Na ≤125 mmol/L).
- All patients should be counseled on avoiding NSAIDs, ACE inhibitors, ARBs, alpha-adrenergic antagonists, and aminoglycoside antibiotics.

ACUTE GENERAL RX

Patients with moderate-volume ascites causing only moderate discomfort may be treated on an outpatient basis with the following diuretic regimen:

1. Spironolactone: Start at 50 to 100 mg/day and titrate up every 3 to 4 days to a maximum dose of 400 mg/day (monotherapy or combination therapy with furosemide).[2]
2. Furosemide: Start at 40 mg/day and titrate up to 160 mg/day maximum (no role for monotherapy). A ratio of 40 mg/day of furosemide to 100 mg/day of spironolactone is an effective strategy in most patients but can modified based on kidney function and electrolytes.[2]
3. Monitor renal function and sodium levels carefully for signs of prerenal azotemia (in patients without edema, goal weight loss is 300 to 500 g/day; in patients with edema, goal weight loss is 800 to 1000 g/day). Furosemide alone is not recommended.[2]
4. Measurement of the urinary sodium level can be helpful to identify noncompliance with dietary sodium restriction and diuretic therapy. Patients excreting more than 78 mmol of sodium/day (24-h urine) and not losing weight likely have nonadherence with low Na diet. Patients with low Na excretion, less than 78 mmol daily, require up titration of diuretics and evaluation of compliance.

Patients with large-volume ascites causing marked discomfort or impairment in activities of daily living may be treated in the outpatient setting with diuretic therapy alone or in combination with large-volume paracentesis.

1. Large-volume paracentesis: Defined as >5L removed during a single paracentesis.
2. Diuretic therapy until loss of fluid is noted (maximum spironolactone 400 mg daily and furosemide 160 mg daily).
   a. No difference in long-term mortality rate was found; however, paracentesis is faster, more effective, and associated with fewer adverse effects.[3]
   b. Patients receiving large-volume paracentesis (>5L) should receive albumin replacement therapy at the dose of 6 to 8 g/L of ascites removed to prevent post-paracentesis circulatory dysfunction (PPCD).[2,6] Patients with renal dysfunction or hyponatremia should receive albumin for lower volumes as well.

Table 2 summarizes primary medical therapy and adjunctive medications used to increase the efficacy of primary therapy in the treatment of ascites.

CHRONIC Rx

- 5% to 10% of patients with large-volume ascites will be refractory to high-dose diuretic treatment.[1] Treatment strategies include repeated large-volume paracentesis with infusion of albumin every 2 to 4 wk or placement of a transjugular intrahepatic portosystemic shunt (TIPS).[3] TIPS evaluation should include echocardiogram, assessment for hepatic encephalopathy (HE), and characterization of liver impairment.
- Long-term albumin administration (40 g weekly) may improve mortality, reduce episodes of HE, and delay accumulation of ascites compared to standard medical therapy.[7] However, more research is needed before recommending the long-term use of albumin in routine management.[2]
- There are limited data on use of nonselective betablockers (NSBBs) in patients with diuretic-resistant ascites. Changes in mean arterial pressure (MAP) should be carefully monitored in patients on NSBBs, and these should be dose-reduced or stopped if substantial decrease in MAP is observed or systolic blood pressure is less than 90 mm Hg.[4]
- Patients known to have ascites should receive a diagnostic paracentesis if they develop any signs of SBP or upon any admission to the hospital even in the absence of these signs.
- Primary prophylaxis for SBP is recommended in patients with ascitic fluid protein <1.5 g/dL along with impaired renal function (creatinine ≥1.2 mg/dL or 106 micromol/L), BUN ≥25 mg/dL or 8.9 mmol/L or Na ≤130 mmol/L, or liver failure (Child-Pugh score ≥9 and bilirubin ≥3 mg/dL or 51 micromol/L).[2]
- Secondary prophylaxis for SBP should be instituted in all patients who were diagnosed with SBP in the form of a daily fluoroquinolone such as ciprofloxacin or norfloxacin, or double-strength trimethoprim-sulfamethoxazole.[2]
- Patients with known ascites who develop gastrointestinal bleeding should receive intravenous ceftriaxone for 7 days to prevent bacterial infections.
- Clinical use of vaptan agents is not currently recommended in cirrhotic patients.
- Oral midodrine 7.5 mg three times daily has been shown to increase urine volume, urine sodium, mean arterial pressure, and survival.[3]
- Peritoneovenous shunts or surgical portosystemic shunts have poor evidence and are not recommended.
- The Automated Low-Flow Ascites pump (not approved in North America) works by transporting small amounts of fluid from the peritoneal cavity to the bladder. Studies have shown improved symptoms and reduced LVP requirements.[3,8]
- Liver transplantation remains definitive management for cirrhosis with refractory ascites.[8] Referral to a transplant-capable center should be discussed.

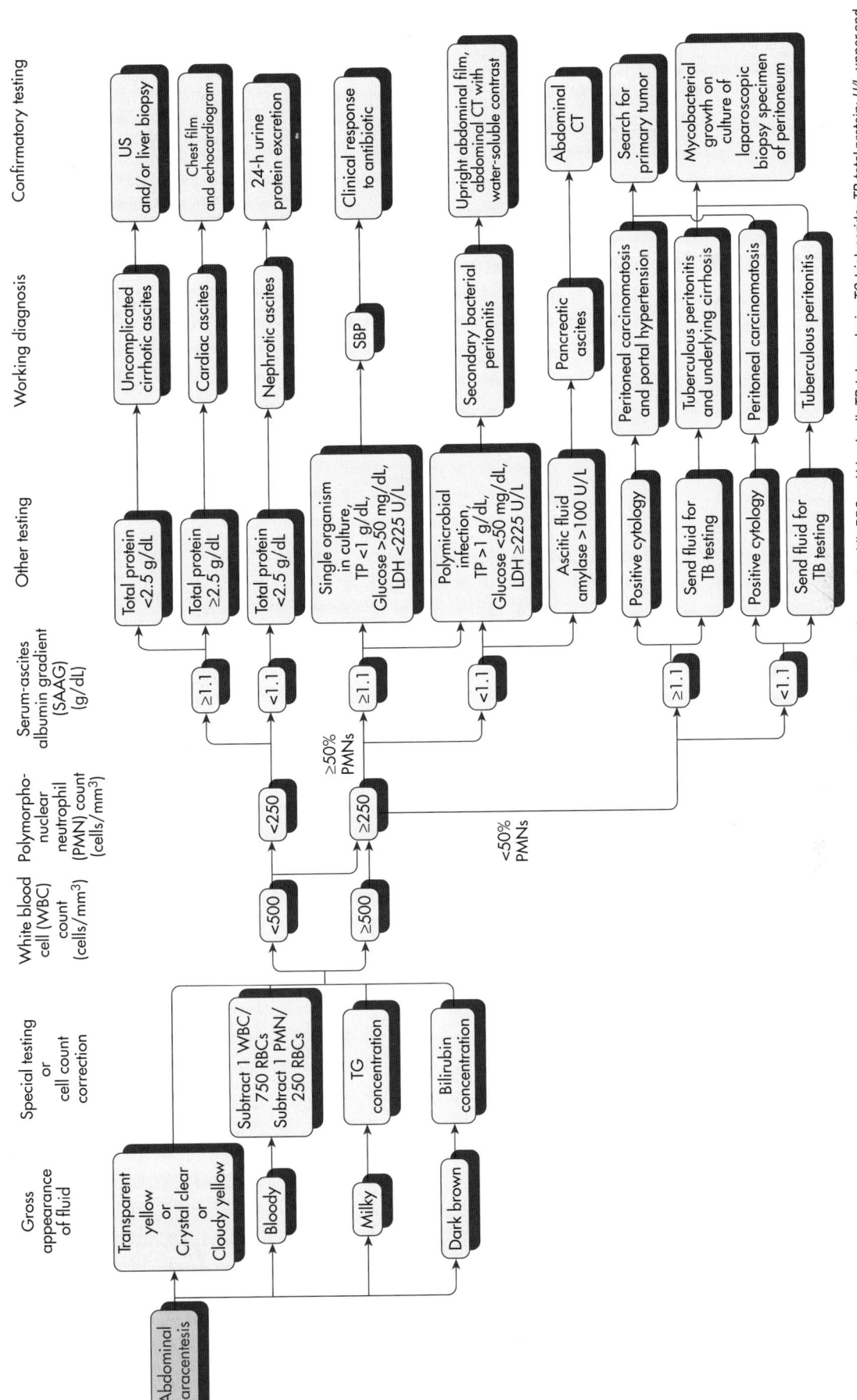

FIG. 3 **Algorithm for the approach to the differential diagnosis of ascites.** *LDH,* Lactic dehydrogenase; *PMN,* polymorphonuclear neutrophil; *RBC,* red blood cell; *TB,* tuberculosis; *TG,* triglyceride; *TP,* total protein; *U/L,* upper and lower; *US,* ultrasound. (From Feldman M et al: *Sleisenger and Fordtran's gastrointestinal and liver disease,* ed 10, Philadelphia, 2016, Elsevier.)

TABLE 2 Primary Medical Therapy and Adjunctive Medications Used to Increase the Efficacy of Primary Therapy in the Treatment of Ascites

Class	Medication	Dosing	Relevant Action	Notes
Diuretics	Spironolactone	400 mg + daily*	Aldosterone receptor antagonist	Primary therapy
	Furosemide	160 mg + daily*	Inhibits Na-K-2Cl symporter	Primary therapy
Vasoconstrictors	Octreotide	300 mcg bid*	Splanchnic vasoconstriction, inhibits RAAS	Also used in combination with midodrine to treat hepatorenal syndrome; given for first 5 days following variceal bleeding to decrease recurrence
	Midodrine	7.5 mg tid*	Inhibits RAAS	Also used in combination with octreotide and albumin to treat hepatorenal syndrome
α2-Agonist	Clonidine	0.075 mg bid*	Inhibits sympathetic outflow, inhibits RAAS	Increases sensitivity to spironolactone
Colloid	Albumin	25 g*	Increased oncotic pressure	Also utilized with large-volume paracentesis and in the treatment of hepatorenal syndrome

*The above doses have been derived from various studies and may not be suitable for all patients. Titration is always recommended.
RAAS, Renin-angiotensin-aldosterone system
From Cameron JL, Cameron AM: *Current surgical therapy,* ed 10, Philadelphia, 2011, Saunders.

TABLE 3 Management of Refractory Ascites

Definitions	Ascites that is not eliminated even with maximum diuretic therapy
	Ascites that is not eliminated because maximum dosages of diuretics cannot be attained, given the development of diuretic-induced complications
Recommended therapy	Total paracentesis + IV albumin (7-9 g/L of ascites removed) if >5 L removed
	Continue with salt restriction and diuretic therapy as tolerated
Alternative therapy	TIPS for patients who require frequent paracenteses (every 1-2 wk) and whose CTP score is ≤11 or MELD <17
Peritoneovenous shunt for patients who are not candidates for TIPS or transplant	

CTP, Child-Turcotte-Pugh; *IV,* intravenous; *MELD,* model for end-stage liver disease; *TIPS,* transjugular intrahepatic portosystemic shunt.
Data from Garcia-Tsao G, Lim JK; Members of the Veterans Affairs Hepatitis C Resource Center Program: Management and treatment of patients with cirrhosis and portal hypertension: recommendations from the Department of Veterans Affairs Hepatitis C Resource Center Program and the National Hepatitis C Program, *Am J Gastroenterol* 104:1802-1829, 2009.
From Vincent JL et al: *Textbook of critical care,* ed 7, Philadelphia, 2017, Elsevier.

- Table 3 summarizes the management of refractory ascites.
- A treatment approach to patients with malignant ascites is described in Fig. E5.

DISPOSITION

- Development of ascites signals a shift to decompensated cirrhosis and close follow-up is required. 2-yr mortality reaches 75% in refractory ascites cases.[3]
- Monitor closely for worsening liver function and development of SBP.

REFERRAL

Referral to hepatology at a transplant-capable center.

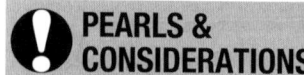

PEARLS & CONSIDERATIONS

COMMENTS

- Prevalence of SBP in patients with ascites ranges between 10% and 30%.[6]

1. Presence of at least 250 neutrophils per cubic millimeter of ascitic fluid is diagnostic; however, ascitic culture should be obtained for every diagnostic paracentesis where SBP is being considered.
2. Gram-negative bacteria such as *E. coli* are the most common isolates.[6]
3. Third-generation cephalosporins are the treatment of choice for most patients. There should be consideration of multidrug resistant organisms (MDRO) in patients with nosocomial infection, critical illness, or recent hospitalization. MDRO treatment may be tailored to local antimicrobiograms.
4. Albumin improves survival in patients with SBP. Antibiotics should be administered with 1.5 g/kg albumin on treatment day 1 and 1.0 g/kg albumin on day 3 to prevent hepatorenal syndrome.[6]
5. For patients diagnosed with SBP, a repeat diagnostic paracentesis may be obtained at 48 h after initiation of antibiotics to assess for response. A decrease of total ascitic polymorphonuclear neutrophil (PMN) count by at least 25% from baseline PMN count is considered a response.[6]
6. By 1 yr post-SBP, 70% of patients have recurrence of SBP and should therefore receive ciprofloxacin 750 mg PO once/wk indefinitely for prophylaxis.[6]

PREVENTION

- Prevention of liver cirrhosis through avoidance of long-term use of alcohol, immunization against hepatitis A and B, and treatment of hepatitis C
- In cirrhotic patients, following a low-sodium diet (<2 g daily)

REFERENCES
Available at eBooks.Health.Elsevier.com.

RELATED CONTENT

Ascites (Patient Information)
Cirrhosis (Related Key Topic)

AUTHORS: **MAYA DEEB, MD** and **TALIA ZENLEA, MD**

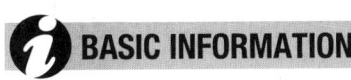

BASIC INFORMATION

DEFINITION

Aspergillosis refers to several forms of a broad range of illnesses caused by infection with *Aspergillus* species. *Aspergillus* species is a ubiquitous mold most commonly found in soil, building materials, and water.

ICD-10CM CODES
B44.0	Invasive pulmonary aspergillosis
B44.1	Other pulmonary aspergillosis
B44.2	Tonsillar aspergillosis
B44.7	Disseminated aspergillosis
B44.81	Allergic bronchopulmonary aspergillosis
B44.89	Other forms of aspergillosis
B44.9	Aspergillosis, unspecified

EPIDEMIOLOGY & DEMOGRAPHICS

INCIDENCE & PREVALENCE:
- *Aspergillus* species are ubiquitous in the environment internationally and occur as a mold found in soil. *Aspergillus fumigatus* is the most common human pathogen.[1]
- *Aspergillus* may cause a variety of illnesses from hypersensitivity pneumonitis to disseminated overwhelming infection in immunosuppressed patients.[2]
- Fig. 1 illustrates the categories of pulmonary aspergillosis.
- Frequently cultured from hospital wards from unfiltered outside air circulating through open windows as well as water sources.
- Reach the patient by airborne conidia (spores) that are small enough (2.5-3 μm) to reach the alveoli on inhalation.

- Can invade the nose, paranasal sinuses, external ear, or traumatized skin.

RISK FACTORS:
- The clinical syndrome depends on the underlying lung architecture, the host's immune response, and the degree of inoculum.
- Incidence of invasive aspergillosis is increasing with advances in the treatment of life-threatening diseases, such as aggressive chemotherapy or bone marrow and solid organ transplantation that are associated with suppression of the immune system. Allogeneic stem cell and lung transplant recipients are at highest risk for invasive pulmonary aspergillosis. Genetic deficiency of the soluble-pattern-recognition receptor known as long pentraxin 3 (PTX3) affects the antifungal capacity of neutrophils and may contribute to the risk of invasive aspergillosis in patients treated with hematopoietic stem-cell transplantation (HSCT).[3]
- Patients with AIDS and a CD4 count <50/mm[3] have an increased susceptibility to invasive aspergillosis, but it is otherwise uncommon in patients with HIV.[4]
- Pandemic influenza A (H1N1) infection may predispose immunocompromised patients to invasive aspergillosis.
- COVID-19 coinfection with invasive pulmonary *Aspergillus* infection has been seen in 20% to 30% of patients with severe acute respiratory distress syndrome (ARDS) requiring intubation and is associated with higher mortality.[5]
- Patients with chronic granulomatous disease are at higher risk for infections with *Aspergillus* species, and it is the most common cause of

infectious death in chronic granulomatous disease (CGD).
- *Aspergillus nidulans* causes mostly invasive infections in patients with chronic granulomatous disease.

ETIOLOGY
- *Aspergillus fumigatus* is the usual cause.
- *Aspergillus flavus* is the second most important species, particularly in invasive disease of immunosuppressed patients and in lesions beginning in the nose and paranasal sinuses. *Aspergillus niger* can also cause invasive human infection.

ALLERGIC FUNGAL SINUSITIS:
- Occurs in patients with history of allergic rhinitis.
- Management involves aerating the sinus and ensuring tissue is not invaded via sinus CT.[2]

ALLERGIC BRONCHOPULMONARY ASPERGILLOSIS (ABPA):
- Symptoms occur most commonly in patients with asthma and cystic fibrosis.
- It is a long-term allergic response to *Aspergillus.*
- Results from an initial type I (immediate hypersensitivity) and type III reactions (immune complexes).
- Underdiagnosed pulmonary disorder in patients with asthma and cystic fibrosis. The reported prevalence in persistently asthmatic patients varies from 1% to 2% and in cystic fibrosis from 2% to 15%.
- Diagnostic criteria for chronic pulmonary aspergillosis are summarized in Table 1.

ASPERGILLOMAS ("FUNGUS BALLS"):
- In the absence of invasion or significant immune response, *Aspergillus* can colonize a

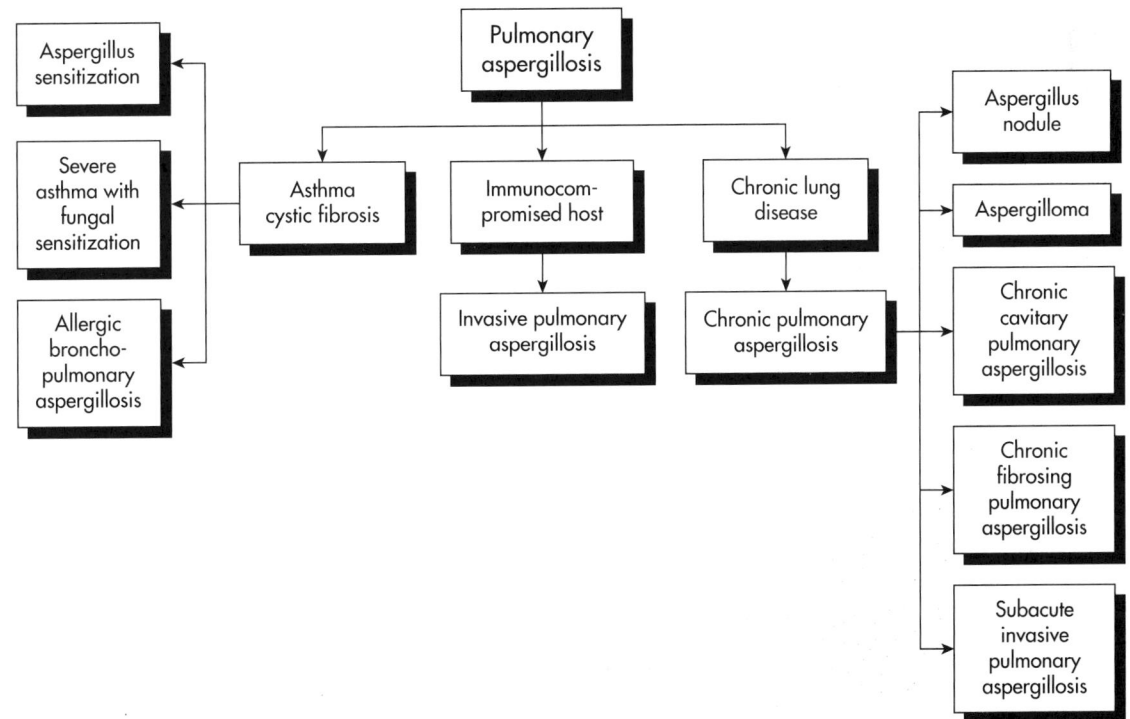

FIG. 1 Categories of pulmonary aspergillosis. (From El-Baba F et al: Pulmonary aspergillosis: what the generalist needs to know, *The American Journal of Medicine* 133(6):668-674, 2020.)

TABLE 1 Diagnostic Criteria for Chronic Pulmonary Aspergillosis

- Thoracic radiological findings consistent with the disease including one or more cavities with or without fungal ball or nodules (CT scan of the chest is preferred over plain films)
- Direct evidence of *Aspergillus* infection (microscopy or culture from biopsy) or an immunological response to *Aspergillus* species (such as elevated serum *Aspergillus* IgG or precipitins, strongly positive serum or bronchoalveolar lavage galactomannan, or *Aspergillus* polymerase chain reaction)
- Exclusion of alternative diagnoses
- Duration of symptoms or radiological changes for at least 3 mo

CT, Computed tomography; *IgG*, immunoglobulin G.
From El-Baba F et al: Pulmonary aspergillosis: what generalists need to know, *The American Journal of Medicine* 133:671-673, 2020.

TABLE 2 Criteria for Classification of Invasive Pulmonary Aspergillosis

Proven invasive pulmonary aspergillosis	Sterile specimen with either direct microscopic identification of hyphae *or* positive *Aspergillus* culture
Probable invasive pulmonary aspergillosis	≥1 host factors: - Prolonged neutropenia defined as <500 neutrophils/mm³ for >10 days - Allogeneic hematopoietic stem cell or solid organ transplant or immunosuppressive therapy - Prolonged corticosteroids at a minimum dose of 0.3 mg/Kg/d for >3 wk *and* ≥1 clinical features: - CT findings consistent with invasive pulmonary aspergillosis such as the "halo sign" or "air-crescent sign" or a cavity *and* Mycological evidence of aspergillosis - Positive *Aspergillus* microscopy or culture from the sputum or BAL, or a positive antigen assay of GM or BDG
Possible invasive pulmonary aspergillosis	≥1 host factors *and* ≥1 clinical features No mycological evidence of aspergillosis

BAL, Bronchoalveolar lavage; *BDG*, beta-D-glucan; *CT*, computed tomography; *gM*, galactomannan.
From El-Baba F et al: Pulmonary aspergillosis: what generalists need to know, *The American Journal of Medicine* 133:671-673, 2020.

preexisting cavity, causing a pulmonary aspergilloma.
- Forms masses of hyphae in a prior pulmonary cavity.
- Patients typically have a history of chronic lung disease, e.g., tuberculosis, sarcoidosis, or emphysema.
- Manifests commonly as hemoptysis.
- Many are asymptomatic.

INVASIVE ASPERGILLOSIS:
- In immunocompromised patients, presents as fever, focal pulmonary infiltrates, nodules, or wedge-shaped opacities.
- Typically a necrotizing bronchopneumonia, ranging from small areas of infiltrate to intensive bilateral hemorrhagic infarction.
- Most common presentation: Unremitting fever and a new pulmonary infiltrate despite broad-spectrum antibiotic therapy in an immuno-suppressed patient.
- Dyspnea and nonproductive cough are common; sudden pleuritic pain and tachycardia, sometimes with a pleural rub, may mimic pulmonary embolism; hemoptysis may also be present.[6]
- Chest radiograph (CXR) may reveal patchy bronchopneumonic, nodular densities,

consolidation, or cavitation. High-resolution CT scan is more sensitive and specific than CXR in neutropenic patients.
- Invasive aspergillosis may occur in the setting of severe influenza infections due to virus-induced respiratory epithelium even among immunocompetent hosts.[7]
- Immunocompromised patients: Invasive pulmonary *Aspergillus* (IPA) generally has an incubation period of around 15 days in neutropenic patients; invasive aspergillosis though, in general, is uncommon in the immunocompetent.[2]
- Criteria for classification of invasive pulmonary aspergillosis are summarized in Table 2.

EXTRAPULMONARY DISSEMINATION:
- Cerebral aspergillosis may occur in persistently immunosuppressed individuals with disseminated disease.[2]
- Abscess formation from direct extension or invasive disease in the sinuses.
- Esophageal or gastrointestinal ulcerations may occur in the immunosuppressed host.
- Fatal perforation of the viscus or bowel infarction may occur.
- Necrotizing skin ulcers (Fig. E2).
- Osteomyelitis (Fig. E3).

- Culture negative endocarditis in patients with abnormal or prosthetic valves who are immunosuppressed.
- Infection of an implantable cardioverter-defibrillator has been reported.[8]

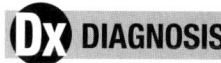 **Dx** **DIAGNOSIS**

DIFFERENTIAL DIAGNOSIS
- Tuberculosis
- Cystic fibrosis
- Carcinoma of the lung
- Eosinophilic pneumonia
- Bronchiectasis
- Sarcoidosis
- Lung abscess

WORKUP
Physical examination and laboratory data

LABORATORY TESTS
ABPA:
- Peripheral blood eosinophilia and an elevated total serum immunoglobulin E (IgE) level.
- Immediate skin test reactivity with *Aspergillus* spp.[2]
- *Aspergillus* serum precipitating antibody.
- Sputum cultures may be positive for *Aspergillus* spp. but are nonspecific.[1]
- Diagnostic criteria for ABPA are summarized in Table 3.

ASPERGILLOMAS:
- Sputum culture
- Serum precipitating antibody

INVASIVE ASPERGILLOSIS:
- Definitive diagnosis requires the demonstration of tissue invasion (i.e., septate, acute angle branching hyphae) or a positive culture from the tissue or fluid obtained by an invasive procedure such as transbronchial biopsy.
- Sputum and nasal cultures: In high-risk patients a positive culture is strongly suggestive of invasive aspergillosis.
- Serology: The *Platelia Aspergillus* ELISA assay detects a circulating fungal antigen, galactomannan. The **galactomannan antigen immunoassay** is often used for diagnosis. Galactomannan is a polysaccharide contained in the cell wall of *Aspergillus*. Its presence in serum or other body fluids, such as samples obtained from bronchoalveolar lavage, is indicative of invasive infection, and it is recommended as an accurate marker for diagnosis in certain patient subpopulations (hematologic malignancy and hematopoietic stem-cell transplantation). The sensitivity of the galactomannan antigen immunoassay can be impaired by antifungal therapy. The β-D glucan assay can also be used to detect early infection but is not specific for *Aspergillus* species.[4]
- False-negative results occur in patients who are receiving antifungal agents other than

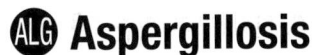

TABLE 3 Diagnostic Criteria for Allergic Bronchopulmonary Aspergillosis

Minimal Essential Diagnostic Criteria of ABPA

Patients with asthma and central bronchiectasis	• Asthma • Central bronchiectasis (inner two thirds of chest CT field) • Immediate cutaneous reactivity to *Aspergillus* • Total serum IgE concentration >417 IU/mL (1000 ng/mL) • Elevated serum IgE—*Aspergillus fumigatus* and/or IgG—*A. fumigatus* (opacities on chest radiograph and serum precipitating antibodies to *A. fumigatus* may be present but are not minimal essential diagnostic criteria)
Patients with asthma (ABPA-seropositive)	Patients with the above criteria 1, 3, 4, 5 (opacities on chest radiograph may be present but are not a minimal essential diagnostic criteria)
Patients with cystic fibrosis	1. Clinical deterioration (increased cough, wheezing, exercise intolerance, increase sputum, decrease in pulmonary function) 2. Immediate cutaneous reactivity to *Aspergillus* or presence of IgE—*A. fumigatus* 3. Total serum IgE concentration ≥1000 IU/mL 4. Precipitating antibodies to *A. fumigatus* or serum IgG—*A. fumigatus* 5. Abnormal chest radiograph (opacities, mucus plugging, or a change from earlier films)

Newly Proposed Diagnostic Criteria

Predisposing conditions	1. Bronchial asthma 2. Cystic fibrosis
Obligatory criteria (both should be present)	1. Type I *Aspergillus* skin test positive (immediate cutaneous hypersensitivity to *Aspergillus* antigen) or elevated IgE levels against *A. fumigatus* 2. Elevated total IgE levels (>1000 IU/mL)*
Other criteria (at least two of three)	1. Presence of precipitating or IgG antibodies against *A. fumigatus* in serum 2. Radiographic pulmonary opacities consistent with ABPA† 3. Total eosinophil count >500 cells/μL in steroid naïve patients (may be historical)

ABPA, Allergic bronchopulmonary aspergillosis; *CT*, computed tomography; *IgE*, immunoglobulin E; *IU*, international units.
*If the patient meets all other criteria, an IgE value <1000 IU/mL may be acceptable.
†The chest radiographic features consistent with ABPA may be transient (i.e., consolidation, nodules, tram-track opacities, toothpaste/finger-in-glove opacities, fleeting opacities) or permanent (i.e., parallel line and ring shadows, bronchiectasis, and pleuropulmonary fibrosis).
From Broaddus VC et al: *Murray & Nadel's textbook of respiratory medicine*, ed 7, Philadelphia, 2022, Elsevier.

fluconazole. The sensitivity of the galactomannan assay for invasive pulmonary aspergillosis is higher in bronchoalveolar lavage fluid than in serum. In patients with risk factors and radiologic findings suggestive of invasive aspergillosis, a positive galactomannan confirms the diagnosis of probable invasive pulmonary aspergillosis.[9]
• Blood cultures: Usually negative (*Aspergillus* is rarely found in the blood).
• Lung biopsy is necessary for definitive diagnosis.

• Biopsy and culture of extrapulmonary lesions.
• Polymerase chain reaction assays may be employed in a case-by-case basis, but their results should be interpreted in conjunction with other diagnostic tests and the clinical context.

IMAGING STUDIES
ABPA:
• CXRs show a variety of abnormalities, from small, patchy, fleeting infiltrates (commonly in the upper lobes) to lobar consolidation or cavitation.
• A majority of patients eventually develop central bronchiectasis.[1]
ASPERGILLOMAS:
• CXR or CT scans usually show the characteristic intracavity mass (Figs. 4 and 5) partially surrounded by a crescent of air.
INVASIVE ASPERGILLOSIS:
• Chest CT scan may reveal cavity formation and the "halo sign" (ground glass opacity surrounding a nodule that is very suggestive of angioinvasive disease). May also see dense nodules, which may cavitate.

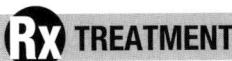 **TREATMENT**

ACUTE GENERAL Rx
ABPA:
• Prednisone (0.5-2 mg/kg/day PO) for 1 to 2 wk, followed by a taper over 2 to 3 mo plus oral itraconazole 5 mg/kg/day up to 400 mg/day with therapeutic drug monitoring for a course of 3 to 6 mo. Alternatives: Voriconazole or posaconazole may be effective.[2]
• If a patient is corticosteroid dependent, prophylaxis for the prevention of *Pneumocystis jiroveci* infection and maintenance of bone mineralization should be considered.
• Bronchodilators and physiotherapy.
• Serial CXR and serum IgE may be useful in guiding treatment.
ASPERGILLOMAS:
• Controversial and problematic; the optimal treatment strategy is unknown.
• Up to 10% of aspergillomas may resolve clinically without overt pharmacologic or surgical intervention.
• Observation for asymptomatic patients.

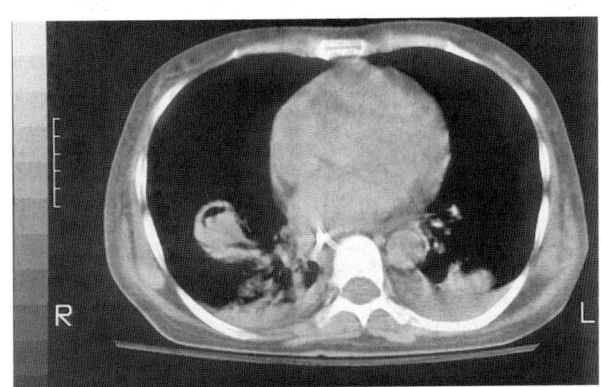

FIG. 4 Computed tomography scan demonstrating an aspergilloma involving the right lower lobe. (From Sellke FW et al: *Sabiston & Spencer surgery of the chest*, ed 9, Philadelphia, 2016, Elsevier.)

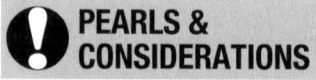
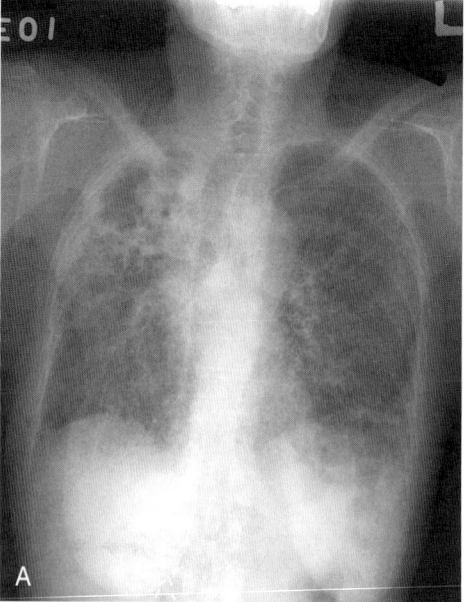

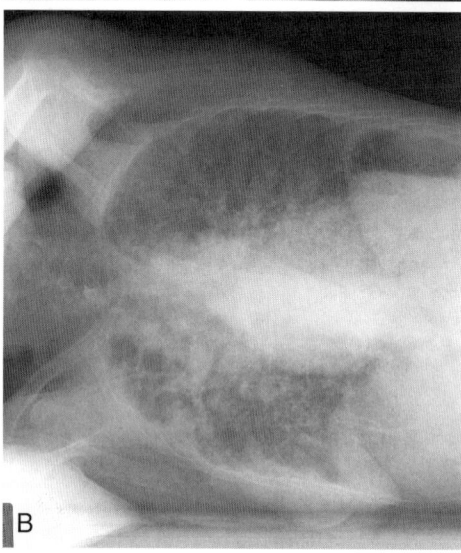

FIG. 5 Posteroanterior **(A)** and decubitus **(B)** chest radiographs demonstrating an aspergilloma within a right upper lobe cavity. The fungus ball "moves" with change in patient position. (From Sellke FW et al: *Sabiston & Spencer surgery of the chest*, ed 9, Philadelphia, 2016, Elsevier.)

- Surgical resection/arterial embolization for those patients with severe hemoptysis or life-threatening hemorrhage.
- For those patients at risk for marked hemoptysis with inadequate pulmonary reserve, consider voriconazole 6 mg/kg IV/PO bid on day 1; then 4 mg/kg IV/PO bid. Isavuconazonium sulfate or itraconazole may also be used as well as transthoracic, intracavitary installation of amphotericin B in poor surgical candidates. (Note: *Aspergillus* now has a higher rate of resistance to itraconazole.)

INVASIVE ASPERGILLOSIS:
- Voriconazole 6 mg/kg IV/PO bid on day 1 followed by 4 mg/kg IV/PO bid. Voriconazole serum concentrations need to be monitored to achieve a target range of 1.0 to 5.5 mg/L (trough on day 4).
- Isavuconazonium sulfate (prodrug of isavuconazole) 372 mg IV/PO three times a day for six doses and then 372 mg IV/PO daily.

- Posaconazole: May be administered as delayed-release tabs (300 mg PO two times on day 1, then 300 mg PO daily) or suspension (200 mg PO four times on day 1, then 400 mg PO twice a day after stabilization of disease) or intravenously (300 mg IV over 90 minutes twice on day 1, then 300 mg IV daily). Posaconazole serum concentrations also may be monitored.
- Posaconazole may also be used as prophylaxis against invasive disease in certain high-risk populations, such as neutropenic patients with acute myeloid leukemia or those with graft versus host disease.

ALTERNATIVE TREATMENT:
- Amphotericin B lipid complex (ABLC) 5 mg/kg IV daily
- Liposomal amphotericin B (L-AMB) 3 to 5 mg/kg IV daily
- Because azoles and echinocandins target different cellular sites, combination therapy

may have additive activity against *Aspergillus* species
- Investigational antifungals in clinical trials include olorofim and fosmanogepix

REFERRAL

To an infectious diseases specialist

⚠ PEARLS & CONSIDERATIONS

- Unlike fluconazole, the potential for drug-drug interactions with voriconazole, isavuconazole, and posaconazole is very high. Azoles may interact with drugs used for chemotherapy or immunosuppression by increasing toxicity and/or by reducing efficacy.
- Azole resistance has appeared in *Aspergillus fumigatus*; the main resistance mechanism is a point mutation of CYP51A, the gene coding

A

I

for 14 alpha-sterol demethylase, the target enzyme of antifungal drugs. Global prevalence of azole resistance in *Aspergillus* is estimated to be approximately 3% to 6%.
- Antifungal susceptibility testing should be considered if there has been extensive prior patient antifungal exposure and/or if there are high rates of local azole resistance.[10]
- Agitation of hospital buildings by renovations or repairs may increase the incidence of *Aspergillus* infections in immunosuppressed individuals.

- Echinocandins should never be used as primary treatment of aspergillosis.
- *Aspergillus* and *Nocardia* species may coinfect.
- Use of antifungal agents in combination is discussed in Box E1.

REFERENCES & SUGGESTED READINGS
Available at eBooks.Health.Elsevier.com

RELATED CONTENT
Aspergillosis (Patient Information)

AUTHORS: **SAJEEV HANDA, MD, SFHM** and **MICHAEL ROSSI, MD**

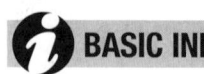

BASIC INFORMATION

DEFINITION
Aspiration pneumonia refers to pulmonary infection of the lower airways and lung parenchyma resulting from entry of colonized oropharyngeal or upper gastrointestinal contents.[1] *Aspiration pneumonia* is considered part of the continuum that also includes community- and hospital-acquired pneumonias.[1] *Chemical pneumonitis* (or *aspiration pneumonitis*) refers to lung injury and inflammation resulting from entry of sterile substances toxic to the lower airways.

SYNONYMS
Pneumonia, aspiration
Aspiration pneumonitis

ICD-10CM CODE
J69.0   Pneumonitis due to inhalation of food and vomit

EPIDEMIOLOGY & DEMOGRAPHICS
INCIDENCE (IN U.S.):
- 7.1 cases per 10,000 people admitted to the hospital[2]
- 30.9 cases per 10,000 people admitted to the hospital >65 yr of age[2]

PREVALENCE (IN U.S.): Unknown (unreliable data)
PREDOMINANT SEX: Slight male predominance[2]
PREDOMINANT AGE: >65 yr
PEAK INCIDENCE: Elderly patients in hospitals or nursing homes[2,3]

PHYSICAL FINDINGS & CLINICAL PRESENTATION
- Symptoms develop within hours to a few days after aspiration event, though anaerobic infections can have a more subacute presentation.
- Clinical presentation ranges from minimal symptoms to fulminant respiratory failure.
- Symptoms can include dyspnea, diffuse wheeze, cough, hypoxia, tachypnea, tachycardia, sputum production, and fever.
- Lung exam may demonstrate wheezes, crackles, or rhonchi.

ETIOLOGY
Complex interaction of etiologies, ranging from chemical (often acid) pneumonitis after aspiration of sterile gastric contents (generally not requiring antibiotic treatment) to bacterial aspiration. Risk factors for aspiration pneumonia include vomiting, decreased consciousness, poor dentition, ineffective cough reflex or glottic closure, and gastroesophageal reflux disease.[4-11] Table 1 and Fig. E1 summarize risk factors for aspiration pneumonia.
COMMUNITY-ACQUIRED ASPIRATION PNEUMONIA:
- Most patients have a mixed infection with aerobic and anaerobic bacteria. The most common bacteria are *Streptococcus pneumoniae, Staphylococcus aureus, Haemophilus influenzae,* and *Enterobacteriaceae.*[12-14]

Anaerobes (*Peptostreptococcus, Fusobacterium nucleatum, Fusobacterium necrophorum, Prevotella,* and *Bacteroides* species) are less frequently isolated.[15]
- High-risk groups: age >65 yr; alcohol use; IV drug use; altered mental status; stroke victims; cardiac arrest; and patients with esophageal disorders, seizures, periodontal disease, or recent dental manipulations.[4-11]

HOSPITAL-ACQUIRED ASPIRATION PNEUMONIA:
- Causative organisms:
  1. Anaerobes listed above, although in many studies gram-negative aerobes (60%) and gram-positive aerobes (20%) predominate[13,16-18]
  2. *E. coli, P. aeruginosa, S. aureus* including MRSA, *Klebsiella, Enterobacter, Serratia, Proteus* spp., *H. influenzae, S. pneumoniae, Legionella,* and *Acinetobacter* spp. (sporadic pneumonias) in two thirds of cases
  3. Fungi, including *Candida albicans,* in <1%[19]
- High-risk groups: Seriously ill hospitalized patients (especially patients with coma, acidosis, alcohol use disorder, uremia, diabetes mellitus, nasogastric intubation, or recent antimicrobial therapy), who are frequently colonized with aerobic gram-negative rods; patients undergoing anesthesia; those with strokes, dementia, or swallowing disorders; patients >65 yr; and those receiving antacids or H_2 blockers, or proton pump inhibitors (but not sucralfate).
- Hypoxic patients receiving concentrated O_2 have diminished ciliary activity, increasing risk for aspiration pneumonia.

DIAGNOSIS

DIFFERENTIAL DIAGNOSIS
- Other necrotizing or cavitary pneumonias (especially tuberculosis, gram-negative pneumonias)
- See "Tuberculosis, Pulmonary"

WORKUP
- Chest x-ray
- Complete blood count (CBC), blood cultures
- Sputum Gram stain and culture
- Consideration of tracheal aspirate or bronchoscopy sample if intubated
- CT of chest if diagnosis is unclear or when suspecting complications

LABORATORY TESTS
- CBC: Leukocytosis often present.
- Sputum Gram stain:
  1. Often useful when carefully prepared immediately after obtaining suctioned or expectorated specimen, examined by experienced observer.
  2. Only specimens with multiple white blood cells and rare or absent epithelial cells should be examined.
  3. Unlike other bacterial pneumonias (e.g., pneumococcal), multiple organisms may be present in aspiration pneumonia.

4. Long, slender rods suggest anaerobes, though these organisms are difficult to isolate due to frequent contamination of sputum samples with oral flora.
5. Sputum from pneumonia caused by acid aspiration may be devoid of organisms.
6. Cultures should be interpreted in light of morphology of visualized organisms.

IMAGING STUDIES
- Chest x-ray may be negative early in the disease course.[20] It often reveals opacities in gravity-dependent lung regions. In an upright patient, opacities commonly affect the basal segments of the lower lobes. In a supine patient, opacities can involve the superior segment of the lower lobes, posterior right upper lobe, or the apicoposterior segment of the left upper lobe (Fig. 2). Chest x-ray can also demonstrate a pattern of diffuse lung involvement characteristic of acute respiratory distress syndrome. (See related content in "Acute Respiratory Distress Syndrome.")
- Aspiration pneumonia of several days' duration (or longer) may reveal necrosis (especially community-acquired anaerobic pneumonias) and even cavitation with air-fluid levels, indicating lung abscess.

TREATMENT

NONPHARMACOLOGIC THERAPY
- Management to prevent repeated aspiration
- Ventilatory support if necessary
- Rehabilitative management: Physical, pulmonary, and dysphagia therapy combined with

TABLE 1   Risk Factors for Dysphagia and Aspiration Pneumonia

Cerebrovascular disease
Ischemic stroke
Hemorrhagic stroke
Subarachnoid hemorrhage
Degenerative neurologic disease
Alzheimer disease
Multiinfarct dementia
Parkinson disease
Amyotrophic lateral sclerosis (motor neuron disease)
Multiple sclerosis
Head and neck cancer
Oropharyngeal malignancy
Oral cavity malignancy
Esophageal malignancy
Other
Scleroderma
Diabetic gastroparesis
Reflux esophagitis
Presbyesophagus
Achalasia

From Vincent JL et al: *Textbook of critical care,* ed 7, Philadelphia, 2017, Elsevier.

appropriate nutrition can reduce length of stay and mortality
- Fig. 3 illustrates a prevention and treatment algorithm for pulmonary aspiration

ACUTE GENERAL Rx

Chemical pneumonitis: Acute aspiration of acidic gastric contents without bacteria may not require antibiotic therapy; initial treatment involves airway maintenance and management of bronchospasm and airway edema. Routine adjunctive treatment with glucocorticoids is not recommended. Empiric antibiotics may be considered in severe cases, but their ongoing use should be reassessed at 48 to 72 hr.[1]

- **Aspiration pneumonia:** Antibiotic selection depends on the site of acquisition (long-term care facility, hospital, community), which modifies risk factors for infection with multidrug-resistant pathogens. Additionally, a history of treatment with broad-spectrum antibiotics in the past 90 days warrants empiric treatment for multidrug-resistant organisms.[21,22]

1. Community-acquired aspiration pneumonia or hospital-acquired cases with low risk of multidrug-resistant pathogens: Ampicillin-sulbactam 1.5 to 3 g every 6 h IV, or amoxicillin-clavulanate PO 875 mg twice daily, or a fluoroquinolone (levofloxacin 750 mg IV or PO) is effective. Clindamycin (450 mg oral qid or 600 mg IV every 8 h) can be added to the other agent when the risk of predominantly anaerobic infection is high.

2. Nursing home aspirations or hospital-acquired aspiration pneumonias with concerns for resistance: Broad-spectrum treatment with piperacillin-tazobactam 4.5 g q8h or 3.375 g q6h, cefepime 2 g q8h, levofloxacin 750 mg IV or PO once daily, imipenem 500 mg q6h or 1 g q8h, or meropenem 1 g q8h. The addition of vancomycin (15 mg/kg q12h IV) or linezolid (600 mg q12h PO or IV) is warranted if MRSA is suspected or known (e.g.,

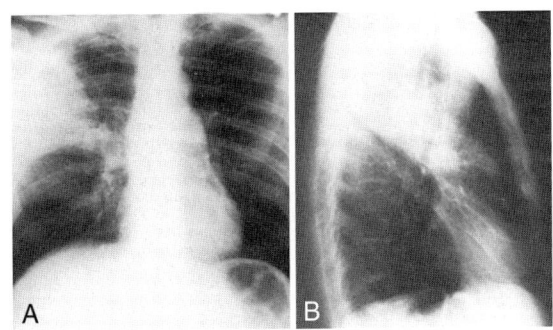

FIG. 2 Anaerobic necrotizing pneumonia following aspiration of oropharyngeal secretions. Multiple, small (<2 cm) radiolucencies are seen throughout the posterior segment of the right upper lobe on the postero-anterior **(A)** and lateral **(B)** projections. (Courtesy Michael Gotway, MD. From Mason RJ et al: *Murray & Nadel's textbook of respiratory medicine,* ed 5, Philadelphia, 2010, Saunders.)

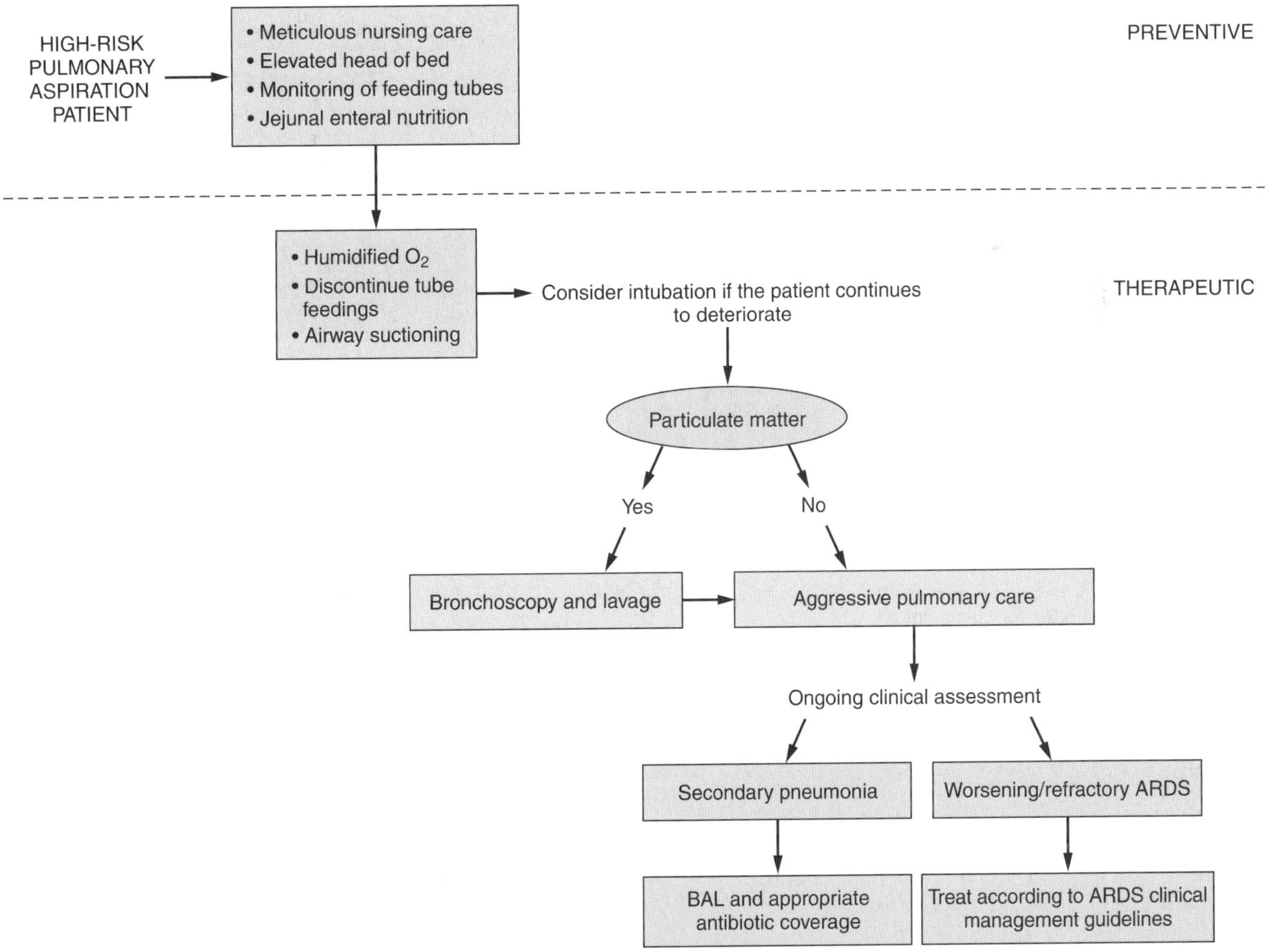

PREVENTIVE

```
HIGH-RISK
PULMONARY  ──▶  • Meticulous nursing care
ASPIRATION       • Elevated head of bed
PATIENT          • Monitoring of feeding tubes
                 • Jejunal enteral nutrition
```

THERAPEUTIC

```
• Humidified O₂
• Discontinue tube   ──▶  Consider intubation if the patient continues
  feedings                 to deteriorate
• Airway suctioning

                          ( Particulate matter )
                         Yes              No

        Bronchoscopy and lavage  ──▶  Aggressive pulmonary care

                          Ongoing clinical assessment

        Secondary pneumonia          Worsening/refractory ARDS

        BAL and appropriate          Treat according to ARDS clinical
        antibiotic coverage          management guidelines
```

FIG. 3 Prevention and treatment algorithm for pulmonary aspiration. *ARDS,* Acute respiratory distress syndrome; *BAL,* bronchoalveolar lavage. (From Newman M et al: *Perioperative medicine,* ed 2, Philadelphia 2022, Elsevier.)

Aspiration Pneumonia 🅐🅛🅖 🅟🅣🅖

BOX 1 Reducing Risk of Aspiration and Aspiration Pneumonia in Older Adults*

Hand Feeding
- Provide a rest period (>30 min) before feeding time.
- Have the patient sit upright at 90 degrees or highest position allowed by medical condition.
- Avoid rushed or forced feeding; feeding by syringe is risky.
- Alternate liquids with solids.
- Recognize the high risks of sedatives, hypnotics, and other psychotropic medications, and try to wean or reduce dosages.
- Speech-language therapist referral: Evaluate patient for possible benefit of chin-down position when swallowing or of adjusting liquid viscosity; thickened liquids of varying types may improve swallowing in some patients (ice cream and Jell-O are considered thin liquids).

Tube Feeding
- *Note:* Both nasogastric and gastrostomy tube feeding may increase aspiration risks.
- Consider continuous feedings rather than intermittent (bolus) feedings.
- Keep backrest elevated at least 30 degrees during feedings, if possible.
- Consider pump-assisted feedings rather than gravity-controlled feedings.
- A gastric residual volume >200 ml during continuous feeding or before intermittent feedings may increase risk (but this remains controversial).[23]
- Prokinetic agents such as metoclopramide or erythromycin may improve feeding tolerance, but are associated with their own serious potential side effects.
- Placing the feeding tube tip beyond the pylorus (jejunostomy, gastrojejunostomy) may reduce aspiration in some patients.
- Using colored dye in tube feeding is contraindicated (it was originally thought that adding coloring to liquid tube feeding formulas would help identify probable feeding aspiration if the dye was found after throat and pulmonary suctioning).[24]

*Most of these suggestions are consensus and expert opinions rather than evidence-based practices.[25-28]
From Fillit HM: Brocklehurst's textbook of geriatric medicine and gerontology, *ed 8, Philadelphia, 2017, Elsevier.*

---

documented nasal or respiratory colonization with MRSA).

a. Knowledge of resident flora in the microenvironment of the aspiration within the hospital is crucial to intelligent antibiotic selection; consult infection control nurses or hospital epidemiologist.

b. Confirmed *Pseudomonas* pneumonia in patients not in septic shock or at high risk of death can be treated with an antipseudomonal beta-lactam agent (piperacillin/tazobactam, cefepime, meropenem) or an antipseudomonal fluoroquinolone pending results of susceptibility testing. In severe cases, empiric two-drug combination therapy with an antipseudomonal beta-lactam agent and an antipseudomonal

fluoroquinolone or an aminoglycoside is recommended. The choice of agents should be guided by the results of drug susceptibility testing when available.

DISPOSITION
Repeat chest x-ray in 6 to 8 wk in most patients.

PREVENTION
For patients with difficulty swallowing thin liquids, adding thickening agents to provide nectar-thick, pudding-thick, and honey-thick fluids is an option. Sitting patients upright when eating (and for some time afterward), chin tucking when swallowing, eating more slowly, and use of various swallowing maneuvers are additional techniques for prevention of aspiration in elderly and debilitated patients (Box 1).

REFERRAL
Consultation with infectious disease and/or pulmonary specialists recommended for patients with respiratory distress, hypoxia, ventilatory support, pneumonia in more than one lobe, necrosis or cavitation on chest x-ray, or for those not clinically responding to antibiotic therapy within 2 to 3 days.

REFERENCES
Available at eBooks.Health.Elsevier.com.

RELATED CONTENT
Aspiration Pneumonia (Patient Information)

AUTHOR: **NARGES ALIPANAH-LECHNER, MD**

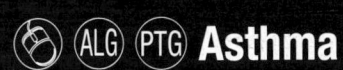
Diseases
and Disorders

I

BASIC INFORMATION

DEFINITION

The National Asthma Education and Prevention Program (NAEPP) guidelines define asthma as "a chronic inflammatory disease of the airways in which many cells and cellular elements play a role: In particular mast cells, neutrophils, eosinophils, T lymphocytes, macrophages, and epithelial cells. In susceptible individuals, this inflammation causes recurrent episodes of coughing (particularly at night or early in the morning), wheezing, breathlessness, and chest tightness. The episodes are usually associated with widespread but variable airflow obstruction that is reversible either spontaneously or as a result of treatment." **Status asthmaticus,** or acute severe asthma, is a refractory state that does not respond to standard therapy such as inhaled beta-agonists or subcutaneous epinephrine. It may persist for several hours.

SYNONYMS

Bronchospasm
Reactive airway disease
Asthmatic bronchitis

ICD-10CM CODES

J45.20	Mild intermittent asthma, uncomplicated
J45.21	Mild intermittent asthma with (acute) exacerbation
J45.22	Mild intermittent asthma with status asthmaticus
J45.30	Mild persistent asthma, uncomplicated
J45.31	Mild persistent asthma with (acute) exacerbation
J45.32	Mild persistent asthma with status asthmaticus
J45.40	Moderate persistent asthma, uncomplicated
J45.41	Moderate persistent asthma with (acute) exacerbation
J45.42	Moderate persistent asthma with status asthmaticus
J45.50	Severe persistent asthma, uncomplicated
J45.51	Severe persistent asthma with (acute) exacerbation
J45.52	Severe persistent asthma with status asthmaticus
J45.901	Unspecified asthma with (acute) exacerbation
J45.902	Unspecified asthma with status asthmaticus
J45.909	Unspecified asthma, uncomplicated
J45.991	Cough variant asthma
J45.998	Other asthma

EPIDEMIOLOGY & DEMOGRAPHICS

- Asthma has been diagnosed in 7.7% of the population in the U.S. Its prevalence is steadily rising among patients older than 65 yr, African Americans, women, and persons living below the poverty level.

- It is estimated that 300 million people have asthma. An increase in prevalence to 400 million is anticipated by 2025.
- It accounts for around 440,000 hospitalizations and 1.8 million emergency department visits yearly in the U.S.
- It was previously more common in children, but given the increase of adult-onset asthma, it is now more common in adults (7.5% of children vs. 7.7% of adults).
- Overall, mortality secondary to asthma has declined in the U.S. to 10.5 per 1 million but has not changed for children ages 1 to 14 yr.
- 50% to 80% of children with asthma develop symptoms before 5 yr of age. Early childhood risk factors for asthma are described in Table 1.
- Box 1 summarizes risk factors for severe and fatal asthma in adults.

PHYSICAL FINDINGS & CLINICAL PRESENTATION

Physical examination findings vary with the stage and severity of asthma and may reveal a normal lung examination. Some degree of wheezing and prolonged expiratory phases of respiration are usually present with persistent or acute disease. Box 2 summarizes signs and symptoms of severe asthma. Physical examination during status asthmaticus may reveal:
- Tachycardia and tachypnea
- Use of accessory respiratory muscles
- Pulsus paradoxus (inspiratory decline in systolic blood pressure >10 mm Hg)
- Absence of wheezing (silent chest) or decreased wheezing can indicate worsening obstruction
- Mental status changes: Generally secondary to hypoxia and hypercapnia and constitute an indication for urgent intubation
- Paradoxical abdominal and diaphragmatic movement on inspiration (detected by palpation over the upper part of the abdomen in a

TABLE 1   Early Childhood Risk Factors for Persistent Asthma

Parental asthma
Allergy:
Atopic dermatitis (eczema)
Allergic rhinitis
Food allergy
Inhalant allergen sensitization
Food allergen sensitization
Severe lower respiratory tract infection:
Pneumonia
Bronchiolitis requiring hospitalization
Wheezing apart from colds
Male gender
Low birthweight
Environmental tobacco smoke exposure
Possible use of acetaminophen (paracetamol)
Exposure to chlorinated swimming pools
Reduced lung function at birth

From Kliegman RM et al: *Nelson textbook of pediatrics,* ed 19, Philadelphia, 2011, Saunders.

semirecumbent position) indicates diaphragmatic fatigue, another sign of impending respiratory crisis

BOX 1   Risk Factors for Severe and Fatal Asthma in Adults

- History of prior nonfatal asthma attack
- Prior intubation
- Female gender
- Age >65 yr
- African American ethnicity
- Obesity
- Tobacco use
- Inhalational drug abuse
- Poorly controlled disease
- Poor recognition of dyspnea and other symptoms
- Steroid dependence
- H1N1 viral infection
- Misuse or lack of proper use of maintenance medications
- Psychiatric illness
- Lack of access to medical care
- Lack of ability to limit triggers (i.e., persistent exposure to pollutants, dust)
- Comorbid heart disease, obesity, and/or diabetes
- Bronchoalveolar lavage predominance of neutrophils, interleukin 8, and matrix metalloproteinase

From Parrillo JE, Dellinger RP: *Critical care medicine, principles of diagnosis and management in the adult,* ed 5, Philadelphia, 2019, Elsevier.

BOX 2   Signs and Symptoms of Severe Asthma

- "Tripoding"—sitting upright and leaning forward
- Diaphoresis
- Use of accessory muscles
- Asynchronous accessory muscle use
- Air trapping and hyperinflation manifesting as decreased inspiratory stroke volume and pulsus paradoxus
- Peak flow <200 L/min and/or <30% predicted*
- FEV1 <1 L/min and/or <20% predicted*
- Evidence of barotrauma:
  - Unilateral diminution in breath sounds
  - Tracheal deviation
  - Thoracic crepitus
- Signs of impending respiratory arrest:
  - Altered mentation
  - Cyanosis
  - Hypoxia
  - Hypercarbia
  - Hemodynamic instability
  - Silent chest

*These values are estimations because both peak expiratory flow rate and forced expiratory volume in 1 second (FEV1) vary with age, gender, and height.
From Parrillo JE, Dellinger RP: *Critical care medicine, principles of diagnosis and management in the adult,* ed 5, Philadelphia, 2019, Elsevier.

ETIOLOGY

- The pathophysiology of asthma involves a complex interaction among various environmental and genetic factors (Figs. E1, E2, and E3). Genetic and phenotypic associations in asthma are described in Box 3.
- Allergic (atopic, extrinsic) asthma is triggered by various aeroallergens or nonallergic (nonatopic) nonspecific (e.g., dust, cigarette smoke, fumes, cold air, exercise) exposures in patients who are prone to develop IgE antibodies in response to various exposures.
- Factors that contribute to worsening asthma control and coexisting conditions are summarized in Table 2.
- A longitudinal epidemiologic cohort study of a prebirth cohort observed that maternal intake of foods commonly considered allergenic (peanut and milk) was associated with a decrease in allergy and asthma in the offspring. No dietary restrictions during pregnancy are therefore recommended for the prevention of allergies or asthma.
- Nonallergic (intrinsic) asthma commonly manifests as adult-onset asthma in response to respiratory tract infection or psychologic stress.
- Occupational exposure to certain organic or nonorganic agents can trigger asthma.
- Dampness and mold contribute to the risk of developing asthma; remediation of these in homes reduces asthma symptoms and medication use in adults.
- Exercise-induced asthma is seen most frequently in adolescents and manifests with bronchospasm after beginning of exercise and improves with discontinuation of exercise.
- Drug-induced asthma is associated with use of NSAIDs, β-blockers, sulfites, and certain foods and beverages.
- There is a strong association of the *ADAM 33* gene with asthma and bronchial hyperresponsiveness. Experimental, genetic, and clinical studies support an important role for Type-2 inflammatory pathways in the pathogenesis of severe asthma. Atopic triggers stimulate Th2 cells to produce IL-5, IL-13, and IL-4, driving IgE synthesis, eosinophilia, and airway changes. IL-5 is felt to be the most specific cytokine in eosinophil regulatory pathways. Nonatopic triggers (e.g., smoke, viruses) also have a vital role in the Type-2 inflammatory pathway. Type-2 Innate Lymphoid Cells (ILC2) produce IL-5, IL-13 through release of Damaged Associated Molecular Patterns (DAMPs) from the respiratory epithelium.
- Damaged airway epithelium also releases innate immunity cytokines known as alarmins (TSLP, IL-25, IL-33). These airway epithelium cytokines initiate multiple Type-2 inflammatory pathways in response to allergen and infection-driven inflammation. IL-33 and IL-25 are known to mainly activate ILC2s. Thymic stromal lipoproteins (TSLP), on the other hand, have been shown to promote antigen-presenting cells (APCs) that lead to the activation of T cells and B cells.

Ⓓⓧ DIAGNOSIS

DIFFERENTIAL DIAGNOSIS

- Postinfectious bronchitis
- Rhinitis with postnasal drip
- Paradoxical vocal fold motion (vocal cord dysfunction)
- Chronic obstructive pulmonary disease (COPD)
- Gastroesophageal reflux disease (GERD)
- Pneumonia and other respiratory tract infections
- Foreign body aspiration (most frequent in younger patients)
- Anxiety disorder
- Interstitial lung disease
- Hypersensitivity pneumonitis
- Heart failure
- Pulmonary embolism

WORKUP

- An algorithm for diagnosing asthma in adults is illustrated in Fig. 4. Diagnosis of asthma requires documentation of airway obstruction and some degree of reversibility.
- For symptomatic adults and children age >5 yr who can perform spirometry, pre- and postbronchodilator spirometry is the recommended test of choice.
- Airflow reversibility is defined as increase in forced expiratory volume in 1 sec (FEV_1 by at least 12% and 200 ml) after inhaling a short-acting bronchodilator.
- The degree of reversibility measured by spirometry correlates with airway inflammation, and patients with a high degree of reversibility have a greater risk of irreversible airflow obstruction in subsequent years.
- For children age <5 yr, spirometry is generally not feasible. Those with asthma symptoms should be treated as having suspected asthma after alternative diagnoses are ruled out.
- Negative spirometry results do not rule out asthma. Patients with high clinical suspicion should undergo bronchial challenge testing with methacholine or other specific agents.
- The clinician should evaluate for environmental causes (e.g., house dust mites, indoor pets) and exposure to other allergens or irritants (e.g., tobacco smoke.)
- In the absence of spirometry, variability of peak flow measurements can be used to diagnose asthma.

After diagnosis, the severity of asthma should be classified during the initial assessment before

BOX 3   Genetic and Phenotypic Associations in Asthma

- **ADAM33:** Gene bronchoconstriction
- **ORMDL3/GSDMB** locus, chromosome 17q21: Childhood onset
- CpG portion of **ACSL3:** Associated with maternal exposure to automobile pollution
- **IL33** on chromosome 9
- **IL2RB** on chromosome 22

From Parrillo JE, Dellinger RP: *Critical care medicine, principles of diagnosis and management in the adult,* ed 5, Philadelphia, 2019, Elsevier.

TABLE 2   Factors That Contribute to Worsening Asthma Control and Coexisting Conditions

Contributing Factor	Proposed Intervention
Tobacco use	Encourage tobacco cessation and assist with both nonpharmacologic and pharmacologic methods to help patients quit smoking; discuss avoidance of secondhand smoke
GERD	Consider empiric therapy for symptomatic GERD Barium swallow or pH probe study to diagnose GERD Impedance study if nonacid reflux is suspected Referral to gastroenterology for evaluation and treatment Consider surgical management for refractory cases
Atopy and allergic rhinitis	Consider empiric therapy with nasal steroids, nasal and oral antihistamines, leukotriene antagonists Consider skin prick testing or specific IgE testing to guide allergen identification and avoidance Referral to allergist or otolaryngologist for evaluation Consider allergen immunotherapy
Nasal polyps and chronic sinusitis	Refer to otolaryngologist for evaluation and treatment Possible surgical intervention for refractory cases Consider aspirin desensitization for patients with nasal polyps and aspirin sensitivity
Vocal cord dysfunction*	Laryngoscopy to diagnose vocal cord dysfunction Referral to speech pathologist for evaluation and treatment
Obesity*	Encourage weight loss Consider bariatric surgery
Obstructive sleep apnea*	Referral for sleep study and initiate therapy for sleep apnea Referral to sleep specialist for complex cases
Psychologic factors*	Evaluate for anxiety and depression

GERD, Gastroesophageal reflux disease; *Ig,* immunoglobulin.
*May coexist with asthma with overlapping symptoms.
From Broaddus VC et al: *Murray & Nadel's textbook of respiratory medicine,* ed 7, Philadelphia, 2022, Elsevier.

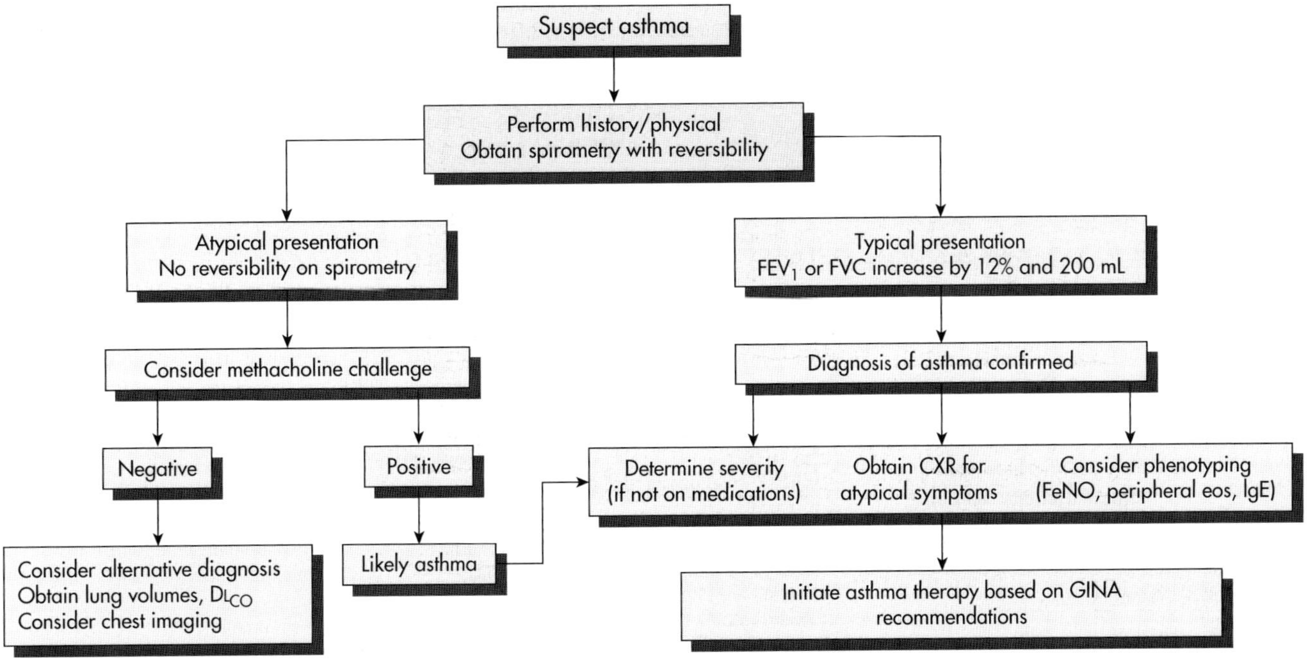

FIG. 4 Algorithm for diagnosing asthma in adults. The diagnosis of asthma is based on a careful personal history, physical examination, and lung function testing. Spirometry should be obtained in every patient in whom asthma is suspected. Other tests are useful when clinical features are atypical and to determine severity and asthma phenotype. *CXR,* Chest radiograph; D_{LCO}, diffusing capacity for carbon monoxide; *eos,* eosinophils; *FeNO,* fraction of exhaled nitric oxide; *FEV₁*, forced expiratory volume in 1 second; *FVC,* forced vital capacity; *GINA,* Global Initiative for Asthma; *IgE,* immunoglobulin E. (From Broaddus VC et al: *Murray & Nadel's textbook of respiratory medicine,* ed 7, Philadelphia, 2022, Elsevier.)

initiating therapy. Patients are divided into four groups based on the severity of their asthma symptoms and number of exacerbations.
- Once therapy is initiated, the emphasis for clinical management should be aimed at achievement of asthma control. The level of asthma control should be used to guide decisions either to maintain or adjust therapy.
- Schedule visits at 2 to 6 wk intervals for patients who are initiating therapy or who require a step up in therapy to achieve or regain asthma control. Schedule visits at 6-12 mo intervals after asthma control is achieved to monitor whether control is maintained. The interval will depend on factors such as the duration of asthma control or the level of treatment required, especially for patients who are on asthma biologic therapy. Consider scheduling visits at 3 mo intervals if step-down therapy is anticipated.

LABORATORY TESTS
- Arterial blood gases (ABGs) can be used during acute bronchospasm in staging the severity of an asthmatic attack:
  1. Mild: Decreased Pao_2 and $Paco_2$, increased pH
  2. Moderate: Decreased Pao_2, normal $Paco_2$, normal pH
  3. Severe: Marked decreased Pao_2, increased $Paco_2$, and decreased pH
- Complete blood count: Leukocytosis with left shift may indicate the existence of bacterial infection. Elevated eosinophils point toward allergic component of asthma.
- Serum IgE and eosinophil levels help guide treatment for patients with severe persistent

asthma and monitor response to treatment in this group.
- Spirometry is recommended at the initial assessment and at least every 1 to 2 yr after treatment is initiated and when the symptoms and peak expiratory flow have stabilized. Spirometry may be performed more frequently, if indicated, based on severity of symptoms or lack of response to treatment.
- Peak expiratory flow rate (PEFR) can be used to assess severity of an acute exacerbation episode. Values should be compared with individual's personal best number (see "asthma action plan").
- Specific allergy testing may be helpful in a subgroup of patients.
- Fractional exhaled nitric oxide (FeNO) can be used to assess airway inflammation and to guide treatment and monitor response.

IMAGING STUDIES
- Chest x-ray: Usually normal, may show evidence of thoracic hyperinflation (e.g., flattening of the diaphragm, increased volume over the retrosternal air space).
- ECG: Tachycardia, nonspecific ST-T wave changes are common during an asthma attack; may also show cor pulmonale, right bundle branch block, right axial deviation, counterclockwise rotation.

Rx TREATMENT

NONPHARMACOLOGIC THERAPY
- Avoidance of triggering factors (e.g., salicylates, sulfites), environmental, or occupational triggers
- Encouragement of regular exercise

- Patient education regarding warning signs of an attack and proper use of medications (e.g., inhalers)
- Assess asthma control with use of validated questionnaires

GENERAL Rx
The 2007 NAEPP Guidelines for the Diagnosis and Management of Asthma and the 2020 Focused Updates to the Asthma Management Guidelines (see Tables 3 to 5) provide treatment algorithms by age groups with a step-up approach based on the severity of symptoms.

An approach to home management of acute asthma is described in Fig. E5. Selected inhaled medications used by patients with asthma are summarized in Table 6.
- Short-acting beta-selective adrenergic agonists (SABAs) administered by inhalation are the most effective therapy for quick relief of asthmatic symptoms. They are recommended for use only as needed for relief of symptoms or before anticipated exposure to known triggers such as exercise. They should not be used as a single agent except for intermittent asthma symptoms.
- When symptoms become more frequent or more severe, step-up treatment with maintenance inhalers is recommended (see Table 3).
- Inhaled corticosteroids (ICSs) are the mainstay of treatment for maintenance therapy.
- Other maintenance treatment options include long-acting beta-agonist (LABA), combination of inhaled corticosteroids and LABA, leukotriene receptor antagonist (LTRA), cromolyn, zileuton, and theophylline.
- There are several corticosteroid/LABA combination inhalers available (fluticasone/

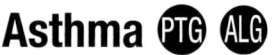
TABLE 3 Stepwise Approach for Managing Asthma in Youths ≥12 Yr and Adults

Treatment	Intermittent Asthma Step 1	MANAGEMENT OF PERSISTENT ASTHMA IN INDIVIDUALS 12+ YR OF AGE				
		Step 2	Step 3	Step 4	Step 5	Step 6^
Preferred	PRN SABA	Daily low-dose ICS and PRN SABA or PRN concomitant ICS and SABA#	Daily and PRN combination low-dose ICS-formoterol#	Daily and PRN combination medium-dose ICS-formoterol#	Daily medium-dose ICS-LABA + LAMA and PRN SABA#	Daily high-dose ICS-LABA + oral systemic corticosteroid + PRN SABA
Alternative		Daily LTRA* and PRN SABA or cromolyn,* or nedocromil,* or zileuton,* or theophylline,* and PRN SABA	Daily medium-dose ICS and PRN SABA or Daily low-dose ICS-LABA, or daily low-dose ICS + LAMA,# or daily low-dose ICS + LTRA,* and PRN SABA or Daily low-dose ICS + theophylline* or zileuton,* and PRN SABA	Daily medium-dose ICS-LABA or daily medium-dose ICS + LAMA, and PRN SABA# or Daily medium-dose ICS + LTRA* or daily medium-dose ICS + theophylline,* or daily medium-dose ICS + zileuton,* and PRN SABA	Daily high-dose ICS + LTRA* or daily high-dose ICS + theophylline,* and PRN SABA	
		Steps 2-4: Conditionally recommend the use of subcutaneous immunotherapy as an adjunct treatment to standard pharmacotherapy in individuals >5 yr of age whose asthma is controlled at the initiation, build up, and maintenance phases of immunotherapy.#			Consider adding Asthma Biologics (e.g., anti-IgE, anti-IL5, anti-IL5R, anti-IL4/IL13)	

EIB, Exercise-induced bronchospasm; *ICS*, inhaled corticosteroid; *LABA*, long-acting beta₂-agonist; *LTRA*, leukotriene receptor antagonist; *prn*, as necessary; *SABA*, inhaled short-acting beta₂-agonist.

*Cromolyn, nedocromil, LTRAs (including zileuton and montelukast), and theophylline were not considered in the 2020 NAEPP update.

**The AHRQ systemic reviews that informed this report did not include studies that examined the role of asthma biologics. Thus this 2020 NAEPP update does not contain specific recommendations for the use of biologics in asthma in Steps 5 and 6.

^Data on the use of LAMA therapy in individuals with severe persistent asthma (Step 6) were not included in the AHRQ systematic review, and thus no recommendation is made.

#Updated based on the 2020 guidelines.

The stepwise approach is meant to assist, not replace, the clinical decision-making required to meet individual patient needs.

If alternative treatment is used and response is inadequate, discontinue it and use the preferred treatment before stepping up.

Zileuton is a less desirable alternative due to limited studies as adjunctive therapy and the need to monitor liver function. Theophylline requires monitoring of serum concentration levels. In step 6, before oral systemic corticosteroids are introduced, a trial of high-dose ICS + LABA + either LTRA, theophylline, or zileuton may be considered, although this approach has not been studied in clinical trials.

Steps 1, 2, and 3 preferred therapies are based on Evidence A; step 3 alternative therapy is based on Evidence A for LTRA, Evidence B for theophylline, and Evidence D for zileuton. Step 5 preferred therapy is based on Evidence B. Step 6 preferred therapy is based on (EPR-2 1997) and Evidence B for omalizumab.

Immunotherapy for steps 2-4 is based on Evidence B for house-dust mites, animal danders, and pollens; evidence is weak or lacking for molds and cockroaches. Evidence is strongest for immunotherapy with single allergens. The role of allergy in asthma is greater in children than in adults.

Clinicians who administer immunotherapy or omalizumab should be prepared and equipped to identify and treat anaphylaxis that may occur.

This information is directly abstracted from the 2007 NAEPP *Expert Panel Report 3: Guidelines for the diagnosis and management of asthma* and is not intended to promote or endorse any of the listed products.

To access the complete 2007 *Expert Panel Report 3: Guidelines for the diagnosis and management of asthma,* go to www.nhlbi.nih.gov/sites/default/files/media/docs/asthsumm.pdf. The "2020 Focused Updates to the Asthma Management Guidelines: a report from the National Asthma Education and Prevention Program Coordinating Committee Expert Panel Working Group" can be found at https://www.nhlbi.nih.gov/sites/default/files/publications/AsthmaManagementGuidelinesReport-2-4-21.pdf

From 2020 Focused Updates to the Asthma Management Guidelines: A Report from the National Asthma Education and Prevention Program Coordinating Committee Expert Panel Working Group. https://www.nhlbi.nih.gov/sites/default/files/publications/AsthmaManagementGuidelinesReport-2-4-21.pdf

salmeterol [Advair], budesonide/formoterol [Symbicort], mometasone/formoterol [Dulera], and ICS/LABA fluticasone furoate 200 mcg and vilanterol 25 mcg inhalation powder [Breo Ellipta]). A large study investigating the safety of LABA and ICS combination inhalers confirmed their long-term safety and demonstrated a reduced risk of exacerbations and improved lung function, when compared with an equivalent dose of ICS alone. A trial[1a] of albuterol–budesonide fixed–dose combination rescue inhaler for asthma revealed that the risk of severe asthma exacerbation was significantly lower with as-needed use of a fixed-dose combination of 180 mcg of albuterol and 160 mcg of budesonide than with as needed use of albuterol alone among patients with un-controlled moderate-to-severe asthma who were receiving a wide range of inhaled glucocorticoid-containing maintenance therapies.

- Long-acting muscarinic antagonists (LAMAs): Studies have shown some degree of benefit when adding a LAMA to ICS + LABA in moderate to severe asthma. The LAMA tiotropium (Spiriva), which has been used for decades as a first-line treatment for COPD, is now approved for the treatment of asthma and is included in the most recent (2020) Global Initiative for Asthma (GINA) guidelines as a possible add-on at step 4. A systematic review including more than 7000 patients demonstrated the use of LAMA compared with placebo as an add-on to inhaled corticosteroids was associated with lower risk of exacerbation. Adding LAMA to a dual LABA-ICS regimen was not shown to reduce exacerbation rates but can improve lung function.

- Triple-therapy combination inhalers (corticosteroid/LABA/LAMA) are also available for the treatment of asthma (fluticasone furoate/vilanterol/umeclidinium [Trelegy Ellipta]). None of these combinations is approved or indicated for the initial treatment of asthma or for acute therapy of asthma symptoms by the Food and Drug Administration (FDA). There is no evidence that one product is more effective than the others.

- Oral corticosteroids are reserved as a last resort for maintenance therapy for recalcitrant cases.

IMMUNOLOGIC TARGETS

- Tezepelumab, a human monoclonal antibody to thymic stromal lymphopoietin (TSLP), is FDA approved as an add-on on therapy for adults and children aged 12 yr and older with severe asthma not controlled by their current asthma regimen.

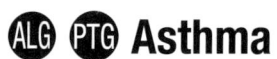

TABLE 4 Stepwise Approach for Managing Asthma in Children 5-11 Yr

Treatment	Intermittent Asthma	MANAGEMENT OF PERSISTENT ASTHMA IN INDIVIDUALS 5-11 YR OF AGE				
	Step 1	Step 2	Step 3	Step 4	Step 5	Step 6
Preferred	PRN SABA	Daily low-dose ICS and PRN SABA	Daily and PRN combination low-dose ICS-formoterol#	Daily and PRN combination medium-dose ICS-formoterol#	Daily high-dose ICS-LABA and PRN SABA	Daily high-dose ICS-LABA + oral systemic corticosteroid and PRN SABA
Alternative		Daily LTRA,* or cromolyn,* or nedocromil,* or theophylline,* and PRN SABA	Daily medium-dose ICS and PRN SABA or Daily low-dose ICS-LABA, or daily low-dose ICS + LTRA, * or daily low-dose ICS + theophylline,* and PRN SABA	Daily medium-dose ICS-LABA and PRN SABA or Daily medium-dose ICS + LTRA* or daily medium-dose ICS + theophylline,* and PRN SABA	Daily high-dose ICS + LTRA* or daily high-dose ICS + theophylline,* and PRN SABA	Daily high-dose ICS + LTRA* + oral systemic corticosteroid or daily high-dose ICS + theophylline* + oral systemic corticosteroid, and PRN SABA
		Steps 2-4: Conditionally recommend the use of subcutaneous immunotherapy as an adjunct treatment to standard pharmacotherapy in individuals > 5 yr of age whose asthma is controlled at the initiation, build up, and maintenance phases of immunotherapy.			Consider omalizumab** #	

EIB, Exercise-induced bronchoconstriction; ICS, inhaled corticosteroid; LABA, long-acting beta$_2$-agonist; LTRA, leukotriene receptor antagonist; prn, as necessary; SABA, inhaled short-acting beta$_2$-agonist.
*Cromolyn, nedocromil, LTRAs (including montelukast), and theophylline were not considered in the 2020 NAEPP update.
**Omalizumab was the only biologic mentioned in the NAEPP 2020 update.
#Updated based on the 2020 guidelines.
The stepwise approach is meant to assist, not replace, the clinical decision-making required to meet individual patient needs.
If alternative treatment is used and response is inadequate, discontinue it and use the preferred treatment before stepping up.
Theophylline is a less desirable alternative due to the need to monitor serum concentration levels.
Step 1 and step 2 medications are based on Evidence A. Step 3 ICS 1 adjunctive therapy and ICS are based on Evidence B for efficacy of each treatment and extrapolation from comparator trials in older children and adults—comparator trials are not available for this age group; steps 4-6 are based on expert opinion and extrapolation from studies in older children and adults. Immunotherapy for steps 2-4 is based on Evidence B for house-dust mites, animal danders, and pollens; evidence is weak or lacking for molds and cockroaches. Evidence is strongest for immunotherapy with single allergens. The role of allergy in asthma is greater in children than in adults. Clinicians who administer immunotherapy should be prepared and equipped to identify and treat anaphylaxis that may occur. This information is directly abstracted from the 2007 NAEPP *Expert Panel Report 3: Guidelines for the diagnosis and management of asthma* and is not intended to promote or endorse any of the listed products.
From 2020 Focused updates to the asthma management guidelines: a report from the National Asthma Education and Prevention Program coordinating committee expert panel working group. https://www.nhlbi.nih.gov/sites/default/files/publications/AsthmaManagementGuidelinesReport-2-4-21.pdf

TABLE 5 Stepwise Approach for Managing Asthma in Children 0-4 Yr

Treatment	Intermittent Asthma	MANAGEMENT OF PERSISTENT ASTHMA IN INDIVIDUALS 0-4 YR OF AGE				
	Step 1	Step 2	Step 3	Step 4	Step 5	Step 6
Preferred	PRN SABA and At the start of RTI: Add short course daily ICS#	Daily low-dose ICS and PRN SABA	Daily medium-dose ICS and PRN SABA	Daily medium-dose ICS-LABA and PRN SABA	Daily high-dose ICS-LABA and PRN SABA	Daily high-dose ICS-LABA + oral systemic corticosteroid and PRN SABA
Alternative		Daily montelukast* or cromolyn,* and PRN SABA		Daily medium-dose ICS + montelukast* and PRN SABA	Daily high-dose ICS + montelukast* and PRN SABA	Daily high-dose ICS + montelukast* + oral systemic corticosteroid and PRN SABA
			For children age 4 yr only, see step 3 and step 4 on Management of Persistent Asthma in Individuals Ages 5-11 Yr diagram.			

ICS, Inhaled corticosteroid; LABA, long-acting beta$_2$-agonist; LTRA, leukotriene receptor antagonist; PRN, as needed; RTI, respiratory tract infection; SABA, inhaled short-acting beta2-agonist;
*Cromolyn and montelukast were not considered for this updated and/or have limited availability for use in the United States. The FDA issued a Boxed Warning for montelukast in March 2020.
#Updated based on the 2020 guidelines.
The stepwise approach is meant to assist, not replace, the clinical decision-making required to meet individual patient needs. If alternative treatment is used and response is inadequate, discontinue it and use the preferred treatment before stepping up.
If clear benefit is not observed within 4-6 wk and patient/family medication technique and adherence are satisfactory, consider adjusting therapy or alternative diagnosis.
Studies on children 0-4 yr are limited. Step 2 preferred therapy is based on Evidence A. All other recommendations are based on expert opinion and extrapolation from studies in other children.
This information is directly abstracted from the 2007 NAEPP *Expert Panel Report 3: Guidelines for the diagnosis and management of asthma* and is not intended to promote or endorse any of the listed products.
From 2020 Focused Updates to the Asthma Management Guidelines: a report from the National Asthma Education and Prevention Program Coordinating Committee Expert Panel Working Group. https://www.nhlbi.nih.gov/sites/default/files/publications/AsthmaManagementGuidelinesReport-2-4-21.pdf

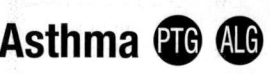

TABLE 6 Selected Inhaled Medications Used by Patients With Asthma

Generic Name	Trade Name*	Dose/Puff	Dose as Puffs	Comments
Beta-Agonist Bronchodilators†				
Albuterol-MDI‡	AccuNeb, Proair HFA, Proventil HFA, Ventolin HFA, Airomir HFA, Salamol HFA	Varies from 90–200 μg	2 puffs as needed for asthma symptoms. Can be repeated every 4 hr. 10–12 puffs in 24 h is the maximum dose. Use of more than 6 puffs/day should prompt medical consultation for asthma control.	All are metered-dose inhalers that deliver a fixed amount of medication per puff.
Albuterol-DPI	Ventolin, Asmasal, Salbulin	100 or 200 μg	1 puff as needed, otherwise same as albuterol MDI.	All are dry powder inhalers that deliver a fixed amount of medication per inhalation.
Albuterol solution	—	Varies from 0.63–5 mg/ml	Inhale while breathing till solution consumed. Need for more than 6 home treatments/day should prompt medical consultation.	This solution is for use with a liquid nebulizer driven by compressed gas. Mix the dose with a volume of sterile normal saline to achieve a nebulizer concentration of 0.63 mg/ml.
Levalbuterol-MDI	Xopenex HFA		Same as albuterol-MDI.	The isolated R-isomer of albuterol. Some studies show superiority to the racemic albuterol found in the MDIs listed above.
Levalbuterol-solution	Xopenex inhalation solution	0.63 mg/ml	Same as albuterol solution.	Nebulizer solution as noted for albuterol above.
Terbutaline-DPI	Bricanyl	250 or 500 μg	Same as albuterol-MDI.	Dry powder inhaler, uses patient generated effort to achieve airflow to disperse and deposit medication.
Terbutaline solution	Bricanyl inhalation solution	2.5 mg/ml	Same as albuterol.	The per dose amount is 2 ml with sterile saline added to achieve the requisite volume for the nebulizer used.
Long-Acting Anticholinergic Bronchodilator for Use in Severe Asthma				
Tiotropium bromide	Spiriva Respimat (MDI)	1.25 μg	2 puffs once/day.	For patients with asthma not controlled by β-agonist and inhaled glucocorticoid treatment.
Inhaled Glucocorticoids				
Beclomethasone	Beclovent, Clenil, Qvar, Asmabec	Comes in both MDI and DPI inhalers with amounts per puff varying from 50–400 μg	Adjust dose to achieve asthma control with a dose of 2 puffs twice/day. The maximum dose is 2 puffs twice daily of the highest strength.	Inhaled glucocorticoid with the longest use record. Although medication is generic, the inhaler type and propellant may be proprietary. Dose adjustments for patients in renal or hepatic failure are not needed.
Budesonide	Budelin, Pulmicort	Inhalers are all DPIs with amounts per dose 100–400 μg. Solution for nebulization is also available with amount of drug per treatment varies between 0.5–1.0 mg	Adjust dose to achieve asthma control with a dose of 2 puffs twice/day. The maximum dose is 2 puffs twice daily of the highest strength.	Dose adjustments for patients in renal or hepatic failure are not needed.
Fluticasone propionate	Flovent, Flixotide	MDIs with 50, 125, 250 μg dose strengths as well as packets for nebulization at 0.25 and 1.0 mg/ml	With MDI, start at low concentration and adjust dose to achieve asthma control with a dose of 2 puffs twice/day. The maximum dose is 2 puffs twice daily of the highest strength. With nebulizer, choose a concentration that gives asthma control when used twice daily.	Dose labels on U.S. marketed inhalers are 44, 110, and 220 μg/puff. The difference is the amount loaded in the metering chamber (outside of U.S.) vs the dose leaving the inhaler (U.S.). Dose adjustments for patients in renal failure not needed. In patients with hepatic failure, patients should be carefully monitored for steroid side effects and dose adjusted appropriately.
Ciclesonide	Alvesco	MDIs delivering 40, 80, or 160 μg	With MDI, start at low concentration and adjust dose to achieve asthma control with a dose of 2 puffs twice/day. The maximum dose is 2 puffs twice daily of the highest strength.	Dose adjustments for patients in renal or hepatic failure are not needed.

TABLE 6 Selected Inhaled Medications Used by Patients With Asthma—cont'd

Generic Name	Trade Name*	Dose/Puff	Dose as Puffs	Comments
Flunisolide	Aerospan	80 μg	Start at 2 puffs twice/day and escalate as needed. 4 puffs twice/day is maximal dose.	Dose adjustments for patients in renal or hepatic failure are not needed.
Mometasone	Asmanex HFA	100 or 200 μg in HFA form; 110 or 220 μg in DPI form	Start with 200 (220) μg once/day (p.m. dosing suggested). Max dose is 800 (880) μg once daily. Titrate dose down as control is achieved.	Dose adjustments for patients in renal failure not needed. In patients with hepatic failure, patients should be carefully monitored for steroid side effects and dose adjusted appropriately.
Combination Inhalers Containing Both IGC and LABA§				
IGC = fluticasone propionate LABA = salmeterol	Advair, Seretide, AirFluSal, Sirdupla	Available as MDIs or DPIs. Each type contains a fixed dose of LABA with varying amounts of IGC. Exact amounts vary by inhaler type.	Start with 1 puff twice daily at the lowest dose of IGC that is effective for asthma control. Titrate up and down as symptom control requires. Max dose is 4 puffs of highest strength per day.	Dose adjustments for patients in renal failure not needed. In patients with hepatic failure, patients should be carefully monitored for steroid side effects and dose adjusted appropriately.
IGC = fluticasone propionate LABA = formoterol	Flutiform	Available only as MDIs. Each strength contains a fixed dose of LABA with varying amounts of IGC.	Start with 2 puffs twice daily at the lowest dose of IGC that is effective for asthma control. Titrate up and down as symptom control requires. Max dose is 4 puffs of highest strength per day.	Dose adjustments for patients in renal failure not needed. In patients with hepatic failure, patients should be carefully monitored for steroid side effects and dose adjusted appropriately. Not recommended for children under 12 yr.
IGC = budesonide LABA = formoterol	DuoResp, Symbicort, Bufoler	Available only as DPIs. Each strength contains a fixed dose of LABA with varying amounts of IGC. Exact amounts vary by inhaler type.	Start with 1 puff twice daily at the lowest dose of IGC that is effective for asthma control. Titrate up and down as symptom control requires. Max dose is 4 puffs of highest strength per day.	Dose adjustments for patients in renal or hepatic failure are not needed.
IGC = budesonide LABA = salmeterol	Busalair	Available only as DPIs. Each strength contains a fixed dose of LABA with varying amounts of IGC. Exact amounts vary by inhaler type.	Start with 1 puff twice daily at the lowest dose of IGC that is effective for asthma control. Titrate up and down as symptom control requires. Max dose is 4 puffs of highest strength per day.	Dose adjustments for patients in renal or hepatic failure are not needed.
IGC = mometasone LABA = formoterol	Dulera	Available only as MDIs. Each strength contains a 5-μg dose of formoterol with varying amounts of IGC. Exact amounts vary by inhaler type.	Start with 1 puff twice daily at the lowest dose of IGC that is effective for asthma control. Titrate up and down as symptom control requires. Max dose is 4 puffs of highest strength per day.	Dose adjustments for patients in renal or hepatic failure are not needed.
IGC = beclomethasone LABA = formoterol	Fostair MDI or DPI or Fostair Inhalation Solution	All contain 6 μg of formoterol with amounts of glucocorticoid varying from 100-200 μg.	Adjust IGC dose to achieve asthma control with a dose of 2 puffs twice/day.	Not available in the U.S.
IGC = fluticasone furoate LABA = vilanterol	Relvar Ellipta or Breo Ellipta	All forms contain 25 μg of vilanterol with amount of glucocorticoid varying from 92-184 μg.	Adjust IGC dose to achieve asthma control with a dose of 2 puffs once/day.	Bronchodilator effect of vilanterol onsets in about 15 min. Dose adjustments for patients in renal failure not needed. In patients with hepatic failure, patients should be carefully monitored for steroid side effects and dose adjusted appropriately.

DPI, Dry powder inhale; *HFA,* hydrofluoroalkane; *IGC,* inhaled glucocorticoid; *LABA,* long-acting β-agonist; *MDI,* metered-dose inhaler.
*Not all products marketing each medication are listed.
†All are short acting with onset of effect 5-10 min and duration of effect 4-8 hr. All patients with asthma should have a short-acting bronchodilator as a rescue inhaler to use for rescue from signs of airway obstruction.
‡The generic names albuterol and salbutamol are synonyms. Albuterol is used in the United States and salbutamol in many other countries.
§LABAs alone should not be used in patients with asthma.
From Goldman L, Shafer AI: *Goldman-Cecil medicine,* ed 26, Philadelphia, 2020, Elsevier.

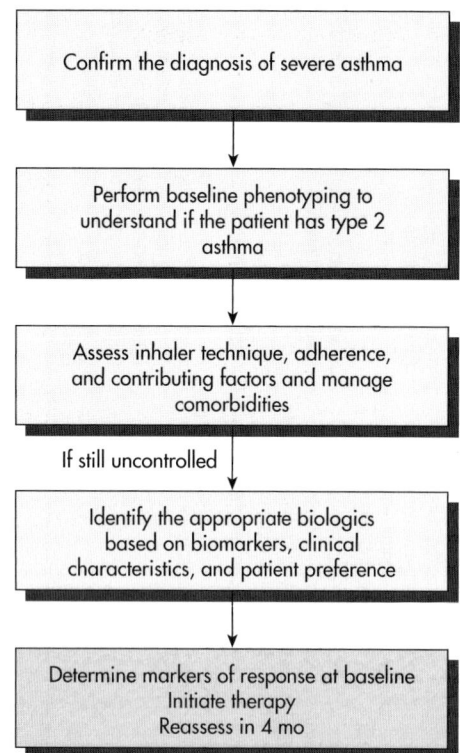

FIG. 6 Recommended process toward initiating biologic therapy. A diagnosis of severe asthma should be confirmed using objective measures of lung function, and evidence for type 2 asthma should be assessed. Before initiating biologic therapy, evaluate for comorbid conditions, alternative diagnoses, and poor inhaler technique or adherence. Measurement of type 2 biomarkers will help select initial therapy. Reassess for clinical response in 4 mo. (From Broaddus VC et al: *Murray & Nadel's textbook of respiratory medicine,* ed 7, Philadelphia, 2022, Elsevier.)

- Dupilumab, a human monoclonal antibody to IL-4 and IL-13, is FDA approved for use in adult and pediatric patients >6 mo with moderate to severe asthma with an eosinophilic phenotype or with oral corticosteroid–dependent asthma.
- Mepolizumab (Nucala), a monoclonal antibody to IL-5, is approved by the FDA as an add-on for patients ≥12 yr with severe eosinophilic asthma that is uncontrolled.
- Reslizumab, another anti-IL-5 monoclonal antibody, has a similar indication for eosinophilic asthma and uses a higher eosinophil cutoff (≥400 μL) based on a greater predictive value for sputum eosinophilia.
- Benralizumab, a monoclonal anti-IL5 receptor alpha antibody, is an additional FDA-approved add-on treatment to consider for patients >12 yr with persistent severe eosinophilic asthma.
- Omalizumab, an anti-IgE monoclonal antibody, is an FDA-approved add-on asthma treatment for moderate to severe persistent asthma in patients 6 yr of age and older with a positive skin test or in vitro reactivity to a perennial aeroallergen and symptoms that are inadequately controlled with inhaled corticosteroids.

BRONCHIAL THERMOPLASTY

Select patients with severe persistent asthma who have failed medical treatment may benefit from bronchial thermoplasty. This requires the insertion of a catheter via bronchoscopy and use of radiofrequency heat to reduce bronchial smooth muscle. Long-term follow-up data showed persistent reduction in asthma exacerbation and fewer ED visits over a period of 5 yr in carefully selected patients. FDA labeling is for "severe persistent asthma inadequately controlled on ICS + LABA."

OTHER MEDICATIONS

- Azithromycin: The AZISAST Trial randomized 109 patients on high-dose ICS/LABA (step 4 or 5 per GINA guidelines) to maintenance therapy with azithromycin or placebo. There was no benefit seen with azithromycin therapy regarding any of the primary outcomes, although a subgroup analysis showed that patients with noneosinophilic asthma had fewer exacerbations. This result suggests azithromycin may be an effective option for the neutrophilic/Th-1 phenotype, but more data are needed.
- Immunosuppressants such as methotrexate can decrease long-term steroid requirements; however, they have significant side effects, and there is no evidence of persistent therapeutic effect after discontinuation. Fig. 6 illustrates a process toward initiating biologic therapy.

SEVERE ASTHMA TREATMENT (ATS/ERS GUIDELINES)

- The American Thoracic Society (ATS) classification of "severe asthma" refers to patients who require high-dose inhaled or near-continuous oral glucocorticoid treatment to maintain asthma control.
- In patients who do not achieve adequate control with the combination of a high-dose inhaled glucocorticoid and LABA, an additional controller medication such as an LTRA or LAMA is recommended.
- For patients with atopic severe asthma who have a serum IgE level of 30 to 700 IU/ml and documented sensitivity to a perennial allergen, adding omalizumab is recommended.
- For patients with severe asthma, frequent exacerbations, and an eosinophilic phenotype despite guideline-based therapy, consider add-on therapy with one of the anti-interleukin (IL)-5 antibodies, mepolizumab, reslizumab, benralizumab, or anti-IL4α receptor antibody dupilumab. Table 7 summarizes FDA-approved biologics for treatment of moderate to severe asthma.
- A decision tree for selecting initial biologic therapy and assessment of response for severe asthma are illustrated in Figs. 7 and 8.
- Bronchial thermoplasty is approved for use in selected adults with severe asthma that is not well controlled with inhaled glucocorticoids and LABAs.
- Potential alternative and experimental therapies include immunomodulatory therapy and macrolide antibiotics.[a]
- In the future, treatments tailored to asthma phenotypes may improve asthma outcomes. Treatment of status asthmaticus is as follows:
1. Oxygen generally started at 2 to 4 L/min by nasal cannula or Venti-Mask at 40% Fio_2; further adjustments are made according to oxygen saturations.
2. Bronchodilators: Initiate treatment with albuterol nebulizer solution (0.63 mg/3 ml, 1.25 mg/3 ml, 2.5 mg/3 ml, or 5.0 mg/ml): 2.5 to 5 mg every 20 min over the first hr, then 2.5 to 10 mg every 1 to 4 hr as needed or 10 to 15 mg/hr continuously. Other useful medications are levalbuterol nebulizer solution (0.31 mg/3 ml, 0.63 mg/3 ml, 1.25 mg/3 ml) and ipratropium nebulizer solution (0.25/ml [0.025%]).
3. Corticosteroids:
   a) Early administration is advised, particularly in patients using steroids at home.
   b) Patients may be started on systemic corticosteroids; methylprednisolone, prednisone, or prednisolone may be used. Dose range is from 40 to 80 mg/day in one or two divided doses, generally given until peak expiratory flow reaches 70% of predicted value.
   c) Generally for corticosteroid courses <1 wk; there is no need to taper the dose.
   d) IV hydration: Judicious use is necessary to avoid heart failure in elderly patients.

---

[a]Recent trials (AMAZES) in patients who have symptomatic asthma despite inhaled maintenance therapy have shown that azithromycin 500 mg 3 times/wk reduced exacerbations and improved quality of life.

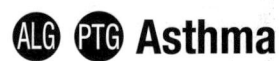

TABLE 7 Summary of FDA-Approved Biologics for Treatment of Moderate to Severe Asthma

Biologic Agent	MOA	Patient Selection	Dosing	Notes
Omalizumab (Xolair) FDA approved in 2003	Humanized IgG1 antibody that binds to the Cε3 domain of free IgE and prevents it from binding to FcεR1	• Age ≥6 yr in the U.S. (≥12 yr in the UK) • IgE: 30-700 IU/ml • Allergic sensitization by skin prick or specific IgE testing	75-375 mg SC per IU every 2-4 wk based on age, weight, and IgE levels	• Highest efficacy in T2-high patients • Efficacy not based on IgE level or eosinophil count • Data from real-world studies demonstrate efficacy when dosed outside accepted weight and IgE levels • Indicated for *moderate to severe* allergic asthma
Mepolizumab (Nucala) FDA approved in 2015	Humanized IgG1 antibody that inhibits IL-5 from binding to the α-subunit of the IL-5 receptor complex on eosinophils	• ≥12 yr • Blood AEC of ≥150 cells/µL at the time of testing or ≥300 cells/µL in the previous yr • ≥300 cells/µL only in the UK	• 100 mg SC every 4 wk • 300 mg SC every 4 wk for EGPA	• Approved for home administration via the autoinjector • In clinic dosing using the lyophilized powder • Only biologic currently approved for EGPA • Demonstrated OCS-sparing effects • Indicated for severe eosinophilic asthma
Reslizumab (Cinqair) FDA approved in 2016	Humanized IgG4 antibody that inhibits IL-5 from binding to the α-subunit of the IL-5 receptor complex expressed on eosinophils	• Age ≥18 yr • Blood AEC ≥400 cells/µL in the previous yr	3 mg/kg IV infusion every 4 wk	Response is better with higher eosinophil counts No data on OCS-sparing effects; SC OCS dosing study was negative Indicated for severe eosinophilic asthma
Benralizumab (Fasenra) FDA approved in 2017	Humanized recombinant IgG1 antibody that binds with high affinity to the α-subunit of the IL-5 receptor	• Age ≥12 yr • Blood AEC ≥300 cells/µL in the previous yr	30 mg SC every 4 wk for the first 3 doses then every 8 wk	• Available for prefilled autoinjector • Results in total depletion of eosinophils • Demonstrated OCS-sparing effects • Indicated for severe eosinophilic asthma
Dupilumab (Dupixent) FDA approved in 2018	Fully human monoclonal antibody to the α-unit of IL-4 receptor; blocks IL-4 and IL-13	• Age ≥12 yr • Moderate to severe asthma • Blood AEC ≥300 cells/µL in the previous yr • FeNO >25 ppb	• 200 mg or 300 mg SC every 2 wk after initial loading dose. No loading dose required for nasal polyps • 200 mg for moderate to severe persistent asthma, 300 mg for atopic dermatitis, nasal polyps and oral steroid-dependent asthma	• Home administration only • Antidrug antibody in 2%-5% patients • Indicated for nasal polyps, atopic dermatitis, and asthma (*moderate to severe* persistent eosinophilic asthma or oral steroid–dependent asthma regardless of T2 markers) • Demonstrated OCS-sparing effects • Exercise caution in patients with baseline eosinophils >1500 cells/µL due to transient elevation of eosinophils for 4 mo after initiation of therapy
Tezepelumab (Tezspire) FDA approved 2021	Human monoclonal antibody anti-TSLP that binds to TSLP	• Adults and children aged 12 yr and older • Severe asthma not controlled by their current asthma regimen	• Administer by subcutaneous injection • Recommended dosage is 210 mg administered once every 4 wk	• Is not available currently for home administration. • Most common adverse reactions (incidence ≥ 3%) are pharyngitis, arthralgia, and back pain.

AEC, Absolute eosinophil count; *EGPA,* eosinophilic granulomatosis with polyangiitis; *FDA,* Food and Drug Administration; *FeNO,* fraction of exhaled nitric oxide; *Ig,* immunoglobulin; *IL,* interleukin; *IU,* international units; *IV,* intravenous; *OCS,* oral corticosteroid; *SC,* subcutaneous.
From Broaddus VC et al: *Murray & Nadel's textbook of respiratory medicine,* ed 7, Philadelphia, 2022, Elsevier.

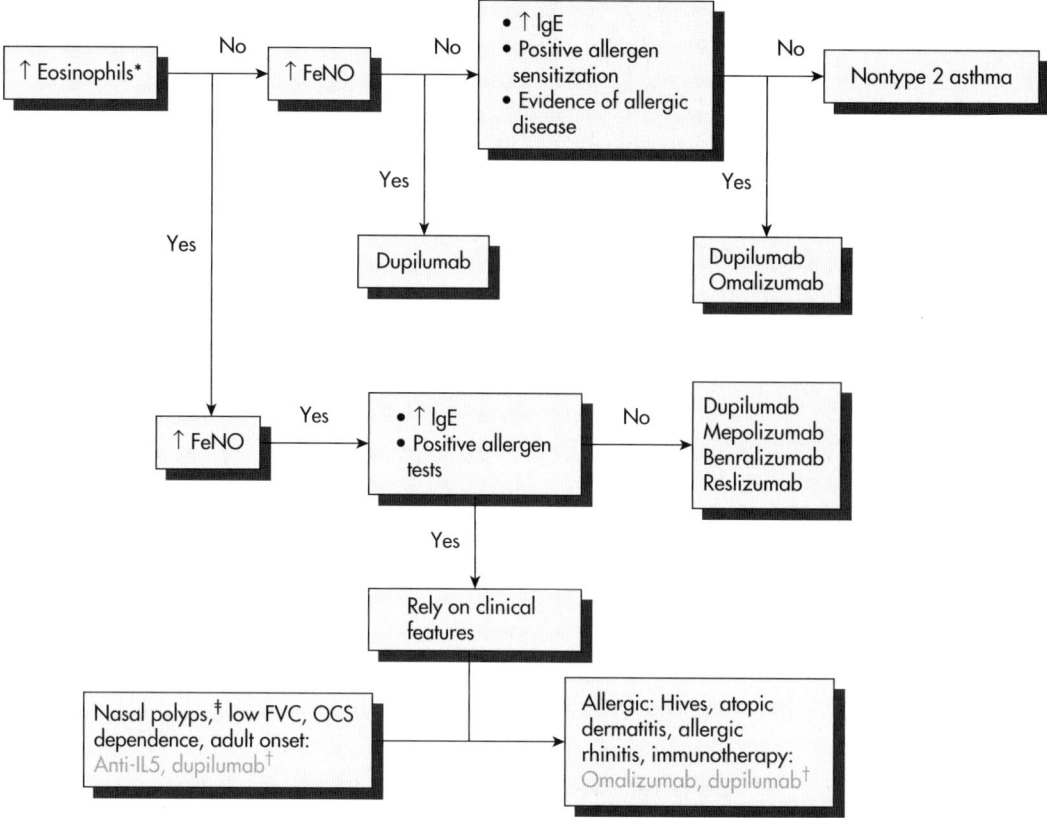

FIG. 7 **Decision tree for selecting initial biologic therapy for severe asthma in patients with type 2 features.** This algorithm is guided by high-quality evidence from clinical trials and supporting data. Medications are listed alphabetically, not in order of preference. Patients should have regular assessment of clinical benefit, and treatment should be adjusted until asthma control is achieved. *Increased eosinophils is defined by blood eosinophil counts >150-300/μL. Dupilumab should not be used for patients with >1500 eosinophils/μL. †At the time of publication, dupilumab is also FDA approved for use in nasal polyps and atopic dermatitis. Omalizumab is also FDA approved for use in chronic urticaria. ‡Nasal polyps predict an enhanced response to these T2 biologics when targeting asthma. The efficacy of each biologic for nasal polyps may differ. *FDA,* U.S. Food and Drug Administration; *FeNO,* fraction of exhaled nitric oxide; *FVC,* forced vital capacity; *IgE,* immunoglobulin E; *OCS,* oral corticosteroid. (From Broaddus VC et al: *Murray & Nadel's textbook of respiratory medicine,* ed 7, Philadelphia, 2022, Elsevier.)

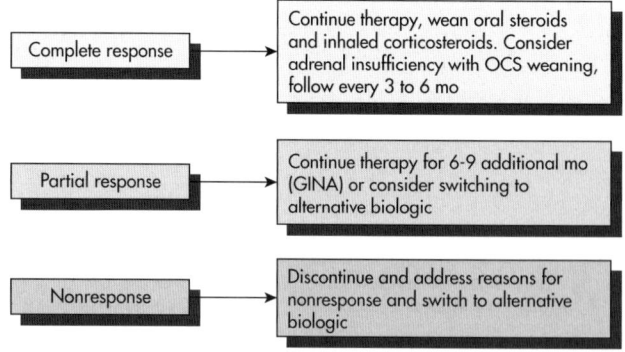

FIG. 8 **Assessing response to biologic therapy.** Before initiating biologic therapy, choose markers of response that will be monitored (e.g., exacerbations, oral corticosteroid use, asthma control, lung function, rescue bronchodilator use, patient comfort, and satisfaction). Most patients will experience at least a partial response to biologic therapy, 10%-15% will have no response, and a small proportion will have a complete response. Assess response continuously and adjust asthma medications and/or biologics based on response. *GINA,* Global Initiative for Asthma; *OCS,* oral corticosteroids. (From Broaddus VC et al: *Murray & Nadel's textbook of respiratory medicine,* ed 7, Philadelphia, 2022, Elsevier.)

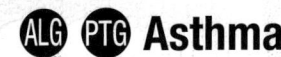

TABLE 8 Summary of Treatment for Life-Threatening Asthma

Treatment	Dose and Frequency	Comments
Oxygen	1-3 L/min by nasal cannula Goal is to maintain oxygen saturation (Spo$_2$) >92% Use heated cascade humidifier to avoid dry air–induced bronchoconstriction	Transient drop in O$_2$ tension with beta-adrenergic therapy Avoid hyperoxia (may be associated with hypercarbia)
Bronchodilators		
Beta$_2$-selective agonists: Albuterol or salbutamol, levalbuterol	*Albuterol:* 2.5-5 mg (0.5-1 ml of 0.5% solution in 5 ml of normal saline) by nebulizer every 20 min for 3 doses total (for optimal delivery, dilute aerosols to a minimum of 3 ml at gas flow of 6-8 L/min), followed by 2.5-10 mg q1-4h as needed, or 10-15 mg/h continuously; titration based on response and severity of symptoms *Albuterol MDI,* delivered with a spacer (each spacer dose takes 1-2 min; 90 μg/puff), 4-8 puffs every 20 min for 4 h, then q4h as needed *Albuterol:* 5-7.5 mg by jet nebulizer (each treatment takes 15-20 min) *Levalbuterol* (0.63 mg/3 ml and 1.25 mg/3 ml nebulizer): 1.25-2.5 mg every 20 min for 3 doses total, then 1.25-5 mg q1-4h as needed, or 5-7.5 mg/h continuous nebulization *Levalbuterol MDI* (45 μg/puff): 4-8 puffs every 20 min for 4 h, followed by q1-4h as needed	Beta$_2$-selective agonists are the cornerstone of therapy Continuous nebulization used for a majority of severely ill patients In study of continuous vs. intermittent therapy in severe exacerbations (excluding life-threatening asthma), no difference noted in pulmonary function improvement or need for hospitalization Lower frequency of side effects with continuous treatment Watch for hypokalemia, tremors, tachycardia, and lactic acidosis Oral or parenteral route: Loss of beta$_2$-selectivity MDI: 4 puffs of albuterol (0.36 mg) = 2.5 mg of albuterol nebulization Levalbuterol 0.63 mg = racemic albuterol 1.25 mg for efficacy and side effects *Intubated patients:* Nebulizers are less efficient in delivering doses to lower airways (6%-10%) than MDIs (11%)
Epinephrine	*Subcutaneous epinephrine* dose for adults: 0.3-0.5 ml of a 1:1000 dilution (1 mg/ml), depending on age and weight; repeat every 20 min for 3 doses total	
Terbutaline	*Subcutaneous terbutaline:* 0.25 mg; repeat every 20 min for 3 doses total	Terbutaline is the parenteral agent of choice in pregnancy For refractory life-threatening asthma: Intravenous epinephrine (high risk for cardiac events, infarction, and arrhythmias) or racemic epinephrine may be considered
Anticholinergics		
Ipratropium (for acute severe asthma warranting visit to emergency department)	*Ipratropium bromide:* 0.5 mg by nebulizer (0.25 mg/ml) every 20 min for 3 doses, then q2-4h as needed *Ipratropium MDI* (0.018 mg/puff): 4-8 puffs per treatment every 20 min for up to 3 h *Combinations:* Albuterol (2.5 mg/3 ml) + ipratropium (0.5 mg/3 ml): 3 ml every 20 min for 3 doses total, then as needed MDI delivering albuterol 90 μg + ipratropium 18 μg: 8 puffs every 20 min for up to 3 h	Ipratropium: Onset of action is slow (20 min), peak effectiveness at 60-90 min, no systemic side effects, improved lung function and reduced recovery time Use a handheld mouthpiece nebulizer (contamination of the ocular area with precipitation of narrow-angle glaucoma may occur if facemask is used for delivery of anticholinergic agent) Ipratropium may be combined with nebulized albuterol dose in the emergency room; no proven benefit shown in hospitalized patients
Corticosteroids: Prednisone, prednisolone, methylprednisolone	40-80 mg/day in 1 or 2 divided doses until peak expiratory flow reaches 70% of predicted or personal bestFEV$_1$ or PEFR <50% Methylprednisolone 40 mg IV q6h or Hydrocortisone 200 mg IV	No advantage of higher doses No advantage of IV therapy over oral if absorption and gut transit are not impaired Total steroid course: 3-10 days, <1 wk; no need to taper steroids Inhaled steroids can be started at any time
Heliox	Helium-oxygen mixture (80-20 or 70-30) Routine use cannot be recommended at this time	Improves O$_2$ and aerosolized medication delivery to distal lung Decreases flow turbulence and resistance Lower gas density facilitates exhalation, reduces air trapping and intrinsic PEEP Improves pulmonary function in subgroup of patients with most severe airflow obstruction
Magnesium sulfate	2 g IV given over 20 min; may repeat Monitor magnesium levels Avoid in renal insufficiency	Bronchodilation from inhibition of the calcium channel and decreased acetylcholine release IV and inhaled or nebulized magnesium sulfate improves pulmonary function in acute severe asthma IV magnesium widely used as adjunct therapy

FEV$_1$, Forced expiratory flow in 1 second; *IV,* intravenous; *MDI,* metered-dose inhaler; *PEEP,* positive end-expiratory pressure; *PEFR,* peak expiratory flow rate.
From Parrillo JE, Dellinger RP: *Critical care medicine, principles of diagnosis and management in the adult,* ed 4, Philadelphia, 2014, Elsevier.

Aggressive IV hydration is not recommended.

e) IV antibiotics are indicated when there is suspicion of bacterial infection (e.g., infiltrate on chest radiograph, fever, or leukocytosis).

f) Intubation and mechanical ventilation are indicated when previous measures fail to produce significant improvement. Table 8 summarizes treatment of life-threatening asthma.

g) Discharge home from the emergency department is appropriate if the FEV_1 or PEF after treatment is 70% or greater of the personal best or predicted value and if there is sustained improvement in lung function and symptoms for at least 1 hr.

Asthma in the workplace[1]:

• Work-related asthma (WRA) encompasses *Occupational Asthma* (OA) defined as asthma caused by a specific agent at the workplace (Tables 9 to 11) and *Work-Exacerbated Asthma* (WEA), which is asthma exacerbated by, but not caused by, nonspecific stimuli in the workplace (Fig. 9).

• OA should be suspected in every adult with new-onset asthma. Although the respiratory symptoms are similar to those encountered in *Non-Work-Related Asthma* (NWRA), in OA their appearance and severity are usually modulated by work exposure. Characteristics of WRA compared with NWRA and OA are summarized in Table 12.

• Advantages and limitations of diagnostic tests for occupational asthma are summarized in Table 13.

REFERRAL

Box 4 describes indications for referral to an asthma specialist.

PEARLS & CONSIDERATIONS

COMMENTS

• The differentiation of asthma from COPD can be challenging. A history of atopy and intermittent, reactive symptoms points toward a diagnosis of asthma, whereas smoking and advanced age are more indicative of COPD. Spirometry is useful in distinguishing asthma from COPD.

• In all asthma patients, it is important to treat or prevent comorbid conditions (e.g., rhinosinusitis, vocal cord dysfunction, gastroesophageal reflux disease). However, despite the presumed association between asthma and GERD, trials of PPIs in patients with poorly controlled asthma did not reveal any beneficial effects.

• According to the 2020 NAEPP guidelines, Steps 3 and 4 had strong recommendations to use daily medium-dose ICS-formoterol not only as maintenance but also for as-needed therapy.

• Inhaled low-dose corticosteroids are the single most effective therapy for adult patients with asthma who require more than an occasional use of SABAs to control their asthma.

• Stepping down inhaled corticosteroids after asthma is well controlled has level A evidence.

• Leukotriene modifiers/receptor agonists represent a reasonable alternative in adults unable or unwilling to use corticosteroids; however, these agents are less effective than monotherapy with inhaled corticosteroids.

• Use of LABAs alone without use of a long-term asthma maintenance medication, such as an inhaled corticosteroid, is contraindicated.

LABAs should also not be used in patients whose asthma is adequately controlled on low- or medium-dose inhaled corticosteroids. Continued use of LABAs may cause down-regulation of the beta-2 receptor with loss of the bronchoprotective effect from rescue therapy with a SABA.

• Patients who remain symptomatic despite inhaled corticosteroids benefit from the addition of LABAs. Trials in patients with poorly controlled asthma despite the use of inhaled glucocorticoids and LABAs have shown that the addition of tiotropium, a long-acting anticholinergic bronchodilator approved for treatment of COPD, increased the time to the first severe exacerbation and provided modest sustained bronchodilation.

• Therapy with systemic corticosteroids accelerates the resolution of acute asthma and reduces the risk of relapse. There is no evidence that doses >50 to 100 mg prednisone equivalent are beneficial.

• In patients with allergies and elevated serum immunoglobulin (Ig) E levels, use of anti-IgE therapy is beneficial.

• Bronchial thermoplasty may be considered in select patients with severe persistent asthma with recurrent exacerbations or ED visits.

• Biologic modifiers of the Th2 immune pathways (neutralizing monoclonal antibodies, receptor antagonists, soluble receptors) as well as epithelial-derived cytokines are potential options for the development of new treatments of severe asthma. Adjunct therapies for bronchospasm are summarized in Table 14.

• The response to treatment for asthma is characterized by wide individual variability. A functional glucocorticoid-induced transcript 1 gene *(GLCCI1)* variant is associated with

---

TABLE 9   Principal Agents Causing Occupational Asthma

AGENT		Occupation or Industry
High-Molecular-Weight Agents		
Cereals, flour	Wheat, rye, barley, buckwheat	Flour mills, bakers, pastry makers
Latex	Proteins from the *Hevea* tree	Health care workers, laboratory technicians
Animals	Mice, rats, cows, seafood	Laboratory workers, farmers, seafood processing
Enzymes	α-Amylase, maxatase, alcalase, papain, bromelain, pancreatin	Baking product production, bakers, detergent production, pharmaceutical industry, food industry
Low-Molecular-Weight Agents		
Isocyanates	Toluene diisocyanate, methylene diphenyldiisocyanate, hexamethylene diisocyanate	Polyurethane production, plastic industry, insulation, molding, spray painting
Metals	Chromium, nickel, cobalt, platinum	Metal refinery, metal alloy production, electroplating, welding
Biocides	Formaldehyde, glutaraldehyde, quaternary ammonium compounds	Health care workers, cleaners
Persulfate salts	Hair bleach	Hairdressers
Acrylates	Cyanoacrylates, methacrylates, diacrylates, and triacrylates	Adhesives, dental and orthopedic materials, sculptured fingernails, printing inks, paints and coatings
Acid anhydrides	Phthalic, trimellitic, maleic, tetrachlorophthalic anhydrides	Epoxy resin workers
Reactive dyes	Reactive black 5, pyrazolone derivatives, vinyl sulfones, carmine	Textile workers, food industry workers
Woods	Red cedar, iroko, obeche, oak, and others	Sawmill workers, carpenters, cabinet and furniture makers

From Broaddus VC et al: *Murray & Nadel's textbook of respiratory medicine,* ed 7, Philadelphia, 2022, Elsevier.

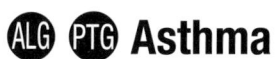

TABLE 10 Frequency of Agents Causing Sensitizer-Induced Occupational Asthma According to a Large European Multicenter Study

HMW Agents	n (%)*	LMW Agents	n (%)*
Flour/grains	369 (31.3)	Isocyanates	206 (17.4)
Latex	36 (3.0)	Persulfate salts	78 (6.6)
Enzymes	26 (2.2)	Metals	42 (3.6)
Storage mites	12 (1.0)	Quaternary ammonium compounds	38 (3.2)
Rodents	11 (0.9)	Acrylate compounds	35 (3.0)
Cow dander	11 (0.9)	Wood dusts	35 (3.0)
Fish and seafood	8 (0.7)	Welding fumes	30 (2.5)
Insects and derived products	6 (0.5)	Cleaning products or disinfectants (NOS)	27 (2.3)
Ornamental plants	6 (0.5)	Epoxy resins	18 (1.5)
Molds	5 (0.4)	Aldehydes	17 (1.4)
Soybean flour	3 (0.2)	Drugs	16 (1.4)
Spices	3 (0.2)	Metalworking fluids	15 (1.3)
Vegetable gums	3 (0.2)	Resins, glues, or paints (NOS)	15 (1.3)
Various plant-derived products	26 (2.2)	Acid anhydrides	11 (0.9)
Various animals and derived products	18 (1.5)	Amines	10 (0.8)
		Colophony	4 (0.3)
Total:	543 (46.5)	Styrene	3 (0.2)
		Reactive dyes	2 (0.2)
		Triglycidyl isocyanurate	2 (0.2)
		Other low-molecular-weight agents (NOS)	21 (17.8)
		Total:	624 (52.9)

HMW, High molecular weight; *LMW*, low molecular weight; *NOS*, not otherwise specified.
*Percentage of total identified agents (*n* = 1167); the causal agent was not precisely identified in 13 subjects.
From Vandenplas O et al: Are high-and low-molecular-weight sensitizing agents associated with different clinical phenotypes of occupational asthma? *Allergy* 74:261-272, 2019.

TABLE 11 Potential Risk Factors for Occupational Asthma

Risk Factor	Evidence	Agents or Settings
Environmental Factors		
High level of exposure	Strong	HMW agents
	Moderate	LMW agents: Platinum salts, acid anhydrides, isocyanates
Cigarette smoking	Moderate	For IgE sensitization: Laboratory animals, snow crab, prawn, salmon, psyllium, green coffee, enzymes, acid anhydrides, platinum, reactive dyes
	Weak	For clinical OA: Laboratory animals, enzymes
Skin exposure	Weak	Isocyanates
Host-Related Factors		
Atopy	Strong	HMW agents
	Weak	LMW agents: Platinum, acid anhydrides
Genetic markers:		
HLA class II alleles	Moderate	LMW agents: Isocyanates, red cedar, acid anhydrides, platinum salts
HMW agents: Laboratory animals, latex
Antioxidant enzymes*	Moderate	Isocyanates
SNPs of alpha-T catenin	Moderate	Isocyanates
TLR4 polymorphisms	Weak	Laboratory animals
IL-4 receptor alpha and IL-13 polymorphisms	Weak	Isocyanates
Preexisting nonspecific bronchial hyperresponsiveness	Moderate	HMW agents: Laboratory animals, flour, latex
Work-related rhinitis	Strong	Laboratory animals
Sex (female)	Weak	Snow crab processors

HLA, Human leukocyte antigen; *HMW*, high molecular weight; *IgE*, immunoglobulin E; *IL*, interleukin; *LMW*, low molecular weight; *OA*, occupational asthma; *SNPs*, single nucleotide polymorphisms, *TLR4*, Toll-like receptor-4.
*Glutathione-S-transferase and N-acetyltransferase.
From Broaddus VC et al: *Murray & Nadel's textbook of respiratory medicine*, ed 7, Philadelphia, 2022, Elsevier.

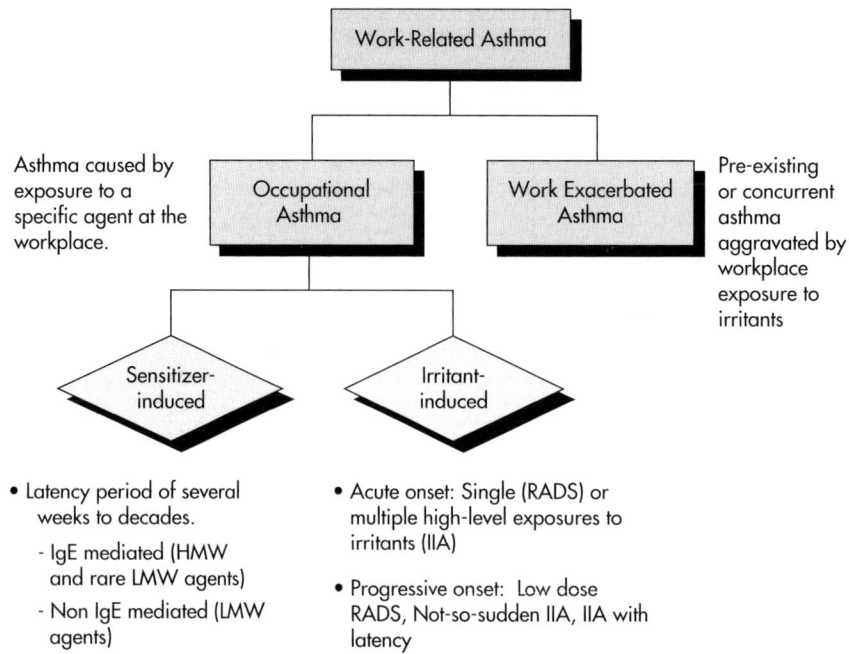

FIG. 9 Categorization of work-related asthma into subsets based on the cause and timing of the asthma. *HMW*, High molecular weight; *IgE*, immunoglobulin E; *IIA*, irritant-induced (occupational) asthma; *LMW*, low molecular weight; *RADS*, reactive airway dysfunction syndrome. (From Broaddus VC et al: *Murray & Nadel's Textbook of Respiratory Medicine* , ed 7, Philadelphia, 2022, Elsevier.)

TABLE 12 Characteristics of Work-Exacerbated Asthma Compared With Non–Work-Related Asthma and Occupational Asthma

Characteristics	Compared With Adults With Non–Work-Related Asthma	Compared With Adults With Occupational Asthma
Sex	Similar,[2,3] or predominance of men in subjects with WEA[4]	Similar,[4] or greater number of women in subjects with WEA[7]
Age	Older[2,3]	Similar or younger[7]
Race	More nonwhite[2]	More nonwhite[7]
Education	Less[2]	N/A
Smoking habits	More likely to have smoked cigarettes[2]	More smokers[4]
Asthma severity	More asthma exacerbations requiring ED visits or hospitalizations in workers with WEA[4] More days with asthma symptoms, more severe asthma based on self-report[2]	Same number of asthma exacerbations requiring ED visits or hospitalizations[8] Greater need of ICS in subjects with WEA[8]
Functional characteristics	Similar FEV$_1$, PC$_{20}$[4]	Less PEF variability when at work in subjects with WEA compared with OA[9] PC$_{20}$ may be lower in subjects with WEA[10]
Airway inflammation	Neutrophilic inflammation inconsistently found depending on the study[5,6]	Less likely to have eosinophilic airway inflammation[6,8]

ED, Emergency department; *FEV$_1$*, forced expiratory volume in 1 second; *ICS*, inhaled glucocorticoids; *N/A*, not applicable; *OA*, occupational asthma; *PC$_{20}$*, provocative concentration of methacholine; *PEF*, peak expiratory flow; *WEA*, work-exacerbated asthma.
From Broaddus VC et al: *Murray & Nadel's textbook of respiratory medicine*, ed 7, Philadelphia, 2022, Elsevier.

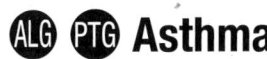
A

Diseases and Disorders

I

TABLE 13 Advantages and Limitations of Diagnostic Tests for Occupational Asthma

Diagnostic Tests	Advantages and Limitations
Assessment of nonspecific bronchial hyperresponsiveness	Simple, low cost Confirms the diagnosis of asthma Low specificity for diagnosis of OA. The absence of airway hyperresponsiveness does not exclude the diagnosis of OA in patients who have been removed from the workplace
Immunologic tests	Easy to perform, low cost Commercial extracts are available (skin prick tests or specific IgE for HMW agents) Measurement of specific IgE available for some LMW agents (anhydrides, acids, isocyanates, aldehydes) but low sensitivity Lack of standardization for most occupational allergens except for latex Can identify the sensitization but not necessarily the disease
PEF monitoring	Low cost Requires workers' collaboration Low adherence (<60%) Possible falsification of results Requires 2 weeks at and away from work (not always possible) Impossible to perform when the worker has been removed from work No standardized method for interpreting the results Interpretation of the results requires experience
Specific inhalation challenges in the laboratory	Confirmation of the diagnosis of OA when test result is positive False-negative test results are possible Costly Available in only a few centers worldwide
Specific inhalation challenges at the workplace	Exclude diagnosis if negative when performed in the usual work conditions Require usual work conditions Costly
Noninvasive measures of airway inflammation	Sputum cell counts • Impossible to falsify • Bring additional evidence to the diagnosis of OA • Costly • Not widely available • Does not allow confirmation or exclusion of the diagnosis of OA by itself Exhaled NO • Easy to perform • Inconsistent results • Difficult to interpret • Affected by many different factors

HMW, High molecular weight; *IgE*, immunoglobulin E; *LMW*, low molecular weight; *NO*, nitric oxide; *OA*, occupational asthma; *PEF*, peak expiratory flow.
From Broaddus VC et al: *Murray & Nadel's textbook of respiratory medicine,* ed 7, Philadelphia, 2022, Elsevier.

BOX 4 Possible Indications for Referral to an Asthma Specialist

- Severe, acute asthma that has caused loss of consciousness, hypoxia, respiratory failure, convulsions, or near death
- Poorly controlled asthma as indicated by admission to a hospital, frequent need for emergency care, need for oral corticosteroids, absence from school or work, disruption of sleep, interference with quality of life
- Severe, persistent asthma requiring step 4 care (consider for patients who require step 3 care)
- Patient <3 yr who requires step 3 or 4 care (consider for patient <3 yr who requires step 2 care)
- Requirement for continuous oral corticosteroids or high-dose inhaled corticosteroids or more than two short courses of oral corticosteroids within 1 yr
- Need for additional diagnostic testing such as allergy skin testing, rhinoscopy, provocative challenge, complete pulmonary function testing, bronchoscopy
- Consideration for immunotherapy
- Need for additional education regarding asthma, complications of asthma and treatment of asthma, problems with adherence to management recommendations, or allergen avoidance
- Uncertainty of diagnosis
- Complications of asthma, including sinusitis, nasal polyposis, aspergillosis, severe rhinitis, vocal cord dysfunction, gastroesophageal reflux

Modified from National Asthma Education and Prevention Program, National Heart, Lung, and Blood Institute: *Expert Panel Report 2: guidelines for the diagnosis and management of asthma,* Bethesda, MD, 1997, National Institutes of Health, NIH publication No 97-4051.

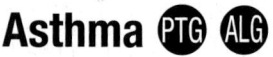

TABLE 14 Adjunct Therapies for Bronchospasm

Nontraditional Therapy for Severe Bronchospasm	Comments
Intravenous beta$_2$-agonists	No data show any benefit in adding IV agent to nebulization Avoid IV isoproterenol owing to danger of myocardial toxicity
Oral or IV leukotriene receptor antagonists (LTRAs): Montelukast 10 mg oral daily, zafirlukast	Rapid bronchodilation in impending respiratory failure Improves pulmonary function within 10 min Oral LTRAs can be added as an adjunct in severe asthma
Noninvasive positive-pressure ventilation (NPPV)	NPPV reduces the need for endotracheal intubation in severe asthma exacerbation
Inhaled nitric oxide (NO) (adding 15 ppm to the inspiratory circuit)	Rapid improvement in ventilated patients with asthma refractory to medical treatment
Omalizumab (anti-IgE antibody)	Role in acute asthma is unstudied Improves asthma control in allergic asthmatics
General anesthetic agents: Isoflurane or halothane anesthesia IV thiopental, IV propofol, IV ketamine	Propofol relaxes the smooth muscles in arteries and veins and has bronchodilator effect
Plasma exchange (during pregnancy) Pumpless extracorporeal carbon dioxide removal Extracorporeal life support (ECLS)	Case reports of adjunct therapies; used as salvage therapy for life-threatening asthma
Glucagon	Rapid smooth muscle relaxant, short half-life; small study report
Nebulized DNase (dornase 2.5 mg via tracheal tube)	Case report of use in pregnant patient with rapid improvement
Bronchial lavage	Anecdotal reports: Exacerbates auto-PEEP, decreases oxygenation

IgE, Immunoglobulin E; *IV,* intravenous; *PEEP,* positive end-expiratory pressure.
From Parrillo JE, Dellinger RP: *Critical care medicine, principles of diagnosis and management in the adult,* ed 4, Philadelphia, 2014, Elsevier.

TABLE 15 Asthma Biomarkers and Associated Phenotypes as Predictors of Response to Specific Therapies

Biomarker	Asthma Phenotype	Predicts
Elevated exhaled nitric oxide (>50 ppb in adults, >35 ppb in children)	T2-high	Response to inhaled steroids
Sputum eosinophils >3%	T2-high	Response to inhaled steroids
Peripheral blood eosinophils (>0.3 × 10^9/L or 300/μL)	T2-high	Response to anti-IL-5 therapy
Elevated total IgE >30 IU	Allergic/T2	Response to omalizumab
Allergy skin tests and elevated specific IgE	Allergic/T2	Response to immunotherapy, omalizumab
Lack of elevated peripheral and sputum eosinophils and low FeNO	T2-low	Response to tiotropium and macrolides (likely to be poor responders to steroids)

FeNO, Fraction of exhaled nitric oxide; *IgE,* immunoglobulin E; *T2,* type 2.
From Broaddus VC et al: *Murray & Nadel's textbook of respiratory medicine,* ed 7, Philadelphia 2022, Elsevier.

substantial decrements in the response to inhaled glucocorticoids in patients with asthma. Another potential cause of the variability in response to treatment is heterogeneity in the role of interleukin-13 expression in the clinical asthma phenotype. Patients with asthma who have a certain biochemical signature are more likely to respond to an anti–interleukin-13 monoclonal antibody than those without such a signature. Identification of genetic variants can eventually lead to personalized asthma treatment. Asthma biomarkers and associated phenotypes as predictors of response to specific therapies are summarized in Table 15. Failure of pharmacologic treatment is often due to uncontrolled comorbid conditions (tobacco, allergic rhinitis, pollutants), poor inhaler technique, or lack of adherence to prescribed medication.

REFERENCES & SUGGESTED READINGS
Available at eBooks.Health.Elsevier.com.

RELATED CONTENT
Asthma (Patient Information)
Asthma-COPD Overlap Syndrome (Related Key Topic)

AUTHORS: **LAREN TAN, MD, MBA** and **DERRICK CLELAND, DO, MPH**

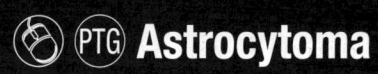
Diseases
and Disorders

I

BASIC INFORMATION

DEFINITION

Astrocytomas are neuroepithelial tumors arising from glial precursor cells called astrocytes. The distinction of different grades of astrocytoma provides important clinical prognostic information (Table 1). According to the World Health Organization (WHO) classification astrocytoma is classified as below based on the histopathology:
- Grade I: Pilocytic astrocytoma
- Grade II: Diffuse astrocytoma
- Grade III: Anaplastic astrocytoma
- Grade IV: Glioblastoma
- Grades III and IV are considered high-grade astrocytomas or malignant

SYNONYM

Astroglial neoplasms

ICD-10CM CODE
C71.9 Malignant neoplasm of brain, unspecified

EPIDEMIOLOGY & DEMOGRAPHICS

- In 2022, there were an estimated 25,050 new cases and 18,280 deaths due to primary central nervous system (CNS) tumors in the U.S.,[1] of which astrocytomas constituted approximately 10% of cases according to the Central Brain Tumor Registry of the United States (CBTRUS).
- The incidence of primary CNS tumor is 6.4 cases per 100,000 persons per yr with age-adjusted death rate of 4.4 per 100,000 population, of which about 50% cases are that of glioblastoma.

PHYSICAL FINDINGS & CLINICAL PRESENTATION

- The presenting symptoms of astrocytoma partly depend on its location and rate of growth.
- Astrocytomas classically present with any one or more of the following features:
  1. Headache (not frequent) are associated with mass effect
  2. New-onset partial or generalized seizures (<50%)
  3. Nausea and vomiting, fatigue, weakness

  4. Focal neurologic deficit (cranial nerve palsy, hemiplegia, ataxia, visual loss, language alteration, etc.)
  5. Change in mood, memory, or mental status
  6. Papilledema (rare)

ETIOLOGY

- No agents have been definitively implicated in the causation of CNS tumors though risk factors can be identified in some patients. Farmers and petrochemical workers have a higher incidence of primary brain tumors, and CNS exposure to ionizing radiation is a known risk factor.
- Different hereditary syndromes are associated with increased risk and high frequency of astrocytoma.
  1. Neurofibromatosis type 1 is associated with increased frequency of astrocytoma.
  2. Inherited syndromes such as Lynch syndrome and Li-Fraumeni syndrome are associated with an increased frequency of malignant gliomas.

GENE AND CHROMOSOMAL ALTERATIONS IN ASTROCYTOMA:

- Alteration in p53, a tumor suppressor encoded by the *TP53* gene on chromosome 17p, plays a key role in the development of at least one third of all grades of astrocytoma. In high-grade astrocytomas, p53 function may be deregulated by alteration of other genes, including amplification of MDM2 or MDM4 and 9p deletions that result in loss of the p14 product of the *CDKN2A* gene.[2]
- Mutations of isocitrate dehydrogenase 1 gene (*IDH1*) occur in a large fraction of grade II and grade III astrocytomas as well as in other gliomas. IDH-mutated tumors have a *better* prognosis compared to IDH-wild type tumors.
- Gliomas can be defined into five molecular groups with the use of three alterations: Mutations in the *TERT* promoter, mutations in *IDH*, and codeletion of chromosome arms 1p and 19q (1p/19q codeletion).[3]

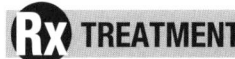 DIAGNOSIS

A provisional diagnosis of astrocytoma is made on clinical grounds and radiographic imaging studies. Tissue pathology is needed to establish the diagnosis and to grade the astrocytoma.

DIFFERENTIAL DIAGNOSIS

The differential diagnosis is vast and includes any cause of headache, seizures, change in mental status, and focal neurologic deficits.

WORKUP

- The imaging modality of choice is contrast-enhanced MRI, which can demonstrate anatomy and pathologic process in detail. Computed tomography (CT) scanning is reserved for patients who are unable or unwilling to get MRI. Biopsy with histological confirmation is required to establish a diagnosis of astrocytoma.
- Stereotactic biopsy under CT or MRI guidance is reserved for tumors that are deeply seated, multicentric tumors, or diffuse nonfocal tumors where surgical resection is not practical. Major objectives of surgical resection are to maximally remove the tumor bulk, reduce tumor-associated mass effect and elevated intracranial pressure, and to provide tissue for pathologic analysis. Surgical resection is carried out in a manner that minimizes the risk to neurological functioning. Surgery can also rapidly reduce the tumor bulk with potential benefits in terms of mass effect, edema, and hydrocephalus.

LABORATORY TESTS

- CBC
- Complete chemistry panel
- Coagulation testing (prothrombin time, partial thromboplastin time)

IMAGING STUDIES

MRI (Fig. 1) is the diagnostic imaging study of choice. MRI with contrast and magnetic resonance angiography are used to locate the margins of the tumor, distinguish vascular masses from tumors, detect low-grade astrocytomas not seen by CT scan, and provide clear views of the posterior fossa.

TREATMENT

ACUTE GENERAL Rx

- Corticosteroids reduce cerebral edema and thus minimize secondary brain injury from cerebral retraction. Usually, dexamethasone is

TABLE 1 Comparison of Astrocytoma Histopathology

	Pilocytic Astrocytoma	Diffuse Astrocytoma	Anaplastic Astrocytoma	Glioblastoma Multiforme
Malignant potential	Benign	Low grade	High grade	Very malignant
Age (approximate)	Children	Third or fourth decade	Fifth decade	Sixth decade
Location	Optic chiasm or hypothalamus > cerebellum > brainstem*	Hemispheres (cortex + white matter)	Hemispheres (cortex + white matter)	Hemispheres (cortex + white matter)
Enhancement	Mild	Mild	Moderate (ring)	Intense
Vasogenic edema	Minimal	Minimal	Moderate	Significant
Calcification	Common	Up to 20%	Occasional	Rare

*It is typically cystic with a mural nodule and located within the posterior fossa—it tends to be solid or lobulated when seen elsewhere.
From Grant LA et al: *Grainger & Allison's diagnostic radiology essentials*, ed 2, Philadelphia, 2019, Elsevier.

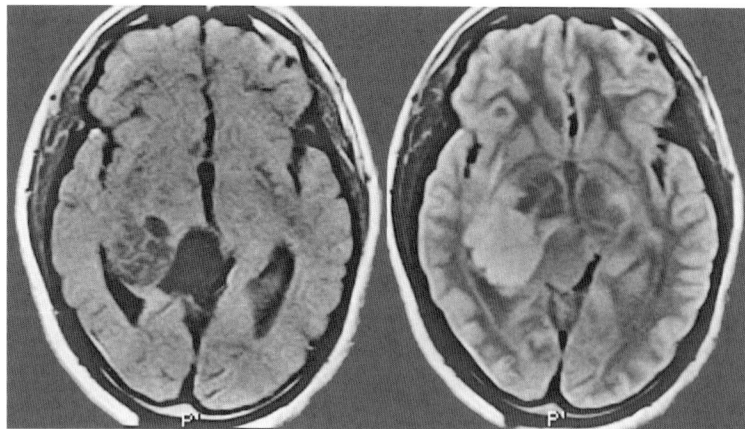

FIG. 1 Magnetic resonance image of a low-grade astrocytoma, demonstrating a hypointense right temporal lesion without contrast enhancement on T1 and hyperintense signal on T2. (From Goetz CG, Pappert EJ: *Textbook of clinical neurology*, Philadelphia, 1999, Saunders.)

started immediately preoperatively in all primary CNS tumors unless CNS lymphoma is suspected and continued in the immediate postoperative period with tapering as quickly as possible.

- If there is increased intracranial pressure and impending herniation, patient should be started on intravenous (IV) mannitol, and mechanical ventilation with hyperventilation should be considered if there is depressed consciousness.
- The use of preoperative prophylactic anticonvulsants is less commonly indicated though the current practice patterns indicate widespread use of levetiracetam or phenytoin.

STAGE-SPECIFIC Rx

- Maximal surgical resection of the tumor, when feasible, is the mainstay of management of astrocytomas. Postoperative adjuvant radiotherapy and chemotherapy approaches are individualized based on pathologic and molecular characteristics of the tumor.
- Grade I astrocytomas are usually indolent, circumscribed tumors. Complete surgical resection is curative for these tumors. If complete surgical resection is not feasible due to tumor location (e.g., tumor in optic pathway, hypothalamus, and in deep midline structures), then asymptomatic patients can be observed in these cases until maximally safe resection is feasible upon progression. Unfortunately, despite aggressive near-total resection, delayed recurrence and eventual malignant transformation are common.
- In grade II astrocytoma, the extent of postoperative residual disease after maximal tumor resection is an important variable for time to first relapse. Postoperative chemotherapy (PCV regimen or temozolomide) concurrent with radiotherapy improves progression-free survival and overall survival.
- In grade III anaplastic astrocytoma, surgical resection followed by postoperative chemotherapy and radiotherapy is routinely used. Recent randomized clinical trials have

established a survival benefit with the use of concurrent chemotherapy (temozolomide or nitrosoureas).

- In grade IV glioblastoma, maximal surgical resection improves median survival. Concurrent temozolomide chemotherapy with radiotherapy followed by further 6 mo of temozolomide chemotherapy improves survival benefit in newly diagnosed patients with the benefit seen mostly in patients whose tumors have MGMT-methylated status.[4] The 2-yr survival in these patients is 16%, and long-term survival is approximately 1%.
- In the case of both recurrent and newly diagnosed glioblastoma, the use of tumor-treatment fields devices in conjunction with the use of temozolomide chemotherapy has demonstrated a survival benefit and is approved by the FDA.[5]

TREATMENT OF RECURRENT DISEASE

- For grade 1 astrocytoma, re-resection should be considered. For patients who have tumors that are not amenable to resection, chemotherapy or radiotherapy can improve recurrence-free survival, although the role of chemotherapy in adults remain controversial.
- For grade 2 astrocytoma, radiation therapy can be considered in the relapsed setting if not given in the adjuvant setting. Data on use of chemotherapy in low-grade gliomas in adults is sparse. Although the results are encouraging, the number of patients treated in these studies is small and there were many methodologic flaws in the studies. For recurrent grade III anaplastic astrocytoma treated with radiation therapy in the past, there is a role for chemotherapy. Nitrosoureas-based regimen and temozolomide have shown efficacy in this setting.
- The combination of irinotecan with bevacizumab or bevacizumab alone has been studied, and median survival is similar with either approach.

- Various targeted therapies are currently being studied in patients with recurrent glioblastoma. The combination of dabrafenib plus trametinib (BRAF and MEK inhibitors) has demonstrated clinical activity in patients with BRAF^{V600E}-mutation–positive recurrent or refractory high-grade glioma and low-grade glioma and was approved by the FDA in this setting.[6]
- Immune checkpoint inhibitors have been evaluated in the recurrent setting, and randomized studies have not shown any survival benefits compared to bevacizumab therapy. However, certain subsets of patients with recurrent glioblastoma multiforme (GBM) have demonstrated survival benefits when used in neoadjuvant approach or in hypermutated tumors.
- Autologous tumor lysate-loaded dendritic cell vaccine (DCVax-L) has been evaluated in addition to standard of care and resulted in statistically significant extension of survival for both newly diagnosed and recurrent GBM patients.[7] Chimeric antigen T-cells (CAR-T) directed against different antigens are being evaluated in patients with recurrent glioma.

PROGNOSIS

- Grade 1 astrocytoma has a good prognosis and is usually cured with surgical resection.
- Grade 2 astrocytoma has a median survival of about 7.5 yr with treatment.
- Grade 3 anaplastic astrocytoma has a median survival of approximately 5 yr. Patients with tumors that have IDH-mutation and 1p/19q codeletion have superior survival compared with patients without deletion.
- Median survival of glioblastoma is approximately 14 mo. Primary glioblastomas are IDH-wild type and account for 90% of cases. Secondary glioblastomas in contrast are IDH-mutated, have typically evolved from low-grade gliomas, and have a much more protracted natural course than the primary cases.

REFERRAL

A multidisciplinary consultation with a neurosurgeon, radiation oncologist, and neuro-oncologist is required to assist in the diagnostic workup and to provide immediate and follow-up treatment.

REFERENCES
Available at eBooks.Health.Elsevier.com.

RELATED CONTENT
Astrocytoma (Patient Information)
Brain Cancer (Patient Information)
Brain Neoplasm, Benign (Related Key Topic)
Brain Neoplasm, Glioblastoma (Related Key Topic)

AUTHOR: **BHARTI RATHORE, MD**

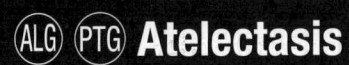
Diseases
and Disorders

I

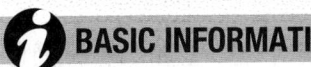 BASIC INFORMATION

DEFINITION

Atelectasis describes collapse of part or all of the lung with resultant volume loss. There are two major types of atelectasis.[1]

- Obstructive atelectasis: Most common and results from a blocked airway (e.g., mucous plug or tumor-obstructing airway) with resorption of the gas in the alveoli distal to the area of obstruction.
- Nonobstructive atelectasis: May result from several nonobstructive etiologies, including external compression from outside the lung (e.g., pleural effusion), abnormalities in surfactant leading to increased tendency for part of the lung to collapse, reduction in size of part of the lung due to scarring, and decreased ventilation of portion of the lung.

ICD-10CM CODE
J98.11   Atelectasis

EPIDEMIOLOGY & DEMOGRAPHICS

- Postoperative patients and patients with lung or chest wall injury are at increased risk of atelectasis.
- Asbestos exposure increases risk for an entity called "rounded atelectasis."
- Occurs frequently in patients receiving mechanical ventilation.
- There is no known racial or sexual predilection for atelectasis.
- Dependent regions of the lung are more prone to atelectasis.

PHYSICAL FINDINGS & CLINICAL PRESENTATION

- Patient may be asymptomatic or may have cough, dyspnea, and decrease in oxygen saturations.
- Physical examination may disclose decreased or absent breath sounds over affected area, with dullness to percussion, decreased fremitus, and decreased vocal resonance.

ETIOLOGY

- Airway obstruction (e.g., endobronchial tumor, a lymph node, foreign bodies, mucous plug)
- Extrinsic bronchial compression (e.g., neoplasms, aneurysms of ascending aorta, enlarged left atrium)
- Pleural disease (e.g., pleural effusion, mesothelioma, rounded atelectasis, pneumothorax)
- Alveolar injury (e.g., toxic fumes, aspiration of gastric contents, infections, acute respiratory distress syndrome)
- Chest wall abnormalities (e.g., trauma, scoliosis, rib fracture, obesity)
- Impaired respiratory mechanics or decreased cough response (e.g., pain, postanesthetic effect, abdominal distention, neuromuscular disease)
- Trauma caused by shear force generated by repetitive expansion and collapse during positive-pressure ventilation (e.g., mechanical ventilation)
- Characteristic rounded atelectasis may be associated with prior asbestos exposure
- Table 1 summarizes anatomic causes of atelectasis

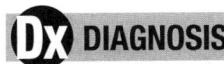 DIAGNOSIS

DIFFERENTIAL DIAGNOSIS

- Neoplasm (bronchogenic carcinoma must be excluded)
- Pneumonia
- Pleural effusion, pulmonary infarction (Fig. E1)
- Abnormalities of brachiocephalic vein and the left pulmonary ligament

WORKUP

- Chest x-ray (Fig. 2)
- Thoracic ultrasonography
- Chest CT scan (prone positioning CT scan with improvement or reduction in atelectasis) may be used to differentiate from other etiology
- Bronchoscopy (in select patients) to assess for endobronchial obstruction

IMAGING STUDIES

- Chest x-ray often suggests the diagnosis.
- Ultrasonography helps differentiate atelectasis from effusion or consolidation.
- Chest CT scan is useful in patients with suspected endobronchial neoplasm or extrinsic bronchial compression. Prone images help differentiate true consolidation from dependent atelectasis.

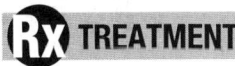 TREATMENT

NONPHARMACOLOGIC THERAPY

- Deep breathing
- Mobilization of the patient: Encouraging out of bed in upright position, ambulation
- Incentive spirometry
- Tracheal suctioning in select patients (e.g., mechanical ventilation and tracheostomy)
- Mechanical airway clearance therapies for improving cough and clearance of secretions from airways:
  1. Positive expiratory pressure (PEP) devices (e.g., Acapella, Aerobika, TheraPEP)
  2. Cough assist devices
  3. Chest physiotherapy with vest therapy, frequencer, or chest wall percussion
- Bronchoscopy might be helpful with mucous plug aspiration, removal of foreign body, or evaluation for endobronchial and peribronchial lesions

ACUTE GENERAL Rx

- Oxygen if indicated
- Positive-pressure breathing (continuous positive airway pressure by face mask, positive end-expiratory pressure for patients on mechanical ventilation)
- Use of mucolytic agents (e.g., acetylcysteine) or hypertonic saline if due to mucous plugging
- Bronchodilator therapy in selected patients
- Pain control in postoperative and trauma cases to facilitate deeper breathing
- Pleural drainage in cases of large effusions, hemothorax, or empyema
- Treatment of atelectasis is summarized in Table 2
- Prevention and treatment of postoperative atelectasis is illustrated in Fig. 3. Perioperative interventions including continuous positive end-expiratory pressure (PEEP) intraoperatively, noninvasive pressure support ventilation following extubation, and early implementation of physical therapy have been shown to reduce the incidence of postoperative atelectasis after thoracic surgery.[2]

CHRONIC Rx

- Mechanical airway clearance therapies.
- If significant endobronchial obstruction, may need to consider debulking of obstruction or possible placement of bronchial stent.
- If external compression (e.g., pleural effusion or mass) is leading to the atelectasis, then need to drain or remove the contributing source of the compression.

TABLE 1   Anatomic Causes of Atelectasis

Cause	Clinical Examples
External compression on the pulmonary parenchyma	Pleural effusion, pneumothorax, intrathoracic tumors, diaphragmatic hernia
Endobronchial obstruction completely obstructing the ingress of air	Enlarged lymph node, tumor, cardiac enlargement, foreign body, mucoid plug, broncholithiasis
Intraluminal obstruction of a bronchus	Foreign body, asthma, granulomatous tissue, tumor, secretions including mucous plugs, bronchiectasis, pulmonary abscess, chronic bronchitis, acute laryngotracheobronchitis, plastic bronchitis
Intrabronchiolar obstruction	Bronchiolitis, interstitial pneumonitis, asthma
Respiratory compromise or paralysis	Neuromuscular abnormalities, osseous deformities, overly restrictive casts and surgical dressings, defective movement of the diaphragm, or restriction of respiratory effort

From Kliegman RM: *Nelson textbook of pediatrics,* ed 21, Philadelphia, 2020, Elsevier.

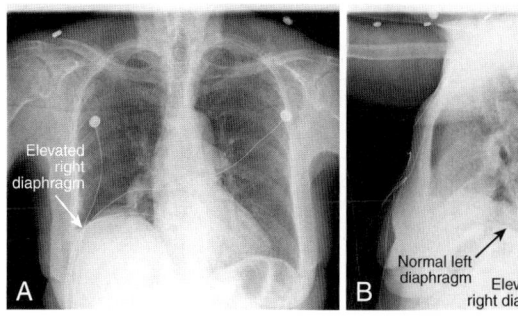

FIG. 2 Atelectasis with elevated diaphragm: An example of volume loss. The right hemidiaphragm in this patient appears elevated on both the posterior-anterior (**A**) and the lateral (**B**) views. Is this the correct interpretation of the x-ray, and if so, what is the cause? Consider the alternative interpretations. A subpulmonic pleural effusion would appear similar, as it would have the same density as liver, heart, and diaphragm and would layer over the diaphragm with the patient upright. This appears less likely in that a meniscus might be seen along the lateral chest wall with a pleural effusion but is not present here. In addition, a pleural effusion occupies space and might be expected to push the heart to the left, whereas in this case the heart may be slightly deviated to the right. Atelectasis of the lower right lung would result in volume loss, pulling the heart and hemidiaphragm into the space normally occupied by the lung. This is consistent with the observed features. An infiltrate in this location could explain the x-ray findings but appears less likely for similar reasons to those cited for effusion. Some simple maneuvers could narrow the differential diagnosis. Chest ultrasound, decubitus x-ray views, or CT could identify an effusion. (From Broder JS: *Diagnostic imaging for the emergency physician,* Philadelphia, 2011, Saunders.)

TABLE 2 Treatment for Atelectasis

Cause of Atelectasis	Treatment
Pleural effusion or pneumothorax	Relieve compression
Mucous plug	Tracheal or bronchoscopic aspiration Continuous positive airway pressure
Foreign body	Bronchoscopic examination
Asthma	Bronchodilator and corticosteroid treatment Recombinant human deoxyribonuclease (off label use) Hypertonic saline with or without bronchodilator
Neuromuscular diseases	Intermittent positive pressure breathing Mechanical insufflator—exsufflator Noninvasive bilevel positive pressure ventilation
Cystic fibrosis	Airway clearance therapies Hypertonic saline with or without bronchodilator

From Kliegman RM: *Nelson textbook of pediatrics,* ed 21, Philadelphia, 2020, Elsevier.

DISPOSITION

Prognosis varies with the underlying etiology.

REFERRAL

- Pulmonary for bronchoscopy to evaluate for obstructing lesion as etiology for atelectasis and for possible removal of foreign body.
- Interventional pulmonology to debulk or remove endobronchial tumor or to place endobronchial stent if indicated.

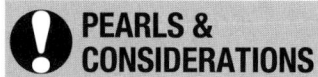

PEARLS & CONSIDERATIONS

COMMENTS

Patients should be educated that frequent changes of position are helpful in clearing secretions. Sitting the patient upright in a chair is recommended to increase both volume and vital capacity relative to the supine position. Adequate pain control and early mobilization are paramount after surgical intervention or rib fractures.

REFERENCES

Available at eBooks.Health.Elsevier.com.

RELATED CONTENT

Atelectasis (Patient Information)

AUTHOR: **LORRIANA E. LEARD, MD**

A

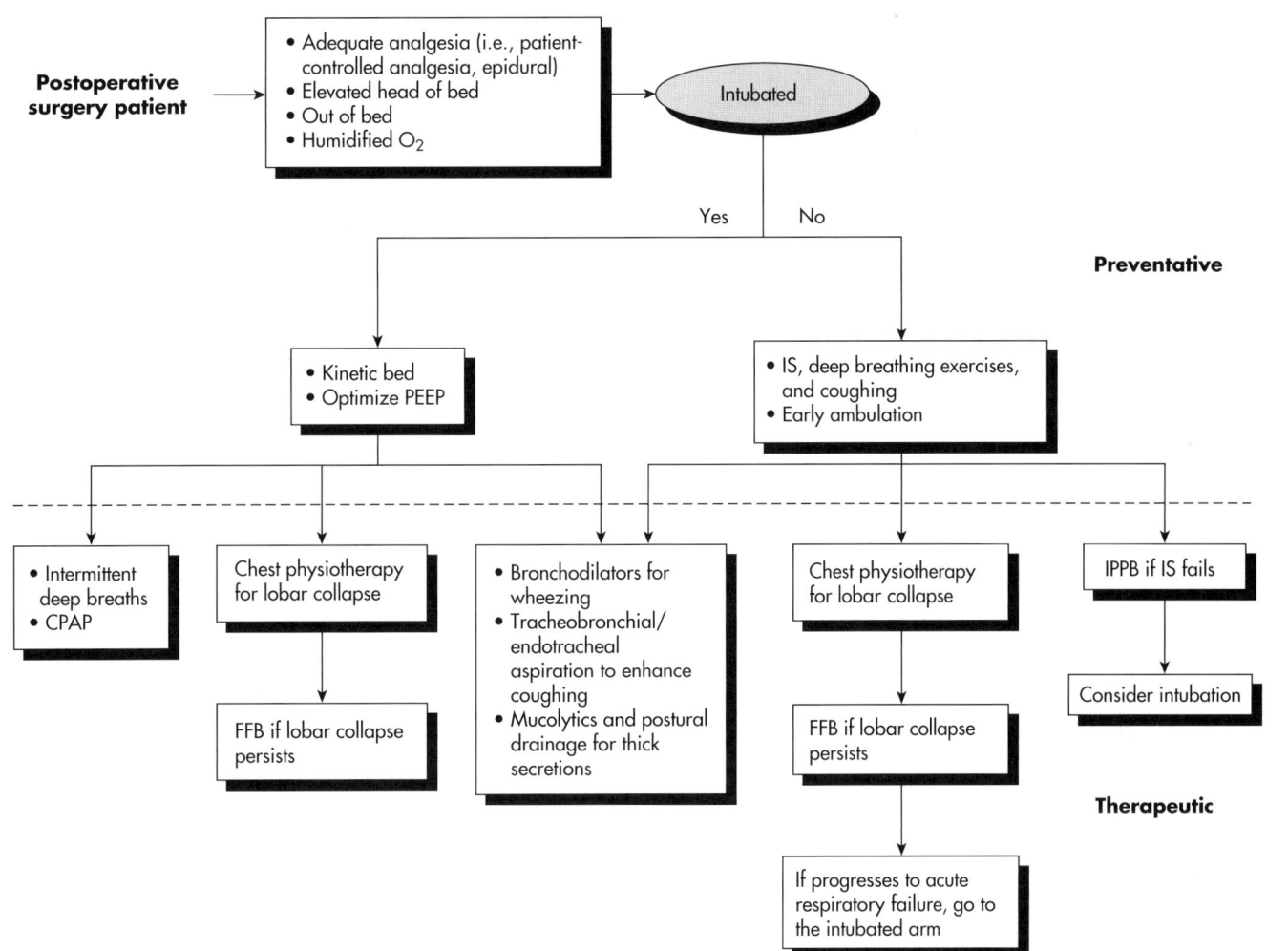

FIG. 3 Prevention and treatment algorithm for postoperative atelectasis. *CPAP,* Continuous positive airway pressure; *FFB,* flexible fiberoptic bronchoscopy; *IPPB,* intermittent positive-pressure breathing; *IS,* incentive spirometry; *PEEP,* positive end-expiratory pressure. (From Newman M et al: *Perioperative medicine,* ed 2, Philadelphia, 2022, Elsevier.)

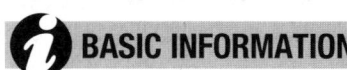

BASIC INFORMATION

DEFINITION

Atopic dermatitis is a chronic inflammatory skin disease characterized by intermittent pruritic eruptions and is associated with a personal and family history of allergic manifestations including food allergies, asthma, and allergic rhino-conjunctivitis (atopy). Box 1 summarizes criteria for atopic dermatitis. Modified criteria for children with atopic dermatitis are described in Box 2. Important and essential features of atopic dermatitis are summarized in Box 3.

SYNONYMS

Eczema
Atopic neurodermatitis
Atopic eczema

ICD-10CM CODES

L20.9   Atopic dermatitis, unspecified
L20.89 Other atopic dermatitis

EPIDEMIOLOGY & DEMOGRAPHICS

- Prevalence is about 30% in most developed nations and exceeds 10% in many countries.
- Approximately 15% to 20% of children and 10% of adults experience atopic dermatitis worldwide.[1]
- About 60% of cases occur in the first year of life with onset occurring most commonly between 3 and 6 mo of age.[2]
- Children with generalized atopic dermatitis are at increased risk of developing asthma and allergic rhinitis, a phenomenon often referred to as the "atopic march."
- General risk factors include female sex, family history of atopy (especially a maternal history of eczema), high latitude (and therefore low sun exposure), and birth order (oldest are at greatest risk).
- Risk factors for developing atopic dermatitis in the first 6 mo of life include African and Asian race/ethnicity, male sex, and greater gestational age at birth.
- Consumption of a Western diet, delivery by cesarean section, exposure to antibiotics prenatally, and colonization with *Clostridium* cluster I are also associated with increased risk and suggest that alternations in the intestinal microbiome may play a role in the development of atopic dermatitis.
- Protective factors include breastfeeding, dog ownership before age 1, and being raised on a farm (i.e., hygiene hypothesis).

PHYSICAL FINDINGS & CLINICAL PRESENTATION

- The clinical characteristics of atopic dermatitis vary depending on age, disease stage, race, or ethnic group, and geographic locations but center around xerosis and pruritus.[1]
- Generally atopic dermatitis presentation can be subdivided into three phases:
  - Acute: Eruption of erythematous papules with serous exudate and crusted erosions
  - Subacute: Dry, scaly, erythematous papules and plaques

- Chronic: Lichenification from repeated scratching

Time course/differences between children and adults

- The lesions are typically on the neck, face, upper trunk, and elbows and knees (extensor surface in younger children and flexural surfaces in older children and adults; Figs. E1 through E6). Atopic dermatitis lesions are usually discrete but vaguely delineated, scaly, and erythematous.
- There is dryness, thickening of the involved areas, discoloration, blistering, and oozing.
- Papular lesions are frequently found in the antecubital and popliteal fossae.
- In children, red scaling plaques are often confined to the cheeks and spare the perioral and perinasal areas (Fig. E7A,B).

BOX 1   Criteria for Atopic Dermatitis

Major criteria
Must have three of the following:
1. Pruritus
2. Typical morphology and distribution
   - Flexural lichenification in adults
   - Facial and extensor involvement in infancy
3. Chronic or chronically relapsing dermatitis
4. Personal or family history of atopic disease (e.g., asthma, allergic rhinitis, atopic dermatitis)

Minor criteria
Must also have three of the following:
- Xerosis
- Ichthyosis, hyperlinear palms, or keratosis pilaris
- IgE reactivity (immediate skin test reactivity, RAST test positive)
- Elevated serum IgE
- Early age of onset
- Tendency for cutaneous infections (especially *Staphylococcus aureus* and HSV)
- Tendency to nonspecific hand/foot dermatitis
- Nipple eczema
- Cheilitis
- Recurrent conjunctivitis
- Dennie-Morgan infraorbital fold
- Keratoconus
- Anterior subcapsular cataracts
- Orbital darkening
- Facial pallor or facial erythema
- Pityriasis alba
- Itch when sweating
- Intolerance to wool and lipid solvents
- Perifollicular accentuation
- Food hypersensitivity
- Course influenced by environmental or emotional factors
- White dermatographism or delayed blanch to cholinergic agents

HSV, Herpes simplex virus; *IgE,* immunoglobulin E; *RAST,* radioallergosorbent test.
From James WD et al: *Andrews' diseases of the skin,* ed 13, Philadelphia, 2020, Elsevier.

BOX 2   Modified Criteria for Children With Atopic Dermatitis

Essential features
1. Pruritus
2. Eczema
   - Typical morphology and age-specific pattern
   - Chronic or relapsing history

Important features
1. Early age at onset
2. Atopy
3. Personal or family history
4. IgE reactivity
5. Xerosis

Associated features
1. Atypical vascular responses (e.g., facial pallor, white dermatographism)
2. Keratosis pilaris, ichthyosis, or hyperlinear palms
3. Orbital or periorbital changes
4. Other regional findings (e.g., perioral changes, periauricular lesions)
5. Perifollicular accentuation, lichenification, or prurigo lesions

IgE, Immunoglobulin E.
From James WD et al: *Andrews' diseases of the skin,* ed 13, Philadelphia, 2020, Elsevier.

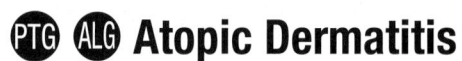
A

Diseases and Disorders

I

BOX 3 Essential, Important, and Associated Features of Atopic Dermatitis

Essential Features
- Pruritus
- Eczema (acute, subacute, chronic)
- Morphology and age-specific patterns
  - Infants and children: Facial, neck, and extensor involvement
  - Any age group: Flexural lesions; sparing of groin
- Chronic or relapsing history

Important Features
- Early age
- Atopy
  - Personal and/or family history of atopic disorders
  - Elevated total serum immunoglobulin E (IgE) or allergen-specific IgE
- Xerosis
- Lichenification

Associated Features
- Atypical vascular responses (e.g., white dermatographism, facial pallor)
- Keratosis pilaris, hyperlinear palms, ichthyosis
- Ocular, periorbital changes
- Other regional findings (perioral, periauricular)
- Perifollicular accentuation, prurigo lesions

- Hertoghe sign: Loss of the outer eyebrow from chronic rubbing.
- Pruritus is the most common and burdensome symptom of atopic dermatitis. Frequent scratching may result in areas of hypopigmentation or hyperpigmentation (more common in black patients).
- In adults, redness and scaling on the dorsal aspect of the hands or about the fingers are the most common expressions of atopic dermatitis; oozing and crusting may be present.
- Secondary skin infections may be present (*Staphylococcus aureus*, dermatophytosis, herpes simplex). *S. aureus* has been shown to colonize 90% of lesions.[4]
- Associated features of atopic dermatitis (atopic stigmata) are summarized in Table 1.

ETIOLOGY
- The pathogenesis of atopic dermatitis is multifactorial, involving immunologic, genetic, and environmental factors that disrupt the epidermis and induce hyperreactivity.
- Epidermal barrier dysfunction and immune dysregulation are key, leading to a cycle of

---

TABLE 1 Associated Features of Atopic Dermatitis (Atopic Stigmata)

Xerosis	<ul><li>Important feature that is present in most patients with AD</li><li>Often most prominent on the lower legs; may be generalized</li><li>Dry skin with fine scale in areas without clinically apparent inflammation</li><li>Typically worse during the winter</li><li>Impaired epidermal barrier function from decreased water content in the stratum corneum leads to easier entry of irritants, which can promote pruritus and initiate an inflammatory response</li></ul>
Ichthyosis vulgaris	<ul><li>Autosomal semidominant disorder with incomplete penetrance caused by mutations in the filaggrin gene *(FLG)*</li><li>~15% of patients with AD have moderate-to-severe ichthyosis vulgaris; conversely, >50% of patients with ichthyosis vulgaris have AD</li><li>Excessive fine, whitish to brown scaling that favors the lower legs (especially the shins) and spares the flexures</li></ul>
Keratosis pilaris	<ul><li>Common condition that affects >40% of patients with AD and ~75% of those with ichthyosis vulgaris</li><li>Onset typically in childhood; may improve after puberty (especially facial involvement)</li><li>Affects the lateral aspect of the upper arms, thighs, and lateral cheeks (especially in children) > trunk and extensor aspects of the distal extremities</li><li>Keratotic follicular papules, often with a rim of erythema or a background of patchy erythema (especially on the cheeks)</li><li>The *keratosis pilaris rubra (KPR)* variant features numerous tiny, "grainlike" follicular papules superimposed on prominent confluent erythema; often widespread on face and ears > trunk & proximal extremities, and tends to persist after puberty; presence of erythema rather than hyperpigmentation differentiates KPR from erythromelanosis follicularis faciei et colli, and a lack of atrophy in KPR differentiates it from keratosis pilaris atrophicans</li><li>Keratolytic agents and topical retinoids are sometimes used to decrease the hyperkeratotic component, but the benefit is limited and these agents can be irritating, especially in AD patients; treatment with vascular lasers (e.g., pulsed dye laser) can sometimes improve associated erythema</li></ul>
Palmar and plantar hyperlinearity	<ul><li>Increased prominence of the palmar and, less often, plantar creases</li><li>Associated with ichthyosis vulgaris and *FLG* mutations</li></ul>
Dennie-Morgan lines	<ul><li>Symmetric, prominent horizontal fold(s) (single or double) just beneath the margin of the lower lid, originating at or near the inner canthus and extending one-half to two-thirds the width of the lid</li></ul>
Periorbital darkening ("allergic shiners")	<ul><li>Skin around the eyes appears gray to violet–brown, while the rest of the facial skin is rather pale</li><li>Periorbital edema and lichenification may also be seen</li></ul>
Anterior neck folds	<ul><li>Horizontal folds across the middle of the anterior neck</li></ul>
Hertoghe sign	<ul><li>Absence or thinning of the lateral eyebrows</li></ul>
White dermographism	<ul><li>Stroking the skin leads to a white streak that reflects excessive vasoconstriction</li><li>Most apparent on the forehead</li><li>Midfacial pallor and a delayed blanch response represent additional manifestations of aberrant vascular reactivity in patients with atopic dermatitis</li></ul>
Follicular prominence	<ul><li>"Goose bump–like" appearance of the skin, most often on the trunk</li><li>More commonly observed in children with darkly pigmented skin</li></ul>

AD, Atopic dermatitis.
From Bolognia J: *Dermatology,* ed 4, 2018, Elsevier.

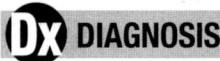

inflammation; filaggrin deficiency, T-lymphocyte proliferation, defective cell immunity, and B-cell immunoglobulin E (IgE) overproduction may all play a significant role.

DIAGNOSIS

DIFFERENTIAL DIAGNOSIS (BOX 4)

- Scabies
- Psoriasis
- Dermatitis herpetiform
- Contact dermatitis
- Photosensitivity
- Seborrheic dermatitis
- Candidiasis, tinea
- Lichen simplex chronicus
- Other: Xerosis, impetigo, Wiskott-Aldrich syndrome, phenylketonuria, ichthyosis, HIV dermatitis, nonnummular eczema, histiocytosis X, malignancies (T-cell lymphoma/mycosis fungoides, Letterer-Siwe disease), graft-versus-host disease, metabolic and nutritional deficiencies (zinc, niacin, pyridoxine deficiencies)
- Table 2 summarizes characteristics and clinical features of disorders in the differential diagnosis of atopic dermatitis

WORKUP (FIG. 8)

Diagnosis is generally based on history and physical examination with the presence of three of the following major features and three minor features.

MAJOR FEATURES:

- Pruritus
- Personal or family history of atopy: Asthma, allergic rhinitis, atopic dermatitis
- Facial and extensor involvement in infants and children
- Flexural lichenification in adults

MINOR FEATURES:

- Elevated IgE
- Eczema-perifollicular accentuation
- Recurrent conjunctivitis
- Ichthyosis
- Nipple dermatitis
- Wool intolerance
- Cutaneous *S. aureus* infections or herpes simplex infections
- Food intolerance
- Hand dermatitis (nonallergic irritant)
- Facial pallor, facial erythema
- Cheilitis
- White dermographism
- Early age of onset (after 2 mo of age)

LABORATORY TESTS

- Laboratory tests are generally not helpful, though 85% of patients have elevated IgE levels.
- Consider skin biopsy only in cases unresponsive to treatment.

TREATMENT

Treatment for atopic dermatitis is based on the clinical stage of disease, the extent of body-surface area involved, age, coexisting conditions, and medications being taken by the patient, the degree to which quality of life is impaired, and the goals of the patient.[1]

NONPHARMACOLOGIC THERAPY

- Proper skin care:
  - Clip nails to decrease abrasion of skin.
  - Moisturize daily with emollients or ceramides, ideally immediately after bathing when the skin is still damp. Severely affected skin can be further hydrated by occlusion with wet dressings.[5]
  - Limit showers to 5 to 10 min with lukewarm water.
  - Use fragrance-free soaps and detergents.
- Bleach baths may be helpful for certain patients.[1]
- Avoidance of triggering factors:
  - Sudden temperature changes or temperature extremes, excessive sunlight, sweating, low humidity in the winter
  - Contact with irritating substance (e.g., wool, cosmetics, some soaps and detergents, tobacco)
  - Foods that provoke exacerbations (e.g., eggs, peanuts, fish, soy, wheat, milk)
  - Stressful situations
  - Allergens and dust
  - Excessive hand washing
  - Very hot, long showers
- Phototherapy in moderation may be effective in resistant cases and typically requires dermatology referral.[6]

ACUTE GENERAL Rx

- Low-potency topical corticosteroids (e.g., 1% to 2.5% hydrocortisone) may be helpful and are generally considered first-line therapy for flares. Recommended use is once or twice daily and applied immediately after bathing before application of emollient. Use intermediate-potency steroids (e.g., triamcinolone, fluocinolone) for more severe cases and limit potent corticosteroids (e.g., betamethasone, desoximetasone, clobetasol) to severe cases.
- Table 3 summarizes relative potencies of topical corticosteroids.
- Crisaborole 2% ointment is a phosphodiesterase type-4 (PDE4) inhibitor modestly effective for short-term treatment of mild to moderate atopic dermatitis, but use can be limited by patient report of discomfort. Cost is also a limiting factor.[7]

BOX 4 Differential Diagnosis of Atopic Dermatitis

Congenital Disorders
- Netherton's syndrome
- Familial keratosis pilaris

Chronic Dermatoses
- Seborrheic dermatitis
- Contact dermatitis (allergic or irritant)
- Nummular eczema
- Psoriasis
- Ichthyoses

Infections and Infestations
- Scabies
- Human immunodeficiency virus-associated dermatitis
- Dermatophytosis

Malignancies
- Cutaneous T cell lymphoma (mycosis fungoides/Sézary syndrome)
- Letterer-Siwe disease

Autoimmune Disorders
- Dermatitis herpetiformis
- Pemphigus foliaceus
- Graft-versus-host disease
- Dermatomyositis

Immunodeficiencies
- Wiskott-Aldrich syndrome
- Severe combined immunodeficiency syndrome
- Hyper-immunoglobulin E syndrome
- Dedicator of cytokinesis 8 (DOCK8)-associated immunodeficiency
- X-linked immune dysregulation, polyendocrinopathy, enteropathy (IPEX) syndrome

Metabolic Disorders
- Zinc deficiency
- Pyridoxine (vitamin B_6) and niacin
- Multiple carboxylase deficiency
- Phenylketonuria

From Leung DYM et al: *Pediatric allergy principles and practice,* ed 4, Philadelphia, Elsevier, 2020.

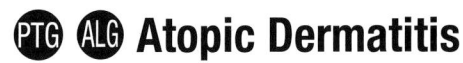

A

TABLE 2   Differential Diagnosis of Atopic Dermatitis (AD)

	Main Age Group Affected	Frequency*	Characteristics and Clinical Features
Other Types of Dermatitis			
Seborrheic dermatitis	Infants	Common	Salmon-red greasy scaly lesions, often on the scalp (cradle cap) and diaper area; generally presents in the first 6 wk of life; typically clears within weeks
Seborrheic dermatitis	Adults	Common	Erythematous patches with yellow, white, or grayish scales in seborrheic areas, particularly the scalp, central face, and anterior chest
Nummular dermatitis	Children and adults	Common	Coin-shaped scaly patches, mostly on legs and buttocks; usually no itch
Irritant contact dermatitis	Children and adults	Common	Acute to chronic eczematous lesions, mostly confined to the site of exposure; history of locally applied irritants is a risk factor; might coexist with AD
Allergic contact dermatitis	Children and adults	Common	Eczematous rash with maximum expression at sites of direct exposure but might spread; history of locally applied irritants is a risk factor; might coexist with AD
Lichen simplex chronicus	Adults	Uncommon	One or more localized, circumscribed, lichenified plaques that result from repetitive scratching or rubbing because of intense itch
Asteatotic eczema	Adults	Common	Scaly, fissured patches of dermatitis overlying dry skin, most often on lower legs
Infectious Skin Diseases			
Dermatophyte infection	Children and adults	Common	One or more demarcated scaly plaques with central clearing and slightly raised reddened edge; variable itch
Impetigo	Children	Common	Demarcated erythematous patches with blisters or honey-yellow crusting
Scabies	Children	Common†	Itchy superficial burrows and pustules on palms and soles, between fingers, and on genitalia; might produce secondary eczematous changes
HIV	Children and adults	Uncommon	Seborrhea-like rash
Keratinization Disorders			
Ichthyosis vulgaris	Infants and adults	Uncommon	Dry skin with fine scaling, particularly on the lower abdomen and extensor areas; perifollicular skin roughening; palmar hyperlinearity; full form (i.e., 2 *FLG* mutations) is uncommon; often coexists with AD
Nutritional Deficiency–Metabolic Disorders			
Zinc deficiency (acrodermatitis enteropathica)	Children	Uncommon	Erythematous scaly patches and plaques, most often around the mouth and anus; rare congenital form accompanied by diarrhea and alopecia
Biotin deficiency (nutritional or biotinidase deficiency)	Infants	Uncommon	Scaly periorofacial dermatitis, alopecia, conjunctivitis, lethargy, hypotonia
Pellagra (niacin deficiency)	All ages	Uncommon	Scaly crusted epidermis, desquamation, sun-exposed areas, diarrhea
Kwashiorkor	Infants and children	Geographic dependent	Flaky scaly dermatitis, swollen limbs with cracked peeling patches
Phenylketonuria	Infants	Uncommon	Eczematous rash, hypopigmentation, blonde hair, developmental delay
Neoplastic Disease			
Cutaneous T-cell lymphoma	Adults	Uncommon	Erythematous pink-brown macules and plaques with a fine scale; poorly responsive to topical corticosteroids; variable itch (in early stages)
Langerhans cell histiocytosis	Infants	Uncommon	Scaly and purpuric dermatosis, hepatosplenomegaly, cytopenias

FLG, Filaggrin gene; *HIV*, human immunodeficiency virus.
*Common = approximately 1/10 to 1/100; uncommon = 1/100 to 1/1000; rare = 1/1000 to 1/10,000; very rare ≤1/10,000.
†Especially in developing countries.
From Kliegman RM: *Nelson textbook of pediatrics,* ed 21, Philadelphia, 2020, Elsevier.

- Oral antihistamines (e.g., hydroxyzine, diphenhydramine) have not been shown to be effective and are generally not recommended. Although the pruritus is not histamine-induced, histamines blockade may be useful for inducing sedation, restful sleep, and prevention of scratching during sleep.
- The topical immunomodulators pimecrolimus and tacrolimus can be used in conjunction with topical corticosteroids and are useful for the face and intertriginous sites, where steroid-induced atrophy may occur. FDA recommends limiting their use for short periods in a specific subset of patients, given concerns about the potential for rare, carcinogenic effects. Pimecrolimus cream 1% has antiinflammatory effects secondary to blockage of activated T-cell cytokine production. Tacrolimus ointment (0.03% or 0.1%) suppresses humoral and cell-mediated immune responses.
- Oral prednisone, intramuscular triamcinolone, psoralen, ultraviolet A light therapy, and Goeckerman regimen are generally reserved for severe cases.
- Cyclosporine, azathioprine, and methotrexate are sometimes tried for recalcitrant disease in adults by physicians who specialize in severe inflammatory skin conditions.[8]
- The monoclonal antibody dupilumab has been shown to be effective in children and adults with moderate to severe atopic dermatitis. It can be used with or without topical steroids and is injected subcutaneously. Cost is a limiting factor.[9]
- The FDA has approved a 1.5% topical cream formulation of the Janus kinase (JAK) inhibitor ruxolitinib for short term noncontinuous chronic treatment of mild to moderate atopic dermatitis in non-immunocompromised patients ≥12 yr old whose disease has not been adequately controlled with other topical drugs. Formulary and cost are significant limiting factors.[10]

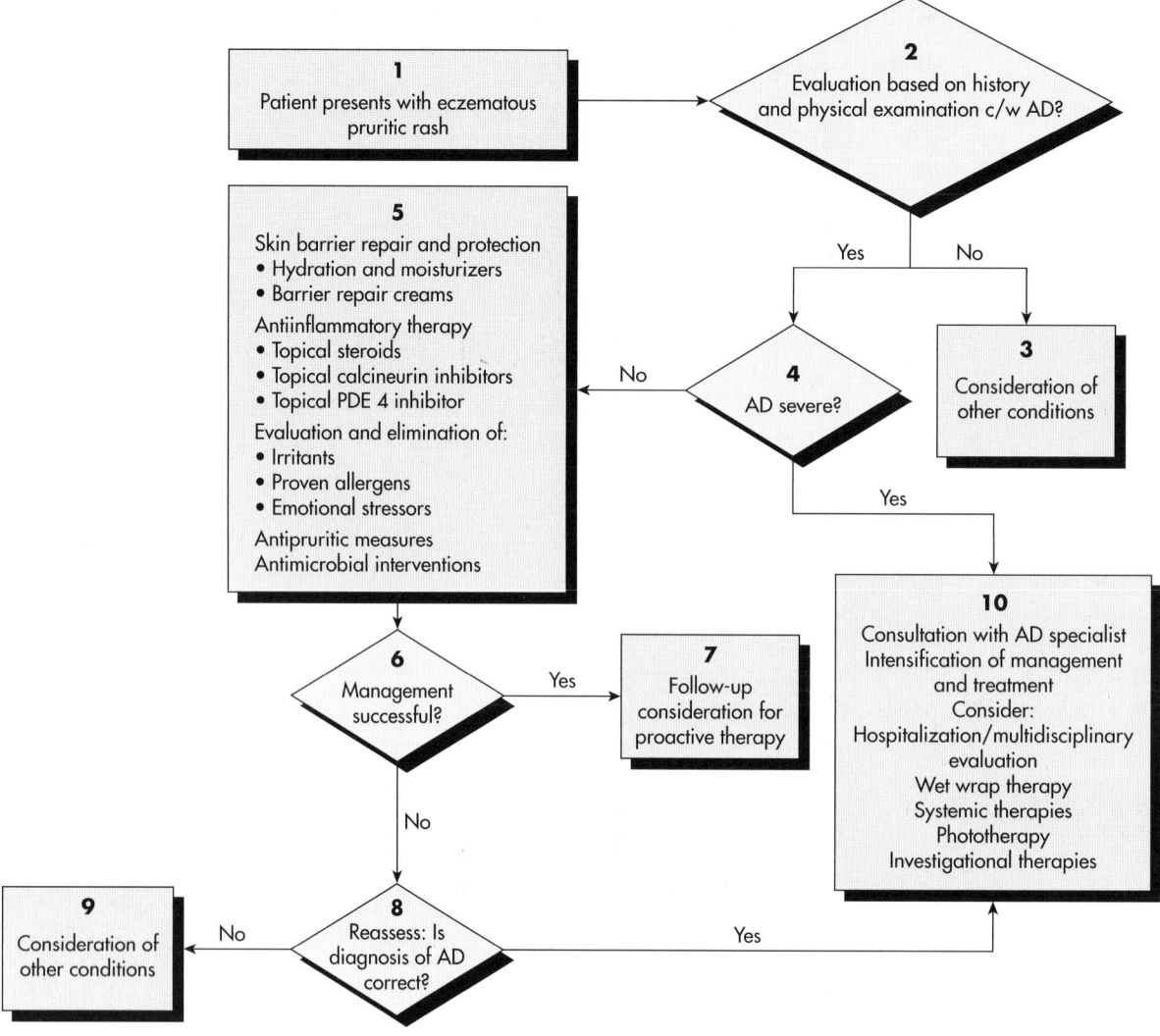

FIG. 8 Clinical algorithm for diagnosis and management of atopic dermatitis *(AD).* (From Leung DYM et al: *Pediatric allergy principles and practice,* ed 4, Philadelphia, 2020, Elsevier.)

TABLE 3   Relative Potencies of Topical Corticosteroids (From Most Potent to Weakest)

Class	Drug	Dosage Form(s)	Strength (%)
I. Very high potency			
	Augmented betamethasone dipropionate	Ointment	0.05
	Clobetasol propionate	Cream, ointment, foam	0.05
	Diflorasone diacetate	Ointment	0.05
	Halobetasol propionate	Cream, ointment	0.05
II. High potency			
	Amcinonide	Cream, lotion, ointment	0.1
	Augmented betamethasone dipropionate	Cream	0.05
	Betamethasone dipropionate	Cream, ointment, foam, solution	0.05
	Desoximetasone	Cream, ointment	0.25
	Desoximetasone	Gel	0.05
	Diflorasone diacetate	Cream	0.05
	Fluocinonide	Cream, ointment, gel, solution	0.05
	Halcinonide	Cream, ointment	0.1
	Mometasone furoate	Ointment	0.1
	Triamcinolone acetonide	Cream, ointment	0.5

Continued

Diseases
and Disorders

I

TABLE 3 Relative Potencies of Topical Corticosteroids (From Most Potent to Weakest)—Cont'd

Class	Drug	Dosage Form(s)	Strength (%)
III-IV. Medium potency			
	Betamethasone valerate	Cream, ointment, lotion, foam	0.1
	Clocortolone pivalate	Cream	0.1
	Desoximetasone	Cream	0.05
	Fluocinolone acetonide	Cream, ointment	0.025
	Flurandrenolide	Cream, ointment	0.05
	Fluticasone propionate	Cream	0.05
	Fluticasone propionate	Ointment	0.005
	Mometasone furoate	Cream	0.1
	Triamcinolone acetonide	Cream, ointment	0.1
V. Lower-medium potency			
	Hydrocortisone butyrate	Cream, ointment, solution	0.1
	Hydrocortisone probutate	Cream	0.1
	Hydrocortisone valerate	Cream, ointment	0.2
	Prednicarbate	Cream	0.1
VI. Low potency			
	Alclometasone dipropionate	Cream, ointment	0.05
	Desonide	Cream, gel, foam, ointment	0.05
	Fluocinolone acetonide	Cream, solution, oil	0.01
VII. Lowest potency			
	Dexamethasone	Cream	0.1
	Hydrocortisone	Cream, ointment, lotion, solution	0.25, 0.5, 1
	Hydrocortisone acetate	Cream, ointment	0.5-1

From Paller AS, Mancini AJ: *Hurwitz clinical pediatric dermatology: a textbook of skin disorders of childhood and adolescence,* ed 5, 2016, Philadelphia, Elsevier.

TABLE 4 Management of Mild, Moderate, and Severe Forms of Atopic Dermatitis

Mild	Moderate	Severe
Bathing and barrier repair*	Bathing and barrier repair*	Bathing and barrier repair*
Avoidance of irritant and allergic triggers	Avoidance of irritant and allergic triggers	Avoidance of irritant and allergic triggers
Intermittent, short-term use of class VI or VII topical steroids ± topical calcineurin inhibitors	Intermittent, short-term use of class III-V topical steroids ± topical calcineurin inhibitors	Class II topical steroids for flares; class III-V topical steroids ± tacrolimus ointment for maintenance
Treatment of superinfection	Treatment of superinfection	Treatment of superinfection
	Oral antihistamines	Oral antihistamines
		Systemic antiinflammatory agents, ultraviolet light therapy

* Barrier repair may be accomplished by application of effective emollients or from barrier-repair agents.
From Paller AS, Mancini AJ: *Hurwitz clinical pediatric dermatology: a textbook of skin disorders of childhood and adolescence,* ed 5, 2016, Philadelphia, Elsevier.

- Antistaphylococcal antibiotics are effective in treating secondary skin infections.
- Table 4 summarizes the management of atopic dermatitis.

DISPOSITION
- Resolution occurs in the majority of patients by adulthood. Seventy percent of patients outgrow AD by puberty.
- Most patients have a course characterized by remissions and intermittent flares.

REFERENCES & SUGGESTED READING
Available at eBooks.Health.Elsevier.com.

RELATED CONTENT
Dermatitis (Patient Information)
Eczema (Patient Information)

AUTHORS: **MATHEW J. LUCAS, MD,** and **ANNA-MARIE TIERNEY, MD**

BASIC INFORMATION

DEFINITION

Atrial fibrillation (AF) is a supraventricular tachyarrhythmia characterized by disorganized and rapid atrial activation and uncoordinated atrial contraction. AF occurs when structural and/or electrophysiologic abnormalities alter atrial tissue to promote abnormal impulse formation and/or propagation. The ventricular rate is dependent on the conduction properties of the atrioventricular (AV) node, which can be influenced by vagal/sympathetic tone, medications, or disease of the AV node.

Multiple classification schemes have been used in the past to characterize AF. The current classification scheme (divided into three major types) used by the American College of Cardiology (ACC)/American Heart Association (AHA) guideline committee is as follows:

- Paroxysmal AF: More than one episode of AF that terminate spontaneously or with intervention within 7 days
- Persistent AF: Episodes of AF that last longer than 7 days
  1. Early-persistent AF: AF that has been continuous for longer than 7 days but fewer than 3 mo
  2. Long-standing persistent AF: AF that has persisted for longer than 1 yr, either because cardioversion has failed or because cardioversion has not been attempted
- Permanent AF: When patient and physician decide to stop pursuing restoring sinus rhythm
- In addition to the previous AF categories, which are mainly defined by episode timing and termination, the ACC/AHA/European Society of Cardiology (ESC) guidelines describe additional AF categories in terms of other characteristics of the patient:
  1. Lone atrial fibrillation (LAF): Generally refers to AF in younger patients without clinical or echocardiographic evidence of cardiopulmonary disease, diabetes, or hypertension
  2. Nonvalvular AF: Atrial fibrillation in the absence of moderate-to-severe mitral stenosis or in the presence of a mechanical heart valve
  3. Secondary AF: Occurs in the setting of a primary condition that may be the cause of the AF, such as acute myocardial infarction, cardiac surgery, pericarditis, myocarditis, hyperthyroidism, pulmonary embolism, pneumonia, or other acute disease. It is considered separately because AF is less likely to recur once the precipitating condition has resolved
  4. Silent AF: Asymptomatic AF diagnosed by an ECG or rhythm strip

SYNONYMS

AF
Paroxysmal atrial fibrillation (PAF)
AFib

ICD-10CM CODES
I48.0	Paroxysmal atrial fibrillation
I48.1	Persistent atrial fibrillation
I48.2	Chronic atrial fibrillation
I48.91	Unspecified atrial fibrillation

EPIDEMIOLOGY & DEMOGRAPHICS

- The prevalence of AF increases with age, from 2% in adults <65 to 9% of those >65 yr old.
- AF affects over 3 million people in the United States. AF is uncommon in infants and children and, when present, almost always occurs in association with structural heart disease.
- The incidence of AF is significantly higher in men than in women in all age groups (1.1% versus 0.8%). AF appears to be more common in whites than in blacks, who may have lower awareness of the disease.
- Stroke due to thromboembolism is the most common and dreaded complication of AF. The rate of ischemic stroke in patients with nonrheumatic AF averages 5% a yr, which is somewhere between 2 and 7× the rate of stroke in patients without AF. The risk of stroke is not due solely to AF; changes in the endothelium and elevated markers of inflammation that may contribute to thrombosis are found in patients with AF, regardless of their rhythm at the time. The attributable risk of stroke from AF is estimated to be 1.5% for those aged 50 to 59 yr, and it approaches 36% for those aged 80 to 89 yr.
- Table 1 summarizes the thromboembolic risk score.

PHYSICAL FINDINGS & CLINICAL PRESENTATION

Clinical presentation is variable:
- Palpitations, dizziness, or light-headedness
- Fatigue, weakness, or impaired exercise tolerance
- Angina
- Dyspnea
- Some patients are asymptomatic
- Cardiac auscultation revealing irregularly irregular rhythm
- Thromboembolic phenomenon such as stroke

ETIOLOGY

- The most frequent change in AF is the loss of atrial muscle mass and atrial fibrosis
- Fibrillation is presumed to be caused by multiple wandering wavelets, usually originating from the pulmonary veins. Both reentrant and focal mechanisms have been proposed. See Fig. 1 for mechanisms of atrial fibrillation. Fig. 2 illustrates an approach to selecting drug therapy for ventricular rate control
- Vascular causes: Hypertensive heart disease
- Valvular heart disease
- Pulmonary causes: Pulmonary embolism, chronic obstructive pulmonary disease, obstructive sleep apnea, carbon monoxide poisoning
- Structural cardiac disease: Hypertrophic cardiomyopathy, congestive heart failure, coronary artery disease, myocardial infarction, congenital heart disease (especially those that lead to atrial enlargement such as atrial septal defect)
- Pericarditis and myocarditis
- Arrhythmias: Atrial tachycardias and atrial flutters have been associated with atrial fibrillation, as has Wolff-Parkinson-White syndrome

- Endocrine: Thyrotoxicosis, hyperthyroidism or subclinical hyperthyroidism, pheochromocytoma, obesity
- Surgery: Both cardiac and noncardiac
- Electrolytes: Hypokalemia, hypomagnesemia
- Systemic stress: Fever, anemia, hypoxia, sepsis, infections (e.g., pneumonia)
- Medications/toxins: Digitalis, adenosine, theophylline, amphetamines, cocaine, antihistamines, alcohol abuse and/or withdrawal, caffeine, steroidal antiinflammatory drugs (SAIDs), nonsteroidal antiinflammatory drugs (NSAIDs). Marine omega-3 fatty acids[1]
- Frequency of vigorous exercise is associated with an increased risk of developing AF in young men and joggers
- Porphyrias have been associated with autonomic dysfunction and increased risk of AF
- Patients with metabolic syndrome, excessive vitamin D intake, or excessive niacin intake have a higher risk of AF

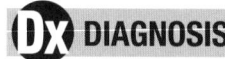 DIAGNOSIS

DIFFERENTIAL DIAGNOSIS

- Multifocal atrial tachycardia
- Atrial flutter
- Frequent atrial premature beats
- Atrial tachycardia
- AV nodal reentry tachycardia (AVNRT)
- Wolff-Parkinson-White syndrome

WORKUP

The evaluation of atrial fibrillation involves diagnosis, determination of the etiology, and classification of the arrhythmia. A minimal evaluation includes a history and physical examination, ECG, transthoracic echocardiogram, and case-specific laboratory work to rule out secondary AF.

LABORATORY TESTS

- Thyroid-stimulating hormone, free T_4
- Serum electrolytes
- Toxicity screen
- CBC count (looking for anemia, infection)
- Renal and hepatic function tests
- D-dimer/CT scan of chest pulmonary embolism protocol (if the patient has risk factors to merit a pulmonary embolism workup)

IMAGING STUDIES

- ECG (Fig. E3)
- Absence of P waves
- Fibrillatory or F waves at the isoelectric baseline with varying amplitude, morphology, and intervals (Fig. 4)
- Irregular ventricular rate
- Echocardiography to rule out structural heart disease (evaluate ventricular size, thickness, and function, atrial size, pericardial disease, and valve function)
- Chest radiography (if pulmonary disease or congestive heart failure [CHF] is suspected)
- Transesophageal echocardiography (TEE): Helpful to evaluate for left atrial thrombus (particularly in the left atrium appendage) to guide cardioversion or ablation (if thrombus is seen, cardioversion should be delayed)

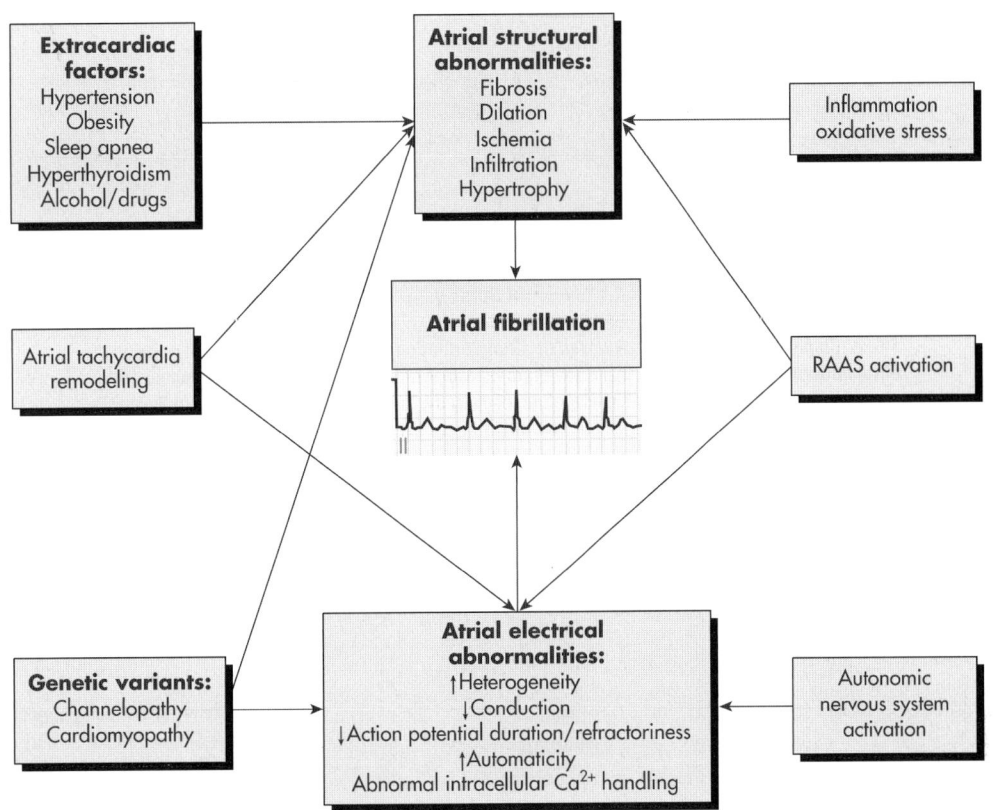

FIG. 1 Mechanisms of atrial fibrillation. Ca^{2+}, Ionized calcium; *RAAS*, renin-angiotensin-aldosterone system. (From Parrillo JE, Dellinger RP: *Critical care medicine, principles of diagnosis and management in the adult,* ed 5, Philadelphia, 2019, Elsevier.)

- CT and MRI: In patients with a positive D-dimer result, chest CT angiogram may be necessary to rule out pulmonary embolus. 3D imaging technologies (CT scan or MRI) are often helpful to evaluate atrial anatomy if AF ablation is planned
- 6-min walk test or exercise test: 6-min walk or exercise testing can help assess the adequacy of rate control. Exercise testing can also exclude ischemia prior to treatment of patients with class Ic antiarrhythmic drugs and can be used to reproduce exercise-induced AF
- Sleep study (if sleep apnea is suspected)
- Holter monitor or event recorder if the diagnosis of AF is in question and to assess AF burden
- Electrophysiologic study: When initiation of AF is secondary to a supraventricular tachycardia, such as AVNRT or Wolff-Parkinson-White syndrome

Rx TREATMENT

ACUTE GENERAL Rx

New-onset AF:

- If the patient is hemodynamically unstable (hypotension, congestive heart failure, or angina), perform synchronized cardioversion after immediate conscious sedation with a rapid short-acting sedative (e.g., midazolam). The ACC/AHA recommendations for cardioversion of atrial fibrillation are summarized in Table 2. The likelihood of cardioversion-related clinical thromboembolism is low in patients with AF lasting <48 h. Patients with AF lasting >2 days have a 5% to 7% risk for clinical thromboembolism if cardioversion

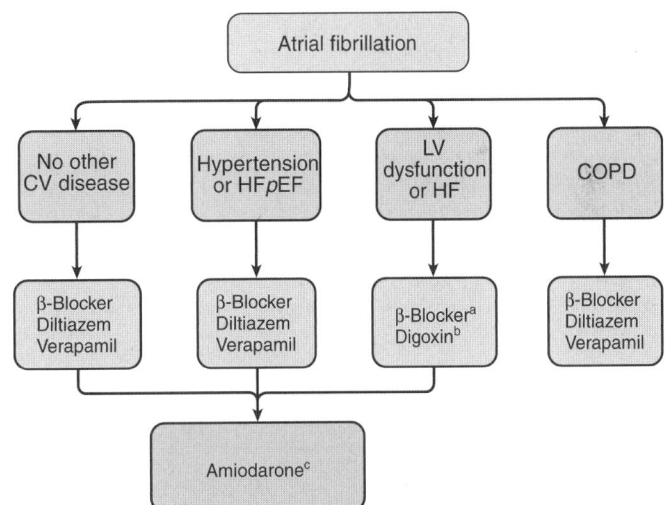

FIG. 2 Approach to selecting drug therapy for ventricular rate control. Drugs are listed alphabetically.
[A]β-Blockers should be instituted after stabilization of patients with decompensated heart failure (HF). The choice of β-blocker (e.g., cardioselective) depends on the patient's clinical condition.
[B]Digoxin is not usually first-line therapy. It may be combined with a β-blocker and/or a nondihydropyridine calcium channel blocker when ventricular rate control is insufficient and may be useful in patients with heart failure.
[C]In part because of concern over its side effect profile, use of amiodarone for chronic control of ventricular rate should be reserved for patients who do not respond to or are intolerant of β-blockers or nondihydropyridine calcium antagonists. *COPD,* Chronic obstructive pulmonary disease; *CV,* cardiovascular; *HF,* heart failure; *HFpEF,* heart failure with preserved ejection fraction; *LV,* left ventricular. (From Parrillo JE, Dellinger RP: *Critical care medicine, principles of diagnosis and management in the adult,* ed 5, Philadelphia, 2019, Elsevier.)

is not preceded by several weeks of anticoagulation therapy. However, if transesophageal echocardiography reveals no atrial thrombus, cardioversion may be performed

safely after therapeutic anticoagulation has been achieved. Alternatively, patients can be safely anticoagulated for approximately 1 mo and then undergo cardioversion without

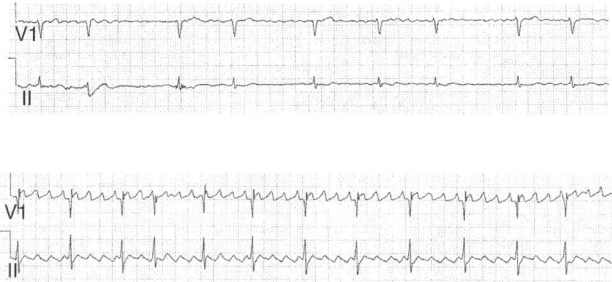

FIG. 4 Comparison between the F waves of atrial fibrillation *(top panel)* **and the flutter waves of atrial flutter** *(bottom panel).* Note that F waves are variable in rate, shape, and amplitude, whereas flutter waves are constant in rate and all aspects of morphology. Shown are leads V1 and II. (From Zipes DP: *Braunwald's heart disease, a textbook of cardiovascular medicine,* ed 11, Philadelphia, 2019, Elsevier.)

transesophageal echocardiogram. Anticoagulant therapy should be continued for at least 1 mo after cardioversion to minimize the incidence of adverse thromboembolic events. It can be stopped after 1 mo as long as AF has not recurred if the patient is deemed low risk of stroke using the congestive heart failure, hypertension, age, diabetes, stroke/TIA, and vascular disease (CHA_2DS_2-VASc) scoring system (see Table 1).

- If the patient is hemodynamically stable, a rate-control strategy is typically pursued initially. ACC/AHA recommendations for pharmacologic rate control of atrial fibrillation are summarized in Table 3.
- Treatment options for rate control include the following:
  1. Diltiazem 0.25 mg/kg (maximum of 25 mg) given intravenously (IV) over 2 min followed by a second dose of 0.35 mg/kg (maximum of 25 mg) 15 min later if the rate is not slowed to <100 beats/min. May then follow with IV infusion 10 mg/hr (range, 5 to 15 mg/hr) to achieve a resting heart rate of <100 beats/min. Onset of action after IV administration is usually within 3 min, with peak effect most often occurring within 10 min. After the ventricular rate is slowed, the patient can be changed to oral diltiazem 60 to 90 mg q4 to 6h. High doses of calcium channel blockers can exacerbate heart failure and thus should be used with caution in patients presenting with symptoms of heart failure or depressed ejection fraction.
  2. Verapamil 2.5 to 5 mg IV initially, then 5 to 10 mg IV 10 min later if the rate is still not slowed to <100 beats/min. After the ventricular rate is slowed, the patient can be changed to oral verapamil 80 to 120 mg q6 to 8h. The main concern is hypotension and heart failure with this medication, and it should not be used in patients with CHF.
  3. Esmolol and metoprolol are beta-blockers available in IV preparations that can be used. High doses of beta-blockers can have negative inotropic effects in heart failure and should be used with caution.
  4. Digoxin is not a potent AV nodal blocking agent and has a potential for toxicity and therefore cannot be relied on for acute control of the ventricular response, but it

TABLE 1 CHA_2DS_2-VASc Score and Associated Increased Annual Risk for Stroke

C	Congestive heart failure	1
H	Hypertension	1
A	Age >75 yr	1
D	Diabetes	1
S	Stroke, TIA	2
V	Vascular disease	1
A	Age 65–74 yr	1
Sc	Sex (female)	1

Total score	Annual risk of stroke
0	0.2%
1	0.6%
2	2.2%
3	3.2%
4	4.8%
5	7.2%
6	9.7%
7	11.2%
8	10.8%
9	12.2%

TIA, Transient ischemic attack.
From Warshaw G et al: *Ham's primary care geriatrics,* ed 7, Philadelphia, 2022, Elsevier.

may be used in conjunction with beta-blockers and calcium channel blockers. It may be a useful adjunct to a beta-blocker in the hypotensive or heart failure patient, which is not infrequent. When used, give 0.5 mg IV loading dose (slow) and then 0.25 mg IV 6 h later. A third dose may be needed after 6 to 8 h; the daily dose varies from 0.125 to 0.25 mg (decrease dosage in patients with renal insufficiency and elderly patients) depending on the heart rate and signs or symptoms of digoxin toxicity. Toxicity is manifested by GI and visual complaints, atrial tachyarrhythmias, heart block, and ventricular tachycardia.
  5. Amiodarone has a class IIa recommendation from the ACC/AHA/ESC for use as a rate-controlling agent for patients who are

intolerant of or unresponsive to other agents, such as patients with heart failure who may otherwise not tolerate diltiazem or metoprolol. Caution should be exercised in those who are not receiving anticoagulation because amiodarone can promote cardioversion, thereby posing a thromboembolic risk.

- AV nodal blocking agents, particularly calcium channel blockers and digoxin, should be avoided in patients with Wolff-Parkinson-White syndrome and AF because, by blocking the AV node, AF impulses may be transmitted exclusively down the accessory pathway, which can result in ventricular fibrillation. If this happens, the patient will require immediate defibrillation. Procainamide, flecainide, or amiodarone can be used instead if Wolff-Parkinson-White syndrome is suspected.
- In the acute setting, pharmacologic cardioversion (e.g., ibutilide, dofetilide) is less commonly used than electrical cardioversion. A major disadvantage with pharmacologic cardioversion is the risk of development of ventricular tachycardia and other serious arrhythmias, especially due to acute prolongation of the QT interval.
- ACC/AHA recommendations for maintenance of sinus rhythm in patients with atrial fibrillation are summarized in Table 4.

CHRONIC THERAPY

- Avoidance of alcohol in patients with suspected excessive alcohol use.
- Treatment of underlying source or cause, if any found.
- Treatment of modifiable risk factors such as obstructive sleep apnea, hypertension, and obesity have been shown to decrease AF burden in patients.
- Per the Atrial Fibrillation Follow-up Investigation of Rhythm Management (AFFIRM) and Rate Control versus Electrical Cardioversion (RACE) trials, either rate control or rhythm control strategies show no difference in composite cardiovascular end points of death, CHF, bleeding, drug side effects, or thromboembolism. However, the more recent Early Treatment of Atrial Fibrillation for Stroke Prevention Trial (EAST-AFNET 4 trial) suggested that an initial rhythm control strategy may result in lower risk

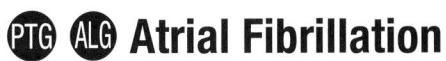

A

I

TABLE 2 ACC/AHA Recommendations for Cardioversion of Atrial Fibrillation

Class	Indication	Level of Evidence
Pharmacologic Cardioversion		
Class I (indicated)	Administration of flecainide, dofetilide, propafenone, or ibutilide is recommended for pharmacologic cardioversion of AF.	A
Class IIa (reasonable)	Administration of amiodarone is a reasonable option for pharmacologic cardioversion of AF.	A
	A single oral bolus dose of propafenone or flecainide ("pill-in-the-pocket") can be administered to terminate persistent AF outside the hospital once treatment has proved safe in the hospital for selected patients without sinus or AV node dysfunction, bundle branch block, QT interval prolongation, the Brugada syndrome, or structural heart disease. Before antiarrhythmic medication is initiated, a beta-blocker or nondihydropyridine calcium channel antagonist should be given to prevent rapid AV conduction in the event atrial flutter occurs.	C
	Administration of amiodarone can be beneficial on an outpatient basis in patients with paroxysmal or persistent AF when rapid restoration of sinus rhythm is not deemed necessary.	C
Class IIb (may be considered)	Administration of quinidine or procainamide might be considered for pharmacologic cardioversion of AF, but the usefulness of these agents is not well established.	C
Class III (not indicated)	Digoxin and sotalol may be harmful when used for pharmacologic cardioversion of AF and are not recommended.	A
	Quinidine, procainamide, disopyramide, and dofetilide should not be started out of the hospital for conversion of AF to sinus rhythm.	B
Direct-Current Cardioversion		
Class I (indicated)	When a rapid ventricular response does not respond promptly to pharmacologic measures for patients with AF with ongoing myocardial ischemia, symptomatic hypotension, angina, or heart failure, immediate R wave–synchronized direct-current cardioversion is recommended.	C
	Immediate direct-current cardioversion is recommended for patients with AF involving preexcitation when very rapid tachycardia or hemodynamic instability occurs.	B
	Cardioversion is recommended in patients without hemodynamic instability when symptoms of AF are unacceptable to the patient. In case of early relapse of AF after cardioversion, repeated direct-current cardioversion attempts may be made after administration of antiarrhythmic medication.	C
Class IIa (reasonable)	Direct-current cardioversion can be useful to restore sinus rhythm as part of a long-term management strategy for patients with AF.	B
	The patient's preference is a reasonable consideration in the selection of infrequently repeated cardioversions for the management of symptomatic or recurrent AF.	C
Class III (not indicated)	Frequent repetition of direct-current cardioversion is not recommended for patients who have relatively short periods of sinus rhythm between relapses of AF after multiple cardioversion procedures despite prophylactic antiarrhythmic drug therapy.	C
	Electrical cardioversion is contraindicated in patients with digitalis toxicity or hypokalemia.	C
Pharmacologic Enhancement of Direct-Current Cardioversion		
Class IIa (reasonable)	Pretreatment with amiodarone, flecainide, ibutilide, propafenone, or sotalol can be useful to enhance the success of direct-current cardioversion and to prevent recurrent AF.	B
	In patients who relapse to AF after successful cardioversion, it can be useful to repeat the procedure after prophylactic administration of antiarrhythmic medication.	C
Class IIb (may be considered)	For patients with persistent AF, administration of beta-blockers, disopyramide, diltiazem, dofetilide, procainamide, or verapamil may be considered, although the efficacy of these agents to enhance the success of direct-current cardioversion or to prevent early recurrence of AF is uncertain.	C
	Out-of-hospital initiation of antiarrhythmic medications may be considered in patients without heart disease to enhance the success of cardioversion of AF.	C
	Out-of-hospital administration of antiarrhythmic medications may be considered to enhance the success of cardioversion of AF in patients with certain forms of heart disease once the safety of the drug has been verified for the patient.	C
Prevention of Thromboembolism in Patients with Atrial Fibrillation Undergoing Cardioversion		
Class I (indicated)	For patients with AF of 48-h duration or longer, or when the duration of AF is unknown, anticoagulation (INR, 2.0-3.0) is recommended for at least 3 wk before and 4 wk after cardioversion, regardless of the method (electrical or pharmacologic) used to restore sinus rhythm.	B
	For patients with AF of more than 48-h duration requiring immediate cardioversion because of hemodynamic instability, heparin should be administered concurrently (unless contraindicated) by an initial intravenous bolus injection, followed by a continuous infusion in a dose adjusted to prolong the activated partial thromboplastin time to 1.5-2× the reference control value. Thereafter, oral anticoagulation (INR, 2.0-3.0) should be provided for at least 4 wk, as for patients undergoing elective cardioversion. Limited data support subcutaneous administration of low-molecular-weight heparin in this indication.	C
	For patients with AF of less than 48-h duration associated with hemodynamic instability (angina pectoris, myocardial infarction, shock, or pulmonary edema), cardioversion should be performed immediately, without delay, for prior initiation of anticoagulation.	C
Class IIa (reasonable)	During the 48 h after onset of AF, the need for anticoagulation before and after cardioversion may be based on the patient's risk of thromboembolism.	C
	As an alternative to anticoagulation before cardioversion of AF, it is reasonable to perform transesophageal echocardiography in search of thrombus in the left atrium or left atrial appendage.	B
	a. For patients with no identifiable thrombus, cardioversion is reasonable immediately after anticoagulation with unfractionated heparin (e.g., initiated by intravenous bolus injection and an infusion continued at a dose adjusted to prolong the activated partial thromboplastin time to 1.5-2× the control value until oral anticoagulation has been established with an oral vitamin K antagonist [e.g., warfarin] as evidenced by an INR ≥2.0).	B

TABLE 2 ACC/AHA Recommendations for Cardioversion of Atrial Fibrillation—cont'd

Class	Indication	Level of Evidence
	Thereafter, continuation of oral anticoagulation (INR, 2.0-3.0) is reasonable for a total anticoagulation period of at least 4 wk, as for patients undergoing elective cardioversion.	B
	Limited data are available to support the subcutaneous administration of a low-molecular-weight heparin in this indication.	C
	b. For patients in whom thrombus is identified by transesophageal echocardiography, oral anticoagulation (INR, 2.0-3.0) is reasonable for at least 3 wk before and 4 wk after restoration of sinus rhythm, and a longer period of anticoagulation may be appropriate even after apparently successful cardioversion because the risk of thromboembolism often remains elevated in such cases.	C
	For patients with atrial flutter undergoing cardioversion, anticoagulation can be beneficial according to the recommendations as for patients with AF.	C

ACC, American College of Cardiology; *AF,* atrial fibrillation; *AHA,* American Heart Association; *AV,* atrioventricular; *INR,* international normalized ratio.
From Zipes DP: *Braunwald's heart disease, a textbook of cardiovascular medicine,* ed 11, Philadelphia, 2019, Elsevier.

TABLE 3 ACC/AHA Recommendations for Pharmacologic Rate Control of Atrial Fibrillation

Class	Indication	Level of Evidence
Class I (indicated)	Measurement of the heart rate at rest and control of the rate with pharmacologic agents (either a beta-blocker or nondihydropyridine calcium channel antagonist, in most cases) are recommended for patients with persistent or permanent AF.	B
	In the absence of preexcitation, intravenous administration of beta-blockers (esmolol, metoprolol, or propranolol) or nondihydropyridine calcium channel antagonists (verapamil, diltiazem) is recommended to slow the ventricular response to AF in the acute setting, exercising caution in patients with hypotension or heart failure.	B
	Intravenous administration of digoxin or amiodarone is recommended to control heart rate in patients with AF and heart failure who do not have an accessory pathway.	B
	In patients who experience symptoms related to AF during activity, the adequacy of heart rate control should be assessed during exercise, adjusting pharmacologic treatment as necessary to keep the rate in the physiologic range.	C
	Digoxin is effective after oral administration to control the heart rate at rest in patients with AF and is indicated for patients with heart failure or left ventricular dysfunction and for sedentary individuals.	C
Class IIa (reasonable)	A combination of digoxin and either a beta-blocker or nondihydropyridine calcium channel antagonist is reasonable to control the heart rate both at rest and during exercise in patients with AF. The choice of medication should be individualized and the dose modulated to avoid bradycardia.	B
	It is reasonable to use ablation of the AV node or accessory pathway to control heart rate when pharmacologic therapy is insufficient or associated with side effects.	B
	Intravenous amiodarone can be useful to control heart rate in patients with AF when other measures are unsuccessful or contraindicated.	C
	When electrical cardioversion is not necessary in patients with AF and an accessory pathway, intravenous procainamide or ibutilide is a reasonable alternative.	C
Class IIb (may be considered)	When the ventricular rate cannot be adequately controlled both at rest and during exercise in patients with AF by a beta-blocker, nondihydropyridine calcium channel antagonist, or digoxin, alone or in combination, oral amiodarone may be administered to control the heart rate.	C
	Intravenous procainamide, disopyramide, ibutilide, or amiodarone may be considered for hemodynamically stable patients with AF involving conduction over an accessory pathway.	B
	When the rate cannot be controlled with pharmacologic agents or tachycardia-mediated cardiomyopathy is suspected, catheter-directed ablation of the AV node may be considered in patients with AF to control the heart rate.	C
Class III (not indicated)	Strict rate control (<80 beats/min at rest or <110 beats/min during 6-min walk) is not beneficial compared to a resting rate <110 beats/min in asymptomatic patients with persistent AF and an ejection fraction >40%, although uncontrolled tachycardia can lead to reversible left ventricular dysfunction over time.	B
	Digitalis should not be used as the sole agent to control the rate of ventricular response in patients with paroxysmal AF.	B
	Catheter ablation of the AV node should not be attempted without a prior trial of medication to control the ventricular rate in patients with AF.	C
	In patients with decompensated heart failure and AF, intravenous administration of a nondihydropyridine calcium channel antagonist may exacerbate hemodynamic compromise and is not recommended.	C
	Intravenous administration of digitalis glycosides or nondihydropyridine calcium channel antagonists to patients with AF and a preexcitation syndrome may paradoxically accelerate the ventricular response and is not recommended.	C

ACC, American College of Cardiology; *AF,* atrial fibrillation; *AHA,* American Heart Association; *AV,* atrioventricular.
From Zipes DP: *Braunwald's heart disease, a textbook of cardiovascular medicine,* ed 11, Philadelphia, 2019, Elsevier.

TABLE 4 ACC/AHA Recommendations for Maintenance of Sinus Rhythm in Patients with Atrial Fibrillation

Class	Indication	Level of Evidence
Class I (indicated)	Before initiation of antiarrhythmic drug therapy, treatment of precipitating or reversible causes of AF is recommended.	C
	Catheter ablation by an experienced operator is useful in selected patients with symptomatic paroxysmal AF who have failed treatment with an antiarrhythmic drug and have a normal or mildly dilated left atrium and normal or mildly reduced left ventricular function.	A
Class IIa (reasonable)	Pharmacologic therapy can be useful in patients with AF to maintain sinus rhythm and to prevent tachycardia-induced cardiomyopathy.	C
	Infrequent, well-tolerated recurrence of AF is reasonable as a successful outcome of antiarrhythmic drug therapy.	C
	Outpatient initiation of antiarrhythmic drug therapy is reasonable in patients with AF who have no associated heart disease when the agent is well tolerated.	C
	In patients with lone AF without structural heart disease, initiation of propafenone or flecainide can be beneficial on an outpatient basis in patients with paroxysmal AF who are in sinus rhythm at the time of drug initiation.	B
	Sotalol can be beneficial in outpatients in sinus rhythm with little or no heart disease, prone to paroxysmal AF, if the baseline uncorrected QT interval is shorter than 460 milliseconds, serum electrolyte values are normal, and risk factors associated with class III drug–related proarrhythmia are not present.	C
	Catheter ablation is a reasonable treatment of symptomatic persistent AF.	A
Class IIb (may be considered)	Catheter ablation may be reasonable for patients with symptomatic paroxysmal AF and significant left atrial dilation or significant left ventricular dysfunction.	A
Class III (not indicated)	Antiarrhythmic therapy with a particular drug is not recommended for maintenance of sinus rhythm in patients with AF who have well-defined risk factors for proarrhythmia with that agent.	A
	Pharmacologic therapy is not recommended for maintenance of sinus rhythm in patients with advanced sinus node disease or AV node dysfunction unless they have a functioning electronic cardiac pacemaker.	C

ACC, American College of Cardiology; *AF,* atrial fibrillation; *AHA,* American Heart Association.
From Zipes DP: *Braunwald's heart disease, a textbook of cardiovascular medicine,* ed 11, Philadelphia, 2019, Elsevier.

of the combined cardiovascular endpoint of death, stroke, or hospitalization. Both approaches require appropriate anticoagulation to reduce stroke risk.

- For patients without symptomatic AF, a rate-control strategy with calcium channel blockers, beta-blockers, or digoxin may be a reasonable option. The RACE 2 trial indicates that a lenient rate control strategy, with a target resting heart rate of <110 beats/min, is noninferior to a strict control strategy, with a target resting heart rate of <80 beats/min and an exercise heart rate of <110 beats/min. Most recent ACC/AHA guidelines, however, recommend targeting a heart rate <80 beats/min over a target of <110 beats/min.
- In patients with symptomatic AF, younger patients, or those with difficult to control heart rate, an attempt should be made to maintain sinus rhythm with antiarrhythmic agents. Options of antiarrhythmic agents include amiodarone, dronedarone (paroxysmal atrial fibrillation only without heart failure), dofetilide, flecainide, propafenone (contraindicated with structural heart disease), or sotalol. The decision of which strategy to follow should be best made in consultation with a cardiologist. Use of dronedarone should be avoided in patients with persistent or permanent atrial fibrillation because of worsened cardiovascular outcomes, especially in those with concomitant symptomatic heart failure (see Fig. 5 for a proposed algorithm to guide maintenance of sinus rhythm).

NONPHARMACOLOGIC THERAPY
- Catheter ablation of AF has become a common procedure for symptomatic drug-refractory or drug-intolerant patients. Sinus rhythm can be maintained long term in the majority of patients with paroxysmal atrial fibrillation (PAF) by circumferential pulmonary vein ablation performed in experienced centers. Established centers have reported success rates of 70% to 85% in patients with paroxysmal AF, but up to 50% of patients may require more than one ablation to achieve success. Complication rates are 4.5% in the largest international survey of hospitals performing this procedure. Success with persistent AF is much lower, with long-term success rates of 40% to 50% in many studies, and such patients often require more than one procedure. The most common techniques used to isolate the pulmonary veins are radiofrequency ablation and cryoballoon ablation, which have shown similar results for patients with PAF.
- Pulmonary vein isolation is being increasingly used to treat AF in patients with heart failure. Trials have shown that pulmonary vein isolation is superior to AV node ablation with biventricular pacing in patients with heart failure who have drug-refractory AF.
- AV nodal ablation with permanent pacemaker implantation may become necessary in some patients in whom rate and rhythm are difficult to control despite drugs and cardioversion, although it is generally used as a therapy of last resort.
- The Cox-Maze III surgical procedure, with its modifications creating electrical barriers to the macroreentrant circuits that are believed to underlie AF, is being performed with good results in some medical centers (preservation of sinus rhythm in 70% to 95% of patients without the use of long-term antiarrhythmic medication). Success rates are higher in paroxysmal than in persistent or permanent atrial fibrillation. Surgical ablation is often used for patients undergoing aortic or mitral valve surgery. As a stand-alone procedure, it is a Class IIb. Some centers perform surgical pulmonary vein isolation similar to this procedure using a mini-thoracotomy or video thoracoscopic "Mini-Maze" approach. Another surgical method is a pericardioscopic approach that allows extensive posterior wall ablation and, when combined with catheter ablation in a "hybrid" approach, has shown promising results for patients with persistent AF.
- It is important to understand that ablation therapy will not eliminate the need to take anticoagulant drugs. Even after ablation, patients with AF face increased risk of thromboembolic events and most electrophysiologists suggest lifelong anticoagulation for patients with elevated stroke risk score. Due to the increasing success rate of ablation, catheter-based therapy is considered the first-line treatment for paroxysmal AF patients intolerant or refractory to one medication or IIa for persistent patients.[2] It remains a IIb indication for patients in long-standing persistent atrial fibrillation.

STROKE PREVENTION
- The decision whether to pursue long-term anticoagulation must be made in light of the patient's risk for a cardioembolic event versus risk for a bleeding event. ACC/AHA recommendations for prevention of thromboembolism in atrial fibrillation are summarized in Table 5. In nonvalvular AF, CHA_2DS_2-VASc has superseded the $CHADS_2$

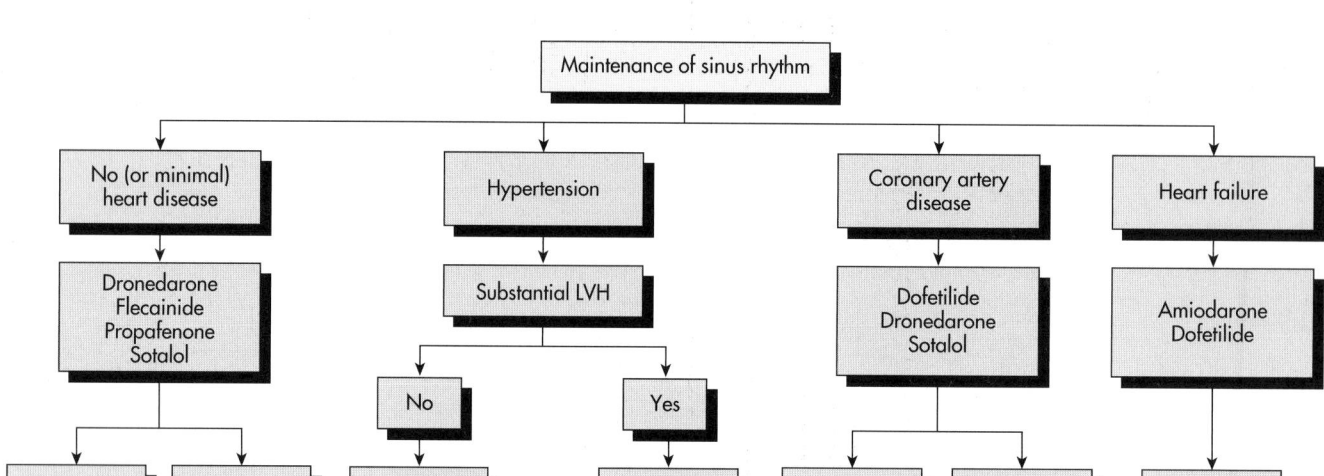

FIG. 5 Therapy to maintain sinus rhythm in patients with recurrent paroxysmal or persistent atrial fibrillation. Drugs are listed alphabetically and not in order of suggested use. The seriousness of heart disease progresses from left to right, and selection of therapy in patients with multiple conditions depends on the most serious condition present. *LVH,* Left ventricular hypertrophy. (From Wann LS et al: 2011 ACCF/AHA/HRS Focused update on the management of patients with atrial fibrillation [updating the 2006 guideline]: a report of the American College of Cardiology Foundation/American Heart Association Task Force on Practice Guidelines, *J Am Coll Cardiol* 57[2]:223-242, 2011.)

scoring system (C = congestive heart failure; H = hypertension; A = age [>75 yr is 2 points]; D = diabetes; S = stroke, transient ischemic attack, or thromboembolic disease [2 points]; V = vascular disease, A = age 65 to 74 yr; and Sc = sex category, with females getting 1 extra point). Patients with a CHA_2DS_2-VASc score of 0 are considered low risk, 1 to 2 are considered moderate risk, and >2 are considered high risk. Per guidelines, patients with a score of 0 do not merit anticoagulation. Patients with a score of 1 can be treated at the discretion of the physician with either aspirin or an oral anticoagulant (warfarin or a novel oral anticoagulant). Anticoagulation with either warfarin or a novel oral anticoagulant is recommended for all men with a $CHADS_2$-VASc score of 2 or above and women with a $CHADS_2$-VASc score of 3 or above. The available direct-acting oral anticoagulants (DOACs) are recommended over warfarin in DOAC-eligible patients with atrial fibrillation.[3]

- Increasing amounts of evidence now show that aspirin likely does not protect a person from stroke in AF and has recently been dropped from most of the ACC/AHA and European Atrial Fibrillation guidelines. Target INR for patients on warfarin with an indication for anticoagulation is 2 to 3 and should be diligently monitored to avoid risk of stroke versus bleeding. Patients with hypertrophic

cardiomyopathy or thyrotoxicosis with AF also have a high risk of stroke and should be anticoagulated irrespective of their $CHADS_2$-VASc score.

- The DOACs include several factor Xa inhibitors (Table 6) and a direct thrombin inhibitor.
  1. Factor Xa inhibitors (apixaban, rivaroxaban, edoxaban) are also effective in reducing stroke and systemic embolism in patients with atrial fibrillation. The Apixaban for Reduction in Stroke and Other Thromboembolic Events in Atrial Fibrillation (ARISTOTLE) trial in patients at high risk for stroke (mean $CHADS_2$ score 2.1) using apixaban, the Rivaroxaban Once Daily Oral Direct Factor Xa Inhibition Compared with Vitamin K Antagonism for Prevention of Stroke and Embolism Trial in Atrial Fibrillation (ROCKET AF) trial using rivaroxaban in patients with $CHADS_2$ score 3.5, and the Effective Anticoagulation with Factor Xa Next Generation in Atrial Fibrillation (ENGAGE-AF) trial using edoxaban in patients with a $CHADS_2$ score of at least 2, showed that these anticoagulants reduce the risk of stroke, systemic embolism, and serious bleeding compared with warfarin. Rivaroxaban showed noninferior efficacy to warfarin in prevention of thromboembolism. Apixaban showed superior stroke reduction, reduced bleeding events, and an overall mortality benefit when compared

with warfarin. Edoxaban showed noninferiority to warfarin with respect to stroke and systemic embolism prevention, with lower rates of bleeding and death from cardiovascular causes, but benefit was limited to patients with moderately impaired renal function. Rivaroxaban and edoxaban are dosed once a day, and apixaban is dosed twice a day. A factor Xa reversal agent, andexanet alfa, has received FDA approval as a reversal for the anticoagulant effect of these agents.
  2. Dabigatran is a direct thrombin inhibitor indicated to reduce the risk of stroke and systemic embolism in patients with nonvalvular atrial fibrillation. In the RE-LY trial of 18,113 patients with mean $CHADS_2$ score of 2.1, dabigatran 110 mg bid was noninferior to warfarin, and 150 mg bid was superior to warfarin in prevention of thromboembolic events. Bleeding risk was similar to that of warfarin for both doses. Idarucizumab has been approved as a dabigatran reversal agent. Onset is immediate, and it provides full reversal for at least 24 h in most patients.

- The decision to anticoagulate should be made irrespective of whether the atrial fibrillation is paroxysmal, persistent, or permanent.
- For patients in whom anticoagulation with warfarin or other anticoagulants is contraindicated due to high bleeding risk (Table 7),

F

BASIC INFORMATION

DEFINITION
Food poisoning is an illness caused by ingestion of food contaminated by bacteria and/or bacterial toxins. A foodborne disease outbreak is defined as two or more cases of a similar illness resulting from ingestion of a common food.

SYNONYMS
Enterotoxln-poisoning
Epidemic vomiting disease

ICD-10CM CODE
A05.9 Bacterial foodborne intoxication, unspecified

EPIDEMIOLOGY & DEMOGRAPHICS
INCIDENCE (IN U.S.):
- CDC estimates that each yr one in six Americans will experience a foodborne illness.
- Approximately 800 foodborne disease outbreaks are reported in the U.S. each year, accounting for approximately 15,000 illnesses, 800 hospitalizations, and 20 deaths. Outbreak-associated foodborne illnesses are only a small subset of the estimated 9.4 million foodborne illnesses that occur annually in the U.S.
- Majority of identifiable causes are bacterial, although more than 250 known diseases can be transmitted through food.

PREDOMINANT AGE: Varies with specific agent.
PEAK INCIDENCE: Varies with specific organism
- Summer: *Staphylococcus aureus, Salmonella, Shigella* spp.
- Summer and fall: *Clostridium botulinum, Vibrio parahaemolyticus.*
- Spring and fall: *Campylobacter jejuni.*
- Winter: *Clostridium perfringens, Yersinia enterocolitica.*

NEONATAL INFECTION: Rare but severe with *Shigella* and *Salmonella* spp.

PHYSICAL FINDINGS & CLINICAL PRESENTATION
- Any combination of GI symptoms and fever. Orthostatic pulse and blood pressure changes should be noted
- Specific organisms suspected on the basis of the incubation period and predominant symptoms (Table 1), although a great deal of overlap exists
  1. Short incubation period (1-6 h): Involve the ingestion of preformed toxin; noninvasive.
     a. *S. aureus:* Nausea, profuse vomiting, and abdominal cramps common; diarrhea possible, but fever uncommon; usually resolves within 24 h; foods implicated in outbreaks include meats, mayonnaise, and cream pastries.
     b. *B. cereus:* Two forms, a short incubation (emetic) form (characterized by vomiting and abdominal cramps in virtually all patients, diarrhea in one third of patients, fever uncommon) and a long incubation (diarrheal) form; illness usually mild, resolves within 12 h; unrefrigerated rice most often implicated as vehicle. Other sources include gravy, meats, stews, vanilla, and sauces.
  2. Moderate incubation period (8-16 h): Involves the in vivo production of toxin; noninvasive.
     a. *C. perfringens:* Severe crampy abdominal pain and watery diarrhea common; fever and vomiting unlikely; symptoms usually resolving within 24 h; outbreaks invariably related to cooked meat or poultry that is allowed to cool without refrigeration; most cases in the fall and winter months. *C. perfringens* is the third most common cause of foodborne illness in the United States.
     b. *B. cereus:* Diarrheal (or long incubation) form most commonly beginning with diarrhea, abdominal cramps, and occasionally vomiting; fever uncommon; usually resolves within 24 h; the responsible food is usually fried rice.
  3. Long incubation period (>16 h): Some toxin-mediated, some invasive.
- Toxin-producing organisms include
  1. *C. botulinum:* Should be considered when a diarrheal illness coincides with or precedes paralysis; severity of illness related to the quantity of toxin ingested; characteristic cranial nerve palsies progressing to a descending paralysis; fever usually absent; usually associated with home-canned foods.
  2. Enterotoxigenic *E. coli* (ETEC): Most common cause of travelers' diarrhea; after 1- to 2-day incubation period, abdominal cramps and copious diarrhea occur; vomiting and fever uncommon; usually resolves after 3 to 4 days; vehicle usually unbottled water or contaminated salad or ice.
  3. Enterohemorrhagic *E. coli* (EHEC): Can cause severe abdominal cramps and watery diarrhea, which may eventually become bloody; bacteria (strain O157:H7) are noninvasive; no fever; illness may be complicated by hemolytic-uremic syndrome; associated with contaminated beef (especially hamburger), unpasteurized milk or juice. Table 2 summarizes the various strains of diarrheagenic *E. coli.*
  4. *V. cholerae:* Varies from a mild, self-limited illness to life-threatening cholera; diarrhea, nausea and vomiting, abdominal cramps, and muscle cramps; no fever; severe cases may progress to shock and death within hours of onset; survivors usually have resolution of symptoms in 1 wk; U.S. cases are either imported or result from ingestion of imported food.
- Invasive organisms include
  1. *Salmonella:* Associated most often with nontyphoidal strains; incubation period generally 12 to 48 h; nausea, vomiting, diarrhea, and abdominal cramps typical; fever possible; outbreaks of gastroenteritis related to contaminated poultry, meat, and dairy products.
  2. *Shigella:* Asymptomatic infection possible, but some with fever and watery diarrhea that may progress to bloody diarrhea and dysentery; with mild illness, usually self-limited, resolves in a few days; with severe illness, may develop complications; transmission usually from person to person but can occur via contaminated food or water.
  3. *C. jejuni:* The most common foodborne bacterial pathogen; incubation period is about 1 day, then a prodrome of fever, headache, and myalgias; intestinal phase marked by diarrhea associated with fever, malaise, and abdominal pain; diarrhea mild to profuse and bloody; usually resolves in about 7 days, but relapse is possible; associated with undercooked meats and poultry, unpasteurized dairy products, and drinking from freshwater streams.
  4. *Y. enterocolitica* and *Y. pseudotuberculosis:* Infrequent causes of enteritis in the United States; children affected more often than adults; fever, diarrhea, and abdominal pain lasting 1 to 3 wk; some with mesenteric adenitis that mimics acute appendicitis; contaminated food or water is usually responsible.
  5. *V. parahaemolyticus:* In the United States, most outbreaks in coastal states or on cruise ships during the summer months; incubation period usually >1 day, followed by explosive watery diarrhea in the majority of cases; nausea, vomiting, abdominal cramps, and headache also common; fever less common; usually resolves by 1 wk; related to ingestion of seafood.
  6. Enteroinvasive *E. coli* (EIEC): A rare cause of disease in the United States; high incidence of fever and bloody diarrhea; may resemble bacillary dysentery.
  7. *V. vulnificus:* May cause serious, often fatal illness in persons with chronic liver disease; GI symptoms usually absent, but fever, chills, hypotension, and hemorrhagic skin lesions possible; patients with liver disease or at increased risk of developing liver disease should avoid eating raw oysters.

ETIOLOGY
- Table 3 describes pathogenic mechanisms in bacterial foodborne disease.
- Classically categorized as either inflammatory (invasive) or noninflammatory.
  1. Noninflammatory: *B. cereus, S. aureus, C. botulinum, C. perfringens, V. cholerae,* enterotoxigenic *E. coli* (ETEC), and enterohemorrhagic *E. coli* (EHEC); toxin-producing organisms that are noninvasive; fecal leukocytes are not seen.
  2. Inflammatory: *Campylobacter,* enteroinvasive *E. coli* (EIEC), *Salmonella, Shigella, V. parahaemolyticus,* and *Yersinia;* cause disease by invasion of intestinal tissue; fecal leukocytes are seen.

TABLE 1 Foodborne Disease Agents and Clinical Presentation

Usual Incubation Periods	Causative Agent	CLINICAL ILLNESS			Epidemiologic and Laboratory Diagnosis
		Fever	Diarrhea	Vomiting	
5 min-6 h (usually <3 h)	Chemical or toxin	Rare	Occasional	Common	Demonstration of toxin or chemical from food or epidemiologic incrimination of food
1-6 h (usually <1 h)	*Staphylococcus aureus* enterotoxin	Rare	Occasional	Profuse	Isolation of organisms in food (>10^5/g)/ vomitus/stool; detection of enterotoxin in food
	Bacillus cereus emetic toxin	Rare	Occasional	Profuse	Isolation of organisms in food (>10^5/g)/ vomitus/stool
6-24 h	*Clostridium perfringens* enterotoxin	Rare	Typical	Occasional	Isolation of organisms or toxin from food (10^5/g) or stools of ill persons, epidemiologic incrimination of food; detection of enterotoxin in food
	B. cereus enterotoxin	Rare	Typical	Occasional	
12-72 h	*Clostridium botulinum*	Clinical syndrome compatible with botulism	Constipation more common		Isolation of organism or toxin from food (10^5/g) or stools; demonstration of toxin in serum or food
16-96 h	*Shigella*	Common	Typical, often bloody	Occasional	Isolation of organism from clinical specimens from two or more ill persons; isolation of organism from epidemiologically implicated food
	Nontyphoidal *Salmonella*	Common	Typical	Occasional	
	Enteroinvasive *E. coli* (EIEC)	Common	Typical, may be bloody	Occasional	
	Enteropathogenic *E. coli* (EPEC)	Occasional	Typical	Occasional	
	Enterotoxigenic *E. coli* (ETEC)	Rare	Typical	Rare	
	Vibrio parahaemolyticus; V. cholerae enterotoxin	Occasional	Typical	Occasional	
1-3 days	Caliciviruses (noroviruses) Rotavirus	Occasional	Typical	Common	Antigen detection (enzyme immunoassay) in stool; immune electron microscopy of stool; detection of viral RNA in stool or vomitus by PCR
1-10 days	*Yersinia*	Uncommon	Typical, severe abdominal pain	Uncommon	Isolation of organisms from food or clinical specimens of ill persons
2-10 days	*Campylobacter jejuni*	Common	Typical, often bloody	Uncommon	Isolation of organisms from food or clinical specimens of ill persons
1-11 days	*Cryptosporidium*	Occasional	Common	Occasional	Demonstration of oocysts in stool or in small bowel biopsy of ill persons; demonstration of organism in epidemiologically implicated food
	Cyclospora	Occasional	Common	Occasional	Demonstration of parasite in stool or in small bowel biopsy of ill persons; demonstration of organism in epidemiologically implicated food
	Giardia intestinalis	Occasional	Common	Occasional	Demonstration of parasite in stool or in small bowel biopsy of ill persons; demonstration of organism in epidemiologically implicated food
2 days-wk	*Bacillus anthracis*	Common	Typical	Frequent	Isolation of organism from blood or contaminated meat
1-7 days	*E. coli* O157:H7 and other Shiga toxin–producing *E. coli*	Uncommon	Typical	Frequent	Isolation of organism from food or stool or identification of toxin in stools of ill persons
3-60 days, usually 7-14	*Salmonella typhi*	Common	Diarrhea or constipation	Uncommon	Isolation of organisms from food or clinical specimens of ill persons
7-21 days	*Brucella* spp.	Common	Common	Rare	Isolation of organisms from blood or bone marrow culture of ill persons; fourfold increase in standard agglutination titer overall several weeks or single titer 1:160 in person with compatible clinical syndrome
1-4 wk	*Giardia lamblia*	Rare	Common	Rare	Stool for ova and parasite examination enzyme immunoassay
2 days-8 wk	*Trichinella spiralis*	Common	Common	Common	Serology, muscle biopsy

PCR, Polymerase chain reaction; *RNA,* ribonucleic acid.
From Cherry JD et al: *Feigin and Cherry's pediatric infectious diseases,* ed 8, Philadelphia, 2019, Elsevier.

Diseases
and Disorders

I

TABLE 2 Diarrheagenic *Escherichia coli*

Strains	Pathogenic Mechanisms	Persons Affected	Clinical Features
DAEC	Diffuse adherence to Hep-2 cells	Children in developing countries	Watery diarrhea (acute) and persistent diarrhea
EAEC	Aggregative adherence to Hep-2 cells	Children in developing countries	Watery diarrhea (acute) and persistent diarrhea
STEC O157:H7 Non-O157:H7 O104:H4*	Shiga toxins 1 and 2	Children and adults Persons who ingest contaminated food, especially hamburger (outbreaks)	Watery diarrhea Bloody diarrhea (classic)
EIEC	Epithelial cell invasion	Children and adults	Watery diarrhea Dysentery
EPEC Typical Atypical	Attaching and effacing Bundle-forming pilus, attachment and effacement lesions or atypical adherence pattern	Children	Watery diarrhea (acute) Persistent diarrhea
ETEC	Heat-labile and/or heat-stable toxin Adherence	Children in developing countries; travelers	Watery diarrhea

DAEC, Diffusely adhering *Escherichia coli; EAEC,* enteroaggregative *E. coli; EIEC,* enteroinvasive *E. coli; EPEC,* enteropathogenic *E. coli; ETEC,* enterotoxigenic *E. coli; STEC,* Shiga toxin–producing *E. coli.*
From Feldman M et al: *Sleisenger and Fordtran's gastrointestinal and liver disease,* ed 10, Philadelphia, 2016, Elsevier.

TABLE 3 Pathogenic Mechanisms in Bacterial Foodborne Disease

Preformed Toxin	Toxin Production in Vivo	Tissue Invasion	Toxin Production and/or Tissue Invasion
Staphylococcus aureus *Bacillus cereus* (short incubation) *Clostridium botulinum*	*Clostridium perfringens* *B. cereus* (long incubation) *C. botulinum* (infant botulism) Enterotoxigenic *Escherichia coli* *Vibrio cholerae* O1 or O139 *V. cholerae* non-O1 Shiga toxin–producing *E. coli*	*Campylobacter jejuni* *Salmonella* *Shigella* Invasive *E. coli*	*Vibrio parahaemolyticus* *Yersinia enterocolitica*

From Mandell GL et al: *Principles and practice of infectious diseases,* ed 6, Philadelphia, 2005, Churchill Livingstone.

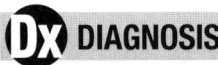

DIAGNOSIS

DIFFERENTIAL DIAGNOSIS

Gastroenteritis caused by viruses (Norwalk, Noro, or rotavirus), parasites *(Amoeba histolytica, Giardia lamblia),* or toxins (ciguatoxins, mushrooms, heavy metals)

LABORATORY TESTS

- Watchful waiting is often the most appropriate option, and ancillary testing is usually not necessary.
- In severe or persistent cases, stool test for fecal leukocytes may help narrow the differential diagnosis.
  1. Send stool for culture and for ova and parasites.
  2. Send stool for *C. difficile* toxin in patients with current or recent antibiotic use.
  3. Note: Some pathogens are not identified on routine stool culture; laboratory should be advised if *Yersinia, C. botulinum, Vibrio,* or enterohemorrhagic *E. coli* (O157:H7) are suspected.
  4. Finding *B. cereus, C. perfringens,* or *E. coli* in stool is of little value, because these may be part of the normal bowel flora.
  5. Stool cultures are positive in less than 40% of cases.
  6. Newer techniques such as polymerase chain reaction (PCR) testing provide a more rapid and reliable determination of specific pathogens.
- If botulism suspected, send food, serum, and stool for toxin assay.
- Blood cultures should be considered for all febrile patients.
- Consider toxic megacolon (identified on plain abdominal sonography).
- Consider sigmoidoscopy to obtain tissue and histology in hospitalized patients with bloody diarrhea.
- Consider lactoferrin measurement if an inflammatory etiology is suspected.

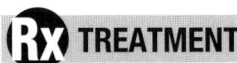

TREATMENT

NONPHARMACOLOGIC THERAPY

Adequate rehydration is the mainstay of therapy.

ACUTE GENERAL Rx

- Most cases of acute infectious diarrhea are viral and antibiotics are not indicated.
- Gastroenteritis caused by the following bacterial organisms requires no antimicrobial treatment: *B. cereus, S. aureus, C. perfringens, V. parahaemolyticus, Yersinia,* and enterohemorrhagic and enteroinvasive *E. coli.*
- The usual cause of travelers' diarrhea is enterotoxigenic *E. coli.* Although usually a self-limited illness, antibiotics can shorten the course in patients with fever or dysentery.
  1. Azithromycin 1000 mg in a single oral dose or
  2. SMX/TMP one DS tab bid for 3 days or
  3. Ciprofloxacin 500 mg PO bid for 3 days
- The mainstay of therapy for cholera is fluid replacement. Antibiotics should be given to decrease shedding and duration of illness.
  1. Doxycycline 300 mg in a single dose or 100 mg PO bid for 3 days
  2. SMX/TMP 1 DS tab bid for 3 days
- Treatment is not indicated for *Salmonella* gastroenteritis. Patients who are at high risk of developing bacteremia may be treated for 48 to 72 h (see "Salmonellosis").
- Although shigellosis tends to be a self-limited illness, antibiotics shorten the course of illness and may limit transmission of the illness (see "Shigellosis").
- Those with moderate or severe *Campylobacter* diarrhea may benefit from treatment.
  1. Azithromycin 500 mg qd for 3 days or
  2. Erythromycin 500 mg PO for 5 days or
  3. Ciprofloxacin 500 mg PO bid for 5 days
- *V. vulnificus* sepsis should be treated with
  1. Doxycycline 100 mg IV bid for 2 wk
  2. Ceftazidime 2 g IV q8h for 2 wk
- For suspected botulism, antitoxin should be administered early (see "Botulism").
- Table 4 summarizes antibiotic therapy for nonsevere infections with common bacterial enteropathogens in immunocompetent adults.

TABLE 4 Antibiotic Therapy for Nonsevere Infections With Common Bacterial Enteropathogens in Immunocompetent Adults

Organism	Recommended Antibiotic(s)	Alternative Antibiotic(s)
***Shigella* Species**		
Shigella infection (non-*dysenteriae;* for *Shigella dysenteriae* type 1, see text)	Ciprofloxacin 500 mg twice daily (or levofloxacin 500 mg daily) × 3 days	Azithromycin 500 mg-1 g daily × 3-5 days TMP/SMX 160 mg/800 mg twice daily, if sensitive, × 3 days
***Salmonella* Species**		
Enterocolitis, uncomplicated	Not usually recommended (see text)	Can consider in areas of high fluoroquinolone quinolone resistance; azithromycin 1 g daily × 5 days
Typhoid and enteric fevers*	Ciprofloxacin 500 mg twice daily (or ofloxacin 400 mg twice daily) × 7-14 days Ceftriaxone 2-3 g IV daily × 7-14 days	
***Campylobacter* Species**		
Campylobacter jejuni	Not usually required Ciprofloxacin 500 mg twice daily × 3 days	Azithromycin 500 mg-1 g × 3-5 days
Yersinia enterocolitica		
Enterocolitis, uncomplicated	Not usually required	An aminoglycoside (parenteral) tetracycline 500 mg 4 times daily × 5 days TMP/SMX 160 mg/800 mg twice daily × 5 days Ciprofloxacin 500 mg twice daily × 5 days Doxycycline 100 mg twice daily × 5 days
Escherichia coli†		
Enterotoxigenic	Endemic disease; usually self-limited, supportive care (see text). Travelers' diarrhea: Ciprofloxacin 500 mg twice daily × 3 days Rifaximin 200 mg 3 times daily × 3 days	Azithromycin 500 mg-1 g daily × 3-5 days TMP/SMX 160 mg/800 mg twice daily, if sensitive, × 3 days
Shiga toxin–producing	Unclear if antibiotics are effective; may be harmful	
***Vibrio* Species**		
Vibrio cholerae	Doxycycline 300 mg × 1 dose	Ciprofloxacin 1 g × 1 dose Azithromycin 1 g × 1 dose Tetracycline 500 mg every 6 h × 3 days
Vibrio parahaemolyticus	Usually not required; no controlled trials	As for *V. cholerae*

*For severe typhoid fever, consider the addition of glucocorticoids (dexamethasone 3 mg/kg × 1, then 1 mg/kg every 6 h × 48 h) to parenteral antimicrobial therapy. Antimicrobial sensitivity testing is required. Fluoroquinolones (e.g., ciprofloxacin) should not be used as empiric therapy in Asia or other areas with high fluoroquinolone resistance.
†Enteropathogenic, enteroaggregative, and diffusely enteroadherent *E. coli* are omitted from this table because these types are defined in research laboratories and are not diagnosed in routine clinical practice. Enteroinvasive *E. coli* presenting as inflammatory diarrhea should be treated empirically as for *Shigella* spp.
TMP/SMX, Trimethoprim/sulfamethoxazole. Note: All antibiotics are administered orally unless otherwise indicated. Recommendations are given for treatment of mild/moderate infections only. Treatments for complicated infections or severely ill, bacteremic, or immunocompromised patients are not listed above and may differ from treatments for mild disease.
From Feldman M et al: *Sleisenger and Fordtran's gastrointestinal and liver disease*, ed 10, Philadelphia, 2016, Elsevier.

CHRONIC Rx
Patients with *Salmonella* infections may become carriers and may require treatment (see "Salmonellosis").

DISPOSITION
- Most infections are self-limited and do not require therapy.
- In immunocompromised host or patient with underlying disease, serious complications are possible.
- Postinfectious syndromes are important with some infections.
  1. Reiter syndrome: *Salmonella, Shigella, Campylobacter, Yersinia* spp.; more common in genetically susceptible host (HLA-B27+)

2. Guillain-Barré syndrome: *Campylobacter* spp.

REFERRAL
If more than a mild illness

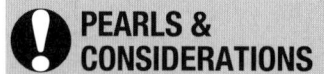 **PEARLS & CONSIDERATIONS**

COMMENTS
- Grossly underreported and undiagnosed
- All cases to be reported to the local health department
- Table E5 summarizes control and prevention measures of foodborne diseases

RELATED CONTENT
Bacterial Food Poisoning (Patient Information)
Salmonellosis (Related Key Topic)
Botulism (Related Key Topic)
Shigellosis (Related Key Topic)

SUGGESTED READINGS
Available at eBooks.Health.Elsevier.com

AUTHOR: **GLENN G. FORT, MD, MPH**

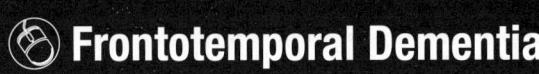
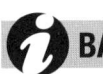 **BASIC INFORMATION**

DEFINITION

Frontotemporal dementia (FTD) is an umbrella term that encompasses three distinct syndromes: Behavioral variant FTD (bvFTD), semantic dementia (SD), and progressive nonfluent aphasia (PNFA). All three syndromes are marked by frontal and/or temporal lobe atrophy; however, they manifest with different clinical presentations. The most common subtype is bvFTD, which is marked by changes in behavior and personality with disinhibition, lack of empathy, and the breaking of social norms. SD is characterized by a loss of word comprehension and meaning, and PNFA presents with agrammatic, nonfluent speech.

SYNONYMS

FTD

FTLD

Frontotemporal lobar degeneration (FTLD) is the term used for the neuropathologic findings seen in the different FTD syndromes.

Pick disease: This term was historically used to refer to FTD. However, it is now strictly a neuropathologic diagnosis for patients found to have Pick bodies at autopsy, as very few diagnoses of FTD are associated with these neuropathologic findings.

ICD-10CM CODES

G31.0   Frontotemporal dementia
G31.01   Pick disease
G31.09   Other frontotemporal dementia

EPIDEMIOLOGY & DEMOGRAPHICS

The current data on epidemiology of FTD are variable due to misdiagnosis and underreporting. The following data are estimations obtained through systematic reviews.

INCIDENCE: The estimated annual incidence is 2.7 to 4.1 per 100,000 persons.

PREVALENCE: The estimated point prevalence is 15 to 22 per 100,000 persons.

PREDOMINANT SEX & AGE: There is a nearly equal distribution by sex, and the average age of presentation is 58 yr.

GENETICS: Approximately 40% of FTD cases have a positive family history, and several genes (Table 1) have been associated with the development of familial FTD. The most common are mutations in *C9ORF72, MAPT,* and *GRN* (Table 2).

PHYSICAL FINDINGS & CLINICAL PRESENTATION

- The early stage of bvFTD is characterized by changes in behavior and personality. Patients display a lack of insight into these changes, and family members may initially think they are suffering a midlife crisis or a new-onset psychiatric disorder. Therefore careful history-taking is required.
- Behavioral changes include disinhibition, impulsivity, distractibility, violation of social norms (such as offensive, insensitive, or inappropriate sexual remarks; inappropriate behaviors; inappropriately explicit or personal conversations; or encroachment on the personal space of others), as well as increased irritability and impulsive criminal behavior (such as shoplifting or violating traffic laws).
- Patients also display decreased ability to empathize with others, insensitivity to the needs and emotions of their loved ones, and detachment in their personal relationships.
- Apathy and inertia are also common symptoms, with possible development of immobility as the disorder progresses.
- Other associated symptoms that may develop are changes in language and speech (verbal aspontaneity, stereotyped phrases, mutism in late stages), repetitive motor movements, or hyperphagia, especially for sweet foods.
- Physical exam findings for bv FTD can include abnormal cognition (e.g., clock drawing test [Fig. 1]), upper and/or lower motor neuron signs, dysarthria, dysphagia, and pseudobulbar affect. Some patients meet criteria for both FTD and amyotrophic lateral sclerosis. This overlap is typically related to a C9ORF72 mutation.
- Although behavioral changes can also occur in the other FTD syndromes SD and PNFA, these two primarily have language deficits that precede the behavioral changes.
  1. SD is characterized by a gradual loss of the knowledge of words, objects, and concepts, with preservation of speech fluency and syntax.
  2. PNFA is characterized by effortful, nonfluent speech, word-finding difficulties, and agrammatism, with preservation of single-word comprehension.

DX DIAGNOSIS

Diagnosis of bvFTD is primarily clinical, with neuroimaging, genetics, and pathology required for further confirmation. In 2011, the International Behavioral Variant FTD Consortium (FTDC) developed revised criteria for the diagnosis of bvFTD (Table 3).

- In summary, six core symptoms that can be seen in bvFTD were identified. The presence of any three is sufficient to diagnose *possible* bvFTD.
- Diagnosis of *probable* bvFTD requires meeting the following three conditions: (1) patient has diagnosed possible bvFTD, (2) significant functional decline, and (3) frontal and/or anterior temporal atrophy/hypoperfusion seen on imaging.

TABLE 1   Clinical, Genetic, and Pathologic Correlations in Frontotemporal Lobar Degeneration

Clinical Presentation	% of FTLD	Associated	Genes	Parkinsonism	MND	IBM PDB	FTLD-tau	FTLD-TDP	FTLD-FUS	FTLD-UPS	FTLD-ni
				COMORBIDITIES				NEUROPATHOLOGIC SUBTYPES			
bvFTD	57%			+	+	+/−	++	++	+	+/−	+/−
		C9orf72	++	+	++		Type B > A		+/−	
		GRN	+	+			Type A			
		MAPT	+	+		+				
		VCP	+/−		+/−	+	Type D			
		CHMP2B	+/−	+/−	+/−				+	
nfvPPA	24%			+	+/−		++	+			
		C9orf72	+							
		GRN	++	+			Type A			
		MAPT	+	+		+				
svPPA	19%			+/−	+/−		+/−	++ (Type C)			
		Rarely genetic								

Number of plus signs (+) signifies relative frequency of the observation; +/− indicates rare observation. *bv,* Behavioral variant; *FTD,* frontotemporal dementia; *FTLD,* frontotemporal lobar degeneration; *FUS,* fused in sarcoma; *IBM,* inclusion body myopathy; *MND,* motor neuron disease; *nfv,* agrammatic or nonfluent variant; *ni,* no inclusions; *PDB,* Paget disease of the bone; *PPA,* primary progressive aphasia; *sv,* semantic variant; *TDP,* TAR DNA-binding protein; *UPS,* ubiquitin-proteasome system.
From Fillit HM: Brocklehurst's textbook of geriatric medicine and gerontology, ed 8, Philadelphia, 2017, Elsevier.

TABLE 2 Gene Mutations Associated With Frontotemporal Dementia

Gene	Chromosome	Protein	Protein Function	Mode of Inheritance	Mutation Frequency in Familial FTD	Mutation Frequency in Sporadic FTD	Age of Onset (Mean, Range)
C9ORF72	9p21.2	Unknown	Unknown	AD	21%	6%	50s (mid 20–80s)
MAPT	17q21.31	Microtubule-associated tau protein	Microtubule stabilization and assembly	AD	6.3%	1.5%	Mid-50s (20–80s)
GRN	17q21.31	Progranulin	Activates signaling cascades for development, inflammation, and wound repair	AD	5%–15%	5%	60s (mid 30–80s)

AD, Autosomal dominant; *FTD,* frontotemporal dementia.
From Deleon J, Miller BL: Frontotemporal dementia. In Daniel CK et al (eds): *Handbook of clinical neurology,* ed 148, Philadelphia, 2018, Elsevier, pp. 409–430.

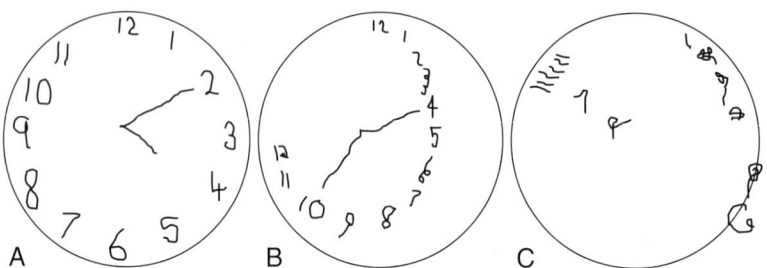

FIG. 1 The clock drawing test. The patient is provided with a circular outline and asked to draw the numbers as they appear on the face of a clock. Once the numbering is complete, the patient is asked to set the hands to a particular time (often "ten past" the hour to test if the patient can suppress the impulse to include the number *10*). **(A)** This drawing demonstrates good planning and use of space. **(B)** This drawing features some impulsiveness because the numbers are drawn out without regard for actual location, and the time "ten past four" is represented by hands pointing to the digits *10* and *4*. Note the perseveration indicated by the extra loops on the digits *3* and *6*. Impulsiveness and perseveration indicate frontal lobe dysfunction. **(C)** This drawing demonstrates gross disorganization, although the patient took several minutes to draw the clock and believed it to be a good representation. (From Stern TA: Massachusetts General Hospital handbook of general hospital psychiatry, ed 7, 2018, Philadelphia, Elsevier.)

- Diagnosis of *definitive* bvFTD can be made only when the patient has possible or probable bvFTD, plus either (1) pathologic evidence of FTLD on biopsy or postmortem or (2) presence of a known causal genetic mutation.

DIFFERENTIAL DIAGNOSIS

- Other neurodegenerative disorders, including Alzheimer disease (AD), Parkinson disease, dementia with Lewy bodies, corticobasal syndrome, progressive supranuclear palsy, and chronic traumatic encephalopathy
- Psychiatric disorders (bipolar disorder, schizophrenia, obsessive-compulsive disorder, depression, personality disorders)
- Spontaneous low intracranial pressure with sagging of the front lobes
- Chronic subdural hematomas, especially frontal
- Central nervous system (CNS) tumors in the prefrontal cortex or compressing the prefrontal cortex
- Metabolic disturbances or nutritional deficiencies (thyroid disease, B_{12} deficiency)
- Substance abuse/toxicities (ethanol, drugs of abuse, heavy metal poisoning)
- Infections (chronic meningitis, HIV-associated dementia, neurosyphilis)

- Cerebrovascular disease (stroke, vascular dementia, lacunar infarctions)
- Autoimmune encephalitis, sarcoidosis

WORKUP

- Careful history-taking with specific attention paid to initial symptoms, time course, progression of symptoms, family history, psychiatric history, and other medical history
- Comprehensive neurologic physical exam to help rule out other CNS etiologies
- Use of the International Behavioral Variant FTD Criteria for diagnosis (Table 3)
- Genetic testing for causal mutations of FTD (*C9ORF72, MAPT,* and *GRN*)
- Medication review (especially drugs that may alter mental status, such as anticholinergics, opiates, benzodiazepines, barbiturates, and neuroleptics)
- Neuropsychologic tests of executive function, memory, and social cognition to rule out other neurodegenerative disorders
- Psychiatric evaluation to rule out psychiatric disorders

LABORATORY TESTS

- CBC, serum electrolytes, glucose, blood urea nitrogen (BUN)/creatinine, liver function tests

- Cerebrospinal fluid (CSF) analysis for infection and measurement of CSF tau and amyloid (which can help differentiate between FTD and AD—not typically measured in clinical practice)
- Vitamin B_{12}, thyroid function tests, HIV, and syphilis screening
- Urine toxicity screen
- In vivo histopathology:
  1. Almost all cases of FTLD have one of the following protein inclusions found on pathologic examination: TAR DNA-binding protein with molecular weight 43 kDa (TDP-43), microtubule-associated protein tau (MAPT), or fused-in-sarcoma protein (FUS).

IMAGING STUDIES

- In general, structural MRI and computed tomography (CT) will show gray matter atrophy in the frontal and/or temporal lobes, anterior cingulate cortex, and insula with variation in distribution between the different FTD subtypes.
  1. Patients with bvFTD specifically will usually show atrophy in the orbitofrontal, anterior cingulate, anterior insular, and anterior temporal cortices.
  2. SD is associated with atrophy in the temporal poles, and PNFA with atrophy in the left perisylvian region.
- A normal MRI scan does not exclude FTD, however, because changes may not be seen in early stages of the disorder. In these cases, PET or SPECT can be used to visualize areas of hypoperfusion/hypometabolism.

℞ TREATMENT

- No disease-modifying drugs currently exist for the treatment of FTD. With advances in the understanding of FTD pathophysiology and genetics, however, new therapies such as antisense oligonucleotides and tau-specific antibodies are being investigated for their efficacy in treating or altering the progression of the syndrome and may see eventual clinical application.
- Current management of FTD is aimed at management of behavioral symptoms through both pharmacologic and nonpharmacologic means.

TABLE 3 International Consensus Criteria for Behavioral Variant FTD

Must be present for any FTD clinical syndrome:
- Shows progressive deterioration of behavior and/or cognition by observation or history

Possible bvFTD
- Three of the features (A-F) must be present; symptoms should occur repeatedly, not just as a single instance:
  - A. Early (3 yr) behavioral disinhibition
  - B. Early (3 yr) apathy or inertia
  - C. Early (3 yr) loss of sympathy or empathy
  - D. Early (3 yr) perseverative, stereotyped, or compulsive/ritualistic behavior
  - E. Hyperorality and dietary changes
  - F. Neuropsychologic profile: Executive function deficits with relative sparing of memory and visuospatial functions

Probable bvFTD
- All the following criteria must be present to meet diagnosis:
  - A. Meets criteria for possible bvFTD
  - B. Significant functional decline
  - C. Imaging results consistent with bvFTD (frontal and/or anterior temporal atrophy on CT or MRI or frontal hypoperfusion or hypometabolism on SPECT or PET)

Definite bvFTD
- Criteria A and either B or C must be present to meet diagnosis:
  - A. Meets criteria for possible or probable bvFTD
  - B. Histopathologic evidence of FTLD on biopsy at post mortem
  - C. Presence of a known pathogenic mutation

Exclusion criteria for bvFTD
- Criteria A and B must both be answered negatively; criterion C can be positive for possible bvFTD but must be negative for probable bvFTD:
  - A. Pattern of deficits is better accounted for by other nondegenerative nervous system or medical disorders
  - B. Behavioral disturbance is better accounted for by a psychiatric diagnosis
  - C. Biomarkers strongly indicative of Alzheimer disease or other neurodegenerative process

Additional features
- Presence of motor neuron findings suggestive of motor neuron disease
- Motor symptoms and signs similar to corticobasal degeneration and progressive supranuclear palsy
- Impaired word and object knowledge
- Motor speech deficits
- Substantial grammatical deficits

bvFTD, Behavioral variant frontotemporal dementia; *CT,* computed tomography; *FTD,* frontotemporal dementia; *FTLD,* frontotemporal lobar degeneration; *MRI,* magnetic resonance imaging; *PET,* positron emission tomography; *SPECT,* single-photon emission computed tomography.
From Rascovsky K et al: Sensitivity of revised diagnostic criteria for the behavioural variant of frontotemporal dementia TT, *Brain* 2011;134:1-22.

NONPHARMACOLOGIC THERAPY
- Due to the impulsivity and the risk for injury seen in bvFTD, discussions with family members about driving, the patient's access to finances, and safety of the physical environment should be conducted early in management.
- For patients with motor symptoms, regular exercise and physical therapy are helpful.
- Speech therapy is helpful for patients with language deficits.
- Diet counseling can aid in prevention of weight gain in patients with hyperphagia.

ACUTE GENERAL Rx
None

CHRONIC Rx
- There are conflicting reports of the efficacy of several medications in the symptomatic treatment of FTD. These include selective serotonin reuptake inhibitors (SSRIs), serotonin and norepinephrine reuptake inhibitors, and antipsychotics.
- SSRIs have the most consensus for their benefit in the management of FTD. They have been shown to help decrease the severity of disinhibition, impulsivity, eating disorders, and repetitive behaviors.
- The use of antipsychotics is controversial, but they are sometimes given to control symptoms of aggression, agitation, and psychosis. However, patients with FTD are also at an increased risk for extrapyramidal side effects due to poorly functioning dopaminergic pathways and thus are usually used only when SSRIs are not successful.

DISPOSITION
- Patients with FTD benefit from having the social support and specialized care offered in dementia-focused care homes and skilled nursing facilities.
- The range and severity of behaviors seen in FTD can put a great burden on family and friends. Education, counseling, and connection with social support or referral to a dementia-focused care home can help reduce caregiver stress.

REFERRAL
Patients who have severe or complex presentations should be referred to a neurologist with expertise in dementia or neurodegenerative disorders.

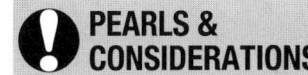

PEARLS & CONSIDERATIONS

FTD is a complex neurologic disorder with a wide variety of presenting symptoms. The most common syndrome seen is bvFTD; therefore patients with gradual-onset changes in personality, disinhibition, and increased impulsivity should be investigated for FTD. Therapy is aimed at management of the behavioral symptoms, most commonly through the use of SSRIs. Social support and dementia-specific care facilities are helpful for both patients and family members.

PATIENT & FAMILY EDUCATION
The Association for Frontotemporal Degeneration (https://www.theaftd.org; 866-507-7222)

SUGGESTED READINGS
Available at eBooks.Health.Elsevier.com.

RELATED CONTENT
Alzheimer Disease (Related Key Topic)
Parkinson Disease (Related Key Topic)
Dementia with Lewy Bodies (Related Key Topic)

AUTHOR: **JOSEPH S. KASS, MD, JD, FAAN**

Frostbite (PTG)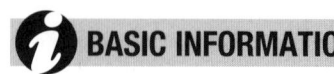

BASIC INFORMATION

DEFINITION
Frostbite represents tissue injury (or death) from freezing and vasoconstriction induced by severe environmental cold exposure.

SYNONYM
Cold-induced tissue injury

ICD-10CM CODES
T35.0 Superficial frostbite involving multiple body regions
T34 Frostbite with tissue necrosis
T345 Frostbite with tissue necrosis of wrist and hand
T34.8 Frostbite with tissue necrosis of ankle and foot
T34.9 Frostbite with tissue necrosis of other and unspecified sites
T35.4 Superficial frostbite involving multiple body regions
T33.9 Superficial frostbite of unspecified sites, initial encounter

EPIDEMIOLOGY & DEMOGRAPHICS
Historically, frostbite was primarily associated with soldiers and adventurers. In recent years, the majority of cases have occurred in urban settings where social disadvantage, physical disability, homelessness, substance use disorder, and psychiatric diseases are the root causes.[1]
- Environmental factors include windchill factor, temperature, duration of exposure, altitude, and degree of wetness. Hands and feet account for >90% of injuries; nose, cheeks, ears, and male genitalia are also more susceptible.[2,3]
- Host factors include psychiatric illness and sedative drugs (especially alcohol, which, in addition to impairing judgment, inhibits shivering and causes cutaneous vasodilation). Other risk factors include immobility, previous frostbite, malnutrition, tobacco use, peripheral neuropathy, peripheral vascular disease, diabetes, exhaustion, and constricting clothing and footwear.[2,3]
- Patients at the extremes of age are at greatest risk, but frostbite is more common in adults between 30 and 49 yr of age with a strong 10:1 male-to-female predominance.[2,3]

PHYSICAL FINDINGS & CLINICAL PRESENTATION
- The frozen part painlessly becomes pale and waxy. Various degrees of tissue destruction similar to that caused by burns are encountered. These are erythema and edema, vesicles and bullae, superficial gangrene, deep gangrene, and injury to muscles, tendons, periosteum, and nerves (Fig. E1). The degree of injury is directly related to the temperature and duration of freezing.
- Frostbite may be classified into four degrees of injury severity or, more practically, into *superficial* (corresponding to first and second degree) and *deep* (corresponding to third and

fourth degree) groups.[4] In both cases, the degree of frostbite can only be accurately determined after rewarming, as initially most frostbite injuries appear similar.
- *Superficial* frostbite involves the skin and subcutaneous tissue. The frozen part is waxy, white (or mottled), and firm but soft and resilient below the surface when gently depressed. After rewarming, there is an initial hyperemia that may be followed by swelling and formation of superficial blisters with clear or milky fluid within 6 to 24 h. There is no ultimate tissue loss.
- *Deep* frostbite extends into the dermis and may involve muscles, nerves, tendons, or bones. The skin may be hard or wooden, without tissue resilience. Nonblanching cyanosis, hemorrhagic blisters, tissue necrosis (Fig. E2), and gangrene may develop. Affected tissue has a poor prognosis and débridement or amputation is generally required.
- Patients initially feel numbness, prickling, and itching. More severe injury can produce paresthesias and stiffness, with burning or throbbing pain upon thawing.

PATHOPHYSIOLOGY
Two phases of tissue injury:
1. The actual *freezing* of the tissues, during which cellular damage is caused by the formation of extracellular ice crystals, which cause osmotic shifts, cellular dehydration, cell membrane lysis, and cell death.[4]
2. The *reperfusion* injury, during which the thawing of damaged endothelial cells releases a cascade of inflammatory mediators (e.g., prostaglandin F, thromboxane A2, bradykinins, histamine), resulting in capillary compression, vascular stasis, progressive ischemic injury, and thrombus formation. These conditions ultimately lead to the destruction of the microcirculation and to cell death.[4]

DIAGNOSIS

DIFFERENTIAL DIAGNOSIS
- Frostnip: A superficial nonfreezing cold injury associated with intense vasoconstriction and characterized by frost forming on the surface of the skin. Transient numbness, tingling, and pallor resolve quickly with warming
- Pernio (chilblains): Self-limited, cold-induced vasculitis associated with purple plaques or nodules, often affecting dorsum of hands and feet; seen with prolonged cold exposure to above-freezing temperatures
- Cold immersion (trench foot): Caused by ischemic injury resulting from sustained, severe vasoconstriction in appendages exposed to wet cold at temperatures above freezing

WORKUP
- Laboratory workup is not indicated unless the patient has systemic hypothermia.
- Early presentation (<24 h from thawing): If there is deep frostbite with potential significant morbidity, perfusion evaluation with magnetic

resonance angiography (MRA) or Tc-99 triple phase scanning should be done emergently in anticipation of potential thrombolysis treatment.[5]
- Late presentation (>24 h from thawing): Noninvasive imaging with MRA or multiphase bone scintigraphy (ideally with single-photon emission computerd tomography/computed tomography [SPECT/CT]) can be used to predict the likely levels of tissue viability for future reconstruction after amputation.[5]

TREATMENT (3 PHASES)

1. FIELD MANAGEMENT[6]
- Prioritize treatment of hypothermia (core body temperature <35° C; 95° F) with systemic and adjunctive rewarming measures if available (e.g., warmed, humidified oxygen, heated intravenous (IV) saline [45° C; 113° F], and warming blankets) before thawing frostbitten extremities.
  1. Shelter patient out of wind and give warm fluids.
- Remove constricting or wet clothing and jewelry from affected digits.
  1. Place cold extremity in a companion's axilla or groin for 10 min, then replace dry gloves/boots.
- Insulate, splint, and elevate affected areas if practical to do so.
  1. Never rub or massage the affected area. Avoid dry heat (e.g., fires and heaters).
- Avoid thawing if there is any risk of refreezing and if possible avoid ambulation on thawed lower extremities (unless only distal toes affected).
- Box 1 describes the Alaska State Guidelines for prehospital treatment of frostbite.[6]

2. REWARMING
- Rapid rewarming (with warm water) limits the freezing injury and yields better outcomes than slow rewarming (e.g., moving to a warmer location).
- Rapid rewarming is achieved by immersing the affected area in a circulating warm water bath with or without a mild antibacterial agent (e.g., chlorhexidine or povidone-iodine) maintained at 37° to 39° C for at least 15 to 30 min up to 1 h, until all tissues are thoroughly rewarmed and pliable with a red-purple color. Active motion during rewarming is advisable; massage is not.[4]
- Administer analgesics during rewarming (ibuprofen and possibly narcotics).[4]

3. POST-THAW TREATMENT
- Tetanus prophylaxis and topical antibiotics if potentially contaminated skin wound.
- Consider systemic antibiotics for patients with significant trauma or signs of infection.
- Débride broken clear vesicles and avoid disrupting intact blisters (especially hemorrhagic ones) unless they are tense or interfere with mobility.
- Topical aloe vera (a potent antiprostaglandin agent) q6h and ibuprofen (a thromboxane

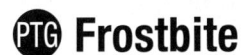

F

I

BOX 1 Alaska State Guidelines for Prehospital Treatment of Frostbite

First Responder/Emergency Medical Technician—I, II, III/Paramedic/Small Bush Clinic
Evaluation and Treatment
A. Anticipate, assess, and treat the patient for hypothermia, if present.
B. Assess the frostbitten area carefully because the loss of sensation may cause the patient to be unaware of soft tissue injuries in that area.
C. Obtain a complete set of vital signs and the patient's temperature.
D. Remove jewelry and clothing, if present, from the affected area.
E. Obtain a patient history, including the date of the patient's last tetanus immunization.
F. If there is frostbite distal to a fracture, attempt to align the limb unless there is resistance. Splint the fracture in a manner that does not compromise distal circulation.
G. Determine whether rewarming the frostbitten tissue can be accomplished in a medical facility. If it can, transport the patient while protecting the tissue from further injury from cold or impacts.
H. If the decision is made to rewarm frostbitten tissue in the field, you should prepare a warm water bath in a container large enough to accommodate the frostbitten tissues without them touching the sides or bottom of the container. The temperature of the water bath should be 99°-102° F (37°-39° C).
   1. Generally, patients with frostbite do not require opiates for pain relief; they occasionally need nonopiate pain medication or anxiolytics. If possible, consult a physician regarding the administration of oral analgesics, such as acetaminophen, ibuprofen, or aspirin. Aspirin or ibuprofen may help improve outcomes by blocking the arachidonic acid pathway.
   2. Immersion injury or frostbite with other associated injuries may produce significant edema and high pain levels. These patients may need opiate pain medications for initial treatment. In this case, advanced life support personnel should administer morphine or other analgesics in accordance with physician-signed standing orders or online medical control.
I. A source of additional warm water must be available.
J. Water should be maintained at approximately at 99°-102° F (37°-39° C) and gently circulated around the frostbitten tissue until the distal tip of the frostbitten part becomes flushed.
K. Pain after rewarming usually indicates that viable tissue has been successfully rewarmed.
L. After rewarming, let the frostbitten tissues dry in the warm air. Do **not** towel dry.
M. After thawing, tissues that were deeply frostbitten may develop blisters or appear cyanotic. Blisters should not be broken and must be protected from injury.
N. Pad between affected digits and bandage affected tissues loosely with a soft, sterile dressing. Avoid putting undue pressure on the affected parts.
O. Rewarmed extremities should be kept at a level above the heart, if possible.
P. Protect the rewarmed area from refreezing and other trauma during transport. A frame around the frostbitten area should be constructed to prevent blankets from pressing directly on the injured area.
Q. Do not allow an individual who has frostbitten feet to walk except when the life of the patient or rescuer is in danger. Once frostbitten feet are rewarmed, the patient becomes nonambulatory.

Mountain Rescue Association: *State of Alaska cold injury guideline,* Juneau, Alaska, 2014, State of Alaska Department of Health and Social Services, pp 30-33. Available at mra.org/wp-content/uploads/2016/05/Alaska-DHSS-EMS-Cold-Injuries-Guidelines-June-2014.pdf.

---

inhibitor) 400 to 600 mg bid to tid (or daily aspirin) can be given until wounds are healed or surgery occurs.
• Thrombolytic therapy[7-12]: May consider if <24 h from thawing in a patient with severe frostbite and evidence of absent perfusion despite full rewarming (i.e., cool skin numb, dusky or blue digits, hemorrhagic blisters and absence of capillary refill by exam or lack of doppler signal in distal pulp). First, evaluate perfusion with angiography (or possibly MRA) to assess for arterial compromise and then administer IV or catheter-directed tissue plasminogen activator (tPA) with use of angiography if perfusion defects are demonstrated. Treatment requires intensive care unit monitoring and concurrent administration of aspirin and heparin in most protocols. Tissue salvage rate appears to correlate with elapsed time to treatment from time of rewarming, and best outcomes are seen within the first 12 h. Although the use of early thrombolytic therapy appears to limit reperfusion injury and reduce subsequent digit amputation, high-quality studies are lacking, and this treatment is not yet U.S. FDA-approved.[13]
• Prior to administering tPA, one must consider the degree of potential disability if affected body parts require eventual amputation, coexisting medical conditions, and the patient understanding the risks of intervention including hemorrhagic stroke and other major bleeding complications.[1]
• Vasodilator therapy: Various vasodilators (NTG, pentoxifylline, phenoxybenzamine, nifedipine, reserpine, and buflomedil) have been tried, with the best evidence favoring prostacyclins (e.g., iloprost, an injectable available in Europe that has is a potent dilator of small-vessel beds and an inhibitor of platelet aggregation). If ilioprost is available, it is easier to administer, has a superior safety profile, has fewer contraindications, and can be managed on a general ward and, potentially, initiated in the field. A small study of Himalayan climbers suggested that it can be beneficial even after the standard 48-h window and perhaps for up to 72 h.[14]
• The Helsinki frostbite management protocol advocates the combined use of tPA and ilioprost to address the thrombotic and vasospastic components of frostbite, respectively.[12,15]
• Daily dressing changes with dry, sterile, noncompressive, and nonadherent dressings. Splint and elevate hands and feet to reduce edema and separate digits with cotton gauze. Avoid any abrasion to limit risk of infection. Excise necrotic tissue.
• Whirlpool hydrotherapy: 1 to 2 times per day for 30 min with warm water (37° C to 39° C), with or without an antiseptic solution if severe edema is present, until there is a clear demarcation of necrotic tissues or evidence of tissue healing.[4]
• Gentle, progressive physical therapy after edema resolves.
• Keep site warm, and avoid all vasoconstrictors, including nicotine. Adjunctive treatments including oral anticoagulation, dextran, sympathectomy, and hyperbaric oxygen are of potential but unproven benefit.[3,4]

DISPOSITION

A majority of patients have long-term residual symptoms, including cold hypersensitivity, neuropathic pain, sensory deficits, hyperhidrosis, secondary Raynaud disease, localized osteoporosis, edema, hair or nail deformities, and (rarely) arthritis. Treatment with tricyclics, gabapentin, calcium channel blockers, botox, and careful protection from further cold exposure may be helpful. Botulinum toxin injections have been administered empirically in highly selected patients to reduce late cold-induced vasospasm and neuropathic pain.[16]

REFERRAL

• Hospitalize for hypothermia or deep frostbite; a burn unit is best.
• Surgical decisions regarding amputation should be deferred until demarcation of viable tissue is clear. Traditionally, this can take 6 to 12 wk by clinical examination. Triple phase Tc-99m bone scan with SPECT/CT in the days after injury can be used to predict level of amputation accurately.[5] Early surgical intervention is indicated if refractory pain, sepsis, or gangrene occurs.

REFERENCES

Available at eBooks.Health.Elsevier.com.

RELATED CONTENT

Frostbite (Patient Information)

AUTHOR: **MICHAEL P. JOHNSON, MD**

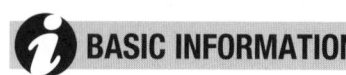

BASIC INFORMATION

DEFINITION

Biliary pain caused by gallbladder dysmotility in the absence of gallstones, sludge, or microlithiasis. It is a diagnosis of exclusion with no evidence of structural disease seen with normal hepatobiliary and pancreatic laboratory and diagnostic imaging modalities.

SYNONYMS

Biliary dyskinesia
Gallbladder dyskinesia
Gallbladder spasm
Acalculous biliary disease
Chronic acalculous cholecystitis
Chronic acalculous
Gallbladder dysfunction
Cystic duct syndrome

ICD-10CM CODE
K82.9   Disease of gallbladder, unspecified

EPIDEMIOLOGY & DEMOGRAPHICS

INCIDENCE: Biliary dyspepsia has an incidence rate of 1% to 6%.
PREVALENCE: 10% to 45% of total population report dyspepsia.
PREDOMINANT SEX & AGE: There is a 3:1 female:male predominance.
RISK FACTORS: There is no consistent relationship to meals or fatty meal intake.

PHYSICAL FINDINGS & CLINICAL PRESENTATION

These patients present with typical biliary pain that fulfills the Rome III criteria:
- Patients present with sporadic epigastric or right upper quadrant pain lasting for 30 min but less than 6 h.
- Episodes are recurrent and occur in sporadic intervals (but not daily).
- The pain is not relieved by bowel movements.
- The pain is not relieved by postural movements.
- The pain is not relieved by antacids.
- The pain builds up to a steady level.
- The pain is severe enough it impedes daily activities and may even require an emergency department visit.

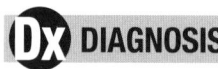

DIAGNOSIS

DIFFERENTIAL DIAGNOSIS
- Primary gallbladder disorders: Gallstones, cholecystitis

- Pancreatobiliary disorders: Cholelithiasis, choledocholithiasis, pancreatitis, pancreatic neoplasm
- Gastrointestinal disorders: Gastroesophageal reflux disorder, peptic ulcer disease, inflammatory bowel disease, irritable bowel syndrome, gastric or esophageal neoplasm
- Metabolic disorders: Obesity, diabetes mellitus
- Cholecystokinin deficiency: Celiac disease

WORKUP

This is a diagnosis of exclusion in a patient with biliary pain. Patients will have normal blood test results and hepatobiliary and pancreatic enzymes, including aspartate aminotransferase (AST), alanine aminotransferase (ALT), alkaline phosphatase (ALP), bilirubin, amylase, and lipase. Imaging, including abdominal ultrasound, is essentially normal without evidence of gallstone or gallbladder sludge pathology.

LABORATORY TESTS

Laboratory tests, including serum AST, ALT, ALP, bilirubin, gamma-glutamyl transferase, amylase, and lipase, are within normal limits.

IMAGING STUDIES

- To exclude gallstone pathology, a transabdominal ultrasound is initial choice for imaging. Transabdominal ultrasound is capable of detecting gallstones up to 3 to 5 mm in size. Patients should fast for at least 8 h before ultrasound to optimize visualization of the gallbladder.
- If gallstones or gallbladder are not found on ultrasound but still suspected, endoscopic ultrasound (EUS) may be used to detect microlithiasis or gallstones smaller than 3 mm.
- Assessing gallbladder emptying through cholecystokinin (CCK)–stimulated cholescintigraphy is essential in the diagnosis. CCK-stimulated cholescintigraphy allows for the calculation of gallbladder ejection fraction (GBEF). Normal GBEF is >38%. Patients with a GBEF <35% to 40% with reproducible pain on CCK stimulation is suggestive of functional gallbladder disorder.

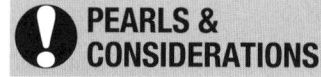

TREATMENT

In patients with appropriate evaluation for suspected functional gallbladder disorder, surgical management with cholecystectomy is the preferred method of treatment.

NONPHARMACOLOGIC THERAPY

Surgical cholecystectomy is the preferred method of treatment. Studies have shown symptomatic relief in up to 98% of patients postcholecystectomy.

ACUTE GENERAL Rx

- Initial management should include adequate analgesic control for abdominal pain.
- Opioid analgesics should be avoided because they may exacerbate symptoms involved in a hypofunctioning gallbladder.

DISPOSITION

Patients with functional gallbladder disorder are often misdiagnosed. These patients require appropriate evaluation to exclude other hepatobiliary etiology. After they are properly diagnosed, these patients have a favorable prognosis after surgical intervention.

COMPLEMENTARY & ALTERNATIVE MEDICINE

Turmeric (Curcuma) has been known to alleviate biliary dyspepsia by stimulating gallbladder contractions.

REFERRAL

- Gastroenterology consultation may be considered to rule out microlithiasis via EUS.
- Surgical consultation should be considered for possible cholecystectomy in select patients.

PEARLS & CONSIDERATIONS

COMMENTS

Functional gallbladder disorder is a diagnosis of exclusion. It is essential that other hepatobiliary pathology be ruled out first. CCK-stimulation scintigraphy showing a reduced GBEF without any other pathology is suggestive of this disorder. Patients fare well with surgical intervention.

RELATED TOPICS

Cholangiocarcinoma (Related Key Topic)
Cholecystitis (Related Key Topic)
Choledocholithiasis (Related Key Topic)
Cholelithiasis (Related Key Topic)

AUTHOR: **FRED FERRI, MD**

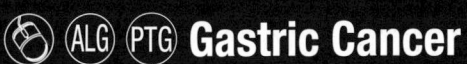

G

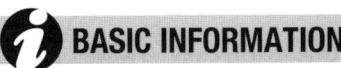 BASIC INFORMATION

DEFINITION

Gastric cancer is an adenocarcinoma arising from the stomach and is histologically subdivided into intestinal and diffuse types; the diffuse type is more common in women and young patients, whereas the intestinal type is predominantly related to environmental factors (smoking; diet high in smoked, salted, and pickled food; nitrates and nitrites) and ethnicity (Asian and Pacific descent).

The classification of gastric adenocarcinoma by depth of invasion is illustrated in Fig. 1.

SYNONYMS

Gastric adenocarcinoma
Stomach cancer
Linitis plastica

ICD-10CM CODES

C16	Malignant neoplasm of stomach
C16.0	Malignant neoplasm of cardia of stomach
C16.1	Malignant neoplasm of stomach
C16.2	Malignant neoplasm of body of stomach
C16.3	Malignant neoplasm of pyloric antrum
C16.5	Malignant neoplasm of lesser curvature of stomach, unspecified
C16.6	Malignant neoplasm of greater curvature of stomach, unspecified
C16.8	Malignant neoplasm of overlapping sites of stomach

EPIDEMIOLOGY & DEMOGRAPHICS

- Gastric cancer is the sixth-commonest cancer worldwide, with an estimated 1,089,103 new cases in 2020. It is the second-leading cause of cancer-related deaths worldwide, with an estimated 768,793 deaths in 2020. Most new cases (70%) occur in developing countries, and Asia accounts for the highest incidence.
- In the U.S., an estimated 26,380 new cases and 11,090 deaths were predicted in 2022.[1]

- The incidence and mortality rate of gastric cancer is 6.7 and 3.4, respectively, per 100,000 persons in the U.S. While the incidence of distal stomach tumors has greatly declined, the incidence of proximal tumors of the cardia and fundus is increasing.
- Gastric cancer is more common in male patients >65 yr.
- The male:female ratio is 3:2.
- Hereditary diffuse gastric cancer (HDGC) has an autosomal-dominant inheritance, and cancer develops at a young age (average age 37 yr). Germline truncating mutations in the tumor-suppressor E-cadherin gene *(CDH1)* are found in up to 50% of these families. It is associated with an 80% lifetime risk of gastric cancer.[2]
- Increased risk of gastric cancer is also seen with Lynch syndrome, familial adenomatous polyposis (FAP), Peutz-Jeghers, juvenile polyposis syndrome, and hyperplastic gastric polyps.

PHYSICAL FINDINGS & CLINICAL PRESENTATION

- Medical history may reveal postprandial fullness, significant weight loss (70% to 80%), nausea/vomiting (20% to 40%), dysphagia (20%), and dyspepsia unrelieved by antacids; epigastric discomfort, usually lessened by fasting and exacerbated by food intake, is also common.
- Epigastric or abdominal mass (30% to 50%), epigastric pain.
- Iron deficiency anemia and hemoccult-positive stools due to tumor bleeding.
- Hard, nodular liver may indicate metastatic disease to the liver.
- Ascites, lymphadenopathy, or pleural effusions may indicate metastases.

ETIOLOGY

- Chronic *Helicobacter pylori* gastritis. Gastric cancer develops in persons infected with *H. pylori* but not in uninfected persons. Persons

with gastric ulcers, nonulcer-related dyspepsia, and gastric hyperplastic polyps are at risk, whereas those with *H. pylori* infection and duodenal ulcer are not at risk. Eradication of *H. pylori* reduces gastric cancer risk.[2]
- Patients with severe gastric atrophy, corpus-predominant gastritis, intestinal metaplasia, and pernicious anemia are at increased risk.
- Tobacco abuse, heavy alcohol consumption.
- Food additives (nitrosamines), smoked foods, occupational exposure to heavy metals, rubber, asbestos.
- Box 1 summarizes risk factors for gastric adenocarcinoma.

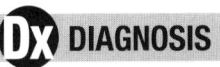 DIAGNOSIS

DIFFERENTIAL DIAGNOSIS

- Gastric lymphoma (5% of gastric malignancies)
- Hypertrophic gastritis
- Peptic ulcer
- Reflux esophagitis

WORKUP

Upper endoscopy (Fig. E2) with biopsy will confirm diagnosis. Endoscopic ultrasonography in combination with PET/computed tomography (CT) scanning and operative lymph node dissection can be used in accurate tumor staging and aids in treatment planning. A general staging and treatment strategy for gastric adenocarcinoma is illustrated in Fig. 3. Table 1 and Fig. 1 describe staging systems for gastric carcinoma.

LABORATORY TESTS

- CBC reveals microcytic anemia.
- Hemoccult-positive stools are detected.
- Chemistry panel can reveal hypoalbuminemia or abnormal liver enzymes in patients with metastasis to the liver.
- Up to 25% of gastric cancers overexpress the HER2/neu receptor, which can be detected

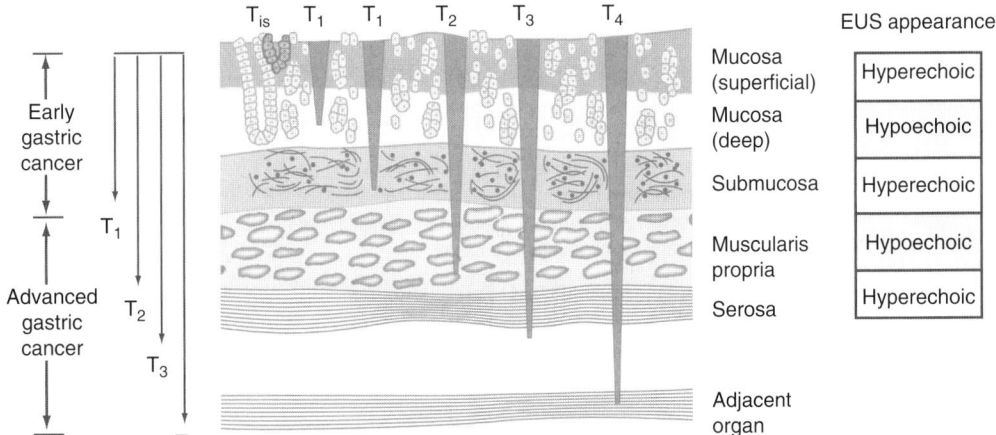

FIG. 1 Classification of gastric adenocarcinoma by depth of invasion (T classification). In the TNM classification, T denotes depth of invasion: T_{is} designates carcinoma in situ; T_1 tumors are confined to the mucosa (T_{1a}) and submucosa (T_{1b}); T_2 tumors invade the muscularis propria but not the serosa; T_3 tumors penetrate the subserosal connective tissue without involving the visceral peritoneum or contiguous structures; and T_4 tumors invade the serosa (visceral peritoneum) and may involve adjacent organs and tissues. In early gastric cancer, the disease is confined to the mucosa and submucosa (T_1), regardless of nodal involvement. (From Feldman M et al [eds]: *Sleisenger and Fordtran's gastrointestinal and liver disease,* ed 10, Philadelphia, 2016, Saunders.)

BOX 1 Risk Factors for Gastric Adenocarcinoma

Definite
H. pylori infection
Chronic atrophic gastritis
Intestinal metaplasia
Dysplasia*
Adenomatous gastric polyps
Cigarette smoking
History of gastric surgery (especially Billroth II)
Genetic factors:
  Family history of gastric cancer (first-degree relative)
  Familial adenomatous polyposis (with fundic gland polyps)
  Hereditary nonpolyposis colorectal cancer
  Peutz-Jeghers syndrome
  Juvenile polyposis

Probable
High salt intake
Obesity (adenocarcinoma of the cardia only)
Snuff tobacco use
History of gastric ulcer
Pernicious anemia
Regular aspirin or other NSAID use (protective)

Possible
Statin use (protective)
Heavy alcohol use
Low socioeconomic status
Ménétrier disease
High intake of fresh fruits and vegetables (protective)
High ascorbate intake (protective)

Questionable
Hyperplastic and fundic gland polyps
Diet high in nitrates
High green tea consumption (protective)

*Surveillance for cancer is recommended in patients with this risk factor.
H. pylori, Helicobacter pylori; *NSAID*, nonsteroidal antiinflammatory drug.
From Feldman M et al (eds): *Sleisenger and Fordtran's gastrointestinal and liver disease,* ed 10, Philadelphia, 2016, Saunders.

TABLE 1 TNM Staging Criteria and Stages for Gastric Carcinoma Based on AJCC Eighth Edition

T Category	T Criteria
$T_x T_0 T_{is} T_1 T_{1a} T_{1b} T_2 T_3 T_4 T_{4a}$	Primary tumor cannot be assessed
	No evidence of primary tumor
	Carcinoma *in situ:* Intraepithelial tumor without invasion of the lamina propria, high-grade dysplasia Tumor invades the lamina propria, muscularis mucosae, or submucosa
	Tumor invades the lamina propria or muscularis mucosae
	Tumor invades the submucosa
	Tumor invades the muscularis propria
	Tumor penetrates the subserosal connective tissue without invasion of the visceral peritoneum or adjacent structures
	Tumor invades the serosa (visceral peritoneum) or adjacent structures
	Tumor invades the serosa (visceral peritoneum)

N Category	N Criteria
$N_x N_0 N_1 N_2 N_3 N_{3a}$	Regional lymph node(s) cannot be assessed
	No regional lymph node metastasis
	Metastasis in one or two regional lymph nodes
	Metastasis in three to six regional lymph nodes
	Metastasis in seven or more regional lymph nodes
	Metastasis in 7-15 regional lymph nodes

M Category	M Criteria
$M_0 M_1$	No distant metastasis
	Distant metastasis

Stage	pT	pN	M
Stage 0	T_{is}	N_0	M_0
Stage IA	T_1	N_0	M_0
Stage IB	$T_1 T_2$	$N_1 N_0$	$M_0 M_0$
Stage IIA	$T_1 T_2 T_3$	$N_2 N_1 N_0$	$M_0 M_0 M_0$
Stage IIB	$T_1 T_2 T_3 T_{4a}$	$N_{3a} N_2 N_1 N_0$	$M_0 M_0 M_0 M_0$
Stage IIIA	$T_2 T_3 T_{4a} T_{4b}$	$N_{3a} N_2 N_1$ or $N_2 N_0$	$M_0 M_0 M_0 M_0$
Stage IIIB	$T_1 T_2 T_3 T_{4a} T_{4b}$	$N_{3b} N_{3b} N_{3a} N_{3a} N_1$ or N_2	$M_0 M_0 M_0 M_0 M_0$
Stage IIIC	$T_3 T_{4a} T_{4b}$	$N_{3b} N_{3b} N_{3a}$ or N_{3b}	$M_0 M_0 M_0$
Stage IV	Any T	Any N	M_1

AJCC, American Joint Committee on Cancer; *TNM*, tumor, node, metastasis.

by immunohistochemistry as a standard practice.

- Mutation-specific predictive genetic testing by polymerase chain reaction for truncating mutations in *CDH1* is recommended in families of patients with familial diffuse cancer because gastric cancer develops in three of every four carriers of a mutant *CDH1* gene. Genetic abnormalities in gastric adenocarcinoma are summarized in Table E2.

IMAGING STUDIES

- Chest and abdomen PET/CT scan to evaluate for metastases.
- Endoscopic ultrasound (EUS) is recommended as part of the staging workup for gastric cancer if there is no evidence of metastatic disease. It provides the most accurate evaluation of the depth of tumor invasion and assessment of perigastric lymph node involvement.

(Rx) TREATMENT

The overall treatment strategy is dependent on tumor stage (early vs. locally advanced vs. metastatic) with surgery being the mainstay of therapy for nonmetastatic cases.

ACUTE GENERAL Rx

- Gastrectomy: Most curable tumors can be removed with adequate margins by subtotal gastrectomy; total gastrectomy is required in proximal cancers or large disease extent. The preferred treatment for lesions arising in the body or antrum of the stomach is a radical distal subtotal resection (Fig. E4), which removes approximately 80% of the stomach, along with the first portion of the duodenum, the gastrohepatic and gastrocolic omenta, and

the nodal tissue adjacent to the celiac axis. Extensive or proximal cancers require a total gastrectomy to achieve an adequate proximal gastric margin (Fig. E5). If total gastrectomy is necessary, a splenectomy is sometimes performed, particularly in gastric cancers of the proximal third of the stomach and tumors of the body near the greater curvature. These cancers are more apt to metastasize to lymph nodes in the splenic hilum that cannot be completely excised without a splenectomy. Routine splenectomy is no longer practiced due to increased complications.

- Laparoscopic distal gastrectomy with extended D2 lymphadenectomy is comparable to open surgery in terms of relapse-free survival for patients with locally advanced gastric cancer and is a potential standard treatment option for locally advanced gastric cancer.[3]

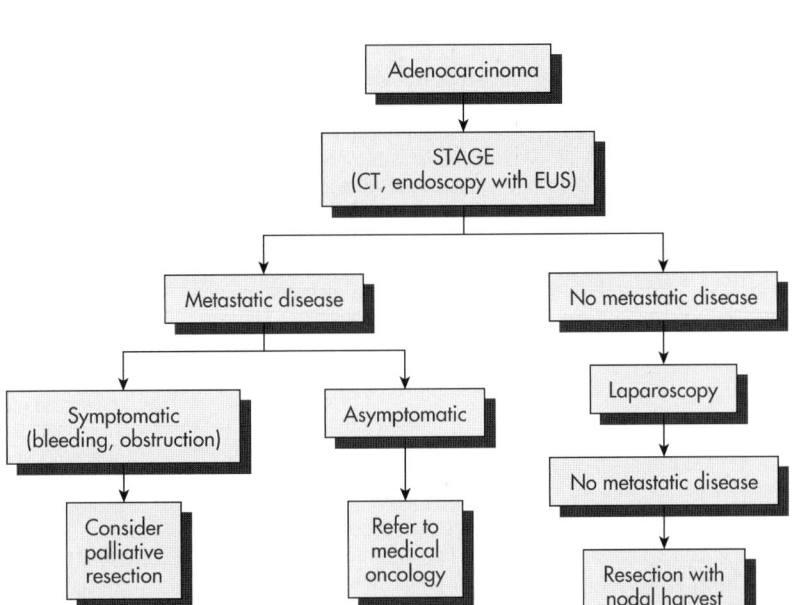

FIG. 3 General staging and treatment strategy for gastric adenocarcinoma. *CT,* Computed tomography; *EUS,* endoscopic ultrasound. (From Townsend CM et al: *Sabiston textbook of surgery,* ed 21, St Louis 2022, Elsevier.)

- In advanced cases, palliative gastrectomy (in cases of major bleeding or obstruction) can be performed. Outlet obstruction can be addressed by performing a gastrojejunostomy or endoscopic stenting.
- Perioperative chemotherapy: In patients with operable, locally advanced, gastric cancer, the use of perioperative chemotherapy can decrease tumor size and downstage while improving progression-free and overall survival. The current standard neoadjuvant regimen is the FLOT (5-fluorouracil [5-FU], leucovorin, oxaliplatin, docetaxel) regimen with three cycles administered before and after resection.[4]
- Similarly, perioperative chemotherapy with oxaliplatin plus S-1 chemotherapy was demonstrated to have better survival than adjuvant CAPOX (capecitabine, oxaliplatin) chemotherapy in a randomized study underscoring the value of perioperative, multimodal approach in these patients.[5]
- Postoperative chemotherapy: For patients who have not received preoperative therapy, modern combination chemotherapy with FOLFOX (5-FU, leucovorin, oxaliplatin) or CAPOX (capecitabine, oxaliplatin) regimens is utilized; radiotherapy is reserved for high-risk patients (positive margins, extracapsular spread) only.
- Recurrent/metastatic cancer: The use of combination chemotherapy in combination with immune checkpoint inhibitor therapy results in improved overall survival. The use of

platinum plus fluoropyrimidine chemotherapy in combination with either pembrolizumab or nivolumab has shown to improve overall survival in randomized trials.[6]
- Patients progressing after first-line chemotherapy derive a survival benefit with the use of taxane chemotherapy in combination with antivascular endothelial growth factor receptor-2 antibody ramucirumab. The oral antimetabolite, trifluridine/tipiracil, has been shown to significantly improve overall survival compared with placebo in heavily pretreated patients with advanced gastric cancer.
- In the subset of patients with gastric cancer expressing *HER2-2/neu* oncogene (20% to 25% cases), the addition of trastuzumab to systemic chemotherapy prolongs overall survival. Improved overall survival rates are seen in patients when treated with trastuzumab deruxtecan (an antibody drug conjugate [ADC]) when compared to conventional salvage chemotherapy approaches.[7]
- Immunotherapy with program death receptor-1 antibodies (nivolumab, pembrolizumab) has been shown to improve survival in previously treated patients with high-MSI tumors.
- Treatment algorithms for newly diagnosed gastric or gastroesophageal junction cancer are illustrated in Figs. E6 and E7.

DISPOSITION
- Median survival rate of metastatic or recurrent gastric carcinoma is 12 to 15 mo overall.
- The 5-yr survival rate for early gastric cancers is >35%.

ⓘ PEARLS & CONSIDERATIONS

COMMENTS
- Gastrectomy patients will need vitamin B_{12} replacement. They are also at risk for dumping syndrome and should be advised to ingest frequent, small meals.
- Prophylactic gastrectomy should be considered in young, asymptomatic carriers of germline truncating *CDH1* mutations who belong to families with highly penetrant heredity diffuse gastric cancer.
- Gastric cancer screening for average-risk patients is not recommended in the U.S.

REFERENCES
Available at eBooks.Health.Elsevier.com.

RELATED CONTENT
Stomach Cancer (Patient Information)

AUTHOR: **RITESH RATHORE, MD**

BASIC INFORMATION

DEFINITION
Gastric outlet obstruction (GOO) is a mechanical obstruction involving the distal stomach or proximal duodenum resulting in delayed gastric emptying. It is not a single entity but rather can be the result of a variety of causes.

SYNONYMS
Pyloric obstruction
Stenosis of the pylorus
GOO

ICD-10CM CODE
K31.5 Obstruction of the duodenum

EPIDEMIOLOGY & DEMOGRAPHICS
INCIDENCE: Accurate statistics on incidence are not available. It is postulated that GOO has decreased over the past several decades due to improved treatment options for peptic ulcer disease, which is historically the leading cause for GOO. More recent data suggest that up to 50% to 80% of new cases are cancer related.[1,2]
RISK FACTORS:
- History of pancreatic or gastric malignancy
- Untreated peptic ulcer disease
- Chronic NSAID use
- *Helicobacter pylori* infection

PHYSICAL FINDINGS & CLINICAL PRESENTATION
- Signs of dehydration (tachycardia, hypotension, dry mucous membranes) are often present.
- Malnutrition may be evident depending on the chronicity of the obstruction.
- Epigastric tenderness may be present.
- Abdominal distention/tympanic mass in epigastric area or left upper quadrant (LUQ).
- Succession splash may be heard with a stethoscope placed on the abdomen while the patient rocks side to side. It has a low sensitivity and is positive if present 3 hr after a meal, which suggests retained gastric contents.
- Sister Mary Joseph nodule (a periumbilical node) or Virchow's node (a left supraclavicular node) may be palpated in the setting of metastatic gastric cancer.

Patients with GOO often present with postprandial nonbilious vomiting, epigastric pain, nausea, easy satiety, and weight loss, though the presentation may differ depending on the cause of the obstruction. Patients with malignancy as the underlying cause often present with a more acute onset of symptoms, whereas those with peptic ulcer disease have more chronic symptoms. Physical examination findings most commonly include signs of dehydration and malnutrition, as well as abdominal tympanic distention and epigastric tenderness.

ETIOLOGY
- Historically, the most common cause of GOO was peptic ulcer disease; however, with the availability of proton pump inhibitors and treatment to eradicate *H. pylori* infection, this has been drastically reduced. Malignancy now accounts for the majority of cases, most frequently pancreatic adenocarcinoma with spread to the duodenum or stomach, or gastric cancer. Other rarer malignant causes include advanced gallbladder carcinoma or cholangiocarcinoma, gastric lymphoma, malignancy of the duodenum, ampullary cancer, and gastric carcinoid.
- Benign causes include peptic ulcer disease, caustic ingestion, stricture and scarring from NSAIDs or postsurgery, acute or chronic pancreatitis, and pancreatic pseudocysts. Rare causes include gastric obstructing polyps, bezoars, or volvulus, Bouveret syndrome (gallstone in the proximal duodenum), congenital annular pancreas, or infiltrative disease from Crohn, amyloid, or tuberculosis. See Table 1.

DIAGNOSIS

Diagnosis is based on clinical presentation, imaging, and often endoscopy with biopsy.

DIFFERENTIAL DIAGNOSIS
It is important to exclude motility causes such as gastroparesis from diabetes, medications, or viral infections. The primary differential diagnosis to be considered in GOO is in determining the causes of the obstruction. See Table 1.

WORKUP
During the initial work up of GOO, it is important assess hydration and nutrition status and to determine the underlying cause. Consider the following:
- Complete blood count, electrolytes, abdominal CT scan, and upper endoscopy

LABORATORY TESTS
Laboratory tests are not diagnostic but should include a complete blood count and electrolytes.
- Electrolytes may reveal evidence of contraction alkalosis and hypokalemia, especially in the setting of repeated vomiting.
- The complete blood count may show evidence of anemia in a patient with underlying malignancy that may become more apparent after fluid replacement.

IMAGING STUDIES
- Abdominal x-rays are often not diagnostic but may reveal a significant gastric bubble.
- CT scan of abdomen (Fig. 1) may reveal gastric distention, mass, and evidence of malignant spread. This should be ordered without oral contrast if upper endoscopy is anticipated.
- Upper endoscopy is usually needed for both diagnostic and therapeutic purposes. This should occur after nasogastric tube placement and suction to remove gastric contents to reduce the chance of aspiration during the procedure. Endoscopy can determine the location and extension of the obstruction and may offer a diagnosis through biopsy.

TREATMENT

The general management of gastric outlet obstruction consists of hydration, correcting metabolic abnormalities, pain management, and alleviating the obstruction.

NONPHARMACOLOGIC THERAPY
- Nothing by mouth (NPO) and nasogastric tube for gastric decompression
- Intravenous fluids using isotonic saline with potassium replacement
- Nutritional support

BENIGN CAUSES
- Management of the obstruction depends on the underlying cause. The following recommendations are for GOO from peptic ulcer disease, the most common benign cause of GOO. Patients with rarer, benign causes of GOO may benefit from some of the following interventions as well but treatment will be more specifically tailored to the underlying cause and decided with consultations from gastroenterology and surgery.
- GOO can be initially managed with 48 to 72 hr of gastric decompression, fluid replacement, correction of metabolic abnormalities, and acid suppression. *H. pylori* infection should be treated if appropriate. If this approach is unsuccessful endoscopic dilation or surgery should be considered.

TABLE 1   Causes of Gastric Outlet Obstruction

Benign	Malignant
Peptic ulcer disease	Pancreatic cancer
Gastric polyps	Gastric cancer
Caustic ingestion	Gallbladder carcinoma
Stricture/scarring from NSAIDs, radiation, postsurgical	Cholangiocarcinoma
	Gastric lymphoma
Acute or chronic pancreatitis	Ampullary cancer
Pancreatic pseudocyst	Duodenum cancer
Bouveret syndrome (gallstone in the proximal duodenum)	Gastric carcinoid
Congenital annular pancreas	
Infiltrative disease (Crohn, amyloid, tuberculosis)	
Bezoars	

NSAID, Nonsteroidal antiinflammatory drug.

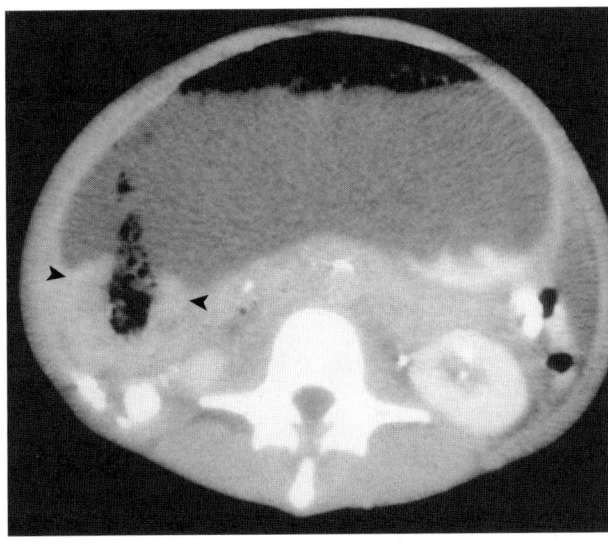

FIG. 1 Gastric outlet obstruction: Cancer of the antrum. A markedly distended stomach with an air-fluid level is seen on computed tomography. In this case, a mass in the distal end of the antrum is apparent *(arrowheads)*. (From Grainger RG et al [eds]: *Grainger & Allison's diagnostic radiology: a textbook of medical imaging,* ed 4, St Louis, 2001, Churchill Livingstone.)

ENDOSCOPIC BALLOON DILATION

Endoscopic balloon dilation (EBD) is most commonly indicated in patients with GOO from peptic ulcer disease. It results in a lasting response in 70% to 80% of patients; however, narrow strictures often need gradual dilations performed in a stepwise fashion over several sessions. Recurrent stenosis requiring two or more dilations is an indication for surgery.

SURGICAL INTERVENTIONS

- The goals of surgery include alleviating the obstruction and suppressing acid secretion.
- Surgical inventions such as laparoscopic antrectomy or distal gastrectomy with vagotomy, vagotomy with drainage via pyloroplasty, and laparoscopic gastrojejunostomy are potential options.

ENDOSCOPIC ULTRASOUND-GUIDED GASTROENTEROSTOMY

Endoscopic ultrasound-guided gastroenterostomy (EUS-GE) is emerging as a potential treatment option for benign (and malignant) GOO and might be associated with fewer adverse effects, fewer recurring symptoms, and decreased need for subsequent interventions compared with other techniques. However, further research is necessary to determine optimal technique and to directly compare the efficacy of EUS-GE with other endoscopic procedures and surgical options.[3,4]

MALIGNANT CAUSES

Management of malignant GOO depends on the type and extent of the underlying malignancy. General therapeutic options include endoscopic stenting, surgical resection or bypass, gastrostomy with possible feeding tube placement, and EUS-GE. Surgery is the treatment of choice when resection can be potentially curative. A laparoscopic approach is recommended based on current guidelines from the American Gastroenterological Association as this results in less blood loss and fewer days of hospitalization.[5] Consultation with gastroenterology, surgery, oncology, and palliative care can guide treatment decisions.

ACUTE GENERAL Rx

- Proton pump inhibitors to decrease gastric secretions
- Antiemetics to treat nausea
- Pain management
- Eradication of *H. pylori* infection, if applicable

CHRONIC Rx

- Avoidance of nonsteroidal anti-inflammatory medications
- Proton pump inhibitors

DISPOSITION

Prognosis depends on the underlying cause of the GOO.

REFERRAL

Gastroenterology should be consulted for initial diagnostic and therapeutic options with consultations from surgery, oncology, and palliative care as needed.

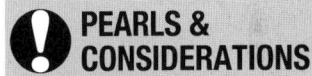

PEARLS & CONSIDERATIONS

COMMENTS

- Malignancy should be considered as the primary cause until proven otherwise.
- All patients, regardless of cause, benefit from a proton pump inhibitor.

REFERENCES
Available at eBooks.Health.Elsevier.com.

RELATED CONTENT

Pancreatic Cancer (Related Key Topic)
Gastric Cancer (Related Key Topic)
Peptic Ulcer Disease (Related Key Topic)
Gallbladder Cancer (Related Key Topic)

AUTHOR: **DANA RICCI CHOFAY, MD**

G

Diseases
and Disorders

I

BASIC INFORMATION

DEFINITION

Gastroesophageal reflux disease (GERD) is a motility disorder characterized primarily by heartburn and caused by the reflux of gastric contents into the esophagus. A current definition is a condition that develops when the reflux of stomach contents causes at least two heartburn episodes per week and/or complications. Table 1 describes a classification system for esophagitis.

SYNONYMS

Peptic esophagitis
Reflux esophagitis
GERD

ICD-10CM CODES
K21.9 Gastroesophageal reflux disease without esophagitis
R12 Heartburn

EPIDEMIOLOGY & DEMOGRAPHICS

- GERD is one of the most prevalent gastrointestinal disorders. It is the most common GI diagnosis recorded during visits to outpatient clinics. From 18% to 28% of adults are affected.
- The estimated prevalence of GERD is 13.3% of the population worldwide and 15.4% in North America. Costs related to GERD in the U.S. are estimated at $10 billion annually.[1]
- Nearly 7% of persons in the United States have heartburn daily, 20% have it monthly, and 60% have it intermittently. Incidence in pregnant women exceeds 80%.
- Nearly 20% of adults use antacids or over-the-counter H_2 blockers at least once a week for relief of heartburn.
- The phenotypic presentations of GERD include nonerosive reflux disease (in 60% to 70% of patients), erosive esophagitis (in 30%), and Barrett esophagus (in 5% to 12%).[1]

PHYSICAL FINDINGS & CLINICAL PRESENTATION

- Physical examination: Generally unremarkable
- Clinical signs and symptoms: Heartburn, dysphagia, sour taste, regurgitation of gastric contents into the mouth

- Chronic cough and bronchospasm
- Chest pain, laryngitis, early satiety, abdominal fullness, and bloating with belching
- Dental erosions in children

ETIOLOGY:
- Incompetent lower esophageal sphincter (LES) (see Fig. E1)
- Medications that lower LES pressure (calcium channel blockers, alpha-adrenergic antagonists, nitrates, theophylline, anticholinergics, sedatives, prostaglandins)
- Foods that lower LES pressure (chocolate, yellow onions, peppermint). Table 2 summarizes modulators of lower esophageal sphincter (LES) pressure
- Tobacco abuse, alcohol, coffee
- Pregnancy
- Gastric acid hypersecretion
- Hiatal hernia (controversial) present in >70% of patients with GERD; however, most patients with hiatal hernia are asymptomatic
- Obesity is associated with a statistically significant increase in the risk for GERD symptoms, erosive esophagitis, and esophageal carcinoma

DIAGNOSIS

DIFFERENTIAL DIAGNOSIS

- Peptic ulcer disease
- Unstable angina
- Esophagitis (from infections such as herpes, *Candida*), medication induced (doxycycline, potassium chloride), eosinophilic esophagitis
- Esophageal spasm (nutcracker esophagus)
- Cancer of esophagus

WORKUP

- Aimed at eliminating the conditions noted in the differential diagnosis and documenting the type and extent of tissue damage (Fig. E2).

Generally, when symptoms of GERD are typical and the patient responds to therapy, there is no need for further diagnostic tests to verify the diagnosis.

- Upper GI endoscopy (Fig. E3) is useful to document the type and extent of tissue damage in persistent GERD and to exclude eosinophilic esophagitis and potentially malignant conditions such as Barrett esophagus. The American College of Physicians recommends endoscopy in the setting of GERD in people with heartburn and alarm symptoms (dysphagia, bleeding, anemia, weight loss, and recurrent vomiting). It is also indicated in people with GERD symptoms that persist despite a therapeutic trial of 4 to 8 wk of bid proton pump inhibitor (PPI) therapy in patients with severe erosive esophagus after a 2-mo course of PPI therapy to assess healing and rule out Barrett esophagus.

LABORATORY TESTS

- 24-hr esophageal pH monitoring with transnasal catheter or a 48-h wireless capsule are sensitive diagnostic tests to assess the degree of acid exposure in the esophagus in patients not responding to acid-reducing therapy; however, they are not practical and generally not done. They are useful in patients with atypical manifestations of GERD, such as chest pain or chronic cough.
- High-resolution esophageal manometry (HRM) is indicated in patients with refractory reflux in whom surgical therapy is planned.
- *Helicobacter pylori* testing is not indicated in GERD.

An upper GI series is useful in patients unwilling to have endoscopy or with medical contraindications to the procedure. It can identify ulcerations and strictures; however, it may miss

---

TABLE 1 Los Angeles Endoscopic Classification System for Esophagitis

Grade A	One or more mucosal breaks confined to folds, ≤5 mm
Grade B	One or more mucosal breaks >5 mm confined to folds but not continuous between the tops of mucosal folds
Grade C	Mucosal breaks continuous between tops of two or more mucosal folds but not the circumferential
Grade D	Circumferential mucosal break

From Feldman M et al: *Sleisenger and Fordtran's gastrointestinal and liver disease*, ed 10, Philadelphia, 2016, Elsevier.

TABLE 2 Modulators of Lower Esophageal Sphincter (LES) Pressure

	Increase LES Pressure	Decrease LES Pressure
Hormones/peptides	Gastrin	CCK
	Motilin	Secretin
	Substance P	Somatostatin
		Vasoactive intestinal peptide
Neural agents	α-Adrenergic agonists	α-Adrenergic antagonists
	β-Adrenergic antagonists	β-Adrenergic agonists
	Cholinergic agonists	Cholinergic antagonists
Foods and nutrients	Protein	Chocolate
		Fat
		Peppermint
Other factors	Antacids	Barbiturates
	Baclofen	Calcium channel blockers
	Cisapride	Diazepam
	Domperidone	Dopamine
	Histamine	Meperidine
	Metoclopramide	Morphine
	Prostaglandin $F_{2\alpha}$	Prostaglandins E_2 and I_2
		Serotonin
		Theophylline

CCK, Cholecystokinin.
From Feldman M et al: *Sleisenger and Fordtran's gastrointestinal and liver disease*, ed 10, Philadelphia, 2016, Elsevier.

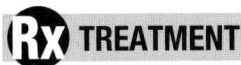

mucosal abnormalities. Only one third of patients with GERD have radiographic signs of esophagitis on an upper GI series.

℞ TREATMENT

NONPHARMACOLOGIC THERAPY

- Lifestyle modifications with avoidance of foods (e.g., citrus- and tomato-based products, onions, spicy foods, carbonated beverages, mint, chocolate, fried foods) and drugs that exacerbate reflux (e.g., caffeine, β-blockers, calcium channel blockers, α-adrenergic agonists, theophylline)
- Avoidance of tobacco and alcohol use
- Elevation of head of bed (4 to 8 in) with blocks
- Avoidance of lying down for at least 2h after eating or drinking, especially after late or large evening meals
- Weight reduction to BMI <25, decreased fat intake
- Avoidance of clothing that is tight around the waist
- A trial in women revealed that adherence to diet and lifestyle changes reduced the risk of GERD to half compared with women who adhered to none[2]

GENERAL Rx

- An empirical 8 wk trial of a PPI given once/day is recommended for patients with classic heartburn and regurgitation but no alarm symptoms. PPIs should be taken 30 to 60 min before a meal because they bind to protein pumps that have been stimulated by meals.[3]
- PPIs (esomeprazole 40 mg qd, omeprazole 20 mg qd, lansoprazole 30 mg qd, rabeprazole 20 mg qd, pantoprazole 40 mg qd, or dexlansoprazole 30 mg) are generally safe, tolerated, and highly effective in most patients (Table E3). Omeprazole and esomeprazole are inhibitors of CYP2C19 and can increase serum concentrations of phenytoin and diazepam. Concomitant use of clopidogrel should also be avoided with omeprazole and esomeprazole. Increased risk of pneumonia has been documented in hospitalized patients. Long-term use of PPIs has been associated with increased risk of osteoporosis, and patients should be warned about an increased risk of fractures with long-term use. Use of PPIs in patients with cirrhosis increases risk of spontaneous bacterial peritonitis and hepatic encephalopathy. Rare side effects of PPIs include acute interstitial nephritis, hypomagnesemia, and QT prolongation.
- H_2 blocker (famotidine 40 mg qhs) can be used but is generally much less effective than PPIs.
- Antacids (may be useful for relief of mild symptoms; however, they are generally ineffective in severe cases of reflux).

- Prokinetic agents (metoclopramide) are indicated only when PPIs are not fully effective. They can be used in combination therapy; however, side effects limit their use.
- Combination of PPE with an agent that reduces esophageal sphincter relaxation (baclofen) plus a neuromodulator (desipramine) may be tried in patients with refractory heartburn before considering surgery.
- For refractory cases: Think first, cut last. Some patients will respond to twice-daily PPIs or as-needed addition of a H_2 receptor blocker at bedtime. However, clinicians should be vigilant for alternative conditions that may be mistaken for GERD (e.g., achalasia).[3] Surgery with Nissen fundoplication (Fig. E4). Potential surgical candidates should have reflux esophagitis documented by esophagogastroduodenoscopy and normal esophageal motility as evaluated by manometry. Surgery generally consists of reduction of hiatal hernia when present and placement of a gastric wrap around the gastroesophageal (GE) junction (fundoplication). Although laparoscopic fundoplication is now widely used, long-term medical therapy is a better choice for most patients who are willing to remain on daily acid-reduction medication. In patients preferring surgical intervention, surgery should not be advised with the expectation that patients with GERD will no longer need to take antisecretory medications or that the procedure will prevent esophageal cancer among those with GERD and Barrett esophagus. Approximately 17.7% of patients who undergo primary laparoscopic antireflux surgery will experience recurrent gastroesophageal reflux requiring long-term medication use or secondary antireflux surgery. Risk factors for recurrence are older age, female sex, and comorbidity.
- Endoscopic radiofrequency heating of the GE junction (Stretta procedure) is a treatment modality for GERD patients unresponsive to traditional therapy. Its mechanism of action remains unclear. Endoscopic gastroplasty (EndoCinch procedure) is also aimed at treating GERD. Initial results appear encouraging; however, long-term studies are needed before recommending these procedures.
- Lifestyle modification must be followed for life because GERD is generally an irreversible condition in most patients.

DISPOSITION:

- Recurrence of reflux is common if treatment is discontinued. Preliminary trials have shown that in patients with severe reflux esophagitis successfully treated with PPI therapy, stopping PPI medication was associated with T lymphocyte–predominant esophageal inflammation and basal cell and papillary hyperplasia without loss of surface cells.

- The majority of patients respond well to therapy. In patients with chronic GERD, long-term outcomes are similar between medical therapy with PPIs and antireflux surgery. Prolonged use of PPIs is associated with increased risk of fractures of hip, wrist, and spine; increased risk of diarrhea from *Clostridium difficile;* pneumonia; and possible iron deficiency from impaired iron absorption. PPIs also block the effects of clopidogrel by inhibiting cytochrome P450 2C19 isozyme. Therefore all PPIs (other than pantoprazole) should be avoided in patients using clopidogrel. H_2 blockers can be used for patients with GERD taking clopidogrel.
- Postsurgical complications occur in nearly 20% of patients (dysphagia, gas, bloating, diarrhea, nausea). Long-term follow-up studies also reveal that within 3 to 5 yr, 52% of patients who had undergone antireflux surgery are taking antireflux medications again.

REFERRAL

- There is a strong and probably causal relation between symptomatic prolonged and untreated GERD, Barrett esophagus, and esophageal adenocarcinoma. GI referral for upper endoscopy is needed when there are concerns about associated peptic ulcer disease, Barrett esophagus, or esophageal cancer.
- Patients with Barrett esophagus should undergo surveillance endoscopy with mucosal biopsy every 2 yr or less because the risk of developing adenocarcinoma of esophagus is at least 30 times greater than that of the general population.
- Testing and treating for *Helicobacter pylori* in patients with GERD has not been shown to improve symptoms.
- All children with dental erosions should be evaluated for GERD.

REFERENCES & SUGGESTED READINGS

Available at eBooks.Health.Elsevier.com.

RELATED CONTENT

Gastroesophageal Reflux Disease (GERD) (Patient Information)
Achalasia (Related Key Topic)
Dysphagia (Related Key Topic)

AUTHOR: **FRED F. FERRI, MD**

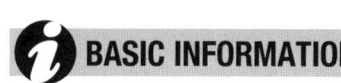
BASIC INFORMATION

DEFINITION

Gestational diabetes mellitus (GDM) is hyperglycemia occurring during the second or third trimester in absence of a pre-pregnancy diagnosis of type 1 or type 2 diabetes.

Screening for gestational diabetes mellitus in asymptomatic pregnant women after 24 wk gestation is a grade B recommendation by the U.S. Preventive Services Task Force (USPSTF). In the U.S., a two-step approach to screening is commonly used and is currently endorsed by the American College of Obstetricians and Gynecologists (ACOG) and the National Institutes of Health (NIH). The International Association of Diabetes in Pregnancy Study Group has recommended a simplified, one-step approach for screening and diagnosing GDM, which has been endorsed by the American Diabetes Association since 2011, with the acknowledgment that the one-step approach increases the prevalence of GDM without clear evidence of benefit. Pregnant women with diabetes mellitus (DM) (gestational or preexisting) are classified according to White classification (Table 1).

SYNONYMS

Gestational diabetes
Diet-controlled gestational diabetes (A1)
Medication-treated gestational diabetes (A2)

ICD-10CM CODES

O24.410	Gestational diabetes mellitus in pregnancy, diet controlled	
O24.414	Gestational diabetes mellitus in pregnancy, insulin controlled	
O24.419	Gestational diabetes mellitus in pregnancy, unspecified control	
O99.810	Abnormal glucose complicating pregnancy	

TABLE 1 White Classification for Pregnant Women With Diabetes (Gestational or Preexisting)

Class	Description
A1	DM diagnosed during pregnancy and controlled by diet
A2	DM diagnosed during pregnancy and requiring medication
B	Insulin-requiring DM diagnosed before pregnancy, age >20 yr, lasting <10 yr
C	Insulin-requiring DM, onset at age 10 - 19 yr, with a duration 10 - 19 yr
D	Onset >10 yr or duration >20 yr, or associated with hypertension or background retinopathy
F	DM with renal disease
H	DM with coronary artery disease
R	DM with proliferative retinopathy
T	DM with renal transplant

DM, Diabetes mellitus.

EPIDEMIOLOGY & DEMOGRAPHICS

INCIDENCE: Approximately 5% of pregnant women in the U.S. will be diagnosed with GDM using the two-step approach and 18% using the one-step approach.

PREDOMINANT SEX & AGE: Women of childbearing age; increased risk is observed in women >35 yr.

RISK FACTORS (BOX 1):
- Overweight or obesity
- Family history of GDM or type 2 diabetes, particularly in first-degree relatives
- Polycystic ovarian syndrome
- Multiple gestation
- Hypertensive disorder of pregnancy or chronic hypertension
- Chronic systemic steroid use
- History of macrosomia in prior pregnancy
- Personal history of abnormal glucose tolerance or GDM in previous pregnancy
- Hispanic, Native American, African American, Asian, or Pacific Islander ethnicity
- Advanced maternal age (over age 35)
- Unexplained perinatal loss or malformation in previous or current pregnancy may be suggestive of preexisting diabetes

GENETICS: Higher rate in women with a family history of GDM or type 2 diabetes in a first-degree relative; specific human leukocyte antigen (HLA) alleles (DR3 or DR4) predispose to the development of DM type 2 after pregnancy.

PHYSICAL FINDINGS & CLINICAL PRESENTATION

Suspect GDM if:
- Fetal size greater than dates on Leopold or increased fundal height measurement
- Ultrasound findings of fetal macrosomia (especially enlarged abdominal circumference) or polyhydramnios
- Marked maternal obesity or weight gain above expected range
- Acanthosis nigricans (as underlying insulin resistance increases risk)
- Symptoms of diabetes
- Glucosuria
- Hemoglobin A1c ≥ 5.7 in the first trimester

ETIOLOGY

During normal pregnancy, several mechanisms contribute to increased insulin resistance. Placental secretion of human placental lactogen (hPL) decreases maternal insulin sensitivity, decreases maternal glucose utilization, and increases lipolysis, all to ensure adequate glucose availability to the growing fetus. Maternal pancreatic beta cells are increased in order to secrete additional insulin to compensate for the increased circulating blood glucose. Insulin resistance is also exacerbated by an increase in maternal adipose deposition, decreased exercise, and increased caloric intake. GDM occurs when maternal insulin secretion cannot meet the increased glucose burden, resulting in carbohydrate intolerance and hyperglycemia.

DIAGNOSIS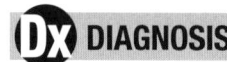

DIFFERENTIAL DIAGNOSIS

Preexisting type 1 or 2 DM not previously diagnosed

WORKUP

- History with focus on personal medical history, prior pregnancy history, and family history
- Routine prenatal examination
- Laboratory evaluation (see the following)

LABORATORY TESTS

- Exclude preexisting diabetes.
- For women with risk factors (see above), order a 1-hr glucose tolerance test at the first prenatal visit, then repeat at 24 to 28 wk if initial screen was normal. If abnormal at intake, consider the probability of undiagnosed preexisting DM or underlying insulin resistance and check hemoglobin A1c. A diagnosis of diabetes is made if a woman meets any of the following criteria: Fasting plasma glucose >126 mg/dl, A1c >6.5%, random plasma glucose >200 mg/dl. The authors consider a first-trimester A1c of ≥5.7 suggestive of preexisting insulin resistance and would be inclined to monitor closely for hyperglycemia.
- Two-step approach:
  1. For screening without risk factors, a 1-hr, nonfasting 50-g oral glucose tolerance test

---

BOX 1 Risk Factors for Gestational Diabetes

Women at greatest risk of gestational diabetes mellitus include those:
- Over 40 yr of age
- With a family history of type 2 diabetes mellitus (first-degree relative with diabetes or a sister with gestational diabetes mellitus)
- Who are overweight (defined as pre-pregnancy body mass index of >35 kg/m²) (moderate risk factor if body mass index 25-35 kg/m²)
- Of racial background including Asian, Middle Eastern, Polynesian, Melanesian or Māori, African American, Indian subcontinent, and Indigenous Australian
- With a previous history of gestational diabetes (moderate risk factor)
- With a previous adverse obstetric outcome such as macrosomia (birth weight more than 4500 g or >90th percentile), shoulder dystocia, or polyhydramnios
- With previously elevated blood glucose level
- With polycystic ovarian syndrome
- On certain medications (e.g., corticosteroids)

From Talley NJ et al: *Essentials of internal medicine,* ed 4, Chatswood, NSW, 2021, Elsevier Australia.

(OGTT) is appropriate. If the result is abnormal (≥130 mg/dl, as defined by Carpenter and Coustan), a 3-hr, 100-g oral glucose tolerance test is performed. The diagnosis of GDM is made if two or more of the following glucose values are met or exceeded:

a. Fasting: 95 mg/dl
b. 1-hr plasma glucose: 180 mg/dl
c. 2-hr plasma glucose: 155 mg/dl
d. 3-hr plasma glucose: 140 mg/dl

1. If one of four values on 3-hr glucose tolerance test is abnormal, consider repeat testing in 1 mo and recommend a low-carbohydrate diet immediately and consultation with a nutritionist. At least one study has demonstrated increased perinatal risk in women with only one of four abnormal values on 3-hr OGTT.

- One-step approach:
  1. Like the two-step, a one-step screening is performed at 24 to 28 wk on all pregnant patients who have not already been diagnosed with diabetes. This is a 2-hr, 75-g oral glucose tolerance test performed after an overnight, 8-hr fast. A diagnosis of GDM is made if one or more of the following values are met or exceeded:
     a. Fasting: ≥92 mg/dl
     b. 1-hr plasma glucose ≥180 mg/dl
     c. 2-hr plasma glucose ≥153 mg/dl
- After pregnancy, women with GDM have an increased risk of developing diabetes during their lifetime. Women with GDM should be screened at or after 6 wk postpartum with a 75-g, 2-hr GTT to diagnose type 2 diabetes using the same criteria as nonpregnant patients. Alternatively, an HgbA1c can be performed at or after 12 wk postpartum.

IMAGING STUDIES

Ultrasound for fetal size is performed in women with GDM. It may be initiated at the time of diagnosis and repeated every 3 to 4 wk if macrosomia is suspected. Clinicians should consider local standards of care.

🅡🅧 TREATMENT

NONPHARMACOLOGIC THERAPY

- Glucose monitoring:
  1. Four times daily: Fasting and 2-hr postprandial (defined as 2 hr after the start of each meal)
  2. Goals: Fasting <95 mg/dl; 2-hr postprandial <120 mg/dl
  3. Can also use 1-hr postprandial goal of <140 mg/dl
- Dietary modifications for glycemic control:
  1. Follow a low-carbohydrate diet; avoid sugar and concentrated sweets; and eat small, frequent meals (three meals with two snacks is often recommended).
  2. Complex carbohydrates should be consumed over simple carbohydrates to prevent glucose fluctuations.
  3. Diet should adequately meet the needs of pregnancy (following sublist) while

restricting carbohydrates to 33% to 40% of daily calories. Caloric needs in pregnancy:
  a. BMI <30: 30 kcal/kg/day
  b. BMI >30: 25 kcal/kg/day
  c. BMI >40: 12 to 14 kcal/kg/day
  4. Regular moderate exercise, defined as 30 min five times per week.
  5. Ongoing nutrition counseling throughout pregnancy.

PHARMACOLOGIC Rx

Initiate if >20% of glucose values are elevated after trial of diet control:

- Insulin: Considered the gold standard in GDM management
  1. There are no randomized controlled trials on insulin regimens, and therapy is largely guided by expert opinion.
  2. Insulin is the only FDA-approved medication for GDM (Pregnancy Class B) and does not cross placenta.
  3. Insulin may be started first line or added when oral medications have failed to achieve glycemic control. The authors consider factors such as the degree of hyperglycemia, obstacles to medication adherence, and gestational age at time of diagnosis (with early-onset diagnosis more likely to progress and require insulin) when initiating therapy. The ADA recommends insulin as first-line pharmacotherapy for GDM, and ACOG (2017) mirrors this recommendation (Level A).
  4. Regardless of insulin regimen initiated, blood glucose values should be reviewed frequently, and the regimen adjusted and customized to optimize each woman's blood glucose levels, using a single agent or combination of long, intermediate, and/or short-acting insulins.
  5. One commonly used regimen:
     a. Insulin 0.7 to 1.0 U/kg/day subcutaneous (based on current pregnant weight), with two thirds of the total daily dose given in the morning and one third of the total daily dose given in the evening.
     b. One third of each dose is given as short-acting insulin and the remaining two thirds as long-acting insulin.
- Oral hypoglycemics:
  1. Oral antidiabetic agents continue to be used in the management of GDM, despite a lack of FDA approval for this indication.
  2. Several recent studies have examined the potential benefits and harms of metformin and glyburide, comparing them with the gold-standard insulin and with each other. Metformin (compared with insulin) has been demonstrated to decrease maternal glucose levels, maternal weight gain, and the risk of gestational hypertension. Evidence grows that it may decrease the risk of preeclampsia as well. Although known to cross the placenta, concerns about the long-term risk in exposed offspring have been mitigated by at least one recent study showing no neurodevelopmental differences with intrauterine exposure to metformin versus insulin. Meanwhile, recent

meta-analyses have demonstrated worse neonatal outcomes with the use of glyburide compared with insulin. With both metformin and glyburide, many women go on to require insulin therapy.
  3. As of 2017, ACOG recommends "in women who decline insulin therapy or for those women whom the obstetrician or obstetric care provider believes the patient will be unable to safely administer insulin, metformin is a reasonable second-line choice" (Level B); while suggesting that glyburide should not be recommended as a first-line agent due to a failure to achieve equivalent outcomes to insulin in most studies (also Level B).
  4. Metformin: Begin at 500 mg PO nightly or bid, and titrate up to a maximum of 2500 mg daily in divided doses.
  5. Glyburide: Begin at 2.5 mg qd, and titrate up to a maximum of 20 mg qd (10 mg bid). Increase dose as needed by 2.5 to 5 mg/wk.

ANTENATAL TESTING

Antepartum testing is recommended for women with pregestational diabetes and gestational diabetes. There is no consensus regarding initiation, frequency, or modality of antepartum testing in gestational diabetes, and this should be guided by local standards.

ONE COMMONLY USED REGIMEN

- Weekly nonstress test/amniotic fluid level beginning at 32 wk or when medications are initiated in women with GDMA2. Less frequent testing or delayed initiation of testing may be considered in women who maintain glycemic control with diet alone (GDMA1), as increased rates of stillbirth have not been observed in these women before 40 wk of gestation.
- Preexisting or poorly controlled diabetes, vascular complications, or concomitant hypertension: Twice weekly NST/AFI beginning at 28 wk. Consider hospital admission to obtain glycemic control.

TIMING AND ROUTE OF DELIVERY

- Women with preexisting diabetes should be induced at 39 wk.
- Women with GDMA2 may also be induced at 39 wk unless otherwise indicated, with decisions regarding induction guided by local standards of care.
- In women with GDMA1, ACOG supports expectant management of up to 40 and 6/7 wk with appropriate antepartum testing.
- Counsel regarding elective cesarean section at or after 39 wk if estimated fetal weight is over 4500 g.
- Consider delivery earlier than 39 wk if poor glycemic control or other medical indications such as growth restriction or preeclampsia.

INTRAPARTUM MANAGEMENT

- Goal is normoglycemia (80 to 120 mg/dl) using insulin and D5 lactated Ringer IV fluid if needed.
- Monitor glucose every 1 to 2 hr in active labor.

- Preparation for shoulder dystocia.
- If on glyburide, discontinue in labor or 12 hr before a scheduled induction.
- If on insulin, consider decreased long-acting insulin by one third to one half before scheduled induction. Most experts recommend holding insulin entirely the morning of a scheduled cesarean delivery.

POSTPARTUM MANAGEMENT

- Class A2: Check fasting blood glucose level before discharge; if abnormal, continue checking at home and schedule early follow-up with primary care physician to confirm diagnosis of DM.
- 6-wk postpartum visit: Screen for impaired glucose tolerance and diabetes with a 75-g, 2-hr glucose tolerance test. Alternatively, an HgbA1c or 3 fasting blood glucose levels may be performed at or after 12 wk postpartum.
- If no evidence of DM, screen annually for DM and counsel on risk factor modification.

REFERRAL

- Nutritionist
- Maternal-fetal medicine
- Diabetes educator
- Nurse care manager, when available

COMPLICATIONS

- Maternal: Preeclampsia, future type 2 DM or GDM, operative delivery
- Fetal: Polyhydramnios, macrosomia, congenital malformations, shoulder dystocia, birth trauma, intrauterine fetal demise
- Neonatal: Hypoglycemia, hypocalcemia, hyperbilirubinemia, polycythemia, perinatal death, respiratory distress, future obesity, and DM

❗ PEARLS & CONSIDERATIONS

- **One-step vs two-step test for diagnosing GDM:** Despite more diagnosis of gestational diabetes with the one-step approach (16.5% for one-step approach, 8.5% for two-step approach), trials have demonstrated no significance between group differences in the risks of the primary outcomes relating to perinatal and maternal complications. Using the one-step approach results in additional fetal testing (including fetal nonstress testing) and additional treatment (including initiation of insulin) with no significant improvement in pregnancy outcomes for the newborn or mother.
- A recent trial comparing lower versus higher glycemic criteria for diagnosis of gestational diabetes revealed that using the lower glycemic criterion (FBS of at least 92 mg per deciliter [≥5.1 mmol per liter], a 1 h level of at least 180 mg per deciliter [≥10.0 mmol per liter], or a 2 h level of at least 153 mg per deciliter [≥8.5 mmol per liter]) did not result in a lower risk or a large-for-gestational-age infant than use of the higher standard glycemic criteria.[1]

- Trials have shown that although treatment of mild gestational DM did not significantly reduce the frequency of a composite outcome that included stillbirth or perinatal death and several neonatal complications, it did reduce the risks of fetal overgrowth, shoulder dystocia, cesarean delivery, and hypertensive disorders.
- Lactation improves maternal glucose metabolism and may prevent or delay the development of type 2 DM following GDM. Higher lactation intensity and longer duration are independently associated with lower 2-yr incidences of DM after a GDM-affected pregnancy.

PREVENTION

Regular exercise, maintenance of ideal body weight, and high-fiber low-glycemic diet

REFERENCE & SUGGESTED READINGS

Available at eBooks.Health.Elsevier.com.

RELATED CONTENT

Gestational Diabetes (Patient Information)
Diabetes Mellitus (Related Key Topic)

AUTHORS: **ELLA STERN, MD,** and **ANTHONY SCISCIONE, DO**

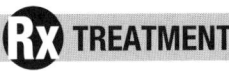

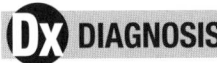 BASIC INFORMATION

DEFINITION

Giardiasis is an intestinal and/or biliary tract infection caused by the noninvasive protozoal parasite *Giardia intestinalis* (also known as *G. lamblia* or *G. duodenalis*). The organism is a widespread zoonotic parasite and frequently contaminates fresh water sources worldwide.

SYNONYMS

Giardiasis
Giardia duodenalis (accepted species name by the CDC)
Giardia intestinalis

ICD-10CM CODE
A07.1   Giardiasis [lambliasis]

EPIDEMIOLOGY & DEMOGRAPHICS

INCIDENCE (IN U.S.):
- Exact incidence unknown. CDC estimates 20,000 cases a yr in the U.S.
- Frequently occurs as waterborne outbreaks in international adoptees, travelers, immunocompromised patients, and those with cystic fibrosis
- *G. lamblia* has been demonstrated in 4% to 7% of submitted stool specimens, making it the most commonly identified intestinal parasite
PREVALENCE (IN U.S.): 4%
PREDOMINANT SEX: Male = female
PREDOMINANT AGE:
- Preschool children, especially if in day care
- 20 to 40 yr of age, especially among sexually active homosexual men (oral-anal contact)
PEAK INCIDENCE:
- Varies with risk factors, outbreaks, but peak onset from early summer through early fall
- All age groups affected
GENETICS: Familial disposition: Patients with common variable immunodeficiency or X-linked agammaglobulinemia are at increased risk of infection

TABLE 1   Symptoms of Giardiasis

Symptom	Frequency (%)
Flatulence	56-74
Anorexia	40-64
Abdominal cramps	55-80
Foul-smelling stool	57-72
Abdominal distention	31
Bloating	55-69
Nausea	58-68
Malaise	84
Diarrhea	89
Belching	30
Weight loss	48-64
Fever	17-28

From Cherry JD et al: *Feigin and Cherry's pediatric infectious diseases,* ed 8, Philadelphia, 2019, Elsevier.

PHYSICAL FINDINGS & CLINICAL PRESENTATION

- More than 70% with one or more intestinal symptoms (diarrhea, flatulence, cramps, bloating, nausea). Table 1 summarizes clinical signs and symptoms of giardiasis
- Incubation period averages 7 to 21 days
- Fever in <30%
- Chronic diarrhea, malabsorption, and weight loss, which can be up to 10% of body weight, are common
- GI bleeding is unusual
- Continuous or intermittent symptoms, lasting for 2 to 4 wk
- Of infected patients, 20% to 25% are asymptomatic and can shed cysts for months

ETIOLOGY

Infection is acquired by ingestion of viable cysts of the organism (Fig. E1), typically in contaminated water or food or by fecal-oral contact. *Giardia* cysts are resistant to chlorination and survive well in cold mountain streams. Fig. E2 illustrates the life cycle of *Giardia duodenalis*.

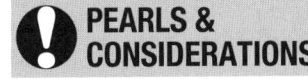 DIAGNOSIS

DIFFERENTIAL DIAGNOSIS

- Other agents of infective diarrhea (amebae, *Salmonella* sp., *Shigella* sp., *Staphylococcus aureus*, *Cryptosporidium*, etc.)
- Noninfectious causes of malabsorption

WORKUP

- Stool specimen (three specimens yield 90% sensitivity) as a saline suspension or duodenal aspirate for microscopic examination to establish diagnosis and exclude other pathogens.
- Immunoassays for *Giardia* sp. Antigens in stool samples such as the direct fluorescent antibody or enzyme-linked immunosorbent assay are now routinely used in most clinical laboratories. These assays are 85% to 98% sensitive and 90% to 100% specific. They are more sensitive than stool microscopy for confirming the diagnosis. They also have a faster turnaround time.

LABORATORY TESTS

Serum albumin, vitamin B_{12} levels, and stool fat test to exclude malabsorption

IMAGING STUDIES

- Not necessary unless biliary obstruction is suspected

- In detection of organism, possible interference by barium in stool from radiographic studies

TREATMENT

NONPHARMACOLOGIC THERAPY

Avoidance of milk products to reduce symptoms of transient lactase deficiency that occur in many patients and can last for weeks to months.

GENERAL Rx

Adult and pediatric (see Table E2):
- Tinidazole: 2-g single dose (50 mg/kg in children over 3 yr of age)
- Alternative regimen: Metronidazole: 250 mg PO tid for 5 to 10 days. Pediatric dose: 5 mg/kg tid × 7 days (metronidazole should be avoided in pregnancy)
- Nitazoxanide: In children aged 12 to 47 mo: 100 mg bid × 3 days. Aged 4 to 11 yr: 200 mg bid × 3 days
- Quinacrine: 100 mg PO tid × 5 to 7 days
- Albendazole: 400 mg PO qd with food × 5 days
- Paromomycin: 25 to 35 mg/kg/day in three doses for 5 to 10 days. Safe for pregnancy

DISPOSITION

Re-infection is possible. Postinfection lactose intolerance is common and is frequently mistaken for recurrent infection.

PEARLS & CONSIDERATIONS

COMMENTS

Travelers to endemic areas (developing world, wilderness areas) should be cautioned to boil drinking water or use water purification tablets (for iodine-containing products, chlorination is not effective). Chronic giardiasis as seen in developing nations can cause delays in growth and development in children due to malabsorption and diarrhea.

SUGGESTED READINGS
Available at eBooks.Health.Elsevier.com.

RELATED CONTENT
Giardiasis (Patient Information)

AUTHOR: **GLENN G. FORT, MD, MPH**

G

Diseases and Disorders

I

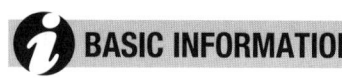

BASIC INFORMATION

DEFINITION

Gonorrhea is a sexually transmitted bacterial infection with a predilection for columnar and transitional epithelial cells. It commonly manifests as urethritis, cervicitis, or salpingitis. Infection may be asymptomatic. It differs between males and females in course, severity, and ease of recognition.

SYNONYMS

Gonococcal urethritis
Gonococcal vulvovaginitis
Gonococcal cervicitis
Gonococcal bartholinitis
GC

ICD-10CM CODES
A54.9	Gonococcal infection, unspecified
O98.211	Gonorrhea complicating pregnancy, first trimester
O98.212	Gonorrhea complicating pregnancy, second trimester
O98.213	Gonorrhea complicating pregnancy, third trimester
O98.219	Gonorrhea complicating pregnancy, unspecified trimester
O98.22	Gonorrhea complicating childbirth
O98.23	Gonorrhea complicating the puerperium
A54.03	Gonococcal cervicitis, unspecified
A54.00	Gonococcal infection of lower genitourinary tract, unspecified

EPIDEMIOLOGY & DEMOGRAPHICS

- The disease is common worldwide, affects both sexes and all ages, especially younger adults; highest incidence is in inner-city areas. Per CDC reports, approximately 1.6 million new cases were found in the U.S. in 2018, with more than half found in young people ages 15 to 24 yr. Gonorrhea is the second most-commonly reported communicable disease.
- Asymptomatic anterior urethral carriage may occur in 12% to 50% of cases in men.
- Asymptomatic in 50% to 80% of cases in women. Most common dissemination is by mucosal passage to fallopian tubes, resulting in pelvic inflammatory disease (PID) in 10% to 15% of infected women. Hematogenous spread may result in septic arthritis and skin lesions. Conjunctivitis rarely occurs but may result in blindness if not rapidly treated. Infection can occur in both men and women in oropharynx and anorectally.
- The World Health Organization (WHO) reported 78 million new cases of gonorrhea worldwide among adults in 2012.

PHYSICAL FINDINGS & CLINICAL PRESENTATION

- Males: Purulent discharge from anterior urethra (Fig. E1), with dysuria appearing 2 to 7 days after infecting exposure. May have rectal infection causing pruritus, tenesmus, and discharge, or may be asymptomatic.
- Females: Initial urethritis or cervicitis may occur a few days after exposure, frequently mild. Infections may be asymptomatic or may not produce recognizable symptoms until complications have occurred. In approximately 20% of cases, uterine invasion occurs after menstrual period with signs and symptoms of endometritis, salpingitis, or pelvic peritonitis. The patient may have purulent discharge or inflamed Skene or Bartholin glands.
- Classic presentation of acute gonococcal PID is fever, abdominal and adnexal tenderness, and, often, absence of purulent discharge. Physical examination may be normal if asymptomatic. Disseminated gonococcal infection (DGI) may manifest with petechial or pustular acral skin lesions (Fig. E2), asymmetric polyarthralgia, tenosynovitis, or oligoarticular septic arthritis. The infection is occasionally complicated by perihepatitis and, rarely, endocarditis or meningitis.

ETIOLOGY

- *Neisseria gonorrhoeae* is also known as gonococcus. Plasmids coding for β-lactamase render some strains resistant to penicillin or tetracycline. There is an increasing frequency of chromosomally mediated resistance to penicillin, tetracycline, fluoroquinolones, and cefoxitin. In the Far East, high-level resistance to spectinomycin is endemic.
- There are a rising number of cases of quinolone-resistant *N. gonorrhoeae* worldwide, with the expected number to rise in the U.S. from importation.
- Men who have sex with men are vulnerable to the emerging threat of antimicrobial-resistant *N. gonorrhoeae*.

DIAGNOSIS

DIFFERENTIAL DIAGNOSIS

- Nongonococcal urethritis (NGU)
- Nongonococcal mucopurulent cervicitis
- *Chlamydia trachomatis*
- *Trichomonas vaginalis*

WORKUP

Diagnosis depends on bacteriologic investigation. Culture and nucleic acid amplification tests (NAAT) are available for the detection of genitourinary infection with *N. gonorrhoeae*.

- NAATs are preferred testing modalities for the detection of genitourinary infection with *N. gonorrhoeae*. The performance of NAATs with respect to overall sensitivity, specificity, and ease of specimen transport is better than that of any other tests available for the diagnosis of gonococcal infections. NAATs should be used to detect gonorrhea except in cases of child sexual assault involving boys and rectal and oropharyngeal infections in prepubescent girls. When evaluating a potential gonorrhea treatment failure, case culture and susceptibility testing might be required. NAATs allow testing of the widest variety of specimen types, including endocervical swabs, vaginal swabs, urethral swabs (men), and urine (from both men and women).
- Culture: Gonorrhea culture on Thayer-Martin medium (organism is fastidious; requires aerobic conditions with increased carbon dioxide atmosphere; incubate ASAP). Culture has a sensitivity of 95% or more for urethral specimens from men with symptomatic urethritis and 80% to 90% for endocervical infection in women. Gram-negative intracellular diplococci are diagnostic in male urethral smears (Fig. E3). There is a false-negative rate of 60% to 70% in female cervical or urethral smears.
  1. Concomitant serologic testing for syphilis for all patients
  2. Concomitant *Chlamydia* testing for all patients
  3. Offer of HIV testing and counseling to all patients

LABORATORY TESTS

- First-catch urine (or genital swab) sample NAAT is the preferred screening and diagnostic test for gonorrhea. These tests have largely replaced collecting culture in many settings where persons are screened for asymptomatic genital infection. These tests are not more sensitive than culture for detecting *N. gonorrhoeae* in cervical or urethral specimen; however, they have specificities >99% and retain sensitivity when used to test voided urine or self-collected vaginal swabs.
- Gonorrhea culture on Thayer-Martin medium (organism is fastidious; requires aerobic conditions with increased carbon dioxide atmosphere; incubate ASAP). Culture has a sensitivity of 95% or more for urethral specimens from men with symptomatic urethritis and 80% to 90% for endocervical infection in women.
- Nonamplified DNA probe tests are less sensitive than culture or NAATs and are not useful in the diagnosis of rectal or pharyngeal infection or for testing urine; however, they are inexpensive, readily available, and offered in many laboratories in combination assays for *C. trachomatis*.
- Concomitant serologic testing for syphilis on all patients.
- Concomitant *Chlamydia* testing on all patients.
- Offer of HIV testing and counseling to all patients.

TREATMENT

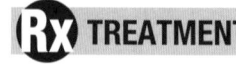

ACUTE GENERAL Rx

For treatment of uncomplicated urogenital, rectal, or pharyngeal gonorrhea, the CDC recommends a single 500-mg IM dose of ceftriaxone. For persons weighing ≥150 kg (300 lbs), a single 1-g IM dose of ceftriaxone should be administered. If chlamydial infection has not been excluded, doxycycline 100 mg orally twice a day for 7 days is recommended. When ceftriaxone cannot be used for treating urogenital or rectal gonorrhea because of cephalosporin allergy, a single 240-mg IM dose of gentamicin, plus a single 2-g

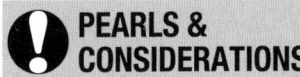
oral dose of azithromycin is an option. Gastrointestinal symptoms, primarily vomiting within 1 hr of dosing, have been reported among 3% to 4% of treated persons. If administration of IM ceftriaxone is not available, a single 800-mg oral dose of cefixime is an alternative regimen. However, cefixime does not provide as high or sustained bactericidal blood levels as does ceftriaxone, and demonstrates limited treatment efficacy for pharyngeal gonorrhea.

When gonococcal expedited partner therapy (provision of prescriptions or medications for the patient to give to a sex partner without the health care provider first examining the partner) is permissible by state law and the partner is unable or unlikely to seek timely treatment, the partner may be treated with a single 800-mg oral dose of cefixime, provided that concurrent chlamydial infection in the patient has been excluded. Otherwise, the partner may be treated with a single 800-mg oral dose of cefixime plus oral doxycycline 100 mg twice daily for 7 days.

In cases of suspected cephalosporin treatment failure, clinicians should obtain relevant clinical specimens for culture and antimicrobial susceptibility testing, consult an infectious disease specialist or STD clinical expert (https://www.stdccn.org/external icon) for guidance in clinical management, and report the case to the CDC through state and local public health authorities within 24 hr. Health departments should prioritize notification and culture evaluation for the patient's sex partner(s) from the preceding 60 days for those with suspected cephalosporin treatment failure or persons whose gonococcal isolates demonstrate reduced susceptibility to cephalosporins.

A test-of-cure is unnecessary for persons with uncomplicated urogenital or rectal gonorrhea who are treated with any of the recommended or alternative regimens. However, for persons with pharyngeal gonorrhea, a test-of-cure is recommended, using culture or nucleic acid amplification tests 7 to 14 days after initial treatment, regardless of the treatment regimen. Because reinfection within 12 mo ranges from 7% to 12%

among persons previously treated for gonorrhea, those who have been treated should be retested 3 mo after treatment, regardless of whether they believe their sex partners were treated. If retesting at 3 mo is not possible, clinicians should retest within 12 mo after initial treatment.

Treatment of arthritis and arthritis-dermatitis syndrome:

- Recommended regimen: Ceftriaxone 1 g IM or IV every 24 hr plus azithromycin 1 g orally as a single dose
- Alternative regimens: Cefotaxime 1 g IV every 8 hr or ceftizoxime 1 g IV every 8 hr *plus* azithromycin 1 g orally in a single dose

PREGNANCY

- Pregnant women infected with *N. gonorrhoeae* in whom chlamydia has been excluded should be treated with ceftriaxone 500 mg IM as a single dose for persons weighing <150 kg (300 lbs) or 1 g of IM ceftriaxone for persons weighing ≥150 kg (300 lbs). If chlamydia has not been excluded, these patients should also receive azithromycin 1 g PO as a single dose. When cephalosporin allergy or other considerations preclude treatment and spectinomycin is not available, consultation with an ID specialist is recommended.

DISPOSITION

- All sexual partners should be identified, examined, tested, and receive presumptive treatment.
- Patients should be counseled to avoid unprotected intercourse with partners for 1 wk after all partners have completed treatment.
- Men or women who have been treated for gonorrhea should be retested in 3 mo because of risk of reinfection. If they are unable to be retested in 3 mo, then they should be retested when they next present to care within 12 mo of their care.

REFERRAL

PID requiring hospitalization, disseminated gonococcal infection

ⓘ PEARLS & CONSIDERATIONS

COMMENTS

- This is a reportable disease.
- The proportion of gonorrhea cases in heterosexual men who are fluoroquinolone resistant (QRNG) has reached 6.7%, an elevenfold increase from 0.6% in 2001. Fluoroquinolone antibiotics are no longer recommended to treat gonorrhea in the U.S.
- The use of azithromycin as the second antimicrobial is preferred over doxycycline in areas of high prevalence of tetracycline resistance.
- The U.S. Preventive Services Task Force (USPSTF) recommends screening for gonorrhea in sexually active females younger than 25 yr and in women 25 and over who are at increased risk for infection (multiple partners, new partner, partner who has concurrent partners). The USPSTF also concludes that the current evidence is insufficient to assess the balance of benefits and harms of screening for gonorrhea in men.
- High-intensity counseling on sexual risk reduction has been shown to reduce sexually transmitted infections (STIs) in primary care and related settings.

SUGGESTED READINGS
Available at eBooks.Health.Elsevier.com.

RELATED CONTENT
Gonorrhea (Patient Information)
Cervicitis (Related Key Topic)
Chlamydia Genital Infections (Related Key Topic)
Pelvic Inflammatory Disease (Related Key Topic)
Urethritis, gonococcal (Related Key Topic)

AUTHORS: **ANTHONY SCISCIONE, DO,** and **ELLA STERN, MD**

Diseases and Disorders

G

I

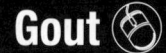

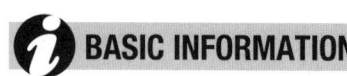 BASIC INFORMATION

DEFINITION

Gout refers to a group of disease states caused by deposition of monosodium urate (MSU) in tissue, resulting from prolonged hyperuricemia. Clinical manifestations of gout include acute and chronic arthritis, soft tissue inflammation, tophus formation, gouty nephropathy, and nephrolithiasis. Untreated hyperuricemia in patients with gout may lead to chronic destructive deforming arthritis.

ICD-10CM CODES
M10	Gout
M10.0	Idiopathic gout
M10.1	Lead-induced gout
M10.2	Drug-induced gout
M10.3	Gout due to impairment of renal function
M10.4	Other secondary gout
M10.9	Gout, unspecified

EPIDEMIOLOGY & DEMOGRAPHICS

PREVALENCE: Self-reported prevalence in the U.S. is estimated at 3.9% of adults.[1] In the U.S., gout has been diagnosed in more than 10 million adults.[2]

PREDOMINANT SEX: Male:female ratio ~4:1. However the prevalence of gout among women has increased in past decade. Compared with men, gout in women is more likely to be associated with diabetes, coronary heart disease, and chronic kidney disease.[3]

PREDOMINANT AGE: 30 to 50 yr in men; >60 yr in women

ETIOLOGY

- Gout is caused by inflammation resulting from MSU crystal deposition. The primary risk factors for MSU deposition are hyperuricemia, although local factors such as temperature, pH, and mechanical stress may play a role. Figs. E1, E2, and E3 illustrate the pathophysiology of gout.
- Hyperuricemia and gout develop from excessive uric acid production, a decrease in the renal excretion of uric acid, or both.
- Primary hyperuricemia results from an inborn error of metabolism and may be attributed to several biochemical defects.
- Secondary hyperuricemia may develop as a complication of acquired disorders (e.g., leukemia) or as a result of the use of certain drugs (e.g., diuretics). Consumption of alcohol, especially beer, increases the risk of gout, and fructose-rich beverage intake is associated with hyperuricemia. Gout promoters and inhibitors are summarized in Table 1.

PHYSICAL FINDINGS & CLINICAL PRESENTATION

ACUTE GOUT:
- Rapid onset of pain and swelling and erythema of a distal joint and/or periarticular soft tissue. Box 1 summarizes clinical pearls in acute gout attacks.
- May present as monoarthritis of any joint. Acute gout of the first metatarsophalangeal (MTP) joint is known as *podagra*.
- 10% to 15% of attacks are polyarticular.

- Spontaneous resolution occurs over days to weeks.

CHRONIC TOPHACEOUS GOUT (FIG. E1):
- Insidious onset of painless arthritis and soft tissue swelling
- Distal small joints characteristic
- May be confused with nodal osteoarthritis
- Box 2 summarizes clinical pearls in chronic gout

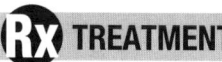 DIAGNOSIS

DIFFERENTIAL DIAGNOSIS OF ACUTE GOUT
- Septic arthritis, cellulitis
- Pseudogout, calcium pyrophosphate crystal deposition disease
- Trauma

DIFFERENTIAL DIAGNOSIS OF CHRONIC GOUT
- Osteoarthritis (OA; especially nodal OA in women)
- Rheumatoid arthritis
- Psoriatic arthritis

Section II describes the differential diagnosis of acute monoarticular and oligoarticular arthritis.

WORKUP
Arthrocentesis and examination of synovial fluid

LABORATORY TESTS
- Uric acid: All patients with gout are hyperuricemic at some time, but during an acute attack the serum uric acid may be normal or low.
- Synovial aspirate: Usually cloudy and markedly inflammatory in nature (elevated white blood cells). Urate crystals in fluid are needle

shaped and strongly negatively birefringent under polarized microscopy[4] (Fig. E5).
- CBC: Neutrophilic leukocytosis often present.
- Inflammatory markers: Erythrocyte sedimentation rate and C-reactive protein often elevated.

IMAGING STUDIES
- Plain radiography for diagnosis and evaluation. No typical findings in early gouty arthritis, but late disease is associated with characteristic punched-out marginal erosions (Fig. E6) and overhanging edges.
- Musculoskeletal ultrasound has been shown to be an effective means of detecting monosodium urate crystal deposition. Ultrasound can differentiate urate crystals that are found on the surface of articular cartilage from CPPD crystals that are seen within the substance of the cartilage (Fig. E7). Double contour sign can be seen.[5]
- Dual-energy computed tomography (DECT) allows for color-coded images and detection of gout deposits and may be beneficial if there is difficulty in establishing the diagnosis.

TREATMENT

TREATMENT OPTIONS FOR ACUTE GOUT (TABLE 2)
- Nonsteroidal antiinflammatory medication (Table 3).
  1. Indomethacin 75 mg bid
  2. Ibuprofen 800 mg tid
  3. Naproxen 500 mg bid
  4. Celecoxib 200 mg bid
- Low-dose colchicine (less toxic, as effective as traditional high-dose colchicine): 1.2 mg PO, followed by 0.6 mg PO 1 h later, then 0.6 mg/day or bid. Dose for renal function.[6]

TABLE 1 Gout Promoters and Inhibitors*

Crystal formation	Seed nucleus (particulate)
	Immunoglobulin
	Phagocytes
	Low temperature
	Low pH
	Cation concentration
	Intraarticular dehydration
	Other (unknown) macromolecules
Triggering the acute flare (local factors)	Rapid change in urate level
	Microcrystal release
	IgG coat (apolipoproteins B, E inhibitory)
	Complement activation (classical, alternate, MAC)
	Inflammasome activation
	Cytokine and chemokine release
	Endothelial activation (e-selectin, ICAM-1, VCAM-1)
	Local trauma
Presence of susceptible phagocytes, mast cells (systemic events)	Surgery, trauma
	Infections, other intercurrent systemic illness
	Alcohol, dietary intake
	Drugs that raise or lower circulating urate level

ICAM-1, Intercellular adhesion molecule 1; *Ig,* immunoglobulin; *MAC,* membrane attack complex; *VCAM-1,* vascular cell adhesion molecule 1.

*A diverse array of proteins and other mediators have been identified on the surfaces of urate crystals. In addition to their proinflammatory effect through opsonizing existing crystals, immunoglobulin M (IgM) and immunoglobulin G (IgG) antibodies may promote crystal formation by providing a stable molecular platform for crystal nucleation and growth. Apolipoproteins are antiinflammatory molecules that coat crystals. The characteristics of the phagocytes encountering the crystals may be crucial; macrophages that are more differentiated are less likely to elicit proinflammatory cytokines.

From Hochberg MC et al: *Rheumatology,* ed 7, Philadelphia, 2019, Elsevier.

- Intraarticular corticosteroid injection (treatment of choice for monoarticular large joint attack): Triamcinolone acetonide 40 mg or equivalent for knee.
- Systemic corticosteroid therapy: Prednisone 40 mg PO for 3 days, then taper over 10 days (limited evidence currently, but studies have shown efficacy).[7]

TREATMENT OF HYPERURICEMIA IN PATIENTS WITH GOUT

The American College of Rheumatology, as well as most international rheumatology guidelines, recommend that every patient with gout who has tophi, more than two attacks of gout per year, chronic kidney disease, or nephrolithiasis be treated with pharmacologic urate-lowering therapy. Serum uric acid should be monitored on a regular basis and urate-lowering therapy intensified until a target of less than 6 mg/dl is reached. In most cases, urate-lowering therapy should be continued for life. Fig. E8 summarizes pharmacologic serum urate–lowering treatment.[1]

The American College of Physicians Guidelines recommends a more conservative approach based on recurrence of symptoms. These guidelines have been criticized for ignoring the progressive nature of gout and perpetuating the well-documented underuse and under-dosing of urate-lowering therapy.

NONPHARMACOLOGIC THERAPY

Lifestyle and dietary modification should always be a component of therapy for patients with gout, but this is rarely effective without concomitant pharmacologic urate-lowering therapy, as dietary modification can lower uric acid only about 1 mg/dl. Recommendations include reducing ingestion of red meat, kidney, liver, yeast extract, shellfish, and overall protein along with restricting alcohol intake. Discontinuation of diuretic therapy may help lower serum uric acid. Women with normal weight and best adherence to dietary approaches to stop hypertension (DASH) diet have a 68% lower risk for gout than women who are overweight or obese and are least adherent to the DASH diet.[3]

PHARMACOLOGIC TREATMENT OF SYMPTOMATIC HYPERURICEMIA

ALLOPURINOL: Allopurinol is very effective and safe when used properly. Correct dosing and patient compliance are essential elements in the prevention of erosive and tophaceous gout. Patients with renal insufficiency are at increased risk for allopurinol hypersensitivity, which manifests as fever, rash, and hepatitis occurring most commonly in the first 3 months of therapy. The rash may progress to life-threatening toxic epidermal necrolysis if not recognized early.

Traditionally, therapy with allopurinol is initiated several weeks after the acute attack has resolved. However, initiation of allopurinol at presentation may improve long-term compliance without reducing the efficacy of acute treatment. The initial dose should be low ($\leq$100 mg/day depending on creatinine clearance) in patients with renal insufficiency and those with very high uric acid levels.[8] High initial doses are associated with increased incidence of allopurinol hypersensitivity. The serum uric acid should be reevaluated after 4 to 6 wk of therapy, and the allopurinol dose adjusted to reduce the serum uric acid to <6 mg/dl. The most common therapeutic dosage of allopurinol is 300 mg/day, but the dose may be increased by 50 to 100 mg every 2 to 3 wk until the target serum uric acid level is achieved. There is evidence that increasing allopurinol doses in patients with renal insufficiency does not result in significant toxicity, but concurrent use with statins and colchicine is associated with a higher incidence of adverse effects. Some authors have reported using doses as high as 800 mg/day without excess toxicity. It is recommended that patients of Han Chinese, Thai, and Korean ancestry be tested for HLA-B*5801 before initiating allopurinol as these individuals are at high risk of allopurinol hypersensitivity if this allele is present.[1]

FEBUXOSTAT: Febuxostat is a xanthine oxidase inhibitor that has been shown to be more potent than allopurinol 300 mg/day for reducing serum uric acid. The chemical structure of febuxostat is different from allopurinol, making cross-reactive allergy unlikely. The metabolism of febuxostat is primarily hepatic, which obviates the need for dose adjustments because of renal insufficiency. Some cases of hepatic toxicity have been reported, and it is recommended that liver function tests be monitored. Febuxostat may help preserve renal function in patients with chronic kidney disease (CKD) but has not been tested in patients with severe renal failure.[1]

The primary indication for febuxostat is demonstrated allergy to allopurinol. The cost of febuxostat may be as much as 40 times that of allopurinol, and there is some evidence suggesting that febuxostat may be associated with higher cardiovascular and all-cause mortality than allopurinol in patients with cardiovascular risk factors. In 2019 the FDA added a boxed warning for increased risk of death with febuxostat.[9]

PROBENECID: Uricosuric agents may be used in patients with good renal function and urinary uric acid <600 mg in a 24-h collection. Probenecid can be used in patients with intolerance to xanthene-oxidase inhibitors. Compliance is poor due to the necessity of taking the drug more often than once daily.[1]

LESINURAD: Lesinurad is a URAT1 and OAT4 inhibitor approved by the FDA in 2015 for gout-associated hyperuricemia unresponsive to xanthine oxidase inhibitor monotherapy, to be taken in combination with a xanthine oxidase inhibitor.[10] This drug was withdrawn in 2019 because of business-related reasons without safety concerns noted.

PEGLOTICASE: Intravenous PEGylated uricase is FDA approved for treatment of severe refractory tophaceous gout. It is a PEGylated recombinant mammalian uricase that rapidly degrades urate when given intravenously. Use is limited by very high cost and potential toxicities, including frequent gout flares and anaphylaxis. Rasburicase is a nonpegylated uricase used in tumor lysis syndrome and is not indicated for gout treatment.[11]

REFERRAL

- Rheumatologist if diagnosis is not clear or therapy is complicated
- Podiatrist for management of pedal complications

⊘ PEARLS & CONSIDERATIONS

- Adherence to a healthful dietary pattern reduces risk of gout. A recent study revealed that women with normal weight and best adherence to the DASH diet (dietary approaches to stop hypertension) had 68% lower risk for gout than did women who were overweight and were nonadherent to the DASH diet.[12]
- The interleukin-1 receptor antagonist anakinra (Kineret) is an effective off-label agent for treatment of gout in complex patients with contraindications to standard therapies. One study found 75% of patients using the biologic saw a partial or complete abatement of symptoms within 4 days.[13]

TABLE 2 Therapeutic Options for Acute Gouty Inflammation

Drug Option	Level of Evidence	Typical Regimens
COX-nonselective NSAIDs	Grade A evidence for each regimen listed	Naproxen, 750-1000 mg/day PO in divided doses for 3 days; then 500-750 mg total daily for 4-7 days Sulindac, 300-400 mg/day in divided doses for 7-10 days Indomethacin, 150-200 mg/day PO in divided doses for 3 days; then 100 mg/day PO in divided doses for 4-7 days
COX-2–selective NSAIDs	Grade A	For example: Celecoxib, 800 mg; then 400 mg on day 1, followed by 400 mg bid for 7 days
Systemic corticosteroids	Grade A evidence for oral prednisolone, 35 mg/day for five or six doses; lower evidence grades for other regimens	Prednisone, 30-60 mg/day for 3 days; then taper every 3 days by 10-15 mg less as a daily dose until discontinuation Oral prednisolone, 35 mg/day for 5-7 days Medrol dose pack (for less severe flares) or to initiate therapy In an NPO patient: • Triamcinolone, 60 mg IM once with additional corticosteroid treatment as needed • Methylprednisolone, 100-150 mg IV for 1-2 days
Intraarticular corticosteroids	Grade C evidence	Particularly useful for flares in a single large joint Triamcinolone acetonide preparations are especially useful Dose titrated to the size of the joint
ACTH	Grade C evidence	25 USP units of synthetic ACTH SC for less severe flares; 40 USP units IM or IV once for more severe flares (including larger joint flares and polyarticular gout) One or two repeated doses of synthetic ACTH at intervals of 12 h are often required with each of these regimens
Oral colchicine	Grade A evidence for FDA-approved regimen	In the U.S: To treat an early acute gout flare: 1.2 mg once followed by 0.6 mg in 1 h and then 12 h later; oral low-dose colchicine at prophylaxis doses until the acute gout flare resolves Outside the U.S: 0.5 mg tid for several days is the EULAR-recommended dosing regimen Oral colchicine treatment of acute gout should be limited to once every 2 wk in those already taking a maintenance low dose of colchicine
Off-label use in U.S: IL-1 antagonism	Grade C for anakinra; grade A for canakinumab	Use of anakinra (e.g., 100 mg/day SC for 3 days) or canakinumab (150 mg SC as single dose) for acute gout flare is not approved by the FDA, but canakinumab is approved by the EMA for this indication

ACTH, Adrenocorticotropic hormone; *bid,* twice a day; *COX,* cyclooxygenase; *EMA,* European Medicines Agency; *EULAR,* European League Against Rheumatism; *FDA,* U.S. Food and Drug Administration; *IL-1,* interleukin-1; *IM,* intramuscularly; *IV,* intravenously; *NPO,* nothing by mouth; *NSAID,* nonsteroidal antiinflammatory drug; *PO,* by mouth; *SC,* subcutaneously; *tid,* three times a day; *USP,* U.S. Pharmacopeia.
From Hochberg MC et al: *Rheumatology,* ed 7, Philadelphia, 2019, Elsevier.

TABLE 3 Treatment of Gout

Acute Gout	Interval Gout	Treatment of Hyperuricemia
NSAIDs (preferred): Indomethacin 50 mg qid or ibuprofen 800 mg tid (or other NSAID in full doses). Contraindicated in patients with renal insufficiency and gastrointestinal disorders. *Or* **Colchicine, oral:** 1.2 mg followed by a second dose of 0.6 mg 1 h later. Contraindicated in patients with renal insufficiency and gastrointestinal disorders *Or* **Intraarticular steroids** (Treatment of choice for large joint monoarthritis): Triamcinolone 40 mg or equivalent for knee *Or* **Systemic steroid therapy** (for patients in whom NSAIDs and colchicine are contraindicated) Prednisone 30-50 mg/day PO or in divided doses. May use lower dose in diabetic or postsurgical patients.	**Colchicine, oral:** 0.6-1.2 mg/day as prophylaxis against recurrent attacks. **NSAIDs may also be used for prophylaxis.** **Hypouricemic agent:** Indicated for patients with recurrent attacks despite prophylaxis, severe hyperuricemia, presence of tophi, urolithiasis, or gouty arthritis **Other:** Weight loss, reduce alcohol (especially beer), diet low in seafood, red meat, organ meat, and fructose	**Colchicine, oral:** 0.6-1.2 mg/day for 4-6 wk before initiating hypouricemic therapy and for several months afterward to prevent recurrent attacks during initiation of hypouricemic therapy *And* **Allopurinol:** Initial dose 100 mg/day in patients with renal insufficiency or very high uric acid levels. Increase dose as needed to attain uric acid less than 6 mg/dl *Or* **Uricosuric agent** (Use only in patients with good renal function and <600 mg uric acid in a 24-h collection): Probenecid, 0.5-1 g bid, or sulfinpyrazone 100 mg tid or qid **Other:** Consider febuxostat for patients allergic to allopurinol and the addition of lesinurad in patients resistant to xanthine oxidase inhibitors. Pegloticase may be useful for selected patients with severe tophaceous gout

bid, Twice a day; *NSAID,* nonsteroidal antiinflammatory drug; *PO,* by mouth; *qid,* four times a day; *tid,* three times a day.

- Do not stop allopurinol during hospitalizations, surgery, or acute attacks unless there is evidence of drug allergy. The dosage of allopurinol should be adjusted in patients with acute kidney injury.

PATIENT & FAMILY EDUCATION

It is essential that patients, families, physicians, and other members of the health care team appreciate the importance of compliance with a daily allopurinol regimen if recurrent flares and progression to chronic arthritis and tophi are to be avoided. Allopurinol should be discontinued only for symptoms suggesting hypersensitivity; otherwise, it should be continued during flares, medical illnesses, and surgical procedures.[14]

REFERENCES

Available at eBooks.Health.Elsevier.com.

RELATED CONTENT

Gout (Patient Information)
Hyperuricemia (Related Key Topic)

AUTHORS: **OMAR KARIM, BS,** and **CAROLINE P. MEEHAN, MD**

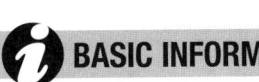
BASIC INFORMATION

DEFINITION

Graves disease is a hypermetabolic state caused by circulating immunoglobulin G (IgG) antibodies that bind to and activate the G-protein–coupled thyrotropin receptor. This activation stimulates follicular hypertrophy and hyperplasia, causing thyroid enlargement as well as increases in thyroid hormone production. It affects the thyroid, ocular muscles, and shin. It is characterized by thyrotoxicosis, diffuse goiter, and infiltrative ophthalmopathy (edema and inflammation of the extraocular muscles and an increase in orbital connective tissue and fat); infiltrative dermopathy characterized by lymphocytic infiltration of the dermis; accumulation of glycosaminoglycans; and occasionally edema.

SYNONYM

Thyrotoxicosis

ICD-10CM CODES
E05.00 Thyrotoxicosis with diffuse goiter without thyrotoxic crisis or storm
E05.01 Thyrotoxicosis with diffuse goiter with thyrotoxic crisis or storm

EPIDEMIOLOGY & DEMOGRAPHICS

INCIDENCE & PREVALENCE: Graves disease is the most common cause of hyperthyroidism. It affects 3% of women and 0.5% of men during their lifetime. There is a slight increased incidence among young African Americans. The annual incidence of Graves disease–associated ophthalmopathy is 16 cases/100,000 women and 3 cases/100,000 men. It is more common in Whites than Asians. Cigarette smoking is a risk factor.
PREDOMINANT AGE: Peak incidence is between 30 and 60 yr.
GENETICS: Patients often report a family history of Hashimoto thyroiditis, Graves disease, or other autoimmune conditions. Increased prevalence of *HLA-B8* and *HLA-DR3* in Whites with Graves disease. Concordance rate is 20% among monozygotic twins.

PHYSICAL FINDINGS & CLINICAL PRESENTATION

- Diffusely enlarged thyroid. Thyroid bruit may be present. Cervical lymphadenopathy also may be present
- Elevated systolic blood pressure with a widened pulse pressure
- Tachycardia, palpitations, tremor, hyperreflexia
- Exophthalmos (50% of patients) (Fig. E1, Fig. E2), lid retraction (lid lag), in which contraction of the levator palpebrae muscles of the eyelids show immobility of the upper eyelid with downward rotation of the eye
- Nervousness, weight loss (weight gain in 10% of patients), heat intolerance, pruritus, muscle weakness, atrial fibrillation
- Increased sweating, brittle nails, clubbing of fingers
- Localized infiltrative dermopathy (1% to 2% of patients) is most frequent over the anterolateral aspects of the legs, commonly over the pretibial area (pretibial myxedema) but can be found at other sites (especially after trauma). It is nonpitting and indurated. It is typically patchy with a peau d'orange appearance to the skin
- Men may have gynecomastia, reduced libido, and erectile dysfunction. Women often have irregular menses

ETIOLOGY

Autoimmune etiology: Thyrotropin receptor antibodies (TRAb) mediated activation of thyroid-stimulating hormone receptor (TSHR). The activity of the thyroid gland is stimulated by the action of T cells, which induce specific B cells to synthesize antibodies against TSHRs in the follicular cell membrane.

DIAGNOSIS

DIFFERENTIAL DIAGNOSIS

- Anxiety disorder
- Premenopausal state
- Thyroiditis
- Other causes of hyperthyroidism (e.g., toxic multinodular goiter, toxic adenoma)
- Other: Metastatic neoplasm, diabetes mellitus, pheochromocytoma

WORKUP

- The diagnosis is made clinically in most instances. The clinical assessment of the patient with Graves orbitopathy is summarized in Table 1.
- The diagnostic workup includes a detailed medical history followed by laboratory and imaging studies and ECG. Patients often present with anxiety, heat intolerance, menstrual dysfunction, increased appetite, and weight loss. Elderly patients can have an atypical presentation (apathetic hyperparathyroidism). For additional information, refer to the topic "Hyperthyroidism."

LABORATORY TESTS

- Increased free thyroxine (T_4) and free triiodothyronine (T_3)
- Decreased thyroid-stimulating hormone
- Measurement of thyroid-stimulating antibodies (TSI) and TRAb
- Table E2 summarizes assays of TSHR antibody nomenclature and indications

IMAGING STUDIES

- 24-h radioactive iodine uptake (RAIU): Increased homogeneous uptake.
- Computed tomography (Fig. E3) or MRI of the orbits (Fig. E4) is useful if there is uncertainty about the cause of ophthalmopathy.

TREATMENT

NONPHARMACOLOGIC THERAPY

- Patient education and discussion of therapeutic options.
- Smoking cessation: Smoking is associated with an increased risk of progression of Graves ophthalmopathy.

ACUTE GENERAL Rx

- Advantages and disadvantages of treatment options for Graves hyperthyroidism are summarized in Table E3.
- Antithyroid drugs (thionamides, ATDs) to inhibit thyroid hormone synthesis or peripheral conversion of T_4 to T_3:
  1. Methimazole or propylthiouracil (PTU) are available. Methimazole is generally preferred because it has a longer half-life, allowing for once-daily dosing. PTU is preferred during pregnancy.
  2. Side effects: Skin rash (3% to 5%), arthralgias, myalgias, granulocytopenia (0.5%); rare side effects: Aplastic anemia, hepatic necrosis (PTU), cholestatic jaundice.
  3. Thionamide antithyroid drug therapy results in a remission in 40% to 50% of patients treated for 12 to 18 mo.
- Radioactive iodine (RAI):
  1. Treatment of choice for patients >21 yr and younger patients who have not achieved remission after 1 yr of ATD therapy.
  2. Contraindicated during pregnancy and lactation.
  3. After radioactive therapy there may be an acute elevation of thyroid antibody titers and exacerbation of ocular symptoms in 15% to 20% of patients.
- Surgery: Near-total thyroidectomy. Indications: Obstructing goiters despite RAI and ATD therapy, patients who refuse RAI and cannot be adequately managed with ATDs, and pregnant women inadequately managed with ATDs. Complications of surgery include hypoparathyroidism (4%) and vocal cord paralysis (1%).
- Adjunctive therapy: Beta-adrenergic receptor blockers (e.g., atenolol 50 to 100 mg/day) to alleviate the beta-adrenergic symptoms of hyperthyroidism (tachycardia, tremor); contraindicated in patients with bronchospasm.
- Graves ophthalmopathy: Methylcellulose eye drops to protect against excessive dryness, sunglasses to decrease photophobia, intraocular and systemic high-dose corticosteroids for severe exophthalmos. Worsening of ophthalmopathy after RAI therapy is often transient and can be prevented by the administration of prednisone. Other treatment options include antiinflammatory and immunosuppressive agents, radiation, and corrective surgical procedures. The administration of the antioxidant selenium (100 μg PO bid) has been recently reported as effective in improving quality of life, reducing ocular involvement, and slowing progression of the disease in patients with mild Graves orbitopathy. Its mechanism of action is believed to be an effect on the oxygen free radicals and cytokines that play a pathogenic role in Graves orbitopathy. Inhibition of the insulin-like growth factor I receptor (IGF-IR) is a new therapeutic strategy to combat the underlying autoimmune etiology of ophthalmopathy.

TABLE 1 Clinical Assessment of Patient With Graves Orbitopathy

SEVERITY MEASURES (USING THE MNEMONIC NO SPECS)

NO SPECS Class	Item	Method
0. **N**o signs or symptoms		
1. **O**nly signs, no symptoms	Lid aperture	With ruler in midline in mm
2. **S**oft tissue involvement	Eyelid and conjunctiva swelling and redness	Inspection, color pictures[a]
3. **P**roptosis	Exophthalmos	Hertel in mm
4. **E**xtraocular muscle involvement	Eye muscle motility Diplopia	Impaired elevation, abduction Subjective grading[b]
5. **C**orneal involvement	Keratitis, ulcer	Fluoresceine
6. **S**ight loss caused by optic nerve involvement	Dysthyroid optic neuropathy (DON)	Visual acuity, color vision, visual fields, optic disc

ACTIVITY MEASURES (USING THE CLINICAL ACTIVITY SCORE [CAS])

Inflammatory Sign	Item	Score
Pain	Spontaneous retrobulbar pain	1
	Pain on up gaze, side gaze, or down gaze	1
Redness	Redness of the eyelids	1
	Redness of the conjunctiva	1
Swelling	Swelling of the eyelids	1
	Swelling of the caruncle and/or plica	1
	Chemosis	1
Maximum CAS Score (assessed momently)		*7*
Impaired function	Increase in proptosis $\geq$2 mm in 1-3 mo	1
	Decrease of $\geq$8 degrees in eye muscle motility in any direction in 1-3 mo	1
		1
	Decrease in visual acuity of more than one line on the Snellen chart (using pinhole) in 1-3 mo	
Maximum CAS Score (assessed over time)		*10*

[a]Color atlas in Dickinson AJ, Perros P: Controversies in the clinical evaluation of active thyroid-associated orbitopathy: use of a detailed protocol with comparative photographs for objective assessment, *Clin Endocrinol (Oxf)* 55:283-303, 2001.
[b]Intermittent diplopia = at awakening or when tired; inconstant diplopia = at extremes of gaze; constant diplopia = in primary or reading position.
CAS, Clinical activity score.
From Melmed S et al: *Williams textbook of endocrinology,* ed 14, Philadelphia, 2020, Elsevier.

Trials with teprotumumab, a human monoclonal antibody inhibitor of IGF-IR, in patients with active, moderate-to-severe ophthalmopathy have shown effectiveness in reducing proptosis.[1]

- Dermopathy and acropachy: Topical corticosteroids are often used but are generally ineffective. Trials using rituximab infusion for dermopathy have shown striking improvement.

CHRONIC Rx

Patients undergoing treatment with ATDs should be seen every 1 to 3 mo until euthyroidism is achieved and every 3 to 4 mo while they are receiving ATDs.

DISPOSITION

- ATDs induce sustained remission in <60% of cases.

- The incidence of hypothyroidism after RAI is >50% within the first yr and 2% per yr thereafter.
- Complications of surgery include hypothyroidism (28% to 43% after 10 yr), hypoparathyroidism (4%), and vocal cord paralysis (1%).
- Successful treatment of hyperthyroidism requires lifelong monitoring for the onset of hypothyroidism or the recurrence of thyrotoxicosis.
- RAI therapy is followed by the appearance or worsening of ophthalmopathy more often than is therapy with methimazole, particularly in patients who are cigarette smokers. It can be prevented with the administration of prednisone 0.5 mg/kg body weight per day starting 2 to 3 days after RAI, continued for 1 mo, then tapered off over 2 mo.

- Mild to moderate ophthalmopathy often improves spontaneously. Severe cases can be treated with high-dose glucocorticoids, orbital irradiation, or both. Orbital decompression may be used in patients with optic neuropathy and exophthalmos (see "Hyperthyroidism").

REFERENCE & SUGGESTED READINGS

Available at eBooks.Health.Elsevier.com.

RELATED CONTENT

Graves Disease (Patient Information)
Hyperthyroidism (Related Key Topic)

AUTHOR: **FRED F. FERRI, MD**

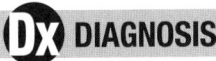

BASIC INFORMATION

DEFINITION

Guillain-Barré syndrome (GBS) is an acute immune-mediated polyradiculoneuropathy (affects nerve roots and peripheral nerves) with predominantly motor involvement. It is the most common cause of acute flaccid paralysis in the Western hemisphere and probably worldwide. By definition, maximal clinical weakness, the clinical nadir, occurs within 4 wk of disease onset. Several variations from the typical presentation of GBS exist (Box 1).

SYNONYMS

GBS
AIDP (acute inflammatory demyelinating polyradiculoneuropathy)
Acute polyneuropathy
Ascending paralysis
Postinfectious polyneuritis

ICD-10CM CODE
G61.0 Guillain-Barré syndrome

EPIDEMIOLOGY & DEMOGRAPHICS

INCIDENCE: 0.81 to 1.9 cases/100,000 persons annually without geographic variation. Incidence increases with age. A slight peak in incidence occurs between late adolescence and early adulthood. A slight male preponderance (3:2) also exists.[1]

PREDISPOSING FACTORS: Viral (HIV, cytomegalovirus [CMV], Epstein-Barr virus [EBV], influenza) and bacterial *(Campylobacter jejuni, Mycoplasma pneumoniae)* infections; systemic illness (Hodgkin lymphoma, immunizations). Major antecedents of GBS are described in Box E2.[2]

PHYSICAL FINDINGS & CLINICAL PRESENTATION

- Symmetric weakness, most commonly involving proximal muscles initially, subsequently involving both proximal and distal muscles; difficulty in ambulating, getting up from a chair, or climbing stairs (Box 3)[3]
- Depressed or absent reflexes bilaterally
- Minimal to moderate glove and stocking paresthesias/dysesthesia/anesthesia or back pain[1]
- Pain (caused by involvement of posterior nerve roots) may be prominent
- Autonomic abnormalities (bradyarrhythmias or tachyarrhythmias, hypotension or hypertension, constipation, urinary retention)[4]
- Respiratory insufficiency (caused by weakness of bulbar/intercostal muscles)
- Facial paresis, ophthalmoparesis, dysphagia (secondary to cranial nerve involvement)
- GBS consists of several clinical variants based on the pattern of clinical involvement and electrophysiologic findings. These include[1]:
  1. AIDP (most common form in Europe and North America)
  2. Acute motor axonal neuropathy (AMAN; most prevalent form in China and Japan)
  3. Acute motor and sensory axonal neuropathy (AMSAN; has more severe sensory involvement and is associated with more severe clinical course and poorer prognosis)
  4. Miller Fisher syndrome (MFS; triad of ophthalmoplegia, ataxia, and areflexia)
  5. Acute pandysautonomia (rapid onset of parasympathetic and sympathetic failure without motor or sensory involvement)
  6. Regional variants (e.g., pharyngeal-cervical-brachial GBS, pure ataxic GBS)

ETIOLOGY

- Unknown, but thought to be caused by infection-induced aberrant immune response.[1]
- Preceding infectious illness 1 to 4 wk before disease onset has been noted. Antecedent events of GBS are summarized in Table 1.[5] The most frequent antecedent infection is *C. jejuni* (associated with 30% of cases of GBS).[6]
- Humoral and cell-mediated immune attack of peripheral nerve myelin, Schwann cells; sometimes with primary axonal involvement.[1]

BOX 1 Classification of Guillain–Barré Syndrome Subtypes and Variants

Common Subtypes
Acute inflammatory demyelinating polyradiculoneuropathy (AIDP)
Acute motor axonal neuropathy (AMAN)
Acute motor-sensory axonal neuropathy (AMSAN)

Rare Variants
Miller-Fisher syndrome
Ataxic variant (acute ataxic neuropathy)
Pharyngeal-cervical-brachial variant
Multiple cranial neuropathy variant
Facial diplegia with paresthesias
Paraparetic variant
Acute pandysautonomia

From Jankovic J et al: *Bradley and Daroff's neurology in clinical practice,* ed 8, Philadelphia, 2022, Elsevier.

BOX 3 Findings Suggesting Guillain-Barré Syndrome

Relative symmetry of symptoms
Mild sensory signs and symptoms
Cranial nerve involvement
Autonomic dysfunction
Absence of fever at onset
Cytoalbuminologic dissociation of cerebrospinal fluid
Typical electrodiagnostic findings
Progression over days to weeks
Recovery beginning 2-4 wk after cessation of progression

From Adams JG: *Emergency medicine: clinical essentials,* Philadelphia, 2013, Saunders.

DIAGNOSIS

DIFFERENTIAL DIAGNOSIS (BOX 4)[5]

- Toxic peripheral neuropathies: Heavy metal poisoning (lead [microcytic anemia], thallium [alopecia], arsenic [typically accompanied by acute GI illness]), medications (vincristine, disulfiram), organophosphate poisoning, hexacarbon (glue sniffer neuropathy)
- Nontoxic peripheral neuropathies: Acute intermittent porphyria, fulminant vasculitic polyneuropathy, infectious (poliomyelitis, diphtheria, Lyme disease, West Nile virus), tick paralysis
- Neuromuscular junction disorders: Myasthenia gravis, botulism, snake envenomation
- Polymyositis and acute necrotizing myopathies
- Metabolic derangements such as hypermagnesemia, hypokalemia, hypophosphatemia
- Acute central nervous system (CNS) disorders such as basilar artery thrombosis with brain stem infarction, brain stem encephalomyelitis, transverse myelitis, or spinal cord compression
- Conversion disorder
- Malingering
- Table 2 differentiates clinical patterns of acute neuromuscular weakness

WORKUP

- Exclude other causes based on clinical history, examination, and laboratory tests.
- Lumbar puncture (may be normal in the first 1 to 2 wk of the illness). Typical findings include elevated cerebrospinal fluid (CSF) protein with few mononuclear leukocytes (albuminocytologic dissociation) in 80% to 90% of patients. Elevated CSF cell counts is an expected characteristic in cases associated with HIV seroconversion.
- Electromyography (EMG)/nerve conduction study (NCS) may be normal in the first 10 to 14 days of the disease. The earliest electrodiagnostic abnormality is prolongation or absence of H-reflexes. NCS evidence of demyelination (prolonged distal latency, conduction velocity slowing, conduction block, temporal dispersion, and prolonged F-waves) in two or more motor nerves confirms diagnosis of AIDP in the appropriate clinical context.

LABORATORY TESTS

- CBC may reveal early leukocytosis with left shift. Electrolytes are tested to exclude metabolic causes of weakness.
- Heavy metal testing; urine porphyria screen; creatine kinase; HIV testing, including tests for HIV seroconversion, especially if CSF demonstrates lymphocytic pleocytosis. MRI of brain and spinal cord with and without contrast may be indicated if diagnosis is uncertain. In GBS, a gadolinium-enhanced MRI of the lumbosacral spine may reveal nerve root enhancement.

TABLE 1 Antecedent Events of Guillain-Barré Syndrome

Antecedent Event	Percentage
Respiratory illness	58
Gastrointestinal illness	22
Respiratory and gastrointestinal illness	10
Surgery	5
Vaccination	3
Other	2
Serologic Evidence of Specific Infectious Agents	
Campylobacter jejuni	
Cytomegalovirus	
Human immunodeficiency virus	
Epstein-Barr virus	
Mycoplasma pneumonia	
Hepatitis A and B	
Zika virus	

From Jankovic J et al: *Bradley and Daroff's neurology in clinical practice,* ed 8, Philadelphia 2022, Elsevier.

- Antibodies against ganglioside GQ1b may be present in up to 90% of patients with MFS. Immunoglobulin G antibodies against ganglioside GM1 may be associated with AMAN. There are no antiganglioside antibodies commonly associated with AIDP.
- In equivocal cases, especially if peripheral nerve vasculitis is a concern, nerve biopsy may aid in confirming a diagnosis of GBS. Sensory nerve biopsy demonstrates segmental demyelination with infiltration of monocytes and T cells into the endoneurium. Axonal loss is commonly seen in sensory nerve biopsy specimens in GBS.

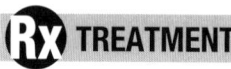 **TREATMENT**

NONPHARMACOLOGIC THERAPY

- Close monitoring of respiratory function (frequent measurements of vital capacity, negative inspiratory force, and tidal volume) and pulmonary toilet should be done because respiratory failure is the major complication in GBS
- Frequent repositioning of patient to minimize formation of pressure sores
- Prevention of venous thromboembolism with antithrombotic stockings as a supplement to pharmacologic venous thromboembolism prevention
- Emotional support and social counseling for patient and family
- Pain control
- Cardiac monitoring to detect arrhythmias
- Physical and occupational therapy once patient is medically stable and able to participate

ACUTE GENERAL Rx

- Option 1: Infusion of IV immunoglobulins (IVIG; 0.4 g/kg/day for 5 days). Always check serum

BOX 4 Differential Diagnostic Considerations in Guillain-Barré Syndrome

Muscle Disorders
- Polymyositis
- Dermatomyositis
- Necrotizing autoimmune myopathy
- Rhabdomyolysis (drugs, toxins, exercise, trauma, metabolic myopathies, etc.)
- Critical illness myopathy

Muscle Membrane Disorders
- Familial periodic paralysis
- Secondary hypokalemic paralysis (thyrotoxicosis, malabsorption, barium salt poisoning, or abuse of diuretics, laxatives, or licorice)

Neuromuscular Junction Disorders
- Myasthenia gravis (myasthenic crisis)
- Botulism
- Drug-induced neuromuscular blockade
- Toxic
  - Organophosphate
  - Nerve gas
  - Tick
  - Black widow spider
  - Snake venoms
- Metabolic
  - Hypermagnesemia (toxemia of pregnancy treated with parenteral magnesium, magnesium-containing antacids, or cathartics)
  - Hypophosphatemia (parenteral hyperalimentation, phosphate-bindings antacids, acute alcohol intoxication, and severe respiratory alkalosis)

Peripheral Nerve and/Root Disorders
- Guillain-Barré syndrome
- Acute intermittent porphyria
- Diphtheritic polyneuropathy
- Critical illness polyneuropathy
- Vasculitic neuropathy
- Heavy metal acute poisoning (thallium, arsenic)
- Diffuse polyradiculopathy
  - Infectious (Lyme, cytomegalovirus [CMV])
  - Inflammatory (sarcoidosis)
  - Neoplastic (solid tumors, lymphomas)

Anterior Horn Cell Disorders
- Acute poliomyelitis (wild-type polio viruses, West Nile virus, enteroviruses)

Spinal Cord Disorders
- Transverse myelitis
- Cord compression (disc herniation, fracture/dislocation, epidural malignancy)
- Cord infarction (anterior spinal artery syndrome)

Brain Stem Disorders
- Central pontine myelinolysis
- Pontine infarct (basilar artery thrombosis)

From Jankovic J et al: *Bradley and Daroff's neurology in clinical practice,* ed 8, Philadelphia, 2022, Elsevier.

IgA levels before infusion to prevent anaphylaxis in IgA-deficient patients.
- Option 2: Early therapeutic plasma exchange (TPE or plasmapheresis: 200 to 250 ml/kg over five sessions every other day), started within 7 days of onset of symptoms, is beneficial in reducing the need for mechanical ventilation in patients with rapidly progressive disease and results in improved rate of recovery. It is contraindicated in patients with cardiovascular disease (recent myocardial infarction [MI], unstable angina), active sepsis, and autonomic dysfunction.
- Both therapies are equally effective and may shorten recovery time by 50%. There is no proven benefit from combining IVIG and plasma exchange. Glucocorticoids are contraindicated.
- Mechanical ventilation may be needed if force vital capacity (FVC) is <12 to 15 ml/kg, vital capacity is rapidly decreasing or is <1000 ml, negative inspiratory force is <20 cm H_2O, PaO_2 is <70, or the patient is having significant difficulty clearing secretions or is aspirating.

CHRONIC Rx

- Ventilatory support may be necessary in 10% to 20% of patients. Adequate fluid/electrolyte support and nutrition are necessary, especially in patients with dysautonomia or bulbar dysfunction.
- Aggressive nursing care to prevent decubitus, infections, fecal impactions, and pressure nerve palsies.
- Monitoring and treatment of autonomic dysfunction (bradyarrhythmias or tachyarrhythmias, orthostatic hypotension, systemic hypertension).

TABLE 2 Clinical Patterns of Acute Neuromuscular Weakness

Cause	Cranial Nerve Involvement	Limb Weakness	Reflexes	Sensory	Autonomic Changes
Guillain-Barré syndrome	Common, facial diplegia	Distal (ascending)	Absent	Common	Possible (20%)
Miller Fisher syndrome	Hallmark: Ophthalmoplegia	Variable hallmark: Ataxia	Absent	Rare	Rare
Myasthenia gravis	Common, ptosis, facial, oculomotor	Proximal (shoulders and thighs)	Normal	Present	Present
Botulism	Symmetric diplopia, ptosis, dysarthria, dysphagia	Descending	Absent or decreased	No	Yes (e.g., ileus, mydriasis, reduced salivation, urinary retention)
Organophosphate poisoning	Bulbar dysfunction, dysarthria, dysphagia	Diffuse	Decreased	Late	Yes (e.g., bradycardia, sialorrhea, bronchorrhea, lacrimation, diarrhea, miosis causing blurry vision)
Brain stem	Common, ocular movement	Crossed findings (face/limbs)	Increased	Common	Rare
Spinal cord	No	Quadriparesis or paraparesis	Decreased then increased	Loss below level	If above thoracic level

From Parrillo JE, Dellinger RP: *Critical care medicine: principles of diagnosis and management in the adult,* ed 5, Philadelphia, 2019, Elsevier.

Diseases and Disorders

I

- Treatment of back pain and dysesthesia with neuropathic pain medications such as tricyclic antidepressants or gabapentin. Opiate narcotics can be used cautiously in the short term but may compound dysautonomia.
- Pharmacologic venous thromboembolism prevention with agents such as heparin (5000 U SC q12h) or enoxaparin (40 mg /day SC) in poorly ambulating and nonambulatory patients.
- Stress ulcer prevention in patients receiving ventilator support.
- Physical and occupational therapy rehabilitation, including supportive devices.

DISPOSITION

- Mortality rate is approximately 3% to 7% worldwide.[1] Causes of death include cardiac arrest, pulmonary embolism, and fulminant infections.
- Complete recovery by 200 days is seen in 80% of patients.[4]
- 65% with incomplete recovery and mild residual symptoms.[4]
- Predictors for poor recovery (inability to walk independently at 1 yr): Age >60 yr, preceding

diarrheal illness, recent CMV infection, fulminant or rapidly progressing course, ventilatory dependence, reduced motor amplitudes (<20% normal), or unexcitable nerves on NCS. Outcomes also may be influenced by complications of medical therapy.[4]
- GBS is a monophasic illness.[1]

REFERRAL

- Neurology to aid in diagnosis and direct treatment
- Pulmonary/critical care for intensive care unit (ICU) management
- Otolaryngology or general surgery for tracheostomy in patients requiring prolonged ventilatory support
- Gastroenterology for percutaneous endoscopic gastrostomy for patients with prolonged inability to obtain nutrition orally

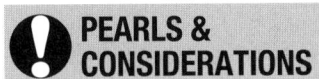 **PEARLS & CONSIDERATIONS**

- GBS is the most common cause of acute flaccid paralysis.

- Close monitoring of ventilatory function with respiratory mechanics (FVC and negative inspiratory force [NIF]) is of paramount importance in all patients with suspected GBS.
- Glucocorticoids are not indicated in GBS and may even slow recovery.
- The association between GBS and common vaccines inspires ongoing debate. A recent study revealed a small increased risk (3 cases per million vaccine doses) of GBS among patients ≥65 yr old following the first dose of the recombinant zoster vaccine (RZV, Shingrix). This risk is numerically similar to GBS risk following actual zoster. There was no excess risk identified after the second doses of the two-dose RZV protocol.[1,7]

REFERENCES
Available at eBooks.Health.Elsevier.com.

RELATED CONTENT
Guillain-Barré Syndrome (Patient Information)

AUTHOR: **LYDIA SHARP, MD**

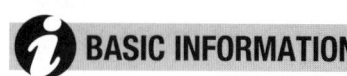
ℹ️ BASIC INFORMATION

DEFINITION

Head and neck squamous cell carcinoma is a malignant disease entity that arises from the epithelium of the mucosal surfaces of the upper aerodigestive tract and accounts for nearly 90% of head and neck cancers. This disease results from exposure to carcinogens and from the accumulation of genetic alterations. The workup and management of these patients depends on the specific subsite of the aerodigestive tract in the head and neck from which the primary tumor arises. These subsites are the oral cavity, oropharynx, nasopharynx, hypopharynx, and larynx. Cutaneous malignancies, thyroid neoplasms, and salivary gland neoplasms also occur in the head and neck but are beyond the scope of this chapter.

SYNONYMS

HNC
Head and neck cancer
HNSCC

ICD-10CM CODES

C00-	Malignant neoplasms of lip, oral cavity,
C14	and pharynx
C30	Malignant neoplasm of nasal cavities, middle ear, and accessory sinuses
C32	Malignant neoplasm of larynx
C77.0	Secondary and unspecified malignant neoplasm of lymph nodes of head, face, and neck

EPIDEMIOLOGY & DEMOGRAPHICS

INCIDENCE:
- U.S. annual incidence of head and neck cancer (90% of which is squamous cell carcinoma) is ~62,000 persons/yr.
- Annual mortality is ~13,000 persons/yr.
- Accounts for ~3% of all cancers in the U.S. and >1.5% of all cancer deaths.
- Head and neck cancer was the seventh most common cancer worldwide in 2018.
- Human papillomavirus (HPV)-associated squamous cell carcinoma of the head and neck accounts for 5% to 20% of all HNSCCs, and 40% to 90% of those that arise in oropharynx.
- Incidence of all forms of HNSCC is on the decline, except oropharyngeal squamous cell carcinoma, which is increasing in incidence, likely related to the rise in human papilloma virus (HPV) associated HNSCC.

PREDOMINANT SEX & AGE: Male:female ratio is approximately 3:1. Risk increases significantly over the age of 40.
PEAK INCIDENCE: Sixth decade of life.
RISK FACTORS: The two most strongly implicated risk factors associated with HNSCC are tobacco and alcohol use. These carcinogens place the entire epithelium of the upper respiratory tract at risk for multiple primary tumors via a process known as field cancerization. More recently, a new subset of HNSCC caused by the HPV has been increasing in prevalence. HPV 16 is the most common genotype detected. Patients are more likely to be white middle-aged men, nonsmokers, with minimal alcohol use and higher socioeconomic status.
GENETICS: Research is ongoing in genetic factors that lead to the development and progression of HNSCC. Tumor-suppressor genes, including *p53*, *NOTCH1*, and *CDKN2A*, among others, have been shown to harbor mutations in patients with HNSCC.

PHYSICAL FINDINGS & CLINICAL PRESENTATION

- Presenting signs and symptoms are related to local effects of the primary tumor, regional spread, metastatic disease, or paraneoplastic phenomena:
  1. Oral cavity, oropharynx, hypopharynx: Painful mass or ulceration (Fig. E1), dysphagia, odynophagia, weight loss
  2. Larynx: Hoarseness, voice change, shortness of breath, stridor
  3. Nasal cavity, paranasal sinus, nasopharynx: Referred otalgia, conductive hearing loss from middle ear effusion, epistaxis, cranial nerve palsies
  4. All sites: Cranial nerve palsies, painless neck mass from regional metastases to cervical lymph nodes. Most common site of distant metastases is the lung, with bone and liver being much less common
- Physical examination: A thorough examination of the head and neck, including cranial nerve examination, otoscopy, inspection and palpation of oral cavity, oropharynx, and neck, and general physical examination:
  1. Concerning examination findings: Unilateral middle ear effusion, ulcerated mass of the oral cavity (Fig. E2) or oropharynx, trismus, painless neck mass

ETIOLOGY

Exposure to carcinogens, including tobacco and alcohol, causes genetic alterations in the epithelium of mucosal surfaces lining the upper aerodigestive tract, leading to malignant transformation of epithelial cells. HPV-associated HNSCC is a direct result of the carcinogenic effects of the virus and is not related to alcohol and tobacco use. Primary nasopharyngeal carcinoma has a weak association with tobacco and alcohol and is endemic to southern China, Southeast Asia, and northern Africa. There is a strong association between Epstein-Barr virus infection and primary nasopharyngeal carcinoma.

🅓🅧 DIAGNOSIS

DIFFERENTIAL DIAGNOSIS

Lymphoma, primary salivary gland malignancy, thyroid malignancy, benign tumors of the upper aerodigestive tract, metastases

WORKUP

- Initial workup includes a full physical examination, indirect and/or direct laryngoscopy, imaging studies of the head and neck as well as the chest and/or body to assess for metastases, laboratory tests as indicated, and referral to a head and neck cancer specialist.
- Additional workup by head and neck cancer specialist:
  1. Flexible fiberoptic laryngoscopy or mirror laryngoscopy
  2. Biopsy of the tumor in office or under anesthesia
  3. Fine-needle aspiration (FNA) and biopsy for patient who presents with a suspicious neck mass
  4. Panendoscopy with biopsy under anesthesia, which may include direct laryngoscopy, esophagoscopy, and/or bronchoscopy

LABORATORY TESTS

CBC, coagulation studies, electrolytes, ECG, liver function tests (albumin, transaminases, alkaline phosphatase), thyroid-stimulating hormone (TSH)

IMAGING STUDIES

- Computed tomography (CT) scan of the neck with contrast: Necessary to evaluate extent of primary tumor and nodal metastases in neck (Fig. E3)
- MRI of head and neck (optional): Useful for nasopharyngeal, infratemporal fossa, temporal bone, parotid, parapharyngeal, skull base, or intracranial involvement
- Chest x-ray examination or CT chest with contrast: To evaluate for lung metastases
- PET/CT (Fig. E4): Highlights areas in the body with increased metabolic uptake. Useful initially to assess extent of primary tumor, location of unknown primary tumor, cervical metastases, distant metastases, and second primary tumors. Can be used to monitor for recurrence in the posttreatment setting

STAGING

Staging is based on the tumor, node, metastasis (TNM) staging system provided by the AJCC (Table 1). Staging varies depending on the head and neck subsite that is involved. Any nodal metastasis in the neck automatically classifies as advanced disease (stage III or IV). Distant metastases place patients at stage IVC. The exception to this is HPV-positive cancer of the oropharynx, in which the most recent staging system allows for a patient to be classified as low as stage II even with cervical nodal metastases given the excellent response to treatment and prognosis for these tumors.

℞ TREATMENT

- Treatment consists of surgery, radiation, chemotherapy, or a combination of any or all of the three modalities. The goal is to use as few modalities as possible to minimize side effects of treatment without compromising oncologic success.
  1. Surgery (Fig. E5): Complete surgical resection of the primary tumor along with

TABLE 1   TNM Staging System for Cutaneous Squamous Cell Carcinoma of the Head and Neck

T: Primary Tumor

T_X	Primary tumor cannot be assessed
T_{is}	Carcinoma in situ
T_1	Tumor <2 cm in greatest dimension
T_2	Tumor ≥2 cm, but <4 cm in greatest dimension
T_3	Tumor ≥4 cm in maximum dimension or minor bone erosion or perineural invasion*
T_4	Tumor with gross cortical bone/marrow, skull base invasion and/or skull base foramen invasion
T_{4a}	Tumor with gross cortical bone/marrow invasion
T_{4b}	Tumor with skull base invasion and/or skull base foramen involvement

N: Regional Lymph Nodes
Clinical N (cN)

N_X	Regional lymph nodes cannot be assessed
N_0	No regional lymph node metastasis
N_1	Metastasis in single ipsilateral lymph node, ≤3 cm in greatest dimension and ENE(−)
N_2	Metastasis in single ipsilateral lymph node, >3 cm but not >6 cm in greatest dimension and ENE(−); or in multiple ipsilateral lymph nodes, none >6 cm in greatest dimension; or in bilateral or contralateral lymph nodes and ENE(−), none >6 cm in greatest dimension and ENE(−)
N_{2a}	Metastasis in single ipsilateral lymph node, >3 cm but no >6 cm in greatest dimension and ENE(−)
N_{2b}	Metastasis in multiple ipsilateral lymph nodes, none >6 cm in greatest dimension and ENE(−)
N_{2c}	Metastasis in bilateral or contralateral lymph nodes, none >6 cm in greatest dimension and ENE(−)
N_3	Metastasis in lymph node, >6 cm in greatest dimension and ENE(−); or metastasis in any node(s) and clinically overt ENE [ENE(+)]
N_{3a}	Metastasis in a lymph node >6 cm in greatest dimension and ENE(−)
N_{3b}	Metastasis in any node(s) and ENE(+)

Pathologic N (pN)

N_X	Regional lymph nodes cannot be assessed
N_0	No regional lymph node metastasis
N_1	Metastasis in single ipsilateral lymph node, ≤3 cm in greatest dimension and ENE(−)
N_2	Metastasis in single ipsilateral lymph node, ≤3 cm in greatest dimension and ENE(+), or >3 cm but not >6 cm in greatest dimension and ENE(−); or metastases in multiple ipsilateral lymph nodes, none >6 cm in greatest dimension and ENE(−); or in bilateral or contralateral lymph nodes, none >6 cm in greatest dimension and ENE(−)
N_{2a}	Metastasis in single ipsilateral lymph node, ≤3 cm in greatest dimension and ENE(+), or a single ipsilateral node >3 cm but not >6 cm in greatest dimension and ENE(−)
N_{2b}	Metastasis in multiple ipsilateral lymph nodes, none >6 cm in greatest dimension and ENE(−)
N_{2c}	Metastasis in bilateral or contralateral lymph nodes, none >6 cm in greatest dimension and ENE(−)
N_3	Metastasis in lymph node, >6 cm in greatest dimension and ENE(−); or in a single ipsilateral node >3 cm in greatest dimension and ENE(+), or multiple ipsilateral, contralateral, or bilateral nodes, any with ENE(+)
N_{3a}	Metastasis in a lymph node >6 cm in greatest dimension and ENE(−)
N_{3b}	Metastasis in a single ipsilateral node >3 cm in greatest dimension and ENE(+), or multiple ipsilateral, contralateral, or bilateral nodes, any with ENE(+)

Note: A designation of *U* or *L* may be used for any N category to indicate metastasis above the lower border of the cricoid *(U)* or below the lower border of the cricoid *(L)*. Similarly, clinical and pathologic ENE should be recorded as ENE(−) or ENE(+).

M: Metastasis

M_0	No distant metastasis
M_1	Present distant metastasis

Staging for Cutaneous Squamous Cell Carcinoma

Stage 0	T_{is}	N_0	M_0
Stage I	T_1	N_0	M_0
Stage II	T_2	N_0	M_0
Stage III	T_3	N_0	M_0
Stage III	T_1	N_1	M_0
Stage III	T_2	N_1	M_0
Stage III	T_3	N_1	M_0
Stage IV	T_1	N_2	M_0
Stage IV	T_2	N_2	M_0
Stage IV	T_3	N_2	M_0
Stage IV	Any T	N_3	M_0
Stage IV	T_4	Any N	M_0
Stage IV	Any T	Any N	M1

*Deep invasion is defined as invasion beyond the subcutaneous fat or >6 mm (as measured from the granular layer of adjacent normal epidermis to the base of the tumor); perineural invasion for T_3 classification is defined as tumor cells within the nerve sheath of a nerve lying deeper than the dermis or measuring ≥0.1 mm in caliper or manifesting with clinical or radiographic involvement of named nerves without skull base invasion or transgression.
ENE, Extranodal extension; *TNM*, tumor, node, metastasis.
From *American Joint Committee on Cancer staging manual*, ed 8, Chicago, 2017, Springer.

unilateral or bilateral neck dissections to remove involved or potentially involved lymph nodes as clinically indicated.

2. Radiation: Allows for easier access to poorly exposed tumors such as those of the larynx, oropharynx, nasopharynx, or hypopharynx. Disadvantages include lengthy, time-intensive treatment course, xerostomia, pain, and higher surgical morbidity if salvage surgery is needed.

3. Chemotherapy: Useful only as an adjuvant to radiation therapy or for palliation. Single-agent cisplatin therapy is widely accepted in the U.S. as a standard for chemoradiation regimens for head and neck cancers of any site. Major toxicities include nausea, vomiting, renal toxicity, ototoxicity, and myelosuppression.

4. Reconstruction: Performed with the goal of optimizing functional and cosmetic outcomes. Options include primary closure, local flaps, regional flaps, skin grafts, and microvascular free flaps from other parts of the body (e.g., radial forearm, fibula, anterolateral thigh, latissimus, etc.).

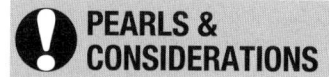

ACUTE GENERAL Rx

- Early-stage disease (stage I or II):
  1. Single-modality treatment with surgery or radiation alone may be appropriate for early-stage head and neck cancer. The choice between one or the other depends on the specific subsite of the head and neck that is involved and the side effects profile for each modality.
  2. Treatment of the potentially involved lymph nodes in the neck with either neck dissection or radiation is controversial and depends on the clinical scenario and the judgment of the treatment team.

- Locoregionally advanced disease (stage III or IV):
  1. In general, these patients have large tumors >4 cm and/or cervical nodal metastases. Treatment typically involves multimodality therapy with either surgery followed by radiation therapy or upfront chemoradiation alone. Depending on the presence of certain adverse pathologic features of the surgical specimen, adjuvant chemoradiation may be necessary. If chemoradiation is the initial treatment modality, surgery may be needed in the adjuvant setting for residual or recurrent disease.
  2. Laryngeal cancers are the exception where select advanced disease with T_3 or N_1 tumors can be managed with single-modality therapy with surgery or radiation alone.
  3. Nasopharyngeal cancer is also an exception. This is not a surgical disease. Managed primarily by radiation to primary site and neck for early-stage disease. Chemoradiation is primary treatment for advanced disease. Surgery is reserved for recurrent or residual disease of primary site or neck following radiation therapy.

- Metastatic disease (stage IVC):
  1. Palliation of symptoms is the primary goal of treatment.

- All patients should be counseled on smoking cessation and avoidance of alcohol.

DISPOSITION

- Prognosis depends on the specific subsite of the head and neck that is involved. Overall 5-yr survival rate for head and neck squamous cell carcinoma is about 55%. This varies with 5-yr survival rates for carcinoma of the lip as high as 89.7% and carcinomas of the hypopharynx as low as ∼30%.

- Patients are followed on a regular basis multiple times a year by a head and neck cancer specialist. After a 5-yr disease-free survival, patients are followed on a yearly basis.

REFERRAL

Referral should be made to an otolaryngologist or oral surgeon who specializes in head and neck cancer.

⬤ PEARLS & CONSIDERATIONS

PREVENTION

- Encourage all patients to cease using tobacco and to limit alcohol consumption.
- Examine the oral cavity and palpate the neck during the annual physical examination. Work up any suspicious masses or lesions.

PATIENT & FAMILY EDUCATION

- https://www.entnet.org/content/head-and-neck-cancer
- http://www.cancer.gov/types/head-and-neck

SUGGESTED READINGS
Available at eBooks.Health.Elsevier.com.

RELATED CONTENT

Laryngeal Carcinoma (Related Key Topic)
Oral Cancer (Related Key Topic)

AUTHOR: **LOUIS F. INSALACO, MD**

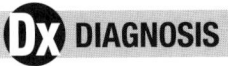
BASIC INFORMATION

DEFINITION

Complete heart block (CHB) is the absence of electrical impulse transmission from the atria to the ventricles when atrioventricular (AV) junction is not physiologically refractory, due to a functional or anatomic impairment of the conduction system, resulting in a bradycardia characterized by AV dissociation. It may be acquired or congenital. CHB can be permanent or reversible. Degenerative changes are the most common cause of CHB.[1]

SYNONYMS

Third-degree AV block
CHB
Complete AV block

ICD-10CM CODE
I44.2 Atrioventricular block, complete

EPIDEMIOLOGY & DEMOGRAPHICS
- The prevalence of CHB is 0.04%.
- The prevalence of CHB increases with age.

PHYSICAL FINDINGS & CLINICAL PRESENTATION

Physical examination may be normal. Cannon A waves may appear in the jugular vein periodically due to the right atrium contracting (against closed tricuspid valve) during ventricular systole. Patients may present with the following clinical manifestations:
- Dizziness, palpitations
- Syncope or presyncope (due to reduced cardiac output)
- Fatigue, shortness of breath, and impaired exercise tolerance
- Mental status changes
- Congestive heart failure
- Angina pectoris
- Some patients may be asymptomatic (e.g., congenital CHB, fast junctional escape rhythm)
- Sudden cardiac arrest

ETIOLOGY
- Fibrosis or sclerosis of the conduction system, Lenègre and Lev diseases[2]
- Acute myocardial infarction (MI)—inferior (14%) or anterior (2%) wall of patients, usually within 24 h
- Drug effect (digitalis, calcium channel blockers, beta-blockers, amiodarone, adenosine)
- Cardiomyopathy and myocarditis (rheumatic fever, diphtheria, viruses, toxoplasmosis, syphilis, COVID-19)
- Bacterial endocarditis with paravalvular abscess formation (e.g., AV endocarditis)
- Infiltrative processes of the myocardium (amyloidosis, sarcoidosis, scleroderma, tumor)[3]
- Metabolic abnormalities (hyperkalemia, hypoxia, hypothyroidism)
- Lyme carditis, rheumatoid nodules, polymyositis, Chagas disease
- Neuromuscular disorders (Becker muscular dystrophy, myotonic muscular dystrophy)
- Congenital (birth from mothers with systemic lupus, large atrial septal defect, and AV canal defects)
- Familial: SCN5 sodium channel mutations have been associated with CHB
- Iatrogenic (cardiac surgery, catheter ablation of arrhythmias, percutaneous coronary intervention). Transcatheter aortic valve implantation (TAVI) is shown to be frequently associated with new conduction abnormalities (2% to 8%); patients with preexisting right bundle branch block are at increased risk of CHB (resolves over time in most patients)
- Paroxysmal due to phase 4 block of the His-Purkinje system

DIAGNOSIS

DIFFERENTIAL DIAGNOSIS
- The differential diagnosis includes lesser degree of AV block, automatic accelerated junctional rhythms, and nonconducted premature atrial contractions.
- The atrial rate must be faster than the ventricular rate (more As than Vs), and the junctional or ventricular rate is regular. Episodes of AV dissociation with an accelerated ventricular or junctional pacemaker overtaking the sinus node can often look like heart block on a single ECG.

WORKUP
- Workup such as routine laboratory tests, cardiac biomarkers, and cardiac imaging should be dictated by the clinical circumstances.
- ECG: Diagnostic of the disease (Figs. 1 and 2):
  1. P waves are present with a regular atrial rate that is faster than the ventricular rate.
  2. P waves are not related to the QRS complexes. The PR intervals are variable.
  3. RR intervals are regular.
  4. QRS complexes may be narrow with a rate of 40 to 60 beats/min (block proximal to His bundle) or wide with a rate of <40 beats/min (block distal to His bundle), depending on the location of the block in the conduction system.
  5. Complete AV block can result from block at the level of AV node, within the His bundle, or distal to it, in the Purkinje system.

TREATMENT

ACUTE GENERAL Rx
- Initial treatment should focus on the hemodynamic stability and symptoms of the patient
- Fig. 3 illustrates the evaluation and management of third-degree AV block
- Consider temporary pacemaker insertion if ventricular escape rate is slow (<40 beats/min) and associated with symptoms or hemodynamic compromise as well as wide QRS escape rhythms, which can be unstable, and QT prolongation above 500 ms, increasing the risk of torsades de pointes ventricular tachycardias
- CHB as a complication of inferior MI usually only requires temporary pacing; however, a CHB as a result of anterior MI often requires permanent pacing (Table 1)
- Acquired CHB usually requires pacing, but patients with congenital CHB often have sufficiently rapid escape rhythm to prevent symptoms and avoid permanent pacemaker implantation
- Withdraw AV-nodal blocking agents if any
- Short-term therapy (until adequate pacing therapy is established):
  1. Vagolytic agents such as atropine may be used to increase the rate of the escape rhythm (for AV nodal level blocks)
  2. Catecholamines such as isoproterenol transiently used for a CHB at any site (use with extreme caution or not at all in patients with coronary artery disease or in patients with digitalis toxicity)
  3. Percutaneous external cardiac pacing (uncomfortable for patients and not always reliably capturing the ventricle)
- Drugs cannot be relied on to increase heart rate (HR) for more than several hours or days without side effects; therefore, temporary or permanent pacemaker insertion is indicated
- Symptomatic CHB in the absence of a condition that is likely to resolve is an American College of Cardiology (ACC)/American Heart Association (AHA)/Heart Rhythm Society (HRS) Class I indication for permanent pacemaker (PPM) placement
- Class I indications for PPM placement in asymptomatic patients according to the ACC/AHA guidelines include[1]:
  1. Patients in sinus rhythm, with documented asystolic pauses greater than or equal to 3.0 sec or an escape rate <40 beats/min, or with an escape rhythm that is below the AV node
  2. Patients with atrial fibrillation and bradycardia with one or more pauses of at least 5 sec or longer
  3. After catheter ablation of the AV junction
  4. If cardiomegaly or left ventricular dysfunction is present with ventricular rates of 40 beats/min or faster
  5. Postoperative CHB that is not expected to resolve
  6. Symptomatic AV block as a consequence of guideline-directed medical therapy for which there is no alternative treatment with strong evidence of therapy benefit (beta-blockers in coronary artery disease [CAD] or heart failure with reduced ejection fraction [HFrEF])
  7. When it is associated with neuromuscular diseases, such as Erb dystrophy (limb-girdle muscular dystrophy), Kearns-Sayre syndrome, myotonic muscular dystrophy, and peroneal muscular atrophy
  8. CHB present during exercise in the absence of myocardial ischemia
- Therapy is directed toward the underlying etiology if there is a reversible source (i.e., IV antibiotics for Lyme disease)

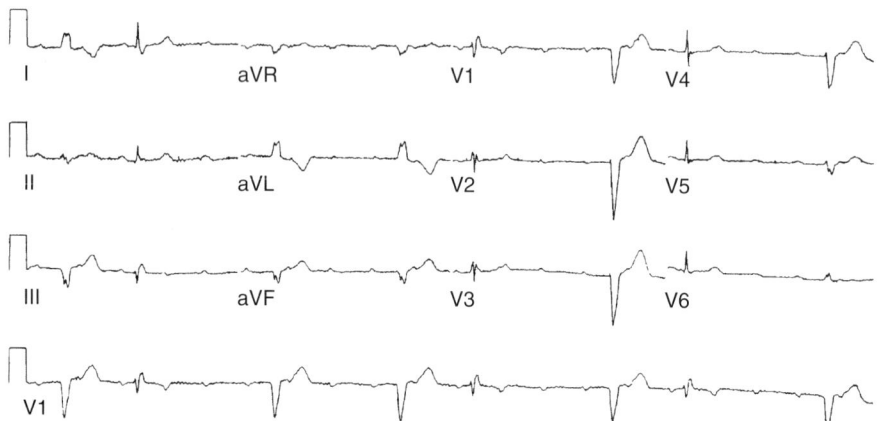

FIG. 1 Third-degree (complete) atrioventricular heart block is characterized by independent atrial (P) and ventricular (QRS) activity. The atrial rate is always faster than the ventricular rate. The PR intervals are completely variable. Some P waves fall on the T wave, distorting its shape. Others may fall in the QRS complex and be "lost." Notice that the QRS complexes are of normal width, indicating that the ventricles are being paced from the atrioventricular junction. (From Goldberger AL [ed]: *Clinical electrocardiography,* ed 5, St Louis, 1994, Mosby.)

FIG. 2 High-grade atrioventricular block. Note that only three P waves conducted to the ventricle in the whole tracing. Conducted P waves were associated with normal PR intervals and right bundle branch block, a finding suggesting infranodal block. All other P waves were blocked, and ventricular escape rhythm with a left bundle branch block pattern is observed. Note that the block is not caused by retrograde concealment in the atrioventricular node or His-Purkinje system from the ventricular escape complexes because the conducted P waves occurred at a short cycle following the escape complexes. *aVF,* Augmented vector foot; *aVL,* augmented vector left; *aVR,* augmented vector right. (From Issa Z et al: *Clinical arrhythmology and electrophysiology,* ed 2, Philadelphia, 2012, Saunders.)

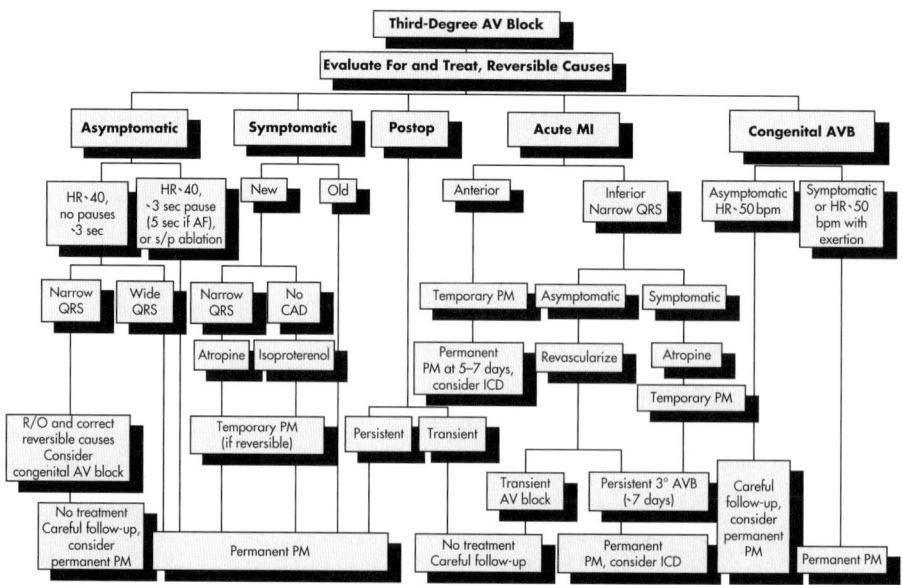

FIG. 3 Evaluation and management of third-degree atrioventricular (AV) block. *AF,* Atrial flutter; *AVB,* atrioventricular block; *bpm,* beats per minute; *CAD,* coronary artery disease; *HR,* heart rate; *ICD,* implantable cardioverter defibrillator; *MI,* myocardial infarction; *PM,* pacemaker; *R/O,* rule out; *s/p,* after. (From Olshansky B et al: *Arrhythmia essentials,* ed 2, Philadelphia, 2017, Elsevier.)

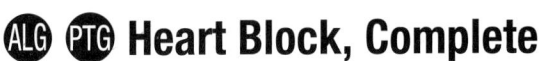
TABLE 1   Indications for Pacing in AV Block

Class I

1. Third-degree or advanced second-degree AV block at any anatomic level associated with any one of the following conditions:
   a. Symptoms (including heart failure) or ventricular arrhythmias attributable to AV block *(Level of Evidence: C)*
   b. Arrhythmias and other medical conditions that require drugs that result in symptomatic bradycardia *(Level of Evidence: C)*
   c. Documented periods of asystole >3.0 sec, any escape rate <40 beats/min, or any escape rhythm below the AV junction (e.g., a wide QRS morphology) in awake, asymptomatic patients in sinus rhythm *(Level of Evidence: C)*
   d. A documented period of asystole >5 sec in awake, asymptomatic patients in atrial fibrillation *(Level of Evidence: C)*
   e. After catheter ablation of the AV junction *(Level of Evidence: C)*
   f. Postoperative AV block that is not expected to resolve after cardiac surgery *(Level of Evidence: C)*
   g. Neuromuscular diseases, such as myotonic muscular dystrophy, Kearns–Sayre syndrome, Erb (limb-girdle) dystrophy, and peroneal muscular atrophy, with or without symptoms of bradycardia *(Level of Evidence: B)*
2. Asymptomatic third-degree AV block at any anatomic site with an average awake ventricular rate >40 beats/min in patients with cardiomegaly or left ventricular dysfunction or if the site of block is below the AV node *(Level of Evidence: B)*
3. Second-degree or third-degree AV block during exercise in the absence of myocardial ischemia *(Level of Evidence: C)*
4. Symptomatic second-degree AV block regardless of type or site of block *(Level of Evidence: B)*

Class IIa

1. Persistent third-degree AV block at any anatomic site with an average ventricular rate >40 beats/min in asymptomatic adult patients in the absence of cardiomegaly *(Level of Evidence: C)*
2. Asymptomatic second-degree AV block at intra- or infra-His levels found at electrophysiologic study *(Level of Evidence: B)*
3. First-degree or second-degree AV block with symptoms similar to those of pacemaker syndrome or hemodynamic compromise *(Level of Evidence: B)*
4. Asymptomatic type II second-degree AV block with a narrow QRS. When type II second-degree AV block occurs with a wide QRS, including isolated right bundle branch block, pacing becomes a Class I recommendation *(Level of Evidence: B)*

Class IIb

1. AV block due to drug use or toxicity when the block is expected to recur even after withdrawal of the drug *(Level of Evidence: B)*
2. Neuromuscular diseases, such as myotonic muscular dystrophy, Kearns–Sayre syndrome, Erb (limb-girdle) dystrophy, and peroneal muscular atrophy with any degree of AV block (including first-degree AV block), with or without symptoms of bradycardia *(Level of Evidence: B)*

Class III

1. Asymptomatic first-degree AV block *(Level of Evidence: B)*
2. Asymptomatic type I second-degree AV block at supra-His (i.e., the AV node) level or another site or not known to be intra- or infra-Hisian by electrophysiologic study *(Level of Evidence: C)*
3. AV block expected to resolve and unlikely to recur (e.g., drug toxicity, Lyme disease, or transient increases in vagal tone or during hypoxia in sleep apnea in the absence of symptoms) *(Level of Evidence: B)*

AV, Atrioventricular.
From Bonow RO et al: *Braunwald's heart disease: a textbook of cardiovascular medicine,* ed 11, Philadelphia, 2019, Saunders.

- Table 2 summarizes the management of complete heart block

CHRONIC Rx

Dual-chamber pacemaker implantation. Patients with a pacemaker need regular follow-up and pacemaker monitoring to ensure proper device functioning. Interest has developed recently in placing the ventricular pacing lead in the His bundle region or left bundle region, which can result in a narrow-paced QRS and may prevent ventricular dyssynchrony associated with traditional RV pacing.[4]

DISPOSITION

- Mortality is highest in the neonatal period in congenital CHB.
- Prognosis is favorable after insertion of a pacemaker and is related to the underlying etiology of complete AV block (e.g., myocardial infarction, cardiomyopathy).
- Nonrandomized studies have shown that PPM insertion improves survival in patients with CHB.

REFERRAL

All patients with CHB should be referred to a cardiologist for consideration of temporary and/or PPM implantation. Patients who receive PPM should be followed routinely every 6 to 12 mo to ensure proper device functioning.

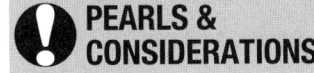 **PEARLS & CONSIDERATIONS**

COMMENTS

- Patients should be instructed to avoid activities that may damage the pacemaker (e.g., contact sports).
- Patients should be followed by cardiologist with routine pacemaker check.
- Pacemaker manufacturers do not recommend any special restrictions regarding proximity to typical household items.
- All pacemaker manufacturers offer pacemakers that are MRI compatible. Older pacemaker models and leads may have a strong relative contraindication for MRI.

- Leadless pacemakers that are implanted directly into the right ventricle using a special delivery system are available for special indications and are primarily used for patients who are at high risk for traditional pacemakers and do not require dual-chamber pacing.
- Some medical procedures, such as lithotripsy, hyperbaric chamber, and electrocautery used during surgery, may require pacemaker programming and testing perioperatively to avoid electromagnetic interference.
- Table E3 describes the five-letter pacemaker code, and Table 4 summarizes common permanent pacemakers.

REFERENCES
Available at eBooks.Health.Elsevier.com.

RELATED CONTENT
Complete Heart Block (Patient Information)

AUTHOR: **ARTEM ASTSATUROV, MD**

TABLE 2 Complete Heart Block Management

Setting	Therapy

Asymptomatic–Acquired	• Rule out reversible causes, including:
	  • Hyperkalemia.
	  • Acute inferior MI.
	  • Digoxin toxicity.
	  • Excess calcium channel blocker therapy.
	  • Lyme disease.
	• If HR <40 beats/min, first-line therapy is a permanent DDD pacemaker.
	• Temporary pacing is indicated if heart rate <40 beats/min.
	• The patient has impaired hemodynamics, and if permanent, pacing cannot be accomplished expeditiously.
	• The CHB has an identifiable and reversible cause, while awaiting recovery.
	• Temporary transvenous pacing must be used with caution in patients with any escape rhythm, particularly if wide QRS complex and slow.
	• Overdrive suppression can occur rapidly.
	• If the rate of escape rhythm >40 beats/min, permanent pacemaker insertion is controversial.
	• Temporary pacing is to be avoided in asymptomatic patients whose ventricular rates are >40 beats/min, especially if the QRS complex is narrow.
	• CHB due to radio frequency ablation of the AV junction to control ventricular response rate in atrial fibrillation requires permanent pacing.
	• May occur even if the patient is asymptomatic from a slow ventricular rate (40 beats/min) that may be quite stable over time.
	• Acquired CHB is associated with a poor short-term prognosis (>50% mortality in the first 6-12 mo after diagnosis).
	• If irreversible, pacing is indicated.

Symptomatic	• A permanent pacemaker is indicated. • Temporary pacing is indicated if permanent pacing cannot be done expeditiously or if CHB has an identifiable and reversible cause (e.g., drug overdose).
Congenital	• Usually associated with a narrow QRS complex with an escape rhythm arising in the AVN. • Patients are usually asymptomatic. • In patients who are asymptomatic, the indications for a pacemaker are controversial. • Patients will need close follow-up, at least annually, for evaluation of symptoms suggesting chronotropic incompetence. • If symptomatic bradycardia, a permanent pacemaker is indicated. • If rate is consistently <50 beats/min and does not increase with exercise (chronotropic incompetence), a permanent pacemaker is indicated.
MI	• If symptomatic bradycardia, a temporary pacemaker is indicated. • If CHB block occurs in the setting of an anterior infarction, permanent pacing is indicated if AVB persists. • CHB in inferior MI is generally in the AVN. • There is usually no need for a permanent pacemaker, as it usually resolves. • If it does not resolve, a permanent pacemaker may be indicated in some cases.
Preoperative	• Permanent pacemaker first, unless the surgery is emergent. • If surgery is emergent, insert a temporary pacemaker preoperative with the plan for a permanent pacemaker after surgery.
Postoperative	• Transcutaneous or temporary transvenous pacing. • A permanent pacemaker is indicated if there is permanent damage to the AV conduction system (e.g., after aortic valve surgery or VSD repair).

AV, Atrioventricular; *AVB,* atrioventricular block; *AVN,* atrioventricular node; *CHB,* complete atrioventricular block; *DDD,* dual chamber; *HR,* heart rate; *MI,* myocardial infarction; *VSD,* ventricular septal defect. From Olshansky B et al: *Arrhythmia essentials,* ed 2, Philadelphia, 2017, Elsevier.

TABLE 4 Common Permanent Pacemakers

Code	Indication	Advantages	Disadvantages
VVI	Intermittent backup pacing; inactive patient	Simplicity; low cost	Fixed rate; risk of pacemaker syndrome
VVIR	Atrial fibrillation	Rate responsive	Requires advanced programming
DDD	Complete heart block	Atrial tracking restores normal physiology	No rate responsiveness; requires two leads and advanced programming
DDDR	Sinus node dysfunction; for rate responsiveness atrioventricular block and need	Universal pacer; all options available by programming	Complexity, cost, programming, and follow-up evaluation

From Marx JA et al: *Rosen's emergency medicine,* ed 8, Philadelphia, 2014, Saunders.

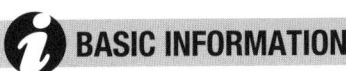
BASIC INFORMATION

DEFINITION

Second-degree heart block or second-degree atrioventricular (AV) heart block is characterized by a failure of one or more, but not all, atrial impulses to conduct to the ventricles. The block may be at any level of the AV conduction system. In both types of second-degree heart block, the sinus rate will continue at regular intervals, resulting in a constant sinus rate. When more than one atrial impulse is present for each ventricular complex, the rhythm may be described as a ratio of the number of atrial impulses to the number of ventricular complexes. Electrocardiographically there are three types of second-degree block:

- Mobitz I (Wenckebach):
  1. Characterized by a progressive prolongation of the PR interval prior to a blocked non-conducted beat and a shorter PR interval after that blocked beat; the conducted impulse will generally be narrow. The cycle may repeat periodically, leading to "grouped beating."
  2. Site of block is usually AV node (proximal to the His bundle).
- Mobitz type II:
  1. Characterized by fixed PR intervals before and after blocked beats and may be associated with a wide QRS morphology (right bundle branch block [RBBB] or left bundle branch block [LBBB] patterns).
  2. Site of block is usually infranodal, especially when QRS is wide.
  3. It has a greater propensity for progressing to third-degree AV block.
- Pure 2:1 conduction patterns cannot be reliably classified as Mobitz type I or type II because there are not enough P waves to characterize prolongation of the PR interval.

SYNONYMS

Wenckebach block (Mobitz type I block)
Mobitz type II block
AV block

ICD-10CM CODES
I44.1   Atrioventricular block, second degree
I45.5   Other specified heart block
Q24.6   Congenital heart block

EPIDEMIOLOGY & DEMOGRAPHICS

Mobitz type I block is more common and may occur in individuals with heightened vagal tone or

as a side effect of medications, such as β-blockers or calcium channel blockers.

PHYSICAL FINDINGS & CLINICAL PRESENTATION

- Patients with Mobitz type I are usually asymptomatic. Patients with either type may feel palpitations or the feeling of "missing a beat." Sudden loss of consciousness without warning (Adams-Stokes attack) can occur in patients with Mobitz type II; however, it is much more common in patients with complete heart block.
- Type I block: There is gradual decrease in the intensity of the first heart sound with widening of the a-c interval in the central venous waveform, ending in a pause, and an a wave not followed by a v wave in the neck along with an irregular pulse.
- Type II block: The first heart sound retains a constant intensity, with intermittent ventricular pauses and a wave not followed by v waves in the neck. There is an irregular pulse for most times with intermittent pauses.

ETIOLOGY

- High vagal tone (young patients, athletes at rest)
- Degenerative changes in the AV conduction system
- Ischemia at the AV nodes (type I with inferior wall myocardial infarction [MI] and type II with anterior wall MI)
- Drugs (digitalis, quinidine, procainamide, adenosine, calcium channel blockers [non-dihydropyridines], β-blockers)
- Cardiomyopathies, collagen vascular diseases, infiltrative diseases (amyloidosis, sarcoidosis, hematochromatosis)
- Myocarditis/endocarditis (infectious, e.g., Lyme disease, Chagas disease; and non-infectious, e.g., systemic lupus erythematosus)
- Hyperkalemia, hypermagnesemia
- Hypothyroidism
- Prior cardiac valve surgery
- Catheter trauma, catheter ablation for arrhythmias

DIAGNOSIS

DIFFERENTIAL DIAGNOSIS

The ECG easily and reliably distinguishes Mobitz type I from Mobitz type II block and from other conduction abnormalities. It should be distinguished from the less common phenomenon of second-degree sinoatrial node exit block.

Mobitz type I block with a normal QRS complex tends to be benign and usually does not progress to more advanced forms of AV conduction within a short period of time because the disease is mostly confined to within the AV node. Mobitz type II block often precedes the development of Adams-Stokes syncope, symptoms are frequent, prognosis is compromised, and progression to third-degree AV block is common and sudden. Thus, type II second-degree AV block with a wide QRS typically indicates diffuse conduction system disease involving even the infranodal His-Purkinje system.[1,2]

WORKUP

ECG, ambulatory monitoring (Holter or external loop recorders) in selected patients

- Mobitz type I (Fig. 1) ECG shows:
  1. Sequential and gradual prolongation of PR interval leading to a nonconducted P wave
  2. Shortened PR interval following the pause as compared with the pre-pause PR interval
  3. Progressive shortening of the R-R interval prior to nonconducted atrial impulse
  4. Usually see "grouped beating" pattern
- Mobitz type II ECG shows (Fig. 2):
  1. Fixed duration of PR interval with constant P-P and R-R intervals
  2. Sudden nonconducted P wave
  3. Abnormal QRS duration or fascicular blocks are common
- In 2:1 AV block (Fig. 3), it cannot be determined based on the 12-lead ECG whether there is Mobitz type I or type II AV block, although a wide QRS complex is suggestive of Mobitz type II:
  1. Administering atropine can improve AV conduction if the AV block is type I or within the AV node; however, if it is infranodal (i.e., type II), the increased sinus rate caused by atropine may worsen the ratio of AV conduction, resulting in worsening bradycardia.
  2. Exercise stress testing may function in the same way as atropine above. If the disease is confined to the AV node, it may improve with exercise, but in cases of Mobitz type II AV block, the degree of AV block will worsen.
  3. Carotid sinus stimulation and other vagal maneuvers may worsen the AV block if it is at the level of the AV node (i.e., Mobitz type I) but will paradoxically improve the ratio of AV conduction by slowing down the sinus rate if it is a Mobitz type II or infranodal AV block.
  4. An algorithm for evaluation of patients with 2:1 AV block is illustrated in Fig. 4.

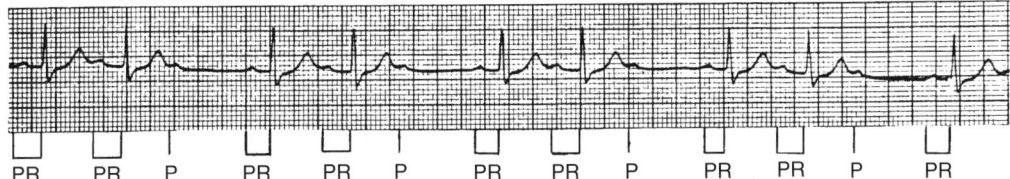

FIG. 1 Wenckebach (Mobitz type I) second-degree atrioventricular block. Notice the progressive increase in PR intervals, with the third P wave in each sequence not followed by a QRS. Wenckebach block produces a characteristically syncopated rhythm with grouping of the QRS complexes (group beating).

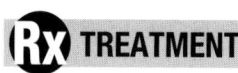
℞ TREATMENT

NONPHARMACOLOGIC THERAPY

Elimination of drugs that may induce AV block such as digoxin, β-blockers, and calcium channel blockers

ACUTE GENERAL Rx

- Treatment is usually not necessary unless the resting heart rate is <40 beats per min (bpm) while awake.
- If symptomatic (e.g., dizziness), atropine 1 mg (may repeat once after 5 min) may be tried to increase AV conduction; if no response, trial of dobutamine or isoproterenol may be helpful prior to insertion of a pacemaker.
- Atropine[1]:
  1. Reduces heart block due to hypervagotonia but not due to AV node ischemia
  2. Does not increase infranodal conduction (third-degree and second-degree AV block that is below the AV node)
  3. Should be used with caution in Mobitz type II AV block due to possible paradoxical decrease in heart rate (as atrial rate increases, AV conduction decreases)
  4. Is ineffective in heart transplantation patients
- If associated with anterior wall MI and wide QRS complex, consider insertion of a temporary pacemaker.
- Indications for permanent pacemaker (PPM) implantation by American College of Cardiology (ACC)/American Heart Association (AHA)/Heart Rhythm Society (HRS) 2019 guidelines[3]:
  1. Second-degree AV block with associated symptomatic bradycardia regardless of the type or site of the block (class I; level of evidence: B)
  2. Second-degree AV block provoked by exercise in the absence of myocardial ischemia (class I; level of evidence: C)
  3. Asymptomatic second-degree AV block at intra- or infra-His levels found at electrophysiologic study (class IIa; level of evidence: B)
  4. First- or second-degree AV block with symptoms similar to those of pacemaker syndrome or hemodynamic compromise (class IIa; level of evidence: B)
  5. Asymptomatic type II second-degree AV block with a wide QRS, including isolated right bundle branch block (class I; level of evidence: B)
  6. PPM is not indicated for asymptomatic type I second-degree AV block at supra-His (AV

Lead V1

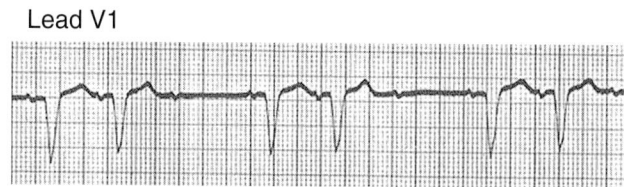

2nd degree AV block (type II) with LBBB

FIG. 2 Mobitz type II atrioventricular (AV) block with left bundle branch block (LBBB). Note the fixed P-P intervals with no change in PR intervals followed by a sudden nonconducted P wave. The LBBB indicates infranodal disease in the His-Purkinje system that is suggestive of Mobitz type II block.

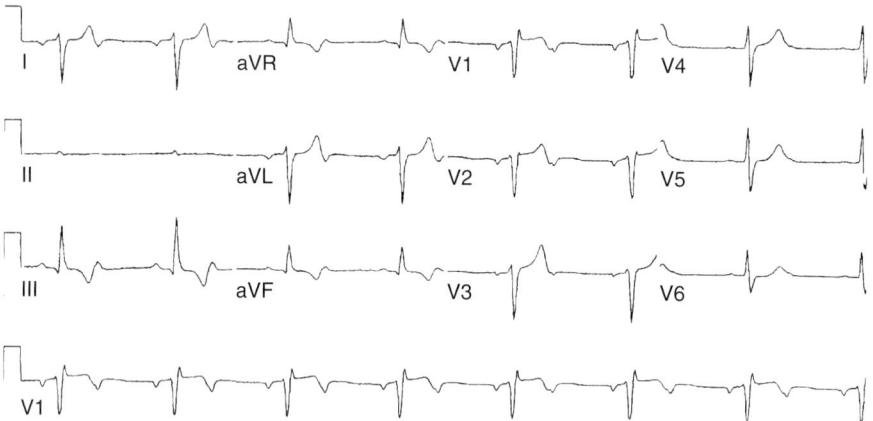

FIG. 3 Second-degree 2:1 atrioventricular block. Notice the short PR interval during conducted complexes and the wide QRS complexes, suggesting block in the His-Purkinje system. (From Issa Z et al: *Clinical arrhythmology and electrophysiology*, ed 2, Philadelphia, 2012, Saunders.)

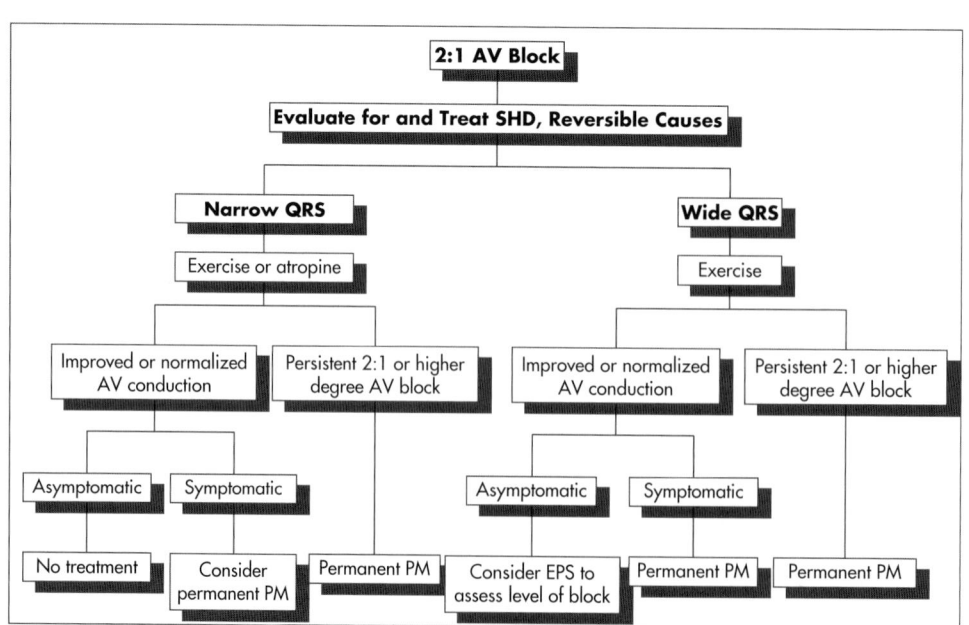

FIG. 4 Evaluation and management of 2:1 AV block. *AV*, Atrioventricular; *EPS*, electrophysiology study; *PM*, pacemaker; *SHD*, structural heart disease (no overt evidence of myocardial, valvular, congenital, or coronary heart disease). (From Olshansky B et al: *Arrhythmia essentials*, ed 2, Philadelphia, 2017, Elsevier.)

node) level or that which is not known to be intra- or infra-Hisian (class III; level of evidence: C)

7. In patients with AV block who have indication for permanent pacing with left ventricular ejection fraction (LVEF) between 36% to 50% and are expected to require ventricular pacing more than 40% of the time, it is reasonable to choose pacing methods that maintain physiologic ventricular activation (e.g., CRT or His bundle pacing) over right ventricular pacing

- Table 1 summarizes the management of Mobitz type I second-degree AV block.
- Table 2 summarizes the management of Mobitz type II second-degree AV block.

DISPOSITION

Prognosis is good with insertion of a pacemaker.

REFERRAL

Referral for pacemaker insertion (see "Acute General Rx")

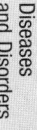

TABLE 1 Mobitz Type I Second-Degree Atrioventricular Block Management

Setting	Therapy

Outpatient— Asymptomatic	• Treadmill testing will help assess chronotropic competence (if this rhythm is not related to myocardial ischemia), as well as enhance AVN conduction, thereby reducing the degree of Wenckebach block (e.g., from 5:4 to 8:7 or producing first-degree AVB only).
	• Holter monitoring can assess the degree and level of AVB and the persistence of the problem during activities of daily living and any diurnal variation.
	• If the QRS duration is wide and Holter monitoring or stress testing suggests infranodal block, an electrophysiology study may help to confirm the level of AVB.
	• If block is demonstrated to be intra- or infra-Hisian, permanent pacemaker implantation is reasonable, even in an asymptomatic patient.
	On occasion, intra-Hisian block can be demonstrated in a patient with a narrow, normal-appearing QRS complex by the production of higher degrees of AV block during treadmill testing with the increase in sinus rate.
	• No therapy.
	  • If not due to reversible cause (e.g., drugs or transient damage to the AV node from Lyme disease) and the QRS duration is normal, as more advanced or complete heart block rarely develops.
	  • There may be increased risk of syncope and symptoms in the future.

Outpatient— Symptomatic	• Some AV nodal blocking drugs (digoxin, β-adrenergic blockers, calcium blockers) may be the cause and should be reduced or stopped, if possible, and then only if severe symptomatic bradycardia occurs.
	• If older or at high risk for structural heart disease, consider an echocardiogram to assess LV function (even if no physical findings are present).
	• If due to a correctable cause such as AV nodal blocking drugs, stop the drug, if possible.
	• If there is a wide QRS or bundle branch block, it is possible that Wenckebach can be due to a block below the AV node (in the His-Purkinje system).
	  • In this case, permanent pacemaker implantation is indicated.
	  • Acutely, intravenous atropine or oral theophylline usually increases conduction through the AV node.
	  • These may paradoxically decrease ventricular rate and increase the degree of block if the block is below the bundle of His.
	• Permanent pacemaker implantation is indicated if symptomatic second-degree AVB is not otherwise correctable.

MI	• Is often reversed during thrombolysis or angioplasty
	• May also appear for the first time concomitantly with these procedures
	• Transient in nature
	• Temporary DDD pacing for the following:
	  • Persistent low heart rate (<40 bpm)
	  • Low cardiac output
	  • Ischemia
	  • Refractory hypotension
	  • Symptoms of light-headedness and dizziness
	• Atropine or theophylline may reverse the block but can cause unwanted tachycardia during drug administration.
	• These drugs are only rarely indicated except at the time of presentation of the patient.
	• Atypical AV block is more common in inferior-posterior MIs due to the Bezold-Jarisch reflex and the effect of increased vagal tone on the AV node.
	  • This is usually transient, and unless there is hemodynamic collapse, there is no need for a temporary pacemaker.
	  • Rarely is there a need for a permanent pacemaker. This is true even if transient third-degree (complete) AV block occurs, as high degrees of block tend to resolve over 5-7 days.
	  • If the AV block does not resolve but the ventricular rate is >40 bpm, no therapy is required if patient is asymptomatic.
	  • If the block does not resolve after 7 days and/or the ventricular rate is <40 or if patient is symptomatic, a permanent pacemaker is indicated.

Preoperative	• Assess drugs given and their need; stop offending drugs that enhance vagal tone, if possible. • If no symptoms, no therapy. • If symptomatic and no reversible causes, provide temporary pacing before surgery. • Need for permanent pacing can be accomplished in the postoperative setting. • Atropine or isoproterenol may be given to increase AV node conduction if symptomatic or hemodynamically significant.
Postoperative	• Rare after CABG but, if it occurs, consider an offending drug or transient ischemia to the AV node. • No therapy is generally needed. • If associated with wide QRS complex, consider block below the His. • If it persists, consider an EP study to assess the level of the block. • If patient is asymptomatic and block is above His, no need for permanent pacemaker. • If patient is symptomatic or block is below the His, permanent pacemaker is indicated. • If the block is associated with valve (especially aortic) surgery, consider direct damage to the AV node. • If persistent, a pacemaker is indicated for symptoms or persistent slow rate (<40 bpm or no increase in rate with exercise).

AV, Atrioventricular; *AVB,* atrioventricular block; *AVN,* atrioventricular node; *bpm,* beats per minute; *CABG,* coronary artery bypass graft; *DDD,* dual-chamber; *EP,* electrophysiology; *LV,* left ventricular; *MI,* myocardial infarction.
From Olshansky B et al: *Arrhythmia essentials,* ed 2, Philadelphia, 2017, Elsevier.

TABLE 2   Mobitz Type II Second-Degree Atrioventricular Block Management

Setting	Therapy

Outpatient—Asymptomatic	• Risk for complete heart block and death is significant (approximately 50%).
	• A dual-chamber permanent pacemaker is recommended as the pacing system of choice. Consider conduction system pacing if high burden of pacing and depressed EF.
	  • Admit the patient for a permanent pacemaker and place on a cardiac monitor.
	  • In the absence of symptoms or progressive (higher-degree AVB), there is no need for a temporary pacemaker before permanent pacemaker implantation.
	  • Avoid atropine.
	  • Evaluate for the presence of underlying cardiac disease, such as infiltrative processes (e.g., amyloid) or MI.

Outpatient—Symptomatic	• Dual-chamber permanent pacemaker implantation is indicated.
	• Admit the patient and place on a cardiac monitor.
	  • If symptomatic or hemodynamically detrimental ventricular bradycardia is present, a temporary pacemaker is indicated if a permanent system cannot be placed expeditiously.
	  • Do not give atropine because this may worsen the AVB and produce a slower ventricular rate.
	  • Exercise, sinus tachycardia, and catecholamines also can worsen the degree of block by enhancing AV nodal conduction and impinging on the refractory period of the His-Purkinje system.

MI	• Place temporary pacemaker.
	  • Mobitz type II second-degree AVB is associated with a high rate of heart failure in this setting.
	  • A permanent pacemaker is indicated if the AVB is persistent because the risk of complete heart block is >50%.
	  • Long-term prognosis may not be improved.
	  • Avoid the use of antiarrhythmic drugs (including lidocaine) in the absence of a pacemaker, unless there is sustained ventricular tachyarrhythmia, as these drugs may worsen the degree of AVB.
	  • Do not give atropine.
	  • Mobitz type II second-degree AVB has a lower (albeit not known with certainty) incidence in the current early revascularization era, but if present or of new onset may improve with time, in rare cases, when persistent, a pacemaker will likely be needed.

Preoperative	• Place permanent pacemaker.
	  • If urgent or emergent surgery, place a temporary pacemaker with the plan for a permanent pacemaker after surgery.
	  • If CABG, epicardial atrial and ventricular wires can be placed, with temporary pacing as standby, until a permanent transvenous pacemaker can be placed.
	   It is best to place the permanent pacemaker after CABG or other cardiac surgery as leads otherwise tend to dislodge.
	  • If endocarditis, temporary pacemaker until infection resolves and after cardiac surgery.
	  • Avoid antiarrhythmic drugs and atropine.

Postoperative	• If bradycardia, temporary pacing (via epicardial wires, if present, after cardiac surgery).
	• Temporary Mobitz type II AV block may resolve after cardiac surgery.
	  • It may be due to trauma near the His-Purkinje system (e.g., with aortic valve surgery, where left bundle branch block is a not-infrequent accompaniment).
	  • Persistent (e.g., more than 3-5 days) Mobitz type II block will require permanent pacing.
	  • No antiarrhythmic drugs should be given unless an adequate backup ventricular pacing is available.
	  • Endocarditis with abscess near the septum can destroy the His-Purkinje system.
	  • Despite surgical repair, permanent pacing will likely be required.
	  • For patients having tricuspid valve replacement, an endocardial lead can occasionally be placed across a porcine bioprosthesis without producing tricuspid regurgitation but should be avoided if there is a mechanical valve.
	  • Tricuspid valve repair (e.g., annuloplasty) should not pose a problem in positioning a right ventricular lead.

AV, Atrioventricular; *AVB,* atrioventricular block; *CABG,* coronary artery bypass graft; *MI,* myocardial infarction.
From Olshansky B et al: *Arrhythmia essentials,* ed 2, Philadelphia, 2017, Elsevier.

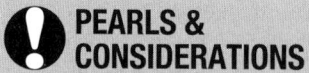

PEARLS & CONSIDERATIONS

COMMENTS

Patients with symptomatic Mobitz type II should be referred for a pacemaker. Asymptomatic patients should be referred if the AV block worsens with exercise and should be followed up routinely for potential development of high-grade AV block.[3]

REFERENCES

Available at eBooks.Health.Elsevier.com.

RELATED CONTENT

Second-Degree Heart Block (Patient Information)

AUTHOR: **ALEEM I. MUGHAL, MD, FHRS**

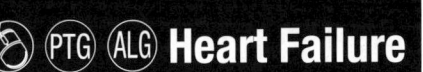
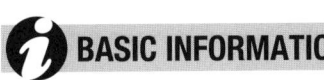 **BASIC INFORMATION**

DEFINITION

Heart failure (HF) is a complex clinical syndrome that can result from any structural or functional cardiac disorder that impairs the ability of the ventricle to fill with or eject blood. The cardinal manifestations of heart failure are dyspnea, fatigue, and fluid retention. The pathophysiology of HF (Fig. E1) is related to progressive activation of the neuroendocrine system to compensate for decreased effective circulating volume (Table 1), leading to total body volume overload and circulatory insufficiency.[1] These events culminate in the development of pulmonary congestion as well as peripheral edema. Specifically, the renin-angiotensin-aldosterone system (RAAS) is implicated; once activated, it can lead to volume expansion (sodium retention) and cardiac fibrosis (mediated through angiotensin II). Another recognized mechanism is disordered adrenergic stimulation as a key component of progression of disease. The term *congestive heart failure* (CHF) usually denotes a volume-overloaded status as a result of HF. Given that not all patients have volume overload at the time of the evaluation, *congestive heart failure* should be distinguished from the broader term *heart failure*.[1]

CLASSIFICATION: The American College of Cardiology/American Heart Association (ACC/AHA) describes the following four stages of HF.[2] This staging model was designed to emphasize the evolution and progression of HF over a continuum and the preventability of HF in at-risk patients.

- Stage A: Patients at high risk (e.g., with hypertension, atherosclerotic disease, diabetes mellitus, metabolic syndrome, cytotoxin, family history) for HF but without structural heart disease or symptoms of HF
- Stage B: Patients with structural heart disease (e.g., left ventricular [LV] dysfunction) but without symptoms of HF
- Stage C: Patients with structural heart disease with prior or current symptoms of HF
- Stage D: Patients with refractory HF requiring specialized interventions

In addition to the ACC/AHA stages described above, the New York Heart Association (NYHA) defines four functional classes of HF designed to describe the symptoms of stage C and D HF.[3] The functional classes are intended to assess the symptoms of HF and may fluctuate with therapy. It should be noted that current guidelines employ the functional classes to aid in determination of appropriate treatment.

- Asymptomatic or symptomatic only at activity levels that would limit normal individuals
- Symptomatic with ordinary exertion (e.g., 2 city blocks or 1 flight of stairs in a faster than usual pace)
- Symptomatic with less than ordinary exertion (e.g., less than 2 city blocks or 1 flight of stairs)
- Symptomatic at rest

Table 2 compares the ACC/AHA and the NYHA classification. Table 3 describes a simplified classification and common clinical characteristics of patients with acute heart failure.

TERMINOLOGY:

- Although HF has traditionally been classified as systolic vs. diastolic, this was dependent on the imaging modality used. With noted variation in the observed systolic function between studies, the ejection fraction serves as a better marker. HF is now categorized into *HF with reduced ejection fraction* (HFrEF) and HF with *preserved ejection fraction* (HFpEF). Other common classifications include right-sided vs. left-sided and high-output vs. low-output.[1] Systolic HF or HFrEF is defined by the presence of impaired contractility of the LV, as measured by ejection fraction (EF) $\leq$40% with clinical signs or symptoms of HF. In contrast, HFpEF has been described as evidence (clinical) of HF with an EF $\geq$50% with or without evidence of diastolic dysfunction. There are two further classifications of HFpEF: HFpEF borderline, used to describe patients with an EF 41% to 49%, and HFpEF improved, used to describe patients who previously had HFrEF with an improvement in their EF.[4]
- Right-sided HF denotes peripheral signs and symptoms of HF without evidence of pulmonary congestion, as opposed to left-sided HF, which typically manifests with pulmonary congestion and subsequent signs and symptoms of right-sided HF.[1] The most common cause of right-sided HF is left-sided HF. High-output HF involves signs and symptoms of HF but features an elevated cardiac output unable to meet the abnormally high metabolic demands of peripheral tissues and is the result of myriad systemic disorders (e.g., systemic arteriovenous fistulas, hyperthyroidism, anemia). The term *acute decompensated HF* (ADHF) refers to worsening of signs or symptoms of HF due to a wide range of causes. Of note, HF is not equivalent to cardiomyopathy or LV dysfunction. These latter terms describe the possible structural or functional reasons for the development of HF, whereas HF is a clinical syndrome characterized by specific symptoms and signs.[1]

SYNONYMS

HF
Congestive heart failure
CHF
Cardiac failure
Cardiogenic shock
Cardiogenic pulmonary edema

ICD-10CM CODES

I50.9	Heart failure, unspecified
I50.20	Unspecified systolic (congestive) heart failure
I50.21	Acute systolic (congestive) heart failure
I50.22	Chronic systolic (congestive) heart failure
I50.23	Acute on chronic systolic (congestive) heart failure
I50.30	Unspecified diastolic (congestive) heart failure
I50.31	Acute diastolic (congestive) heart failure
I50.32	Chronic diastolic (congestive) heart failure
I50.33	Acute on chronic diastolic (congestive) heart failure
I50.40	Unspecified combined systolic (congestive) and diastolic (congestive) heart failure
I50.41	Acute combined systolic (congestive) and diastolic (congestive) heart failure
I50.42	Chronic combined systolic (congestive) and diastolic (congestive) heart failure
I50.43	Acute on chronic combined systolic (congestive) and diastolic (congestive) heart failure

EPIDEMIOLOGY & DEMOGRAPHICS

- There is variability in the reported demographics of HF due to heterogeneous definitions and classifications of HF. Incidence rate is lowest among white women and highest among black men. African Americans have the highest risk for HF of the demographic groups with blacks having a higher 5-yr mortality rate than whites.[1]
- The lifetime risk of developing HF is 20% for Americans $\geq$40 yr of age.
  1. In the U.S., HF incidence has largely remained stable over the past several decades, with >650,000 new HF cases diagnosed annually.[2]
  2. Based on NHANES data, from 2013 to 2016, an estimated 6.2 million Americans $\geq$20 yr of age had HF. This represents an increase from an estimated 5.7 million U.S. adults with HF from 2009 to 2012.[5]
  3. Projections show that the prevalence of HF will increase 46% from 2012 to 2030, resulting in >8 million people $\geq$18 yr of age with HF.[6]
  4. There has been an increase in the prevalence of HF in the population over time. This is primarily due to improved treatment of hypertension and valvular and coronary disease, allowing patients to survive an early death only to later develop HF.[6]
- HF is primarily a condition of the elderly. Approximately 80% of patients hospitalized with HF are older than 65 yr. HF is the most common inpatient diagnosis in the U.S. for patients aged >65 yr.[6]
- HF incidence increases with age, rising from approximately 20 per 1000 individuals 65 to 69 yr to >80 per 1000 individuals among those >85 yr. Before age 75, the incidence of HF is higher in males, but both sexes are equally affected after this age cutoff.[5]
- In the U.S., 809,000 hospital discharges and 2.3 million ED visits/physician visits were associated with HF in 2016, which is a decline compared with 1.02 million hospital discharges in 2006.[5,6]
- Prevalence: 6.2 million persons in the U.S. and an estimated 26 million persons worldwide. The prevalence of HF is rising, especially in the elderly, particularly due to aging of the population and improved survival from other conditions.[5]
- The estimated (direct and indirect) cost of HF in the U.S. was >$40 billion in 2012, with over

TABLE 1 Compensatory Mechanisms in Heart Failure

Compensatory Response	Stimuli	Beneficial Effects	Adverse Effects	Potential Pharmacologic Interventions
Renin-angiotensin system activation	↓ CO/BP ↓ Renal blood flow ↑ β-adrenergic activity	Maintain vital organ perfusion through vasoconstriction and sodium retention	↑ Afterload → worsened LV function Adverse LV remodeling (apoptosis, myocyte hypertrophy)	ACE inhibitors ARBs
Adrenergic activation	↓ CO/BP	↑ CO through ↑ in heart rate and contractility ↑ BP	↑ Ischemia ↑ Afterload → worsened LV function ↑ LVEDP → pulmonary congestion Adverse LV remodeling (apoptosis, myocyte hypertrophy)	β-adrenergic blocking agents
Renal salt and water retention	↑ Antidiuretic hormone ↑ Norepinephrine ↑ Angiotensin II ↑ Aldosterone ↓ Renal blood flow	↑ Preload → ↑ Stroke volume and CO	Pulmonary and systemic congestion Adverse LV remodeling	Diuretics Aldosterone inhibitors ACE inhibitors, ARBs β-adrenergic blocking agents
↑ Natriuretic peptide secretion	Volume expansion (atrial stretch)	Diuresis Natriuresis Partial inhibition of renin-angiotensin system and norepinephrine	None known	Natriuretic peptides

ACE, Angiotensin-converting enzyme; *ARB*, angiotensin receptor blocker; *BP*, blood pressure; *CO*, cardiac output; *LV*, left ventricular; *LVEDP*, left ventricular end-diastolic pressure.
From Sellke FW et al: *Sabiston & Spencer surgery of the chest,* ed 9, 2016, Elsevier.

TABLE 2 American College of Cardiology/American Heart Association (ACC/AHA) Stages of Heart Failure (HF) Compared to the New York Heart Association (NYHA) Functional Classification

ACC/AHA Stages		NYHA Functional Classification	
A	At high risk for HF but without structural heart disease or symptoms of HF	None	
B	Structural heart disease but without signs or symptoms of HF	I	No limitation of physical activity Ordinary physical activity does not cause symptoms of HF
C	Structural heart disease with prior or current symptoms of HF	I	No limitation of physical activity Ordinary physical activity does not cause symptoms of HF
		II	Slight limitation of physical activity Comfortable at rest, but ordinary physical activity results in symptoms of HF
		III	Marked limitation of physical activity Comfortable at rest, but less than ordinary activity causes symptoms of HF
D	Refractory HF requiring specialized interventions	IV	Unable to carry on any physical activity without symptoms of HF, or symptoms of HF at rest

From Zipes DP: *Braunwald's heart disease, a textbook of cardiovascular medicine,* ed 11, Philadelphia, 2019, Elsevier.

half of these costs spent on hospitalizations. The mean cost of HF-related hospitalizations is $23,077 per patient and is higher when HF was a secondary rather than the primary diagnosis.[5]

- HFrEF and HFpEF each make up about half of the overall HF burden. Of hospitalized HF events, half are in patients with HFrEF and the other half in patients with HFpEF.[7]
- The presence of ADHF services as an important juncture in the progression of HF, indicative of a worsening clinical course with increased risk of mortality and rehospitalization. An average hospitalization length for HF in the United States ranges around 4 to 5 days but carries a 1-yr mortality rate of ~30%, over threefold of an increase from chronic, stable HF that does not require hospitalization.[8,9]

RISK FACTORS: Several conditions are associated with an increased risk of developing heart failure. If these are identified and treated appropriately, it may be possible to delay, if not prevent, the onset of HF.[4]

- Hypertension: The incidence of HF is higher in patients with higher blood pressures, older age of the hypertensive patient, and in patients who have been hypertensive for longer.
- Diabetes mellitus: The incidence of HF is increased in patients with diabetes mellitus, independent of the presence of structural heart disease.
- Metabolic syndrome: Appropriately treating hypertension, diabetes mellitus, and dyslipidemia can decrease the incidence of HF.
- Atherosclerotic disease: Patients with atherosclerotic disease are likely to develop HF.

PHYSICAL FINDINGS & CLINICAL PRESENTATION

The clinical and physical exam findings should be given the highest priority when determining the diagnosis of HF. These signs and symptoms are dependent on the severity of disease, precipitant factors, comorbid conditions, and whether the HF symptoms are predominantly right-sided or left-sided. Clues in the patient's history when evaluating HF are summarized in Table 4.

- Common clinical manifestations are[2]:
  1. Dyspnea on exertion, that can progress to dyspnea at rest, caused by increasing pulmonary vascular congestion
  2. Orthopnea, caused by increased venous return in the recumbent position and further elevated pulmonary venous pressure
  3. Paroxysmal nocturnal dyspnea (PND) resulting from multiple factors including increased venous return in the recumbent position, decreased Pa_{O_2}, and decreased adrenergic stimulation of myocardial function during sleep
  4. Nocturnal angina resulting from increased myocardial oxygen demand (secondary to increased venous return in the recumbent position causing increased preload) in patients with concomitant coronary artery disease (CAD)

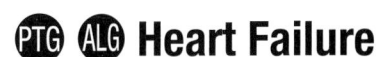
TABLE 3 Simplified Classification and Common Clinical Characteristics of Patients With Acute Heart Failure

Clinical Classification	Symptom Onset	Triggers	Signs and Symptoms	Clinical Assessment	Course
Decompensated heart failure	Usually gradual	Noncompliance, ischemia, infections	Peripheral edema, orthopnea, dyspnea on exertion	SBP: Variable CXR: Often clear despite elevated filling pressures	Variable, high rehospitalization rate
Acute hypertensive heart failure	Usually sudden	Hypertension, atrial arrhythmias, ACS	Dyspnea (often severe), tachypnea, tachycardia, rales common	SBP: High (>180/100 mm Hg) CXR with pulmonary edema Hypoxemia common	High acuity, but patient often responds quickly to therapy with vasodilators, noninvasive ventilation Postdischarge mortality is low
Cardiogenic shock	Variable	Progression of advanced HF or major myocardial insult (e.g., large AMI, acute myocarditis)	End-organ hypo-perfusion; oliguria, confusion, cool extremities	SBP: Low or low normal LV function usually severely depressed RV dysfunction common Laboratory evidence of end-organ dysfunction (renal, hepatic)	High inpatient mortality Poor prognosis unless readily reversible cause or mechanical support, transplantation

ACS, Acute coronary syndrome; *AMI,* acute myocardial infarction; *CXR,* chest x-ray film; *LV,* left ventricular; *RV,* right ventricular; *SBP,* systolic blood pressure.
From Zipes DP: *Braunwald's heart disease, a textbook of cardiovascular medicine,* ed 11, Philadelphia, 2019, Elsevier.

Diseases and Disorders

I

5. *Cheyne-Stokes respiration* (alternating phases of apnea and hyperventilation) caused by prolonged circulation time from lungs to brain as a result of impaired cardiac output
6. Fatigue, lethargy, and decreased functional capacity resulting from low cardiac output and hypoperfusion of peripheral tissues
7. Table 5 summarizes common presenting symptoms and signs of decompensated heart failure
- Physical examination (Table 6)[2]:
  1. Fine pulmonary crackles, wheezes, tachypnea, hypoxia (due to elevated pulmonary pressures). Crackles may be absent in chronic and longstanding high pulmonary venous pressure because it allows for lymphatic drainage in the lungs to increase
  2. Tachycardia and narrowed pulse pressure (due to increased sympathetic tone)
  3. S3 gallop, paradoxic splitting of S2, jugular venous distention, peripheral edema in dependent tissues, congestive hepatomegaly, ascites, and hepatojugular reflux (due to volume overload)
  4. Perioral and peripheral cyanosis, decreased capillary refill, pulsus alternans, and cool extremities (due to decreased cardiac output)
- Six common clinical presentations identified by European Society of Cardiology of Acute Heart Failure Syndromes[10]:
  1. ADHF presenting with hypertension (SBP >160): The hypertension leads to increased afterload causing pulmonary vascular congestion
  2. Worsening or decompensation of chronic HF
  3. Flash pulmonary edema
  4. Cardiogenic shock
  5. Acute coronary syndrome (ACS) and ADHF
  6. Isolated RV failure

TABLE 4 Using the Medical History to Assess the Heart Failure Patient

Symptoms Associated With HF Include:

Fatigue
Shortness of breath at rest or during exercise
Dyspnea
Tachypnea
Cough
Diminished exercise capacity
Orthopnea
Paroxysmal nocturnal dyspnea
Nocturia
Weight gain/weight loss
Edema (of extremities, scrotum, or elsewhere)
Increasing abdominal girth or bloating
Abdominal pain (particularly if confined to right upper quadrant)
Loss of appetite or early satiety
Cheyne-Stokes respirations (often reported by family rather than patient)
Somnolence or diminished mental acuity

Historical Information Helpful in Determining if Symptoms Are Caused by HF

A past history of HF
Cardiac disease (e.g., coronary artery disease, valvular or congenital disease, previous myocardial infarction)
Risk factors for heart failure (e.g., diabetes, hypertension, obesity)
Systemic illnesses that can involve the heart (e.g., amyloidosis, sarcoidosis, inherited neuromuscular diseases)
Recent viral illness or history of HIV infection or Chagas disease
Family history of HF or sudden cardiac death
Environmental and/or medical exposure to cardiotoxic substances
Substance abuse
Noncardiac illnesses that could affect the heart indirectly, including high-output states (e.g., anemia, hyperthyroidism, arteriovenous fistulas)

HIV, Human immunodeficiency virus.
From Zipes DP: *Braunwald's heart disease, a textbook of cardiovascular medicine,* ed 11, Philadelphia, 2019, Elsevier.

- Each of these scenarios may require different therapies to effectively stabilize and treat the patient

Acute precipitants of HF decompensation include noncompliance with salt restriction or medications (most common cause), any acute systemic illness, infection, arrhythmias (e.g., atrial fibrillation), ischemia or infarction, uncontrolled hypertension, new medications, negative inotropic agents such as calcium channel blockers/antiarrhythmic agents), nonsteroidal antiinflammatory drugs (NSAIDs), renal dysfunction, toxins (e.g., ethanol and anthracyclines), surgery, or valvular catastrophe.[10]

ETIOLOGY

LEFT VENTRICULAR FAILURE: The dichotomy of whether HF occurs in the setting of preserved or reduced LV systolic function plays an important role in treatment strategies. Patients with HFpEF may have significant abnormalities in active relaxation and passive stiffness of the LV as well

TABLE 5 Common Presenting Symptoms and Signs of Decompensated Heart Failure

Symptoms	Signs
Predominantly Related to Volume Overload	
Dyspnea (exertional, paroxysmal nocturnal dyspnea, orthopnea, or at rest), cough, wheezing	Rales, pleural effusion
Foot and leg discomfort	Peripheral edema (legs, sacral)
Abdominal discomfort/bloating; early satiety or anorexia	Ascites/increased abdominal girth; right upper quadrant pain or discomfort; hepatomegaly/splenomegaly; scleral icterus
	Increased weight
	Elevated jugular venous pressure, abdominojugular reflux
	Increasing S_3, accentuated P_2
Predominantly Related to Hypoperfusion	
Fatigue	Cool extremities
Altered mental status, daytime drowsiness, confusion, or difficulty concentrating	Pallor, dusky skin discoloration, hypotension
Dizziness, presyncope, or syncope	Pulse pressure (narrow)
	Proportional pulse pressure (low)
Other Signs/Symptoms of Acute Heart Failure	
Depression	Orthostatic hypotension (hypovolemia)
Sleep disturbances	S_4
Palpitations	Systolic/diastolic cardiac murmurs

From Zipes DP: *Braunwald's heart disease, a textbook of cardiovascular medicine,* ed 11, Philadelphia, 2019, Elsevier.

TABLE 6 Physical Findings of Heart Failure

Tachycardia
Extra beats or irregular rhythm
Narrow pulse pressure or thready pulse*
Pulses alternans*
Tachypnea
Cool and/or mottled extremities*
Elevated jugular venous pressure
Dullness and diminished breath sounds at one or both lung bases
Rales, rhonchi, and/or wheezes
Apical impulse displaced leftward and/or inferiorly
Sustained apical impulse
Parasternal lift
Third and/or fourth heart sound (either palpable and/or audible)
Tricuspid or mitral regurgitant murmur
Hepatomegaly (often accompanied by right upper quadrant discomfort)
Ascites
Presacral edema
Anasarca*
Pedal edema
Chronic venous stasis changes

*Indicative of more severe disease.
From Zipes DP: *Braunwald's heart disease, a textbook of cardiovascular medicine,* ed 11, Philadelphia, 2019, Elsevier.

as valvular disease. HfrEF denotes poor pump function.[10]
- Abnormal LV systolic function:
  1. CAD (acute or chronic ischemia, myocardial infarction [MI], LV aneurysm), the most common cause of cardiomyopathy in the U.S., comprising 50% to 75% of HF patients.
  2. Increased afterload or pressure overload (severe hypertension, aortic stenosis)
  3. Increased preload or volume overload (mitral regurgitation, aortic regurgitation)
  4. Cardiomyopathy: Idiopathic, infiltrative (nonischemic)
  5. Infectious (Chagas, myocarditis)
  6. Infiltrative (amyloidosis, sarcoidosis, hemochromatosis)
  7. Toxins (ethanol, cocaine, anthracyclines)
  8. Tachycardia induced (e.g., with atrial fibrillation)
- Preserved LV systolic function (Table 7)[11]:
  1. Impaired relaxation (myocardial ischemia, diabetes mellitus, metabolic syndrome)
  2. Tachyarrhythmia (featuring reduced diastolic filling time)
  3. Restrictive cardiomyopathy (myocardial stiffness, such as hypereosinophilic syndrome, amyloidosis, hemochromatosis)
  4. High cardiac output (thiamine deficiency, anemia, thyrotoxicosis, arteriovenous malformations)
  5. Increased afterload (uncontrolled hypertension, aortic stenosis, hypertrophic obstructive cardiomyopathy)
  6. Hypervolemia (oliguric renal failure, iatrogenic)

RIGHT VENTRICULAR FAILURE:
- Left-sided HF
- Chronic hypoxemic pulmonary disease
- Valvular heart disease (mitral stenosis or regurgitation)
- Pulmonary embolism
- Primary pulmonary hypertension
- Right-to-left shunts that cause systemic hypoxemia (e.g., large patent foramen ovale and tetralogy of Fallot)
- Left-to-right shunts that cause volume overload (e.g., atrial and ventricular septal defects)
- Bacterial endocarditis (right-sided)
- Right ventricular infarction

ⒹⓍ DIAGNOSIS

DIFFERENTIAL DIAGNOSIS
- COPD, asthma
- Cirrhosis
- Nephrotic syndrome
- Venous insufficiency
- Pulmonary embolism
- ARDS (adult respiratory distress syndrome)
- Pneumonia, flu, and COVID-19
- Heroin overdose

WORKUP
- ACC/AHAA guidelines for initial and serial evaluation of heart failure are summarized in Table 8.
- Blood work (to diagnose potentially reversible causes, identify comorbidities, and assess disease severity)[2]:
  1. CBC (to evaluate for anemia, infections), urinalysis, blood urea nitrogen (BUN), creatinine, electrolytes (worsening hyponatremia is a marker of disease severity and is associated with higher mortality rates), liver enzymes (hepatic congestion), thyroid function (especially in the elderly or patients with comorbid atrial fibrillation or known thyroid disease).
  2. Fig. 2 illustrates the use of biomarkers in HF. B-type natriuretic peptide (BNP) is a cardiac neurohormone secreted from the ventricles in response to elevated LV end-diastolic pressure. While the sensitivity is low in asymptomatic patients, low BNP level has a negative predictive value up to 90% in symptomatic patients. An elevated BNP correlates with severity of disease and parallels closely morbidity and mortality outcome measures. N-terminal-pro-BNP (NT-pro-BNP) is the cleavage remnant of BNP. It has a longer half-life and is renally cleared, making it susceptible to alterations in renal function. A level of <300 pg/ml has an age-independent 98% negative predictive value. There are new data to suggest that BNP screening and early intervention with risk factor modification in patients at risk of developing heart failure may prevent development of left ventricular dysfunction (class IIa recommendation). Natriuretic peptide biomarkers are also useful (class IA recommendation) both for diagnosis in patients presenting with dyspnea and for prognosis in patients with acute decompensated heart failure and chronic heart failure. Measurement of baseline levels of natriuretic peptide biomarkers on

TABLE 7 Mechanisms/Factors Contributing to the Pathophysiology of Heart Failure With Preserved Ejection Fraction

Cardiovascular

LV Structure

Concentric remodeling, LV hypertrophy

LV Function

Diastolic dysfunction: Abnormal relaxation, decreased recoil, abnormal filling, decreased distensibility, increased diastolic pressure
Systolic dysfunction: Abnormal midwall and long-axis shortening, decreased twist
Hemodynamic load
Increased afterload and filling load
Heterogeneity
Dyssynergy, dyssynchrony
Left atrial structure and function
Increased LA volume and stiffness, decreased LA reservoir function, passive conduit function and active booster pump function
Ischemia
Subendocardial and microvascular disease, impaired coronary, pulmonary, and peripheral flow reserve
Rate and rhythm abnormalities
Chronotropic incompetence, atrial fibrillation, supraventricular tachycardia
Vascular dysfunction
Arterial stiffening, endothelial dysfunction

Cardiomyocyte

Abnormal calcium homeostasis ($\uparrow$ diastolic calcium or $\downarrow$ rate of calcium reuptake $\rightarrow$ incomplete or impaired relaxation)
Sarcolemmal calcium channels (Na^+/Ca^{2+} exchanger and calcium pump)
Sarcoplasmic reticulum Ca^{2+}ATPase (SERCA) abundance and function
Proteins modifying SERCA activity: Phospholamban, calmodulin, calsequestrin abundance, and phosphorylation state
Sarcoplasmic reticulum calcium release channels
Energetics ($\downarrow$ ATP or $\uparrow$ ADP slows actin-myosin cross-bridge release)
ADP/ATP ratio, ADP and P_i concentration, phosphocreatine shuttle function
Proteins regulating cross-bridge formation and calcium sensitivity
Troponin C: Calcium binding
Troponin I: Phosphorylation state
Cytoskeletal proteins
Microtubules (increased density) $\rightarrow$ $\uparrow$ diastolic stiffness
Titin isoforms ($\uparrow$ noncompliant isoform and phosphorylation state) $\rightarrow$ $\uparrow$ diastolic stiffness

Extracellular Matrix

Collagen structure, geometry, content, collagen I/III ratio
Collagen homeostasis, synthesis, postsynthetic processing, posttranslational crosslinking, degradation
Basement membrane proteins
Bioactive proteins and peptides: MMP/TIMP, SPARC, TGF-β
Fibroblast structure, function, phenotype
Myofibroblast transdifferentiation

Extra Cardiac

Extrinsic forces (RV-LV interaction and pericardial constraint)
Peripheral muscle and ergoreflex dysfunction
Pulmonary hypertension (secondary to chronic pulmonary venous hypertension)
Neurohormonal activation
Comorbid conditions (renal dysfunction, anemia, chronic lung disease)

ADP, Adenosine diphosphate; *ATP,* adenosine triphosphate; *LA,* left atrium; *LV,* left ventricle; *RV,* right ventricle; *SPARC,* secreted protein, acidic and rich in cysteine [osteonectin]; *TGF,* transforming growth vector.
From Mann DL et al: *Braunwald's heart disease,* ed 10, Philadelphia, 2015, Elsevier.

admission to the hospital is useful to establish a prognosis in acutely decompensated HF, and predischarge natriuretic peptide level can be useful to establish a postdischarge prognosis. There are insufficient data to recommend natriuretic peptide biomarker–guided therapy or serial measurements for the purpose of reducing hospitalization or deaths. ACC/AHA/HFSA guidelines for the use of biomarkers in HF are summarized in Table 9.

3. Cardiac biomarkers may be elevated if ischemia is the precipitant factor. However, slight elevations are very common and may not always be due to obstructive coronary artery disease. These elevations could be due to subendocardial ischemia (due to increased end-diastolic pressure resulting in decreased perfusion) and necrosis, or cardiomyocyte damage from the inflammatory cytokines or oxidative stress. Impaired renal function is very common, and decreased clearance of the biomarkers can contribute to their elevation. Therefore these elevations should be interpreted in the context of the clinical setting. Despite that, in patients with acute decompensated heart failure (ADHF), a positive cardiac troponin test (from whatever mechanism) is associated with worse prognosis.

4. Screening for dyslipidemia and glucose intolerance, which are risk factors for CAD.
5. If hemochromatosis is suspected (specifically in Northern European patients), consider checking a transferrin saturation and ferritin level.
6. Consider HIV testing in high-risk patients and COVID-19 testing in all patients.

- Electrocardiogram (ECG)[2]:
  1. Look for signs of prior MI, chamber enlargement, hypertrophy, heart block, arrhythmia, and evidence of pericardial effusion.
  2. More than 25% of patients with HF have some form of intraventricular conduction abnormality that manifests as an increased QRS duration. The most common pattern seen is left bundle-branch block.
- Chest x-ray (Fig. 3)[2]:
  1. Evaluate for pulmonary venous congestion, pulmonary edema, pleural effusion, cardiomegaly, chamber dilation, and Kerley B lines.
- Echocardiography[2]:
  1. Plays a critical diagnostic role in patients with HF and is useful in assessment of systolic, diastolic function in addition to assessment of valvular structure and function.
- Exercise stress testing[2]:
  1. May be useful in evaluating concomitant ischemic etiologies and assessment of degree of disability in stable compensated patients.
- Cardiac catheterization[2]:
  1. Left heart catheterization can help to identify coronary artery disease as a cause of HF. Right heart catheterization can help to evaluate intracardiac filling pressures, estimates of valvular areas, presence of intracardiac shunts, and calculation of hemodynamic properties such as cardiac output, systemic vascular resistance, and pulmonary artery wedge pressure to further guide management.
- Cardiac MRI[2]:
  1. Useful modality in accurately estimating EF (with less variability than conventional 2D echocardiography). MRI is also useful in excluding pericardial disease, identifying infiltrative disease, and assessing viability in cases of HF caused by underlying ischemic heart disease.

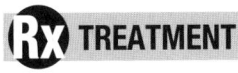 **TREATMENT**

(Fig. 4)

NONPHARMACOLOGIC GENERAL MEASURES

- Assess the etiology and severity of disease. Educate the patient and family about the nature of the disorder. Assess the home setting and if patient has social support to ensure compliance, especially for patients with dementia.
- Identify and correct precipitating factors (e.g., increased sodium load, medication noncompliance, ischemia, infections, anemia, thyrotoxicosis) and address lifestyle modification

TABLE 8 ACC/AHA Guidelines for Initial and Serial Evaluation of Heart Failure

Class		Level of Evidence
Indication: History, Physical Examination, and Risk Scoring		
I	A Thorough history and physical examination should be obtained/performed in patients presenting with HF to identify cardiac and noncardiac disorders or behaviors that might cause or accelerate the development or progression of HF.	C
	In patients with idiopathic DCM, a three-generational family history should be obtained to aid in establishing the diagnosis of familial DCM.	C
	Volume status and vital signs should be assessed at each patient encounter. This includes serial assessment of weight, as well as estimates of jugular venous pressure and the presence of peripheral edema or orthopnea.	B
IIa	Validated multivariable risk scores can be useful to estimate subsequent risk of mortality in ambulatory or hospitalized patients with HF.	C
Indication: Diagnostic Tests and Biomarkers (also see below)		
I	Initial laboratory evaluation of patients presenting with HF should include complete blood count, urinalysis, serum electrolytes (including calcium and magnesium), blood urea nitrogen, serum creatinine, glucose, fasting lipid profile, liver function tests, and thyroid-stimulating hormone.	C
	Serial monitoring, when indicated, should include serum electrolytes and renal function.	C
	A 12-lead ECG should be performed initially on all patients presenting with HF.	C
	In ambulatory patients with dyspnea, measurement of BNP or N-terminal pro-B-type natriuretic peptide (NT-proBNP) is useful to support clinical decision making regarding the diagnosis of HF, especially in the setting of clinical uncertainty, and measurement of BNP or NT-proBNP is useful for establishing prognosis or disease severity in chronic HF.	A
IIa	Screening for hemochromatosis or HIV is reasonable in select patients who present with HF.	C
	Diagnostic tests for rheumatologic diseases, amyloidosis, or pheochromocytoma are reasonable in patients presenting with HF in whom there is a clinical suspicion of these diseases.	C
	BNP-guided or NT-proBNP—guided HF therapy can be useful to achieve optimal dosing of GDMT in select, clinically euvolemic patients followed in a well-structured HF disease management program.	B
IIb	The usefulness of serial measurement of BNP or NT-proBNP to reduce hospitalization or mortality in patients with HF is not well established. The measurement of other clinically available tests, such as biomarkers of myocardial injury or "fibrosis," may be considered for additive risk stratification in patients with chronic HF.	B
Indication: Noninvasive Cardiac Imaging		
I	Patients with suspected or new-onset HF, or those presenting with acute decompensated HF, should undergo a chest radiograph to assess heart size and pulmonary congestion and to detect alternative cardiac, pulmonary, and other diseases that may cause or contribute to the patient's symptoms.	C
	A two-dimensional echocardiogram with Doppler should be performed during initial evaluation of patients presenting with HF to assess ventricular function, size, wall thickness, wall motion, and valve function.	C
	Repeat measurement of EF and measurement of the severity of structural remodeling are useful to provide information in patients with HF who have had a significant change in clinical status; who have experienced or recovered from a clinical event; who have received treatment, including GDMT, that might have had a significant effect on cardiac function; or who may be candidates for device therapy.	C
IIa	Noninvasive imaging to detect myocardial ischemia and viability is reasonable in patients presenting with de novo HF who have known CAD and no angina, unless the patient is not eligible for revascularization of any kind.	C
	Viability assessment is reasonable in select situations when planning revascularization in HF patients with CAD.	B
	Radionuclide ventriculography or MRI can be useful to assess LVEF and volume when echocardiography is inadequate.	C
	MRI is reasonable when assessing myocardial infiltrative processes or scar burden.	B
III: No benefit	Routine repeat measurement of LV function assessment in the absence of clinical status change or treatment interventions should not be performed.	B
Indication: Invasive Evaluation		
I	Invasive hemodynamic monitoring with a pulmonary artery catheter should be performed to guide therapy in patients who have respiratory distress or clinical evidence of impaired perfusion in whom the adequacy or excess of intracardiac filling pressures cannot be determined from clinical assessment.	C
IIa	Invasive hemodynamic monitoring can be useful for carefully selected patients with acute HF who have persistent symptoms despite empiric adjustment of standard therapies and (a) whose fluid status, perfusion, or systemic or pulmonary vascular resistance is uncertain; (b) whose systolic pressure remains low, or is associated with symptoms, despite initial therapy; (c) whose renal function is worsening with therapy; (d) who require parenteral vasoactive agents; or (e) who may need consideration for mechanical circulatory support or transplantation.	C
	When ischemia may be contributing to HF, coronary arteriography is reasonable for patients eligible for revascularization.	C
	Endomyocardial biopsy can be useful in patients presenting with HF when a specific diagnosis is suspected that would influence therapy.	C
III: No benefit	Routine use of invasive hemodynamic monitoring is not recommended in normotensive patients with acute decompensated HF and congestion with symptomatic response to diuretics and vasodilators.	B
III: Harm	Endomyocardial biopsy should not be performed in the routine evaluation of patients with HF.	C

ACC, American College of Cardiology; *AHA,* American Heart Association; *BNP,* B-type natriuretic peptide; *CAD,* coronary artery disease; *DCM,* dilated cardiomyopathy, *ECG,* electrocardiogram; *EF,* ejection fraction; *GDMT,* guideline-directed medical therapy; *HIV,* human immunodeficiency virus; *LV,* left ventricle; *LVEF,* left ventricular ejection fraction; *MRI,* magnetic resonance imaging.
From Zipes DP: *Braunwald's heart disease, a textbook of cardiovascular medicine,* ed 11, Philadelphia, 2019, Elsevier.

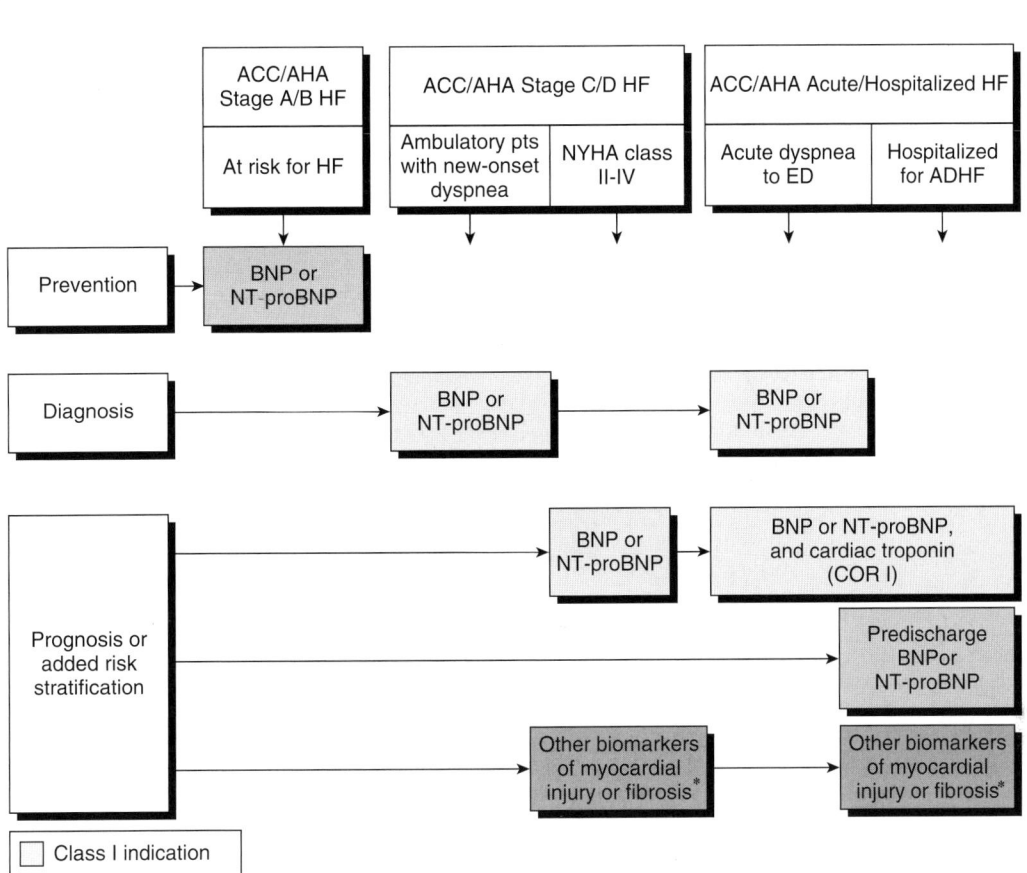

FIG. 2 Indications for the use of biomarkers in heart failure. *Other biomarkers of injury or fibrosis include soluble ST2 receptor, galectin-3, and high-sensitivity troponin. *ACC,* American College of Cardiology; *AHA,* American Heart Association; *ADHF,* acute decompensated heart failure; *BNP,* B-type natriuretic peptide; *COR,* class of recommendation; *ED,* emergency department; *HF,* heart failure; *NT-proBNP,* N-terminal pro-B-type natriuretic peptide; *NYHA,* New York Heart Association; *pts,* patients. (Modified from Yancy CW et al: 2017 ACC/AHA/HFSA focused update of the 2013 ACCF/AHA guideline for the management of heart failure: a report of the American College of Cardiology/American Heart Association Task Force on Clinical Practice Guidelines and the Heart Failure Society of America, *J Am Coll Cardiol* 70[6]:776, 2017. In Zipes DP: *Braunwald's heart disease, a textbook of cardiovascular medicine,* ed 11, Philadelphia, 2019, Elsevier.)

TABLE 9 ACC/AHA/HFSA Guidelines for Use of Biomarkers in Heart Failure

Class		Level of Evidence
Biomarkers for Prevention of HF		
IIa	For patients at risk of developing HF, natriuretic peptide biomarker–based screening can be useful to prevent the development of left ventricular dysfunction (systolic or diastolic) or new-onset HF.	B-R
Biomarkers for Diagnosis		
I	In patients presenting with dyspnea (acute or chronic), measurement of natriuretic peptide biomarkers is useful to support a diagnosis or exclusion of HF.	A
Biomarkers for Prognosis or Added Risk Stratification		
I	Measurement of BNP or NT-proBNP is useful for establishing prognosis or disease severity in chronic HF.	A
I	Measurement of baseline levels of natriuretic peptide biomarkers and/or cardiac troponin on admission to the hospital is useful to establish a prognosis in acutely decompensated HF.	A
IIa	During an HF hospitalization, a predischarge natriuretic peptide level can be useful to establish a postdischarge prognosis.	B-NR
IIb	In patients with chronic HF, measurement of other clinically available tests, such as biomarkers of myocardial injury or fibrosis, may be considered for additive risk stratification.	B-NR

ACC, American College of Cardiology; *AHA,* American Heart Association; *BNP,* B-type natriuretic peptide; *HF,* heart failure; *HFSA,* Heart Failure Society of America; *NT-proBNP,* N-terminal pro-B-type natriuretic peptide.
From Zipes DP: *Braunwald's heart disease, a textbook of cardiovascular medicine,* ed 11, Philadelphia, 2019, Elsevier.

(e.g., smoking and alcohol cessation, weight reduction, avoiding use of nonsteroidal anti-inflammatory drugs [NSAIDs]). Anemia is common in patients with HF. In patients with NYHA class II and III symptoms and iron deficiency, IV iron replacement may be reasonable to improve functional status and quality of life (class IIb recommendation).[12,13] Treatments with erythropoiesis-stimulating agents (ESAs) have not shown improved clinical outcomes in patients with systolic HF and mild-to-moderate anemia and are thus not recommended.[14]

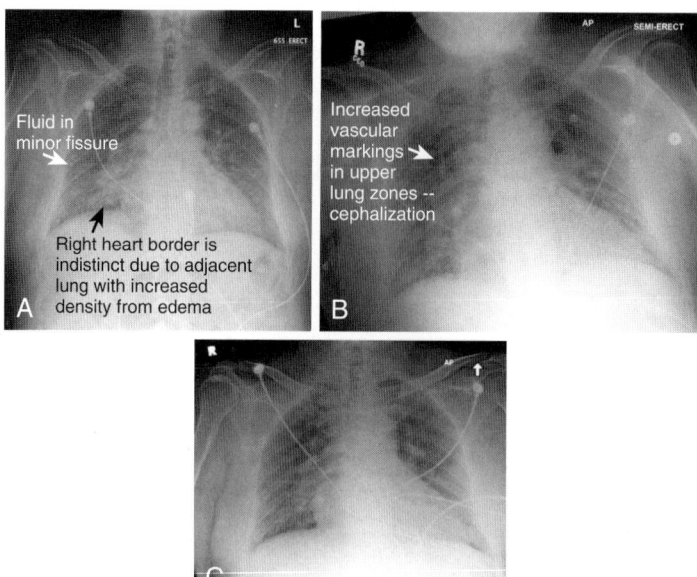

FIG. 3 Congestive heart failure. Mild left ventricular hypertrophy with restricted filling, ejection fraction >55%, and no pericardial effusion. This 63-yr-old man with coronary artery disease, chronic renal insufficiency, and diastolic heart failure (ejection fraction >55%) presented multiple times for dyspnea (**A, B,** and **C,** first through third clinical presentations). Each of these three radiographs shows signs of moderate pulmonary edema. The diaphragms and costophrenic angles are clear, suggesting no pleural effusion. The right heart border in all three images is indistinct because of interstitial edema in these locations. Portions of the left heart border are also indistinct. The upper lung fields have a hazy appearance indicating mild edema. Fluid is visible in the minor fissure on all three images. Does the similarity of these radiographs mean that edema is not the cause of the patient's dyspnea? No, he simply presented with pulmonary edema on all three occasions. (From Broder JS: *Diagnostic imaging for the emergency physician,* Philadelphia, 2011, Saunders.)

Table 10 describes ACC/AHA guidelines for treating patients at high risk for development of heart failure.

- Review list of medications and discontinue the ones that can contribute to HF (e.g., NSAIDs, antiarrhythmic drugs, calcium channel blockers, thiazolidinediones).[2]
- Dietary sodium restriction of <2 g/day is commonly recommended to patients with HF and is endorsed by many guidelines.[2]
- Restrict fluid intake to <2 L/day in patients with hyponatremia.[2]
- Caloric supplementation should be provided to patients with advanced HF with weight loss and muscle wasting due to cardiac cachexia. Weight loss may reflect cachexia caused by the higher total energy expenditure associated with HF compared with that of healthy sedentary subjects. The diagnosis of cardiac cachexia independently predicts a worse prognosis.[10]
- For patients with coexisting obstructive sleep apnea, continuous positive airway pressure (CPAP) may be reasonable after polysomnography (class IIb recommendation).[2]
- Exercise training (or regular physical activity) is recommended as safe and effective for patients with class I to III HF who are able to participate to improve functional status (class I recommendation). Cardiac rehabilitation is unfortunately an underused preventive measure, although it has been shown to reduce morbidity and mortality. Intensive cardiac rehabilitation can be useful in clinically stable patients with HF to improve functional capacity, exercise duration, health-related quality of life, and mortality (class IIa

recommendation). Home-based cardiac rehabilitation is also an equally effective alternative if patients cannot participate in regular cardiac rehabilitation.[2]
- Pneumococcal vaccination, annual influenza vaccination.[2]
- ACC/AHA guidelines for treatment of asymptomatic left ventricular systolic dysfunction are summarized in Table 11.

TREATMENT OF ADHF

- Four phases in treatment of ADHF:
  1st phase: Initial stabilization and management (Table 12)
  2nd phase: Inpatient hospital care (Table 13)
  3rd phase: Early discharge planning and care
  4th phase: Early post-discharge care
- 1st phase: Initial stabilization and management
- Short-term goals: Hemodynamic stabilization, stabilization of respiratory status, symptom relief, optimization of tissue perfusion, and recognition of more immediately life-threatening conditions (e.g., arrhythmias, valvular catastrophe, MI, cardiac tamponade). Initial therapy of ADHF is contingent on appropriate determination of clinical scenario.[1]
- Management as per clinical scenario:
  1. ADHF-associated hypertension: Goal is afterload reduction and decrease of systemic hypervolemia. Mode of treatment: Diuresis (IV loop diuretics) and vasodilators (acutely nitrates and morphine followed by treatment with ACE inhibitors or angiotensin receptor blockers [ARBs]).
  2. Worsening or decompensation of chronic HF (HFrEF or HFpEF): Goal is control of

volume status. Treatment is accomplished with vasodilators and diuretics.[10]
  3. Flash pulmonary edema: Goal is afterload reduction (vasodilators such as nitrates acutely), respiratory status stabilization, and diuresis (IV loop diuretics). Rate control can be initiated in patients with atrial fibrillation or tachyarrhythmias as it may improve cardiac filling and function.[10]
  4. Cardiogenic shock: Goal is hemodynamic stabilization. Treatment consists of inotropes + vasopressors ± mechanical circulatory support ± emergent revascularization if indicated.[10]
  5. ACS and ADHF: Goal is hemodynamic stabilization + emergent restoration of coronary perfusion. See "Acute Coronary Syndrome".
  6. Isolated RV failure: Goals are identification of etiology: (1) Valvular, (2) pulmonary hypertension, and (3) primary RV failure secondary to ischemia. Treatment: Depends on etiology, either corrective surgery vs. treatment of pulmonary hypertension (endothelin antagonists, calcium channel blockers, phosphodiesterase inhibitors) vs. coronary reperfusion therapies.[10]

ACUTE PHARMACOLOGIC TREATMENTS:

- Vasodilators (Table 14) are appropriate in most patients with ADHF (contraindicated in cardiogenic shock and severe aortic stenosis).
  1. Nitroglycerin (0.4 to 0.8 mg sublingually every 3 to 5 min, or by intravenous infusion starting at 0.2 to 0.4 mcg/kg/min with subsequent up titration) may be administered in the emergency setting until relative hypotension ensues. Nitrates are

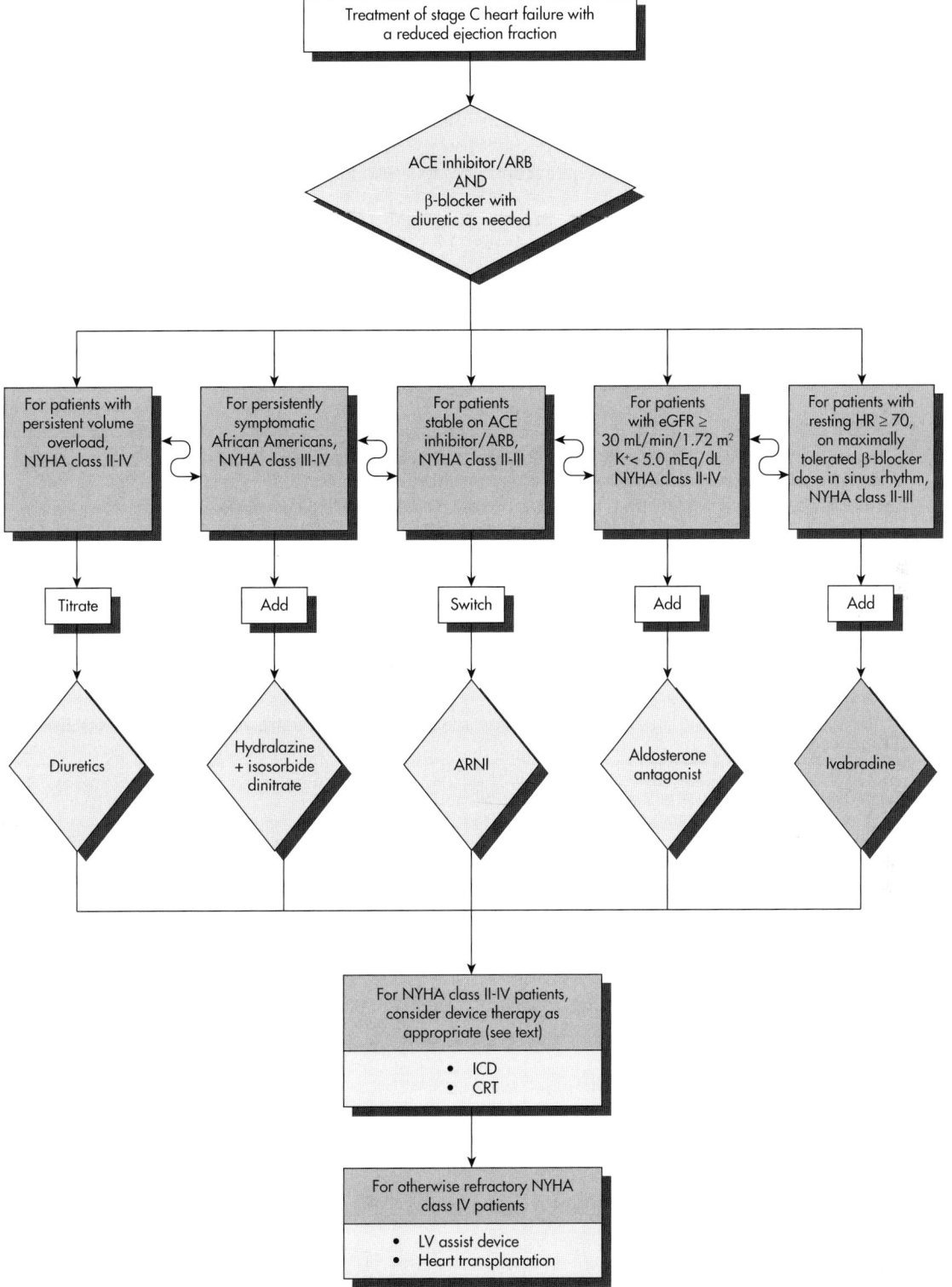

FIG. 4 General approach to heart failure. Stage C heart failure with a reduced ejection fraction. Evidence-based, guideline-directed medical therapy. *ACE*, angiotensin-converting enzyme; *ARB*, angiotensin-receptor blocker; *ARNI*, angiotensin receptor-neprilysin inhibitor; *CRT*, cardiac resynchronization therapy; *eGFR*, estimated glomerular filtration rate; *HR*, heart rate; *ICD*, implantable cardiovascular-defibrillator; *LV*, left ventricular; *MRA*, mineralocorticoid receptor antagonist; *NYHA*, New York Heart Association; *SGLT2i*, sodium glucose cotransporter 2 inhibitor. (Adapted from Yancy CW, Januzzi JL, Jr. et al: 2017 ACC Expert Consensus Decision Pathway for optimization of heart failure treatment: answers to 10 pivotal issues about heart failure with reduced ejection fraction: a report of the American College of Cardiology Task Force on Expert Consensus Decision Pathways, *J Am Coll Cardiol* 71:201-230, 2018. In Goldman L, Shafer AI: *Goldman-Cecil medicine,* ed 26, Philadelphia, 2019, Elsevier.)

H

Diseases
and Disorders

I

TABLE 10 ACC/AHA Guidelines for Treating Patients at High Risk of Developing Heart Failure (Stage A)

Class	Indication	Level of Evidence
I	Hypertension and lipid disorders should be controlled in accordance with contemporary guidelines to lower the risk of HF.	A
I	In patients at increased risk, stage A, the optimal blood pressure in those with hypertension should be less than 130/80 mm Hg.	B-R
I	Other conditions that may lead to or contribute to HF, such as obesity, diabetes mellitus, tobacco use, and known cardiotoxic agents, should be controlled or avoided.	C
II	For patients at risk of developing HF, natriuretic peptide biomarker–based screening followed by team-based care, including a cardiovascular specialist optimizing GDMT, can be useful to prevent the development of left ventricular dysfunction (systolic or diastolic) or new-onset HF.	B-R

ACC, American College of Cardiology; *AHA*, American Heart Association; *GDMT*, guideline-directed medical therapy; *HF*, heart failure.
From Zipes DP: *Braunwald's heart disease, a textbook of cardiovascular medicine,* ed 11, Philadelphia, 2019, Elsevier.

TABLE 11 ACC/AHA Guidelines for Treatment of Asymptomatic Left Ventricular Systolic Dysfunction (Stage B)

Class	Indication	Level of Evidence
I	In all patients with a recent or remote history of MI or ACS and reduced EF, ACE inhibitors should be used to prevent symptomatic HF and reduce mortality. In patients intolerant of ACE inhibitors, ARBs are appropriate unless contraindicated.	A
	In all patients with a recent or remote history of MI or ACS and reduced EF, evidence-based β-blockers should be used to reduce mortality. β-blockade and ACE inhibition should be used in all patients with a recent or remote history of MI regardless of EF or presence of HF.	B
	In all patients with a recent or remote history of MI or ACS, statins should be used to prevent symptomatic HF and cardiovascular events.	A
	Blood pressure should be controlled in accordance with clinical practice guidelines for hypertension to prevent symptomatic HF.	A
	ACE inhibitors should be used in all patients with a reduced EF to prevent symptomatic HF.	A
	β-blockers should be used in all patients with a reduced EF to prevent symptomatic HF.	C
IIa	To prevent sudden death, placement of an ICD is reasonable in patients with asymptomatic ischemic cardiomyopathy who are at least 40 days post-MI, have an LVEF of 30% or less, are on appropriate medical therapy, and have reasonable expectation of survival with a good functional status for more than 1 yr.	B
III: Harm	Nondihydropyridine calcium channel blockers with negative inotropic effects may be harmful in asymptomatic patients with low LVEF and no symptoms of HF after MI.	B

ACC, American College of Cardiology; *ACE*, angiotensin-converting enzyme; *ACS*, acute coronary syndrome; *AHA*, American Heart Association; *ARB*, angiotensin receptor antagonist; *EF*, ejection fraction; *HF*, heart failure; *ICD*, implantable cardioverter-defibrillator; *LVEF*, left ventricular ejection fraction; *MI*, myocardial infarction.
From Zipes DP: *Braunwald's heart disease, a textbook of cardiovascular medicine,* ed 11, Philadelphia, 2019, Elsevier.

TABLE 12 ACC/AHA Guidelines for Treatment of Symptomatic Left Ventricular Systolic Dysfunction (Stage C)

Class	Indication	Level of Evidence
	Nonpharmacologic Interventions	
I	Patients with HF should receive specific education to facilitate HF self-care.	B
	Exercise training (or regular physical activity) is recommended as safe and effective for patients with HF who are able to participate to improve functional status.	A
IIa	Cardiac rehabilitation can be useful in clinically stable patients with HF to improve functional capacity, exercise duration, HRQOL, and mortality.	B
	Sodium restriction is reasonable for patients with symptomatic HF to reduce congestive symptoms.	C
	Continuous positive airway pressure (CPAP) can be beneficial to increase LVEF and improve functional status in patients with HF and sleep apnea.	B
	Pharmacologic Interventions	
I	Measures listed as class I recommendations for patients in stages A and B are recommended where appropriate.	A, B, C
	GDMT should be the mainstay of pharmacologic therapy for HFrEF.	A
	Diuretics	
I	Diuretics are recommended in patients with HFrEF who have evidence of fluid retention, unless contraindicated, to ameliorate symptoms.	C
	Angiotensin-Converting Enzyme Inhibitors/Adrenergic Receptor Blockers	
I	ACE inhibitors are recommended in patients with HFrEF and current or previous symptoms, unless contraindicated, to reduce morbidity and mortality.	A
	ARBs are recommended in patients with HFrEF with current or previous symptoms who are ACE inhibitor–intolerant, unless contraindicated, to reduce morbidity and mortality.	A
IIa	ARBs are a reasonable choice to reduce morbidity and mortality as alternatives to ACE inhibitors for first-line therapy in patients with HFrEF, especially in those already taking ARBs for other indications, unless contraindicated.	A
IIb	Addition of an ARB may be considered in persistently symptomatic patients with HFrEF who are already being treated with an ACE inhibitor and a β-blocker in whom an aldosterone antagonist is not indicated or tolerated.	A
III: Harm	Routinely combining an ACE inhibitor, an ARB, and an aldosterone antagonist.	C

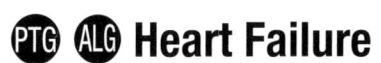

H

I

TABLE 12 ACC/AHA Guidelines for Treatment of Symptomatic Left Ventricular Systolic Dysfunction (Stage C)—cont'd

Class	Indication	Level of Evidence
	β-Blockers	
I	Use of one of the three β-blockers proven to reduce mortality (i.e., bisoprolol, carvedilol, and sustained-release metoprolol succinate) is recommended for all patients with current or previous symptoms of HFrEF, unless contraindicated, to reduce morbidity and mortality.	A
	Aldosterone Receptor Antagonists	
I	Aldosterone receptor antagonists (or mineralocorticoid receptor antagonists) are recommended in patients with NYHA class II-IV and LVEF of ≤35%, unless contraindicated, to reduce morbidity and mortality.	A
I	Aldosterone receptor antagonists are recommended to reduce morbidity and mortality after an acute MI in patients with LVEF of ≤40% who develop symptoms of HF or who have a history of diabetes mellitus, unless contraindicated.	B
III: Harm	Inappropriate use of aldosterone receptor antagonists is potentially harmful because of life-threatening hyperkalemia or renal insufficiency when serum creatinine is >2.5 mg/dl in men or >2.0 mg/dl in women (or estimated glomerular filtration rate <30 ml/min/1.73 m²), and/or potassium >5.0 mEq/liter.	B
	SGLT-2 Inhibitors	
I	In patients with symptomatic chronic HFrEF, SGLT2 inhibitors are recommended to reduce hospitalization for HF and cardiovascular mortality, irrespective of the presence of type 2 diabetes.	A
IIa	In patients with HFmrEF (LVEF 41%-49%), SGLT2 inhibitors can be beneficial in decreasing HF hospitalizations and cardiovascular mortality.	B
	Hydralazine and Isosorbide Dinitrate	
I	The combination of hydralazine and isosorbide dinitrate is recommended to reduce morbidity and mortality for patients self-described as African Americans with NYHA class III-IV HFrEF receiving optimal therapy with ACE inhibitors and β-blockers, unless contraindicated.	A
IIa	A combination of hydralazine and isosorbide dinitrate can be useful to reduce morbidity or mortality in patients with current or previous symptomatic HFrEF who cannot be given an ACE inhibitor or ARB because of drug intolerance, hypotension, or renal insufficiency, unless contraindicated.	B
	Digoxin	
IIa	Digoxin can be beneficial in patients with HFrEF, unless contraindicated, to decrease hospitalizations for HF.	B
	Anticoagulation	
I	Patients with chronic HF with permanent/persistent/paroxysmal atrial fibrillation and an additional risk factor for cardioembolic stroke (history of hypertension, diabetes mellitus, previous stroke or transient ischemic attack, or ≥75 yr of age) should receive chronic anticoagulant therapy.	A
I	The selection of an anticoagulant agent (warfarin, dabigatran, apixaban, or rivaroxaban) for permanent/persistent/paroxysmal atrial fibrillation should be individualized on the basis of risk factors, cost, tolerability, patient preference, potential for drug interactions, and other clinical characteristics, including time in the international normalized ratio therapeutic range if the patient has been taking warfarin.	C
IIa	Chronic anticoagulation is reasonable for patients with chronic HF who have permanent/persistent/paroxysmal atrial fibrillation but no additional risk factor for cardioembolic stroke.	B
III: No benefit	Anticoagulation is not recommended in patients with chronic HFrEF without atrial fibrillation, a previous thromboembolic event, or a cardioembolic source.	B
	Statins	
III: No benefit	Statins are not beneficial as adjunctive therapy when prescribed solely for HF.	A
	Omega-3 Fatty Acids	
IIa	Omega-3 PUFA supplementation is reasonable to use as adjunctive therapy in patients with NYHA class II-IV symptoms and HFrEF or HFpEF, unless contraindicated, to reduce mortality and cardiovascular hospitalizations.	B
	Drugs of Unproven Value or That May Cause Harm	
III: No benefit	Nutritional supplements as treatment for HF are not recommended in patients with current or previous symptoms of HFrEF.	B
	Hormonal therapies other than to correct deficiencies are not recommended for patients with current or previous symptoms of HFrEF.	C
III: Harm	Drugs known to adversely affect the clinical status of patients with current or previous symptoms of HFrEF are potentially harmful and should be avoided or withdrawn whenever possible (e.g., most antiarrhythmic drugs, most calcium channel blocking drugs [except amlodipine], NSAIDs, or thiazolidinediones).	B
	Long-term use of infused positive inotropic drugs is potentially harmful for patients with HFrEF, except as palliation for patients with end-stage disease who cannot be stabilized with standard medical treatment (see recommendations for stage D).	C
	Calcium Channel Blockers	
III: No benefit	Calcium channel blocking drugs are not recommended for routine therapy in patients with HFrEF.	A

ACC, American College of Cardiology; *ACE,* angiotensin-converting-enzyme; *AHA,* American Heart Association; *ARB,* angiotensin-receptor blocker; *GDMT,* guideline-directed medical therapy; *HF,* heart failure; *HFpEF,* heart failure with preserved ejection fraction; *HFrEF,* heart failure with reduced ejection fraction; *HRQOL,* health-related quality of life; *LVEF,* left ventricular ejection fraction; *MI,* myocardial infarction; *NYHA,* New York Heart Association; *NSAID,* nonsteroidal antiinflammatory drug; *PUFA,* polyunsaturated fatty acid.
Adapted from Mann DL et al: *Braunwald's heart disease,* ed 10, Philadelphia, 2015, Elsevier and updated to include ACC/AHA/HFSA 2022 guidelines.

contraindicated after use of phosphodiesterase inhibitors such as sildenafil due to risk of hypotension.[10]

2. Sodium nitroprusside (0.1 to 0.2 mcg/kg/min as an intravenous infusion) is a potent vasodilator with balanced venous and arteriolar effects that usually requires hemodynamic monitoring with an arterial line and may precipitate coronary steal and thiocyanate toxicity (elevated risk in renal failure).[10]

3. When given intravenously, loop diuretics have an immediate vasodilator effect that provides clinical relief of symptoms before diuresis begins. Due to gut edema and unpredictable patterns of absorption, oral formulation may become less effective. Therefore intravenous formulation should be used in the acute setting.[10] Studies showed no difference in outcome when using bolus dosing vs. continuous IV

TABLE 13 ACC/AHA Recommendations for the Hospitalized Patient With Heart Failure (HF)

Class	Indication	Level of Evidence*
I	Thorough history and physical examination to evaluate for adequacy of systemic perfusion, volume status, contribution of precipitating factors and/or comorbidities, and whether HF is associated with preserved ejection fraction.	C
	Concentrations of B-type natriuretic peptide (BNP) or N-terminal pro-B-type natriuretic peptide (NT-proBNP) to evaluate dyspnea if the contribution of heart failure is not known.	A
	Acute coronary syndrome should be promptly identified by electrocardiogram and cardiac troponin testing, and treated, as appropriate to the overall condition and prognosis of patient.	C
	Oxygen therapy should be administered to relieve symptoms related to hypoxemia.	C
	Improve systemic perfusion in patients who present with rapid decompensation and hypoperfusion associated with decreasing urine output and other manifestations of shock.	C
	Treatment of significant fluid overload with intravenous loop diuretics. The diuretic dose should be titrated to relieve symptoms and to reduce extracellular fluid volume excess.	B, C
	Monitor the effects of therapy with careful measurement of fluid intake and output; vital signs; body weight, and symptoms of systemic perfusion and congestion.	C
	Intensify the diuretic regiment when the diuresis is inadequate to relieve congestion.	C
	Intravenous inotropic or vasopressor drugs should be administered to maintain systemic perfusion and preserve end-organ performance in patients with clinical evidence of hypotension associated with hypoperfusion and elevated cardiac filling pressures.	C
	Invasive hemodynamic monitoring to guide therapy in patients who are in respiratory distress or with clinical evidence of impaired perfusion if filling pressures cannot be determined from clinical assessment.	C
	Medications should be reconciled and adjusted as appropriate on admission to and discharge from the hospital.	C
	Maintenance treatment with oral therapies known to improve outcomes (ACE inhibitors or ARBs and β-blocker therapy) in the absence of hemodynamic instability or contraindications.	C
	Initiation of treatment with oral therapies known to improve outcomes (ACE inhibitors or ARBs and β-blocker therapy) in stable patients prior to hospital discharge.	B
	During transition from intravenous to oral diuretic therapy, patient should be monitored carefully for supine and upright hypotension, worsening renal function, and HF signs/symptoms.	C
	Comprehensive written discharge instructions for patients and their caregivers is strongly recommended.	C
	Postdischarge systems of care, if available, should be used to facilitate the transition to effective outpatient care.	B
IIa	Urgent cardiac catheterization and revascularization in patients with acute HF with known or suspected acute myocardial ischemia due to occlusive coronary disease when there are signs and symptoms of inadequate systemic perfusion and revascularization is likely to prolong meaningful survival.	C
	Intravenous nitroglycerin, nitroprusside, or nesiritide for patients with evidence of severely symptomatic fluid overload in the absence of systemic hypotension.	C
	Ultrafiltration for patients with refractory congestion not responding to medical therapy.	B
IIb	Intravenous inotropic drugs (dopamine, dobutamine, or milrinone) for patients presenting with documented severe systolic dysfunction, low blood pressure, and evidence of low cardiac output, with or without congestion, to maintain systemic perfusion and preserve end-organ performance.	C
III	Use of parenteral inotropes in normotensive patients with acute decompensated HF without evidence of decreased organ perfusion.	B
	Routine use of invasive hemodynamic monitoring in normotensive patients with acute decompensated HF and congestion with symptomatic response to diuretics and vasodilators.	B

ACC, American College of Cardiology; *ACE,* angiotensin-converting enzyme; *AHA,* American Heart Association; *ARB,* angiotensin-receptor blocker.
*See guidelines text for definition of level of evidence categories.
From Zipes DP: *Braunwald's heart disease, a textbook of cardiovascular medicine,* ed 11, Philadelphia, 2019, Elsevier.

infusion.[15] Administration of smaller doses of short-acting loop diuretics multiple times daily is preferable to a single large dose because the kidneys can avidly reabsorb sodium after the initial diuresis. However, if a certain dose is not adequate to force diuresis, the dose, rather than the frequency, should be increased until a single effective dose is reached; more frequent doses can be added as needed. Therefore monitoring of urine output, renal function, and electrolytes is key. The addition of a distal tubule inhibitor such as metolazone 30 min prior to loop diuretic dosing has a synergistic effect and often enhances diuresis because it inhibits sodium reabsorption in the distal segment in the face of increased sodium delivery from the loop. Diuretics should be used with caution in patients with aortic stenosis.

- Inotropic agents are used for temporary hemodynamic support in cardiogenic shock, but they have not been shown to improve survival. Many of these agents have serious associated adverse events including myocardial necrosis and malignant arrhythmias.[16]
  1. Dobutamine (starting at 2.5 to 5 mcg/kg/min) can be used for inotropic support but is associated with increased myocardial oxygen demand and cardiac arrhythmias and may result in hypotension from decreased systemic vascular resistance.
  2. Milrinone (37.5 to 75 mcg/kg loading dose, followed by 0.375 to 0.75 mcg/kg/min) can be used as a vasodilator and inotropic agent, but is associated with increased oxygen demand and cardiac arrhythmias, and may result in hypotension from decreased systemic vascular resistance.
- Renal replacement therapy or ultrafiltration (can be used as an alternative to pharmacologic diuresis in ADHF when renal function is significantly compromised).[2]
- ACE inhibitors or ARBs, if part of a patient's chronic medication regimen, should be continued in the absence of hypotension, acute renal failure, or hyperkalemia.[10]
- β-blockers, if part of a patient's chronic medication regimen, may be continued or reduced in dosage in mild exacerbations of HF but should be discontinued in patients with hypotension or those requiring inotropic support. β-blockers should not be initiated in patients who are not on chronic β-blocker therapy until euvolemia is achieved unless used for rate control.[10]

TABLE 14 Intravenous Vasoactive Agents for Treatment of Acute Heart Failure

Intravenous Medication	Initial Dose	Effective Dose Range	Comments
Vasodilators			
Nitroglycerin; glyceryl trinitrate	20 μg/min	40-400 μg/min	Hypotension, headache Tolerance with continuous use after 24 h
Isosorbide dinitrate	1 mg/h	2-10 mg/h	Hypotension, headache Tolerance with continuous use within 24 h
Nitroprusside	0.3 μg/kg/min	0.3-5 μg/kg/min (usually <4 μg/kg/min)	Caution in patients with active myocardial ischemia Hypotension; cyanide side effects (nausea, dysphoria); thiocyanate toxicity; light sensitive
Nesiritide	2 μg/kg bolus with 0.010-0.030 μg/kg/min infusion*	0.010-0.030 μg/kg/min[†]	Uptitration: 1 μg/kg bolus, then increase infusion rate by 0.005 μg/kg/min no more frequently than every 3 h, up to maximum of 0.03 μg/kg/min Hypotension, headache (less than with organic nitrates)
Inotropes			
Dobutamine	1-2 μg/kg/min	2-20 μg/kg/min	For inotropy and vasodilation; hypotension, tachycardia, arrhythmias; ?mortality
Dopamine	1-2 μg/kg/min	2-4 μg/kg/min	For inotropy and vasodilation; hypotension, tachycardia, arrhythmias; ?mortality
	4-5 μg/kg/min	5-20 μg/kg/min	For inotropy and vasoconstriction; tachycardia, arrhythmias; ?mortality
Milrinone	25-75 μg/kg bolus over 10-20 min* followed by infusion	0.10-0.75 μg/kg/min	For vasodilation and inotropy; hypotension, tachycardia, arrhythmias; renal excretion; ?mortality
Enoximone[††]	0.25-0.75 mg/kg	1.25-7.5 μg/kg/min	For vasodilation and inotropy; hypotension, tachycardia, arrhythmias; ?mortality
Levosimendan[††]	12-24 μg/kg bolus over 10 min followed by infusion	0.5-2.0 μg/kg/min	For vasodilation and inotropy; active metabolite present for ~84 hr; hypotension, tachycardia, arrhythmias; ?mortality
Epinephrine		0.05-0.5 μg/kg/min	For vasoconstriction and inotropy; tachycardia, arrhythmias, end-organ hypoperfusion; ?mortality
Norepinephrine		0.2-1.0 μg/kg/min	For vasoconstriction and inotropy; tachycardia, arrhythmias, end-organ hypoperfusion; ?mortality

*Some clinicians do not administer a bolus dose to decrease the risk of hypotension. Bolus not recommended in patients with hypotension.

[†]Lower doses have also been effective in some small studies.

[††]Not approved for use in all countries.

From Zipes DP: *Braunwald's heart disease, a textbook of cardiovascular medicine,* ed 11, Philadelphia, 2019, Elsevier.

- Morphine sulfate can cause venodilation and thus reduce cardiac preload. It may be used to reduce patient work of breathing and anxiety, but recent retrospective studies have suggested increased incidence of mechanical ventilation and in-hospital mortality in patients who received morphine.[10]
- If ADHF with preserved EF is suspected, therapy is usually aimed at relief of symptoms and correction of any potential precipitating etiologies (e.g., tachycardia, hypertension, ischemia). Treatment generally involves diuretics to reduce pulmonary congestion with caution to not overdiurese given the need for elevated filling pressures in these patients to ensure adequate stroke volume and cardiac output. Nitrates may be useful in providing symptomatic relief but may precipitate hypotension. Ventricular rate should be controlled in the presence of atrial fibrillation, which, at rapid rates, is poorly tolerated in patients with impaired diastolic filling. Negative inotropic agents such as β-blockers and calcium channel blockers can be used with caution.[2] ACC/AHA/HSFA guidelines for treatment of patients with stage C HF and preserved left ventricular ejection fraction are summarized in Table 15.
- Nesiritide (recombinant brain natriuretic protein) does not reduce morbidity or mortality (ASCEND-HF trial).[17]
- 2nd phase: Inpatient hospital care.

1. This phase of treatment includes further diuresis and stabilization of volume status (Table 16). The patient should be carefully brought to euvolemia with daily volume status and electrolyte monitoring. The patient should also be transitioned to oral diuretics when stabilized. While inpatient, the patient should have his/her medical and device management optimized with the therapies discussed later.
- 3rd phase: Early discharge planning and care.
1. The patient should be transitioned to oral diuretics and be placed on optimum outpatient maintenance therapy. If the patient was on IV inotropic therapy, oral regimens should be adjusted while these infusions are tapered off. Prolonged physiologic effects of these IV inotropic agents after their discontinuation before discharge may mask the inadequate diuretic regimen and intolerance to the vasodilator doses. This can result in readmission, especially with milrinone due to its long half-life that can be further prolonged by the common coexisting impaired renal function. Therefore it may be recommended that patients who received inotropic infusions remain hospitalized for at least 48 h after inotropic agents are discontinued and optimize the oral regimen.
- 4th phase: Early post-discharge care.
1. The patient will require reevaluation and constant monitoring in order to avoid

another episode of ADHF. Emphasis should be placed on importance of compliance with instructions regarding dietary restrictions and daily body weight monitoring. Early follow-up should be scheduled as well as outpatient electrolyte monitoring if required after medication adjustments.

CHRONIC TREATMENT OF HFREF: The goals of HF therapy are clinical improvement followed by stabilizing, slowing, or even reversing deterioration in myocardial function, and ultimately a reduction in risk of morbidity (including hospitalization rates) and mortality.[2]

- ACE inhibitors[18]:
1. Reduce morbidity and mortality.
2. Produce both venous and arterial vasodilation acutely, thereby reducing both preload and afterload.
3. Potential mechanism of long-term benefit is attenuation of RAAS activation and decreased myocardial remodeling and fibrosis.
4. Used as first-line therapy for asymptomatic LV dysfunction (LVEF <40%) and symptomatic systolic HF (ACC/AHA grades A to D).
5. Therapy should be initiated at low doses to prevent hypotension and rapidly titrated to higher doses as tolerated.
6. Contraindications to the use of ACE inhibitors are renal insufficiency (creatinine clearance <30 ml/min), bilateral renal artery stenosis, hyperkalemia, hypotension, or adverse reactions (e.g., angioedema).

TABLE 15 ACC/AHA/HFSA Guidelines for Treatment of Patients With Stage C Heart Failure and Preserved Left Ventricular Ejection Fraction (HFpEF)

Class	Indication	Level of Evidence
I	Systolic and diastolic blood pressure should be controlled in accordance with published clinical practice guidelines to prevent morbidity.	B
	Diuretics should be used for relief of symptoms due to volume overload.	C
IIa	Coronary revascularization is reasonable in patients with coronary artery disease in whom symptoms (angina) or demonstrable myocardial ischemia is judged to be having an adverse effect on symptomatic heart failure.	C
	Management of atrial fibrillation according to published clinical practice guidelines is reasonable to improve symptomatic heart failure.	C
	The use of β-blocking agents, ACE inhibitors, and ARBs in patients with hypertension is reasonable to control blood pressure.	C
IIb	In appropriately selected patients with HFpEF (with EF $\geq$45%, elevated BNP levels or heart failure admission within 1 yr, estimated glomerular filtration rate >30 ml/min, creatinine <2.5 mg/dl, potassium <5.0 mEq/L), aldosterone receptor antagonists might be considered to decrease hospitalizations.	B-R
IIb	The use of ARBs might be considered to decrease hospitalizations.	B
III: No benefit	The routine use of nitrates or phosphodiesterase-5 inhibitors to increase activity or quality of life in patients with HFpEF is ineffective.	B-R
III: No benefit	Routine use of nutritional supplements is not recommended.	C

ACC, American College of Cardiology; *ACE,* angiotensin-converting enzyme; *AHA,* American Heart Association; *ARB,* angiotensin receptor blocker; *BNP,* B-type (brain) natriuretic peptide; *HFSA,* Heart Failure Society of America.
From Zipes DP: *Braunwald's heart disease, a textbook of cardiovascular medicine,* ed 11, Philadelphia, 2019, Elsevier.

TABLE 16 Therapeutic Approaches for Volume Management in Acute Heart Failure (AHF)

Severity of Volume Overload	Diuretic	Dose (mg)	Comments
Moderate	Furosemide, or	20-40, or up to 2.5 times oral dose	IV administration preferable in symptomatic patients
	Bumetanide, or	0.5-1.0	Titrate dose according to clinical response.
	Torsemide	10-20	Monitor Na$^+$, K$^+$, creatinine, BP
Severe	Furosemide, or	40-160, or 2.5 times oral dose 5-40 mg/h infusion	Intravenously
	Bumetanide, or	1-4/0.5-2 mg/h infusion (max, 2-4 mg/h, limit 2-4 h)	Bumetanide and torsemide have higher oral bioavailability than furosemide, but IV administration preferable in AHF.
	Torsemide	20-100/5-20 mg/h	
	Ultrafiltration	200-500 ml/h	Adjust ultrafiltration rate to clinical response; monitor for hypotension; consider hematocrit sensor.
Refractory to loop diuretics	Add HCTZ, *or*	25-50 twice daily	Combination with loop diuretic may be better than very high dose of loop diuretics alone.
	Metolazone, *or*	2.5-10 once daily	Metolazone more potent if creatinine clearance <30 ml/min
	Chlorothiazide, *or*	250-500 mg IV 500-1000 mg PO	
	Spironolactone	25-50 once daily	Spironolactone best choice if patient not in renal failure and normal or low serum K$^+$, although may not be very potent
In case of alkalosis	Acetazolamide	0.5	Intravenously
Refractory to loop diuretics and thiazides	Add dopamine (renal vasodilation), *or* dobutamine or milrinone (inotropic agent) Ultrafiltration, or hemodialysis if coexisting renal failure		

BP, Blood pressure; *IV,* intravenous; *HCTZ,* hydrochlorothiazide; *PO,* by mouth.
From Zipes DP: *Braunwald's heart disease, a textbook of cardiovascular medicine,* ed 11, Philadelphia, 2019, Elsevier.

- ARBs[19]:
  1. Receptor antagonists to the angiotensin II receptor.
  2. Clinical trials have not shown any superiority compared to ACE inhibitors in patients with systolic HF (LVEF <40%).
  3. Reserved for patients who are ACE inhibitor intolerant.
  4. Combination therapy with ARBs and ACE inhibitors is generally not recommended.
  5. Have a similar contraindication profile to ACE inhibitors. Routine combined use of an ACE inhibitor, ARB, and aldosterone antagonist is potentially harmful for patients with HFrEF.

- Angiotensin receptor–neprilysin inhibitor (ARNI) (valsartan/sacubitril)[20,21]:
  1. Neprilysin is an enzyme that degrades natriuretic peptides, bradykinin, adrenomedullin, and other vasoactive peptides.
  2. In a randomized controlled trial (PARADIGM-HF)[20] that compared valsartan/sacubitril with enalapril in symptomatic patients with HFrEF tolerating an adequate dose of either ACE inhibitor or ARB, the ARNI

reduced the composite end point of cardiovascular death or HF hospitalization significantly, by 20%. Additionally, in another randomized controlled trial (PIONEER—HF),[21] in HFrEF patients hospitalized with decompensated HF, initiation of valsartan/sacubitril caused a greater reduction in NT-proBNP concentration than enalapril. Rates of adverse effects did not significantly differ between the two groups.

3. In patients with chronic symptomatic HFrEF NYHA class II or III who tolerate an ACE inhibitor or ARB, replacement by an ARNI is recommended to further reduce morbidity and mortality (class I).

4. ARNI should not be administered concomitantly with ACE inhibitors or within 36 h of the last dose of an ACE inhibitor (class III: Harm).

5. ARNI should not be administered to patients with a history of angioedema (class III: Harm).

6. ARNI has not shown additional benefit over ARB in patients with preserved ejection fraction and is not indicated in this group of patients.

- Beta-adrenergic blockers (β-blockers)[22-24]:
  1. Reduce morbidity and mortality. Such benefits observed with bisoprolol (CIBIS II trial),[22] metoprolol succinate (MERIT-HF trial),[23] and carvedilol (COPERNICUS trial).[24]
  2. Benefit is believed to be conferred by blockade of sympathetic effects of neurohormonal stimulation due to HF.
  3. Are considered first-line therapy for symptomatic patients with systolic HF (NYHA class ≥II and LVEF <35%).
  4. Only carvedilol, bisoprolol, and metoprolol succinate (long acting) have been approved for the medical treatment of chronic HF; these agents are generally started in patients judged to be euvolemic and dosage is to be slowly up titrated as tolerated.
  5. Adverse effects include worsening HF (due to negative inotropic effects), fatigue, dizziness, bradycardia, hypotension, and bronchospasm.

- Aldosterone receptor antagonists[25-27]:
  1. Reduce morbidity and mortality.
  2. Indicated in patients with NYHA class II-IV HF, with LVEF ≤35%, already treated with ACE inhibitors and β-blockers without significant renal insufficiency or hyperkalemia. Patients with NYHA class II should have a history of prior cardiovascular hospitalization or elevated plasma natriuretic peptide levels to be considered for aldosterone receptor antagonists. Creatinine should be ≤2.5 mg/dl in men or ≤2.0 mg/dl in women (or estimated glomerular filtration rate >30 ml/min/1.73 m^2), and potassium should be <5.0 mEq/L. They are also indicated for post-MI patients with EF ≤40% who have either symptomatic HF or diabetes mellitus.
  3. Spironolactone may cause gynecomastia, galactorrhea, and hyperkalemia (especially in patients with baseline renal insufficiency or type 4 renal tubular acidosis). It has been

best studied in chronic HF with NYHA class III to IV symptoms (RALES study).[25]

  4. Eplerenone is associated with fewer endocrine side effects and has especially been studied in post myocardial infarction left ventricular dysfunction (EPHESUS trial)[26] and in chronic systolic HF with only class II symptoms (EMPHASIS-HF trial).[27]
  5. Inappropriate use of aldosterone receptor antagonists is potentially harmful because of life-threatening hyperkalemia or renal insufficiency when serum creatinine is >2.5 mg/dl in men or >2.0 mg/dl in women (or estimated glomerular filtration rate <30 ml/min/1.73 m^2), and/or potassium >5.0 mEq/L.

- Diuretics[28]:
  1. They are used to maintain euvolemia and to improve symptoms as discussed previously.
  2. Although data on diuretic efficacy are limited, a meta-analysis of a few small trials found that they were associated with reduction in mortality as well as reduced hospitalization for HF.
  3. Of note, loop diuretics with better bioavailability, such as torsemide and bumetanide, may be used in diuretic-resistant patients but are generally more expensive.
  4. The ADVOR trial[28a] revealed that the addition of acetazolamide, a carbonic anhydrase inhibitor that reduces proximal tubular sodium, to loop diuretics can improve the efficiency of loop diuretics and lead to faster decongestion in patients with acute decompensated heart failure with volume overload.

- Combination of isosorbide dinitrate and hydralazine[29]:
  1. Cause venous (nitrates) and arteriolar (hydralazine) vasodilation resulting in decreased preload and afterload.
  2. The combination of hydralazine and isosorbide dinitrate is recommended to reduce morbidity and mortality for patients self-described as African Americans with NYHA class III to IV HFrEF receiving optimal therapy with ACE inhibitors and β-blockers, unless contraindicated.
  3. A combination of hydralazine and isosorbide dinitrate can be useful to reduce morbidity or mortality in patients with current or prior symptomatic HFrEF who cannot be given an ACE inhibitor or ARB because of drug intolerance, hypotension, or renal insufficiency, unless contraindicated.
  4. Adverse effects of nitrates include hypotension, headaches, and tolerance as well as reflex tachycardia and lupus-like syndrome with hydralazine.

- Digoxin[30]:
  1. Positive inotropic and negative chronotropic drug that works by inhibition of the sodium-potassium transmembrane exchange pump and through its vagomimetic action.
  2. Commonly used in patients with concomitant atrial fibrillation.
  3. Has been shown to reduce HF-related hospitalizations but does not confer any

mortality benefit (DIG trial).[30] However, there is evidence suggesting that digoxin may actually have an effect on survival that varies with the serum digoxin level; survival was improved when the level was between 0.5 and 0.8 ng/ml (most often in men) and significantly worsened when it was ≥1.2 ng/ml and >0.9 mg/ml in women.
  4. Caution must be used in patients with abnormal renal function to avoid digoxin toxicity and life-threatening arrhythmia. Avoid hypokalemia because potassium competes with digoxin on the same site of the Na^+-K^+-ATPase pump.

- I$_f$ channel inhibitor (ivabradine)[31]:
  1. Ivabradine is a new therapeutic agent that selectively inhibits the I$_f$ current in the sinoatrial node, providing heart rate reduction.
  2. Ivabradine can be beneficial to reduce HF hospitalization for patients with symptomatic (NYHA class II-III) stable chronic HFrEF (LVEF ≤35%) who are receiving guideline-directed therapy, including a β-blocker at maximum tolerated dose, and who are in sinus rhythm with a heart rate of 70 bpm or greater at rest (class IIa).

- Sodium-Glucose Cotransporter 2 (SGLT2) Inhibitor[32-36]:
  1. SGLT2 inhibitors are known to lower blood sugar in patients with type 2 diabetes mellitus. However, they also possess properties associated with natriuresis, decreased fluid retention and edema, decreased RAAS activation, decreased sympathetic nervous system, reduced inflammation, and reduced oxidative stress. Thus, they are associated with improved cardiac structure and function (decreased preload, reduced remodeling/fibrosis, improved systolic function). They are also associated with improved endothelial function and overall improved vascular function.
  2. Currently used SGLT2 inhibitors include empagliflozin, canagliflozin, dapagliflozin, and ertugliflozin.
  3. Dapagliflozin has been shown to reduce cardiovascular deaths and hospitalizations in patients with NYHA class II, III or IV HF (LVEF ≤40%) regardless of the presence or absence of diabetes (DAPA-HF).[33]
  4. Empagliflozin has been shown to reduce heart failure hospitalizations and cardiovascular deaths in patients with HF with both reduced ejection fraction (EMPEROR-Reduced)[34] and preserved ejection fraction (EMPEROR-Preserved).[35]
  5. According to the new heart failure guidelines, in patients with symptomatic chronic HFrEF (EF≤40%), SGLT2i are now recommended to reduce hospitalization for HF and cardiovascular mortality, irrespective of the presence of type 2 diabetes (class I recommendation).[2] In patients with HFrEF, the new guidelines support the combination use of ARNI, β-blocker, MRA, and SGLT2 inhibitor as a new therapeutic standard.

TABLE 17 ACCF/AHA Guidelines for Cardiac Resynchronization Therapy (CRT)

Class	Indication	Level of Evidence
I	CRT is indicated for patients who have LVEF of 35% or less, sinus rhythm, LBBB with QRS duration of 150 msec or greater, and NYHA Class II, III, or ambulatory IV symptoms on GDMT.	A for NYHA Class III/IV B for Class II
IIa	CRT can be useful for patients who have LVEF of 35% or less, sinus rhythm, non-LBBB pattern with QRS duration of 150 msec or greater, and NYHA Class III/ambulatory Class IV symptoms on GDMT.	A
	CRT can be useful for patients who have LVEF of 35% or less, sinus rhythm, LBBB with QRS duration of 120-149 msec, and NYHA Class II, III, or ambulatory IV symptoms on GDMT.	B
	CRT can be useful in patients with atrial fibrillation and LVEF of 35% or less on GDMT if (a) the patient requires ventricular pacing or otherwise meets CRT criteria and (b) atrioventricular nodal ablation or pharmacologic rate control will allow near-100% ventricular pacing with CRT.	B
	CRT can be useful for patients on GDMT who have LVEF of 35% or less and are undergoing placement of new or replacement device with anticipated requirement for significant (>40%) ventricular pacing.	C
IIb	CRT may be considered for patients who have LVEF of 35% or less, sinus rhythm, non-LBBB pattern with QRS duration of 120-149 msec, and NYHA Class III/ambulatory Class IV on GDMT.	B
	CRT may be considered for patients who have LVEF of 35% or less, sinus rhythm, non-LBBB pattern with QRS duration of 150 msec or greater, and NYHA Class II symptoms on GDMT.	B
	CRT may be considered for patients who have LVEF of 30% or less, ischemic etiology of HF, sinus rhythm, LBBB with QRS duration of 150 msec or greater, and NYHA Class I symptoms on GDMT.	C
III: No benefit	CRT is not recommended for patients with NYHA Class I or II symptoms and non-LBBB pattern with QRS duration less than 150 msec.	
	CRT is not indicated for patients whose comorbidities and/or frailty limit survival with good functional capacity to less than 1 yr.	

ACCF, The American College of Cardiology Foundation; *AHA*, American Heart Association; *GDMT*, guideline-directed medical therapy; *LBBB*, left bundle-branch block; *LVEF*, left ventricular ejection fraction; *NYHA*, New York Heart Association.
From Zipes DP: *Braunwald's heart disease, a textbook of cardiovascular medicine,* ed 11, Philadelphia, 2019, Elsevier.

6. In patients with mildly reduced EF of 41-49% (HFmrEF), SGLT2i may be beneficial in reducing hospitalization for HF and cardiovascular mortality (class IIa recommendation).[2]
- Cardiac resynchronization therapy (CRT)[37]:
  1. Improves morbidity and mortality rates in selected patients.
  2. The presence of a bundle-branch block or other intraventricular conduction delay (IVCD) can cause ventricular dyssynchrony, which induces regional loading disparities and reduces the efficiency of ventricular contraction, thereby further impairing the systolic function of a failing ventricle.
  3. CRT is indicated for patients who have LVEF ≤35%, sinus rhythm, left bundle-branch block with a QRS duration of 150 ms or greater, and NYHA class II, III, or ambulatory IV symptoms on guideline-directed medical therapy. CRT is NOT indicated in patients whose functional status and life expectancy are limited predominantly by chronic noncardiac conditions. Life expectancy should be >1 yr.
  4. In the appropriate subset of patients, CRT in addition to optimal medical therapy has been shown in numerous clinical trials to improve symptoms by at least one NYHA class, improve 6-min walk distance and quality of life, reduce rate of HF-related hospitalization, and reduce rate of all-cause and cardiovascular mortality.
  5. ACC/AHA guidelines for cardiac resynchronization therapy are summarized in Table 17.
- Implantable cardioverter-defibrillators (ICDs)[2,38]:
  1. Sudden cardiac death (SCD) is a common cause of death in patients with HF in both ischemic and nonischemic cardiomyopathies. Ventricular tachycardia (VT) degenerating into ventricular fibrillation (VF) is the culprit in the majority of patients with SCD, although bradyarrhythmias do also occur with less frequency.
  2. ICD therapy is recommended for primary prevention of SCD to reduce total mortality in selected patients with nonischemic dilated cardiomyopathy or ischemic heart disease at least 40 days post-MI with LVEF ≤35% and NYHA class II or III symptoms on chronic guideline-directed medical therapy, who have reasonable expectation of meaningful survival for >1 yr.
  3. Patients with HF who survive an episode of sudden cardiac arrest or experience sustained VT in the presence of LVEF <35% are at high risk for future arrhythmic events and SCD and obtain a mortality benefit from ICD placement for secondary prevention, with or without adjunctive therapies such as antiarrhythmic drugs, radiofrequency ablation, surgery, or transplant.
  4. ACC/AHA guidelines for indications for implantable cardioverter-defibrillators are summarized in Table 18.
- In the absence of an indication (e.g., atrial fibrillation), routine use of anticoagulation is currently not recommended in patients with HF. Even with the increased risk for LV thrombus formation in dilated cardiomyopathy and subsequent thromboembolization, data are conflicting about benefits of antithrombotic (antiplatelet or anticoagulant) therapy for primary prevention to reduce thromboembolic events or mortality in patients with systolic HF who are in sinus rhythm (SOLVD, V-HeFT, SAVE, HELAS, and WASH trials). It may be reasonable to consider anticoagulation for secondary prevention in patients with HF who had a prior thromboembolic event; however, risks and benefits should be carefully assessed.
- Antiplatelet agents are recommended for patients with concomitant CAD.
- Statins are not beneficial as adjunctive therapy when prescribed solely for the diagnosis of HF in the absence of other indications for their use.
- Calcium channel blocking drugs are not recommended as routine treatment for patients with HFrEF.
- Omega-3 polyunsaturated fatty acid supplementation is reasonable to use as adjunctive therapy in patients with NYHA class II to IV symptoms and HFrEF or HFpEF, unless contraindicated, to reduce mortality and cardiovascular hospitalizations.
- Percutaneous coronary intervention (PCI) or surgical revascularization should be considered in patients with HF and significant CAD who are revascularization candidates.
- In general, quadruple therapy, if tolerated, is recommended as foundational therapy. If all four therapies (ARNI, β-blocker, MRA, SGLT2 inhibitor) are initiated simultaneously at low doses, all pathways are blocked to some degree, and this results in rapid improvement of mortality and health status as well as rapid

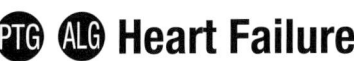

H

TABLE 18 ACCF/AHA Guidelines for Indications for Implantable Cardioverter-Defibrillators (ICDs)

Class	Indication	Level of Evidence
I	ICD therapy is recommended for primary prevention of SCD in selected patients with HFrEF at least 40 days post-MI with LVEF less than 35% and NYHA Class II or III symptoms receiving chronic GDMT, who are expected to live more than 1 yr.	A
I	ICD therapy is recommended for primary prevention of SCD in selected patients with HFrEF at least 40 days post-MI with LVEF less than 30% and NYHA Class I symptoms receiving GDMT, who are expected to live more than 1 yr.	B
IIa	To prevent SCD, placement of ICD is reasonable in patients with asymptomatic ischemic cardiomyopathy who are at least 40 days post-MI, have an LVEF of 30% or less, are on appropriate medical therapy, and have reasonable expectation of survival with a good functional status for more than 1 yr.	B
IIb	ICD therapy to prevent SCD in patients with nonischemic cardiomyopathy who are at least 40 days post-MI, have LVEF less than 35%, with NYHA Class II or III symptoms while undergoing chronic optimal medical therapy, and have reasonable expectation of survival for more than 1 yr with good functional status.	B
	Usefulness of implantation of ICD is of uncertain benefit to prolong meaningful survival in patients with high risk of non-SCD, as predicted by frequent hospitalizations, advanced frailty, or comorbidities such as systemic malignancy or severe renal dysfunction.	B

HFrEF, Heart failure with reduced ejection fraction; *MI,* myocardial infarction; *SCD,* sudden cardiac death; see Table 17 for other abbreviations.
From Zipes DP: *Braunwald's heart disease, a textbook of cardiovascular medicine,* ed 11, Philadelphia, 2019, Elsevier.

Diseases and Disorders

I

TABLE 19 ACC/AHA Guidelines for Treatment of Patients With End-Stage Heart Failure (Stage D)

Class	Indication	Level of Evidence
	Nonpharmacologic Interventions	
IIa	Fluid restriction (1.5-2 L/day) is reasonable in stage D, especially in patients with hyponatremia.	B
	Inotropic Support	
I	Until definitive therapy (e.g., coronary revascularization, MCS, heart transplantation) or resolution of the acute precipitating problem, patients with cardiogenic shock should receive temporary IV inotropic support to maintain systemic perfusion and preserve end-organ performance.	C
IIa	Continuous IV inotropic support is reasonable as "bridge therapy" in patients with stage D refractory to GDMT and device therapy who are eligible for and awaiting MCS or cardiac transplantation.	B
IIb	Short-term, continuous IV inotropic support may be reasonable in those hospitalized patients presenting with documented severe systolic dysfunction who present with low blood pressure and significantly depressed cardiac output, to maintain systemic perfusion and preserve end-organ performance.	B
	Long-term, continuous IV inotropic support may be considered as palliative therapy for symptom control in select patients with stage D despite optimal GDMT and device therapy who are not eligible for either MCS or cardiac transplantation.	B
III: Harm	Long-term use of either continuous or intermittent, IV parenteral positive inotropic agents, in the absence of specific indications or for reasons other than palliative care, is potentially harmful in the patient with HF.	B
	Use of parenteral inotropic agents in hospitalized patients without documented severe systolic dysfunction, low blood pressure, or impaired perfusion, and evidence of significantly depressed cardiac output, with or without congestion, is potentially harmful.	B
	Mechanical Circulatory Support (MCS)	
IIa	MCS is beneficial in carefully selected patients with stage D HFrEF in whom definitive management (e.g., cardiac transplantation) or cardiac recovery is anticipated or planned.	B
	Nondurable MCS, including the use of percutaneous and extracorporeal ventricular assist devices (VADs), is reasonable as a "bridge to recovery" or "bridge to decision" for carefully selected patients with HFrEF with acute, profound hemodynamic compromise.	B
	Durable MCS is reasonable to prolong survival for carefully selected patients with stage D HFrEF.	B
	Cardiac Transplantation	
I	Evaluation for cardiac transplantation is indicated for carefully selected patients with stage D HF despite GDMT, device, and surgical management.	C

ACC, American College of Cardiology; *AHA,* American Heart Association; *GDMT,* Guideline-directed medical therapy; *HF,* heart failure; *HFrEF,* heart failure with reduced ejection fraction; *IV,* intravenous.
From Zipes DP: *Braunwald's heart disease, a textbook of cardiovascular medicine,* ed 11, Philadelphia, 2019, Elsevier.

reduction of HF hospitalizations. Some therapies offer further incremental benefit with increased doses (particularly ARNI and β-blocker), so if a patient tolerates quadruple therapy, doses can be increased to maximally tolerated doses.
- The following drugs can be added in selected patients in the absence of contraindications:
  1. Aldosterone antagonists improve survival in NYHA class II with LVEF <30% or NYHA class III-IV with EF <35%. Kidney function should be stable with eGFR ≥30 ml/min and potassium <5 mEq/L.
  2. Combination of hydralazine with a nitrate in patients (particularly African Americans) with a reduced EF.
  3. Digoxin reduces hospitalizations for HF and controls HR in atrial fibrillation. It can also help control symptoms.

CHRONIC TREATMENT OF HFPEF:
- To date, there is a relative dearth of clinical trials examining effective chronic treatment strategies in this subset of patients with HFpEF. Current therapies are mainly for symptomatic relief. ACC/AHA guidelines for treatment of patients with end-stage heart failure are summarized in Table 19.
- Therapy mainly centers on relief of volume overload with judicious diuretic use, treatment of ischemia via coronary revascularization (Table 20), management of atrial fibrillation, controlling heart rate and blood pressure to prevent acute decompensation, and restriction

TABLE 20 ACC/AHA Guidelines for Surgical/Percutaneous/Transcatheter Interventional Treatments of Heart Failure

Class	Indication	Level of Evidence
I	Coronary artery revascularization via CABG or percutaneous intervention is indicated for patients (HFpEF and HFrEF) on GDMT with angina and suitable coronary artery anatomy, especially for a left main artery stenosis (>50%) or left main–equivalent disease.	C
IIa	CABG to improve survival is reasonable in patients with mild to moderate LV systolic dysfunction (EF 35%-50%) and significant (≥70% diameter stenosis) multivessel CAD or proximal left anterior descending coronary artery stenosis when viable myocardium is present in the region of intended revascularization.	B
	CABG or medical therapy is reasonable to improve morbidity and cardiovascular mortality for patients with severe LV dysfunction (EF <35%), HF, and significant CAD.	B
	Surgical aortic valve replacement is reasonable for patients with critical aortic stenosis and a predicted surgical mortality of no greater than 10%.	B
	Transcatheter aortic valve replacement after careful candidate consideration is reasonable for patients with critical aortic stenosis who are deemed inoperable.	B
IIb	CABG may be considered with the intent of improving survival in patients with ischemic heart disease with severe LV systolic dysfunction (EF <35%) and operable coronary anatomy whether or not viable myocardium is present.	B
	Transcatheter mitral valve repair or mitral valve surgery for functional mitral insufficiency is of uncertain benefit and should only be considered after careful candidate selection and with a background of GDMT.	B
	Surgical reverse remodeling or LV aneurysmectomy may be considered in carefully selected patients with HFrEF for specific indications, including intractable HF and ventricular arrhythmias.	B

ACC, American College of Cardiology; *AHA*, American Heart Association; *CABG*, coronary artery bypass grafting; *CAD*, coronary artery disease; *EF*, ejection fraction; *GDMT*, guideline-directed medical therapy; *HF*, heart failure; *HFpEF*, heart failure with preserved ejection fraction; *HFrEF*, HF with reduced ejection fraction; *LV*, left ventricle.
From Mann DL et al: *Braunwald's heart disease*, ed 10, Philadelphia, 2015, Elsevier.

of sodium and fluid to prevent volume overload.
- Recently, SGLT2 inhibitors have emerged as a promising option for patients with HFpEF, conferring a mortality benefit and reduced hospitalizations.[35] According to the new heart failure guidelines, in patients with HFpEF, SGLT2 inhibitors can be beneficial in decreasing cardiovascular mortality and in decreasing HF hospitalization (class IIa recommendation).[2]
- Diuretics should be used for relief of symptoms due to volume overload in patients with HFpEF.
- The use of β-blocking agents, ACE inhibitors, and ARBs in patients with hypertension is reasonable to control blood pressure in patients with HFpEF.
- The use of ARBs might be considered to decrease hospitalizations for patients with HFpEF.
- Aldosterone antagonists may be used in appropriate patients with HFpEF (EF >45%, elevated BNP or HF admission in the past year, potassium <5.0 mEq/L, estimated glomerular filtration rate >30 and creatinine <2.5 mg/dl) to decrease hospitalizations (class IIb recommendation).
- Routine use of nitrates or phosphodiesterase-5 inhibitors to increase activity or quality of life in patients with HFpEF is not recommended as there is no benefit.
- There is no evidence to support routine use of nutritional supplements, and they are not recommended for patients with HFpEF.
- Surgical options (Table 21) for contributing critical aortic stenosis, constrictive pericarditis, and hypertrophic cardiomyopathy (HCM) should be entertained in appropriate patients.
- In patients with comorbidities including anemia, hypertension, and sleep apnea, the following recommendations are made:
  1. Intravenous iron replacement in patients with NYHA class II and III HF and iron deficiency (ferritin <100 ng/ml or 100 to 300 ng/ml with transferrin saturation <20%) to improve functional status and quality of life (class IIb recommendation).
  2. Titration of medical therapy to attain systolic blood pressure <130 mm Hg is recommended in patients with HFrEF and hypertension, as well as in patients with HFpEF and persistent hypertension after treatment of volume overload (class I recommendation).
  3. A formal sleep assessment should be obtained in patients with NYHA class II to IV HF with suspicion of sleep-disordered breathing. Continuous positive airway pressure should be used in patients with HF and obstructive sleep apnea to improve sleep quality and daytime sleepiness (class IIb recommendation).

DISPOSITION
- Coordination of care (Table 22) is essential in patients with chronic heart failure.
- Annual mortality of systolic HF ranges from 10% in stable patients with mild symptoms to 50% in patients with NYHA class IV disease (a mortality rate rivaling some malignancies). The Seattle Heart Failure Model provides an accurate estimate of 1-, 2-, and 3-yr survival before and after different therapies. This model can be useful to assess the need for LV assist device implantation or urgent transplantation. The calculator is available online at http://depts.washington.edu/shfm/.
- Cardiac transplantation has a 5-yr survival rate of ∼70% and represents a viable option in selected patients. Fig. E5 describes an algorithm for evaluation of potential heart transplant recipient.[39]
- The use of an LV assist device (LVAD) in patients with advanced HF can result in a clinically meaningful survival benefit and improve quality of life in patients who are not candidates for cardiac transplantation.[39,40] There are two approved uses of LVADs specifically as a bridge to transplant and as destination therapy. There are two major categories of LVAD pulsatile flow devices vs. continuous flow devices. Continuous flow devices are associated with increased survival as destination therapy as compared to medically managed controls (REMATCH trial).[41]

REFERENCES
Available at eBooks.Health.Elsevier.com.

RELATED CONTENT
Heart Failure (Patient Information)

AUTHORS: **SHILPA VIJAYAKUMAR, MD,** and **ARAVIND RAO KOKKIRALA, MD, FACC**

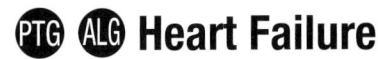
TABLE 21 Surgery for Management of Heart Failure (HF): Guideline Recommendations

2016 ESC Guidelines for the Diagnosis and Treatment of Acute and Chronic Heart Failure
Recommendations for Myocardial Revascularization in Patients With Chronic HF

- Myocardial revascularization is recommended when angina persists despite antiangina drugs; *class I, level of evidence A.*
  The choice between CABG and PCI should be made by the heart team after careful review.
  CABG is recommended for patients with angina and significant LM or LM-equivalent stenosis to improve prognosis.
  CABG is recommended for patients with HFrEF, significant CAD (LAD or multivessel disease), and LVEF <35%.

2014 ACC/AHA/AATS/PCNA/SCAI/STS Focused Update of the Guideline for the Diagnosis and Management of Patients With Stable Ischemic Heart Disease*

- A heart team approach to revascularization is recommended in patients with diabetes mellitus and complex multivessel CAD; *class 1, level of evidence C.*
- CABG is generally recommended in preference to PCI to improve survival in patients with diabetes mellitus and multivessel CAD for which revascularization is likely to improve survival (3-vessel CAD or complex 2-vessel CAD involving the proximal LAD); *class 1, level of evidence B.*

2014 AHA/ACC Guideline for the Management of Patients With Valvular Heart Disease†
Indications for Aortic Valve Surgery in Aortic Stenosis (as) With Left Ventricular Dysfunction

- AVR is recommended for asymptomatic patients with severe AS and LVEF <50%; *class I, level of evidence B.*
- AVR is reasonable in symptomatic patients with low-flow/low-gradient severe AS with reduced LVEF with a low-dose dobutamine stress study that shows an aortic velocity ≥4.0 m/sec or mean pressure gradient ≥40 mm Hg with a valve area of ≤1.0 cm²; *class IIa, level of evidence B.*
- AVR is reasonable for patients with moderate AS who are undergoing other cardiac surgery; *class IIa, level of evidence C.*
- TAVR is recommended in patients who meet an indication for AVR for AS and who have a prohibitive surgical risk and post-TAVR survival >12 mo; *class I, level of evidence B.*
- TAVR is a reasonable alternative to surgical AVR in patients who meet an indication for AVR and who have a high surgical risk; *class IIa, level of evidence B.*

Indications for Aortic Valve Surgery in Aortic Regurgitation (AR) With LV Dysfunction

- AVR is recommended for symptomatic patients with severe AR; *class I, level of evidence B.*
- AVR is indicated for patients with severe AR and LV systolic dysfunction; *class I, level of evidence B.*

Indications for Mitral Valve Surgery in Functional Mitral Regurgitation (MR)

- Mitral valve surgery is reasonable for patients with chronic severe functional MR who are undergoing CABG or AVR; *class IIa, level of evidence C.*
- Mitral valve surgery may be considered for severely symptomatic patients (NYHA Class III/IV) with chronic severe functional MR; *class IIb, level of evidence B.*
- Mitral valve repair may be considered for patients with chronic moderate functional MR who are undergoing other cardiac surgery; *class IIb, level of evidence C.*

ESC/EACTS Guidelines on the Management of Valvular Heart Disease (Version 2012)‡
Indications for Mitral Valve Surgery in Chronic Secondary Mitral Regurgitation (MR)

- Surgery is indicated in patients with severe MR undergoing CABG and LVEF >30%; *class I, level of evidence C.*
- Surgery should be considered in patients with moderate MR undergoing CABG; *class IIa, level of evidence C.*
- Surgery should be considered in symptomatic patients with severe MR, LVEF <30%, option for revascularization, and evidence of viability; *class IIa, level of evidence: C.*
- Surgery may be considered in patients with severe MR, LVEF >30%, who remain symptomatic despite optimal medical management (including CRT if indicated) and have low comorbidity, when revascularization is not indicated; *class IIb, level of evidence C.*

AATS, American Association for Thoracic Surgery; *ACC*, American College of Cardiology; *AHA*, American Heart Association; *AS*, aortic stenosis; *AVR*, aortic valve replacement; *CABG*, coronary artery bypass grafting; *CAD*, coronary artery disease; *CRT*, cardiac resynchronization therapy; *EACTS*, European Association for Cardio-Thoracic Surgery; *ESC*, European Society of Cardiology; *HFrEF*, heart failure with reduced ejection fraction; *LAD*, left anterior descending coronary artery; *LM*, left main coronary artery; *LV*, left ventricle; *LVEF*, left ventricular ejection fraction; *NYHA*, New York Heart Association; *PCI*, percutaneous coronary intervention; *PCNA*, Preventive Cardiovascular Nurses Association; *SCAI*, Society for Cardiovascular Angiography and Interventions; *STS*, Society of Thoracic Surgeons; *TAVR*, transcatheter aortic valve replacement.

*Fihn SD et al: 2014 ACC/AHA/AATS/PCNA/SCAI/STS focused update of the guideline for the diagnosis and management of patients with stable ischemic heart disease: a report of the American College of Cardiology/American Heart Association Task Force on Practice Guidelines, and the American Association for Thoracic Surgery, Preventive Cardiovascular Nurses Association, Society for Cardiovascular Angiography and Interventions, and Society of Thoracic Surgeons, *Circulation* 130:1749-1767, 2014.
†Nishimura RA et al: 2014 AHA/ACC guideline for the management of patients with valvular heart disease, *J Thorac Cardiovasc Surg* 148:E1-E132, 2014.
‡Vahanian A et al: Guidelines on the management of valvular heart disease (version 2012), *Eur Heart J* 33:2451-2496, 2012.
From Zipes DP: *Braunwald's heart disease, a textbook of cardiovascular medicine*, ed 11, Philadelphia, 2019, Elsevier.

TABLE 22 Coordinating Care for Patients With Chronic Heart Failure

Class	Indication	Level of Evidence
I	Effective systems of care coordination with special attention to care transitions should be deployed for every patient with chronic HF that facilitate and ensure effective care that is designed to achieve GDMT and prevent hospitalization.	B
	Every patient with HF should have a clear, detailed, and evidence-based plan of care that ensures the achievement of GDMT goals, effective management of comorbid conditions, timely follow-up with the health care team, appropriate dietary and physical activities, and compliance with secondary prevention guidelines for cardiovascular disease. This plan of care should be updated regularly and made readily available to all members of the patient's health care team.	C
	Palliative and supportive care is effective for patients with symptomatic advanced HF to improve quality of life.	B

GDMT, Guideline directed medical therapy; *HF*, heart failure.
From Mann DL et al: *Braunwald's heart disease*, ed 10, Philadelphia, 2015, Elsevier.

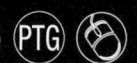
BASIC INFORMATION

DEFINITION

Heat exhaustion and heat stroke are part of a continuum of heat-related illness, and unless factors leading to heat exhaustion are corrected swiftly, affected patients can progress to heat stroke.

- **Heat exhaustion:** An illness resulting from prolonged, heavy activity in a hot environment with subsequent dehydration, electrolyte depletion, and rectal temperature >37.8° C (100° F) but ≤40° C (104° F).
- **Heat stroke:** A life-threatening heat illness characterized by extreme hyperthermia (core temperature >40° C [104.0° F]), dehydration, multiorgan failure, and neurologic manifestations. Heat stroke can be further subdivided into "exertional heat stroke" occurring in generally healthy individuals undergoing strenuous physical activity in warm conditions and "nonexertional heat stroke" often seen in elderly and/or debilitated patients with impaired thermal regulations due to illness or medications (see "Etiology").

SYNONYMS

Heat illness
Hyperthermia

ICD-10CM CODES
T67.5 Heat exhaustion, unspecified
T67.0 Heatstroke and sunstroke
T67.1 Heat syncope
T67.2 Heat cramp
T67.3 Heat exhaustion, anhydrotic
T67.6 Heat fatigue, transient

EPIDEMIOLOGY & DEMOGRAPHICS

INCIDENCE (IN U.S.): Incidence of heat stroke is approximately 20 cases/100,000 population.
PREDOMINANT AGE: Heat exhaustion and stroke occur more frequently in elderly patients, especially those taking diuretics or medications that impair heat dissipation (e.g., phenothiazines, anticholinergics, antihistamines, β-blockers). Table 1 describes factors predisposing to serious heat illness.

PHYSICAL FINDINGS & CLINICAL PRESENTATION

HEAT EXHAUSTION:
- Generalized malaise, weakness, headache, muscle and abdominal cramps, nausea, vomiting, hypotension, tachycardia.
- Rectal temperature is usually normal.
- Sweating is usually present.

HEAT STROKE:
- Neurologic manifestations (seizures, tremor, hemiplegia, coma, psychosis, other bizarre behavior)
- Evidence of dehydration (poor skin turgor, sunken eyeballs)
- Tachycardia, hyperventilation
- Skin is hot, red, and flushed
- Sweating is often (not always) absent, particularly in elderly patients

- Classic heat stroke generally develops slowly over days and occurs predominantly in older persons and in those with chronic illness. Clinically heat stroke can be divided into three phases: A hyperthermic neurologic acute phase, a hematologic-enzymatic phase (peaking 24 to 48 h after the event), and a late renal-hepatic phase (if clinical symptoms are sustained for 96 h or longer).[1] Exertional heat stroke is more common in young, healthy persons; has a more rapid onset; and is associated with higher core temperatures. Table 2 compares classic and exertional heat stroke. Box 1 summarizes organ dysfunction seen in patients with heat stroke

ETIOLOGY

- Exogenous heat gain (increased ambient temperature)
- Increased heat production (exercise, infection, hyperthyroidism, drugs)

TABLE 1 Factors Predisposing to Serious Heat Illness

Individual Factors

Lack of acclimatization
Low physical fitness
Excessive body weight
Dehydration
Advanced age
Young age

Health Conditions

Inflammation and fever
Viral infection
Cardiovascular disease
Diabetes mellitus
Gastroenteritis
Rash, sunburn, and previous burns to large areas of skin
Seizures
Thyroid storm
Neuroleptic malignant syndrome
Malignant hyperthermia
Sickle cell trait
Cystic fibrosis
Spinal cord injury

Drugs

Anticholinergic properties (atropine)
Antiepileptic (topiramate)
Antihistamines
Glutethimide (Doriden)
Phenothiazines
Tricyclic antidepressants
Amphetamines, cocaine, "ecstasy"
Ergogenic stimulants (e.g., ephedrine, ephedra)
Lithium
Diuretics
β-Blockers
Ethanol

Environmental Factors

High temperature
High humidity
Little air motion
Lack of shade
Heat wave
Physical exercise
Heavy clothing
Air pollution (nitrogen dioxide)

From Goldman L, Schafer AI: *Goldman's Cecil medicine,* ed 24, Philadelphia, 2012, Saunders.

- Impaired heat dissipation (high humidity, heavy clothing, neonatal or elderly patients, drugs [phenothiazines, anticholinergics, antihistamines, butyrophenones, amphetamines, cocaine, alcohol, β-blockers])
- Diuretics, laxatives
- In infants a major risk factor is confinement in a closed car
- Fig. E1 describes an algorithm of the pathophysiology of heat stroke

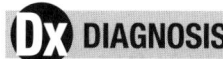 DIAGNOSIS

DIFFERENTIAL DIAGNOSIS

- Infections (meningitis, encephalitis, sepsis)
- Head trauma
- Epilepsy
- Thyroid storm
- Acute cocaine intoxication
- Malignant hyperthermia
- Heat exhaustion can be differentiated from heat stroke by the following:
  1. Essentially intact mental function and lack of significant fever in heat exhaustion
  2. Mild or absent increases in creatine phosphokinase (CPK), aspartate aminotransferase (AST), lactate dehydrogenase (LDH), and alanine aminotransferase (ALT) in heat exhaustion

WORKUP

- Heat stroke: Comprehensive history, physical examination, and laboratory evaluation
- Heat exhaustion: In most cases, laboratory tests not necessary for diagnosis

LABORATORY TESTS

Laboratory abnormalities may include the following:
- Elevated blood urea nitrogen (BUN), creatinine, hematocrit
- Hyponatremia or hypernatremia, hyperkalemia or hypokalemia
- Elevated LDH, AST, ALT, CPK, bilirubin
- Lactic acidosis, respiratory alkalosis (from hyperventilation)
- Myoglobinuria, hypofibrinogenemia, fibrinolysis, hypocalcemia

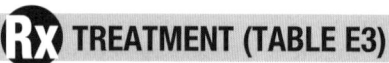 TREATMENT (TABLE E3)

- Treatment of heat exhaustion consists primarily of placing the patient in a cool, shaded area and providing rapid hydration and salt replacement.
  1. Fluid intake should be at least 2 L q4h in patients without history of congestive heart failure.
  2. Salt replacement can be accomplished by using one-quarter teaspoon of salt or two 10-grain salt tablets dissolved in 1 L of water.
  3. If intravenous (IV) fluid replacement is necessary, young athletes can be given normal saline IV (3 to 4 L over 6 to 8 h); in elderly patients, consider using D5$\frac{1}{2}$ NS IV

TABLE 2 Comparison of Classic and Exertional Heat Stroke

Patient Characteristics	Classic	Exertional
Age	Young children or elderly	15-55 yr
Health	Chronic illness	Usually healthy
Fever	Unusual	Common
Prevailing weather	Frequent in heat waves	Variable
Activity	Sedentary	Strenuous exercise
Drug use	Diuretics, antidepressants, anticholinergics, phenothiazines	Ergogenic stimulants or cocaine
Sweating	Often absent	Common
Acid-base disturbances	Respiratory alkalosis	Lactic acidosis
Acute renal failure	Uncommon	Common ($\approx 15\%$)
Rhabdomyolysis	Uncommon	Common ($\approx 25\%$)
CK	Mildly elevated	Markedly elevated (500-1000 U/L)
ALT, AST	Mildly elevated	Markedly elevated
Hyperkalemia	Uncommon	Common
Hypocalcemia	Uncommon	Common
DIC	Mild	Marked
Hypoglycemia	Uncommon	Common

ALT, Alanine aminotransferase; *AST,* aspartate aminotransferase; *CK,* creatine kinase; *DIC,* disseminated intravascular coagulation.
From Goldman L, Schafer AI: *Goldman's Cecil medicine,* ed 24, Philadelphia, 2012, Saunders.

with the rate titrated to cardiovascular status.
- Patients with heat stroke should undergo rapid cooling.
  1. Remove the patient's clothes and place the patient in a cool and well-ventilated room.
  2. If patient is unconscious, position on his or her side and clear the airway. Protect airway and augment oxygenation (e.g., nasal O_2 at 4 L/min to keep oxygen saturation $>90\%$).
  3. Monitor body temperature every 5 min. Measurement of the patient's core temperature with a rectal probe is recommended. The goal is to reduce the body temperature to 39° C (102.2° F) in 30 to 60 min. Advantages, disadvantages, and efficacy of various cooling methods are described in Table E4.
  4. Spray the patient with a cool mist and use fans to enhance airflow over the body (rapid evaporation method).
  5. Immersion of the patient in ice water, stomach lavage with iced saline solution, IV administration of cooled fluids, and inhalation of cold air are advisable only when the means for rapid evaporation are not available. Immersion in tepid water (15° C [59° F]) is preferred over ice water immersion to minimize risk of shivering.
  6. Use of ice packs on axillae, neck, and groin is controversial because they increase peripheral vasoconstriction and may induce shivering.
  7. Antipyretics are ineffective because the hypothalamic set point during heat stroke is normal despite the increased body temperature.
  8. Intubate a comatose patient, insert a Foley catheter, and start nasal O_2. Continuous ECG monitoring is recommended.
  9. Insert at least two large-bore IV lines and begin IV hydration with normal saline (NS) or Ringer lactate.
  10. Draw initial laboratory studies: Electrolytes, CBC, blood urea nitrogen, creatinine, AST, ALT, CPK, LDH, glucose, prothrombin time (international normalized ratio), partial thromboplastin time, platelet count, Ca^{2+}, lactic acid, and arterial blood gases.
  11. Treat complications as follows:

BOX 1 Organ Dysfunction Seen in Patients With Heat Stroke

Encephalopathy
Rhabdomyolysis
Acute renal failure
Acute respiratory distress syndrome
Myocardial injury
Hepatocellular injury
Intestinal ischemia and infarction
Pancreatic injury
Hemorrhagic complication (e.g., disseminated intravascular coagulation)

From Adams JG et al: *Emergency medicine, clinical essentials,* ed 2, Philadelphia, 2013, Elsevier.

a. Hypotension: Vigorous hydration with normal saline or Ringer lactate
b. Convulsions: Diazepam 5 to 10 mg IV (slowly)
c. Shivering: Chlorpromazine 10 to 50 mg IV
d. Acidosis: Use bicarbonate judiciously (only in severe acidosis)
- Observe for evidence of rhabdomyolysis and hepatic, renal, or cardiac failure and treat accordingly.

DISPOSITION

Most patients recover completely within 48 h. Central nervous system injury is permanent in 20% of cases. Mortality rate can exceed 30% in patients with prolonged and severe hyperthermia. Delayed access to cooling is the leading cause of morbidity and mortality in persons with heat stroke.

REFERENCE
Available at eBooks.Health.Elsevier.com.

RELATED CONTENT

Heat Exhaustion and Heat Stroke (Patient Information)
Acute Kidney Injury (Related Key Topic)
Rhabdomyolysis (Related Key Topic)

AUTHOR: **FRED F. FERRI, MD**

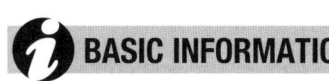
ℹ️ BASIC INFORMATION

DEFINITION

Abnormal uterine bleeding (AUB) is a broad term for variations in normal menses. Normal duration of menstrual flow is 5 days, with normal menstrual cycles lasting 21 to 35 days. Heavy menstrual bleeding with normal cycles, historically called menorrhagia, is a large volume of menstrual blood loss quantified as >80 ml per cycle. Bleeding also may be prolonged, intermenstrual, frequent, and irregular. This language replaces prior terms such as *metrorrhagia* (bleeding between cycles); *polymenorrhea* (menses <21 days apart); and *oligomenorrhea* (menses >35 days apart).[1-3]

The PALM-COEIN classification of AUB was adopted in 2011 to standardize terminology and reflect etiology: *P*olyp, *A*denomyosis, *L*eiomyoma, *M*alignancy and hyperplasia, *C*oagulopathy, *O*vulatory dysfunction, *E*ndometrial, *I*atrogenic, and *N*ot yet classified. The PALM-COEIN terminology is used to classify the etiology of the bleeding; for instance, AUB-P would refer to AUB due to polyps.[1-4]

SYNONYMS

Menorrhagia
Menometrorrhagia
Dysfunctional uterine bleeding
Irregular menstrual cycle

ICD-10CM CODES
N92.0   Excessive and frequent menstruation with regular cycle
N92.1   Excessive and frequent menstruation with irregular cycle
N92.2   Excessive menstruation at puberty
N92.4   Excessive bleeding in the premenopausal period
N92.6   Irregular menstruation, unspecified

EPIDEMIOLOGY & DEMOGRAPHICS

INCIDENCE: AUB occurs in 10% to 15% of reproductive-age patients, 5% of emergency room visits in nonpregnant patients, 30% of office visits, and 70% of gynecologic consults.[2,3]
PREVALENCE: 9% to 14%[1]
PREDOMINANT SEX & AGE: Females ages 13 to 50, with peak in adolescence and perimenopausal periods.[1]
RISK FACTORS: Genetic predisposition, anticoagulation treatment, obesity, endocrinopathies, autoimmune disease, liver disease, renal disease, and sex hormone secreting tumors.
GENETICS: Hereditary coagulopathy (most commonly von Willebrand disease or platelet dysfunction disorders) can be seen in 20% of women with heavy menstrual bleeding and can present in adolescents with prior undiagnosed coagulopathy. This can lead to hospitalization in up to 19% of affected women.[1,3]

PHYSICAL FINDINGS & CLINICAL PRESENTATION HISTORY

Age, age at menarche or menopause, menstrual bleeding patterns, severity of bleeding, pain, underlying medical conditions, surgical history, medications, family history, hirsutism, acne, symptoms of thyroid dysfunction or other endocrinopathies[1-4]

- If heavy bleeding since menarche, screen for signs and symptoms of hemostatic disorder, including postpartum hemorrhage, surgery-related bleeding, bleeding from dental work, easy bruising, epistaxis, and frequent gum bleeding[3]
- Physical examination: Weight, hirsutism, acne, thyroid nodules, signs of insulin resistance (acanthosis nigricans), signs of bleeding disorder (petechiae, ecchymoses, pallor, swollen joints), pelvic examination including external, speculum, and bimanual examinations

ETIOLOGY

- PALM-COEIN
- Additional etiologies: Pregnancy/miscarriage; atrioventricular (AV) malformations; cervical/endometrial infections; foreign body, such as intrauterine device (IUD) malposition; use of hormones; anticoagulation medications; severe kidney or liver disease; thyroid disorder[3-4]

🅓🆇 DIAGNOSIS

DIFFERENTIAL DIAGNOSIS

In addition to the PALM-COEIN classification, it is also important to consider etiologies as listed earlier, including urinary and GI tract sources.

Differential diagnosis of AUB can be further narrowed by age.
- AUB in 13- to 18-yr-olds is most commonly caused by anovulation due to immature or dysregulation of hypothalamic-pituitary-ovarian axis as a function of normal physiology. This also can be when coagulopathy disorders are first identified.[1,3]
- AUB in 19- to 39-yr-olds is most commonly due to pregnancy or structural issues such as polyps or fibroids, and cancer is relatively rare in this age range.[1,3]
- AUB in 40-yr-old and older commonly is due to ovulation changes with perimenopause, but cancer has increased incidence in this age range.[1,3]

WORKUP

- History and physical examination
- Laboratory, pathology, and imaging studies

LABORATORY TESTS

- Pregnancy test
- CBC
- Thyroid-stimulating hormone (TSH)

- Wet prep and cervical cultures (*Chlamydia trachomatis* and *Neisseria gonorrhoeae*) if indicated
- Pap smear if indicated
- Targeted screening for bleeding disorders if suspected
- Endometrial sampling by endometrial biopsy or hysteroscopic sampling for women >45 yr or <45 yr with indication such as history of unopposed estrogen (polycystic ovary syndrome, obesity), failed medical management, or persistent abnormal bleeding
- Iron studies if anemia is suspected

IMAGING STUDIES

- Pelvic ultrasound. Transvaginal ultrasound provides better assessment than transabdominal and is preferred.
- Sonohysterography or hysteroscopy if ultrasound is not adequate or further evaluation of the cavity is required, especially to assess for intracavitary lesions; superior to ultrasonography in detection of intracavitary lesions.
- MRI if needed for surgical planning or further evaluation of structural abnormality.

🆁🆇 TREATMENT

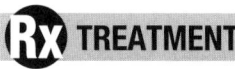

ACUTE GENERAL Rx

First-line therapy for acute AUB without known bleeding disorders is hormonal management, such as oral progestins, high-dose combined oral contraceptive pills, IV estrogen, tranexamic acid. Blood transfusion as indicated. Surgical management includes dilation and curettage, endometrial ablation (Fig. E1), uterine artery embolization, or hysterectomy (Table 1).[1-4] A comparison of effective reduction of blood loss with each treatment modality is summarized in Table 2.

CHRONIC Rx

- Combined hormonal contraceptives (pill, transdermal patch, vaginal ring) in a cyclic or continuous regimen
- Progesterone intrauterine device
- Oral progesterone
- Gonadotropin-releasing hormone analogue
- Elagolix (GnRH agonist) was FDA approved in 2020 for heavy premenstrual bleeding associated with uterine fibroids. Currently it is not recommended for use >24 mo due to concern for bone density loss
- Nonsteroidal antiinflammatory drugs
- Tranexamic acid

SURGICAL MANAGEMENT

- Need for surgical intervention depends on stability of patient, bleeding severity, contraindication to medical management, or lack of response to medical management
- Dilation and curettage

TABLE 1 Pros and Cons of Different Hysterectomy Methods

	Pros	Cons
Total abdominal hysterectomy (TAH)	Cervix is removed; therefore no further need for smears and no further risk of cervical malignancy (thus particularly suitable for those with a history of abnormal cytology) Good access to ovaries	Increased surgical morbidity
Subtotal abdominal hysterectomy	Fewer complications than TAH (↓ bleeding, ↓ infection, ↓ bladder injury, ↓ ureteric damage) Good access to ovaries	Risk of cervical cancer remains as before
Vaginal hysterectomy	May be lower incidence of bladder and bowel injury in straightforward cases (compared with abdominal hysterectomy) No painful abdominal wound	Limited ovarian access Contraindicated with: • Large uterus • Restricted uterine mobility • Limited vaginal space • Adnexal pathology • Cervix flush with vagina

From Magowan BA: *Clinical obstetrics and gynecology,* ed 4, Philadelphia, 2019, Elsevier.

TABLE 2 Reduction of Menstrual Blood Loss With Treatment

Agent Used	Decrease in Menstrual Blood Loss (%)
EACA	47
AMCA	44-54
NSAID	21-50
Oral contraceptives	52
Levonorgestrel IUD at 3, 6, and 12 mo	82, 88, 96
Endometrial ablation	Up to 100; 68%-78% of patients achieve normal menses
Hysterectomy	100

AMCA, Tranexamic acid; *EACA,* ε-aminocaproic acid; *IUD,* intrauterine device; *NSAID,* nonsteroidal antiinflammatory drug.
From Gershenson DM et al: *Comprehensive gynecology,* ed 8, Philadelphia, 2022, Elsevier.

• Hysteroscopic resection of uterine pathology including endometrial polyps and submucosal leiomyoma
• Myomectomy
• Endometrial ablation
• Uterine artery embolization
• Hysterectomy

REFERRAL
• Refer to gynecologist if:
  1. Unresponsive to initial hormonal management
  2. Concern for a structural etiology or malignancy

3. Endometrial sampling reveals endometrial hyperplasia or malignancy. Resampling is necessary with progestin therapy for hyperplasia. If endometrial hyperplasia associated with complex glands or atypia, consultation with gynecologist is warranted due to high degree of progression to malignancy

REFERENCES
Available at eBooks.Health.Elsevier.com.

RELATED CONTENT
Heavy Menstrual Bleeding (Menorrhagia) (Patient Information)
Abnormal Uterine Bleeding (Related Key Topic)

AUTHORS: **LEAH SAYLOR, DO,** and **NIMA R. PATEL, MD, MS**

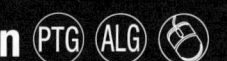
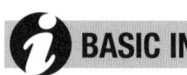 **BASIC INFORMATION**

DEFINITION
Infection of the human gastric mucosa with the organism *Helicobacter pylori,* a spiral-shaped gram-negative organism with unique features that allow it to survive in the hostile gastric environment.

SYNONYMS
H. pylori infection
Previously known as *Campylobacter*

ICD-10CM CODE
B96.81   *Helicobacter pylori [H. pylori]* as the cause of diseases classified elsewhere

EPIDEMIOLOGY & DEMOGRAPHICS
H. pylori is the most common chronic bacterial infection in human beings, probably affecting 50% of the Earth's population in all age groups, as well as 30% to 40% of the U.S. population. In developing nations, infection is acquired at an earlier age and occurs more frequently (70% prevalence in Africa).

CLINICAL PRESENTATION
- *H. pylori* causes histologic gastritis in all affected individuals. The majority of cases are asymptomatic and unlikely to proceed to serious consequences.
- *H. pylori* is a causative agent in peptic ulcer disease (PUD), gastric adenocarcinoma, and gastric mucosa–associated lymphoid tissue lymphoma, as well as a risk factor for iron deficiency anemia and likely chronic idiopathic thrombocytopenic purpura. It may manifest with the signs and symptoms of these disorders, including abdominal pain, bloating, anorexia, and early satiety. Fig. 1 describes association of *H. pylori* infection and disease states.
- "Alarm symptoms" that should prompt more immediate and aggressive workup include weight loss, dysphagia, protracted nausea or vomiting, anemia, melena, and palpable abdominal mass, particularly in older individuals.

ETIOLOGY
- Route of acquisition is unknown but is presumed to be person to person by fecal-oral or possibly oral-oral transmission.
- The majority of cases are acquired in childhood. Socioeconomic status and living conditions in childhood affect risk of acquisition of infection. These factors include housing density, number of siblings, overcrowding, sharing a bed, and lack of running water.
- Iatrogenic transmission has been documented.
- *H. pylori* does not invade gastroduodenal tissue, but disrupts the mucous layer, causing the underlying mucosa to be more vulnerable to acid peptic damage.
- It is unclear what differentiates the subset of patients with *H. pylori* who go on to develop ulcers or cancer.

Dx DIAGNOSIS

DIFFERENTIAL DIAGNOSIS
- Infection with *H. pylori* should be considered in the face of PUD, gastric cancer, gastritis, and gastric mucosa–associated lymphoid tissue (MALT) lymphoma.
- *H. pylori* should be considered in the differential diagnosis of upper GI tract disease, along with nonulcer dyspepsia, reflux esophagitis, biliary tract disease, gastroparesis, pancreatitis, ischemic bowel, and unexplained iron deficiency anemia.

WORKUP
- Workup is indicated in patients with active PUD, a history of documented peptic ulcer, or gastric MALT lymphoma, as well as those with immune thrombocytopenic purpura (ITP), and otherwise unexplained iron deficiency. The role of routine screening in high-risk populations is not clear. However, numerous studies suggest that *H. pylori* eradication is protective against progression of premalignant gastric lesions. Consider testing those starting long-term NSAID, low-dose aspirin, or proton pump inhibitor (PPI) therapy. Routine identification and treatment of *H. pylori* in cases of nonulcer dyspepsia, gastroesophageal reflux disease (GERD), and in asymptomatic individuals in populations at high risk for gastric cancer is considered controversial. There is insufficient evidence to advocate screening in asymptomatic first-degree relatives of gastric cancer patients. A test-and-treat strategy may be used in patients younger than 55 with uncomplicated dyspepsia who have no alarm symptoms.
- Results of testing must be interpreted in relation to the individual patient's likelihood of *H. pylori* infection based on demographic risk factors. In the U.S. population, increased probability of infection exists in African Americans, Hispanics/Latinos, immigrants from developing nations, patients with poor socioeconomic status, Native Americans from Alaska, and persons >50 yr.
- Routine screening for *H. pylori* is not indicated in asymptomatic patients who are at low risk of infection.
- Infected patients with functional dyspepsia often benefit from treatment and should be evaluated for *H. pylori*.

LABORATORY TESTS
- Testing may be invasive or noninvasive depending on the need for endoscopy for other indications. There is no indication for endoscopy solely to diagnose *H. pylori*.
- Tests for *H. pylori* are differentiated as active or passive. Active tests provide direct evidence that *H. pylori* infection is currently present and include urea breath testing and stool antigen testing. Passive testing, which includes all serologic testing for *H. pylori,* detects the presence of antibodies to the organism. It is limited by its inability to distinguish between active current infection and prior infection that has resolved.
- Tests that use urease as a marker (urea breath and stool antigen tests and biopsy for urease activity) may result in false-negative results in patients taking antibiotics, bismuth, or antisecretory therapy, as well as those with active ulcer bleeding. Patients should be off antibiotics for 4 wk and off protein pump inhibitors for 2 wk before urea breath or stool antigen testing.

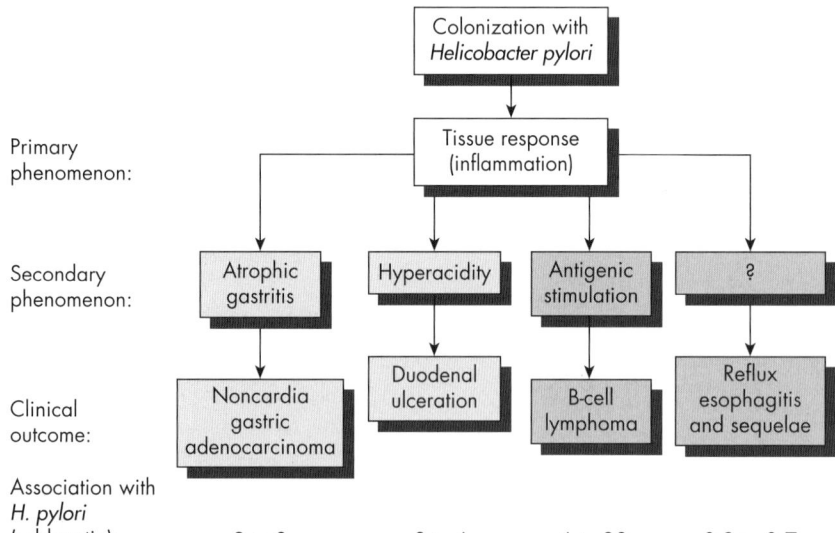

FIG. 1 Association of *Helicobacter pylori* colonization and disease states. After *H. pylori* acquisition, virtually all persons develop persistent colonization that lasts for life. Colonization induces tissue responses termed *chronic gastritis.* This process affects gastric physiology, including glandular structure, acid secretion, and antigen processing, which in turn affect disease risk. Colonization with *H. pylori* increases the risk for certain diseases (duodenal ulcer, gastric ulcer, noncardiac gastric adenocarcinoma, and B-cell lymphomas) but appears to decrease the risk for gastroesophageal reflux disease and its complications, including Barrett esophagus, and adenocarcinoma of the esophagus or gastric cardia. (From Mandell GL et al: *Principles and practice of infectious diseases,* ed 7, Philadelphia, 2010, Churchill Livingstone.)

- When diagnostic endoscopy is indicated (for suspicion or follow-up of PUD or gastric MALT), antral biopsy should be tested for urease activity. If urease testing is likely to show a false-negative result because of recent PPI, bismuth, or antibiotic use, or active ulcer bleeding, the sample should undergo histologic examination.
- In cases in which biopsy is not indicated, urea breath testing or stool antigen testing is indicated to evaluate for active infection. Urea breath testing is slightly more expensive than stool antigen testing, but both costs are in the modest range. Choice can be made based on patient preference and availability. The sensitivities and specificities of these two tests are similar (>90%), but sensitivity may be reduced in the face of active upper GI bleed or recent PPI use.
- Serologic testing should be avoided, although it may be useful in low-risk patients in areas with low prevalence to confirm lack of infection. In this situation, positive results should be confirmed with an active testing method.

⒭ⓧ TREATMENT

ACUTE GENERAL Rx

- Test only patients whom you intend to treat if positive (see "Workup"). At this time, the value of eradicating *H. pylori* infection has been clearly demonstrated in patients with PUD or gastric MALT lymphoma.
- The optimal antibiotic regimen remains undefined. In addition to efficacy, side effects, cost, and ease of administration must be considered.
- Due to increasing resistance to clarithromycin, decisions regarding appropriate regimens should take into account local rates of clarithromycin resistance, as well as any prior macrolide exposure for the patient. Clarithromycin resistance can be assumed to be >15% in the U.S. unless local resistance information is available.
- The following regimens may be considered for first-line therapy:
  1. Quadruple therapy: PPI (esomeprazole 20 mg, lansoprazole 30 mg, pantoprazole 40 mg, omeprazole 40 mg, or rabeprazole 20 mg, all given bid), with twice-daily clarithromycin (500 mg), amoxicillin (1 g bid), and metronidazole 500 mg bid for 10 to 14 days.
  2. Bismuth quadruple therapy: PPI twice daily (see earlier) combined with bismuth subsalicylate (Pepto-Bismol and others) 262 or 525 mg four times daily, as well as tetracycline (500 mg qid) and metronidazole (250 mg qid or 500 mg tid-qid) for 10 to 14 days. This is now recommended as first-line therapy in areas of high clarithromycin resistance and in patients with penicillin allergy.
- Fixed-dose combinations of omeprazole, amoxicillin, rifabutin (Talicia), and others are now available for treatment of *H. pylori* infection in adults. They may improve compliance, but cost and formulary are significant limiting factors.
- Rifabutin triple therapy (rifabutin, amoxicillin, and PPI is also available as an alternative option for first-line empiric treatment.
- Vonoprazan (a potassium-competitive acid blocker) has been FAD approved for *H. pylori* treatment in combination with amoxicillin (Voquezna Dual Pak) and with amoxicillin and clarithromycin (Voquezna Triple Pak).
- Current guidelines recommend extended treatment of 10 to 14 days.
- Recent guidelines suggest multiple other regimens that can be considered based on local resistance patterns and patient's allergy profile.
- Prior exposure to a macrolide or metronidazole, for any reason, is associated with increased resistance. A preferable regimen would include medications to which the patient has not been previously exposed.
- Diarrhea and abdominal cramping are commonly observed with many of the regimens. (Probiotics may diminish this effect.) Other side effects may include a metallic taste with metronidazole or clarithromycin, neuropathy, seizures, and disulfiram-like reaction with metronidazole, diarrhea with amoxicillin, photosensitivity with tetracycline, and *Clostridium difficile* infection with any antibiotic exposure. Bismuth may cause black stool and constipation. Tetracycline is contraindicated in pregnant patients.
- 20% of patients may not respond to initial therapy. It is important to reinforce compliance. Second-line therapy should avoid antibiotics used in initial treatment and should include either bismuth-containing quadruple therapy or levofloxacin-containing triple therapy (regardless of local clarithromycin resistance patterns). When possible, management of those who do not respond to two courses of therapy should be guided by antimicrobial sensitivity testing (endoscopy with biopsy for cultures and sensitivity).

CHRONIC Rx

- It is essential to document clearance of infection after the completion of treatment.

Repeat testing is generally performed 1 mo after completion of antibiotics and at least 2 wk after cessation of PPI therapy.
- Active tests such as urea breath test and stool antigen testing should be used. They are equally accurate in confirming eradication, and either may be used depending on availability and patient preference.
- Serology does not reliably revert to undetectable levels after treatment and should not be used to determine eradication.

DISPOSITION

Consider further evaluation in patients with recurrent symptoms after appropriate treatment.

REFERRAL

- Patients with gastric MALT lymphoma should be followed by a gastroenterologist and oncologist with expertise in the care of lymphoid neoplasms.
- Patients with dyspepsia who have tested positive for *H. pylori* and failed two courses of treatment should be referred for endoscopy and biopsy for culture and sensitivity.

❗ PEARLS & CONSIDERATIONS

- It remains unclear whether *H. pylori* eradication reduces the risk of progression to gastric cancer.
- Outcomes in PUD and gastric MALT lymphoma are improved with treatment of associated *H. pylori* infection.
- Tests that provide direct evidence of active *H. pylori* infection (urea breath and stool antigen testing) are preferred. These may result in false-negative results in patients taking antibiotics, bismuth, or antisecretory agents, which should be stopped at an appropriate time interval before testing.
- Be aware of high-risk populations in low-prevalence settings, including immigrants from Mexico, South America, Southeast Asia, and Eastern Europe.

SUGGESTED READINGS

Available at eBooks.Health.Elsevier.com.

RELATED CONTENT

Helicobacter pylori Infection (Patient Information)
Gastritis (Related Key Topic)
Peptic Ulcer Disease (Related Key Topic)

AUTHOR: **FRED F. FERRI, MD**

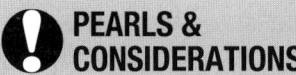

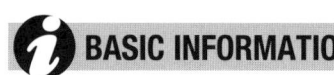

BASIC INFORMATION

DEFINITION
Hemochromatosis is an autosomal recessive disorder that disrupts the body's regulation of iron and is characterized by increased accumulation of iron in various organs (adrenals, liver, pancreas, heart, testes, kidneys, pituitary) and eventual dysfunction of these organs if not treated appropriately.

SYNONYMS
Bronze diabetes
Hereditary hemochromatosis (HH)

ICD-10CM CODES
E83.110 Hereditary hemochromatosis
E83.111 Hemochromatosis due to repeated red blood cell transfusions
E83.118 Other hemochromatosis
E83.119 Hemochromatosis, unspecified

EPIDEMIOLOGY & DEMOGRAPHICS
INCIDENCE: In whites, approximately 1/385 persons.
PREDOMINANT SEX & AGE: Generally diagnosed in men in their fifth decade. Diagnosis in females is generally not made until 10 to 20 yr after menopause.
GENETICS: Most common genetic disorder in North European ancestry. It affects 1 in every 150 to 220 persons of Northern European descent. Homozygosity for the *C282Y* mutation is now found in approximately 5/1000 persons of European descent.

PHYSICAL FINDINGS & CLINICAL PRESENTATION
- In earlier stages, patients completely asymptomatic and diagnosed due to abnormal laboratory tests
- Hepatic dysfunction leading to hepatomegaly, fibrosis, and eventually cirrhosis
- Noninflammatory arthropathy (Fig. E1)
- Gonadal insufficiency leading to loss of libido and testicular atrophy
- Diabetes mellitus: Risk greater in patients with family history
- Iron-induced cardiac disease resulting in cardiomyopathy, heart failure, and arrhythmias
- Skin pigmentation

ETIOLOGY
- Hemochromatosis results from a failure in the regulation of the key liver-derived iron regulatory hormone hepcidin to respond to increasing iron stores. Hemochromatosis is caused by several genetic disorders, the majority of which result in loss-of-function mutations in regulatory components of hepcidin synthesis[1]. The majority of the patients diagnosed with hemochromatosis have mutation in the *HFE* gene and are either homozygous for the *C282Y* mutation *(C282Y/C282Y)* or compound heterozygote for the *C282Y* mutation and either the mutation *H63D (C282Y/H63D)* or less commonly the *S65C (C282Y/S65C)*.

- The remainder of the patients are classified as non–*HFE*-associated hemochromatosis.

DIAGNOSIS

DIFFERENTIAL DIAGNOSIS
- Hereditary anemias with defect of erythropoiesis
- Cirrhosis, chronic liver disease, porphyria cutanea tarda
- Repeated blood transfusions
- Table 1 summarizes hereditary causes of iron overload

WORKUP
Medical history, physical examination, and laboratory evaluation should be focused on affected organ systems (see "Physical Findings & Clinical Presentation"). Fig. 2 outlines evaluation for possible hereditary hemochromatosis in an individual with negative family history. Liver biopsy is the gold standard for diagnosis; it reveals iron deposition in hepatocytes, bile ducts, and supporting tissues.

LABORATORY TESTS
Hemochromatosis may be characterized by elevations in serum transferrin saturation, ferritin levels, or hematologic measures. Since iron-related laboratory measurements vary, a sustained elevation must be documented on multiple occasions.[1]
- Transferrin saturation is the best screening test. Values >45% have a sensitivity of 94% in men and 73% in women for detection of *C282Y* homozygosity and are an indication for further testing.
- Elevated serum ferritin (about 300 mcg/L in men and above 200 mcg/L in women) has a sensitivity of 88% in men and 57% in women[1] and is good evidence of iron overload, but other causes like chronic inflammatory conditions, malignancy, and so forth need to be ruled out as ferritin is also an acute phase reactant.
- Genotypical screening for *C282Y* and *H63D* mutation in *HFE* gene should be done in patients with high transferrin saturation, elevated ferritin, or both.
- Liver biopsy (Fig. E3) is the gold standard but is not needed in somebody who has a persistently elevated transferrin saturation, elevated ferritin, or both.
- Hepatic iron index can help differentiate between various causes of iron overload.
- Elevated aspartate aminotransferase, alanine aminotransferase, and alkaline phosphatase are seen.
- Hyperglycemia is common in advanced stages.
- Endocrine abnormalities (decreased testosterone, luteinizing hormone, follicle-stimulating hormone) are noted.
- Table 2 describes laboratory findings in patients with hereditary hemochromatosis.

IMAGING STUDIES
Routine radiologic imaging is not needed. MRI (Fig. E4) may show low signal intensity in the liver and can be used to estimate hepatic iron concentration. Liver elastography is useful to estimate the degree of fibrosis.

TREATMENT

The goal of therapy is the removal of excess iron and maintaining it at a normal or near-normal level. Phlebotomy is first-line treatment. The goal is to reduce serum ferritin to 50 to 100 mg/ml. Box 1 summarizes the treatment of *HFE*-related hereditary hemochromatosis.

NONPHARMACOLOGIC THERAPY
Phlebotomy is the treatment of choice.

ACUTE GENERAL Rx
- The timing and frequency of phlebotomy needs to be individualized for each patient.
- For patients with heavy iron overload, twice-weekly phlebotomies should be started. In most patients, weekly phlebotomy is adequate.
- The effectiveness of treatment is monitored by periodic ferritin measurement. The goal is to bring ferritin level below 50 ng/ml.
- Patients with iron overload due to transfusion-dependent anemias may not tolerate phlebotomy. For these patients, iron chelation may be needed.
- The chelating agent deferoxamine has to be given daily as a 9- to 12-h IV or subcutaneous infusion, and compliance is difficult.
- The oral chelating agent deferasirox (Exjade) is effective but should not be used in patients with high-risk myelodysplastic syndrome because it can cause renal impairment, hepatic impairment, or GI hemorrhage, which can be fatal.

CHRONIC Rx
After the ferritin has been brought to <50 ng/ml, phlebotomy is needed on an as-needed basis to keep the ferritin at that level.

DISPOSITION
- Serum ferritin measurement is the most useful prognostic indicator of disease severity.
- Prognosis is good if phlebotomy is started early (before onset of cirrhosis or diabetes mellitus); women can have the full phenotypic expression of the disease, including cirrhosis, and also should be aggressively treated.

REFERRAL
For liver biopsy if diagnosis is uncertain

PEARLS & CONSIDERATIONS

COMMENTS
- Persons who are homozygous for the *HFE* gene mutation *C282Y* comprise 85% to 90% of phenotypically affected individuals. Patients who are heterozygous for both *C282Y* and *H63D* generally do not have clinically evident

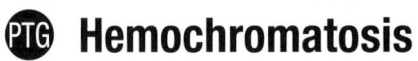
TABLE 1 Hereditary Iron Overload Disorders

Disorder	Gene, Chromosome Location	Inheritance	Plasma Transferrin Saturation	Plasma Ferritin	Iron Deposition Sites	Clinical Manifestations
Hereditary hemochromatosis, HFE-associated (type 1; OMIM235200)	HFE, 6p21	Autosomal recessive	Early increase; >45%	Later increase after third decade of life	Parenchymal iron overload affecting hepatocytes, heart, pancreas, other organs	Liver and heart disease, diabetes, gonadal failure, arthritis, skin pigmentation
Hereditary hemochromatosis, TFR2-associated (type 3; OMIM604250)	TFR2, 7q22	Autosomal recessive	Early increase; >45%	Later increase after third decade of life	Parenchymal iron overload affecting hepatocytes, heart, pancreas, other organs	Liver and heart disease, diabetes, gonadal failure, arthritis, skin pigmentation
Juvenile hemochromatosis, hemojuvelin-associated (type 2A; OMIM 602390)	HJV, 1q21	Autosomal recessive	Early increase; >45%	Increased by second decade of life	Parenchymal iron overload affecting hepatocytes, heart, pancreas, other organs	As for hereditary hemochromatosis, but liver involvement less prominent
Juvenile hemochromatosis, hepcidin-associated (type 2B; OMIM613313)	HAMP, 19q13	Autosomal recessive	Early increase; >45%	Increased by second decade of life	Parenchymal iron overload affecting hepatocytes, heart, pancreas, other organs	As for hereditary hemochromatosis, but liver involvement less prominent
Hemochromatosis, DMT1-associated (OMIM 206100)	SCL11A2, 12q13	Autosomal recessive	Early increase; >45%	Normal to moderately elevated	Hepatic iron overload, predominantly in hepatocytes	Severe microcytic anemia, liver dysfunction
Atransferrinemia (OMIM 209300)	TF, 3q22	Autosomal recessive	No plasma transferrin	Increased	Parenchymal iron overload affecting hepatocytes, heart, pancreas; no iron stores in bone marrow or spleen	Transfusion-dependent iron-deficiency anemia, growth retardation, poor survival
Aceruloplasminemia (OMIM 604290)	CP, 3q24-q25	Autosomal recessive	Decreased	Increased	Marked iron accumulation in basal ganglia, liver, pancreas	Diabetes, progressive neurologic disease, retinal degeneration
Hemochromatosis, ferroportin-associated, with impaired iron export (type 4A; OMIM606069)	SLC40A1, 2q32	Autosomal dominant	Remains normal or low	Early increase	Predominantly macrophage iron deposition	None
Hemochromatosis, ferroportin-associated, with hepcidin resistance (type 4B; OMIM606069)	SLC40A1, 2q32	Autosomal dominant	Early increase; >45%	Early increase	Parenchymal iron overload affecting hepatocytes, heart, pancreas, other organs	Similar to HFE-associated hemochromatosis

From Hoffman R et al: *Hematology: basic principles and practice,* ed 7, Philadelphia, 2018, Elsevier.

disease unless coexisting factors (e.g., excessive alcohol intake) are present.

- Patients with hemochromatosis and serum ferritin levels <1000 ng/ml are unlikely to have cirrhosis. Liver biopsy to screen for cirrhosis may be unnecessary in such patients.
- Cirrhotic patients must be periodically monitored (ultrasound or computed tomography scan) because of their increased risk of hepatocellular carcinoma.
- HFE gene testing for C282Y mutation is a cost-effective method of screening relatives of patients with hereditary hemochromatosis. The American College of Gastroenterology recommends genotyping persons who have abnormal iron screening tests and first-degree relatives of those identified with C282Y homozygosity.
- Established cirrhosis, hypogonadism, destructive arthritis, and insulin-dependent diabetes mellitus secondary to hemochromatosis cannot be reversed with repeated phlebotomy, but their progress can be slowed.
- In patients who are heterozygous for C282Y or H63D mutation, clinically meaningful iron overload does not develop.

- Screening for hepatocellular carcinoma is reserved for those with hereditary hemochromatosis and cirrhosis.

REFERENCE
Available at eBooks.Health.Elsevier.com.

RELATED CONTENT
Hemochromatosis (Patient Information)

AUTHOR: **FRED F. FERRI, MD**

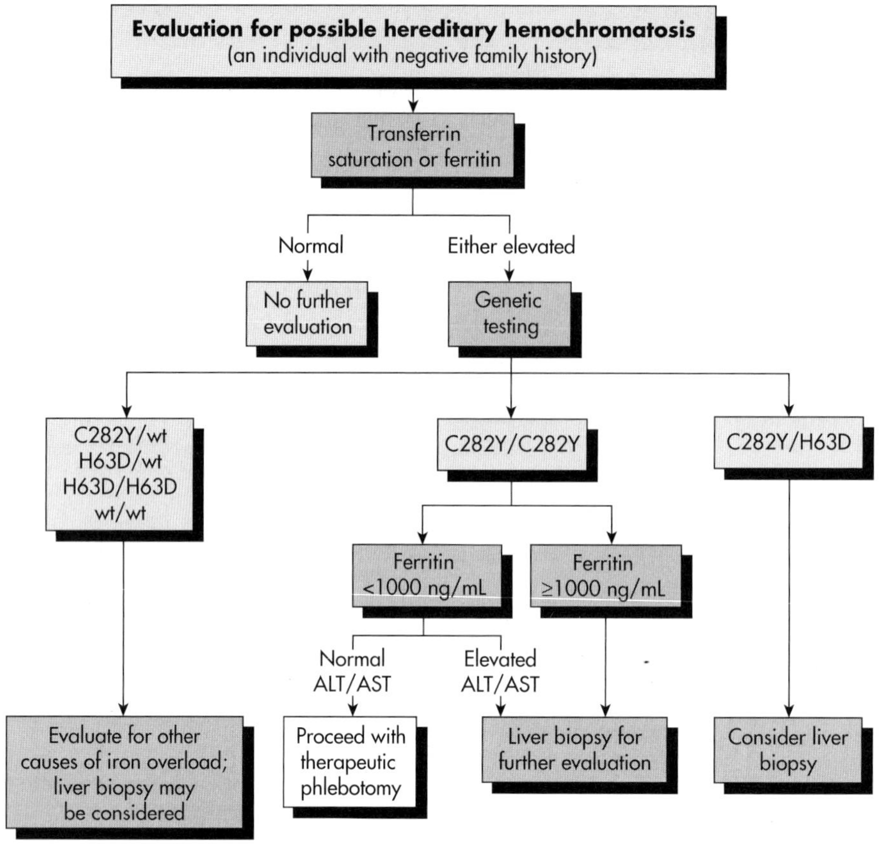
Evaluation for possible hereditary hemochromatosis
(an individual with negative family history)
Transferrin saturation or ferritin
Normal
Either elevated
No further evaluation
Genetic testing
C282Y/wt
H63D/wt
H63D/H63D
wt/wt
C282Y/C282Y
C282Y/H63D
Ferritin <1000 ng/mL
Ferritin ≥1000 ng/mL
Normal ALT/AST
Elevated ALT/AST
Evaluate for other causes of iron overload; liver biopsy may be considered
Proceed with therapeutic phlebotomy
Liver biopsy for further evaluation
Consider liver biopsy

FIG. 2 Proposed algorithm for diagnosis and management of hereditary hemochromatosis. *ALT,* Alanine aminotransferase; *AST,* aspartate aminotransferase; *wt,* wild-type (normal). (From Goldman L, Schafer AI: *Goldman-Cecil medicine,* ed 26, Philadelphia, 2019, Elsevier.)

TABLE 2 Laboratory Findings in Patients With Hereditary Hemochromatosis

		PATIENTS WITH HEREDITARY HEMOCHROMATOSIS	
Measurements	**Normal Subjects**	**Asymptomatic**	**Symptomatic**
Blood (Fasting)			
Serum iron level (μg/dl)	60-180	150-280	180-300
Serum transferrin level (mg/dl)	220-410	200-280	200-300
Transferrin saturation (%)	20-45	45-100	80-100
Serum ferritin level (ng/ml)			
Men	20-200	150-1000	500-6000
Women	15-150	120-1000	500-6000
Genetic (*HFE* Mutation Analysis)			
C282Y/C282Y	wt/wt[‡]	*C282Y/C282Y*	*C282Y/C282Y*
*C282Y/H63D**	wt/wt	*C282Y/H63D*	*C282Y/H63D*
Liver			
Hepatic iron concentration			
μg/g dry weight	300-1500	2000-10,000	8000-30,000
μmol/g dry weight	5-27	36-179	140-550
Hepatic iron index[†]	<1	1 to >1.9	>1.9
Liver histology			
Perls Prussian blue stain	0, 1+	2+ to 4+	3+, 4+

*Compound heterozygote.

[†]Calculated by dividing the hepatic iron concentration (in μmol/g dry weight) by the age of the patient (in years). With the increased use of genetic testing in patients with iron overload, the specificity of the hepatic iron index has diminished.

[‡]wt/wt: Wild type (normal).

From Goldman L, Schafer AI: *Goldman's Cecil medicine,* ed 24, Philadelphia, 2012, Saunders.

BOX 1 Treatment of *HFE*-Related Hereditary Hemochromatosis

Perform phlebotomy of 500 ml (1 unit) of whole blood weekly unless the hematocrit value drops below 37%.

Check the transferrin saturation and ferritin levels at 2- to 3-mo intervals to monitor response (optional).

When the iron stores are depleted (ferritin 50 to 100 ng/ml and transferrin saturation <50%), proceed to maintenance phlebotomy of 1 unit of whole blood every 2-3 mo. Aim to keep the transferrin saturation <50%; if successful, the ferritin level should remain between 50 and 100 ng/ml.

From Feldman M et al: *Sleisenger and Fordtran's gastrointestinal and liver disease*, ed 10, Philadelphia, 2016, Elsevier.

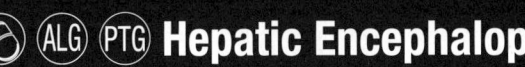
Diseases and Disorders

I

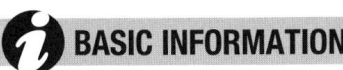 BASIC INFORMATION

DEFINITION

Hepatic encephalopathy is a neuropsychiatric syndrome occurring in patients with severe impairment of liver function and consequent accumulation of toxic products not metabolized by the liver. It is characterized by gradual impairment of the ability to perform mental tasks and to react to external stimuli. Fig. 1 illustrates the hepatic encephalopathy grades in acute liver failure. *Minimal hepatic encephalopathy* refers to patients with hepatic cirrhosis and mild cognitive impairment, but no history of overt encephalopathy.

SYNONYMS

Hepatic coma
Portal systemic encephalopathy
HE

ICD-10CM CODES
G92	Toxic encephalopathy
G93.40	Encephalopathy, unspecified
G93.41	Metabolic encephalopathy
K70.40	Alcoholic hepatic failure without coma
K70.41	Alcoholic hepatic failure with coma
K72.0	Acute and subacute hepatic failure
K72.00	Acute and subacute hepatic failure without coma
K72.01	Acute and subacute hepatic failure with coma
K72.1	Chronic hepatic failure
K72.10	Chronic hepatic failure without coma
K72.11	Chronic hepatic failure with coma
K72.9	Hepatic failure, unspecified
K72.90	Hepatic failure, unspecified without coma
K72.91	Hepatic failure, unspecified with coma
K91.82	Postprocedural hepatic failure

EPIDEMIOLOGY & DEMOGRAPHICS

INCIDENCE & PREVALENCE: Hepatic encephalopathy occurs in >40% of all cases of cirrhosis.

PHYSICAL FINDINGS & CLINICAL PRESENTATION

Hepatic encephalopathy can be classified by clinical stages described in Table 1. Other widely used scales are the four score criteria and the West Haven criteria. The West Haven criteria for grading hepatic encephalopathy is as follows:
- Grade (0): No abnormalities noted
- Grade (1): Unawareness (mild), euphoria or anxiety, shortened attention span, impairment of calculation ability, lethargy, or apathy
- Grade (2): Disorientation to time, obvious personality change, inappropriate behavior
- Grade (3): Somnolence to stupor, responsiveness to stimuli, gross disorientation, bizarre behavior
- Grade (4): Coma

The physical examination in hepatic encephalopathy varies with the stage and may reveal the following abnormalities:
- Skin: Jaundice, palmar erythema, spider angiomata, ecchymosis, dilated superficial periumbilical veins (caput medusae) in patients with cirrhosis
- Eyes: Scleral icterus, Kayser-Fleischer rings (Wilson disease)
- Breath: Fetor hepaticus
- Chest: Gynecomastia in men with chronic liver disease
- Abdomen: Ascites, small nodular liver (cirrhosis), tender hepatomegaly (congestive hepatomegaly)
- Rectal examination: Hemorrhoids (portal hypertension), guaiac-positive stool (alcoholic gastritis, bleeding esophageal varices, peptic ulcer disease, bleeding hemorrhoids)
- Genitalia: Testicular atrophy in males with chronic liver disease
- Extremities: Pedal edema from hypoalbuminemia
- Neurologic: Flapping tremor (asterixis), obtundation, coma with or without decerebrate posturing

ETIOLOGY
- Hepatic encephalopathy is thought to be caused mainly by accumulation of unmetabolized ammonia. The shunting of ammonia into the systemic circulation results in neuronal dysfunction leading to hepatic encephalopathy
- Precipitating factors in patients with underlying cirrhosis (upper gastrointestinal bleeding, hypokalemia, hypomagnesemia, analgesic and sedative drugs, sepsis, alkalosis, increased dietary protein)
- Acute fulminant viral hepatitis
- Drugs and toxins (e.g., isoniazid, acetaminophen, diclofenac and other NSAIDs, statins, methyldopa, loratadine, propylthiouracil, lisinopril, labetalol, halothane, carbon tetrachloride, erythromycin, nitrofurantoin, troglitazone, herbal products, flavocoxid)
- Reye syndrome
- Shock and/or sepsis
- Fatty liver of pregnancy
- Metastatic carcinoma, hepatocellular carcinoma
- Other: Autoimmune hepatitis, ischemic venoocclusive disease, sclerosing cholangitis, heat stroke, amebic abscesses

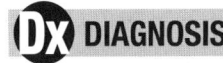 DIAGNOSIS

DIFFERENTIAL DIAGNOSIS
- Delirium caused by medications or illicit drugs
- Cerebrovascular accident, subdural hematoma
- Meningitis, encephalitis
- Hypoglycemia
- Uremia
- Cerebral anoxia
- Hypercalcemia
- Metastatic neoplasm to brain
- Alcohol withdrawal syndrome/Wernicke-Korsakoff syndrome
- Hyponatremia
- Postictal state

WORKUP
Hepatic encephalopathy should be considered in any patient with cirrhosis who presents with neuropsychiatric manifestations. Exclude other etiologies with comprehensive history (obtained from patient, relatives, and others), physical examination, and laboratory and imaging studies. A pertinent history should include exposure to hepatitis, ethanol intake, drug history, exposure to toxins, IV drug abuse, measles or influenza with aspirin use (Reye syndrome), and history of carcinoma (primary or metastatic). Minimal hepatic encephalopathy may not be obvious on clinical examination but can be detected with neurophysiologic and neuropsychiatric testing.

LABORATORY TESTS
- Alanine aminotransferase, aspartate aminotransferase, bilirubin, alkaline phosphatase, glucose, calcium, electrolytes, blood urea nitrogen, creatinine, albumin
- Complete blood count, platelet count, prothrombin time, partial thromboplastin time
- Serum and urine toxicology screen in suspected medication or illegal drug use
- Blood and urine cultures, urinalysis

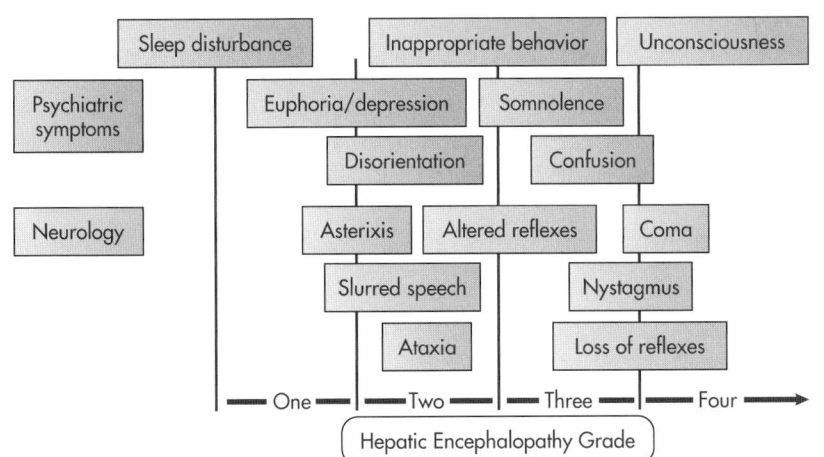

FIG. 1 Hepatic encephalopathy grade in acute liver failure. (From Parrillo JE, Dellinger RP: *Critical care medicine: principles of diagnosis and management in the adult*, ed 4, Philadelphia, 2014, Elsevier.)

Hepatic Encephalopathy PTG ALG

TABLE 1 Clinical Stages of Hepatic Encephalopathy

Stage	Asterixis	EEG Changes	Clinical Manifestations
I (prodrome)	Slight	Minimal	Mild intellectual impairment, disturbed sleep-wake cycle
II (impending)	Easily elicited	Usually generalized	Drowsiness, confusion, coma/inappropriate behavior, disorientation, mood swings
III (stupor)	Present if patient cooperative	Grossly abnormal slowing of rhythm	Drowsy, unresponsive to verbal commands, markedly confused, delirious, hyperreflexia, positive Babinski sign
IV (coma)	Usually absent	Appearance of delta waves, decreased amplitudes	Unconscious, decerebrate or decorticate response to pain present (stage IVA) or absent (stage IVB)

EEG, Electroencephalogram.
From Fuhrman BP et al: *Pediatric critical care,* ed 4, Philadelphia, 2011, Saunders.

TABLE 2 Managing Precipitants of Portosystemic Encephalopathy

Precipitant	Management
Volume depletion	Commonly from diuretics. Correct with IV albumin and stop diuretics
Infection	Treat specific infection. If SBP, give antibiotics and IV albumin
Renal failure and electrolyte imbalance	Identify cause and correct
Alcohol	Cease and manage withdrawal
Sedatives	Cease
Portosystemic shunt (TIPS)	Lactulose or rifaximin
Hepatocellular carcinoma	Specific management; see section on liver tumors
Protein load, including GI bleed	Endoscopy and management of portal hypertensive bleed. Dietary protein restriction is rarely required and should not be chronically commenced to avoid malnutrition
Constipation	Lactulose

GI, Gastrointestinal; *IV,* intravenous; *SBP,* spontaneous bacterial peritonitis; *TIPS,* transjugular intrahepatic portosystemic shunt.

- Venous ammonia level. Measurement of serum ammonia level is useful in the evaluation of acute liver failure because levels correlate with the severity of encephalopathy and elevated levels are predictive of severe encephalopathy and cerebral edema. It is not useful for the evaluation or screening of hepatic encephalopathy in patients with chronic liver disease because it can neither rule in nor rule out hepatic encephalopathy, and levels do not correlate with the degree of encephalopathy
- Arterial blood gases

IMAGING STUDIES

CT scan or MRI of the brain may be useful in selected patients to exclude other etiologies when diagnosis is unclear.

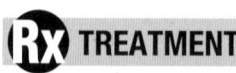 **TREATMENT**

NONPHARMACOLOGIC THERAPY

- Identification and treatment of precipitating factors (Table 2).
- Restriction of protein intake is ill-advised and not necessary since normal protein intake does not appear to exacerbate hepatic encephalopathy.

ACUTE GENERAL Rx

The approach to patients with high grade hepatic encephalopathy is shown in Fig. 2. Table 3 summarizes the management of fulminant hepatic failure.
Reduction of colonic ammonia production:

- Lactulose 25 ml twice daily initially; dose is subsequently adjusted depending on clinical response to achieve production of three bowel movements daily. IV ornithine aspartate should be considered for those not responding to lactulose.
- The oral antibiotic rifaximin (550 mg PO bid) is effective in reducing the risk of recurrent hepatic encephalopathy in patients with cirrhosis and preventing post TIPS hepatic encephalopathy. It can be taken with lactulose, and the combination of lactulose and rifaximin is superior to lactulose alone in reversing hepatic encephalopathy. Rifaximin has also been shown to be effective in improving psychometric performance and health-related quality of life in patients with minimal hepatic encephalopathy. It is well tolerated but expensive.[1]
- Probiotics (e.g., one capsule containing 112.5 billion viable lyophilized bacteria tid) might also be beneficial in altering gut flora to reduce ammonia production.

Treatment of cerebral edema:

- Cerebral edema is often present in patients with acute liver failure, and it accounts for nearly 50% of deaths. Monitoring intracranial pressure by epidural, intraparenchymal, or subdural transducers and treatment of cerebral edema with mannitol (100 to 200 ml of 20% solution [0.3 to 0.4 g/kg of body weight]) given by rapid IV infusion are helpful in selected patients (e.g., potential transplantation patients).
- Fig. 3 illustrates the management of a sustained rise in intracranial pressure in liver failure.
- Dexamethasone and hyperventilation (useful in head injury) are of little value in treating cerebral edema from liver failure.

CHRONIC Rx

- Avoidance of any precipitating factors (e.g., high-protein diet, medications).
- Consideration of liver transplantation in selected patients with progressive or recurrent encephalopathy (Box 1). Liver transplantation remains the only curative therapeutic option.

DISPOSITION

Prognosis varies with the underlying etiology of the liver failure and the grade of encephalopathy (generally good for grades 1 or 2; poor for grades 3 or 4). Without proper therapy, the survival rate at 1 yr is 42% and decreases to 23% at 3 yr.

REFERRAL

The early stages of hepatic encephalopathy can be managed in the outpatient setting, whereas stages III or IV require hospital admission.

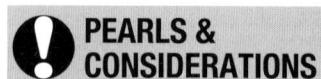 **PEARLS & CONSIDERATIONS**

COMMENTS

- Trials have shown that adding IV albumin to lactulose may improve outcomes in severe hepatic encephalopathy by reducing oxidative stress through reduction of levels of circulating cytokines and endotoxins.
- Long-acting benzodiazepines should not be used to treat anxiety and sleep disorders in patients with cirrhosis, as they may precipitate encephalopathy.

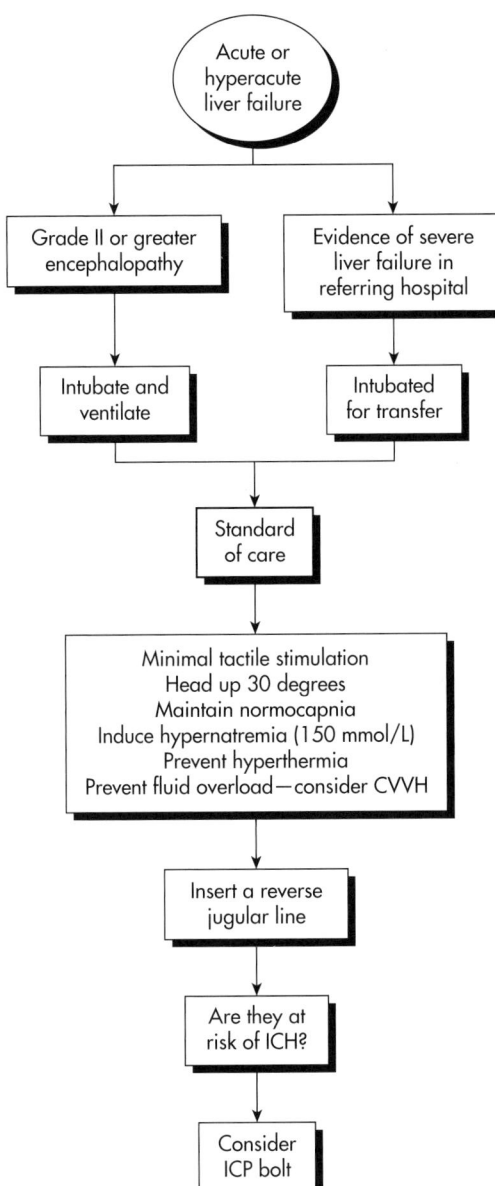

FIG. 2 Initial management of patient with high-grade encephalopathy. *CVVH*, Continuous venovenous hemofiltration; *ICH*, intracranial hypertension; *ICP*, intracranial pressure. (From Parrillo JE, Dellinger RP: Critical care medicine: principles of diagnosis and management in the adult, ed 5, Philadelphia, 2019, Elsevier.)

TABLE 3 Management of Fulminant Hepatic Failure

No sedation except for procedures
Minimal handling
Enteric precautions until infection ruled out
Monitor:
1. Heart and respiratory rate
2. Arterial BP, CVP
3. Core/toe temperature
4. Neurologic observations
5. Gastric pH (>5.0)
6. Blood glucose (>4 mmol/L)
7. Acid-base
8. Electrolytes
9. PT, PTT
Fluid balance:
1. 75% maintenance
2. Dextrose 10%-50% (provide 6-10 mg/kg/min)
3. Sodium (0.5-1 mmol/L)
4. Potassium (2-4 mmol/L)
Maintain circulating volume with colloid/FFP coagulation support only if required
Drugs:
1. Vitamin K
2. H$_2$ antagonist
3. Antacids
4. Lactulose
5. N-acetylcysteine for acetaminophen toxicity
6. Broad-spectrum antibiotics
7. Antifungals
Nutrition:
1. Enteral feeding (1-2 g protein/kg/day)
2. PN if ventilated

BP, Blood pressure; *CVP*, central venous pressure; *FFP*, fresh frozen plasma; *PN*, parenteral nutrition; *PT*, prothrombin time; *PTT*, partial thromboplastin time.
From Fuhrman BP et al: *Pediatric critical care,* ed 4, Philadelphia, 2011, Saunders.

- Patients not responding to supportive therapy should be evaluated for liver transplantation.
- Not all patients with cirrhosis develop hepatic encephalopathy. It has been shown that 40% of persons with cirrhosis and minimal hepatic encephalopathy do not develop overt hepatic encephalopathy in long-term follow-up. There are genetic factors associated with development of hepatic encephalopathy in patients with cirrhosis.

Genetic analyses have shown that glutaminase TACC and CACC haplotypes are linked to the risk for overt hepatic encephalopathy.

REFERENCE & SUGGESTED READINGS
Available at eBooks.Health.Elsevier.com.

RELATED CONTENT

Encephalopathy (Patient Information)
Cirrhosis (Related Key Topic)
Hepatic Encephalopathy (Related Key Topic)

AUTHOR: **FRED F. FERRI, MD**

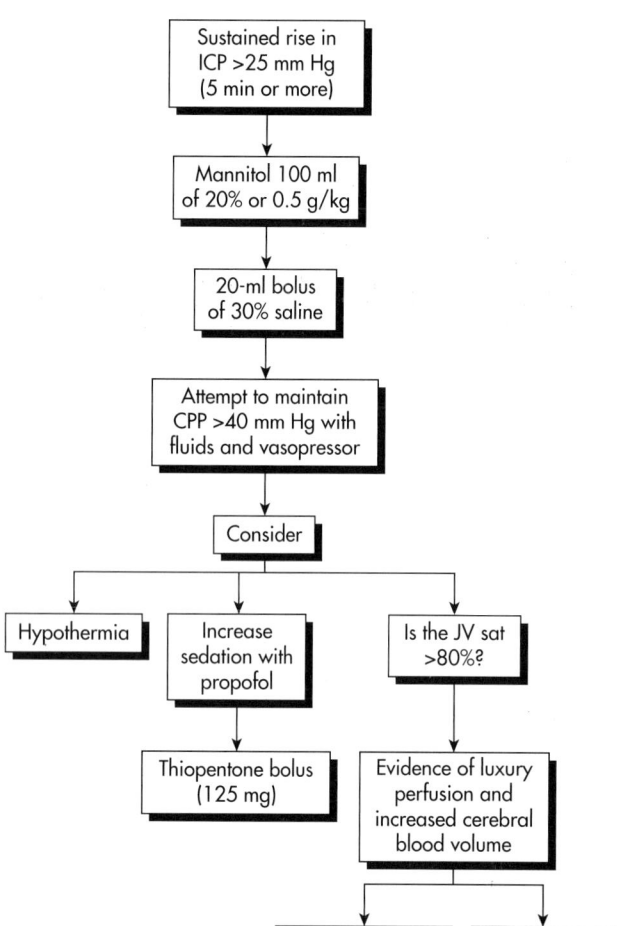

FIG. 3 Management of a sustained rise in intracranial pressure. *CPP,* Cerebral perfusion pressure; *ICP,* intracranial pressure; *JV,* jugular venous; *Sats,* saturation. (From Parrillo JE, Dellinger RP: *Critical care medicine: principles of diagnosis and management in the adult,* ed 5, Philadelphia, 2019, Elsevier.)

BOX 1   Various Prognostic Criteria Used for Liver Transplantation in Patients With Fulminant Hepatic Failure

King's College Criteria
Acetaminophen overdose:
- Arterial pH <7.3 (irrespective of grade of encephalopathy) or
- PT >100 sec (INR >6.5)
- Serum creatinine >3.4 mg/dl (>300 μmol/L)
- Patients with grade III and IV hepatic encephalopathy
Nonacetaminophen liver injury:
- PT >100 sec (INR >6.5) (irrespective of grade of encephalopathy) or any three of the following variables:
  1. Age <10 or >40 yr
  2. Non-A, non-B hepatitis, halothane hepatitis, idiosyncratic drug reactions
  3. Jaundice >7 days before onset of encephalopathy
  4. Serum bilirubin 17.4 mg/dl (300 μmol/L)
  5. PT >50 sec

Cliché Criteria
Factor V <20% in persons <30 yr or both of the following:
- Factor V <30% in patients >30 yr
- Grade III or IV encephalopathy

Serum Gc Globulin Levels
Decreasing Gc levels due to dying hepatocytes

Serum α-Fetoprotein Level
Serial increase from day 1 to day 3 has shown correlation with survival

Liver Biopsy
70% necrosis is discriminant of 90% mortality

From Vincent JL et al: *Textbook of critical care,* ed 6, Philadelphia, 2011, Saunders.

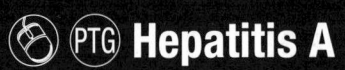

BASIC INFORMATION

DEFINITION

Hepatitis A is generally an acute self-limiting infection of the liver by an enterically transmitted picornavirus, hepatitis A virus (HAV). Infection may range from asymptomatic to fulminant hepatitis.

SYNONYMS

Infectious hepatitis
Short incubation hepatitis
Type A hepatitis
HAV (hepatitis A virus)

ICD-10CM CODES
B15.0   Hepatitis A with hepatic coma
B15.9   Hepatitis A without hepatic coma

EPIDEMIOLOGY & DEMOGRAPHICS

INCIDENCE:
- Hepatitis A occurs worldwide, affecting 1.4 million people annually and accounting for 20% to 40% of cases of viral hepatitis in the U.S. It is the most common cause of viral hepatitis worldwide.
- The seroprevalence increases with age, ranging from 10% in individuals aged <5 yr to 74% in those aged >50 yr.
- In the U.S., average disease rate was ~15 cases/100,000 persons/yr before routine vaccination of all children in certain states. The incidence after 2005 is about 1 case/100,000. There were 18,846 reported cases in the U.S. in 2019.
- The incidence is relatively higher in some regions in the U.S., including Arizona, Alaska, California, Idaho, Nevada, New Mexico, Oklahoma, Oregon, South Dakota, and Washington.
- At-risk groups include:
  1. Residents and staff of group homes
  2. Children and employees of day care centers
  3. People who engage in oral–anal contact, regardless of sexual orientation
  4. IV drug abusers
  5. Travel to endemic areas
  6. Areas of overcrowding, poor sanitation, inadequate sewage treatment

PREVALENCE:
- Approximately three fourths of the U.S. population has serologic evidence of prior infection.
- Anti-HAV prevalence has an inverse relation to income and household size.

PREDOMINANT SEX: None, except higher infection rates seen in men who have sex with men who engage in oral–anal contact.

PREDOMINANT AGE & PEAK INCIDENCE:
- In areas of high rates of hepatitis A, virtually all children are infected while younger than 10 yr, but disease is rare.
- In areas of moderate rates of hepatitis A, disease occurs in late childhood and young adults.
- In areas of low rates of hepatitis A, most cases occur in young adults.

INCUBATION PERIOD: Averages 30 days (15 to 50)

PHYSICAL FINDINGS & CLINICAL PRESENTATION

- Infection with HAV may have acute or subacute presentation, icteric or anicteric. Severity of illness seems to increase with age (90% of infection in children aged <5 yr may be subclinical).
- The incubation period of HAV is 2 to 6 wk.
- A preicteric, prodromal phase of approximately 1 to 14 days; 15% no apparent prodrome. Symptoms are usually abrupt in onset and may include anorexia, fatigue, malaise, nausea, vomiting, fever, headache, and mild abdominal pain.
- Less common symptoms are chills, myalgias, arthralgias, upper respiratory symptoms, constipation, diarrhea, pruritus, urticaria.
- Jaundice occurs in >70% of patients. Patients older than 30 yr are more likely than younger individuals to have jaundice.
- The icteric phase is preceded by dark urine.
- Bilirubinuria is typically followed a few days later by clay-colored stools and icterus.

PHYSICAL EXAMINATION

- Jaundice: Peaks in severity 2 wk after onset
- Hepatomegaly
- Splenomegaly
- Cervical lymphadenopathy
- Evanescent rash
- Petechiae
- Cardiac arrhythmias

COMPLICATIONS

- Cholestasis
- Fulminant hepatitis
- Arthritis
- Myocarditis
- Optic neuritis
- Transverse myelitis
- Thrombocytopenic purpura
- Aplastic anemia
- Red cell aplasia
- Henoch-Schönlein purpura
- Immunoglobulin A (IgA) dominant glomerulonephritis

ETIOLOGY

- Caused by HAV, a 27-nm, nonenveloped, icosahedral, positive-stranded ribonucleic acid (RNA) virus.
- Transmission is fecal-oral route, from person to person. Transmission occurs with close contact or with food- or water-borne outbreaks with inadequately purified water or cooked foods. Recent outbreaks have involved green onions and tomatoes.
- Parenteral transmission is considered rare.
- Vertical transmission has also been reported.

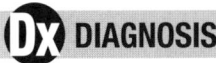 DIAGNOSIS

DIFFERENTIAL DIAGNOSIS

- Other hepatitis virus (B, C, D, E): Characteristics of the main hepatitis viruses are described in Table 1. Serology and polymerase chain reaction (PCR) test results are summarized in Table 2.
- Infectious mononucleosis
- Cytomegalovirus infection
- Herpes simplex virus infection
- Leptospirosis
- Brucellosis
- Drug-induced liver disease
- Ischemic hepatitis
- Autoimmune hepatitis

WORKUP

- IgM antibody specific for HAV
- Liver function tests; ALT and AST elevations are sensitive for liver damage but not specific for HAV
- Elevated erythrocyte sedimentation rate (ESR)
- CBC; may find mild lymphocytosis

LABORATORY TESTS

- Diagnosis confirmed by IgM anti-HAV; it is detectable in almost all infected patients at presentation and remains positive for 3 to 6 mo.
- A fourfold rise in titer of total antibody (IgM and IgG) to HAV confirms acute infection.

TABLE 1   Characteristics of the Main Hepatitis Viruses

	HAV	HBV	HCV	HDV	HEV
Family	Picornavirus	Hepadnavirus	Flavivirus	Incomplete	Calicivirus
Nucleic acid	RNA	DNA	RNA	RNA	RNA
Diameter (nm)	27	42	32	36	34
Incubation period (weeks)	2-6	6-24	2-26	6-9	2-10
Spread					
Feces	Yes	No	No	No	Yes
Blood	Uncommon	Yes	Yes	Yes	No
Sexual	Uncommon	Yes	Uncommon	Yes	?
Vertical	No	Yes	Uncommon	Yes	No
Chronic infection	No	Yes	Yes	Yes	No
Vaccine	Available	Available	Nil	Nil	Nil

HAV, Hepatitis A virus; *HBV,* hepatitis B virus; *HCV,* hepatitis C virus; *HDV,* hepatitis D virus; *HEV,* hepatitis E virus.
From Cameron P, et al. *Textbook of adult emergency medicine,* ed 5, 2019, Australia, Elsevier.

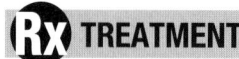

- HAV detection in stool and body fluids by electron microscopy.
- HAV RNA detection in stool, body fluids, serum, and liver tissue.
- ALT and AST usually more than 8 times normal in acute infection.
- Bilirubin usually 5 to 15 times normal.
- Alkaline phosphatase minimally elevated, but higher level in cholestasis.
- Albumin and prothrombin time are generally normal; if elevated, they may herald hepatic necrosis.
- Fig. 1 illustrates the typical course of hepatitis A.

IMAGING STUDIES
- Rarely useful
- Sonogram (fulminant hepatitis)

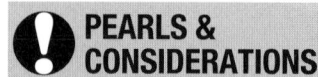

TREATMENT
- Usually self-limited
- Supportive care
- Those with fulminant hepatitis may require hospitalization and treatment of associated complications
- Activity as tolerated
- Advise to avoid alcohol and hepatotoxic drugs
- Patients with fulminant hepatitis should be assessed for liver transplantation

CHRONIC Rx
No chronic HAV and no chronic carrier state. The majority of patients have resolution of symptoms and liver abnormalities within 3 mo.

DISPOSITION
- Follow-up as outpatient.

- Most patients recover within 3 mo of infection, although 5% to 10% of patients will experience a relapse in the first 6 mo.
- HAV is a self-limited infection and does not cause chronic hepatitis.

REFERRAL
- To a hepatologist if severe, fulminant hepatitis develops
- To a transplant surgeon if liver transplant becomes a consideration for fulminant hepatitis and liver failure

PEARLS & CONSIDERATIONS

- All cases of hepatitis A should be reported to the public health authorities because foodborne or water-borne outbreaks may occur, and public health efforts (mass vaccination or immunoglobulin therapy) may prevent secondary cases.
- Hepatitis A is a common illness in internationally traveled and developing countries. Pretravel vaccination is strongly recommended for travelers who are HAV susceptible. Table 3 summarizes recommendations for preexposure use of hepatitis A virus vaccine. Updated dosage recommendations are described in Table 4.
- Handwashing is important because the hepatitis A virus may survive for up to 4 hr on the fingertips.
- There have been significant recent outbreaks of hepatitis A in the U.S. In 2016 to 2019 there was an increase of cases by 294% vs. cases in 2013 to 2015. This was mostly among the homeless, IV drug abusers, men having sex with men, and individuals who consumed certain imported food items.

PREVENTION
- Improvement in hygiene and sanitation
- Heating food
- Avoidance of water and foods from endemic area

PASSIVE IMMUNIZATION
- Immunoglobulin provides protection against HAV through passive transfer of antibody.
- Preexposure prophylaxis indicated for people traveling to endemic areas with immune globulin (Ig 0.02 or 0.06 ml/kg given IM) who have not received or cannot receive the hepatitis A vaccine before departure. The lower dose is effective for up to 3 mo, and the higher dose is effective for up to 5 mo.
- Postexposure prophylaxis (PEP): For individuals with a recent exposure to hepatitis A who have not received the vaccine, postexposure prophylaxis is warranted with either immunoglobulin (Ig 0.02 ml/kg given IM) or a single dose of the hepatitis A vaccine within 2 wk of the exposure. For healthy persons ages 12 mo to 40 yr of age, a single dose of the hepatitis A vaccine should be given. Children <12 mo, adults >40 yr of age, and persons who have chronic liver disease and

TABLE 2 Diagnostic Blood Tests: Serology and Viral Polymerase Chain Reaction

HAV	HBV	HCV	HDV	HEV
Acute/Active Infection				
Anti-HAV IgM (+)	Anti-HBc IgM (+)	Anti-HCV (+)	Anti-HDV IgM (+)	Anti-HEV IgM (+)
Blood PCR positive*	HBsAg (+)	HCV RNA (+) (PCR)	Blood PCR positive	Blood PCR positive*
	Anti-HBs (−)		HBsAg (+)	
	HBV DNA (+) (PCR)		Anti-HBs (−)	
Past Infection (Recovered)				
Anti-HAV IgG (+)	Anti-HBs (+)	Anti-HCV (+)	Anti-HDV IgG (+)	Anti-HEV IgG (+)
	Anti-HBc IgG (+)†	Blood PCR (−)	Blood PCR (−)	Blood PCR (−)
Chronic Infection				
N/A	Anti-HBc IgG (+)	Anti-HCV (+)	Anti-HDV IgG (+)	N/A
	HBsAg (+)	Blood PCR (+)	Blood PCR (−)	
	Anti-HBs (−)		HBsAg (+)	
	PCR (+) or (−)		Anti-HBs (−)	
Vaccine Response				
Anti-HAV IgG (+)	Anti-HBs (+)	N/A	N/A	N/A
	Anti-HBc (−)			

HAV, Hepatitis A virus; *HBc*, hepatitis B core; *HBs*, hepatitis B surface; *HBsAg*, hepatitis B surface antigen; *HBV*, hepatitis B virus; *HCV*, hepatitis C virus; *HDV*, hepatitis D virus; *HEV*, hepatitis E virus; *Ig*, immunoglobulin; *N/A*, not applicable; *PCR*, polymerase chain reaction.

*Research tool.

†Still poses a risk for reactivation.

From Kliegman RM: *Nelson textbook of pediatrics*, ed 21, Philadelphia, 2020, Elsevier.

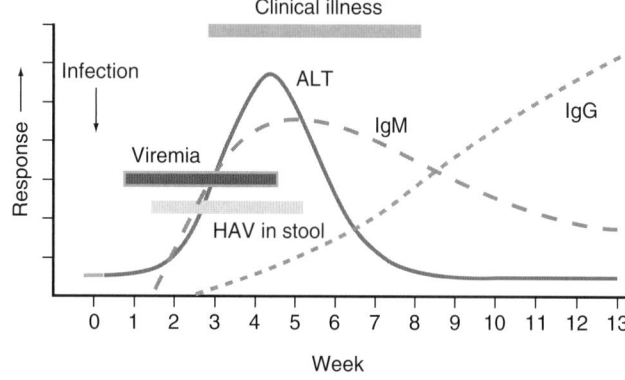

FIG. 1 Immunologic, virologic, and biochemical events during the course of a typical hepatitis A virus (HAV) infection. *ALT,* Alanine transaminase; *IgG,* immunoglobulin G; *IgM,* immunoglobulin M. (From Cherry JD et al: *Feigin and Cherry's pediatric infectious diseases,* ed 8, Philadelphia, 2019, Elsevier.)

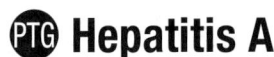

TABLE 3 Recommendations for Routine Preexposure Use of Hepatitis A Virus Vaccine

Group	Comments
Children	Vaccine should be given to all children at age 1 yr (12-23 mo).* Vaccination of children 2-18 yr may also be warranted.†
International travelers‡	IG may be given in addition to or instead of vaccine; children <12 mo should receive IG.
Close contacts of newly arriving international adoptees Men who have sex with men	All persons who anticipate close personal contact (e.g., household contact or regular babysitter) during the first 60 days after arrival Includes adolescents
Illicit drug users	Includes adolescents
Persons with chronic liver disease, such as those with hepatitis B or C	Increased risk of fulminant hepatitis A with HAV infection
Persons receiving clotting factor concentrates	
Persons who work with HAV in research laboratory settings	

HAV, Hepatitis A virus; *IG,* immunoglobulin.
*Hepatitis A vaccine is not licensed for children <12 mo.
†States and communities with existing vaccination programs for children aged 2 to 18 yr are encouraged to maintain these programs. Catch-up vaccination for this age group may be warranted elsewhere in the context of ongoing outbreaks among children.
‡Persons traveling to Canada, Western Europe, Japan, Australia, or New Zealand are at no greater risk than in the U.S.
From Bennett JE et al: *Mandell, Douglas, and Bennett's principles and practice of infectious diseases,* ed 8, Philadelphia, 2015, Saunders.

TABLE 4 Indications and Updated Dosage Recommendations for GamaSTAN S/D Human Immune Globulin for Preexposure and Postexposure Prophylaxis Against Hepatitis A Infection

Indication	Updated Dosage Recommendation
Preexposure prophylaxis	
Up to 1 mo of travel	0.1 ml/kg
Up to 2 mo of travel	0.2 ml/kg
2 mo of travel or longer	0.2 ml/kg (repeat every 2 mo)
Postexposure prophylaxis	0.1 ml/kg

From Kliegman RM et al: *Nelson textbook of pediatrics,* ed 21, Philadelphia, 2020, Elsevier.

who are immunocompromised should receive immunoglobulin.

ACTIVE IMMUNIZATION

- There are several inactivated and attenuated hepatitis vaccines; only the inactivated vaccines are currently available for use, and they have been found to be safe and highly immunogenic: HAVRIX or VAQTA. These can be used in adults and children older than 12 mo. They are given as a two-dose regimen 6 mo to 1 yr apart. A combined hepatitis A and hepatitis B vaccine called TWINRX is also available.
- Protective antibody levels were reached in 94% to 100% of adults 1 mo after the first dose; similar results have been found for children and adolescents.
- Theoretic analyses of antibody levels estimate duration of immunity to be 10 to 20 yr.
- Vaccine should be considered for persons who are at risk. Those traveling to or working in endemic areas, men who have sex with men, illegal drug users, persons with chronic liver disease, and children in areas with high rates of hepatitis A infection.
- The Advisory Committee on Immunization Practices recommends routine hepatitis A vaccination for all children beginning at 12 to 23 mo of age. Simultaneous administration of MMR and HCPA vaccines is recommended for infants aged 6 to 11 mo traveling internationally. The travel-related dose for infants aged 6 to 11 mo should not be counted towards the routine two-dose series.

SUGGESTED READINGS
Available at eBooks.Health.Elsevier.com.

RELATED CONTENT
Hepatitis A (Patient Information)

AUTHOR: **GLENN G. FORT, MD, MPH**

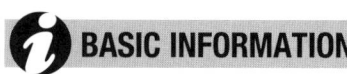

BASIC INFORMATION

DEFINITION

Hepatitis B is an infection of the liver parenchymal cells caused by the hepatitis B virus (HBV).

SYNONYMS

Serum hepatitis
Long incubation (30 to 180 days) hepatitis HBV
HBV

ICD-10CM CODES
B16	Acute hepatitis B
B16.0	Acute hepatitis B with delta-agent with hepatic coma
B16.1	Acute hepatitis B with delta-agent without hepatic coma
B16.2	Acute hepatitis B without delta-agent with hepatic coma
B16.9	Acute hepatitis B without delta agent and without hepatic coma
B18.0	Chronic viral hepatitis B with delta-agent
B18.1	Chronic viral hepatitis B without delta-agent
B19.1	Unspecified viral hepatitis B
B19.10	Unspecified viral hepatitis B without hepatic coma
B19.11	Unspecified viral hepatitis B with hepatic coma

EPIDEMIOLOGY & DEMOGRAPHICS

INCIDENCE:
- In U.S. overall incidence is ~1.1 cases/100,000.
- Much higher incidence in Europe (~1 million new cases annually) and in areas of high endemicity.
- In the U.S., transmission is mainly horizontal (percutaneous and mucous membrane exposure to infectious blood and other body fluids [e.g., sexual transmission, either homosexual or heterosexual]); also from needle sharing among drug abusers; occupational exposure to contaminated blood and blood products; persons receiving transfusions of blood and blood products; and hemodialysis patients.
NOTE: Improved screening of blood and blood products has greatly reduced, although not eliminated, the risk of posttransfusion HBV infection.
- In areas of high endemicity, transmission is largely vertical (perinatal): HBV exists in the blood and body fluids. Perinatal transmission from HBsAg-positive mothers is as high as 90% unless immunoprophylaxis is given.

PREVALENCE:
- An estimated 296 million people have chronic hepatitis B, of whom 221 million live in low- and middle-income countries.[1] North America, Western Europe, and Australia are areas of low prevalence, <2%. In the U.S. an estimated 800,000 to 2.2 million people have chronic HBV infection. About two-thirds of them are unaware that they are infected.

- Africa, Asia, and the Western Pacific region are areas of high prevalence, ≥8%.
- Southern and Eastern Europe have intermediate rates, 2% to 7%.
- Chronically infected persons, those with positive HBsAg for >6 mo, represent the major source of infection.
- As many as 95% of infants and children aged <5, who typically have subclinical acute infection, will become chronic HBV carriers.
- Adults are more likely to have clinically evident acute infection, but only 1% to 5% will develop chronic infection.
- ~0.1% of patients with acute infection will develop fulminant acute hepatitis resulting in death.

PREDOMINANT SEX:
- Predominant in males because of increased intravenous (IV) drug abuse, homosexuality.
- Females more commonly terminate in chronic carrier state.

PREDOMINANT AGE: 20 to 45 yr

PEAK INCIDENCE: 30 to 45 yr of age, at rates of 5% to 20%

GENETICS: Neonatal infection:
- Rare in the U.S.
- High (up to 90%) in areas of high endemicity (only 5% to 10% of perinatal infections occur in utero).

PHYSICAL FINDINGS & CLINICAL PRESENTATION

- The incubation period of HBV infection is 4 to 24 wk. HBV infection presents as acute hepatitis in a minority of patients
- Patients often present with nonspecific symptoms
- Profound malaise (Fig. E1)
Many asymptomatic cases
- Prodrome:
  1. 15% to 20% serum sickness (urticaria, rash, arthralgia) during early HBsAg
  2. HBsAg-Ab complex disease (polyarteritis nodosa–arthritis, arteritis, glomerulonephritis)
- Hepatomegaly (87%) with right upper quadrant (RUQ) tenderness:
  1. Hepatic punch tenderness
  2. Splenomegaly: Rare (10% to 15%)
- Jaundice (30% of patients), dark urine, with occasional pruritus
- Variable fever (when present, generally precedes jaundice and rapidly declines following onset of icteric phase)
- Spider angiomata: Rare; resolves during recovery
- Rare polyarteritis nodosa, cryoglobulinemia

ETIOLOGY

- Caused by HBV (42-nm hepadnavirus with an outer surface coat [HBsAg], inner nucleocapsid core [HBcAg; HBeAg]; DNA polymerase; and partially double-stranded DNA genome). There are eight genotypes (A to H) based on nucleotide sequence. The prevalence of each genotype varies widely.
- Transmission by parenteral route (needle use, tattooing, ear piercing, acupuncture, transfusion

of blood and blood products, hemodialysis, sexual contact), perinatal transmission.
- Infection may result from contact of infectious material with mucous membranes and open skin breaks (e.g., HBV is stable and can be transmitted from toothbrushes, utensils, razors, baby toys, assorted medical equipment [respirators, endoscopes]).
- Oral intake of infectious material may result in infection through breaks in the oral mucosa.
- Food or water are virtually never found to be sources of HBV infection.
- Infection occurs primarily in liver, where necrosis probably results from cytotoxic T-cell response, direct cytopathic effect of HBcAg (core antigen), high-level HBsAg (surface antigen) expression, or coinfection with delta (D) hepatitis virus (RNA delta core within HBsAg envelope).
- Recovery (>90%):
  1. Fulminant hepatitis occurring in <1% (especially if coinfected with hepatitis D); 80% fatal
  2. Unusual (5%) prolonged acute disease for 4 to 12 mo, with recovery
  3. Overall fatality increases with age and viral inoculation (e.g., transfusions)
- Chronic hepatitis B (CHB) infection (1% to 2%), four phases:
  1. Immune-tolerant phase: A highly replicative/low-inflammatory phase in which HBV DNA levels are high (typically >1 million IU/ml), alanine aminotransferase (ALT) levels are normal, and biopsy samples have minimal signs of significant inflammation or fibrosis.
     a. This phase can persist for years, especially in those infected prenatally. More than 90% of perennial infection develop into chronic infection.
     b. With age there is a likely transformation to an HBeAg-positive immune-active phase.
  2. HBeAg-positive immune-active phase: Elevated ALT and HBV DNA levels in conjunction with liver injury (≥20,000 IU/ml). Median age of onset is 30 yr in those infected at a young age. Biopsy will show moderate to severe inflammation or fibrosis.
  3. Inactive CHB phase: HBV DNA levels are low or undetectable (<2000 IU/ml), ALT levels are normal, and anti-HBe is present. Biopsy shows minimal necroinflammation but variable fibrosis.
  4. HBeAg-negative immune reactivation phase: Elevated ALT and elevated HBV DNA (≥2000 IU/ml). Biopsy will show moderate to severe necroinflammation and fibrosis.
- Table 1 summarizes causes of hepatitis flares in patients with CHB.
- The most feared complications of CHB are cirrhosis and hepatocellular carcinoma (HCC), which kill more than 300,000 people/yr globally. One quarter to one third of patients will go on to develop these complications. The risk of developing HCC appears to be greatest among individuals with the highest serum levels of HBV DNA.

TABLE 1 Causes of Hepatitis Flares in Patients With Chronic Hepatitis B

Cause of Flare	Comment
Spontaneous	Factors that precipitate viral replication are unclear
Immunosuppressive therapy	Flares are often observed during withdrawal of the agent; preemptive antiviral therapy is required
Antiviral therapy for HBV	
Interferon	Flares are often observed during the second to third mo of therapy in 30% of patients; may herald virologic response
Nucleoside analog	
During treatment	Flares are no more common than with placebo
Drug-resistant HBV	Severe consequences can occur in patients with advanced liver disease
On withdrawal	Flares are caused by the rapid reemergence of wild-type HBV; severe consequences can occur in patients with advanced liver disease
HIV treatment	Flares can occur as a result of the direct toxicity of HAART or with immune reconstitution; HBV increases the risk of antiretroviral drug hepatotoxicity
Genotypic variation	
Precore and core promoter mutants	Fluctuations in serum ALT levels are common with precore mutants
Superinfection with other hepatitis viruses	May be associated with suppression of HBV replication

ALT, Alanine aminotransferase; *HAART,* highly active antiretroviral therapy; *HBV,* hepatitis B virus; *HIV,* human immunodeficiency virus.
From Feldman M et al (eds): *Sleisenger and Fordtran's gastrointestinal and liver disease,* ed 10, Philadelphia, 2016, Saunders.

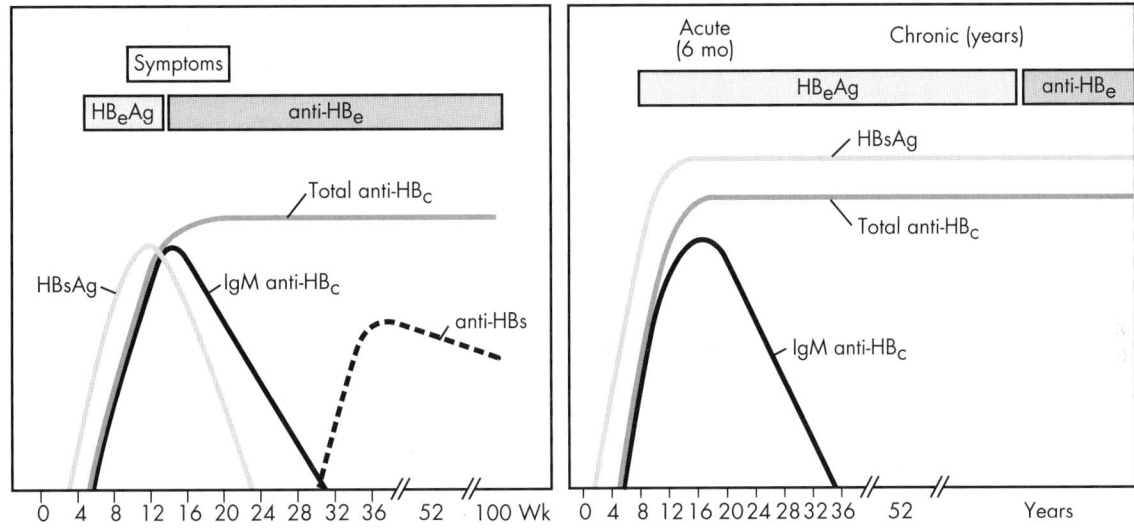

FIG. 2 Typical course of hepatitis B. *Left,* Typical course of acute hepatitis B. *Right,* Chronic hepatitis B. *HBc,* Hepatitis B core; *HBe,* hepatitis B early; *HBeAg,* hepatitis B early antigen; *HBs,* hepatitis B surface; *HBsAg,* hepatitis B surface antigen; *IgM,* immunoglobulin M. (From Mandell GL et al: *Principles and practice of infectious diseases,* ed 7, Philadelphia, 2010, Saunders.)

DX DIAGNOSIS

DIFFERENTIAL DIAGNOSIS

- Acute disease confused with other viral hepatitis infections (A, C, D, E).
- Any viral illness producing systemic disease and hepatitis (e.g., yellow fever, Epstein-Barr virus (EBV), cytomegalovirus (CMV), HIV, rubella, rubeola, coxsackie B, adenovirus, herpes simplex or zoster).
- Nonviral causes of hepatitis (e.g., leptospirosis, toxoplasmosis, alcoholic hepatitis, drug-induced [e.g., acetaminophen, INH], toxic hepatitis [carbon tetrachloride, benzene]).

WORKUP

- Acute serum specimen for hepatitis B serology (HBsAg, HBsAb, HBcAb, HBeAg, HBeAb), HBDNA by polymerase chain reaction (PCR)
- Life function tests (LFTs)
- CBC
- Liver biopsy: Rarely indicated for diagnosis of fulminant viral hepatitis, chronic hepatitis, cirrhosis, carcinoma

LABORATORY TESTS

- Diagnosis of acute HBV infection is best confirmed by immunoglobulin M (IgM) HBcAb in acute or early convalescent serum or by HBDNA by PCR.
  1. Generally, IgM present during onset of jaundice
  2. Coexisting HBsAg
- HBsAg and IgG-HBcAb during acute jaundice are strongly suggestive of remote HBV infection and another cause for current illness (Fig. 2).
- HBsAb alone is suggestive of immunization response.
- With recovery, HBeAg is rapidly replaced by HBeAb in 2 to 3 mo, and HBsAg is replaced by HBsAb in 5 to 6 mo.
- In chronic HBV hepatitis, HBsAg and HBeAg are persistent without corresponding Ab.
- In chronic carrier state, HBsAg is persistent, but HBeAg is replaced by HBeAb.

- HBcAb develops in all outcomes.
- HBeAg correlation with highest infectivity; appearance of HBeAb heralds recovery.
- LFTs:
  1. ALT and AST: Usually more than eight times normal (often 1000 U/L) at onset of jaundice (minimal acute ALT/aspartate aminotransferase [AST] rises often followed by chronic hepatitis or hepatocellular carcinoma).
  2. Bilirubin: Variably elevated in icteric viral hepatitis.
  3. Alkaline phosphatase: Minimally elevated (one to three times normal) acutely.
- Albumin and prothrombin time:
  1. Generally normal
  2. If abnormal, possible harbinger of impending hepatic necrosis (fulminant hepatitis)
- White blood cell (WBC) and erythrocyte sedimentation rate (ESR): Generally normal.

IMAGING STUDIES

- Sonogram to document rapid reduction in liver size during fulminant hepatitis or mass in hepatocellular carcinoma
- FibroScan (transient elastography): A noninvasive specialized ultrasound test to quantify liver fibrosis without liver biopsy

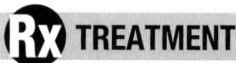 **TREATMENT**

NONPHARMACOLOGIC THERAPY

- Symptomatic treatment as necessary
- Activity as tolerated
- High-calorie diet preferred; often best tolerated in morning

ACUTE GENERAL Rx

- In most cases of acute HBV infection, no treatment is necessary; >90% of adults will spontaneously clear infection.
- Hospitalization advisable for any patient in danger from dehydration caused by poor oral intake, whose prothrombin time (PT) is prolonged, who has rising bilirubin level >15 to 20 µg/dl, or who has any clinical evidence of hepatic failure. Table 2 summarizes indications for prompt or urgent treatment of hepatitis B.
- IV therapy needed (rarely) for hydration during severe vomiting.
- Avoid hepatically metabolized drugs.
- No therapeutic measures are beneficial.
- Steroids not shown helpful.

CHRONIC Rx

- Treatment of chronic HBV infection is dependent on which phase the patient is found to be in:
  1. Therapy is warranted for patients in immune-active CHB stage (HBeAg negative or HBeAg positive) to decrease the risk of liver-related complications. Treatment options include:
  2. Nucleoside analogues:
     a. Entecavir: A nucleotide analogue. Dose 0.5 to 1 mg/day, suppresses HBV DNA replication and improves liver inflammation and fibrosis.
     b. Tenofovir disoproxil: 300 mg/day, is another nucleotide analogue. A newer formulation, tenofovir alafenamide (Vemlidy) 25 mg/day, has less renal and bone toxicity in long-term use.
     c. Other nucleotide agents: Lamivudine, telbivudine, and adefovir are less frequently used due to issues of resistance.
     d. Cure rates with nucleotide agents are between 1% and 12%, and thus most patients will require treatment indefinitely but are considered first line of therapy.
  3. Pegylated interferon alfa:
     a. Pegylated interferon 2a: 180 µg subcutaneously weekly for 48 wk. This will lead to seroconversion rates of 20% to 30% (HBeAg to anti-HBe), and 65% of patients will have HBV DNA <2000 IU/ml off therapy, but cure rates remain low at 3% to 7% and has significant side effects: Bone marrow suppression and exacerbation of existing neuropsychiatric symptoms, including depression. Candidates for interferon therapy should not have significant psychiatric disease, cardiac disease, cytopenia, seizure disorder, autoimmune disease, or pregnancy.
  4. Therapy is not warranted in adults with immune-tolerant CHB. LFTs should be checked every 6 mo to look for conversion to immune-active or inactive status.
     a. Therapy may be warranted for select adults >40 with normal ALT and elevated HBV DNA (≥1 million IU/ml) with liver biopsy showing significant necroinflammation or fibrosis.
  5. HBeAg-positive adults without cirrhosis who seroconvert to anti-HBe on therapy with entecavir or tenofovir disoproxil can discontinue treatment after a period of treatment consolidation.
  6. It is recommended that patients receive indefinite therapy with entecavir or tenofovir disoproxil if HBeAg-negative immune-active CHB is present, unless there is a competing rationale for treatment discontinuation.
  7. Adults with compensated cirrhosis and low levels of viremia (<2000 IU/ml) should be treated with entecavir or tenofovir disoproxil to reduce the risk of decompensation, regardless of ALT level.

DISPOSITION

- Follow-up as outpatient
- Acute disease: Infection will resolve (defined as clearance of hepatitis B surface antigen within 6 mo) in 90% of adult patients
- Rare fatalities (fulminant hepatitis)
- Possible chronic carrier state, cirrhosis, hepatocellular carcinoma

TABLE 2 Indications for Prompt or Urgent Treatment of Hepatitis B

	Indications	Preferred Agent	Principal Supportive Data
Cirrhosis*			
Decompensated	Clinical stabilization; minimizing risk for recurrence after transplant	Entecavir (0.5 mg) or tenofovir (300 mg)[†]	Open label; multiple large case series
Borderline compensated	Forestalling disease progression; avoidance of transplantation	As above	Undefined
Well compensated	As above	As above	Randomized controlled trials
Acute Liver Failure			
HBV reactivation	Minimizing further liver injury; reducing risk of recurrence after liver transplantation, if needed	Entecavir (0.5 mg) or tenofovir (300 mg)[†]	Open label with comparison with historical controls
Severe acute hepatitis	Minimizing further liver injury and enhancing full recovery	Consider lamivudine or telbivudine[‡]	Small case series

HBV, Hepatitis B virus.

*It has been the author's (RP) practice to use maintenance antiviral therapy for all hepatitis B surface antigen (HBsAg)-positive patients with cirrhosis to prevent reactivation of hepatitis B.

[†]Daily dose should be adjusted according to the patient's renal function, as indicated in the manufacturer's recommendations.

[‡]Either agent can be used if the anticipated duration of therapy is ≤6 mo.

From Feldman M et al: *Sleisenger and Fordtran's gastrointestinal and liver disease,* ed 10, Philadelphia, 2016, Elsevier.

- Cure of HBV is an unrealistic goal for most patients with chronic infection because only a few patients will become HBsAb with current treatment modalities
- Without intervention, deaths from chronic hepatitis B are expected to peak at 1.14 million by 2035[1]

REFERRAL

To infectious disease specialist and gastroenterologist for consultation regarding fulminant hepatitis or prolonged cholestasis, for cases of uncertain etiology, or for treatment of CAH

🅵 PEARLS & CONSIDERATIONS

- The American Association for the Study of Liver Diseases (AASLD) recommends that in men infected with hepatitis B, liver cancer screening begin at age 40 and in women infected with hepatitis B, liver cancer screening begin at age 50
- Other high-risk groups for the development of liver cancer include persons born of Asian/ Pacific Islander descent, persons born in

Africa, persons coinfected with hepatitis C, hepatitis D, or HIV, and persons with a family history of liver cancer and individuals with cirrhosis

COMMENTS

- Virus and HBsAg in high titers in blood for 1 to 7 wk before jaundice and for a variable time thereafter.
- Screening (HBV surface antigen [HBsAg], HBV core antigen antibody, antibody to HBsAg) should be offered to high-risk groups.
- Transmission is possible during entire period of HBsAg (and especially during HBeAg) in serum.
- Universal precautions should be followed for all contacts with blood or secretions/excretions contaminated with blood.
- Antiviral therapy is recommended in pregnancy to reduce perinatal transmission if HBsAg positive and HBV DNA >200,000 IU/ml. Can use tenofovir disoproxil, lamivudine, or telbivudine. Tenofovir may be preferred because it has a better resistance profile, and there are more safety data in pregnant women with hepatitis B. Fig. 3 describes an algorithm

for the treatment of hepatitis B surface antigen (HBsAg)-positive mothers during pregnancy.
- Preventing before exposure:
  1. Lifestyle changes.
  2. Meticulous testing of blood supply (although some chronically infected, infectious donors are HBsAg negative).
  3. Sterilization via steam or hypochlorite.
  4. Hepatitis B vaccine for high-risk groups given intramuscularly (IM) in deltoid to induce HBsAb (response should be confirmed) is protective (>90% effective). Yeast-derived HBsAg vaccines include: Recombivax HB (10 mcg HBsAg/ml) and Engerix-B (20 μg HBsAg/ml), each as a three-dose series over 6 mo. An alternative vaccine is the two-dose hepatitis B virus vaccine (HEPLISAV-B) that uses a novel immunostimulatory adjuvant for use in adults ≥18 yr old, administered at 0 and 1 mo.
  5. Recommendation for universal childhood immunization with doses at birth, 1 mo, and 6 mo.
  6. The U.S. Advisory Committee on Immunization Practices has recommended universal hepatitis B vaccination for adults between the ages of 19 and 59 years and has liberalized the recommendation for vaccination of adults who are 60 yr or older with risk factors for hepatitis B. The committee has also proposed universal one-time hepatitis B screening for all adults (>18 yr).[1]
- Prevention after exposure:
  1. HBV hyperimmune globulin (HBIG) (0.06 ml/ kg IM) given immediately after needlestick, within 14 days of sexual exposure, or at birth, followed by HBV vaccination. A second dose of HBIG is given in 28 days for those refusing vaccine or vaccine nonresponders.
  2. Standard immune globulin: Nearly as effective as HBIG.
- Preventive therapy with entecavir or tenofovir disoproxil for patients who test positive for HBsAg and are undergoing chemotherapy may reduce the risk for HBV reactivation and HBV-associated morbidity and mortality.
- Hepatitis B prophylaxis is described in Section V.
- Table 3 summarizes interpretation of serologic markers and serum DNA in hepatitis B.
- The U.S. Preventive Services Task Force (USPSTF) recommends screening for hepatitis B infection in adolescents and adults of high risk. Patients at high risk include the following:
  1. People born in countries or area with HBV prevalence ≥2%
  2. People who were not vaccinated at birth and were both in the U.S. to parents who were born in countries or areas with prevalence >8%
  3. HIV-positive people

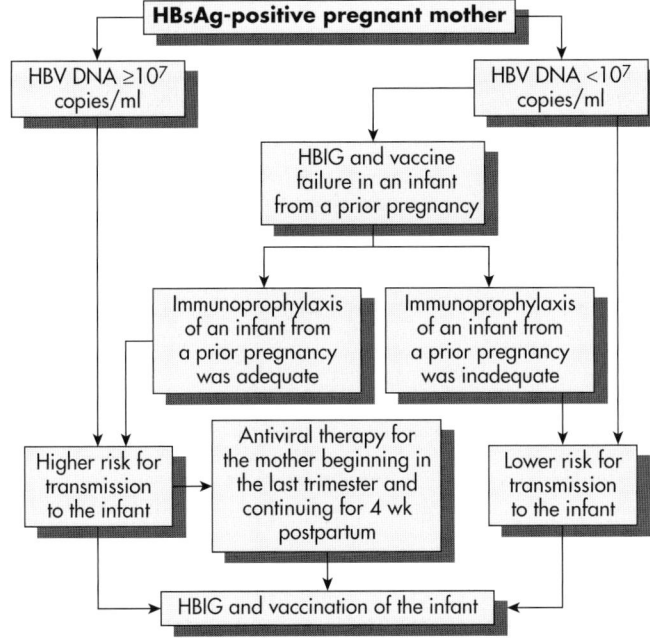

FIG. 3 Algorithm for the treatment of hepatitis B surface antigen (HBsAg)-positive mothers during pregnancy. The goal of treatment in highly viremic mothers is to lower the serum HBV DNA level by several $\log_{10}$ IU/ml by the time of delivery to minimize the chance of newborn infection. The choice of antiviral agent is less important if treatment of the mother is not needed long term. In the event that the treatment needs to be continued after delivery, the patient should be started on a high-genetic-barrier drug initially or switched to one immediately after delivery. See text for further details about drug selection. *DNA,* Deoxyribonucleic acid; *HBIG,* hepatitis B immune globulin; *HBV,* hepatitis B virus. (From Feldman M et al. [eds]: *Sleisenger and Fordtran's gastrointestinal and liver disease,* ed 10, Philadelphia, 2016, Saunders.)

TABLE 3   Interpretation of Serologic Markers and Serum DNA in Hepatitis B

	HBsAg	HBeAg	Anti-HBc IgM	Anti-HBc IgG	Anti-HBs	Anti-HBe	HBV DNA*
Acute hepatitis	+	+/−	+				+
Acute hepatitis, window period			+				
Recovery from acute hepatitis			+	+	+	+/−	
Chronic hepatitis	+	+					+
Chronic hepatitis (precore mutant)	+					+	+
Inactive carrier	+					+/−	
Vaccinated					+		

anti-HBc IgG, Hepatitis B core antibody (IgG type); *anti-HBc IgM*, hepatitis B core antibody (IgM type); *anti-HBe*, hepatitis B early antibody; *anti-HBs*, hepatitis B surface antibody; *DNA*, deoxyribonucleic acid; *HBeAg*, hepatitis Be antigen; *HBsAg*, hepatitis B surface antigen; *HBV DNA*, hepatitis B viral DNA.
*HBV DNA >10^5 copies/ml.
From Andreoli TE et al: *Andreoli and Carpenter's Cecil essentials of medicine*, ed 8, Philadelphia, 2010, Saunders.

4. Intravenous-drug users
5. Men who have sex with men
6. People who live in households with, or have sex with, HBV-positive people

REFERENCE & SUGGESTED READINGS
Available at eBooks.Health.Elsevier.com.

RELATED CONTENT
Hepatitis B (Patient Information)

AUTHOR: **GLENN G. FORT, MD, MPH**

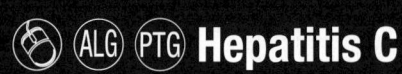

H

 BASIC INFORMATION

DEFINITION

Hepatitis C is a liver parenchymal infection caused by hepatitis C virus (HCV).

SYNONYM

Transfusion-related non-A, non-B hepatitis

ICD-10CM CODES
B17.1	Acute hepatitis C
B17.10	Acute hepatitis C without hepatic coma
B17.11	Acute hepatitis C with hepatic coma
B18.2	Chronic viral hepatitis C
B19.20	Unspecified viral hepatitis C without hepatic coma
B19.21	Unspecified viral hepatitis C with hepatic coma

EPIDEMIOLOGY & DEMOGRAPHICS

Hepatitis C infection is the most common chronic blood-borne infection in the U.S. About 3% of baby boomers test positive for the virus. The CDC now in 2022 recommends:
- One-time, routine, opt out HCV testing for all individuals aged 18 or older (I,B)
- One-time HCV testing should be performed for all persons <18 yr with activities, exposures, or conditions or circumstances associated with an increased risk of HCV infection (I,B).
- Prenatal HCV testing as part of routine prenatal care is recommended with each pregnancy (I,B).
- Periodic repeat HCV testing should be offered to all persons with activities, exposures, or conditions or circumstances associated with an increased risk of HCV exposure (IIa,C).
- Annual HCV testing is recommended for all persons who inject drugs, for HIV infected men who have unprotected sex with men, and all men who have sex with men taking pre-exposure prophylaxis (PrEP) (IIa,C).
- Regardless of age or setting prevalence, all persons with risk factors should be tested for hepatitis C with periodic testing while risk factors persist.
- Any person who requests hepatitis C testing should receive it, regardless of disclosure risk, because many persons might be reluctant to disclose stigmatizing risk.

The U.S. Preventive Services Task Force (USPSTF) recommends screening of all adults 18 to 79 yr for hepatitis C infection.

INCIDENCE: HCV infects more than 185 million individuals worldwide. Approximately 20% of patients chronically infected with HCV progress to cirrhosis.
- 150,000 new cases/yr (37,500 symptomatic; 93,000 later chronic liver disease; 30,700 cirrhosis). The incidence of acute HCV has declined substantially over the past 30 yr (from 7.4/100,000 to 0.7/100,000).
- ~9000 of these ultimately die of HCV infection; most common (40%) cause of nonalcoholic liver disease in the United States.

PREVALENCE (IN U.S.):
- Overall prevalence of anti-HCV antibody is 1% to 1.2% (an estimated 2.7 million persons nationwide).
- Highest prevalence in hemophiliacs transfused before 1987 and users of injection drugs, 72% to 90%. Over past 30 yr, blood transfusion as a risk factor declined from 15% of cases to 1.9%.
- Among low-risk groups, prevalence 0.6%.

PREDOMINANT SEX: Slight male predominance.
PREDOMINANT AGE: Highest prevalence in 30- to 49-yr age group (65%).
PEAK INCIDENCE:
- 20 to 39 yr of age.
- African Americans and Whites have similar incidence of acute disease; Hispanics have higher rates.
- Prevalence is substantially higher among non-Hispanic Blacks than among non-Hispanic Whites.

GENETICS: Neonatal infection is rare; increased risk with maternal HIV-1 coinfection.

PHYSICAL FINDINGS & CLINICAL PRESENTATION
- Symptoms usually develop 7 to 8 wk after infection (range of 2 to 26 wk), but 70% to 80% of cases are subclinical.
- 10% to 20% report acute illness with jaundice and nonspecific symptoms (abdominal pain, anorexia, malaise).
- Fulminant hepatitis may rarely occur during this period.
- After acute infection, 15% to 25% have complete resolution (absence of HCV RNA in serum, normal alanine aminotransferase [ALT]).
- Progression to chronic infection is common, 50% to 84%. 74% to 86% have persistent viremia; spontaneous clearance of viremia in chronic infection is rare. 60% to 70% of patients will have persistent or fluctuating ALT levels; 30% to 40% with chronic infection have normal ALT levels.
- 15% to 20% of those with chronic HCV will develop cirrhosis over a period of 20 to 30 yr; in most others, chronic infection leads to hepatitis and varying degrees of fibrosis. Table 1 summarizes factors associated with progression of hepatic fibrosis in patients with chronic HCV infection. Table 2 describes factors associated with cirrhosis in persons with hepatitis C infection.
- 0.4% to 2.5% of patients with chronic infection develop hepatocellular carcinoma (HCC).
- 25% of patients with chronic infection continue to have an asymptomatic course with normal liver function tests (LFTs) and benign histology.
- In chronic HCV infection, extrahepatic sequelae include a variety of immunologic and lymphoproliferative disorders (e.g., cryoglobulinemia, membranoproliferative glomerulonephritis, and possibly Sjögren syndrome, autoimmune thyroiditis, polyarteritis nodosa, aplastic anemia, lichen planus, porphyria cutanea tarda, B-cell lymphoma, others).
- Direct antiviral treatment should be initiated without delay in patients with clinically significant extrahepatic manifestations of chronic HCV infection. Studies have shown a close link between treatment-induced, sustained viral clearance and a low risk of extrahepatic manifestations of HCV infection.[1]
- Fig. 1 illustrates the natural history of HCV infection.

ETIOLOGY
- Caused by HCV (single-stranded RNA flavivirus). HCV genotype 1 accounts for about 75% of HCV in the U.S. Genotypes 2 and 3 account for about 20% to 25% of infections, genotype 4 for 6%, and genotypes 5 and 6 for about 1%.
- Most HCV transmission is parenteral.

TABLE 1 Factors Associated With Progression of Hepatic Fibrosis in Patients With Chronic Hepatitis C Virus Infection

Established	Possible	Not Associated
Age >40 yr	Increased hepatic iron concentration	Viral genotype
Alcohol consumption	Male gender	Viral load
Hepatitis B virus coinfection	Serum ALT level	
HIV coinfection		
Immunosuppressed state		
Insulin resistance		
Marijuana use		
Obesity		
Schistosomiasis		
Severe hepatic necroinflammation		
Smoking		
White race		

ALT, Alanine aminotransferase; *HIV,* human immunodeficiency virus.
From Feldman M et al (eds): *Sleisenger and Fordtran's gastrointestinal and liver disease,* ed 10, Philadelphia, 2016, Saunders.

TABLE 2 Factors Associated With Cirrhosis in Persons With Hepatitis C Infection

Factor	Impact	Comment
Environmental		
Alcohol use	+4	The importance of minimal alcohol ingestion (<20 g/day) has not been established
Host		
HIV infection	+4	Increasingly important as HIV-related survival improves; may be masked by competing mortality
HBV infection	+3	Strong effect when HBsAg positive; relatively uncommon
Age	+4	Strong effect; increases as low as 40 yr. Hard to distinguish from infection duration
Body mass index	+2	Associated with metabolic syndrome
Duration of HCV infection	+3	Cirrhosis is rare before 10 yr
HLA type	+1?	HLA B54 is correlated with increased risk of cirrhosis; DRB1*0301 with lack of cirrhosis
Viral		
Quasispecies complexity	+1	Cross-sectional studies cannot assess causality, and complexity may be confounded by duration of infection
HCV genotype 1	+1?	Genotype 1b in some, but not other studies, could be confounded by longer duration of 1b infections
Quantitative measures of viremia (serum or plasma HCV RNA level)	+2	Not always detected or lost in multivariate analysis of age or HIV

HCV, Hepatitis C virus; *HIV*, human immunodeficiency virus; *HLA*, human leukocyte antigen; *RNA*, ribonucleic acid.
From Bennett JE et al: *Mandell, Douglas, and Bennett's principles and practice of infectious diseases*, ed 8, Philadelphia, 2015, Saunders.

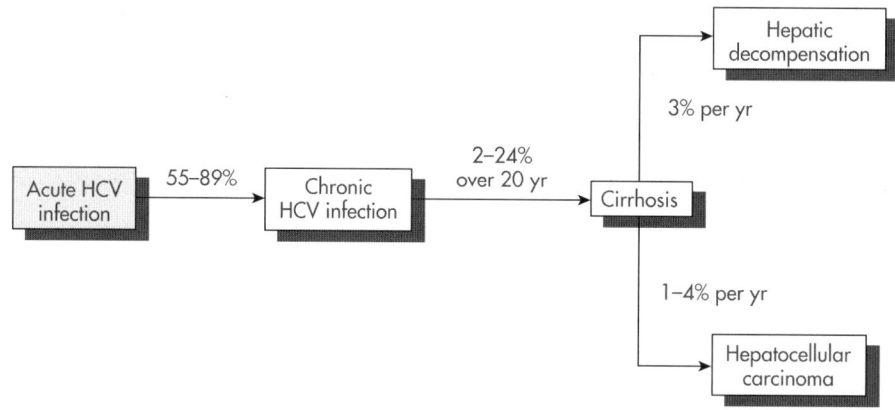

FIG. 1 Natural history of HCV infection. Hepatic decompensation includes ascites, hepatic encephalopathy, variceal hemorrhage, hepatorenal syndrome, or hepatic synthetic dysfunction. *HCV*, Hepatitis C virus. (From Feldman M et al [eds]: *Sleisenger and Fordtran's gastrointestinal and liver disease*, ed 10, Philadelphia, 2016, Saunders.)

- In the United States, advances in screening of blood and blood products have made transfusion-related HCV infection rare (the risk is estimated to be 0.001% per unit transfused).
- Injecting-drug use accounts for most HCV transmission in the United States (60% of newly acquired cases, 20% to 50% of chronically infected persons).
- Occupational needlestick exposure from an HCV-positive source has a seroconversion rate of 1.8% (range 0% to 7%).
- Nosocomial transmission rates (from surgery and procedures such as colonoscopy and hemodialysis) are extremely low.
- Sexual transmission and maternal-fetal transmission are infrequent (estimated at 5%).
- No identifiable risk in 40% to 50% of community-acquired hepatitis C, but snorting of cocaine by shared use of straw or rolled-up paper has been identified as a risk factor because it causes microscopic bleeding of nasal mucosa.
- HCV infection may stimulate production of cytotoxic T lymphocytes and cytokines (INF-γ), which probably mediate hepatic necrosis.

🄓🅧 DIAGNOSIS

DIFFERENTIAL DIAGNOSIS

- Other hepatitis viruses (A, B, D, E).
- Other viral illnesses producing systemic disease (e.g., yellow fever, Epstein-Barr virus, cytomegalovirus, HIV, rubella, rubeola, coxsackie B, adenovirus, herpes simplex virus, herpes zoster virus).
- Nonviral hepatitis (e.g., leptospirosis, toxoplasmosis, alcoholic hepatitis, drug-induced hepatitis [acetaminophen, isoniazid], toxic hepatitis).

WORKUP

- Acute hepatitis C antibody, viral genotyping, viral titers.
- LFTs, CBC.
  NOTE: ALT is an easy and inexpensive test to monitor infection and efficacy of therapy. However, ALT levels may fluctuate or even be normal in active or chronic infection and even with cirrhosis, and ALT may remain elevated even after clearance of viremia.
- Liver biopsy with histologic staging had been the gold standard for assessing the degree of

disease activity and the likelihood of disease progression and also to help rule out other causes of liver disease but is less used with advent of newer technologies
- Transient elastography (FibroScan) is a noninvasive specialized ultrasound assessment that quantifies liver fibrosis and corresponds it to the equivalent in the METAVIR scoring system traditionally used in liver biopsies. It is being increasingly used in place of liver biopsy in most institutions.

LABORATORY TESTS

- Diagnosis of acute hepatitis C is often by exclusion, because it takes 6 wk to 12 mo to develop anti-HCV antibody (70% positive by 6 wk, 90% positive by 6 mo).
- Diagnostic tests include serologic assays for antibodies and molecular tests for viral particles.
  1. Enzyme immunoassay is the test for anti-HCV antibody:
     a. The current version can detect antibody within 4 to 10 wk after infection.
     b. False-negative rate in low-risk populations is 0.5% to 1%.

c. False negatives also occur in immune-compromised persons, HIV-1, renal failure, HCV-associated essential mixed cryoglobulinemia.

d. False positives in autoimmune hepatitis, paraproteinemia, and persons with no risk factors.

- The recombinant immunoblot assay that was previously recommended as a follow-up to positive antibody test is no longer available. The CDC now recommends that anyone who tests positive for HCV antibodies receive a follow-up HCV RNA test.
- Qualitative and quantitative HCV RNA tests using polymerase chain reaction (PCR): Lower limit of detection is <43 IU/ml.
- Used to confirm viremia and to assess response to treatment.
- Qualitative PCR useful in patients with negative enzyme immunoassay in whom infection is suspected.
- Quantitative tests use either branched-chain DNA or reverse transcription PCR; the latter is more sensitive.
- Viral genotyping can distinguish among genotypes 1, 2, 3, 4, 5, and 6, which is helpful in choosing therapy; most of these tests use PCR. Genotypes 1, 2, 3, and 4 predominate in the United States and Europe (genotype 1 is especially common in North America [60% to 75% of hepatitis C infections in the United States]).
- FibroSure score uses a combination of six serum markers of liver function plus age and sex in a patented algorithm to generate a measure of fibrosis and necroinflammatory activity in the liver as a quantitative surrogate marker for the corresponding METAVIR scoring system.
- LFTs: ALT and AST may be elevated to more than eight times normal in acute infection; in chronic infection ALT may be normal or fluctuate.
- Bilirubin may be 5 to 10 times normal.
- Albumin and prothrombin time generally normal; if abnormal, may be harbinger of impending hepatic necrosis.
- WBC and erythrocyte sedimentation rate (ESR) are generally normal.
- HIV testing. Infection with HCV is seen in 15% to 30% of individuals with HIV infection due to shared risk factors.
- All patients infected with HCV should be tested for hepatitis B. HBV vaccination is recommended for susceptible individuals, because HBV reactivation may occur during treatment of HCV with direct-acting antiviral therapy.

IMAGING STUDIES

- Transient elastography (FibroScan) to quantify liver fibrosis as an absolute score. Some insurance companies use this score as a basis to determine eligibility for treatment.
- Sonogram: Rapid liver size reduction during fulminant hepatitis or mass in HCC.

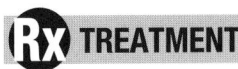 **TREATMENT**

NONPHARMACOLOGIC THERAPY

Activity and diet as tolerated; avoid saw palmetto and green tea leaf herbs.

ACUTE GENERAL Rx

- Supportive care.
- Avoid hepatically metabolized drugs.

CHRONIC Rx

Response to therapy is influenced by HCV genotype. Recommendations for the treatment of hepatitis C in adults are changing constantly as new therapies come to the market. The advent of direct-acting antiviral agents (DAAs) has drastically changed treatment options and improved cure rates to >95%. The most up-to-date guidance is available at the website www.hcvguidelines.org. The following is a brief summary of the guidelines based on genotype. Newer agents containing fixed-dose combinations of DAA drugs have been approved for HCV infections caused by any of the six major HCV genotypes in patients without cirrhosis or with compensated cirrhosis. These agents are Mavyret (combination of glecaprevir, an HCV NS3/4A protease inhibitor; and pibrentasvir, an NS5A inhibitor) and Vosevi (combination of the NS5B nucleotide polymerase inhibitor sofosbuvir, the NS5A inhibitor velpatasvir, and the NS3/4A protease inhibitor voxilaprevir). Both agents are approved for use in treatment-experienced patients, and Mavyret is also approved for treatment-naïve patients. Currently, these treatment regimens are expensive and are covered by most insurance plans.

Genotype 1a: Options for treatment-naïve patients without cirrhosis, listed by level of evidence:
- Daily fixed-dose combination of glecaprevir (300 mg)/pibrentasvir (120 mg) (Mavyret) for 8 wk. Rating: Class I, Level A.
- Daily fixed-dose combination of ledipasvir (90 mg)/sofosbuvir (400 mg) (Harvoni) for 12 wk. Rating: Class I, Level A. (Can also use this regimen for only 8 wk for patients who are non-Black, HIV-uninfected, and whose HCV RNA level is <6 million IU/ml. Rating: Class I, Level B.)
- Daily fixed-dose combination of sofosbuvir (400 mg)/velpatasvir (100 mg) (Epclusa) for 12 wk. Rating: Class I, Level A.
- Alternative regimen: Daily fixed-dose combination of elbasvir (50 mg)/grazoprevir (100 mg) (Zepatier) for 12 wk and in those who do not have baseline NS5A RAVs (amino acid substitutions at 28, 30, 31, or 93 that confer resistance to elbasvir). Rating: Class I, Level A.

Genotype 1a: Options for treatment-naïve patients with compensated cirrhosis:
- Daily fixed-dose combination of glecaprevir (300 mg)/pibrentasvir (120 mg) [Mavyret] for 8 wk. Rating: Class I, Level B. Use 12 wk if HIV–hepatitis C coinfected.
- Daily fixed-dose combination of ledipasvir (90 mg)/sofosbuvir (400 mg) [Harvoni] for 12 wk. Rating: Class I, Level A.
- Daily fixed-dose combination of sofosbuvir (400 mg)/velpatasvir (100 mg) [Epclusa] for 12 wk. Rating: Class I, Level A.
- Alternative: Daily fixed-dose combination of elbasvir (50 mg)/grazoprevir (100 mg) [Zepatier] and in those in whom no baseline NS5A RAVs for elbasvir are detected for 12 wk. Rating: Class I, Level A.

Genotype 1b: Treatment-naïve patients without cirrhosis:
- Daily fixed-dose combination of elbasvir (50 mg)/grazoprevir (100 mg) [Zepatier] for 12 wk. Rating: Class I, Level A.
- Daily fixed-dose combination of glecaprevir (300 mg)/pibrentasvir (120 mg) [Mavyret] for 8 wk. Rating: Class I, A. Use 12 wk if HIV–hepatitis C coinfected.
- Daily fixed-dose combination of ledipasvir (90 mg)/sofosbuvir (400 mg) [Harvoni] for 12 wk. Rating: Class I, Level A. (Can treat for 8 wk in patients who are non-Black, HIV-uninfected, and whose HCV RNA level is <6 million IU/ml. Class I, Level B.)
- Daily fixed-dose combination of sofosbuvir (400 mg)/velpatasvir (100 mg) [Epclusa] for 12 wk. Rating: Class I, Level A.

Genotype 1b: Treatment-naïve patients with compensated cirrhosis:
- Daily fixed-dose combination of elbasvir (50 mg)/grazoprevir (100 mg) [Zepatier] for 12 wk. Rating: Class I, Level A.
- Daily fixed-dose combination of glecaprevir (300 mg)/pibrentasvir (120 mg) [Mavyret] for 8 wk. Rating: Class I, Level B. Use 12 wk if HIV–hepatitis C coinfected.
- Daily fixed-dose combination of ledipasvir (90 mg)/sofosbuvir [Harvoni] for 12 wk. Rating: Class I, Level A.
- Daily fixed-dose combination of sofosbuvir (400 mg)/velpatasvir (100 mg) [Epclusa] for 12 wk. Rating: Class I, Level A.

Genotype 2: Treatment-naïve regimens without cirrhosis:
- Daily fixed-dose combination of glecaprevir (300 mg)/pibrentasvir (120 mg) [Mavyret] for 8 wk. Rating: Class I, Level A.
- Daily fixed-dose combination of sofosbuvir (400 mg)/velpatasvir (100 mg) [Epclusa] for 12 wk. Rating: Class I, Level A.

Genotype 2: Treatment-naïve patients with compensated cirrhosis:
- Daily fixed-dose combination of sofosbuvir (400 mg)/velpatasvir (100 mg) [Epclusa] for 12 wk. Rating: Class I, Level A.
- Daily fixed-dose combination of glecaprevir (300 mg)/pibrentasvir (120 mg) for 8 wk. Rating: Class I, Level B. Use 12 wk if HIV–hepatitis C coinfected.

Genotype 3: Treatment-naïve patients without cirrhosis:
- Daily fixed-dose of glecaprevir (300 mg)/pibrentasvir (120 mg) for 8 wk. Rating: Class I, Level A.
- Daily fixed-dose combination of sofosbuvir (400 mg)/velpatasvir (100 mg) [Epclusa] for 12 wk. Rating: Class I, Level A.

Genotype 3: Treatment-naïve patients with compensated cirrhosis:
- Daily fixed-dose combination of glecaprevir (300 mg)/pibrentasvir (120 mg) [Mavyret] for 8 wk. Rating: Class I, Level B.
- Daily fixed-dose combination of sofosbuvir (400 mg)/velpatasvir (100 mg) [Epclusa] for patients without baseline NS5A RAS Y93H for velpatasvir for 12 wk. Rating: Class I, Level A.

- Alternative regimens:
  1. Daily fixed-dose combination of sofosbuvir (400 mg)/velpatasvir (100 mg) with weight-based ribavirin for patients with baseline NS5A RAS Y93H for velpatasvir for 12 wk. Rating: IIa, Level A.
  2. Daily fixed-dose combination of sofosbuvir (400 mg)/velpatasvir (100 mg) [Epclusa]/voxilaprevir (100 mg) for patients with baseline NS5A RAS Y93H for velpatasvir for 12 wk. Rating: Class IIa, Level B.

Genotype 4: Treatment-naïve patients without cirrhosis:

- Daily fixed-dose combination of glecaprevir (300 mg)/pibrentasvir (120 mg) [Mavyret] for 8 wk. Rating: Class I Level A.
- Daily fixed-dose combination of sofosbuvir (400 mg)/velpatasvir (100 mg) [Epclusa] for 12 wk. Rating: Class I, Level A.
- Daily fixed-dose combination of elbasvir (50 mg)/grazoprevir (100 mg) [Zepatier] for 12 wk. Rating: Class I, Level A.
- Daily fixed-dose combination of ledipasvir (90 mg)/sofosbuvir (400 mg) [Harvoni] for 12 wk. Rating: Class I, Level A.

Genotype 4: Treatment-naïve patients with compensated cirrhosis:

- Daily fixed-dose combination of sofosbuvir (400 mg)/velpatasvir (100 mg) [Epclusa] for 12 wk. Rating: Class I, Level A.
- Daily fixed-dose combination of glecaprevir (300 mg)/pibrentasvir (120 mg) [Mavyret] for 8. Rating: Class I, Level B. Use 12 wk if HIV–hepatitis C coinfected.
- Daily fixed-dose combination of elbasvir (50 mg)/grazoprevir (100 mg) [Zepatier] for 12 wk. Rating: Class IIa, Level B.
- Daily fixed-dose combination of ledipasvir (90 mg)/sofosbuvir (400 mg) [Harvoni] for 12 wk. Rating: Class IIa, Level B.

Genotypes 5 and 6: Treatment-naïve patients with and without compensated cirrhosis:

- Daily fixed-dose combination of glecaprevir (300 mg)/pibrentasvir (120 mg) [Mavyret] for 8 wk Rating: Class I, Level A. Use 12 wk if HIV–hepatitis C coinfected.
- Daily fixed-dose combination of sofosbuvir (400 mg)/velpatasvir (100 mg) [Epclusa] for 12 wk. Rating: Class I, Level B.
- Daily fixed-dose combination of ledipasvir (90 mg)/sofosbuvir (400 mg) [Harvoni] for 12 wk. Rating: Class IIa, Level B.

Drug interactions can be significant with these regimens (https://www.hep-druginteractions.org/). With DAA regimens, viral loads are measured at 4 wk into the therapy to monitor success and at the end of therapy. A final viral load is measured 12 wk after completing the treatment, and, if undetectable, the patient is considered to have a sustained virologic response (SVR), which equates to a cure.

For *patients with decompensated cirrhosis,* there are also guidelines per genotype as well (https://www.hcvguidelines.org/). Treatment is based on genotype and whether the patient is able to use ribavirin or is ribavirin ineligible. A regimen exists for patients with decompensated cirrhosis and genotype 1 to 6 in whom prior sofosbuvir or NS5A inhibitor–based treatment failed: Ledipasvir (90 mg)/sofosbuvir (400 mg) [Harvoni] with low initial dose of ribavirin (600 mg; increase as tolerated) for 24 wk (IIc) or sofosbuvir (400 mg)/velpatasvir (100 mg) [Epclusa] with weight-based ribavirin for 24 wk (IIc).

Determination of cirrhosis: Liver biopsy is not required. A patient is presumed to have cirrhosis if they have a FIB-4 Score >3.25 or any of the following findings from a previously performed test:

- Transient elastography indicating cirrhosis (e.g., FibroScan stiffness >12.5 kPA)
- FibroSure score >0.58 warrants treatment by most insurers. A score of 0.72 to 0.74 equals to a stage 3 METAVIR and >0.74 stage 4 cirrhosis
- Clinical evidence of cirrhosis (liver nodularity and/or splenomegaly on imaging, platelet <150,000/mm^3
- Prior liver biopsy showing cirrhosis

$$FIB - 4\,Score = \frac{Age\ (Years) \times AST\ Level\ (U/L)}{Platelet\ count\ (10^9/L) \times \sqrt{ALT\left(\frac{U}{L}\right)}}$$

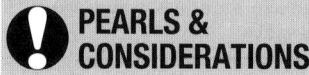

Fibrosis-4 (FIB-4) Calculator

In 2017, a new salvage regimen was approved: Once-daily Vosevi (fixed-dose combination of 100-mg voxilaprevir (HCV NS3/4A protease inhibitor) plus 400-mg sofosbuvir and 100-mg velpatasvir. Eligible patients include:

- Genotypes 1, 2, 3, 4, 5, or 6 in patients previously treated with a regimen containing an NS5A inhibitor for 12 wk (NOTE: In clinical trials, prior experience with NS5A inhibitors included daclatasvir, elbasvir, ledipasvir, ombitasvir, or velpatasvir.)
- Genotype 1a or 3 in patients previously treated with sofosbuvir without an NS5A inhibitor for 12 wk. (NOTE: In clinical trials, prior treatment experience included sofosbuvir with or without any of the following: Peginterferon alfa/ribavirin, ribavirin, HCV NS3/4A protease inhibitors: Boceprevir, simeprevir, or telaprevir.)
- Liver transplantation:
  1. Hepatitis C is the main indication for liver transplantation in the United States.
  2. It is the only option for patients with deteriorating HCV-related cirrhosis and for some patients with HCC.
  3. Recurrent infection occurs in almost all patients with progressive fibrosis and cirrhosis; as many as 20% progress to cirrhosis within 5 yr posttransplant.
  4. There are regimens to treat HCV infection in post–liver transplant patients and will depend on whether patient is treatment naïve or experienced, genotype, and whether patient has compensated or decompensated cirrhosis.

DISPOSITION

- The absence of HCV RNA in blood 12 wk after completion of treatment is considered a cure. There is no need to check HCV antibodies because they will remain positive indefinitely.
- SVR after treatment among HCV-infected persons at any stage of fibrosis is associated with reduced HCC.
- Periodic abdominal ultrasonography for HCC screening (with or without alpha-fetoprotein testing) every 6 mo is recommended in patients with cirrhosis even after obtaining virologic cure.

REFERRAL

- To a hepatologist or infectious disease specialist for treatment for hepatitis C in patients who have been previously treated or for treatment failures with DAA agents.
- To a transplant surgeon for consideration of liver transplant if indicated.

❗ PEARLS & CONSIDERATIONS

- More rapid progression of disease in persons who drink alcohol regularly, persons of advanced age at time of infection, and those coinfected with other viruses (HIV, hepatitis B). All persons with identified HCV infection should receive a brief alcohol screening and intervention as clinically indicated.
- Regression of cirrhosis has been demonstrated after antiviral therapy in some patients with chronic hepatitis C. Regression is associated with decreased disease-related morbidity and improved survival.
- The presence of interleukin (IL)-28B and human leukocyte antigen (HLA) class II is independently associated with spontaneous resolution of HCV infection, and single nucleotide polymorphism IL-28B and DQB1*03:01 may explain ~15% of spontaneous resolution of HCV infection.
- In 2021 the FDA-approved Epclusa (sofosbuvir and velpatasvir) to treat hepatitis C in children 6 yr and older or weighing at least 37 lbs (17 kg) with any of the six genotypes without cirrhosis or with mild cirrhosis. Epclusa with ribavirin was approved in the same population for severe cirrhosis.

REFERENCE & SUGGESTED READINGS

Available at eBooks.Health.Elsevier.com.

RELATED CONTENT

Hepatitis C (Patient Information)

AUTHOR: **GLENN G. FORT, MD, MPH**

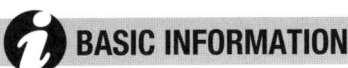

BASIC INFORMATION

DEFINITION
Hepatocellular carcinoma (HCC) is a malignant neoplasm of the hepatocytes.

SYNONYMS
Hepatoma
HCC

EPIDEMIOLOGY & DEMOGRAPHICS
HCC is the seventh most common cancer worldwide (~905,000 new cases/yr) and the second most common cause of cancer deaths (~830,000 deaths/yr). Incidence varies worldwide:
Incidence:
- 85% of patients with hepatocellular carcinoma have cirrhosis
Prevalence:
- Areas with high rates of hepatitis B and C (East Asia, sub-Saharan Africa) have highest incidence
Predominant Sex:
- Male:female ratios are between 2:1 and 4:1
Peak Incidence:
- Fifth and sixth decades in Western countries, earlier in areas with perinatal transmission of hepatitis B
- Incidence has grown in the U.S. due to chronic hepatitis C, increasing nonalcoholic fatty liver disease (NAFLD), metabolic syndrome, obesity, and diabetes mellitus
  1. During the past two decades, the incidence in the U.S. doubled and HCC is the fastest rising cause of cancer-related deaths in the U.S.
  2. In 2022, an estimated 41,260 new cases and 30,520 deaths occurred in the U.S.[1] The incidence in the U.S. is expected to increase to 56,200 cases by 2030.
  3. The greatest proportional increase has been among Hispanics and whites between 45 and 60 yr of age.
  4. The mean age of diagnosis is approximately 65 yr.
Risk Factors:
  1. Chronic hepatitis B infection accounts for 50% of all cases and most childhood cases
  2. Chronic hepatitis C infection markers are found in 80% to 90% of patients with HCC in Japan and 30% to 50% in the U.S.
  3. Cirrhosis from other causes: Alcoholic liver disease, nonalcoholic steatohepatitis, primary biliary cirrhosis, hemochromatosis, α1-antitrypsin deficiency, and autoimmune hepatitis
  4. Hepatotoxins: Aflatoxin B1
  5. Systemic diseases affecting the liver: Tyrosinemia
  6. Obesity and diabetes mellitus

PHYSICAL FINDINGS & CLINICAL PRESENTATION
- One third of patients are asymptomatic.
- Abdominal pain may be the initial presentation.
- Signs of underlying cirrhosis and portal hypertension are often present.

- Previously compensated cirrhosis with new ascites, encephalopathy, jaundice, or bleeding.
- Paraneoplastic syndromes (hypoglycemia, erythrocytosis, hypercalcemia, severe diarrhea, dermatomyositis) may be present. Box 1 summarizes paraneoplastic syndromes associated with hepatocellular carcinoma.
- Table 1 summarizes symptoms and signs of hepatocellular carcinoma.

DIAGNOSIS

DIFFERENTIAL DIAGNOSIS
- Metastatic cancers to liver
- Intrahepatic cholangiocarcinoma
- Benign liver neoplasms (adenomas, focal nodular hyperplasia, and hemangiomas)
- Focal fatty infiltration

WORKUP
- History regarding risk factors
- Physical examination with attention to signs of chronic liver disease
- Laboratory evaluation and imaging studies
- Imaging studies: Ultrasound for initial testing; 3-phase CT scan or dynamic contrast-enhanced MRI

LABORATORY TESTS
- Liver function tests.
- α-Fetoprotein (AFP) levels can be elevated in 70% of patients. An AFP level >400 ng/ml is highly suggestive of HCC; however, elevations may not be seen in up to 40% of patients with small lesions (1 to 2 cm).
- Paraneoplastic syndromes associated with HCC may cause hypercalcemia, hypoglycemia, and polycythemia.
- Elevated serum HBV DNA level (≥10,000 copies/ml) is a strong risk predictor of HCC independent of HBeAg, serum aminotransferase level, and liver cirrhosis.

BOX 1 Paraneoplastic Syndromes Associated With Hepatocellular Carcinoma

Carcinoid syndrome
Hypercalcemia
Hypertension
Hypertrophic osteoarthropathy
Hypoglycemia
Neuropathy
Osteoporosis
Polycythemia (erythrocytosis)
Polymyositis
Porphyria
Sexual changes—isosexual precocity, gynecomastia, feminization
Thyrotoxicosis
Thrombophlebitis migrans
Watery diarrhea syndrome

From Feldman M et al: *Sleisenger and Fordtrans' gastrointestinal and liver disease,* ed 10, Philadelphia, 2016, Elsevier.

IMAGING STUDIES
Ultrasound (US), CT scan (Fig. E1), or MRI. Ultrasound is most commonly used as a screening test for HCC in high-risk patients every 6 mo. Fig. E2 shows a laparoscopic view of a cirrhotic liver with a nodular hepatoma.

The following imaging modalities are recommended based on US findings:
- Hepatic lesion <1 cm needs to be followed with a repeat US every 3 mo to ensure the lesion does not change in size. If stable for 24 mo, the interval for US can be increased to every 6 mo.
- Hepatic lesion >1 cm needs further confirmatory imaging with either a CT scan or an MRI scan. If the chosen imaging modality shows characteristics typical of HCC (hypervascular in the arterial phase with washout in the portal venous or delayed phase) the diagnosis of HCC is confirmed with no need for additional diagnostic testing or biopsy. If the imaging modality is inconclusive or atypical for HCC, then the alternate imaging test must be performed. If the second imaging modality is also inconclusive, an image-guided biopsy is recommended.

BIOPSY: Percutaneous biopsy under ultrasound or CT scan is obtained in the event that imaging studies are nondiagnostic or atypical for HCC, or if no cirrhosis is present. Negative biopsy results should be followed and the hepatic nodule reassessed every 3 to 6 mo until it is no longer seen, enlarges, or shows diagnostic characteristics.

SCREENING: Screening high-risk patients with US every 6 mo is currently recommended to identify early-stage HCC.[2] The use of AFP in addition to US increases detection rate but also increases false-positive results. The use of AFP alone should be discouraged due to limited sensitivity and specificity. Patients on transplant waiting lists should be regularly screened for

TABLE 1 Symptoms and Signs of Hepatocellular Carcinoma

Symptom	Frequency (%)
Abdominal pain	59-95
Weight loss	34-71
Weakness	22-53
Abdominal swelling	28-43
Nonspecific GI symptoms	25-28
Jaundice	5-26
Sign	
Hepatomegaly	54-98
Ascites	35-61
Fever	11-54
Splenomegaly	27-42
Wasting	25-41
Jaundice	4-35
Hepatic bruit	6-25

GI, Gastrointestinal.
From Feldman M et al: *Sleisenger and Fordtran's gastrointestinal and liver disease,* ed 10, Philadelphia, 2016, Elsevier.

HCC because in the U.S. the development of HCC gives increased priority for liver transplantation. Screening for HCC is recommended in the following groups:

- Hepatitis B carriers (HBsAg positive): Asian males >40 yr, Asian females >50 yr, all cirrhotic hepatitis B carriers, family history of HCC and North American blacks/Africans older than age 20 yr
- Cirrhosis (nonhepatitis B): Hepatitis C, alcoholic cirrhosis, hemochromatosis, primary biliary cirrhosis, and possibly α1-antitrypsin deficiency, autoimmune hepatitis, and nonalcoholic steatohepatitis

STAGING: The commonly used Barcelona Clinic Liver Cancer (BCLC) staging system includes patient performance status, cancer symptoms, number and size of nodules, and liver function.[3,4] The TNM staging classification is described in Table 2.

Treatment is determined according to stage (Fig. 3):

- Early stage (A): Asymptomatic single tumor 5 cm or 3 nodules, each ≤3 cm
- Intermediate stage (B): Patients with tumors that exceed early criteria but do not yet show cancer-related symptoms, vascular invasion, or metastases
- Advanced stage (C): Patients with mild cancer-related symptoms and/or vascular invasion or extrahepatic spread
- End-stage (D): Patients with advanced, symptomatic disease

℞ TREATMENT

- Treatment options for hepatocellular carcinoma are summarized in Table 3. Fig. 4 describes a treatment algorithm for HCC.
- Early stage: Curative treatment (surgical resection or liver transplantation).
- Patients who have a single lesion can be offered surgical resection if they are noncirrhotic or have cirrhosis with well-preserved liver function, normal bilirubin, and no significant portal hypertension.
- Liver transplantation is an effective option for patients with HCC corresponding to the Milan criteria (Table 4). Living donor transplantation can be offered for HCC if the waiting time is expected to be long. Local ablation is safe and effective therapy for patients who cannot undergo resection or as a bridge to transplantation. With these options, survival at 5 yr ranges from 50% to 70%.
- Radiofrequency ablation (RFA) is used in patients with early HCC who are not surgical candidates, and very high local control rates at 2 yr are obtained (>90%), but eventual recurrence rates can approach 70% at 5 yr.
- Intermediate stage: Transarterial chemoembolization (TACE) is recommended as first-line, noncurative therapy for nonsurgical patients with large/multifocal HCC who do not have vascular invasion or extrahepatic spread. More recently, transarterial use of selective internal radiation therapy (SIRT) with yttrium-90 radiolabeled glass microspheres is an alternative to traditional TACE approaches in this setting. Median survivals exceed 2 yr.
- Advanced stage: Multiple options for advanced HCC have been approved recently including targeted therapy, antiangiogenic therapy, and immunotherapy.[3,4]
- First-line therapy:
  1. Sorafenib and lenvatinib are oral multikinase inhibitors, which are both approved as standard first-line therapy options.[5]
  2. In untreated patients, the checkpoint inhibitor atezolizumab combined with antiangiogenic antibody bevacizumab resulted in better overall and progression-free survival outcomes than sorafenib.[6] Also, the checkpoint inhibitor sintilimab combined with bevacizumab biosimilar improved overall survival in Chinese patients with unresectable HCC.
  3. More recently, dual immunotherapy with the combination of tremelimumab and durvalumab has demonstrated improved survival in first-line treatment of patients with unresectable HCC.[7]
- Second-line therapy:
  1. In previously treated patients, the oral multikinase inhibitors regorafenib and cabozantinib have shown improved survival.
  2. Also, in previously treated patients, the immune checkpoint inhibitors nivolumab and pembrolizumab have demonstrated improved survival outcomes. In addition, the combination of ipilimumab and nivolumab received accelerated approval in patients previously treated with sorafenib.
  3. The antiangiogenic antibody ramucirumab has demonstrated improved survival in HCC patients previously treated with sorafenib.

DISPOSITION

- For resectable HCC, the 5-yr survival after liver transplantation is 50% to 70% and 30% to 50% with surgical resection. For unresectable HCC, the overall prognosis is poor.
- Tumor size is an independent prognostic factor for resected small HCC (≤50 mm in diameter). Patients with tumors of 0 to 35 mm diameter have a better 60-mo HCC specific survival rate than do those with larger tumors (36 to 50 mm).
- In the U.S. the 5-yr overall survival rate for HCC is approximately 10%.

TABLE 2 Hepatocellular Carcinoma TNM Staging Classification and Milan Criteria for Liver Transplantation

T STAGE	
T_x	The primary tumor is not assessable
T_0	No tumor is present
T_1	A single tumor (of any size) without blood vessel invasion
	T_{1a}: Solitary tumor <2 cm (greatest dimension) without vascular invasion
	T_{1b}: Solitary tumor >2 cm (greatest dimension) without vascular invasion
T_2	A single tumor >2 cm *with* vascular invasion or multiple tumors (none >5 cm)
T_3	Multiple tumors, any more >5 cm
T_4	Tumor(s) invading a major branch of the portal or hepatic vein with direct invasion of adjacent organs including the diaphragm (other than gallbladder) or with perforation of the visceral liver peritoneum
N stage	
N_x	The lymph nodes are not assessable
N_0	There is no regional nodal involvement
N_1	There is regional nodal involvement
M stage	
M_0	There is no distant tumor spread
M_1	There is distant tumor spread

Milan criteria for liver transplantation

1 tumor ≤5 cm in diameter, or

Up to 3 tumors ≤3 cm in diameter

+ No vascular invasion

+ No extrahepatic disease

Note

The tumor/node/metastasis (TNM) staging classification does not consider the background liver function, which is often impaired in cirrhosis and will affect treatment options and prognosis. Other staging systems consider both disease extent and liver function, but have not been compared accurately against one another:

- Barcelona Clinic Liver Cancer (BCLC) system
- Cancer of the Liver Italian Program (CLIP) system
- Okuda system

From Grant LA: *Grainger & Allison's diagnostic radiology essentials*, ed 2, Philadelphia, 2019, Elsevier.

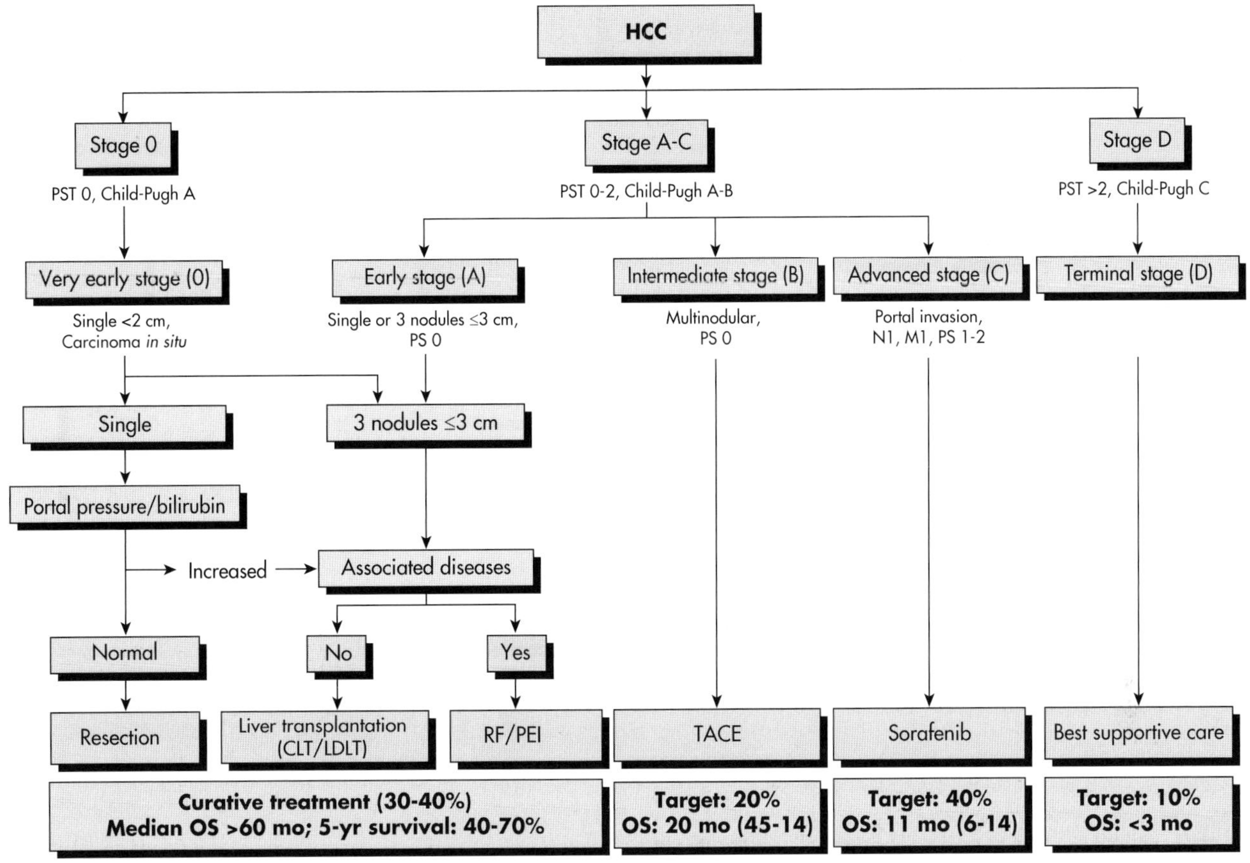

Diseases and Disorders

I

```
                                    ┌─────────┐
                                    │   HCC   │
                                    └─────────┘
        ┌───────────────────────────────┼───────────────────────────────┐
  ┌──────────┐                    ┌──────────┐                      ┌──────────┐
  │ Stage 0  │                    │Stage A-C │                      │ Stage D  │
  └──────────┘                    └──────────┘                      └──────────┘
PST 0, Child-Pugh A          PST 0-2, Child-Pugh A-B           PST >2, Child-Pugh C
```

```
  ┌──────────────────┐   ┌──────────────┐  ┌─────────────────────┐ ┌─────────────────┐ ┌─────────────────┐
  │Very early stage(0)│   │Early stage(A)│  │Intermediate stage(B)│ │Advanced stage(C)│ │Terminal stage(D)│
  └──────────────────┘   └──────────────┘  └─────────────────────┘ └─────────────────┘ └─────────────────┘
  Single <2 cm,         Single or 3 nodules ≤3 cm,  Multinodular,    Portal invasion,
  Carcinoma in situ             PS 0                    PS 0          N1, M1, PS 1-2
```

Resection	Liver transplantation (CLT/LDLT)	RF/PEI	TACE	Sorafenib	Best supportive care
Curative treatment (30-40%) **Median OS >60 mo; 5-yr survival: 40-70%**			**Target: 20%** **OS: 20 mo (45-14)**	**Target: 40%** **OS: 11 mo (6-14)**	**Target: 10%** **OS: <3 mo**

Single → Portal pressure/bilirubin → Increased → Associated diseases → No / Yes

3 nodules ≤3 cm → Associated diseases

Normal → Resection

FIG. 3 Updated Barcelona Clinic Liver Cancer staging system and treatment strategy, 2011. *CLT,* Cadaveric liver transplantation; *HCC,* hepatocellular carcinoma; *PEI,* percutaneous ethanol injection; *LDLT,* living donor liver transplant; *RF,* radiofrequency ablation; *TACE,* transarterial chemoembolization. (From Grant LA: *Grainger & Allison's diagnostic radiology essentials,* ed 2, Philadelphia, 2019, Elsevier.)

TABLE 3   Treatment Options for Hepatocellular Carcinoma

Treatment Modality	Comments
Surgical resection	Curative but limited to noncirrhotic patients and cirrhotic patients without portal hypertension
Liver transplantation	Successful in selected patients with limited disease; requires lifelong immunosuppression
Radiofrequency ablation or ethanol injection	Potentially curative for small tumors, including multiple tumors
Transarterial chemoembolization (TACE) or Y90 brachytherapy	Prolongs survival in unresectable tumors if hepatic function is preserved; not curative
Immunotherapy	Checkpoint inhibitors improve survival in both untreated and treated patients
Targeted molecular therapies	Sorafenib and lenvatinib improve patient survival in previously untreated patients. Regorafenib and cabozantinib improve patient survival in previously treated patients
Antiangiogenic therapy	Bevacizumab in combination with immunotherapy improves survival

REFERRAL

Multidisciplinary gastrointestinal cancer team comprised of gastroenterology, transplant surgery, surgical oncology, interventional radiology, medical oncology, and radiation oncology

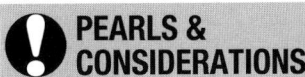

PEARLS & CONSIDERATIONS

- Universal hepatitis B vaccination in children in endemic areas has been shown to decrease the incidence of HCC.
- Treatment of patients with chronic hepatitis B–associated cirrhosis with lamivudine

reduces the incidence of HCC. Treatment with entecavir in chronic hepatitis B-HCC can improve hepatic function and MELD score.
- Treatment with interferon-based therapy in patients with noncirrhotic hepatitis C reduces risk of HCC in patients demonstrating a sustained viral response.
- HCC screening is recommended in high-risk patients because curative therapies are available only for small and early HCC.
- Patients diagnosed with HCC with an AFP >1000 are at increased risk for recurrence after transplantation regardless of tumor size.

- Low-dose daily aspirin use has been associated with less progression of liver disease in patients with chronic hepatitis B or C and lower HCC risk in those patients.[8]

REFERENCES

Available at eBooks.Health.Elsevier.com.

RELATED CONTENT

Liver Cancer (Patient Information)

AUTHOR: **BHARTI RATHORE, MD**

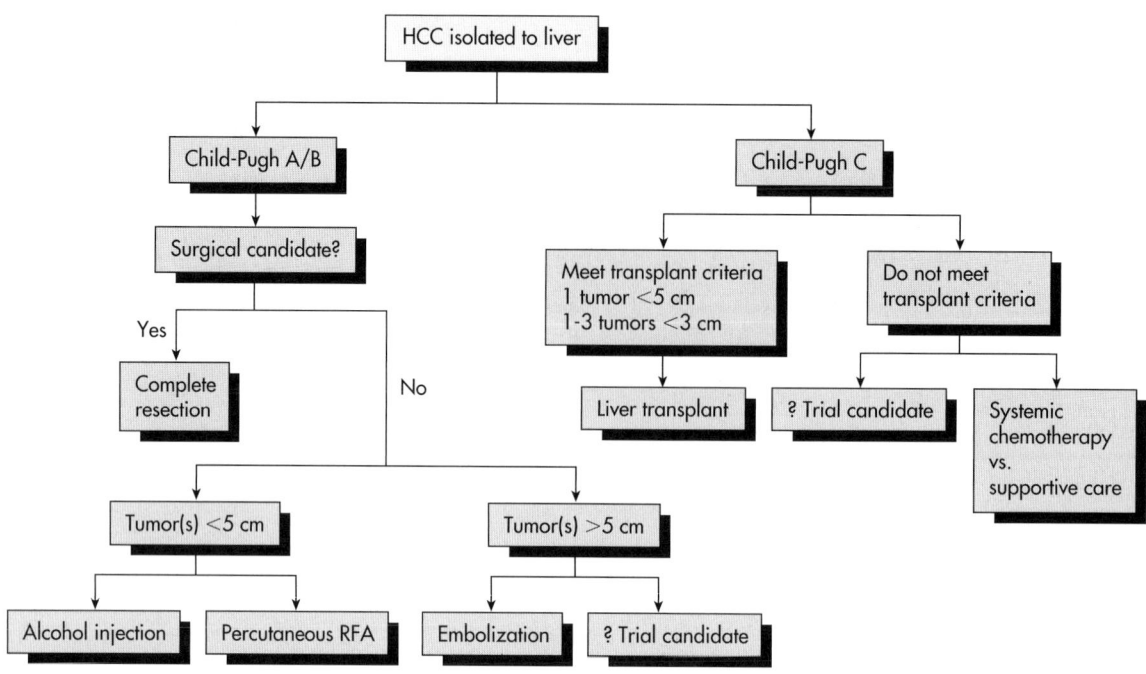

FIG. 4 Treatment algorithm for hepatocellular carcinoma (HCC). *RFA,* Radiofrequency ablation. (From Bruix J, Sherman M: AASLD: Management of hepatocellular carcinoma: an update, *Hepatology* 53(3):1020-1022, 2011.)

TABLE 4 Milan Criteria of Eligibility for Liver Transplantation

Presence of a tumor ≤5 cm in diameter in patients with single hepatocellular carcinomas

Or

≤3 Tumor nodules, each 3 cm or less in diameter, in patients with multiple tumors

From Cameron JL, Cameron AM: *Current surgical therapy,* ed 10, Philadelphia, 2011, Saunders.

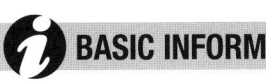

BASIC INFORMATION

DEFINITION

Hereditary breast and ovarian cancer syndrome (HBOC) patients carry a significant cancer-associated alteration in the *BRCA1* and/or *BRCA2* gene. These genetic mutations can confer a heightened risk of malignancy in the breast, ovary, fallopian tube, and peritoneum in women and an elevated risk of prostate and breast cancer in men. Additionally, the risk of pancreatic cancer and skin cancer are elevated for both men and women. Another condition, Lynch syndrome or hereditary nonpolyposis colorectal cancer (HNPCC), is associated with an increased risk of endometrial cancer and ovarian cancer in women and cancer of the colon, stomach, pancreas, and small bowel in both women and men. Patients with Lynch syndrome carry significant pathogenic alterations in one of five genes, as noted below.

The cancer risk to those who test positive for these genetic mutations is significantly greater than the cancer risk associated with those who test negative—both in the general population and in those patients with a personal and/or family cancer history. Frequently, a cancer that is associated with a heritable genetic mutation presents at a younger age than that seen in the general population can be a relatively rarer type of cancer and/or affect multiple same-side family members. Identifying carriers can significantly reduce the morbidity and mortality of the patient and close family members.

SYNONYMS

HBOC
Hereditary breast and ovarian cancer syndrome
Lynch syndrome/hereditary nonpolyposis colorectal cancer (HNPCC)
Hereditary cancer syndrome

ICD-10CM CODES
Z15.01	Genetic susceptibility to malignant neoplasm of breast
Z15.02	Genetic susceptibility to malignant neoplasm of ovary
Z80.3	Family history of malignant neoplasm of breast
Z80.41	Family history of malignant neoplasm of ovary
Z80.49	Family history of malignant neoplasm of other genital organs (uterus, vagina, for example)
Z84.81	Family history of carrier of genetic disease

EPIDEMIOLOGY & DEMOGRAPHICS

INCIDENCE: Overall, an estimated 6% to 10% of gynecologic cancers are heritable. Approximately 7% to 10% of the estimated 276,480 (American Cancer Society 2020 estimate) new breast cancer cases annually are likely to be associated with heredity. Inherited pathogenic *BRCA 1, 2* mutations account for an estimated 11% to 15% of the estimated 21,750 (American Cancer Society 2020 estimate) annual new ovarian cancer cases. Less than 1% of the general population has a pathogenic mutation in the *BRCA 1* or *2* gene. As noted above, Lynch syndrome–associated mutations increase ovarian and uterine cancer as well as colorectal (up to 5% of colorectal cancers are considered heritable), pancreatic, and gastric cancers. This article will, however, focus on gynecologic disease. Tables 1 and 2 summarize genes associated with hereditary breast and ovarian cancer predisposition.

PREDOMINANT SEX & AGE: Although females are predominantly affected, males who carry deleterious mutations in *BRCA 1, 2* are at a significantly higher risk for cancer. Both sexes can transmit the altered gene to their offspring.

RISK FACTORS: *BRCA1* and *BRCA2* mutations can generate a greater risk of breast cancer than other well-established factors such as increased breast density, history of atypical ductal or lobular hyperplasia, nulliparity, obesity, and family history.

Up to 37% of breast cancer patients and 100% of ovarian/tubal/peritoneal cancer patients are at risk for hereditary breast and ovarian cancer syndrome.

Hereditary breast and ovarian cancer syndrome (HBOC):
- Individuals with *BRCA1*, *BRCA2* mutations (Fig. 1)
- Red flags (not an exhaustive list) for possible HBOC include personal or family history of:
  1. Personal breast cancer diagnosed at ≤45 yr old
  2. Triple-negative breast cancer (ER-, PR-, Her2-)
  3. Ovarian cancer: Very important factor (mostly papillary serous)
  4. Male breast cancer
  5. Two primary breast cancers
  6. Ashkenazi Jewish ancestry
  7. Breast cancer with ≥2 relatives with an HBOC-associated cancer (breast, ovary, prostate, pancreatic cancers)
  8. A previously identified HBOC mutation

TABLE 1 Genes Associated With Hereditary Breast Cancer Predisposition

Gene	Syndrome	Relative Risk of BC	BC Risk by Age 80 Yr	Associated Cancers
High Penetrance				
BRCA1	HBOC	~15-30	70%	Ovarian, other
BRCA2	HBOC	~10-20	70%	Ovarian, pancreatic, prostate, other
p53	Li-Fraumeni syndrome	100	50% by 60 yr	Soft tissue sarcoma, osteosarcoma, brain tumors, adrenocortical carcinoma, leukemia, other
PTEN	Cowden syndrome	No reliable estimate	70%-80%	Thyroid (follicular and rarely papillary) endometrial, genitourinary, other
	Bannayan-Riley-Ruvalcaba syndrome			
	Proteus			
	Proteus-like syndrome			
STK11	Peutz-Jeghers syndrome	No reliable estimate	30% by age 60	Small intestine, colorectal, uterine, testicular and ovarian sex chord tumors, other
CDH1	Hereditary diffuse gastric carcinoma	~3.25	39%	Lobular breast, diffuse gastric, other
Lower or Moderate Penetrance				
ATM (heterozygote)	Ataxia-telangiectasia in homozygotes	~3	30	Undefined in heterozygotes
CHK2 (CHEK2)	Li-Fraumeni variant	1.5-3	20%-30%	Undefined
PALB2	None known	5	~40	Undefined in heterozygotes

BC, Breast cancer; HBOC, hereditary breast and ovarian cancer syndrome.
From Niederhuber JE: *Abeloff's clinical oncology*, ed 6, Philadelphia, 2020, Elsevier.

9. Two or more close relatives with breast cancer, one of whom was diagnosed at age 50 or younger
10. Three or more HBOC-associated cancers at any age

GENETICS: The transmission pattern is autosomal dominant. A child whose father or mother has a *BRCA* mutation has a 50% chance of inheriting that genetic mutation.

NOTE:
- One half of *BRCA* carriers inherit the mutation from their father.
- Early onset of cancer may be a more important red flag than the number of affected family members, especially if the number of family members is small to begin with.
- Testing criteria (Tables 3 and 4), as per National Comprehensive Cancer Network (NCCN) guidelines, may differ from the red flags noted previously.
- Family history extends to first-, second-, and third-degree relatives.
- Consider Lynch syndrome–associated cancers (e.g., colorectal, gastric, brain, pancreas, small bowel, skin, ureter, renal pelvis, GI polyps), as Lynch syndrome is also associated with ovarian and uterine (endometrial) cancer.
- *BRCA* stands for BReast CAncer.

1. The majority (84%) of the approximately 7% of breast cancers and 14% of ovarian cancers that result from a heritable mutation are due to a *BRCA1* (52%) and *BRCA2* (32%) gene mutation.
2. By age 70, in comparison to the 7.3% risk of breast cancer in the general population, or approximately double that risk if one has an affected first-degree relative, *BRCA1* and *BRCA2* mutation carriers have up to an 87% reported risk of developing breast cancer. As opposed to a general-population risk of 2% for developing a second breast primary within 5 yr of the initial diagnosis, women with HBOC mutations have a 12% to 27% risk. This risk climbs to a reported 50% (*BRCA2*) and up to 64% (*BRCA1*) by age 70.
3. By age 70, in contrast to the 0.7% risk of ovarian cancer in the general population, there is a reported risk of up to 27% to 63% for *BRCA2* and *BRCA1* mutation carriers, respectively. The risk for ovarian cancer within 10 yr of a breast cancer diagnosis is 6.8% (*BRCA2*) to 12.7% (*BRCA1*) as opposed to a general-population risk of less than 1.0%.
4. Men with HBOC have an up to tenfold increased risk for breast cancer and a more than twofold increase in prostate cancer in comparison to the general-population risk. In men, the *BRCA2* mutation increases this cancer risk more than the *BRCA1* mutation. In fact, the breast cancer risk for a male with a *BRCA2* mutation is up to 80 times the risk seen in the general population.
5. Both men and women have an elevated risk (up to sevenfold) for pancreatic cancer (*BRCA2* >1) and for melanoma (2.5-fold increase with *BRCA2* + *status*).
6. Ashkenazi Jewish ancestry is associated with founder mutations 187delAG (*BRCA1*), 5382insC (*BRCA1*), and 6174delT (*BRCA2*), which confer a significantly elevated risk for breast and ovarian cancer. As opposed to the 1 in 400 risk in the general population, 1 in 40 individuals of Ashkenazi Jewish descent have a *BRCA 1* or *2* mutation.

Lynch Syndrome (Hereditary Nonpolyposis Colorectal Cancer - HNPCC):
- Individuals with *MLH1, MSH2, MSH6, PMS2, EPCAM* mutations.
- By age 70, Lynch syndrome carriers have—in addition to an increased risk for colorectal, gastric, hepatobiliary, urinary tract, small bowel, brain, skin, and pancreatic cancers— up to an approximately twentyfold increase in ovarian cancer (4% to 12% risk vs. the general-population risk of 0.7%) and up to an approximately fortyfold increase in uterine cancer (25% to 60+% risk vs. the general-population risk of 1.6%).
- The previously listed genes and others (e.g., *PTEN, TP53, CDH1, STK11*) that are found less frequently are considered high-penetrance genes, as they can increase the relative risk of their respective syndromes by greater than four- to fivefold.
- Other, more moderate-penetrant genes (e.g., *CHEK2, ATM, PALB2, BRIP1, RAD51C,*

TABLE 2 Genes Associated With Hereditary Ovarian Cancer Predisposition

Gene	Syndrome	Relative Risk of OC	OC Risk by Age 80 Yr	Associated Cancers
High Penetrance				
BRCA1	Hereditary breast ovarian cancer syndrome	~50	~40%	Breast, other
BRCA2	Hereditary breast ovarian cancer syndrome	~8	11%-26%	Breast, pancreas, prostate, other
MLH1 *MSH2* *MSH6* *PMS2* *EPCAM*	Lynch syndrome	~4	~20%	Colon Uterine Stomach Small intestine Urinary tract Pancreatic Possible other sites
Lower or Moderate Penetrance				
RAD51C	None	~5	~6%	Undefined Autosomal recessive Fanconi anemia
RAD51D	None	~12	~14%	Undefined Autosomal recessive Fanconi anemia

OC, Ovarian cancer.
From Niederhuber JE: *Abeloff's clinical oncology,* ed 6, Philadelphia, 2020, Elsevier.

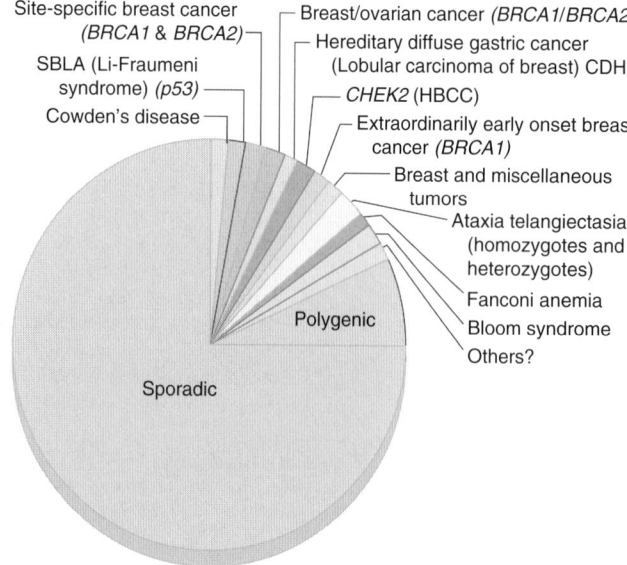

FIG. 1 Schematic depicting heterogeneity in breast cancer. *HBCC*, Hereditary breast and colorectal cancer; *SBLA*, sarcoma, breast and brain tumors, leukemia, laryngeal and lung cancer, and adrenal cortical carcinoma. (From Goldman L, Schafer AI: *Goldman's Cecil medicine,* ed 24, Philadelphia, 2012, Saunders.)

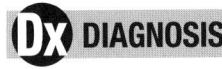

TABLE 3 Testing Criteria for Breast Ovarian Cancer Syndrome*

Individual from a family with a known deleterious *BRCA1* or *BRCA2* gene mutation

Personal history of breast cancer plus one or more of the following:

- Diagnosed at ≤45 yr of age
- Diagnosed at ≤50 yr of age with
  - An additional breast cancer primary
  - At least one close blood relative with breast cancer at any age
  - At least one close relative with pancreatic cancer
  - At least one close relative with prostate cancer
  - An unknown or limited family history
- Diagnosed at age 60 with
  - Triple-negative breast cancer
- Diagnosed at any age with
  - At least one close blood relative with breast cancer before 50 yr of age
  - At least two close blood relatives with breast cancer at any age
  - At least one close blood relative with pancreatic cancer
  - At least two close blood relatives with prostate cancer
  - A close female blood relative with ovarian cancer
  - An individual of ethnicity associated with a higher mutation frequency
- Personal history of ovarian cancer
- Personal history of male breast cancer
- Personal history of prostate cancer at any age with a close relative with breast, ovarian, or pancreatic cancer at any age
- Personal history of pancreatic cancer and Ashkenazi Jewish ancestry
- Family history meeting any of the above criteria

See NCCN guidelines for the most up-to-date and detailed description for counseling and testing.

*For more detailed information, see the National Comprehensive Cancer Network (NCCN) guidelines.
From Disaia PJ et al: *Clinical gynecologic oncology*, ed 9, Philadelphia, 2017, Elsevier.

TABLE 4 National Comprehensive Cancer Network (NCCN) Guidelines for Recommending Genetic Testing for *BRCA1* or *BRCA2* Mutations*

Personal history of breast cancer and one or more of the following:

- Diagnosed at age ≤45 yr
- Diagnosed with at least two breast cancer primaries (bilateral, separate ipsilateral), the first at age 50 yr
- Diagnosed at age ≤50 yr with one or more close relatives[†] with breast cancer (prostate or pancreatic) at any age
- Diagnosed with triple-negative breast cancer at age ≤60 yr
- Diagnosed at any age with one or more close relatives with breast cancer at age ≤50 yr
- Diagnosed at any age with two or more close relatives at any age
- Diagnosed at any age with one or more close relatives with invasive ovarian cancer (including fallopian tube and primary peritoneal) at any age
- Diagnosed at any age with two or more close relatives with pancreatic and/or prostate cancer
- Having a close male relative with breast cancer at any age

*Individuals with a limited or unknown family history may have an underestimated probability of a familial gene mutation detection.
[†]Close relative pertains to first-, second-, or third-degree blood relatives on the same side (either maternal or paternal) of the family.
From Disaia PJ et al: *Clinical gynecologic oncology*, ed 9, Philadelphia, 2017, Elsevier.

RAD51D), that is, those that are associated with a two- to fourfold increase in the relative risk of cancer, should be considered when assessing risk and ordering genetic tests.

- More than 12 known gene mutations are associated with an elevated risk for breast cancer, and a similar number are associated with an elevated risk for ovarian cancer. As such, screening for *BRCA1, BRCA2* alone will miss these mutations.
- In addition to established deleterious mismatch repair gene mutations, gene alterations that are categorized in the literature as emerging risk mutations are also associated with hereditary gynecologic and other cancers.

PHYSICAL FINDINGS & CLINICAL PRESENTATION

- Present at a younger age
- Bilaterality more likely
- Multiple primaries in one individual

ETIOLOGY

Hereditary cancers are typically due to a tumor suppression gene mutation that interferes with DNA repair thus allowing an otherwise potentially avoidable cancer to develop. This is distinct from familial cancers in which there is no isolated gene mutation. Such cancers appear in the family more frequently than that which would be statistically seen in the general population. Non-genetic factors such as lifestyle habits and environmental influences contribute to cancer risk as well.

DX DIAGNOSIS

DIFFERENTIAL DIAGNOSIS

- General (sporadic) population or familial basis for the cancer in question—when the genetic testing is negative.
- Hereditary cancer is more likely to present at a younger age, to span a number of generations, to affect more family members than would be expected (if a large enough family), be associated with a suspicious familial pattern, and to include some rarer (ovary, male breast cancer, pancreatic cancer, for example) presentations.

In addition to the more common syndromes listed previously, consider Cowden *(PTEN)*, Peutz-Jeghers *(STK11)*, Li-Fraumeni *(TP53)*, and others (Table 5).

WORKUP

Family history questionnaire (revisited during subsequent visits), patient and family interviews, genetic counseling/risk assessment (including tools such as Tyrer-Cuzick/Gail/Claus models), and tailored cancer screening and genetic testing. Tablet-based intake questionnaires and computer algorithms are increasingly being used to identify at-risk patients.

LABORATORY TESTS

- A simple blood or saliva sample drawn in the office or a lab, after informed consent, is needed. This specimen should be sent to a reliable laboratory recognized nationally for its genetic cancer testing accuracy (technologic and interpretative), reporting format, and the support staff ability and availability for consultation, office counseling, and testing integration. Look for a laboratory that has published peer-reviewed data and has an accurate classification methodology that relies on an extensive database. Realize that these labs are not FDA approved and that CLIA certification, while needed, relies on just in-house data. Remember also that most patients get tested only once in their lifetime, and so accuracy is imperative. Update testing should be offered as appropriate and available.
- Options include:
  1. Syndrome specific (limited): For example, HBOC-*BRCA* testing (including large rearrangement detection); Lynch syndrome; founder mutation testing (187delAG, 5382insC, 6174delT)—Ashkenazi Jewish population (occasionally recommended as the first test for this population); single-site testing (if a previously identified gene mutation is known in the family); cancer specific, for example, breast cancer panel—*BRCA 1, 2* with/without reflex to broader panel (i.e., sequential testing).
  2. Comprehensive panel testing: Can include HBOC syndrome (*BRCA1, BRCA2*), Lynch syndrome (*MLH1, MSH2, MSH6, PMS2,*

H

I

Diseases and Disorders

Hereditary Breast and Ovarian Cancer

TABLE 5 Summary of Syndromes With Malignant Manifestations Associated With Breast and Ovarian Cancer

Syndrome	Breast Cancer	Ovarian Cancer	Endometrial Cancer	Colon Cancer	Other types of cancer
Hereditary breast and ovarian cancer	X	X			Pancreatic, prostate, and melanoma
Lynch		X	X	X	Gastric, ureteral, biliary, pancreatic, glioblastoma, renal pelvis
Li-Fraumeni	X			X	Sarcomas, brain, adrenocortical
Cowden	X		X	X	Benign mucocutaneous lesions, thyroid, gastrointestinal hamartomas
Peutz-Jeghers	X	X		X	Cervical adenoma malignum, gastrointestinal hamartomas, pancreatic, gastric, small bowel
Hereditary diffuse gastric cancer	X				Gastric, colorectal

Data from National Comprehensive Cancer Network. Breast Cancer: NCCN Evidence Blocks. Version 2.2019. NCCN Clinical Practice Guidelines in Oncology [after login]. Fort Washington, PA: NCCN; 2019 and Hampel H et al: A practice guideline from the American College of Medical Genetics and Genomics and the National Society of Genetic Counselors: referral indications for cancer predisposition assessment. Guideline Development Group, American College of Medical Genetics and Genomics Professional Practice and Guidelines Committee, and National Society of Genetic Counselors Practice Guidelines Committee, *Getet Med* 17:70-87, 2015. In American College of Obstetricians and Gynecologists, Committee Opinion, Number 793, December 2019.

EPCAM), Li-Fraumeni (*TP53*), Cowden (*PTFN*), Peutz-Jeghers (*STK11*), *PALB2, CHEK2, ATM, BRIP1, RAD51C*, and others [upward of 30+ genes]).

- Choice of the test is generally based on personal/family history, although thoroughness of the risk assessment may be limited by attempting to choose a gene test based on history/phenotype alone.
- Comprehensive panel testing has been shown to increase mutation detection. It can aid in test selection when patients qualify for more than one syndrome/cancer-specific test, and it can be used to capture a potentially broader view of risk. There may be a concern, however, for detecting and managing discovered mutations that are not clinically actionable at that time.
- Categories of results include (1) positive or negative (or more nuanced categories) for a deleterious mutation or (2) a genetic variant of uncertain significance, in which a cancer risk is not yet established or ruled out. Genetic testing companies will notify the ordering provider as to an update in category, as new data becomes available. It is critical that the classification of these variants is accurate.

IMAGING STUDIES

Screening transvaginal pelvic ultrasonography, annual mammography, annual MRI (when breast cancer risk is 20% or more based on Tyrer-Cuzick or other breast cancer risk screening models)

TREATMENT & RISK REDUCTION

- Heightened surveillance, judicious chemoprevention, and prophylactic surgery have been associated with improved outcomes.
- Surveillance includes patient breast awareness, clinician and self-breast exam, mammography, MRI, transvaginal ultrasonography, and CA-125 blood testing, for example.

- Chemopreventive approaches have been shown to reduce the risk of ovarian cancer by up to 60% (with an oral contraceptive) and risk of contralateral breast cancer by as much as 53% (with tamoxifen).
- In HBOC patients, prophylactic total mastectomy can reduce the risk of breast cancer by 90%, and a bilateral salpingo-oophorectomy, after childbearing or by age 40, can reduce the risk of ovarian cancer by up to 96% and the risk of breast cancer by up to 68%.
- Consider preimplantation genetic diagnosis in conjunction with in vitro fertilization.

REFERRAL

If services are needed beyond one's practice or comfort level, consider consulting with knowledgeable genetic counselors, gynecologists, gynecologic oncologists, breast surgeons, and gastroenterology specialists, among others.

PEARLS & CONSIDERATIONS

- Be vigilant. Be motivated by the risks: Women with these mutations are approximately 10 times more likely to develop breast cancer and 20 to 30 times more likely to develop ovarian cancer. **Look for red flags during every encounter**, regardless of the patient's chief complaint or scheduled visit type and inquire and regularly update information about the patient's personal and family history of cancer. Consider that approximately 10% of general practice patients have a significant family history. Supply a printed family history questionnaire. Always consider your patient's cancer risk, especially when charting a new treatment course or planning a surgical procedure. Oftentimes, a more comprehensive approach should be taken if a patient proves to be a mutation carrier.
- Adjust the age at which screening/treatment is initiated and the frequency of the visits depending on the age of the youngest affected

family member, the at-risk cancer site, and the carrier status of the patient.

- Encourage input from the patient during the screening, workup, follow-up, and treatment.
- Recommend that the patient verify any questionable family history, collect appropriate family documentation/testing, and involve her family in the process. This involvement can include advising, counseling, and testing for close relatives.
- Focus counseling and testing (if appropriate) those family member(s) who, if tested, would render genetic testing of progeny/other family members less necessary. Testing an affected family member is oftentimes the most appropriate, efficient, cost-effective, and informative approach.
- Genetic testing can more accurately predict risk and enable a more tailored management approach than relying on one's family history alone. Be mindful that there may be other, although as yet unidentified, mutations at the root of one's patient's personal or family cancer history. Thus periodic update testing, as appropriate, is paramount.
- Refer to your professional societies and the NCCN for screening and surveillance/imaging/treatment guidelines. Don't hesitate to engage the assistance of a genetic counselor, gynecologist, oncologist, breast surgeon, and/or a gastroenterologist during this initial phase and, subsequently, as needed.
- Involve other appropriate specialists in the patient's short- and long-term care depending on the at-risk anatomic systems.
- Remember that *BRCA1*- and *BRCA2*-positive men are at a significantly higher risk for breast and prostate cancer, as well as skin and pancreatic cancer.
- Consider prophylactic bilateral (nerve- and nipple-sparing, if appropriate) mastectomy and bilateral salpingo-oophorectomy in high-risk patients.
- Encourage high-risk patients to complete childbearing at a younger age and consider, as appropriate, subsequent prophylactic bilateral

salpingo-oophorectomy and menopause hormone therapy options.

- Recommend prophylactic bilateral salpingectomy for at-risk premenopausal patients during any other surgical procedure—once childbearing is complete. Consider assistive reproductive options, as appropriate.
- Genetic information cannot be used as the basis for a "preexisting condition" with regard to health insurance or employment, according to federal and state laws. However, it may play a role with respect to life insurance, disability insurance, and long-term care insurance.
- While insurance coverage generally is available, panel testing reimbursement may occasionally be challenged. Vocalize and document your support of the appropriate testing and management, with both your patient and her or his insurance company. Enlist the assistance of your local professional society, as needed.
- There may be a medical-legal risk if a failure to identify and/or genetically counsel or test a high-risk patient and/or her family results in a delay in the diagnosis or worsened prognosis of breast or ovarian cancer. The provider, laboratory, and the insurance company/

employer may have legal exposure for failing to order testing, for providing inaccurate results, or for denial of coverage, respectively.
- Being aware of a patient's cancer risk facilitates initiation of those preventive screenings and management strategies that have been shown to reduce the likelihood of cancer and improve early cancer detection rates. This can be of tremendous benefit both for the patient and family.

PREVENTION

Consider appropriate screening and surveillance (awareness/physical exam by patient and health care provider, imaging studies, diagnostic procedures/lab studies, counseling, and genetic testing) as well as prophylactic surgery and chemopreventive measures. Reassess at each subsequent office visit.

A new blood test (Galleri) designed to detect and locate up to 50 different cancers in asymptomatic patients using DNA sequencing to uncover abnormal cell-free DNA methylation patterns has been recently introduced on the market. This may serve to identify those larger groups of nongenetic cancers allowing earlier

evaluation and treatment and ideally a better prognosis.

PATIENT & FAMILY EDUCATION

Always encourage patients to revisit their personal and family history and to update this information with all of their health care providers and their family members. Recommend that patients initiate discussions with their family members and other health care providers in an ongoing effort to reduce their and their loved ones' risk of heritable cancer.

Refer to NCCN guidelines (www.nccn.org) and national specialty society recommendations.

SUGGESTED READINGS
Available at eBooks.Health.Elsevier.com.

RELATED CONTENT
Breast Cancer (Related Key Topic)
Lynch Syndrome (Related Key Topic)
Ovarian Cancer (Related Key Topic)

AUTHOR: **DAVID I. KURSS, MD, FACOG, NCMP**

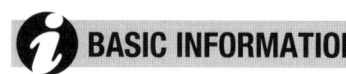
BASIC INFORMATION

DEFINITION

Herpes simplex is a viral infection caused by the herpes simplex virus (HSV). HSV-1 is associated primarily with oral infections, and HSV-2 causes mainly genital infections. However, either type can infect any site. After the primary infection, the virus enters the nerve endings in the skin directly below the lesions and ascends to the dorsal root ganglia, where it remains in a latent stage until it is reactivated.

SYNONYMS

Genital herpes
Herpes labialis
Herpes gladiatorum
Herpes digitalis
Oral herpes

ICD-10CM CODES

A60	Anogenital herpesviral (herpes simplex) infections
A60.04	Herpesviral vulvovaginitis
B00	Herpesviral (herpes simplex) infections
B00.1	Herpesviral vesicular dermatitis
B00.82	Herpes simplex myelitis
B00.9	Herpesviral infection, unspecified
P35.2	Congenital herpesviral (herpes simplex) infection

EPIDEMIOLOGY & DEMOGRAPHICS

- More than 85% of adults have serologic evidence of HSV-1 infection. The seroprevalence of adults with HSV-2 in the U.S. is 25%; however, only approximately 20% of these persons recall having symptoms of HSV infection.
- Most cases of eye or digital herpetic infections are caused by HSV-1.
- Worldwide, more than 400 million persons have genital herpes caused by HSV-2. In the U.S., 1 in 5 adults is infected with HSV-2, and 1 million new infections occur yearly.
- Frequency of recurrence of HSV-2 genital herpes is higher than HSV-1 oral labial infection.
- The frequency of recurrence is lowest for oral labial HSV-2 infections.
- The incidence of complications from herpes simplex (e.g., herpes encephalitis) is highest in immunocompromised hosts.
- Male circumcision significantly reduces the incidence of HSV-2.

PHYSICAL FINDINGS & CLINICAL PRESENTATION

PRIMARY INFECTION:

- Symptoms occur from 3 to 7 days after contact (respiratory droplets, direct contact).
- Constitutional symptoms include low-grade fever, headache and myalgias, regional lymphadenopathy, and localized pain.
- Pain, burning, itching, and tingling last several hours.
- Grouped vesicles, usually with surrounding erythema, appear and generally ulcerate or crust within 48 h (Fig. E1).

- The vesicles are uniform in size (differentiating it from herpes zoster vesicles, which vary in size). Scattered erosions covered with exudate may be noted on genitals (Fig. E2).
- During the acute eruption the patient is uncomfortable; involvement of lips and inside of mouth (Fig. E1) may make it unpleasant for the patient to eat; urinary retention may complicate involvement of the genital area.
- Lesions generally last from 2 to 6 wk and heal without scarring.

RECURRENT INFECTION:

- Generally caused by alteration in the immune system; fatigue, stress, menses, local skin trauma, and exposure to sunlight are contributing factors.
- The prodromal symptoms (fatigue, burning and tingling of the affected area) last 12 to 24 h.
- A cluster of lesions generally evolves within 24 h from a macule to a papule and then vesicles surrounded by erythema; the vesicles coalesce and subsequently rupture within 4 days, revealing erosions covered by crusts.
- The crusts are generally shed within 7 to 10 days, revealing a pink surface.
- The most frequent location of the lesions is on the vermilion border of the lips (HSV-1), the penile shaft or glans penis and the labia (HSV-2), buttocks (seen more frequently in women), fingertips (herpetic whitlow), and trunk (may be confused with herpes zoster).
- Rapid onset of diffuse cutaneous herpes simplex (eczema herpeticum) may occur in certain atopic infants and adults. It is a medical emergency, especially in young infants, and should be promptly treated with acyclovir.
- Herpes encephalitis, meningitis, and ocular herpes can occur in patients with immunocompromised status and occasionally in normal hosts.

ETIOLOGY

HSV-1 and HSV-2 are both DNA viruses.

DIAGNOSIS

DIFFERENTIAL DIAGNOSIS

- Impetigo
- Behçet syndrome
- Coxsackie virus infection
- Syphilis
- Stevens-Johnson syndrome
- Herpangina
- Aphthous stomatitis
- Varicella
- Herpes zoster

WORKUP

Diagnosis is based on clinical presentation. Laboratory evaluation confirms diagnosis.

LABORATORY TESTS

- Direct immunofluorescent antibody slide tests provide a rapid diagnosis.
- Viral culture is the most definitive method for diagnosis; results are generally available in 1 or 2 days. The lesions should be sampled

during the vesicular or early ulcerative stage; cervical samples should be taken from the endocervix with a swab.
- Pap smear will detect HSV-infected cells in cervical tissue from women without symptoms.
- Serologic tests for HSV: Immunoglobulin (Ig) G and IgM serum antibodies. Antibodies to HSV occur in 50% to 90% of adults. The presence of IgM or a fourfold or greater rise in IgG titers indicates a recent infection (convalescent sample should be drawn 2 to 3 wk after the acute specimen is drawn).
- Tzanck smear is a readily available test that will demonstrate multinucleated giant cells. However, it is not a highly sensitive test.

TREATMENT

- Herpes Genitalis: Because no cure exists for herpes genitalis, treatment is focused on reducing the number of recurrences through suppressive therapy and on promoting rapid healing when a recurrence is present. In addition, treatment aims to reduce infectivity by reducing viral shedding and to reduce complications, such as urinary retention and aseptic meningitis. Tables 1 and 2 summarize antiviral chemotherapy for HSV infection.
- Herpes Labialis: Antiviral therapy shortens the duration of discomfort/pain, hastens healing, and reduces viral shedding, thereby reducing dissemination of HSV. Treatment should be initiated ideally in the prodromal stage and no later than 48 h from the onset of lesions to obtain maximal clinical effect. Oral antiviral agents for herpes labialis include aciclovir, famciclovir, and valaciclovir, and they are superior to topical antiviral agents. Topical acyclovir, penciclovir, and docosanol are optional treatments for recurrent herpes labialis, but they are less effective than oral treatments.

DISPOSITION

Most patients recover from the initial episode or recurrences without complications; immunocompromised hosts are at risk for complications (e.g., disseminated herpes simplex infection, herpes encephalitis).

REFERRAL

- Hospital admission in patients with herpes encephalitis or herpes meningitis and in immunocompromised hosts with diffuse herpes simplex infection
- Ophthalmology referral in patients with suspected ocular herpes

PEARLS & CONSIDERATIONS

COMMENTS

- Provide patient education regarding transmission of HSV.
- Condom use offers significant protection against HSV-1 infection in susceptible women.

TABLE 1 Topical and Oral Antiviral Medications Used for Herpes Simplex Virus Infections*

Drug	Formulation	Regimen	Indication/Comment
Topical			
Acyclovir	5% cream (2 g, 5 g)	Apply 5 times/day	Recurrent HL; A: ≥12 yr; 4 days; Rx
	5% ointment (15 g, 30 g)	Apply 6 times/day	Initial GH, localized HSV; A: Adults; 7 days; Rx
Penciclovir	1% cream (1.5 g, 5 g)	Apply q2h (awake)	Recurrent HL; A: ≥12 yr; 4 days; Rx
Docosanol	10% cream (2 g)	Apply 5 times/day	HL; A: ≥12 yr; treat until healed; OTC
Oral (all Rx)			
Acyclovir	200-mg capsule		A: ≥2 yr
	400-mg, 800-mg tablet		
	200-mg/5-ml susp		
		200 mg 5 times/day	Initial GH; 10 days
		200 mg 5 times/day	Recurrent GH; 5 days
		400 mg 2 times/day	Suppression, recurrent GH; up to 12 mo, then reevaluate
Famciclovir	125-, 250-, 500-mg tablet		A: ≥18 yr
		1500-mg single dose	Recurrent HL
		1000 mg 2 times/day	Recurrent GH; 1 day
		250 mg 2 times/day	Suppression, recurrent GH; up to 12 mo
Valacyclovir	500-mg, 1-g caplet		A: Adults and ≥12 yr for HL
		1 g 2 times/day	Initial GH; 10 days
		500 mg 2 times/day	Recurrent GH; 3 days
		500 mg-1 g once daily	Suppressive GH
		2 g 2 times/day	HL; 1 day; both adults and children ≥12 yr

*Approved indications and regimens listed; often used off-label.
A, Approved; *GH,* genital herpes; *HL,* herpes labialis; *HSV,* herpes simplex virus; *OTC,* over-the-counter; *Rx,* by prescription.
From Paller AS, Mancini AJ: *Hurwitz clinical pediatric dermatology: a textbook of skin disorders of childhood and adolescence,* ed 5, Philadelphia, 2016, Elsevier.

TABLE 2 Antiviral Treatment for Herpes Simplex Virus in the Nonpregnant Patient

Indication	ANTIVIRAL AGENT		
	Valacyclovir	**Acyclovir**	**Famciclovir**
First clinical episode	1000 mg bid, 7–10 days	400 mg tid; or 200 mg five times/day, 7–10 days	250 mg tid, 7–10 days
Recurrent episodes	1000 mg daily, 5 days; or 500 mg bid, 3 days	800 mg bid, 5 days; or 800 mg tid, 2 days	125 mg bid, 5 days 500 mg once then 250 mg bid, 2 days; 1000 mg bid, 1 day
Daily suppressive	1000 mg daily (≥10 recurrences/yr) or 500 mg daily (≤9 recurrences/yr)	400 mg bid	250 mg bid

bid, Twice per day; *tid,* three times per day.
Data from Workowski KA, Bolan GA, Centers for Disease Control and Prevention: Sexually transmitted diseases treatment guidelines, 2015, *MMWR Recomm Rep* 64(RR-03):1-137, 2015; Gershenson DM et al: *Comprehensive Gynecology,* ed 8, Philadelphia, 2022, Elsevier.

- Patients should be instructed on the use of condoms for sexual intercourse and on avoiding kissing or sexual intercourse until lesions are crusted. Pericoital application of tenofovir gel, an antiretroviral vaginal gel, has also been shown to reduce the risk of HSV-2 in women. This may be useful in regions of the world where use of condoms is shunned.
- Patients should also avoid contact with immunocompromised hosts or neonates while lesions are present.
- Proper handwashing techniques should be explained.
- Patients with herpes gladiatorum (cutaneous herpes in athletes involved in contact sports) should be excluded from participation in active sports until lesions have resolved.
- Many new HSV-2 infections are asymptomatic. Since HSV-2 antibody tests have become commercially available, an increasing number of persons have learned that they have genital herpes through serologic testing. Persons with asymptomatic HSV-2 infection shed virus in the genital tract less frequently than persons with symptomatic infection, but much of the difference is attributable to less frequent genital lesions because genital lesions are accompanied by frequent viral shedding. The U.S. Preventive Services Task Force (USPSTF) recommends against routine serologic screening for genital HSV infection in asymptomatic adolescents and adults, including those that are pregnant.
- Suppressive treatment of HSV-2 infection lowers the incidence of genital lesions by 70% to 80% but cuts the rate of HSV-2 transmission to uninfected partners by only 50%.

- Pregnancy: Antiviral prophylaxis with acyclovir is recommended from 36 wk of gestation until delivery in women with a history of genital herpes. Elective cesarean delivery should be performed in laboring patients with active lesions to decrease the risk of neonatal herpes.
- Trials involving investigational herpes simplex vaccine have found it to be effective in preventing HSV-1 genital disease and infection, but not in preventing HSV-2 disease or infection.

RELATED CONTENT

Genital Herpes (Patient Information)
Oral Herpes (Patient Information)

AUTHOR: **FRED F. FERRI, MD**

ℹ️ BASIC INFORMATION

DEFINITION

Herpes zoster is a disease caused by reactivation of the varicella-zoster virus, with spread of the virus alone from the sensory nerve to the dermatome. After the primary infection (chickenpox), the virus becomes latent in the dorsal root ganglia and reemerges when there is a weakening of the immune system (as a result of disease or advanced age). Over 90% of the adult U.S. population is latently infected with varicella zoster virus. Reactivation of latent varicella zoster virus (VZV) produces the clinical syndrome herpes zoster (shingles), which manifests as a unilateral eruption along a single dermatome and is usually preceded by prodromal pain and paresthesia. The eruption lasts around 7 to 10 days and progresses from erythematous macules and papules to vesicles, then pustules, and finally crusts over.

SYNONYMS

Shingles
HZ

ICD-10CM CODES

B02	Herpes zoster
B02.0	Zoster encephalitis
B02.1	Zoster meningitis
B02.30	Zoster ocular disease, unspecified
B02.31	Zoster conjunctivitis
B02.32	Zoster iridocyclitis
B02.33	Zoster keratitis
B02.34	Zoster scleritis
B02.39	Other herpes zoster eye disease
B02.7	Disseminated zoster
B02.8	Zoster with other complications
B02.9	Zoster without complications

EPIDEMIOLOGY & DEMOGRAPHICS

- Herpes zoster occurs during the lifetime of 10% to 20% of the population. There are approximately 1 million cases annually in the U.S. The incidence of herpes zoster has increased fourfold over the past six decades.
- There is an increased incidence in immunocompromised patients (chemotherapy, radiotherapy, immunosuppression due to corticosteroids, AIDS, DM, malignancy), the elderly (most common after age 60) (Fig. 1), and children who acquired chickenpox when younger than 2 mo.

PHYSICAL FINDINGS & CLINICAL PRESENTATION

- Pain generally precedes skin manifestation by 3 to 5 days and is generally localized to the dermatome that will be affected by the skin lesions.
- Constitutional symptoms are often present (malaise, fever, headache).
- The initial rash consists of erythematous maculopapules generally affecting one dermatome (thoracic region in majority of cases [Fig. 2]). Typically, the rash does not cross the midline. Some patients (<30%) may

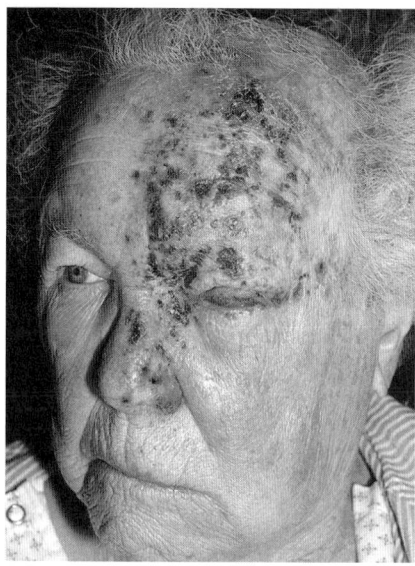

FIG. 1 Herpes zoster, involvement of the V1 dermatome. (From James WD et al: *Andrews' diseases of the skin: clinical dermatology,* ed 12, Philadelphia, 2016, Elsevier.)

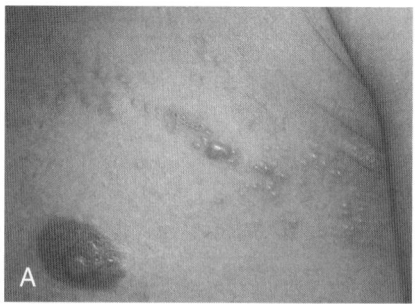
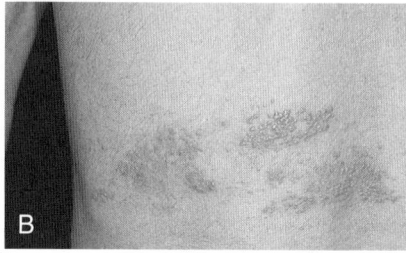

FIG. 2 A and B, Herpes zoster lesions in T3 distribution. (From Swartz MH: *Textbook of physical diagnosis,* ed 7, Philadelphia, 2014, Saunders.)

have scattered vesicles outside the affected dermatome. In rare cases the rash can be generalized (Fig. E3).
- The initial maculopapules evolve into vesicles and pustules by the third or fourth day.
- The vesicles have an erythematous base (Fig. E4), are cloudy, of various sizes (a distinguishing characteristic from herpes simplex, in which the vesicles are of uniform size), and may have a classic appearance of grouped vesicles (Fig. 5).
- The vesicles subsequently become umbilicated and then form crusts that generally fall off within 3 wk; scarring may occur.

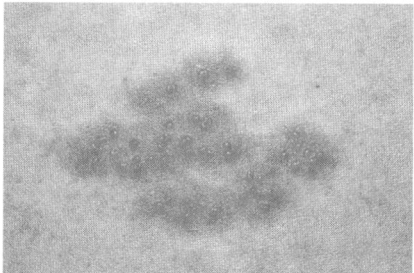

FIG. 5 Herpes zoster. Classic appearance of grouped vesicles. (From White GM, Cox NH [eds]: *Diseases of the skin: a color atlas and text,* ed 2, St Louis, 2006, Mosby.)

- Pain during and after the rash is generally significant. Postherpetic neuralgia occurs after herpes zoster in approximately one third of patients aged 60 yr and older and can persist for months or years.
- Secondary bacterial infection with *Staphylococcus aureus* or *Streptococcus pyogenes* may occur.
- Regional lymphadenopathy may occur.
- Herpes zoster may involve the trigeminal nerve (most frequent cranial nerve involved); involvement of the first division of the trigeminal nerve is known as "herpes zoster ophthalmicus" and can result in blindness. The appearance of blisters on the tip of the nose (Hutchinson sign) is a common manifestation of herpes zoster ophthalmicus. Involvement of the geniculate ganglion can cause facial palsy and a painful ear, with the presence of vesicles on the pinna and external auditory canal (Ramsay Hunt syndrome).
- Pain typical of herpes zoster in the absence of cutaneous lesions, known as "Zoster sine herpete," is rare.

ETIOLOGY

Reactivation of varicella virus (human herpes virus III)

🅍 DIAGNOSIS

DIFFERENTIAL DIAGNOSIS

- Rash: Herpes simplex and other viral infections, contact dermatitis
- Pain from herpes zoster: May be confused with acute myocardial infarction, pulmonary embolism, pleuritis, pericarditis, renal colic

WORKUP

The diagnosis of herpes zoster is usually made by the characteristic dermatomal presentation.

LABORATORY TESTS

Laboratory tests are generally not necessary. In cases where the clinical diagnosis is not obvious, PCR testing for varicella zoster virus has high sensitivity and specificity. It is readily available and results can usually be obtained in less than 24 h. Other laboratory studies for diagnosis of herpes zoster include viral culture, DFA, and serologic testing.

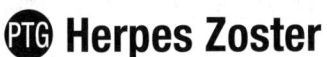

H

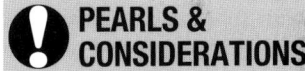 TREATMENT

NONPHARMACOLOGIC THERAPY

- Wet compresses (using Burow solution or cool tap water) applied for 15 to 30 min 5 to 10 times a day may be useful to break vesicles and remove serum and crust. Then carefully pat dry.
- Care must be taken to prevent any secondary bacterial infection by keeping cutaneous lesions clean and dry.

ACUTE GENERAL RX[1]

- Aciyclovir, valacyclovir, and famciclovir are guanosine analogs that are phosphorylated by thymidine kinase to a triphosphate form that inhibits viral deoxyribonucleic acid (DNA) polymerase. The oral bioavailability of the antivirals determines the number of daily administrations. Patient compliance tends to decrease as the number of daily administrations increases. Oral antiviral agents can shorten the disease course and help prevent postherpetic neuralgia. They can decrease acute pain, inflammation, and vesicle formation when treatment is begun within 72 hr of onset of rash. Treatment options are:
  1. Valacyclovir 1000 mg tid for 7 days
  2. Famciclovir 500 mg tid for 7 days
  3. Acyclovir 800 mg 5 times daily for 7 to 10 days

  Acyclovir-resistant VZV infections have been reported in immunocompromised patients (i.e., acquired immune deficiency syndrome [AIDS], transplant patients). In these cases, foscarnet (given intravenously 40 mg/kg three times daily) can be used as an alternative.
- The role of corticosteroids in herpes zoster is controversial. Many physicians prescribe them to improve rash healing and reduce pain severity; however, a Cochrane review failed to show sufficient evidence to support the use of corticosteroids for the prevention of postherpetic neuralgia. Corticosteroids can be considered in older patients within 72 hr of clinical presentation or if new lesions are still appearing if there are no contraindications to their use. Initial dose is prednisone 60 mg/day decreased by 5 mg/day until finished.
- Immunocompromised patients and patients with herpes zoster complicated by CNS

involvement should be treated with IV acyclovir 10 to 15 mg/kg q8h in 1-hr infusions for 7 days, with close monitoring of renal function and adequate hydration; vidarabine (continuous 12-hr infusion of 10 mg/kg/day for 7 days) is also effective for treatment of disseminated herpes zoster in immunocompromised hosts.
- Patients with AIDS and transplant recipients may develop acyclovir-resistant varicella-zoster; these patients can be treated with foscarnet (40 mg/kg IV q8h) continued for at least 10 days or until lesions are completely healed.
- **Postherpetic neuralgia (PHN):** Pain management is especially difficult with conventional analgesics in zoster patients who develop PHN. Calcium channel $\alpha2$-δ ligands (gabapentin and pregabalin), tricyclic antidepressants, opioids, topical lidocaine, selective serotonin and norepinephrine reuptake inhibitors (duloxetine and venlafaxine), and topical capsaicin have been shown to reduce the pain associated with PHN. Of these medications, only gabapentin, pregabalin, 5% lidocaine patch, and 8% capsaicin patch have been approved by the Food and Drug Administration (FDA) specifically for the treatment of PHN. Adding gabapentin to an antiviral in patients with acute herpes zoster appears to significantly reduce the incidence of PHN. Gralise, a once-daily medication for the treatment of postherpetic neuralgia, is an extended-release form of gabapentin that not only has been shown to significantly decrease PHN pain scores but may also be associated with fewer side effects than its immediate-release counterpart. FDA has also approved Horizant, gabapentin enacarbil, for the once-daily therapy of PHN.

DISPOSITION

- The incidence of postherpetic neuralgia (defined as pain that persists more than 90 days after onset of rash) increases with age (<30% by age 40 yr, >70% by age 70 yr); antivirals reduce the risk of postherpetic neuralgia.
- Incidence of disseminated herpes zoster is increased in immunocompromised hosts (e.g., 15% to 50% of patients with active Hodgkin disease).

- Immunocompromised hosts are also more prone to neurologic complications (encephalitis, myelitis, cranial and peripheral nerve palsies, acute retinal necrosis). The mortality rate is 10% to 20% in immunocompromised hosts with disseminated zoster.
- Motor neuropathies occur in 5% of all cases of zoster; complete recovery occurs in >70% of patients.
- Rates of HZ recurrence are more frequent than previously reported and are comparable to rates of first HZ occurrence in immunocompetent individuals.

REFERRAL

- Hospitalization for IV acyclovir in patients with disseminated herpes zoster.
- Patients with herpes zoster ophthalmicus should be referred to an ophthalmologist.
- Consultation with an otolaryngologist is advisable in patients with Ramsey Hunt syndrome.
- Vaccination: In the absence of the herpes zoster vaccine, persons who live to 85 yr of age have a 50% risk of herpes zoster. Immunocompetent adults ≥50 yr (including those who have already received Zostavax) are appropriate candidates for recombinant varicella zoster virus vaccine (Shingrix). It consists of two doses 2 to 6 mo apart and is preferred over Zostavax for herpes zoster prevention. Adults who are VZV seronegative (never had varicella) should be immunized against varicella with two doses of varicella vaccine (Varivax). Despite its efficacy and safety, use of this vaccine remains low (<8% of potential recipients).

⚠ PEARLS & CONSIDERATIONS

REFERENCE & SUGGESTED READING
Available at eBooks.Health.Elsevier.com.

RELATED CONTENT
Shingles (Patient Information)
Postherpetic Neuralgia (Related Key Topic)
Ramsey Hunt Syndrome (Related Key Topic)

AUTHOR: **FRED F. FERRI, MD**

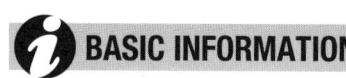
BASIC INFORMATION

DEFINITION

High-altitude sickness refers to a spectrum of cerebral and pulmonary syndromes related to hypoxemia that occurs following rapid ascent to high altitudes in unacclimatized individuals. Common acute high-altitude illnesses include high-altitude headache (HAH), acute mountain sickness (AMS), high-altitude cerebral edema (HACE), and high-altitude pulmonary edema (HAPE).

SYNONYMS

Altitude sickness
High-altitude headache (HAH)
Acute mountain sickness (AMS)
High-altitude pulmonary edema (HAPE)
High-altitude cerebral edema (HACE)

ICD-10CM CODES
T70.2 Other and unspecified effects of high altitude
W94 Exposure to high and low air pressure and changes in air pressure

EPIDEMIOLOGY & DEMOGRAPHICS

- Millions of people worldwide are at risk of developing altitude sickness annually.
- 80% of people who ascend rapidly to high altitudes develop HAH.[1]
- AMS affects approximately 25% of individuals ascending rapidly to an altitude of 2000 m (6500 ft) and 60% to 80% of people ascending to 4500 m (14,750 ft).[2]
- The incidence of HACE is reported to be 0.5% to 1% at elevations in excess of 4500 m (14,750 ft).[3]
- HACE is often complicated by concomitant HAPE.
- The incidence of HAPE is reported to be 2% at 3000 m (10,000 ft) and 4% at 4500 m (14,750 ft).[4]

- AMS and HACE affect men and women equally.
- Studies suggest that climbers with a prior history of HAPE have a roughly 60% chance of recurrence if they ascend to the same elevation at the same rate.[5,6]

PHYSICAL FINDINGS & CLINICAL PRESENTATION (TABLE 1)

High Altitude Headache (HAH)
- Headache that develops within 24 hr of ascent.
- Bilateral, frontal or frontotemporal, dull or pressing quality.
- Mild to moderate intensity and aggravated by exertion, movement, straining, coughing, or bending.
- May be worse when lying down.
- Headache resolves within 8 hr of descent.
- HAH should resolve with analgesics and/or 10 to 15 min of supplementary oxygen.[1]
- Difficult to distinguish from headaches secondary to dehydration.

Acute Mountain Sickness (AMS)
- AMS is thought to be a progression of HAH.[1]
- Occurs within 6 to 12 hr after rapid ascent to 2500 m (8000 ft) in 10% to 25% of unacclimatized persons.[2]
- Headache is the most common symptom. Often worse when lying down which may exacerbate sleep disturbance.
- Dizziness and light-headedness.
- Nausea, vomiting, and loss of appetite.
- Fatigue.
- Sleep disturbance from an exaggerated hyperventilatory phase of periodic respiration in response to hypoxemia and alkalosis.[1]
- The Lake Louise AMS Score has been developed to standardize the diagnosis and severity of AMS in research studies.[7]
- AMS can evolve into HAPE and HACE.
- Retinal hemorrhages can be present from increased blood flow or breakdown in the blood-retinal barrier.[1]

- Supplemental oxygen may be used as a temporizing treatment and to support the clinical diagnosis.

High Altitude Cerebral Edema (HACE)
- Usually presents several days after AMS, 24 to 72 hr after elevation gain.[7]
- Headache, nausea, vomiting, mild fever, confusion, irritability, drowsiness, stupor, hallucinations, seizures, and paralysis.
- Truncal ataxia and encephalopathy.
- Coma and death from brain herniation may develop within hours of the first symptoms.

High Altitude Pulmonary Edema HAPE
- Typically occurs 2 to 4 days after ascent to more than 3000 m (10,000 ft); note that HAPE is not always preceded by AMS symptoms.[2]
- It can occur at a lower elevation in patients with pulmonary hypertension.
- Dyspnea out of proportion to the level of exertion, loss of stamina.
- Dry cough or cough with frothy rust- or pink-tinged sputum.
- Chest tightness.
- Tachycardia, tachypnea.
- Rales on auscultation, cyanosis.

ETIOLOGY

- As altitude increases, the atmospheric pressure and partial pressure of oxygen (PO2) decrease. Although the percentage of oxygen in the air remains the same, the decreased partial pressure reduces the oxygen available in the alveoli and the diffusion gradient across the alveoli into the blood. This can result in hypoxemia.
- Competing drives to hyperventilate in response to low oxygen saturation and to hypoventilate due to low partial pressure of carbon dioxide (PCO2) lead to periodic respiration, which can dramatically disturb sleep exacerbating other symptoms.
- Increased cerebral blood flow and the loss of autoregulation of intracranial pressure may contribute to increased cerebral vascular

---

TABLE 1 Clinical Characteristics of High-Altitude Illnesses

	HAH	Mild AMS	Moderate to Severe AMS	HACE
			CLINICAL CLASSIFICATION	
Symptoms	Headache only	Headache plus one more symptom (nausea/vomiting, fatigue/lassitude, dizziness, or difficulty sleeping) All symptoms of mild severity	Headache plus one or more symptoms (nausea/vomiting, fatigue/lassitude, dizziness, or difficulty sleeping) Symptoms of moderate to severe intensity	±Headache Worsening of symptoms seen in moderate to severe AMS
LL-AMS score*	1-3, headache only	2-4	5-15	
Physical signs	None	Possible peripheral edema	Possible peripheral edema	Ataxia Altered mental status peripheral edema
Findings	None	Possible mild altitude adjusted desaturation	Slightly increased body temperature Slight altitude adjusted desaturation Widened A-a gradient Elevated ICP White matter edema (CT, MRI)	HAPE common: Positive chest radiograph, rales, dyspnea at rest Altitude adjusted desaturation Elevated ICP White matter edema (CT, MRI)

AMS, Acute mountain sickness; *CT*, computed tomography; *HACE*, high-altitude cerebral edema; *HAH*, high-altitude headache; *HAPE*, high-altitude pulmonary edema; *ICP*, intracranial pressure; *LL-AMS*, Lake Louise AMS; *MRI*, magnetic resonance imaging.
*The self-reported Lake Louise AMS score.
From Auerbach P: *Wilderness medicine, expert consult, premium edition—enhanced online features and print*, Philadelphia, 2012, Saunders.

permeability and subsequent brain edema (HACE).

- Hypobaric hypoxia can trigger elevated pulmonary pressures, resulting in protein-rich, hemorrhagic exudates into the lung alveoli due to a breakdown in the pulmonary blood-gas barrier (HAPE).
- The body responds to low oxygen partial pressures through a process of acclimatization that takes place over days to weeks (see "Comments").

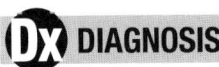 DIAGNOSIS

Made by clinical presentation and physical exam findings.

DIFFERENTIAL DIAGNOSIS

- Dehydration
- Carbon monoxide poisoning
- Hypothermia
- Infection
- Substance abuse
- Congestive heart failure
- Pulmonary embolism
- Cerebrovascular accident
- Box 1 summarizes the differential diagnosis of high-altitude illnesses

WORKUP

Typically, the diagnosis is self-evident after history and physical examination. Subsequent laboratory tests and imaging studies help monitor cardiopulmonary and central nervous system status in patients admitted to the intensive care unit for pulmonary and/or cerebral edema. In patients with HAPE occurring at lower altitudes (< 2500 m [8000 ft]), an evaluation of preexisting pulmonary hypertension or an intracardiac shunt should be considered. Pulse oximetry that does not return to normal on descent can be helpful to evaluate severity of HAPE and follow its resolution.

LABORATORY TESTS

Not useful for initial diagnosis, unless to rule out an alternative diagnosis.

IMAGING STUDIES

- Chest x-ray showing Kerley B-lines and patchy edema

- CT scan of the head showing diffuse or patchy edema
- MRI of the head showing characteristic intense T2 signal in the white matter

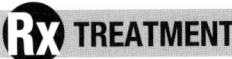 TREATMENT

NONPHARMACOLOGIC THERAPY

- Stop the ascent to allow acclimatization or initiate descent until symptoms have resolved.
- Patient with AMS can stay at the same altitude and may ascend once symptoms resolve.
- If AMS symptoms recur or fail to resolve after 2 to 3 days, descent is indicated.[2]
- Descent is mandatory for all persons with HACE or HAPE and should be initiated immediately with development of symptoms of HACE or HAPE. Symptoms of HACE and HAPE may quickly worsen and incapacitate the patient, which can turn a relatively easy descent into a logistically complicated rescue requiring substantial resources.
- Supplemental oxygen is used for treatment of severe AMS, HAPE, and HACE.
- Portable hyperbaric bags are useful if available at the site and can temporize a difficult situation to allow descent.
- Adequate hydration is key for AMS of any severity.

ACUTE PHARMACOLOGIC PROPHYLAXIS AND THERAPY

- Nonsteroidal antiinflammatory drugs (e.g., ibuprofen 600 mg every 6 hr, beginning 6 hr before ascending) are often used for prophylaxis of traditional altitude sickness and in treating headaches in AMS. However, trials have shown that ibuprofen is slightly inferior to acetazolamide for acute mountain sickness prevention and should not be recommended over acetazolamide for rapid ascent.[8] Headache that does not resolve after treatment with NSAIDs is concerning, and patients should not ascend further and should consider descent until it improves.
- Acetazolamide 125 to 250 mg PO twice daily is the preferred agent and has been effective for both prevention and acute therapy in patients with AMS and HACE.[9]
- Dexamethasone is also effective in reducing symptoms of AMS and can be used as an

alternative to acetazolamide in individuals who are intolerant to acetazolamide (sulfa allergy). It should be added to acetazolamide in patients with HACE.[10]
- Dexamethasone initial dose of 8 mg PO/IM/IV followed by 4 mg PO every 6 hr is used in patients with severe AMS, HAPE, or HACE.[11]
- Nifedipine 10 mg sublingual followed by long-acting nifedipine 30 mg bid is used for patients with HAPE who cannot descend immediately. Salvage therapy in absence of supplemental oxygen and descent also includes phosphodiesterase-5 inhibitors (sildenafil or tadalafil), which decrease pulmonary artery pressure.[12]
- Table 2 summarizes recommended medications for the prevention and treatment of altitude sickness.

CHRONIC THERAPY

Prevention is the most prudent therapy. Recommendations include:
- Slow, staged ascent to avoid altitude sickness.
- Start the ascent below 2500 meters (8000 ft).
- Ascend 300 m/day (1000 ft/day).
- Spend two nights at the same altitude every 3 days.
- Sleep at lower heights than the altitude climbed ("climb high, sleep low").
- Limiting extreme exertion on arrival at a new higher elevation for 24 hr may also decrease the likelihood of AMS.
- Box 2 summarizes field treatment of high-altitude illness.

DISPOSITION

- AMS typically improves over a period of 2 to 3 days if altitude is unchanged or possibly much quicker if altitude is reduced.
- HAPE is the most common cause of death among patients with altitude illnesses. Aggressive treatment with descent (or hyperbaric therapy if unable to descend) and oxygen are warranted.[6]
- More than 60% of patients with HAPE will have recurrence of symptoms on subsequent climbs.[5,6]
- In HACE, neurologic deficits may persist for weeks but eventually resolve. If coma occurs, prognosis is poor.

REFERRAL

Cardiology and neurology referrals are made in patients with pulmonary edema and central nervous system findings, respectively.

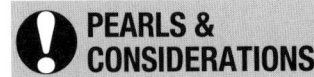 PEARLS & CONSIDERATIONS

COMMENTS

- Acclimatization is the process in which an individual who normally resides at low altitudes adapts to hypobaric hypoxia to improve tolerance and performance at higher altitudes. These mechanisms include:
  1. An increase in respiratory rate and tidal volume. This hyperventilation decreases

---

BOX 1   Differential Diagnosis of High-Altitude Illnesses

Acute mountain sickness and high-altitude cerebral edema	Dehydration, exhaustion, viral or bacterial infection, alcohol hangover, hypothermia, carbon monoxide poisoning, migraine, hyponatremia, hypoglycemia, diabetic ketoacidosis, CNS infection, transient ischemic attack, arteriovenous malformation, stroke, seizures, brain tumors, ingestion of toxins or drugs, acute psychosis
High-altitude pulmonary edema	Asthma, bronchitis, pneumonia, mucus plugging (secondary to previous), idiopathic hyperventilation syndrome, pulmonary embolism, heart failure, myocardial infarction

From Auerbach P: *Wilderness medicine, expert consult, premium edition—enhanced online features and print,* Philadelphia, 2012, Saunders.

TABLE 2 Recommended Medications for the Prevention and Treatment of Altitude Sickness

Medication	Indication	Route	Dose
Acetazolamide	Prevention of AMS, HACE	Oral	62.5 mg or 125 mg twice per day Pediatrics: 2.5 mg/kg every 12 hr
	Treatment of AMS*	Oral	250 mg twice per day Pediatrics: 2.5 mg/kg every 12 hr
Dexamethasone	Prevention of AMS, HACE	Oral	2 mg every 6 hr or 4 mg every 12 hr Pediatrics: Should not be used for prophylaxis
	Treatment of AMS, HACE	Oral, IV, IM	AMS: 4 mg every 6 hr HACE: 8 mg once then 4 mg every 6 hr Pediatrics: 0.15 mg/kg/dose every 6 hr
Nifedipine	Prevention of HAPE	Oral	30 mg SR version every 12 hr, or 20 mg of SR version every 8 hr
	Treatment of HAPE	Oral	30 mg SR version every 12 hr, or 20 mg of SR version every 8 hr
Tadalafil	Prevention of HAPE	Oral	10 mg twice per day
Salmeterol	Prevention of HAPE	Inhaled	125 µg twice per day†

AMS, Acute mountain sickness; HACE, high-altitude cerebral edema; HAPE, high-altitude pulmonary edema; IM, intramuscular; IV, intravenous; SR, sustained release.

*Acetazolamide can also be used at this dose as an adjunct to dexamethasone in HACE treatment, but dexamethasone remains the primary treatment for that disorder.

†Should not be used as monotherapy and should only be used in conjunction with oral medications.

From Goldman L, Shafer AI: *Goldman-Cecil Medicine*, ed 26, Philadelphia, 2019, Elsevier.

BOX 2 Field Treatment of High-Altitude Illness

High-Altitude Headache and Mild Acute Mountain Sickness
- Stop ascent, rest, acclimatize at same altitude
- Symptomatic treatment as necessary with analgesics and antiemetics
- Consider acetazolamide, 125 to 250 mg bid, to speed acclimatization
- OR descend 500 m (1640 ft) or more

Moderate to Severe Acute Mountain Sickness
- Low-flow oxygen, if available
- Acetazolamide, 125 to 250 mg bid, with or without dexamethasone, 4 mg PO, IM, or IV q6h
- Hyperbaric therapy
- OR immediate descent

High-Altitude Cerebral Edema
- Immediate descent or evacuation
- Oxygen, 2 to 4 L/min
- Dexamethasone, 8 mg PO, IM, or IV, then 4 mg q6h
- Hyperbaric therapy

High-Altitude Pulmonary Edema
- Minimize exertion and keep warm
- Immediate descent or hyperbaric therapy
- Oxygen, 4 to 6 L/min until improving, then 2 to 4 L/min
If above unavailable, one of the following:
- Nifedipine, 30 mg extended release q12h
- Sildenafil 50 mg q8h
- Tadalafil 10 mg q12h
- β-agonists may be helpful

Periodic Breathing
- Acetazolamide, 62.5 to 125 mg at bedtime as needed

From Auerbach P: *Wilderness medicine, expert consult, premium edition—enhanced online features and print*, Philadelphia, 2012, Saunders.

---

4. Cerebral vasodilation to increase blood flow to the brain.
5. Rise in hemoglobin. This process can take a week to occur in response to the need for improved oxygen delivery and can take several weeks for a meaningful increase in hemoglobin to occur.

- Adaptation to altitude is different from acclimatization and refers to physiologic differences in permanent residents at high altitude (e.g., an increased oxygen diffusion capacity and very elevated hemoglobin levels).
- Risk calculators exist for predicting acute mountain sickness that incorporate history of altitude illness, speed of ascent, and altitude reached.[13]
- Risk factors for the development of altitude sicknesses are:
  1. Rapid ascent
  2. Previous history of altitude sickness
  3. Strenuous exertion on arrival
  4. Obesity
  5. Male gender
  6. Alcohol consumption
  7. Chronic obstructive pulmonary disease (COPD)
- Physical fitness is not protective against nor fully predictive of high-altitude illness.
- Special consideration should be made for patients with chronic medical conditions prior to high-altitude travel. Specifically, patients who are at high risk for severe hypoxemia, impaired ventilatory response, pulmonary vascular changes, or complications from existing conditions at high altitude.[14]
- Medical contraindications to travel above 2500 m include[14]:
  1. Advanced COPD (FEV1 <30% of predicted value), restrictive lung disease (TLC <50% predicted value) or requirement for continuous oxygen therapy
  2. Pulmonary hypertension (systolic PAP >60 mm Hg)
  3. Sickle cell disease
  4. Poorly controlled seizure disorder
  5. Untreated, high-risk cerebrovascular abnormality
  6. Acute exacerbation of pre-existing medical conditions
- Acetazolamide is useful in COPD patients to lessen the risk of severe high-altitude symptoms but patients with moderate-to-severe COPD should be advised to avoid vacations to high altitude.[15]

REFERENCES
Available at eBooks.Health.Elsevier.com.

RELATED CONTENT
Altitude Sickness (Patient Information)

AUTHORS: **EUGENE CARRAGEE, MD, STEPHANIE SUTTER, MD,** and **JEFFREY W. SALL, PHD, MD**

arterial carbon dioxide improving alveolar oxygenation, even at extreme altitudes.
2. An early increase in heart rate and stroke volume to improve oxygen delivery via increased cardiac output. After 1 wk, both parameters decrease secondary to diuresis and lower catecholamine levels.

3. Pulmonary hypertension develops in response to hypoxemia, resulting in improvement of the ventilation-perfusion mismatch (versus response to hypoxemic pulmonary vasoconstriction) but may be maladaptive and lead to the development of HAPE.

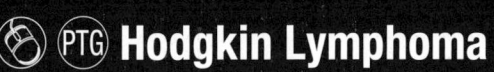
Diseases
and Disorders

I

BASIC INFORMATION

DEFINITION

Hodgkin lymphoma is a malignant disorder arising from germinal center B cells and characterized histologically by the presence of multinucleated giant cells (Reed-Sternberg cells) in a mixed inflammatory background.

ICD-10CM CODES

C81.90 Hodgkin lymphoma, unspecified, unspecified site
C81.00 Nodular lymphocyte predominant Hodgkin lymphoma, unspecified site
C81.10 Nodular sclerosis classical Hodgkin lymphoma, unspecified site
C81.20 Mixed cellularity classical Hodgkin lymphoma, unspecified site
C81.30 Lymphocyte depleted classical Hodgkin lymphoma, unspecified site
C81.79 Other classical Hodgkin lymphoma, extranodal and solid organ sites
C81.90 Hodgkin lymphoma, unspecified, unspecified site
C81.91 Hodgkin lymphoma, unspecified, lymph nodes of head, face, and neck
C81.92 Hodgkin lymphoma, unspecified, intrathoracic lymph nodes
C81.93 Hodgkin lymphoma, unspecified, intra-abdominal lymph nodes
C81.94 Hodgkin lymphoma, unspecified, lymph nodes of axilla and upper limb
C81.95 Hodgkin lymphoma, unspecified, lymph nodes of inguinal region and lower limb
C81.96 Hodgkin lymphoma, unspecified, intrapelvic lymph nodes
C81.97 Hodgkin lymphoma, unspecified, spleen
C81.98 Hodgkin lymphoma, unspecified, lymph nodes of multiple sites
C81.99 Hodgkin lymphoma, unspecified, extranodal and solid organ sites

EPIDEMIOLOGY & DEMOGRAPHICS

- There is a bimodal age distribution (15 to 34 yr and >50 yr).
- Incidence is 2.6 in 100,000 cases; >8800 new cases of Hodgkin lymphoma diagnosed annually in the U.S.
- Concordance for Hodgkin lymphoma in identical twins suggests that a genetic susceptibility underlies Hodgkin lymphoma in young adulthood.
- There is association between certain HLA haplotypes, especially HLA-A1.
- There is an increased risk in smokers and HIV-infected individuals.

PHYSICAL FINDINGS & CLINICAL PRESENTATION

- Painless palpable lymphadenopathy is the most common presenting symptom.
- The most common site of involvement is the neck region.
- Fever and night sweats: Fever in a cyclical pattern (days or weeks of fever alternating with afebrile periods) is known as Pel-Ebstein fever.
- Unexplained weight loss, generalized malaise.
- Persistent, nonproductive cough.
- Lymph node pain associated with alcohol ingestion often because of heavy eosinophil infiltration of the tumor sites is relatively uncommon.
- Generalized pruritus.
- Hepatosplenomegaly.
- Other: Superior vena cava syndrome, spinal cord compression (rare), erythema nodosum (very rare), ichthyosis (very rare).

ETIOLOGY

- Evidence implicating Epstein-Barr virus remains controversial.
- Cigarette smoking has also been implicated.
- Many recent studies reveal that the malignant Hodgkin/Reed-Sternberg cells are pre-apoptotic germinal center B cells that acquire genomic perturbations that prevent their effective elimination and create the microenvironment of ineffective immune reaction that sustains their survival.

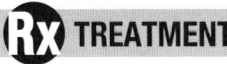 DIAGNOSIS

DIFFERENTIAL DIAGNOSIS

- Non-Hodgkin lymphoma
- Sarcoidosis and other rare nonmalignant lymphadenopathies (e.g., Kikuchi-Fujimoto disease, Castleman disease)
- Infections (e.g., cytomegalovirus, Epstein-Barr virus, toxoplasmosis, HIV, tuberculosis)
- Drug reaction

WORKUP

Diagnosis is confirmed by lymph node biopsy. The World Health Organization classifies Hodgkin lymphoma into two groups: Classic Hodgkin lymphoma (CHL; 95%) and nodular lymphocyte-predominant Hodgkin lymphoma (NLPHL; 5%). Classic Hodgkin lymphoma has four main histologic subtypes based on the type of immune infiltrate surrounding the Hodgkin/Reed-Sternberg cells, but they do not have major clinical or prognostic relevance: Nodular sclerosis (Fig. E1), mixed cellularity (Fig. E2), lymphocyte rich, and lymphocyte depleted. NLPHL is a separate disease with differing histopathologic and clinical characteristics, and specific therapy more resembling non-Hodgkin lymphomas.

Nodular sclerosis occurs mainly in young adulthood, whereas the mixed cellularity type is more prevalent after age 50 yr. Table 1 summarizes key features of Hodgkin lymphomas.

Staging: Table 2 describes the Ann Arbor/Cotswold staging classification.

Proper staging requires the following:
- Detailed history (with documentation of "B symptoms") and physical examination
- Excisional biopsy with histologic, immunophenotypic and immunohistochemical analysis
- Laboratory evaluation (complete blood count, erythrocyte sedimentation rate [ESR], blood urea nitrogen, creatinine, liver function tests, albumin, lactate dehydrogenase, HIV test), immunophenotypic markers
- Positron emission tomography (PET)/computed tomography (CT) scan of the chest, abdomen, and pelvis
- Unilateral bone marrow biopsy in selected patients (rarely indicated)

Box 1 summarizes recommended staging procedures for Hodgkin lymphoma.

℞ TREATMENT

ACUTE GENERAL Rx

The main therapeutic modality includes chemotherapy with or without radiotherapy depending on stage and other risk factors (Table 3). Patients are generally assigned to one of the three risk groups: Early favorable (stage 1 or 2 without risk factors), early unfavorable (stage 1 or 2 with risk factors), or advanced (stage 3 or 4). In general, chemotherapy plus involved-site radiotherapy is standard treatment for early favorable or unfavorable Hodgkin lymphoma; chemotherapy alone may be appropriate for many patients. Chemotherapy (Table 4) is used for advanced stage disease with radiotherapy in selected patients, mainly in those with bulky disease.

Most oncologists use the combination of doxorubicin, bleomycin, vinblastine, and dacarbazine (ABVD). ABVD does not cause infertility or stem cell damage and can be used in patients with HIV infection. The four drugs comprising ABVD are administered intravenously, on day 1 and 15 of 28-day cycles, which are typically not delayed for asymptomatic cytopenias.

Patients with early favorable CHL (i.e., stage 1 or 2 with fewer than three nodal sites of involvement, no B symptoms, bulky or extranodal disease, and baseline ESR <50) can be treated with two cycles of ABVD followed by 20 Gy of involved-field radiation therapy. Extending chemotherapy or increasing radiation dose does not improve outcomes, although radiation therapy has been replaced by additional cycles of chemotherapy in some trials.

Patients with early unfavorable Hodgkin lymphoma (stage 1 or 2 with the aforementioned risk factors) typically receive four cycles of ABVD plus involved-site radiotherapy to 30 Gy. Extended chemotherapy alone, in the absence of bulky disease, is an alternative approach, especially in younger women who may have increased risk of breast cancer after radiation therapy. The risk of disease recurrence is higher in patients who receive chemotherapy alone, but there may be no difference in overall survival.

Advanced-stage CHL is typically treated with one of the three regimens: ABVD, dose-escalated bleomycin, etoposide, doxorubicin hydrochloride (Adriamycin), cyclophosphamide, vincristine (Oncovin), procarbazine and prednisone (BEACOPP), or BV-AVD. ABVD is typically given as six monthly cycles, though patients who achieve a complete metabolic response on a restaging PET-CT performed after two cycles may omit further

TABLE 1 Key Features of Histologic Subtypes of Hodgkin Lymphoma

Lymphoma (% of Cases)	Demographics, Clinical Presentation	Morphology	Cell Surface Markers
Nodular sclerosis (70%)	M = F, <30 yr with mediastinal mass, occasional spleen or lung involvement; 40% have B symptoms; most patients present with stage II disease	Broad bands of collagen, nodules of lymphoid tissue with aggregates of HRS cells and lacunar cells, multinucleated variants	CD15, CD30, CD45-EBV in 1%-40%
Mixed cellularity (20%)	M > F; median age, 38 yr; peripheral lymphadenopathy common, spleen, BM; B symptoms common; patients often stage III or IV	Classic HRS cells in mixture of lymphocytes, plasma cells, eosinophils, histiocytes	CD15, CD30, CD45-EBV in 75%
Lymphocyte-rich (~5%)	M > F, older age; peripheral lymphadenopathy; B symptoms rare; most patients with stage I or II disease	Scattered classic HRS cells among numerous small lymphocytes; nodular growth pattern	CD15, CD30; Oct2 and BOB.1 vary; J-chain absent; EBV in 40%-75%
Lymphocyte depleted (<1%)	M > F; median age, 30-37 yr; B symptoms, advanced stage common; associated with HIV; poor prognosis	Classic HRS cells common with paucity of background lymphocytes; pleomorphic HRS cells mimic sarcoma	CD15, CD30, CD45-EBV positive in HIV-affected patients
Nodular, lymphocyte predominant (NLPHL, 5%)	M > F, 30-50 yr, with peripheral lymphadenopathy	Mononuclear cells with convoluted nuclei (popcorn or L&H cells) loosely aggregated in nodules of small B cells	CD45, CD20, bcl-6, J-chain, Oct-2, BOB.1, EBV absent in LP cells

BM, Bone marrow; *CHL,* classical Hodgkin lymphoma; *EBV,* Epstein-Barr virus; *F,* female; *HIV,* human immunodeficiency virus; *HRS,* Hodgkin Reed-Sternberg; *L&H,* lymphocytic and histiocytic; *LP,* lymphoplasmacytic; *M,* male.
From McPherson RA, Pincus MR: *Henry's clinical diagnosis and management by laboratory methods,* ed 23, St Louis, 2017, Elsevier.

TABLE 2 Cotswold-Modified Ann Arbor Staging System for Hodgkin Lymphoma

Stage	Criteria
I	Disease affecting a single lymph node region or lymphoid structure (e.g., spleen, thymus, Waldeyer ring)
II	Disease affecting two or more discrete lymph node regions confined to the same side of the diaphragm
III	Disease affecting two or more discrete lymph node regions or lymphoid structures on both sides of the diaphragm
IV	Disease that has spread to one or more extranodal sites (that do not meet the criteria for E) or extralymphatic structure including involvement of the bone marrow, liver, or lungs
Designation	**Criteria**
A	Absence of B symptoms[a]
B	Presence of B symptoms[a]
S	Involvement of the spleen
E	Single extranodal site or involvement of an extranodal site that is contiguous to an involved nodal region
X	Bulky disease as defined as >1/3 mediastinum at its widest part or a nodal mass >10 cm at its greatest diameter

[a]B symptoms: Constitutional symptoms including night sweats, fevers, or weight loss (>10% over 6 mo).
From Hoffman R et al: *Hematology, basic principles and practice,* ed 7, Philadelphia, 2018, Elsevier.

bleomycin, continuing with four cycles of AVD. BEACOPP is an intensified regimen consisting of bleomycin, etoposide, doxorubicin, cyclophosphamide, vincristine, procarbazine, and prednisone. It results in better initial tumor control, but the long-term survival may not significantly differ from ABVD, and the rate of complications is higher (including 3% rate of treatment-related death, secondary leukemias, and universal infertility).

BV-AVD is a combination of brentuximab vedotin (a CD30-targeting antibody-drug conjugate) and doxorubicin, vinblastine, and dacarbazine. In patients with previously untreated stage III or IV classic Hodgkin lymphoma,[1] this regimen provides improved modified progression-free survival compared with ABVD, although with higher rates of neutropenia and neuropathy.

- Recommendations for the primary treatment of Hodgkin lymphoma outside of clinical trials are described in Table 5.
- Patients who experience recurrent or refractory disease typically receive second-line (salvage) chemotherapy followed by consolidative autologous stem cell transplantation, although in some cases radiation therapy can be used.
- Patients who experience recurrent Hodgkin lymphoma after second-line treatment can receive further effective treatment using targeted immunotherapy.
- Brentuximab vedotin is an anti-CD30 antibody drug conjugate associated with an overall response rate of 75% in relapsed/refractory Hodgkin lymphoma. It can also be used as a maintenance therapy for high-risk patients undergoing autologous stem cell transplantation.
- Checkpoint inhibitors are monoclonal antibodies targeting the programmed death 1 (PD-1) molecule (present on T cells) or its ligands (present on Hodgkin/Reed-Sternberg cells). This group includes agents such as nivolumab and pembrolizumab, which are both approved for treatment of relapsed/refractory Hodgkin lymphoma. The overall response rate to nivolumab among patients with Hodgkin lymphoma who relapsed after autologous stem cell transplant and posttransplant brentuximab vedotin was 65%. The overall response rate to pembrolizumab among patients with Hodgkin lymphoma relapsing after ≥3 lines of therapy was 69%.

DISPOSITION

- Classic Hodgkin lymphoma is cured in >95% of patients with early favorable disease, about 85% of those with early unfavorable disease, and 75% to 80% of those with advanced-stage disease.
- Stage is the principal prognostic factor, although in advanced-stage disease, the International Prognostic Score can further stratify prognosis (Table 6)
- Unlike escalated BEACOPP, ABVD is not associated with a risk of leukemia.
- Mediastinal irradiation increases the risk of subsequent cardiac disease, including valvular and pericardial disease, accelerated coronary artery disease, and conduction abnormalities.

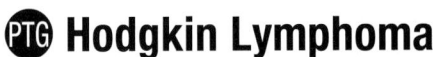

H

BOX 1   Recommended Staging Procedures for Hodgkin Lymphoma

The following staging procedures are recommended for the initial workup of Hodgkin lymphoma:
1. Adequate surgical biopsy reviewed by an experienced hematopathologist
2. Cytologic examination of any effusion in selected cases
3. Detailed history, with attention to the presence or absence of systemic symptoms, and a careful physical examination, emphasizing node chains, size of the liver and spleen, and inspection of Waldeyer ring
4. Routine laboratory tests: Complete blood cell count, erythrocyte sedimentation rate, liver and kidney function tests, and HIV serology
5. Neck, chest, and abdominal CT imaging fused with 18-fluorodeoxyglucose (FDG) PET scan (Fig. E3)

From Goldman L, Schafer AI: *Goldman's Cecil medicine*, ed 24, Philadelphia, 2012, Saunders.

TABLE 3   Standard Treatment Approach According to Prognostic Group

Early-favorable HL	Combined modality therapy • 2-4 cycles of chemotherapy followed by involved-field radiotherapy
Early-unfavorable HL (intermediate-stage)	Combined modality therapy • 4-6 cycles of chemotherapy followed by involved-field radiotherapy
Advanced HL	Extensive chemotherapy • 6 cycles of chemotherapy ± consolidation with localized radiotherapy

HL, Hodgkin lymphoma.
From Hoffman R et al: *Hematology, basic principles and practice*, ed 7, Philadelphia, 2018, Elsevier.

TABLE 4   Standard Chemotherapy Regimens for the Treatment of Advanced Hodgkin Lymphoma

Regimen	Drugs	Route	Schedule
ABVD	Doxorubicin 25 mg/m^2	IV	Day 1 and 15
	Bleomycin 10 mg/m^2	IV	Day 1 and 15
	Vinblastine 6 mg/m^2	IV	Day 1 and 15
	Dacarbazine 375 mg/m^2	IV	Day 1 and 15
			Every 28 days
BEACOPP (escalated)	Bleomycin 10 mg/m^2	IV	Day 8
	Etoposide 200 mg/m^2	IV	Day 1-3
	Doxorubicin 35 mg/m^2	IV	Day 1
	Cyclophosphamide 1250 mg/m^2	IV	Day 1
	Vincristine 1.4 mg/m^2	IV	Day 8
	Procarbazine 100 mg/m^2	PO	Days 1-7
	Prednisolone 40 mg/m^2	PO	Days 1-14
	G-CSF	SC	From day 8
			Every 21 days

ABVD, Adriamycin (doxorubicin), bleomycin, vinblastine, dacarbazine; *BEACOPP*, bleomycin, etoposide, Adriamycin (doxorubicin), cyclophosphamide, Oncovin (vincristine), procarbazine, and prednisone; *G-CSF*, granulocyte colony-stimulating factor; *IV*, intravenous; *PO*, by mouth; *SC*, subcutaneous.
From Hoffman R et al: *Hematology, basic principles and practice*, ed 7, Philadelphia, 2018, Elsevier.

• Radiation therapy increases the risk of developing secondary solid tumors, especially breast cancer in women younger than age 30 yr.
• Table 7 describes potential late complications of Hodgkin lymphoma treatment and appropriate clinical responses and preventive strategies during survivorship phase.

REFERRAL

• To surgery for lymph node biopsy
• Fertility clinic for sperm banking
• Hematology/oncology
• Radiation oncology, in selected cases

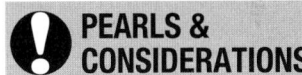 **PEARLS & CONSIDERATIONS**

COMMENTS

• Young male patients should consider sperm banking before the initiation of therapy even though the risk of infertility with ABVD is low. Symptomatic males, particularly with advanced stage Hodgkin lymphoma, may have disease-related oligospermia at diagnosis.
• Chemotherapy with or without involved-field radiotherapy should be the standard treatment for Hodgkin lymphoma with early-stage disease. Chemotherapy is the standard of care for advanced stage.
• After failure of ABVD therapy, more than 60% of patients who have had a relapse and about 30% of patients with initially refractory lymphoma can be cured with subsequent therapy.
• Classic Hodgkin lymphoma has the highest rate of response to immunotherapy with checkpoint inhibitors among all human cancers. These treatments are actively investigated for first-line therapy.

REFERENCE & SUGGESTED READINGS

Available at eBooks.Health.Elsevier.com.

RELATED CONTENT

Hodgkin Lymphoma (Patient Information)

AUTHOR: **ADAM J. OLSZEWSKI, MD**

TABLE 5 Recommendations for the Primary Treatment of Hodgkin Lymphoma Outside of Clinical Trials

Group	Stage	Recommendation
Early favorable	CS I-II A, no RFs	2 cycles ABVD + ISRT (20 Gy) (or 3-4 cycles or ABVD alone)
Early unfavorable	CS I-II A/B + RFs	4-6 cycles ABVD ±30 Gy for nonbulky disease 4-6 cycles ABVD + 30 Gy for bulky disease
Advanced stages	CS IIB + RFs, CS III A/B, CS IV A/B	6 cycles ABVD (deescalated to AVD among patients with negative PET after 2 cycles); 6 cycles BV-AVD BEACOPP-escalated *or* BEACOPP-14 ± RT, 20-30 Gy for residual tumor (PET positive) and/or bulky disease

ABVD regimen, doxorubicin, vinblastine, bleomycin, and dacarbazine; *BEACOPP-baseline* regimen, bleomycin, etoposide, doxorubicin, cyclophosphamide, vincristine, procarbazine, and prednisone; *BEACOPP-escalated* regimen, bleomycin, etoposide, doxorubicin, cyclophosphamide, vincristine, procarbazine, prednisone, and G-CSF; *BEACOPP-14* regimen, bleomycin, etoposide, doxorubicin, cyclophosphamide, vincristine, procarbazine, prednisone, and G-CSF; *BV-AVD*, brentuximab, vedotin, doxorubicin, vinblastine, and dacarbazine; *CS*, clinical stage; *IF*, involved field; *ISRT*, involved-site radiation therapy; *MOPP* regimen, mechlorethamine, Oncovin (vincristine), procarbazine, and prednisone; *PET*, positron emission tomography; *RF*, risk factors; *RT*, radiation therapy; *Stanford V* regimen, nitrogen mustard, doxorubicin, vinblastine, bleomycin, vincristine, etoposide, and prednisone.

TABLE 6 International Prognostic Score (IPS) for Advanced Hodgkin Lymphoma

No. of Prognostic Factors	% of patients	5-yr FFP (%)	5-yr OS (%)
0-1 (low-risk)	29	79	90
2-3 (intermediate-risk)	52	64	80
4-7 (high-risk)	19	47	59

Risk factors: (1) serum albumin <4 g/dl; (2) hemoglobin <10.5 g/dl; (3) male sex; (4) stage IV disease by Ann Arbor classification; (5) age ≥45 yr; (6) white cell count ≥15,000/mm^3; and (7) absolute lymphocyte count <600/mm^3 or <8% of all white blood cells

FFP, Freedom from progression; *OS*, overall survival.
From Hoffman R et al: *Hematology, basic principles and practice*, ed 7, Philadelphia, 2018, Elsevier.

TABLE 7 Potential Late Complications of Hodgkin Lymphoma Treatment and Appropriate Clinical Responses and Preventive Strategies

Risk/Problem	Incidence/Response
Dental caries	Neck or oropharyngeal irradiation can cause decreased salivation. Patients should have careful dental care follow-up and should make their dentist aware of the previous irradiation.
Hypothyroidism	Thyroid irradiation during curative therapy for Hodgkin lymphoma leads to hypothyroidism in >50% of patients. All patients whose TSH level becomes elevated should be treated with lifelong thyroxine replacement in doses sufficient to suppress TSH levels to low normal. This is also necessary to ensure that the radiation-damaged thyroid is not subjected to long-term stimulation by thyroid-stimulating hormone, which can increase the risk of thyroid neoplasm.
Infertility	ABVD is not known to cause permanent gonadal toxicity, although oligospermia for 1-2 yr after treatment is common. Direct or scatter radiation to gonadal tissue can cause infertility, amenorrhea, or premature menopause, but this seldom occurs with the current fields used for the treatment of Hodgkin lymphoma. Thus with the current chemotherapy regimens and radiation fields used, most patients will not develop these problems. In general, after treatment, women who continue menstruating are fertile, but men require semen analysis to provide a specific answer. High-dose chemoradiotherapy and hematopoietic stem cell transplantation almost always cause permanent infertility in both genders, although some young women occasionally recover fertility.
Impaired immunity to infections	Hodgkin lymphoma and its treatment can lead to lifelong impairment of full immunity to infection. All patients should be given annual influenza immunization and pneumococcal immunization every 5 yr. Patients whose spleen has been irradiated or removed should also be immunized against meningococcal types A and C and *Haemophilus influenzae* type B. As for all adults, diphtheria, tetanus, and COVID-19 immunizations should be kept up-to-date.
Secondary neoplasms	Although uncommon, certain secondary neoplasms occur with increased frequency in patients who have been treated for Hodgkin lymphoma. These include acute myelogenous leukemia, thyroid, breast, lung, and upper gastrointestinal carcinoma and melanoma, and cervical carcinoma in situ. It is appropriate to screen for these neoplasms for the rest of the patient's life because they might have lengthy induction periods. Women who undergo breast irradiation before age 30 benefit from intensified breast cancer screening using MRI.

ABVD, Adriamycin, bleomycin, vinblastine, dacarbazine; *MRI*, magnetic resonance imaging; *TSH*, thyroid-stimulating hormone.
From Abeloff MD: *Clinical oncology*, ed 3, Philadelphia, 2004, Saunders.

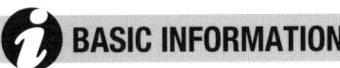

BASIC INFORMATION

DEFINITION

The human immunodeficiency virus (HIV) is a retrovirus that is responsible for causing acquired immunodeficiency syndrome (AIDS). HIV infection does not necessarily mean a person has AIDS. Table 1 summarizes surveillance case definition for HIV.

SYNONYMS

HIV
AIDS: The result of progressive HIV infection in which a person has a weakened immune system and meets specific diagnostic criteria (See "Acquired Immunodeficiency Syndrome" in Section I and Table 2.)

ICD-10CM CODE

B20 Human immunodeficiency virus (HIV) disease

EPIDEMIOLOGY & DEMOGRAPHICS (IN U.S.)

- An estimated 1.2 million people in the United States are infected with HIV, and approximately 14% of them do not know they are infected.[1]
- Worldwide each year, an estimated 1.3 million persons living with HIV become pregnant. The vast majority of pregnant persons living with HIV reside in low- and middle-income countries with limited access to anti-viral therapy (ART) and in the absence of ART, 15% to 30% of infants born to persons with HIV acquire HIV antenatally or perinatally, with additional transmission during breast feeding.[1a]
- There are ~38,000 new HIV diagnoses each year, according to the Centers for Disease Control and Prevention (CDC).[1]
- Incidence is highest among gay, bisexual, and other men who have sex with men (MSM) and African American/Black and Hispanic/Latino populations.

PREDOMINANT RISK GROUPS:

- Gay, bisexual, and other MSM is the group most affected by HIV.
- MSM account for approximately two thirds of all new diagnoses each year, according to the CDC.[1]
- HIV disproportionately affects MSM of younger age and African American/Black and Hispanic/Latino background.
- Heterosexual transmission accounts for ~25% of new HIV diagnosis. Injection drug use accounts for ~6% to 7%.
- Table 3 summarizes risk factors associated with sexual transmission of HIV.

RACIAL DATA:

- African American/Black individuals account for >40% of all new HIV diagnoses despite being 12% of the U.S. population.[1]
- Hispanics/Latinos account for >25% of all new HIV diagnoses despite being 18% of the U.S. population.

GENETICS:

Familial Disposition

Individuals with deletions in the *CCR5* gene are immune from infection with macrophage tropic virus (the predominant virus in sexual transmission).[2] Other genetic variants may contribute to rapid progression or long-term control of the virus once infected. One in 300 individuals infected with HIV is an "elite controller," which means they are able to maintain a normal CD4 count and undetectable viral load through immune control.[3]

Congenital Infection

- Fewer than 100 children a year <13 yr receive a diagnosis of perinatally acquired HIV, according to the CDC.[4]
- No specific congenital abnormalities are associated with HIV infection, although there is a higher risk of spontaneous abortion and low birth weight.

Neonatal Infection

- May occur during delivery or via breastfeeding.
- Typically asymptomatic.
- All pregnant women should be tested for HIV and, if positive, take anteretrovirals (ARVs).[5]

PHYSICAL FINDINGS & CLINICAL PRESENTATION

- Signs and symptoms are variable with stage of disease (Fig. 1).

TABLE 2 Surveillance Definitions of AIDS-Defining Conditions

Opportunistic Infections:
- *Pneumocystis jiroveci (carinii)*
- *Mycobacterium avium* complex
- *Mycobacterium tuberculosis*
- Toxoplasmosis
- Candidiasis: Esophageal and systemic
- Histoplasmosis
- Cryptococcosis
- Cryptosporidiosis and isosporiasis
- Leishmaniasis
- Cytomegalovirus disease
- Recurrent bacterial infections (≥2 episodes/yr)

Lymphomas

Kaposi Sarcoma

Cervical Cancer

AIDS Dementia Syndrome

Wasting Syndrome

AIDS, Acquired immunodeficiency syndrome.
From Hoffman R et al: *Hematology: basic principles and practice*, ed 7, Philadelphia, 2018, Elsevier.

TABLE 3 Risk Factors Associated With Sexual Transmission of HIV

Sexually transmitted infections
    Ulcerative or nonulcerative diseases
Genital tract inflammation
HIV disease
    Higher viral loads
    Lower CD4+ levels
    Acute HIV infection
    Lack of effective antiretroviral therapy
    Lack of heterozygosity or homozygosity for the inactivating 32-base pair deletion in the chemokine receptor gene *(CCR5)*
Anatomic factors
    Lack of circumcision
    Cervical ectopy
    Leukocytospermia
    Hormonal contraception
Sexual practices
    Receptive anal intercourse
    Sexual activity during menses
    Bleeding during intercourse (disruption of vaginal mucosa through trauma)
    Lack of barrier protection
HIV viral features
    Syncytium formation
    Certain viral clades

From Bennett JE et al: *Mandell, Douglas, and Bennett's principles and practice of infectious diseases*, ed 8, Philadelphia, 2015, Saunders.

TABLE 1 Surveillance Case Definition for HIV Infection in Adults and Adolescents (Age >13 yr)

Stage	Laboratory Evidence	Clinical Evidence
Stage 1	Laboratory confirmation of HIV infection and CD4+ T-lymphocyte count of ≥500 cells/μL or CD4+ T-lymphocyte percentage of ≥29%[a]	No AIDS-defining condition (see Table 2)
Stage 2	Laboratory confirmation of HIV infection and CD4+ T-lymphocyte count of 200-499 cells/μL or CD4+ T-lymphocyte percentage of 14%-28%[a]	No AIDS-defining condition (see Table 2)
Stage 3	Laboratory confirmation of HIV infection and CD4+ T-lymphocyte count of <200 cells/μL or CD4+ T-lymphocyte percentage of <14%[a]	Documentation of an AIDS-defining condition with laboratory confirmation of HIV infection (see Table 2)
Stage unknown	Laboratory confirmation of HIV infection and no information on CD4+ T-lymphocyte count or percentage	No information on presence of an AIDS-defining condition

[a]The CD4+ T-lymphocyte percentage is a percentage of the total lymphocyte count.
AIDS, Acquired immunodeficiency syndrome.
From Hoffman R et al: *Hematology: basic principles and practice*, ed 7, Philadelphia, 2018, Elsevier.

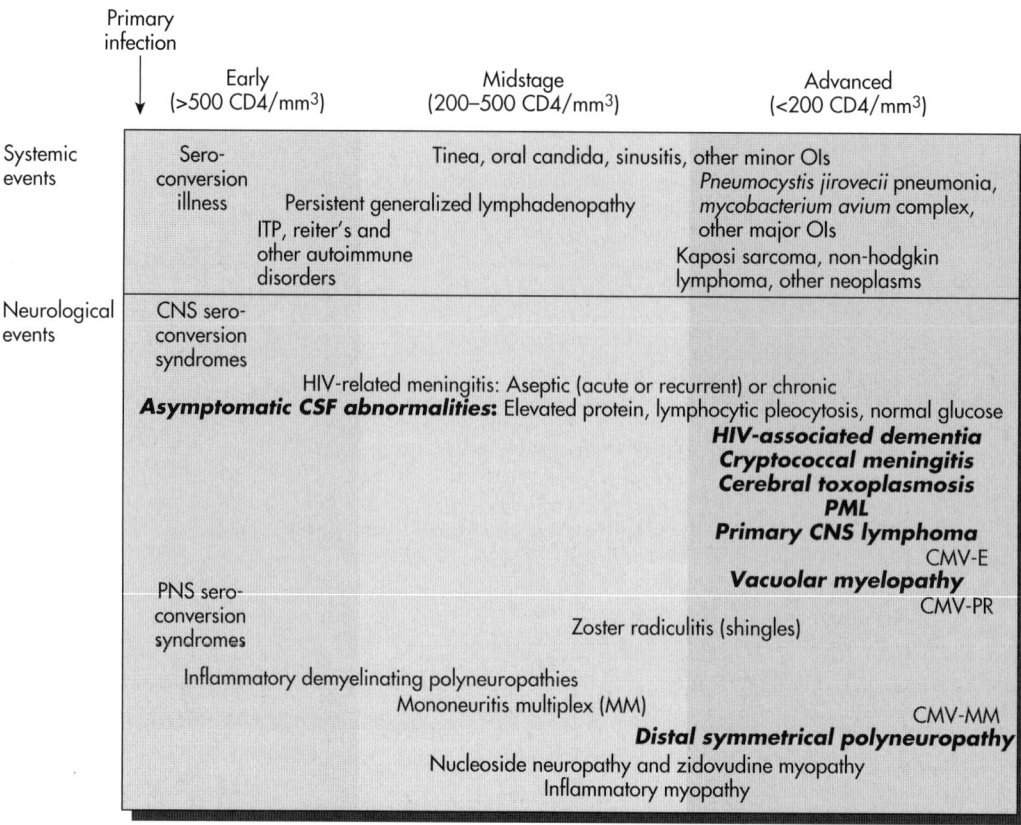

FIG. 1 Systemic and neurologic events in human immunodeficiency virus (HIV) infection. Temporal sequence is approximate and indicates the increasing risk of systemic and neurologic complications as HIV infection advances. *CMV-E,* Cytomegalovirus encephalitis; *CMV-PR,* CMV polyradiculitis; *CNS,* central nervous system; *CSF,* cerebrospinal fluid; *ITP,* idiopathic thrombocytopenic purpura; *OIs,* opportunistic infections; *PML,* progressive multifocal leukoencephalopathy; *PNS,* peripheral nervous system. (From Jankovic J et al: *Bradley and Daroff's neurology in clinical practice,* ed 8, Philadelphia, 2022, Elsevier.)

- Acute HIV infection (0 to 3 mo, usually within several weeks)[6]:
  1. Causes a self-limited mononucleosis-like illness in 50% to 80% of individuals, characterized by fever, sore throat, lymphadenopathy, headache, and a rash resembling roseola. Individuals may also be asymptomatic.
  2. In a minority of acute cases, aseptic meningitis, Bell palsy, or peripheral neuropathy may occur.
  3. Opportunistic infections such as thrush or *Pneumocystis jiroveci* pneumonia (PJP) may occur.
- Chronic HIV infection is usually characterized by a prolonged asymptomatic "latent" phase without symptoms followed by nonspecific symptoms of lymphadenopathy, fatigue, weight loss, diarrhea, and skin changes, including seborrheic dermatitis, localized herpes zoster, and/or fungal infection.
- Advanced disease is characterized by AIDS-associated diseases, including infections and malignancies (see specific disorders). Anemia may be multifactorial (Table 4).
- HIV infection in women may be associated with lower levels of viral load at comparable degrees of immunosuppression when compared with men. Furthermore, women may, on average, have higher CD4 counts at the time of HIV diagnosis.

- Another special consideration in women infected with HIV is the high incidence of human papillomavirus (HPV) coinfection and risk for cervical cancer. HIV-positive women should be screened for cervical cancer at time of initial HIV diagnosis and annually thereafter if Pap testing is normal.[7] If the results of three consecutive Pap tests are normal, then follow-up testing can occur every 3 yr. HPV vaccination is also recommended in men and women 9 to 26 yr who are HIV positive (three doses at 0, 1 to 2, and 6 mo). For adults aged 27 to 45 yr, clinicians should discuss and may consider HPV vaccination in persons who are most likely to benefit.
- Coinfection with HIV and hepatitis C virus (HCV) is common because of similar transmission risk. Hepatitis C is most commonly transmitted by contaminated needles or blood exposure. HCV can be transmitted sexually, but the risk is low. Patients with HIV and HCV progress faster to cirrhosis. Patients may already have signs of advanced liver disease at the time of diagnosis.

ETIOLOGY

- HIV is a single-stranded ribonucleic acid (RNA) retrovirus (Fig. E2) that is categorized as type 1 or 2.
- HIV-1 was derived from transmission of a simian immunodeficiency virus (SIV) from

chimpanzees in Central Africa; HIV-2 was derived from an SIV found in sooty mangabey monkeys from West Africa.[8]
- HIV-1 is the predominant pathogenic retrovirus in human populations; HIV-2 has limited distribution (primarily West Africa) and tends to progress less rapidly than HIV-1. HIV-2 should be considered in individuals from West Africa or whose sexual partners are from West Africa.
- HIV is transmitted by sexual contact, shared needles, blood transfusion, or from mother to child during pregnancy, delivery, or breastfeeding.
- Primary target of infection: CD4 lymphocytes.

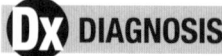 **DIAGNOSIS**

DIFFERENTIAL DIAGNOSIS

- Acute HIV infection: Often diagnosed or confused with mononucleosis or other respiratory viral infections.
- Late symptoms: Similar to those produced by other wasting/chronic illnesses such as neoplasms, tuberculosis (TB), disseminated fungal infection (such as *Candida*), malabsorption, or depression.
- HIV-related encephalopathy: Confused with Alzheimer disease or other causes of chronic dementia (cognitive impairment in HIV infection is described in another chapter in Section

TABLE 4 Etiology of Anemia in Human Immunodeficiency Virus

TABLE 4 Etiology of Anemia in Human Immunodeficiency Virus

HIV Related

HIV Infection
- Anemia of chronic disease
- Blunted production/response to erythropoietin
- Suppression of CFU-GEMM (HIV/inflammatory cytokines)

Neoplasms Infiltrating BM

Non-Hodgkin lymphoma, KS, Hodgkin lymphoma

Infections of the BM
- Parvovirus B19
- Atypical mycobacteria (MAI/MAC)
- *Mycobacterium* tuberculosis
- *Histoplasma*
- CMV

Medications Causing Decreased Production	Medications Causing Hemolysis
• RT inhibitors	• Indinavir
• Ganciclovir	• Bactrim and Dapsone in G6PD deficiency
• Bactrim	
• Amphotericin B	

HIV Unrelated
- B$_{12}$ and/or folic acid deficiencies
- Iron deficiency caused by chronic blood loss

BM, Bone marrow; *CFU-GEMM*, colony-forming unit–granulocyte, erythrocyte, macrophage, megakaryocyte; *CMV*, cytomegalovirus; *G6PD*, glucose-6-phosphate dehydrogenase; *KS*, Kaposi sarcoma; *MAC*, mycobacterium avium complex; *MAI*, mycobacterium avium-intracellulare; *RT*, reverse transcriptase.
From Hoffman R et al: *Hematology: basic principles and practice*, ed 7, Philadelphia, 2018, Elsevier.

I); myelopathy and neuropathy possibly resembling other demyelinating diseases such as multiple sclerosis.
- Direct central nervous system (CNS) involvement: Manifests as encephalopathy, myelopathy, or neuropathy in advanced cases. Table 5 summarizes neuromuscular syndromes in HIV infection.
- Renal failure, rheumatologic disorders (Table 6), thrombocytopenia, or cardiac abnormalities (Table E7) may be seen in association with HIV-1.

WORKUP

Diagnosis is established by testing for HIV-1 or HIV-2 antibodies in the blood. The CDC recommends routine testing for patients in all health care settings unless the patient declines (opt-out screening). This includes routine testing of pregnant women. It is also recommended that separate written consent should no longer be required, although by law this is being addressed on a state-by-state basis. Generally, all persons aged 13 to 64 yr should undergo HIV testing at least once and more frequently (at least once a year) if risk factors.[9] For individuals who may be at higher risk (e.g., men who are having sex with multiple other men), 3 to 6 mo is recommended.

An FDA-approved at-home rapid HIV screening test is available. It uses swabs of oral fluids from upper and lower gums. A positive test requires confirmatory testing. Clinicians should be aware of the "window period" (i.e., an antibody test may take up to 3 mo to become "reactive" in a person with newly acquired HIV infection).

LABORATORY TESTS

HIV antibodies are detected by a two-step technique:
- An initial screening test (i.e., either an antibody/antigen test or an antibody test).
- Confirmation of an initial positive screening test with more specific assays. The classic confirmatory test is the Western blot, but other modalities may be used. Fig. 3 illustrates the laboratory diagnosis of HIV infection.
- Screening antibody tests generally measure HIV-1 and HIV-2 antibodies. Confirmatory tests will generally differentiate between HIV-1 and HIV-2 as well. However, commercial viral load assays (HIV RNA polymerase chain reaction [PCR]) are specific only for HIV-1 in the United States.
- Fourth-generation antibody/antigen tests can detect the "p24" antigen, which is present early in HIV infection and can be used to diagnose HIV earlier than previous generations. An HIV RNA PCR still should be sent if acute HIV infection is suspected.
- Baseline viral resistance testing (e.g., genotype) is recommended for all newly diagnosed patients with HIV to guide choice of antiretroviral therapy (ART).
- The CD4 count and HIV viral load (e.g., HIV RNA PCR) should be measured in all patients.
- The CD4 count is a marker of current immune status. Table 8 describes the World Health Organization (WHO) immunologic classification for established HIV infection.
- The HIV RNA PCR (viral load) is predictive of disease progression.

TABLE 5 Neuromuscular Syndromes in Human Immunodeficiency Virus Type 1 Infection

Diagnosis	Disease Stage	Clinical Features	Diagnostic Studies	Treatment
AIDP CIDP	Early > late	Weakness more than sensory loss	CSF: ↑ WBCs ↑↑ Protein NCS: Demyelination	Early: IVIG, steroids, plasmapheresis Late: Consider ganciclovir/foscarnet
MM	Early or late	Multiple painful mononeuropathies	NCS: Multifocal axonal neuropathy Biopsy: Inflammation/vasculitis CMV	Early: None Late: Steroids/cyclophosphamide Ganciclovir/foscarnet
Nucleoside Neuropathy	Any stage	Distal sensory loss Neuropathic pain	NCS: Distal axonopathy Increased serum lactate	Nucleoside withdrawal
DSPN	Late	Distal sensory loss Neuropathic pain	NCS: Distal axonopathy	NSAIDs, capsaicin AED, tricyclics
PP	Late	Progressive flaccid paraparesis, urinary dysfunction, LS pain	CSF: Increased WBCs (PMNs), CMV PCR+	Ganciclovir/foscarnet Cidofovir
DILS	Late	Sjögren syndrome, distal motor and sensory loss, pain	NCS: Axonal neuropathy Biopsy: CD8+ T cells, HIV-1	Zidovudine/ART Steroids
Zidovudine Myopathy	Any stage	Proximal weakness Myalgias	EMG: ± irritative Biopsy: Ragged red fibers	Zidovudine withdrawal
Polymyositis	Any stage	Proximal weakness Myalgias	EMG: ± irritative Biopsy: Inflammatory infiltrates	Steroids, IVIG Immunosuppressants
ALS-like	Late	Weakness, dysphagia	EMG: Neurogenic	ART

AED, Antiepileptic drug; *AIDP*, acute inflammatory demyelinating polyneuropathy; *ALS*, amyotrophic lateral sclerosis; *ART*, antiretroviral therapy; *CIDP*, chronic inflammatory demyelinating polyneuropathy; *CMV*, cytomegalovirus; *CSF*, cerebrospinal fluid; *DILS*, diffuse infiltrative lymphocytosis syndrome; *DSPN*, distal sensory polyneuropathy; *EMG*, electromyography; *IVIG*, intravenous immunoglobulin; *LS*, lumbosacral; *MM*, mononeuritis multiplex; *NCS*, nerve conduction studies; *NSAID*, nonsteroidal antiinflammatory drug; *PCR*, polymerase chain reaction; *PMNs*, polymorphonuclear leukocytes; *PP*, progressive polyradiculopathy; *WBCs*, white blood cells.
From Bennett JE et al: *Mandell, Douglas, and Bennett's principles and practice of infectious diseases*, ed 8, Philadelphia, 2015, Saunders.

TABLE 6 Rheumatic Diseases Associated With or Occurring in Patients With HIV Infection

Unique to HIV Infection
1. Diffuse infiltrative lymphocytosis syndrome
2. HIV-associated arthritis
3. Zidovudine-associated myopathy
4. Painful articular syndrome

Encountered in HIV-Infected Patients
1. HIV-associated reactive arthritis
2. Polymyositis
3. Psoriatic arthritis
4. Polyarteritis nodosa
5. Giant cell arteritis
6. Hypersensitivity angiitis
7. Granulomatosis with polyangiitis
8. Henoch-Schönlein purpura
9. Behçet's disease
10. Infectious arthritis (bacterial, fungal)

Ameliorated by HIV Infection but Worsening or Reappearing With IRIS
1. Rheumatoid arthritis
2. Systemic lupus erythematosus
3. Sarcoidosis

IRIS, Immune reconstitution inflammatory syndrome.
From Firestein GS et al: *Firestein & Kelley's textbook of rheumatology,* ed 11, Philadelphia, 2021, Elsevier.

- Rapid serologic tests have been increasingly used and are useful in specific settings: Occupational exposures, pregnant women in labor without previous testing, and patients in high seroprevalence areas (for immediate results). Specimens are either blood or saliva and results are given within 1 to 20 min. Although sensitivity is high (99%), false-positive tests are more common in low seroprevalence populations. Thus, all positive results must be confirmed with standard serology.
- Early during infection (i.e., acute HIV infection), standard antibody tests may be negative ("window period"). The fourth-generation antibody/antigen test reduces this window period. The standard for diagnosing HIV during acute infection is by testing for HIV RNA (viral load).
- Table 9 compares the WHO and CDC staging systems.

🆁🆇 TREATMENT

NONPHARMACOLOGIC THERAPY
Maintenance of adequate nutrition

ACUTE GENERAL Rx
Acute management of opportunistic infections and malignancies (see "AIDS-associated disorders," "Pneumonia, *Pneumocystis jiroveci (carinii);*" "Cryptococcosis;" "Tuberculosis, Pulmonary;" "*Cryptosporidium* Infection;" "Toxoplasmosis;" etc., elsewhere in this text)

CHRONIC Rx
All HIV-infected patients should be considered for ART regardless of CD4 cell count. The benefit of ART is well established in preventing progression to AIDS and associated opportunistic infections. Furthermore, individuals who are on ART and undetectable are highly unlikely to transmit HIV to others (i.e., "Treatment as Prevention"). Identifying individuals with HIV as soon as possible and prescribing ART is the basis of effective public health approaches to addressing HIV. Updated guidelines are available for further recommendiates.[10]

- Therapy is strongly recommended for all patients with established HIV infection regardless of the CD4 count. Most people with chronic HIV infection are asymptomatic. ART is recommended regardless of CD4 cell counts. The recommendations are due to the safety and benefit of newer antivirals in preventing AIDS and decreasing both morbidity and mortality. Earlier treatment may also help reduce transmission of the virus to others due to reductions in viral loads.
- ART generally consists of using a three-drug regimen to treat HIV infection. Classes of antiretrovirals include[11]:
  1. Nucleoside/nucleotide reverse transcriptase inhibitor (NRTI): Zidovudine (AZT), lamivudine (3TC), emtricitabine (FTC), tenofovir disoproxil fumarate (TDF), tenofovir alafenamide (TAF), and abacavir (ABC).
  2. Protease inhibitors (PI): Lopinavir/ritonavir, atazanavir, fosamprenavir, darunavir, saquinavir, and tipranavir. These PIs may be "boosted" by ritonavir or cobicistat to increase levels.
  3. Nonnucleoside reverse transcriptase inhibitors (NNRTI): Nevirapine, efavirenz, etravirine, doravirine, or rilpivirine.
  4. Integrase inhibitors (II): Raltegravir, elvitegravir, bictegravir, dolutegravir, and cabotegravir.
  5. Fusion inhibitors: Enfuvirtide (T-20). This drug is administered through subcutaneous injections and is only used as part of a salvage regimen for individuals who have failed multiple other regimens.
  6. CCR5 inhibitors: Maraviroc. Before using this drug, a viral trophism assay should be checked to determine if the virus uses the CCR5 coreceptor to infect cells. If the virus uses the CXCR4 coreceptor, this drug will not be effective.
  7. Postattachment inhibitors: Ibalizumab. Blocks CD4 receptors that HIV needs to enter cells with.
  8. Attachment inhibitors: Fostemsavir. Binds to the gp120 protein on the outer surface of HIV, preventing HIV from entering CD4 cells.
- Adding a fourth drug to the three-drug regimen does not improve viral suppression or outcomes and is not recommended. Treatment interruptions based upon CD4 responses appear harmful in recent comparative studies versus standard continuous treatment protocols and should be avoided. Antiretroviral

regimens for initial therapy are summarized in Table 10.
- Typical dosing regimen consists of two NRTIs and either an NNRTI, PI, or II. IIs are now the preferred third drug because of tolerability. Data support inclusion of lamivudine or emtricitabine as one of the two NRTIs.
- Two-drug regimens with specific antiretroviral medications may be an option in certain situations. Dolutegravir/lamivudine is the preferred option in appropriate clinical situations in which it is preferable to avoid other NRTIs such as abacavir and tenofovir-based regimens. Dolutegravir/lamivudine is not recommended for individuals with a higher viral load (>500,000 copies/ml), hepatitis B virus (HBV) and HIV coinfection, or when results of genotypic resistance testing are unavailable.
- Individuals with drug-resistant HIV may be on more complex and atypical regimens. Consultation with an HIV specialist is recommended.

Standard NRTIs include:
- Tenofovir disoproxil fumarate/emtricitabine 1 tablet once daily. Individuals with underlying renal dysfunction or requiring other nephrotoxic agents may be at increased risk of renal toxicity while taking tenofovir. TDF may also be associated with reductions in bone mineral density.
- Tenofovir alafenamide/emtricitabine 1 tablet once daily. TAF is a newer formulation of TDF with less nephrotoxicity and bone mineral density effects but may lead to increased weight gain. Both TDF/FTC and TAF/FTC are recommended components of the initial regimen (with a "backbone" medication). TDF should be avoided in patients with a creatinine clearance (CrCl) <60 ml/min. TAF should be avoided in patients with a CrCl <30 ml/min.
- Abacavir/lamivudine 1 tablet once daily. Abacavir may be associated with increased risk of myocardial infarction. Before using this drug, individuals should be checked for human leukocyte antigen (HLA)-B*5701. Individuals with this allele are at higher risk of serious hypersensitivity reactions, and this drug should be avoided.
- Zidovudine/lamivudine 1 tablet twice daily. Once widely prescribed; now rarely used due to lower efficacy compared with tenofovir-emtricitabine; zidovudine is associated with lipoatrophy and anemia, as well as GI and CNS side effects.

Standard backbone regimens include:
- Integrase inhibitors: (these are now considered first line):
  1. Bictegravir (50 mg once daily): Fixed-dose combination of bictegravir with the NRTIs TAF and FTC.
  2. Dolutegravir (50 mg once daily): Fixed-dose combination of dolutegravir and the NRTIs abacavir and lamivudine for once-daily treatment of HIV-1 infection. HLA-B*5701 should be checked first.
  3. Elvitegravir: Given with cobicistat (booster) and tenofovir/emtricitabine in a fixed-dose combination.

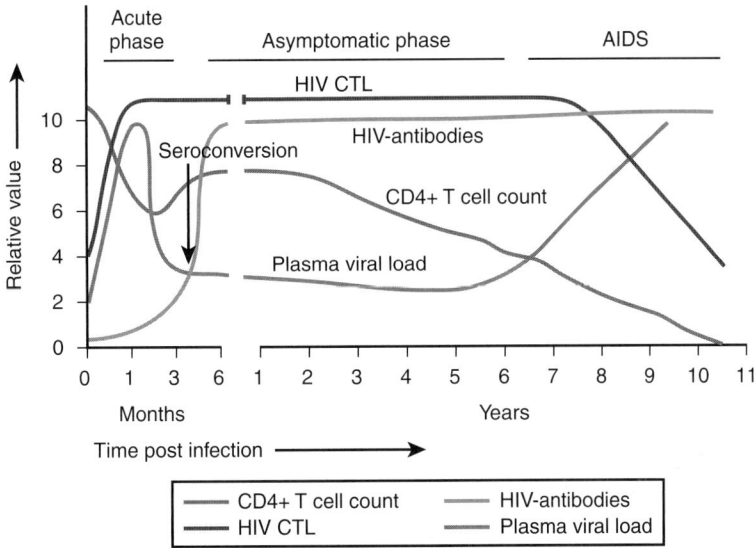

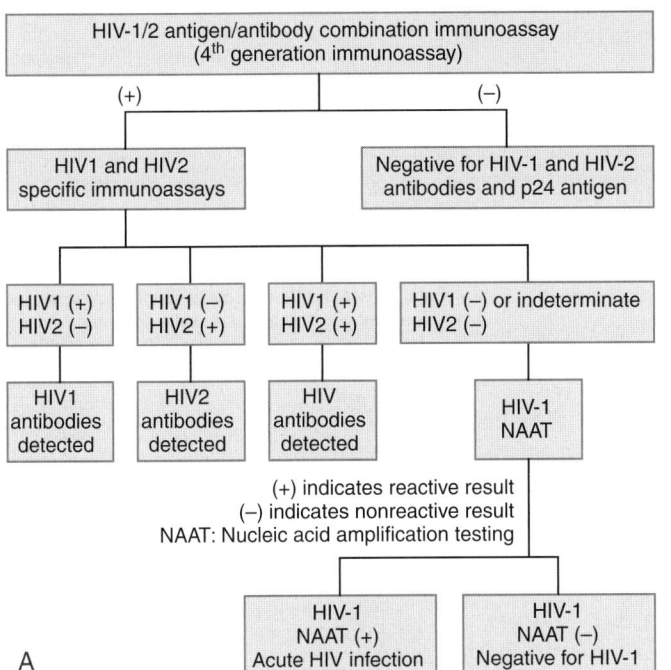

HIV-1/2 antigen/antibody combination immunoassay
(4th generation immunoassay)

(+)   (−)

HIV1 and HIV2 specific immunoassays   Negative for HIV-1 and HIV-2 antibodies and p24 antigen

| HIV1 (+) HIV2 (−) | HIV1 (−) HIV2 (+) | HIV1 (+) HIV2 (+) | HIV1 (−) or indeterminate HIV2 (−) |

| HIV1 antibodies detected | HIV2 antibodies detected | HIV antibodies detected | HIV-1 NAAT |

(+) indicates reactive result
(−) indicates nonreactive result
NAAT: Nucleic acid amplification testing

| HIV-1 NAAT (+) Acute HIV infection | HIV-1 NAAT (−) Negative for HIV-1 |

A

1. Screen with an HIV-1/2/p24 antibody/antigen assay. If negative, chances of an established HIV-1 or HIV-2 infection are low.
2. Test screen positive samples with immunoassay that differentiates between HIV-1 and HIV-2.
3. Specimens with a reactive screen and negative or indeterminate for HIV-1/HIV-2 differentiation need to be confirmed by HIV-1 NAAT.
    1. A reactive HIV-1 NAAT result and a nonreactive HIC-1/HIV-2 antibody differentiation immunoassay are consistent with laboratory evidence of acute HIV-1 infection.
    2. A reactive HIV-1 NAAT result and indeterminate HIV-1/HIV-2 antibody differentiation immunoassay indicate a false positive on the initial screen immunoassay.
    3. A negative HIV-1 NAAT results and nonreactive or indeterminate HIV-1/HIV-2 antibody differentiation immunoassay result are consistent with a false positive result on the initial screening immunoassay.
4. Laboratories should use this same testing algorithm, beginning with the antigen/antibody combination screen immunoassay, with serum or plasma specimens submitted for testing after a reactive result from any rapid HIV test.
5. No further testing is required for specimens that are nonreactive on the initial screening immunoassay.
6. Inconsistent or conflicting results should be investigated with follow-up testing on a newly collected specimen.

FIG. 3 Laboratory diagnosis of human immunodeficiency virus (HIV) infection. *AIDS,* Acquired immunodeficiency syndrome; *CTL,* cytotoxic T lymphocytes; *DNA,* deoxyribonucleic acid; *RNA,* ribonucleic acid. (From McPherson RA, Pincus MR: *Henry's clinical diagnosis and management by laboratory methods,* ed 23, Philadelphia, 2017, Elsevier.)

Assay	Comments

Prognosis/Monitoring Treatment

HIV viral load

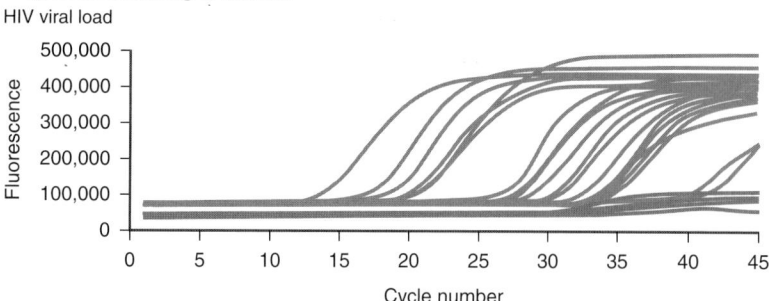

- The same method should be used for monitoring individual patients to minimize technical variation in HIV blood levels.
- HIV viral load testing is used to
  - Diagnose acute retroviral syndrome before seroconversion develops.
  - Assess prognosis and progression of HIV disease.
  - Guide antiretroviral therapy.
  - Define a baseline level so that response to therapy can be measured.
  - Monitor response to therapy.
- Greater than 0.5 log (threefold) change in blood HIV load is considered clinically significant.
- Genotypic assays are helpful in antiretroviral-naive patients for initial assessment of treatment options. Genotyping is also useful for patients who develop virologic failure with rising HIV viral load during highly active antiretroviral therapy, and need guidance for treatment modification.
- Genotyping detects changes in the nucleic acid sequence of the relevant HIV1 gene and identifies drug resistance by detecting mutations in the HIV1 genome that lead to specific amino acid substitutions in the HIV1 RT or protease enzymes.

Genotypic HIV assays

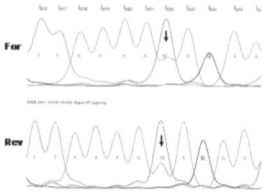

Resistance-associated reverse transcriptase (RT) mutation K103N
Resistance to nevirapine and efavirenz

Phenotypic assays

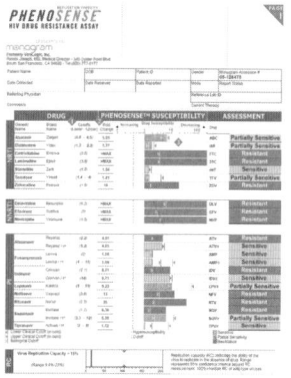

- Phenotypic assays amplify RT and protease genes from the patient's HIV predominant quasi-species virus RNA or proviral DNA. These amplicons are then inserted into a laboratory virus that lacks the genes, creating a hybrid virus. The hybrid virus is then propagated in cell culture, and its ability to propagate in the presence of varying concentrations of the anti-HIV agent is measured. Results are expressed as concentrations of drug required to inhibit 50% of growth (IC50) compared with a wild-type control strain.

Virtual phenotypes

B

- The patient's HIV genotype is compared with a database containing many known HIV drug-resistant and susceptible genotypes to predict the patient's response to therapy.

FIG. 3 cont'd

Assay	Comments
Immune Status	

Immune Status

CD4 cell counts
(% CD4 and absolute number)

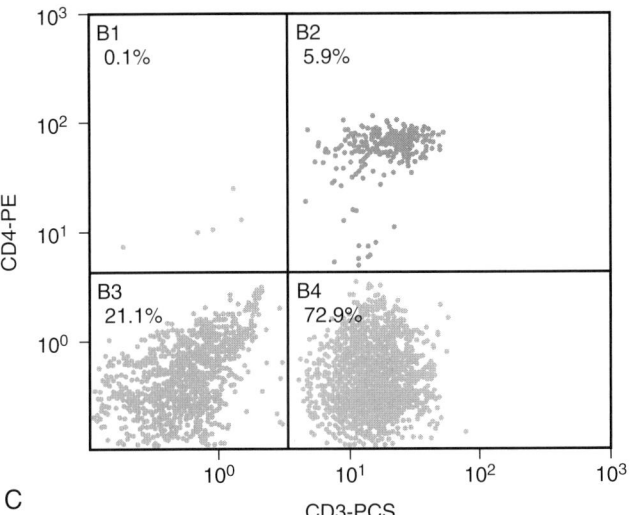

C

- CD4 cell count and CD4/CD8 ratio are used to
  - Stage HIV disease.
  - Help establish the risk of specific HIV-associated infectious or neoplastic complications.
  - Determine the need for prophylaxis against opportunistic infections.
  - Determine the need for and response to antiretroviral therapy.

FIG. 3 cont'd

TABLE 8 World Health Organization Immunologic Classification for Established HIV Infection

HIV-Associated Immunodeficiency	AGE-RELATED CD4 VALUES			
	<11 mo (% CD4+)	12-35 mo (% CD4+)	36-59 mo (% CD4+)	>5 yr (Absolute No/mm^3 or % CD4+)
None or not significant	>35	>30	>25	>500
Mild	30-35	25-30	20-25	350-500
Advanced	25-29	20-24	15-19	200-349
Severe	<25	<20	<15	<200 or <15%

From Bennett JE et al: *Mandell, Douglas, and Bennett's principles and practice of infectious diseases,* ed 8, Philadelphia, 2015, Saunders.

TABLE 9 Comparison of WHO and CDC Staging Systems*

WHO Stage[†]	WHO T-Lymphocyte Count and Percentage[‡]	CDC Stage[§]	CDC T-Lymphocyte Count and Percentage
Stage 1 (HIV infection)	CD4+ T-lymphocyte count of ≥500 cells/mm^3	Stage 1 (HIV infection)	CD4+ T-lymphocyte count of ≥500 cells/mm^3 or CD4+ T-lymphocyte percentage of ≥29
Stage 2 (HIV infection)	CD4+ T-lymphocyte count of 350-499 cells/mm^3	Stage 2 (HIV infection)	CD4+ T-lymphocyte count of 200-499 cells/mm^3 or CD4+ T-lymphocyte percentage of 14-28
Stage 3 (advanced HIV disease [AHD])	CD4+ T-lymphocyte count of 200-349 cells/mm^3	Stage 2 (HIV infection)	CD4+ T-lymphocyte count of 200-499 cells/mm^3 or CD4+ T-lymphocyte percentage of 14-28
Stage 4 (acquired immunodeficiency syndrome [AIDS])	CD4+ T-lymphocyte count of <200 cells/mm^3 or CD4+ T-lymphocyte percentage of <15	Stage 3 (AIDS)	CD4+ T-lymphocyte count of <200 cells/mm^3 or CD4+ T-lymphocyte percentage of <14

*For reporting purposes only.

[†]Among adults and children aged ≥5 yr.

[‡]Percentage applicable for stage 4 only.

[§]Among adults and adolescents (ages ≥13 yr). CDC also includes a fourth stage, stage unknown; laboratory confirmation of HIV infection but no information on CD4+ T-lymphocyte count or percentage and no information on AIDS-defining conditions.

CDC, Centers for Disease Control and Prevention; *WHO,* World Health Organization.

From Bennett JE et al: *Mandell, Douglas, and Bennett's principles and practice of infectious diseases,* ed 8, Philadelphia, 2015, Saunders.

TABLE 10 Which Antiretroviral Regimen to Choose for Initial Therapy

Preferred Regimens	Comments
Integrase inhibitor-based regimen Bictegravir/TAF/FTC	Use abacavir only in individuals who are HLA-B*5701 negative. Dolutegravir/3TC should not be used in individuals with HIV RNA >500,000 copies/ml, HBV coinfection, or in whom ART is to be started before the results of HIV genotypic resistance testing for reverse transcriptase or HBV testing are available.
Dolutegravir + TDF/FTC or TAF/FTC Dolutegravir/ABC/3TCDolutegravir/3TC PI-based regimen Darunavir/r or Darunavir/c (once daily) + TDF/FTC or TAF/FTC	Use if there is a concern for drug resistance.
Preferred regimen for pregnant women ABC/3TC or TDF/FTC plus raltegravir or darunavir/r or atazanavir/r	TDF should be avoided in renal impairment.

Alternative Regimens	Comments
INSTI-based regimens Raltegravir + TDF/FTC or TAF/FTC Elvitegravir/cobicistat/TDF/FTC Elvitegravir/cobicistat/TAF/FTC RAL + ABC/3TC	
NNRTI-based regimens (in alphabetical order) DOR/TDF/3TC or DOR + TAF/FTC EFV/TDF/FTC or EFV + TAF/FTC RPV/TDF/FTC or RPV/TAF/FTC	EFV should not be used with caution in the first trimester of pregnancy or in women trying to conceive. NVP should not be used in patients with moderate to severe hepatic impairment (Child-Pugh B or C). Should not be used in women with pretreatment CD4 >250 cells/mm^3 or men with CD4 >400 cells/mm^3.
PI-based regimens (in alphabetical order) ATV/r or ATV/c + TDF/FTC or TAF/FTC DRV/c or DRV/r + ABC/3TC	ABC should not be used in patients who test positive for HLA-B*5701. Use with caution in patients with high risk of cardiovascular disease or with pretreatment HIV. RNA >100,000 copies/ml. Once-daily LPV/r is not recommended in pregnant women.

3TC, Lamivudine; *ABC*, abacavir; *ART*, antiretroviral therapy; *ATV*, atazanavir; *DOR*, doravirine; *DRV*, darunavir; *EFV*, efavirenz; *FPV*, fosamprenavir; *FTC*, emtricitabine; *HLA*, human leukocyte antigen; *INSTI*, integrase strand transfer inhibitor; *LPV*, lopinavir; *MRV*, maraviroc; *NNRTI*, nonnucleoside reverse transcriptase inhibitor; *NVP*, nevirapine; *PI*, protease inhibitor; *r*, low dose ritonavir; *RAL*, raltegravir; *RNA*, ribonucleic acid; *RPV*, rilpivirine; *TAF*, tenofovir alafenamide; *TDF*, tenofovir disoproxil fumarate. The following combinations in the recommended list are available as fixed-dose combination formulations: ABC/3TC, EFV/TDF/FTC, LPV/r, TDF/FTC, RPV/TDF/FTC, and ZDV/3TC.

Modified from DHHS Panel on Antiretroviral Guidelines for Adults and Adolescents: Guidelines for the use of antiretroviral agents in adults and adolescents with HIV. Washington, DC: Department of Health and Human Services.

4. Raltegravir (400 mg twice a day). Has a lower barrier to resistance, and other IIs should be considered first.
- NNRTIs:
1. Efavirenz 600 mg daily: Should be used in caution in women in the first trimester or those who are contemplating pregnancy.
2. Rilpivirine: Given with tenofovir and emtricitabine as part of a fixed-dose combination.
3. Nevirapine 200 mg two times a day: Avoid with CD4 count >250 in men and >350 cells/mm^3 in women because of the risk of hepatitis. Rarely used.
4. Etravirine 200 mg two times a day: This drug is generally used in patients for whom other regimens have failed. Etravirine retains activity in many patients who have developed resistance against efavirenz and nevirapine.
- PIs (ritonavir boosted):
1. Darunavir and ritonavir (800 mg and 100/day): This is considered a preferred PI regimen within the U.S. Department of Health and Human Services (DHHS) guidelines with either tenofovir disoproxil fumarate or TAF and emtricitabine.
2. Atazanavir and ritonavir (300 mg and 100 mg) 2 tablets a day: Lower pill burden but use with caution with acid-reducing agents (can alter absorption).
3. Lopinavir and ritonavir (200 mg/50 mg) 2 tablets twice a day (or 4 tablets once a day): Most likely to cause diarrhea and has the greatest negative effect on triglyceride levels; less commonly used.
4. Fosamprenavir and ritonavir (700 mg and 100 mg) 2 tablets twice a day (or 4 tablets once a day): Cannot take fosamprenavir with sulfa allergy; less commonly used.
5. Saquinavir and ritonavir: Saquinavir is no longer recommended for initial treatment of any patient and should be prescribed only in consultation with a specialist.
- All these drugs have their own unique, as well as class-specific, side effects and require careful follow-up to achieve optimal antiviral effects. Compliance with the drug regimen and tolerance of common side effects are critically important to maintain drug efficacy. Antiviral response should be monitored by baseline HIV viral load and CD4 count and repeat measurement at 2 and 4 wk into treatment and then periodically (every 3 to 6 mo) to ensure viral suppression.
- All patients should have genotypic resistance testing upon entry into medical care and before initiation of ART.
- In experienced patients, an antiretroviral regimen should be constructed based on past antiretroviral use and the results of genotypic or phenotypic testing.
- Patients with a CD4 count <200/mm^3 should be given preventive therapy for PJP (Table 11).
- Evaluation of chronic diarrhea in patients with HIV is described in the "Acquired Immunodeficiency Syndrome" topic in Section I.
- Criteria for discontinuing and restarting opportunistic infection prophylaxis for adults and adolescents with HIV infection is described in Table 12.
- HIV infection in a pregnant woman poses special challenges and considerations. Appropriate and timely ART given to mother and newborn has been shown to dramatically reduce the risk of perinatal transmission of HIV. The goal of therapy is to achieve an undetectable viral load. For HIV-infected pregnant women who are already receiving ART: (1) Continue therapy if suppressing viral replication, but avoid use of efavirenz in the first trimester (substitution is recommended in the first trimester); (2) if viremia on therapy, genotypic testing is recommended. For HIV-infected pregnant women who have never received ART: (1) All women should start on ART as soon as possible. Most antiretrovirals are safe in pregnancy; however, efavirenz should be avoided because of possible teratogenicity (Class D), DDI and D4T should be avoided (potential of lactic acidosis), and some protease inhibitors may be dose-altered in pregnancy. Nevirapine should not be initiated in an antiretroviral-naive pregnant patient with CD4 counts >250 cells/mm^3 because of the risk of hepatotoxicity. (2) Women who do not

TABLE 11 Criteria for Discontinuing and Restarting Opportunistic Infection Prophylaxis for Adults and Adolescents With Human Immunodeficiency Virus Infection

Opportunistic Infection	Criteria for Discontinuing Primary Prophylaxis	Criteria for Restarting Primary Prophylaxis	Criteria for Discontinuing Secondary Prophylaxis/Chronic Maintenance Therapy	Criteria for Restarting Secondary Prophylaxis/Chronic Maintenance Therapy
Pneumocystis pneumonia (PJP)	CD4+ count >200 cells/mm³ for >3 mo in response to ART	CD4+ count <200 cells/mm³	CD4+ count increased from <200 cells/mm³ to >200 cells/mm³ for ≥3 mo in response to ART If PJP is diagnosed when CD4+ count >200 cells/mm³, prophylaxis should probably be continued for life regardless of CD4+ count rise in response to ART	CD4+ count <200 cells/mm³, or if PCP recurred at a CD4+ count >200 cells/mm³
Toxoplasma gondii encephalitis (TE)	CD4+ count >200 cells/mm³ for >3 mo in response to ART	CD4+ count <100-200 cells/mm³	Successfully completed initial therapy, remain asymptomatic of signs and symptoms of TE, and CD4+ count >200 cells/mm³ for >6 mo in response to ART	CD4+ count <100 cells/mm³
Microsporidiosis	Not applicable	Not applicable	No signs and symptoms of nonocular microsporidiosis and CD4+ count >200 cells/mm³ for >6 mo in response to ARTPatients with ocular microsporidiosis should be on therapy indefinitely regardless of CD4+ count	No recommendation
Disseminated Mycobacterium avium complex (MAC) disease	CD4+ count >100 cells/mm³ for ≥3 mo in response to ART	CD4+ count <50 cells/mm³	If fulfill the following criteria Completed ≥12 mo therapy, and no signs and symptoms of MAC, and have sustained (≥6 mo) CD4+ count >100 cells/mm³ in response to ART	CD4+ count <50 cells/mm³
Bartonellosis	Not applicable	Not applicable	If fulfill the following criteria Received 3-4 mo of treatment CD4+ count >200 cells/mm³ for ≥6 mo Certain specialists would discontinue therapy only if Bartonella titers have also decreased by fourfold	No recommendation
Mucosal candidiasis	Not applicable	Not applicable	If used, reasonable to discontinue when CD4+ count >200 cells/mm³	No recommendation
Cryptococcal meningitis	Not applicable	Not applicable	If fulfill the following criteria Completed course of initial therapy Remain asymptomatic of cryptococcosis CD4+ count ≥200 cells/mm³ for >6 mo in response to ART Certain specialists would perform a lumbar puncture to determine if cerebrospinal fluid is culture and antigen negative before stopping therapy	CD4+ count <100 cells/mm³
Histoplasma capsulatum infection	If used, CD4+ count >150 cells/mm³ for 6 mo on ART	For patients at high risk for acquiring histoplasmosis, restart at CD4+ count ≤150 cells/mm³	If fulfill the following criteria Received itraconazole for ≥1 yr. Negative blood cultures CD4+ count >150 cells/mm³ for ≥6 mo in response to ART Serum Histoplasma antigen <2 units	CD4+ count ≤150 cells/mm³
Coccidioidomycosis	If used, CD4+ count ≥250 cells/mm³ for ≥6 mo	If used, restart at CD4+ count <250 cells/mm³	**Only for patients with focal coccidioidal pneumonia:** Clinically responded to ≥12 mo of antifungal therapy CD4+ count >250 cells/mm³ Receiving ART Suppressive therapy should be continued indefinitely, even with increase in CD4+ count on ART for patients with diffuse pulmonary, disseminated, or meningeal diseases	No recommendation
Cytomegalovirus retinitis	Not applicable	Not applicable	CD4+ count >100 cells/mm³ for >3-6 mo in response to ART. Therapy should be discontinued only after consultation with an ophthalmologist, taking into account magnitude and duration of CD4+ count increase, anatomic location of the lesions, vision in the contralateral eye, and the feasibility of regular ophthalmologic	No recommendation

Continued

TABLE 11 Criteria for Discontinuing and Restarting Opportunistic Infection Prophylaxis for Adults and Adolescents With Human Immunodeficiency Virus Infection—cont'd

Opportunistic Infection	Criteria for Discontinuing Primary Prophylaxis	Criteria for Restarting Primary Prophylaxis	Criteria for Discontinuing Secondary Prophylaxis/Chronic Maintenance Therapy	Criteria for Restarting Secondary Prophylaxis/Chronic Maintenance Therapy
Isospora belli infection	Not applicable	Not applicable	monitoring. Routine (every 3 mo) ophthalmologic follow-up is recommended for early detection of relapse or immune restoration uveitis. Sustained increase in CD4+ count to >200 cells/mm^3 for >6 mo in response to ART and without evidence of *I. belli* infection	No recommendation

ART, Antiretroviral therapy.

Modified from Centers for Disease Control and Prevention: Guidelines for prevention and treatment of opportunistic infections in HIV-infected adults and adolescents. Recommendations from CDC, the National Institutes of Health, and the HIV Medicine Association of the Infectious Disease Society of America, *MMWR* 58(RR-4), 2009.

TABLE 12 Prophylaxis to Prevent First Episode of HIV-Related Opportunistic Disease

Pathogen	Indication	First Choice	Alternative
Pneumocystis jiroveci pneumonia (PJP, previously referred to as *Pneumocystis carinii*, PCP)	CD4+ count <200 cells/mm^3 or oropharyngeal candidiasis. CD4+ <14% or history of AIDS-defining illness. CD4+ count >200 but <250 cells/mm^3 if monitoring CD4+ count every 1-3 mo is not possible	Trimethoprim-sulfamethoxazole (TMP-SMX) double-strength PO daily; *or* single-strength daily	TMP-SMX 1 double-strength PO 3 times weekly; *or* dapsone 100 mg PO daily or 50 mg PO bid; *or* aerosolized pentamidine 300 mg via Respirgard II nebulizer every month; *or* atovaquone 1500 mg PO daily
Toxoplasma gondii encephalitis	*Toxoplasma* IgG–positive patients with CD4+ count <100 cells/mm^3. Seronegative patients receiving PCP prophylaxis not active against toxoplasmosis should have *Toxoplasma* serology retested if CD4+ count declines to <100 cells/mm^3. Prophylaxis should be initiated if seroconversion occurred	TMP-SMX, 1 double-strength PO daily	TMP-SMX 1 double-strength PO 3 times weekly; *or* TMP-SMX 1 single-strength PO daily; *or* dapsone 50 mg PO daily + pyrimethamine 50 mg PO weekly + leucovorin 25 mg PO weekly; *or* dapsone 200 mg PO weekly + pyrimethamine 75 mg PO weekly + leucovorin 25 mg PO weekly
Mycobacterium tuberculosis infection (TB) (treatment of latent TB infection or LTBI)	(1) Diagnostic test for LTBI, no evidence of active TB, and no prior history of treatment for active or latent TB (2) Diagnostic test for LTBI, but close contact with a person with infectious pulmonary TB and no evidence of active TB (3) A history of untreated or inadequately treated healed TB (i.e., old fibrotic lesions) regardless of diagnostic tests for LTBI and no evidence of active TB	Isoniazid (INH) 300 mg PO daily or 900 mg PO twice weekly for 9 mo—both plus pyridoxine 25 mg PO daily; *or* for persons exposed to drug-resistant TB, selection of drugs after consultation with public health authorities	Rifampin (RIF) 600 mg PO daily × 4 mo; or rifabutin (dosage depends on ART regimen). Be careful of drug interactions with these medications (PIs and NNRTIs). Isoniazid (15 mg/kg rounded up to the nearest 50 or 100 mg; 900 mg maximum) and rifapentine (10-14.0 kg 300 mg; 14.1-25.0 kg 450 mg; 25.1-32.0 kg 600 mg; 32.1-49.9 kg 750 mg; ≥50.00 kg 900 mg maximum) once weekly for a total of 3 mo
Disseminated *Mycobacterium avium* complex (MAC) disease	CD4+ count <50 cells/mm^3—after ruling out active MAC infection	Azithromycin 1200 mg PO once weekly; *or* clarithromycin 500 mg PO bid; *or* azithromycin 600 mg PO twice weekly	RFB 300 mg PO daily (dosage adjustment based on drug-drug interactions with antiretroviral therapy); rule out active TB before starting RFB
Streptococcus pneumoniae infection	CD4+ count >200 cells/mm^3 and no receipt of pneumococcal vaccine in the past 5 yr. CD4+ count <200 cells/mm^3—vaccination can be offered. In patients who received polysaccharide pneumococcal vaccination (PPV) when CD4+ count <200 cells/mm^3 but has increased to >200 cells/mm^3 in response to antiretroviral therapy	A single dose of PCV13 followed by a single dose of PPSV23 at least 8 wk later. A second dose of PPSV23 should be given 5 yr after the initial PPSV23 dose	
Influenza A and B virus infection	All HIV-infected patients	Inactivated influenza vaccine 0.5 ml IM annually	
Histoplasma capsulatum infection	CD4+ count ≤150 cells/mm^3 and at high risk because of occupational exposure or live in a community with a	Itraconazole 200 mg PO daily	

TABLE 12 Prophylaxis to Prevent First Episode of HIV-Related Opportunistic Disease—cont'd

Pathogen	Indication	First Choice	Alternative
Coccidioidomycosis	hyperendemic rate of histoplasmosis (>10 cases/100 patient-yr) Positive IgM or IgG serologic test result in a patient from a disease-endemic area; and CD4+ count <250 cells/mm^3	Fluconazole 400 mg PO daily itraconazole 200 mg PO bid	
Varicella-zoster virus (VZV) infection	*Preexposure prevention:* Patients with CD4+ count ≥200 cells/mm^3 who have not been vaccinated, have no history of varicella or herpes zoster, or who are seronegative for VZV Note: Routine VZV serologic testing in HIV-infected adults is not recommended. *Postexposure—close contact with a person who has active varicella or herpes zoster* For susceptible patients (those who have no history of vaccination or of either condition, or are known to be VZV seronegative)	*Preexposure prevention:* Primary varicella vaccination (Varivax), 2 doses (0.5 ml SC) administered 3 mo apart. If vaccination results in disease because of vaccine virus, treatment with acyclovir is recommended *Postexposure therapy:* Varicella-zoster immune globulin (VariZIG) 125 IU per 10 kg (maximum of 625 IU) IM, administered within 96 h after exposure to a person with active varicella or herpes zoster Note: As of June 2007, VariZIG can be obtained only under a treatment IND (1-800-843-7477, FFF Enterprises).	VZV-susceptible household contacts of susceptible HIV-infected persons should be vaccinated to prevent potential transmission of VZV to their HIV-infected contacts. Alternative postexposure therapy: Postexposure varicella vaccine (Varivax) 0.5 ml SC × 2 doses, 3 mo apart if CD4+ count >200 cells/mm^3; *or* preemptive acyclovir 800 mg PO 3×/ day for 5 days These two alternatives have not been studied in the HIV population
Human papillomavirus (HPV) infection	Women aged 11-26 yr. Men aged 11-26 yr	HPV quadrivalent vaccine 0.5 ml IM mo 0, 2, and 6	
Hepatitis A virus (HAV) infection	HAV-susceptible patients with chronic liver disease or who are injection-drug users, or men who have sex with men. Certain specialists might delay vaccination until CD4+ count >200 cells/mm^3	Hepatitis A vaccine 1 ml IM ×2 doses—at 0 and 6-12 mo IgG antibody response should be assessed 1 mo after vaccination; nonresponders should be revaccinated	
Hepatitis B virus (HBV) infection	All HIV patients without evidence of prior exposure to HBV should be vaccinated with HBV vaccine, including patients with CD4+ count <200 cells/mm^3. *Patients with isolated anti-HBc:* Consider screening for HBV DNA before vaccination to rule out occult chronic HBV infection	Hepatitis B vaccine IM (Engerix-B 20 μg/ ml or Recombivax HB 10 μg/ml) at 0, 1, and 6 mo anti-HBs should be obtained 1 mo after completion of the vaccine series.	Some experts recommend vaccinating with 40-μg doses of either vaccine
	Vaccine nonresponders: Defined as anti-HBs <10 IU/ml 1 mo after a vaccination series For patients with low CD4+ count at the time of first vaccination series, certain specialists might delay revaccination until after a sustained increase in CD4+ count with antiretroviral therapy	Revaccinate with a second vaccine series	Some experts recommend revaccinating with 40-μg doses of either vaccine

AIDS, Acquired immunodeficiency syndrome; *ART,* antiretroviral therapy; *HB,* hepatitis B; *Ig,* immunoglobulin; *IM,* intramuscular; *IND,* investigational new drug; *NNRTI,* nonnucleoside analog reverse transcriptase inhibitor; *PI,* protease inhibitors; *PO,* by mouth; *RFB,* rifabutin.
Modified from Centers for Disease Control and Prevention: Guidelines for prevention and treatment of opportunistic infections in HIV-infected adults and adolescents: recommendations from CDC, the National Institutes of Health, and the HIV Medicine Association of the Infectious Disease Society of America, *MMWR* 58(RR-4), 2009.

need ART for their own health should also initiate three-drug therapy but may do so at the end of the first trimester.
- Preferred ART medications during pregnancy include:
  1. NRTIs: TDF/FTC, TDF/3TC, or ABC/3TC
  2. INSTI: Raltegravir; dolutegravir can be used after the first trimester; limited data with bictegravir. Elvitegravir should not be used in pregnancy because of inadequate drug concentrations.
  3. PIs: ATV/r or DRV/r
- ART should continue through the baby's birth. Zidovudine should also be given intravenously to the woman at the time of labor if the woman has an HIV RNA >1000 copies/ml or there is a concern for poor adherence, regardless of whether it is an existing

component of her three-drug regimen. In women with viral loads persistently >1000 copies/ml despite appropriate ART, cesarean section may further lower risk of transmission. For women with HIV RNA <1000 copies/ml zidovudine (AZT) should also be given to the newborn for the first 6 wk of life. If HIV RNA levels are >1000 copies/ml, infants should receive combination ART, which may include zidovudine, lamivudine, and nevirapine for 6 wk. Mothers should completely avoid nursing.

DISPOSITION
- Ongoing care consisting of frequent medical evaluations and monitoring of CD4 counts and HIV viral loads.

- Long-term care focused on providing up-to-date ART and prophylaxis of PJP and other opportunistic infections, as well as early detection of complications.
- Ongoing assessment for cardiovascular risk and other primary prevention interventions.
- Screening for hepatitis A, B, and C. Treatment when indicated. Drugs such as TDF and lamivudine have activity against both HIV and hepatitis B and may be used in patients with coinfection.
- Vaccinations including hepatitis A and B (when susceptible), pneumococcus (PCV13 and PPSV23), tetanus/diphtheria/pertussis, meningococcal, and influenza. COVID-19 vaccination is also safe to administer at all CD4 cell counts. Box 1 summarizes vaccinations in HIV-positive adults.

BOX 1   Vaccination in HIV-Positive Adults

Generally Avoid
- Bacille Calmette-Guérin (BCG)
- Oral polio
- Oral typhoid

Avoid if CD4+ Cells <200
- Yellow fever
- Measles
- Varicella-zoster virus (VZV)

Give Routinely
- Tetanus/diphtheria (or Tdap)
- Hepatitis A/B
- *Streptococcus pneumoniae*
- *Haemophilus influenzae* type B (Hib)
- Meningococcal
- Influenza, yearly

Give if Indicated for Travel
- Typhoid Vi
- Meningococcal
- Polio, inactivated polio vaccine (IPV)
- Rabies
- Japanese encephalitis
- Tick-borne encephalitis

From Auerbach P: *Wilderness medicine, expert consult, premium edition—enhanced online features and print*, Philadelphia, 2012, Saunders.

- Yearly screening for other sexually transmitted infections (chlamydia, gonorrhea, and syphilis). This includes trichomonas in women and extragenital testing for chlamydia and gonorrhea (i.e., pharyngeal and rectal) in MSM.
- Consideration of AIDS (lymphomas, HPV) and non-AIDS related (screening for general population, age-specific cancers).

REFERRAL

To a physician knowledgeable and experienced in the management of HIV infection and its complications. According to 2018 CDC surveillance data, only 78% of patients are linked to care within 30 days after diagnosis, and a sustained viral suppression is achieved in only 55% to 60% of persons (and a smaller percentage of infected adolescents and young adults) with diagnosed HIV.[12]

PREVENTION

- TDF/FTC or TAF/FTC may be used as pre-exposure prophylaxis (PrEP). Individuals who are HIV negative may take TDF/FTC or TAF/FTC once a day to prevent HIV infection. TDF/FTC as PrEP has been demonstrated to be effective in MSM, heterosexuals, and injection drug users. Importantly, TAF/FTC as PrEP has been shown to be effective in MSM and transwomen but not for cisgender women. Individuals on PrEP should be monitored every 3 mo for renal dysfunction, HIV status, other STIs, and adherence. The FDA has approved Apretude, an intramuscular extended-release (ER) formulation of the integrase strand transfer inhibitor (INSTI) cabotegravir (CAB-LA) for use every 2 mo to prevent sexually acquired HIV-1 infection in at-risk adolescents and adults. Recent trials have shown that CAB-LA is superior to daily oral TDF-FTC in preventing HIV infection among MSM and transgender women.
- Postexposure prophylaxis (PEP) is an effective prevention intervention for individuals exposed to HIV infection, either occupationally or through a sexual exposure. PEP should be taken within 72 h of an exposure and continued for 28 days. Baseline HIV status, renal function, hepatitis B/C, and liver function should be assessed. The recommended first-line regimen is TDF/FTC or TAF/FTC once daily plus raltegravir 400 mg PO twice daily or dolutegravir 50 mg once daily. The FDA has approved Cabenuva, an extended-release formulation of cabotegravir copackaged with an extended-release formulation of rilpivirine. As a once-monthly IM regimen for adults with HIV-1 infection who are virologically suppressed (HIV-1 RNA <50 copies/mL) on a stable antiretroviral regimen without history of treatment failure and without resistance to either drug.

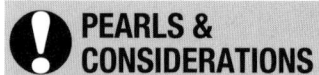

PEARLS & CONSIDERATIONS

COMMENTS

- ART should be initiated in all HIV-infected individuals regardless of CD4 cell counts.
- ART in combination with avoidance of breastfeeding and elective cesarean section in women with viremia reduces risk for mother-to-child transmission.

REFERENCES & SUGGESTED READINGS

Available at eBooks.Health.Elsevier.com.

RELATED CONTENT

Human Immunodeficiency Virus (HIV) Infection (Patient Information)
Acquired Immunodeficiency Syndrome (Related Key Topic)

AUTHOR: **PHILIP A. CHAN, MD, MS**

H

Diseases
and Disorders

I

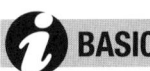

BASIC INFORMATION

DEFINITION

Hydronephrosis, Greek for "water inside the kidney," is an anatomic dilation of the collecting system of the kidneys (renal pelvis and/or calyces). When combined with ureteric dilation, the term hydroureteronephrosis is used. *Hydronephrosis is a structural finding, not a specific diagnosis, and is not synonymous with obstruction.*[1,2] Etiologically, hydronephrosis can result from obstruction to antegrade urine flow (kidney>ureter/s>bladder>urethra), retrograde reflux of urine across the ureterovesical junction (vesicoureteral reflux), or simply too much urine for ureters to handle (as in pathologic diuresis states).

SYNONYMS

Pelviectasis
Caliectasis
Pelvocaliectasis
Pyelocaliectasis

ICD-10CM CODES

N13.1   Hydronephrosis with ureteral stricture, not elsewhere classified
N13.2   Hydronephrosis with renal and ureteral calculous obstruction
N13.30   Unspecified hydronephrosis
N13.39   Other hydronephrosis
Q62.0   Congenital hydronephrosis
Q62.11   Hydronephrosis with ureteropelvic junction obstruction

EPIDEMIOLOGY & DEMOGRAPHICS

Prevalence derived from multiple autopsy series ranges from 2% to 4%,[3] with subjects ranging from neonates to geriatric patients. Antenatal hydronephrosis is one of the most common findings in prenatal ultrasound scans, affecting up to 5% of pregnancies, with 30% to 40% persisting postnatally.[4] Of these, 40% will resolve spontaneously. Hydronephrosis in children is often caused by congenital and structural abnormalities of the kidneys and ureters, such as ureteropelvic junction obstruction or vesicoureteral reflux. Hydronephrosis in adults is often a result of obstruction of one or both kidneys, usually caused by stones, tumors, infections, and trauma. Stones are the most common cause of upper urinary tract obstruction.[2,3] In adults 20 to 60 yr old, hydronephrosis is more common in women, secondary to pregnancy/gynecologic causes. During pregnancy, physiologic hydronephrosis (more commonly on the right) occurs in up to 90% of cases, is often asymptomatic, and typically resolves postpartum. In older patients (age >60 yr), obstruction from prostate enlargement and obstruction from malignancy are the most common causes.[1,2]

CLINICAL PRESENTATION

Hydronephrosis may present as an asymptomatic, incidental finding during imaging performed for another purpose. Symptoms often indicate an element of obstruction. Presentation depends on etiology (obstruction, reflux), degree of obstruction (complete or partial), duration (acute or chronic), anatomic factors (unilateral or bilateral; intrinsic or extrinsic to the ureter), underlying comorbidities (diabetes mellitus, immunocompromised, postoperative states, etc.) and presence of superimposed urinary tract infection.

HISTORY:
- Pain is usually present along the flank, with radiation toward the ipsilateral groin or lower abdominal quadrant. If onset Is sudden and severe, consider a ureteral stone. Ureteral stone also should be a differential for males presenting with penile/ipsilateral testicular pain and benign genital examination/scrotal ultrasound. If pain is induced by diuresis (e.g., following consumption of alcohol), consider ureteropelvic junction obstruction (Dietl crisis). When obstruction is subacute to chronic, symptoms may be vague, less intense, or absent, and may wax and wane in severity (colic). Extrinsic compression (e.g., malignancy-associated compression of ureters or retroperitoneal fibrosis) usually has a more insidious onset compared with intrinsic obstruction (e.g., ureteral stone or blood clot).
- Nausea and vomiting are typically associated with acute obstruction, usually from an intrinsic process.
- Oliguria/anuria may occur with complete, bilateral obstruction, or with an obstructed solitary kidney.
- Urinary symptoms are often absent unless there is an associated condition, including urinary tract infection, distal ureteral stone, or urinary retention. These voiding symptoms include dysuria, urinary urgency, and, frequency, pelvic pressure, and discomfort.

- Hematuria may indicate a stone, urinary tract infection, or malignancy.
- The site of obstruction can relate to the presentation, with upper tract obstruction frequently presenting with flank pain, whereas lower tract obstruction is often associated with obstructive voiding symptoms.

PHYSICAL EXAMINATION: A complete physical examination is warranted but may not be helpful in the assessment of hydronephrosis. Special attention should be paid to the following:
- Blood pressure.
- Palpable abdominal mass: Rare, except in children or thin patients with massive hydronephrosis. Costovertebral angle tenderness is typically not a reliably present (or absent) finding. An enlarged, often percussible bladder is the most common lower abdominal "mass."
- Complete genitourinary and pelvic examinations:
  1. Pelvic examination will assess for pelvic masses or pelvic organ prolapse, which is rarely associated with ureteral obstruction.
  2. Digital rectal examination will assess for prostatic abnormality or rectal mass.
  3. Genital examination (bedside or via cystoscopy) may show meatal stenosis/urethral stricture disease.
  4. Residual urine volume may demonstrate incomplete emptying of the bladder. Residual urine volume can be evaluated indirectly by bedside ultrasonography or directly by bladder catheterization.

ETIOLOGY

Hydronephrosis can be caused by extrinsic or intrinsic factors relative to the urinary tract (Table 1). Causes may be grouped as congenital or acquired.

TABLE 1   Hydronephrosis: Differential Diagnoses

Obstructive

Intrinsic to the urinary tract	*Ureter:* Ureteropelvic junction obstruction, ureterovesical junction obstruction, stricture, tumor, ureterocele, stone, blood clot, sloughed papilla, infection, hyperplastic polyp
	Bladder: Malignancy, stone, bladder neck obstruction, urine retention, neurogenic lower urinary tract dysfunction
	Prostate: Benign prostatic enlargement, prostatitis, abscess, prostate malignancy
	Urethra: Stricture, stone, diverticulum, malignancy, posterior urethral valves, phimosis
Extrinsic to the urinary tract	**Reproductive system:** *Uterus:* Pregnancy, prolapse, fibroids, malignancy *Ovary:* Malignancy, cyst, abscess **Vascular system:** *Aneurysm:* Abdominal aorta, iliac vessel *Aberrant vessels:* Ureteropelvic junction *Venous:* Retrocaval ureter, ovarian vein syndrome **Gastrointestinal system:** Inflammatory bowel disease, GI malignancy, abscesses, cysts **Diseases of the retroperitoneum:** Retroperitoneal fibrosis Retroperitoneal malignancy (primary or metastatic deposits) Hematoma Lymphocele Iatrogenic injury

Nonobstructive

	Vesicoureteral reflux
	Extrarenal pelvis
	Pyelonephritis
	Pathologic diuresis (diabetes insipidus, postobstructive diuresis)

GI, Gastrointestinal.

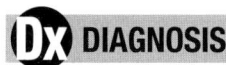
DIAGNOSIS

DIFFERENTIAL DIAGNOSIS

Diagnostic workup depends on age, acuity of presentation, associated symptoms, and if hydronephrosis was diagnosed incidentally.

LABORATORY TESTS[1]

- Evaluation of kidney function: Blood urea nitrogen and creatinine. If azotemia is present, bilateral obstruction or unilateral obstruction of a solitary kidney is present.
- Electrolyte abnormalities: Hyponatremia or hypernatremia, hyperkalemia, and low bicarbonate concentration. Calculation of fractional excretion of sodium (FeNa) or FEUrea can help provide clues to etiology of acute kidney injury.[1]
- Urinalysis and sediment examination: White blood cells, red blood cells, or bacteria in the appropriate setting (e.g., infection, stones). Urine microscopy facilitates crystal identification, which may suggest urinary stone disease. The sediment may be normal in obstructive renal disease.
- Urine culture: Urinalysis or presentation suggests urinary tract infection.

IMAGING STUDIES[2]

- Ultrasound is an excellent initial screening test, especially for children and pregnant women, with evaluation of the kidneys, portions of the ureters, bladder wall, bladder volume, and contour of the collecting system and ureters. Point-of-care ultrasound provides early, rapid imaging and aids patient triage and justification for additional imaging.[5] Ultrasound is >90% sensitive and specific for hydronephrosis. Although not definitive, the absence of ureteral jets on ultrasound may be an indirect sign of obstruction (Fig. E1).
- Abdominal plain film or KUB (kidney, ureter, and bladder) x-rays have limited diagnostic value unless conducted with ultrasound and may demonstrate radiopaque kidney or ureteral stones.
- Abdominal CT scan without intravenous contrast medium localizes sites of obstruction (Figs. E2 and E3), especially if a ureteral calculus is the cause of obstruction. A normal ureteral width by unenhanced CT is 2 to 3 mm wide in adults. If kidney function is normal, CT urography (without and then with contrast, and with delayed images of the ureters), provides anatomic information and is the modality of choice for assessment of upper tract tumors or incidental hydronephrosis.

- MRI is an alternative to CT that provides detail but cannot directly detect a stone. Severely impaired renal function may preclude gadolinium administration. MRI may be used when other tests are inconclusive or contraindicated (e.g., pregnancy, chronic kidney disease, radiocontrast media allergy).
- Antegrade or retrograde ureterogram/pyelogram is an invasive procedure used when CT or MRI scans with radiocontrast media are contraindicated (e.g., contrast allergy, renal impairment).
- Voiding cystourethrography (VCUG) establishes vesicoureteral reflux and bladder neck or urethral obstruction.
- Radioisotope renography (diuretic renography, Tc-99m MAG3 renogram) is a functional procedure that provides differential renal function and determines presence of clinically significant obstruction.[1]

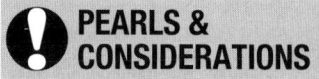
TREATMENT[2,3]

ACUTE GENERAL Rx

- Analgesics (NSAIDs vs. opioid analgesics, based on clinical situation), antiemetics, and fluids for treatment of pain, nausea, and vomiting
- Antibiotics for urinary tract infection/pyelonephritis
  Specific management:
- Management depends on presence of obstruction, etiology, and location of hydronephrosis. Prompt treatment of infection and relief of obstruction prevent long-term loss of kidney function. Chronic renal obstruction from any cause may produce permanent functional deterioration. Renal recovery depends on duration and severity of obstruction.
- General principles include the following:
  1. Routine outpatient evaluation for hydronephrosis is appropriate in asymptomatic or minimally symptomatic patients with no infection, electrolyte derangements, or acute kidney injury.
  2. Surgical treatment is aimed at relieving obstruction when hydronephrosis is associated with urinary tract infection, acute kidney injury, uncontrollable pain, or nausea and vomiting. Surgical treatment is also indicated with complete urinary obstruction from a bilateral obstructing process or unilateral obstruction in a solitary kidney.
  3. Urethral catheter or suprapubic catheter placement is indicated for bladder outlet obstruction. Monitor patients for

postobstructive diuresis after relief of obstruction.
  4. Ureteral stenting is carried out for decompression of one or both kidneys. Percutaneous nephrostomy tubes are an alternative to stenting and may be required in the setting of extrinsic ureteral compression or when ureteral stenting is not possible or fails.

REFERRAL

Prompt referral is paramount in the setting of severe symptoms, infection, or impaired renal function.

- Urology for diagnostic and/or therapeutic procedures (pediatric urologist for antenatal or postnatal hydronephrosis)
- Oncology for diagnosed neoplasm
- Gynecology for pregnancy or if female pelvic anatomy is involved
- Nephrology for electrolyte/acid-base disturbances

PEARLS & CONSIDERATIONS

COMMENTS

- Hydronephrosis is not a primary disorder, and an underlying etiology must be sought.
- Children often have congenital causes; adults generally have acquired intrinsic or extrinsic causes.
- There are obstructive and nonobstructive causes of hydronephrosis. Further evaluation can be performed without specialty consultation with a CT urogram, magnetic resonance urogram, or diuretic renogram.
- Prompt renal decompression is critical when hydronephrosis is associated with infection, severe kidney injury, and/or electrolyte abnormalities.

PREVENTION

Timely and appropriate management of acute kidney obstruction prevents long-term kidney damage. Hydronephrosis may persist after relief of the obstructing cause.

REFERENCES & SUGGESTED READINGS

Available at eBooks.Health.Elsevier.com.

AUTHORS: **DEEPANSH DALELA, MD,** and **DAVID A. LEAVITT, MD**

BASIC INFORMATION

DEFINITION

Hypercholesterolemia refers to a blood cholesterol measurement ≥200 mg/dl.

SYNONYMS

Hyperlipidemia
Hypercholesteremia
Dyslipidemia
Type II familial hyperlipoproteinemia

ICD-10CM CODE

E78.0 Pure hypercholesterolemia

EPIDEMIOLOGY & DEMOGRAPHICS

- More than 105 million (37% of) adults in the U.S. have total blood cholesterol levels higher than 200 mg/dl. Of this group, more than 36 million adults have extremely high-risk cholesterol levels over 240 mg/dl (13%).
- For men over the age of 20, approximately 48% of White men, 45% of Black men, and 50% of Hispanic men have high blood cholesterol.
- For women over the age of 20, approximately 50% of White women, 42% of Black women, and 50% of Hispanic women have hypercholesterolemia.
- Prevalence of hypercholesterolemia increases with age.
- According to National Health and Nutrition Examination Survey (NHANES) data approximately 47% of adults had at least one of three risk factors for cardiovascular disease—uncontrolled high blood pressure, uncontrolled high levels of low-density lipoproteins (LDL) cholesterol, or current smoking.

PHYSICAL FINDINGS & CLINICAL PRESENTATION

- A detailed medication history should be performed because some medications may affect lipid levels (e.g., thiazides, corticosteroids, β-blockers, and estrogens).
- The physical examination should include measurements of body mass index and blood pressure (BP), thyroid and liver assessments, and examining peripheral pulses including carotids for bruits.
- Physical findings, particularly in the familial forms may include:
  1. Tendon xanthomas
  2. Xanthelasma
  3. Arcus corneae
  4. Arterial bruits (young adulthood)

ETIOLOGY

PRIMARY:

- Genetics
- Obesity
- Dietary intake

SECONDARY:

- Hypothyroidism
- Diabetes mellitus (DM)
- Nephrotic syndrome

- Obstructive liver disease: Hepatoma, extrahepatic biliary obstruction, primary biliary cirrhosis
- Alcohol or tobacco use
- Dysgammaglobulinemia (multiple myeloma, systemic lupus erythematosus)
- Drugs: Oral contraceptives, progesterone, corticosteroids, thiazide diuretics, β-blockers, androgenic steroids, retinoic acid derivatives, protease inhibitors

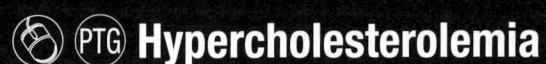 **DIAGNOSIS**

DIFFERENTIAL DIAGNOSIS

- Always consider underlying secondary causes for the elevated cholesterol.
- Patients with very high LDL cholesterol usually have genetic forms of hypercholesterolemia (see "Hyperlipoproteinemia, Primary"). Early detection of these cases and family testing to identify similarly affected relatives is important.
- Metabolic syndrome:
  1. A constellation of lipid and nonlipid risk factors of a metabolic origin
  2. Diagnosed when three or more of the following are present: Abdominal obesity (waist circumference >40 in for men and >35 in for women); fasting triglycerides >150 mg/dl; HDL <40 mg/dl in males and <50 mg/dl in females; systolic BP >130 mm Hg and diastolic BP >85 mm Hg; fasting glucose >110 mg/dl

WHO SHOULD BE SCREENED:

- The American Association of Clinical Endocrinologists (AACE) recommends screening of patients >20 yr of age for elevated cholesterol every 5 yr, males >45 yr and females >55 yr of age every 1 to 2 yr, and >65 yr of age every yr up to 75 yr of age regardless of coronary artery disease (CAD) risk status. Patients above 75 yr of age with multiple CAD risk factors should continue to get screened annually.
- The United States Preventive Services Task Force (USPSTF) supports routine screening for men aged >35 yr and women aged >45 yr by measurement of nonfasting total and HDL cholesterol alone.
- In 2010 the USPSTF recommended routine screening for overweight and obese persons aged <20 yr.
- In 2011, American College of Cardiology (ACC)/American Heart Association (AHA) recommended screening for hypertriglyceridemia by a nonfasting measurement. A nonfasting level of <200 mg/dl is commensurate with an optimal level of <100 mg/dl, and no further testing is required. However, a nonfasting level of >200 mg/dl warrants further testing with a fasting lipid profile.

LABORATORY TESTS

- Obtain a lipid profile. A fasting lipid panel has been traditionally preferred over a nonfasting lipid profile; however, this recommendation has come into question, and expert consensus statements from Canada and Europe

recommend nonfasting lipid testing as the new standard for lipid measurement. In nonfasting patients, triglyceride levels ≥175 mg/dl should be considered elevated as compared with <150 mg/dl for fasting panels. Fasting lipid panels are preferred for patients with triglycerides over 400 mg/dl.

- Lipoprotein(a) [Lp(a)]: Current U.S. guidelines suggest that Lp(a) may be used as a "risk-enhancing factor" to support statin prescription, in concert with other factors and shared decision-making, among primary prevention patients aged 40 to 75 yr with an estimated 10-yr risk for atherosclerotic cardiovascular disease (ASCVD) of 5.0% to 19.9%.[1]
- Perform a workup for secondary causes if clinically indicated, such as thyroid-stimulating hormone, metabolic profile, liver function tests (LFTs), and fasting glucose.

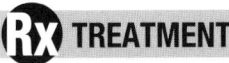 **TREATMENT**

NONPHARMACOLOGIC THERAPY

- First-line treatment: Dietary therapy can result in 5% to 15% reduction in LDL cholesterol level
- Composition of the **TLC diet:**
  1. Total fat 25% to 30% of total calories
  2. Polyunsaturated fat up to 10% of total calories
  3. Monounsaturated fat up to 20% of total calories
  4. Saturated fats <7% of total calories
  5. Carbohydrate 50% to 60% of total calories
  6. Protein 15% of total calories
  7. No more than 200 mg/day of cholesterol
  8. Fiber 20 to 30 g/day
- Increased physical activity: Encourage 30 min of moderately intense physical activity, four to six times a wk (e.g., brisk walking, riding stationary bike, water aerobics)
- Maintenance of a healthy weight
- Avoidance of tobacco products
- Counseling on CAD risk factors (Table 1)
- Plant-based diets (including stanol-containing margarines, oat bran, and nuts) have shown effectiveness in controlling lipids

ACUTE GENERAL Rx

No acute treatment needed

TABLE 1 Risk Factors for Heart Disease

1. Cigarette smoking
2. Hypertension (BP ≥140/90 mm Hg or on medications)
3. Low HDL cholesterol (<40 mg/dl)*
4. Family history of premature CHD (<55 yr in first-degree male relative or <65 yr in first-degree female relative)
5. Age (men ≥45 yr, women ≥55 yr)

*HDL cholesterol >60 mg/dl counts as a negative risk factor; its presence removes one risk factor from the total count.
BP, Blood pressure; *CHD*, congenital heart disease; *HDL*, high-density lipoprotein cholesterol.

H

Diseases and Disorders

I

BOX 1 2013 ACC/AHA Summary of Key Recommendations for the Treatment of Blood Cholesterol to Reduce ASCVD Risk in Adults

A. Heart-healthy lifestyle habits should be encouraged for all individuals
B. The appropriate intensity of statin therapy should be initiated or continued
  1. Clinical ASCVD*
    a. Age 75 yr or less and no safety concerns: High-intensity statin (class I, level A)
    b. Age 75 yr or safety concerns: Moderate-intensity statin (class I, level A)*
  2. Primary prevention: Primary LDL-C 190 mg/dl or greater
    a. Rule out secondary causes of hyperlipidemia (class I, level B)
    b. Age 21 yr or older: High-intensity statin (class I, level B)
    c. Achieve at least a 50% reduction in LDL-C (class IIa, level B)
    d. LDL-C lowering nonstatin therapy may be considered to further reduce LDL-C (class IIb, level C)
  3. Primary prevention: Diabetes, 40 to 75 yr of age, and LDL-C 70 to 189 mg/dl
    a. Moderate-intensity statin (class I, level A)
    b. Consider high-intensity statin when 7.5% or greater 10-yr ASCVD risk using the Pooled Cohort Equations (class IIa, level B)‡
  4. Primary prevention: No diabetes, 40 to 75 yr of age, and LDL-C 70 to 189 mg/dl
    a. Estimate 10-yr ASCVD risk using the Risk Calculator based on the Pooled Cohort Equations in those *not* receiving a statin; estimate risk every 4 to 6 yr (class I, level B)
    b. To determine whether to initiate a statin, engage in a clinician-patient discussion of the potential for ASCVD risk reduction, adverse effects, drug-drug interactions, and patient preferences
    c. Reemphasize heart-healthy lifestyle habits and address other risk factors (class IIa, level C)
      i. 7.5% or greater 10-yr ASCVD risk: Moderate- or high-intensity statin (class I, level A)
      ii. 5% to 7.5% 10-yr ASCVD risk: Consider moderate-intensity statin (class IIa, level B)
      iii. Other factors may be considered: LDL-C 160 mg/dl or greater, family history of premature ASCVD, hs-CRP 2.0 mg/L or greater, CAC score 300 Agatston units or greater, ABI less than 0.9, or lifetime ASCVD risk (class IIb, level C)
  5. Primary prevention when LDL-C is less than 190 mg/dl and age is less than 40 or more than 75 yr, or less than 5% 10-yr ASCVD risk
    a. Statin therapy may be considered in selected individuals (class IIb, level C)
  6. Statin therapy is not routinely recommended for individuals with NYHA class II-IV heart failure or who are receiving maintenance hemodialysis
C. Regularly monitor adherence to lifestyle and drug therapy with lipid and safety assessments
  1. Assess adherence, response to therapy, and adverse effects within 4 to 12 wk following statin initiation or change in therapy (class I, level A)
    a. Measure a fasting lipid panel (class I, level A)
    b. Do not routinely monitor ALT or CK unless symptomatic (class IIa, level C)
    c. Screen and treat type 2 diabetes according to current practice guidelines. Heart-healthy lifestyle habits should be encouraged to prevent progression to diabetes (class I, level B)
    d. Anticipated therapeutic response: Approximately 50% or greater reduction in LDL-C from baseline for high-intensity statin and 30% to 50% for moderate-intensity statin (class IIa, level B)
      i. Insufficient evidence for LDL-C or non–HDL-C treatment targets from RCTs
      ii. For those with unknown baseline LDL-C, an LDL-C less than 100 mg/dl was observed in RCTs of high-intensity statin therapy
    e. Less than anticipated therapeutic response:
      i. Reinforce improved adherence to lifestyle and drug therapy (class I, level A)
      ii. Evaluate for secondary causes of hyperlipidemia if indicated (class I, level A)
      iii. Increase statin intensity, or if on maximally tolerated statin intensity, consider addition of nonstatin therapy in selected high-risk individuals (class IIb, level C)§
    f. Regularly monitor adherence to lifestyle and drug therapy every 3 to 12 mo once adherence has been established. continue assessment of adherence for optimal ASCVD risk reduction and safety (class I, level A)
D. In individuals intolerant of the recommended intensity of statin therapy, use the maximally tolerated intensity of statin (class I, level B). If there are muscle or other symptoms, establish that they are related to the statin (class IIa, level B)

*Clinical ASCVD includes acute coronary syndromes, history of MI, stable or unstable angina, coronary or other arterial revascularization, stroke, TIA, or peripheral arterial disease presumed to be of atherosclerotic origin.
‡These factors may include primary LDL-C of 160 mg/dl or greater or other evidence of genetic hyperlipidemias; family history of premature ASCVD with onset at less than 55 yr of age in a first-degree male relative or at less than 65 yr of age in a first-degree female relative; hs-CRP 2 mg/L or greater; CAC score 300 Agatston units or greater or 75th percentile or greater for age, sex, and ethnicity; ABI less than 0.9; or lifetime risk of ASCVD. Additional factors that might aid in individual risk assessment could be identified in the future.
§High-risk individuals include those with clinical ASCVD, an untreated LDL-C 190 mg/dl or greater, suggesting genetic hypercholesterolemia, or individuals with diabetes 40 to 75 yr of age and LDL-C 70 to 189 mg/dl.
ABI, Ankle brachial index; ACC, American College of Cardiology; AHA, American Heart Association; ALT, alanine transaminase; ASCVD, atherosclerotic cardiovascular disease; CAC, coronary artery calcium; CK, creatine kinase; hs-CRP, high sensitivity C-reactive protein; LDL-C, low-density lipoprotein cholesterol; MI, myocardial infarction; NYHA, New York Heart Association; RCTs, randomized clinical trials; TIA, transient ischemic attack.
From 2013 ACC/AHA guideline on the treatment of blood cholesterol to reduce atherosclerotic cardiovascular risk in adults: a report of the American College of Cardiology/American Heart Association Task Force on Practice Guidelines, J Am Coll Cardiol 63(25 Pt B):2889-2934, 2014.

TABLE 2 Atherosclerotic Cardiovascular Disease

1. Coronary heart disease: Acute coronary syndromes, history of myocardial infarction, stable or unstable angina, coronary or other arterial revascularization
2. Stroke or transient ischemic attack
3. Peripheral arterial disease

CHRONIC Rx

• Box 1 summarizes the key recommendations for the treatment of blood cholesterol to reduce ASCVD risk in adults.
• The guidelines identify four high-risk groups that benefit from statin therapy:
  1. Patients with clinical ASCVD (Table 2, Fig. 1)
  2. LDL ≥190 mg/dl
  3. DM aged 40 to 75 yr and LDL 70 to 189 mg/dl
  4. 10-yr risk for ASCVD ≥7.5% and LDL 70 to 189 mg/dl
• The 10-yr risk of ASCVD is calculated with the risk calculator available at http://my.americanheart.org/cvriskcalculator.
• ASCVD events are reduced by using the maximum tolerated statin intensity in the aforementioned groups shown to benefit the most (Tables 3 and 4).

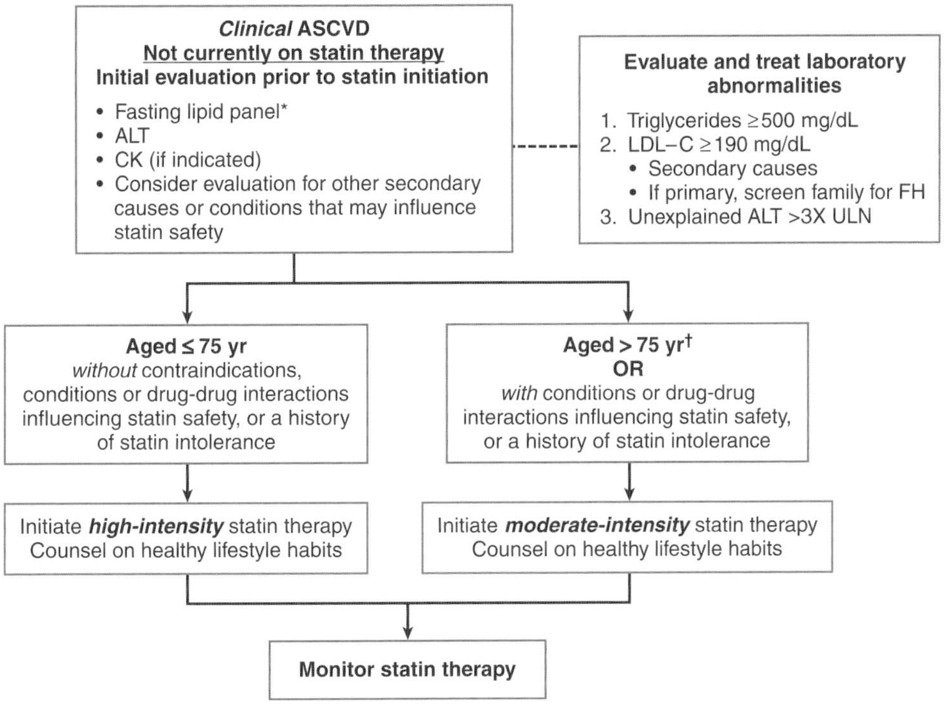

H

I

Clinical ASCVD
Not currently on statin therapy
Initial evaluation prior to statin initiation

- Fasting lipid panel*
- ALT
- CK (if indicated)
- Consider evaluation for other secondary causes or conditions that may influence statin safety

Evaluate and treat laboratory abnormalities

1. Triglycerides ≥500 mg/dL
2. LDL–C ≥190 mg/dL
   - Secondary causes
   - If primary, screen family for FH
3. Unexplained ALT >3X ULN

Aged ≤ 75 yr
without contraindications, conditions or drug-drug interactions influencing statin safety, or a history of statin intolerance

Aged > 75 yr†
OR
with conditions or drug-drug interactions influencing statin safety, or a history of statin intolerance

Initiate **high-intensity** statin therapy
Counsel on healthy lifestyle habits

Initiate **moderate-intensity** statin therapy
Counsel on healthy lifestyle habits

Monitor statin therapy

FIG. 1 Initiating statin therapy in individuals with clinical ASCVD. *Fasting lipid panel is preferred. In a nonfasting individual, a nonfasting non–HDL-C >220 mg/dl may indicate genetic hypercholesterolemia that requires further evaluation or a secondary etiology. If nonfasting triglycerides are >500 mg/dl, a fasting lipid panel is required. †It is reasonable to evaluate the potential for ASCVD benefits and for adverse effects and to consider patient preferences in initiating or continuing a moderate- or high-intensity statin in individuals with ASCVD >75 yr of age. *ALT,* Alanine transaminase; *ASCVD,* atherosclerotic cardiovascular disease; *CK,* creatine kinase; *FH,* familial hypercholesterolemia; *HDL-C,* high-density lipoprotein cholesterol; *LDL-C,* low-density lipoprotein cholesterol; *ULN,* upper limit of normal. (Modified from Stone NJ et al: 2013 ACC/AHA guideline on the treatment of blood cholesterol to reduce atherosclerotic cardiovascular risk in adults: a report of the American College of Cardiology/American Heart Association Task Force on Practice Guidelines, *J Am Coll Cardiol,* 2013. In Mann DL et al: *Braunwald's heart disease,* ed 10, Philadelphia, 2015, Elsevier.)

TABLE 3 Statin Benefit Groups and Recommended Therapy

Statin Benefit Group	High Intensity	Moderate Intensity	Additional Testing
Clinical ASCVD	Yes	Consider†	None
Primary LDL-C >190 mg/dl	Yes	Consider†	None
Diabetes without ASCVD and 10-yr risk ≥7.5%*	Yes	Consider†	None
Diabetes without ASCVD and 10-yr risk <7.5%*	Consider‡	Yes	Case-by-case
Primary prevention and 10-yr risk ≥7.5%*	Consider‡	Yes	Case-by-case
Primary prevention and 10-yr risk <7.5%*	Consider‡	Consider‡	Case-by-case

*Based on Pooled Cohort Risk Equations.
†If age >75 yr or not candidate for high intensity.
‡If abnormal high-sensitivity C-reactive protein, coronary artery calcium, ankle-brachial index, lifetime risk.
ASCVD, Atherosclerotic cardiovascular disease; *LDL-C,* low-density lipoprotein cholesterol.
From Boyden TF et al: Implementing new guidelines in the management of blood cholesterol, *Am J Med* 127:705, 2014.

- Additional factors such as C-reactive protein >2 mg/L, primary LDL >160, genetic hyperlipidemias, family history of premature coronary heart disease (CHD), ankle-brachial index <0.9, and coronary artery calcium score (CAD) assessed with computed tomography may be used in patients who are not in one of four statin benefit groups and for whom a decision to initiate statin therapy is otherwise unclear. Statins are generally beneficial in patients at intermediate risk and selected patients with borderline risk who have a calcium score that is 100 or higher or who are in

- the 75th percentile or higher for their age, sex, and race. Statins should also be considered in persons with scores of 1 to 99, particularly if they are age 55 yr or older.
- Percent reduction in LDL cholesterol is used as a guide to compliance and adherence to therapy in the 2018 AHA/ACC Revised Clinical Practice Guidelines (Fig. 2). Studies have shown that compared with less-intensive LDL-C lowering, more intensive lowering reduces all-cause mortality and cardiovascular mortality; patients with higher baseline LDL-C have greater benefit.

- Moderate-intensity statin therapy should be continued for individuals >75 yr of age for secondary prevention. However, factors such as comorbidities, safety, and priorities of care should be considered before initiating statins for primary prevention of ASCVD.
- Adherence to lifestyle and to statin therapy should be reiterated with patients before the addition of a nonstatin drug.
- High-risk patients with a suboptimal response to statins who are unable to tolerate a recommended intensity or who are completely statin intolerant may benefit from the addition

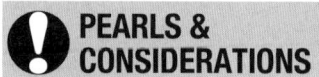

TABLE 4 High-, Moderate-, and Low-Intensity Statin Therapy*

Statin Therapy	DAILY DOSE		
	High Intensity[†] ↓LDL-C ≥50%	Moderate Intensity[‡] ↓LDL-C 30<50%	Low Intensity[§] ↓LDL-C <30%
Atorvastatin	(40[‖])-80 mg	10 (20) mg	
Rosuvastatin	20 (40) mg	(5) 10 mg	
Simvastatin		20-40 mg[¶]	10 mg
Pravastatin		40 (80) mg	10-20 mg
Lovastatin		40 mg	20 mg
Fluvastatin		80 mg (Fluvastatin XL)	20-40 mg
Fluvastatin		40 mg**	
Pitavastatin		2-4 mg	1 mg

*Individual responses to statin therapy varied in randomized, controlled trials and vary in clinical practice. A less-than-average response may have a biologic basis. Statins and dosages in bold were reduced in major cardiovascular events in randomized, controlled trials. Statins and doses in italics were approved by the FDA but were not tested in randomized, controlled trials.

[†]Daily dose decreases LDL-C levels by an average of ≥50%.

[‡]Daily dose decreases LDL-C levels by an average of 30 to <50%.

[§]Daily dose decreases LDL-C levels by an average of <30%.

[‖]Evidence from 1 randomized, controlled trial only; down-titration if patient is unable to tolerate atorvastatin, 80 mg.

[¶]Although simvastatin, 80 mg, was evaluated in randomized, controlled trials, the FDA recommends against initiation of or titration to 80 mg of simvastatin because of increased risk for myopathy and rhabdomyolysis.

**Twice daily.

FDA, U.S. Food and Drug Administration; *LDL-C*, low-density lipoprotein cholesterol; *XL*, extended-release.

Reprinted with permission of the authors: Stone NJ et al: 2013 ACC/AHA guideline on the treatment of blood cholesterol to reduce atherosclerotic cardiovascular risk in adults: a report of the American College of Cardiology/American Heart Association Task Force on Practice Guidelines, *J Am Coll Cardiol* 63(25, Part B):2889-2934, 2014.

of a nonstatin cholesterol-lowering agent such as ezetimibe and/or Protein Convertase Subtilisin/Kexin 9 (PCSKS 9) inhibitor to reduce risk for major cardiovascular events.[2] Combination therapies for LDL are summarized in Table 5.

- Ezetimibe inhibits cholesterol absorption in the intestine, whereas statins inhibit cholesterol production primarily in the liver. Ezetimibe is not as effective as most statins, but will reduce LDL by 15% to 22%. It can reduce the risk of heart attacks and strokes when taken alongside a statin, but there is little evidence it can do this if used on its own.
- PCSK9 binds to LDL receptors on hepatocytes, promotes receptor degradation, and prevents LDL-C clearance from the circulation thereby increasing serum concentrations of LDL-C. PCSK9 monoclonal antibody inhibitors alirocumab (Praluent), evolocumab (Repatha), and inclisiran (Leqvio), a PCSK9-directed small interfering RNA, are currently indicated as adjunct to diet and maximally tolerated statin therapy for the treatment of adults with heterozygous familial hypercholesterolemia or clinical atherosclerotic cardiovascular disease, who require additional lowering of LDL cholesterol. PCSK9 inhibitors lower risk for ischemic cardiovascular events in persons with stable CAD and elevated atherogenic lipoproteins despite statin therapy. These medications are administered by subcutaneous injection and are expensive.
- The management of metabolic syndrome includes weight reduction, increased physical activity, and treatment of hypertension, elevated triglycerides, and low HDL cholesterol.
- According to recent studies, each 40 mg/dl reduction in LDL cholesterol by statin therapy confers a 20% reduction in ASCVD. In other words, a relative risk reduction of 30% in ASCVD by moderate-intensity therapy and 45% by high-intensity therapy has been approximated.
- Recent trials have shown that bempedoic acid, an inhibitor of ATP citrate lyase, reduces LDL cholesterol. The addition of bempedoic acid to maximally tolerated statin therapy did not lead to a higher incidence of overall adverse events than placebo and led to significant lowering of LDL cholesterol.
- Recent trials have shown that bempedoic acid, an inhibitor of ATP citrate lyase, reduces LDL cholesterol. The addition of bempedoic acid to maximally tolerated statin therapy did not lead to a higher incidence of overall adverse events than placebo and led to significant lowering of LDL cholesterol.
- Table 6 summarizes oral drugs affecting lipoprotein metabolism.

DISPOSITION & FOLLOW-UP

- Baseline LFT testing should be done before initiation of statin therapy and as clinically indicated thereafter.
- Creatine kinase level monitoring is not recommended unless a patient reports muscle weakness or myalgias.
- Statin therapy should be monitored by repeating a lipid profile within 4 to 12 wk after initiation of therapy.

- Counseling about behavioral lifestyle changes and risk factors for CHD should be provided at every follow-up visit.
- Adverse effects of statin-associated diabetes vary by statin intensity: One excess case of diabetes per 1000 treated individuals with moderate-intensity statin and three excess cases of diabetes per 1000 treated individuals with high-intensity statin per year has been reported. Myopathy and hemorrhagic stroke incidence is around one excess case per 10,000 treated individuals.
- Per new guidelines, those who develop diabetes during statin therapy should be advised to continue moderate to high intensity statins to reduce their risk of ASCVD events and should adhere to a heart-healthy diet, engage in physical activity, cease tobacco use, and maintain a healthy body weight (Table 6).
- Regarding choice of statin, Atorvastatin and Rosuvastatin are preferred in most patients with moderate to high; hypercholesterolemia for patients on simvastatin with moderate to high. Maintain patients on 80 mg daily of simvastatin only if they have been taking this dose for 12 or more mo without evidence of muscle toxicity. Do not start new patients on simvastatin 80 mg. Place patients who do not meet their LDL goal on simvastatin 40 mg on alternative LDL-C-lowering treatment(s) to reach goal.

REFERRAL

Patients with rare lipid disorders, hyperlipoproteinemias, patients resistant to treatment, on complex regimens, and with evidence of disease progression despite treatment should be referred to a lipid specialist.

PEARLS & CONSIDERATIONS

COMMENTS

- New features in the 2018 clinical practice guidelines compared to the 2013 guidelines support the addition of nonstatin medications (ezetimibe or PCSK9 inhibitors) to statin therapy for secondary prevention in patients at very high risk. In primary prevention, a clinical patient risk discussion is strongly recommended before a decision is made about statin treatment. Among intermediate-risk patients, identification of risk-enhancing factors and coronary calcium testing is recommended when considering the use of a statin.
- Familial hypercholesterolemia (FH) is characterized by elevated cholesterol concentrations early in life. Untreated FH is associated with premature cardiovascular disease in adulthood. Screening can detect FH in children, and lipid-lowering treatment in childhood can reduce lipid concentrations in the short term, with little evidence of harm. A 20-yr follow-up study of statin therapy has shown that initiation of statin therapy during childhood in patients with FH slows the progression of carotid

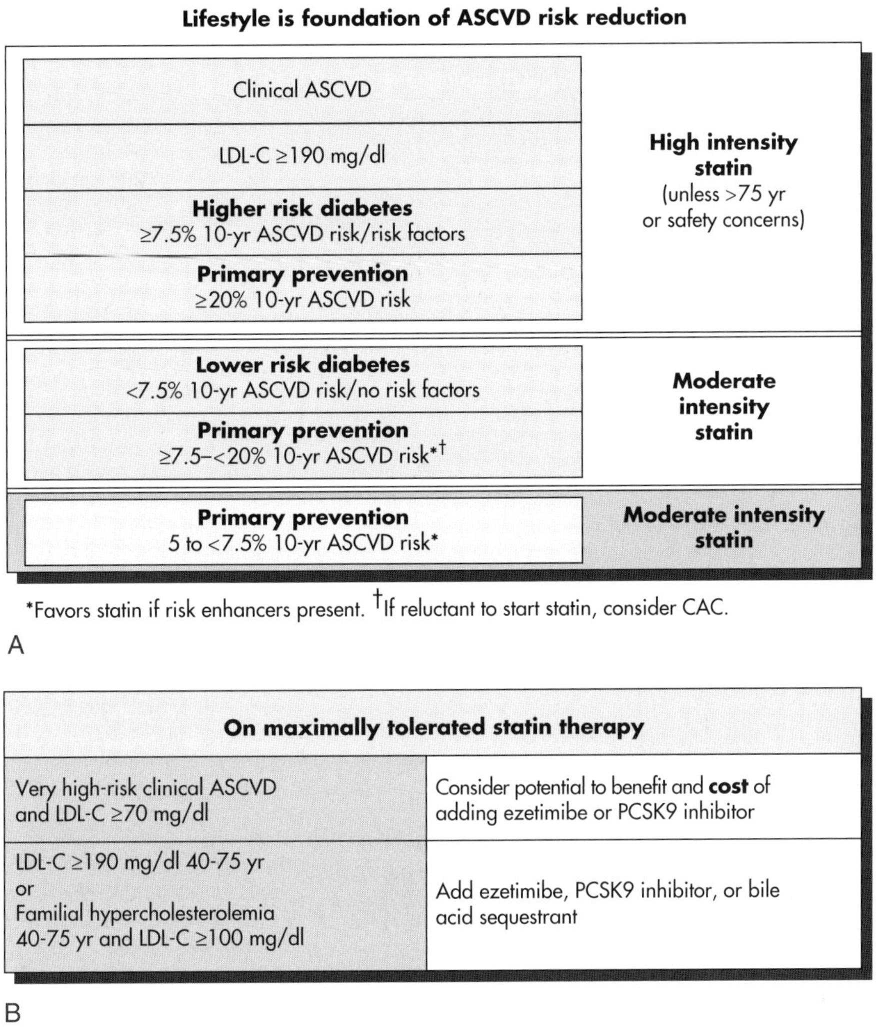

Lifestyle is foundation of ASCVD risk reduction

Clinical ASCVD	**High intensity statin** (unless >75 yr or safety concerns)
LDL-C ≥190 mg/dl	
Higher risk diabetes ≥7.5% 10-yr ASCVD risk/risk factors	
Primary prevention ≥20% 10-yr ASCVD risk	
Lower risk diabetes <7.5% 10-yr ASCVD risk/no risk factors	**Moderate intensity statin**
Primary prevention ≥7.5–<20% 10-yr ASCVD risk*†	
Primary prevention 5 to <7.5% 10-yr ASCVD risk*	**Moderate intensity statin**

*Favors statin if risk enhancers present. †If reluctant to start statin, consider CAC.

A

On maximally tolerated statin therapy	
Very high-risk clinical ASCVD and LDL-C ≥70 mg/dl	Consider potential to benefit and **cost** of adding ezetimibe or PCSK9 inhibitor
LDL-C ≥190 mg/dl 40-75 yr or Familial hypercholesterolemia 40-75 yr and LDL-C ≥100 mg/dl	Add ezetimibe, PCSK9 inhibitor, or bile acid sequestrant

B

FIG. 2 A and **B,** Summary of 2018 ACC/AHA cholesterol guideline recommendations for statin and nonstatin therapy. Background color denotes class and level of evidence: Green = Class I (strong) recommendation; yellow = Class IIa (reasonable) recommendation; blue = Grade A (high) level of evidence; orange = Grade B (moderate) level of evidence. *ASCVD,* Atherosclerotic cardiovascular disease; *CAC,* coronary artery calcium; *LDL-C,* low-density lipoprotein cholesterol. (From Goldman L, Shafer AI: *Goldman's Cecil medicine*, ed 26, St Louis, 2019, Elsevier.)

TABLE 5 Combination Therapies for LDL

Statin plus ezetimibe	Ezetimibe added to a statin may further reduce LDL by 20% or more and reduce triglycerides by 7%-13%. The combination provides equivalent LDL reduction to a fourfold increase in statin dose. Daily ezetimibe added to a low-dose statin given 2-3 times/wk can improve tolerance. Combination pills containing statin and ezetimibe are available. Most common side effects reflect those of the individual drugs. Combination ezetimibe and simvastatin has been shown to decrease cardiovascular events in patients with renal disease and acute coronary syndrome.
Statin and PCSK9 inhibitors	This combination is the most effective known treatment for hypercholesterolemia. There are no known negative interactions between these two therapies. This combination reduces CHD events more than statin alone.
Statin plus bile acid sequestrants	Bile acid sequestrants in combination with statins further decrease LDL from 24% to 60%. Cholestyramine and colestipol can interfere with the absorption of statins. Colesevelam does not affect statin absorption. The statin-colesevelam combination is not ideal for patients with high triglycerides but may be useful in those with type 2 diabetes mellitus because colesevelam reduces glycemia.
Statin plus niacin	Adding niacin to a statin can lower LDL by 10% to 20%, in addition to beneficial effects on triglycerides. When used in combination with a statin, the maximum dose of niacin should be 2000 mg/day. This combination in subjects with already low LDL levels did not reduce CHD events.
Bile acid sequestrants plus niacin	Before the availability of statins, bile acid sequestrants plus niacin were used to lower LDL in high-risk patients. The availability of colesevelam and extended-release niacin has made this combination tolerable for many patients who are unable to use statins.
Ezetimibe plus bile acid sequestrants	Ezetimibe inhibits cholesterol absorption, and sequestrants enhance cholesterol excretion through conversion to bile acids. The combination can have additive effects. This combination is useful for patients who cannot take statins.

CHD, Coronary heart disease; *LDL,* low-density lipoprotein; *PCSK9,* proprotein convertase subtilisin/kexin type 9.
From Melmed S et al: *Williams textbook of endocrinology,* ed 14, St Louis, 2019, Elsevier.

TABLE 6 Drugs Affecting Lipoprotein Metabolism

Drug Class	Agents and Daily Doses	Lipid/Lipoprotein Effects	Side Effects	Contraindications
HMG-CoA reductase inhibitors (statins)	Lovastatin (10-40 mg) Pravastatin (10-80 mg) Simvastatin† (5-80 mg) Fluvastatin (20-40 mg) Atorvastatin (10-80 mg) Rosuvastatin (5-40 mg) Pitavastatin (2-4 mg)	LDL↓ 20%-60% HDL↑ 5%-15% TG↓ 7%-30%	Myalgias, myositis Increased liver enzymes New-onset diabetes (with intensive therapy) Unproven concerns about memory loss	Active or chronic liver disease Pregnancy Concomitant use of certain drugs*
Bile acid sequestrants	Colestipol (5-20 g) Colesevelam‡ (2.6-3.8 g) Cholestyramine (4-16 g)	LDL↓ 15%-30% HDL↑ 3%-5% TG No change or increase	Gastrointestinal distress, constipation, drug interaction, hypertriglyceridemia Decreased absorption of fat-soluble vitamins	TG >300 mg/dl GI motility disorder
Omega-3 fatty acids	Fish oils (4-6 g)	TG↓ 45% HDL↑ 13%	Increased bleeding time Nausea	Caution with anticoagulant therapy
Nicotinic acid	Immediate release (niacin) (1.5-3 g) Extended release (Niaspan) (1-2 g)	LDL↓ 5%-25% HDL↑ 15%-35% TG↓ 20%-50%	Flushing Hyperglycemia Hyperuricemia (or gout) Upper GI distress Hepatotoxicity	Chronic liver disease Severe gout Diabetes Peptic ulcer disease Pregnancy/lactation
Fibric acids	Gemfibrozil (600 mg bid) Fenofibrate (45-145 mg)	LDL↓ 5%-20% HDL↑ 10%-20% TG↓ 20%-50%	Dyspepsia Gallstones Myopathy (especially with concomitant use of gemfibrozil and statins)	Severe renal disease (dose adjustment for fenofibrate) Severe hepatic disease Caution with statins Can worsen LDL cholesterol
Ezetimibe (cholesterol absorption inhibitor)	Ezetimibe (10 mg)	LDL↓ 18% HDL↑ 1% TG↓ 8%	Abdominal pain; myalgias	Liver disease Avoid with resins and fibrates

*Cyclosporine, macrolide antibiotics, various antifungal agents, and cytochrome P-450 inhibitors (fibrates and niacin should be used with appropriate caution).
†Dosages of simvastatin 80 mg are no longer recommended. Potential interactions with amlodipine and ranolazine warrant doses ≤2 mg daily.
‡Colesevelam reduces glucose and A1c ~0.5% and has been approved for treatment of diabetes with dyslipidemia.
GI, Gastrointestinal; *HDL*, high-density lipoprotein; *HMG-CoA*, 3-hydroxy-3-methylglutaryl coenzyme A; *LDL*, low-density lipoprotein; *TG*, triglyceride.
Modified from The National Cholesterol Education Program, *JAMA* 285:2486, 2001. In Boyden TF et al: Implementing new guidelines in the management of blood cholesterol, *Am J Med* 127:705, 2014.

intima media thickness and reduces the risk of cardiovascular disease in adulthood.

- The American Academy of Pediatrics (AAP) guideline (*Pediatrics* 122:198, 2008) recommends consideration toward pharmacologic treatment for children with LDL >190 mg/dl or >160 mg/dl if other risk factors are present.
- *HDL cholesterol efflux capacity* refers to the ability of HDL to accept cholesterol from macrophages, which is a key step in reverse cholesterol transport. It is inversely associated with the incidence of cardiovascular events and may be a useful biomarker when added to traditional risk factors.

- There are currently no pharmacologic therapies approved to reduce Lp(a) and ASCVD risk. Although PCSK9 monoclonal antibodies reduce Lp(a), they are not approved for use among individuals who meet LDL cholesterol targets. Niacin modestly reduces Lp(a) but may not further reduce ASCVD risk in addition to statins.[3,4]

REFERENCES & SUGGESTED READINGS

Available at eBooks.Health.Elsevier.com.

RELATED CONTENT

High Cholesterol (Patient Information)
Coronary Artery Disease (Related Key Topic)
Hyperlipoproteinemia, Primary (Related Key Topic)
Statin-Induced Muscle Syndrome (Related Key Topic)

AUTHOR: **FRED F. FERRI, MD**

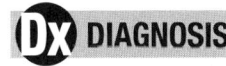
BASIC INFORMATION

DEFINITION

Hypercoagulable state is an inherited or acquired condition associated with an increased risk of thrombosis. A classification of hypercoagulable states is described in Table 1.

SYNONYM

Thrombophilia

ICD-10CM CODES
D68.5 Primary thrombophilia
D68.6 Other thrombophilia
D68.8 Other specified coagulation defects
D68.9 Coagulation defect, unspecified

EPIDEMIOLOGY & DEMOGRAPHICS

INCIDENCE, PREVALENCE, PREDOMINANT SEX AND AGE: See Table 2. Significant variations in the prevalence rates and thrombotic risks for hypercoagulable states are reported. This may reflect geographic variation in the prevalence of genetic defects, different populations, or the presence of other unidentified thrombophilic risk factors. When thrombosis occurs, it is often associated with an acquired risk factor (e.g., surgery, pregnancy, oral contraceptive [OC] use).

RISK FACTORS: Family history of thrombosis, increasing age, tobacco use, immobility, surgery, prior history of deep vein thrombosis (DVT) pregnancy, hormone replacement therapy, trauma, connective tissue disease, underlying malignancy, medications (megestrol acetate, tamoxifen, oral contraceptives). Potential prothrombotic states are summarized in Table 3.

PHYSICAL FINDINGS & CLINICAL PRESENTATION

- Inherited thrombophilia is usually associated with VTE, most commonly DVT[1]
- Some acquired thrombophilias are associated with arterial thrombosis[1]
- Pregnancy complications[1]
- Medical conditions associated with increased risk of thrombosis

ETIOLOGY

- Thrombosis is often a multifactorial process with genetic, environmental, and acquired factors. Table E4, Table E5, Table E6, and Table E7 describe causes of acquired and inherited deficiencies in antithrombin, protein C, and protein S.
- All thrombotic factors ultimately lead to blood flow stasis, endothelial damage, or change in blood constituents to cause thrombosis. These

three components of thrombosis are known as the Virchow triad.
- Thrombotic risk increases with use of OCs or hormone replacement therapy (HRT) and during the pregnancy/postpartum period.[1]
- Adverse pregnancy outcomes may be caused by thrombosis of the uteroplacental circulation.

DIAGNOSIS

DIFFERENTIAL DIAGNOSIS

INHERITED: Factor V Leiden (FVL) mutation[2-4]:
- Autosomal-dominant mutation with low penetrance
- Causes activated protein C resistance (APCR); 90% of APCR is caused by FVL mutation

TABLE 3 Potential Prothrombotic States

Congenital

Deficiency of anticoagulants
AT-III, protein C or protein S, plasminogen
Resistance to cofactor proteolysis
Factor V Leiden
High levels of procoagulants
Prothrombin 20210 mutation
Damage to endothelium

Acquired

Obstruction to flow indwelling lines
Pregnancy
Polycythemia/dehydration
Immobilization
Injury
Trauma, surgery, exercise
Inflammation
IBD, vasculitis, infection, Behçet syndrome
Hypercoagulability
Malignancy
Antiphospholipid syndrome
Nephrotic syndrome
Oral contraceptives L-Asparaginase

Rare Other Entities

Congenital dysfibrinogenemia
Acquired
Paroxysmal nocturnal hemoglobinuria
Thrombocythemia
Vascular grafts

AT-III, Antithrombin III; *IBD,* inflammatory bowel disease.
From Kliegman RM et al: *Nelson textbook of pediatrics,* ed 19, Philadelphia, 2011, Saunders.

TABLE 1 Classification of Hypercoagulable States

Hereditary	Mixed	Acquired
Loss of Function		
Antithrombin deficiency	Hyperhomocysteinemia	Previous venous thromboembolism
Protein C deficiency	Obesity	Pregnancy, puerperium
Protein S deficiency	Cancer	
		Drug-induced:
		Heparin-induced thrombocytopenia
		Prothrombin complex concentrates
		L-Asparaginase
		Hormonal therapy
Gain of Function		
Factor V Leiden	Postoperative	
Prothrombin FII G20210A	Myeloproliferative disorders	
Elevated factor VIII, IX, or XI		

From Hoffman R et al: *Hematology: basic principles and practice,* ed 7, Philadelphia, 2018, Elsevier.

TABLE 2 Hypercoagulable Conditions

	Prevalence in General Population (%)	Prevalence in Population with Thrombosis (%)	A/V Events	Relative Risk of Thrombosis
FVL mutation	5% of whites; rare in nonwhites	12%-40%	V	Heterozygous: 3-7; homozygous: 80
Prothrombin G20210A mutation	3% of whites; rare in nonwhites	6%-18%	V	3
AT deficiency	0.02%	1%-3%	V	20-50
PC deficiency	0.2%-0.4%	3%-5%	V	7-15
PS deficiency	0.03%-0.1%	1%-5%	V	5-11
Antiphospholipid antibody syndrome	1%-2%	5%-21%	V + A	2-11

A, Arterial; *AT,* antithrombin; *FVL,* factor V Leiden; *PC,* protein C; *PS,* protein S; *V,* venous.

Diseases and Disorders

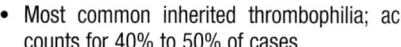

- Most common inherited thrombophilia; accounts for 40% to 50% of cases
- Risk of VTE is sevenfold greater in heterozygous carriers compared with noncarriers; however, the risk increases to 30-fold in heterozygous carriers who use OCP compared with noncarriers who do not use OCP
- Risk of VTE is increased 100-fold in homozygous women who use OCP
- May be associated with cardiovascular disease in select high-risk subgroups

Prothrombin G20210A mutation[5-8]:

- Autosomal-dominant mutation with low penetrance
- OC use in heterozygous carriers is associated with a sixfold increased risk of VTE compared with noncarriers not using OCs
- May be associated with cardiovascular disease in select high-risk subgroups and young patients with ischemic stroke
- Causes increased mRNA accumulation and protein synthesis, leading to elevated prothrombin plasma concentrations

Protein C, protein S, antithrombin (AT) deficiency[5,9]:

- Autosomal-dominant inheritance; many mutations identified for each of these conditions
- Decreased level (type I deficiency) or abnormal function (type II deficiency)
- First episode of thrombosis is usually in young adults

Protein C and protein S[9,10]:

- Homozygous condition is very rare; usually associated with lethal thrombosis in infancy
- Associated with warfarin-induced skin necrosis, which occurs secondary to depletion of vitamin K–dependent anticoagulant factors sooner than procoagulant factors in the first few days of therapy

AT deficiency[10]:

- Most thrombogenic of the inherited thrombophilias; 50% lifetime risk of thrombosis.
- Homozygous condition is very rare, probably not compatible with normal fetal development.
- Arterial thrombosis can occur rarely.
- Can cause heparin resistance.

Other possible causes: Non-0 blood group, dysfibrinogenemia, elevated thrombin-activatable fibrinolysis inhibitor, elevated factor IX and factor XI levels

ACQUIRED: Antiphospholipid antibody syndrome (APS)[10]:

- Most common cause of acquired thrombophilia
- Can present as arterial or venous thrombosis, recurrent pregnancy loss, and adverse pregnancy outcomes
- Thromboembolic events occur in up to 30% of population; high risk of recurrent thrombosis (up to 70% reported)
- See "Antiphospholipid Antibody Syndrome" for more information

Conditions associated with increased risk of thrombosis:

- Prior thrombosis
- Trauma
- Medical illness: Heart failure, respiratory failure, infection, diabetes mellitus, obesity, nephrotic syndrome, inflammatory bowel disease
- Chronic hemolysis–paroxysmal nocturnal hemoglobinuria, atypical hemolytic uremic syndrome, sickle cell anemia
- Pregnancy (sixfold increased risk of VTE), postpartum, OC use (fourfold increased risk, higher risk with third-generation OCs), transdermal contraceptive patch, HRT (twofold increased risk), tamoxifen, raloxifene
- Immobilization, travel
- Surgery (especially orthopedic), central venous catheters
- Hyperviscosity syndromes
- Myeloproliferative neoplasms
- Malignancy: Disease or treatment related
- Heparin-induced thrombocytopenia and thrombosis
- Smoking

WORKUP

- History (presence of conditions or use of medications predisposing to thrombosis, family history of thrombosis), physical examination, laboratory tests, imaging studies. Routine investigations to evaluate a patient with thrombosis are summarized in Box 1.
- Age-appropriate cancer screening.
- No consensus exists regarding screening for thrombophilia; few cost-effectiveness or outcomes data are available. Thrombophilia screening is probably overused, as results usually do not change management.[1]
- Thrombophilia screening is not recommended for primary prevention of VTE; some advocate testing prior to OC use or pregnancy in women with a strong family history of thrombosis or thrombophilia.[1,11,12] Box 2 summarizes recommendations regarding when to perform a thrombophilia screen. Essential tests for thrombophilia screening are described in Box 3.
- Screening not recommended if VTE was associated with an identified risk factor. A possible exception is thrombosis associated with pregnancy, the postpartum period, or with OC use.[1,11,12]
- Reasonable to pursue workup for VTE with weak triggers, a strong family history, and female family members of childbearing age; consider testing for FVL, prothrombin G20210A mutation, protein C, protein S, and AT deficiency. Consider testing for APS if extensive DVT or pulmonary embolism (PE).[1,11,12]
- Unprovoked VTE:
  1. Screen individuals for APCR, prothrombin G20210A mutation, protein C, protein S, AT deficiency, and APS if any of the following are present: <50 yr of age at first episode of thrombosis + strong family history of thrombosis or female family member of childbearing age, thrombosis in unusual anatomic location (cerebral veins or splanchnic veins; if splanchnic veins, consider testing as well for myeloproliferative neoplasms [MPN] and paroxysmal nocturnal hemoglobinuria [PNH]).[1]
  2. Screen all others for APS.[1]
- Arterial thrombosis: Screen for APS.[1]
- NOTE: Routine screening for factor VIII level or hyperhomocysteinemia is not recommended.[10]

TIMING OF WORKUP:

- Ideally >2 wk after discontinuation of vitamin K antagonists (VKA) and >2 days after discontinuation of direct oral anticoagulant (DOAC) (except for APS, which requires prolonged anticoagulation).[1]
- NOTE: Acute thrombosis, anticoagulation, pregnancy, and many medical conditions can affect the results and must be considered in the timing and interpretation of the workup.[1,12]

BOX 1 Routine Investigations to Evaluate a Patient With Thrombosis

Test	Abnormality	Diagnostic Information
Complete blood count	Elevated hematocrit Increased white count Increased platelet count Leukopenia Thrombocytopenia	Myeloproliferative disorder (e.g., essential thrombocythemia, polycythemia vera); may be found in paroxysmal nocturnal hemoglobinuria; if associated with heparin administration, consider heparin-induced thrombocytopenia
Blood film	Leukoerythroblastic changes	Underlying neoplasm invading bone marrow
Liver function tests	Abnormal tests	May point to malignancy
Renal function	Impaired renal function	Assess prior to anticoagulation with heparin, low-molecular-weight heparin or new oral anticoagulants
Urinalysis	Proteinuria	Nephrotic syndrome; may be associated with venous thromboembolism or renal vein thrombosis
PT and aPTT	Prolonged PT and aPTT	To enable safe anticoagulation to proceed if required Need to exclude lupus anticoagulant

From Hoffman R et al: *Hematology: basic principles and practice,* ed 7, Philadelphia, 2018, Elsevier.

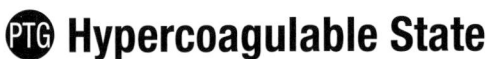
BOX 2 When to Perform a Thrombophilia Screen

Clinical Scenario
- First episode of unprovoked venous thromboembolism in individuals younger than 40 yr of age
- Thrombosis in an unusual site (e.g., cerebral or mesenteric thrombosis)
- Two or more first-degree relatives with unprovoked thrombosis
- Three or more early pregnancy losses, or one or more fetal deaths after 10 wk gestation

BOX 3 Essential Tests for Thrombophilia Screening

- Basic coagulation screen
  1. International normalized ratio (INR): To exclude warfarin effect—warfarin will lower protein C and S levels
  2. Activated partial thromboplastin time (aPTT): To exclude heparin effect—heparin will lower antithrombin levels
- Functional assay for antithrombin (with heparin to detect type II defects)
- Functional assay for protein C
- Functional assay for protein S (immune assays for total and free protein S)
- APC resistance assay: With genetic test for factor V Leiden for confirmation of abnormal results
- Genetic test for *FIIG 20210A* gene mutation
- Anticardiolipin and β_2-glycoprotein-1 antibodies (IgG and IgM) and lupus anticoagulant assay

LABORATORY TESTS

- Initial workup: CBC with peripheral smear, electrolytes, calcium, creatinine, blood urea nitrogen (BUN), liver function tests, prothrombin time/partial thromboplastin time, prostate-specific antigen (in men aged >50 yr), urinalysis.[10]
- NOTE: Genetic counseling and written informed consent should be obtained before genetic testing. Abnormal nongenetic tests should be repeated after 6 wk to decrease false-positive results.[13]
- APC-resistance assay tests for factor V Leiden mutation. Presence of lupus anticoagulant causes false positives. Follow-up positive result with a confirmatory genetic test.[10]
- Prothrombin G20210A mutation testing.[10]
- AT, protein C, and protein S deficiency: Functional assays are initial tests, then follow up positive result with antigenic assay to determine the type of deficiency. Note that antigenic assays for protein S should measure free and total levels. The functional assays for protein C and S deficiency testing may be falsely low in the presence of APCR or elevated factor VIII level and falsely high if lupus anticoagulant is present.[10]
- APS: Any one of the following found elevated on two occasions at least 12 wk apart: Lupus anticoagulant, anticardiolipin antibodies (IgG/IgM isotype), or anti–B_2-glycoprotein-I antibodies (IgG/IgM isotype).[10]

IMAGING STUDIES

Chest radiograph and other tests as appropriate to diagnose thrombosis and rule out associated conditions

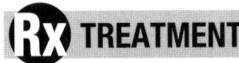 **TREATMENT**

NONPHARMACOLOGIC THERAPY

OC/HRT use and smoking should be avoided.[1]

PROPHYLAXIS

- Prophylactic anticoagulation in high-risk situations.[1]
- Patients with AT deficiency may benefit from antithrombin concentrates in high-risk situations.[14]
- Pregnancy prophylaxis: Timing and intensity of therapy are based on the patient's risk (genetic or acquired defect and clinical history). Women with thrombophilia and recurrent adverse pregnancy outcomes may benefit from prophylaxis with heparin (low-molecular-weight heparin most commonly used) and low-dose aspirin.[11]

ACUTE GENERAL Rx

Initial therapy is the same as for individuals with and without thrombophilia, with exceptions for protein C, AT, and APS deficiency as detailed in the following:

Venous thrombosis:
- DOACs such as Xa inhibitors (rivaroxaban and apixaban) have been FDA-approved for treatment in acute DVT and are currently recommended as first-line therapy. They have been found to be noninferior to warfarin, appear easier to use with fewer drug interactions, and have a trend toward less major bleeding.[15]
- In patients unable to take DOACs, begin low-molecular-weight heparin (LMWH) and warfarin simultaneously. Continue heparin for at least 5 days and until international normalized ratio (INR) is therapeutic for 2 consecutive days; continue warfarin for at least 3 mo. Aim for INR of 2 to 3. Unfractionated heparin (UH) or fondaparinux (factor Xa inhibitor) may be used as alternatives to LMWH. LMWH is preferred over UH (except in patients with massive pulmonary embolism, increased risk of bleeding, or renal failure) because of equivalent or superior effectiveness and a better safety profile.
- Thrombophilia is not associated with a higher risk of recurrent VTE during warfarin therapy, with the exception of cancer patients in whom LMWH for 3 to 6 mo is associated with lower rates of recurrence than warfarin therapy.[15]
- In pregnancy, anti-coagulate with heparin throughout pregnancy and for at least 6 wk postpartum. Minimum duration of anticoagulation should be 6 mo. LMWH is preferred over UH. Warfarin may be used postpartum.[9]
- Consider thrombolysis or thrombectomy in patients with massive pulmonary embolism or large proximal lower extremity DVT.[15]

Protein C deficiency:
- Warfarin-induced skin necrosis: Discontinue warfarin, give vitamin K, and start heparin anticoagulation. Consider protein C replacement with protein C concentrate or fresh frozen plasma. Warfarin may be restarted at a low dose (2 mg daily for 3 days and increase by 2 to 3 mg daily until target INR is reached). Continue heparin for at least 5 days and until warfarin-induced anticoagulation is achieved.

AT deficiency:
- AT concentrates may be used if difficulty achieving anticoagulation (heparin resistance), severe thrombosis, or recurrent thrombosis despite adequate anticoagulation.[9]

APS:
- Warfarin is superior to rivaroxaban in patients with APS. The RAPS trial randomized patients with triple positive APS to receive either rivaroxaban or warfarin and found significantly higher rates of thrombosis in the rivaroxaban group. A subsequent trial noted increased endogenous thrombin potential (a marker of less effective anticoagulation) in APS patients switched to rivaroxaban following initial VKA therapy compared to those continued on warfarin. This study was not powered to assess clinical efficacy. If a patient with triple positive APS is on DOAC, it is recommended to transition them to VKA therapy.[15]

Arterial thrombosis:
- Anticoagulation and evaluation for thrombolysis or surgery

CHRONIC Rx

- Optimal duration of anticoagulation remains unknown. Length of therapy may be individualized by assessing the risk of recurrence. Residual thrombosis (on ultrasonography) or elevated D-dimer levels after completion of anticoagulation are associated with an increased risk of recurrence. With these findings, consider prolonging anticoagulation.

TABLE 8 Management of Women With a History of Venous Thrombosis During Pregnancy and the Puerperium

Clinical History	Thrombophilia	Antepartum	Postpartum[a]
Prior VTE due to a transient risk factor	No	Surveillance	Yes
Prior VTE due to pregnancy or estrogens	Yes or no	Prophylactic LMWH	Yes
Prior idiopathic VTE	Yes or no	Prophylactic LMWH	Yes
Recurrent VTE	Yes or no	Treatment dose LMWH	Resume long-term anticoagulation
No prior VTE Positive family history	Antithrombin deficiency; homozygous FII G20210A; or Factor V Leiden; or dual heterozygosity for both mutations	Prophylactic or intermediate dose LMWH	Yes

LMWH, Low-molecular-weight heparin; *VTE,* venous thromboembolism.
[a]Postpartum prophylaxis involves a 6-wk course of prophylactic doses of LMWH or dose-adjusted warfarin (target INR: 2.0 to 3.0).
From Hoffman R et al: *Hematology: basic principles and practice,* ed 7, Philadelphia, 2018, Elsevier.

- Must consider risk and benefit; risk of major bleeding 2% to 3% annually in general population on anticoagulation but higher in the elderly (7% to 9% per yr). Long-term anticoagulation is usually not indicated given the low risk of recurrent thrombosis for most conditions and the bleeding risk associated with anticoagulation.
- Indefinite anticoagulation considered if any of the following:
  1. Life-threatening thrombosis or thrombosis at an unusual site
  2. More than a single genetic defect
  3. Presence of AT deficiency or APS
  4. Unprovoked DVT or PE with low bleeding risk
  5. >1 Provoked DVT or PE with low bleeding risk
- Patients with active cancer may benefit from indefinite anticoagulation.

DISPOSITION
Depends on underlying condition

REFERRAL
Hematology, maternal-fetal medicine, obstetric medicine

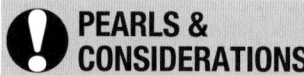
PEARLS & CONSIDERATIONS

COMMENTS
- Women with thrombophilic defects but no prior history of venous thromboembolism, or family history of the same, likely do not require antepartum prophylaxis or postpartum treatment, but definitive data are lacking. A summary of these recommendations is provided in Table 8.

- DOACs and warfarin therapy effectively reduce the risk of recurrent VTE; when therapy is discontinued VTE risk increases.
- Warfarin is preferred over DOAC for triple positive APS patients based on the data showing rivaroxaban to be inferior to warfarin in this population.[15]
- Previous episode of VTE is a major risk factor for recurrence regardless of the presence of thrombophilia. Risk is greatest in the first 2 yr after thrombosis. 40% of all patients with unprovoked VTE have recurrence within 5 yr.[1]
- Genetic risk factors for thrombosis in nonwhites remain largely unknown.
- Interpreting workup: Many medical conditions cause acquired abnormalities.
  1. Acute thrombosis may be associated with lupus anticoagulant, increased anticardiolipin antibodies, and elevated factor VIII levels[10]
     a. Heparin therapy: Antithrombin levels decrease by up to 30%; can affect lupus anticoagulant testing depending on available assay[10]
     b. Warfarin therapy: Cannot measure protein C and protein S (levels and function decrease); antithrombin levels may increase; can affect lupus anticoagulant testing
     c. Acute thrombosis: Antithrombin level, protein C, and protein S levels may be falsely lowered[10]
  2. Protein C, protein S, and antithrombin levels decrease with surgery, liver disease, disseminated intravascular coagulation, and chemotherapy. Protein C level also decreases with severe infection but levels increase with age and hyperlipidemia. Protein S and antithrombin levels also decrease with nephrotic syndrome, pregnancy, and estrogen therapy (HRT, OCs)[10]

  3. APCR is increased with pregnancy, estrogen therapy (HRT, OCs), and certain cancers; elevated factor VIII level and antiphospholipid antibodies can cause APCR[10]

PREVENTION
Evidence is equivocal in regard to the effectiveness of compression stockings in preventing post-thrombotic syndrome.

PATIENT & FAMILY EDUCATION
National Blood Clot Alliance
120 White Plains Road, Suite 100
Tarrytown, NY 10591
www.stoptheclot.org/contact.htm
National Collaborative Outreach Project of the Blood Clot Outreach Program at the Hemophilia and Thrombosis Center University of North Carolina at Chapel Hill
www.clotconnect.org/about-clot-connect/about
Factor V Leiden Resources
www.fvleiden.org/resources/index.html
APS Foundation of America, Inc.
P.O. Box 801
LaCrosse, WI 54602-0801
www.apsfa.org/

REFERENCES
Available at eBooks.Health.Elsevier.com.

RELATED CONTENT
Thrombophilia (Patient Information)
Antiphospholipid Antibody Syndrome (Related Key Topic)
Deep Vein Thrombosis (Related Key Topic)
Pulmonary Embolism (Related Key Topic)

AUTHORS: **NIRAV HARIBHAKTI, MD, PHARMD,** and **JOHN L. REAGAN, MD**

BASIC INFORMATION

DEFINITION

Hyperemesis gravidarum refers to a severe and persistent form of nausea and vomiting in pregnancy. While no precise criteria exist to define hyperemesis, it may be characterized by at least a 5% weight loss from prepregnancy weight, dehydration, ketonuria, and electrolyte imbalance. Typical onset occurs at week 4 to 8 of pregnancy, continuing through week 14 to 16 of pregnancy.

ICD-10CM CODES
O21.0   Mild hyperemesis gravidarum
O21.1   Hyperemesis gravidarum with metabolic disturbance

EPIDEMIOLOGY & DEMOGRAPHICS

INCIDENCE: 0.3% to 3% of pregnancies
RISK FACTORS: Women with increased placental mass, including molar pregnancy or multiple gestation, family history or personal history of hyperemesis gravidarum, prior miscarriage, nulliparity, young age, hyperthyroidism, gastrointestinal disorders, vestibular disease, motion sickness, long interpregnancy interval, and supertaster status. Alcohol use, smoking, and anosmia may be protective. A female fetus increases the risk by 1.27-fold.
GENETICS: A genetic predisposition may exist; hyperemesis gravidarum is more common among first-degree relatives of those diagnosed with the condition, and certain placental protein gene variants associated with hyperemesis have been identified.

PHYSICAL FINDINGS & CLINICAL PRESENTATION

- Weight loss of more than 5% from pregravid weight
- Symptoms: Nausea, vomiting, spitting, enhanced olfactory senses, food and/or fluid intolerance, lethargy
- Signs: Poor skin turgor, dry mucous membranes, hypotension, tachycardia
- Complications include inadequate caloric and nutritional intake, dehydration, and electrolyte abnormalities, including hyponatremia, hypocalcemia, hypokalemia, and, in severe cases, hypochloremic metabolic acidosis or Wernicke encephalopathy from thiamine deficiency. Severe hyperemesis gravidarum also has been shown to correlate with higher rates of anxiety and depression

ETIOLOGY

Unknown, but likely multifactorial. Theories include interactions between hCG and the thyroid, gestational hyperestrogenemia, and gastric dysrhythmias.

DIAGNOSIS

DIFFERENTIAL DIAGNOSIS

- Gastrointestinal conditions: Gastroenteritis, gastroparesis, biliary tract disease, hepatitis, intestinal obstruction, peptic ulcer disease, appendicitis, inflammatory bowel disease
- Genitourinary tract conditions: Pyelonephritis, nephrolithiasis
- Metabolic disease: Hyperthyroidism, hyperparathyroidism, diabetic ketoacidosis, cannabinoid hyperemesis syndrome, porphyria, adrenal insufficiency
- Neurologic conditions: Pseudotumor cerebri, vestibular lesions, migraines, tumors of the central nervous system, cyclic vomiting syndrome
- Miscellaneous: Drug toxicity or intolerance, psychogenic
- Pregnancy-related conditions: Acute fatty liver of pregnancy, preeclampsia

WORKUP

Diagnosis is one of exclusion. History and physical examination along with laboratory tests to rule out other causes of vomiting should be performed.

LABORATORY TESTS

- BMP may reveal hyponatremia, hypokalemia, low serum urea.
- Urinalysis may show elevated specific gravity, ketonuria, or proteinuria.
- Liver enzymes (ALT typically more elevated than AST, both usually reaching only two to three times the upper limit of normal).
- Serum bilirubin (<4 mg/dl).
- Serum amylase or lipase (up to $5\times$ greater than normal).
- CBC may show an increase in hematocrit from volume depletion.
- Magnesium and calcium may be low.
- TSH and free T_4 (transient hyperthyroidism occurs in two thirds of women with hyperemesis gravidarum; this is biochemical hyperthyroidism that usually resolves by 18 wk of gestation; testing and treatment should not be undertaken without additional clinical evidence of intrinsic thyroid disease).

IMAGING STUDIES

- Ultrasound to evaluate for multiple gestation or molar pregnancy
- If the patient is having associated pain, a right upper quadrant ultrasound may be indicated to evaluate biliary tract disease

TREATMENT

NONPHARMACOLOGIC THERAPY

- Prevention with prenatal vitamins before conception
- Avoidance of foods and smells that trigger nausea
- Ginger (200 to 500 mg q8h)
- Protein-heavy meals
- Frequent small meals, every 1-2 hr
- Reassurance and support, in some cases intensive cognitive-behavioral therapy

ACUTE GENERAL Rx

- Pyridoxine (vitamin B_6) 10 to 25 mg PO q8h
- Doxylamine 12.5 to 25 mg qhs
- Pyridoxine (10 mg)/doxylamine (10 mg) combination, starting with 2 tablets qhs and adding an additional 1 tablet every A.M. and 1 tablet every P.M. if needed
- Antiemetics including promethazine, prochlorperazine, metoclopramide, and ondansetron have been shown to be generally safe and effective in improving pregnancy outcome
- Corticosteroids (methylprednisolone, prednisone) may be considered after 10 wk of gestation
- IV fluid and electrolyte administration if evidence of deficiency is found
- Thiamine prior to dextrose administration to avoid Wernicke encephalopathy
- Restart oral intake gradually no less than 48 hr after vomiting has stopped

CHRONIC Rx

- If unable to tolerate oral intake, consider replacing with enteral or parenteral feeding
- Repeated IV fluid and electrolyte replacement can be conducted through outpatient visits

COMPLEMENTARY & ALTERNATIVE MEDICINE

- Supportive psychotherapy
- Acupuncture
- Acupressure with use of a wrist band

DISPOSITION

- Infants born from pregnancies complicated by hyperemesis may have a higher risk of being small for gestational age or low birth weight than those not; however, this may be limited to infants of women who have experienced significant weight loss in the setting of hyperemesis.
- Women with hyperemesis gravidarum should be counseled that they have a higher risk than other women of developing similar symptoms in future pregnancies.

PEARLS & CONSIDERATIONS

COMMENTS

Nausea and vomiting in early pregnancy are associated with psychosocial morbidity.

SUGGESTED READINGS
Available at eBooks.Health.Elsevier.com.

RELATED CONTENT
Hyperemesis Gravidarum (Patient Information)

AUTHORS: **T. CAROLINE BANK, MD**, and **MARWAN MA'AYEH, MD**

Hyperglycemic Hyperosmolar Syndrome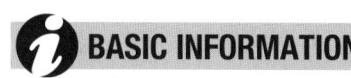

BASIC INFORMATION

DEFINITION

Hyperglycemic hyperosmolar syndrome (HHS) is a life-threatening complication of diabetes mellitus characterized by marked hyperglycemia, dehydration, electrolyte derangements, and hyperosmolality with or without mental obtundation, all in the absence of significant ketoacidosis.

SYNONYMS

HHS
Hyperosmolar hyperglycemic syndrome
Diabetic hyperosmolar syndrome
Hyperglycemic hyperosmolar nonketotic syndrome
Hyperglycemic hyperosmolar nonketotic coma
Hyperosmolar hyperglycemic state
Nonketotic hyperosmolar syndrome

ICD-10CM CODES

E08.00	Diabetes mellitus due to underlying condition with hyperosmolarity without nonketotic hyperglycemic-hyperosmolar coma (NKHHC)
E08.01	Diabetes mellitus due to underlying condition with hyperosmolarity with coma
E09.00	Drug or chemical induced diabetes mellitus with hyperosmolarity without nonketotic hyperglycemic-hyperosmolar coma (NKHHC)
E09.01	Drug or chemical induced diabetes mellitus with hyperosmolarity with coma
E11.00	Type 2 diabetes mellitus with hyperosmolarity without nonketotic hyperglycemic-hyperosmolar coma (NKHHC)
E11.01	Type 2 diabetes mellitus with hyperosmolarity with coma
E13.00	Other specified diabetes mellitus with hyperosmolarity without nonketotic hyperglycemic-hyperosmolar coma (NKHHC)
E13.01	Other specified diabetes mellitus with hyperosmolarity with coma

EPIDEMIOLOGY & DEMOGRAPHICS

HHS is a rare condition that most commonly affects patients with type 2 diabetes mellitus. Approximately 20% of patients have no history of diabetes.[1] Older adults with new-onset diabetes or those who have poorly controlled type 2 diabetes and are predisposed to extracellular fluid volume depletion (dehydration) are at increased risk for HHS. Social and racial-ethnic disparities are remarkable with Black race/ethnicity and lower income individuals at heightened risk of HHS.[2] Mortality from HHS is estimated at 5% to 20%, a greater mortality rate than for diabetic ketoacidosis. Prognosis is determined by several factors, including age, degree of dehydration, and presence of other comorbidities.

PHYSICAL FINDINGS & CLINICAL PRESENTATION[1]

- Polyuria, polydipsia, weight loss, weakness
- Mental status changes that can range from full alertness to coma
- Focal neurologic signs (e.g., hemiplegia, hemianopsia) or seizures (focal or generalized), aphasia, visual hallucinations
- Symptoms of coexisting illnesses or comorbidities that may have precipitated the event
- Signs of extracellular fluid volume depletion, including dry mucous membranes, poor skin turgor, sunken eyes, hypotension, and tachycardia
- Normothermia or hypothermia despite the presence of infection, due to peripheral vasodilation

ETIOLOGY

HHS can be precipitated by various conditions[1]:
- Infection is the most common precipitant (especially pneumonia, urinary tract infections, and COVID-19)
- Insulin deficiency (undiagnosed diabetes, inadequate insulin, or medication nonadherence)
- Inflammatory conditions (e.g., acute pancreatitis, acute cholecystitis)
- Ischemia/infarction (e.g., myocardial infarction, stroke, bowel ischemia)
- Kidney failure
- Severe dehydration (e.g., burns, heat stroke)
- Drugs (e.g., steroids, thiazides, beta blockers, atypical antipsychotics, sympathomimetics including cocaine, alcohol, and pentamidine)

A relative insulin deficiency provides enough insulin to inhibit ketogenesis but is insufficient to inhibit hepatic gluconeogenesis and glycogenolysis or to promote peripheral glucose uptake, resulting in consequent hyperglycemia. With underlying illness, counterregulatory hormone excess leads to further blood glucose elevation. The resultant extreme hyperglycemia leads to osmotic diuresis.[3,4] If adequate hydration is not maintained, dehydration and worsening renal function ensue. In patients with inadequate fluid intake due to altered thirst mechanisms or the inability to access fluids, as may be seen in older adults, the risk of severe dehydration further increases. Diminished renal filtration further impairs glucose excretion, thus exacerbating the hyperglycemia, dehydration, and hyperosmolality and increasing the risk for cardiovascular collapse.

DIAGNOSIS

DIFFERENTIAL DIAGNOSIS

- Diabetic ketoacidosis

- Stroke (especially in older adults with neurologic abnormalities)
- Hypovolemic or septic shock
- Encephalopathy

WORKUP

After an initial history is obtained, perform a physical examination that includes immediate evaluation of airway, breathing, circulation, mental status, volume status, and signs suggestive of a precipitating event, including infection, myocardial infarction, or stroke.

LABORATORY TESTS

- Hyperglycemia: Blood glucose >600 mg/dl (Box 1)[5]
- Serum osmolality: Usually >320 mOsm/kg
- Complete metabolic panel: Serum creatinine, blood urea nitrogen (BUN), electrolytes, glucose
- Serum sodium: May be low, normal, or high. Hyperglycemia increases plasma osmolality that translocates intracellular water to the extracellular compartment, decreasing serum sodium. Serum sodium can be corrected by adding 1.6 mmol/L to the measured serum sodium level for every 100 mg/dl increase in serum glucose >100 mg/dl and <400 mg/dl, and then increase the sodium level by 4 mmol/L for each glucose increment of 100 mg/dl above 400 mg/dl.[6] Marked osmotic diuresis induced by hyperglycemia may cause the serum sodium level to be normal or high
- Serum potassium and phosphate: Total body potassium and phosphate deficits typically occur due to urinary losses from osmotic diuresis. However, these levels may be acutely normal or high due to extracellular shift secondary to insulin deficiency and hyperosmolality
- Anion gap and serum lactate: Anion gap may be normal or elevated in the setting of lactic acidosis
- Arterial blood gas: pH >7.30
- Serum and urine ketones: Negative or small
- Serum bicarbonate: >15 mmol/L
- Hemoglobin A1c (if not performed in past 3 mo)
- Complete blood count with differential. May indicate presence of underlying infection [leukocytosis >25,000 mm³], inflammatory condition, hemoconcentration. A leukocytosis of 10,000 to 15,000 mm³ is expected from the stress of illness alone[1]
- Urinalysis, urine/sputum/blood cultures as indicated based on physical exam findings to evaluate the precipitating illness and other comorbidities

---

BOX 1 Diagnostic Testing Criteria for Patients With Hyperglycemic Hyperosmolar State[5]

Glucose higher than 600 mg/dl
Normal pH (classically, however, patients are often mildly acidotic)
No significant ketosis*
Serum osmolarity
- >320 mOsm/L with any mental status changes, *or*
- >350 mOsm/L

*Serum acetoacetate is often present, typically an absent or low β-hydroxybutyrate level.

From Adams JG et al (eds): *Emergency medicine: clinical essentials,* ed 2, Philadelphia, 2013, Saunders.

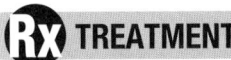
IMAGING STUDIES

Electrocardiogram (ECG), chest radiograph, and other imaging studies as indicated to evaluate the precipitating causes

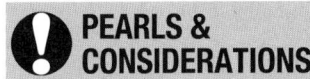 **TREATMENT**

ACUTE GENERAL Rx[1,3,4]

Aggressive fluid resuscitation, intravenous insulin, and electrolyte correction are the mainstays of treatment. The initial goal of HHS treatment includes restoring the water deficit with intravenous fluids. This will help to normalize the plasma hyperosmolality, improve renal perfusion and insulin resistance, reduce the counterregulatory hormone release, and eventually correct hyperglycemia. Selecting the appropriate type of fluid is important to prevent complications related to dysnatremia. Improper management of plasma sodium concentration and plasma osmolality during treatment of HHS has been associated with the life-threatening complication of cerebral edema.

AGGRESSIVE INTRAVENOUS FLUID REPLACEMENT: Due to trivial ketonemia and the insulin sensitivity of most HHS patients, initial treatment is intravenous fluid alone without insulin. Insulin used prior to intravenous hydration or early in resuscitation risks a precipitous drop in serum osmolality. In the absence of cardiac compromise or end-stage renal disease, infuse 0.9% normal saline (NS) at an initial rate of 1 L/h for the first hour. This is then followed by adjustments in the rate of infusion based on electrolyte values and hemodynamics. A lower rate of 250 to 500 ml/h may be adequate in the absence of severe dehydration. If the corrected serum sodium is elevated, 0.45% NS may be infused instead. Reassess corrected sodium needs by frequent checks and calculation. Recommended sodium decline is 0.5 mmol/L/h and should not surpass 10 to 12 mmol/L per day. Use measured or calculated osmolality to guide the rate of fluid resuscitation for gradual normalization of osmolality. Recommended serum osmolality decline is 3 mOsm/kg per hour. Once serum glucose decreases to 300 mg/dl, change the intravenous fluid to 5% dextrose with 0.45% NS at 150 to 250 ml/h.

INSULIN: Once glucose is no longer significantly improving with fluids alone, reassess patient's fluid status and initiate intravenous insulin. Administer initial bolus of intravenous regular insulin 0.1 units/kg followed by 0.1 units/kg per hour infusion or a continuous infusion of 0.14 units/kg per hour without initial bolus. If serum glucose declines by less than 50 to 75 mg/dl in the first hour, increase the insulin infusion rate every hour until a decline is noted. Once the serum glucose reaches 300 mg/dl, decrease the insulin infusion rate to 0.02 to 0.05 units/kg per hour to maintain serum glucose between 200 and 300 mg/dl until resolution of HHS.

POTASSIUM REPLACEMENT: Insulin therapy shifts potassium intracellularly, frequently causing hypokalemia. If serum potassium at presentation is between 3.3 and 5.2 mmol/L, infuse 20 to 30 mmol of potassium chloride (KCl) with each liter of intravenous fluid to maintain serum potassium between 4 and 5 mmol/L. If the serum potassium concentration at presentation is <3.3 mmol/L, replace potassium by administering KCl infusion at 20 to 30 mmol/h, and withhold insulin until the serum potassium concentration is >3.3 mmol/L. If the serum potassium at presentation is >5.2 mmol/L, monitor serum potassium level every 2 h without intravenous potassium supplementation.

PHOSPHORUS AND MAGNESIUM REPLACEMENT:
- Phosphorus and magnesium replacement are not routinely recommended. There are no studies of the utility of phosphate administration during treatment of HHS. Very low phosphorus levels may limit adenosine triphosphate (ATP) generation, thus limiting adequate diaphragm function. In patients with cardiac dysfunction, respiratory depression, or anemia and serum phosphate <1 mg/dl, add 20 to 30 mmol/L potassium phosphate to intravenous fluids.
- Monitor serum glucose hourly and serum electrolytes, BUN, and creatinine every 2 to 4 h until resolution of HHS.

TRANSITION TO SUBCUTANEOUS INSULIN: Normalization of serum osmolality and mental status indicates resolution of HHS. At this point, a transition to subcutaneous insulin should be performed. Overlap the initiation of subcutaneous intermediate- or long-acting insulin and discontinuation of intravenous insulin by 2 to 4 h to ensure adequate insulin levels and prevent rebound hyperglycemia. In patients with a known history of diabetes, their home insulin regimen may be initiated if adequate prior to presentation. In patients with poorly controlled diabetes, the subcutaneous insulin dose can be determined based on their stable insulin drip requirement. Insulin-naive patients may be started on basal-bolus insulin therapy either by calculation of total daily dose of 0.5 to 0.8 units/kg (split as half-basal and half-bolus; administer one third total bolus for each meal) or by their individual stable insulin drip requirements. Further subcutaneous insulin dose titration is based on subsequent blood glucoses. Resolution of glucotoxicity and inciting condition(s) will decrease insulin requirements. The underlying infection/inflammatory condition or precipitating event must be adequately treated.

CHRONIC THERAPY: Most patients will need insulin at discharge, at least short term. Patients whose diabetes was previously well controlled on oral agents may resume oral therapy after blood glucose stabilization by insulin.

DISPOSITION

Most patients require treatment in an emergency care setting, such as the intensive care unit or in a step-up facility.

PEARLS & CONSIDERATIONS

COMMENTS

- When patients with end-stage renal disease experience development of HHS, special management considerations are needed.[7] Aggressive fluid resuscitation is unnecessary in anuric end-stage renal disease patients, because most patients cannot produce the osmotic diuresis associated with normal kidney function. Note that urinary potassium and phosphorus losses will not occur, thereby limiting the need for supplementation. Lower continuous insulin infusion rates are required in patients with end-stage renal disease because of decreased insulin clearance. Hemodialysis is typically delayed until serum glucoses are corrected. Precipitous decreases in serum glucose from insulin administration and hemodialysis may result in rapid shifts in tonicity, predisposing cerebral edema.
- Education of the patient, family, and caregivers at long-term care facilities regarding optimal glycemic control, limiting modifiable risk factors for HHS, and prevention of dehydration is paramount.

REFERENCES
Available at eBooks.Health.Elsevier.com.

AUTHOR: **JESSICA E. SHILL, MD**

BASIC INFORMATION

DEFINITION

Abnormal elevation of serum potassium (K^+) concentration. It is associated with either normal or altered total body stores of potassium. Normal serum K^+ is 3.5 to 5.0 milliequivalents per liter (mEq/L). Hyperkalemia is defined as being mild (5.1 to 6.0 mEq/L), moderate (6.0 to 7.0 mEq/L), and severe (>7.0 mEq/L). Serum K^+ >7 mEq/L can lead to significant hemodynamic and neurologic consequences. Levels of K^+ >8.5 mEq/L can cause respiratory paralysis or cardiac arrest and can be rapidly fatal if untreated.

SYNONYM

Hyperpotassemia

ICD-10CM CODE
E87.5 Hyperpotassemia

EPIDEMIOLOGY & DEMOGRAPHICS

INCIDENCE & PREVALENCE[1,2]:
- Overall incidence and prevalence of hyperkalemia in the general population is unknown.
- Rarely detected in the general population, hyperkalemia is encountered in only 2.6% of Emergency Department visits and 3.5% of hospital admissions.
- Chronic kidney disease (CKD) patients have the highest prevalence of hyperkalemia, at approximately 10%. Increased risk depends on the present underlying conditions, including end-stage kidney disease (ESKD), acute kidney injury (AKI), cardiovascular disease (CVD), diabetes mellitus (DM), metabolic acidosis (especially nonanion gap acidosis), and medications such as renin-angiotensin-aldosterone system inhibitors (RAASi), mineralocorticoid receptor antagonists (MRA), and other potassium-sparing diuretics.
- The prevalence of an ICD-10 diagnosis for hyperkalemia was 14.6%.

PREDOMINANT SEX & AGE[1]:
- More common with increasing age due to increased prevalence of etiologic factors such as CKD, DM, CVD, and concomitant use of medications that predispose to hyperkalemia.
- Lower socioeconomic groups also have an increased prevalence, where monitoring of drug therapy and control of DM and hypertension are often inadequate.

RISK FACTORS[3]: Usually multifactorial, associated with various combinations of kidney failure (often oliguric), potassium supplementation, drugs that impair kidney potassium excretion, and movement of potassium out of cells due to hyperglycemia or inorganic metabolic acidosis.

Primary risk factor is CKD, especially if glomerular filtration rate (GFR) is <15 to 20 ml/min per 1.73 m^2, more commonly associated with diabetes mellitus types 1 and 2 or urinary tract obstruction with nephropathy (especially if there is interstitial nephritis).

Medications associated with hyperkalemia:

- Potassium-sparing diuretics (e.g., spironolactone, triamterene, amiloride, eplerenone, finerenone)
- NSAIDs
- ACE inhibitors (ACEIs)
- Angiotensin II type 1 receptor blockers (ARBs)
- Angiotensin receptor Neprilysin inhibitor (ARNI)
- Direct renin inhibitors
- Calcineurin inhibitors (cyclosporine, tacrolimus, and voclosporin)
- Pentamidine
- Digoxin toxicity, particularly in CKD patients
- Trimethoprim-containing medications
- Heparin
- Ketoconazole
- Metyrapone
- β-blockers
- Succinylcholine
- Penicillin
- Herbs
- Dietary Salt substitutes

RISK FACTORS:
- Male sex
- Not Black
- DM
- CVD
- Congestive heart failure (CHF)
- AKI
- CKD
- Metabolic acidosis (hyperchloremic, nonanion gap)
- Urinary obstruction
- Total Parenteral Nutrition

GENETICS: Syndromes associated with hyperkalemia include:
- Pseudohypoaldosteronism type 1 (autosomal recessive)
- Pseudohypoaldosteronism type 2 (autosomal dominant; familial hyperkalemic hypertension, i.e., Gordon syndrome):
  1. Rare inherited form of hyperkalemia characterized by hypertension, hyperchloremic metabolic acidosis, and hyperkalemia with normal GFR
  2. Sequence variants of several genes that are involved in renal tubular sodium, potassium, or chloride transport
  3. All forms respond to treatment with thiazide-like diuretics
- Hyperkalemic periodic paralysis (autosomal dominant)
  1. Genetic sequence variant resulting in flaccid, generalized weakness and hyperkalemia
- Glomerulopathy with fibronectin deposits (autosomal dominant)
  1. Unknown genetic variant that produces proteinuria, hypertension, and type 4 renal tubular acidosis (RTA)
- Disorders of steroid metabolism and mineralocorticoid receptors:
  1. 21-hydroxylase deficiency with low aldosterone level
  2. Aldosterone synthase deficiency with low aldosterone level

  3. Congenital mineralocorticoid (aldosterone) receptor defect (exceedingly rare)
- Congenital hypoaldosteronism (autosomal recessive):
  1. Genetic variant associated with low aldosterone and salt wasting
  2. Increased serum ratio of 18-hydroxycorticosterone to aldosterone
- Nephronophthisis:
  1. Manifestations include bilaterally enlarged kidneys, inflammatory portal fibrosis, and development of ESKD
- Disorders of chloride homeostasis (autosomal recessive):
  1. Genetic variant causing isolated hyperchlorihidrosis with excessive salt-wasting in sweat resulting in severe hyponatremic dehydration and hyperkalemia

PHYSICAL FINDINGS & CLINICAL PRESENTATION[4]

Most patients presenting with hyperkalemia are asymptomatic, with the abnormal laboratory parameter discovered inadvertently. Symptoms, when present, are nonspecific and primarily related to neuromuscular or cardiac dysfunction.
- Muscle paralysis
- Dyspnea
- Palpitations
- Chest pain
- Nausea or vomiting
- Paresthesias

Aside from bradycardia, the physical exam usually does not alert the examiner to a diagnosis of hyperkalemia. Flaccid paralysis and/or depressed or absent deep tendon reflexes may be detected.

ETIOLOGY (TABLE 1)

- Total body potassium content is approximately 3200 mEq and is primarily an intracellular ion (predominantly in muscle cells) with only 2% (70 mEq) residing in the extracellular space.
- Potassium is maintained in a narrow range of normal (3.8 to 5.0 mEq/L) by redundant and highly efficient homeostatic mechanisms that simultaneously control internal potassium ion redistribution while regulating net potassium excretion. When a defect occurs in one or both of these two processes, a net rise in extracellular potassium occurs, resulting in hyperkalemia.
- The kidney is responsible for regulation of potassium reabsorption and excretion (95%). Kidney failure or failure of tubular potassium secretion are the typical reasons for hyperkalemia.
- CKD is the most important predisposing condition for hyperkalemia due to a reduction of glomerular filtration. Patients with progressive CKD should consume a potassium-restricted diet. Low-sodium intake may be compensated by an increase in salt-substitute (containing potassium chloride) intake that may inadvertently increase potassium intake. AKI is commonly accompanied by hyperkalemia.

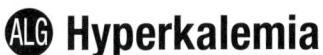

TABLE 1   Causes of Hyperkalemia

High Intake of K$^+$ Ions

- Only if there is also a disorder leading to a low rate of excretion of K$^+$ ions

Shift of K$^+$ Ions Out of Cells

- Tissue breakdown (e.g., crush trauma, rhabdomyolysis, tumor lysis), exhausting exercise, after seizures, status epilepticus
- Na/K-ATPase problem
  1. Tissue hypoxia
  2. Lack of a stimulus (e.g., lack of insulin [e.g., patients with DKA], inhibition of insulin release by α-adrenergic surge, use of nonselective β-blockers)
  3. Inhibition of Na/K-ATPase (e.g., by drugs, e.g., digoxin)
- α-Adrenergic surge (causing inhibition of the release of insulin or a direct effect to cause a shift of K$^+$ ions out of cells)
- Hyperosmolality (e.g., administration of mannitol)
- Metabolic acidosis due to acids that cannot be transported on the monocarboxylic acid cotransporter (e.g., HCl, citric acid)
- Increase K$^+$ efflux from cells (administration of succinylcholine, fluoride intoxication)
- Hereditary causes (e.g., hyperkalemic periodic paralysis)

Diminished K$^+$ Ion Loss in the Urine

- *Advanced chronic renal insufficiency*
- *Drugs that interfere with renal K$^+$ ion excretion*
  1. Drugs that cause acute renal failure or acute interstitial nephritis
  2. Drugs that interfere with the renin–angiotensin–aldosterone axis (e.g., nonsteroidal anti-inflammatory drugs, direct renin blockers, ACE inhibitors, angiotensin receptor blockers)
  3. Drugs that inhibit aldosterone synthesis (e.g., heparin, ketoconazole)
  4. Aldosterone receptor blockers (e.g., spironolactone, eplerenone)
  5. Drugs that block ENaC in the CDN (e.g., amiloride, trimethoprim)
  6. Drugs the interfere with activation of ENaC via proteolytic cleavage (e.g., nafamostat mesylate)
- *Diminished electrogenic reabsorption of Na$^+$ ions in the CDN*
  1. Very low delivery of Na$^+$ ions to the CDN
  2. Some patients with hyporeninemic hypoaldosteronism
  3. Low levels of aldosterone (e.g., Addison's disease)
  4. Genetic disorders involving the aldosterone receptor or ENaC (type I pesudohypoaldosteronism)
- *Increased electroneutral reabsorption of Na$^+$ ions in DCT or CDN*
  1. Increased reabsorption of Na$^+$ and Cl$^-$ ions in the DCT (e.g., familial hypertension with hyperkalemia [WNK 4 or WNK1 mutations]), drugs (e.g., calcineurin inhibitors), and some patients with diabetic nephropathy and hyporeninemic hypoaldosteronism
  2. Increased electroneutral reabsorption of Na$^+$ and Cl$^-$ ions in the CDN due to increased parallel activity of pendrin and NDCBE (e.g., some patients with hyporeninemic hypoaldosteronism)

ACE, Angiotensin-converting enzyme; *Cl,* chloride; *CDN,* cortical distal nephron; *DCT,* distal convoluted tubule; *DKA,* diabetic ketoacidosis; *ENaC,* epithelial sodium channels; *K,* potassium; *Na,* sodium; *NDCBE,* sodium-driven chloride/bicarbonate exchanger.
From Kamel SK, Halpertin ML: *Fluid, electrolyte, and Acid-Base Physiology,* ed 5, Philadelphia, 2017, Elsevier.

Hyperkalemia in AKI may originate from or be exacerbated by a potassium load from increased tissue breakdown that may occur with rhabdomyolysis, gastrointestinal bleeding, or blood transfusions with outdated blood. These processes can often result in the development of severe and life-threatening hyperkalemia.

- DM with insulin deficiency and/or hypertonicity with hyperglycemia.
- CVD, especially myocardial infarctions, left ventricular hypertrophy, and CHF, are often associated with various pharmacologic interventions that may induce or worsen hyperkalemia. CVD in association with CKD contributes to the development of hyperkalemia.
- RAASi, potassium-sparing diuretic administration, or digoxin in association with CKD may produce hyperkalemia in up to 10% of treated individuals vs. 2% of non-CKD patients. In

patients at risk for hyperkalemia, dual RAASi therapy should not be used.
- β_2-receptor blockers, digoxin, heparin: The potassium elevation is generally small with mild increase, from 0.2-0.5 mEq/L.
- CHF. Hyperkalemia risk is strongly associated with stage of CKD and use of spironolactone, especially in addition to a RAASi medication.

DX DIAGNOSIS

DIFFERENTIAL DIAGNOSIS

Hyperkalemia develops through three mechanisms: Impaired cellular potassium redistribution, decreased renal potassium secretion, and increased potassium intake. In the presence of normal renal and adrenal function, it is difficult to ingest sufficient potassium to become hyperkalemic. Consequently, hyperkalemia is rarely seen in people without advanced CKD, unless

supervening factors are present. The differential diagnosis is listed in Table 2.

WORKUP

Figs. 1, E2, and E3 illustrate a clinical approach to hyperkalemia. The following steps should be followed in the workup of hyperkalemia:

- Rule out pseudohyperkalemia: An in vitro phenomenon caused by mechanical release of potassium from cells during phlebotomy or specimen processing. This may be encountered with severe leukocytosis (>70,000/cm^3), thrombocytosis (platelet count >500,000 cm^3), prolonged fist-clenching during phlebotomy, and use of a small-bore needle. The diagnosis is made when serum K$^+$ exceeds the plasma K$^+$ by >0.5 mEq/L (>0.5 mmol/L). Contamination with potassium-EDTA in some specimen tubes can spuriously increase plasma potassium, and the diagnostic clue is a low plasma calcium concentration.
- If there is no predisposition for hyperkalemia, repeat laboratory testing before treatment is undertaken.
- ECG for electrocardiographic signs of hyperkalemia. ECG changes may not follow a classical progression pattern, described below:
  1. Early ECG changes are seen with serum K$^+$ of 5.5 to 6.5 mEq/L: Peaked T waves (Fig. 4), especially in precordial leads; shortened QT interval; and variable ST segment depression.
  2. Serum K$^+$ >6.5 mEq/L: Widening QRS complex with intraventricular conduction delay (QRS >120 milliseconds that does not meet the criteria for right or left bundle branch block).
  3. Serum K$^+$ >7 mEq/L: Decreased P wave amplitude with increased PR interval and development of bradycardia (atrioventricular node block).
  4. Serum K$^+$ >8.0 mEq/L: Absence of P waves and progressive widening of QRS that merges with T wave (sine wave), followed by ventricular fibrillation or asystole.

In hemodialysis patients with hyperkalemia, T wave tenting was nonpredictive of serum potassium, especially in older adults and in patients with DM. There have even been case reports of severe hyperkalemia with no ECG changes.

- Examine for the symptoms or physical findings of hyperkalemia and order basic studies:
  1. ECG
  2. CBC and platelet count
  3. Basic metabolic profile with a calculated estimated GFR (eGFR) (CKD alone should not develop hyperkalemia until eGFR is <20 to 25 ml/min per 1.73 m^2)
  4. Urine potassium and sodium concentrations
  5. Depending on history and results of initial laboratory testing, the following treatments may be indicated:
     a. Serum glucose concentration to rule out hypertonicity
     b. Digoxin level, as applicable

TABLE 2 Differential Diagnosis of Hyperkalemia

- Pseudohyperkalemia
- Cellular redistribution from intra- to extracellular space
  1. Mineral acid acidosis (not endogenous organic acidosis)
     a. Hyperkalemia inhibits ammoniagenesis, reducing net acid secretion and compounding metabolic acidosis
  2. Hypertonicity (hyperglycemia, sucrose, mannitol)
  3. DM: Insulin deficiency
  4. Hyperkalemic periodic paralysis
  5. Beta$_2$-adrenergic antagonists
  6. Alpha-adrenergic agonists
  7. Drugs
     a. Glucagon
     b. Digoxin overdose
     c. Aminocaproic acid-A
     d. Tetrodotoxin
     e. Succinylcholine
  8. Rebound after labile
  9. Extreme exercise
  10. Crush and tissue injury
     a. Rhabdomyolysis
     b. Hemolysis
     c. Tumor lysis syndrome
- Decreased renal excretion
  1. CKD
     a. Use of nonsteroidal antiinflammatory drugs (NSAIDs)
  2. ESKD
  3. Type 4 renal tubular acidosis
     a. Diabetes mellitus
     b. Obstructive nephropathy
     c. Amiloride
     d. Trimethoprim
     e. Pentamidine
     f. Succinylcholine (muscle depolarizing anesthetic)
     g. Volume depletion
     h. HIV infections
- Excess intake (rare except in advanced CKD or ESKD)
  1. Salt substitute (typically, KCl)
  2. Potassium-enriched foods (melons, citrus juice, raw coconut juice [44.3 mmol/L], Noni juice [56 mmol/L])
  3. Riverbed clay (red clay) very enriched, with 100 mEq K/100 g clay
- Mineralocorticoid deficiency (Addison disease)
  1. Hypoaldosteronism: Primary or secondary
  2. HIV infection
- Defect of tubular function or voltage defect resulting in hyperkalemia and hypertension:
  1. Genetic
     a. Pseudohyperaldosteronism type 2
- Also known as familial hyperkalemic hypertension or Gordon syndrome
  1. Acquired
     a. Calcineurin inhibitors (tacrolimus and cyclosporine)

CKD, Chronic kidney disease; *DM*, diabetes mellitus; *ESKD*, end-stage kidney disease; *KCl*, potassium chloride.

c. Arterial or venous blood gas, if acidosis is suspected
d. Urinalysis with microscopy
e. Serum cortisol and aldosterone levels after other common causes are ruled out
f. Serum uric acid and phosphorus concentration to rule out tumor lysis syndrome
g. Serum creatinine phosphokinase (CPK), calcium, and phosphorus measurements for rhabdomyolysis

- Accurate assessment of kidney function by eGFR or calculated GFR to define AKI or CKD stage and risk of hyperkalemia and acid-base status, especially if a hyperchloremic, nonanion gap metabolic acidosis is present.
- Hyperchloremic, nonanion gap metabolic acidosis associated with hyperkalemia is usually a type 4 RTA, with hyporeninemic hypoaldosteronism, which is common with urinary tract outlet obstruction, diabetic kidney disease, and acute or chronic kidney disorders involving the tubules.
- Determine presence of a renal origin for hyperkalemia using the urine potassium concentration as renal or endogenous vs. exogenous, with nephrology consultation as required.

LABORATORY TESTS

- Serum electrolytes, blood urea nitrogen, and creatinine
- Urinalysis and urine protein–creatinine ratio
- Serum and plasma potassium levels
- Serum and urine creatinine levels
- Cortisol level
- Aldosterone level
- 18-Hydroxycorticosterone level

IMAGING STUDIES

- Ultrasound of the kidneys and bladder
- Computed tomography scan of the kidneys, ureters, and bladder

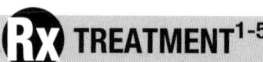 TREATMENT[1-5]

- The treatment of severe hyperkalemia requires three tasks carried out in close succession:
  I. Reverse any electrocardiographic changes caused by the hyperkalemia to prevent a fatal arrhythmia (calcium)
  II. Redistribute potassium into cells (insulin, albuterol, and sodium bicarbonate when there is metabolic acidosis)
  III. Removal of the potassium from the body (sodium polystyrene sulfonate, zirconium cyclosilicate, patiromer, or dialysis)
- Supportive measurements such as fluids, pacing, and pressors do not work in the setting of hyperkalemia. In acute, severe, life-threatening hyperkalemia, the approach is divided into two components. First, stabilize the myocardium to prevent a fatal arrhythmia. Giving intravenous (IV) calcium is cardioprotective in the setting of hyperkalemia, commonly reversing all hyperkalemic ECG changes within seconds of administration. However, it does not decrease the potassium levels; therefore other therapies are needed to reduce the potassium level.
- Before giving calcium, make sure digoxin toxicity is not present, as calcium administration can be fatal in the face of digoxin-induced hyperkalemia.
- Treatment intensity is directly related to the rapidity with which hyperkalemia developed, absolute potassium level, and evidence for toxicity by symptoms, neuromuscular examination, and ECG changes. The more rapid the rise in potassium, the higher the level; the more severe the cardiotoxicity depicted by the ECG changes, the more aggressive the therapy should be.

NONPHARMACOLOGIC THERAPY

- The mainstay of therapy should be educating the patient and the family regarding a low-potassium diet (<3 g/day), as well as providing a list of high-potassium foods to avoid.

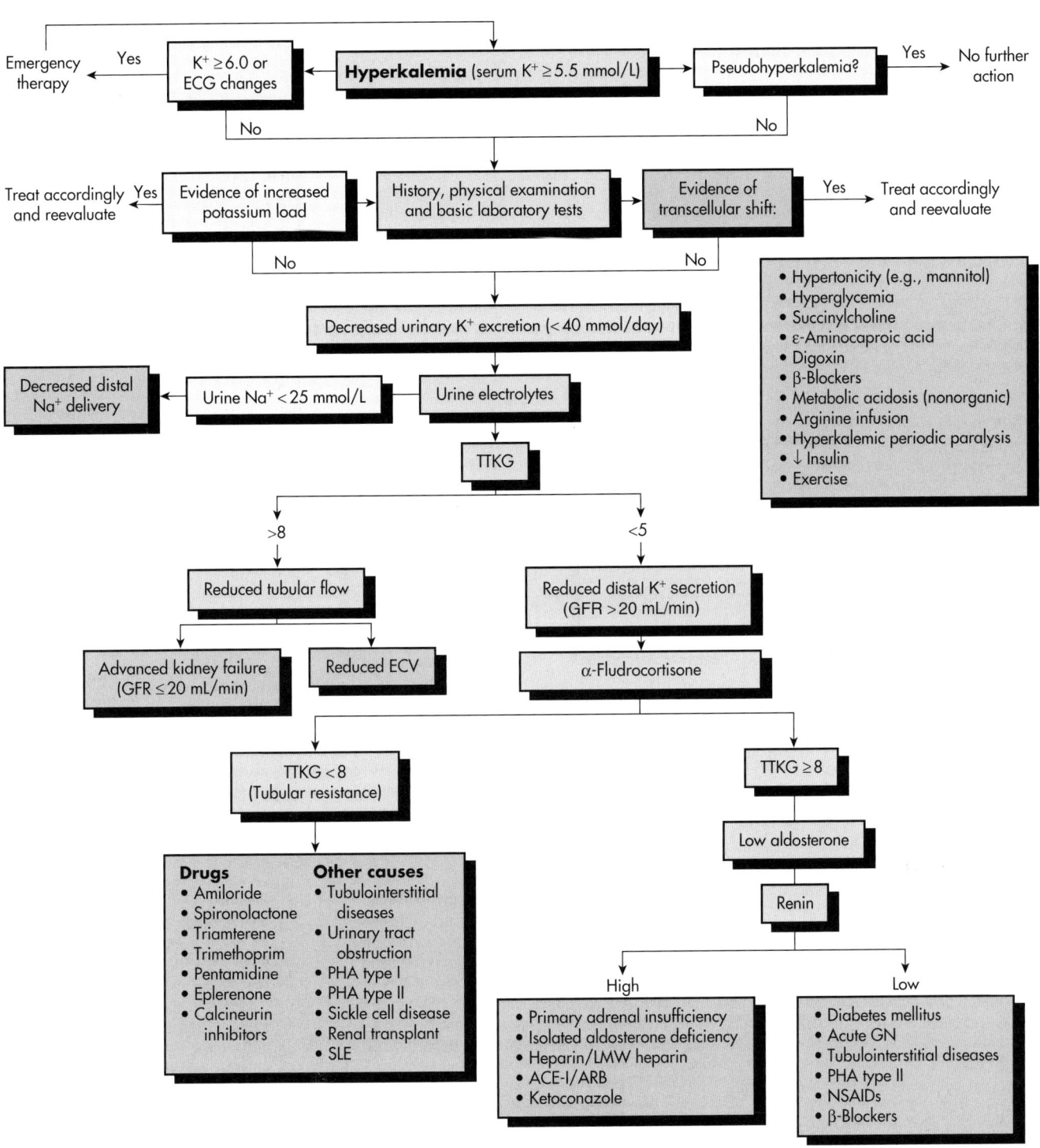

FIG. 1 Clinical approach to hyperkalemia. *ACE-I,* Angiotensin-converting enzyme inhibitor; *ARB,* angiotensin II type 1 receptor blocker; *CCD,* cortical collecting duct; *ECG,* electrocardiogram; *ECV,* effective circulatory volume; *GFR,* glomerular filtration rate; *GN,* glomerulonephritis; *HIV,* human immunodeficiency virus; *K,* potassium; *LMW heparin,* low-molecular-weight heparin; *Na,* sodium; *NSAID,* nonsteroidal antiinflammatory drug; *PHA,* pseudohypoaldosteronism; *SLE,* systemic lupus erythematosus; *TTKG,* transtubular potassium gradient. (From Skorecki K et al: *Brenner & Rector's the kidney,* ed 10, Philadelphia, 2016, Elsevier.)

- Maintaining adequate extracellular fluid volume and prevention of volume depletion, which limits potassium excretion by the kidney.
- Increasing patient awareness of hyperkalemia including use of educational tools facilitating communication about hyperkalemia (e.g., https://www.kidney.org/atoz/content/what-hyperkalemia).

ACUTE GENERAL Rx

In patients with severe hyperkalemia, treatment (Fig. 5) is as follows:[6,7]
- IV calcium (Fig. 6) to ameliorate cardiac toxicity (if not digoxin toxic).
  1. 10% calcium gluconate or calcium chloride (gluconate preferred).

  2. 10 ml of 10% solution IV over 10 min (repeat in 5 min if not effective or arrhythmia recurs).
- Identify and remove sources of potassium intake.
- IV glucose and insulin infusion to enhance cellular uptake of potassium.

Diseases and Disorders

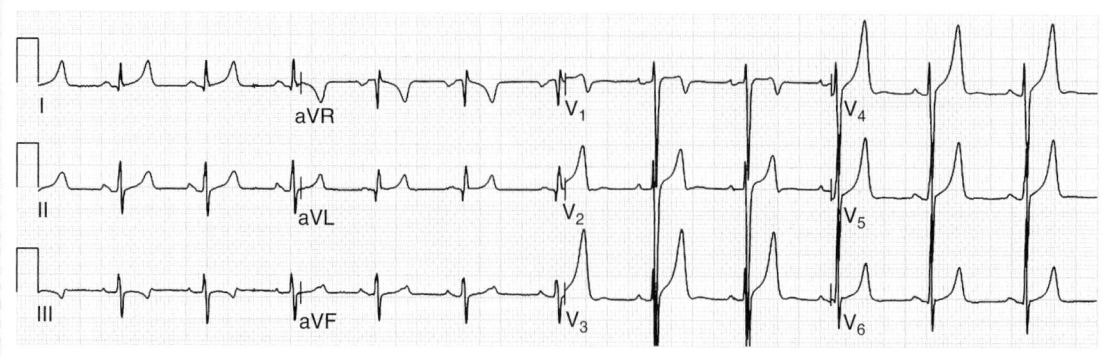

FIG. 4 Tall peaked T waves with hyperkalemia. This 12-lead electrocardiogram shows the tented T waves that are commonly seen in mild to moderate degrees of hyperkalemia. Tented T waves of hyperkalemia need not be tall, although in this case they are. *aVF,* Augmented vector foot; *aVL,* augmented vector left; *aVR,* augmented vector right. (From Olshansky B et al: *Arrhythmia essentials,* ed 2, Philadelphia, 2017, Elsevier.)

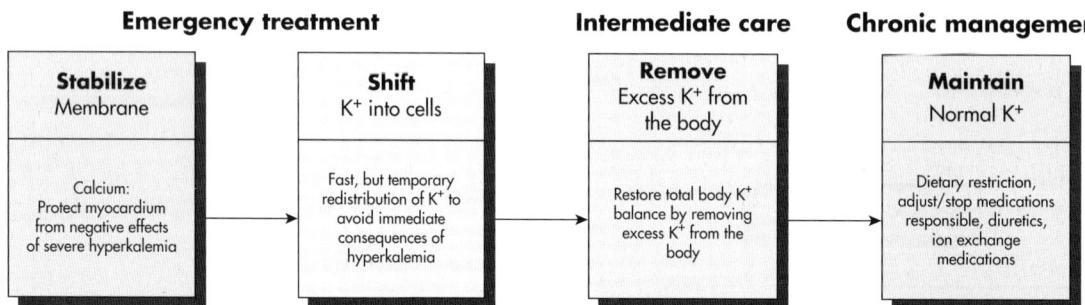

FIG. 5 Management of hyperkalemia. Here is the approach to managing severe hyperkalemia. During emergency treatment, the immediate concern is to stabilize the membranes to protect the myocardium from the negative effects of severe hyperkalemia by administering calcium gluconate. In the next few minutes, the priority is to shift potassium (K^+) into the cells with a fast but temporary redistribution of K^+ to avoid immediate consequences of hyperkalemia. This is accomplished with insulin and β2-adrenergic receptor agonists. In the following hours to days, intermediate care is focused on removing the K^+ from the body and restoring total K^+ balance with potassium binders, loop diuretics or dialysis. Sodium bicarbonate may be used to shift K^+ into cells when metabolic acidosis is the cause of hyperkalemia. Once total body K^+ balance is achieved, attempts to identify the underlying cause follow and developing long-term management plans including a low-potassium diet, discontinuation, or modification of RAAS inhibitors, and the use of the newer potassium binders.

1. Make sure to closely monitor glucose every hour for several hours for hypoglycemia, especially in patients with advanced CKD.
- Correct severe acidosis with IV sodium bicarbonate.
- Consider beta-adrenergic agonist therapy (e.g., nebulized albuterol, 10 mg via Venturi mask). Preferred over alkali therapy in patients with CKD.
- Increase potassium excretion with administration of loop diuretic IV or cation-exchange medications mentioned previously.
  1. Medications that increase potassium excretion in addition to IV saline and loop diuretics, such as an aldosterone analogue (e.g., 9-alpha fludrocortisone acetate [Florinef]) in patients with hyporeninemia or hypoaldosteronism or patients with hyperkalemia who have solid organ transplant and are on calcineurin inhibitor (CNI).
- Emergency dialysis for refractory hyperkalemia, defined as ongoing hyperkalemia unresponsive to conservative measures.
- After correction of hyperkalemia, long-term management should be initiated to maintain normal potassium. Measures include dietary potassium restriction, adjusting/stopping medications associated with hyperkalemia, and/or administration of newer ion exchange resins such as sodium zirconium cyclosilicate and patiromer. The use of sodium polystyrene sulfate has greatly decreased due to lack of data demonstrating consistent efficacy and because newer agents are available (i.e., patiromer and zirconium cyclosilicate).

CHRONIC Rx

In the presence of a moderate elevation of potassium and no ECG abnormalities:
- Correct origin of increased potassium (e.g., inhibited excretion or increased intake)
- Increase potassium excretion with a diuretic or potassium ion exchange medication (Table 3).
  1. Sodium polystyrene sulfonate (SPS) is a polymeric cation-exchange resin (dose: 15 to 30 g up to four times daily).
     a. Sodium ion exchanger and is nonselective for potassium, also having affinity for calcium and magnesium ions.
     b. Lacking long-term use studies, with only one small 7-day randomized clinical study performed.
     c. Short-term efficacy is inconsistent with variable onset of action (hours to days).
     d. Reported adverse events include intestinal ischemia and colonic necrosis (rare, 16 or 23 events per 1000 person-yr). FDA added warning label to SPS regarding concomitant use of sorbitol (historically used to prevent constipation) and the risk of colonic necrosis and other serious gastrointestinal adverse events. Concomitant use of sorbitol with SPS is currently not recommended.
     e. Long-term use can result in hypocalcemia and hypomagnesemia, and levels should be monitored intermittently.
     f. Medications can potentially bind other medications, so should not be taken for 3 h before or after dosing.
  2. Patiromer is a nonreabsorbed oral calcium-containing potassium-binding polymer suspension (dose: 8.4 to 25.2 g daily).
     a. Shown to lower serum potassium in hyperkalemia associated with diabetic nephropathy and CHF on RAASi.
     b. Calcium is the ion exchanger (not sodium), and it can form calcium carbonate in the colon and affect absorption of some medications, especially

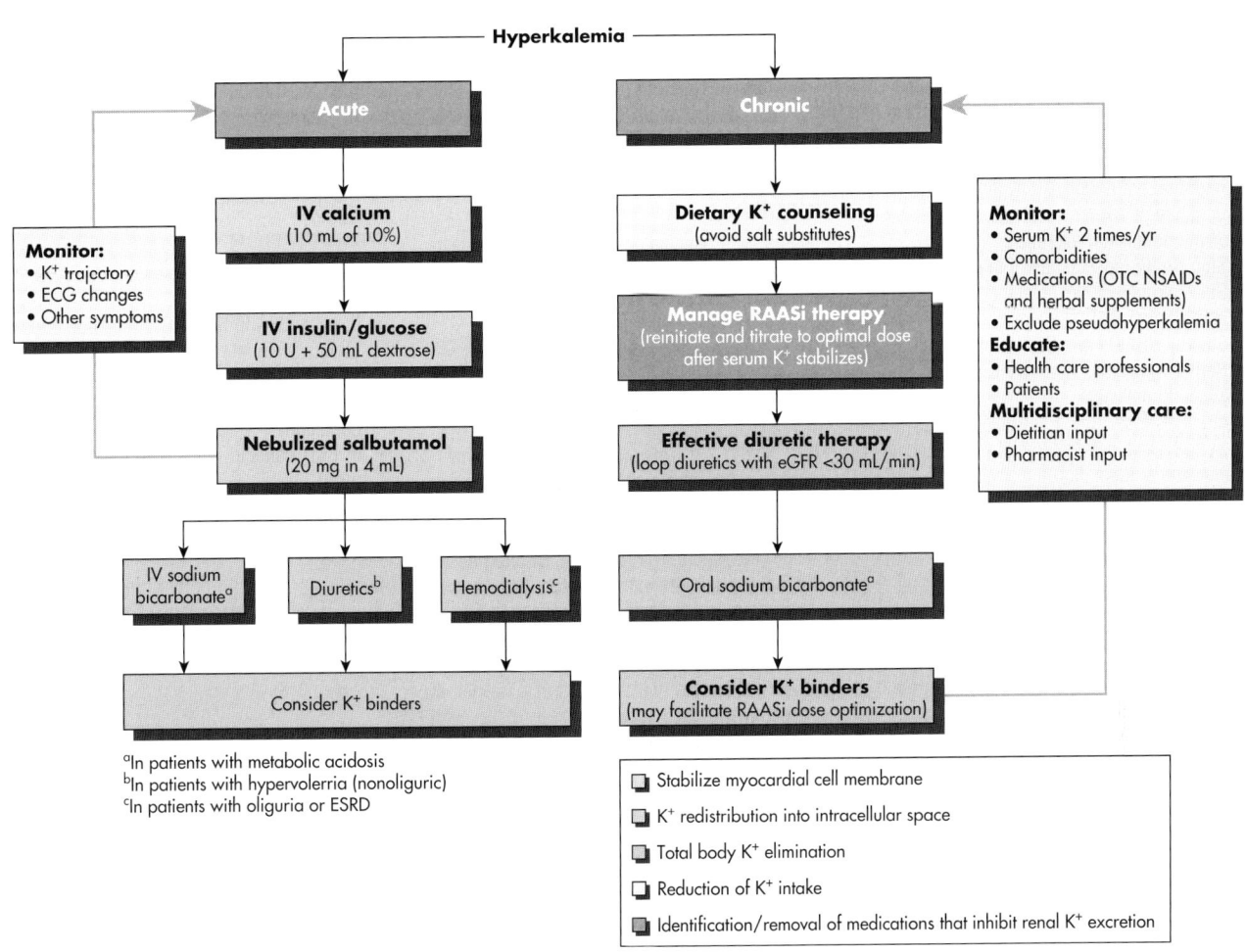

FIG. 6 Algorithm for treatment of hyperkalemia. Treatment options for the management of acute and chronic hyperkalemia. In patients with acute hyperkalemia, intravenous *(IV)* calcium reduces membrane excitation in cardiac tissue within 1 to 3 min, while insulin and b-agonists redistribute potassium *(K+)* to the intracellular space (30 to 60 min) but do not reduce total body K+. b-Agonists have a short duration of effect (2 to 4 h), and glucose must be administered with insulin to prevent hypoglycemia. Sodium bicarbonate use, which promotes K+ elimination through increased urinary K+ excretion, is limited to patients with metabolic acidosis, and effective diuretic therapy depends on residual kidney function. Hemodialysis increases total K+ elimination and may be used for resistant acute hyperkalemia. *ECG,* Electrocardiography; *eGFR,* estimated glomerular filtration rate; *ESRD,* end-stage renal disease; *NSAIDs,* nonsteroidal antiinflammatory drugs; *OTC,* over-the-counter; *RAASi,* renin-angiotensin-aldosterone system inhibition. (From Palmer BF et al: Clinical management of hyperkalemia, *Mayo Clin Proc* 96(3):749, 2021.)

TABLE 3   Available Potassium Ion Exchange Resins

	Sodium Polystyrene Sulfonate	Patiromer	Sodium Zirconium Cyclosilicate
Dosage	15-30 g One to four times daily	8.4 g, 16.8 g, or 25.2 g Once daily	10 g, 3 times daily for up to 48 h; then 5 g every other day to 15 g daily
Counterion	Sodium	Calcium	Sodium
Average daily sodium load	1500-12,000 mg	0 mg	400-2400 mg
Concomitant dose separation with other oral medications	3-h separation	3-h separation	2-h separation

ciprofloxacin, levothyroxine, and metformin. Administer at least 3 h before or after all oral medications.
c. Can bind magnesium and may be associated with hypomagnesemia. Magnesium monitoring is recommended with long-term use.

3. Sodium zirconium cyclosilicate is a non-absorbed inorganic polymer that selectively exchanges potassium for sodium and hydrogen ions (Initial dose: 10 g, three times daily for up to 48 h. Subsequent dose: 5 g every other day to 15 g daily for long-term use).

a. Sodium is the exchanged ion and may be associated with sodium overload if large doses are used for a prolonged time.
b. Agent is taken at least 2 h before or after all oral medications.
Patiromer and sodium zirconium cyclosilicate are much more palatable and predictable, and

efficacy has been demonstrated in clinical trials compared to SPS. The use of the newer potassium binders is often limited by the formularies available to some patients depending on their insurance, often leaving SPS as the only viable choice.

Management of nonurgent hyperkalemia:
- Discontinue or reduce medications that interfere with potassium excretion.
  1. Stop RAASi (special care if in combination)
  2. Stop spironolactone, eplerenone, amiloride, and triamterene
  3. Stop all NSAIDs and COX-2 inhibitors
  4. Herbal medicine: Stop Chan su and Noni juice, if applicable
  5. Modify CNI therapy, if feasible
- Prescribe a low-potassium diet (70 mEq/day).
- Administer a loop diuretic or thiazide (CNI-induced hyperkalemia).
- If serum bicarbonate is <22 mmol/L, administer sodium bicarbonate tablets (650 mg tablet [7.8 mmol per tablet]) or Shohl solution (sodium citrate [1 mmol per ml] 3 to 60 ml twice per day).
- Patiromer or sodium zirconium cyclosilicate avoids use of SPS for chronic hyperkalemia.
  1. Neither agent is used for severe/urgent hyperkalemia.
- Continuation of a RAASi may be possible when using patiromer or sodium zirconium cyclosilicate.

DISPOSITION
- Patients with acute symptomatic hyperkalemia with ECG changes should be admitted to a hospital in a monitored bed/intensive care unit.

- Asymptomatic patients with no ECG changes can be treated as outpatients and educated extensively regarding a low-potassium diet, with close follow-up including a repeat potassium in 24 to 48 h, depending on the severity, and one week later.

REFERRAL
Patients with associated hypertension, proteinuria, CKD, or persistent hyperkalemia should be referred to a nephrologist for evaluation.

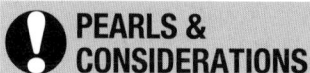 **PEARLS & CONSIDERATIONS**

COMMENTS
- Rule out hemolysis of blood samples.
- If a spurious result is suspected, repeat the test.
- Rule out pseudohyperkalemia, defined as an in vitro phenomenon in which the ex vivo serum potassium level in the specimen tube is elevated, but the in vivo plasma potassium is in the normal range.
- Risk associated with comparable levels of hyperkalemia is higher in individuals with normal kidney function compared to those with CKD.
- Do not administer IV calcium or insulin/dextrose if no ECG changes for hyperkalemia are seen.
- Provide education regarding avoidance of rich potassium-containing foodstuffs and encourage dietary restriction of potassium (avoid salt substitutes).

- Evaluate for urinary obstruction, especially in patients with diabetes (neurogenic bladder) and in older men (prostatic hypertrophy).
- After diagnosis, treatment and resolution of hyperkalemia, RAASi should be reinitiated if medically indicated prior.

PREVENTION
- Avoid combination therapies of an ARB, ACEI, or direct renin inhibitor.
- In patients with type 4 RTA, provide education about avoiding potassium-containing foodstuffs, avoiding travel to areas where such foods are common, and avoiding volume depletion.
- In CKD patients or patients with type 4 RTA, avoid using salt substitutes that contain potassium chloride.

PATIENT & FAMILY EDUCATION
Education regarding potassium content of foods is of practical importance. A certified renal nutritionist should review the patient's medical records for potential dietary interventions and provide necessary education.

REFERENCES
Available at eBooks.Health.Elsevier.com.

RELATED CONTENT
Chronic Kidney Disease (Related Key Topic)

AUTHORS: **PRIYASHA SURI, MD,** and **NELSON KOPYT, DO**

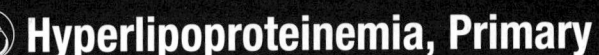
BASIC INFORMATION

DEFINITION

- Primary hyperlipoproteinemia is a group of genetic disorders of the lipid transport proteins in the blood that manifests as abnormally elevated levels of cholesterol, triglycerides, or both in the serum of affected patients.
- Usually defined as total cholesterol, low-density lipoprotein (LDL), triglycerides, or lipoprotein A levels above 90th percentile or high-density lipoprotein (HDL) or apo A-1 levels below the 10th percentile for the general population. Fig. E1 illustrates the structure of lipoproteins. Plasma lipoprotein composition is described in Table E1.

SYNONYM

Hyperlipidemia

ICD-10CM CODES

E78.0	Pure hypercholesterolemia
E78.2	Mixed hyperlipidemia
E78.1	Pure hyperglyceridemia
E78.4	Other hyperlipidemia
E78.3	Hyperchylomicronemia

EPIDEMIOLOGY & DEMOGRAPHICS

INCIDENCE: The most common types are lipoprotein A excess, hypertriglyceridemia, and combined hyperlipidemia.
- Incidence of heterozygous familial hypercholesterolemia: 1:500
- Incidence of homozygous familial hypercholesterolemia: 1:1 million
- Familial hypercholesterolemia: Autosomal dominant disorder
- Familial combined hyperlipidemia: Possibly an autosomal dominant disorder
- Multifactorial predilection: Apparent in majority of affected individuals

GENETICS:
- Familial lipoprotein lipase deficiency: Autosomal recessive, resulting in an elevation in the plasma chylomicrons and triglycerides
- Familial apoprotein CII deficiency: Autosomal recessive, resulting in increased serum chylomicrons, very low-density lipoprotein (VLDL), and hypertriglyceridemia
- Familial type 3 hyperlipoproteinemia: Single-gene defect requiring contributory factors to manifest
- Familial hypercholesterolemia: Autosomal dominant defect of the LDL receptor, resulting in an elevated serum cholesterol level and normal triglycerides. HoFH is the most severe form of the disease. LDL levels can reach over 500 mg/dl and can cause death in childhood
- Familial hypertriglyceridemia: Common, autosomal dominant defect resulting in elevated VLDL and triglycerides
- Multiple lipoprotein–type hyperlipidemia: Autosomal dominant, manifesting as isolated hypercholesterolemia, isolated hypertriglyceridemia, or hyperlipidemia
- Polygenic hypercholesterolemia: Multifactorial
- Polygenic hyperalphalipoproteinemia: Autosomal dominant or polygenic, causing an elevated HDL
- A classification of lipoprotein disorders and their clinical findings and management are summarized in Table 2

PHYSICAL FINDINGS & CLINICAL PRESENTATION

- Familial lipoprotein lipase deficiency: Recurrent bouts of abdominal pain in infancy, eruptive xanthomas, hepatomegaly, splenomegaly, lipemia retinalis
- Familial apoprotein CII deficiency: Occasional eruptive xanthomas
- Familial type 3 hyperlipoproteinemia: Xanthoma striata palmaris or tuberoeruptive xanthomas, xanthelasmas, arterial bruits at a young age, gangrene of the lower extremities at a young age
- Familial hypercholesterolemia: Tendon xanthomas, arcus corneae, xanthelasma
- Familial hypertriglyceridemia: Associated obesity; eruptive xanthomas (Fig. E2) can develop with exacerbations

ETIOLOGY

- Genetic defects causing lipid abnormalities
- Environmental influences, including diet, drugs, and alcohol intake

DIAGNOSIS

DIFFERENTIAL DIAGNOSIS

Secondary causes of hyperlipoproteinemias:
- Hypothyroidism
- Diabetes mellitus
- Pancreatitis
- Autoimmune hyperlipoproteinemia
- Nephrotic syndrome
- Biliary obstruction; Table E3 describes the differential diagnosis of hyperlipidemia and dyslipidemia

WORKUP

- Family history for premature cardiac disease
- Personal history of recurrent pancreatitis
- Detailed physical examination

LABORATORY TESTS

- Standard lipid profile; Table 4 summarizes laboratory findings in lipid disorders
- If normal, further testing with measurement of lipoprotein A, apo B, and apo A-1
- Lipoprotein electrophoresis and ultracentrifugation (for phenotypic classification)
- Workup for secondary causes: Thyroid-stimulating hormone, fasting glucose, liver function, renal function, urinary protein

TREATMENT

NONPHARMACOLOGIC THERAPY

- Cornerstone of treatment: Dietary therapy
  1. TLC diet (**t**herapeutic **l**ifestyle **c**hanges): See "Hypercholesterolemia" topic

- Risk factor reduction includes smoking cessation, treatment of hypertension, exercise
- Familial lipoprotein lipase deficiency and familial apoprotein CII deficiency: Fat-free diet
- Remainder of cases, except those with polygenic hyperalphalipoproteinemia: Fat- and cholesterol-restricted diets
- Nonpharmacologic interventions can include LDL apheresis and liver transplantation

ACUTE GENERAL Rx

No acute treatment is needed.

CHRONIC Rx

- Medications commonly used to treat hyperlipidemias are summarized in Table 5. Table 6 differentiates statins based on potency.
- Familial lipoprotein lipase deficiency, polygenic hyperalphalipoproteinemia, or familial apoprotein CII deficiency: No chronic drug therapy.
- Familial type 3 hyperlipoproteinemia: Usually responds well to secondary causes being treated and diet therapy; if not, fibric acids may be tried.
- Familial hypercholesterolemia: Statins, bile acid sequestrants, or niacin. Ezetimibe and proprotein convertase subtilisin/Kexin type 9 (PCSK9 inhibitors) can be added to statins to achieve LDL goals.[1] PCSK9 binds to LDL receptors on hepatocytes, promote receptor degradation, and prevent LDL-C clearance from the circulation thereby increasing serum concentrations of LDL-C. PCSK9 monoclonal antibody inhibitors alirocumab (Praluent), evolocumab (Repatha), and inclisiran (Leqvio), a PCSK9-directed small interfering RNA, are currently indicated as adjunct to diet and maximally tolerated statin therapy for the treatment of adults with heterozygous familial hypercholesterolemia or clinical atherosclerotic cardiovascular disease, who require additional lowering of LDL cholesterol. PCSK9 inhibitors lower risk for ischemic cardiovascular events in persons with stable CAD and elevated atherogenic lipoproteins despite statin therapy. These medications are administered by subcutaneous injection and are expensive.
- Familial hypertriglyceridemia: Fibric acids (fenofibrate), niacin, omega-3 PUFA-containing fish oil capsules. Icosapent ethyl, a highly purified eicosapentaenoic acid ester, has been shown to lower triglyceride levels and cardiovascular risk in patients with hypertriglyceridemia. Icosapent ethyl (Vascepa) is indicated as an adjunct to diet to relieve triglyceride levels in adult patients with severe (≥500 mg/dl) hypertriglyceridemia. It is also indicated as an adjunct to maximally tolerated statin therapy to reduce the risk of myocardial infarction, stroke, coronary revascularization and unstable angina requiring hospitalization in adult patients with elevated triglyceride levels (≥150 mg/dl) and established cardiovascular disease or diabetes mellitus and two or more additional risk factors for cardiovascular disease.

TABLE 2   Disorders of Lipids: Clinical Findings and Management

Disorder	Xanthomas	Cardiovascular	Gastrointestinal	Neurologic	Ophthalmologic	Other Findings	Management
Type I	Eruptive, tendinous, xanthelasmas	None	Acute abdomen, hepatosplenomegaly, pancreatitis	None	Lipemia retinalis, retinal vein occlusion	Diabetes, lipemic plasma	Diet, plasmapheresis
Type II	Planar, especially intertriginous, tendinous, tuberous	Generalized atherosclerosis	None	None	Arcus cornea	None	Type IIa: Bile acid sequestrants, statins, niacin, fish oil Type IIb: Statins, niacin, fibrate
Type III	Planar, especially palmar, tuberous	Atherosclerosis	None	None	None	Abnormal glucose tolerance, hyperuricemia	Statins, fibrate
Type IV	Eruptive, tuberous	Atherosclerosis	Acute abdomen, hepatosplenomegaly, pancreatitis	None	Lipemia retinalis	Obesity	Statins, fibrate, niacin
Type V	Eruptive, tuberous	Atherosclerosis	Acute abdomen, hepatosplenomegaly, pancreatitis	None	Lipemia retinalis	Obesity, hyperinsulinemia	Niacin, fibrate
Tangier	Macular rash, foam cells in biopsies	Atherosclerosis	Acute abdomen, hepatosplenomegaly	Peripheral neuropathy	Corneal infiltration	Enlarged orange tonsils, lymphadenopathy	
Apolipoprotein A-I and C-III deficiency	Planar and tendon xanthomas, foam cells in biopsies	Atherosclerosis	Normal	Normal	Corneal clouding	None	
HDL deficiency with planar xanthomas	Planar xanthomas, foam cells in biopsies	Atherosclerosis	Hepatomegaly	Normal	Corneal opacity	None	

HDL, High-density lipoprotein.
From Paller AS, Mancini AJ: *Hurwitz clinical pediatric dermatology: a textbook of skin disorders of childhood and adolescence,* ed 5, 2016, Elsevier.

- Multiple lipoprotein–type hyperlipidemia: Drug therapy aimed at the predominant lipid abnormality noted.
- Recent data suggest in patients with lipoprotein abnormalities that treatment goals should be based on non-HDL cholesterol rather than LDL cholesterol.
- The FDA has approved mipomersen and lomitapide in patients with homozygous familial hypercholesterolemia already taking maximum doses of other lipid-lowering drugs. Both medicines are hepatotoxic and very expensive.
- Recent trials with bempedoic acid, an inhibitor of adenosine triphosphate citrate lyase that lowers LDL cholesterol, have shown to significantly lower LDL when bempedoic acid was added to maximally tolerated statin therapy. The FDA has recently approved bempedoic acid for use alone (Nexletol) and in a fixed-dose combination with ezetimibe (Nexlizet) as an adjunct to diet and maximally tolerated statin therapy in adults with heterozygous familial hypercholesterolemia or established ASCVD who require additional LDL-C lowering.

DISPOSITION
- Those with polygenic hyperalphalipoproteinemia: Excellent prognosis for longevity
- Those with familial hypercholesterolemia, familial type 3 hypercholesterolemia, or multiple lipoprotein–type hyperlipidemia: Even with aggressive treatment, at high risk for accelerated atherosclerosis and coronary artery disease

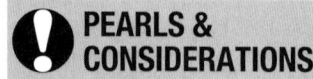 **PEARLS & CONSIDERATIONS**

COMMENTS
- Patient information is available through the American Heart Association.

- Lipid-lowering drug therapy is recommended for children $\geq$10 yr whose LDL-C levels remain extremely elevated after 6 mo to 1 yr of dietary modification. Drug therapy also can be considered for children with LDL-C levels of $\geq$190 mg/dl.

REFERENCE & SUGGESTED READINGS
Available at eBooks.Health.Elsevier.com.

RELATED CONTENT
Hypercholesterolemia (Related Key Topic)

AUTHOR: **FRED F. FERRI, MD**

TABLE 4   Laboratory Findings in Lipid Disorders

Disorder	Inheritance	OMIM No.	Prevalence	Cholesterol	Triglycerides	VLDL	Chylomicrons	LDL	HDL	Serum	Cause
Type I a: Familial hyperchylomicronemia	AR	239600, 246650, 615947	1/million	↑	↑↑↑	↑	↑	↓	↓↓↓	Creamy top	a. Deficiency from mutations in lipoprotein lipase; *LMF1*; *GPIHBP1*
b: Familial apoprotein C2 or A-V deficiency		207750, 133650									b. Deficient ApoC-2 or ApoA-5 (see Type V)
c: —		118830									c. LP lipase inhibitor in blood
Type II a: Familial hypercholesterolemia	AD	143890, 144010, 603776	1 in 500 for heterozygotes	↑	NI or ↑	↑	NI	↓	↓	Clear	LDL receptor defect in 60%-80%; *APOB*, *PCSK9*, each <5%
	AR	603813									*LDLRAP1*
b: Familial combined hyperlipidemia	AD, AR	144250	1 in 100							Clear	Polygenic; Decreased LDL receptor and ApoB-100 dysfunction
Type III Familial dysbetalipoproteinemia	AR	107741	1 in 10,000	↑	↑	↑	↑	↓	NI	Turbid	ApoE-2 synthesis
Type IV Familial hypertriglyceridemia	AD	144600	1 in 100	↑	NI ↑	↑	NI	↓	↓↓	Turbid	Renal disease, diabetes
Type V	AR	144650	Very rare	↑	↑↑↑	↑	↑	↓	↓↓↓	Creamy top, turbid bottom	Apo A-V (ApoA-5) deficiency

AD, Autosomal dominant; *Apo*, apolipoprotein; *AR*, autosomal recessive; *HDL*, high-density lipoprotein; *LDL*, low-density lipoprotein; *LP*, lipoprotein; *NI*, normal; *OMIM*, Online Mendelian Inheritance in Man; *VLDL*, very low-density lipoprotein; ↑, increased; ↓, decreased.

From Paller AS, Mancini AJ: *Hurwitz clinical pediatric dermatology: a textbook of skin disorders of childhood and adolescence*, ed 5, 2016, Elsevier.

Diseases and Disorders

I

TABLE 5 Drugs Used to Treat Hyperlipidemia

Class and Drugs Available	Dosage	Major Lipoprotein Decreased	Mechanism
HMG-CoA Reductase Inhibitors			
Rosuvastatin	5-40 mg/day	LDL	Decrease cholesterol synthesis; increase LDL receptor–mediated removal of LL
Atorvastatin	10-80 mg/day		
Simvastatin	5-40 mg/day		
Lovastatin	10-80 mg/day		
Pravastatin	10-40 mg/day		
Fluvastatin	20-80 mg/day		
Pitavastatin	1-4 mg//day		
PCSK9 Inhibitors			
Evolocumab	140 mg SC q2 wk or 420 mg SC monthly	LDL	Prevent degradation of the LDL receptor
Alirocumab	75-150 mg SC q2 wk		
Intestinal Cholesterol Absorption Inhibitor			
Ezetimibe	10 mg/day	LDL	Inhibits cholesterol absorption
Bile Acid Sequestrants			
Cholestyramine	4-12 g bid	LDL	Increase sterol excretion and LDL clearance
Colestipol	5-15 g bid		
Colesevelam	3.75-4.375 g/day		
Fibric Acid Derivatives			
Gemfibrozil	600 mg bid	VLDL (LDL)	Decrease VLDL production; enhance LPL action
Fenofibrate[a]	30-200 mg/day		
Omega-3 Fatty Acids			
Lovaza (1-g capsule contains EPA and DHA)	4 g/day	VLDL	Inhibit VLDL production
Vascepa (1-g capsule contains EPA)	4 g/day		
Epanova (1-g capsule contains EPA and DHA free fatty acids)	2-4 g/day		
Nicotinic Acid			
Niacin (crystalline)	1-3 g/day	VLDL (LDL)	Decrease VLDL production; enhance LPL action
Niaspan (extended-release niacin)	500-2000 mg/day		
ApoB Antisense Oligonucleotide			
Mipomersen	200 mg weekly SC injection	VLDL, LDL, Lp(a)	Inhibits synthesis of apolipoprotein B
Microsomal Triglyceride Transfer Protein Inhibitor			
Lomitapide	5-60 mg/day	VLDL, LDL, Lp(a)	Inhibits microsomal triglyceride transfer protein

bid, Twice a day; *DHA,* docosahexaenoic acid; *EPA,* highly concentrated ethyl esters of eicosapentaenoic acid; *HMG-CoA,* 3-hydroxy-3-methylglutaryl coenzyme A; *LDL,* low-density lipoproteins; *Lp(a),* lipoprotein(a); *LPL,* lipoprotein lipase; *PCSK9,* proprotein convertase subtilisin/kexin type 9; *q,* every; *SC,* subcutaneously; *VLDL,* very low-density lipoprotein.
[a]There are several different preparations of fenofibrate with different doses.
From Melmed S et al: *Williams textbook of endocrinology,* ed 14, St Louis, 2019, Elsevier.

TABLE 6 High-, Moderate-, and Low-Intensity Statin Therapy

High Intensity	Moderate Intensity	Low Intensity
Daily dose lowers LDL on average by approximately ≥50%[a]:	Daily dose lowers LDL on average, by approximately 30% to <50%[a]:	Daily dose lowers LDL, on average, by <30%[a]:
Rosuvastatin 20-40 mg	Rosuvastatin 5-10 mg	Simvastatin 10 mg
Atorvastatin 40-80 mg	Atorvastatin 10-20 mg	Lovastatin 20 mg
	Simvastatin 20-40 mg	Pravastatin 10-20 mg
	Lovastatin 40 mg	Fluvastatin 20-40 mg
	Pravastatin 40-80 mg	Pitavastatin 1 mg
	Fluvastatin 40 mg bid	
	Pitavastatin 2-4 mg	

bid, Twice a day; *LDL,* low-density lipoprotein cholesterol.
[a]Note that individual responses vary.
Data from Robinson JG et al: ACC/AHA guideline on the treatment of blood cholesterol to reduce atherosclerotic cardiovascular risk in adults: a report of the American College of Cardiology/American Heart Association Task Force on Practice Guidelines, *J Am Coll Cardiol* 63:2889-2934, 2014.

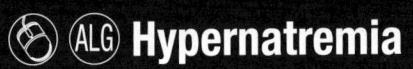

BASIC INFORMATION

DEFINITION

Hypernatremia is a clinical disorder that results from net water deficit (i.e., dehydration). It is identified when the serum sodium concentration (S_{Na}) exceeds the upper limit of the normal range (145 mEq/L). Hypernatremia does not reflect the net total body sodium content or extracellular fluid volume status. Consequently, patients with hypernatremia may be hypovolemic, hypervolemic, or normovolemic.

SYNONYMS

Hyperosmolality
Hypertonicity
High serum sodium concentration
Dehydration hyponatremia

ICD-10CM CODES
E87.0   Hyperosmolality and/or hypernatremia
E86.0   Dehydration/Volume Depletion

EPIDEMIOLOGY & DEMOGRAPHICS

The prevalence of hypernatremia varies based on the defined population and clinical setting. In the outpatient setting, hypernatremia occurs at the extremes of age. The prevalence among adults is 0.7% while prevalence among elderly is 2.6%.[1] Almost 60% of cases develop in hospitalized patients, and approximately 80% of these cases occur in intensive care units.[2]

Among noncritical hospitalized patients, the prevalence of hypernatremia is 0.2% to 2.5%.[2,3] The incidence is greater in critically ill and older adult patients, and the prevalence ranges from 10% to 26% in the hospitalized population.[2,3] The severity of hypernatremia correlates with mortality.[2] In patients with COVID-19, hypernatremia is noted in as high as 10%, and these patients have a two-fold increased risk of death.[2,4]

RISK FACTORS:
- Age >60 yr
- Sex
- Acute kidney injury on admission
- Altered mental status
- Mechanical ventilation
- Enteral tube feeding
- Negative fluid balance
- Hyperglycemia
- Hypertonic solution administration (e.g., bicarbonate or mannitol)
- Hypokalemia
- Hypercalcemia
- Underlying polyuric disorders

PHYSICAL FINDINGS & CLINICAL PRESENTATION
- Symptoms generally correlate with severity of hypernatremia, how rapidly hypernatremia developed (Figs. 1 and 2), and the underlying cause.

Hypernatremia

Is hypernatremia acute?

- Short time course
- Usually due to Na+ gain

- >48 hours
- Usually due to water deficit

Yes

No

- Danger: Intracranial hemorrhage
- Therapy: Rapid lowering of P_{Na} if severe symptoms

- Danger: Cerebral edema if P_{Na} is lowered rapidly
- Therapy: Fall in P_{Na} not to exceed 8 mmol/L/24 hr

FIG. 1 Emergencies associated with hypernatremia. The emergencies in patients with acute hypernatremia are caused by brain cell shrinkage and resultant rupture of blood vessels, leading to focal intracerebral and subarachnoid hemorrhages. The danger in the patient with chronic hypernatremia is a rapid and large fall in the PNa, which results in brain cell swelling and possibly brain herniation. (From Kamel SK, Halpertin ML: *Fluid, electrolyte, and acid-base physiology,* ed 5, Philadelphia 2017, Elsevier.)

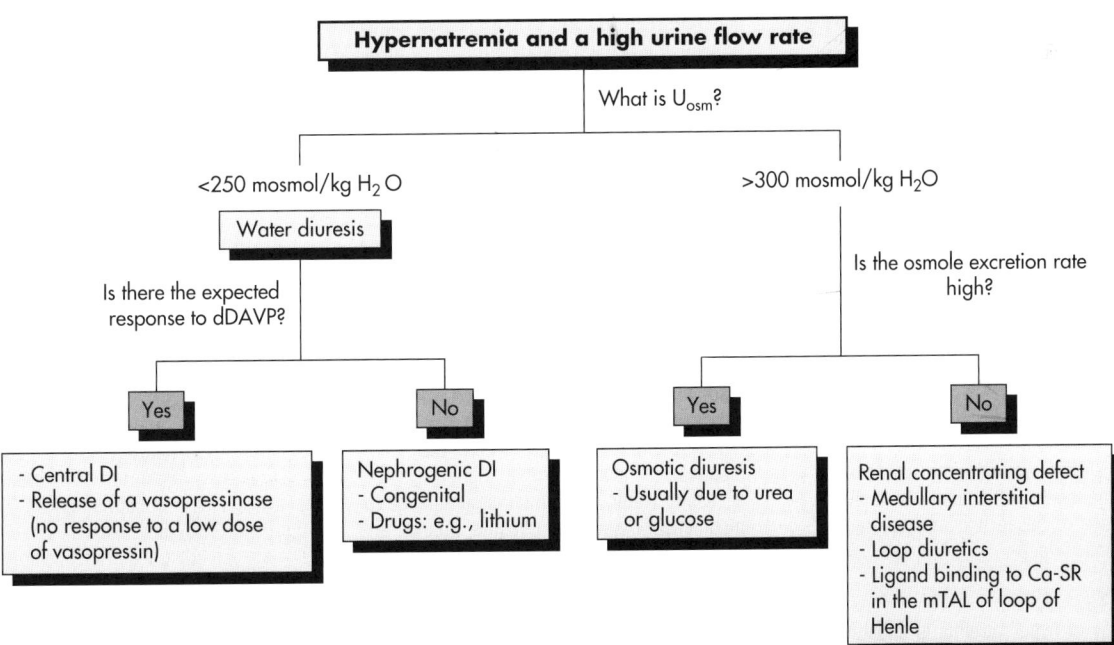

FIG. 2 Hypernatremia with a high urine flow rate. The first step is to determine whether the water loss is caused by a water diuresis or an osmotic diuresis, or whether there is a renal concentrating defect. The principal tools are assessment of the U_{osm} (urine osmolality) and calculation of the osmole excretion rate. In a patient with central diabetes insipidus *(DI)* or a water diuresis caused by the release of a vasopressinase, U_{osm} should rise to a value that is higher than the P_{osm} (plasma osmalality) in response to the administration of deamino-D-arginine vasopressin *(dDAVP)*. If not, nephrogenic DI is the basis of the water diuresis. A value of the U_{osm} that is higher than 300 mosmol/kg H_2O suggests that the basis of hypernatremia is an osmotic diuresis if the osmole excretion rate is appreciably higher than 1000 mosmol/day or a renal concentrating defect if the osmole excretion rate is not high. Examples of ligand binding to the calcium sensing receptor *(Ca-SR)* in the medullary thick ascending limb *(mTAL)* of the loop of Henle include calcium ions in a patient with hypercalcemia, cationic drugs (e.g., gentamicin, cisplatin). (From Kamel SK, Halpertin ML: *Fluid, electrolyte, and acid-base physiology,* ed 5, Philadelphia 2017, Elsevier.)

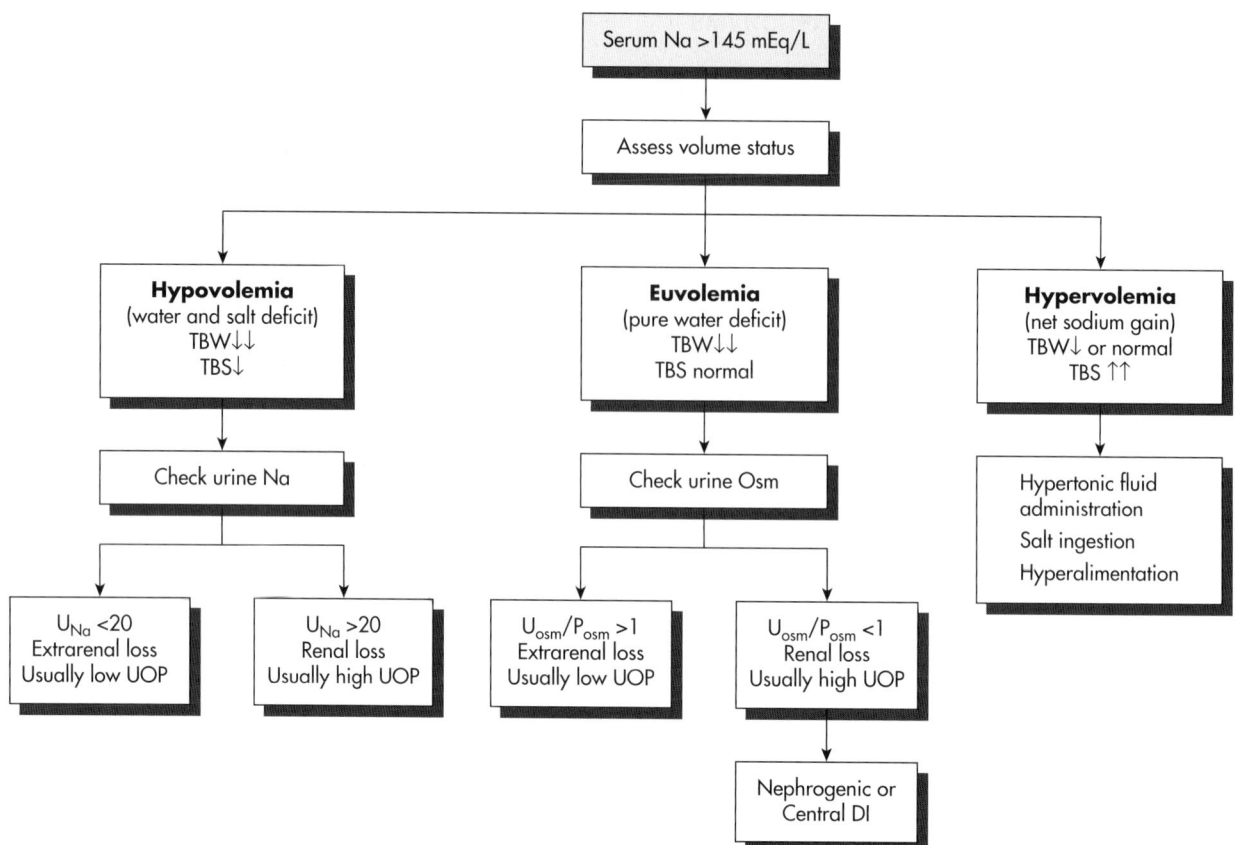

FIG. 3 Diagnostic approach to hypernatremia. *DI,* Diabetes insipidus; *Na, sodium; Osm,* osmolality; *TBS,* total body salt; *TBW,* total body water; *UOP,* urine output; U_{osm}, urine osmolality; P_{osm}, plasma osmolality. (Adapted from Gilbert SJ, Weiner DE: *National Kidney Foundation primer on kidney disease,* ed 6, Philadelphia, 2017, Saunders.)

- In mild hypernatremia, symptoms can include generalized muscle weakness, fatigue, restlessness, anorexia, nausea, and vomiting.[5]
- With severe hypernatremia, symptoms can begin with lethargy and irritability and progress to confusion, seizures, and rarely, coma.[5]
- In extreme scenarios, particularly in infants, hypernatremia-induced brain cell shrinkage can lead to intracranial bleeding from vascular stretching.[6,7]
- Polydipsia and polyuria may be present in certain types of hypernatremia, such as with diabetes insipidus (DI).[6]
- Key elements of the history should focus on respective fluid and water intake and loss, urine output, insensible losses, thirst response, and accessibility to water and fluids.[6]
- Clinicians should evaluate the extracellular fluid volume status of patients to facilitate determination of cause and management of hypernatremia (Fig. 3).

ETIOLOGY

- The etiology of hypernatremia is understood through the Edelman equation (refer to "Hyponatremia"). S_{Na} closely approximates the ratio of total exchangeable body (TB) cations (sodium and potassium, $TB_{Na} + TB_K$) to total body water (TBW).[8]
- Serum [Na] = S_{Na} = $(TB_{Na} + TB_K)/TBW$.[8]

- Hypernatremia is the result of net water deficit or excessive sodium intake.[8] Renal water regulation and thirst stimuli are the key physiologic components that prevent hypernatremia and maintain homeostasis.[8]
- To prevent hypernatremia, water is retained and urine is concentrated by the kidneys under the influence of antidiuretic hormone or arginine vasopressin (AVP). Impairment of AVP secretion, reduction of the corticomedullary concentration gradient, or inability of AVP to stimulate water reabsorption leads to excessive renal water loss and hypernatremia.[8]
- Elevated plasma osmolality from hypernatremia triggers the hypothalamic thirst response.[8] If water intake exceeds water loss or net solute gain, hypernatremia is avoided.[8] Hypernatremia develops when the thirst response is impaired or when there is a lack of access to water, a common circumstance for mechanically ventilated patients, infants, and older adults who may have cognitive impairment(s) and physical limitation(s).[7,8]

Hypernatremia can be classified in the following manner:
- Excessive water loss[1]
  1. GI losses
     a. Vomiting or nasogastric losses
     b. Ileostomy
     c. Pancreaticobiliary fistula
     d. Diarrhea
     e. Laxatives

  2. Renal losses[1]
     a. Osmotic diuresis
        (1) Osmotic diuretics (mannitol, sorbitol, glycine)
        (2) Glucosuria (hyperglycemia, SGLT2 inhibitor administration)
        (3) Urea diuresis (e.g., steroid use, high-protein diet, hypercatabolic state)
        (4) Postobstructive and post–acute tubular necrosis (post-ATN) diuresis
     b. Water diuresis[1,9]
        (1) Central diabetes insipidus (CDI)
            (a) Genetic
                i. Autosomal dominant
                ii. Autosomal recessive
            (b) Acquired (e.g., posttrauma, iatrogenic, craniopharyngioma, metastatic cancers, encephalitis)
            (c) Sarcoidosis
            (d) Langerhans cell histiocytosis
            (e) Eosinophilic granulomatosis
        (2) Nephrogenic diabetes insipidus (NDI)[10]
            (a) Genetic
                i. Arginine vasopressin receptor 2 *(AVPR2)* or aquaporin 2 *(AQP2)* gene sequence variants
                ii. Autosomal dominant polycystic kidney disease

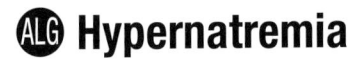

iii. Familial hypocalciuric hypercalcemia from renal calcium–sensing receptor mutation
  (b) Acquired
    i. Chronic kidney disease
    ii. Post-ATN diuresis
    iii. Hypokalemia
    iv. Hypercalcemia (diverse causes)
    v. Drugs (e.g., lithium, amphotericin, ifosfamide, demeclocycline)
    vi. Gestation (increased placental vasopressinase)
- Impaired water intake[6]
  1. Adipsia or hypodipsia
     a. Septo-optic dysplasia
     b. Craniopharyngioma
  2. Impaired access to water
     a. Mechanical ventilation
     b. Dementia
     c. Cognitive impairment
- Excessive sodium intake[6]
  1. Hypertonic saline or sodium bicarbonate administration
  2. Salt tablet excess ingestion
  3. Saltwater drowning

An alternative classification based on extracellular fluid volume status is presented in Table 1.

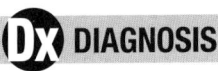

DIAGNOSIS

DIFFERENTIAL DIAGNOSIS

Hypernatremia is a clinical result of net water deficit as a result of dehydration.[11] Conversely, volume depletion occurs as a result of net loss of total body sodium and water that reduces the extracellular fluid and intravascular volumes.[11,12] The combination of dehydration and volume depletion has management implications. For example, normovolemic hypernatremia is caused by pure water loss, and the appropriate volume of water replacement is adequate treatment.[12,13] This strategy is not appropriate in hypovolemic hypernatremia because volume electrolytes (sodium and potassium) and water losses also require replacement.[12,13]

WORKUP

- Workup: Detailed history and physical examination. Historical features that reveal volume depletion and/or dehydration are critical and include a family history of DI and medication or drug use that enhances renal water excretion.[13]
- Hospitalized patients: Frequent monitoring of cumulative fluid intake and fluid losses is mandatory. The most common cause is replacement of total net fluid loss with 0.9% saline.[6,12]
- Hypernatremia in adults: Usually develops from net water loss and inability to access water (e.g., altered mentation, mechanical ventilation).[6] If access to water is not restricted, etiologies that impair thirst center function should be considered.
- In the presence of polyuria, the underlying etiology should be sought.

LABORATORY TESTS[8]

- Serum chemistry: Serial S_{Na} measurements based on clinical scenario (e.g., 2 to 12 h). Frequent monitoring maintains the correction rate of S_{Na} at recommended levels. Derangements of other electrolyte and renal parameters frequently accompany hypernatremia.
- Urine osmolality (U_{osm}): With a normal hypothalamic-pituitary-kidney axis, a plasma osmolality (P_{osm}) elevation of $\geq 1\%$ induces AVP secretion and increases urine concentration (U_{osm} exceeds P_{osm}, typically >600 to 700 mOsm/kg). Accordingly, U_{osm} distinguishes central or nephrogenic DI from the presence of extrarenal water loss.
  1. Low U_{osm} (<300 mOsm/kg) suggests hypernatremia from CDI or NDI. After an initial diagnostic workup is conducted, differentiation between CDI and NDI is required (see "Diabetes Insipidus" chapter).
  2. High U_{osm} typically occurs from extrarenal water losses.
- Urine sodium (U_{Na}) and urine potassium (U_K): U_{Na} assists in the determination of intravascular volume (see Fig. 3). The sum of U_{Na} and U_K quantify urine electrolyte-free water clearance to guide therapy, as explained later. Electrolyte-free water has no effective osmolality (tonicity) at equilibrium and is water composed of no electrolytes with or without urea. Urinary parameters should be monitored every 12 to 24 h until S_{Na} is adequately corrected.

TREATMENT

- Treatment of hypernatremia requires replacement of the existing water deficit and of ongoing daily electrolyte-free water losses.
- Volume replacement generally precedes replacement of water deficit.
- A stepwise approach to the therapy of hypernatremia is depicted in Fig. 4.
  1. Step 1: Determine rate of S_{Na} correction.[5,13]
     a. Although the exact risk is unknown, overcorrection of chronic hyponatremia (>48 h) may induce serious neurologic consequences, namely cerebral edema.
     b. Based on clinical data from infants and critically ill adults, chronic hypernatremia should not be corrected faster than 10 to 12 mEq/L/day, or an average of 0.5 mEq/L/h. This rate would apply to most nonhospitalized older adult patients because hypernatremia develops over several days.
     c. In rare individuals with acute hypernatremia (e.g., intentional or accidental massive sodium ingestions), the S_{Na} may be rapidly corrected (within 24 h) to

- Step 1: Identify rate of correction.
- Step 2: Calculate free water deficit.

$$\text{Water deficit} = \text{TBW} \left[\frac{\text{Current } S_{Na} - \text{Desired } S_{Na}}{\text{Desired } S_{Na}} \right]$$

- Step 3: Choose fluid replacement regimen.

$$\text{Change in } S_{Na} = \frac{\text{Infusate Na} - \text{Current } S_{Na}}{\text{TBW} + 1}$$

- Step 4: Assess ongoing water losses.
  - Urinary water losses estimated by free water clearance

$$C_{\text{electrolyte-free}} = V \left[1 - \frac{U_{Na} + U_K}{S_{Na}} \right]$$

  - Insensible water losses approximately 15-20 mL/kg/day
- Step 5: Determine underlying cause.

FIG. 4 Approach to treatment of hypernatremia. $C_{\text{electrolyte-free}}$, Electrolyte-free water clearance; *Na*, sodium; S_{Na}, serum sodium; *TBW*, total body water; U_K, urine potassium; U_{Na}, urine sodium; *V*, urine volume. (Adapted from Gilbert SJ, Weiner DE: *National Kidney Foundation primer on kidney disease,* ed 6, Philadelphia, 2017, Saunders.)

normal S_{Na} levels. The rate of correction should be no less than 0.25 mmol/h, as prolonged hypernatremia is associated with mortality risk.

2. Step 2: Calculate free water deficit[6,8]
   a. Free water deficit is the volume of free water required to correct the current S_{Na} to the target S_{Na}. This is estimated by the Adrogué-Madias formula:
      (1) Water deficit = TBW × [(Current S_{Na}/Target S_{Na}) – 1].
   b. For the preceding formula, TBW is the estimated TBW. TBW estimates are 50% to 60% of lean body weight in men and women. Target S_{Na} is the S_{Na} that should be achieved in a 24-h period as determined in Step 1.

3. Step 3: Choose fluid replacement regimen[6,8]
   a. With a pure water deficit, the water deficit of Step 2 should be replaced by enteral water or intravenous D_5W.
   b. When possible, the enteral route should be used during hydration therapy to avoid rapid glucose water infusions that may induce hyperglycemia and produce an osmotic diuresis. This pathophysiologic sequence may occur, as D_5W infusion rates are increased to greater than 300 ml/h.
   c. The rate of water replacement (ml/h) is obtained by dividing the calculated water deficit volume by 24 h. It is essential that the ongoing rate of water loss (e.g., urine losses, stool losses) be addressed simultaneously.
   d. Because hypovolemia is present in more than 50% of cases of hypernatremia, concurrent volume replacement with

isotonic fluid should be administered (0.9% sodium chloride or lactated Ringer's solution, as required). An alternative strategy is to use a single infusion of 0.45% saline solution that replaces salt and water along with potassium deficits. For example, 1 L of 0.45% NaCl adds 500 ml of water and 500 ml of 0.9% NaCl to the TBW.
   e. The change in S_{Na} with 1 L of a particular replacement fluid can be predicted by the Adrogué-Madias formula:
      (1) Change in S_{Na} = ($Na_{Infusate}$ – current S_{Na}) / (TBW + 1).
   f. This formula applies to the one-time administration of a 1-L infusate with a sodium concentration ($Na_{Infusate}$). $Na_{Infusate}$ concentrations for 0.45% saline, 0.9% saline, and 3% saline are 77, 154, and 513 mEq/L, respectively.

4. Step 4: Assess ongoing water losses[6,8]
   a. Ongoing daily water losses (skin, stool, and respiratory tract) must be calculated and treated simultaneously. Failure to account for these losses leads to an undercorrection of hypernatremia.
   b. Urinary losses are estimated by the electrolyte-free water clearance equation shown in Fig. 4.
   c. Insensible water losses can be estimated as 15 to 20 ml/kg/day.

Evaluate for any underlying cause of hypernatremia and treat accordingly. If hypernatremia occurs with hypervolemia, use loop diuretics to remove excess sodium.[8] However, diuretic therapy will also increase water losses that must be accounted for.

Repeat Steps 1 to 4 until S_{Na} is reduced to approximately 140 to 145 mEq/L.

The preceding method represents guidance based on classical estimating equations and periodic monitoring of clinical parameters and is key to achievement of the target S_{Na}.

DISPOSITION

Management of hypernatremia generally warrants inpatient admission because patients have underlying conditions that impair the thirst response.

REFERRAL

Nephrology consultation for management of hypernatremia and evaluation of underlying causes is appropriate. Endocrinology consultation may be warranted if DI is suspected.

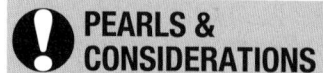

PEARLS & CONSIDERATIONS

COMMENTS

- Hypernatremia is a water-deficit problem associated with impaired thirst and/or inability to obtain water.
- Hypernatremia has morbid consequences, including mortality.
- Hypernatremia may present with hypovolemia, and the latter is usually treated first.
- The S_{Na} correction rate includes determination of the water deficit plus ongoing water losses.

REFERENCES

Available at eBooks.Health.Elsevier.com

AUTHORS: **LALATHAKSHA KUMBAR, MD,** and **RUCHI JALOTA SAHOTA, MD**

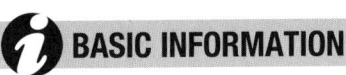 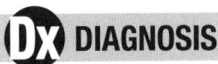

H

Diseases
and Disorders

BASIC INFORMATION

DEFINITION

Hyperparathyroidism is an endocrine disorder caused by excessive secretion of parathyroid hormone (PTH) from the parathyroid glands. Autonomous production of PTH resulting in hypercalcemia defines primary hyperparathyroidism. Secondary hyperparathyroidism occurs when the parathyroid glands appropriately increase PTH production in response to low calcium or vitamin D states. Primary hyperparathyroidism is the focus of this section.

ICD-10CM CODES
E21.0	Primary hyperparathyroidism
E21.1	Secondary hyperparathyroidism, not elsewhere classified
E21.2	Other hyperparathyroidism
E21.3	Hyperparathyroidism, unspecified
N25.81	Secondary hyperparathyroidism of renal origin

EPIDEMIOLOGY & DEMOGRAPHICS

INCIDENCE: 66 cases/100,000 person-year in women and 25 cases/100,000 person-year in men in the United States.[1] Although malignancy is the most common cause of hypercalcemia in hospitalized patients, primary hyperparathyroidism is the most common cause of hypercalcemia in the outpatient setting.[2]

PREVALENCE: Varies by country and race with ~23 cases/10,000 women and 8.5 cases/10,000 men in the United States.[1]

PREDOMINANT SEX & AGE: Higher prevalence in women (female:male ratio 4:1)[3] and peaks in the early postmenopausal year.[4]

PHYSICAL FINDINGS & CLINICAL PRESENTATION

The majority of patients with primary hyperparathyroidism are asymptomatic. Diagnosis is usually considered in patients after an incidental discovery of elevated calcium or PTH levels on biochemical screening or during the evaluation for decreased bone mass.

The development of symptoms varies with severity and rapidity of disease progression and reflects both the hypercalcemia and hyperparathyroid components of the disease process. Symptoms associated with hypercalcemia (Table 1) are as follows[2,3,5]:

- Cardiovascular: Hypertension, shortened QT interval, bradycardia, arrhythmia, valvular calcification, left ventricular hypertrophy, and increased mean carotid intima-media thickness
- GI: Anorexia, nausea, vomiting, constipation, abdominal pain, peptic ulcer disease, and pancreatitis
- Genitourinary (GU): Nephrolithiasis (15% to 20%), nephrocalcinosis, renal insufficiency, polydipsia, polyuria, nocturia, nephrogenic diabetes insipidus, and renal tubular acidosis
- Musculoskeletal: Weakness, myopathy, bone pain, osteopenia, osteoporosis, gout, pseudogout, chondrocalcinosis, osteitis fibrosa cystica, and subperiosteal bone resorption
- Central nervous system: Confusion, anxiety, fatigue, difficulty concentrating, lethargy, obtundation, depression, and coma
- Other: Pruritus, metastatic calcifications, band keratopathy

ETIOLOGY

- Regulators of PTH secretion are illustrated in Fig. 1. Most cases of primary

hyperparathyroidism are sporadic.[3] Hyperparathyroidism can be associated with rare familial conditions in <10%, such as multiple endocrine neoplasia (MEN-1 and MEN-2), familial hyperparathyroidism–jaw tumor syndrome, familial isolated hyperparathyroidism, and neonatal severe hyperparathyroidism.[2] Higher prevalence of hyperparathyroidism is noted with head and neck irradiation, chronic low calcium or vitamin D status, and lithium therapy.[6]

- Pathologic characteristics include adenoma (80%),[3] hyperplasia (15% to 20%),[3] or carcinomas (<1%).[7]

DIAGNOSIS

DIFFERENTIAL DIAGNOSIS

- Primary hyperparathyroidism:
  1. Adenoma (80%)
  2. Hyperplasia (15% to 20%)
  3. Carcinomas (<1%)
- Secondary hyperparathyroidism (Box 1) precipitated by conditions that result in hypocalcemia:
  1. Renal calcium loss (i.e., medication: Loop diuretics and hypercalciuria)
  2. Calcium deficiency
  3. Vitamin D deficiency
  4. Malabsorption
  5. Chronic kidney disease (most common)[2]
  6. Pseudohypoparathyroidism (PTH resistance)
  7. Inhibition of bone resorption (i.e., bisphosphonates and denosumab)
- Other causes of hypercalcemia (Table 2) include:

TABLE 1 Signs and Symptoms of Primary Hyperparathyroidism

Target Organ or System	Symptoms	Comments
Renal	Nephrolithiasis, nephrocalcinosis, polyuria, polydipsia, renal insufficiency	15%-20% of patients have kidney stones
Skeletal	Fragility fractures	Unrelated to significant trauma
	Osteopenia/osteoporosis	Cortical bone > trabecular bone (distal third of radius most affected)
	Bone pain	Common
	Osteitis fibrosa cystica	Rare, but may occur with advanced disease, characterized by bone pain and multiple skeletal deformities, including salt and pepper appearance of the skull, bone cysts, and brown tumors of bone
Neuromuscular	Proximal muscle weakness, muscular atrophy, gait disturbance	Rare
	Easy fatigability, generalized weakness	Common
Gastrointestinal	Gastroesophageal reflux, constipation, abdominal pain, peptic ulcer disease	Common / Rare
	Nausea, vomiting, acute pancreatitis	Rare, can be seen in cases of severe hypercalcemia
Neuropsychiatric	Fatigue, depression, anxiety, emotional lability, sleep disturbances, lethargy, memory loss, inability to concentrate, mental status change, psychosis, obtundation, and coma	Often reported
	Rare, can be seen with severe hypercalcemia	
Cardiovascular	Exacerbation of hypertension, valvular disease, myocardial calcifications, premature atherosclerosis, left ventricular hypertrophy, shortened QT interval, conduction abnormalities, and heart block	Conflicting data on improvement of cardiac parameters after parathyroidectomy

From Townsend CM et al: *Sabiston textbook of surgery,* ed 21, St Louis, 2022, Elsevier.

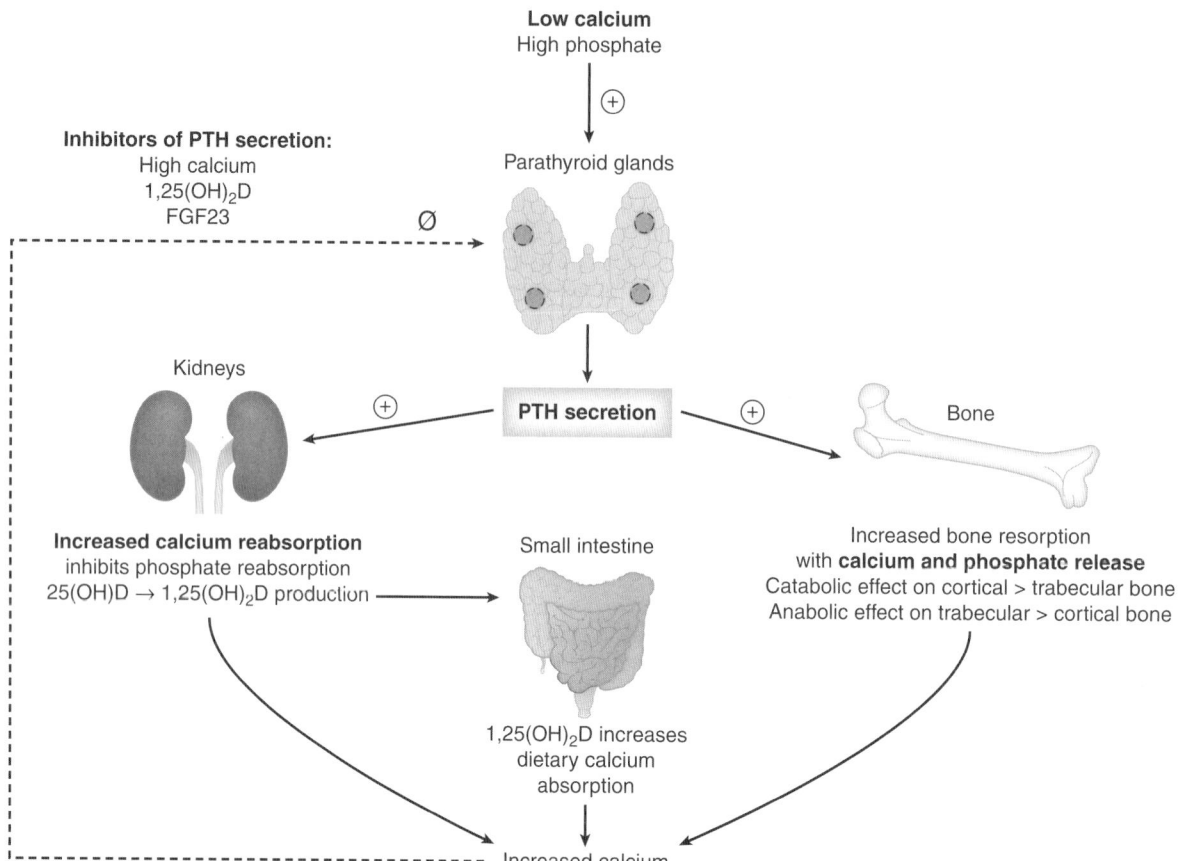

FIG. 1 Regulators of parathyroid hormone (PTH) secretion and PTH effects on calcium homeostasis. *FGF23,* Fibroblast growth factor 23; *25(OH)D,* 25-hydroxyvitamin D; *1,25(OH)₂D,* 1,25-dihydroxyvitamin D. (From Townsend CM et al: *Sabiston textbook of surgery,* ed 21, St Louis, 2022, Elsevier.)

BOX 1   Causes of Secondary Hyperparathyroidism

- Chronic renal failure
- 25-Hydroxyvitamin D deficiency
- Malabsorption syndromes
  Celiac disease
  Cystic fibrosis
  Short gut syndrome
  Bariatric procedures
- Medications
  Lithium
  Diuretics (e.g., hydrochlorothiazide, furosemide)
- Metabolic abnormalities
  Hypermagnesemia
  Hyperphosphatemia
- Congenital disorders
  Transient neonatal hyperparathyroidism
  DiGeorge syndrome

From Townsend CM et al: *Sabiston textbook of surgery,* ed 21, St Louis, 2022, Elsevier.

1. Medications: Thiazide diuretics, lithium therapy
2. Vitamin D intoxication, milk-alkali syndrome
3. Vitamin A toxicity
4. Familial hypocalciuric hypercalcemia (FHH)
5. Renal failure (tertiary hyperparathyroidism)
6. Thyrotoxicosis
7. Granulomatous disorders (e.g., sarcoidosis)
8. Malignancy (e.g., lung cancer, lymphoma, multiple myeloma, and bone metastasis)
9. Prolonged immobilization

WORKUP (TABLE 3)

- Typically, primary hyperparathyroidism is confirmed with an elevated serum calcium and PTH level.
  1. Two measurements of serum calcium are required for the confirmation of hypercalcemia. Total calcium should be corrected for low albumin using the formula: Corrected calcium = serum calcium + 0.8 × 4 − serum albumin. If a reliable laboratory is available, ionized calcium should be considered, especially in conditions associated with acid-base disturbances or low albumin states. Patients with primary hyperparathyroidism can also present with normal calcium levels (normocalcemic primary hyperparathyroidism).
  2. The serum intact PTH level is the best test to evaluate the etiology of hypercalcemia. PTH is elevated or in the high normal range (i.e., inappropriately normal for an elevated calcium state) in primary hyperparathyroidism.
- Other causes of hypercalcemia should be ruled out. These are typically associated with low PTH levels. Exceptions include lithium use and FHH.
  1. Review medication history to determine lithium, thiazide, vitamin D, or calcium intake.

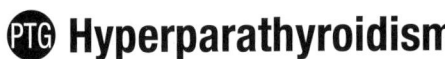

TABLE 2   Causes of Hypercalcemia

Endocrine	Primary hyperparathyroidism
	Tertiary hyperparathyroidism
	Familial hypocalciuric hypercalcemia
	Hyperthyroidism
Malignancy	Tumors producing PTHrP (SCC of lung, bladder cancer, renal cell cancer)
	Osteolytic bone metastasis
	Hematologic malignancies (lymphoma, leukemia, multiple myeloma)
Granulomatous disease	Sarcoidosis
	Tuberculosis
	Fungal infection
Medications	Calcium
	Thiazide diuretics
	Lithium
	Vitamin A and D intoxication
	Milk alkali syndrome
Miscellaneous	Paget and other bone diseases with prolonged immobilization

PTHrP, Parathyroid hormone–related peptide; *SCC,* squamous cell carcinoma.
From Townsend CM et al: *Sabiston textbook of surgery,* ed 21, St Louis, 2022, Elsevier.

TABLE 3   Evaluation of Patients With Suspected or Confirmed Primary HPT

Tests	Comments
Laboratory Tests	
Serum total calcium	Baseline laboratory tests for diagnosis of primary HPT and to rule out the most common causes of secondary HPT
Intact PTH	
Creatinine, GFR	
25-Hydroxyvitamin D	
Ionized calcium	For patients with normocalcemic primary HPT
Albumin	If low, calculate corrected calcium (mg/dl) = (0.8 [4.0-patient's albumin (g/dl)] + total calcium (mg/dl)
Serum phosphate	Low in approximately 50% of patients with primary HPT
Alkaline phosphatase	Marker of bone turnover, indicates extent of bone disease
Urine Tests	
24-H urine calcium and creatinine	Screen for increased risk of kidney stones and for familial hypocalciuric hypercalcemia
If urine calcium <100 mg/24 h, calculate CCCR	CCCR = (24-h calcium urine/calcium serum)/(24-h creatinine urine/creatinine serum)
Imaging	
DXA	Measurements of bone mineral density at the lumbar spine, hip femoral neck, and distal radius
Abdominal imaging for kidney stones or nephrocalcinosis	Plain abdominal x-ray, abdominal ultrasound, or noncontrast CT
Vertebral spine assessment	Plain x-ray, CT, or DXA
Genetic Testing	
Indications	Patients with pHPT less than 40 yr with multigland disease and patients with a family history of pHPT or syndromes associated with pHPT

CCCR, Calcium creatinine clearance ratio; *CT,* computed tomography; *DXA,* dual-energy x-ray absorptiometry; *GFR,* glomerular filtration rate; *HPT,* hyperparathyroidism; *pHPT,* primary hyperparathyroidism; *PTH,* parathyroid hormone.

2. Check 24-h urine calcium: Creatinine to rule out FHH. Urine calcium is very low (<100 mg), and calcium clearance/creatinine clearance ratio is <0.01 in FHH. PTH can be normal or high in FHH.

3. Consider PTH-related peptide (PTHrP) to evaluate hypercalcemia related to malignancies and 1,25-hydroxyvitamin D to assess hypercalcemia secondary to granulomatous diseases or lymphomas.

4. Multiple myeloma and bone metastasis can also result in a high calcium state and therefore must be appropriately evaluated.
- Rule out other causes of elevated PTH (i.e., secondary hyperparathyroidism). Serum calcium is typically low or low-normal in secondary hyperparathyroidism.
  1. Check calcium and 25-hydroxyvitamin D to rule out deficiency states.
  2. Check serum creatinine to assess renal function and 24-h urine calcium and creatinine to evaluate renal calcium loss.

LABORATORY TESTS

- Serum calcium (ionized or corrected calcium): Normal or elevated in primary hyperparathyroidism
- Serum phosphorus: Low or low-normal in primary hyperparathyroidism
- PTH: Elevated or high-normal in primary hyperparathyroidism
- Serum creatinine and estimated glomerular filtration rate (GFR)
- 24-h urine calcium and creatinine
- 25-hydroxyvitamin D, 1,25-hydroxyvitamin D, PTHrP levels
- ECG may reveal shortening of the QT interval secondary to severe hypercalcemia (>12 mg/dl)

IMAGING STUDIES (TABLE 4)

- Parathyroid localization with technetium-99m sestamibi (Fig. E2 and Fig E3) can identify potential adenomas to help with surgical planning.[8] The inferior parathyroid glands are more commonly ectopic and can be found anywhere from the angle of the mandible to the pericardium. The most common ectopic location for an inferior gland is within the thymus (Fig. 4)
- Parathyroid ultrasound (Fig. 5, Fig E6), dynamic (4D) CT, and MRI are also used to localize the parathyroid adenoma.[8]
- Bone mineral density (BMD) imaging of the spine, hip, and forearm (distal third of radius) is recommended for all patients with hyperparathyroidism to assess the risk for osteoporosis and fragility fractures. Plain radiographic abnormalities are illustrated in Fig. E7 and Fig. E8. Cortical bone loss (i.e., distal one third radius) is greater than trabecular bone loss (i.e., hip and spine) in hyperparathyroidism.[9]
- Renal ultrasound can be considered to assess asymptomatic renal stones.

(Rx) TREATMENT

Modality of treatment depends on disease progression and which patients are more likely to suffer end-organ effects of hyperparathyroidism or benefit the most from surgery. Fig. 9 illustrates an algorithm for managing persistent or recurrent hyperparathyroidism.

- Surgery is the only definitive treatment for symptomatic primary hyperparathyroidism. Surgery can normalize calcium levels,

TABLE 4 Characteristics of Preoperative Imaging Studies in Patients With Hyperparathyroidism

Imaging	Imaging Findings	Sensitivity, Ppv	Advantages	Limitations	Updates
US	Hypoechoic nodule with well-defined hypervascular echogenic capsule	76%, 93%	Noninvasive, inexpensive, can be performed rapidly by the surgeon with simultaneous evaluation of the thyroid	Unable to see ectopic mediastinal, retroesophageal, or retropharyngeal glands; decreased sensitivity in multigland disease and small glands; thyroid nodules and lymph nodes can cause false-positives	US elastography
Sestamibi-SPECT	Increased focal uptake and prolonged retention of the technetium-99m sestamibi	79%, 90%	Detects ectopic and posterior glands; lower radiation than 4D-CT, operator-independent	Long duration of time for the exam; more expensive than US and 4D-CT, radiation exposure; decreased sensitivity for multigland disease and small glands; false-positives (lymph nodes, thyroid tissue, granulomatous disease)	PET scanning with various radiopharmaceuticals under investigation
4D-CT	Soft tissue nodule with peaked enhancement in arterial phase and washout in venous phase with polar vessel	81%-89%, 93%	Rapid acquisition time, superior anatomic information, superior sensitivity than other techniques, more successful in localizing small adenomas and multigland disease	High radiation dose, intravenous contrast use, some contrast artifact in neck veins can occur	Protocols with fewer phases or less contrast, to diminish radiation and contrast dose
MRI	Homogeneous or marbled appearance with high intensity on T2-weighted images, intermediate to low intensity on T1-weighted images	43%-94%	No radiation, contrast not necessary, superior anatomic information	Expensive, long duration of study acquisition, cannot use in patients with metal implants, low specificity	Dixon fat suppression method
[18]F-fluorocholine PET/CT	Focal tracer uptake	93%, 90%	Decreased radiation and acquisition time compared to some sestamibi protocols, higher sensitivity	Limited data on new tracer, limited availability	Ability to differentiate between parathyroid adenoma and hyperplasia preoperatively based on maximal standardized uptake values

CT, Computed tomography; *4D-CT,* four-dimensional CT; *MRI,* magnetic resonance imaging; *PET/CT,* positron emission tomography/CT; *SPECT,* single photon emission CT; *US,* ultrasound.
From Townsend CM et al: *Sabiston textbook of surgery,* ed 21, St Louis, 2022, Elsevier.

decrease the risk for kidney stones, improve BMD and fracture risk, and enhance quality-of-life measures. Established indications for parathyroidectomy in patients with primary hyperparathyroidism are summarized in Box 2. Indications for parathyroidectomy in patients with secondary and tertiary hyperparathyroidism are described in Box 3.

1. Surgical approaches include:
   a. Minimally invasive parathyroidectomy has increased in popularity.[8] The surgeon will identify and remove the abnormal gland that was identified on preoperative imaging. This technique has limited dissection and has improved recovery time. Intraoperative monitoring of PTH level is done to ensure the removal of the abnormal gland. Fall of PTH level by 50% and into the normal range is expected within 15 to 30 min after removal of the abnormal gland.[3]
   b. Bilateral neck exploration under general anesthesia is the traditional surgical approach. All parathyroid glands are identified and compared. An experienced endocrine surgeon cures >95% of patients undergoing bilateral neck exploration. Potential complications include transient and permanent hypocalcemia secondary to hypoparathyroidism and recurrent laryngeal nerve injury.

- Medical management:
  1. Because inadequate calcium and vitamin D status stimulates PTH, it is not necessary to significantly restrict calcium and vitamin D intake. Vitamin D replacement safely improves vitamin D level and decreases PTH level without significantly increasing serum calcium level and urinary calcium excretion. Repletion of vitamin D is recommended in patients whose levels are <30 mg/dl (75 mmol/L).[6] Dietary calcium intake should be approximately 1000 mg/day.
  2. Encourage physical activity because immobilization increases bone resorption.
  3. Recommend adequate hydration (at least 2 L) to minimize the risk of nephrolithiasis.
  4. For patients who are not surgical candidates or who refuse surgery, pharmacologic options are available. The choice of pharmacologic agents is dependent on the desired goal.

- Cinacalcet (Sensipar) is an oral calcimimetic agent that activates the calcium-sensing receptor in the parathyroid gland. It decreases PTH production and subsequently normalizes

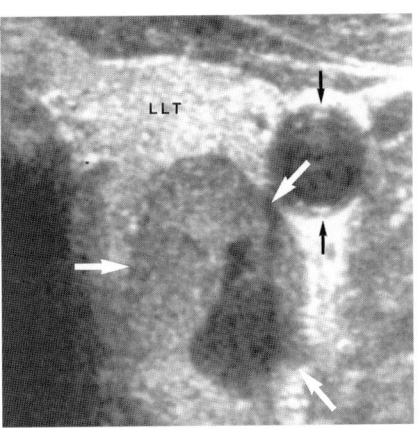

FIG. 5 High-resolution ultrasonography of the left lobe of the thyroid (LLT) anterior to a parathyroid adenoma *(white arrows).* There is a small area of cystic degeneration within the posterior aspect of the adenoma. Carotid artery *(black arrows).* (From Adam A et al: *Grainger & Allison's diagnostic radiology,* ed 5, London, 2007, Churchill Livingstone. In Grant LA: *Grainger & Allison's diagnostic radiology essentials,* ed 2, London, 2019, Elsevier.)

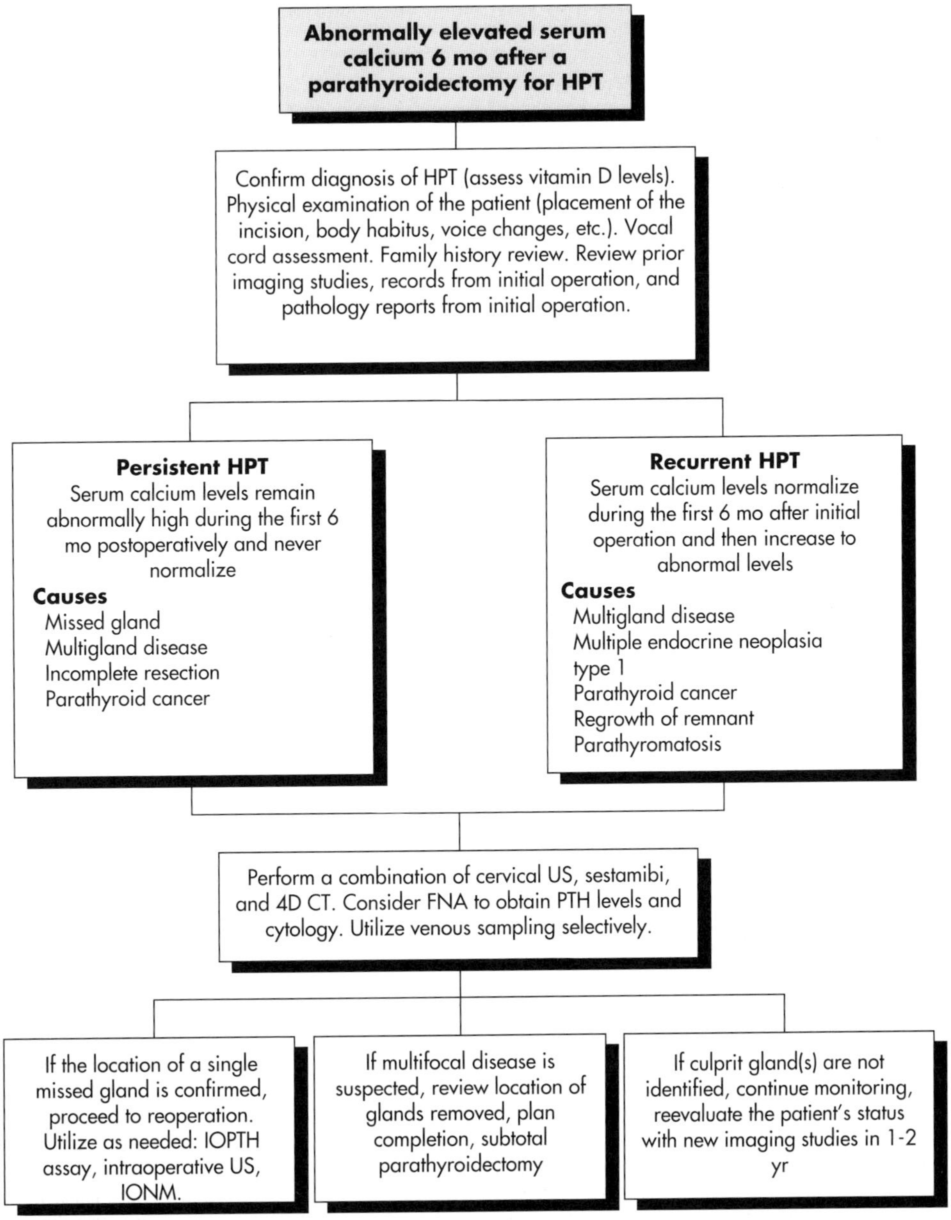

Abnormally elevated serum calcium 6 mo after a parathyroidectomy for HPT

↓

Confirm diagnosis of HPT (assess vitamin D levels). Physical examination of the patient (placement of the incision, body habitus, voice changes, etc.). Vocal cord assessment. Family history review. Review prior imaging studies, records from initial operation, and pathology reports from initial operation.

Persistent HPT
Serum calcium levels remain abnormally high during the first 6 mo postoperatively and never normalize

Causes
Missed gland
Multigland disease
Incomplete resection
Parathyroid cancer

Recurrent HPT
Serum calcium levels normalize during the first 6 mo after initial operation and then increase to abnormal levels

Causes
Multigland disease
Multiple endocrine neoplasia type 1
Parathyroid cancer
Regrowth of remnant
Parathyromatosis

↓

Perform a combination of cervical US, sestamibi, and 4D CT. Consider FNA to obtain PTH levels and cytology. Utilize venous sampling selectively.

If the location of a single missed gland is confirmed, proceed to reoperation. Utilize as needed: IOPTH assay, intraoperative US, IONM.

If multifocal disease is suspected, review location of glands removed, plan completion, subtotal parathyroidectomy

If culprit gland(s) are not identified, continue monitoring, reevaluate the patient's status with new imaging studies in 1-2 yr

FIG. 9 Algorithm for managing persistent or recurrent hyperparathyroidism (HPT). *4D CT,* Four-dimensional computed tomography; *FNA,* fine-needle aspiration; *IONM,* intraoperative neurophysiologic monitoring; *IOPTH,* intraoperative parathyroid hormone; *PTH,* parathyroid hormone; *sestamibi,* technetium (^{99m}Tc) sestamibi imaging; *US,* ultrasonography. (From Cameron JL, Cameron AM: *Current surgical therapy,* ed 12, Philadelphia, 2017, Elsevier.)

BOX 2   Established Indications for Parathyroidectomy in Patients With Primary Hyperparathyroidism

- All symptomatic patients (renal, bone, neurocognitive, or neuropsychiatric symptoms)
- Serum calcium >1 mg/dl above the upper limit of normal
- Age <50 yr
- BMD T score <−2.5 (osteoporosis) or significant reduction in BMD
- Vertebral compression fracture on spine imaging
- Impaired renal function with GFR <60 ml/min
- Nephrolithiasis or nephrocalcinosis
- Hypercalciuria with increased stone risk (urine calcium >400 mg/24 h)
- When active surveillance and routine long-term follow-up is not a good option

From Townsend CM et al: *Sabiston textbook of surgery,* ed 21, St Louis, 2022, Elsevier.

BOX 3   Indications for Parathyroidectomy in Patients With Secondary and Tertiary Hyperparathyroidism

Indications for Parathyroidectomy in Patients With Secondary Hyperparathyroidism (SHPT)
SHPT refractory to medical therapy:
- Parathyroid hormone >1000 pg/ml
- Calcium × phosphorus product >55

Renal osteodystrophy
Calciphylaxis
Other retractable symptoms, including uremic pruritus, persistent anemia, bone pain, muscle pain, abdominal pain, fatigue, and weakness

Indications for Parathyroidectomy in Patients With Tertiary Hyperparathyroidism
Severe hypercalcemia (calcium >12.5 mg/dl)
Persistent hypercalcemia ≥2 yr after renal transplantation, associated with:
- Decline in renal function, without graft rejection
- Nephrolithiasis
- Progressive bone disease
- Pancreatitis

From Cameron JL, Cameron AM: *Current surgical therapy,* ed 12, Philadelphia, 2017, Elsevier.

or decreases serum calcium levels, without significant BMD changes.[9] It is indicated for the treatment of severe hypercalcemia in patients with primary hyperparathyroidism who are unable to undergo surgery. It is also indicated for the treatment of secondary hyperparathyroidism associated with chronic kidney disease and for hypercalcemia associated with parathyroid carcinoma.

- Agents such as bisphosphonates (e.g., alendronate, zoledronate) that inhibit bone resorption and increase BMD should be considered when improvement in BMD is the primary goal in patients with hyperparathyroidism.
- Medical monitoring is recommended for asymptomatic primary hyperparathyroidism. Majority of patients do not manifest disease progression during observation. However, one third of asymptomatic patients progressed over a 15-yr follow-up.[10]
  1. Indications for medical monitoring:
     a. Clinically asymptomatic and >50 yr old
     b. Serum calcium level only mildly elevated (<1 mg/dl above upper limit normal)
     c. GFR >60 ml/min and no nephrolithiasis or nephrocalcinosis
     d. No evidence of osteoporosis
     e. Medically unfit for surgery or refusing surgery
- Symptoms should be assessed regularly. Serum calcium, creatinine, and GFR should be checked annually and DXA performed at three sites every 1 to 2 yr or vertebral fracture assessment of the spine is clinically indicated (e.g., height loss, back pain).[11]

ACUTE GENERAL Rx

Severe and/or symptomatic hypercalcemia may require hospitalization, especially if serum calcium >12 mg/dl. Acute management of hypercalcemia includes:
- Vigorous hydration with IV normal saline (2 to 4 L/day). Fluid status must be monitored in patients with cardiac dysfunction or renal insufficiency to avoid fluid overload. Loop diuretics are often administered to increase calcium excretion or in patients who have risk of volume overload.[12]

- Bisphosphonates can effectively decrease calcium levels. Zoledronate (4 mg IV over 15 min) or pamidronate (60 to 90 mg IV over 4 h) are both effective. Onset of action is 24 to 48 h.
- Calcitonin (4 units/kg IM/SC every 12 h) may be used with bisphosphonates to achieve a more rapid reduction of calcium levels. Onset of action is within hours; however, efficacy is limited to 48 h.
- Denosumab, a human monoclonal antibody that binds RANK ligand, also has been used in patients with severe hypercalcemia and parathyroid carcinoma because it lowers serum calcium and bone turnover. Unlike bisphosphonates, no dose adjustment is needed for patients with renal dysfunction.[12]

ⓘ PEARLS & CONSIDERATIONS

COMMENTS

- Parathyroidectomy should be considered for all patients with symptomatic hyperparathyroidism. Surgery also should be considered in older adults with reasonable life expectancy because fracture risk is lower with parathyroidectomy than with nonoperative management.[13] If surgery is contraindicated or not desired, cinacalcet and bisphosphonates can be used.
- Asymptomatic patients can be monitored with serial calcium, creatinine, estimated glomerular filtration rate, and BMD measurements. Disease progression may result in surgery.
- Most patients can be managed medically by limiting factors that result in hypercalcemia (e.g., dehydration, immobilization, thiazide diuretics) and maintaining normal calcium and vitamin D intake.
- Patients with osteopenia and high fracture risk may require antiresorptive therapy such as bisphosphonates.
- Patients with nephrolithiasis and elevated serum calcium should be evaluated for primary hyperparathyroidism. A study of U.S. veterans with kidney stones revealed hypoparathyroidism in 38% of hypercalcemic patients, and 26% of these patients underwent parathyroidectomy within 2 yr after their kidney stone episode.[14]

REFERENCES
Available at eBooks.Health.Elsevier.com.

RELATED CONTENT
Hyperparathyroidism (Patient Information)

AUTHORS: **DIANELYS MENDEZ, MD,** and **VICKY CHENG, MD**

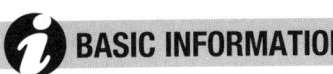
Diseases
and Disorders

I

BASIC INFORMATION

DEFINITION

Hypersensitivity pneumonitis (HP) is an inflammatory lung disease caused by the inhalation of an antigen to which the patient is sensitized and hyperresponsive.

SYNONYMS

HP
Extrinsic allergic alveolitis (EAA)
Bird fancier's lung
Farmer's lung
Malt worker's lung
"Ventilation" pneumonitis
Maple bark-stripper's lung
Sauna taker's lung
Hot tub lung

ICD-10CM CODES
J67.x Hypersensitivity pneumonitis due to specific organic dusts
J67.9 Hypersensitivity pneumonitis due to unspecified organic dust

EPIDEMIOLOGY & DEMOGRAPHICS

- Estimates of the prevalence and incidence of HP vary considerably and depend on the definition and methods used to establish the diagnosis.
- Clinical presentation depends on the intensity of exposure, environmental conditions, and genetic risk factors that remain poorly understood.
- More than 300 causative agents have been identified, and the number continues to grow.
- Causative agents in residential and occupational exposures include birds, mold, humidifiers, fountains, steam irons, dry sausage molds, moldy cheese, contaminated wood, biofilm contained within wind instruments (e.g., trombone, saxophone), and organic and inorganic chemicals, including metalworking fluids.
- It is likely that genetic factors are involved that result in an exaggerated lung response to an offending agent. The major histocompatibility complex is the most studied thus far.

PHYSICAL FINDINGS & CLINICAL PRESENTATION

- Presentation is heterogeneous and, until recently, was classified by the clinical presentation as acute, subacute, or chronic HP based on the intensity, frequency, and duration of antigen exposure and symptoms.[1]
  1. Acute HP: Fever, chills, malaise, cough, and dyspnea that occur within 4 to 8 h of an intense exposure. This flulike syndrome improves in 24 to 48 h and can be mistaken for an acute respiratory infection.
  2. Subacute HP: Progressive dyspnea and cough that occurs after weeks or months of sustained low-level exposure or recurrent exposure to an offending antigen.

  3. Chronic HP: Progression of subacute HP, with chronic, progressive dyspnea and cough, fatigue, and weight loss, over months or years of low-level exposure to an offending agent.
- Because these clinical presentations are not consistently associated with outcomes, HP is currently classified as fibrotic or nonfibrotic.[2]
- Physical examination findings include inspiratory crackles and squeaks on lung auscultation, hypoxemia, cyanosis, possibly fever, and clubbing.

ETIOLOGY

- Numerous environmental agents, both at home and in occupational settings.
- Common sources of antigens: "Moldy" hay, silage, grain, or vegetables; bird droppings or feathers (including those found commonly in down pillows, blankets, and upholstered furniture); low–molecular-weight chemicals (e.g., isocyanates); pharmaceutical products.
- Fig. E1 illustrates the pathogenesis of hypersensitivity pneumonitis.

DIAGNOSIS
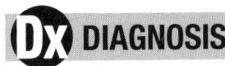

DIFFERENTIAL DIAGNOSIS

See Table 1 for differential diagnosis at different stages of HP. Table 2 summarizes typical features and the differential diagnosis of hypersensitivity pneumonitis.

WORKUP (FIG. 2)

- Establishing the diagnosis of HP and identifying the offending exposure has treatment and prognostic implications. The diagnosis of HP is based on a combination of exposure history, radiographic findings, bronchoalveolar lavage (BAL), and histologic features.[2]
- Major diagnostic criteria:
  1. **Exposure:** Compatible clinical features (cough and dyspnea) in the setting of an environmental exposure known to cause HP, temporal relation between exposure

TABLE 1 Stages of Hypersensitivity Pneumonitis

Acute Stages	Chronic Stages
Allergic bronchopulmonary aspergillosis	Idiopathic pulmonary fibrosis (IPF)
	Bronchiectasis
	Chronic bronchitis
Pulmonary embolism	Nonspecific interstitial pneumonia (NSIP)
Asthma	
Aspiration pneumonia	Connective tissue–related lung disease
Bacterial pneumonia	Sarcoidosis
Fungal or mycobacterial pneumonia	
Bronchiolitis obliterans–organizing pneumonia	
Eosinophilic pneumonia	
Churg-Strauss syndrome	
Wegener granulomatosis	

and disease, clinical improvement with antigen avoidance. Detailed occupational, hobby, and home exposure history is required, along with a high index of suspicion. Questions should address environmental exposure to grain dusts; animal handling; food processing; cooling towers; fountains; metal-working fluids; symptom improvement away from exposure; pets (particularly birds); hobbies involving chemicals, feathers, or fur; organic dusts; presence of humidifiers, dehumidifiers, or hot tubs/saunas; leaking or flooding indoors; visible fungal growth in living or working environment; and feather pillows, bedding, or upholstered furniture. Common causes of hypersensitivity pneumonitis are summarized in Table 3. In up to 50% of patients the specific offending exposure may remain unidentified.

2. **Radiographic:** A typical or compatible HP pattern on high-resolution computed tomography scan (HRCT). Features of small airway disease, including mosaic attenuation, a three-density pattern of normal lung, ground-glass opacity, air trapping, and centrilobular nodules. Findings most often are present with an upper lobe predominance. Fibrosis, including septal thickening, traction bronchiectasis, and honeycombing, may be present and often spares the lower lobes.

3. **BAL:** Lymphocytosis >30%. Bronchoscopy with BAL provides useful supportive data in the diagnosis of HP. Usually reveals intense lymphocytosis (typically T cells >40%) of predominantly CD8+ suppressor cells.

4. **Histologic:** A typical or probable HP pattern on transbronchial biopsy or surgical lung biopsy. Poorly formed nonnecrotizing granulomas, giant cells, chronic bronchiolocentric inflammation, airway-centered interstitial fibrosis, absence of alternative diagnosis. In chronic HP, fibrosis can resemble usual interstitial pattern with fibroblastic foci or a nonspecific interstitial pneumonia pattern.

- HP must be suspected in patients presenting with cough, dyspnea, fever, and malaise. A thorough exposure history and an HRCT of the chest are the two most useful tests to make the diagnosis.[3] BAL lymphocytosis supports the diagnosis. Surgical lung biopsy is especially helpful to achieve a confident diagnosis when HRCT shows a usual interstitial pneumonia pattern.

LABORATORY TESTS

- Serum precipitin test for immunoglobulin G (IgG) antibodies against offending antigen have a sensitivity and specificity of 83% and 68%, respectively. Asymptomatic patients may have IgG antibodies in serum. HP may occur without a positive precipitin test. When positive, precipitins indicate that the patient has been exposed to the antigen during his or

TABLE 2 Typical Features and Differential Diagnosis of Hypersensitivity Pneumonitis

	Nonfibrotic	Fibrotic
Time course of presentation and inciting antigen exposure	1. Acute symptom onset 2. Exposure to antigen 3. Temporal relation of symptoms to exposure usually recognized 4. Chronic presentations are less common	1. Chronic, insidious symptom onset 2. Inciting antigen may not be recognized 3. Unclear relation between exposure and symptoms
Symptoms	1. Cough, dyspnea at rest and/or with exertion 2. Systemic symptoms including fever, chills, myalgias	1. Dyspnea on exertion 2. Cough, typically nonproductive
Physical examination	1. Fever, tachypnea, hypoxemia 2. Crackles on chest exam 3. Inspiratory musical squeaks/squawks 4. May have normal exam	1. Inspiratory Velcro crackles 2. Inspiratory musical squeaks/squawks 3. Hypoxemia on exertion 4. May have normal exam
HRCT chest imaging	1. Diffuse ground-glass opacities 2. Centrilobular nodules 3. Bronchovascular distribution 4. Mosaic attenuation ± air trapping on expiratory imaging 5. Mixed interstitial (ground-glass opacities or high-attenuation areas) and obstructive (mosaic changes or low-attenuation areas), i.e., "headcheese" sign	1. May have similar findings as acute HP, but also: a. Fibrosis—reticulation, traction bronchiectasis or bronchiolectasis, honeycombing
Bronchoalveolar lavage fluid analysis	1. Lymphocytosis (lack of this finding does not exclude HP)	1. Lymphocytosis less common (lack of this finding does not exclude HP)

Histopathologic findings	1. Neutrophilic and lymphocytic infiltrates involving bronchioles and alveolar interstitium
	2. Poorly formed granulomas
	3. Lymphocytic bronchiolitis
	4. Foci of organizing pneumonia
		1. Features seen in acute HP, plus:
		   a. Peribronchiolar fibrosis
		   b. Interstitial fibrosis ± bridging features
		   c. UIP-like pattern with honeycombing and fibroblastic foci

Differential diagnosis	1. Viral, atypical pneumonia
	2. CTD-ILD
	3. Drug reaction
	4. Inhalational fever (e.g., organic dust toxic syndrome)
	5. Toxic fume inhalation
	6. Asthma
	7. Sarcoidosis
	8. Mycobacterial infection
	9. Aspiration pneumonitis
	10. Bronchiolitis obliterans
	11. Organizing pneumonia
	12. Acute fibrinous and organizing pneumonia
	13. Granulomatous-lymphocytic interstitial lung disease
		1. Other ILD:
		   a. CTD-ILD
		   b. NSIP
		   c. IPF
		2. Sarcoidosis
		3. Familial ILD
		4. Pleuroparenchymal fibroelastosis

CTD, Connective tissue disease; *HP,* hypersensitivity pneumonitis; *HRCT,* high-resolution computed tomography; *ILD,* interstitial lung disease; *IPF,* idiopathic pulmonary fibrosis; *NSIP,* nonspecific interstitial pneumonitis.
From Broaddus VC et al: *Murray & Nadel's textbook of respiratory medicine,* ed 7, Philadelphia, 2022, Elsevier.

her life. Further exploration to determine if any particular antigen is the cause of the disease is warranted.

- Lactate dehydrogenase (LDH) is increased and tends to decrease with improvement.
- Pulmonary function tests: Restrictive ventilatory pattern is typically seen. Decreased FEV1, decreased forced vital capacity, decreased total lung capacity, decreased diffusing capacity, and decreased static compliance.
- Arterial blood gases show mild hypoxemia (worsens with exercise) and A-a gradient shows slight increase.
- The role for controlled inhalation provocation test using aerosolized materials of the suspected causative agent has not been established.

IMAGING STUDIES

- Chest x-ray examination: Nonspecific; may be normal in early stages.
- High-resolution chest CT scan (Fig. 3): May vary with stage of disease but often includes features of small airway disease, including mosaic attenuation, a three-density pattern of normal lung, ground-glass opacity, air trapping, and centrilobular nodules. Findings most often are present with an upper lobe predominance. The chronic stage may reveal honeycombing, air trapping, and traction bronchiectasis.

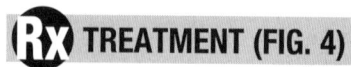 **TREATMENT (FIG. 4)**

NONPHARMACOLOGIC THERAPY

- Identification and complete avoidance of exposure to the offending antigen is the cornerstone of treatment. Avoidance can lead to resolution of acute and subacute HP, as well as to stability and improved survival in chronic HP.[4]

ACUTE GENERAL Rx

- Corticosteroids accelerate initial recovery for acute and subacute HP, but may have no effect long term (from a controlled study in farmer's lung).[5]

H

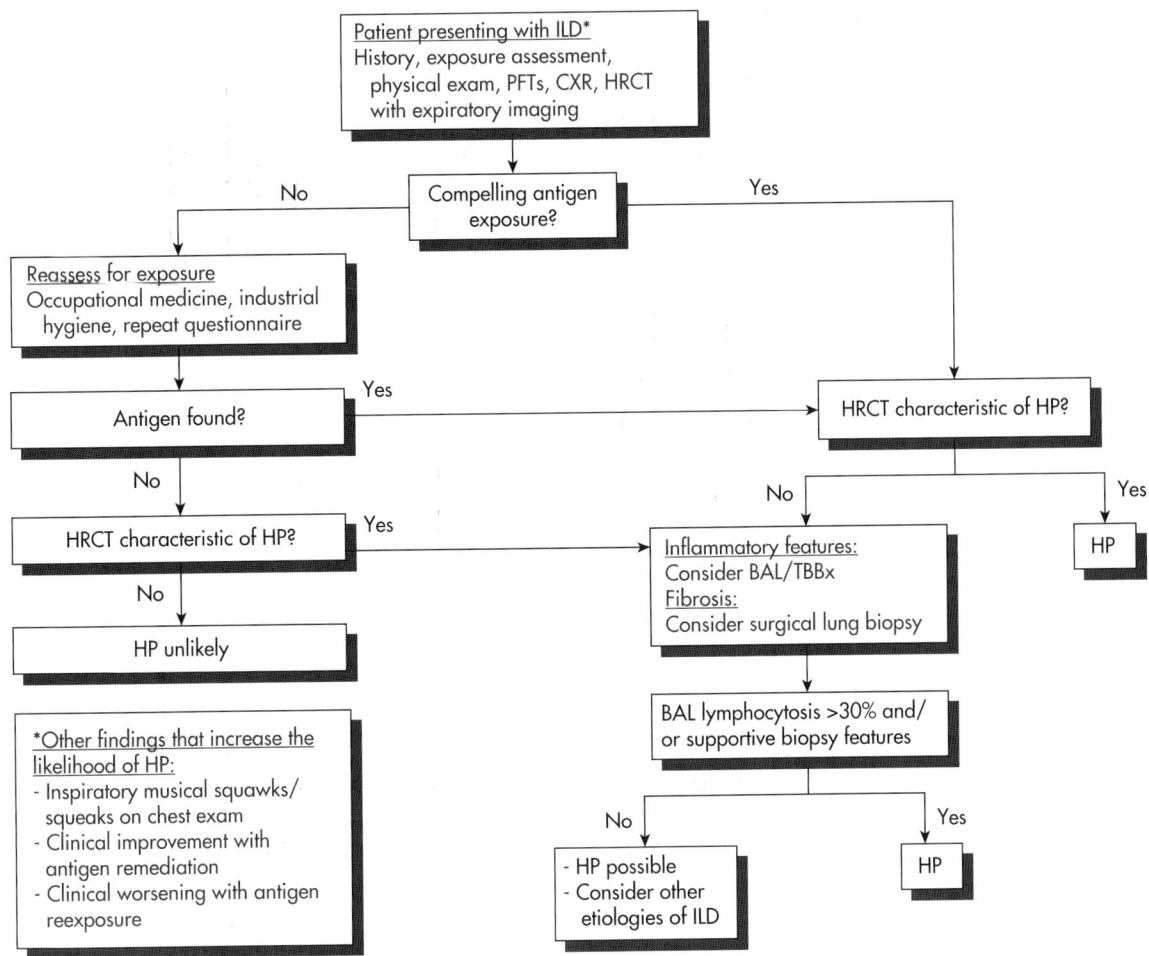

FIG. 2 Approach to the diagnosis of hypersensitivity pneumonitis (HP). The diagnostic HP approach requires thorough exposure evaluation, exclusion of alternative etiologies, and multidisciplinary evaluation. The first and most crucial step in determining the likelihood of diagnosis is characterizing the occupational and environmental exposure by a comprehensive history and/or exposure questionnaire. Because the identification of the inciting antigen source and mitigation are critical, referral to an occupational medicine specialist or industrial hygienist may be helpful, especially when a more detailed investigation is needed. The combination of the clinical context, exposure history, and chest high-resolution computed tomography (HRCT) pattern inform the degree of diagnostic certainty: Confident vs. working diagnosis vs. unlikely. For patients with a working diagnosis, on a case-by-case basis and in the setting of multidisciplinary discussion, further testing including bronchoalveolar lavage (BAL)/transbronchial biopsy (TBBx) and/or surgical lung biopsy may be considered. After the HP diagnosis is made, if not previously done in a patient with suspected HP, removal of the inciting antigen and careful reevaluation for possible ongoing reexposure are vital. CXR, Chest radiograph; ILD, interstitial lung disease; PFTs, pulmonary function tests. (From Broaddus VC et al: *Murray & Nadel's textbook of respiratory medicine*, ed 7, Philadelphia, 2022, Elsevier.)

- Prednisone 0.5 mg/kg for 1 to 2 wk then tapered over 4 wk.

CHRONIC Rx

- For subacute and chronic HP, steroid-sparing immunosuppression with mofetil mycophenolate or azathioprine, which are better tolerated than prednisone, should be considered for maintenance treatment.[6] Although there are no randomized controlled trials, a retrospective study showed that treatment with either agent was associated with a 4% improvement in DLCO at 1 yr.[7]
- Once the offending antigen exposure has been remediated, and there is improvement or stabilization of symptoms and pulmonary function tests, consider gradual tapering off of immunosuppression.
- For chronic HP with progressive fibrosis despite antigen avoidance and immunosuppression,

switching to or adding antifibrotic therapy could be considered. Nintedanib and pirfenidone, medications with antifibrotic and antiinflammatory properties, have been shown to slow the progression of progressive fibrosing interstitial lung disease in randomized clinical trials.[8,9] Nintedanib has FDA approval.

DISPOSITION/PROGNOSIS

Prognosis is good for patients with acute or subacute HP, especially if the offending antigen is identified. In bird-related hypersensitivity pneumonitis, the amount of household avian dust predicts prognosis.[10] Antigen avoidance alone or with immunosuppression can lead to improvement

- Prognosis is worse for patients with chronic HP; approximately 25% die within 5 yr in a cohort of pigeon breeders' lung disease. Chronic HP is associated progressive

pulmonary fibrosis, development of pulmonary hypertension, and right heart failure. Honeycombing on HRCT and clubbing indicate advanced disease with poor survival.

REFERRAL

- Pulmonologist: To identify potential exposures and educate patient on its avoidance, establish the diagnosis in multidisciplinary conference and develop a treatment and monitoring strategy.
- Thoracic surgeon: For surgical lung biopsy.
- Lung transplant center: To consider lung transplant candidacy. Patients with chronic HP who undergo lung transplant have excellent survival, reported at 89% at 5 yr in a single-center series; better than survival after lung transplant for IPF.[11] HP can recur in the transplanted lung with exposure to the offending antigen.

TABLE 3 Common Causes of Hypersensitivity Pneumonitis (HP)

Disease	Antigen	Scenario/Source
Microbes		
Farmer's lung	Thermophilic actinomycetes, *Faeni rectovirgula*	Moldy hay, silage, grain
Humidifier lung	*Thermoactinomyces vulgaris, T. sacchari, T. candidus*	Contaminated forced air systems, water reservoirs
Hot tub lung	*Mycobacterium* avian complex spp.	Contaminated hot tubs
Wind instrument lung	*Fusarium* spp., *Penicillium* spp., *M. chelonae*, *Candida* spp., *Cryptococcus* spp.	Contaminated trombone, bagpipe, saxophone
Metalworking fluid lung	*M. immunogenum*, *Pseudomonas* spp.	Aerosolized metalworking fluid
Summer-type HP	*Trichosporum cutaneum*	Contaminated old houses
Mushroom worker's lung	*T. sacchari*	Mushroom compost
Suberosis	*T. viridis, Aspergillus fumigatus, Pseudomonas* spp.	Cork molds
Esparto lung	*Aspergillus fumigatus*	Moldy *Stipa tenacissima* grass
Woodworker's lung	*Alternaria* spp. wood dusts	Moldy oak, cedar, mahogany
Animal Proteins		
Pigeon breeder's lung	Pigeon droppings, feathers, serum	Pigeons, domestic and environmental
Bird fancier's lung	Avian droppings, feathers, serum	Parakeets, budgerigars, love birds, cockatiels, chickens
Duvet lung	Avian feathers	Pillows, duvets, sleeping bags stuffed with feathers
Animal handler's lung	Rats, gerbils	Urine, pelts, serum, proteins
Bat lung	Bat proteins	Bat droppings
Chemical Sensitizers		
Chemical worker's lung	Isocyanates	Spray paints, polyurethane foams, glues
Epoxy resin lung	Phthalic anhydride	Heated epoxy resin
Pauli's reagent alveolitis	Sodium diazobenzene sulfate	Laboratory reagent

From Broaddus VC et al: *Murray & Nadel's textbook of respiratory medicine*, ed 7, Philadelphia, 2022, Elsevier.

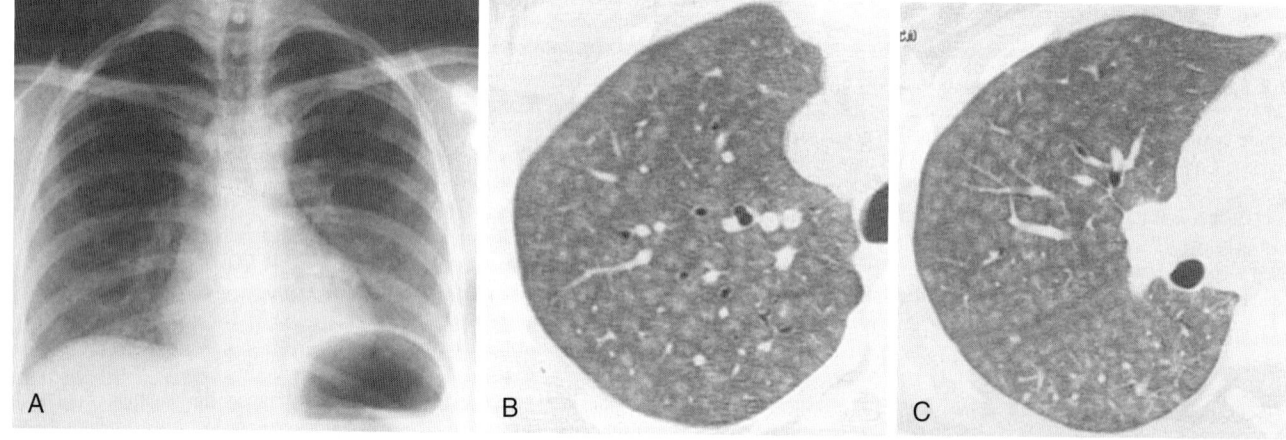

FIG. 3 Nonfibrotic hypersensitivity pneumonitis. (A) Chest x-ray examination of a patient with hypersensitivity pneumonitis shows diffuse poorly defined nodular opacities. **(B)** High-resolution computed tomography (HRCT; 1.5-mm thin section) image through the lung of the same patient shows profuse centrilobular ground-glass opacity nodules. **(C)** HRCT scan of a different patient with bird breeder's lung shows diffuse ground-glass attenuation with reticular opacities and centrilobular ground-glass opacity nodules. (From Broaddus VC et al: *Murray & Nadel's textbook of respiratory medicine*, ed 7, Philadelphia, 2022, Elsevier.)

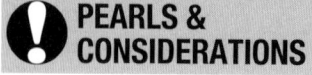 **PEARLS & CONSIDERATIONS**

- HP occurs more frequently in nonsmokers than smokers.

- Chronic HP may be difficult to distinguish from IPF. Diagnosis often made in the lung explant at the time of transplant.

REFERENCES
Available at eBooks.Health.Elsevier.com.

RELATED CONTENT
Hypersensitivity Pneumonitis (Patient Information)
Interstitial Lung Disease (Related Key Topic)

AUTHOR: **AIDA VENADO, MD, MAS**

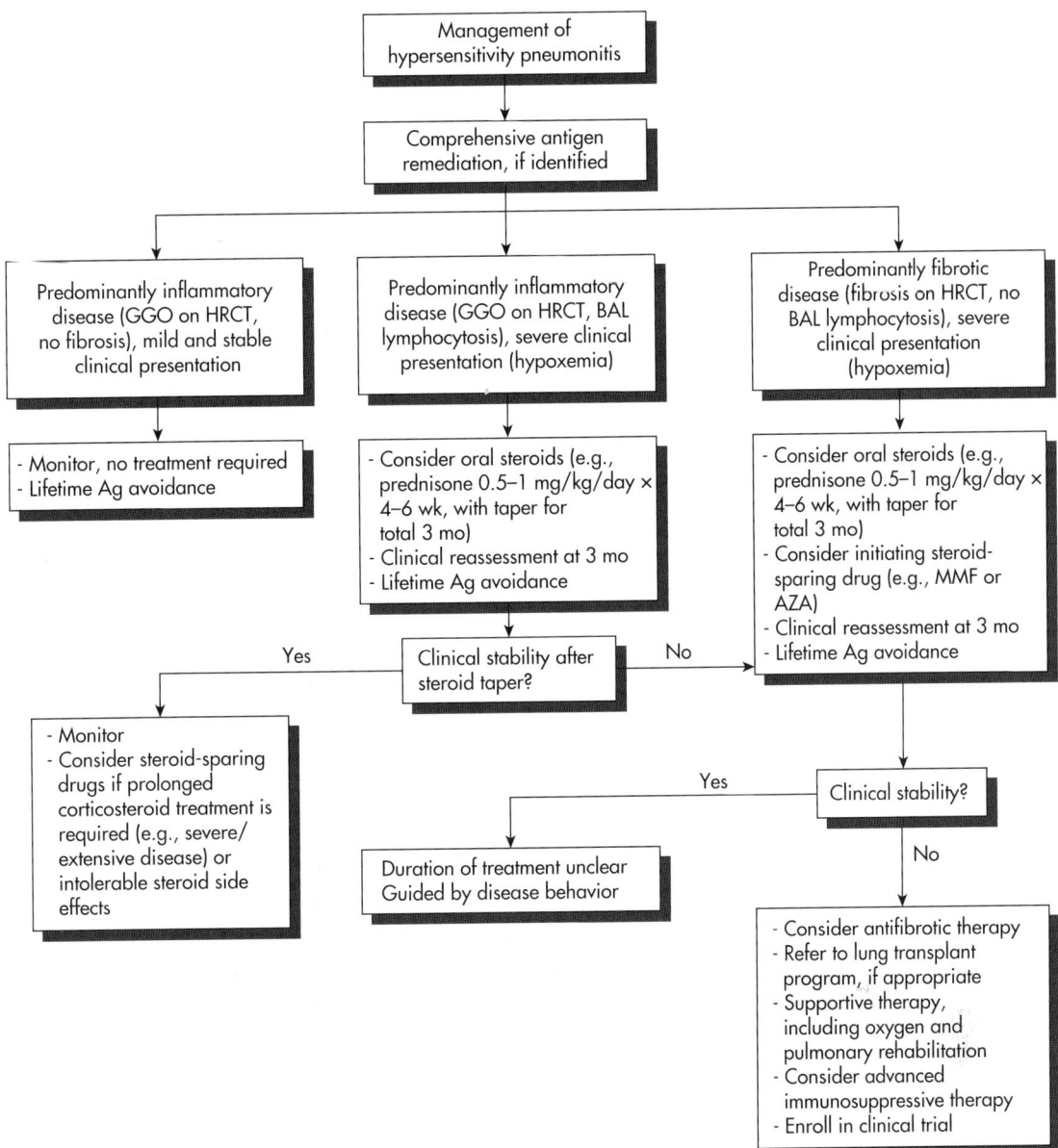

FIG. 4 Approach to the management of hypersensitivity pneumonitis (HP). Pharmacologic therapy is often initiated when clinically significant disease progression is recognized despite comprehensive inciting antigen remediation or avoidance. Initial treatment is often with systemic corticosteroids in the form of prednisone with a tapering schedule. Patients require monitoring and management of corticosteroid adverse reactions as well as assessment for clinical, physiologic, and/or radiographic response before considering coadministering and/or transition to corticosteroid-sparing agents. The multidisciplinary approach to HP includes symptom management, supplemental oxygen for hypoxemic patients, pulmonary rehabilitation, smoking cessation, appropriate vaccinations, referral for lung transplant evaluation if indicated, treatment of comorbid conditions, and palliative/end-of-life care. *Ag,* Antigen; *AZA,* azathioprine; *BAL,* bronchoalveolar lavage; *GGO,* ground-glass opacity; *HRCT,* high-resolution computed tomography; *MMF,* mycophenolate mofetil. (From Broaddus VC et al: *Murray & Nadel's textbook of respiratory medicine,* ed 7, Philadelphia, 2022, Elsevier.)

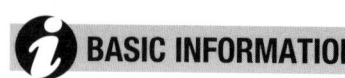
BASIC INFORMATION

DEFINITION

Normal blood pressure (BP) in adults can be defined as systolic BP <120 mm Hg and diastolic BP <80 mm Hg. Elevated BP is defined as systolic BP between 120 and 129 mm Hg or diastolic BP <80 mm Hg. Hypertension (HTN) can be divided into (1) stage 1: Systolic BP from 130 to 139 mm Hg or diastolic BP from 80 to 89 mm Hg and (2) stage 2: Systolic BP ≥140 mm Hg or diastolic BP ≥90 mm Hg. This definition is based on accurate measurements and average of ≥2 readings on ≥2 occasions.

SYNONYMS

HTN
Essential hypertension
Idiopathic hypertension
High BP

ICD-10CM CODES

I10	Essential (primary) hypertension
I15.0	Renovascular hypertension
I15.1	Hypertension secondary to other renal disorders
I15.2	Hypertension secondary to endocrine disorders
I15.8	Other secondary hypertension
I15.9	Secondary hypertension, unspecified
O10.919	Unspecified pre-existing hypertension complicating pregnancy, unspecified trimester
I67.4	Hypertensive encephalopathy

EPIDEMIOLOGY & DEMOGRAPHICS

- In the U.S., 50% of people aged 60 to 69 yr and ~75% of people >70 yr of age are affected by HTN. Worldwide, it is estimated that 41% of people ages 35 to 70 yr have HTN, and only 46.5% of them are aware of it.
- Peak prevalence increases with age and is highest among non-Hispanic Black adults in the U.S.
- HTN is linked with a higher risk of heart attack, stroke, heart failure, and kidney disease.

PHYSICAL FINDINGS & CLINICAL PRESENTATION

Physical examination may be entirely within normal limits, except for the presence of elevated BP. A proper initial physical examination on a hypertensive patient should include the following:

- The BP should be measured with an appropriately sized cuff (bladder of the cuff should cover at least two thirds of the circumference of the arm) and taken in both arms (the higher of the readings being used). Table 1 describes BP cuff size and error in measurement.
- The BP should be measured twice on each visit and separated by at least 1 to 2 min to allow the return of trapped blood.
- The patient should be seated in a calm environment for at least 5 min with the arm in which BP is measured rested on support level with the heart.

- Postural BP change should always be recorded in the elderly to diagnose postural hypotension. This is assessed by taking BP in supine (after 5-min rest) and standing (after 2 min) positions. A drop of ≥20 mm Hg in systolic, a drop of ≥10 mm Hg diastolic BP, or symptoms of cerebral hypoperfusion is suggestive of postural (orthostatic) hypotension.
- A diagnosis of HTN may be established if the BP is markedly elevated (>180/110 mm Hg) or has evidence of end organ damage; otherwise such a diagnosis should wait until BP is found elevated on >2 readings on >2 different occasions.
- Nonoffice (home, workplace, 24-h ambulatory) BP determination to establish the pattern of HTN (sustained, "white coat," or "masked" HTN) in selected patients.
- Measure heart rate, height, weight, body mass index, and waist circumference.
- Some general clinical clues for when to screen for secondary HTN include:
  1. Severe or resistant HTN
  2. An acute rise in BP developing in a patient with previous stable BP
  3. Age less than 30 yr, nonobese, non-Black with no family history of HTN
  4. Sudden onset or accelerated HTN
  5. Age of onset before puberty. If above is suspected, additional tests for secondary HTN should be done, including renin, aldosterone, cortisol levels, 24-h urine metanephrines, and serum catecholamines
- Physical examination should include searching for secondary causes, and sequelae of HTN.
- Examine skin for the presence of café-au-lait spots (neurofibromatosis), uremic appearance (renal failure), and violaceous striae (Cushing syndrome).
- Perform careful funduscopic examination; check for papilledema, retinal exudates, hemorrhages, arterial narrowing, arteriovenous compression.
- Examine neck for carotid bruits, distended neck veins, and enlarged thyroid gland.
- Perform extensive cardiopulmonary examination: Check for a laterally displaced point of maximal intensity, an S3 or S4, and valvular murmurs.
- Palpate abdomen for renal masses (pheochromocytoma, polycystic kidneys), and auscultate for bruit over the aorta and renal arteries.
- Examine arterial pulses (dilated or absent femoral pulses and BP greater in upper extremities than lower extremities suggest aortic coarctation).
- Look for truncal obesity (Cushing syndrome) and pedal edema (congestive heart failure [CHF]).
- Table 2 provides a guide to evaluation of identifiable causes of HTN.
- Table 3 summarizes clinical clues to guide the investigation in young patients with hypertension that has a potentially hereditary cause.

ETIOLOGY

- Essential (primary) HTN (85%)
- Drug induced or drug related (5%)
  1. NSAIDs
  2. Oral contraceptives
  3. Corticosteroids
- Renal HTN (5%)
  1. Renal parenchymal disease (3%)
  2. Renovascular HTN (RVH) (<2%)
- Endocrine (<2%) (Table 4)
  1. Primary aldosteronism (at least 5%)
  2. Pheochromocytoma (0.2%)
  3. Cushing syndrome and long-term steroid therapy (0.2%)
  4. Hyperparathyroidism or thyroid disease (0.2%)
- Coarctation of the aorta (0.2%)
- Causes of secondary hypertension are summarized in Box 1

DIAGNOSIS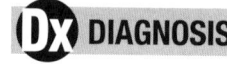

WORKUP

- The objective for the initial evaluation of HTN is to establish the diagnosis and stage of HTN. Table 5 summarizes initial laboratory evaluation of the hypertensive patient.

TABLE 1 Blood Pressure Cuff Size and Error in Measurement*

	ARM CIRCUMFERENCE		
Cuff Bladder Size	28 cm or less	29-42 cm	43 cm or more
Regular (12 × 23 cm)	Accurate	Overestimates SBP by 4-8 mm Hg DBP by 3-6 mm Hg	Overestimates SBP by 16-17 mm Hg DBP by 10-11 mm Hg
Large (15 × 33 cm)	Underestimates SBP by 2-3 mm Hg DBP by 1-2 mm Hg	Accurate	Overestimates SBP by 5-7 mm Hg DBP by 2-4 mm Hg
Thigh (18 × 36 cm)	Underestimates SBP by 5-7 mm Hg DBP by 1-3 mm Hg	Underestimates SBP by 5-7 mm Hg DBP by 2-4 mm Hg	Accurate

DBP, Diastolic blood pressure reading; SBP, systolic blood pressure reading.

*Overestimation means that hypertension may be diagnosed in someone with normal blood pressure; underestimation means that the blood pressure reading may be normal in someone who actually has high blood pressure. See text for further discussion.

From McGee S et al: Evidence-based physical diagnosis, ed 4, Philadelphia, 2018, Elsevier.

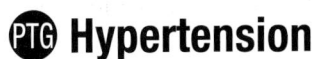
TABLE 2 Guide to Evaluation of Identifiable Causes of Hypertension

Suspected Diagnosis	Clinical Clues	Diagnostic Testing
Chronic kidney disease	Estimated GFR <60 ml/min/1.73 m² Urine albumin-to-creatinine ratio ≥30 mg/g	Renal sonography
Renovascular disease	New elevation in serum creatinine, marked elevation in serum creatinine with ACEI or ARB, drug-resistant hypertension, flash pulmonary edema, abdominal, or flank bruit	Renal sonography (atrophic kidney), CT or MR angiography, invasive angiography
Coarctation of the aorta	Arm pulses > leg pulses, arm BP > leg BP, chest bruits, rib notching on chest radiography	MR angiography, TEE, invasive angiography
Primary aldosteronism	Hypokalemia, drug-resistant hypertension	Plasma renin and aldosterone, 24-h urine aldosterone and potassium after oral salt loading, adrenal vein sampling
Cushing syndrome	Truncal obesity, wide and blanching purple striae, muscle weakness	1 mg dexamethasone-suppression test, urinary cortisol after dexamethasone, adrenal CT
Pheochromocytoma	Paroxysms of hypertension, palpitations, perspiration, and pallor; diabetes	Plasma metanephrines, 24-h urinary metanephrines and catecholamines, abdominal CT or MR imaging
Obstructive sleep apnea	Loud snoring, large neck, obesity, somnolence	Polysomnography

ACEI, Angiotensin-converting enzyme inhibitor; *ARB,* angiotensin receptor blocker; *BP,* blood pressure; *CT,* computed tomography; *GFR,* glomerular filtration rate; *MR,* magnetic resonance; *TEE,* transesophageal echocardiography.
From Goldman L, Schafer AI: *Goldman's Cecil medicine,* ed 24, Philadelphia, 2012, Saunders.

TABLE 3 Clinical Clues to Guide the Investigation in Young Patients With Hypertension That Has a Potentially Hereditary Cause

Specific Conditions	Possible Causes of Familial Hypertension	Clinical Clues
Catecholamine-Producing Tumors		
Pheochromocytoma/paraganglioma	Familial cases are responsible for <30% of cases, including MEN2A and MEN2B, von Hippel-Lindau disease, neurofibromatosis, and familial paraganglioma syndromes (SDH complex mutations)	Paroxysmal palpitations, headaches, diaphoresis, pale flushing; syndromic features of any of the associated disorders
Neuroblastomas (adrenal)	1%-2% of neuroblastomas are familial	
Aortic or renovascular lesions		
Coarctation of the aorta	Overrepresented in families but no familial distribution	Asymmetry between upper- and lower-extremity BP, radial-formal pulse delay; associated with Turner syndrome, Williams syndrome, and bicuspid aortic valve
Renal artery stenosis caused by fibromuscular dysplasia or inherited arterial wall lesions	<10% familial with AD pattern	Abnormal renal vascular imaging results; vascular disease in the carotid territory at an early age; common in neurofibromatosis and Williams syndrome; also present in tuberous sclerosis, Ehlers-Danlos syndrome, and Marfan syndrome
Parenchymal kidney disease GN	Alport disease (X-linked, AR, or AD), familial IgA nephropathy (AD with incomplete penetrance)	Proteinuria, hematuria, low eGFR
PKD	ADPKD type 1 or 2, ARPKD	Multiple renal cysts (as few as three in patients under 30 yr)
Adrenocortical disease	AD chimeric fusion of the 11β-hydroxylase and aldosterone synthase genes	Cerebral hemorrhages at young age, cerebral aneurysms; mild hypokalemia; high plasma aldosterone, low renin
Glucocorticoid-remediable aldosteronism (familial hyperaldosteronism type I)		
Familial hyperaldosteronism	AD; unknown defect	Severe type 2 hypertension in early adulthood; high plasma aldosterone, low renin; no response to glucocorticoid treatment
Familial hyperaldosteronism type III	AD; unknown defect	Severe hypertension in childhood with extensive target-organ damage; high plasma aldosterone, low renin; marked bilateral adrenal enlargement
Congenital adrenal hyperplasia	AR mutations in 11β-hydroxylase or 21-hydroxylase	Hirsutism, virilization; hypokalemia and metabolic alkalosis; low plasma aldosterone and renin
Monogenic Primary Renal Tubular Defects		
Gordon syndrome	AD mutations of *KLHL3, CUL3, WNK1,* and *WNK4;* AR mutations of *KLHL3*	Hyperkalemia and metabolic acidosis with normal renal function
Liddle syndrome	AD mutations of the epithelial sodium channel	Hypokalemia and metabolic alkalosis; low plasma aldosterone and renin
Apparent mineralocorticoid excess	AD mutation in 11β-hydroxysteroid dehydrogenase type 2	Hypokalemia and metabolic alkalosis; low plasma aldosterone and renin
Geller syndrome	AD mutation in the mineralocorticoid receptor AD mutations in the phosphodiesterase E3A enzyme	Hypokalemia and metabolic alkalosis; low plasma aldosterone and renin; increased BP during pregnancy or exposure to spironolactone
Hypertension-brachydactyly syndrome		
Unknown mechanisms		
Hypertension-brachydactyly syndrome	AD	Short fingers (small phalanges) and short stature; brain stem compression from vascular tortuosity in the posterior fossa
Essential Hypertension		
	Polygenic	When obesity or metabolic syndrome is present, the likelihood of essential hypertension is higher

AD, Autosomal dominant; *ADPKD,* autosomal dominant polycystic kidney disease; *AR,* autosomal recessive; *ARPKD,* autosomal recessive polycystic kidney disease; *BP,* blood pressure; *eGFR,* estimated glomerular filtration rate; *GN,* glomerulonephritis; *IgA,* immunoglobulin A; *MEN,* multiple endocrine neoplasia; *PKD,* polycystic kidney disease; *SDH,* succinate dehydrogenase.
From Skorecki K et al: *Brenner and Rector's the kidney,* ed 10, Philadelphia, 2016, Elsevier.

TABLE 4 Adrenocortical Causes of Hypertension

Low Renin and High Aldosterone
Primary Aldosteronism
1. Aldosterone-producing adenoma (APA)—30% of cases
2. Bilateral idiopathic hyperplasia (IHA)—60% of cases
3. Primary (unilateral) adrenal hyperplasia—2% of cases
4. Aldosterone-producing adrenocortical carcinoma—<1% of cases
5. Familial hyperaldosteronism (FH)
   a. FH type I (*CYP11B1/CYP11B2* germline chimeric gene)—<1% of cases
   b. FH type II (APA or IHA; germline *CLCN2* mutations—<6% of cases
   c. FH type III (germline *KCNJ5* mutations)—<1% of cases
   d. FH type IV (germline *CACNA1H* mutations)—<0.1% of cases
6. Ectopic aldosterone-producing adenoma or carcinoma—<0.1% of cases

Low Renin and Low Aldosterone
1. Congenital adrenal hyperplasia
   a. 11β-Hydroxylase deficiency
   b. 17α-Hydroxylase deficiency
2. Deoxycorticosterone-producing tumor
3. Primary cortisol resistance
4. Apparent mineralocorticoid excess (AME)/11β-HSD 2 deficiency
   a. Genetic
   b. Type 1 AME
   c. Type 2 AME
5. Acquired
   a. Licorice or carbenoxolone ingestion (type 1 AME)
   b. Cushing syndrome (type 2 AME)

Cushing Syndrome
1. Exogenous glucocorticoid administration—most common cause
2. Endogenous
   a. ACTH-dependent—85% of cases
      1) Pituitary
      2) Ectopic
   b. ACTH-independent—15% of cases
      1) Unilateral adrenal disease (adenoma or carcinoma)
      2) Bilateral adrenal disease
         a) Bilateral adenoma
         b) Macronodular hyperplasia
         c) Primary pigmented nodular adrenal disease (rare)

ACTH, Corticotropin; *HSD,* hydroxysteroid dehydrogenase.
From Melmed S et al: *Williams textbook of endocrinology,* ed 14, 2019, Elsevier.

- Gather office and nonoffice BP readings, assess presence of target organ damage (TOD), assess the level of global cardiovascular disease risk, and produce a plan for individualized monitoring and therapy.
- Patient counseling and education should be prominent features of the initial evaluation.
- Pertinent history:

BOX 1 Causes of Secondary Hypertension

Endocrine causes
Epinephrine excess
Aldosterone excess
Thyroid disease
Pregnancy
Vascular causes
Coarctation of the aorta
Renal artery stenosis
Atherosclerosis (smokers, diabetes mellitus, advancing age)
Renal disease
Inherited
Inflammation—glomerulonephritis
Diabetes mellitus
Drug reactions
Renal tumors (renal cell carcinoma, reninoma)
Medication-induced
NSAIDs
Corticosteroids
Analgesics
Ethanol
Cyclosporine (ciclosporin)
SSRIs
Oral contraceptives
Malignancy-related
Skin lesions such as endothelinomas
PTH- and PTHRP-producing cancers
Anti–VEGF-related cancer treatment
Adrenal tumors
Multiple endocrine neoplasia

NSAIDs, Nonsteroidal antiinflammatory drugs; *PTH,* parathyroid hormone; *PTHRP,* parathyroid hormone–related protein; *SSRI,* selective serotonin reuptake inhibitor; *VEGF,* vascular endothelial growth factor.
From Talley NJ et al: *Essentials of internal medicine,* ed 4, Chatswood, NSW, 2021, Elsevier Australia.

1. Age of onset of HTN, previous antihypertensive therapy
2. Family history of HTN, stroke, cardiovascular disease
- Diet, salt intake, caffeine, alcohol, drugs (e.g., oral contraceptives, NSAIDs, decongestants, steroids).
- Occupation, lifestyle, pain, socioeconomic status, psychologic factors.
- Other cardiovascular risk factors: Hyperlipidemia, obesity, diabetes mellitus.
- Symptoms of secondary HTN:
  1. Headache, palpitations, excessive perspiration (possible pheochromocytoma)
  2. Weakness, polyuria (consider hyperaldosteronism)
  3. Claudication of lower extremities (seen with coarctation of aorta)
  4. Loud snoring, daytime somnolence, morning confusion (may warrant evaluation for sleep apnea)

LABORATORY TESTS
- Routine laboratory tests recommended before initiating therapy include:
  1. Urinalysis with microscopic evaluation; for signs of glomerulopathy
  2. Basic metabolic panel and calcium; for signs of kidney damage, hypokalemia (primary

aldosteronism and Cushing syndrome), hypercalcemia (hyperparathyroid)
3. CBC
4. Screening for coexisting diseases that may adversely affect prognosis; hemoglobin A_{1c} or fasting glucose level, serum lipid panel
5. Optional tests include measurement of urinary albumin or albumin/creatinine ratio

IMAGING STUDIES
- ECG: Check for presence of left ventricular hypertrophy (LVH) with strain pattern.
- Renal duplex ultrasonography, CT angiography or magnetic resonance angiography of the renal arteries in suspected renovascular hypertension (renal artery stenosis) may be considered.

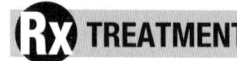 **TREATMENT**

NONPHARMACOLOGIC THERAPY
Lifestyle modifications (the initial treatment of hypertension should focus on lifestyle modifications [Table 6]):
- Weight loss if overweight (target body mass index [BMI] <25).
- Limit alcohol intake to 1 oz of ethanol per day (<2 drinks/day) in men or 0.5 oz (<1 drink/day) in women.
- Regular aerobic exercise (at least 30 min/day on most days).
- Reduce sodium intake to <100 mmol/day (<1.5 g of sodium/day).
- Maintain adequate dietary potassium (>3500 mg/day) intake in patients with normal kidney function.
- Smoking cessation.
- The BP reduction seen ranges from 2 to 20 mm Hg, most significant with substantial weight loss and the implementation of the Dietary Approaches to Stop Hypertension (DASH) eating plan, which relies on a diet high in fruits and vegetables, moderate in low-fat dairy products, and low in animal protein but with substantial amount of plant protein from legumes and nuts.

ACUTE GENERAL Rx
- Multiple recent consensus documents regarding BP goals and when to initiate treatment have been published. Antihypertensive medications are summarized in Table 7. Antihypertensive choices in the setting of cardiovascular comorbidity are described in Table 8.
  1. For low-risk adults (no ASCVD or 10-yr CVD risk <10%) with stage 1 hypertension, management should start with nonpharmacologic therapy. If BP remains uncontrolled after 3 to 6 mo, then consider starting pharmacologic therapy.[1]
  2. For adults with confirmed hypertension and known cardiovascular disease (CVD) or 10-yr atherosclerotic cardiovascular disease (ASCVD) event risk of 10% or higher, a BP target of less than 130/80 mm Hg is recommended.[2]

TABLE 5 Initial Laboratory Evaluation of the Hypertensive Patient to Investigate the Presence of Comorbid Conditions, Secondary Causes, or Established Target-Organ Damage

Test	Clinical Usefulness
Serum creatinine (and estimated glomerular filtration rate)	Assessment of renal function. Identifies parenchymal kidney disease as a possible secondary cause as well as established TOD.
Serum potassium	Low potassium (of renal origin) suggests mineralocorticoid excess (primary or secondary), glucocorticoid excess, Liddle syndrome. High potassium with normal renal function suggests Gordon syndrome. Low levels raise caution about the use of thiazides and loop diuretics. High levels preclude the use of ACEIs, ARBs, renin inhibitors, and potassium-sparing diuretics.
Serum sodium	If high, suggests primary aldosteronism. If low, alerts to the need to avoid thiazide diuretics.
Serum bicarbonate	If high, suggests aldosterone excess (primary or secondary). If low with normal renal function, suggests Gordon syndrome (with high potassium) or primary hyperparathyroidism (with high calcium).
Serum calcium	If high, suggests primary hyperparathyroidism.
Serum glucose	Identifies prediabetes or diabetes. In the appropriate setting, suggests glucocorticoid excess, pheochromocytoma, or acromegaly.
Lipid profile	Identifies hyperlipidemia.
Hemoglobin/hematocrit	If high, in the absence of other hematologic abnormalities or underlying lung disease, suggests sleep apnea.
Urinalysis*	Proteinuria and hematuria identify a possible secondary cause (glomerulonephritis). Proteinuria can also be a marker of TOD.
Electrocardiogram	Identifies left ventricular hypertrophy, old myocardial infarction, or other ischemic changes. Identifies conduction abnormalities that may preclude the use of β-blockers or nondihydropyridine CCBs.

The most recent guidelines do not recommend blood urea nitrogen (BUN) measurement alone.
ACEI, Angiotensin-converting enzyme inhibitor; *ARB*, angiotensin receptor blocker; *CCB*, calcium channel blocker; *TOD*, target-organ damage.
*Some organizations recommend screening microalbuminuria as a more sensitive tool to identify early renal injury.
From Skorecki K et al: *Brenner and Rector's the kidney*, ed 10, Philadelphia, 2016, Elsevier.

TABLE 6 Effects of Lifestyle Modifications on Blood Pressure

Lifestyle Modification	Specifics	Level of Evidence	Approximate Reduction in Systolic Blood Pressure
Weight loss	Maintain BMI <25 kg/m²	A	5-20 mm Hg per 10 kg weight loss
Physical activity	At least 30 min per day	A	~5 mm Hg
Reduce salt intake	Limit sodium to 2.4 g per day	A	~5 mm Hg
Heart-healthy diet, such as DASH	Low-fat diet with fruits and vegetables	A	~11 mm Hg
Potassium supplementation	Preferably as part of dietary modification	A	~4 mm Hg
Stop smoking		A	1-6 mm Hg
Moderation of alcohol consumption	Limit alcohol to ≤2 drinks/day for men and ≤1 drink/day for women	A	~4 mm Hg

A, Supported by one or more high quality randomized trials; *BMI*, body mass index, *DASH*, Dietary Approaches to Stop Hypertension.
Modified from Whelton PK, Carey RM, Aronow WS, et al: 2017 ACC/AHA/AAPA/ABC/ACPM/AGS/APhA/ASH/ASPC/NMA/PCNA Guideline for the Prevention, Detection, Evaluation, and Management of High Blood Pressure in Adults: a report of the American College of Cardiology/American Heart Association Task Force on Clinical Practice Guidelines, *J Am Coll Cardiol* 71:e127-e248, 2018. In Warshaw G et al: *Ham's primary care geriatrics*, ed 7, Philadelphia, 2022, Elsevier.

3. For adults with confirmed hypertension without additional markers of increased CVD risk, a BP target of less than 130/80 mm Hg may be reasonable.
- In addition, initiation of therapy recommendations is as follows:

1. Use of BP-lowering medication is recommended for primary prevention of CVD in adults with no history of CVD and with an estimated 10-yr ASCVD risk <10% and stage 2 HTN.

2. Use of BP-lowering medications is recommended for secondary prevention of recurrent CVD events in patients with clinical CVD and for primary prevention in adults with an estimated 10-yr ASCVD risk of 10% or higher and stage 1 HTN.
3. Initiate antihypertensive drug therapy with two first-line agents of different classes for adults with stage 2 HTN and BP more than 20/10 mm Hg higher than their target.
4. Patients with diabetes mellitus and chronic kidney disease are considered high risk.
5. In the general non-Black population, preferred initial agents are thiazide-type diuretics, angiotensin-converting enzyme inhibitors (ACEI), calcium channel blockers (CCBs), or angiotensin receptor blockers (ARBs). ACEI or ARBs are preferred initial agents in diabetics and those with chronic kidney disease (CKD) in this population.[3]
6. Preferred initial agents in the Black population (including diabetics) are thiazide-type diuretics or CCBs.
7. When selecting drugs, try to give once per day dosages to improve compliance. Also consider the cost of the medication, metabolic and subjective side effects, and drug-drug interactions.
- The major advantages and limitations of each class of drugs are described as follows:
  1. Thiazide diuretics:
     a. Advantages: Inexpensive, once-daily dosing. Useful in edematous states, CHF, chronic renal disease, elderly patients (decreased incidence of hip fractures in elderly patients)
     b. Disadvantages: Significant adverse metabolic effects (hypokalemia), increased risk of cardiac arrhythmias, sexual dysfunction, gout flares, possible adverse effects on lipids and glucose levels
  2. β-Blockers:
     a. Advantages: Ideal in hypertensive patients with ischemic heart disease or status post myocardial infarction (MI); favored in hyperkinetic, young patients (resting tachycardia, wide pulse pressure, hyperdynamic heart) and stable CHF patients
     b. Disadvantages: Adverse effect on quality of life (increased incidence of fatigue, depression, impotence), bronchospasm, hypoglycemia, peripheral vascular disease, adverse effects on lipids, masking of signs and symptoms of hypoglycemia in diabetics
  3. Calcium antagonists:
     a. Advantages: Helpful in hypertensive patients with ischemic heart disease. Generally favorable effect on quality of life; can be used in patients with bronchospastic disorders, renal disease, peripheral vascular disease, metabolic disorders, and salt sensitivity. CCBs' BP-lowering effect is independent of Na^+ intake.

TABLE 7 Antihypertensive Drugs

Drug Class	Mechanism of Action	Possible Adverse Effects
Thiazide-like diuretics Chlorthalidone Hydrochlorothiazide Indapamide	Inhibit sodium and chloride reabsorption in the kidney, reducing intravascular volume and peripheral vascular resistance	Volume depletion hypotension, hyponatremia, hypokalemia, hypomagnesemia, hyperuricemia (gout), hyperglycemia, renal impairment
Potassium-sparing diuretics Triamterene Spironolactone		
Angiotensin-converting enzyme inhibitors (ACE inhibitors) Benazepril Captopril Fosinopril Lisinopril Ramipril	Inhibits ACE, interfering with conversion of angiotensin I to angiotensin II, reducing vasoconstriction	Hyperkalemia (with impaired renal function), cough, angioedema, rash, renal impairment, altered taste
Angiotensin II receptor blockers (ARB) Candesartan Irbesartan Losartan Valsartan	Antagonizes angiotensin II AT1 receptors, reducing vasoconstriction	Hyperkalemia, renal impairment Do not use an ACE inhibitor and an ARB simultaneously
Beta-Blockers		Sinus bradycardia, heart block, fatigue, bronchospasm, hyperglycemia, confusion. Not recommended as first-line agents unless the patient has ischemic heart disease or heart failure
Beta₁ Selective Metoprolol	Selectively antagonizes β-1 adrenergic receptors	
Dual acting Carvedilol Labetalol	Antagonizes α-1, β-1, and β-2 adrenergic receptors	
Calcium channel blockers—Nondihydropyridines Diltiazem Verapamil	Prolong AV node refractory period and have negative inotropic effect; less effective as vasodilators	Sinus bradycardia, heart block, heart failure, rash, GERD, constipation, gingival hyperplasia
Calcium channel blockers—Dihydropyridines Amlodipine Felodipine Nicardipine Nifedipine	Inhibit calcium influx, relaxing vascular smooth muscle and decreasing peripheral resistance causing vasodilation with little or no negative effect upon cardiac contractility or AV nodal conduction	Peripheral edema
Alpha-adrenergic agonists, centrally acting Methyldopa Clonidine	Stimulates α-2 adrenergic receptors centrally	Sedation, dry mouth, constipation. Avoid in older adults because of central nervous system adverse effects
Alpha₁ selective adrenergic antagonists, peripherally acting Doxazosin Prazosin Terazosin	Antagonizes peripheral α-1 adrenergic receptors	Orthostatic hypotension. Consider in patients with benign prostatic hypertrophy

GERD, Gastroesophageal reflux disease.
From Warshaw G et al: *Ham's primary care geriatrics,* ed 7, Philadelphia, 2022, Elsevier.

TABLE 8 Antihypertensive Choice in the Setting of Cardiovascular Comorbidity

COMPELLING INDICATION	DIURETIC	BB	ACEI	ATRA	CCB	ALDO ant
Heart failure	✔	✔	✔	✔		✔
Post myocardial infarction		✔	✔			✔
High risk of coronary artery disease	✔	✔	✔		✔	
Diabetes	✔	✔	✔	✔	✔	
Chronic kidney disease			✔	✔		
Recurrent stroke prevention	✔		✔			

ACEI, Angiotensin-converting enzyme inhibitor; *ALDO ant,* aldosterone antagonist; *ATRA,* angiotensin II receptor antagonist, *BB,* beta-adrenoceptor antagonist; *CCB,* calcium-channel blocker.
From Talley NJ et al: *Essentials of internal medicine,* ed 4, Chatswood, NSW, 2021, Elsevier Australia.

b. Disadvantages: Diltiazem and verapamil should be avoided in patients with CHF caused by systolic dysfunction because of their negative inotropic effects; pedal edema may occur with nifedipine and amlodipine; constipation can be severe in elderly patients receiving verapamil. CCB-related edema is positional in nature and improves with lying position; additional strategies include switching CCB classes, reducing dosage, giving the medication later in the day, and adding a venodilator (nitrates, an ACE, or an ARB); diuretics may improve edema, but at the expense of a reduction in plasma volume.

4. ACE inhibitors:
   a. Advantages: First-line therapy for patients with left ventricular dysfunction, helpful in prevention of diabetic renal disease; effective in decreasing LVH, and remodeling.
   b. Disadvantages: Dry cough is a frequent side effect (5% to 20% of patients); hyperkalemia may occur in patients with diabetes or severe renal insufficiency; hypotension may occur in volume-depleted patients; increased risk of renal failure in patients with renal artery stenosis; contraindicated in pregnancy.

5. ARBs:
   a. Advantages: Well tolerated, favorable impact on quality of life; useful in patients unable to tolerate ACE inhibitors because of persistent cough and in CHF and diabetic patients; single daily dose. An episode of renal insufficiency with ACE inhibitors does not rule out future therapy with an ARB unless high-grade bilateral renal artery stenosis exists.
   b. Disadvantages: Hypotension may occur in volume-depleted patients; hyperkalemia; risk of renal failure in renal artery stenosis; contraindicated in pregnancy.

6. Alpha-adrenergic blockers:
   a. Advantages: No adverse effect on blood lipids or insulin sensitivity; helpful in benign prostatic hypertrophy.
   b. Disadvantages: Postural hypotension, sedation; syncope can be avoided by giving an initial low dose at bedtime. Generally considered third- or fourth-line agent.

7. Central alpha-antagonists:
   a. Oral clonidine mainstay of therapy for hypertensive urgencies because of the ease of administration and relative safety.
   b. Transdermal clonidine; useful in management of labile HTN, the hospitalized patient who cannot take medications by mouth, and patients subject to early-morning BP surges. At equivalent doses, transdermal clonidine is more apt to precipitate salt and water retention than is the case with oral clonidine.
   c. Dose beyond 0.4 mg causes fatigue, sedation, dry mouth, salt and water retention, and rebound HTN upon abrupt termination of the medication.

8. Combined α- and β-adrenergic receptor blockers:
   a. Labetalol, nebivolol, and carvedilol: Use is reserved to treat complicated hypertensive patient when an antihypertensive effect beyond β-blockade is sought. IV labetalol is used for hypertensive emergencies. Carvedilol is shown to have less adverse effect on glycemic control than metoprolol and to reduce urinary protein excretion in hypertensive diabetic patients.

9. Direct-acting smooth muscle relaxant: Hydralazine
   a. Advantages: Beneficial in Black patients when used with isosorbide dinitrate.
   b. Disadvantages: May lead to reflex tachycardia, worsening ischemia (best used with nitrates), at higher doses or with renal failure can lead to a reversible drug-induced lupus.

10. Renin inhibitors: Newest class of antihypertensives (Aliskiren):
    a. Advantages: Generally well tolerated; once-daily dosing; can be used alone or in combination with other antihypertensive agents (avoid combining with ACE inhibitors or ARBs given increase of hyperkalemia).
    b. Disadvantages: Contraindicated in pregnancy; should not be used in patients with impaired renal function; excessive cost; paucity of cardiovascular outcomes data showing benefit.

TREATMENT OF RENOVASCULAR HYPERTENSION: The therapeutic approach varies with the cause of the renovascular hypertension (RVH) (refer to "Renal Artery Stenosis" for additional information).

- Young patients with fibromuscular dysplasia refractory to medical therapy can be treated with percutaneous transluminal renal angioplasty (PTRA).
- Medical therapy is advisable in elderly patients with atheromatous RVH; useful agents are:
  1. β-Blockers: Highly effective in patients with elevated plasma renin
  2. ACE inhibitors: Highly effective; however, should be avoided in patients with bilateral renal artery stenosis or with a solitary kidney and renal artery stenosis
  3. Diuretics: Often used in combination with ACE inhibitors
- Surgical revascularization: A recent trial revealed that renal-artery stenting does not confer a significant benefit with respect to the prevention of clinical events when added to comprehensive, multifactorial medical therapy in people with atherosclerotic renal-artery stenosis and hypertension or CKD.

HTN DURING PREGNANCY:
- HTN complicates 5% to 12% of all pregnancies.
- The American Obstetrical Committee defines BP of 130/80 mm Hg as the upper limit of normal at any time during pregnancy.
- A rise of 30 mm Hg systolic or 15 mm Hg diastolic is also considered abnormal regardless of the absolute values obtained.
- Hypertension during pregnancy can be from chronic HTN, gestational HTN, preeclampsia or preeclampsia superimposed on chronic HTN. It is important to distinguish the etiology because the risk to mother and fetus is much greater in preeclampsia. In pregnant women with mild chronic hypertension, a strategy of targeting a blood pressure of less than 140/90 mm Hg is associated with better pregnancy outcomes than a strategy of reserving treatment only for severe hypertension, with no increase in the risk of small-for-gestational-age birth weight.[3a]
- Treatment of chronic HTN during pregnancy is as follows:
  1. Initial treatment with conservative measures (proper nutrition, limited physical activity).
  2. When drug therapy is necessary, initiation of methyldopa, hydralazine, labetalol, or nifedipine is preferred. Table 9 summarizes

TABLE 9 Drugs Used to Treat Hypertension in Pregnancy

Drug	Starting Dose	Maximum Dose	Comments
Acute Treatment of Severe Hypertension			
Hydralazine	5-10 mg IV every 20 min	20 mg*	Avoid in cases of tachycardia and persistent headaches
Labetalol	20-40 mg IV every 10-15 min	220 mg*	Avoid in women with asthma or congestive heart failure
Nifedipine	10-20 mg PO every 30 min	50 mg*	Avoid in case of tachycardia and palpitations
Long-Term Treatment of Hypertension			
Methyldopa	250 mg bid	4 g/day	
Labetalol	100 mg bid	2400 mg/day	
Nifedipine	10 mg bid	120 mg/day	
Thiazide diuretic	12.5 mg bid	50 mg/day	

bid, Twice daily; *IV*, intravenous.
*If desired blood pressure levels are not achieved, switch to another drug.
From Gabbe SG: *Obstetrics*, ed 6, Philadelphia, 2012, Saunders.

drugs used to treat hypertension in pregnancy.

3. ACE inhibitors can cause fetal and neonatal complications; their use should be avoided in pregnancy.

4. The safety of CCBs remains unclear.

5. Diuretics should be used only if there is a specific reason for initiating and maintaining their use (e.g., HTN associated with severe fluid overload or left ventricular dysfunction).

MALIGNANT HTN, HYPERTENSIVE EMERGENCIES, AND HYPERTENSIVE URGENCIES:
Definitions:

- Malignant HTN occurs with HTN when there are grades III and IV retinopathy (exudates, hemorrhages, and papilledema).
  1. The rate of BP rise is a critical factor in the development of malignant HTN.
  2. Complications and mortality rates are much higher in malignant HTN compared with essential HTN.
  3. Requires immediate BP reduction (not necessarily into normal ranges) to prevent or limit target organ disease.
- Hypertensive emergencies occur when the BP elevation is >180 mm Hg systolic and/or >120 mm Hg diastolic without evidence of new or progressive organ dysfunction. It requires rapid lowering of BP to prevent end-organ damage.
- Hypertensive urgencies are BP elevations >180 mm Hg systolic and/or >120 mm Hg diastolic with end-organ damage that should be corrected within 24 h of presentation.
  1. Most clinicians suggest lowering the BP to <160 mm Hg/<100 mm Hg or to a level no more than 30% lower than the patient's baseline BP.

Therapy: The choice of therapeutic agents varies with the cause. IV medications are preferred in hypertensive emergencies.

- Nitroprusside is the drug of choice in hypertensive encephalopathy, HTN and intracranial bleeding, malignant HTN, HTN and heart failure, dissecting aortic aneurysm (used in combination with propranolol); its onset of action is immediate. Because it is metabolized to cyanide, patients should be carefully monitored for toxicity (mental status changes, acidemia).
- Fenoldopam is a vasodilator agent useful for the short-term (up to 48 h) management of severe HTN when rapid but quickly reversible reduction of BP is required. It should be avoided in patients with glaucoma.
- Other commonly used agents are the IV CCBs nicardipine and clevidipine (useful for urgent treatment of HTN in the ICU or operating room),

the β-blocker esmolol (useful in aortic dissection or postoperative HTN), labetalol (combined β-adrenergic and α-blocker useful in patients with coronary disease), phentolamine (useful for catecholamine-related emergencies), IV nitroglycerin (used in patients with cardiac ischemia and hypertensive crisis), and hydralazine (used for hypertensive emergencies in pregnancy).

- Table 10 summarizes IV medications useful in hypertensive crisis.

The following are important points to remember when treating hypertensive emergencies:

- Introduce a plan for long-term therapy at the time of the initial emergency treatment.
- Agents that reduce arterial pressure can cause the kidney to retain sodium and water; therefore, the judicious administration of diuretics should accompany their use.
- The initial goal of antihypertensive therapy is not to achieve a normal BP, but rather to gradually reduce the BP; cerebral hypoperfusion may occur if the mean BP is HTN in patients with CKD.

HTN MANAGEMENT IN THE NEUROLOGIC-NEUROSURGICAL ICU:

- Guidelines for BP management in the most common conditions treated in the neurologic-neurosurgical intensive care unit are summarized in Table 11.

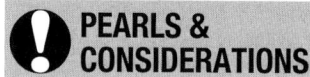

PEARLS & CONSIDERATIONS

COMMENTS

- "Masked hypertension" refers to the detection of HTN with home or ambulatory monitoring. Up to 40% of patients with BP less than 140/90 mm Hg in the office may have masked hypertension. Automated BP monitors are useful to screen for masked HTN.
- "White coat hypertension" is defined as an elevated BP during medical office examination, whereas BP is in the normal range while at home. Its prevalence is as high as 30% among patients with an elevated BP in the office. These patients are at increased risk for overt HTN.
- For patients with HTN, every 20/10 mm Hg increase in BP doubles the risk of cardiovascular events.
- Most patients will require at least two medications for BP control.
- If BP is greater than 20/10 mm Hg above goal, therapy should be initiated with two drugs.
- Resistant HTN: HTN is considered resistant if the BP cannot be reduced below target levels

in patients who are compliant with an optimal triple-drug regimen that includes a diuretic. Terms *refractory* and *resistant* are used interchangeably. Causes include pseudohypertension, measurement artifact, medication nonadherence, volume overload, and secondary HTN.

1. Pseudohypertension in elderly: Hardened and sclerotic artery is not compressible; hence, falsely elevates BP measurement artifact.
2. Measurement artifact: BP taken incorrectly (small cuff, improper support).

- Renal sympathetic denervation: A blinded trial did not show a significant reduction of systolic BP in patients with resistant hypertension 6 mo after renal artery denervation as compared with a sham control.[4]
- Barriers to BP control: System issues, provider issues, patient issues, and behavior issues. The rate at which physicians adopt recommended changes based on evidence-based findings can be quite slow and has been properly described as "clinical inertia."
- Indications for specialist referral for patients with HTN are described in Table 12.
- U.S. guidelines for the treatment of HTN recommend the following[2]:
  1. Use of BP-lowering medication for secondary prevention in patients with cardiovascular disease and average SBP ≥130 mm Hg or DBP ≥80 mm Hg, and for primary prevention in adults with an estimated 10-yr ASCVD risk of >10% and an average SBP ≥130 mm Hg or DBP ≥80 mm Hg.
  2. In patients with no history of cardiovascular disease and an estimated 10-yr ASCVD risk <10%, BP-lowering medication is recommended for those with an average SBP ≥140 mm Hg or an average DBP ≥90 mm Hg.

REFERENCES
Available at eBooks.Health.Elsevier.com.

RELATED CONTENT
High Blood Pressure (Patient Information)
High Blood Pressure—Child (Patient Information)
Eclampsia (Related Key Topic)
Pheochromocytoma (Related Key Topic)
Preeclampsia (Related Key Topic)
Renal Artery Stenosis (Related Key Topic)

AUTHOR: **TANIA B. BABAR, MD**

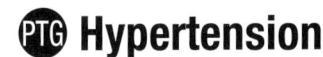

TABLE 10 Treatment of Hypertensive Crisis: Intravenous Medications

Drug Name and Mechanism of Action	Indications/Advantages/Dose	Disadvantages/Adverse Effects/Metabolism Cautions
Sodium Nitroprusside Nitric oxide compound; vasodilation of arteriolar and venous smooth muscle Increases cardiac output by decreasing afterload	Useful in most hypertensive emergencies Onset of action immediate, duration of action 1-2 min Dose: 0.25 µg/kg/min Maximum dose: 8-10 µg/kg/min	Contraindicated in high-output cardiac failure, congenital optic atrophy. Anemia and liver disease at risk of cyanide toxicity: Acidosis, tachycardia, change in mental status, almond smell on breath. Risk of thiocyanate toxicity with renal disease: Psychosis, hyperreflexia, seizure, tinnitus. Cautious use with increased intracranial pressure. Do not use maximum dose for >10 min. Crosses the placenta.
Nitroglycerin Directly interacts with nitrate receptors on vascular smooth muscle Primarily dilates venous bed Decreases preload	Use with symptoms of cardiac ischemia, perioperative hypertension in cardiac surgery Initial dose: 5 µg/min Maximum dose: 100 µg/min	Contraindicated in angle-closure glaucoma, increased intracranial pressure. Blood pressure decreased secondary to decreased preload, cardiac output—avoid when cerebral or renal perfusion compromised. Caution with right ventricular infarct.
Labetalol β- and α-Adrenergic blockade α:β-Blocking ratio is 1:7	Onset of action 2-5 min, duration 3-6 h Bolus 20 mg, then 20-80 mg every 10 min for maximum dose 300 mg Infuse at 0.5-2 mg/min	Avoid in bronchospasm, bradycardia, congestive heart failure, greater than first-degree heart block, second/third trimester pregnancy. Use caution with hepatic dysfunction, inhalational anesthetics (myocardial depression). Enters breast milk.
Esmolol Cardioselective β1-adrenergic blocking agent	Use with aortic dissection Use during intubation, intraoperative, and postoperative hypertension Onset of action 60 sec, duration 10-20 min, 200-500 µg/kg/min for 4 min, then infuse 50-300 µg/kg/min	See labetalol. Not dependent on renal or hepatic function for metabolism (metabolized by hydrolysis in red blood cells).
Fenoldopam Postsynaptic dopamine-1 agonist; decreases peripheral vascular resistance; 10 times more potent than dopamine as vasodilator	May be advantageous in kidney disease, increases renal blood flow, increases sodium excretion, no toxic metabolites Initial dose: 0.1 µg/kg/min, with titration every 15 min No bolus	Contraindicated in glaucoma (may increase intraocular pressure) or allergy to sulfites; hypotension, especially with concurrent β-blocker. Check serum potassium every 6 h. Concurrent acetaminophen may significantly increase blood levels. Dose-related tachycardia.
Hydralazine Primarily dilates arteriolar vasculature	Primarily used in pregnancy/eclampsia Dose: 10 mg every 20-130 min; maximum dose 20 mg Decreases blood pressure in 10-20 min Duration of action 2-4 h	Reflex tachycardia; give β-blocker concurrently. May exacerbate angina. Half-life 3 h, affects blood pressure for 100 h. Depends on hepatic acetylation for inactivation.
Phentolamine α-Adrenergic blockade	Used primarily to treat hypertension from excessive catecholamine excess (e.g., pheochromocytoma) Dose: 5-15 mg Onset of action 1-2 min, duration 3-10 min	β-Blockade is generally added to control tachycardia or arrhythmias. As in all catecholamine excess states, β-blockers should never be given first, as the loss of β-adrenergically mediated vasodilation will leave α-adrenergically mediated vasoconstriction unopposed and result in increased pressure.
Nicardipine Dihydropyridine calcium channel blocker; inhibits transmembrane influx of calcium ions into cardiac and smooth muscle	Onset of action 10-20 min, duration 1-4 h Initial dose: 5 mg/h to maximum of 15 mg/h	Avoid with congestive heart failure, cardiac ischemia. Adverse effects include tachycardia, flushing, headache.
Clevidipine Short-acting dihydropyridine calcium channel antagonist	Initial dose: 1 mg/h; can be increased to 21 mg/h	Reduces blood pressure without affecting cardiac filling pressures or causing reflex tachycardia.
Enalaprilat Angiotensin-converting enzyme inhibitor	Onset of action 15-20 min, duration 12-24 h Dose: 1.25-5 mg every 6 h	Response not predictable, with high renin states may see acute hypotension. Hyperkalemia in setting of reduced glomerular filtration rate. Avoid in pregnancy.
Trimethaphan Nondepolarizing ganglionic blocking agent; competes with acetylcholine for postsynaptic receptors	Used in aortic dissection Dose: 0.5-5 mg/min	Does not increase cardiac output. No inotropic cardiac effect. Disadvantages include parasympathetic blockade, resulting in paralytic ileus and bladder atony and development of tachyphylaxis after 24-96 h of use.

From Vincent JL et al: *Textbook of critical care*, ed 7, Philadelphia, 2017, Elsevier.

H

Diseases and Disorders

I

TABLE 11   Guidelines for Blood Pressure Management in the Most Common Conditions Treated in the Neurologic-Neurosurgical Intensive Care Unit

Diagnosis	Recommendation
Acute ischemic stroke	Establish and maintain BP <185/110 mm Hg before receiving intravenous thrombolysis
	Keep <180/105 mm Hg if thrombolysis
	Treat only BP >220/120 mm Hg if no thrombolysis
	Keep <180/105 mm Hg following endovascular clot retrieval
Intracerebral hemorrhage	Keep SBP <180 and MAP <130 mm Hg
	(ideal SBP <160 mm Hg)
Subarachnoid hemorrhage	Keep SBP <160 mm Hg before aneurysm treated
	Do not lower BP after aneurysm treated
Traumatic brain injury	Keep adequate MAP to maintain CPP 60-70 mm Hg
	Suggested SBP goals: >100 mm Hg (ages 50-69 yr) or >110 mm Hg (ages 15-49 yr)

BP, Blood pressure; *CPP*, cerebral perfusion pressure; *MAP*, mean arterial pressure; *SBP*, systolic blood pressure.
From Jankovic J et al: *Bradley and Daroff's neurology in clinical practice*, ed 8, Philadelphia 2022, Elsevier.

TABLE 12   Indications for Specialist Referral for Patients With Hypertension

Urgent Treatment Needed
Accelerated hypertension (severe hypertension with grade III-IV retinopathy)
Particularly severe hypertension (>220/120 mm Hg)
Impending complications (e.g., transient ischemic attack, left ventricular failure)
Possible Underlying Cause
Any clue in history or examination of a secondary cause (e.g., hypokalemia with increased or high-normal plasma sodium)
Elevated serum creatinine
Proteinuria or hematuria
Sudden onset or worsening of hypertension
Young age (any hypertension <20 yr; needing treatment <30 yr)
Therapeutic Problems
Multiple drug intolerances
Multiple drug contraindications
Persistent nonadherence or nonconcordance
Special Situations
Unusual blood pressure variability
Possible white coat hypertension
Hypertension in pregnancy

From Floege J et al: *Comprehensive clinical nephrology*, ed 4, Philadelphia, 2010, Saunders.

BASIC INFORMATION

DEFINITION

Hyperthyroidism is a hypermetabolic state resulting from excess thyroid hormone. Thyrotoxicosis is a general term for excess circulating and tissue hormone levels.

SYNONYM

Thyrotoxicosis

ICD-10CM CODES
E05.00	Thyrotoxicosis with diffuse goiter without thyrotoxic crisis or storm
E05.01	Thyrotoxicosis with diffuse goiter with thyrotoxic crisis or storm
E05.10	Thyrotoxicosis with toxic single thyroid nodule without thyrotoxic crisis or storm
E05.11	Thyrotoxicosis with toxic single thyroid nodule with thyrotoxic crisis or storm
E05.20	Thyrotoxicosis with toxic multinodular goiter without thyrotoxic crisis or storm
E05.21	Thyrotoxicosis with toxic multinodular goiter with thyrotoxic crisis or storm
E05.30	Thyrotoxicosis from ectopic thyroid tissue without thyrotoxic crisis or storm
E05.31	Thyrotoxicosis from ectopic thyroid tissue with thyrotoxic crisis or storm
E05.40	Thyrotoxicosis factitia without thyrotoxic crisis or storm
E05.41	Thyrotoxicosis factitia with thyrotoxic crisis or storm
E05.80	Other thyrotoxicosis without thyrotoxic crisis or storm
E05.81	Other thyrotoxicosis with thyrotoxic crisis or storm
E05.90	Thyrotoxicosis, unspecified without thyrotoxic crisis or storm
E05.91	Thyrotoxicosis, unspecified with thyrotoxic crisis or storm
E06.2	Chronic thyroiditis with transient thyrotoxicosis

EPIDEMIOLOGY & DEMOGRAPHICS

INCIDENCE & PREVALENCE:
- Hyperthyroidism affects 2% of women and 0.2% of men in their lifetimes.
- Toxic multinodular goiter usually occurs in women >55 yr and is more common than Graves disease in the elderly.

PHYSICAL FINDINGS & CLINICAL PRESENTATION

- Patients with hyperthyroidism generally present with tachycardia, tremor, hyperreflexia, anxiety, irritability, emotional lability, panic attacks, heat intolerance, sweating, increased appetite, diarrhea, weight loss, menstrual dysfunction (oligomenorrhea, amenorrhea). Presentation may be different in elderly patients (see the following).
- Patients with Graves disease may present with exophthalmos, lid retraction, and lid lag (Graves ophthalmopathy). The following signs and symptoms of ophthalmopathy may be present: Blurring of vision, photophobia, increased lacrimation, double vision, and deep

orbital pressure. Clubbing of fingers associated with periosteal new bone formation in other skeletal areas (Graves acropachy) and pretibial myxedema may also be noted.
- Clinical signs of hyperthyroidism in the elderly may be masked by manifestations of coexisting disease (e.g., new-onset atrial fibrillation, exacerbation of congestive heart failure).

ETIOLOGY (TABLE 1)

- Graves disease (diffuse toxic goiter): 80% to 90% of all cases of hyperthyroidism
- Toxic multinodular goiter (Plummer disease)
- Toxic adenoma
- Iatrogenic and factitious
- Transient hyperthyroidism (subacute thyroiditis, Hashimoto thyroiditis)
- Rare causes: Hypersecretion of thyroid-stimulating hormone (TSH) (e.g., pituitary neoplasms), struma ovarii, ingestion of large amount of iodine in a patient with preexisting thyroid hyperplasia or adenoma (Jod-Basedow phenomenon), hydatidiform mole, carcinoma of thyroid, amiodarone therapy

DX DIAGNOSIS

DIFFERENTIAL DIAGNOSIS

- Anxiety disorder
- Pheochromocytoma
- Metastatic neoplasm
- Diabetes mellitus
- Premenopausal state

TABLE 1 Causes of Hyperthyroidism

I. Excessive TSH-Receptor Stimulation

Graves disease (TRAb)
Pregnancy-associated transient hyperthyroidism (hCG)
Trophoblastic disease (hCG)
Familial gestational hyperthyroidism (mutant TSH receptor)
TSH-producing pituitary adenoma

II. Autonomous Thyroid Hormone Secretion

Multinodular toxic goiter (somatic mutations)
Solitary toxic thyroid adenoma (somatic mutation)
Congenital activating TSH-receptor mutation (genomic mutation)

III. Destruction of Follicles With Release of Hormone

Subacute de Quervain thyroiditis (virus infection)
Painless thyroiditis/postpartum thyroiditis (hashitoxicosis—autoimmune)
Acute thyroiditis (bacterial infection)
Drug-induced thyroiditis (amiodarone, interferon-γ)

IV. Extrathyroidal Sources of Thyroid Hormone

Iatrogenic overreplacement with thyroid hormone
Excessive self-administered thyroid medication
Food and supplements containing excessive thyroid hormone
Functional thyroid cancer metastases
Struma ovarii

hCG, Human chorionic gonadotropin; *TRAb,* thyrotropin-receptor antibodies; *TSH,* thyroid-stimulating hormone (thyrotropin).
From Melmed S et al: *Williams textbook of endocrinology,* ed 14, St Louis, 2019, Elsevier.

WORKUP

Suspected hyperthyroidism requires laboratory confirmation and identification of its etiology because treatment varies with cause. A detailed medical history will often provide clues to the diagnosis and etiology of the hyperthyroidism. Fig. 1 describes a diagnostic approach to suspected hyperthyroidism.

LABORATORY TESTS

- Elevated free thyroxine (T_4)
- Elevated free triiodothyronine (T_3): Generally not necessary for diagnosis
- Low TSH (unless hyperthyroidism is a result of the rare hypersecretion of TSH from a pituitary adenoma). Serum TSH is the best test for diagnosis of thyrotoxicosis
- Thyroid autoantibodies useful in selected cases to differentiate Graves disease from toxic multinodular goiter (absent thyroid antibodies)

IMAGING STUDIES

- 24-h radioactive iodine uptake (RAIU) is useful to distinguish hyperthyroidism from iatrogenic thyroid hormone synthesis (thyrotoxicosis factitia) and from thyroiditis (Box 1).
- An overactive thyroid shows increased uptake, whereas a normal underactive thyroid (iatrogenic thyroid ingestion, painless or subacute thyroiditis) shows normal or decreased uptake.
- The RAIU results also vary with the etiology of the hyperthyroidism:
  1. Graves disease: Increased homogeneous uptake
  2. Multinodular goiter: Increased heterogeneous uptake
  3. Hot nodule: Single focus of increased uptake
- RAIU is also generally performed before the therapeutic administration of radioactive iodine to determine the appropriate dose.

RX TREATMENT

NONPHARMACOLOGIC THERAPY

Patient education regarding thyroid disease and discussion of the therapeutic options. Avoidance of strenuous physical exercise, caffeine, and tobacco in patients with uncontrolled thyrotoxicosis. Patients should be informed that radioiodine, antithyroid drugs, and surgery are all reasonable treatment options for hyperthyroidism. It is crucial for the physician to have a detailed discussion with the patient about the benefits and risks relative to lifestyle, patients' values, and coexisting conditions.

ACUTE GENERAL Rx

ANTITHYROID DRUGS (THIONAMIDES): Propylthiouracil (PTU) and methimazole inhibit thyroid hormone synthesis by blocking production of thyroid peroxidase (PTU and methimazole) or inhibit peripheral conversion of T_4 to T_3 (PTU). Methimazole is favored by most endocrinologists because of the potential for hepatic failure

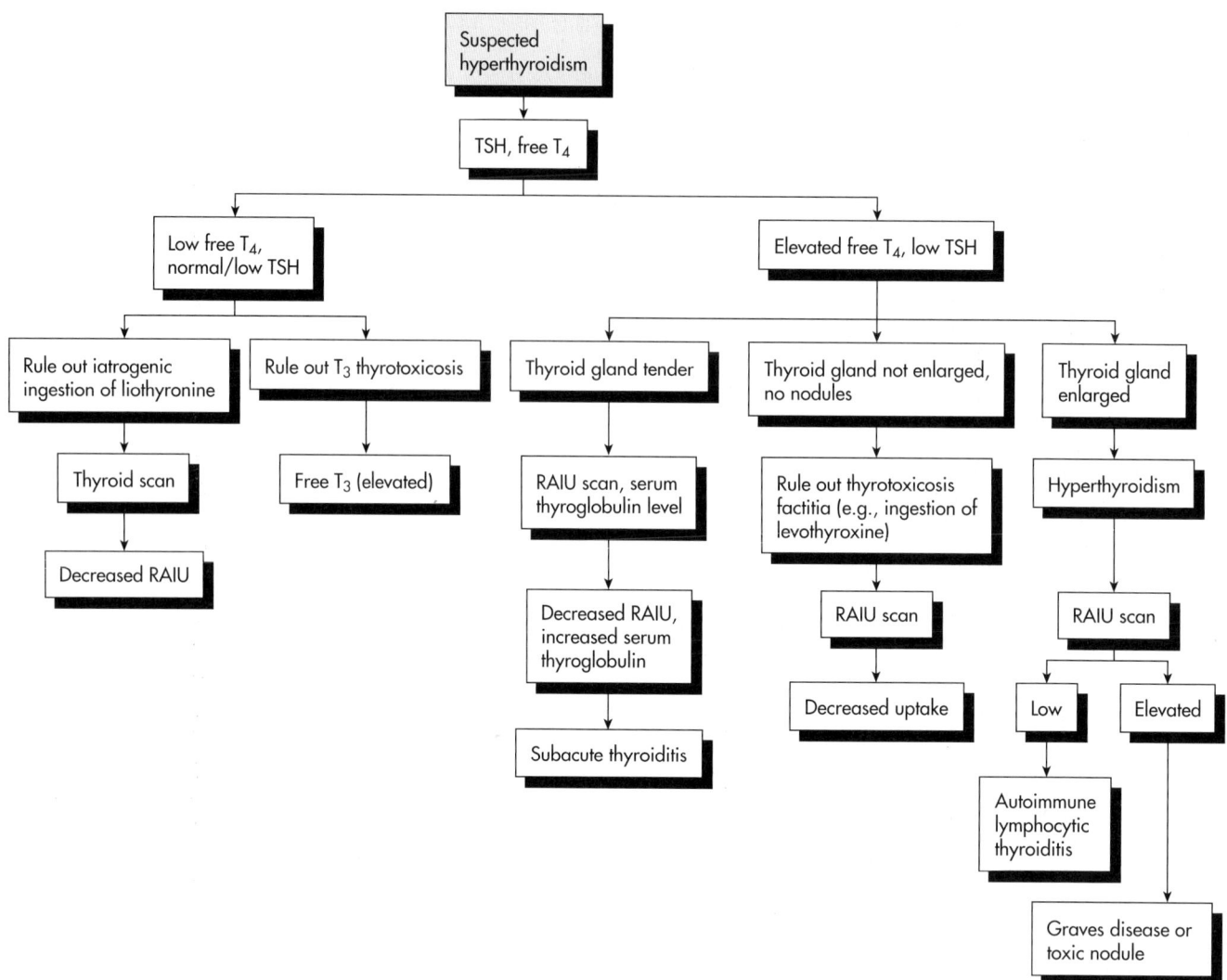

FIG. 1 Hyperthyroidism. *RAIU*, Radioactive iodine uptake; *TSH*, thyroid-stimulating hormone.

BOX 1   Differentiation of Causes of Hyperthyroidism According to Pattern of Radionucleotide Uptake

Reduced Uptake	Generalized Increased Uptake	Focal Increased Uptake
• Thyroiditis • Exogenous thyroxine • Iodine loading • Ectopic thyroid hormone secretion (struma ovarii)	• Graves' disease • Excess thyroid-stimulating hormone stimulation	• Toxic multinodular goiter • Hyperfunctioning adenoma

From Talley NJ et al: *Essentials of internal medicine*, ed 4, Chatswood, NSW, 2021, Elsevier Australia.

---

with PTU. PTU is preferred in pregnant women during the first trimester because methimazole has been associated with aplasia cutis and with choanal and esophageal atresia. CBC and differential should be obtained before their use.

- Dosage: Methimazole 15 to 30 mg/day given as a single dose; PTU 50 to 100 mg PO q8h.
- Antithyroid drugs can be used as the primary form of treatment or as adjunctive therapy before radioactive therapy or surgery or afterward if the hyperthyroidism recurs.
- Side effects: Skin rash (3% to 5% of patients), arthralgias, myalgias, granulocytopenia (0.5%). Rare side effects are aplastic anemia, hepatic necrosis from PTU, cholestatic jaundice from methimazole.
- When antithyroid drugs are used as primary therapy, they are usually given for 6 to 18 mo; prolonged therapy may cause hypothyroidism.

Monitor thyroid function every 2 mo for 6 mo, then less frequently.

- The use of antithyroid drugs before radioiodine therapy is best reserved for patients in whom exacerbation of hyperthyroidism after radioactive iodine therapy is hazardous (e.g., elderly patients with coronary artery disease or significant coexisting morbidity). In these patients the antithyroid drug can be stopped 2 days before radioactive iodine therapy, resumed 2 days later, and continued for 4 to 6 wk.

RADIOIODINE THERAPY (RADIOACTIVE IODINE [RAI; ¹³¹I]):

- RAI is the treatment of choice for patients age >21 yr and younger patients who have not achieved remission after 1 yr of antithyroid drug therapy. RAI is also used in hyperthyroidism caused by toxic adenoma or toxic multinodular goiter.
- Contraindicated during pregnancy (can cause fetal hypothyroidism) and lactation. Pregnancy should be excluded in women of childbearing age before RAI is administered.
- A single dose of RAI is effective in inducing a euthyroid state in nearly 80% of patients.

- There is a high incidence of post-RAI hypothyroidism (>50% within first yr and 2%/yr thereafter); these patients should be frequently evaluated for the onset of hypothyroidism. There is a modest but significant excess risk for thyroid cancer and excess mortality risk for breast cancer and other solid cancer with RAI treatment.[1]

SURGICAL THERAPY (SUBTOTAL THYROIDECTOMY):

- Indicated in obstructing goiters, in any patient who refuses RAI and cannot be adequately managed with antithyroid medications (e.g., patients with toxic adenoma or toxic multinodular goiter), and in pregnant patients who cannot be adequately managed with antithyroid medication or develop side effects to them. Thyroidectomy can also be considered as primary therapy in refractory cases of amiodarone-induced hyperthyroidism. Thyroidectomy is not indicated for low RAIU hyperthyroidism.
- Patients should be rendered euthyroid with antithyroid drugs before surgery.
- Complications of surgery include hypothyroidism (28% to 43% after 10 yr), hypoparathyroidism, and vocal cord paralysis (1%).
- Most patients should be started on replacement doses of levothyroxine (1.7 mcg/kg/day) before discharge from hospital.
- Hyperthyroidism recurs after surgery in 10% to 15% of patients.

ADJUNCTIVE THERAPY: Propranolol alleviates the beta-adrenergic symptoms of hyperthyroidism; initial dose is 20 to 40 mg PO q6h; dosage is gradually increased until symptoms are controlled. Major contraindications to propranolol are congestive heart failure and bronchospasm. Diagnosis and treatment of thyrotoxic storm are also discussed in Section I.

CHRONIC Rx

- Patients undergoing treatment with antithyroid drugs should be seen every 1 to 3 mo until euthyroidism is achieved and every 3 to 4 mo while they remain on antithyroid therapy. After treatment is stopped, periodic monitoring of thyroid function tests with TSH is recommended every 3 mo for 1 yr, then every 6 mo for 1 yr, then annually.

- Orbital decompression surgery can be used to correct Graves orbitopathy. The administration of the antioxidant selenium (100 mcg PO bid) has been recently reported as effective in improving quality of life, reducing ocular involvement, and slowing progression of the disease in patients with mild Graves orbitopathy. Its mechanism of action is believed to be an effect on the oxygen free radicals and cytokines that play a pathogenic role in Graves orbitopathy.

DISPOSITION

Successful treatment of hyperthyroidism requires lifelong monitoring for the onset of hypothyroidism or the recurrence of thyrotoxicosis.

REFERRAL

- Endocrinology referral is recommended at the time of initial diagnosis and during treatment.
- Surgical referral in selected patients (see "Surgical Therapy").
- Hospitalization of all patients with thyrotoxic storm.

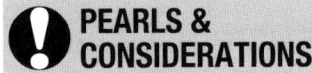 **PEARLS & CONSIDERATIONS**

COMMENTS

- Elderly hyperthyroid patients may have only subtle signs (weight loss, tachycardia, fine skin, brittle nails). This form is known as *apathetic hyperthyroidism* and manifests with lethargy rather than hyperkinetic activity. An enlarged thyroid gland may be absent. Coexisting medical disorders (most commonly cardiac disease) may also mask the symptoms. These patients often have unexplained congestive heart failure, worsening of angina, or new-onset atrial fibrillation resistant to treatment. See the topic "Graves Disease" for additional information on diagnosis and treatment.
- **Subclinical hyperthyroidism** is defined as a normal serum-free thyroxine and free triiodothyronine levels with a TSH level suppressed below the normal range and usually undetectable. Prevalence in the general population is 1% to 2%. These patients usually do not present with signs or symptoms of overt hyperthyroidism. Subclinical hyperthyroidism is

associated with an increased risk of atrial fibrillation and heart failure in older adults. Treatment options include observation or a therapeutic trial of low-dose antithyroid agents for 6 mo to attempt to induce remission. The American Thyroid Association and the American Association of Clinical Endocrinologists recommend treatment of patients with TSH levels <0.1 mIU if they are older than 65 or have associated comorbidities (osteoporosis, heart failure).

- ***Thyrotoxic periodic paralysis (TPP)*** is a hyperthyroidism-related hypokalemia and muscle-weakening condition resulting from a sudden shift of potassium into cells. Many patients do not have other symptoms of hyperthyroidism. Typical presentation involves an Asian adult male with acute fatigue and muscle weakness initially presenting in the lower extremities. Physical examination reveals decreased deep tendon reflexes, hypertension, and tachycardia. ECG often reveals U waves, high QRS voltage, and first-degree atrioventricular block. Additional laboratory testing reveals normal acid-base state, hypokalemia with low urinary potassium excretion (spot urinary potassium concentration <20 mEq/L from potassium shift into cells), hypophosphatemia, hypophosphaturia, and hypercalciuria. Electromyography during attacks shows low-amplitude compound muscle action potential of the tested muscle. Therapy consists of cautious potassium supplementation (increased risk of rebound hyperkalemia). Use of nonselective β-blockers (e.g., propranolol) to counteract hyperadrenergic activity, which may be causing TPP, may also be useful.

REFERENCE & SUGGESTED READINGS

Available at eBooks.Health.Elsevier.com.

RELATED CONTENT

Hyperthyroidism (Patient Information)
Graves Disease (Related Key Topic)
Thyrotoxic Storm (Related Key Topic)

AUTHOR: **FRED F. FERRI, MD**

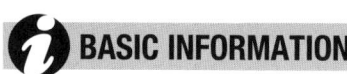

BASIC INFORMATION

DEFINITION

Hypoglycemia refers to abnormally low blood glucose levels in circulating plasma. It is defined as a glucose value <70 mg/dl (3.9 mmol/L). "Serious hypoglycemia" refers to values <54 mg/dl (3.0 mmol/L). "Severe hypoglycemia" is any glucose value necessitating external assistance to correct it. "Reactive hypoglycemia" refers to symptoms of hypoglycemia with plasma glucose value >70 mg/dl. A multitude of scenarios can lead to this potentially fatal condition.[1]

SYNONYMS

Glycopenia
Low blood glucose
Low blood sugar
HG

ICD-10CM CODES

E10.641	Type 1 diabetes mellitus with hypoglycemia with coma
E10.649	Type 1 diabetes mellitus with hypoglycemia without coma
E11.641	Type 2 diabetes mellitus with hypoglycemia with coma
E11.649	Type 2 diabetes mellitus with hypoglycemia without coma
E13.641	Other specified diabetes mellitus with hypoglycemia with coma
E13.649	Other specified diabetes mellitus with hypoglycemia without coma
E16.1	Other hypoglycemia
E16.2	Hypoglycemia, unspecified

EPIDEMIOLOGY & DEMOGRAPHICS

- Most commonly seen in patients with diabetes mellitus (DM)[1,2]
- More common in type 1 DM. Estimated that glucose levels may be as low as 50 to 60 mg/dl ~10% of the time in type 1 DM.[1,3]
- Although less prevalent than type 1, absolute cases of hypoglycemia is higher in patients with type 2 DM because of the significantly larger population of people with type 2 DM. Rates of severe hypoglycemic episodes in type 1 DM range from 115 to 320 episodes/100 patient years, whereas rates for type 2 DM range from 35 to 70 episodes/100 patient years.[2,3]
- Elderly adults with DM are at higher risk of hypoglycemia because of alterations in adaptive physiologic responses to low glucose levels. In addition, this patient population has comorbidities, including cognitive and functional decline, that interfere with rapid identification and response to hypoglycemic episodes. Elderly patients are more likely to be hospitalized for insulin-related hypoglycemia than younger cohorts.[2]

PHYSICAL FINDINGS & CLINICAL PRESENTATION[1]

- Symptoms are often nonspecific.

- Early symptoms include sweating, pallor, anxiety, palpitations, hunger, and tremor.
- Late symptoms with lower plasma glucose levels include seizures, altered mental status, and coma.
- Profound or prolonged hypoglycemic episodes can cause irreversible brain injury, cardiopulmonary arrest, and death.
- Older adults may present with atypical symptoms: Nausea, unsteadiness, falls, or transient ischemia that can delay diagnosis.[2]

ETIOLOGY (BOX 1)

- Systemic glucose balance and effects of circulating hormones on endogenous production and use of glucose are described in Table 1. Physiologic responses to decreasing plasma glucose concentrations are summarized in Table 2.
- Medications are the most common cause of hypoglycemia.[1,2]
- Most common causes include hyperinsulinemia due to therapeutic treatment with exogenous insulin and/or insulin secretagogues (sulfonylureas [SU] and meglitinides [MG]). Can also be exacerbated by medication use without proper exogenous glucose intake or increased insulin sensitivity due to weight loss.[2]
- Alcohol use leading to lack of endogenous glucose production[1,2]
- Critical illness
  1. Organ failure (hepatic, cardiac, or renal)

TABLE 1 Systemic Glucose Balance[a] and Effects of Circulating Hormones on Endogenous Production and Use of Glucose

	HORMONAL EFFECTS		
Source of Glucose Influx or Efflux	Insulin	Glucagon	Epinephrine
Glucose Influx into the Circulation			
Exogenous glucose delivery			
Endogenous glucose delivery			
In liver: Glycogenolysis and gluconeogenesis	↓	↑	↑
In kidneys: Gluconeogenesis	↓		↑
Glucose Efflux Out of the Circulation			
Ongoing brain glucose utilization			
Variable glucose utilization by other tissues (e.g., muscle fat, liver, kidneys)	↑		↓

[a]Total glucose influx = total glucose efflux.
From Melmed S et al: *Williams textbook of endocrinology,* ed 14, Philadelphia, 2019, Elsevier.

TABLE 2 Physiologic Responses to Decreasing Plasma Glucose Concentrations

Response	Glycemic Threshold[a] (mmol/L [mg/dl])	Physiologic Effects	Role in Prevention or Correction of Hypoglycemia (Glucose Counterregulation)
↓ Insulin	4.4-4.7 (80-85)	↑ R_a (↓ R_d)	Primary glucose regulatory factor, first defense against hypoglycemia
↑ Glucagon	3.6-3.9 (65-70)	↑ R_a	Primary glucose counterregulatory factor, second defense against hypoglycemia
↑ Epinephrine	3.6-3.9 (65-70)	↑ R_a, ↓ R_c	Involved, critical when glucagon is deficient, third defense against hypoglycemia
↑ Cortisol and growth hormone	3.6-3.9 (65-70)	↑ R_a, ↓ R_c	Involved, not critical
Symptoms	2.8-3.1 (50-55)	↑ Exogenous glucose	Prompt behavioral defense (food ingestion)
↓ Cognition	<2.8 (50)	—	(Compromises behavioral defense)
↓ Brain glucose metabolism	<2.8 (50)	—	—

[a]Arterialized venous, not venous, plasma glucose concentrations.
R_a, Rate of glucose appearance, glucose production by the liver and kidneys; R_c, rate of glucose clearance by insulin-sensitive tissues; R_d, rate of glucose disappearance, glucose utilization by insulin-sensitive tissues such as skeletal muscle (no direct effect on central nervous system glucose utilization).
From Melmed S et al: *Williams textbook of endocrinology,* ed 14, Philadelphia, 2019, Elsevier.

BOX 1   Causes of Hypoglycemia

Postprandial Hypoglycemia (Reactive)
- Postoperative rapid gastric emptying (alimentary hyperinsulinism)
- Fructose intolerance
- Galactosemia
- Leucine intolerance
- Idiopathic

Fasting Hypoglycemia
- Overuse of glucose
- Elevated insulin levels
- Exogenous insulin (therapeutic, factitious)
- Oral hypoglycemic (therapeutic, factitious)
- Islet cell disorders (adenoma, nesidioblastosis, cancer)
- Excessive islet cell function (prediabetes, obesity)
- Antibodies to endogenous insulin
- Normal to low insulin levels
- Ketotic hypoglycemia
- Hypermetabolic state (sepsis)
- Rare extrapancreatic tumors
- Carnitine deficiency

Underproduction of Glucose
- Hormone deficiencies (growth hormone, glucagon, hypoadrenalism)
- Enzyme disorders
- Glycogen metabolism (glycogen phosphorylase, glycogen synthetase)
- Hexose metabolism (glucose-6-phosphatase, fructose-1,6-biphosphatase)
- Glycolysis, Krebs cycle (phosphoenolpyruvate carboxykinase, pyruvate carboxylase, malate dehydrogenase)
- Alcohol and probably other drugs
- Liver disease (cirrhosis, fulminant hepatic failure)
- Severe malnutrition

From Jankovic J et al: *Bradley and Daroff's neurology in clinical practice,* ed 8, Philadelphia, 2022, Elsevier.

2. Sepsis (urinary tract infection and pneumonia common sources in elderly population)
- Hormone deficiency (cortisol, glucagon, and epinephrine)
- Endogenous hyperinsulinism (insulinoma, functional β-cell disorders, insulin autoimmune hypoglycemia)
- Rare fatal episodes thought to be secondary to ventricular arrhythmias

DX DIAGNOSIS[1]

Characterized by Whipple triad:
- Symptoms potentially explained by hypoglycemia
- Low blood glucose levels during the symptoms
- Relief of symptoms with administration of glucose or glucagon

DIFFERENTIAL DIAGNOSIS

Hypoglycemic symptoms in the presence of normal plasma glucose levels (>70 mg/dl) point to other etiologies: Postprandial syndrome, stroke, sepsis, seizure/postictal state, cardiac disease, psychiatric disease, metabolic disorders (hyperthyroidism, pheochromocytoma), drug intoxication.[1]

WORKUP

- If Whipple triad is positive, the next step is to consider a patient's medical status.[1]
- Iatrogenic factors are the most common causes of hypoglycemia in hospitalized patients (review the NPO status, timing of feeding,

glucose-lowering medications, and interactions between medications).[1]
- Detailed history, including past medical history, a thorough medication history, and timing of hypoglycemia (in regard to meals and medications).
- Special attention should be given to chronic diseases that can precipitate hypoglycemia such as chronic renal disease with a glomerular filtration rate <60.[2]

LABORATORY TESTS

- An algorithm for recognition and evaluation of hypoglycemia is described in Fig. E1.
- If the cause is not apparent after a thorough history, the following is appropriate:

FASTING

If symptoms witnessed when fasting, with verified low blood glucose levels, consider the following laboratory tests: Plasma glucose, β-hydroxybutyrate (BHOB), insulin, C-peptide, proinsulin, screen for SU and MG metabolites.[1]

POSTPRANDIAL

- Plasma glucose, insulin, C-peptide, and proinsulin before ingestion of the meal and every 30 min thereafter for 5 h.[1]
- Only evaluate the samples drawn when glucose levels are <60 mg/dl.
- If a patient has a presentation consistent with Whipple triad, then measure SU, MG, and antibodies to insulin.[1]

72-H FAST[1]:
- Collect blood specimens for measurement of plasma glucose, insulin, C-peptide, proinsulin,

and BHOB every 6 h until the glucose concentration is <60 mg/dl.
- Increase frequency of sampling to every 1 to 2 h.
- Insulin, C-peptide, and proinsulin are only relevant in those specimens in which the plasma glucose concentration is <60 mg/dl.
- The fast should be ended when any of the following occurs:
  1. The plasma glucose concentration is <45 mg/dl.
  2. The patient has symptoms or signs of hypoglycemia.
  3. 72 h has elapsed.
  4. The plasma glucose concentration is <55, and Whipple triad has been documented on a prior occasion.
- Insulin antibodies are also measured but do not need to be measured during the hypoglycemic state.

IMAGING STUDIES[1]

If hypoglycemia is suspected secondary to an insulinoma or malignancy, transabdominal ultrasound (US), computed tomography scan, or endoscopic US can be used to help with diagnosis as well as for staging purposes.

RX TREATMENT
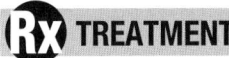

NONPHARMACOLOGIC THERAPY[1]

- Recognition of signs and symptoms, and self-monitoring of blood glucose, are especially important in insulin-deficient patients.
- Avoiding drugs that can exacerbate condition (e.g., alcohol) if it occurs on repeated occasions.
- Bedtime snacks if hypoglycemia occurs at night.
- In situations caused by tumor etiologies (e.g., islet cell, insulinoma, and nonislet cell), definitive treatment may require surgical removal.

PHARMACOLOGIC THERAPY[1,4]

- Treating the underlying etiology that exacerbates hypoglycemia (e.g., infection, proper diabetic regimen, proper diabetic diet)
- Fast-acting carbohydrates (e.g., glucose tablets, hard candy, intravenous [IV] dextrose infusion)
- Pure glucose (dextrose) if caused by insulin secretagogue in addition with α-glucosidase inhibitor
- In severe hypoglycemia with seizure activity, 25 g of 50% dextrose IV or 0.5 to 1.0 mg intramuscular/subcutaneous glucagon
- In persistent hypoglycemia after IV dextrose, therapy think sulfonylurea overdose or insulin pump malfunction. If an insulin pump is present, remove it. If sulfonylurea overdose is suspected, treat with IV dextrose infusion and octreotide 50 to 100 µg every 6 to 12 h for adults and 1 to 2 µg/kg every 6 to 12 h.[4]
- Fig. 2 describes a management algorithm for hypoglycemia

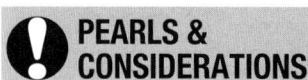
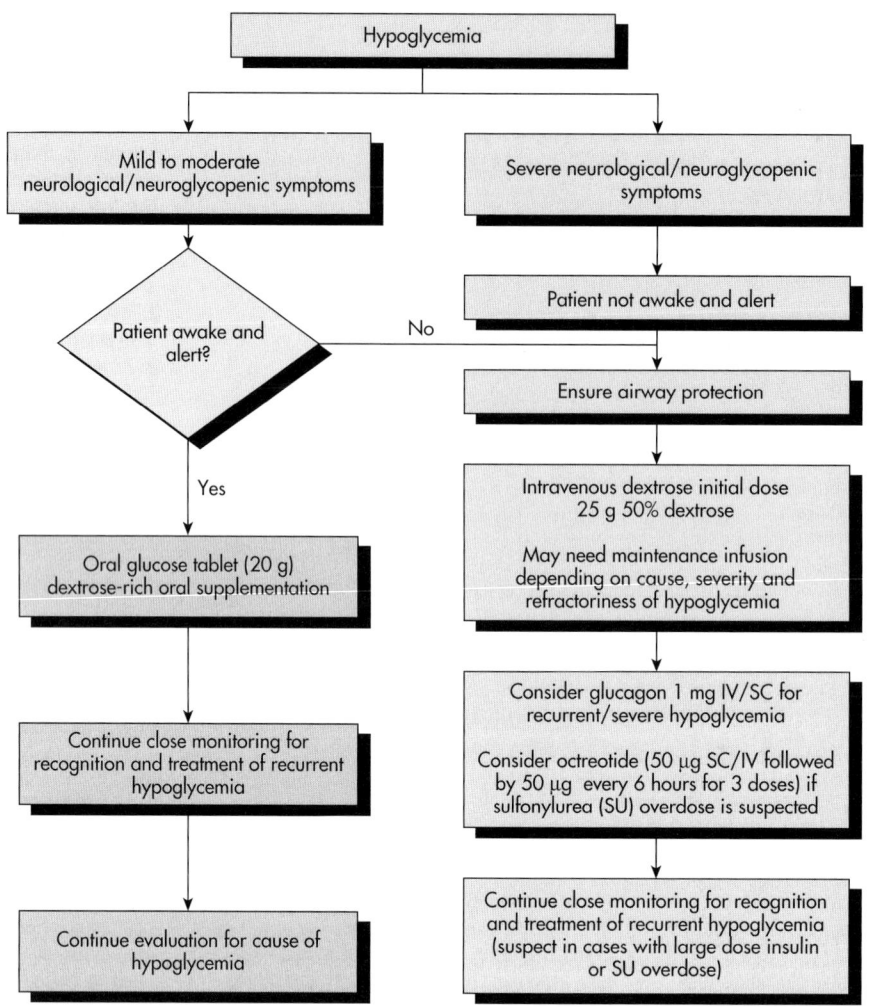

FIG. 2 Management of hypoglycemia. *IV*, Intravenous; *SC*, subcutaneous. (From Vincent JL et al: *Textbook of critical care,* ed 7, Philadelphia, 2017, Elsevier.)

REFERRAL

- Most scenarios of hypoglycemia can be managed by primary care physicians by adjusting medications.
- If the cause is not clear, then endocrinology referral is recommended.
- Severe symptomatic hypoglycemia needs emergent treatment.

PEARLS & CONSIDERATIONS

- Hypoglycemia can cause severe morbidity and death if not dealt with promptly and effectively.

- Hypoglycemia is very common in patients with DM, especially type 1 DM, and most commonly it is a side effect of medications.
- Elderly patients with DM are at higher risk for serious hypoglycemic episodes and can initially present with atypical symptoms.
- In patients who are hospitalized, the etiology is often multifactorial.
- Clinically important hypoglycemia is uncommon in nondiabetic patients, and evaluation for a hypoglycemic disorder in these patients should only occur if the Whipple triad is met.
- Pediatric hypoglycemia: A classification of hypoglycemia in infants and children is summarized in Table E3.

REFERENCES

Available at eBooks.Health.Elsevier.com.

RELATED CONTENT

Diabetes Mellitus (Related Key Topic)
Insulinoma (Related Key Topic)

AUTHORS: **BENJAMIN E. HOOK, MD,** and **MARCIN BYRA, DO**

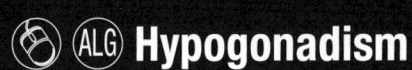
Diseases and Disorders

I

BASIC INFORMATION

DEFINITION

Male hypogonadism is a clinical syndrome involving subnormal testosterone levels and/or impaired sperm production due to dysfunction at one or both levels of the hypothalamic-pituitary-testicular axis.

SYNONYM

Testicular dysfunction

ICD-10CM CODES
E23.0 Hypopituitarism
E23.1 Drug-induced hypopituitarism
E29   Testicular dysfunction
E29.1 Testicular hypofunction
E29.8 Other testicular dysfunction
E29.9 Testicular dysfunction, unspecified
E89.3 Postprocedural hypopituitarism

EPIDEMIOLOGY & DEMOGRAPHICS

INCIDENCE: Hypogonadism is the most common clinical disorder of the testis. Incidence is unclear due to the many possible underlying factors, nonspecificity of symptoms, and questions relating to the adequacy of a diagnostic serum total testosterone threshold.

PREVALENCE: Prevalence of hypogonadism increases with aging, obesity, diabetes mellitus, and other comorbidities. The average decrease in serum total testosterone levels in aging men is 1% to 2% per yr. Prevalence rises to 23% among men in their 70s. However, in population-based surveys of community-dwelling middle-aged and older males, prevalence of hypogonadism is approximately 6%.

RISK FACTORS: These are many and include genetic abnormalities; the aging process; pituitary and testicular lesions and disorders; medications; drug abuse; HIV disease; acute illnesses; chronic cardiac, hepatic, renal, and pulmonary diseases; cancer; ionizing radiation; chemotherapy; obesity; and malnutrition.

GENETICS: Genetic abnormalities underlie a number of hypogonadal disorders including Klinefelter syndrome, Noonan syndrome, hemochromatosis, Kallmann syndrome, and Prader-Willi syndrome.

PHYSICAL FINDINGS & CLINICAL PRESENTATION

Sexual (Specific):
- Decrease in frequency of erections
- Erectile dysfunction
- Decrease in libido
- Decreased fertility
- Small or shrinking testes
- Gynecomastia
- Diminished sexual hair
- Hot flushes and sweats

Neuropsychologic (Less Specific):
- Depression
- Inability to concentrate
- Diminished motivation and vitality
- Decrease in self-confidence
- Diminished energy and stamina

- Sleep disturbances

Physical Features and Findings:
- Diminished capacity for physical activity
- Decrease in physical endurance and performance
- Diminished muscle mass and strength
- Increase in body fat
- Decrease or loss of axillary and pubic hair and decrease in shaving frequency
- Fine wrinkling over the lateral aspects of the face
- Breast enlargement with or without tenderness
- Change in consistency and decrease in size of testes

- Fragility fractures
- Anemia

ETIOLOGY

- The importance of a careful history and examination cannot be overstated to determine the etiology of possible hypogonadism. Primary hypogonadism is a result of a decrease in testicular testosterone secretion and/or a decrease in spermatogenesis with an associated increase in gonadotropin levels as in Klinefelter syndrome, cryptorchidism, and following orchitis, testicular trauma, chemotherapy, and irradiation. The causes of primary hypogonadism are summarized in Table 1.

TABLE 1 Causes of Primary Hypogonadism

Common Causes	Uncommon Causes
Androgen Deficiency and Impairment of Sperm Production	
Congenital or Developmental Disorders	
Klinefelter syndrome (XXY) and variants	Myotonic dystrophy
	Uncorrected cryptorchidism
	Noonan syndrome
	Bilateral congenital anorchia
	Polyglandular autoimmune syndrome
	Testosterone biosynthetic enzyme defects
	CAH (TART)
	Complex genetic syndromes
	Down syndrome
	LH receptor mutation
Acquired Disorders	
Bilateral surgical castration or trauma	Orchitis
Drugs (spironolactone, ketoconazole, abiraterone, enzalutamide, alcohol, chemotherapy agents)[a]	
Ionizing radiation	
Systemic Disorders	
Chronic liver disease (hepatic cirrhosis)[a,b]	Malignancy (lymphoma, testicular cancer)
Chronic kidney disease[a,b]	Sickle cell disease[b]
Aging[b]	Spinal cord injury
	Vasculitis (polyarteritis)
	Infiltrative disease (amyloidosis, leukemia)
Isolated Impairment of Sperm Production or Function	
Congenital or Developmental Disorders	
Cryptorchidism	Myotonic dystrophy
Varicocele	Sertoli cell–only syndrome
Y chromosome microdeletions	Primary ciliary dyskinesia
	Down syndrome
	FSH receptor mutation
Acquired Disorders	
Orchitis	Environmental toxins
Ionizing radiation	
Chemotherapy agents	
Thermal trauma	
Systemic Disorders	
Acute febrile illness	Spinal cord injury
Malignancy (testicular cancer, Hodgkin disease)[b]	
Idiopathic azoospermia or oligozoospermia	

[a]Functional causes that are potentially reversible with discontinuation of offending medication, or with liver or renal transplantation.
[b]Combined primary and secondary hypogonadism.
CAH, Congenital adrenal hyperplasia; *FSH,* follicle-stimulating hormone; *LH,* luteinizing hormone; *TART,* testicular adrenal rest tumor.
From Melmed S et al: *Williams textbook of endocrinology,* ed 14, Philadelphia, 2019, Elsevier.

- Secondary hypogonadism is due to hypothalamic-pituitary dysfunction, which results in a decrease in testosterone levels and/or spermatogenesis with gonadotropin levels that are subnormal or inappropriately within the normal range. Table 2 summarizes causes of secondary hypogonadism.

- Combined primary and secondary hypogonadism is a result of deficits at both the level of the hypothalamic-pituitary axis and testes with variable gonadotropin levels depending upon the predominance of the level of the defect.

TABLE 2 Causes of Secondary Hypogonadism

Common Causes	Uncommon Causes
Androgen Deficiency and Impairment of Sperm Production	
Congenital or Developmental Disorders	
Constitutional delayed puberty	CHH due to genetic mutations
Hemochromatosis	CHH, idiopathic (IHH)
	Kallmann syndrome
	Congenital adrenal hypoplasia
	Isolated LH deficiency, LHβ mutations
	Complex genetic syndromes
Acquired Disorders	
Hyperprolactinemia[a]	Hypopituitarism
Opioids[a]	
Androgenic anabolic steroids, progestins, estrogen excess[a]	
GnRH agonist or antagonist[a]	
	Pituitary or hypothalamic tumor
	Surgical hypophysectomy, pituitary or cranial irradiation
	Vascular compromise, traumatic brain injury
	Granulomatous or infiltrative disease
	Infection
	Pituitary stalk disease
	Lymphocytic or autoimmune hypophysitis
	Acquired IHH
Systemic Disorders	
Glucocorticoid excess (Cushing syndrome)[a,b]	Chronic systemic illness[a,b]
Chronic organ failure[a,b]	Spinal cord injury
Chronic liver disease (hepatic cirrhosis), chronic kidney disease, chronic lung disease, chronic heart failure[a]	Transfusion-related iron overload (β-thalassemia)[a]
Chronic systemic illness[a,b]	Sickle cell disease
Type 2 diabetes mellitus[a]	Cystic fibrosis
Malignancy[a]	
Rheumatic disease (rheumatoid arthritis)[a]	
HIV disease[a]	
Starvation,[b] malnutrition,[b] eating disorders, endurance exercise[a]	
Morbid obesity, obstructive sleep apnea[a]	
Acute and critical illness[a]	
Aging (comorbid illnesses associated with aging)[a,b]	
Isolated Impairment of Sperm Production or Function	
Congenital or Developmental Disorders	
	Congenital adrenal hyperplasia (21-hydroxylase deficiency, 11β-hydroxylase deficiency)
	Isolated FSH deficiency, FSHβ mutations
Acquired Disorders	
Testosterone, androgenic anabolic steroids	Androgen- or hCG-secreting tumors
Malignancy (Hodgkin disease, testicular cancer)[b]	Hyperprolactinemia

[a]Functional causes that are potentially reversible or treatable with discontinuation of offending medication, treatment of underlying cause of gonadotropin suppression or organ transplantation.
[b]Combined primary and secondary hypogonadism.
CHH, Congenital hypogonadotropic hypogonadism; *FSH,* follicle-stimulating hormone; *GnRH,* gonadotropin-releasing hormone; *hCG,* human chorionic gonadotropin; *HIV,* human immunodeficiency virus; *IHH,* idiopathic hypogonadotropic hypogonadism; *LH,* luteinizing hormone.
From Melmed S et al: *Williams textbook of endocrinology,* ed 14, Philadelphia, 2019, Elsevier.

🅓🅧 DIAGNOSIS (FIG. 1)

DIFFERENTIAL DIAGNOSIS

Hypogonadotropic or Secondary Hypogonadism:
- Pituitary dysfunction: Hypopituitarism, functioning or nonfunctioning pituitary tumor, lymphocytic hypophysitis, infiltrative disease as with sarcoidosis, hemochromatosis, and histiocytosis X
- Hyperprolactinemia: Prolactinoma, medication-related, chronic kidney disease
- Genetic: Kallmann syndrome with anosmia, Prader-Willi syndrome with morbid obesity
- Acute and chronic illnesses; malnutrition; emotional disorders; HIV; sleep apnea; aging; malignancies; obesity; and renal, hepatic, pulmonary, and cardiac diseases
- Opioids, central nervous system (CNS): Active medications, glucocorticoid excess, and GnRH analogues (androgen deprivation therapy)

Hypergonadotropic or Primary Hypogonadism:
- Genetic: Klinefelter syndrome, Noonan syndrome, myotonic dystrophy
- Gonadal damage due to drugs, alcohol, radiation, chemotherapy, trauma
- Congenital anorchia (vanishing testis syndrome)
- Cryptorchidism
- Mumps orchitis, HIV orchitis
- Diabetes mellitus
- Hodgkin disease
- Aging

Combined primary and Secondary Hypogonadism:
- Hemochromatosis, sickle cell disease, thalassemia
- Alcoholism, glucocorticoid therapy, aging
- Chronic cardiac, hepatic, renal, pulmonary diseases, and HIV disease

WORKUP

- Determine the presence or absence of male hypogonadism on the basis of history, clinical manifestations and findings, and documentation of consistently low serum total testosterone levels and/or abnormal seminal fluid analysis.
- Morning serum total testosterone levels should be measured on at least two or three occasions for confirmation of diagnosis and when necessary followed by measurement of serum free or bioavailable testosterone.
- Serum follicle-stimulating hormone (FSH) and luteinizing hormone (LH) levels are measured to determine whether hypogonadism is primary, secondary, or a result of combined defects of the hypothalamic-pituitary axis and testis. The cause of testosterone deficiency should be definitively determined before initiation of testosterone replacement therapy.
- Hormonal assessment of gonadal status should not be done during an acute or subacute illness.

LABORATORY TESTS

- Serum total testosterone is tightly bound to sex hormone binding globulin (SHBG) and weakly bound to circulating albumin. 0.5% to 3% of serum total testosterone is unbound or free.

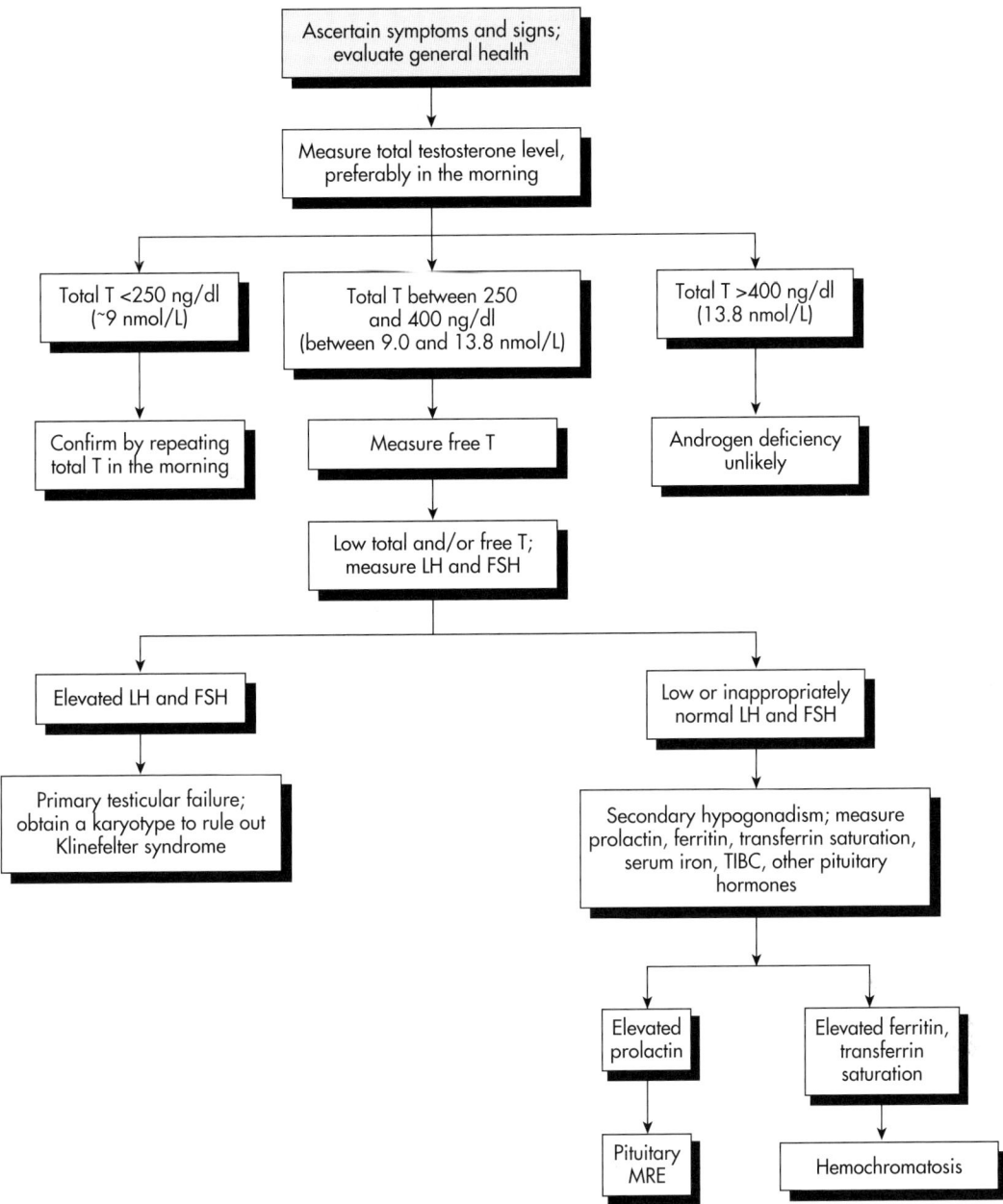

FIG. 1 Algorithm showing an approach for the diagnostic evaluation of adult men suspected of having androgen deficiency. *FSH,* Follicle-stimulating hormone; *LH,* luteinizing hormone; *MRE,* magnetic resonance elastography; *T,* testosterone; *TIBC,* total iron-binding capacity. (From Shalender B, Shehzad B: Diagnosis and treatment of hypogonadism in men, *Best Pract Res Clin Endocrin* 25:251-270, 2011.)

- Liquid chromatography tandem mass spectrometry assays for total serum testosterone are more accurate than immunoassays.
- Bioavailable testosterone refers to unbound testosterone plus the testosterone that is loosely bound to albumin.
- Free testosterone, if necessary, is best measured by equilibrium dialysis or centrifugal ultrafiltration.
- An SHBG measurement is helpful in determining the adequacy or normality of a serum total testosterone measurement. Conditions that lower SHBG include obesity, protein-losing states, androgens, hypothyroidism, and familial SHBG deficiency. Increases in SHBG occur in those with hyperthyroidism,

hepatitis, cirrhosis, and HIV disease, aging, and by estrogens.
- The lower limit of normal for serum total testosterone in a healthy young male is approximately 240 to 950 ng/dl and a low-normal serum free testosterone in a young normal male is 5 to 20 ng/dl. Serum total testosterone in a healthy young male ranges from 300 to 1000 ng/dl and normal free testosterone ranges from 5 to 20 ng/dl.
- Serum total testosterone levels can vary from day to day, and there is a diurnal rhythm in young normal males with morning levels that are higher by approximately 20% to 25% as compared with levels in the afternoon.

- In elderly males, the diurnal rhythm is diminished with levels approximately 10% lower in the afternoon as compared with morning levels.
- Serum FSH and LH measurements are important in delineating primary, secondary, and combined hypogonadism.
- Hypogonadal symptoms are more likely to be seen in those with total serum testosterone levels of less than 230 ng/dl for young normal males. Serum total testosterone levels of <150 ng/dl are unequivocally low.
- Transient suppression of total serum testosterone may occur during acute illness, in males that are being treated with glucocorticoid, in those taking opiates or CNS-active medications, in those with malnutrition or

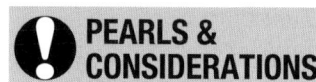

poor eating habits, and during excessive physical exercise.

- Quantity and quality of sperm counts and activity can vary in a significant way for a variety of reasons. Therefore, in assessing fertility, seminal fluid analysis should be done on two or more occasions, each separated by 2 or more wk, and on semen collected within an hour of ejaculation after more than 2 days of abstinence.
- Depending on the clinical picture and examination, other studies may be necessary, including a karyotype analysis, for example, for Klinefelter syndrome, or serum prolactin measurement for patients with possible hyperprolactinemia, which may be drug-induced, related to a prolactinoma, or to chronic renal disease.

IMAGING STUDIES

In males with severe androgen deficiency with low serum gonadotropin levels, increased serum prolactin levels, hypopituitarism, severe headaches, and visual defects, an MRI of the pituitary would be appropriate. In males with hypogonadism and a history of fractures, dual energy x-ray absorptiometry measurements of spine and hip should be obtained to further delineate the status of the skeletal system.

Rx TREATMENT

Testosterone replacement therapy is indicated when patients have symptoms and signs of hypogonadism and serum testosterone levels that are consistently subnormal with levels of <250 ng/dl. The goal of replacement therapy is to restore serum testosterone levels to within the normal range of values and to have a positive effect on the constellation of hypogonadal symptoms and signs. Subnormal spermatogenesis, if present in such patients, is not affected by testosterone therapy. In patients with hypogonadotropic or secondary hypogonadism, chorionic gonadotropin and/or GnRH therapy can optimize spermatogenesis, whereas, generally in patients with primary hypogonadism, subnormal spermatogenesis and infertility are irreversible. The treatment of adult male hypogonadism is summarized in Table 3.

NONPHARMACOLOGIC THERAPY

- Weight reduction, especially when it appears to be a major factor underlying male hypogonadism
- Discontinuation of anabolic steroids, CNS-active medications, and narcotic abuse
- Surgery or radiation therapy for patients with a pituitary functioning or nonfunctioning tumor with visual field abnormality and headaches who are not candidates for further medical therapy or have been unsuccessfully treated with medication
- Surgery indicated for chronic gynecomastia and, occasionally, in cases with recent-onset gynecomastia that has not responded to testosterone replacement therapy

CHRONIC Rx

Testosterone formulations:

- Parenteral testosterone preparations: Testosterone enanthate (generic) and testosterone cypionate (Depo-Testosterone and generic) 150 to 200 mg are injected intramuscularly every 2 wk. Following injections, there are appreciable fluctuations in serum testosterone, with levels rising within the first several days and a subsequent decrease to normal and in some cases to below normal at the end of the 2 wk. As a result of the varying levels of testosterone, patients may have related symptoms. Adjustments in dose and dosing interval may help to alleviate the serum fluctuations and clinical symptoms. Testosterone undecanoate (AUEFD-ENDO) is an injectable depot formulation FDA-approved for male hypogonadism. The recommended dosage is 750 mg injected intramuscularly at 0 and 4 wk, and then every 10 wk thereafter.
- Topical testosterone preparations:
  1. Testosterone adhesive patch (Androderm) delivers 2.5 or 5 mg of testosterone when applied nightly to the back, abdomen, upper arms, or thighs. Serum testosterone levels rise to within normal range in a few hours after application and, thereafter, are relatively stable. Daily doses of up to 10 mg may be necessary.
  2. Testosterone 1% gels (AndroGel and Testim). AndroGel is available in 2.5 g and 5 g gel units that deliver 2.5 mg and 5 mg of testosterone, respectively. The gel is applied daily in the morning by hand over the shoulder, upper arms, or abdomen. Adjustments in dose to 7.5 g or 10 g of gel may be necessary to optimize serum testosterone levels. AndroGel (1.62%) pump is also available for daily application. Testim is available in 5-g and 10-g tubes and with morning applications over the shoulders or arms delivers 5 mg and 10 mg of testosterone, respectively. Both AndroGel and Testim provide relatively stable serum testosterone levels. Two new transdermal formulations, Fortesta and Axiron, are now available and are applied daily by metered dose pumps. With these preparations, care is necessary to avoid skin-to-skin contact exposure with others.
- Testosterone pellets: 3 to 6 pellets of testosterone each containing 75 mg of testosterone are surgically inserted subcutaneously every 3 to 6 mo and provide relatively stable serum testosterone levels.
- Testosterone undecanoate (Jatenzo) is an oral testosterone formulation approved for patients with hypogonadism associated with structural or genetic etiologies, and it is not indicated in men with age-related hypogonadism.

RISKS & ADVERSE EFFECTS

- Contraindications to testosterone therapy include prostate cancer, breast cancer, chronic obstructive pulmonary disease, untreated obstructive sleep apnea, congestive heart failure, and polycythemia. Relative contraindications include severe benign prostatic

hyperplasia, hematocrit ≥50% at baseline, sleep apnea, and severe congestive heart failure.
- Patients on chronic testosterone therapy need to be followed carefully with prostate and prostate-specific antigen assessments and hematocrit measurements for possible excessive induction of erythrocytosis, initially at 3 to 6 mo and at regular intervals thereafter. Table 4 summarizes monitoring during testosterone treatment.
- Current testosterone use for 6 mo or shorter is associated with 63% higher risk for venous thromboembolism (VTE). VTE risk peaks during the first 6 mo and declines to 25% thereafter.

REFERRAL

Endocrinology for full endocrine and metabolic assessment and therapy. Urology for further assessment and follow-up of the prostate and for evaluation and therapy of erectile dysfunction. Neurosurgery for evaluation and possible surgery for a pituitary lesion. Plastic surgery for chronic gynecomastia. Reproductive endocrinology for those with an infertility problem.

❶ PEARLS & CONSIDERATIONS

COMMENTS

- Do not screen men "routinely" for hypogonadism. Screening men with nonspecific symptoms of hypogonadism (e.g., decreased energy) is also not recommended. Screening should be limited to men with specific signs and symptoms of hypogonadism.
- Male hypogonadism is an important and frequently encountered problem that requires a complete medical history, examination, and hormonal assessment to determine whether a patient has hypogonadism and requires testosterone replacement therapy. Treated patients need to be seen on a regular basis to avoid possible testosterone adverse effects. Patients requiring testosterone replacement should have testosterone, prostate specific antigen, and hematocrit levels monitored.
- Trials to evaluate the effects of testosterone treatment in older men revealed that in symptomatic men 65 yr of age or older, raising testosterone concentrations for 1 yr from moderately low to the mid-normal range had a moderate benefit with respect to sexual function and some benefit with respect to mood and depressive symptoms but no benefit with respect to vitality or walking distance.
- Controversy exists regarding the safety of testosterone replacement therapy following reports of increased risk of cardiovascular events. However, a recent trial among men with androgen deficiency dispensed testosterone prescriptions revealed lower risk of cardiovascular outcomes over a median follow-up of 3.4 yr.
- Clinical trials have also demonstrated that testosterone replacement in men with low testosterone increases volumetric bone mineral density and estimated bone strength more in trabecular than peripheral bone and more in the spine than the hip.

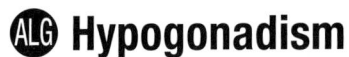

TABLE 3 Treatment of Adult Male Hypogonadism

Formulation	Dosage	Advantages	Disadvantages
Treatment of Androgen Deficiency			
Formulations Available in the United States			
Parenteral Testosterone Esters			
Testosterone enanthate or cypionate, IM injections	*Adults:* 150-200 mg IM every 2 wk or 75-100 mg IM every wk 50 mg, 75 mg, or 100 mg SC by autoinjector *Prepubertal boys:* 50-100 mg monthly or 25-50 mg every 2 wk, increasing to 50-100 mg every 2 wk and then to adult replacement dosage over 2-4 yr or until spontaneous pubertal development occurs	Extensive clinical use Inexpensive with self-injection Some dose flexibility	IM injections, discomfort Symptomatic fluctuation of T concentrations (supraphysiologic after injection to low normal or low before next injection) Frequent IM injections to reduce fluctuations of T concentrations More erythrocytosis than with transdermal T
Testosterone undecanoate, IM injections	750 mg at 0 and 4 wk, then every 10 wk	Less frequent IM injections Maintenance of normal T concentrations for a longer duration No apparent fluctuations in symptoms	REMS: Slow, deep IM injection in clinic (no self-injection); 30-min observation for potential POME and anaphylaxis IM injections, discomfort Large-volume injection (3 ml) Self-injection not possible Rarely, cough immediately after injection Prolonged maintenance of T level after discontinuation if adverse effects develop
Transdermal Testosterone			
Testosterone patch (nonscrotal)	2 or 4 mg (one patch) or 6 mg (one 2-mg plus one 4-mg patch) applied daily over nonpressure areas	Low- to mid-normal physiologic T concentrations Mimics normal circadian variation when applied nightly No injections Less erythrocytosis than with parenteral T Rapid withdrawal of T replacement if adverse effects occur	Frequent skin irritation Low-normal T concentrations: Two patches may be needed Skin adhesion poor with excessive sweating Daily application More expensive than parenteral T
Testosterone gels and solution	*1% T gel:* 5-10 g of gel (containing 50-100 mg of T) applied daily over shoulders or upper arms; available in foil sachets of 2.5 or 5.0 g (containing 25 or 50 mg of T, respectively), or a tube of 5 g (containing 50 mg of T) *1.62% T gel:* 20.25-81.00 mg (containing 20.25-81.00 mg of T) applied daily to shoulders or upper arms; available in 20.25- and 40.50-mg packets (containing 20.25 and 40.50 mg of T, respectively) or metered-dose pump delivering 12.5 mg per pump depression *2% gel:* 40-70 mg (containing 40-70 mg of T) applied daily to inner thighs; available in a metered-dose pump delivering 10 mg per pump depression *2% solution:* 30-120 mg applied to underarms; available in a metered-dose pump applicator delivering 30 mg per pump depression	Low- to high-normal steady-state physiologic T concentrations No injections Little skin irritation Dose flexibility Rapid withdrawal of T replacement if adverse effects occur For 1.62% or 2% gel: Less gel amount in more concentrated formulations Less gel amount in more concentrated formulations For 2% solution: Absorption of solution not affected by deodorant or antiperspirant Absorption of solution not affected by deodorant or antiperspirant	Potential for contact transfer of T to women or children Daily application More expensive than parenteral T, especially with higher doses Moderately high DHT concentrations One formulation has a musk odor and another is associated with stickiness or skin dryness Slight skin irritation in some men Solution may drip under arms
Transbuccal testosterone	30-mg tablet applied between cheek and gum two times daily	Mid-normal steady-state physiologic T concentrations No injections, patch or gel application, or their associated disadvantages Rapid withdrawal of T replacement if adverse effects occur	Twice-daily application Gum irritation or inflammation Altered or bitter taste High learning curve for proper application; requires careful instruction or poor acceptability occurs Tablets may be difficult to remove or may fall off prematurely No dose flexibility Moderately high DHT concentrations More expensive than parenteral T

Continued

TABLE 3 Treatment of Adult Male Hypogonadism—cont'd

Formulation	Dosage	Advantages	Disadvantages
Testosterone nasal gel	11 mg (delivering 1.1 mg of T) three times daily (every 6-8 hr) for a total daily dose of 33 mg (delivering 3.3 mg of T) daily Available in a metered-dose pump that delivers 5.5 mg (delivering 0.55 mg of T) per pump depression	No injections No interaction with sympathomimetic nasal decongestants	Thrice-daily administration Learning curve for proper administration Fluctuation in T concentrations from lower- to upper-normal range after administration No nose blowing or sniffing for 1 hr after administration Discontinue with severe rhinitis Nasal irritation Not recommended with other intranasal drugs or chronic nasal conditions
Testosterone pellets	2-6 pellets (each 3.2 mm diameter × 9 mm in length pellet containing 75 mg of T, for a total of 150-450 mg of T delivered) implanted SC every 3-6 mo (usually 3-4 mo)	Maintenance of normal T concentrations for a longer duration	Requires surgical incision Extrusion, bleeding, and infection can occur uncommonly Large number of pellets Not easily removed; fibrosis may occur Lack of ability for rapid withdrawal of T replacement if adverse effects occur Infrequent use
Oral testosterone undecanoate	40-80 mg PO with meals twice a day to three times daily	Oral administration is convenient for many	Twice- or thrice-daily administration Variable T concentrations and clinical responses Requires administration with meal High DHT concentrations

Testosterone Formulations Available Outside the United States

Formulation	Dosage	Advantages	Disadvantages
Testosterone-in-adhesive matrix patch	Two patches (delivering 4.8 mg of T per day) applied every 2 days	Low- to mid-normal physiologic T concentrations Duration 2 days No injections	Some skin irritation Two patches needed

Treatment to Initiate and Maintain Sperm Production in Men with Hypogonadotropic Hypogonadism

Initially to Stimulate Testosterone and Potentially Sperm Production

Formulation	Dosage	Advantages	Disadvantages
hCG	500-2000 IU given SC two to three times weekly to maintain serum T concentrations within the normal range for 6-12 mo	Effective in stimulating endogenous T production In men with acquired and some men with partial congenital hypogonadotropic hypogonadism, sperm production may be stimulated with hCG treatment alone SC injections easier than IM injections (smaller needle, injection not as deep) Less fluctuation in T concentrations compared with IM T ester injections No injection, patch, or buccal tablet	Injections two to three times weekly Expensive Higher doses needed in men with concomitant primary testicular disease (e.g., cryptorchidism) Breast tenderness or gynecomastia secondary to high estradiol production by testes May require dilution Occasional burning sensation with injection Ineffective in primary hypogonadism

Added to hCG to Stimulate Sperm Production

Formulation	Dosage	Advantages	Disadvantages
FSH Human menopausal gonadotropin, human FSH, or recombinant human FSH	After 6-12 mo of hCG treatment alone resulting in normal T concentrations, add FSH 75-300 IU given SC three times weekly for an additional 6-12 mo or longer	Effective in stimulating sperm production in men with hypogonadotropic hypogonadism	Injections three times weekly Extremely expensive, prohibitive cost for most Breast tenderness or gynecomastia secondary to high estradiol production by testes May require dilution Occasional burning sensation with injection In men with concomitant primary testicular disease (e.g., cryptorchidism), stimulation of spermatogenesis is not likely

To Stimulate Testosterone and Sperm Production

Formulation	Dosage	Advantages	Disadvantages
GnRH	5-25 ng/kg SC every 2 hr by programmable infusion pump for 6-12 mo	Effective in stimulating both endogenous T and sperm production	GnRH not readily available Requires pump use and management, usually in a specialized center Expensive Infrequently used except at certain sites Rarely, local irritation, infection

DHT, Dihydrotestosterone; *FSH*, follicle-stimulating hormone; *GnRH*, gonadotropin-releasing hormone; *hCG*, human chorionic gonadotropin; *IM*, intramuscular; *PO*, orally; *POME*, potential pulmonary oil microembolism; *REMS*, Risk Evaluation and Mitigation Strategy; *SC*, subcutaneous; *T*, testosterone.
From Melmed S et al: *Williams textbook of endocrinology*, ed 14, Philadelphia, 2019, Elsevier.

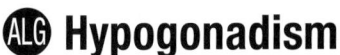

TABLE 4 Monitoring During Testosterone Treatment

Parameter	Timing	Further Management
Measures of Efficacy		
Symptoms and signs of androgen deficiency	At baseline, after 3-12 mo, and then yearly	Continue testosterone treatment in men with clinical improvement and no adverse effects. Consider discontinuing testosterone treatment in men if no clinical improvement.
BMD	For men at high risk for fracture, BMD before treatment; for men with osteoporosis or minimal-trauma fracture, BMD after 1-2 yr	Institute appropriate treatment for men with osteoporosis, including calcium and vitamin D.
Serum testosterone	*Testosterone ester injection:* After 3-6 mo, measured midway between injections or at end of dosing interval (if androgen deficiency symptoms are present at that time) *Testosterone patch:* After 3-4 wk, at 8-10 hr after application *Testosterone gel:* After 2 wk, at any time after application *Buccal testosterone:* After 4-6 wk, at any time after application (preferably in the morning) *Testosterone pellets:* At end of dosing interval *Oral testosterone undecanoate:* After 1 wk, at 3-5 hr after oral dose *Testosterone undecanoate injection:* At end of dosing interval	Adjust dose or dosing interval to achieve serum testosterone concentrations in the mid-normal range.
Adverse Effects		
Hematocrit	At baseline, after 3-6 mo, and then yearly	If hematocrit is >54%, stop or reduce dosage of testosterone until hematocrit declines to normal and reinitiate testosterone at a lower dosage. Investigate for a hypoxic condition such as obstructive sleep apnea or chronic lung disease.
PSA level, with or without DRE (using shared decision making, i.e., if a patient desires prostate cancer screening after discussion of risks and benefits of PSA screening and monitoring), in men >50 yr (>40 if risk factors for prostate cancer)	At baseline, after 3-6 mo, and then according to accepted guidelines	Urologic evaluation with any of the following: • Confirmed PSA >4 ng/ml any time during testosterone treatment • PSA increase >1.4 ng/ml within 12 mo of testosterone treatment • Palpable abnormality (nodule or induration) on DRE • Worsening of lower urinary tract symptoms (e.g., IPSS score >19)
Obstructive sleep apnea (snoring, witnessed apnea, daytime somnolence, unexplained erythrocytosis, worsening hypertension or edema)	At baseline, after 3-12 mo, and then yearly	Evaluate for obstructive sleep apnea or adjustment of CPAP settings. Evaluate for other causes of hypoxia.
Formulation-specific adverse effects	At baseline, after 3-6 mo, and then yearly	Discontinue and switch to another formulation.
Testosterone ester injections	Discomfort, bleeding, or hematoma with IM injections Fluctuations in energy, mood, libido Allergy to oil vehicle (rare)	Reinstruct on the self-injection site technique. Consider shortening the injection interval if the nadir testosterone level is low.
Testosterone patch	Skin irritation Adhesion to skin	Coadministration of corticosteroid cream may reduce skin irritation.
Testosterone gel	Contact transfer to others Skin dryness at site of application	Reinstruct on washing hands and covering application area after gel dries or showering 4-6 hr after application, avoiding prolonged skin-to-skin contact of application site with women and children.
Buccal testosterone tablets	Gum irritation or inflammation Poor adhesion to gums Altered or bitter taste	Reinstruct on proper application and reassure to complete an adequate trial with the correct technique.
SC testosterone pellets	Pellet extrusion Implantation-site infection, bleeding, fibrosis	Reimplant pellets. Treat infection with appropriate drainage and antibiotics.

BMD, Bone mineral density; *CPAP,* continuous positive airway pressure; *DRE,* digital rectal examination; *IM,* intramuscular; *IPSS,* International Prostate Symptom Score; *PSA,* prostate-specific antigen; *SC,* subcutaneous.
From Melmed S et al: *Williams textbook of endocrinology,* ed 14, Philadelphia, 2019, Elsevier.

SUGGESTED READINGS
Available at eBooks.Health.Elsevier.com.

AUTHOR: **JOSEPH R. TUCCI, MD, FACP, FACE**

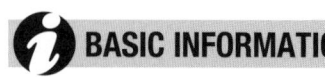

BASIC INFORMATION

DEFINITION

An osmole is a solute that attracts water across a semipermeable membrane. Tonicity or effective osmolality refers to the direction of water flux with plasma water as the referent solution. Net water flow into the central nervous system (CNS) from plasma is a hypotonic state and from the CNS to plasma is a hypertonic state. Solutes that rapidly equilibrate between intracellular fluid (ICF) and extracellular fluid (ECF) compartments are ineffective osmoles because no net water movement between compartments occurs.

Hyponatremia is defined as a measured plasma or serum sodium concentration (S_{Na}) less than the lower limit of normal (<130 to 135 mmol/L). Since clinical manifestations of hyponatremia are due to hypotonicity, appropriate clinical management depends on distinguishing the majority of patients with hypotonic hyponatremia from those who are hypertonic or isotonic. Isotonic hyponatremia, also known as pseudohyponatremia, is due solely to a laboratory artifact (vide infra). The reader should be aware that some textbooks still incorrectly use the term "pseudohyponatremia" to refer to hypertonic hyponatremia. Hyponatremia is used synonymously with hypotonic hyponatremia in this chapter. References to pseudohyponatremia and hypertonic hyponatremia are specifically identified by these terms.

SYNONYMS

Low serum sodium concentration
Hypo-osmolality

ICD–10CM CODE

E87.1 Hypo-osmolality and hyponatremia

EPIDEMIOLOGY & DEMOGRAPHICS

PREVALENCE: The prevalence of hyponatremia varies widely according to setting and population age. In the general U.S. population dataset of the National Health and Nutrition Examination Survey (NHANES), the overall prevalence was 1.72%.[1] One study of emergency department patients reported a prevalence of 2.3% in patients 16 to 21 yr old and 16.9% in patients >80 yr. Following surgery for traumatic hip fracture, the incidence of moderate (<135 mmol/L) and severe (<130 mmol/L) postoperative hyponatremia was 27% (95% CI, 21.7% to 32.5%) and 9% (95% CI, 5.7% to 12.8%), respectively. The prevalence was reported at approximately 8% in stable, older outpatients and 18% to 20% in sick or frail populations. The overall incidence at or during hospital admission is comparable. Higher rates are noted in patients admitted for congestive heart failure (CHF) or cirrhosis and in older adult patients admitted for fragility fractures.
PREDOMINANT SEX & AGE: Prevalence of hyponatremia was significantly higher in women in the NHANES dataset (2.09%; $P = 0.004$) and increased with age.[1]
RISK FACTORS: In NHANES, hyponatremia was more common in participants with hypertension,

diabetes, coronary artery disease, stroke, chronic obstructive pulmonary disease, cancer, and psychiatric disorders, and less common in participants with no comorbidities (1.04%; $P <0.001$).[1] A significant risk of death was associated with hyponatremia in unadjusted (hazard ratio [HR], 3.61; $P <0.001$) and adjusted Cox models (HR 2.43; $P <0.001$). The incidence in outpatients who were using thiazide diuretics was 15.1%, with a HR of 4.95 (95% CI, 4.12 to 5.96). Reported frequencies of hyponatremia in outpatients taking selective serotonin reuptake inhibitors or selective norepinephrine reuptake inhibitors varied widely, between 0.5% and 32%.
GENETICS: The hyponatremic disorder referred to as nephrogenic syndrome of inappropriate antidiuresis (SIAD), is caused by rare familial gain-of-function sequence variants of the V2 vasopressin receptor (V2R) gene. Activation of variant receptors located in the renal collecting duct produces overt hyponatremia in infancy.[2]

PHYSICAL FINDINGS & CLINICAL PRESENTATION

- Critical history includes detailed assessment of fluid consumption and diet, gastrointestinal and insensible losses of fluid and electrolytes, urine outputs, and changes in weight, medication use, and behavior or cognition. Recent medical procedures involving irrigation of tissue beds (e.g., transurethral prostatectomy or hysteroscopy with endometrial resection), participation in marathons or other strenuous endurance exercise, or attendance at "rave" parties where illicit use of 3,4-methylenedioxy-methamphetamine (MDMA, or ecstasy) is common should be noted.[3] Comorbid conditions that increase the risk of hyponatremia include malignancy, CNS or pulmonary disease, adrenal insufficiency, CHF, liver disease, and nephrotic syndrome.
- The etiology of hyponatremia may affect the clinical presentation directly and/or by its effect on the extracellular fluid volume (ECFV) and exchangeable Na (TB_{Na}). Hypovolemia and hypervolemia (respectively, decreased or increased total ECFV and TB_{Na}) are identified by conventional clinical criteria (including clinical exam demonstrating edema, ascites, and pulmonary congestion and hemodynamic variables) but specifically does not refer to intravascular volume. If available, vector bioimpedance analysis has been shown to further increase accuracy.[4] Specific manifestations of the precipitating cause or underlying diseases may be evident (e.g., fever and delirium following the use of MDMA, stigmata of alcoholism or malnutrition, fever and/or localizing symptoms related to pneumonia or other pulmonary disease, or headaches and visual field defects from an intracranial mass).
- Neurologic symptoms predominate as the direct clinical manifestations of hyponatremia, mainly due to astrocyte swelling. Compensatory processes that reduce cerebral edema by extrusion of electrolytes, amino acids, and carbohydrates from brain cells take 24 hr to become fully active and up to 7 days to reach completion. Therefore patients who develop

hyponatremia over less than 24 to 48 hr have the highest degree of brain swelling, the most severe neurologic symptoms, and greatest risk of permanent or fatal brain injury. Postpubertal, premenopausal women appear to undergo cerebral compensation more slowly, placing them at greater risk from acute hyponatremia.[5]
- Acute hyponatremia may result in nausea and malaise as S_{Na} approaches 130 mmol/L or less. Headache, lethargy, obtundation, neurogenic pulmonary edema, and/or seizures may occur when S_{Na} is <120 mmol/L. In the most severe cases, death from brain stem herniation can occur.[6]
- Chronic hyponatremia rarely presents with life-threatening clinical manifestations. However, subtler neurologic disturbances such as ataxia, short-term memory deficits, fatigue, lethargy, and nausea have been commonly reported. Muscular weakness and elevated creatine kinase and even rhabdomyolysis may occur. Chronic hyponatremia has also been associated with increased risk of falls, fractures, and osteoporosis in older patients. In addition, hyponatremia has been associated with increased risk of cardiovascular complications and mortality in a diverse group, including older outpatients, general hospital-admitted patients, and patients admitted for stroke, subarachnoid hemorrhage, CHF, cirrhosis, pneumonia, hip fracture, and liver transplantation.[7-9]

ETIOLOGY

- Hypotonic hyponatremia: The S_{Na} after correction for hyperglycemia (or the effects of exogenous effective osmoles such as mannitol or sorbitol) closely approximates the ratio of exchangeable total body cations (sodium and potassium, $TB_{Na} + TB_K$) to total body water (TBW).[10]
  1. Serum $[Na] = S_{Na} = (TB_{Nae} + TB_{Ke})/TBW$
  2. The term *exchangeable* means that sodium or potassium ions can easily enter or exit from their compartment(s), respectively, which are the ECF and ICF spaces. TB_{Na} is the main determinant of ECF volume, and TB_K is the principal determinant of ICF volume.
  3. Hypotonic hyponatremia results from a decrease of the numerator, increase of the denominator, or both.
- ECFV depletion (disproportionately greater decrease of TB_{Na} and/or TB_K than TBW)
  1. Gastrointestinal losses with intake of hypotonic fluids
  2. Renal losses (diuresis, tubulopathies) with intake of hypotonic fluid
  3. Cerebral salt wasting
- Normovolemic hyponatremia (normal ECFV and TB_{Na})[3]
  1. SIAD (see "Syndrome of Inappropriate Antidiuresis")
  2. Medications (thiazide diuretics, selective and nonselective serotonin reuptake inhibitors, narcotics, MDMA/ecstasy, carbamazepine, cyclophosphamide, nicotine,

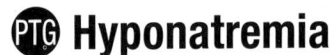
Diseases and Disorders

I

desmopressin, phenothiazines, terlipressin)
3. Pain, nausea, stress
4. Marathon running or other endurance exercise[11]
5. Primary polydipsia
6. Solute-limited water excretion (tea-and-toast diet, beer potomania)
7. Adrenal insufficiency
8. Reset osmostat
9. Severe potassium deficiency with normal total body sodium
- Hypervolemic hyponatremia (disproportionately greater increase in TBW than increased TB_{Na}) is associated with decreased effective arterial blood volume.
  1. Nephrotic syndrome
  2. Cirrhosis
  3. Congestive heart failure

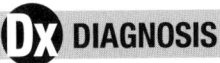 DIAGNOSIS

DIFFERENTIAL DIAGNOSIS

- **Pseudohyponatremia:** This is a laboratory artifact of decreasing prevalence and magnitude, rarely lowering falsely the S_{Na} by more than 5 mEq/L. Since it is an in vitro, not an in vivo phenomenon, no net water movement into the CNS occurs.[12] Serum osmolality is normal in pseudohyponatremia *only* if the other determinants of calculated serum osmolality are normal (i.e., serum concentrations of glucose and blood urea nitrogen [BUN]). Many clinicians misunderstand this and incorrectly diagnose pseudohyponatremia whenever they encounter low S_{Na} with "normal" serum osmolality (275 to 295 mOsm/L) as measured by freezing point depression with a low S_{Na}. By far, the most common cause for this situation is the combination of hypotonic hyponatremia with an elevated serum glucose or BUN. The more reliable method for diagnosing pseudohyponatremia is to calculate the serum osmolal gap, normally less than 10 mOsm/kg H_2O.
  1. Serum osmolal gap (mOsm/kg H2O) = Lab-measured S_{Osm} − Calculated-S_{Osm}
  2. Calculated-S_{Osm} = [2 × S_{Na} (mmol/L) + BUN (mg/dl)/2.8 + Glucose (mg/dl)/18 + Ethanol (mg/dl)/4.6]
  3. This calculated difference increases to abnormal values when the serum sodium used to compute calculated osmolality is artifactually low.
  4. Note that BUN and ethanol are ineffective osmoles that do not alter S_{Na}, while glucose is an effective osmole that shifts water from ICF to ECF and lowers S_{Na} by approximately 1.6 mEq/L for each increase of 100 mg/dl.
  5. Normally, the plasma solid (protein and lipid) phase occupies approximately 7% of plasma volume. S_{Na} is reported as milliequivalents (mEq) of sodium per liter of plasma. Consequently, certain pathologic conditions (severe hypertriglyceridemia, lipoprotein-X, and paraproteinemias) associated with an increased solid phase may artifactually reduce S_{Na} measurements

because the volume of water, and therefore the number of sodium ions per volume of plasma, is reduced, despite a normal concentration of sodium in plasma water. When pseudohyponatremia is suspected, measurement of S_{Na} by direct ion-selective electrode potentiometry of undiluted plasma (e.g., by blood gas analyzer), which measures plasma water sodium concentration, is recommended.[12]

- **Hypertonic hyponatremia:** Small solutes such as glucose (in absence of insulin), mannitol, and sorbitol accumulate to higher concentrations in the ECF than in the ICF and shift water from the ICF to the ECF compartment. Since the ICF has a very low sodium concentration (10 to 15 mmol/L), S_{Na} is diluted and hyponatremia occurs. With hyperglycemia, a decrease in S_{Na} of 1.6 mmol/L occurs for each increment of serum glucose of 100 mg/dl.[13]

WORKUP

- Fig. E1 illustrates the initial steps in the clinical approach to the patient with hyponatremia.
- A diagnostic approach to the patient with chronic hyponatremia is described in Fig. E2.
- A comprehensive history should include details of medication use, drug abuse, psychiatric disorders, exercise habits, prior S_{Na} measurements, diet, external fluid losses, volume and composition of oral and intravenous (IV) fluid intake, and any suggestion of disorders associated with hyponatremia (e.g., disorders of the lungs, CNS, heart, kidney, liver, or adrenal gland; malignancies; diabetes mellitus; nausea; vomiting; pain; or stress).
- Comprehensive physical examination including careful review of vital signs, weight, intake and outputs; evidence of increased ECFV (e.g., edema, ascites, pulmonary congestion, or pleural effusions), volume contraction, and evidence of comorbid diseases listed previously (e.g., abnormal pulmonary, neurologic or cardiovascular exam, or hepatomegaly).

LABORATORY TESTS

- Serum glucose to adjust for dilutional effect on S_{Na}
- Serum potassium: Potassium is the principal intracellular cation. Because S_{Na} = (TB_{Na} + TB_K)/TBW, decreases in TB_K lower S_K and S_{Na}.[10]
- Random urine osmolality and 24-hr urine volume: U_{osm} <100 mOsm/kg H_2O usually indicates appropriate suppression of antidiuretic hormone (ADH), suggesting diagnoses of solute-limited water excretion, primary polydipsia, or a reset osmostat (if S_{Na} is below the patient's altered setpoint). U_{osm} ≥100 mOsm/kg H_2O generally indicates that ADH is present. However, U_{osm} approximately 300 mOsm/kg is frequently encountered in patients using loop diuretics regardless of ADH level, and even higher osmolality can be seen during osmotic diuresis. The latter is characterized by total urine osmolar excretion >900 mOsm/day. However, in both cases urinary ([Na] +

[K]) equals approximately 60 to 90 mmol/L, resulting in significant electrolyte-free water (EFW) loss.
- Random urine sodium (U_{Na}), and urine potassium (U_K). U_{Na} <20 mmol/L: Stimulation of the renin angiotensin aldosterone system due to decreased ECFV or decreased effective arterial blood volume. Urine potassium losses should be calculated replaced during therapy.
- Specific testing for comorbid diseases listed previously as clinically indicated (e.g., fasting morning cosyntropin-stimulated serum cortisol level and brain natriuretic peptide).

IMAGING STUDIES

Not routinely required. Computed tomography or magnetic resonance imaging may be indicated in the presence of specific symptoms, a diagnosis of an associated etiology, or an evaluation of an associated delirium coincident with acute hyponatremia.

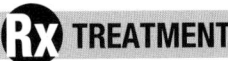 TREATMENT

NONPHARMACOLOGIC THERAPY

Hyponatremic patients excrete less EFW than they ingest or receive. Moderate fluid restriction (10 to 15 ml/kg) is indicated while patients are hyponatremic, especially if EFW excretion remains impaired. Diets high in protein, sodium, and potassium increase urine osmolar load and increase free water excretion.

ACUTE GENERAL Rx

- Acute (hypotonic) hyponatremia is defined as developing in less than 48 hr. Changes in brain cell volume in patients with hyponatremia are illustrated in Fig. E3. Acute hyponatremia results in larger increases in brain water content than equivalent changes in S_{Na} due to lack of brain cell adaptation to hypotonicity. Consequently, correction of acute hyponatremia is a medical emergency and mandates an increase in S_{Na} of 4 to 6 mmol/L within the initial 1 to 3 hr of therapy, depending on severity of symptoms and acuity of S_{Na} elevation. Iatrogenic cases, classically children or premenopausal women receiving perioperative hypotonic fluids, are fortunately rare now. These circumstances can present with headache or nausea prior to the onset of severe symptoms and require emergent correction (Fig. 4). Acute hyponatremia is rare in patients with high ECFV.
- Controlled increases of S_{Na} at a rapid rate nearly always require hypertonic saline: Recommended rate of correction in severe acute hyponatremia is an increase in S_{Na} of 4 to 6 mmol/L in the first hour. Consultation with a nephrologist or other expert clinician in the management of severe acute hyponatremia should be undertaken. In normovolemic patients, furosemide 20 to 40 mg IV may be used concurrently with hypertonic saline to prevent complications of acute ECFV expansion, although the additional loss of EFW may result in more rapid increases in S_{Na}.
- Regardless of type of treatment, acute hyponatremia requires monitoring in an intensive

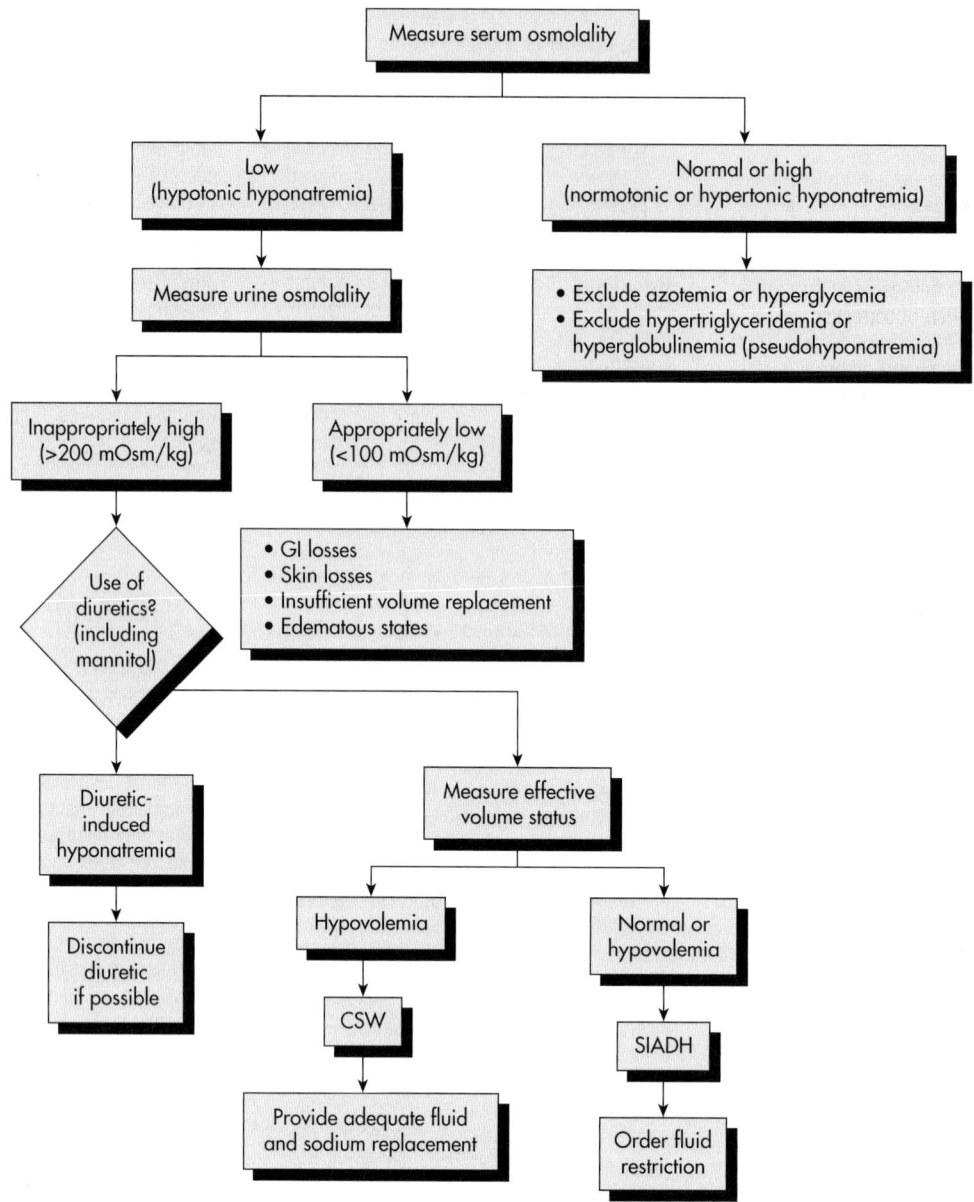

FIG. 4 Algorithm for the diagnosis and management of hyponatremia in critically ill neurologic patients. *CSW,* Cerebral salt-wasting; *GI,* gastrointestinal; *SIADH,* syndrome of inappropriate secretion of antidiuretic hormone. (From Jankovic J et al: *Bradley and Daroff's neurology in clinical practice,* ed 8, Philadelphia, 2022, Elsevier.)

care setting with frequent measurements of S_{Na}, urine volume, and U_{osm} until patients are neurologically stable and S_{Na} approaches the lower normal range.

CHRONIC Rx

- Chronic hyponatremia develops over 48 h or more: Prevention of cerebral edema occurs via adaptive loss of intracellular electrolytes and organic osmolytes (i.e., beta taurine, myoinositol, and others). Consequently, the risk for cerebral edema is minimized while the risk of overly rapid correction of the S_{Na} increases. Precipitous increases of the S_{Na} can result in osmotic demyelination syndrome.[14] A recommended target for correction of hyponatremia in this setting is 6 to 8 mmol/L per day.[7-9]
- Hypovolemia with chronic hyponatremia: Usual clinical practice is administration of

0.9% saline to restore ECFV. The direct effect of isotonic solutions on S_{Na} is negligible. However, eventual reestablishment of euvolemia can be expected to suppress ADH and may trigger rapid increases in S_{Na} accompanied by high urinary EFW loss, at which point administration of desmopressin (DDAVP) may prevent overly rapid correction of chronic hyponatremia.[15,16] Regardless of volume status, administration of DDAVP with quantitatively determined volumes of D_5W to lower S_{Na} back to safe concentrations following overly rapid correction has been shown to prevent or reverse osmotic demyelination syndrome.[17]
- Overcorrection of S_{Na}: Risk of overly rapid correction is greatest for hyponatremic patients with low solute intake (tea-and-toast diets or beer potomania). These patients have U_{osm} <100 mOsm/kg H_2O with ADH

suppression. Reflex administration of IV saline is contraindicated: 1 L of IV 0.9% saline (308 mOsm/L) supplies an osmolar load sufficient for excretion in 3 to 6 L of hypotonic urine in the absence of ADH. The preferred treatment of this situation is fluid restriction and dietary supplementation to supply appropriate quantities of protein and electrolytes. If needed, small quantities of 0.9% saline can be given quantitatively to augment oral intake. If rapid urinary water loss occurs during treatment of hyponatremia (i.e., >200 ml/h for 2 or more h), urine output may be therapeutically blunted by DDAVP to prevent overcorrection of S_{Na}.
- The treatment of normovolemic patients is covered in detail in the "Syndrome of Inappropriate Antidiuresis" and is only briefly reviewed here.[2] The goal of therapy in these patients is to reduce TBW in a controlled

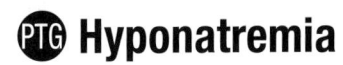

fashion maintaining TB_{Na} and TB_K. Some patients with chronic normovolemic hyponatremia (e.g., drug-induced etiologies or primary polydipsia) have self-limited abnormalities and primarily require monitoring to prevent excessively rapid correction. Active therapy as described later can be started to shorten the hospital stay or if the offending drug cannot be discontinued. If required, DDAVP can be administered intermittently to temporarily block further losses of free water to slow the overall rate of correction. If overcorrection occurs, oral and/or IV hypotonic fluids may be quantitatively administered to actively lower the serum sodium actively.[14-16] Other disorders may only slowly resolve the condition and require more active therapy as delineated in "Syndrome of Inappropriate Antidiuresis," consisting of either a direct V2 receptor antagonist or a loop diuretic combined with replacement of electrolytes lost during diuresis.

DISPOSITION
- Patients with symptomatic or severe hyponatremia require monitoring in an intensive care unit setting until the S_{Na} is stabilized at a safe level. Periodic monitoring of serum sodium, urine volume, and urine osmolality and electrolytes is required, with adjustments in therapy as outlined previously as needed.
- Potential contributing causes should be evaluated and treated appropriately.
- Risk of recurrence depends primarily on the nature of the underlying disorders present. Hypovolemic hyponatremia (e.g., diarrhea- or diuretic-induced electrolyte and water losses) or drug-induced SIAD generally do not recur if the offending medication is discontinued or if

gastrointestinal losses are not chronic. Older patients with solute-limited diuresis due to low electrolyte and protein intake may be resistant to major changes in diet. However, the oral administration of NaCl tablets and/or protein supplements may be salutary.[18] Oral urea (available in the U.S. as a "medical food supplement") has been successfully used as therapy, but should be initiated in collaboration with a nephrologist or endocrinologist.[19] In addition to disease-specific management, incurable conditions (e.g., chronic CNS or pulmonary disease, CHF, or cirrhosis) may require lifelong fluid restriction (10 to 15 ml/kg/day), high protein and electrolyte diets as tolerated, and periodic monitoring of the S_{Na} to reduce the risk of recurrent hyponatremia.

REFERRAL
- Referral to specialists in nephrology, endocrinology, and/or critical care medicine are recommended in cases of severe or symptomatic hyponatremia. Expertise is required to establish appropriate rates of correction of S_{Na} and monitor and adjust therapeutic regimens to achieve target S_{Na}.
- Outpatient referral to nephrology or endocrinology may be required to facilitate the treatment of patients with mild, chronic, or recurrent hyponatremia.

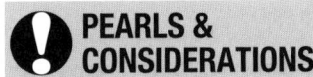

COMMENTS
PREVENTION: Well-meaning family members, friends, news media, and health care providers

often encourage patients who have chronic kidney disease or those who are prescribed diuretics to drink large amounts of water. When these patients consume more free water than they excrete, hyponatremia develops. Similarly, participants in marathons or other high-intensity endurance activities may ingest large volumes of water that more than offset losses, thereby self-inducing acute hyponatremia. Patients at risk for hyponatremia should have a specific fluid prescription that avoids both extremes. Conversely, patients with diarrheal losses or those who develop decreased ECFV from diuretics must be informed that intake of water or other hypotonic fluids alone will produce hyponatremia but will not effectively restore ECFV. Sodium, potassium, and water intake are all required for resolution of hyponatremia. Safe, outpatient correction of ECFV requires the consumption of electrolyte-containing tablets, powders, and solutions that are now widely promoted for adults. By contrast, originally available sports drinks have high sugar content but relatively low quantities of electrolytes and may be inadequate for electrolyte replacement.

REFERENCES
Available at eBooks.Health.Elsevier.com.

RELATED CONTENT
Syndrome of Inappropriate Antidiuresis (Related Key Topic)

AUTHOR: **MARK D. FABER, MD, MACM**

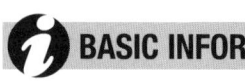
BASIC INFORMATION

DEFINITION

A decrease in parathyroid hormone (PTH) secretion or function results in hypoparathyroidism. In **primary hypoparathyroidism,** absence or dysfunction of the parathyroid gland results in inadequate PTH secretion and subsequent hypocalcemia and hyperphosphatemia. Surgical hypoparathyroidism is the most common etiology, followed by autoimmune disorders.[1] Individuals with autoimmune polyglandular syndrome 1 typically present in childhood/adolescence with candidiasis, hypoparathyroidism, and adrenal insufficiency. Impaired function of PTH (i.e., PTH resistance) can also cause hypocalcemia and hyperphosphatemia, but the measured PTH level is elevated in this circumstance. A maternally transmitted mutation in the *GNAS1* gene results in PTH resistance (i.e., pseudohypoparathyroidism). It is associated with characteristic features that include developmental delay, short stature, round facies, and short 4th metacarpal known as Albright hereditary osteodystrophy (AHO). Paternal transmission manifests with AHO without PTH resistance (i.e., pseudohypoparathyroidism; Table 1). **Secondary hypoparathyroidism,** a condition in which PTH levels are low in response to hypercalcemic states, is discussed in Section IV (see hypercalcemia discussion in the "Calcium" topic).

ICD-10CM CODES
E20.0	Idiopathic hypoparathyroidism
E20.1	Pseudohypoparathyroidism
E20.8	Other hypoparathyroidism
E20.9	Hypoparathyroidism, unspecified
E89.2	Postprocedural hypoparathyroidism
P71.4	Transitory neonatal hypoparathyroidism

EPIDEMIOLOGY & DEMOGRAPHICS

The incidence and prevalence of primary hypoparathyroidism depends on the etiology of the condition. Estimated prevalence in the U.S. is between 23 and 37 cases per 100,000 person-yr.[2] Postoperative hypoparathyroidism is the most common etiology (75%).[1] This occurs in the setting of thyroid or parathyroid surgery as a result of removal of, or vascular compromise of, the parathyroid glands during surgery. Transient hypoparathyroidism (<6 mo) can be as high as 83% postoperatively, but permanent dysfunction (>6 mo) is less common (4.6%).[1] Autoimmune disorders are the second most common cause of hypoparathyroidism in adults. Autoimmune polyglandular syndrome type I is reported to have an incidence worldwide of 1:1,000,000.[3] Genetic causes constitute <10% of cases of hypoparathyroidism.[4]

PHYSICAL FINDINGS & CLINICAL PRESENTATION

The symptoms of hypoparathyroidism are primarily related to hypocalcemia. The presentation of symptoms varies with the severity and duration of illness. Acute manifestations are characterized by neuromuscular irritability such as seizures and laryngospasms.[5] The severity of which depends on the rate of change in calcium, degree of hypocalcemia, and variability among patients. Prolonged QT interval is the classic cardiovascular manifestation of hypocalcemia.[4] Delirium and cognitive impairment are the most common reported psychiatric symptoms.[6] Chronic hypoparathyroidism can affect multiple organ systems, including renal, skeletal, neurologic, neuropsychiatric, and immune system.[7] Basal ganglia calcifications are a classic manifestation of chronic hypoparathyroidism and likely due to elevated CA × P product and/or elevated phosphorus itself.[4] Stage 3 to 5 chronic kidney disease and kidney stones are common renal complications of chronic hypoparathyroidism.[8,9] Table 2 lists the acute and chronic manifestations of hypoparathyroidism.

In addition to the hypocalcemia-related symptoms, syndromes associated with hypoparathyroidism have distinct clinical findings. Conditions associated with hypoparathyroidism include[2]:
- Autoimmune polyglandular syndrome type 1: Mucocutaneous candidiasis and adrenal insufficiency
- DiGeorge syndrome: Dysmorphic facies, cleft palate, short stature, cognitive delay
- Pseudohypoparathyroidism: Developmental delay, short stature, round face, short fourth metacarpal (Albright hereditary osteodystrophy)
- Hypoparathyroidism-retardation-dysmorphism syndrome: Growth retardation, microcephaly, microphthalmia, small hands and feet, abnormal teeth
- Hypoparathyroidism-deafness-renal dysplasia syndrome: Sensorineural deafness
- Kearns-Sayre syndrome: Paralysis of eye muscles and pigmentary retinopathy

ETIOLOGY

There are several etiologies of hypoparathyroidism[2,3,10]:
- Postoperative hypoparathyroidism; most common cause (75% of cases)
- Destruction of the parathyroid glands:
  1. Autoimmune polyglandular syndrome type 1
  2. Radiation to the neck
  3. Infiltrative diseases (e.g., metastatic carcinoma, Wilson disease, hemochromatosis, amyloidosis, thalassemia, granulomatous disease)
- Developmental defects of the parathyroid glands:
  1. Isolated hypoparathyroidism
  2. Branchial dysembryogenesis (DiGeorge syndrome)
  3. Hypoparathyroidism-retardation-dysmorphism syndrome
  4. Hypoparathyroidism-deafness-renal dysplasia syndrome
  5. Mitochondrial dysfunction associated with hypoparathyroidism
     a. Kearns-Sayre syndrome
     b. Mitochondrial encephalomyopathy with lactic acidosis and stroke-like episodes (MELAS) syndrome
     c. Mitochondrial trifunctional protein (MTP) deficiency syndrome
- Functional and secretory defects of the parathyroid glands:
  1. Activating mutation of the calcium-sensing receptor alters the set point of the receptor and decreases PTH secretion
  2. Activating antibodies to calcium-sensing receptor alters the set point of the receptor and decreases PTH secretion
  3. PTH resistance (i.e., target organs unresponsive to PTH action)
     a. Pseudohypoparathyroidism (PHP): Heterogeneous disorder presenting in childhood characterized by hypocalcemia, hyperphosphatemia, and elevated PTH levels. Table 3 summarizes the various types of PHP
     b. Hypermagnesemia and hypomagnesemia

DIAGNOSIS

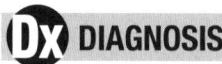

DIFFERENTIAL DIAGNOSIS
- Secondary hypoparathyroidism as a result of hypercalcemia.
- Other conditions associated with hypocalcemia. These conditions are usually associated with an elevated PTH hormone level.

WORKUP
- Hypoparathyroidism is characterized by hypocalcemia and hyperphosphatemia as a result of inadequate PTH secretion.
  1. Two measurements of serum calcium are required for the confirmation of hypocalcemia. Total calcium should be corrected for low albumin utilizing the formula:

TABLE 1 Types of Hypoparathyroidism

Type	Calcium	PO₄	PTH	Comments
Hypoparathyroidism	↓	↑	↓	Surgical removal (most common cause)
Pseudohypoparathyroidism	↓	↑	Ø↑	End-organ resistance to parathyroid hormone and Albright hereditary osteodystrophy
Pseudo-pseudohypoparathyroidism	Normal	Normal	Normal	Only Albright hereditary osteodystrophy

PO₄, Phosphate; *PTH,* parathyroid hormone.
Adapted from Weissleder R et al: *Primer of diagnostic imaging,* ed 5, St Louis, 2011, Mosby.

TABLE 2 Acute and Chronic Manifestations of Hypoparathyroidism

Organ System	Acute and Chronic Manifestations
Cardiovascular	Hypotension Bradycardia Impaired cardiac contractility Prolonged QTc Torsade de pointes/arrhythmias Cardiomyopathy/congestive heart failure ST, QS, T-wave changes on electrocardiography suggestive of myocardial infarction Increased risk of ischemic heart disease and all cardiovascular outcomes in nonsurgical hypoparathyroidism
Dental	Dental aplasia or hypoplasia Failure of tooth eruption Enamel hypoplasia Defective root formation Severe dental caries
Dermatologic	Dry, rough, puffy, coarse skin Brittle hair with hair loss Brittle nails with transverse grooves
Immune	Increased risk of infection, particularly urinary tract infection
Neurologic and neuromotor	Seizures, most commonly tonic-clonic or focal motor, although atypical absence or akinetic seizures also described Spikes and bursts of high-voltage, paroxysmal slow waves on electroencephalogram Basal ganglia and other brain calcifications Extrapyramidal or cerebellar dysfunction
Neuromuscular	Fatigue Neuromuscular irritability Perioral/extremity numbness/tingling Muscle cramping with carpal/pedal spasms or generalized muscle contractions Bronchospasm and laryngospasm Chvostek sign Trousseau sign
Neuropsychiatric	Reduced quality of life Depression Bipolar disease Delirium Cognitive impairment Irritability Depression/anxiety Psychosis
Ophthalmologic	Papilledema Cataract (primarily posterior subcapsular)
Renal	Hypercalciuria Nephrocalcinosis Nephrolithiasis Renal insufficiency and renal failure
Skeletal	Elevated bone density compared with healthy, age-matched controls Markedly reduced bone remodeling

From Cusano N, Bilezikian JP: Signs and symptoms of hypoparathyroidism, *Endocrinol Metab Clin North Am* 47(4):759-770, 2018.

Corrected calcium = measured calcium + [(4 − albumin) × 0.8]. If a reliable laboratory is available, ionized calcium should be considered especially in conditions associated with acid-base disturbances or low albumin states.

2. Serum phosphorus is usually high-normal or elevated in primary hypoparathyroidism.
3. Serum intact PTH (iPTH) level, second- or third-generation immunoassay,[9] is the single best test to evaluate the etiology of hypocalcemia. Typically, PTH is low or inappropriately normal in primary hypoparathyroidism and elevated in most other conditions associated with low calcium levels. However, PTH is also elevated in disorders associated with impaired PTH function (i.e., pseudohypoparathyroidism). Genetic studies as indicated if medical or family history is suggestive of disease.

The diagnosis is established by concurrent measurements of ionized calcium or corrected calcium that is within the lower limit of normal range and low or undetectable levels of PTH on two separate occasions at least 2 wk apart.[9]

LABORATORY TESTS
- Total and ionized calcium: Low in hypoparathyroidism
- PTH: Low in hypoparathyroidism and high in PTH resistance states like pseudohypoparathyroidism
- Phosphorus: High-normal or high in hypoparathyroidism
- Magnesium: Both hypomagnesemia and hypermagnesemia can cause hypoparathyroidism
- Serum creatinine
- 25-hydroxyvitamin D and 1,25-hydroxyvitamin D levels
- 24-h urine calcium and creatinine to evaluate the risk for renal stones
- ECG should be considered. Hypocalcemia is associated with prolonged QT interval, rarely ST-segment elevations

IMAGING STUDIES
- Renal ultrasonography to detect the presence of nephrocalcinosis and renal stones
- Soft tissue calcifications may be noted on plain x-rays (Fig. E1)
- Skull x-ray for basal ganglia and other intracerebral calcifications[11]

TABLE 3 Types of Pseudohypoparathyroidism (PHP)

Disorder	Urinary cAMP Response to PTH	Urinary PO$_4$ Response to PTH	Other Hormonal Resistance	AHO	Pathophysiology
PHP type 1A	Decreased	Decreased	Yes	Yes	G$_s\alpha$ mutation
Pseudo-PHP	Normal	Normal	No	Yes	G$_s\alpha$ mutation
PHP type 1B	Decreased	Decreased	No	No	*GNAS1* imprinting mutations
PHP type 1C	Decreased	Decreased	Yes	Yes	G$_s\alpha$ activity normal
PHP type 2	Normal	Decreased	No	No	Vitamin D deficiency or myotonic dystrophy in some cases

AHO, Albright hereditary osteodystrophy; *cAMP*, cyclic adenosine monophosphate; *GNAS1*, portion of the *GNAS* complex locus encoding; G$_s\alpha$, α-subunit of the stimulatory G protein; *PO$_4$*, phosphate; *PTH*, parathyroid hormone.
From Melmed S et al: *Williams textbook of endocrinology*, ed 12, Philadelphia, 2011, Saunders.

Rx TREATMENT

NONPHARMACOLOGIC THERAPY

Diet:
- Consumption of calcium-enriched food (i.e., dairy)
- Restriction of phosphate intake (i.e., commercially prepared foods)

Parathyroid autotransplantation:
- Hypoparathyroidism and subsequent hypocalcemia are common problems after neck exploration for total or near-total thyroidectomy or parathyroidectomy. In cases where there is concern for postoperative hypoparathyroidism, parathyroid autotransplantation of one or two parathyroid glands into the forearm or sternocleidomastoid muscle should be performed to prevent postoperative hypoparathyroidism.

PHARMACOLOGIC THERAPY

The mainstay of treatment for primary hypoparathyroidism is pharmacologic therapy with calcium and vitamin D supplementation. The goals of therapy are to control symptoms and minimize complications of therapy. The aim should be to achieve a low-normal serum calcium level (8.0 to 8.5 mg/dl), high-normal serum phosphorus level, calcium-phosphorus product <55 mg^2/dl^2, normal magnesium level, 24-h urinary calcium <300 mg/day, and 25-hydroxyvitamin D >20 to 30 ng/ml.[10]
- Vitamin D:
  1. There are several vitamin D preparations available on the market, but the treatment of choice for patients with primary hypoparathyroidism is calcitriol. It is an active metabolite that does not require hydroxylation in the liver or kidney and therefore bypasses the PTH-mediated 1-α hydroxylation defect that occurs with hypoparathyroidism.
  2. Calcitriol 0.25 to 1 ug once or twice daily is usually required to correct hypocalcemia and improve symptoms. Its maximal effect is seen after 10 h and it lasts for 2 to 3 days.
  3. High doses of Vitamin D2 (ergocalciferol) or Vitamin D3 (cholecalciferol) may also be used.
- Calcium:
  1. Calcium carbonate or calcium citrates are common oral agents used for treatment of hypocalcemia associated with hypoparathyroidism. Calcium carbonate contains 40% elemental calcium, and calcium citrate contains 21% elemental calcium. Calcium carbonate requires an acidic environment for effective absorption, and as a result, it must be taken with food. Its effectiveness is decreased with concomitant use of H$_2$ blockers or proton pump inhibitors. Calcium citrate does not require an acidic environment for effective absorption.
  2. Start with a dose of 500 to 1000 mg of elemental calcium two to three times daily and adjust the dose for a desired calcium in the low-normal range. As much as 9 g of calcium have been required on occasion.[4]
- Magnesium:
  1. Hypocalcemia is difficult to correct without normalizing magnesium levels.
  2. Magnesium sulfate IV 2 g over 20 min followed by 1 g/h infusion can be considered in severe deficiency states. Milder deficiencies can be managed with oral magnesium 100 mg three times a day.
- Thiazide diuretics:
  1. Thiazide diuretics (25 to 100 mg daily) decrease urine calcium excretion and decrease kidney stones. They should be considered in individuals with urine calcium >250 mg/day.[10] Thiazide diuretics should not be used in patients with autoimmune polyendocrine syndrome type 1 with adrenal insufficiency and autosomal dominant hypoparathyroidism type 1 with Bartter syndrome.[9]
- Phosphate binders:
  1. Usually used when phosphate above 6.5 mg/dL[12]
- PTH replacement:
  1. The REPLACE study has demonstrated the efficacy of injectable synthetic human PTH (1-84) in decreasing urinary calcium excretion and serum phosphorus and maintaining serum calcium in the normal range with reduced requirements for calcium and vitamin D supplementation.[11]
  2. PTH (1-84, Natpara, an 84-amino acid single-chain polypeptide identical to native parathyroid hormone) is the first FDA-approved product for use in the treatment of hypoparathyroidism as an adjunct to calcium and vitamin D. PTH (1-84) is recommended for patients who are not well controlled on conventional therapy alone, who have gastrointestinal tract disorder associated with malabsorption, those taking high doses of supplementation, or those with continuous symptomatology despite treatment with above therapies.[13] PTH (1–84) is given as a once daily subcutaneous injection with dose ranging from 25 to 100 mcg daily.

ACUTE GENERAL Rx

Severe and/or symptomatic hypocalcemia requires hospitalization. Acute management of hypocalcemia includes:
- Telemetry monitoring for arrhythmias associated with severe hypocalcemia
- IV infusion of 10% calcium gluconate (93 mg of elemental calcium/10 ml) in 50 ml of 5% dextrose over 15 to 30 min, followed by an infusion of 0.5 to 1.5 mg/kg/h until calcium levels are in the low-normal range[4]

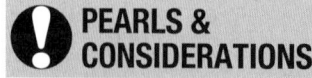 PEARLS & CONSIDERATIONS

COMMENTS

- The mainstay of treatment for primary hypoparathyroidism is calcitriol and calcium supplementation to maintain a goal serum calcium level in the low-normal range. IV calcium should be considered if calcium <7.0 mg/dl.
- PTH (1-84) should be considered in patients who are not well controlled on conventional therapy.
- Treatment of hypothyroidism is commonly associated with hypercalciuria, nephrocalcinosis, nephrolithiasis, and renal insufficiency. It is recommended to target blood calcium levels to the lower end of the normal range in order to reduce hypercalciuria. Urinary calcium levels should also be monitored periodically.
- Hypomagnesemia causes functional, reversible parathyroid hypofunction. Magnesium levels should be assessed and appropriately replaced in all patients with hypocalcemia before a low PTH level is attributed to hypoparathyroidism.
- In patients undergoing neck exploration, consideration should be given to the parathyroid glands. Auto transplantation of one or more parathyroid glands should be considered when appropriate to prevent postoperative hypoparathyroidism.

REFERENCES

Available at eBooks.Health.Elsevier.com.

AUTHORS: **DIANELYS MENDEZ, MD,** and **VICKY CHENG, MD**

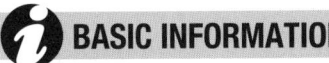 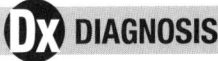

H

I

BASIC INFORMATION

DEFINITION

Hypopituitarism (from the Latin *pituita,* meaning "phlegm") is the deficiency of one or more of the hormones of the anterior or posterior pituitary gland resulting from diseases of the hypothalamus or pituitary gland. Panhypopituitarism indicates the loss of all the pituitary hormones but is often used in clinical practice to describe patients deficient in growth hormone (GH), gonadotropins, corticotropin, or thyrotropin in whom posterior pituitary function remains intact.

SYNONYMS

Panhypopituitarism
Pituitary insufficiency

ICD-10CM CODES
E23.0 Hypopituitarism
E23.1 Drug-induced hypopituitarism
E89.3 Postprocedural hypopituitarism

EPIDEMIOLOGY & DEMOGRAPHICS

Incidence of 4.2 cases/100,000 persons

PHYSICAL FINDINGS & CLINICAL PRESENTATION

Symptoms depend on type of onset, number and severity of hormone deficiencies, their target organs, and age of onset (Table 1). Physiologic regulators of pituitary hormone secretion are summarized in Table 2.
- Mass effect of a pituitary tumor can cause headaches and visual disturbances (typically as bitemporal hemianopsia).
- Rhinorrhea.
- Corticotropin deficiency:
  1. Fatigue and weakness, no appetite, abdominal pain, nausea, vomiting, failure to thrive in children, and hyponatremia. If the onset is abrupt, hypotension and shock.

- Thyrotropin deficiency:
  1. Fatigue and weakness, weight gain, cold intolerance, anemia, constipation
  2. Bradycardia, hung-up reflexes, pretibial edema, change in voice, and hair loss
- Gonadotropin deficiency:
  1. Loss of libido, erectile dysfunction, amenorrhea, hot flashes, dyspareunia, infertility, gynecomastia, decreased muscle mass, and anemia
- GH deficiency:
  1. Growth retardation in children
  2. Easy fatigue, hypoglycemia
  3. Lean mass is reduced and fat mass is increased, leading to obesity
  4. Decreased bone mineral density, increased low-density lipoprotein cholesterol, obesity, increased inflammatory cardiovascular markers (interleukin-6 and C-reactive protein)
- Hyperprolactinemia:
  1. Galactorrhea, hypogonadism, inability to lactate after delivery
  2. Posterior pituitary (vasopressin; antidiuretic hormone [ADH] deficiency): Diabetes insipidus with polyuria, polydipsia, nocturia, hypotension, and dehydration

ETIOLOGY

It can be congenital or acquired:
- Congenital: Mutations in transcription factors produce multiple hormonal deficiencies. Mutations in genes produce single hormonal deficiency.
- Acquired (Table 3): The result of destruction of pituitary cells caused by:
  1. Pituitary apoplexy: Hemorrhage or infarction of the pituitary gland. Predisposing factors include diabetes mellitus, anticoagulation therapy, head trauma, and radiation therapy. Sheehan syndrome: Postpartum necrosis, a rare complication after pregnancy.

2. Infiltrative disease, including sarcoidosis, hemochromatosis, histiocytosis X, Wegener granulomatosis, lymphocytic hypophysitis, and infection of the pituitary (tuberculosis, mycosis, syphilis).
3. Primary empty sella syndrome: Flattening of the pituitary gland caused by extension of the subarachnoid space and filling of cerebrospinal fluid into the sella turcica.
4. Pituitary tumors: Classified by size (microadenomas, <10 mm; macroadenomas, >10 mm) and function. Prolactin-secreting tumors and nonfunctioning tumors account for the majority of pituitary adenomas.
5. Suprasellar tumors: Craniopharyngiomas are the most common.

DIAGNOSIS

The diagnosis of hypopituitarism is suspected by clinical history and physical findings and is established by blood tests to confirm the presence of hormone deficiency.

DIFFERENTIAL DIAGNOSIS

The differential diagnosis is as outlined under "Etiology."

WORKUP

Includes baseline determination of each anterior pituitary hormone followed by dynamic provocative stimulation tests, radiograph imaging, and formal visual field testing. Table 4 summarizes testing for assessment of anterior pituitary function.

LABORATORY TESTS

- Corticotropin deficiency:
  1. The presence of a 9:00 A.M. cortisol level >20 mcg/dl or <4 mcg/dl usually confirms sufficiency or deficiency, respectively.
  2. Corticotropin stimulation test using 250 mcg of corticotropin given intravenous (IV) and measuring serum cortisol before and 30 and 60 min after administration. A normal response is an increase in serum cortisol level >20 mcg/dl.
  3. With pituitary disease these test results may be indeterminate, and more dynamic testing such as an insulin-tolerance or metyrapone test may be necessary.
- Thyrotropin deficiency:
  1. Thyroid-stimulating hormone (TSH) and free T_4 measurements
  2. Primary hypothyroidism shows elevated TSH with low free T_4. Secondary hypothyroidism shows normal or low TSH with low free T_4 and low T_3 resin uptake.
- Gonadotropin deficiency:
  1. Follicle-stimulating hormone (FSH), luteinizing hormone (LH), estrogen, and testosterone measurements.
  2. In men, hypogonadotropic hypogonadism is seen with low testosterone levels and normal or low FSH and LH levels (ideally measured at 9:00 A.M. because of diurnal

TABLE 1 Clinical Effects of Pituitary Hormone Deficiencies

In panhypopituitarism, all are combined, although diabetes insipidus (ADH deficiency) is often absent

Hormone	Context	Symptoms and Signs
ACTH	Acute	Fatigue, weakness, hypotension, weakness, vomiting
	Chronic	As in Addison disease, except lack of pigmentation, electrolyte disturbance and hypovolemia Hypoglycemia, weight loss
TSH	Children	Growth retardation
	Adults	As for primary hypothyroidism, thyroid atrophy
GH	Children	Growth retardation, increased adiposity
	Adults	↓ Exercise capacity, ↓ lean mass, ↑ fat mass, ↑ cardiovascular risk
Gonadotropins	Children	Failure of sexual maturation, lack of pubertal growth spurt
	Men	As for primary hypogonadism, testicular atrophy, infertility
	Women	Secondary amenorrhea, infertility, osteoporosis
Prolactin	Women	Failure of lactation
Vasopressin (ADH)		Polyuria, dilute urine, thirst, nocturia, hypernatremia

ACTH, Adrenocorticotropic hormone; *ADH,* antidiuretic hormone; *GH,* growth hormone, *TSH,* thyroid-stimulating hormone.
From Talley NJ et al: *Essentials of internal medicine,* ed 4, Chatswood, NSW, 2021, Elsevier Australia.

TABLE 3 Causes of Acquired Pituitary Insufficiency

Traumatic
- Surgical resection
- Radiation damage
- Traumatic brain injury

Infiltrative/Inflammatory
- Primary hypophysitis
- Lymphocytic
- Granulomatous
- Xanthomatous
- Secondary hypophysitis
- Sarcoidosis
- Langerhans cell histiocytosis
- Infections
- Granulomatosis with polyangiitis
- Takayasu disease
- Hemochromatosis

Infections
- Tuberculosis
- *Pneumocystis jirovecii* infection
- Fungal (histoplasmosis, aspergillosis)
- Parasites (toxoplasmosis)
- Viral (cytomegalovirus)

Vascular
- Pregnancy related
- Aneurysm
- Apoplexy
- Diabetes
- Hypotension
- Arteritis
- Sickle cell disease

Neoplastic
- Pituitary adenoma
- Parasellar mass
- Rathke cyst
- Dermoid cyst
- Meningioma
- Germinoma
- Ependymoma
- Glioma
- Craniopharyngioma
- Hypothalamic hamartoma, gangliocytoma
- Pituitary metastatic deposits
- Hematologic malignancy
- Leukemia
- Lymphoma

Functional
- Nutritional
- Caloric restriction
- Malnutrition
- Excessive exercise
- Critical illness
- Acute illness
- Chronic renal failure
- Chronic liver failure
- Hormonal
- Hyperprolactinemia
- Hypothyroidism
- Drugs
- Anabolic steroids
- Glucocorticoid excess
- GnRH agonists
- Estrogen
- Dopamine
- Somatostatin analog
- Thyroid hormone excess

GnRH, Gonadotropin-releasing hormone.
Modified from Kaiser U, Ho KKY: Pituitary physiology and diagnostic evaluation. In Melmed S et al (eds): *Williams textbook of endocrinology,* ed 13, Philadelphia, 2016, Elsevier; and Kliegman RM: *Nelson textbook of pediatrics,* ed 21, Philadelphia, 2020, Elsevier, Table 8.5, p. 193.

rhythm). Check free testosterone if patient is obese.
3. In premenopausal women with amenorrhea, low estrogen with normal or low FSH and LH levels is typically seen.
- GH deficiency:
  1. Insulin-induced hypoglycemia stimulation test using 0.1 to 0.15 unit/kg regular insulin given IV and measuring GH 30, 60, and 120 min after administration. A normal response is a GH level >3 mcg/dl. This test is contraindicated in seizure disorder or ischemic heart disease.
  2. Combination of GH-releasing hormone plus arginine is an alternative test, with a diagnostic threshold of 9 mcg/L.
  3. Because the relation between serum insulin-like growth factor (IGF)-1 and GH levels blurs with age, a normal serum IGF-1 does not exclude the diagnosis in older adults.
- Hyperprolactinemia: Prolactin levels may be elevated in prolactin-secreting pituitary adenomas.
- Vasopressin deficiency:
  1. Urinalysis shows low specific gravity.
  2. Urine osmolality is low.
  3. Serum osmolality is high.
  4. Fluid deprivation test over 18 h with inability to concentrate the urine.
  5. Serum vasopressin level is low.
  6. Electrolytes may show hyponatremia and exclude hyperglycemia.

IMAGING STUDIES
- Imaging is the first step in identifying an underlying cause.
- MRI (Fig. E1) is more sensitive than computed tomography (CT) in visualizing the pituitary fossa, sella turcica, optic chiasm, pituitary stalk, and cavernous sinuses. It is also more sensitive in detecting pituitary microadenomas. CT with contrast can be used if MRI is not available.
- Surveillance scan at baseline and 12 mo thereafter depending on protocol and clinical symptoms.

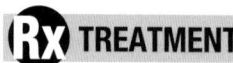 **TREATMENT**

Three-fold: Removing underlying cause (surgery or radiation), treating hormonal deficiencies, and addressing any other repercussions from deficiency. Table 5 summarizes replacement therapy for adult hypopituitarism.

NONPHARMACOLOGIC THERAPY
- IV fluid resuscitation, correction of electrolyte and metabolic abnormalities with potassium bicarbonate, and oxygen therapy.
- Transsphenoidal surgery for tumors causing specific symptoms.
- Radiation or stereotactic radiosurgery ("gamma knife") for medically unresponsive, surgically unresectable tumors and tumors for which other modalities are contraindicated. It is both safe and effective for recurrent or residual pituitary adenomas.

ACUTE GENERAL Rx
Acute situations such as adrenal crisis or myxedema coma can occur in untreated hypopituitarism and should be treated accordingly with IV corticosteroids (e.g., hydrocortisone 100- to 250-mg bolus followed by hydrocortisone 100 mg IV q6h for 24 h) and levothyroxine (e.g., 5-8 mcg/kg IV over 15 min, then 100 mcg IV q24h).

CHRONIC Rx
Treatment is lifelong:
- Adrenocorticotropic hormone (ACTH) deficiency: Hydrocortisone 10 mg orally (PO) every morning and 5 mg PO every evening or prednisone 5 mg PO every morning and 2.5 mg PO every evening. Dexamethasone or prednisone is often preferred because of longer duration of action.
- LH and FSH deficiency:
  1. In men, testosterone enanthate or propionate 200 to 300 mg intramuscular (IM) every 2 to 3 wk, or transdermal testosterone scrotal patches can be tried.
  2. In women who are not interested in fertility, conjugated estrogen 0.3 to 1.25 mg/day and held the last 5 to 7 days of each mo with the addition of medroxyprogesterone 10 mg/day given during days 15 to 25 of the normal menstrual cycle. In those who have secondary hypogonadism and wish to become pregnant, pulsatile gonadotropic-releasing hormone may be of benefit.
- TSH deficiency: Levothyroxine 0.05 to 0.2 mg/day. Only free thyroxine should be used to monitor appropriate dosing to maintain thyroxine level in the mid to upper half of normal range.
- GH deficiency (Fig. 2):
  1. GH replacement in children is universally accepted.
  2. GH replacement in adults is not generally recommended and requires careful consideration of each individual case. It may have effects on quality of life, body composition, bone density, and cardiovascular risk factors.
  3. Side effects of replacement include peripheral edema, arthralgia, and headaches.
  4. Usual GH dose is between 0.2 and 0.4 mg, determined by the age and sex of a patient and increments of 0.1 mg every 2 to 4 wk until serum IGF-1 is in the upper part of the normal range. Young adults and women taking estrogen require a higher dose.
- ADH deficiency:
  1. Desmopressin (DDAVP) 10 to 20 mcg by intranasal spray or 0.05 to 0.1 mg PO bid is used in patients with diabetes insipidus.
  2. Vasopressin: 5 to 10 U given IM or subcutaneous q6h.

DISPOSITION
- Hormone replacement therapy is adjusted according to serum hormone monitoring.
- If untreated can lead to adrenal crisis, severe hyponatremia and hypothyroidism, metabolic abnormalities, and death.

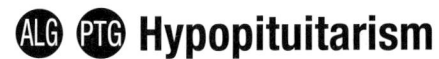

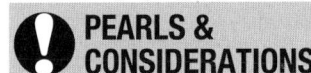

TABLE 4 Assessment of Anterior Pituitary Function

Test	Dose	Normal Response	Side Effects
ACTH			
Insulin tolerance	0.1-0.15 U/kg IV	Peak cortisol response >18 µg/dl, or increase by 7 µg/dl	Sweating, palpitation, tremor
Metyrapone	Oral administration of 30 mg/kg at 11 P.M.	Peak 11-DOC ≥7 µg/dl Peak cortisol ≤7 µg/dl Peak ACTH >75 pg/ml	Nausea, insomnia, adrenal crisis
CRH stimulation	100 µg IV	Peak ACTH ≥ two-fold to four-fold Peak cortisol ≥20 µg/dl or ↑ ≥7 µg/dl	Flushing
ACTH stimulation	250 µg IV or IM or 1 µg IV	Peak cortisol ≥20 µg/dl	Rare
TSH			
Serum T$_4$ (free T$_4$) Total T$_3$ TSH—third generation TRH stimulation	200-500 µg IV	Peak TSH ≥2.5-fold or ↑ ≥5-6 mU/L (females), ↑ ≥2-3 mU/L (males)	Flushing, nausea, urge to micturate
PRL			
Serum PRL TRH stimulation	200-500 µg IV	PRL ≥2.5-fold	Flushing, nausea, urge to micturate
LH/FSH			
Serum LH and FSH Serum testosterone GnRH stimulation	100 µg IV	Elevated in menopause and in men with primary testicular failure 300-900 ng/ml (age-adjusted normal ranges) LH ≥ two-fold to three-fold, or by 10 IU/L FSH 1.5-2-fold, or by 2 IU/L	Rare
GH			
Insulin tolerance	0.1-0.15 U/kg	GH peak >5 µg/L	Sweating, palpitation, tremor
Glucagon	1-1.5 mg IM	GH peak >3 µg/L	Nausea, headaches
L-Arginine plus GHRH	0.5 g/kg (max 30 g) IV over 30 min	Peak GH >9 µg/L	Nausea
GHRH	1 µg/kg		Flushing

ACTH, Adrenocorticotropic hormone; *CRH,* corticotropin-releasing hormone; *11-DOC,* 11-deoxycorticosterone; *FSH,* follicle-stimulating hormone; *GH,* growth hormone; *GHRH,* growth hormone–releasing hormone; *GnRH,* gonadotropin-releasing hormone; *IM,* intramuscular; *IV,* intravenous; *LH,* luteinizing hormone; *PRL,* prolactin; *T$_3$,* triiodothyronine; *T$_4$,* thyroxine; *TSH,* thyroid-stimulating hormone; *TRH,* thyrotropin-releasing hormone.
From Melmed S et al: *Williams textbook of endocrinology,* ed 14, Philadelphia, 2019, Elsevier.

TABLE 5 Replacement Therapy for Adult Hypopituitarism[a]

Deficient Hormone	Treatment
ACTH	Hydrocortisone, 10-20 mg/day in divided doses Cortisone acetate, 15-25 mg/day in divided doses
TSH	l-Thyroxine, 0.05-0.2 mg/day according to T$_4$ levels
FSH/LH	*Males:* Testosterone enanthate, 200 mg IM every 2-3 wk Testosterone undecanoate, 1000 mg IM every 3-6 mo Testosterone skin patch, 2.5-5.0 mg/day—can increase dose up to 7.5 mg/day Testosterone gel, 5-10 g/day (delivering 50-100 mg/day) For fertility: hCG three times weekly, or hCG + FSH or menopausal gonadotropin or GnRH *Females (nonoral route is recommended):* Estradiol skin patch, 4-8 mg, twice weekly Estradiol gel Conjugated estrogen, 0.65 mg/day Micronized estradiol, 1 mg/day Estradiol valerate, 1-2 mg Piperazine estrone sulfate, 1.25 mg All of the estrogens are administered with progesterone or progestin sequentially or in combination if uterus present For fertility: Menopausal gonadotropin and hCG or GnRH
GH	*Adults:* Somatotropin, 0.2-1.0 mg/day SC *Children:* Somatotropin, 0.02-0.05 mg/kg/day
Vasopressin	Intranasal desmopressin, via rhinal tube, 5-20 µg twice daily Oral DDAVP, 300-600 µg/day, usually in divided doses

[a]Doses shown should be individualized and reassessed during stress, surgery, or pregnancy.
ACTH, Adrenocorticotropic hormone; *DDAVP,* desmopressin acetate; *FSH,* follicle-stimulating hormone; *GH,* growth hormone; *GnRH,* gonadotropin-releasing hormone; *hCG,* human chorionic gonadotropin; *IM,* intramuscularly; *LH,* luteinizing hormone; *SC,* subcutaneously; *T$_4$,* thyroxine; *TSH,* thyroid-stimulating hormone.
From Melmed S et al: *Williams textbook of endocrinology,* ed 14, Philadelphia, 2019, Elsevier.

- Complications: Visual deficit, adrenal crisis, susceptibility to infection and other stressors.
- Prognosis: Stable patients have a favorable prognosis with replacement hormone therapy. Patients with acute decompensation are in critical condition with a high mortality rate.

REFERRAL

Consultation with an endocrinologist and neurosurgeon for surgical treatment

PEARLS & CONSIDERATIONS

- All patients sustaining moderate to severe head injury should undergo assessment of anterior pituitary function during the acute phase and at 6 mo.
- IGF-1 can be used as a marker of GH deficiency.
- All tests of GH secretion are more likely to give false-positive results in obese patients.
- The GH axis is the most vulnerable to the effects of radiotherapy; doses as low as 18 Gy in children have caused GH deficiency.
- Sequence of hormonal disruption: GH secretion then gonadotropin secretion. TSH and adrenocorticotropic hormone secretion are somewhat resistant.

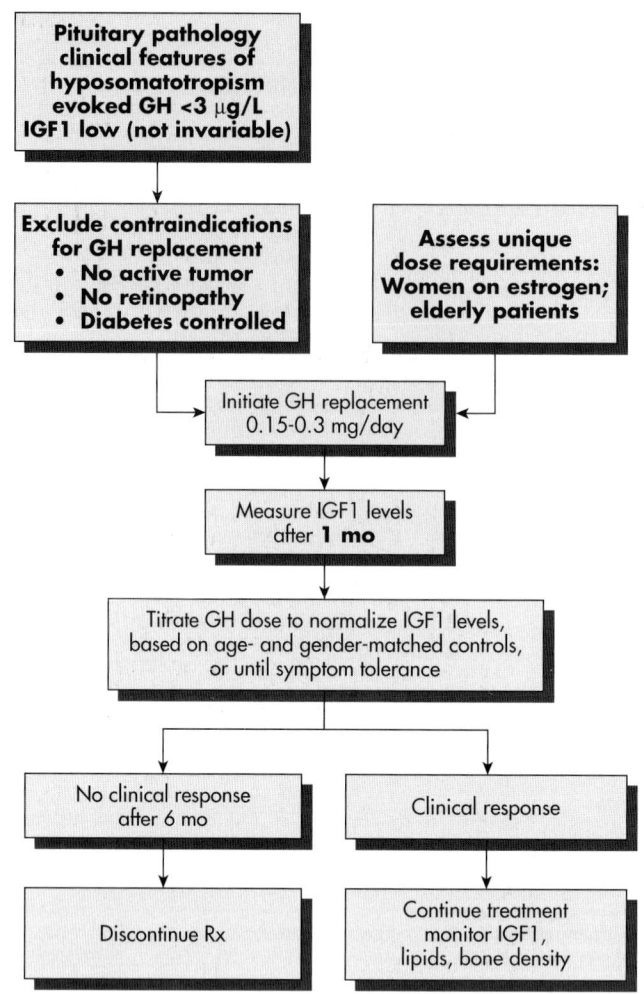

FIG. 2 Management of somatotropin deficiency in adults. Patients older than 60 yr require lower maintenance doses. Women receiving oral estrogen require higher doses than those receiving transdermal estrogen preparations. *GH,* Growth hormone; *IGF1,* insulin-like growth factor 1; *Rx,* treatment. (From Melmed S et al: *Williams textbook of endocrinology,* ed 14, Philadelphia, 2019, Elsevier.)

- Thyroxine supplementation increases the rate of cortisol metabolism and can lead to adrenal crisis, so corticosteroids should be replaced first.
- All patients receiving glucocorticoid replacement therapy should wear proper identification stating the need for this therapy.
- Stress doses of corticosteroids are indicated before surgery or for any medical emergency (e.g., sepsis, acute myocardial infarction).
- Antidiuretic hormone deficiency may be masked if there is ACTH deficiency with symptoms only appearing when cortisol has been replaced.

COMMENTS
- Mineralocorticoid replacement is not necessary in secondary adrenal insufficiency because the renin-angiotensin-aldosterone system is unaffected by pituitary failure.
- Patients with adult-acquired GH deficiency must meet at least two criteria before replacement therapy: A poor GH response to at least two standard stimuli and hypopituitarism from pituitary or hypothalamic damage. The criteria are different in children in whom GH is required for normal growth.

- Prevention of acute decompensation can be accomplished by reminding patients to increase the dose of hydrocortisone in response to stress.
- Medical therapy should precede surgical therapy.

RELATED CONTENT
Hypopituitarism (Patient Information)

AUTHOR: **FRED F. FERRI, MD**

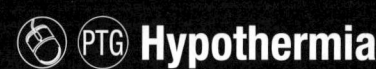
BASIC INFORMATION

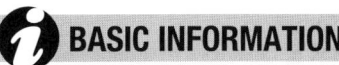

DEFINITION

Hypothermia is a rectal temperature $<35°$ C ($95.8°$ F). "Accidental hypothermia" is an unintentionally induced decrease in core temperature in the absence of preoptic anterior hypothalamic conditions.

ICD-10CM CODES

R68.0 Hypothermia, not associated with low environmental temperature
T68 Hypothermia

EPIDEMIOLOGY & DEMOGRAPHICS

- Hypothermia occurs most frequently in the following groups: Alcoholics; homeless; learning-impaired; patients with cardiovascular, cerebrovascular, or pituitary disorders; those using sedatives or tranquilizers; and elderly patients.
- >700 persons in the U.S. die from hypothermia annually.

PHYSICAL FINDINGS & CLINICAL PRESENTATION

The clinical presentation varies with the severity of hypothermia. Shivering may be absent if body temperature is $<33.3°$ C ($92°$ F) or in patients taking phenothiazines.

Hypothermia may masquerade as cerebrovascular accident, ataxia, or slurred speech, or the patient may appear comatose or clinically dead. Signs of hypothermia are summarized in Box 1.

Physiologic stages of hypothermia (Table 1):
- Stage HT I: Mild hypothermia (typical core temperature 32.2° C to 35 °C [90° F to 95° F]): Arrhythmias, ataxia
- Stage HT II: Moderate hypothermia (core temperature 28° C to 32.2° C [82.4° F to 90° F]):
  1. Progressive decrease of level of consciousness, pulse, cardiac output, and respiration
  2. Fibrillation, dysrhythmias (increased susceptibility to ventricular tachycardia)
  3. Elimination of shivering mechanism for thermogenesis
- Stage HT III: Severe hypothermia (core temperature $\leq28°$ C to 24° C [82.4° F to 75° F]):
  1. Absence of reflexes or response to pain
  2. Decreased cerebral blood flow, decreased CO_2
  3. Increased risk of ventricular fibrillation or asystole
  4. Vital signs present
- Stage IV: No vital signs (core temperature $<24°$ C [75° F])

ETIOLOGY

Exposure to cold temperatures for a prolonged period. Contributing factors include:
- Drugs: Ethanol, phenothiazines, sedative-hypnotics
- Skin disorders: Extensive burns, severe psoriasis, exfoliative dermatitis

- Metabolic disorders: Hypopituitarism, hypothyroidism, hypoadrenalism
- Neurologic abnormalities: Stroke, head trauma, acute spinal cord transection, impaired shivering
- Other: Lack of acclimatization, aggressive fluid resuscitation, sepsis, heat stroke treatment
- Table 2 summarizes factors predisposing to hypothermia

DIAGNOSIS

DIFFERENTIAL DIAGNOSIS

- It is crucial to determine an accurate core temperature measurement. Advantages and considerations of various methods to determine core temperature are summarized in Table 3. Core temperature is best monitored with an esophageal probe. Rectal and bladder temperature generally lag behind core temperatures during the rewarming process
- Cerebrovascular accident
- Myxedema coma
- Drug intoxication
- Hypoglycemia

LABORATORY TESTS

- Metabolic and respiratory acidosis are usually present.
  1. When blood cools, the arterial pH increases, oxygen tension (Po_2) increases, and the pCO_2 falls. Temperature correction factors for arterial blood gas specimens are summarized in Box 2.
  2. Blood gas analyzers warm the blood to 37° C ($98.6°$ F), increasing the partial pressure of dissolved gases, resulting in higher oxygen and carbon dioxide levels and a lower pH than the patient's actual values. A decrease in K^+ initially, then an increase in K^+ with increasing hypothermia; extreme hyperkalemia indicates a poor prognosis.

BOX 1 Signs of Hypothermia

Head, Eye, Ear, Nose, Throat
- Mydriasis
- Decreased corneal reflexes
- Extraocular muscle abnormalities
- Erythropsia
- Flushing
- Facial edema
- Epistaxis
- Rhinorrhea
- Strabismus

Cardiovascular
- Initial tachycardia
- Subsequent tachycardia
- Arrhythmias
- Decreased heart tones
- Hepatojugular reflux
- Jugular venous distention
- Hypotension
- Peripheral vasoconstriction

Respiratory
- Initial tachypnea
- Adventitious sounds
- Bronchorrhea
- Progressive hypoventilation
- Apnea

Gastrointestinal
- Ileus
- Constipation
- Abdominal distention or rigidity
- Poor rectal tone
- Gastric dilation in neonates or in adults with myxedema
- Vomiting

Genitourinary
- Anuria
- Polyuria
- Oliguria
- Testicular torsion

Neurologic
- Depressed level of consciousness
- Ataxia
- Dysarthria
- Amnesia
- Anesthesia

- Areflexia
- Poor suck reflex
- Hypoesthesia
- Antinociception
- Initial hyperreflexia
- Hyporeflexia
- Central pontine myelinolysis

Psychiatric
- Impaired judgment
- Perseveration
- Mood changes
- Peculiar "flat" affect
- Altered mental status
- Paradoxical undressing
- Neuroses
- Psychoses
- Suicide
- Organic brain syndrome
- Anorexia nervosa
- Depression
- Apathy
- Irritability

Musculoskeletal
- Increased muscle tone
- Shivering
- Rigidity or pseudo-rigor mortis
- Paravertebral spasm
- Opisthotonos
- Compartment syndrome

Dermatologic
- Erythema
- Pallor
- Cyanosis
- Icterus
- Scleral edema
- Ecchymosis
- Edema
- Pernio
- Frostnip
- Frostbite
- Panniculitis
- Cold urticaria
- Necrosis
- Gangrene

From Auerbach P: *Wilderness medicine, expert consult premium edition—enhanced online features and print*, Philadelphia, 2012, Saunders.

TABLE 1 Hypothermia: Stages and Associated Clinical Manifestations

Stage	CORE TEMPERATURE °F	CORE TEMPERATURE °C	Clinical Manifestations
Normothermia	98.6	37.0	
Mild hypothermia	95.0	35.0	Cold diuresis, maximal shivering
	93.0	33.8	Ataxia, poor judgment, J wave
	91.0	32.7	Amnesia, blood pressure difficult to measure
Moderate hypothermia	89.0	31.6	Stupor, pupils dilated
	87.0	30.5	Shivering ceases
	85.0	30.0	Cardiac arrhythmias, insulin inactive
	82.0	27.8	Unconsciousness, ventricular fibrillation likely
	80.0	26.6	No muscle reflexes
Profound hypothermia	78.0	25.5	Acid-base disturbances, no response to pain
	75.0	23.8	Pulmonary edema, hypotension
	73.0	22.7	No corneal reflexes
	66.0	18.8	Heart standstill
	62.0	16.6	Isoelectric electrocardiogram
	57.6	14.2	Lowest infant survival from accidental hypothermia
	48.2	9.0	Lowest adult survival from accidental hypothermia

From Goldman L, Shafer AI: *Goldman-Cecil medicine*, ed 26, Philadelphia, 2019, Elsevier.

TABLE 2 Factors Predisposing to Cold Injury

Individual Factors

Inadequate clothing and shelter
Lean and low body fat
Low physical fitness
Prior exhaustive physical exercise
Advanced age
Young age
Black race (men and women)

Health Conditions

Burns
Diabetes mellitus
Hypoglycemia
Neurologic lesions
Dementia
Hypoadrenalism, hypopituitarism, hypothyroidism
Prior frostbite or trench foot
Raynaud phenomenon
Sickle cell trait
Trauma
Spinal cord injury

Drugs

Alcohol
Anesthetics
Antidepressants
Antithyroid agents
Sedatives and narcotics

Environmental Factors

Cold temperatures
High air motion
Rain and immersion
Skin contact with metal and fuels
Repeated cold exposure
Physical fatigue
Immobility
High-altitude and low-oxygen-tension environments

From Goldman L, Shafer AI: *Goldman-Cecil medicine*, ed 26, Philadelphia, 2019, Elsevier.

- Hematocrit increases (caused by hemoconcentration), decreasing leukocytes and platelets (caused by splenic sequestration).
- Blood viscosity, increased clotting time.

IMAGING STUDIES

- Chest x-ray: Generally not helpful; may reveal evidence of aspiration (e.g., intoxicated patient with aspiration pneumonia).
- ECG: Prolonged PR, QT, and QRS segments, depressed ST segments, inverted T waves, atrioventricular block, and hypothermic J waves (Osborne waves) may appear at temperatures less than 33.0° C (91.4° F); characterized by notching of the junction of the QRS complex and ST segments (Fig. 1).

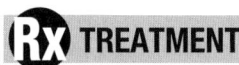 **TREATMENT**

NONPHARMACOLOGIC THERAPY

- The first critical step in management of accidental hypothermia is initiating passive external rewarming by removing wet clothing and covering the patient with insulating material.
- Specific treatment of hypothermia varies with the following:
  1. Degree of hypothermia
  2. Existence of concomitant diseases (e.g., cardiovascular insufficiency)
  3. Patient's age and medical condition (e.g., elderly; debilitated patients vs. young, healthy patients)
- General measures:
  1. Secure an airway before warming all unconscious patients; precede endotracheal intubation with oxygenation (if possible) to minimize the risk of arrhythmias during the procedure.
  2. Peripheral vasoconstriction may impede placement of a peripheral intravenous catheter; consider femoral venous access as an alternative to the jugular or subclavian sites to avoid ventricular stimulation.
  3. A Foley catheter should be inserted, and urinary output should be monitored and maintained >0.5 to 1 ml/kg/h with intravascular volume replacement.
  4. Box 3 summarizes measures for preparing hypothermic patients for transport.

ACUTE GENERAL Rx

- Continuous ECG monitoring of patients is recommended. Ventricular arrhythmias can be treated with bretylium; lidocaine is generally ineffective, and procainamide is associated with an increased incidence of ventricular fibrillation in hypothermic patients.
- Correct severe acidosis and electrolyte abnormalities.
- Hypothyroidism, if present, should be promptly treated (see "Myxedema Coma").
- If clinical evidence suggests adrenal insufficiency, administer IV methylprednisolone.
  In patients unresponsive to verbal or noxious stimuli or with altered mental status, 100 mg of thiamine, 0.4 mg of naloxone, and 1 ampule of 50% dextrose may be given.
  Warm (104° F to 113° F [40° C to 45° C]), humidified oxygen should also be given if available.
- Specific treatment:
  1. Mild hypothermia (rectal temperature <32.3° C [90° F]): Passive external rewarming is indicated. Place the patient in a warm room (temperature >21° C [69.8° F]), and cover with insulating material after gently removing wet clothing; recommended rewarming rates vary between 0.5° C/h and 20° C/h (32.9° F/h and 68° F/h) but should not exceed 0.55° C/h (32.99° F/h) in elderly persons.
  2. Moderate to severe hypothermia:
     a. Active core rewarming
        (1) Delivery of heat by way of fluids: Warm gastrointestinal irrigation (with saline enemas and by nasogastric tube); IV fluids (usually D_5NS without potassium) warmed to 104° F to 107.6° F (40° C to 42° C), peritoneal dialysis with dialysate heated to 40.5° C to 42.5° C (104.9° F/h to 108.5° F/h).
        (2) Inhalation of heated, humidified oxygen (warmed to 40° C [104° F]) increases core temperature by 1° C (1.8° F) per h and decreases evaporative heat loss from respiration.
  3. Active external rewarming: Immersion in a bath of warm water (40° C to 41° C); active external rewarming may produce shock because of excessive peripheral vasodilation. Ideal candidates are previously healthy, young patients with acute immersion hypothermia.

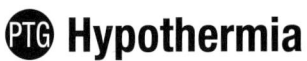

TABLE 3 Core Temperature Measurements

Type	Advantages	Considerations
Rectal	Convenient	Insert 15 cm (6 in)
	Continuous monitoring	Lags during transition from cooling to rewarming
		Falsely elevated with peritoneal lavage
		Falsely low if probe is in cold feces or when lower extremities are frozen
Esophageal	Convenient	Insert 24 cm (9.5 in) below larynx
	Continuous monitoring	Tracheal misplacement
		Aspiration
		Falsely elevated with heated inhalation
Tympanic	Approximates hypothalamic temperature via internal carotid artery	Probe: Tympanic membrane perforation; canal hemorrhage Infrared: Unreliable; cerumen effect
Bladder	Convenient	Unreliable
	Continuous monitoring	Falsely elevated with peritoneal lavage
		Falsely low with cold diuresis

From Auerbach P: *Wilderness medicine, expert consult premium edition—enhanced online features and print*, Philadelphia, 2012, Saunders.

BOX 2 Temperature Correction Factors for Arterial Blood Gas Specimens*

ABG Component Correction Factor
$pH + 0.015 (37 - T_c)$
$Pao_2 - 0.072 (37 - T_c) \times Pao_2$
$Paco_2 - 0.044 (37 - T_c) \times Paco_2$

Example
A patient presents with a core temperature of 32° C with the following ABG values: pH 7.12, $Paco_2$ 52 mm Hg, and Pao_2 52 mm Hg. Corrections for temperature are as follows:
$pH = 7.12 + [0.015 (37 - 32)] = 7.195$
$Pao_2 = 52 - [0.072 (37 - 32) \times 52] = 33.28$ mm Hg
$Paco_2 = 52 - [0.044 (37 - 32) \times 52] = 40.56$ mm Hg
These corrections also may be used for hyperthermia.

*Arterial blood gas values not corrected for temperature in significantly hypothermic patients yield falsely low pH and falsely elevated $Paco_2$ and Pao_2 values.
From Parrillo JE, Dellinger RP: *Critical care medicine, principles of diagnosis and management in the adult*, ed 5, Philadelphia, 2019, Elsevier.

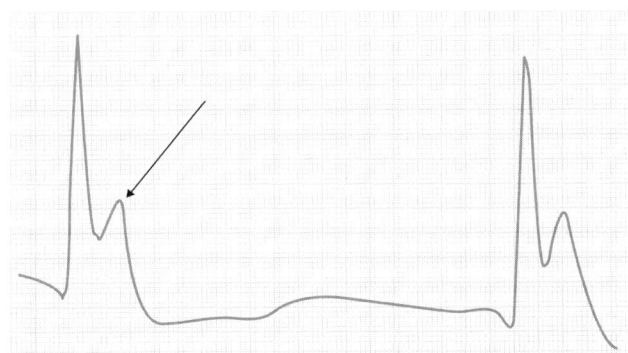

FIG. 1 J (Osborne) wave. (From Goldman L: *Goldman-Cecil medicine*, ed 26, Philadelphia, 2020, Elsevier.)

BOX 3 Preparing Hypothermic Patients for Transport

1. The patient must be dry. Gently remove or cut off wet clothing and replace it with dry clothing or a dry insulation system. Keep the patient horizontal, and do not allow exertion or massage of the extremities.
2. Stabilize injuries (i.e., the spine; place fractures in the correct anatomic position). Open wounds should be covered before packaging.
3. Initiate heated intravenous infusions (IVs) if feasible; bags can be placed under the patient's buttocks or in a compressor system. Administer a fluid challenge.
4. Active rewarming should be limited to heated inhalation and truncal heat. Insulate hot water bottles in stockings or mittens, and then place them in the patient's axillae and groin.
5. The patient should be wrapped. Begin building the wrap by placing a large plastic sheet on the available surface (floor, ground), and on it place an insulated sleeping pad. A layer of blankets, a sleeping bag, or bubble wrap insulating material is laid over the sleeping pad. The patient is then placed on the insulation. Heating bottles are put in place along with IVs, and the entire package is wrapped layer over layer, with the plastic as the final closure. The patient's face should be partially covered, but a tunnel should be created to allow access for breathing and monitoring.

From Auerbach P: *Wilderness medicine, expert consult premium edition—enhanced online features and print*, Philadelphia, 2012, Elsevier.

4. Extracorporeal blood warming with cardiopulmonary bypass appears to be an efficacious rewarming technique in young, otherwise healthy persons.
5. Patients with cardiac instability and those in cardiac arrest should be transported to a center capable of providing extracorporeal membrane oxygenation (ECMO) unless other conditions (e.g., trauma) require transport to a closer facility.

SUGGESTED READING
Available at eBooks.Health.Elsevier.com.

RELATED CONTENT
Hypothermia (Patient Information)

AUTHOR: **FRED F. FERRI, MD**

H

Diseases and Disorders

I

Hypothyroidism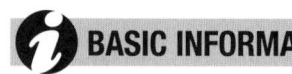

ℹ️ BASIC INFORMATION

DEFINITION
Hypothyroidism is a disorder caused by the inadequate secretion of thyroid hormone.

SYNONYM
Myxedema

ICD-10CM CODES
E00.9 Congenital iodine-deficiency syndrome, unspecified
E02 Subclinical iodine-deficiency hypothyroidism
E03.0 Congenital hypothyroidism with diffuse goiter
E03.1 Congenital hypothyroidism without goiter
E03.2 Hypothyroidism due to medicaments and other exogenous substances
E03.3 Postinfectious hypothyroidism
E03.8 Other specified hypothyroidism
E03.9 Hypothyroidism, unspecified
E89.0 Postprocedural hypothyroidism

EPIDEMIOLOGY & DEMOGRAPHICS
INCIDENCE & PREVALENCE: 1.5% to 2% of women and 0.2% of men. Overall, about 1 in 300 persons in the U.S. has hypothyroidism.
PREDOMINANT AGE: Incidence of hypothyroidism increases with age; among persons older than 60 yr, 6% of women and 2.5% of men have laboratory evidence of hypothyroidism (thyroid-stimulating hormone [TSH] more than twice normal level).

PHYSICAL FINDINGS & CLINICAL PRESENTATION
- Hypothyroid patients generally present with the following signs and symptoms: Fatigue, lethargy, weakness, constipation, weight gain, cold intolerance, muscle weakness, slow speech, slow cerebration with poor memory
- Skin: Dry, coarse, thick, cool, sallow (yellow color caused by carotenemia); nonpitting edema in skin of eyelids and hands (myxedema) secondary to infiltration of subcutaneous tissues by a hydrophilic mucopolysaccharide substance (Fig. E1, *A* and *B*)
- Hair: Brittle and coarse; loss of outer third of eyebrows
- Face: Dulled expression, thickened tongue, thick and slow-moving lips
- Thyroid gland: May or may not be palpable (depending on the cause of the hypothyroidism)
- Heart sounds: Distant, possible pericardial effusion
- Pulse: Bradycardia
- Neurologic: Delayed relaxation phase of the deep tendon reflexes, cerebellar ataxia, hearing impairment, poor memory, peripheral neuropathies with paresthesia
- Musculoskeletal: Carpal tunnel syndrome, muscular stiffness, weakness

ETIOLOGY (TABLE 1)
- Primary hypothyroidism (thyroid gland dysfunction): The cause of >90% of the cases of hypothyroidism
  1. Hashimoto thyroiditis is the most common cause of hypothyroidism after age 8 yr
  2. Idiopathic myxedema (nongoitrous form of Hashimoto thyroiditis)
  3. Previous treatment of hyperthyroidism (radioiodine therapy, subtotal thyroidectomy)
  4. Subacute thyroiditis
  5. Radiation therapy to the neck (usually for malignant disease)
  6. Iodine deficiency or excess
  7. Drugs (lithium, paraaminosalicylate, sulfonamides, phenylbutazone, amiodarone, thiourea). Box E1 summarizes medications that may cause iatrogenic hypothyroidism.
  8. Congenital (approximately one case per 2000 to 4000 live births)
  9. Prolonged treatment with iodides
- Secondary hypothyroidism: Pituitary dysfunction, postpartum necrosis, neoplasm, infiltrative disease-causing deficiency of TSH
- Tertiary hypothyroidism: Hypothalamic disease (granuloma, neoplasm, or irradiation causing deficiency of thyrotropin-releasing hormone)
- Tissue resistance to thyroid hormone: Rare

🅳🅧 DIAGNOSIS

DIFFERENTIAL DIAGNOSIS
- Depression
- Dementia from other causes
- Systemic disorders (e.g., nephrotic syndrome, congestive heart failure, amyloidosis)

LABORATORY TESTS (TABLE 2)
- TSH, free T_4, thyroid peroxidase antibodies (TPOAB)
- Increased TSH: TSH may be normal if patient has secondary or tertiary hypothyroidism, is receiving dopamine or corticosteroids, or the level is obtained after severe illness
- Decreased free T_4 in hypothyroidism, normal free T_4 in subclinical hypothyroidism
- Other common laboratory abnormalities: Hyperlipidemia, hyponatremia, and anemia
- Increased antimicrosomal and antithyroglobulin antibody titers: Useful when autoimmune thyroiditis is suspected as the cause of the hypothyroidism. The American Thyroid Association recommends treatment of pregnant patients with subclinical hypothyroidism and antithyroid peroxidase (anti-TPO) antibody positivity
- Fig. 2 describes a strategy for the laboratory evaluation of patients with suspected hypothyroidism

🆁🅧 TREATMENT

NONPHARMACOLOGIC THERAPY
Patients should be educated regarding hypothyroidism and its possible complications. Patients should also be instructed about the need for lifelong treatment and monitoring of their thyroid abnormality. Patients should also be informed about potential drug and food interactions. Levothyroxine is best taken with water on an empty stomach 60 min before breakfast or at bedtime 3 h after last meal.

ACUTE GENERAL Rx
Start replacement therapy with levothyroxine (L-thyroxine) 25 to 100 μg/day, depending on the patient's age and the severity of the disease. Physiologic combinations of L-thyroxine plus liothyronine do not offer any objective advantage over L-thyroxine alone. The levothyroxine dose may be increased every 6 to 8 wk, depending on the clinical response and serum TSH level. Elderly patients and patients with coronary artery disease should be started with 12.5 to 25 μg/day (higher doses may precipitate angina). The average maintenance dose of levothyroxine is 1.7 μg/kg/day (100 to 150 μg/day in adults). The elderly may require <1 μg/kg/day, whereas children generally require higher doses (up to 3 to 4 μg/kg/day). Pregnant patients also have increased requirements. Estrogen therapy may also increase the need for thyroxine. Women with hypothyroidism should increase their levothyroxine dose by approximately 30% as soon as pregnancy is confirmed. Close monitoring of serum thyrotropin levels and adjustment of levothyroxine dose to maintain a TSH level of a <2.5 mU/L before conception and during the first trimester and a TSH level of 4.0 mU/L as upper limit during the second and third trimester. Table E3 summarizes conditions that alter levothyroxine requirements.

CHRONIC Rx
- Periodic monitoring of TSH level is an essential part of treatment. Patients should be evaluated initially with office visit and TSH levels every 6 to 8 wk until the patient is clinically euthyroid and the TSH level is normalized. The frequency of subsequent visits and TSH measurement can then be decreased to every 6 to 12 mo. Pregnant patients should be checked every trimester.
- For monitoring therapy in patients with central hypothyroidism, measurement of serum free thyroxine (free T_4 level) is appropriate and should be maintained in the upper half of the normal range.

REFERRAL
Admission to the hospital intensive care unit is recommended in all patients with myxedema coma. Additional information on the diagnosis and treatment of this life-threatening complication of hypothyroidism is available under "Myxedema Coma" in Section I.

❗ PEARLS & CONSIDERATIONS

COMMENTS
- **Subclinical hypothyroidism** occurs in as many as 20% of elderly patients and is

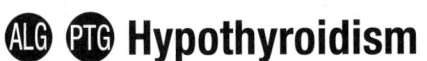

H

Diseases
and Disorders

I

TABLE 1 Causes of Hypothyroidism

Primary Hypothyroidism

Acquired

- Hashimoto thyroiditis
- Iodine deficiency (endemic goiter)
- Drugs blocking synthesis or release of T_4 (e.g., lithium, ethionamide, sulfonamides, iodide)
- Drug-induced thyroid destruction (e.g., interferon alpha, interleukin 2, tyrosine kinase inhibitors, blockers of CTLA4 or PD1)
- Amiodarone (reversible or permanent)
- Goitrogens in foodstuffs or as endemic substances or pollutants
- Thyroid infiltration (amyloidosis, hemochromatosis, sarcoidosis, Riedel struma, cystinosis, scleroderma)
- Postablative thyroiditis due to ^{131}I, surgery, or therapeutic irradiation for nonthyroidal malignancy
- Transient hypothyroidism following painless thyroiditis (including postpartum) or painful subacute thyroiditis

Congenital

- Iodide transport or utilization defect (NIS or pendrin mutations)
- Iodotyrosine dehalogenase deficiency
- Organification disorders (TPO deficiency or dysfunction)
- Defects in thyroglobulin synthesis or processing
- Thyroid agenesis or dysplasia
- TSH receptor defects
- Thyroidal G_s protein abnormalities (pseudohypoparathyroidism type 1a)
- Idiopathic TSH unresponsiveness

Consumptive Hypothyroidism

- Rapid destruction of thyroid hormone due to D3 expression in large hemangiomas or hemangioendotheliomas

Defects of Thyroxine to Triiodothyronine Conversion

- Selenocysteine insertion sequence–binding protein 2 (SECISBP2) defect

Central Hypothyroidism

Acquired

- Pituitary origin (secondary)
- Hypothalamic disorders (tertiary)
- Bexarotene (retinoid X receptor agonist)
- Dopamine or severe illness

Congenital

- TSH deficiency or structural abnormality
- TSH receptor defect

Resistance to Thyroid Hormone

- Generalized
- "Pituitary" dominant

NIS, Sodium-iodide symporter; *TPO,* thyroid peroxidase; *TSH,* thyroid-stimulating hormone (thyrotropin).
From Melmed S et al: *Williams textbook of endocrinology,* ed 14, Philadelphia, 2019, Elsevier.

TABLE 2 Laboratory Evaluation of Patients With Suspected Hypothyroidism or Thyroid Enlargement[a]

TSH, Free T4	TPOAb	Diagnosis
TSH >10 mU/L		
Low	+	Primary hypothyroidism due to autoimmune thyroid disease
Low-normal	+	Primary "subclinical" hypothyroidism (autoimmune)
Low or low-normal	−	Recovery from systemic illness
		External irradiation, drug-induced, congenital hypothyroidism
		Iodine deficiency
		Seronegative autoimmune thyroid disease
		Rare thyroid disorders (amyloidosis, sarcoidosis, etc.)
		Recovery from subacute granulomatous thyroiditis
Normal	+, −	Consider TSH or T_4 assay artifacts
Elevated	−	Thyroid hormone resistance
		Blockade of T_4 to T_3 conversion (amiodarone) or a congenital 5′-deiodinase deficiency
		Consider assay artifacts
TSH 5-10 mU/L		
Low, low-normal	+	Early primary autoimmune hypothyroidism
Low, low-normal	−	Milder forms of nonautoimmune hypothyroidism (see earlier)
		Central hypothyroidism with impaired TSH bioactivity
Elevated	− (+)	Consider thyroid hormone resistance
		T_4 to T_3 conversion blockade (e.g., amiodarone)
TSH 0.5-5 mU/L		
Low, low-normal	− (+)	Central hypothyroidism
		Salicylate or phenytoin therapy
		Desiccated thyroid or T_3 replacement
TSH <0.5 μU/L		
Low, low-normal	− (+)	"Post-hyperthyroid" hypothyroidism (^{131}I or surgery)
		Central hypothyroidism
		T_3 or desiccated thyroid excess
		Following excess levothyroxine withdrawal

TgAb, Antithyroglobulin antibody; *TPOAb,* thyroid peroxidase autoantibody; *TSH,* thyroid-stimulating hormone (thyrotropin); +, present; −, not present.
[a]Initial tests: Serum TSH, serum free T_4, TPO, or TgAb.
From Melmed S et al: *Williams textbook of endocrinology,* ed 14, Philadelphia, 2019, Elsevier.

characterized by an elevated serum TSH and a normal free T_4 level. Subclinical hypothyroidism is not associated with typical symptoms of overt hypothyroidism.[1] Subclinical hypothyroidism can progress to overt hypothyroidism, especially if antithyroid antibodies are present.

It is associated with an increased risk of coronary heart disease events and mortality, particularly in those with a TSH concentration of 10 mU/L or greater. Treatment is individualized and controversial. Some trials have shown that levothyroxine provides no apparent benefit in older persons (≥80 yr of age) with subclinical hypothyroidism. The management of subclinical hypothyroidism should be individualized on the basis of TSH level, comorbid conditions, risk factors, and patient preference. In general, replacement therapy is recommended by most physicians for patients with serum TSH >10 mU/L and with presence of goiter or thyroid autoantibodies or patient has risk factors. Subclinical thyroid dysfunction is not associated with cognitive decline or dementia and treatment of subclinical thyroid dysfunction is unlikely to improve cognitive function.[2]

- ***Congenital hypothyroidism*** is a pediatric disorder with an observed prevalence of one in 2000 to 4000 live births in the U.S. Screening is conducted in all newborns in all states and accomplished by measuring TSH from dried

whole blood spots collected on a newborn by heel stick within the first 24 to 48 hr of life. Currently 14 states perform a routine second screen at approximately 2 wk of age. A two-screen approach is preferred because retrospective analysis found that 20% of congenital hypothyroidism cases were in infants who had normal TSH on the first screen but elevated TSH concentrations on the second screen.

- Switching among FDA-approved generic levothyroxine preparations in patients with stable doses and normal TSH levels is safe and not associated with changes in TSH.[3]

REFERENCES & SUGGESTED READINGS
Available at eBooks.Health.Elsevier.com.

RELATED CONTENT
Hypothyroidism (Patient Information)
Myxedema Coma (Related Key Topic)

AUTHOR: **FRED F. FERRI, MD**

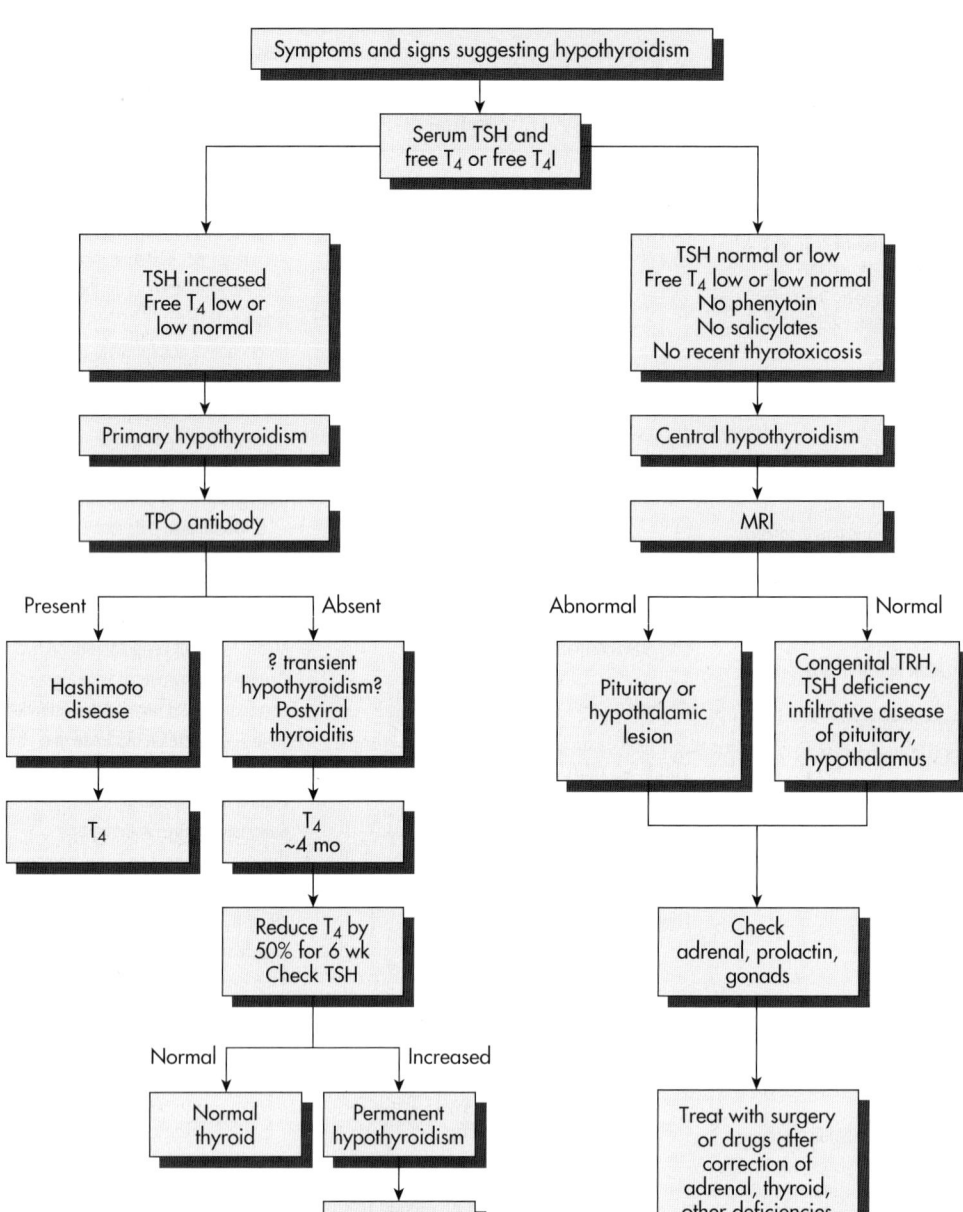

FIG. 2 Strategy for the laboratory evaluation of patients with suspected hypothyroidism. The principal differential diagnosis is between primary and central hypothyroidism. The serum thyrotropin (TSH) concentration is the critical laboratory determination that in general allows recognition of the cause of the disease. An exception is the individual with a recent history of thyrotoxicosis (and suppressed TSH) in whom a low free thyroxine (T_4) level may be associated with a reduced TSH level for several months after relief of the thyrotoxicosis. In patients with primary hypothyroidism, the absence of thyroid peroxidase (TPO) antibodies raises a possible diagnosis of transient hypothyroidism following an undiagnosed episode of subacute or postviral thyroiditis. In such patients, a trial of levothyroxine in reduced dosage after 4 mo may reveal recovery of thyroid function, thus avoiding permanent levothyroxine replacement. *MRI,* Magnetic resonance imaging; *TRH,* thyrotropin-releasing hormone; $T_4I,$ thyroxine index. (From Melmed S et al: *Williams textbook of endocrinology,* ed 14, Philadelphia, 2019, Elsevier.)

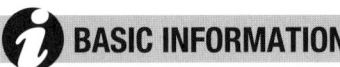 BASIC INFORMATION

DEFINITION
Idiopathic pulmonary fibrosis (IPF) is a specific form of chronic, progressive, fibrosing interstitial pneumonia with a histologic pattern of usual interstitial pneumonia (UIP) occurring in the absence of an identifiable cause of lung injury. Clinically, it is characterized by progressive parenchymal scarring and loss of pulmonary function.

SYNONYMS
Cryptogenic fibrosing alveolitis
IPF
Pulmonary fibrosis
Usual interstitial pneumonia

ICD-10CM CODE
J84.112 Idiopathic pulmonary fibrosis

EPIDEMIOLOGY & DEMOGRAPHICS
- Incidence: 7 to 16 cases/100,000 persons/yr in the U.S.
- Clinically IPF affects >50,000 people in the U.S. and accounts for 20% to 30% of interstitial lung diseases. It is the most common idiopathic interstitial pneumonia.
- Most commonly presents in sixth and seventh decades.
- More common in men than women.
- More common in current and past smokers.
- No distinct geographic distribution.
- No clear racial predilection.

GENETICS:
- Familial forms account for 3% to 25% of cases. Genetic variants include mutations in surfactant protein C and telomerase as well as polymorphisms of the *MUC5B* gene.

PHYSICAL FINDINGS & CLINICAL PRESENTATION
- Most present with gradual onset (>6 mo) of exertional dyspnea and nonproductive cough. Progressive dyspnea is usually the most prominent symptom. Cough affects up to 80% of patients with IPF and is frequently disabling.
- Fine bibasilar inspiratory crackles, "Velcro-like crackles" in >80% of patients, with progression up the lung fields as disease advances.
- Clubbing is found in 25% to 50% of patients.
- Cyanosis and right heart failure (cor pulmonale) may occur late in the disease course.
- There are no extrapulmonary findings beyond clubbing and signs of right heart failure.
- Fever and wheezing are rare and suggest an alternative diagnosis.

ETIOLOGY
- Unknown. Fig. 1 illustrates a proposed pathogenetic sequence in IPF.
- Cigarette smoking, environmental exposures, gastroesophageal reflux, and microaspiration have been associated with IPF.
- Aberrant tissue repair and fibrosis are believed to play a greater role in the pathogenesis than generalized inflammation. Immune system activation and increased vascular permeability contribute to the underlying pathology.

DIAGNOSIS

DIFFERENTIAL DIAGNOSIS
- Occupational exposures (e.g., asbestos) may cause pneumoconiosis with a UIP pattern
- Connective tissue diseases (e.g., rheumatoid arthritis [RA], systemic sclerosis) can cause a UIP pattern
- Chronic hypersensitivity pneumonitis (HP)
- Idiopathic fibrotic nonspecific interstitial pneumonia (NSIP)
- Drug-induced interstitial lung disease
- Desquamative interstitial pneumonia (DIP)
- Respiratory bronchitis–interstitial lung disease (RB-ILD)
- Pleuroparenchymal fibroelastosis
- NOTE: IPF is considered a diagnosis of exclusion

WORKUP
It is critical to establish a confident diagnosis to distinguish IPF from other diseases with better prognosis and different treatment. Multidisciplinary discussion with pulmonology, radiology, and pathology is encouraged as standard of care to decide if a surgical lung biopsy is necessary and to reach consensus on the diagnosis.[1]
- Laboratory tests: There are no specific laboratory tests for IPF; however, IPF requires excluding connective tissue disease-associated interstitial lung disease. Thus, serologic testing is recommended. Antinuclear antibodies, rheumatoid factor, and anticyclic citrullinated peptide are helpful to exclude RA, in which UIP is the most common pattern.[2]

IMAGING STUDIES
- Chest x-ray shows bilateral reticular opacities most prominent in the periphery and lower lobes. Fig. 2 is a chest x-ray showing diffuse bilateral lower lung predominant reticular opacities in a patient with IPF.
- High-resolution computed tomography scan (HRCT) of the chest (Fig. 3) is the most useful diagnostic test. HRCT can show one of four radiographic patterns.
  1. UIP: Lower lobe and peripheral predominant honeycombing, reticulation, and traction bronchiectasis. Mild ground-glass opacities (GGO) could be present in areas of fibrosis. It predicts histologic UIP and precludes the need for surgical lung biopsy.
  2. Probable UIP: Same as UIP, but without honeycombing. When the pretest probability is high—severe traction bronchiectasis in a patient of male sex, >60 yr—it predicts histologic UIP in >90% of cases.[3]
  3. Indeterminate for UIP: Lower lobe and peripheral predominant subtle reticulation, with or without mild GGO. The pattern does not suggest a specific etiology.
  4. Alternative diagnosis: Findings suggestive of another etiology such as mosaic attenuation, air trapping, predominant GGO, consolidation, nodules, cysts, a peribronchovascular, perilymphatic, or upper/mid lung predominant distribution, pleural plaques, etc.
- Surgical lung biopsy: Obtained by video-assisted thoracoscopy or open thoracotomy in carefully selected patients when the radiographic pattern is indeterminate for UIP, and the diagnosis remains unclear. It can show one of four patterns.
  1. UIP: Normal lung with patchy, mostly subpleural or paraseptal, areas of dense fibrosis with distortion (e.g., microscopic honeycombing), fibroblastic foci, and no features to suggest other diagnosis. Establishes IPF diagnosis in the absence of a radiographic alternative diagnosis.

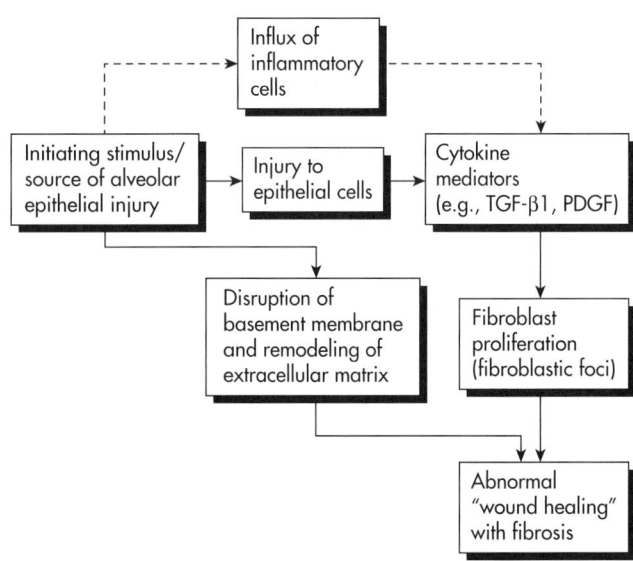

FIG. 1 Proposed pathogenetic sequence in idiopathic pulmonary fibrosis. *Dotted lines* indicate that although there is an influx of inflammatory cells, this is not thought to be a primary component of pathogenesis. *PDGF,* Platelet-derived growth factor; *TGF-β1,* transforming growth factor-β1. (From Weinberger SE: *Principles of pulmonary medicine,* ed 7, Philadelphia, 2019, Elsevier.)

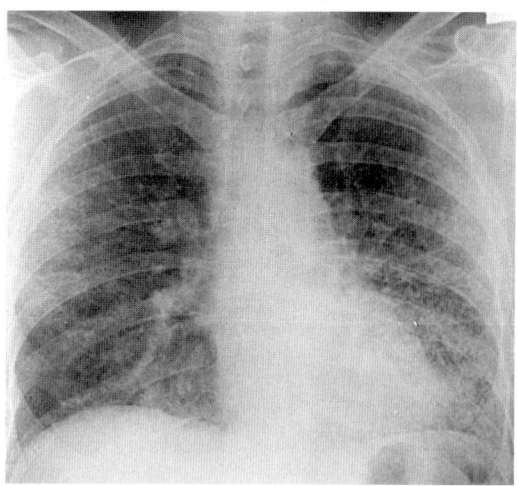

FIG. 2 Chest radiograph shows diffuse bilateral lower lung predominant reticular opacities in a patient with idiopathic pulmonary fibrosis (IPF). (From Mason RJ: *Murray & Nadel's textbook of respiratory medicine,* ed 5, Philadelphia, 2010, Saunders.)

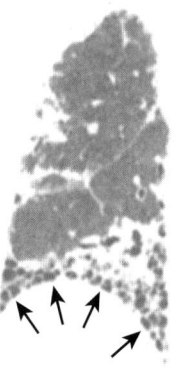
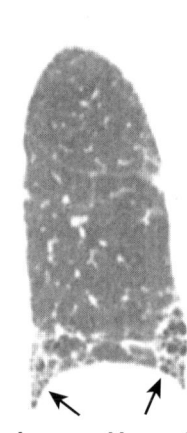

FIG. 3 Pulmonary fibrosis, honeycombing, and a usual interstitial pneumonia (UIP) pattern in idiopathic pulmonary fibrosis (IPF). Coronal high-resolution computed tomography reconstruction shows honeycombing *(arrows)* with a basal and subpleural predominance. This is typical of a UIP pattern. (From Webb WR et al: *Fundamentals of body CT,* ed 4, Philadelphia, 2015, Saunders.)

TABLE 1 Summary of Histologic Findings for Immunologic Lung Diseases

Disease	Histology
Granulomatous	
Foreign body, inorganic dust	Simple granuloma
Hypersensitivity pneumonitis	Poorly formed granulomas, peribronchiolar lymphoplasmacytic infiltrate, organizing pneumonia
Infections	
Tuberculosis	Caseating granulomas
Sarcoidosis	Noncaseating granulomas in a lymphangitic pattern
Granulomatous Vasculitides	
Wegener granulomatosis	Necrotizing granulomas involving vasculature
Churg-Strauss syndrome	Necrotizing granulomas involving vasculature
Eosinophilic pneumonias	Granulomas with eosinophilic predominance; interstitial edema
Histiocytosis X	Granulomas with Langerhans cells
Alveolitic	
Drug-associated injury	Interstitial edema with inflammatory cells
Goodpasture syndrome	Linear staining of basement membrane with anti-IgG antibodies typically seen on renal biopsy; interstitial edema with inflammatory cells
Idiopathic Interstitial Pneumonias	
Idiopathic pulmonary fibrosis	Peripheral lobular fibrosis with less involvement of the centrilobular region, and fibroblastic foci in the interface of both
Desquamative interstitial pneumonia	Accumulation of macrophages in the alveolar spaces
Idiopathic nonspecific interstitial pneumonia	Alveolar septa diffusely thickened with inflammation and fibrosis. Preserved architecture
Acute interstitial pneumonia	Diffuse alveolar damage with thickened fibrotic interstitium; proliferating fibroblasts
Respiratory bronchiolitis–associated interstitial lung disease	Macrophages infiltrating distal bronchioles
Organizing pneumonia	Alveolar filling with polypoid plugs of granulation tissue that can contain inflammatory cells.
Lymphocytic interstitial pneumonia	Diffuse thickening of alveolar septa with lymphocytes forming lymphoid aggregates with germinal centers
Idiopathic pleuroparenchymal fibroelastosis	Diffuse alveolar damage with fibrosis

Modified from Sellke FW et al: *Sabiston & Spencer surgery of the chest,* ed 9, Philadelphia, 2016, Elsevier; and Jones et al: Histopathologic approach to the surgical lung biopsy in interstitial lung disease. In: Collard HR, Richeldi L (eds): *Interstitial lung disease,* Philadelphia, 2018, Elsevier, pp. 141-155.

2. Probable UIP: Same as UIP but the extent is insufficient to exclude other diagnoses. Establishes IPF diagnosis in combination with radiographic probable UIP.
3. Indeterminate for UIP: Some features of UIP but with features suggesting another cause of UIP or an alternative diagnosis. Establishes IPF diagnosis in combination with a radiographic UIP pattern.
4. Alternative diagnosis: Features of other diseases. Excludes IPF. Table 1 summarizes histologic findings for immunologic diseases.

- Transbronchial lung biopsy with a molecular classifier (Envisia) has a specificity of 88% and sensitivity of 70% compared to diagnosis from pathology review, with 84% positive and 77% negative predictive value for UIP.[4] Its use could be considered when avoiding the risk of surgical lung biopsy is preferred.
- Pulmonary function tests show a restrictive pattern and reduced diffusing capacity.
- Six-min walk test may show reduced exercise tolerance and/or exertional hypoxia.

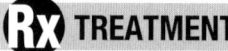 **TREATMENT**

- Two FDA-approved oral medications have similar proven efficacy in slowing disease progression, but neither restores normal lung parenchyma nor improves quality of life. Both are associated with substantial side effects.[5]
1. Pirfenidone is an antifibrotic medication without a known mechanism of action. It is taken three times a day with food. Its major side effects are nausea, abdominal discomfort, and photosensitivity. Liver function tests (LFTs) must be monitored.[6]
2. Nintedanib is a tyrosine kinase inhibitor taken twice daily. Its major side effect is diarrhea, which often resolves. LFTs also need to be followed.[7]

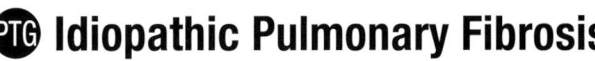

BOX 1 Guidelines for Lung Transplantation for Interstitial Lung Disease

Timing of Referral

Referral should be made at time of diagnosis, even if a patient is being initiated on therapy, for histopathologic UIP or radiographic evidence of a probable or definite UIP pattern.

Abnormal lung function: FVC <80% predicted or DLCO <40% predicted.

Any form of pulmonary fibrosis with one of the following in the past 2 yr:

- Relative decline in FVC 10%
- Relative decline in DLCO 15%
- Relative decline in FVC 5% in combination with worsening of respiratory symptoms or radiographic progression

Supplemental oxygen requirement either at rest or on exertion.

For inflammatory ILDs, progression of disease (either on imaging or pulmonary function) despite treatment.

For patients with connective tissue disease or familial pulmonary fibrosis, early referral is recommended as extrapulmonary manifestations may require special consideration.

Timing of Listing

Any form of pulmonary fibrosis with one of the following in the past 6 mo despite appropriate treatment:

- Absolute decline in FVC >10%
- Absolute decline in DLCO >10%
- Absolute decline in FVC >5% with radiographic progression.

Desaturation to <88% on 6-min walk test or >50 m decline in 6-min walk test distance in the past 6 mo.

Pulmonary hypertension on right heart catheterization or two-dimensional echocardiography (in the absence of diastolic dysfunction).

Hospitalization because of respiratory decline, pneumothorax, or acute exacerbation.

FVC, Forced vital capacity; *DLCO,* diffusion of carbon monoxide; *ILDs,* interstitial lung diseases; *UIP,* usual interstitial pneumonia.
From Leard LE et al: Consensus document for the selection of lung transplant candidates: an update from the International Society for Heart and Lung Transplantation, *J Heart Lung Transpl* S1053-2498(21):02407-4, 2021.

- Additional new therapies are being investigated and are in phase I, II, and III trials.
- The combination of prednisone, azathioprine, and *N*-acetylcysteine was associated with increased mortality in a randomized clinical trial and is contraindicated.
- Treatment includes supportive care (pulmonary rehabilitation, supplemental oxygen, influenza and pneumococcal vaccination), referral for lung transplant consideration, and palliative care.[8]
- Gabapentin (up to 1800 mg/day) acts on airway nerves and is effective for cough, though side effects of sedation and fatigue may limit its use.[9] Other options include benzonatate, guaifenesin with codeine, and menthol lozenges. If postnasal drip or gastroesophageal reflux could be contributing to cough, it is reasonable to treat them.
- Treatment of asymptomatic gastroesophageal reflux may be reasonable given association between pulmonary fibrosis and reflux or microaspiration.

- Lung transplantation is the only therapy shown to prolong survival in IPF. Guidelines for transplantation in patients with interstitial lung disease, including IPF, are summarized in Box 1.[10] (See chapter on "Lung Transplantation.") Posttransplant 5-yr survival for IPF patients is approximately 50% to 60%. Median survival time is longer after bilateral lung transplantation than single lung transplantation but is associated with more complications during the first yr.[11]
- Acute exacerbation of IPF, defined as worsening dyspnea (<1 mo), the presence of new opacities on chest imaging, and the lack of evidence of infection, has a yearly incidence of 7% to 32%. Progressive respiratory failure may require mechanical ventilation; however, a palliative care approach is often chosen instead. Treatment for exacerbations typically includes high-dose corticosteroids and broad-spectrum antibiotics, although the efficacy of this approach is unproven and questionable.[12]

DISPOSITION

- Spontaneous remissions do not occur, although long periods of stability can occur.
- Natural history includes progressive loss of pulmonary function. Predictors of poor outcome include older age, male gender, moderately to severely reduced forced vital capacity (FVC) and diffusion of carbon monoxide (DLCO), and development of pulmonary hypertension.
- There is an increased risk of lung cancer.
- Mean survival after the diagnosis of biopsy-confirmed IPF is 3 to 5 yr, although with new therapies available, survival is less defined.
- Lung transplantation is the only therapy shown to prolong survival.
- Respiratory failure is the most common cause of death.

REFERRAL

- To pulmonologist, with review in multidisciplinary discussion to establish confident diagnosis.
- Referral for participation in clinical trials.
- Early referral to a lung transplant center for evaluation.
- Late-stage management should include palliative care referral.

⚠ PEARLS & CONSIDERATIONS

- The course is progressive, with a high mortality. The most common cause of death in IPF is respiratory failure.
- Critical to differentiate IPF from other interstitial lung diseases because prognosis and treatment approaches differ.
- Two oral therapies have been shown to slow disease progression are available. Additional novel treatments are being investigated.
- Patients with IPF should be referred early for consideration of lung transplantation.

REFERENCES
Available at eBooks.Health.Elsevier.com.

RELATED CONTENT
Idiopathic Pulmonary Fibrosis (Patient Information)
Interstitial Lung Disease (Related Key Topic)

AUTHOR: **AIDA VENADO, MD, MAS**

Diseases and Disorders

I

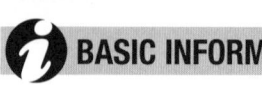 **BASIC INFORMATION**

DEFINITION

Immune thrombocytopenic purpura (ITP) is an autoimmune disorder in which antibody-coated or immune complex–coated platelets are destroyed prematurely, resulting in peripheral thrombocytopenia.[1] The autoantibodies may also affect megakaryocytes and impair platelet production. In primary ITP, the thrombocytopenia is isolated, whereas in secondary ITP, the condition is associated with other disorders (e.g., systemic lupus erythematosus [SLE], HIV, chronic lymphocytic leukemia [CLL], lymphoma). Distinguishing ITP from other causes of thrombocytopenia is very important because ITP requires a different approach to treatment rather than addressing the underlying causes in other types of thrombocytopenia.

SYNONYMS

ITP
Immune thrombocytopenia

ICD-10CM CODE
D69.3 Immune thrombocytopenic purpura

EPIDEMIOLOGY & DEMOGRAPHICS

INCIDENCE: Primary ITP occurs in 1 to 6/100,000 adults/yr.[2]
PREVALENCE: In the U.S., 8/100,000 in children and 12/100,000 in adults.[3] Given ITP is often a chronic condition, prevalence significantly exceeds incidence.
PREDOMINANT SEX: 72% of patients >10 yr are female; among children, males are more commonly affected.[2]
PREDOMINANT AGE: Children ages 1 to 6 yr and young women (70% are <40 yr). New onset of ITP after age 60 yr is uncommon; comprehensive workup for secondary ITP may be required.

PHYSICAL FINDINGS & CLINICAL PRESENTATION

The presentation of ITP is different in children and adults:
- Children generally present with sudden onset of bruising and petechiae from severe thrombocytopenia.
- In adults, the presentation is insidious; a history of prolonged purpura may be present. Many patients are diagnosed incidentally based on automated laboratory tests that now routinely include platelet counts. Bleeding may be present in up to two thirds of patients.
- Fatigue is a common symptom and often correlates with platelet count.
- The physical examination may be entirely normal.
- Patients with severe thrombocytopenia may have petechiae, purpura, epistaxis, or heme-positive stool from gastrointestinal bleeding. Life-threatening bleeding is uncommon and generally confined to patients with platelets <10,000/mm³.
- Splenomegaly is unusual; its presence should alert to the possibility of other etiologies of thrombocytopenia.

- The presence of dysmorphic features (skeletal anomalies, auditory abnormalities) may indicate a congenital disorder as the cause of the thrombocytopenia.

ETIOLOGY

Increased platelet destruction is caused by autoantibody targets to platelet-membrane antigens, particularly antibodies against platelet GPIIb/IIIa or GPIb/IX.[4] The spleen has a major role in ITP by producing autoantibodies in the white pulp and removing autoantibody-coated platelets in the red pulp. Production of antibodies could be triggered either by immunogenicity of membrane glycoproteins (GPs) on the platelet surface or by external factors such as infections or medications. Reduced platelet lifespan due to clearance is the predominant cause of thrombocytopenia.

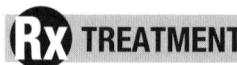 **DIAGNOSIS**

DIFFERENTIAL DIAGNOSIS
- ITP is a diagnosis of exclusion.
- Falsely low platelet count due to aggregation (resulting from ethylenediaminetetraacetic acid [EDTA]-dependent or cold-dependent agglutinins). Platelet count is corrected by using heparin or citrate anticoagulated tube.
- Variety of infections, including viral infections (e.g., HIV, hepatitis C, Epstein-Barr virus causing mononucleosis, cytomegalovirus, *H. pylori,* SARS-CoV-2, rubella).
- Drugs commonly implicated are heparin (heparin-induced thrombocytopenia [HIT]), quinidine, antibiotics (linezolid, vancomycin, sulfonamides, rifampin), platelet inhibitors (tirofiban, abciximab, eptifibatide), cimetidine, NSAIDs, thiazide diuretics, antirheumatic agents (gold salts, penicillamine), and many chemotherapeutic agents (cyclosporine, fludarabine, carboplatin, oxaliplatin).
- Hypersplenism resulting from liver disease.
- Myelodysplastic and lymphoproliferative disorders.
- Pregnancy.
- Hypothyroidism.
- SLE, rheumatoid arthritis, antiphospholipid syndrome.
- Microangiopathic processes include thrombotic thrombocytopenic purpura (TTP), hemolytic-uremic syndrome (HUS), and disseminated intravascular coagulation (DIC).
- Congenital thrombocytopenia (e.g., Fanconi syndrome, May-Hegglin anomaly, Bernard-Soulier syndrome).
- Evans syndrome is a rare autoimmune disorder characterized by autoimmune hemolytic anemia (AIHA) and immune thrombocytopenia (ITP).

LABORATORY TESTS
- CBC, platelet count, and peripheral smear: Platelets are decreased. The peripheral smear should show large platelets and no schistocytes (Fig. E1). Red blood cells and white blood cells have a normal morphology. Unless the patient has been bleeding, the hemoglobin level and leukocyte count should be normal.

- Reticulated platelets (RPs) are the youngest circulating platelets, analogous to the relationship between reticulocytes and mature red blood cells. RPs can be quantified by flow cytometry or with an automated measurement called the "immature platelet fraction" (IPF) can be used to aid in diagnosis of ITP, if the clinical picture is unclear.[5] The IPF is typically elevated in thrombocytopenia caused by peripheral consumption/destruction (e.g., ITP), and it is usually normal in production defects such as bone marrow failure syndromes.
- Additional tests may be ordered to exclude other causes of the thrombocytopenia when clinically indicated (e.g., HIV screening test, antinuclear antibody [ANA], thyroid-stimulating hormone [TSH] [hypothyroidism and hyperthyroidism can cause thrombocytopenia], liver enzymes, hepatitis C Ab).
- Direct assay of platelet-bound antibodies has an estimated positive predictive value of only 80% to 83%. A negative test cannot be used to rule out the diagnosis.
- Bone marrow aspiration and biopsy are recommended in adults older than >60 yr if there is evidence of immature cells on peripheral smear or persistent neutropenia. Biopsy in an ITP patient shows a normal to increased number of megakaryocytes; other hemopoietic lineages are normal.

IMAGING STUDIES

CT scan of abdomen/pelvis in patients with splenomegaly to exclude other disorders causing thrombocytopenia

Rx TREATMENT

NONPHARMACOLOGIC THERAPY
- Minimize activity to prevent injury or bruising (e.g., contact sports should be avoided).
- Stop any potentially offending drugs (see "Etiology"). Avoid medications that increase the risk of bleeding (e.g., aspirin and other NSAIDs).

ACUTE GENERAL Rx
- Treatment varies with the platelet count, patient's age, and bleeding status. The goal of therapy is to provide a safe platelet count to prevent clinically important bleeding. For newly diagnosed patients with minimal bleeding, treatment consists of corticosteroids vs. observation when platelet counts are <30,000 /mm³ and hospital admission when platelet counts are <20,000 /mm³ (Fig. E2).
- Outpatient observation and frequent monitoring of platelet count are needed in asymptomatic established ITP patients with platelet counts >20,000/mm³.
- Oral prednisone: 1 mg/kg/day for 1 to 2 wk followed by gradual taper is the most common initial regimen. Prolonged courses (>6 wk) of prednisone are not recommended. Response rates range from 50% to 75%, and most responses occur within the first 3 wk.[6]

- IV methylprednisolone: 30 mg/kg/day (maximum dose of 1 g/day for 2 or 3 days) infused over 20 to 30 min plus IV immunoglobulin (1 g/kg/day for 2 or 3 days).
- Pulse-dose oral dexamethasone: Given at a dose of 40 mg/day for 4 consecutive days when given for three to four cycles every 4 wk results in a high response rate (80% to 85%) and has been shown to have fewer side effects when compared to longer courses of prednisone.[7] A meta-analysis of nine randomized trials revealed no major increase in efficacy but confirmed less toxicity and faster increases in platelet counts using high-dose dexamethasone.[8]
- Continuation of corticosteroids is limited by long-term complications associated with its use (osteoporosis, weight gain, opportunistic infections, emotional lability, avascular necrosis).
- Infusion of platelets should only be given to patients with life-threatening hemorrhage or those undergoing emergent surgery.
- IV immunoglobulin (typically 1 to 2 g/kg in divided doses) is used in two settings: Corticosteroid-refractory patients and pregnant patients. It rapidly increases platelet count in nearly 80% of patients, but its effect is transient.
- Anti-D immunoglobulin, a pooled IgG product derived from the plasma of Rh(D)-negative donors, is also effective. It can be given only to patients who are Rh(D) positive with hemoglobin >8 mg/dl, and the usual dose is 50 to 75 mcg/kg.
- Rituximab, a monoclonal antibody directed against the CD20 antigen, is used as a second-line agent. Usual dose is 375 mg/m^2 weekly ×4 wk.
- Splenectomy is considered a subsequent option in case of rituximab failure. Previously, it was considered in adults with platelet count <20,000/mm^3 after 6 wk of medical treatment or after 6 mo if more than 10 to 20 mg/day of prednisone is still required to maintain a platelet count >30,000/mm^3. In children, splenectomy is generally reserved for persistent thrombocytopenia (>1 yr) and clinically significant bleeding. Appropriate immunizations (pneumococcal vaccine in adults and children, *Haemophilus influenzae* vaccine, meningococcal vaccine in children) should be administered earlier than 2 wk before planned splenectomy. Post-splenectomy vaccinations should be performed in all cases.
- Additional second-line agents are thrombopoietin receptor agonists (TPO-RA), azathioprine, cyclosporin A, cyclophosphamide, danazol, dapsone, mycophenolate mofetil, and *Vinca* alkaloids. A recent trial of mycophenolate mofetil addition to a glucocorticoid for first-line treatment of ITP regulated in a greater response and a lower risk of refractory or relapsed ITP, but with somewhat decreased quality of life.[9]
- Romiplostim, a recombinant fusion protein, and the oral TPO-RA eltrombopag are effective in increasing platelet count in adult patients with chronic ITP refractory to corticosteroids and/or splenectomy.[10]
- Fostamatinib is an inhibitor of the enzyme spleen tyrosine kinase (Syk). Syk plays an important role in phagocytosis of FcγR-mediated signal transduction and inflammatory propagation.[11] It received FDA approval of chronic ITP in adults who had an insufficient response to previous treatment including corticosteroids, intravenous immunoglobulin (IVIG), splenectomy, and/or a TPO-RA (10). The recommended initial dose is 100 mg PO twice daily. It can be increased to 150 mg twice daily if the platelet count has not responded to at least 50,000/mm^3 at 1 mo.
- Preliminary trials with rilzabrutinib, an oral, reversible covalent inhibitor of Bruton's tyrosine kinase have shown that it may increase platelet counts in patients with ITP by means of a dual mechanism of action: Decreased macrophage-mediated platelet destruction and reduced production of pathogenic autoantibodies.[11,12]

PREGNANCY Rx

- No treatment is required when platelet count is >30,000/mm^3 or higher until 36 wk gestation, or earlier in case of premature labor.
- Oral corticosteroids and IVIG.
- Refractory ITP may require splenectomy in the second trimester.

DISPOSITION

- More than 80% of children have a complete remission within 8 wk.
- In adults, the course of the disease is chronic; only 5% of adults have spontaneous remission. However, majority of adults will reach stable, safe platelet count.
- The principal cause of death from ITP is intracranial hemorrhage (1% of children, 5% of adults).

REFERENCES & SUGGESTED READINGS

Available at eBooks.Health.Elsevier.com

AUTHORS: **MINESH NANDI, MD, IMRAN PUTHAWALA, MD,** and **PATAN GULTAWATVICHAI, MD**

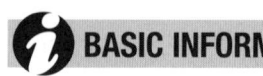

BASIC INFORMATION

DEFINITION

Urinary incontinence is the involuntary leakage of urine.

SYNONYM

Urinary incontinence

ICD-10CM CODES	
N39.3	Stress incontinence (female) (male)
N39.41	Urgency urinary incontinence
N39.46	Mixed incontinence
N39.49	Disorder of urinary system, unspecified
R32	Unspecified urinary incontinence
R39.81	Functional urinary incontinence

EPIDEMIOLOGY & DEMOGRAPHICS

INCIDENCE/PREVALENCE: In the general population between the ages of 15 and 64, 1.5% to 5% of men and 25% to 57% of women have urinary incontinence[1]. The incidence among young women is 25%[2]; middle-aged and postmenopausal women is 44% to 57%[1]; and older women is 75%.[3]

CLINICAL, PSYCHOLOGICAL, & SOCIAL IMPACT

- Fewer than 50% of women living with incontinence in the U.S. consult health care professionals for care, resulting in significant physical and psychological limitations.[4] Many women choose to turn to home remedies, commercially available absorbent materials, and supportive aids. As the incontinence worsens, many women become depressed, limit social interaction, refrain from sexual intimacy, and become homebound. It is estimated that $19.5 billion in direct costs is spent annually on incontinence in the U.S.[5] Urinary incontinence contributes to approximately 6% of nursing home admissions in the older population, leading to a cost of $3 billion per yr. With aging populations around the world, this cost is dramatically increasing every year.

MAJOR TYPES OF INCONTINENCE

The continence mechanisms are complex and include multiple levels of control: Central and peripheral nervous systems (Fig. E1), the detrusor muscle, the urethra, and pelvic floor muscles. Dysfunction at any of these levels can lead to incontinence.

- **Stress urinary incontinence (SUI)** (Table 1) is the involuntary loss of urine with effort or physical exertion, or with any activity that increases intraabdominal pressure (sneezing, coughing, etc.). The most common risk factors are parity and obesity. Table 2 summarizes typical symptom differences in stress and urge incontinence. SUI may be demonstrated with a simple cough stress test during examination. The cotton swab test can determine the degree of urethral mobility, which may be helpful in determining which type of surgical procedure to perform, but this test is not useful for diagnosing SUI.

1. **Intrinsic sphincter deficiency (ISD)** is the most severe form of SUI and indicates a urethra that cannot remain closed even at rest. On urodynamic testing, this is diagnosed with a maximal urethral closure pressure <20 cm H_2O and leak point pressure <60 cm H_2O.
- **Urgency urinary incontinence (UUI)** is the involuntary loss of urine associated with urgency, a sudden compelling desire to pass urine that is difficult to defer. The diagnosis is often made clinically based on patient's report of symptoms but may also be associated with involuntary detrusor contractions on urodynamic investigation. May be idiopathic or neurogenic.
- **Overactive bladder (OAB)** is described as a constellation of symptoms, including urgency, with or without urgency urinary incontinence, usually with urinary frequency and nocturia. It should be distinguished from excessive fluid intake and must exclude urinary tract infection.

Can occur in up to 27% of men and up to 43% of women.
- **Mixed urinary incontinence** is the involuntary leakage of urine associated with urgency and with physical exertion, effort, sneezing or coughing.
- **Overflow incontinence** is the leakage of urine resulting from urinary retention with resultant overflow or spilling of the urine. Causes include hypotonic bladder resulting from age, neurologic conditions such as diabetes or spinal cord injury, prior surgery, drug effects (e.g., intravesical Botox), or fecal impaction. It may also be caused by obstruction at the bladder neck and urethra, such as from prior anti-incontinence surgery, pelvic organ prolapse, urethral stenosis, or detrusor-sphincter dyssynergia.
- **Functional urinary incontinence** is the involuntary leakage of urine resulting from chronic cognitive, functional, or mobility impairments. This is a diagnosis of exclusion and

---

TABLE 1 Surgical Treatment of Stress Incontinence

Abdominal retropubic urethropexy (suspension)
Marshall-Marchetti-Krantz
Burch operation

Sling procedure:
Pubovaginal (bladder neck) sling
Autologous:
Rectus abdominis fascia
Tensor fascia lata
Anterior vaginal wall sling
Allograft (cadaveric fascia lata fascia)
Xenograft:
Porcine dermis
Small intestinal submucosa
Synthetic mesh (polypropylene)
Tension-free midurethral sling (polypropylene):
Retropubic
Transobturator
Single incision

Urethral-bulking agents:
Carbon-coated zirconium beads
Calcium hydroxyapatite
Cross-linked polydimethylsiloxane

From Lipshultz LI et al: *Urology and the primary care practitioner,* ed 3, Philadelphia, 2008, Elsevier.

TABLE 2 Typical Symptom Differences in Stress and Urge Incontinence

Symptom	Stress Incontinence	Urge Incontinence
Leakage with exertion, cough, sneeze, activity	Yes	No
Leakage with sensation or urgency	No	Yes
Frequency, nocturia	No	Yes
Large volume urine loss	No	Yes
Leakage with running water, key in the door	No	Yes
Leakage with position change from sitting to standing	Possible	Yes
Leakage while recumbent	No	Possible
History of childhood bedwetting	No	Yes

From Gershenson DM et al: *Comprehensive gynecology,* ed 8, Philadelphia, 2022, Elsevier.

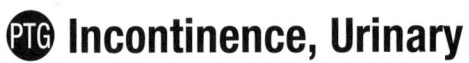
may be cured by improving the patient's functional status, treating comorbidities, changing medications, and reducing environmental barriers.

- **Extraurethral urinary incontinence** is leakage that bypasses the urethral meatus (i.e., vesicovaginal fistula or ectopic ureter).

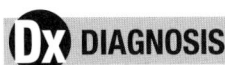 **DIAGNOSIS**

HISTORY

- Because many women are hesitant to bring up symptoms of incontinence, these symptoms should be elicited through simple screening (Tables 3 and 4). Lower urinary tract symptoms are summarized in Table 5.
- History of present illness, psychosocial factors, congenital disorders, access issues for the physically challenged, neurologic disorders, and medication use are coexistent disorders that may affect the urinary tract.
- Urinary incontinence may be characterized by frequency of incontinence episodes, severity, and extent of bother.
- Voiding diary to assess total voided volume, frequency of micturition, mean volume voided, largest single volume, diurnal distribution, and nature and severity of incontinence.
- Assessments of the severity of symptoms and goals for treatment are important parts of the history.

WORKUP

- General physical examination:
  1. Confounding conditions including mobility issues. Comorbid conditions that can cause or contribute to urinary incontinence in elderly patients are summarized in Table 6. Table 7 describes medications that can cause or contribute to urinary incontinence
  2. Neuromuscular deficits (gait of the patient)
- Pelvic exam:
  1. Concurrent pelvic organ prolapse
  2. Vaginal discharge
  3. Estrogen status
  4. Pelvic floor strength assessment
  5. Neurologic examination to assess sacral nerves with anal wink and bulbocavernosus reflex
- Rectal examination to assess sphincter tone and stool impaction
- Simple cough stress test
- Urethral hypermobility
- Postvoid residual check with bladder scan or catheter to exclude retention
- 3-day bladder diary to assess frequency, timing, and volume of voids

LABORATORY TESTS

It is important to rule out urinary tract infection and microscopic hematuria with urinalysis and/or culture prior to more invasive testing for other causes for incontinence.

SPECIALIZED STUDIES

- **Urodynamic testing:** Measures different facets of urine storage and evacuation; usually necessary only if basic office evaluation does not elicit the cause of incontinence, if incontinence is persistent despite treatments, or if there are confounding contributors to incontinence including prior surgery
  1. Simple cystometrogram: Graph of bladder and abdominal pressures related to fluid volume during filling/storage/voiding to assess sensation and capacity; also assesses presence of detrusor contractions, whether voluntary or involuntary
  2. Uroflowmetry and pressure-flow studies: Measure the mechanisms of bladder emptying and rate of urine flow

---

TABLE 3 Recommendations for Urinary Incontinence (UI) Screening

Organization	Target Population	Recommendation	Level of Evidence/Grade of Recommendation/Rationale
USPSTF	All older adults	Screen for UI as part of an overall prevention recommendations for older adults	Not provided
Women's Preventive Services Initiative	All women	Screen annually for UI	Weak; detect UI before it significantly affects women's lives
World Health Organization	All older persons	Routinely check for UI in older women and men	Rationale: At least half of women with UI do not report this issue to their general practitioner
ACOVE	All persons age ≥75 yr	1. During an initial evaluation, all persons should have documentation of the presence or absence of UI 2. During annual evaluations, all persons should have documentation of the presence or absence of UI	N/A

ACOVE, Assessing Care of Vulnerable Elderly; *USPSTF,* US Preventive Services Task Force.
From Warshaw G et al: *Ham's primary care geriatrics,* ed 7, Philadelphia, 2022, Elsevier.

TABLE 4 Screening Questions for Incontinence

Type of Incontinence	Question	Psychometrics
Any	• "Have you had any problems with bladder or urine control?" • "Do you ever leak urine when you don't want to?"	Kappa 0.8 (95% CI, 0.3-0.9) Percentage agreement 90% (95% CI, 84-95%)
Stress incontinence	• "Do you ever leak urine coughing, sneezing, lifting, walking, or running?"	Positive LR 2.2 (95% CI, 1.6-3.2) Negative LR 0.39 (95% CI, 0.25-0.61) Sensitivity 0.86 (95% CI, 0.79-0.90) Specificity 0.60 (95% CI, 0.51-0.68) Posttest probability decreases with age (from 87-42%)
Urge incontinence	• "Do you experience such a strong and sudden urge to void that you leak before reaching the toilet?"	Positive LR 4.2 (95% CI, 2.3-7.6) Negative LR 0.48 (95% CI, 0.36-0.62) Sensitivity 0.75 (95% CI, 0.68-0.81) Specificity 0.77 (95% CI, 0.69-0.84) Posttest probability increases with age (from 52-91%)

CI, Confidence interval; *LR,* likelihood ratio (likelihood that a given test result would be expected in a patient with the target disorder compared with the likelihood that the same result would be expected in a patient without the target disorder).
From Warshaw G et al: *Ham's primary care geriatrics,* ed 7, Philadelphia, 2022, Elsevier.

TABLE 5 Lower Urinary Tract Symptoms

Symptom	Description
Urgency	Compelling, often sudden need to void that is difficult to defer.
Urge incontinence	Leakage preceded by/associated with urgency. Common precipitants include running water, hand washing, going out in the cold, even the sight of the garage or trying to unlock the door when returning home. The need to "rush to the toilet" and length of time one can forestall an urgency episode are less useful symptoms because they reflect cognition, mobility, toilet availability, and sphincter control, as well as bladder function.
Stress incontinence	Leakage with effort, exertion, sneezing, or coughing. Leakage may be provoked by minimal or no activity when there is severe sphincter damage. Leakage coincident with cough, laugh, sneeze, or physical activity suggests failure of sphincter mechanisms. Leakage that occurs seconds after the activity, especially if difficult to stop, suggests a cough-induced uninhibited detrusor contraction.
Mixed incontinence	Presence of both urgency and stress UI symptoms. Patients vary in the predominance, severity, and/or bother of urge versus stress leakage.
Overactive bladder	Symptom syndrome (not a specific pathologic condition) consisting of urgency, frequency, and nocturia, with or without urge incontinence.
Frequency	Complaint of needing to void too often during the day, as defined by the patient.
Nocturia	Complaint of waking at night one or more times to void. If these voids are associated with UI, the term *nocturnal enuresis* may be used.
Slow (weak) stream	Perception of reduced urine flow, usually compared with previous performance.
Hesitancy	Difficulty in initiating voiding, resulting in a delay in the onset of voiding after the individual feels ready to pass urine.
Straining	Muscular effort either to initiate, maintain, or improve the urinary stream.
Intermittent stream	Sensation that the bladder is not empty after voiding.
Postvoid dribbling	Small amounts/drops of urine after voiding has stopped. More common in men.

UI, Urinary incontinence.
From Warshaw GA et al: *Ham's primary care geriatrics*, ed 7, Philadelphia 2022, Elsevier.

3. Urethral mechanism and pressure studies
4. Electromyography: Studies the neuromuscular activity of pelvic muscles and striated urethral sphincter during filling and micturition
- **Cystourethroscopy:** Procedure that can be done in the office or the operating room. An endoscope is inserted into the urethra to view the inside of the bladder and urethra. This procedure is not routinely used to evaluate incontinence unless hematuria is present or prior pelvic surgery is noted on history

IMAGING STUDIES

- Usually ordered only if history and/or physical findings suggest other, less common causes of incontinence (i.e., genitourinary fistula) or if microscopic hematuria is present.
- Renal ultrasound may be used to assess for hydronephrosis.
- CT urogram may be used to assess upper tract abnormalities, congenital anomalies, genitourinary fistula, and microscopic hematuria etiologies.

🆁🆇 TREATMENT

- Fig. 2 illustrates a treatment algorithm for stress, urge, and mixed incontinence.
- The recommended approach to urinary incontinence is a stepped care plan first offering noninvasive behavioral modifications such as bladder training, weight loss, and fluid management. Fig. E3 summarizes the diagnosis and treatment of overactive bladder.
- **Pelvic floor muscle training,** including Kegel exercises, often augmented with biofeedback or electrical stimulation, is an important component of first-line therapy for stress, urge, and mixed incontinence. Women should

perform 45 to 50 exercises per day to achieve good results (60% to 85% reduction in incontinence if biofeedback is also used).
- **Local estrogen** may have some benefit in decreasing urinary incontinence.[6] Systemic estrogen therapy does not appear to be effective in treatment or prevention of incontinence.
- **Pharmacotherapy** is usually reserved for urgency urinary incontinence (Table 8):
  1. Antimuscarinic (anticholinergic) medications: Block parasympathetic muscarinic receptors (detrusor M2/M3 receptors) to inhibit involuntary detrusor contractions:
     a. Agents available: Darifenacin, fesoterodine, oxybutynin (available orally and as a transdermal patch), solifenacin, tolterodine, and trospium
     b. Efficacy: Shown to improve symptoms and continence but only modestly compared with placebo
     c. Side effects: High rates of discontinuation due to side effects, most often dry mouth and constipation. May also exacerbate urinary retention, blurred vision, dyspepsia, and impaired cognitive function, with some studies now showing an association with dementia if used for >2 yr; contraindicated in narrow-angle glaucoma
     d. Of note, trospium may have a lower risk of cognitive impairment given the size of the molecule as it is less likely to cross the blood-brain barrier
  2. Beta-agonists: Stimulate β3-adrenergic receptor in the detrusor muscle to cause relaxation and increase bladder capacity
     a. Agents available: Mirabegron, vibegron
     b. Efficacy: Significant reductions in urgency incontinence in randomized trials
     c. Side effects: Mirabegron: Tachycardia, hypertension, headache, and diarrhea (similar to placebo); not recommended

in uncontrolled hypertension. Vibegron: Has not been associated with blood pressure elevations. Its most common side effects are headaches and nasopharyngitis.
  3. The combination of anticholinergic drug and a beta3 agonist may be more effective than either drug alone in patients who do not respond to monotherapy.
  4. OnabotulinumtoxinA (Botox A) (Table 9): Inhibits the presynaptic release of acetylcholine from motor neurons at the neuromuscular junction to paralyze the muscle; given by cystoscopic intravesical injection every 6 to 12 mo.
     a. Efficacy: Similar rates of improvement seen when compared with antimuscarinic medications, but more women reporting complete resolution of urgency urinary incontinence with Botox A; third-line treatment due to adverse effects
     b. Adverse effects: Urinary retention or incomplete bladder emptying (5% requiring catheterization) and urinary tract infections (33%)
- **Peripheral tibial nerve stimulation** (see Table 9): 30-min session of tibial nerve stimulation once per week for 12 wk followed by a customized maintenance plan to treat OAB. Compared with placebo, pooled success rate was 60% in a guideline published by American Urological Association; fewer adverse events noted when compared with antimuscarinic medication.
- **Sacral neuromodulation** (see Table 9): Stimulation of bladder and pelvic floor nerves to treat OAB, UUI, and idiopathic urinary retention. The mechanism is unknown. The procedure occurs in a two-stage process: First the electrode is placed near S3 to determine if symptoms are improved by 50%; if so, then

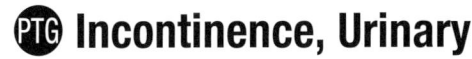
TABLE 6 Comorbid Conditions That Can Cause or Contribute to Urinary Incontinence in Frail Older Adults

Conditions	Comments	Implications for Management
Comorbid Medical Illnesses		
Diabetes mellitus	Poor control can cause polyuria and precipitate or exacerbate incontinence; also associated with increased likelihood of urgency incontinence and diabetic neuropathic bladder	Better control of diabetes can reduce osmotic diuresis and associated polyuria, improve incontinence
Degenerative joint disease	Can impair mobility and precipitate urgency UI	Optimal pharmacologic and nonpharmacologic pain management can improve mobility, toileting ability
Chronic pulmonary disease	Associated cough can worsen stress UI	Cough suppression can reduce stress incontinence and cough-induced urgency UI
Congestive heart failure Lower extremity venous insufficiency	Increased nighttime urine production can contribute to nocturia and UI	Optimizing pharmacologic management of congestive heart failure, sodium restriction, support stockings, leg elevation, and late afternoon dose of rapid-acting diuretic may reduce nocturnal polyuria, associated nocturia, nighttime UI
Sleep apnea	May increase nighttime urine production by increasing production of atrial natriuretic peptide	Diagnosis and treatment of sleep apnea, usually with continuous positive airway pressure devices, may relieve UI, reduce nocturnal polyuria and associated nocturia
Severe constipation and fecal impaction	Associated with "double" incontinence (urine and fecal)	Appropriate use of stool softeners Adequate fluid intake and exercise Disimpaction if necessary
Neurologic and Psychiatric Conditions		
Stroke	Can precipitate urgency UI and, less often, urinary retention; also impairs mobility	UI after acute stroke often resolves with rehabilitation; persistent UI should be further evaluated. Regular toileting assistance essential for those with persistent mobility impairment
Parkinson disease	Associated with urgency UI; also causes impaired mobility and cognition in late stages	Optimizing management may improve mobility, improve UI. Regular toileting assistance essential for those with mobility and cognitive impairment in late stages
Normal-pressure hydrocephalus	Presents with UI, along with gait and cognitive impairments	Patients presenting with all three symptoms should be considered for brain imaging to rule out this condition; may improve with a ventricular-peritoneal shunt
Dementia (Alzheimer, multiinfarct, others)	Associated with urgency UI; impaired cognition and apraxia interfere with toileting and hygiene	Regular toileting assistance essential for those with mobility and cognitive impairment in late stages
Depression	May impair motivation to be continent; may also be a consequence of incontinence	Optimizing pharmacologic and nonpharmacologic management of depression may improve UI Discontinuation or modification of drug regimen
Medications		
Functional Impairments		
Impaired mobility, impaired cognition	Impaired cognition and/or mobility due to a variety of conditions (listed above) and others can interfere with ability to toilet independently and can precipitate UI	Regular toileting assistance essential for those with severe mobility and/or cognitive impairment
Environmental Factors		
Inaccessible toilets Unsafe toilet facilities No contrasting color between toilet and seat Caregivers unavailable for toileting assistance	Frail, functionally impaired persons require accessible and safe toilet facilities and, in many cases, human assistance to be continent	Environmental alterations may be helpful; supportive measures such as pads may be necessary if caregiver assistance not regularly available

UI, Urinary incontinence.
From Fillit HM: *Brocklehurst's textbook of geriatric medicine and gerontology*, ed 8, Philadelphia, 2017, Elsevier.

next the pulse generator is implanted. Evidence suggests 70% of women experience significant improvement in their symptoms with sacral neuromodulation.
- **Augmentation cystoplasty:** Older procedure that was used before introduction of sacral neuromodulation in patients with poorly compliant bladders who were at risk for upper tract deterioration, completed by using a gastrointestinal segment.
- **Devices:**

1. Continence pessaries: For women with SUI who wish to defer or avoid surgery; helps increase urethral resistance during increased intraabdominal pressure.
2. Over-the-counter vaginal or urethral inserts: Disposable devices used to support the urethra, especially in women with situational stress incontinence (i.e., only when exercising); however, urethral inserts have been associated with a high rate of urinary tract infection.

- **Surgery:** Indicated for women with SUI without symptom control after conservative management or as first-line treatment in appropriately counseled women who decline more conservative treatment:
1. Synthetic slings are the most common primary surgical treatment for SUI. Cure rates of 62% to 98% have been reported in a recent systematic review:
   a. Transvaginal/retropubic: Trocars are passed through the retropubic space

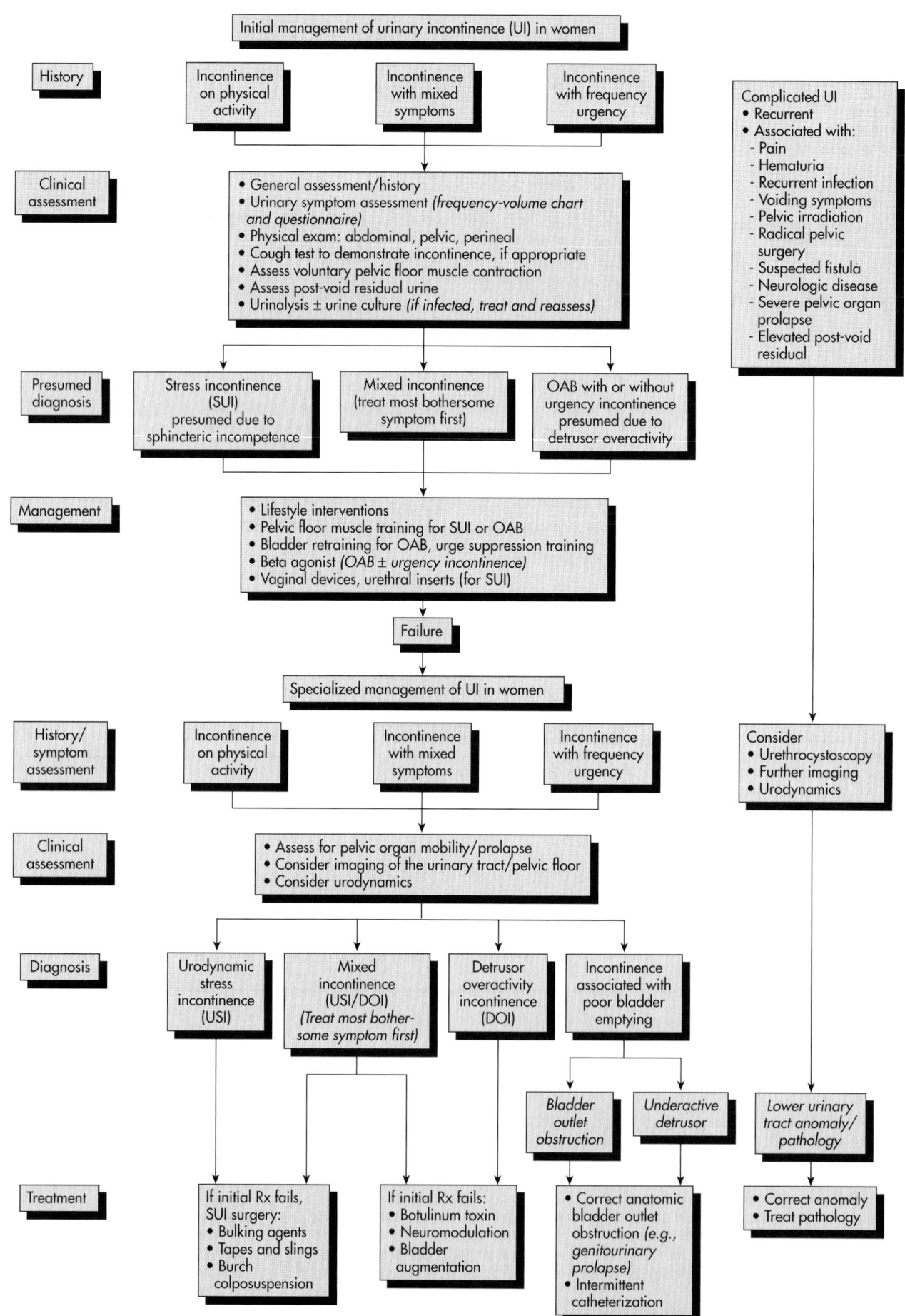

FIG. 2 Summary treatment algorithm for stress, urge, and mixed incontinence. (From Gershenson DM et al: *Comprehensive gynecology,* ed 8, Philadelphia, 2022, Elsevier.)

TABLE 7 Medications That Can Cause or Contribute to Urinary Incontinence in Frail Older Adults

Medications	Effects on Continence
α-Adrenergic agonists	Increased smooth muscle tone in urethra and prostatic capsule may precipitate obstruction, urinary retention, related symptoms
α-Adrenergic antagonists	Decreased smooth muscle tone in urethra may precipitate stress urinary incontinence in women
Angiotensin-converting enzyme inhibitors	Cause cough that can exacerbate UI
Anticholinergics	May cause impaired emptying, urinary retention, and constipation, which can contribute to UI; may cause cognitive impairment, reduce effective toileting ability
Calcium channel blockers	May cause impaired emptying, urinary retention, and constipation, which can contribute to UI; may cause dependent edema, which can contribute to nocturnal polyuria
Cholinesterase inhibitors	Increase bladder contractility, may precipitate urgency UI
Diuretics	Cause diuresis and precipitate UI
Lithium	Polyuria due to diabetes insipidus
Opioid analgesics	May cause urinary retention, constipation, confusion, immobility, all of which can contribute to UI
Psychotropic drugs Sedatives Hypnotics Antipsychotics Histamine-1 receptor antagonists	May cause confusion and impaired mobility and precipitate UI; anticholinergic effects; confusion
Selective serotonin reuptake inhibitors	Increase cholinergic transmission, may lead to urinary UI
Others—gabapentin, glitazones, nonsteroidal antiinflammatory drugs	Can cause edema, which can lead to nocturnal polyuria and cause nocturia and nighttime UI

UI, Urinary incontinence.
From Fillit HM: *Brocklehurst's textbook of geriatric medicine and gerontology,* ed 8, Philadelphia, 2017, Elsevier.

from the midurethra to the abdomen (or vice versa). Short-term cure rates range from 73% to 82%, according to a 2009 Cochrane meta-analysis, with de novo urgency in approximately 6% of patients.

b. Transobturator: Trocars are passed from the vagina behind the ischium (or vice versa), with similar cure rates as the retropubic slings.

c. Single-incision slings: Only one vaginal incision is needed beneath the urethra; ends of the sling are secured in the internal obturator muscle. A trial comparing mini-slings with midurethral slings revealed that single-incision mini-slings were noninferior to standard midurethral slings with respect to patient-recorded success at 15 mo, and the percentage of patients reporting success remained similar in the two groups at the 36-mo follow-up.[7]

2. Autologous fascial slings: Usually considered second line after the failure of synthetic slings due to length and morbidity of the operation. Cure rates estimated to be 50% to 75% depending on definition of cure.

3. Cadaveric slings: Usually second line; use has declined more recently because of concerns with early failure and declining success rate over time. Cure rates of 74%

TABLE 8 Pharmacologic Treatment for Urgency Urinary Incontinence

Indication(s)	Agent	Comments
Urgency UI OAB Urgency predominant–stress UI	All agents	With baseline average UI episodes/day of 1.6 to 5.3, mean reduction in episodes/day with placebo 1.08 (95% CI, 0.86-1.30); vs. IR formulations 1.46 (1.28, 1.64), and ER formulations 1.78 (1.61, 1.94). Head-to-head comparison trials of agents of limited quality
Antimuscarinics	Oxybutynin Immediate release (IR) 2.5-5 mg three to four times daily Extended release (ER, Ditropan XL) 5-20 mg once daily Topical patch (Oxytrol) 3.9-mg patch applied twice weekly Topical gel (Gelnique) 3% (84 mg, pump) and 10% (100 mg, sachet) once daily	Highest rate of dry mouth with immediate release, lowest with topical forms Application site rash in ~15% with patch
	Tolterodine IR (Detrol) 1-2 mg one tab twice daily ER (Detrol LA) 2-4 mg once daily	
	Fesoterodine (Toviaz) 4-8 mg once daily	Prodrug of tolterodine
	Darifenacin (Enablex) 7.5-15 mg once daily	Constipation
	Solifenacin (VESIcare) 5-10 mg once daily	
	Trospium IR (Sanctura) 20 mg once to twice daily ER (Sanctura XR) 60 mg daily	Must be given on empty stomach
	β-3 agonist	
Urgency UI OAB	Mirabegron (Myrbetriq) 25-50 mg once daily	ADEs include hypertension; use with caution in patients with hypertension. Use with caution with metoprolol and digoxin

ADEs, Adverse drug effects; *OAB*, overactive bladder; *UI*, urinary incontinence.
From Warshaw G et al: *Ham's primary care geriatrics,* ed 7, Philadelphia, 2022, Elsevier.

TABLE 9 Minimally Invasive Treatment for Refractory Urge Urinary Incontinence

Treatment	Method	Efficacy/Level of Evidence	Comments
Botulinum toxin	Injection in detrusor during cystoscopy	Can reduce UI with a slightly higher cure compared with antimuscarinics, although with a greater risk of urinary retention (Level of Evidence = B)	Patients must be willing to do self-catheterization because of the risk of urinary retention Optimal dosing for specific patient groups such as older women is uncertain
Sacral nerve modulation	Percutaneous implantation of a trial electrode at the S3 sacral root, which is connected to an external stimulator. Patients responding to the trial have a permanent lead with a pacemaker-like energy source implanted		Anticipated newer MRI-compatible models will end need to explant stimulators before imaging
Percutaneous tibial nerve stimulation		Very small trials only	Patients unlikely to see efficacy before 6 weeks of treatment Limited coverage by insurance

MRI, Magnetic resonance imaging; *UI,* urinary incontinence.
From Warshaw G et al: *Ham's primary care geriatrics,* ed 7, Philadelphia, 2022, Elsevier.

at 12 to 23 mo and 80% at 48 mo or greater.
4. Retropubic urethropexy (i.e., Burch procedure [open abdominal or laparoscopic]): A large meta-analysis estimated cure rates to be 82% at 12 to 23 mo and 73% at 48 mo or longer for open procedures.
- **Bulking agents:** For treatment of stress incontinence, without hypermobility or in poor surgical candidates:
  1. Available agents: Carbon-coated zirconium beads, calcium hydroxyapatite, cross-linked polydimethylsiloxane
  2. Effectiveness: Relatively noninvasive but less effective than surgical intervention; cure rate at 63% to 80% at 1 yr
- Treatment for urinary retention and overflow incontinence focuses on reversal of modifiable factors and drainage of urine from the bladder:
  1. Clean intermittent self-catheterization
  2. Sacral neuromodulation

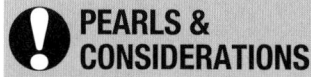

PEARLS & CONSIDERATIONS

COMMENTS
- Weight loss and exercise are helpful for urinary incontinence in obese women. Overweight and obese women with urinary incontinence also have a high prevalence of monthly fecal incontinence (16% found to be associated with low dietary fiber intake after adjustment for other known risk factors for fecal incontinence).
- Transient causes of urinary incontinence in the elderly are described in Table 10.
- Other forms of incontinence:
  1. Nocturnal enuresis: Loss of urine occurring during sleep; can occur as idiopathic or neurogenic
  2. Postvoid dribble: A postsphincteric collection of urine seen with urethral diverticulum; can be idiopathic
  3. Extraurethral incontinence: Enterovesical, urethral; also known as *fistula*
- Conditions that predispose to surgical failure: Advanced age, prior failed incontinence surgery, concurrent detrusor instability, abnormal perineal electromyography, pelvic radiation.
- The Women's Preventive Services Initiative (WPSI) recommends screening women for urinary incontinence annually.

REFERENCES & SUGGESTED READINGS
Available at eBooks.Health.Elsevier.com.

TABLE 10 Transient Causes of Urinary Incontinence (DIAPPERS)

D	Delirium/AMS state
I	Infection, urinary (symptomatic)
A	Atrophic urethritis/vaginitis
P	Pharmaceuticals (diuretics, and so on)
P	Psychological, especially depression
E	Endocrine (hypercalcemia, hypokalemia, glycosuria)
R	Restricted mobility
S	Stool impaction

AMS, Altered mental status.
From Floege J et al: *Comprehensive clinical nephrology,* ed 4, Philadelphia, 2010, Saunders.

RELATED CONTENT
Urinary Incontinence (Patient Information)
Pelvic Organ Prolapse (Related Key Topic)

AUTHORS: **ASHLEY HODGES, MD,** and **ANTHONY SCISCIONE, DO**

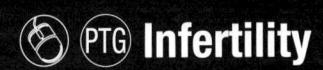

I

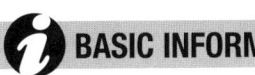 BASIC INFORMATION

DEFINITION

Infertility in a reproductive-age couple is defined as the inability to conceive after unprotected intercourse for ≥ 1 yr. When a female is greater than 35 yr of age, an evaluation is recommended after 6 mo without successful pregnancy. Earlier evaluation at any age is warranted with preexisting symptoms or medical conditions.

SYNONYM

Sterility

ICD-10CM CODES

N46	Male infertility
N46.8	Other male infertility
N46.9	Male infertility, unspecified
N97.0	Female infertility associated with anovulation
N97.1	Female infertility of tubal origin
N97.2	Female infertility of uterine origin
N97.8	Female infertility of other origin
N97.9	Female infertility, unspecified
O09.00	Supervision of pregnancy with history of infertility, unspecified trimester
O09.01	Supervision of pregnancy with history of infertility, first trimester
O09.02	Supervision of pregnancy with history of infertility, second trimester
O09.03	Supervision of pregnancy with history of infertility, third trimester
Z31.81	Encounter for male factor infertility in female patient

EPIDEMIOLOGY & DEMOGRAPHICS

PREVALENCE: One in eight reproductive age couples experience infertility. This prevalence is consistent in all developed countries, and there is evidence that it is historically stable. Infertility affects 8.8% of U.S. women aged 15 to 49 years and approximately 12.7% of reproductive age women seek treatment for infertility each year.[1,2]
PREDOMINANT SEX & AGE: By definition this is a diagnosis of reproductive age couples. Infertility increases with aging in both males and females, but more dramatically in women (Table 1). Male factor is responsible in nearly 40% of couples, and the female factor is responsible in approximately 50% of couples. The remainder of the cases are either combined male and female, or unexplained infertility, meaning a clear cause is not identified.
PEAK INCIDENCE: The incidence of infertility increases with age. Subtle decreases in female

TABLE 1   Types of Infertility

Type	Prevalence
Female factor infertility	40%-55%
Male factor infertility	25%-40%
Both male and female factor infertility	10%-30%
Unexplained infertility	25%

From Talley NJ et al: *Essentials of internal medicine,* ed 4, Chatswood, NSW, 2021, Elsevier Australia.

fertility start as early as age 30. The rate of infertility increases dramatically after age 37, and unassisted pregnancies become extremely uncommon as women reach the mid-40s. There is also a subtle, but still detectable, decrease in male fertility that may start as early as age 30.
RISK FACTORS: Aging is among the most common risk factors, predominantly among females, although there is evidence that aging affects male fertility as well. Women are increasingly deferring pregnancy due to the lack of a partner or career. Tubal factor infertility can be a result of endometriosis, prior tubal surgery, prior ruptured appendix, or sexually transmitted diseases such as chlamydia and gonorrhea. Ovulatory dysfunction is most commonly caused by polycystic ovarian syndrome (PCOS). Other causes of ovulatory dysfunction include hypothalamic dysfunction, thyroid disorders, hyperprolactinemia, and extremes of weight, particularly obesity. Male factor infertility may be idiopathic or due to trauma, infection, varicocele, obstruction, hypothalamic dysfunction, or exposure to environmental toxins. Smoking is the most common lifestyle choice that impairs fertility.

PHYSICAL FINDINGS & CLINICAL PRESENTATION

- Age
- Previous fertility, particularly if no pregnancy has occurred in another relationship despite absence of contraception
- Absence of secondary sexual characteristics

- Abnormal uterine bleeding or absent or irregular menstruation
- Clinical signs of androgen excess: Hirsutism, acne, alopecia
- Abnormal pelvic exam: Enlarged uterus, adnexal masses, pelvic/abdominal tenderness
- History of urologic surgery in male or trauma to testes

ETIOLOGY

- Female factor:
  1. Advanced age
  2. Tubal factor: Pelvic inflammatory disease, endometriosis, prior pelvic surgery, history of ruptured appendicitis, prior elective sterilization
  3. Anatomic: Uterine fibroids, polyps, intrauterine adhesions, congenital uterine anomalies
  4. Oligo-/anovulation: Most frequently due to polycystic ovarian syndrome (PCOS), but also due to thyroid abnormalities, hyperprolactinemia, nonclassic congenital adrenal hyperplasia, or hypothalamic dysfunction
- Male factor (Table 2):
  1. Abnormal semen analysis
  2. Elective sterilization
- Idiopathic: Both male and female

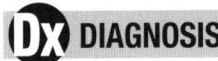 DIAGNOSIS

WORKUP

- Confirmation of ovulation: History of regular menstrual cycles, mid-luteal serum

TABLE 2   Causes of Male Infertility

Cause	Examples
Hypogonadism	
Isolated impairment of sperm production or function	
Androgen deficiency and impaired sperm production	
Androgen resistance	
Disorders of Sperm Transport	
Genital tract obstruction	Congenital bilateral absence of the vas deferens, cystic fibrosis, other congenital defects, vasectomy, postinfectious fibrosis, Young syndrome
Accessory gland dysfunction	Androgen deficiency or resistance, infection or inflammation, antisperm antibodies (immunologic)
SNS dysfunction	Autonomic neuropathy, sympatholytic drugs, sympathectomy, retroperitoneal or abdominopelvic surgery, spinal cord injury or disease, vasovasostomy
Ejaculatory Dysfunction	
Premature or retarded ejaculation	
Retrograde ejaculation	Prostatectomy, bladder neck surgery, autonomic neuropathy, SNS dysfunction
Reduced ejaculation	Androgen deficiency or resistance, SNS dysfunction, ureteral abnormalities
Coital Disorders	
Erectile dysfunction	
Defects in coital technique	Infrequent intercourse (<once weekly), poor timing in relation to ovulation, premature withdrawal of penis

SNS, Sympathetic nervous system.
From Melmed S et al: *Williams textbook of endocrinology,* ed 14, Philadelphia, 2019, Elsevier.

progesterone, basal body temperature testing, urinary luteinizing hormone predictor kits
- Complete transvaginal pelvic ultrasound
- Ovarian reserve testing: Anti-Müllerian hormone, follicle-stimulating hormone (FSH), and estradiol obtained on cycle day 2, 3, or 4 and antral follicle count
- Fallopian tube evaluation: Hysterosalpingogram (HSG) (Fig. E1) or sonohysterosalpingogram
- Uterine cavity evaluation: HSG, saline infusion sonohysterography, hysteroscopy, or 3D ultrasound of uterus
- Male factor: Semen analysis

LABORATORY TESTS

- Semen analysis, using Kruger strict morphology. Abstain 2 to 5 days prior to test.
- FSH and estradiol collected cycle day 2, 3, or 4 and anti-Müllerian hormone as a measure of ovarian reserve.
- Mid-luteal progesterone (ideally 7 days prior to expected menses). Given variability of serum progesterone measurements throughout the day and absence of a reliable threshold, most practitioners use clinical criteria to diagnose ovulatory dysfunction.
- Thyroid-stimulating hormone (TSH).
- In patients with oligo- or anovulation: Prolactin, testosterone, 17-hydroxyprogesterone.

IMAGING STUDIES

- Day 2 or 3 transvaginal pelvic ultrasound to assess uterine or adnexal abnormalities and to count the number of small antral follicles (2 to 9 mm) as a measure of ovarian reserve. If oligo- or anovulatory, to assess for polycystic-appearing ovary
- Hysterosalpingogram (early follicular phase after menses complete but before ovulation, typically between days 5 and 12 of the menstrual cycle)
- Also used for imaging of uterine cavity: Saline infusion sonohysterography, 3D ultrasound of uterus, hysteroscopy

℞ TREATMENT[3]

Once the patient presents for evaluation, testing should be completed as quickly as possible, ideally within one menstrual cycle. The couple should follow up with the evaluating provider once all testing is completed, and treatment should be initiated as abnormalities are found.

ACUTE GENERAL Rx

- Fertility preservation options among females are summarized in Table E3.
- Oligo- or anovulation should be treated with ovulation induction agents, such as aromatase inhibitors or clomiphene citrate. A recent multicenter trial found that aromatase inhibitors achieved higher live birth rates than clomiphene citrate.[4] Historically, clomiphene citrate has been used, but a very well done randomized controlled trial convincingly demonstrated that letrozole is superior in patients with PCOS.[5] Far less commonly, ovulatory dysfunction is the result of hypothalamic

dysfunction. In these patients, once hypothalamic or pituitary abnormalities are excluded with MRI, ovulation can be achieved using injectable gonadotropins.
- Tubal factor infertility may be treated surgically if mild, and if the female patient is young and can afford the time to attempt pregnancy over multiple menstrual cycles. If the patient is older or if the tubal pathology is moderate to severe, in vitro fertilization (IVF) is recommended. Indications for IVF are summarized in Box 1.
- Uterine anatomic abnormalities such as submucosal fibroids, polyps, intrauterine adhesions, or septate uterus should be corrected if they are identified. Fibroids that do not impact the uterine cavity probably do not interfere with fertility. Removal of intramural or subserosal fibroids is reserved for situations in which these cause distortion of the uterine cavity or bothersome symptoms such as excessive vaginal bleeding, pain, or pressure.
- Male infertility: Referral to urologist for complete evaluation. Fertility preservation options for males are summarized in Table E4. If semen analysis is severely abnormal, the following laboratory testing is recommended: Testosterone, FSH, estradiol, luteinizing hormone, TSH and prolactin, karyotype and Y-chromosome microdeletion.
  1. Mild male factor infertility may be treated with intrauterine insemination (IUI), but severe male factor will usually require assisted reproductive technologies (ART) with intracytoplasmic sperm injection (ICSI) in the laboratory, where sperm is injected directly into the oocyte.[6] Some men may require epididymal aspiration or testicular biopsy to obtain sperm for IVF/ICSI. Donor sperm may be necessary in cases of azoospermia due to testicular failure, if male partner has a genetic disorder, or if couple is unable to proceed with IVF/ICSI.
  2. Fig. 2 illustrates an algorithm for the evaluation and management of men with oligoasthenoteratospermia.
- Unexplained infertility can be treated empirically using superovulation with clomiphene

---

BOX 1 Indications for In Vitro Fertilization

Blocked or absent fallopian tubes
Low sperm counts or absent sperm (azoospermia requiring TESE)
Advanced reproductive age
Endometriosis
Unexplained infertility unresponsive to IUI therapy
Screening for aneuploid embryos and/or genetic disease
Fertility preservation

IUI, Intrauterine insemination; *TESE*, testicular sperm extraction.
From Gershenson DM et al: *Comprehensive gynecology*, ed 8, Philadelphia, 2022, Elsevier.

---

citrate, aromatase inhibitors, or gonadotropins combined with intrauterine insemination with partner's or donor sperm. Most providers recommend using an oral ovulation induction agent with insemination as a first-line superovulatory agent because it is inexpensive. After three cycles, approximately 30% of couples will conceive. After 3 to 4 cycles, few couples will be successful, and it is recommended to move forward with IVF. There is evidence suggesting that moving to IVF after 3 mo of clomiphene citrate and intrauterine insemination shortens the time interval to achieving pregnancy.[7] A randomized trial in women with unexplained infertility revealed ovarian stimulation with letrozole resulted in a significantly lower frequency of multiple gestation but also a lower frequency of live birth, as compared with gonadotropin but not as compared with clomiphene.
- Donor egg or embryo may be required in cases of premature ovarian insufficiency or due to age factor. Some couples may elect to pursue adoption.
- For LGBTQ couples, many family building options are available, including IUI or IVF utilizing donor sperm, donor oocytes, donor embryo, and/or gestational carrier, depending on the needs of the couple.

DISPOSITION

- Most couples will achieve a pregnancy, provided that they are willing to proceed with treatment including ovulation induction, superovulation, IUI, IVF, or gamete donation.
- Adoption is also a worthwhile and viable possibility for couples unable to conceive.

COMPLEMENTARY & ALTERNATIVE MEDICINE

Acupuncture is widely used by women being treated for infertility. Limited data suggest some benefit, with possible mechanisms of action including increasing blood flow to the uterus and/or ovaries. Despite these studies, it is unproven whether acupuncture definitely improves IVF outcomes. Patients may additionally benefit from the stress relief that acupuncture provides.

REFERRAL

Couples should be referred to a reproductive endocrinologist once the complexity of treatment exceeds the comfort level of the provider, whether a family physician, internist, or general gynecologist. Complex ovulation and superovulation induction and ART are best managed by a board-certified reproductive endocrinologist.

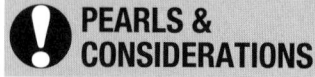 **PEARLS & CONSIDERATIONS**

COMMENTS

- The incidence of heterotopic pregnancy in patients who have undergone ART is more common compared with an unassisted conception. Identification of a patient with ultrasound-proved intrauterine pregnancy

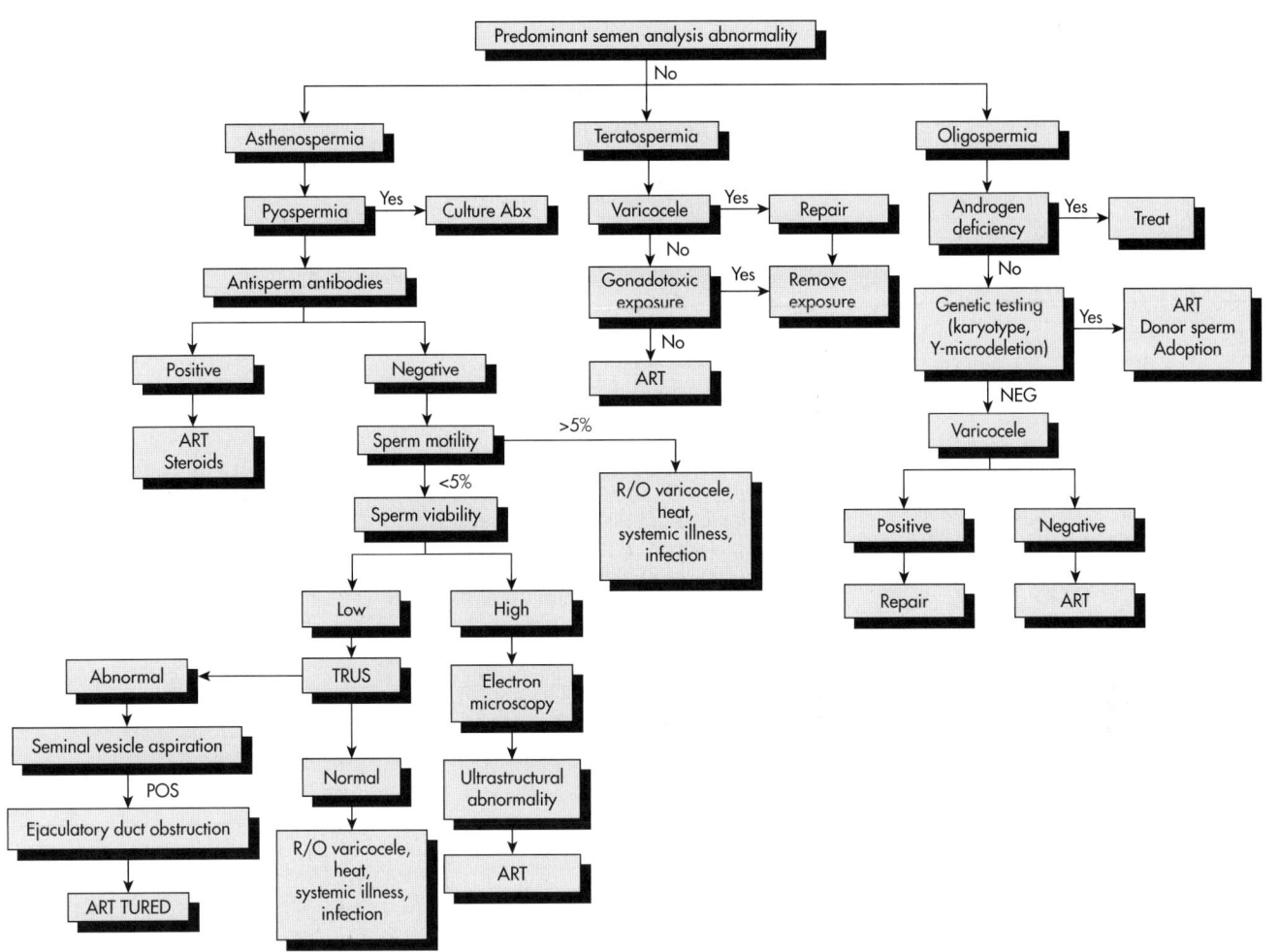

FIG. 2 Algorithm for the evaluation and management of men with oligoasthenoteratospermia. *Abx*, Antibiotics; *ART*, assisted reproductive technology; *NEG*, negative; *POS*, positive; *R/O*, rule out; *TRUS*, transrectal ultrasound; *TURED*, transurethral resection of the ejaculatory ducts. (From Bach PV, Schlegel PN: Male infertility. In *Yen and Jaffe's reproductive endocrinology*, ed 8, Philadelphia, 2019, Elsevier, p 586.)

who used ART to conceive should NOT necessarily exclude the possibility of an ectopic gestation.
- Single-embryo transfer is recommended in the vast majority of IVF cycles to reduce the rate of multiple gestation and subsequent risks to fetus and mother.
- Preimplantation genetic testing for monogenic/single-gene defects (PGT-M) or preimplantation genetic testing for chromosomal structural rearrangement (PGT-SR) is used in selected IVF cycles when one or both parents has one or more known genetic abnormalities or chromosomal rearrangements to test embryos for these specific genetic abnormalities prior to implantation.
- Preimplantation genetic testing for aneuploidy (PGT-A) is used in IVF cycles to screen embryos for aneuploidy prior to implantation.

PREVENTION
- Techniques that reduce the incidence of pelvic inflammatory disease, such as condom use, can reduce pelvic adhesions that are associated with tubal factor infertility.
- Women should be made aware of the fact that delaying pregnancy into the later reproductive years reduces the likelihood for successful pregnancy. Many women are cryopreserving oocytes or embryos for future use.
- Oocyte, embryo, or sperm cryopreservation is recommended for patients undergoing gonadotoxic chemotherapy or radiation treatment as a means of fertility preservation. Ovarian tissue cryopreservation can be used for patients who do not have time to undergo ovarian stimulation. Prepubertal testicular tissue cryopreservation may also be performed under a research protocol. All patients should be referred to a reproductive endocrinologist before planned treatment to discuss fertility preservation options.

PATIENT & FAMILY EDUCATION
Patient support groups such as *Resolve* (https://www.resolve.org) are available to help couples during evaluation and treatment of infertility, which can be extraordinarily stressful.

REFERENCES
Available at eBooks.Health.Elsevier.com.

RELATED CONTENT
Infertility (Patient Information)
Amenorrhea (Related Key Topic)
Pelvic Inflammatory Disease (Related Key Topic)
Polycystic Ovary Syndrome (Related Key Topic)

AUTHOR: **EMELIA ARGYROPOULOS BACHMAN, MD, FACOG**

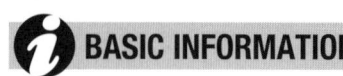

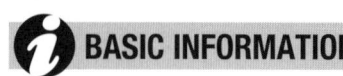 BASIC INFORMATION

DEFINITION

Inflammatory anemia, also known as anemia of chronic disease (ACD), refers to the impaired production of erythrocytes associated with chronic inflammatory states, such as cancer, chronic infection, or autoimmune diseases. Recent data have connected inflammatory anemia with severe, acute inflammation, such as critical illness, or with milder but persistent inflammatory signals that occur in obesity, aging, and kidney failure.[1] It is a disorder of iron homeostasis (Table 1) promoted by hepcidin-25 in response to an inflammatory condition.

SYNONYMS

Anemia of chronic disease
ACD
Anemia, inflammatory

ICD-10CM CODES

D63.8 Anemia in chronic diseases classified elsewhere
D63.0 Anemia in neoplastic disease
D64.8 Anemia, unspecified

EPIDEMIOLOGY & DEMOGRAPHICS

PREVALENCE:

- Second-most prevalent anemia after iron deficiency anemia:
  1. Around 11% of men and 10% of women ages 65 to 85 yr
  2. >20% of adults older than 85 yr

PATHOPHYSIOLOGY (FIG. 1)

Iron is carried in the bloodstream shelled by a hollow protein called transferrin (<0.2% of total iron body content) or at the core of hemoglobin in red blood cells (RBCs; 60% of total iron body content). It is mainly stored (15% to 30% of total iron body content) inside the liver, spleen, and skeletal muscle as ferritin and in lysosomes as hemosiderin. The rest of the body iron content is trapped in skeletal muscle myoglobin and mitochondrial cytochromes. In clinical practice, ferritin is a surrogate for iron stores, and total iron binding capacity (TIBC) is a surrogate for transferrin and iron carrying capacity.

Cells involved in the response to inflammation cause the release of cytokines, such as interleukin 6 (IL-6), which stimulates hepatic release of hepcidin. Hepcidin is a circulating protein that blocks ferroportin, an iron channel responsible for the exit of iron from enterocytes (and thus gastrointestinal absorption) and macrophages (which accumulate iron from engulfed senescent blood cells). IL-1 and tumor necrosis factor (TNF)-alpha stimulate interferon-gamma release by marrow stromal cells, which in turn suppress the erythroid response to erythropoietin (EPO). In chronic kidney disease, ACD is a consequence of decreased production of EPO and decreased renal clearance of hepcidin. The low availability of serum iron causes iron deficiency in the bone marrow compartment and decreased reticulocyte levels.

CLINICAL PRESENTATION

- Generalized symptoms include fatigue, shortness of breath, and weakness.
- It is important to consider other complaints if the underlying diagnosis is unknown, such as weight loss (malignancy, chronic infections, connective tissue diseases), anorexia, nausea, paresthesias, pleuritic chest pain, weight gain (chronic kidney disease [CKD]), diarrhea, bloody stools, abdominal pain, oral ulcers (IBD), and fevers (HIV, chronic infections).
- Physical findings may include pallor, lymphadenopathy, signs of connective tissue diseases (malar rash, sclerodactyly), palpable or visible masses, and localized findings for infection or malignancy.

ETIOLOGY

- Malignancy
- CKD (patients with CKD stage IV [glomerular filtration rate [GFR] <30 ml/min] should be screened for ACD)
- Congestive heart failure [CHF] (ACD is the main cause of anemia in CHF patients)
- Chronic infections
- Anemia of critical illness (develops within days)
- Connective tissue diseases

TABLE 1 Suspected Causes of Anemia of Chronic Disease

Shortened erythrocyte survival
Block in reuse of iron by erythrocyte
Direct inhibition of erythropoiesis
Relative deficiency of erythropoietin

From Hoffman R et al: *Hematology, basic principles and practice,* ed 7, Philadelphia, 2018, Elsevier.

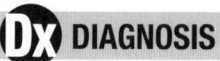 DIAGNOSIS

Isolated ACD:
- CBC with differential: Normocytic, normochromic, moderate (Hb rarely <8 g/dl) anemia
- Hypoproliferative anemia (low reticulocyte index; corrected reticulocyte count <2%)

Iron studies:
- Low iron concentration as in IDA (iron deficiency anemia)
- Normal/high ferritin (>35 mg/dl) in ACD as it is an acute phase reactant (Fig. 2)
- Low/normal TIBC (as opposed to IDA) and low transferrin saturation (as in IDA)
- Normal soluble transferrin receptor (sTfR, high in IDA)

Combined ACD/IDA:
- If normal to high ferritin, sTfR/log ferritin ratio <1 defines isolated ACD, and ratio >2 defines combined IDA/ACD

DIFFERENTIAL DIAGNOSIS

- Liver injury (increases ferritin):
  1. Iron deficiency anemia:
     a. Other causes of normocytic anemia or microcytic anemia (Table 2)
     b. Red blood cell loss or destruction:
        (1) Acute blood loss
        (2) Hypersplenism
        (3) Hemolysis
     c. Decreased red blood cell production:
        (1) Primary causes:
            (a) Bone marrow hypoplasia or aplasia
            (b) Myeloproliferative disease
            (c) Pure red blood cell aplasia
     d. Secondary causes:
        (1) Chronic renal failure
        (2) Liver disease
        (3) Endocrine deficiency states
        (4) Sideroblastic anemia

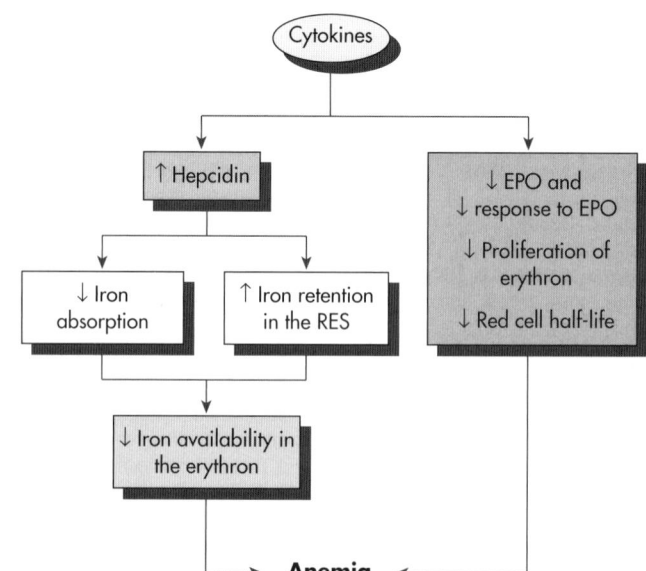

FIG. 1 Pathophysiologic factors associated with the development of anemia of chronic disease. *EPO,* Erythropoietin; *RES,* reticuloendothelial system. (From Hoffman R et al: *Hematology, basic principles and practice,* ed 7, Philadelphia, 2018, Elsevier.)

I

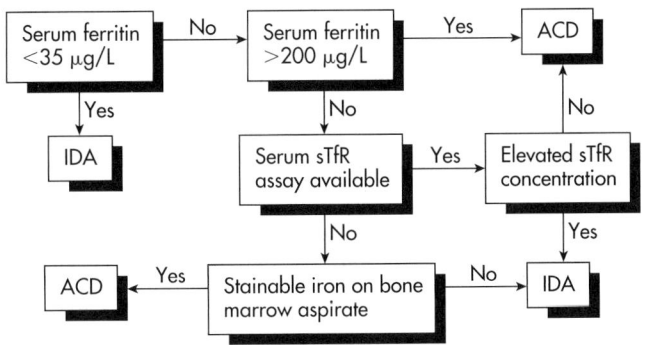

FIG. 2 Differential diagnosis of anemia with low serum iron. *ACD*, Anemia of chronic disease; *IDA*, iron deficiency anemia; *sTfR*, soluble transferrin receptor.

TABLE 2 Laboratory Features in Microcytic Hypochromic Anemias

	Serum Iron	Serum TIBC	% Saturation	MARROW % Sideroblasts	Iron Stores	Serum Ferritin	ZPP	Hb A$_2$	Hb F
Iron deficiency	↓	↑	↓	↓	↓	↓	↑	N-↓	N
β-Thalassemia trait	N (↑)	N	N	N	N-↑	N-↑	N	↑	N-↑
ACD	↓	N-↓	↓	↓	N-↑	N-↑	↑	N	N
Sideroblastic anemia	↑	↓	↑	↑	↑	↑	↑ (↓)	N	N-↑

ACD, Anemia of chronic disease; *Hb*, hemoglobin; *N*, normal; *TIBC*, total iron-binding capacity; *ZPP*, zinc protoporphyrins; ↓, decreased; ↑, increased.
From McPherson RA, Pincus MR: *Henry's clinical diagnosis and management by laboratory methods*, ed 23, Philadelphia, 2017, Elsevier.

WORKUP

CBC, reticulocyte count, peripheral smear (Fig. E3), iron level, ferritin, TIBC. Table 3 summarizes characteristic findings in inflammatory anemia. Characteristic bone marrow findings of increased iron stores in stromal histiocytes and impaired erythroid iron incorporation are shown in Fig. E4.

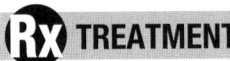 **TREATMENT**

Treat the underlying disorder/disease.

ACUTE GENERAL Rx

- The treatment of inflammatory anemia is directed primarily at treatment of underlying conditions, which can improve symptoms and facilitate hemoglobin recovery.
- Packed RBC (PRBC) transfusion is usually reserved for severe anemia (with Hb level <7 g/dl or <8 g/dl in patients with cardiac disease), especially if complicated with ongoing bleeding.

CHRONIC Rx

- Erythropoiesis-stimulating agents (ESA) (epoetin alfa and darbepoetin alfa) are FDA approved for use in patients with anemia resulting from:
  1. Chronic kidney disease
  2. Chemotherapy

- A 1998 study, the Normal Hematocrit Cardiac Trial (NHCT), showed a nonsignificant increase in the combined endpoint death and nonfatal myocardial infarction in patients with goal hematocrit of 33% versus 27%. Subsequent studies (CHOIR, CREATE, and TREAT) showed that higher doses and higher hematocrit targets were associated with increased cardiovascular events.
- ESA dose should be individualized for each patient, and the lowest sufficient dose to reduce PRBC transfusions should be used.[2] A hemoglobin target of ~10 g% is widely accepted. Iron deficiency should be ruled out before ESA is started. After starting ESA therapy, ASH/ASCO guidelines recommend periodic monitoring of iron status. When there is no or suboptimal response to oral therapy, parenteral iron therapy should be considered before concluding that a patient is nonresponsive to iron therapy.
- The hepcidin–ferroportin axis is the target of development of novel agents of which the most promising are hypoxia-induced factor modulators. Hypoxia-inducible factor (HIF) is a transcription factor that promotes expression of erythropoietin. HIF is upregulated by inhibition of PHD. Small molecule inhibitors of

prolyl hydroxylase domain dioxygenases (HIF-PHI [prolyl hydroxylase inhibitor]) stimulate the production of endogenous erythropoietin and improve iron metabolism.[3] The clinical development of three oral agents targeting this axis—daprodustat, roxadustat, and vadadustat—has now completed randomized clinical development.
- Among patients with CKD undergoing dialysis, the oral hypoxia-inducible factor prolyl hydroxylase inhibitors (HIF-PHI) daprodustat was noninferior to ESAs regarding the change in the hemoglobin level from baseline and cardiovascular outcomes.
- Additionally, among patients with CKD and anemia who were not undergoing dialysis, daprodustat was noninferior to darbepoetin alfa with respect to the change in the hemoglobin level from baseline and with respect to cardiovascular outcomes.

REFERENCES

References
Available at eBooks.Health.Elsevier.com.

AUTHOR: **DONNY V. HUYNH, MD**

TABLE 3 Laboratory Characteristics of ACD, IDA, and IDA With Inflammation

	Anemia of Chronic Disease (ACD)	Iron Deficiency Anemia (IDA)	IDA With Inflammation
Mean corpuscular volume (MCV)	72-100 fl	<85 fl	<100 fl
Mean corpuscular hemoglobin concentration (MCHC)	<36 g/dl	<32 g/dl	<32 g/dl
Serum iron	Decreased	Decreased	Decreased
Serum total iron-binding capacity (TIBC)	Typical below mid-normal range	Elevated	Less than upper limit of normal range
Transferrin saturation*	2%-20%	<15% (usually <10%)	<15%
Serum ferritin	>35 μg/L	<35 μg/L	>35 μg/L, <200 μg/L
Serum soluble transferrin receptor concentration (sTfR)	Normal (may be increased if serum ferritin >200 μg/L)	Increased	Increased
TfR index (sTfR/log ferritin)	<1	>2	>2
Hepcidin	High	Low	Normal
Stainable iron in bone marrow	Present	Absent	Absent

*Serum iron/TIBC * 100.

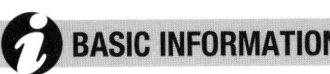

BASIC INFORMATION

DEFINITION

Inflammatory myopathies are idiopathic diseases of muscle characterized clinically by muscle weakness and pathologically by inflammation and muscle fiber breakdown. They may be further classified as dermatomyositis (DM), immune-mediated necrotizing myopathy, polymyositis (PM), antisynthetase syndrome, and inclusion body myositis (IBM).[1] See separate topics on "Inclusion Body Myositis" and "Necrotizing Autoimmune Myopathy" for details regarding these topics.

SYNONYMS

Immune-mediated myopathies
Idiopathic inflammatory myopathies
Myositis syndromes
Polymyositis
Dermatomyositis
IMM

ICD-10CM CODES

M33.02	Juvenile dermatopolymyositis with myopathy
M33.12	Other dermatopolymyositis with myopathy
M33.20	Polymyositis, organ involvement unspecified
M33.22	Polymyositis with myopathy
M33.90	Dermatopolymyositis, unspecified, organ involvement unspecified
M33.92	Dermatopolymyositis, unspecified with myopathy

EPIDEMIOLOGY & DEMOGRAPHICS

Inflammatory myopathies are the largest group of potentially treatable myopathies in children and adults.
DM:
- Occurs in children and in adults (bimodal age peak)
- Average age at diagnosis is 40 to 60 yr in adults, 4 to 14 yr in children[2]
- More common in females than in males (2:1)[2]
- Incidence: 9.54 to 32.74:100,000[2]
- Dermatomyositis is associated with a higher risk of cancer, especially in those older than age 50 yr[3]
PM:
- Occurs mostly in adults, very rare in children[4]
- Average age at diagnosis is over 20 yr[4]
- More common in females[4]
- Least common inflammatory myopathy[4]
- Exact incidence unknown
Antisynthetase syndrome:
- Associated with antibodies against aminoacyl transfer RNA synthetases[5]
- More common in women[5]
- Average age at diagnosis is 48 yr[5]

PHYSICAL FINDINGS & CLINICAL PRESENTATION

- Most patients have a subacute onset over weeks to months.

- Pattern is typically symmetric proximal muscle weakness involving the proximal limbs (shoulder and pelvic girdles).
- Weakness of neck flexion and extension is common.
- Difficulty getting up from a chair, climbing stairs, reaching for objects above head, or combing hair.
- Distal muscle involvement and ocular involvement are uncommon.
- Sensation is preserved.
- Reflexes may be preserved or diminished.
- Dysphagia and dysphonia result from involvement of striated muscle of the pharynx and proximal esophagus.
- Esophageal dysmotility is common in DM.
- Respiratory failure from associated pulmonary fibrosis.
- Cardiac conduction abnormalities can be seen with DM.
- Systemic autoimmune disease occurs frequently in PM and rarely in DM.
- Skin findings in DM:
  1. Heliotrope rash on the upper eyelids
  2. Erythematous rash on the face
  3. May also involve the back and shoulders (shawl sign), neck and chest (V-shape), knees (Fig. E1), and elbows
  4. Photosensitivity
  5. Gottron papules (violaceous papules overlying dorsal interphalangeal or metacarpophalangeal areas, elbow or knee joints)
  6. Nail cracking, thickening, and irregularity (Fig. E2) with periungual telangiectasia
  7. Associated with increased risk of interstitial lung disease
- Antisynthetase syndrome is associated with:
  1. Interstitial lung disease[5]
  2. Arthritis[5]
  3. Raynaud phenomenon[5]
  4. Mechanic's hands (dry, cracked skin on hands)[5]

ETIOLOGY

Mechanisms of muscle fiber damage in myositis are illustrated in Fig. E3.
DM: Complex, immune-mediated microangiopathy. Adaptive immune response via humorally mediated complement attack
PM: Unknown:
- Cell-mediated immune major histocompatibility-I (MHC-1) process directed against muscle fibers is likely, given biopsy features.

DIAGNOSIS

- The diagnosis of each subtype of inflammatory myopathy is based on clinical history, pattern of muscle involvement, electromyographic findings, muscle biopsy (Table E1), and presence of certain antibodies.
  1. Myopathic pattern of muscle weakness.
  2. Characteristic rash in DM.
  3. Electromyography (EMG) shows myopathic (small-amplitude, short-duration, polyphasic) motor potentials with early recruitment.

4. Majority of patients have "irritable" features (fibrillations and positive sharp waves) on EMG.
5. See "Laboratory Tests."
6. Biopsy is required for diagnosis and should confirm inflammation before treatment is started. Table 2 describes histologic features of idiopathic inflammatory myopathies. In idiopathic inflammatory myopathies, myopathic features (variation in fiber size, fiber splitting, fatty replacement of muscle tissue, and increased endomysial connective tissue) should be seen in addition to:
   a. DM: Perifascicular atrophy, membrane attack complex (MAC) deposition along capillaries
   b. PM: Endomysial infiltrates composed of CD8+ T cells and macrophages invading nonnecrotic muscle fibers that express MHC-I antigen

DIFFERENTIAL DIAGNOSIS (TABLE E3)

- IBM
- Muscular dystrophies
- Amyloid myoneuropathy
- Amyotrophic lateral sclerosis
- Myasthenia gravis
- Eaton-Lambert syndrome
- Drug-induced myopathies (e.g., quinidine, NSAIDs, penicillamine, HMG-CoA-reductase inhibitors)
- Diabetic amyotrophy
- Guillain-Barré syndrome
- Hyperthyroidism or hypothyroidism
- Lichen planus
- Amyopathic DM (rash without weakness)
- DM sine rash (weakness with characteristic biopsy, but no rash)
- Systemic lupus erythematosus (SLE)
- Contact atopic or seborrheic dermatitis
- Psoriasis

LABORATORY TESTS

- Creatine kinase (CK) is the most sensitive muscle enzyme test for muscle breakdown.
- CK is typically elevated (5 to 50× normal) in active PM.
- CK may be normal or only slightly elevated in DM.
- Aldolase, aspartate aminotransferase, alanine aminotransferase, alkaline phosphatase, and lactate dehydrogenase (LDH) may be elevated.
- Anti-Jo-1 antibodies are seen in myositis with associated interstitial lung disease but are not specific for either DM or PM.
- Myositis-specific and myositis-associated autoantibodies in adult polymyositis and dermatomyositis and juvenile dermatomyositis are summarized in Table E4.
- DM: Anti-MDA-5, anti-Mi-2, anti-TIF-1, and anti-NXP2 (implicated in cancer-associated dermatomyositis).
- PM: Antisynthetase antibodies associated with interstitial lung disease, arthritis, fever, and "mechanic's hands."

TABLE 2 Histologic Features of Idiopathic Inflammatory Myopathies

Feature	Dermatomyositis	Polymyositis	Inclusion Body Myositis
Necrosis of muscle fibers	+	+	+
Variation in fiber diameter	+	+	+
Regeneration of muscle fibers	+	+	+
Proliferation of connective tissue	+	+	+
Infiltration of mononuclear cells*	+	+	+
Perivascular and perimysial inflammation	+	−/+	−/+
Endomysial inflammation	−/+	+	+
Perifascicular atrophy	+	−	−
Abnormally dilated capillaries	+	−/+	−
Reduced capillary density	+	−/+	−
Deposition of complement on vessel walls	+	−/+	−
Microinfarcts	+	−	−
Invasion of nonnecrotic fibers by cytotoxic T lymphocytes and macrophages	−	+	+
Expression of major histocompatibility complex class I on muscle fibers	−/+	+	+
Rimmed vacuoles with amyloid deposits and tubulofilaments†	−	−	+
Angulated or atrophic and hypertrophic fibers	−	−	+
Ragged red or cytochrome oxidase–negative fibers	−	−	+

*Inflammation is absent in a small proportion of polymyositis and dermatomyositis biopsies.
†Also seen in chronic neurogenic conditions and distal myopathies.
From Firestein GS et al: *Kelley's textbook of rheumatology*, ed 9, Philadelphia, 2013, Saunders, Elsevier.

- Electrolytes, thyroid-stimulating hormone, Ca, and Mg should be evaluated to exclude other causes of weakness.
- Check ECG for cardiac involvement.

IMAGING STUDIES

- Chest x-ray is used to rule out pulmonary involvement. If suspicious for pulmonary interstitial disease, a high-resolution computed tomography scan of the chest may be helpful.
- Radiography is an efficient means of identifying and characterizing soft-tissue calcinosis (Fig. E4).
- Although MRI arguably has greater diagnostic value than electromyography or serum enzyme measurements in cases of suspected idiopathic inflammatory myopathy, MRI findings have not been formalized as a diagnostic criterion for idiopathic inflammatory myopathy. The acceptance of MRI as a diagnostic

tool in myositis may be inhibited by the high cost and the need for more reliable and validated methods of summarizing the findings of MRI. MRI evaluation before biopsy, however, has become routine at many tertiary care centers. Fascial disease is manifested on MRI by fascial or perifascial hyperintensity on fluid-sensitive sequences. The edema-like signal in the deep subcutis may accompany fasciitis and can indicate associated panniculitis.
- Video fluoroscopy or barium swallow study to look for upper esophageal dysfunction in patients with dysphagia and DM.
- Table E5 summarizes affected organs and their evaluation in inflammatory muscle disease.

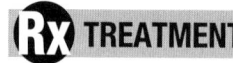 **TREATMENT**

Goal: Maintain function, minimize disease/iatrogenic sequelae

NONPHARMACOLOGIC THERAPY

- Sun-blocking agents with SPF 15 or greater for skin protection in patients with DM
- Physical therapy beneficial for gait training and increasing muscle tone and strength
- Occupational therapy assists with activities of daily living
- Speech therapy to monitor patients with swallowing dysfunction

ACUTE GENERAL Rx

- Corticosteroids are the mainstay of therapy. Start prednisone 0.7 to 1 mg/kg per day, up to a maximum dose of 60 mg/day. If severe disease, can give methylprednisolone 1 g intravenous (IV) daily for 3 to 5 days before starting prednisone. Continue until muscle strength improves. Begin tapering by 5 to 10 mg/mo. Consider every-other-day prednisone treatment at same dose (may decrease side effects).[6]
- Consider IV immunoglobulin (IVIG) if patient fails to improve on prednisone, or muscle enzymes begin rising when tapering off prednisone. See "Chronic Rx" for specific dosage.
- Hydroxychloroquine can be used to treat the cutaneous lesions of DM.
- A treatment algorithm for adult patients with inflammatory myopathies is illustrated in Fig. 5.

CHRONIC Rx

- Chronic prednisone therapy may be needed for years, but other immunosuppressive ("steroid-sparing") agents may be added early to decrease long-term steroid side effects.
- Azathioprine starting with 50 g daily, titrating to 100 mg/day after 1 week to goal of 2 mg/kg/day.[6]
- Methotrexate 5 to 7.5 mg weekly, increased by 2.5 mg/wk to total of 25 mg/wk; consider intramuscular dosing if PO is ineffective. Use cautiously in patients with interstitial lung disease due to possible pulmonary fibrosis.
- IV immunoglobulin 2 g/kg total dose over 2 to 5 days.
- IV cyclophosphamide 0.5 to 1 g/m^2 monthly for 6 mo is preferred to oral dosing for refractory cases. However, oral dosing of cyclophosphamide is 1 to 2 mg/kg per day PO or 2 to 4 mg/kg per day in conjunction with prednisone.[6]
- Cyclosporine A: Initial dose 2.0 to 2.5 mg/kg bid; long-term maintenance is lowest effective dose.
- Mycophenolate mofetil 500 mg PO bid, titrate to 1500 mg PO bid over 1 to 2 mo.[6]

DISPOSITION

- 20% to 30% of patients achieve clinical remission with treatment.[6]
- In patients with residual weakness, deficits typically remain stable over long-term follow-up.
- 10% experience recurrent disease.
- Serum CK often returns to normal before symptoms improve.

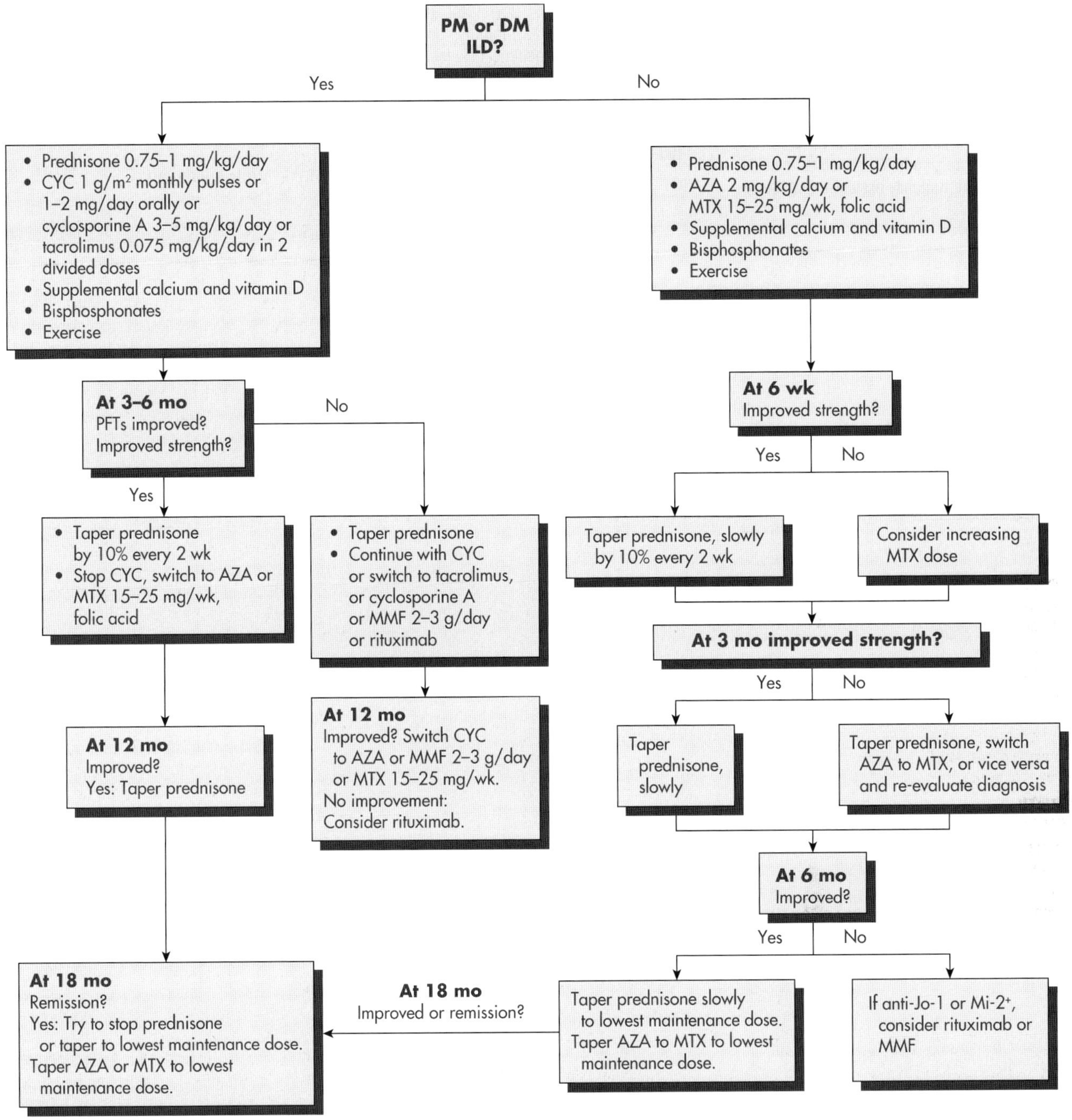

PM or DM ILD?

Yes / No

Yes →

- Prednisone 0.75–1 mg/kg/day
- CYC 1 g/m² monthly pulses or 1–2 mg/day orally or cyclosporine A 3–5 mg/kg/day or tacrolimus 0.075 mg/kg/day in 2 divided doses
- Supplemental calcium and vitamin D
- Bisphosphonates
- Exercise

No →

- Prednisone 0.75–1 mg/kg/day
- AZA 2 mg/kg/day or MTX 15–25 mg/wk, folic acid
- Supplemental calcium and vitamin D
- Bisphosphonates
- Exercise

At 3–6 mo
PFTs improved?
Improved strength?

No →

Yes ↓

- Taper prednisone by 10% every 2 wk
- Stop CYC, switch to AZA or MTX 15–25 mg/wk, folic acid

- Taper prednisone
- Continue with CYC or switch to tacrolimus, or cyclosporine A or MMF 2–3 g/day or rituximab

At 12 mo
Improved?
Yes: Taper prednisone

At 12 mo
Improved? Switch CYC to AZA or MMF 2–3 g/day or MTX 15–25 mg/wk.
No improvement: Consider rituximab.

At 6 wk
Improved strength?

Yes / No

Taper prednisone, slowly by 10% every 2 wk

Consider increasing MTX dose

At 3 mo improved strength?

Yes / No

Taper prednisone, slowly

Taper prednisone, switch AZA to MTX, or vice versa and re-evaluate diagnosis

At 6 mo
Improved?

Yes / No

Taper prednisone slowly to lowest maintenance dose. Taper AZA to MTX to lowest maintenance dose.

If anti-Jo-1 or Mi-2⁺, consider rituximab or MMF

At 18 mo
Remission?
Yes: Try to stop prednisone or taper to lowest maintenance dose. Taper AZA or MTX to lowest maintenance dose.

At 18 mo
Improved or remission?

FIG. 5 Treatment algorithm for adult patients with polymyositis (PM) or dermatomyositis (DM). *AZA,* Azathioprine; *CYC,* cyclophosphamide; *ILD,* interstitial lung disease; *MMF,* mycophenolate mofetil; *MTX,* methotrexate; *PFT,* pulmonary function test; *SC,* subcutaneous. (From Firestein GS et al: *Firestein & Kelley's textbook of rheumatology,* ed 11, Philadelphia, 2021, Elsevier.)

- During exacerbations, enzymes may rise before clinical symptoms appear.
- Poor prognostic indicators include delay in diagnosis, older age, recalcitrant disease, malignancy, interstitial pulmonary fibrosis, dysphagia, leukocytosis, fever, and anorexia.
- Infection, malignancy, and cardiac and pulmonary dysfunction are the most common causes of death.

REFERRAL

Neurology or rheumatology referral should be made to help establish the diagnosis and implement treatment.

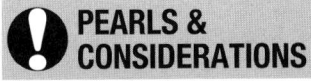 **PEARLS & CONSIDERATIONS**

- Do not implement treatment before muscle biopsy.
- When assessing response to treatment, clinical muscle strength is more important than muscle enzyme tests.
- The concern for malignancies (ovary, lung, breast, GI) associated with DM is legitimate and merits screening in patients older than age 40 at time of diagnosis and every 2 to 3 yr thereafter.

- No association exists between juvenile DM and malignancy.
- Overlap syndrome refers to patients with DM who also meet criteria for a connective tissue disorder (e.g., rheumatoid arthritis, scleroderma, SLE).
- In any patient taking steroids, closely monitor for:
  1. Diabetes or glucose intolerance (2-h oral glucose tolerance test)
  2. Osteopenia/osteoporosis (DEXA scan q6mo)
  3. Cataracts (yearly ophthalmologic appointment)

4. Hypertension
5. Psychiatric side effects including depression or psychosis
6. Poor sleep
7. Peptic ulcer disease (prescribe H_2 antagonist or proton pump inhibitor)

- Clinical and immune response features can be used for categorizing heterogeneous myositis syndromes and mutually exclusive and stable phenotypes and are useful for predicting clinical signs and symptoms, associated environmental and genetic risk factors, and responses to therapy and prognosis.

REFERENCES

Available at eBooks.Health.Elsevier.com.

RELATED CONTENT

Dermatomyositis and Polymyositis (Patient Information)
Inclusion Body Myositis (Related Key Topic)
Necrotizing Autoimmune Myopathy (Related Key Topic)

AUTHOR: **LYDIA SHARP, MD**

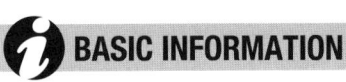

I

Diseases
and Disorders

I

BASIC INFORMATION

DEFINITION

Interstitial lung disease (ILD) is a heterogenous group of disorders, characterized by varying patterns of lung inflammation and fibrosis. The term "ILD" arises from the histological appearance that the interstitium is abnormal, although the alveoli, airways, blood vessels, lymphatic vessels, and pleura are often altered as well.[1] ILDs are classified as either arising from an identified cause or idiopathic.[2] A clinical classification of the interstitial lung diseases is summarized in Table 1.

SYNONYMS

Interstitial pulmonary disease
ILD
Diffuse parenchymal lung disease (DPLD)
Interstitial pneumonia
Pulmonary fibrosis

ICD-10CM CODES
J84.17	Other interstitial pulmonary diseases with fibrosis in diseases classified elsewhere
J84.89	Other specified interstitial pulmonary diseases
J84.9	Interstitial pulmonary disease, unspecified
J84.115	Respiratory bronchiolitis interstitial lung disease
J84.848	Other interstitial lung diseases of childhood

EPIDEMIOLOGY & DEMOGRAPHICS

INCIDENCE & PREVALENCE: Incidence varies widely with type of ILD. The most common ILDs are sarcoidosis, cryptogenic organizing pneumonia, and idiopathic pulmonary fibrosis. The prevalence of these syndromes varies widely across different populations as defined by age, gender, and race. The overall prevalence of ILD is estimated to be up to 76.0 cases per 100,000 people in Europe and 74.3 cases per 100,000 in the U.S.[3]

PREDOMINANT SEX & AGE: Some ILDs are more common in women, such as those resulting from autoimmune diseases, also known as connective tissue disorders.[4] Lymphangioleiomyomatosis (LAM) occurs almost exclusively in premenopausal women. ILDs caused by occupational exposures are more common in men. Most ILDs occur in people >50 yr; however, sarcoidosis most often presents in younger populations.

RISK FACTORS: Common identifiable risk factors include environmental exposures such as down, mold, silicone, and asbestos; reactions to drugs such as chemotherapeutic agents, tyrosine kinase inhibitors, amiodarone, and nitrofurantoin; radiation therapy; connective tissue disease including rheumatoid arthritis, scleroderma, and myositis; and pathologic acid reflux. Both tobacco and drug use can cause ILD. Some individuals have increased genetic susceptibility to developing ILD from impaired cellular repair mechanisms, such as telomere shortening.

TABLE 1 Clinical Classification of the Interstitial Lung Diseases

Connective Tissue Diseases

Scleroderma
Polymyositis-dermatomyositis
Systemic lupus erythematosus
Rheumatoid arthritis
Mixed connective tissue disease
Ankylosing spondylitis

Treatment-Related or Drug-Induced Diseases

Antibiotics (nitrofurantoin, sulfasalazine)
   Antiarrhythmics (amiodarone, tocainide, propranolol)
Antiinflammatories (gold, penicillamine)
Anticonvulsants (Dilantin)
Chemotherapeutic agents (mitomycin C, bleomycin, busulfan, cyclophosphamide, chlorambucil, methotrexate, azathioprine, BCNU [carmustine], procarbazine)
Therapeutic radiation
Oxygen toxicity
Narcotics

Primary and Idiopathic Diseases

Sarcoidosis
Primary pulmonary Langerhans cell histiocytosis (eosinophilic granuloma)
Amyloidosis
Pulmonary vasculitis
Gaucher disease
Niemann-Pick disease
Hermansky-Pudlak syndrome
Neurofibromatosis
Lymphangioleiomyomatosis
Tuberous sclerosis
Idiopathic pulmonary fibrosis
Nonspecific interstitial pneumonia
Cryptogenic organizing pneumonia
Respiratory bronchiolitis ILD or desquamative interstitial pneumonia
Acute interstitial pneumonia
Lymphocytic interstitial pneumonia
Pleuroparenchymal fibroelastosis
Bone marrow transplantation
Eosinophilic pneumonia
Alveolar proteinosis
Alveolar microlithiasis
Metastatic calcification

Occupational and Environmental Diseases

Inorganic

Silicosis
Asbestosis
Hard-metal pneumoconiosis
Coal worker's pneumoconiosis
Berylliosis
Talc pneumoconiosis
Siderosis (arc welder)
Stannosis (tin)

Organic (hypersensitivity pneumonitis)

Bird breeder's lung
Farmer's lung

ILD, Interstitial lung disease.
Modified from Mason RJ: *Murray & Nadel's textbook of respiratory medicine,* ed 5, Philadelphia, 2010, Saunders.

PHYSICAL FINDINGS & CLINICAL PRESENTATION

- Shortness of breath (especially with exertion)
- Cough (dry)
- Tachypnea
- Bibasilar end-inspiratory dry crackles

- Pulmonary hypertension
- Cyanosis
- Clubbing

Hallmarks of ILD include restriction of lung volumes and reduced diffusing capacity. The restrictive process can result from different abnormalities depending on the type of ILD including acute and subacute inflammatory changes, which are potentially reversible, and fibrosis, which is largely irreversible. Diffusion abnormalities can result from loss of functional capillaries from fibrosis, emphysema, or pulmonary hypertension.

- Specific changes may be seen:
  1. Granulomatous: Accumulation of T lymphocytes, macrophages, and epithelioid cells into granulomas in lung parenchyma
  2. Inflammation and fibrosis: Injury to epithelium causes inflammation; if chronic, inflammation spreads to interstitium and vascular areas

ETIOLOGY

The lungs are constantly exposed to potentially noxious stimuli from environmental and occupational exposures, smoking, drugs, radiation, autoimmune disease, pathologic acid reflux, etc. Lung injury leads to regeneration, repair, or remodeling responses that can result in restoration of normal tissue, inflammation, or fibrosis. Alveolar epithelial damage from repeated injuries promotes migration of inflammatory cells into the lungs. If regeneration or repair of the epithelium fails, remodeling occurs.[5] A fibrotic milieu promotes proliferation of fibroblasts and collagen deposition.

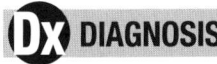 **DIAGNOSIS**

DIFFERENTIAL DIAGNOSIS

- Heart failure
- Pneumonia: Viral, bacterial, mycobacterial, fungal, and pneumocystis
- Pulmonary embolism
- COPD
- Pulmonary hypertension
- Vasculitis
- Metastatic malignancy manifesting as lymphangitic carcinomatosis
- Conditions associated with nonspecific interstitial pneumonitis pattern are summarized in Table 2

WORKUP

- Establishing a confident ILD diagnosis, as well as the type of ILD, which has treatment and prognostic implications, requires identifying clinical, radiographic, and histologic patterns of lung injury.
- Multidisciplinary discussion (MDD), which is considered the standard of care to diagnose ILD, includes a pulmonologist, radiologist, and pathologist. Detailed exposure history, exam findings, pulmonary function tests (PFT), laboratory tests, and high-resolution computed tomography (HRCT) scan of the chest are reviewed. If a confident diagnosis remains

TABLE 2 Conditions Associated With Nonspecific Interstitial Pneumonitis Pattern

Autoimmune connective tissue diseases

Chronic hypersensitivity pneumonitis

Infection (e.g., viral or atypical bacterial)

Inherited or acquired immunodeficiency

Drug toxicity

Idiopathic

From Broaddus VC et al: *Murray & Nadel's textbook of respiratory medicine*, ed 7, Philadelphia, 2022, Elsevier.

unclear, surgical lung biopsy should be considered and then reviewed in MDD. Fig. 1 illustrates the approach to ILD diagnosis.

- PFTs most often show restriction, characterized by decreased total lung capacity (TLC) and forced vital capacity (FVC) due to reduced lung compliance caused by alveolar wall thickening or filling of alveolar spaces as a result of inflammation and fibrosis. Inflammation, fibrosis, emphysema, and pulmonary vascular alterations can lead to impaired gas exchange, measured by the diffusing capacity of carbon monoxide (DLCO). FEV_1/FVC is usually normal or increased because lung stiffness keeps small airways open, although some conditions (e.g., sarcoidosis, hypersensitivity pneumonitis) may cause small airway obstruction and air trapping.
- Bronchoscopy with bronchoalveolar lavage (BAL) can show increased lymphocytes in chronic hypersensitivity pneumonitis and sarcoidosis, increased eosinophils in eosinophilic pneumonia, and can exclude infection.
- Bronchoscopic transbronchial biopsy is of limited utility. Cryobiopsy may yield sufficient tissue when done by experienced operators. Surgical lung biopsy provides sufficient tissue for diagnosis in >90% of cases. Histologic patterns of lung injury and their ILD associations are summarized in Tables 3 and 4 and illustrated in Figs. E2 and E3.

LABORATORY TESTS

- ABGs may be normal or show respiratory alkalosis and widened Aa gradient.
- Serologic tests can identify autoimmune features and connective tissue diseases: Antinuclear antibodies, rheumatoid factor, anticyclic citrullinated peptide, SS-A, SS-B, Scl-70, RNA pol III, RNP, myositis panel, creatinine kinase, aldolase. Antineutrophil cytoplasmic antibodies or antibasement membrane antibodies should be obtained if vasculitis is suspected.
- Serum precipitins are of limited utility to investigate exposures associated with hypersensitivity pneumonitis.
- Angiotensin-converting enzyme testing (ACE levels) in sarcoidosis is of unclear value.
- Laboratory findings in the interstitial lung diseases are summarized in Table 5.

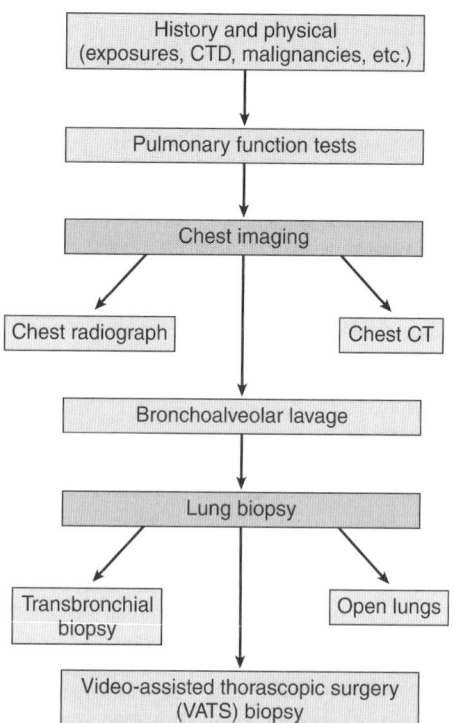

FIG. 1 Algorithm for the approach to a patient with interstitial lung disease. *CT,* Computed tomography; *CTD,* connective tissue disease. (From Sellke FW et al: *Sabiston & Spencer surgery of the chest,* ed 9, Philadelphia, 2016, Elsevier.)

IMAGING STUDIES

- Chest x-ray may appear normal or show opacities, often in a reticular pattern.
- HRCT is necessary to evaluate the radiographic pattern of lung injury. It can demonstrate consolidation, ground glass opacity, reticulation, traction bronchiectasis, fibrosis, air trapping, and cysts. It also may identify pulmonary artery enlargement in patients with pulmonary hypertension. Table 6 summarizes radiographic features of ILDs.
- Echocardiography is useful to evaluate cardiac size and function, and to screen for pulmonary hypertension, which can complicate advanced ILD.

🆁🅧 TREATMENT

NONPHARMACOLOGIC THERAPY

- Avoidance of tobacco and occupational exposures
- The mainstay of therapy is to identify the cause of the lung injury and completely avoid it, e.g., discontinue offending drugs or remove environmental exposures. Avoidance alone may be sufficient to reverse acute and subacute inflammation.

ACUTE GENERAL Rx

- Pharmacologic treatment varies significantly depending on the type of ILD; thus it is essential to try to correctly classify the type of ILD. Steroids and other immunosuppressants are beneficial for inflammatory conditions, such as hypersensitivity pneumonitis and connective tissue disease, but should be avoided in idiopathic pulmonary fibrosis. Please see specific chapters on Asbestosis, Cryptogenic Organizing Pneumonia, Eosinophilic Granulomatosis With Polyangiitis, Eosinophilic Pneumonia, Hypersensitivity Pneumonitis, and Idiopathic Pulmonary Fibrosis that discuss specific treatment regimens.
- For patients with acute or subacute inflammation demonstrated by consolidation or ground glass opacity in HRCT, immunosuppression with steroids or steroid-sparing agents, such as mofetil mycophenolate and azathioprine, could expedite improvement. While steroids often cause rapid improvement, their multiple side effects may limit their prolonged use. Patients should be closely monitored with PFTs to assess the ILD trajectory. If there is improvement or stabilization after 4 to 12 wk of steroids, the dose should be tapered. If the patient's condition declines as steroids are weaned, starting mofetil mycophenolate or azathioprine for maintenance may allow steroid tapering. If patients are at high risk for steroid-induced side effects, mofetil mycophenolate or azathioprine monotherapy could be considered from the beginning.
- For patients with scleroderma-associated ILD and those with other progressive fibrosing ILDs, nintedanib added to immunosuppression or monotherapy should be considered. Nintedanib is a tyrosine kinase inhibitor with antifibrotic and antiinflammatory properties that lowers the annual rate of FVC decline compared to placebo.[6,7]

TABLE 3 Histologic Patterns in the Interstitial Lung Diseases and Their Disease Associations

Histologic Patterns	Clinical Associations
Usual interstitial pneumonia	Idiopathic pulmonary fibrosis; connective tissue diseases (uncommon); asbestosis; chronic hypersensitivity pneumonitis; chronic aspiration pneumonia; chronic radiation pneumonitis; Hermansky-Pudlak syndrome
Nonspecific interstitial pneumonia	Idiopathic; connective tissue diseases; drugs; AIDS
Diffuse alveolar damage	Acute interstitial pneumonia (Hamman-Rich syndrome); acute respiratory distress syndrome (ARDS); drugs (cytotoxic agents, heroin, paraquat, ethchlorvynol, aspirin); toxic gas inhalation; radiation therapy; oxygen toxicity; connective tissue disease; infections
Organizing pneumonia	Cryptogenic organizing pneumonia; organizing stage of diffuse alveolar damage; drugs (amiodarone, cocaine); infections; connective tissue diseases
Desquamative interstitial pneumonia/ respiratory bronchiolitis	Cigarette smoking; idiopathic DIP of childhood
Lymphocytic interstitial pneumonia	Idiopathic; hypogammaglobulinemia; autoimmune diseases, including Hashimoto thyroiditis, lupus erythematosus, primary biliary cirrhosis, Sjögren syndrome, myasthenia gravis, chronic active hepatitis; AIDS; allogeneic bone marrow transplantation
Eosinophilic pneumonia	Idiopathic acute and chronic; tropical filarial eosinophilia; parasitic infections; allergic bronchopulmonary aspergillosis; allergic granulomatosis of Churg and Strauss; hypereosinophilic syndrome; AIDS
Alveolar proteinosis	Pulmonary alveolar proteinosis; acute silicosis; aluminum dust; AIDS; myeloproliferative disorder
Diffuse alveolar hemorrhage	
with capillaritis	Wegener granulomatosis; microscopic polyangiitis; systemic lupus erythematosus; polymyositis; scleroderma; rheumatoid arthritis; mixed connective tissue disease; lung transplantation; drugs (retinoic acid, propylthiouracil, Dilantin); Behçet disease; cryoglobulinemia; Henoch-Schönlein purpura; pauci-immune glomerulonephritis; immune complex glomerulonephritis
without capillaritis	Idiopathic pulmonary hemosiderosis; systemic lupus erythematosus; Goodpasture syndrome; diffuse alveolar damage; pulmonary venoocclusive disease; mitral stenosis; lymphangioleiomyomatosis
Amyloid deposition	Primary amyloidosis; multiple myeloma; lymphocytic interstitial pneumonia
Granuloma	Sarcoidosis; hypersensitivity pneumonitis; pulmonary Langerhans cell histiocytosis; silicosis; intravenous talcosis; berylliosis; lymphocytic interstitial pneumonia; infections

AIDS, Acquired immunodeficiency syndrome; *DIP,* desquamative interstitial pneumonia.
Modified from Mason RJ: *Murray & Nadel's textbook of respiratory medicine,* ed 5, Philadelphia, 2010, Saunders.

TABLE 4 Histologic Patterns of Interstitial Lung Disease

Acute lung injury
1. Diffuse alveolar damage
2. Organizing pneumonia
3. Acute fibrinous and organizing pneumonia
Consolidation of alveolar spaces
1. Eosinophilic pneumonia
2. Desquamative interstitial pneumonia
3. Pulmonary alveolar proteinosis
Interstitial fibrosis
1. Usual interstitial pneumonia
2. Nonspecific interstitial pneumonia (fibrosing NSIP)
Interstitial inflammation
1. Nonspecific interstitial pneumonia (cellular NSIP)
2. Lymphocytic interstitial pneumonia
3. Hypersensitivity pneumonitis

From Broaddus VC et al: *Murray & Nadel's textbook of respiratory medicine,* ed 7, Philadelphia, 2022, Elsevier.

CHRONIC GENERAL Rx

- Supplemental oxygen in patients with hypoxemia is beneficial to support physical activity and prevent development of pulmonary hypertension. Patients with interstitial disease should receive long-term oxygen therapy for severe resting hypoxemia and ambulatory oxygen for severe exertional desaturation.[8]

- Pulmonary rehabilitation improves exercise tolerance and strength in patients with ILD.[9]
- Lung transplant should be considered in appropriate patients (see chapter on Lung Transplant).[10]

DISPOSITION

The prognosis is highly variable and depends on the cause, severity of illness, and initial response to treatment.

REFERRAL

- Pulmonary referral for workup and management
- Surgical referral for biopsy
- Referral for lung transplant evaluation

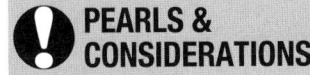

PEARLS & CONSIDERATIONS

COMMENTS

- In ILD evaluation, it is important to obtain a thorough history of tobacco and drug use, prior medications, workplace and environmental exposures, and pets, as well as to conduct a complete review of systems, including signs and symptoms that might suggest an underlying connective tissue disease.
- Establishing the specific type of ILD is essential for both management and prognosis.

PREVENTION

- Proper industrial hygiene, including use of necessary respiratory protective equipment, is important, as well as close monitoring of patients receiving medications with known pulmonary toxicity.
- Symptoms of an ILD in the setting of an autoimmune condition need to be evaluated thoroughly.

REFERENCES
Available at eBooks.Health.Elsevier.com.

RELATED CONTENT
Asbestosis (Related Key Topic)
Cryptogenic Organizing Pneumonia (Related Key Topic)
Eosinophilic Granulomatosis With Polyangiitis (Related Key Topic)
Eosinophilic Pneumonia (Related Key Topic)
Hypersensitivity Pneumonitis (Related Key Topic)
Idiopathic Pulmonary Fibrosis (Related Key Topic)
Interstitial Pulmonary Disease (Patient Information)
Sarcoidosis (Related Key Topic)

AUTHOR: **AIDA VENADO, MD, MAS**

TABLE 5 Radiographic Features of the Interstitial Lung Diseases

Feature	Diseases
Upper zone–predominant disease	Radiation pneumonitis; neurofibromatosis; chronic sarcoidosis; pulmonary Langerhans cell histiocytosis; silicosis; chronic hypersensitivity pneumonitis; chronic eosinophilic pneumonia; ankylosing spondylitis; nodular rheumatoid arthritis; berylliosis; drug induced (amiodarone, gold, BCNU [carmustine]); radiation
Increased lung volumes	Lymphangioleiomyomatosis; chronic sarcoidosis; chronic pulmonary Langerhans cell histiocytosis; tuberous sclerosis; neurofibromatosis
Radiographic honeycomb lung	Idiopathic pulmonary fibrosis; connective tissue disease; asbestosis; drug induced; lymphocytic interstitial pneumonia; chronic aspiration pneumonia; hemosiderosis; Hermansky-Pudlak syndrome; alveolar proteinosis
Pneumothorax	Pulmonary Langerhans cell histiocytosis; lymphangioleiomyomatosis; tuberous sclerosis; neurofibromatosis, IPF
Kerley B lines	Lymphangitic carcinomatosis; lymphangioleiomyomatosis; left atrial hypertension (mitral valve disease, venoocclusive disease); lymphoma; amyloidosis
Lymphadenopathy	Sarcoidosis; lymphoma; lymphangitic carcinomatosis; lymphoid interstitial pneumonia; berylliosis; amyloidosis; Gaucher disease
Pleural disease	Lymphangitic carcinomatosis; connective tissue disease; asbestosis (pleural calcification); lymphangioleiomyomatosis (chylous effusion); drug induced (nitrofurantoin, radiation); sarcoidosis
Eggshell calcification of lymph nodes	Silicosis; sarcoidosis; radiation

IPF, Idiopathic pulmonary fibrosis.
From Mason RJ: *Murray & Nadel's textbook of respiratory medicine,* ed 5, Philadelphia, 2010, Saunders.

TABLE 6 Laboratory Findings in the Interstitial Lung Diseases

Finding	Diseases
Leukopenia	Sarcoidosis; connective tissue disease; lymphoma; drug induced
Leukocytosis	Systemic vasculitis; hypersensitivity pneumonitis; lymphoma
Eosinophilia	Eosinophilic pneumonia; sarcoidosis; systemic vasculitis; drug induced (sulfa, methotrexate)
Thrombocytopenia	Sarcoidosis; connective tissue disease; drug induced; Gaucher disease; idiopathic pulmonary fibrosis
Hemolytic anemia	Connective tissue disease; sarcoidosis; lymphoma; drug induced; idiopathic pulmonary fibrosis
Normocytic anemia	Diffuse alveolar hemorrhage syndromes; connective tissue disease; lymphangitic carcinomatosis
Urinary sediment abnormalities	Connective tissue disease; systemic vasculitis; drug induced
Hypogammaglobulinemia	Lymphocytic interstitial pneumonia
Hypergammaglobulinemia	Connective tissue disease; sarcoidosis; systemic vasculitis; idiopathic pulmonary fibrosis; asbestosis; silicosis; lymphocytic interstitial pneumonia; lymphoma
Serum autoantibodies	Rheumatoid arthritis, scleroderma, inflammatory myopathies (dermatomyositis, polymyositis, immune-mediated necrotizing myopathy), mixed connective tissue disease, Sjogren syndrome, systemic lupus erythematosus
Serum immune complexes	Idiopathic pulmonary fibrosis; lymphocytic interstitial pneumonia; systemic vasculitis; connective tissue disease; pulmonary Langerhans cell histiocytosis
Serum angiotensin-converting enzyme	Sarcoidosis; hypersensitivity pneumonitis; silicosis; acute respiratory distress syndrome; Gaucher disease
Antibasement membrane antibody	Goodpasture syndrome
Antineutrophil cytoplasmic antibody	Systemic vasculitis

Adapted from Mason RJ: *Murray & Nadel's textbook of respiratory medicine,* ed 5, Philadelphia, 2010, Saunders.

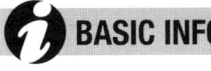
BASIC INFORMATION

DEFINITION
Classified into two broad categories:
1. Acute interstitial nephritis (AIN):
   a. Decrease in kidney function resulting from delayed hypersensitivity immune-mediated injury; most often drug-induced
   b. Characterized on kidney biopsy by edema and leukocyte infiltration of the renal interstitium and tubules *(tubulitis)*, which classically spares glomeruli and blood vessels
2. Chronic interstitial nephritis:
   a. Final common pathway of many chronic kidney diseases (CKD) including diabetic kidney disease, hypertensive kidney disease, unresolved AIN, chronic obstruction, high-grade vesicoureteral reflux, and chronic bacterial infections
   b. Characterized on renal biopsy by interstitial fibrosis with mononuclear leukocyte infiltration and tubular atrophy

SYNONYMS
Acute tubulo-interstitial nephritis
Contracted kidney
Cirrhosis of the kidney
Granular kidney
Renal sclerosis

ICD-10CM CODES
N05.8	Unspecified nephritic syndrome with other morphologic changes
N05.9	Unspecified nephritic syndrome with unspecified morphologic changes
N10	Acute tubulo-interstitial nephritis
N11	Chronic tubulo-interstitial nephritis
N11.8	Other chronic tubulo-interstitial nephritis
N11.9	Chronic tubulo-interstitial nephritis, unspecified
N12	Tubulo-interstitial nephritis, not specified as acute or chronic
N14	Drug- and heavy metal-induced tubulo-interstitial and tubular conditions
N15	Other renal tubulo-interstitial diseases
N16	Renal tubulo-interstitial disorders in diseases classified elsewhere
N17.8	Other acute kidney failure

EPIDEMIOLOGY & DEMOGRAPHICS
PREVALENCE:
- Prevalence of AIN is significantly underestimated.
- AIN is found in 0.5% to 2.6% of all kidney biopsies, but prevalence may be as high as 12.9% to 18.6% in patients who have had biopsy for acute kidney injury (AKI) of unknown etiology.
DEMOGRAPHICS:
- Increased incidence in older adults attributed to reduced glomerular filtration rate (GFR), immune-mediated dysfunction, increasing medication use, and comorbidities.[1]
- Median age at presentation is 65 yr.
RISK FACTORS:
- Advanced age (>65 yr)

- Volume depletion
- Underlying kidney disease
- Congestive heart failure
- Diabetes
- HIV infection

PHYSICAL FINDINGS & CLINICAL PRESENTATION[2-4]
SIGNS AND SYMPTOMS:
- For AIN, the most common presentation is an asymptomatic elevation of serum creatinine and blood urea nitrogen (BUN) levels. When advanced, AIN is associated with nonspecific symptoms of AKI from any cause:
  1. Malaise
  2. Anorexia
  3. Nausea and vomiting
  4. Oliguria or polyuria
  5. Hematuria
  6. Flank pain
- Classic triad (fever, maculopapular rash, and eosinophilia) is present in only 5% to 10% of cases[1-3]:
  1. If present, the rash is usually a truncal maculopapular morbilliform eruption.
  2. Triad is characteristic of methicillin-related AIN; this antibiotic has not been prescribed in the U.S. for 4 decades.
- A small minority present with tubulo-interstitial nephritis and uveitis (TINU) syndrome. The uveitis may be symptomatic or subclinical and may develop before, during, or after kidney injury. Adolescent females are most often affected by TINU.[1]
- For chronic interstitial nephritis, there may be a subacute to protracted rise in serum creatinine without obvious symptomatology that is classified as unspecified CKD.

ETIOLOGY
ACUTE INTERSTITIAL NEPHRITIS:
- **Drug-induced:** Accounts for 70% of cases, and more than 150 agents have been implicated.[4] AKI usually develops 10 to 14 days after exposure to the drug but may develop earlier when there has been prior drug exposure.
  1. Antibiotics (beta-lactams, sulfonamides, rifampin, fluoroquinolones)
  2. Nonsteroidal antiinflammatory drugs (NSAIDs), including selective cyclooxygenase-2 (COX-2) inhibitors
  3. Proton pump inhibitors and H_2 blockers (primarily cimetidine)
  4. Loop diuretics (furosemide, bumetanide) and thiazide diuretics
  5. Antineoplastic agents
  6. Anticonvulsants
  7. Allopurinol (particularly common cause of drug rash or reaction with eosinophilia and systemic symptoms [DRESS] with AIN)
  8. Immunotherapy with checkpoint pathway inhibitors
  9. 5-aminosalicylates (mesalamine)
- **Infection** (10% to 15%): Systemic or localized to genitourinary system.
  1. Bacteria: *Streptococci, Corynebacterium diphtheriae, legionellae, Yersinia, Mycobacteria* spp., *Mycoplasma, rickettsiae, E. coli*

  2. Viruses: *Cytomegalovirus, Epstein–Barr virus, Orthohantavirus,* hepatitis C virus, herpes simplex virus-1 and -2, Human immunodeficiency virus-1, Rubulavirus (mumps), human polyomavirus-1 (BK) and -2 (JC), Influenza A virus
  3. Other: *Treponema pallidum, Toxoplasma gondii, Babesia* species
- **Other Causes** (15% to 20%)[1,2]:
  1. Idiopathic (10%)
- Immune disorders: Systemic lupus erythematosus, Sjögren syndrome, small-vessel vasculitides, autoimmune pancreatitis
- Neoplastic disorders (multiple myeloma)
- Drug reaction with eosinophilia and systemic symptoms (DRESS) syndrome
- Immunoglobulin G4 (IgG4)-related disease
- Hypocomplementemic tubulointerstitial nephritis
CHRONIC INTERSTITIAL NEPHRITIS:
- Metabolic diseases (urate nephropathy, hypercalcemic nephropathy, hypokalemic nephropathy, oxalate nephropathy)
- Sarcoidosis
- Heavy metals
- Chronic urinary tract obstruction
- Aristolochic acid
- Diabetic kidney disease
- Hypertensive kidney disease
- Chronic pyelonephritis
- Drugs: Indinavir, cisplatin, tacrolimus, cyclosporine, lithium
OVERLAP OF ACUTE & CHRONIC INTERSTITIAL NEPHRITIS: Some metabolic processes and autoimmune disorders can present either as acute or chronic interstitial nephritis. For example, oxalate nephropathy can present as acute interstitial nephropathy in the setting of ethylene glycol ingestion or chronic interstitial nephritis in cases of bariatric surgery and high oxalate-containing diet.

DIAGNOSIS

DIFFERENTIAL DIAGNOSIS
Other causes of AKI or CKD include acute tubular necrosis, atheroembolic disease, glomerulonephritis, hypertensive nephrosclerosis, prerenal azotemia, obstructive nephropathy, and renal vascular disease.

WORKUP
- Diagnosis is typically recognized by the temporal relationship between onset and resolution of AKI with use and discontinuation of a known culprit drug.
- Gold standard for diagnosis is kidney biopsy. This procedure is reserved for clinical situations with an unclear diagnosis, when removal of the offending agent does not result in improvement or influences medical care, or when steroid initiation is being considered.

LABORATORY TESTS
- No single laboratory test has sufficient positive or negative predictive value to diagnose interstitial nephritis.

- Diagnosis is based on clinical history, urine and serum abnormalities, and clinical course.[3,5]

URINE TESTS:
- Urine eosinophils: Historical marker of AIN. Eosinophiluria is not sensitive or specific enough to establish AIN and occurs more frequently in noninterstitial kidney disorders.[6]
- Urinalysis: Sterile pyuria, microhematuria, glucosuria, and proteinuria usually <300 mg/dl.
  1. Urine protein < 1 g in 24 h
  2. Microscopic hematuria (less than 50%)
  3. FeNa > 1%
- Nephrogenic diabetes insipidus, especially in chronic tubulointerstitial disease.
- Urine sediment analysis: Leukocytes, leukocyte casts, red cells, and tubular epithelial cells (Fig. E1). However, a bland urine sediment can also be seen in interstitial nephritis, especially if chronic. A lack of pyuria does not exclude AIN. Additionally, granular casts may be noted when tubulitis is present.[3]

BLOOD TESTS
- Serum chemistry profile: Elevated BUN, elevated creatinine, low serum phosphorus, and low serum urate concentrations may be present.
- Complete blood count with differential findings include the following:
  1. Eosinophilia: Not sensitive; if present, this finding greatly increases clinical suspicion for a systemic drug reaction. Eosinophilia may also occur in other causes of AKI including cholesterol emboli, vasculitis, and hematologic or solid organ malignancy.
- Hemoglobin level that is disproportionately low compared to degree of AKI, attributed to loss of interstitial erythropoietin-producing cells.
- If drug-related AIN is not suspected, laboratory testing for infection, vasculitis, and autoimmune disorders is warranted depending on the clinical context.
- Low complements and elevated serum total IgG and/or IgG4 levels or hypergammaglobulinemia in patients with immunoglobulin G4 (IgG4)-related disease or hypocomplementemic interstitial nephritis.

IMAGING STUDIES
Gallium scintigraphy (gallium-67 scan), positron emission tomography, and computed tomography have been used to evaluate AIN in patients. These tests may distinguish between AIN and other forms of AKI in patients who are not candidates for kidney biopsy.[3]

KIDNEY BIOPSY[3,7]
Critical to diagnosis of interstitial nephritis in patients with broad differential diagnosis of AKI. Biopsy findings include the following (Fig. E2):
- Predominant lymphocytic and monocytic infiltrate.
- Eosinophils suggestive of drug-induced AIN.
- Tubulitis (renal tubular invasion by inflammatory cells) compatible with AIN.
- Early inflammation with edema may transition to fibrosis with tubular atrophy as disorder becomes chronic.
- Granuloma formation implies infectious origin of AIN, especially in regions where the infectious etiologies described earlier are endemic. Necrotizing granulomas typically seen in fungal infections and tuberculosis.

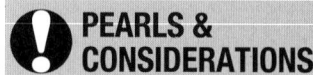
Rx TREATMENT

NONPHARMACOLOGIC THERAPY
Largely supportive; removal of offending agent, if known, will resolve 60% of cases.

ACUTE GENERAL Rx
- Maintain adequate hydration and urine output.
- Identify and treat infection(s).
- Avoid nephrotoxins and medications that impair renal blood flow.
- Uveitis in TINU syndrome may be asymptomatic. An ophthalmologic exam is recommended in idiopathic AIN.
- Retrospective studies and anecdotal literature have shown that steroid treatment initiated within 7 days of diagnosis may reduce the requirement for long-term dialysis in patients with drug-induced AIN who have not responded to drug withdrawal alone.[8] Steroids are the basis of treatment in idiopathic AIN, AIN associated with systemic disease, and TINU. Regimens vary. Some include an initial steroid pulse of methylprednisolone, 250 to 500 mg for 3 consecutive days, followed by prednisone 1 mg/kg.[8] Alternative regimen: Prednisone 1 mg/kg with no intravenous steroid pulse, with tapering over 4 to 6 wk; prolonged steroid tapering does not improve outcomes. Steroids are not administered to patients with significant kidney fibrosis on histologic examination.
- Cyclophosphamide, cyclosporine, and mycophenolate mofetil are anecdotal therapies for steroid-resistant disease. Mycophenolate mofetil has the most evidence for use as a steroid-sparing agent if AKI recurs when steroids are tapered or discontinued, or when adverse effects from steroid therapy occur.

CHRONIC Rx
- Limit exposure to known nephrotoxic agents
- Medication dosage adjustments by glomerular filtration rate
- Rigorous control of blood pressure, diabetes, and cholesterol
- Treat causes of chronic obstructive uropathy

DISPOSITION
With AIN:
- Complete recovery with return to baseline creatinine occurs in 60% to 65% of cases.[4]
- Partial recovery is seen in 10% to 20%.[4]
- Irreversible damage in 5% to 10%.[4]
- Relapse is common with repeated exposure to offending agents.

REFERRAL
Renal consultation is often required when diagnosis is unclear, biopsy is required, or there is treatment-resistant disease.

PEARLS & CONSIDERATIONS

COMMENTS
Drug-induced AIN occurs primarily when the offending agent is initiated within the preceding 30 days of diagnosis. The most common drug classes are beta-lactam antibiotics, NSAIDs, and proton pump inhibitors. In contrast to acute tubular necrosis, which is often associated with oliguria, early AIN may be associated with polyuria. Therefore, a high index of suspicion in this clinical setting is critical for establishing early diagnosis.

PREVENTION
Use known offending agents with care, especially in older adults and persons with known underlying kidney disease.

PATIENT & FAMILY EDUCATION
www.nlm.nih.gov/medlineplus/ency/article/000464.htm.

REFERENCES
Available at eBooks.Health.Elsevier.com

RELATED CONTENT
Interstitial Nephritis (Patient Information)

AUTHORS: **SANDEEP SOMAN, MD,** and **HAMMOOD AHMED, MD**

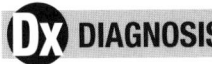

BASIC INFORMATION

DEFINITION

Anemia is defined as a hemoglobin level 2 standard deviations below normal for age and sex. Iron deficiency anemia is anemia resulting from inadequate iron supplementation or excessive blood loss.

SYNONYMS

Anemia
Iron deficiency

ICD-10CM CODES

D50.0	Iron deficiency anemia secondary to blood loss (chronic)
D50.8	Other iron deficiency anemias
D50.9	Iron deficiency anemia, unspecified
099.019	Anemia complicating pregnancy, unspecified trimester

EPIDEMIOLOGY & DEMOGRAPHICS

- Dietary iron deficiency occurs often in infants as a result of unsupplemented milk diets. It is also commonly seen in women during their reproductive yr, as a result of heavy menstrual periods, and during pregnancy (increased demand).
- Iron deficiency is the most common nutritional deficiency worldwide.
- The prevalence of iron deficiency is greatest among toddlers ages 1 to 2 yr (7%) from inadequate intake and female individuals ages 12 to 49 yr (9%-16%) from menstrual losses.
- The prevalence of iron deficiency is 2% in adult men, 9% to 12% in non-Hispanic White women, and 20% in Black and Mexican American women.
- GI cancer is diagnosed in 10% of elderly patients with iron deficiency anemia.

PHYSICAL FINDINGS & CLINICAL PRESENTATION

- Most patients have normal examination results.
- Skin pallor and conjunctival pallor may be present.
- Signs and symptoms specific for iron deficiency are koilonychias, pica, pagophagia, blue sclera, glossitis, and angular stomatitis (Fig. E1).
- Patients with severe anemia can have palpitations, headache, weakness, dizziness, and easy fatigability.

ETIOLOGY

- Blood loss from GI or menstrual bleeding (genitourinary blood loss less often the cause)
- Dietary iron deficiency (rare in adults)
- Poor iron absorption in patients with gastric or small-bowel surgery
- Repeated phlebotomy
- Increased requirements (e.g., during pregnancy)
- Other: Traumatic hemolysis (abnormally functioning cardiac valves), idiopathic pulmonary hemosiderosis (iron sequestration in pulmonary macrophages), paroxysmal nocturnal hemoglobinuria (intravascular hemolysis)
- The most common cause worldwide is hookworm infection

DIAGNOSIS

DIFFERENTIAL DIAGNOSIS

- Anemia of chronic disease
- Sideroblastic anemia
- Thalassemia trait
- Lead poisoning

WORKUP

Diagnostic workup consists primarily of laboratory evaluation. Table 1 describes laboratory studies differentiating the most common microcytic anemias. Most patients with iron deficiency anemia are asymptomatic in the early stages. With progressive anemia, the major symptoms are fatigue, dizziness, exertional dyspnea, pagophagia (ice eating), and pica. Patient history may also suggest GI blood loss (melena, hematochezia, hemoptysis).

LABORATORY TESTS

- Laboratory results vary with the stage of deficiency.
- Absent iron marrow stores and decreased serum ferritin are the initial abnormalities.
- Decreased serum iron and increased total iron-binding capacity (TIBC) are the next abnormalities.
- Hypochromic microcytic anemia is present with significant iron deficiency.
- Peripheral smear in patients with iron deficiency generally reveals microcytic hypochromic red blood cells (Fig. E2) with a wide area of central pallor, anisocytosis, and poikilocytosis when severe.
- Laboratory abnormalities consistent with iron deficiency are low serum ferritin level, increased RBC distribution width with values generally >15, low mean corpuscular volume, low mean corpuscular hemoglobin, increased TIBC, and low serum iron.
- In patients diagnosed with iron deficiency anemia, a GI workup including an upper endoscopy and colonoscopy is recommended to look for source of iron loss.

TREATMENT

The goal of therapy is to supply sufficient iron to correct the low hemoglobin and replenish iron stores.

NONPHARMACOLOGIC THERAPY

Patients should be instructed to consume foods that contain large amounts of iron, such as liver, red meat, and legumes.

ACUTE GENERAL Rx

- Iron supplementation will result in reticulocytosis and will generally increase hemoglobin levels by 0.5 to 1 g per wk.
- Treatment consists of ferrous sulfate 325 mg PO daily for 3 to 6 mo. Doses higher than 325 mg/day are poorly tolerated. Calcium supplements can decrease iron absorption; therefore these medications should be staggered. Supplemental vitamin C can increase oral absorption.
- Parenteral iron therapy is reserved for patients with poor tolerance, noncompliance with oral preparations, or malabsorption. Indications for intravenous iron therapy are summarized in Table 2.
- Transfusion of packed RBCs is indicated in patients with severe symptomatic anemia.

CHRONIC Rx

Patients should be instructed to continue their iron supplements for at least 6 mo or longer to correct depleted body iron stores.

TABLE 1 Laboratory Studies Differentiating the Most Common Microcytic Anemias

Study	Iron Deficiency Anemia	α or β Thalassemia	Anemia of Chronic Disease
Hemoglobin	Decreased	Decreased	Decreased
MCV	Decreased	Decreased	Normal-decreased
RDW	Increased	Normal	Normal-increased
RBC	Decreased	Normal-increased	Normal-decreased
Serum ferritin	Decreased	Normal	Increased
Total Fe binding capacity	Increased	Normal	Decreased
Transferrin saturation	Decreased	Normal	Decreased
FEP	Increased	Normal	Increased
Transferrin receptor	Increased	Normal	Increased
Reticulocyte hemoglobin concentration	Decreased	Normal	Normal-decreased

Fe, Ferritin; *FEP,* free erythrocyte protoporphyrin; *MCV,* mean corpuscular volume; *RBC,* red blood cell; *RDW,* red cell distribution width. From Kliegman RM et al: *Nelson textbook of pediatrics,* ed 19, Philadelphia, 2011, Saunders.

Diseases and Disorders

TABLE 2　Indications for Intravenous Iron Therapy

Accepted Indications

- Oral iron intolerance
- Oral iron refractoriness, including iron refractory iron deficiency anemia (IRIDA)
- Need for a quick recovery, e.g., severe anemia of pregnancy
- Chronic bleeding not manageable with oral iron
- Concurrently with erythropoiesis-stimulating agents in chronic kidney disease
- Gastrointestinal disorders (inflammatory bowel disease, acute flares)
- Substitution for blood transfusions when not accepted by patient

Novel Proposed Indications

- Iron deficiency in chronic heart failure
- Perioperative anemia (transfusion sparing strategy)
- Anemia of chronic kidney disease before treatment with erythropoiesis-stimulating agents
- Persistent anemia after erythropoiesis-stimulating agents in cancer patients on chemotherapy

From Goldman L, Shafer AI: *Goldman-Cecil medicine,* ed 26, Philadelphia, 2019, Elsevier.

TABLE 3　Responses to Iron Therapy in Iron Deficiency Anemia

Time After Iron Administration	Response
12-24 hr	Replacement of intracellular iron enzymes; subjective improvement; decreased irritability; increased appetite
36-48 hr	Initial bone marrow response; erythroid hyperplasia
48-72 hr	Reticulocytosis, peaking at 5-7 days
4-30 days	Increase in hemoglobin level
1-3 mo	Repletion of stores

From Kliegman RM et al: *Nelson textbook of pediatrics,* ed 19, Philadelphia, 2011, Saunders.

TABLE 4　Differential Diagnosis of Microcytic Anemia That Fails to Respond to Oral Iron

Poor compliance (true intolerance of iron is uncommon)

Incorrect dose or medication

Malabsorption of administered iron

Ongoing blood loss including gastrointestinal, menstrual, and pulmonary

Concurrent infection or inflammatory disorder inhibiting the response to iron

Concurrent vitamin B_{12} or folate deficiency

Diagnosis other than iron deficiency:

- Thalassemias
- Hemoglobin C and E disorders
- Anemia of chronic disease
- Lead poisoning
- Sickle thalassemias, hemoglobin SC disease
- Rare microcytic anemias

SC, Sickle cell.
From Kliegman RM et al: *Nelson textbook of pediatrics,* ed 19, Philadelphia, 2011, Saunders.

DISPOSITION

- Most patients respond rapidly to iron supplementation with improvement in CBC and general well-being (Table 3). GI side effects from oral iron therapy are common and may require decreased dosage to once every other day or to change to parenteral iron.
- A differential diagnosis of microcytic anemia that fails to respond to oral iron is described in Table 4.

REFERRAL

GI referral for evaluation of GI malignancy is recommended in all patients with iron deficiency and suspected GI blood loss.

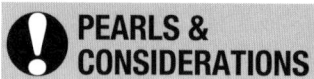 **PEARLS & CONSIDERATIONS**

COMMENTS

- Iron deficiency may impair aerobic performance and worsen symptoms in patients with heart failure. Treatment with intravenous iron in patients with chronic heart failure and iron deficiency has been shown to improve symptoms, quality of life, and functional capacity.
- If the diagnosis of iron deficiency anemia is made, locating the suspected site of iron loss is mandatory.

RELATED CONTENT

Algorithm for Diagnosis of Anemias (Algorithm in Section III)
Anemia (Patient Information)

AUTHOR: **FRED F. FERRI, MD**

BASIC INFORMATION

DEFINITION

Irritable bowel syndrome (IBS) is a chronic functional disorder manifested by alteration in bowel habits and recurrent abdominal pain and bloating. IBS is a symptom complex influenced by a variety of physiologic determinants from gut to brain and back. The ROME IV criteria for diagnosis of IBS are:

- Patient has recurrent abdominal pain ≥1 day per wk, on average, in the previous 3 mo, with an onset ≥6 mo before diagnosis.
- Abdominal pain is associated with at least two of the following three symptoms:
  1. Pain related to defecation
  2. Change in frequency of stool
  3. Change in form (appearance) of stool
- Patient has none of the following warning signs:
  1. Age ≥50 yr, no previous colon cancer screening, and presence of symptoms
  2. Recent change in bowel habit
  3. Evidence of overt GI bleeding (e.g., melena or hematochezia)
  4. Nocturnal pain or passage of stool
  5. Unintentional weight loss
  6. Family history of colorectal cancer or inflammatory bowel disease
  7. Palpable abdominal mass or lymphadenopathy
  8. Evidence of iron deficiency anemia on blood testing
  9. Positive test for fecal occult blood
- The criteria must be fulfilled for at least the past 3 mo with symptom onset at least 6 mo before the diagnosis.
- Table 1 subtypes IBS by predominant stool pattern.

SYNONYMS

Irritable colon
Spastic colon
IBS

ICD-10CM CODES
K58   Irritable bowel syndrome
K58.9 Irritable bowel syndrome without diarrhea
K58.0 Irritable bowel syndrome with diarrhea

EPIDEMIOLOGY & DEMOGRAPHICS

- IBS is the most common functional bowel disorder. An estimated 15 million people in the U.S. have IBS.
- IBS occurs in 7% to 21% of the general population of industrialized countries and is responsible for >50% of gastrointestinal (GI) referrals. Worldwide adult prevalence is 12%. Incidence increases during adolescence and peaks in third and fourth decades of life.
- Female:male ratio is 2:1. Peak prevalence is from 20 to 39 yr of age.
- Nearly 50% of patients have psychiatric abnormalities, with anxiety disorders being most common.

PHYSICAL FINDINGS & CLINICAL PRESENTATION

- The clinical presentation of IBS consists of abdominal pain and abnormalities of defecation, which may include loose stools, usually after meals and in the morning, alternating with episodes of constipation.
- Physical examination is generally normal.
- Nonspecific abdominal tenderness and distention may be present.

ETIOLOGY

- Unknown, believed to be multifactorial. Fig. 1 illustrates a biopsychologic model of IBS pathophysiology.
- Associated pathophysiology includes altered GI motility, alteration in gut flora, and increased gut sensitivity.
- Risk factors: Anxiety, depression, personality disorders, history of childhood sexual abuse, and domestic abuse in women.

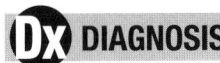

DIAGNOSIS

DIFFERENTIAL DIAGNOSIS

- Inflammatory bowel disease (IBD)
- Diverticulitis
- Colon malignancy
- Endometriosis
- Peptic ulcer disease
- Biliary liver disease
- Chronic pancreatitis
- Constipation caused by medications (opiates, calcium channel blockers, anticholinergics)
- Diarrhea caused by medications (metformin, colchicine, proton pump inhibitors, antacids, antibiotics)
- Small-bowel overgrowth
- Celiac disease

TABLE 1   Subtyping Irritable Bowel Syndrome by Predominant Stool Pattern

- IBS with constipation (IBS-C)—hard or lumpy stools* ≥25% and loose (mushy) or watery stools† ≥25% of bowel movements‡
- IBS with diarrhea (IBS-D)—loose (mushy) or watery stools† ≥25% and hard or lumpy stool* ≥25% of bowel movements‡
- Mixed IBS—hard or lumpy stools* ≥25% and loose (mushy) or watery stools† ≥25% of bowel movements‡
- Unsubtyped IBS (IBS unclassified)—insufficient abnormality of stool consistency to meet criteria for IBS with constipation, diarrhea, or mixed‡

*Bristol Stool Form Scale 1-2 (separate hard lumps like nuts [difficult to pass] or sausage-shaped but lumpy).
†Bristol Stool Form Scale 6-7 (fluffy pieces with ragged edges, a mushy stool or watery, no solid pieces, entirely liquid).
‡In the absence of use of antidiarrheals or laxatives.
IBS, Irritable bowel syndrome.
Adapted from Sayuk GS, Gyawali CP: Irritable bowel syndrome: modern concepts and management options, *Am J Med* 128(8):817-827, 2015.

- Parasites
- Lymphoma of GI tract
- Pelvic floor dyssynergia

WORKUP

Diagnostic workup (Table 2) is aimed primarily at excluding the conditions listed in the differential diagnoses. A step-wise approach is critical. It is important to identify red flags of other diseases, such as weight loss, rectal bleeding, onset in patients >50 yr, fever, nocturnal pain, and family history of malignancy or IBD. Additional red flags include abnormal examination (e.g., mass, enlarged lymph nodes, stool positive for occult blood, muscle wasting) and abnormal laboratory values (anemia, leukocytosis, abnormal chemistry).

LABORATORY TESTS

- Blood work is generally normal. CBC is reasonable to evaluate for anemia. The presence of anemia should alert to the possibility of a colonic malignancy or IBD.
- Other reasonable tests include C-reactive protein, tissue transglutaminase antibody (rule out celiac disease), and TSH (rule out thyroid abnormalities).
- Fecal calprotectin level is useful to differentiate IBS from inflammatory bowel disease in patients who have IBS with diarrhea or with both diarrhea and constipation. Fecal calprotectin levels less than 40 mcg/g exclude IBD in patients with IBS.
- Testing of stool for ova and parasites should be considered only in patients with chronic diarrhea. Evaluation of stool for *Clostridium difficile* may be helpful in patients with predominant diarrhea symptoms who have recently taken antibiotics.

IMAGING STUDIES

- Imaging studies (e.g., flat and upright abdominal radiograph, small-bowel series, sonogram or CT of abdomen and pelvis) are normal and not necessary for diagnosis.
- Lower endoscopy is generally normal except for the presence of some spasms. Colonoscopic imaging should be performed only in persons who have alarm features to rule out organic disease and in persons older than 50 yr to screen for colorectal cancer.

TREATMENT

NONPHARMACOLOGIC THERAPY

- The patient should be encouraged to maintain an adequate fiber intake and to eliminate foods that aggravate symptoms. Avoidance of caffeine, dairy products, fatty foods, and dietary excesses is also helpful. Several clinical trials have shown that a diet low in fermentable oligosaccharides, disaccharides, monosaccharides, and polyols (FODMAPs) improves symptoms in nearly 70% of patients with IBS.[1a]
- Cognitive-behavioral therapy is also recommended, particularly in younger patients, because psychosocial stressors are important

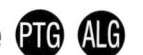
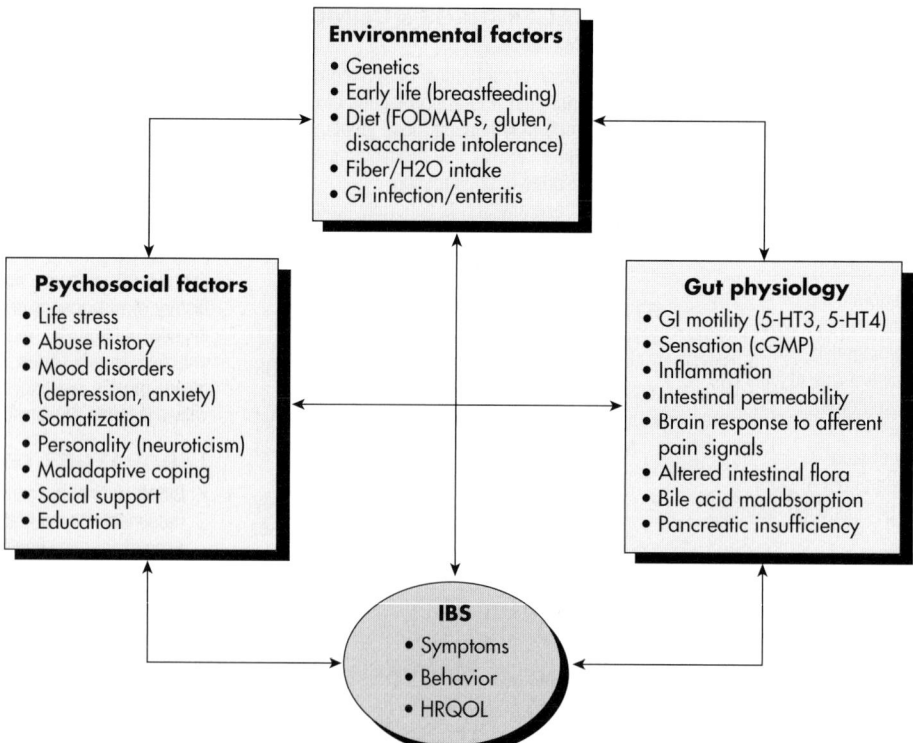

FIG. 1 A biopsychosocial model of irritable bowel syndrome pathophysiology. Irritable bowel syndrome is thought to be a multifactorial disorder, deriving from a potential multitude of etiopathogenic factors, including environmental, psychological, and physiologic factors. This model highlights the complex, often bidirectional interplay of these factors in the experience of irritable bowel syndrome symptoms. *cGMP,* Cyclic guanosine monophosphate; *5-HT3,* serotonin type 3; *5-HT4,* serotonin type 4; *FODMAPS,* fermentable oligosaccharides, disaccharides, monosaccharides, and polyols; *GI,* gastrointestinal; *H20,* water; *HRQOL,* health-related quality of life; *IBS,* irritable bowel syndrome. (Modified from Sayuk GS, Gyawali CP: Irritable bowel syndrome: modern concepts and management options, *Am J Med* 128(8):817-827, 2015.)

triggers of IBS. Reassurance that the disorder is benign and education about trigger avoidance and stress management are important.
- Importance of regular exercise and adequate fluid intake should be stressed.
- Fig. E2 illustrates the management of IBS.

GENERAL Rx
- The mainstay of treatment of IBS is diet. A FODMAP diet has been proven effective. Fiber is helpful for relief of constipation but not for relief of pain. Because symptoms are chronic, the use of laxatives should generally be avoided.
- Soluble fiber (psyllium) is more effective in symptom relief than insoluble fiber (bran). Fiber supplementation with psyllium 1 tbsp bid or calcium polycarbophil (FiberCon) 2 tablets one to four times daily followed by 8 oz of water may be necessary in some patients.
- Patients should be instructed that there might be some increased bloating on initiation of fiber supplementation, which should resolve within 2 to 3 wk. It is important that patients take these fiber products on a regular basis and not only as needed. Fiber is not effective in patients with diarrhea-predominant IBS and may worsen symptoms in these patients.
- Patients who appear anxious can benefit from use of sedatives or selective serotonin

reuptake inhibitors (SSRIs). Tricyclic antidepressants in low doses are also effective in some patients with diarrhea-predominant IBS.
- C-2 chloride channel activators: Lubiprostone (Amitiza) is a chloride channel activator that stimulates chloride-rich intestinal fluid secretion and accelerates small intestine and colonic transmit time. It may be effective in chronic constipation-predominant IBS unresponsive to conventional treatment. Usual dose is 8 to 24 mcg bid with food. Side effects include headache and nausea.
- Linaclotide (Linzess) is a guanylate cyclase-C (GC-C) agonist FDA approved for IBS with constipation. It stimulates secretion of chloride and bicarbonate into the intestinal lumen, mainly through activation of the CFTR ion channel, resulting in increased intestinal fluid and accelerated transit. Usual dose for IBS is 290 mcg 30 min before eating. The most common adverse effects are diarrhea, abdominal pain, flatulence, and abdominal distension.
- Tenapanor (Ibsrela) is an FDA-approved sodium/hydrogen exchanger 3 (NHE3) for twice daily oral treatment of IBS with constipation in adults. Its mechanism of action involves decreasing absorption of sodium, increasing osmotic secretion of water into the gut, shortening intestinal transit time, and softening stool consistency.[1]

- Loperamide is effective for diarrhea. Alosetron, a serotonin type-3 receptor antagonist previously withdrawn because of severe constipation and ischemic colitis, has been reintroduced with limited availability. It is indicated only for women with severe chronic diarrhea-predominant IBS unresponsive to conventional therapy and not caused by anatomic or metabolic abnormality. Starting dose is 1 mg qd.
- Eluxadoline (Viberzi) is an FDA-approved μ-opioid receptor agonist and Δ-opioid receptor antagonist for IBS with diarrhea. It decreases muscle contractility, inhibits water and electrolyte secretion, and increases rectal sphincter tone. Usual dose is 100 mg PO bid taken with food.
- Alterations in gut flora have been identified as potentially contributing to IBS (84% of IBS patients have an abnormal lactulose breath test, suggesting small-intestinal bacterial overgrowth). Rifaximin, a gut-selective antibiotic, has been used in recent trials to eradicate bacterial overgrowth (70% eradication rate). A dose of 400 mg tid for 10 days was reported effective in improving IBS symptoms up to 10 wk after discontinuation of therapy. Until additional evidence is available, use of rifaximin or other antibiotics in IBS should be reserved for patients with proven bacterial overgrowth.

TABLE 2 Irritable Bowel Syndrome Treatment Strategy: A Way Forward

1. Evaluation
   a. Consider conditions that mimic IBS (e.g., celiac disease, microscopic colitis, bile acid diarrhea, pancreatic insufficiency, carbohydrate intolerances, medication side effects, postsurgical neoanatomy)
   b. Assess for the presence of alarm symptoms
   c. Evaluate for symptom triggers (e.g., stressors, diet)
   d. Explore presence of other functional GI (e.g., functional dyspepsia) and non-GI disorders (e.g., fibromyalgia), psychiatric comorbidity, and drug intolerances
   e. Understand previous IBS treatment experiences
2. Selection of treatment approach
   a. Predicated on symptom severity and dominant symptoms
   b. Symptom severity (intensity, bother, effects on quality of life)
      i. Mild symptoms, intermittent symptoms, low symptom burden: Symptomatic or peripheral therapy
      ii. Moderate symptoms: Centrally acting neuromodulators, especially if symptomatic therapy does not provide adequate benefit
      iii. Severe symptoms and those with comorbidities (non-GI functional disorders, psychiatric): Both centrally acting neuromodulators and peripheral therapy
         a. Concurrent affective disorders need to be managed
         b. Other central therapies (cognitive and behavioral therapy, hypnosis, stress reduction) may need to be considered
   c. Dominant symptoms (diarrhea, constipation, pain, other GI symptoms)
      i. Constipation predominant
         a. Laxatives, fiber
         b. Novel agents (linaclotide, lubiprostone)
      ii. Diarrhea predominant
         a. Antidiarrheals
         b. Alosetron
         c. Address dysbiosis (rifaximin, probiotics)
         d. Diet (low FODMAP)
         e. Bile binders (cholestyramine, colesevelam)
         f. Disaccharidases (lactase)
      iii. Pain predominant
         a. Antidepressants (TCAs and SNRIs preferred)
         b. Linaclotide when constipation present
         c. Avoid narcotics
3. Education and therapeutic alliance
   a. Inform patient about etiopathogenesis
   b. Reaffirm legitimacy of diagnosis; allay concerns about organic disease
   c. Provide information about support organizations (International Foundation for Functional Gastrointestinal Disorders)

FODMAP, Fermentable oligosaccharides, disaccharides, monosaccharides, and polyols; *GI,* gastrointestinal; *IBS,* irritable bowel syndrome; *SNRI,* serotonin-norepinephrine reuptake inhibitor; *TCA,* tricyclic antidepressant.

- Antispasmodics-anticholinergics (e.g., dicyclomine, hyoscyamine) are often used, but efficacy data from clinical trials are inconclusive.
- Probiotics: Bifidobacteria and some combinations of probiotics have shown some limited efficacy. Lactobacilli do not appear to be effective for the treatment of IBS. Additional data showing efficacy is needed before probiotics can be endorsed for treatment of IBS.
- Antidepressants: SSRIs are more effective than placebo for relief of global IBS symptoms.

DISPOSITION
More than 60% of patients respond successfully to treatment over the initial 12 mo; however, IBS is a chronic, relapsing condition and requires prolonged therapy.

REFERRAL
GI referral is recommended in patients with rectal bleeding, fever, nocturnal diarrhea, anemia, weight loss, or onset of symptoms >40 yr. Consultation is also necessary if specialized diagnostic procedures such as endoscopy are necessary.

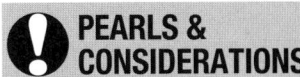 **PEARLS & CONSIDERATIONS**

COMMENTS
- Patients should be educated regarding maintenance of a high-fiber diet and elimination of stressors, which can precipitate attacks of IBS. They should be reassured that their condition does not lead to cancer.
- Recent drug efforts (alosetron, tegaserod) are aimed at serotonergic receptors in the gut because most of the serotonin in the body is found in the GI tract and is believed to be involved in the mediation of visceral sensation and motility.
- Cognitive-behavioral therapy is effective in the treatment of patients with IBS and should be considered as part of the armamentarium against this disorder.
- Some patients with IBS but without celiac disease show symptom improvement on a wheat-free diet. A 2- to 3-wk trial of wheat avoidance may be reasonable in patients with treatment-resistant IBS.
- Fecal microbiota transplantation (FMT) delivered via upper endoscopy seems to be efficacious in improving symptoms in all IBS subtypes in early clinical trials.

REFERENCES & SUGGESTED READINGS
Available at eBooks.Health.Elsevier.com

RELATED CONTENT
Irritable Bowel Syndrome (Patient Information)

AUTHOR: **FRED F. FERRI, MD**

I

Diseases and Disorders

I

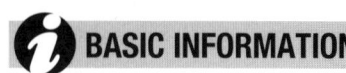
BASIC INFORMATION

DEFINITION
Ischemic colitis (IC) is tissue damage and inflammation of the large intestine due to a reduction in blood flow.

SYNONYMS
Intestinal ischemia
Colonic ischemia
IC

ICD-10CM CODES
K51.50	Left-sided colitis without complications
K51.51	Left-sided colitis with complications
K51.511	Left-sided colitis with rectal bleeding
K51.512	Left-sided colitis with intestinal obstruction
K51.513	Left-sided colitis with fistula
K51.514	Left-sided colitis with abscess
K51.518	Left-sided colitis with other complication
K51.519	Left-sided colitis with unspecified complications
K52.3	Indeterminate colitis
K55.0	Acute vascular disorders of intestine
K55.031	Focal (segmental) acute (reversible) ischemia of large intestine
K55.032	Diffuse acute (reversible) ischemia of large intestine
K55.039	Acute (reversible) ischemia of large intestine, extent unspecified
K55.9	Vascular disorder of intestine, unspecified

EPIDEMIOLOGY & DEMOGRAPHICS
INCIDENCE: IC is the most common type of intestinal ischemia, with an overall age- and sex-adjusted annual incidence of 15.6 to 17.7 per 100,000 person-yr. Those under 40 yr had an incidence of 1.1 per 100,000, while those over 80 yr had incidence rates of 107 per 100,000.[1]

PREDOMINANT SEX & AGE:
- More common among older patients (60s to 70s)
- Female predominance

RISK FACTORS:
- Older age
- Atherosclerotic disease, with associated disease processes such as diabetes, hypertension, and hyperlipidemia
- Abdominal Aortic Aneurysm Repair: There is an overall higher incidence IC after AAA repair, and it was higher in open repair compared to endovascular repair
- Atrial fibrillation
- Chronic constipation: Possible mechanism is increased intraluminal pressure resulting in decreased blood flow to the mucosa, thus resulting in ischemic attacks
- Hypercoagulable state
- Sickle cell disease
- Hypoalbuminemia
- Shock and hypotension
- Infection (cytomegalovirus (CMV), E. coli)

- Iatrogenic: Prescription drugs include oral contraceptives, bowel preparation for colonoscopy, and vasopressors[2]
- Lifestyle: Illicit drug use, such as cocaine use, can result in IC, with most changes on the right side.[2] A total of 27% recreational triathletes, 20% marathon runners, and 87% ultramarathon runners tested positive for fecal occult blood, with accounts of IC developing in high endurance runners[3]

PHYSICAL FINDINGS & CLINICAL PRESENTATION
Classic presentation of IC is of an elderly patient presenting with sudden crampy abdominal pain and hematochezia within the first 24 h. Pain secondary to large bowel ischemia is often not as severe as pain associated with small bowel ischemia. Associated symptoms include the urge to defecate accompanying the developing abdominal pain.[2]

On physical exam, the initial abdominal exam may be normal. However, the patient may also have peritoneal signs in severe illness or bowel perforation, and there may be associated hypotension and tachycardia. On rectal exam, there will be guaiac positive stool.

ETIOLOGY
GENERAL:
- A reduction in blood flow, usually sudden, to a segment of the bowel causes inadequate oxygenation that would be necessary for normal cellular metabolism.
- Overall, the superior mesenteric artery provides blood flow from the duodenum to the mid transverse color, while the inferior mesenteric artery supplies blood to the remaining part of the colon and superior rectum. Particularly affected are the watershed regions of the colon (Fig. E1), which have limited collateral circulation (splenic flexure aka Grifith point and sigmoid colon aka Sudeck point).
- Medical and surgical conditions associated with ischemic colitis are summarized in Box 1.

SPECIFIC:
- Nonocclusive disease (20%):
  1. Hypoperfusion: Cardiac failure, septic shock, hemorrhagic shock, hemodialysis, or any other condition that can cause hypotension
  2. Iatrogenic: Drugs (especially constipation-inducing). Medications associated with ischemic colitis are summarized in Box 2
  3. Colonic obstruction: Colon cancer, constipation, volvulus, bowel obstruction
  4. Long-distance running or other endurance sports
- Occlusive disease (80%):
  1. Arterial: Thrombus/emboli (Fig. E2), cholesterol emboli, small vessel disease (atherosclerosis, diabetes, vasculitis, rheumatoid arthritis, radiation, amyloidosis), trauma
  2. Surgical: Aortic aneurysm repair, cardiac catheterization, cardiopulmonary bypass, colectomy, endoscopy, renal transplant
  3. Venous: Mesenteric venous thrombosis, hypercoagulable state, sickle cell disease, pancreatitis, portal hypertension, lymphocytic phlebitis

---

BOX 1 Medical and Surgical Conditions Associated With Ischemic Colitis

Cardiovascular/Pulmonary
Atherosclerosis*
Atrial fibrillation
Chronic obstructive pulmonary disease
Hypertension

Gastrointestinal
Constipation
Diarrhea
Irritable bowel syndrome

Low Flow State
Septic shock
Congestive heart failure
Hemorrhagic shock
Hypotension

Surgery
Abdominal surgery
Aortic surgery
Cardiovascular surgery

Invasive Interventions
Postendovascular abdominal manipulations (e.g., chemoembolization)
Postcolonoscopy

Metabolic/Rheumatoid
Diabetes mellitus
Dyslipidemia
Rheumatoid arthritis
Systemic lupus erythematosus

Miscellaneous
Hypercoagulable states†
Sickle cell disease
Long-distance running

*For example, ischemic heart disease, cerebrovascular disease, peripheral vascular disease.
†Antiphospholipid syndrome, factor V Leiden deficiency, protein C and S deficiency.
From Cameron JL, Cameron AM: *Current surgical therapy*, ed 12, Philadelphia, 2017, Elsevier.

BOX 2 Drugs Associated With Ischemic Colitis

Constipation-inducing drugs (opioids and nonopioids)
Immunomodulator drugs (anti-TwNFα, type 1 interferon-α, type 1 interferon-β)
Chemotherapeutic drugs (e.g., Taxanes)
Cocaine and methamphetamines
Female hormones
Oral contraceptive medications
Antibiotics
Pseudoephedrine
Serotoninergic (e.g., Alosetron, Sumatriptan)
Diuretics

From Cameron JL, Cameron AM: *Current surgical therapy*, ed 12, Philadelphia, 2017, Elsevier.

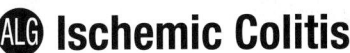

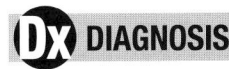 **DIAGNOSIS**

DIFFERENTIAL DIAGNOSIS

- Infectious colitis (e.g., *Clostridium difficile, Salmonella, Shigella*)
- Inflammatory bowel disease, inflammatory bowel syndrome, celiac disease
- Small bowel ischemia
- Constipation
- Diverticulitis
- Bowel obstruction
- Pancreatitis
- Appendicitis
- Malignancy
- Radiation enteritis

WORKUP

The clinical presentation is often vague and can be variable from patient to patient. A high index of suspicion must be maintained in any patient presenting with abdominal pain and bloody stool, especially if they are elderly or have risk factors. In addition to the physical exam, the following are key to confirming the diagnosis:
- Laboratory studies
- Computed tomography (CT)
- Lower endoscopy

LABORATORY TESTS

- General:
  1. CBC: Leukocytosis
  2. Comprehensive metabolic panel
  3. Liver function panel
- Specific markers: There are no specific laboratory tests for ischemic colitis. However, elevated levels of certain markers suggest inadequate global perfusion:
  1. Lactate
  2. Lactate dehydrogenase
  3. Creatine kinase (CK)
  4. Amylase
- Infectious workup: Stool studies, parasite testing, virus panel
- Coagulation studies
- Type and screen

IMAGING STUDIES

- Abdominal CT with contrast: Although findings can be nonspecific, the value of CT is in distinguishing ischemic colitis from nonischemic causes of abdominal pain. It also can assess the degree of ischemia and gauge the need for surgical intervention. It may identify arterial emboli or venous obstruction. Specific findings suggestive of ischemic colitis include, but are not limited to, intestinal wall thickening, thumbprinting, pericolonic stranding, and peritoneal free fluid or free air. Pneumatosis (the presence of gas in the colonic wall), portal venous gas, and the presence of megacolon usually indicate severe disease requiring immediate surgical intervention.
- Abdominal radiograph: Should be used in critical patients who are too unstable for a CT scan to look for gas formation in the bowel wall or free air in the abdomen suggestive of perforation.

- Lower endoscopy: This is the gold standard for confirming diagnosis of ischemic colitis in the stable patient. In the absence of peritoneal signs, colonoscopy is the test of choice on an unprepared colon to evaluate the degree of ischemia. If ischemia is suspected, lower endoscopy should be performed within the first 24 to 48 h. In most cases, visual inspection of the colonic wall will confirm the diagnosis and dictate the need for conservative versus surgical management. However, endoscopy should not be performed in patients with acute peritonitis or evidence of irreversible ischemic damage on CT. There is a risk of perforation.[2]

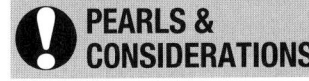 **TREATMENT**

- Treatment depends on the severity of disease and the specific etiology of colonic ischemia. However, the mainstay of therapy consists of optimizing blood flow to ischemic regions of bowel and removing any potential exacerbating factors. Initial care consists of aggressive intravenous (IV) crystalloid resuscitation, bowel rest, and broad-spectrum antibiotics with aerobic and anaerobic coverage. A treatment algorithm is illustrated in Fig. 3.
- In mild cases where patients are hemodynamically stable and do not have signs of peritonitis, colonoscopy should be performed. Patients with nonviable bowel seen on endoscopy require immediate operative intervention. However, the remainder of patients should be managed medically. Consider the use of a nasogastric tube in patients with abdominal distention or signs of ileus or bowel obstruction with parenteral nutrition for those who need prolonged bowel rest. Avoid vasoconstrictive medications as these can exacerbate colonic hypoperfusion; however, do not withhold their use in clinically unstable patients. Monitor signs of adequate end organ perfusion (e.g., mental status, abdominal pain, urine output). Management of underlying causes (e.g., heart failure, vascular disease, sepsis) should be considered.
- In severe cases not responding to supportive therapy, where patients are exhibiting acute peritonitis, sepsis, hypotension, or pain out of proportion to clinical exam, surgical abdominal exploration is warranted. Resection of gangrenous segments of bowel may be necessary. Colonoscopy should be avoided in these patients.[2,4]

NONPHARMACOLOGIC THERAPY

- Open or laparoscopic abdominal exploration to identify necrotic bowel. Box 3 summarizes indications for surgical intervention in patients with ischemic colitis.
  1. Bowel prep should not be given due to risk of perforation or toxic dilation[4]
  2. Bowel resection may be indicated in severe colitis
  3. Repeat surgical exploration normally is performed within 12 to 24 h, especially after colonic resection, to assess the

viability of colonic tissue and state of the anastomosis. Intraoperative infrared angiography based on IV injection of indo cyanine green (Fig. E4) can be used as an adjunct for decisions of whether to resect in determining margins and the integrity of intestinal anastomoses
  4. Primary anastomosis after colonic resection is contraindicated in certain cases (e.g., presence of aortic or iliac grafts; or when tissue is too friable for stable anastomosis)
- Nasogastric (NG) tube for bowel decompression if ileus or obstruction is present and bowel rest with possible necessity for parenteral nutrition.

ACUTE GENERAL Rx

- Supportive care:
  1. IV fluids
  2. Bowel rest
  3. Broad-spectrum antibiotics (aerobic and anaerobic coverage)
  4. Pain control
- Anticoagulation (not indicated in nonocclusive ischemia but may be considered in proven arterial occlusion or mesenteric vein thrombosis)

CHRONIC Rx

- Avoid overly aggressive hypertension treatment.
- Avoid dehydration.
- Avoid extreme exercise.

DISPOSITION

- Overall prognosis for ischemic colitis is dependent upon location of disease, comorbidities, and whether surgery was required.
- Most cases of acute ischemic colitis are nongangrenous and resolve completely with medical care in 1 to 2 days.
- The need for surgery in more severe cases portends a worse prognosis and is associated with increased morbidity and mortality. Any risk factors for ischemic colitis should be identified and mitigated as much as possible.
- Follow-up colonoscopy or imaging should be used to evaluate for structure or resolution of the colitis.

REFERRAL

Prompt general surgery consultation is indicated in patients with the following:
- Hemodynamic instability and peritoneal signs on examination
- CT showing signs of bowel infarction or perforation
- Endoscopy showing nonviable bowel or peritoneal signs

PEARLS & CONSIDERATIONS

COMMENTS

Ischemic colitis typically occurs in older patients who have multiple comorbidities. A high index of suspicion should be maintained for patients with

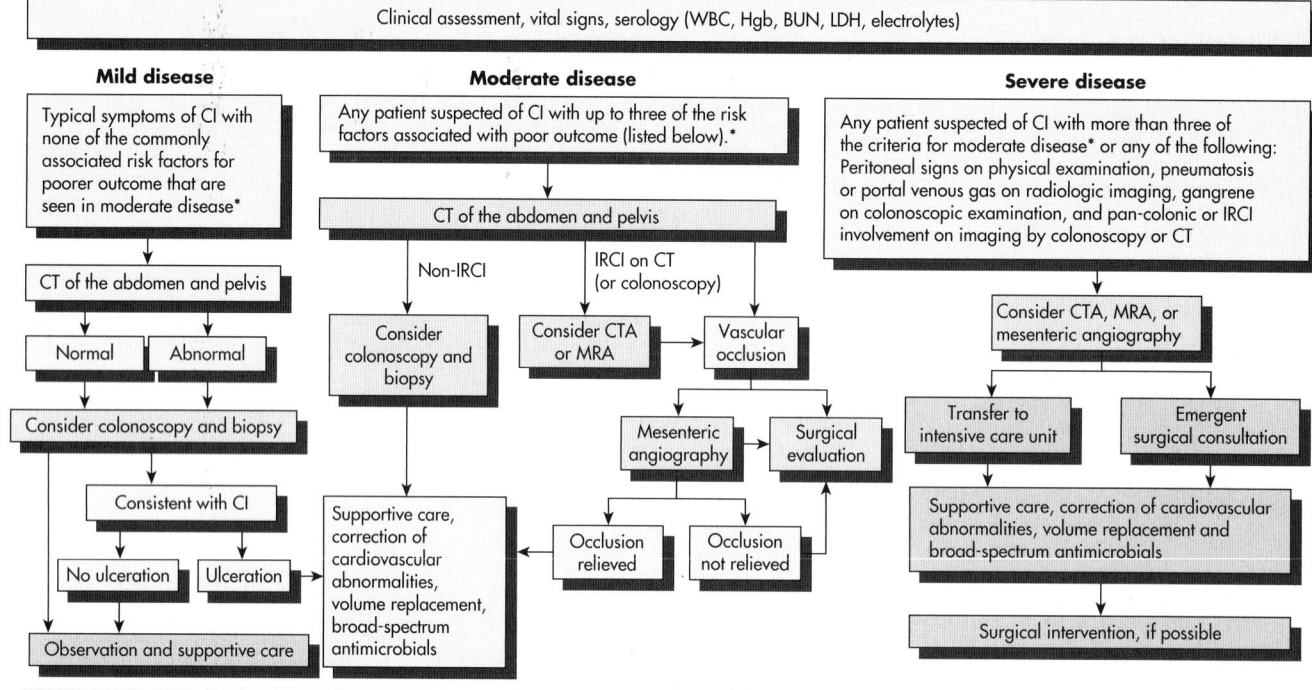

Algorithm for the management of patients suspected of having colon ischemia

Clinical assessment, vital signs, serology (WBC, Hgb, BUN, LDH, electrolytes)

Mild disease

Typical symptoms of CI with none of the commonly associated risk factors for poorer outcome that are seen in moderate disease*

↓

CT of the abdomen and pelvis

↓ ↓

Normal | Abnormal

↓

Consider colonoscopy and biopsy

↓

Consistent with CI

↓ ↓

No ulceration | Ulceration

↓

Observation and supportive care

Moderate disease

Any patient suspected of CI with up to three of the risk factors associated with poor outcome (listed below).*

↓

CT of the abdomen and pelvis

↓ Non-IRCI   ↓ IRCI on CT (or colonoscopy)

Consider colonoscopy and biopsy | Consider CTA or MRA → Vascular occlusion

↓   ↓   ↓

                          Mesenteric angiography → Surgical evaluation

                          ↓   ↓

                          Occlusion relieved | Occlusion not relieved

Supportive care, correction of cardiovascular abnormalities, volume replacement, broad-spectrum antimicrobials

Severe disease

Any patient suspected of CI with more than three of the criteria for moderate disease* or any of the following: Peritoneal signs on physical examination, pneumatosis or portal venous gas on radiologic imaging, gangrene on colonoscopic examination, and pan-colonic or IRCI involvement on imaging by colonoscopy or CT

↓

Consider CTA, MRA, or mesenteric angiography

↓ ↓

Transfer to intensive care unit | Emergent surgical consultation

↓

Supportive care, correction of cardiovascular abnormalities, volume replacement and broad-spectrum antimicrobials

↓

Surgical intervention, if possible

*Risk factors associated with poor outcome: Male gender, hypotension (SBP <90 mm Hg), tachycardia (HR >100 beats per min), abdominal pain without rectal bleeding, BUN >20 mg/dl, Hgb <12 g/dl, LDH >350 U/l, serum sodium <136 mEq/l (mmol/l), WBC >15 × 10⁹/cmm

FIG. 3 Colon ischemia algorithm. Diagnosis and treatment of colon ischemia *(CI)* based upon disease severity. *BUN,* Blood urea nitrogen; *CT,* computed tomography; *CTA,* computed tomography angiography; *Hgb,* hemoglobin; *IRCI,* isolated right-colon ischemia; *LDH,* lactate dehydrogenase; *MRA,* magnetic resonance angiography; *MRI,* magnetic resonance imaging; *WBC,* white blood cell count. (From Brandt LJ et al: ACG clinical guideline: epidemiology, risk factors, patterns of presentation, diagnosis, and management of colon ischemia [CI], *Am J Gastroenterol* 110:18-44, 2015. In Goldman L, Shafer AI: *Goldman-Cecil medicine,* ed 26, Philadelphia, 2019, Elsevier.)

BOX 3   Indications for Surgical Intervention in Patients With Ischemic Colitis

Acute
Peritonitis
Bowel perforation
Bowel necrosis
Fulminant colitis
Massive hemorrhage
Sepsis

Chronic
Intractable symptoms (abdominal pain, bloody diarrhea, etc.) lasting >2 wk
Recurrent sepsis
Chronic colitis
Ischemic stricture
Malnutrition from protein-losing enteropathy

From Cameron JL, Cameron AM: *Current surgical therapy,* ed 12, Philadelphia, 2017, Elsevier.

recent endovascular procedures. These patients require close outpatient follow-up and management by a primary care provider.

PREVENTION
Avoid overly aggressive hypertension treatment, dehydration, and extreme exercise.

REFERENCES
Available at eBooks.Health.Elsevier.com.

RELATED CONTENT
Mesenteric Venous Thrombosis (Related Key Topic)
Acute Mesenteric Ischemia (Related Key Topic)

AUTHORS: **DIANA X. ZHOU, MD,** and
THOMAS M. TRIPLETT, MD

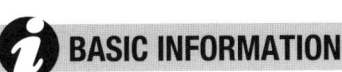

BASIC INFORMATION

DEFINITION

- A common form of vascular liver disease
- Occurs when a severe systemic disturbance leads to decreased perfusion to the liver resulting in tissue hypoxia

SYNONYMS

Hypoxic hepatitis
Shock liver
Ischemic hepatopathy
Hepatic necrosis

ICD-10CM CODES

K75.89 Other specified inflammatory liver disease
K76.2   Central hemorrhagic necrosis of liver

EPIDEMIOLOGY & DEMOGRAPHICS

Occurs worldwide
INCIDENCE:
- Less than 1% on the inpatient medical wards
- Incidence is higher (2.5%) in intensive care unit

PREVALENCE:
- Recognized as most frequent cause of acute liver injury
- 57% of patients with liver enzymes >1000 IU/L have ischemic hepatitis
- Prevalence up to 10% in the intensive care setting

PREDOMINANT AGE:
- Can occur in all ages
- Most common in elderly

PEAK INCIDENCE: Highest in the cardiac care units

RISK FACTORS:
- Most common is cardiovascular disease
- Chronic heart failure
- Cirrhosis

GENETICS: No genetic predisposition

PHYSICAL FINDINGS & CLINICAL PRESENTATION

- Altered mental status may be present due to decreased cerebral perfusion.
- Other symptoms are often masked by the overall disease state.
- Hepatic synthetic function is usually preserved in ischemic hepatitis.

ETIOLOGY

- Cardiac disease is the most common (Fig. E1)
- This includes myocardial infarction, arrhythmias, cardiac tamponade, and cardiogenic shock
- Majority of patients have markedly increased cardiac filling pressures
- Respiratory failure and sepsis are the second and third most common
- Hypovolemic shock from hemorrhage, dehydration, and heat stroke
- Hypotension (only 1 in 2 patients have documented low blood pressures)
- See Box 1 for a brief summary of the different causes of ischemic hepatitis

DIAGNOSIS

DIFFERENTIAL DIAGNOSIS (BOX 2)

- Acute viral hepatitis
- Autoimmune hepatitis
- Drug-induced liver injury
- Other toxins and medications (i.e., acetaminophen toxicity)

WORKUP

- Diagnosed by laboratory parameters and the clinical context of a hospitalized patient.
- Workup is directed at identifying the predisposing cause.
- Liver biopsy is not required.
- Histology shows centrilobular (zone 3) necrosis with preservation of the hepatic architecture.
- Necrosis can extend to the midzonal hepatocytes in the setting of prolonged ischemia.

LABORATORY TESTS

- Extremely elevated aminotransferase levels, often exceeding 200 times the upper limit of normal.
- Aspartate aminotransferase (AST) and alanine aminotransferase (ALT) rapidly rise after the ischemic insult.
- They peak within 1 to 3 days.
- They usually return to normal within 7 to 10 days if the initial ischemic insult is resolved.
- Lactate dehydrogenase (LDH) level is extremely elevated.
- ALT/LDH ratio of less than 1.5 is suggestive.
- Prothrombin time can be slightly prolonged.
- The serum bilirubin can be mildly increased.
- Serum bilirubin peaks after the aminotransferases peak.
- Increased blood urea nitrogen and creatinine levels from acute tubular necrosis and renal dysfunction.

IMAGING STUDIES

Imaging is not required for the diagnosis.

TREATMENT

NONPHARMACOLOGIC THERAPY

Management is directed at treating the underlying illness causing the systemic disturbance.

ACUTE GENERAL Rx

- Hemodynamic resuscitation
- Inotropic agents for cardiogenic shock
- Intravenous fluid resuscitation with or without vasoconstrictors for septic or hypovolemic shock
- Blood transfusions if hypovolemic shock from blood loss
- These measures optimize hepatic perfusion and resolve tissue hypoxia
- There is no role for *N*-acetylcysteine administration

CHRONIC Rx

- Ensure stability of underlying illness
- No specific liver-directed therapy

BOX 1 Causes of Ischemic Hepatitis

Cardiovascular disease (most common): Cardiogenic shock
Respiratory failure
Sepsis/septic shock
Hypovolemic shock: Hemorrhage, volume depletion
Hypotension

BOX 2 Common Differentials of Ischemic Hepatitis

Acute viral hepatitis (e.g., hepatitis A, hepatitis B)
Autoimmune hepatitis
Toxins (e.g., herbal supplements)
Medications (e.g., acetaminophen)

DISPOSITION

- Most commonly a self-limited and benign condition if promptly managed.
- Occasionally associated with significant mortality.
- Prognosis is determined by the severity of the underlying illness. In-hospital mortality associated with ischemic hepatitis is roughly 50%.
- Patients with underlying chronic heart failure or cirrhosis have worse outcomes.
- Other poor prognostic factors include persistently elevated aminotransferase and multiorgan failure.

REFERRAL

- Referral to a hepatologist is not required once illness is resolved.
- Referral is appropriate if patient has underlying cirrhosis.

PEARLS & CONSIDERATIONS

COMMENTS

- Have a high index of suspicion for this diagnosis in a hospitalized patient with severe systemic illness and significantly elevated AST and ALT.
- Use ALT/LDH ratio to aid in the diagnosis.
- Do not be alarmed if bilirubin continues to rise after AST and ALT peak.
- Hypotension is often not documented or not present at all.
- Patients with significantly elevated liver enzymes should be evaluated for occult heart failure.

PREVENTION

Ensure stability of comorbidities (e.g., cardiac disease)

AUTHOR: **FRED FERRI, MD**

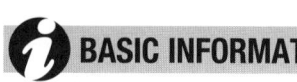 **BASIC INFORMATION**

DEFINITION

Benign neonatal hyperbilirubinemia or physiologic jaundice represents a normal, transient increase in bilirubin levels observed in almost all newborn infants. Due to an imbalance in bilirubin production and elimination, it appears after 24 h of age, and usually resolves by approximately 2 to 3 wk of age in full-term infants. Hyperbilirubinemia is pathologic if: (1) observed in the first 24 hr of age; (2) the total serum bilirubin (TSB) level is >95th percentile on the Bhutani nomogram in infants born at $\geq$35 wk gestational age (GA); (3) the bilirubin level is increasing by > 5 mg/dl/day or >0.2 mg/dl/h; or (4) jaundice persists beyond 2 to 3 wk of age in full-term infants. Most neonates present with physiologic hyperbilirubinemia, but a subset of infants will develop severe hyperbilirubinemia warranting treatment.

SYNONYMS

Neonatal jaundice
Physiologic jaundice
Pathologic jaundice

ICD 10-CM CODES
P58.9 Neonatal jaundice due to excessive hemolysis, unspecified
P59.0 Neonatal jaundice associated with preterm delivery
P59.3 Neonatal jaundice from breast milk inhibitor
P59.9 Neonatal jaundice, unspecified

EPIDEMIOLOGY & DEMOGRAPHICS

Fig. 1 illustrates the metabolism of bilirubin in the neonatal period. Transient neonatal hyperbilirubinemia is an almost universal condition, and approximately 60% of term and 80% of preterm infants develop jaundice in the first wk of life. However, the current incidence of severe hyperbilirubinemia and bilirubin encephalopathy is unknown. Past studies have estimated that approximately 2% of term or late preterm infants experience a TSB > 20 mg/dl while less than 1% experience a TSB >25 mg/dl. Acute bilirubin encephalopathy can occur in infants with untreated severe hyperbilirubinemia, with an estimated risk of 2% to 10% for infants with a TSB >30 mg/dl.
Risk factors for severe hyperbilirubinemia:
- Predischarge TSB or transcutaneous bilirubin measurement in the high-risk or high-intermediate-risk zone
- Lower GA
- Exclusive breastfeeding with suboptimal intake
- Clinical jaundice observed in the first 24 h of life
- Isoimmune hemolytic disease
- Previous sibling with jaundice
- Phototherapy before discharge
- Cephalohematoma or significant bruising
- Trisomy 21
- Macrosomic infant of a diabetic mother
- East Asian race

Risk factors for hyperbilirubinemia neurotoxicity:
- GA < 38 wk; risk increases with prematurity
- Isoimmune hemolytic disease, G6PD deficiency, or other hemolytic condition
- Sepsis
- Albumin <3.0 mg/dl
- Significant clinical instability in previous 24 h

PHYSICAL FINDINGS & CLINICAL CHARACTERISTICS

Clinically, hyperbilirubinemia manifests as jaundice, which is defined as yellowing of the skin, sclera, and mucous membranes. Jaundice is typically seen when the TSB level exceeds 5 mg/dl. Biochemically, hyperbilirubinemia is defined as an increase in TSB as a result of an elevated indirect serum bilirubin. Often, infants are asymptomatic. Common historical factors include poor feeding, exclusive breastfeeding, decreased urine and stool output.

ETIOLOGY

Pathologic jaundice or severe hyperbilirubinemia most commonly results from one of the mechanisms noted in Table 1.

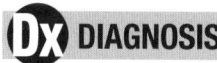 **DIAGNOSIS**

DIFFERENTIAL DIAGNOSIS

Physiologic jaundice, conjugated hyperbilirubinemia/cholestasis

WORKUP

The American Academy of Pediatrics recommends that all infants be assessed for jaundice at least every 12 h following delivery until discharge, and that the TcB or TSB should be measured between 24 and 48 h after birth or before discharge if that occurs earlier. Fig. E2 illustrates a schematic approach to the diagnosis of neonatal jaundice.

LABORATORY TESTS

Infant cord blood can be sent for direct antibody testing, blood type, and Rh determination. When measuring a TSB, a screening direct or conjugated bilirubin measurement should be obtained. A CBC, smear, reticulocyte count, and comprehensive metabolic panel can also be helpful in determining the etiology and evaluating illness severity.

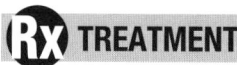 **TREATMENT**

NONPHARMACOLOGIC THERAPY

Lactation support can decrease the likelihood of severe hyperbilirubinemia, mothers should breastfeed 8 to 12 times per day to aid milk supply. Supplementing breastfeeding with formula is also an option.

ACUTE GENERAL Rx

The ultimate goal of recognizing and treating hyperbilirubinemia is to prevent bilirubin neurotoxicity. Phototherapy is a mainstay of treatment and should be initiated when the TSB is at or above phototherapy threshold based on the infant's age, gestational age, and presence or absence of neurotoxic risk factors. Phototherapy can be considered when the bilirubin level is within 2 to 3 points from threshold, though the

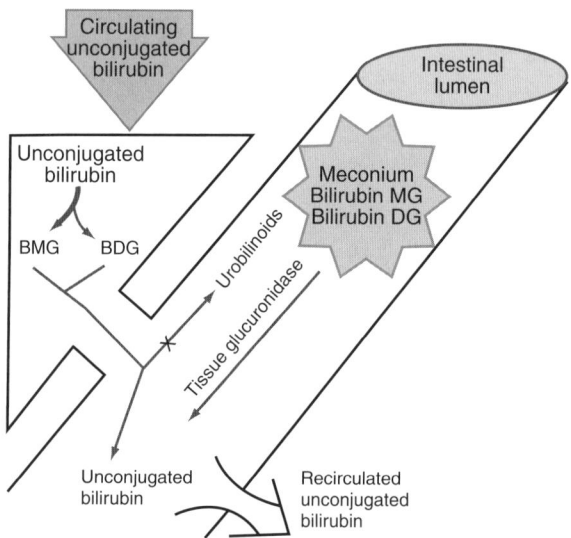

FIG 1 Metabolism of bilirubin in the neonatal period. Neonatal production rate of bilirubin is 6-8 mg/kg/24 h (in contrast to 3-4 mg/kg/24 h in adults). Water-insoluble bilirubin is bound to albumin. At the plasma-hepatocyte interface, a liver membrane carrier (bilitranslocase) transports bilirubin to a cytosolic binding protein (ligandin or Y protein, now known to be glutathione *S*-transferase), which prevents back-absorption to plasma. Bilirubin is converted to bilirubin monoglucuronide (*BMG*). Neonates excrete more BMG than adults. In the fetus, conjugated lipid-insoluble BMG and bilirubin diglucuronide (*BDG*) must be deconjugated by tissue β-glucuronidases to facilitate placental transfer of lipid-soluble unconjugated bilirubin across the placental lipid membranes. After birth, intestinal or milk-containing glucuronidases contribute to the enterohepatic recirculation of bilirubin and possibly to the development of hyperbilirubinemia. (From Kliegman, RM: *Nelson textbook of pediatrics*, ed 21, Philadelphia, 2020, Elsevier.)

TABLE 1 Etiologies of Pathologic Jaundice

Increased Bilirubin Production	Decreased Bilirubin Clearance	Increased Enterohepatic Circulation
Isoimmune hemolytic disease (mother/ infant blood group incompatibility)	Hypoalbuminemia	Breast milk jaundice
Inherited red blood cell membrane defect	Decreased ligandin	Breastfeeding failure/inadequate breastfeeding jaundice
Hemoglobinopathies	Prematurity	Ileus
Enzyme deficiencies	Small for gestational age	Intestinal obstruction
Hematomas	Crigler-Najjar type I and II	
Birth Trauma	Gilbert Syndrome	
Sepsis	Hypothyroidism	
Macrosomic infants of diabetic mothers (due to polycythemia or excess bruising)		

risk of overtreatment for the infant and family should be considered. Exposing the infant as much as possible and covering their eyes results in the most efficient decline in bilirubin levels. Supportive care in the form of maintaining adequate enteral hydration and thermoregulation is important. Initiation of phototherapy should be guided based on hour-specific bilirubin levels and infant risk factors. A clear consensus is lacking for the discontinuation of phototherapy, but most recent guidelines suggest that discontinuing phototherapy is an option when the TSB has decreased by at least 2 mg/dl below the hour-specific threshold at the initiation of phototherapy. The timing of rebound testing after phototherapy discontinuation should be guided by the infant's risk level for rebound hyperbilirubinemia. Exchange transfusion is infrequent but is indicated in any infant with acute bilirubin encephalopathy and should be considered when TSB reaches the exchange transfusion threshold.

DISPOSITION

Prognosis and outcomes in treated infants are excellent. Rates of kernicterus, a preventable cause of cerebral palsy, are low and bilirubin induced neurotoxicity be prevented with adequate screening and treatment.

REFERRAL

Consider consultation with a neonatologist if the TSB rises > 0.5 mg/dl/h or if the infant falls within 2 mg/dl of the exchange transfusion threshold.

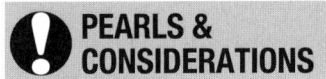

PEARLS & CONSIDERATIONS

COMMENTS

All newborns should undergo a risk assessment for hyperbilirubinemia prior to discharge. Physical assessment of jaundice alone is an unreliable predictor of TSB. The infant's age in hours and associated risk factors should be used to evaluate and manage treatment decisions. Less commonly, neonatal jaundice is the result of conjugated (direct) hyperbilirubinemia, also known as *cholestasis*. Conjugated hyperbilirubinemia is defined as a conjugated bilirubin concentration >1.0 mg/dl when the TSB is ≤ 5 mg/dl or >20% of TSB when the TSB is >5 mg/dl. It is always considered pathologic and deserves a separate evaluation and treatment.

PREVENTION

Preventing hyperbilirubinemia begins with an early assessment of risk factors for each infant. If the maternal antibody screen is positive or unknown, the infant should have a direct antiglobulin (DAT) and the infant's blood type should be determined as soon as possible. Providing early feeding support is important, as adequate intake plays a critical role in preventing hyperbilirubinemia.

SUGGESTED READINGS

Available at eBooks.Health.Elsevier.com

AUTHORS: **AMY SLOANE, MD,** and **TIMOTHY NELIN, MD**

J

Diseases and Disorders

I

Jaundice in the Adult Patient

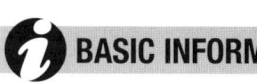 BASIC INFORMATION

DEFINITION
Jaundice is a yellowish discoloration of the sclera, skin, and mucous membranes resulting from deposition of bilirubin in the tissue, which occurs in the presence of an excessive amount of bilirubin in the bloodstream. Clinically detectable jaundice in adults is a serum bilirubin of 2.5 to 3 mg/dl.

SYNONYM
Icterus

ICD-10CM CODE
R17 Unspecified jaundice

EPIDEMIOLOGY & DEMOGRAPHICS
The prevalent causes of jaundice by age and sex:
- Young adulthood (for either sex): Viral hepatitis, Gilbert disease
- Middle adulthood (for either sex): Drug-induced hepatitis and cirrhosis
- Middle-aged and older men: Alcoholic liver disease, pancreatic cancer, hepatoma, primary hemochromatosis
- Women: Primary biliary cirrhosis, chronic active hepatitis, choledocholithiasis, carcinoma of the gallbladder

PHYSICAL FINDINGS & CLINICAL PRESENTATION
Presentation can vary from an incidental finding to acute and life-threatening. History and physical examination give important clues to the underlying condition.
Key history of present illness findings:
- Duration of jaundice
- Associated symptoms: Abdominal pain, fever, nausea, malaise, pruritus, chills, changes in urine and stool color, arthralgias, myalgias, rash, anorexia and/or weight loss
Key social history/exposure findings:
- Alcohol use, injection of illicit drugs, tattoos, use of hepatotoxic medication or herbal products, blood transfusions, unprotected sex, ingestion of shellfish, travel, occupational exposure to toxins
Key medical history findings:
- Prior abdominal/biliary surgery, prior episodes of jaundice, prior diagnosis of hepatitis B or C, inflammatory bowel disease
Key physical findings:
- Vital sign abnormalities: Fever, hypotension, tachycardia
- Signs of acute disease: Abdominal tenderness, splenomegaly, abdominal mass, encephalopathy, Murphy sign
- Signs of chronic liver disease: Palmar erythema, spider angiomas/nevi, bruising, gynecomastia, testicular atrophy, ascites, weight loss, Kayser-Fleischer rings (Wilson), caput medusa, internal hemorrhoids, scleral icterus, hepatic hydrothorax, Dupuytren contractures, muscle wasting

ETIOLOGY
Disruption in any of the three phases of bilirubin metabolism can lead to jaundice:

- Prehepatic phase: An increase in heme degradation products from red blood cell (RBC) catabolism, ineffective erythropoiesis, or breakdown of muscle myoglobin and cytochromes; leads to indirect (unconjugated) hyperbilirubinemia
- Intrahepatic phase: Destruction of the hepatocytes or disruption of either of the two separate biochemical processes that conjugate bilirubin in the hepatocyte; may lead to indirect (unconjugated) or direct (conjugated) hyperbilirubinemia
- Posthepatic phase: Blockage of the release of water-soluble bilirubin from the hepatobiliary system, preventing excretion into the stool or urine or recycling within the gut flora; leads to direct (conjugated) hyperbilirubinemia

(Dx) DIAGNOSIS

DIFFERENTIAL DIAGNOSIS
Prehepatic causes:
- Hemolytic processes (e.g., sickle cell disease, spherocytosis, thalassemia, G6PD, immune hemolysis, hemolytic uremic syndrome [HUS], microangiopathic hemolytic anemia [MAHA], paroxysmal nocturnal hemoglobinuria [PNH]), ineffective erythropoiesis (e.g., thalassemia, folate, severe iron deficiency), or large hematoma reabsorption
Intrahepatic causes:
- If unconjugated hyperbilirubinemia: Enzyme metabolism disorders (Gilbert disease, Crigler-Najjar syndrome), drugs that alter the enzymatic pathways such as rifampin, isoniazid, and probenecid
- If conjugated hyperbilirubinemia: Intrahepatic cholestasis caused by:
  1. Viruses: Hepatitis A, B, and C; Epstein-Barr (EBV), hemorrhagic viruses (yellow fever, Ebola)
  2. Other infections: Bacteria (leptospirosis, MAI), parasites (schistosomiasis, malaria, amebiasis), fungal (Blastomyces, Histoplasma)
  3. Alcohol: Alcoholic hepatitis, alcoholic cirrhosis
  4. Autoimmune: Primary biliary cirrhosis, primary sclerosing cholangitis, autoimmune hepatitis
  5. Hepatotoxic drug-induced: Acetaminophen (most common), antibiotics (amoxicillin-clavulanate [most common], sulfamethoxazole-trimethoprim, ciprofloxacin, isoniazid [INH]), cardiovascular drugs (statins, amiodarone), central nervous system agents (valproate, phenytoin, chlorpromazine), antineoplastic drugs (tyrosine kinase inhibitors, tumor necrosis factor inhibitors, methotrexate), tumor necrosis factor inhibitors, steroids (estrogenic or anabolic), NSAIDs, valproic acid, some herbals such as kava, ma huang, and off-market weight-loss supplements
  6. Hereditary/metabolic: Sickle cell disease and other RBC dyscrasias, hemochromatosis, Wilson disease, Dubin-Johnson and Rotor syndromes, α-antitrypsin deficiency,

glycogen storage disease, NASH (nonalcoholic steatohepatitis), porphyria, benign recurrent intrahepatic cholestasis
  7. Systemic diseases invading liver: Sarcoidosis, amyloidosis, hemochromatosis, tuberculosis, Mycobacterium avium intracellulare
  8. Other: Cirrhosis, sepsis, total parenteral nutrition, intrahepatic cholestasis of pregnancy, graft-versus-host disease, environmental toxins, benign postoperative state
Posthepatic causes:
- Intrinsic or extrinsic obstruction of the biliary system:
  1. Blockage within hepatobiliary tree: Strictures, cholangiocarcinoma, gallbladder cancer, carcinoma of ampulla of Vater, infection (e.g., cytomegalovirus [CMV], Cryptosporidium in patients with AIDS, parasites), choledocholithiasis
  2. Blockage outside of hepatobiliary tree: Pancreatitis, pancreatic carcinoma, pancreatic pseudocyst, lymphoma
- Pseudojaundice: Not related to bilirubin but rather resulting from excessive ingestion of foods containing beta carotene (e.g., carrots, melons, squash)

WORKUP
1. History, physical examination, and first-line lab tests can often clarify diagnosis. Fig. 1 describes a clinical approach to jaundice.
   Table 1 summarizes the differential diagnosis of critical and emergent diagnoses in patients with jaundice.

LABORATORY TESTS
- First-line tests:
  1. Serum total and direct bilirubin
  2. Urinalysis
  3. Liver function tests (aspartate aminotransferase [AST], alanine transaminase [ALT], gamma-glutamyl transpeptidase [GGTP], alkaline phosphatase), CBC, liver synthetic function (albumin, prothrombin time [PT], partial thromboplastin time [PTT]), pancreatic function (amylase, lipase)
- If serum total bilirubin and direct bilirubin are elevated and urine is positive for bilirubin, consider intrahepatic or posthepatic process. If serum total bilirubin is elevated but direct bilirubin is normal (unconjugated hyperbilirubinemia) and urine is negative for bilirubin, consider prehepatic or intrahepatic processes
Additional tests if diagnosis unclear:
- Screen for hepatitis A, B, and C; if still unclear, then consider following options based on history and physical
- Other viruses: EBV, CMV
- Autoimmune disorders: Antimitochondrial antibody (elevated in primary biliary cirrhosis); antismooth muscle antibody, antinuclear antibodies (ANA; elevated in autoimmune hepatitis); antinuclear cytoplasmic antibody (elevated in primary sclerosing cholangitis)
- Ceruloplasmin (elevated in Wilson disease)
- Alpha-1 antitrypsin deficiency (elevated in cirrhosis and emphysema)

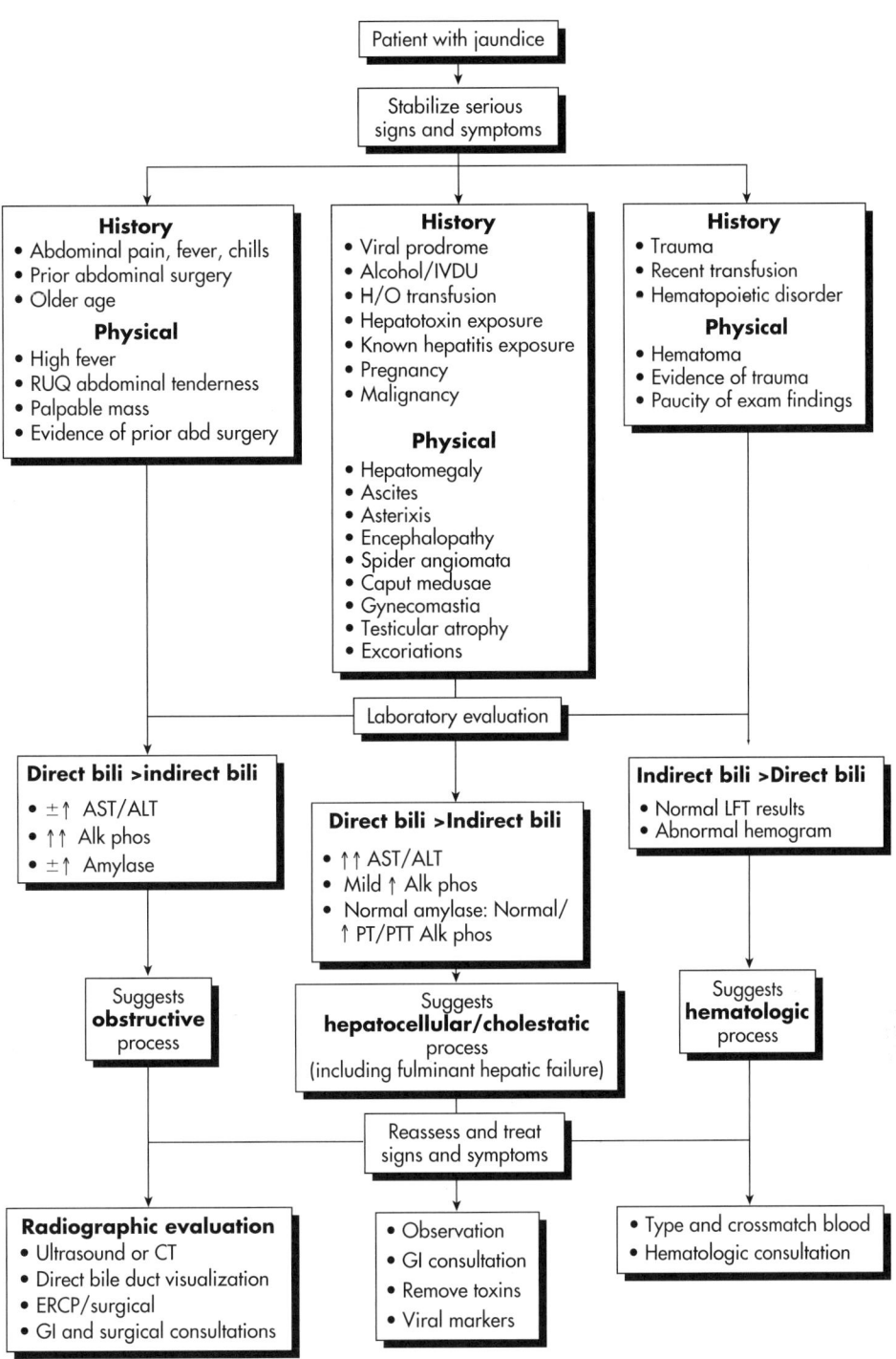

FIG. 1 Management of the patient with jaundice. *Alk phos,* Alkaline phosphatase; *ALT,* alanine aminotransferase; *AST,* aspartate aminotransferase; *bili,* bilirubin; *CT,* computed tomography; *ERCP,* endoscopic retrograde cholangiopancreatography; *GI,* gastrointestinal; *H/O,* history of; *IVDU,* intravenous drug use; *LFT,* liver function test; *PT,* prothrombin time; *PTT,* partial thromboplastin time; *RUQ,* right upper quadrant. (From Marx AJ et al: *Rosen's emergency medicine: concepts and clinical practice,* ed 7, Philadelphia, 2010, Elsevier.)

- Ferritin, Fe saturation (elevated in hemochromatosis)
- Blood smear (RBC dyscrasias)
- Diagnosis of exclusion: Gilbert syndrome
- Liver biopsy: Essential in diagnosis of chronic hepatitis. Can be used for diagnosis of liver masses but carries a substantial risk

IMAGING STUDIES
- Abdominal ultrasound: First-line study (Figs. E2 and E3) may be completed bedside, most sensitive for proximal biliary tract disease; presence of dilated ducts hints at an extrahepatic process.

- Abdominal computed tomography (CT): Often necessary to elucidate more information on liver, pancreas, and distal biliary system.
- Endoscopic retrograde cholangiopancreatography: Rarely necessary for diagnostics. Refer to GI consultant.

TABLE 1 Jaundice: Differential Diagnosis of Critical and Emergent Diagnoses

System	Critical	Emergent	Nonemergent
Hepatic	Fulminant hepatic failure	Hepatitis of any cause with confusion, bleeding, or coagulopathy	Hepatitis with normal mental status, normal vital signs, and no active bleeding
	Toxin	Wilson disease	
	Virus	Primary biliary cirrhosis	
	Alcohol	Autoimmune hepatitis	
	Ischemic insult	Liver transplant rejection	
	Reye syndrome	Infiltrative liver disease	
		Drug induced (isoniazid, phenytoin, acetaminophen, ritonavir, halothane, sulfonamides)	
		Toxin ingestion or exposure	
Biliary	Cholangitis	Bile duct obstruction (stone, inflammation, stricture, neoplasm)	
Systemic	Sepsis	Sarcoidosis	Posttraumatic hematoma resorption
	Heatstroke	Amyloidosis	Total parenteral nutrition
		Graft-versus-host disease	
Cardiovascular	Obstructing AAA	Right-sided congestive heart failure	
	Budd-Chiari syndrome	Veno-occlusive disease	
	Severe congestive heart failure		
Hematologic-oncologic	Transfusion reaction	Hemolytic anemia	Gilbert syndrome
		Massive malignant infiltration	Physiologic neonatal jaundice
		Inborn error of metabolism	
		Pancreatic head tumor	
		Metastatic disease	
Reproductive	Preeclampsia or HELLP syndrome	Hyperemesis gravidarum	
	Acute fatty liver of pregnancy		Cholestasis of pregnancy

AAA, Abdominal aortic aneurysm; *HELLP,* hemolysis, elevated liver enzymes, low platelets.
From Marx JA et al: *Rosen's emergency medicine,* ed 8, Philadelphia, 2014, Saunders.

- Percutaneous transhepatic cholangiography: Rarely necessary for diagnostics. Refer to GI or surgical consultant.
- Magnetic resonance cholangiopancreatography: Noninvasive visualization of bile and pancreatic ducts. Refer to GI consultant.
- Endoscopic ultrasound: Used for characterization and, if needed, biopsy of any focal lesions found within biliary tree and/or pancreas. Refer to GI consultant.
- Liver elastography: Can be done via ultrasound, CT, and MRI to predict the stage of hepatic fibrosis.

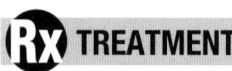 **TREATMENT**

NONPHARMACOLOGIC THERAPY
Depends on underlying cause of the jaundice and clinical stability of the patient. Generally, obstructive causes require surgical treatment, while nonobstructive causes require medical treatment.

ACUTE GENERAL Rx
Acute, life-threatening illness (e.g., cholecystitis or ascending cholangitis) requires prompt diagnosis with basic labs and bedside diagnostics, with early surgical and GI consultation in conjunction. Suspicious medications should be stopped. Initiate medical management of symptoms with analgesia, intravenous (IV) fluids, correction of coagulopathies, and consideration of antibiotics. *N-*Acetylcysteine can be given for acetaminophen overdose.

CHRONIC Rx
Reversible causes must be ruled out first—suspicious medications and EtOH must be discontinued. Consider GI consult for management of many intrahepatic diseases, such as treatment of hepatitis B or C, Wilson disease with penicillamine, hemochromatosis with phlebotomy, or for stent insertion with ERCP for posthepatic obstruction. Consider surgical consult for resection of pancreatic masses, cholecystectomy, etc.

Symptomatic pruritus may be treated with cholestyramine for bilirubin binding or with antihistamines to decrease the itch reflex. Ursodiol may be used to treat primary biliary cirrhosis and for gallstone prevention/dissolution.

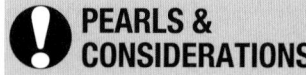 **PEARLS & CONSIDERATIONS**

COMMENTS
- Heed the warning of unstable vital signs to diagnose life-threatening illness; early collaboration with surgical and gastroenterology colleagues is helpful in complex patient care scenarios.
- Careful history and physical examination, basic labs, and prompt bedside imaging frequently lead to accurate diagnosis.
- Very high serum bilirubin (>15 mg/dl) is most likely to be seen in cirrhosis. Watch for hepatorenal syndrome in these patients.

RELATED CONTENT
Jaundice (Patient Information)

AUTHORS: **ALLA GOLDBURT, MD, PAOLO G. PACE, MASc, MD,** and **MINTA PATEL, MD**

BASIC INFORMATION

DEFINITION

Junctional rhythm is an abnormal cardiac rhythm originating in the His bundle or atrioventricular (AV) node. This diagnosis includes three distinct entities based on rate[1]:

1. Junctional Bradycardia has a rate below 40 bpm.
2. Junctional escape rhythm has a rate of 40 to 60 bpm.
3. Accelerated junctional rhythm has a rate of 60 to 100 bpm.
4. Junctional ectopic tachycardia (JET) has a rate of >100 bpm.

SYNONYMS

Junctional escape rhythm
Accelerated junctional rhythm
Junctional ectopic tachycardia (JET)
Nodal rhythm disorder
Ectopic rhythm disorder
Junctional premature depolarization

ICD-10CM CODE
I49.2 Junctional premature depolarization

EPIDEMIOLOGY & DEMOGRAPHICS

INCIDENCE: Junctional rhythm occurs more commonly in children because of higher vagal tone (13% of 10- to 13-yr-old boys, 45% of 7- to 10-yr-old children, and 19% of infants have junctional rhythm during sleep). Endurance athletes have a 20% incidence of junctional rhythm, for a similar reason.[2]

PREVALENCE: Junctional Ectopic tachycardia (JET) is a rare cause of supraventricular tachycardia. It is rare in the pediatric population and even less common in adults. On the contrary, junctional rhythm is common although the prevalence is not well defined.[1,3–6]

RISK FACTORS: Conduction system disease, heart block, digitalis intoxication, heart surgery, endocarditis.[1]

GENETICS: Family history can be found in almost half of patients with JET, and in some patients it is associated with maternal lupus anti-SSA and anti-SSB.[5] ACE deletion polymorphism has been related to increased risk of JET.[4]

PHYSICAL FINDINGS & CLINICAL PRESENTATION

ESSENTIAL HISTORY:

- Previous history of syncope, presyncope, lightheadedness.
- Drugs, especially digoxin. Amount taken, time of ingestion. The digestion time is especially important because the serum digoxin level ideally should be measured at least 6 h after ingestion to ensure accuracy. Obtain a thorough medication history to determine if any recent additions or dosing changes were made. Presence of renal failure can result in higher or even toxic serum levels of digoxin. Hypokalemia renders cardiac tissue more susceptible to the effects of digoxin and should be promptly corrected in the event of digoxin

toxicity. Other medications such as beta-blockers and nondihydropyridine calcium channel blockers may also result in a junctional escape rhythm primarily by causing atrioventricular (AV) block.[1,7,8,9]

SYMPTOMS:
- Light-headedness
- Syncope
- Palpitations
- Symptoms associated with digitalis intoxication: Gastrointestinal symptoms such as anorexia, nausea, vomiting, and abdominal pain. Neurologic manifestation such as lethargy, fatigue, delirium, confusion, weakness. Visual changes: Alteration in color vision, diplopia, photophobia, decreased visual acuity.[7]

PHYSICAL EXAMINATION:
- Vital signs
- Look for evidence of hypoperfusion and end organ dysfunction
- Cannon A-waves on examination of the jugular pulse.

ETIOLOGY

Junctional tachycardia can occur as a primary arrhythmia (usually in children-JET), secondary to digitalis intoxication or catecholamine intoxication, or in the setting of injury to the His bundle (e.g., after valve surgery, abscess, sarcoidosis, myocarditis, ischemia).[6]

DIAGNOSIS

DIFFERENTIAL DIAGNOSIS

- AVNRT (atrioventricular nodal reentrant tachycardia)[3,10]
- AVRT (atrioventricular reentrant tachycardia)[3,10]

- Accelerated idioventricular rhythm, in the case of junctional rhythm with aberrant conduction[3,10]
- Fig. 1 illustrates arrhythmias originating in the atrioventricular node

WORKUP

- Vital signs
- 12-lead ECG (Figs. E2 and 3). The rhythm is almost perfectly regular, and the QRS complex is generally narrow and similar to the complex seen during sinus rhythm. Retrograde P waves with a very short interval from QRS to P wave can be seen[3,4]
- History of cardiac surgery, fevers, drug ingestion[6]

LABORATORY TESTS
- Serum digoxin concentration
- Serum potassium concentration
- Creatinine and blood urea nitrogen (BUN) to assess renal function
- Troponin
- Serum antibody testing for Lyme disease, if junctional escape rhythm is associated with AV block[1]

IMAGING STUDIES
Echocardiogram

TREATMENT

Junctional tachycardia may be a marker for a serious underlying condition such as digitalis toxicity, post cardiac surgery, endocarditis, hypokalemia, or myocardial ischemia. Underlying conditions should be sought and corrected accordingly.[4,6,7,10] Amiodarone seems to be the most effective pharmacologic agent. Ivabradine,

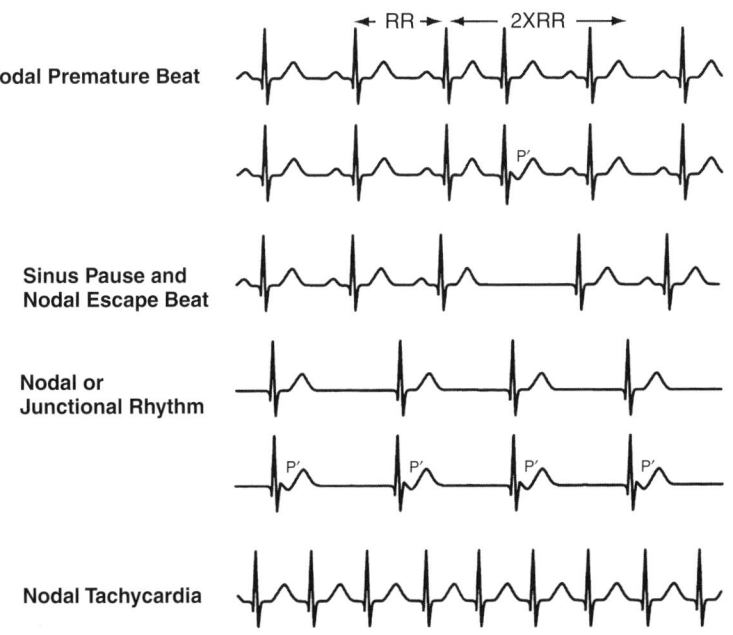

FIG. 1 Arrhythmias originating in the atrioventricular node. (From Park MK: *Park's pediatric cardiology for practitioners*, ed 6, Philadelphia, 2014, Elsevier.)

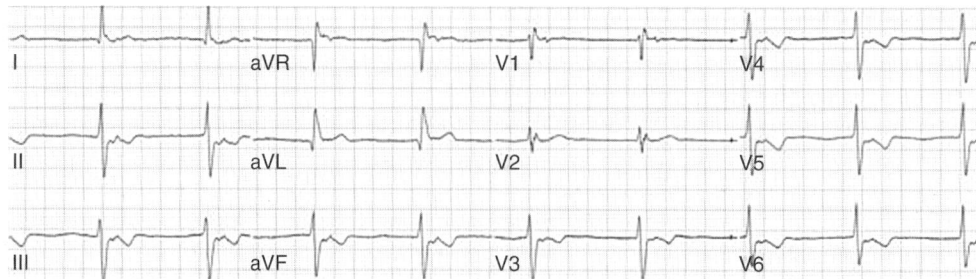

FIG. 3 **Junctional rhythm with retrograde P waves that are negative in the inferior leads.** *aVF,* Augmented vector foot; *aVL,* augmented vector left; *aVR,* augmented vector right. (From Parrillo JE, Dellinger RP: *Critical care medicine: principles of diagnosis and management in the adult,* ed 4, Philadelphia, 2014, Elsevier.)

nifekalant, and landiolol may have roles in suppressing JET.[6,11,12]

NONPHARMACOLOGIC THERAPY

- Junctional escape rhythm in the setting of sinus arrest or complete heart block without reversible cause necessitates permanent pacemaker implantation.[13]
- Junctional ectopic tachycardia can be treated with antiarrhythmics or radiofrequency ablation.[14]

ELECTROPHYSIOLOGY STUDY: The origin of this tachycardia is within the His bundle or AV node, and it can be diagnosed definitively by intracardiac recordings. Junctional rhythm most frequently takes the form of escape rhythms in the presence of sinus node dysfunction or AV nodal block, which can be diagnosed on electrophysiology (EP) study. These escape rhythms usually have a QRS morphology identical to that seen during sinus rhythm. In such cases there is no P wave before the QRS complexes. The P waves can occur simultaneously with the QRS complexes; more commonly, they are retrograde. When the junctional rhythm is faster than 100 beats/min, it is called junctional tachycardia.[14]

ACUTE GENERAL Rx

The mainstay of managing nonparoxysmal junctional tachycardia is to correct the underlying abnormality. Withholding digitalis when junctional tachycardia is the only clinical manifestation of toxicity is usually adequate. If, however, ventricular arrhythmias or high-grade heart block are observed, then treatment with digitalis-binding agents may be indicated.[6-8,13]

DISPOSITION

Admit to cardiac telemetry if symptomatic. Consider specialty referral to cardiac electrophysiology.

REFERRAL

Refer to cardiologist.

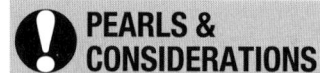

PEARLS & CONSIDERATIONS

COMMENTS

- Junctional rhythm often is observed in patients with AV dissociation, which can lead to atrial contraction against closed atrioventricular valves, resulting in cannon-A waves. This wave will cause pulsation in the neck and abdomen, headache, cough, jaw pain, and possible hypotension.[13]
- The presence of a slow (30-40 bpm) and perfectly regular rhythm in a patient with atrial fibrillation often indicates junctional rhythm with complete heart block.[15]

PREVENTION

N/A

REFERENCES

Available at eBooks.Health.Elsevier.com.

RELATED CONTENT

Digoxin Overdose (Related Key Topic)
Sick Sinus Syndrome (Related Key Topic)
Heart Block, Complete (Related Key Topic)
Heart Block, Second-Degree (Related Key Topic)

AUTHOR: **JAVIER BALDA, MD**

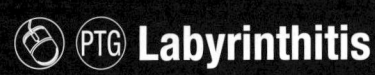

L

I

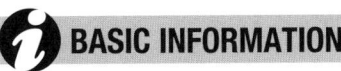 **BASIC INFORMATION**

DEFINITION

Labyrinthitis is an acute vestibular syndrome resulting from inflammation of the membranous labyrinth of the inner ear.[1] Symptoms include acute onset of dizziness with either hearing loss or tinnitus in association with nausea or vomiting, gait instability, nystagmus, and head-motion intolerance that lasts days or weeks.[2] Vestibular neuritis or neuronitis is often used interchangeably with labyrinthitis because of the clinical presentation is so similar. However, vestibular neuritis does not result in hearing loss and is due to inflammation of the vestibular nerve without membranous labyrinth involvement.

SYNONYMS

Acute labyrinthitis
Acute vestibular neuronopathy
Vestibular neuronitis
Vestibular neuritis
Viral neurolabyrinthitis

ICD-10CM CODES
H81.23 Vestibular neuronitis, bilateral
H83.01 Labyrinthitis, right ear
H83.02 Labyrinthitis, left ear
H83.03 Labyrinthitis, bilateral
H83.09 Labyrinthitis, unspecified ear

EPIDEMIOLOGY & DEMOGRAPHICS

INCIDENCE (IN U.S.): Incidence of labyrinthitis specifically (as opposed to vestibular neuritis) is not known
PREDOMINANT AGE: Any

PHYSICAL FINDINGS & CLINICAL PRESENTATION

CLINICAL PRESENTATION:
- Acute-onset dizziness with hearing loss or tinnitus
- Nausea or vomiting
- Gait instability
- Nystagmus
- Head-motion intolerance
- Duration of symptoms: Days to weeks
- During the first day, the patient usually has difficulty focusing the eyes because of spontaneous nystagmus.

- Usually has benign course with complete recovery within 1 to 3 mo, although older patients may have intractable dizziness that persists for many months.

PHYSICAL FINDINGS:
Nystagmus: spontaneous unidirectional horizontal-torsional nystagmus that attenuates with fixation and whose fast phase beats away from the affected side and intensifies when looking in the direction of the fast phase and diminishes when looking away.[3]
No skew deviation on Alternate Cover Test.

The presence of skew deviation is a very specific finding for a brain stem lesion rather than a peripheral cause of acute vestibulopathy.
Corrective saccade on head impulse test (HIT)
- Nausea
- Vomiting
- Vertigo worsening with head movement
- Abnormal caloric electronystagmography (ENG) tests
- Hearing loss in the affected ear or ears
- Normal otoscopic examination typically
- Normal elemental neurologic examination aside from elements related to vestibulopathy such as nystagmus and a positive head thrust test

ETIOLOGY

Symptoms often preceded for 1 to 2 wk by a viral-like illness. Labyrinthitis may be either bacterial or viral and may be either tympanogenic (i.e., resulting from spread of infection into the inner ear from the middle ear, antrum, or petrous apex), meningogenic, or hematogenic from encephalitis or brain abscess. The round window membrane is considered the most likely pathway of inflammatory mediators from the middle to the inner ear that subsequently give rise to labyrinthitis.

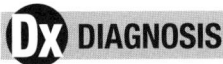 **DIAGNOSIS**

DIFFERENTIAL DIAGNOSIS
- Acute labyrinthine ischemia (ischemic stroke of the labyrinthine artery)
- Labyrinthine fistula
- Benign paroxysmal positional vertigo
- Ménière disease
- Cholesteatoma
- Drug-induced vestibulocochlear nerve damage

- Vestibulocochlear nerve (cranial nerve VIII) tumor
- Head trauma
- Vertebrobasilar stroke
- Dehiscence of the superior semicircular canal

WORKUP

Physical examination should include the following elements[3]:
- Otoscopic examination
- HINTS Plus Exam to distinguish patients with an acute vestibular syndrome due to peripheral cause from those with brain stem stroke:
  1. Head Impulse Test: A test of the vestibuloocular reflex (VOR) performed as follows: "Standing in front of the patient, the examiner holds the patient's head by each side, instructs the patient to maintain focus on the examiner's nose and to keep the head and neck loose. Then the examiner quickly turns the patient's head approximately 10 to 20 degrees, using a lateral to center motion. The normal (individuals with normal vestibular function) response is that the patient's focus stays locked on the examiner's nose. The presence of a corrective saccade (the eyes move with the head, then snap back in a fast corrective movement to the examiner's nose) is a positive test (abnormal VOR), which generally indicates a peripheral process, usually vestibular neuritis. The absence of a corrective saccade in an acute vestibular syndrome is consistent with a stroke. If an acutely dizzy patient with an acute vestibular syndrome does not have nystagmus, it is unlikely to be vestibular and, therefore, the HIT should not be used."[3]
  2. Nystagmus: Spontaneous unidirectional horizontal-torsional nystagmus that attenuates with fixation indicates a peripheral direction-changing gaze-evoked nystagmus or nystagmus that is pure torsional or vertical should be considered central in origin.[3]
  3. Test of skew deviation with Alternative Cover Test: "With the patient looking directly at the examiner's nose, the examiner alternately covers the right eye, then the left eye, and continues alternating back and forth, approximately every 2 seconds. In patients with skew deviation, each time the covered eye is uncovered, there is a

TABLE 1	Acute Vestibular Syndrome Oculomotor Physical Findings		
Oculomotor Examination Component	**Peripheral (Usually Vestibular Neuritis)**	**Central (Usually Posterior Circulation Stroke)**
Nystagmus (neural gaze and gaze to the right and left)	Dominantly horizontal, direction-fixed, beating away from the affected side	Direction-changing horizontal or dominantly vertical and/or torsional, then central[a] (often mimics peripheral)
Test of skew (alternate cover test)	Normal vertical eye alignment (i.e., no skew deviation)	Often mimics peripheral; if skew deviation is present then central[b]
HIT	Unilaterally abnormal toward the affected side (presence of a corrective saccade)	Usually bilaterally normal (no corrective saccade)

NOTE: Strokes in the AICA territory may produce a unilaterally HIT that mimics vestibular neuritis, but hearing loss is usually present as a clue. If a patient has bilaterally abnormal HIT, this is also suspicious for a central lesion if nystagmus is present (AICA stroke or Wernicke's syndrome).
[a]Inferior branch vestibular neuritis presents with down-beat-torsional nystagmus in a patient with an AVS should be considered to be central (a stroke).
[b]Skew deviation evident by bedside alternate cover testing is rare in peripheral vestibular cases; its presence should be considered to be central (a stroke, often in the brain stem).
From Edlow JA. A new approach to the diagnosis of acute dizziness in adult patients, *Emerg Med Clin North Am* 34(4):717-742, 2016.

slight vertical correction. One side corrects upward and the other corrects downward. The amplitude of correction is small—1 to 2 mm; therefore, it is key for the examiner to focus on one eye (either one), rather than following the uncovered eye. A normal response is no vertical correction, and an abnormal response should be considered a stroke in patients with an acute vestibular syndrome." [2]

4. Test of hearing (the Plus): Loss of hearing could indicate either labyrinthitis (if the rest of the examination is consistent with a peripheral etiology) or can be part of an anterior inferior cerebellar artery (AICA) stroke syndrome (if the rest of the examination suggests a central etiology).

- General neurologic examination, focusing on cranial nerves, including hearing, cerebellar testing, and long-tract signs. Because a lateral medullary stroke (Wallenberg syndrome) can present with an acute vertigo (with accompanying dysarthria, dysphagia, or hoarseness and may have a Horner's syndrome and decreased ipsilateral facial pain and temperature sensation and contralateral decreased body pain and temperature sensation without any weakness or loss of light touch sensation), it is important to test the cranial nerves carefully.
- Gait testing: Patients who cannot walk independently are unsafe for discharge and are more likely to have a stroke as a cause of their acute vestibular syndrome. Patient with cerebellar dysfunction may have truncal ataxia without abnormalities on finger to nose or rapid alternating movement testing. Patients too symptomatic to walk can be assessed for truncal ataxia by asking them to sit upright on the stretcher without holding onto the side rails.[2]

LABORATORY TESTS

- Routine laboratory tests are generally not helpful.
- If there is a history of significant emesis, check electrolytes, blood urea nitrogen, and creatinine.

IMAGING STUDIES

- Imaging studies are usually not useful but are relied on to evaluate for stroke as a cause of acute vestibular syndrome.
  1. CT is a poor test for posterior circulation stroke.
  2. MRI with diffusion-weighted imaging, misses 10% to 20% of strokes in the first 24 to 48 h of an acute vestibular syndrome patient.
- Therefore, in patients with an acute vestibular syndrome, the physical examination leads to a correct diagnosis more frequently than imaging.
- MRI of the brain with and without contrast with fine cuts through the internal auditory canal is indicated if there is an abnormal cranial nerve examination, headache, concern for stroke, or suspicion of cranial nerve VIII nerve tumor.
- Head CT with fine cuts through temporal bones is indicated if there is a history of trauma or suspicion of cholesteatoma.

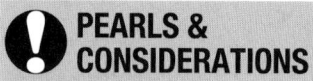 **TREATMENT**

NONPHARMACOLOGIC THERAPY

- Reassurance
- Initial bed rest, then encourage increase in activity as tolerated
- Vestibular rehabilitation

ACUTE GENERAL Rx

- Treatment options include antiemetics such as promethazine or ondansetron; vestibular suppressants such as the antihistamines meclizine or diphenhydramine; the anticholinergic scopolamine; and the benzodiazepines diazepam or lorazepam. These medications should be continued for only a few days during the acute phase. These medications should be used with caution in the elderly. Methylprednisolone 100 mg/day for 3 days, with slow taper is sometimes used but has not shown benefit in hastening recovery.
- Valacyclovir has not been shown to be helpful.

CHRONIC Rx

- No specific pharmacologic chronic therapy. Meclizine should not be used chronically.
- Vestibular rehabilitation is useful for patients with persistent symptoms.

DISPOSITION

Usually does not require hospital admission unless the patient is unable to tolerate oral intake of liquids

REFERRAL

- Refer if symptoms persist or neurologic abnormalities are present.
- Consider vestibular rehabilitation

ⓘ PEARLS & CONSIDERATIONS

COMMENTS

Labyrinthitis is a term that usually implies peripheral vestibulopathy associated with hearing loss. The term *vestibular neuronitis* is typically used when hearing is not affected. Despite this technical distinction, many physicians use these terms interchangeably.

HINT Plus Exam is useful in patients with an acute vestibular syndrome to determine whether the lesion is peripheral or possibility due to a stroke.

REFERENCES
Available at eBooks.Health.Elsevier.com

RELATED CONTENT

Labyrinthitis (Patient Information)
Benign Paroxysmal Positional Vertigo (Related Key Topic)
Vestibular Neuronitis (Related Key Topic)

AUTHOR: **JOSEPH S. KASS, MD, JD, FAAN**

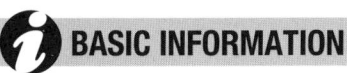

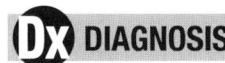 **BASIC INFORMATION**

DEFINITION

Lactose intolerance is the insufficient concentration of lactase enzyme, leading to fermentation of malabsorbed lactose by intestinal bacteria with subsequent production of intestinal gas and various organic acids, manifesting clinically with diarrhea, abdominal pain, flatulence, or bloating after lactose intake. Lactose malabsorption occurs when a substantial amount of lactose is not absorbed in the intestine. Lactase deficiency is defined as brush-border lactase activity that is markedly reduced relative to the activity observed in infants.

SYNONYMS

Lactose malabsorption
Lactase deficiency
Milk intolerance
Carbohydrate malabsorption

ICD-10CM CODES
E73.9 Lactose intolerance, unspecified
E73.8 Other lactose intolerance

EPIDEMIOLOGY & DEMOGRAPHICS

- Nearly 50 million people in the U.S. have partial or complete lactose intolerance. There are racial differences, with <25% of White adults being lactose intolerant but >85% of Asian Americans and >60% of African Americans having some form of lactose intolerance.
- There are geographic variations: Highest in Asians (up to 90%), lowest in northern Europeans (approximately 10%), intermediate in southern Europeans and Middle Eastern populations (up to 40%).

PHYSICAL FINDINGS & CLINICAL PRESENTATION

- Abdominal tenderness and cramping, bloating, flatulence
- Diarrhea
- Symptoms are directly related to the osmotic pressure of substrate in the colon and occur ~2 h after ingestion of lactose
- Physical examination: May be entirely within normal limits

ETIOLOGY

- Before it can be absorbed, lactose is cleared to glucose and galactose by the enzyme lactase in the brush border of the small intestine. If the amount of lactase is marginal or its expression is left, lactose intolerance will result.
- Congenital lactase deficiency: Common in premature infants; rare in term infants and generally inherited as a chromosomal recessive trait.
- Secondary lactose intolerance: Usually a result of injury of the intestinal mucosa (Crohn disease, viral gastroenteritis, AIDS enteropathy, cryptosporidiosis, Whipple disease, sprue).
- Acquired primary lactase deficiency (adult-type hypolactasia OMIM #223100) is the most common form of lactase deficiency worldwide. The decline in lactase activity is a multifactorial process that is regulated at the gene transcription level and leads to decreased biosynthesis, retardation of intracellular transport, or maturation of the enzyme lactase-phlorizin hydrolase.

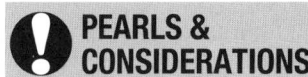 **DIAGNOSIS**

DIFFERENTIAL DIAGNOSIS

- Inflammatory bowel disease
- Irritable bowel syndrome
- Pancreatic insufficiency
- Nontropical and tropical sprue
- Cystic fibrosis
- Diverticular disease
- Bowel neoplasm
- Laxative abuse
- Celiac disease
- Parasitic disease (e.g., giardiasis)
- Viral or bacterial infections

WORKUP

- A detailed dietary history is essential in the evaluation of patients with suspected carbohydrate malabsorption.
- The diagnosis can usually be made on the basis of the history and improvement with dietary manipulation.
- Diagnostic workup may include confirming the diagnosis with hydrogen breath test and excluding other conditions listed in the differential diagnosis that may also coexist with lactase deficiency.

LABORATORY TESTS

- Laboratory evaluation may not be necessary in patients with significant history.
- Lactose breath hydrogen test: A rise in breath hydrogen >20 ppm within 90 min of ingestion of 50 g of lactose is positive for lactase deficiency. This test is positive in 90% of patients with lactose malabsorption. Common causes of false-negative results are recent use of oral antibiotics or recent high colonic enema. Fig. E1 illustrates the role of symptoms in determining the clinical importance of lactose malabsorption.
- The lactose tolerance test is an older and less accurate testing modality (20% rate of false-positive and false-negative results). The patient is administered an oral dose of 1 to 1.5 g of lactose/kg body weight. Serial measurement of blood glucose level on an hourly basis for 3 h is then performed. The test is considered positive if the patient develops intestinal symptoms and the blood glucose level rises <20 mg/dl above the fasting baseline level.
- Diarrhea associated with lactase deficiency is osmotic in nature with an osmotic gap and a pH <6.5.

IMAGING STUDIES

Imaging studies are generally not indicated. A small bowel series may be useful in patients with significant malabsorption.

TREATMENT

NONPHARMACOLOGIC THERAPY

Management consists of reducing lactose exposure by avoiding milk and milk-containing products or using milk in which the lactose has been prehydrolyzed with lactase. A lactose-free diet generally results in prompt resolution of symptoms. Lactose is primarily found in dairy products but may be present as an ingredient or component of common foods and beverages. Possible sources of lactose include breads, candies, cold cuts, dessert mixes, cream soups, bologna, commercial sauces and gravies, chocolate, drink mixes, salad dressings, and medications. Labels should be read carefully to identify sources of lactose.

ACUTE GENERAL Rx

- Addition of lactase enzyme supplement (Lactaid tablets, Dairy Ease) before the ingestion of milk products may prevent symptoms in some patients. However, it is not effective for all lactose-intolerant patients.
- Lactose-intolerant patients must ensure adequate calcium intake. Calcium supplementation is recommended to prevent osteoporosis.

CHRONIC Rx

Patient education regarding foods high in lactose, such as milk, cottage cheese, or ice cream, is recommended.

DISPOSITION

Clinical improvement with restriction or elimination of milk products

REFERRAL

GI referral for endoscopic procedures if concomitant GI disorders are suspected

PEARLS & CONSIDERATIONS

COMMENTS

- There is great variability in signs and symptoms in patients with lactose intolerance depending on the degree of lactase deficiency. Most individuals with presumed lactose malabsorption can tolerate 12 to 15 g of lactose or up to 12 oz of milk daily without symptoms.
- Nondairy synthetic drinks (e.g., Coffee-Mate) and use of rice milk are generally well tolerated.

RELATED CONTENT

Lactose Intolerance (Patient Information)

AUTHOR: **FRED F. FERRI, MD**

L

Diseases and Disorders

I

Lead Poisoning 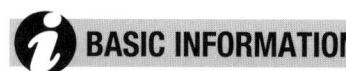 (PTG)

BASIC INFORMATION

DEFINITION
Lead is a potent, pervasive neurotoxicant. Lead poisoning refers to multisystem abnormalities resulting from excessive lead exposure.

SYNONYM
Plumbism

ICD-10CM CODES
T56.0X1A	Toxic effect of lead and its compounds, accidental (unintentional), initial encounter
T56.0X1D	Toxic effect of lead and its compounds, accidental (unintentional), subsequent encounter
T56.0X1S	Toxic effect of lead and its compounds, accidental (unintentional), sequela
T56.0X2A	Toxic effect of lead and its compounds, intentional self-harm, initial encounter
T56.0X2D	Toxic effect of lead and its compounds, intentional self-harm, subsequent encounter
T56.0X2S	Toxic effect of lead and its compounds, intentional self-harm, sequela
T56.0X3A	Toxic effect of lead and its compounds, assault, initial encounter
T56.0X3D	Toxic effect of lead and its compounds, assault, subsequent encounter
T56.0X3S	Toxic effect of lead and its compounds, assault, sequela
T56.0X4A	Toxic effect of lead and its compounds, undetermined, initial encounter
T56.0X4D	Toxic effect of lead and its compounds, undetermined, subsequent encounter
T56.0X4S	Toxic effect of lead and its compounds, undetermined, sequela

EPIDEMIOLOGY & DEMOGRAPHICS
- Lead poisoning is most common in children ages 1 to 5 yr (17,000 cases/100,000 persons). The highest rates are among Blacks, those with low income, and urban children.
- In 1991 the Centers for Disease Control and Prevention (CDC) lowered the definition of a safe blood lead level to <10 mcg/dl of whole blood (a blood lead level of 25 mcg/dl was considered acceptable before 1991).
- It is estimated that >15% of preschoolers in the U.S. have a blood lead level >15 mcg/dl.

PHYSICAL FINDINGS & CLINICAL PRESENTATION
- Findings vary with the degree of toxicity (Table 1). Examination may be normal in patients with mild toxicity.
- Myalgias, irritability, headache, and general fatigue may be present initially.
- Abdominal cramping, constipation, weight loss, tremor, paresthesias and peripheral neuritis, seizures, and coma may occur with severe toxicity.
- Motor neuropathy is common in children with lead poisoning; learning disorders are also frequent.

ETIOLOGY
Chronic, repeated exposure to paint containing lead, plumbing, storage of batteries, pottery, or lead soldering. Concentration of lead is generally highest in lead-based paint on exterior surfaces. Among interior surfaces, windows are most likely to have the highest lead content. Table 2 summarizes common sources of lead.

DIAGNOSIS

DIFFERENTIAL DIAGNOSIS
- Polyneuropathies from other sources
- Anxiety disorder, attention deficit disorder
- Malabsorption, acute abdomen
- Iron deficiency anemia

WORKUP
Laboratory screening: All U.S. children should be considered to be at risk for lead poisoning and should be screened routinely starting at age 1 yr for low-risk children and age 6 mo for high-risk children. Lead poisoning risk assessment questions to be asked between 6 months and 6 years are summarized in Table 3.

LABORATORY TESTS
- Venous blood lead level: Normal level, <5 mcg/dl; levels of 50 to 70 mcg/dl, indicative of moderate toxicity; levels >70 mcg/dl, associated with severe poisoning
- Mild anemia with basophilic stippling on peripheral smear
- Elevated zinc protoporphyrin levels or free erythrocyte protoporphyrin level
- An increased body burden of lead with previous high-level exposure in patients with occupational lead poisoning can be demonstrated by measuring the excretion of lead in urine after premedication with calcium ethylenediaminetetraacetic acid (EDTA) or another chelating agent

IMAGING STUDIES
- Imaging studies are generally not necessary.
- A plain abdominal film can visualize lead particles in the gut.
- "Lead lines" may be noted on x-ray films of long bones.

TABLE 2   Sources of Lead

Paint chips
Dust
Soil
Parent's or older child's occupational exposure (auto repair, smelting, construction, remodeling, plumbing, gun/bullet exposure, painting, e-scrap)
Glazed ceramics
Herbal remedies (e.g., Ayurvedic medications)
Home remedies including antiperspirants, deodorants (litargirio)
Jewelry (toys or parents')
Stored battery casings (or living near a battery smelter)
Lead-based gasoline
Moonshine alcohol
Mexican candies; Ecuadorian chocolates
Indoor firing ranges
Retained bullet fragments
Imported spices (svanuri marili, zafron, kuzhambu)
Lead-based cosmetics (kohl, surma)
Lead plumbing (water)
Imported foods in lead-containing cans
Imported toys
Home renovations
Antique toys or furniture

From Kliegman RM: *Nelson's textbook of pediatrics*, ed 21, Philadelphia, 2020, Elsevier.

TABLE 1   Serum Lead Levels and Symptoms

Level (μg/dl)	SYMPTOMS Adults	SYMPTOMS Children
10	None	Decreased IQ
		Decreased hearing
		Decreased growth
20	Increased protoporphyrin	Decreased nerve conduction velocity
	No symptoms	Increased protoporphyrin
30	Increased blood pressure	Decreased vitamin D metabolism
	Decreased hearing	
40	Peripheral neuropathies	Decreased hemoglobin synthesis
	Nephropathy	
	Infertility (men)	
50	Decreased hemoglobin synthesis	Lead colic
70	Anemia	Anemia
		Encephalopathy
		Nephropathy
100	Encephalopathy	Death

IQ, Intelligence quotient.
From Marx JA et al: *Rosen's emergency medicine*, ed 8, Philadelphia, 2014, Saunders.

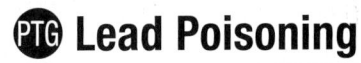
Diseases and Disorders

I

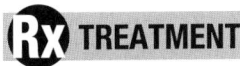 TREATMENT

NONPHARMACOLOGIC THERAPY

- Provide adequate amounts of calcium, iron, zinc, and protein in patient's diet.
- Family education on sources of lead exposure and potential adverse health effects.

ACUTE GENERAL Rx

- The use of chelation in cases of acute lead poisoning is guided by the patient's clinical status and the blood lead level. For children with blood levels of 10 to 19 mcg/dl, the CDC recommends nonpharmacologic interventions (see "Nonpharmacologic Therapy").
- For children with blood levels between 20 and 44 mcg/dl, the CDC recommendations

TABLE 3 Lead Poisoning Risk Assessment Questions to Be Asked Between 6 Months and 6 Years

Does the child live in or regularly visit a home built before 1950?

Does the child spend any time in a building built before 1978 with recent or ongoing painting, repair work, remodeling, or damage?

Is there a brother, sister, housemate, playmate, or community member being followed or treated (or even rumored to be) for lead poisoning?

Does the child live with an adult whose job or hobby involves exposure to lead (e.g., lead smelting and automotive radiator repair)?

Does the child live near an active lead smelter, battery recycling plant, or other industry likely to release lead?

Does the family use home remedies or pottery from another country?

From Marcdante KJ et al: *Nelson essentials of pediatrics*, ed 9, Philadelphia, 2023, Elsevier.

include case management by a qualified social worker, clinical management, environmental assessment, and lead hazard control. Chelation therapy should be considered in children with refractory blood lead levels.
- Chelation therapy (Table 4) is indicated in children with blood lead levels >45 mcg/dl.
- Succimer (DMSA) 10 mg/kg PO q8h for 5 days then q12h for 2 wk can be used in patients with levels between 45 and 70 mcg/dl.
- Edetate calcium disodium (EDTA) and dimercaprol (BAL) are effective in patients with severe toxicity.
- Use of both EDTA and DMSA is indicated in children with blood levels >70 mcg/dl.
- D-Penicillamine (Cuprimine) also can be used for lead poisoning, but it is not FDA approved for this condition.

CHRONIC Rx

- Reduce exposure, remove any potential lead sources.
- Correct iron deficiency and any other nutritional deficiencies.
- Recheck blood lead level 7 to 21 days after chelation therapy.

DISPOSITION

Patients with mild to moderate toxicity generally improve without any residual deficits. The presence of encephalopathy at diagnosis is a poor prognostic sign. Residual neurologic deficits may persist in these patients. Chelation therapy seems to slow the progression of renal insufficiency in patients with mildly elevated body lead burden.

REFERRAL

If exposure to lead is work related, it should be reported to the Office of the United States Occupational Safety and Health Administration (OSHA). Follow-up testing is mandatory in all patients after an abnormal screening blood lead level.

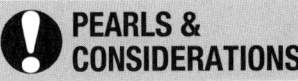 PEARLS & CONSIDERATIONS

COMMENTS

- Even blood lead concentrations as low as 5 to 10 mcg/dl are inversely associated with children's IQ scores at age 3 and 5 yr. A recent study evaluating long-term ramifications of childhood lead exposure revealed that childhood lead exposure was associated with lower cognitive function and socioeconomic status at age 38 yr, with declines in IQ, and downward social mobility.
- Screening of household members of affected individuals is recommended.
- In children with blood lead levels of >45 mg/dl, treatment with succimer does not improve scores on tests of cognition, behavior, or neuropsychological function.
- Lead toxicity may delay growth and pubertal development in girls.
- Low-level environmental lead exposure may accelerate progressive renal insufficiency in patients without diabetes who have chronic renal disease. Repeated chelation therapy may improve renal function and slow the progression of renal failure.

SUGGESTED READINGS
Available at eBooks.Health.Elsevier.com.

RELATED CONTENT
Lead Poisoning (Patient Information)

AUTHOR: **FRED F. FERRI, MD**

TABLE 4 Chelators*

Chelator	Dose	Indications	Contraindications
Deferoxamine	15 mg/kg/h up to 24 h (titrate up slowly because of hypotension)	Iron level >500 g/dl or systemic symptoms	
Dimercaprol (British anti-Lewisite [BAL])	Lead encephalopathy: 75 mg/m² deep IM injection every 4 h for 5 days in children or 4 mg/kg every 4 h for adults Arsenic (severe): No established regimen; consider 3 mg/kg IM every 4 h for 48 h; then twice daily for 7-10 days Mercury: 5 mg/kg IM first; then 2.5 mg/kg every 12-24 h	Lead level >70 g/dl or encephalopathy Arsenic: Symptomatic patient with known exposure Mercury: Inorganic	Peanut allergy Organic mercury poisoning
CaNa₂EDTA	1500 mg/m²/day continuous IV infusion 50 mg/kg/day or 1000 mg/m²/day in 2-4 divided doses for up to 5 days if less severe symptoms	Lead: Given after first dose of BAL for blood lead level above 70 g/dl or encephalopathy	
Succimer (DMSA)	10 mg/kg q8h × 5 days; then q12h for 14 days	Lead level of 45-69 g/dl Arsenic: If tolerated orally for subacute and chronic toxicity Mercury: Acute and chronic	
D-Penicillamine	25 mg/kg q6h × 5 days	Lead level of 45-69 g/dl, succimer not tolerated Arsenic: Only if BAL and DMSA are unavailable Mercury: If BAL and DMSA are unavailable or not tolerated	Penicillin allergy
DMPS (investigational)	5 mg/kg/dose IM q6-8h day 1, q8-12h day 2, q12-24h day 3 and until 24-h urine is <50 μg/L	Lead (chronic) Arsenic Mercury	

DMPS, 2,3-Dimercapto-1-propanesulfonic acid; *EDTA*, edetate calcium disodium; *IM*, intramuscular; *IV*, intravenous; *q*, every.
*Indications for chelation and dosing regimens may change. Consult with a toxicologist or poison control center for the most up-to-date recommendations.
From Marx JA et al: *Rosen's emergency medicine*, ed 8, Philadelphia, 2014, Saunders.

Liver Abscess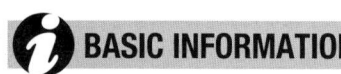

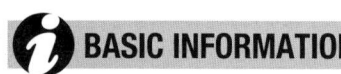

BASIC INFORMATION

DEFINITION

Liver abscess is a necrotic infection of the liver usually classified as pyogenic or amebic.

SYNONYMS

Pyogenic hepatic abscess
Amebic hepatic abscess

ICD-10CM CODE
K75.0   Abscess of liver

EPIDEMIOLOGY & DEMOGRAPHICS

INCIDENCE: Incidence of pyogenic liver abscess is 2.3 cases per 100,000 population.
PREVALENCE (WORLDWIDE): Amebic liver abscess is more common than pyogenic liver abscess.
PREVALENCE (IN U.S.): Pyogenic liver abscess is more common than amebic liver abscess.
PREDOMINANT SEX & AGE: More common in men than women; male/female ratio of 2:1; most common in fourth to sixth decades of life.

PHYSICAL FINDINGS & CLINICAL PRESENTATION

- Fever, chills, and sweats
- Weakness/malaise
- Anorexia with weight loss
- Nausea, vomiting, and diarrhea
- Cough with pleuritic chest pain
- Right upper quadrant abdominal pain
- Hepatomegaly
- Splenomegaly
- Jaundice
- Pleural effusions, rales, and friction rubs may be present
- Most abscesses occur on the right lobe of the liver

ETIOLOGY

- Pyogenic liver abscess is usually polymicrobial (*Klebsiella pneumoniae* [43%], *Escherichia coli* [33%], *Streptococcus* spp. [37%], *Pseudomonas aeruginosa*, *Proteus* spp., *Bacteroides* spp. [24%], *Fusobacterium* spp., *Actinomyces* spp., gram-positive anaerobes, and *Staphylococcus aureus*).
- Pyogenic liver abscess occurs from:
  1. Biliary disease with cholangitis (accounts for approximately 40% to 60%).
  2. Gallbladder disease with contiguous spread to the liver.
  3. Diverticulitis or appendicitis with spread via the portal circulation.
  4. Hematogenous spread via the hepatic artery, though uncommon; if a solitary organism is isolated, a distant source of hematogenous seeding should be sought.
  5. Penetrating wounds.
  6. Cryptogenic.
  7. Infection by way of portal system (portal pyemia).
  8. No causes found in approximately half of cases.
  9. Incidence increased in patients with diabetes and metastatic cancer.
  10. Table 1 summarizes underlying etiology and bacteriology of liver abscesses.
- Amebic hepatic abscess is caused by the parasite *Entamoeba histolytica*. Amebiasis is usually due to fecal-oral contamination and invades the intestinal mucosa, gaining entry into the portal system to reach the liver. Amebic abscess occurs in 3% to 7% of patients with amebiasis.
- A comparison of pyogenic and amebic liver abscess is summarized in Table 2.
  Box 1 describes pearls for amebic liver abscesses. The abscess is usually solitary (85%) and in the right lobe (72%).

DIAGNOSIS

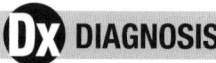

The diagnosis of liver abscess requires a high index of suspicion after a detailed history and physical examination. Imaging studies and microbiologic, serologic, and percutaneous techniques (e.g., aspiration) confirm the presence of a liver abscess.

DIFFERENTIAL DIAGNOSIS

- Cholangitis
- Cholecystitis

TABLE 1 Underlying Etiology and Bacteriology

Etiology	Bacteriology
Biliary, benign	*Escherichia coli* *Klebsiella* spp. *Enterococcus*
Biliary, malignant	*Pseudomonas* spp. Multiply resistant GN aerobes VRE Yeast
Diverticulitis/appendicitis	GN aerobes *Bacteroides fragilis*
Severe cholecystitis	See "Biliary, benign" *Clostridium perfringens* *Bacteroides* spp.
Subcutaneous abscess	*Staphylococcus* spp. MRSA
Endocarditis	*Enterococcus* spp. *Staphylococcus* spp.
Cryptogenic	Anaerobes

GN, Gram-negative; *MRSA*, methicillin-resistant *Staphylococcus aureus*; *VRE*, vancomycin-resistant *Enterococcus*.
From Cameron JL, Cameron AM: *Current surgical therapy*, ed 10, Philadelphia, 2011, Saunders.

TABLE 2 Features of Bacterial and Amebic Abscesses

	Demographics	Risk Factors	Symptoms	Laboratory Findings	Radiographic Features	Diagnosis	Treatment
Bacterial liver abscess	50-70 yr Male = female	Recent bacterial infection, biliary obstruction, diabetes mellitus	Fevers, chills, malaise, anorexia, diarrhea, cough, pleuritic chest pain, RUQ pain	Leukocytosis, anemia, elevated alkaline phosphatase and bilirubin, low albumin, positive blood cultures (50%)	Multifocal (50%), usually right lobe, irregular margins	Aspirate (70%-80% positive)	Percutaneous drainage and antibiotics
Amebic liver abscess	18-50 yr Male > female	Alcohol intake, HLA-DR3, oral and anal sex, contaminated enema apparatus, travel to or living in an endemic area	Fever, RUQ pain, hepatic tenderness, anorexia, weight loss, uncommon to have colitis	Leukocytosis, no eosinophilia, mild anemia, elevated alkaline phosphatase, elevated ESR, positive serology	Single abscess (80%), usually right lobe, wall enhancement seen on CT scan with IV contrast	Aspirate (trophozoites rarely seen) can rule out superimposed bacterial infection, positive serology and risk factors	Metronidazole and iodoquinol

CT, Computed tomography; *ESR*, erythrocyte sedimentation rate; *HLA*, human leukocyte antigen; *IV*, intravenous; *RUQ*, right upper quadrant.
From Goldman L, Schafer AI: *Goldman-Cecil medicine*, ed 26, Philadelphia, 2019, Elsevier.

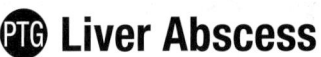

BOX 1   Pearls for Amebic Liver Abscesses

- Only 10%-20% of patients with amebic liver abscess have a history of diarrhea.
- Treat the intestinal infection to prevent relapse of amebic liver abscess. Failure to use luminal amebicidal agents after metronidazole in cases of amebic abscess results in a 10% relapse rate.
- Failure to show response to antiamebic medication requires evaluation for polymicrobial infection with bacteria.
- Amebic abscess usually responds clinically to antimicrobial therapy in 3-7 days, although imaging takes several months to show resolution.
- Percutaneous drainage is rarely required.

From Cameron JL, Cameron AM: *Current surgical therapy,* ed 10, Philadelphia, 2011, Saunders.

- Diverticulitis
- Appendicitis
- Perforated viscus
- Mesentery ischemia
- Pulmonary embolism
- Pancreatitis

WORKUP

- The workup of a liver abscess should focus on differentiating between amebic and pyogenic causes.
- Features suggesting an amebic cause include travel to an endemic area, single abscess rather than multiple abscesses, subacute onset of symptoms, and absence of conditions predisposing to pyogenic liver abscess, as highlighted under "Etiology."
- Laboratory studies are not specific but are useful as adjunctive tests.
- Imaging studies cannot differentiate between the two, and bacteriologic cultures may be sterile in 50% of the cases.

LABORATORY TESTS

- Complete blood count: Leukocytosis
- Liver function tests: Alkaline phosphatase is most commonly elevated (95% to 100%); aspartate transaminase (AST) and alanine transaminase (ALT) elevated in 50% of cases; elevated bilirubin (28% to 30%); decreased albumin
- Prothrombin time (INR): Prolonged (70%)
- Blood cultures: Positive in 50% of cases
- Aspiration (50% sterile)
- Stool samples for *E. histolytica* trophozoites (positive in 10% to 15% of amebic liver abscess cases)
- Serologic testing for *E. histolytica* should be done on all patients, but it is important to remember that it does not differentiate acute from old infections

IMAGING STUDIES

- Ultrasound (80% to 100% sensitivity in detecting abscesses) shows round or oval hypoechogenic mass (Fig. E1, A).
- CT scan is more sensitive in detecting hepatic abscesses and contiguous organ extension and is the imaging study of choice (Fig. E1, B, and Fig. E2).
- Chest x-ray: Abnormal in 50% of the cases, may reveal elevated right hemidiaphragm, subdiaphragmatic air-fluid levels, pleural effusions, and consolidating infiltrates.

- Most liver abscesses are single; however, multiple liver abscesses can occur with systemic bacteremia.

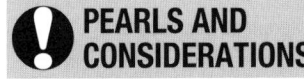 **TREATMENT**

NONPHARMACOLOGIC THERAPY

- The management of pyogenic liver abscess differs from that of amebic liver abscess.
- Medical management is the cornerstone of therapy in amebic liver abscess, whereas early intervention in the form of surgical therapy or catheter drainage and parenteral antibiotics is the rule in pyogenic liver abscess greater than 3 cm. Smaller abscesses (<3 cm) can generally be treated with broad-spectrum antibiotics.

ACUTE GENERAL Rx

- Percutaneous drainage under CT or ultrasound guidance is essential in the treatment of pyogenic liver abscesses.
- Aspiration of hepatic amebic abscesses is not required unless there is no response to treatment or a pyogenic cause is being considered.
- Empiric broad-spectrum antibiotics are recommended initially until culture results are available. Common choices include:
  1. Metronidazole (500 mg IV q8h) plus ceftriaxone or levofloxacin.
  2. Monotherapy with a beta-lactam/beta-lactamase inhibitor, such as piperacillin/tazobactam (4.5 g q6h), ticarcillin-clavulanate (3.1 g q4h), or ampicillin-sulbactam (3 g q6h).
  3. Monotherapy with a carbapenem, such as imipenem (500 mg IV q6h), meropenem (1 g q8h), or ertapenem (1 g daily).
  4. Duration of antibiotic treatment is usually 4 to 6 wk with IV antibiotics used for the first 1 to 2 wk or until a favorable clinical response, followed thereafter with oral antibiotics (e.g., metronidazole 500 mg PO q8h plus ciprofloxacin 500 mg PO q12h).
  5. Third-generation cephalosporins should not be used as single agents for empiric therapy because of risk of the emergence of beta-lactamase–producing bacteria.
- Antibiotic coverage for amebic liver abscesses includes:
  1. Metronidazole 750 mg PO tid for 10 days or tinidazole.

2. Eradication of the coexistent intestinal infection with paromomycin for 10 days.

CHRONIC Rx

- If fever persists for 2 wk despite percutaneous drainage and antibiotic therapy as outlined under "Acute General Rx," or if there is failure of aspiration or failure of percutaneous drainage, surgery is indicated.
- In patients not responding to intravenous antibiotics and percutaneous drainage, hepatic artery antibiotic infusion can be considered.
- In patients with evidence of metastatic disease that is causing biliary obstruction, a gastroenterology consultation for endoscopic retrograde cholangiopancreatography and stenting should be considered.

DISPOSITION

- Most patients with pyogenic liver abscesses defervesce within 2 wk of treatment with antibiotics and drainage.
- No randomized controlled studies have evaluated the optimal duration of antibiotic therapy for pyogenic liver abscess. Typical duration of antibiotic therapy is at least 4 to 6 wk.
- Pyogenic liver abscess cure rates using percutaneous drainage and antibiotics have been reported to be between 88% and 100%.
- Mortality rate of untreated pyogenic liver abscess is nearly 100%.
- Most patients with amebic liver abscesses defervesce within 4 to 5 days of treatment.
- Amebic liver abscess mortality rate is <1% unless complications occur (see "Comments").
- Follow-up imaging should be used to monitor response to therapy; continue treatment until CT scan shows complete or near-complete resolution of cavity.

REFERRAL

Infectious disease, gastroenterology, interventional radiology, and general surgical consultations are recommended in any patient with hepatic abscess.

⚠ PEARLS AND CONSIDERATIONS

COMMENTS

- Complications of pyogenic and amebic liver abscesses include:
  1. Pleuropulmonary extension, resulting in empyema, abscess, and fistula formation
  2. Peritonitis
  3. Purulent pericarditis
  4. Sepsis
- Amebic liver abscesses complicate amebic colitis in nearly 10% of cases.

RELATED CONTENT

Liver Abscess (Patient Information)
Amebiasis (Related Key Topic)

AUTHOR: **FRED F. FERRI, MD**

BASIC INFORMATION

DEFINITION
While there is no agreed upon definition, Long COVID refers to a heterogenous group of symptoms persisting for 12 or more wk after the initial infection with SARS-COV-2 that cannot be explained by an alternative diagnosis.

SYNONYMS
Post-Acute Sequelae of COVID-19 (PASC)
Post COVID-19 Condition
Long-Haul COVID

ICD 10-CM CODE
U09.9   Post COVID-19 condition, unspecified

EPIDEMIOLOGY & DEMOGRAPHICS
INCIDENCE: As many as 50% of survivors of acute SARS-COV-2 infection experience persistent, variable symptoms more than 30 days post-acute infection; as many as 1 in 3 self-report symptoms 3 mo post-acute infection
PREVALENCE: Unknown, though ranging in the millions in the U.S. and UK
PREDOMINANT SEX & AGE: Female, ages 35 to 69
RISK FACTORS: Prior hospitalization for COVID-19 infection, working in health care, high BMI, presence of one or more activity-limiting health conditions

PHYSICAL FINDINGS & CLINICAL PRESENTATION
Manifestations of Long COVID may be multisystemic, though one system may predominate, mild to severe in their presentation, and may persist 12 wk or more and up to 2 yr. Symptoms and exam findings may include but are not limited to:
- Pulmonary findings such as cough, wheeze, tachypnea, altered or increased work of breathing, breathing pattern disorder, and shortness of breath, which may continue following the acute viral infection
- Cardiovascular symptoms such as chest pain, chest pressure, and palpitations
- Neurologic symptoms such as headache, memory and concentration difficulties, cognitive impairment, "brain fog", anosmia, ageusia or dysgeusia, and neuropathy; mental health changes like depression and anxiety, poor sleep
- Autonomic dysregulation resulting in orthostatic hypotension, dizziness, frequent nausea and gastrointestinal disturbance, and hyperalgesia
- Allergic symptoms such as conjunctivitis, rash, pruritus
- Functional impairment in tasks of daily living, generalized fatigue, exercise intolerance (as determined by chronotropic incompetence, for example), or post-exertional symptom exacerbation (PESE) or malaise (PEM)

ETIOLOGY
Given the heterogenous presentation of Long COVID, the pathophysiology, while unknown, is likely multifactorial and may differ among patients with different comorbidities or risk factors. Possible mechanisms include cellular injury, immune dysfunction due to autoimmunity or chronic inflammation, viral persistence, and unmasking or exacerbation of other comorbidities, such as primary pulmonary disease or heart failure.

DIAGNOSIS

DIFFERENTIAL DIAGNOSIS
Diagnosis relies upon a multisystemic appraisal. Long COVID should be considered in those with new or newly worsened features of pulmonary, cardiovascular, neurologic, autonomic, rheumatologic, or psychiatric disease following the acute period of SARS-COV-2 infection. However, Long COVID is a diagnosis of exclusion, and alternative etiologies of presenting symptoms should be ruled out prior to diagnosis. Additionally, providers should be careful of anchoring bias given the prevalence of prior COVID-19 infections.

WORKUP
- Workup should be tailored to individual and predominant symptoms, accounting for the identification of alternative, treatable etiologies, such as asthma, for example
- Obtaining a full history and physical exam, including full neurologic, cognitive, and psychiatric assessment is essential to characterizing disease onset, frequency, intensity and impact on daily functions
- Other initial assessments may include obtaining an EKG, rest and ambulatory pulse oximetry, PFTs, ambulatory cardiac monitoring, and tilt table testing

LABORATORY TESTS
Consider CBC, CMP, TFT, B12, ANA, ESR, CRP, and D-dimer when clinically appropriate if concerned for VTE

IMAGING STUDIES
Consider chest x-ray, high-resolution chest CT, transthoracic echocardiogram

TREATMENT

NONPHARMACOLOGIC THERAPY
- Those experiencing new pulmonary, cardiac, autonomic, and functional impairments may benefit from cardiac, pulmonary, and general physical rehabilitation.
- Other symptom specific forms of rehabilitation, such as olfactory training, may be available to those with anosmia and other sensory deficits.
- Autonomic symptoms, like orthostatic hypotension, may improve with compression stockings, as well as lifestyle management to avoid and manage triggers.
- Behavioral health measures, such as counseling for mood disorders and sleep, should also play a role in the treatment of Long COVID when indicated.

ACUTE GENERAL Rx
- There are no known treatments for Long COVID.
- Acute treatment is symptom dependent; no one specific pharmacologic therapy is indicated for those suspected to have Long COVID.
- Vaccination against SARS-COV-2 may have a modest to no effect on symptom intensity. Vaccination has not been shown to worsen symptoms in those with Long COVID.

CHRONIC Rx
Similar to acute treatment, there are no disease-specific therapy recommendations for the management of Long COVID.

DISPOSITION
There are no reliable predictors of duration of symptoms, though most patients may expect to improve or recover within 3 to 12 mo. Symptoms may plateau for long periods, fluctuate, or be retriggered by emotional or physical stress, but time could potentially be shortened via engagement with pulmonary, cardiac, and physical rehabilitation.

REFERRAL
Specialty referral should be tailored to specific concerns regarding symptom management. Primary care providers should serve as coordinators of a multidisciplinary approach to management, although some health care networks have also developed dedicated Long COVID clinics that may also serve as entry points for coordination of care. Physical Medicine and Rehabilitation (PM&R) providers have served at the forefront of providing support and care of those patients with functional impairments due to Long COVID.

PEARLS & CONSIDERATIONS

- The best guide to improvement is subjective patient feelings of symptomatic remission.
- No one individual's therapeutic needs and expectations of recovery are the same.
- Benefits of full SARS-COV-2 vaccination should be discussed with all patients without contraindications.

PREVENTION
Vaccination against SARS-COV-2 should be recommended for those without contraindications to prevent COVID-19 and its sequelae, such as long COVID.

PATIENT & FAMILY EDUCATION
https://www.cdc.gov/coronavirus/2019-ncov/long-term-effects/index.html

SUGGESTED READINGS
Available at eBooks.Health.Elsevier.com

AUTHORS: **YOSEPH A. ALDRAS, MD,** and **JENNIE E. JOHNSON, MD**

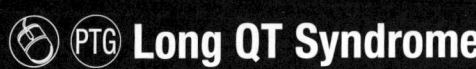

L

Diseases and Disorders

I

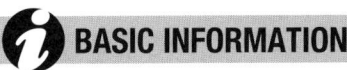 **BASIC INFORMATION**

DEFINITION

Long QT syndrome (LQTS) is a disorder of myocardial repolarization characterized by a prolongation of the QT interval on the ECG associated with an increased risk of developing life-threatening ventricular arrhythmias, most commonly torsades de pointes (a specific type of polymorphic ventricular tachycardia), which may lead to ventricular fibrillation and sudden cardiac death (SCD). This syndrome may be either genetic or acquired.

SYNONYMS

LQTS
Congenital forms:
Jervell and Lange-Nielsen syndrome (associated with deafness)
Romano-Ward syndrome (associated with normal hearing)

ICD-10CM CODE
I45.81 Long QT syndrome

EPIDEMIOLOGY & DEMOGRAPHICS

- Congenital LQTS is thought to account for >3000 deaths in childhood per year in the United States.
- The prevalence of congenital LQTS is at least 1 in 2000 live births (based on genotype/phenotype positive infants). The incidence of genotype positive/phenotype negative is higher, close to 1 in 1000 births.
- Incidence of LQTS is thought to be between 1:2500 and 1:10,000 in the general population, although it has been difficult to estimate because of incomplete penetrance. Congenital form associated with deafness is autosomal recessive (Jervell and Lange-Nielsen syndrome) and is less common than the autosomal dominant form as well as more severe.[1]
- Congenital form associated with normal hearing (Romano-Ward syndrome) is autosomal dominant. Although inheritance of LQTS is autosomal dominant, female predominance has often been observed and has been attributed to an increased susceptibility to cardiac arrhythmias in women. LQTS is more likely to express itself before puberty in males and after puberty in females.
- Multiple LQTS genes have been identified to date. However, as clinical genetic testing evolves, some previously associated LQTS-susceptibility genes have been reconsidered as unlikely to be causative for congenital LQTS. Three LQTS genes account for more than 80% of congenital LQTS.
- Mortality rate is estimated to be about 1% per year.
- Multiple mutations causing congenital LQTS have been described. The most common types of LQTS are described in Table 1.

PHYSICAL FINDINGS & CLINICAL PRESENTATION

- Palpitations, presyncope.
- Syncope suggestive of cardiac/arrhythmic origin (not vasovagal syncope).
- Resuscitated sudden cardiac arrest.
- Seizure (often, patients with LQTS are misdiagnosed with epilepsy).
- Family history of LQTS, but a family history of SCD has not been proved to be a risk factor for SCD in patients with LQTS.
- Abnormal ECG (prolonged QT) in asymptomatic relatives of known case.
- Prolonged QTc interval on average among patients with genetically confirmed LQTS is approximately 470 ms. In general the 99th percentile QTc values are 460 ms (prepuberty), 470 ms in postpubertal males, and 480 ms in postpubertal females.
- In case of congenital LQTS the presentation of syncope or SCD is typically triggered by exercise and swimming in LQT1 patients (45% cases, mutation in KCNQ1 gene); in LQT2 (25% to 40% cases, mutation in KCNH2 gene) patients by emotion, pregnancy, or noise; and patients with LQT3 (5% to 10% cases, mutation in SCN5A) are at highest risk of events when at rest or asleep.[2]

ETIOLOGY

- Cardiac repolarization abnormality
- Congenital cause (hundreds of mutations on more than 10 genes have been identified)
- Most of the gene mutations affect function of ion channels leading to prolonged repolarization (i.e., sodium and potassium channels resulting in either increased Na^+ influx or decreased K^+ efflux). These mutations prolong depolarization and predispose the patient to torsades de pointes.
- Acquired causes:
  1. Drugs (Table E2): Dofetilide, ibutilide, bepridil, quinidine, procainamide, sotalol, amiodarone, ranolazine, disopyramide, phenothiazines and antiemetic agents (droperidol, domperidone), tricyclic antidepressants, antipsychotics (quetiapine, ziprasidone, iloperidone), citalopram, antihistamines, quinolones, azithromycin, astemizole or cisapride given with ketoconazole or erythromycin, clarithromycin, and antimalarials, particularly among patients with asthma or those using potassium-lowering medications; also common in patients receiving methadone.
  2. Electrolyte abnormalities, commonly hypokalemia, hypomagnesemia, hypocalcemia (especially in patients with malabsorption syndrome)
  3. Liquid protein diet
  4. Central nervous system lesions
  5. Structural heart disease (heart failure, diastolic dysfunction, myocardial ischemia, and left ventricular hypertrophy)
  6. Hypothyroidism
  7. Bradyarrhythmias

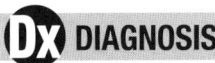 **DIAGNOSIS**

DIFFERENTIAL DIAGNOSIS

- See "Syncope."

TABLE 1 Common Types of Long QT (LQT) Syndrome

	LQT1	LQT2	LQT3
Pathophysiology			
Gene	KCNQ1 (KvLQT1)	KCNH2 (formerly "HERG")	SCN5A
Protein	$K_v7.1$	$K_v11.1$	$Na_v1.5$
Ionic current	Decreased I_{Ks}	Decreased I_{Kr}	Increased late I_{Na}
Clinical presentation			
Incidence of cardiac events	63%	46%	18%
Incidence of SCD	4%	4%	4%
Arrhythmia triggers	Emotional/physical stress (swimming, diving)	Emotional stress, arousal (alarm clock, telephone), rest, postpartum period	Sleep/rest
ECG	Broad-based T wave	Low-amplitude, bifid T wave	Long isoelectric ST segment
QT response to exercise	Attenuated QTc shortening and an exaggerated QTc prolongation during early and peak exercise	Normal QT during exercise but with exaggerated QT hysteresis	Supernormal QT shortening
Management			
Exercise restriction	+++	++	?
Response to beta-blockers	+++	+++	?
Potassium supplement	+	++	+
Left cervicothoracic sympathectomy	++	++	++
Response to mexiletine	+	+	++

From Issa Z et al: *Clinical arrhythmology and electrophysiology*, ed 2, Philadelphia, 2012, Saunders.

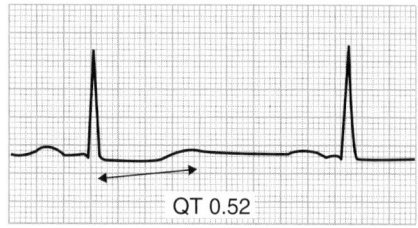

A

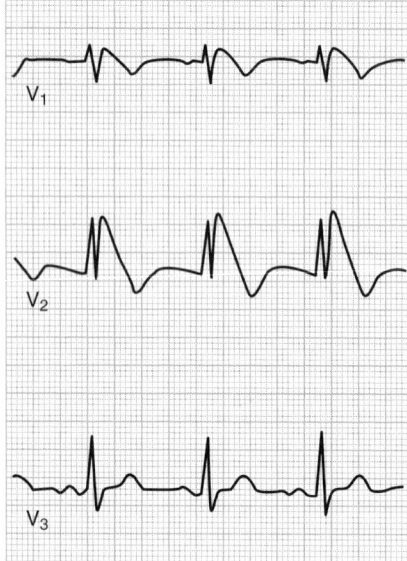

B

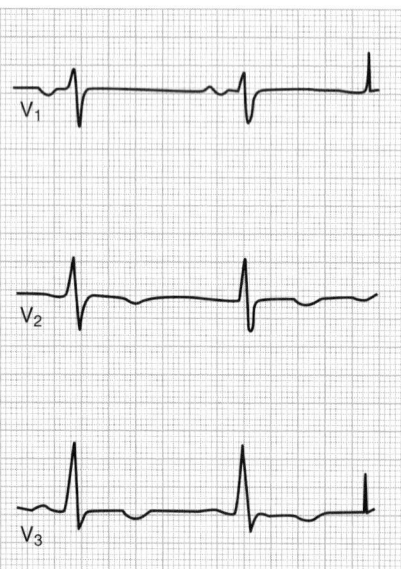

C

FIG. 1 Sinus rhythm electrocardiogram findings in three genetic sudden death syndromes.
A, QT prolongation during sinus rhythm in a patient with long QT syndrome. **B,** ST elevation in V_1 and V_2 in a patient with Brugada syndrome. **C,** T wave inversion in V_1-V_3 in a patient with arrhythmogenic ventricular dysplasia. (From Goldman L, Schafer AI: *Goldman's Cecil medicine,* ed 24, Philadelphia, 2012, Saunders.)

- Brugada syndrome, arrhythmogenic right ventricular dysplasia, and LQTS are major causes of genetic sudden death syndromes (Fig. 1).
- Catecholaminergic Polymorphic Ventricular Tachycardia (CPVT).

Diagnostic criteria for the congenital LQTS as per 2013 HRS Guidelines[3]:

LQTS is diagnosed:

- In the presence of a LQTS risk score $\geq$3.5 (Table E3) in the absence of a secondary cause for QT prolongation and/or
- In the presence of an unequivocally pathogenic mutation in one of the LQTS genes or
- In the presence of a QT interval corrected for heart rate using Bazett formula (QTc) $\geq$500 ms in repeated 12-lead electrocardiogram (ECG) and in the absence of a secondary cause for QT prolongation
- LQTS can be diagnosed in the presence of a QTc between 480 and 499 ms in repeated 12-lead ECGs in a patient with unexplained syncope in the absence of a secondary cause for QT prolongation and in the absence of a pathogenic mutation

WORKUP

Cardiology referral is recommended for all cases. Genetic analysis is an essential step for risk stratification of patients with congenital prolonged QT and is important for identification of potential mutation carriers within the proband family. There is evidence for gene-specific triggers of events and therapeutic efficacy. Molecular screening should become part of the routine clinical management of LQTS.

In relatives of known patients with LQTS or in young patients with syncope:

- Stress test may prolong the QT interval or cause T-wave alternans.
- Valsalva maneuver: May prolong the QT interval or cause T-wave alternans.
- Prolonged ECG monitoring with various stimulations aimed at increasing catecholamines and assess for QT prolongation (perform in a setting that can provide resuscitation with α- and β-antagonists readily available).
- Epinephrine-induced prolongation of the QT interval (epinephrine infusion QT stress test).
- Genetic analysis:
  1. *LQT1* locus of *KCNQ1* potassium channel gene.
  2. *LQT2* locus of *KCNH2 (formerly "HERG")* potassium channel gene.
  3. *LQT3* locus of *SCN5A* sodium channel gene.
  4. These three variants account for >80% of all genotyped LQTS patients, whereas the remaining genes are responsible for a minority of cases.
- Risk stratification for each genetic variant on the basis of gender and QTc: Groups are defined on the basis of the probability of the first cardiac event (syncope, cardiac arrest, or sudden death) before age 40 yr or before therapy.[2] Specific mutations, depending on type, location, and degree, may confer a high risk even if the ECG abnormalities are mild. Clinically, QT interval duration was the strongest predictor of risk for cardiac events; a QTc

exceeding 500 ms identifies patients with the highest risk.

1. High risk (>50% of cardiac event): QTc $\geq$500 ms and LQT1 or LQT2, or male with LQT3.
2. Moderate risk (30% to 50%): QTc <500 ms in male with LQT3 or in female with LQT2 or LQT3, and female with LQT3 with QTc $\geq$500 ms.
3. Low risk (<30%): QTc <500 ms and LQT1 or male LQT2 with QTc <500 ms.
4. Prophylactic treatment should be considered in all patients with moderate or high risk for cardiac events based on the above risk stratification scheme (Table E4).

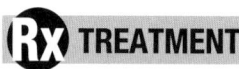 ## TREATMENT

NONPHARMACOLOGIC THERAPY

- Physical activity and LQTS.
  1. LQT1 patients experience 90% of lethal events under physical and emotional stress. Swimming and diving should be avoided or performed under supervision. In patients with LQT2 and LQT3, children and adolescents can resume participation in physical education classes, and adults should be encouraged to stay physically active.[4]
  2. In atheletes diagnosed with LQTS who wish to participate in competitive sports, shared decision making with a LQTS specialist should be performed.
  3. Regarding competitive athletics for individuals with congenital LQTS, there is a difference of opinion between the 2015 AHA/ACC Scientific Statement on Eligibility and the Disqualification Recommendations for Competitive Athletes, which allows participation in competitive events and training sessions dependent on availability of automated external defibrillator (AED).[4] In contrast, previous European guidelines advise precautionary restriction from competitive sports in these situations.
- Implantation of an implantable cardioverter-defibrillator (ICD) in the vast majority of LQTS patients is not necessary, and most patients with LQTS (90% or more in LQTS expert centers) do not need and should not receive an ICD. (5) Consider ICD placement in following situations (Table 5)[5]:
  1. Survivors of sudden cardiac arrest without a reversible cause
  2. In patients with LQTS-associated sudden cardiac arrest while compliant with beta-blocker therapy
  3. In patients with recurrent cardiac syncope in spite of β-blockers and left cardiac sympathetic denervation
- ICD is never indicated based solely on the family history, as it is not a personal risk factor for the patient with LQTS.

PHARMACOLOGIC THERAPY

- All patients with LQTS and a history of syncope, seizures, or resuscitated SCA should be treated with a β-blocker.

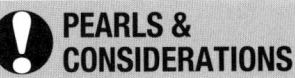

TABLE 5 Management of Patients With Long QT Syndrome

Type of Syndrome	Management	Indication
Congenital	β-blockers	Asymptomatic patients, symptomatic patients (who do not have bronchospasm)
	Cervicothoracic sympathectomy	Refractory symptoms, especially in pediatric patients
	Cardiac pacing	Refractory symptoms associated with bradycardia, pauses
	Implantable cardioverter-defibrillator	Cardiac arrest, refractory syncope, prophylaxis for moderate- to high-risk patients for cardiac events
Acquired	Elimination of causative drug or condition	All patients
	Magnesium sulfate	Nonsustained ventricular tachycardia, torsades de pointes (even with a normal serum magnesium concentration)
	Administration of potassium (to keep serum K$^+$ >4.5 mEq/L)	Serum K$^+$ <4.5 mEq/L
	Maneuvers to increase heart rate (cardiac pacing, isoproterenol)	Bradycardia, arrhythmias refractory to magnesium sulfate

K$^+$, Potassium.
Adapted from Crawford MH et al (eds): *Cardiology,* ed 2, St Louis, 2004, Mosby.

- β-blockers, chiefly propranolol and nadolol, are an initial therapy of choice—there are differential responses to β-blocker therapy among different genetic variants; especially effective among LQT1 or LQT2 patients. Studies showed the efficacy of β-blockers with an overall mortality <2% over a mean follow-up exceeding 5 yr.
- In patients with LQT3, mexiletine shortens the QTc and, increasingly, combination therapy with propranolol and mexiletine is utilized in these patients.
- In the 20% to 30% of patients who continue to have symptoms on a β-blocker, the main options are either left cardiac sympathetic denervation (LCSD) or the prophylactic implantation of an ICD.
- In patients with frequent ICD shocks or in those with high risk for SCD where ICD placement cannot be performed, cardiac pacing and/or LCSD may be indicated.
- In patients with recurrent syncope and/or aborted cardiac arrest despite combined ICD and β-blocker, LCSD as adjunctive therapy can be performed.[6]
- For patients with LQTS who continue to receive appropriate ICD shocks or who have a high-risk phenotype but prefer to avoid an ICD, potassium retention strategies are implemented, regardless of the underlying LQTS genotype.[2]
- Correctable factors including electrolyte disorders—hypokalemia and hypomagnesemia—and avoidance of precipitating drugs that may further prolong the QT interval is mandatory. A complete list of drugs that can potentially prolong QT may be found at www.crediblemeds.org/.[7]

- For patients with acquired form and torsades de pointes, IV magnesium and atrial or ventricular pacing are initial choices.
- Table 4 summarizes management of patients with LQTS.

PROGNOSIS

- In carefully treated patients, mortality is around 0.5% to 1% over 20 yr.
- The timing and frequency of syncope, QTc prolongation, and gender are predictive of risk for aborted cardiac arrest and SCD during adolescence. Higher risk is present in those with one or two or more episodes of syncope in the last 10 yr compared with those with no syncopal episodes, those with QTc >530 ms, and males ages 10 to 12 yr.

PEARLS & CONSIDERATIONS

COMMENTS

- Family history should be assessed for a history of sudden death and other deaths that may have occurred as manifestations of LQTS (e.g., sudden infant death, drowning, and loss of consciousness while driving).
- ICDs are an important component of therapy, but most LQTS patients do not need and should not receive an ICD based only on LQTS diagnosis.
- Propranolol and nadolol are considered superior to metoprolol for prevention of arrhythmias in LQTS.

RELATED CONTENT

Long QT Syndrome (Patient Information)
Torsades de Pointes (Related Key Topic)

REFERENCES

Available at eBooks.Health.Elsevier.com.

AUTHOR: **ARTEM ASTSATUROV, MD**

Diseases and Disorders

L

I

Lung Abscess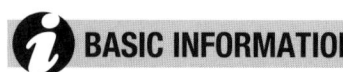

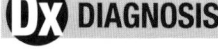 BASIC INFORMATION

DEFINITION

A lung abscess is an infection of the lung parenchyma resulting in necrosis and cavity formation.

SYNONYM

Pulmonary abscess
Abscess, lung

ICD-10CM CODES
A06.5   Amebic lung abscess
J85.1   Abscess of lung with pneumonia
J85.2   Abscess of lung without pneumonia

EPIDEMIOLOGY & DEMOGRAPHICS

INCIDENCE:
- The exact incidence is unknown; however, it has significantly decreased with the advent of antibiotics.
- Lung abscess is more common in the elderly because of an increased risk of periodontal disease and dysphagia.

RISK FACTORS (TABLE 1):
- Alcohol use disorder
- Seizure disorders
- Cerebrovascular disorders with dysphagia
- Head trauma
- Substance use disorders
- General anesthesia
- Esophageal disorders (e.g., scleroderma, esophageal carcinoma)
- Poor oral hygiene
- Poor cough reflex
- Obstructive lung neoplasm
- Bronchiectasis
- Obstructive foreign body

PHYSICAL FINDINGS & CLINICAL PRESENTATION

Symptoms are generally insidious, occurring over weeks to months
- Fever
- Cough
- Sputum production (purulent with foul odor)
- Pleuritic chest pain
- Hemoptysis
- Dyspnea
- Malaise, fatigue, and weakness
Physical exam findings
- Tachycardia and tachypnea

- Poor dentition
- Dullness to percussion, whispered pectoriloquy, and bronchophony
- Amphoric breath sounds (low-pitched sound of air moving across a large open cavity)

ETIOLOGY

- Aspiration is the most common cause of lung abscess, with periodontal disease being a major predisposing factor.[1]
- Septic emboli, superinfection of a pulmonary infarct, or extension from an adjacent mediastinal or subphrenic abscess could result in lung abscess formation.
- Lung abscesses are most often caused by anaerobic microorganisms *(Peptostreptococci, Bacteroides* species, *Fusobacterium, Prevotella)* and microaerophilic streptococci such as *Streptococcus milleri, Streptococcus anginosus, and Streptococcus mitis.*[2]
- They frequently are polymicrobial with an anaerobic infection mixed with aerobic or facultative anaerobic organisms *(S. aureus, E. coli, K. pneumoniae, P. aeruginosa).*
- Nonbacterial pathogens include parasitic organisms *(Paragonimus westermani, Entamoeba histolytica)* and fungi *(Aspergillus, Cryptococcus, Histoplasma, Blastomyces,* and *Coccidioides* spp.)
- Lung abscesses in immunocompromised hosts are commonly due to Gram-negative bacilli but can include many organisms including *Nocardia, Legionella micdade, Rhodococcus equi, mycobacteria,* and *fungi.*
- Lung necrosis caused by community strains (USA 300 strain) of methicillin-resistant *Staphylococcus aureus* (MRSA) in adolescents and young adults following an acute influenza infection can be quite fulminant.
- Multiresistant *Klebsiella pneumoniae* has been isolated from lung abscesses in Taiwan.[3]

DIAGNOSIS

Lung abscess may be classified as primary or secondary.[1]
- *Primary lung abscess* refers to abscess formation in immunocompetent hosts; usually a result of aspiration.
- *Secondary lung abscess* refers to abscess formation in individuals with immunodeficiency

or those with a preexisting pulmonary condition (e.g., lung cancer, bronchiectasis).
Lung abscess may be defined as acute or chronic.
- Acute lung abscess denotes symptoms being present for less than 6 wk.
- Chronic lung abscess denotes symptoms being present for longer than 6 wk.

DIFFERENTIAL DIAGNOSIS

The differential diagnosis for cavitary lung lesions can be separated into infectious and noninfectious causes.
INFECTIOUS:
- Bacterial (anaerobic, aerobic, facultative anaerobes, mycobacteria)
- Fungal (histoplasmosis, coccidioidomycosis, blastomycosis, aspergillosis, cryptococcosis, zygomycetes)
- Parasitic (amebiasis, echinococcosis)
NONINFECTIOUS:
- Malignancy (primary lung carcinoma, metastatic lung disease, lymphoma)
- Vasculitis (granulomatosis with polyangiitis)
- Septic emboli
- Bronchiectasis
- Obstructive mass or foreign body

WORKUP

- The workup of a patient with lung abscess attempts to elicit a primary or secondary cause.
- Routine blood tests are not specific in diagnosing lung abscesses.
- Most diagnoses are made from imaging studies.
- Bacteriologic, fungal, and parasitic studies are necessary to diagnose a specific pathogen.

LABORATORY TESTS

- CBC with leukocytosis
- Bacteriologic studies:
  1. Sputum Gram stain and culture (commonly contaminated by oral flora).
  2. Fiberoptic bronchoscopy with bronchial brushings and/or bronchial washings is commonly performed in those who have failed standard therapy and in immunocompromised individuals to rule out opportunistic infections. Of note, caution should be taken when performing bronchoalveolar lavage or biopsies of the cavity as this could cause spillage of abscess material.[2]
  3. Percutaneous transthoracic aspiration may also be used to identify an organism, especially when located adjacent to the pleura.
  4. Blood cultures in those with sepsis or septic shock.
  5. If a pleural effusion is present, performing a thoracentesis may provide an uncontaminated specimen to isolate the causative organism of the neighboring abscess.

IMAGING STUDIES

- The diagnosis of lung abscess can be made by chest x-ray demonstrating a cavitary lesion with an air-fluid level.

TABLE 1   Risk Factors for Aspiration Pneumonia and Lung Abscess

Increased bacterial inoculum	Periodontal disease, gingivitis, tonsillar or dental abscess, drugs that decrease gastric acidity
Impairment of consciousness	Drugs, alcohol, general anesthesia, metabolic encephalopathy, coma, shock, cerebrovascular accident, cardiopulmonary arrest, seizures, surgery, trauma
Impairment of cough and gag reflexes	Vocal cord paralysis, intratracheal anesthesia, endotracheal tube, tracheostomy, myopathy, myelopathy, other neurologic disorders
Impairment of esophageal function	Diverticula, achalasia, strictures, disorders of gastrointestinal motility, neoplasm, tracheoesophageal fistula, pseudobulbar palsy
Emesis	Nasogastric tube, gastric dilation, ileus, intestinal obstruction

From Cohen J, Powderly WG: *Infectious diseases,* ed 2, St Louis, 2004, Mosby.

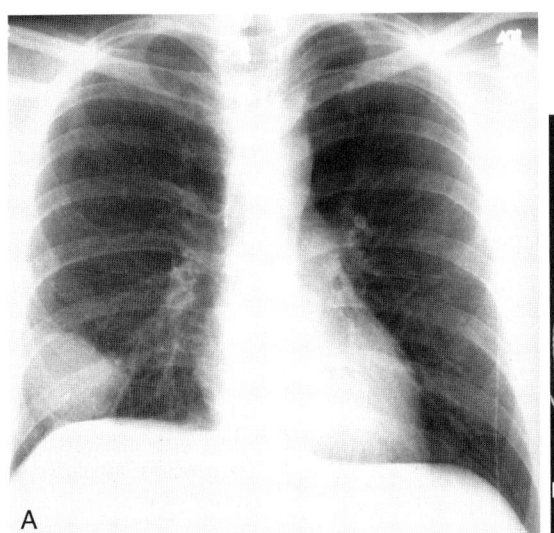
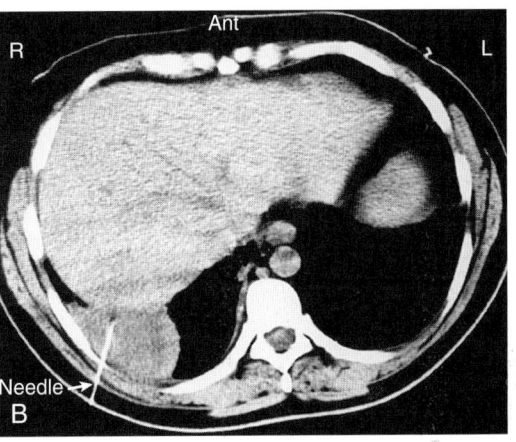
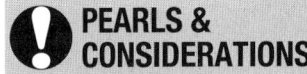

FIG. 1 Lung abscess. On a chest radiograph, a lung abscess may look to be a solid, rounded lesion **(A),** or, if it has a connection with the bronchus, there may be an air-fluid level in a thick-walled cavitary lesion. CT scanning **(B)** can be used to localize the lesion and to place a needle for drainage and aspiration of contents for culture. (From Mettler FA [ed]: *Primary care radiology,* Philadelphia, 2000, Saunders.)

- Lung abscesses are most commonly found in the posterior segment of the right upper lobe or the superior segment of the lower lobes (the dependent regions of the lung when supine).
- Chest CT scan can help to localize and size the lesion. In addition, it can assist in differentiating lung abscesses from other pathologic processes (e.g., tumor, empyema, infected bulla) (Fig. 1).
- Transthoracic echocardiogram may be indicated to rule out vegetations/endocarditis if imaging is suggestive of septic emboli.

Rx TREATMENT

NONPHARMACOLOGIC THERAPY

- Oxygen therapy.
- The efficacy of airway clearance maneuvers including postural drainage and chest percussion is less established and holds a risk of abscess rupture.

ACUTE GENERAL Rx

Antibiotics are the mainstay of treatment and are largely empiric due to the difficulty in isolating anaerobes on culture. Regimens should include combination of a beta-lactam/beta-lactamase inhibitor or a carbapenem.[2]

- Piperacillin/tazobactam 3.375 g IV q6h in aspiration pneumonia with lung abscess.
- Ceftriaxone 1 to 2 g IV q24h plus metronidazole 500 mg IV q8h.
- Clindamycin can be used and is more effective for anaerobic lung abscess than penicillin alone. Dose: 900 mg IV q8h until improved, then 300 to 600 mg PO q6h. (However, other regimens are often preferred to decrease risk of *C. difficile*.)
- Penicillin 1 to 2 million units IV q4h until improvement (afebrile, decreased phlegm production), followed by penicillin VK 500 mg PO q6h for 2 to 3 wk but often up to 6 to 8 wk

and can be given with metronidazole doses of 7.5 mg/kg IV q6h, followed by PO 500 mg bid to 4×per day dosing as an alternative to clindamycin.

- Penicillin should not be used alone because many mouth flora anaerobes now produce penicillinase enzymes.
- Metronidazole should not be used alone because it is not active against microaerophilic streptococci and some anaerobic cocci.
- Other alternatives are ampicillin/sulbactam and carbapenems such as imipenem and meropenem.

Duration of antibiotic therapy ranges from weeks to months. This largely depends on clinical and radiographic improvement.

CHRONIC Rx

- Bronchoscopy to assist with drainage and/or diagnosis is indicated in patients who fail to respond to antibiotics. Evaluating the airways is important if there is concern for an underlying malignancy or foreign body obstruction.
- Surgery is indicated in rare cases (~10%) in patients with complications of lung abscess (see "Comments").[1]

DISPOSITION

- Majority of patients fully recover with the use of antibiotics alone.
- Complications of lung abscesses include:
  1. Empyema
  2. Massive hemoptysis
  3. Pneumothorax
  4. Bronchopleural fistula
  5. Hepatobronchial fistula
  6. Brain abscess
  7. Bronchiectasis
- Mortality from lung abscess is approximately 15% to 20%.[4]
- Despite appropriate therapy, mortality may be as high as 75% in immunocompromised

patients, those with bronchial obstruction, or those with large abscesses (>6 cm).

REFERRAL

- Pulmonary and infectious disease consultation is recommended if a lung abscess is present.
- An interventional radiologist may be able to perform drainage and obtain cultures if indicated.

! PEARLS & CONSIDERATIONS

COMMENTS

- It is essential to choose antibiotics with good anaerobic coverage.
- Cases refractory to antibiotics are usually the result of:
  1. Large cavity size (>6 cm)
  2. Recurrent aspiration
  3. Thick-walled cavities
  4. Obstructive lesion (e.g., lung mass or foreign body)
  5. Empyema formation
  6. Resistant organisms or other organisms such as mycobacterium, fungi, or parasites that are not covered by current therapy
- Percutaneous transthoracic tube drainage, endoscopic drainage or surgery may be indicated if the patient is not improving with antibiotic therapy.[5,6]

REFERENCES

Available at eBooks.Health.Elsevier.com.

RELATED CONTENT

Lung Abscess (Patient Information)
Aspiration Pneumonia (Related Key Topic)

AUTHOR: **NISHA H. GIDWANI, MD**

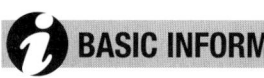 **BASIC INFORMATION**

DEFINITION

Primary lung neoplasms are malignancies arising from lung tissue. The two different major subtypes are non–small cell lung cancer (NSCLC, 85% of all lung cancers; squamous cell carcinoma, adenocarcinoma, and large cell carcinoma) and small cell lung cancer (SCLC, 15% of all lung cancers).

ADENOCARCINOMA: Represents 35% to 40% of lung carcinomas; frequently located in mid-lung and periphery; initial metastases are to lymphatics; frequently associated with peripheral scars; adenocarcinoma is described as preinvasive, minimally invasive, or invasive.

SQUAMOUS CELL: Represents 20% to 30% of lung cancers; central location; metastasis by local invasion; frequent cavitation and obstructive phenomena.

SMALL CELL: Represents 15% of lung carcinomas; central location; metastasis through lymphatics; associated with lesion of the short arm of chromosome 3; high cavitation rate.

LARGE CELL: Represents 10% to 15% of lung carcinomas; frequently located in the periphery; metastasis to central nervous system and mediastinum; rapid growth rate with early metastasis.

LEPIDIC-PREDOMINANT PATTERN (BRONCHOALVEOLAR): Represents 5% of lung carcinomas; frequently located in the periphery; may be bilateral; initial metastasis through lymphatic, hematogenous, and local invasion; no correlation with cigarette smoking; cavitation rare.

SYNONYM

Lung cancer

ICD-10CM CODES

C34.10	Malignant neoplasm of upper lobe, unspecified bronchus or lung
C34.11	Malignant neoplasm of upper lobe, right bronchus or lung
C34.12	Malignant neoplasm of upper lobe, left bronchus or lung
C34.2	Malignant neoplasm of middle lobe, bronchus or lung
C34.30	Malignant neoplasm of lower lobe, unspecified bronchus or lung
C34.31	Malignant neoplasm of lower lobe, right bronchus or lung
C34.32	Malignant neoplasm of lower lobe, left bronchus or lung
C34.80	Malignant neoplasm of overlapping sites of unspecified bronchus and lung
C34.81	Malignant neoplasm of overlapping sites of right bronchus and lung
C34.82	Malignant neoplasm of overlapping sites of left bronchus and lung
C34.90	Malignant neoplasm of unspecified part of unspecified bronchus or lung
C34.91	Malignant neoplasm of unspecified part of right bronchus or lung
C34.92	Malignant neoplasm of unspecified part of left bronchus or lung

EPIDEMIOLOGY & DEMOGRAPHICS

- Lung cancer is responsible for >30% of cancer deaths in males and >25% of cancer deaths in females. It is the second-most common cancer in the world (slightly fewer cases than breast cancer) and is by far the leading cause of cancer-related death globally.
- Tobacco smoke is implicated in 90% of cases; of these, secondhand smoke is responsible for approximately 20% of cases.
- In the U.S., there were an estimated 236,740 new cases of lung cancer and 130,180 deaths from lung cancer in 2022.[1] Worldwide, the estimated number of new cases and deaths in 2020 was 2.2 million and 1.8 million, respectively.
- From 1990 through 2013 the percentage of patients with non–small cell lung cancer who never smoked rose from 8% to 16%, raising concerns about environmental carcinogens.
- Coincident with the decrease in smoking rates and the introduction of lung cancer low-dose CT screening, as well as the introduction of newer immunotherapy treatments, the mortality from lung cancer in the U.S. continues to decrease.[2] However, death rates among African Americans continue to be disproportionately higher.

PHYSICAL FINDINGS & CLINICAL PRESENTATION (TABLES 1 AND 2)

- Weight loss, fatigue, fever, anorexia, dysphagia
- Cough, hemoptysis, dyspnea, wheezing
- Chest, shoulder, and bone pain
- Paraneoplastic syndromes (see Table 3):
  1. Lambert-Eaton myasthenic syndrome: Myopathy involving proximal muscle groups
  2. Endocrine manifestations: Hypercalcemia, ectopic adrenocorticotropic hormone secretion, syndrome of inappropriate excretion of adrenocorticotropic hormone (SIADH)
  3. Neurologic: Subacute cerebellar degeneration, peripheral neuropathy, cortical degeneration
  4. Musculoskeletal: Polymyositis, clubbing, hypertrophic pulmonary osteoarthropathy
  5. Hematologic or vascular: Migratory thrombophlebitis, marantic thrombosis, anemia, thrombocytosis, or thrombocytopenia

TABLE 1   Presenting Symptoms With Bronchogenic Carcinoma

Symptoms	Patients (%)
Cough	45-75
Weight loss	8-68
Dyspnea	37-58
Hemoptysis	27-57
Chest pain	27-49
Hoarseness	2-18

From Midthun DE, Jett JR: Clinical presentation of lung cancer. In: Pass HI et al, (eds): *Lung cancer: principles and practice*, Philadelphia, 1996, Lippincott-Raven, p. 422.

6. Cutaneous: Acanthosis nigricans, dermatomyositis
- Pleural effusion (10% of patients), recurrent pneumonias (from obstruction), localized wheezing
  Superior vena cava syndrome: Obstruction of venous return of the superior vena cava is most commonly caused by bronchogenic carcinoma or metastasis to paratracheal nodes.
  1. The patient usually reports headache, nausea, dizziness, visual changes, syncope, and respiratory distress.
  2. Physical examination reveals distention of thoracic and neck veins, edema of face and upper extremities, facial plethora, and cyanosis.
  3. *Horner syndrome:* Constricted pupil, ptosis, facial anhidrosis caused by spinal cord damage between C8 and T1 because of a superior sulcus tumor (bronchogenic carcinoma of the extreme lung apex).
  4. *Pancoast tumor:* A superior sulcus tumor associated with ipsilateral Horner syndrome and shoulder pain.

ETIOLOGY

- Tobacco abuse: The molecular pathology of smoking-related lung cancer is illustrated in Fig. 1. The chance of developing lung cancer for a 40-pack-yr persistent smoker is 20 times that of someone who never smoked.
- Environmental agents (e.g., radon) and industrial agents (e.g., ionizing radiation, asbestos, nickel, uranium, vinyl chloride, chromium, arsenic, coal dust).
- Lung cancer susceptibility and risk increased in inherited cancer syndromes caused by germline mutations in p53, retinoblastoma, and epidermal growth factor receptor *(EGFR)* genes.
- Fig. E2 illustrates the multistep cellular carcinogenesis in lung cancer.

TABLE 2   Expanded Clinical Evaluation

Symptoms Elicited In History

Constitutional—weight loss >10 lb
Musculoskeletal—focal skeletal pain
Neurologic—headaches, syncope, seizures, extremity weakness, recent change in mental status

Signs Found on Physical Examination

Lymphadenopathy (>1 cm)
Hoarseness
Superior vena cava syndrome
Bone tenderness
Hepatomegaly (>13 cm span)
Focal neurologic signs, papilledema
Soft tissue mass

Routine Laboratory Tests

Hematocrit <40% in males
Hematocrit <35% in females
Elevated alkaline phosphatase, γ-glutamyl transferase, aspartate aminotransferase, calcium

From Broaddus VC et al: *Murray & Nadel's textbook of respiratory medicine*, ed 7, Philadelphia, 2022, Elsevier.

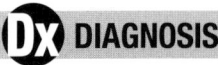

Dx DIAGNOSIS

DIFFERENTIAL DIAGNOSIS

- Pneumonia
- Tuberculosis (TB)
- Metastatic carcinoma to the lung
- Lung abscess
- Granulomatous disease
- Carcinoid tumor
- Sarcoidosis
- Benign lesions that simulate thoracic malignancy:
  1. Lobar atelectasis: Pneumonia, chronic inflammatory disease, allergic bronchopulmonary aspergillosis
  2. Multiple pulmonary nodules: Septic emboli, Wegener granulomatosis, sarcoidosis, rheumatoid nodules, fungal disease, multiple pulmonary atrioventricular fistulas
  3. Mediastinal adenopathy: Sarcoidosis, lymphoma, primary TB, fungal disease, silicosis, pneumoconiosis, drug-induced (e.g., phenytoin, trimethadione)
  4. Pleural effusion: Congestive heart failure, pneumonia with parapneumonic effusion, TB, viral pneumonitis, ascites, pancreatitis, collagen-vascular disease

WORKUP

- The workup generally includes chest computed tomography (CT), positron-emission tomographic (PET) scan, and tissue biopsy. Molecular testing for treatable oncogenic alterations should be performed to further classify NSCLC. Common immunohistochemical markers used in the diagnosis of lung tumors are summarized in Table 4. Table 5 describes common molecular alterations in lung tumors.
- Additional lab tests include CBC, serum chemistry studies.
- Diagnosis and staging of lung cancer should be performed simultaneously to minimize invasive testing.

LABORATORY TESTS

Various modalities are available to obtain a tissue diagnosis:

- Biopsy of any suspicious lymph nodes (e.g., supraclavicular or mediastinal node).
- Flexible fiberoptic bronchoscopy: Brush and biopsy specimens are obtained from any visualized endobronchial lesions. The use of a gene-expression classifier has a high sensitivity across different lesion sizes, locations, stages, and cell type of lung cancer. The combination of the classifier plus bronchoscopy has a sensitivity of >85%. In intermediate-risk patients with a non-diagnostic bronchoscopic examination, a negative classifier score provides support for a more conservative diagnostic approach.
- Transbronchial needle aspiration: Done with a special needle passed through the bronchoscope; this technique is useful to sample mediastinal masses or paratracheal lymph nodes.
- Transthoracic fine-needle aspiration biopsy with fluoroscopic or CT scan guidance to evaluate peripheral pulmonary nodules.
- Endobronchial ultrasound (EBUS) guided biopsy and staging is now routinely used to evaluate suspected mediastinal and hilar nodes.

TABLE 3 Paraneoplastic Syndromes Associated With Bronchogenic Carcinoma

Syndrome	Cell Type	Mechanism
Hypertrophic pulmonary osteoarthropathy and clubbing	All types	Unknown
Hyponatremia	SCLC most common; may be any type	SIADH, ectopic antidiuretic hormone production by tumor
Hypercalcemia	Usually squamous cell	Bone metastases, osteoclast-activating factor, parathyroid hormone–like hormone, prostaglandins
Cushing syndrome	Usually SCLC	Ectopic ACTH production
Lambert-Eaton myasthenic syndrome	Usually SCLC	Voltage-sensitive calcium channel antibodies in >75%; affects presynaptic neuronal calcium channel activity
Other neuromyopathic disorders	SCLC most common; may be any type	Antineuronal nuclear antibodies, also known as anti-Hu; others unknown
Thrombophlebitis	All types	Unknown

ACTH, Adrenocorticotropic hormone; *SCLC,* small cell lung cancer; *SIADH,* syndrome of inappropriate secretion of antidiuretic hormone.
Adapted from Andreoli TE et al: *Andreoli and Carpenter's Cecil essentials of medicine,* ed 8, Philadelphia, 2010, Saunders.

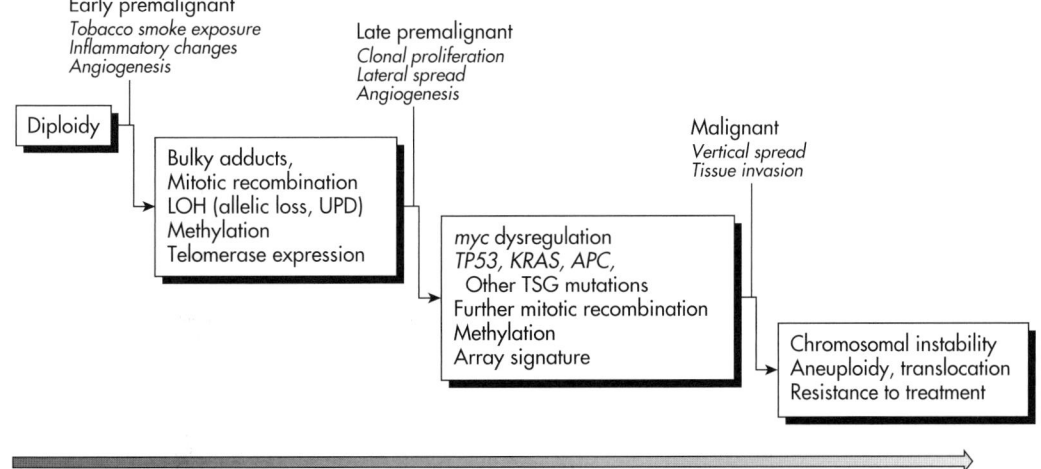

Phases of Molecular Carcinogenesis, Lung

FIG. 1 The molecular pathology of smoking-related lung cancer begins with the direct interaction between metabolites of carcinogenic polyaromatic hydrocarbons in cigarette smoke with host DNA. This creates bulky adducts that affect DNA repair and create transcription errors. The result is a wide range of genomic losses, gains, translocations, and point mutations that account for the high degree of molecular heterogeneity in lung tumors with diverse physiologic effects. *LOH,* Loss of heterozygosity; *TSG,* tumor suppressor gene; *UPD,* uniparental disomy. (From Niederhuber JE: *Abeloff's clinical oncology,* ed 6, Philadelphia, 2020, Elsevier.)

TABLE 4 Common Immunohistochemical Markers Used in the Diagnosis of Lung Tumors

Diagnosis	Positive Immunohistochemical Markers
Squamous cell carcinoma	Cytokeratin (CK) cocktail (e.g., AE1/AE3)
	p63
	p40
	CK5/6
	CK7 in up to 30%
Adenocarcinoma, including adenocarcinoma in situ or minimally invasive adenocarcinoma, nonmucinous	CK cocktail
	CK7
	TTF-1
	Napsin A
In situ and invasive mucinous adenocarcinoma	CK cocktail
	CK7
	CK20
	cdx-2
	TTF-1 rare
Large cell neuroendocrine carcinoma	CK cocktail
	TTF-1
	CD56
	Chromogranin A
	Synaptophysin
Carcinoid tumor	CK cocktail
	TTF-1 (weaker than in high-grade neuroendocrine tumors)
	CD56
	Chromogranin A
	Synaptophysin
Atypical carcinoid tumor	CK cocktail (tends to be patchy)
	TTF-1 (weaker than in high-grade neuroendocrine tumors)
	CD56
	Chromogranin A
	Synaptophysin
Common differential diagnoses:	
• Colonic adenocarcinoma	CK20+/CK7−
• Lung, breast, pancreatobiliary, upper gastrointestinal adenocarcinoma	CK7+/CK20−
• Urothelial carcinoma	CK7+/CK20+
• Prostatic adenocarcinoma	CK7−/CK20−
• Mesothelioma	Calretinin, WT1, CK5/6
• Malignant melanoma	S-100, HMB-45, Melan-A

From Niederhuber JE: *Abeloff's clinical oncology*, ed 6, Philadelphia, 2020, Elsevier.

- Mediastinoscopy and anteromedial sternotomy in suspected tumor involvement of the mediastinum.
- Pleural biopsy in patients with pleural effusion.
- Thoracentesis of pleural effusion and cytologic evaluation of the obtained fluid may confirm diagnosis.

IMAGING STUDIES
- Chest x-ray (Fig. 3): The radiographic presentation often varies with the cell type. Presence of pleural effusion, lobar atelectasis, and mediastinal adenopathy can occur in any cell type.
- CT scan of the chest (Fig. 4) can evaluate mediastinal and pleural extension. The chest CT should include liver and adrenal glands (common sites of metastases). CT or MRI of brain should be considered in a patient presenting with neurologic symptoms (e.g., headaches, vision disturbances).
- PET with ^{18}F-fluorodeoxyglucose (^{18}F-FDG) (Fig. E5) is superior to CT in detecting mediastinal and distant metastases in NSCLC. It is useful for preoperative staging of NSCLC.
- The use of PET-CT (Fig. E6) for preoperative staging of NSCLC reduces both the total number of thoracotomies and the number of futile thoracotomies.

STAGING
After confirmation of diagnosis, patients should undergo staging:
- In NSCLC, the TNM staging system is used (Table 6). Both stage I (no lymph node involvement) and stage II (ipsilateral bronchopulmonary/hilar lymph nodes or T_3 tumor) include localized tumors for which surgical

TABLE 5 Examples of Common Molecular Alterations in Lung Tumors

Diagnosis	Common Molecular Alterations
Squamous preneoplasia	LOH—3p, 9p21, 8p21–23, aneuploidy, methylation
Atypical adenomatous hyperplasia	LOH—3p, 9p, aneuploidy
	K-ras codon 12 mutation
Adenocarcinoma	p53 mutation
	p16 mutation/inactivation
	K-Ras (42%); smokers more common
	EGFR overexpression (40%)
	EGFR mutation
	Her2/neu, COX-2 overexpression
Squamous cell carcinoma	p53 mutation
	p16 inactivation
	Allelic loss 3p
	EGFR overexpression (80%)
Large cell carcinoma	K-Ras, p53, loss p16
Large cell neuroendocrine carcinoma	p53
	bcl-2 overexpression
	Rb mutation
	3p21, FHIT, 3p22-24, 5q21,9p21
Small cell carcinoma	Rb mutation (80+%)
	p53 mutation 50%-80%
	BCL-2 expression
	3p21, FHIT, 3p22-24, 5q21,9p21

COX-2, Cyclooxygenase 2; *EGFR*, epidermal growth factor receptor; *LOH*, loss of heterozygosity.
From Niederhuber JE: *Abeloff's clinical oncology*, ed 6, Philadelphia, 2020, Elsevier.

resection is the preferred treatment. Stage III is subdivided into III$_A$ (potentially resectable) and III$_B$/III$_C$ (unresectable). Stage IV indicates metastatic disease with stage IV$_A$ referring to intrathoracic metastases or pleural involvement or single extrathoracic metastasis. Stage IV$_B$ includes tumors with multiple extrathoracic metastases.
- In SCLC, the staging system developed by the Veterans Administration Lung Cancer Study Group is used. It contains two stages:
  1. Limited-stage disease: Confined to the regional lymph nodes and to one hemithorax (excluding pleural surfaces), which can be included in a single radiation portal
  2. Extensive-stage disease: Spread beyond the confines of limited-stage disease
- Pretreatment staging procedures for lung cancer patients, in addition to complete history and physical examination, generally include the following tests:
  1. Laboratory evaluation: Complete blood count, complete metabolic panel; arterial blood gases and pulse oximetry in selected cases

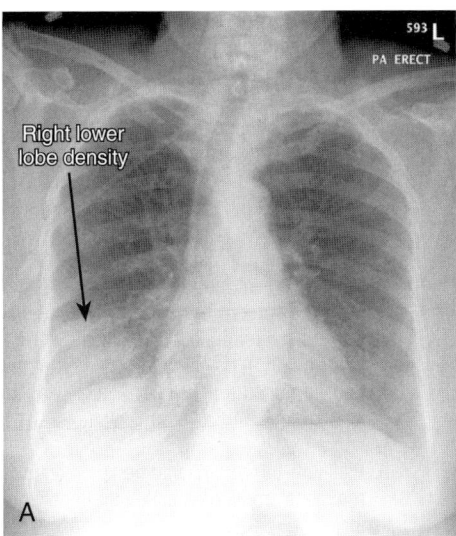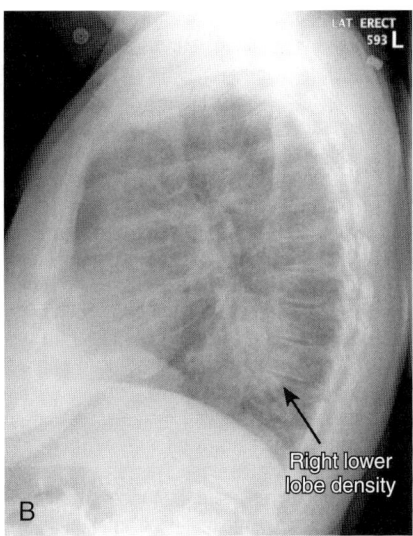

FIG. 3 Lung neoplasm, primary. Lung mass presenting with hemoptysis. **A,** Posterior-anterior (PA) chest x-ray. **B,** Lateral chest x-ray. This 83-yr-old female presented with hemoptysis of a quarter-sized clot. Her posterior-anterior chest x-ray shows a rounded right lower lobe density. On the lateral view, this is visible in the retrocardiac space. This density measures 7.6 cm in diameter. Pneumonia, neoplasm, or abscess could have this appearance on chest x-ray. Computed tomography was performed to further delineate the pathology (see Fig. 5). (From Broder JS: *Diagnostic imaging for the emergency physician,* Philadelphia, 2011, Saunders.)

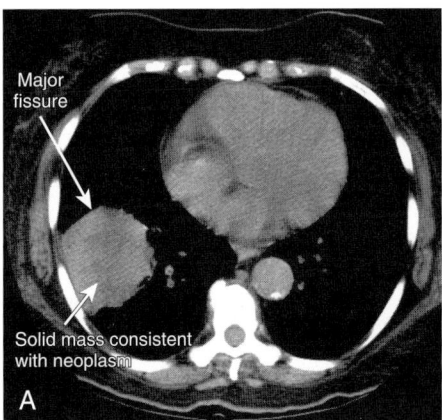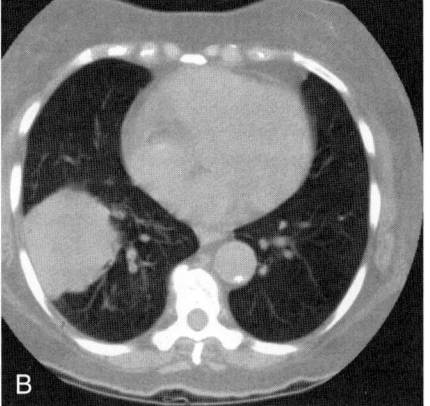

FIG. 4 Lung neoplasm, primary. Lung mass presenting with hemoptysis. Same patient as in Fig. 3. Noncontrast computed tomography was performed (contrast was withheld as a consequence of the patient's renal dysfunction) and shows a 6 x 6 cm round lesion abutting the oblique fissure (also called the major fissure) and lateral chest wall. **A,** Soft tissue windows. **B,** Lung windows. On soft tissue windows the center appears slightly darker, indicating lower density that may represent central necrosis. If IV contrast had been given, an area of necrosis would have failed to enhance. Infection or infarction is technically possible, but a pulmonary neoplasm is the most likely explanation for this lesion. Biopsy showed this to be a moderately differentiated squamous cell carcinoma. (From Broder JS: *Diagnostic imaging for the emergency physician,* Philadelphia, 2011, Saunders.)

2. Biopsy of any accessible suspect lesions
3. Pulmonary function studies
4. CT scan of chest and PET scan: Trials have shown a reduction in futile thoracotomies for patients who undergo preoperative PET assessment in addition to conventional workup
5. Mediastinoscopy or anterior mediastinotomy in patients being considered for curative lung resection. Newer technologies in preoperative staging include endoscopic bronchial ultrasonography and esophageal ultrasonography to guide biopsies
6. MRI brain to assess for metastases

Rx TREATMENT

NONPHARMACOLOGIC THERAPY
- Nutritional support
- Avoidance of tobacco and other substances toxic to the lungs
- Supplemental oxygen

ACUTE GENERAL Rx
Non–Small Cell Carcinoma: *(Tables 7 and 8)*
1. Surgical resection is standard in patients with operable NSCLC (stage I or II) who are surgical candidates. This represents approximately 15% to 30% of diagnosed

cases. Lobectomy is the traditional standard surgical approach. Lesser resections including sublobar resections are now deemed equivalent in appropriate cases with smaller or peripheral tumors or in patients with marginal pulmonary reserve.[3] A recent trial[3a] revealed that in patients with NSCLC with a tumor size of 2 cm or less and pathologically confirmed node-negative disease in the hilar and mediastinal lymph nodes, sublobar resection is not inferior to lobectomy with respect to disease-free interval.
2. Stereotactic ablative radiotherapy is a reasonable option for patients with localized NSCLC who are not surgical candidates.[4] Multimodality treatment guidelines are summarized in Table 9.
3. Preoperative evaluation includes cardiac status and pulmonary function assessment. Pneumonectomy is possible if the patient has a preoperative $FEV_1 = 2$ L or if the maximal voluntary ventilation is >50% of predicted capacity. Individuals with FEV_1 >1.5 L are suitable for lobectomy without further evaluation unless there is evidence of interstitial lung disease or undue dyspnea on exertion. In that case, carbon dioxide diffusion in the lung (DLCO) should be measured. If the DLCO is <80% predicted normal, the individual may not be clearly operable.
4. Conventional radiotherapy fails to durably control the primary lung tumor in nearly 70% of patients and 2-yr survival is less than 40%. Stereotactic body radiation (SBRT) uses several highly focused radiation beams to deliver total higher doses of radiotherapy (in high doses in 3 to 5 fractions) and is much more effective than conventional radiotherapy, with a local control rate equivalent to that with surgery in inoperable early-stage lung cancer.
5. Preoperative chemotherapy plus immunotherapy has been utilized in patients with larger primary tumors and involved mediastinal nodes (stages IB- IIIA) who are being considered for surgery and demonstrated to improve pathological complete response rates and disease-free survival in patients. A recent trial[4a] in patients with resectable NSCLC revealed that neoadjuvant nivolumab plus chemotherapy results in significantly longer event-free survival and a higher percentage of patients with a pathological complete response than chemotherapy alone. The addition of nivolumab to neoadjuvant chemotherapy did not increase the incidence of adverse events or impede the feasibility of surgery.
6. Postoperative adjuvant chemotherapy with doublet regimens significantly increases 5-yr survival (69% vs. 54%) in patients with completely resected stage II-IIIA NSCLC. For stage I NSCLC there may be some patients (tumors >4 cm) who benefit from adjuvant chemotherapy. In addition, postoperative adjuvant immunotherapy followed by 1 yr of checkpoint inhibitor

TABLE 6 TNM Stage Groups for Non–Small Cell Lung Cancer

Stage	T	N	M
Stage 0	T_{is}	N_0	M_0
Stage I$_{A1}$	T_{mi} or T_{1a}	N_0	M_0
Stage I$_{A2}$	T_{1b}	N_0	M_0
Stage I$_{A3}$	T_{1c}	N_0	M_0
Stage I$_B$	T_{2a}	N_0	M_0
Stage II$_A$	T_{2b}	N_0	M_0
Stage II$_B$	T_{1a-c}	N_1	M_0
	T_{2a-b}	N_1	M_0
	T_3	N_0	M_0
Stage III$_A$	T_{1a-c}	N_2	M_0
	T_{2a-b}	N_2	M_0
	T_3	N_1	M_0
	T_4	N_{0-1}	M_0
Stage III$_B$	T_{1a-c}	N_3	M_0
	T_{2a-b}	N_3	M_0
	T_{3-4}	N_2	M_0
Stage III$_C$	T_{3-4}	N_3	M_0
Stage IV$_A$	Any T	Any N	M_{1a-1b}
Stage IV$_B$	Any T	Any N	M_{1c}

TNM, Tumor, node, metastases.

therapy (atezolizumab) has shown improvement in survival over chemotherapy alone. An algorithm for selecting patients with stage I NSCLC for postoperative adjuvant chemotherapy is outlined in Fig. 7.

7. Postoperative adjuvant targeted therapy with EGFR inhibitor osimertinib in patients with EGFR-mutated, resected stage IB-IIIA NSCLC conveys a major survival benefit when administered with or without chemotherapy use.

- Treatment of unresectable NSCLC:
  1. Radiotherapy alone can be used primarily for treatment of central nervous system metastases, skeletal metastases, and superior vena cava syndrome.
  2. In unresectable stage 3 disease, concurrent chemotherapy and thoracic radiotherapy, followed by maintenance immunotherapy with checkpoint inhibitor durvalumab (in responding patients), is the standard therapeutic approach with a 5-yr survival rate of 43%.
  3. Chemotherapy, targeted therapy, and immune checkpoint inhibitor therapy are the mainstays of treatment for relapsed or metastatic NSCLC. Initial stratification is done based on pathology (squamous vs. nonsquamous cancers), presence of driver mutations (e.g., *EGFR, ALK, ROS1, BRAF, MET, RET, KRASC-G12C,* and *NTRK* mutations in adenocarcinomas), and expression of programmed death receptor ligand-1 (PD-L1). Table 10 summarizes selected NSCLC oncogenes and targeted therapy.

4. The current approach in advanced NSCLC without driver mutations relies on using the PD-L1 score to generate recommendations for immunotherapy alone (PD-L1 score >50%), combination chemotherapy and immunotherapy (PD-L1 score 1% to 49%), or chemotherapy alone (PD-L1 score 0%).

5. Platinum-based chemotherapy doublet regimens are recommended for fit patients including platinum plus pemetrexed for nonsquamous cancers, whereas for squamous cancers taxane plus carboplatin, cisplatin plus vinorelbine, and gemcitabine plus cisplatin are utilized with none being clearly superior to the others. The addition of bevacizumab to chemotherapy results in significant survival benefit in nonsquamous cancers.

TABLE 7 Summary of Current Treatment Strategies for Non–Small Cell Lung Cancer

Stage	Surgery	Chemotherapy	Radiotherapy	Chemoradiotherapy	Comments
IA and IB	First line	Adjuvant—tumors $\geq$4 cm	First line*	No	Role of adjuvant chemotherapy for stage IB not clearly defined but should be considered in tumors $\geq$4 cm in size and/or high-risk features (vascular invasion, visceral pleural involvement)
IIA and IIB	First line	Adjuvant	No	No	5-yr survival improvement with adjuvant chemotherapy about 5%
T3 due to multiple tumor nodules same lobe	Lobectomy to resect primary and satellite nodules				
T3 due to chest wall invasion	En bloc resection				
Superior sulcus tumors					Neoadjuvant chemoradiotherapy improves survival in this subset of stage IIB
IIIA	First line for N0-1	Adjuvant treatment in completely resected IIIA	Neoadjuvant or adjuvant in the setting of N2 nodes	First line for unresectable N2 disease Followed by consolidation immunotherapy	Combined chemotherapy $\pm$ radiotherapy followed by surgery is feasible in select N2 disease, but more data are needed to recommend routinely
IIIB and IIIC	No	No	No	First line Followed by consolidation immunotherapy	
IV	No	First line: Systemic therapy[†]: • Chemotherapy • Targeted therapy • Immunotherapy • Chemotherapy and immunotherapy	Radiotherapy is used for palliation only	No	All stage IV adenocarcinomas should have mutational analysis, including *EGFR, ALK*-fusion, *ROS1,* and *KRAS* All stage IV NSCLC should be tested for PD-L1

*SBRT for patients who are medically unfit or who refuse surgery.

[†]First-line therapy in stage IV NSCLC is selected based on (1) histology: pemetrexed for nonsquamous cell, gemcitabine for squamous cell, and bevacizumab is approved as an adjunct to chemotherapy in the first-line setting in patients with nonsquamous histology and no other contraindications; (2) presence of molecular target guides first-line therapy; (3) PD-L1 expression >50% used to select patients eligible for first-line pembrolizumab.

From Broaddus VC et al: *Murray & Nadel's textbook of respiratory medicine,* ed 7, Philadelphia, 2022, Elsevier.

TABLE 8 Targeted Therapy for Metastatic NSCLC With Molecular Target

Biomarker	First-Line Therapy	Second-Line Therapy	Promising Therapies
EGFR mutations	Erlotinib Gefitinib Afatinib Osimertinib	Osimertinib (after first- or second-generation TKI if T790M)	
ALK-fusion	Crizotinib Alectinib Ceritinib	Lorlatinib Brigatinib	
ROS1	Crizotinib Entrectinib		Repotrectinib
BRAF		Dabrafenib/trametinib	
RET-fusions			LOXO-292 BLU-667
MET exon 14 mutation		Crizotinib	Capmatinib Savolitinib Tepotinib
HER2 dysregulation			Trastuzumab* Ado-trastuzumab*
KRAS^{G12C} mutation			AMG510 MRTX849

*Off-label use.
From Broaddus VC et al: *Murray & Nadel's textbook of respiratory medicine*, ed 7, Philadelphia, 2022, Elsevier.

TABLE 9 Summary of Multimodality Guidelines

Stage Level of Evidence	Surgery	Adjuvant Therapy	Radiation	Chemotherapy
I	Yes	No	No	No	1B—Surgical resection 1B—Against postoperative chemotherapy 1A—Against postoperative radiation therapy
II	Yes	Yes	No	Yes	1B—Surgical resection 1A—Postoperative chemotherapy 2A—Against postoperative radiation therapy
IIIA					
(N2-occult)	Yes	Yes	May be considered	Yes	1A—Adjuvant chemo 2C—Adjuvant radiation
(N2-discrete)	Yes	No	Yes	Yes	1A—Definite or induction followed by surgery
			(Definitive or induction recommended)		1C—Against primary resection followed by adjuvant therapy
IIIB	No	No	Yes	Yes	1A—Definitive concurrent
(N2, N3)			(Definitive concurrent)		1A—Against induction followed by surgery

From Sellke FW et al: *Sabiston & Spencer surgery of the chest*, ed 9, 2016, Philadelphia, Elsevier.

6. Single-agent immune checkpoint inhibitors approved for first line use in patients with PD-L1 score >50% include pembrolizumab, atezolizumab, and cemiplimab.[5] Inhibitors approved for use in combination with doublet chemotherapy include pembrolizumab and atezolizumab. The dual immunotherapy combination with ipilimumab and nivolumab is also an approved option in patients with PD-L1 score >1% while short-course chemotherapy plus this dual immunotherapy can be used in patients independent of PD-L1 score status.[6] Recently, the combination of chemotherapy plus durvalumab and tremelimumab immunotherapy has also been shown to improve survival in metastatic patients.[7]

7. Tyrosine kinase inhibitors that target activating driver mutations are used as initial and/or subsequent therapy in patients whose adenocarcinomas that harbor such mutations:

a. EGFR mutations (20% to 25% cases) are more commonly detected in never or light smokers and in Asian patients. Gefitinib, erlotinib, afatinib, osimertinib, and dacomitinib are oral EGFR inhibitors that have showed impressive responses and improvements in median overall survival to the range of 30 mo. Currently, first-line therapy with the oral inhibitor osimertinib is the preferred option based on updated data demonstrating median overall survival of 36 mo.[9] EGFR exon 20 insertion mutations (which do not respond to oral EGFR inhibitors) can now be treated with the recently approved bispecific EGFR/c-met antibody amivantamab.

b. Oncogenic fusion genes consisting of EML4 and anaplastic lymphoma kinase (ALK) are present in 4% to 5% of cases and can be treated with oral inhibitors crizotinib, ceritinib, alectinib, brigatinib, or lorlatinib.

c. Approximately 2% of adenocarcinomas have genetic rearrangements involving the ROS1 protooncogenic receptor tyrosine kinase (ROS1), and these patients can be treated with the oral inhibitors crizotinib and ceritinib.

d. Approximately 2% of adenocarcinomas harbor the BRAF V600E mutation, and these patients can be treated with the combination of oral BRAF/MEK inhibitor (dabrafenib plus trametinib) therapy.

e. Mutations leading to MET exon 14 skipping are found in 3% to 4% of patients with advanced non–small cell lung cancer. The FDA has approved the oral inhibitors capmatinib and tepotinib for the treatment of adult patients with NSCLC harboring this specific MET mutation.

f. RET (rearranged during transfection) rearrangements occur in 1% to 2% of unselected NSCLC cases and are commonly found in patients who have never smoked or are minimal smokers. The oral inhibitors selpercatinib and pralsetinib are now approved in patients with RET fusion-positive NSCLC who were previously treated with platinum-based chemotherapy and who had never undergone treatment.

g. NTRK fusions are clinically targetable and have been identified to be the predominant drivers of growth in <1% of advanced lung cancers. The treatment of patients with NTRK fusion-positive cancers with a first-generation TRK inhibitor, such as larotrectinib or entrectinib, is associated with high response rates but eventual development of resistance.

h. KRAS G12C mutations occur in 13% of patients with advanced NSCLC. The FDA approved the oral inhibitor sotorasib based on activity in previously treated patients who had received chemotherapy and/or immunotherapy.[9]

L

Diseases and Disorders

I

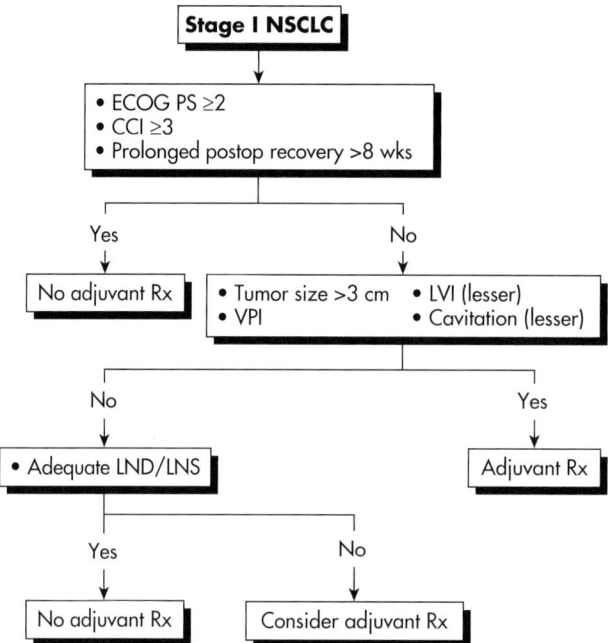

FIG. 7 Algorithm for selecting patients with stage I non–small cell lung cancer *(NSCLC)* **for postoperative adjuvant chemotherapy.** *CCI,* Charlson Comorbidity Index; *ECOG PS,* Eastern Cooperative Oncology Group Performance Status; *LND,* mediastinal lymph node dissection; *LNS,* systematic mediastinal lymph node sampling; *LVI,* lymphovascular invasion; *Rx,* treatment; *VPI,* visceral pleural invasion. (From Niederhuber JE: *Abeloff's clinical oncology,* ed 6, Philadelphia, 2020, Elsevier.)

TABLE 10   Selected Non–Small Cell Lung Cancer Oncogenes and Targeted Therapy

Oncogene Alteration	Incidence (%)	Clinical Relevance	Treatment
BRAF			
Mutation	1-3	V600E mutation: Most common, equal association with smokers and nonsmokers May be mechanism of acquired EGFR TKI resistance	Dabrafenib plus trametinib
EGFR (ErbB1, HER1)			
Mutation	13-50	Exon 19 deletion and Exon 21-point mutation are the most common Predominantly adenocarcinoma and nonsmokers; up to 50% frequency in Asians	TKI: Gefitinib, erlotinib, afatinib, osimertinib
EML4-ALK			
Fusion	3-7	Most frequent in adenocarcinomas, nonsmokers, men, and younger patients	Nonspecific TKI: Crizotinib, ceritinib, alectinib, brigatinib
Her2/neu (ErbB2)			No approved therapy
Mutation	2-6	Mostly adenocarcinomas and nonsmokers	
Amplification	23	Mechanism of resistance to EGFR TKI	
KRAS			
Mutation	5-30	Mostly adenocarcinomas and smokers May contribute to resistance to ALF, BRAF, and PI3K inhibitors	No approved therapy
MET			No approved therapy
Mutation	<5		
Amplification	21	Mechanism of resistance to EGFR TKI	
PIK3CA			No approved therapy
Mutation	<10	Frequently occurs in association with other mutations; more common in squamous cell	
Amplification	5-43	Mechanism of resistance to EGFR TKI	
PTEN			
Mutation	1.7-10	Associated with PI3K activation, resistance to EGFR TKI, and sensitivity to PI3K inhibitors More frequent in squamous cell	
Loss of function	4-21	Associated with PI3K activation, resistance to EGFR TKI, and sensitivity to PI3K inhibitors More frequent in squamous cell	
RET fusion gene	1-2	Mostly adenocarcinomas and nonsmokers	No approved therapy
ROS1 fusion gene	2	Mostly adenocarcinomas, nonsmokers, and younger patients	TKI: Crizotinib
VEGF			Monoclonal antibodies: Bevacizumab VEGFR TKI

BRAF, v-Raf murine sarcoma viral oncogene homolog B1; *EGFR,* epidermal growth factor receptor; *EML4-ALK,* echinoderm microtubule-associated protein-like 4 anaplastic lymphoma kinase; *ERBB,* avian erythroblastosis oncogene B; *Her2,* human epidermal growth factor receptor 2; *KRAS,* Kirsten Rat sarcoma viral oncogene homolog; *MET,* mesenchymal-epithelial transition; *PIK3CA,* phosphoinositide-3-kinase catalytic alpha polypeptide; *PTEN,* phosphatase and tensin homolog; *RET,* rearranged during transfection; *ROS1,* reactive oxygen species 1; *TKI,* tyrosine kinase inhibitor; *VEGF,* vascular endothelial growth factor; *VEGFR,* vascular endothelial growth factor receptor.
From Sellke FW et al: *Sabiston & Spencer surgery of the chest,* ed 9, 2016, Philadelphia, Elsevier.

L

I

TABLE 11   Lung Cancer Screening Recommendations

Asymptomatic patients age 55-77 yr	>30 pack-yr	Current smoker or quit <15 yr	Annual screening with low-dose CT
Asymptomatic patients >77 yr	<30 pack-yr	Quit smoking >15 yr ago	Low-dose CT screening should not be performed
Patients with comorbidities that adversely influence their ability to tolerate treatment of early-stage screen-detected lung cancer or that substantially limit their life expectancy			Low-dose CT screening should not be performed

CT, Computed tomography.
From Warshaw G et al: *Ham's primary care geriatrics*, ed 7, Philadelphia, 2022, Elsevier.

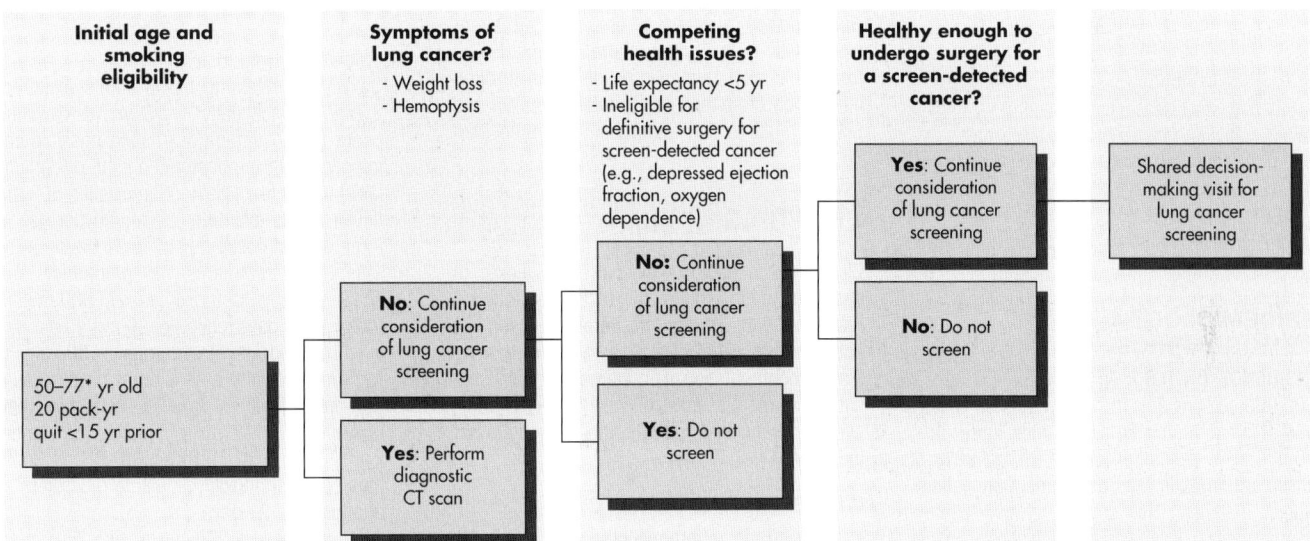

FIG 8   Algorithm for considering patient eligibility for lung cancer. *Centers for Medicare and Medicaid Services eligibility criteria. *CT,* computed tomography. (Modified from Broaddus VC et al: *Murray & Nadel's textbook of respiratory medicine*, ed 7, Philadelphia 2022, Elsevier.)

8. Early initiation of palliative care focusing on management of symptoms, psychosocial support, and assistance with decision making in patients with metastatic NSCLC leads to improved quality of life, longer survival, and less use of aggressive end-of-life care.

SMALL CELL LUNG CANCER:
- Limited-stage disease: Standard treatments include thoracic radiotherapy and chemotherapy (cisplatin and etoposide).
- Extensive-stage disease: Standard combination chemotherapy regimens include platinum plus etoposide or platinum plus irinotecan. The addition of the PD-1 antibody atezolizumab or durvalumab to standard first-line chemotherapy has been proven to improve overall survival and is considered a standard approach in current practice.
- Prophylactic cranial irradiation for patients in complete remission to decrease the risk of central nervous system metastasis.
- Despite high initial response rates, most patients eventually relapse. Topotecan or irinotecan may be an option for these patients. Immune checkpoint inhibitors have demonstrated survival benefit in SCLC patients who have failed standard therapies. Lurbinectedin, a selective inhibitor of oncogenic transcription, is now approved for patients who developed disease progression after first-line therapy.[10]

DISPOSITION
- The 5-yr survival of patients with resectable NSCLC (stages I-III) is approximately 30%. The 5-yr survival for stage 4 patients is increasing, with survival rates in the 25% range reported in current trials with the use of targeted therapy and immunotherapy.
- Median survival time in patients with limited-stage disease SCLC is 15 mo; in patients with extensive-stage SCLC, it is in the range of 12 mo.
- Among patients with metastatic NSCLC, early palliative care results in longer survival and significant improvements in both quality of life and mood.
- Population-level mortality from NSCLC in the United States fell sharply from 2013 to 2016, and survival after diagnosis improved substantially. Reduction in incidence along with modern treatment advances are likely explanations for the reduction in mortality observed.

⚠ **PEARLS & CONSIDERATIONS**

Screening with use of low-dose computed tomography (LDCT) for detection of lung cancer among persons with a heavy history of smoking increases the percentage of lung cancer cases that are diagnosed in stage 1 and reduces mortality from lung cancer. The National Lung Screening Trial (NLST) showed that lung cancer screening with LDCT resulted in a 20% reduction in lung cancer mortality.[11] New guidelines (Table 11 and Fig. 8) recommend annual LDCT for those who are current or former smokers ages 50 to 77 yr with a smoking history threshold of 20 pack years. Screening should be discontinued once a person has not smoked for 15 yr or develops a health problem that substantially limits life expectancy or the ability or willingness to have curative lung surgery.

REFERENCES
Available at eBooks.Health.Elsevier.com.

RELATED CONTENT
Lung Cancer (Patient Information)
Lung Cancer Screening (Patient Information)
Horner Syndrome (Related Key Topic)
Lambert-Eaton Myasthenic Syndrome (Related Key Topic)
Paraneoplastic Syndromes (Related Key Topic)
Superior Vena Cava Syndrome (Related Key Topic)

AUTHOR: **RITESH RATHORE, MD**

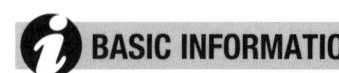

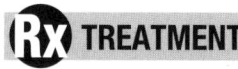 **BASIC INFORMATION**

DEFINITION

Lyme disease is a multisystem inflammatory disorder caused by the transmission of a spirochete, *Borrelia burgdorferi,* via the bite of infected *Ixodes* ticks, taking 36 to 48 h for a tick to take a blood meal and transmit the infecting organism to the host. Table E1 summarizes the Centers for Disease Control and Prevention (CDC) Lyme disease surveillance case definition.

SYNONYMS

Bannwarth syndrome (Europe)
Acrodermatitis chronica atrophicans

ICD-10CM CODES

A69.20	Lyme disease, unspecified
A69.21	Meningitis due to Lyme disease
A69.22	Other neurologic disorders in Lyme disease
A69.23	Arthritis due to Lyme disease
A69.29	Other conditions associated with Lyme disease

EPIDEMIOLOGY & DEMOGRAPHICS

INCIDENCE (IN U.S.): In the U.S., 4.4 cases/100,000 persons; it is the most common vector-borne infection in the U.S., with more than 30,000 new cases reported each yr. 90% of cases are found in Massachusetts, Connecticut, Rhode Island, New York, New Jersey, Pennsylvania, Minnesota, Wisconsin, and California. The area of transmission in the U.S. is expanding farther into the South and upper Northeast (Fig. E1). The disease also occurs in Europe and Asia with a different *Ixodes* tick vector. Table E2 summarizes principal vector ticks and spirochetes associated with Lyme borreliosis.

PREDOMINANT SEX: Male = female
PREDOMINANT AGE: Median age of 28 yr
PEAK INCIDENCE: May to November

PHYSICAL FINDINGS & CLINICAL PRESENTATION

Lyme disease may present in the following stages (Table E3):
- *Early localized stage (incubation period 3 to 30 days):* Early Lyme disease, erythema migrans (EM); skin rash, often at site of tick bite (the CDC has defined EM rash as an expanding red macule or papule that must reach at least 5 cm in size, with or without central clearing); target lesions from ECM can be found in 60% to 80% of localized infections; possible fever, myalgias 3 to 32 days after tick bite
- *Early disseminated stage (incubation period 3 to 6 wk):* Days to weeks later; multiorgan system involvement, including central nervous system (CNS) with aseptic meningitis–type picture or Bells palsy, joints (arthritis or arthralgias), cardiac including varying degrees of heart block; related to dissemination of spirochete
- *Late stage (incubation period month to year):* Month to year after tick exposure; affects central and peripheral nervous system, cardiac, joints

Common presenting signs and symptoms include:
- EM (Fig. E2). Most patients with EM (about 80%) have a single lesion, but the bacteria can disseminate hematogenously to other sites in the skin and result in often smaller erythema migrans lesions (Figs. E3 and E4).
- Lymphadenopathy, neck pains, pharyngeal erythema, myalgias, hepatosplenomegaly.
- Patients will complain of malaise, fatigue, lethargy, headache, fever/chills, neck pain, myalgias, back pain.

ETIOLOGY

B. burgdorferi transmitted from bite of an *Ixodes* tick (mostly in the nymph stage but can also be from adult ticks). Human infection occurs through inoculation of spirochetes in infected saliva and usually requires tick attachment for more than 36 hr.

DX **DIAGNOSIS**

Clinical presentation, exposure to ticks in endemic area, and diagnostic testing for antibody response to *B. burgdorferi.* Serologic testing at early stages is usually negative; therefore, in early stage, documentation of erythema migrans lesion with a compatible epidemiologic history is sufficient for diagnosis, and laboratory testing is not indicated.

DIFFERENTIAL DIAGNOSIS
- Chronic fatigue/fibromyalgia
- Acute viral illnesses
- Babesiosis
- Human granulocytic anaplasmosis

WORKUP

Serologic testing is the principal means of laboratory diagnosis of Lyme disease. Current recommendations include using a sensitive enzyme immunoassay (EIA) or immunofluorescence assay, followed by a Western immunoblot assay for specimens yielding positive or equivocal results.

LABORATORY TESTS
- ELISA testing and if positive or equivocal then followed by a Western blot immunoglobulin M (IgM) and IgG (Table E4). A Western blot IgM assay is positive if two of three bands present. The Western blot IgG is positive if five of ten bands present.
- An alternative serologic test is the VlsE C6 ELISA (enzyme-linked immunosorbent assay) (C6 peptide), which detects an IgG response earlier and may be more sensitive than the ELISA, but its specificity is lower than the two-tier testing method.
- In 2019, the FDA cleared several Lyme assays allowing for an EIA serology test rather than the Western Blot assay as the second test in the Lyme disease testing algorithm.
- Early disease often is difficult to diagnose serologically, secondary to slow immune response.
- Culturing of skin lesions (EM) and polymerase chain reaction (PCR) of synovial fluid or

cerebrospinal fluid can also give the diagnosis of active infection.
- Fig. 5 is an algorithm for the diagnosis and treatment of arthritis associated with Lyme disease.

IMAGING STUDIES
- ECG
- Echocardiogram if conduction abnormalities are present with cardiac involvement
- Computed tomography scan, MRI of brain in patients with CNS involvement

Rx **TREATMENT**

Early localized Lyme disease:
- Doxycycline 100 mg bid in adults (children: 2 mg/kg twice daily if ≥8 yr) [doxycycline offers the advantage of treating possible co-infection with the bacterial agents of ehrlichiosis] for 10 to 14 days or amoxicillin 500 mg tid for adults (children: 50 mg/kg per day in three divided doses) for 14 to 21 days.
- Alternative treatments for pregnancy and children ≤8 yr: Cefuroxime axetil 500 mg bid for 14 to 21 days (children: 30 mg/kg per day in two divided doses), azithromycin 500 mg PO for 7 to 10 days but should **not** be used as a first-line agent, as it is less effective than doxycycline and amoxicillin. NOTE: The American Academy of Pediatrics (AAP Red Book) now considers doxycycline safe regardless of age for up to 21 days.
- A single dose of 200 mg doxycycline given within 72 h of removing an engorged *Ixodes* tick can significantly reduce the risk of development of Lyme disease in endemic areas and is reasonable prophylaxis in nonpregnant adults and children ≥8 yr old.

Early disseminated and late persistent infection:
- 28 days of treatment is often prescribed, although recent evidence supports treating patients with a 14-day course of oral doxycycline for early neurologic Lyme disease in ambulatory patients. Doxycycline and ceftriaxone appear equally effective for acute disseminated Lyme disease.
- Arthritis: 28 days of doxycycline or amoxicillin plus probenecid.
- Neurologic involvement requires parenteral antibiotics. Those who fail to respond should be treated with IV ceftriaxone or cefotaxime.
- Ceftriaxone 2 g/day IV for 21 to 28 days; alternative: Cefotaxime 2 g q8h IV; alternative: Penicillin G 5 million U qid.
- Cardiac involvement: IV ceftriaxone or cefotaxime plus cardiac monitoring.
- Prolonged treatment with IV or PO antibiotic therapy for up to 90 days did not improve symptoms more than placebo.

Post–Lyme disease syndrome:
- Presence of disabling symptoms such as fatigue, malaise, diffuse pains, and poor concentration, which may be due to an exuberant host inflammatory response even in patients who have received proper antibiotic treatment
- Antibiotics are not indicated. Antibiotic treatment of patients with persistent unexplained

DIAGNOSIS AND TREATMENT OF LYME ARTHRITIS

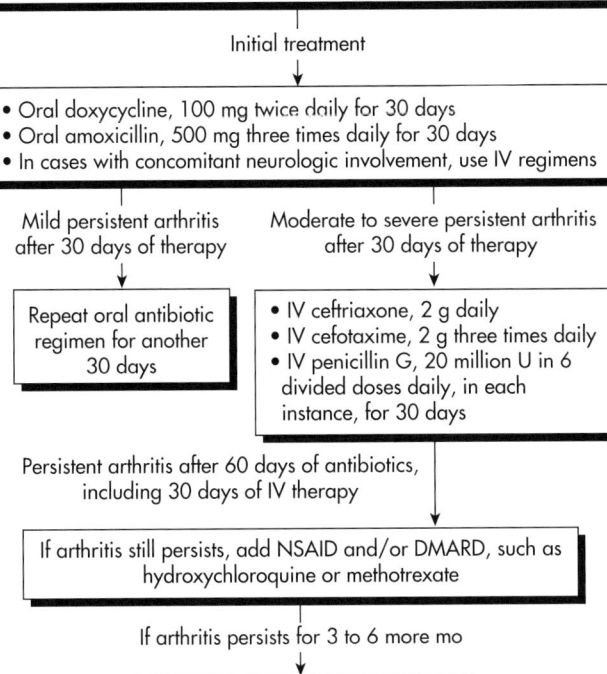

FIG. 5 **Algorithm for the diagnosis and treatment of arthritis associated with Lyme disease.** *DMARD,* Disease-modifying antirheumatic drug; *DNA,* deoxyribonucleic acid; *ELISA,* enzyme-linked immunosorbent assay; *Ig,* immunoglobulin; *IV,* intravenous; *NSAID,* nonsteroidal antiinflammatory drug; *PCR,* polymerase chain reaction. (From Hochberg MC: *Rheumatology,* ed 7, Philadelphia, 2019, Elsevier.)

symptoms despite previous antibiotic treatment of Lyme disease provides little, if any, benefit and carries significant risk
• Supportive care

DISPOSITION
• The patient often needs careful follow-up and supportive care for the arthralgia-neuritis symptoms.
• 10% to 20% of treated patients may have lingering symptoms of fatigue, disrupted sleep, and musculoskeletal complaints.

Repeat episodes of EM in appropriately treated patients are due to reinfection and not to relapse.

REFERRAL
• To a neurologist if significant neurologic complications (meningitis, myelitis, ophthalmoplegia, Bell palsy)
• To a cardiologist if the patient develops evidence of cardiac conduction disturbances or pericarditis

! PEARLS & CONSIDERATIONS

• A physician diagnosis of classic EM in an endemic region of Lyme disease is sufficient to make a definitive diagnosis.
• In some patients with Lyme disease, nonspecific complaints such as headache, fatigue, and arthralgia may persist for months after appropriate (and ultimately successful) antibiotic treatment. Long-term antibiotic treatment does not provide additional beneficial effects.
• There is no evidence of current or previous *Borrelia burgdorferi* infection in most patients evaluated at university-based Lyme disease referral centers. Psychiatric comorbidity and other psychologic factors are prominent in the presentation and outcome of some patients who inaccurately ascribe longstanding symptoms to "chronic Lyme disease."
• It is important to realize that one tick bite can transmit Lyme disease *and* the bacterial agents of either ehrlichiosis or babesiosis (protozoan parasite), or even both, and these latter agents require separate serologic testing and possibly therapy. *Ehrlichiosis* is treated with doxycycline, but *Babesia* would require a different therapy. Powassan virus can also be transmitted by the *Ixodes* tick bite and causes an encephalitis seen in eastern Canada and northcentral, northeastern, and upper midwestern United States. Cases have been increasing.
• Tick bite protection: EPA-registered insect repellents containing DEET, picaridin, IR3535, oil of lemon eucalyptus (OLE), para-menthane-3,8-diol (PMD), or 2-undecanone can prevent ticks from attaching when applied and can last for several hours. OLE and PMD products cannot be used on children under 3 yr of age.

SUGGESTED READINGS
Available at eBooks.Health.Elsevier.com.

RELATED CONTENT
Lyme Disease (Patient Information)

AUTHOR: **GLENN G. FORT, MD, MPH**

Lymphedema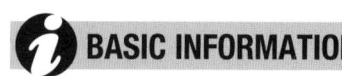

BASIC INFORMATION

DEFINITION
A primary role of the lymphatic system is to transport proteins from the interstitium to the heart. When the transport capacity of the lymphatic system is reduced, proteins accumulate in the interstitium. Accumulated proteins attract water, which creates a high protein swelling in the subcutaneous tissues called lymphedema. Lymphedema can be classified as primary or secondary (Box 1).

SYNONYM
Elephantiasis

ICD-10CM CODES
I89.0 Lymphedema, not elsewhere classified
I97.2 Postmastectomy lymphedema syndrome
Q82.0 Hereditary lymphedema

EPIDEMIOLOGY & DEMOGRAPHICS
PRIMARY LYMPHEDEMA:
- Found in 1.1/100,000 people aged <20 yr
- Females outnumber males 3.5:1
- Incidence peaks between ages 12 and 16 (puberty)

SECONDARY LYMPHEDEMA: See specific etiology in the following

PHYSICAL FINDINGS & CLINICAL PRESENTATION
Lymphedema is a slow-onset, progressive disease characterized by an asymmetric, inflammatory swelling, traveling distal to proximal, that can affect any body part including limbs, trunk, head/neck, and genitals (Fig. E1). Box 2 summarizes lymphedema staging from the International Society of Lymphology.
STAGE 0: LATENCY:
- Decreased lymphatic system transport capacity due to primary or secondary etiology
- Subjective complaints of affected body part feeling heavy or achy
- No objective findings, no apparent swelling
STAGE I: REVERSIBLE:
- Edema is observable, soft, pitting, and reversible with elevation.
- No secondary skin changes are present.
STAGE II: SPONTANEOUSLY IRREVERSIBLE:
- Skin becomes more firm/fibrotic, therefore less pitting.
- Edema does not reverse to normal with elevation.
- Possibility of infections (cellulitis), wounds, or weeping (lymphorrhea).

STAGE III: ELEPHANTIASIS:
- Skin becomes very firm/fibrotic, therefore nonpitting.
- Evidence of substantial skin changes (e.g., papillomas, lobules, "peau d' orange").

ETIOLOGY
Lymphedema is caused by a reduction in lymphatic system transport and is classified into primary and secondary forms.
PRIMARY LYMPHEDEMA:
- Occurs when the lymphatic system does not mature properly during fetal development
  1. Aplasia
  2. Hypoplasia
  3. Hyperplasia
- Can be familial, genetic, or hereditary
- Lymphedema congenital: Symptoms present at birth (Fig. 2)
- Lymphedema praecox: Symptoms onset before the age of 35 (commonly during puberty)
- Lymphedema tardum: Symptoms onset at the age of 35 or after
SECONDARY LYMPHEDEMA:
- Occurs secondary to a disruption or obstruction of the lymphatic system caused by:
  1. Filariasis (number one cause worldwide)
  2. Lymph node surgery/radiation due to cancer (number one cause in the U.S.)
  3. Other: Chronic venous insufficiency (CVI), deep vein thrombosis (DVT), infection, surgery/trauma, lipedema, and obesity

DIAGNOSIS

- Lymphedema is primarily a clinical diagnosis made on the basis of past medical history and objective findings that distinguish it from other causes of chronic edema.
- A Stemmer sign is often used to identify lymphedema (inability to pick up or pinch a fold of skin at the base of the second toe or finger).
- When physical examination is inconclusive, other available imaging tests can help make the diagnosis (see "Imaging Studies").

BOX 1 Classification of lymphedema

Primary lymphedema
- Congenital lymphedema (Milroy disease)
- Lymphedema praecox
- Lymphedema tarda

Syndromes associated with primary lymphedema
- Yellow nail syndrome
- Turner syndrome
- Noonan syndrome
- Pes cavus
- Phakomatosis pigmentovascularis
- Distichiasis-lymphedema
- Emberger syndrome
- WILD syndrome
- Hypotrichosis-telangiectasia-lymphedema syndrome

Cutaneous disorders sometimes associated with primary lymphedema
- Yellow nails
- Hemangiomas
- Xanthomatosis and chylous lymphedema
- Congenital absence of nails

Secondary lymphedema
- Postmastectomy lymphedema
- Melphalan isolated limb perfusion
- Malignant occlusion with obstruction
- Extrinsic pressure
- Factitial lymphedema
- Postradiation therapy
- Following recurrent lymphangitis/cellulitis
- Lymphedema of upper limb in recurrent eczema
- Granulomatous disease
- Rosaceous lymphedema
- Primary amyloidosis

Complications of lymphedema
- Cellulitis of lymphedema
- Elephantiasis nostra verrucosa
- Ulceration
- Lymphangiosarcoma

From James WD et al: *Andrews' diseases of the skin*, ed 12, Philadelphia, 2016, Elsevier.

BOX 2 Lymphedema Staging

Stage 0: Latent
- Impaired lymphatic function
- No evident edema; subclinical
- May last months or years before progression

Stage I: Spontaneously Reversible
- Early accumulation of protein-rich fluid
- Pitting edema
- Subsides with elevation

Stage II: Spontaneously Irreversible
- Accumulation of protein-rich fluid
- Pitting edema progresses to fibrosis
- Does not resolve with elevation alone

Stage III: Lymphostatic Elephantiasis
- Nonpitting
- Significant fibrosis
- Trophic skin changes

From International Society of Lymphology: The diagnosis and treatment of peripheral edema: 2009 consensus document of the International Society of Lymphology, *Lymphology* 42(2):51-60, 2009.

- Nutritional therapy (reducing the amount of proteins ingested) is ineffective in the treatment of lymphedema.

PHARMACOLOGIC THERAPY
No drugs have been shown to be beneficial in the treatment of lymphedema. Diuretics in particular have not been found to be effective in removing proteins from lymphedematous quadrants and may promote the development of volume depletion.

SURGERY
Surgery for lymphedema has been proven largely unsuccessful and should not be considered before CDT. Surgical procedures are divided into two types:
- Physiologic procedures: Those performed to improve lymph node drainage (e.g., anastomoses of the lymph system with the venous system, lymph node transplant).
- Excisional or debulking procedures: Those performed to excise the subcutaneous tissue (e.g., Charles procedure [Fig. E4], Thompson procedure, the modified Homans procedure [Fig. E5], and liposuction). Liposuction-circumferential suction-assisted lipectomy represents a newly proposed method to reduce morbidity involved in the traditional excisional techniques.

PEARLS & CONSIDERATIONS
- Lymphedema is a chronic, generally incurable but very manageable condition that requires lifelong care and attention along with psychosocial support.
- Children and adolescents (along with parents and adults) should be encouraged to pursue a normal life, participating in school activities and sports (preferably noncontact, such as swimming).
- Infections such as cellulitis should be treated promptly.
- If the etiology is filariasis caused by the parasites *Wuchereria bancrofti* or *Brugia malayi*, treatment is diethylcarbamazine citrate 5 mg/kg in divided doses for 3 wk.
- Patients with lymphedema commonly manifest psychiatric comorbidities as a result of their disease, such as anxiety; depression; adjustment problems; and difficulty in vocational, domestic, or social domains.
- Lymphedema can be complicated in rare cases by development of lymphangiosarcomata or other cutaneous malignancies.
- Gene therapy to develop new lymphangiosis in the affected body parts is a potential clinical remedy in the future.

SUGGESTED READING
Available at eBooks.Health.Elsevier.com.

RELATED CONTENT
Lymphedema (Patient Information)

AUTHORS: **FRANK G. FORT, MD, FACS, RPHS,** and **KATHRYN TAYLOR ANILOWSKI, MS, PT, CLT-LANA**

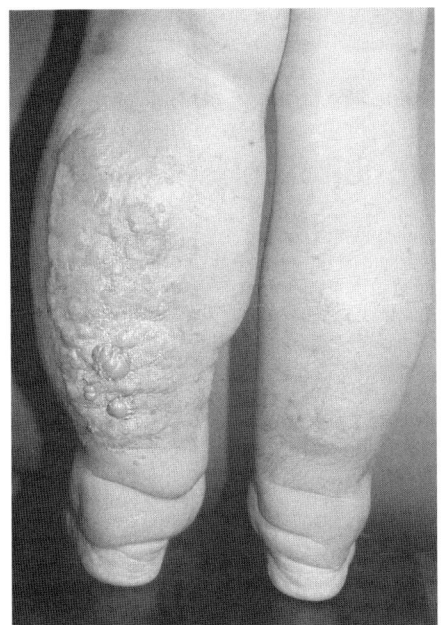

FIG. 2 Milroy disease. (Courtesy of Dr. Lawrence Lieblich. In James WD et al: *Andrews' diseases of the skin,* ed 12, Philadelphia, 2016, Elsevier.)

DIFFERENTIAL DIAGNOSIS
Other causes of edema that should be ruled out before treatment for lymphedema include cardiac, renal, hepatic, and thyroid dysfunction.

WORKUP
A detailed history and physical examination should help exclude most of the differential diagnoses.

LABORATORY TESTS
- Blood urea nitrogen, creatinine, liver function tests, albumin, urine analysis, and thyroid function tests are obtained to exclude possible systemic causes of edema.
- Genetic testing may be practical in defining a specific hereditary syndrome with a discrete gene mutation such as lymphedema distichiasis *(FOXC2),* Milroy disease *(VEGFR-3),* Meige disease, or Klippel-Trenaunay-Weber syndrome.

IMAGING STUDIES
- Lymphoscintigraphy: Diagnostic image of choice for lymphedema (if needed)
- Indocyanine green (ICG) fluorescent lymphography: Can now be used to identify sentinel nodes, to demonstrate superficial lymph channels and functional lymphatics, to indicate treatment pathways, and to confirm the effectiveness of therapeutic techniques
- MRI: Primarily used in tumor diagnosis
- Duplex ultrasound: Determines venous involvement in the edema
- Computed axial tomography (CAT): Distinguishes between fatty tissue and accumulations of protein-rich fluids
- Lymphography: Phased out in favor of less invasive techniques

Rx TREATMENT

NONPHARMACOLOGIC THERAPY
- Complete decongestive therapy (CDT) is backed by longstanding research and experience as the primary treatment of choice for lymphedema in both children and adults (Fig. E3). It should be delivered by a certified lymphedema therapist (CLT). CDT involves a two-phase treatment program:
  1. Phase 1—Reduce tissue congestion of affected body part with daily treatments:
     a. Manual lymph drainage
     b. Skin care
     c. Compression wrapping of limb
     d. Decongestive exercises
  2. Phase 2—Maintain decongestion with home maintenance program:
     a. Daily use of elastic and inelastic compression garments that are properly fitted according to circumference and length to prevent lymphedema from returning.
     b. Compression is graduated; most of the compression is distal with decreasing compression in the stocking proximally.
     c. Different knits and compression classes are available for different stages of lymphedema.
     d. Choices of garments include below-the-knee stockings, thigh-high stockings, pantyhose, sleeves, bras, and truncal garments.
- Massage (or any modality that increases blood flow) can have negative effects on lymphedema by increasing vasodilation. Therefore it is contraindicated on the lymphedematous quadrants.
- Compression pumps have not been found to be effective in removing proteins from lymphedematous quadrants.

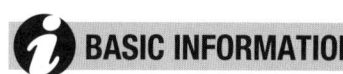
BASIC INFORMATION

DEFINITION

Malabsorption is the diminished intestinal absorption of dietary nutrients. The majority of malabsorption is due to either congenital or acquired defects in the membrane transport system, absorption, and brush border processing in the intestinal epithelium.

SYNONYM

Maldigestion

ICD-10CM CODES

K90.4	Malabsorption due to intolerance, not elsewhere classified
K90.89	Other intestinal malabsorption
K90.9	Intestinal malabsorption, unspecified
K91.2	Postsurgical malabsorption, not elsewhere classified

EPIDEMIOLOGY & DEMOGRAPHICS

PREDOMINANT SEX & AGE: More common in females, with a mean age of 40
RISK FACTORS:
- Excessive alcohol consumption
- History of celiac disease
- History of irritable bowel disease
- Intestinal surgery

GENETICS: HLA-DQ2 present in 95% of celiac disease

PHYSICAL FINDINGS & CLINICAL PRESENTATION

- Most commonly nonspecific symptoms such as abdominal flatulence and distention are seen.
- Due to the osmotic load from maldigestion/malabsorption, watery diarrhea may be present. In the case of fat digestive disorder, steatorrhea ensues.
- Weight loss is very common, but many patients are able to compensate by increased caloric load. Diffuse disease often has much more pronounced weight loss.
- Chronic protein malabsorption can cause hypoalbuminemia, leading to edema and ascites.
- Both microcytic and macrocytic anemia can result from micronutrient deficiency (iron/B_{12}). These patients can be pale and present with fatigue.
- Bleeding disorders from vitamin K deficiency can lead to ecchymosis, melena, and hematuria.
- Vitamin D deficiency can lead to bone disorders. Secondary hyperparathyroidism can be a presenting feature.
- Electrolyte and vitamin deficiency can lead to neurologic disorders such as ataxia, weakness, and neuropathy, and may have positive Chvostek or Trousseau sign.
- Autoimmune disease-specific dermatologic findings such as alopecia, pellagra, erythema nodosum, pyoderma gangrenosum, cheilosis, glossitis, and aphthous ulcers may be present.
- Cardinal clinical features of specific malabsorptive disorders are summarized in Table 1.

ETIOLOGY

- Can be congenital or acquired.
- Disease-specific etiology. Mechanisms of malabsorption, malabsorbed substrates, and representative causes are summarized in Table 2.

DIAGNOSIS

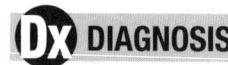

DIFFERENTIAL DIAGNOSIS

- Crohn disease
- Celiac disease

TABLE 1   Cardinal Clinical Features of Specific Malabsorptive Disorders

Disorder	Cardinal Clinical Features
Adrenal insufficiency	Skin darkening, hyponatremia, hyperkalemia
Amyloidosis	Renal disease, nephrotic syndrome, cardiomyopathy, neuropathy, carpal tunnel syndrome, macroglossia, hepatosplenomegaly
Bile acid deficiency	Ileal resection or disease, liver disease
Carcinoid syndrome	Flushing, cardiac murmur
Celiac disease	Variable symptoms: Dermatitis herpetiformis, alopecia, aphthous mouth ulcers, arthropathy, neurologic symptoms, and (life-threatening) malnutrition; elevated liver biochemical test levels, mild iron deficiency
Crohn disease	Arthritis, aphthous mouth ulcers, episcleritis, uveitis, pyoderma gangrenosum, erythema nodosum, abdominal mass, fistulas, perianal fistulae, primary sclerosing cholangitis (PSC), laboratory signs of inflammation
CF	Chronic sinopulmonary disease, meconium ileus, distal intestinal obstruction syndrome (DIOS), elevated sweat chloride
Cystinuria, Hartnup disease	Kidney stones, dermatosis
Diabetes mellitus	Long history of diabetes and diabetic complications
Disaccharidase deficiency	Bloating and cramping, intermittent diarrhea
GI fistulas	Previous intestinal surgery or trauma, Crohn disease
Glucagonoma	Migratory necrolytic erythema, enlarged gallbladder
Hyperthyroidism, hypothyroidism	Symptoms and signs of thyroid disease
Hypogammaglobulinemia	Recurrent infections
Intestinal ischemia	Other ischemic organ manifestations; abdominal pain with eating (chronic mesenteric ischemia)
Lymphoma	Enlarged mesenteric or retroperitoneal lymph nodes, abdominal mass, abdominal pain, fever
Mastocytosis	Urticaria pigmentosum, peptic ulcer
Mycobacterium avium complex infection	AIDS
Pancreatic insufficiency	History of pancreatitis, abdominal pain, or alcoholism; large-volume fatty, oily stools; passage of orange oil
Parasitic infection	History of travel to endemic areas
PBC	Jaundice, itching
Scleroderma	Dysphagia, inability to open the mouth widely, Raynaud phenomenon, skin tightening
SIBO	Previous intestinal surgery, motility disorder (scleroderma, pseudo-obstruction), small intestinal diverticula, strictures
Tropical sprue	History of travel to endemic area
Tuberculosis	Specific history of exposure, living in or travel to endemic area, immunosuppression, abdominal mass or intestinal obstruction, ascites
Whipple disease	Lymphadenopathy, fever, arthritis, cerebral symptoms, heart murmur (pulmonary valve), oculomasticatory myorhythmia
ZES	Peptic ulcers, diarrhea

AIDS, Acquired immunodeficiency syndrome; *CF,* cystic fibrosis; *GI,* gastrointestinal; *PBC,* primary biliary cholangitis; *SIBO,* small intestinal bacterial overgrowth; *ZES,* Zollinger-Ellison syndrome.
From Feldman M et al: *Sleisenger and Fordtran's gastrointestinal and liver disease,* ed 10, Philadelphia, 2016, Elsevier.

TABLE 2 Mechanisms of Malabsorption, Malabsorbed Substrates, and Representative Causes

Pathophysiologic Mechanism	Malabsorbed Substrate(s)	Representative Causes
Maldigestion		
Conjugated bile acid deficiency	Fat Fat-soluble vitamins Calcium Magnesium	Hepatic parenchymal disease Biliary obstruction SIBO with bile acid deconjugation Ileal bile acid malabsorption CCK deficiency
Pancreatic insufficiency	Fat Protein Carbohydrate Fat-soluble vitamins Vitamin B_{12} (cobalamin)	Congenital defects Chronic pancreatitis Pancreatic tumors Inactivation of pancreatic enzymes (e.g., ZES)
Reduced mucosal digestion	Carbohydrate Protein	Congenital defects Acquired lactase deficiency Generalized mucosal disease (e.g., celiac disease, Crohn disease)
Intraluminal consumption of nutrients	Vitamin B_{12} (cobalamin)	SIBO Helminthic infections (e.g., *Diphyllobothrium latum* infection)
Malabsorption		
Reduced mucosal absorption	Fat Protein Carbohydrate Vitamins Minerals	Congenital transport defects Generalized mucosal diseases (e.g., celiac disease, Crohn disease) Previous intestinal resection or bypass Infections Intestinal lymphoma
Decreased transport from the intestine	Fat Protein	Intestinal lymphangiectasia Primary Secondary (e.g., solid tumors, Whipple disease, lymphomas) Venous stasis (e.g., from heart failure)
Other Mechanisms		
Decreased gastric acid and/or intrinsic factor secretion	Vitamin B_{12}	Pernicious anemia Atrophic gastritis Previous gastric resection
Decreased gastric mixing and/or rapid gastric emptying	Fat Calcium Protein	Previous gastric resection Autonomic neuropathy
Rapid intestinal transit	Fat	Autonomic neuropathy Hyperthyroidism

CCK, Cholecystokinin; *SIBO,* small intestinal bacterial overgrowth; *ZES,* Zollinger-Ellison syndrome.
From Feldman M et al: *Sleisenger and Fordtran's gastrointestinal and liver disease,* ed 10, Philadelphia, 2016, Elsevier.

- Hartnup disease
- Chronic pancreatitis
- Pancreatic insufficiency
- Cystic fibrosis
- Short bowel syndrome
- Neoplasm
- Abetalipoproteinemia
- Lactose intolerance
- Small intestine bacterial overgrowth
- Chronic atrophic gastritis
- Zollinger-Ellison syndrome
- Chronic cholestasis
- Cirrhosis

WORKUP

- A detailed history including alcohol consumption and surgical history as well as autoimmune disease can help diagnose the underlying disease. It is important to screen for anemia and electrolyte abnormalities due to malabsorption.
- Table E3 summarizes malabsorptive diseases or conditions in which noninvasive tests can establish malabsorption or provide a diagnosis.

LABORATORY TESTS

- CBC, serum iron, vitamin B_{12}, and folate to detect for anemia.
- **Prothrombin time:** Elevated prothrombin time can suggest vitamin K deficiency.
- **Fat malabsorption:** The gold standard is the 72-h stool elastase or fat collection. More than 6/g day in the stool is pathologic. This test can be cumbersome, so other options are available. Sudan III stain and acid steatocrit tests are qualitative measures of steatorrhea. Serologic testing for celiac disease should be considered as well.
- **Carbohydrate malabsorption:** Carbohydrate malabsorption leads to fermentation of the undigested carbohydrates by intestinal bacteria.
- The urinary D-xylose test for carbohydrate absorption in the small intestine. After loading with D-xylose, urinary D-xylose levels are measured. Low levels suggest intestinal malabsorption.
- Lactose intolerance can be tested by the lactose tolerance test or the breath test. The lactose tolerance test measures blood glucose after lactose administration. Development of symptoms or inadequate increase in blood sugar is indicative of lactose intolerance. H_2/CO_2 breath tests using specific forms of carbohydrates can detect malabsorption as well.
- **Protein malabsorption:** Protein malabsorption is likely due to small intestinal bacterial overgrowth or protein gastroenteropathies. Alpha-1 antitrypsin clearance or 99mTc-albumin gamma camera scintigraphy may aid in this diagnosis.
- **Pancreatic insufficiency:** Fecal elastase and chymotrypsin levels can distinguish from pancreatic and intestinal causes.
- **Vitamin deficiency:** It is important to assess serum vitamin B_{12} and methylmalonic acid levels. Schilling test is rarely used but can be useful in some cases.
- **Bile acid malabsorption:** Quantitative stool bile acid measurement is the preferred method of diagnosis. SeHCAT test (selenium homocholic acid taurine test) is another option but less likely used.
- **Bacterial overgrowth:** This can be detected with endoscopic jejunal aspirate culture or a less invasive hydrogen breath test.
- Table 4 summarizes useful laboratory tests for evaluating patients with suspected malabsorption and for establishing possible nutrient deficiencies.

IMAGING STUDIES

- Abdominal ultrasound can identify thickened small bowel wall
- Endoscopy for visualization and biopsy
- Small bowel follow through
- Abdominal computed tomography/MRI
- Endoscopic retrograde cholangiopancreatography/magnetic resonance cholangiopancreatography/endoscopic ultrasound for identification of pancreatic abnormalities
- Capsule endoscopy

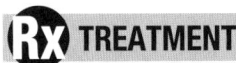 **TREATMENT**

Involves identification and treatment of the underlying illness, treatment of diarrhea, and nutritional repletion

NONPHARMACOLOGIC THERAPY

- A gluten-free diet in patients with celiac disease. Avoidance of lactose-containing product in lactose intolerance.
- Avoidance of caffeine and high sugar containing compounds has been found to decrease diarrhea in some cases.

ACUTE GENERAL Rx

- Control of the underlying disease should be primary goal.
- It is also essential to control any volume and electrolyte abnormalities that might exist.

TABLE 4   Useful Laboratory Tests for Patients With Suspected Malabsorption and for Establishing Possible Nutrient Deficiencies

Test	Comment(s)
Blood Cell Count	
Hematocrit, hemoglobin	Decreased in iron, vitamin B_{12}, and folate malabsorption or with blood loss
Mean corpuscular hemoglobin or mean corpuscular volume	Decreased in iron malabsorption; increased in folate and vitamin B_{12} malabsorption
White blood cells, differential	Decreased in vitamin B_{12} and folate malabsorption; low lymphocyte count in lymphangiectasia
Biochemical Tests (Serum)	
TGs	Decreased in severe fat malabsorption
Cholesterol	Decreased in bile acid malabsorption or severe fat malabsorption
Albumin	Decreased in severe malnutrition, lymphangiectasia, protein-losing enteropathy
Alkaline phosphatase	Increased in calcium and vitamin D malabsorption (severe steatorrhea); decreased in zinc deficiency
Calcium, phosphorus, magnesium	Decreased in extensive small intestinal mucosal disease, after extensive intestinal resection, or in vitamin D deficiency
Zinc	Decreased in extensive small intestinal mucosal disease or intestinal resection
Iron, ferritin	Decreased in celiac disease, in other extensive small intestinal mucosal diseases, and with chronic blood loss
Other Serum Tests	
Prothrombin time	Prolonged in vitamin K malabsorption
β-Carotene	Decreased in fat malabsorption from hepatobiliary or intestinal diseases
Immunoglobulins	Decreased in lymphangiectasia, diffuse lymphoma
Folic acid	Decreased in extensive small intestinal mucosal diseases, with anticonvulsant use, in pregnancy; may be increased in SIBO
Vitamin B_{12}	Decreased after gastrectomy, in pernicious anemia, terminal ileal disease, SIBO, and infection with *Diphyllobothrium latum*
Methylmalonic acid	Markedly elevated in vitamin B_{12} deficiency
Homocysteine	Markedly elevated in vitamin B_{12} or folate deficiency
Citrulline	May be decreased in destructive small intestinal mucosal disease or intestinal resection
Stool Tests	
Fat	Qualitative or quantitative increase in fat malabsorption
Elastase, chymotrypsin	Decreased concentrations and output in exocrine pancreatic insufficiency
pH	Less than 5.5 in carbohydrate malabsorption

SIBO, Small intestinal bacterial overgrowth; *TGs,* thyroglobulins.
From Feldman M et al: *Sleisenger and Fordtran's gastrointestinal and liver disease,* ed 10, Philadelphia, 2016, Elsevier.

CHRONIC Rx

- Control of chronic diarrhea with loperamide should be one of the goals in a chronic malabsorptive state.
- Correction of volume and electrolyte disturbance with oral rehydration therapy should be made a priority.
- Bile acid conjugates can decrease steatorrhea in some cases.
- Pancreatic insufficiency is typically treated with a low-fat diet and exogenous pancreatic enzymes.
- Teduglutide-homolog of GLP-2 has been shown to increase absorptive surface area in short bowel syndrome.
- Periodic DEXA scans are indicated in chronic malabsorption in the setting of vitamin D deficiency.

- Oral supplementation with vitamins and minerals is important, sometimes requiring parenteral therapy.

REFERRAL

- Gastroenterology consultation can help in diagnosis when initial laboratory testing is unclear.
- Nutrition consultation can help patients with diet modification to alleviate symptoms.

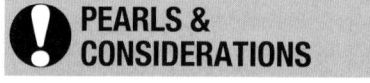 **PEARLS & CONSIDERATIONS**

COMMENTS

- Malabsorption should be considered a sign of an underlying disease.

- Treatment should focus on treating the underlying disorder.
- Nutrient and volume repletion should be priority in any treatment plan of malabsorption.

RELATED CONTENT

Celiac Disease (Related Key Topic)
Crohn Disease (Related Key Topic)
Cystic Fibrosis (Related Key Topic)
Irritable Bowel Syndrome (Related Key Topic)
Lactose Intolerance (Related Key Topic)
Chronic Pancreatitis (Related Key Topic)
Short Bowel Syndrome (Related Key Topic)
Small Bowel Intestinal Bacterial Overgrowth (Related Key Topic)
Ulcerative Colitis (Related Key Topic)

AUTHOR: **FRED F. FERRI, MD**

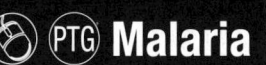

BASIC INFORMATION

DEFINITION

Malaria is a protozoan disease caused by intra-erythrocytic protozoa of the genus *Plasmodium* and transmitted by female *Anopheles* spp. mosquitoes. It is endemic throughout most of the tropics and is characterized by hectic fever and often presents with classic malarial paroxysm. Five species of genus *Plasmodium* usually infect humans (Table 1):

- *P. falciparum*
- *P. vivax*
- *P. malariae*
- *P. ovale*
- *P. knowlesi*

SYNONYMS

Periodic fever
Tertian malaria
Quartan malaria
Tropical splenomegaly

ICD-10CM CODES

B50.9 *Plasmodium falciparum* malaria, unspecified
B51.9 *Plasmodium vivax* malaria without complications
B52.9 *Plasmodium malariae* malaria without complications
B53.0 *Plasmodium ovale* malaria
B53.8 Other parasitologically confirmed malaria, not elsewhere classified
B54 Unspecified malaria

EPIDEMIOLOGY & DEMOGRAPHICS

GLOBAL:

- Approximately 219 million cases in 2018 in more than 100 countries (Fig. E1)
- Approximately 405,000 deaths in 2018, with more than 80% of the deaths occurring in children of sub-Saharan Africa
- Three billion people live in malaria-endemic areas

U.S.:

- 2078 cases reported to the Centers for Disease Control and Prevention (CDC) in the U.S. in 2017 (Fig. E2). In the majority of reported cases, U.S. civilians who acquired infection abroad had not adhered to a chemoprophylaxis regimen that was appropriate for the country in which they acquired malaria
- More than 50% of the reported cases in the U.S. are *P. falciparum*. On average, there are six deaths per year in the U.S.
- Most infections limited to:
  1. Immigrant population
  2. Returned travelers or troops from endemic area
- Occasionally, transmission through exposure to infected blood product or shared intravenous needles by users of injection drugs
- Congenital transmission possible
- Local mosquito-borne transmission reported
- Competent mosquito vectors present
  1. *A. albimanus* in Eastern U.S.
  2. *A. freeborni* in Western U.S.

GEOGRAPHIC DISTRIBUTION:

- *P. falciparum:* Sub-Saharan Africa, Papua New Guinea, Solomon Islands, Haiti, Indian subcontinent
- *P. vivax:* Central America, South America, North Africa, Middle East, Indian subcontinent
- *P. ovale:* West Africa
- *P. malariae:* Worldwide
- *P. knowlesi:* Southeast Asia

PARASITE LIFE CYCLE (FIG. E3):

- Human infection begins when a female anopheline mosquito bites (only female anopheline mosquito takes blood meal) and inoculates plasmodial sporozoites into bloodstream. The bite usually occurs between dusk and dawn.
- The sporozoites then travel to the liver and invade the hepatocytes.
- In the hepatocytes, the sporozoites mature to tissue schizonts or become dormant hypnozoites.

- The tissue schizonts amplify the infection by producing a large number of merozoites (10,000 to 30,000).
- Each merozoite is capable of invading an RBC and can establish the asexual cycle of replication in RBCs.
- Asexual cycles produce and release 24 to 32 merozoites at the end of 48- or 72-h (*P. malariae*) cycles.
- The hypnozoites are only found in relapsing malaria *P. vivax* or *P. ovale* and may remain dormant for up to 5 yr.
- Eventually some intraerythrocytic parasites develop into gametocytes. Male and female gametocytes are taken up by a female anopheline mosquito with a blood meal where they fertilize in the mosquito gut to produce a diploid zygote that matures to an ookinete; haploid sporozoites are generated that migrate to the salivary gland of the mosquito to infect another human.

PHYSICAL FINDINGS & CLINICAL PRESENTATION

- Fever is the hallmark of malaria, known as malarial paroxysm, initially daily until synchronization of infection after several weeks, when fever may occur every other day (tertian) in *P. vivax, P. ovale,* or *P. falciparum* malaria or every third day (quartan) in *P. malariae* malaria. Table 2 describes the WHO criteria for severe malaria.
- Classic malarial paroxysm characterized by:
  1. Cold stage: Abrupt onset of cold feeling associated with rigors, shakes
  2. Hot stage: High fever ($\sim 40^\circ$ C; 104° F) associated with restlessness
  3. Sweating stage: Patient defervesces
- Nonspecific symptoms are:
  1. Headache
  2. Cough
  3. Myalgia
  4. Vomiting
  5. Diarrhea
  6. Jaundice

TABLE 1 Characteristics of the *Plasmodium* Species Responsible for Human Malaria

Characteristic	SPECIES				
	P. falciparum	*P. vivax*	*P. ovale*	*P. malariae*	*P. knowlesi*
Incubation period in days (range)	12 (8-25)	14 (8-27)	17 (15 to ≥18)	28 (15 to ≥40)	11 (9 to >12)
Periodicity of febrile attacks (hours)	None	48	48	72	24
Earliest appearance of gametocytes (days)	10	3	?	?	?
Relapse	No	Yes	Yes	No	No
Duration of untreated infection (years)	1-2	1.5-4	1.5-4	3-50	?
RBC preference	Younger cells (but can invade cells of all ages)	Reticulocytes	Reticulocytes	Older cells	?
Characteristic morphology	Ring forms	Schüffner dots	Schüffner dots	Normal-sized cells	Ring forms
	Multiply infected cells	Enlarged RBCs	Enlarged RBCs	Band or rectangular forms of trophozoites	Occasional multiply infected cells
	Banana-shaped gametocytes				Band forms

RBC, Red blood cell.
From Cherry JD et al: *Feigin and Cherry's textbook of pediatric infectious diseases,* ed 8, Philadelphia, 2019, Elsevier.

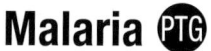

TABLE 2 World Health Organization Criteria for Severe Malaria, 2000

Impaired consciousness
Prostration
Respiratory distress
Multiple seizures
Jaundice
Hemoglobinuria
Abnormal bleeding
Severe anemia
Circulatory collapse
Pulmonary edema

From Kliegman RM et al: *Nelson textbook of pediatrics*, ed 19, Philadelphia, 2011, Saunders.

- *P. falciparum:*
  1. Most pathogenic of the four species.
  2. Rapidly progresses to high-level parasitemia.
  3. Important cause of the fatal malaria.
  4. Classic malarial paroxysm is usually absent.
  5. Incubation period after exposure is 12 days (range: 9 to 60 days).
  6. Cytoadherence and resetting of RBCs play central role in pathogenesis.
  7. The sequestration of RBCs in vital organs leads to fatal complications.
  8. Cerebral malaria is a feared complication.
  9. Invades erythrocytes of all ages.
  10. Lacks hypnozoites (intrahepatic stage), does not relapse.
  11. Blood smear usually shows ring form only.
  12. Pigment color is black.
  13. Banana-shaped gametocytes; if seen in blood, smear is diagnostic.
  14. Chloroquine resistance is widely present.
- *P. vivax:*
  1. Known as tertian malaria: Fever occurs every other day.
  2. Duffy blood-group antigen FYA- or FYB-related receptor is needed for attachment to RBC.
  3. FyFy phenotype (most West African) individuals are resistant to *P. vivax* malaria.
  4. Incubation period after exposure is 14 days (range: 8 to 27 days).
  5. Hypnozoites may cause relapse of infection after years.
  6. Infects mainly reticulocytes.
  7. Irregularly shaped large rings and trophozoites, enlarged RBCs, and Schüffner dots are seen in peripheral blood smear.
  8. Pigment color is yellow-brown.
  9. *P. vivax* from Papua New Guinea has reduced sensitivity to chloroquine.
  10. Primaquine is needed to eradicate the hypnozoites.
- *P. ovale:*
  1. Also known as tertian malaria; fever occurs every other day.

2. Occurs mainly in tropical Africa.
3. Incubation period after exposure is 14 days (range: 8 to 27 days).
4. Hypnozoites may cause relapse of infection.
5. Infects mainly reticulocytes.
6. Infected RBC is seen as enlarged, oval shape containing large ring or trophozoites with Schüffner dots.
7. Pigment color is dark brown.
8. Primaquine needed to eradicate the hypnozoites.
9. No chloroquine resistance has been encountered.
- *P. malariae:*
  1. Known as quartan malaria; fever occurs every third day.
  2. Common cause of chronic malarial infection.
  3. May persist for 20 to 30 yr after leaving the endemic area.
  4. Worldwide distribution.
  5. Incubation period after exposure is 30 days (range: 16 to 60 days).
  6. Lacks hypnozoites (intrahepatic stage).
  7. May persist in blood for many years if treated inadequately.
  8. Chronic infection may cause soluble immune-complex, resulting in nephritic syndrome.
  9. Infects mainly mature RBCs.
  10. Band or rectangular forms of trophozoites are commonly seen in peripheral blood smear.
  11. Pigment color is brown-black.
- *Cerebral malaria:*
  1. Feared complication of *P. falciparum* infection.
  2. Mortality is ~20%.
  3. Pathogenesis is poorly understood.
  4. Ischemia as a result of sequestration of parasites or cytokines induced by parasite toxin(s) is the key debate.
  5. Seizure and altered mental status leading to coma are cardinal manifestation.
  6. Hypoglycemia, lactic acidosis, and elevated circulating tumor necrosis factor alpha (TNF-α) may be present.
  7. CSF studies: No increase of WBC count or protein, raised lactate concentrate, and increased opening pressure, especially in children, may be present.

DX DIAGNOSIS

DIFFERENTIAL DIAGNOSIS
- Typhoid fever
- Dengue fever
- Yellow fever
- Viral hepatitis
- Influenza
- Brucellosis
- Urinary tract infection
- Leishmaniasis
- Trypanosomiasis
- Rickettsial diseases
- Leptospirosis
- Table 3 summarizes the differential diagnosis of uncomplicated malaria

WORKUP
- Clinical diagnosis is notoriously inaccurate.
- Demonstration of malarial parasites in blood smear is essential.
- Newer molecular diagnostic techniques (polymerase chain reaction, rapid diagnostic tests) are promising (Table 4).

LABORATORY TESTS
- The thick and thin blood film is required to identify malarial parasites (Fig. E4). A Giemsa-stained film of the patient's peripheral blood should be examined for parasites as soon as possible.
- The thick smears are more sensitive and primarily used to detect the presence of parasites.
- The thin smears are used for species differentiation and parasite density estimation.
- A patient who is suspected of having malaria but who has no parasite seen in blood smears should have blood smears repeated every 12 to 24 h for 3 consecutive days.

PREPARATION OF BLOOD SMEAR:
- Must be prepared from fresh blood obtained by pricking the finger.
- The thin smear is fixed in methanol before staining.
- The thick smear is stained unfixed.
- The smear should be stained with a 3% Giemsa solution (pH of 7.2) for 30 to 45 min.
- The parasite density should be estimated by counting the percentage of RBCs infected, not the number of parasites, under an oil immersion lens on thin film.

COMMON ERRORS IN READING MALARIAL SMEARS:
- Platelets overlying an RBC
- Misreading artifacts as parasites
- Concern about missing a positive slide

MOLECULAR DIAGNOSIS OF MALARIA:
- Rapid diagnostic tests (RDT):
  1. Employ immunochromatographic lateral flow technology for antigen detection.
  2. Thus far only one RDT has been FDA approved: BinaxNOW Malaria test kit.
  3. This kit is based on antigens histidine-rich protein-2 (HRP-2) and aldolase.
  4. For *P. falciparum*: Sensitivity 95% and specificity 94%.
  5. For *P. vivax*: Sensitivity 69% and specificity 100%.
- Limitations of the BinaxNOW Malaria test:
  1. Not approved for mixed infections.
  2. Should not be used for *P. malariae* and *P. ovale* as data are limited.
  3. Positive test must be confirmed by microscopy.
  4. Negative results require confirmation by thick and thin smears.
  5. This test cannot be used to monitor therapy as antigen persists after the elimination of the parasite, causing false positives.
- Other diagnostic tests available include:
  1. Tagged monoclonal antibodies for malaria antigen detection.
  2. Nucleic acid amplification and detection: Polymerase chain reaction (PCR) can detect

TABLE 3 Differential Diagnosis of Uncomplicated Malaria*

	Symptoms	Physical Examination	Laboratory Tests	Geography
Malaria	Fever Nonspecific myalgias, arthralgias, malaise, nausea, vomiting	Hepatomegaly Splenomegaly	Malaria smear positive Thrombocytopenia Hyperbilirubinemia	Primarily tropical areas
Viral syndromes (flu, pneumonia, early gastroenteritis)	Fever Nonspecific myalgias, arthralgias, malaise Nausea, vomiting	Lymphadenopathy	Low white cell count, lymphocyte predominant	Worldwide, frequently seen in local epidemics
Bacterial pneumonia	Fever Productive cough	Tachypnea Increased respiratory effort (intercostal and subcostal recession, use of accessory muscles) Crepitations (rales) Decreased oxygen saturation (<90%)	Leukocytosis	Worldwide
Meningitis (bacterial or viral)	Fever Altered mental status	Neck stiffness	Concomitant parasitemia uncommon in bacterial meningitis WBCs in CSF (>5-10/μl, or >10 times higher than the predicted CSF WBC count[†])	Worldwide
Dengue	Retro-orbital pain Pain/tenderness of the extraocular eye muscles, particularly on extreme lateral gaze	Skin rash develops in at least 50% by day 2-3	Leukopenia Thrombocytopenia	Less common in sub-Saharan Africa
Leptospirosis	Fever, headache, dry cough, shaking, chills, nausea, vomiting, diarrhea, muscle pain, abdominal pain	Muscle tenderness (myositis), conjunctivitis, hepatosplenomegaly	Elevated creatinine kinase, abnormal urine sediment, proteinuria, normal to elevated WBC counts	Worldwide distribution Association with freshwater exposure
Typhus	High fever, dry cough, low back pain, headache, nausea, vomiting, abdominal pain, diarrhea, nausea, chills, delirium, photophobia, myalgia	Rash begins on the chest and spreads to the rest of the body (except the palms of the hands and soles of the feet) The early rash is a light rose color and fades when pressed Later, the rash becomes dull and red and does not fade People with severe typhus may also develop petechiae	Anemia Thrombocytopenia Twofold to fivefold elevation of liver enzymes	Worldwide distribution, murine typhus (Rickettsia typhi) seen in areas of poor hygiene and cold temperatures Epidemic typhus (Rickettsia prowzekii) associated with exposure to rat fleas or rat feces
Viral hemorrhagic fevers	Fever, bleeding diathesis, malaise, fatigue, myalgias, headache, vomiting, diarrhea, hypotension, shock	Flushing of the face and chest, frank bleeding, ecchymoses, renal failure, edema	Cytopenias seen early in illness with elevated WBC seen in late disease, coagulation abnormalities	Worldwide distribution and caused by several families of RNA viruses

*Individual patients may have more than one diagnosis.
[†]Predicted CSF WBC count/μl = CSF RBC count × (peripheral blood WBC count ÷ peripheral blood RBC count).
CSF, Cerebrospinal fluid; *RBC,* red blood cell; *RNA,* ribonucleic acid; *WBC,* white blood cell.
From Ryan ET: *Hunter's tropical medicine and emerging infectious diseases,* ed 10, Philadelphia, 2020, Elsevier.

parasites down to a level of one to five parasites per microliter of blood. PCR can detect mixed species infection and is now considered the gold standard for diagnosis.
3. Fluorescence microscopy with acridine orange or other staining.
4. Dark field microscopy.

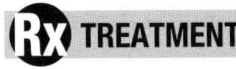 **TREATMENT**

NONPHARMACOLOGIC THERAPY
ANTIMOSQUITO MEASURES:
- Eradication of mosquito breeding places by chemical spray
- Use of mosquito nets properly in the endemic areas
- Use of protective clothing
- Use of insect spray (permethrin), mosquito coils, or repellents such as diethyltoluamide

(DEET). For adults, DEET (30% to 50%) is generally protective for at least 4 hr. For smaller children, use DEET at ≤20% concentration

ACUTE GENERAL Rx
A definitive diagnosis of malaria is essential for specific antimalarial chemotherapy.
UNCOMPLICATED CHLOROQUINE-SENSITIVE PLASMODIUM VIVAX, PLASMODIUM OVALE, OR PLASMODIUM MALARIAE (NON-FALCIPARUM MALARIA):
- Chloroquine:
  1. Adults: 600 mg base (= 1000 mg salt) orally immediately, followed by 300 mg base (= 500 mg salt) orally at 6, 24, and 48 h.
  2. Children: 10 mg base/kg orally immediately, followed by 5 mg base/kg orally at 6, 24, and 48 h.
  3. Maximum total dose: 1500 mg base (= 2500 mg salt).

  4. An alternative agent is hydroxychloroquine (Plaquenil): 620 mg base (= 800 mg salt) orally immediately, followed by 310 mg base (= 400 mg salt) orally at 6, 24, and 48 h.
- In the case of *P. vivax* and *P. ovale*, treatment with primaquine 15 mg daily for 14 days is needed to eradicate the exoerythrocytic forms, especially the hypnozoites responsible for relapses.
- G6PD should be measured before primaquine is given. Primaquine is not recommended for those who are glucose-6-phosphate dehydrogenase deficient, because primaquine can cause hemolysis and even death in G6PD-deficient persons. Normal G6PD levels must be documented before using primaquine for either chemoprophylaxis or treatment.
- Chloroquine-resistant *P. vivax* has been documented; in that case use quinine sulfate

TABLE 4 Malaria Rapid Diagnostic Tests Available in the U.S.[a]

RDT Name	Malaria Antigen Target	Malaria Species Detected	Sensitivity	Comment
BinaxNOW	HRP-2 and aldolase	P. falciparum, P. vivax, P. malariae, and P. ovale	94% for P. falciparum 84% for non-P. falciparum 87% for pure P. vivax infections 62% for pure P. ovale and P. malariae infections	Sensitivity increased to 96% for pure P. falciparum infection Overall specificity of 99% FDA-approved for use in the U.S.
ParaSight F	HRP-2	P. falciparum	96.5%-100% in Kenya when >60 parasites/μL, lower with less parasitemia 40% in travelers when <50 parasites/μL, >93% when >100 parasites/μL	Antigen persists for 6-7 days 6 in 11.9%-20% of subjects whose blood smears had cleared Not FDA approved for use in the U.S.
ICT Malaria Pf/Pv	HRP-2 and aldolase	P. falciparum and P. vivax	97% for P. falciparum 44% for P. vivax	Specificity of 90% for P. falciparum Specificity of 100% for P. vivax Not FDA-approved for use in the U.S.
OptiMAL-IT	LDH	P. falciparum, P. vivax, P. malariae, and P. ovale	85%-95%; decreased with lower parasite density	Specificity of 100% P. falciparum, 75%-85% for P. vivax Not FDA approved for use in the U.S.
Clearview	LDH	P. falciparum, P. vivax, P. malariae, and P. ovale	93% specificity of 100%, with sensitivities of 99%, 90.0%, 86%, and 60%, respectively, for P. falciparum, P. vivax, P. malariae, and P. ovale	Specificity of 100% for P. falciparum, 99% for P. vivax, 90% for P. malariae, and 60% for P. ovale Not FDA-approved for use in the U.S.

[a]Direct microscopy should be performed where available with a negative RDT, given higher false-negative rates with low parasitemia, and when severe malaria is suspected.
FDA, Food and Drug Administration; *HRP-2,* histidine-rich protein-2; *ICT,* immunochromatographic diagnostic test; *LDH,* lactate dehydrogenase; *RDT,* rapid diagnostic test.
From Cherry JD et al: *Feigin and Cherry's textbook of pediatric infectious diseases,* ed 8, Philadelphia, 2019, Elsevier.

(10 mg/kg) plus either tetracycline or doxycycline or clindamycin for 7 days.

UNCOMPLICATED FALCIPARUM MALARIA OR SPECIES NOT IDENTIFIED:
- Chloroquine can be used cautiously for falciparum malaria acquired in chloroquine-sensitive areas (chloroquine is more rapidly effective than quinine).
- For uncomplicated *P. falciparum,* an oral artemisinin combination therapy (ACT), is recommended by the CDC as the first-line agent. While there are numerous ACT combinations, the only ACT approved in the U.S. is artemether-lumefantrine (Coartem), which is not widely available. Do not delay therapy in trying to obtain it; use another first-line agent. Dosage for adults: 4 tablets artemether-lumefantrine (20/120 mg) as a single dose, then 4 tablets again after 8 h, then 4 tablets q12h for 2 days (take with food). Can cause prolongation of QT interval. Not recommended in infants <5 kg. Dose dependent on weight in children:
  1. 5 to 15 kg: 1 tablet (20/120 mg) as a single dose, then 1 tablet again after 8 h, then 1 tablet q12h for 2 days
  2. 16 to 25 kg: 2 tablets (40/240 mg) as a single dose, then 2 tablets again after 8 h, then 2 tablets q12h for 2 days
  3. 26 to 35 kg: 3 tablets (60/360 mg) as a single dose, then 3 tablets again after 8 hr, then 3 tablets q12h for 2 days
  4. >35 kg: Treat as adult
- Atovaquone-proguanil (Malarone): 250 mg atovaquone/100 mg proguanil: 4 adult tabs PO once a day for 3 days with food. Pediatric dosage: Pediatric tablets (62.5 mg atovaquone/25 mg proguanil) are used based on weight:
  1. 5 to 8 kg: 2 pediatric tabs PO once daily for 3 days

  2. 9 to 10 kg: 3 pediatric tabs PO once daily for 3 days
  3. 11 to 20 kg: 1 adult tab PO once daily for 3 days
  4. 21 to 30 kg: 2 adult tabs PO once daily for 3 days
  5. 31 to 40 kg: 3 adult tabs PO once daily for 3 days
  6. >40 kg: 4 adult tabs PO once daily for 3 days
- Another first-line option for treatment in adults is oral quinine sulfate 10 mg (salt)/kg (usually 650 mg) q8h for 3 to 7 days plus doxycycline 100 mg PO bid, both for 7 days. Pediatric dosage: Quinine sulfate 10 mg/kg PO tid plus clindamycin 20 mg/kg per day divided tid, both for 7 days.
- Table 5 summarizes some treatment guidelines for severe *Plasmodium falciparum* malaria.

ALTERNATIVES:
- Quinine sulfate plus clindamycin 900 mg tid for 7 days in adults.
- Mefloquine 750 mg PO, then 500 mg PO 6 to 12 h later in adults.
- Atovaquone-proguanil (Malarone) or quinine sulfate plus doxycycline can be used when species is unknown. Artemether-lumefantrine is also recommended by the World Health Organization (WHO) for treatment of unknown species, but in U.S. is approved only for *P. falciparum,*
- Other ACT combinations not yet available in the U.S: Artesunate-amodiaquine, artesunate-mefloquine, artesunate-sulfadoxine-pyrimethamine, dihydroartemisinin-piperaquine, artesunate-pyronaridine tetraphosphate.

NOTE: Parasitemia may paradoxically rise in the first 24 to 36 h and is not an indication of treatment failure.

SEVERE FALCIPARUM MALARIA:
- It is a medical emergency; intensive care is preferred. Features of complicated malaria are summarized in Table 6.
- Measurement of blood glucose, lactate, ABG is important.
- IV quinidine gluconate 10 mg salt/kg loading dose (maximum 600 mg) in normal saline (NS); infuse slowly over 1 to 2 h, followed by continuous infusion of 0.02 mg/kg/min until patient can swallow.
- Need to monitor ECG for observation of QT interval as can prolong. Also need to monitor blood pressure and glucose to avoid hypoglycemia.
- Alternatively, IV artesunate: 2.4 mg/kg IV at hour 0, then at 12 and 24 h followed by 2.4 mg/kg once daily. If <20 kg use 3.0 mg/kg per dose. This medication is now FDA approved and commercially available for the initial treatment of severe malaria in children and adults regardless of the infecting species of malaria parasite. It has shown reduced mortality compared to parenteral quinine in clinical trials in patients with severe malaria in Asia and Africa.
- Plasmapheresis is an option for parasitemia >30% or in pregnant women and in elderly with severe malaria.

NOTE: WHO recommends IV artesunate as the treatment of choice for severe malaria in adults and children in area of low transmission. Data on children in high-transmission regions are limited, and WHO recommends treatment with artesunate, artemether, or quinine.

MULTIDRUG-RESISTANT MALARIA:
- Mefloquine 1250 mg as a single dose, *or*
- Halofantrine 500 mg every 6 h for 3 doses, repeat same course after 1 wk
- Combination therapy usually preferred

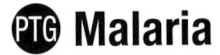
M

TABLE 5 Treatment Guidelines for Severe *Plasmodium falciparum* Malaria

Drug	Dose	Comments

Artemisinin compounds
Artesunate
Artemether
	2.4 mg/kg IV bolus at 0, 12, 24 hr, then daily until patient is able to transition to the following oral regimen:
	1. Artemether + lumefantrine: Tablets containing 20 + 120 mg, 40 + 240 mg of artemether and lumefantrine, respectively
	  • Adults ≥35 kg: 80 + 480 mg twice daily for 3 days
	  • Children:
	    • 5 to <15 kg: 20 + 120 mg twice daily for 3 days
	    • 15 to <25 kg: 40 + 240 mg twice daily for 3 days
	    • 25 to <35 kg: 60 + 360 mg twice daily for 3 days
	2. Artesunate + amodiaquine: A fixed-dose combination tablet containing 25 + 67.5 mg, 50 + 135 mg, 100 + 270 mg of artesunate and amodiaquine, respectively
	  • Adults ≥36 kg, 200 + 540 mg daily for 3 days
	  • Children:
	    • 4.5 to <9 kg: 25 + 67.5 mg daily for 3 days
	    • 9 to <18 kg: 50 + 135 mg daily for 3 days
	    • 18 to <36 kg: 100 + 270 mg daily for 3 days
	3. Dihydroartemisinin (DHA) + piperaquine (PPQ): Tablets containing 20 + 160 mg, 40 + 320 mg of DHA and PPQ, respectively
	  • Adults:
	    • 36 to <75 kg: 120 + 960 mg daily for 3 days
	    • ≥75 kg: 160 + 1280 mg daily for 3 days (no data on dose recommendation >100 kg)
	  • Children
	    • 5 to <7 kg: 10 + 80 mg daily for 3 days
	    • 7 to <13 kg: 20 + 160 mg daily for 3 days
	    • 13 to <24 kg: 40 + 320 mg daily for 3 days
	    • 24 to <36 kg: 80 + 640 mg daily for 3 days
	4. Artesunate or quinine PO to complete 7 days plus doxycycline, 100 mg PO bid × 7 days
	5. Artesunate or quinine PO to complete 7 days plus clindamycin, 20 mg base/kg/d PO, tid × 7 days
	Initial dose: 3.2 mg/kg IM (anterior tight); maintenance dose: 1.6 mg/kg IM daily until patient is able to transition to oral regimen as described earlier for artesunate
		Artesunate has "investigational new drug" status in the U.S. and is available only on request to the CDC (770-488-7788). Eligibility requirements include inability to take oral medications, high levels of parasitemia, clinical evidence of severe malaria, intolerance of or contraindication to quinidine, failure of quinidine therapy, and lack of rapid access to quinidine. Where available, artesunate rectal suppositories (10 mg/kg) may be used in children <5 yr of age if IV or IM administration is not possible. Doxycycline is contraindicated in children <8 yr of age and in pregnancy. Atovaquone/proguanil is packaged in the U.S. in fixed-dose combination tablets of 250 mg atovaquone/100 mg proguanil for adults and 62.5 mg atovaquone/25 mg proguanil for children. Safety of atovaquone/proguanil in pregnancy has not been established.

Cinchona Alkaloid Regimens Quinine dihydrochloride	20 mg salt/kg IV or IM on admission, then 10 mg/kg q8h. Can be given IM if IV administration is not possible. One of the following drugs should also be given concurrently: 1. ACT as listed earlier. 2. Doxycycline as listed earlier. If patient unable to take PO, give 100 mg IV q12h and switch to PO when possible. Avoid rapid IV administration. 3. Clindamycin as listed earlier. If patient unable to take PO, give 10 mg base/kg loading dose IV followed by 5 mg base/kg IV q8h and switch to PO when possible. Avoid rapid IV administration.	The infusion rate of IV quinine should be rate controlled and not exceed 5 mg salt/kg/h. The drug is usually diluted in 5% dextrose and infused over 4 h. IV quinine is not available in the U.S. When administering IM, the dose should be split and diluted to a concentration of 60-100 mg/kg and delivered to each thigh. Reduce the quinine dose by one third (to 10 mg salt/kg q12h) after 48 h in patients with severe renal and/or hepatic dysfunction. Doxycycline is contraindicated in children <8 yr old and in pregnancy.
Quinidine gluconate	6.25 mg base/kg (= 10 mg salt/kg) IV on admission over 1-2 h, then 0.0125 mg base/kg min (= 0.02 mg salt/kg per min) continuous infusion. An alternative regimen is 15 mg base/kg (= 24 mg salt/kg) loading dose IV infused over 4 hr, followed by 7.5 mg base/kg (= 12 mg salt/kg) infused over 4 h q8h, starting 8 h after the loading dose. A second drug should be given concurrently as listed earlier for quinine.	The loading dose should be omitted if the patient received >40 mg/kg quinine in the preceding 48 h or mefloquine in the previous 12 h. Reduce the dose by one third after 48 h in patients with severe renal and/or hepatic dysfunction.

ACT, Artemisinin combination therapy; *bid,* twice a day; *CDC,* Centers for Disease Control and Prevention; *IM,* intramuscular; *IV,* intravenous; *PO,* by mouth; *q,* every; *tid,* thrice a day.
From Vincent JL et al: *Textbook of critical care,* ed 7, Philadelphia, 2017, Elsevier.

DISPOSITION

RISK FACTORS FOR FATAL MALARIA:
• Failure to take chemoprophylaxis
• Delay in seeking medical care
• Misdiagnosis

COMPLICATIONS OF MALARIA:
• Anemia

• Acidosis
• Hypoglycemia
• Respiratory distress
• Disseminated intravascular coagulation
• Blackwater fever
• Renal failure
• Shock

REFERRAL
• To an infectious disease specialist or travel medicine expert for severe malaria complications
• To an intensive care specialist if severe cerebral malaria or other major organ failure develops

TABLE 6   Features of Complicated Malaria

Physical Findings	Laboratory Investigations
Impaired consciousness/unrousable coma (Blantyre Coma Score ≤2) (children > adults) Prostration (unable to walk or sit up) Failure to feed Convulsions (more than 2 in 24 h) (children > adults) Acidotic breathing (children > adults) Shock (systolic blood pressure <70 mm Hg in adults, <50 mm Hg in children) Clinical jaundice + evidence of another organ dysfunction (adults > children) Abnormal spontaneous bleeding Pulmonary edema (radiologic evidence) (adults > children)	Hypoglycemia (<2.2 mmol/L or 40 mg/dl) (children > adults) Metabolic acidosis (plasma bicarbonate <15 mmol/L) (children > adults) Severe anemia (hemoglobin <5 g/dl, PCV <15%) (children > adults) Hemoglobinuria Hyperparasitemia (>2%, or 100,000/μl in low transmission setting, >5%, or 250,000/μl in high-transmission settings) Hyperlactatemia (>5 mmol/L) Renal impairment (creatinine >265 μmol/L) (adults > children)

PCV, Packed cell volume.
From Ryan ET: *Hunter's tropical medicine and emerging infectious diseases,* ed 10, Philadelphia, 2020, Elsevier.

- All malaria cases are mandated to be reported to local and state health departments by health care providers or laboratory staff

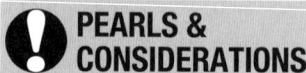

PEARLS & CONSIDERATIONS

HOST RESPONSE
- The specific immune response to malaria confers protection from high-level parasitemia and disease but not from infection.
- Asymptomatic parasitemia without illness (premunition) is common among adults in endemic areas.
- Immunity is specific for both the species and the strain of infecting malarial parasites.
- Immunity to all strains is never achieved.
- Normal spleen function is an important host factor because of immunologic as well as filtering functions of the spleen.
- Both humoral and cellular immunity is necessary for protection.
- Polyclonal increase in serum level of immunoglobulin G (IgG), IgM, and IgA occurs in immune individuals.
- Antibody to antigenically variant protein PfEMP1 is important for protection in case of *P. falciparum* malaria.
- Passively transferred IgG from immune individuals has been shown to be protective.
- Maternal antibody confers relative protection of infants from severe disease.
- Genetic disorders (sickle cell disease, thalassemia, and G6PD deficiency) confer protection from death because parasites are unable to grow efficiently in low-oxygen tensions, thus preventing high-level parasitemias.
- Individuals deficient of Duffy factor in RBCs are resistant to infection by *P. vivax.*
- Nonspecific defense mechanisms, such as cytokines (TNF-α, IL-1, -6, -8), also play an important role in protection, causing fever (temperatures of 40° C [104° F] damage mature parasites) and other pathologic effects.

PREVENTION OF MALARIA: Medications are available for the prophylaxis of malaria and will vary depending on level of chloroquine resistance in a given area (Table 7).

AREAS FREE OF CHLOROQUINE-RESISTANT *P. FALCIPARUM* MALARIA: Chloroquine 300 mg base (500 mg chloroquine phosphate) PO/wk. Start 1 wk prior to arrival in malaria area, then weekly while there and for 4 wk on leaving malaria area. Pediatric dose: 8.3 mg/kg (5 mg/kg base). Alternatives for adults include atovaquone-proguanil (Malarone): 1 adult tablet per day starting 1 to 2 days prior to arriving in malaria area, then daily while there and then for 7 days daily on leaving malaria area. For children, atovaquone-proguanil pediatric tablets based on weight:
- 11 to 20 kg: 1 pediatric tablet
- 21 to 30 kg: 2 pediatric tablets
- 31 to 40 kg: 3 pediatric tablets
- 40 kg: 1 adult tablet

AREAS WITH CHLOROQUINE-RESISTANT *P. FALCIPARUM* MALARIA:
- Atovaquone-proguanil (Malarone): Dosing as previously
- Mefloquine 250 mg (228 mg base) PO/wk, starting 1 wk before arriving in malaria area, weekly while there and then weekly for 4 wk on return. In children, mefloquine dose is based on weight:
  1. <15 kg: 5 mg/kg
  2. 16 to 19 kg: ¼ adult dose
  3. 20 to 30 kg: ½ adult dose
  4. 31 to 45 kg: ¾ adult dose
  5. >45 kg: Adult dose
- Doxycycline 100 mg PO/day for adults and children aged >8. Start 1 to 2 days before travel, daily while in malaria area, and then daily for 4 wk on return.
- Tafenoquine (Arakoda, Krintafel) is a long-acting primaquine analog FDA approved in two different strengths: 300-mg single dose for antimalarial therapy (Krintafel) for acute *P. vivax* or *P. ovale* infection, coadministered on the first or second day of chloroquine therapy; and 200-mg dose as chemoprophylaxis (Arakoda): Loading dose is 200 mg once/day for 3 days. Maintenance dose is 200 mg once/wk starting 7 days after last loading dose, terminal dose is 200 mg once (7 days after last maintenance dose). G6PD levels should be measured with tafenoquine.

SPECIAL CONSIDERATIONS:
- Long-term visitors or travelers.

- Children aged <12 yr.
- Immunocompromised host.
- Pregnant women: Chloroquine and mefloquine are safe in pregnancy but not atovaquone-proguanil. A recent trial revealed that the burden of malaria in pregnancy was significantly lower among adolescent girls or women who received intermittent preventive treatment with dihydroartemisinin-piperaquine than among those who received sulfadoxine-pyrimethamine, and monthly treatment with dihydroartemisinin-piperaquine was superior to three-dose dihydroartemisinin-piperaquine with regards to several outcomes. Avoid doxycycline and primaquine.
- An increasing number of areas in southeast Asia have mefloquine-resistant malaria, including Cambodia, Thailand, and Vietnam. Therefore, in specific regions of these countries, mefloquine cannot be used for prophylaxis or treatment.

PREVENTION OF RELAPSE:
- Treatment of *P. vivax* requires the clearing of asexual parasites, but relapse can be prevented only if dormant hypnozoites are cleared from the liver (a treatment termed "radical cure").
- The recommended treatment to prevent relapse of *Plasmodium vivax* malaria is primaquine at a total dose of 3.5 mg per kilogram of body weight. A recent trial[2] revealed that the administration of primaquine, a total dose of 7.0 mg per kg had higher efficacy in preventing relapse of *P. vivax* malaria than a total dose of 3.5 mg per kg through day 168.
- Tafenoquine, slowly eliminated, single dose 8-aminoquinoline is effective in significantly lowering the risk of *P. vivax* recurrence in patients with phenotypically normal GG PD activity.

VACCINATION:
- Mosquirix (RTS,S), a recombinant protein-based vaccine, is approved to use in children to prevent malaria in Africa. It showed an efficacy of about 30% in babies 6 to 12 wk old and about 46% in babies 5 to 17 mo old.
- New DNA-based vaccines are in development.
- A long-acting monoclonal antibody CIS43LS was shown to prevent malaria for up to 4 to 36 wk after controlled infection.[1]

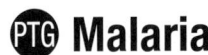

M

TABLE 7 Drug Regimens Used for Prevention of Malaria

Drug	Adult Dosage	Pediatric Dosage	Comments
Chloroquine-Sensitive Areas			
Chloroquine phosphate (drug of choice)	500 mg salt (300 mg base) orally once/wk	8.3 mg/kg salt (5 mg/kg base) once/wk, up to adult dose of 300 mg base	Begin 1-2 wk before exposure, continue during exposure, and continue for 4 wk after exposure May be used in pregnant women
Hydroxychloroquine sulfate	400 mg salt (310 mg base) orally once/wk	6.5 mg/kg salt (5 mg/kg base) orally once/wk	Begin 1-2 wk before exposure, continue during exposure, and continue for 4 wk after exposure An alternative to chloroquine for use only in areas with chloroquine-sensitive malaria
Chloroquine-Resistant Areas			
Atovaquone-proguanil	250 mg/100 mg (1 tablet) daily	5-8 kg: Pediatric tablet daily 9-10 kg: Pediatric tablet daily 11-20 kg: 1 Pediatric tablet daily 21-30 kg: 2 Pediatric tablets daily 31-40 kg: 3 Pediatric tablets daily >40 kg: 1 Adult tablet daily	Begin 1-2 days before exposure, continue during exposure, and continue for 7 days after exposure Pediatric tablets contain 62.5 mg atovaquone and 25 mg proguanil hydrochloride See text for contraindications
Mefloquine	250 mg salt (228 mg base) orally once/wk	≤9 kg: 5 mg/kg salt (4.6 mg/kg base) orally once/wk 10-19 kg: Tablet orally once/wk 20-30 kg: Tablet orally once/wk 31-45 kg: Tablet orally once/wk >45 kg: 1 Tablet orally once/wk	Begin 1-2 wk before exposure, continue during exposure, and continue for 4 wk after exposure
Or			
Doxycycline	100 mg daily	2.2 mg/kg/day up to 100 mg/day	Begin 1-2 days before exposure, continue during exposure, and for 4 wk after exposure; not to be used in children >8 yr or pregnant women
Or			
Alternative			
Primaquine	52.6 mg salt (30 mg base) orally daily	0.8 mg/kg salt (0.5 mg/kg base) up to adult dose orally daily	Begin 1-2 days before exposure, continue during exposure, and continue for 7 days after exposure Contraindicated in people with G6PD deficiency, in pregnancy, and during lactation Prophylaxis to areas principally with *P. vivax*
Tafenoquine (Krintafel)	300 mg tab once		Prevention of relapse of *P. vivax* 300 mg once

G6PD, Glucose-6-phosphate dehydrogenase.
From Cherry JD et al: *Feigin and Cherry's textbook of pediatric infectious diseases,* ed 8, Philadelphia, 2019, Elsevier.

MALARIA INFORMATION:
- Prevent malaria for up to 4 to 36 wk after controlled infection
  CDC Travelers' Health, CDC Travelers' Health Hotline (877) 394-8747; CDC Travelers' Health Fax (888) 232-3299
- CDC Malaria Epidemiology (770) 488-7788; internet:http://www.cdc.gov

- Table E8 summarizes sources for malaria prophylaxis, diagnosis, and treatment recommendations
- Box E1 describes useful malaria vocabulary

REFERENCES & SUGGESTED READINGS
Available at eBooks.Health.Elsevier.com.

RELATED CONTENT
Malaria (Patient Information)

AUTHOR: **GLENN G. FORT, MD, MPH**

Malignant Hyperthermia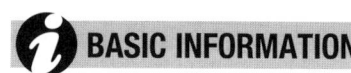

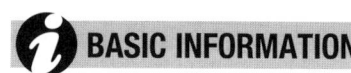 BASIC INFORMATION

DEFINITION

Malignant hyperthermia (MH) is a rare life-threatening subclinical myopathy that can manifest clinical symptoms in MH-susceptible (MHS) individuals after exposure to triggering medications. These drugs include halogenated anesthetic gases, such as halothane, isoflurane, sevoflurane, and desflurane, as well as the depolarizing neuromuscular blocking agent succinylcholine.[1-11] When given to genetically susceptible individuals, these agents may cause a hypermetabolic crisis. Initial signs include hypercarbia or rising end-tidal carbon dioxide (ETCO$_2$) levels in ventilated patients, tachypnea, and tachycardia, with subsequent hyperthermia, acidemia, arrhythmias, or skeletal muscle rigidity.[1-3,6,8-10,12,13] Clinical presentation may be variable, especially during surgery and general anesthesia. Mortality has recently been reported to be 1.4% to 5%, down from 70% in the past, likely due to the prevalence of intraoperative temperature and ETCO$_2$ monitoring, reduced use of succinylcholine, and the use of dantrolene for treatment.[8,10,14]

SYNONYMS

Anesthesia-related hyperthermia
Hyperpyrexia, malignant
Hyperthermia, malignant
Malignant hyperpyrexia
MHS
MH

ICD-10CM CODES

T88.3XXA	Malignant hyperthermia due to anesthesia
T88.3XXA	Initial encounter
T88.3XXD	Subsequent encounter
T88.3XXS	Sequelae
Z15.89	Malignant hyperthermia susceptibility
Z84.89	Family history of malignant hyperthermia
Z87.898	History of malignant hyperthermia

EPIDEMIOLOGY & DEMOGRAPHICS

Malignant hyperthermia results from a biochemical cascade within the skeletal muscle tissue of MHS individuals following exposure to one or more "triggering" medications, including halogenated volatile anesthetics and the skeletal muscle relaxant, succinylcholine. This is due to excessive release of sarcoplasmic calcium, which occurs because of a genetic anomaly.[2,6-10,12,14-16] The result is a hypermetabolic and prolonged contractile state, with subsequent serious morbidity and possible mortality, especially without prompt diagnosis and treatment. A recent study comparing human muscle fiber mitochondria from non-MHS patients to those from MHS patients found that mitochondria from MHS patients displayed anatomic and physiologic differences when exposed to halothane, while the non-MHS fibers did not.

All ethnic groups are at risk. MH susceptibility is associated with, although distinct from, central core, multiminicore disease, and King-Denborough syndrome.[6,7,12]

PREVALENCE: In the general population, the prevalence of MHS is estimated to be between 1:2000 to 1:3000.[3,8,10,12] In family cohorts of patients who are susceptible, the prevalence of susceptibility ranges from 1:200 to 1:5000 due to incomplete penetrance and variable expressivity.[3,8,10,12]

PREDOMINANT SEX & AGE: MH male to female ratio is 2:1.[8,10,15] Children account for up to half of cases.[8,10]

PEAK INCIDENCE: Among patients undergoing general anesthesia, the incidence is approximately 1:100,000, considerably lower than its estimated prevalence.[8-10]

RISK FACTORS:

- Preoperatively, the patient and family history is used to evaluate the risk of MH and other myopathies. It is important to note that previous exposure to triggering agents with no sequelae does not exclude the possibility of a future MH crisis since half of afflicted patients may have had a prior uneventful exposure to a triggering agent.[3,4,6,10,12,17]
- Patients with other *RYR1* abnormalities, such as central core myopathy, multiminicore disease (*RYR1* or *SELENON*), or King-Denborough syndrome though not true MHS, should not receive succinylcholine or volatile anesthetics.[4,6-12,15]
- Increased muscle mass, especially in body-builders, appears to be an independent predictor of increased susceptibility to, recurrence of, and death from MH episodes. This finding is independent of the increased incidence in males noted above.[15]
- Patients with dystrophinopathies such as Duchenne and Becker muscular dystrophy, enzymopathies of skeletal muscle such as McArdle disease, statin-induced myopathy, or exercise- and heat-induced rhabdomyolysis, may develop rhabdomyolysis when exposed to these agents, especially succinylcholine.[6,8,12]
  1. This pathophysiology, though different from that of MH, may result in similar signs and symptoms.
  2. However, it is important to understand that dantrolene is unlikely to be of value in treating these causes of rhabdomyolysis.

GENETICS:

- Three genes have been associated with MH susceptibility (*RYR1*, *CACNA1S*, and *STAC3*), which are inherited in an autosomal dominant pattern or may arise de novo.[4,6,8,10,12]
- In an evolving field of study, a multitude of variants have been recognized as being functionally characterized to MH susceptibility (MHS).[2,4,6-10,12]
  1. The most common are mutations leading to MH susceptibility involving *RYR1* that encodes the ryanodine receptor-Ca^{2+} release channel of skeletal muscle sarcoplasmic reticulum.
  2. A *CACNA1S* mutation causes another form.
  3. Other types are less common and in some cases (a *CACNA2D* mutation and *RYR1*) may interact.

4. However, the genetic basis of MH susceptibility may be unknown and unrelated to the three known genes.

PHYSICAL FINDINGS & CLINICAL PRESENTATION[2,3,8,10,13,18]

- Within minutes to hours after a triggering agent is administered, the patient may develop hypercarbia or tachycardia.
- Manifestations of increased skeletal muscle metabolism include increased CO$_2$ production, leading to elevated mixed venous and arterial pCO$_2$, and an elevated ETCO$_2$.
- Hyperthermia or a rapidly increasing temperature is often a later finding as a result of hypermetabolism and is present in more than 50% of MH events. Higher core body temperature correlates with increased morbidity.
- Blood pressure response is variable as effects of sympathetic stimulation and peripheral vasodilatation due to metabolic by-products are balanced.
- Rhabdomyolysis, a condition of skeletal muscle injury and necrosis, is associated with an increased creatine kinase (CK), observed myoglobinuria (if a urinary catheter is present), and subsequent acute renal failure or DIC (disseminated intravascular coagulation) may develop.
- Masseter muscle rigidity in the context of succinylcholine use can be present. However, it may be unrelated to MHS, particularly if it is mild and not associated with generalized rigidity, and it is transient, terminating within minutes of succinylcholine dissipation.
- The skin may be erythematous initially, progressing to a mottled, cyanotic appearance.
- Arrhythmias may develop in the setting of hyperkalemia. The most common is tachyarrhythmia.
- Box 1 summarizes the findings consistent with MH.[2,3,8,10,13]

ETIOLOGY

Approximately 50% of cases of MH susceptibility (MHS) are inherited primarily related to variants of *RYR1* or *CACNA1S*; the remainder are presumed to be the result of a new mutations.[2,4,6,8,9,12] The majority of the mutations, either inherited or de novo, are on chromosome 19 encoding the ryanodine receptor gene *RYR1* (19q13.1, with at least 35 variants).[6-9,12,14] The result is the abnormality of skeletal muscle calcium homeostasis and susceptibility to MH, with significant clinical variability due to incomplete penetrance and variable expressivity.

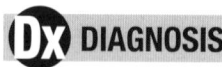 DIAGNOSIS

DIFFERENTIAL DIAGNOSIS[3,8]

- Exertional heatstroke
- MH symptomology following excessive heat exposure to a MHS patient who did not receive a triggering agent
- Neuroleptic malignant syndrome
- Fever
- Thyrotoxicosis
- Pheochromocytoma

BOX 1 Positive Findings Consistent With Malignant Hyperthermia (MH)

History of recent exposure to trigger agent, including volatile anesthetic agents or succinylcholine
    Family or personal history of MH susceptibility
    Total body rigidity
    Inappropriately elevated (38.8° C [101.8° F]) or rapidly increasing temperature (>1.5° C [34.7° F] over 5 min)
    Inappropriate tachypnea
    Profuse sweating
    Mottled, cyanotic skin
    Dark urine, urine dipstick testing shows a positive result from blood without red cells in the sediment and no hemolysis
    Unexplained, excessive bleeding
    Unexplained ventricular tachycardia or fibrillation
    Inappropriate hypercarbia (venous $Paco_2$ >65 mm Hg, arterial $Paco_2$ >55 mm Hg) if the patient is receiving positive-pressure ventilation or is spontaneously breathing with greater than normal minute ventilation
    Arterial base excess more negative than −8 mEq/L
    Arterial pH <7.25
    Potassium concentration >6 mEq/L
    Creatine kinase >10,000 IU/L

From Fuhrman BP et al: *Pediatric critical care*, ed 4, Philadelphia, 2011, Saunders.

- Central nervous system infection or space-occupying lesion
- MDMA (Ecstasy), cocaine, alcohol withdrawal, or amphetamine use
- Serotonin syndrome
- Adverse reaction to monoamine oxidase inhibitors or anticholinergic drug
- Strychnine poisoning
- Sepsis
- Drug withdrawal
- Rhabdomyolysis
- Transfusion reactions

WORKUP[3,8,10]

- MH can often be distinguished from other causes of hyperthermia based on a history of exposure to a triggering agent.
- A rapid rise in ETCO₂ with no change in minute ventilation under anesthesia, especially in the setting of tachycardia, should prompt consideration of MH until proven otherwise.
- A Clinical Grading Scale (CGS) evaluates several clinical criteria (rigidity, muscle breakdown, respiratory acidosis, temperature, cardiac involvement, family history, and other indicators such as base excess) and can be used to rank the qualitative likelihood of an event representing malignant hyperthermia.[4,8,13]

LABORATORY TESTS[3,8,10,11,13,16]

Considerations for laboratory testing fall into three scenarios:
- In the acute setting, electrolytes, creatine kinase, arterial blood gas, and urine myoglobin.
- Once the diagnosis is presumptive, it is important to monitor serial lab data including:
  1. Blood gases
  2. Electrolytes, especially potassium and creatinine
  3. Creatine kinase
  4. Urine myoglobin
  5. Coagulation studies to evaluate for DIC

- If hyperthermia is less acute or the presentation atypical, thyroid function studies, CBC, toxicology screen, and plasma fractionated metanephrines or 24-h urine fractionated metanephrines and catecholamines may be useful. Treatment should not be delayed while these labs are pending.

IMAGING STUDIES

A CT scan of the head may be obtained to evaluate for a space-occupying lesion if clinically indicated. Imaging should never delay prompt treatment of strongly suspected MH.

SUSCEPTIBILITY TESTING:

- Testing for MH susceptibility involves genetic evaluation or the in vitro muscle contracture test.
  1. The in vitro muscle contracture test is considered the gold standard and involves placing a muscle biopsy specimen in a bath of caffeine or halothane. Significant muscle contraction is 97% to 99% sensitive for MH susceptibility, with a specificity of 78% to 94%.[8] Testing can be expensive since it is performed only in a few sites in the U.S. and must be performed on fresh tissue sample(s).[8]
  2. Genetic testing, while noninvasive, has a sensitivity of <50%. Testing can be costly and prohibitive depending on insurance reimbursement and laboratory fees.[4,8]
  3. Generally, a positive contracture test leads to genetic testing, unless there is a positive family history, in which case the patient may choose genetic testing directly.
- Testing for MHS can be performed preoperatively in patients deemed to be at risk or those with a personal or family history of anesthesia-induced complications suggestive of MH.
  1. Depending on the wishes of the patient and/or family following a thorough history and counseling, a decision to proceed with anesthesia and surgery without prior testing

may be reasonable. If possible, the case should be scheduled as the first case in the room with the plan to avoid volatile agents or succinylcholine.
  2. In such a case, the patient should be counseled that forgoing testing may place them at risk if an intubation is required in an emergency setting, succinylcholine is used unknowingly, and the patient truly has MHS.
- After an acute event, the patient should be advised to undergo susceptibility testing to confirm the diagnosis and the need to test other immediate family members at risk. If positive, the patient should be given a letter and wear a medical alert bracelet.

Rx TREATMENT

NONPHARMACOLOGIC THERAPY[3,8]

The patient should be cooled to 38° C (100.4° F). This can be accomplished with ice packs to the axillae and groin, a cooling blanket, a fan with cool mist, or chilled IV fluids. In extreme situations, partial extracorporeal bypass or iced peritoneal lavage have proven helpful.
- Frequent evaluation of core temperature, hemodynamics, and gas exchange are imperative.

ACUTE GENERAL RX (SEE BOX 2)[3,8,10,11]

- Notify the surgeon to stop surgery immediately. Discontinue all triggering agents and switch to nontriggering agents if surgery must be continued.
- Call for help! Management of MH requires multiple personnel for various tasks.
- Request the facility's MH cart and have someone call MHAUS (Malignant Hyperthermia Association of the U.S.).
- Hyperventilate with 100% oxygen at flows of 10 L/min to flush volatile anesthetics and decrease ETCO₂. Insert charcoal filters, if available, into the inspiratory and expiratory limb of the breathing circuit to further absorb agent.
- Administer dantrolene as a rapid IV bolus at a dose of 2.5 mg/kg through a large bore catheter. Repeat every five minutes until an observable decrease is seen in muscle rigidity, tachycardia, or ETCO₂; a total dose greater than 10mg/kg may be required, especially in patients with greater muscle mass.
- Initiate cooling measures. Apply ice to the axilla, groin, or head.
- Up to 25% of patients will have recrudescence of their symptoms, on average 13 h after the initiation of MH. Dantrolene, 1mg/kg IV every 4 to 6 h or by continuous infusion at 0.1 to 0.3 mg/kg/hr IV, is recommended for at least 24 to 48 h after an event. Additional boluses may be needed for breakthrough signs.
- Call ICU to arrange for continued observation. Place additional lines in the patient as necessary including an arterial line. Send and order serial labs for close monitoring.

BOX 2   Management of an Acute Malignant Hyperthermia Episode in the Intensive Care Unit

1. Administer high-flow 100% oxygen via a nonrebreathing mask and consider endotracheal intubation.
2. For ventilated patients, administer an FiO_2 of 1.0 and increase minute ventilation to control $PaCO_2$.
3. Administer dantrolene (2.5 mg/kg intravenously) and repeat until acidosis and muscle rigidity have resolved. Repeat dantrolene (1 mg/kg) every 6 h.
4. Initiate cooling with ice packs in the axillae and groin; decrease room temperature; use hypothermia blankets, iced intravenous saline solution, and lavage body cavities with cold saline solution if temperature is greater than 39° C (102.2° F). Stop cooling when core temperature falls to 38° C (100.4° F).
5. Correct metabolic acidosis with sodium bicarbonate (1 to 2 mEq/kg initially), and give subsequent doses based on base excess and body weight.
6. Administer calcium chloride (10 mg/kg) or calcium gluconate (100 to 200 mg/kg) for cardiotoxicity associated with hyperkalemia.
7. Give regular insulin (0.1 U/kg) and glucose (0.3 to 0.5 g/kg) to correct hyperkalemia if severe.
8. Administer lidocaine (1 mg/kg) to treat ventricular arrhythmias. Consider amiodarone (5 mg/kg IV) for refractory, stable ventricular tachycardia. Do not delay defibrillation or cardiopulmonary resuscitation if indicated for cardiovascular instability.
9. Maintain urine output of 2 ml/kg/hr with aggressive cold fluid administration, furosemide (0.5 to 1 mg/kg), and additional mannitol (0.25 to 0.3 g/kg) if needed.
10. Consider quantitative end-tidal CO_2 monitoring.
11. Monitor core temperature (pulmonary artery, esophageal temperature probe, rectal probe).
12. Place arterial catheter for invasive blood pressure monitoring and frequent blood sampling. Consider central venous catheter and/or pulmonary artery catheter if indicated by cardiovascular instability.
13. Repeat blood gases and electrolytes until these normalize. Repeat CK at least every 6 hours while the patient is in ICU and then daily until CK returns to normal. Assess glucose, clotting, hepatic, and renal functions. Repeat lactic acid measurement after each dantrolene administration.
14. Consider hemodialysis if indicated.
15. Consider intensive care monitoring for at least 24 h after MH episode or after recrudescence of MH.
16. Refer the patient for muscle caffeine-halothane contracture testing and consider genetic testing. Pursue a pathologic diagnosis for other occult myopathies.

From Fuhrman BP et al: *Pediatric critical care*, ed 4, Philadelphia, 2011, Saunders.

- Recently, one study suggested that in at least one MH model involving the RyR receptor, dantrolene treatment may be ineffective in the setting of insufficient levels of cytoplasmic Mg^{++}. MgATP hydrolysis, a process that normally increases Mg^{++} during contraction, by itself may be insufficient to raise the Mg^{++} concentration in the setting of low resting Mg^{++} levels, thereby preventing dantrolene from being effective.
- Aggressive hydration with forced diuresis and alkalization of the urine should be instituted for rhabdomyolysis. Observe closely for the development of compartment syndrome, renal failure, and DIC. Use of calcium channel blockers should be avoided since the combination with dantrolene may produce profound hyperkalemia and significantly depress cardiac function.

CHRONIC RX[3,8,10]

- MH is an acute disease, resolving in 24 to 48 h with appropriate treatment.
- The MHS patient should be aware that exercise in excessive heat and/or humidity could trigger an episode of MH without exposure to a pharmacologic triggering agent.
- The patient as well as immediate family members should be advised to undergo susceptibility testing.

- The patient should be given a letter by his/her anesthesiologist and wear a medical alert bracelet.

DISPOSITION

After MH crisis, patients should be admitted to the intensive care unit for at least 24 h where close monitoring and supportive care can be maximized.[8,10]

REFERRAL

Anesthesiology, cardiology, nephrology, and hematology consultation as appropriate. After the acute event, a genetics consult may be warranted to facilitate testing.[8,10]

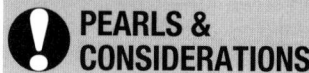 **PEARLS & CONSIDERATIONS**

COMMENTS

- MH is a life-threatening condition that requires prompt recognition to minimize illness, end-organ damage, and/or death.
- Family or personal history of problems with general anesthesia in the past are clues to susceptibility and should prompt careful preoperative evaluation.
- Prophylactic dantrolene is no longer recommended for known MHS patients undergoing general anesthesia with nontriggering agents.

PATIENT & FAMILY EDUCATION

- The patient and his/her family should be made aware of the diagnosis so that they can provide information to the anesthesiologist and other intraoperative caregivers when undergoing any type of surgery or procedure under sedation.
- The patient should be given a letter that can be shown to future caregivers.
- A medical alert bracelet should be recommended.

REFERENCES

Available at eBooks.Health.Elsevier.com.

AUTHORS: **SARA PARK, MD** and **EDWARD SUH, MD, MPH**

ⓘ BASIC INFORMATION

DEFINITION

Mastitis is local painful inflammation of the breast that may or may not be accompanied by infection, flulike symptoms, and abscess formation.

ICD-10CM CODES
N61 Inflammatory disorders of breast
O91.12 Abscess of breast associated with the puerperium
O91.22 Nonpurulent mastitis associated with the puerperium

EPIDEMIOLOGY & DEMOGRAPHICS

- Mastitis is the most common cause of inflammatory breast disease, and most cases are related to lactation (puerperal mastitis).
  1. Nonpuerperal cases of mastitis can affect either the periareolar (periductal) region or peripheral breast tissue.
  2. Periductal mastitis (PM, also known as duct ectasia) is most common in younger, reproductive-age women. The majority of those affected are active smokers.
- In lactating mothers, mastitis typically occurs in the first 3 mo of the postpartum period (74% to 95% of cases).
- When severe, mastitis can lead to a breast abscess (5% to 11%) or septicemia.
- Delayed diagnosis and treatment of lactational mastitis can lead to discontinuation of breast-feeding, breast tissue damage, or recurrence.
- In younger, nonlactating women, infection often presents as periductal mastitis and is caused by inflamed milk ducts near the nipple.
- Granulomatous mastitis (GM) is a rarer form of benign inflammation of the breast and also most commonly occurs in reproductive-age women. It generally affects the breast peripherally.
- Mastitis also can occur in infancy when there is breast hypertrophy from maternal hormones, called neonatal mastitis (NM).
  1. Approximately 50% of neonates with mastitis will develop an abscess.

PREVALENCE: Lactational mastitis occurs in up to 33% of mothers
PREDOMINANT SEX & AGE: Females of reproductive age
RISK FACTORS:
- Previous mastitis
- Milk stasis and missed feedings, or extended periods between feedings such as when an infant begins to sleep through the night
- History of oversupply
- Cracked, fissured, or sore nipples
- Primiparity and infant attachment difficulties
- Cleft lip or palate or short frenulum in infant
- Use of manual breast pump
- Foreign material: Breast implants, nipple piercings
- Rapid weaning
- Smoking (periductal mastitis)
- Obesity (periductal mastitis)
- Conditions that impair immunity (peripheral or granulomatous mastitis): Diabetes, steroid use, rheumatoid arthritis

PHYSICAL FINDINGS & CLINICAL PRESENTATION

- Warmth, redness, noncyclic tenderness in breast
- Unilateral or bilateral
- Malaise, myalgias, fevers, chills, nausea
- Decreased milk output
- Breast is hard and swollen in a wedge-shaped area
- Lactational mastitis tends to be found in the breast periphery, whereas nonlactational mastitis tends to be peri- or sub-areolar
- In PM, breast mass near nipple with retraction or discharge
  1. Can present simultaneously with abscess or even mammary duct fistula
- In GM, enlarged axillary lymph nodes or sinus tract formation

ETIOLOGY

- In lactational mastitis, infection occurs as a result of milk stasis and irritation of the milk ducts due to local immune response to milk proteins.
- Bacterial infection of subcutaneous tissue due to breaks in skin.
- Most commonly, *Staphylococcus aureus;* less common, *S. epidermidis,* group A beta-hemolytic streptococci, *S. pneumoniae, Escherichia coli, Candida albicans, Mycobacterium tuberculosis.* Up to 40% are polymicrobial.
- GM results from inflammation with epithelioid histiocytes and multinucleated giant cells and can be caused by etiologies like tuberculosis, sarcoidosis, foreign body reaction, parasitic and mycotic infections, or idiopathic.
- Periductal mastitis occurs following inflammation around nondilated subareolar ducts and often can progress to abscess formation. Peripheral abscesses can result from trauma, usually in the setting of comorbid conditions impairing immunity such as diabetes or use of immunosuppressive medications.
- Neonatal mastitis caused by *S. aureus* or gram-negative enteric bacteria.

ⒹⓍ DIAGNOSIS

DIFFERENTIAL DIAGNOSIS

- Engorgement, plugged duct (Table 1)
- Breast abscess
- Inflammatory or other breast cancer (3% of women diagnosed with breast cancer are lactating)
- Paget disease of breast
- Mastitis as a symptom of hyperprolactinemia or galactorrhea
- GM can be manifestation of systemic disease (sarcoidosis, Wegener granulomatosis, giant cell arteritis [GCA], polyarteritis nodosa, tuberculosis [TB], syphilis)

WORKUP

- History and clinical exam with thorough breast exam are generally sufficient for diagnosis.
  1. Be sure to address time, course, and duration of symptoms as well as breast history, including lactation, recent trauma, and prior treatment
  2. Physical exam should include special attention to inflammatory changes and their location, skin changes, assessment of nipple for skin changes and discharge, axillary or supraclavicular adenopathy, and presence or absence of breast mass
- Recurrent mastitis should include workup for underlying breast disease.

LABORATORY TESTS

- Simple lactational mastitis requires no milk culture or laboratory studies.
- Obtain midstream sample of milk for culture and sensitivities in refractory mastitis or in methicillin-resistant *S. aureus*-suspected cases.
- CBC and blood cultures in toxic-appearing patients.
- In abscess formation, culture of drainage or aspirate fluid.
- Inpatient intravenous antibiotics may be necessary in severe cases or recalcitrant to outpatient treatment.
- Gram stain and culture indicated in infant mastitis.

IMAGING STUDIES

- Not necessary unless refractory mastitis or abscess suspected.
  1. An abscess generally presents as a hypoechoic mass on ultrasound.
- In the context of a discrete mass on exam, age-appropriate breast imaging starting with ultrasound (US) (Fig. E1) is recommended to exclude carcinoma.
- In PM, US should be performed.
- In GM, mammogram and US-guided fine needle aspiration (FNA) are standard.

TABLE 1 Comparison of Findings of Engorgement, Plugged Duct, and Mastitis

Characteristics	Engorgement	Plugged Duct	Mastitis
Onset	Gradual, immediately	Gradual, after feedings	Sudden, after 10 days postpartum
Site	Bilateral	Unilateral	Usually unilateral
Swelling and heat	Generalized	May shift/little or no heat	Localized red, hot, and swollen
Body temperature	<38.4° C; 101.1° F	<38.4° C; 101.1° F	>38.4° C; 101.1° F
Systemic symptoms	Feels well	Feels well	Flulike symptoms

From Lawrence RA, Lawrence RM: *Breastfeeding: a guide for the medical profession,* ed 5, St Louis, 1999, Mosby.

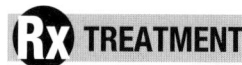

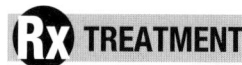 TREATMENT

NONPHARMACOLOGIC THERAPY

- Mainstay of therapy is effective milk removal through continued breastfeeding or pumping. Patient should be encouraged to continue breastfeeding her infant(s) throughout her treatment unless otherwise indicated.
- Consider referral to a certified lactation consultant to improve breastfeeding technique.
  1. Positioning the infant with its chin pointed towards the affected area can help to drain the affected area.
- Warm compresses, increased fluid intake, good nutrition, and rest.
- In abscess formation (10% of women who are treated for bacterial mastitis), surgical drainage or needle aspiration is necessary, followed by antibiotic therapy based on sensitivities of culture.
- In PM, aspiration or incision and drainage of abscesses should be performed, followed by culture of aspirate to guide antibiotic selection. If applicable, smoking cessation should be encouraged.

ACUTE GENERAL Rx

- NSAIDs and analgesics (e.g., acetaminophen, ibuprofen). There is insufficient evidence to support or refute the effectiveness of antibiotic therapy.
- Patients should be asked about history of penicillin allergy and history of methicillin-resistant *S. aureus* infection, either in herself or members of her household. Common antibiotic regimens include:
- No history of MRSA (methicillin-resistant *S. aureus*):
  1. Penicillinase-resistant antibiotic: Dicloxacillin 250 mg 4×/day for 7 days
  2. Cephalexin 500 mg 4×/day for 10 to 14 days
  3. Inpatient: Nafcillin or oxacillin 2 g intravenous (IV) q4h
  4. Erythromycin may be used in patients allergic to penicillin
- Suspected MRSA or high-risk penicillin allergy:
  1. Trimethoprim/sulfamethoxazole 160 mg/800 mg 2×/day for 10 to 14 days; should not be used when breastfeeding healthy infants <2 mo or compromised infants
  2. Clindamycin 300 mg 4×/day for 10 to 14 days
  3. Inpatient: Vancomycin 1 g IV q12h
- Women should be reassured that antibiotics and antiinflammatory medicines are safe for her infant(s).
- If no clinical response to antibiotics, MRSA or abscess should be considered. Again, if abscess is suspected or symptoms do not resolve with empiric antibiotic treatment, imaging should be performed to exclude other pathology. A biopsy should be performed based on imaging results.
- Antibiotic treatment in patients with abscesses should continue for up to 10 days following aspiration or incision and drainage, and antibiotic choice should be guided by culture results.
- Oxytocin nasal spray if letdown reflex disturbed.
- Consider treatment for candidal infection if *bilateral* symptoms and infant with thrush. Both infant and mother will require treatment.
  1. Topical clotrimazole for mother and oral nystatin for infant, with careful washing of all pacifiers and nipples
  2. If resistant to topical treatment, can consider oral fluconazole; however, data in breastfeeding are limited
  3. Onset of candida infection can follow antibiotic treatment for presumed mastitis
- Infant mastitis typically is treated in an inpatient setting with parenteral antibiotics based on results of Gram stain.
- Most PM cases are treated adequately with a combination of antibiotics including anaerobic coverage (supported by culture results if available), needle aspiration/incision, and drainage. In recurrent cases, surgical removal of diseased ducts may be needed, which may necessitate referral to an experienced breast surgeon.
- If antibiotic and NSAID treatment for GM fails, immunosuppressive drugs (steroids, methotrexate) can be used. Surgical management is not recommended due to associated slow wound healing.

CHRONIC Rx

- No evidence proving benefit of prophylactic antibiotics to prevent lactational mastitis
- In GM, systemic corticosteroids or wide surgical resection

DISPOSITION

- Most women with mastitis can be treated with antibiotics on an outpatient basis.
- Criteria for admission include:
  1. Signs of sepsis or hemodynamic instability
  2. Rapidly progressing infection
  3. Immunocompromised status
- If admission is necessary, the infant should be admitted with her to allow for continued breastfeeding.

COMPLEMENTARY & ALTERNATIVE MEDICINE

- Complementary therapies not assessed in prospective studies: *Belladonna, Phytolacca, Chamomilla,* sulfur, *Bellis perennis,* mupirocin, fucidic acid ointment, antisecretory factor, nisin
- Several strains of lactobacilli have shown promise as probiotic agents that might be useful in treating mastitis, including *L. fermentum* and *L. salivarius*. These results should be replicated before this approach is adopted widely

REFERRAL

- Refer to surgeon for severe PM or significant lactational abscess that does not resolve with conservative measures

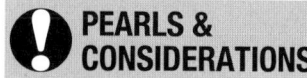 PEARLS & CONSIDERATIONS

COMMENTS

- Early recognition and treatment is important to prevent complications such as breast abscesses, sepsis, and early weening.
- 25% of breastfeeding mothers with one episode of mastitis stop breastfeeding.
- Patients may experience a temporary decrease in milk supply that should improve once she begins to recover and as long as she continues to breastfeed or adequately express.
- Increasing incidence of MRSA mastitis.
- Lactational mastitis is a risk factor for vertical transmission of infections (i.e., HIV-1, cytomegalovirus, measles, hepatitis B and C).
- When reassessing refractory nonlactational mastitis, the most important consideration is the possibility of cancer.
- Nonlactational mastitis can be a manifestation of systemic disease.
- GM mimics breast cancer both clinically and radiologically (>50% of reported cases are initially mistaken for carcinoma). This includes FNA, which is sometimes interpreted as malignant.

SUGGESTED READINGS

Available at eBooks.Health.Elsevier.com.

RELATED CONTENT

Lactational Mastitis (Patient Information)
Mastitis (Patient Information)
Breast Abscess (Related Key Topic)
Fibrocystic Breast Disease (Related Key Topic)

AUTHORS: **ANTHONY SCISCIONE, DO,** and **ERIN BISHOP, MD**

BASIC INFORMATION

DEFINITION
Medical marijuana or medical cannabis refers to the use of the unprocessed *Cannabis sativa* plant, part of the plant, or extracts from the plant as medical therapy to treat disease or alleviate symptoms.

SYNONYMS
Medical cannabis
Cannabinoids—biologically active compounds that activate the cannabinoid receptors. They may be derived from the plant or be synthetic.
CBD—cannabinol
THC—Δ^9-tetrahydrocannabinol

ICD-10CM CODES
F12.9	Cannabis use, unspecified
Z02.79	Encounter for issue of other medical certificate
Z79.899	Other long-term (current) drug therapy

BACKGROUND
- Medical use of marijuana has been restricted since classification as a Schedule I substance by the Controlled Substance Act in 1970.[1]
- First medical marijuana law (MML) was enacted in California in 1996, allowing for use of medical cannabis despite lack of Food and Drug Administration (FDA) testing for safety and efficacy.[1]
- As of February 2022, medical use of marijuana is permitted at the state level for 37 states, 3 territories, and the District of Columbia.[1]
- Cannabis is the second most commonly used recreational drug worldwide after alcohol.[2]
  1. In 2019, 48.2 million Americans >12 yr old (18% of the U.S. population) reported any marijuana use at least once in the past year.[3]
  2. In 2018, 2% of the U.S. population reported medical marijuana use.
  3. Of 2014 marijuana smokers, 6.2% used medical marijuana only, and 3.6% used medical and recreational marijuana.[4]
  4. Residents of medical marijuana states were 1.3 times more likely to use medical marijuana in 2015 compared to 2013.[5]

MECHANISM OF ACTION
- Cannabinoids elicit their effects by interacting with cannabinoid receptors in various central nervous system (CNS) locations, eliciting diverse CNS and peripheral nervous system (PNS) effects (Box 1).
- Primarily bind to CB1 G-protein-coupled receptors in the basal ganglia, hippocampus, cortex, and cerebellum, eliciting antinociception, locomotor, and psychoactive effects.
- Marijuana contains >400 plant-derived compounds, >60 classified as cannabinoids, with the major phytocannabinoids being cannabidiol (CBD) and Δ^9-tetrahydrocannabinol (THC).

FORMULATIONS
Research has demonstrated a wide range of THC and CBD concentrations in various formulations, with frequent inaccurate labelling.
- Cigarettes
- Tinctures
- Capsules
- Vaporization cartridges
- Purified cannabinoids butane hash oil (BHO)
- Supercritical fluid extracts (SFEs or "dabs")
- Buccal sprays
- Edibles
- Lozenges
- Transdermal patches

INDICATIONS
- Variable evidence for treatment of:
  1. Chronic pain
  2. Chemotherapy-induced nausea/vomiting
  3. HIV-related anorexia
  4. Glaucoma
  5. Anxiety
  6. Multiple sclerosis (MS)
  7. Seizures
- Marijuana has not been FDA approved as safe and effective for any indication and remains a Schedule I drug.
- However, there are phytocannabinoids and synthetic phytocannabinoid analogs that have received FDA approval.
  1. Dronabinol and Nabilone (synthetic THC analogs) are schedule II FDA approved medications for AIDS-associated anorexia and chemotherapy-induced nausea, respectively.[6]
  2. Purified cannabidiol oral solution (Epidiolex) is FDA approved for seizures associated with Dravet or Lennox-Gastaut syndrome.
- Qualifying diagnoses for certification for prescription medical marijuana vary by state, but typically include:
  1. Cancer
  2. Glaucoma
  3. HIV/AIDS
  4. Hepatitis C
  5. Cachexia
  6. Severe, debilitating, chronic pain
  7. Severe nausea
  8. Seizures
  9. Severe muscle spasms
  10. Crohn disease
  11. Alzheimer disease
  12. PTSD
  13. Sickle cell disease

EFFICACY
- There is published evidence demonstrating that marijuana improves noncancer-related pain, chemotherapy-induced nausea and vomiting, and spasticity in multiple sclerosis.[6,7]
  1. A 2011 systematic review of randomized controlled trials (RCTs) demonstrated statistically significant improvement in pain scores for noncancer-related chronic pain in 15 of 18 trials with no serious adverse effects.[7]
  2. A 2015 systematic review and meta-analysis showed improved response in nausea and vomiting compared to placebo (OR 3.82).[8]
  3. A 2018 systematic review demonstrated a decrease in nausea and vomiting following chemotherapy (RR 3.60 compared to placebo), improved spasticity with MS (RR 1.45 compared to placebo), and a modest benefit with primarily neuropathic pain (RR 1.37 compared to placebo) with frequent adverse effects including psychosis, "feeling high," and somnolence (number needed to harm = 5 to 8).[9]
     a. No statistically significant improvement was noted in acute pain.
  4. A Cochrane review in 2013 found no statistically significant weight gain with dronabinol in HIV/AIDS patients, and multiple RCTs have identified megestrol acetate as superior to dronabinol for weight gain in cancer patients.[10]
  5. A 2020 systematic review and meta-analysis showed extremely limited evidence for benefits for Crohn disease and ulcerative colitis, with only three RCTs all showing no improvement of marijuana over placebo.[11]
  6. In 2019, a systematic review determined that there was sufficient evidence from five reviews that cannabinoids may be effective for multiple sclerosis symptoms of pain and/or spasticity.[8,12]
  7. In a study of 54,000 adults in 37 states with medical cannabis access, more than half reported that cannabis use led to less use of other analgesics both opioid and nonopioid and one quarter to one third reported that cannabis use led to less use of physical therapy or cognitive-behavioral therapy.[12a]

RISKS OF USE
- Marijuana use has been demonstrated to impair short-term memory consolidation, reaction time, and concept formation, and to increase incidence of road traffic accidents, ataxia, euphoria, disorientation, dry mouth, somnolence, and, at high doses, psychosis, panic, and paranoia.
- Marijuana has been shown to worsen preexisting anxiety, depression, and schizophrenia. It should be used with caution, particularly in combination with other drugs with similar effects.[13]
- Meta-analyses demonstrate increased respiratory symptoms of cough, sputum production, and wheeze with smoking marijuana; however, there was no statistical difference in pulmonary function.
- Medical marijuana does have drug–drug interactions, and adverse effects can be potentiated by other medications. In particular, concomitant use of other medications such as opiates and benzodiazepines should be avoided as it could lead to somnolence and respiratory suppression.[13]
- Acute marijuana intoxication is associated with reversible changes in P and T waves and ST segments (pseudo-Wellens syndrome).

M

BOX 1 Acute Effects of Marijuana

Relaxation, euphoria, jocularity
Jitteriness, anxiety, paranoia, panic
Depersonalization, subjective time-slowing
Dizziness, sensation of floating
Impaired coordination and balance
Impaired memory and judgment
Conjunctival injection, decreased salivation
Urinary frequency
Tachycardia
Systolic hypertension and postural hypotension
Bradycardia, hypotension
Increased appetite and thirst
Decreased intraocular pressure
Analgesia
Auditory and visual illusions or hallucinations
Psychosis

From Jankovic J et al: *Bradley and Daroff's neurology in clinical practice*, ed 8, Philadelphia, 2022, Elsevier.

- Medical marijuana should be stored away from children given the risk of toxic ingestion.

PRESCRIBING

- Marijuana remains classified as a schedule I drug under the Controlled Substance Act of 1970.
- However, the Justice Department declared it would not prosecute any physician who recommends medical marijuana for a legitimate medical indication in a state where it has been legalized.[1]
- Medical marijuana card (MMC)
  1. MMC allows a patient to possess a certain amount of marijuana for medical use and not be prosecuted for possession of marijuana.
  2. To obtain an MMC, a patient must obtain physician certification confirming a clinical indication for medical marijuana.
  3. With an MMC, the patient can go to a licensed medical marijuana compassion center (dispensary), which will dispense a dose and formulation of medical marijuana appropriate for the patient's medical condition.
  4. Physicians do not prescribe the dose or formulation of medical marijuana.
- To certify a patient for a medical marijuana card, physicians must
  1. Complete a Department of Health certification form.
  2. Forms vary by state, but typically consist of a single-page form indicating a qualifying diagnosis that is to be signed by the physician. Complete and document a full medical history and physical exam.
  3. Explain the risks, benefits, and side effects of medical marijuana.

  4. Continue an ongoing role on the patient's health care team.
  5. Maintain accurate medical records and documentation of the patient's clinical indication for medical marijuana.
- Some states require additional physician training and registration with the state medical marijuana program prior to being able to certify patients.
- Physicians are under no obligation to issue medical marijuana certifications.

❗ PEARLS & CONSIDERATIONS

- Medical marijuana has been shown to improve noncancer-related pain, chemotherapy-induced nausea and vomiting, and spasticity in multiple sclerosis.
  1. Qualifying diagnoses (may vary from state to state) for a medical marijuana card include
     a. Cancer
     b. Glaucoma
     c. HIV/AIDS
     d. Hepatitis C
     e. Cachexia
     f. Debilitating chronic pain
     g. Severe nausea
     h. Seizures
     i. Severe muscle spasms
     j. Crohn disease
     k. Alzheimer disease
     l. PTSD
     m. Sickle cell disease.
  2. Adverse effects include increased incidence of road traffic accidents and

pulmonary and cognitive side effects. At high doses, psychosis, panic, and paranoia can occur.

Hospitals may also have specific restrictions and policies regarding medical marijuana for inpatient stays.

- Medical marijuana laws and regulations permit patients to use medical marijuana if certified by a physician but vary by state.
  1. Physician certification involves documentation that a patient has a qualifying clinical condition.
  2. A medical marijuana card entitles a patient or designated caregiver to possess a given amount of marijuana and therefore will not be prosecuted for possession of marijuana.
  3. Medical marijuana can be obtained at state regulated medical marijuana compassion centers (dispensaries). Compassion centers obtain marijuana from licensed cultivators and offer a variety of formulations that are regulated by the state.
  4. There is no FDA oversight of the compassion centers.
- Physicians do not prescribe the dose or formulation of medical marijuana.
- Physicians are under no obligation to issue medical marijuana certifications.
- Emergency department (ED) visits attributable to inhaled cannabis are more frequent than those attributable to edible cannabis, although the latter is associated with more acute psychiatric visits and more ED visits than expected.

PATIENT & FAMILY EDUCATION

- Patients must possess a valid state-issued ID and apply for a state medical marijuana card.
- Patients can obtain medical marijuana from compassion centers without a medical marijuana card but could then be prosecuted for possession of marijuana.
- Patients should be aware that concomitant use of other medications such as opiates and benzodiazepines should be avoided as it could lead to somnolence and respiratory suppression.
- Patients should store medical marijuana away from children given the risk of toxic ingestions.

REFERENCES
Available at eBooks.Health.Elsevier.com

RELATED CONTENT
Pain Management in Chronic Pain (Related Key Topic)
Chemotherapy-Induced Nausea and Vomiting (Related Key Topic)

AUTHOR: **SETH CLARK, MD, MPH, FASAM**

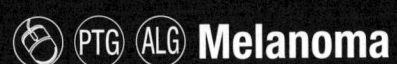

M

 BASIC INFORMATION

DEFINITION

Melanoma is a skin neoplasm arising from the malignant degeneration of melanocytes. It is classically subdivided in four types (Table 1):
1. Superficial spreading melanoma
2. Nodular melanoma
3. Lentigo maligna melanoma
4. Acral lentiginous melanoma

SYNONYMS

Malignant melanoma
Cutaneous malignant melanoma

ICD-10CM CODES

C43.30	Malignant melanoma of unspecified part of face
C43.31	Malignant melanoma of nose
C43.4	Malignant melanoma of scalp and neck
C43.51	Malignant melanoma of anal skin
C43.52	Malignant melanoma of skin of breast
C43.59	Malignant melanoma of other part of trunk
C43.8	Malignant melanoma of overlapping sites of skin
C43.9	Malignant melanoma of skin, unspecified
D03.8	Melanoma in situ of other sites
D03.9	Melanoma in situ, unspecified

EPIDEMIOLOGY & DEMOGRAPHICS

- In 2021, 106,000 new melanoma cases were diagnosed in the U.S. and over 7000 people died of this disease.
- Melanoma is more common in men.
- Melanoma is much more common in Whites (17.2 per 100,000 White men) than in African Americans (1 per 100,000 African American men). Increased risk of developing melanomas is found in patients with fair skin, red hair, light eyes, abundance of freckles, atypical moles, or large amount of moles (>50). A personal history of any skin cancer or a family history of melanoma also increases the risk.
- Melanoma is the leading cause of death from skin cancer. Although it represents <10% of all skin cancers, it accounts for at least 70% of deaths related to skin cancer.
- The median age at diagnosis is 53 yr.
- Individuals with high recreational/intermittent sun exposure, history of blistery sunburns in childhood or adolescence, and exposure to artificial ultraviolet radiation from use of tanning beds have a higher risk for developing melanoma.
- Superficial spreading melanoma occurs most often in young adults on sun-exposed areas.
- Acral lentiginous melanoma is most often found in Asian Americans and African Americans and is unrelated to sun exposure.
- 8% to 10% of melanomas arise in people with a family history of the disease.

PHYSICAL FINDINGS & CLINICAL PRESENTATION

Variable depending on the subtype of melanoma:
- Superficial spreading melanoma is most often found on the lower legs, arms, and upper back. It may have a combination of many colors or may be uniformly brown or black.
- Nodular melanoma can be found anywhere on the body, but it most frequently occurs on the trunk on sun-exposed areas. It has a dark-brown or red-brown appearance and can be dome shaped (or pedunculated). Lesions are frequently misdiagnosed because they may resemble a blood blister or hemangioma (Fig. E1) and may also be amelanotic.
- Lentigo maligna melanoma is generally found in older adults in areas continually exposed to the sun and frequently arising from lentigo maligna (Hutchinson freckle) or melanoma in situ. It might have a complex pattern and variable shape; color is more uniform than in superficial spreading melanoma.
- Acral lentiginous melanoma frequently occurs on soles, subungual mucous membranes, and palms (sole of the foot is the most prevalent site). Unlike other types of melanoma, it has a similar incidence in all ethnic groups.
- The warning signs that the lesion may be a melanoma can be summarized with the ABCDE mnemonic (Table E2):
  A: Asymmetry (e.g., lesion is bisected and halves are not identical)
  B: Border irregularity (uneven, ragged border) (Fig. E2)
  C: Color variegation (presence of various shades of pigmentation)
  D: Diameter enlargement (>6 mm)
  E: Evolving (mole changing in size, shape, or color, or mole that differs visibly from surrounding moles ["ugly duckling" sign])

ETIOLOGY

- Ultraviolet light is the most important cause of malignant melanoma.
- There is a modest increase in melanoma risk in patients with small nondysplastic nevi and a much greater risk in those with dysplastic lesions.
- The *CDKN2A* gene, residing at the 9p21 locus, is often deleted in patients with familial melanoma.
- A mutated signal transduction molecule, v-raf murine sarcoma viral oncogene homolog B *(BRAF),* has been identified in 40% to 60% of patients with melanoma.

TABLE 1 Histologic Subtypes of Cutaneous Melanoma

	Frequency	Location	Characteristics	Morphology
Superficial spreading melanoma	70% Women > men	Lower extremities	Slow radial growth phase	Flat during early phase, macule or papule
Nodular melanoma	15%-30%	Trunk, head	Rapid vertical growth	Papule or nodule

Continued

TABLE 1 Histologic Subtypes of Cutaneous Melanoma—cont'd

	Frequency	Location	Characteristics	Morphology
Lentigo maligna 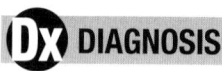	10%-15% More common in the elderly	Face, neck, arms Chronically sun-damaged skin	Slow radial growth, confirmed to the epidermis for many years	Large macule, arises in a preexisting nevus
Acral lentiginous	<5% More common in Asians and African Americans	Soles, palms Beneath nail beds (subungual)	Slow radial growth phase with vertical phase later on	Large dark patch, arising in a preexisting lesion

Ⓓⓧ DIAGNOSIS

DIFFERENTIAL DIAGNOSIS

- Dysplastic nevi
- Solar lentigo
- Vascular lesions
- Blue nevus
- Basal cell carcinoma
- Seborrheic keratosis

WORKUP

- Dermoscopy (use of an instrument that shines polarized light on skin surfaces and magnifies skin lesions) can increase the accuracy in diagnosing melanoma by 10% to 27%.
- Any suspicious lesion should be biopsied. Perform excisional biopsy with elliptical excision that includes 1 to 2 mm of normal skin surrounding the lesion and extends to the subcutaneous tissue; incisional punch biopsy is sometimes necessary in surgically sensitive areas (e.g., digits, nose). It is essential that the size of the specimen be adequate to determine the histologic depth of penetration, which is known as the Breslow depth.
- Sentinel lymph node excision (SLNE) is the most important staging and potentially prognostic procedure for patients with melanoma. It should be considered in patients with intermediate (1 to 4 mm) melanomas or high-risk skin tumors to obtain information regarding a patient's subclinical lymph node status with minimal morbidity. The National Comprehensive Cancer Network (NCCN) recommends that SLNE be discussed with and offered to patients classified as stage IB or II, and should be

considered for patients with stage IA melanoma and "adverse" features that might portend a higher risk of sentinel node tumor thickness of 0.8 mm or more with the presence of ulceration. SLNE involves the use of radiologic lymphoscintigraphy to map lymphatic drainage from the site of the primary melanoma to the first sentinel lymph node in the region. When properly performed, if the sentinel node is negative, the remaining lymph nodes in the region will not have metastases in more than 98% of cases. If the sentinel nodes are negative, no additional regional surgery is recommended. The staging of intermediate thickness (1.2 to 3.5 mm) primary melanomas, according to the results of sentinel node biopsy, provides important prognostic information and identifies patients with nodal metastases whose survival can be prolonged by immediate lymphadenectomy.

- The staging system for melanoma adapted by the American Joint Committee on Cancer (AJCC) can be found in Table 3.

LABORATORY TESTS

The pathology report should indicate the following:
- Tumor thickness (Breslow microstage).
- Tumor depth: The depth of invasion is the most important histologic prognostic parameter in evaluating the primary tumor.
- Mitotic rate: Tabulated as mitoses per square millimeter in the dermal part of the tumor in which most mitoses are identified.
- Radial growth rates vs. vertical growth rate: Radial growth phase describes the growth of

melanoma within the epidermis and along the dermal-epidermal junction.
- Tumor infiltrating lymphocytes have a strong predictive value in vertical growth phase melanomas and are defined as brisk, nonbrisk, or absent.
- Histologic regression: Characterized by the absence of melanoma in the epidermis and dermis flanked on one or both sides by melanoma.
- Reverse-transcription polymerase chain reaction assay for tyrosine messenger RNA is a useful marker for the presence of melanoma cells. It is performed on sentinel lymph node biopsy and is useful for detection of submicroscopic metastases.

Ⓓⓧ TREATMENT (FIG. 3)

- Initial excision of the melanoma
- Reexcision of the involved area after histologic diagnosis: The margins of reexcision depend on the Breslow depth.
  1. For melanoma in situ, margin should be 5 mm.
  2. For melanomas with Breslow depth up to 1 mm, the recommended surgical margin is 1 cm.
  3. For melanomas of tumor thickness >1 mm and <4 mm, 2-cm excision margin is recommended.
  4. For melanomas >4 mm, a 2 cm margin is recommended.
- Sentinel lymph node excision is recommended in all patients with melanoma greater than 1 mm in depth or ulcerated melanomas greater than 0.8 mm.

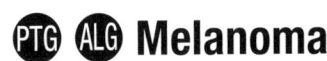
TABLE 3   The TNM Classification for Melanoma Adapted by the American Joint Committee on Cancer (AJCC, 8th edition)

T Classification	Thickness	Ulceration Status/Mitoses
T_{is} (in situ)	n/a	n/a
T_1	<1.0 mm	Unknown or unspecified
T_{1a}	<0.8 mm	Without ulceration
T_{1b}	0.8-1.0 mm	With/without ulceration
T_2	>1.0-2.0 mm	Unknown or unspecified
T_{2a}	>1.0-2.0 mm	Without ulceration
T_{2b}	>1.0-2.0 mm	With ulceration
T_3	>2.0-4.0 mm	Unknown or unspecified
T_{3a}	>2.0-4.0 mm	Without ulceration
T_{3b}	>2.0-4.0 mm	With ulceration
T_4	>4.0 mm	Unknown or unspecified
T_{4a}	>4.0 mm	Without ulceration
T_{4b}	>4.0 mm	With ulceration

Regional Nodes (N)	Number of Nodes	Presence of In-Transit, Satellite, and/or Microsatellite Metastases
N_0	0	None
N_1	One tumor-involved node or any number of in-transit, satellite, and/or microsatellite metastases with no tumor-involved nodes	
N_{1a}	One clinically occult (sentinel biopsy detected)	No
N_{1b}	One clinically detected	No
N_{1c}	No regional node	Yes
N_2	Two or three tumor-involved nodes or any number of in-transit, satellite, and/or microsatellite metastases with one tumor-involved node	
N_{2a}	Two or three clinically occult (sentinel biopsy detected)	No
N_{2b}	Two or three, at least one clinically detected	No
N_{2c}	One clinically occult or clinically detected	Yes
N_3	Four or more tumor-involved nodes or any number of in-transit, satellite, and/or microsatellite metastases with two or more tumor-involved nodes, or any number of matted nodes without or with in-transit, satellite, and/or microsatellite metastases	
N_{3a}	Four or more clinically occult (sentinel biopsy detected)	No
N_{3b}	Four or more, at least one of which was clinically detected, or the presence of any number of matted nodes	No
N_{3c}	Two or more clinically occult or clinically detected and/or presence of any number of matted nodes	Yes

M Category	Anatomic Site	LDH Level
M_0	No distant metastases	n/a
M_1	Evidence of distant metastases	
M_{1a}	Distant metastasis to skin, soft tissue including muscle, and/or nonregional lymph node	$M_{1a}(0)$: Normal $M_{1a}(1)$: Elevated
M_{1b}	Distant metastasis to lung with or without M_{1a} sites of disease	$M_{1b}(0)$: Normal $M_{1b}(1)$: Elevated
M_{1c}	Distant metastasis to non-CNS visceral sites with or without M_{1a} or M_{1b} sites of disease	$M_{1c}(0)$: Normal $M_{1c}(1)$: Elevated
M_{1d}	Distant metastasis to CNS with or without M_{1a}, M_{1b}, or M_{1c} sites of disease	$M_{1d}(0)$: Normal $M_{1d}(1)$: Elevated

CNS, Central nervous system; *LDH,* lactic dehydrogenase; *TNM,* tumor, nodes, metastases.

- Complete lymph node dissection is recommended for patients who present with palpable lymph nodes at the time of diagnosis.
- Adjuvant therapy:
  1. Ipilimumab, an antibody that blocks cytotoxic T-lymphocyte–associated antigen 4 (CTLA-4), improves survival in stage III high-risk resected melanoma but is associated with significant immune adverse events.
  2. Immune checkpoint PD-1 (programmed death receptor-1) antibodies, nivolumab, and pembrolizumab have demonstrated superiority to ipilimumab in patients with resected high-risk stage III melanoma and are considered the standard of care.
  3. The combination regimen of BRAF inhibitor and MEK inhibitor (dabrafenib plus trametinib) has shown improved relapse-free survival in resected BRAF V600-mutant stage III melanoma and is another option for these patients.
- Advanced or metastatic disease:
  1. The use of immune checkpoint inhibitors has improved overall survival in patients with previously treated or untreated metastatic melanoma irrespective of BRAF mutation status. Monotherapy with the PD-1 inhibitors nivolumab or pembrolizumab has been approved for the treatment of metastatic melanoma in treatment-naïve patients and also in cases of progression after initial therapy with ipilimumab.
  2. Combination immunotherapy with the use of nivolumab and ipilimumab in previously untreated patients with unresectable or metastatic melanoma and those with brain metastasis has shown to improve survival compared to monotherapy with either ipilimumab or nivolumab. Common immune-mediated toxicity seen with the use of the combination includes dermatitis, colitis, hepatitis, and hypophysitis. High-grade toxicity with treatment discontinuation is seen in 50% of patients.
  3. In patients who carry the V600E *BRAF* mutation, the combination of oral BRAF inhibitors and oral MEK inhibitors improves overall survival in patients with previously untreated melanoma. Three such combination regimens (vemurafenib plus cobimetinib; dabrafenib plus trametinib; and encorafenib plus binimetinib) are approved by the FDA for use in this setting. Targeted therapy is useful in patients with rapidly growing melanoma with *BRAF* mutations, but resistance appears in almost all patients, with a median progression-free survival of 15 to 18 mo. High-risk patients with brain metastases appear to have response rates of 40% to 50%.
  4. The combination of atezolizumab (PD-L1 checkpoint inhibitor), cobimetinib (MEK inhibitor), and vemurafenib (BRAF inhibitor) has been shown to improve progression-

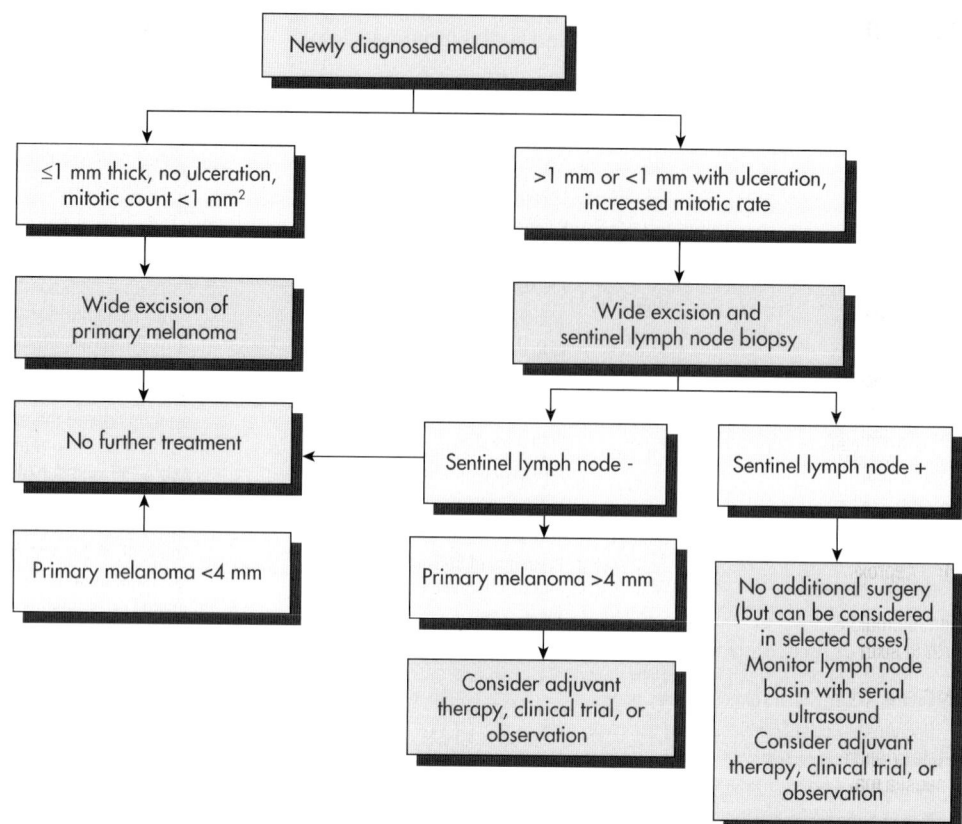

FIG. 3 Treatment algorithm for newly diagnosed melanoma. (From Goldman L, Schafer AI: *Goldman-Cecil medicine,* ed 26, Philadelphia, 2019, Elsevier.)

free survival compared with placebo in patients with *BRAF* mutated advanced melanoma and is likely to be another option in this setting.

5. The relativity trial has shown that the inhibition of two immune checkpoints, LAG-3 and PD-1, with relatlimab and nivolumab combination provides a greater benefit with regard to progression-free survival than inhibition of PD-1 alone in patients with previously untreated metastatic or unresectable melanoma.[1]

6. Adaptive cell therapy with tumor-infiltrating lymphocytes (TILs) have shown promising responses. In a recent phase 3 trial[1a] in patients with advanced melanoma progression-free survival was significantly longer among those who received TIL therapy then among those who received ipilimumab.

• Patients with a history of melanoma should be followed up with skin examinations every 6 mo or sooner if patient detects any new lesions; the assessments usually consist of medical history, physical examination, laboratory values, and chest radiograph.

DISPOSITION

• Prognosis varies with the stage of the melanoma. The 5-yr survival related to thickness is as follows: <0.76 mm, 99% survival; 0.6 to 1.49 mm, 85%; 1.5 to 2.49 mm, 84%; 2.5 to 3.9 mm, 70%; >4 mm, 44%.

• The 5-yr survival in patients with distant metastasis was historically <10% but is improving with current therapeutic options and is now >20% and with combination immunotherapy is approaching 50%.[2]

• Treatment of advanced disease consists (in addition to surgical excision and lymph node dissection) of chemotherapy, immunotherapy, and radiation therapy. Nivolumab combined with ipilimumab has shown clinically meaningful activity in melanoma metastatic to the brain.

REFERENCES & SUGGESTED READINGS
Available at eBooks.Health.Elsevier.com.

RELATED CONTENT
Melanoma (Patient Information)

AUTHOR: **MARIA CONSTANTINOU, MD**

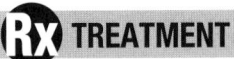
Diseases and Disorders

I

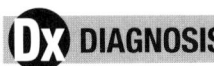 BASIC INFORMATION

DEFINITION

Ménière disease is a syndrome characterized by recurrent vertigo with fluctuating hearing loss, tinnitus, and fullness in the ear.

SYNONYMS

Endolymphatic hydrops
Lermoyez syndrome
Idiopathic endolymphatic hydrops

ICD-10CM CODES

H81.01 Ménière disease, right ear
H81.02 Ménière disease, left ear
H81.03 Ménière disease, bilateral
H81.09 Ménière disease, unspecified ear

EPIDEMIOLOGY & DEMOGRAPHICS

INCIDENCE (IN U.S.): Approximately 190/100,000 persons
PREDOMINANT SEX: Female:male ratio of 1.3:1
PEAK INCIDENCE: Fourth to sixth decade of life

PHYSICAL FINDINGS & CLINICAL PRESENTATION

- Hearing may be unilaterally decreased.
- Pallor, sweating, and nausea may occur during a severe attack.
- Usually the patient develops a sensation of fullness and pressure along with decreased hearing and tinnitus in a single ear.
- The patient typically experiences severe vertigo, which peaks within minutes, then slowly subsides over hours.
- May see spontaneous nystagmus on examination.
- Persistent sense of disequilibrium for days is typical after an acute episode.
- May have vestibulopathy demonstrable with a positive head thrust test.

ETIOLOGY

- Unknown; viral, autoimmune, and genetic causes have been suggested.
- Endolymphatic hydrops is the postmortem histologic hallmark. Endolymphatic hydrops may create cytochemical changes that disturb endolymphatic fluid homeostasis, leading to spiral ganglion cell death.

DX DIAGNOSIS

Proposed guidelines by the American Academy of Otolaryngology-Head and Neck Surgery (AAO-HNS) for diagnosis and severity of Ménière disease (Box E1).

DIFFERENTIAL DIAGNOSIS

- Acoustic neuroma
- Migrainous vertigo
- Multiple sclerosis
- Autoimmune inner ear syndrome
- Otitis media
- Vertebrobasilar disease
- Labyrinthitis

WORKUP

- Diagnosis is primarily made by history, although further diagnostic tests may help support the diagnosis. Guidelines to define Ménière disease are described in Table 1.
- Audiogram may show sensorineural hearing loss with lower frequencies primarily affected. Hearing loss may recover either partially or completely after an attack. Recurrent attacks may lead to a persistent and progressive sensorineural hearing loss.
- Electronystagmography may show peripheral vestibular deficit.
- Both vestibular-evoked myogenic potential (VEMP) studies and electrocochleography (ECoG) have low sensitivity and specificity for Ménière disease and are not clinically useful.

LABORATORY TESTS

No laboratory serologic test is specific for Ménière disease. A thyroid panel, glucose, hemoglobin A1C, antinuclear antibodies, urinalysis, chemistry panel, RPR, Lyme disease antibodies, and allergy testing can be ordered to screen for other disorders such as thyroid or autoimmune diseases, diabetes, otorenal syndrome, syphilis, Lyme disease, and allergy-mediated Ménière disease.

IMAGING STUDIES

- MRI to rule out acoustic neuroma or other retrocochlear lesion, especially if cerebellar or CNS dysfunction is present.
- Recent efforts have shown a role for MRI with intratympanic gadolinium.

RX TREATMENT

NONPHARMACOLOGIC THERAPY

Limit activity during attacks.

ACUTE GENERAL Rx

- Prochlorperazine 5 to 10 mg PO q6h or 25 mg PO bid
- Promethazine 12.5 to 25 mg PO q4 to 6h
- Diazepam 5 to 10 mg IV/PO for acute attack
- Meclizine 25 mg q6h
- Scopolamine patch

CHRONIC Rx

- Diuretics such as furosemide, hydrochlorothiazide, or acetazolamide.
- Lifestyle modification recommendations include salt restriction and avoidance of caffeine.
- For refractory cases, intratympanic gentamicin injections to the affected ear; endolymphatic sac surgery.

DISPOSITION

- Patients are usually followed by an neurotologist or ENT specialist.
- Usual course of disease consists of alternating attacks and remissions.
- Majority of patients can be managed medically. Of all patients, 10% to 30% will undergo surgical intervention for persistent incapacitating vertigo.

REFERRAL

To an otolaryngologist for surgical intervention if attacks persist despite medical therapy

REFERENCES & SUGGESTED READINGS

Available at eBooks.Health.Elsevier.com.

RELATED CONTENT

Ménière Disease (Patient Information)

AUTHOR: **JOSEPH S. KASS, MD, JD, FAAN**

TABLE 1 Guidelines to Define Ménière Disease

Definition	Symptoms
Certain Ménière disease	Histopathologic confirmation
Definite Ménière disease	≥2 definitive spontaneous episodes of vertigo 20 min to 12 hr Audiometrically documented low- to medium-frequency sensorineural hearing loss in one ear, defining the affected ear on at least one occasion before, during, or after one of the episodes of vertigo Fluctuating aural symptoms (hearing, tinnitus, or fullness) in the affected ear Not better accounted for by another vestibular diagnosis
Probable Ménière disease	One definite episode of vertigo Audiometrically documented hearing loss on at least one occasion Tinnitus or aural fullness in the treated ear Other causes excluded
Possible Ménière disease	Episodic vertigo without documented hearing loss, or sensorineural hearing loss (SNHL) fluctuating or fixed, with disequilibrium but nonepisodic Other causes excluded

Meningioma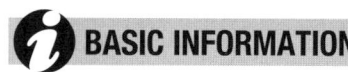

BASIC INFORMATION

DEFINITION

Meningiomas are generally slow-growing tumors arising from arachnoid cells of the arachnoid villi; 90% are benign.

ICD-10CM CODE
D32.0 Benign neoplasm of cerebral meninges

EPIDEMIOLOGY & DEMOGRAPHICS

INCIDENCE: 7.92/100,000 persons/yr but increases with age. Most common primary type of central nervous system tumor, and most common nonmalignant primary central nervous system tumor.[1]
PREDOMINANT SEX & AGE: Female:male ratio of almost 3:1 (in ages 35 to 54) in the brain and up to 6:1 in the spinal cord; 1:1 in childhood.[1]
PEAK INCIDENCE: Males: Sixth decade, females: Seventh decade, incidence increases with age, dramatic increase in incidence after age 65; rare in childhood.[1]
RISK FACTORS: Ionizing radiation results in increased incidence and a shorter latency period. Neurofibromatosis type 2 (NF2) is an autosomal dominant genetic disorder that predisposes to multiple intracranial tumors. Approximately half of all individuals with NF2 have meningiomas, most of which are intracranial.[2] Studies have suggested a link between hormonal factors and development of meningioma, specifically estrogen exposure. Multiple prospective cohort studies have also found an association between higher body mass index and meningioma, possibly relating to increased levels of circulating estrogen through increased adipose tissue. At present, there is no conclusive evidence to support a causal relationship with cell phone usage and subsequent development of meningioma.[1]
GENETICS: Meningiomas may be isolated or found in association with other genetic diseases, such as NF2 and familial meningioma. Other genetic conditions associated with increased incidence of meningioma include BAP1 tumor predisposition syndrome, Rubinstein-Taybi syndrome, multiple endocrine neoplasia, type 1, Gorlin syndrome, Cowden syndrome 1, Werner syndrome, and familial meningiomatosis. Approximately half of meningiomas have allelic losses involving the NF2 and DAL-1 genes. Allelic losses of chromosomes 1p, 2p, 6q, 9q,

10q, 14q, 17p, and 18q may be associated with histologic progression. Genome-wide association studies (GWAS) have discovered two genomic variants associated with increased meningioma risk in genes for MLLT10 and possibly RIC8A. Further, GWAS analysis also demonstrates an association between longer telomere length and increased risk of meningiomas.[3]

PHYSICAL FINDINGS & CLINICAL PRESENTATION

- Neurologic symptoms vary with location and size (Table 1); meningiomas can arise from the dura at any site, although they most commonly occur within the skull and at sites of dural reflection (i.e., the cerebral convexities and the falx). Other less common locations include the sphenoid wing, olfactory groove, and optic nerve sheath.[4]
- The presence of focal symptoms such as vision loss, hearing loss, or mental status change depend on the site of origin and the time course of growth.
- Most common presentation is with a focal or generalized seizure or gradually worsening neurologic deficit. Seizures are present preoperatively in 30% to 40%.[5]
- Typically slow growing and asymptomatic; many meningiomas are asymptomatic and/or discovered incidentally on a neuroimaging study or at autopsy.

ETIOLOGY

- Meningiomas are thought to arise from a multistep progression of genetic changes.
- Mutations of the NF2 gene on chromosome 22 are found in patients with neurofibromatosis type 2 and >50% of sporadic meningiomas. This gene is thought to act as a tumor suppressor gene; the protein product, merlin, is also involved in cytoskeletal organization.[2]
- DAL-1, located on chromosome 18p, is another tumor suppressor gene that has been identified in a subset of the approximately 40% of sporadic meningiomas with neither the NF2 gene mutations nor allelic loss of chromosome 22q.[2-3]
- Cranial radiation may be responsible for some cases following an appropriate latency period from 10 to 20 yr. Meningiomas that result from radiation are generally more aggressive.[5]
- The link with steroid hormones and their receptors is suggested by the increase in growth

rate and/or development of meningiomas during pregnancy, increased incidence in women who use postmenopausal hormones, and in association with breast carcinomas.[4]

DIAGNOSIS

DIFFERENTIAL DIAGNOSIS

Other well-circumscribed intracranial tumors that involve the dura or subdural space:
- Acoustic schwannoma (typically at the pontocerebellar junction)
- Ependymoma, lipoma, and metastases within spinal cord
- Metastatic disease from lymphoma/adenocarcinoma
- Inflammatory disease such as sarcoidosis and Wegener granulomatosis
- Infections such as tuberculosis

WORKUP

Imaging studies with CT or MRI, followed by surgical removal with histologic confirmation

LABORATORY TESTS

According to the World Health Organization (WHO) classification, there are nine benign histologic variants (accounting for 90% of all meningiomas) and four variants associated with increased recurrence and rates of metastasis. 80% of meningiomas are classified as benign meningiomas or WHO grade I.[6]

IMAGING STUDIES

- Cranial CT scanning or MRI can detect and determine the extent of meningiomas (Fig. 1). CT can show hyperostosis and/or intratumoral calcifications. MRI with contrast (Fig. 2) is the imaging modality of choice to demonstrate the dural origin of the tumor in most cases, with

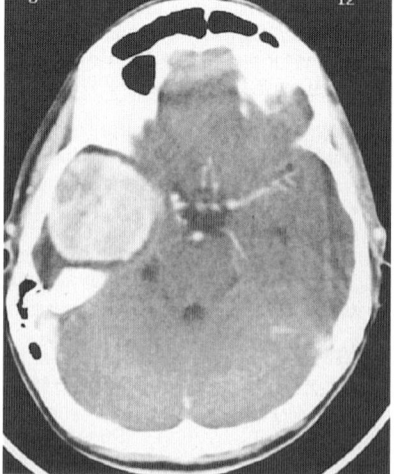

FIG. 1 Contrast-enhanced computed tomography scan demonstrates a large contrast-enhancing right sphenoid wing meningioma. (From Specht N [ed]: *Practical guide to diagnostic imaging*, St Louis, 1998, Mosby.)

TABLE 1 Locations and Presentations of Meningiomas

Location	Presenting Manifestation
Parasagittal	Urinary incontinence, dementia, gradual paraparesis, seizures
Lateral convexity	Variable depending on structures compressed, including slow hemiparesis, speech abnormalities
Olfactory groove	Anosmia, visual disturbance, dementia, Foster-Kennedy syndrome
Suprasellar	Hormonal failure, bitemporal hemianopsia, optic atrophy
Sphenoid ridge	Extraocular nerve paresis, exostoses, proptosis, seizures

From Goetz CG, Pappert EJ: *Textbook of clinical neurology*, Philadelphia, 1999, Saunders.

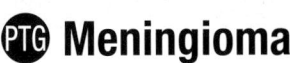

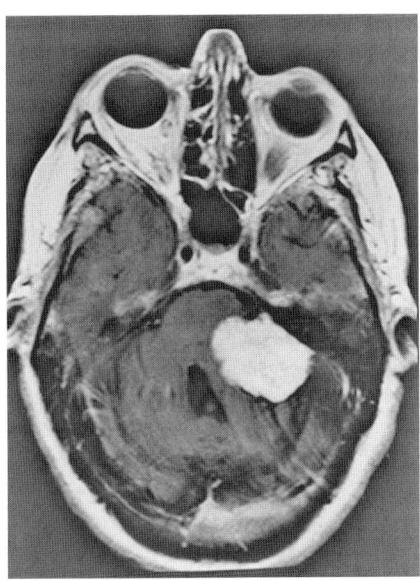

FIG. 2 Magnetic resonance imaging picture of a posterior fossa meningioma, demonstrated an extra-axial homogeneously contrast-enhanced mass arising from the tentorium and compressing the cerebellar hemisphere. (From Goetz CG, Pappert EJ: *Textbook of clinical neurology*, Philadelphia, 1999, Saunders.)

the characteristic "tail" sign that tracks along the dura outside brain parenchyma.[7]
- On nonenhanced scans, meningiomas are typically isodense or slightly hyperdense to brain and are homogeneous in appearance. They show homogeneous contrast enhancement; gadolinium can facilitate imaging of smaller additional lesions that are missed on unenhanced images.[7]
- Indistinct margins, marked edema, mushroom-like projections from tumor, brain parenchymal infiltration, and heterogeneous enhancement are suggestive of more aggressive behavior.[7]
- Positron emission tomography (PET) scan may help in predicting the aggressiveness of the tumor and the potential for recurrence, but it is not used routinely.[7]

Rx TREATMENT

Primary management depends on signs or symptoms, age of patient, and location and size of tumor. Observation may be appropriate if tumors are discovered incidentally and/or if growth is indolent and unlikely to cause symptoms.[8]

PHARMACOLOGIC THERAPY
- Although a variety of chemotherapeutic agents have been studied, there is no established effective systemic therapy.[8]

- In 2020, the CEVOREM trial in France, a Phase 2 trial, demonstrated efficacy in treating recurrent meningioma with everolimus (an mTOR inhibitor) and octreotide (a somatostatin agonist).[9]
- Inhibition of hormone receptors, such as progesterone, estrogen, and androgen, has failed to demonstrate clinical benefit.[8]
- Treatment with molecularly targeted approaches, such as angiogenesis inhibition, is currently under study.

NONPHARMACOLOGIC THERAPY
- The mainstay of treatment for meningiomas remains surgical removal. Complete resection is usually attempted when feasible. After total excision, recurrence rates of 0% to 20% have been observed, while 20% to 50% of patients recur within 5 yr of a subtotal resection.[8]
- Active surveillance to monitor for tumor recurrence is important in higher grade tumors.
- Radiation therapy is the only validated form of adjuvant therapy and may be beneficial in patients with incomplete resections or inoperable tumors. Stereotactic radiosurgery can provide local control with more limited toxicity.[8]

ACUTE GENERAL Rx
- For lesions that cause significant mass effect, steroids are sometimes used to decrease brain edema.
- Anticonvulsants are used if the patient presents with seizures.

CHRONIC Rx
- Prophylactic use of anticonvulsants is not recommended in patients without a history of seizures.
- There are limited data on the efficacy of traditional chemotherapy, and the evidence is largely anecdotal. The most extensively evaluated agents are hydroxyurea, mifepristone (RU486), and interferon alfa-2b. Recently, somatostatin analogs and mTOR inhibitors have been evaluated in multicenter clinical trials, primarily in malignant recurrent meningiomas.[8]

DISPOSITION
- Estimated surgical mortality is 7%. Significant morbidity and mortality can be observed in meningiomas with otherwise favorable pathology secondary to unfavorable location (e.g., skull base). 10-yr relative survival is 80.4% in the cerebral meninges vs. 93.2% in spinal meninges.[10-11]
- Long-term outcome varies based on pathology, tumor grade, location, and completeness of resection. 10-yr relative survival for nonmalignant meningioma is 81.5%, with highest survivability in the youngest age

group. 10-yr relative survival for malignant meningioma is 53.5%, with similar age-based effects.[7]
- Most incidentally discovered meningiomas remain asymptomatic and have a slow rate of growth. Calcified tumors may be less likely to progress than noncalcified ones.
- Meningiomas may recur after surgical resection or progress to a higher grade. Risk factors for recurrence include multiple allelic chromosomal losses, local brain invasion, high rate of mitosis, and highly anaplastic features.[12]

REFERRAL
- Neurosurgical consultation for all cases
- Neurology, radiation oncology, and oncology consults depending on presence of other sequelae or in the setting of recurrence

PEARLS & CONSIDERATIONS

COMMENTS
- Many meningiomas are discovered incidentally; most are benign and remain asymptomatic. A first follow-up MRI should be performed 3 to 6 mo after the tumor is identified to rule out an atypical meningioma with rapid growth.
- "Dural tail," which is the thickening of the dura adjacent to the mass, is a classic finding on neuroimaging studies.
- Individuals with neurofibromatosis type 2 are at high risk to develop meningiomas.

PATIENT & FAMILY EDUCATION
- Meningioma Mommas: meningiomamommas.com
- Meningioma Support and Patient Information Group
- National Brain Tumor Society
- Meningioma Online Support Group: braintrust.org/meningioma.html

REFERENCES
Available at eBooks.Health.Elsevier.com.

RELATED CONTENT
Meningioma (Patient Information)

AUTHORS: **LILY C. PHAM, MD** and **NATHAN CLARKE, MD**

M

Diseases and Disorders

I

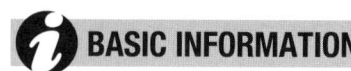
BASIC INFORMATION

DEFINITION

Bacterial meningitis is an inflammation of meninges with increased intracranial pressure, and pleocytosis or increased WBCs in cerebrospinal fluid (CSF) secondary to bacteria in the pia-subarachnoid space and ventricles, leading to neurologic sequelae and abnormalities.

SYNONYMS

Spinal meningitis
Bacterial meningitis

ICD-10CM CODES
G00.9 Bacterial meningitis, unspecified
G00.8 Other bacterial meningitis
G01   Meningitis in bacterial diseases classified elsewhere

EPIDEMIOLOGY & DEMOGRAPHICS

INCIDENCE (IN U.S.): 1.3 to 2.0 cases/100,000 persons; 1.2 million cases per year in the world; 135,000 deaths annually worldwide. The rate of bacterial meningitis declined dramatically in the U.S. starting in the early 1990s with the introduction of the *Haemophilus influenzae* type b (Hib) vaccine and in 2000 with the introduction of the conjugate pneumococcal vaccine.
PREDOMINANT SEX: Male = female
PREDOMINANT AGE: All ages, neonate to geriatric

PHYSICAL FINDINGS & CLINICAL PRESENTATION

- Fever
- Headache
- Neck stiffness, nuchal rigidity, meningismus
- Altered mental state, lethargy
- Vomiting, nausea
- Photophobia
- Seizures
- Coma; lethargy, stupor
- Rash: Petechial and purpuric lesions (Fig. E1) associated with meningococcal infection, purpura fulminans
- Myalgia
- Cranial nerve abnormality (unilateral)
- Papilledema
- Dilated, nonreactive pupil(s)
- Posturing: Decorticate/decerebrate
- Physical examination findings of Kernig sign and Brudzinski sign (Fig. E2) in adults with meningitis are often seen later in the course of disease and may not be helpful in determining early meningeal inflammation

ETIOLOGY

The bacterial etiology of meningitis depends on the age of the patient. *Neisseria meningitidis* is now more common than *Haemophilus influenzae* as a cause of bacterial meningitis in children as well as adults, and streptococci (*Streptococcus pneumoniae*) are still common causes of community-acquired bacterial meningitis. *H. influenzae* is the cause of >30% of cases of meningitis (usually in infants and children <6 yr of age). It is associated with sinusitis, otitis media.

- Neonates: Group B *Streptococcus*, gram-negative rods such as *E. coli*, *Listeria monocytogenes*
- Infants ≥1 mo and <3 mo: Group B streptococci (40%), gram-negative rods (30%), *Streptococcus pneumoniae* (14%), and *Neisseria meningitidis* (12%)
- Infants ≥3 mo and <3 yr:
  1. *S. pneumoniae* (45%)
  2. *N. meningitidis* (34%)
  3. *S. agalactiae* (group B streptococci) (11%)
  4. *H. influenzae*
  5. *E. coli*
- Ages ≥3 yr and <10 yr:
  1. *S. pneumoniae* (47%)
  2. *N. meningitidis* (32%)
- Ages ≥10 yr and <19 yr
  1. *N. meningitidis* (55%)
  2. *S. pneumoniae*
- Adults: *S. pneumoniae*, *N. meningitidis*, and *Streptococcus agalactiae* (third most common cause in adults)
- *Listeria monocytogenes* is uncommon in the general population but is often seen in older adults and in those with cell-mediated immune deficiencies
- People with HIV/AIDS are at increased risk for invasive meningococcal disease (IMD)

DIAGNOSIS

An algorithm for early management of suspected bacterial meningitis is illustrated in Fig. 3. Lumbar puncture should be performed as soon as possible. Key elements to diagnosis are CSF evaluation and CT scan or MRI if the patient is in a coma or has focal neurologic deficits, pupillary abnormalities, or papilledema. Tables 1 and 2 describe tests of CSF in patients with suspected CNS infection.

DIFFERENTIAL DIAGNOSIS (BOX E1)

- Endocarditis, bacteremia
- Intracranial tumor
- Lyme disease
- Brain abscess
- Partially treated bacterial meningitis
- Medications
- SLE
- Seizures
- Acute mononucleosis
- Other infectious meningitides
- Neuroleptic malignant syndrome
- Subdural empyema
- Subarachnoid hemorrhage (Table 3)
- Rocky Mountain spotted fever

WORKUP

CSF examination (Table 4):
- Opening pressure >100 to 200 mm Hg
- WBC usually >1000/mm³
- Neutrophilic predominance: >80%
- Gram stain of CSF: Positive in 60% to 90% of patients
- CSF protein: >50 mg/dl

- CSF glucose: <40 mg/dl
- Culture: Positive in 65% to 90% of cases
- Multiplex PCR assay for detection of *S. pneumoniae*, *H. influenza*, *N. meningitidis*, and *L. monocytogenes* offer 100% sensitivity and 98% specificity

LABORATORY TESTS

Blood culturing, WBC with differential, and CSF examination (see "Workup")

IMAGING STUDIES

- Guidelines from the Infectious Society of America recommend CT of brain before lumbar puncture in patients presenting with:
  1. A high clinical suspicion for subarachnoid hemorrhage
  2. New focal neurologic deficit
  3. Papilledema
  4. Seizures within a week
  5. Altered mental status
  6. History of central nervous system disease (e.g., tumor, stroke)
  7. Immunodeficiency
  8. Age 60 or older

TREATMENT

Empiric therapy (Table 5) is necessary with IV antibiotic treatment if patient has purulent CSF fluid at time of lumbar puncture, is asplenic, or has signs of DIC/sepsis pending Gram stain and culture results. Try to obtain blood and CSF cultures before starting antimicrobial therapy, but do not delay therapy if obtaining them is not possible. If CT scan is indicated (see "Imaging Studies" for indications) it should not delay empiric antibiotic therapy. Therapy after Gram stain pending cultures is recommended for the following:

- Neonates: Ampicillin: 200 to 400 mg/kg per day divided q6 to 8 hr plus ceftazidime with or without gentamicin: 7.5 mg/kg IV in three divided doses
- 1 to 23 mo: Vancomycin: 60 mg/kg per day IV (maximum up to 4 g/day) divided in four doses plus third-generation cephalosporin: Ceftriaxone: 100 mg/kg (maximum dose 4 g/day) in one or two divided doses or cefotaxime: 300 mg/kg per day IV (maximum dose of 12 g/day) in three or four divided doses
- Children: Vancomycin: 60 mg/kg per day IV (maximum dose 4 g/day) in four divided doses plus third-generation cephalosporin: Ceftriaxone 100 mg/kg per day IV (maximum 4 g/day) or cefotaxime: 300 mg/kg IV (maximum dose of 12 g/day) in three or four divided doses
- Adults: Vancomycin: 15 to 20 mg/kg IV every 8 to 12 hr plus third-generation cephalosporin: Ceftriaxone: 2 g IV q12h or cefotaxime: 2 g IV q4 to 6 hr. For adults over 50 yr of age also add ampicillin 2 g IV every 4 hr to cover *Listeria*
- Immunocompromised patients: Vancomycin *plus* ampicillin *plus* either cefepime 2 g IV every 8 hr to cover *Pseudomonas* or meropenem 2 g IV q8h for adults, which also covers *Pseudomonas*

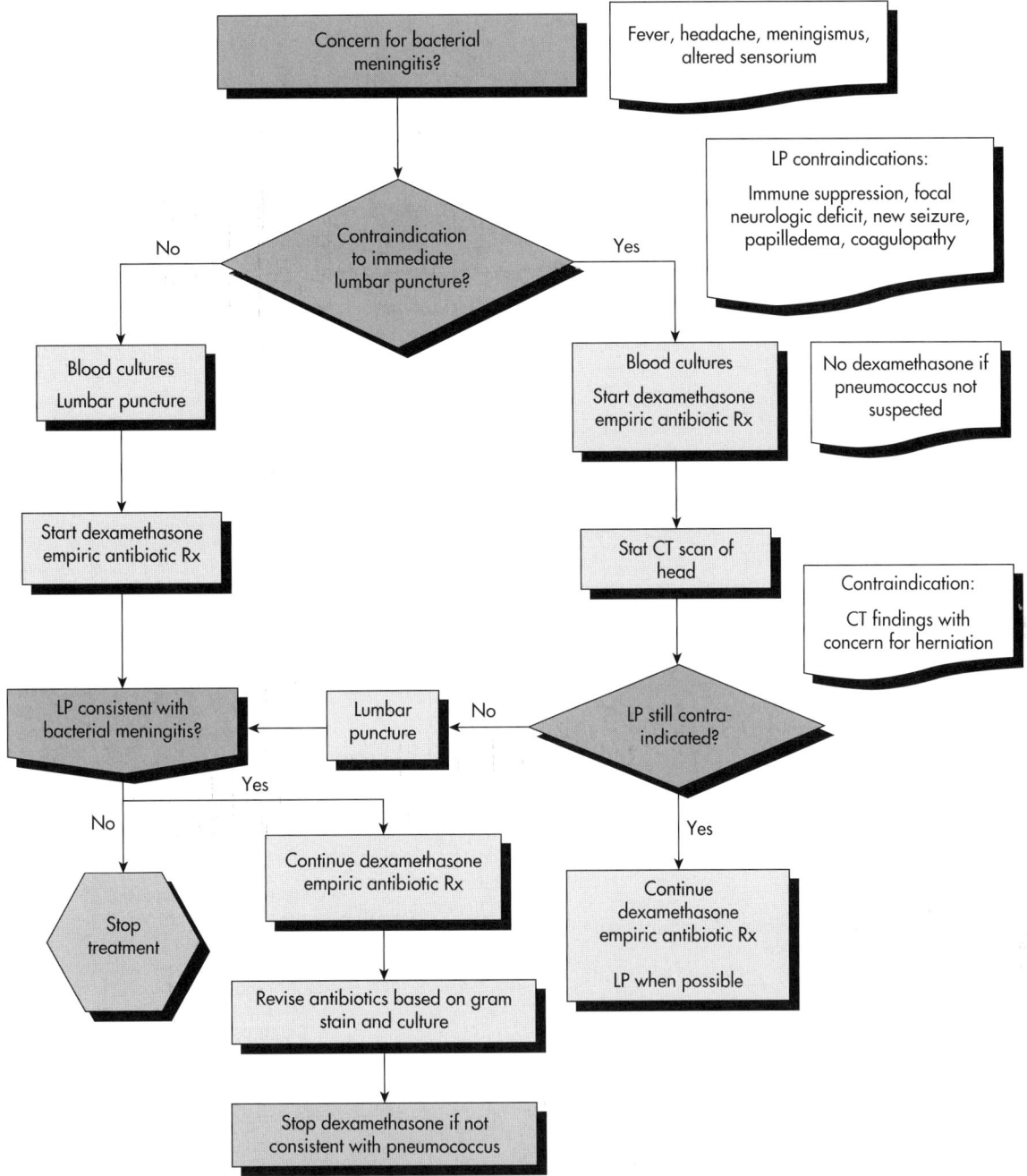

FIG. 3 Algorithm for early management of suspected bacterial meningitis including when to suspect the diagnosis, when imaging prior to lumbar puncture is appropriate, and when to initiate and discontinue empiric antibiotics and adjuvant dexamethasone. *CT,* Computed tomography; *LP,* lumbar puncture; *Rx,* treatment. (Based on Tunkel AR et al: Practice guidelines for the management of bacterial meningitis, *Clin Infect Dis* 39:1267-1284, 2004; and additional information from Hasbun R et al: Computed tomography of the head before lumbar puncture in adults with suspected meningitis, *N Engl J Med* 345:1727-1733, 2001; Glimåker M et al: Adult bacterial meningitis: earlier treatment and improved outcome following guideline revision promoting prompt lumbar puncture, *Clin Infect Dis* 60:1162-1169, 2015; and Brouwer MC et al: Corticosteroids for acute bacterial meningitis, *Cochrane Database Syst Rev* 12(9):CD004405, 2015.)

Use of corticosteroids in adults:
• Dexamethasone 0.15 mg/kg q6h for first 4 days of therapy should be used for adults in developed countries with known or suspected bacterial meningitis. Decreased mortality and neurologic sequelae (hearing loss, etc.) are seen with adjunct therapy in patients with pneumococcal meningitis but not other pathogens. The benefit of dexamethasone is less clear in developing countries with high HIV

prevalence and malnutrition or with delayed clinical presentations.
• Dexamethasone also benefits children with Hib meningitis if given at the same time or before the first dose of the antibiotic: 0.15 mg/kg per dose q6h for 2 to 4 days. The use and benefit of corticosteroids in children with suspected or pneumococcal or meningococcal meningitis to prevent neurologic sequelae is

not as clear and should be individualized after analysis of risk and benefits.

DISPOSITION

Bacterial meningitis is a reportable disease that needs to be reported to local health authorities. Droplet precautions should be used for first 24 hr of therapy for suspected or confirmed *N. meningitidis* infection.

Meningitis, Bacterial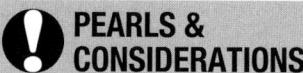

TABLE 1 Tests of Cerebrospinal Fluid in Patients With Suspected Central Nervous System Infection

Routine Tests

White blood cell count with differential

Red blood cell count[a]

Glucose concentration[b]

Protein concentration

Gram stain

Bacterial culture

Selected Specific Tests Based on Clinical Suspicion

Viral culture[c]

Smears and culture for acid-fast bacilli

Venereal Disease Research Laboratory (VDRL)

India ink preparation

Cryptococcal polysaccharide antigen

Fungal culture

Antibody tests (IgM or IgG, or both)[d]

Nucleic acid amplification tests (e.g., polymerase chain reaction)[e]

Cytology[f]

Flow cytometry

[a]Should be checked in the first and last tubes; in patients with a traumatic tap, there should be a decrease in the number of red blood cells with continued flow of cerebrospinal fluid (CSF). See text for the formula for determining whether the numbers of CSF red blood cells and white blood cells are consistent with a traumatic tap.
[b]Compare with serum glucose drawn just before lumbar puncture.
[c]Yield of viral culture may be low.
[d]May be useful for specific causes of meningitis and encephalitis.
[e]Most useful for specific viral causes of encephalitis and causes of chronic meningitis.
[f]In patients with suspected malignancy.
From Bennett JE et al: *Mandell, Douglas, and Bennett's principles and practice of infectious diseases*, ed 8, Philadelphia, 2015, Saunders.

TABLE 3 Acute Bacterial Meningitis and Subarachnoid Hemorrhage

Finding	Frequency (%)
Acute Bacterial Meningitis	
Neck stiffness	84
Fever	66-97
Altered mental status	55-95
Kernig or Brudzinski sign	61
Focal neurologic signs	9-37
Seizures	5-28
Petechial rash	3-52
Subarachnoid Hemorrhage	
Neck stiffness	21-86
Seizures	7-32
Altered mental status	29-64
Focal neurologic findings	10-36
Fever	6
Preretinal hemorrhage	4

Diagnostic standard: For *meningitis*, cerebrospinal fluid pleocytosis and microbiologic or postmortem data supporting bacterial meningitis; for *subarachnoid hemorrhage*, computed tomography or lumbar puncture.
From McGee S: *Evidence-based physical diagnosis*, ed 4, Philadelphia, 2018, Elsevier.

REFERRAL

- To a neurologist if persistent neurologic sequelae develop after bacterial meningitis
- To an infectious disease consultant if a patient has recurrent bacterial meningitis; such patients deserve a workup for an anatomic (CSF dural leak) or immunologic defect (complement defect, hyposplenism, immunoglobulin deficiency)

⚠ PEARLS & CONSIDERATIONS

COMMENTS

- Patients with bacterial meningitis often require ICU care either to manage complications evident on presentation or for monitoring for any complications that may subsequently develop during their course. Criteria for admission to an ICU are summarized in Table 6.
- Nosocomial bacterial meningitis may result from invasive procedures (e.g., placement of ventricular catheters, lumbar puncture, craniotomy, spinal anesthesia). Treatment of this different spectrum of microorganisms requires empirical antimicrobial therapy with vancomycin plus either cefepime, ceftazidime, or meropenem. In cases of basilar skull fracture, effective empirical antimicrobial therapy consists of vancomycin plus a third-generation cephalosporin.
- False-positive elevations of CSF where blood cell counts can be found after traumatic lumbar puncture or in patients with intracerebral or subarachnoid hemorrhage in which RBCs and WBCs are introduced into the subarachnoid space. In those instances, the following formula should be used as a correction factor for the true WBC count in the presence of CSF RBCs:

$$\text{Adjusted WBC in CSF} = \text{Actual WBC in CSF} - \frac{\text{WBC in blood} \times \text{RBC in CSF blood}}{\text{RBC in blood}}$$

In the previous equation, the amount being subtracted is the predicted CSF WBC that would occur if all the CSF WBCs were the result of blood contamination.

TABLE 2 Bacterial Meningeal Pathogens and Their Diagnostic Tests

Organism	Blood	Cerebrospinal Fluid
Streptococcus pneumoniae	Culture	Gram stain: Gram-positive diplococci in pairs Culture Meningitis/encephalitis panel
Listeria monocytogenes	Culture	Gram stain: Gram-positive rods Culture Meningitis/encephalitis panel
Neisseria meningitides	Culture	Gram stain: Gram-negative diplococcus Culture
Haemophilus influenzae type b	Culture	Gram stain: Gram-negative coccobacillus Culture Meningitis/encephalitis panel
Mycobacterium tuberculosis		20-30 mL for AFB stain and culture; PCR
Treponema pallidum	RPR/VDRL; MHA-TPA; FTA-ABS; TPPA	VDRL (nontraumatic tap)
Coxiella burnetii	Acute and convalescent serologies	
Brucella spp.	Culture: Acute and convalescent serologies	Gram stain: Gram-negative coccobacillus Culture
Borrelia spp.	ELISA → if equivocal or +, then IgG and IgM WB (follow CDC guidelines for + WB)	Antibody index: Anti-*Borrelia* IgG in CSF/anti-*Borrelia* IgG in serum to total IgG in CSF/total IgG in serum
Leptospira spp.	Acute and convalescent serologies (MAT only done in reference labs, ELISA and lateral flow dipstick less sensitive and specific) Culture: Special media; may need to keep for 8-12 wk	Culture: Special media, fastidious

AFB, Acid-fast bacilli; *CDC*, Centers for Disease Control and Prevention; *CSF*, cerebrospinal fluid; *ELISA*, enzyme-linked immunosorbent assay; *FTA-ABS*, fluorescent treponemal antibody absorbed; *Ig*, immunoglobulin; *MAT*, microscopic agglutination test; *MHA-TPA*, microhemagglutination assay–*Treponema* antibody absorption test; *PCR*, polymerase chain reaction; *RPR*, rapid plasma reagin test; *TPPA*, *Treponema pallidum* particle agglutination; *VDRL*, Venereal Disease Research Laboratory test; *WB*, Western blot test.
From Jankovic J et al: *Bradley and Daroff's neurology in clinical practice*, ed 8, Philadelphia, 2022, Elsevier.

TABLE 4   Cerebrospinal Fluid Findings in Various Central Nervous System Disorders

CONDITION	PRESSURE (CM H_2O)	LEUKOCYTES (CELLS/μL)	PROTEIN (mg/dL)/ GLUCOSE (mg/dL)	COMMENTS
Normal	10-20	<5; 60-70% lymphocytes, 30-40% monocytes, 1-3% neutrophils	20-45/>50% of serum glucose	WBC up to 10-20 cells/μL can be normal in neonates
Acute bacterial meningitis	Usually elevated (>25)	>100; usually thousands; PMNs predominate	100-500/usually <40 or <40% of serum glucose	Organisms may be seen on Gram stain and recovered by culture
Partially treated bacterial meningitis	Normal or elevated	1-10,000; PMNs usual but mononuclear cells may predominate if pretreated for extended period	>100/depressed or normal	Pretreatment may render CSF sterile, but bacteria may be detected by PCR
Tuberculous meningitis	Usually elevated; may be low because of CSF block in advanced stages	10-500; PMNs early but lymphocytes and monocytes predominate later	100-500; may be higher in presence of CSF block/ usually <50	Acid-fast smear and culture or mycobacteria PCR may be positive. Adenine deaminase can be used to aid in the diagnosis
Fungal	Usually elevated	10-500; PMNs early; mononuclear cells predominate later	20-500/usually <50	Organisms may be seen on smear, in culture, or by India ink preparation, and antigen may be positive in cryptococcal disease
Viral meningitis or meningoencephalitis	Normal or slightly elevated	10-1,000; PMNs early; mononuclear cells predominate later	<50/normal or depressed	Viruses may be detected by PCR
Abscess (parameningeal infection)	Normal or elevated	0-100 PMNs unless rupture into CSF	20-200/normal	Profile may be completely normal

CSF, Cerebrospinal fluid; *PCR*, polymerase chain reaction; *PMNs*, polymorphonuclear leukocytes.
From Marcdante KJ et al: *Nelson essentials of pediatrics*, ed 9, Philadelphia 2023, Elsevier.

TABLE 5   Empiric Treatment of Suspected Bacterial Meningitis in Adults[a,1,2,3,4]

Host Factors to Consider	
	Age >50 yr? Risk for *Listeria monocytogenes* and aerobic gram-negative rods
	Immune suppression? Includes host defects (e.g., HIV, alcoholism, lymphoma) and treatment-related (e.g., posttransplant, corticosteroids)
	Health care–associated? Includes trauma, postneurosurgical, shunt- or ventriculostomy-related
	Life-threatening penicillin/β-lactam allergy? Aztreonam or fluoroquinolone alternatives for gram-negative rods; trimethoprim-sulfamethoxazole an alternative for *L. monocytogenes*

Host	Likely Pathogens	Empiric Therapy	Additional Considerations
Age 15-50 yr without Immune Suppression	*Streptococcus pneumoniae, Neisseria meningitidis,* group B β-hemolytic streptococci	Vancomycin + third-generation cephalosporin[b]	Adjuvant dexamethasone Consider rifampin if high rates of cephalosporin-resistant *S. pneumoniae*
Age ≥50 yr without Immune Suppression	*S. pneumoniae, N. meningitidis,* group B β-hemolytic streptococci, *L. monocytogenes,* aerobic gram-negative rods	Vancomycin + ampicillin + third-generation cephalosporin[b]	Adjuvant dexamethasone Consider rifampin if high rates of cephalosporin-resistant *S. pneumoniae*
Immune Suppression	*S. pneumoniae, N. meningitidis,* group B β-hemolytic streptococci, *L. monocytogenes, Staphylococcus aureus,* aerobic gram-negative rods including *Pseudomonas aeruginosa*	Vancomycin + ampicillin + cefepime or meropenum[c]	Adjuvant dexamethasone Consider rifampin if high rates of cephalosporin-resistant *S. pneumoniae*
Health Care–Associated: Trauma, Postneurosurgical, or Shunt-Associated[c]	*S. aureus,* coagulase-negative staphylococci, aerobic gram-negative rods including *P. aeruginosa*	Vancomycin + ceftazidime or cefepime or meropenem[c]	Dexamethasone not indicated Consider rifampin for staphylococci Consider intrathecal therapy for shunt-/ventriculostomy-associated infection
Health Care–Associated: Basilar Skull Fracture	*S. pneumoniae, Haemophilus influenzae,* group A β-hemolytic streptococci	Vancomycin + third-generation cephalosporin[b]	Adjuvant dexamethasone Consider rifampin if high rates of cephalosporin-resistant *S. pneumoniae*

HIV, Human immunodeficiency virus.
[a]Age older than 15 yr.
[b]Third-generation cephalosporin: Ceftriaxone 2 g q12h or cefotaxime 2 g q4-6h.
[c]Dosing of other agents (modified for renal insufficiency): Vancomycin targeted to vancomycin trough levels of 15-20 μg/ml; ampicillin 2 g q4h; ceftazidime 2 g q8h; cefepime 2 g q8h; meropenem 2 g q8h.
[1]van de Beek D et al: Community-acquired bacterial meningitis, *Nat Rev Dis Primers* 2, 16074, 1-20, 2016.
[2]Thigpen MC et al for the Emerging Infections Programs Network: Bacterial meningitis in the United States, 1998-2007, *N Engl J Med* 364(21):2016-2025, 2011.
[3]Tunkel AR et al: Practice guidelines for the management of bacterial meningitis, *Clin Infect Dis* 39(9):1267-1284, 2004.
[4]Tunkel AR et al: 2017 Infectious Diseases Society of America's clinical practice guidelines for health care-associated ventriculitis and meningitis, *Clin Infect Dis* 64(6):e34-e65, 2017.
From Parrillo JE, Dellinger RP: *Critical care medicine, principles of diagnosis and management in the adult*, ed 5, Philadelphia, 2019, Elsevier.

TABLE 6 Major Complications of Bacterial Meningitis Requiring ICU Level of Care for Monitoring and Management[1,2,3,4,5]

Type of Complication	Etiologies, Prevalence	Management Strategies
Neurologic Complications		
Increasing intracranial pressure	Brain edema, 6%-10%	Strategies: Osmotic diuresis, intracranial pressure monitoring, head of bed elevation, prophylactic lumbar drain Glycerol and hypothermia not beneficial and may result in higher mortality
Hydrocephalus	Communicating hydrocephalus, 3%-8% Obstructive hydrocephalus uncommon	Repeated lumbar puncture, lumbar drain, ventriculostomy
Focal neurologic deficits	Arterial infarct or vasculitis, 10%-15% Venous infarction, 3%-5% Hearing loss, 14%-30% Cranial nerve deficits, especially eighth nerve, 15%-30% Hemorrhage, <1% Brain abscess, subdural empyema <1%	Radiographic studies to look for focal intracranial complications Administer dexamethasone for suspected pneumococcal meningitis to decreases risk of hearing loss
Seizures	Multiple etiologies, 14%-33%	Continuous EEG monitoring, antiepileptic agents Prophylactic antiepileptic agents not routinely recommended
Agitation	Common	Careful sedation
Other Complications		
Hyponatremia	Up to 25%-30%	? Hypertonic saline solution Presence of hyponatremia did not affect outcome
Sepsis and cardiorespiratory failure	38%	Hemodynamic support, mechanical ventilation
Pneumonia	17%, most often with *Streptococcus pneumoniae*	Ventilatory support

EEG, Electroencephalographic.

[1]van de Beek D et al: Community-acquired bacterial meningitis, *Nat Rev Dis Primers* 2(16074):1-20, 2016.
[2]Bijlsma MW et al: Community-acquired bacterial meningitis in adults in the Netherlands, 2006-2014: a prospective cohort study, *Lancet Infect Dis* 16(3):339-347, 2016.
[3]Durand ML et al: Acute bacterial meningitis in adults: review of 493 episodes, *N Engl J Med* 328(1):21-28, 1993.
[4]Tunkel AR et al: Practice guidelines for the management of bacterial meningitis, *Clin Infect Dis* 39(9):1267-1284, 2004.
[5]Brouwer MC et al: What's new in bacterial meningitis, *Intensive Care Med* 42(3):415-417, 2016.
From Parrillo JE, Dellinger RP: *Critical care medicine, principles of diagnosis and management in the adult*, ed 5, Philadelphia, 2019, Elsevier.

PREVENTION

- Prevention of meningitis can be achieved through chemoprophylaxis of close contacts (household members and anyone exposed to oral secretions).
- Effective medications are rifampin 10 mg/kg PO bid for 2 days or ceftriaxone 250 mg IM single dose in patients older than age 12; 125 mg IM if age 12 or younger.
- Ciprofloxacin 500 mg for prevention of *Neisseria* meningitis can be given to patients older than 18 yr who cannot tolerate rifampin to eradicate pharyngeal colonization.
- Menactra: A protein-conjugate vaccine against serogroup A, C, Y, W-135 capsular polysaccharides is available for adults (up to 55 yr) and children older than 2 yr.
- Two new vaccines for *Neisseria* meningitis serogroup B (MenB) are now available: Bexsero and Trumenba. The FDA has also recently licensed MenQuadfi, a quadrivalent polysaccharide conjugate vaccine that uses tetanus toxoid as a protein carrier for prevention of *Neisseria meningitidis* serogroups A, C, W, and Y in persons >2 yr old.
- Children with cochlear implants are at increased risk of developing bacterial meningitis.
- Patients on eculizumab (Soliris) are at high risk for invasive meningococcal disease and should receive Menactra and a MenB vaccine and may need lifelong antibiotic prophylaxis as well.

SUGGESTED READINGS
Available at eBooks.Health.Elsevier.com.

RELATED CONTENT
Meningitis (Patient Information)
Meningitis, viral (Related Key Topic)
Meningitis, fungal (Related Key Topic)

AUTHOR: **GLENN G. FORT, MD, MPH**

🛈 BASIC INFORMATION

DEFINITION

Viral meningitis is an acute febrile illness with signs and symptoms of meningeal irritation, usually with a lymphocytic pleocytosis of the cerebrospinal fluid (CSF) and negative CSF bacterial stains and cultures.

SYNONYMS

Aseptic meningitis
Viral meningitis

ICD-10CM CODES
A87.8   Other viral meningitis
A87.9   Viral meningitis, unspecified

EPIDEMIOLOGY & DEMOGRAPHICS (TABLE 1)

INCIDENCE (IN U.S.): 11 cases/100,000 persons; leads to 26,000 to 42,000 hospitalizations per year
PREDOMINANT SEX: Male = female
GENETICS: Those with abnormal humoral immunity and agammaglobulinemia have associated difficulty with viral clearance

PHYSICAL FINDINGS & CLINICAL PRESENTATION

- Fever
- Headache
- Nuchal rigidity
- Photophobia
- Myalgias
- Vomiting
- Rash

ETIOLOGY

- Enterovirus: 85% to 95% of all cases. Most common are coxsackieviruses and echoviruses
- Parechoviruses
- Mumps virus
- Measles
- Arboviruses from mosquitoes: Eastern equine encephalitis (EEE), West Nile, St. Louis
- Herpes: HSV-1, HSV-2, VZV, HHV-6, and HHV-7
- Acute HIV
- Lymphocytic choriomeningitis virus
- Adenovirus
- Cytomegalovirus (CMV) and Epstein-Barr virus (EBV)
- Other arthropod-borne viruses: Powassan virus
- Influenza A and B virus
- Box E1 summarizes etiologic agents, factors, and diseases associated with aseptic meningitis

🅳🅧 DIAGNOSIS

The diagnostic approach is similar to that for bacterial meningitis (see "Meningitis, Bacterial"); the foremost need is to rule out bacterial meningitis with CSF evaluation. Presentation may be similar to that of meningitis with bacterial involvement.

DIFFERENTIAL DIAGNOSIS

- Bacterial meningitis
- Meningitis secondary to Lyme disease, tuberculosis (TB), syphilis, amebiasis, leptospirosis
- Rickettsial illnesses: Rocky Mountain spotted fever
- Migraine headache
- Medications
- Systemic lupus erythematosus (SLE)
- Acute mononucleosis/EBV
- Seizures
- Carcinomatous meningitis

WORKUP

CSF examination:
- Usually shows pleocytosis
- Lymphocytic predominance (neutrophils in early stages)
- Opening pressure: 200 to 250 mm Hg H_2O ($\leq$250 mm/H_2O)
- WBC: 100 to 1,000 mm^3
- Increased CSF protein (<200 mg/dl)
- Slightly decreased or normal CSF glucose (>45 mg/dl)
- Negative Gram stain, cultures, CIE, latex agglutination
- Viral cultures or serologic testing may be diagnostic
- Polymerase chain reaction (PCR) for HSV or enterovirus (which could shorten duration of antibiotic treatment and hospitalization if bacterial meningitis was suspected); multiplex or panel-based PCR tests that test for multiple viruses and bacteria at the same time in a single CSF sample are available. CSF PCR diagnosis of viral nervous system disease is summarized in Table 2.
- Antibody detection in CSF for diagnosis of West Nile virus meningitis

LABORATORY TESTS

CBC with differential, blood culturing, and CSF examination (see "Workup")

IMAGING STUDIES

CT scan or MRI: If cerebral edema, focal neurologic findings develop

🅡🅧 TREATMENT

- No specific antiviral therapy for most viruses. Treatment is supportive unless herpes simplex virus (HSV) is detected, which would be treated with IV acyclovir: 10 to 12.5 mg/kg q8h in adults for 14 to 21 days. Pediatric dose: 10 to 15 mg/kg q8h in children <12 yr and 20 mg/kg q8h in neonatal herpes.
- Empiric antibiotics may be given until CSF cultures exclude bacterial meningitis.

DISPOSITION

Viral meningitis is almost always an uncomplicated illness that will resolve; however, relapsing headache, myalgia, and weakness may occur for 2 to 3 wk after onset of symptoms.

❗ PEARLS & CONSIDERATIONS

- Enteroviruses are the most common cause of viral meningitis and are transmitted by fecal-oral route and less commonly by the respiratory route. They are more common in summer and fall mos. From 2000 to 2005, the most common serotypes were coxsackieviruses A9, B5, and B1 and echoviruses 6, 9, 13, 18, and 30.

TABLE 1   Epidemiology of Acute Viral Meningitis

			EPIDEMIOLOGIC FACTORS*	
Season	Patient's Age (yr)	Patient's Sex	Risk Factor	Suggested Viral Agent
Summer-fall	Infant	—	Infected mother	Coxsackievirus B
	1-15	—	Swimming pools, closed communities	Enteroviruses
			Geographic area: California, southeastern U.S.	California serogroup virus
Winter	1-15	—	School exposure	Varicella virus, measles virus
		Male:female 3:1		Mumps virus
	16-21	—	College exposure	Measles virus
		Male:female 3:1		Mumps virus
				Epstein-Barr virus (mononucleosis)
	Any	—	Mice, rats, hamsters	Lymphocytic choriomeningitis virus
	Adults	—	Varicella-zoster	Varicella-zoster virus
Any	Any	—	Immunocompromise	Adenovirus
		—	Acquired immunodeficiency syndrome	Human immunodeficiency virus

*Epidemiologic factors are suggestive but should not be used to exclude diagnoses in individual cases.
From Gorbach SI: *Infectious diseases*, ed 2, Philadelphia, 1998, Saunders.

TABLE 2 CSF PCR Diagnosis of Viral Nervous System Disease

Virus	Sensitivity	Specificity
Adenovirus	Unknown	
Dengue	Unknown	
Enterovirus	>95% (meningitis), <10% for AFM with EV-D68 or <25% with neuroinvasive EV-A71	>95%
Herpesviruses		
HCMV	100% in immunocompromised	High
	>60% in congenital CMV infection	High
EBV	98.5% as tumor marker in HIV patients with primary CNS lymphoma	Unknown
HSV-1 and -2	>95%	>95%
HHV-6	Unknown	Unknown
VZV	>95%	>95%
HIV	HIV RNA present at all stages	High
HTLV I and II	75%	98.5%
Influenza	Unknown but > culture	Unknown
Japanese encephalitis virus	Unknown (higher early)	High
JC virus	50%-90% in PML, lower copy # in more immunocompetent pts	98%
LCMV	Unknown	Unknown
Mumps	Unknown	High
Measles	Unknown	High
Parvovirus B-19	80%	Unknown
Rabies	90%	High
WNV	70% (higher early)	High
SARS-CoV2	Unknown, likely low (nasopharyngeal RT-PCR high acutely)	High
ZIKV	Unknown (congenital ZIKV syndrome)	High

AFM, Acute flaccid myelitis; *CNS,* central nervous system; *CSF,* cerebral spinal fluid; *EBV,* Epstein-Barr virus; *HCMV,* human cytomegalovirus; *HHV,* human herpesvirus; *HSV,* herpes simplex virus; *HTLV,* human T-cell lymphotropic virus; *LCMV,* lymphocytic choriomeningitis virus; *PCR,* polymerase chain reaction; *PML,* progressive multifocal leukoencephalopathy; *RT-PCR,* reverse transcription polymerase chain reaction; *VZV,* varicella-zoster virus; *WNV,* West Nile virus; *ZIKV,* Zika virus.
From Jankovic J et al: *Bradley and Daroff's neurology in clinical practice,* ed 8, Philadelphia 2022, Elsevier.

• Herpes simplex type 2 (HSV-2) can be a cause of a primary episode of meningitis and also be a cause of recurrent episodes of lymphocytic meningitis. HSV-2 meningitis presents most often without a history of genital herpes or genital symptoms. Recurrent aseptic meningitis, also known as Mollaret disease, is predominantly caused by HSV-2 infection.

SUGGESTED READINGS
Available at eBooks.Health.Elsevier.com.

RELATED CONTENT
Meningitis (Patient Information)
Meningitis, Bacterial (Related Key Topic)

AUTHOR: **GLENN G. FORT, MD, MPH**

Diseases
and Disorders

I

BASIC INFORMATION

DEFINITION

Menopause is the permanent cessation of menstrual periods for 1 yr or permanent cessation of ovulation after lost ovarian activity without any other obvious pathologic or physiologic cause. It is the reproductive stage of life marked by waxing and waning estrogen levels followed by decreasing ovarian function. Primary ovarian insufficiency (previously also referred to as premature ovarian failure) and no menstrual periods may also occur because of depletion of ovarian follicles before the age of 40 yr and is considered to be abnormal.

SYNONYMS

Change of life
Climacteric ovarian failure

ICD-10CM CODES
E28.310	Symptomatic premature menopause
E28.319	Asymptomatic premature menopause
N95.1	Menopausal and female climacteric states
N95.8	Other specified menopausal and perimenopausal disorders
Z78.0	Asymptomatic menopausal state

EPIDEMIOLOGY & DEMOGRAPHICS

- Average age of menopause in the U.S. is 51 yr.
- Age at which menopause occurs is primarily genetically determined.
- Smokers experience menopause an average of 1.5 yr earlier than nonsmokers.
- The menopausal transition, or perimenopause, begins on average 4 yr before the last menstrual period, which is usually in a woman's mid- to late-40s.
- Approximately 70% of middle-aged women experience vasomotor symptoms (hot flashes, night sweats, or both).

PHYSICAL FINDINGS & CLINICAL PRESENTATION

- Menopausal vasomotor symptoms (VMS, hot flashes, flushes): Night sweats, cardiovascular disease, coronary artery disease, atherosclerosis, headaches, tiredness, and lethargy; vasomotor symptoms typically begin around entry into the menopausal transition and tend to continue well after the final menstrual period. The median duration of hot flashes has been reported as 4 yr in some studies and in others, 10.2 yr, but the length of hot flashes was largely dictated by how early they began in the perimenopause. Variations in duration of hot flashes also may vary between racial/ethnic groups.
- Either complete cessation of menses or a period of irregular cycles and diminished or heavier bleeding
- Atrophic vaginitis, which can cause burning, itching, bleeding, dyspareunia
- Osteoporosis
- Osteopenia
- Psychological dysfunction:

1. Anxiety
2. Depression
3. Insomnia
4. Nervousness
5. Irritability
6. Inability to concentrate
7. Sleep disturbance
- Sexual changes, decreased libido, dyspareunia
- Urinary incontinence

ETIOLOGY

- The most common etiology: Physiologic, caused by depleted granulosa and theca cells that fail to react to endogenous gonadotropins, producing less estrogen; decreased negative feedback in the hypothalamic pituitary access, increased follicle-stimulating hormone (FSH), and increased luteinizing hormone (LH), which leads to stromal cells that continue to produce androgens as a result of the LH stimulation.
- Surgical castration.
- Other factors that contribute to menopause can be family history of early menopause, cigarette smoking, blindness, abnormal chromosomal karyotype (Turner syndrome, gonadal dysgenesis), precocious puberty, and left-handedness.

DIAGNOSIS

DIFFERENTIAL DIAGNOSIS

- Primary ovarian insufficiency
- Asherman syndrome
- Hypothalamic dysfunction
- Hyper or hypothyroidism
- Pituitary tumors
- Adrenal abnormalities
- Ovarian abnormalities
- Polycystic ovarian syndrome
- Pregnancy
- Ovarian neoplasm
- Tuberculosis of the endometrium

WORKUP

- Physical examination, height, weight, blood pressure, breast examination, and pelvic examination are needed.
- If the clinical picture is highly suggestive of menopause, reassurance or hormone replacement therapy such as estrogen can be prescribed to help with menopausal symptoms (after appropriate counseling). If all symptoms resolve, then a diagnosis essentially has been made. Before estrogen is prescribed, however, a complete history and physical examination are needed. If a patient has an estrogen-dependent malignancy, unexplained abnormal uterine bleeding, a history of thrombophlebitis, or acute liver disease, estrogen therapy is contraindicated.
- Progesterone challenge test: Medroxyprogesterone 10 to 20 mg PO or progesterone 100 mg IM to induce withdrawal bleeding. If no withdrawal bleeding is obtained, a hypoestrogenic state is assumed to be present.
- Assess risk for coronary artery disease, osteoporosis, cigarette smoking, personal history, history of breast cancer, liver disease, active coagulation disorder, or any unexplained vaginal bleeding.

LABORATORY TESTS

- No laboratory tests may be indicated if the patient fulfills clinical criteria of menopause at an anticipated average age.
- The possibility of pregnancy must always be excluded in a woman with new onset amenorrhea by a serum hCG.
- FSH, LH, and estrogen levels: Markedly elevated FSH and markedly depressed estrogen level constitute laboratory diagnosis of ovarian failure; LH only if polycystic ovarian disease is to be ruled out in a younger patient. It is not necessary to obtain an FSH if the patient fulfills the clinical criteria for menopause. Similarly, since estradiol levels vary during the menstrual cycle, estradiol levels are rarely necessary or informative.
- Anti-Müllerian hormone (produced by the granulosa cells) will demonstrate a decrease.
- TSH to rule out thyroid dysfunction and prolactin level if patient has symptoms of galactorrhea and if suspicion of pituitary adenoma exists.
- A general chemistry profile to check for any systemic diseases.
- Pap smear per standard guidelines, endometrial biopsy, or dilation and curettage in patients who have had irregular periods or intermenstrual or postmenopausal bleeding.
- Mammogram as recommended by American Congress of Obstetricians and Gynecologists for preventative care.
- For women under the age of 40, a complete evaluation for abnormal uterine bleeding is suggested.

IMAGING STUDIES

- Per standard protocols, CT scan or MRI of sella if pituitary tumor is suspected
- Bone density studies if high-risk condition for osteoporosis exists
- Pelvic ultrasound to check endometrial stripe as determined by clinical history (i.e., in the setting of postmenopausal bleeding)

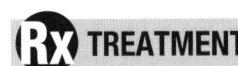 TREATMENT

NONPHARMACOLOGIC THERAPY

- A balanced diet: Low in fat, with total fat intake being <30% of calories; total calories sufficient to maintain body weight or produce weight loss if that is desired
- Avoidance of smoking, excessive alcohol or caffeine intake, and spicy foods (if they trigger hot flashes)
- Exercise: Weight-bearing exercise for osteoporosis prevention
- Kegel exercises for strengthening the pelvic floor
- Adequate calcium intake: 1,200 mg of calcium daily (total diet plus supplement) and 800 IU of vitamin D daily in patients with osteoporosis.

Many patients, however, do not need additional supplementation if getting adequate calcium and vitamin D from dietary intake and sun exposure
- Change in the ambient temperature (may ameliorate hot flashes and reduce night sweats)
- Vitamin E
- Vaginal lubricants to help with the dyspareunia attributable to vaginal dryness (e.g., Replens, K-Y Jelly, or Gyne-Moistrin cream)

ACUTE GENERAL Rx

Vasomotor symptoms are best managed with systemic hormone therapy given in the lowest dose and for the shortest period possible. Estrogen replacement in symptomatic patients can be administered in a variety of forms, including oral estrogen and transdermal estrogen patch. The lowest effective dose should be prescribed.
- Examples of oral estrogen include:
  1. Conjugated estrogens: Start with 0.3 mg daily and increase to 1.25 mg daily depending on symptoms.
  2. Estradiol: Start with 0.5 mg daily and increase up to 2 mg daily.
  3. Esterified estrogens: Start with 0.3 to 1.25 mg daily.
  4. Estropipate: Start with 0.75 to 3.0 mg daily.
  5. Esterified estrogen/testosterone combination: Give 1.25 mg and methyltestosterone 2.5 mg (Estratest) and esterified estrogen 0.625 mg and methyltestosterone 1.25 mg (Estratest HS [half-strength]). May improve sexual enjoyment and libido.
- If the patient has had a hysterectomy for benign disease, estrogen alone is sufficient. In patients who have an intact uterus, progestin is critical to prevent endometrial hyperplasia associated with unopposed estrogen, which is protective against endometrial cancer. Progestins can be prescribed as continual daily dose or cyclic fashion. Most commonly prescribed progestins include medroxyprogesterone acetate 2.5 mg, 5 mg, and 10 mg; Prometrium 100 mg, 200 mg, and 400 mg; and Aygestin 5 mg. Continuous hormone replacement therapy is preferred because after time the patient should be amenorrheic. Patients should be counseled that they may experience some irregular spotting for the first 6 to 9 mo after starting hormone replacement therapy. Cyclic therapy will cause withdrawal bleeding.
- Combination oral preparations Femhrt, Prefest, Prempro, Activella, Premphase are commonly used. However, the U.S. Preventive Services Task Force recommends against the use of combined estrogen and progestin for the prevention of chronic conditions such as cardiovascular disease in postmenopausal women.
- The combination of conjugated estrogen and bazedoxifene is approved for the treatment of moderate to severe vasomotor symptoms associated with menopause and also for prevention of postmenopausal osteoporosis in women with an intact uterus.

- Transdermal patches can be either estradiol (Estraderm, Vivelle, FemPatch) 0.025 to 0.1 mg applied twice weekly or Climara 0.025 to 0.1 mg used once a week. With these preparations, progesterone should be used in a similar fashion. Apply CombiPatch twice weekly (combination estrogen and progesterone) or Climara Pro once per wk (one patch).
- Vaginal estrogen creams can be used; these should be reserved for local therapy of atrophic vaginitis. Minimal systemic absorption does occur; however, blood levels are unpredictable. Usual dose 0.5 to 2 g intravaginally daily, cyclically 3 wk on and 1 wk off. When symptoms improve, once to twice weekly is adequate maintenance.
- Vagifem estradiol vaginal tablets. Initial dosage: One Vagifem tablet, inserted vaginally, daily for 2 wk. Maintenance dose: One Vagifem tablet, inserted vaginally, twice weekly.
- Femring vaginal ring delivering the equivalent of 0.5 mg/day inserted every 3 mo or Estring 0.0075 mg/day.
- EstroGel 0.06% (estradiol gel). One pump (1.25 g/day) applied to one arm from wrist to shoulder.
- The FDA contraindications to menopause hormone therapy include the following diseases and disorders: Active liver disease; current, past, or suspected breast cancer; active or recent anterior thromboembolic disease; cardiac disease (angina, myocardial infarction); known or suspected estrogen-sensitive malignant conditions; known hypersensitivity to the active substance of the therapy or to any of the excipients; porphyria cutanea tarda; previous idiopathic or current venous thromboembolism; undiagnosed genital bleeding; untreated hypertension; untreated endometrial hyperplasia.
- For women in whom estrogen is contraindicated or for those who do not wish to take estrogen, the following regimens can be used:
  1. Serotonin reuptake inhibitors, especially in women with menopausal mood disorders
  2. Depo-Provera 150 mg IM every month (may be helpful in alleviating hot flashes)
  3. Clonidine 0.05 to 0.15 mg PO daily (questionable efficacy) or transdermal clonidine patch
  4. Bellergal-S (questionable efficacy)
  5. Nonhormonal therapies for vasomotor symptoms are summarized in Box 1
- Tibolone significantly improves vasomotor symptoms, libido, and vaginal lubrication. Not available in the U.S.

CHRONIC Rx

Hormone replacement therapy should be used only for the short term unless benefits outweigh the risks of long-term use. Following the results of the Women's Health Initiative (WHI), the FDA has instituted a "black box" warning on postmenopausal hormone replacement products, suggesting that the lowest dose should be used for the shortest period of time. This necessitates a considered counseling session with patients contemplating hormone replacement prior to the

initiation of therapy and then on a periodic basis after that, usually at least on a yearly basis.

DISPOSITION

If treated, the patient should have resolution of her symptoms and reduced incidence of osteoporosis. Hormonal and osteoporosis treatments available and approved for use in postmenopausal women are summarized in Box 2.

Lifelong medical supervision is necessary to monitor adequacy of treatment and prevention of complications. This should include regular Pap smears in accordance with the American Society for Colposcopy and Cervical Pathology (ASCCP) guidelines until the age of 65, pelvic examinations, breast examinations, mammography, and endometrial sampling of any type of abnormal bleeding. If untreated, the vasomotor symptoms will eventually dissipate; however, this may take several years in a small percentage of women. Some women who are in their 80s have experienced hot flashes. Urogenital atrophy will continue to worsen. Osteoporosis and coronary artery disease risks will increase with every passing year.

REFERRAL

Most menopausal women are managed by their gynecologists. However, this condition can be managed adequately by a primary care physician who has an interest in treating menopausal women.

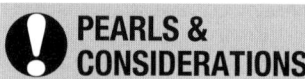

PEARLS & CONSIDERATIONS

COMMENTS

- Short-term risks of hormone replacement therapy (HT) include an eighteenfold increased rise for cholecystitis, three-and-a-half-fold risk of a thrombo-cardiac event in the first year, and possible increased risk of stroke and myocardial infarction.
- Results of the WHI study found that for every 10,000 women taking HT (combination of both estrogen and progesterone) for 1 yr (10,000 person-yr), seven more would have coronary events, eight would have more strokes, eight would have more pulmonary emboli, and eight would have earlier breast cancer than would 10,000 women taking a placebo. Benefits of

---

BOX 1   Nonhormonal Therapies for Vasomotor Symptoms

Antidepressants (SSRIs/SNRIs)
Gabapentin
Clonidine
Isoflavones, red clover, black cohosh
Cognitive behavior therapy
Acupuncture
Stellate ganglion block

SNRI, selective norepinephrine reuptake inhibitor; *SSRI,* selective serotonin reuptake inhibitor.
From Gershenson DM et al: *Comprehensive Gynecology,* ed 8, Philadelphia, 2022, Elsevier.

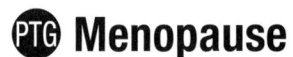

BOX 2 Hormonal and Osteoporosis Treatments: Available and Approved for Use in Postmenopausal Women

Estrogens
Oral
CEE, 0.3, 0.45, 0.625, 0.9, 1.25, and 2.5 mg
Piperazine estrone sulfate, equivalent of 0.625, 1.25, and 2.5 mg
Esterified, 0.3, 0.625, 0.9, 1.25, and 2.5 mg
Micronized estradiol, 0.5, 1, and 2 mg

Transdermal
Estradiol patches, 0.014, 0.025, 0.0375, 0.05, 0.75, and 0.10 mg/day
Estradiol gels, 0.25 to 1.5 mg/day various brands
Estradiol spray, 1.53 mg/day

Vaginal
Cream, CEE (0.0625%), estradiol (0.01%)
Estradiol ring, 2 mg: release for atrophy 7.5 µg/day for 3 mo
Estradiol acetate ring for vasomotor symptoms: 50 to 100 µg/day for 3 mo
Estradiol hemihydrate (tablet) 10 µg: 1 tablet per day for 2 wk, then twice/wk
Estradiol soft gel inset, 4 µg and 10 µg: daily use for 2 wk, then twice/wk

Parenteral
Intramuscular injections should be avoided

Progestins
Oral
Medroxyprogesterone acetate, 2.5, 5, and 10 mg
Norethindrone acetate, 5 mg
Micronized progesterone, 100 and 200 mg

Vaginal
Micronized progesterone, 100 mg
Progesterone gel, 4% and 8%

Combinations
Oral
CEE + MPA (0.625 mg) + MPA (2.5 or 5 mg)
CEE + MPA (0.3 mg + MPA, 1.5 mg)
Micronized estradiol (1 mg) + norethindrone, acetate (0.5 mg); or 0.5 mg with 0.1 orethindrone acetate
Micronized estradiol (1 mg) + 0.5 mg drospirenone; or 0.5 mg estradiol and 0.25 mg drospirenone
Ethinyl estradiol (5 µg), norethindrone acetate (1 mg or 2.5 µg), and 0.5 mg norethindrone acetate
CEE + bazedoxifene (SERM), 0.45 + 20 mg/day
Micronized estradiol (1 mg) + micronized progesterone (100 mg) in single tablet

Transdermal
Patch, 0.05 mg estradiol with 140 µg or 250 µg norethindrone acetate
Patch, 0.045 mg estradiol with levonorgestrel 0.015 mg

Androgens
Oral
Esterified estrogen and methyl testosterone (0.625/1.25 mg and 1.25/2.5 mg)

Transdermal
Patch, 150 µg/300 µg, approved outside the United States

Other nonhormonal products
Ospemifene (SERM), 60 mg/day for vulvovaginal atrophy
Paroxetine (SSRI), 7.5 mg/day for vasomotor symptoms

Medications for osteoporosis
Bisphosphonates
Alendronate, 5 and 10 mg daily; 35 and 70 mg weekly
Risedronate, 5 mg; 35 mg weekly
Ibandronate, 150 mg monthly and 3I mg IV every 3 mo
Zoledronic acid 5 mg once yearly
Etidronate, 200 mg (intermittent)

Selective estrogen receptor modulators (SERMs)
Raloxifene, 60 mg

Others for osteoporosis
Tibolone, 2.5 mg (not approved in the United States)
Denosumab, 60 mg subcutaneously every 6 mo
Human parathyroid hormone 1-34; 20 µg subcutaneously daily
Romosozumab 105 mg × 2 (prefilled syringes) subcutaneously once/mo

CEE, Conjugated equine estrogens; *IV,* intravenously; *MPA,* medroxyprogesterone acetate.
From Gershenson DM et al: *Comprehensive Gynecology,* ed 8, Philadelphia, 2022, Elsevier.

HT were six fewer cases of colorectal cancer and five fewer hip fractures per 10,000 women.

- HT should not be initiated or continued for the primary or secondary prevention of coronary heart disease.
- Estrogen-replacement therapy should only be prescribed for patients with sufficient menopausal symptoms that impact the patient's quality of life.
- Interestingly, women who start hormone therapy early in menopause may have cardiac and other benefits. A recent trial showed that oral estradiol therapy was associated with less progression of subclinical atherosclerosis (measured as change in carotid-artery intima media thickness [CIMT]) than with placebo when therapy was initiated within 6 yr after menopause but not when it was initiated 10 or more yr after menopause. Estradiol had no significant effect on cardiac CT measures of atherosclerosis in either postmenopause stratum.

SUGGESTED READINGS
Available at eBooks.Health.Elsevier.com.

RELATED CONTENT
Menopause (Patient Information)
Hot Flashes (Related Key Topic)
Osteoporosis (Related Key Topic)

AUTHORS: **SHANICE AKOTO, MD, MPH,** and **RACHEL WRIGHT HEINLE, MD, FACOG**

M

Diseases and Disorders

I

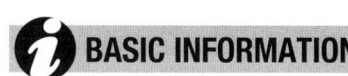

BASIC INFORMATION

DEFINITION

Malignant mesothelioma is a neoplasm originating from the mesothelial surfaces of the pleural (80%) or peritoneal cavities (20%). The three major histologic subtypes are: Epithelial (most common), sarcomatous, and mixed (epithelial/sarcomatous).

SYNONYM

Malignant mesothelioma

ICD-10CM CODES
C45.0 Mesothelioma of pleura
C45.1 Mesothelioma of peritoneum
C45.2 Mesothelioma of pericardium
C45.7 Mesothelioma of other sites
C45.9 Mesothelioma, unspecified

EPIDEMIOLOGY & DEMOGRAPHICS

- Associated with asbestos exposure with a latency of 20 to 50 yr.
- About 3000 new cases annually are diagnosed in the U.S. with an incidence of one to three cases per 100,000 population depending on occupational asbestos exposure.
- More common in men (5:1).

Family members of exposed workers have a higher risk due to cleaning of contaminated clothes but incidence in the U.S. has leveled off due to regulation of asbestos use.

- Incidence of mesothelioma increases with age; median age at presentation is >70 yr.
- More than 8 million persons in the U.S. are at risk because of prior asbestos exposure.

PHYSICAL FINDINGS & CLINICAL PRESENTATION

- Dyspnea
- Nonpleuritic chest pain
- Fever, weight loss, sweats, fatigue, loss of appetite
- Dysphagia, superior vena cava syndrome, Horner syndrome in advanced stages
- Auscultation may reveal unilateral loss of breath sounds
- Dullness on percussion may be present

ETIOLOGY

- Asbestos exposure (>70% of patients).
- Other reported potentially causal factors include prior radiation therapy and extravasated Thorotrast, zeolite, and erionite fibers.
- Mutations of BRCA1-associated protein 1 (BAP1) cyclin-dependent kinase inhibitor 2A gene *(CDKN2A)* have been causally linked to development of mesothelioma.

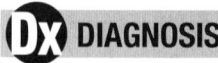 DIAGNOSIS

DIFFERENTIAL DIAGNOSIS

Metastatic adenocarcinomas (from lung, breast, ovary, kidney, stomach, prostate)

WORKUP

- Contrast-enhanced CT of the chest and upper abdomen is recommended as the initial method of investigation.[1]
- Staging evaluation (Box 1) includes complete history (including occupational history), physical examination, and testing to determine potential operability (CT, bone scan, pulmonary function tests [PFTs]).
- Thoracoscopy, pleuroscopy, and open-lung biopsy are useful in obtaining adequate tissue samples for diagnosis.
- Pulmonary function tests.
- PET-CT scan (Figs. E1 and E2) is performed only in patients considered candidates for surgery to determine resectability.

- Staging: The tumor, node, metastasis (TNM) system categorizes mesothelioma in stages I to IV similar to that used for non-small cell lung cancer.

LABORATORY TESTS

- Diagnostic thoracentesis is generally insufficient for diagnosis because pleural effusions may only reveal atypical mesothelial cells.
- Immunohistochemistry is useful to distinguish adenocarcinoma from epithelial malignant mesothelioma (mesotheliomas are generally carcinoembryonic antigen negative and cytokeratin positive).
- Thrombocytosis and anemia may be found on initial laboratory evaluation.

BOX 1 International Mesothelioma Interest Group (IMIG) Staging System

T: Primary Tumor and Extent
T_1:
a. Tumor limited to ipsilateral parietal pleura, including mediastinal and diaphragmatic pleura; no involvement of the visceral pleura
b. Tumor involving the ipsilateral parietal pleura, including mediastinal and diaphragmatic pleura; scattered foci or tumor also involving the visceral pleura
T_2 Tumor involving each of the ipsilateral pleural surfaces (parietal, mediastinal, diaphragmatic pleura); scattered foci or tumor also involving the visceral pleura:
a. Involvement of diaphragmatic muscle
b. Confluent visceral pleura (including the fissures) or extension of tumor from visceral pleura into the underlying pulmonary parenchyma
T_3 Locally advanced but potentially resectable tumor; tumor involving all the ipsilateral pleural surfaces (parietal, mediastinal, diaphragmatic, and visceral pleura) with at least one of the following features:
a. Involvement of the endothoracic fascia
b. Extension into mediastinal fat
c. Solitary, complete resectable focus or tumor extending into the soft tissues of the chest wall
d. Nontransmural involvement of the pericardium
T_4 Locally advanced, technically nonresectable tumor; tumor involving all the ipsilateral pleural surfaces (parietal, mediastinal, diaphragmatic, and visceral pleura) with at least one of the following features:
a. Diffuse extension or multifocal mass of tumor in the chest wall, with or without associated rib destruction
b. Direct transdiaphragmatic extension of the tumor to the peritoneum
c. Direct extension of tumor to the contralateral pleura
d. Direct extension of tumor to one or more mediastinal organs
e. Direct extension of tumor into the spine
f. Tumor extending through the internal surface of the pericardium with or without a pericardial effusion or tumor involving the myocardium

N: Lymph Nodes
N_x Regional lymph nodes cannot be assessed
N_0 No regional lymph node metastases
N_1 Metastases in ipsilateral bronchopulmonary or hilar lymph nodes
N_2 Metastases in the subcarinal or the ipsilateral mediastinal lymph nodes, including the ipsilateral internal mammary nodes
N_3 Metastases in contralateral mediastinal, contralateral internal mammary, ipsilateral, or contralateral supraclavicular scalene lymph nodes

M: Metastases
M_x Presence of distant metastases cannot be assessed
M_0 No (known) metastasis
M_1 Distant metastasis present

Stage Grouping
  I. a. $T_{1a}N_0M_0$
      b. $T_{1b}N_0M_0$
  II. $T_2N_0M_0$
  III. Any T_3M_0, any N_1M_0, any N_2M_0
  IV. Any T_4, any N_3, any M_1

From Sellke FW et al: *Sabiston & Spencer surgery of the chest,* ed 9, Philadelphia, 2016, Elsevier.

Diseases and Disorders

I

BOX 2 Therapeutic Options for Malignant Pleural Mesothelioma

Single-Modality Therapy
- Debulking surgery (pleurectomy/decortication or extrapleural pneumonectomy)
- Radiation (external beam, brachytherapy)
- Chemotherapy (single- or double-agent approach: Doxorubicin, cyclophosphamide, cisplatinum; gemcitabine, pemetrexed, and cisplatin)

Multimodality Therapy
- Surgery and adjuvant radiation
- Surgery and adjuvant chemotherapy
- Surgery and adjuvant chemoradiotherapy

Innovative Therapies Under Investigation
- Intracavitary lavage with hyperthermic chemotherapy
- Photodynamic therapy
- Gene therapy
- Angiogenesis
- Immunogenic therapy

From Sellke FW et al: *Sabiston & Spencer surgery of the chest,* ed 9, Philadelphia, 2016, Elsevier.

- Soluble mesothelin levels have been demonstrated to track with ongoing systemic therapy, but its clinical utility has not been validated.
- Serum osteopontin levels (when available) can also be used to distinguish persons with exposure to asbestos who do not have cancer from those with exposure to asbestos who have pleural mesothelioma. Higher levels are correlated with a poorer prognosis.

IMAGING STUDIES
- Chest radiographs may reveal pleural plaques (Fig. E3) or calcifications in the diaphragm.
- CT scans of the chest and abdomen, bone scan, and PET scan are used to assess the stage of disease.

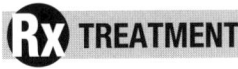 **TREATMENT**

GENERAL Rx
- Treatment is guided by staging, histologic subtype, and the patient's functional status.[1,2]
- Box 2 summarizes therapeutic options for malignant pleural mesothelioma.
- Operable patient (epithelial type, no positive nodes, confined to pleura, adequate PFTs): The two surgical techniques for therapeutic intervention are:
  1. Decortication (pleurectomy).
  2. Extrapleural pneumonectomy (EPP).
  3. With EPP, patients are eligible to be treated with either preoperative or postoperative radiation therapy to improve local control.
  4. Postoperative chemotherapy with cisplatin and pemetrexed and subsequent external-beam radiation are used with limited success.
- Inoperable patient (elderly patient, extensive disease, sarcomatous or mixed histology type, poor PFTs):
  1. Chemotherapy is administered to improve survival; supportive care is a standard option.

2. Combined modality therapies (radiation therapy, chemotherapy, and biologics) have also been used to reduce both local and distant recurrences.
3. First-line chemotherapy options include the combination of cisplatin and pemetrexed with or without additional bevacizumab (antiangiogenic agent).[3] Patients with progressive cancer after initial chemotherapy can often be treated with single-agent chemotherapy (gemcitabine or vinorelbine).
4. The FDA has approved the combination of dual immunotherapy with ipilimumab and nivolumab as first-line therapy in advanced mesothelioma based on a 14% improvement in 2-yr overall survival and a 4-mo improvement in median overall survival for the intent to treat population.[4]
5. The FDA has approved for first-line treatment for malignant pleural mesothelioma (MPM) patients a device called NovoTTF-100L, which is based on the delivery of specific electric frequencies (tumor treating fields [TTFs]) in combination with chemotherapy, to interfere with cancer cell proliferation. The reported median overall survival was 18.2 mo with no increase in systemic toxicity among patients treated with this approach.[5]
6. Improvement in survival has been shown with use of immune checkpoint inhibitors targeting the programmed death-1 (PD-1) pathway (pembrolizumab, durvalumab, nivolumab with or without ipilimumab) in patients previously treated with chemotherapy alone.
7. Intrapleural instillation of cisplatin or biologics (e.g., interferons, interleukin-2) is generally limited to very early disease because it can penetrate to only a very limited depth of the tumor and there is a propensity of the pleural space to become progressively obliterated with advancing disease.
8. Among nonmetastatic patients who underwent nonradical lung-sparing surgery

and chemotherapy, the use of radical hemithoracic radiotherapy (RHR) to the involved pleural cavity was associated with a 2-yr survivor of 58% versus 28% in patients receiving palliative radiotherapy.[6] However, there was a major increase in pulmonary toxicity with the use of RHR.
- In advanced stages, radiation therapy is often used for palliation of local chest pain.
- Obliteration of the pleural space (pleurodesis) with instillation of talc or tetracycline into the pleural cavity is done in the treatment of recurrent symptomatic pleural effusions.
- Several biomarkers have been evaluated extensively in mesothelioma management.[7]
  1. Serum mesothelin is not sensitive or specific for diagnostic purposes, but serial measurements during chemotherapy can be useful as a monitoring tool.
  2. Recent data reveal that plasma fibulin-3 levels can distinguish healthy persons with exposure to asbestos from patients with mesothelioma. In conjunction with effusion fibulin-3 levels, plasma fibulin-3 levels can further differentiate mesothelioma effusions from other malignant and benign effusions.

DISPOSITION
- The overall prognosis of malignant mesothelioma is dismal, with a median survival of 8 mo. The 5-yr overall survival is better for patients with lower stages: Localized (20%), regional (12%), and distant (8%).
- Patients who receive trimodality therapy (surgery, radiation therapy, systemic therapy) have improved survivals of ∼18 mo; however, less than 10% of cases fit in this category.
- In the U.S., age-adjusted mortality has been reduced from almost 14 deaths per 1 million persons in 2000 to 11 deaths per 1 million in 2015.[1]

⚠ PEARLS & CONSIDERATIONS

- Patients with early disease should be referred to treatment centers specializing in multidisciplinary therapy before attempts are made to obliterate the pleural space with pleurodesis.
- Patients with advanced or resected disease should be treated with appropriate combination chemotherapy as listed previously.

REFERENCES
Available at eBooks.Health.Elsevier.com.

RELATED CONTENT
Mesothelioma (Patient Information)
Asbestosis (Related Key Topic)

AUTHOR: **BHARTI RATHORE, M.D.**

Migraine Headache 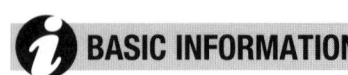 PTG

BASIC INFORMATION

DEFINITION

Migraine headaches are recurrent severe headaches that either are preceded by a focal neurologic symptom (migraine with aura), occur independently without preceding focal neurologic symptoms (migraine without aura), or have atypical presentations (migraine variants). The migraine aura (Box 1) typically is characterized by visual or sensory symptoms that develop over 5 to 60 min. If the aura includes unilateral motor weakness, the migraine is referred to as hemiplegic. In migraine with and without aura, the headache is typically moderate to severe, unilateral, pulsatile, made worse with head movement, and associated with nausea and vomiting, photophobia, and phonophobia. Migraines that occur ≥15 days every mo for ≥3 mo are known as chronic; otherwise, they are referred to as episodic. *Status migrainosus* (SM) is a complication of migraine with debilitating pain and associated symptoms lasting for more than 72 hours. The most common triggers are stress and sleep disruption.[1a]

ICD-10CM CODES

G43.909	Migraine, unspecified, not intractable, without status migrainosus
G43.1	Migraine with aura (classical migraine)
G43.0	Migraine without aura (common migraine)
G43.2	Status migrainosus
G43.3	Complicated migraine

EPIDEMIOLOGY & DEMOGRAPHICS

INCIDENCE: Increases from infancy, peaks during the third decade of life, then decreases. It is the second leading cause of years lived with disability worldwide for all ages and the leading cause in woman aged 16 to 49 yr.[1b]

PREVALENCE (IN U.S.): Migraine is the third-most prevalent disease in the world. Globally, it is estimated to affect 1 billion people, and it has an estimated 1-yr prevalence of approximately 12% in the general population.[1] It affects approximately 39 million people in the U.S.[2-3]

PREDOMINANT SEX: Female:male ratio of about 3:1.[3]

PREDOMINANT AGE: Peak prevalence between ages of 18 and 49.

GENETICS: Familial predisposition: More than 50% of migraine sufferers have an affected family member.[1]

- Autosomal-dominant transmission for some rare migraine variants (familial hemiplegic migraine, cerebral autosomal-dominant arteriopathy with subcortical infarcts and leukoencephalopathy [CADASIL]); familial hemiplegic migraines have been associated with calcium channelopathy, sodium channelopathy, and Na^+/K^+-ATPase dysfunction.

PHYSICAL FINDINGS & CLINICAL PRESENTATION

- Normal between episodes
- Normal for migraine without aura
- Focal motor or sensory abnormalities (Fig. E1) possible for migraine with aura or migraine variants
- Common aura types include scintillating scotoma, bright zigzags (fortifications), and other visual distortions (Fig. E2) such as macropsia or micropsia (enlargement or shrinkage of objects) that often cross visual fields. Homonymous visual disturbance, sensory phenomena such as hemibody paresthesia, speech disturbances, or hemiparesis (familial or sporadic hemiplegic migraine) also can occur independently or associated with visual symptoms

ETIOLOGY

The pathophysiology of migraines is not clearly understood, although the primary neuronal event results in a trigeminovascular reflex causing neurogenic inflammation. Calcitonin-gene related peptide (CGRP) is released by the trigeminal ganglion and binds receptors around meningeal vessels leading to inflammation. Serotonin, substance P, and nitric oxide also play a role, but the exact mechanism is unknown. Cortical spreading depressions are likely responsible for the aura.[4]

DIAGNOSIS

- Migraine without aura:[5]
- Five attacks fulfilling criteria
- Headache attacks lasting 4 to 72 h
- Headache has at least two of the following characteristics:
  1. Unilateral location
  2. Pulsating quality
  3. Moderate or severe pain intensity
  4. Aggravation or causing avoidance of routine physical activity
- At least one of the following during headache:
  1. Nausea and/or vomiting
  2. Photophobia and phonophobia
- Migraine with typical aura:[5]
- At least two attacks
- Aura consisting of at least one of the following, but no motor weakness:

1. Fully reversible visual symptoms, including positive and/or negative features
2. Fully reversible sensory symptoms, including positive and/or negative features
3. Fully reversible dysphasic speech disturbance
- At least two of the following:
  1. Homonymous visual symptoms and/or unilateral sensory symptoms
  2. At least one aura symptom develops gradually over >5 min and/or different aura symptoms occur in succession over >5 min
  3. Each symptom lasts between 5 and 60 min
- A migraine occurring during or within 60 min of the aura

DIFFERENTIAL DIAGNOSIS

- A diagnosis of migraine is possible only after five recurrent episodes.
- The first or the worst headache should always be investigated, and the differential includes headaches from all secondary causes.
- Headache red flags can be remembered by the mnemonic SSNOOP5:
  1. S: Systemic symptoms of fever, weight loss
  2. S: Secondary risk factors of immunosuppression from any cause, cancer
  3. N: Neurologic deficits, altered consciousness
  4. O: Onset is sudden, abrupt, split second thunderclap
  5. O: Older, age >50 for new-onset headache should be worked up for giant cell arteritis
  6. P: Pattern: Change in headache pattern
  7. P: Pregnancy
  8. P: Positional or postural
  9. P: Papilledema
  10. P: Precipitation with Valsalva maneuver or exertion
- Section II describes the differential diagnosis of headaches. Table 1 compares tension-type and migraine headaches.
- Useful mnemonic for migraine is POUND: Pulsatile, One day in duration, Unilateral, Nausea/vomiting, Disabling.

WORKUP

- In general, no additional investigation is needed with recurrent, typical attacks with usual age of onset, family history, and a normal physical examination.
- Fundus examination is important to evaluate for the possibility of optic disk edema, which would suggest a secondary cause of headache such as idiopathic intracranial hypertension (IIH).
- If there is an unusual presentation, headache with red flags, and/or unexpected findings on examination, investigation for other causes is required.

LABORATORY TESTS

Lumbar puncture for history of abrupt-onset headaches and uncertain diagnosis of migraine

IMAGING STUDIES

- Imaging should be done in patients with any of the red flags for secondary headache, such as

BOX 1 Auras of Migraine

Sensory phenomena
  Special senses
    Visual, olfactory, auditory, gustatory
  Paresthesias, especially lips and hand
Motor deficits
  Hemiparesis, hemiplegic
Neuropsychologic changes
Aphasia
Perceptual impairment, especially for size, shape, and time
Emotional and behavioral
  Anxiety, depression, irritability, (rarely) hyperactivity

From Kaufman DM et al: *Kaufman's clinical neurology for psychiatrists*, ed 8, Philadelphia, 2017, Elsevier.

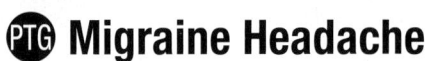

TABLE 1 Comparison of Tension-Type and Migraine Headaches

	Tension-Type	Migraine
Location	Bilateral	Hemicranial*
Nature	Dull ache	Throbbing*
Severity	Slight–moderate	Moderate–severe
Associated symptoms	None	Nausea, hyperacusis, photophobia
Behavior	Continues working	Seeks seclusion
Effect of alcohol	Reduces headache	Worsens headache

*In approximately half of patients, at least at onset.
From Kaufman DM et al: *Kaufman's clinical neurology for psychiatrists*, ed 8, Philadelphia, 2017, Elsevier.

described by the SSNOOP5 mnemonic (see "Differential Diagnosis" above).
- MRI brain with and without contrast is the imaging modality of choice for almost all headache types, although CT head without contrast may be used in the acute setting to evaluate for subarachnoid hemorrhage or other causes of acute intracranial hemorrhage.

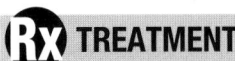 **TREATMENT**

Consider the use of a headache log/diary to identify triggers of headaches, record efficacy of treatments, and track history of headaches.

NONPHARMACOLOGIC THERAPY
- Avoid any identifiable provoking factors: Caffeine, tobacco, and alcohol may trigger attacks, as may dietary or other environmental precipitants (less common).
- Avoid emotional stressors and minimize variations in daily routine with regular sleep, meals, and exercise.
- Relaxation training, behavioral therapy, and biofeedback. Trials have shown that among young persons with chronic migraine, the use of cognitive-behavioral therapy (CBT) plus amitriptyline results in greater reductions in days with headaches and migraine-related disability compared with use of headache education plus amitriptyline;[6] however, overall evidence is mixed.[7]
- Trials in patients with migraine without aura have shown that acupuncture may be associated with long-term reduction in migraine recurrence.[8]

ACUTE ANALGESIC Rx
- Many oral agents are ineffective because of poor absorption from migraine-induced gastric stasis. Nonoral route of administration should be selected in patients with severe nausea or vomiting.
- NSAIDs such as ketorolac, ibuprofen, and naproxen, or combination analgesics, may be used first line for mild migraine headaches.[1,9]
- Barbiturate-containing compounds should be avoided because they are potentially addictive and promote medication overuse headaches.
- Opioids are not effective for treating patients with migraine headaches and should not be used.

ACUTE ABORTIVE Rx
- Triptans (subcutaneous [SC], PO, and intranasal) are the drug class of choice for abortive

therapy. Meta-analysis suggests that 10 mg rizatriptan, 40 mg eletriptan, and 12.5 mg almotriptan are most effective. Sumatriptan may also be given, especially in combination with an NSAID, like naproxen. Early administration improves effectiveness. Triptans are relatively contraindicated in heart disease and hemiplegic migraine.[1,9]
- Gepants (rimegepant, atogepant ubrogepant): Small-molecule CGRP antagonists newly approved for acute migraine abortive therapy, especially when triptans are ineffective or contraindicated. There have been no clear cardiac risks with this class.[1,9]
- Ditans (lasmiditan): 5HT1-F agonist newly approved for acute migraine abortive therapy, especially when triptans are ineffective or contraindicated. There have been no clear cardiac risks with this class. Patients should not drive for 8 h after taking due to concern for somnolence.[1,9-10]
- IV antiemetics (prochlorperazine, metoclopramide, chlorpromazine) may be used in addition to triptans. Acute dystonic reactions, QT prolongation, and akathisia are rare side effects. These are generally not used as monotherapy.
- Ergotamine, ergotamine combinations (PO/PR), and dihydroergotamine (DHE 45) (SC, IV, IM, intranasal) have well-documented efficacy against migraines. DHE is usually administered in combination with an antiemetic drug (Table 2) but cannot be given within 24 h of a triptan.
- IV dexamethasone may be used to prevent recurrence but should not be used frequently due to risk for toxicity.
- Greater and lesser occipital nerve blocks may also be performed to alleviate pain in the acute setting. These injections may be combined with auriculotemporal, supraorbital, and supratrochlear nerve block to achieve anesthesia in the area of perceived pain.

PROPHYLAXIS Rx
- Prophylactic treatment is generally indicated when headaches are disabling more than 6 days of the month, less than 5 days per month but significantly disabling, or when symptomatic treatments are contraindicated or not effective. All prophylaxes should be maintained for at least 3 mo before deeming the medication a failure.[11]
- Well-established options for prophylactic treatment include β-blockers (propranolol, timolol, atenolol, metoprolol), tricyclic antidepressants (amitriptyline, nortriptyline), and the

antiepileptic drugs topiramate and sodium divalproate (valproic acid).
- CGRP monoclonal antibodies: A new class of injectable drugs that target the CGRP molecule or its receptor. There are currently four FDA-approved drugs in this class, erenumab (Aimovig, once-a-month injection), fremanezumab (Ajovy, once-a-month or quarterly injection), galcanezumab (Emgality, once-a-month injection), and eptinezumab (Vyepti, quarterly infusion), with more under study. These drugs can be used first line for episodic and chronic migraine but are usually used after failure of oral prophylactic treatment.[1,11]
- Gepants (rimegepant): Small-molecule CGRP antagonist newly approved for acute migraine abortive therapy as well as prophylaxis.
- Less-established options include calcium channel blockers, selective norepinephrine serotonin reuptake inhibitors, memantine, and other antiepileptic medications.
- Supraorbital transcutaneous electrical stimulation has been approved by the FDA for prophylaxis of episodic migraine and is widely available with a prescription in Europe and North America.
- For prevention of headaches in adult patients with chronic migraines only (≥15 headache days/mo for ≥3 mo), onabotulinum toxin A (Botox) injections are the only approved therapy.

DISPOSITION
With advancing age, many patients will have sustained reduction in frequency of migraine headaches.

REFERRAL
To neurologist if uncertain about diagnosis or treatment not effective

⚠ PEARLS & CONSIDERATIONS
- Migraines that change in character or headaches that are different from the patient's typical ones need to be reevaluated.
- Long-term and frequent use of analgesic medications can result in medication overuse or rebound headaches. Early initiation of prophylactic medication is key.
- Avoid use of narcotics, barbiturates, and benzodiazepines because they are habit forming. Narcotics and barbiturates also promote medication overuse headaches.
- Migraine with aura is associated with an increase in stroke and thromboembolism risk and is a relative contraindication to the use of combined oral contraceptives in women.

REFERENCES
Available at eBooks.Health.Elsevier.com.

RELATED CONTENT
Migraine Headache (Patient Information)

AUTHOR: **ANJALI SUNDARAMOORTHY, DO**

TABLE 2 Abortive and Analgesic Therapy for Migraine*

Drug	Route	Dose
Triptans (Serotonin Agonists)		
Sumatriptan	Subcutaneous	6 mg, repeat in 2 hr (max 2 doses/day)
Sumatriptan	Oral	25 mg, 50 mg, 100 mg, repeat in 2 hr (max 200 mg/day)
Sumatriptan	Nasal spray	5 mg, 20 mg, repeat in 2 hr (max 40 mg/day)
Zolmitriptan	Oral	1.25, 2.5 mg, 5 mg, repeat in 2 hr (max 10 mg/day)
Zolmitriptan	Nasal spray	5 mg, repeat in 2 hr (max 10 mg/day)
Zolmitriptan	Orally disintegrating tab	2.5, 5 mg, repeat in 2 hr (max 10 mg/day)
Naratriptan	Oral	1 mg, 2.5 mg, repeat in 4 hr (max 5 mg/day)
Rizatriptan	Oral	5 mg, 10 mg, repeat in 2 hr (max 30 mg/day)
Almotriptan	Oral	6.25 mg, 12.5 mg, may repeat in 2 hr (max 25 mg/day)
Eletriptan	Oral	20 mg, 40 mg, may repeat in 2 hr (max 80 mg/day)
Frovatriptan	Oral	2.5 mg, may repeat in 2 hr (max 7.5 mg/day); may also be used for mini prophylaxis
Gepants (CGRP antagonists)		
Rimegepant	Orally disintegrating tab	75 mg, only once per 24 hours
Ubrogepant	Oral	50 mg, 100 mg, may repeat in 2 hr (max 200 mg/day)
Ditans (5HT1-F agonists)		
Lasmiditan	Oral	50 mg, 100 mg, 200 mg (once in 24 hours)
Ergotamine Preparations		
Ergotamine and caffeine	Oral	2 tablets, may repeat 1 tab q30 min (max 6/day)
Ergotamine and caffeine	Rectal	1 suppository, repeat in 1 hr (max 2/day)
Ergotamine	Sublingual	1 tablet, repeat in 1 hr (max 2/day)
Dihydroergotamine	Intramuscular	0.5-1.0 mg, repeat twice at 1-hr intervals (max 3 mg/attack)
	Subcutaneous	
	Intravenous	
	Nasal spray	
Isometheptene + dichloralphenazone + acetaminophen	Oral	1 to 2 capsules, repeat in 4 hr (max 8/day)
Nonsteroidal Antiinflammatory Drugs		
Acetaminophen + (should not be used alone)	Oral	2 tablets, repeat in 6 hr (max 8/day aspirin + caffeine)
Naproxen	Oral	550-750 mg, repeat in 1 hr (max 3 times/wk)
Meclofenamate	Oral	100-200 mg, repeat in 1 hr (max 3 times/wk)
Flurbiprofen	Oral	50-100 mg, repeat in 1 hr (max 3 times/wk)
Ibuprofen	Oral	200-300 mg, repeat in 1 hr (max 3 times/wk)
Antiemetics		
Promethazine	Oral	50-125 mg
	Intramuscular	No clear benefit in migraine, may be used
Prochlorperazine	Oral	1-25 mg
	Rectal	2.5-25 mg (suppository)
	Intramuscular/intravenous	5-10 mg, good evidence for strong benefit
Chlorpromazine	Oral	10-25 mg
	Rectal	50-100 mg (suppository)
	Intravenous	Up to 35 mg, use with monitoring, some evidence for good benefit
Trimethobenzamide	Oral	250 mg
	Rectal	200 mg
Metoclopramide	Oral	5-10 mg
	Intramuscular	10 mg
	Intravenous	5-10 mg
Dimenhydrinate	Oral	50 mg

*For side effects and contraindications, consult the manufacturer's drug insert before prescribing any of these drugs.
CGRP, Calcitonin-gene related peptide.
Modified from Wiederholt WC: *Neurology for non-neurologists,* ed 4, Philadelphia, 2000, Saunders.

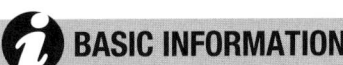

BASIC INFORMATION

DEFINITION

Significant cognitive impairment in the absence of dementia with preserved activities of daily living (ADLs). Mild cognitive impairment (MCI) is an intermediate state between normal cognitive function and dementia. The main distinctions between MCI and mild dementia are that in the latter, more than one cognitive domain is invariably involved and substantial interference with daily life is evident.

SYNONYMS

Mild neurocognitive disorder
MCI

ICD-10CM CODE
G31.84 Mild cognitive impairment, so stated

EPIDEMIOLOGY & DEMOGRAPHICS

INCIDENCE: 12 to 15 cases per 1000 person/yr age $\geq$65
51 to 77 cases per 1000 person/yr age $\geq$75
PREVALENCE: 15% to 25% in those older than age 70
PREDOMINANT SEX & AGE: Male, age $\geq$75
PEAK INCIDENCE: In the elderly
RISK FACTORS: Male sex, age, lower socioeconomic status, lower educational level, vascular risks (diabetes, obesity, cerebrovascular attack [CVA], myocardial infarction [MI], hypertension [HTN]), obstructive sleep apnea, depression, sedentary lifestyle.
GENETICS: *APOE4* genotype
- Various pathways result in amyloid accumulation and deposition in pre-Alzheimer presenting as MCI

CLINICAL PRESENTATION

- Subjective memory problems, preferably corroborated by another person.
- Preserved functional status (ADLs).
- Normal general thinking and reasoning skills.
- Subtypes of MCI include amnestic (mainly involves memory loss) vs. nonamnestic with involvement of other cognitive domains (single domain vs. multiple domains).
- Domains affected in MCI include memory, visuospatial skills, learning, language, attention, and executive function.
- Olfactory dysfunction may be associated with amnestic MCI and progression to Alzheimer dementia.

ETIOLOGY

Neurodegenerative, vascular, traumatic, depression, or due to underlying medical condition

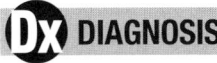

DIAGNOSIS

DIFFERENTIAL DIAGNOSIS

- Age-associated memory impairment (AAMI)
- Delirium
- Dementia
- Depression
- "Reversible" cognitive impairment:
  1. Medication related (anticholinergics)
  2. Hypothyroidism
  3. Vitamin B$_{12}$ deficiency
- Reversible central nervous system (CNS) conditions:
  1. Subdural hematoma
  2. Normal pressure hydrocephalus

WORKUP

HISTORY:
- Focus on specific cognitive deficits and impairment with emphasis on time course of deficits.
- Review all medications that may impact cognition (i.e., anticholinergics).
- Rule out depression and delirium.
- Perform functional assessment.
- Additional history from family members or caregivers is important.
- Assess vascular risks.
- Evaluate sleep issues and pain
- Assess how cognitive concerns affect day to day life.

PHYSICAL EXAM:
- Check blood pressure
- Neurologic exam to rule out reversible CNS causes of cognitive impairment
- Gait and balance assessment
- Cardiovascular exam

COGNITIVE FUNCTION TESTING:
- Mental status testing using brief cognitive assessment tool (MOCA [Montreal Cognitive Assessment] or SLUMS [St. Louis University Mental Status] or others) followed by neuropsychologic testing if appropriate for specific deficits in cognitive domains. MOCA may be a better tool in identifying and following MCI with higher sensitivity to monitor cognitive decline in longitudinal monitoring. Neuropsychologic testing longitudinally for the first couple of years can help to determine stability vs. progression. It can establish a baseline for future testing of cognition and can help to rule out concurrent factors that impact cognition.

LABORATORY TESTS

- CBC
- Comprehensive metabolic profile
- Thyroid-stimulating hormone
- Vitamin B$_{12}$
- Syphilis testing
- HIV testing

IMAGING STUDIES

- Imaging should be performed with focal neurologic deficits, rapid progression and symptoms, or atypical presentations.
- Computed tomography (CT) imaging can detect most reversible CNS conditions leading to cognitive impairment.
- MRI is preferred and further evaluates vascular, infectious, neoplastic, and inflammatory conditions.

TREATMENT

- There is insufficient evidence to recommend use of cholinesterase inhibitors for MCI. They are not approved for treating MCI, have shown little efficacy in altering progression to dementia, and can have significant side effects.
- Consider treatment with these medications only if memory complaints appear to be significantly affecting day-to-day quality of life in individual patients or in amnestic subtypes of MCI after risk-versus-benefit discussion with patient and family.

NONPHARMACOLOGIC THERAPY

- Role of cognitive rehabilitation to target specific deficits.
- Regular dental exams and good dental hygiene should be encouraged. Significant periodontal disease is associated with MCI.
- Caregiver education and counseling.
- Multicomponent physical and mental exercises to maintain cognition should be recommended. Daily physical activity, at least 30 min on most days, has been shown to be beneficial in maintaining cognition. Reading and group discussion can also be beneficial.
- Cognition can improve in those with obstructive sleep apnea who become compliant with continuous positive airway pressure (CPAP).
- Alcohol consumption in excess can worsen cognition.
- Aids and strategies for memory impairment are summarized in Box 1.

DISPOSITION

- Progression to Alzheimer at the rate of 5% to 15% per year.
  1. Risk factors for progression to dementia include presence of vascular risk factors, significant cognitive impairment, depression, hearing loss, loss of smell, and presence of extrapyramidal signs.
- Mortality of those with MCI is twice that of those without MCI.
- Two- to threefold increase in risk of nursing home placement in those with MCI.

COMPLEMENTARY & ALTERNATIVE MEDICINE

- No clear indications for antioxidants, and studies in humans are inconclusive. Over-the-counter herbs and supplements for memory should be discouraged, since they do not have any good evidence to prove efficacy and can have interactions and significant side effects. These agents are not FDA approved for MCI.

REFERRAL

Consider referral to a memory specialist if more than just memory is involved or for further evaluation of specific deficits.

M

Diseases and Disorders

I

BOX 1   Aids and Strategies for Memory Impairment

External
Reminders by Others
Tape recorder or portable voice organizer
Notes written by hand or entered into smartphone calendar

Time Reminders
Alarm clock, phone call, smartphone app
Personal organizer or diary
Calendar or wall planner
Orientation board

Place Reminders
Labels
Codes (colors, symbols)

Person Reminders
Name tags
Clothes that offer a cue

Organizers
Lists
Personal organizer or diary
Numbered series of reminders
Items grouped for use
Calendar and event alarm on smartphone or tablet

Internal
Mental retracing of events
Visual imagery
Alphabet searching
Associations to what is already recalled
Rehearsal
First-letter mnemonics
Chunking or grouping of items

From Jankovic J et al: *Bradley and Daroff's neurology in clinical practice*, ed 8, Philadelphia, 2022, Elsevier.

- MCI becomes clinically relevant when quality of life is affected such as problems making financial decisions and problems with personal day-to-day interactions.
- Depression should be ruled out prior to making a diagnosis of MCI since it is highly prevalent in the elderly.
- Anticholinergic medication use should be evaluated carefully prior to making a diagnosis of MCI.

PREVENTION
Patients with MCI should be counseled on strategies to prevent progression to dementia. They should remain physically and mentally active, have a well-balanced diet, continue activities that are socially engaging, reduce stress in their lives, and aggressively pursue treatment of vascular risk factors.

PATIENT & FAMILY EDUCATION
- Patients with MCI typically have poor retention and rapid loss of newly learned information.
- For additional information for patients, families, and clinicians: Alzheimer's Association (https://www.alzheimers.org).

AUTHORS: **BIRJU B. PATEL, MD,** and **N. WILSON HOLLAND, MD**

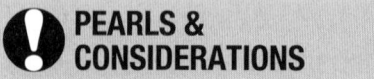

PEARLS & CONSIDERATIONS

COMMENTS
- Patients with MCI usually report short-term memory concerns such as misplacing things, not remembering names of people, word-finding difficulties, forgetting day-to-day tasks, not being able to read a book, or not being able to follow a conversation.
- Women with MCI are higher risk for progression to dementia than men.

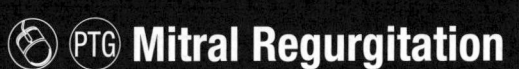

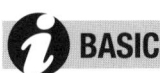 **BASIC INFORMATION**

DEFINITION

Mitral regurgitation (MR) is retrograde blood flow into the left atrium resulting from any part of an incompetent mitral valve apparatus. This condition may cause left ventricular (LV) failure, as well as increased left atrial and pulmonary pressures leading to pulmonary hypertension and right-sided heart failure.

SYNONYMS

Mitral insufficiency
MR

ICD-10CM CODES
I34.0	Nonrheumatic mitral (valve) insufficiency
I05.1	Rheumatic mitral insufficiency
I05.9	Mitral valve disease, unspecified
I05.2	Rheumatic mitral stenosis with insufficiency
Q23.3	Congenital mitral insufficiency

EPIDEMIOLOGY & DEMOGRAPHICS

Mitral regurgitation is a common valvular abnormality occurring in about 10% of the total population. The incidence of MR has increased over the past 30 yr. However, this may be due to increasing availability of echocardiography leading to MR diagnosis rather than to an actual increase in the prevalence of this condition.

PHYSICAL FINDINGS & CLINICAL PRESENTATION

Heart sounds:
- Diminished S1 as valve leaflets fail to coapt properly
- Widely split S2 as A2 occurs earlier because of decreased LV ejection time
- Presence of an S3 as a result of increased flow into a dilated LV caused by severe MR with systolic impairment

Heart murmurs:
- Holosystolic, high-pitched, "blowing" murmur is most easily audible at apex with radiation to base, left axilla, or back. There is a poor correlation between the intensity of the systolic murmur and the degree of regurgitation. However, an early diastolic to mid-diastolic rumble (pseudomitral stenosis) suggests severe MR. The murmur of acute MR may be short and unimpressive. This is because the sudden volume overload increases left atrial and pulmonary venous pressures leading to pulmonary congestion and hypoxia, whereas decreased blood delivery to the tissues with concomitant decrease in LV systolic pressure limits the pressure gradient driving MR to early systole.
- Hyperdynamic apex, sometimes with palpable LV lift and apical thrill.
- Symptomatic patients with MR generally present with the following:
  1. Symptoms suggestive of heart failure (fatigue, dyspnea, orthopnea, paroxysmal nocturnal dyspnea, edema)
  2. Hemoptysis (caused by pulmonary hypertension)
  3. Atrial fibrillation

ETIOLOGY

Primary MR:
- Idiopathic myxomatous degeneration of the mitral valve, mitral valve prolapse (most common cause of MR in industrialized countries)[1].
- Papillary muscle dysfunction or rupture (typically as a result of an inferior wall myocardial infarction)
- Ruptured chordae tendineae
- Infective endocarditis
- Calcified mitral valve annulus
- Rheumatic valvulitis (may be combined with mitral stenosis; common in developing countries)
- Systemic lupus erythematosus (Libman-Sacks endocarditis)
- Drugs: Fenfluramine, dexfenfluramine, pergolide, cabergoline
- Congenital cleft valve
- Ischemic MR due to papillary muscle dysfunction from multivessel coronary artery disease (CAD)

Secondary MR:
- Hypertrophic cardiomyopathy
- LV dilation (e.g., secondary to dilated cardiomyopathy)

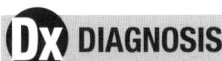 **DIAGNOSIS**

DIFFERENTIAL DIAGNOSIS

- Hypertrophic cardiomyopathy
- Tricuspid regurgitation
- Aortic stenosis
- Aortic sclerosis
- Ventricular septal defect
- Atrial septal defect

WORKUP

- Diagnostic workup consists of echocardiography, ECG, and chest radiograph; cardiovascular magnetic resonance (CMR) and cardiac catheterization are sometimes needed to confirm severity of the disease.
- Recent studies suggest that in patients with severe asymptomatic MR, normal LV function and elevations of brain natriuretic peptide (BNP) >105 pg/ml have an independent and additive prognostic value that may identify high-risk patients and aid in the selection of patients for early surgery.

IMAGING STUDIES

- Echocardiography (Fig. 1): TTE is the initial imaging modality of choice, with TEE performed if insufficient or discordant information is obtained from TTE. Findings include dilated left atrium, hyperdynamic left ventricle, erratic motion of the leaflet in patients with ruptured chordae tendineae, and color flow Doppler with evidence of MR. The most important aspect of the echocardiographic examination is the quantification of the severity of MR (Table 1). A vena contracta width $\geq$0.7 cm, a regurgitant volume $\geq$60 ml, regurgitant orifice area $\geq$0.40 cm^2 by PISA (proximal isovelocity surface area), and systolic pulmonary vein flow reversal are all echocardiographic criteria of severe MR

- Chest x-ray:
  1. Left atrial enlargement, LV enlargement
  2. Possible pulmonary congestion, although most often normal
- ECG:
  1. Left atrial enlargement
  2. LV hypertrophy
  3. Atrial fibrillation
- Cardiac catheterization: To confirm severity of MR, or to rule out presence of coronary artery disease in patients being evaluated for surgical replacement
- Can consider cardiac MRI in cases where echocardiography is limited or LV function/dimensions are borderline, or when clinical condition and echocardiographic findings are discordant

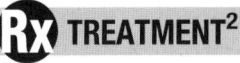 **TREATMENT**[2]

NONPHARMACOLOGIC THERAPY

- Salt restriction
- Surgical repair or replacement (see the following)

ACUTE GENERAL Rx

- Medical: Medical therapy is primarily directed toward treatment of the etiology or complications (e.g., atrial fibrillation, ischemic heart disease, infective endocarditis, hypertension, and heart failure).
  1. The utility of afterload reduction to decrease the regurgitant fraction and increase cardiac output depends upon the etiology of MR. In acute MR, intravenous vasodilators (such as sodium nitroprusside or nicardipine) has shown some utility. This afterload reduction can also be achieved by intra-aortic balloon counter pulsation. Long-term use of guideline directed medical therapy for heart failure, while it does not slow the progression of MR, should be implemented when other indications such as hypertension and LV dysfunction are present.
  2. Control ventricular response in atrial fibrillation when rapid ventricular response is present. Use anticoagulants if atrial fibrillation occurs. Note that current guidelines do not consider atrial fibrillation in patients with MR "valvular" and nonvitamin K anticoagulation agents may be used for stroke prophylaxis.
  3. Diuresis and achieving a euvolemic state may significantly decrease the degree of functional MR caused by volume overload and heart failure.
- Surgery: Surgery is the only definitive treatment for MR. Although no randomized trial of mitral valve repair vs. replacement exists, repair is favored over replacement[3] in degenerative mitral valve disease due to its lower perioperative risk, improved event-free survival, freedom from complications of prosthetic valves, and better postoperative LV function. It is a class I indication in patients with the following diagnoses (Fig. 2):

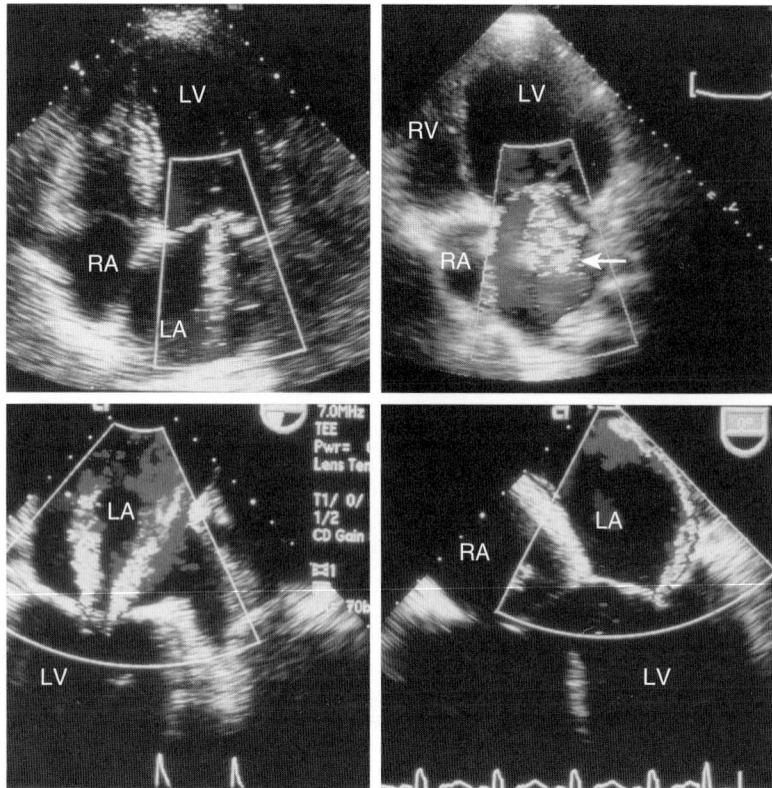

FIG. 1 Mitral regurgitation. Four panels depicting varying degrees of mitral regurgitation; the two top panels are apical four-chamber transthoracic views showing, on the left, mild mitral regurgitation and, on the right, moderate to severe mitral regurgitation. On the left, note the relatively narrow jet directed from the tips of the mitral valve toward the posterior left atrial wall. On the right, note the larger jet, filling approximately 40% of the left atrial cavity. The two bottom panels are transesophageal echocardiograms. On the left, note the mitral regurgitation occurring in two discrete jets and, on the right, the highly eccentric jet, which courses along the extreme lateral wall of the left atrium. *LA,* Left atrium; *LV,* left ventricle; *RA,* right atrium; *RV,* right ventricle. (From Zipes DP et al [eds]: *Braunwald's heart disease,* ed 7, Philadelphia, 2005, Saunders.)

TABLE 1 Mitral Regurgitation Severity*

	I (Mild)	II (Moderate)	III (Moderate)	IV (Severe)
MR = jet (%LA)	<15	15-30	35-50	>50
Spectral Doppler	Faint	—	—	Dense
Vena contracta	<3 mm	—	—	≥7 mm
Pulmonary vein flow	S >D	Normal to systolic blunting	Systolic blunting	Systolic reversal
RV (ml)	<30	30-44	45-59	≥60
ERO (cm2)	<0.2	0.2-0.29	0.3-0.39	≥0.40
PISA	Small	—	—	Large

D, Antegrade flow in diastole; *ERO,* effective regurgitant orifice; *%LA,* percentage of left atrial area encompassed by the MR jet with color flow Doppler; *MR,* mitral regurgitation; *PISA,* proximal isovelocity surface area; *RV,* regurgitant volume; *S,* antegrade flow in systole.

*For some parameters, the observation is valid at the extremes of MR severity and there may be marked overlap in intermediate (grades II, III) MR. In these instances, no value is presented.

From Zipes DP et al (eds): *Braunwald's heart disease,* ed 7, Philadelphia, 2005, Saunders.

1. Acute severe MR
2. Symptomatic patients with severe primary MR irrespective of LV systolic function. Asymptomatic patients with severe primary MR and LV systolic dysfunction (LVEF ≤60%) or progressive dilation (LVESD ≥40 mm)
• Surgery is a class IIa (reasonable) recommendation in:

1. Severe MR with new-onset atrial fibrillation, even if asymptomatic
2. Asymptomatic severe MR with pulmonary hypertension (≥50 mm Hg at rest or ≥60 mm Hg during exercise)
3. Asymptomatic severe MR secondary to flail leaflet[4].
4. Asymptomatic severe MR with normal LV systolic function (LVEF ≥60% and

LVESD ≤40 mm) in whom the likelihood of successful repair without residual MR is >95% and operative mortality is <1%
• Surgery is a class IIb recommendation in symptomatic patients (New York Heart Association [NYHA] class III to IV) with severe MR with severe LV dysfunction or dilation (LVEF <30% or LV at end-systole >55 mm, respectively) in whom LV dysfunction is not the primary cause for the MR as well as functional MR where it is secondary to LV dysfunction.
• Quantitative grading of MR is a powerful predictor of the clinical outcome of asymptomatic MR. In general, patients with regurgitant orifice areas of ≥40 mm² should be considered for prompt surgery, whereas those with orifices between 20 and 39 mm² can be followed closely.
• Percutaneous mitral valve repair methods are continually being investigated. The MitraClip is a catheter-delivered clip that grasps and approximates the edges of the mitral leaflets at the origin of the regurgitant jet. This device is FDA approved for use in patients with significant symptomatic degenerative or primary MR (>3+) who are too high risk for surgery. Transcatheter edge-to-edge repair in severely symptomatic patients with primary severe MR and high or prohibitive surgical risk has a class IIa indication. In 2019, the FDA expanded approval for symptomatic secondary or functional MR. In patients with HF and moderate-to-severe or severe secondary MR who remained symptomatic despite GDMT, TEER was safe, provided a durable reduction in MR, reduced the rate of HFH, and improved survival, quality of life, and functional capacity compared with GDMT alone through 36 months.[5] Secondary analysis of the COAPT data showed presence of moderate to severe tricuspid regurgitation (TR) worsened clinical outcomes and should be considered when selected patients for this minimally invasive therapy vs. surgical repair.[6]
• Ischemic MR has been a source of controversy as to whether moderate or greater MR should be fixed at the time of revascularization with coronary artery bypass graft surgery (CABG). Mitral valve repair can be considered at the time of CABG in moderate MR, and mitral valve repair is reasonable for severe MR (class IIa) in the presence of a basal aneurysm or dyskinesis, significant leaflet tethering due to wall motion abnormalities, and moderate-to-severe LV remodeling (LV end-diastolic diameter >65 mm).

DISPOSITION

Prognosis is generally good unless there is significant impairment of LV function or significantly elevated pulmonary artery pressures. Most patients remain asymptomatic for many yr (average interval from diagnosis to onset of symptoms is 16 yr). In patients with chronic severe MR, MR is commonly progressive, with onset of other symptoms or LV dysfunction within 6 to 10 yr. However, surgery should be advised well before the onset of symptoms in

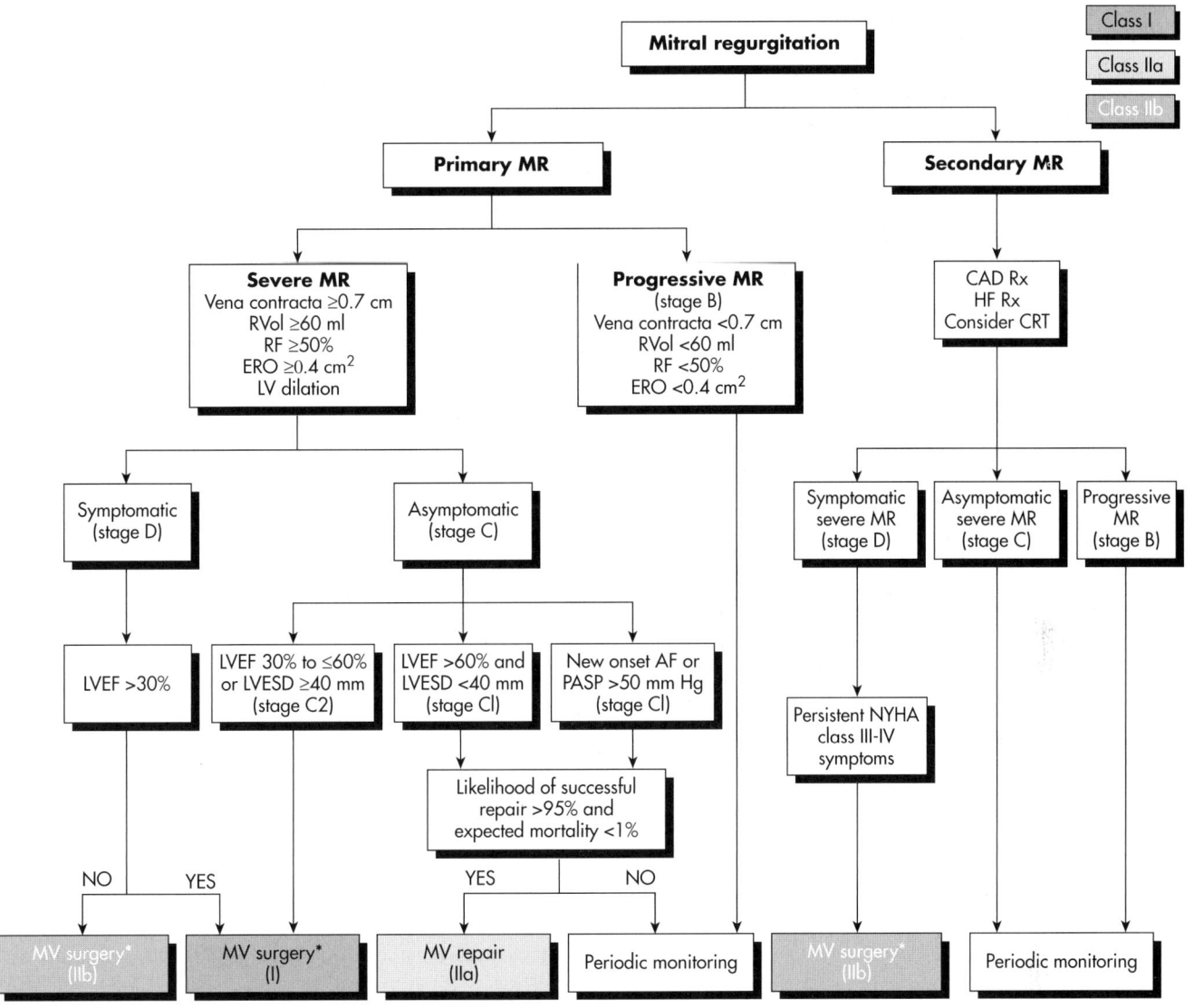

FIG. 2 Indications for surgery for MR. *Mitral valve repair is preferred over MVR when possible. *AF,* Atrial fibrillation; *CAD,* coronary artery disease; *CRT,* cardiac resynchronization therapy; *ERO,* effective regurgitant orifice; *HF,* heart failure; *LV,* left ventricle; *LVEF,* left ventricular ejection fraction; *LVESD,* left ventricle end-systolic dimension; *MR,* mitral regurgitation; *MV,* mitral valve; *MVR,* mitral valve replacement; *NYHA,* New York Heart Association; *PASP,* pulmonary artery systolic pressure; *RF,* regurgitant fraction; *RVol,* regurgitant volume; *Rx,* therapy. (From Nishimura RA et al: ACC/AHA focused update of valvular heart disease guideline, *J Am Coll Cardiol* 70:254-289, 2017.)

case of worsening LVEF and LV systolic dimensions and presence of pulmonary hypertension or atrial fibrillation, all of which are poor prognostic signs.

REFERRAL

- Surgical referral in selected patients (see "Acute General Rx"). Emergency surgery is usually necessary in patients with acute MR caused by ruptured papillary muscle or chordae tendineae after myocardial infarction.
- Mitral valve repair can also be accomplished with percutaneous implantation of a MitraClip device in patients who are too high risk for surgery.

PEARLS & CONSIDERATIONS

COMMENTS

- Although vasodilators and other agents should be used to treat hypertension in patients with severe MR, there is no evidence that they will delay the need for eventual valve surgery, which is the definitive treatment for severe MR.
- In 2007, the AHA guidelines for prevention of infectious endocarditis were revised and routine antibiotic prophylaxis to undergo

dental or other invasive procedures is no longer recommended, unless the patient has had prior endocarditis.

REFERENCES

Available at eBooks.Health.Elsevier.com.

RELATED CONTENT

Mitral Regurgitation (Patient Information)

AUTHORS: **MOHAMED A. ABDELAZEEM, MD,** and **UYEN T. LAM, MD**

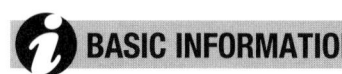

BASIC INFORMATION

DEFINITION

Mitral stenosis is a narrowing of the mitral valve orifice that prevents proper opening during diastole and obstruction of blood flow from the left atrium to the left ventricle. Due to thickening of the leaflets there is restricted movement. The obstruction leads to increased pressure in the left atrium, pulmonary vasculature, and the right side of the heart. The cross section of a normal orifice measures 4 to 6 cm^2. Symptoms usually develop with exercise when the orifice measures <2.5 cm^2, and symptoms may develop at rest when the orifice is <1.5 cm^2.

SYNONYM

MS

ICD-10CM CODES
I05.0	Rheumatic mitral stenosis
I05.2	Rheumatic mitral stenosis with insufficiency
I34.2	Nonrheumatic mitral (valve) stenosis
Q23.2	Congenital mitral stenosis

EPIDEMIOLOGY & DEMOGRAPHICS

- The predominant cause of mitral stenosis is rheumatic heart disease; however, the occurrence of mitral valve stenosis has decreased worldwide over the past 30 yr (particularly in developed countries) as a result of declining incidence of rheumatic fever due to appropriate antibiotic use.
- There remains a high prevalence of rheumatic heart disease in developing countries.
- Rheumatic heart disease has a predilection for the mitral valve, aortic valve, and to some extent the tricuspid valve.
- The incidence of MS is higher in women (2:1 female:male ratio).
- Outbreaks of rheumatic fever in the United States are due to increased virulence of a streptococcal strain or enhanced immigration from where rheumatic heart disease is prevalent.

PHYSICAL FINDINGS & CLINICAL PRESENTATION

PHYSICAL FINDINGS "Mitral facies" that are pinkish-purple patches on the cheek due to low cardiac output and vasoconstriction usually indicate severe MS. Loud first heart sound (S1) caused by delayed valve closure preceded by an opening snap and rapid rising left ventricular (LV) pressure. A low-pitched rumbling diastolic murmur is heard best at the apex. The intensity of the murmur is not related to the severity of the stenosis, but the duration is holodiastolic in severe MS. An opening snap (OS) caused by tensing of the valve leaflets after the cusps have opened completely. The OS follows S2 by 0.03 to 0.14 sec, and the shorter the S2 to OS interval, the more severe the MS, due to the increasing left atrial pressures. A diastolic thrill may be palpable at the apex, especially with the patient in the left lateral recumbent position. A left parasternal heave secondary to right ventricular (RV) hypertrophy and pulmonary hypertension. An accentuated P2 and/or a soft, early diastolic decrescendo murmur (Graham Steell murmur) caused by pulmonary regurgitation may be present in patients with pulmonary hypertension (not specific for mitral stenosis).

SYMPTOMS & PRESENTATION

- Dyspnea is the most common symptom, along with fatigue and decreased exercise capacity. These symptoms occur due to an inability to increase cardiac output, especially with exercise, and elevated pulmonary capillary wedge pressures, with resultant increase in pulmonary artery pressures. The stages of mitral stenosis are summarized in Table 1.
- Pregnancy in females with advanced MS may be poorly tolerated due to the 50% increase in cardiac output that occurs in pregnancy. This can often be the initial presentation of symptoms in a previously asymptomatic patient.
- Acute pulmonary edema may occur after an increase in flow across the mitral valve secondary to an increase in cardiac output or heart rate (exertion, tachyarrhythmias, fever, anemia, pregnancy etc.).
- Paroxysmal nocturnal dyspnea (PND) and orthopnea secondary to elevated left atrial pressure may occur.
- Hemoptysis can be present secondary to rupture of thin-walled dilated bronchial veins due to an abrupt increase in left atrial pressure.
- Chest pain can be caused by RV pressure overload and/or concomitant coronary artery disease in up to 15% of patients.
- Hoarseness due to the enlargement of the left atrium compressing the recurrent laryngeal nerve.

COMPLICATIONS

- Pulmonary hypertension that results from chronically elevated pulmonary capillary wedge pressures can lead to RV dysfunction and signs and symptoms of right heart failure (hepatomegaly, pulsatile liver, peripheral edema, ascites). This is sometimes referred to the "second stenosis" of mitral stenosis.
- Atrial fibrillation is more prevalent in patients with more severe MS, increasing age, and other valvular abnormalities.
- The left ventricle is typically "protected" in mitral stenosis and exists in a low-pressure state; however, rheumatic MS often coexists with mitral regurgitation and occasionally with aortic valve dysfunction, both of which can cause LV dysfunction.

TABLE 1 Stages of Mitral Stenosis

Stage	Definition	Valve Anatomy	Valve Hemodynamics	Hemodynamic Consequences	Symptoms
A	At risk for MS	Mild valve doming during diastole	Normal transmitral flow velocity	None	None
B	Progressive MS	Rheumatic valve changes with commissural fusion and diastolic doming of the mitral valve leaflets Planimetered MVA >1.5 cm^2	Increased transmitral flow velocities MVA >1.5 cm^2 Diastolic pressure half-time <150 m sec	Mild to moderate LA enlargement Normal pulmonary pressure at rest	None
C	Asymptomatic severe MS	Rheumatic valve changes with commissural fusion and diastolic doming of the mitral valve leaflets Planimetered MVA ≤1.5 cm^2 (MVA ≤1 cm^2 with very severe MS)	MVA ≤1.5 cm^2 (MVA ≤1 cm^2 with very severe MS) Diastolic pressure half-time ≥150 msec (Diastolic pressure half-time ≥220 msec with very severe MS)	Severe LA enlargement Elevated PASP >30 mm Hg	None
D	Symptomatic severe MS	Rheumatic valve changes with commissural fusion and diastolic doming of the mitral valve leaflets Planimetered MVA ≤1.5 cm^2	MVA ≤1.5 cm^2 (MVA ≤1 cm^2 with very severe MS) Diastolic pressure half-time ≥150 msec (Diastolic pressure half-time ≥220 msec with very severe MS)	Severe LA enlargement Elevated PASP >30 mm Hg	Decreased exercise tolerance Exertional dyspnea

The transmitral mean pressure gradient should be obtained to determine the full hemodynamic effect of the MS and usually is >5 to 10 mm Hg in severe MS; however, because of the variability of the mean pressure gradient with heart rate and forward flow, it has not been included in the criteria for severity.

LA, Left atrium; *MS*, mitral stenosis; *MVA*, mitral valve area; *PASP*, pulmonary artery systolic pressure.

From Mann DL et al: *Braunwald's heart disease*, ed 10, Philadelphia, 2015, Elsevier.

- Systemic embolic events are caused by left atrial thrombi. These are associated with atrial fibrillation 80% of the time, since mitral stenosis leads to left atrial enlargement, which is a predisposing factor for atrial arrhythmias.

RADIOGRAPHIC & HEMODYNAMIC FINDINGS

- Prominent A wave on the pulmonary capillary wedge pressure tracing. This is analogous to the prominent A wave seen in systemic venous pressure tracings with tricuspid stenosis.
- Straightening of the left heart border seen on chest radiography indicative of left atrial enlargement.
- Fig. 1 shows schematic representations of LV, aortic, and left atrial pressures, showing normal relationships and alterations with mild and severe MS.

ETIOLOGY

- Rheumatic fever (RF) is the predominant cause of MS. RF causes thickening of the leaflet tips, commissure fusion, and chordal shortening and fusion. This leads to the classic doming of the leaflets in diastole due to fusion of the leaflet tips at the commissures. Rheumatic fever involves the leaflet tips first with progression toward the annulus. This is opposite of mitral annular calcification, which typically starts in the annulus and proceeds out to the leaflet tips, leading to mitral stenosis in severe cases.
- An atrial septal defect associated with rheumatic mitral stenosis is termed *Lutembacher syndrome*.
- Parachute valve, a congenital defect, has the usual two mitral leaflets, but the chordae, instead of diverging to insert into two papillary muscles, converge into one major papillary muscle, which allows little mobility of the leaflets, as in cor triatriatum (heart with three atria), in which there is a thin membrane that obstructs the pulmonary vein flow and simulates mitral stenosis.
- Less common causes are severe mitral annular calcification usually seen in end-stage renal disease patients, endomyocardial fibroelastosis, malignant carcinoid syndrome, systemic lupus erythematosus, Whipple disease, Fabry disease, rheumatoid arthritis, 3,4-methylenedioxy-methamphetamine (MDMA) use, and significant age-related changes.
- Medications: Ergot alkaloids (methysergide and ergotamine).

DX DIAGNOSIS

DIFFERENTIAL DIAGNOSIS

Causing similar symptoms of LV inflow obstruction.
- Left atrial myxoma
- Ball valve thrombus
- Other valvular abnormalities (e.g., tricuspid stenosis, mitral regurgitation)
- Atrial septal defect

IMAGING STUDIES

- Echocardiography (Fig. 2):

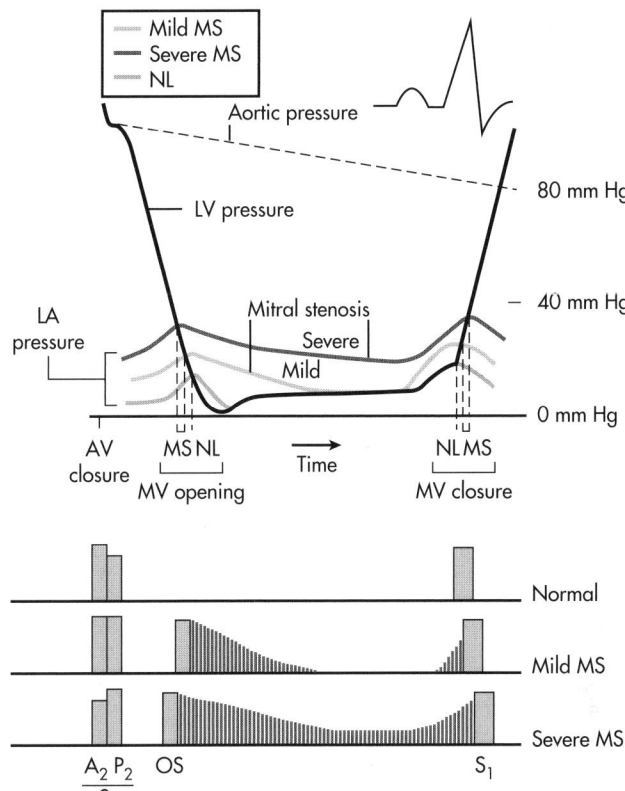

FIG. 1 Schematic representation of left ventricular *(LV)*, aortic, and left atrial *(LA)* pressures, showing normal relationships and alterations with mild and severe mitral stenosis *(MS)*. Corresponding classic auscultatory signs of MS are shown at the bottom. The higher left atrial V wave of severe MS causes earlier pressure crossover and earlier mitral valve *(MV)* opening, leading to a shorter time interval between aortic valve *(AV)* closure and the opening snap *(OS)*. The higher left atrial end-diastolic pressure with severe MS also results in later closure of the mitral valve. With severe MS, the diastolic rumble becomes longer and there is accentuation of the pulmonic component *(P₂)* of the second heart sound *(S₂)* in relation to the aortic component *(A₂)*. *NL,* Normal limits. (From Zipes DP: *Braunwald's heart disease, a textbook of cardiovascular medicine,* ed 11, Philadelphia, 2019, Elsevier.)

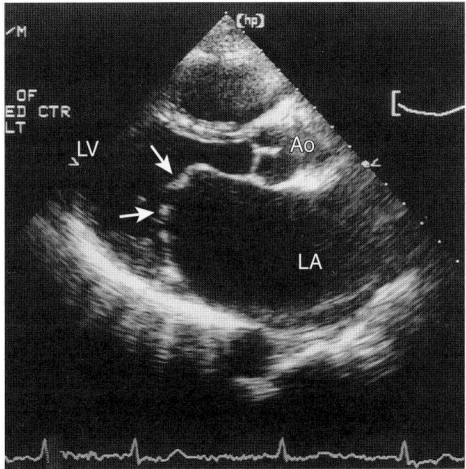

FIG. 2 Mitral stenosis. Parasternal long-axis view of a patient with mitral stenosis and a pliable noncalcified mitral valve leaflet. Note the "doming" motion of the mitral valve leaflets *(arrows)*. Valves with these morphologic features are excellent candidates for percutaneous balloon valvotomy. *Ao,* Aorta; *LA,* left atrium; *LV,* left ventricle. (From Zipes DP et al [eds]: *Braunwald's heart disease,* ed 7, Philadelphia, 2005, Saunders.)

1. Two-dimensional echocardiogram can be used to measure valve area by direct planimetry or calculate it by the Doppler pressure half-time method (this may be inaccurate in patients with concomitant diastolic dysfunction, atrial septal defects, or aortic insufficiency, and those who recently have undergone mitral valvuloplasty), or the continuity equation can be used to calculate the valve area. It also can

be measured using the proximal isovelocity surface area method. A valve area ≤ 1.5 cm^2 is consistent with severe MS (and ≤ 1.0 cm^2 with very severe MS). The transmitral gradient can also be calculated. A mean gradient of >10 mm Hg indicates severe MS, a gradient of 5 to 10 mm Hg is consistent with moderate MS, and 0 to 5 mm Hg is consistent with mild MS or no MS.

2. M-Mode echocardiography will also show a markedly diminished E-to-F slope of the anterior mitral valve leaflet during diastole. There can be loss of the "A-wave" due to increased left atrial pressure or the presence of associated atrial fibrillation. There is also fusion of the commissures, resulting in "doming" of the leaflets during diastole.

3. Grading of leaflet thickness, mobility, calcification, and subvalvular thickening (Wilkins score) with a score of 0 to 4 for each characteristic can predict hemodynamic results and outcome of balloon mitral valvuloplasty (a low score of less than 8 is favorable for balloon valvuloplasty and a high score is unfavorable). A score above 8 would favor a surgical approach. In addition, mitral regurgitation that is greater than mild would preclude a balloon mitral valvuloplasty procedure.

4. Doppler echocardiography can be used to assess for pulmonary hypertension and to give an estimate of the pulmonary artery systolic pressure at rest and with exercise.

5. Patients with known mitral stenosis: A follow-up echocardiography is recommended to assess for pulmonary artery pressures and valve gradient, and to determine the optimal timing of surgical or percutaneous intervention. According to the 2020 American Heart Association/American College of Cardiology (AHA/ACC) focused valve guideline, echocardiogram is recommended every year for very severe MS with mitral valve area <1.0 cm^2, every 1 to 2 yr with severe MS with mitral valve area ≤ 1.5 cm^2, and every 3 to 5 yr with progressive MS with mitral valve area >1.5 cm^2.[1]

- Chest x-ray examination:
  1. Straightening of the left cardiac border caused by enlarged left atrium
  2. Left atrial enlargement on lateral chest x-ray examination
  3. Prominence of pulmonary arteries that indicates pulmonary hypertension
  4. Possible pulmonary congestion and edema (Kerley B lines)
- ECG:
  1. RV hypertrophy; right axis deviation caused by pulmonary hypertension
  2. Left atrial enlargement (broad, biphasic P waves in lead V1 and duration of P-waves >0.11 sec in lead II); this is termed "P-mitrale"
  3. Atrial fibrillation
- Cardiac catheterization:
  1. Measurement of pulmonary artery pressure and transmitral pressure gradients at rest

TABLE 2 Approaches to Mechanical Relief of Mitral Stenosis

Approach	Advantages	Disadvantages
Closed surgical valvotomy	Inexpensive Relatively simple Good hemodynamic results in selected patients Good long-term outcome	No direct visualization of valve Only feasible with flexible, noncalcified valves Contraindicated with MR grade higher than 2+ Surgical procedure with general anesthesia
Open surgical valvotomy	Visualization of valve allows directed valvotomy Concurrent annuloplasty for MR is feasible	Best results with flexible, noncalcified valves Surgical procedure with general anesthesia
Valve replacement	Feasible in all patients regardless of extent of valve calcification or severity of MR	Surgical procedure with general anesthesia Effect of loss of annular-papillary muscle continuity on LV function Prosthetic valve Chronic anticoagulation
Balloon mitral valvotomy	Percutaneous approach Local anesthesia Good hemodynamic results in selected patients Good long-term outcome	No direct visualization of valve Only feasible with flexible noncalcified valves Contraindicated with MR grade higher than 2+

LV, Left ventricular; *MR*, mitral regurgitation.
From Zipes DP: *Braunwald's heart disease, a textbook of cardiovascular medicine*, ed 11, Philadelphia, 2019, Elsevier.

or with exercise (supine biking or raising weights with arms while lying supine)
2. Measurement of transmitral flow and calculation of the valve area
3. Is not routinely recommended for the evaluation of MS but is useful when the echocardiographic findings are non-diagnostic or discrepant with the clinical scenario
4. Cardiac catheterization in addition to echocardiography can be used to monitor the hemodynamics during a balloon mitral valvuloplasty procedure

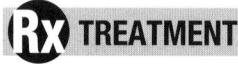 **TREATMENT**

NONPHARMACOLOGIC THERAPY
Decrease level of activity in symptomatic patients, and salt restriction if pulmonary congestion is present.

ACUTE GENERAL Rx
- Medical:
  1. Anticoagulation for the prevention of systemic embolic events in patients with MS and:
     a. Atrial fibrillation: In patients with atrial fibrillation and rheumatic mitral stenosis, anticoagulation with a vitamin K antagonist with a goal international normalized ratio (INR) of 2.5 is indicated. Further study is needed to establish the efficacy of direct oral anticoagulants (DOACs) in this setting
     b. Prior embolic event
  2. Documented left atrial thrombus or left atrial appendage thrombus
  3. Ventricular rate control (to increase diastolic filling period) with β-blockers, non-dihydropyridine calcium channel blockers,

or digitalis and aggressive treatment of tachyarrhythmias.
4. Treat congestive heart failure with loop diuretics and sodium restriction.
5. Antibiotic prophylaxis to prevent recurrent rheumatic fever is usually not indicated unless there is presence of high-risk features such as prior endocarditis, prosthetic heart valves, valvulopathy of the transplanted heart, and certain cases of cyanotic congenital heart disease.
6. Physical activity and exercise. Patients with mild MS in sinus rhythm with a peak pulmonary artery pressure <50 mm Hg can participate in all competitive sports. Patients with moderate MS and in sinus rhythm or atrial fibrillation with a peak pulmonary artery pressure of <50 mm Hg can participate in low to moderate static and dynamic sports. Patients in sinus rhythm with severe MS should not participate in any competitive sports. Patients in atrial fibrillation with any degree of MS and on anticoagulation should avoid all competitive sports.
7. Mild to moderate MS may be tolerated in pregnancy with medical therapy alone.
- Table 2 summarizes approaches to mechanical relief of mitral stenosis.
- Percutaneous mitral balloon commissurotomy (PMBC) is the therapy of choice for symptomatic patients with severe MS (valve area ≤ 1.5 cm^2) with a favorable valvuloplasty score (Table 3), minimal or no mitral regurgitation, and no left atrial thrombus. PMBC is reasonable for asymptomatic patients with very severe MS (mitral valve area ≤ 1.0 cm^2) and favorable valve morphology in the absence of left atrial thrombus or moderate to severe MR (class IIa indication). PMBC is also considered the procedure of choice in

TABLE 3 Wilkins Score for Assessing Appropriateness of Percutaneous Balloon Mitral Commissurotomy

Grade	Mobility	Thickening	Calcification	Subvalvular Thickening
1	Highly mobile valve with only leaflet tips restricted	Leaflets near normal in thickness (4-5 mm)	A single area of increased echocardiographic brightness	Minimal thickening just below the mitral leaflets
2	Leaflet mid and base portions have normal mobility	Midleaflets normal, considerable thickening of margins (5-8 mm)	Scattered areas of brightness confined to leaflet margins	Thickening of chordal structures extending to one-third of the chordal length
3	Valve continues to move forward in diastole, mainly from the base	Thickening extending through the entire leaflet (5-8 mm)	Brightness extending into the midportions of the leaflets	Thickening extended to distal third of the chords
4	No or minimal forward movement of the leaflets in diastole	Considerable thickening of all leaflet tissue (>8-10 mm)	Extensive brightness throughout much of the leaflet tissue	Extensive thickening and shortening of all chordal structures extending down to the papillary muscles

Sum of the four items ranges between 4 and 16. With a score of 8 or less, percutaneous balloon mitral valvuloplasty is likely to be successful. If the score is more than 8, surgery is recommended.
From Townsend CM et al: *Sabiston textbook of surgery*, ed 21, St Louis, 2022, Elsevier.

TABLE 4 ACC/AHA Guidelines for Intervention for Mitral Stenosis (MS)

Class	Indication	LOE
I	PMBC for symptomatic patients with severe MS (MVA $\leq$1.5 cm^2, stage D) and favorable valve morphology in the absence of contraindications.	A
	Mitral valve surgery in severely symptomatic patients (NYHA Class III/IV) with severe MS (MVA $\leq$1.5 cm^2, stage D) who are not high risk for surgery and who are not candidates for or failed previous PMBC.	B
	Concomitant mitral valve surgery for patients with severe MS (MVA $\leq$1.5 cm^2, stages C or D) undergoing other cardiac surgery.	C
IIa	PMBC is reasonable for asymptomatic patients with very severe MS (MVA $\leq$1 cm^2, stage C) and favorable valve morphology in the absence of contraindications.	C
	Mitral valve surgery is reasonable for severely symptomatic patients (NYHA class III/IV) with severe MS (MVA $\leq$1.5 cm^2, stage D) provided there are other operative indications.	C
IIb	PMBC may be considered for asymptomatic patients with severe MS (MVA $\leq$1.5 cm^2, stage C) and favorable valve morphology who have new onset of AF in the absence of contraindications.	C
	PMBC may be considered for symptomatic patients with MVA $\geq$1.5 cm^2 if there is evidence of hemodynamically significant MS during exercise.	C
	PMBC may be considered for severely symptomatic patients (NYHA class III/IV) with severe MS (MVA $\leq$1.5 cm^2, stage D) who have suboptimal valve anatomy and are not candidates for surgery or at high risk for surgery.	C
	Concomitant mitral valve surgery may be considered for patients with moderate MS (MVA, 1.6-2.0 cm^2) undergoing other cardiac surgery.	C
	Mitral valve surgery and excision of the left atrial appendage may be considered for patients with severe MS (MVA $\leq$1.5 cm^2, stages C and D) who have had recurrent embolic events while receiving adequate anticoagulation.	C

LOE, Level of evidence; *MVA,* mitral valve area; *NYHA,* New York Heart Association; *PMBC,* percutaneous mitral balloon commissurotomy.
From Nishimura R et al: 2013 AHA/ACCF guideline for valvular heart disease: a report of the American College of Cardiology Foundation/American Heart Association Task Force on Practice Guidelines, *J Am Coll Cardiol* 63:e57-e185, 2014.

pregnant women with rheumatic MS and in New York Heart Association (NYHA) class III to IV heart failure and/or unresponsive to adequate medical treatment. In addition, it may be considered for severely symptomatic (NYHA class III/IV) patients with very severe MS (mitral valve area $\leq$1.5 cm^2) who are not candidates for surgery or are at high risk for surgery, even if they have suboptimal valve anatomy (class IIb indication). Regular follow-up is needed after PMBC because restenosis may occur. Repeat intervention can be performed as long as valve anatomy remains favorable; however, there is usually more fibrosis and deformation of the valve with subsequent procedures. The approximate frequency of repeat intervention is 10% at 7 yr.

- Mitral valve surgery is indicated for patients with moderate to severe symptomatic MS when PMBC is not available or is contraindicated (valvuloplasty score $\leq$8) or the valve is calcified, when MR is more than mild, when left atrial thrombus is present, and when the surgical risk is acceptable. The surgical approaches include closed mitral valvotomy, open valvotomy and repair (preferred), and mitral valve replacement when repair is not possible.
- Table 4 summarizes guidelines for intervention for mitral stenosis.

PROGNOSIS
- Prognosis is generally good except in patients with chronic pulmonary hypertension.
- Operative mortality rates for mitral valve replacement are 1% to 5% at most institutions.

REFERENCES
Available at eBooks.Health.Elsevier.com.

RELATED CONTENT
Mitral Stenosis (Patient Information)

AUTHORS: **DANA PRICE, MD,** and **ARAVIND RAO KOKKIRALA, MD, FACC**

Mitral Valve Prolapse (PTG)

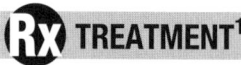 BASIC INFORMATION

DEFINITION
Mitral valve prolapse (MVP) is the bulging of one or both of the mitral valve leaflets ≥2 mm above the annular plane into the left atrium during systole. MVP syndrome refers to a constellation of MVP and associated symptoms (e.g., autonomic dysfunction, palpitations) or other physical abnormalities (e.g., pectus excavatum).

SYNONYMS
MVP
Mitral click murmur syndrome
Barlow syndrome

ICD-10CM CODES
I34.1 Nonrheumatic mitral (valve) prolapse
I34.0 Nonrheumatic mitral (valve) insufficiency

EPIDEMIOLOGY & DEMOGRAPHICS
- MVP is the leading cause of organic mitral regurgitation (MR).
- MVP can be found by echocardiogram in 2.4% of the general population with some studies suggesting that it is more common in women than in men.
- Increased incidence is seen with autoimmune thyroid disorders, Ehlers-Danlos syndrome, Marfan syndrome, osteogenesis imperfecta, pseudoxanthoma elasticum, pectus excavatum, anorexia nervosa, and bulimia.
- Compared to men, women with MVP have less posterior prolapse (22% vs. 31%), less flail (2% vs. 8%), more leaflet thickening (32% vs. 28%), and less frequent severe mitral regurgitation (MR) (10% vs. 23%).
- Although MVP is more common in women than men, men more often develop severe regurgitation requiring surgical intervention.

PHYSICAL FINDINGS & CLINICAL PRESENTATION
- The most common auscultatory finding in cardiac examination is a non-ejection mid to late systolic click best heard at the apex. When the valve prolapses, it gets caught by the subvalvular structures, causing an abrupt halt that creates the click. It is caused by degeneration of the valve resulting in an abnormal ratio between the length of the mitral apparatus and left ventricle (LV) during contraction.
- If regurgitation is present, a crescendo mid to late systolic murmur may be heard that worsens with standing and Valsalva maneuver.
- Timing of click within the cardiac cycle varies with loading conditions within the left ventricle (i.e., may occur earlier with standing or Valsalva and later with squatting or expiration).
- May be associated with small anteroposterior chest diameter, scoliosis, pectus excavatum, or low BMI.
- Most patients with MVP are asymptomatic; symptoms, if present, consist primarily of chest pain, palpitations, fatigue, dyspnea, and anxiety.

- Neurologic abnormalities (e.g., transient ischemic attack [TIA] or stroke) are rare.
- A spectrum of arrhythmias, mainly paroxysmal supraventricular tachycardia and atrial and ventricular premature beats, etc. is also observed with mitral valve prolapse. There is also an increased association with Wolff-Parkinson-White syndrome and QT prolongation.

ETIOLOGY
- Myxomatous degeneration of connective tissue within mitral valve, usually involving multiple leaflet segments (e.g., Barlow disease). In contrast, fibroelastic deficiency of single leaflet segment (usually the middle scallop of the posterior leaflet) develops in elderly patients.
- Congenital deformity of mitral valve and supportive structures.
- Secondary to other disorders of connective tissue such as Ehlers-Danlos, Marfan, or pseudoxanthoma elasticum. Association with other connective tissue disorders suggests that MVP results from defective embryogenesis in cells of mesenchymal origin.

(Dx) DIAGNOSIS

DIFFERENTIAL DIAGNOSIS
- Other valvular abnormalities (especially MR)
- Anxiety or panic disorders
- Pulmonary embolism
- Atypical chest pain

WORKUP
- Medical history and physical examination with increased suspicion in patients with other findings of connective tissue disorder.
- Two- or three-dimensional echocardiography in patients with a systolic click or murmur on careful auscultation.
- Cardiac MRI is an emerging tool for the evaluation and diagnosis of MVP but has not yet been independently validated. However, MRI should be considered because it may be helpful in accurately quantifying the amount of mitral regurgitation when present. ECG is most often normal but may show nonspecific ST-T wave changes, prolonged QT interval, prominent Q waves, or early repolarization with J-point elevation in young patients.

IMAGING STUDIES
Echocardiography (Fig. 1) shows one or more leaflets prolapsing >2 mm into the left atrium during systole in a long axis view. Mitral leaflets may be thickened (>5 mm) with myxomatous degeneration. MR is typically present but may only occur during late systole or with exertion. If moderate or severe MR is present, findings of dilated left atrium, LV dilation and/or dysfunction, and elevated estimated RV systolic pressure may also be present. There is an increased incidence of secundum-type atrial septal defects (ASDs) in

patients with MVP are readily identified by echocardiography.

(Rx) TREATMENT[1]

NONPHARMACOLOGIC THERAPY
Avoidance of stimulants (e.g., caffeine, nicotine) in patients with palpitations. Sometimes reassurance is sufficient to reduce the severity of symptoms in many patients.

ACUTE GENERAL Rx
Beta-blockers may be used in symptomatic patients (e.g., palpitations, chest pain) to decrease the heart rate and contractility, thus potentially decreasing the stretch on the prolapsing valve leaflets.

CHRONIC Rx
Monitoring for complications:
- MR (most common complication); on rare occasion may occur acutely due to rupture of chordae tendineae.
- Routine echocardiographic monitoring is indicated at the following intervals with patients with evidence of mitral regurgitation:
  1. Stage B with mild regurgitation: Every 3 to 5 yr
  2. Stage B with moderate regurgitation: Every 1 to 2 yr

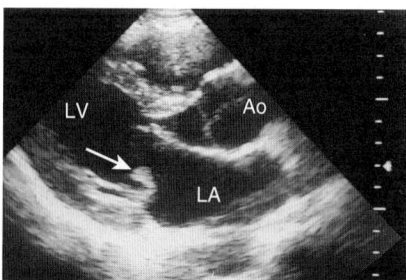
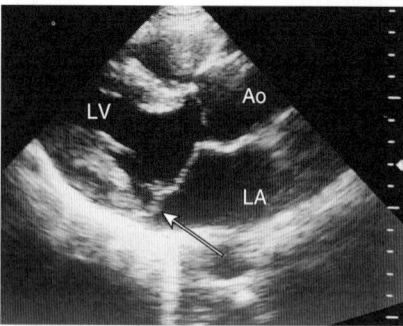

FIG. 1 Mitral valve prolapse. Parasternal long-axis view in diastole *(top)* and systole *(bottom)* in a patient with mitral valve prolapse and myxomatous changes. In the *upper panel,* note the open mitral valve and the diffuse thickening of the posterior mitral valve leaflet *(arrow).* The lower panel was recorded in systole. Note that both leaflets prolapse behind the plane of the mitral valve annulus. The prolapse of the posterior leaflet is somewhat more prominent *(arrow). Ao,* Aorta; *LA,* left atrium; *LV,* left ventricle. (From Zipes DP et al [eds]: *Braunwald's heart disease,* ed 7, Philadelphia, 2005, Saunders.)

TABLE 1   Predictors of Clinical Outcome in Mitral Valve Prolapse

Predictor	Survival	Valve Surgery	Arrhythmias or Sudden Death	Endocarditis
Age	+++	+++	−	−
Gender	++	++	−	−
Leaflet thickness or redundancy	+++	+++	++++	++++
Severity of mitral regurgitation	++++	++++	++++	++++
Systolic click	+	−	−	−
Left ventricular dilation	+	++++	++	−
Left atrial dilation	−	++	+	−

Symbols indicate the relative predictive value of each variable for the listed clinical outcomes on a scale of no predictive value (−) to strongly predictive (++++).
From Bonow RO et al: *Braunwald's heart disease: a textbook of cardiovascular medicine,* Philadelphia, 2012, Saunders.

3. Stage C1 (asymptomatic severe MR without LV dysfunction): Every 6 to 12 mo
- Bacterial endocarditis (risk is three to eight times that of the general population); higher risk in patients with concomitant regurgitation. However, routine antibiotic prophylaxis is not recommended.
- TIA or stroke caused by embolic phenomena (from fibrin and platelet thrombi) in patients with thickened leaflets; risk in young patients is <0.05% per yr. If present, aspirin (75 to 325 mg) is indicated for secondary prevention.
- Cardiac arrhythmias with the vast majority being supraventricular and benign.
- Sudden death (rare); most often associated with acute flail leaflets or caused by ventricular arrhythmias associated with other structural heart disease.
- The incidence of complications of MVP is very low (<1% per yr). Table 1 lists variables that are predictors of favorable clinical outcome in mitral valve prolapse.

Major predictors of outcomes were moderate or severe MR and depressed ejection fraction (EF); minor predictors were LA diameter 40 mm or greater, flail leaflet, atrial fibrillation, and age 50 yr or older.

SURGICAL REFERRAL

Surgical referral may be necessary in patients who develop progressive MR with surgical indications as per guidelines for valvular heart disease (see topic on "Mitral Regurgitation").

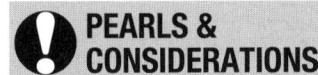 **PEARLS & CONSIDERATIONS**

COMMENTS

- Recent studies suggest that the prevalence of MVP and its propensity to cause symptoms and serious complications have been overestimated in the past.

- The relationship between MVP syndrome and sudden cardiac death is unclear. The best evidence suggests that there is only a slight risk in subsets of patients with MVP who have severe MR, severe valvular deformity, complex ventricular arrhythmias, QT prolongation, and a history of syncope.
- Asymptomatic patients with MVP and mild or no MR can be evaluated clinically every 3 to 5 yr. High-risk patients (those with symptoms, arrhythmias, or significant regurgitation) should undergo a follow-up examination once a year.
- In 2007, the AHA guidelines for prevention of infectious endocarditis were revised, and prophylactic antibiotics are no longer recommended for patients with MVP without previous endocarditis.

PATIENT & FAMILY EDUCATION

www.themitralvalve.org

REFERENCES

Available at eBooks.Health.Elsevier.com.

RELATED CONTENT

Mitral Valve Prolapse (Patient Information)

AUTHORS: **MOHAMED A. ABDELAZEEM, MD,** and **UYEN T. LAM, MD**

M

Diseases and Disorders

I

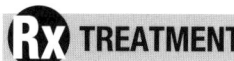

BASIC INFORMATION

DEFINITION
Molluscum contagiosum (MC) is a DNA poxvirus characterized by discrete skin lesions with central umbilication. It predominantly affects children.

SYNONYM
MC

ICD-10CM CODE
B08.1 Molluscum contagiosum

EPIDEMIOLOGY & DEMOGRAPHICS
- Peak occurrence ranges from 2 to 5 years, with an estimated overall prevalence of 2.8% among children.
- The disease tends to occur in epidemics, characteristically targeting childcare centers, swimming pools, and schools.
- Molluscum contagiosum spreads by auto-inoculation, scratching, or touching a lesion.
- It usually occurs in young children. It is also common in sexually active adults and patients with HIV infection.
- Incubation period varies between 4 and 8 wk.
- Spontaneous resolution in immunocompetent patients can occur after several months.

PHYSICAL FINDINGS & CLINICAL PRESENTATION
- The characteristic lesions appear as flesh-colored, domed papules with central umbilication that may present anywhere on the body surface, including the genitalia in sexually active individuals. The individual lesion appears initially as a small (2 to 3 mm), flesh-colored, firm, smooth-surfaced papule with subsequent central umbilication. Lesions are frequently grouped (Fig. 1). The size of each lesion generally varies from 2 to 6 mm in diameter.
- Typical distribution in children involves the face, extremities, and trunk. Mucous membranes are spared.
- Distribution in adults generally involves pubic and genital areas (Figs. E2 and E3).
- Severe, diffuse involvement may be seen in patients with immunosuppression, including human immunodeficiency virus (HIV) infection.
- Erythema and scaling at the periphery of the lesions may be present as a result of scratching or hypersensitivity reaction.
- Lesions are not present on the palms and soles.

ETIOLOGY
Viral infection of epithelial cells caused by a poxvirus, molluscum contagiosum

DIAGNOSIS

Diagnosis is usually established by the clinical appearance of the lesions (distribution and central umbilication). A magnifying lens can be used to observe the central umbilication. If necessary, the diagnosis can be confirmed by removing a typical lesion with a curette and examining the content on a slide after adding potassium hydroxide and gentle heating. Staining with toluidine blue will identify viral inclusions.

DIFFERENTIAL DIAGNOSIS
- Verruca plana (flat warts): No central umbilication, not dome shaped, irregular surface, can involve palms and soles
- Herpes simplex: Lesions become rapidly umbilicated
- Varicella: Blisters and vesicles are present
- Folliculitis: No central umbilication, presence of hair piercing the pustule or papule
- Cutaneous cryptococcosis in AIDS patients: Budding yeasts will be present on cytologic examination of the lesions
- Basal cell carcinoma: Multiple lesions are absent
- Cellulitis

WORKUP
Careful examination of the papules

LABORATORY TESTS
Generally not indicated in children.
- Dermoscopy to confirm the presence of the characteristic amorphous, lobular, yellow central umbilication
- Methylene blue smear preparation to identify molluscum bodies
- Histopathology to identify eosinophilic intracellular inclusion bodies (Henderson–Paterson bodies)

These investigations are required only when the diagnosis is in doubt.

Screening for other sexually transmitted diseases is recommended in all cases of genital molluscum contagiosum.

TREATMENT

GENERAL Rx
- Therapy is individualized depending on number of lesions, immune status, and patient's age and preference.
- Observation for spontaneous resolution is reasonable in patients with few, small, non-irritated, and nonspreading lesions. In patients with limited disease, MC frequently resolves in months without scarring.
- Genital lesions should be treated in all sexually active patients.
- Liquid nitrogen cryotherapy.
- Carbon dioxide laser.
- Curettage after pretreatment of the area with combination prilocaine 2.5% with lidocaine 2.5% cream (EMLA) for anesthesia is useful for treatment of a few lesions. Curettage should be avoided in cosmetically sensitive areas because scarring may develop.
- Treatments with liquid nitrogen therapy in combination with curettage are effective in older patients who do not object to some discomfort.
- Application of cantharidin 0.7% to individual lesions covered with clear tape will result in blistering over 24 hr and possible clearing without scarring. This medication should be avoided on facial lesions.
- Other treatment measures include use of imiquimod cream or tretinoin 0.025% gel or 0.1% cream at bedtime, daily use of salicylic acid (Occlusal) at bedtime, and use of laser therapy.
- Trichloroacetic acid peel generally repeated every 2 wk for several weeks is useful in immunocompromised patients with extensive lesions.

PEARLS & CONSIDERATIONS

COMMENTS
Genital molluscum contagiosum in children may be indicative of sexual abuse.

RELATED CONTENT
Molluscum Contagiosum (Patient Information)

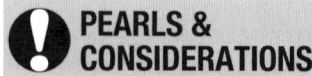

AUTHOR: **FRED F. FERRI, MD**

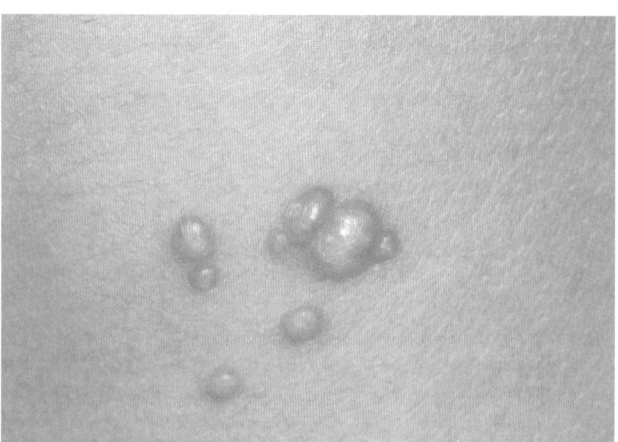

FIG. 1 Grouped molluscum. (From Kliegman RM et al: *Nelson textbook of pediatrics,* ed 19, Philadelphia, 2011, Saunders.)

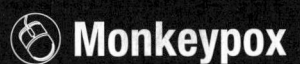
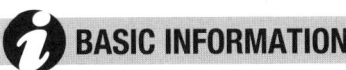 **BASIC INFORMATION**

DEFINITION

Monkeypox is a linear double-strand DNA virus approximately 250 kb in size and is of the family *Poxviridae*, subfamily *Cordopoxvirinae*, genus *Orthopoxvirus*, and species *monkeypox* (Table 1). The virus is considered a zoonotic disease first identified in laboratory monkeys in the 1950s. The natural hosts of monkeypox virus include rope squirrels, tree squirrels, Gambian pouched rats, and African dormice. In the U.S. it is commonly found in prairie dogs. There are two main clades of monkeypox that have been identified: clade I (formerly Central African clade) and clade 2 (formerly West African clade), with the latter being the more severe form of the virus.

SYNONYMS

MPX
MPXV
Monkey pox
Monkey pox virus

ICD 10-CM CODE

B04   Monkeypox

EPIDEMIOLOGY & DEMOGRAPHICS

INCIDENCE: The first case in the current outbreak was diagnosed in a[1] traveler to the UK from Nigeria in May 2022.
PREVALENCE: Over 41,000 cases globally and 15,000 cases in the U.S. as of August 2022

PREDOMINANT SEX & AGE: Males: Can affect any age group but typically seen in sexually active individuals
RISK FACTORS: MSM, multiple sex partners, anonymous sex, LGBTQ+ community, close intimate contact with someone who has confirmed monkeypox, or coming into contact with bedding, towels, clothing, etc., that has been in contact with an infected person
GENETICS: Uncertain, but viral tropism appears to occur downstream of virus binding and entry into the cell.

PHYSICAL FINDINGS & CLINICAL PRESENTATION

- Patients can be asymptomatic during the incubation period, which can last from 3 to 17 days, and the illness typically lasts from 2 to 4 weeks.
- Lesions can be firm, rubbery, deep-seated, with an umbilication at the center, and are purulent-filled. The 2022 outbreak has demonstrated variations in the classical monkeypox appearance, including rashes that[2] can be disseminated or localized to lesions. Lesions can occur in the mouth, throat, anorectal region, palms and soles of the hands and feet, and can be found on extremities and the trunk (Fig. 1).
- Rectal symptoms have been noted, such as bloody or purulent stool and rectal pain.
- Patients can develop fever, chills, malaise, myalgias, headache, and lymphadenopathy (Fig. E2).
- Rashes sometimes are present or absent.

- Respiratory symptoms have been described, including sore throat, congestion, and cough.
- The lesions usually evolve together and progress through four stages, which include macular, papular, vesicular, and pustular before scabbing, and lesions are considered healed and noncontagious when scabs fall off and a new layer of skin has replaced the lesion.

ETIOLOGY

- Caused by the monkeypox virus and by coming into contact with individuals who have active monkeypox lesions or their bedding, towels, and clothing.
- Other modes of transmission include coming into contact with infected wildlife (Fig. E3).
- The virus gains access to the body by entering through the oropharynx, nasopharynx, or intradermal routes. Once entry is gained, the virus replicates at the site of inoculation and makes copies of itself within the cell cytoplasm upon hijacking cellular machinery; it does not enter the cell nucleus. The virus then spreads to lymph nodes and other bodily organs (Fig. E4).

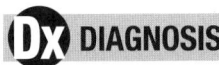 **DIAGNOSIS**

DIFFERENTIAL DIAGNOSIS (TABLE 2)

- Smallpox
- Syphilis (primary and secondary)
- Bacterial skin infection (cellulitis, impetigo, etc.)
- Herpes simplex virus

TABLE 1   Genera and Species of the Family Poxviridae, Subfamily Chordopoxvirinae, That Affect Humans

Genus and Species	Geographic Distribution	Other Infected Animals	Reservoir
Orthopoxvirus			
Variola	Eradicated (formerly worldwide)	Humans	None
Monkeypox	Africa (United States)*	Humans, primates, zoo animals, prairie dogs	Squirrels, dormice, Gambian giant rat, hedgehog, jerboa, opossum, woodchuck
Cowpox	Western Eurasia	Humans, cats, cows, elephants, gerbils, rats, okapi, zoo animals	Rodents (bank voles, long-tailed field mouse)
Vaccinia	Worldwide	Humans, cows, buffalo, rabbits, pigs	Most likely rodents
Parapoxvirus			
Bovine papular stomatitis	Worldwide	Humans, cows	Unknown (cows?)
Orf (contagious ecthyma, contagious pustular dermatitis)	Worldwide	Humans, sheep, goat, Artiodactyla, other ruminants	Unknown (sheep? goats?)
Pseudo-cowpox (paravaccinia, milker's nodule)	Worldwide	Humans, cows	Unknown (cows?)
Parapoxvirus of seals	Worldwide	Humans, seals	Unknown (seals?)
Parapoxvirus of reindeer	Finland	Humans, reindeer	Unknown
Molluscipoxvirus			
Molluscum contagiosum	Worldwide	Humans	Humans
Yatapoxvirus			
Tanapox	Africa	Humans, rodents	Mosquitoes(?), rodents(?)
Yabapox	Africa	Humans, primates	Unknown (primates?)
Yaba monkey tumor	Africa	Primates	Unknown

*Import of monkeypox to the United States with Gambian giant rats.
Adapted from Damon IK: Poxviruses. In Knipe DM, Howley PM (eds): *Field's virology*. Philadelphia, Lippincott Williams & Wilkins, 2007, pp 2948-2975; Essbauer S et al: Zoonotic poxviruses, *Vet Microbiol* 229-236, 2009; and Breman JG: Poxviruses. In Strickland GT (ed.): *Hunter's tropical medicine*, ed 8. Philadelphia, Saunders, 2000, pp 207-210.

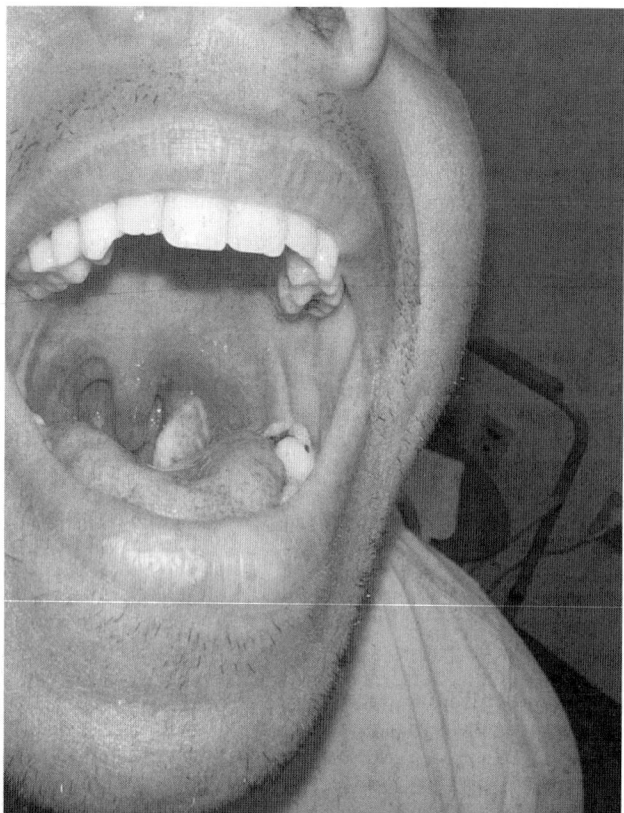

FIG. 1 Left and right tonsils with overlying purulent exudates. The left tonsil has extensive purulence, and the right tonsil has early development of lesions. (Image courtesy of Glenn Fort, MD, MPH, and Frank Sanchez, MD, MBA.)

TABLE 2 Differential Diagnosis of Monkeypox, Smallpox, and Chickenpox

Variable	Monkeypox	Smallpox	Chickenpox
Incubation period, days	7-17	7-17	12-14
Prodrome period, days	1-4	2-4	0-2
Symptom			
Fever, severity	Moderate	Severe	Mild or none
Malaise, severity	Moderate	Moderate	Mild
Headache, severity	Moderate	Severe	Mild
Lymphadenopathy, severity	Moderate	None	None
Lesions			
Depth (diameter in mm)	Superficial to deep (4-6)	Deep (4-6)	Superficial (2-4)
Distribution	Centrifugal (mainly)	Centrifugal	Centripetal
Evaluation	Homogeneous rash	Homogeneous rash	Heterogeneous rash
Time to desquamation, days	14-21	14-21	6-14
Frequency of lesions on palms or soles of feet	Common	Common	Rare

- Varicella
- Molluscum contagiosum
- Disseminated cryptococcal infection
- Disseminated gonococcal infection
- Scabies
- Drug eruptions
- Contact dermatitis/atopic dermatitis
- Measles

WORKUP

- The CDC has established case definitions for monkeypox to guide clinicians encountering suspected patients (Table 3).
- This includes suspecting a case in a patient who has developed a new rash or had contact with someone who had similar symptoms, is part of a high-risk population (MSM, LGBTQ+, sex

worker), or has traveled to an endemic region and developed symptoms within 21 days.
- If there is high clinical suspicion of a monkeypox diagnosis given the above information, it is advised that individuals undergo testing and receive treatment.

LABORATORY TESTS

- Detection of *Orthopoxvirus* DNA by polymerase chain reaction testing of a clinical specimen.
- Detection of *Orthopoxvirus* using immunohistochemical or electron microscopy testing methods.
- Detection of monkeypox virus DNA by polymerase chain reaction testing or next-generation sequencing of a clinical specimen.
- Isolation of monkeypox virus in culture from a clinical specimen.
- Demonstration of detectable levels of anti-*Orthopoxvirus* IgM antibody 4 to 56 days after rash onset.
- If superimposed bacterial infection is suspected, blood cultures and CBC can help determine if sepsis is occurring.

IMAGING STUDIES

- CT head if encephalitis suspected, although this is a rare complication. Lymphadenopathy can be a prominent but nonspecific feature detected. Cutaneous lesions may be seen.
- MRI can show monkeypox encephalitis, with findings being diffuse edema with increased FLAIR signal in the thalamus, parietal cortex, and meningeal enhancement may be present. Other sites can be visualized as well, including the internal rectal wall.

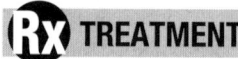 **TREATMENT**

ACUTE GENERAL Rx

- Typically, monkeypox infection is a self-limiting disease.
- Tecovirimat, aka "Tpoxx," antiviral medication
  1. 600 mg Q12 for 14 days PO, IV 200mg Q12, Tx can be shorter depending on clinical course
- Pre-/postexposure prophylaxis
  1. Vaccination can either be given as preexposure prophylaxis or postexposure prophylaxis, if it is given as postexposure prophylaxis, it is recommended to be given with 4 to 14 days of exposure to lessen disease severity and duration.
  2. Two vaccines are available in the U.S.: Jynneos and ACAM2000.
  3. ACAM200 is a live replication competent smallpox vaccine used only in a select group of patients and is associated with more adverse effects. Use of this vaccine is contraindicated in immunosuppressed populations.
  4. Modified Vaccinia Ankara (MVA) Jynneos is a live attenuated nonreplicating vaccinia virus given in two doses that are spaced 28 days apart and injected into the triceps of the arm. Recently, the CDC has recommended switching the site of injection to

TABLE 3 Centers for Disease Control and Prevention Case Definition for Monkeypox

CRITERIA FOR CLASSIFICATION

Clinical Criteria	Epidemiologic Criteria	Laboratory Criteria

• Rash (macular, papular, vesicular, or pustular; generalized or localized; discrete or confluent)
• Fever (subjective or measured temperature of ≥99.3°F [≥37.4°C])
• Other signs and symptoms:
  1. Chills and/or sweats
  2. Headache
  3. Backache
  4. Lymphadenopathy
  5. Sore throat
  6. Cough
  7. Shortness of breath
	• Exposure* to an exotic wild mammalian pet[†] obtained on or after April 15, 2003, with clinical signs of illness (e.g., conjunctivitis, respiratory symptoms, and/or rash)
	• Exposure* to an exotic or wild mammalian pet[†] with or without clinical signs of illness that has been in contact with either a mammalian pet[§] or a human with monkeypox
	• Exposure[¶] to a suspect, probable, or confirmed human case of monkeypox
		• Isolation of monkeypox virus in culture
		• Demonstration of monkeypox virus DNA by polymerase chain reaction testing of a clinical specimen
		• Demonstration of virus morphologically consistent with an *Orthopoxvirus* by electron microscopy in the absence of exposure to another *Orthopoxvirus*
		• Demonstration of presence of *Orthopoxvirus* in tissue using immunohistochemical testing methods in the absence of exposure to another *Orthopoxvirus*

CASE CLASSIFICATION

Suspect Case	Probable Case	Confirmed Case
• Meets one of the epidemiologic criteria, AND • Fever or unexplained rash, AND • Two or more signs or symptoms with onset of first sign or symptoms <21 days after last exposure meeting epidemiologic criteria	• Meets one of the epidemiologic criteria, AND • Fever, AND • Vesicular-pustular rash with onset of first sign or symptom <21 days after last exposure meeting epidemiologic criteria, OR • If rash is present but the type is not described, demonstrates elevated levels of IgM antibodies reactive with *Orthopoxvirus* between at least days 7–56 after rash onset**	• Meets one of the laboratory criteria

Exclusion Criteria

• An alternative diagnosis can fully explain the illness,[‡] OR
• The case was reported on the basis of primary or secondary exposure to an exotic or wild mammalian pet or a human (see epidemiologic criteria) subsequently determined not to have monkeypox, provided other possible epidemiologic exposure criteria are not present, OR
• A case without a rash does not develop a rash within 10 days of onset of clinical symptoms consistent with monkeypox.[§§]
• The case is determined to be negative for nonvariola generic *Orthopoxvirus* by polymerase chain reaction testing of a well-sampled rash lesion by the approved Laboratory Response Network (LRN) protocol, OR
• The case is determined to have undetectable levels of IgM antibody during the period 7-56 days after rash onset.[¶¶]

*Includes living in a household, petting or handling, or visiting a pet-holding facility (e.g., pet store, veterinary clinic, pet distributor).
[†]Includes prairie dogs, Gambian giant rats, and rope squirrels.
[§]Includes living in a household or originating from the same pet-holding facility as another animal with monkeypox.
[¶]Includes skin-to-skin or face-to-face contact.
**Levels of circulating IgM antibody reactive with *Orthopoxvirus* antigen are determined by enzyme-linked immunosorbent assay (ELISA) and reported as optical density (OD) values. Values greater than three standard deviations above the mean OD of six independent negative controls are considered "elevated." IgM antibody levels may be elevated in persons who have been recently (within 1 year) vaccinated for smallpox.
[‡]Factors that might be considered in assigning alternative diagnoses include the strength of the epidemiologic exposure criteria for monkeypox, the specificity of the diagnostic test, and the compatibility of the clinical presentation and course of illness for the alternative diagnosis
[§§]If possible, obtain convalescent-phase serum specimen from these patients.
[¶¶]The optimal timing of specimen collection for determination of IgM levels is between days 7 and 56 post–rash onset. However, elevated levels of IgM antibodies may be detectable before day 7 or after day 56 post–rash onset; therefore a negative result during this phase should not be interpreted to indicate an absence of monkeypox infection.

intradermally in the forearm to allow for a much lower volume injected than the subcutaneous route, in order to provide more vaccine to the population.

5. Tpoxx can be used for postexposure prophylaxis in patients unable to receive vaccination.
6. Trifluridine Ophthalmic Solution (Viroptic): Q4 hours for 7 to 10 days has been used off-label for ocular complications due to monkeypox.

DISPOSITION

Patients usually have a self-limiting course, and recover completely without any long-term sequelae. Scarring has been noted following some lesions. Mortality has been estimated to be 1% to 4% with common causes of death being bacterial superinfection of lesions.

REFERRAL

• To the local/state Department of Health with suspected cases and vaccination
• Infectious diseases consultant for guidance on oral therapy and vaccination

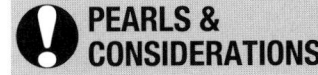
PEARLS & CONSIDERATIONS

COMMENTS

• Be sure to inquire about sexual and travel history, as this information will help significantly in guiding the clinician to the correct diagnosis.
• Be aware that there is considerable overlap with common rashes and sexually transmitted infections, such as syphilis.
• There are now cases that have involved children, likely through skin-to-skin contact with infected individuals.

INFECTION PREVENTION AND CONTROL

• Individuals with monkeypox should quarantine from others until all lesions have scabbed and fallen off and a new layer of skin has grown over the lesion(s); this can be anywhere from 2 to 4 wk.
• Vaccination with the Jynneos vaccine is recommended for all men who have sex with men.

- The World Health Organization recommends consistent condom use during any sexual activity for 12 wk following recovery.
- Individuals with monkeypox should also quarantine from their pets as there have been recent reports of pets becoming infected with monkeypox from their owners.
- Standard precautions are advised when interacting with infected patients, which includes gowns, gloves, and protective eyewear.
- Infected patients who are hospitalized should be placed in a single room with a private restroom.

PATIENT & FAMILY EDUCATION

- Avoid close intimate contact with individuals suspected of monkeypox infection and their clothing, bed coverings, and surfaces that have been exposed to their lesions.
- Patients with multiple sex partners and individuals of the LGBTQ+ community appear to be affected in higher proportions than other individuals (over 90% of cases in the 2022 outbreak); however, this is a disease that can affect all populations.

- The role of sexual transmission of monkeypox virus is still being evaluated.

SUGGESTED READINGS
Available at eBooks.Health.Elsevier.com

AUTHORS: **FRANK SANCHEZ, MD, MBA,** and **GLENN FORT, MD, MPH**

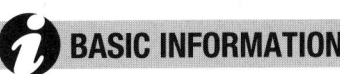

BASIC INFORMATION

DEFINITION

MGUS is a premalignant disorder characterized by the clonal expansion of plasma cells or lymphoplasmacytic cells. It is typically detected incidentally when patients undergo testing with serum or urine protein electrophoresis.[1] The term "monoclonal gammopathy of undetermined significance" (MGUS) is defined by the presence of a serum monoclonal (M) protein less than 3 g/dl and clonal plasma cells less than 10% in the bone marrow. In addition, there must be no evidence of end organ dysfunction such as renal insufficiency, anemia, hypercalcemia, or bony lesions on skeletal surveys (Table 1).

SYNONYMS

MGUS
Non-IgM MGUS
IgM MGUS
Light chain MGUS
Monoclonal gammopathy of unknown significance

ICD-10CM CODE
D47.2 Monoclonal gammopathy of undetermined significance (MGUS)

EPIDEMIOLOGY & DEMOGRAPHICS

INCIDENCE: In the U.S., the estimated age-adjusted incidence of MGUS is higher in men than in women. The annual incidence of MGUS in men is 120 per 100,000 at age 50 yr and increases to 530 per 100,000 at age 80 yr, whereas the incidence for women is 60 per 100,000 at age 50 yr and 370 per 100,000 at age 80 yr.[2]

PREVALENCE: MGUS is associated with increasing age; approximately 3.2% of persons older than 50 yr and 5.3% of persons older than 70 yr have an elevated M protein level without end organ dysfunction.[3] Studies have shown that at clinical diagnosis, MGUS is most likely to have been present undetected for a median duration of more than 10 yr. The prevalence of MGUS is also higher in African Americans. In one study, there was an almost twofold to threefold increase in prevalence among the African American population compared with the Caucasian population.

PREDOMINANT SEX & AGE: The median age at diagnosis is about 70 yr. Prevalence is higher in men than in women at any given age.

RISK FACTORS: Race (African American), older age, male sex, exposure to pesticides, and family history of MGUS or other plasma cell disorders have been associated with a higher risk of MGUS.[4] The cumulative risk of progression into multiple myeloma or related disorders is approximately 1% per yr. A variety of disorders (Table 2) are also associated with monoclonal gammopathy.

PHYSICAL FINDINGS & CLINICAL PRESENTATION

- MGUS typically is detected after a routine blood test reveals an elevated total protein concentration and is a common finding in medical practice.
- Patients are asymptomatic.
- Physical exam is normal.

ETIOLOGY

- The mechanism is unknown, and most cases are sporadic. The causes of malignant transformation of MGUS into multiple myeloma is still not well understood. Genetic predisposition, cytokine release, and bone marrow angiogenesis may play a role in the progression of MGUS into multiple myeloma.
- Characterized by a rearrangement of immunoglobulin genes resulting in the production of a monoclonal protein.

DIAGNOSIS

DIFFERENTIAL DIAGNOSIS

- Smoldering myeloma (Table E3)
- Multiple myeloma
- Waldenström agammaglobulinemia
- Secondary monoclonal gammopathies
  1. Chronic liver disease
  2. Rheumatologic diseases
  3. Chronic myelomonocytic leukemia
  4. Chronic neutrophilic leukemia
  5. Lichen myxedematosus
- Pyoderma gangrenosum
- AL amyloidosis
- Idiopathic Bence Jones proteinuria

LABORATORY TESTS

- Protein studies with serum free light chain assay
- Serum protein electrophoresis (Fig. E1): IgG most common, followed by IgM and IgA
- 24-hour urine protein excretion and urine electrophoresis
- Serum and urine immunofixation
- Determination of serum free light chain ratio (kappa and lambda free light chains)
- Hemoglobin
- Serum calcium and creatinine
- Examination of the bone marrow aspirate only when clinically indicated. It is not necessary in MGUS patients with low-risk fractures (no end organ damage. Ig gammopathy less than 1.5 g/dl, normal serum free light chain ratio)

IMAGING STUDIES

- Skeletal survey
- Bone mineral density at baseline (MGUS is associated with increased risk of osteoporosis)

TREATMENT

- Risk stratification per IMWG consensus[5]:
  1. Low risk: Serum M protein <1.5 g/dl, IgG subtype, normal genetics, free light chain ratio between 0.26 and 1.65. Absolute risk of progression (ARP) at 20 yr is 5%.
  2. Low-intermediate risk: Any 1 factor abnormal. ARP at 20 yr is 21%.
  3. High-intermediate risk: Any 2 factors abnormal. ARP at 20 yr is 37%.
  4. High risk: More than 3 factors abnormal. ARP at 20 yr is 58%.
- Follow-up by risk category: Patients with MGUS should be tested again within 4 to 6 mo from the time of first diagnosis to exclude evolving multiple myeloma. Those with low-risk MGUS can be followed up every 1 to 2 yr, whereas those with intermediate- or high-risk MGUS need to be followed up at least annually for life or until they develop a life-expectancy-threatening condition.
- Reevaluation consists of:
  1. Serum protein electrophoresis with immunofixation
  2. 24-hour urine protein excretion
  3. Serum free light chain assessment:
     a. Complete blood count
     b. Serum creatinine and calcium
     c. Careful history and physical examination to look for signs and symptoms known to evolve from MGUS

DISPOSITION

- Annual risk of progression to malignancy depends on type of M protein[6,7]:
  1. Non-IgM MGUS: 1% per yr
  2. IgM MGUS: 1.5% per yr
  3. Light-chain MGUS: 0.3% per yr
- Non-IgM and light-chain MGUS tend to progress to myeloma or amyloidosis
- IgM MGUS tends to progress to Waldenström macroglobulinemia
- Risk of infection (bacterial and viral) is twofold compared with healthy controls
- Increased risk of mortality from bacterial infections

REFERRAL

To hematologist/oncologist for evaluation

PEARLS & CONSIDERATIONS

- Approximately 55% of 70-yr-old patients diagnosed as having MGUS have had the condition for more than 10 yr.
- Most patients with MGUS should be monitored every 6 to 12 mo for signs and symptoms of progression to a malignancy.
- There is no indicated treatment for asymptomatic MGUS.
- A decision-making pathway in the diagnosis and management of peripheral neuropathy with MGUS is illustrated in Fig. E2.
- Some patients can develop monoclonal gammopathy of renal (MGRS) or neurologic significance (MGNS), and treatment sometimes is indicated in these cases.[8,9]
  1. MGRS is typically associated with non-IgM MGUS and should be proven by a kidney biopsy. Treatment should follow myeloma or amyloidosis-targeted regimens.

TABLE 1   Disease Definitions for the Monoclonal Gammopathies: MGUS and Related Disorders

Type of Monoclonal Gammopathy	Premalignancy With a Low Risk of Progression (1%-2% per yr)	Premalignancy With a High Risk of Progression (10% per yr)	Malignancy
IgG and IgA (non-IgM) monoclonal gammopathies*	**Non-IgM MGUS** All 3 criteria must be met: Serum monoclonal protein <3 g/dl Clonal bone marrow plasma cells <10%, and absence of end-organ damage such as hypercalcemia, renal insufficiency, anemia, and bone lesions (CRAB) that can be attributed to the plasma cell proliferative disorder	**Smoldering multiple myeloma** Both criteria must be met: Serum monoclonal protein (IgG or IgA) ≥3 g/dl and/or clonal bone marrow plasma cells ≥10%, and absence of end-organ damage such as lytic bone lesions, anemia, hypercalcemia, or renal failure that can be attributed to a plasma cell proliferative disorder	**Multiple myeloma** All 3 criteria must be met except as noted: Clonal bone marrow plasma cells ≥10% Presence of serum and/or urinary monoclonal protein (except in patients with true nonsecretory multiple myeloma), and evidence of end-organ damage that can be attributed to the underlying plasma cell proliferative disorder, specifically Hypercalcemia: Serum calcium >11.5 mg/dl or renal insufficiency: Serum creatinine >2 mg/dl or estimated creatinine clearance <40 ml/min Anemia: Normochromic, normocytic with a hemoglobin value of >2 g/dl below the lower limit of normal or a hemoglobin value <10 g/dl Bone lesions: Lytic lesions or severe osteopenia attributed to a plasma cell proliferative disorder or pathologic fractures
IgM monoclonal gammopathies	**IgM MGUS[†]** All 3 criteria must be met: Serum IgM monoclonal protein of any level Normal bone marrow and absence of end-organ damage such as anemia, constitutional symptoms, hyperviscosity, lymphadenopathy, or hepatosplenomegaly that can be attributed to the underlying lymphoproliferative disorder	**Smoldering Waldenström macroglobulinemia** Both criteria must be met: Serum IgM monoclonal protein of any level and/or bone marrow lymphoplasmacytic infiltration of any level, and no evidence of anemia, constitutional symptoms, hyperviscosity, lymphadenopathy, or hepatosplenomegaly that can be attributed to the underlying lymphoproliferative disorder	**Waldenström macroglobulinemia** All criteria must be met: IgM monoclonal gammopathy of any level, and any level of bone marrow lymphoplasmacytic infiltration (usually intratrabecular) by small lymphocytes that exhibit plasmacytoid or plasma cell differentiation and a typical immunophenotype (e.g., surface IgM+, CD5+/−, CD10−, CD19+, CD20+, CD23−) that satisfactorily excludes other lymphoproliferative disorders, including chronic lymphocytic leukemia and mantle cell lymphoma Evidence of anemia, constitutional symptoms, hyperviscosity, lymphadenopathy, or hepatosplenomegaly that can be attributed to the underlying lymphoproliferative disorder. Presence of the *MYD88* L265P mutation **IgM myeloma** All criteria must be met: Symptomatic monoclonal plasma cell proliferative disorder characterized by a serum IgM monoclonal protein regardless of size Presence of 10% plasma cells on bone marrow biopsy Presence of lytic bone lesions related to the underlying plasma cell disorder and/or translocation t(11;14) on fluorescence in situ hybridization
Light-chain monoclonal gammopathies	**Light-chain MGUS** All criteria must be met: Abnormal FLC ratio (<0.26 or >1.65) Increased level of the appropriate involved light-chain (increased kappa FLC in patients with ratio >1.65 and increased lambda FLC in patients with ratio <0.26) No immunoglobulin heavy-chain expression on immunofixation Clonal bone marrow plasma cells <10%, and absence of end-organ damage such as hypercalcemia, renal insufficiency, anemia, and bone lesions (CRAB) that can be attributed to the plasma cell proliferative disorder	**Idiopathic Bence Jones proteinuria** All criteria must be met: Urinary monoclonal protein on urine protein electrophoresis ≥500 mg/24 hr and/or clonal bone marrow plasma cells ≥10% No immunoglobulin heavy-chain expression on immunofixation Absence of end-organ damage such as hypercalcemia, renal insufficiency, anemia, and bone lesions (CRAB) that can be attributed to the plasma cell proliferative disorder	**Light-chain multiple myeloma[†]** Same as multiple myeloma except no evidence of immunoglobulin heavy-chain expression

CRAB, Hypercalcemia, renal failure, anemia, and bone disease; *FLC*, free light chain; *Ig*, immunoglobulin; *MGUS*, monoclonal gammopathy of undetermined significance.

* Occasionally patients with IgD and IgE monoclonal gammopathies have been described and will be part of this category as well.

[†]Note that conventionally IgM MGUS is considered a subtype of MGUS, and similarly light-chain multiple myeloma is considered as a subtype of multiple myeloma. Unless specifically distinguished, when the terms MGUS and multiple myeloma are used in general, they include IgM MGUS and light-chain multiple myeloma, respectively.

Modified from Rajkumar SV et al: Advances in the diagnosis, classification, risk stratification, and management of monoclonal gammopathy of undetermined significance: implications for recategorizing disease entities in the presence of evolving scientific evidence, *Mayo Clin Proc* 85:945-948, 2010.

TABLE 2 Diseases Associated With Monoclonal Gammopathy

Plasma cell and related disorders	MGUS Solitary plasmacytoma: Bone Soft tissue Multiple myeloma Waldenström macroglobulinemia Primary amyloidosis	
Lymphoid disorders	Non-Hodgkin lymphoma	Monoclonal protein observed in CLL (>20% of cases with IgM, ≈50% with IgG, light chains also observed), extranodal marginal zone lymphomas (>30% of cases and correlated with BM involvement), follicular, mantle cell, and diffuse large B-cell lymphomas also reported with serum M proteins as has AITL
	Hodgkin lymphoma	Rare but reported
	Castleman disease	<2% with monoclonal gammopathy
Other hematologic disorders	Acquired von Willebrand disease	IVIG more effective than factor concentrate in increasing factor VIII coagulant and VWF levels
	Gaucher disease	Observed in 25% in one study; M protein declined after splenectomy
	Pernicious anemia, pure RBC aplasia, hereditary spherocytosis, MPD, MDS	
Connective tissue disorders	SLE	IgG, IgM, and IgA have been observed, no difference in disease activity or outcome
	Inclusion body myositis	80% with IgG M protein
	Polymyositis, RA, scleroderma	
Neurologic disorders	POEMS syndrome	Most have M-protein of λ light chain
	Peripheral neuropathy	Most common is IgM In half, IgM protein binds to myelin-associated glycoprotein Size of M protein not correlated with severity of neuropathy Treatment with Waldenström macroglobulinemia regimens
	Myasthenia gravis, ALS, Alzheimer disease	
Dermatologic disorders	Schnitzler syndrome	Neutrophilic urticarial dermatitis, monoclonal IgM protein, and two of: Lymphadenopathy, fever, hepatosplenomegaly, joint pain, increased ESR, increased neutrophils, or abnormal bone imaging
	Scleredema	
	Pyoderma gangrenosum	Frequently an IgA protein
Infections	HIV	Both IgG and IgM M proteins observed
	HCV	M protein present in up to 10% of patients
Immunosuppression	Renal transplant	In children CMV infection associated with M protein
	Liver and heart transplant	Most patients with posttransplant lymphoproliferative disorders have M proteins
	BM transplant	Observed in both autologous and allogeneic transplants Appearance of M protein correlated with GVHD
Renal dysfunction	AL amyloidosis Monoclonal fibrillary glomerulonephritis Immunotactoid glomerulonephritis Cryoglobulinemic glomerulonephritis Light-chain proximal tubulopathy Crystal storing histiocytosis Crystal globulin glomerulonephritis Monoclonal immunoglobulin deposition disease Proliferative glomerulonephritis and monoclonal immunoglobulin deposition	Biopsy advised if acute kidney injury (AKI) stage 3, estimated glomerular filtration rate (eGFR) <60 ml/min and >2 ml/min/yr decline, proteinuria >1 g/24 hr, albumin/creatinine ratio >30, Fanconi syndrome Consider biopsy if AKI stage 1 or 2, eGFR <60 ml/min and <2 ml/min/yr decline, albumin/creatinine ratio 3:30 and eGFR >60 ml/min, hematuria, and eGFR <60 ml/min, evidence of light chain proteinuria Defer biopsy if stable eGFR, bland urinalysis, no evidence of light chain proteinuria

AITL, Angioimmunoblastic T-cell lymphoma; *ALS,* amyotrophic lateral sclerosis; *BM,* bone marrow; *CLL,* chronic lymphocytic leukemia; *CMV,* cytomegalovirus; *ESR,* erythrocyte sedimentation rate; *GVHD,* graft-versus-host disease; *HCV,* hepatitis C virus; *HIV,* human immunodeficiency virus; *Ig,* immunoglobulin; *IVIG,* intravenous immunoglobulin; *MDS,* myelodysplastic syndrome; *MGUS,* monoclonal gammopathy of uncertain significance; *MPD,* myeloproliferative disorder; *POEMS,* polyneuropathy, organomegaly, endocrinopathy, monoclonal gammopathy, and skin changes; *RA,* rheumatoid arthritis; *RBC,* red blood cell; *SLE,* systemic lupus erythematosus; *VWF,* von Willebrand factor.

From Hoffman R et al: *Hematology: basic principles and practice,* ed 7, Philadelphia, 2018, Elsevier.

2. MGNS is associated with IgM MGUS and should be sensory, bilateral, symmetrical, and length dependent. Nerve conductions studies should show demyelination, and anti-MAG antibodies can be positive in 50% of the cases. Treatment should follow Waldenström macroglobulinemia–targeted regimens.

REFERENCES & SUGGESTED READINGS

Available at eBooks.Health.Elsevier.com.

AUTHOR: **JORGE J. CASTILLO, MD**

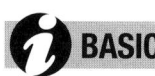
BASIC INFORMATION

DEFINITION

Infectious mononucleosis (IM) is a symptomatic infection most commonly caused by Epstein-Barr virus (EBV) and characterized by a classic triad of fever, tonsillar pharyngitis, and lymphadenopathy (predominantly cervical).[1] Fatigue is also a very common finding. IM was first coined in 1920 to describe a syndrome characterized as an acute infectious process accompanied by atypical large peripheral blood lymphocytes.

SYNONYMS

Mononucleosis
EBV
Kissing disease

ICD-10CM CODES
B27	Infectious mononucleosis
B27.0	Gamma herpesviral mononucleosis
B27.1	Cytomegaloviral mononucleosis
B27.8	Other infectious mononucleosis
B27.9	Infectious mononucleosis

EPIDEMIOLOGY & DEMOGRAPHICS

INCIDENCE (IN U.S.): 500 cases/100,000 persons/yr; worldwide, approximately 90% lifetime prevalence by age 30 yr.
PREDOMINANT SEX: Incidence is the same but occurs earlier in females.
PREDOMINANT AGE: Symptomatic infection most common between the ages of 15 and 24 yr. The age at which primary EBV infection is acquired is potentially increasing in developed countries.[2]

Young children rarely develop clinical signs of IM. Infection during childhood is more common in lower socioeconomic groups and may vary by geographic location or social factors, such as crowding, sharing a bedroom, maternal education, day care attendance, and school catchment area.

PHYSICAL FINDINGS & CLINICAL PRESENTATION

- Following an incubation period of 4 to 7 wk, there are two common presentations.[1-3] The first presentation represents the prodromal period with gradual onset of fever, chills, malaise, and anorexia for several days. This is followed by the second presentation of the classic triad of pharyngitis, fever, and lymphadenopathy. These patients often report the worst sore throat of their life. Pharyngitis (Fig. E1) is typically the most severe symptom and is characterized by white tonsillar exudates that may spread to the tongue. Up to half of patients may have palatal petechiae.
- Lymphadenopathy (nonnecrotic) can be diffuse, but most commonly occurs in both the anterior and posterior triangles of the neck.
- Splenomegaly may be palpable, most commonly during the second week of illness. Most patients have some degree of splenomegaly on ultrasound assessment. Hepatomegaly with some degree of hepatitis is also

common. In 75% of cases there is some increase in alanine aminotransferase (ALT).[3]
- Rash (Fig. E2) is uncommon but will occur in nearly all patients who receive ampicillin or amoxicillin due to a transient penicillin hypersensitivity.
- IM is usually a self-limited illness (2 to 4 wk), but symptoms of malaise and fatigue may last months before resolving.[1]
- At times, IM can present as fever and adenopathy without pharyngitis.
- Although acute complications may be severe, they are uncommon and tend to resolve completely. Reported complications include cholestatic liver disease, chronic hepatitis, or even liver failure; hemolytic anemia; splenic rupture; or airway compromise.[3,4]
- Splenic rupture is rare, with an incidence rate <1%, but it is the most feared.[4] It should be suspected in anyone with confirmed or suspected IM who presents with acute abdominal or chest pain. Most cases occur in the first 3 wk of symptoms.
- Airway compromise, as evidenced by stridor, cyanosis, and/or tachypnea, is reported in 1% to 3% of cases and is an indication for hospitalization.
- Systemic corticosteroids are indicated for treating those at risk or with impending airway

obstruction, and usually lead to improvement in 12 to 36 hr. Acute tonsillectomy may be pursued if steroids are not sufficient to mitigate the risk for obstruction.[5]
- Late complications may include lymphoproliferative cancers (Burkitt lymphoma and Hodgkin lymphoma), multiple sclerosis, rheumatoid arthritis, and chronic active EBV infection (CAEBV).[3]
- EBV may also cause hemophagocytic disease, alternatively referred to as EBV-associated hemophagocytic lymphohistiocytosis (EBV-HLH), characterized by fever, splenomegaly, and cytopenias with high ferritin and soluble CD25.
- Box 1 and Table 1 summarize the features of IM in immunocompetent patients.

ETIOLOGY

The most common cause of IM (90%) is primary infection with EBV.[1] Cytomegalovirus (CMV) is the most common cause of the other 10% of IM, but CMV infection often occurs in infancy or early childhood and is minimally symptomatic. Other causes include human herpes virus-6, herpes simplex virus-1, and HIV. Primary EBV infection during childhood also often causes few or no symptoms; persistent fatigue and recurrent/persistent fevers are the most common reasons

---

BOX 1 Summary of Features of Infectious Mononucleosis (IM) in Immunocompetent Patients

Epstein-Barr virus (human herpesvirus-4)
Pathophysiology
- Virus enters through oropharyngeal epithelial and lymphoid cells.
- Virus attaches to CD21 on B cells.
- Viral antigens—viral capsid antigen (VCA), early antigen (EA), Epstein-Barr nuclear antigen (EBNA)—are produced and elicit antibody production.

Humoral Immune Response
- Immunoglobulin (Ig)M against VCA rises during incubation and prodrome, falls over few weeks to months.
- IgG against VCA rises during incubation, decreases during convalescence, remains detectable for life.
- Antibodies to EA rise 2-3 wk after onset of illness, then fall.
- Antibodies to EBNA rise during convalescence, detectable for life.

Cellular Immune Response
- T cells activated during second week of illness.
- CD8-positive cytotoxic T cells kill infected B cells.
- Natural killer cells kill infected B cells.
- Some resting memory B cells remain latently infected.

Clinical Features
- 4- to 7-wk incubation period
- Vague onset of symptoms
- Fever, sore throat, lymphadenopathy
- Adolescents, young adults more often symptomatic than younger children

Laboratory Features
- Leukocytosis with absolute lymphocytosis and atypical lymphocytes
- Transient monocytosis
- Relative and absolute neutropenia early on
- Mild thrombocytopenia in half of cases
- Hemolytic anemia in 1%-3% of cases, often with anti-I specificity
- Elevated transaminases in 85%-100% of cases, but clinical jaundice rare
- Spot test is simple, rapid, specific, based on agglutination of horse red blood cells (RBCs)
- Heterophil antibody (HA) test is based on differential absorption of IM-specific HA by beef RBC stroma and guinea pig kidney

From McPherson RA, Pincus MR: *Henry's clinical diagnosis and management by laboratory methods,* ed 23, Philadelphia, 2017, Elsevier.

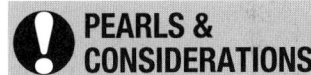
TABLE 1   Clinical Manifestations of Infectious Mononucleosis in Children and Adults

Sign or Symptom	FREQUENCY (%)		
	Age <4 yr	Age 4-16 yr	Adults (Range)
Lymphadenopathy	94	95	93-100
Fever	92	100	63-100
Sore throat or tonsillopharyngitis	67	75	70-91
Exudative tonsillopharyngitis	45	59	40-74
Splenomegaly	82	53	32-51
Hepatomegaly	63	30	6-24
Cough or rhinitis	51	15	5-31
Rash	34	17	0-15
Abdominal pain or discomfort	17	0	2-14

From Hoffman R et al: *Hematology, basic principles and practice*, ed 7, Philadelphia, 2018, Elsevier.

parents bring symptomatic children to medical care.

EBV infects epithelial cells and resting B cells of the oropharynx. It is then found in saliva, making it transmittable through coughing, sharing drink/food, and kissing; thus the pseudonym "kissing disease." IM is more prevalent during adolescence when these types of close contact increase. How it is transmitted in younger children is less clear.

EBV levels peak during the active phase of infection but can persist in the oropharynx for up to 18 mo. Transmission may also occur sexually because EBV can be isolated in cervical epithelial cells and male seminal fluid. It has also been shown to be transmitted by blood transfusion, solid organ transplantation, or hematopoietic cell transplantation.

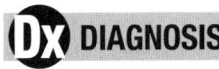 **DIAGNOSIS**

DIFFERENTIAL DIAGNOSIS
- Heterophile-negative IM caused by CMV
- Bacterial and viral causes of pharyngitis
- Toxoplasmosis
- Acute retroviral syndrome of HIV, lymphoma

WORKUP[2]
Initial testing consists of heterophile antibody (monospot) and CBC with differential. Fig. 3 illustrates the serologic evaluation of patients with clinical symptoms of acute IM and atypical lymphocytosis.

LABORATORY TESTS
- About 85% of patients with EBV-related IM will have a positive heterophile antibody test, making it the best initial test for diagnosis of EBV infection (sensitivity of 71% to 90% for

diagnosing IM). However, the test has a 25% false-negative rate in the first week of illness because the amount of heterophile antibody may not be above the limit for detection early in the disease. A negative test should be repeated if clinical suspicion is high; negative results are common in patients symptomatic for <2 wk and children <4 yr. False-positive heterophile antibody tests have been reported in other acute infections, autoimmune diseases, and cancer.
- About 10% of patients will have a persistently negative heterophile antibody test. In this event, further testing may be pursued with EBV viral capsid antigen (VCA) IgG and IgM antibody testing, as well as EBV nuclear antigen (EBNA) antibodies for staging of infection. Early diagnosis in monospot-negative cases may be made by isolating IgM to the VCA, which is usually positive during the acute illness and disappears after 4 to 6 wk. If the monospot test remains negative (without evidence of acute infection with antibody testing) for 8 wk, alternative diagnoses should be considered. The monospot usually remains positive for 3 to 6 mo but can last >1 yr.
- Increased white blood count (WBC) is common, with a relative lymphocytosis and neutropenia. Atypical lymphocytes (Fig. E4) are the hallmark of IM but are not pathognomonic. Mild thrombocytopenia is common. A falling hematocrit may signal splenic rupture or severe immune-mediated hemolytic anemia. Elevated hepatocellular enzymes and cryoglobulins occur in many cases.

IMAGING STUDIES
Chest x-ray may rarely show infiltrates. An elevated left hemidiaphragm may occur in cases of splenic rupture.

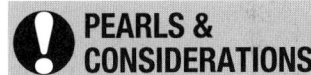 **TREATMENT**

NONPHARMACOLOGIC THERAPY
- No specific treatment exists; focus is on supportive care and symptomatic relief with analgesics, antipyretics, and hydration. Supportive rest is advocated by some, but the effect on outcome is not clear. Prolonged rest may result in deconditioning, which may contribute to further fatigue.
- Splenectomy if rupture occurs; transfusions for severe anemia or thrombocytopenia.

GENERAL Rx
- There is no role for antiviral agents such as acyclovir in the management of IM.

CHRONIC Rx
CAEBV is treated with hematopoietic cell transplantation.

DISPOSITION
Eventual resolution of all symptoms is the rule.

PEARLS & CONSIDERATIONS

COMMENTS
- Contact sports should be avoided during the first month of illness because splenic rupture can occur during this time, even in the absence of clinically detectable splenomegaly.[3]
- Between 30% and 75% of college freshmen are seronegative for EBV. Each year nearly 20% of susceptible persons become infected, and up to 50% of these persons develop IM.
- Pharmacologic therapy, including corticosteroids, is not indicated in mild illness or for symptomatic relief. Use of corticosteroids is controversial because they may impair clearance of the viral load.
- The use of steroids, however, (Fig. 5), should be considered in patients who have severe acute complications, such as thrombocytopenia, hemolytic anemia, or impending airway obstruction.

REFERENCES
Available at eBooks.Health.Elsevier.com.

RELATED CONTENT
Mononucleosis (Patient Information)
Epstein-Barr Virus Infection (Related Key Topic)

AUTHOR: **RUSSELL J. MCCULLOH, MD**

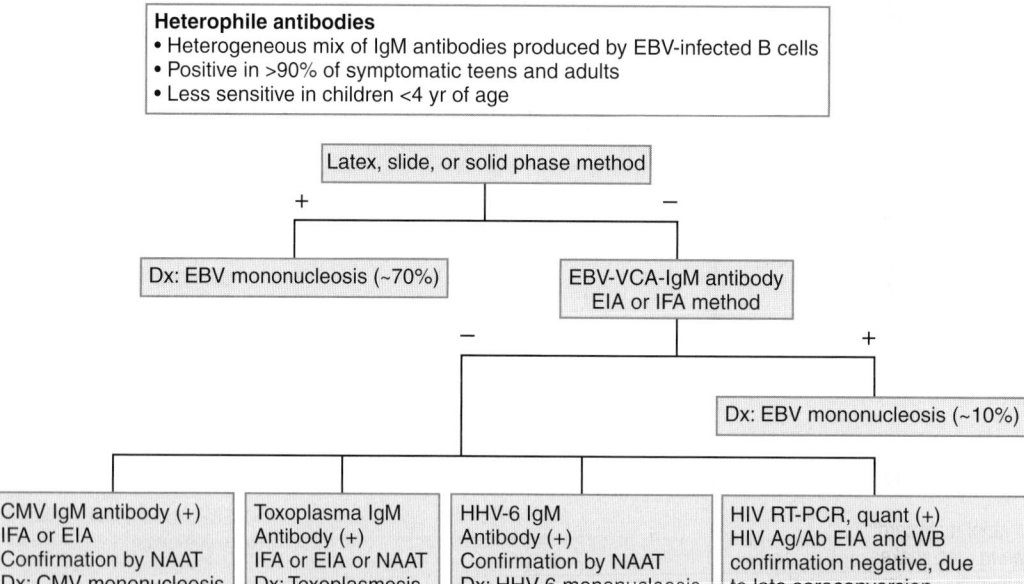

FIG. 3 Serologic evaluation of patients with clinical symptoms of acute infectious mononucleosis and atypical lymphocytosis. *Ab,* Antibody; *Ag,* antigen; *CMV,* cytomegalovirus; *Dx,* diagnosis; *EBV,* Epstein-Barr virus; *EIA,* enzyme immunoassay; *HHV-6,* human herpesvirus 6; *HIV,* human immunodeficiency virus; *IFA,* immunofluorescent assay; *IgM,* immunoglobulin M; *NAAT,* nucleic acid amplification testing; *quant,* quantitative; *RT-PCR,* reverse transcriptase polymerase chain reaction; *VCA,* viral capsid antigen; *WB,* Western blot. (From McPherson RA, Pincus MR: *Henry's clinical diagnosis and management by laboratory methods,* ed 23, Philadelphia, 2017, Elsevier.)

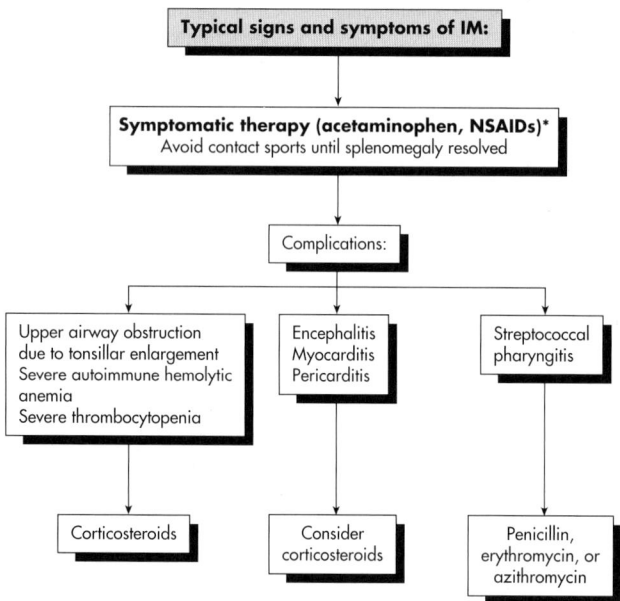

FIG. 5 Algorithm for management of infectious mononucleosis. *IM,* Infectious mononucleosis; *NSAID,* nonsteroidal antiinflammatory drug.
*Consider corticosteroids in moderate/severe cases.

BASIC INFORMATION

DEFINITION

Multifocal atrial tachycardia (MAT) is a supraventricular tachyarrhythmia (rate greater than 100 beats per minute) with organized atrial activity, showing P waves having at least three or more different morphologies and irregular P-P, P-R, and R-R intervals. MAT is differentiated from atrial fibrillation by discrete P wave depolarizations and an isoelectric baseline between P waves.

SYNONYMS

MAT
Chaotic atrial rhythm
Multiform atrial rhythm
Chronic atrial tachycardia
Repetitive multifocal paroxysmal atrial tachycardia
Multifocal ectopic atrial tachycardia
The term *wandering pacemaker* or multifocal atrial rhythm is used for a similar arrhythmia associated with heart rates less than 100 bpm.

ICD-10CM CODE
I47.1 Supraventricular tachycardia

EPIDEMIOLOGY & DEMOGRAPHICS

Estimated prevalence in hospitalized patients is 0.05% to 0.37%.[1] Right atrial hypertension and distention (from secondary pulmonary hypertension from advanced chronic obstructive pulmonary disease [COPD] or left ventricular dysfunction) potentially cause MAT.[2] The average age of onset is 70 yr of age.

The entity is usually associated with underlying pulmonary disease with right atrial electromechanical delay (60% of cases);[1] the arrhythmia has been identified in up to 20% of patients hospitalized for acute respiratory failure.[3] COPD is present in approximately 55% of patients with MAT, and significant lung disease is associated in roughly 60% of cases, including pneumonia, pulmonary embolism, hypoxia, hypercapnia, and acidosis.

MAT has been identified in patients with coronavirus disease 2019; however, it was not associated with increased mortality.[4]

MAT may also be seen in patients with heart failure, valvular heart disease, pulmonary hypertension, and hypomagnesemia. These patients are in general quite ill and have an in-hospital mortality rate of 40% to 60% from pulmonary, cardiac, and/or other serious diseases.

PHYSICAL FINDINGS & CLINICAL PRESENTATION

Symptoms:
• Palpitations
• Light-headedness
• Presyncope and/or syncope are rare
• Symptoms of the underlying pulmonary disease, if applicable
• Physical findings associated with the underlying pulmonary disease, if applicable
• Most episodes do not cause hemodynamic compromise; however, it can lead to decompensation if there is coexisting advanced cardiac disease (i.e., severe multivessel obstructive coronary artery disease or decompensated heart failure)
• High heart rates associated with MAT can sometimes worsen systemic oxygenation or exacerbate heart disease if there is coexisting pulmonary or cardiac disease, respectively

ETIOLOGY

• Exact mechanism is unknown; however, there are two leading theories:
  1. Atrial pacemaker activity arises from different atrial locations. This is supported by variable P waves and PR intervals.
  2. A single focus with different exit pathways or abnormalities in intraatrial conduction.
• Potentially caused by right atrial hypertension and distention such as that found in pulmonary hypertension (from advanced COPD) or left ventricular dysfunction.
• Also seen in other circumstances; therefore atrial distention may not be a universal mechanism.
• Exacerbated by underlying pulmonary disease (COPD, hypoxia, pulmonary embolism, pneumonia), cardiac disease, hypercarbia, acidosis, electrolyte disturbances (hypokalemia and hypomagnesemia).
• Other associations:
  1. Drugs like isoproterenol, aminophylline, and theophylline
  2. Chronic renal failure (15% of patients with MAT has chronic renal failure)
  3. Sepsis and recent surgery

DIAGNOSIS

DIFFERENTIAL DIAGNOSIS

• Atrial fibrillation (no discernable P waves; up to 55% of patients with MAT will develop atrial fibrillation, MAT can degenerate into atrial fibrillation)
• Atrial flutter with variable atrioventricular conduction (regular P-P intervals; MAT has variable P-P intervals)
• Sinus tachycardia with frequent premature atrial contractions (PACs) or ventricular premature beats (regular P-P intervals)
• Paroxysmal atrial tachycardia

WORKUP

• ECG (Fig. 1)
• Chest x-ray examination
• Pulmonary function tests
• Electrolytes
• Arterial blood gases

TREATMENT

• Correction and/or improvement in the underlying pulmonary or metabolic dysfunction if possible (e.g., electrolyte repletion if associated with hypomagnesemia and/or hypokalemia).[5]
• Correction of oxygenation and acid-base disorders.
• Avoid drugs such as theophylline, isoproterenol, etc.
• Intravenous magnesium infusion may occasionally be helpful even in patients with normal magnesium levels.
• Calcium channel blockers: Verapamil may be effective acutely and chronically and is often used as first line in patients with preserved left ventricular function *if there are symptoms related to tachycardia.*
• β-Blockers (metoprolol is relatively cardioselective) can be used if not contraindicated by obstructive lung disease, acute heart failure, hypotension, hypersensitivity, heart block, or sinus node dysfunction.
• If the arrhythmia is asymptomatic, it can be left untreated.
• Direct current cardioversion is ineffective.
• Antiarrhythmics are ineffective.
• Anticoagulation is currently not indicated, although some recent studies have linked frequent atrial ectopy on ambulatory monitoring with stroke risk
• No significant role for catheter ablation; however, in extreme cases of refractory MAT in symptomatic patients who cannot tolerate medical therapy or in MAT resistant to medical therapy, atrioventricular nodal ablation with pacemaker implantation has been performed.
• Table E1 summarizes the treatment of multifocal atrial tachycardia.

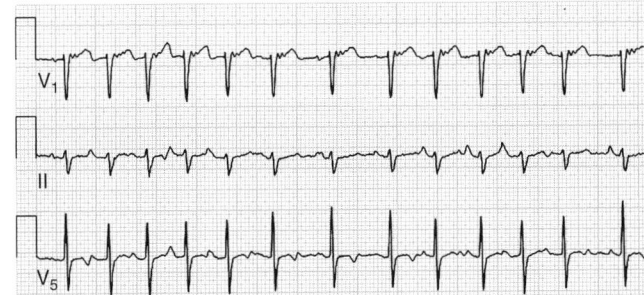

FIG. 1 Multifocal atrial tachycardia (MAT). This three-lead rhythm strip (leads II, V₁, and V₅) shows an irregularly irregular narrow QRS complex rhythm. However, unlike in atrial fibrillation, each QRS complex is preceded by discrete, conducted P waves. There are at least three different P wave morphologies and PR intervals, consistent with MAT. (From Olshansky B et al: *Arrhythmia essentials,* ed 2, Philadelphia, 2017, Elsevier.)

REFERENCES

Available at eBooks.Health.Elsevier.com.

AUTHOR: **VYBHAV JETTY, MD, MHA**

Diseases and Disorders

I

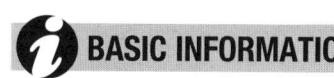

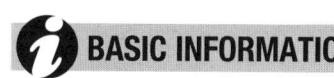

BASIC INFORMATION

DEFINITION

Multiple endocrine neoplasia (MEN) refers to a group of heritable genetic syndromes characterized by the development of specific groups of tumors of the endocrine glands.

SYNONYMS

MEN I: Wermer syndrome
MEN IIA: Sipple syndrome

ICD-10CM CODES

E31.2	Multiple endocrine neoplasia [MEN] syndromes
E31.20	Multiple endocrine neoplasia [MEN] syndrome, unspecified
E31.21	Multiple endocrine neoplasia [MEN] syndrome type I
E31.22	Multiple endocrine neoplasia [MEN] syndrome type IIA
E31.23	Multiple endocrine neoplasia [MEN] syndrome type IIB

EPIDEMIOLOGY & DEMOGRAPHICS [1,2]

INCIDENCE:
- MEN I: 25 in 10,000
- MEN II: 1 in 30,000

PREVALENCE:
- MEN I: 1/30,000
- MEN II: 1/35,000 (predominantly MEN IIA)

RISK FACTORS: Family history of MEN syndrome, although it can also occur sporadically

GENETICS:
- MEN I: Autosomal-dominant mutation in MEN1 tumor-suppressor gene[1]
- MEN IIA and MEN IIB: Autosomal-dominant mutations in RET proto-oncogene[2]

PHYSICAL FINDINGS & CLINICAL PRESENTATION

- Patients may present due to screening or may present with a MEN-associated tumor. Tumors are found incidentally due to biochemical abnormalities or to symptoms.
- MEN I (PPP [pituitary, pancreas, parathyroid])[3,4]
  1. Diagnostic criteria generally include two MEN-associated tumors, one tumor in a patient with a family history, or positive genetic testing
  2. Primary hyperparathyroidism (parathyroid adenoma or hyperplasia) is the most common manifestation and can cause hypercalcemia (urolithiasis, GI disturbance, bone pain, neuropsychiatric disturbances) and also affect bone density
  3. Pancreatic neuroendocrine tumors cause symptoms related to their secretory properties or metastases
     a. Gastrinoma: Peptic ulcers, diarrhea, esophageal symptoms (see "Gastrinoma")
     b. Insulinoma: Hypoglycemic symptoms upon fasting and after exercise (see "Insulinoma")
     c. Glucagonoma: Necrolytic migratory erythema (a blistering skin lesion), diabetes/glucose intolerance, weight loss

     d. VIPoma: Diarrhea, hypokalemia, decreased gastric acid
     e. Somatostatinoma: Hyperglycemia, cholelithiasis, diarrhea, abdominal pain, weight loss
     f. Nonfunctioning tumors can metastasize (frequently to the liver), a frequent cause of death in MEN I
  4. Pituitary tumors may cause compressive symptoms, such as visual field defects or hypopituitarism (see "Pituitary Adenoma"). Hormonal secretion may also cause symptoms.
     a. Prolactinoma (most common pituitary tumor in MEN I): Menstrual irregularities, hypogonadism, gynecomastia, and/or galactorrhea (see "Prolactinoma")
     b. Somatotroph adenomas (producing growth hormone): Gigantism or acromegaly (frontal bossing, increased shoe/hat size, hyperglycemia, hyperhidrosis) depending on patient age (see "Acromegaly")
     c. Corticotroph adenomas (producing adrenocorticotropic hormone): Cushingoid features such as weight gain, moon facies, hyperglycemia, bone loss, proximal muscle weakness, hypertension, hypokalemia (see "Cushing Disease and Syndrome")
     d. Nonfunctioning (nonsecretory) tumors
  5. Other manifestations: Carcinoid tumors, collagenomas, angiofibromas, meningiomas, lipomas
- MEN IIA:[5,6]
  1. Medullary thyroid carcinoma (MTC) is a tumor of the thyroid's calcitonin-secreting C cells. It can present with a neck mass, as well as flushing and diarrhea due to elevated calcitonin levels.
  2. Primary hyperparathyroidism: See "MEN I." Less aggressive in "MEN IIA."
  3. Pheochromocytoma is an adrenal tumor producing catecholamines, which can lead to life-threatening hypertensive crises.
- MEN IIB:[5,6]
  1. MTC
  2. Pheochromocytoma
  3. Oral mucosal neuromas

ETIOLOGY

Tumor development facilitated by the previously described genetic mutations (Table E1).

DIAGNOSIS

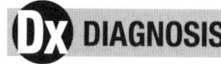

DIFFERENTIAL DIAGNOSIS

Tumors associated with MEN may occur sporadically.

WORKUP

- MEN I: Note that opinions vary regarding the aggressiveness and frequency of screening for MEN-associated tumors. Fig. E1 illustrates an algorithm for screening and management of MEN1 syndromes.
  1. Genetic testing: Offered to patients meeting MEN I clinical criteria or to patients in whom

there is high suspicion, as well as to first-degree relatives of MEN I patients.
  2. Hyperparathyroidism screening: Parathyroid hormone (PTH) and calcium annually.
  3. Pancreatic tumor screening: Annual pancreas imaging (endoscopic ultrasonography, computed tomography [CT], or MRI) and annual biochemical testing (glucose, gastrin, vasoactive intestinal peptide [VIP], glucagon, insulin, pancreatic polypeptide, chromogranin A). Notably, Gallium-68 DOTATATE PET-CT is an exciting new tool for neuroendocrine tumor localization, though it is not typically utilized in screening at this time.
  4. Pituitary tumor screening: Insulin-like growth factor 1 (IGF-1) and prolactin annually and pituitary MRI every 3 to 5 yr.
  5. Carcinoid tumor screening: Chest CT or MRI every 2 yr.
- MEN IIA:
  1. Genetic testing: At-risk members of families with known RET mutations should undergo screening for the specific mutation. Patients with MTC should have genetic testing of the tumor and genetic testing based on results. Cutaneous lichen amyloidosis (a skin finding) should prompt testing; Hirschsprung disease may also prompt testing.[2]
  2. Hyperparathyroidism screening: PTH and calcium annually
  3. Pheochromocytoma: Plasma catecholamines and metanephrines annually for screening, age to begin depending on specific mutation; CT and MRI may localize; I-123 and PET (possibly including gallium-68 DOTATATE PET-CT) also helpful for localization.[7]
  4. MTC screening: Depends on risk category; physical exam, neck ultrasound, and calcitonin level yearly; carcinoembryonic antigen may also be indicated.[5,6]
- MEN IIB:
  1. Genetic testing: See "MEN IIA"
  2. Pheochromocytoma: See "MEN IIA"
  3. MTC screening: Although there may be a role for monitoring, prophylactic thyroidectomy is typically performed early

LABORATORY TESTS

See "Workup."

IMAGING STUDIES

See "Workup."

TREATMENT

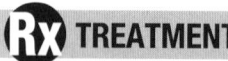

No therapy available at this time to reverse the underlying genetic cause. Treatment (both medical and surgical) focuses on tumor prevention and management.

NONPHARMACOLOGIC THERAPY

- MEN I:[3,4]
  1. For hyperparathyroidism, surgical parathyroidectomy is indicated in patients with

significant hypercalcemia, osteoporosis, renal disease, or nephrolithiasis or found to be at high risk for nephrolithiasis. Hyperparathyroidism may be treated surgically with parathyroidectomy.
2. Pituitary tumors may be surgically excised via transsphenoidal approach; notably, medical therapy is first line for prolactinoma.
3. Pancreatic tumor treatment is extremely variable. Gastrinoma is frequently complicated by duodenal metastases, which are difficult to treat surgically, so treatment choice varies between centers. Ulcers caused by gastrinoma may require endoscopic or surgical management. Surgery is preferred for insulinoma, VIPoma, and glucagonoma. Nonfunctioning tumors may be treated surgically depending on tumor size and location. Conservative management for insulinoma may involve frequent carbohydrate intake. Cytotoxic chemotherapy and tyrosine kinase inhibitors are options for patients with metastatic disease. Peptide receptor radionucleotide therapy (PRRT) is an emerging and exciting therapeutic modality for metastatic disease.
• MEN IIA:
1. MTC is generally treated surgically. Prophylactic thyroidectomy is considered based on genetic mutation. Almost all children with MEN IIA will require thyroidectomy (screening as previously described). Patients should undergo ultrasound and total thyroidectomy with cervical lymph node dissection. Extent of further neck dissection depends on metastases and may be guided by calcitonin levels. A more palliative surgical approach is considered in the setting of advanced disease.[5,6]
2. Hyperparathyroidism: Resection of only enlarged glands with intraoperative PTH monitoring is preferred.
3. Pheochromocytoma is treated surgically. Unilateral adrenalectomy is preferred, although many patients will develop a contralateral pheochromocytoma. Preoperative blood pressure control with alpha blockade is key. If present, pheochromocytoma must be removed before thyroidectomy.[7]
• MEN IIB:
1. MTC: Prophylactic thyroidectomy offered in childhood.[5,6]
2. Pheochromocytoma: See "MEN IIA."

ACUTE GENERAL Rx

• MEN I:[3,4]
1. Hyperparathyroidism causes hypercalcemia that may be treated with intravenous (IV) hydration, diuretics, and bisphosphonates. Early vitamin D repletion prevents

bone destruction postoperatively due to the "hungry bone syndrome."
2. Gastrinoma may lead to peptic ulcers requiring IV proton-pump inhibitor (PPI).
3. Supportive care (glucose for hypoglycemia caused by insulinoma; fluids and electrolytes for hypovolemia caused by diarrhea from VIPoma or gastrinoma) is required.
• MEN IIA:
1. Hyperparathyroidism: See "MEN I."
2. Pheochromocytoma: Preoperative blood pressure control is key; alpha blockers are first line. Phenoxybenzamine irreversibly blocks alpha adrenergic receptors; doxazosin may also be helpful. Calcium channel blockers can be utilized. There is concern that unopposed beta blockade may allow for alpha-medicated vasoconstriction.[7]
• MEN IIB:
1. Pheochromocytoma: See "MEN IIA."

CHRONIC Rx

• MEN I:[3,4]
1. Hyperparathyroidism may be amenable to agonists of the calcium-sensing receptor (cinacalcet), although surgery is preferred in patients who meet surgical criteria and are operative candidates.
2. Pancreatic tumors may benefit from medical therapy.
   a. Gastrinoma: PPI or H2 antagonists, somatostatin agonists (such as octreotide)
   b. Insulinoma: Diazoxide or somatostatin agonists
   c. Glucagonoma and VIPoma: Somatostatin agonists
3. Adjunctive medical therapy can be considered for pituitary tumors, although surgical treatment is first-line with the exception of prolactinoma (for which dopamine agonists are first line). Radiation therapy and/or medical therapy are considered in cases of incomplete resection or regrowth.
   a. Prolactinoma: Dopamine agonists (bromocriptine or cabergoline). Temozolomide is a chemotherapeutic agent for refractory cases.
   b. Somatotroph adenoma: Somatostatin or dopamine agonists, growth hormone receptor antagonist
   c. Corticotroph adenoma: Antiadrenal agents, adrenal enzyme blocker (such as ketoconazole), somatostatin or dopamine agonists, glucocorticoid receptor blockers
• MEN II A:
1. Hyperparathyroidism: See "MEN I."
2. MTC: Tyrosine kinase inhibitors and chemotherapy may help treat metastatic disease.

After thyroidectomy, levothyroxine is indicated (thyroid-stimulating hormone suppression not required).[5,6]
• MEN IIB
MTC: See "MEN II A."

DISPOSITION

Most workup can be done as an outpatient (multidisciplinary team); inpatient stays may be required due to acute complications or for surgical procedures.

COMPLEMENTARY & ALTERNATIVE MEDICINE

MEN is unlikely to be amenable to this.

REFERRAL

Patients with MEN should be followed by a multispecialty team, including endocrinologists, endocrine surgeons, and genetic counselors.

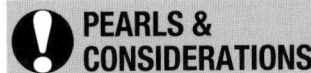

PEARLS & CONSIDERATIONS

COMMENTS

MEN is a group of genetic syndromes that requires close monitoring and intervention to prevent and treat tumor development, as well as genetic counseling of patients and family members.

PREVENTION

Prevention focuses on screening for MEN in persons at risk and early identification of MEN-associated tumors.

PATIENT & FAMILY EDUCATION

• American Multiple Endocrine Neoplasia Support: https://www.amensupport.org/
• Association for Multiple Endocrine Neoplasia Disorders: https://www.amend.org.uk/

REFERENCES

Available at eBooks.Health.Elsevier.com.

RELATED CONTENT

Acromegaly (Related Key Topic)
Cushing Disease and Syndrome (Related Key Topic)
Gastrinoma (Related Key Topic)
Hyperparathyroidism (Related Key Topic)
Insulinoma (Related Key Topic)
Pheochromocytoma (Related Key Topic)
Pituitary Adenoma (Related Key Topic)
Prolactinoma (Related Key Topic)
Thyroid Carcinoma (Related Key Topic)

AUTHORS: **HARIKRASHNA B. BHATT, MD,** and **RUSSELL E. BRATMAN, MD**

Diseases and Disorders

I

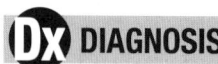

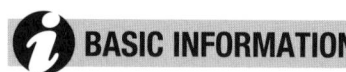 **BASIC INFORMATION**

DEFINITION

Multiple myeloma (MM) is a plasma cell neoplasm characterized by production of a monoclonal protein in the blood or urine and clonal proliferation of malignant plasma cells in the bone marrow leading to end-organ dysfunction.

The transition from normal cells to genomic instability is not well understood, but current evidence suggests that antigenic stimulation may be a key factor (Fig. E1). Diagnostic criteria for the diagnosis of MM were updated by the International Myeloma Working Group (IMWG) in 2014 and require the following:

- Presence of ≥10% plasma cells on examination of the bone marrow (or biopsy of a tissue with monoclonal plasma cells) and any one or more of the following myeloma-defining events[2]:
  1. End-organ damage (calcium elevation, renal insufficiency, anemia, or bone lesions [CRAB criteria])
  2. Clonal bone marrow plasma cell percentage ≥60%
  3. Involved: Uninvolved serum free light ratio ≥100
  4. >1 focal lesion on MRI studies

SYNONYM

MM

ICD-10CM CODES

C90.00 Multiple myeloma not having achieved remission
C90.01 Multiple myeloma in remission
C90.02 Multiple myeloma in relapse

EPIDEMIOLOGY & DEMOGRAPHICS

INCIDENCE:
- 5 cases/100,000 persons (African Americans are affected twice as frequently as Whites, males more than females).
- MM is the second most common hematologic malignancy and accounts for 10% of all cases.
- Estimated 34,470 new cases and 12,640 deaths occurred in 2022 in the U.S.[1]

PREDOMINANT AGE: The peak incidence is in the seventh decade at a median age of 69 yr old.

PHYSICAL FINDINGS & CLINICAL PRESENTATION

Patients present with one or more of the following:
- Back or thoracic bone pain or pathologic fractures caused by osteolytic lesions
- Anemia and fatigue with bone marrow infiltration
- Recurrent infections due to impaired neutrophil function and immunoglobulin deficiency
- Nausea and vomiting caused by constipation and uremia
- Delirium resulting from hypercalcemia
- Neurologic complications due to spinal cord or nerve root compression
- Purpura, epistaxis from thrombocytopenia

- Paresthesias, weight loss, generalized weakness

Dx DIAGNOSIS

DIFFERENTIAL DIAGNOSIS

- Metastatic carcinoma to bone marrow
- Lymphoma, non-Hodgkin
- Bone neoplasms (e.g., sarcoma)
- Monoclonal gammopathy of undetermined significance
- Primary amyloidosis
- Waldenström macroglobulinemia

- Table 1 compares diagnostic criteria for multiple myeloma, myeloma variants, and monoclonal gammopathy of unknown significance (MGUS)

LABORATORY TESTS

- The evaluation of patients with multiple myeloma is summarized in Table 2.
- Normochromic, normocytic anemia; rouleaux formation on peripheral smear (Fig. E2).
- Hypercalcemia is present in 15% of patients at diagnosis.
- Elevated blood urea nitrogen, creatinine, uric acid, and total protein.

TABLE 1 Diagnostic Criteria for Multiple Myeloma, Myeloma Variants, and Monoclonal Gammopathy of Unknown Significance

Monoclonal Gammopathy of Undetermined Significance (MGUS) or Monoclonal Gammopathy, Unattributed/Unassociated (MG[u])
M protein in serum <30 g/L
Bone marrow clonal plasma cells <10%
No evidence of other B-cell proliferative disorders
No myeloma-related organ or tissue impairment (no end-organ damage, including bone lesions)

Asymptomatic Myeloma (Smoldering Myeloma)
M protein in serum >30 g/L and/or bone marrow clonal plasma cell ≥10%-60%
No related organ or tissue impairment (no end-organ damage, including bone lesions) or symptoms

Symptomatic Multiple Myeloma (MM)
M protein in serum and/or urine[a]
Bone marrow (clonal) plasma cells[a] or plasmacytoma
Related organ or tissue impairment (end-organ damage, including bone lesions)
Clonal bone marrow plasma cell percentage ≥60%
Involved: Uninvolved serum free light ratio ≥100
>1 focal lesion on MRI studies

Solitary Plasmacytoma of Bone
No M protein in serum and/or urine[b]
Single area of bone destruction caused by clonal plasma cells
Bone marrow not consistent with MM
Normal skeletal survey (and MRI of spine and pelvis if done)
No related organ or tissue impairment (no end-organ damage other than solitary bone lesion)[b]

Nonsecretory Myeloma
No M protein in serum and/or urine with immunofixation
Bone marrow clonal plasmacytosis ≥10% or plasmacytoma
Related organ or tissue impairment (end-organ damage, including bone lesions)

Extramedullary Plasmacytoma
No M protein in serum and/or urine[c]
Extramedullary tumor of clonal plasma cells
Normal bone marrow
Normal skeletal survey
No related organ or tissue impairment (end-organ damage including bone lesions)

Multiple Solitary Plasmacytomas (Recurrent or Not)
No M protein in serum and/or urine[d]
More than one localized area of bone destruction or extramedullary tumor of clonal plasma cells that may be recurrent
Normal bone marrow
Normal skeletal survey and MRI of spine and pelvis if done
No related organ or tissue impairment (no end-organ damage other than the localized bone lesions)

Myeloma-Related Organ or Tissue Impairment (End-Organ Damage)
Calcium levels increased: Serum calcium >0-25 mmol/L above the upper limit of normal or >2-75 mmol/L
Renal insufficiency: Creatinine >173 mmol/L
Anemia: Hemoglobin 2 g/dl below the lower limit of normal or hemoglobin <10 g/dl
Bone lesions: Lytic lesions or osteoporosis with compression fractures (MRI or CT may clarify)
Other: Symptomatic hyperviscosity, amyloidosis, recurrent bacterial infections (more than two episodes in 12 mo)

CT, Computed tomography; *MRI,* magnetic resonance image.
[a]If flow cytometry is performed, most plasma cells (>90%) will show a neoplastic phenotype.
[b]A small M component may sometimes be present.
[c]A small M component may sometimes be present.
[d]A small M component may sometimes be present.
From Hoffman R et al: *Hematology: basic principles and practice,* ed 7, Philadelphia, 2018, Elsevier.

M

I

TABLE 2 Evaluation of Patients With Multiple Myeloma

Evaluation for Diagnosis
Evaluation for Monoclonal Protein

Serum protein electrophoresis, immunofixation
Quantitative immunoglobulin by nephelometric method
24-H urine collection for electrophoresis and Bence Jones protein assessment and immunofixation
Serum free light chain and ratio

Evaluation for Clonal Plasma Cells

Bone marrow aspirate and biopsy for histology
Clonality by immunostaining or flow cytometry by κ/λ staining
Fine-needle aspiration of plasmacytoma if indicated

Evaluation for End-Organ Damage

Hemogram to detect anemia
Chemistry panel for renal function and calcium
Radiologic evaluation: Skeletal survey
PET-CT or MRI as indicated for bone lesions or extramedullary disease

Evaluation for Risk Stratification

β_2-Microglobulin and serum albumin for ISS stage
Cytogenetics and fluorescence in situ hybridization on bone marrow sample
LDH
C-reactive protein

Other Investigations for Selected Patients

Abdominal fat pad or rectal biopsy for amyloid
Solitary lytic lesion biopsy
Serum viscosity if IgM component or high IgA levels or serum M component >7 g/dl
Immunofixation for IgD or IgE in select cases

CT, Computed tomography; *Ig*, immunoglobulin; *ISS*, International Staging System; *LDH*, lactate dehydrogenase; *MRI*, magnetic resonance imaging; *PET*, positron emission tomography.
From Hoffman R et al: *Hematology: basic principles and practice*, ed 7, Philadelphia, 2018, Elsevier.

- Urine protein immunoelectrophoresis: Proteinuria from overproduction and secretion of free monoclonal kappa or lambda chains (Bence Jones protein).
- Serum protein immunoelectrophoresis: Monoclonal protein (M spike) on immunoelectrophoresis in approximately 75% of patients (Fig. E3); decreased levels of normal immunoglobulins (Ig).
  1. The increased immunoglobulins are generally IgG (70%) and IgA (20%).
  2. Approximately 5% to 10% of patients have only increased light chains in the urine by electrophoresis (light chain MM).
  3. A small percentage (<2%) of patients have nonsecretory MM but have other evidence of the disease (e.g., positive bone marrow examination).
- Abnormally elevated or decreased kappa:lambda ratios suggest the presence of monoclonal light chain proteins.
- Bone marrow biopsy demonstrating plasma cells >10%.
- Elevated serum beta 2-microglobulin indicates high tumor mass and advanced stage.
- Elevated serum lactate dehydrogenase at diagnosis is associated with a poor prognosis.

- Patients may present with abnormal chromosomes (Table E3) identified by fluorescence in situ hybridization (FISH). High-risk patients (<25% of patients at diagnosis) have any of the following:
  1. Deletion 17p
  2. Translocation 4;14
  3. Translocation 14;16
  4. Translocation 14;20
  5. Gain of chromosome 1q21

IMAGING STUDIES

Imaging modalities for disease assessment in myeloma are summarized in Table 4. X-ray films often demonstrate punched-out lytic lesions or osteoporosis (Figs. E3, E4, E5, and E6). Computed tomography (CT) can identify rib involvement and differentiate it from osteoporotic and traumatic fractures (Fig. E7). MRI is the preferred technique for suspected spinal compression or soft tissue plasmacytomas. Bone scans may not be useful because MM lesions are not blastic. PET scans are used for detection of osseous and extraosseous disease.

STAGING

Table 5 describes the Revised International Staging System (R-ISS) for MM that incorporates traditional laboratory parameters and high-risk chromosomal abnormalities detected by FISH on bone marrow samples.[3] This system classifies patients into three risk groups (high, intermediate, and standard). Risk stratification in MM is summarized in Tables 6 and 7.

Rx TREATMENT

NONPHARMACOLOGIC THERAPY

Prevention of renal failure with adequate hydration and avoidance of nephrotoxic agents and dye contrast studies.

ACUTE GENERAL Rx

- Treatment strategy depends on the transplant eligibility of the patient.[4,5]
- Transplant-eligible patients receive 3 to 6 mo of induction chemotherapy with triplet regimens such as the RVD regimen (bortezomib, lenalidomide, and dexamethasone) or the CyBorD regimen (cyclophosphamide, bortezomib, and dexamethasone). Quadruplet regimens include the addition of daratumumab, a monoclonal antibody targeting CD38, and can be used in select transplant-eligible and ineligible myeloma patients.[5] Upon achieving a partial response, these patients undergo stem cell collection followed by high-dose melphalan chemotherapy and autologous SCT.
- Early use of ASCT has demonstrated a continued improvement in progression-free survival but no consistent overall survival benefit.
- Patients with high-risk features (high R-ISS stage, poor cytogenetics, extramedullary disease) should undergo ASCT subsequently, which can be safely performed in most centers in fit patients up to age 75 yr.

- Patients typically receive maintenance chemotherapy with either lenalidomide and/or bortezomib after ASCT for at least 2 yr or until disease progression.
- In transplant-ineligible patients, induction chemotherapy can be identical to that offered transplant-eligible patients but can be dose modified to allow for better tolerability.[4] Less aggressive regimens can be considered, including:
  1. Lenalidomide and dexamethasone
  2. Bortezomib and dexamethasone
- Relapsed myeloma: If the relapse occurs more than 6 mo after conventional therapy is stopped, the initial chemotherapy regimen can be reinstituted. Options can include[6]:
  1. Second- or third-generation proteasome inhibitors (carfilzomib and ixazomib).
  2. Immunomodulatory drugs (thalidomide, pomalidomide).
  3. The monoclonal antibodies elotuzumab (targeting signaling lymphocytic activation molecule F7 [SLAMF7]), daratumumab, and isatuximab.
  4. The histone deacetylase (HDAC) inhibitor panobinostat is also approved in this setting.
  5. The nuclear protein transport inhibitor selinexor can be used alone or in combination with other agents.[7]
  6. The B-cell maturation antigen (BCMA)–targeted antibody drug conjugate (ADC) belantamab-mafodotin was approved for relapsed and refractory myeloma.
  7. Idecabtagene vicleucel, a chimeric antigen receptor therapy (CAR T-cell therapy) targeting BCMA, is approved for relapsed and refractory myeloma that has progressed after four or more prior lines of therapy.[8]
- ASCT can be considered as salvage therapy in patients who had stem cells cryopreserved early in the course of the disease, as this approach has been studied leading to similar survival compared to up-front transplantation.
- Asymptomatic/smoldering myeloma: Approximately 15% of patients are recognized incidentally and present without significant symptoms. The rate of progression of smoldering MM to symptomatic disease is 10% per yr for the initial 5 yr, decreasing to 5% for the next 5 yr, and decreasing further to 1.5% per yr thereafter. Patients are considered high risk if they have two of the following criteria:
  1. Bone marrow plasmacytosis ≥20%
  2. Involved:uninvolved serum-free light chain ratio ≥20
  3. Monoclonal protein ≥2 g/dl
- Lenalidomide alone or lenalidomide plus dexamethasone has demonstrated an improvement in progression-free survival in treatment of high-risk smoldering myeloma.

CHRONIC Rx

- Management of infections:
  1. Common causative bacterial agents are *Streptococcus pneumoniae* and *Haemophilus influenzae*.

TABLE 4   Imaging Modalities for Disease Assessment in Myeloma

	Use	Sensitivity/Specificity	False-Negatives	False-Positives
Bone scan	• For diagnostic screening, except for multiple myeloma	Varies	• Pure osteolytic lesions	• Trauma • Inflammation • Benign tumor • Healing
X-ray	• Can clarify nonspecific findings on bone scan • Assesses risk of fracture • Possible follow-up of tumor response, but evidence of response takes considerable time to appear	Low sensitivity	• Low disease burden • Osteopenia	• Trauma • Inflammation • Benign tumor • Healing
CT	• For anatomic detail in axial skeleton • Possible follow-up of tumor response, but role is still undefined	High sensitivity	• Low disease burden	• Trauma • Inflammation • Benign tumor • Healing
MRI	• Detection of spinal cord compression • Can help distinguish benign from malignant vertebral compression fracture • Possible follow-up of tumor response, but role is still undefined	High sensitivity and specificity	• Lesion only in cortex	• Edema
PET scan	• May eventually become first-line screening test for bone metastases • Possible follow-up of tumor response, but role is still undefined	High specificity	• Lesion only in cortex	• After chemotherapy
Bone density	• Measure osteoporosis • Response to bisphosphonates	High specificity and sensitivity		• Age-related osteoporosis

CT, Computed tomography; *MRI,* magnetic resonance imaging; *PET,* positron emission tomography.
From Hoffman R et al: *Hematology: basic principles and practice,* ed 7, Philadelphia, 2018, Elsevier.

TABLE 5   Revised International Staging System (R-ISS) for Multiple Myeloma Staging System

Stage	Criteria
I	ALL of the following: • Serum β-2 microglobulin <3.5 mg/L • Serum albumin >3.5 mg/dl • No high-risk chromosomal abnormalities by FISH • Normal LDH level
II	• Fitting neither stage I nor III
III	• Serum β-2 microglobulin >5.5 mg/L *AND* either elevated LDH *OR* high-risk chromosomal abnormalities by FISH [(del 17(p) and/or translocation t(14;16) and/or translocation t(4;14)]

FISH, Fluorescence in situ hybridization; *LDH,* lactate dehydrogenase.

TABLE 6   Risk Stratification in Multiple Myeloma

Investigations Recommended for Risk Stratification

Serum albumin and β₂-microglobulin to determine ISS stage
Bone marrow examination for t(4;14), t(14;16), and del(17p) on identified PCs by FISH
LDH
Immunoglobulin type: IgA
Histology: Plasmablastic disease or plasma cell leukemia

Additional Investigations for Risk Stratification

Cytogenetics
Gene expression profiling
Labeling index
MRI/PET scan
DNA copy number alteration by CGH/SNP array

CGH/SNP, Comparative genomic hybridization/single-nucleotide polymorphism; *DNA,* deoxyribonucleic acid; *FISH,* fluorescence in situ hybridization; *IgA,* immunoglobulin A; *ISS,* International Staging System; *LDH,* lactate dehydrogenase; *MRI,* magnetic resonance imaging; *PC,* plasma cell; *PET,* positron emission tomography.
From Hoffman R et al: *Hematology: basic principles and practice,* ed 7, Philadelphia, 2018, Elsevier.

2. Prophylactic therapy against *Pneumocystis jiroveci* with trimethoprim-sulfamethoxazole in patients receiving high-dose corticosteroid regimens.
3. Patients should be vaccinated against *S. pneumoniae,* influenza, shingles, COVID-19, and *H. influenzae.*
4. Prophylactic therapy against herpes zoster with acyclovir is required for patients receiving proteosome inhibitors or monoclonal antibodies.

• Hypercalcemia is aggressively treated with intravenous fluids, bisphosphonates, and corticosteroids. Monthly bisphosphonate use with pamidronate or zoledronate or the RANK-ligand inhibitor denosumab provides significant protection against skeletal complications and improves the quality of life of patients.
• Thromboprophylaxis: Risk assessment followed by aspirin prophylaxis for low/standard risk or low-molecular-weight heparin (LMWH), warfarin, or direct oral anticoagulant for high-risk cases.
• Pain control with analgesics, including narcotics, or radiation for painful bone lesions.
• Surgical stabilization of pathologic fractures as well as vertebroplasty or kyphoplasty for selected vertebral lesions.
• Anemia is treated with erythropoietin.

DISPOSITION

• In patients presenting at an age <60 yr, the 10-yr survival is approximately 30% and median length of survival after diagnosis is now 7 to 8 yr. Prognosis is better in patients with indolent or smoldering myeloma. Median survival time is approximately 10 yr in persons

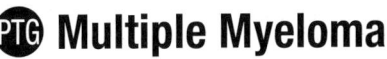

TABLE 7 Standard Risk Factors for Multiple Myeloma and the Revised International Staging System

Prognostic Factor	Criteria
ISS Stage	
I	Serum β_2-microglobulin <3.5 mg/L, serum albumin $\geq$3.5 g/dl
II	Not ISS stage I or III
III	Serum β_2-microglobulin $\geq$5.5 mg/L
CA by iFISH	
High risk	Presence of del(17p) and/or translocation t(4;14) and/or translocation t(14;16)
Standard risk	No high-risk CA
LDH	
Normal	Serum LDH below the upper limit of normal
High	Serum LDH above the upper limit of normal
A New Model for Risk Stratification for MM R-ISS stage	
I	ISS stage I and standard-risk CA by iFISH and normal LDH
II	Not R-ISS stage I or III
III	ISS stage III and either high-risk CA by iFISH or high LDH

CA, Chromosomal abnormalities; *iFISH*, interphase fluorescence in situ hybridization; *ISS*, International Staging System; *LDH*, lactate dehydrogenase; *MM*, multiple myeloma; *R-ISS*, Revised International Staging System.
From Greipp PR et al: International staging system for multiple myeloma, *J Clin Oncol* 23:3412, 2005. In Hoffman R et al: *Hematology: basic principles and practice,* ed 7, Philadelphia, 2018, Elsevier.

with no lytic bone lesions and a serum myeloma protein concentration <3 g/dl.

- Adverse outcome is seen with increased beta-2 microglobulin, low serum albumin, circulating plasma cells, plasmablastic features in bone marrow, increased plasma cell labeling index, and poor cytogenetics [t (4;14) or t (14;16) translocation, deletion 17p].

- Tandem transplantation (two successive ASCT) improves survival among patients who do not have a very good partial response after ASCT or have high-risk features.
- Phase 1 trials in relapsed or refractory MM with teclistamab, a T-cell–redirecting bispecific antibody that targets both CD3 expressed on the surface of T cells and B-cell maturation antigen expressed on the surface of myeloma cells, has shown a high rate of deep and durable response in patients with triple-class–exposed relapsed or refractory multiple myeloma. Cytopenias and infections were common.[9]

REFERRAL

To hematologist for management of disease, and bone marrow transplant specialist for transplantation options and management

REFERENCES

Available at eBooks.Health.Elsevier.com.

RELATED CONTENT

Multiple Myeloma (Patient Information)

AUTHOR: **BHARTI RATHORE, MD**

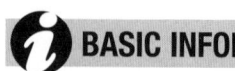 **BASIC INFORMATION**

DEFINITION

Multiple sclerosis (MS) is a chronic, predominantly autoimmune demyelinating disease of the central nervous system (CNS), characterized by subacute neurologic deficits correlating with CNS lesions (typical for MS in location, shape, and orientation) separated in time (typically at least 1 mo) and space, and excluding other possible disease.[1-3]

An MS relapse is defined as an acute to subacute (peaking over hours to days) onset of neurologic dysfunction (typically focal) lasting at least 24 h, and caused by inflammatory CNS demyelination. Relapses can be symptomatic or asymptomatic, the latter of which are represented by new enhancing MRI lesions without correlating symptoms.

Active subtypes include:
- **Relapsing-remitting MS (RRMS)** (85%): Relapses followed by complete or near-complete recovery over weeks to months (rarely beyond 6 mo), 50% to 85% of which later evolve to secondary progressive MS.[2-3]
- **Primary progressive MS (PPMS)** (10% to 15%): Progressive worsening of neurologic disability from the onset, with rare distinct relapses.[2-3]
- **Secondary progressive MS (SPMS):** Progressive worsening of neurologic disability over at least 1 yr with few or no distinct relapses, from a prior course consistent with RRMS.
  - Progressive-relapsing or relapsing-progressive courses can be incorporated into definitions of PPMS or SPMS, respectively.
- **Clinically isolated syndrome (CIS):** An initial, isolated clinical event lasting at least 24 h and typical for MS relapse, but not yet meeting criteria for dissemination in time and space. Correlating demyelinating lesions on MRI are associated with 60% to 80% risk of developing a second relapse (and therefore, MS) within several years, vs. 20% without the presence of typical MS lesions on MRI.[2-3] The definition for RRMS is met when another distinct relapse occurs or when MRI demonstrates new lesions typical for MS.[2,4]
- **Radiologically isolated syndrome (RIS):** The presence of CNS lesions on MRI that meet the diagnostic imaging criteria for MS, without correlating symptoms or symptoms typical for MS. Approximately 50% develop MS within 10 years.[1,2]
- **Solitary sclerosis:** Characterized by isolated or minimal CNS demyelinating lesion(s) with associated progressive neurologic morbidity similar to that in progressive MS, without any clinical or radiologic evidence of new MS-type lesions.[2]

Rare MS variants include:
- **Marburg variant:** Characterized by acute onset and a fulminant, often malignant course (severe disability or death can occur within a year of initial symptoms). MRI reveals tumefactive (tumor-like) demyelinating lesion(s) with extensive edema. Pathology shows severe inflammation with extensive necrosis. May also involve the peripheral nerves.[5]
- **Baló's concentric sclerosis:** Has a monophasic and rapidly progressive course. Neuroimaging and pathology show alternating rings of high- and low-signal intensity (on MRI) representing demyelination and intact myelination, resembling an onion bulb.[5] More common in those of Chinese and Filipino descents.
- **Schilder's disease (myelinoclastic diffuse sclerosis):** Onset is typically in childhood with 1 to 2 large, confluent lesions. Usually progresses to involve widespread, bilateral regions of the CNS, and has variable course and prognosis.[6-7] Etiology is unclear but may have a possible association with preceding infectious illness.

SYNONYMS

MS
Disseminated sclerosis

ICD-10CM CODE
G35 Multiple sclerosis

EPIDEMIOLOGY & DEMOGRAPHICS

PREVALENCE: More common in people raised in northern latitudes and in certain genetic clusters.[1] Global prevalence of MS is estimated to be around 36 per 100,000 people ($\sim$3 million people).[8] There are currently nearly 1 million people living with MS in the United States.[9]

PREDOMINANT SEX & AGE: Female:male ratio is approximately 3:1.[1]

PEAK INCIDENCE: Most common permanently disabling disorder of the central nervous system in young adults.[1] Two thirds of patients have incidence between 20 and 40 yr; mean age of onset is 30 yr. Ranges from infancy to 70 yr.[10]

RACE: Although more common in White people of Northern European descent, MS has been demonstrated to occur across most races and ethnic backgrounds. Recent studies suggest up to 47% higher risk of MS in Black vs. White women in the United States. Hispanic, Asian, and Native American populations have demonstrated lower incidence of MS thus far, compared to White and Black populations. Features of MS that have been more commonly associated with Black patients (compared to White patients) include transverse myelitis, vision loss from optic neuritis, earlier progression to disability, and higher lesion burden. Hispanic patients may also more frequently have optic neuritis and transverse myelitis, as well as younger age of disease onset and more severe disease course. Asian patients may have higher rates of optic nerve and spinal cord involvement.[11]

GENETICS: Frequency of MS in dizygotic twins and siblings is 3% to 5%, and 30% to 50% in monozygotic twins. $\sim$200 genes have been identified that contribute to the risk of developing MS.[1] Most common associations include human leukocyte antigen classes I and II (*DRB1*1501, DQA1*0102, DQB1*0602*), (*DRB1*0405-DQA1*0301-DQB1*0302* in the Mediterranean population). A notable epigenetic interaction between vitamin D and the main MS-linked *HLA-DRB1*1501* allele has been elucidated. Conversely, *HLA-A*02* has been associated with a reduced odds of developing MS.[12]

PHYSICAL FINDINGS & CLINICAL PRESENTATION

Findings depend on the location of the CNS lesion(s) and may include the following:
- Common: Nonspecific complaints such as fatigue (most common, with 80% lifetime prevalence), blurred vision, diplopia, vertigo, falls, hemiparesis, paraparesis, monoparesis, numbness, paresthesias, ataxia, cognitive impairment, depression, anxiety, pseudobulbar affect (involuntary crying or laughing out of context), sexual dysfunction, and bowel/bladder dysfunction
- Visual abnormalities: Horizontal nystagmus, visual field deficits, Marcus Gunn pupil (i.e., relative afferent papillary defect—normal consensual light reflex; however, when swinging a flashlight from the unaffected eye to the affected eye, direct light causes paradoxical pupillary dilation in the affected eye), sixth nerve palsy, internuclear ophthalmoplegia (paresis of the adducting eye on conjugate lateral gaze with simultaneous horizontal nystagmus of the abducting eye) (Fig. 1)
- Corticospinal tract(s) involvement: Transverse myelitis, upper motor neuron signs such as spasticity (particularly leg spasms at night or after prolonged immobility), hyperreflexia, clonus, extensor plantar responses, tonic spasms, upper motor neuron pattern of weakness
- Sensory involvement: May include partial or full dermatomal loss of pain and temperature, loss of vibration (common) and position sense, temperature dysregulation, thoracic band of sensory loss, paresthesias, trigeminal neuralgia

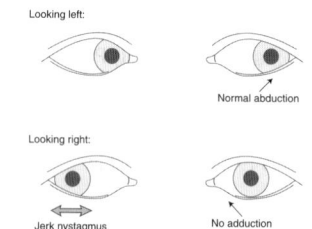

FIG. 1 Internuclear ophthalmoplegia. When the patient in the figure looks to the left (*top row*), both eyes move normally, but when the patient looks to the right (*bottom row*), the left eye fails to adduct ("weak" medial rectus) and the contralateral eye develops a jerk nystagmus. The finding is named for the side with weak adduction (i.e., in this example, a *left* internuclear ophthalmoplegia), and the lesion is in the *ipsilateral* medial longitudinal fasciculus (i.e., *left* medial longitudinal fasciculus in this example). See the text. (From McGee S: *Evidence-based physical diagnosis*, ed 4, Philadelphia, 2018, Elsevier.)

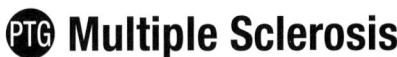

- Ataxia: Intention tremor, dysmetria, dysdiadochokinesis, titubation, inability to tandem gait
- Bladder dysfunction: Detrusor hyperreflexia (urge incontinence), urinary frequency, flaccidity (neurogenic bladder), and dyssynergia (bladder contracts against a closed sphincter)
- **Lhermitte sign:** Flexion of the neck elicits an electrical sensation extending down the spine and occasionally into the extremities, due to involvement of the posterior cervical spinal cord[2,13]
- **Uhthoff phenomenon:** Transient recurrence or worsening of preexisting neurologic deficits with small elevations in core body temperature (e.g., during exercise or warm bathing)[2]

ETIOLOGY

Likely multifactorial, with evidence for autoimmunity (autoreactive T and B lymphocytes), environmental factors (low sunlight exposure, vitamin D deficiency, smoking, obesity, shift work), and genetics (Mendelian and epigenetic). Environmental risk factors during childhood include exposure to certain viruses (e.g., Epstein-Barr virus and human herpes virus 6), low ultraviolet light exposure, and month of birth (higher in spring).[1,14]

DX DIAGNOSIS

- **MS:** Based on the revised 2017 McDonald criteria[2] (Table 1).
- **RRMS:** See Table 1.
- **PPMS:** Insidious progression of neurologic disability for at least 1 yr, independent of disability associated with clinical relapse(s), with at least two of the following: (1) evidence of positive cerebrospinal fluid (CSF)-specific oligoclonal bands (OCBs), and (2) MRI evidence of at least one brain or (3) at least two spinal cord MS-like lesions.[3]
- **MRI diagnostic criteria for dissemination in space:** At least one T_2-hyperintense lesion in at least two of the following regions: Periventricular, cortical or juxtacortical, infratentorial, spinal cord.[2]
- **MRI and CSF diagnostic criteria for dissemination in time:** (1) Presence of both gadolinium-enhancing and nonenhancing lesions on a single MRI; (2) presence of new T_2-hyperintense or enhancing lesion(s) on a subsequent MRI; (3) at least two CSF-specific OCBs.[2]

DIFFERENTIAL DIAGNOSIS[15] (TABLE 2)

- **Autoimmune:** Acute disseminated encephalomyelitis (ADEM), postvaccination encephalomyelitis, neuromyelitis optica spectrum disorder (NMOSD), myelin oligodendrocyte glycoprotein antibody disease (MOGAD), antiphospholipid antibody syndrome, autoimmune glial fibrillary acidic protein (GFAP) astrocytopathy
- **Degenerative:** Amyotrophic lateral sclerosis, primary lateral sclerosis, cerebral autosomal dominant arteriopathy with subcortical infarcts

and leukoencephalopathy (CADASIL), multisystem atrophy
- **Genetic:** Fabry disease, Wilson disease, spinocerebellar ataxia, hereditary spastic paraparesis
- **Hematologic:** Lymphoma, histiocytosis, thrombotic thrombocytopenic purpura
- **Infectious:** Lyme disease, neurosyphilis, HIV, tropical spastic paraparesis (human T-lymphotropic virus type 1 or HTLV-1), progressive multifocal leukoencephalopathy (PML, caused by the JC virus), Listeria, Whipple disease (*Tropheryma whipplei*), acute flaccid myelitis, chronic meningitis, CNS tuberculosis, or fungal disease
- **Inflammatory:** Systemic lupus erythematosus, vasculitis, neurosarcoidosis, Sjögren syndrome, Guillain-Barré syndrome, Behçet disease, celiac disease
- **Toxic/Nutritional/Metabolic:** Vitamin B_{12} deficiency, copper deficiency, nitrous oxide toxicity, inherited leukodystrophies, central pontine myelinolysis
- **Mitochondrial:** Leber hereditary optic neuropathy; mitochondrial encephalopathy, lactic acidosis, and stroke-like episodes (MELAS)
- **Neoplasms:** CNS lymphoma, metastases, paraneoplastic disease, gliomatosis cerebri
- **Vascular:** Susac syndrome, subcortical infarcts, Binswanger disease, amyloid angiopathy, cavernous or arteriovenous malformation, cerebral venous sinus thrombosis

DIAGNOSTIC STUDIES (TABLE 3)

- Lumbar puncture to evaluate for presence of CSF-specific OCBs (Fig. 2), for cases that are atypical, and to evaluate for mimics of MS. Typical CSF abnormalities (Table 4) may include elevated protein (>100 mg/dl), mild pleocytosis, and elevated CSF-specific immunoglobulin G (IgG) synthesis rate. 70% of clinically definite MS (CDMS) demonstrate elevated CSF-specific IgG synthesis and 90% demonstrate CSF-specific OCBs[2] (serum protein electrophoresis should be sent to the lab simultaneously with CSF for both of these tests). False-positive results for IgG synthesis, and rarely for positive OCBs, can be seen in

CNS infections, parainfectious processes, vasculitis, and CNS lymphoma.
- Serum: CBC with differential, comprehensive metabolic panel, liver function tests (LFTs), vitamin B_{12}, copper, 25-OH vitamin D_3.

TABLE 1 Summary of Revised 2017 McDonald Criteria for Diagnosis of Multiple Sclerosis

RRMS/Clinical Attacks	Clinical Lesions	Paraclinical Testing Needed
2	2	None
2	1	MRI dissemination in space *or* a second clinical attack at a different CNS site
1	2	MRI dissemination in time *or* CSF-specific oligoclonal bands
1	1	1. Additional clinical attack at a different CNS site or MRI dissemination in space 2. MRI dissemination in time or CSF-specific oligoclonal bands

Evidence of clinical lesions by physical examination or evoked potentials.
CNS, Central nervous system; *CSF*, cerebrospinal fluid; *MRI dissemination in space*, ≥1 T2 lesions in 2 of the 4 typical areas for MS lesions—periventricular, juxtacortical, infratentorial, or spinal cord; *MRI dissemination in time*, a new lesion at follow-up MRI at any time, or presence of both an enhancing and nonenhancing lesion at any time; *RRMS*, relapsing-remitting multiple sclerosis.

TABLE 2 Conditions That Can Be Mistaken for Multiple Sclerosis and Other Diseases of Myelin

Vascular Disease
Small-vessel cerebrovascular disease
Vasculitis
CADASIL
Antiphospholipid antibody syndrome

Structural Lesions
Craniocervical junction, posterior fossa, or spinal tumors
Cervical spondylosis or disc herniation
Chiari malformation or syrinx

Degenerative Diseases
Hereditary myelopathy
Spinocerebellar degeneration

Infections
HTLV-1 infection
HIV myelopathy or HIV-related cerebritis
Neuroborreliosis (e.g., Lyme disease)
John Cunningham (JC) JC virus/progressive multifocal leukoencephalopathy
Neurosyphilis

Other Inflammatory Conditions
Systemic lupus erythematosus
Sjögren syndrome
Sarcoidosis

Monofocal or Monophasic Demyelinating Syndromes
Neuromyelitis optica spectrum disorder
Acute disseminated encephalomyelitis

Other Conditions
Hashimoto thyroiditis with or without encephalopathy
Nonspecific MRI abnormalities related to migraine, aging, or trauma

CADASIL, Cerebral autosomal dominant arteriopathy with subcortical infarcts and leukoencephalopathy; *HIV*, human immunodeficiency virus; *HTLV*, human T-cell lymphotropic virus; *MRI*, magnetic resonance imaging.
From Goldman L, Schafer AI: *Goldman's Cecil medicine*, ed 24, Philadelphia, 2012, Saunders.

TABLE 3 Comparison of Sensitivity of Laboratory Testing in Multiple Sclerosis

	VER	BAER	SSEP	OCB	MRI
Clinically definite multiple sclerosis	80%-85%*	50%-65%	65%-80%	85%-95%	90%-97%

*Numbers show the percentage of patients with abnormal study results.
BAER, Brain stem auditory evoked response; *MRI,* magnetic resonance imaging; *OCB,* oligoclonal band; *SSEP,* somatosensory evoked potential; *VER,* visual evoked response.
From Jankovic J et al: *Bradley and Daroff's neurology in clinical practice,* ed 8, Philadelphia, 2022, Elsevier.

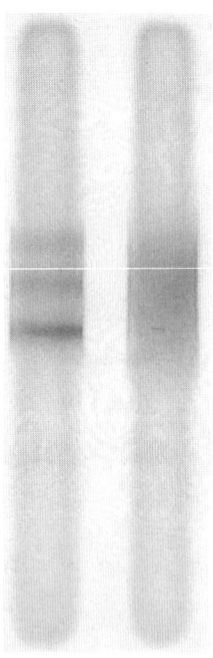

FIG. 2 Electrophoresis of CSF of a patient with multiple sclerosis *(left),* compared to the CSF of someone with no central nervous system inflammatory disease *(right),* shows three distinct, horizontal oligoclonal bands. (From Kaufman DM et al: *Kaufman's clinical neurology for psychiatrists,* ed 9, Philadelphia, 2023, Elsevier.)

TABLE 4 Cerebrospinal Fluid Abnormalities in Multiple Sclerosis

	Albumin	IgG/TP	IgG/Albumin	IgG Index	Oligoclonal Banding of Ig
Clinically definite multiple sclerosis	23%	67%	60%-73%	70%-90%	85%-95%
Normal controls	3%	—	36%	3%	7%*

*Other neurologic disease.
IgG/TP, Immunoglobulin G value/total protein.
From Jankovic J et al: *Bradley and Daroff's neurology in clinical practice,* ed 8, Philadelphia, 2022, Elsevier.

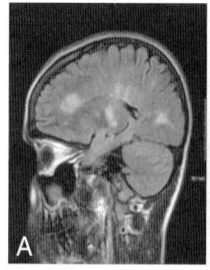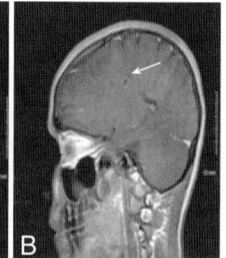

FIG. 3 Multiple sclerosis. (A) Sagittal fluid-attenuated inversion recovery image magnetic resonance scan shows multiple lesions in corpus callosum, "Dawson fingers" (periventricular fingerlike lesions oriented toward the ventricles), along with ovoid and punctuate lesions in the deep white matter. **(B)** Gadolinium-enhanced scan shows an enhancing lesion *(arrow).*

- Consider in the proper clinical setting: AQP4-IgG (to diagnose neuromyelitis optica), MOG-IgG, antinuclear antibody (ANA), ACE (a test with low specificity and sensitivity for sarcoidosis), antineutrophil cytoplasmic antibodies, antiphospholipid and anticardiolipin antibodies, Sjögren antibodies, thyroid stimulating hormone (TSH), free T_4, peripheral blood smear, very-long-chain fatty acids, arylsulfatase A, lactate, pyruvate, urine organic acids, plasma amino acids.
- Consider optical coherence tomography (OCT) or evoked potentials (visual, somatosensory, and brain stem auditory evoked response).

IMAGING
MRI of the brain with and without gadolinium contrast Fig. 3 is recommended in all cases. MRI with and without contrast of the cervical (Fig. E4) and thoracic spines should also be performed, if possible, to assess for spinal cord lesions. MRI assesses for both acute and chronic lesions, as well as for atrophy, and should be repeated at least annually for disease surveillance and monitoring of disease-modifying therapy (DMT) efficacy. A normal MRI of the brain does not definitively exclude early MS but makes it extremely unlikely.[4]

🅡🅧 TREATMENT

NONPHARMACOLOGIC THERAPY
Patient education regarding disease characteristics, treatment options, risks and benefits of treatment, and prognosis. Often, patients need to incorporate intermittent rest periods on a daily basis and when physically active (for energy conservation), and avoid exposure to heat, which typically worsens symptoms (but not the disease).

Recommend physical therapy for new or worsening weakness, incoordination, or spasticity.

ACUTE GENERAL RX (TABLE 5)
For relapses: High-dose intravenous (IV) or oral methylprednisolone (1 g/day for 3 to 5 days).[16] A proton pump inhibitor and insulin sliding scale should be simultaneously administered to prevent gastrointestinal ulcers and treat steroid-induced hyperglycemia.

The Optic Neuritis Treatment Trial showed worse outcomes in optic neuritis after oral methylprednisolone compared with intravenous.[17] However, the COPOUSEP trial published in 2015 demonstrated nearly equivalent efficacy in improvement of symptoms and/or full recovery between 1000 mg daily for 3 days of oral and IV methylprednisolone in all types of relapses. High-dose corticosteroids do not alter long-term outcomes of the disease, but instead accelerate recovery from symptoms of the current relapse.[17-18]

Plasma exchange can be considered for steroid-refractory cases.[19]

CHRONIC Rx
- Most FDA-approved disease-modifying therapies (DMTs) are approved for use only in relapsing forms of MS (which include CIS, RRMS, and active SPMS—or SPMS with relapses). Ocrelizumab and mitoxantrone are the first FDA-approved DMTs for use in PPMS and SPMS, respectively.
- **Injectable DMTs**: These medications include the first generation of MS drugs (interferons and glatiramer acetate), which have a low risk of side effects but modest efficacy in preventing future relapses. Ofatumumab is a newer injectable DMT with high efficacy but higher risk of side effects than the older injectable DMTs.
  1. **Interferons:** Include interferon beta-1a (intramuscular injection [IM Avonex, dose of 30 mcg once per wk; IM Plegridy, starting

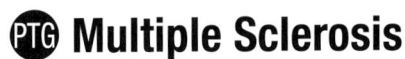

TABLE 5 Approved Medications for Multiple Sclerosis

Generic (Brand) Name and Mode of Administration	Indications(s)	Side Effects	Chemical Structure
Glatiramer acetate, Copaxone Daily SQ injection	To reduce relapse frequency in patients with relapsing-remitting multiple sclerosis (MS) and patients who have experienced a first clinical episode and have MRI features consistent with MS	Injection site reactions, lipoatrophy with prolonged use	Synthetic polymer
IM IFN-β-1a, Avonex Weekly IM injection	To slow accumulation of physical disability and decrease frequency of clinical exacerbations in patients with relapsing forms of MS and patients who have experienced a first clinical episode and have MRI features consistent with MS	Flulike symptoms, injection site reactions, neutropenia, anemia, liver function test abnormalities	Interferon beta-1 alpha
SC IFN-β-1a, Rebif Three times per wk SQ injections	To slow accumulation of physical disability and decrease frequency of clinical exacerbations in relapsing forms of MS	Flulike symptoms, injection site reactions, neutropenia, anemia, liver function test abnormalities	Interferon beta-1-alpha
IFN-β-1b, Betaseron Every other day SQ injections	To reduce the frequency of clinical exacerbations in patients with relapsing forms of MS and patients who have experienced a first clinical episode and have MRI features consistent with MS	Flulike symptoms, injection site reactions, neutropenia, anemia, liver function test abnormalities	Interferon beta-1-beta
Fingolimod, Gilenya Daily oral tablet	To reduce frequency of clinical exacerbations and delay accumulation of physical disability in patients with relapsing forms of MS	Risk of herpes virus infections, bradycardia, macular edema, and changes on pulmonary function test.	Sphingosine-1-phosphate receptor blocker
Natalizumab, Tysabri Monthly IV infusions	As monotherapy for relapsing forms of MS; to delay accumulation of physical disability and reduce frequency of clinical exacerbations	PML brain infection (risk 1:1,000)	α4-integrin adhesion molecule blocker
Mitoxantrone, Novantrone IV chemotherapy	To reduce neurologic disability and/or the frequency of clinical relapses in secondary (chronic) progressive, progressive relapsing or worsening relapsing-remitting MS	Cardiomyopathy, increased risk of secondary lymphoid malignancies	Cytotoxic chemotherapy; synthetic antineoplastic anthracenedione
Teriflunomide, Aubagio Daily oral tablet	To reduce frequency of relapses in relapsing-remitting MS	Hepatotoxicity, bone marrow suppression, peripheral neuropathy	Pyrimidine synthesis inhibitor
Dimethyl fumarate, Tecfidera Twice daily capsule	To reduce frequency of relapses in relapsing-remitting MS	Flushing, gastrointestinal side effects, lymphopenia	Dimethyl fumarate
Ocrelizumab, Ocrevus Every-6-mo infusion	To reduce frequency of relapses in relapsing-remitting MS; slows progression in primary progressive MS	Infusion reactions; risk of infection	B-cell antibody
Cladribine 2 wk of oral pills/yr	To reduce frequency of relapses in relapsing-remitting MS	Potential cancer risk; risk of infection	Purine synthesis modulator

IV, Intravenous; *MRI,* magnetic resonance imaging; *MS,* multiple sclerosis.
From Jankovic J et al: *Bradley and Daroff's neurology in clinical practice,* ed 8, Philadelphia, 2022, Elsevier.

dose of 63 mcg uptitrated over 1 mo to 125 mcg every 2 wk; subcutaneous (SC) Rebif, dose of 22 or 44 mcg three times per wk]) and **interferon beta-1b** (SC Betaseron, SC Extavia; doses of 0.25 mg every other day). Involve a complex and multifactorial mechanism of action, including increased expression of antiinflammatory mediators and downregulated expression of proinflammatory cytokines. Side effects can include fatigue, flulike symptoms, injection site reactions such as skin necrosis, depression, hepatotoxicity, seizures, anemia, leukopenia, thrombocytopenia, and thrombotic microangiopathy. CBC with differential, LFTs, and thyroid function tests should be obtained before initiating and regularly monitored during

treatment (initially every 3 mo for 6 mo, then annually).
2. **Glatiramer acetate** (SC Copaxone, SC Glatopa; doses of 20 mg daily or 40 mg three times per wk): Synthetic protein that simulates myelin basic protein and shifts T cells from the proinflammatory Th1 to regulatory Th2 profile. Common side effects include injection site reactions (such as lipoatrophy and skin necrosis) and brief postinjection reactions such as flushing, chest tightness, tachycardia, and dyspnea; no laboratory monitoring is needed.
3. **Ofatumumab** (SC Kesimpta; dose of 20 mg weekly for 3 wk, no injection for 1 wk, then 20 mg per mo): Anti-CD20 monoclonal antibody injectable. Side effects can include injection site reactions, headache, hepatitis

B virus (HBV) reactivation, low immunoglobulins, and increased risk of infections (especially upper respiratory tract infections [URIs]). Before initiating and during treatment, obtain CBC with differential (including lymphocyte subsets), LFTs, immunoglobulins, and HBV and JC virus antibodies. Live or live-attenuated vaccinations should be administered at least 1 mo before starting treatment.
- **Oral DMTs:** These medications are newer and more efficacious than the initial injectable DMTs in preventing MS relapses, but carry a higher risk of serious side effects and infections. Review the patient's general risk of infections before starting any oral DMT.
1. Fingolimod (Gilenya; dose of 0.5 mg daily), siponimod (Mayzent; starting dose of

0.25 mg daily, titrated up to 1 to 2 mg daily over 4 to 5 days), ozanimod (Zeposia; starting dose of 0.23 mg uptitrated over 1 wk to 0.92 mg daily), or ponesimod (Ponvory; starting dose of 2 mg uptitrated over 2 wk to 20 mg daily): Mechanism of action involves sphingosine-1-phosphate receptor modulation and lymphocyte sequestration. Side effects can include diarrhea, headache, back pain, abdominal pain, cough, hepatotoxicity, bradycardia with the first dose (requiring cardiac monitoring and ECG for at least 8 h after administration), arrhythmia, orthostatic hypotension, hypertension, pancytopenia, macular edema (requiring ophthalmologic exam at baseline, at 3 mo, and annually thereafter for those with history of diabetes or uveitis), increased risk of infections (including PML, cryptococcal meningitis, herpes simplex virus [HSV] encephalitis, disseminated VZV), posterior reversible encephalopathy syndrome (PRES), increased risk of skin cancers (requiring regular skin examinations), and reduced pulmonary function. Before initiating treatment, obtain baseline HSV, JC virus, and VZV serologies, CBC with differential, LFTs, macular OCT, and possibly CYP2C9 genotype (if considering siponimod); monitor CBC with differential and LFTs every 3 to 6 mo during treatment. Live or live-attenuated vaccinations should be administered at least 1 mo before starting treatment.

2. **Teriflunomide** (Aubagio; dose of 14 mg daily): Reversible inhibitor of pyrimidine synthesis (enzyme dihydroorotate dehydrogenase). Side effects can include headache, nausea, diarrhea, hypertension, alopecia, peripheral neuropathy, paresthesias, severe hepatotoxicity, hypersensitivity reactions (anaphylaxis, angioedema, Stevens-Johnson syndrome, toxic epidermal necrolysis, drug reaction with eosinophilia and systemic symptoms [DRESS]), and interstitial lung disease. Patients should avoid becoming pregnant while on teriflunomide (pregnancy category X). Serum levels can be measured, and the drug can be eliminated by a course of activated charcoal or cholestyramine. Before initiating treatment, check baseline blood pressure, CBC with differential, LFTs, and tuberculosis (TB) test; monitor monthly LFTs for the first 6 mo, and CBC and LFTs every 3 to 6 mo during treatment.

3. **Dimethyl fumarate** (Tecfidera; starting dose of 120 mg twice daily for 2 wk, then 240 mg twice daily), **diroximel fumarate** (Vumerity; starting dose of 231 mg twice daily for 1 wk, then 462 mg twice daily), or **monomethyl fumarate** (Bafiertam; starting dose of 95 mg twice daily for 1 wk, then 190 mg twice daily): Inhibit transcription of nuclear factor-κB (NF-κB; in the nuclear factor erythroid 2–related factor 2 [Nrf-2] pathway). Side effects can include nausea, abdominal discomfort (can be reduced with use of H2 blockers or proton pump inhibitors), pruritus, and flushing (can be reduced with concurrent use of aspirin and taking with food)—especially during the first month—and rarely, lymphopenia, with increased risk of infections such as PML. Before initiating treatment, check CBC with differential, LFTs, VZV and JC virus antibodies; monitor CBC with differential and LFTs every 3 to 6 mo during treatment.

4. **Cladribine** (Mavenclad; total dose of 3.5 mg/kg administered orally in two short courses 1 yr apart): A purine antimetabolite that inhibits DNA synthesis and depletes both T and B lymphocytes. FDA-approved for use in relapsing forms of MS, except for CIS. Side effects can include hematologic toxicity, alopecia, increased risk of infections, increased risk of malignancy, weight loss, and hepatic injury. Pregnancy should be avoided during treatment and for at least 6 mo after the last dose, and breastfeeding is contraindicated during treatment days and for 10 days after the last dose. It is also contraindicated in patients who are immunocompromised, have active chronic infections, or have cancer. CBC with differential, TB test, and viral serologies (e.g., HIV, VZV, HSV, hepatitis B and C, JC virus) should be checked before initiating treatment and monitored regularly during treatment. Live or live-attenuated vaccinations should be administered at least 1 mo before starting treatment.

- **IV DMTs:** These are generally the newest and most efficacious for preventing MS relapses. They consequently also carry a higher risk of serious side effects and infections. Live or live-attenuated vaccinations should be administered at least 1 mo before starting treatment with any of these.

1. **Natalizumab** (Tysabri; dose of 300 mg monthly): A humanized monoclonal antibody that binds to the lymphocyte surface protein α4-integrin, which inhibits binding to VCAM-1 and, therefore, movement of lymphocytes across the bloodstream. It has been associated with a *higher* risk of PML than other immunomodulatory therapies. Testing for JC virus antibody (along with CBC with differential and LFTs) should be done every 6 mo because conversion to a positive antibody occurs at increased frequency while on this drug. If positive, PML is still rare, but the risk increases with increased length of therapy (>2 yr), history of chemotherapy or prior immunosuppression, and high level of JC virus antibodies. Other potential serious side effects can include infusion reactions, HSV and other infections, hepatotoxicity, and thrombocytopenia.

2. **Ocrelizumab** (Ocrevus; dose of 600 mg every 6 mo, with the first dose divided as 300 mg given 2 wk apart): Humanized monoclonal antibody to CD20+ B cells. FDA-approved for use in PPMS as well as all relapsing forms of MS. Side effects can include leukopenia, low immunoglobulins, infusion reactions, increased risk of infections (upper and lower respiratory tract infections, UTI, HSV, skin infections), HBV reactivation, and possibly an increased risk of breast cancer. Before starting treatment, obtain baseline CBC with differential, immunoglobulins, TB test, and viral serologies, including HBV, HCV, VZV, HSV, HIV, and JC virus. Monitor CBC with differential (including lymphocyte subsets), immunoglobulins, HBV, and JC virus antibodies 1 to 2 times per yr. This medication is contraindicated in patients with history of active HBV infection.

3. **Alemtuzumab** (Lemtrada; dose of 12 mg daily for 5 days, then 12 mg daily for 3 days 1 yr later): Anti-CD52 humanized monoclonal antibody and second-line therapy for patients who have failed at least two FDA-approved MS therapies. FDA-approved for use in relapsing forms of MS, except for CIS. Side effects can include the development of autoimmune conditions (34% developed autoimmune thyroid disorders), cytopenias, hepatotoxicity, infusion reactions, stroke, arterial dissection, hemophagocytic lymphohistiocytosis (HLH), bleeding or clotting disorders such as immune thrombocytopenic purpura (ITP) and TTP, pneumonitis, Goodpasture disease, increased risk of certain cancers, and increased risk of infections including PML. Only available through a restricted access program. It is contraindicated in patients who are immunocompromised or have chronic active infections. Requires monthly monitoring of CBC with differential (including lymphocyte subsets), LFTs, TSH, renal function tests, and urinalysis until at least 4 yr after the last course, and HSV prophylaxis for at least 2 mo after each dose.

4. **Mitoxantrone** (Novantrone; 12 mg/m^2 every 3 mo for 2 yr): An antineoplastic anthracenedione (DNA-reactive agent) that inhibits B-cell, T-cell, and macrophage proliferation and impairs antigen presentation. FDA-approved for use in SPMS, progressive-relapsing MS, and worsening RRMS; however, now used very infrequently. Potential serious side effects include secondary acute myeloid leukemia, neutropenia, and cardiotoxicity (CHF). Is contraindicated if baseline neutrophil count <1,500 cells/mm^3 and hepatic impairment (due to reduced clearance). Requires initial evaluation and regular monitoring (prior to each dose) of CBC with differential, LFTs, ECG, echocardiogram (for left ventricular ejection fraction), and pregnancy test if relevant (pregnancy category D).

- Symptomatic therapy:
1. **Gait dysfunction:** Initial management should be referral to physical therapy, use of ankle-foot orthoses (for footdrop), and/or mobility aids. Dalfampridine (Ampyra) is a potassium channel blocker that is FDA-approved to improve walking speed (objectively measured by a timed 25-ft walk

test) in patients with MS; its use is contra-indicated in patients with epilepsy.

2. **Spasticity:** Initial management should be twice-daily stretching exercises and referral to physical therapy. Can next consider baclofen (starting dose of 10 mg twice daily) or tizanidine (starting dose of 2 mg nightly; requires monitoring of liver enzymes). For severe spasticity not responsive to these medications, dantrolene (starting dose of 25 mg daily; requires monitoring of liver enzymes) or diazepam (average daily dose of 15 mg) may be tried. Onabotulinum toxin type A injection can be used for focal intractable spasticity. Intrathecal baclofen pump can be used for generalized intractable spasticity. Acute worsening of spasticity may be caused by infections such as UTI, injury, recent surgery, or colder temperatures.[20]

3. **Urge incontinence and retention:** Obtain urinalysis and post-void residual bladder ultrasound. Recommend fluid restriction at night, scheduled voiding, and avoidance of caffeine and alcohol. Incontinence can be initially treated with anticholinergic/muscarinic therapy such as oxybutynin, trospium, tolterodine, or solifenacin. Mirabegron is a beta-3 agonist indicated for treatment of neurogenic detrusor overactivity (overactive or neurogenic bladder). Urinary retention can be treated with tamsulosin. In both cases, UTI or bladder infection should be ruled out. Intermittent catheterization, intradetrusor onabotulinum toxin A injections, and neuromodulation (tibial nerve stimulation) are more advanced options for severe neurogenic bladder symptoms and require management by a urologist.[21]

4. **Dysesthesias:** Can treat with carbamazepine (200 mg twice daily), oxcarbazepine (starting dose of 300 mg daily), gabapentin (starting dose of 300 mg daily), or pregabalin (starting dose of 50 mg daily).

5. **Fatigue:** Initial management should involve medication review, depression screening, evaluating for underlying sleep disorder, energy conservation strategies, exercise program, and weight loss for obesity. Can next consider medical management with amantadine (100 mg twice daily), modafinil (starting dose of 100 mg every morning), or a stimulant such as methylphenidate.

6. **Tremor:** Can treat with clonazepam (starting dose of 0.5 mg daily), propranolol (starting dose of 20 to 40 mg twice daily), or gabapentin (starting dose of 300 mg daily).

7. **Cognitive impairment:** Can objectively screen with the Symbol Digit Modalities Test, if available. Assess for other causes of cognitive impairment, such as neurodegenerative disease, depression, fatigue, disordered sleep, and polypharmacy. Recommend conservative strategies, such as the use of checklists, reminders, diaries, and calendars, and regular physical exercise and social activity.

8. **Depression and anxiety:** Refer for cognitive-behavioral therapy. Consider starting a selective serotonin reuptake inhibitor (SSRI) or serotonin norepinephrine reuptake inhibitor (SNRI). Distinguish between depression and pseudobulbar affect, which is treated with dextromethorphan/quinidine (Nuedexta).

DISPOSITION

Most patients have complete or near-complete recovery weeks to months after a relapse, even without acute treatment with high-dose steroids. Typically, two relapses occur in RRMS patient per year (75% will have >1 relapse). Although the rate of disease progression is highly variable, there is higher risk of greater long-term disability with higher relapse rate during the first 2 to 5 yr, poor recovery from initial relapses, older age of onset, involvement of multiple systems, male sex, African American, and primary progressive disease.

DMTs have significantly improved since their introduction, and the current treatment goal is no relapses and no disease progression on imaging.

REFERRAL

- Referral to a neurologist is highly recommended. Referral to an MS specialist should be considered in cases of poor response to initial therapy and/or if there is concern about complications of therapies.

- Referrals for physical, speech, and occupational therapy for motor, sensory, and speech symptoms.
- Referral to a mental health provider and/or psychiatrist for depression/anxiety.
- Referral to neuropsychology for cognitive impairment symptoms.
- Referral to urology if bladder-sphincter dyssynergia is possible, if symptoms are not responsive to first-line medications, or in case of complications such as recurrent UTI, hematuria, renal impairment, hydronephrosis, or stress incontinence.

⚠ PEARLS & CONSIDERATIONS

- Pseudorelapse, which is a recurrence of symptoms from a prior relapse (either symptomatic or asymptomatic), may occur with heat, exercise, fatigue, fever, or infections (urinary tract infections are common in patients with MS). Symptoms should subside within 24 h after elimination of the trigger; if symptoms persist, consider obtaining MRI to rule out a new symptomatic relapse.
- Pseudoprogression is the insidious progression of neurologic disability due to factors unrelated to MS pathogenesis, typically that of other comorbidities (degenerative joint disease, neurodegenerative disease, etc.).
- Headache, fever, altered mental status, CSF pleocytosis, or recurrent relapses over days to weeks raises concern for CNS infection or ADEM.

REFERENCES
Available at eBooks.Health.Elsevier.com.

RELATED CONTENT
Multiple Sclerosis (Patient Information)
Neuromyelitis Optica Spectrum Disorder (Related Key Topic)
Optic Neuritis (Related Key Topic)

AUTHORS: **NATASHA CHOUDHURY, MD,** and **COREY ELAM GOLDSMITH, MD, FAAN**

BASIC INFORMATION

DEFINITION

Myasthenia gravis (MG) is an autoimmune disorder affecting postsynaptic neuromuscular transmission, most commonly mediated by antibodies directed against the nicotinic acetylcholine receptor (AChR) of the neuromuscular junction. Anti-AChR antibodies cause a decrease in functional postsynaptic ACh receptors, resulting in fatigable weakness. A small percentage of MG patients lack AChR antibodies, and a subset of these patients possess antibodies against muscle-specific tyrosine kinase (MuSK) or low-density lipoprotein receptor–related protein 4 (LRP4), which both affect pre- and postsynaptic function of the neuromuscular junction.[1,2] Finally, a portion of AChR antibody-negative myasthenia patients do not possess any detectable antibodies, and this group of patients is appropriately termed "seronegative." A classification of MG is described in Table 1.

SYNONYM

MG

ICD-10CM CODES
G70.00	Myasthenia gravis without (acute) exacerbation
G70.01	Myasthenia gravis with (acute) exacerbation
P94.0	Transient neonatal myasthenia gravis

EPIDEMIOLOGY & DEMOGRAPHICS

INCIDENCE (IN U.S.): 8 to 10 cases annually per 1 million persons. It is the most common disorder of neuromuscular junction transmission.
PREVALENCE (IN U.S.): 150 to 250 cases per 1 million persons.
PREDOMINANT SEX: Females are affected more often than males (3:2) in adults; they are equally affected in the elderly.
PEAK INCIDENCE: Female, second to third decades; male, sixth to eighth decades.
GENETICS: Increased frequency of HLA-B8, DR3.

PHYSICAL FINDINGS & CLINICAL PRESENTATION

- The hallmark of MG is weakness worsened with exercise and improved with rest.
- Generalized weakness involving proximal muscles, the diaphragm, and neck extensors is common.
- Weakness is confined to eyelids and extraocular muscles in approximately 15% of patients (Figs. 1, E2, 3, and Box 1). This is referred to as ocular myasthenia gravis.
- Bulbar symptoms of ptosis, diplopia, dysarthria, and dysphagia are common.
- Reflexes, sensation, and coordination remain normal.

ETIOLOGY

An antibody-mediated decrease in nicotinic AChRs in the postsynaptic neuromuscular junction results in defective neuromuscular transmission and subsequent muscle weakness and fatigue. Early-onset MG is associated with *HLA-B8.1*, whereas late-onset MG is associated with *HLA-DQB1, HLA-DQA1,* and *HLA-DRB1.*[3]

Some myasthenia gravis patients present with MuSK or LRP4 antibodies instead of AChR antibodies. The MuSK antibody is present in about 40% to 50% of the subset of individuals who lack the AChR antibody, and the LRP4 antibody is present in a fraction of the remainder.[1] Both MuSK and LRP4 antibodies interrupt the process of AChR aggregation at the neuromuscular junction. Anti-MuSK patients have a similar syndrome to AChR MG, although they may have more bulbar weakness, facial tongue and proximal muscle atrophy, and either lack of or paradoxic response to pyridostigmine. Anti-LRP4 patients generally have milder symptoms that favor ocular findings. However, serious cases can still yield severe clinical symptoms.[1] Both MuSK and LRP4 antibody MG have not been shown to have any association with thymoma.[4]

Less than 10% of myasthenia gravis patients are seronegative for AChR, MuSK, and LRP4 antibodies. This syndrome is termed *seronegative myasthenia gravis* and presents with a higher proportion of entirely ocular symptoms. Generally, this group of patients responds well to classic MG therapies, including pyridostigmine, steroids, immunosuppression, and thymectomy.

Serologic and clinical presentation of myasthenia gravis subgroups are summarized in Table 2.

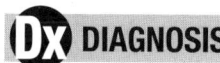 DIAGNOSIS

DIFFERENTIAL DIAGNOSIS

Lambert-Eaton myasthenic syndrome, botulism, medication-induced myasthenia, chronic progressive external ophthalmoplegia, congenital myasthenic syndromes, thyroid disease, basilar meningitis, intracranial mass lesion with cranial neuropathy, Miller-Fisher variant of Guillain-Barré syndrome

WORKUP

- Edrophonium (Tensilon) test (Fig. E4): Useful in MG patients with ocular symptoms, although uncommonly used now. Cardiac monitoring and atropine ready at the bedside are essential.
- Patients with MG may also have a positive ice-pack test (Fig. E5).
- Repetitive nerve stimulation: Successive stimulation shows decrement of muscle action

---

TABLE 1 Osserman Classification Used by the Myasthenia Gravis Foundation of America to Standardize Clinical Symptoms[1]

Class I	Any ocular muscle weakness
Class II	Ocular muscle weakness of any severity, MILD limb weakness
Class IIa	Predominantly limb and/or axial muscle weakness
Class IIb	Predominantly bulbar and/or respiratory muscle weakness
Class III	Ocular muscle weakness of any severity, MODERATE weakness of other muscles
Class IIIa	Predominantly limb and/or axial muscle weakness
Class IIIb	Predominantly bulbar and/or respiratory muscle weakness
Class IV	Ocular muscle weakness of any severity, SEVERE weakness of other muscles
Class IVa	Predominantly limb and/or axial muscle weakness
Class IVb	Predominantly bulbar and/or respiratory muscle weakness
Class V	Intubation with or without mechanical ventilation

[1]Jaretzki A et al: Myasthenia gravis: recommendations for clinical research standards. Task Force of the Medical Scientific Advisory Board of the Myasthenia Gravis Foundation of America, *Neurology* 55:16-23, 2000.
From Parrillo JE, Dellinger RP: *Critical care medicine: principles of diagnosis and management in the adult,* ed 5, Philadelphia, 2019, Elsevier.

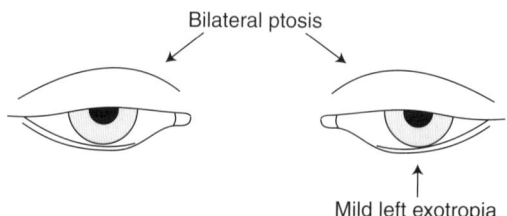

FIG. 1 Myasthenia gravis. Myasthenia gravis may mimic any ocular disorder causing diplopia, although most often it mimics weakness of the superior rectus muscle or medial rectus muscle (i.e., difficulty with sustained elevation or adduction of the eye, respectively). Clues to the diagnosis of myasthenia gravis are associated ptosis, fluctuating course, and normal pupils. (From McGee S: *Evidence-based physical diagnosis,* ed 4, Philadelphia, 2018, Elsevier.)

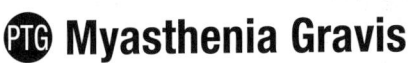

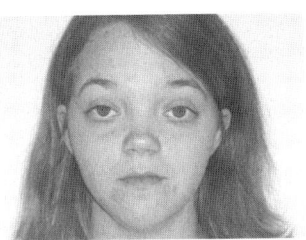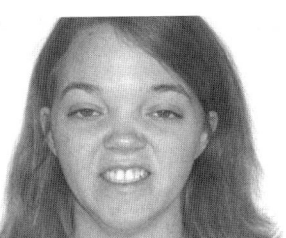

FIG. 3 Typical myasthenic facies. At rest *(left)*, there is slight bilateral lid ptosis, which is partially compensated by asymmetric contraction of the frontalis muscle, raising the right eyebrow. During attempted smile *(right)*, there is contraction of the medial portion of the upper lip and horizontal contraction of the corners of the mouth without the natural upward curling, producing a "sneer." (From Jankovic J et al: *Bradley and Daroff's neurology in clinical practice,* ed 8, Philadelphia 2022, Elsevier.)

BOX 1   Ocular Findings in Myasthenia Gravis

1. Weakness usually involves one or more ocular muscles without overt pupillary abnormality.
2. Weakness is typically variable, fluctuating, and fatigable.
3. Ptosis that shifts from one eye to the other is virtually pathognomonic of MG.
4. With limited ocular excursion, saccades are superfast, producing ocular "quiver."
5. After downgaze, upgaze produces lid overshoot ("lid twitch")
6. Pseudo-internuclear ophthalmoplegia—limited adduction, with nystagmoid jerks in abducting eye.
7. In asymmetric ptosis, covering the ptotic eye may relieve contraction of the opposite frontalis.
8. Passively lifting a ptotic lid may cause the opposite lid to fall: "Enhanced ptosis" or "curtain sign."
9. Edrophonium may improve only some of several weak ocular muscles; others may actually become weaker.
10. Edrophonium may relieve asymmetric ptosis and produce retraction of the opposite lid from frontalis contraction.
11. The opposite lid may droop further as the more involved lid improves after edrophonium.
12. Cold applied to the eye may improve lid ptosis: "Ice-pack test" (see Fig. E5).

From Jankovic J et al: *Bradley and Daroff's neurology in clinical practice,* ed 8, Philadelphia, 2022, Elsevier.

potential in clinically weak muscle; may be negative in up to 50%.
- Single-fiber electromyography: Highly sensitive; abnormal in up to 95% of patients.
- Serum AChR antibodies MuSK and/or LRP4 antibodies.

LABORATORY TESTS
- Forced vital capacity (FVC) is the most useful test for assessing neuromuscular respiratory status. Patients with an FVC of <20 ml/kg are at high risk of respiratory failure and should be monitored in an ICU setting. Although the decision of when to intubate is a clinical one, FVC falling below 10 to 15 ml/kg generally requires intubation.
- CT scan with contrast of anterior chest to look for thymoma (about 10% of patients) or thymic hyperplasia (about 80% of patients). Prevalence increases with age.
- Thyroid-stimulating hormone and free T$_4$ to rule out thyroid disease.

(Rx) TREATMENT

NONPHARMACOLOGIC THERAPY
- Patient education to facilitate recognition of worsening symptoms and impress need for medical evaluation at onset of clinical deterioration
- Avoidance of selected drugs (Table 3) known to provoke exacerbations of MG (β-blockers, aminoglycoside and quinolone antibiotics, penicillamine, interferons, class I antiarrhythmics [procainamide, quinidine, etc.])
- Prompt treatment of infections, diet modification, and speech evaluation with dysphagia

ACUTE GENERAL RX (TABLE E4)
- Symptomatic treatment with acetylcholinesterase inhibitors:
  1. Pyridostigmine 30 to 60 mg PO q4 to 6h initially; onset of effect is 30 min, duration 4 h. May be titrated up to 120 mg every 4 h. GI upset is common with higher doses and may respond to hyoscyamine.

- Immunosuppressive treatment with corticosteroids is first-line treatment, and is often transitioned to a nonsteroidal immunosuppressive agent such as azathioprine or mycophenolate to avoid the significant side effects of long-term steroid use:
  1. Prednisone initiated at 10 to 20 mg daily titrated by 5-mg increments to effect or dose of 1 mg/kg/day with improvement in 2 to 4 wk and maximal response by 3 to 6 mo.
  2. Azathioprine initiated at 50 mg daily titrated to 2 to 3 mg/kg/day with clinical effect in 6 to 12 mo. Azathioprine is not recommended in patients with no thiopurine methyltransferase activity.
  3. Mycophenolate mofetil 500 mg twice a day titrated to 2 g/day with clinical effect in 3 to 6 mo, but can be up to 12 mo.
- Targeted immunotherapy for myasthenia gravis allows quicker and more effective treatment with fewer side effects. Multiple new therapies are currently being researched and/or in clinical trials, including Fc receptor inhibitors, complement inhibitors, IL-6 inhibitors, chimeric antigen receptor (CAR) and chimeric autoantibody receptor (CAAR) T cell therapy, and hematopoietic stem cell transplantation.[5] A current list of some alternative agents is below:
  1. Efgartigimod alfa given at 10 mg/kg for 4 wk in weekly infusions with clinical effect within 1 mo. This drug is an Fc receptor inhibitor that promotes IgG degradation and was approved by the FDA in 2021. Further research is needed to determine the long term benefit of this drug, but it can be considered as a glucocorticoid-sparing bridge until slower-acting agents such as azathioprine and mycophenolate take effect.[6]
  2. Ravulizumab initiated as IV infusion at 2.4-3 g (weight based) followed by 3-3.6 g (weight based) 2 wk after loading dose, followed by every 8 wk afterwards. This drug is a human monoclonal antibody that binds complement C5 similar to eculizumab but with a more convenient dosing schedule. It was FDA approved for AChR antibody positive patients in 2022.[7]
  3. Eculizumab initiated at 900 mg IV weekly for four doses, then 1200 mg on the 5th wk and every 2 wk afterwards. Like ravulizumab, this drug is a complement inhibitor approved for adult patients who are acetylcholine-antibody positive and have severe symptoms despite current immunotherapy use.
  4. Cyclosporine initiated at 5 mg/kg/day with clinical effect within 1 to 2 mo. Note a faster onset of effect than azathioprine or mycophenolate, but also a less tolerable side effect profile due to concerns for renal toxicity and drug interactions.
  5. Tacrolimus initiated at 0.1 mg/kg/day divided into two doses then titrated to plasma concentration of 7 to 8 ng/ml with clinical effect within 6 to 12 mo. This drug is

TABLE 2   Serologic and Clinical Presentation of Myasthenia Gravis Subgroups[1-8]

	AChR Antibody	MuSK Antibody	LRP4 Antibody	Striated Muscle Antigens Titin Antibody RyR Antibody	Age at Onset Sex	Clinical Findings	Response to Therapy	Response to Thymectomy	Prognosis
Ocular MG	50%-75%	None	None	None	Older Male	Ocular	Good	Good	Good (but 50% can develop generalized MG in 2 yr)
Early-onset generalized MG	80%-85% (high titer)	None	None	None-rare	<50 yr	General	Rarely needs immuno-suppression	Good	Less severe Low mortality
Late-onset generalized MG	None-rare	None	None	50% 54% titin 33% RyR	≥50 yr	General	Often requires immuno-suppression	Poor	Severe
Thymomatous-associated MG	Positive, nearly 100% (low titer)	None	None	95% 50% titin 47% RyR	Ranges: Older but <40 yr if RyR	General If RyR: Ocular, bulbar, respiratory weakness	Often requires immuno-suppression	Fair	RyR: Invasive, malignant thymoma Severe Higher mortality
Generalized MG MuSK positive	None	100%	None	None	Younger female	Facial, bulbar, neck, respiratory weakness paraspinal, esophageal muscles	Poor response to AChE inhibitors	Poor (no thymic changes)	Severe, progressive course
Generalized MG LRP4 positive	None	None	100%	None	Younger female	General	Good	Not enough data	Fair
MG with thymic hyperplasia	89%	None	None	None	Younger female	General	Good	Good	Good
ACh antibody negative	Negative	Negative	Negative	Present	Younger female	General	Poor		Fair

ACh, Acetylcholine; *AChE,* acetylcholinesterase; *AChR,* acetylcholine receptor; *MG,* myasthenia gravis; *MuSK,* muscle-specific tyrosine kinase; *LRP4,* low-density lipoprotein receptor-related protein 4; *RyR,* ryanodine receptor.

[1]Romi F et al: Myasthenia gravis patients with ryanodine receptor antibodies have distinctive clinical features, *Eur J Neurol* 14:617-620, 2007.
[2]Romi F et al: Myasthenia gravis: clinical, immunological, and therapeutic advances, *Acta Neurol Scand* 111:134-141, 2005.
[3]Akaishi T et al: Response to treatment of myasthenia gravis according to clinical subtype, *BMC Neurol* 16:225, 2016.
[4]Gilhus NE, Verschuuren JJ: Myasthenia gravis: subgroup classification and therapeutic strategies, *Lancet Neurol* 14:1023-1036, 2015.
[5]Hong Y et al: Autoantibody profile and clinical characteristics in a cohort of Chinese adult myasthenia gravis patients, *J Neuroimmunol* 298:51-57, 2016.
[6]Gilhus NE et al: Myasthenia gravis-autoantibody characteristics and their implications for therapy, *Nat Rev Neurol* 12:259-268, 2016.
[7]Roberts PF et al: Thymectomy in the treatment of ocular myasthenia gravis, *J Thorac Cardiovasc Surg* 122:562-568, 2001.
[8]Rivner MH et al: Clinical features of LRP4/agrin-antibody-positive myasthenia gravis: a multicenter study, *Muscle Nerve* 62(3):333-343, 2020. Available from https://doi.org/10.1002/mus.26985.
From Parrillo JE, Dellinger RP: *Critical care medicine: principles of diagnosis and management in the adult*, ed 5, Philadelphia, 2019, Elsevier.

better tolerated than cyclosporine but still has potential for serious side effects.

6. Rituximab initiated at 1 g every 2 wk for two doses, OR 375 mg/m[2] weekly for four doses. Generally used in refractory MG or earlier in MuSK antibody MG. Redosing interval varies per protocol and by clinical response of the patient.

• Plasmapheresis and IV immunoglobulin (IVIG) are short-term options for immunotherapy during an exacerbation. There is no significant difference in efficacy between IVIG and plasmapheresis.[8]

• Mechanical ventilation is lifesaving in the setting of a myasthenic crisis. Consider elective intubation if forced vital capacity is <10 to 15 ml/kg.

• Fig. E6 illustrates a flowchart for the management of myasthenic crisis.

SURGICAL Rx

• In thymomatous MG, thymectomy is indicated in all patients. If the tumor cannot be surgically resected, chemotherapy can be considered for prevention of local invasion and symptom relief.

• For nonthymomatous AChR-antibody positive MG, thymectomy improves clinical outcomes and reduces the need for steroids sustained over at least a 5-yr period. Surgical referral should be considered in patients <60 yr old without significant medical comorbidities even if no frank thymic tissue is seen on imaging, especially if they are refractory to therapy.[9,10]

• MuSK and LRP4 myasthenia are not associated with thymic pathology and generally thymectomy is not beneficial for these patients.[11]

TABLE 3 Medications to Avoid in Myasthenia Gravis[1]

Medications to Avoid	Examples	Recommendation for Avoidance	Mechanism of Weakness
Antibiotics			
Aminoglycosides	Gentamycin Streptomycin	Contraindicated	Blocks ACh receptor, prevents release of ACh
	Tobramycin Amikacin	Less likely problematic	
Antimalarials	Quinine Chloroquine	Contraindicated	Presynaptic blockage of voltage-dependent sodium channels and postsynaptic potentiation of depolarization
Macrolides	Erythromycin, Tetracycline Azithromycin	Relative	Affects presynaptic transmission
Fluoroquinolones	Moxifloxacin Ciprofloxacin Levofloxacin Ofloxacin	FDA black box warning	Unknown
Ketolide	Telithromycin	FDA black box warning	Unknown
	Polymyxins	Contraindicated	Presynaptic and postsynaptic effects
Cardiovascular			
Antiarrhythmics	Procainamide Propafenone	Contraindicated	Decreases the release of ACh Sodium influx blocker
β-Blockers	Propranolol Atenolol Ophthalmic timolol	Relative	Unclear—may be at the neuromuscular junction or muscle membrane
Calcium channel blocker	Verapamil Amlodipine	Relative	Presynaptic and postsynaptic blockade of L-type calcium channels
Anticonvulsants			
	Phenytoin	Relative	Depressed postsynaptic response to ACh; inhibition of calcium channel; increase in muscle membrane threshold
	Carbamazepine	Relative	Triggers immune response
	Gabapentin	Relative	Binds voltage-gated calcium channel
Chemotherapeutic Agents			
	Doxorubicin Etoposide Cisplatin	Relative	Unknown
Others			
	Interferon	Relative	Autoantibody production
Neuromuscular blocking agents	Atracurium Cisatracurium Vecuronium	Relative	Blocks ACh receptors
Statins		Relative	Unknown
Corticosteroids		Relative	Direct blocking of ACh receptor through ionic channels
Botulinum toxin		Contraindicated	Impairs synaptic transmission
Magnesium		Relative	Impairs synaptic transmission
Penicillamine		Contraindicated	Binds the ACh receptor; induces antibodies to receptor

ACh, Acetylcholine; *FDA,* Food and Drug Administration.
[1]Ahmed A, Simmons Z: Drugs which may exacerbate or induce myasthenia gravis: a clinician's guide, *Internet J Neurol* 10:1-8, 2008.
From Parrillo JE, Dellinger RP: *Critical care medicine: principles of diagnosis and management in the adult,* ed 5, Philadelphia, 2019, Elsevier.

DISPOSITION
Course of disease is highly variable. Mortality rate has decreased from 75% to 4.5% over the past four decades.

REFERRAL
- Referral to a general neurologist or neuromuscular specialist is appropriate.
- Surgical referral for thymectomy in selected cases (see "Surgical Rx").

⦸ PEARLS & CONSIDERATIONS
- Sustained upward or lateral gaze and arm abduction for 120 sec may be necessary to elicit subtle signs on examination.
- Myasthenic patients can worsen rapidly and warrant careful observation during an exacerbation or when ill.

REFERENCES
Available at eBooks.Health.Elsevier.com.

RELATED CONTENT
Myasthenia Gravis (Patient Information)

AUTHORS: **MITCHELL POWELL, MD,** and **LYDIA SHARP, MD**

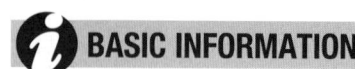
BASIC INFORMATION

DEFINITION

Myelodysplastic syndromes (MDSs) are a group of acquired clonal disorders of hematopoietic stem cells characterized by altered differentiation and proliferation. Presenting features include peripheral blood cytopenias and bone marrow hypercellularity with morphologic abnormalities, which reflects underlying ineffective hematopoiesis with inadequate maturation.

CLASSIFICATION

- Earlier classification systems for MDS have included the French-American-British (FAB) classification (1997), the 1997 World Health Organization (WHO) classification, and the 2008 modified WHO classification.
- Currently, the revised 2016 WHO classification is in clinical use (Table 1).

SYNONYMS

MDS
Preleukemia

ICD-10CM CODES
D46.9 Myelodysplastic syndrome, unspecified
D46.C Myelodysplastic syndrome with isolated del(5q) chromosomal abnormality
D46.Z Other myelodysplastic syndromes

EPIDEMIOLOGY & DEMOGRAPHICS

INCIDENCE (IN U.S.): Approximately 4 new cases/100,000 persons per yr. An estimated 30,000 new cases are diagnosed annually in the U.S. The true incidence is likely to be higher because of incomplete case assessment and underreporting of MDS in cancer registries, and it may be close to 75 per 100,000 among persons over the age of 70 years.[1]

PREDOMINANT AGE: More common in elderly patients; median age about 70 years

PHYSICAL FINDINGS & CLINICAL PRESENTATION

- Patients often present with fatigue due to anemia.
- Patients can present with thrombocytopenia and leukopenia.
- Skin pallor, mucosal bleeding, and ecchymosis may be present.
- Fever, infection, and dyspnea are common.

ETIOLOGY

Normal human aging is the most important risk factor for development of MDS due to progressive acquisition of somatic mutations by the hematopoietic stem cells throughout the human life span. Exposure to radiation, chemotherapeutic agents, benzene, or other organic compounds is also associated with myelodysplasia. Table 2 describes predisposing factors and epidemiologic associations of patients with MDS. MDS is

---

TABLE 1 2016 World Health Organization Classification of the Adult Myelodysplastic Syndromes

Name	Dysplastic Lineages	Cytopenias*	Ring Sideroblasts as % of Marrow Erythroid Elements	BM and PB Blasts	Cytogenetics by Conventional Karyotype Analysis
MDS with single lineage dysplasia (MDS-SLD)	1	1 or 2	$<15\%/<5\%^{\dagger}$	BM $<5\%$, PB $<1\%$, no Auer rods	Any, unless fulfills all criteria for MDS with isolated del(5q)
MDS with multilineage dysplasia (MDS-MLD)	2 or 3	1-3	$<15\%/<5\%^{\dagger}$	BM $<5\%$, PB $<1\%$, no Auer rods	Any, unless fulfills all criteria for MDS with isolated del(5q)
MDS With Ring Sideroblasts (MDS-RS)					
MDS-RS with single lineage dysplasia (MDS-RS-SLD)	1	1 or 2	$\geq15\%/\geq5\%^{\dagger}$	BM $<5\%$, PB $<1\%$, no Auer rods	Any, unless fulfills all criteria for MDS with isolated del(5q)
MDS-RS with multilineage dysplasia (MDS-RS-MLD)	2 or 3	1-3	$\geq15\%/\geq5\%^{\dagger}$	BM $<5\%$, PB $<1\%$, no Auer rods	Any, unless fulfills all criteria for MDS with isolated del(5q)
MDS with isolated del(5q)	1-3	1-2	None or any	BM $<5\%$, PB $<1\%$, no Auer rods	del(5q) alone or with 1 additional abnormality except -7 or del(7q)
MDS With Excess Blasts (MDS-EB)					
MDS-EB-1	0-3	1-3	None or any	BM 5%-9% or PB 2%-4%, no Auer rods	Any
MDS-EB-2	0-3	1-3	None or any	BM 10%-19% or PB 5%-19% or Auer rods	Any
MDS, Unclassifiable (MDS-U)					
With 1% blood blasts	1-3	1-3	None or any	BM $<5\%$, PB $= 1\%$,[‡] no Auer rods	Any
With single lineage dysplasia and pancytopenia	1	3	None or any	BM $<5\%$, PB $<1\%$, no Auer rods	Any
Based on defining cytogenetic abnormality	0	1-3	$<15\%^{\S}$	BM $<5\%$, PB $<1\%$, no Auer rods	MDS-defining abnormality
Refractory cytopenia of childhood	1-3	1-3	None	BM $<5\%$, PB $<2\%$	Any

*Cytopenias defined as hemoglobin <10 g/dl; platelet count $<100 \times 10^9$/L; and absolute neutrophil count $<1.8 \times 10^9$/L. Rarely, MDS may present with mild anemia or thrombocytopenia above these levels. PB monocytes must be $<1 \times 10^9$/L.
[†]If SF3B1 mutation is present.
[‡]1% PB blasts must be recorded on at least 2 separate occasions.
[§]Cases with $\geq15\%$ ring sideroblasts by definition have significant erythroid dysplasia and are classified as MDS-RS-SLD.
From Arber DA et al: The 2016 revision to the World Health Organization classification of myeloid neoplasms and acute leukemia, *Blood* 127(20):2391-2405, 2016.

extremely rare in pediatric age group but if does arise in patients <18 years of age, work up for inherited or congenital disorders should be sought. With recent advances in genomic sequencing technologies, some individuals with or without cytopenias are found to have somatic clonal mutations which in some cases go on to develop MDS or AML. The understanding regarding these potential premalignant conditions (ICUS, CHIP, CCUS) including factors that determine progression continues to evolve. Up to 40 genes that affect specific functional pathways are mutated in MDS, with 90% of patients having at least one mutation and a median of two to three mutations detected per patient. The most common mutations occur in genes involved in RNA splicing (*SF3B1, SRSF2, U2AF1,* and *ZRSR2*), epigenetic modification (*TET2, ASXL1,* and *DNMT3A*), regulators of signal transduction (*NRAS* and *JAK2*), and transcription factors (*RUNX1* and *TP53*). An increasing number of germline mutations (RUNX1, GATA2, DDX41, etc) are also being identified which are shown to be associated with a familial syndrome with inherited predisposition of developing MDS.

TABLE 2 Predisposing Factors and Epidemiologic Associations of Patients With Myelodysplastic Syndrome

Heritable

Constitutional Genetic Disorders

Trisomy 8 mosaicism
Familial monosomy 7
Down syndrome (trisomy 21)
Neurofibromatosis 1
Germ cell tumors [embryonal dysgenesis del(12p)]

Congenital Neutropenia

Kostmann syndrome
Shwachman-Diamond syndrome

DNA Repair Deficiencies

Fanconi anemia
Ataxia-telangiectasia
Bloom syndrome
Xeroderma pigmentosum
Pharmacogenomic polymorphisms (GSTq1-null)

Acquired

Senescence

Mutagen Exposure

Alkylator therapy (chlorambucil, cyclophosphamide, melphalan, N-mustards)
Topoisomerase II inhibitors (anthracyclines)
β Emitters (32p)
Autologous stem cell transplantation
Environmental/occupational (benzene)
Tobacco
Aplastic anemia
Paroxysmal nocturnal hemoglobinuria

DNA, Deoxyribonucleic acid.
From Hoffman R et al: *Hematology, basic principles and practice,* ed 7, Philadelphia, 2018, Churchill Livingstone.

Dx DIAGNOSIS

DIFFERENTIAL DIAGNOSIS

- Hereditary dysplasias (e.g., Fanconi anemia, Diamond-Blackfan syndrome)
- Vitamin B_{12}/folate deficiency
- Copper deficiency
- Exposure to toxins (drugs, alcohol, chemotherapy)
- Renal failure
- Irradiation
- Autoimmune disease
- Paroxysmal nocturnal hemoglobinuria

WORKUP

Diagnostic workup includes laboratory evaluation and bone marrow examination (Fig. E1). Cytogenetic analysis (Box E1) by conventional metaphase karyotyping or by MDS FISH assessment should be performed in patients with MDS. Next-generation sequencing (NGS) can be performed on bone marrow to provide additional information on mutations. Genes recurrently mutated in myelodysplastic syndrome are summarized in Table 3. Physical examination, medical history, and laboratory tests aiding in diagnosis of MDS are described in Table 4. Key features of the major myelodysplastic syndromes are summarized in Table 5.

The 2016 WHO classification of myeloid neoplasms is now used to classify MDS and is broadly categorized into the following subtypes: MDS with dysplasia, MDS with ring sideroblasts (MDS-RS), MDS with excess blasts (MDS-EB), and MDS unclassifiable (MDS-U).

TABLE 3 Genes Recurrently Mutated in Myelodysplastic Syndrome

Gene	Frequency (%)	Notes
Splicing Factors		
SF3B1	20-30	Strong association with RARS
SRSF2	10-15 (MDS) 40 (CMML)	Enriched in CMML
U2AF1	5-12	Association with del(20q)
Epigenetic Modifiers		
TET2	20-30 (MDS) 40-50 (CMML)	Enriched in CMML Mutually exclusive with IDH
DNMT3A	8-13	
ASXL1	10-20 (MDS) 30-40 (CMML)	Enriched in CMML
EZH2	5-10 (MDS) 20-30 (CMML)	Enriched in CMML May be functionally involved in 7q−
IDH1/2	<5	More frequent in AML
ATRX	Rare	Associated with acquired thalassemia
Transcription Factors		
RUNX1	10-15	Can be somatic or germline
GATA2	Rare	Mostly germline
ETV6	<5	Can be somatic or germline
TP53	10-12	Association with complex karyotype, therapy-related disease
Kinases and Receptors		
JAK2	<5	Enriched in RARS-T
NRAS	5-10	Seen in progression to AML
CBL	<5	Enriched in JMML
PTPN11	<5	More common in JMML
BRAF	Rare	Also seen in hairy cell leukemia
Cohesin Complex		
STAG2	5-10	Cohesin class mutations enriched in high-risk MDS and secondary AML
RAD21	<5	
SMC3	<2	
SMC1A	<2	
GCPR Complex		
GNAS	Rare	Mutations recently described in wide range of hematologic malignancies, including MDS
GNB1	Rare	

AML, Acute myeloid leukemia; *CMML,* chronic myelomonocytic leukemia; *GCPR,* G-coupled protein receptor; *IDH,* isocitrate dehydrogenase; *JMML,* juvenile myelomonocytic leukemia; *MDS,* myelodysplastic syndrome; *RARS,* refractory anemia with ring sideroblasts; *RARS-T,* RARS with thrombocytosis.
From Hoffman R et al: *Hematology, basic principles and practice,* ed 7, Philadelphia, 2018, Elsevier.

From Hoffman R et al: *Hematology, basic principles and practice,* ed 7, Philadelphia, 2018, Churchill Livingstone.

TABLE 4 Physical Examination, Medical History, and Laboratory Tests Aiding in Diagnosis of Myelodysplastic Syndrome

Medical History
- Duration of symptoms
- History of blood disease
- History of exposure to occupational toxins or cytotoxic agents
- Medication history
- Alcohol intake
- Comorbid conditions
- Family history of hematological disorders

Physical Examination
- Pallor
- Petechiae
- Purpura
- Bruising
- Tachypnea
- Signs of infection
- Splenomegaly

Laboratory Testing
- Complete blood count with a manual differential
- Reticulocyte count
- Vitamin B_{12} and folate levels
- Consider methylmalonic acid and red blood cell folate levels
- Iron, total iron-binding capacity, and ferritin level
- Thyroid-stimulating hormone level
- Lactate dehydrogenase
- Antinuclear antibody
- Coombs test and haptoglobin
- Serum erythropoietin level
- Human leukocyte antigen (histocompatibility antigens) typing in appropriate patients
- Paroxysmal nocturnal hemoglobinuria screen

Bone Marrow Testing
- Hematopathology
- Percentage of blasts on 200 cell aspirate differential
- Presence or absence of Auer rods
- Percentage of cellularity of bone marrow biopsy
- Iron stain on aspirate (ringed sideroblasts)
- Iron stain on biopsy (storage)
- Dysplastic features (% and number of dysplastic lineages)
- Cytogenetics (karyotype of 20 metaphase cells)
- Fluorescent in situ hybridization
- Flow cytometry (not useful for quantitation)

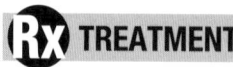 **TREATMENT**

NONPHARMACOLOGIC THERAPY
- Packed red blood cell (PRBC) transfusions in patients with severe symptomatic anemia
- Platelet transfusions in patients with severe thrombocytopenia or those with bleeding episodes

ACUTE GENERAL Rx
- The initial focus of MDS therapy involves stratification of patients into very-low-, low-, intermediate-, high-, and very-high-risk states using the well-defined and validated revised International Prognostic Scoring System (IPSS-R). This was developed from an evaluation of 7012 patients and utilizes five major variables for evaluating clinical outcomes: Cytogenetic risk groups, marrow blast percentage, and depth of cytopenias (hemoglobin, platelet, and absolute neutrophil count levels, respectively). New prognostic systems incorporating molecular mutations into the IPSS (IPSS-Molecular or IPSS-M) are available (Published June 12, 2022, *NEJM Evid* 2022; 1 (7) although it is not widely adopted yet. The WHO classification has also recently been updated to distinguish patients with defining genetic abnormalities (SF3B1, deletion 5q or TP53) from morphologically defined subtypes.
- Although the current WHO diagnostic classification (5th edition) distinguishes MDS from AML based on the percentage of blasts (MDS, <20% blasts and AML ≥ 20% blasts), MDS with >10% blasts could be treated similarly to AML.

Fig. 2 and Table 6 summarize a treatment approach for MDS.
- Very-low- and low-risk patients are treated with supportive care or growth factors.
- Intermediate-, high-, and very-high-risk patients are offered treatment with hypomethylating agents (HMAs) along with supportive care.
- The only potentially curative treatment for MDS is hematopoietic cell transplantation (HCT). All patients with higher risk MDS (and selected low risk patients with poor risk molecular features) should be referred for consideration of HCT soon after diagnosis. Older age should not preclude HCT as a reduced intensity conditioning HCT has been shown to offer better survival in patients with higher risk MDS compared to HMAs or best supportive care.
- Erythropoietin (10,000 to 60,000 units/wk) or pegylated erythropoietin (200 to 500 mg every 1 to 3 wk) is used in patients with symptomatic anemia. Responses with increase in hemoglobin and decreased transfusion requirements are achieved typically in patients who have serum erythropoietin levels <500 U/L and adequate iron stores.
- Luspatercept is a recombinant fusion protein that binds transforming growth factor β superfamily ligands to reduce SMAD2 and SMAD3 signaling. It was evaluated in patients with very-low-risk to intermediate-risk MDS with ring sideroblasts (often associated with SF3B1 variant) who had been receiving regular PRBC transfusions and was found to achieve transfusion independence in 38% patients versus 13% receiving placebo. It is particularly useful for anemia either refractory to erythropoietin stimulating agents (ESA) or unlikely to respond to ESA.
- DNA methyltransferase inhibitors: Azacitidine, a pyrimidine nucleoside analogue of cytidine, has been shown to improve the quality of life for patients and to prolong overall survival. Decitabine, another nucleoside analogue, has also been FDA approved for patients with MDS. These agents may also be useful in preventing the transition of MDS to AML.
- The fixed-dose oral combination of decitabine and cedazuridine was approved by FDA on July 2020 for adult patients with intermediate -1, intermediate-2, and high risk MDS, including those with previously treated and untreated, de novo, and secondary MDS. This was based on two open-label randomized cross over trials which demonstrated a CR rate of 18-21% and median duration of CR of 7.5 – 8.7 months.
- Immunomodulators: Lenalidomide, an immunomodulatory agent, reduces PRBC transfusion dependence in low-risk, non-5q deletion MDS patients but with increased hematologic adverse events. It can also reduce transfusion requirements and reverse cytologic and cytogenetic abnormalities in patients who have 5q deletion MDS.
- Additionally, lenalidomide augments erythropoietin receptor signaling in vitro and improves hemoglobin response significantly when used in combination with erythropoietin in patients with lower-risk, non-del(5q) MDS.
- Thrombopoietin receptor agonists are often avoided in MDS patients with excess blasts (except in palliative settings) in view higher rates of transformation to AML in clinical trials.
- Results of chemotherapy are generally disappointing. AML-style combination chemotherapy regimens generally induce a complete response in only a minority of patients, and the average duration of response is <1 yr.
- Myeloid growth factors (granulocyte colony-stimulating factor [G-CSF], granulocyte-macrophage colony-stimulating factor [GM-CSF]) are used in patients with severe neutropenias and high infection risk. Additionally, these provide a synergistic effect when used in combination with erythropoietin in terms of improvement in the hemoglobin levels.

CHRONIC Rx
- Monitor for infections, bleeding, and complications of anemia.
- Supportive measures include PRBC transfusions and erythropoietin for anemia, platelet transfusions for severe thrombocytopenia, and antimicrobials to treat opportunistic infections.
- Iron overload from frequent PRBC transfusions (>50 to 100 PRBC units) should prompt the use of iron chelation therapy with a view to improve survival.

DISPOSITION
- The 5-yr overall survival is approximately 30%. Median overall survival rates are best for patients with refractory anemia (56 mo), refractory anemia with ring sideroblasts (48 mo), and deletion 5q subtype (32 mo). The International Prognostic Scoring System (IPSS) for MDS is summarized in Tables 7 and E8. Table 9 describes survival based on IPSS.

TABLE 5 Diagnostic Criteria for Myelodysplastic Syndrome

A. Presence of at Least One Unexplained Cytopenia for at Least 6 Mo[a]

Hemoglobin <11 g/dl, *or*

Absolute neutrophil count <1.5 × 10^9/L, *or*

Platelet count <100 × 10^9/L

***plus* B. Presence of One or More MDS-Qualifying Criteria:**

>10% dysplasia in one or more hematopoietic lineage, *or*

5%-19% blasts in bone marrow, *or*

MDS-defining cytogenetic abnormality, such as:

t(1;3)(p36.3;q21.1)	t(2;11)(p21;q23)	inv(3)(q21;q26.2)
t(3;21)(q26.2;q22.1)	−5 or del(5q)	t(6;9)(p23;q34)
−7 or del(7q)		del(9q)
del(11q)	t(11;16)(q23;p13.3)	del(12p) or t(12p)
−13 or del(13q)	i(17q) or del(17p)	idic(X)(q13)

***plus* C. Exclusion of Alternative Diagnoses**

AML (i.e., <20% blasts, and no t(8;21), inv(16), t(16;16), t(15;17), or erythroleukemia) or *ALL*

Other hematologic diseases (aplastic anemia, PNH, LGL, lymphoma, myelofibrosis, and other MPN)

Viral infections (HIV, EBV, parvovirus)

Nutritional deficiencies (iron, copper, B_{12}, folate)

Medications (methotrexate, azathioprine, isoniazid, cytotoxic chemotherapy)

Alcohol or other toxins

Autoimmune diseases (SLE, Felty syndrome, ITP, autoimmune hemolytic anemia)

Congenital disorders (Diamond-Blackfan anemia, Shwachman-Diamond syndrome, Fanconi anemia, and others)

ALL, Acute lymphoblastic leukemia; *AML,* acute myeloid leukemia; *EBV,* Epstein-Barr virus; *HIV,* human immunodeficiency virus; *ITP,* immune thrombocytopenic purpura; *LGL,* large granular lymphocyte leukemia; *MDS,* myelodysplastic syndrome; *MPN,* myeloproliferative neoplasm; *PNH,* paroxysmal nocturnal hemoglobinuria; *SLE,* systemic lupus erythematosus.
[a]Diagnosis can be made earlier than 6 mo if no other cause is apparent for cytopenias, or there are excess blasts or an MDS-defining cytogenetic abnormality.
From Hoffman R et al: *Hematology, basic principles and practice,* ed 7, Philadelphia, 2018, Elsevier.

- Long-term remission rates in young patients with allogeneic stem cell transplantation approach 40% to 50%.
- The risk of transformation to AML varies with cytogenetics and bone marrow blast percentage.

REFERRAL

- Hematology referral for all patients
- Bone marrow transplant evaluation for stem cell transplant eligibility as a potentially curative modality

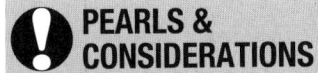

PEARLS & CONSIDERATIONS

COMMENTS

- Somatic point mutations in *TP53, EZH2, ETV6, RUNX1,* and *ASXL1* are predictors of poor overall survival in patients with MDS independent of established risk factors. Patients with cytogenetic abnormalities associated with poor prognosis should be considered for upfront allogeneic stem cell transplantation.
- Many younger patients who respond to immunosuppressive therapy with drugs such as antithymocyte globulin and cyclosporine have clonal expansions of cytotoxic $CD8^+$ T cells that suppress normal hematopoiesis, as well as expansion of $CD4^+$ helper T cell subsets that promote and sustain autoimmunity.
- Nearly 50% of the deaths that result from MDS are the result of cytopenias associated with bone marrow failure.

SUGGESTED READINGS

Available at eBooks.Health.Elsevier.com.

RELATED CONTENT

Myelodysplastic Syndrome (Patient Information)

AUTHOR: **KAPIL S. MELEVEEDU, MD**

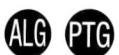

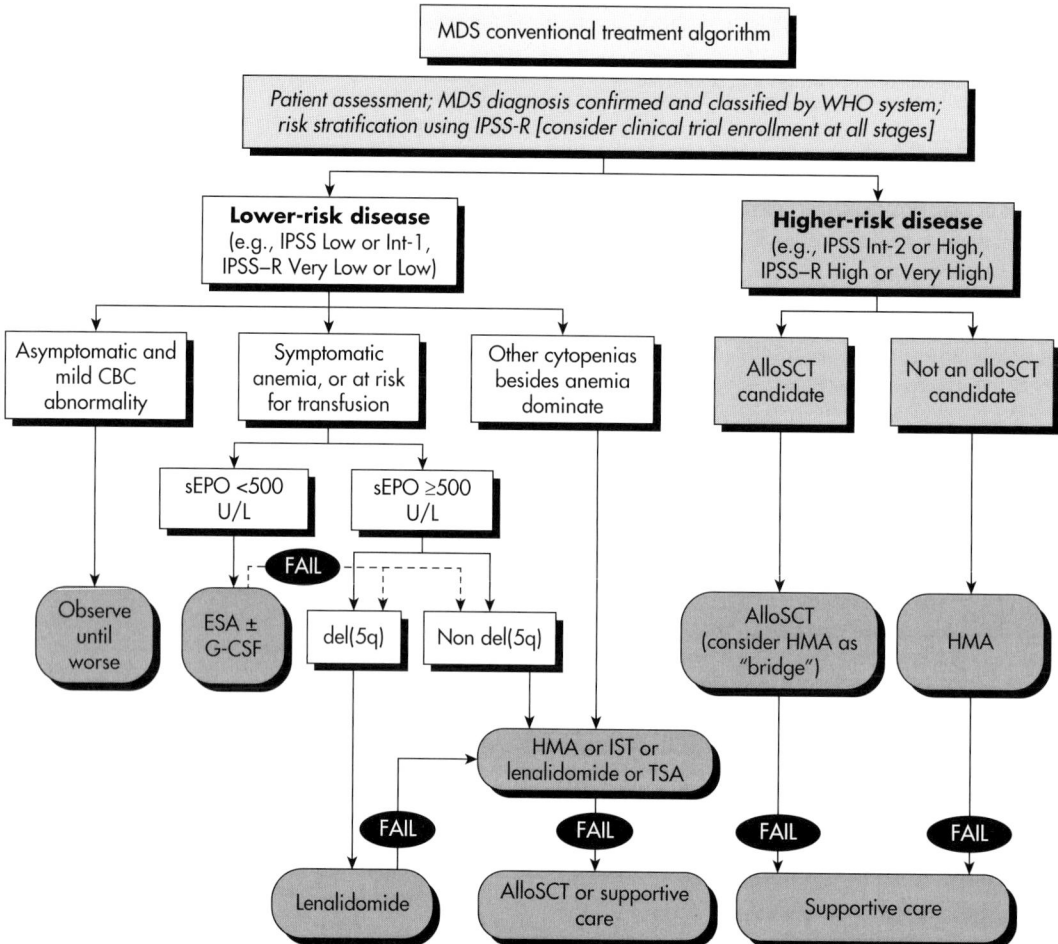

FIG. 2 A suggested treatment algorithm for myelodysplastic syndrome (*MDS*), described further in the text and in Table 6. Risk assessment has traditionally been based on the International Prognostic Scoring System (*IPSS*) (and more recently the IPSS-R), but that is likely to change with the advent of new prognostic scoring systems and molecular markers. IPSS-R intermediate-risk disease may follow the track for lower- or higher-risk disease. Disease classification should use the 2016 World Health Organization (*WHO*) system. Clinical trial enrollment should be considered at each step. Some clinicians would proceed to lenalidomide without a trial of an *ESA* if del(5q) is present, even if the serum erythropoietin level is less than 500 U/L. *alloSCT,* Allogeneic stem cell transplantation; *CBC,* complete blood count; ESA, erythropoiesis-stimulating agent (epoetin or darbepoetin—off-label uses); *G-CSF,* granulocyte colony-stimulating factor (e.g., filgrastim or tbo-filgrastim); *HMA,* hypomethylating agent (azacitidine or decitabine); *IPSS-R,* revised International Prognostic Scoring System; *IST,* immunosuppressive therapy (antithymocyte globulin with cyclosporine A or tacrolimus—off-label uses); *SCT,* stem cell transplantation; *sEPO,* serum erythropoietin level; *TSA,* thrombopoiesis-stimulating agent (e.g., eltrombopag, romiplostim—off-label uses). (From Niederhuber JE: *Abeloff's clinical oncology,* ed 6, Philadelphia, 2020, Elsevier.)

TABLE 6　Available Therapies for Myelodysplastic Syndromes in the U.S. and Preferred Dosage Regimen[a]

1. Erythropoiesis-stimulating agents (should hold if hemoglobin $\gg$ 10 g/dl)
   a. Epoetin alfa 20-60,000 mIU/wk subcutaneously; dose can be adjusted every 1-2 mo depending on response; or
   b. Darbepoetin alfa 200-300 μg subcutaneously every 1-2 wk or 500 μg subcutaneously every 3 wk; or
   c. Epoetin alfa as per (a) plus G-CSF (filgrastim) 0.5 μg /kg subcutaneously 1-3 times per wk (pegfilgrastim is commonly substituted in the U.S., but data are absent, and splenic rupture and leukemoid reactions are risks)
2. Iron chelation therapy
   a. Deferoxamine (starting dose ∼20 mg/kg/day; a typical effective dose for an adult is 6 g/day subcutaneously or intravenously, administered by infusion pump over 8-16 h daily); or
   b. Deferasirox, tablet for oral suspension 20-30 mg/kg/day orally once daily oral tablet, 14-28 mg/kg/day, adjust as tolerated and according to efficacy.
   c. Deferiprone (L1) is available outside the U.S., but is only approved for thalassemia in the U.S. and is a weaker chelator than the other two and cytopenias can be problematic
3. Lenalidomide: 10 mg orally once daily for 21-28 days per 28-day cycle (dose reduction due to cytopenias is commonly required)
4. Azacitidine: 75 mg/m^2/day subcutaneously or intravenously for 7 days, repeat every 28 days; "weekend-sparing" schedules may also be effective
5. Decitabine: 15 mg/m^2/dose over 3-4 h intravenously every 8 h × 9 doses (= 3 days); or 20 mg/m^2/day intravenously over 1-2 h daily × 5 consecutive days; repeat every 4-6 wk
6. Immunosuppression: Equine ATG per aplastic anemia regimens (e.g., 40 mg/kg/day × 4 days intravenously, after test dose), with corticosteroids to prevent serum sickness, with or without cyclosporine A or tacrolimus
7. Miscellaneous therapies such as antifibrinolytics (aminocaproic acid, tranexamic acid) and androgens (danazol) can be useful in some cases.

ATG, Antithymocyte globulin; *G-CSF,* granulocyte colony-stimulating factor.
[a]Consult the package insert in each case. Only azacitidine, lenalidomide, and decitabine are approved by the U.S. Food and Drug Administration for myelodysplastic syndrome–related indications in the U.S.
From Niederhuber JE: *Abeloff's clinical oncology,* ed 6, Philadelphia, 2020, Elsevier.

TABLE 7　1997 International Prognostic Scoring System for Myelodysplastic Syndromes (IPSS)

Variable	SCORE			
	0	0.5	1	1.5
Marrow blasts (%)	<5	5-10	–	11-20
Karyotype	Good	Intermediate	Poor	–
Cytopenias	0-1	2-3	–	–

From Hoffman R et al: *Hematology, basic principles and practice,* ed 7, Philadelphia, 2018, Elsevier.

TABLE 9　Survival Based on International Prognostic Scoring System for Myelodysplastic Syndromes (Percent)

IPSS Risk Group	# Patients	2 Yr	5 Yr	10 Yr	15 Yr
Low	267 (33%)	85	55	28	20
Intermediate-1	314 (38%	70	35	17	12
Intermediate-2	179 (22%)	30	8	0	–
High	56 (7%)	5	0	–	–

IPSS, International Prognostic Scoring System.
From Hoffman R et al: *Hematology, basic principles and practice,* ed 7, Philadelphia, 2018, Elsevier.

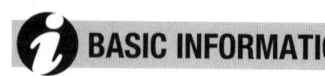
BASIC INFORMATION

DEFINITION

Myocardial infarction (MI) is a clinical syndrome characterized by symptoms of myocardial ischemia, persistent electrocardiographic (ECG) changes, and release of biomarkers of myocardial necrosis resulting from an insufficient supply of oxygenated blood to an area of the heart. MI may be classified as ST-segment elevation MI (STEMI) and non–ST-segment elevation MI (NSTEMI) depending on the ECG findings on MI presentation. Acute coronary syndrome (ACS) refers to acute myocardial ischemia without myocardial necrosis (unstable angina) and myocardial necrosis and infarction (NSTEMI or STEMI). According to the European Society of Cardiology/American College of Cardiology guidelines, the following criteria for acute evolving or recent MI (NSTEMI and STEMI) satisfies the diagnosis:

- Detection of the rise and/or fall of cardiac biomarker values (preferably cardiac troponin [cTn]) with at least one value above the 99th percentile upper reference limit and with at least one of the following:
  1. Symptoms of ischemia
  2. Development of pathologic Q waves in the ECG
  3. Imaging evidence of new loss of viable myocardium or a new regional wall motion abnormality
  4. Identification of an intracoronary thrombus by angiography or autopsy pathologic findings of acute MI
  5. Electrocardiogram criteria:
     a. STEMI:
        (1) New, or presumed new, significant ST-T changes or new left bundle branch block (LBBB) in appropriate clinical setting
        (2) New ST elevation at the J-point in at least 2 contiguous leads of $\geq$2 mm (0.2 mV) in men or $\geq$1.5 mm (0.15 mV) in women in leads V2 to V3 and/or of $\geq$1 mm (0.1 mV) in another contiguous chest leads or the upper limb leads
     b. NSTEMI:
        (1) New ST-segment depression $\geq$0.5 mV (0.5 mm) and T-wave abnormalities

New generation troponin assays are extremely sensitive to small changes in serum troponin levels at the cost of diagnostic specificity for MI related to plaque rupture or erosion.

Universal classification of acute MI:

- Type 1: Spontaneous MI related to ischemia due to a primary coronary event such as plaque erosion and/or rupture, fissuring, or dissection.
- Type 2: MI secondary to ischemia, other than coronary artery disease, due to either increased oxygen demand or decreased supply (e.g., coronary endothelial dysfunction, coronary artery spasm, coronary embolism, anemia, arrhythmias, respiratory failure, hypertension with/without left ventricular hypertrophy [LVH], or hypotension).

Also, in critically ill patients or in patients undergoing major noncardiac surgery, elevated values of cardiac biomarkers may appear due to the direct toxic effects of endogenous or exogenous high circulating catecholamine levels.

- Type 3: Sudden unexpected cardiac death, including cardiac arrest, often with symptoms suggestive of myocardial ischemia, accompanied by presumed new ST elevation, new left bundle branch block, or evidence of fresh thrombus in a coronary artery by angiography and/or at autopsy, or death occurring before blood samples could be obtained or at a time before the appearance of cardiac biomarkers in the blood.
- Type 4a: MI associated with percutaneous coronary intervention. Elevation of cTn >5× percentile of upper reference limit (URL) in patients with normal baseline value, or a rise of cTn >20% if the baseline values are stable and are stable or falling. In addition to either symptoms of ischemia, new ischemic ECG changes or new LBBB, or angiographic loss of a patent coronary artery, persistent slow or no-flow, or embolization, or imaging of new wall motion abnormality.
- Type 4b: MI associated with stent thrombosis as documented by angiography or at autopsy in the setting of myocardial ischemia and with a rise/fall of cardiac biomarker values.
- Type 5: MI associated with coronary artery bypass grafting. Elevation of cardiac biomarker values >10× 99% URL in patients with normal baseline cTn values, in addition to either new pathologic Q waves or new LBBB, or new native coronary artery occlusion or imaging of new abnormal wall motion abnormality.
- Myocardial Infarction With Nonobstructive Coronary Arteries (MINOCA): It is defined as acute myocardial infarction in the absence of obstructive coronary artery disease. Conditions like Takotsubo cardiomyopathy, spontaneous coronary artery dissection, coronary artery spasm, microvascular dysfunction, and pulmonary embolism come under this novel category.

SYNONYMS

MI
ST-elevation MI
Heart attack
Acute myocardial infarction
AMI
Coronary thrombosis
Coronary occlusion

ICD-10CM CODES
I21.01	ST elevation (STEMI) myocardial infarction involving left main coronary artery
I21.02	ST elevation (STEMI) myocardial infarction involving left anterior descending coronary artery
I21.09	ST elevation (STEMI) myocardial infarction involving other coronary artery of anterior wall
I21.11	ST elevation (STEMI) myocardial infarction involving right coronary artery
I21.19	ST elevation (STEMI) myocardial infarction involving another coronary artery of inferior wall
I21.21	ST elevation (STEMI) myocardial infarction involving left circumflex coronary artery
I21.29	ST elevation (STEMI) myocardial infarction involving other sites
I21.3	ST elevation (STEMI) myocardial infarction of unspecified site
I21.4	Non-ST elevation (NSTEMI) myocardial infarction
I22.0	Subsequent ST elevation (STEMI) myocardial infarction of anterior wall
I22.1	Subsequent ST elevation (STEMI) myocardial infarction of inferior wall
I22.2	Subsequent non-ST elevation (NSTEMI) myocardial infarction
I22.8	Subsequent ST elevation (STEMI) myocardial infarction of other sites
I22.9	Subsequent ST elevation (STEMI) myocardial infarction of unspecified site

EPIDEMIOLOGY & DEMOGRAPHICS

INCIDENCE & PREVALENCE (IN U.S.):

- According to data from National Health and Nutrition Examination Survey (NHANES) 2013 to 2016 (National Heart, Lung, and Blood Institute [NHLBI] tabulation), cardiovascular disease prevalence excluding hypertension was 9% (24.3 million in 2016).
- In 2013 in the U.S., coronary heart disease alone caused $\approx$1 of every 7 deaths. In 2013, 370,213 Americans died of coronary heart disease. Each year, an estimated 660,000 Americans have a new coronary attack (defined as first hospitalized myocardial infarction or coronary heart disease death), and 305,000 have a recurrent attack. It is estimated that an additional 160,000 silent myocardial infarctions occur each year. Approximately every 34 sec, one American has a coronary event, and approximately every 1 min 24 sec, an American will die of one.
- Community incidence rates as well as mortality rates from STEMI have declined over the past decade, whereas those for NSTEMI have increased. At present, STEMI comprises approximately 30% to 40% of MI presentations. In-hospital mortality (approximately 5% to 6%) and 1-yr mortality (approximately 7% to 18%). The most common cause of death in adults over the age of 40 is myocardial infarction. A heart attack takes the life of >1,500,000 people each year in the U.S.
- Modifiable risk factors such as hypertension, diabetes, and cigarette smoking have recently declined, although hyperlipidemia has shown no significant change, and obesity has steadily increased.
- Tobacco use remains the second-leading cause of total deaths and disability. The percentage of adults who reported current cigarette use declined from 24.1% in 1998 to 15.5% in 2016. Still, almost one third of

coronary heart disease deaths are attributable to smoking and exposure to secondhand smoke. Patients with first acute MI were found to have an almost threefold increase in cigarette smoking from 2002 to 2009. Cigarette smoking is associated with endothelial dysfunction, prothrombotic defects, and increased oxidative stress.

- It is more prevalent in males between the ages of 45 and 65 yr old; there is no predominant sex differential after the age of 65.
- Women comprised 30% of STEMI patients. They experience more lethal and severe first acute MIs than men regardless of comorbidity, previous angina, or age. Studies have suggested that women are less likely to receive reperfusion therapy, have longer reperfusion times, are often given the standard of care treatment within 24 hr of presentation, and have higher risk of bleeding with antithrombotic therapy.
- At least one fourth of all MIs are clinically unrecognized. Approximately 23% of patients with STEMI in the U.S. have diabetes mellitus, and three quarters of all deaths among patients with diabetes mellitus are related to coronary artery disease. Diabetes mellitus is associated with higher short- and long-term mortality after STEMI. In the CRUSADE (Can Rapid risk stratification of Unstable angina patients Suppress ADverse outcomes with Early implementation of the ACC/AHA guidelines) trial, 7% of eligible patients did not receive reperfusion therapy. The most important factor for not providing reperfusion therapy in eligible patients was increasing age.
- 6% to 15% of MIs are not associated with obstructive coronary disease or angiography.[1]

PHYSICAL FINDINGS & CLINICAL PRESENTATION

The clinical presentation of myocardial infarction is usually based on a history of substernal pressure–type chest pain radiated to the neck, lower jaw, left arm, or mid-back lasting 20 min or more that is not completely relieved by sublingual nitroglycerin. The pain may not be severe. Some patients may present with atypical symptoms such as nausea/vomiting, shortness of breath, fatigue, palpitations, and diaphoresis. The elderly in particular may present with dizziness or syncope. The patients who tend to present with atypical symptoms are more likely to be women, diabetic patients, or elderly patients and less frequently receive reperfusion therapy and other evidence-based therapies than patients with a typical chest pain presentation. Records show that up to 30% of patients with STEMI present with atypical symptoms.

Physical findings:

- Skin may be diaphoretic and exhibit pallor (because of decreased oxygen).
- Rales may be present at the bases of lungs (indicative of heart failure [HF]).
- Cardiac auscultation may reveal an apical systolic murmur caused by mitral regurgitation

from papillary muscle dysfunction; S3 or S4 may also be present.
- Up to 10% of patients may present with acute pulmonary edema and/or cardiogenic shock.
- Physical examination may be completely normal.

ETIOLOGY

- Coronary atherosclerosis and plaque rupture
- Coronary artery spasm
- Coronary embolism (caused by infective endocarditis, rheumatic heart disease, intracavitary thrombus, atrial fibrillation)
- Periarteritis and other coronary artery inflammatory diseases
- Dissection into coronary arteries (aneurysmal or iatrogenic or spontaneous)
- Anomalous origin of coronary artery, especially interarterial (aorta and pulmonary artery) course of coronary artery
- MI with normal coronaries: More frequent in younger patients and cocaine addicts. The risk of acute MI is increased by a factor of 24 during the 60 min after the use of cocaine in persons who are otherwise at relatively low risk. Most patients with cocaine-related MI are young, nonwhite, male cigarette smokers without other risk factors for coronary heart disease and who have a history of repeated cocaine use. Blood and urine toxicology screen for cocaine is recommended in all young patients who present with acute MI
- Hypercoagulable states, increased blood viscosity (polycythemia vera and autoimmune diseases such as systemic lupus, antiphospholipid syndrome)

DX DIAGNOSIS

DIFFERENTIAL DIAGNOSIS

The various causes of myocardial ischemia are described along with the differential diagnosis of chest pain.

LABORATORY TESTS

- Electrocardiogram (Fig. 1): A 12-lead ECG should be performed and shown to an experienced emergency physician within 10 min of emergency department (ED) arrival for all patients with chest discomfort (or anginal equivalent) or other symptoms suggestive of MI. Table 1 and Table 2 describe ECG findings in myocardial infarction. If the initial ECG is not diagnostic for MI but the patient remains symptomatic and there is a high clinical suspicion for MI, serial ECGs at 5- to 10-min intervals or continuous 12-lead ST-segment monitoring should be performed to detect the potential development of ST deviation. In patients with inferior STEMI, right-sided ECG leads should be obtained to look for ST elevation suggestive of right ventricular (RV) infarction. The joint ESC/ACCF/AHA committee for the definition of MI established the definition for the diagnosis of ST-elevation MI, which is considered to be present when there is an

ST-segment elevation in two contiguous leads, ≥ 2 mm for men and ≥ 1.5 mm for women in precordial leads and/or ≥ 1 mm in limb leads. ST-segment elevation is measured at 0.08 sec after the J point (the junction between the end of the QRS and the beginning of the ST segment). In addition, ST depression in >2 precordial leads (V1 to V4) may indicate transmural posterior injury; multilead ST depression with coexistent ST elevation in lead aVR has been described in patients with left main or proximal left anterior descending artery involvement.
- New or presumably new LBBB at presentation occurs infrequently, may interfere with ST-elevation analysis. Thus consider MI only if clinically appropriate.
- Diagnosing new STEMI in patients with old left bundle branch block could be challenging. Sgarbossa and colleagues emphasized that concordant 1 mm ST-segment elevation in any lead with a positive QRS deflection or discordant ST-segment elevation >5 mm in any lead with negative QRS deflection suggest STEMI.
- New ST-segment depression ≥ 0.5 mV (0.5 mm) and T-wave abnormalities suggest NSTEMI. ECG findings alone, without laboratory results, are sufficient to diagnose STEMI; therefore treatment should not be delayed until biomarkers are available.
- Cardiac troponin levels: Cardiac-specific troponin T (cTnT) and cardiac-specific troponin I (cTnI) are generally indicative of myocardial injury with increases in serum levels of >99th percentile of a normal reference population. Detection of a rise and fall pattern of the measurements is essential to the diagnosis of AMI. The rise may occur relatively early after muscle damage (3 to 6 hr), peak at 12 to 16 hr, and may be present for several days after MI (up to 7 days for cTnI and more than 14 days for cTnT). Earlier peaking and rapid decline of cardiac enzymes may present in light of successful revascularization (Fig. 2). cTnT or cTnI tests can be falsely positive for myocardial infarction in patients with renal failure, heart failure, myocarditis, aortic dissection, and pulmonary embolism. Recently, highly sensitive troponin assays (hs-cTnI, hs-cTnT) have also been developed to facilitate an early diagnosis of AMI. Most patients can be diagnosed with AMI within the first 2 to 3 hr of presentation. However, an initial negative high-sensitivity troponin at the time of presentation is not sensitive enough to completely rule out AMI. MI can be excluded in most patients by 6 hr of presentation, and guidelines suggest serial samples be obtained every 3 to 6 hr after an initial sample if there is a high degree of suspicion for AMI(1&2).
- Troponin is the preferred marker for the diagnosis of myocardial necrosis. A single high-sensitivity assay for cardiac troponin (hs-cTnT) concentration below the limit of detection in combination with a nonischemic ECG may successfully rule out an MI in patients presenting to EDs with possible emergency

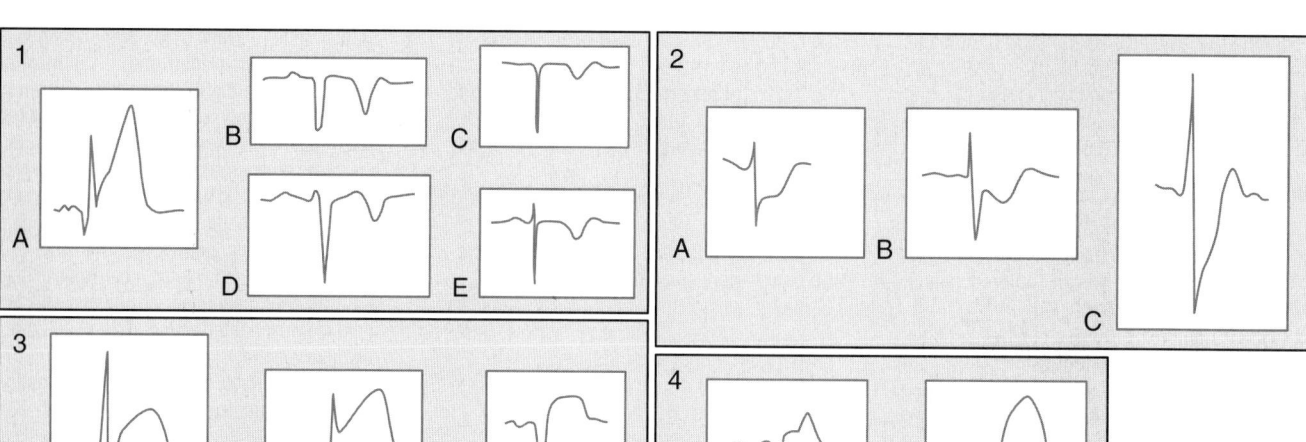

FIG. 1 Electrocardiographic findings of acute myocardial infarction (AMI). (1) T-wave abnormalities of AMI. *A,* Prominent "hyperacute" T wave. *B* through *E,* T-wave inversions of non–ST-segment elevation MI (NSTEMI). (2) ST-segment depression. *A,* Flat. *B,* Downsloping. *C,* Upsloping. (3) ST-segment elevation. *A,* Convex ST-segment elevation. *B,* Obliquely straight ST-segment elevation. *C,* Convex ST-segment elevation. (4) Pathologic Q waves. *A,* Pathologic Q wave of completed myocardial infarction. *B,* Simultaneous ST-segment elevation with pathologic Q wave 2 hr into the course of ST-segment elevation MI (STEMI). (From Vincent JL et al: *Textbook of critical care,* ed 6, Philadelphia, 2011, Saunders.)

TABLE 1 Leads Showing Abnormal Electrocardiographic Findings in Myocardial Infarction.

	Limb Leads	Precordial Leads
Lateral	I, aVL	V5, V6
Anterior		V1, V2, V3
Anterolateral	I, aVL	V2-V6
Diaphragmatic	II, III, aVF	
Posterior		V1-V3*

aVF, Augmented vector foot; *aVL,* augmented vector left.

* None of the leads is oriented toward the posterior surface of the heart. Therefore in posterior infarction, changes that would have been present in the posterior surface leads will be seen in the anterior leads as a mirror image (e.g., tall and slightly wide R waves in V1 and V2, comparable to abnormal Q waves, and tall and wide, symmetric T waves in V1 and V2).

From Park MK: *Park's pediatric cardiology for practitioners,* ed 6, Philadelphia, 2014, Elsevier.

acute coronary syndrome.[2] Because troponins need 7 to 14 days to be cleared by the kidneys, they are not sensitive enough to detect a recurrent MI within days from the initial MI. CK-MB isoenzyme can be useful in such circumstances (see Fig. 2).

- CK-MB isoenzyme is also a useful marker for MI if troponin levels are not available. It is released in the circulation in amounts that correlate with the size of the infarct. An increased CK-MB value for the diagnosis of MI is defined as a measurement above the 99th percentile of the upper reference limit. CK-MB can be detected within 3 to 8 hr of the onset of chest pain, peak at 12 to 24 hr, and return to baseline levels within 24 to 48 hr.

IMAGING STUDIES

Imaging studies such as a high-quality portable chest X-ray, transthoracic echocardiography, and a contrast chest computed tomography (CT) scan should be used to differentiate MI from aortic dissection, pulmonary embolism, and other intrathoracic causes of chest pain (i.e., pneumonia and pneumothorax) in patients for whom this distinction is initially unclear, or to assess for complications of AMI such as pulmonary edema. Transthoracic echocardiography may provide evidence of focal wall motion abnormalities and facilitate triage in patients with ECG findings that are difficult to interpret.

RISK ASSESSMENT

For STEMI patients, TIMI (Thrombolysis in Myocardial Infarction) risk index, TIMI risk score (30-day outcomes), and GRACE (Global Registry of Acute Coronary Events) risk score (6-mo outcomes) are commonly available risk assessment models. In the TIMI risk score for STEMI, the mean 30-day mortality was 6.7%. It is composed of eight baseline variables. The risk score showed a >40-fold graded increase in mortality, with scores ranging from 0 to >8 (P <0.0001); 30-day mortality was 0.1% among patients with a score of 0, 2.25 with a score of 5, and >8.8% among patients with a score of 8 or greater. The higher the score, the higher the 30-day mortality rate. The variables are divided between historic, exam, and presentation:

HISTORIC:
- Age 65 to 74 (2 points), >75 (3 points)
- Diabetes/HTN or angina (1 point)

EXAM:
- Systolic blood pressure (SBP) <100 mm Hg (3 points)
- Heart rate >100 bpm (2 points)
- Killip 2 to 4 (2 points)
- Weight <67 kg (1 point)

PRESENTATION:
- Anterior ST elevation or LBBB (1 point)
- Time to reperfusion >4 hr (1 point)

For NSTEMI patients, TIMI risk score (14-day outcomes) and GRACE (Global Registry of Acute Coronary Events) risk score (in hospital outcomes) are available. See variables for TIMI risk score below.
- Age ≥65 yr
- Presence of ≥3 risk factors for CAD
- Known CAD (coronary artery stenosis ≥50%)
- Aspirin use in the past 7 days
- ≥2 episodes of angina within 24 hr
- ST changes ≥0.05 mV
- Positive cardiac enzymes

In TIMI score for the NSTEMI patients, each variable scores one point. The risk score of 6 to 7 carries estimated major acute coronary event (MACE) rate of 41% during 14 days of post-MI. Risk assessment is a continuous process that should be repeated throughout hospitalization and at time of discharge.

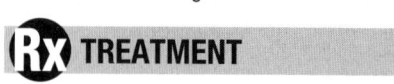 **TREATMENT**

NONPHARMACOLOGIC THERAPY

- Limit patient's activity: Bed rest with bedside commode for the initial 12 to 24 hr. If the patient remains stable, gradually increase.

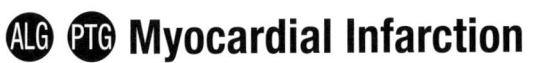
TABLE 2 Electrocardiographic Manifestations of Myocardial Infarction

ST Elevation
Electrocardiographic Manifestations of Acute Myocardial Ischemia (in the Absence of Left Bundle Branch Block)
New ST elevation at the J point in two contiguous leads with the following cut points:
- $\geq$0.1 mV in all leads (except V2-V3)
- In leads V2-V3 the following cut points apply:
  - $\geq$0.2 mV in men $\geq$40 yr
  - $\geq$0.25 mV In men <40 yr
  - $\geq$0.15 mV in women

ST Depression and T Wave Changes
- New horizontal or downsloping ST depression $\geq$0.05 mV in two contiguous leads
- T-wave inversion $\geq$0.1 mV in two contiguous leads with a prominent R wave or R/S ratio >1

Electrocardiographic Manifestations of Ischemia in the Setting of Left Bundle Branch Block

Electrocardiographic Criterion	Points
ST-segment elevation $\geq$1 mm and concordant with the QRS complex	5
ST-segment depression $\geq$1 mm in lead V1, V2, or V3	3
ST-segment elevation $\geq$5 mm and discordant with the QRS complex	2

A score of $\geq$3 had a specificity of 98% for acute MI

Electrocardiographic Changes Associated with Previous Myocardial Infarction (in the Absence of Left Ventricular Hypertrophy and Left Bundle Branch Block)
Any Q wave in leads V2-V3 $\geq$0.02 sec or a QS complex in leads V2 and V3
Q wave $\geq$0.03 sec and $\geq$0.1-mV deep or QS complex in leads I, II, aVL, aVF, or V4-V6 in any 2 leads of a contiguous lead grouping (I, aVL; V1-V6; II, III, aVF)
R wave $\geq$0.04 sec in V1-V2 and R/S $\geq$1 with a concordant positive T wave in absence of a conductions defect.

aVF, Augmented vector foot; *aVL,* augmented vector left; *MI,* myocardial infarction.

- Diet: Nothing by mouth until stable, then clear liquids as tolerated to advance gradually to a diet tailored to the patient's comorbidities (i.e., diabetes, hypertension, heart failure, hyperlipidemia, renal failure, chronic obstructive pulmonary disease [COPD], etc.).
- Patient education to decrease the risk of subsequent cardiac events, counseling on smoking cessation, dietary restrictions, regular exercise, and medication compliance should be initiated when the patient is medically stable.

ACUTE GENERAL Rx
- Fig. 3 shows a treatment algorithm for STEMI. Assessment and treatment algorithm for non–ST-segment MI is described in Fig. 4. Rationale of the treatment of a patient with STEMI is based on "time is muscle." Therefore all communities should create and maintain a regional system of STEMI care that includes assessment and continuous quality improvement of EMS and hospital-based activities. A 12-lead ECG must be done by EMS personnel at the site of first medical contact (FMC).
- Reperfusion therapy should be administered to all eligible patients with STEMI with symptom onset within 12 hr. Indications for primary angioplasty and comparison with fibrinolytic therapy are described in Table 3. Primary PCI is the recommended method of reperfusion when it can be performed in a timely fashion by experienced operators with an ideal FMC-to-device time system goal of 90 min or less.

- In the absence of contraindications, fibrinolytic therapy (Table 4) should be administered to patients with STEMI at non–PCI-capable hospitals when the anticipated FMC-to-device time at a PCI-capable hospital exceeds 120 min because of unavoidable delays. Door-in door-out time (DIDO) for fibrinolytic therapy should be less than 30 min. If more than 30 min delay, transfer the patient to a PCI-capable hospital.
- Among STEMI patients who were treated with fibrinolytics, patients with >50% ST-segment resolution on EKG were at much lower risk for cardiac-related mortality compared with those with <50% resolution at 30 days.
- PCI is superior to thrombolytic therapy and is the standard of care. It is effective and generally results in more favorable outcomes than thrombolytic therapy.
- Primary PCI should be performed in patients with STEMI and persistent ischemic symptoms and who have contraindications to fibrinolytic therapy, irrespective of the time delay from FMC, or in patients with cardiogenic shock or acute severe HF irrespective of time delay from myocardial infarction (MI) onset, first medical contact to balloon time is <90 min or door to balloon/door to needle time is <1 hr, symptoms onset was >3 hr ago and when diagnosis of STEMI in doubt. Coronary stents (drug-eluting or bare-metal) are useful in patients with STEMI (3,4,5 &6).
- The question of culprit vessel vs. complete revascularization during PCI has been brought

up since the stent technology was applied to the management of STEMI. The most recent clinical trials (CuLPRIT, PRAMI, and DANAMI3-PRIMULTI [FFR-driven revascularization]) appear to favor complete revascularization in the setting of STEMI. However, CULPRIT-SHOCK trial showed culprit vessel only PCI associated with 9.5% absolute reduction in the rate of death or renal replacement therapy at 30 days compared to multivessel PCI in acute MI patients with cardiogenic shock. One-yr outcomes did not show significant difference in mortality between two groups. Korea Acute Myocardial Infarction-National Institutes of Health (KAMIR-NIH) Registry data showed better outcomes with multivessel PCI in cardiogenic shock patients compared to culprit vessel-only PCI. Thus multivessel PCI should be reserved for few selective patients.
- For patients presenting to a non–PCI-capable hospital, rapid assessment should be done of (1) the time from onset of symptoms, (2) the risk of complications related to STEMI, (3) the risk of bleeding with fibrinolysis, (4) the presence of shock or severe HF, and (5) the time required for transfer to a PCI-capable hospital and a decision about administration of fibrinolytic therapy reached. Because the effectiveness of thrombolytics is time dependent, these agents should ideally be administered either in the field or within 30 min of the patient's arrival to the emergency department (door-to-needle time).
- Fibrinolytic therapy: If tissue plasminogen activator (t PA) or reteplase is used, anticoagulants, such as heparin, are given to increase the likelihood of patency in the infarct-related artery for 48 hr and preferably for the duration of the index hospitalization, up to 8 days. In patients receiving fibrinolysis for STEMI, treatment with enoxaparin is superior to treatment with unfractionated heparin for 48 hr but is associated with an increase in major bleeding episodes. In patients receiving streptokinase or APSAC, heparin after thrombolysis is not indicated because it does not offer any additional benefit and can result in increased bleeding complications. Tenecteplase and reteplase are comparable with accelerated infusion recombinant t-PA in terms of efficacy and safety but are more convenient because they are administered by bolus injection. Lanoplase and heparin bolus plus infusion are as effective as tPA with regard to mortality rate, but the rate of intracranial hemorrhage is significantly higher.
- Absolute contraindications to thrombolytic therapy (Table 5) include history of intracranial hemorrhage, known intracranial malignant neoplasm or arteriovenous malformation, ischemic stroke within 3 mo (except acute ischemic stroke within 4.5 hr), suspected aortic dissection, active bleeding or bleeding diathesis (except menses), significant closed head or facial trauma within 3 mo, intracranial or intraspinal surgery within 2 mo, or severe uncontrolled hypertension (unresponsive to therapy). For streptokinase, this applies to prior treatment within 6 mo.

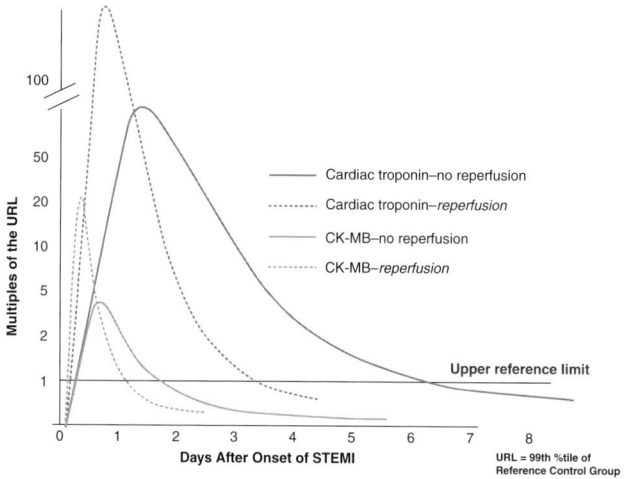

FIG. 2 Trends of troponin and CK-MB following revascularization in MI. *CK-MB*, Creatine kinase-MB; *STEMI*, ST-segment elevation myocardial infarction; *URL*, upper reference limit. (Modified from Shapiro BP, Jaffe AS: Cardio biomarkers. In Murphy JG, Lloyd MA [eds]: *Mayo Clinic cardiology: concise textbook*, ed 3, Rochester, MN, 2007, Mayo Clinic Scientific Press, and New York, 2007, Informa Healthcare USA. Used with permission of Mayo Foundation for Medical Education and Research.)

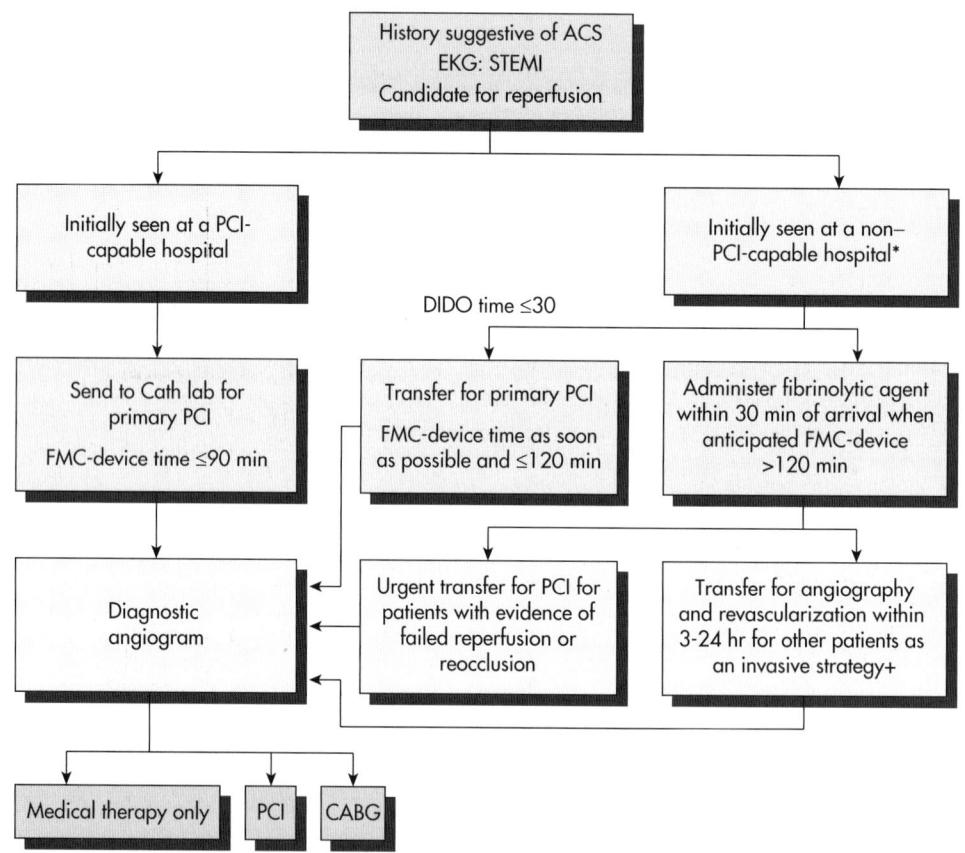

FIG. 3 Reperfusion therapy for patients with STEMI. *Patients with cardiogenic shock or severe heart failure initially seen at a non–PCI-capable hospital should be transferred for cardiac catheterization and revascularization as soon as possible, irrespective of time delay from MI onset. +Angiography and revascularization should not be performed within the first 2 to 3 hr after administration of fibrinolytic therapy. *ACS*, Acute coronary syndrome; *CABG*, coronary artery bypass graft; *Cath*, catheterization; *DIDO*, door-in to door-out; *EKG*, electrocardiogram; *FMC*, first medical contact; *MI*, myocardial infarction; *PCI*, percutaneous coronary intervention; *STEMI*, ST-elevation myocardial infarction. (Modified from O'Gara PT et al: 2013 ACCF/AHA guideline for the management of ST-elevation myocardial infarction, *JACC* 61(4):e78-e140, 2013.)

- Relative contraindications: History of chronic severe, poorly controlled hypertension, SBP >180 mm Hg, diastolic blood pressure (DBP) >110 mm Hg, history of prior ischemic stroke more than 3 mo, dementia, known intracranial pathology, traumatic or prolonged cardiopulmonary resuscitation (CPR) (>10 min), major surgery <3 wk, recent internal bleeding within 2 to 4 wk, noncompressible vascular punctures, pregnancy, active peptic ulcer, oral anticoagulant therapy. After the administration of thrombolytics, immediate transfer to a PCI-capable facility is advisable without waiting for lytic results.
- Transfer to a PCI-capable hospital: Immediate transfer for STEMI patients who develop cardiogenic shock or acute severe HF, irrespective of the time delay from MI onset.

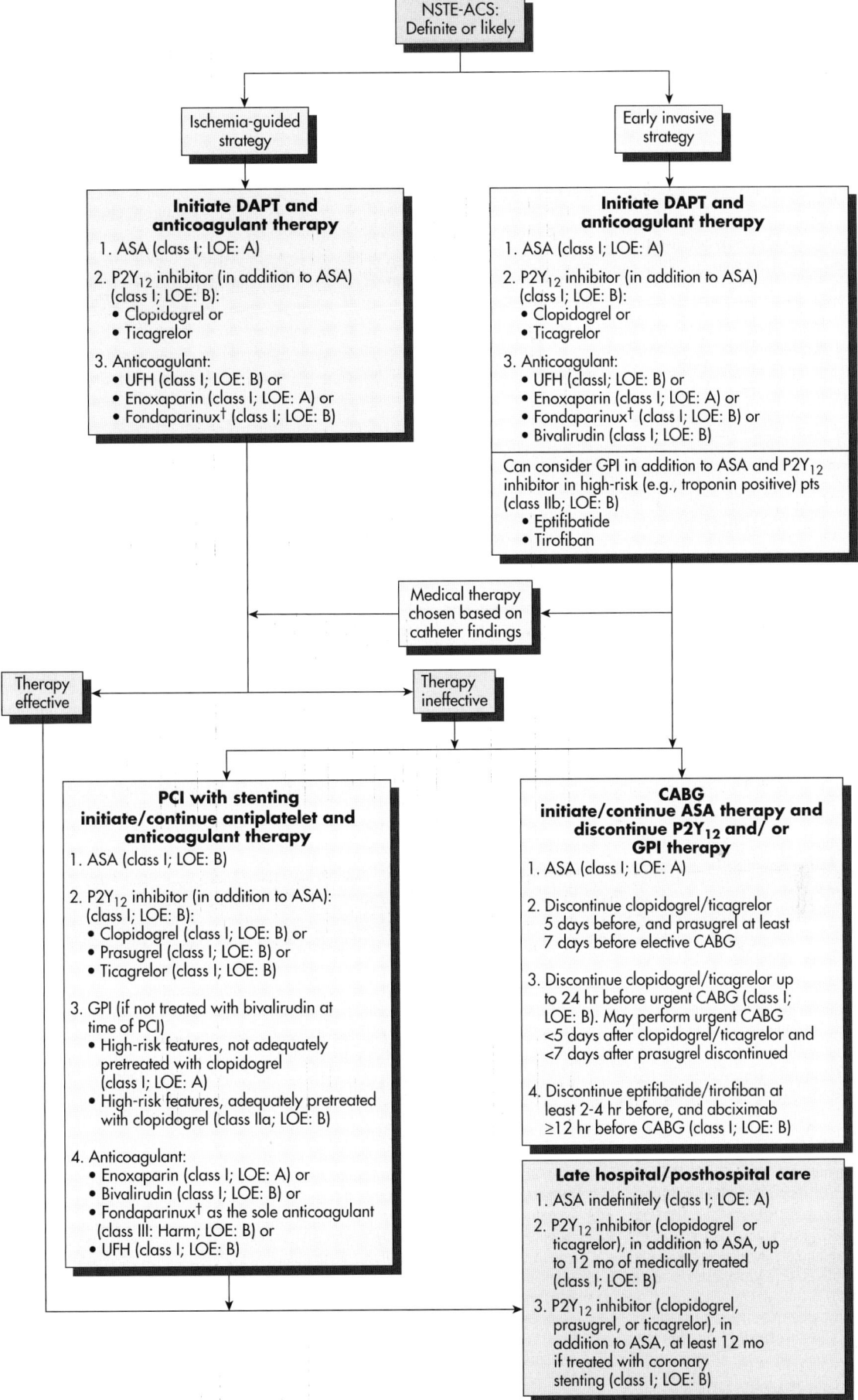

FIG. 4 Algorithm for management of patients with definite or likely non–ST-elevation acute coronary syndromes (*NSTE-ACS*). †In patients who have been treated with fondaparinux (as upfront therapy) who undergo percutaneous coronary intervention (PCI), an additional anticoagulant with anti-IIa activity should be administered at the time of PCI because of the risk of catheter thrombosis. *ASA,* Acetylsalicylic acid (aspirin); *CABG,* coronary artery bypass grafting; *DAPT,* dual-antiplatelet therapy; *GPI,* glycoprotein inhibitor; *LOE,* level of evidence; *pts,* patients; *UFH,* unfractionated heparin. (From Amsterdam EA et al: 2014 AHA/ACC guideline for the management of patients with non–ST-elevation acute coronary syndromes: a report of the American College of Cardiology/American Heart Association Task Force on Practice Guidelines, *J Am Coll Cardiol* 64:e139-228, 2014. In Zipes DP: *Braunwald's heart disease, a textbook of cardiovascular medicine,* ed 11, Philadelphia, 2019, Elsevier.)

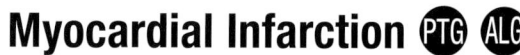
TABLE 3 Indications for Primary Angioplasty and Comparison With Fibrinolytic Therapy

Indications

Alternative recanalization strategy for ST segment elevation or LBBB acute MI within 12 hr of symptom onset (or >12 hr if symptoms persist)

Cardiogenic shock developing within 36 hr of ST segment elevation/Q wave acute MI or LBBB acute MI in patients >75 yr old who can be revascularized within 18 hr of shock onset

Recommended only at centers performing >200 PCI/yr with backup cardiac surgery and for operators performing <75 PCI/yr

Advantages of Primary PCI

Higher initial recanalization rates

Reduced risk of intracerebral hemorrhage

Less residual stenosis; less recurrent ischemia or infarction

Usefulness when fibrinolysis contraindicated

Improvement in outcomes with cardiogenic shock

Disadvantages of Primary PCI (Compared With Fibrinolytic Therapy)

Access, advantages restricted to high-volume centers, operators

Longer average time to treatment

Greater dependence on operators for results

Higher system complexity, costs

LBBB, Left bundle branch block; *MI,* myocardial infarction; *PCI,* percutaneous coronary intervention (includes balloon angioplasty, stenting).
From Goldman L, Schafer AI: *Goldman's Cecil medicine,* ed 24, Philadelphia, 2012, Saunders.

TABLE 4 Dosing Regimens of Commonly Used Thrombolytic Agents

Thrombolytic Agents	Dosing Regimen
t-PA (alteplase)	15 mg bolus IV, followed by 0.75 mg/kg body weight (not to exceed 50 mg) over 30 min, followed by 0.5 mg/kg (not to exceed 35 mg) over 60 min
r-PA (reteplase)	Two 10-U IV boluses, given 30 min apart
TNK–t-PA (tenecteplase)	Single bolus IV 0.5 mg/kg (dose rounded to the nearest 5 mg, ranging from 30 to 50 mg)
Streptokinase	1.5 million U IV over 60 min

IV, Intravenous; *PA,* plasminogen activator; *r-PA,* recombinant plasminogen activator; *TNK–t-PA,* tenecteplase tissue plasminogen activator; *t-PA,* tissue plasminogen activator; *U,* units.
From Andreoli TE et al: *Andreoli and Carpenter's Cecil essentials of medicine,* ed 8, Philadelphia, 2010, Saunders.

Urgent transfer if the patient demonstrates evidence of failed reperfusion or reocclusion after fibrinolytic therapy.

- Coronary angiography should not be performed within the first 2 to 3 hr after administration of fibrinolytic therapy.
- Coronary artery bypass graft (CABG): Urgent CABG is indicated in patients with STEMI and coronary anatomy not amenable to PCI who have ongoing or recurrent ischemia, cardiogenic shock, severe HF, or other high-risk features. CABG is recommended in patients with STEMI at time of operative repair of mechanical defects. Box 1 summarizes CABG in patients with MI.
- Therapeutic hypothermia should be started as soon as possible in comatose patients with STEMI and out-of-hospital cardiac arrest caused by ventricular fibrillation (VF) or pulseless ventricular tachycardia, including patients who undergo primary PCI.
- Immediate angiography and PCI when indicated should be performed in resuscitated out-of-hospital patients.

- The use of mechanical circulatory support is reasonable in patients with STEMI who are hemodynamically unstable and require urgent CABG.
- For NSTEMI patients, immediate invasive strategy (within 2 hr) recommended in patients with refractory angina, signs or symptoms of congestive heart failure or new or worsening ischemic mitral regurgitation, hemodynamic instability, recurrent angina or ischemia at rest or with low level activities despite intensive medical therapy and sustained ventricular tachycardia or ventricular fibrillation.
- Early invasive strategy (<24 hr) for NSTEMI patients recommended if GRACE risk for more than 140, dynamic ST changes on EKG and temporal change in troponin levels.
- NSTEMI patient with low-risk TIMI score (0 or 1) and/or low GRACE score (<109) and/or troponin-negative female patients can benefit from ischemia-guided strategy. Fibrinolytic therapy is contraindicated in NSTEMI patients.

- Medical therapy should be initiated immediately in the emergency department for all MI patients. This includes:
1. Routine measures
   a. Oxygen: Supplemental oxygen should be administered to patients with arterial oxygen desaturation (SaO_2 less than 90%). No benefit has been demonstrated to supplemental oxygen in patients with normal SaO_2.
   b. Nitroglycerin: Increase oxygen supply by reducing coronary vasospasm and decrease oxygen consumption by reducing ventricular preload. Patients with ongoing ischemic discomfort should receive sublingual nitroglycerin every 5 min for a total of three doses, after which an assessment should be made about the need for intravenous nitroglycerin. Intravenous nitroglycerin is indicated for relief of ongoing ischemic discomfort, control of hypertension, or management of pulmonary congestion. Nitrates should not be administered to patients whose systolic blood pressure is <90 mm Hg or ≥30 mm Hg below baseline or severe bradycardia (<50 beats/min), tachycardia (>100 beats/min), or suspected RV infarction. Nitrates should not be administered to patients who have received a phosphodiesterase inhibitor for erectile dysfunction within the last 24 hr (48 hr for tadalafil).
   c. Adequate analgesia: Morphine sulfate 2 to 4 mg intravenous (IV) initially with increments of 2 to 8 mg IV at 5- to 10-min intervals can be given for severe pain unrelieved by nitroglycerin. Morphine can reduce the catecholamine surge caused by anxiety and pain, particularly in patients with anterior myocardial infarctions, which in turn can reduce heart rate and pulmonary capillary wedge pressure (PCWP), the increased cardiac workload and oxygen demand, leading to decreased ischemia and pulmonary congestion. Hypotension from morphine can be treated with careful IV hydration with saline solution. If sinus bradycardia accompanies hypotension, use atropine (0.5 to 1.0 mg IV q5min prn to a total dose of 2.5 mg). Respiratory depression caused by morphine can be reversed with naloxone 0.8 mg. Morphine sulfate and nitroglycerine should be avoided in patients with RV involvement who usually present with bradycardia and hypotension. Pain management in these cases should be provided preferentially with meperidine 25 to 50 mg intravenously q4h, in combination with Phenergan 12.5 mg to prevent nausea and/or vomiting. Blood pressure support with normal saline solution is of critical importance to maintain adequate hemodynamics until optimal revascularization is accomplished.

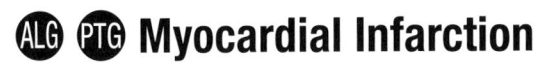
TABLE 5 Contraindications to and Cautions in the Use of Fibrinolytics for Treating ST-Elevation Myocardial Infarction*

Absolute Contraindications

Any previous intracranial hemorrhage
Known structural cerebral vascular lesion (e.g., arteriovenous malformation)
Known malignant intracranial neoplasm (primary or metastatic)
Ischemic stroke within 3 mo *except* acute ischemic stroke within 4.5 hr
Suspected aortic dissection
Active bleeding or bleeding diathesis (excluding menses)
Significant closed-head or facial trauma within 3 mo
Intracranial or intraspinal surgery within 2 mo
Severe uncontrolled hypertension (unresponsive to emergency therapy)
For streptokinase, previous treatment within the previous 6 mo

Relative Contraindications

History of chronic, severe, poorly controlled hypertension
Significant hypertension at initial evaluation (SBP >180 mm Hg or DBP >110 mm Hg)†
History of previous ischemic stroke >3 mo
Dementia
Known intracranial pathology not covered in Absolute Contraindications
Traumatic or prolonged (>10 min) cardiopulmonary resuscitation
Major surgery (<3 wk)
Recent (within 2 to 4 wk) internal bleeding
Noncompressible vascular punctures
Pregnancy
Active peptic ulcer
Oral anticoagulant therapy

DBP, Diastolic blood pressure; *MI,* myocardial infarction; *SBP,* systolic blood pressure.
*Viewed as advisory for clinical decision making and may not be all-inclusive or definitive.
†Could be an absolute contraindication in low-risk patients with MI.
From O'Gara PT et al: 2013 ACCF/AHA guideline for the management of ST-elevation myocardial infarction: a report of the American College of Cardiology Foundation/American Heart Association task force on practice guidelines, *J Am Coll Cardiol* 61:e78, 2013. In Zipes DP: *Braunwald's heart disease, a textbook of cardiovascular medicine,* ed 11, Philadelphia, 2019, Elsevier.

BOX 1 CABG in Patients With Acute MI

Class I
1. Emergency CABG is recommended in patients with acute MI in whom (1) primary PCI has failed or cannot be performed, (2) coronary anatomy is suitable for CABG, and (3) persistent ischemia of a significant area of myocardium at rest or hemodynamic instability refractory to nonsurgical therapy is present.
2. Emergency CABG is recommended in patients undergoing surgical repair of a postinfarction mechanical complication of MI, such as ventricular septal rupture, mitral valve insufficiency because of papillary muscle infarction or rupture, or free wall rupture.
3. Emergency CABG is recommended in patients with cardiogenic shock and who are suitable for CABG irrespective of the time interval from MI to onset of shock and time from MI to CABG.
4. Emergency CABG is recommended in patients with life-threatening ventricular arrhythmias (believed ischemic in origin) in the presence of left main stenosis greater than or equal to 50% or three-vessel CAD.

Class IIa
1. The use of CABG is reasonable as a revascularization strategy in patients with multivessel CAD with recurrent angina or MI within the first 48 hr of STEMI presentation as an alternative to a more delayed strategy.
2. Early revascularization with PCI or CABG is reasonable for selected patients older than 75 yr of age with ST-segment elevation or left bundle branch block who are suitable for revascularization irrespective of the time interval from MI to onset of shock.

Class III
1. Emergency CABG should not be performed in patients with persistent angina and a small area of viable myocardium who are stable hemodynamically.
2. Emergency CABG should not be performed in patients with no reflow (successful epicardial reperfusion with unsuccessful microvascular reperfusion).

From Hillis LD et al: 2011 ACCF/AHA guideline for coronary artery bypass graft surgery: a report of the American College of Cardiology Foundation/American Heart Association task force on practice guidelines, *J Am Coll Cardiol* 58:e123-e210, 2011. In Parrillo JE et al: *Critical care medicine, principles of diagnosis and management in the adult,* ed 5, Philadelphia, 2019, Elsevier.

d. Aspirin 162 to 325 mg PO should be crushed and chewed to enhance drug absorption and delivery. It should be given as soon as possible and continued indefinitely at 81 mg daily. Depending on the clinical and ECG findings, if the patient is suspected to have a coronary anatomy that needs CABG rather than PCI, aspirin should be continued. P2Y12 receptor antagonists should be avoided (except cangrelor) because they increase the perioperative bleeding risk; on-pump surgery should be deferred for at least 24 hr after clopidogrel and ticagrelor. Off-pump surgery might be considered within 24 hr of clopidogrel or ticagrelor if the benefits of revascularization outweigh the risk of bleeding. However, if the coronary artery disease is likely to benefit from PCI alone, then a loading dose of clopidogrel 600 or 300 mg or ticagrelor 180 mg PO or prasugrel 60 mg should be given as early as possible and no later than 1 hr after PCI. P2Y12 receptor antagonist should be continued for at least 1 yr after acute coronary syndrome or after primary PCI. Prasugrel showed significant net clinical benefit (MACE vs. bleeding complications) only in patients with MI who underwent revascularization. It shouldn't be given for non-revascularized patients. Ticagrelor or clopidogrel can be given in patients with MI with or without catheter-based revascularization. Cangrelor is the newest direct-acting P2Y12 platelet receptor inhibitor. It has a similar chemical structure to ATP, with a half-life of 3 to 6 min. It is given IV as a bolus plus 120 min of infusion at the time of primary PCI in patients who are naïve to P2Y12 receptor antagonists. It was approved by the FDA in 2015 after the CHAMPION PHOENIX trial. Clopidogrel and prasugrel should be started after its infusion is finished. The ticagrelor loading dose can be given during the infusion. Considering rapid onset action and clearance, cangrelor can be started in the emergency room at the time of high-risk acute myocardial infarction diagnosis irrespective surgical or catheter-based revascularization.

2. In patients receiving fibrinolytics only or balloon angioplasty without stent, P2Y12 antagonists can be given for as little as 14 days. Clopidogrel is recommended for postfibrinolytic patients.

3. Unfractionated heparin (UFH) is recommended in all patients with NSTEMI and STEMI (fibrinolysis or invasive revascularization). UFH infusion should not exceed more than 48 hr after PCI or fibrinolysis in the absence of an ongoing indication due to risk of heparin-induced thrombocytopenia. NSTEMI patients who underwent ischemia-guided therapy, low-molecular- weight

heparin (LMWH) showed better MACE outcomes compared with UFH. The benefit was not significant in revascularized patients. Bivalirudin was associated with lower MACE and bleeding events in STEMI patients compared with UFH. However, it increased the risk of stent thrombosis. In NSTEMI patients who are undergoing PCI, LMWH, bivalirudin, and UFH are acceptable.

4. Beta-adrenergic blocking agents should generally be given to all patients who do not exhibit evidence of shock. Table 6 summarizes recommendations for β-blocker therapy for STEMI. β-blockers are useful to reduce myocardial oxygen consumption and prevent tachyarrhythmias. Early IV beta blockage (in the initial 24 hr) followed by institution of an oral maintenance regimen is also effective in reducing recurrent infarction and ischemia. Oral β-blockers should be initiated in the first 24 hr in patients with MI who do not have any of the following: Signs of HF, evidence of a low-output state, sinus tachycardia, increased risk for cardiogenic shock, or other contraindications for its use (bradycardia, PR interval more than 0.24 sec, second- or third-degree heart block, active asthma, or reactive airways disease).

5. They should be continued during and after hospitalization for all patients with MI and with no contraindications to their use for at least 2 yr. Patients with initial contraindications to the use of β-blockers in the first 24 hr after MI should be reevaluated to determine their subsequent eligibility. It is reasonable to administer intravenous β-blockers at the time of presentation to patients with MI and no contraindications to their use who are hypertensive or have ongoing ischemia.

6. In patients with acute MI, treatment with drug-eluting stents is associated with decreased mortality rates and a reduction in the need for repeated revascularization procedures compared with treatment including bare-metal stents.

7. Gp IIb/IIIa inhibitors in the era of DAPT therapy and primary PCI have failed to show benefit with "upstream" treatment. Abciximab might be useful in the presence of large thrombus burden during primary PCI. For patients receiving bivalirudin as the primary anticoagulant, routine adjunctive use of GP IIb/IIIa inhibitors is not recommended but may be considered as adjunctive or "bail-out" therapy in selected cases. In patients with acute coronary syndrome with high-risk features and not adequately pretreated with P2Y12 inhibitors, it is useful to administer GP IIb/IIIa inhibitors at the time of PCI.

CHRONIC Rx

- Discharge medications in all patients with MI (unless contraindicated) should include antiischemic medications (e.g., nitroglycerin, β-blocker), lipid-lowering agents, and

TABLE 6 Recommendations for β-Blocker Therapy for ST-Elevation Myocardial Infarction (STEMI)

Recommendation	COR	LOE
Oral β-blockers should be initiated in the first 24 hr in patients with STEMI who do not have any of the following:	I	B
Signs of heart failure or evidence of a low-output state		
Increased risk for cardiogenic shock*:		
• Age >70 yr		
• Systolic blood pressure <120 mm Hg		
• Sinus tachycardia >110 beats/min or heart rate <60 beats/min		
• Increased time since the onset of symptoms of STEMI		
Other relative contraindications to use of oral β-blockers:		
• PR interval longer than 0.24 sec		
• Second- or third-degree heart block		
• Active asthma or reactive airways disease		
β-blockers should be continued during and after hospitalization for all patients with STEMI and no contraindications to their use.	I	B
Patients with initial contraindications to the use of β-blockers in the first 24 hr after STEMI should be reevaluated to determine their subsequent eligibility.	I	C
It is reasonable to administer IV β-blockers at initial encounter to patients with STEMI and no contraindications to their use who are hypertensive or have ongoing ischemia.	IIa	B

COR, Class of recommendation; *IV,* intravenous; *LOE,* level of evidence.
*The greater the number of risk factors present, the higher the risk for development of cardiogenic shock.
Modified from O'Gara PT et al: 2013 ACCF/AHA guideline for the management of ST-elevation myocardial infarction: a report of the American College of Cardiology Foundation/American Heart Association task force on practice guidelines, *J Am Coll Cardiol* 61:e78, 2013. In Zipes DP: *Braunwald's heart disease, a textbook of cardiovascular medicine,* ed 11, Philadelphia, 2019, Elsevier.

antiplatelet therapy (aspirin and/or P2Y12 antagonists).

- Aspirin, 81 mg PO daily, but should be continued indefinitely unless not tolerated (e.g., GI bleed). In MI patients, clopidogrel 75 mg PO daily; ticagrelor, 90 mg bid, or prasugrel, 10 mg PO daily, can be combined with aspirin and should be continued without interruption for a minimum of 12 mo after drug-eluting stent placement; however, aspirin should be continued indefinitely. In cases of high bleeding risk or significant overt bleeding, consider discontinuation of P2Y12 inhibitor after 6 mo (Fig. 5). Combining P2Y12 antagonists with aspirin reduces risk for repeat myocardial infarction and stent thrombosis. If there is an elective surgical intervention pending, it is recommended to defer the surgery until completion of the full course of the P2Y12 antagonist treatment. Duration dual antiplatelet therapy in high-bleeding-risk (HBR) patients is debatable. Many randomized controlled trials support single antiplatelet therapy 1 or 3 mo after PCI in HBR acute coronary syndrome populations.

- Angiotensin-converting enzyme inhibitors (ACEIs) should be started within the first 24 hr of MI to all patients having MI with anterior infarction, pulmonary congestion, or LV EF <40%, in the absence of hypotension. They reduce LV dysfunction and dilation and slow the progression to HF during and after acute MI. Angiotensin receptor blockers (ARBs) should be given to patients who have indication but are intolerant of ACEIs. IV formulations of ACEIs should not be given within the first

24 hr of STEMI due to risk of hypotension. ARBs offer no advantage over ACEIs and should be considered only in patients who are intolerant to ACEIs.

1. ACEIs may be stopped in patients without complications and no evidence of LV dysfunction after 6 to 8 wk.
2. ACEIs should be continued indefinitely in patients with impaired LV function (EF <40%) or clinical HF.

- Long-term aldosterone antagonist therapy should be prescribed for post-MI patients without significant renal dysfunction (creatinine ≤2.5 mg/dl in men and ≤2.0 mg/dl in women) or hyperkalemia who are already taking an ACEI, a β-blocker, and have LV EF <40% with symptomatic HF or diabetes.

- In late 2018, American College of Cardiology (ACC) recommended LDL goal of <70 mg/dl for secondary prevention of atherosclerotic cardiovascular disease. Goal should further be reduced to <55mg/dl in patients with existing atherosclerotic vascular disease and familial hypercholesterolemia. High-intensity statins (atorvastatin 40 to 80 mg or rosuvastatin 20 to 40 mg) should be started as early as possible in all patients with MI regardless of lipid panel, not only for their lipid-lowering effects, but also their antiinflammatory properties (JUPITER trial), which can stabilize the ruptured plaque. Atorvastatin 80 mg can be used (PROVE IT-TIMI 22 and MIRACL trials). IMPROVE-IT trial showed adding ezetimibe to statin treatment could decrease recurrent MI and ischemic stroke in MI patients. FDA also approved two PCSK9 (proprotein convertase

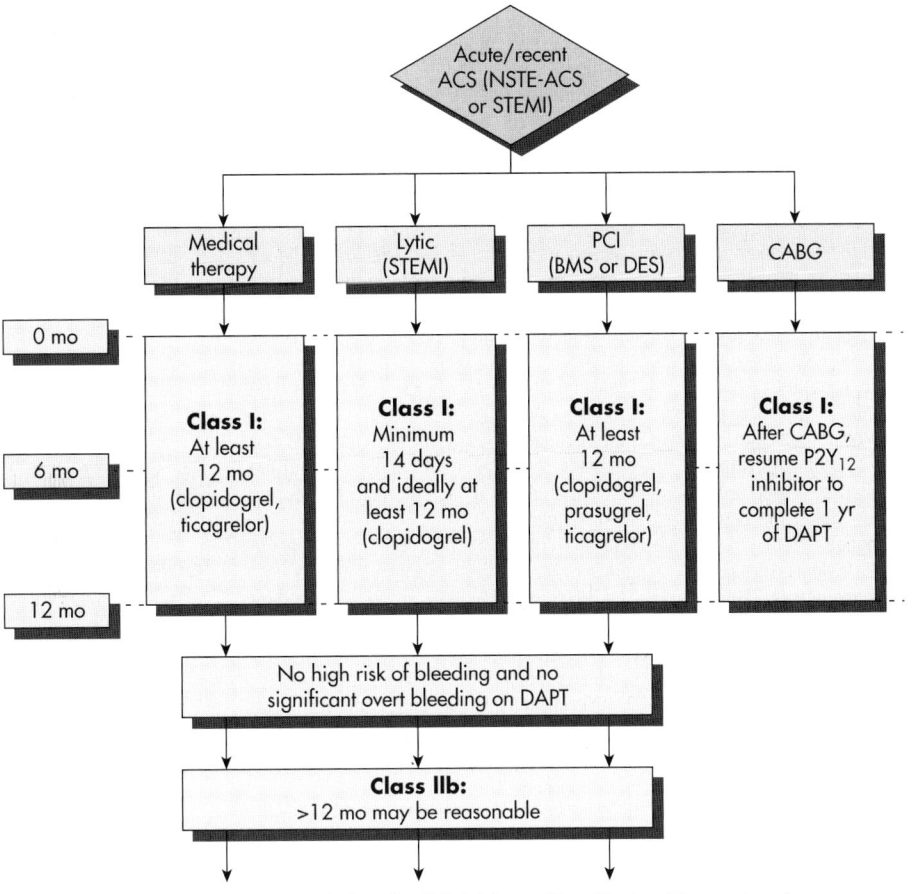

FIG. 5 ACC/AHA guideline recommendation for duration and choice of antiplatelet agent in patients with recent acute coronary syndrome (ACS), including STEMI aspirin therapy is generally continued indefinitely post-ACS. In patients treated with dual-antiplatelet therapy (DAPT) after DES implantation who have a high risk of bleeding (e.g., use of oral anticoagulant therapy, major intracranial surgery) or develop significant overt bleeding, discontinuation of P2Y12 inhibitor therapy after 6 mo for ACS may be reasonable. The optimal duration of prolonged DAPT is not established. *BMS,* Bare-metal stent; *CABG,* coronary artery bypass grafting; *DES,* drug-eluting stent; *lytic,* fibrinolytic therapy; *NSTE-ACS,* non–ST-elevation acute coronary syndrome; *PCI,* percutaneous coronary intervention; *STEMI,* ST-elevation myocardial infarction. (Modified from Levine GN et al: 2016 ACC/AHA guideline focused update on duration of dual antiplatelet therapy in patients with coronary artery disease, *J Am Coll Cardiol* 68(10):1082-115, 2016. In Zipes DP: *Braunwald's heart disease, a textbook of cardiovascular medicine,* ed 11, Philadelphia, 2019, Elsevier.)

subtilisin/kexin type 9) inhibitors (alirocumab and evolocumab) for heterozygous familial hypercholesterolemia patients who are receiving maximally tolerated statins or patients with clinical atherosclerotic cardiovascular disease who require lowering LDL levels. Newer 2018 lipid guidelines suggested starting PCSK9 inhibitor in very high-risk atherosclerotic cardiovascular disease patients who did not meet the LDL goal on high intensity statin and ezetimibe. One should always consider adding ezetimibe to high intensity statin prior to initiation of PCSK9 inhibitor due to cost issues. A fasting lipid panel should be checked during the first 24 hr of hospital course, and the intensive therapy can be stepped down if appropriate. Inclisiran, evinacumab and bempedoic acid are reasonable non–statin therapy alternatives in patients who are unable to tolerate statin and reach target LDL levels.

- In diabetic patients, HbA1c goal should be aimed at below or around 7.0% to reduce micro- and macrovascular complications. Oral hypoglycemic agents GLP1 (glucagon-like peptide) agonist (liraglutide) and SGLT2

(sodium-glucose cotransporter) inhibitor (empagliflozin) showed significant mortality benefit in type 2 diabetic patients with history of CAD.
- ACC/AHA 2017 hypertension guidelines recommend initiation of blood pressure (BP)-lowering medications in patients with clinical CVD and an average SBP $\geq$130 mm Hg or a DBP $\geq$80 mm Hg for goal BP of <130/80.

COMPLICATIONS OF MI

- Cardiogenic shock: Emergent revascularization with either PCI or CABG is the recommended treatment.
- Sustained ventricular tachycardia: Implantable cardioverter-defibrillator therapy (ICD) is indicated before discharge in patients who develop sustained ventricular tachycardia/ventricular fibrillation more than 48 hr after STEMI, provided the arrhythmia is not due to transient or reversible ischemia, reinfarction, or metabolic abnormalities.
- Pacing in MI: Temporary pacing is indicated for symptomatic bradyarrhythmias unresponsive to medical treatment and after revascularization. AV block and bradyarrhythmias in the

setting of inferior wall MI are usually transient, will not require long-term pacing, and usually resolve within 2 to 4 wk of the event. On the contrary, AV block and bradyarrhythmias or new LBBB in the presence of an anterior wall MI is usually a sign of severe disruption of the bundle of His and often requires a permanent pacemaker.
- Pericarditis after MI: Post-MI pericarditis can occur early after MI. Dressler syndrome is an autoimmune inflammatory reaction to myocardial antigen after myocardial infarction. Symptoms of pericarditis usually occur 2 to 3 wk after myocardial infarction. Aspirin is recommended for treatment of pericarditis after MI. Glucocorticoids and nonsteroidal antiinflammatory drugs are potentially harmful for treatment of pericarditis after STEMI.
- Severe mitral regurgitation from papillary muscle rupture (1%), interventricular septum rupture (0.2%), and free wall rupture (1% to 3%) are the three major mechanical complications that can occur after acute myocardial infarction. Echocardiogram is helpful in diagnosing papillary muscle rupture, ventricular septal rupture, and free wall rupture. Right

heart catheterization is needed to show "step-up" in oxygen saturation at the level of right ventricle. Emergent surgical repair is the treatment of choice for ventricular free wall rupture, intraventricular septum rupture, and papillary muscle rupture.

EVALUATION OF POST-MI PATIENTS

- Noninvasive testing for ischemia should be performed before discharge to assess the presence and extent of inducible ischemia in patients with STEMI who have not had coronary angiography and do not have high-risk clinical features for which coronary angiography would be warranted. It might be considered before discharge to evaluate the functional significance of a noninfarct artery stenosis previously identified at angiography and/or before discharge to guide the post-discharge exercise prescription.
- Assessment of LV function: LV ejection fraction should be measured in all patients with STEMI. Echocardiography to rule out presence of mural thrombi in patients suspected of having an extensive infarction (more common with anterior wall MI); contrast echocardiography is added if mural thrombus is suspected.
  1. Assessment of risk for sudden cardiac death: Patients with an initially reduced LV ejection fraction, <40%, who are possible candidates for implantable cardioverter-defibrillator therapy should undergo reevaluation of LV ejection fraction at 90 days (or 42 days if no revascularization was performed). ICD is recommended when LVEF remains <35% in the presence of NYHA class II or III heart failure, or in patients with LVEF <30% regardless of symptoms, if the life expectancy is >1 yr.
- Cardiac rehabilitation/secondary prevention programs are recommended for patients with STEMI.

DISPOSITION

The prognosis after MI depends on multiple factors:
- New bundle branch block, Mobitz II second-degree block, and third-degree heart block adversely affect outcome.
- Size of infarct: The larger it is, the higher the post-MI mortality rate. Significant myocardial stunning with subsequent improvement of ventricular function occurs in most patients after anterior MI. A lower level of creatine

kinase, an estimate of the extent of necrosis, is independently predictive of recovery of function.
- Site of infarct: Inferior wall MI carries a better prognosis than anterior wall MI; however, patients with inferior wall MI and right ventricular involvement have a high risk for arrhythmic complications and cardiogenic shock.
- Ejection fraction after MI: The lower the LV ejection fraction, the higher the mortality rate after MI. The risk of death is higher in the first 30 days after MI among patients with LV dysfunction, HF, or both.
- Presence of post-MI angina indicates a high mortality rate.
- Performance on low-level exercise test: The presence of ST-segment changes during the test is a predictor of high mortality rate during the first year.
- Presence of pericarditis during the acute phase of MI increases mortality rate at 1 yr.
- The Killip classification is an independent predictor of all-cause 30-day mortality:
  1. Killip class I include individuals with no clinical signs of HF. Mortality rate is 6%.
  2. Killip class II includes individuals with rales or crackles in the lungs, S3 gallop, and elevated jugular venous pressure. Mortality rate is 17%.
  3. Killip class III describes individuals with frank acute pulmonary edema. Mortality rate is 38%.
  4. Killip class IV describes individuals in cardiogenic shock or hypotension (measured as systolic blood pressure <90 mm Hg) and evidence of peripheral vasoconstriction (oliguria, cyanosis, or sweating). Mortality rate is 67%.
- Self-reported moderate alcohol consumption in the year before acute MI is associated with reduced 1-yr mortality rate.
- Discharge medication in patients with MI should include lipid-lowering agents. Statins may also lower vascular inflammation and damage by mechanisms other than reduction of low-density lipoprotein cholesterol. Early initiation of statin treatment in patients with acute MI is associated with reduced 1-yr mortality rate.
- Additional poor prognostic factors include cigarette smoking, history of hypertension or prior MI, presence of ST-segment depression in acute MI, older age, diabetes mellitus, and

female sex (especially women >50 yr). Lammintausta and Fonarow reported that single men and women who live alone have a 60% to 70% greater risk of a heart attack. Furthermore, the study showed >160% increase in the risk of sudden death in these groups when compared to people who are married or live with family.
- Renal disease, even mild, as assessed by the estimated glomerular filtration rate, is a major risk factor for cardiovascular complications after MI.
- Although black patients with MI have worse outcomes than their white counterparts, these differences did not persist after adjustment for patient factors and site of care.

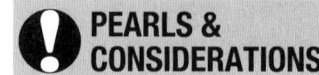

❗ PEARLS & CONSIDERATIONS

COMMENTS

- Approximately 1.5 million patients undergo PCI in the U.S. each year. Depending on local practices and the diagnostic criteria used, 5% to 30% of these patients have evidence of a periprocedural MI.
- The 12-lead ECG has low sensitivity for the detection of MI if the culprit lesion is in the left circumflex artery (LCX). If the initial 12-lead ECG is not diagnostic and high clinical suspicion for acute coronary syndrome exists, it is reasonable to obtain additional posterior chest leads (V7 to V9) to detect LCX occlusion.
- Triad of hypotension, elevated jugular venous pressure, and clear lungs are suggestive of RV infarction in patients with inferior AMI. Administration of nitroglycerin is contraindicated due to hypotension. IV fluids, inotropic support, and early reperfusion are the mainstays of treatment.

REFERENCES
Available at eBooks.Health.Elsevier.com.

RELATED CONTENT
Heart Attack (Patient Information)
Acute Coronary Syndrome (Related Key Topic)
Angina Pectoris (Related Key Topic)
Coronary Artery Disease (Related Key Topic)

AUTHOR: **MAHESWARA SATYA GANGADHARA RAO GOLLA, MD**

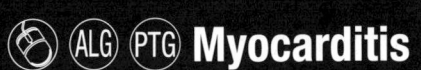

BASIC INFORMATION

DEFINITION
Myocarditis broadly refers to inflammatory disease of the heart muscle (myocardium). Disease severity may range from benign and self-limiting illness to severe, acute decompensation requiring intensive care. Myocarditis may result from exposure to a variety of infectious and noninfectious triggers.

ICD-10CM CODES
I40.0	Infective myocarditis
I40.1	Isolated myocarditis
I40.8	Other acute myocarditis
I40.9	Acute myocarditis, unspecified
A39.52	Meningococcal myocarditis
B26.82	Mumps myocarditis
B33.22	Viral myocarditis
B58.81	Toxoplasma myocarditis
D86.85	Sarcoid myocarditis
I01.2	Acute rheumatic myocarditis
I09.0	Rheumatic myocarditis
I41	Myocarditis in diseases classified elsewhere
I51.4	Myocarditis, unspecified

EPIDEMIOLOGY & DEMOGRAPHICS
- Myocarditis is often underdiagnosed.
- The incidence of focal myocarditis reported at autopsy is 1% to 9% in asymptomatic patients and 50% in patients infected with HIV.
- Myocarditis is the third leading cause of sudden unexpected death (as high as 8% to 9%), especially in competitive athletes. Approximately 1% to 5% of patients that test positive for viral infections may develop myocarditis.

PHYSICAL FINDINGS & CLINICAL PRESENTATION
- Clinical symptoms are heterogeneous, ranging from asymptomatic to severe forms resulting in cardiogenic shock and arrhythmias.
- The most common presentations in patients are new onset heart failure (<6 mo), chest pain, and arrhythmias, which include sinus tachycardia as well as atrial and ventricular premature contractions.
- Chest pain, especially pleuritic and positional, presents when the pericardium is involved.
- Persistent tachycardia may be present, out of proportion to fever.
- Bradyarrhythmia and new-onset unexplained heart block may also occur both in infectious (e.g., Lyme disease) and in immune-mediated forms of myocarditis.
- Faint S_1, S_3, and S_4 gallops on auscultation are important signs of impaired ventricular function.
- Murmur of functional mitral regurgitation and functional tricuspid regurgitation caused by severe left ventricular and right ventricular dilation.
- Pericardial friction rub if associated with pericarditis as in the clinical syndrome of myopericarditis.
- Patients may present with a history of a recent flu-like syndrome or nonspecific viral prodrome (fever, arthralgias, malaise, fatigue). Children often have a more fulminant presentation than adults. Difficulty breathing is the most common presentation of pediatric myocarditis.
- Congestive heart failure (CHF) symptoms that usually manifest with fatigue and decreased exercise capacity and appetite.
- Signs of biventricular failure (hypotension, hepatomegaly, peripheral edema, distention of neck veins, S_3 sounds, and pulmonary edema).
- Presyncope or syncope can occur secondary to ventricular arrhythmias.
- Sudden cardiac death from ventricular tachycardia/ventricular fibrillation mediated by inflammation and/or a scar, which sets up a reentry-mediated pathway for ventricular arrhythmias.
- Acute coronary syndrome, which can occur due to local coronary spasm and inflammation and can present on ECG as acute injury pattern or ischemic changes.

ETIOLOGY
- Infection:
  1. Viral (adenovirus, parvovirus B19, hepatitis C virus [HCV], Coxsackie B virus, cytomegalovirus, enterovirus, poliovirus, mumps, HIV, and Epstein-Barr virus, etc.). Viruses are the most common cause of myocarditis in developed countries. In the 1980s and 1990s, enteroviruses and adenoviruses were frequently associated with myocarditis and dilated cardiomyopathy. In the past 20 yr, however, other viruses such as HCV, parvovirus B19, herpesvirus 6 (HH6), and HIV have emerged as the significant pathogens (Box E1)
  2. Bacterial (*Staphylococcus aureus, Clostridium perfringens*, diphtheria, mycoplasma, Mycobacterium tuberculosis, and any severe bacterial infection)
  3. Mycotic *(Candida, Mucor, Aspergillus, Blastomyces, Histoplasma)*
  4. Parasitic (*Trypanosoma cruzi*—most common worldwide, *Trichinella, Echinococcus, Amoeba, Toxoplasma*)
  5. Rickettsia rickettsii
  6. Spirochetal *(Borrelia burgdorferi*—Lyme carditis)
- Rheumatic fever
- Systemic lupus erythematosus
- Granulomatosis with polyangiitis
- Giant cell arteritis and Takayasu arteritis
- Drugs and medications (e.g., cocaine, emetine, doxorubicin, sulfonamides, isoniazid, methyldopa, amphotericin B, tetracycline, phenylbutazone, lithium, 5-fluorouracil, phenothiazines, interferon-alfa, nivolumab, ipilimumab, tricyclic antidepressants, cyclophosphamides, smallpox vaccination)
- Toxins (carbon monoxide, ethanol, diphtheria toxin, lead, arsenicals)
- Systemic and collagen-vascular disease (scleroderma, sarcoidosis, celiac disease, Sjögren syndrome, Kawasaki syndrome, etc.)
- Celiac disease: Two reports from Italy suggest that celiac disease, which is often clinically unsuspected, accounts for as many as 5% of patients with autoimmune myocarditis or idiopathic DCM
- Radiation
- Postpartum status
- Post–stem cell transplantation
- Hypersensitivity reactions from insect bites, such as bee and wasp bites; from snake bites; and from tetanus toxoid
- Vaccines

DIAGNOSIS (TABLE 1)

DIFFERENTIAL DIAGNOSIS
- Ischemic cardiomyopathy and nonischemic cardiomyopathies, including dilated idiopathic cardiomyopathy
- Acute coronary syndrome
- Valvular heart disease
- Infiltrative diseases of the myocardium, such as sarcoidosis, amyloidosis, hemochromatosis, and Chagas disease

The differential diagnosis of chest pain is described in Section II.

WORKUP
- Medical history: The clinical presentation of myocarditis is nonspecific and can consist of fatigue, palpitations, dyspnea, precordial discomfort, and myalgias.
- Diagnostic workup includes chest X-ray, ECG, laboratory evaluation, echocardiogram, cardiac catheterization, cardiac MRI, and endomyocardial biopsy (in selected patients on the basis of the likelihood of finding specific treatable disorders such as giant cell myocarditis). Of note, endomyocardial biopsy has a sensitivity of only 10% to 35% using standard histologic criteria. This is due to variability in interpretation and sampling error.

LABORATORY TESTS
- Elevated cardiac troponin is suggestive of myocarditis in patients with clinically suspected myocarditis. Troponin I specificity is 89%; sensitivity is 34% to 53%. Elevated troponin aids in diagnosis but does not confer a prognostic value. A normal level does not rule out the diagnosis
- Increased creatine kinase (CK) (with elevated MB fraction, lactate dehydrogenase), and aspartate aminotransferase from myocardial necrosis
- Elevation of cardiac troponin I or T is more common than CK-MB elevation in patients with biopsy-proven myocarditis
- The elevations of cardiac troponin I were correlated with a short duration (typically less than 1 mo) of CHF symptoms, indicating that the majority of myocardial necrosis occurs early in the disease course
- Persistent elevations of cardiac biomarkers are indicative of ongoing myocardial necrosis
- BNP or NT-proBNP is recommended if patient has heart failure symptoms

TABLE 1 Expanded Criteria for Diagnosis of Myocarditis

Suggestive of myocarditis:	2 positive categories
Compatible with myocarditis:	3 positive categories
High probability of being myocarditis:	all 4 categories positive

(Any matching feature in category = positive for category)

Category I: Clinical Symptoms
- Clinical heart failure
- Fever
- Viral prodrome
- Fatigue
- Dyspnea on exertion
- Chest pain
- Palpitations
- Presyncope or syncope

Category II: Evidence of Cardiac Structural or Functional Perturbation *in the Absence* of Regional Coronary Ischemia
- Echocardiography evidence
- Regional wall motion abnormalities
- Cardiac dilation
- Regional cardiac hypertrophy
- Troponin release
- High sensitivity ($>$0.1 ng/ml)
- Positive indium In 111 antimyosin scintigraphy
- Normal coronary angiography *or*
- Absence of reversible ischemia by coronary distribution on perfusion scan

Category III: Cardiac Magnetic Resonance Imaging
- Increased myocardial T2 signal on inversion recovery sequence
- Delayed contrast enhancement after gadolinium-DTPA infusion

Category IV: Myocardial Biopsy—Pathologic or Molecular Analysis
- Pathology findings compatible with Dallas criteria
- Presence of viral genome by polymerase chain reaction or in situ hybridization

DTPA, Diethylenetriamine penta-acetic acid.

- Increased erythrocyte sedimentation rate and C-reactive protein (nonspecific but may be of value in following the progress of the disease and the response to therapy)
- Increased white blood cell count (also nonspecific). An increase in eosinophils can be seen with parasitic infections
- Viral titers (acute and convalescent)
- Cold agglutinin titer, antistreptolysin O titer, blood cultures when appropriate
- Lyme disease antibody titer
- RPR, VDRL
- Histology on endomyocardial biopsy may reveal histiocytic and mononuclear cellular infiltrates, fulfilling the Dallas criteria, which were developed by a panel of cardiac pathologists as a working standard to define the disease; active myocarditis is defined as "an inflammatory infiltrate of the myocardium with necrosis and/or degeneration of adjacent myocytes not typical of the ischemic damage associated with coronary artery disease"
- Based on the European Society of Cardiology Working Group on Myocardial and Pericardial Diseases, immunohistochemical criteria of myocarditis are abnormal inflammatory infiltrates defined as $>$14 leukocytes/mm^2 including up to 4 monocytes/mm^2 with the presence of $>$7 CD^3 positive T lymphocytes/mm^2

- A novel microRNA (the human homologue hsa-mir-Chr8:96) has been reported useful to distinguish patients with myocarditis from those with myocardial infarction[1]

IMAGING STUDIES

- Chest X -ray: Enlargement of cardiac silhouette with or without pulmonary congestion may be present.
- ECG: May be normal or show nonspecific findings. Sinus tachycardia with nonspecific ST-T wave changes unless there is concomitant pericarditis in which the ECG changes are more specific; intraventricular conduction defects and bundle branch blocks are uncommon in typical viral myocarditis but are common manifestations in cardiac sarcoid and idiopathic giant cell myocarditis. The presence of Q waves or left bundle branch block was associated with higher rates of death or transplantation in some patients.
- Lyme disease and diphtheria can cause varying degrees of heart block.
- Changes mimicking acute myocardial infarction (regional ST elevations and Q waves) can occur with focal necrosis from myocarditis.

- Echocardiogram:
  1. The most useful test in detecting decreased ventricular function in suspected myocarditis even when subclinical.
  2. Acute severe myocarditis is associated with left ventricular systolic dysfunction with decreased ejection fraction.
  3. The systolic dysfunction is generally global but may be regional or segmental as in the case of focal myocarditis.
  4. Exercise-induced wall motion abnormalities may also be seen. This is usually due to microvascular dysfunction.
  5. Abnormal tissue Doppler signal can provide additional evidence for the presence of myocarditis.
  6. The echocardiogram can also be helpful with diagnosing coexisting pericardial involvement (for example, with the presence of a pericardial effusion).
  7. The spheroid dysfunctional ventricle in acute myocarditis tends to remodel to the more normal elliptical shape over several months.
- Cardiac catheterization and angiography:
  1. To rule out coronary artery disease. Coronary angiography is most commonly normal with evidence of minimal or no coronary artery disease.
- Endomyocardial biopsy.
  1. A right ventricular endomyocardial biopsy can confirm the diagnosis, although a negative biopsy result does not exclude myocarditis owing to the low sensitivity of this test. Recent studies have shown that myocardial biopsy may be unnecessary because immunosuppression therapy based on biopsy results is generally ineffective. However, if idiopathic giant cell myocarditis is suspected, biopsy can confirm this diagnosis, and immunosuppression therapy is indicated in this patient cohort.
- Cardiac MRI (Fig. E1):
  1. Can be used to detect myocardial edema and myocyte injury in myocarditis.
  2. Increased focal or global signal intensity can be used to calculate an edema ratio. Edema in the absence of necrosis or scar represents reversible injury and thus can predict functional recovery.
  3. Late gadolinium enhancement (LGE) and the presence of increased focal and global myocardial contrast enhancement relative to skeletal muscle.
  4. Any combination of two of the above has a sensitivity and specificity of 76% and 96%, with 85% diagnostic accuracy, and is the gold standard for diagnosis of myocarditis, as opposed to routine biopsy.
  5. Cardiac MRI has demonstrated that myocarditis tends to start as a focal process and becomes a more global process over time, with the extent of myocardial enhancement correlating with clinical status and left ventricular function.
  6. The pattern of LGE is different from that in ischemic cardiomyopathy. LGE in myocarditis tends to involve the epicardium with

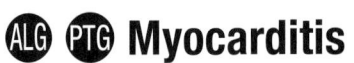

variable extension into the mid myocardium and sparing of the endocardium. This is in contrast to ischemic injury, which involves endocardium first with extension outward.
- Indium-111-labeled antimyosin antibody scintigraphy is positive in myocarditis with a sensitivity of up to 65%.

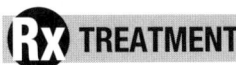 **TREATMENT**

NONPHARMACOLOGIC THERAPY
- Supportive care is the first line of therapy for patients with myocarditis.
- Restrict physical activity (to decrease cardiac work). Bed rest is advisable during viremia.
- Avoid heavy use of alcohol.
- Nonsteroidal antiinflammatory drugs (NSAIDs) should be avoided in patients with HF generally, given the risk of HF exacerbation and possible risk of increased mortality. NSAIDs in the lowest required dose are reserved for patients with perimyocarditis in whom LV function is normal and who have prominent chest pain from pericarditis.

ACUTE GENERAL Rx
- Treat the underlying cause (e.g., use specific antibiotics for bacterial infection, management of autoimmune disease).
- Treat congestive heart failure (CHF) with diuretics, angiotensin-converting enzyme inhibitors (ACE inhibitors), and salt restriction. A beta-blocker may be added once clinical stability has been achieved. In patients with myocarditis associated with severe left ventricular dysfunction, major treatment decisions such as referral for heart transplant, left ventricular assist device, and with implantable cardioverter-defibrillator (ICD) implantation should be deferred for 3 to 6 mo when feasible to allow for improvement with optimal medical therapy.
- Patients who are left with an LVEF $\leq$35% despite optimal medical therapy for 3 to 6 mo, and who have good functional status with prognosis >1 yr, will benefit from primary prevention therapy with ICD implantation as in patients with ischemic cardiomyopathy and other nonischemic cardiomyopathies.
- Antiarrhythmics if needed for ventricular arrhythmias. When antiarrhythmic therapy is necessary, options include amiodarone, dofetilide, and, in patients without class IV HF, cautious use of beta-blockers or calcium channel blockers. ICD implantation for secondary prevention in patients who have life-threatening ventricular arrhythmias and have good functional status with prognosis >1 yr.
- Complete heart block and/or symptomatic bradycardia are indications for pacing during the acute phase of myocarditis but are usually

transient. Permanent pacing is typically not required.
- Management of heart failure with reduced ejection fraction in following the AHA/ACC guidelines in order to decrease mortality.
- Anticoagulation is indicated in patients with evidence of systemic embolism or presence of acute left ventricular thrombus. Standard criteria for anticoagulation for atrial fibrillation should also be applied.
- Mechanical assist devices such as intra-aortic balloon pumps, Impella device, and left ventricular assist device (LVAD) if low output heart failure or cardiogenic shock persists despite medical therapy.
- Cardiac transplantation in patients with chronic or acute fulminant myocarditis with intractable cardiomyopathy and persistent CHF.
- Corticosteroid use is contraindicated in early infectious myocarditis. It is the treatment of choice in patients with immune-checkpoint inhibitor related myocarditis. Steroids also may be indicated in select patients with intractable CHF, severe systemic toxicity, severe life-threatening arrhythmias, and when it is the treatment for the underlying etiology as below.
- Immunosuppressive drugs (prednisone with cyclosporine/Cytoxan or azathioprine) do not have any significant effect on the prognosis of myocarditis and should not be used in the routine treatment of patients with myocarditis. Immunosuppression may have a role in the treatment of myocarditis from systemic autoimmune disease (e.g., lupus, scleroderma); in idiopathic giant cell myocarditis, sarcoidosis, or myocarditis caused by hypersensitivity reactions; or in severe hemodynamic compromise.
- Observational data suggest that patients with giant cell myocarditis treated with certain immunosuppressive regimens have improved survival compared with patients who do not receive immunosuppressive treatment.
- In patients with ongoing viral genomic expression, preliminary data suggest that treatment with interferons may improve both symptoms and left ventricular function when compared with standard heart failure therapy.
- IV immunoglobulins have been studied, but because of lack of efficacy data, at present there is no indication for their use except in some pediatric cases or those refractory to immunosuppressive therapy.
- Improved cardiac function and arrhythmias have been reported in patients with celiac disease and myocarditis or DCM following a gluten-free diet with or without immunosuppressive therapy, but controlled data are lacking.
- In patients who develop myocarditis following the first dose of a COVID-19 mRNA vaccine, we

suggest that the second dose be deferred in most cases; it is reasonable for such individuals to choose to receive a second dose once the episode has completely resolved if the risk of severe COVID-19 is high. Individuals with a history of resolved myocarditis or pericarditis unrelated to COVID-19 vaccination can receive an mRNA vaccine. Of note, myocarditis secondary to COVID-19 vaccine is typically mild in severity with a trend towards normalization of left ventricular systolic function within 6 mo in preliminary observational studies.[2,3]
- A treatment algorithm for patients with myocarditis is described in Fig. E2.

DISPOSITION
- The natural history of myocarditis is illustrated in Fig. E3. Most patients with acute myocarditis and mild cardiac involvement have a partial or a full clinical recovery. In some cases, however, the process may continue subclinically with eventual progression to a cardiomyopathy. Therefore all patients with myocarditis should be followed up at least initially at intervals of 1 to 3 mo, depending on their initial severity of illness. Of those with advanced cardiac dysfunction, 33% will have residual cardiac dysfunction, and 25% may progress to cardiac transplantation or death.
- Prognosis is best for patients with fulminant lymphocytic myocarditis (severe hemodynamic compromise, rapid onset of symptoms, or high fever). These patients tend to have complete recovery with total resolution of myocarditis on repeat biopsy.
- In contrast, patients with giant cell myocarditis have an extremely poor prognosis with a median survival of <6 mo, and most require cardiac transplantation.
- In patients with immune-checkpoint inhibitor related myocarditis, regardless of the severity of presentation, the patient should not be rechallenged with immunotherapy.
- The American Heart Association recommends 3 to 6 mo abstinence from competitive sports after myocarditis[4]

REFERRAL
Consider heart transplant if intractable CHF develops.

REFERENCES
Available at eBooks.Health.Elsevier.com.

RELATED CONTENT
Myocarditis (Patient Information)

AUTHORS: **DANA PRICE, MD,** and **ARAVIND RAO KOKKIRALA, MD, FACC**

M

Diseases and Disorders

I

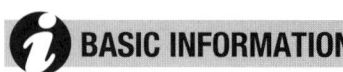
BASIC INFORMATION

DEFINITION

Narcolepsy is a chronic neurologic sleep disorder characterized by excessive daytime sleepiness and dysregulation of rapid eye movement (REM) sleep. It is the second most common cause of disabling daytime sleepiness after obstructive sleep apnea. Symptoms of REM sleep dysregulation include cataplexy, sleep paralysis, and hallucinations during the transition between wake and sleep. A short REM latency, poor nocturnal sleep, and REM behavior disorder are frequently observed. A hypocretin (orexin) deficiency has been noted in certain types of narcolepsy due to cellular destruction of the posterolateral hypothalamus.[1-3] The international classification of diseases (ICD-10) codes are summarized in Table 1.

SYNONYMS

Hypersomnia of central origin
Narcolepsy with cataplexy (Type I)
Narcolepsy-cataplexy syndrome (Type I)
Narcolepsy with hypocretin deficiency (Type I)
Narcolepsy without cataplexy (Type II)
Narcolepsy without hypocretin deficiency (Type II)
Gélineau syndrome

ICD-10CM CODES

G47.411 Narcolepsy with cataplexy
G47.419 Narcolepsy without cataplexy

EPIDEMIOLOGY & DEMOGRAPHICS

INCIDENCE:[1,4]: 0.74/100,000 persons/yr (Type I)
  1.34/100,000 persons/yr (Type II)—the true incidence is unknown
PREVALENCE: 25 to 100/100,000 (Type I)
  65.4/100,000 (Type II)
PREDOMINANT SEX: Males and females are equally affected
PREDOMINANT AGE: Primary peak 15 to 25 years of age
  Secondary peak 35 to 45 years of age
  Range: 10 to 55 years of age
RISK FACTORS: Hypothalamic lesions (tumor, demyelinating plaque, etc), head injury, history of meningitis or encephalitis, family history of narcolepsy, vascular malformations, neurosarcoidosis, stroke, and obesity[3,5-7]
GENETICS:[6]:
- Associated with human leukocyte antigen (HLA) subtypes, specifically, *DQB1*0602,* which is present in 95% of patients with cataplexy and 96% of patients with hypocretin deficiency. Of note, approximately 20% of the general population may also be positive for HLA-DQB1*0602.
- Risk of narcolepsy increases 20 to 40 times if a family member is affected.
- Monozygotic twin concordance rate is 17% to 36%, thus indicating an incomplete penetrance and suggesting an environmental factor in the disease process.

PHYSICAL FINDINGS & CLINICAL PRESENTATION[7]

- An overwhelming urge to sleep with chronic hypersomnia may occur during the day (Table 2).
- Cataplexy occurs in 60% to 100% of patients with narcolepsy and is reported as a partial or complete loss of voluntary muscle control with preserved consciousness that is precipitated by a strong emotion, more commonly with laughter. This is the most specific symptom and is considered pathognomonic for narcolepsy type I.[1]
- Hypnagogic (wake to sleep) or hypnopompic (sleep to wake) hallucinations have been reported in 60% to 80% of patients with narcolepsy.
- Sleep paralysis, defined as loss of muscle tone during the transition between sleep and wakefulness, occurs in 60% to 80% of patients with narcolepsy. It may occur with hallucinations and can be interrupted by sensory stimuli.
- Only about one third of patients will have all four symptoms of narcolepsy: Chronic daytime sleepiness, cataplexy, hypnagogic hallucinations, and sleep paralysis.
- Fragmented sleep is seen in 60% to 80% of narcolepsy patients and can often be mistaken for insomnia or other intrinsic sleep disorder.
- Other symptoms that have been reported in narcolepsy include automatic behavior or semipurposeful movements in 40% of patients and memory disturbances in 50% of patients.
- The clinical presentation of narcolepsy with cataplexy in children and adolescents may be different from that of adults (Table E3). Children may present with prolonged nocturnal sleep or paradoxically may present with hyperactive behavior, insomnia, and bizarre hallucinations. Children may present with characteristic *cataplectic facies* (facial weakness with tongue protrusion) not associated with emotion, or cataplexy may be manifested with perioral dystonic movements (Fig. E1).[8]

ETIOLOGY

The loss of hypocretin/orexin signaling, genetic factors, and brain lesions are presently identified factors in the development of narcolepsy. Molecular mimicry is also thought to play a role.
HYPOCRETIN/OREXIN:
- Loss of hypocretin-1 and hypocretin-2 (also known as orexin-A and orexin-B) producing neurons in the lateral hypothalamus.[2-3]
- Human cerebrospinal fluid (CSF) levels of hypocretin-1 are low (<110 pg/ml) to undetectable in narcoleptics with cataplexy.

TABLE 1 International Classification of Sleep Disorders: Definitions and Pathophysiology

Condition	Diagnostic Criteria*	Pathophysiology
Type 1 narcolepsy	Presence of two or more of the following: Cataplexy, positive MSLT, and low CSF hypocretin-1	Hypocretin deficiency 98% HLA-DQB1*06:02
Type 2 narcolepsy	Positive MSLT; most often with no or unclear cataplexy	Unknown, heterogenous ~16% Hypocretin deficiency ~40% HLA-DQB1*0602
Secondary narcolepsy	As above, but due to neurologic conditions	With or without hypocretin deficiency, various disorders
Idiopathic hypersomnia	No cataplexy, no SOREMPs during the MSLT	Unknown, likely heterogeneous

*Abnormal Multiple Sleep Latency Test (MSLT): Sleep latency ≤8 min, ≥2 sleep-onset REM periods (SOREMPs), including a nocturnal SOREMP. For details, see *International Classification of Sleep Disorders*, ed 3. (American Academy of Sleep Medicine: *International classification of sleep disorders*, ed 3, Darien, IL, 2014, American Academy of Sleep Medicine).
CSF, Cerebrospinal fluid; *HLA,* human leukocyte antigen; *REM,* rapid eye movement.
From Kryger M et al: *Principles and practice of sleep medicine,* ed 6, Philadelphia, 2017, Elsevier.

TABLE 2 Major Clinical Features of Narcolepsy

Major Manifestations	
Excessive sleepiness	100%
Cataplexy	70%
Sleep paralysis	25%-50%
Hypnagogic/hypnopompic hallucinations	20%-40%
Disturbed night sleep	70%-80%
Automatic behavior	20%-40%

From Jankovic J et al: *Bradley and Daroff's neurology in clinical practice,* ed 8, Philadelphia, 2022, Elsevier.

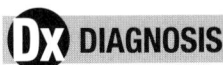
- Narcolepsy without cataplexy may have a different etiology due to the fact that CSF hypocretin levels are usually normal in these patients, which implies that there may be a completely separate mechanism in these patients, or it may result from a less extensive loss of hypocretin neurons or impaired signaling.

SECONDARY ETIOLOGIES:
- Central nervous system lesions including tumors, vascular malformations, and strokes have all been reported to cause secondary narcolepsy.
- Direct injury to the hypocretin neurons or their projections is the most likely cause of secondary narcolepsy due to central nervous system lesions.
- Narcolepsy has been reported in genetic syndromes, including Prader-Willi syndrome, Coffin-Lowry syndrome, and Niemann-Pick disease type C, as well as demyelinating and paraneoplastic syndromes (anti-Ma).[5-6,9]

Dx DIAGNOSIS

DIFFERENTIAL DIAGNOSIS
Excessive daytime somnolence:[7]
- Idiopathic hypersomnia with long or short sleep time
- Inadequate sleep hygiene
- Behaviorally induced insufficient sleep syndrome
- Central or obstructive sleep apnea (sleep-disordered breathing)
- Circadian rhythm disorder
- Psychiatric disorders (especially depression)
- Diencephalic lesions
- Drug or alcohol abuse or withdrawal
- Hypothyroidism
- Increased intracranial pressure
- Traumatic brain injury
- Kleine-Levin syndrome
- Autism
- Autosomal dominant cerebellar ataxia, deafness, and narcolepsy
- Seizures
- Neurodegenerative diseases
Cataplexy:[7]
- Seizures
- Periodic paralysis
- Recurrent isolated sleep paralysis
- Cardiovascular insufficiency
- Psychogenic (multiple causes)
- Lesions of the hypothalamus or brain stem

WORKUP
- Because persistent hypersomnia can occur with many conditions, it is important to rule out other sleep disorders.
- Narcolepsy is often diagnosed by clinical history. The Epworth Sleepiness Scale is very useful in determining the degree of excessive daytime sleepiness (Table 4). A modified Epsworth Sleepiness Scale for children and adolescents is described in Table 5.
- The medical history should include questions regarding severity of daytime hypersomnia while also evaluating for sleep-disordered

---

TABLE 4   Epworth Sleepiness Scale

How likely are you to doze off or fall asleep in the following situations, in contrast to just feeling tired? This refers to your usual way of life in recent time. Even if you have not done some of these things recently, try to work out how they would have affected you. Use the following scale to choose the most appropriate number for each situation.
0 = Would never doze
1 = Slight chance of dozing
2 = Moderate chance of dozing
3 = High chance of dozing

Situation	Chance of Dozing
Sitting and reading	
Watching TV	
Sitting and inactive in a public place (theater or meeting)	
As a passenger in a car for an hour without a break	
Lying down to rest in the afternoon when circumstances permit	
Sitting and talking to someone	
Sitting quietly after lunch (without alcohol)	
In a car, while stopped for a few minutes in traffic	
Total	

From Johns MW: A new method for measuring daytime sleepiness: the Epworth Sleepiness Scale, *Sleep* 14:540-545, 1991.

TABLE 5   Epworth Sleepiness Scale for Children and Adolescents

Scale
0 = Would never fall asleep
1 = Slight chance of falling asleep
2 = Moderate chance of falling asleep
3 = High chance of falling a sleep

Activities	Score
Sitting and reading	
Sitting and watching TV or a video	
Sitting in a classroom at school during the morning	
Sitting and riding in a car or bus for about half an hour	
Lying down to rest or nap in the afternoon	
Sitting and talking to someone	
Sitting quietly by yourself after lunch	
Sitting and eating a meal	

Modified from Janssen KC et al: Validation of the Epworth sleepiness scale for children and adolescents using Rasch analysis, *Sleep Med* 33:30-35, 2017.

---

breathing, transient muscle weakness triggered by emotion, hallucinations while falling asleep or upon awakening, and inability to move after awakening. The clinical evaluation should also address symptoms of seizures and paraneoplastic disorders while also asking about previous stroke or genetic disorders. A detailed family history is imperative. Hypothalamic dysfunction such as unexplained weight gain, endocrine abnormalities, circadian dysrhythmias, and autonomic nervous system problems may provide useful insight.[9]
- A thorough examination including a detailed neurologic examination should be performed.
- Nocturnal polysomnography followed by a multiple sleep latency test (MSLT) remains the gold standard for the diagnosis of narcolepsy. The mean sleep latency should be ≤8 minutes with two or more SOREMPs (sleep onset REM periods). A drug screen should also be performed to rule out pharmacologic modulations of sleep. Actigraphy is also recommended before the sleep study to ensure adequate sleep was achieved and improve the reliability of test results. Medications that affect sleep should be briefly held before the sleep study (if safe to do so).[7]

LABORATORY TESTS
CSF hypocretin (if cataplexy is present but the MSLT is negative)
HLA testing [DQB1*0602] (optional)

Rx TREATMENT

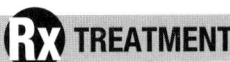

Narcolepsy can be treated with a combination of behavioral and pharmacologic approaches.[10-11] Examples of initial treatment packages for adults are summarized in Table 6.

NONPHARMACOLOGIC THERAPY

Avoidance of over-the-counter drugs and illicit drugs, optimal sleep hygiene, scheduled daily naps and caffeine intake, and psychosocial support can be used for symptoms of excessive daytime somnolence. However, non-pharmacologic therapy is typically not sufficient for treatment of narcolepsy alone but is often used as adjunct therapy with medications.

PHARMACOLOGIC THERAPY (TABLES 7, E8, AND 9)

For excessive daytime somnolence:[11]
- Sodium oxybate: A central nervous system depressant that can be used for the treatment of cataplexy and REM-related symptoms; 2.25 to 4.5 g PO at bedtime followed by another 2.25 to 4.5 g in 2.5 to 4 h.
- Combination of calcium, magnesium, potassium, and sodium oxybates is a new formulation.
- Modafinil 200 to 400 mg orally (PO) every morning or divided bid
- Armodafinil 150 or 250 mg PO as a single dose in the morning
- Methylphenidate IR 10 to 15 mg PO bid to tid initially
- Methylphenidate LA 18 to 54 mg every morning or divided bid

- Dextroamphetamine 10 to 60 mg daily
- Pitolisant: Initial dose is 8.9 mg (two 4.45 mg tablets) taken once daily on waking; the first FDA-approved histamine-3 (H3) receptor antagonist/inverse agonist for narcolepsy
- Solriamfetol: Initial dose is 75 mg daily but can be increased to 150 mg daily

For cataplexy:[10-11]
- Sodium oxybate: A central nervous system depressant that can be used for the treatment of cataplexy and rapid eye movement (REM) related symptoms; 2.25 to 4.5 g at bedtime followed by another 2.25 to 4.5 g in 3 to 4 h
- Combination of calcium, magnesium, potassium, and sodium oxybates is a new formulation
- Fluoxetine 20 mg/day initially
- Sertraline 25 mg/day initially
- Venlafaxine 37.5 mg/day initially
- Clomipramine 25 mg/day initially
- Protriptyline 5 mg tid initially
- Imipramine 25 to 50 mg/day initially
- Desipramine 10 mg bid initially
- Atomoxetine 40 mg/day initially
- Pitolisant: Initial dose is 8.9 mg (two 4.45 mg tablets) taken once daily on waking; the first FDA-approved H3 receptor antagonist/inverse agonist for narcolepsy

DISPOSITION

This is a chronic sleep disorder that can be successfully managed with medications and lifestyle adjustments.

REFERRAL

Because of the complexity of this disorder and its ever-changing management and treatment, patients should be referred to centers or programs with highly trained sleep specialists with expertise caring for these patients, especially if sodium oxybate (Xyrem or Xywav) therapy is needed.

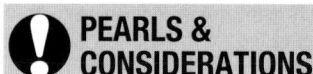

PEARLS & CONSIDERATIONS

Many patients with narcolepsy report the onset of symptoms beginning in childhood to early adulthood, with a long delay of actual diagnosis on the order of 10 to 15 years. Typically, excessive daytime sleepiness is the initial symptom, followed by REM dysregulation (e.g., cataplexy, sleep paralysis, hypnagogic/hypnopompic hallucinations). Patients with narcolepsy also have higher than expected incidence of other sleep disorders, including obstructive sleep apnea, periodic limb movements of sleep, and REM sleep behavior disorder.[10]

TABLE 6 Examples of Initial Treatment Packages for Adults

General Measures

Avoid shifts in sleep schedule
Avoid heavy meals and alcohol intake
Regular timing of nocturnal sleep: 10:30 P.M. to 7 A.M.
Naps: Strategically timed naps if possible (e.g., 15 min at lunchtime, 15 min at 5:30 P.M.)

Medications for Sleepiness

The effects of stimulant medications vary widely among patients. The dosing and timing of medications should be individualized to optimize performance. Additional doses, as needed, may be suggested for periods of anticipated sleepiness.

Modafinil* 100-200 mg (taken when waking up in the morning) and 100-200 mg at lunchtime *or* sodium oxybate[†] at bedtime: Dosage must start low at 2.25 g taken twice while in bed (at bedtime and 2.5-4 hr after bedtime); increase to total dosage of 5-6 g within 2-4 wk. This initial dose is usually ineffective, so increase to 3 g at bedtime and 3 g approximately 2.5-4 hr after bedtime if tolerated. Depending on response, dosage can be increased to as high as 9 g total nightly dose. Do not increase above 9 g because of risk of serious side effects during sleep. It may take more than 2 mo for daytime symptoms to improve, and cataplexy may improve faster than excessive daytime sleepiness. If the patient is already taking a daytime stimulant, it may be possible to reduce the stimulant dose or to discontinue it once a therapeutic dosage of sodium oxybate has been reached.

Methylphenidate 5 mg (three or four tablets; 10 mg when waking up; 5 mg 30 min before lunch; 5 mg near 3 P.M.; better action is always obtained if the drug is taken on an empty stomach) or 20 mg SR in the morning (on an empty stomach)

If Persistent Difficulties

Modafinil 200 mg in the morning and 200 mg at lunch (total daily dosage, 400 mg) *or* add sodium oxybate (GHB) at bedtime: Dosage must start low as indicated above.

Methylphenidate (SR): 20 mg in the morning; 5 mg after noon nap; 5 mg at 4 P.M. *or* possibly (more in teenagers) atomoxetine: Start at 0.5 mg/kg within 1 wk to appropriate dosage of 1-1.2 mg/kg taken in the morning

If No Response

Dextroamphetamine sulfate: 15 mg on awakening; 5 mg afternoon nap; 5 mg at 3:30 or 4 P.M. (or 15 mg at awakening and 15 mg after noon nap)

Medications for Cataplexy[‡]

Sodium oxybate (see above)
Venlafaxine 150-300 mg
Fluoxetine 20-60 mg
Duloxetine 60 mg

If No Response

Clomipramine 75-125 mg, *or* viloxazine 150-200 mg, *or* imipramine 75-125 mg

---

*Modafinil works best in naive subjects. It should be the drug of first choice in children and adults.
[†]Response to sodium oxybate is slow.
[‡]Medications may be taken in the evening near bedtime (sodium oxybate, clomipramine, imipramine), only in the morning (fluoxetine), or in the morning and at lunchtime (viloxazine, venlafaxine). The only medications specifically approved for use in narcolepsy by the Food and Drug Administration are modafinil and sodium oxybate.
SR, Sustained-release tablet.
From Kryger M et al: *Principles and practice of sleep medicine,* ed 6, Philadelphia, 2017, Elsevier.

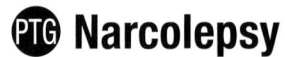

TABLE 7 Narcolepsy Drugs Currently Available

Drug	Usual Dosage* (All Drugs Administered Orally)
Treatment of EDS	
Stimulants[i]	
Modafinil	100-400 mg/day
Sodium oxybate	6-9 g/day (divided in two doses)
Methylphenidate	10-60 mg/day
Atomoxetine	10-25 mg/day
Dextroamphetamine	5-60 mg/day
Methamphetamine	20-25 mg/day
Treatment of Auxiliary Effects (e.g., Cataplexy)	
Sodium oxybate (gamma-hydroxybutyrate)	6-9 g/day (divided in two doses)
Antidepressants	
Without Atropinic Side Effects	
Venlafaxine XR	75-300 mg/day
Fluoxetine	20-60 mg/day
Viloxazine	50-200 mg/day
Duloxetine	60 mg/day
With Atropinic Side Effects	
Protriptyline	2.5-20 mg/day
Imipramine	25-200 mg/day
Clomipramine	25-200 mg/day
Desipramine	25-200 mg/day

*On occasion, depending on clinical response, the dose may be outside the usual dosage range.

[i]Most stimulants should be administered in divided doses, commonly in the morning and at lunchtime. This is recommended for amphetamines and modafinil. Methylphenidate has a fast elimination rate, so the slow-release (SR) formula may be helpful in the morning (e.g., 20 mg SR). If it is administered by 5-mg increments, the usual timing of methylphenidate administration is every 3 to 4 h until 3 P.M.

EDS, Excessive daytime somnolence.

From Kryger M et al: *Principles and practice of sleep medicine,* ed 6, Philadelphia, 2017, Elsevier.

COMMENTS

Narcolepsy is a rare disorder that is under-diagnosed. The average time from onset of symptoms to diagnosis is 5 to 15 years. Cataplexy is specific for narcolepsy, but other symptoms of REM dysregulation, including sleep paralysis and hypnagogic or hypnopompic hallucinations, can occur even in normal patients. SOREM or REM periods on an MSLT may occur as a result of sleep deprivation or withdrawal from REM-suppressing drugs. Actigraphy and a review of medications are recommended to further evaluate.

REFERENCES

Available at eBooks.Health.Elsevier.com.

RELATED CONTENT

Narcolepsy (Patient Information)

AUTHOR: **ANNISE WILSON, MD**

TABLE 9 Treatment Options for Narcolepsy in the Pediatric Population

Symptom	Management Options[a,b]	Suggested Dosages in Pediatric Patients
Excessive daytime sleepiness	Sodium oxybate: U.S. FDA approved for ≥7 years of age Methylphenidate (>6 years of age) Amphetamines (>3 years of age) Modafinil/armodafinil (>17 years of age) Atomoxetine (>6 years of age)	Sodium oxybate: 2-6 g Methylphenidate: 10-40 mg Dextroamphetamine: 5-40 mg Modafinil: 100-400 mg, Armodafinil: 50-250 mg Atomoxetine: 10-25 mg
Cataplexy	Sodium oxybate (≥7 years of age) Atomoxetine Venlafaxine Clomipramine Imipramine Protriptyline Fluoxetine Sertraline Citalopram	Venlafaxine: 37.5-150 mg Clomipramine: 10-75 mg Fluoxetine: 20-40 mg, Citalopram: 10-40 mg
General	Nonbehavioral interventions: Scheduled naps Well-designed exercise program Career counseling Personalized psychological support	

[a]The most recent systematic review of the literature by the American Academy of Sleep Medicine supports the use modafinil and sodium oxybate to treat narcolepsy in the pediatric population at a conditional strength of recommendation.

[b]Only traditional stimulants and sodium oxybate are approved therapies for pediatric narcolepsy.

FDA, U.S. Food and Drug Administration.

From Kryger M et al: *Principles and practice of sleep medicine,* ed 7, Philadelphia, 2023, Elsevier.

Nasopharyngeal Carcinoma

ℹ️ BASIC INFORMATION

DEFINITION

Nasopharyngeal carcinoma (NPC) is an epithelial carcinoma originating in the nasopharynx and has a clinical behavior distinct from other head and neck carcinomas.

SYNONYM

Nasopharynx cancer
NPC

ICD-10CM CODE

C11.9 Malignant neoplasm of nasopharynx, unspecified

EPIDEMIOLOGY & DEMOGRAPHICS

- NPC is an uncommon cancer that is endemic to east and southeast Asia (70% of cases). In 2020, there were an estimated 133,354 new cases and 80,008 deaths globally.[1]
- Incidence rate of 3 per 100,000 population in China and 0.4 per 100,000 in Caucasian population. Its incidence is decreasing steadily in the endemic regions in Asia.
- Incidence is higher in males (2.5 times than females).

RISK FACTORS:
- Epstein-Barr virus (EBV) infection
- Tobacco smoking
- Alcohol consumption
- Family history
- Consumption of preserved foods
- Poor oral hygiene

GENETICS:
- Human leukocyte antigen (HLA) genes residing at the major histocompatibility complex (MHC) region on chromosome 6p21 have been widely recognized as major risk loci conferring nasopharyngeal carcinoma risk.
- Genomic changes involved in the development of NPC include: Multiple loss-of-function mutations in the NFkB–negative regulators, recurrent genetic lesions such as loss of the CDKN2A/CDKN2B locus, CCND1 amplification, TP53 mutation, and mutations in the PI3K/MAPK signaling pathways.[2]

CLINICAL PRESENTATION

- Chronically blocked or stuffy nose
- Recurrent epistaxis and bloody rhinorrhea
- Hearing impairment and tinnitus
- Headache
- Ear pain
- Palpable neck adenopathy
- Cranial nerve palsies

ETIOLOGY

- Pathologic subtypes of squamous NPC are keratinizing, nonkeratinizing, and basaloid types. The keratinizing subtype accounts for less than 20% of cases worldwide and is seen in nonendemic areas. The nonkeratinizing subtype constitutes most cases in endemic areas (>95%) and is predominantly associated with Epstein-Barr virus (EBV) infection.
- Persistent EBV infection in genetically mutated epithelial cells and the proliferation of infected cells lead to tumorigenic transformation.[3,4] Chronic exposure of the nasopharyngeal mucosa to environmental carcinogens increases DNA damage and leads to somatic genetic changes in the nasopharyngeal epithelial cells. EBV infection in turn facilitates inactivation of a variety of cancer-related genes. During tumor development, acquired mutations of regulatory factors in the NF-κB signaling pathway alter the activity of additional cancer-related genes. Mutations in the MHC class I genes, PI3K/MAPK pathways as well as somatic mutations of TP53 and RAS genes may be at play in the development of tumor recurrence and metastasis.

Dx DIAGNOSIS

DIFFERENTIAL DIAGNOSIS

- Nasal polyps
- Nasopharyngeal lymphoma
- Nasopharyngeal sarcoma

WORKUP

- Direct nasopharyngoscopy by ear, nose, throat (ENT) physician followed by biopsy (Fig. E1) and imaging studies (Fig. E2)

LABORATORY TESTS

- Complete blood count
- Comprehensive chemistry panel
- Circulating cell-free EBV DNA is a biomarker for nasopharyngeal carcinoma. Pretreatment plasma EBV-DNA levels may add to the prognostic value of conventional TNM staging systems (Table E1)

IMAGING STUDIES

- CT or MRI of the head and neck; MRI is better than CT for soft-tissue extent assessment and retropharyngeal nodal detection.
- PET/CT is used to assess for detection of distant metastasis and for detection of residual cancer after completion of therapy.

Rx TREATMENT

The mainstay of therapy is not surgery but concurrent chemotherapy and radiation therapy. Both adjuvant chemotherapy and to a lesser extent neoadjuvant chemotherapy are routinely utilized after and before chemoradiotherapy in the clinical setting.[5]

NONPHARMACOLOGIC THERAPY

- Surgery is utilized for diagnostic biopsies and for neck dissection in the setting of residual neck lymphadenopathy after completion of definitive chemoradiotherapy.
- Supportive care with gastrostomy tube nutrition is often required to maintain nutritional and hydration status during treatment.

ACUTE GENERAL Rx

- Intensity modulated radiotherapy (IMRT) with concurrent every 3-wk cycles of cisplatin and 5-fluorouracil chemotherapy is a standard approach in patients with locoregionally advanced NPC. Adjuvant chemotherapy with cisplatin and gemcitabine is routinely administered with improved overall survival through reduction of distant metastases.
- Neoadjuvant (induction) chemotherapy with a multiagent chemotherapy regimen prior to definitive chemoradiotherapy has been shown to improve survival but with increased hematologic and gastrointestinal toxicity in a recent meta-analysis of seven randomized controlled trials involving 2311 patients.[6]
- In recurrent or metastatic disease, the addition of immune checkpoint inhibitor camrelizumab to chemotherapy has demonstrated an improvement in progression-free survival and has the potential to change standard practice on maturity of data.[7]
- Besides systemic chemotherapy and anti-epidermal growth factor receptor inhibitor (EGFR) approaches, the use of single-agent immune checkpoint inhibitors (pembrolizumab, nivolumab, camrelizumab) has demonstrated significant antitumor efficacy in patients with recurrent or metastatic disease.[8]
- Significant supportive care with nutrition, hydration, and mucositis management (especially pain control) is required.
- Posttherapy rehabilitation with swallowing therapy, dental care, endocrinology care, and lymphedema care are often required.

DISPOSITION

- Early stage disease patients typically have a good outcome (5-yr survival 60% to 75%), whereas stage 4 patients have a poor outcome (5-yr survival <40%).

REFERRAL

- Diagnosis is usually confirmed by biopsy performed by otorhinolaryngology physician.
- Referrals include to medical oncology, radiation oncology, dietitian, and gastroenterology.

❗ PEARLS & CONSIDERATIONS

- Analysis of EBV DNA in plasma samples has been found to be useful in screening for early asymptomatic cases. NPC was detected significantly earlier and outcomes were better in participants who were identified by screening compared to those in a historical cohort.[3]
- Higher pretreatment, mid-treatment, and posttreatment EBV DNA levels have been significantly correlated with poor outcomes for patients afflicted with NPC.[4]

REFERENCES

Available at eBooks.Health.Elsevier.com.

RELATED CONTENT

Head and Neck Squamous Cell Carcinoma (Related Key Topic)

AUTHOR: **RITESH RATHORE, MD**

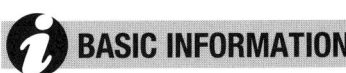
Diseases
and Disorders

I

BASIC INFORMATION

DEFINITION

Necrotizing fasciitis (NF) is a rapidly spreading bacterial infection of the deep fascia, with associated inflammation, leading to necrosis of subcutaneous tissue planes. This infection can occur in wounds from trauma or surgical wounds or can be spontaneous or idiopathic. There are two clinical types, both of which carry a high rate of morbidity and mortality.

SYNONYMS

NF
Soft tissue gangrene
Flesh-eating bacteria
Fournier gangrene
Hemolytic streptococcal gangrene

ICD-10CM CODE
M72.6   Necrotizing fasciitis

EPIDEMIOLOGY & DEMOGRAPHICS

INCIDENCE: Invasive group A *Streptococcus* infection occurs at a rate of 3.5 cases per 100,000 persons, with a case fatality rate of around 24%.
PREDOMINANT SEX: Male > female.
PREDOMINANT AGE: 6 to 50 yr; less common in children.

PHYSICAL FINDINGS & CLINICAL PRESENTATION

CLINICAL TYPES OF NECROTIZING FASCIITIS:
- Type I: Necrotizing fasciitis: At least one anaerobic species is isolated in conjunction with one or more facultative anaerobic species, such as streptococci (not group A), *and* members of the *Enterobacteriaceae* (gram-negative rods)
- Anaerobic bacteria, most commonly *Bacteroides* or *Peptostreptococcus* spp.
- *Enterobacteriaceae*: *Escherichia coli*, *Klebsiella* spp., *Proteus* spp., *Enterobacter* spp.
- Usually associated with diabetes or peripheral vascular disease
- Example of type I: Fournier gangrene of the perineum
- Type II: Necrotizing fasciitis: Group A *Streptococcus* is isolated alone or in combination with other bacteria, most likely *Staphylococcus aureus*. Also known as hemolytic streptococcal gangrene

1. Example of type II: Invasive group A *Streptococcus*, associated with virulence factors type 1 and type 3 M protein

EXAMPLES OF NECROTIZING FASCIITIS:
- Fournier gangrene: Aggressive type I infection of the perineum usually caused by penetration of the gastrointestinal or urethral mucosa by enteric organisms. It can rapidly spread to involve the scrotum, penis, and abdominal wall or gluteal muscles, causing gangrene. Use of sodium-glucose cotransporter-2 (SGLT2) inhibitors in diabetics has been associated with Fournier gangrene.
- Clostridial cellulitis: Caused by *Clostridium perfringens* associated with local trauma or surgery and crepitus caused by gas production; generally noted in the skin, with deeper tissues generally spared.

PHYSICAL FINDINGS

Minor skin trauma, toxic-appearing patient:
- Open skin wound
- Severe pain at injury or surgical site
- Fever, confusion, weakness, diarrhea
- Early skin erythema, quickly spreading in hours to days
- Skin redness changes to purple discoloration
- Gangrenous skin changes may develop
- Loosening of skin and subcutaneous skin in association with deep fascial necrosis (Fig. E1). "Woody" induration and crepitus of involved area are characteristics
- Muscle involvement, thrombosis of blood vessels, and myonecrosis may develop
- Bullae and gas formation at site

ETIOLOGY

- NF usually arises from skin damage or trauma. Risk is increased with presence of comorbidities (diabetes mellitus, cancer, liver disease, immunosuppression, use of SGLT2 inhibitors)
- Polymicrobial: Mixture of anaerobes and aerobic enteric gram-negative rods
- Group A streptococci (*S. pyogenes*)
- *S. aureus*
- *C. perfringens*
- *Bacteroides fragilis*
- *Vibrio vulnificus*
- Methicillin-resistant *S. aureus* (MRSA), especially community-acquired MRSA

DIAGNOSIS

DIFFERENTIAL DIAGNOSIS
- Cellulitis
- Pyomyositis

- Gas gangrene
- A classification of necrotizing skin, soft tissue, and muscle infections is described in Table 1

WORKUP

- Diagnosis of necrotizing fasciitis generally requires incision and probing. In patients with necrotizing fasciitis, there is no resistance to probing subcutaneously, and there is fascial plane involvement. Fig. E2 is an algorithm for assessment and treatment of suspected necrotizing fasciitis.
- Laboratory tests:
  1. The laboratory risk indicator for necrotizing fasciitis (LRINEC) consists of the following six variables (Table 2). When present, the reported positive predictive value is 92%: CBC with differential (leukocytosis [white blood count >15,000], anemia [Hb <13.5]), elevated C-reactive protein (≥15 mg/dl), hyponatremia (sodium <135 mEq/L), elevated creatinine (>1.6 mg/dl), hyperglycemia (glucose >180 mg/dl).
  1. Cultures of skin, soft tissue, or debrided tissue, aerobically and anaerobically. Blood cultures are positive in 60% of patients with type II infections and 20% with type I infections.
- Imaging:
  1. Radiographs may show subcutaneous gas in fascial planes.
  2. Computed tomography (CT) or MRI may be helpful because they can detect gas in the tissues. MRI with contrast is more sensitive than CT.

TREATMENT

- Aggressive surgical debridement of involved necrotic tissues is essential *as soon as possible* to reduce mortality.
- Fasciotomies of extremities may be necessary.
- Immediate start of empiric antibiotics:
  1. Type I: Vancomycin, daptomycin, or linezolid plus piperacillin/tazobactam; a carbapenem (such as imipenem, meropenem, or doripenem); and third-generation cephalosporin + metronidazole or a fluoroquinolone plus metronidazole (ceftriaxone) are reasonable choices pending cultures. Empiric clindamycin may also be added to suppress toxin production by staphylococci and streptococci. It is important to always have anaerobic coverage. Use the highest dosages possible for age and CrCl.

TABLE 1 Classification of Necrotizing Skin, Soft-Tissue, and Muscle Infections

Disease	Bacteriology	Comments
Necrotizing Cellulitis		
Clostridial cellulitis	*Clostridium perfringens*	Local trauma, recent surgery; fascial/deep muscle spared
Nonclostridial cellulitis	Mixed: *Escherichia coli, Enterobacter, Peptostreptococcus* spp., *Bacteroides fragilis*	Diabetes mellitus predisposes; produces foul odor
Meleney synergistic gangrene	*Staphylococcus aureus*, microaerophilic streptococci	Rare infection; postoperative; slowly expanding, indolent, ulceration in superficial fascia
Synergistic necrotizing cellulitis	Mixed aerobic and anaerobic, including *B. fragilis, Peptostreptococcus* spp.	Diabetes mellitus predisposes; variant of necrotizing fasciitis type I; involves skin, muscle, fat, and fascia
Necrotizing Fasciitis		
Type I	Mixed aerobic and anaerobic; staphylococci, *B. fragilis, E. coli,* group A streptococci, *Peptostreptococcus* spp., *Prevotella, Porphyromonas* spp., *Clostridium* spp.	Usually requires a breach in the mucous membrane layer either through surgery or penetrating injuries or from chronic medical conditions such as diabetes, peripheral vascular disease, malignancy, and anal fissures
Type II	Group A streptococci	Increasing in frequency and severity since 1985; very high mortality; often begins at site of nonpenetrating minor trauma such as a bruise or muscle strain but often no identified precursor
		Predisposing factors: Blunt/penetrating trauma, varicella (chickenpox), intravenous drug abuse, surgical procedures, childbirth, nonsteroidal antiinflammatory drug use
Myonecrosis		
Clostridial myonecrosis	*Clostridium* spp.	Predisposing factors: Deep/penetrating injury, bowel and biliary tract surgery, improperly performed abortion and retained placenta, prolonged rupture of the membranes, and intrauterine fetal demise or missed abortion in postpartum patients. Recurrent gas gangrene occurs at sites of previous gas gangrene
Streptococcal myonecrosis	Streptococci	
Special Type of Necrotizing Soft-Tissue Infection		
Fournier gangrene	Polymicrobial, with *E. coli* the predominant aerobe and *Bacteroides* the predominant anaerobe. Other microflora: *Proteus, Staphylococcus,* Enterococcus, aerobic and anaerobic *Streptococcus, Pseudomonas, Klebsiella,* and *Clostridium*	Necrosis of the scrotum or perineum that starts with scrotal pain and erythema and rapidly spreads onto anterior abdominal wall and gluteal muscle. It is more often seen in diabetics and can be associated with trauma

From Vincent JL et al: *Textbook of critical care,* ed 6, Philadelphia, 2011, Saunders.

2. Type II: For group A *Streptococcus*, give intravenous (IV) penicillin G, 4 million U q4h in patients who weigh >60 kg with clindamycin, 600 to 900 mg IV q8h.
   a. Clindamycin has the added effect of suppressing toxin production. If MRSA is suspected, add vancomycin, daptomycin, or linezolid.
- Intravenous gammaglobulin (IVIG): 1 g/kg on day 1 and 0.5 g/kg on days 2 and 3 neutralizes circulating streptococcal toxins and has been shown beneficial in severe forms of invasive group A streptococcal infections, although data are not definitive.
- For *Vibrio vulnificus* use doxycycline plus ceftazidime; for *Aeromonas hydrophila* use doxycycline plus ciprofloxacin.
- Hyperbaric oxygen evaluation as an adjunct to surgery and IV antibiotics.

SUGGESTED READINGS

Available at eBooks.Health.Elsevier.com.

AUTHOR: **GLENN G. FORT, MD, MPH**

TABLE 2 Laboratory Risk Indicator for Necrotizing Fasciitis (LRINEC)[a]

Variable	Points
CRP >150 mg/L	4
Leukocytosis	1
WBC count between 15,000 and 25,000/mm^3	2
WBC count >25,000/mm^3	
Anemia	1
Hgb between 11 and 13.5 g/dl	2
Hgb <11 g/dl	
Hyponatremia	2
Na <135 mmol/L	
Renal insufficiency	2
Cr >1.6 mg/dl	
Serum glucose >180 mg/dl	1

Cr, Creatinine; *CRP,* C-reactive protein; *Hgb,* hemoglobin; *WBC,* white blood cell.

[a]LRINEC score <6 points is considered low risk for necrotizing soft tissue infection but does not rule out the diagnosis. High clinical suspicion for necrotizing soft tissue infection warrants surgical debridement, irrespective of LRINEC score.

From Spec A et al: *Comprehensive review of infectious diseases,* Philadelphia, 2019, Elsevier.

Nephrotic Syndrome 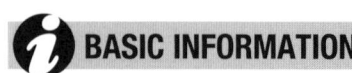 (ALG) (PTG)

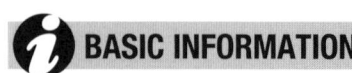

BASIC INFORMATION

DEFINITION

Nephrotic syndrome is characterized by heavy proteinuria (usually defined as >3.5 g/24 h), hypoalbuminemia, hyperlipidemia, lipiduria, and edema. Nephrotic-range proteinuria involves urine protein excretion of >3.5 g/24 h without other features of the nephrotic syndrome. Proteinuria, primarily in the form of albuminuria, can have many causes that share a common mechanism of glomerular injury, the most common being diabetes, focal segmental glomerulosclerosis, membranous nephropathy, minimal change disease, and amyloidosis. Though less common, disorders that are classically categorized under the nephritic syndrome may also lead to nephrotic-range proteinuria.[1]

ICD-10CM CODES
N04.9 Nephrotic syndrome with unspecified morphologic changes
N04.0 Nephrotic syndrome with minor glomerular abnormality
N04.1 Nephrotic syndrome with focal and segmental glomerular lesions
N04.2 Nephrotic syndrome with diffuse membranous glomerulonephritis
N04.3 Nephrotic syndrome with diffuse mesangial proliferative glomerulonephritis
N04.4 Nephrotic syndrome with diffuse endocapillary proliferative glomerulonephritis
N04.5 Nephrotic syndrome with diffuse mesangiocapillary glomerulonephritis
N04.6 Nephrotic syndrome with dense deposit disease
N04.7 Nephrotic syndrome with diffuse crescentic glomerulonephritis
N04.8 Nephrotic syndrome with other morphologic changes

EPIDEMIOLOGY & DEMOGRAPHICS

- Among children (especially <6 yr), the most common causes of nephrotic syndrome (NS) are the following: Minimal change disease (MCD) (75% of pediatric cases), focal and segmental glomerulosclerosis (FSGS) (7% to 20% of cases).[2]
  1. Variation in incidence of NS depending on country of origin, or ethnicity, with proportions ranging from 1.15 to 16.9 per 100,000 children. Incidence is highest among children of south Asian ancestry.[1]
  2. Incidence of steroid resistance ranges from 2.1% to 27.3% and varies by country of origin.[2]
  3. African American children are more likely to have biopsy-proven focal and segmental glomerulosclerosis (FSGS, 42% to 72%) and have highest proportion with progression to ESRD compared with European Americans. In South Asian children, FSGS is reported less commonly at 15% to 39%.[3]
  4. Minimal change disease (MCD) (75% of pediatric cases).
  5. Focal and segmental glomerulosclerosis (FSGS) (7% to 20% of cases).
- In adults, diabetes is the most frequent cause of nephrotic syndrome, followed by membranous nephropathy and FSGS. FSGS is also the most common primary (nonsystemic) cause of nephrotic-range proteinuria and is more common in persons of African ancestry.[1,4,5]
- Membranous nephropathy is the second most common primary cause of nephrotic syndrome in adults.
  1. FSGS is more common in persons of African ancestry.
  2. Membranous nephropathy is more common in White patients.

PHYSICAL FINDINGS & CLINICAL PRESENTATION[1,2]

- Patients commonly present with lower extremity and/or periorbital edema, and weight gain.
- Ascites and anasarca may occur.
- Hypercoagulability is a potential clinical manifestation.
- Patients are at higher risk for infections due to urinary immunoglobulin loss.

ETIOLOGY

Disorders that exclusively affect the basement membrane or podocyte generally have a noninflammatory pathology and lead to proteinuria as primarily albuminuria, the hallmark of glomerular disease.[1-4]

Traditionally, the clinical correlate to this pathologic schema has been a subdivision of patients into those with a nephrotic vs. those with a nephritic presentation. Nephritic disorders have subnephrotic proteinuria, low glomerular filtration rates, and hematuria. Nephrotic disorders have greater proteinuria, often normal glomerular filtration rates, and lack hematuria. While generally true, this schema may cause diagnostic confusion because nephritic disease may present with nephrotic-range proteinuria, especially earlier in the disease course before glomerular filtration is substantially reduced. It is better to categorize these disorders as nephrotic, with a noninflammatory urine sediment (i.e., proteinuria without casts or cellular elements) vs. nephritic, with an inflammatory sediment (i.e., proteinuria plus red blood cell [RBC] casts and/or dysmorphic RBCs).[2]

Fig. 1 details the clinical breakdown. In this chapter, we focus on primary diseases that present with a noninflammatory sediment (MCD, FSGS, membranous nephropathy, and amyloidosis) and on primary disorders with inflammatory sediment that are often with nephrotic-range

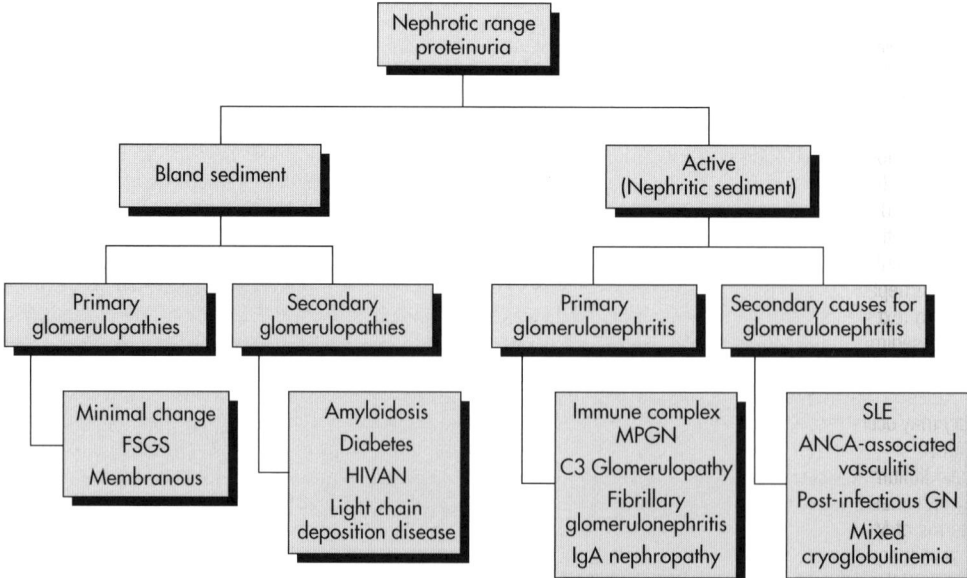

FIG. 1 An approach to nephrotic-range proteinuria. *ANCA,* Antineutrophil cytoplasmic antibody; *C3,* complement component 3; *FSGS,* focal and segmental glomerulosclerosis; *GN,* glomerulonephritis; *IgA,* immunoglobulin A; *HIVAN,* HIV-associated nephropathy; *MPGN,* membranoproliferative glomerulonephritis; *SLE,* systemic lupus erythematosus.

TABLE 1 Important Clinical, Serologic, and Pathologic Features of Selected Diseases Causing Nephrotic Syndrome

Disease	Important Clinical Features	Serologic Features	Pathologic Features
Minimal change disease	Rapid onset with heavy proteinuria and rapid remission with therapy. True steroid resistance is rare and should prompt repeat biopsy to rule out FSGS.	Complements are normal.	Light microscopy (LM) shows completely normal kidney architecture. Immunofluorescence microscopy: Normal. Electron microscopy (EM): Diffuse podocyte effacement.
Primary FSGS	Often heavier proteinuria and low serum albumin and edema. Tip lesion subtype and collapsing FSGS often have more explosive onset. Sediment usually bland, but RBCs can be seen. Usually no cellular casts.	Complements are normal.	LM: Only one glomerulus need show features of FSGS to make diagnosis. Immunofluorescence microscopy: Often devoid of immunoglobulin, although IgM can be seen. EM: Often has diffuse podocyte effacement.
Secondary FSGS	Proteinuria is often subnephrotic, or if nephrotic, serum albumin levels are maintained. Minimal edema.	HIV and parvovirus infection can cause phenotype identical to idiopathic collapsing FSGS.	LM: Often shows evidence of glomerulomegaly. EM: Foot process effacement is less diffuse.
Primary membranous nephropathy	Often seen in older White patients. More likely than other forms of nephrotic syndrome to be associated with thrombotic complications. Sediment: Bland. RBCs can be found, although RBC casts are usually found.	Serum antiphospholipase A2 receptor antibodies are found in 70% of patients with idiopathic primary membranous nephropathy. Antineutral endopeptidase antibodies are found in a minority of others.	LM: Characterized by thickening of the GBM; "spikes" can be seen on silver stain. Immunofluorescence microscopy: C3 and IgG noted in granular pattern. Newer techniques stain for antiphospholipase A2 receptor antibody in situ. EM: Associated with subepithelial deposits.
Secondary membranous nephropathy	Associated with malignancy, lupus, syphilis, hepatitis B and C, medications (gold, captopril, penicillamine, etc.).	Notable for the absence of antiphospholipase A2 antibodies. ANA, hepatitis B, HCV serologies are helpful. RPR can be sent in context of appropriate history.	Morphology is exactly the same except when examined by EM. On high power, one sees both subendothelial and mesangial deposits in addition to classic subepithelial deposits.
Amyloidosis	Often found with massive proteinuria. Kidney size is enlarged. Bland sediment.	UPEP, SPEP, serum free light chains may be positive. The UPEP will show glomerular proteinuria, which can help differentiate from myeloma kidney.	LM: Often notable for nodular pattern. Diagnosis can be made by staining using Congo red or thioflavin T. Immunofluorescence microscopy: Antibody use can differentiate AA from AL amyloid. EM: Shows characteristic random 10-nm fibrils.
Diabetes	Often associated with nephrotic-range proteinuria in the setting of retinopathy. Kidney sizes are preserved.	No specific serologic tests are positive.	LM: Nodular pattern often seen, thickened GBM.
MPGN	Often associated with nephrotic-range proteinuria with a "nephritic" sediment. RBC casts often seen along with dysmorphic RBC.	C3 and C4 are often low in immune complex MPGN. Immune complex GN warrants checking SPEP and UPEP, as gammopathy is associated with MPGN. Hepatitis B, HCV, ANA, and cryoglobulins are also warranted. C3 alone is low in dense deposit disease and C3 glomerulonephritis, which may prompt specific tests for complement dysregulation.	The key point here is to look at the IF. If immunofluorescence shows both immunoglobulin and complement deposition, the diagnosis is immune complex MGPN. If only complement, the diagnosis is most likely C3 glomerulopathy (either dense deposit disease or C3 glomerulonephritis).

ANA, Antinuclear antibody; *C3*, complement component 3; *FSGS*, focal and segmental glomerulosclerosis; *GBM*, glomerular basement membrane; *GN*, glomerulonephritis; *HCV*, hepatitis C virus; *Ig*, immunoglobulin; *MPGN*, membranoproliferative glomerulonephritis; *RBC*, red blood cell; *RPR*, rapid plasma reagin; *SPEP*, serum protein electrophoresis; *UPEP*, urine protein electrophoresis.

proteinuria, such as membranoproliferative glomerulonephritis (MPGN). The evaluation of nephritic syndrome is noted by worsening glomerular filtration in the setting of proteinuria and hematuria. Important points regarding the most common etiologies of nephrotic syndrome are detailed in the following text (Table 1).

- MCD has a bland urine sediment with abrupt onset of disease and abrupt remission.
  1. Proteinuria may exceed 20 g daily.
  2. Acute kidney injury may occur in severe NS associated with MCD.
  3. NSAID use, chronic lithium ingestion, viral infections, and lymphomas are associated with secondary forms of MCD.
- FSGS, primary and secondary: Primary FSGS, possibly caused by an autoimmune triggered circulating permeability factor, typically manifests with full nephrotic syndrome and requires immunosuppressive therapy.

1. FSGS is more prevalent in persons of African ancestry.[3,6]
2. Secondary FSGS is caused by a known etiology, including heroin use, sickle cell disease, scarring of any kind from prior injury, obesity, low nephron mass, HIV, etc. Most cases of secondary FSGS are associated with lower levels of proteinuria (often subnephrotic), higher serum albumin levels, and less edema (e.g., HIV-associated nephropathy is an important exception and is associated with heavy proteinuria and rapid progression if untreated). Distinguishing between primary and secondary FSGS is important therapeutically. Many forms of glomerular injury can produce morphologic features of FSGS, and worsening proteinuria attributable to secondary FSGS generally portends worse outcomes.[3,6]

- Membranous nephropathy may be primary or secondary. Primary membranous nephropathy is due to in situ deposition of antibodies directed against a glomerular antigen. In 70% or more cases, the epitope is identified as phospholipase A2 receptor. A second, less common epitope is thrombospondin type-1 domain-containing 7A (THSD7A). Secondary membranous nephropathy is often due to infection (e.g., hepatitis B, malaria, schistosomiasis, syphilis), autoimmune disease (e.g., systemic lupus erythematosus [SLE]), medications (e.g., D-penicillamine, gold), and malignancies. Distinguishing between the two subtypes is important for management.[5,7,8]
- Kidney amyloidosis is frequently due to aberrantly folded immunoglobulin light chains (AL amyloid) or serum amyloid A protein (AA amyloid associated with chronic inflammation), and other less common amyloid-types. Kidney

size is often enlarged, and proteinuria may be massive. On histology, ongo red staining detects amyloid proteins.[9]

- Diabetic nephropathy occurs most commonly in diabetics with longstanding diabetes, uncontrolled diabetes, and hypertension. The correlation between retinopathy, proteinuria, and diabetic nephropathy is well established in patients with type 1 diabetes. The relationship is less well established in type 2 diabetes, and absence of retinopathy does not preclude a diagnosis of diabetic nephropathy.
- MPGN usually has immune complex deposition with complement or alternate complement system activation without immune complex formation (e.g., C3 glomerulopathy). The prior classification of types 1, 2, and 3 MPGN is obsolete, and a pathophysiologic scheme is used now. Common causes are infections (e.g., hepatitis C), autoimmune disorders (e.g., SLE), disorders of the alternative complement pathway (C3 glomerulopathy), or dysproteinemias (e.g., monoclonal gammopathies). Distinguishing between these possibilities guides therapy. Urinary sediment often contains dysmorphic erythrocytes and erythrocyte casts and is also associated with heavy proteinuria.[10]

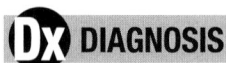 **DIAGNOSIS**

DIFFERENTIAL DIAGNOSIS

- Other conditions that present with edema (congestive heart failure, cirrhosis, protein-losing enteropathy, severe malnutrition)
- Glomerulonephritis from disorders commonly associated with inflammatory urinary sediment and glomerular inflammation

WORKUP

Serum creatinine, and blood urea nitrogen, 24-h urine protein collection and urinary sediment examination.[1,11] Abnormalities in any of the these tests should prompt nephrology consultation.

- Serologic testing may include urine and serum electrophoresis, HIV, hepatitis B surface antigen, hepatitis C virus (HCV) antibody, and antinuclear antibody (ANA). As urinary sediment examination is not 100% sensitive in ruling out an inflammatory process, C3 and C4 can be checked, as complement levels are often low in many inflammatory glomerulonephritides and often low in MPGN.
  1. Depending on practice patterns, these tests are used selectively before or, in some cases, after biopsy to better define an etiology.
- Antiphospholipase A2 receptor antibody (anti-PLA2R) titer. Elevated titers are found in primary membranous nephropathy and less commonly in secondary membranous nephropathy. With treatment, patients may develop immunologic remission (decreasing anti-PLA2R titers) prior to a clinical remission based on urine proteinuria. Monitoring titers during the treatment course may guide

treatment duration and limit toxic side effects of therapy.[4,5,11,12]

- Kidney biopsy is performed in most instances unless there is a contraindication to biopsy or the disease is diagnosed through serologic testing (IE anti-PLA2R antibody) or other organ biopsy (IE fat pad or bone marrow in amyloidosis).

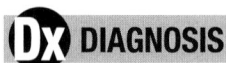 **TREATMENT**

NONIMMUNOSUPPRESSIVE THERAPY

- Control of proteinuria is key to treating progressive kidney disease. Nearly all trials of nondiabetic chronic kidney disease demonstrate that reducing proteinuria improves renal survival. ACE inhibitors (ACEIs) or angiotensin II type 1 receptor blockers (ARBs) should be used at maximally tolerated doses.[1,11]
  1. The exception is MCD, where proteinuria reduction may rapidly occur during therapy.
  2. Nondihydropyridine calcium channel blockers (verapamil, diltiazem) can be used in lieu of ACEIs or ARBs when these agents are contraindicated.
- For proteinuria >1 g per day, the target blood pressure is <125/75 mm Hg.
- With the exception of MCD, patients with nephrotic-range proteinuria and hyperlipidemia should be treated with HMG-CoA synthetase inhibitors (statins).
- Although some patients with nephrotic syndrome are hypercoagulable (particularly those with membranous nephropathy), the role of prophylactic anticoagulation is controversial and not well defined. For patients with membranous nephropathy and serum albumin levels <2.0 g/dl, anticoagulation should be considered if bleeding risk is low.[2,11]

- Low sodium diet (<2 g daily) with diuretics.
- Diuretic resistance is common due to gut wall edema and hypoalbuminemia. More bioavailable diuretics (bumetanide, torsemide) may increase urine output better than furosemide. Thiazide diuretics can be added to loop agents to augment diuresis.
- Loop diuretics should be dosed at least on a twice-daily basis.

IMMUNOSUPPRESSIVE THERAPY

Important terms in dealing with the management of nephrotic-range proteinuria due to primary glomerular diseases are listed in Table 2. First-line therapies for each disease are highlighted in the following.[11]

- MCD: First-line therapy in adults is prednisone (1 mg/kg per day to a maximum of 80 mg per day) for a minimum of 4 wk and maximum of 16 wk. Steroids are tapered over 6 mo for favorable responses. Second-line options include cyclophosphamide and/or calcineurin inhibitors. Newer, randomized controlled trial data from studies of children reveal efficacy of rituximab in steroid-dependent patients with recurrent relapsing MCD. Consequently, rituximab may become a reasonable option for patients who do not respond to conventional therapy.[12]
- FSGS: Primary FSGS is often treated with high-dose prednisone (maximum, 80 mg daily in adults) tapered over 6 mo. Alternative regimens include low-dose prednisone with cyclosporine. Mycophenolate mofetil (MMF) has also been used in primary FSGS. Treatment of secondary FSGS is based on arresting the underlying cause and nonspecific therapy with an ACEI or ARB, blood pressure control, weight loss, and dietary protein restriction. Immunosuppression is avoided.[11]
- Membranous nephropathy: Acceptable treatments include alternating months of

TABLE 2 Important Definitions in Dealing With Treatment of Primary Nephrotic Syndrome

Definition	Adults	Children
Complete remission	Reduction in proteinuria to <0.3 g/24 hr	<4 mg/m² per hr on at least 3 occasions within 7 days and serum albumin >3.5 g/dl
Partial remission	Reduction in proteinuria between 0.3 g/24 hr and 3.5 g daily with ≥50% decrease in proteinuria from baseline	Disappearance of edema, increase in serum albumin >3.5 g/dl, and persistent proteinuria >4 mg mg/m² per hr or >100 mg/m² per hr
Relapse*	Increase in proteinuria to >3.5 g daily after 1 mo of complete or partial remission	Urine dipstick 3+ or proteinuria >40 mg/m² per hr occurring on 3 days within 1 wk
Steroid dependent*	Two consecutive relapses occurring during therapy or within 14 days of completing therapy	Two relapses of proteinuria within 14 days after stopping or during alternate-day steroid therapy
Steroid resistant*	Persistence of proteinuria without significant reduction despite prednisone therapy at 1 mg/kg for 16 wk	Persistence of proteinuria despite prednisone therapy at 60 mg/m² for 4 wk

*These definitions only truly apply to diseases such as minimal change disease and focal and segmental glomerulosclerosis (FSGS).
Adapted from Cattran DC et al: Cyclosporine in idiopathic glomerular disease associated with the nephrotic syndrome: workshop recommendations, *Kidney Int* 72(12):1429-1447, 2007, and *KDIGO clinical practice guidelines for glomerulonephritis.*

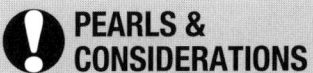
N

cyclophosphamide and steroids, calcineurin inhibitors with low-dose steroids or without steroids, and rituximab. Therapy for secondary membranous nephropathy is directed at treating the underlying cause (malignancy, SLE, etc.).[11]

- Amyloidosis, diabetes, and immune complex MPGN: Treatment is specific for the underlying disorder. In rapidly progressive HCV-related MPGN, immunosuppressive therapy with rituximab or glucocorticoids and cyclophosphamide can be administered during direct-acting antiviral therapy.[11]
- MPGN: A reclassification of MPGN highlights alternative complement cascade activation (C3 glomerulonephritis) as etiologic. MPGN is considered immune complex mediated or complement mediated by immunofluorescent microscopy. Treatment may now involve agents (e.g., eculizumab) that inhibit the complement cascade. Prior nontargeted approaches (e.g., steroids) for MPGN have been largely unsuccessful, except in selected pediatric cases.[11,13]

REFERRAL

Nephrology consultation is recommended for all cases of nephrotic syndrome.

PEARLS & CONSIDERATIONS

- Albuminuria generally implies that glomerular disease is present. The urine protein electrophoresis defines the type(s) of proteins excreted: Albumin, immunoglobulins, and tubular.
- Massive proteinuria (>20 g daily) is rarely encountered with inflammatory glomerulonephritis and generally indicates MCD, FSGS, membranous nephropathy, or amyloidosis.
- Partial remissions and steroid resistance are rarely seen in primary minimal change disease. These circumstances require repeat kidney biopsy because FSGS is often revealed.
- Proteinuria is quantitated by a 24-h urine collection with evaluation of urinary creatinine excretion to document adequacy of collection. Spot collections have not been validated for heavy proteinuria or patients with rapidly changing creatinine values. A spot urine protein:creatinine ratio directly obtained from the 24-h collection defines the relationship between spot and true ratios for therapeutic monitoring.

- Most noninflammatory processes progress slowly. If a sediment without RBC casts is detected with a rapidly increasing serum creatinine and heavy proteinuria, the differential is relatively narrow:
  1. MCD with acute tubular necrosis or acute interstitial nephritis that may occur with NSAID administration[7]
  2. Any form of nephrotic syndrome associated with acute tubular necrosis
  3. Bilateral renal vein thrombosis superimposed on nephrotic syndrome
  4. Myeloma cast nephropathy
  5. Collapsing FSGS from lupus, HIV infection, bisphosphonate therapy, or thrombotic microangiopathy[3,6]

REFERENCES AND SUGGESTED READINGS
Available at eBooks.Health.Elseviver.com.

RELATED CONTENT

Nephrotic Syndrome (Patient Information)

AUTHOR: **RUPALI AVASARE, MD**

Diseases and Disorders

I

Neuroleptic Malignant Syndrome

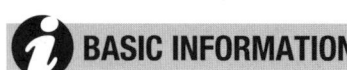 **BASIC INFORMATION**

DEFINITION

Neuroleptic malignant syndrome (NMS) is a rare but potentially life-threatening disorder characterized by hyperthermia, muscular rigidity, autonomic dysfunction, and depressed/fluctuating levels of arousal that evolve over 24 to 72 h.[1] This occurs as an idiosyncratic adverse reaction to medications that affect the central dopaminergic system, usually D2 receptors blockade.[2]

SYNONYMS

NMS
Neuroleptic-Induced Acute Dystonia [3]

ICD-10CM CODE

G21.0 Malignant neuroleptic syndrome

EPIDEMIOLOGY & DEMOGRAPHICS

INCIDENCE: 0.02% to 0.03%[4] (reduced incidence with newer antipsychotics)
0.2 to 3.2% incidence in patients receiving neuroleptics[5]
PREVALENCE: Meta-analysis yielded an overall estimate of 0.991/1000 [6]
PREDOMINANT SEX: 50% more likely to be males[7]
PREDOMINANT AGE: Most likely to occur in young adulthood[7]

RISK FACTORS:

- History of intake of dopamine antagonists, e.g., typical and atypical antipsychotics (typical antipsychotics are more likely to cause NMS). NMS is most often seen after initial administration or a dosage change, higher doses, or parenteral treatment[2]
- Dehydration, high external temperature, or physical restraint[2]
- Prior history of an NMS episode or a personal and/or family history of catatonia is a risk factor for developing NMS[10]
- Withdrawal of a dopaminergic agonist[11]

GENETICS: A1 allele carriers of DRD2 gene are at 10.5 times higher risk of having NMS[8]
CYP2D6 gene variants leads to lower metabolism of neuroleptics predisposing to NMS[9]

PHYSICAL FINDINGS & CLINICAL PRESENTATION

- Syndrome typically begins abruptly while the patient is taking therapeutic (not toxic) dosages of neuroleptics. NSM can develop within hours to days after an exposure to a causative agent.[1]
- Muscle rigidity (hypertonia, cogwheeling, or "lead pipe" rigidity). It can be generalized, symmetric, and could vary from a mild increase in tone to extreme generalized body rigidity, such as opisthotonos. Focal increases of muscular tone can also be present in the form of blepharospasm, oculogyric crisis, or trismus. Nystagmus, dysphagia, dysarthria, or aphonia can also be present as a result of increased muscular tone.[2]
- Hyperthermia (38.6° to 42.3° C [101.48° to 108.14° F], usually <40° C [104° F]) without major fluctuations or chills[2]
- Dysautonomia: Diaphoresis, tachycardia, tachypnea, labile blood pressure (hypertension or postural hypotension), sialorrhea, skin pallor, urinary incontinence[1]
- AMS: Agitation, catatonia, fluctuating consciousness, obtundation

ETIOLOGY

- Exact etiology is unknown, but it has been suggested that sudden and marked dopamine receptor blockade in nigrostriatal, hypothalamic, mesolimbic, and mesocortical pathways leads to clinical manifestations seen in NMS[9]
- Calcium mediated disruption of musculoskeletal system is another theorized etiology of NMS[2]
  1. All antipsychotics are known to cause NMS, although different neuroleptic drugs have different potencies for inducing NMS
  2. Typical neuroleptics:
     a. High potency: Haloperidol
     b. Medium potency: Chlorpromazine, fluphenazine
     c. Low potency: Levomepromazine, loxapine

TABLE 1 Clinical Features of Serotonin Toxicity, Neuroleptic Malignant Syndrome, and Anticholinergic Syndrome

	Anticholinergic Toxicity	Neuroleptic Malignant Syndrome	Serotonin Syndrome	Adrenergic Toxicity
Tempo	Rapid onset	Slow onset (1-3 days)	Rapid onset (min-h)	
Mental state:	+++	+++	+ (late stage)	+
1. Confusion	+++	Akathisia	+++	+++
2. Agitation/restlessness	+	++ (severe)		
3. Coma				
Motor system:	+	++	—	—
1. Bradykinesia	+	+	+++	+++
2. Tremor		++ (lead pipe)	+	—
3. Rigidity		0	++	—
4. Hypertonia		—	+++	+++
5. Hyperreflexia		—	+++ (LL > UL)	++
6. Clonus (ankle/eye)		—	+	—
7. Myoclonus			+ (rare)	++
8. Seizures				
Autonomic system:[a,b]	—	+++		—
1. Instability	++	Labile (systolic blood pressure >30 mm Hg above baseline)	+	++
2. Hypertension	++		+	+++
3. Tachycardia	—	Labile (>30 beats/min above baseline)	+++	++
4. Diaphoresis	+++[c]	+++	++	++
5. Hyperthermia		+++	++	
Others:	—	+++	++	++
1. Rhabdomyolysis	++	—	+++	++
2. Mydriasis				

[a]These features are nonspecific and do not assist in differentiating among syndromes.
[b]Mechanism is excess serotonin.
[c]Mechanism is inability to sweat and unopposed dopamine centrally, leading to dysregulation. +: mild, ++: moderate, +++: severe, —: not affected.
LL, Lower limbs; *UL,* upper limbs.

3. Atypical neuroleptics:
   a. Low potency: Risperidone, olanzapine, clozapine, quetiapine
- NMS has also been associated with non-antipsychotic agents with antidopaminergic activity such as metoclopramide, promethazine, tetrabenazine, droperidol, diatrizoate, and amoxapine[1]

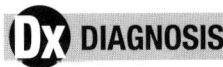 **DIAGNOSIS**

DIFFERENTIAL DIAGNOSIS[1]
- Infectious: Encephalitis, meningitis, brain abscess, rabies, tetanus, sepsis
- Metabolic: Pheochromocytoma, thyrotoxicosis, rhabdomyolysis, AKI
- Toxic: Substances of abuse (ecstasy, phencyclidine), heavy metals (lead, arsenic), lithium, salicylates
- Drug-induced (Table 1): Serotonin syndrome, malignant hyperthermia, drug withdrawal, or overdose, lithium toxicity.
- Environmental: Heatstroke, spider envenomation
- Neuropsychiatric: Catatonia, acute psychosis with agitation, status epilepticus, Parkinsonism
- Table E2 summarizes the differential diagnosis of neuroleptic malignant syndrome

WORKUP
A careful and thorough drug history should be obtained. There is a significant overlap in the features of NMS and serotonin syndrome. The major difference is the presence of hyperreflexia in NMS and myoclonus in serotonin syndrome.

LABORATORY TESTS[2]
- Creatine phosphokinase (CPK) (sensitivity 0.71)
- Urinary myoglobin
- CBC with differential
- Comprehensive metabolic panel
- Arterial blood gas
- Drug levels
- Urinalysis
- Cerebrospinal fluid (CSF) Studies

IMAGING STUDIES
CT Head or MRI Brain.
CSF studies and imaging may be considered to evaluate for other possible differentials.[2]

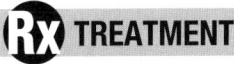 **TREATMENT**

NONPHARMACOLOGIC THERAPY
- Stop all neuroleptic drugs[2] and reinstitute any recently discontinued dopaminergic agonists[11]
- Remember that metoclopramide is also an antidopaminergic drug that must be discontinued and avoided.
- Respiratory and nutritional support as required.

- Careful fluid balance monitoring with adequate hydration[11] (intravenous in severe cases).
- Active cooling[2] (e.g., cooling blanket and antipyretics).
- Skilled nursing care is necessary to prevent decubitus ulcers in bed-confined patients.

ACUTE GENERAL Rx
- Bromocriptine, a dopamine receptor agonist, is the mainstay of therapy for patients with NMS. Initial dose of 2.5 mg is given PO q8h-12h and is increased by 2.5 mg/day until clinical improvement is seen or up to a maximum of 45mg/day. The drug should be continued for at least 10 days after the syndrome has been controlled and then tapered slowly.[1]
- Dantrolene, which blocks calcium efflux from the sarcoplasmic reticulum of skeletal muscles, inhibits the excessive muscle contractions that generate myoglobinemia. Initially, patients can be given a bolus of 1 to 2.5 mg/kg followed by 1mg/kg IV q6 up to a maximum dose of 10mg/kg/day. After 2 to 3 days, patients may be given the drug orally (25 to 600 mg/day in divided doses). Oral dantrolene therapy (50 to 600 mg/day) may be continued for several days afterward.
- Amantadine, an N-Methyl-D-aspartate (NMDA) receptor antagonist with possible dopaminergic properties, can be administered orally at doses of 100 to 200 mg PO bid for moderate to severe cases. As an adjunctive treatment, it has been shown to reduce mortality in comparison to supportive therapy alone.
- IV benzodiazepines (e.g., diazepam 2 to 10 mg, with total daily dose of 10 to 60 mg) to relax muscles and control agitation.
- Electroconvulsive therapy may be beneficial in pharmacologically refractory cases.[12] Succinylcholine should not be used because it may cause hyperkalemia and cardiac arrhythmias in patients with rhabdomyolysis or dysautonomia.

CHRONIC Rx
- Respiratory care, nutritional support, and physical therapy may be required in more severe cases.
- Appropriate therapy would be required in patients with persistent neuropsychiatric sequelae of NMS (e.g., antidepressants for depression, cognitive-behavioral therapy for cognitive deficits, rehabilitation for contractures).

DISPOSITION
- Mortality rate is currently up to 10% despite therapeutic measures.[1] Serious sequelae may occur in a further 20%. Majority of the patients recover completely within 2 to 14 days.[1]
- Rhabdomyolysis is the most common complication. Other complications include

acute kidney injury, respiratory failure, pneumonia, and sepsis.[2]
- Causes of death include arrhythmias, disseminated intravascular coagulation (DIC), cardiovascular, respiratory, or renal failure.[1]
- Factors adversely affecting mortality are increased age, acute respiratory failure, renal failure, and core temperature >104° F (40° C).
- Patients should be monitored closely for future complications of pharmacologic therapy.

REFERRAL
If the patient's condition is critical, it is preferable to treat the patient in a medical/neurologic ICU.

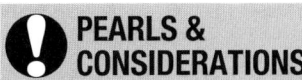 **PEARLS & CONSIDERATIONS**

COMMENTS
Early detection and diagnosis lead to a more favorable outcome. Refer to recent consensus diagnostic criteria as a guide. Treatment is a medical emergency.

Sudden withdrawal from dopaminergic agents (such as those used in Parkinson disease) may lead to "levodopa withdrawal syndrome" that presents with similar clinical manifestations.

Patients with dementia with Lewy bodies have increased susceptibility to neuroleptic malignant syndrome.
Prevention[13]:
- Conservative use of antipsychotics with slow titration
- Avoidance of risk factors (dehydration, exhaustion, agitation)
- Do not withdraw dopaminergic medications rapidly
- Monitoring of vital signs, temperature, and volume status
- If necessary, antipsychotic rechallenge should not be attempted for at least 2 wk after the resolution of NMS

PATIENT & FAMILY EDUCATION:
- Patients and family should be thoroughly counseled about the syndrome and educated to look for initial signs and symptoms of NMS.
- Patients should be consented for further medication use after a clear explanation of the risk-benefit analysis.[13]
- Avoidance of preventable risk factors (dehydration, high temperature).

REFERENCES
Available at eBooks.Health.Elsevier.com.

AUTHORS: **AHMAD MUMTAZ, MD,** and **FARIHA JAMAL, MD**

N

Diseases and Disorders

I

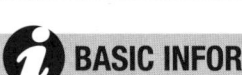
BASIC INFORMATION

DEFINITION
Neuromyelitis optica spectrum disorder (NMOSD) is an uncommon autoimmune inflammatory demyelination disorder of the central nervous system (CNS). It is a clinical syndrome defined by predilection to affect particular regions of the CNS: Specifically the optic nerve, spinal cord (typically with longitudinally extensive transverse myelitis), and some areas of the brain including periependymal regions (most strikingly the area postrema). The clinical syndrome is further subdivided into seropositive NMOSD (AQP4-IgG+ - 80% of patients) and seronegative NMOSD (MOG-IgG+, negative for both AQP4-IgG and MOG-IgG, or unknown serologic status).[1]

SYNONYMS
NMOSD
Neuromyelitis Optica (NMO)
Devic's Disease

ICD 10-CM CODE
G36.0   Neuromyelitis optica [Devic]

EPIDEMIOLOGY & DEMOGRAPHICS
INCIDENCE:
- Wide variety of estimated incidence, ranging from 0.037 per 100,000 in Australia and New Zealand to 0.73 per 100,000 in Afro-Caribbean region.[2]

PREVALENCE:
- Wide variety of estimated prevalence, ranging from 0.7 per 100,000 in Australia and New Zealand to 10 per 100,000 in Afro-Caribbean region.[2]
- In the U.S., the estimated prevalence was 13 per 100,000 in Black Americans and 4 per 100,000 in White Americans.[3]

PREDOMINANT SEX & AGE:
- Median age of onset is 40 years old.[4]
- 10:1 female to male (seropositive AQP4-IgG+)
- 1:1 and 1:2 female to male (seronegative AQP4-IgG+)[5]

PEAK INCIDENCE:
- Peak incidence appears to be in the African and Afro-Caribbean populations.

RISK FACTORS:
- Other autoimmune diseases including systemic lupus erythematosus.[4]

GENETICS: Though presently not well understood, there has been postulated a genetic predisposition towards NMOSD. Specifically relevant to seropositive NMOSD, associations with AQP4-IgG seropositivity and HLA-DRB1*03 (DR3) in French and Brazilian populations and HLA-DPB1*0501 in Japanese and Chinese populations have been described.[6]

PHYSICAL FINDINGS & CLINICAL PRESENTATION
Findings depend on the location of the CNS lesion(s) and may include the following:
- Common: Nonspecific complaints such as fatigue (most common, with 80% lifetime prevalence), blurred vision, diplopia, vertigo, falls, hemiparesis, paraparesis, monoparesis, numbness, paresthesias, ataxia, cognitive impairment, depression, anxiety, pseudobulbar affect (involuntary crying or laughing out of context), sexual dysfunction, and bowel/bladder dysfunction
- Optic neuritis: Unilateral or bilateral
- Corticospinal tract(s) involvement: Transverse myelitis often involving three or more segments of the spinal cord, upper motor neuron signs such as spasticity (particularly leg spasms at night or after prolonged immobility), hyperreflexia, clonus, extensor plantar responses, tonic spasms, upper motor neuron pattern of weakness
- Area postrema syndrome: Intractable hiccupping and/or vomiting (occurs in up to 60% of patients during their disease course)
- Brainstem syndromes including combinations of cranial nerve palsies, weakness, sensory loss, and ataxia.
- Diencephalic syndromes: Narcolepsy, thalamic/hypothalamic-mediated dysfunction
- Sensory involvement: May include partial or full dermatomal loss of pain and temperature, loss of vibration (common) and position sense, temperature dysregulation, thoracic band of sensory loss, paresthesias, trigeminal neuralgia
- Bladder dysfunction: Due to spinal cord involvement.

ETIOLOGY
As AQP4 is expressed in the central nervous system most abundantly on the foot processes of astrocytes, seropositive NMOSD should be understood as an antibody-mediated astrocytopathy. In a clinical relapse, accumulation of AQP4-IgG stimulates an inflammatory response mediated by such factors as complement activation and interleukins such as interleukin-6 (IL-6), leading to the influx of granulocytes. This cascades into a substantial local inflammatory response, leading to bystander damage of local cells and cell products such as myelin or axons themselves. On the other hand, MOG-IgG associated NMOSD is more clearly demyelinating, with some histopathologic studies bearing features similar to type II MS pattern demyelinating lesions.[6] The specifics of non-MOG-IgG seronegative NMOSD pathophysiology are less well understood.

DIAGNOSIS

DIFFERENTIAL DIAGNOSIS
OPTIC NEURITIS:
- Inflammatory: MS, sarcoidosis, granulomatosis with polyangiitis, lupus, Sjögren syndrome, acute disseminated encephalomyelitis, paraneoplastic (CRMP-5, CV-2), autoimmune optic neuropathy, autoimmune glial fibrillary acidic protein (GFAP) astrocytopathy
- Infectious: Neurosyphilis, tuberculosis (TB), Lyme disease, HIV, cytomegalovirus, herpes simplex virus, varicella-zoster virus, Epstein-Barr virus, West Nile virus, dengue fever, Bartonella henselae, Rickettsia spp., Toxocara spp., Q fever, histoplasmosis, toxoplasmosis, helminths, periorbital infections
- Ischemic: Anterior and posterior ischemic optic neuropathies, diabetic papillopathy, branch or central retinal artery or vein occlusion
- Drugs and toxins: Arsenic, methanol, ethambutol, cyclosporine, etc.
- Mitochondrial: Leber hereditary optic neuropathy, other mitochondrial

TRANSVERSE MYELITIS:
- Multiple sclerosis
- Acute demyelinating encephalomyelitis (where TM tends to be monophasic)
- Autoimmune syndromes: systemic lupus, Sjögren syndrome, antiphospholipid antibody syndrome, sarcoidosis, and paraneoplastic conditions, which can be progressive or relapsing.
- Infectious causes of myelitis include HIV, syphilis, varicella zoster (associated with shingles), human T-cell leukemia virus type 1, Lyme disease, COVID-19, arboviruses such as West Nile virus (typically causing a poliomyelitis-type acute flaccid paralysis), or enteroviruses (typically causing acute flaccid paralysis mainly in children).

WORKUP
NMOSD remains a clinical diagnosis, supported by serologic studies for the antibodies and/or characteristic MRI findings (Box 1).

LABORATORY TESTS
- AQP4-IgG (serum)
- MOG-IgG (serum)
- Consider antinuclear antibody (ANA), angiotensin-converting enzyme (ACE; a test with low specificity and sensitivity for sarcoidosis), antineutrophil cytoplasmic antibodies, antiphospholipid and anticardiolipin antibodies, Sjögren antibodies, thyroid-stimulating hormone (TSH), free T_4
- Lumbar puncture to evaluate for elevated protein (>100 mg/dl), pleocytosis (often with neutrophilic or eosinophilic predominance in NMOSD). Oligoclonal bands (OCBs) can be seen in NMOSD but much less commonly than in multiple sclerosis. Evaluate for other causes of transverse myelitis.
- Serum: Complete blood count (CBC) with differential, comprehensive metabolic panel, liver function tests (LFTs), vitamin B_{12}, copper, 25-OH vitamin D_3
- In some cases, optical coherence tomography can be helpful, which may demonstrate thinning of the retinal nerve fiber layer and ganglion cell inner plexiform layer.

IMAGING STUDIES
Magnetic resonance imaging (MRI) of the brain and spinal cord with and without contrast is recommended in all cases. There are some imaging patterns to recognize in NMOSD:
- In the spinal cord, transverse myelitis is most frequently longitudinally extensive (that is, a single lesion involving three or more vertebral

BOX 1 2015 International Consensus Diagnostic Criteria for NMOSD

Diagnostic criteria for NMOSD with AQP4-IgG
1. At least one core clinical characteristic
2. Positive test for AQP4-IgG using best available detection method (cell-based assay strongly recommended)
3. Exclusion of alternative diagnoses

Diagnostic criteria for NMOSD without AQP4-IgG or NMOSD with unknown AQP4-IgG status
1. At least two core clinical characteristics occurring as a result of one or more clinical attacks and meeting all of the following requirements:
   a. At least one core clinical characteristic must be optic neuritis, acute myelitis with LETM, or area postrema syndrome
   b. Dissemination in space (two or more different core clinical characteristics)
   c. Fulfillment of additional MRI requirements, as applicable
2. Negative tests for AQP4-IgG using best available detection method, or testing unavailable
3. Exclusion of alternative diagnoses

Core clinical characteristics
1. Optic neuritis
2. Acute myelitis
3. Area postrema syndrome: episode of otherwise unexplained hiccups or nausea and vomiting
4. Acute brainstem syndrome
5. Symptomatic narcolepsy or acute diencephalic clinical syndrome with NMOSD-typical diencephalic MRI lesions
6. Symptomatic cerebral syndrome with NMOSD-typical brain lesions

Additional MRI requirements for NMOSD without AQP4-IgG and NMOSD with unknown AQP4-IgG status
1. Acute optic neuritis: requires brain MRI showing (a) normal findings or only nonspecific white matter lesions, OR (b) optic nerve MRI with T2-hyperintense lesion or T1-weighted gadolinium enhancing lesion extending over 1/2 optic nerve length or involving optic chiasm
2. Acute myelitis: requires associated intramedullary MRI lesion extending over at least three contiguous segments (LETM) OR at least three contiguous segments of focal spinal cord atrophy in patients with history compatible with acute myelitis
3. Area postrema syndrome: requires associated dorsal medulla/area postrema lesions
4. Acute brainstem syndrome: requires associated periependymal brainstem lesions

segments), though shorter segment lesions can occur in a minority of cases.
- In the optic nerve, >50% of the length of the nerve is commonly involved, with a preference for the posterior portion. Optic chiasm may be involved. Bilateral optic nerve involvement is less common (Fig. 1).
- In the brain, there is preferential involvement of the periependymal regions, including diencephalic and periventricular tissue. Involvement of the area postrema is especially characteristic. Lesions can occur elsewhere in both the supratentorial and infratentorial compartments, but these are less specific.

Rx TREATMENT

NONPHARMACOLOGIC THERAPY

Patient education regarding disease characteristics, treatment options, risks and benefits of treatment, and prognosis. Often, patients need to incorporate intermittent rest periods on a daily basis and when physically active (for energy conservation), and avoid exposure to heat, which typically worsens symptoms (but not the disease).

Recommend physical therapy for new or worsening weakness, incoordination, or spasticity.

ACUTE GENERAL Rx

- Given the potential for significant morbidity associated with acute NMOSD relapses, early recognition and intervention are considered important.
- For acute relapses or worsening, treat with 1 gram of methylprednisolone intravenously (IVMP) for 3-5 days.

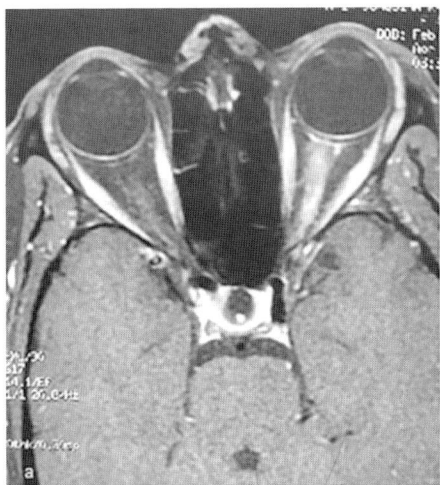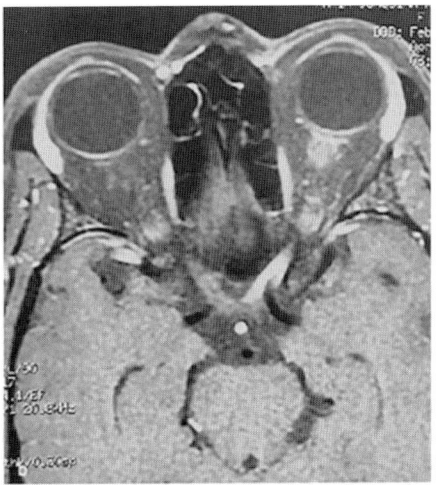

FIG. 1 Axial T1-weighted contrast-enhanced image of the orbital (**A**) and intracranial (**B**) segments of the left optic nerve. Note involvement of greater than 50% of the length of the optic nerve as well as the involvement of the intracranial segment and optic chiasm. (From Lana-Peixoto MA et al: Neuromyelitis optica spectrum disorder associated with dengue virus infection, *J Neuroimmunol* 318:53-55, 2018. Figure 2.)

TABLE 1   Drugs With Phase II/III Trials in NMOSD

DRUGS WITH PHASE II/III TRIALS IN NMOSD			
Name	**Mechanism of Action**	**Dose and Delivery**	**Side Effects/Monitoring**
Eculizumab[10]	Inhibits the terminal complement protein C5 and prevents its cleavage into C5a, which is pro-inflammatory, and C5b, which coordinates the formation of membrane cytolytic attack complex.	900 mg intravenously weekly for the first 4 doses starting on day 1, followed by 1200 mg every 2 weeks starting at week 4	−Approved for AQP4-IgG positive NMOSD −Increased infections with leukopenia and lymphopenia −Increased risk of infection with encapsulated bacteria, especially *Neisseria meningitidis* (meningococcal vaccination is mandatory before starting treatment)
Inebilizumab[11]	Binds to the B-cell surface antigen CD19 targeting B cells and CD19+ plasmablasts	300 mg administered intravenously on days 1 and 15 every 6 months	−Approved for AQP4-IgG positive NMOSD −Lymphopenia, reduced immunoglobulin levels −Increased infections
Satralizumab[12-13]	Binds to membrane-bound and soluble IL-6 receptors, preventing IL-6 from binding and inhibiting the IL-6 signaling pathways involved in inflammation	120 mg subcutaneously at weeks 0, 2, and 4 and every 4 weeks thereafter	−Approved for AQP4-IgG positive NMOSD −Leukopenia, increased infections
Rituximab[9]	Binds to the B-cell surface antigen CD20 surface expressed on B-lymphocytes	375 mg/m^2 intravenously every week for 4 weeks, then 6-month interval dosing (alternatively, 2 doses of 1,000 mg with 2 weeks interval)	Extralabel use for NMOSD

Adapted from Mora Cuervo DL et al: Immunobiology of neuromyelitis optica spectrum disorders, *Curr Opin Neurobiol* 76(102618):102618, 2022. Table 1.

- Plasma exchange (PLEX) should be considered in those who do not respond briskly to IVMP. This strategy has been found to significantly reduce the likelihood of residual deficits.[7]

CHRONIC Rx

- Chronic immunomodulation is indicated in most cases.
- Chronic steroids, azathioprine, mycophenolate mofetil, intravenous immunoglobulins,[8] and rituximab[9] can be used, especially for seronegative NMOSD.
- For seropositive (AQP4-IgG +) NMOSD, there are FDA approved therapies. In choosing between these therapies, a variety of factors should be considered including dosing frequency, comorbidities, and risk of opportunistic infections (Table 1).
    1. Eculizumab[10]
    2. Inebilizumab[11]
    3. Satralizumab[12]

DISPOSITION

- NMOSD, like MS, follows a relapsing clinical course in the vast majority of cases.
- Disability is largely accrued over time as a direct consequence of damage sustained during relapses. In cases of untreated seropositive NMOSD at 5 years after onset, more than 40% of patients are blind in at least one

eye, nearly 25% require assistance to walk, and mortality is close to 10%.[4]

REFERRAL

- Timely referral to a neurologist is critical. Given the prospect of significant residual deficits, a multidisciplinary approach to mitigating disability is advisable.
- Consider consultation with physical therapy/occupational therapy/speech therapy, neuro-ophthalmology, PM&R, and urology as well as engaging the services of social work.

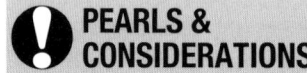

PEARLS & CONSIDERATIONS

COMMENTS

- NMOSD is a relapsing inflammatory autoimmune disorder of the central nervous system with preferential involvement of the optic nerve, spinal cord, and periependymal regions of the brain including the area postrema.
- Each relapse can result in permanent disability. Prompt recognition and treatment for relapses should be adopted, with steroids and early consideration for escalation to plasma exchange.

- Chronic preventative immunomodulation plays an important role in reducing the frequency of relapses and thus reducing disability. There are presently three FDA approved medications for seropositive (AQP4-IgG +) NMOSD with many more in development, and effective options including rituximab can be utilized for seronegative (MOG-IgG +, dual negative, or serologic status unknown) NMOSD.

PATIENT & FAMILY EDUCATION

Multiple organizations exist to spread awareness, fund research, and support patients with NMOSD. Among these are the Siegel Rare Neuroimmune Association (https://wearesrna.org/), the Sumaira Foundation (https://www.sumairafoundation.org/), and the Guthy-Jackson Charitable Foundation (https://guthyjacksonfoundation.org/).

REFERENCES

Available at eBooks.Health.Elsevier.com.

RELATED CONTENT

Optic Neuritis (Related Key Topic)
Multiple Sclerosis (Related Key Topic)
Transverse Myelitis (Related Key Topic)

AUTHOR: **MICHAEL Z. MOORE, MD**

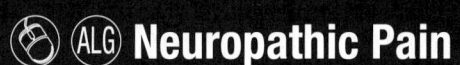
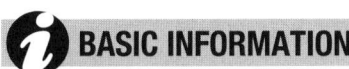 BASIC INFORMATION

DEFINITION

Neuropathic pain is not itself a disease but rather a symptom that is associated with multiple different diseases and localizations within the nervous system. Thus, it is not enough to define its presence without searching for a cause. It is defined as the sensation derived from the abnormal discharges of impaired or injured neural structures in either the peripheral or central nervous system. Descriptors include:

- Hyperesthesia: Heightened sensitivity to non-painful stimuli (e.g., light touch)
- Hyperalgesia: Heightened sensitivity to painful stimuli (e.g., pinprick), or reduced threshold to feel pain
- Allodynia: Pain provoked by a stimulus that is not normally painful
- Paresthesias: Abnormal sensations, typically "tingling" or "prickling," present with or without any tactile stimulation

SYNONYM

Neuralgia

ICD-10CM CODES
B02.29	Postherpetic neuralgia
G50.0	Trigeminal neuralgia
G58.0	Intercostal neuropathy
G58.7	Mononeuritis multiplex
G58.8	Other specified mononeuropathies
G58.9	Mononeuropathy, unspecified
G61.9	Inflammatory polyneuropathy, unspecified
G62.0	Drug-induced polyneuropathy
G62.1	Alcoholic polyneuropathy
G62.9	Polyneuropathy, unspecified
G63.2	Diabetic polyneuropathy
G63.5	Polyneuropathy in systemic connective tissue disease
G63.8	Polyneuropathy in other diseases classified elsewhere
G79.2	Neuralgia and neuritis
G89.0	Central pain syndrome
M79.2	Neuralgia and neuritis, unspecified

EPIDEMIOLOGY & DEMOGRAPHICS

- Estimates of the prevalence of neuropathic pain in the general population range from 1.6% to 8.2%[1]
- Demographics vary widely depending on etiology, for example:
  1. Postherpetic neuralgia: Affects elderly, pain seen in almost 100% of cases
  2. AIDS: 30% of patients affected
  3. Diabetes mellitus: 20% to 24% affected (prevalence rates vary, increasing with longer disease duration); most diabetic neuropathy is painless (although, given the prevalence of diabetes and diabetic neuropathy, it is a common cause of neuropathic pain)
  4. Fabry disease: Affects mostly children, pain in 81% to 90% of patients

PHYSICAL FINDINGS & CLINICAL PRESENTATION

- History: Important for localization and diagnosis[1-2]
  1. Quality (description) of neuropathic pain: Burning, hot or cold, "icy hot," "pins and needles," stinging, lancinating, sharp, shooting
  2. Distribution of symptoms may aid in localization (i.e., "stocking-glove" symptoms in generalized neuropathy, numbness in a peripheral nerve territory in focal neuropathy or dermatome in radiculopathy)
  3. Generalized small fiber neuropathy: Dysesthesias without numbness common, but many etiologies (e.g., diabetes) cause both small and large fiber dysfunction
  4. Large fiber neuropathy (LFPN): Coexisting numbness, hyporeflexia, or weakness may be seen, usually worse distally
  5. Nerve root: Coexisting neck or low back pain that radiates along a specific dermatome; most common cause is structural compression
  6. Spinal cord symptoms: Coexisting spasticity, bowel or bladder involvement, sensory level
  7. Prior history of thalamic stroke in central thalamic pain syndrome (Dejerine-Roussy syndrome)
  8. Family history may suggest a genetic cause
- Examination: See Table 1. Table 2 describes joint involvement in neuropathic arthropathy. Fig. E1 illustrates a diagnostic approach to neuropathic pain. Fig. E2 shows a neuropathic ankle

ETIOLOGY & LABORATORY EVALUATION (TABLE 3)

- Metabolic: Diabetes mellitus; malnutrition and alcoholism; vitamin B_{12} deficiency; thiamine deficiency; porphyria; Fabry disease
- Vascular: Prior stroke usually in the thalamus, peripheral nerve vasculitis
- Inflammatory: Autoimmune diseases (systemic vasculitides, systemic lupus erythematosus, Sjögren syndrome, etc.), acute inflammatory demyelinating polyneuropathy

TABLE 1   Examination

Exam Finding	Localization
Pinprick/temperature loss alone	Small fibers only
Pinprick/temperature loss + vibratory/proprioceptive loss	Small and large fibers
Sensory loss and motor dysfunction worse distally than proximal	Large fiber neuropathy
Sensory loss and motor dysfunction along single nerve distribution	Single nerve
Sensory loss and motor dysfunction along multiple single nerves	Multiple mononeuropathies (i.e., mononeuropathy multiplex)
Motor and sensory loss involving multiple nerves belonging to specific region of brachial or lumbar plexus	Plexopathy
Sensory loss along dermatome with multiple myotomal muscles affected	Nerve root lesion
Asymmetric sensory loss without weakness and pseudoathetosis	Dorsal root ganglion
Vibratory/proprioceptive loss without pinprick/temperature loss	Dorsal column dysfunction (from compressive lesion, B_{12} deficiency, or tabes dorsalis from neurosyphilis)
Sensory level with weakness below the level of lesion and long tract signs (spasticity/Babinski sign)	Spinal cord lesion
Hemisensory hyperalgesia	Contralateral thalamus

TABLE 2   Joint Involvement in Neuropathic Arthropathy

Disease	Site of Involvement
Diabetes mellitus	Midtarsal, metatarsophalangeal, tarsometatarsal
Syringomyelia	Shoulder, elbow, wrist
Amyloidosis	Knee, ankle
Congenital sensory neuropathy	Knee, ankle, intertarsal, metatarsophalangeal
Tabes dorsalis	Knee, hip, ankle
Leprosy	Tarsal, tarsometatarsal

From Hochberg MC et al: *Rheumatology*, ed 5, St Louis, 2011, Mosby.

Diseases and Disorders

I

TABLE 3 Clinical Presentation and Laboratory Findings

Neuropathy Type	Predisposition	Examination Findings	EMG/NCS	Laboratory Analysis
Idiopathic small fiber PN	Age >50	Strength: Normal Reflexes: Normal Pos/vib: Normal Pain/temp: Decreased distally	Normal	Serum studies: Normal Skin biopsy: Abnormal Sudomotor studies: Abnormal
Diabetic PN	Long-standing disease, family history	Strength normal to reduced, sensation reduced distally	Abnormal	Abnormal glucose tolerance: High fasting glucose
Inherited PN	Family history	Pes cavus, hammer toes, reduced reflexes, sensation reduced distally	Abnormal	Genetic studies may be abnormal, other studies normal
Familial amyloid PN	Family history	Pain/temp loss, reduced reflexes, orthostasis	Abnormal if large fibers affected; also carpal tunnel syndrome	Transthyretin genetic study
Acquired amyloid PN	Monoclonal gammopathy	Pain/temp loss, reduced reflexes, orthostasis	Abnormal if large fibers affected; also carpal tunnel syndrome	SPEP, UPEP, immunofixation abnormal
Fabry disease	Age, renal failure, strokes	Normal; possible reduced pain/temp sensation	Normal	α-Galactosidase levels in cultured fibroblasts
PN + mixed connective tissue disease	History of lupus, rheumatoid arthritis, Sjögren syndrome	Reduced reflexes and distal sensation	Abnormal	ANA, RF, SS-A/SS-B may be abnormal
Peripheral nerve vasculitis	Asymmetric disease	Multiple peripheral nerves involved	Abnormal	ANA, RF, SS-A/SS-B, ANCA, cryoglobulins may be abnormal
Paraneoplastic neuropathy	Lung cancer risk factors, chemical exposures	Asymmetric sensory loss, pseudoathetosis, relatively preserved strength	Abnormal	Anti-Hu
Sarcoidosis	Pulmonary sarcoid	Multiple mononeuropathies	Abnormal	Abnormal biopsy, elevated serum ACE, CXR abnormal
Arsenic	Pesticides, copper smelting	Reduced reflexes and distal sensation	Abnormal	Elevated arsenic in plasma, urine, and hair
HIV	Multiple partners, unprotected sex, IV drug abuse, blood transfusion	Variable, but most often reduced reflexes and distal sensation	Abnormal if large fibers involved	HIV antibody

ACE, Angiotensin-converting enzyme; ANA, antibody to nuclear antigens; ANCA, antineutrophil cytoplasmic antibodies; CXR, chest x-ray; EMG, electromyography; HIV, human immunodeficiency virus; IV, intravenous; NCS, nerve conduction studies; PN, polyneuropathy; Pos, position sensation; RF, rheumatoid factor; SPEP, serum protein electrophoresis; SS-A, Sjögren syndrome A; SS-B, Sjögren syndrome B; Temp, temperature sensation; UPEP, urine protein electrophoresis; Vib, vibration sensation.
Adapted from Mendell JR, Sahenk Z: Painful sensory neuropathy, *N Engl J Med* 348(13):1243, 2003.

(classically presents with ascending weakness without numbness although pain is also a common feature), chronic inflammatory demyelinating polyneuropathy, sarcoidosis, multiple sclerosis
- Infiltrative: Amyloidosis, paraproteinemias (e.g., monoclonal gammopathy of uncertain significance [MGUS] associated neuropathy)
- Infectious: Postviral (brachial neuritis), HIV/AIDS, herpes simplex virus (HSV), varicella-zoster virus (VZV; postherpetic neuralgia), Lyme disease, leprosy (thickened nerves and skin lesions), syphilis
- Neoplastic and paraneoplastic-carcinomatous infiltration of nerve/nerve root, anti-Hu
- Drugs/toxins: History of exposure to alcohol, chemotherapeutic agents (paclitaxel, vincristine), isoniazid, metronidazole, or heavy metals (thallium, arsenic)
- Peripheral neuropathies frequently associated with pain are summarized in Box E1

ⒹⓍ DIAGNOSIS

LABORATORY TESTS
- Fasting blood glucose
- 2-h oral glucose tolerance test (OGTT)
- Vitamin B_{12} level

- If B_{12} level normal: Serum methylmalonic acid and homocysteine levels
- Serum erythrocyte sedimentation rate (ESR), antinuclear antibodies (ANA), Sjögren syndrome (SS)-A and SS-B, c-ANCA, p-ANCA
- RPR or FTA-ABS
- Serum ACE level (sarcoid)
- HIV antibody
- Serum protein electrophoresis (SPEP), urine protein electrophoresis (UPEP), immunofixation
- Urine and stool protoporphyrins, if porphyria is suspected clinically
- Hu antibody: Can be seen in both small cell and non–small cell lung cancers, may be positive without evidence of lung cancer
- Lumbar puncture: Protein elevation, oligoclonal bands, cerebrospinal fluid (CSF)/serum IgG index

ELECTROPHYSIOLOGY STUDIES
- Electrophysiologic testing (electromyography with nerve conduction studies): May be normal in small fiber neuropathies or central nervous system (CNS) lesion, but is often abnormal in large fiber neuropathies
- Quantitative sensory testing: Abnormal in small and large fiber neuropathy

- Evoked potentials (only if suspicion for spinal cord lesion)

PATHOLOGY STUDIES
- Nerve biopsy is occasionally useful in selected cases, particularly when vasculitis, sarcoidosis, or amyloid neuropathy are in the differential.
- Skin biopsy for intraepidermal nerve fiber (IENF) density may be useful for small fiber neuropathy when other studies are normal.
- Rectal or abdominal fat pad biopsy may show amyloid deposition in systemic amyloidosis.

IMAGING STUDIES
Based on localization:
- MRI (with and without contrast):
  1. Of the brain to exclude thalamic pathology if symptoms and signs are consistent with thalamic lesion (hemibody pain)
  2. Of the spinal cord and nerve roots to exclude structural, inflammatory, neoplastic, or infectious causes
  3. Of the lumbar spine to evaluate for arachnoiditis
- If MRI cannot be performed, consider:
  1. Computed tomography (CT) of the brain for thalamic pathology

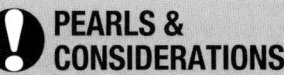
N

2. CT myelography of the spinal cord to evaluate for structural/neoplastic disease, but only if clinical signs of spinal or nerve root compromise are present

(Rx) TREATMENT

NONPHARMACOLOGIC THERAPY

- Counseling should be initiated at the beginning of therapy to address psychologic issues exacerbating physiologic pain. It needs to also be emphasized that the goal of therapy is to reduce and not necessarily eliminate the pain[3]
- Weight-bearing exercise (>4 h a week), t'ai chi, and massage therapy, especially in cases of chronic neck and low back pain but also in painful neuropathy[4]
- Optimization of glucose control
- Cognitive-behavioral therapy
- Percutaneous electrical nerve stimulation (TENS unit)
- Dorsal column spinal cord stimulation—FDA approved for treatment of peripheral diabetic neuropathy pain[4]

ACUTE GENERAL Rx

- Treatment of the underlying cause if possible will help slow or prevent worsening.
- Medications may reduce or alleviate pain but do not affect numbness.
- General neuropathic pain:[3-6]
- Antiepileptics:
  1. Pregabalin has the best level of evidence: Begin 50 mg PO tid, increase slowly to 100 to 200 mg PO tid.
  2. Gabapentin: Begin 300 mg PO qd, advance to 300 mg PO tid by the end of the first wk. Effective dose: Higher than 1600 mg/day. Max dose: 1200 mg PO tid.
  3. Sodium channel blockers: Sodium valproate, oxcarbazepine, lamotrigine, and lacosamide can be tried as second line agents.[3]
- Antidepressants:

1. Tricyclic antidepressants (TCAs): Nortriptyline preferred over amitriptyline (fewer anticholinergic side effects with nortriptyline). Begin 25 mg PO qd in adults, or 10 mg qd in elderly. Increase dose by 25 mg every week as tolerated until usual maximal effective dose of 150 mg/day.
2. Duloxetine: Begin 30 mg daily, increase to 60 to 120 mg daily. Duloxetine is effective in diabetic neuropathy, postherpetic neuropathy, and chemotherapy-induced painful peripheral neuropathy.
3. Venlafaxine and desvenlafaxine
- Analgesics: When first and second-line agents are ineffective, opioids are sometimes used but are overall not recommended and there is no benefit in their long-term use in neuropathic pain.[3]
- Topical anesthetics:
  1. 5% lidocaine patch, apply to area of pain, max three patches every 12 h.
  2. Isosorbide dinitrate spray.
  3. Capsaicin cream and patches are inconsistent in their ability to relieve pain and may exacerbate it. A capsaicin 8% patch is approved specifically for postherpetic neuralgia and is applied for 60 min under medical supervision.
- Procedural/surgical: This option is considered mostly when the patient suffers from pain secondary to spinal cord or cauda equina injury. Procedures should be considered only when all other therapeutic modalities have failed. In addition, the patient should be cautioned that surgical procedures may not result in pain relief and may be associated with significant morbidity and even mortality.
  1. Dorsal root rhizotomy
  2. Nerve blocks
  3. Spinal cord stimulator

DISPOSITION

Prognosis depends on multiple factors, including:
- Etiology of pain

- Treatment of any underlying condition
- Initiation of appropriate (often multiple) therapeutic modalities
- Patient compliance with prescribed regimen

Most care is accomplished in the outpatient setting, except when surgery is required.

REFERRAL

- Pain clinic
- Neurology
- Psychiatry
- Psychology
- Physiatry
- Anesthesiology (nerve blocks)
- Neurosurgery if considering surgical management

(!) PEARLS & CONSIDERATIONS

- Factitious disorder and malingering frequently manifest with pain complaints. These are diagnoses of exclusion and require negative evaluation for organic etiologies before diagnosis is made.
- Peripheral neuropathy in diabetics increases the risk of foot ulceration by sevenfold. Abnormal results in monofilament testing and vibratory perception (alone or in combination with the appearance of the feet, ulceration, and ankle reflexes) are the most helpful sign for the detection of LFPN.

RELATED TOPIC

Trigeminal neuralgia (Related Key Topic)

AUTHOR: **COREY ELAM GOLDSMITH, MD, FAAN**

REFERENCES

Available at eBooks.Health.Elsevier.com.

Diseases
and Disorders

I

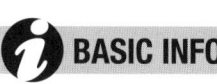 **BASIC INFORMATION**

DEFINITION

- Nonalcoholic *fatty liver disease* (NAFLD) is a spectrum of diseases based on histopathologic findings and representing a morphologic rather than a clinical diagnosis (Fig. 1). It is liver disease occurring in patients who do not abuse alcohol and manifesting histologically by mononuclear cells and/or polymorphonuclear cells, hepatocyte ballooning, and spotty necrosis. Nonalcoholic steatohepatitis (NASH) is a subset of NAFLD. Patients with NASH have progressive disease that can result in fibrosis and cirrhosis. A diagnosis of NAFLD is contingent on the following factors:
  1. Alcohol consumption in amounts less than those considered hepatotoxic.
  2. Absence of serologic evidence of other hepatic diseases or disorders.
  3. Liver biopsy showing predominant macrovesicular steatosis or steatohepatitis.
- NAFL is defined as ≥5% hepatic steatosis without evidence of hepatocellular injury or fibrosis.
- NASH is ≥5% hepatic fibrosis with inflammation and hepatocellular injury with or without fibrosis.
- *NASH cirrhosis* is the presence of cirrhosis with current or past evidence of steatosis.

SYNONYMS

Nonalcoholic steatohepatitis (NASH)
NAFLD
Fatty liver hepatitis
Diabetes hepatitis
Alcohol-like liver disease
Laënnec disease

ICD-10CM CODE

K76.0 Fatty (change of) liver, not elsewhere classified

EPIDEMIOLOGY & DEMOGRAPHICS

- NAFLD affects 30% of the adult general population in the U.S.
- Increased prevalence in obese persons (57% to 74%), type 2 diabetes mellitus, and hyperlipidemia (primarily hypertriglyceridemia).
- Most common cause of abnormal liver test results in adults in the United States (accounts for up to 90% of cases of asymptomatic alanine aminotransferase (ALT) elevations).
- NAFLD is more prevalent in men than women.
- NAFLD is more prevalent in the Hispanic population.
- Approximately 20% of patients with NAFLD have NASH, and 10% to 30% of patients with NASH have NASH cirrhosis.

PHYSICAL FINDINGS & CLINICAL PRESENTATION

- Most patients are asymptomatic.
- Patients may report a sensation of fullness or discomfort on the right side of the upper abdomen.
- Nonspecific complaints of fatigue or malaise may be reported.
- Hepatomegaly (Table 1) is generally the only positive finding on physical examination.
- Acanthosis nigricans may be found in children.

ETIOLOGY

- Metabolic syndrome and insulin resistance are the most reproducible factors in the development of NAFLD and accumulation of triglycerides within the liver. High baseline and continuously increasing fasting insulin levels are independent determinants for future development of NAFLD. The transition from NAFLD to NASH is poorly understood; there may be a genetic component. The presence of the I48M variant of PNPLA3 increases risk for

TABLE 1 Symptoms, Signs, and Laboratory Features of Nonalcoholic Fatty Liver Disease

Symptoms	Signs	Laboratory Features
Common		
None (48%-100% of patients)	Hepatomegaly	2- to 4-fold elevation of serum ALT and AST levels AST/ALT ratio <1 in most patients Serum alkaline phosphatase level slightly elevated in one third of patients Normal serum bilirubin, serum albumin, and prothrombin time Elevated serum ferritin level
Uncommon		
Vague right upper quadrant pain Fatigue Malaise	Splenomegaly Spider telangiectasias Palmar erythema Ascites	Low-titer (<1:320) antinuclear antibodies

ALT, Alanine aminotransferase; *AST,* aspartate aminotransferase.
From Feldman M et al: *Sleisenger and Fordtran's gastrointestinal and liver disease,* ed 10, Philadelphia, 2016, Elsevier.

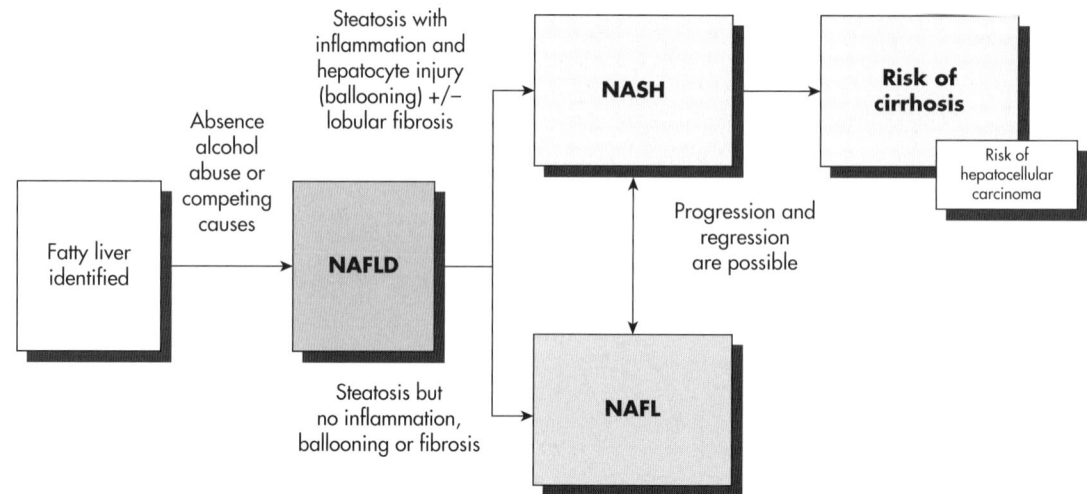

FIG. 1 Relationship between fatty liver, NAFLD, NAFL, and NASH. *NAFL,* Nonalcoholic fatty liver; *NAFLD,* nonalcoholic fatty liver disease; *NASH,* nonalcoholic steatohepatitis. (From Budd J, Cusi K: Nonalcoholic fatty liver disease: what does the primary care physician need to know? *Am J Med* 133:536-543, 2020.)

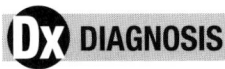
and severity of NAFLD. Genetic polymorphism (TM6SF2) also increases NAFLD risk.
- Risk factors are obesity (especially truncal obesity), diabetes mellitus, hyperlipidemia.

Dx DIAGNOSIS

DIFFERENTIAL DIAGNOSIS
- Alcohol-induced liver disease (a daily alcohol intake of 20 g in females and 30 g in males [three 12-oz beers or 12 oz of wine] may be enough to cause alcohol-induced liver disease)
- Viral hepatitis
- Autoimmune hepatitis
- Toxin- or drug-induced liver disease
- Box 1 summarizes the various causes of fatty liver disease

WORKUP
Diagnosis is usually suspected on the basis of hepatomegaly, asymptomatic elevations of transaminases, or "fatty liver" on sonogram of abdomen in obese patients with little or no alcohol use. Fig. E2 and Fig. 3 illustrate algorithms for the diagnostic approach to NAFLD. Transient elastography is a noninvasive imaging modality that can be used to screen for the development of hepatic fibrosis (Fig 4). In obese patients newer "XL" FibroScan machines are more accurate. Liver biopsy can confirm diagnosis and provide prognostic information. It should be considered in patients with suspected advanced liver fibrosis (presence of obesity or type 2 diabetes, aspartate aminotransferase [AST]:ALT ratio 1, age 45 yr). NAFLD activity score on liver biopsy is described in Table 2. The FIB-4 score can screen noninvasively for clinically significant fibrosis. It is derived from AGG, ALT, and AST levels and platelet count and can be obtained using online calculators. Patients with low-risk FIB-4 scores (<1.3) can be followed routinely in primary care. Patients with FIB-4 scores between 1.3 to 2.67 are considered to be at intermediate risk for fibrosis and should undergo transient elastography scan. Patients with FIB-4 scores >2.67 are considered high risk for fibrosis and should be referred to a hepatologist.[1]

LABORATORY TESTS
- Elevated ALT, AST: AST:ALT ratio is usually <1, but can increase as fibrosis advances. In advanced fibrosis AST to ALT ratio is >1 and platelet count is low.

- Negative serology for infectious hepatitis; generally normal gamma-glutamyl transpeptidase and serum alkaline phosphatase.
- Hyperlipidemia (primarily hypertriglyceridemia) may be present.
- Elevated glucose levels may be present.
- Prolonged prothrombin time, hypoalbuminemia, and elevated bilirubin may be present in advanced stages.
- Elevated serum ferritin and increased transferrin saturation may be found in up to 10% of patients; however, hepatic iron index and hepatic iron level are normal.
- Antismooth muscle antibodies and antinuclear antibodies at low titer are not uncommon.

IMAGING STUDIES
- Ultrasound generally reveals diffuse increase in echogenicity as compared with that of the kidneys; computed tomography (CT) scan reveals diffuse low-density hepatic parenchyma. The sensitivity of ultrasound and CT scan for detection of fat in liver is over 90% if hepatic steatosis exceeds 33%.
- Occasionally patients may have focal rather than diffuse steatosis, which may be misinterpreted as a liver mass on ultrasound or CT (Fig. E5); use of MRI in these cases will identify focal fatty infiltration.
- Vibration-controlled elastography (FibroScan) can also be used to evaluate noninvasively for hepatic fibrosis and to further stratify patients and is more cost effective than MRI.[1a]

Rx TREATMENT

NONPHARMACOLOGIC THERAPY
- Weight reduction in all obese patients. The American Gastroenterological Association recommends that the initial target weight loss be 10% of baseline weight at a rate of 1 to 2 lb (0.45 to 0.90 kg) per week. The Mediterranean diet reduces fat intake and enables weight loss. A diet with fish may slow fatty liver disease progression in patients who also consume meat.[1b] Fresh fish consumption is associated with increases in short-chain fatty acids, unconjugated bile acids, and increases in intestinal faecalibacterium which may improve hepatic steatosis.[1c]
- Increase physical activity. Vigorous and moderate exercise are equally effective in reducing intrahepatic triglyceride content, the effect being largely mediated by weight loss.
- Alcohol has a deleterious effect on NAFLD and should be avoided.

ACUTE GENERAL Rx
- There are no drugs currently approved by FDA for NAFLD. Medications to control hyperlipidemia (e.g., fenofibrates for elevated triglycerides) and hyperglycemia (e.g., pioglitazone, insulin, metformin) can lead to improvement in abnormal liver test results.
- A 3-yr trial with pioglitazone (30 mg/day), an insulin-sensitizing thiazolidinedione, revealed that pioglitazone treatment was associated with long-term metabolic and histologic

---

BOX 1   Causes of Fatty Liver Disease

Acquired Metabolic Disorders
Diabetes mellitus
Dyslipidemia
Kwashiorkor and marasmus
Obesity
Rapid weight loss
Starvation
Cytotoxic and Cytostatic Drugs
L-Asparaginase
Azacitidine
Bleomycin
Cisplatin
5-Fluorouracil
Methotrexate
Tetracyclines (inhibit mitochondrial beta oxidation)
Other Drugs and Toxins
Amiodarone
Camphor
Chloroform
Cocaine
Ethanol
Ethyl bromide
Estrogens
Glucocorticoids
Griseofulvin
Highly active antiretroviral therapy (zidovudine, stavudine, didanosine)
Lycopodium serratum (Jin Bu Huan, an herbal supplement)
Nifedipine
Nitrofurantoin
Nonsteroidal antiinflammatory drugs (piroxicam, ibuprofen, indomethacin, sulindac)

Tamoxifen
Valproic acid
Metals
Antimony
Barium salts
Chromates
Mercury
Phosphorus
Rare earth metals of low atomic number
Thallium compounds
Uranium compounds
Inborn Errors of Metabolism
Abetalipoproteinemia
Familial hepatosteatosis
Galactosemia
Glycogen storage disease
Hereditary fructose intolerance
Homocystinuria
Systemic carnitine deficiency
Tyrosinemia
Weber-Christian syndrome
Wilson disease
Surgical Procedures
Biliopancreatic diversion
Extensive small bowel resection
Jejunoileal bypass
Miscellaneous Conditions
Industrial exposure to petrochemicals
Inflammatory bowel disease
Jejunal diverticulosis with bacterial overgrowth
Partial lipodystrophy
Total parenteral nutrition

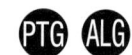
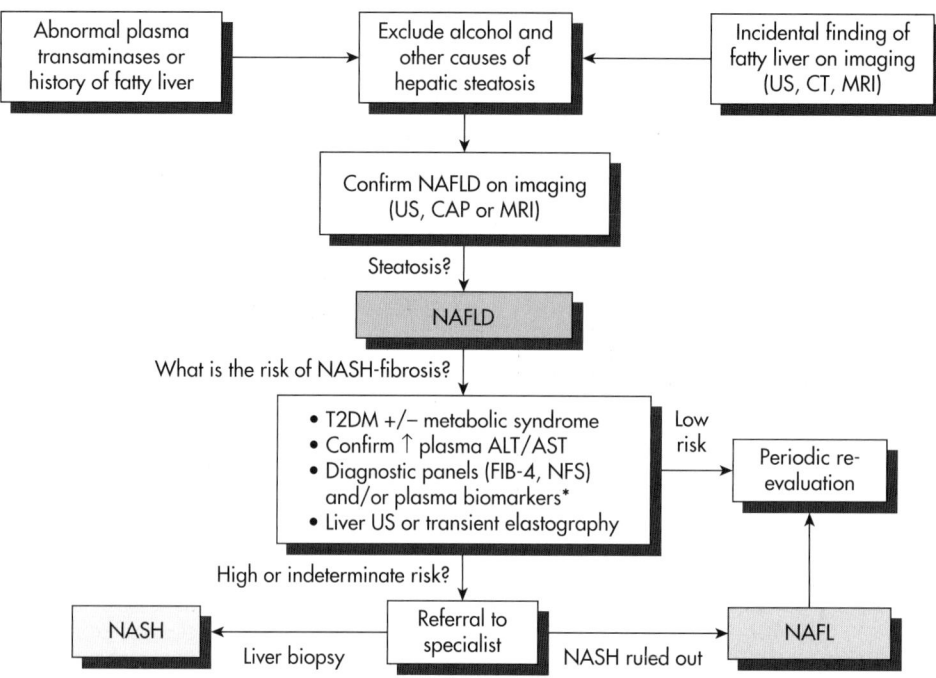

FIG. 3 Diagnosis of NAFLD, NAFL, and NASH. *ALT,* Alanine aminotransferase; *AST,* aspartate aminotransferase; *CAP,* controlled attenuation parameter; *CT,* computed tomography; *MRI,* magnetic resonance imaging (used largely in research settings); *NAFL,* nonalcoholic fatty liver; *NAFLD,* nonalcoholic fatty liver disease; *NASH,* nonalcoholic steatohepatitis; *NFS,* NAFLD fibrosis score; *T2DM,* type 2 diabetes mellitus; *US,* liver ultrasound. *Plasma biomarkers: several commercial ones are available and others are in development.[2-9] (From Budd J, Cusi K: Nonalcoholic fatty liver disease: what does the primary care physician need to know? *Am J Med* 133:536-543, 2020.)

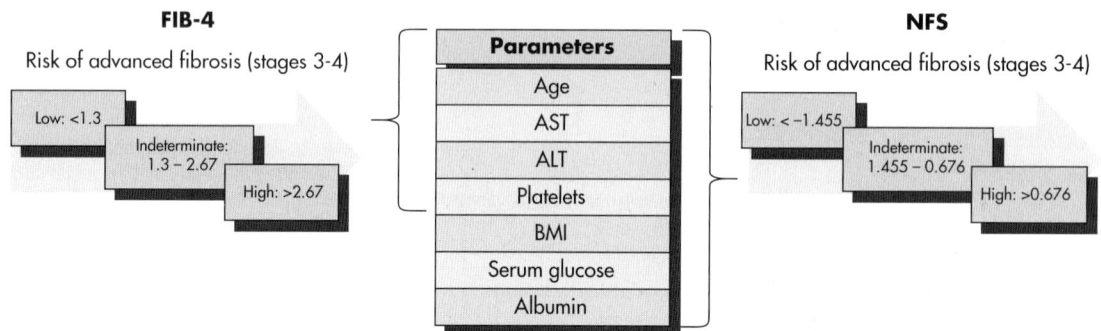

FIG. 4 Parameters and interpretation of FIB-4 and NFS for establishing the risk of advanced fibrosis (stages 3-4). *ALT,* Alanine aminotransferase; *AST,* aspartate aminotransferase; *BMI,* body mass index; *FIB-4,* fibrosis-4 score; *NFS,* NAFLD fibrosis score. (From Budd J, Cusi K: Nonalcoholic fatty liver disease: what does the primary care physician need to know? *Am J Med* 133:536-543, 2020.)

improvement in patients with prediabetes or type 2 diabetes mellitus and NASH. These results suggest that NASH progression may be halted, and the natural history of the disease may be modified with the use of pioglitazone in patients with prediabetes or type 2 diabetes mellitus.[1] Glucagon-like peptide-1 receptor agonists (GLP-1RA) like liraglutide have shown modest improvement in reduction of plasma aminotransferase and steatosis.

DISPOSITION

- Patients with pure steatosis on liver biopsy generally have a relatively benign course.
- The presence of steatohepatitis or advanced fibrosis on liver biopsy is associated with a worse prognosis.

REFERRAL

Liver transplantation should be considered in patients with decompensated, end-stage disease; however, in these patients there may be a recurrence of NAFLD posttransplantation.

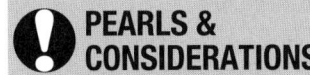 **PEARLS & CONSIDERATIONS**

COMMENTS

- NAFLD is closely associated with metabolic disorders, even in nonobese, nondiabetic subjects. It can be considered an early predictor of metabolic disorders, particularly in the normal-weight population. The presence of metabolic syndrome is a strong predictor of NAFLD.

- NAFLD is associated with an increased risk of incident cardiovascular disease that is independent of the risk conferred by traditional risk factors and components of the metabolic syndrome.
- 10% of patients with NASH have progression to advanced fibrosis. Most common in patients older than 50, ALT > twice normal, body mass index >28, triglycerides >150 mg/dl.
- Statins are not contraindicated in patients with NASH and should be considered in hypercholesterolemic patients.
- A recent trial has shown that daily aspirin use is associated with reduced risk for fibrosis progression in patients with NAFLD.[1]

REFERENCES & SUGGESTED READINGS

Available at eBooks.Health.Elsevier.com.

RELATED CONTENT

Fatty Liver (Patient Information)

AUTHOR: **FRED F. FERRI, MD**

TABLE 2 NAFLD Activity Score on a Liver Biopsy Specimen

Steatosis	
5%	1
5%-33%	2
33%-66%	3
Ballooning	
None	0
Few	1
Many	2
Lobular Inflammation	
Mild	1
Moderate	2
Severe	3
Total Score	
0-2	Likely not NASH
3-4	Intermediate
5-8	Likely NASH

NAFLD, Nonalcoholic fatty liver disease; *NASH,* nonalcoholic steatohepatitis.
From Feldman M et al: *Sleisenger and Fordtran's gastrointestinal and liver disease,* ed 10, Philadelphia, 2016, Elsevier.

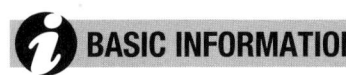
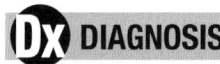 BASIC INFORMATION

DEFINITION

Non-Hodgkin lymphoma (NHL) is a heterogeneous group of malignancies of the lymphoreticular system. There are approximately 60 different NHL subtypes.[1] The WHO classification of lymphomas is summarized in Fig. 1.

SYNONYM

NHL

ICD-10CM CODES

C85.90	Non-Hodgkin lymphoma, unspecified, unspecified site
C85.91	Non-Hodgkin lymphoma, unspecified, lymph nodes of head, face, and neck
C85.92	Non-Hodgkin lymphoma, unspecified, intrathoracic lymph nodes
C85.93	Non-Hodgkin lymphoma, unspecified, intra-abdominal lymph nodes
C85.94	Non-Hodgkin lymphoma, unspecified, lymph nodes of axilla and upper limb
C85.95	Non-Hodgkin lymphoma, unspecified, lymph nodes of inguinal region and lower limb
C85.96	Non-Hodgkin lymphoma, unspecified, intrapelvic lymph nodes
C85.97	Non-Hodgkin lymphoma, unspecified, spleen
C85.98	Non-Hodgkin lymphoma, unspecified, lymph nodes of multiple sites
C85.99	Non-Hodgkin lymphoma, unspecified, extranodal and solid organ sites

EPIDEMIOLOGY

- Seventh most common neoplasm in the U.S. (>80,000 new cases annually).[2] Incidence increases with age; majority of patients are older than 60 yr of age.
- In the U.S. and Europe, diffuse large B-cell lymphoma (DLBCL) is the most common subtype (30% of the cases), and follicular lymphoma (FL) is the second most common subtype (25% of the cases).[3]
- In patients with HIV, NHL is the most common tumor (followed by Kaposi sarcoma). DLBCL accounts for 80% to 90% of the cases.[4]
- Factors associated with an increased risk of non-Hodgkin lymphoma are summarized in Box 1.

PHYSICAL FINDINGS & CLINICAL PRESENTATION

- Patients often present with lymphadenopathy.
- Approximately one third of the NHL involve extranodal sites, which can result in unusual presentations (e.g., gastrointestinal tract involvement can simulate peptic ulcer disease).
- Presence of B symptoms like unexplained weight loss, fever, fatigue, and night sweats are seen typically in aggressive lymphomas.
- Aggressive lymphomas have acute or subacute presentation with increasing size of the mass and B symptoms.
- Indolent lymphomas have a more chronic course, with asymptomatic lymphadenopathy and/or slowly progressive cytopenias.

- Hepatomegaly and splenomegaly may be present.
- Cough, dyspnea can occur with bulky mediastinal involvement.

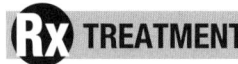 DIAGNOSIS

DIFFERENTIAL DIAGNOSIS

- Hodgkin lymphoma
- Viral infections (e.g., mononucleosis)
- Metastatic carcinoma
- Autoimmune conditions
- Sarcoidosis

WORKUP

Initial laboratory evaluation may be entirely normal. Elevated serum LDH may be seen in aggressive lymphoma or in indolent lymphoma with high disease burden. In cases of highly aggressive NHL (e.g., Burkitt lymphoma), spontaneous tumor lysis syndrome (TLS) may be seen, characterized by hyperkalemia, hyperuricemia, hypocalcemia, hyperphosphatemia, and acidosis. TLS can be life threatening and is considered a medical emergency. Acute management includes aggressive IV fluid repletion and/or rasburicase. Proper staging of NHL includes the following:

- A thorough history and physical examination.
- Excisional or incisional surgical biopsy is preferred. Image-guided core needle biopsies may be acceptable in patients without peripheral adenopathy. Fine needle aspirates are not adequate for precise lymphoma subclassification. Laparoscopic lymph node biopsy or mediastinoscopy can be used on an outpatient basis for most patients with intraabdominal or mediastinal lymphoma, respectively.
- Tissue biopsy with histologic, immunophenotypic, and genetic studies interpretation. Major molecular alterations in non-Hodgkin lymphomas are summarized in Table 1.
- Routine laboratory evaluation (complete blood count, flow cytometry in selected circumstances, urinalysis, LDH, blood urea nitrogen, creatinine, serum calcium, uric acid, liver function tests, serum protein electrophoresis).
- HIV and hepatitis B testing. HTLV-1 testing is encouraged in peripheral T-cell lymphomas (especially in Japanese, Caribbean, and South American patients).[5]
- Bone marrow evaluation (aspirate and biopsy) in selected patients (Fig. E2).
- Fluorine-18 fluorodeoxyglucose (FDG) positron emission tomography (PET) integrated with CT (Fig. E3) has emerged as a tool for staging, response evaluation, and posttreatment surveillance in patients with aggressive subtypes of NHL.
- CT scan of chest, abdomen, and pelvis with IV contrast in selected patients.
- Depending on the histopathology, the results of the previous studies, and the planned therapy, some other tests may be performed.
- Lumbar puncture is needed in some patients with aggressive NHL, and most patients with HIV-associated NHL, to evaluate for CNS involvement by lymphoma.

- The evaluation of a new patient with non-Hodgkin lymphoma is summarized in Table 2.

CLASSIFICATION

For clinical approach, NHL is subdivided into indolent, aggressive, and highly aggressive disease.

STAGING

The Ann Arbor staging system that was initially developed for Hodgkin lymphoma (HL) was revised as the Lugano criteria and remains the current standard; but unlike HL, NHL does not spread predictably via lymphatic channels to contiguous nodal regions, so stage is only one of multiple contributors to prognosis (Table 3). Disease subtype has greater therapeutic implications in NHL than in Hodgkin lymphoma. Fig. 4 illustrates a diagnostic algorithm outlining the steps in classification of B-cell lymphomas composed of cells of small to intermediate size.

TREATMENT

ACUTE GENERAL Rx

The therapeutic regimen varies with specific lymphoma subtype and pathologic stage. Following are the commonly used therapeutic modalities:

INDOLENT NHL:

- Deferment of therapy and careful observation in asymptomatic patients with low volume (burden) disease.
- Local radiotherapy for stage I disease, depending on location of disease.
- Rituximab, an anti-CD20 monoclonal antibody, with or without chemotherapy is used in patients with symptomatic or progressive disease.
- The addition of rituximab to chemotherapy is generally well tolerated and has increased response and survival rates in NHL patients. Patients who received rituximab, cyclophosphamide, doxorubicin, vincristine, and prednisone (R-CHOP) had higher response rates (96% vs. 90%) with a better 2-yr overall survival rate (95% vs. 90%) than patients who received CHOP without rituximab.[6] Similarly, patients who received rituximab, cyclophosphamide, vincristine, and prednisone (R-CVP) had higher response rates (81% vs. 57%) and better overall survival at 4 yr (83% vs. 77%) than patients who were treated with CVP without rituximab.[7]
- In a phase III noninferiority study, the combination of bendamustine and rituximab was associated with better progression-free survival rates than R-CHOP (70 vs. 31 mo) with fewer toxic effects.[8] Subset analyses showed better progression-free survival in patients with follicular lymphoma, mantle cell lymphoma, and lymphoplasmacytic lymphoma.
- The combination of obinutuzumab and chemotherapy followed by obinutuzumab maintenance was approved by the FDA in previously untreated patients with follicular lymphoma based on a randomized study, in

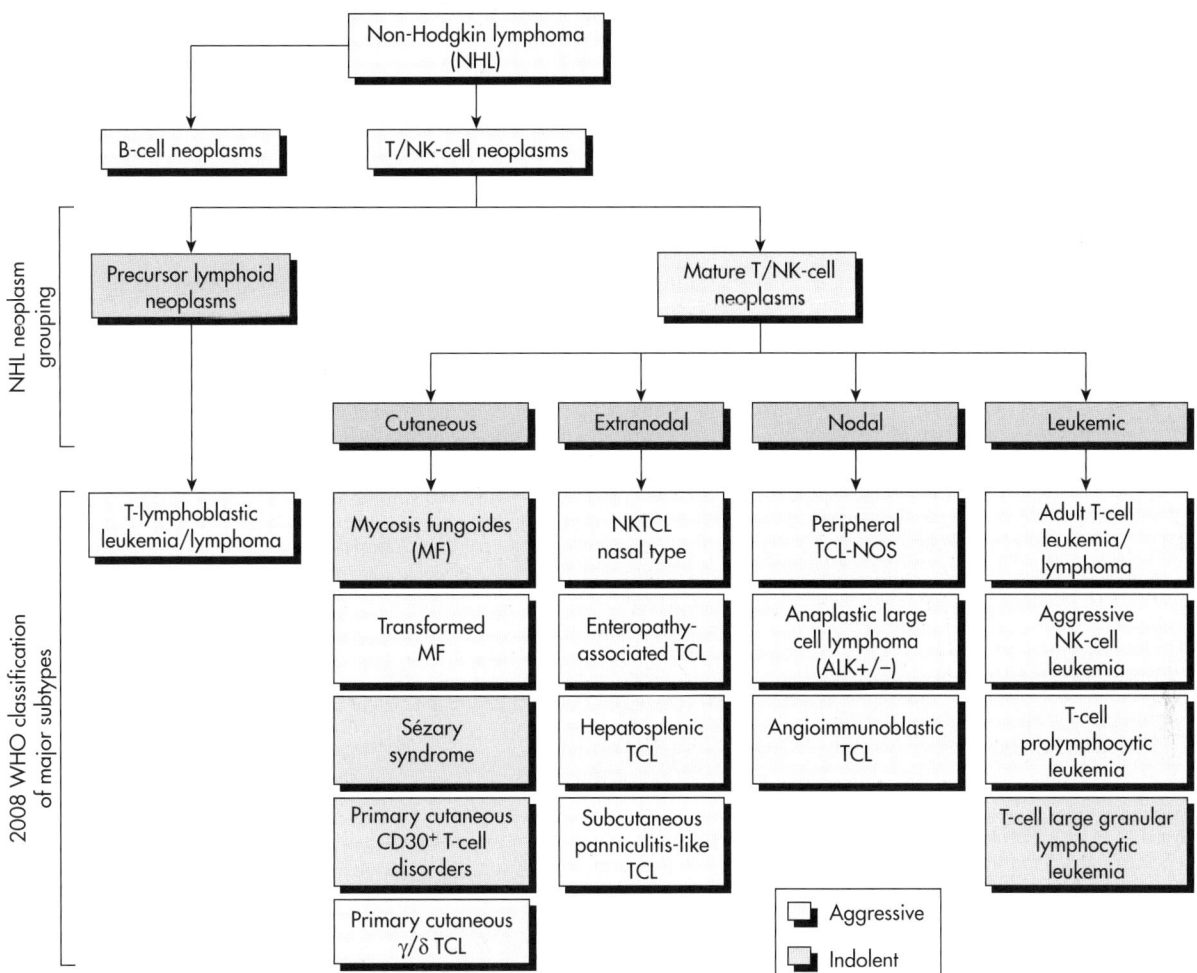

FIG. 1 World Health Organization (WHO) classification of the mature T-cell neoplasms. *NK,* Natural killer; *NKTCL,* nasal NK/T-cell lymphoma; *NOS,* not otherwise specified; *TCL,* T-cell lymphoma; *WHO,* World Health Organization. (From Hoffman R et al: *Hematology: basic principles and practice,* ed 7, Philadelphia, 2018, Elsevier.)

BOX 1   Factors Associated With an Increased Risk of Non-Hodgkin Lymphoma

Immunosuppression, acquired
    after solid-organ or hematopoietic stem
    cell transplantation
    HIV/AIDS
Congenital immunodeficiency syndromes
Increasing age (waning immunity)
Previous history of HL or NHL
Family history of NHL
Drugs
    Methotrexate
    TNF-α inhibitors
Occupational exposures
    Herbicides, pesticides, wood dust,
        epoxy glue, organic solvents
    Farming, forestry, painting, carpentry,
        tanning

From Niederhuber JE: *Abeloff's clinical oncology,* ed 6, Philadelphia, 2020, Elsevier.

which obinutuzumab and chemotherapy were associated with longer median progression-free survival than rituximab and chemotherapy.[9]
- Combination regimens containing cytarabine such as R-CHOP alternating with R-DHAP or the NORDIC regimen are used for the frontline treatment of aggressive mantle cell lymphoma.[10] Bendamustine and rituximab, R-CHOP, and lenalidomide and rituximab are less aggressive regimens for mantle cell lymphoma.[8,11,12] Mantle cell lymphoma can have indolent or aggressive clinical behavior.
- Maintenance rituximab after rituximab-containing regimens has been associated with better progression-free survival rates than observation in follicular and mantle cell lymphoma.[13] However, its practice has been impacted by the COVID-19 pandemic given the association between rituximab use and the development of severe COVID-19 infection and decreased responses to vaccination.

- *H. pylori*–associated gastric marginal zone lymphoma can be treated with a course of antibiotics. For persistent cases after eradication or for *H. pylori*–negative cases, radiotherapy is highly effective.
- Splenic marginal zone lymphoma is typically treated with rituximab. Splenectomy can be performed for symptomatic splenomegaly.
- Rituximab or chemoimmunotherapy regimens can be used in patients with advanced stage extranodal, splenic, or nodal marginal zone lymphoma.[14]
- The oral BTK inhibitor ibrutinib is FDA-approved for the treatment of patients with mantle cell lymphoma, lymphoplasmacytic lymphoma, and marginal zone lymphoma.[15-17] Acalabrutinib and zanubrutinib, second-generation BTK inhibitors, have been approved for relapsed mantle cell lymphoma.[18,19] Zanubrutinib has been approved for lymphoplasmacytic lymphoma and marginal zone lymphoma.[20,21]

TABLE 1 Major Molecular Alterations in Non-Hodgkin Lymphomas

NHL Histologic Type	Alteration	Cases Affected (%)	Proto-Oncogene Involved	Mechanism of Proto-Oncogene Activation	Proto-Oncogene Function
Lymphoplasmacytic lymphoma	MYD88 L265P mutation	95	MYD88	Activation	B-cell signaling
Follicular lymphoma	t(14;18)(q32;q21)	90	BCL-2	Transcription deregulation	Negative regulator of apoptosis
Mantle cell lymphoma	t(11;14)(q13;q32)	70	BCL-1/cyclin D1	Transcription deregulation	Cell cycle regulator
MALT lymphoma	t(11;18)(q21;q21)	50	API₂/MLT	Fusion protein	API₂ has antiapoptotic activity
	t(1;14)(p22;q32)		BCL-10	Transcription deregulation	Antiapoptosis
Diffuse large B-cell lymphoma	der(3)(q27)	35	BCL-6	Transcription deregulation	Transcriptional repressor required for GC formation
	t(14;18)(q32;q21)	15	BCL-2	Transcription deregulation	Negative regulator of apoptosis
	t(8;14)(q24;q32)	10	MYC	Transcription deregulation	Transcription factor regulating cell proliferation and growth
Burkitt lymphoma	t(8;14)(q24;q32)	80	MYC	Transcription deregulation	Transcription factor regulating cell proliferation and growth
	t(2;8)(p11;q24)	15	MYC		
	t(8;22)(q24;q11)	5	MYC		
Anaplastic large T-cell lymphoma	t(2;5)(p23;q35)	60	NPM/ALK	Fusion protein	ALK is a tyrosine kinase
	Locus 6p25.3	30	DUSP22/IRF4	Tumor suppressor	Inhibit T-cell lymphomagenesis in ALK negative ALCL
	inv(3)(q26q28)	8	TBL1XR1/TP63	Inhibit apoptosis	Inhibit apoptosis in ALK negative ALCL

GC, Gastric cancer; *MALT*, mucosa-associated lymphoid tissue; *NHL*, non-Hodgkin lymphoma.
From Niederhuber JE: *Abeloff's clinical oncology*, ed 6, Philadelphia, 2020, Elsevier.

TABLE 2 Evaluation of a New Patient With Non-Hodgkin Lymphoma

Evaluation	Mandatory	As Indicated
Confirm diagnosis	Adequate biopsy reviewed by experienced hematopathologists	Immunophenotyping with immunohistochemistry +/− flow cytometry; Cytogenetics/molecular studies
General overview and risks of therapy	History and physical examination; Complete blood cell count; Chemistry screen (including liver and renal function studies); HIV serology; Hepatitis B serologies	Blood coagulation studies; EBV serology and PCR assay; Hepatitis C serology; HTLV-1 serology; Serum electrolytes, uric acid; Assessment of cardiac ejection fraction; Pregnancy testing in women; Discussion of fertility issues
Prognostic categorization	Serum lactate dehydrogenase; Serum albumin	Erythrocyte sedimentation rate; Serum β2-microglobulin
Anatomic disease	Chest, abdominal, and pelvic CT with contrast enhancement	Ultrasonography; FDG-PET/CTMRI
Occult sites of involvement		Unilateral bone marrow biopsy with aspirate; Lumbar puncture with flow cytometry of CSF; Biopsy of suspicious sites; Blood flow cytometry

CSF, Cerebrospinal fluid; *CT*, computed tomography; *EBV*, Epstein-Barr virus; *FDG-PET*, fluorodeoxyglucose-18–labeled positron emission tomography; *HIV*, human immunodeficiency virus; *MRI*, magnetic resonance imaging; *PCR*, polymerase chain reaction.
From Niederhuber JE: *Abeloff's clinical oncology*, ed 6, Philadelphia, 2020, Elsevier.

- The oral PI3K inhibitors idelalisib and copanlisib and the EZH2 inhibitor tazemetostat have been FDA-approved for the treatment of relapsed follicular lymphoma.[22-24]
- The PI3K inhibitor umbralisib had its FDA approval withdrawn in June 2022 due to safety concerns. It was formerly approved for use in previously treated marginal zone lymphoma (at least one prior therapy) and follicular lymphoma (at least three prior therapies).
- The proteasome inhibitor bortezomib and the immunomodulating agent lenalidomide are FDA-approved for the treatment of relapsed mantle cell lymphoma but are less preferred than BTK inhibitors.
- CAR T-cell therapy has been approved for relapsed or refractory follicular lymphoma (axicabtagene ciloleucel and tisagenlecleucel)[25,26] and mantle cell lymphoma (brexucabtagene autoleucel).[27]
- Stem cell transplantation (autologous or allogeneic) may confer long-term disease control in multiple relapsed or refractory disease.
- Table 4 summarizes chemotherapy regimens in indolent lymphomas.

AGGRESSIVE NHL: The most common aggressive NHL is DLBCL. The 5-yr overall survival rate is 60%. The addition of rituximab against CD20 B-cell lymphoma to the CHOP regimen (R-CHOP) increased the complete response rate and prolonged overall survival in patients with DLBCL, based on randomized controlled trials, without clinically significant increase in toxicity.[28-30] R-CHOP has shown to be safe and effective in patients with HIV-associated NHL.[31]

Most common regimens used in DLBCL include:
- Three to four cycles of R-CHOP followed by involved-field radiotherapy, or four to six cycles of R-CHOP alone are appropriate approaches in patients with localized DLBCL.
- Six cycles of R-CHOP are appropriate in patients with advanced-stage DLBCL.
- The antibody-drug conjugate targeting CD79b polatuzumab vedotin, in combination with R-CHP, has emerged as an option for the

TABLE 3 Non-Hodgkin Lymphoma: Lugano Staging Classification

Stage	Features
I	Involvement of a single lymph node region or lymphoid structure (e.g., spleen, thymus, Waldeyer ring), or a single extranodal location without nodal involvement (IE)
II	Involvement of two or more lymph node regions on the same side of the diaphragm or limited nodal disease with limited contiguous extranodal involvement (IIE)
III	Involvement of lymph node regions or structures on both sides of the diaphragm
IV	Involvement of diffuse or noncontiguous extranodal site(s)

From Niederhuber JE: *Abeloff's clinical oncology,* ed 6, Philadelphia, 2020, Elsevier.

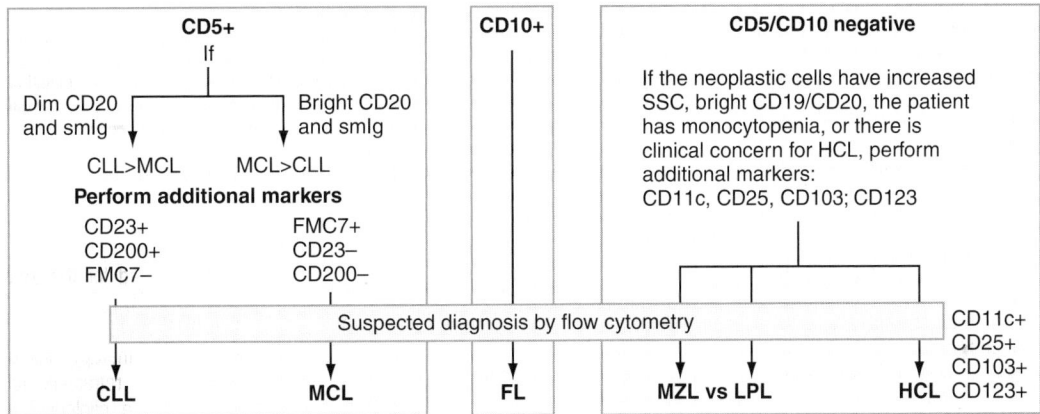

FIG. 4 This diagnostic algorithm outlines the steps in classification of B-cell lymphomas composed of cells of small to intermediate size. *BL,* Burkitt lymphoma; *CLL,* chronic lymphocytic leukemia; *FL,* follicular lymphoma; *HCL,* hairy cell leukemia; *IgM,* immunoglobulin M; *IHC,* immunohistochemistry; *LPL,* lymphoplasmacytic lymphoma; *MBL,* monoclonal B-cell lymphocytosis; *MCL,* mantle cell lymphoma; *MZL,* marginal zone lymphoma; *SmIg,* surface immunoglobulin; *SSC,* scleroderma and systemic sclerosis. (From McPherson RA, Pincus MR: *Henry's clinical diagnosis and management by laboratory methods,* ed 23, Philadelphia, 2017, Elsevier.)

treatment of previously untreated diffuse large B-cell lymphoma.[32] FDA potential approval is planned for April 2023.
- For patients with double-hit (defined as harboring rearrangement of MYC, BCL-2, and/ or BCL-6), HIV-associated and primary mediastinal large cell lymphoma, R-EPOCH (infusional etoposide, doxorubicin, and vincristine, along with cyclophosphamide, prednisone, and rituximab) is preferred over R-CHOP.[33]

- Granulocyte-colony stimulating factor (e.g., filgrastim) may be effective in reducing the risk of febrile neutropenia in patients over 65 yr with aggressive lymphoma undergoing chemotherapy.

TABLE 4 Chemotherapy Regimens in Lymphomas

BR (Every 28 Days)
- Bendamustine 90 mg/m^2 on days 1 and 2
- Rituximab 375 mg/m^2 IV on day 1

CVP-R (Every 21 Days)
- Cyclophosphamide 750 mg/m^2 IV on day 1
- Vincristine 1.4 mg/m^2, up to a maximal dose of 2 mg IV, on day 1
- Prednisone 40 mg/m^2 daily PO on days 1-5
- Rituximab 375 mg/m^2 IV day 1

R-CHOP (Every 21 Days)
- Cyclophosphamide 750 mg/m^2 IV on day 1
- Doxorubicin 50 mg/m^2 IV on day 1
- Vincristine 1.4 mg/m^2, up to a maximal dose of 2 mg IV, on day 1
- Prednisone 100 mg daily PO on days 1-5
- Rituximab 375 mg/m^2 IV on day 1

R-EPOCH (Every 21 Days)
- Rituximab 375 mg/m^2 IV on day 0 or 1 of each therapy cycle
- Doxorubicin 10 mg/m^2 IV per day on days 1-4
- Vincristine 0.4 mg/m^2 IV per day on days 1-4 (dose not capped)
- Etoposide 50 mg/m^2 IV per day on days 1-4
- Cyclophosphamide 750 mg/m^2 IV on day 5
- Prednisone 60 mg/m^2 PO twice daily on days 1-5

R-Hyper-CVAD (Every 21 Days)[36]

Cycles 1, 3, 5, and 7
- Rituximab 375 mg/m^2 IV on day 1
- Cyclophosphamide (with mesna) 300 mg/m^2 IV over 3 h every 12 h on days 2-4 (total 6 doses)
- Vincristine 1.4 mg/m^2 (maximum 2 mg) IV on days 5 and 12
- Doxorubicin 16.6 mg/m^2 IV by continuous infusion on days 5-7
- Dexamethasone 40 mg/day PO/IV on days 2-5 and days 12-15

Cycles 2, 4, 6, and 8
- Rituximab 375 mg/m^2 IV on day 1
- Methotrexate 200 mg/m^2 IV over 2 h, followed by 800 mg/m^2 IV continuous infusion over 22 h on day 2
- Leucovorin 50 mg PO starting 12 h after completion of methotrexate infusion, followed by 15 mg PO every 6 h for 8 dosed until the methotrexate level is less than 0.1 μM/L
- Cytarabine 3000 mg/m^2 IV over 2 h every 12 h on days 3 and 4 (4 doses total)

Rituximab Monotherapy
- Rituximab 375 mg/m^2 weekly for 4 wk

R^2 (every 28 days)
- Rituximab 375 mg/m^2 weekly for 4 wk, then every 28 days until cycle 5 (8 doses total)
- Lenalidomide 20 mg PO daily, 21 days on and 7 days off, for 12 cycles

From Hoffman R et al: *Hematology, basic principles and practice,* ed 7, Philadelphia, 2018, Elsevier.

- Treatment with high-dose chemotherapy and autologous bone marrow transplant: Compared with conventional chemotherapy, increases overall survival in patients with chemotherapy-sensitive relapsed DLBCL.
- Chimeric antigen receptor T-cell therapy agents (axicabtagene ciloleucel, tisagenlecleucel, and lisocabtagene maraleucel) have been FDA approved for patients with relapsed or refractory diffuse large B-cell lymphoma after two prior lines of chemotherapy.[34-36]
- Axicabtagene ciloleucel and lisocabtagene maraleucel have been FDA-approved for patients with relapsed or refractory diffuse large B-cell lymphoma within 12 mo of first-line chemoimmunotherapy or relapse after first-line chemoimmunotherapy and are not eligible for hematopoietic stem cell transplant due to comorbidities or age.[37,38]

- The anti-CD79 antibody drug conjugate polatuzumab vedotin in combination with bendamustine and rituximab[39]; the selective inhibitor of nuclear export selinexor[40]; the anti-CD19 monoclonal antibody tafasitamab in combination with lenalidomide[41]; and loncastuximab tesirine[42] have been FDA approved for the treatment of relapsed and/or refractory diffuse large B-cell lymphoma.

HIGHLY AGGRESSIVE NHL: The most common high-grade NHL subtype is Burkitt lymphoma (BL). BL affects younger patients than DLBCL and is common in HIV-infected individuals. Regimens more intensive than R-CHOP are needed to cure patients with high-grade NHL. The most used multi-agent regimens include hyper-CVAD, CODOX-M/IVAC, and dose-adjusted EPOCH, usually in combination with rituximab.[43-45] The 5-yr survival approximates 75%.

DISPOSITION

- Patients with indolent NHL in the rituximab era experience long survival despite the lack of curative potential of chemoimmunotherapy. Patients with aggressive NHL may achieve a cure with chemoimmunotherapy. Chimeric antigen receptor T-cell therapy agents have emerged as a novel therapeutic option for relapsed and refractory indolent and aggressive B-cell NHL.
- Prognostic factors include the lymphoma subtype, age of patient, and extent of disease. Table 5 describes the International Prognostic Index (IPI) for aggressive lymphomas.[46] Studies of the IPI in the modern era incorporating the anti-CD20 monoclonal antibody rituximab show an overall improved prognosis with 33% of the highest-risk patients alive 5 yr from diagnosis and 96% in the lowest risk.

TABLE 5 Clinical Prognostic Indexes

International Prognostic Index (IPI) for Aggressive Lymphomas[1]

Risk Group	IPI Score[a]	CR Rate (%)	5-Yr OS Rate (%)
Low	0, 1	87	73
Low intermediate	2	67	51
High intermediate	3	55	43
High	4, 5	44	26

Follicular International Prognostic Index (FLIPI)[2]

Risk Group	FLIPI Score[b]	Distribution (%)	5-Yr OS Rate (%)
Low	0-1	36	90.6
Intermediate	1-2	37	77.6
Poor	≥3	27	52.5

Mantle Cell International Prognostic Index (MIPI)[3]

Risk Group	MIPI Score[c]	Distribution (%)	Median Survival Rate
Low	0-3	44	Not reached
Intermediate	4-5	35	51 mo
High	6-11	21	29 mo

CR, Complete response; *OS*, overall survival.

[a]One point is given for the presence of each of the following characteristics: Age older than 60 yr, elevated serum lactate dehydrogenase (LDH) level, Eastern Cooperative Oncology Group performance status ≥2, Ann Arbor stage III or IV, and more than two extranodal sites.

[b]One point is given for the presence of each of the following characteristics: Age older than 60 yr, elevated serum LDH level, hemoglobin level <12 g/dl, Ann Arbor stage III or IV, and number of nodal sites ≥5.

[c]Points are based on age, ECOG performance status, white blood cell count, and serum LDH level.

[1]The International Non-Hodgkin's Lymphoma Prognostic Factors Project: A predictive model for aggressive non-Hodgkin's lymphoma, *N Engl J Med* 329:987-994, 1993.

[2]Solal-Celigny P et al: Follicular lymphoma international prognostic index, *Blood* 104:1258-1265, 2004.

[3]Hoster E et al: A new prognostic index (MIPI) for patients with advanced-stage mantle cell lymphoma, *Blood* 111:558-565, 2008.
From Niederhuber JE: *Abeloff's clinical oncology*, ed 6, Philadelphia, 2020, Elsevier.

- Patients who present with HIV-related NHL and low CD4+ cell count have a poor prognosis (median duration of survival is 15 to 34 mo). Despite therapeutic advances, the management of HIV-associated lymphomas is challenging due to potential pharmacologic interactions and increased risk of infectious complications. It is important to optimize the CD4 cell count during treatment. Referral to an HIV specialist is recommended.

REFERENCES
Available at eBooks.Health.Elsevier.com.

RELATED CONTENT
Non-Hodgkin Lymphoma (Patient Information)

AUTHORS: **LUIS MALPICA, MD,** and **JORGE J. CASTILLO, MD**

N

Diseases and Disorders

I

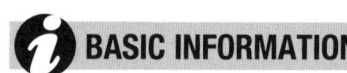
i BASIC INFORMATION

DEFINITION

Normal pressure hydrocephalus (NPH) is a syndrome of symptomatic hydrocephalus in the setting of normal cerebrospinal fluid (CSF) pressure. Ventricular expansion results in compression of brain parenchyma and stretching of the corticospinal and other tracts of the internal capsule (Fig. E1). The classic clinical triad of NPH includes gait disturbance, cognitive decline, and incontinence.

SYNONYMS

Hydrocephalus, Normal pressure
NPH
Occult hydrocephalus
Extraventricular obstructive hydrocephalus
Chronic hydrocephalus

ICD-10CM CODES
G91.2   Normal pressure hydrocephalus
G91.8   Other hydrocephalus

EPIDEMIOLOGY & DEMOGRAPHICS

INCIDENCE: The exact incidence is not known. In one study the incidence was found to be 5.5/100,000, but it may account for up to 5% of dementia in the U.S. Hospital discharge data suggest approximately 11,500 new cases diagnosed annually (may be overestimated). The prevalence of NPH was found to be 21.9/100,000 ($\sim$ 0.22%) in one study but also may be as high as 14% among extended care facility patients.
PREDOMINANT SEX: Males = females
PREDOMINANT AGE: NPH is more common with increasing age. In one study of 1238 patients who had undergone a head CT and neuropsychiatric evaluation, 0.2% of patients between 70 and 79 had probable NPH, and 5.9% of those 80 yr old and older had probable NPH.[1]

PHYSICAL FINDINGS & CLINICAL PRESENTATION[2]

- Gait difficulty (Fig. E2): A "magnetic" gait, in which patients have difficulty initiating ambulation. The gait may be broad-based and shuffling, with the appearance that the feet are stuck to the floor. Difficulty with turns may also be seen.
- Cognitive decline: Mental slowing, forgetfulness, and inattention, typically without agnosia, aphasia, or other cortical disturbances.
- Incontinence: Initially may have urinary urgency; incontinence later develops. Fecal incontinence also occasionally occurs. In one prospective study of 55 consecutive patients with idiopathic NPH, nocturia was the most common symptom, urge incontinence was the most bothersome, and 100% had detrusor overactivity on urodynamic studies.[3]
- *Gegenhalten* (paratonia or involuntary resistance with passive movement) or other frontal lobe signs may be seen.

ETIOLOGY

- Approximately 50% of cases are idiopathic; the prevailing thought is that these cases are due to either increased CSF production or reduced absorption.
- The remaining cases are secondary to a variety of causes, including prior subarachnoid hemorrhage, meningitis, head trauma, or intracranial surgery.
- Symptoms are presumed to result from stretching of cortical, limbic, and thalamo-cortical fibers that lie near the ventricles as dilation occurs.

Dx DIAGNOSIS

DIFFERENTIAL DIAGNOSIS

- Vascular dementia
- Alzheimer disease with extrapyramidal features
- Cognitive impairment in the setting of Parkinson disease or parkinsonism-plus syndromes
- Dementia with Lewy bodies
- Frontotemporal dementia
- Cervical spondylosis with cord compromise in the setting of degenerative dementia
- HIV-associated dementia
- Chronic bifrontal subdural hematomas
- Table E1 differentiates MRI findings between hydrocephalus and atrophy

WORKUP

Alternate causes of cognitive complaints, gait abnormalities, and urinary complaints are very common, and workup should include investigation for alternative explanations. Gait problems occur in 20% of individuals over 75 and is associated with the development of dementia.[4]

Large-volume lumbar puncture should be performed with assessment of improvement in gait.[2] Speed of walking 30 feet and number of steps when turning should be evaluated. Improvement in gait after a high volume lumbar puncture is highly correlated with shunt responsiveness.[5]

- Measurement of CSF outflow resistance by an infusion test or CSF pressure monitoring is sometimes used to help predict surgical outcome. External lumbar drainage (ELD) is being used more commonly and can be done over a period of 1 to 3 days at special centers that specialize in evaluating patients with adult hydrocephalus.

LABORATORY TESTS

- CSF should be sent for routine fluid analysis to exclude other pathologies.
- CSF biomarkers may be useful in excluding Alzheimer disease (e.g., Tau/A-beta 42). However, such biomarker tests are not used in routine clinical practice yet.

IMAGING STUDIES

- CT scan or MRI (Fig. 3) can be used to document ventriculomegaly. The distinguishing feature of NPH is ventricular enlargement out of proportion to sulcal atrophy (Fig. E4), and typically the frontal horn ratio (Evans index) exceeds 0.30.[2,6] An algorithm for evaluation of patients with enlarged ventricles is described in Fig. 5.
- MRI has advantages over CT, including better ability to visualize structures in the posterior fossa, visualize transependymal CSF flow (seen as periventricular T2 FLAIR hyperintensity), and document extent of white matter lesions. On MRI a flow void in the aqueduct and third ventricle ("jet sign"), thinning and elevation of the corpus callosum on sagittal images, rounding of the frontal horns, and a pattern known as *disproportionately enlarged subarachnoid space hydrocephalus* (DESH) may be seen. DESH is characterized by narrow CSF space at the high convexity/midline areas and enlarged sylvian fissures and is associated with a good response to CSF shunting.[7] MRI time-resolved 2D phase contrast imaging with velocity encoding can also be used to visualize CSF flow.
- Isotope cisternography and dynamic MRI studies have not been shown to be superior in predicting shunt outcome.

Rx TREATMENT

- There is no evidence that NPH can be effectively treated with medications. CSF diversion via a ventriculoperitoneal (VP) shunt is a definitive treatment.[8] Fig. 6 illustrates an algorithm for selection of patients for VP shunt.

NONPHARMACOLOGIC THERAPY

Response to VP shunting is variable. Some patients (variable depending on series reported) show significant improvement from shunting; however, effectiveness of shunting has never been demonstrated in a randomized controlled trial. Gait is most likely to improve as well as urinary symptoms, but cognitive symptoms are less likely to improve.[8]

- Factors that may predict positive outcome with surgery:
  1. NPH caused by prior trauma, subarachnoid hemorrhage, or meningitis
  2. History of mild impairment in cognition <2 yr duration
  3. Presence of gait abnormality
  4. Onset of gait abnormality before cognitive decline
  5. Imaging demonstrates hydrocephalus without sulcal enlargement, including normal-size sylvian fissures and cortical sulci, and absent or mild white matter lesions
  6. Transependymal CSF flow visualized on MRI
  7. Large-volume tap or ELD produces dramatic but temporary relief of symptoms
  8. High *normal* opening pressure
- Factors that may predict negative outcome with surgery:
  1. Extensive white matter lesions or diffuse cerebral atrophy on MRI
  2. Moderate to severe cognitive impairment
  3. Onset of cognitive impairment before gait disorder
  4. History of alcohol abuse

ACUTE GENERAL Rx

Shunting in selected patients

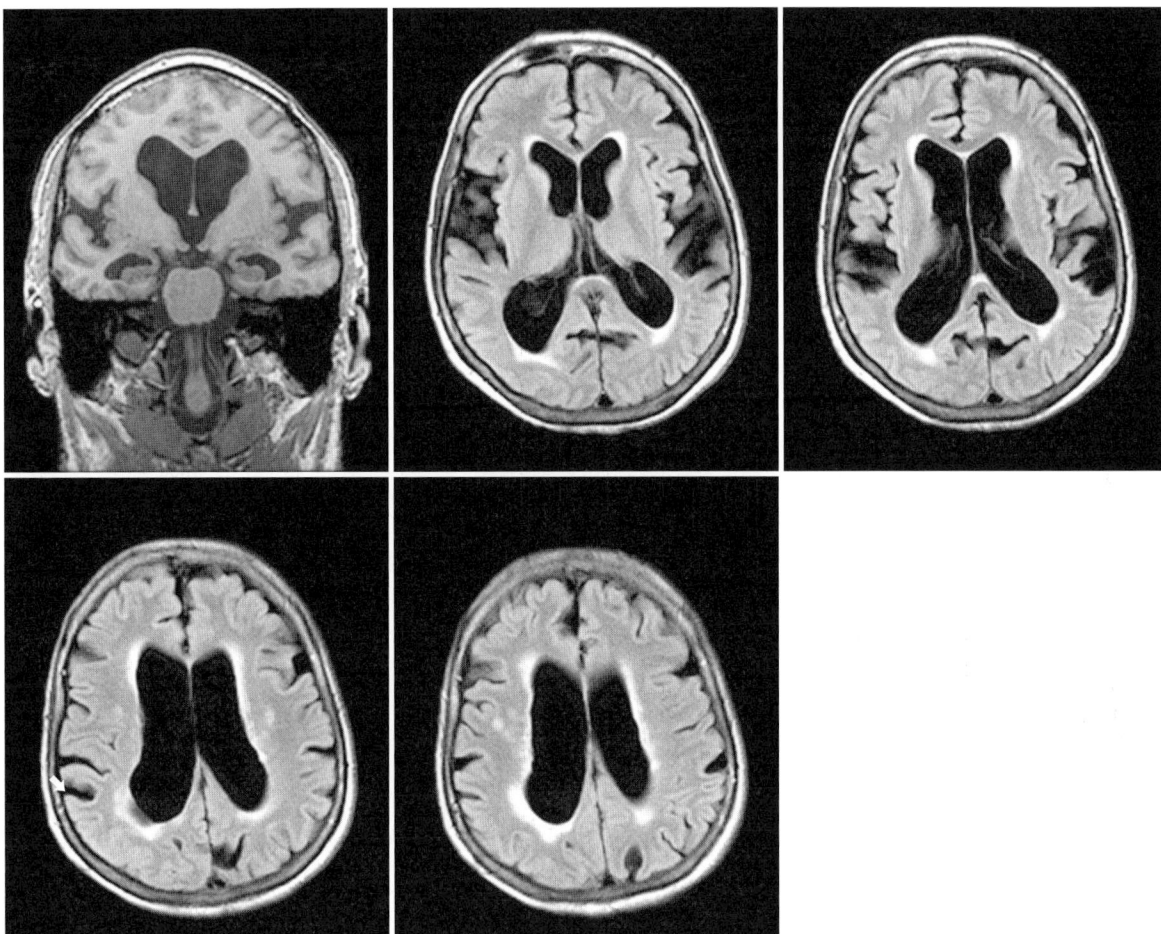

FIG. 3 *Top row: Left image* reveals enlargement of the sylvian fissures and crowding at the apex consistent with disproportionately enlarged subarachnoid space hydrocephalus. *Middle and right images* demonstrate ventricular enlargement and transependymal flow seen in normal pressure hydrocephalus (NPH). *Bottom row:* Entrapped sulci seen in NPH (*white arrow*). (From Jankovic J et al: *Bradley and Daroff's neurology in clinical practice,* ed 8, Philadelphia, 2022, Elsevier.)

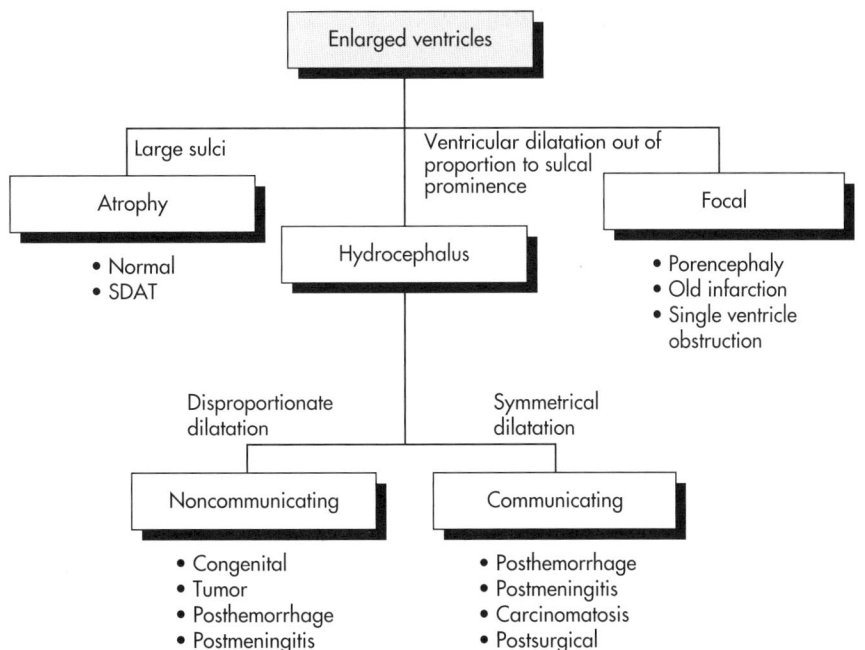

FIG. 5 Radiographic differential diagnosis of enlarged ventricles. *SDAT,* Senile dementia of the Alzheimer type. (From Weissleder R et al: *Primer of diagnostic imaging,* ed 5, St Louis, 2011, Mosby.)

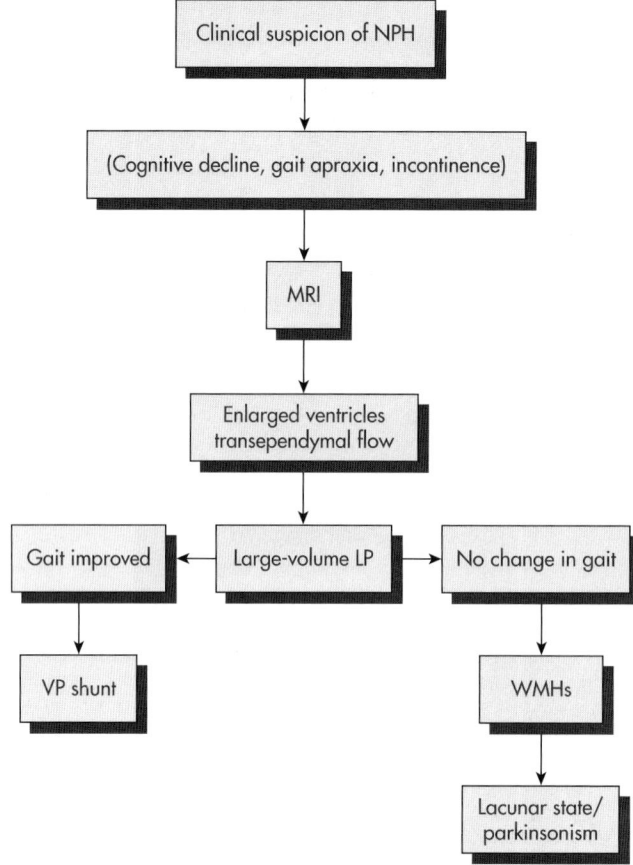

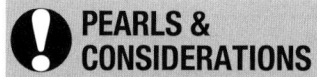

FIG. 6 An algorithm for selection of patients for ventriculoperitoneal (VP) shunt. Patients with the clinical triad undergo FLAIR MRI. If communicating hydrocephalus is found without excessive atrophy and with transependymal absorption, then a large volume of cerebrospinal fluid is removed, and the changes in the gait observed over several days. In those with improvement in gait, a VP shunt is done. Patients with white-matter changes in the deep white matter probably have lacunar state. Those with white matter changes compatible with microvascular disease most likely have lacunar state or parkinsonism. *FLAIR,* Fluid-attenuated inversion recovery; *LP,* lumbar puncture; *MRI,* magnetic resonance imaging; *NPH,* normal-pressure hydrocephalus; *WMHs,* white matter hyperintensities. (From Jankovic J et al: *Bradley and Daroff's neurology in clinical practice,* ed 8, Philadelphia, 2022, Elsevier.)

DISPOSITION
Symptoms of NPH may progress over time. Prompt diagnosis may improve chances for treatment success.

REFERRAL
Patients should be referred to a neurologist with experience in evaluating NPH followed by a neurosurgeon for shunting in appropriate patients.

ⓘ PEARLS & CONSIDERATIONS

Each of the cardinal symptoms of NPH is commonly seen in the elderly and occurs in multiple disease processes; therefore differential diagnoses should always be considered carefully.

REFERENCES
Available at eBooks.Health.Elsevier.com.

RELATED CONTENT
Normal Pressure Hydrocephalus (Patient Information)

AUTHOR: **COREY ELAM GOLDSMITH, MD, FAAN**

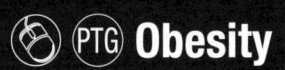
 BASIC INFORMATION

DEFINITION

Obesity refers to having an excess amount of body fat in relation to lean body mass, or a body mass index (BMI) of ≥ 30 kg/m^2. Overweight is defined as BMI of 25 to 29.9 kg/m^2, and morbid obesity refers to adults with a BMI ≥ 40 kg/m^2. BMI is used as a surrogate measure of obesity. Weight classification by BMI is summarized in Table 1. Abdominal obesity is defined as waist circumference >102 cm (40 in) in men and >88 cm (35 in) in women.

ICD-10CM CODES

E66.01	Morbid (severe) obesity due to excess calories
E66.09	Other obesity due to excess calories
E66.1	Drug-induced obesity
E66.2	Morbid (severe) obesity with alveolar hypoventilation
E66.8	Other obesity
E66.9	Obesity, unspecified
O99.210	Obesity complicating pregnancy, unspecified trimester
O99.211	Obesity complicating pregnancy, first trimester
O99.212	Obesity complicating pregnancy, second trimester
O99.213	Obesity complicating pregnancy, third trimester
O99.214	Obesity complicating childbirth
O99.215	Obesity complicating the puerperium

EPIDEMIOLOGY & DEMOGRAPHICS

- The World Health Organization first recognized obesity as a worldwide epidemic in 1997. As of 2005, 1.6 billion adults worldwide were classified as overweight, 400 million of whom were obese. It is predicted that the combination of overweight and obesity will soon eclipse public health issues such as malnutrition and infectious diseases as the most significant cause of poor health.
- Worldwide, data from the Global Burden of Disease Study from 1980 to 2013 indicate the prevalence of adult obesity has increased from 28.8% to 36.9% in men and 29.8% to 38% in women. The prevalence of childhood and adolescent obesity has also substantially increased.
- Based on U.S. NHANES data from 2011 to 2012, the prevalence of abdominal obesity was 54%. It is estimated that by 2023, 2 in every 5 adults and 1 in every 4 children in the U.S. will be categorized as obese.
- Obesity is the most common health problem in women of reproductive age. Obesity before pregnancy is disproportionately prevalent among women who identify as American Indian and Alaska Native (40%), non-Hispanic Black (39%), or Hispanic (32%), as compared with those who identify as non-Hispanic White (26%) or non-Hispanic Asian (10%).[1]
- The present cost of obesity in the U.S. population is estimated at $100 billion annually.

Approximately two thirds of people living in the U.S. are overweight, which is the highest percentage in the world.

- For persons with a BMI ≥ 30 kg/m^2, all-cause mortality is increased by 50% to 100% above that of persons with BMI in the range of 20 to 25 kg/m^2.
- Obesity is an independent risk factor for cardiovascular disease (CVD), type 2 diabetes, hypertension, cancer (particularly colon, prostate, breast, and gynecologic malignancies), sleep apnea, degenerative joint disease, thromboembolic disorders, digestive tract diseases (gallstones), and dermatologic disorders.
- Significant morbidity and risk of death are projected to begin in young adulthood, resulting in $>100,000$ excess cases of coronary heart disease (CHD) by 2035, even with the most modest projection of future obesity.
- When children enter kindergarten, 12.4% are obese, and another 14.9% are overweight. Data show that incident obesity between the ages of 5 and 14 yr is more likely to have occurred at younger ages.[2]
- Obesity in adolescence is significantly associated with increased risk of incident severe obesity in adulthood, with variations by sex and race/ethnicity. Overweight or obese adults who were obese as children have increased risk of type 2 DM, dyslipidemia, hypertension, and carotid artery atherosclerosis.
- Obesity is a major preventable cause of death and disability in the U.S. (the other is tobacco).
- Extensive data indicate that weight loss can reverse or arrest the harmful effects of obesity.
- In 2013 nearly 180,000 bariatric surgery procedures were performed in the U.S. Of these procedures 42% were laparoscopic sleeve gastrectomy, 34% were Roux-en-Y gastric bypass, and 15% were laparoscopic adjustable gastric banding.

PHYSICAL FINDINGS & CLINICAL PRESENTATION

- Physical examination should assess the degree and distribution of body fat, signs of secondary causes of obesity, and obesity-related comorbidities.

- Increased waist circumference is apparent. Excess abdominal fat is clinically defined as a waist circumference >40 in (>102 cm) in men and >35 in (>88 cm) in women (in Asian men and women, >36 in and >33 in, respectively). Central obesity is a risk factor for mortality even among individuals with normal BMIs.
- Symptoms associated with hypertension, coronary artery disease (CAD), and diabetes (e.g., polyuria, polydipsia, acanthosis nigricans, retinopathy, and neuropathy) may be present.
- Obesity is associated with cardiac hypertrophy, diastolic dysfunction, and decreased aortic compliance, which are independent predictors of cardiovascular risk.
- Joint pain and swelling are associated with degenerative joint disease secondary to obesity.
- The physical exam and ECG often underestimate the presence and extent of cardiac dysfunction in obese patients. Jugular venous distention and hepatojugular reflux may not be seen, and heart sounds are frequently distant.
- A large quantity of fluid is present in the interstitial space of adipose tissue, as the interstitial space is $\sim 10\%$ of the tissue wet weight. This excess fluid in this compartment, if redistributed into the circulation, can have negative repercussions in obese individuals with heart failure. Obese individuals have higher cardiac output and a lower total peripheral resistance than do lean individuals, and obesity is associated with persistence of elevated cardiac filling pressure during exercise.
- Obesity predisposes to heart failure through several different mechanisms: Increased total blood volume, increased cardiac output, left ventricular hypertrophy (LVH), left ventricular diastolic dysfunction, and adipositas cordis (excessive epicardial fat and fatty infiltration of the myocardium).

ETIOLOGY

- The pathophysiology of obesity is complex and poorly understood, but includes social, nutritional, physiologic, psychological, and genetic factors (Table 2).

TABLE 1 Weight Classification by BMI

Weight Classification	Obesity Class	BMI (KG/M2) Europeans	BMI (KG/M2) Asians	Risk of Obesity-Related Diseases
Underweight		<18.5	<17.5	Increased
Normal weight		18.5-24.9	17.5-22.9	Normal
Overweight		25.0-29.9	23.0-27.4	Increased
Obesity	I	30.0-34.9	27.5-32.4	High
	II	35.0-39.9	32.5-37.5	Very high
Extreme obesity (polysarcia)	III	≥ 40.0	≥ 37.5	Extremely high

BMI, Body mass index.
From Melmed S et al: *Williams textbook of endocrinology,* ed 14, Philadelphia, 2020, Elsevier.

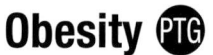
TABLE 2 Gene Mutations Associated With Obesity

Gene	Effect	Action on	Inheritance	Linked To
Leptin/leptin receptor	Appetite stimulant	Hypothalamus	Autosomal recessive	Severe childhood obesity
Ghrelin receptor	Appetite stimulant	Hypothalamus	Autosomal recessive	Short stature and obesity
Melanocortin 4 receptor	Appetite inhibitor	Hypothalamus	Autosomal dominant	Increased fat mass, insulin resistance
Proopiomelanocortin (POMC)	Appetite inhibitor	Melanocortin 4 receptor in hypothalamus	Autosomal recessive	Severe early onset obesity by age 1 and excessive eating caused by insatiable hunger
Neuropeptide Y (NPY)	Appetite stimulant	Hypothalamus	Autosomal recessive	Hypertension, high low-density lipoprotein cholesterol, triglycerides, increased food intake and hunger

From Townsend CM et al: *Sabiston textbook of surgery*, ed 21, St Louis, 2022, Elsevier.

- Environmental factors such as a sedentary lifestyle and chronic ingestion of excess calories can cause obesity.
- Obesity may be related to genetic factors, which are thought to be polygenic. Genetic studies with adopted children have demonstrated that they have similar BMIs to their biologic parents but not their adoptive parents. Twin studies also demonstrate a genetic influence on BMI.
- Secondary causes of obesity can result from medications (antipsychotics, steroids, and protease inhibitors being common ones) and neuroendocrine disorders (like Cushing syndrome and hypothyroidism).
- Box 1 summarizes medical conditions associated with severe obesity.

DIAGNOSIS

- BMI will establish the diagnosis of obesity. BMI is defined as the adult's weight in kilograms divided by the square of his or her height—and is closely correlated with total body fat content.
- BMI values can categorize patients into three classes of obesity:
  1. Class I (mild): BMI of 30.0 to 34.9 kg/m²
  2. Class II (moderate): BMI of 35.0 to 39.9 kg/m²
  3. Class III (severe): BMI of ≥40 kg/m²
- Although BMI is commonly used to define obesity, it is not a highly accurate indicator of body fat composition in children, who are undergoing rapid changes in height, or in bodybuilders or athletes who have large amounts of muscle tissue.
- Waist circumference or waist-hip ratio is indicative of visceral adipose tissue/intra-abdominal fat, which may be more deleterious than overall overweight or obesity.

DIFFERENTIAL DIAGNOSIS

It is important to evaluate obese patients for secondary medical causes of obesity. Hypothalamic disorders, hypothyroidism, Cushing syndrome, insulinoma, depression, and drugs (corticosteroids, antidepressants, second-generation antipsychotics,

BOX 1 Medical Conditions Associated With Severe Obesity

Cardiovascular
Hypertension
Sudden cardiac death myocardial infarction
Cardiomyopathy
Venous stasis disease
Deep venous thrombosis
Pulmonary hypertension
Right-sided heart failure
Pulmonary
Obstructive sleep apnea
Hypoventilation syndrome of obesity
Asthma
Metabolic
Metabolic syndrome (abdominal obesity, hypertension, dyslipidemia, insulin resistance)
Type 2 diabetes
Hyperlipidemia
Hypercholesterolemia
Nonalcoholic steatotic hepatitis (NASH) or nonalcoholic fatty liver disease (NAFLD)
Gastrointestinal
Gastroesophageal reflux disease
Cholelithiasis
Musculoskeletal
Degenerative joint disease
Lumbar disk disease
Osteoarthritis
Ventral hernias
Genitourinary
Stress urinary incontinence
End-stage renal disease (secondary to diabetes and hypertension)
Gynecologic
Menstrual irregularities
Skin/Integumentary System
Fungal infections
Boils, abscesses
Oncologic
Cancer of the thyroid, prostate, esophagus, kidney, stomach, colon, rectum, gallbladder, pancreas, female cancers of the breast, ovaries, cervix, and endometrium
Neurologic/Psychiatric
Pseudotumor cerebri
Depression
Low self-esteem
Stroke
Social/Societal
History of physical abuse
History of sexual abuse
Discrimination for employment
Social discrimination

From Townsend CM et al: *Sabiston textbook of surgery*, ed 21, St Louis, 2022, Elsevier.

sulfonylureas, and HIV protease inhibitors) can cause obesity. In children, certain genetic conditions, such as Prader-Willi syndrome, are associated with obesity.

WORKUP

History should be obtained regarding weight change, family history of obesity, and eating and exercise behavior. Assessment for eating disorders and depression should be made. Attention should be directed to the use of nutritional supplements, over-the-counter medications, hormones, diuretics, and laxatives. The workup of an obese patient typically requires laboratory work to assess for risks and complications as well as to rule out underlying causative medical conditions.

LABORATORY TESTS

- Obese patients should be assessed for medical consequences of their obesity by screening for metabolic syndrome. This includes measurement of fasting lipid profile, blood pressure, and waist circumference and screening for diabetes or prediabetes (oral glucose tolerance test, fasting glucose, or hemoglobin A1C).
- Polycythemia might warrant screening for sleep apnea. Liver function tests should be obtained to screen for hepatic steatosis.
- In the proper clinical setting, thyroid function studies and dexamethasone suppression testing will exclude hypothyroidism and Cushing syndrome as underlying causes of obesity. If insulinoma is suspected, the patient will need to undergo a 72-hr fast to confirm hypoglycemia with inappropriate insulin secretion.
- Obesity is associated with changes in the ECG, including a reduction in voltage and nonspecific ST-T changes that may interfere with diagnosis of LVH or CAD.

IMAGING STUDIES

- Several methods are available for determining or calculating total body fat but offer no significant advantage over the BMI. These include measurement of total body water, total body potassium, bioelectrical impedance, and dual-energy x-ray absorptiometry.
- Buoyancy testing is an accurate method for determining total body fat composition.

OTHER STUDIES

Obesity increases the risk of obstructive sleep apnea, which, in turn, increases the risks of hypertension, cardiac arrhythmias, CVD, stroke, and heart failure. Therefore one should have a low threshold to screen obese patients for obstructive sleep apnea via sleep study/polysomnography.

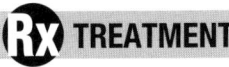

TREATMENT

The National Heart, Lung, and Blood Institute (NHLBI) developed guidelines for selecting treatment strategies for overweight and obese patients based on BMI and comorbidities. They recommend a combination of dietary management, physical activity management, and behavior therapy for anyone with a BMI ≥25 or with a high-risk waist circumference and two or more obesity-associated comorbidities. Pharmacotherapy should be considered for patients with a BMI ≥30 or ≥27 with comorbidities.

Bariatric surgery is indicated for patients with a BMI ≥35 with comorbidities and for any patient with a BMI ≥40 (Table 3).

NONPHARMACOLOGIC THERAPY

- The cornerstones for weight management and reduction are calorie restriction, exercise, and behavioral modification. Assessment of patient's willingness to make changes must be evaluated, as treatment is more likely to succeed in motivated patients.
- The NHLBI guidelines recommend an initial diet to produce a calorie deficit of 500 to 1000 kcal/day. This has been shown to reduce total body weight by an average of 8% over 3 to 12 mo.
- These guidelines recommend the use of a food diary to focus on dietary substitutes.
- Thirty min of moderate-intensity activity on 5 or more days of the wk results in health benefits for obese individuals. Moreover, several studies indicate that 60 to 80 min of moderate to vigorous physical activity may provide additional benefit.
- Increased physical activity without caloric restriction (minimal or no weight loss) can reduce abdominal (visceral) adipose tissue and improve insulin resistance.
- The key features of the standard behavioral modification program include goal setting, self-monitoring, stimulus control (modification of one's environment to enhance behaviors that will support weight management), cognitive restructuring (increased awareness of perceptions of oneself and one's weight), and prevention of relapse (weight regain).
- Mammalian sleep is closely integrated with the regulation of energy balance. Trials have shown that the amount of human sleep contributes to the maintenance of fat-free body mass at times of decreased energy intake. Lack of sufficient sleep may compromise the efficacy of typical dietary interventions for weight loss and related metabolic risk reduction.

ACUTE GENERAL Rx

- According to the NHLBI *Guidelines on the Identification, Evaluation, and Treatment of Overweight and Obesity in Adults* and the U.S. Food and Drug Administration (FDA), pharmacotherapy is indicated for:
  1. Obese patients with a BMI ≥30
  2. Overweight patients with a BMI of ≥27 and concomitant obesity-related risk factors or diseases, such as hypertension, diabetes, or dyslipidemia
- Pharmacologic treatment options include:
  1. Gastrointestinal lipase inhibitors: Orlistat is the only drug available for long-term treatment of obesity. It blocks the digestion and absorption of ingested dietary fat. It is a reversible inhibitor of pancreatic, gastric, and carboxyl ester lipases and phospholipase A2, which are required for the hydrolysis of dietary fat in the gastrointestinal tract. Side effects include flatulence, fecal incontinence, cramps, and oily spotting. There can also be impairment of absorption of fat-soluble vitamins (A, D, E, K) and beta-carotene. Oxalate-associated acute kidney injury and rare severe liver injury have also been reported.

TABLE 3 Weight-Loss Treatment Guidelines From the National Heart, Lung, and Blood Institute*

Treatment	BMI				
	25.0-26.9	27.0-29.9	30.0-34.9	35.0-39.9	>40.0
Diet, physical activity, behavioral therapy, or all three	Yes	Yes	Yes	Yes	Yes
Pharmacotherapy†		In patients with obesity-related diseases	Yes	Yes	Yes
Surgery‡				In patients with obesity-related diseases	Yes

*Data are from https://www.nhlbi.nih.gov/science/obesity-nutrition-and-physical-activity. These guidelines are generally consistent with those from the American Heart Association, the American Medical Association, the American Diabetic Association, the Obesity Society (Practical Guide), the American Diabetes Association, the American Academy of Family Physicians, the American College of Sports Medicine, and the American Cancer Society. *BMI* denotes body mass index, calculated as the weight in kilograms divided by the square of the height in meters.

†Pharmacotherapy should be considered only in patients who are not able to achieve adequate weight loss with available conventional lifestyle modifications and who have no absolute contraindications for drug therapy.

‡Bariatric surgery should be considered only in patients who are unable to lose weight with available conventional therapy and who have no absolute contraindications for surgery.

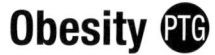

2. C serotonin agonists: Lorcaserin is a selective serotonin agonist that acts centrally to reduce appetite, aiding weight loss. Adverse effects include headache, upper respiratory infections, dizziness, and nausea. While there is little evidence of serotonin-associated cardiac valvular disease or pulmonary hypertension (as seen with nonselective serotonergic agonists fenfluramine and dexfenfluramine), long-term data is currently limited.

3. Sympathomimetic medications: Phentermine and diethylpropion are currently approved for short-term treatment of obesity. They reduce food intake by causing early satiety. Side effects include increased blood pressure and increased pulse. They are Schedule IV drugs with a potential for abuse. Other sympathomimetic drugs that have been removed from the market due to concerns about cardiovascular safety are sibutramine, phenylpropanolamine, and ephedrine.

4. Antidepressants: While not FDA-approved for treatment of obesity alone, bupropion and fluoxetine are antidepressants that have been associated with modest weight loss. The FDA has recently approved a fixed-dose combination of bupropion with the opioid receptor antagonist naltrexone. It is called Contrave and approved for use as an adjunct to diet and exercise in patients with BMI $\geq$30 kg/m^2 or a BMI $\geq$27 kg/m^2 and one or more weight-related comorbidities (e.g., diabetes, hypertension, dyslipidemia).

5. Antiepileptic drugs: Zonisamide and topiramate (also used in migraine therapy) have been associated with weight loss in clinical trials but are not currently FDA-approved for treatment of obesity alone.

6. Diabetes drugs: While not FDA-approved for treatment of obesity alone, metformin and pramlintide (synthetic human amylin) have been associated with weight loss in the treatment of individuals with diabetes. The GLP-1 receptor agonist liraglutide (Victoza) is now FDA approved at a higher dose as Saxenda for chronic weight management in adults with BMI $\geq$30 or a BMI $\geq$27 with a weight-related comorbidity such as hypertension, dyslipidemia, or diabetes. Semaglutide (Ozempic, Rybelsus) plus lifestyle intervention is associated with clinically relevant reduction in body weight in adults with overweight or obesity.[3] In adolescents with obesity, a trial of once-weekly semaglutide plus lifestyle intervention resulted in a mean change in BMI of 16.1% with semaglutide vs. 0.6% with placebo after 68 weeks.[3a]

CHRONIC Rx

- According to the NHLBI guidelines, surgical intervention is an option for selected patients with clinically severe obesity (a BMI $\geq$40 or a BMI $\geq$35 with comorbid conditions), when patients are at high risk for obesity-associated morbidity or death, and when

---

BOX 2 Patient Requirements for Bariatric Surgery

1. Patients with a BMI of 40 kg/m^2 or greater are potential candidates for bariatric surgery.
2. Patients with a BMI of 35 to 40 kg/m^2 with significant obesity-related comorbidity are also potential candidates for bariatric surgery.
3. Patients with a history of dieting.
4. Patients with no recent substance abuse.
5. Patients should be evaluated by a multidisciplinary team that includes a dietitian and psychologic evaluation before surgery.

From Cameron JL, Cameron AM: *Current surgical therapy,* ed 12, Philadelphia, 2017, Elsevier.

BOX 3 Preoperative Evaluation and Postoperative Care

Before the Clinic Visit
Documented, medically supervised diet
Counseling and referral from the primary care physician
Reading a comprehensive written brochure and/or attendance at a seminar regarding operative procedures, expected results, and potential complications
Initial Clinic Visit
Group presentation on information in the booklet
Group presentation on preoperative and postoperative nutritional issues by the nutritionist
Individual assessment by the surgeon's team
Individual counseling session with the surgeon
Individual counseling session with the nutritionist
Screening blood tests
Subsequent Events/Evaluations
Full psychological assessment and evaluation as indicated
Medical specialist evaluations as indicated
Insurance approval for coverage of the procedure
Screening flexible upper endoscopy as indicated
Screening ultrasound of the gallbladder (if present)
Arterial blood gas analysis as indicated
Subsequent Clinic Visits
Counseling session with the surgeon (including selection of the date for surgery)
Education session with the nurse educator
Preoperative evaluation by the anesthesiologist
Final paperwork by the preadmissions center

From Townsend CM et al: *Sabiston textbook of surgery,* ed 21, St Louis, 2022, Elsevier.

---

less invasive methods of weight loss have failed. Box 2 summarizes patient requirements for bariatric surgery. Preoperative evaluation and postoperative care are described in Box 3

- Eligible patients should also be at an acceptable risk for surgery, well informed, and motivated.
- Restrictive surgeries limit the amount of food the stomach can hold and slow the rate of gastric emptying. These include Roux-en-Y gastric bypass (RYGB), vertical banded gastroplasty (VSG), laparoscopic adjustable silicone gastric banding (LAGB), and endoscopic sleeve gastroplasty (ESG). RYGB combines creation of a small gastric pouch with a modest intestinal or small bowel bypass to produce weight loss through both restrictive and malabsorptive means. A traditional RYGB consists of transection of a small (15-ml) proximal gastric pouch along the lesser curvature of the stomach from the larger gastric segment, combined with a modest (encompassing 60 to 150 cm) intestinal bypass. The Roux-en-Y configuration allows biliopancreatic secretions and digestive juices to pass through the bile duct into the duodenum and then merge with the alimentary stream passing down from the stomach at the Y-type connection. The lengths of both the Roux and biliopancreatic limbs can be varied to produce more malabsorption. Most weight is lost in the first year. Approximately 80% of patients typically experience weight stabilization, usually slightly above weight nadir, approximately 3 yr after surgery. The remaining 20% of patients slowly regain excess weight over longer-term follow-up and risk regaining much of the lost weight. VSG (Fig. E1) is now the most commonly performed major bariatric procedure. This operation restricts intake via a 70% vertical gastric resection, creating a long and narrow tubular gastric reservoir with no intestinal bypass. LAGB is an inflatable silicone prosthetic device that is placed around the top portion of the stomach, just below the esophagus (Fig. E2) and restricts the upper stomach size to a small volume. The band is attached to a reservoir, with a port placed under the skin on the abdominal wall, and the inner lining of the band is a balloon that is adjustable by the addition or removal of saline from the reservoir port. Inflation of the band increases the restriction of gastric outlet size and food flow.

Band slippage is the most common LAGB complication. Other potential complications include port or tubing malfunction, stomal obstruction, band erosion, pouch dilation, and port infection. Gastric necrosis of the stomach wall is a rarer late complication that results from ischemia caused by a combination of gastric prolapse—the part of the stomach below the band herniates up through the device—and pressure from the band. Less commonly used are biliopancreatic diversion (BPD) and BPD with duodenal switch (BPDDS) procedures (Fig. E3), which result in an extreme degree of malabsorption and are reserved for the treatment of "superobese" patients. BPD combines a partial, subtotal gastrectomy and a very long Roux-en-Y anastomosis with a short common channel for nutrient absorption. With this procedure, patients can eat much larger quantities of food and still achieve and maintain weight loss. Disadvantages include higher postoperative surgical risks, loose and foul-smelling stools, intestinal ulcers, anemia, vitamin and mineral deficiencies, and possible protein-calorie malnutrition. Because of these potential problems, patients who undergo BPD require lifelong dietary supplementation and close follow-up monitoring.[4] ESG is a relatively new procedure. Larger trials will determine its long-term efficacy and safety.[5] In ESG the endoscopist places transmural gastric sutures to restrict gastric volume and delay gastric emptying. This endoscopic procedure is reversible and avoids complications associated with more invasive procedures. Complications of bariatric surgery are summarized in Box E4.

- Gastric bypass has better outcomes than gastric band procedures for long-term weight loss, type 2 diabetes control and remission, hypertension, and hyperlipidemia.[6] These procedures have benefits that include lower perioperative mortality rate, a quicker recovery period, and no malabsorption issues. However, they are not as effective as gastric bypass for weight reduction and comorbidity improvement.
  1. Malabsorptive surgeries reduce nutrient absorption by shortening the length of small intestine. These include jejunoileal bypass and the duodenal switch operation (DS).
  2. Restrictive malabsorptive bypass procedures combine the elements of gastric restriction and selective malabsorption. These include Roux-en-Y gastric bypass (considered the gold standard because of its high level of effectiveness and durability) and biliopancreatic diversion. These procedures have higher rates of comorbidity improvement than restrictive surgeries but can be complicated by malabsorption and nutritional deficiencies.
- Compared with usual care, bariatric surgery is associated with reduced number of cardiovascular deaths and lower incidence of cardiovascular events and cancer mortality[7] in obese adults. A study on bariatric surgery patients demonstrated a significant reduction in long-term cardiovascular events. Ten-yr follow-up estimated relative risk reductions

ranging from 18% to 79% according to the Framingham risk score, and 8% to 62% with the PROCAM risk score.
- A long-term observational study of obese patients with type 2 diabetes showed that bariatric surgery was associated with higher diabetes remission rates and fewer complications than usual care. Remission of type 2 DM occurs in 60% to 80% of patients 2 yr after surgery and persists in about 30% of patients 15 yr after Roux-en-Y gastric bypass.
- Liposuction is removal of fat by aspiration after injection of physiologic saline. This technique reduces the subcutaneous fat but has failed to improve insulin sensitivity or risk factors for CHD.
- Fluid filled, space-occupying intragastric balloons (IGBs) can also be used for weight loss. They are inserted endoscopically and left in place for 6 months. Volume can be adjusted endoscopically. Weight loss is as much as 10% of body weight. Weight gain after removal is an issue as only 74% of IGB patients were able to maintain more than 40% of weight loss during treatment in a recent study.[8]
- The Maestro Rechargeable System is a subcutaneously implanted device FDA approved for weight loss in adults with a BMI of 40 to 45 or with a BMI of $\geq$35 and at least one obesity-related comorbidity. It utilizes high-frequency electrical pulses to block vagus nerve signals between the brain and stomach. It is less effective than bariatric surgery for weight loss. The list price for the Maestro system exceeds $15,000.
- The AspireAssist device is FDA approved for weight loss in adults $\geq$22 yr old with a BMI of 35 to 55. It requires the insertion of a PEG tube endoscopically and pulled through a percutaneous incision. Thirty min after a meal, the patient attaches a connector to it and drains a portion of their stomach content into a toilet. The tube is then flushed with potable water. The connector stops working after 115 cycles (6 wk) and is replaced at a follow-up appointment. Estimated cost for procedure and follow-ups are $13,000 for the first yr.
- Plenity is a hydrogel formulation of cellulose and citric acid available in capsules taken 20 to 30 min before lunch or dinner with 500 ml of water. The hydrogel particles hydrate up to 100 times their original weight in the stomach to create a feeling of fullness. The matrix is then digested and broken down in the colon and eliminated in the feces. Plenity is available by prescription for patients with a BMI of 25 to 30 kg/m^2 regardless of comorbidities.

DISPOSITION
- The incidence of venous thromboembolism in the upper tertile of BMI was 2.42 times that of the lowest BMI tertile. Obese patients have a higher incidence of postoperative thromboembolic events when undergoing noncardiac surgery.
- Obesity may be associated with higher rates of postoperative pulmonary complications and poor wound healing.

- Weight-stable obese subjects have an increased risk of arrhythmias and sudden death even in the absence of cardiac dysfunction.
- Obesity and the cardiac autonomic nervous system are intrinsically related. A 10% increase in body weight is associated with a decline in parasympathetic tone accompanied by a rise in mean heart rate. Conversely, a 10% weight loss in severely obese patients is associated with significant improvement in autonomic nervous system cardiac modulation, including decreased heart rate and increased heart rate variability.
- Postmortem Determinants of Atherosclerosis in Youth (PDAY) study data provided convincing evidence that obesity in adolescents and young adults accelerates the progression of atherosclerosis decades before the appearance of clinical manifestations.
- Obesity accelerates the progression of native coronary atherosclerosis and after coronary artery bypass grafting.
- In older adults, obesity is associated with protection against hip fracture, but this protective effect on bone status does not offset the extensive array of potential adverse effects on conditions common in the older population.
- A 3-yr trial comparing midterm effects of bariatric surgery on patients with obesity and hypertension revealed Roux-en-Y gastric bypass (RYGB) is an effective strategy for midterm blood pressure control and hypertension remission, with fewer medications required in patients with hypertension and obesity.[8]
- A study on the effects of diet vs. gastric bypass on metabolic function in type 2 diabetes revealed that the metabolic benefits of gastric bypass surgery and diet are similar and related to weight loss itself, with no evident clinically important effects independent of weight loss.[9] A 10-yr trial in obese diabetic patients comparing bariatric surgery versus medical treatment for promoting remission and preventing diabetes-related complications revealed that surgery patients had fewer diabetes-related complications but more digestive and metabolic complications.[9,10]

REFERRAL
Obesity is commonly seen in the primary care setting. If pharmacologic therapy is considered, consultation with physicians specializing in obesity and experienced with the use of the drug is recommended. In addition, consultation with nutritionists and behavioral therapists is helpful. A consultation with general surgery is indicated in patients being considered for surgical intervention.

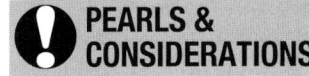

PEARLS & CONSIDERATIONS

COMMENTS
- Enhanced weight-loss counseling helps about one third of obese patients achieve long-term,

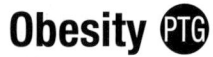

clinically meaningful weight loss. Adults can lose 1 to 2 lbs (0.45 to 0.9 kg) per wk by consuming 500 to 1000 fewer calories per day.
- The NHLBI launched the Obesity Education Initiative in January 1991. The overall purpose of the initiative is to help reduce the prevalence of overweight along with the prevalence of physical inactivity to reduce the risk of CHD and overall morbidity and mortality rates from CHD.
- Brown adipose tissue represents a natural target for the modulation of energy expenditure. The presence of brown adipose tissue in humans may be quantified with the use of 18F-fluorodeoxyglucose PET-computed tomography (CT). The amount of brown adipose tissue is inversely correlated with BMI, suggesting a potential role of brown adipose tissue in adult human metabolism.
- Obesity, glucose intolerance, and hypertension in childhood are strongly associated with increased rates of premature death from endogenous causes in this population.
- Recent trials have shown that among persons living in a controlled setting, calories alone account for the increase in fat. Protein affected energy expenditure and storage of lean body mass but not body fat storage.
- Data are lacking for the role of pharmacotherapy and bariatric surgery in the elderly population.

PREVENTION
- Prevention of overweight and obesity involves both increasing physical activity and dietary modification to reduce caloric intake.

- There is compelling evidence that prevention of weight regain in formerly obese individuals requires 60 to 90 min of moderate-intensity activity or lesser amounts of vigorous intensity activity.
- Moderate-intensity activity of approximately 45 to 60 min per day, or 1.7 physical activity level (PAL), is required to prevent the transition to overweight or obesity. For children, even more activity time is recommended.
- Clinicians can help guide patients to develop personalized eating plans and help them recognize the contributions of fat, concentrated carbohydrates, and large portion sizes.
- Clinicians must work with patients to modify other risk factors such as tobacco use, high glycemic intake, and elevated blood pressure to prevent the long-term chronic disease sequelae of obesity. Generally lower carbohydrate, moderate fat intake, with stable protein and energy intake results in higher energy expenditure during weight-loss maintenance.[6]
- Regular screening of body weight and BMI measurements at routine office visits can help identify early weight gain.
- Among obese adolescents, the most rapid weight gain occurs between 2 and 6 yr of age. Most children who are obese at that age are obese in adolescence.[6]
- A clinical practice guideline for the evaluation from the American Academy of Pediatrics[11] for evaluating and managing children and adolescents with obesity recommends the following:
  1. Any child ≥2 yr old with BMI ≥85th percentile should undergo a comprehensive history and physical, including examinations of mental-behavioral health, social determinants of health, blood pressure, and age-appropriate blood work (e.g., lipids, ALT, HbA1c).
  2. The mainstay of management is intensive health behavior and lifestyle treatment (IHBLT), an in-person, family-based program requiring at least 26 hours of face-to-face time during 3 to 12 months.
  3. Pharmacotherapy can be used as an adjunct to IHBLT for selected teens ≥12 yr old. Medications (metformin, orlistat, glucagon-like peptide-1 receptor agonists, topiramate) should be chosen based on indications, benefits, and risks.
  4. Evaluation for metabolic and bariatric surgery should be considered for teens ≥13 yr old with severe obesity (BMI ≥120% of the 95th percentile) and clinically significant co-morbidities.

PATIENT & FAMILY EDUCATION
Information can be obtained on the American Obesity Association website (http://www.obesity.org/) and the American Medical Association website (https://www.ama-assn.org/).

REFERENCES & SUGGESTED READINGS
Available at eBooks.Health.Elsevier.com.

RELATED CONTENT
Obesity, Female (Patient Information)
Obesity, Male (Patient Information)
Obesity, Child (Patient Information)

AUTHOR: **FRED F. FERRI, MD**

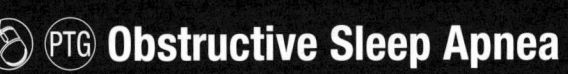

BASIC INFORMATION

DEFINITION

Sleep apnea refers to repetitive episodes of reduction or cessation of inspiratory airflow during sleep, usually associated with episodes of hypoxemia or physiologic arousal. Inspiratory airflow limitation is due to some combination of upper airway collapse and loss or instability of ventilatory drive. When sleep apnea is primarily due to upper airway collapse, it is referred to as obstructive sleep apnea (OSA); when it is predominantly due to loss of ventilatory drive, it is referred to as central sleep apnea (CSA; Fig. 1). This chapter will focus on OSA.

OSA is clinically defined and classified using the apnea-hypopnea index (AHI), the number of apneas or hypopneas occurring per hour of sleep (Table 1).

SYNONYMS

Sleep-disordered breathing

Sleep-disordered breathing refers to a broader category of sleep breathing problems that includes OSA, CSA, elevated apnea-hypopnea index (AHI) regardless of symptoms, hypoventilation syndromes, and the interaction of these with other respiratory conditions such as chronic obstructive pulmonary disease (COPD). Obstructive sleep apnea syndrome (OSAS)

The concept of sleep apnea syndrome refers to an elevated AHI in the presence of symptoms such as excessive daytime sleepiness or nocturnal choking and gasping. OSA is diagnosed with AHI ≥15 regardless of symptoms.
Obstructive sleep apnea–hypopnea syndrome (OSAHS)

ICD-10CM CODES
G47.30 Sleep apnea, unspecified
G47.31 Primary central sleep apnea
G47.33 Obstructive sleep apnea (adult) (pediatric)
G47.37 Central sleep apnea in conditions classified elsewhere
G47.39 Other sleep apnea
P28.3   Primary sleep apnea of newborn

EPIDEMIOLOGY & DEMOGRAPHICS

- OSA is an increasingly common disease worldwide, rising in prevalence in conjunction with obesity.
- Latest estimates suggest nearly one third of U.S. adults ages 30 to 69 yr have some degree of sleep-disordered breathing, and nearly 15% have moderate or severe OSA.[1]
- Risk of OSA increases with age, male sex, postmenopausal status, and obesity and other features of the metabolic syndrome. Age and obesity appear to have a powerful interaction.
- Due to the very high prevalence in the general population, clinicians should retain a high index of suspicion for OSA in patients who may not fit the stereotype of the OSA patient. Factors such as chronic nasal congestion, tonsillar hypertrophy, conditions affecting upper airway tone, and unfavorable craniofacial and upper airway anatomy can predispose patients of any weight or sex to OSA. Family history may give an indication that some of these risk factors are present.
- OSA in pregnant patients is less common than in the general population but is not rare; one recent meta-analysis estimated prevalence (AHI ≥5) at 15%.[2] OSA prevalence in pregnancy increases with gestational age and is also higher in older mothers. In premenopausal women, obesity is the most significant risk factor for OSA.
- Prevalence in the general pediatric population is estimated to be 1% to 6%, but may be higher in obese adolescents.[3]

PHYSICAL FINDINGS & CLINICAL PRESENTATION

The clinical presentation of sleep apnea varies by etiology and subtype (Table 2). Cardinal symptoms of OSA include loud snoring, nocturnal choking or gasping, frequent awakenings from sleep, and feeling unrestored or excessively sleepy during the day, even if sleeping an adequate amount of time.

Some patients may have no symptoms at all, even with severe OSA, or symptoms only noted by the bed partner. Often, the patient may not associate systemic symptoms with sleep symptoms.

NOCTURNAL SYMPTOMS:
- Snoring (especially when loud, habitual, and bothersome to others, most sensitive symptom)[4]
- Witnessed apneas (often interrupting snoring and end with a snort)
- Awakening with gasping, choking, or smothering sensations (most specific indicator)[4]
- Restless sleep
- Frequent awakenings

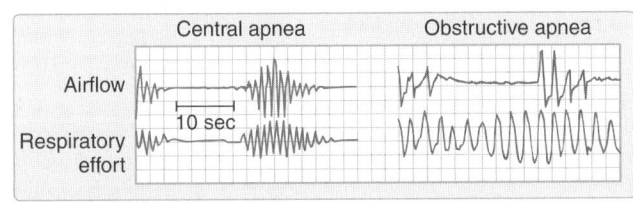

FIG. 1 Central and obstructive sleep apnea: The relationship between airflow and respiratory effort in central and obstructive apnea. During central apnea, cessation of airflow occurs without associated ventilatory effort. Respiratory effort is present during an obstructive apnea. (From Wellman A, White DP: Central sleep apnea and periodic breathing. In Kryger M, Dement W [eds]: *Principles and practice of sleep medicine,* ed 5, Philadelphia, 2011, Saunders, pp. 1140-1152.)

TABLE 1 Definitions

Apnea
- An event lasting ≥10 sec characterized by ≥90% reduction from pre-event baseline in oronasal thermistor airflow. An apnea is scored as:
  - Obstructive, if there is continued or increasing respiratory effort throughout the event
  - Central, if respiratory effort is absent throughout the entire event
  - Mixed, if effort is initially absent, then resumes in the latter part of the event
- There is no minimum desaturation or microarousal requirement for scoring of an apnea.

Hypopnea
- An event lasting ≥10 sec characterized by a ≥30% reduction from pre-event baseline in peak nasal pressure inspiratory airflow which is associated with (definitions vary by sleep lab and insurer):
  - Definition 1A: Either a ≥3% reduction in arterial SpO_2 pre-event baseline or a microarousal (most commonly used definition by the AASM and most U.S. sleep labs)
  - Definition 1B: A ≥4% reduction in arterial SpO_2 from pre-event baseline value (definition required by Medicare)

Respiratory Event–Related Arousal (RERA)
- A sequence of breaths lasting ≥10 sec that does not meet criteria for apnea or hypopnea, which is characterized by increasing respiratory effort or inspiratory flattening of the nasal pressure flow signal leading to a microarousal.

Hypoventilation
- An increase in arterial Pco_2 to >55 mm Hg for ≥10 min or an increase in arterial Pco_2 ≥10 mm Hg above awake supine values to >50 mm Hg for ≥10 min

Metrics of Severity
Apnea-Hypopnea Index: Average number of apneas plus hypopneas per hour of sleep.
Respiratory Disturbance Index: Average number of apneas plus hypopneas plus RERAs per hour of sleep.

Consensus Definitions of Severity in Adults
Normal: <5 episodes/hr
Mild sleep apnea: ≥5 and <15 episodes/hr
Moderate sleep apnea: ≥15 and <30 episodes/hr
Severe sleep apnea: ≥30 episodes/hr

Adapted from Broaddus C et al: *Murray and Nadel's textbook of respiratory medicine,* ed 7, Philadelphia, 2022, Saunders.

TABLE 2 Clinical Characteristics of Patients With Sleep Apnea

CENTRAL		
Nonhypercapnic	**Hypercapnic**	**Obstructive**
Insomnia	Daytime sleepiness Morning headache	Daytime sleepiness
Mild intermittent snoring	Snoring	Prominent snoring
Awakenings (choking/dyspnea)	Respiratory failure	Witnessed apneas/gasping
Normal body habitus	Normal or obese	Commonly obese
	Polycythemia	Upper airway narrowing
	Cor pulmonale	

From Kryger M et al: *Principles and practice of sleep medicine*, ed 7, Philadelphia, 2023, Elsevier.

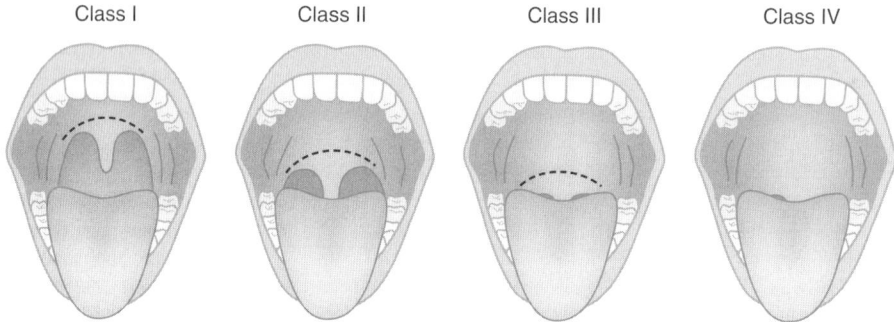

Class I   Class II   Class III   Class IV

FIG. 2 Mallampati classification. Visualized with the patient in the sitting position, head held in a neutral position, mouth wide open, tongue protruding to the maximum, without phonation. Class I is characterized by direct visualization of the soft palate, uvula, palatine tonsils, and pillars. Classification increases until only the hard palate is visible (class IV). (From Townsend CM Jr et al: *Sabiston textbook of surgery*, ed 19, Philadelphia, Elsevier, 2012.)

- Insomnia (particularly trouble with sleep maintenance)
- Restless legs syndrome (RLS)
- Nocturia
- Gastroesophageal reflux disease (GERD)
- Night sweats

DAYTIME SYMPTOMS:
- Excessive daytime sleepiness (a commonly used instrument is the Epworth Sleepiness Scale; a score $\geq$10 suggests abnormal sleepiness)
- Unrefreshing sleep regardless of duration
- Daytime fatigue
- Morning headache (improving within a few hours of waking, fairly specific for OSA) [4]
- Dry mouth or throat on awakening
- Mental fog, or problems with memory, concentration, and cognitive function
- Depressed mood
- Anxiety, irritability, or short temper
- Chronic pain or fibromyalgia-like symptoms
- Inattentiveness or, in children, attention-deficit/hyperactivity disorder (ADHD) symptoms
- Decreased libido, or erectile dysfunction in men

HISTORICAL FINDINGS AND ASSOCIATED CONDITIONS:
- Weight gain (in one study, a 10% increase in weight over 4 yr predicts a sixfold increase in the likelihood of developing an AHI $\geq$15)[5]
- Chronic nasal congestion (often with allergic triad in children)

- Cardiovascular, cerebrovascular, and metabolic disease
  1. In pregnant women, this includes history of hypertensive diseases of pregnancy, gestational diabetes, and advanced maternal age
- Motor vehicle accidents or occupational accidents
- Family history of OSA (odds increase with each additional close family member)
- Conditions affecting shape or compensatory tone of the airway:
  1. Neuromuscular disorders (e.g., demyelinating diseases, amyotrophic lateral sclerosis [ALS], muscular dystrophy, severe cervical spondylosis)
  2. Hypermobility syndromes (e.g., Marfan, Ehlers-Danlos)
  3. Disorders affecting craniofacial development (cleft palate, Down syndrome)
  4. OSA should always be suspected in patients with Down syndrome
- OSA may cause or exacerbate comorbid sleep disorders, most commonly insomnia and RLS. These may be the presenting complaints. Known associations between neuroendocrine abnormalities and major sleep conditions are summarized in Table E3.

OBJECTIVE FINDINGS:
- Obesity
- Neck circumference of $\geq$43 cm (17 in) in men and $\geq$38 cm (15 in) in women[6]

1. OSA is more likely at lower body mass index (BMI) and neck circumference in Asian populations
- Tonsillar hypertrophy: In many pediatric patients and the occasional adult patient, identification of enlarged tonsils can prompt referral for curative tonsillectomy
- Low-hanging soft palate (i.e., a high Mallampati classification; Fig. 2)
- Signs of nasal congestion (e.g., turbinate hypertrophy, severely deviated nasal septum)
- Retrognathia or micrognathia (often associated with dental crowding and overbite/overjet; Fig. E3)
- Scalloping of the edge of the tongue (evidence of tongue too large for oral cavity; Fig. E3)

The STOP-BANG Questionnaire (Fig. 4) and the Berlin Questionnaire are widely used and well-validated screening instruments that summarize some of the most common signs, symptoms, and associated conditions. These can be helpful in developing a clinic protocol for referral.

ETIOLOGY

During sleep, the wakefulness drive to breath is absent, leading to an unmasking of predisposition to upper airway collapse. Ventilatory instability or low arousal threshold can cause obstructive apneas to occur in sequential or repetitive fashion.
- Mechanical loads resulting in narrowing of upper airway (Fig. E5)

The STOP-BANG Questionnaire

Snoring	Do you snore loudly (louder than talking or loud enough to be heard through closed doors)?
Tired	Do you often feel tired, fatigued, or sleepy during the daytime?
Observed	Has anyone observed you stop breathing during your sleep?
Blood pressure	Do you have or are you being treated for high blood pressure?
BMI	Body mass index >35?
Age	Age over 50 yr old?
Neck circumference	Neck circumference greater than 40 cm?
Gender	Gender male?

FIG. 4 The STOP-BANG Questionnaire. High risk of obstructive sleep apnea is indicated by answering YES to ≥5 questions OR answering YES to ≥2 more of the STOP questions (the first 4 questions) plus YES to at least one of the following: Male gender, body mass index *(BMI)* ≥35, neck circumference ≥40 cm (16 inches). Intermediate risk is YES to ≥3 questions. (Adapted from Kryger M et al: *Atlas of clinical sleep medicine,* ed 2, Philadelphia, 2014, Saunders.)

1. Obesity (likely mediated by lingual fat deposition)
2. Size and position of maxilla, mandible, palate, and other craniofacial properties
3. Adenotonsillar hypertrophy
4. Fluid overload
5. Inflammation (e.g., allergies, GERD, local tissue trauma from snoring)
- Impairment of compensatory neuromuscular or central nervous system activity
  1. Neuromuscular disorders or metabolic disorders
  2. Diminished airway muscle activity/reflexes (may be exacerbated by local trauma due to snoring and reflux)
  3. Instability or impairment of ventilatory drive
  4. Low arousal threshold

DX DIAGNOSIS

DIFFERENTIAL DIAGNOSIS

Consider other causes of sleepiness, fatigue, or paroxysmal awakenings. A systematic approach can involve considering other sleep disorders and then considering nonsleep-related causes. Other etiologies that should not be missed:
- Decompensated heart failure or arrhythmia, or cardiac ischemia presenting with paroxysmal nocturnal dyspnea
- Decompensated COPD or asthma presenting as above or with nocturnal cough

- If reports of sleepiness, fatigue, or exertional intolerance are relatively abrupt, consider an undetected cardiac or pulmonary event

Sleep disorders likely to mimic OSA
- Primary snoring
- Central sleep apnea (especially in patients with heart failure or on opioids)
- Obesity hypoventilation syndrome (OHS, 90% of cases coexist with OSA, but 10% of cases can be seen in absence of OSA, risk increases with BMI, particularly ≥40)

Sleep disorders likely to cause sleepiness and fatigue (often comorbid with OSA, but can independently explain sleepiness as well)
- Insufficient sleep
- Insomnia
- Restless legs syndrome (RLS is exacerbated by untreated OSA)
- Circadian rhythm disorder
- Shift work sleep disorder

Less common sleep disorders that may cause sleepiness
- Narcolepsy (but OSA must be ruled out or treated prior to diagnosis)
- Idiopathic hypersomnia
- Parasomnias (includes sleep walking, sleep eating, REM behavior disorder)
- Periodic limb movement disorder

Nonsleep-related disorders likely to cause nocturnal symptoms or abrupt awakening
- Alcohol use, particularly heavy or close to bed time

- Nocturnal gastroesophageal reflux
- Asthma
- Anxiety or panic disorder
- Benign prostatic hyperplasia
- Nocturnal seizures (not common, but important to consider)

Nonsleep-related disorders likely to cause fatigue or sleepiness
- Medication side effects (particularly when several centrally acting agents are combined, consider over-the-counter sleep aids also)
- Iron deficiency (even in absence of anemia or RLS)
- Mood disorders (antidepressants, antipsychotics, anxiolytics can also cause hypersomnia)
- Hypothyroidism
- Anemia
- Traumatic brain injury
- Neurologic conditions (e.g., Parkinson disease, multiple sclerosis, dementia)
- Connective tissue diseases or chronic pain
- Other advanced systemic illness or malignancy

WORKUP
SAFETY:
- All patients with suspected OSA should be screened for drowsiness while driving, recent motor vehicle accidents, or "close calls" while driving.
- An occupational history focused on professional operation of vehicles or other modes of transportation, long commute times, operation

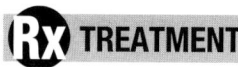
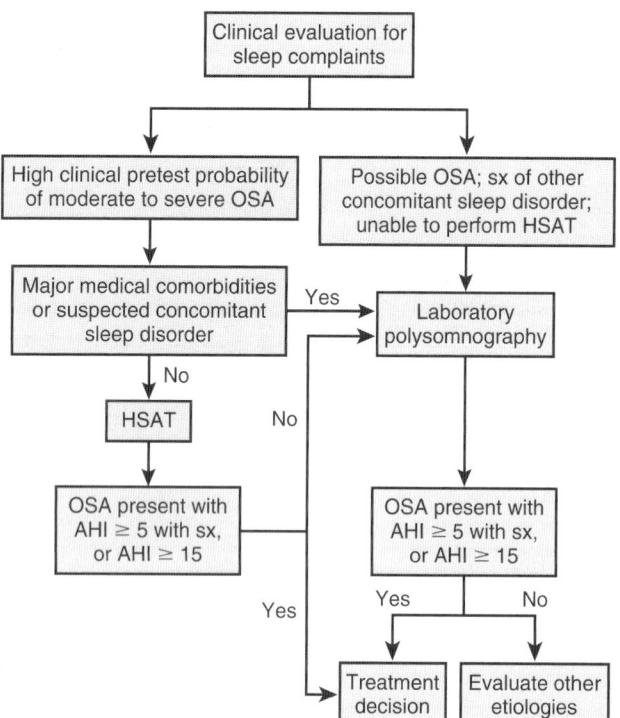

FIG. 6 Approach to the diagnosis of obstructive sleep apnea (OSA). An ambulatory pathway for patients with symptomatic moderate to severe OSA without other major comorbidities is shown in *blue*. Patients with a lower pretest probability of OSA or who are suspected of having another sleep disorder are recommended for evaluation in the laboratory-based pathway in *orange*. *AHI,* Apnea-hypopnea index; *HSAT,* home sleep apnea testing. (From Broaddus C et al: *Murray and Nadel's textbook of respiratory medicine*, ed 7, Philadelphia, 2022, Saunders.)

of heavy machinery, or other occupations where falling asleep on the job might have catastrophic effects is essential.[7]
- A thorough review of prescribed and recreational substances should be performed, including alcohol, opioids, muscle relaxants, other sedatives, and centrally acting medications.

DIAGNOSTIC EVALUATION (SEE FIG. 6)
- OSA is confirmed by nocturnal polysomnography (PSG), which is the gold standard for diagnosis, or home sleep apnea testing (HSAT). Particularly in the wake of the COVID-19 pandemic, HSAT has become a more reasonable option in many circumstances.
- PSG is recommended for occupational screening (e.g., pilots, train operators, commercial drivers).
- PSG is optimal for suspected mild OSA (e.g., in a young adult patient without other comorbidities) because it may detect more subtle respiratory events than HSAT and can accurately quantify total sleep time (rather than simply time in bed).
- HSAT is best used as an alternative to PSG in cases where clinical suspicion is high for moderate or severe OSA and there are no comorbidities that might influence sleep testing. Referral to a sleep specialist or PSG should be considered when there is comorbid COPD, heart failure, neuromuscular

weakness, or a suspected hypoventilation syndrome, or if there is concern for another nonrespiratory sleep disorder requiring PSG such as narcolepsy, severe insomnia, or parasomnias.
- HSAT is not yet approved for routine pediatric testing.
- Diagnosis of OSA in adults is made using a combination of AHI and symptoms:
  1. Mild: ≥ 5 to <15 respiratory events per hour (with symptoms or comorbidities)
  2. Moderate: ≥ 15 to <30 respiratory events per hour
  3. Severe: ≥ 30 respiratory events per hour
- Note that formal diagnosis of mild OSA requires the presence of symptoms (including those noted by the bed partner) or presence of a comorbidity such as hypertension, excessive daytime sleepiness, heart attack, heart failure, stroke, mood disorders or insomnia, or impaired cognition.
- The respiratory disturbance index (RDI) includes additional respiratory events (RERAs, see Table 1) that are not captured in the AHI. Using the more sensitive RDI for diagnosis instead of the AHI may be most appropriate in sleepy, symptomatic patients.
- In children, the thresholds for severity of OSA are lower compared to adults.

LABORATORY TESTS
- CBC to look for anemia or erythrocytosis
- Ferritin and iron panel if RLS or anemia (or other relevant CBC abnormality) is present

- Thyroid studies if thyroid dysfunction is suspected
- Bicarbonate level on basic metabolic panel can serve as a surrogate marker for chronic hypercapnia and can be used to stratify risk for OHS as an alternative or additional diagnosis; bicarbonate <27 in a patient with BMI <35 has high negative predictive value for OHS.
- Arterial blood gas testing if hypercapnia needs to be ruled out
- Cardiac and pulmonary testing as guided by history and symptomatology

Rx TREATMENT

ACUTE GENERAL Rx
- Avoid alcohol for 4 to 6 h before bedtime.
- Avoid narcotics, muscle relaxants, and sedating medications.

CHRONIC Rx
- Weight loss
  1. Most patients with OSA will benefit from weight loss. Weight loss by any modality is effective for reducing the severity of OSA, and sufficient weight loss can be curative in some patients.[8,9]
  2. Exercise without weight loss may improve OSA,[5] and lifestyle interventions reduce OSA in proportion to weight loss.[8]
  3. Medication-assisted weight loss should be considered.[8,10,11] Many patients with OSA who are overweight or obese will have comorbidities that can guide selection of a weight loss agent.
  4. Bariatric surgery leads to improvement or resolution of OSA for most patients, in addition to improvements in metabolic syndrome outcomes.
- Positive airway pressure (PAP)
  1. Continuous positive airway pressure (CPAP) is the first-line and most effective therapy for OSA (Fig. 7). It delivers a constant airway pressure that serves as a pneumatic splint relieving upper airway obstruction.[12] Most new devices sold today can be in autotitrating CPAP mode (auto-CPAP or APAP), which increases or decreases the level of pressure in response to change in airflow, vibratory snoring, or changes in circuit pressure. This allows for prescription of APAP immediately after diagnostic PSG or HSAT, with titration of pressures done at home.
  2. Other methods of delivering positive pressure include bilevel positive airway pressure (BPAP).[12] In addition to delivering expiratory positive airway pressure (EPAP, equivalent to CPAP), BPAP also delivers a higher inspiratory positive airway pressure (IPAP). BPAP may be used for certain patients with hypoventilation syndromes, or occasionally in the treatment of OSA where CPAP is not well-tolerated.
- Oral appliance
  1. Mandibular advancement devices fit over the teeth like a mouthguard while engaging

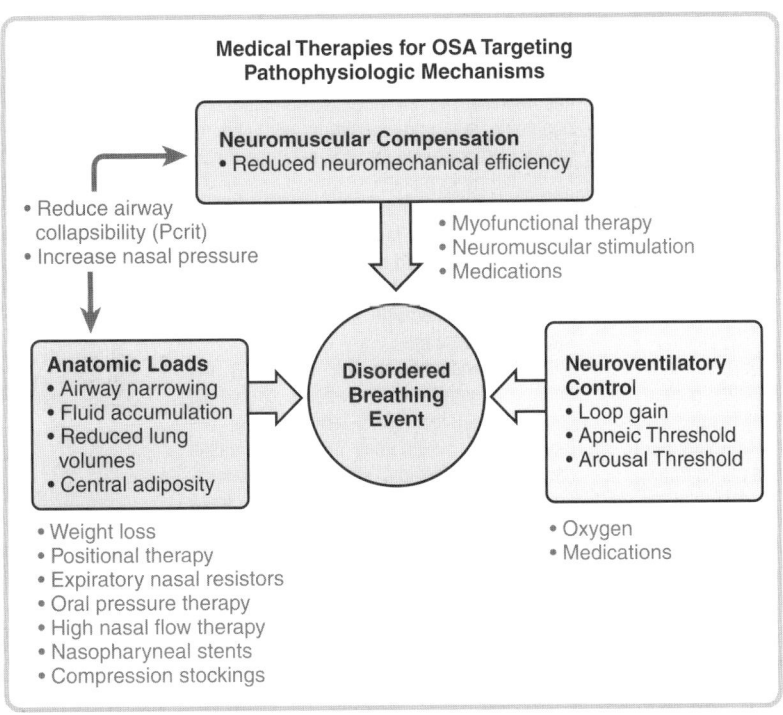

Medical Therapies for OSA Targeting Pathophysiologic Mechanisms

Neuromuscular Compensation
• Reduced neuromechanical efficiency

• Reduce airway collapsibility (Pcrit)
• Increase nasal pressure

• Myofunctional therapy
• Neuromuscular stimulation
• Medications

Disordered Breathing Event

Anatomic Loads
• Airway narrowing
• Fluid accumulation
• Reduced lung volumes
• Central adiposity

Neuroventilatory Control
• Loop gain
• Apneic Threshold
• Arousal Threshold

• Weight loss
• Positional therapy
• Expiratory nasal resistors
• Oral pressure therapy
• High nasal flow therapy
• Nasopharyneal stents
• Compression stockings

• Oxygen
• Medications

FIG. 7 Therapies for obstructive sleep apnea *(OSA)* stratified by mechanism. Traditional therapies such as continuous positive airway pressure (CPAP) use nasal pressure to overcome anatomic loads. By contrast, upper airway surgery and weight loss reduce anatomic loads (measured as airway collapsibility, *Pcrit*). Therapeutic strategies that address impairments in neuromuscular function and neuroventilatory control are less well established, but include myofunctional therapies, neuromuscular stimulation, use of medications to modulate tone or increase arousal threshold, and supplemental oxygen. (Adapted from Kryger M et al: *Principles and practice of sleep medicine,* ed 6, Philadelphia, 2017, Elsevier.)

BOX 1 Surgical Treatment Options

Nasal Surgery
Nasal septoplasty
Inferior turbinate reduction
Adenoidectomy
Nasal tumor or polyp resection
Nasal valve reconstruction

Palatal Surgery
Palatal radiofrequency ablation
Pillar implants
Injection snoreplasty
Tonsillectomy
Uvulopalatopharyngoplasty/Z-palatoplasty
Transpalatal advancement pharyngoplasty

Hypopharyngeal Surgery
Lingual tonsillectomy
Partial midline glossectomy
Tongue base radiofrequency ablation
Mandibular osteotomy and genioglossal advancement
Hyoid myotomy and suspension
Tongue-suspension suture
Maxillomandibular osteotomy and advancement

From Flint PW et al: *Cummings otolaryngology, head and neck surgery,* ed 7, Philadelphia, 2021, Elsevier.

the maxillary and mandibular dental arches, inducing protrusion of the mandible and more favorable positioning of the tongue and other airway structures. They are most effective for the treatment of mild to moderate OSA, and tend to work better in those with retrognathia, supine OSA, and lower BMI. Although CPAP is more efficacious,

this advantage may be offset by inferior compliance relative to oral appliance, resulting in similar effectiveness. There is no overall difference between oral appliances and CPAP with respect to improvement in blood pressure, daytime sleepiness, or quality of life.[13] Severely hypoxemic patients or patients requiring

rapid treatment should be treated with CPAP.
• Surgical treatment (Box 1):
  1. Presurgical planning may involve several visits to identify specific anatomic areas of narrowing (nasal, pharyngeal, tongue base, hypopharynx) and select the appropriate surgery. See details that are listed below. Sometimes, these surgeries may be performed in combination or in sequence.
  2. Adenotonsillectomy is often curative for children with OSA and also for select adults with tonsillar hypertrophy.
  3. Uvulopalatopharyngoplasty, which involves resection of the uvula and soft palate.
  4. Maxillomandibular advancement surgery involves osteotomies of the maxilla and mandible to allow the entire lower face to be projected forward, creating a more favorable configuration for the soft tissues and dilators of the oropharynx.[14]
  5. Hypoglossal nerve stimulation (HGNS) involves surgical placement of an implant in the upper chest, connected to the hypoglossal nerve, which helps recruit lingual muscles, reducing pharyngeal collapsibility and decreasing upper airway resistance. Operation of the device requires nightly activation by the patient with a remote control.
  6. Palatal implant surgery and maxillary expansion for high-arched palates are other surgical options.

7. Nasal septoplasty/turbinectomy could be considered for patients with severe anatomic deformities or chronic nasal congestion refractory to medical therapy.

- Other treatments:
  These treatments are generally best used as adjunctive strategies or used in mild cases with patients seeking to avoid devices and surgery.
  1. Optimal treatment of allergic rhinitis, including nasal irrigation, nasal steroids, antihistamines, and modifications to environment.
  2. Side sleeping will reduce OSA in many patients. In well-selected patients, guided by PSG or HSAT results, positional therapy may even be a first line choice. Body pillows, wedge pillows, physical or electronic position trainers, or other devices can be helpful.
  3. Nasal EPAP devices are one-way expiratory valves worn over the nose. Resistance to exhalation at the nose generates positive airway pressure, reducing apneas.
  4. Myofunctional therapy, a set of upper airway exercises to reduce snoring and apneas, can be suggested to motivated patients as an adjunctive therapy.
  5. Orthodontic treatment may be an option in children.

DISPOSITION

- Patients should be counseled on risks of untreated sleepiness, particularly when it comes to driving. Short-term prognosis for excessive daytime sleepiness and snoring is good with regular use of CPAP.
- Problems with tolerance of CPAP at initiation are common but surmountable. Scheduled follow-up to assess CPAP usage and to address problems proactively is necessary.
- Mask fit, claustrophobia, nasal congestion, and the habitual nature of the therapy are common barriers to care.
- CPAP machines provide daily usage reports logging hours of use and estimating AHI on treatment (Fig. E8). In most U.S. practice settings, the durable medical equipment company supplying the CPAP device can provide these reports on request and provide assistance with troubleshooting issues related to CPAP comfort or equipment malfunction.
- Residual excessive sleepiness (RES) despite adequate treatment of OSA should prompt consideration of alternative causes. Modafinil or armodafinil can be considered for treatment once other causes are ruled out and are first-line medications for RES. Solriamfetol is a dopamine and norepinephrine reuptake inhibitor FDA approved for RES, although it may be limited by formulary.

- If central sleep apnea is diagnosed, evaluate for underlying heart failure or opioid use, and treat underlying heart failure as appropriate or reduce opioid use to the extent possible. Consult sleep medicine to determine if PAP therapy is indicated.

- Although evidence on the matter is not entirely straightforward, patients should be counseled on likely long-term risks of untreated OSA, which may include increased risks of hypertension, stroke, heart failure, arrhythmia, cognitive impairment, and others (Fig. E9).
  1. Observational studies show strong association between increasing OSA severity, vascular events, and early mortality. These studies have long follow-up times, on the order of 10 yr or longer, and inflection points in mortality curves do not appear until late into the observation period.[15]
  2. Randomized controlled trials (RCTs) have failed to show that CPAP reduces incident cardiovascular events in those with moderate to severe OSA.[15] Critiques of these studies include low adherence to CPAP (3 h/night), the necessity of excluding excessively sleepy patients for ethical reasons, selection of composite outcomes (obscuring effectiveness in preventing stroke), and insufficient follow-up time (follow-up times on the order of 3 to 5 yr).
  3. RCT evidence supports improvement in mood and quality of life with CPAP.

REFERRAL

- HSAT and APAP can lower barriers to care and for some patients enable diagnosis and treatment initiation entirely at home.
- Referral to sleep medicine may be helpful when ruling out other sleep disorders, evaluating SDB in the setting of advanced cardiopulmonary or neuromuscular disease, or when seeking CPAP alternatives.
- Sleep psychologists can be consulted for CPAP desensitization or motivational interviewing approaches to improve adherence.

- Referral to medical weight management or bariatric surgery should be considered for obese patients with OSA.
- Surgical referral to otolaryngology should be considered for children with adenotonsillar hypertrophy and for adults who are unresponsive to weight loss and CPAP therapy.
- Referral to a qualified dentist for treatment with an oral appliance is a good alternative to CPAP for those with uncomplicated mild to moderate OSA.

❗ PEARLS & CONSIDERATIONS

- OSA is a common disorder that is highly prevalent and underdiagnosed. OSA should be considered in patients of every age, gender, and weight status. Prevalence is particularly high in patients with the metabolic syndrome.
- An atypical presentation of a common disorder will still be common. Symptoms such as mental fog, nocturia, night sweats, insomnia, and mood disturbances can be useful in prompting diagnostic evaluation.
- An occupational and driving history is a key component of the sleep history. In most situations, the greatest short-term morbidity from untreated OSA is due to excessive daytime sleepiness leading to motor vehicle and occupational accidents.
- Allow the presence or absence of significant symptoms to guide treatment recommendations in borderline and mild cases.
- Weight loss by any modality can lead to improvement of OSA and should be discussed as part of treatment.
- The single most effective therapy for OSA is CPAP, with quieter and more comfortable masks and machines developed over the last decade. Adjustments to equipment settings and behavioral therapies can be employed to improve patient acceptance.
- There are alternatives to CPAP, including oral appliances and well-established surgical treatments for OSA.

REFERENCES

Available at eBooks.Health.Elsevier.com.

AUTHORS: **DAVID CLAMAN, MD,** and **ALEXANDER GOMEZ, MD**

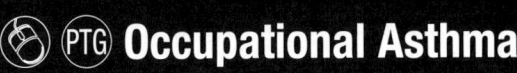

BASIC INFORMATION

DEFINITION

The National Institute for Occupational Safety and Health (NIOSH) defines occupational asthma (OA), or work-related asthma (WRA), as "asthma triggered by an exposure at work." Additionally, the same triggers can lead to "work-exacerbated asthma (WEA)" in which someone previously diagnosed with asthma has worsening symptoms due to an occupational exposure.[1] The American College of Chest Physicians further classifies this form of asthma as either "sensitizer-induced OA" in which a patient becomes sensitized to a specific substance at work, or "irritant-induced OA" caused by inhalation of an irritant at work[2] (Fig. 1). There have been hundreds of triggers, around ~600, identified to date that have been linked to occupational asthma. These triggers are categorized by either low or high molecular weight and as either sensitizers or irritants.[3]

SYNONYM

Asthma, occupational

ICD-10CM CODES

J45.909	Occupational asthma Industrial asthma Environmental asthma
J67.8	Mill-workers' asthma Woodworkers' asthma Bakers' asthma Cheese-makers' asthma Feather asthma Flour asthma Red-cedar asthma Sawdust asthma
J68.8	Silo-workers' asthma Meat wrapper asthma
J45.998	Isocyanate-induced asthma Platinum asthma Printers' asthma
J68.3	Chemical-induced asthma
J66.0	Cotton-dust asthma
J69.8	Detergent asthma
J45.20	Hay asthma
J60	Miner's asthma
J66.8	Tea-makers' asthma

EPIDEMIOLOGY & DEMOGRAPHICS

According to the NIOSH, 17% of asthma developed in adulthood is attributed to work-related exposures. Among those with known asthma, a median prevalence of 22% experience work-exacerbated asthma, and it has been reported as high as 58% in some studies. Males and females are equally affected; however, there has been a higher prevalence documented among those who are Black, American Indian/Alaska Native, or of Puerto Rican descent.[4]

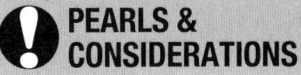

DIAGNOSIS (Fig. 1)

WORKUP

The workup and testing for diagnosing occupational asthma overlaps with asthma (e.g., pulmonary function tests [PFTs], methacholine testing, skin prick testing, etc.); however, the occupational history and the temporal association of symptoms allow for delineating between the two (as illustrated in Fig. 1). Specific inhalation challenge (SIC) testing, skin prick testing, and serologic testing (e.g., antigen specific immunoglobulin E testing) can be utilized to isolate the antigens(s) in question and can be tailored such that they mimic the patient's possible work exposures; samples can also be obtained directly from the patient's work site for more accurate testing. Serial tests (e.g., peak expiratory flow rates, PFTs, methacholine testing, etc.) should also be performed following removal from the work site or exposures, for a minimum of two weeks, to determine if symptoms and testing markers improve with avoidance of triggers.[5] Recent studies have shown that change in nonspecific bronchial hyperresponsiveness (NSBH) (e.g., two- to threefold decrease in concentration of methacholine causing 20% decrease in FEV_1) and associated increase in sputum eosinophils (>3% pre-/post-SIC) are the most specific tests (97% when combined; 90% sputum testing alone) for diagnosing OA, whereas serial peak expiratory flow and change in NSBH (at/off work) are the most sensitive tests (92%) for diagnosing OA.[6]

TREATMENT

NONPHARMACOLOGIC THERAPY

As seen with traditional asthma, the most important nonpharmacologic treatment for OA or WEA is to avoid the trigger or irritant once it is identified. Avoidance of triggers can occur by changing the patient's work environment by limiting activities that may relate to the exposure or by having the patient wear a respirator that can prevent inhalation of various antigens. However, if the exposure is severe enough such that adjustments are unable to be made to the working environment, it is advisable for the patient to switch careers, if feasible. It should be noted that within the AHRQ review performed in 2005 better outcomes were observed among those who changed careers compared to those who did not.[2] Overall treatment of OA and WEA should focus on optimization of asthma treatment while simultaneously limiting exposure(s).

CHRONIC Rx

The treatment for OA and WEA does not differ from other forms of asthma and should be treated utilizing a similar stepwise approach.

PEARLS & CONSIDERATIONS

COMMENTS

- Key history taking that focuses on the temporal association of asthmatic symptoms as they may relate to various occupations, especially if asthma is diagnosed in adulthood.
- If OA or WEA is suspected, it is advisable for clinicians to review the Association of Occupational and Environmental Clinics (AOEC) Exposure Code List, which can be accessed at: http://www.aoec.org/tools.htm. Thus allowing physicians to better isolate the antigen(s) of interest for more specific clinical testing to occur.[7]

REFERENCES
Available at eBooks.Health.Elsevier.com.

RELATED CONTENT
Asthma (Related Key Topic)

AUTHORS: **LAREN TAN, MD, MBA,** and **DERRICK CLELAND, DO, MPH**

O

Diseases and Disorders

I

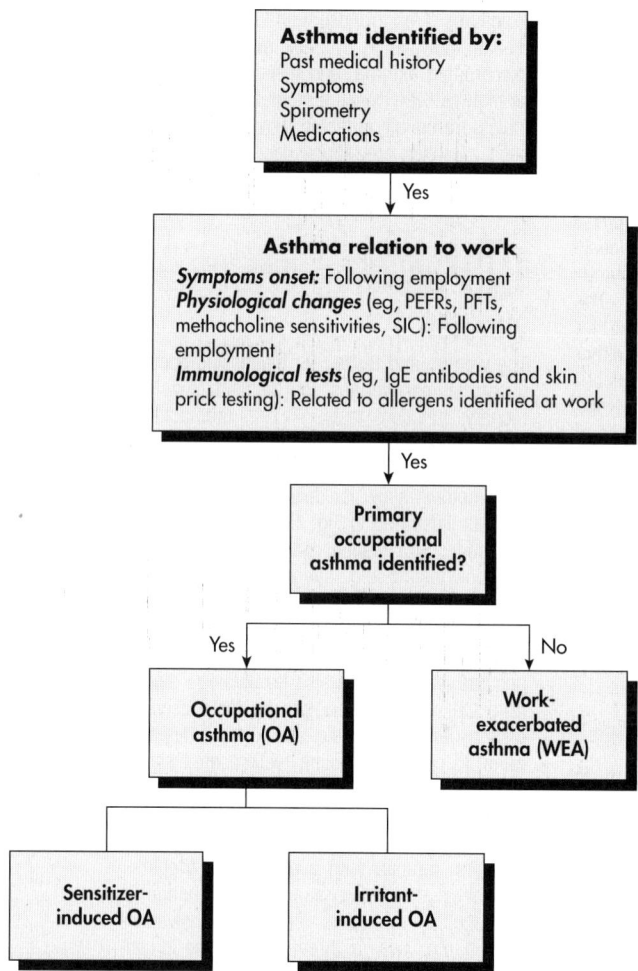

FIG. 1 Diagnostic algorithm for occupational asthma. *IgE,* Immunoglobulin E; *PEFRs,* peak expiratory flow recordings; *PFTs,* pulmonary function tests; *SIC,* specific inhalation challenge. (Adapted from Tarlo SM et al: Diagnosis and management of work-related asthma: American College of Chest Physicians Consensus Statement [published correction appears in *Chest* 134(4):892], *Chest* 134(3 Suppl):1S-41S, 2008. https://doi.org/10.1378/chest.08-0201.)

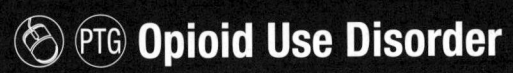

O

 BASIC INFORMATION

DEFINITION

- Opioid use disorder (OUD) is defined as a cluster of cognitive, behavioral, and physiologic symptoms in which the individual continues use of opiates despite significant opiate-induced problems. Opiate use disorder is a chronic, relapsing disorder characterized by repeated self-administration that usually results in opiate tolerance, withdrawal, and compulsive drug use. Tolerance is the need to increase dose to achieve the same effect. Dependence may occur with or without the physiologic symptoms of tolerance and withdrawal.
- There are four stages of addiction:
  1. Stage I, acute drug effects: Rewarding effects of drug result from neurobiologic changes in response to the acute drug use. Duration varies from hours to days.
  2. Stage II, transformation to addiction: Associated with changes in neuronal function that accumulate with repeated administration and diminish over days or weeks after discontinuation of drug use.
  3. Stage III, relapse after extended periods of abstinence: Precipitated by an incubation of cue-induced craving (people, places, and things as triggers) and priming (relapse precipitated by drug exposure).
  4. Stage IV, end-stage addiction: Vulnerability to relapse endures for years and results from prolonged changes at the cellular level.
- Pseudoaddiction: Undertreatment of pain resulting in "opiate-seeking" behaviors such as "doctor shopping" and multiple emergency department visits. These behaviors disappear with adequate treatment of pain.

SYNONYMS

Opioid dependence
OUD
Opiate addiction
Opiate abuse
Narcotic addiction
Narcotic abuse
Substance use disorder

ICD-10CM CODES
F11.10	Opioid abuse, uncomplicated
F11.120	Opioid abuse with intoxication, uncomplicated
F11.121	Opioid abuse with intoxication delirium
F11.122	Opioid abuse with intoxication with perceptual disturbance
F11.129	Opioid abuse with intoxication, unspecified
F11.14	Opioid abuse with opioid-induced mood disorder
F11.150	Opioid abuse with opioid-induced psychotic disorder with delusions
F11.151	Opioid abuse with opioid-induced psychotic disorder with hallucinations
F11.159	Opioid abuse with opioid-induced psychotic disorder, unspecified
F11.181	Opioid abuse with opioid-induced sexual dysfunction
F11.182	Opioid abuse with opioid-induced sleep disorder
F11.188	Opioid abuse with other opioid-induced disorder
F11.19	Opioid abuse with unspecified opioid-induced disorder

EPIDEMIOLOGY & DEMOGRAPHICS

INCIDENCE: It is estimated that more than 2.5 million Americans have an opioid use disorder.
PREVALENCE:
- Each year, U.S. retail pharmacies dispense over 170 million prescriptions for opioid pain relievers. Commonly used opioids are summarized in Box 1.
- The percentage of eighth-, tenth-, and twelfth-graders who have used heroin has more than doubled since the late 1990s. This increase has largely been attributed to decreased price and increased purity in the last decade. In 2019, 1.6 million Americans older than 12 yr were estimated to have OUD.[1]
- After plateauing in 2018 to 2019, opioid overdose deaths increased sharply in the past 3 years with the majority attributed to illicitly manufactured fentanyl.[1]
- The Drug Enforcement Administration and Centers for Disease Control and Prevention has issued nationwide alerts identifying fentanyl, particularly illicitly manufactured fentanyl, as a threat to public health and safety. Illicitly manufactured fentanyl is pharmacologically similar to pharmaceutical fentanyl but is unlawfully produced in clandestine laboratories and obtained via illicit drug markets; it also includes fentanyl analogs. Fentanyl is a synthetic opioid 50 to 100 times more potent than morphine and approved for the management of surgical/postoperative pain, severe chronic pain, and breakthrough cancer pain.
- In the U.S., approximately 10 million adults are prescribed long-term opioid therapy (LTOT) for chronic pain despite inadequate evidence of long-term benefit and growing evidence of harm.

PREDOMINANT SEX: Males abuse opioids more commonly than females, with a male:female ratio of 3:1 for heroin and 1.5:1 for prescription opiates.
PEAK INCIDENCE: The majority of new abusers of opiates are <26 yr.
RISK FACTORS:
- Family history
- Prior history of addiction
- Psychiatric disorders

GENETICS:
- Genetic epidemiologic studies suggest a high degree of heritable vulnerability for opioid dependence.
- Gene polymorphism for dopamine receptor/transporters, opioid receptors, serotonin receptors/transporters, proenkephalin, and catechol-*O*-methyltransferase all appear to be associated with vulnerability to opioid dependence. Future interventions for opiate dependence may include medications identified through genetic research.

PHYSICAL FINDINGS & CLINICAL PRESENTATION

- Physical examination is often noncontributory.
- Small-sized pupils may be the only observable sign of use because only mild tolerance develops for miosis. Acute effects of opioid agonists are summarized in Box 2.
- Scars or tracks from chronic IV use may be visible over the veins of the arms, hands, ankles, neck, and breasts.
- Inflamed nasal mucosa or respiratory wheezing may be apparent in patients who are snorting heroin or OxyContin.

BOX 1 Commonly Used Opioids

Agonist
  Camphorated tincture of opium (paregoric)
  Morphine
  Meperidine (Demerol)
  Methadone
  Fentanyl
  Hydromorphone (Dilaudid)
  Oxycodone
  Hydrocodone
  Propoxyphene (Darvon)
  Heroin
Antagonist
  Naloxone (Narcan)
  Naltrexone
Mixed Agonist–Antagonist
  Pentazocine (Talwin)
  Butorphanol (Stadol)
  Buprenorphine (Buprenex)

From Jankovic J et al: *Bradley and Daroff's neurology in clinical practice,* ed 8, Philadelphia, 2022, Elsevier.

BOX 2 Acute Effects of Opioid Agonists

"Rush"
Euphoria or dysphoria
Drowsiness, "nodding"
Analgesia
Nausea, vomiting
Miosis
Dryness of the mouth
Sweating
Pruritus
Cough suppression
Respiratory depression
Hypothermia
Postural hypotension
Constipation
Biliary tract spasm
Urinary retention

From Jankovic J et al: *Bradley and Daroff's neurology in clinical practice,* ed 8, Philadelphia, 2022, Elsevier.

BOX 3 Symptoms and Signs of Opioid Withdrawal

Drug craving
Anxiety, irritability
Lacrimation
Rhinorrhea
Yawning
Sweating
Mydriasis
Myalgia, muscle spasms
Piloerection
Anorexia, nausea, vomiting
Diarrhea
Abdominal cramps
Productive coughing
Hot flashes
Fever
Tachycardia
Tachypnea
Hypertension
Erection, orgasm

From Jankovic J et al: *Bradley and Daroff's neurology in clinical practice,* ed 8, Philadelphia, 2022, Elsevier.

BOX 4 Commonly Used Psychostimulants

Dextroamphetamine
Methamphetamine
Ephedrine
Pseudoephedrine
Methylphenidate (Ritalin)
Pemoline (Cylert)
Phenmetrazine (Preludin)
Phentermine
3,4-Methylenedioxymethamphetamine (MDMA, "Ecstasy")
Cocaine
Cathinone, methcathinone

From Jankovic J et al: *Bradley and Daroff's neurology in clinical practice,* ed 8, Philadelphia, 2022, Elsevier.

- Patients in withdrawal may have more dramatic findings such as tachycardia, hypertension, fever, piloerection (goose flesh), mydriasis, lacrimation, central nervous system (CNS) arousal, irritability, and repeated yawning. Box 3 summarizes symptoms and signs of opioid withdrawal. In patients with sympathetic overactivity and panic attacks, use of CNS stimulants (Box 4), such as amphetamines or cocaine, should also be ruled out.
- Although gastrointestinal symptoms of nausea, vomiting, and abdominal pain are common in opioid withdrawal, other causes such as gastroenteritis, pancreatitis, peptic ulcer disease, and intestinal obstruction need to be ruled out.
- The history may provide relevant information in making the diagnosis. Significant findings may include:
  1. A long history of opioid self-administration, typically by the IV or intranasal route but sometimes through smoking as well.

TABLE 1 CAGE-AID

1. Have you ever tried to Cut down on your alcohol or drug use?
2. Do you get Annoyed when people comment about your drinking or drug use?
3. Do you feel Guilty about things you have done while drinking or using drugs?
4. Do you need an Eye-opener to get started in the morning?

Two or more questions answered in the affirmative require further assessment. *AID,* Adapted to include drugs.
From Bowman S et al: Reducing the health consequences of opioid addiction in primary care, *Am J Med* 126:565-571, 2013.

2. Polysubstance use. Intoxication by drugs other than narcotics (e.g., benzodiazepines, barbiturates) should be ruled out in unconscious patients.
3. A high incidence of non-opioid-related psychiatric disorders (>80%).
4. History of problems at work, school, or relationships associated with drug use.
5. History of legal problems associated with drug use, such as arrest for possession, robbery, or prostitution.
6. History of interpersonal violence (as perpetrator or victim).
7. History of physical problems such as skin infections, phlebitis, endocarditis, or liver diseases attributable to acetaminophen toxicity (Vicodin/Percocet) or viral hepatitis. Hepatitis C is the most prevalent blood-borne pathogen. It is present in approximately 90% of opiate-dependent people and is often spread by sharing IV drug paraphernalia or snorting devices. There is also a higher incidence of HIV infection.

ETIOLOGY

Opioid use disorder is a biopsychosocial disorder. Pharmacologic, social, genetic, and psychodynamic factors interact to influence abusive behaviors. Pharmacologic factors are especially prominent in opiate addiction because these drugs are strong reinforcing agents due to their euphoric effects and their ability to reduce anxiety and increase self-esteem and the patient's subjective feelings of improved ability to cope with daily challenges.

🅳🅧 DIAGNOSIS

DIFFERENTIAL DIAGNOSIS

- Psychiatric disorders (e.g., anxiety, depression, bipolar disorder).
- Acute medical illness (e.g., hypoglycemia, seizure disorder, sepsis, renal or hepatic insufficiency) may mimic opiate withdrawal symptoms.

WORKUP

The history is the most important part of the workup. A single-question screening test ("How many times in the past year have you used an illegal drug or used a prescription

TABLE 2 Drug Abuse Screening Test (DAST-10)

1. Have you used drugs other than those required for medical reasons?
2. Do you abuse more than one drug at a time?
3. Are you unable to stop using drugs when you want to?
4. Have you ever had blackouts or flashbacks as a result of drug use?
5. Do you ever feel bad or guilty about your drug use?
6. Does your spouse (or parents) ever complain about your involvement with drugs?
7. Have you neglected your family because of your use of drugs?
8. Have you engaged in illegal activities in order to obtain drugs?
9. Have you ever experienced withdrawal symptoms (felt sick) when you stopped taking drugs?
10. Have you had medical problems as a result of your drug use (e.g., memory loss, hepatitis, convulsions, bleeding)?

Two or more questions answered in the affirmative require further assessment.
From Bowman S et al: Reducing the health consequences of opioid addiction in primary care, *Am J Med* 126:565-571, 2013.

TABLE 3 CRAFFT Screening Tool for Adolescents

1. Have you ever ridden in a Car driven by someone (including yourself) who was high or had been using alcohol or drugs?
2. Do you ever use alcohol or drugs to Relax, feel better about yourself, or fit in?
3. Do you ever use alcohol or drugs while you are by yourself Alone?
4. Do you ever Forget things you did while using alcohol or drugs?
5. Do your Family or Friends ever tell you that you should cut down on your drinking or drug use?
6. Have you ever gotten into Trouble while you were using alcohol or drugs?

Two or more questions answered in the affirmative require further assessment.
From Bowman S et al: Reducing the health consequences of opioid addiction in primary care, *Am J Med* 126:565-571, 2013.

medication for nonmedical reasons?") should be incorporated in the medical history. Useful screening tools for OUD are the CAGE-AID (Table 1), the DAST-10 (Table 2), and the CRAFFT (Table 3). The CAGE-AID has a sensitivity of 70% and a specificity of 85% when two questions are answered in the affirmative. The DAST-10 can discriminate between current users versus former users. The CRAFFT is a useful screening tool for adolescents. A CRAFFT score of 2 or higher is optimal for identifying any problem (sensitivity 76%, specificity 94%), any disorder (sensitivity 80%, specificity 86%), and drug dependence (sensitivity 92%, specificity 80%).
- Observation of opioid withdrawal is indicative of opioid addiction.

- Observation of purposeful behaviors such as complaints and manipulations directed at getting more drugs and anxiety during withdrawal is suggestive of opioid addiction.
- Screen blood and urine for opioid metabolites.
- Screen for communicable diseases: HIV, hepatitis B and hepatitis C, tuberculosis.
- Screen for endocarditis in patients with newly diagnosed murmurs.

LABORATORY TESTS
- Urine and serum toxicology screen
- Complete blood count
- Chemistries (alanine aminotransferase, aspartate aminotransferase, serum creatinine): Elevated liver function test (LFT) results may be from viral hepatitis or acetaminophen toxicity
- Hepatitis screen: If hepatitis C antibody positive, follow up with hepatitis C polymerase chain reaction (viral load) even in patients with normal LFTs
- HIV
- PPD

IMAGING STUDIES
Generally not helpful in routine diagnosis and treatment. Consider echocardiography in patients with heart murmurs and liver sonography or CT scan in patients with elevated LFTs or who are positive for hepatitis C or B (increased risk of hepatocellular carcinoma).

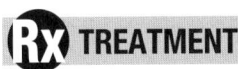 **TREATMENT**

NONPHARMACOLOGIC THERAPY
- Brief counseling interventions during a visit with their primary care physician or OB/GYN have proved efficacious in motivating patients for treatment
- Therapeutic communities (residential)
- 12-step or other self-help groups (e.g., Alcoholics Anonymous, Narcotics Anonymous)
- Relapse prevention (counseling)
- Opioid prevention education (Table 4)

ACUTE GENERAL Rx
- Medical withdrawal (not overdosed). Opioid withdrawal alone is not recommended for

TABLE 4 Basic Components of Opioid Overdose Prevention Education Curriculum

1. Know the signs of an opioid overdose (e.g., unresponsive, limp, slow, shallow breathing, pale or clammy, fingernails or lips turning blue, gurgling).
2. Call 911.
3. Administer rescue breathing.
4. Administer naloxone if no response and Emergency Medical Services has not yet arrived.
5. Stay with the person until help arrives.

From Bowman S et al: Reducing the health consequences of opioid addiction in primary care, *Am J Med* 126:565-571, 2013.

treatment of opioid use disorder in most patients because of increased risk of overdose death and infectious disease (e.g., HIV through IV drug use) following detoxification.
- Short- (30 days) or long-term (30 to 180 days) protocols.
- Buprenorphine (opioid partial agonist) or methadone (opioid agonist) is initiated in tapering doses.
- CDC guidelines advise naloxone coprescription to patients with a history of overdose, substance use disorder, and concurrent benzodiazepine use as well as patients using higher doses of opioids (defined as at least 50 mg of morphine [or equivalent]). Every state in the U.S. now has a naloxone access law that allows an individual to obtain naloxone without a personal prescription. Laws also grant civil and criminal immunity to laypersons who administer naloxone.
- Clonidine 0.1 mg bid to tid can be used to minimize autonomic symptoms (sweating) and craving.
- Nonsteroidal antiinflammatory drugs for body and muscle aches.
- The anticholinergic dicyclomine can be used to minimize gastrointestinal hyperactivity.
- Nonbenzodiazepine hypnotics, low-dose atypical antipsychotics (e.g., quetiapine), or low-dose tricyclic antidepressants are effective for promoting adequate sleep.
- Psychosocial supports tailored to patient needs should be offered as an adjunct to medical treatment.

CHRONIC Rx
Opioid antagonist treatment:
- Buprenorphine/naloxone is the preferred first-line treatment. Methadone is an alternative in certain populations.
- Naltrexone: Does not stabilize neuronal circuitry like partial or full opioid agonists and generally results in poor outcomes, much like Antabuse for alcohol.
- Opioid partial agonist therapy: Buprenorphine (Suboxone, Bunavail).
- Opioid agonist therapy: Methadone.
- NOTE: Buprenorphine and methadone are both metabolized by the cytochrome P-450 3a4 and 2d6 I isoenzyme pathways. Prescribers should be aware of multiple possible drug interactions. Methadone and buprenorphine produce similar improvements during opioid withdrawal, although buprenorphine is associated with less sedation and respiratory depression. To avoid precipitating more intense withdrawal, buprenorphine should be initiated 12 to 18 h after the last administration of opioids in patients who misuse shorter-acting opioids (48 h in patients who are receiving long-acting drugs such as methadone), with initial doses of 4 to 8 mg.[2]

PATIENT SELECTION FOR BUPRENORPHINE OR METHADONE
- Appropriate patients for buprenorphine office-based treatment:

1. Patients interested (highly motivated) in treatment
2. Have no major contraindications (see following)
3. Can be expected to be reasonably compliant with treatment
4. Understand the benefits and risks of buprenorphine treatment
5. Willing to follow safety precautions
- Less likely to be appropriate for office-based treatment:
1. Have comorbid dependence on benzodiazepines or other CNS depressants (including ethylene alcohol)
2. Have significant untreated psychiatric comorbidities
3. Have active or chronic suicidal or homicidal ideation or attempts
4. Have multiple previous treatments with frequent relapses
5. Have poor response to previous treatment with buprenorphine
6. Have significant medical complications (e.g., hepatic insufficiency, bacterial endocarditis, active tuberculosis)
- Methadone maintenance: Narcotic treatment program (clinic setting) indications:
1. Evidence of opiate addiction >1 yr
2. Two failed previous treatment attempts
3. Patients not appropriate for office-based treatment
4. Eligible without active "use" if prior methadone maintenance patient within previous 2 mo
5. Pregnancy

DISPOSITION
- Opioid addiction is a chronic, relapsing disease
- High rate of relapse after "detox"
- Relapse potential after medically supervised withdrawal from methadone:
1. 90% after 1 yr stable in treatment
2. 80% after 3 yr stable in treatment
3. 70% after 5 yr stable in treatment
- Postmarketing surveillance indicates that the diversion and abuse of prescription opioid medications increased between 2002 and 2010 and plateaued or decreased between 2011 and 2013. These findings suggest that the U.S. may be making some progress in controlling the abuse of opioid analgesics.[2]

REFERRAL
Refer to addiction medicine specialist or narcotic treatment program when the neurobiologic disease of opioid addiction is identified.

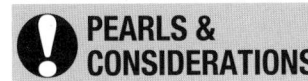 **PEARLS & CONSIDERATIONS**

COMMENTS
- Detoxification is contraindicated during pregnancy. Methadone maintenance has been the gold standard for the pregnant opioid-addicted patient regardless of the duration of the addiction or prior treatment attempts. The use

of buprenorphine in pregnancy is associated with a lower risk of adverse neonatal outcomes than methadone use; however, the risk of adverse maternal outcomes is similar among persons who receive buprenorphine and those who receive methadone.[3]

- Breastfeeding is encouraged in mothers on methadone maintenance. The American Academy of Pediatrics statement regarding "Transfer of Drugs and Other Chemicals into Human Milk" has placed methadone into the "usually compatible with breastfeeding" group based on the assumption that maternal urine is monitored to detect use of illicit drugs. The U.S. Department of Health and Human Services also recommends that mothers on methadone be encouraged to breastfeed.
- When a physician identifies a patient as a "drug seeker," it is imperative that the physician avoid abruptly stopping the opioid prescription because this will often result in the patient's buying the drugs illegally. These patients should be counseled and referred for treatment.
- Patients on methadone or buprenorphine who have pain resulting from an acute injury will need pain medication in addition to their daily dose of methadone or buprenorphine. They will require higher than usual doses of pain medications because of opioid receptor blockade attributable to their methadone or buprenorphine use.
- Opioid-dependent patients have a lower pain threshold resulting from hyperalgesia caused by the long-term use of opioids.

PREVENTION

Education is the hallmark of prevention:
- School drug prevention education programs.
- Educate children about their family medical history, including diseases of addiction.
- Address childhood psychiatric disorders to prevent self-medicating.
- Educate patients on nonopioid analgesics for pain management.

Opioid overdose:
- Naloxone (Narcan) is a competitive mμ-opioid receptor antagonist in the brain and is effective for opioid overdose. It is available for IM/IV and intranasal administration. It begins

---

TABLE 5   Organizations Providing Referral Information for Patients

Organization	Resources/Website
Substance Abuse and Mental Health Services Administration (SAMHSA)	Opioid treatment program directory: www.dpt2.samhsa.gov/treatment/.
Physicians who provide buprenorphine	Buprenorphine physician and treatment program locator: www.samhsa.gov/medication-assisted-treatment/treatment/buprenorphine.
Pain Action	Chronic pain management materials for patients: www.painaction.com/.
Substance abuse treatment facilities	Substance Abuse treatment facility locator: http://dasis3.samhsa.gov/.
Harm Reduction Coalition	Local risk reduction resources and programs, overdose prevention education, and naloxone prescribing information: www.harmreduction.org/.
Narcotics Anonymous (NA)	General information and meeting information for NA, a 12-step program modeled after Alcoholics Anonymous: www.na.org/.

From Bowman S et al: Reducing the health consequences of opioid addiction in primary care, *Am J Med* 126:565-571, 2013.

to reverse respiratory depression, sedation, and hypotension 2 to 5 min after IM administration and 1 to 2 min after IV administration. Treatment of opioid overdose is summarized in Box 5.

PATIENT & FAMILY EDUCATION

- Stigma of addictions and treatment often interferes with good treatment.
- Family needs to be educated so they can support the patient's efforts.
- Encourage family meeting with addiction specialist, counselor.
- Recommend support groups for family members. Table 5 identifies organizations providing referral information for patients.

Recommendations for integrating risk reduction strategies for addressing opioid misuse in the primary care setting are summarized in Table E6.
- Physicians should also offer reliant immunizations to people with OUD, including hepatitis A and B and TDAP and consider referral to syringe service programs.[1]

REFERENCES & SUGGESTED READINGS
Available at eBooks.Health.Elsevier.com.

RELATED CONTENT
Drug Use Disorder (Patient Information)
Opioid Overdose (Related Key Topic)

AUTHOR: **FRED F. FERRI, MD**

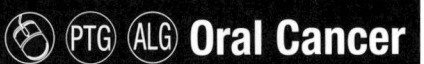

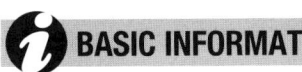 **BASIC INFORMATION**

DEFINITION

Oral cancers refer to malignant transformation of the oral tissues usually preceded by a process of sequential dysplastic changes leading to the development of squamous carcinoma. Oral squamous cell cancers (OSCC) include oral cavity cancers (lip, floor of mouth, buccal mucosa, anterior tongue, gingivae, hard palate, retromolar trigone), oropharynx cancers (base of tongue, tonsils, soft palate, pharyngeal walls), and hypopharynx cancers (pyriform sinus, postcricoid area, posterior pharyngeal wall).

SYNONYMS

Head and neck cancer
Oral malignant neoplasm
OSCC

ICD-10CM CODES

C01	Malignant neoplasm of base of tongue
C03	Malignant neoplasm of gum
C04	Malignant neoplasm of floor of mouth
C05	Malignant neoplasm of palate
C06	Malignant neoplasm of other and unspecified parts of mouth
C09	Malignant neoplasm of tonsil
C10	Malignant neoplasm of oropharynx
C11	Malignant neoplasm of nasopharynx
C12	Malignant neoplasm of piriform sinus
C13	Malignant neoplasm of hypopharynx
C14	Malignant neoplasm of other and ill-defined sites of lip, oral cavity and larynx
C14.0	Malignant neoplasm of pharynx, unspecified
C14.2	Malignant neoplasm of Waldeyer ring
C14.8	Malignant neoplasm of overlapping sites of lip, oral cavity and pharynx

EPIDEMIOLOGY & DEMOGRAPHICS

INCIDENCE & PREVALENCE:

- In 2022, there were an estimated 54,000 new cases and 11,230 deaths in the U.S.[1]
- The incidence of oral cancers linked to alcohol and tobacco use has declined in the U.S. and other developed countries, whereas those linked to the human papillomavirus (HPV), primarily HPV type 16, have increased for cancers in the tonsils and base of tongue.[2] Differences between the traditional nonhuman papillomavirus–associated vs. HPV-associated oropharyngeal squamous cell carcinoma are summarized in Table 1.
- In Asian countries where chewing betel nut is customary, oral cancer accounts for up to 40% of cancers in some regions.

PREDOMINANT SEX & AGE: The ratio of oral cancer in males:females is 2.5:1 in the U.S. Black males have a higher early incidence in the 50-yr to 60-yr age group, but with increasing age, White men predominate.

RISK FACTORS (FIG. 1): The following factors are implicated in the development of oral cancer:
- Tobacco use
- HPV infection (primarily types 16 and 18)
- Alcohol
- Immune deficiency
- Radiation
- Betel nut consumption
- Solar radiation

GENETICS: The genes that are critically altered in OSCC include *TP53*, the retinoblastoma family, *p16* and cyclin *D1*. The *TP53, CCND1,* and *CDKN2A* genes are established cancer genes in HPV-negative cancers.[3] *TP53* and the genes encoding the Rb family are established cancer genes in HPV-positive cancers. Signaling pathways that are involved in the pathogenesis of oral cancers include that of the human epidermal receptor (HER) family, vascular endothelial growth factor (VEGF) receptor, and signal transducer and activator of transcription 3 (STAT 3). The tumor suppressor gene *TP53* is frequently mutated in HPV-negative tumors.

PHYSICAL FINDINGS & CLINICAL PRESENTATION

- Specific patient complaints may include the following: Oral ulcers or mass, choking, difficulty breathing, dysphagia, odynophagia, voice hoarseness, globus sensation, otalgia, ear or nose stuffiness, hemoptysis, trismus, neck mass, and pain in the head/neck region.
- Generalized symptoms and signs may include weight loss, fatigue, anorexia, altered mood, and sleep.
- Clinically, oral cancers can present as:
  1. Erythroplakia (flat red patch); can mimic inflammatory or traumatic lesions
  2. Leukoplakia (white patch; Fig. E2)
  3. Raised lesion
  4. Ulcerated lesion
  5. Warty lesion or growth

DIAGNOSIS

DIFFERENTIAL DIAGNOSIS

- Oral leukoplakia
- Invasive fungal infections
- Chancre of early syphilis and gumma of tertiary syphilis
- Chronic ulcer
- Metastatic or locally invading cancers from sinuses or other sites of the body

WORKUP

- Primary workup includes either biopsy or fine-needle aspiration (FNA) of the presenting lesion or suspected neck lymph node for histopathologic analysis. HPV assessment with p16 immunohistochemical staining and confirmatory in situ hybridization (ISH) testing is performed when indicated for oropharynx primary tumors.
- Detailed examination of the oral cavity, pharynx, larynx, neck, ears, nose, and cranial nerves should be performed.
- Laryngoscopy and examination under anesthesia are commonly performed.
- Pretreatment evaluation of tumor size, the extent of invasion, and the presence or absence of regional lymph node metastases is critical for planning treatment.
- Laboratory workup can include complete blood count, complete chemistry panel, and thyroid function.
- Staging workup includes CT or MRI imaging of the head and neck and a chest X-ray. If locoregional or advanced disease is a consideration, a PET scan is typically completed.

TABLE 1 Differences Between the Traditional Nonhuman Papillomavirus–Associated Versus Human Papillomavirus–Associated Oropharyngeal Squamous Cell Carcinoma

Variables	Traditional Non–HPV-Associated OPSCC	HPV-Associated OPSCC
Demographics	Older (age $\geq$60 yr); male:female = 3:2	Younger (age 40-60 yr); male:female = 3:1, Caucasians
Risk profile	Tobacco, alcohol	Minimal/no addiction habit, epidemiologic correlation with sexual history
Molecular biology	p16 inactivation, p53 mutation, higher mutation rates and genetic instability	p16 overexpression, wild-type p53, lower mutation rates
Pathology	Keratinizing SCC, well to moderate to poorly differentiated	Nonkeratinizing SCC, poorly differentiated
Clinical presentation	Less bulky nodes	Small/unknown primary with bulky, cystic, or multiple nodes
Prognosis	Guarded, 5-yr survivals ~40%-60%	Good, 5-yr survivals ~80%-90%
Prognostic variables	T- and N-category, margin, ENE, smoking	T-category, five or more metastatic nodes, margins (?)
Mode of recurrence	Locoregional recurrence more frequent	Locoregional recurrence infrequent, distant metastasis predominant mode

ENE, Extracapsular extension; *HPV,* human papillomavirus; *OPSCC,* oropharyngeal squamous cell carcinoma; *SCC,* squamous cell carcinoma.

From Flint PW et al: *Cummings otolaryngology, head and neck surgery,* ed 7, Philadelphia, 2021, Elsevier.

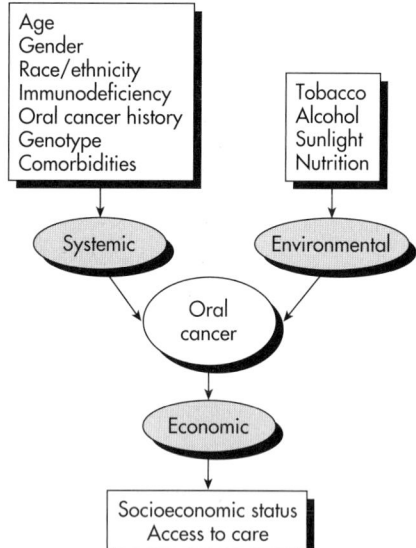

FIG. 1 Risk model for oral cancer. Oral cancer is a multifactorial disease process that includes systemic, environmental, and economic effects. The interplay of these variables ultimately leads to the incidence of this disease. The multifactorial nature of oral cancer should be addressed in the assessment of a patient's risk. (From Jones DL, Rankin KV: Oral cancer and associated risk factors. In Cappelli D, Mobley C [eds]: *Prevention in clinical oral health care,* St Louis, 2008, Elsevier, pp. 68-77.)

- The tumor, node, and metastasis (TNM) system is used for staging of OSCC and is subdivided according to primary tumor sites: (1) lip and oral cavity, (2) pharynx.

℞ TREATMENT

- Fig. 3 illustrates a management algorithm for squamous cell carcinoma of the oropharynx.
- Surgery, radiation therapy, and chemotherapy are treatment modalities involved in the treatment plan for OSCC.
- The use of supportive and special therapeutic modalities such as nutritional therapy including feeding gastrostomy, speech and swallowing therapy, reconstructive surgery, and speech prosthesis is required often.
- For treatment purposes OSCC are classified as early (T1 or T2 lesions), locoregional (T3 to T4 or any N), or metastatic (M1) stages. Site-specific TNM staging is done as per the primary tumor site (e.g., oral cavity, oropharynx, hypopharynx, etc.).
- After staging completion, the initial treatment considerations include:[4,5]
  1. Determination of primary tumor resectability (resectable vs. unresectable)
  2. Management of neck nodes
  3. Intent of radiation therapy (curative vs. palliative)
  4. Need for organ preservation
  5. Need for reconstructive surgery
  6. Need for chemotherapy
  7. HPV status of tumor

- Localized tumors (stage I or II) can be approached by initial surgical resection or definitive radiotherapy. Locoregionally advanced tumors (stage III and localized IV) that are resectable are typically approached by upfront surgery followed by adjuvant radiation and/or chemotherapy. Unresectable patients are typically treated with definitive chemotherapy and radiotherapy. Patients with distant metastatic disease are treated with systemic chemotherapy, while locally recurrent tumors can be approached with either surgery or chemotherapy or both.
- Surgery is typically associated with less long-term morbidity than radiation therapy. Surgical therapy traditionally involved wide-exposure approaches (mandibulotomy, trans-pharyngeal access). Newer surgical techniques allow tumor resection through the mouth. Recently, transoral robotic surgery (TORS) has been developed to improve access to oropharyngeal squamous cell carcinomas with excellent oncologic outcomes.[6]
  1. Acute surgical complications can include infection, bleeding, aspiration, wound breakdown, fistula, and flap loss.
  2. Surgical procedures can cause functional deficits in speech and swallowing, but these adverse effects can be minimized by appropriate reconstruction and prostheses.
  3. Recent randomized trial data results have demonstrated equivalent results with sentinel lymph node biopsy vs. neck dissection in early (T1 to T2) oral cancer cases.
- Definitive radiation therapy is reserved for patients who cannot tolerate surgery or for whom surgical resection would result in particularly severe functional impairment.
  1. Radiation therapy can include external beam radiation and brachytherapy.
  2. Radiation therapy side effects include mucositis, radiation dermatitis, loss of taste, dysphagia, dental caries and decay, and xerostomia.
  3. Late complications can include skin/soft tissue atrophy and fibrosis, osteoradionecrosis, and trismus.
- Systemic chemotherapy can be administered alone or in combination with radiotherapy, depending on the disease stage. Agents typically used include cisplatin, carboplatin, 5-fluorouracil, taxanes, and the epidermal growth factor receptor (EGFR) antibody cetuximab.
- For locally advanced OSCC, the combination of cisplatin and radiotherapy is the regimen of choice. Recent reports have demonstrated similar outcomes with standard every-3-wk administered cisplatin and lower doses of once-weekly administered cisplatin, but with lower toxicity rates.[7] Cetuximab was demonstrated to be inferior to cisplatin when used concurrently with radiotherapy in patients with locally advanced HPV-positive oral cancers. In selected patients with large primary tumors or bulky nodal disease, neoadjuvant chemotherapy may be utilized prior to chemo-radiotherapy administration.

- Patients who have metastatic cancers or unresectable locoregional recurrences usually are treated with systemic chemotherapy.
- Front-line chemoimmunotherapy with a regimen consisting of platinum plus 5-fluorouracil chemotherapy in combination with the checkpoint inhibitor, pembrolizumab has been demonstrated to be a superior regimen in patients with recurrent or metastatic head and neck cancer.[8] Alternatively, doublet chemotherapy regimens (platinum plus either 5-fluorouracil or platinum plus taxane) can be combined with the EGFR–targeting antibody cetuximab in this setting.
- In patients who have not received checkpoint inhibitor therapy previously, nivolumab and pembrolizumab have been shown to improve survival outcomes after failure of first-line chemotherapy.
- The negative predictive value of posttreatment PET imaging in patients with locally advanced cancer who have been treated with chemo-radiotherapy is 98% to 99%.

DISPOSITION

- Prognosis depends on the staging and resectability of the primary tumor as well as on patient performance status.
- Tumor HPV status is a strong and independent prognostic factor for survival among patients with base of tongue and oropharyngeal cancer.

REFERRAL

Referral to multidisciplinary head and neck cancer team consisting of ENT or head/neck surgeon, radiation oncologist, medical oncologist, speech therapy, and dietitian.

❗ PEARLS & CONSIDERATIONS

COMMENTS

- Oral cavity cancer is the sixth most common cancer globally.
- Biopsy with HPV-status assessment is the key for accurate diagnosis.
- Posttreatment rehabilitation and surveillance is important.

PREVENTION

- Encourage patients to stop using any type of tobacco and drinking alcohol.
- Examine oral cavities at annual checkups and work up suspicious lesions.

REFERENCES
Available at eBooks.Health.Elsevier.com.

RELATED CONTENT
Mouth Cancer (Patient Information)

AUTHOR: **RITESH RATHORE, MD**

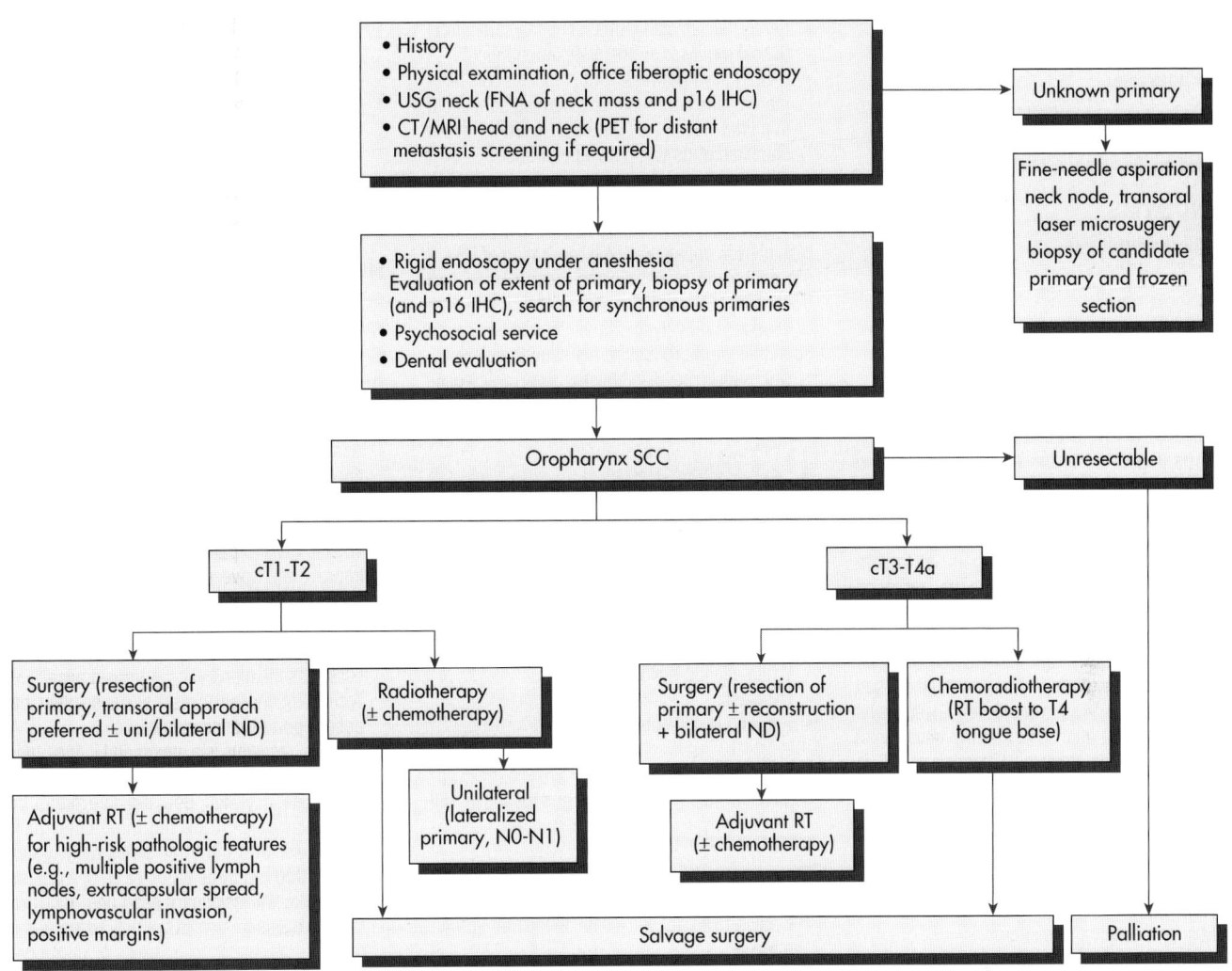

FIG. 3 Management algorithm for squamous cell carcinoma *(SCC)* of the oropharynx. *CT*, Computed tomography; *cT#*, clinical tumor stage; *FNA*, fine-needle aspiration; *IHC*, immunohistochemistry; *MRI*, magnetic resonance imaging; *ND*, neck dissection; *PET*, positron emission tomography; *RT*, radiotherapy; *USG*, ultrasonography. (From Flint PW et al: *Cummings otolaryngology, head and neck surgery,* ed 7, Philadelphia, 2021, Elsevier.)

Oral Hairy Leukoplakia 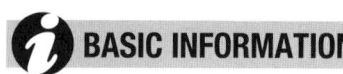 (PTG)

BASIC INFORMATION

DEFINITION
Oral hairy leukoplakia (OHL) is a painless, white, nonremovable, plaque-like lesion typically located on the lateral aspect of the tongue.

SYNONYMS
Oral hairy leukoplakia
OHL

ICD-10CM CODE
K13.3 Hairy leukoplakia

EPIDEMIOLOGY & DEMOGRAPHICS
INCIDENCE & PREVALENCE: Epstein-Barr virus (EBV) is implicated in the etiology of OHL, and the incidence of EBV seroprevalence is high in individuals who are HIV seropositive. OHL may also occur in other immunosuppressed individuals, for example, organ transplant recipients, as well as individuals receiving systemic or inhaled steroids.[1]
RISK FACTORS: OHL is usually found in HIV-seropositive individuals but may also be identified in smokers and other immunocompromised patients, such as transplant recipients (particularly renal and bone marrow transplants) and patients taking steroids.[2] Diagnosis of OHL is an indication to test for HIV.

PHYSICAL FINDINGS & CLINICAL PRESENTATION
- Varying morphology and appearance (Fig. E1), which may change daily.
- May be unilateral or bilateral.
- White plaques can be small with fine, vertical corrugations on the lateral margin of the tongue (Fig. 2). The plaques from OHL are adherent to the tongue surface (in contrast to candidal plaques, which may be easily scraped off).
- Irregular surface; may have prominent folds or projection, occasionally markedly resembling hairs.
- May spread to cover the entire dorsal surface or spread onto the ventral surface of the tongue where the lesions usually appear flat.

- Rarely, lesions can manifest on the soft palate, buccal mucosa, or posterior oropharynx.
- Usually asymptomatic, but some patients have mouth pain, soreness, or a burning sensation; impaired taste, or difficulty eating; others complain of its unsightly appearance.[3]

ETIOLOGY
EBV is implicated in the etiology of OHL. It likely results from unchecked lytic replication of EBV in the epithelium of keratinized cells. OHL differs from most EBV-related diseases in that infection is predominantly lytic rather than latent, with abundant virus production resulting in cell lysis.

OHL should be differentiated from oral leukoplakia, which is a potentially premalignant condition.

DIAGNOSIS

DIFFERENTIAL DIAGNOSIS
- Oral homogenous/nonhomogeneous leukoplakia
- *Candida albicans*
- Lichen planus
- Idiopathic leukoplakia
- White sponge nevus
- Dysplasia
- Squamous cell carcinoma

WORKUP
Requires physical examination and testing for HIV

LABORATORY TESTS
The *provisional* diagnosis is clinical and based on:
- Visual inspection
- Inability to scrape the lesion off the tongue with a blade
- Failure to respond to antifungal therapy
The *presumptive* diagnosis requires biopsy and histologic demonstration of:
- Epithelial hyperplasia with hairs
- Absence of inflammatory cell infiltrate
The *definitive* diagnosis requires:
- In situ hybridization of histologic or cytologic specimens revealing EBV DNA *or*
- Electron microscopy of specimens revealing herpes-like particles

- Measurement of the DNA content in cells of oral leukoplakia may be used to predict the risk of oral carcinoma
- NOTE: Specimens obtained from lesions may demonstrate hyphae of *Candida albicans,* which may coexist and potentiate EBV-induced OHL[3]

TREATMENT

NONPHARMACOLOGIC THERAPY
OHL is usually asymptomatic and requires no specific therapy. It may resolve spontaneously and is generally benign in HIV-seropositive patients.

ACUTE GENERAL Rx
- Antiretroviral therapy (ART) has considerably changed the frequency of oral lesions caused by opportunistic infections in HIV-seropositive individuals.
- Topical retinoids (0.1% vitamin A) may improve the appearance of OHL-affected oral surfaces through their dekeratinizing and immunomodulation effects; however, they are expensive, and prolonged use may result in a burning sensation over the treated area.
- Topical podophyllin resin 25% solution has been reported to induce resolution.
- Surgical excision and cryotherapy may help, but the lesions may recur.
- High-dose acyclovir 800 mg five times per day, valacyclovir 1000 mg three times daily, famciclovir 500 mg three times daily, ganciclovir 1000 mg three times daily, or foscarnet 40 mg/kg intravenous three times daily will cause lesions to resolve but only temporarily.[3]

REFERRAL
Referral to ENT or oral surgeon for biopsy of tongue to confirm diagnosis.

PEARLS & CONSIDERATIONS

- OHL may be the presenting sign of patients infected with HIV who are unaware of their status.
- The incidence has decreased significantly in the era of antiretroviral therapy.

REFERENCES
Available at eBooks.Health.Elsevier.com.

RELATED CONTENT
Acquired Immunodeficiency Syndrome (Related Key Topic)
Oral Hairy Leukoplakia (Patient Information)
Epstein-Barr Virus Infection (Related Key Topic)
Human Immunodeficiency Virus (Related Key Topic)

AUTHORS: **SAJEEV HANDA, MD, SFHM,** and **ANNA HARDESTY, MD**

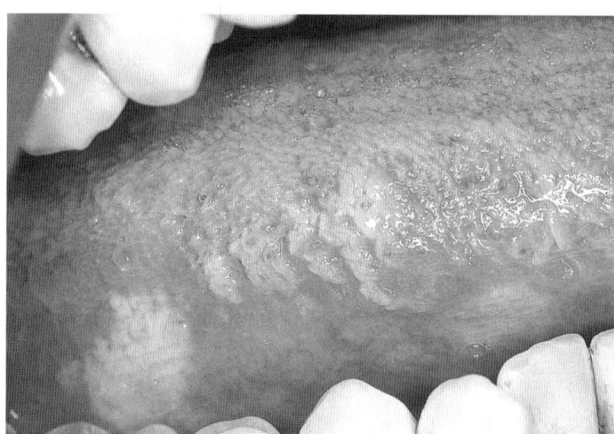

FIG. 2 Oral hairy leukoplakia along the lateral tongue margin is characterized by vertically corrugated keratotic ridges. (From Flint PW et al: *Cummings otolaryngology, head and neck surgery,* ed 7, Philadelphia, 2021, Elsevier.)

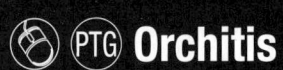

O

 BASIC INFORMATION

DEFINITION

Orchitis is an inflammatory process (usually infectious) involving the testicles. Infection may be viral or bacterial and can be associated with infection of other male sex organs (prostate, epididymis, or bladder) or lower urogenital tract or sexually transmitted diseases often via hematogenous spread. Common causes are:

- Viral: Mumps—20% postpubertal; Coxsackie B virus
- Bacterial: Pyogenic via spread from involving epididymis; bacteria include *Escherichia coli*, *Klebsiella pneumoniae*, *P. aeruginosa*, *Staphylococcus*, *Streptococcus* or *Rickettsia*, *Brucella* spp.; in sexually active men: *Neisseria gonorrhoeae* and *Chlamydia trachomatis*
- Other:
  1. Viral—HIV-associated, Cytomegalovirus (CMV), Zika
  2. Fungi
     a. Cryptococcosis
     b. Histoplasmosis
     c. *Candida*
     d. Blastomycosis
     e. Syphilis
  3. *Mycobacterium tuberculosis* and *M. leprae*
  4. Parasitic causes: Toxoplasmosis, filariasis, schistosomiasis
- Table 1 describes a classification of epididymitis and orchitis based on etiology

SYNONYMS

Epididymo-orchitis
Testicular infection
Testicular inflammation

ICD-10CM CODES
N45.9 Orchitis, epididymitis, and epididymo-orchitis without abscess
A54.1 Gonococcal orchitis
A56.1 Chlamydial orchitis
N51.1 Mumps orchitis

EPIDEMIOLOGY & DEMOGRAPHICS

PREDOMINANT SEX: Male
PREDOMINANT ORGANISM: The leading cause of viral orchitis is mumps. The mumps virus rarely causes orchitis in prepubertal males but involves one or both testicles in nearly 30% of postpubertal males.

PHYSICAL FINDINGS & CLINICAL PRESENTATION

- Testicular pain, unilateral or bilateral swelling
- May have associated epididymitis, prostatitis, fever, scrotal edema, erythema, cellulitis
- Inguinal lymphadenopathy
- Acute hydrocele (bacterial)
- Rare development: Abscess formation, pyocele of scrotum, testicular infarction
- Spermatic cord tenderness may be present
- Granulomatous

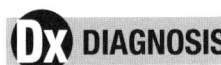 **DIAGNOSIS**

Clinical presentation as described previously with possible history of acute viral illness or concomitant epididymitis

DIFFERENTIAL DIAGNOSIS

- Epididymo-orchitis-gonococcal
- Autoimmune disease
- Vasculitis
- Epididymitis
- Mumps, with or without parotitis
- Neoplasm
- Hematoma
- Spermatic cord torsion
- Behçet disease

LABORATORY TESTS

- CBC with differential
- Urinalysis
- Viral titer—mumps. Mumps immunoglobulin M (IgM) will be detectable after 5 days of onset of clinical mumps and remain positive for up to 4 wk. A reverse-transcriptase polymerase chain reaction (RT-PCR) on serum or buccal or oral swab is another option
- Urine culture for mumps virus
- Ultrasound of testicle to rule out abscess
- Urine nucleic acid amplification tests (NAATs) for *Neisseria gonorrhoeae* and *Chlamydia trachomatis*

IMAGING STUDIES

Ultrasound if abscess suspected

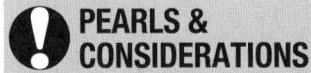 **TREATMENT**

- Dependent on cause
- Viral (mumps): Observation; bed rest, ice packs, analgesics, and a scrotal sling for support may provide some relief of discomfort that accompanies mumps orchitis
- Bacterial: Empiric antibiotic treatment with parenteral antibiotic treatment until pathogen identified:
  1. Ceftriaxone 500 mg IM as a single dose for persons weighing <150 kg (300 lb), 1 g of IM ceftriaxone for persons weighing ≥150 kg (300 lb) plus doxycycline (100 mg PO bid for 10 days), in men <35 yr old to cover *Neisseria gonorrhoeae* and *Chlamydia trachomatis*. In men who have sex with men or men >35 yr old: Levofloxacin 500 to 750 mg IV/PO qd for 10 to 14 days *or* ampicillin-sulbactam *or* third-generation cephalosporin or piperacillin/tazobactam
- Surgery for abscess, pyogenic process

DISPOSITION

Follow-up for evidence of recurrence, hypogonadism, and infertility may be needed with bilateral orchitis.

REFERRAL

- To a urologist if surgical drainage is needed
- To an endocrinologist if hypogonadism develops
- To a fertility specialist if infertility develops

(!) **PEARLS & CONSIDERATIONS**

Consider tuberculous orchitis if symptoms fail to respond to standard antibacterial therapy, even in the absence of chest radiographic evidence of pulmonary tuberculosis.

SUGGESTED READING
Available at eBooks.Health.Elsevier.com

RELATED CONTENT

Orchitis (Patient Information)
Epididymitis (Related Key Topic)
Mumps (Related Key Topic)

AUTHOR: **GLENN G. FORT, MD, MPH**

TABLE 1 Classification of Epididymitis and Orchitis

Acute Epididymitis or Epididymo-Orchitis	Granulomatous Epididymitis or Orchitis	Viral Orchitis
Neisseria gonorrhoeae	*Mycobacterium tuberculosis*	Mumps
Chlamydia trachomatis	*Treponema pallidum*	Enteroviruses
Escherichia coli		
Streptococcus pneumoniae		
Klebsiella spp.	*Brucella* spp.	
Salmonella spp.	Sarcoid	
Other urinary tract pathogens	Fungal	
Idiopathic	Parasitic	
	Idiopathic	

From Cohen J, Powderly WG: *Infectious diseases*, ed 2, St Louis, 2004, Mosby.

BASIC INFORMATION

DEFINITION

Orthostatic hypotension (OH) is defined as the presence of at least one of the following:
- Decrease in systolic blood pressure by ≥20 mm Hg *or*
- Decrease in diastolic blood pressure by ≥10 mm Hg, within 3 min of standing
It is a physical sign that requires further investigation to discern its underlying etiology.

Recent studies have shown that blood pressure measurements within 1 min might be more useful in predicting fractures, falls, and other adverse events and that for most patients, assessment within 1 min of standing rather than waiting for 3 min may be sufficient.[1]

SYNONYMS

Postural hypotension
OH

ICD-10CM CODE
I95.1 Orthostatic hypotension

EPIDEMIOLOGY & DEMOGRAPHICS

- The incidence of OH is increased in older people. Surveys have shown OH to be present in approximately 20% of adults over 65 yr of age.
- Also, higher incidence noted in those with diseases associated with autonomic dysfunction (e.g., Parkinson disease, diabetes mellitus).
- OH may cause up to 30% of all syncopal events in the elderly, and OH is associated with an increased risk of heart failure among those aged 45 to 55 yr and an increased risk of cardiovascular disease and all-cause mortality among those aged 55 yr and older.
- OH can be a common cause and/or a contributor to hospitalization in older adult patients.[2]
- There is an association between orthostatic hypotension and cognitive dysfunction among older adults.

PHYSICAL FINDINGS & CLINICAL PRESENTATION

- Symptoms may include dizziness, lightheadedness, syncope, visual and auditory disturbances, weakness, diaphoresis, pallor, and nausea.
- OH may be asymptomatic, especially in older hypertensive patients with autonomic dysfunction. These patients tend to have systolic hypertension when seated or supine.
- Associated with increased autonomic activity during meals (from increased splanchnic blood flow), exercise, prolonged standing, and hot weather.
- Supine and nocturnal hypertension in patients with OH may indicate an underlying autonomic dysfunction.

ETIOLOGY

- There are two main mechanisms for OH: Autonomic dysfunction and volume depletion.

- Normal response: Assumption of an upright posture results in the pooling of approximately 500 ml of blood in the lower extremities due to gravity and decreased venous return, decreased cardiac output, and decreased arterial pressure. The consequent increase in sympathetic tone due to increased carotid baroreceptor activity causes arterial and venous constriction as well as positive inotropic and chronotropic effects, thereby limiting the fall in upright blood pressure. Peripheral vasoconstriction is also mediated by increased activity of the renin-angiotensin system and decreased activity of atrial natriuretic factor.
- Autonomic dysfunction: Impairment of the baroreceptor reflex, as in central (such as Parkinson disease) or peripheral autonomic dysfunction (such as diabetes) and aging, may cause OH because decreased blood pressure cannot be counteracted by the aforementioned regulatory mechanisms.
- Volume depletion: May be caused by diuretics, vomiting, hemorrhage, and hyperglycemia. Mechanism of OH in these patients is similar to what is described earlier, with failure of the regulatory mechanisms kicking in.

DIAGNOSIS

DIFFERENTIAL DIAGNOSIS (BOX 1)

Common:
- Medications: Antihypertensives, antidepressants (tricyclics), antipsychotics (phenothiazines), alcohol, narcotics, barbiturates, insulin, nitrates, PDE-5 inhibitors, alpha-adrenergic antagonists
- Reduced intravascular volume (hemorrhage, dehydration, hyperglycemia, hypoalbuminemia)
- Postprandial effect (especially in the elderly)
- Vasovagal syncope
- Deconditioning
- Central autonomic dysfunction (Parkinson disease)
- Peripheral autonomic dysfunction (diabetes mellitus, Guillain-Barré syndrome)
Uncommon:
- Central autonomic dysfunction (Shy-Drager syndrome)
- Postganglionic autonomic dysfunction: Impaired norepinephrine release
- Autoimmune autonomic dysfunction: Nicotinic acetylcholine receptor autoantibodies
- Paraneoplastic autonomic dysfunction: Anti-Hu antibodies (in small-cell lung cancer)
- Postural tachycardia syndrome (POTS): Usually occurs in young women; an abnormally large increase in heart rate is observed in the upright position, caused by increased venous pooling from autonomic dysfunction of the lower extremities, but blood pressure is not affected because of an excess of plasma norepinephrine
- Impaired cardiac output (myocardial infarction, aortic stenosis, arrhythmias)
- Cerebrovascular accident

- Adrenal insufficiency
- Deconditioning
- Carotid sinus hypersensitivity
- Anxiety, panic attacks
- Seizures
- Sepsis
- Idiopathic

WORKUP

- Obtain a detailed history including medication list, recent history of potential volume loss, medical history of congestive heart failure, malignancy, diabetes and alcoholism, evidence on history and physical examination of parkinsonism, ataxia, peripheral neuropathy, or dysautonomia.[3]
- In assessing patients for orthostatic hypotension, blood pressure measurement changes going from supine to standing are more sensitive than going from sitting to standing.[4]
- Measure supine blood pressure after the patient has been resting comfortably. The duration of time that the patient should spend supine and standing when measuring orthostatic hypotension is controversial. Limited

---

BOX 1 Differential Diagnosis of Orthostatic Hypotension

Autonomic Disorders
Pure autonomic failure
Multiple system atrophy
Familial dysautonomia
Dopamine β-hydroxylase deficiency
Baroreflex failure
Secondary autonomic neuropathies
Hypovolemia Disorders
Hemorrhage or plasma loss
Overdiuresis
Overdialysis
Idiopathic hypovolemia
Endocrinologic disorders
Addison disease
Hypoaldosteronism
Pheochromocytoma
Renovascular hypertension
Vascular insufficiency
Varicose veins
Absent venous valves
Arteriovenous malformations
Vasodilator excess
Mastocytosis (histamine, prostaglandin D_2)
Hyperbradykininism (bradykinin)
Carcinoid (bradykinin)
Hypermagnesemia
Paroxysmal autonomic syncope
Glossopharyngeal syncope
Micturition syncope
Carotid sinus syncope
Swallow syncope
Cough syncope
Bezold-Jarisch reflex activation
Miscellaneous
Drugs and toxins
Stokes-Adams attacks
Gastrectomy
Hypokinesia, weightlessness, bed rest

From Jankovic J et al: *Bradley and Daroff's neurology in clinical practice*, ed 8, Philadelphia, 2022, Elsevier.

evidence supports having the patient remain supine for 5 to 10 min before obtaining the supine blood pressure, followed by blood pressure measurement within 1 min of standing and again after 3 min of standing. The blood pressure cuff must be held at the level of the right atrium; holding the cuff below this level will result in a 5 to 10 mm Hg underestimation of blood pressure.
- Thorough neurologic examination should be performed.

LABORATORY TESTS
- Hemoglobin and hematocrit
- Consider blood urea nitrogen/creatinine if suspecting dehydration as the cause
- ECG if suspecting underlying cardiac cause
- Consider when treatable causes of OH have been ruled out:
  1. Blood pressure and heart rate monitoring with a tilt-table test
  2. Plasma norepinephrine measurements (to distinguish postganglionic from preganglionic autonomic dysfunction)
  3. Other methods, which use the Valsalva maneuver or measure sweating as indirect means of evaluating the autonomic nervous system

IMAGING STUDIES
None

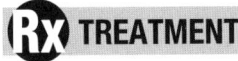 **TREATMENT**

NONPHARMACOLOGIC THERAPY[4]
- Patient education (leg crossing, prolonged sitting before first standing in the morning, avoid excessive straining and hot baths)
- High-salt diet (e.g., bouillon cubes); caution if history of heart failure
- Liberal fluid intake
- Take needed antihypertensive medications at different times of the day
- Raise the head of the bed at night
- Compression stockings (to include splanchnic circulation)
- Multiple low-carbohydrate meals to avoid postprandial OH
- Avoid large carbohydrate loads and excess alcohol consumption

ACUTE GENERAL Rx
- Correction of volume status and impairment of cerebral perfusion.
- Review medication list and attempt to eliminate those potentially contributing to OH.

CHRONIC Rx
- Fludrocortisone: 0.1 mg/day (may combine with an alpha-1 agonist to lower the dose of each); monitor for electrolyte disturbances and supine hypertension
- Midodrine (alpha-1 agonist): 10 mg three times a day; monitor for supine hypertension
- Erythropoietin (consider if anemic)
- Caffeine (for postprandial hypotension)
- Table 1 summarizes management of orthostatic hypotension in older adults.

OTHER TREATMENTS
- Pyridostigmine (enhances renal sodium reabsorption): 0.2 to 0.6 mg/day (not U.S. Food and Drug Administration [FDA] approved for this indication)
- Octreotide: 300 to 600 mg/day (not FDA approved for this indication)
- Indomethacin (prostaglandin inhibitor)
- DDAVP (experimental)
- Droxidopa (used for patients with autonomic dysfunction to increase the availability of norepinephrine) has been FDA approved for treatment of adults with symptomatic neurogenic orthostatic hypotension caused by primary autonomic failure or nondiabetic autonomic neuropathy

⊘ PEARLS & CONSIDERATIONS

COMMENTS
- The presence of OH should always trigger a search for an underlying etiology.
- OH is diagnosed by observing changes in blood pressure, not heart rate.
- Volume depletion should cause an increased heart rate on standing; a lack of heart rate response in this setting suggests autonomic dysfunction.
- Pharmacotherapy with mineralocorticoids may require concomitant potassium replenishment and monitoring for hypertension.
- Evidence to support the efficacy of pharmacologic interventions to treat OH, including midodrine, is limited.
- The etiology of OH is often multifactorial in older patients, but increased susceptibility to volume depletion due to decreased baroreceptor reflexes frequently contributes. Chronic vitamin D deficiency is associated with the development of OH.
- Intensive blood pressure control did not increase injurious falls compared with controls among community-dwelling older adults

TABLE 1 Management of Orthostatic Hypotension in Older Adults

Identify and treat correctable causes.

Reduce or eliminate drugs causing orthostatic hypotension.

Avoid situations that may exacerbate orthostatic hypotension.
- Standing motionless
- Prolonged recumbency
- Large meals
- Hot weather
- Hot showers
- Straining at stool or with voiding
- Isometric exercise
- Ingesting alcohol
- Hyperventilation
- Dehydration

Raise the head of the bed to a 5- to 20-degree angle.

Wear waist-high, custom-fitted, elastic stockings and an abdominal binder.

Participate in physical conditioning exercises.

Participate in controlled postural exercises using the tilt table.

Avoid diuretics and eat salt-containing fluids (unless congestive heart failure is present).

Drug therapy:
- Caffeine
- Fludrocortisone
- Midodrine
- Desmopressin
- Erythropoietin

From From Fillit HM: *Brocklehurst's textbook of geriatric medicine and gerontology,* ed 8, Philadelphia, 2017, Elsevier.

participating in the Systolic Blood Pressure Intervention Trial (SPRINT).
- The physical examination of patients with dizziness, gait disturbance, and/or falls should include an assessment for OH. OH is an independent predictor of unexplained falls in older adults.
- Because OH may be asymptomatic, physical examination of those at risk must include assessment of blood pressure in both the supine and upright positions.

AUTHOR: **HUSSAIN R. KHAWAJA, MD, FACP**

REFERENCES
Available at eBooks.Health.Elsevier.com.

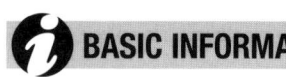

ⓘ BASIC INFORMATION

DEFINITION
Osteomyelitis is an acute or chronic infection of the bone secondary to the hematogenous or contiguous source of infection or direct traumatic inoculation, which is usually bacterial.

SYNONYM
Bone infection

ICD-10CM CODES
M86	Osteomyelitis
M86.0	Acute hematogenous osteomyelitis
M86.1	Other acute osteomyelitis
M86.2	Subacute osteomyelitis
M86.3	Chronic multifocal osteomyelitis
M86.6	Other chronic osteomyelitis
M86.9	Osteomyelitis, unspecified

EPIDEMIOLOGY & DEMOGRAPHICS
PREDOMINANT SEX: Male > female
PREDOMINANT AGE: All ages

PHYSICAL FINDINGS & CLINICAL PRESENTATION
HEMATOGENOUS OSTEOMYELITIS:
- Usually occurs in tibia/fibula (children)
- Localized inflammation: Often secondary to trauma with accompanying hematoma or cellulitis
- Abrupt fever
- Lethargy
- Irritability
- Pain in involved bone
VERTEBRAL OSTEOMYELITIS:
- Usually hematogenous
- Fever: 50%
- Localized pain/tenderness. Back pain is the most common initial symptom (86% of cases)
- Neurologic defects: Motor/sensory (sensory loss, weakness, radiculopathy)
CONTIGUOUS OSTEOMYELITIS:
- Direct inoculation
- Associated with trauma, fractures, surgical fixation
- Chronic infection of skin/soft tissue
- Fever, drainage from surgical site
CHRONIC OSTEOMYELITIS:
- Bone pain
- Sinus tract drainage, nonhealing ulcer
- Chronic low-grade fever
- Chronic localized pain

ETIOLOGY
- MSSA: Methicillin-sensitive *Staphylococcus aureus*
- MRSA: Methicillin-resistant *S. aureus*
- *Pseudomonas aeruginosa*
- *Enterobacteriaceae*
- *Streptococcus pyogenes*
- Enterococcus
- Mycobacteria

- Fungi
- Coagulase-negative staphylococci
- *Salmonella* (in sickle cell disease)

ⒹⓍ DIAGNOSIS

DIFFERENTIAL DIAGNOSIS
- Gaucher disease
- Bone infarction
- Charcot joint
- Fracture

WORKUP
- Erythrocyte sedimentation rate (ESR), C-reactive protein: Nondiagnostic but if significantly elevated they increase the pretest probability of osteomyelitis and can be useful in monitoring therapeutic response
- Blood culturing, CBC with differential
- Bone culture. A culture of a biopsy specimen has a significantly higher overall diagnostic yield than does a blood culture. Bone samples should be cultured for aerobic and anaerobic bacteria and for fungi
- Pathologic evaluation of bone biopsy for acute/chronic changes consistent with necrosis or acute inflammation
- Polymerase chain reaction (PCR) analysis of specimens obtained by means of biopsy or puncture may be useful for organisms that are difficult to identify (anaerobic bacteria, *Bartonella* sp., *Kingella kingae*); however, broad-range PCR has suboptimal sensitivity and specificity due to contamination and may not provide sufficient information on the susceptibility of the microorganisms to antibiotics

IMAGING STUDIES
- Bone radiograph examination (Fig. E1): Initial study but not sensitive in early osteomyelitis as may not show changes for as much as 2 wk
- MRI with and without contrast (Fig. E2): Most accurate imaging study. CT only if patient has contraindication to MRI
- Triple-phase technetium-99m bone scan (Fig. F3) when MRI is unavailable or contra-indicated. Typically positive within a few days after onset of symptoms but accuracy is lower than that of MRI
- Gallium scan (Ga-67) scintigraphy with single-photon emission CT (SPECT) has higher accuracy than bone scan but is less sensitive for detection of epidural abscess in vertebral osteomyelitis
- Indium-111–labeled leukocyte scintigraphy scan; low sensitivity (<20%) for vertebral osteomyelitis
- Positron emission tomography (PET) scanning with ^{18}F-fluorodeoxyglucose has high accuracy (similar to MRI) and is useful in patients with metallic implants
- Table 1 summarizes imaging findings in osteomyelitis

ⓇⓍ TREATMENT

- Surgical debridement in biopsy-positive cases will guide direction for antibiotic therapy. This will vary with type of osteomyelitis. Duration of therapy is usually 4 to 6 wk for acute osteomyelitis; chronic osteomyelitis may need a longer course of medication
- Orthopedic hardware should be removed if possible
- *S. aureus* (MSSA): Cefazolin IV, nafcillin IV, vancomycin IV (in patient allergic to penicillin)
- *S. aureus* (MRSA): Vancomycin IV, linezolid IV or PO, daptomycin IV
- *Streptococcus* spp: Ceftriaxone, IV penicillin G in sensitive species
- *P. aeruginosa:* Cefepime, imipenem/cilastatin, or meropenem
- *Enterobacteriaceae:* Ceftriaxone or ertapenem
- Anaerobes: Clindamycin, piperacillin-tazobactam, cefotetan, or metronidazole
- Table 2 summarizes antimicrobial therapy for selected microorganisms in osteomyelitis. A retrospective analysis revealed that in diabetic foot osteomyelitis adjunctive rifampin is associated with improved amputation-free survival
- Hyperbaric oxygen therapy: May be useful in chronic osteomyelitis
- Wound-assisted vacuum device may help closure of wound
- Surgical debridement of all devitalized bone and tissue
- Immobilization of affected bone (plaster, traction) if bone is unstable
- Recommended antibiotic therapy for osteomyelitis in children is summarized in Table E3

DISPOSITION
Acute hematogenous osteomyelitis usually resolves without recurrence or long-term complications, but contiguous focus osteomyelitis, bone infections from open fractures, or osteomyelitis frequently recurs.

REFERRAL
- To an orthopedic surgeon if chronic osteomyelitis with need for bone debridement, bone grafting, or stabilization of infected tissue adjacent to a bone fracture
- To an infectious disease specialist for appropriate treatment for difficult-to-treat or recalcitrant infections
- To a hyperbaric oxygen chamber service for nonhealing, chronic osteomyelitis

❗ PEARLS & CONSIDERATIONS

- Chronic osteomyelitis is one of the most challenging infections to treat; the high failure rate is a consequence of poor vascular supply, nondistensible bone tissue, and limited penetration of bone tissue.

TABLE 1 Imaging Findings in Osteomyelitis

	Plain Radiograph	CT	MRI	NM
Acute	Minimal findings. Soft-tissue swelling may be seen	Not useful	Bone marrow edema can occur as early as 24-48 h, seen as low T1, and high T2 signal	May show increased uptake, but takes a few days
Subacute	Lucent or sclerotic lesion, periosteal reaction, soft-tissue swelling	Cortical and marrow abnormalities including abscess, periosteal reaction, soft-tissue edema, and abscess	Bone marrow changes, cortical abnormalities seen as thickening, bone abscess, periosteal reaction, increased T2 signal in soft tissues, abscess formation. Postgadolinium T1W sequences outline abscess cavities clearly	Three-phase bone scintigram, indium-111 WBC scan and combined studies are useful, especially to assess multifocal involvement. PET-CT generally not used in this context, but may be useful in exceptional circumstances
Chronic	Bone sclerosis, cortical thickening, sequestrum and cloaca, bone destruction, resorption, and deformities	Much better than plain radiographs to demonstrate cloaca and sequestrum, periosteal new bone formation, and abscess	Better soft-tissue and bone marrow resolution to demonstrate medullary and cortical changes, sequestra and cloaca well demonstrated, useful to outline soft-tissue abscess, and sinus tracts	Generally useful if there is a problem with diagnosis. Combined WBC and bone marrow scintigram is useful. May highlight multiple sites of involvement

CT, Computed tomography; *MRI,* magnetic resonance imaging; *NM,* nuclear medicine; *PET,* positron emission tomography; *WBC,* white blood cell.
From Grant LA: *Grainger & Allison's diagnostic radiology essentials,* ed 2, Philadelphia, 2019, Elsevier.

TABLE 2 Antimicrobial Therapy for Selected Microorganisms in Chronic Osteomyelitis in Adults

Microorganism	First Choice*	Alternative Choice
Methicillin/oxacillin/nafcillin-sensitive staphylococci	Nafcillin sodium or oxacillin sodium 1.5-2 g IV q4h for 4-6 wk *or* cefazolin 1-2 g IV q8h for 4-6 wk	Vancomycin 15 mg/kg IV q12h for 4-6 wk
Methicillin/oxacillin/nafcillin-resistant staphylococci (MRSA)	Vancomycin[†] 15 mg/kg IV q12h for 4-6 wk *or* daptomycin 6 mg/kg IV q24h	Linezolid 600 mg PO/IV q12h *or* levofloxacin[†] 500-750 mg PO/IV daily, plus rifampin 600-900 mg PO for 6 wk if susceptible to both drugs
Penicillin-sensitive streptococci	Aqueous penicillin G 20 epto^6 U/24 h IV either continuously or in six equally divided daily doses *or* ceftriaxone 1-2 g IV q24h *or* cefazolin 1-2 g IV q8h for 4-6 wk	Vancomycin 15 mg/kg IV q12h for 4-6 wk
Enterococci	Aqueous crystalline penicillin G 20×10^6 U/24 h IV either continuously or in six equally divided daily doses *or* ampicillin sodium 12 g/24 h IV either continuously or in six equally divided daily doses; the addition of gentamicin sulfate 1 mg/kg IV or IM q8h for 1-2 wk is *optional*	Vancomycin[†] 15 mg/kg IV q12h; the addition of gentamicin sulfate 1 mg/kg IV or IM q8h for 1-2 wk is *optional*
Enterobacteriaceae	Ceftriaxone 1-2 g IV q24h for 4-6 wk or ertapenem 1 g IV q24h	Ciprofloxacin 500-750 mg PO q12h for 4-6 wk or levofloxacin 500-750 mg PO q24h
Pseudomonas aeruginosa	Cefepime 2 g IV q12h, meropenem 1 g IV q8h, or imipenem 500 mg IV q6h for 4-6 wk	Ciprofloxacin 750 mg PO q12h for 4-6 wk or ceftazidime 2 g IV q8h

IM, Intramuscular; *IV,* intravenous; *MRSA,* methicillin-resistant *Staphylococcus aureus; PO,* by mouth.
*Antimicrobial selection should be based on in vitro sensitivity data, as well as allergies, intolerances, and drug interactions in individual patients.
[†]Doses shown are based on normal renal and hepatic function and may need to be adjusted or serum levels monitored (vancomycin).

- Parenteral antibiotics are usually chosen initially, but oral fluoroquinolones have good bone penetration and may be used in stable patients. A recent trial comparing oral versus IV antibiotics for bone and joint infections found that oral antibiotic therapy is not inferior to IV antibiotic therapy when used during the first 6 wk for complex orthopedic infections.
- The optimal duration of therapy for vertebral osteomyelitis is unclear. Trials comparing 6 wk to 12 wk of antibiotic treatment in pyogenic vertebral osteomyelitis showed similar cure rates (91%) in both groups.

SUGGESTED READINGS
Available at eBooks.Health.Elsevier.com.

RELATED CONTENT
Osteomyelitis (Patient Information)

AUTHOR: **GLENN G. FORT, MD, MPH**

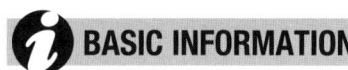

BASIC INFORMATION

DEFINITION

Osteoporosis is a skeletal disorder characterized by a progressive loss of bone mass and a decline in bone density and quality that results in increased bone fragility and a higher fracture risk. Poor bone mass acquisition during adolescence and bone loss during the sixth decade of life are the main processes responsible for osteoporosis. The various types are as follows:

PRIMARY OSTEOPOROSIS: Primary osteoporosis is the loss of bone mass due to aging and decreased gonadal function, not to any other chronic illness.

- Idiopathic osteoporosis: Unknown pathogenesis; may occur in children and young adults.
- Type I osteoporosis (postmenopausal women): Occurs after menopause due to an abrupt decline in estrogen production. It is characterized by accelerated and disproportionate trabecular bone loss and is associated with fractures of the spine, hip, and wrist.
- Type II osteoporosis (involutional): Occurs in both men and women aged >70 yr due to the progressively negative balance between bone formation and resorption. It is characterized by both trabecular and cortical bone loss and associated with fractures of the spine, long bones, and hip.

SECONDARY OSTEOPOROSIS: Secondary osteoporosis is bone loss due to another chronic condition such as thyroxine excess, hyperparathyroidism, malignancies, gastrointestinal disease, medications, renal failure, and connective tissue diseases (see "Differential Diagnosis").

ICD-10CM CODES
M81.0	Age-related osteoporosis without current pathological fracture
M81.4	Drug-induced osteoporosis
M81.5	Idiopathic osteoporosis
M81.6	Localized osteoporosis

EPIDEMIOLOGY & DEMOGRAPHICS

PREVALENCE (IN U.S.):
- Affects more than 10 million people in the U.S.
- Annual incidence of osteoporotic fractures exceeds 1.5 million in the U.S. (70% women)
- Twice as common in women than in men
- Health care costs in excess of $17 billion annually
- Health inequities in screening and treatment: Black women are less likely to be screened for osteoporosis and receive fewer prescriptions for osteoporosis treatment after diagnosis when compared with white women

RISK FACTORS:
- Female sex
- Postmenopausal state
- Advanced age
- Small body frame, low body weight (<58 kg)
- White or Hispanic ancestry
- Sedentary lifestyle
- Nulliparity
- Calcium deficiency
- Previous low-trauma fracture

- Parental history of hip fracture
- Tobacco use
- Excess alcohol use (>3 drinks per day)
- Long-term glucocorticoid use
- Chronic disease states; e.g., primary ovarian insufficiency, diabetes mellitus, androgen deficiency, inflammatory bowel disease, hyperthyroidism, hypercortisolism

PHYSICAL FINDINGS & CLINICAL PRESENTATION

- Most commonly asymptomatic.
- Insidious and progressive development of dorsal kyphosis *(dowager's hump),* loss of height, and skeletal pain typically associated with fracture; reduced gait speed or grip strength; other physical findings related to other conditions with associated increased risk for osteoporosis such as nodular thyroid, hepatic enlargement, jaundice, cushingoid features (see "Risk Factors" and Boxes 1 and 2).

ETIOLOGY

Normal bone turnover involves balance between process of bone resorption and bone formation. Osteoclasts resorb bone, and osteoblasts secrete bone matrix for building bone. In postmenopausal women, rate of bone turnover increases after loss of ovarian function, leading to progressive bone loss.

Several fracture risk calculation tools have been developed. Clinical risk factors used in the World Health Organization Fracture Risk Assessment Tool (WHO FRAX) 10-yr fracture risk calculator are summarized in Box 3.

Dx DIAGNOSIS

DIFFERENTIAL DIAGNOSIS
- Malignancy (multiple myeloma, lymphoma, leukemia, metastatic carcinoma)
- Primary hyperparathyroidism
- Osteomalacia
- Paget disease
- Osteogenesis imperfecta: Types I, III, and IV

SCREENING
- History and physical examination with appropriate evaluation for risk factors and secondary

---

BOX 1 Major Clinical Risk Factors for Osteoporotic Fracture

- Age
- Gender
- Previous fragility fracture
- Glucocorticoid therapy
- History of falls
- Family history of hip fracture
- Other causes of secondary osteoporosis
- Low body mass index
- Smoking
- High alcohol intake

From Hochberg MC: *Rheumatology,* ed 7, Philadelphia, 2019, Elsevier.

BOX 2 Causes of Secondary Osteoporosis

- Endocrine
  1. Hypogonadism in either sex, including untreated, premature menopause and treatment with aromatase inhibitors or androgen deprivation therapy
  2. Hyperthyroidism
  3. Hyperprolactinemia
  4. Cushing disease
  5. Diabetes
- Gastrointestinal
  1. Celiac disease
  2. Inflammatory bowel disease
  3. Chronic liver disease
  4. Chronic pancreatitis
  5. Other causes of malabsorption
- Rheumatologic
  1. Rheumatoid arthritis
  2. Other inflammatory arthropathies
- Hematologic
  1. Multiple myeloma
  2. Hemoglobinopathies
  3. Systemic mastocytosis
  4. Chronic heparin treatment
- Respiratory
  1. Cystic fibrosis
  2. Chronic obstructive pulmonary disease
- Metabolic
  1. Homocystinuria
- Chronic renal disease
- Immobility

From Hochberg MC: *Rheumatology,* ed 7, Philadelphia, 2019, Elsevier.

BOX 3 Clinical Risk Factors Included in the FRAX Case-Finding Algorithm

- Age (50-90 yr)
- Sex
- Weight (in kilograms) and height (in centimeters). Body mass index is automatically computed from height and weight
- Previous fragility fracture (yes/no)
- Parental history of hip fracture (yes/no)
- Current tobacco smoking (yes/no)
- Long-term use of oral glucocorticoids (over 3 mo) (yes/no)
- Rheumatoid arthritis (yes/no)
- Alcohol consumption of 3 or more units daily (yes/no)
- Other causes of secondary osteoporosis (yes/no): Includes type 1 diabetes, osteogenesis imperfecta, longstanding untreated hyperthyroidism, hypogonadism or premature menopause (<45 yr), chronic malnutrition, malabsorption, chronic liver disease

From World Health Organization: WHO risk fracture assessment tool. www.sheffield.ac.uk/FRAX/. From Hochberg MC: *Rheumatology,* ed 7, Philadelphia, 2019, Elsevier.

causes. Medications associated with osteoporosis are summarized in Table 1. Investigations for secondary osteoporosis are summarized in Box 4.

- WHO guidelines for the diagnosis of osteoporosis are based on bone mineral density (BMD) measurements of the hip or spine in g/cm² and are reported as a T score.
- Dual-energy x-ray absorptiometry (DEXA) is the gold standard for screening and monitoring changes in BMD due to excellent precision, widespread availability, low cost, and minimal radiation exposure.
- DEXA (Fig. 1) is indicated in all women 65 yr and older and in postmenopausal women younger than 65 yr of age who are at risk for fracture (e.g., weight <127 lbs, parental history of hip fracture, use of medications that cause bone loss, current smoking, excessive alcohol use, rheumatoid arthritis, or presence of diseases that cause bone loss). Clinical indications for bone densitometry are summarized in Table 2. Causes of erroneous bone mineral density measures by DEXA in the lumbar spine are summarized in Table 3.
- FRAX questionnaire (Fig. 2): Use of FRAX calculator (www.sheffield.ac.uk/FRAX/) is proposed by the U.S. Preventive Services Task Force (USPSTF) to determine the need for screening in women between the ages of 50 and 64. If the FRAX 10-yr major osteoporotic risk is greater than or equal to 9.3%, the USPSTF recommends screening with DEXA scan.
- Currently, routine testing in men for osteoporosis is not recommended unless there are clinical manifestations of low bone mass.
- Recommendations as to when to repeat bone density testing should be based on initial T scores (Fig. 3). Data from the Study of Osteoporotic Fractures indicates that in women with normal bone density or mild osteopenia, repeat testing might not be necessary for another 10 to 15 yr. For women with moderate osteopenia, a screening interval of 3 to 5 yr may be appropriate. For women with advanced bone loss/osteoporosis, testing every 1 to 2 yr is recommended.

TABLE 1 Medications Associated With Osteoporosis

System	Medication
Endocrine	Aromatase inhibitors (e.g., anastrozole)
	Excess thyroxine replacement
	Glucocorticoids
	Gonadotropin-releasing hormone agonists
	Ovarian-suppressing drugs (e.g., medroxyprogesterone acetate)
	Thiazolidinediones
	SGLT2 inhibitors
Gastrointestinal	Proton pump inhibitors
Hematologic	Heparin
	Warfarin
Infectious disease	Antiretroviral therapy
Immunosuppressant	Cyclosporine
	Cytotoxic drugs
	Tacrolimus
Neurologic	Anticonvulsants—phenytoin, phenobarbital, carbamazepine
Psychiatric	Selective serotonin reuptake inhibitors
Renal	Loop diuretics (e.g., furosemide)

From Hochberg MC: *Rheumatology*, ed 7, Philadelphia, 2019, Elsevier.

BOX 4 Investigations for Secondary Osteoporosis in Older People With Low-Trauma Fractures or Low Bone Mineral Density

CBC
ESR or CRP
Biochemical profile: Including renal function, adjusted serum calcium, and alkaline phosphatase
Thyroid function tests
Serum testosterone, sex hormone–binding globulin, LH, FSH (men)
Serum and urine electrophoresis (vertebral fractures)
Serum 25OHD and PTH

From Fillit HM: *Brocklehurst's textbook of geriatric medicine and gerontology*, ed 8, Philadelphia, 2017, Elsevier.

LABORATORY TESTS (BOX 5)

- CMP
- CBC
- TSH
- 24-hr urinary calcium levels and 26-hydroxyvitamin D level may be helpful in evaluating for secondary causes of osteoporosis
- Consider celiac panel and serum protein electrophoresis

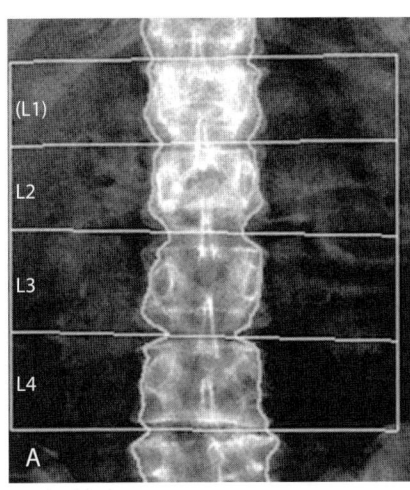
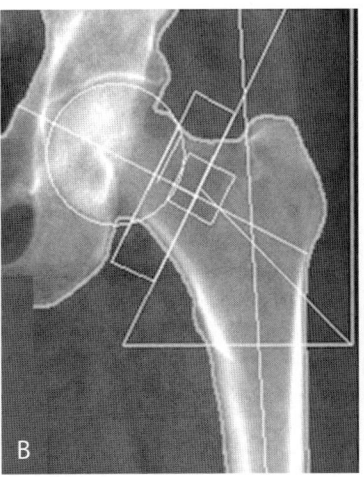
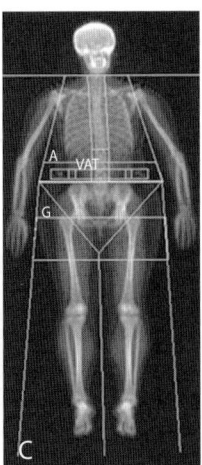

FIG. 1 Dual-energy x-ray absorptiometry (DEXA) provides "areal" bone mineral density (BMD) (g/cm²) and is currently the gold standard for diagnosis of osteoporosis by bone densitometry (World Health Organization definition T score −2.5 or below) in **(A)** posteroanterior lumbar spine (L1 through L4) or **(B)** hip (femoral neck or total). **C,** DEXA of the whole body can provide information on total and regional BMD and body composition (fat and muscle mass). Recent additional parameters measured are android A/gynoid G ratio and visceral adipose tissue (VAT). (From Pope TL et al: *Musculoskeletal imaging*, ed 2, Philadelphia, 2014, Saunders.)

TABLE 2 Clinical Indications for Bone Densitometry

All postmenopausal women <65 yr who have one or more additional risk factors for osteoporosis (besides menopause)

All women >65 yr regardless of additional risk factors

To document reduced bone density in patients with vertebral abnormalities or osteopenia on radiographs

Estrogen-deficient women at risk for low bone density who are considering use of estrogen or an alternative therapy, if bone density would influence the decision

Women who have been receiving estrogen replacement therapy for prolonged periods or to monitor the efficacy of a therapeutic intervention or interventions for osteoporosis

To diagnose low bone mass in people treated with glucocorticoids

To document low bone density in people with asymptomatic primary or secondary hyperparathyroidism

From Firestein GS et al: *Firestein & Kelley's textbook of rheumatology,* ed 11, Philadelphia, 2021, Elsevier.

TABLE 3 Causes of Erroneous Bone Mineral Density Measures by DEXA in the Lumbar Spine

Overestimation of Bone Mineral Density

Extraneous calcification (lymph nodes, aorta)

Degenerative disk and spine disease (osteophytes)

Ankylosing spondylitis

Vertebral fracture

Sclerotic metastases

Vertebral hemangioma

Overlying metal artifacts (navel rings)

Surgical interventions (metallic rods, spinal fusion)

Vertebroplasty

Paget disease

Treatment with strontium ranelate

Underestimation of Bone Mineral Density

Laminectomy

DEXA, Dual-energy x-ray absorptiometry.
From Pope TL et al: *Musculoskeletal imaging,* ed 2, Philadelphia, 2014, Saunders.

- Biochemical markers of bone remodeling may be useful to predict rate of bone loss and/or follow therapy response. Specific biochemical markers (listed below) are followed to document response to therapy.
  1. High-turnover osteoporosis: High levels of resorption markers (lysyl pyridinoline, deoxy lysyl pyridinoline, n-telopeptide of collagen cross-links, C-telopeptide of collagen cross-links) and formation markers (osteocalcin and bone-specific alkaline phosphatase); indicates accelerated bone loss responding best to antiresorptive therapy
  2. Low or normal-turnover osteoporosis: Normal or low levels of the markers of resorption and formation (see "high-turnover osteoporosis" listed previously); no accelerated bone loss; responds best to drugs that enhance bone formation

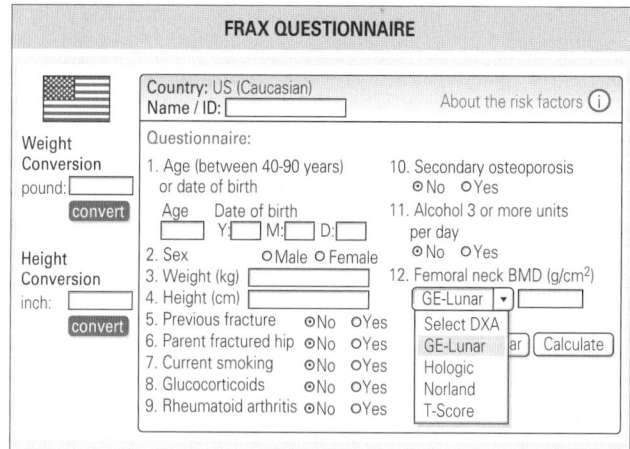

FIG. 2 FRAX questionnaire. (From Hochberg MC: *Rheumatology,* ed 7, Philadelphia, 2019, Elsevier.)

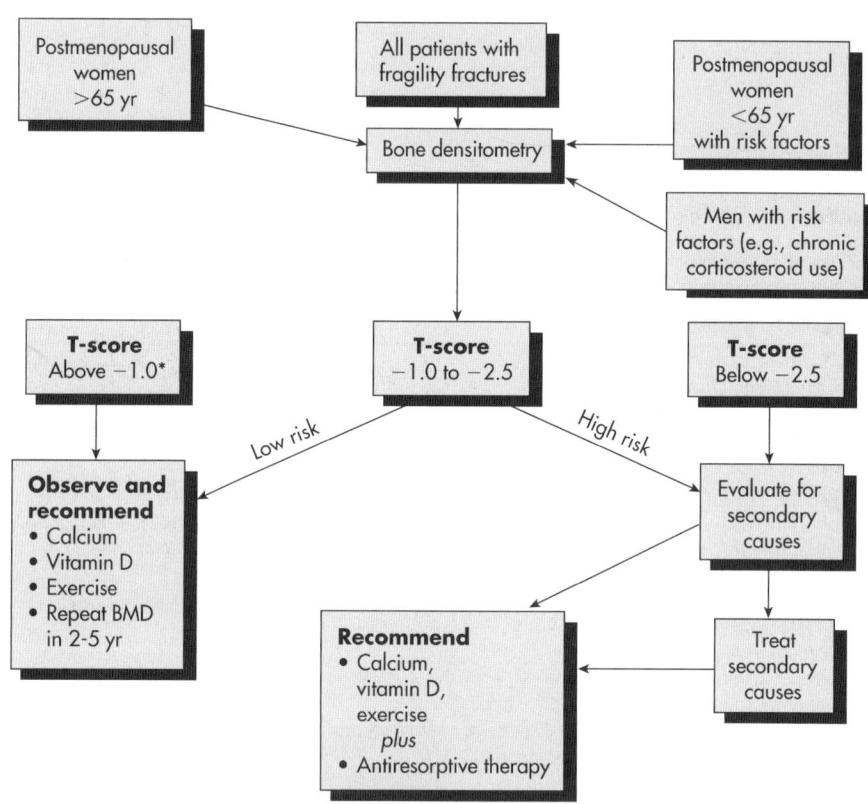

*Patients with fragility fractures and a T-score above −1.0 should be evaluated for other causes of pathologic fracture.

FIG. 3 Diagnosis and management of osteoporosis.

IMAGING STUDIES

- Bone mineral density (BMD) determination (see "Workup") should be performed on all women with determined risk factors and/or associated secondary causes. Criteria for the diagnosis of osteoporosis based on measurement of bone density and T score are summarized in Table 4.
  1. Normal: BMD <1 SD below the young adult reference mean
  2. Osteopenia: BMD 1 to 2.5 SD below the young adult reference mean
  3. Osteoporosis: BMD >2.5 SD below the young adult reference mean
- For patients undergoing treatment: The frequency of BMD monitoring is controversial and many experts recommend that clinicians should not monitor BMD during the initial 5-yr drug treatment period because no studies have proven that such monitoring improves fracture outcomes.
  1. X-ray exam of appropriate part of skeleton (Figs. 4 and 5) is indicated to evaluate clinical osteoporotic fracture only.

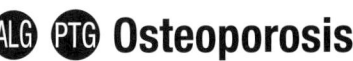

BOX 5 Recommended Laboratory Investigations for Individuals With Osteoporosis

Recommended screening in all patients
- Serum calcium, albumin, phosphorus *, †, ‡, §
- Serum creatinine *, †, ‡, §
- Liver function tests *
- Bicarbonate *
- Complete blood count *
- 24-hr urinary calcium level *, †, ‡, §
- 25-hydroxyvitamin D level *, †, ‡, §
- Thyroid-stimulating hormone level *, †, ‡, §

Other testing, if appropriate
- Biochemical markers of bone turnover *, †, ‡, §
- Cortisol levels *, ‡
- Protein electrophoresis *, †, §
- Parathyroid hormone level *, §

*American Association of Clinical Endocrinologists guidelines.
‡U.S. Surgeon General's report.
†National Osteoporosis Foundation Physician's Guide.
§American College of Obstetricians and Gynecologists.
From Hochberg MC: *Rheumatology,* ed 7, Philadelphia, 2019, Elsevier.

TABLE 4 Diagnostic Categories for Osteoporosis Based on World Health Organization Criteria

Category	Definition
Normal	BMD not more than 1 SD below the young adult mean value
Low bone mass (osteopenia)	BMD lying between 1 and 2.5 SD below the young adult mean value
Osteoporosis	BMD more than 2.5 SD below the young adult mean value

BMD, Bone mineral density; *SD,* standard deviation.
From World Health Organization data, 1994. In Hochberg MC: *Rheumatology,* ed 7, Philadelphia, 2019, Elsevier.

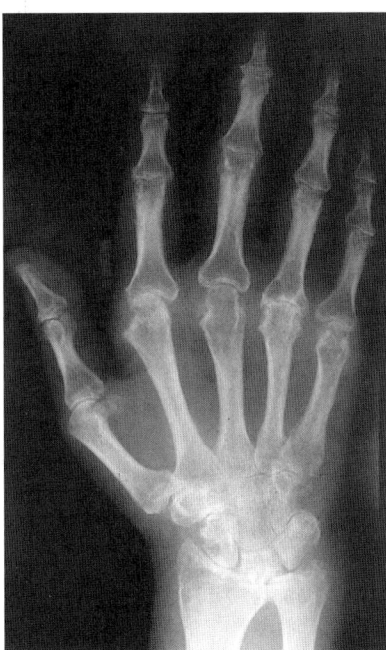

FIG. 4 Regional osteoporosis. Hand radiograph in early rheumatoid arthritis (RA) shows periarticular osteopenia at the metacarpophalangeal and interphalangeal joints, with joint space narrowing and juxtaarticular erosions. The periarticular osteopenia is the earliest radiographic feature of RA and is related to hyperemia, synovial inflammation, and local cytokines that stimulate osteoclastic bone resorption. (From Pope TL et al: *Musculoskeletal imaging,* ed 2, Philadelphia, 2015, Saunders.)

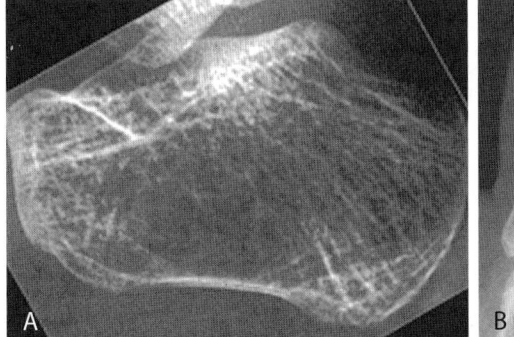
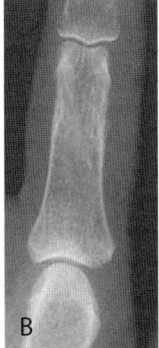

FIG. 5 General osteoporosis. Radiographic features include reduced radiographic density (osteopenia) with reduction in the number of trabeculae, which may be destroyed completely, and the bone cortex becomes thinned as evident in the lateral radiograph of the calcaneus **(A)** and radiograph of the phalanx **(B)**. When these features are present, bone densitometry using dual-energy x-ray absorptiometry (DEXA) should be suggested. (From Pope TL et al: *Musculoskeletal imaging,* ed 2, Philadelphia, 2015, Saunders.)

Rx TREATMENT

When to treat:
- Osteoporosis criteria met based on DEXA measurements of BMD
- History of hip or vertebral fracture
- Osteopenia on DEXA + 10-yr FRAX score of greater than or equal to 3% at hip or greater than or equal to 20% of major osteoporotic fracture

NONPHARMACOLOGIC THERAPY

Prevention:
- Identification and minimization of risk factors
- Appropriate diagnosis and treatment of secondary causes
- Behavioral modification: Proper nutrition, physical activity (specifically weight-bearing activity), fracture prevention strategies, fall risk reduction

ACUTE GENERAL Rx

- Vitamin D supplement: 600 IU/day for persons 19 to 70 yr of age and 800 IU/day for persons 71 yr and older. Recommended supplementation of calcium and vitamin D is summarized in Table 4.
- Calcium supplement: The recommended dietary intake of calcium for women 19 to 50 yr of age and men 19 to 70 yr of age is 1000 mg/day; women older than age 50 and men older than age 70 require 1200 mg/day. Calcium intake above 2500 mg/day (2000 mg/day in persons >50 yr of age) should be avoided. Consumption of calcium-rich foods and beverages is the preferred approach to ensuring adequate calcium intake.[1]
- Oral bisphosphonates (alendronate, risedronate): Decrease bone resorption by attenuating osteoclast activity. They are first-line therapy for the treatment of most patients with osteoporosis, with proven efficacy to reduce fracture risk. The bisphosphonates differ in binding affinity, dose frequency, and route of administration. To facilitate absorption, most oral bisphosphonates are taken on an empty stomach with a full glass of

water. Patients are instructed to remain in a sitting or standing position for 30 to 60 min. Contraindications include esophageal disorders, inability to remain standing for 30 to 60 min after taking the medication, chronic kidney disease, and Roux-en-Y gastric bypass procedures. Adverse side effects include gastroesophageal reflux disease, esophagitis, transient hypocalcemia, musculoskeletal pain, renal impairment, ocular side effects, jaw necrosis, and atypical femur fracture.

- Biologic agents: Denosumab is a human monoclonal antibody that inhibits osteoclast formation and prevents resorption for treatment of postmenopausal osteoporosis. It is used as a second-line pharmacologic treatment to reduce the risk of fractures in postmenopausal females diagnosed with primary osteoporosis who have contraindications to or experience adverse effects of biphosphonates.[2] Dosage is 60 mg subcutaneously every 6 mo. Romosozumab is a monoclonal antibody that increases bone formation and decreases bone resorption by binding to sclerostin. It may be considered for patients who are at high risk for fracture and cannot tolerate any other osteoporotic therapies. Dosage is two consecutive subcutaneous injections (105 mg each) for a total dose of 210 mg once monthly. It should not be used in patients who have had a myocardial infarction or stroke in the past yr.
- Zoledronic acid: A bisphosphonate given by IV infusion over at least 15 min, 5 mg once per yr may be used in patients who are unable to tolerate oral bisphosphonates. It is contraindicated in patients with acute renal failure.
- Teriparatide is a recombinant human parathyroid hormone used for postmenopausal women with osteoporosis who are at high risk for fracture, especially vertebral fractures. It is also used in men with primary or hypogonadal osteoporosis who are at high risk of fracture. It is administered by injection 20 mcg daily, subcutaneously into the thigh or abdominal wall. Use for more than 2 yr is not recommended. It stimulates bone formation and reduces the risk of fracture but may increase the risk of stroke in older women with osteoporosis. Common side effects include headaches, myalgia, hypercalcemia, and

TABLE 5 Effect of Major Treatment Options on the Risk of Vertebral, Nonvertebral, and Hip Fractures

	Vertebral Fractures	Nonvertebral Fractures	Hip Fractures
Alendronate	A	A	A
Etidronate	A	ND	ND
Risedronate	A	A	A
Raloxifene	A	ND	ND
Strontium ranelate	A	A	(A)
Teriparatide	A	A	ND
Denosumab	A	A	A
Zoledronate *	A	A	A
Ibandronate *	A	(A)	ND
Calcium and vitamin D *	ND	A	A

A indicates evidence from randomized, controlled trials and/or meta-analysis; *(A)* reflects that a beneficial effect on fracture risk was found only in post hoc subgroup analysis; *ND* indicates that fracture reduction has not been demonstrated.
From Fillit HM: *Brocklehurst's textbook of geriatric medicine and gerontology*, ed 8, Philadelphia, 2017, Elsevier.

hypercalciuria. Trials involving abaloparatide, a selective activator of the parathyroid hormone type 1 receptor, have also shown reduced risk of new vertebral and nonvertebral fractures in postmenopausal women with osteoporosis. Use of teriparatide is followed by a biphosphonate upon its discontinuation in females with primary osteoporosis and a very high risk of fractures.[2]
- Estrogen prescription drugs or raloxifene should not be prescribed to treat women with osteoporosis.

CHRONIC Rx

- Lifelong attention to behavior modification (nutrition, physical activity, fracture prevention strategies) and compliance with pharmacologic intervention. Recommendations include weight-bearing and muscle-strengthening exercises, smoking cessation, reduced alcohol intake, and adoption of fall prevention strategies.
- There is little evidence to guide physicians about long-term bisphosphonate therapy. The decision to continue drug therapy beyond 5 yr should reflect reassessment of risk and benefit. The risks of atypical fracture of the femur and osteonecrosis of the jaw (ONJ)[2] increase after 5 yr of bisphosphonate use[2]. It is

reasonable to consider a drug holiday in postmenopausal women who are not at high fracture risk after 3 yr (IV) to 5 yr (oral) of bisphosphonate therapy. Continued treatment may be advisable in those at highest risk.
- Continuing need to eliminate high-risk factors when possible and to optimally manage secondary causes of osteoporosis.

DISPOSITION

Goals for diagnosis and treatment include identification of women at risk; initiation of lifelong preventive measures for all women; institution of treatment modalities that will result in a decrease in fracture risk; and reduction of morbidity, mortality, and unnecessary institutionalization, thereby improving quality of independent life and productivity. Table 5 summarizes the effect of major treatment options on the risk of vertebral, nonvertebral, and hip fractures.

AUTHORS: **SYDNEY FORD, MD, MPH,** and **RACHEL WRIGHT HEINLE, MD, FACOG**

REFERENCES
Available at eBooks.Health.Elsevier.com

BASIC INFORMATION

DEFINITION

Otitis externa refers to a variety of conditions causing inflammation and/or infection of the external auditory canal (and/or auricle and tympanic membrane).[1] There are six subgroups of otitis externa:

- Acute localized otitis externa (furunculosis)
- Acute diffuse bacterial otitis externa (i.e., "swimmer ear")
- Chronic otitis externa
- Eczematous otitis externa
- Fungal otitis externa (otomycosis)
- Invasive or necrotizing (malignant) otitis externa

SYNONYM

See "Definition."

ICD-10CM CODES
H60.90	Unspecified otitis externa, unspecified ear
H60.2	Malignant otitis externa
H60.3	Other infective otitis externa
H60.5	Acute otitis externa, non-infective
H60.8	Other otitis externa

EPIDEMIOLOGY & DEMOGRAPHICS[2]

INCIDENCE (IN U.S.):
- Among the most common disorders
- An estimated 10% of people develop external otitis during their lifetime
- Affects 3% to 10% of patients seeking otologic care

PREVALENCE (IN U.S.):
- Diffuse otitis externa is most often seen in swimmers and in hot, humid climates, conditions that lead to water retention in the ear canal. In the U.S., 44% of AOE-related healthcare visits occur June to August[1]
- Necrotizing otitis externa is more common in elderly, diabetics, and immunocompromised patients[3]

PREDOMINANT SEX: None
PREDOMINANT AGE:
- Occurs at all ages; however, incidence is highest during childhood and decreases with age[1]
- Necrotizing otitis externa: Typically occurs in elderly: Mean age >65 yr[3]

PHYSICAL FINDINGS & CLINICAL PRESENTATION

The two most common symptoms are otalgia, ranging from pruritus to severe pain exacerbated by motion (e.g., chewing), and otorrhea. Patients may also experience aural fullness and hearing loss due to swelling and occlusion of the canal. More intense symptoms may occur with bacterial otitis externa, with or without fever, and lymphadenopathy (anterior to tragus).[1] Findings unique to specific forms of the infection include:

- Acute localized otitis externa (furunculosis)[1]:
  1. Occurs from infected hair follicles, usually in the outer third of the ear canal, forming pustules and furuncles
  2. Furuncles are superficial and pointing or deep and diffuse
- Impetigo[1]:
  1. In contrast to furunculosis, this is a superficial spreading infection of the ear canal that may also involve the concha and the auricle
  2. Begins as a small blister that ruptures, releasing straw-colored fluid that dries as a golden crust
- Erysipelas[1]:
  1. Caused by group A streptococcus (Streptococcus pyogenes [GAS])
  2. May involve the concha and canal
  3. May involve the dermis and deeper tissues
  4. Area of cellulitis, often with severe pain
  5. Fever, chills, malaise
  6. Regional adenopathy
- Eczematous or seborrheic otitis externa[1]:
  1. Stems from a variety of dermatologic problems that can involve the external auditory canal
  2. Severe itching, erythema, scaling, crusting (Fig.E1), and fissuring possible
- Acute diffuse otitis externa (swimmer ear)[1]:
  1. Begins with itching and a feeling of pressure and fullness in the ear that becomes increasingly tender and painful
  2. Mild erythema and edema of the external auditory canal, which may cause narrowing and occlusion of the canal (Fig. E2), leading to hearing loss
  3. Minimal serous secretions, which may become profuse and purulent
  4. Tympanic membrane may appear dull and infected
  5. Usually absence of systemic symptoms such as fever, chills
- Otomycosis[1]:
  1. Chronic superficial infection of the ear canal and tympanic membrane
  2. In primary fungal infection, major symptom is intense itching
  3. In secondary infection (fungal infection superimposed on bacterial infection), major symptom is pain
  4. Fungal growth of variety of colors
- Chronic otitis externa[1]:
  1. Dry and atrophic canal
  2. Typically lack of cerumen
  3. Itching, often severe, and mild discomfort rather than pain
  4. Occasionally mucopurulent discharge
  5. With time, thickening of the walls of the canal, causing narrowing of the lumen
- Necrotizing otitis externa (also known as malignant otitis externa). Typically seen in older patients with diabetes or in patients who are immunocompromised[3]
  1. Redness, swelling, and tenderness of the ear canal
  2. Classic finding of granulation tissue on the floor of the canal and the bone–cartilage junction
  3. Small ulceration of necrotic soft tissue at bone–cartilage junction
  4. Most common symptoms: Pain (often severe) and otorrhea
  5. Lessening of purulent drainage as infection advances
  6. As the infection advances, osteomyelitis of the base of the skull and temporomandibular joint osteomyelitis can develop
  7. Facial nerve palsy often the first and only cranial nerve defect
  8. Possible involvement of other cranial nerves

ETIOLOGY[1]

- Box 1 summarizes common pathogens in otitis externa
- Acute localized otitis externa: *Staphylococcus aureus*
- Impetigo:
  1. *S. aureus* including MRSA
  2. *Streptococcus pyogenes* (GAS)
- Erysipelas: GAS
- Eczematous otitis externa:
  1. Seborrheic dermatitis
  2. Atopic dermatitis
  3. Psoriasis
  4. Neurodermatitis
  5. Lupus erythematosus
- Acute diffuse otitis externa:
  1. Swimming
  2. Hot, humid climates
  3. Tightly fitting hearing aids
  4. Use of ear plugs
  5. *Pseudomonas aeruginosa*
  6. *S. aureus* including MRSA
- Otomycosis:
  1. Prolonged use of topical antibiotics and steroid preparations
  2. Uncontrolled diabetes mellitus can contribute to risk
  3. *Aspergillus* (80% to 90%)
  4. *Candida*
- Chronic otitis externa: Persistent low-grade infection and inflammation
- Necrotizing otitis externa (NOE)[3]:
  1. Complication of persistent otitis externa
  2. Typically starts in the external auditory canal and spreads to the stylomastoid

BOX 1 Common Pathogens in Otitis Externa

Gram-negative Organisms
Pseudomonas aeruginosa
Pseudomonas spp. Nov. "otitidis"
Proteus mirabilis
Serratia marcescens

Gram-positive Organisms
Staphylococcus aureus
Staphylococcus epidermidis
Corynebacterium auris
Enterococcus faecalis

Fungi and Yeasts
Aspergillus fumigatus
Candida albicans
Candida parapsilosis

From Cherry JD et al: *Feigin and Cherry's pediatric infectious diseases,* ed 8, Philadelphia, 2019, Elsevier.

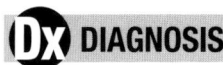

foramen, then to the mastoid tip and the jugular foramen. Finally, it extends to the petrous apex and the middle cranial fossa
3. *P. aeruginosa*
4. High index of suspicion for atypical organisms (MRSA) in patients without diabetes

Dx DIAGNOSIS

DIFFERENTIAL DIAGNOSIS

- Acute otitis media
- Bullous myringitis
- Mastoiditis
- Foreign bodies
- Neoplasms
- Contact dermatitis
- Eczema
- Ramsey-Hunt syndrome
- Seborrhea
- Otomycosis
- Referred pain
- Table 1 describes the differential diagnosis of painful external ear and auditory canal disorders

WORKUP

Thorough history and physical examination, including pneumatic otoscopy if available

LABORATORY TESTS

- Cultures from the canal are usually not necessary unless the condition does not respond to treatment.

- Leukocyte count normal or mildly elevated.
- Erythrocyte sedimentation rate is often quite elevated in malignant otitis externa.

IMAGING STUDIES

- Computed tomography scan (Fig. E3) is the best technique for defining bone involvement and extent of disease in malignant otitis externa.
- MRI is slightly more sensitive in evaluation of soft tissue changes and intracranial extension of infection.
- Gallium scans are more specific than bone scans in diagnosing NOE.
- Follow-up scans are helpful in determining efficacy of treatment. note: Expert opinion supports history and physical examination as the best means of diagnosis. Persistent pain that is constant and severe should raise the question of NOE (particularly in the elderly, diabetics, and immunocompromised patients).

Rx TREATMENT

NONPHARMACOLOGIC THERAPY

- Cleansing and debridement of the ear canal with cotton swabs and hydrogen peroxide or other antiseptic solution allows a more thorough examination of the ear.
- If the canal lumen is edematous and too narrow to allow adequate cleansing, a cotton wick or gauze strip inserted into the canal serves as a conduit for topical medications to be drawn into the canal. Usually remove wick after 2 days.
- Local heat is useful in treating deep furunculosis.
- Incision and drainage is indicated in treatment of superficial pointing furunculosis.

ACUTE GENERAL Rx

Topical medications:
- An acidifying agent such as 2% acetic acid (Vosol) inhibits growth of bacteria and fungi.
- Topical antibiotics (in the form of otic or ophthalmic solutions) or antifungals, often in combination with an acidifying agent and a steroid preparation. Direct application of topical agents to the infected site is a key element in the treatment of external otitis regardless of severity. Proper installation of eardrops entails tilting the head toward the opposite shoulder, pulling the superior aspect of the auricle upward, and filling the ear canal with drops. In young children, the earlobe should be pulled downward to fill the canal.
- The ideal antibiotic regimen should have coverage against the most common pathogens, *S. aureus* and *P. aeruginosa*.
- Side effect profile can also influence choice of treatment. Ototoxicity is the most important concern with aminoglycoside drugs, including neomycin, tobramycin, and gentamicin. Aminoglycosides are a significant potential source for iatrogenic hearing loss and balance dysfunction, particularly in the presence of tympanic membrane perforation. Allergic contact dermatitis is commonly associated with neomycin when used for prolonged courses. Topical fluoroquinolones can cause local irritation.
- The following are some of the available preparations:
  1. Neomycin otic solutions and suspensions:
     a. With polymyxin-B-hydrocortisone (Cortisporin)
     b. With hydrocortisone-thonzonium (Coly-Mycin S)
  2. Polymyxin-B-hydrocortisone (Otobiotic)
  3. Quinolone otic solutions:
     a. Ofloxacin 0.3% solution (Floxin Otic)
     b. Ciprofloxacin 0.3% with hydrocortisone (Cipro HC)
  4. Quinolone ophthalmic solutions:
     a. Ofloxacin 0.3% (Ocuflox)
     b. Ciprofloxacin 0.3% (Ciloxan)
  5. Aminoglycoside ophthalmic solutions:
     a. Gentamicin sulfate 0.3% (Garamycin)
     b. Tobramycin sulfate 0.3% (Tobrex)
     c. Tobramycin 0.3% and dexamethasone 0.1% (TobraDex)
  6. Chloramphenicol 0.5% otic solution or 0.25% ophthalmic solution (Chloromycetin)
  7. Gentian violet (methylrosaniline chloride 1%, 2%)
  8. Antifungals:
     a. Amphotericin B 3% (Fungizone lotion)
     b. Clotrimazole 1% solution (Lotrimin)
     c. Tolnaftate 1% (Tinactin)
- Topical preparations should be applied qid (bid for quinolones, antifungals), generally for

TABLE 1 Differential Diagnosis of Painful External Ear and Auditory Canal Disorders

Disorder	Clinical Features
Acute otitis externa	Diffuse redness, swelling, and pain of the canal with greenish to whitish exudate; often very tender pinna
Malignant otitis externa	Rapidly progressive, severe swelling and redness of pinna, which may be laterally displaced
Dermatitis	
Eczema	History of atopy, presence of lesions elsewhere; lesions are scaly, red, pruritic, and weeping
Contact	History of cosmetic use or irritant exposure; lesions are scaly, red, pruritic, and weeping
Seborrhea	Scaly, red, papular dermatitis; scalp may have thick, yellow scales
Psoriasis	History or presence of psoriasis elsewhere; erythematous papules that coalesce into thick, white plaques
Cellulitis	Diffuse redness, tenderness, and swelling of the pinna
Furuncles	Red, tender papules in areas with hair follicles (distal third of the ear canal)
Infected periauricular cyst	Discrete, palpable lesions; history of previous swelling at same site; cellulitis may develop, obscuring cystic structure
Insect bites	History of exposure; lesions are red, tender papules
Herpes zoster	Painful, vesicular lesions in the ear canal and tympanic membrane in the distribution of cranial nerves V and VII
Perichondritis	Inflammation of the cartilage, usually secondary to cellulitis
Tumors	Palpable mass, destruction of surrounding structures
Foreign body	Foreign body may cause secondary trauma to the ear canal or become a nidus for an infection of the ear canal
Trauma	Bruising and swelling of external ear; there may be signs of basilar skull fracture (cerebrospinal fluid otorrhea, hemotympanum)

From Kliegman RM: *Nelson textbook of pediatrics*, ed 21, Philadelphia, 2020, Elsevier.

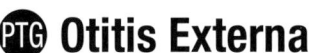

BOX 2 Considerations if Acute Otitis Externa Fails to Respond to Initial Ototopical Therapy

- Self-instrumentation trauma
- Malignant external otitis
- Contact dermatitis
- Failure to adhere to preventive measures (such as avoidance of water exposure)
- Improper administration of ototopical therapy
- Immunosuppression: Diabetes, prior radiotherapy
- Inadequate penetration of ototopical therapy due to copious debris or thickened canal skin
- Misdiagnosis: Canal cholesteatoma or keratosis obturans, autoimmune condition, mycobacterial infection, malignancy
- Resistance of involved organism to ototopical therapy choice

From Flint PW et al: *Cummings otolaryngology, head and neck surgery*, ed 7, Philadelphia, 2021, Elsevier.

TABLE 2 Complications of Acute and Chronic Otitis Externa

Complication	Description	Treatment
Cellulitis/perichondritis/chondritis	Extension of infection into soft tissues and cartilage of the auricle	Oral administration of antibiotics with adequate coverage of *Pseudomonas* species
Malignant otitis externa	Extension of infection beyond the EAC into soft tissue, mastoid and skull base; can evolve into temporal bone osteomyelitis	Underlying metabolic or immune abnormality to be addressed; culture-directed antibiotic therapy; typically requires a prolonged (6-wk) course of antipseudomonal antibiotic
Medial canal fibrosis	Fibrous scar of the medial EAC; a sequela of COE	Surgical treatment with canalplasty vs. lateral graft tympanoplasty; bone-anchored hearing device if surgery is not indicated
Perforation of the tympanic membrane	Often seen in the setting of fungal OE	Elimination of infection; tympanoplasty if spontaneous repair does not occur

COE, Chronic otitis externa; *EAC*, external auditory canal; *OE*, otitis externa.
From Flint PW et al: *Cummings otolaryngology, head and neck surgery*, ed 7, Philadelphia, 2021, Elsevier.

3 days after cessation of symptoms (average 10-14 days total).
Systemic antibiotics:
- Reserved for when the infection has spread beyond the ear canal.
- Treatment usually for 10 days with ciprofloxacin 750 mg q12h or ofloxacin 400 mg q12h, or with antistaphylococcal agent (e.g., dicloxacillin or cephalexin 500 mg q6h). Use Bactrim or clindamycin when MRSA suspected or cultured at one DS twice a day instead of cephalexin or dicloxacillin. For malignant otitis externa (due to *Pseudomonas aeruginosa* in >90% of cases), effective agents are meropenem 1 g intravenous (IV) q8h or

ciprofloxacin 400 mg IV q12h or 750 mg PO q12h or cefepime 2 g q12h.
Treatment for NOE:
- Combined oral quinolones with topical quinolones for 4 to 6 wk may be sufficient for initial therapy.[3]
- IV antipseudomonals with or without aminoglycosides are appropriate in refractory cases.[3]
- Local debridement.
Pain control:
- May require NSAIDs or opioids
- Topical corticosteroids to reduce swelling and inflammation

CHRONIC Rx
- Patients prone to recurrent infections should try to identify and avoid precipitants to infection.
- Swimmers should try tight-fitting ear plugs or tight-fitting bathing caps and remove all excess water from the ears after swimming.
- Treat underlying systemic diseases and dermatologic conditions that predispose to infection.
- Hearing aids should be removed nightly and regularly cleaned.

DISPOSITION
- Inadequate treatment of otitis externa may lead to NOE and mastoiditis.
- Considerations if acute otitis externa fails to respond to initial ototopical therapy are summarized in Box 2.
- Complications of acute and chronic otitis externa are summarized in Table 2.

REFERRAL
To an otolaryngologist:
- NOE
- Treatment failure
- Severe pain

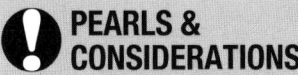 **PEARLS & CONSIDERATIONS**

Otitis externa varies in severity from a mild irritation of the external acoustic canal (swimmer ear) that resolves spontaneously by simply removing the offending agent (stay out of freshwater or wear ear plugs when swimming) to a life-threatening infection with the risk of intracranial extension, gram-negative bacterial meningitis, and severe neurologic impairment with multiple cranial neuropathy. Do not miss severe malignant otitis externa in patients who are diabetic, elderly, or immunocompromised.

REFERENCES
Available at eBooks.Health.Elsevier.com.

RELATED CONTENT
Otitis Externa (Patient Information)

AUTHOR: **LYNN C. FULLENKAMP, MD, JD**

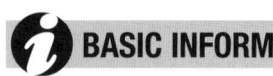

BASIC INFORMATION

DEFINITION

Acute otitis media (AOM) is defined by infected middle ear fluid resulting in moderate to severe bulging of the tympanic membrane (TM) or new onset of otorrhea not due to acute otitis externa. Table 1 summarizes otitis media definitions and terminology. Care should be taken to differentiate AOM from serous otitis media, which involves noninfected middle ear fluid that does not result in bulging of the TM. Serous otitis media does not require antibiotic treatment.[1,2]

SYNONYMS

Acute suppurative otitis media
Purulent otitis media
Acute otitis media
AOM

ICD-10CM CODES

H65.3   Chronic mucoid otitis media
H66.0   Acute suppurative otitis media
H66.4   Suppurative otitis media, unspecified
H66.9   Otitis media, unspecified
H66.1   Chronic tubotympanic suppurative otitis media
H66.2   Chronic atticoantral suppurative otitis media

EPIDEMIOLOGY & DEMOGRAPHICS

INCIDENCE (IN U.S.):
- Affects patients of all ages but is largely a disease of infants and young children
- Affects approximately 80% of all children by age 5 yr
- Occurs three or more times in one third of all children by age 3 yr
- Costs associated with otitis media exceed $5 billion, with 40% of the costs occurring from patients ages 1 to 3 yr
- One of the most common indications for antibiotic prescription among children

PEAK INCIDENCE:
- AOM occurs at all ages but is most prevalent between 6 and 24 mo of age.
- A second peak in incidence occurs between 4 and 6 yr of age.
- AOM is most frequent in the fall, winter, and early spring (coincident with peak respiratory virus prevalence in the community).
- Incidence of infection declines with age; AOM is seen infrequently in adults.

RISK FACTORS:
- Daycare attendance
- Limited or no breastfeeding
- Tobacco smoke exposure
- Pacifier use
- Craniofacial anomalies
- Immune globulin G (IgG) or subclass deficiencies

PHYSICAL FINDINGS & CLINICAL PRESENTATION[3]
- Moderate to severe bulging of the TM.
- Fluid in the middle ear along with signs and symptoms of local inflammation.

1. Erythema with diminished light reflex (Fig. E1)
- As infection progresses, middle ear exudation occurs (exudative phase); the exudate rapidly changes from serous to purulent (suppurative phase).
- Retraction and poor mobility of the TM ensues, and the TM begins to bulge.
- At any time during the suppurative phase, the TM may rupture, releasing the middle ear contents (otorrhea).
- Erythema of the TM without other abnormalities is not a diagnostic criterion for acute otitis media (AOM) because it may occur with any inflammation of the upper respiratory tract, crying, or nose blowing.
- Symptoms[1]:
  1. Rapid- or recent-onset otalgia, ranging from slight discomfort to severe, is the most common presenting symptom.
  2. Hearing loss while middle ear fluid is present.
  3. Otorrhea (if TM has ruptured).
  4. Systemic symptoms such as fever, listlessness, irritability, decreased appetite, vomiting, and diarrhea are common. Although vertigo, facial swelling, nystagmus, tinnitus, lethargy, and facial nerve palsies can occur as rare complications of AOM; these symptoms should prompt consideration of an alternate diagnosis.
  5. Table 2 summarizes symptom scoring systems designed to aid in diagnosis.
- After an episode of AOM:
  1. Persistence of effusion for weeks or months (called secretory, serous, or nonsuppurative otitis media)
  2. Fever and otalgia usually absent
  3. Hearing loss possible (10 to 50 dB, with predominant involvement of the low frequencies)
  4. Manifestations of the sequelae and complications of otitis media are summarized in Table E3

ETIOLOGY
- Most common etiology is a viral upper respiratory tract infection, which causes inflammation and dysfunction of the eustachian tube and transient aspiration of nasopharyngeal secretions into the middle ear (Fig. 2). Bacterial colonization from the nasopharynx in conjunction with eustachian tube dysfunction leads to infection.
- May occasionally develop as a result of hematogenous spread or by direct invasion from the nasopharynx.
- Conjugated pneumococcal vaccination of children has resulted in decreases in *Streptococcus pneumoniae* causing AOM.
- Most common bacterial pathogens[4,5]:
  1. *Haemophilus influenzae* is now the most common causative pathogen of AOM in children.
  2. *S. pneumoniae* causes up to half of cases and is the least likely of the major pathogens to resolve without treatment.
  3. *Moraxella catarrhalis.*

Of increasing importance, infection caused by penicillin-nonsusceptible *S. pneumoniae* (MIC >0.1 mg/ml), ranging from 8% to 34%. About 50% of PNSSP isolates are penicillin-intermediate (MIC 0.1 to 2.0 mg/ml).
- Group A streptococci is associated with higher rates of TM perforation than AOM caused by other pathogens.
- Viral pathogens:
  1. Respiratory syncytial virus (RSV)
  2. Rhinovirus
  3. Adenovirus
  4. Influenza
- Others:
  1. *Mycoplasma pneumoniae*
  2. *Chlamydia trachomatis*
  3. *Streptococcus pyogenes* (Latin America)

DIAGNOSIS

DIFFERENTIAL DIAGNOSIS
- Otitis externa
- Otitis media with effusion (OME): An algorithm for distinguishing between acute otitis media and otitis media with effusion is illustrated in Fig. 3
- Referred pain from mouth, nasopharynx, or throat
- Section II describes the differential diagnosis of earache

WORKUP (TABLE 4)

Thorough otoscopic examination. AOM is a visual diagnosis based on viewing the tympanic membrane. Adequate visualization of the tympanic membrane may require removal of cerumen and debris from the external ear canal.
- Tympanometry
  1. Measures compliance of the tympanic membrane and middle ear pressure
  2. Detects the presence of fluid, but cannot determine whether the fluid is infected
- Acoustic reflectometry
  1. Measures sound waves reflected from the middle ear
  2. Is useful in infants >3 mo
  3. Increased reflected sound correlated with the presence of effusion, but cannot determine whether the fluid is infected

LABORATORY TESTS
- Tympanocentesis.
  1. Not necessary in most cases because the microbiology of middle ear effusions has been shown to be extremely consistent
  2. May be indicated in:
     a. Patients who do not respond to treatment in 72 hr or those who experience multiple treatment failures
     b. Immunocompromised patients
- Cultures of the nasopharynx are not helpful.
- Blood counts (generally unnecessary) usually reveal leukocytosis with polymorphonuclear elevation.
- Plain mastoid radiographs (generally unnecessary) reveal haziness in the periantral cells that may extend to entire mastoid.

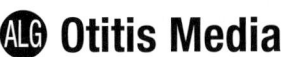

TABLE 1 Otitis Media Definitions and Terminology

Preferred Term	Definition	Comment
Otitis media (OM)	Inflammation of the middle ear without reference to etiology or pathogenesis	Nonspecific umbrella term for any condition associated with middle ear inflammation
Acute otitis media (AOM)	Rapid onset of signs and symptoms of inflammation in the middle ear	Diagnosed when there is moderate to severe bulging of the ear drum; mild bulging of the ear drum and recent (<48 h) onset of ear pain or intense erythema of the ear drum; or acute ear discharge unrelated to otitis externa (inflammation of the external ear canal)*
Recurrent AOM (rAOM)	≥3 well-documented and separate AOM episodes in the preceding 6 mo or ≥4 episodes in the preceding 12 mo with >1 episode in the past 6 mo	Children without persistent MEE tend to have a good prognosis and often improve spontaneously; children with persistent MEE have a poorer prognosis and might benefit from ventilation tubes
Otitis media with effusion (OME)	Fluid in the middle ear without signs or symptoms of acute ear infection	Diagnosed by one or more of the following: Reduced ear drum mobility on pneumatic otoscopy, reduced ear drum mobility on tympanometry, opaque ear drum or a visible air-fluid interface behind the ear drum on otoscopy
Chronic OME	OME persisting for ≥3 mo from date of onset (if known) or from date of diagnosis (if onset is unknown)	Chronic OME has much lower rates of spontaneous resolution compared to OME of new onset or following an episode of AOM
Chronic suppurative otitis media (CSOM)	Chronic inflammation of the middle ear and mastoid mucosa with a nonintact ear drum (perforation or ventilation tube) and persistent ear discharge	No consensus on duration of ear discharge needed for diagnosis, with recommendations ranging from 2 wk to at least 3 mo
Middle ear effusion (MEE)	Fluid in the middle ear from any cause	MEE is present with both OME and AOM and might persist for weeks or months after the signs and symptoms of AOM resolve

*The degree of bulging does not reflect AOM severity. Severe AOM is defined as having moderate-to-severe ear pain, ear pain for at least 48 h, or temperature 39° C or higher.
From Flint PW et al: *Cummings otolaryngology, head and neck surgery,* ed 7, Philadelphia, 2021, Elsevier.

TABLE 2 Acute Otitis Media Symptom Scoring Systems Designed to Aid in Diagnosis

3-Item Otitis Media Score (OM-3)	Ear Treatment Group Symptom Questionnaire (ETG-5)	Acute Otitis Media Faces Scale (AOM-FS)	Otoscopic Severity Scale (OS-8)	Acute Otitis Media Severity of Symptom Scale (AOM-SOS)	Otitis Media Clinical Severity Index (OM-CSI) 30-Point Scale[a]	Otitis Media Clinical Severity Index (OM-CSI) 10-Point Scale[a]
Physical suffering	Ear pain	Seven facial expressions ranging from no problem to extreme problem	Eight categories of TM inflammation[b]	Ear pain	Ear pain	Ear pain
Emotional distress	Fever			Ear tugging	Fever	Fever
Limitation of activities	Irritability			Irritability	Irritability	Irritability
	Appetite			Decreased play	Fever at examination	Fever at examination
	Sleep quality			Decreased appetite	TM erythema	TM erythema
				Difficulty sleeping	TM mobility	TM mobility
				Fever	TM position	TM position
					Effusion color	Effusion color
					Otorrhea	Otorrhea

TM, Tympanic membrane.
[a]The 30-point scale used a 2- to 5-point Likert scale and the 10-point scale used a 2- to 3-point Likert scale.
[b]0 = normal; 1 = erythema only; 2 = erythema, air-fluid level, clear fluid; 3 = erythema, complete effusion, no opacification; 4 = erythema, opacification with air-fluid level or air bubbles, no bulging; 5 = erythema, complete effusion, opacification, no bulging; 6 = erythema, bulging rounded doughnut appearance of the tympanic membrane; 7 = erythema, bulging, complete effusion and opacification with bulla formation.
From Cherry JD et al: *Feigin and Cherry's pediatric infectious diseases,* ed 8, Philadelphia, 2019, Elsevier.

- CT or MRI may be indicated if serious complications are suspected (meningitis, brain abscess, severe mastoiditis).

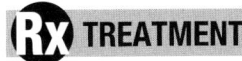 **TREATMENT**

ACUTE GENERAL Rx
- Hydration, avoidance of irritants (e.g., tobacco smoke, air pollution, bottle feeding), nasal decongestants, cool mist humidifier, and oral ibuprofen or acetaminophen. Topical procaine or lidocaine preparations (if available) are an alternative to oral analgesics for children ≥2 yr but should not be used in children with tympanic membrane perforation.[3]

- Antibiotics: See section on 'Complementary & Alternative Medicine Therapies'.

SURGICAL Rx
- There is no evidence to support the routine use of myringotomy, but in severe cases it provides prompt pain relief and accelerates resolution of infection.
- Purulent secretions retained in the middle ear can lead to increased pressure that may lead to spread of infection to contiguous areas. Myringotomy to decompress the middle ear is sometimes necessary to avoid complications such as mastoiditis, facial nerve paralysis, labyrinthitis, meningitis, and brain abscess.

CHRONIC Rx
- Among children 6 to 35 mo of age with recurrent acute otitis media, the rate of episodes of acute otitis media during a 2-yr period is not significantly lower with tympanostomy-tube placement than with medical management, however myringotomy and tympanostomy tube placement for persistent or recurrent middle ear effusion unresponsive to medical therapy can be considered if fluid has persisted for ≥3 mo if bilateral or ≥6 mo if unilateral.
- Adenoidectomy, with or without tonsillectomy, often is advocated for treatment of recurrent otitis media, although evidence for this procedure is controversial.

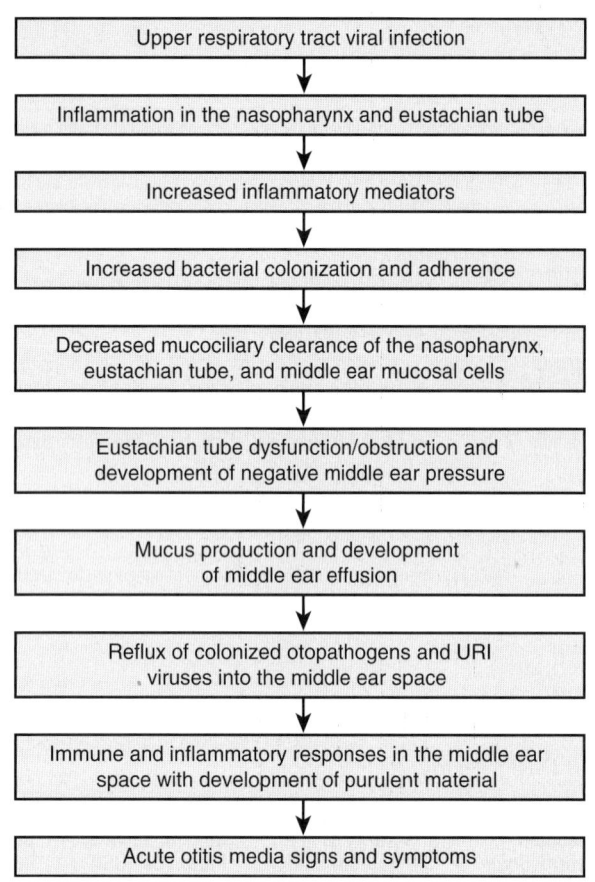

FIG. 2 Pathogenesis of virus-induced acute otitis media. *URI,* Upper respiratory infection. (From Cherry JD et al: *Feigin and Cherry's pediatric infectious diseases,* ed 8, Philadelphia, 2019, Elsevier.)

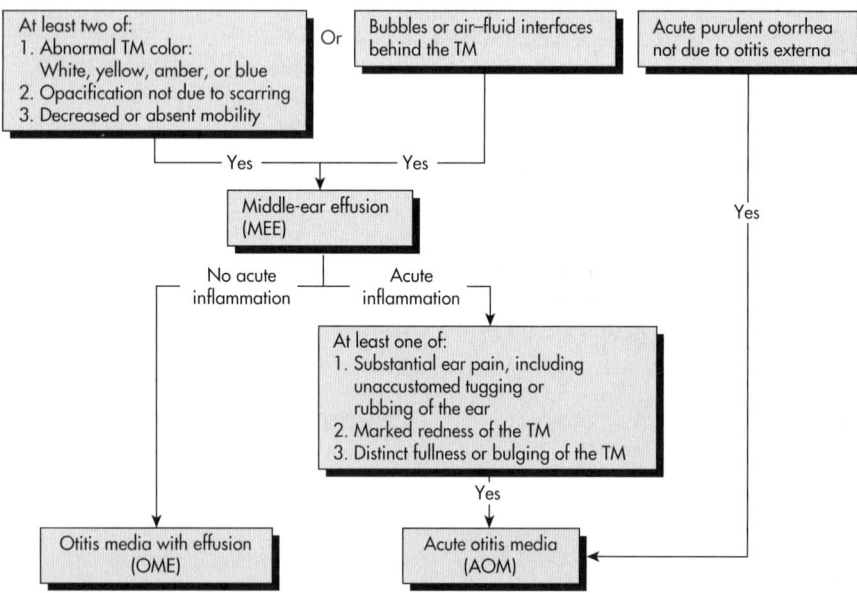

FIG. 3 Algorithm for distinguishing between acute otitis media and otitis media with effusion. *TM,* tympanic membrane. (From Kliegman RM: *Nelson textbook of pediatrics,* ed 21, Philadelphia, 2020, Elsevier.)

- Long-term complications include tympanic membrane perforations, cholesteatoma, tympanosclerosis, ossicular necrosis, toxic or suppurative labyrinthitis, hearing loss, and intracranial suppuration.

DISPOSITION

Patients can be treated at home as outpatients with the rare exception of patients with evidence of local suppurative complications (e.g., meningitis, acute mastoiditis, brain abscess, cavernous sinus, or lateral sinus thrombosis).

COMPLEMENTARY & ALTERNATIVE MEDICINE THERAPIES[6]:

- Xylitol and vitamin intake may help prevent further otitis media.[7]
- Biologically based therapies such as botanical extracts can be used if there is no perforation (all prepared in an olive oil base) and can be a reasonable complement during observation period or with the wait-and-see approach.
  1. Calendula
  2. Hypericum perforatum homeopathic preparation—can help with pain[7]
  3. Lavendar
  4. Vitamin E oil
- Manipulative methods have also been used by those properly trained in osteopathic manipulation and chiropractic techniques. Osteopathy requires weekly treatment for 3 wk and is an adjunct to other treatment modalities. Chiropractic techniques: Little is published and there are currently no randomized controlled trials on PubMed.
- Chinese medicine has shown promising results but demands further research.[7]
  Antimicrobials:
  Note: Most uncomplicated cases of AOM resolve spontaneously, without complications. Studies have demonstrated limited therapeutic benefit from antibiotic therapy. Watchful waiting is appropriate for children who look well, can be comforted with supportive care, and are old enough to easily evaluate. Children <24 mo with bilateral AOM should receive antibiotic therapy. Children with severe signs or symptoms (moderate or severe otalgia or otalgia for ≥48 h or temperature ≥39° C) should also receive antibiotic therapy. Fig. E4 illustrates an algorithm for management of acute otitis media in pediatric populations.
  When opting to use antibiotic therapy[2,4,8-10]:
- Amoxicillin has been used for years as first line treatment of AOM but because of increased prevalence of AOM caused by beta-lactamase strains of *H. influenzae* and *M. catarrhalis* some expert clinicians now recommend amoxicillin-clavulanate for initial treatment.
- Treatment failure is defined by lack of clinical improvement of signs or symptoms after 3 days (72 h or greater) of therapy.
- With treatment failure (if using amoxicillin), in the absence of an identified etiologic pathogen, therapy should be redirected to cover:
  1. Drug-resistant *S. pneumoniae*
  2. β-lactamase–producing strains of *H. influenzae* and *M. catarrhalis*
- Agents fulfilling these criteria include amoxicillin/clavulanate, second-generation (e.g., cefuroxime axetil, cefaclor) or third-generation (e.g., oral cefdinir or cefpodoxime or IM ceftriaxone) cephalosporins. Cefaclor, cefixime, loracarbef, and ceftibuten should be avoided given their limited activity against pneumococci.
- Cross-resistance between TMP/SX and macrolides and the β-lactams exists; therefore

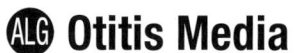
TABLE 4 Diagnostic Modalities for Otitis Media

Modality	Description	Comment
Signs and symptoms (obtained by history)	Includes ear-specific symptoms (ear pain, hearing loss), nonspecific symptoms (nausea, irritability, sleep disturbance, anorexia), and signs (fever, vomiting)	The hallmark of AOM and OME are ear pain and hearing loss, respectively, but signs and symptoms alone have poor diagnostic accuracy
Symptom severity scales	Parent-reported measures of AOM severity using categoric responses or a faces scale	Not useful for AOM diagnosis, but can be used to rate severity, follow the course of disease, and assess outcomes
Otoscopy	Visual examination of the ear canal and tympanic membrane with an otoscope	Bulging tympanic membrane is characteristic of AOM; opaque or cloudy tympanic membrane is characteristic of OME
Pneumatic otoscopy	Examination of the middle ear using an otoscope to create an air-tight (hermetic) seal in the ear canal and then gently squeezing (or releasing) the attached rubber bulb to change the pressure in the ear canal and observe the tympanic membrane	A normal tympanic membrane moves briskly with applied pressure, but the movement is minimal or sluggish when there is fluid in the middle ear; no motion is observed if tympanic membrane is not intact
Otomicroscopy	Examination of the ear canal and tympanic membrane using the binocular, otologic microscope to obtain a magnified view with good depth perception	Primary use is to assess tympanic membrane abnormalities (atrophy, sclerosis, retraction pockets) and to help distinguish surface findings from middle ear pathology
Tympanometry	An objective measure of middle ear function that requires an air-tight seal in the ear canal. Tympanometry provides a graph showing how energy admitted to the ear canal is reflected back to an internal microphone while the canal pressure is varied from negative to positive (pressure admittance function) and can be performed with a portable (handheld) unit or a desktop machine	If the middle ear is filled with fluid, tympanic membrane vibration is impaired and the result is a flat, or nearly flat, tracing. If the middle ear is filled with air but at a higher or lower pressure than the surrounding atmosphere, the peak on the graph will be shifted in position based on the pressure (to the left if negative, to the right if positive)
Acoustic reflectometry	Uses a transducer and microphone at the entrance of the ear canal, without an air-tight seal, to measure how much sound is reflected off the tympanic membrane	Higher reflectivity levels indicate a greater probability of effusion, but unlike tympanometry it only assesses the probability of effusion and cannot measure middle ear function
Computed tomography	An imaging procedure, using ionizing radiation, to create a detailed scan of the temporal bone	Useful in surgical planning for CSOM but not useful for primary diagnosis of AOM, OME, or CSOM

AOM, Acute otitis media; *CSOM,* chronic suppurative otitis media; *OME,* otitis media with effusion.
From Flint PW et al: *Cummings otolaryngology, head and neck surgery,* ed 7, Philadelphia, 2021, Elsevier.

patients who do not respond to amoxicillin are more likely to have infections resistant to TMP/SMX and macrolides.
- Fluoroquinolones are not indicated as first- or second-line therapy for AOM and should be avoided in young children due to risks of musculoskeletal effects and limited dosing guidance and limited availability of oral suspension compounds or compounding pharmacies.
- Treatment should be modified according to cultures and sensitivities when available.
- Treatment course is 10 days for children <2 yr and those with severe symptoms, 7 days for children age 2 to 5 yr, and 5 to 7 days for children ≥6 yr.
- Follow-up should be tailored to clinical improvement and concern for neurocognitive developmental delays in at-risk children. Standard follow-up of all cases is no longer recommended.
- Antibiotic prophylaxis to reduce the frequency of AOM episodes in children with recurrent AOM is not recommended.

- Table E5 summarizes suggested antibiotics for treatment of otitis media and for patients who have failed first-line antibiotic treatment.

REFERRAL
- To otorhinolaryngologist in cases of:
  1. Medical treatment failure
  2. An uncertain diagnosis; adults with one or more episodes of AOM should be referred for evaluation to rule out an underlying process (e.g., malignancy)
  3. Any of the above-mentioned acute and chronic complications

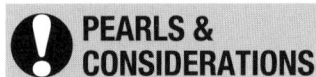 **PEARLS & CONSIDERATIONS**

COMMENTS
- Otoscopic findings are critical for accurate AOM diagnosis.[11]

- AOM microbiology has changed with use of pneumococcal conjugate vaccine (PCV13).
- Antibiotics are modestly more effective than no treatment but cause adverse effects in 4% to 10% of children.
- Most antibiotics have comparable clinical success.

PREVENTION
- Vaccinate against common pathogens.
- Breastfeed and bottle-feed infants in an upright position.
- Avoid irritants (e.g., tobacco smoke).

REFERENCES
Available at eBooks.Health.Elsevier.com.

AUTHOR: **KATHERINE ELIZABETH MCGRAW, MD**

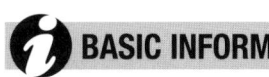

BASIC INFORMATION

DEFINITION

Ovarian cancer is not one disease, but a constellation of distinct cancer subtypes classified according to their tissue of origin. About 90% of tumors are epithelial ovarian cancers, 5% are germ cell tumors, and 5% are sex cord-stromal tumors. A classification of ovarian epithelial tumors is summarized in Table E1.

SYNONYMS

Epithelial ovarian cancer
Germ cell tumor
Sex cord stromal tumor
Ovarian tumor of low malignant potential
Ovarian malignancy

ICD-10CM CODES

C56.9	Malignant neoplasm of unspecified ovary
C56.1	Malignant neoplasm of right ovary
C56.2	Malignant neoplasm of left ovary

EPIDEMIOLOGY & DEMOGRAPHICS

INCIDENCE: Ovarian cancer ranks fifth in cancer deaths among biologic females and is the leading cause of gynecologic cancer–related deaths. There are 10.6 cases/100,000 persons and ~19,880 new cases annually. Lifetime risk for developing ovarian cancer is 1.1%. The rate of diagnosis of ovarian cancer has been slowly declining over the past 20 yr.[1]
PREVALENCE: Median age at time of diagnosis: 63 yr

RISK FACTORS:
- Low parity
- Delayed childbearing
- Smoking
- Polycystic ovary syndrome
- Endometriosis
- High-fat diet
- Lynch II syndrome (nonpolyposis colon cancer, endometrial cancer, breast cancer, and ovarian cancer clusters in first- and second-degree relatives)
- Breast-ovarian familial cancer syndrome
- Site-specific familial ovarian cancer
- The **strongest** risk factors are advancing age and family history of ovarian and breast cancer
- Factors that **decrease** the risk of ovarian cancer include previous pregnancy, oral contraceptive pill use, hysterectomy, tubal ligation, or salpingectomy
- Table 2 summarizes risk and protective factors for ovarian cancer

GENETICS: The greatest risk factors of ovarian cancer are a family history and associated genetic syndromes. More than 90% of inherited ovarian malignancies are associated with BRCA1 and BRCA2 mutations. BRCA mutations interact with and affect DNA repair proteins. The estimated lifetime risk of ovarian cancer for patients with either of these mutations is 65% to 74%.
Genetic counseling is recommended for certain patients, including those with:
- Epithelial ovarian cancer at any age

- Breast cancer diagnosed at age 45 yr or younger
- Breast cancer with two distinct and sequential primaries, the first one diagnosed at age 50 yr or younger
- Breast cancer that is triple-negative and diagnosed at age 60 yr or younger
- Breast cancer at any age, with at least one close relative diagnosed at age 50 yr or younger
- Breast cancer diagnosed at any age, with two or more close relatives with breast cancer; one close relative with epithelial ovarian cancer; or two close relatives with pancreatic cancer or aggressive prostate cancer
- Breast cancer, with a close male relative at any age who has breast cancer
- Breast cancer and Ashkenazi Jewish ancestry
- A family with a known deleterious BRCA1 or BRCA2 mutation

PHYSICAL FINDINGS & CLINICAL PRESENTATION

- Patients with ovarian cancer commonly present with nonspecific symptoms. A recent study revealed that at the time of diagnosis 72% of women had at least one symptom and 32% had two or more symptoms (Table 3). The most common presenting symptoms were abdominal or pelvic pain (31%) and bloating or a sensation of abdominal fullness (26%).[2]
- 60% present with advanced disease
- Abdominal fullness, early satiety, dyspepsia
- Pelvic pain, back pain, constipation
- Pelvic or abdominal mass (Table 4)
- Lymphadenopathy (inguinal)

TABLE 2 Risk and Protective Factors for Ovarian Cancer

Increased Risk	Protective
Lifestyle and diet factors	Lifestyle and diet factors
Aging	Soy intake
Obesity	Flavonoids
Tall stature	High calcium
Animal fat intake	Sun exposure
α-linolenic acid	Adequate sleep
Dairy foods	Metformin
Lactose product	
Cigarette use	
Diabetes mellitus	
Reproductive factors	Reproductive factors
Menopausal hormone therapy	Oral contraceptive
Menopausal age	Breastfeeding
Infertility	Tubal sterilization
Polycystic ovarian syndrome	Salpingectomy
Endometriosis	Hysterectomy
Pelvic inflammatory disease	Parity
Genetic factors	

From Niederhuber JE: *Abeloff's clinical oncology*, ed 6, Philadelphia, 2020, Elsevier.

- Sister Mary Joseph nodule (umbilical mass)

ETIOLOGY

- Can be inherited as site-specific familial ovarian cancer (two or more first-degree relatives have ovarian cancer)
- Breast-ovarian cancer syndrome (clusters of breast and ovarian cancer among first- and second-degree relatives)
- Lynch syndrome
- There is no contributory family history and an unknown etiology in the majority of ovarian cancer cases

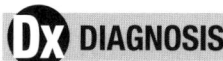

DIAGNOSIS

DIFFERENTIAL DIAGNOSIS

- Primary peritoneal cancer mesothelioma
- Benign ovarian tumor
- Functional ovarian cyst
- Endometriosis
- Ovarian torsion
- Pelvic kidney
- Pedunculated uterine fibroid

TABLE 3 Symptoms in Ovarian Cancer

Symptom	% of patients
Pain (late symptom)	50-60
Abdominal swelling (persistent bloating)	50-65
Anorexia	20
Nausea and vomiting	20
Weight loss	15
Abnormal vaginal bleeding	15
Frequency	10
Malaise	5
Change in bowel habit	5
Virilization	Rare
Precocious puberty	Rare

From Magowan BA: *Clinical obstetrics & gynecology*, ed 4, London, 2019, Elsevier.

TABLE 4 Signs of Ovarian Cancer

Sign	% of patients
Pelvic mass	70-80
Abdominal mass	60-70
Ascites	30-40
Pleural effusion	10-15
Hepatomegaly	<5
Cervical lymphadenopathy	<5

From Magowan BA: *Clinical obstetrics & gynecology*, ed 4, London, 2019, Elsevier.

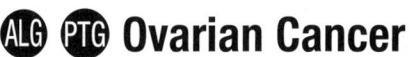
O

Diseases
and Disorders

I

- Primary cancer from breast, gastrointestinal tract, or other pelvic organ metastasized to the ovary

WORKUP

- Definitive diagnosis made at laparotomy; epithelial ovarian cancer most common type of ovarian cancer (90% of ovarian cancer cases)
- Careful physical and history, including family history
- Exclusion of nongynecologic etiologies
- Observation of small cystic masses in premenopausal women for regression for 2 mo
- FIGO classification of ovarian carcinoma is described in Table 5
- Referral to specialists who have extensive training and experience in treating ovarian cancer significantly increases survival after an ovarian cancer diagnosis

LABORATORY TESTS

- CBC.
- Chemistry profile including liver tests and calcium (to evaluate for paraneoplastic syndrome).
- CA-125 or lysophosphatidic acid level. Use of these tests for annual screening is controversial, and most experts warn against universal screening with this marker. Only about 50% of early-stage ovarian cancers will be associated with elevated CA-125. Additionally, false elevations may occur with uterine leiomyoma, endometriosis, pregnancy, and intra-abdominal infections. The PLCO cancer screening trial revealed that annual screening based on CA-125 and vaginal ultrasound is ineffective, and diagnostic follow-up of false positives resulted in a 15% serious complication rate.
- Consider the following laboratory tests: Human chorionic gonadotropin, inhibin, alpha-fetoprotein, neuron-specific enolase, and lactate dehydrogenase.
- A panel of three serum biomarkers (apolipoprotein A-1 [ApoA-1], transthyretin [TTR], and transferrin [TF]) has been reported useful in distinguishing normal samples from early-stage ovarian cancer with a sensitivity of 84% and normal samples from late-stage ovarian cancer with a sensitivity of 97%.
- BRCA1/2 testing is recommended for all women with ovarian cancer.

IMAGING STUDIES

- Ultrasound
- Chest x-ray examination
- Computed tomography or MRI of abdomen and pelvis help evaluate extent of disease (Fig. E1)
- Mammogram

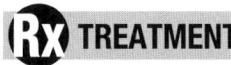 TREATMENT

NONPHARMACOLOGIC THERAPY

Virtually all cases of ovarian cancer involve surgical exploration. This includes:
- Abdominal cytology
- Total abdominal hysterectomy and bilateral salpingo-oophorectomy (except when fertility preservation is desired and the disease is the early stage)
- Omentectomy
- Diaphragm sampling
- Selective lymphadenectomy (pelvic and para-aortic nodes)
- Primary cytoreduction with a goal of residual tumor diameter <2 cm
- Bowel surgery, splenectomy if needed to obtain optimal (<2 cm) cytoreduction
- Conventional treatment includes surgical debulking (cytoreduction) followed by chemotherapy. However, patients with low-grade, well-differentiated stage I ovarian cancer do not benefit from adjuvant chemotherapy

ACUTE GENERAL Rx

- Optimal cytoreduction (debulking) is generally followed by chemotherapy (except in some early-stage disease [stage I without high-risk features is treated with surgery alone]).
- Cisplatin-based combination chemotherapy is used for stage II or greater, 6-mo treatment. Compared with IV paclitaxel plus cisplatin, IV paclitaxel plus intraperitoneal cisplatin and paclitaxel improves survival rates in patients with optimally debulked stage III ovarian cancer.
- Chemotherapy regimens continue to change as research continues. Bevacizumab, a humanized antivascular endothelial growth factor monoclonal antibody, has been shown to be effective in improving progression-free survival in women with ovarian cancer. Trials using bevacizumab during and up to 10 mo after carboplatin and paclitaxel chemotherapy have shown prolongation of the median progression-free survival by about 4 mo in patients with advanced epithelial ovarian cancer.
- Antibody drug conjugates in conjunction with VEG-F inhibitors such as bevacizumab are a promising new area of study that is currently under investigation for treatment of patients who are resistant to platinum-based chemotherapy. This area remains under investigation.[3]
- PARP inhibitors are up-and-coming chemotherapeutic agents that have been used for maintenance therapy and have been shown to improve progression-free survival among patients with platinum-sensitive high-grade serous cancers. PARP inhibitors work by pharmacologically inhibiting the enzyme poly (ADP-ribose) polymerase. Three PARP inhibitors are currently U.S. Food and Drug Administration approved for different indications. Olaparib, an oral polymerase inhibitor, was approved in 2014 and has shown

TABLE 5 Staging of Ovarian Carcinomas*

Stage	Characteristics
I	Tumor confined to the ovaries
IA	Growth limited to one ovary (capsule intact); no tumor on ovarian surface; no malignant cells in the ascites or peritoneal washings
IB	Tumor limited to both ovaries (capsule intact); no tumor on ovarian surface; no malignant cells in the ascites or peritoneal washings
IC	Tumor limited to one or both ovaries
1C1	Surgical spill
1C2	Capsule ruptured before surgery or tumor on ovarian surface
1C3	Malignant cells in the ascites or peritoneal washings
II	Tumor involves one or both ovaries with pelvic extension
IIA	Extension or metastases to the uterus or fallopian tubes
IIB	Extension to other pelvic intraperitoneal tissues
III	Tumor involving one or both ovaries with cytologically or histologically confirmed spread to the peritoneum outside the pelvis or metastasis to the retroperitoneal lymph nodes
IIIA1	Positive retroperitoneal lymph nodes only (cytologically or histologically proved)
IIIA1 (i)	Metastasis up to 10 mm in greatest dimension
IIIA1 (ii)	Metastasis more than 10 mm in greatest dimension
IIIA2	Microscopic extrapelvic (above the pelvic brim) peritoneal involvement with or without positive retroperitoneal lymph nodes
IIIB	Macroscopic peritoneal metastasis beyond the pelvis up to 2 cm in greatest dimension, with or without metastasis to the retroperitoneal lymph nodes
IIIC	Macroscopic peritoneal metastasis beyond the pelvis more than 2 cm in greatest dimension, with or without metastasis to the retroperitoneal lymph nodes (includes extension of tumor to capsule of liver and spleen without parenchymal involvement of either organ)
IV	Distant metastases excluding peritoneal metastases
IVA	Pleural effusion with positive cytology
IVB	Parenchymal metastases and metastases to extraabdominal organs (including inguinal lymph nodes and lymph nodes outside of the abdominal cavity)

*According to the International Federation of Gynecology and Obstetrics (FIGO), 2014.
Berek, JS, Renz, M, Kehoe, S, Kumar, L, Friedlander, M. Cancer of the ovary, fallopian tube, and peritoneum: 2021 update. *Int J Gynecol Obstet.* 2021;155(Suppl. 1):61-85. https://doi.org/10.1002/ijgo.13878.

antitumor activity in patients with high-grade serous ovarian cancer with or without *BRCA1* and *BRCA2* germline mutations. Rucaparib was approved in 2016 to treat high-grade serous cancers with *BRCA1* and *BRCA2* germline or somatic mutations. Lastly, niraparib was approved in 2017 for use in high-grade serous cancers with or without *BRCA1* and *BRCA2* mutations.

- Second-look surgery when chemotherapy is complete generally is no longer recommended because this has not been shown to improve survival.
- In most cases, neoadjuvant (presurgical) chemotherapy has no advantage over post-surgical initiation of chemotherapy. However, some trials have shown that neoadjuvant chemotherapy followed by interval debulking surgery is not inferior to debulking surgery followed by chemotherapy as a treatment option for patients with bulky stage IIIC or IV ovarian carcinoma. Complete resection of all macroscopic disease, whether performed as primary treatment or after neoadjuvant chemotherapy, remains the objective whenever cytoreductive surgery is performed.

CHRONIC Rx

- If CA-125 is increasing, this may indicate recurrent disease. However, routine monitoring of CA-125 at every visit does not improve survival and should be reserved for addressing specific clinical concerns.
- Physical and pelvic examinations recommended every 2 to 4 mo for 2 yr, every 3 to 6 mo during third yr, then annually after 5 yr.
- Annual Pap smear.
- A treatment approach algorithm for recurrent ovarian cancer is illustrated in Fig. 2.

- A recent randomized trial of cytoreductive surgery for relapsed ovarian cancer revealed that in women with recurrent ovarian cancer, cytoreductive surgery followed by chemotherapy results in longer overall survival than chemotherapy alone. Secondly, cytoreductive surgery should be considered an appropriate option in properly selected patients if it can be performed by experienced surgeons in centers of excellence.[4]

DISPOSITION

- Overall 5-yr survival rates remain low because of the preponderance of late-stage disease:
  1. Stage I and II: 80% to 100%
  2. Stage III: 15% to 20%
  3. Stage IV: 5%
- Younger patients (<50 yr) in all stages have a considerably better 5-yr survival than older patients (40% vs. 15%).
- Among women with high-grade serous ovarian cancer, *BRCA2* mutation, but not *BRCA1* deficiency, is associated with improved survival, improved chemotherapy response, and genome instability compared with *BRCA* wild-type.
- Among patients with invasive epithelial ovarian cancer (EOC), having a germline mutation in *BRCA1* or *BRCA2* is associated with improved 5-yr overall survival. *BRCA2* carriers have the best prognosis.

PEARLS & CONSIDERATIONS
COMMENTS

- The U.S. Preventive Services Task Force has concluded that current evidence does not show any mortality benefit to routine screening for ovarian cancer with transvaginal ultrasonography or single-threshold serum CA-125

testing and that the harms of such screening are at least moderate. This recommendation applies to asymptomatic women who are not known to have a high-risk hereditary cancer syndrome.
- Oral contraceptives reduce the risk of ovarian cancer by 40% to 50%. The greatest risk reduction is present after ≥15 yr of oral contraceptive use.
- Patients at high risk for developing ovarian cancer (*BRCA1*/*BRCA2* gene mutation, hereditary nonpolyposis colorectal cancer syndrome) should consider prophylactic salpingo-oophorectomy after childbearing is complete. Prophylactic bilateral salpingo-oophorectomy reduces ovarian cancer by 80%. It is recommended by age 35 to 40 yr for *BRCA1* carriers and by age 45 for *BRCA2* carriers. If surgery is declined, the National Comprehensive Cancer network guidelines recommend intensive surveillance with pelvic and abdominal sonogram and serum CA-125 every 6 mo starting at age 35 or 10 yr earlier than cancer diagnosis in family member.

REFERENCES & SUGGESTED READINGS
Available at eBooks.Health.Elsevier.com.

RELATED CONTENT
Ovarian Cancer (Patient Information)
Ovarian Neoplasm, Benign (Related Key Topic)

AUTHORS: **LAUREN DAVIS RIVERA, MD, MSEd, MD,** and **SUDESHNA CHAATTERJEEE-PAER, MD**

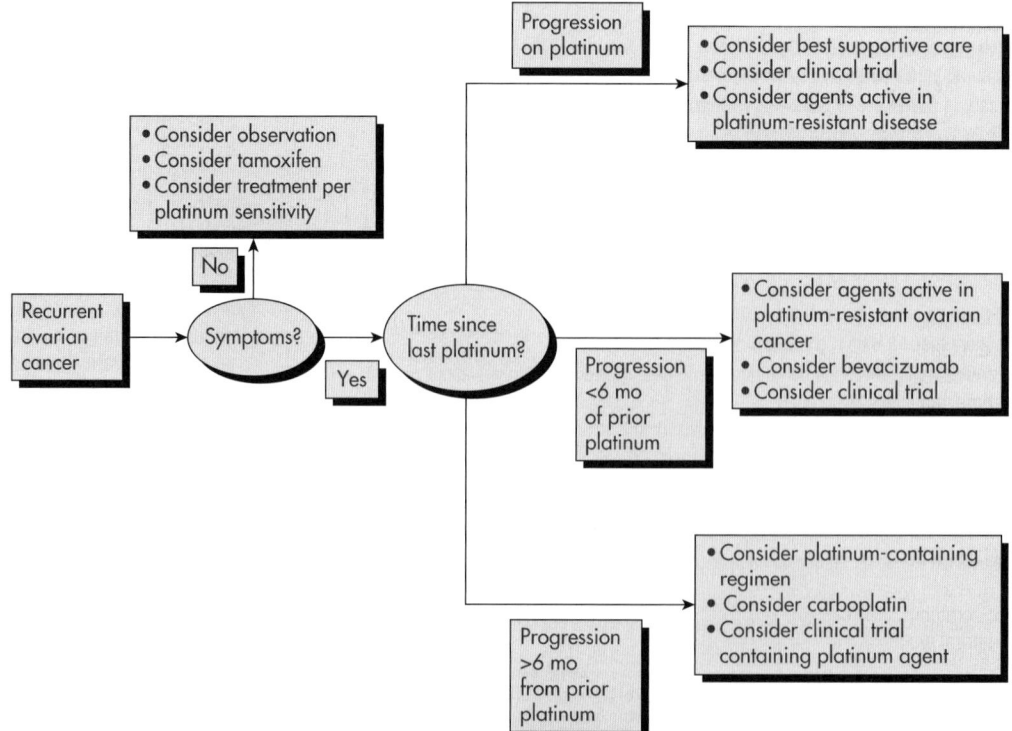

FIG. 2 Treatment approach algorithm for recurrent ovarian cancer. (From Niederhuber JE: *Abeloff's clinical oncology,* ed 6, Philadelphia, 2020, Elsevier.)

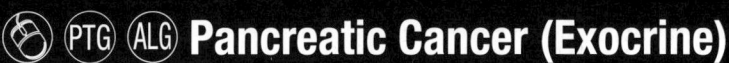
BASIC INFORMATION

DEFINITION

Pancreatic cancer is an adenocarcinoma derived from pancreatic duct epithelium. Pancreatic intraepithelial neoplasia (PIN) refers to microscopic premalignant lesions in the pancreatic ducts that then undergo stepwise progression from low grade to high grade with accumulating genetic alterations. Intraductal papillary mucinous neoplasms (IPMN) are precursors to pancreatic cancer with a 25% overall risk of invasive cancer especially in lesions arising from the main pancreatic duct.

ICD-10CM CODES
C25.9	Malignant neoplasm of pancreas, unspecified
C25.0	Malignant neoplasm of head of pancreas
C25.1	Malignant neoplasm of body of pancreas
C25.2	Malignant neoplasm of tail of pancreas
C25.3	Malignant neoplasm of pancreatic duct

EPIDEMIOLOGY & DEMOGRAPHICS

INCIDENCE:
- In 2022, it is estimated that there were 62,210 new cases and 49,830 deaths in the U.S.[1] It is the third-leading cause of cancer-related death in the U.S.
- Majority of patients present with advanced disease, and <20% patients present with potentially resectable tumors. At the time of diagnosis after symptoms develop 50% of patients have stage IV disease and an additional 35% have stage III disease.[2]

PREDOMINANT SEX:
- The male:female ratio is 2:1.

PREDOMINANT AGE:
- Median age at diagnosis is 71 yr.

PHYSICAL FINDINGS & CLINICAL PRESENTATION

Presenting symptoms are generally related to location[3]:
- Jaundice (60% to 70% of pancreatic cancers are located in the head of the pancreas)
- Dull abdominal pain or vague abdominal discomfort
- Weight loss
- Anorexia/change in taste, asthenia
- Nausea
- Uncommonly: Depression, gastrointestinal bleeding, acute pancreatitis (from obstruction of the pancreatic duct), back pain
- Trousseau syndrome may be the initial presentation in some patients
- Table 1 summarizes demographic features and presenting symptoms in pancreatic cancer patients

PHYSICAL FINDINGS
- Icterus
- Excoriations from scratching pruritic skin
- Cachexia and temporal wasting
- Ascites
- Hepatomegaly

ETIOLOGY

Unknown, but several conditions have been associated with pancreatic cancer[3]:
- Smoking
- Alcoholism
- Genetics: Up to 20% of patients have a family history of the disease
- Genetic syndromes and associated genes: Hereditary pancreatitis (PRSS1, SPINK1), Peutz-Jeghers syndrome (STK11[LKB1]), familial atypical multiple mole and melanoma syndrome (p16), hereditary breast and ovarian cancer syndromes (BRCA1, BRCA2, PALB2), ataxia telangiectasia (ATM), and Li-Fraumeni syndrome (P53)
- Gallstones
- Diabetes mellitus (present in at least 50% of patients with pancreatic cancer): New-onset diabetes after age 50 years confers a G- to S-fold increased risk for pancreatic ductal adenocarcinoma.[2]
- Chronic pancreatitis
- Diet rich in animal fat
- Occupational exposure: Oil refining, paper manufacturing, chemical industry
- Overweight or obesity during early adulthood is associated with a greater risk of pancreatic cancer and a younger age of disease onset. Obesity at an older age is associated with a lower overall survival in patients with pancreatic cancer
- There are four major driver genes for pancreatic cancer: KRAS, CDKN2A, TP53, and SMAD4. KRAS mutation and alterations in CDKN2A are early events in pancreatic cancer tumorigenesis
- Table 2 summarizes nongenetic and genetic risk factors for pancreatic cancer

DIAGNOSIS

DIFFERENTIAL DIAGNOSIS
- Common duct cholelithiasis
- Cholangiocarcinoma
- Common duct stricture
- Sclerosing cholangitis
- Primary biliary cirrhosis
- Autoimmune pancreatitis
- Drug-induced cholestasis (e.g., phenothiazines)
- Other pancreatic tumors (islet cell tumor, cystadenocarcinoma, epidermoid carcinoma, sarcomas, lymphomas)

WORKUP
- Initial laboratory testing includes complete blood count, comprehensive chemistry panel.
- The bile duct antigen CA 19-9 is not useful for screening but is utilized for risk assessment after surgical resection, detecting recurrence, and therapeutic monitoring in patients undergoing systemic therapy.[4]
- All patients diagnosed with pancreatic cancer should undergo risk assessment for underlying cancer-associated hereditary syndromes. Germline genetic testing for cancer susceptibility should be considered even if family history is unremarkable.

Routine Laboratory Tests	% Abnormal
Alkaline phosphatase	80
Bilirubin	55
Total protein	15
Amylase	15
Hemoglobin	60

IMAGING STUDIES
- Multidetector helical computed tomography (CT) (Fig. E1) with intravenous (IV) administration of contrast is the imaging procedure of choice for initial evaluation.
- Endoscopic ultrasonography (Fig. E2) is useful when the diagnosis is strongly suspected and tissue is required for diagnostic purposes. Fine-needle aspiration biopsy combined with

TABLE 1 Demographic Features and Presenting Symptoms and Signs in Patients With Unresectable (Palliated) and Resectable (Resected) Pancreatic Cancer

	Palliated (N = 256)	Resected (N = 512)
Demographic Features		
Age, average (yr)	64.0	65.8
Men/women	57%/43%	55%/45%
Race	91% white	91% white
Symptoms and Signs (%)		
Abdominal pain	64	36*
Jaundice	57	72*
Weight loss	48	43
Nausea/vomiting	30	18*
Back pain	26	2*

*P = 0.001 vs. palliated group.
From Feldman M et al: Sleisenger and Fordtran's gastrointestinal and liver disease, ed 10, Philadelphia, 2016, Elsevier.

TABLE 2 Nongenetic and Genetic Risk Factors for Pancreatic Cancer

Variable	Risk Increase
Nongenetic Risk Factors	
Chronic pancreatitis	13.3
New-onset type 2 diabetes	7.9
Long-standing diabetes mellitus	2.0
Obesity	2.0
Smoking	1.8
Alcohol abuse	1.2
Non–O blood group	1.3
Genetic Syndrome and Associated Genes	
Familial pancreatic cancer (unknown gene)	
One first-degree relative	9
Three first-degree relatives	32
Familial adenomatous polyposis *(APC)*	4.5-6
Breast and ovarian cancer syndrome *(BRCA1, BRCA2, PALB2)*	2-3.5
Peutz-Jeghers syndrome *(STK11/LKB1)*	132
Hereditary pancreatitis *(PRSS1, SPINK1)*	69
Familial atypical multiple mole melanoma pancreatic carcinoma syndrome *(P16INK4A/CDKN2A)*	47
Lynch syndrome *(MLH1, MSH2, MSH6, PMS2, EPCAM)*	8.6
Cystic fibrosis *(CFTR)*	3.5
Ataxia-telangiectasia *(ATM)*	Unknown
Genetic Polymorphisms	
ABO	1.3
NR5A2	1.3
TERT	1.2
PDX1	1.2
BCAR1, CTRB1, CTRB2	1.5
ZNRF3	1.2
LINC00673	1.3
ETAA1	1.1
TP63	1.1
SUGCT	1.1

From Niederhuber JE: *Abeloff's clinical oncology*, ed 6, Philadelphia, 2020, Elsevier.

endoscopic ultrasonography is the preferred modality for evaluation of cystic or mass lesions to determine malignancy.
- Endoscopic retrograde cholangiopancreatography (ERCP, Fig. E3) is useful in patients with jaundice needing an endoscopic stent to relieve obstruction.
- PET scans are of limited value in pancreatic cancer and are not part of standard management.

Noninvasive Imaging	% Abnormal
Abdominal ultrasonography	60
Abdominal CT scan (with contrast) (Fig. E4)	90
Abdominal MRI scan	90
Invasive Imaging	**% Abnormal**
ERCP	90
CT scan or ultrasonography-guided needle aspiration cytology	90-95

STAGING

2018 AJCC eighth edition of staging system for pancreatic cancer

PRIMARY TUMOR (T):

T_X	Primary tumor cannot be assessed
T_0	No evidence of primary tumor
T_1	Tumor <2 cm
T_2	Tumor >2 cm and <4 cm
T_3	Tumor >4 cm
T_4	Tumor involves celiac axis or superior mesenteric artery (unresectable primary)

LYMPH NODES (N):

N_0	No regional lymph nodes
N_1	Metastasis in 1-3 regional lymph nodes
N_2	Metastasis in >4 regional lymph nodes

DISTANT METASTASES (M):

M_X	Presence of distant metastasis cannot be assessed
M_0	No distant metastasis
M_1	Distant metastasis

STAGING GROUPS:

I_A	T_1, N_0, M_0
I_B	T_2, N_0, M_0
II_A	T_3, N_0, M_0
II_B	T_{1-3}, N_1, M_0
III	$T_{1-3}, N_2, M_0 T_4$, any N, M_0
IV	Any T, any N, M_1

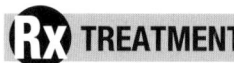 **TREATMENT**

Treatment sequencing strategies are summarized in Fig. 5 and Table 3.
- The overall treatment strategy is guided by the tumor resectability status and the patient's functional status. Pancreatic cancer (exocrine) is initially classified as resectable, borderline resectable, unresectable, and metastatic.[3]
- Palliative therapeutic ERCP with metal or plastic stents is performed for biliary decompression.

RESECTABLE DISEASE

Surgery:
- Classification of resectability of pancreatic cancer per the National Comprehensive Cancer Network and Surgical Oncology Expert Consensus Statement is summarized in Table 4.
- Curative pancreaticoduodenectomy (Whipple procedure) for pancreatic head and neck tumors is feasible in only 10% to 20% of patients (solitary lesion <5 cm, no locoregional invasion). Surgical mortality rate can be up to 5%. Distal pancreatectomy ($+/-$ splenectomy) is used for pancreatic body or tail tumors.
- Due to the complexity of surgery and risk for significant morbidity and mortality, current guidelines recommend that pancreatic resections be carried out in centers that perform at least 15 to 20 cases annually. High-volume institutions are associated with higher negative-margin status and higher 5-yr survival rates, and that patients are more likely to receive multimodality therapy at these centers.[5]

ADJUVANT THERAPY

- Adjuvant chemotherapy has been demonstrated to improve postoperative survival in multiple randomized trials and is considered the standard of care in patients with resected cancers.
- Single agent 5-fluorouracil (5-FU) or gemcitabine is reserved for patients with older age or borderline performance status and results in median overall survival in the 20-mo range.

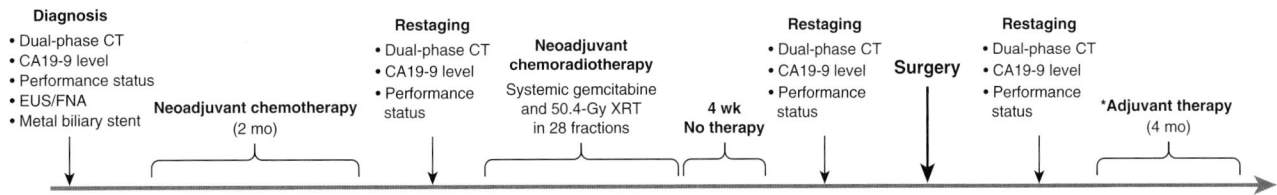

A
*Systemic therapy alone (FOLFIRINOX, gem-nab) is being considered by many clinicians because of the efficacy of these regimens in advanced disease and the challenges of delivering FOLFIRINOX in the adjuvant setting after such a large operation.
**Surgery is typically performed in the fifth week after the completion of XRT.
***Patients are restaged during postop week six if their recovery has been uncomplicated; however, there is no need to restage if recovery is complicated and the patient is not a suitable candidate to receive further systemic therapy.

B
*The benefit of further postoperative/adjuvant systemic therapy after a more prolonged induction phase is being questioned, especially in those patients of advanced age or when postoperative recovery is slow.

FIG. 5 Schematic representation of treatment sequencing in **(A)** resectable and **(B)** borderline resectable pancreatic cancer (PC). *CA 19-9*, Cancer antigen 19-9; *CT*, computed tomography; *EUS*, endoscopic ultrasound scan; *FNA*, fine-needle aspiration; *FOLFIRINOX*, 5-fluorouracil, leucovorin, irinotecan, and oxaliplatin; *gem-nab*, gemcitabine/nab-paclitaxel; *XRT*, external radiotherapy. (From Cameron JL, Cameron AM: *Current surgical therapy*, ed 12, Philadelphia, 2017, Elsevier.)

TABLE 3 Comparison of Treatment Sequencing Strategies for Patients With Pancreatic Cancer (Outside of a Clinical Trial)

Stage	NCCN	MCW
Resectable	• Surgery • Restaging • Adjuvant therapy ($+/-$ chemoradiotherapy; 6 mo)	• Neoadjuvant chemoradiotherapy (5.5 wk)* • Restaging • Surgery • Restaging • Adjuvant therapy (4 mo)
Borderline resectable	• Neoadjuvant therapy (regimen not specified) • Restaging • Surgery • Restaging • Consider adjuvant therapy	• Neoadjuvant chemotherapy (2 mo) • Restaging • Neoadjuvant chemoradiotherapy (5.5 wk) • Restaging • Surgery • Restaging • Adjuvant therapy (4 mo)
Locally advanced	• Chemotherapy • Restaging • Chemoradiotherapy in selected patients	• Chemotherapy (minimum 4 mo) • Restaging • Chemoradiotherapy • Restaging • Surgery in highly selected patients
Metastatic	• Systemic therapy • Clinical trial	• Systemic therapy • Clinical trial

NOTE: Clinical trials are preferred in all patients with pancreatic cancer (regardless of stage of disease) who have a performance status acceptable for treatment.
FOLFIRINOX, 5-fluorouracil, leucovorin, irinotecan, and oxaliplatin; *gem-nab*, gemcitabine/nab-paclitaxel; *MCW*, Medical College of Wisconsin; *NCCN*, National Comprehensive Cancer Network.
*Systemic therapy alone (FOLFIRINOX, gem-nab) is being considered by many clinicians because of the efficacy of these regimens in advanced disease and the challenges of delivering FOLFIRINOX in the adjuvant setting after such a large operation.
From Cameron JL, Cameron AM: *Current surgical therapy*, ed 12, Philadelphia, 2017, Elsevier.

The combination of gemcitabine and capecitabine (GEMCAP) results in median overall survival of 28-mo range.
• The use of the modified FOLFIRINOX (5-FU, oxaliplatin, and irinotecan) regimen is the standard of care in patients with adequate performance status (ECOG 0-1) results in striking outcomes with reported median overall survival of 54 mo.[6] Adjuvant use of gemcitabine and nab-paclitaxel is potentially useful, but a clear survival benefit has not been demonstrated.

• Adjuvant radiotherapy is controversial and is best limited to patients with poor risk features, margin-positive status, multiple involved nodes, or extranodal extension.

NEOADJUVANT THERAPY

• In patients with resectable and borderline-resectable pancreatic cancer, the use of upfront combination chemotherapy, and possibly chemoradiotherapy, has been shown to lead to improved resectability and survival outcomes.[7] Both FOLFIRINOX and gemcitabine-based regimens are routinely used in this setting.

RECURRENT/METASTATIC DISEASE

• In patients with metastatic disease, accepted upfront chemotherapy treatment approaches have demonstrated improvement in survival outcomes. Acceptable chemotherapy regimens for locally advanced and metastatic disease are summarized in Table 5.
• Options can include gemcitabine alone, combination regimen consisting of 5-fluorouracil, leucovorin, irinotecan, and oxaliplatin (FOLFIRINOX), or the combination of nab-paclitaxel plus gemcitabine. Multiagent regimens have an improved survival outcome compared with single-agent therapy. Liposomal irinotecan in combination with infusional 5-fluorouracil is now also approved in the setting of progressive disease.
• Maintenance therapy with the PARP inhibitor olaparib (after systemic chemotherapy) in germline *BRCA* mutated pancreatic cancer improves progression-free survival.[8]
• Poor survival outcomes are seen in patients with poor performance status, significant weight loss, and with liver metastases.

TABLE 4 Classification of Resectability of Pancreatic Cancer per the National Comprehensive Cancer Network and Surgical Oncology Expert Consensus Statement

Resectability Status	Criteria
Resectable	• No distant metastases • No radiographic evidence of SMV and portal vein abutment, distortion, tumor thrombus, or venous encasement • Clear fat planes around the celiac axis, hepatic artery, and SMA

Borderline resectable	• For tumors of the head or uncinate process:
	  1. Solid tumor contact with the SMV or portal vein of >180 degrees with contour irregularity of the vein or thrombosis of the vein but with suitable vessel proximal and distal to the site of involvement, allowing for safe and complete resection and vein reconstruction
	  2. Solid tumor contact with the IVC
	  3. Solid tumor contact with the common hepatic artery without extension to the celiac axis or hepatic artery bifurcation, allowing for safe and complete resection and reconstruction
	  4. Solid tumor contact with the SMA ≤180 degrees
	  5. Solid tumor contact with variable anatomy (e.g., accessory right hepatic artery, replaced right hepatic artery, replaced common hepatic artery, and the origin of replaced or accessory artery), and the presence and degree of tumor contact should be noted if present, as it may affect surgical planning
	• For tumors of the body or tail:
	  1. Solid tumor contact with the celiac axis of ≤180 degrees
	  2. Solid tumor contact with the celiac axis >180 degrees without involvement of the aorta and with an intact and uninvolved gastroduodenal artery, thereby permitting a modified Appleby procedure (although some members of the consensus committee preferred this criterion to be in the unresectable category)

Unresectable/locally advanced	• Head of pancreas or uncinate lesions:
	  1. Solid tumor contact with the SMA >180 degrees
	  2. Solid tumor contact with the celiac axis >180 degrees
	  3. Solid tumor contact with the first jejunal SMA branch
	  4. Unreconstructable SMV or portal vein because of tumor involvement or occlusion (can be because of tumor or bland thrombus)
	  5. Contact with the most proximal draining jejunal branch into the SMV
	• Body and tail lesions:
	  1. Solid tumor contact of >180 degrees with the SMA or celiac axis
	  2. Solid tumor contact with the celiac axis and aortic involvement
	  3. Unreconstructable SMV or portal vein because of tumor involvement or occlusion (can be because of tumor or bland thrombus)
	• For all sites:
	  1. Distant metastases
	  2. Metastases to lymph nodes beyond the field of resection

Metastatic	• Any presence of distant metastases

IVC, Inferior vena cava; *SMA,* spinal muscular atrophy; *SMV,* superior mesenteric vein.
From Niederhuber JE: *Abeloff's clinical oncology,* ed 6, Philadelphia, 2020, Elsevier.

TABLE 5 Acceptable Chemotherapy Regimens for Locally Advanced and Metastatic Disease[a]

Locally Advanced or Unresectable	Metastatic Disease
Options for patients with good performance status: • FOLFIRINOX • Gemcitabine + albumin bound-paclitaxel • Gemcitabine + erlotinib • Gemcitabine + capecitabine • Gemcitabine + cisplatin (especially in patients with *BRCA1/2* mutation and/or family history) • Capecitabine single agent • CI 5-FU • Fixed-dose gemcitabine/docetaxel/capecitabine (GTX regimen) • Fluoropyrimidine + oxaliplatin • Chemotherapy (any of above) followed by chemoradiation or SBRT • Chemoradiation or SBRT	Options for patients with good performance status: • FOLFIRINOX (category 1) • Gemcitabine + albumin bound-paclitaxel (category 1) • Gemcitabine + erlotinib (category 1) • Gemcitabine (category 1) • Gemcitabine + capecitabine • Gemcitabine + cisplatin (especially in patients with *BRCA1/2* mutation and/or family history) • Fixed-dose gemcitabine/docetaxel/capecitabine (GTX regimen) (category 2B) • Fluoropyrimidine + oxaliplatin (category 2B)
Options for patients with poor performance status: • Gemcitabine • Capecitabine • CI 5-FU	Options for patients with poor performance status: • Gemcitabine (category 1) • Capecitabine (category 2B) • CI 5-FU (category 2B)

CI, Continuous infusion; *FOLFIRINOX,* 5-FU, irinotecan, oxaliplatin; *5-FU,* 5-fluorouracil; *GTX,* gemcitabine, docetaxel, capecitabine; *SBRT,* stereotactic body radiation therapy.
[a]Level of recommendation is based on National Comprehensive Cancer Network (NCCN) Guidelines. Category 1 is based on high-level evidence with uniform NCCN consensus that the intervention is appropriate. Category 2B is based on lower level evidence with NCCN consensus that the intervention is appropriate.
From Niederhuber JE: *Abeloff's clinical oncology,* ed 6, Philadelphia, 2020, Elsevier.

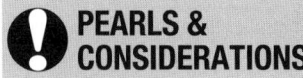
TABLE 6 Risk Factors for Pancreatic Cancer

Risk Factor	Relative Increase in Risk
High Risk (>10-fold)	
FAMMM	13- to 47-fold
Hereditary pancreatitis	50- to 83-fold
Peutz-Jeghers syndrome	132-fold
Three or more first-degree relatives with PC	14- to 32-fold
Moderate Risk (5- to 10-fold)	
Two first-degree relatives with PC	4- to 6.4-fold
Cystic fibrosis	5.3-fold
Chronic pancreatitis	2- to 19-fold
BRCA2 mutation carrier	3.5- to 10-fold
PALB2 mutation carrier	6-fold
Low Risk (<5-fold)	
Cigarette smoking	1.5- to 3-fold
Alcohol consumption	None to 1.2-fold
Obesity	None to 1.7-fold
Diabetes mellitus	1.3- to 2.6-fold
One first-degree relative with PC	3-fold
BRCA1 mutation carrier	None to 2-fold
Familial adenomatous polyposis	4-fold
Li-Fraumeni syndrome	2-fold
Lynch syndrome	2- to 8-fold

FAMMM, Familial atypical multiple-mole melanoma; *PC,* pancreatic cancer.
From Niederhuber JE: *Abeloff's clinical oncology,* ed 6, Philadelphia, 2020, Elsevier.

TABLE 7 Recommendations for Screening

HRIs to Consider for Screening
FAMMM patients with *CDKN2A*
Patients with hereditary pancreatitis
Patients with hereditary PJS
Three or more first-, second-, or third-degree relatives with PC with at least one being a first-degree relative
Two or more first-degree relatives with PC
BRCA1, BRCA2, or *PALB2* mutation carriers with at least one first- or second-degree relative with PC

Age to Start Screening
Age 45-50 yr *or* 15 yr before age of earliest occurrence of PC in the family (whichever is earliest)
Consider age 30 yr for patients with PJS

FAMMM, Familial atypical multiple-mole melanoma; *HRI,* high-risk individual; *PC,* pancreatic cancer; *PJS,* Peutz-Jeghers syndrome.
From Niederhuber JE: *Abeloff's clinical oncology,* ed 6, Philadelphia, 2020, Elsevier.

- Combined chemoradiotherapy can be utilized in the case of patients with locally advanced but unresectable cases and confers a modest improvement in median overall survival.

DISPOSITION

Adjuvant postoperative chemotherapy has a significant survival benefit in patients with resected pancreatic cancer.

- Adjuvant chemotherapy with FOLFIRINOX regimen significantly delays the development of recurrence and results in median survival of approximately 54 mo.
- The role of radiotherapy in the adjuvant setting is best restricted to patients who have a high risk for locoregional recurrence.

PEARLS & CONSIDERATIONS

COMMENTS

- Risk factors for pancreatic cancer and recommendations for screening of individuals at risk are summarized in Tables 6 and 7. New-onset diabetes (NOD) after age 50 yr confers a sixfold to eightfold increased risk for sporadic (nonfamilial) pancreatic ductal adenocarcinoma (PDAC) in the 3 yr after diagnosis. About 20% of patients with PDAC have NOD, and about 1% of patients with NOD will be diagnosed with PDAC in the 3 yr after NOD.[9]
- The U.S. Preventive Services Task Force (USPSTF) recommends against routine screening for pancreatic cancer in asymptomatic adults since it found no evidence that screening is effective in reducing mortality rates. There is potential for significant harm because of the low prevalence of pancreatic cancer, limited accuracy of available screening tests, invasive nature of diagnostic tests, and poor outcome of treatment.
- Alcohol consumption, specifically liquor consumption of more than three drinks per day, increases pancreatic cancer mortality independent of smoking.
- Patients should be referred for pancreatic cancer surgery to high-volume medical centers that perform at least 15 to 20 cases a yr.

REFERENCES
Available at eBooks.Health.Elsevier.com.

RELATED CONTENT
Pancreatic Cancer (Patient Information)

AUTHOR: **RITESH RATHORE, MD**

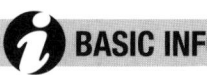 **BASIC INFORMATION**

DEFINITION

- Acute pancreatitis is an inflammatory process of the pancreas with intrapancreatic activation of enzymes that may also involve peripancreatic tissue and/or remote organ systems. The diagnosis of acute pancreatitis requires at least two of the following criteria: Serum amylase or lipase ≥3 times normal, abdominal pain consistent with pancreatitis, and radiographic findings (CT or MRI) of acute pancreatitis.
- The Ranson scoring system for acute pancreatitis is described in Boxes 1 and 2.
- The **Revised Atlanta Criteria** (Box 3) uses early prognostic signs, organ failure, and local complications to define disease severity:
  1. **Mild pancreatitis:** No organ failure, no local or systemic complications, pancreatitis typically resolves in first week
  2. **Moderate pancreatitis:** Transient organ failure (≤48 h) *or* local complications (e.g., pancreatic necrosis, peripancreatic fluid collections, peripancreatic necrosis) *or* exacerbation of comorbid disease
  3. **Severe pancreatitis:** Persistent organ failure (>48 h)
- The **BALI Score** evaluates only four variables:
  1. BUN ≥25 mg/dl
  2. Age ≥65 yr
  3. LDH ≥300 U/L
  4. Interleukin-6 level ≥300 pg/ml
- These measurements are taken at admission and at 48 h. Mortality is >25% for a score of 3 and exceeds 50% with a score of 4.
- **Severe acute pancreatitis (SAP)** is diagnosed by the presence of any of the following four criteria:
  1. Organ failure with one or more of the following: Shock (systolic blood pressure <90 mm Hg), pulmonary insufficiency (Pao$_2$ ≤60 mm Hg), renal failure (serum creatinine >2 mg/dl after rehydration), and gastrointestinal bleeding (>500 ml/24 h)
  2. Local complications such as necrosis, pseudocyst, or abscess
  3. At least three of the Ranson criteria (see Boxes 1 and 2) *or*
  4. At least eight of the Acute Physiology and Chronic Health Evaluation II (APACHE II) criteria

ICD-10CM CODES
K85.0	Idiopathic acute pancreatitis
K85.1	Biliary acute pancreatitis
K85.2	Alcohol-induced acute pancreatitis
K 85.3	Drug-induced pancreatitis
K85.6	Other acute pancreatitis
K85.9	Acute pancreatitis, unspecified

EPIDEMIOLOGY & DEMOGRAPHICS

- The incidence of pancreatitis is increasing in the U.S. Admissions for acute pancreatitis have increased dramatically, and acute pancreatitis was the number-one GI-related cause for admission across U.S. hospitals in 2012. There are >270,000 cases of acute pancreatitis reported annually in the U.S., with 40%+ resulting from gallstone disease (most common cause) and 30% caused by alcohol consumption.
- Incidence in urban areas is twice that of rural areas (20/100,000 persons in urban areas).
- 20% of patients have necrotizing pancreatitis; the remainder have interstitial, or edematous, pancreatitis.
- Drugs are responsible for less than 5% of all cases of acute pancreatitis.

PHYSICAL FINDINGS & CLINICAL PRESENTATION

- Epigastric tenderness and guarding, often radiating to the back; pain usually developing suddenly, reaching peak intensity within 10 to 30 min, severe and lasting several hours without relief. Rarely, some patients can have painless severe pancreatitis
- Nausea and vomiting (up to 90% of cases)
- Hypoactive bowel sounds (from ileus)
- Tachycardia, shock (from decreased intravascular volume)
- Confusion (from metabolic disturbances)
- Fever (SIRS response or infection when pancreatic necrosis is present)
- Decreased breath sounds (pleural effusions) or rales (atelectasis, acute respiratory distress syndrome [ARDS])
- Jaundice (from obstruction or compression of biliary tract)
- Ascites (from tear in pancreatic duct, leaking pseudocyst)
- Palpable abdominal mass (pseudocyst, phlegmon, abscess, carcinoma)
- Evidence of hypocalcemia (Chvostek sign, Trousseau sign)
- Evidence of retroperitoneal bleeding (hemorrhagic pancreatitis):
  1. Ecchymosis around the umbilicus **(Cullen sign)**
  2. Ecchymosis involving the flanks **(Grey Turner sign)**
- Tender subcutaneous nodules (caused by subcutaneous fat necrosis)

ETIOLOGY

- The most common causes of acute pancreatitis are gallstones (40% of cases) and excessive alcohol consumption (30% of cases). Alcohol-related pancreatitis is most common after long term (>10 yr of heavy drinking). The pathophysiology of severe acute pancreatitis is illustrated in Fig. 1
- Hypertriglyceridemia (usually >1000 mg/dl) from any cause
- Drugs (e.g., thiazides, furosemide, corticosteroids, tetracycline, estrogens, valproic acid, metronidazole, azathioprine, methyldopa, pentamidine, ethacrynic acid, procainamide, amiodarone, sulindac, nitrofurantoin, ACE inhibitors, danazol, cimetidine, piroxicam, gold, ranitidine, sulfasalazine, isoniazid, acetaminophen, cisplatin, didanosine, opiates, erythromycin, metformin, GLP-1 receptor agonists, incretin mimetics)
- Abdominal trauma
- Surgery
- Endoscopic retrograde cholangiopancreatography (ERCP), especially with manipulation of the pancreatic duct
- Infections (predominantly viral)
- Peptic ulcer (penetrating duodenal ulcer)
- Pancreas divisum (congenital failure to fuse of dorsal or ventral pancreas)
- Idiopathic
- Pregnancy
- Vascular (vasculitis, ischemic)

BOX 1 Ranson Prognostic Criteria for Nongallstone Pancreatitis

- At presentation
  1. Age >55 yr
  2. Blood glucose level >200 mg/dl
  3. White blood cell count >16,000 cells/mm^3
  4. Lactate dehydrogenase level >350 IU/L
  5. Aspartate aminotransferase level >250 IU/L
- After 48 h of admission
  1. Hematocrit*: Decrease >10%
  2. Serum calcium level <8 mg/dl
  3. Base deficit >4 mEq/L
  4. Blood urea nitrogen level: Increase >5 mg/dl
  5. Fluid requirement >6 L
  6. Pao$_2$ <60 mm Hg
- Ranson score ≥3 defines severe pancreatitis.

*Compared with admission value.
From Townsend CM et al: *Sabiston textbook of surgery,* ed 21, St Louis, 2022, Elsevier.

BOX 2 Ranson Prognostic Criteria for Gallstone Pancreatitis

At presentation
- Age >70 yr
- Blood glucose level >220 mg/dl
- White blood cell count >18,000 cells/mm^3
- Lactate dehydrogenase level >400 IU/L
- Aspartate aminotransferase level >250 IU/L

After 48 h of admission
- Hematocrit*: Decrease >10%
- Serum calcium level <8 mg/dl
- Base deficit >5 mEq/L
- Blood urea nitrogen level: Increase >2 mg/dl
- Fluid requirement >4 L
- Pao$_2$: Not available

Ranson score ≥3 defines severe pancreatitis.

*Compared with admission value.
From Townsend CM et al: *Sabiston textbook of surgery,* ed 21, St Louis, 2022, Elsevier.

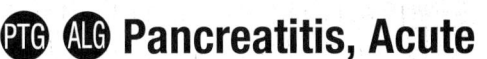

BOX 3 Atlanta Criteria for Acute Pancreatitis

Organ Failure, as Defined by
Shock (systolic blood pressure <90 mm Hg)
Pulmonary insufficiency (Pa_{O_2} <60 mm Hg)
Renal failure (creatinine level >2 mg/dl after fluid resuscitation)
Gastrointestinal bleeding (>500 ml/24 h)

Systemic Complications
Disseminated intravascular coagulation (platelet count ≤100,000)
Fibrinogen <1 g/L
Fibrin split products >80 μg/dl
Metabolic disturbance (calcium level ≤7.5 mg/dl)

Local Complications
Necrosis
Abscess
Pseudocyst
Severe pancreatitis is defined by the presence of any evidence of organ failure or a local complication.

From Townsend CM et al: *Sabiston textbook of surgery,* ed 21, St Louis, 2022, Elsevier.

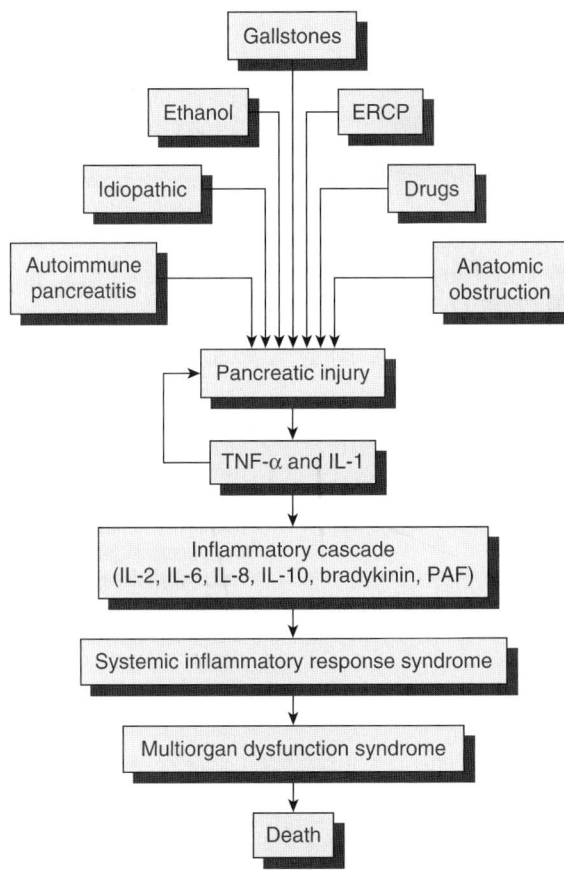

FIG. 1 Pathophysiology of severe acute pancreatitis. The local injury induces the release of tumor necrosis factor-alpha (TNF-α) and interleukin-1 (IL-1). Both cytokines produce further pancreatic injury and amplify the inflammatory response by inducing the release of other inflammatory mediators, which cause distant organ injury. This abnormal inflammatory response is responsible for the mortality seen during the early phase of acute pancreatitis. *ERCP,* Endoscopic retrograde cholangiopancreatography; *PAF,* platelet-activating factor. (From Townsend CM et al: *Sabiston textbook of surgery,* ed 21, St Louis 2022, Elsevier.)

- Hypercalcemia
- Pancreatic carcinoma (primary or metastatic)
- Renal failure
- Hereditary pancreatitis, such as in patients with cystic fibrosis
- Immunoglobulin G subclass 4 (IgG4) disease
- Occupational exposure to chemicals: Methanol, cobalt, zinc, mercuric chloride, creosol, lead, organophosphates, chlorinated naphthalenes

- Others: Scorpion venom, obstruction at ampulla region (neoplasm, duodenal diverticula, Crohn disease, rarely celiac disease), hypotensive shock, autoimmune pancreatitis
- Causes of acute pancreatitis in pediatric patients are summarized in Table E1

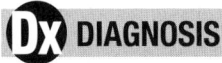 DIAGNOSIS

DIFFERENTIAL DIAGNOSIS
- PUD
- Acute cholangitis, biliary colic
- High intestinal obstruction
- Early acute appendicitis
- Diabetic ketoacidosis
- Pneumonia (basilar)
- Myocardial infarction (inferior wall)
- Renal colic
- Ruptured or dissecting aortic aneurysm
- Mesenteric ischemia

LABORATORY TESTS
Pancreatic enzymes:
- Amylase is increased, usually elevated in the initial 3 to 5 days of acute pancreatitis. Iso-amylase determinations (separation of pancreatic cell isoenzyme components of amylase) are useful in excluding occasional cases of salivary hyperamylasemia. The use of isoamylase rather than total serum amylase reduces the risk of erroneously diagnosing pancreatitis and is preferred by some as initial biochemical test in patients suspected of having acute pancreatitis.
- Urinary amylase determinations are useful to diagnose acute pancreatitis in patients with lipemic serum, to rule out elevated serum amylase caused by macroamylasemia, and to diagnose acute pancreatitis in patients whose serum amylase is normal.
- Serum lipase levels are elevated in acute pancreatitis; the elevation is less transient than serum amylase and more sensitive in patients with alcoholic pancreatitis. Concomitant evaluation of serum amylase and lipase does not improve diagnostic accuracy of acute pancreatitis. Serial measurements have limited usefulness because levels are not predictors of severity. Elevated serum trypsin levels are diagnostic of pancreatitis (in absence of renal failure).
- Serum C-reactive protein is an excellent laboratory marker of severity; a level >150 mg/dl at 48 h is associated with severe pancreatitis.
- Rapid measurement of urinary trypsinogen-2 (if available) is useful in the emergency department as a screening test for acute pancreatitis in patients with abdominal pain; a negative dipstick test for urinary trypsinogen-2 rules out acute pancreatitis with a high degree of probability, whereas a positive test indicates need for further evaluation.
- Interleukin-6 level: Worse prognosis with level ≥300 pg/ml.

ADDITIONAL TESTS
- CBC: Reveals leukocytosis; hematocrit (Hct) may be initially increased as a result of

- hemoconcentration; decreased Hct may indicate hemorrhage or hemolysis.
- Blood urea nitrogen (BUN) is increased because of dehydration. Serial BUN measurements are the most valuable lab test for predicting mortality during the initial 48 h.
- Elevation of serum glucose in a previously normal patient correlates with the degree of pancreatic malfunction and may be related to increased release of glycogen, catecholamines, and glucocorticoid release and decreased insulin release.
- Liver profile: Aspartate aminotransferase (AST) and lactate dehydrogenase (LDH) are increased as a result of tissue necrosis; bilirubin and alkaline phosphatase may be increased from common bile duct obstruction. A threefold or greater rise in serum alanine aminotransferase concentrations is an excellent indicator (95% probability) of biliary pancreatitis.

- Serum calcium is decreased because of saponification, precipitation, and decreased parathyroid hormone response.
- Arterial blood gases: Pao_2 may be decreased as a result of ARDS, pleural effusion(s); pH may be decreased as a result of lactic acidosis, respiratory acidosis, and renal insufficiency.
- Serum electrolytes: Potassium may be increased from acidosis or renal insufficiency; sodium may be increased from dehydration.

IMAGING STUDIES

- Abdominal plain films are useful initially to distinguish other conditions that may mimic pancreatitis (perforated viscus). They may reveal localized ileus (sentinel loop), pancreatic calcifications (chronic pancreatitis), blurring of left psoas shadow, dilation of transverse colon, calcified gallstones.

- Chest x-ray may reveal elevation of one or both diaphragms, pleural effusions, basilar infiltrates, or platelike atelectasis.
- Abdominal ultrasonography is useful in detecting gallstones (sensitivity of 60% to 70% for detecting stones associated with pancreatitis). Its availability and noninvasive nature make it the initial imaging study of choice; its major limitation is the presence of distended bowel loops overlying the pancreas.
- CT scan (Fig. 2) is less sensitive than ultrasound in identifying gallstones and exposes the patient to risk of contrast-induced nephropathy. It is, however, superior to ultrasonography in identifying pancreatitis and defining its extent, and it also plays a role in diagnosing pseudocysts (they appear as a well-defined area surrounded by a high-density capsule); gastrointestinal fistulization or infection of a pseudocyst can also be identified by the presence of gas within the pseudocyst. Sequential contrast-enhanced CT is useful for detection of pancreatic necrosis. The severity of pancreatitis can also be graded by CT scan (Table 2). (A = normal pancreas, B = enlarged pancreas [1 point], C = pancreatic and/or peripancreatic inflammation [2 points], D = single peripancreatic collection [3 points], E = at least two peripancreatic collections and/or retroperitoneal air [4 points]. Percentage of pancreatic necrosis <30% [2 points], 30% to 50% [4 points], >50% [6 points]. The CT severity index is calculated by adding grade points to points assigned for percentage of necrosis.)
- Magnetic resonance cholangiopancreatography (MRCP) has >90% sensitivity for choledocholithiasis and can identify other anatomic abnormalities.
- Endoscopic ultrasonography (EUS) is a minimally invasive test that provides high-resolution imaging of the pancreas. It is useful to identify anatomic abnormalities of the pancreas and has good sensitivity and specificity for small gallstones (≤5 mm).
- ERCP indications: Useful to perform biliary sphincterotomy and stone removal in the presence of a retained bile duct stone seen on imaging. The role and timing of ERCP in patients with acute biliary pancreatitis has been controversial. Guidelines from the American College of Gastroenterology suggest that urgent ERCP (within 24 h of admission) is indicated in patients with biliary pancreatitis who have concurrent acute cholangitis, but it is not needed in most patients who do not have evidence of ongoing biliary obstruction.

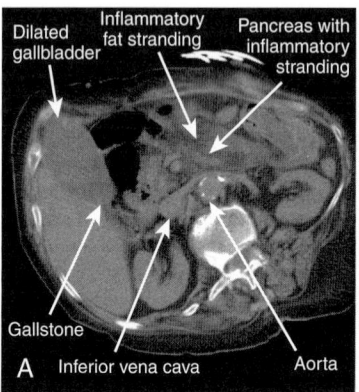 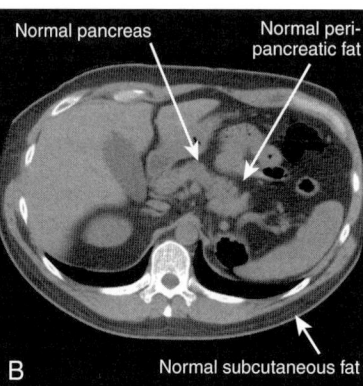

FIG. 2 Gallstone pancreatitis and normal pancreas for comparison, axial computed tomography without contrast. A, Gallstone pancreatitis CT. A dilated gallbladder is visible with a hyperdense dependent lesion consistent with a gallstone. The region of the pancreas shows significant inflammatory stranding. In this patient the pancreas lies just anterior to the left renal vein, which can be seen crossing anterior to the aorta and entering the inferior vena cava. **B,** A normal pancreas is visible. This pancreas is surrounded by uninflamed fat, which is dark (nearly black). Compare this normal fat with normal subcutaneous fat. (From Broder JS: *Diagnostic imaging for the emergency physician,* Philadelphia, 2011, Saunders.)

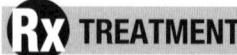 **TREATMENT**

NONPHARMACOLOGIC THERAPY

- Bowel rest with avoidance of liquids or solids during the acute illness. Limited data suggest that early feeding in patients with acute pancreatitis does not seem to increase adverse events and, for patients with mild to moderate pancreatitis, may reduce length of hospital stay.

TABLE 2 Computed Tomography (CT) Severity Index Score for Pancreatitis*

Grade†	CT Findings	Score
A	Normal pancreas	0
B	Focal or diffuse enlargement of the pancreas, contour irregularities, heterogeneous attenuation, no peripancreatic inflammation	1
C	Grade B plus peripancreatic inflammation	2
D	Grade C plus a single fluid collection	3
E	Grade C plus multiple fluid collections or gas	4
Percent Necrosis Present on CT		
0		
<33		
33-50		
>50		

*Severity Index Score = Grade score + Percent necrosis score. Maximum score = 10; severe disease = 6 or higher.
†Severity of the acute inflammatory process.
From Adams JG et al: *Emergency medicine: clinical essentials,* ed 2, Philadelphia, 2013, Elsevier.

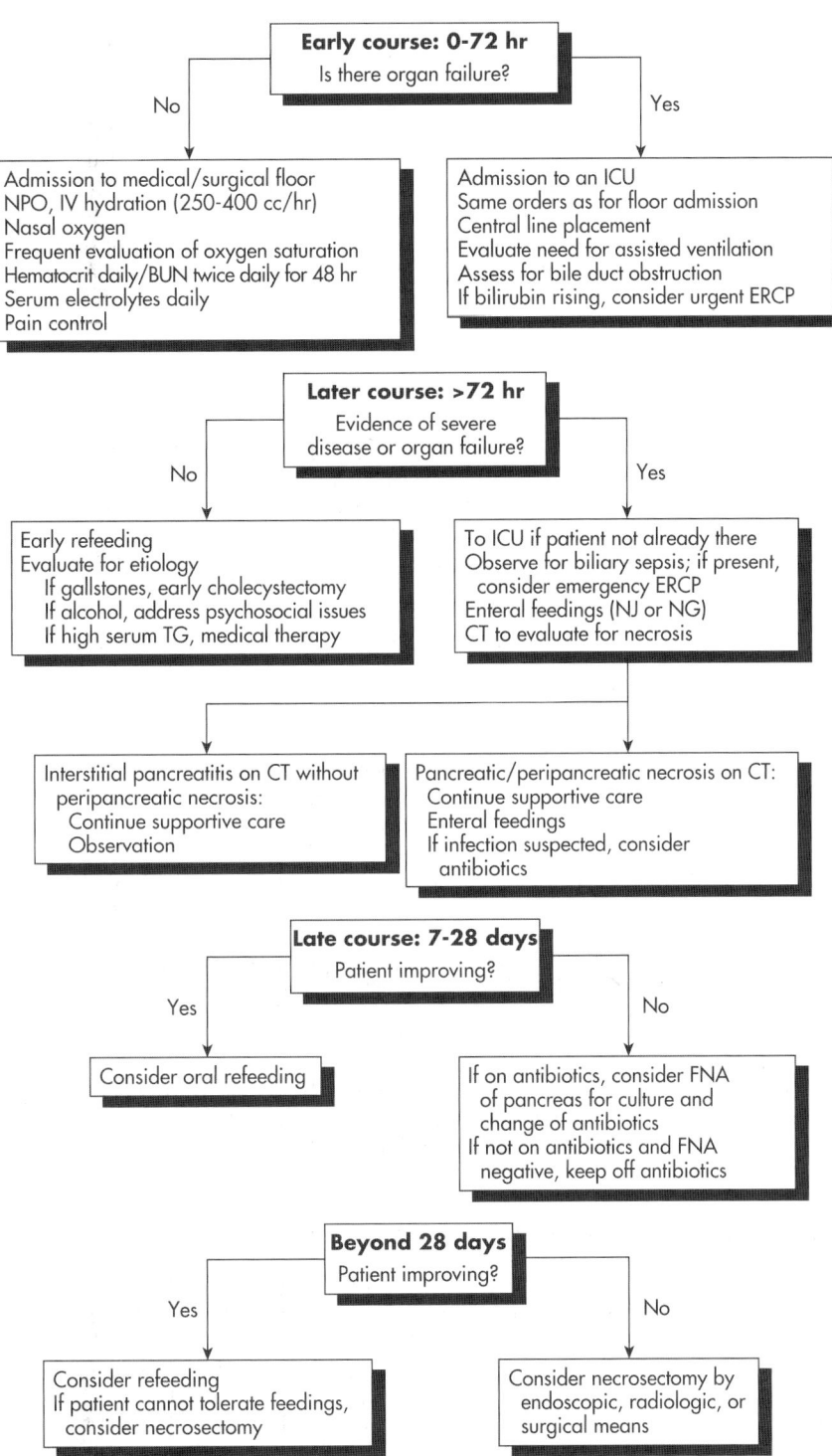

FIG. 3 Algorithm for the management of acute pancreatitis at various stages in its course. *NJ,* Nasojejunal. (From Feldman M et al: *Sleisenger and Fordtran's gastrointestinal and liver disease,* ed 10, Philadelphia, 2016, Elsevier.)

- Avoidance of alcohol and any drugs associated with pancreatitis.

ACUTE GENERAL Rx
GENERAL MEASURES:
- Assess severity of pancreatitis.
- An algorithm for the management of acute pancreatitis is described in Fig. 3.

- Maintain adequate intravascular volume with IV hydration. The ideal quantity of fluid resuscitation has been controversial. Traditionally aggressive fluid resuscitation (250 to 500 ml/h) with isotonic crystalloids was regarded as critical in managing acute pancreatitis, unless cardiac or renal disease precluded it. Recent trials have show that

moderate fluid resuscitation results in similar clinical outcomes as did aggressive resuscitation with less fluid overload.[1]
- Patient should remain NPO until clinically improved, stable, and hungry. Enteral feedings are preferred over total parenteral nutrition if supplemental nutrition is necessary. Enteral nutrition reduces mortality, multiple organ

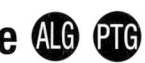

failure, systemic infections, and operative interventions more than total parenteral nutrition does in patients with acute pancreatitis. Parenteral nutrition may be necessary in patients who do not tolerate enteral feeding or in whom an adequate infusion rate cannot be reached within 2 to 4 days. The American Gastroenterological Association recommends that oral feedings be started within 24 h of admission in patients with mild to moderate pancreatitis. A recent trial revealed that patients started on a low-fat diet on admission were discharged about 5 days earlier than patients in whom feeding was delayed.

- Nasogastric suction is useful only in severe pancreatitis to decompress the abdomen in patients with ileus.
- Control pain: IV hydromorphone or fentanyl. Meperidine and morphine are also commonly used narcotics for pain control, although morphine has been shown to increase sphincter of Oddi pressure and has delayed metabolite clearance in patients with concomitant renal failure.
- Correct metabolic abnormalities (e.g., replace calcium and magnesium as necessary).
- Prophylactic antibiotics are not recommended, regardless of the severity or presence of pancreatic necrosis.
- An algorithm for the management of acute pancreatitis at various stages is described in Fig. 3.

SPECIFIC MEASURES:
- Pancreatic or peripancreatic infection develops in 30% of patients with pancreatic necrosis. The use of antibiotics is justified if the patient has evidence of septicemia, pancreatic abscess, or pancreatitis caused by biliary calculi with concomitant cholangitis. Their use should generally be limited to 5 to 7 days to prevent development of fungal superinfection. Appropriate empiric antibiotic therapy should penetrate pancreatic necrosis. Options include a carbapenem alone (due to anaerobic coverage) or a quinolone, ceftazidime, or cefepime, combined with an enteric anaerobic agent such as metronidazole. CT-guided fine-needle aspiration (FNA) can be performed to culture the infected necrosis and tailor antibiotic therapy. If sampling of infected necrosis occurs and is sterile, antibiotics should be discontinued
- Surgical therapy has a limited role in acute pancreatitis; it is indicated in the following:
  1. Gallstone-induced pancreatitis: Cholecystectomy when acute pancreatitis subsides. However, randomized trials have shown that patients with mild gallstone pancreatitis can undergo cholecystectomy safely during the first 48 h of hospitalization
  2. Perforated peptic ulcer
  3. Necrotizing pancreatitis with infected necrotic tissue is associated with an elevated rate of complications and increased risk of death. Traditional treatment has been open necrosectomy; surgical necrosectomy induces a

proinflammatory response and is associated with a high complication rate. Recent trials have shown that a step-up approach consisting of percutaneous drainage followed, if necessary, by minimally invasive retroperitoneal necrosectomy may have a lower rate of complications and death. A recent trial did not show superiority of immediate drainage over postponed drainage with regard to complications in infected necrotizing pancreatitis. Endoscopic transgastric necrosectomy, a form of natural orifice transluminal endoscopic surgery, has been shown in recent trials to be effective in reducing the proinflammatory response as well as reducing complications
- Identification and treatment of complications:
  1. **Pseudocyst:** Round or spheroid collection of fluid, tissue, pancreatic enzymes, and blood
     a. Diagnosed by CT scan or sonography.
     b. Treatment: Pancreatic pseudocysts can be drained surgically or endoscopically. The endoscopic approach is preferable when the patient's anatomy is suitable and an experienced endoscopist is available. CT scan or ultrasound-guided percutaneous drainage (with a pigtail catheter left in place for continuous drainage) can be used, but the recurrence rate is high; the conservative approach is to reevaluate the pseudocyst (with CT scan or sonography) after 6 to 7 wk and surgically drain it if the pseudocyst has not decreased in size.
     c. Generally, pseudocysts <5 cm in diameter are reabsorbed without intervention, whereas those >5 cm require surgical intervention after the wall has matured.
  2. **Phlegmon:** Represents pancreatic edema. It can be diagnosed by CT scan or sonography. Treatment is supportive as it usually resolves spontaneously
  3. **Pancreatic abscess:** Diagnosed by CT scan (presence of air in the retroperitoneum); Gram staining and cultures of fluid obtained from guided percutaneous aspiration usually identify bacterial organism. Therapy is surgical (or catheter) drainage and IV antibiotics (carbapenem is the drug of choice)
  4. **Pancreatic ascites:** Usually caused by leaking of pseudocyst or tear in pancreatic duct. Paracentesis reveals very high amylase and lipase levels in the pancreatic fluid; ERCP may demonstrate the lesion. Treatment is surgical correction if exudative ascites from severe pancreatitis does not resolve spontaneously
  5. **Abdominal compartment syndrome:** Caused by intraabdominal leakage of fluids from volume resuscitation or ascites. Diagnosed with sustained intraabdominal pressure >20 mm Hg with new-onset organ failure

  6. **Gastrointestinal bleeding:** Caused by alcoholic gastritis, bleeding varices, stress ulceration, or disseminated intravascular coagulation (DIC)
  7. **Renal failure:** Caused by hypovolemia, resulting in oliguria or anuria, cortical or tubular necrosis (shock, DIC), or thrombosis of renal artery or vein
  8. **Hypoxia:** Caused by ARDS, pleural effusion, or atelectasis
  9. **Vascular:** Splenic, portal, or superior mesenteric vein thrombosis; pseudoaneurysm

THERAPY OF UNCOMMON FORMS OF PANCREATITIS
- **Autoimmune pancreatitis (AIP):** Fibroinflammatory disease characterized by an IgG4 lymphoplasmacytic infiltrate. It is a variant of chronic pancreatitis and has been associated with other autoimmune disorders (e.g., primary sclerosing cholangitis, Sjögren syndrome). The inflammatory process is generally responsive to corticosteroid therapy. Older men aged 60 to 70 yr are primarily affected. Patients present with abdominal pain, weight loss, anorexia, and obstructive jaundice. IgG4 levels are elevated. Radiographically on CT, the pancreas is diffusely enlarged, with a characteristic smooth, capsulelike rim ("sausage pancreas"). Features of type 1 and type 2 autoimmune pancreatitis are summarized in Table 3. Type II autoimmune hepatitis (idiopathic duct-centric chronic pancreatitis) is associated with inflammatory bowel disease and not related to IgG4 cell deposition.
- **Hypertriglyceridemic pancreatitis (HTGP):** IV insulin therapy is the cornerstone of immediate treatment, with supplemental IV glucose infusion if the serum glucose levels are not elevated. IV heparin was previously used as well, but its effectiveness has come into question. Antihyperlipidemic agents (fibrates) should be initiated as adjuvant therapy as soon as possible for long-term control. Beneficial results have been reported with early (within 48 h) initiation of apheresis with therapeutic plasma exchange when there is concomitant hypocalcemia, lactic acidosis, or other signs of organ dysfunction.

DISPOSITION
Prognosis varies with the severity of pancreatitis; overall mortality rate in acute pancreatitis is 5% to 10%. Prognostic criteria for acute pancreatitis are described in Table 4.

REFERRAL
- Hospitalization is indicated in moderate to severe cases of pancreatitis.
- Surgical consultation is needed in suspected gallstone pancreatitis, perforated peptic ulcer, or presence of necrotic or infected foci. Acute pancreatitis can generally be attributed to gallstones when patients have both abnormal

TABLE 3 Features of Type 1 and Type 2 Autoimmune Pancreatitis

Feature	Type 1	Type 2
Histology	Lymphoplasmacytic infiltration Dense periductal infiltrate without damage to ductal epithelium Storiform fibrosis Obliterative phlebitis Abundant (>10 cells/HPF) IgG4-positive cells Fibroinflammatory process may extend to peripancreatic region	Periductal lymphoplasmacytic and neutrophilic infiltration Destruction of the duct epithelium by neutrophils (granulocytic epithelial lesion [GEL]) Obliterative phlebitis is rare No IgG4-positive cells
Average age at presentation	60-70 yr	40-50, but may present in young adults and even children
Gender predominance	Male	Equal
Usual clinical presentations	Obstructive jaundice (75%) Acute pancreatitis (15%)	Obstructive jaundice (50%) Acute pancreatitis (33%)
Pancreatic imaging	Diffuse pancreatic enlargement (40%) Focal pancreatic enlargement (60%)	Diffuse pancreatic enlargement (15%) Focal pancreatic enlargement (85%)
IgG4	Level elevated in serum (~2/3 of patients) Positive in staining of involved tissues	Not associated
Other organ involvement	Biliary strictures Pseudotumors Kidney Lung Others Retroperitoneal fibrosis Sialoadenitis	Not associated
Associated diseases	See above (other organ involvement)	IBD
Long-term outcome	Frequent relapses	Rare or no relapse

HPF, High power field; IBD, inflammatory bowel disease; IgG4, immunoglobulin G, subclass 4.
From Feldman M et al: Sleisenger and Fordtran's gastrointestinal and liver disease, ed 10, Philadelphia, 2016, Elsevier.

TABLE 4 Prognostic Criteria for Acute Pancreatitis

Ranson Criteria*	Simplified Glasgow Criteria†	Computed Tomography Criteria‡
On admission: Age >55 yr WBC >16,000/μL AST >250 U/L LDH >350 U/L Glucose >200 mg/dl 48 h after admission: Hematocrit decrease by >10 BUN increase by >5 mg/dl Ca²⁺ <8 mg/dl Arterial Po₂ <60 mm Hg Base deficit >4 mEq/L Fluid sequestration >6 L	Within 48 h of admission: Age >55 yr WBC >15,000/μL LDH >600 U/L Glucose >180 mg/dl Albumin <3.2 g/dl Ca²⁺ <8 mg/dl Arterial Po₂ <60 mm Hg BUN >45 mg/dl	Normal Enlargement Pancreatic inflammation Single fluid collection Multiple fluid collection

AST, Aspartate aminotransferase; BUN, blood urea nitrogen; LDH, lactate dehydrogenase; WBC, white blood cells.
*Three or more Ranson criteria predict a complicated clinical course. Data from Ranson JH et al: Prognostic signs and nonoperative peritoneal lavage in acute pancreatitis, Surg Gynecol Obstet 143:209-219, 1976.
†Data from Blamey SL et al: Prognostic factors in acute pancreatitis, Gut 25:1340, 1984.
‡Grades A and B represent mild disease with no risk of infection or death. Grade C represents moderately severe disease with a minimal likelihood of infection and essentially no risk of mortality. Grades D and E represent severe pancreatitis with an infection rate of 30% to 50% and mortality rate of 15%. Data from Balthazar EJ et al: Acute pancreatitis value of CT in establishing prognosis, Radiology 174:331, 1990.
From Goldman L, Ausiello D (eds): Cecil textbook of medicine, ed 24, Philadelphia, 2012, Saunders.

liver enzymes and gallstones (or sludge) on imaging. Such patients should consider cholecystectomy before discharge to prevent recurrent pancreatitis.
• Gastroenterology consultation in severe or recurrent pancreatitis, when ERCP is needed for gallstone pancreatitis, or when the cause of pancreatitis is unclear.

• Consider intensive care unit transfer for patients who require aggressive fluid resuscitation and are at risk of volume overload from cardiac or renal causes. Similarly, consider transfer for patients with developing ARDS, patients with abdominal compartment syndrome (with surgical consultation), and those who require apheresis.

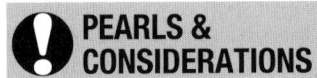 **PEARLS & CONSIDERATIONS**

• Acute pancreatitis is the most common major complication of ERCP. NSAIDs are potent inhibitors of phospholipase A₂, cyclooxygenase, and neutrophil-endothelial interactions, which play an important role in the pathogenesis of

acute pancreatitis. Preliminary trials show that among patients at high risk for post-ERCP pancreatitis, rectal indomethacin (given as two 50-mg indomethacin suppositories administered immediately after ERCP) significantly reduced the incidence of post-ERCP pancreatitis.
• Pancreatic stent placement decreases the risk of post-ERCP pancreatitis.
• Statins reduce risk for pancreatitis in adults. Fibrates do not affect risk for pancreatitis other than in patients with hypertriglyceridemia-induced pancreatitis.
• Diabetes mellitus may develop from extensive pancreatic necrosis.

REFERENCE & SUGGESTED READINGS
Available at eBooks.Health.Elsevier.com.

RELATED CONTENT
Acute Pancreatitis (Patient Information)

AUTHOR: **DAVID J. LUCIER, Jr, MD, MBA, MPH**

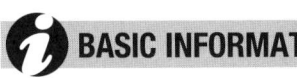

BASIC INFORMATION

DEFINITION

- A **panic attack** is a relatively brief, sudden episode of intense fear or apprehension, often associated with a sense of impending doom and various uncomfortable and disquieting physical and/or cognitive symptoms.[1] Panic attacks may be unexpected ("out of the blue") or expected (i.e., triggered by a particular object or situation). Panic attacks may be present in a variety of different anxiety-related disorders (e.g., phobias, social anxiety, obsessive-compulsive disorder) and other mental disorders (e.g., depression, substance use, PTSD, and psychosis).
- **Panic disorder** is diagnosed after at least one uncued panic attacks have occurred followed by at least 1 mo (or more) of significant concern about future attacks, worry about their implications, or a major change in behavior related to these attacks. The criteria for diagnosis of panic disorder are summarized in Table E1.
- **Agoraphobia** is anxiety about, and avoidance of, places or situations in which the ability to escape is perceived to be limited or embarrassing or in which help might not be available in the event of having a panic attack. Starting with DSM-5, agoraphobia is considered a disorder separate from panic disorder (Table E2), though the two can occur comorbidly.

SYNONYMS

Anxiety attacks
Fear attacks
Ataque de nervios (Latin America), "soul loss" (Cambodia)
Fearful spells

ICD-10-CM CODES	
F41.0	Panic disorder
F40.0	Agoraphobia
DSM-5-TR CODES	
300.01	Panic disorder
300.22	Agoraphobia

EPIDEMIOLOGY & DEMOGRAPHICS[2-6]

INCIDENCE: 1% to 1.7% 1-mo incidence of panic attacks
PREVALENCE:
- 15% to 20% lifetime prevalence of one or more panic attacks.
- Panic disorder is much less common, with a lifetime prevalence of 3.8%; the chronicity of panic disorder is reflected in a similar 1-yr prevalence rate of 2.4%.
- Agoraphobia with or without panic disorder is relatively rare; lifetime prevalence of 2.5% and 0.2% to 0.8% 1-yr prevalence of agoraphobia without panic disorder.
- Lower rates of panic disorder are reported among Latinos, African Americans, Caribbean blacks, and Asian Americans (DSM-5).
- Estimates of panic disorder prevalence for Asian, African, and Latin American countries are lower (0.2% to 1.7%).

- During the SARS-CoV-2 pandemic in 11 countries, the incidence of panic disorder was 3%; the prevalence was 13.7%.[5]
PREDOMINANT SEX:
- Panic disorder and agoraphobia twice as common in women
- Panic disorder with comorbid agoraphobia three times as common in women
PREDOMINANT AGE:
- Age of onset is typically late adolescence to mid-30s. Onset earlier in males (24 yr) than females (28 yr). Some may experience onset later in life.
- Onset after age 45 yr is rare and should raise suspicion of different etiology.
PEAK INCIDENCE:
- Chronic condition with a waxing and waning course.
- Bimodal incidence peaks noted, with the first peak between ages 15 and 24 yr and second peak between ages 35 and 44 yr.
RISK FACTORS[1]:
- Environmental triggers: Adverse childhood, recent separation and loss, long-lasting stressful events; smoking.
- Temperamental: Negative affect, anxiety sensitivity, and harm avoidance. Severe separation anxiety in childhood may precede the panic disorder.
GENETICS[6-8]:
- Risk of developing panic disorder in first-degree relatives of individuals with panic disorder is four to seven times that of general population.
- Findings in twin studies: Heritability estimates for panic disorder range from 28% to 50%.

PHYSICAL FINDINGS & CLINICAL PRESENTATION

Panic disorder:
- Presents either with a panic attack or worries related to anticipation of a future panic attack or its implications.
- Typical presentation: Unexpected, untriggered, and recurrent episodes of intense anxiety and fear with associated physiologic changes (e.g., palpitations, sweating, tremulousness, shortness of breath, chest pain, gastrointestinal distress, faintness, derealization, paresthesia). This is accompanied by associated worry of dying, heart attack, stroke, passing out, losing control, or losing one's mind. Panic attacks are often described as "the most terrifying" episode an individual has experienced.
- Individuals with panic disorder are more likely to present to the emergency department or primary care physician following a panic attack. Often, complaining of physical symptoms such as chest pain, palpitations, dizziness, or difficulty breathing. Thirty percent of patients presenting with chest pain have panic disorder; 10% of patients with comorbid panic attacks and non-cardiac chest pain may develop panic disorder. In a recent study of 1327 patients reporting non-cardiac chest pain, 77.1% had visited the emergency department following a panic attack.[4,5,9]

Agoraphobia:
- Rare complaints to physician. May manifest in missed office visits or tardiness. Patients may request home visits or telephone care.
- Fear or anxiety about situations or activities such as the following:
  1. Crowded public areas (stores [particularly checkout lines]), public transportation, flying, church)
  2. Individual interactions (hairdresser, dentist, meetings)
  3. Driving (especially if alone, far from home, over bridges, through tunnels, on highways, or on isolated roads)
- This fear is a result of the belief that he or she might experience a panic attack and would be unable to exit readily. Patients may also experience fear of other symptoms, beyond the paniclike symptoms, such as falling or incontinence.
- On exposure to or anticipation of exposure to feared situations, significant anxiety occurs. Anxiety may generate somatic symptoms that trigger a full- or limited-symptom panic attack. Patients believe that escape from these situations reduces the alarming symptoms, thus reinforcing future avoidance. In actuality, symptom relief stems from adrenaline breaking down in the body after approximately 20 min.

ETIOLOGY

Hypotheses (NOTE: There are sufficient data to support each model. Models are not mutually exclusive.):
- Central dysregulation of autonomic arousal (typically localized to the locus ceruleus); similar symptoms may be chemically induced with yohimbine, caffeine, or cholecystokinin.
- Cognitive overreaction (i.e., "catastrophic misinterpretation") to relatively mild or benign physiologic cues that then triggers a genuine autonomic cascade and further misinterpretations.
- Dysfunction of a central suffocation alarm mechanism; some signs of compensated respiratory alkalosis. Can be experimentally induced with sodium lactate or carbon dioxide.

DIAGNOSIS

DIFFERENTIAL DIAGNOSIS

Medical conditions:
- Endocrinopathies:
  1. Hyperthyroidism
  2. Hyperparathyroidism
  3. Pheochromocytoma
  4. Carcinoid tumor
- Cardiac and respiratory diseases:
  1. Arrhythmias
  2. Myocardial infarction
  3. Chronic obstructive pulmonary disease
  4. Asthma
  5. Mitral valve prolapse
  6. Pulmonary embolism
- Metabolic:
  1. Hypoglycemia
  2. Electrolyte imbalances
  3. Porphyria

P

Diseases and Disorders

I

- Seizure disorders: Ictal fear happens with simple partial seizures of meso-temporal lobe origin and lasts for seconds to minutes. May evolve to a focal seizure with impaired awareness.
- Substance- or medication-induced anxiety disorder: Therapeutic (theophylline, steroids), intoxication (cocaine, amphetamine, caffeine, diet pills, cannabis) or withdrawal (alcohol, barbiturates, benzodiazepines).
- Psychiatric disorders (NOTE: Panic attacks are common in a variety of psychiatric disorders. Panic disorder could be conceptualized as a phobia of the somatic sensations or situations that have become paired with panic attacks.):
  1. Phobias (e.g., specific phobia or social phobia). Note that fear of going on a plane because of crashing would be a specific phobia, whereas fear of going on a plane because one is then trapped and worries about panic is more suggestive of panic disorder with comorbid agoraphobia
  2. Obsessive-compulsive disorder (cued by exposure to the object of the obsession)
  3. Posttraumatic stress disorder (cued by recall of a trauma)
  4. Generalized anxiety disorder (cued by excessive worry)
  5. Somatic symptom disorder (cued by more persistent anxiety and somatic symptoms)

WORKUP

- Emergency presentation: Cardiac, respiratory, or neurologic symptoms
- History and physical examination to rule out a concomitant medical or substance-related condition

NOTE: Panic disorder and agoraphobia are not diagnoses of exclusion, but exclusion of other conditions is usually required.

LABORATORY TESTS

- Thyroid profile
- Electrolyte measures, including calcium
- Toxicology screen
- ECG
- Acute cases: Possible monitoring and cardiac enzymes to rule out arrhythmia or ischemia

IMAGING STUDIES

- For temporal lobe dysfunction (e.g., temporal lesions or as ictal or interictal manifestation of temporal lobe focal seizures): Brain CT scan or MRI or an electroencephalogram in some patients
- Holter monitor to rule out occult or episodic arrhythmias
- Chest x-ray, arterial blood gases, or pulmonary function tests if respiratory compromise suspected

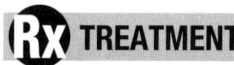 **TREATMENT**

NONPHARMACOLOGIC THERAPY

- Recent systematic review of RCTs demonstrate that cognitive-behavioral therapy (CBT)

and short-term psychodynamic therapy are reliable first-line psychotherapies.[10]
- Cognitive-behavioral therapy (CBT), in particular panic control treatment (PCT), is generally very effective, with strongest results for cognitive restructuring (i.e., challenging catastrophic misinterpretations of somatic symptoms), in vivo or imaginal exposures (i.e., exposure to panic triggers in a controlled graded hierarchical fashion from least to most difficult with the goal of habituation and extinction of the fear response), and interoceptive exposures (i.e., repeated recreation and management of feared somatic sensations via activities such as chair spinning, straw breathing, and hyperventilation).[11,12]
- CBT effect sizes are equal to or larger than for pharmacotherapy, attrition rates are lower, and relapse rates are lower. Treatment may take several sessions spread over weeks and may require referral to a behavioral specialist. CBT has been shown to be the most effective intervention for panic disorder with or without agoraphobia across treatment sites. CBT may also be effectively delivered online (e.g., iCBT).[13]
- A recent dismantling study of cognitive-behavioral therapy components for panic disorder suggests that interoceptive exposure and a face-to-face setting were associated with better treatment efficacy whereas muscle relaxation and virtual reality exposure were associated with significantly lower efficacy.[14]

ACUTE GENERAL Rx

- Benzodiazepines, particularly clonazepam and alprazolam: Highly effective in the acute setting, although long-term use is contraindicated for effective outcome and due to addictive potential.
- Low-dose clonazepam for patients with rare panic attacks and asymptomatic periods (0.25 to 0.5 mg PO or sublingually PRN).
- Start patient on selective serotonin reuptake inhibitor (SSRI) or similar agent and taper patient off benzodiazepine by wk 2 to 3.

CHRONIC Rx

- Preferred pharmacologic agents: Antidepressants with a significant serotonin reuptake inhibitory action. Generally, start at low dose and titrate upward. Minimum treatment duration is 6 to 8 mo, but many patients need to take medications indefinitely. These medications should not be discontinued abruptly; they should be tapered due to withdrawal effects including rebound anxiety.
  1. SSRIs: Sertraline (50 to 200 mg/day), citalopram (20 to 60 mg/day), escitalopram (5 to 30 mg/day), fluoxetine (5 to 60 mg/day), fluvoxamine (50 to 300 mg/day) and paroxetine (10 to 60 mg/day)
  2. Imipramine (100 to 300 mg/day)
  3. SNRIs: Venlafaxine (37.5 to 225 mg/day)

- Combination CBT plus SSRI has shown good long-term effects and is somewhat better than antidepressants or CBT alone. Combination CBT plus benzodiazepine does not provide any added benefit and may undermine CBT (interoceptive and in vivo exposures may be less effective if the benzodiazepine is completely controlling the anxiety).

DISPOSITION

- Typical course is chronic but with significant waxing and waning (common to have long periods of remission).
- Presence of agoraphobia associated with a more chronic course.
  Findings with long-term follow-up studies: 6 to 10 yr after treatment some 30% are in remission, 40% to 50% have improved with residual symptoms, and the remainder are either unchanged or worse.[14,15]

REFERRAL

- For patients who do not respond to an SSRI, CBT is the preferred treatment.

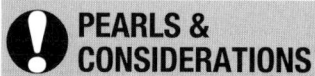 **PEARLS & CONSIDERATIONS**

- Patient and family education is an important first step in the management of panic disorder. Psychoeducation provides more adaptive explanations for the benign somatic sensations paired with panic. Presentation of genetic information and explanation of the nonthreatening nature of the physiology of each of the symptoms the patient experiences serve as a good start to allay fears and reduce stigma. It may also ensure compliance with treatment.
- Resumption of avoided activities or situations is a positive prognostic sign and may promote further therapeutic gains. Patients should be encouraged to resume such activities after treatment is stabilized.
- Additional types of interventions such as mindfulness meditation through programs like Mindfulness Based Stress Reduction (MBSR) may be helpful in treating panic disorder and agoraphobia.
- The therapist's adherence to the treatment protocol and the therapeutic alliance established during the first session predict a better outcome for the long-term success of CBT for panic disorder with or without comorbid agoraphobia.

REFERENCES

Available at eBooks.Health.Elsevier.com.

RELATED CONTENT

Panic Disorder (Patient Information)

AUTHORS: **PERLA M. ROMERO GÓMEZ, MD,** and **JOHN DENNINGE, MD, PHD**

BASIC INFORMATION

DEFINITION

Paraneoplastic syndromes are a group of disorders caused by either an abnormal immune response to malignancy or as a result of hormonal or other soluble factors produced by these malignancies. They often affect areas of the body distant from the site of the original tumor or metastases, which contrasts with syndromes that are direct complications of tumor invasion, compression, or metastasis (e.g., superior vena cava syndrome). Findings and symptoms are specific to each syndrome. Paraneoplastic syndromes can affect multiple organ systems and remain a challenging diagnostic entity.

ICD-10CM CODES
E22.2 Syndrome of inappropriate secretion of antidiuretic hormone
E83.5 Disorders of calcium metabolism
G13.0 Paraneoplastic neuromyopathy and neuropathy
G13.1 Other systemic atrophy primarily affecting central nervous system in neoplastic disease
G73.1 Lambert-Eaton syndrome in neoplastic disease
G73.3 Myasthenic syndromes in other diseases classified elsewhere

EPIDEMIOLOGY & DEMOGRAPHICS
- Paraneoplastic syndromes may affect as many as 8% of cancer patients.[1]
- See Table 1 for epidemiology of each syndrome.

PHYSICAL FINDINGS & CLINICAL PRESENTATION

Hypercalcemia of malignancy:
- Nausea/vomiting
- Constipation
- Abdominal pain
- Anorexia
- Hypertension
- Fatigue
- Altered mental status (from confusion to coma)
- Depression/anxiety
- Polyuria
- Acute kidney injury
- Bone pain

Syndrome of inappropriate antidiuretic hormone (SIADH):
- Headache
- Weakness
- Anorexia
- Nausea, vomiting
- Memory impairment, irritability, restlessness, seizures
- Obtundation or coma may be seen with hyponatremia <125 mEq/L

Cushing syndrome:
- Muscle weakness
- Rapid weight gain
- Centripetal fat distribution, progressing to obesity; limbs are often spared or wasted

- Characteristic "moon facies" resulting from accumulation of fat deposition in the cheeks
- Skin atrophy, easy bruising, and purple abdominal striae due to skin fragility
- Hyperpigmentation, notably in sun-exposed areas
- Menstrual irregularity, mild hirsutism in women
- Hypertension
- Depression, anxiety, irritability[1]

Paraneoplastic thrombocytosis:
- Thrombosis
- Nausea, vomiting
- Paresthesias, visual disturbances, headache

Paraneoplastic erythrocytosis:
- Erythroderma
- Postshower (aquagenic) pruritus
- Plethora

Paraneoplastic glomerulonephritis:
- Renal failure: Oliguric or anuric
- Malaise
- Nausea, vomiting

Paraneoplastic Neurologic Syndromes (Table 2 and Table 3):[2]

Paraneoplastic cerebellar degeneration (PCD):
- May develop prodrome of dizziness, nausea, vomiting
- Ataxia
- Diplopia
- Dysphagia, dysarthria

Lambert-Eaton myasthenic syndrome (LEMS):
- Gradual onset of symmetric proximal muscle weakness and fatigability; lower extremity

involvement is more common. Uniquely, strength improves after exercise.
- Hyporeflexia may also be improved after exercise.
- Mild bulbar dysfunction, although respiratory failure can occur late in the disease process.
- Dysautonomia, especially erectile dysfunction.

Myasthenia gravis (MG):
- Ocular symptoms: Ptosis and diplopia
- Weakness of facial muscles, notably with fatigable chewing
- Weakness of neck extensor and flexor muscles; proximal and distal extremities may also be involved
- May progress to involve muscles of respiration and respiratory crisis

Opsoclonus myoclonus syndrome (OMS):
- Truncal ataxia and unsteady gait
- Involuntary and conjugate gaze rapid eye movements (opsoclonus)
- Muscle twitching (myoclonus)
- Other symptoms: Irritability, sleep disturbance, dysarthria or mutism

Limbic encephalitis (LE):
- Insidious mood or psychiatric changes; hallucinations
- Short-term memory loss
- Hyperthermia or somnolence if hypothalamic involvement
- Seizures occur in up to half of patients

Paraneoplastic dermatologic and rheumatologic syndromes:
- Acanthosis nigricans
- Dermatomyositis (DM)
- Necrolytic migratory erythema

TABLE 1 Epidemiology of Each Paraneoplastic Syndrome

Condition	Prevalence	Risk Factors
Hypercalcemia of malignancy	Up to 20% of all cancer patients	Squamous cell cancers (lung, head, and neck), breast, kidney, bladder, and ovarian cancers, lymphoma
Syndrome of inappropriate antidiuretic hormone (SIADH)	Up to 2% of all cancer patients. Found in 10%-45% of SCLC patients	SCLC
Cushing syndrome	Approximately 2% of all cancer patients (50% of these are SCLC)	SCLC, pituitary adenoma, benign and malignant adrenal tumors, carcinoid tumors
Limbic encephalitis (LE)	Less than 1%	SCLC, testicular germ cell tumor, breast cancer, ovarian teratoma
Paraneoplastic cerebellar degeneration	Less than 1%	SCLC, Hodgkin lymphoma, breast cancer
Lambert-Eaton myasthenic syndrome (LEMS)	3% of SCLC patients	SCLC, prostate cancer, lymphoma
Paraneoplastic thrombocytosis	5%-20% of patients with solid tumors	Lung, colorectal, mesothelioma
Paraneoplastic erythrocytosis	4% of patients	Renal cell carcinoma, hepatocellular carcinoma
Paraneoplastic glomerulonephritis	2%-4% of patients	Hodgkin lymphoma, thymoma, prostate cancer
Myasthenia gravis (MG)	15% of thymoma patients	Thymoma
Opsoclonus myoclonus syndrome (OMS)	Less than 1%	SCLC, breast cancer, ovarian teratoma in adults; neuroblastoma in children

SCLC, Small cell lung cancer.

TABLE 2 Paraneoplastic Syndromes

Syndrome	Tumor	Associated Antibodies
Cerebellar Degeneration	SCLC	Anti-Hu
	Gynecologic	Anti-Yo
	Breast	Anti-Ri
	Lymphoma	Anti-CV2
Faciobrachial Dystonic Seizures	Metastases	Anti-LGI1
	SCLC	Anti-VGCC
Lambert-Eaton Myasthenic Syndrome	SCLC	
Limbic Encephalitis	SCLC	Anti-Hu
	Testes	Anti-Ma
	Breast	Anti-Amphiphysin
	Ovarian teratoma	Anti-NMDA receptor
	Thymoma	Anti-VGKC
	Metastases	Anti-GAD
		Anti-LGI1
Opsoclonus-Myoclonus	Neuroblastoma	Anti-Ri
	SCLC	
	Breast	
Sensory Neuronopathy	SCLC	Anti-Hu
Stiff-Person Syndrome	SCLC	Anti-GAD
	Breast	Anti-Amphiphysin
	Thymoma	

GAD, Glutamic acid decarboxylase; *LGI1*, leucine-rich glioma inactivated-1; *NMDA*, N-methyl-D-aspartate; *SCLC*, small cell lung cancer; *VGCC*, voltage-gated calcium channel; *VGKC*, voltage-gated potassium channel.
From Kaufman DM et al: *Kaufman's clinical neurology for psychiatrists*, ed 9, Philadelphia, 2023, Elsevier.

TABLE 3 Paraneoplastic Syndromes of the Nervous System

Classical
Limbic encephalitis
Encephalomyelitis
Cerebellar degeneration
Opsoclonus-myoclonus
Sensory neuronopathy
Gastrointestinal pseudoobstruction/autonomic neuropathy
Lambert–Eaton myasthenic syndrome
Inflammatory myopathy
Nonclassical
Brain stem encephalitis
Stiff-person syndrome
Motor neuron disease
Necrotizing myelopathy
Optic neuropathy/retinopathy
Acute sensorimotor neuropathy
Chronic sensorimotor neuropathy
Myasthenia gravis
Autoimmune Encephalitides
NMDAR encephalitis
AMPAR encephalitis

AMPAR, Alpha-amino-3-hydroxy-5-methyl-4-isoxazolepropionic acid receptor; *NMDAR*, anti-N-methyl-D-aspartate receptor.
From Swaiman KF: *Swaiman's pediatric neurology, principles and practice*, ed 6, 2017, Elsevier.

- Hypertrophic osteoarthropathy
- Leukocytoclastic vasculitis
- Paraneoplastic pemphigus
- Polymyalgia rheumatica
- Sweet syndrome (acute febrile neutrophilic dermatosis)
- Sign of Leser-Trélat (explosive onset of multiple seborrheic keratoses)

ETIOLOGY

Paraneoplastic endocrine syndromes are caused by ectopic production of bioactive substances (e.g., hormones or peptides) that lead to metabolic derangements:[3]

- **Hypercalcemia of malignancy:**
  1. *Humoral hypercalcemia of malignancy (HHM):* Due to production of parathyroid hormone-related peptide (PTHrP). Accounts for 80% of hypercalcemia of malignancy cases. Most common in lung (Table 4) and breast cancer (also seen in renal, bladder, ovarian cancer, and lymphoma).
  2. *Other etiologies of hypercalcemia of malignancy:* 1,25-dihydroxyvitamin D production from increased 1α-hydroxylase activity causes hypercalcemia in Hodgkin and non-Hodgkin lymphomas.
  3. *Osteolytic activity:* 20% of hypercalcemia of malignancy cases. Tumor cells produce local factors that stimulate osteoclast activation, resulting in increased bone resorption. This is seen in multiple myeloma and in some cases of lymphoma where there is bone marrow infiltration.
  4. *True ectopic parathyroid hormone (PTH):* Rare. Thyroid and nonthyroid tumors can also produce PTH, leading to hypercalcemia.[4]

TABLE 4 Hypercalcemia of Malignancy

Cancer	Frequency (%)	Mechanism
Lung	35	PTHrP
		Local osteolysis
Breast	25	PTHrP
		Local osteolysis
Head and neck	6	PTHrP
Renal	3	PTHrP
		Local osteolysis
Multiple myeloma	15	PTHrP (rare)
		Local osteolysis
		1,25-Dihydroxyvitamin D
Prostate	7	Local osteolysis
Lymphoma	15	1,25-Dihydroxyvitamin D
		PTHrP

PTHrP, Parathyroid hormone-related protein.
From Skorecki K et al: *Brenner and Rector's the kidney*, ed 10, Philadelphia, 2016, Elsevier.

- **SIADH:** Ectopic production of antidiuretic hormone (ADH) (arginine vasopressin, atrial natriuretic peptide) by tumor cells leads to inappropriately concentrated urine and natriuresis.
- **Cushing syndrome:** Ectopic adrenocorticotropic hormone (ACTH) promotes excess production of cortisol and other glucocorticoids from the adrenal glands, which do not respond to normal HPA feedback.
- **Paraneoplastic erythrocytosis**: Mediated by inappropriate production of erythropoietin (EPO) and is associated most with renal cell carcinoma and hepatocellular carcinoma.
- **Paraneoplastic thrombocytosis**: Overproduction of inflammatory cytokines, especially interleukin-6, which induces thrombopoietin (TPO) mRNA expression and protein synthesis in the liver. Unlike secondary (reactive) thrombocytosis, TPO levels are not elevated.[5]
- **Paraneoplastic glomerulonephritis**: Acute renal failure in the setting of newly diagnosed malignancy that is not explained by direct tumor involvement of the kidneys or genitourinary system. Diseases include minimal change disease, rapidly progressive glomerulonephritis, focal segmental glomerulonephritis, immunoglobulin A nephropathy, and membranous nephropathy.
- **Paraneoplastic neurologic syndromes (PNS):** Due to immune cross-reactivity between tumor cells and components of the nervous system. Tumor-directed antibodies (onconeural antibodies) are produced by the patient in response to a developing cancer. These onconeural antibodies and associated onconeural antigen-specific T lymphocytes attack components of the nervous system because of antigenic similarity (molecular

TABLE 5 Diagnostic Criteria for Paraneoplastic Neurologic Syndromes

Definite Paraneoplastic Neurologic Syndromes
- A classical syndrome and cancer that develops within 5 yr of the diagnosis of the neurologic disorder
- A nonclassical syndrome that resolves significantly after cancer treatment without concomitant immunotherapy provided that the syndrome is not susceptible to spontaneous remission
- A nonclassical syndrome with onconeural antibodies (well characterized or not) and cancer that develops within 5 yr of the diagnosis of the neurologic disorder
- A neurologic syndrome (classical or not) with well-characterized onconeural antibodies (anti-Hu, Yo, CV2, Ri, Ma2, or amphiphysin) and no cancer

Possible Paraneoplastic Neurologic Syndromes
- A classical syndrome, no onconeural antibodies, no cancer, but at high risk to have an underlying tumor
- A neurologic syndrome (classical or not) with partially characterized onconeural antibodies and no cancer
- A nonclassical syndrome, no onconeural antibodies, and cancer present within 2 yr of diagnosis

From Swaiman KF et al: *Swaiman's pediatric neurology: principles and practice*, ed 6, Philadelphia, 2017, Elsevier.

BOX 1 Evaluation and Diagnosis of Paraneoplastic Syndromes

- Characterize abnormality; obtain laboratory studies, imaging, and biopsy, as necessary.
- Carefully elicit any additional symptoms and signs.
- Eliminate common causes.
- If there is no obvious etiology, consider a paraneoplastic syndrome.
- If signs and symptoms are consistent with a paraneoplastic syndrome, undertake a search for an unknown primary cancer or recurrence or progression of a known primary tumor.
- Screening should include a careful physical examination with breast, gynecologic, and prostate evaluations; basic hematology, chemistry, and urine studies; chest radiograph; and mammography.
- Computed tomography (CT) of the chest, abdomen and pelvis, or positron emission tomography/CT is indicated if there are any suspicious symptoms, signs, or laboratory abnormalities. Antibody testing for paraneoplastic neurologic syndromes and/or skin biopsy should be performed as indicated.
- Consider treatment of cancer and/or appropriate palliative treatment, including immunosuppressive therapy for paraneoplastic symptoms when possible.

mimicry). Diagnostic criteria for paraneoplastic neurologic syndromes are summarized in Table 5.
- **LE, PCD, LEMS, MG, OMS:** Cross-reactive autoantibodies against various components of the central and peripheral nervous system.

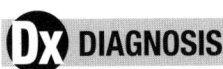 **DIAGNOSIS**

DIFFERENTIAL DIAGNOSIS
- **Hypercalcemia of malignancy:** Primary hyperparathyroidism, familial hypocalciuric hypercalcemia, excess calcium intake, vitamin D toxicity, chronic granulomatous disorders, thiazide diuretics, rhabdomyolysis. It is important to differentiate between HHM and osteolytic causes of malignancy-associated hypercalcemia because prognosis and response to treatment differ
- **SIADH:** Hypovolemic hyponatremia, volume overload, reset osmostat, adrenal insufficiency, hypothyroidism, psychogenic polydipsia, central nervous system disturbances including stroke, hemorrhage, infection, and trauma.
- **Cushing syndrome:** Excess glucocorticoid administration, pituitary adenoma, benign or malignant adrenal tumors

- **Paraneoplastic thrombocytosis:** Reactive thrombocytosis from iron deficiency anemia, infection, inflammation, essential thrombocythemia
- **Paraneoplastic erythrocytosis:** Polycythemia vera, secondary polycythemia from smoking, high-affinity hemoglobinopathies, or chronic hypoxia (e.g., severe chronic obstructive pulmonary disease)
- **Paraneoplastic glomerulonephritis:** Renal failure from intrinsic injury from nephrotoxic agents (e.g., chemotherapy), postrenal failure from bladder obstruction, or rarely direct metastatic invasion from a primary tumor
- **LE, PCD, LEMS, MG, OMS:** Multiple sclerosis, stroke, meningitis, encephalitis, neurodegenerative diseases, myelitis, mixed connective tissue disease

WORKUP
- History and physical examination. Box 1 summarizes the evaluation and diagnosis of paraneoplastic syndromes.[6]
- Age-appropriate cancer screening
- Chest-abdomen-pelvis computed tomography (CT)
- Paraneoplastic neurologic syndromes: Lumbar puncture, PET, EEG, EMG

LABORATORY TESTS
Hypercalcemia of malignancy:
- Serum calcium and albumin levels to measure corrected calcium (HHM more common when serum Ca^{2+} >13 mg/dl)
- Ionized serum calcium
- PTH (low to normal)
- PTHrP (elevated)
- $1,25(OH)_2D$ levels (if the above values are inconclusive)
- Serum protein electrophoresis, urine protein electrophoresis, serum free light chain assay

SIADH:
- Serum (corrected for glucose) and urine sodium (serum sodium <135 mEq/L or urine sodium >40 mEq/L)
- Serum and urine osmolality (serum osm <280 mOsm/kg of water and/or urine osm >100 mOsm/kg of water)

Cushing syndrome:
- Initial testing: Low-dose dexamethasone suppression test, late-night salivary cortisol, 24-h urinary free cortisol excretion.
- Once diagnosis is confirmed: High-dose dexamethasone suppression tests can help to distinguish Cushing syndrome (pituitary hypersecretion of ACTH) from patients with ectopic ACTH production.
- Potassium and glucose should be monitored closely due to increased risk of hypokalemia and hyperglycemia.
- **LE:** Anti-Hu, anti-Ma2, anti-CRMP5, anti-LGI1, anti-AMPAR, anti-mGluR5, cerebrospinal fluid (CSF) analysis, anti-N-methyl-D-aspartate receptor, anti–gamma-aminobutyric acid AR (anti-GABA-AR), anti-GABA-BR
- **PCD:** Anti-Yo, anti-Tr, anti-Hu, anti-Ma, anti-Ri, anti-CV2, anti-VGCC, anti-mGluR1, CSF analysis
- **LEMS:** Anti-VGCC (P/Q), CSF analysis
- **MG:** Anti-AChR, anti-MuSK, CSF analysis
- **Paraneoplastic thrombocytosis:** CBC, liver panel, iron panel, *JAK2* mutation, *CALR* mutation, *MPL* mutation
- **Paraneoplastic erythrocytosis:** CBC, EPO level, *JAK2* mutation, peripheral blood smear
- **Paraneoplastic glomerulonephritis:** Basic metabolic panel, urinalysis, urine protein to creatinine ratio, 24-h urine protein collection, urine sediment analysis

IMAGING STUDIES[7]
- **Hypercalcemia of malignancy:** CT imaging to evaluate for breast lesion, lung mass, or lymphadenopathy
- **SIADH:** CT imaging to evaluate for brain or lung mass
- **Cushing syndrome:** CT scan, MRI, or octreotide scan
- **LE, PCD, LEMS, MG:** CT chest, FDG-PET scan, MRI
- **Paraneoplastic erythrocytosis:** CT renal mass protocol or renal ultrasound to evaluate for renal cell carcinoma

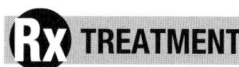 **TREATMENT**

NONPHARMACOLOGIC THERAPY

Hypercalcemia of malignancy:
- Treatment of underlying malignancy, either surgical resection or chemotherapy/radiation of identified tumors
- Fluid resuscitation, typically with initial 1 L bolus of isotonic saline followed by 200 to 300 ml/h to achieve euvolemia, followed by maintenance hydration

SIADH:
- Surgical resection of identified tumors
- Fluid restriction
- Maintain adequate dietary protein and salt intake
- **Cushing syndrome:** Surgical resection of identified tumors

LE, PCD, LEMS, MG
- Intravenous immunoglobulin
- Plasma exchange

ACUTE GENERAL Rx

Hypercalcemia of malignancy:
- Aggressive fluid hydration with normal saline to promote renal calcium excretion
- Bisphosphonates, either pamidronate or zoledronic acid intravenous infusions (treatment side effects are renal dysfunction and osteonecrosis of the jaw)
- Calcitonin weight-based dosing, although tachyphylaxis occurs after 48 h of administration
- Loop diuretics if concurrent heart failure or renal failure
- Corticosteroids in cases of myeloma and lymphoma
- Hemodialysis in severe cases[8]

SIADH:
- If patient develops seizure or obtundation in cases of severe hyponatremia, then sodium replacement with hypertonic saline (3%) is indicated
- Sodium should be corrected at a rate less than 8 mEq/L in any 24-h period to decrease chances of osmotic demyelination syndrome. Desmopressin, free water, and/or nephrology

consultation may be required for an overly rapid correction[9]

Cushing syndrome:
- Diuretics and antihypertensive agents for blood pressure and volume status management

CHRONIC Rx

- Chronic treatment is centered on treatment of the underlying malignancy
- **Hypercalcemia of malignancy:**
  1. Bisphosphonate therapy every 4 wk in cases of bone metastasis
  2. Chronic calcitonin use can be considered
  3. Denosumab, a monoclonal antibody that inhibits osteoclastic bone resorption by blocking RANKL from binding to osteoclastic RANK receptors, can be used in patients refractory to bisphosphonate therapy
- **SIADH:**
  1. Demeclocycline and vasopressin receptor antagonists (vaptans: Conivaptan and tolvaptan, although tolvaptan should not be used for longer than 30 days and should be avoided in patients with liver disease)
  2. Cessation of any possible causative medications
  3. Oral salt tablets if dietary salt intake insufficient
- **Cushing syndrome:** If surgery contraindicated, consider inhibition of adrenal enzymes with ketoconazole, mitotane, metyrapone
- **LE/PCD:** Glucocorticoids, cyclophosphamide, rituximab
- **LEMS:** Pyridostigmine, azathioprine, glucocorticoids
- **MG:** Pyridostigmine, azathioprine, cyclosporine, mycophenolate, rituximab
- **Paraneoplastic thrombocytosis:** Consider prophylactic low-molecular-weight heparin or aspirin if no contraindications exist, siltuximab (antibody against interleukin-6)

DISPOSITION

Specific to each condition; however, humoral hypercalcemia of malignancy carries a poor overall prognosis with 30-day mortality of 50%.

REFERRAL

Oncology, endocrinology, neurology, nephrology

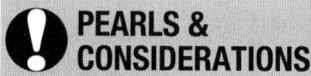 **PEARLS & CONSIDERATIONS**

COMMENTS

- Signs or symptoms of a paraneoplastic syndrome may manifest prior to the identification of a malignancy.
- If paraneoplastic syndrome is suspected, a thorough workup for a tumor is indicated.
- With treatment of the primary tumor, the clinical effects of hypercalcemia of malignancy, SIADH, and Cushing syndrome may improve or resolve.
- Neurologic paraneoplastic syndromes can have long-term effects due to permanent central nervous system or peripheral nervous system damage. Tumor detection can also be difficult as these immune-mediated syndromes may also be keeping the tumor in check.
- New neurologic deficits after starting a checkpoint inhibitor (e.g., PD-1 inhibitor) may indicate drug-induced autoimmunity rather than a paraneoplastic syndrome.[10]

PREVENTION

- Smoking cessation
- Age-appropriate cancer screening

PATIENT & FAMILY EDUCATION

In conditions with autoimmune etiology (LE, PCD, LEMS, MG, OMS), symptoms may not improve even if the tumor is identified and treated, as damage to the nervous system may be sustained or permanent.

REFERENCES

Available at eBooks.Health.Elsevier.com.

AUTHORS: **PRANAVI SANKA, MD,** and **JOHN L. REAGAN, MD**

BASIC INFORMATION

DEFINITION

Idiopathic Parkinson disease (PD) is a progressive neurodegenerative synucleinopathy defined by bradykinesia plus either resting tremor or rigidity.

SYNONYMS

PD
Paralysis agitans

ICD-10CM CODES

G20	Parkinson disease
G21.1	Other drug-induced secondary parkinsonism
G21.11	Neuroleptic-induced parkinsonism
G21.2	Secondary parkinsonism due to other external agents
G21.3	Postencephalitic parkinsonism
G21.4	Vascular parkinsonism
G21.8	Other secondary parkinsonism
G21.9	Secondary parkinsonism, unspecified

EPIDEMIOLOGY & DEMOGRAPHICS

PREVALENCE:
- It is the second most common neurodegenerative disease worldwide and is found in every country.[1]
- Affects more than 1 million people in North America at 0.3% of the population and 1% of people over the age of 60. Prevalence increases with age.
- In those aged >70 yr, 700/100,000 are affected.
- Lifetime risk of PD is 2% in men and 1.3% in women.

PHYSICAL FINDINGS & CLINICAL PRESENTATION

- Prodromal symptoms during 3 yr before patients receive a diagnosis of PD include problems with working, lifting heavy objects, and balance.[1a]
- Tremor (Figs. E1 and 2)—typically a resting tremor with a frequency of 4 to 6 Hz that is often first noted in the hand as a pill-rolling tremor (thumb and forefinger). Can also involve the leg and lip. Tremor improves with purposeful movement. Usually starts asymmetrically.
- Rigidity (Fig. E3)—increased muscle tone that persists throughout the range of passive movement of a joint. Rigidity, like resting tremor, is usually asymmetric at onset.
- Akinesia/bradykinesia (Figs. E4 and 5)—slowness in initiating movement and decrement with repeated movements.
- Postural instability—tested by "pull test." Ask patient to stand in place with back to examiner. Examiner pulls patient back by the shoulders, and proper response would be to take no steps back or very few steps back without falling. Retropulsion is a positive test, as is falling straight back. Postural instability is usually mild early in the disease course but can be significant in later stages. If falls and postural reflexes are greatly impaired early on, then consider other disorders, such as progressive supranuclear palsy (PSP).
- Masked facies (hypomimia) (Fig. 6)—face seems expressionless, giving the appearance of depression. Decreased blink; often there is excess drooling.
- Gait disturbance.
- Stooped posture, decreased arm swing.
- Difficulty initiating the first step; small shuffling steps that increase in speed (festinating gait) (Fig. E7). Steps become progressively faster and shorter while the trunk inclines further forward.
- Other complaints and findings early on include handwriting becoming smaller (micrographia) and voice becoming softer and often "gruffer" (hypophonia).
- Nonmotor symptoms in PD include neuropsychiatric (depression, apathy, impulse control disorders, hallucinations), cognitive, dysautonomia (especially orthostatic hypotension, sexual dysfunction, and anosmia), and sensory abnormalities. These symptoms also may be subject to fluctuations during "on" vs. "off" states.
- Common premotor symptoms of PD include constipation, anosmia, depression, and REM sleep behavior disorder (Table 1).

ETIOLOGY

- Most cases are sporadic. Age is the most common risk factor, although a combination of both environmental and genetic factors likely contributes to disease expression.
- Both pesticides and drinking well water are factors correlated with a higher incidence of PD.
- 10% to 15% have a genetic etiology. Several different genes have been identified; these include the parkin gene (a significant cause of early-onset autosomal recessive PD), *LRRK2* (the most common cause of familial and sporadic parkinsonism associated with later onset of PD), and *PINK1* (associated with early-onset PD).[1]

DIAGNOSIS

- A clinical diagnosis usually can be made based on a comprehensive history and physical examination. The cardinal signs used to diagnose PD are (mnemonic = ART):
  1. **A**kinesia/bradykinesia—slowing and decrement of movement
  2. **R**igidity, of the cogwheel type
  3. **T**remor (resting, typically 4 to 6 Hz)
- Diagnostic criteria require bradykinesia plus either resting tremor or rigidity plus at least two supporting criteria and absence of absolute exclusion criteria and absence of red flags.[2]
  1. Supporting criteria: Clear benefit of dopaminergic therapy, presence of levodopa-induced dyskinesia, rest tremor, presence of hyposmia, or cardiac sympathetic denervation on MIBG scintigraphy.
  2. Absolute exclusion criteria: No response to high-dose levodopa therapy, cerebellar abnormalities, downward vertical supranuclear gaze palsy, frontotemporal dementia symptoms early in the disease process, only lower limb involvement >3 yr, cortical sensory loss, progressive aphasia, or alternative diagnosis. These findings would suggest another diagnosis.
  3. Red flags: Severe autonomic failure or rapid progression of gait impairment in the first 5 yr, early bulbar involvement, inspiratory respiratory dysfunction, early recurrent falls, contractures, or bilateral symmetric parkinsonism. These findings would suggest another diagnosis.

DIFFERENTIAL DIAGNOSIS

- Multiple system atrophy (MSA): Distinguishing features include early autonomic dysfunction (including urinary incontinence, orthostatic hypotension, and erectile dysfunction), parkinsonism, cerebellar signs, and normal cognition.
- Dementia with Lewy bodies (DLB): Parkinsonism with concomitant dementia; patients often have early hallucinations and fluctuations in level of alertness and mental status.
- Corticobasal syndrome (CBD): Often begins asymmetrically with apraxia, cortical sensory loss in one limb, and, sometimes, alien limb phenomenon.
- Progressive supranuclear palsy (PSP): Tends to have axial rigidity greater than appendicular (limb) rigidity. These patients have early and severe postural instability. Hallmark is supranuclear gaze palsy that usually involves vertical gaze (especially downward) before horizontal.
- Essential tremor: Bilateral postural and action tremor.
- Secondary (acquired) parkinsonism (Box 1):
  1. Iatrogenic: Many, including any of the neuroleptics and antipsychotics. The high-potency D_2-blocker neuroleptics are most likely to cause parkinsonism. Metoclopramide can also cause parkinsonism. Abuse of methamphetamine has been linked to risk of PD
  2. Postinfectious parkinsonism: Von Economo encephalitis
  3. Chronic traumatic encephalopathy (dementia pugilistica): Parkinsonism and dementia after repeated head trauma
  4. Toxins (e.g., MPTP, manganese, carbon monoxide)
  5. Cerebrovascular disease: "Vascular parkinsonism" (basal ganglia infarcts); often lower limbs (especially gait) affected more than upper extremities
  6. Red flags suggesting a diagnosis other than PD are summarized in Box 2

WORKUP

- Identification of clinical signs and symptoms associated with PD (see "Physical Findings"), and elimination of conditions that may mimic it

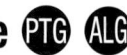
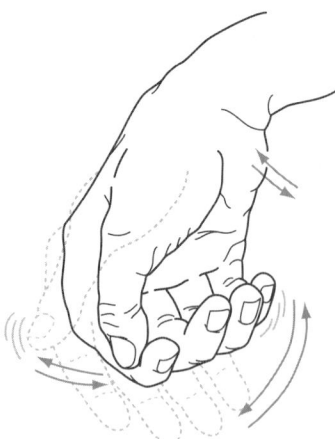

FIG. 2 *Resting tremor*—a cardinal feature of Parkinson disease—consists of a relatively slow (4 to 6 Hz) to-and-fro flexion movement of the wrist, hand, thumb, and fingers most apparent when patients sit comfortably. Its similarity to rolling a pill or a coin between the thumb and index finger gave rise to the description "pill-rolling" tremor. The tremor is exaggerated or sometimes apparent only when patients are anxious. (From Kaufman DM et al: *Kaufman's clinical neurology for psychiatrists,* ed 9, Philadelphia, 2023, Elsevier.)

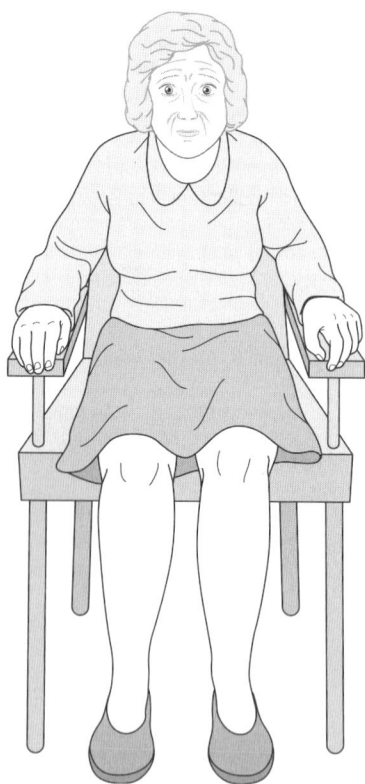

FIG. 5 Parkinson disease patients typically sit motionless with their legs uncrossed and their feet flat. Their arms remain on the chair or in their lap and rarely participate in normal gestures or repositioning movements. They do not shift their weight from one hip to another or make any unnecessary movements. (From Kaufman DM et al: *Kaufman's clinical neurology for psychiatrists,* ed 9, Philadelphia, 2023, Elsevier.)

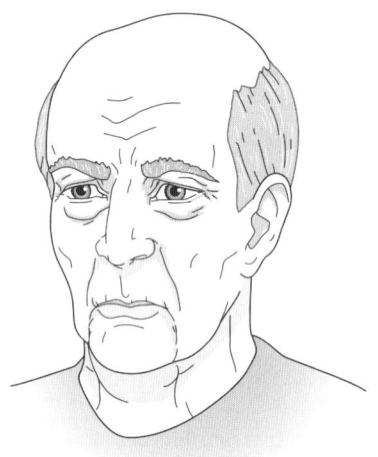

FIG. 6 Compared to normal individuals of the same age, Parkinson disease patients blink less frequently, show less facial expression, and move their head less frequently. Neurologists have called patients' facial appearance a "stare" or "masked facies" (Latin, face or countenance). Even when subtle, the masked face gives the appearance of apathy or depression. (From Kaufman DM et al: *Kaufman's clinical neurology for psychiatrists,* ed 9, Philadelphia, 2023, Elsevier.)

with a comprehensive history and physical examination.
- Routine genetic testing is not recommended.
- Can evaluate for response to carbidopa/levodopa (C/L) to differentiate PD from other causes of parkinsonism such as PSP, MSA, CBD.

IMAGING STUDIES

- MRI of the head may sometimes distinguish between idiopathic PD and other conditions that present with signs of parkinsonism (see "Differential Diagnosis").
- Dopamine transporter imaging (DaTscan with [123I]β-CIT SPECT) evaluates the level of dopamine in the striatum and can be used to confirm parkinsonism in atypical cases. Normally there is dopamine reuptake in the caudate and putamen that can light up to look like a comma. If there is poor reuptake in the putamen as seen in PD, only the caudate lights up, similar to a period on imaging. DaTscan is approved to distinguish essential tremor from parkinsonism but cannot distinguish between different causes of parkinsonism.[2] Interpretation can be tricky, and routine use is not recommended at this time.

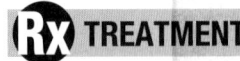 TREATMENT

NONPHARMACOLOGIC THERAPY

- Physical therapy (to help with exercise and help in evaluation of safe equipment to use), speech therapy, swallow evaluation. A safe, practical, and reasonable exercise regimen should be encouraged.[3,4]
- Avoidance of drugs that can induce or worsen parkinsonism: Neuroleptics (especially high potency), certain antiemetics (prochlorperazine, trimethobenzamide), metoclopramide, nonselective MAO inhibitors (MAO-Is) (may induce hypertensive crisis), reserpine, methyldopa.

ACUTE GENERAL Rx

- Levodopa is the gold standard, but patients <65 can be started on agonists if preferred.[5]
- It is appropriate to initiate pharmacotherapy when required by symptoms. Fig. 8 describes treatment of motor symptoms in patients with parkinsonism.
- Motor complications do develop during the course of the disease and likely reflect the combination of disease progression and the side effects of dopaminergic medications.

CHRONIC Rx

- Levodopa therapy:
  1. The gold standard is levodopa with a peripheral dopa decarboxylase inhibitor (carbidopa) to minimize side effects (nausea, light-headedness, postural hypotension).[5,6] The combination of the two drugs is marketed under the trade name Sinemet. Levodopa therapy has been found to reduce morbidity and mortality in PD patients.
  2. Usual starting dose is 25/100 mg (C/L) tid 1 h before (or after) meals. Typically better effect before meals, but lower side effects when taken with protein-rich meals.
  3. Controlled-release (Sinemet CR), extended-release (Rytary), infusion (Duopa), and

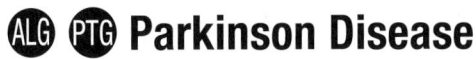
TABLE 1 Sleep and Night Problems in Parkinson Disease and Suggested Management

Problem	Potential Diagnosis	Proposed Management
Frequent Nocturia (± Two Episodes/Night)		
Normal volumes	Sleep apnea syndrome	Check for sleep apnea and treat appropriately
Small volumes, poor stream	Prostatism	Refer to urologist
Small volumes, good stream	Parkinsonism: associated nocturia	Intranasal desmopressin, oral amitriptyline, or transdermal rotigotine patch; if detrusor instability: oxybutynin, tolterodine, Myrbetriq
		Decrease evening fluid intake; empty bladder before bed; avoid evening dosing with diuretics, antihypertensives, or vasodilators; have a urinal at the bedside table
Difficulty Initiating Sleep		
Early in the evening	Too early lights-off	Switch off lights later
	Anxiety or behavioral insomnia	Sleep hygiene; treat anxiety
		Evening melatonin, eszopiclone, doxepin
With restlessness	Restless legs syndrome	Check for low ferritin; remove antidepressant drugs; if the diagnosis is uncertain, consider polysomnography with leg monitoring; try gabapentin, pregabalin or opiates, such as tramadol, if not confused
Late in the night	Altered circadian cycle	Sleep hygiene; decrease levodopa/dopamine agonists in the evening
		Melatonin 1-2 h before the desired bedtime
Late in night, hypomanic	Assess for impulse control disorder	Decrease dopamine agonists; keep on levodopa monotherapy; close neuropsychologic follow-up
Difficulty Resuming Sleep		
With cramps, muscle pain, slowness	Nocturnal bradykinesia	Immediate-release levodopa with a glass of water during awakenings
		Continuous drug delivery (ropinirole transdermal patch; pramipexole or extended-release ropinirole; apomorphine infusion; intrajejunal levodopa-carbidopa infusion)
		Satin bed sheets to aid movement in bed
With restlessness	Restless legs syndrome	Similar to nocturnal bradykinesia treatment
With anxiety	Anxious disorder	Evening antidepressants (mirtazapine, doxepin, paroxetine)
With low mood	Depressive disorder	Treat the depression
Nightmares, Agitation		
Confused at night when awake	Hallucinations, psychosis, confusion	Remove or reduce the evening dose of dopamine agonist or antidepressant; assess for sleep apnea;
		Antipsychotics (quetiapine, clozapine)
Kicks, shouts, slaps	REM sleep behavior disorders	Secure the bed environment; discontinue antidepressant; assess likelihood of sleep apnea (video-PSG before treating)
		Melatonin, 3-9 mg in the evening, clonazepam, 0.5-2 mg in the evening
Daytime Sleepiness		
Falls asleep unexpectedly	Sleep attack	Check for possible sedating drugs (e.g., dopamine agonists) and remove or change them; warn patient not to drive
Falls asleep more often than before		Consider the Epworth Sleepiness Score; ask about associated hallucinations; consider PSG and MSLT
		Treat sleep apnea if severe
		Decrease/stop the dopamine agonist during daytime, and other sedative drugs
		Caffeine, modafinil, methylphenidate

MSLT, Multiple Sleep Latency Test; *PSG,* polysomnography; *REM,* rapid eye movement.
From Kryger M et al: *Principles and practice of sleep medicine,* ed 7, Philadelphia, 2023, Elsevier.

inhaled (Inbrija) preparations are also available, but their use should be supervised by a neurologist.

4. Stalevo (combination Sinemet and entacapone, a COMT inhibitor). Useful for patients with motor fluctuations (wearing off); has no role in treating patients with early PD.

5. Duopa (C/L), administered by a 16-h infusion to the jejunum through either a nasojejunal tube (short-term) or PEG-J tube (long-term), is used for treating motor fluctuations in patients with advanced PD.

6. Inbrija (levodopa inhalation powder) is used to treat "off" periods in patients taking C/L, but does not replace taking regular C/L. It works quickly and is easy to carry. It cannot be used if an MAO-I was used in the past 2 wk.

7. Treatment of levodopa-related motor complications in PD are summarized in Fig. 9.

- Dopamine receptor agonists (ropinirole, pramipexole, rotigotine) are not as potent as levodopa, but they are often used as initial treatment in younger patients in an attempt to delay the onset of complications (dyskinesias, motor fluctuations) associated with levodopa therapy.[5,6] In general, they cause more side effects than levodopa, including nausea, vomiting, light-headedness, peripheral edema, confusion, and somnolence. They can also cause impulse control behaviors such as hypersexuality, binge eating, and compulsive shopping and gambling. Presence of these must be assessed at each visit as the appearance of these side effects is often under-reported and their consequences can be severe. Dopamine agonists also can be associated with a prolonged withdrawal syndrome.
  1. Ropinirole: Initial dose is 0.25 mg tid but must be titrated over the course of 4 wk to 1 mg tid and then may be increased by 1.5 mg/wk to a maximum of 24 mg/day. An extended-release formulation is also available.
  2. Pramipexole: Initial dose is 0.125 mg tid but must be titrated over the course of weeks to 1.5 to 4.5 mg/day in three doses. An extended-release formulation is also available.
  3. Rotigotine: 2 mg to 6 mg/24 h as transdermal patch.
  4. Apomorphine: A dopamine agonist used for acute, intermittent treatment of unpredictable "off" episodes with advanced Parkinson disease.

- COMT inhibitors (entacapone, opicapone, and tolcapone) are used as adjunct to levodopa therapy to treat end-of-dose wearing off.

- MAO-B inhibitors can be used as monotherapy early in the disease or as adjunctive therapy in later stages; they have been shown to have milder symptomatic benefit than dopamine agonists or levodopa.[5,6] They are well tolerated and easy to titrate. Concurrent use of stimulants and sympathomimetics should be avoided. Certain food restrictions may apply.
  1. Rasagiline: Initial dose is 0.5 mg/day, then 1 mg/day. The ADAGIO study suggests that 1 mg rasagiline may have disease-modifying benefits, but results must be interpreted with caution.
  2. Selegiline: Usual dose, 5 mg bid with breakfast and lunch. Has amphetamine by-product, so has mild stimulant-like effects, which can be beneficial in some patients.
  3. Safinamide: FDA approved as add-on therapy for C/L that reduces "off time" and increases "on time" with fewer dyskinesias. Starting dose is 50 mg/day for 2 wk, which can be increased if needed to 100 mg/day.

- Istradefylline is the first FDA-approved adenosine A 2A receptor agonist for use as an adjunct to C/L in adults with PD experiencing "off" episodes.

- Amantadine (unclear mechanism of action, but reported to modulate the dopamine and glutamate systems in the CNS) can be used alone early in the disease. Later in the disease, it is especially useful in the treatment of dyskinesias. Dosage is 100 mg tid (titrate weekly from 100 mg daily). Must adjust for elderly and renal impairment. The most notable side effect, especially in the elderly, is confusion. Extended-release amantadine (Gocovri) may have fewer side effects.

- Anticholinergic agents are only helpful in treating tremor but may be more effective than levodopa for tremor in some circumstances. They can also be used to treat drooling in patients with PD. Potential side effects include constipation, urinary retention, memory impairment, and hallucinations. They should be avoided in the elderly.
  1. Trihexyphenidyl: Initial dose, 1 mg PO tid
  2. Benztropine: Usual dose, 0.5 to 1 mg daily or bid

- Treatment of nonmotor symptoms:[3] Nonmotor symptoms such as depression, anxiety, irritability, dementia, psychosis, constipation, urinary and sexual dysfunction, sleep disturbances such as REM behavior disorder, decreased sense of smell, and impulsive behavior, among others, often cause a great deal of distress for patients and caretakers alike. Treatable symptoms should be addressed pharmacologically using medications appropriate for elderly patients sensitive to antidopaminergic medications.

- Psychosis: Dopamine agonists and anticholinergics can cause hallucinations, so adjustment of these medications should be the first step. Pimavanserin (Nuplazid) is FDA approved for the treatment of PD psychosis and has been shown effective for the treatment of hallucinations and delusions associated with PD psychosis. The medication is an inverse agonist of $5-HT_{2A}$ and $5-HT_{2C}$ receptors without any evidence of dopamine blockade.

- PD dementia: Rivastigmine (Exelon), a cholinesterase inhibitor available both orally and transdermally as a patch (with few GI side effects), is approved to treat not only Alzheimer disease but also PD dementia.

- There are monoclonal antibody therapies against alpha synuclein in the pipeline to help with treatment of motor symptoms and cognitive symptoms in PD.

Treatment of motor symptoms of Parkinson disease

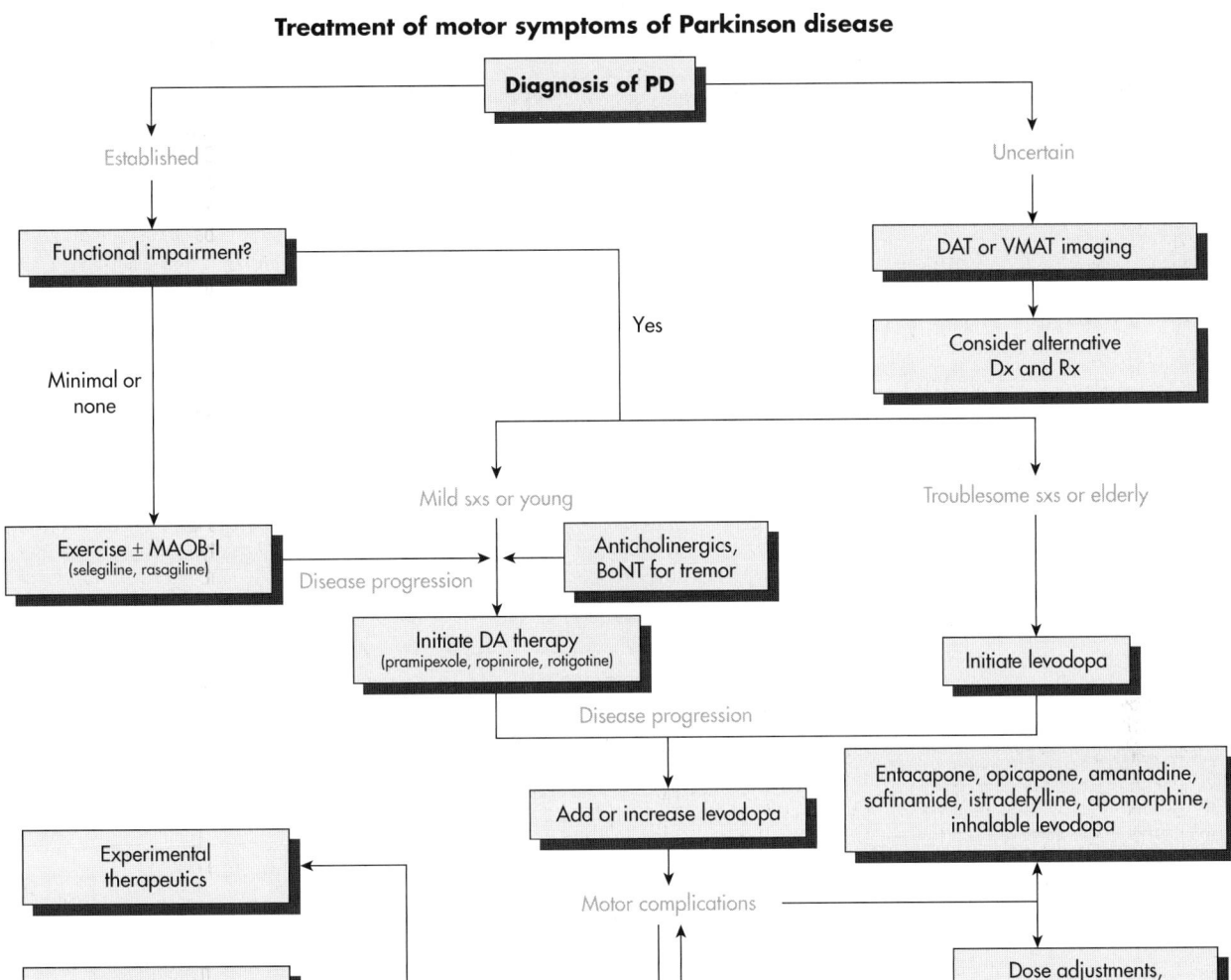

FIG. 8 Treatment of motor symptoms of Parkinson disease. Algorithm for the treatment of Parkinson disease (PD). *BoNT,* Botulinum neurotoxin; *DA,* dopamine agonist; *DAT,* dopamine transporter; *DBS,* deep brain stimulation; *Dx,* diagnosis; *FUS,* focused ultrasound; *MAOB-1,* monoamine oxidase inhibitor type 1; *MAOI,* monoamine oxidase inhibitor; *Rx,* treatment; *VMAT2,* vesicular monoamine transporter 2. (From Jankovic J et al: *Bradley and Daroff's neurology in clinical practice,* ed 8, Philadelphia, 2022, Elsevier.)

SURGICAL OPTIONS (BOX 3)

- Pallidal (globus pallidus interna) and subthalamic deep-brain stimulation (subthalamic nucleus) are currently the surgical options of choice for patients with advanced PD; similar improvement in motor function and adverse effects have been reported after either procedure.[7-9] Subthalamic targets have the benefit of possible medication lowering compared to pallidal targets. Compared with ablative procedures, DBS has the advantage of being reversible and adjustable. Thalamic DBS may be useful for refractory tremor. It improves the cardinal motor symptoms, extends medication "on" time, and reduces motor fluctuations during the day. In general, patients are likely to benefit from this therapy if they show a clear response to levodopa.

Therefore, when considering DBS, patients should be evaluated for motor response to levodopa by stopping levodopa overnight and evaluating motor response before and after a dose of levodopa.

- Focused ultrasound (FUS) is an imaging-guided method for creating therapeutic lesions in dead-brain structures, including the subthalamic nucleus. FUS subthalamotomy in one hemisphere improved motor features of PD in selected patients with asymmetric signs.[10] At 3 mo, patients who were most likely to benefit were younger, had lower motor severity scores, or had higher dyskinesia scores.[11] Longer and larger trials are required to determine the effect and safety of FUS in persons with Parkinson disease. DBS is currently favored over FUS as it can be

continually reprogrammed to account for worsening disease and does not cause a permanent lesion.

- Surgery is often limited to patients with disabling, medically refractory problems, and patients must still have a good response to L-dopa to undergo surgery. Yet for many patients, earlier stimulation might provide an improved motor benefit before disability from other symptoms has occurred and should be considered at an earlier stage of PD. DBS results in decreased dyskinesias, fluctuations, rigidity, and tremor.

DISPOSITION

PD usually follows a slowly progressive course leading to disability over the course of several years. However, every patient will progress

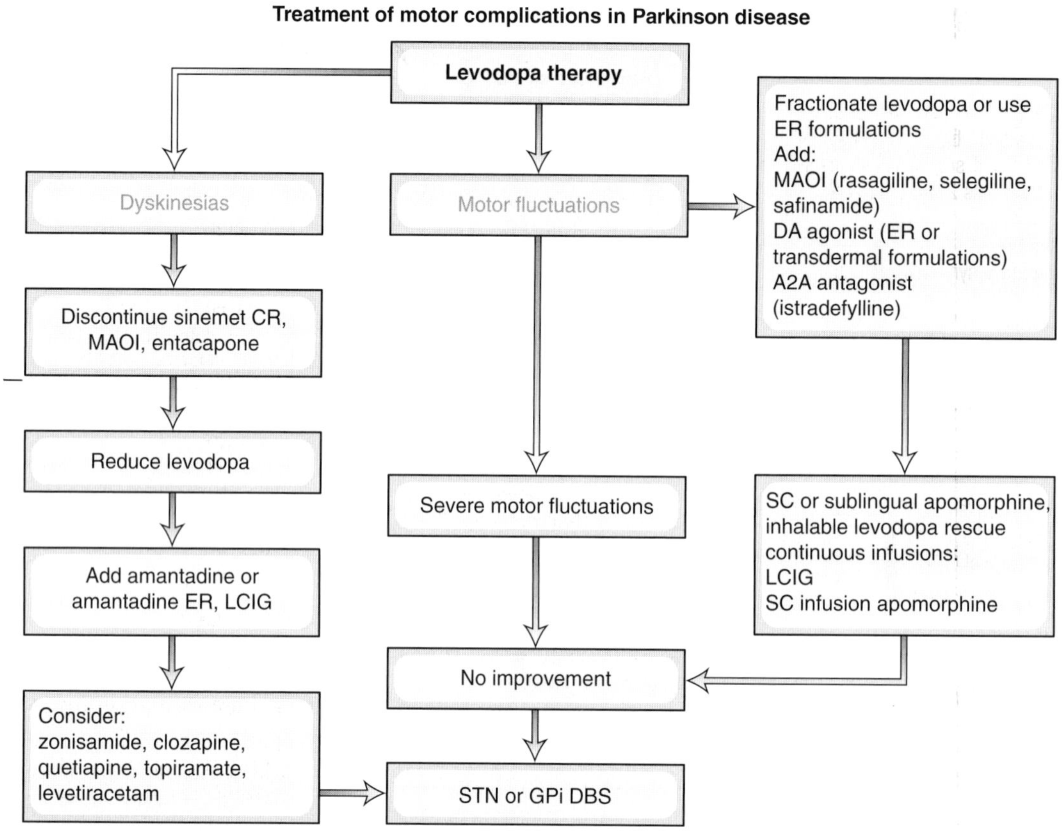

Treatment of motor complications in Parkinson disease

Levodopa therapy

Dyskinesias

Discontinue sinemet CR, MAOI, entacapone

Reduce levodopa

Add amantadine or amantadine ER, LCIG

Consider: zonisamide, clozapine, quetiapine, topiramate, levetiracetam

Motor fluctuations

Fractionate levodopa or use ER formulations
Add:
MAOI (rasagiline, selegiline, safinamide)
DA agonist (ER or transdermal formulations)
A2A antagonist (istradefylline)

Severe motor fluctuations

SC or sublingual apomorphine, inhalable levodopa rescue continuous infusions:
LCIG
SC infusion apomorphine

No improvement

STN or GPi DBS

FIG. 9 **Treatment of levodopa-related motor complications in Parkinson disease.** *A2A,* Adenosine A2A receptor; *COMTI,* catechol-o-methyl-transferase inhibitor; *CR,* controlled release; *DA,* dopamine agonist; *DBS,* deep brain stimulation; *ER,* extended release; *GPi,* globus pallidus interna; *LCIG,* levodopa-carbidopa infusion gel; *MAOI,* monoamine oxidase inhibitor; *SC,* subcutaneous; *STN,* subthalamic nucleus. (From Jankovic J et al: *Bradley and Daroff's neurology in clinical practice,* ed 8, Philadelphia, 2022, Elsevier.)

BOX 3 Ablative and Stimulation Procedures for Parkinson Disease

Ablative procedures
Thalamotomy
Pallidotomy
Subthalamotomy
Deep brain stimulation (DBS) procedures
Thalamus (Vim nucleus)
Globus pallidus pars interna (Gpi)
Subthalamic nucleus (STN)
Restorative procedures
Fetal cell transplantation
Stem cell transplantation

From Warshaw G et al: *Ham's primary care geriatrics,* ed 7, Philadelphia, 2022, Elsevier.

individually, and patients should be reassured that this diagnosis does not, by definition, result in being either wheelchair or bed bound.

REFERRAL
- Neurology consultation is recommended at initial diagnosis of PD.
- Exercise is important for all patients with PD.
- Participation in outpatient physical and speech therapy program is recommended for patients with moderate to advanced disease.
- Neuropsychiatry in patients considering DBS.

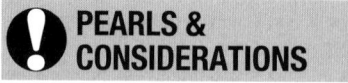

PEARLS & CONSIDERATIONS

- Asymmetry of symptoms at onset is typical of PD and therefore very useful in distinguishing PD from other causes of parkinsonism.
- Although resting tremor is a common presenting symptom, up to 25% of patients with idiopathic PD do not have classic resting tremor.
- PD patients can have mouth tremor, but head tremors are commonly seen with essential tremor.

REFERENCES
Available at eBooks.Health.Elsevier.com.

RELATED CONTENT
Parkinson Disease (Patient Information)

AUTHOR: **COREY ELAM GOLDSMITH, MD, FAAN**

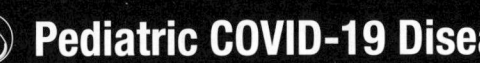
Diseases
and Disorders

I

 **BASIC INFORMATION**

DEFINITION

Coronavirus disease 2019 (COVID-19) is an infectious disease caused by a coronavirus discovered in 2019 named severe acute respiratory syndrome coronavirus 2 (SARS-CoV-2).

SYNONYMS

Multisystem inflammatory syndrome in children (MIS-C)

ICD10-CM CODES

U07.1	COVID-19
J12.82	Pneumonia due to coronavirus disease 2019
M35.81	Multisystem inflammatory syndrome (MIS)
Z20.822	Contact with and (suspected) exposure to COVID-19
Z86.16	Personal history of COVID-19

EPIDEMIOLOGY & DEMOGRAPHICS

- The emergence of COVID-19 is the third coronavirus outbreak in humans since 2000; included are the 2002 severe acute respiratory syndrome coronavirus (SARS-CoV) and 2012 Middle East respiratory syndrome coronavirus (MERS-CoV).
- The incubation period of COVID-19 ranges from 2 to 14 days with a median of 5 days.
- Acute pneumonia caused by SARS-CoV-2 was first identified in December 2019. The primary cluster was connected with a seafood and live animal market in Wuhan City, the capital of Hubei Province, in China.
- In March 2020, COVID-19 was declared a pandemic by the World Health Organization (WHO).
- In late April/early May 2020, the United Kingdom National Health Service and the Centers for Disease Control and Prevention (CDC) issued public health advisories highlighting a multisystem inflammatory syndrome in children (MIS-C).
- Throughout the COVID-19 pandemic, many variants are known to cause disease globally. Significant variants of interest include the delta and omicron (including BA.5) variants.
- As of August 2022, over 14 million children had tested positive for COVID-19 in the U.S., representing 18.4% of all cases.
- Approximately 150,000 pediatric admissions with confirmed COVID-19 were reported from August 2020 to August 2022. Similar to the adult population, a third of children hospitalized for COVID-19 require intensive care unit (ICU) admission. Up to 0.1% of COVID-19 cases in children result in mortality.

ROUTE OF TRANSMISSION

- Exposure to COVID-19 occurs via three primary mechanisms:
  1. Airborne inhalation of fine droplets and aerosol particles (including during medical "aerosol-generating procedures").
  2. Deposition of droplets and particles on exposed mucous membranes (mouth, nose, eyes).
  3. Touching mucous membranes with contaminated (virus-containing) hands.
- Transmission may occur through fomites, but this is markedly less efficient than the primary mechanisms described earlier.
- Vertical transmission of COVID-19 is thought to be rare. Data suggest that neonates born to people with COVID-19 are at increased risk for admission to the neonatal intensive care unit. Current evidence suggests that breast milk is not a source of COVID-19 infection.

INCIDENCE:

- Children of all ages can get COVID-19. Males and females are equally affected.
- By February 2022, approximately 75% of children and adolescents (ages 0 to 17 yr) in the U.S. were seropositive for SARS-CoV-2.
- Children from underrepresented racial and ethnic groups appear to be disproportionately affected by acute COVID-19 and COVID-19–associated hospitalizations and deaths, perhaps related to social determinants of health.

RISK FACTORS:

- Underlying conditions are associated with higher rates of hospitalization and ICU admission.
- The most common underlying conditions are obesity, chronic lung disease/asthma, developmental delay, congenital heart disease, and sickle cell disease.
- Almost one third of hospitalized children with SARS-CoV-2 infection required ICU admission or invasive mechanical ventilation.

PHYSICAL FINDINGS & CLINICAL PRESENTATION

ACUTE COVID-19 INFECTION:

- The clinical spectrum of SARS-CoV-2 infections in children ranges from asymptomatic to life-threatening.
- Signs/symptoms include:
  1. Most frequent: Fever and/or cough.
  2. Less frequent: Fatigue, headache, myalgia, nasal congestion, rhinorrhea, anosmia, ageusia (loss of taste), sore throat, stridor, shortness of breath, abdominal pain, diarrhea, nausea, vomiting, or decreased oral intake.
- Children with severe COVID-19 may present with acute respiratory failure, myocarditis, shock, acute renal failure, coagulopathy, and multisystem organ failure.
- Laboratory evidence: Lymphocytosis *or* lymphopenia, mildly elevated inflammatory markers (C-reactive protein [CRP], erythrocyte sedimentation rate [ESR], procalcitonin), mildly elevated liver enzymes.
- Radiographic evidence:
  1. Chest x-ray: Unilateral or bilateral opacities.
  2. Chest computed tomography (CT): Unilateral or bilateral ground-glass opacities and consolidation with surrounding halo sign.

MULTISYSTEM INFLAMMATORY SYNDROME IN CHILDREN (MIS-C):

- MIS-C is a serious delayed complication of COVID-19 infection. In most studies, there was a lag of several weeks between the peak of COVID-19 cases within communities and the rise of MIS-C cases.
- Most MIS-C cases have occurred in older children (≥5 yr of age) and adolescents who were previously healthy. Black and Hispanic children appear to be disproportionally affected.
- Signs/symptoms include fever, abdominal pain, vomiting, diarrhea, skin rash, mucocutaneous lesions, hypotension, and shock.
- Laboratory evidence: Elevated inflammatory markers (CRP, ESR, procalcitonin), elevated markers of cardiac damage (troponin, brain natriuretic peptide [BNP]).
- Cardiac dysfunction on echocardiogram.
- Over 50% of children with MIS-C require ICU admission.

ETIOLOGY

The WHO has classified SARS-CoV-2 as a new betacoronavirus that infects humans. Bats are the suspected natural reservoir of SARS-CoV-2.

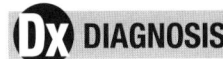 **DIAGNOSIS**

DIFFERENTIAL DIAGNOSIS

ACUTE COVID-19 INFECTION:

- Influenza virus, parainfluenza virus, adenovirus, respiratory syncytial virus, rhinovirus, human metapneumovirus, non-COVID-19cc coronavirus, and other known viral respiratory infections
- Atypical organisms: *Mycoplasma pneumoniae*, chlamydia pneumonia, and legionellosis
- Bacterial pneumonia
- Streptococcal pharyngitis
- Viral and bacterial gastrointestinal infections

MIS-C:

- Kawasaki disease or Kawasaki disease shock syndrome
- Toxic shock syndrome
- Myocarditis or heart failure
- Macrophage activation syndrome
- Hemophagocytic lymphohistiocytosis

WORKUP

ACUTE COVID-19 INFECTION:

- Laboratory studies:
  1. SARS-CoV-2 polymerase chain reaction (PCR) on upper and/or lower respiratory secretions. Rapid antigen test using nasal swab can detect viral proteins but with less sensitivity than PCR.
  2. CBC, complete metabolic panel (CMP), inflammatory markers (CRP, ESR, procalcitonin).
- Chest x-ray, chest CT (used sparingly and only for hospitalized children with specific clinical indications).

MIS-C:

- Laboratory studies:
  1. SARS-CoV-2 PCR or antigen testing; serologic testing if available.

2. Inflammatory markers: CRP, ESR, fibrinogen, procalcitonin, D-dimer, ferritin, lactic acid dehydrogenase (LDH), interleukin-6 (IL-6), neutrophil and lymphocyte count, and albumin.
3. Markers of cardiac injury: Troponin and BNP.
- Due to frequent association with cardiac involvement, echocardiogram and electrocardiogram are recommended to evaluate myocardial function, coronary arteries, and cardiac rhythm.

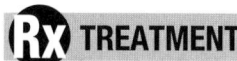 **TREATMENT**

ACUTE COVID-19 INFECTION:
- Children with mild disease usually recover at home with supportive care and appropriate isolation guidelines.
- Mainstay of hospital-based treatment is supportive care: Fluid resuscitation, inotropic support, respiratory support (including prone positioning for severe hypoxemia), and (rarely) extracorporeal membrane oxygenation (ECMO).
- Remdesivir is the only FDA-approved treatment of COVID-19 in children. It is available for use in high-risk, nonhospitalized patients within 7 days of symptom onset; high-risk hospitalized patients; or children with severe and/or critical disease.
- The National Institutes of Health Panel on COVID-19 has provided recommendations on specific therapies:
  1. Dexamethasone has been shown to be beneficial in children with COVID-19 who require high-flow oxygen, noninvasive ventilation, invasive mechanical ventilation, or ECMO.
  2. For patients who do not have improvement in oxygenation within 24 hr after initiation of dexamethasone, baricitinib or tocilizumab may be considered.
  3. Paxlovid (ritonavir-boosted nirmatrelvir) may be used in high-risk, nonhospitalized children within 5 days of symptom onset.
  4. There is insufficient evidence to recommend for or against usage of anti-SARS-CoV-2 monoclonal antibody products in children (such as bebtelovimab, bamlanivimab plus etesevimab, or casirivimab plus imdevimab), but may be considered on a case-by-case basis for nonhospitalized children who are at high risk for severe disease.
  5. The use of convalescent plasma is *not recommended* for the pediatric population, unless considered on a case-by-case basis in consultation with an infectious disease specialist.
- Antibacterial therapy is reasonable if there is a concern for a superimposed bacterial pneumonia.
- Vaccination to prevent severe COVID-19 disease is now available for adults and for children 6 mo and older.

MIS-C:
- Mainstay is supportive care: Fluid resuscitation, inotropic support, respiratory support, and (rarely) ECMO.
- Antiinflammatory treatments, including intravenous immunoglobulin (IVIG) and steroids, have been used with success as a first-line therapy. IL-1 antagonists have also been used in refractory cases.
- Aspirin therapy is recommended if coronary arteries are involved.
- Thrombosis prophylaxis is often used, given the hypercoagulability associated with MIS-C.

DISPOSITION
- Most children infected with COVID-19 experience mild, self-limiting illness.
- The duration of hospitalization is usually less than 7 days. Of the patients requiring intensive care, the majority recover well.
- Except for rare situations, a test-based strategy is no longer recommended to determine when an individual with a COVID-19 infection is no longer infectious.
- Patients recovering from MIS-C who had significant myocardial involvement require pediatric cardiology follow-up.

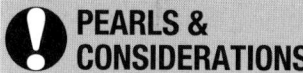 **PEARLS & CONSIDERATIONS**

- SARS-CoV-2 enters human cells through the ACE2 receptor, which is highly expressed on type II alveolar epithelial cells, myocardial cells, proximal tubule cells of the kidney, enterocytes of the small intestine, neurons in the brain, and vascular endothelial cells. This may explain the multiple organ involvement.
- During times of high community spread of COVID-19, face mask wearing (excluded are children under age 2 yr), frequent handwashing, routine cleaning/disinfecting of frequently touched surfaces, and maintaining social distancing lower the risk of transmission.
- During aerosol-generating procedures in patients with COVID-19, current guidelines recommend that clinicians wear gowns, gloves, N95 masks, and eye protection and place patients in negative-pressure rooms whenever possible.
- The benefits of getting vaccinated markedly outweigh the small risk of vaccine-related myocarditis. The mRNA vaccines (Pfizer-BioNTech and Moderna) have been linked with myocarditis; boys and men between the ages of 16 and 29 yr have a higher risk. The risk of myocarditis is between 2 and 5 times higher after SARS-CoV-2 infection than after vaccination.
- Maternal vaccination with two doses of mRNA vaccine is associated with a reduced risk of hospitalization for COVID-19, including for critical illness, among infants younger than 6 mo of age.[1]

REFERENCE & SUGGESTED READINGS

Available at eBooks.Health.Elsevier.com.

AUTHORS: **DANIEL CHILCOTE, MD,** and **MARGARET PRIESTLEY, MD**

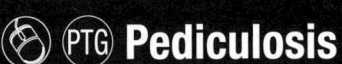
BASIC INFORMATION

DEFINITION

Pediculosis is lice infestation. Humans can be infested with three kinds of lice: *Pediculus capitis* (head louse), *Pediculus corporis* (body louse), and *Phthirus pubis* (pubic, or crab, louse).[1] Lice inject saliva into the skin and feed on human blood, causing local inflammation.[2] They deposit eggs (nits) on hair shafts (head lice and pubic lice) and along the seams of clothing (body lice). Nits remain firmly attached and hatch within 7 to 10 days. Lice are obligate human parasites and cannot survive away from their hosts for longer than 7 to 10 days.[2]

SYNONYM

Lice

ICD-10CM CODES

B85.0	Pediculosis due to *Pediculus humanus capitis*
B85.1	Pediculosis due to *Pediculus humanus corporis*
B85.2	Pediculosis, unspecified
B85.3	Phthiriasis
B85.4	Mixed pediculosis and phthiriasis
Z11.8	Screening for head lice
Z20.7	Exposure to head lice
Z83.1	Family history of lice
Z86.19	History of lice

EPIDEMIOLOGY & DEMOGRAPHICS

- There are 6 to 12 million cases of head lice in the United States annually in children between ages 3 and 11, with infection more common in females.[1]
- Head lice affect children of all socioeconomic levels. Risk factors include sharing hair care items and attending day care. Frequency of hair washing, brushing, and hair length do not modify risk of infestation.[3]
- Risk factors for body lice include poor hygiene, homelessness, and crowded living conditions. Unlike head and pubic lice, body lice can transmit disease.[1]
- Pubic lice in a child, including infestation of the eyelashes, may indicate sexual abuse.[1,4]
- Pubic lice are usually spread during sexual intercourse, are most common in adolescents and young adults, and diagnosis should prompt additional STI evaluation.[1,4]
- Pets are not implicated in the transmission of lice.

PHYSICAL FINDINGS & CLINICAL PRESENTATION

- Infections may be asymptomatic. However, pruritis is the most common symptom, caused by hypersensitivity to lice saliva and fecal material. Secondary bacterial infections may develop from excoriation sores from scratching (Fig. 1).[2,3]
- Nits can be identified by examining hair shafts (Fig. E2) in cases of head and pubic lice or on clothing (Fig. 3) in instances of body lice.[1-4]

- Head lice are most frequently found on the nape of the neck and behind the ears.[2]
- Lymphadenopathy may be present (cervical adenopathy with head lice, inguinal lymphadenopathy with pubic lice).[3]
- Pubic lice may affect the hair around the anus.[1]

ETIOLOGY

Lice are most commonly transmitted by close personal contact and less commonly by use of contaminated objects (e.g., combs, clothing, bed linen, hats). Lice cannot jump or fly.[1-4]

DIAGNOSIS

DIFFERENTIAL DIAGNOSIS

- Seborrheic dermatitis
- Scabies
- Eczema
- Other: Pilar casts, trichonodosis (knotted hair), monilethrix (beaded hair)
- Table 1 describes the differential diagnosis of nits

WORKUP

Diagnosis is made by seeing live, adult lice (Fig. 4), which are typically 1 to 3 mm in length, as nits alone may be hatched or nonviable. Using bright light, a magnifying glass, and a fine-toothed comb can aid in diagnosis.[2]

LABORATORY TESTS

Wood's light examination is useful to screen a large number of children: Live nits fluoresce, empty nits have a gray fluorescence, and nits with unborn lice reveal white fluorescence.

TREATMENT

ACUTE GENERAL Rx

The following products are available for treatment of head and pubic lice. Generally, body lice can be treated with nonpharmacologic therapies. Because head and pubic lice present minimal

health risk, therapy should prioritize safety and cost. Side effects of topical therapy include pruritis, erythema, and mild burning. These side effects do not indicate treatment failure and do not necessitate retreatment. Additionally, clinicians should heed local resistance patterns, and if patients fail standard therapy, consultation with an infectious disease specialist may be beneficial.

- Permethrin is available over the counter (1% permethrin [Nix]) or by prescription (5% permethrin [Elimite]). It should be applied to damp hair and rinsed out after 10 min. Repeat application is generally not necessary in patients with head lice, but if required, it is most efficacious when performed 9 days after first treatment. Permethrin is nontoxic and FDA approved for use in children >2 mo old. Resistance to permethrin is widespread.[2,3]
- Pyrethrin with piperonyl butoxide applied and washed off after 10 min.
- Malathion, an organophosphate, is effective in head lice, but is available by prescription only. It is applied to dry hair but is not commonly used due to its malodor, risk of flammability, and prolonged application time (8 to 12 h). It is contraindicated in children <2 yr old.[2-3]
- Spinosad is a topical suspension applied to dry hair for 10 min, then rinsed out. Its application may be repeated 7 days later if live lice are seen. It is more effective than permethrin, but more expensive. It is safe for use in pregnant persons (category B—no evidence of risk in humans) and in children >6 mo old.[2-3]
- Benzyl alcohol lotion 5% (Ulesfia) is a prescription-only, FDA-approved treatment of head lice in patients >6 mo old. The lotion is applied to dry hair and left on for 10 min. Treatment must be repeated after 7 days because the drug is not ovicidal.[2-3]
- Eyelash infestation can be treated with the application of ophthalmic-grade, prescription petroleum jelly rubbed into the eyelashes 2 to 4 times a day for 10 days.
- In patients with resistance to 1% permethrin cream rinse, a 10-day course of trimethoprim-sulfamethoxazole (TMP-SMX) 8 mg/kg/day in

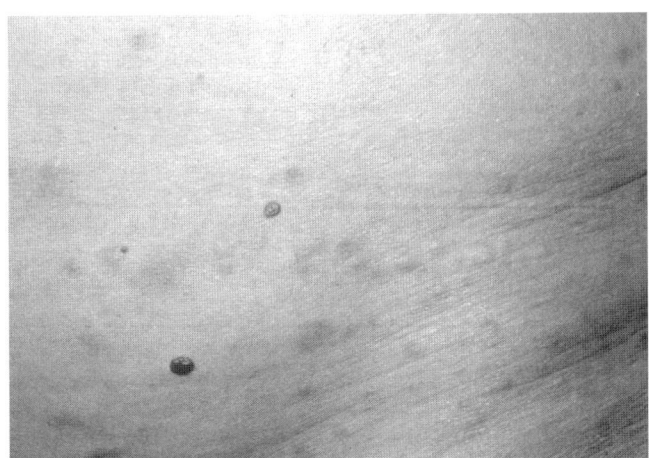

FIG. 1 Pediculosis corporis. (From Micheletti RG et al: *Andrews' diseases of the skin, clinical atlas,* ed 2, Philadelphia, 2023, Elsevier.)

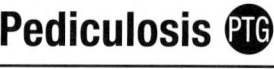

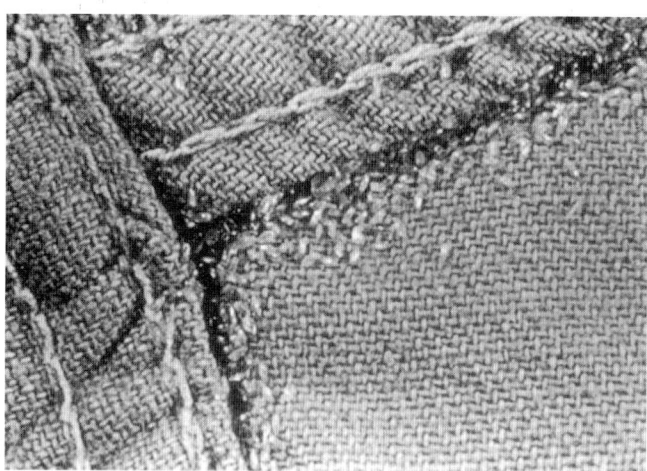

FIG. 3 Pediculosis; nits in clothing. (From Micheletti RG et al: *Andrews' diseases of the skin, clinical atlas,* ed 2, Philadelphia, 2023, Elsevier.)

TABLE 1 Differential Diagnosis of Nits

Diagnosis	Comment
Nits	Firmly adherent to hair shaft; not easily removed with fingers
Seborrheic dermatitis (dandruff)	Diffuse scalp scaling; scales occasionally adhere to hair but easy to remove; scalp erythema may be present
Hair casts	Keratin protein that encircles hair shaft; easily removed
Piedra	Fungal infection of hair; firm nodules attached to hair shafts, white or black in color
Psoriasis	Thick silvery scales, often present overlying red plaques on the scalp
Hair products	Hairspray, mousse, gel

From Paller AS, Mancini AJ: *Hurwitz clinical pediatric dermatology, a textbook of skin disorders of childhood and adolescence,* ed 5, Philadelphia, 2016, Elsevier.

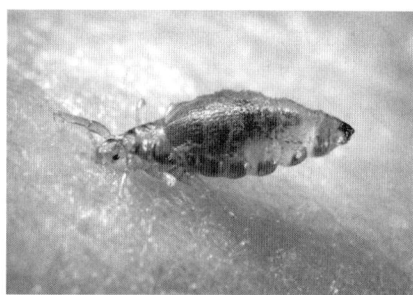

FIG. 4 Body louse, *Pediculus humanus* **var.** *corporis,* **as it was obtaining a blood meal from human host.** (Courtesy Public Health Image Library, Centers for Disease Control and Prevention. From Vincent JL et al: *Textbook of critical care,* ed 6, Philadelphia, 2011, Saunders.)

divided doses is an effective treatment for head lice infestation, especially for eyelash infestations with *Phthirus pubis.* However, the risk of Stevens-Johnson syndrome should be weighed against the minimal health risk posed by lice, especially in the setting of other efficacious regimens.[2]

- Ivermectin, an antiparasitic drug, given as an oral dose of 250 to 400 mcg/kg of body weight on days 1 and 9, is effective for head lice resistant to other treatments. Ivermectin should not be used in children <15 kg given risk of neurotoxicity. Ivermectin 0.5% lotion is FDA approved as a single-use topical treatment for head lice in patients >6 mo, but may be cost prohibitive.[2,3]

COMPLEMENTARY & ALTERNATIVE MEDICINE

- Wet combing is a widely recommended but unproven adjunctive therapy.
- Personal items such as combs and brushes should be soaked in hot water for 15 to 30 min. Clothing, towels, and bed linens used in the 48 h prior to treatment should be washed in hot water (>130 °F [>54.4 °C]), and then dried for 10 min at the hottest setting. Items that cannot be washed should be sealed in a plastic bag for 2 wk.
- Vacuuming floors and furniture is recommended, but excessive, costly household cleaning is not needed.
- Gaseous pesticides are toxic and should not be used.

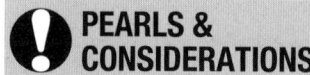

PEARLS & CONSIDERATIONS

COMMENTS

- Given the low risk of classroom transmission, the American Academy of Pediatrics does not support exclusion from school because of head lice.[2]
- Close contacts and household members should also be examined for the presence of lice.
- Patients with pubic lice should notify their sexual contacts. Sexual partners within the last month should be treated.
- Finding nits without live, adult lice, especially >0.25 inches from the scalp, suggests past infection.
- Lice-removal companies may be helpful for some families, but no studies exist comparing efficacy of professional vs. home removal.

REFERENCES

Available at eBooks.Health.Elsevier.com

RELATED CONTENT

Lice (Patient Information)

AUTHORS: **EILEEN EVERLY, MD,** and **LEORA LIEBERMAN, MD**

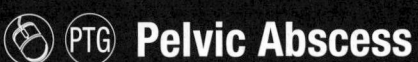

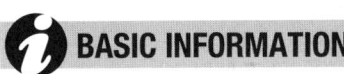 **BASIC INFORMATION**

DEFINITION

Pelvic abscess is an acute or chronic infection, most commonly involving the pelvic viscera. Treatment requires directed therapy including broad-spectrum antimicrobials and, if medical therapy fails, surgical intervention. There are four categories based on etiologic factors:
- Ascending infection, spreading from cervix through endometrial cavity to adnexa, forming a tuboovarian complex
- Infection occurring in the puerperium, which spreads to the adnexa from the endometrium or myometrium by a hematogenous or lymphatic route
- Abscess complicating pelvic surgery
- Involvement of the pelvic viscera as a result of spread from contiguous organs, such as appendicitis or diverticulitis

SYNONYMS

Tuboovarian abscess (TOA)
Vaginal cuff abscess

ICD-10CM CODES
K63.0	Abscess of intestine
K65.1	Peritoneal abscess
K68.11	Postprocedural retroperitoneal abscess
K68.12	Psoas muscle abscess
K68.19	Other retroperitoneal abscess
N70.93	Salpingitis and oophoritis, unspecified
N70.0	Acute salpingitis and oophoritis
N70.1	Chronic salpingitis and oophoritis

EPIDEMIOLOGY & DEMOGRAPHICS

INCIDENCE:
- 34% of hospitalized patients with pelvic inflammatory disease
- <1% of patients undergoing hysterectomy, most frequently with vaginal approach
- Peak incidence between 15 and 40 yr

RISK FACTORS: Same risk factors as for pelvic inflammatory disease, although in 30% to 50% of patients there is no prior history of salpingitis before abscess forms.

PHYSICAL FINDINGS & CLINICAL PRESENTATION
- Abdominal or pelvic pain (90%)
- Fever or chills (50%)
- Abnormal bleeding (21%)
- Vaginal discharge (28%)
- Nausea (26%)
- Up to 60% to 80% present without fever or leukocytosis; absence of these findings should not exclude diagnosis

ETIOLOGY
- Mixed flora of anaerobes, aerobes, and facultative anaerobes, such as *Escherichia coli*, *Bacteroides fragilis*, *Prevotella* spp., aerobic streptococci, and *Peptococcus* and *Peptostreptococcus* spp.

- *Neisseria gonorrhoeae* and *Chlamydia* are the major etiologic bacteria in cervicitis and salpingitis but are rarely found in abscess cavity cultures.
- In elderly patients consider diverticular disease.

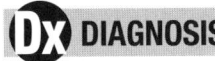 **DIAGNOSIS**

DIFFERENTIAL DIAGNOSIS
- Pelvic neoplasms, such as ovarian tumors and leiomyomas.
- Ovarian torsion.
- Inflammatory masses involving adjacent bowel or omentum, such as ruptured appendicitis or diverticulitis.
- Pelvic hematomas, as may occur after cesarean section or hysterectomy.
- Ectopic pregnancy.

LABORATORY TESTS
- CBC with differential
- Aerobic as well as anaerobic cultures of cervix, blood, urine, sputum, peritoneal cavity (if entered), and abscess cavity before starting antibiotics
- Pregnancy test in patients of reproductive age

IMAGING STUDIES
- Sonogram: Noninvasive, inexpensive study to confirm diagnosis, estimate size of abscess, and monitor response to therapy; sensitivity >90%
- CT scan: Used for both diagnosis and therapy (CT-guided drainage) (Fig. E1)
  1. Useful where sonogram provides insufficient information, as with intraabdominal abscesses
  2. Success rate with CT-guided abscess drainage: Unilocular, 90%; multilocular, 40%

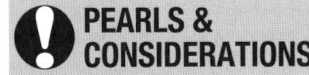 **TREATMENT**

Major concerns:
- Desire for future fertility
- Likelihood of rupture of abscess, with resulting peritonitis, septic shock, and morbid sequelae

ACUTE GENERAL Rx
- Clinical quandary is whether patient requires immediate surgical intervention (uncertain diagnosis or suspicion of rupture) or management with IV antibiotics, reserving surgery for those with inadequate clinical response (e.g., 48 to 72 hr of therapy, with persistent fever or leukocytosis, increasing size of mass, or suspicion of rupture). Laparoscopic surgery should be reserved for experienced surgeons and in cases of unruptured pelvic abscess.
- Surgery indicated in poor response to medical therapy. Early surgery may be needed in those with large adnexal masses (>8 cm), or in immunocompromised patients.

- Antibiotic combinations:
  1. Cefotetan 2 g IV q12h or cefoxitin 2 g IV q6h or ampicillin-sulbactam 3 g IV q6h plus doxycycline 100 mg PO or IV q12h
  2. For penicillin allergic patients: Clindamycin 900 mg IV q8h plus gentamicin either 3 to 5 mg/kg q24h or loading dose 2 mg/kg IV/IM loading dose plus maintenance dose 1.5 mg/kg q8h
- During medical management, high index of suspicion for acute rupture, such as acute worsening of abdominal pain or new-onset tachycardia and hypotension, mandating immediate surgical intervention after patient stabilization.
- Surgical options:
  1. Laparoscopy with drainage and irrigation.
  2. CT-guided drainage (interventional radiology)
  3. Transvaginal colpotomy (abscess must be midline, dissect rectovaginal septum, and be adherent to vaginal fornix)
  4. Laparotomy, including total abdominal hysterectomy with bilateral salpingo-oophorectomy or unilateral salpingo-oophorectomy
  5. Evidence of ruptured tuboovarian abscess is a surgical emergency

DISPOSITION
- Of patients treated with medical therapy alone, pregnancy rate is 25%. Of patients treated with both medical and laparoscopic surgical management, pregnancy rate is between 32% and 63%. Pregnancy rate decreases with recurrent episodes.
- No response in 30% to 40%; can be treated with either CT-guided drainage or surgical intervention, keeping in mind that unilateral adnexectomy may give equal chance of cure versus hysterectomy, yet preserve reproductive potential.

REFERRAL
If patient has a tuboovarian abscess, refer to gynecologist.

⚠ PEARLS & CONSIDERATIONS

COMMENTS
- If *Actinomyces* species is isolated from culture, treatment with penicillin is required for an extended period (6 wk to 3 mo).
- Most common cause of preventable death: Physician delay in diagnosis.

RELATED CONTENT
Pelvic Abscess (Patient Information)
Pelvic Inflammatory Disease (Related Key Topic)

AUTHORS: **ELLA STERN, MD,** and **MARWAN MA'AYEH, MD**

P

Diseases
and Disorders

I

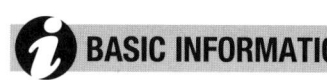
BASIC INFORMATION

DEFINITION

Pelvic inflammatory disease (PID) is infection and inflammation of the female upper genital tract (including uterus, fallopian tubes, ovaries, and/or pelvic peritoneum) unrelated to pregnancy or surgical intervention. PID can be classified as acute ($\leq$30 days' duration), subclinical, or chronic (>30 days' duration).

SYNONYMS

PID
Endometritis
Salpingitis
Oophoritis
Adnexitis
Pelvic peritonitis
Pyosalpinx
Tuboovarian abscess
TOA

ICD-10CM CODES

A18.17	Tuberculous female pelvic inflammatory disease
A52.76	Syphilitic pelvic inflammatory disease
A54.2*	Gonococcal pelviperitonitis and other gonococcal genitourinary infections
A54.24	Gonococcal female pelvic inflammatory disease
A56.1*	Chlamydial infection of pelviperitoneum and other genitourinary organs
A56.11	Chlamydial female pelvic inflammatory disease
A56.19	Other chlamydial genitourinary infection
N70*	Salpingitis and oophoritis
N70.0*	Acute salpingitis and oophoritis
N70.01	Acute salpingitis
N70.02	Acute oophoritis
N70.03	Acute salpingitis and oophoritis
N70.1*	Chronic salpingitis and oophoritis
N70.11	Chronic salpingitis
N70.12	Chronic oophoritis
N70.13	Chronic salpingitis and oophoritis
N70.9*	Salpingitis and oophoritis, unspecified
N70.91	Salpingitis, unspecified
N70.92	Oophoritis, unspecified
N70.93	Salpingitis and oophoritis, unspecified
N71*	Inflammatory disease of uterus, except cervix
N71.0	Acute inflammatory disease of uterus
N71.1	Chronic inflammatory disease of uterus
N71.9	Inflammatory disease of uterus, unspecified
N72	Inflammatory disease of cervix uteri
N73*	Other female pelvic inflammatory diseases
N73.0	Acute parametritis and pelvic cellulitis
N73.1	Chronic parametritis and pelvic cellulitis
N73.2	Unspecified parametritis and pelvic cellulitis
N73.3	Female acute pelvic peritonitis
N73.4	Female chronic pelvic peritonitis
N73.5	Female pelvic peritonitis, unspecified
N73.6	Female pelvic peritoneal adhesions (postinfective)
N73.8	Other specified female pelvic inflammatory diseases
N73.9	Female pelvic inflammatory disease, unspecified
N74	Female pelvic inflammatory disorders in diseases classified elsewhere

*Indicates nonbillable codes.

EPIDEMIOLOGY & DEMOGRAPHICS

INCIDENCE & PREVALENCE: Pelvic inflammatory disease is most often diagnosed in young, sexually active women. The incidence of PID is difficult to ascertain given its broad diagnostic criteria, its propensity to be missed as a diagnosis, and the challenges with follow-up due to patients seeking urgent or emergent care for this condition. The Centers for Disease Control and Prevention estimates 1 million new cases of PID are diagnosed yearly. The incidence may be rising given recent sharp increases in sexually transmitted diseases (STDs) associated with PID in the United States. PID has long-term health risks for women, including recurrent infection, chronic pelvic pain, pelvic adhesive disease, and tubal disease resulting in ectopic pregnancy and infertility.

RISK FACTORS:
- Sexually active adolescent and young women
- History of PID
- Prior chlamydial or gonorrheal infection
- Multiple or new sexual partners within past 12 mo
- Sexual partner diagnosed with sexually transmitted infection (STI)
- Nonuse of barrier contraception

PHYSICAL FINDINGS & CLINICAL PRESENTATION
- Pelvic or lower abdominal pain
- Abnormal vaginal discharge
- Abnormal uterine bleeding
- Postcoital bleeding
- Dysuria
- Dyspareunia
- Fever
- Nausea and vomiting (suggestive of peritonitis)

PHYSICAL FINDINGS
- Fever
- Abnormal vaginal discharge
- Cervical friability
- Cervical motion tenderness
- Uterine tenderness
- Adnexal tenderness
- Adnexal mass
- Right upper quadrant tenderness (perihepatitis, Fitz-Hugh-Curtis syndrome [Fig. E1]): 5% to 10% of PID cases may develop right upper quadrant pain, pleuritic pain, and tenderness in the right upper quadrant when the liver is palpated. The pain may radiate to the shoulder or into the back. Liver transaminase levels may be elevated.

NOTE: Women with PID may be asymptomatic and/or have a benign physical examination.

ETIOLOGY

PID occurs as a result of ascending infection from the lower genital tract. Infections are often polymicrobial, and although gonorrheal and chlamydial infections are commonly implicated in the development of PID, fewer than 50% of women test positive for these organisms. This is likely due in part to increased STI screening efforts. PID may also arise in the setting of organisms associated with normal vaginal flora such as:
- *Bacteroides fragilis*
- *Escherichia coli* and other enteric gram-negative rods
- *Gardnerella vaginalis*
- *Haemophilus influenzae*
- *Streptococcus agalactiae*

Rarer infectious causes include the following: *Mycoplasma hominis, Ureaplasma urealyticum, Mycoplasma genitalium* (a concern because of antibiotic resistance), *Mycobacterium tuberculosis* (an important cause in developing countries), and cytomegalovirus (CMV).

(Dx) DIAGNOSIS

Diagnosis of PID is made when a sexually active female has clinical or pathologic evidence of upper genital tract infection and inflammation, which includes any cervical motion tenderness, uterine tenderness, or adnexal tenderness. Box 1 summarizes the Centers for Disease Control and Prevention (CDC) criteria for diagnosing PID. Although no single test or measure reliably diagnoses the spectrum of disorders that comprise PID, a clinical diagnosis of symptomatic PID has a positive predictive value of 65% to 90%:
- Providers should maintain a low threshold for diagnosis and treatment of PID given significant long-term health risks associated with the disease, especially if untreated
- The CDC suggests that women with risk factors, abdominal or pelvic pain, and any pelvic tenderness (cervical, uterine, and/or adnexal) be treated for PID
- Definitive criteria for diagnosis of PID include:
  1. Laparoscopic abnormalities consistent with PID
  2. Histopathologic evidence of endometritis in women with clinical suspicion for PID
  3. Transvaginal sonography or other imaging techniques showing thickened, fluid-filled tubes with or without free pelvic fluid or tuboovarian complex or Doppler studies indicative of pelvic infection such as tubal hyperemia

However, requiring the aforementioned criteria before empiric treatment would not only lead to underdiagnosis and treatment but also delay treatment and lead to unnecessary morbidity.
- Supportive criteria for that enhance diagnostic specificity of PID include:
  1. Oral temperature >38.3° C (>101° F)
  2. Abnormal cervical mucopurulent discharge or cervical friability
  3. Predominance of white blood cells (WBCs) on saline microscopy of vaginal fluid

BOX 1 Centers for Disease Control and Prevention Guidelines for Diagnosis of Acute Pelvic Inflammatory Disease: Clinical Criteria for Initiating Therapy

Minimum criteria
Empirical treatment of PID should be initiated in sexually active young women and others at risk for STIs if the following minimum criteria are present and no other causes(s) for the illness can be identified:

Lower abdominal tenderness *or*

Adnexal tenderness *or*

Cervical motion tenderness

Additional criteria for diagnosing PID
Oral temperature >38° C (100.4° F)

Abnormal cervical or vaginal discharge (mucopurulent)

Presence of abundant WBCs on microscopy of vaginal secretions

Elevated erythrocyte sedimentation rate

Elevated C-reactive protein

Laboratory documentation of cervical infection with *Neisseria gonorrhoeae* or *Chlamydia trachomatis*

Definitive criteria for diagnosing PID
Histopathologic evidence of endometritis on endometrial biopsy

Transvaginal sonography or MRI showing thickened fluid-filled tubes, with or without free pelvic fluid or tuboovarian complex

Laparoscopic abnormalities consistent with PID

Although initial treatment can be made before bacteriologic diagnosis of *C. trachomatis* or *N. gonorrhoeae* infection, such a diagnosis emphasizes the need to treat sex partners.

MRI, Magnetic resonance imaging; *PID,* pelvic inflammatory disease; *STIs,* sexually transmitted infections; *WBCs,* white blood cells.
From Gershenson DM et al: *Comprehensive gynecology,* ed 8, Philadelphia, 2022, Elsevier.
Data from Workowski KA, Bolan GA, Centers for Disease Control and Prevention: Sexually transmitted diseases treatment guidelines, 2015, *MMWR Recomm Rep* 64(RR-03):1-137, 2015.

4. Elevated acute inflammatory markers (erythrocyte sedimentation rate [ESR] or C-reactive protein)
5. Neisseria gonorrhoeae or Chlamydia trachomatis infection

DIFFERENTIAL DIAGNOSIS
- Appendicitis
- Ectopic pregnancy
- Intrauterine/other pregnancy
- Ovarian cyst
- Adnexal torsion
- Endometriosis
- Urinary tract infection (cystitis or pyelonephritis)

WORKUP
- History: As in risk factors and clinical presentation, previously
- Physical examination: As in physical findings, previously

LABORATORY TESTS
- Wet mount: Clue cells, increased WBCs
- Gram stain of endocervical exudate: >30 polymorphonuclear cells per high-power field correlates with chlamydial or gonococcal infection
- Endocervical cultures for *N. gonorrhoeae* and *C. trachomatis*
- CBC: Leukocytosis

- Human chorionic gonadotropin to rule out intrauterine or ectopic pregnancy
- Elevated acute phase reactants: ESR >15 mm/h, C-reactive protein
- HIV and rapid plasma reagin, with consideration for other STI screening such as hepatitis B surface antigen, hepatitis C Ab (HIV increases incidence of tuboovarian abscess [TOA])
- Fallopian tube aspirate or peritoneal exudate culture if laparoscopy or drainage of TOA performed
- Endometritis on endometrial biopsy if performed

IMAGING STUDIES
Ultrasonography is commonly used to assess for PID and can be used to determine inpatient vs. outpatient treatment by presence or absence of TOA. Findings include:
- Thick-walled adnexal mass with heterogenous or cystic contents suggestive of abscess
- Dilated fallopian tubes (note that normal fallopian tubes are rarely identified on ultrasonography)
- "Cogwheel sign" indicating thickened fallopian tube walls
- Heterogenous fluid within the endometrium Computed tomography or MRI scan may be useful to better characterize adnexal masses and/or rule out other pathology, such as appendicitis or renal calculus. Choice of

imaging modality will depend on clinical suspicion, logistical access, and associated cost.

PROCEDURES
Endometrial biopsy that reveals endometritis may support a diagnosis of PID. Laparoscopy has been utilized as a gold standard for diagnosing PID, but due to the invasive nature of this procedure and the risks and costs associated, it is rarely indicated as a diagnostic tool.

Rx TREATMENT

Primary management of PID is medical, with broad-spectrum antibiotics administered in an outpatient setting. Inpatient treatment should be initiated when:
- Surgical emergency is not excluded (such as acute appendicitis, ruptured ectopic pregnancy, or ovarian torsion)
- Severe illness, nausea or vomiting, or temperature >38.5° C (>101.3° F)
- TOA (Fig. E2) is present
- Patient is unable or unwilling to complete outpatient treatment (including medication regimen and clinical follow-up)
- Outpatient treatment fails to improve symptoms in 48 to 72 h
- Pregnancy, immunodeficiency, or other complicating medical condition exists
Evidence-based guidelines recommended by the CDC for acute PID are as follows:

INPATIENT REGIMENS
Recommended parenteral regimens
- Ceftriaxone 1 g intravenous (IV) q24h *PLUS* doxycycline 100 mg oral (PO) or IV q12h *PLUS* metronidazole 500 mg IV q12h *OR*
- Cefotetan 2 g IV q12h *PLUS* doxycycline 100 mg PO or IV q12h *OR*
- Cefoxitin 2 g IV q6h *PLUS* doxycycline 100 mg PO or IV q12h *OR*
Alternative parenteral regimen
- Ampicillin/sulbactam 3 g IV q6h *PLUS* doxycycline 100 mg PO or IV q12h.
- Clindamycin 900 mg IV q8h *PLUS* gentamicin loading dose IV or intramuscular (IM) (2 mg/kg of body weight), followed by a maintenance dose (1.5 mg/kg) q8h. Single daily dosing (3 to 5 mg/kg) can be substituted.
- When clinical improvement is apparent based on symptoms, physical exam, and laboratory criteria, antibiotics may be transitioned from IV to PO with doxycycline PO and metronidazole PO or clindamycin PO (depending on the regimen selected) administered to complete 14 days of total antibiotic therapy. If a patient does not improve despite use of a recommended antibiotic regimen, further workup and potential procedural intervention are warranted.

OUTPATIENT REGIMENS (BOX 2)
Recommended IM/PO regimens
- Ceftriaxone 500 mg IM in a single dose *PLUS* doxycycline 100 mg PO bid for 14 days *PLUS* metronidazole 500 mg PO bid for 14 days *OR*

BOX 2 Centers for Disease Control and Prevention Recommendations for Ambulatory Management of Acute Pelvic Inflammatory Disease

---

Ceftriaxone, 250 mg IM, single dose
or
Cefoxitin, 2 g IM, single dose, and probenecid, 1 g PO administered concurrently in a single dose
or
Other parenteral third-generation cephalosporin (e.g., ceftizoxime, cefotaxime)
plus
Doxycycline, 100 mg PO bid for 14 days
with or without
Metronidazole, 500 mg PO bid for 14 days

bid, Twice daily; *IM,* intramuscularly; *PO,* per os (orally).
From Gershenson DM et al: *Comprehensive gynecology,* ed 8, Philadelphia, 2022, Elsevier.
Modified from Workowski KA, Bolan GA, Centers for Disease Control and Prevention: Sexually transmitted diseases treatment guidelines, 2015, *MMWR Recomm Rep* 64(RR-03):1-137, 2015.

- Cefoxitin 2 g IM in a single dose and probenecid 1 g PO administered concurrently in a single dose *PLUS* doxycycline 100 mg PO bid for 14 days *PLUS* metronidazole 500 mg PO bid for 14 days *OR*
- Other third-generation cephalosporin (ceftizoxime or cefotaxime) *PLUS* doxycycline 100 mg PO bid for 14 days *PLUS* metronidazole 500 mg PO bid for 14 days

Alternative intramuscular/oral regimen if the patient has a cephalosporin allergy

- Levofloxacin 500 mg PO daily *PLUS* metronidazole 500 mg PO bid for 14 days
- Moxifloxacin 400 mg PO daily for 14 days (preferred if *M. genitalium*)
- Azithromycin 500 mg IV daily for 1 to 2 doses followed by 250 mg PO daily for 7 days or in combination with metronidazole 500 mg PO tid for 12 to 14 days

Due to quinolone-resistant *N. gonorrhoeae,* antimicrobial susceptibility testing should be performed if a culture is positive for gonorrhea in a patient with a cephalosporin allergy. If the isolate is quinolone-resistant, consultation with an infectious disease specialist is recommended.

TREATMENT CONSIDERATIONS

- Antimicrobials should include coverage against *N. gonorrhoeae* and *C. trachomatis* even if these organisms are not identified on culture.
- Women should avoid sexual activity until they and their sexual partners have been adequately treated and symptoms have resolved.
- TOA may require drainage, which may be accomplished by interventional radiology via aspiration or placement of a drain, or by a gynecologist via vaginal or laparoscopic means. Recurrent/persistent TOAs may be managed by total abdominal hysterectomy with bilateral salpingo-oophorectomy after acute treatment of infection.
- Treatment of PID in women with intrauterine devices (IUDs) does not include/require removal of the device unless there is no clinical improvement after 48 to 72 hr of treatment with an approved regimen. IUDs rarely serve as a source for PID, especially >3 wk after insertion.
- Sexual partners of patients diagnosed with PID or other STIs should be evaluated and treated appropriately. In the setting of PID, treat all sexual partners within 60 days of onset of symptoms. Some states allow for expedited partner therapy (EPT), such that a woman's provider is able to supply her with enough medication to treat herself and her partner(s).
- Treatment of chronic PID may be aimed at a different spectrum of microbes and should be tailored appropriately.

DISPOSITION

- Given the risk of reinfection, all women should be retested for gonorrhea and chlamydia 3 mo after treatment.
- Follow-up includes confirmation of partner treatment, education on use of barrier contraception, and risks of PID and long-term sequelae, including:
  1. Recurrent PID
  2. Chronic pelvic pain
  3. Fallopian tube damage that leads to infertility and/or ectopic pregnancy
  4. Fitz-Hugh-Curtis syndrome
  5. Potential risk for cancer: Limited studies have suggested a small association between PID and ovarian, endometrial, and colon cancer

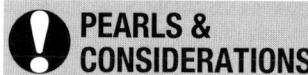

❗ PEARLS & CONSIDERATIONS

COMMENTS

- Maintain a low threshold for the diagnosis and treatment of PID given the risks for progression to severe infection and to significant and chronic medical and reproductive complications.
- Most patients are candidates for outpatient therapy, but inpatient hospitalization is recommended in select cases.
- Use only CDC-recommended treatment regimens unless contraindicated due to severe patient allergy; in such cases, check local susceptibilities of suspected pathogen.
- Offer HIV and other STI screening to all women with suspected or diagnosed PID.
- IUDs may be retained unless women have failed to improve with 48 to 72 h of treatment.
- Treat sexual partners of women with PID, with EPT if possible.
- Counsel patients on abstinence until they and their partners have completed treatment.
- Test for reinfection with gonorrhea and chlamydia 3 mo after treatment.

PREVENTION

Women aged <25 yr and/or participating in high-risk sexual behavior should be screened annually for gonorrhea and chlamydia; studies have shown such screening to reduce cases of PID by >50%. The importance of minimizing partner exposures and using barrier contraception (either alone or in conjunction with another method) should also be emphasized.

SUGGESTED READINGS
Available at eBooks.Health.Elsevier.com

RELATED CONTENT
Pelvic Inflammatory Disease (Patient Information)
Chlamydia Genital Infections (Related Key Topic)
Gonorrhea (Related Key Topic)
Pelvic Abscess (Related Key Topic)

AUTHORS: **COURTNEY PFEUTI, MD,** and **GRETCHEN MAKAI, MD**

ℹ BASIC INFORMATION

DEFINITION

Peptic ulcer disease (PUD) is an ulceration in the stomach (Table 1) or duodenum resulting from an imbalance between mucosal protective factors and various mucosal damaging mechanisms (see "Etiology").

SYNONYMS

PUD
Duodenal ulcer (DU)
Gastric ulcer (GU)

ICD-10CM CODES

K25.3	Acute gastric ulcer without hemorrhage or perforation
K25.7	Chronic gastric ulcer without hemorrhage or perforation
K26.3	Acute duodenal ulcer without hemorrhage or perforation
K26.7	Chronic duodenal ulcer without hemorrhage or perforation
K27.0	Acute peptic ulcer, site unspecified, with hemorrhage
K27.1	Acute peptic ulcer, site unspecified, with perforation
K27.2	Acute peptic ulcer, site unspecified, with both hemorrhage and perforation
K27.3	Acute peptic ulcer, site unspecified, without hemorrhage or perforation
K27.4	Chronic or unspecified peptic ulcer, site unspecified, with hemorrhage
K27.5	Chronic or unspecified peptic ulcer, site unspecified, with perforation
K27.6	Chronic or unspecified peptic ulcer, site unspecified, with both hemorrhage and perforation
K27.7	Chronic peptic ulcer, site unspecified, without hemorrhage or perforation
K27.9	Peptic ulcer, site unspecified, unspecified as acute or chronic, without hemorrhage or perforation
P78.82	Peptic ulcer of newborn
Z87.11	Personal history of peptic ulcer disease

EPIDEMIOLOGY & DEMOGRAPHICS

- *Incidence*: 250,000 to 500,000 (200,000-400,000 duodenal; 50,000-100,000 gastric) annually; duodenal ulcer/gastric ulcer ratio is 4:1.
- *Anatomic location:* <90% of duodenal ulcers occur in the first portion of the duodenum; gastric ulcers occur most frequently in the lesser curvature near the incisura angularis.

PHYSICAL FINDINGS & CLINICAL PRESENTATION

- Epigastric pain is the most frequently reported symptom of PUD. The pain is typically improved with food or antacids and worsened by fasting.
- Physical examination is often unremarkable.
- Patient may have epigastric tenderness, tachycardia, pallor, hypotension (from acute or chronic blood loss), nausea and vomiting (if pyloric channel is obstructed), board-like abdomen and rebound tenderness (if perforated, Fig. E1), and hematemesis or melena (with a bleeding ulcer). Box 1 describes key symptoms and signs of peptic ulcer.

ETIOLOGY

Often multifactorial. The following are common mucosal damaging factors:
- *Helicobacter pylori* infection. *H. pylori* is the major cause of PUD. It is found in more than 70% of patients with duodenal ulcers and gastric ulcers in the U.S. Rates are much higher (>90%) in other parts of the world.

Eradication of *H. pylori* markedly reduces peptic ulcer recurrence.
- Medications (NSAIDs, glucocorticoids). Risk factors for development of NSAID-related ulcers are described in Box 2.
- Incompetent pylorus or lower esophageal sphincter
- Bile acids
- Impaired proximal duodenal bicarbonate secretion
- Decreased blood flow to gastric mucosa
- Acid secreted by parietal cells and pepsin secreted as pepsinogen by chief cells
- Cigarette smoking
- Alcohol

BOX 2 Risk Factors for Development of NSAID-Related Ulcers

Definite
Advanced age
History of ulcer
Concomitant corticosteroid therapy
Concomitant anticoagulation therapy
High doses of NSAIDs
Serious systemic disorders
Possible
Concomitant infection with *Helicobacter pylori*
Cigarette smoking
Consumption of alcohol

From Andreoli TE et al: *Andreoli and Carpenter's Cecil essentials of medicine,* ed 8, Philadelphia, 2010, Saunders.

TABLE 1 Gastric Ulcer Types

Type	Location	Acid Level
I	Lesser curve at incisura	Low to normal
II	Gastric body with duodenal ulcer	Increased
III	Prepyloric	Increased
IV	High on lesser curve	Normal
V	Anywhere	Normal, NSAID-induced

NSAID, Nonsteroidal antiinflammatory drug.
From Townsend CM et al: *Sabiston textbook of surgery,* ed 21, St Louis, 2022, Elsevier.

BOX 1 Key Symptoms and Signs of Peptic Ulcer

Uncomplicated Ulcer
No symptoms ("silent ulcer" in up to 40% of cases)
Epigastric pain
Pain may radiate to the back, thorax, other parts of abdomen (cephalad most likely, caudad least likely)
Pain may be nocturnal (most specific), "painful hunger" relieved by food, or continuous (least specific)
Nausea
Vomiting
Heartburn (mimics or associated with gastroesophageal reflux)

Complicated Ulcer
Acute perforation
Severe abdominal pain
Shock
Abdominal board-like rigidity (and rebound and other signs of peritoneal irritation)
Free intraperitoneal air
Hemorrhage
Hematemesis and/or melena
Hemodynamic changes, anemia
Previous history of ulcer symptoms (80%)
Gastric outlet obstruction
Satiation, inability to ingest food, eructation
Nausea, vomiting (and related disturbances)
Weight loss

From Goldman L, Schafer AI: *Goldman's Cecil medicine,* ed 24, Philadelphia, 2012, Saunders.

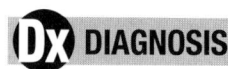

DIAGNOSIS

DIFFERENTIAL DIAGNOSIS

- Gastroesophageal reflux disease
- Cholelithiasis syndrome
- Pancreatitis
- Gastritis
- Nonulcer dyspepsia
- Neoplasm (gastric carcinoma, lymphoma, pancreatic carcinoma)
- Angina pectoris, myocardial infarction, pericarditis
- Dissecting aneurysm
- Other: High small-bowel obstruction, pneumonia, subphrenic abscess, early appendicitis

WORKUP

Comprehensive history and physical exam to exclude other diagnoses. Diagnostic modalities include endoscopy or upper GI series. Endoscopy is preferred and remains the gold standard for diagnosis of PUD. The presence of a mucosal break ≥5 mm in the stomach or duodenum confirms the diagnosis. An algorithm for evaluation, treatment, and surveillance of a patient with gastric ulcer is illustrated in Fig. 2.

LABORATORY TESTS

- Routine laboratory evaluation is usually unremarkable.
- Anemia may be present in patients with significant GI bleeding.
- *H. pylori* testing by endoscopic biopsy, urea breath test, or stool antigen test (*H. pylori* stool antigen) is recommended:
  1. The urea breath test documents active infection (sensitivity and specificity >90%). The patient ingests a small amount of urea labeled with carbon 13 or carbon 14. If urease is present (produced by the organism), the urea is hydrolyzed and the patient exhales labeled carbon dioxide that is then collected and measured. Use of proton pump inhibitors (PPIs) within 2 wk of the urea breath test may interfere with test results.
  2. Stool antigen test is an ELISA that identifies *H. pylori* antigen in a stool specimen through a polyclonal anti–*H. pylori* antibody. It is as accurate as the urea breath test for diagnosis of active infection and follow-up evaluation of patients treated for *H. pylori*. A negative result on the stool antigen test 6 wk after completion of therapy identifies

patients in whom eradication of *H. pylori* was successful.
  3. Serologic testing for antibodies to *H. pylori* is easy and inexpensive; however, the presence of antibodies demonstrates previous but not necessarily current infection. Antibodies to *H. pylori* can remain elevated for months to years after infection has cleared; therefore antibody levels must be interpreted in light of the patient's symptoms and other test results (e.g., PUD seen on upper GI series).
  4. Histologic evaluation of endoscopic biopsy samples is considered by many the gold standard for accurate diagnosis of *H. pylori* infection. However, detection of *H. pylori* depends on the site and number of biopsy samples, the method of staining, and experience of the pathologist.
- Additional laboratory evaluation is indicated only in specific cases (e.g., amylase level in suspected pancreatitis, serum gastrin level in suspected Zollinger-Ellison [ZE] syndrome).

IMAGING STUDIES

- Conventional upper GI barium studies (rarely performed) identify ~70% to 80% of PUD;

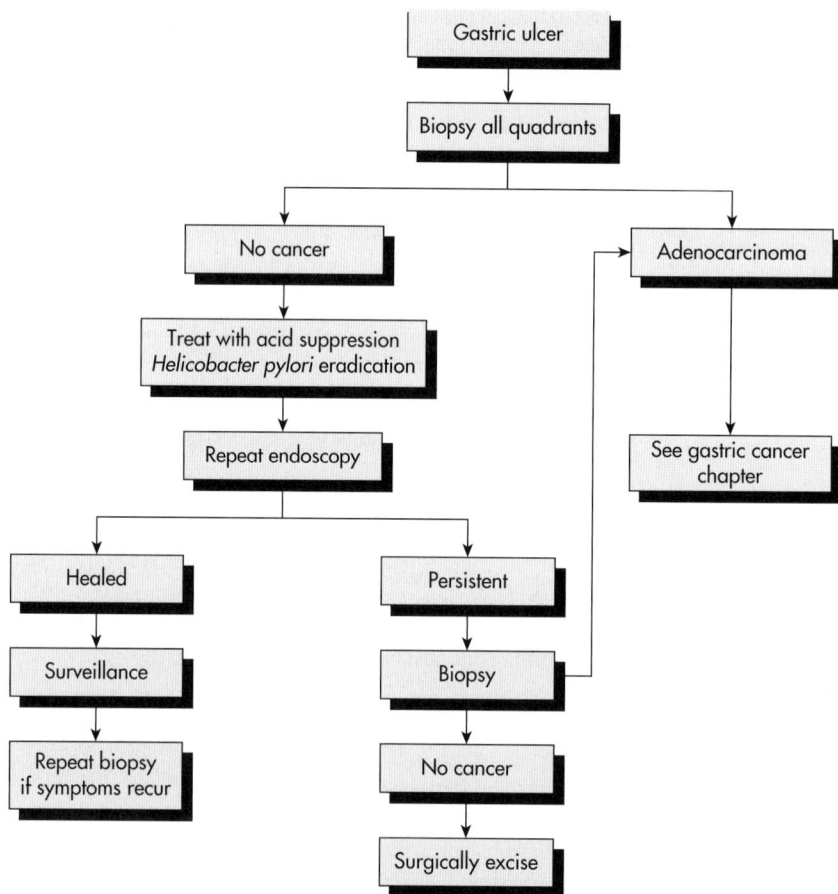

FIG. 2 Algorithm for evaluation, treatment, and surveillance of a patient with a gastric ulcer. (From Townsend CM et al: *Sabiston textbook of surgery,* ed 21, St Louis, 2022, Elsevier.)

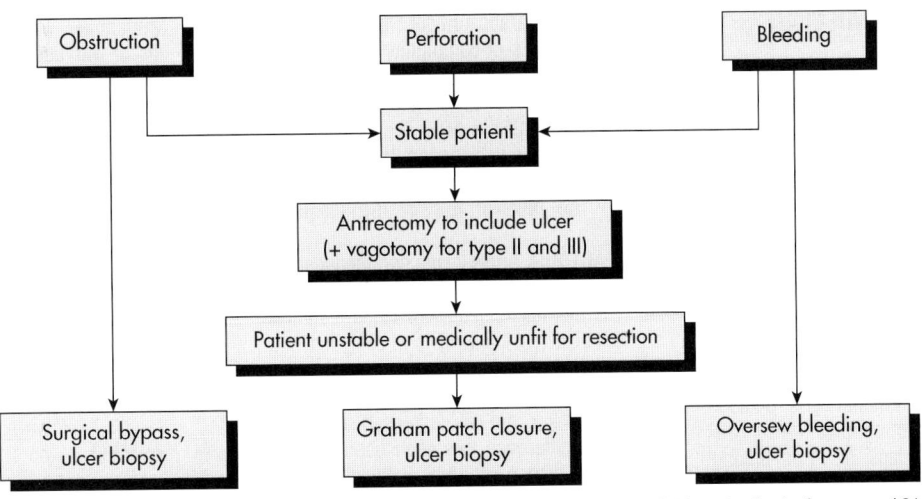

FIG. 3 Algorithm for the management of complicated gastric ulcer disease. (From Townsend CM et al: *Sabiston textbook of surgery*, ed 21, St Louis, 2022, Elsevier.)

accuracy can be increased to ~90% by using double contrast.
- Abdominal CT is helpful when suspecting perforating PUD (sensitivity >95%).

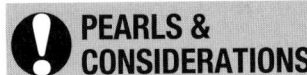 **TREATMENT**

NONPHARMACOLOGIC THERAPY
- Stop smoking; smoking increases the risk of PUD, decreases the healing rate, and increases the frequency of recurrence.
- Avoid NSAIDs and alcohol.
- Special diets have been proved unrelated to ulcer development and healing; however, avoid foods that cause symptoms.

ACUTE GENERAL Rx
Eradication of *H. pylori,* when present, can be accomplished with various regimens (see "*Helicobacter pylori* Infection").
PUD patients testing negative for *H. pylori* should be treated with antisecretory agents:
- H_2-Receptor antagonists (H$_2$RAs): Famotidine and nizatidine are effective; they are usually given in split dose or at nighttime.
- PPIs: Can also induce rapid healing; they are usually given 30 min before meals.
Antacids and sucralfate are also effective agents for the treatment and prevention of PUD.
- Glycopyrrolate, an anticholinergic drug, is available as a generic 2-mg tablet and as an oral disintegrating tablet (ODT) to reduce symptoms of peptic ulcer by decreasing volume, and acidity of gastric secretions. Formulary, and cost are limiting factors of the oral disintegrating tablet.

CHRONIC Rx
Maintenance therapy in peptic ulcer patients is indicated in the following situations:
- Persistent smokers
- Recurrent ulcerations
- Long-term treatment with NSAIDs, glucocorticoids
- Elderly or debilitated patients
- Aggressive or complicated ulcer disease (e.g., perforation, hemorrhage)
- Asymptomatic bleeders

DISPOSITION
- The recurrence rate for untreated PUD is ~60% (>70% in smokers). Treatment decreases the recurrence rate by nearly 30%.
- Patients with recurrent ulcers should be retreated for an additional 8 wk and then placed on maintenance therapy with H$_2$RAs, PPIs, sucralfate, or antacids.
- An ulcer is considered refractory to treatment if healing is not evident after 8 wk for duodenal ulcers and 12 wk for gastric ulcers. In these patients, maximum acid inhibition (e.g., esomeprazole 40 mg bid) is preferred over continued therapy with standard antiulcer therapy.
- An algorithm for the management of complicated gastric ulcer disease is illustrated in Fig. 3.
- Eradication of *H. pylori* (when present) is indicated in all patients. A negative stool antigen test for *H. pylori* 6 wk after treatment accurately confirms cure of *H. pylori* infection with reasonable sensitivity in initially seropositive healthy subjects.
- Screening for ZE syndrome should also be considered in patients with multiple recurrent ulcers; in patients with ZE, the serum gastrin level is >1000 pg/ml and the basal acid output is usually >15 mEq/hr.
- Surgery for refractory ulcers is now only rarely performed; it consists of highly selective vagotomy for duodenal ulcers or ulcer removal with antrectomy or hemigastrectomy without vagotomy for gastric ulcers.

REFERRAL
- GI referral for patients requiring endoscopy
- Surgical referral for patients with nonhealing ulcers despite appropriate medical therapy

! PEARLS & CONSIDERATIONS

COMMENTS
- Patients with gastric ulcers should generally have repeat endoscopy after 8 to 12 wk of antisecretory therapy to document healing and test exfoliative cytology for gastric carcinoma. Patients with duodenal ulcers and those with low-risk gastric ulcers, such as young patients on NSAIDs, generally do not require endoscopic surveillance.
- After endoscopic treatment of bleeding peptic ulcers, bleeding recurs in up to 20% of patients. PPI administration intravenously by continuous infusion substantially reduces the risk of recurrent bleeding. High-dose intravenous (IV) esomeprazole (80 mg IV bolus followed by 8 mg/hr infusion over 72 hr) given after successful endoscopic therapy to patients with high-risk peptic ulcer bleeding has been reported to reduce recurrent bleeding at 72 hr and to maintain sustained clinical benefits for up to 30 days.
- Among low-dose aspirin recipients who had peptic ulcer bleeding, continuous aspirin therapy may increase the risk for recurrent bleeding.

RELATED CONTENT
Peptic Ulcer (Patient Information)
Helicobacter pylori Infection (Related Key Topic)

AUTHOR: **FRED F. FERRI, MD**

BASIC INFORMATION

DEFINITION

Performance-enhancing drugs (PEDs) are substances used by individuals, typically recreational and professional athletes, to improve body aesthetics and potentially their performance. Commonly used agents include hormones with anabolic properties (Table 1), such as insulin, insulin-like growth factor-1 (IGF-1), growth hormone (GH), erythropoietin, diuretics, levothyroxine, aromatase inhibitors, clomiphene, selective estrogen receptor modulators (SERMs), gamma-hydroxybutyrate, and stimulants.[1,2] The focus of this chapter will be the hormonal PEDs, particularly androgenic-anabolic steroids (AAS), the most frequently used class of PEDs among weightlifters and athletes, GH, and insulin.[3]

SYNONYMS

PED
Anabolic steroids

ICD-10CM CODES

F55.3	Abuse of steroids or hormones; or F55.0 Abuse of nonpsychoactive substances
F55.8	Abuse of other nonpsychoactive substances
F15.10	Other stimulant abuse, uncomplicated

EPIDEMIOLOGY & DEMOGRAPHICS

INCIDENCE: The CDC reported that 3.2% of high school students had taken AAS at least once without a doctor's prescription.[4]
PREVALENCE: A global meta-analysis of AAS demonstrated a lifetime prevalence of 3.3%, with a higher prevalence in men than women (6.4% vs. 1.6%), with a higher rate among recreational athletes (18.4%) than professional athletes (13.3%).[5]

Field et al[6] found that 12% of adolescent boys and 8% of girls reported use of some type of product to improve strength, gain muscle mass,

TABLE 1 Performance-Enhancing Hormones

Anabolic Androgenic Steroids
17β-Esters of testosterone (cypionate, enanthate, heptylate, propionate, undecanoate, buciclate)
17α-Alkyl derivatives of testosterone (methyltestosterone, fluoxymesterone, oxandrolone, stanozolol)
19-Nortestosterone (nandrolone)
17β-Esters of 19-nortestosterone (decanoate, phenpropionate)
19-Norandrostenedione
19-Norandrostenediol
Tetrahydrogestrinone
Peptide hormones
Growth hormone
Insulin-like growth factor 1
Insulin
Erythropoietin

From Melmed S et al: *Williams textbook of endocrinology*, ed 14, Philadelphia, 2019, Elsevier.

or improve appearance. About 5% of high school athletes and 24% of community gym members report using GH and 12% of male weightlifters use GH or IGF-1.
PREDOMINANT SEX & AGE: The average age of onset of androgen use appears to be in the early 20s,[3] although use is common among teenagers.[6] The ratio of use in men:women is >50:1.[7,8]
RISK FACTORS: Adolescents and teenagers are at increased risk for use of PED because of their nature of risk-taking behaviors, experimentation, and lack of insight into long-term complications.[9] Athletes in certain sports such as football, baseball, basketball, wrestling, gymnastics, and weight training are at increased risk.[10] No significant difference has been seen in racial/ethnic prevalence of AAS use.[7] Substance abuse and mental health disorders are more common in those with AAS dependence. In a study of 223 men entering a drug treatment program, it was found that men using opioids used AAS more than men using other drugs (25% vs. 5%).[11] In another study, 50% of users dependent on AAS met *Diagnostic and Statistical Manual of Mental Disorders-IV* (DSM-IV) criteria for lifetime history of opioid dependence or abuse.[11] AAS use also has been linked to alcohol use.[12] In an online survey of 492 male bodybuilders, AAS use was associated with higher odds of psychopathic traits.[13]

PHYSICAL FINDINGS & CLINICAL PRESENTATION

AAS abuse may be suspected in men who present with gynecomastia, decreased testicular size, hair loss, sexual dysfunction, acne, infertility, and a muscular appearance. Women who have AAS abuse may present with a muscular appearance, male-pattern baldness, menstrual irregularity, decreased voice pitch, and acne. GH results in increased fat mass with abdominal obesity and decreased lean body mass, and patients may have decreased aerobic capacity.[3] Athletes abusing insulin may present with increased weight, despite physical training, or hypoglycemic events.

ADVERSE EFFECTS

- AAS abuse can affect multiple organ systems (Table 2), which include the following[3]:
  1. Cardiovascular: Dyslipidemia, cardiomyopathy, conduction abnormalities, hypertension
  2. Neuroendocrine: Hypothalamic-pituitary suppression leading to hypogonadism, gynecomastia
  3. Neuropsychiatric: Major mood disorders (mania or hypomania, depression), aggression, AAS dependence
  4. Hematologic: Coagulation abnormalities, polycythemia
  5. Hepatic: Inflammatory and cholestatic effects
  6. Renal: Renal failure secondary to rhabdomyolysis, focal segmental glomerulosclerosis
  7. Other reported effects include premature epiphyseal closure, tendon rupture, acne,

and striae. Infectious complications can occur with use of contaminated needles or products obtained on the black market.
- GH abuse can lead to systemic adverse effects such as edema, cardiomyopathy, glucose intolerance or diabetes mellitus, excessive sweating, myalgias, arthralgias, and carpal tunnel syndrome.[3]
- Use of insulin may result in hypoglycemia, which can lead to coma and death if left untreated.
- Erythropoietin increases plasma viscosity and red cell mass and thereby results in increased risk of thromboembolic events, cardiovascular events, hypertension, stroke, and death.[3]

ETIOLOGY

AAS:
- AAS are synthesized from structural modifications of the testosterone molecule. The

TABLE 2 Side Effects of Anabolic Androgenic Steroids

Cardiovascular
Cardiomyopathy
Lipid disorders (decreased HDL, increased LDL)
Increased platelet aggregation
Increased hematocrit
Elevated blood pressure
Cosmetic
Gynecomastia
Acne
Hair loss
Cutaneous striae
Reproductive-Endocrine
Libido changes
Subfertility
In Males
Testicular atrophy
Impaired spermatogenesis
Erectile dysfunction
Prostate diseases
In Females
Hirsutism
Breast atrophy
Voice deepening
Virilization (clitoromegaly)
Menstrual disturbances
Hepatic
Cholestasis
Steatosis
Tumors
Hepatocellular adenoma and carcinoma
Hepatic angiosarcoma and cholangiocarcinoma
Psychologic
Aggression
Mood swings
Anxiety
Psychosis
Irritability
Dependence
Withdrawal
Depression
Injection Related
Infection
Bruising
Fibrosis
Injection site pain

HDL, High-density lipoprotein; LDL, low-density lipoprotein.
From Melmed S et al: *Williams textbook of endocrinology*, ed 14, Philadelphia, 2019, Elsevier.

synthetic derivatives differ in their affinity for the androgen receptor, metabolism and duration of action, and anabolic effects.[3]
- The commonly used AAS are testosterone, dihydrotestosterone, boldenone, trenbolone, parenteral 19-nortestosterone derivatives such as nandrolone, and oral 17-α-alkylated androgens such as stanozolol.[3,14]
- Testosterone increases muscle mass and maximal voluntary strength, increases net oxygen delivery to the tissue by increasing red cell mass and tissue capillarity, and improves neuromuscular transmission.[3]
- Testosterone derivatives promote increase in nitrogen concentration in muscle, which results in an anabolic state, preserve muscle mass, and prohibit muscle breakdown by inhibiting the binding of glucocorticoids to muscle.[9]
- Testosterone effects on mood and aggression promote more intense training in athletes.[9]

GH:
- GH, or somatotropin, is an amino acid protein involved in skeletal and organ growth, lipolysis, and regulation of lean body mass.[15]
- Use of GH in GH-deficient individuals stimulates lipolysis and fatty acid oxidation to provide energy during the fasting state, spares protein oxidation, increases lean body mass, and decreases fat mass.[3]
- A meta-analysis of 11 studies showed improvement in body composition including increased lean body mass and decreased fat mass but no significant change in muscle strength or aerobic exercise capacity in healthy young subjects who administered GH.[16]
- There is little evidence that the use of supraphysiologic GH improves physical performance.[3,15]

Insulin:
- Insulin, with glucose, as a PED is primarily anecdotal but is possible because of its wide availability and affordability.
- It is thought to be used to enhance recovery after a heavy workout through increasing glucose and amino acid transport into human muscles[3] and thus stimulating protein synthesis to promote muscle anabolism.[17]
- It can also help endurance athletes through lipogenesis and inhibiting the release of free fatty acids, which are muscle fuel.[3]

Erythropoietin:
- Erythropoietin is a glycoprotein hormone that binds to red cell progenitor receptors to activate the JAK-2 signaling pathway, promote red cell production, and increase red cell mass.[3]
- Erythropoietin-stimulating agents (ESAs) increase oxygen delivery to the muscle.
- ESAs are most often used in endurance sports, such as cycling, triathlons, long-distance running, and cross-country skiing.[18]

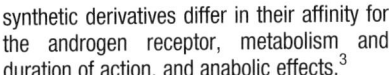

DIAGNOSIS

DIFFERENTIAL DIAGNOSIS
- Hyperprolactinemia: Elevated prolactin resulting in hypogonadism
- Acromegaly: GH-secreting pituitary adenoma
- Insulinoma: Rare tumor secreting insulin

WORKUP
Use of the biologic passport has recently been adapted in the detection of AAS use. The biologic passport is based on the concept that an individual's serum and urine hormones do not change significantly over time.[19] Baseline and follow-up laboratory testing are done to monitor the hormonal levels. Use of athlete biologic passport has also been studied for use in detection of GH.[20]

LABORATORY TESTS
- AAS
  1. Hemoglobin and hematocrit: Increased
  2. Serum total and free testosterone: Suppressed
  3. Serum luteinizing hormone and follicular-stimulating hormone: Suppressed
  4. Sperm count: Low
  5. Urinary ratio of testosterone glucuronide to epitestosterone glucuronide ($>4{:}1$)[9]
  6. The ratio of carbon 13 (13C) to carbon 12 (12C) in urinary metabolites of testosterone using isotope ratio mass spectrometry[21]
- GH
  1. Measurement of the variants of GH (isoforms) secreted by the pituitary gland: Increase in the ratio of recombinant/pituitary 22-kDA isoforms. Test must be done within 12 to 24 h of the last dose.[22]
  2. Measurement of the downstream products: IGF-1 and procollagen type III amino-terminal propeptide (P-III-NP). Test can be done up to 7 days.[22]
- Erythropoietin-stimulating agents
  1. Total hemoglobin mass and hematocrit
  2. Reticulocyte count
  3. Urine electrophoresis to detect recombinant erythropoietin[3]

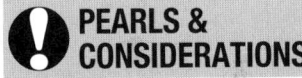

TREATMENT

NONPHARMACOLOGIC THERAPY
- Management of AAS abuse is based on the patient's willingness to quit. If the patient is not willing or ready to quit, the patient should be informed of the side effects of continued use.
- For those who use AAS for less than a year, many have spontaneous recovery of the hypothalamic-pituitary axis in 1 to 3 mo and normalization of sperm concentrations within 12 to 16 mo after cessation.[23]

ACUTE GENERAL Rx
- For increased hematocrit and hemoglobin caused by erythropoietin or AAS abuse, therapeutic phlebotomy can be used along with cessation of use of the abused substance.
- Hypoglycemia caused by insulin abuse can be treated with oral or intravenous glucose or administration of glucagon intramuscularly.

CHRONIC Rx
- Prescription of intramuscular testosterone at dosage of up to twice the usual replacement dosage with taper to a physiologic dosage over several months has been done to convince men to quit AAS use and avoid severe AAS withdrawal in the process.[14]
- A trial of clomiphene or human chorionic gonadotropin (hCG) therapy to increase testosterone concentrations and spermatogenesis may be considered for those who desire fertility, especially for men who use AAS for more than a year.[24,25]

REFERRAL
- Referral for treatment of users with associated mood disorder and alcohol or illicit drug use.[14]
- Individuals with AAS dependence may have "muscle dysmorphia" or depression related to AAS withdrawal, which may require psychotherapy interventions such as cognitive behavioral therapy.[26]
- Peer-led programs such as ATLAS (Adolescents Training and Learning to Avoid Steroids) for male athletes and ATHENA (Athletes Targeting Healthy Exercise & Nutrition Alternatives) for female athletes.[15]

PEARLS & CONSIDERATIONS

PREVENTION
- Early education and discussion with youth and athletes.
- Educational programs such as ATLAS and ATHENA have been shown effective in preventing substance abuse.[15]

PATIENT & FAMILY EDUCATION
- Maintaining an open dialogue and understanding the motive behind the use of PED are a few suggestions to address PED use.[9]
- Educating the athletes against the use of PEDs and discussing the side effects of PEDS also have been suggested.[9]

REFERENCES
Available at eBooks.Health.Elsevier.com.

AUTHORS: **BENYAMIN FARAHVASH, MD,** and **VICKY CHENG, MD**

P

Diseases and Disorders

I

ℹ️ BASIC INFORMATION

DEFINITION

Acute pericarditis is the inflammation (or infiltration) of the pericardium. The pericardium is a rigid, avascular fibrous sac with both visceral and richly innervated parietal layers where fluid resides for lubrication. It is characterized by at least two of the following four criteria:[1] (1) Chest pain, (2) specific electrocardiographic changes, (3) pericardial friction rub, and (4) new or worsening pericardial effusion.

ICD-10CM CODES

I30.0	Acute nonspecific idiopathic pericarditis
I30.1	Infectious pericarditis
I30.8	Other forms of acute pericarditis
I30.9	Acute pericarditis, unspecified
I31.0	Chronic adhesive pericarditis
I31.1	Chronic constrictive pericarditis
I31.3	Pericardial effusion (noninflammatory)
I31.9	Diseases of pericardium, unspecified (tamponade)
I31.2	Hemopericardium

EPIDEMIOLOGY & DEMOGRAPHICS

- Most common form of pericardial disease worldwide
- Observed in 0.1% to 0.2% of hospitalized patients and accounts for 5% of emergency room admissions for chest pain[2]
- Recurrence rate as high as 20% to 30% of cases, while 50% of recurrent pericarditis cases persist
- Four definitions: Acute (<4 to 6 wk), incessant (>4 to 6 wk), recurrent (after symptom-free interval), and chronic (>3 mo)

PHYSICAL FINDINGS & CLINICAL PRESENTATION (TABLE 1)

- Chest pain: Characteristically sharp, pleuritic, positional (improved by sitting up and leaning forward).
- Pericardial rub: A triphasic (ventricular systole, early diastole, atrial contraction), scratchy sound best heard at the lower left sternal border is pathognomonic. Unlike pleural friction rub, the rub of pericarditis is not affected by respiration.
- Pericardial effusion: Beck triad (hypotension, elevated jugular venous pressure, and muffled heart sounds) suggests pericardial tamponade.

ETIOLOGY (TABLE 2)

- In developed countries, viral and idiopathic etiologies are the most common.[3]
- Viral causes can include common gastrointestinal or respiratory flulike illnesses, whereas Parvovirus B19, Epstein-Barr, and HIV are also quite common precipitants.[4]
- The novel coronavirus SARS-CoV-2, as well as its vaccines, have been rarely associated with pericarditis.

- Tuberculosis accounts for 80% to 90% of pericarditis in developing countries, with a high prevalence in HIV-positive patients.
- Neoplastic etiologies (7% to 13%) are typically of lung, breast, esophageal, hematologic, and melanoma origin.
- Autoimmune syndromes (3% to 4%) include systemic lupus erythematosus and rheumatoid arthritis, Sjögren syndrome, sarcoidosis, scleroderma.
- Drug-induced: Procainamide, hydralazine, phenytoin, isoniazid, rifampin, doxorubicin, mesalamine, adalimumab, immune checkpoint inhibitors.
- Radiation-induced pericarditis prevalence is improving, with better radioprotective techniques. Morbidity is closely related to the radiation dose due to damage of capillary endothelial cells, lymphatic stenosis or occlusion.
- Metabolic: Uremia, myxedema, anorexia nervosa.
- Postcardiac injury syndrome: Post-pericardiotomy, postpacemaker lead placement, postcatheter ablation, post-CPR, post-PCI, perimyocardial infarction, or Dressler syndrome.

🅓🅧 DIAGNOSIS

DIFFERENTIAL DIAGNOSIS

- Angina pectoris and acute coronary syndrome
- Myopericarditis, perimyocarditis, Takotsubo stress cardiomyopathy syndrome
- Dissecting aortic aneurysm
- Pulmonary and thoracic causes: Thromboembolism, infarction, pneumothorax, pneumonia with pleurisy, costochondritis
- Gastrointestinal causes: Hepatitis, cholecystitis, GERD, esophageal spasm or rupture
- Box 1 summarizes the differential diagnosis of pericardial effusion by etiology

WORKUP (TABLE 3)

Table 4 summarizes an initial approach to acute pericarditis. Diagnosis of pericarditis requires at least two of the four following clinical criteria:
- Typical pleuritic chest pain
- Pericardial friction rub
- Suggestive ECG changes (diffuse concave ST segment elevation, PR depression in all leads except for AVR where there is elevation)
- New or worsening pericardial effusion

LABORATORY TESTS

Initial laboratory tests may determine severity of inflammation and acuity of patient's condition, while also guiding workup and treatment timeline:[5]
- Inflammatory markers: Erythrocyte sedimentation rate, (high-sensitivity) C-reactive protein (CRP), and complete blood count with differential
- Cardiac biomarkers (troponin T and I) suggest myocardial involvement
- Basic metabolic profile

Additional lab studies:
- HIV
- PPD/QuantiFERON-TB Gold
- Antinuclear antibody, rheumatoid factor
- TSH
- Routine viral studies are not indicated since they are low yield

PERICARDIAL FLUID & TISSUE SAMPLING

Indications for pericardiocentesis are:
- Tamponade physiology
- Moderate to large pericardial effusion with symptoms, or refractory to medical therapy
- Suspicion of a neoplastic, bacterial, or tuberculous process
- Evidence of constrictive or effusive-constrictive pericarditis

---

BOX 1   Major Differential Diagnosis of Pericardial Effusion by Etiology

Noninfectious
- Malignancy (usually metastatic)
- Myocardial infarction associated (Dressler syndrome)
- Uremia
- Myxedema (rare cause of tamponade physiology)
- Trauma (penetrating or nonpenetrating)
- Chylopericardium
- Acute idiopathic
- Rheumatic fever
- Collagen vascular disease (systemic lupus erythematosus, rheumatoid arthritis, scleroderma, Wegener granulomatosis)
- Postsurgical (cardiac and intrathoracic)
- Drug induced (procainamide, hydralazine, phenytoin, doxorubicin, isoniazid)

Infectious
- Viral (coxsackievirus, echovirus, mumps, adenovirus, hepatitis, human immunodeficiency virus)
- Bacterial (pneumococcus, *Streptococcus*, *Staphylococcus*)
- Tuberculous
- Fungal (histoplasmosis, coccidiomycosis, *Candida*, particularly in immunosuppressed patients)

From Niederhuber JE: *Abeloff's clinical oncology*, ed 6, Philadelphia, 2020, Elsevier.

TABLE 1 Manifestations of Pericarditis

SYMPTOMS

Chest pain (worsened if lying down or with inspiration)
Dyspnea
Malaise
Patient assumes sitting position

SIGNS

Nonconstrictive

Fever
Tachycardia
Friction rub (accentuated by inspiration, body position)
Enlarged heart by percussion and x-ray examination
Distant heart sounds

Tamponade

As above, plus:
Distended neck veins
Hepatomegaly
Pulsus paradoxus (>10 mm Hg with inspiration)
Narrow pulse pressure
Weak pulse, poor peripheral perfusion

Constrictive

Distended neck veins
Kussmaul sign (inspiratory increase in jugular venous pressure)
Distant heart sounds
Pericardial knock
Hepatomegaly
Ascites
Edema
Tachycardia

From Marcdante KJ et al: *Nelson essentials of pediatrics*, ed 9, Philadelphia, 2023, Elsevier.

- Pericardiocentesis is for diagnostic and therapeutic purposes. The pericardial fluid should be analyzed for RBC, WBC, Gram stain, culture, cytology, glucose, pH, LDH, and protein. In select cases, consider checking triglyceride for chylopericardium, adenosine deaminase (ADA), or PCR for tuberculosis
- Pericardial biopsy can be performed for cases of recurrent pericardial effusion when pericardial fluid analysis does not reveal etiology, and especially if malignancy or tuberculosis is suspected

IMAGING STUDIES

- ECG (Fig. 1): Changes in the ECG reflect inflammation of the epicardium, because the parietal pericardium is electrically inert. The ECG changes are staged as follows:
  1. Stage I (Acute phase): Hours to few days. PR-segment depression in all leads except aVR (where PR elevation is seen) and diffuse concave ST-segment elevations
  2. Stage II (Intermediate phase): Seen in first wk with return of PR and ST segments to baseline
  3. Stage III (Intermediate): T-wave inversion in leads previously showing ST-segment elevation
  4. Stage IV (Late phase): Normalization of the ECG or indefinite persistence of T-wave inversions

TABLE 2 Etiology of Pericarditis and Pericardial Effusion

IDIOPATHIC (PRESUMED VIRAL) INFECTIOUS AGENTS

Bacterial

Group A streptococci
Staphylococcus aureus
Pneumococcus, meningococcus*
*Haemophilus influenzae**
Mycobacterium tuberculosis

Viral†

Coxsackievirus (group A, B)
Echovirus
Mumps
Influenza
Epstein-Barr
Cytomegalovirus

Fungal

Histoplasma capsulatum
Coccidioides immitis
Blastomyces dermatitidis
Candida

COLLAGEN VASCULAR-INFLAMMATORY AND GRANULOMATOUS DISEASES

Rheumatic fever
Systemic lupus erythematosus (idiopathic and drug-induced)
Rheumatoid arthritis
Kawasaki disease
Scleroderma
Mixed connective tissue disease
Inflammatory bowel disease
Sarcoidosis
Vasculitis

TRAUMATIC

Cardiac contusion (blunt trauma)
Penetrating trauma
Postpericardiotomy syndrome
Radiation

CONTIGUOUS SPREAD

Pleural disease
Pneumonia
Aortic aneurysm (dissecting)

METABOLIC

Hypothyroidism
Uremia
Chylopericardium

NEOPLASTIC

Primary
Contiguous (lymphoma)
Metastatic
Infiltrative (leukemia)

OTHER ETIOLOGIC DISORDERS/FACTORS

Drug reaction
Pancreatitis
After myocardial infarction
Thalassemia
Central venous catheter perforation
Heart failure
Hemorrhage (coagulopathy)

*Infectious or immune complex.
†Common (viral pericarditis or myopericarditis is probably the most common cause of acute pericarditis in a previously normal host).
From Kliegman RM et al (eds): *Practical strategies in pediatric diagnosis and therapy*, ed 2, Philadelphia, 2004, Saunders. In Marcdante KJ et al: *Nelson essentials of pediatrics*, ed 9, Philadelphia, 2023, Elsevier.

- Echocardiogram is used to evaluate for pericardial effusion (present in 50%-60% of patients) (Fig. E2). Echocardiogram can help exclude STEMI (through absent wall motion abnormality) and support the diagnosis of constrictive pericarditis or tamponade. Echocardiogram is also recommended for guidance for pericardiocentesis.
- Chest x-ray: Performed to rule out abnormalities of the mediastinum or lung fields. Cardiac silhouette may appear enlarged when pericardial effusion accumulates over ≥200 ml of fluid (Fig. E3). Calcifications around the heart may be seen with chronic constrictive pericarditis.
- Computed tomography: Evaluation of associated pleuropulmonary and extra thoracic diseases and pericardial calcifications.
- Cardiac MRI (Fig. E4) is recommended in patients with elevated troponin I or T and can also be helpful in cases of chronic constrictive pericarditis and malignancy.

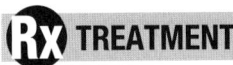

Rx TREATMENT

NONPHARMACOLOGIC THERAPY

- Physical activity should be restricted until pain resolves, and inflammatory markers, ECG, and echocardiogram normalize.
- Athletes should avoid competitive activity for 3 mo at a minimum. Exercise intensity, HR >100 bpm, and shear stress on pericardium are thought to worsen inflammation. With myocardial involvement (positive troponin), athletic activity must be avoided for at least 6 mo.
- Patient education should be provided of potential warning signs of complications such as cardiac tamponade, recurrent pericarditis (which can occur in up to one third of patients), and chronic constrictive pericarditis.

ACUTE GENERAL Rx

- High-dose aspirin (750 to 1000 mg tid) or NSAIDs (e.g., ibuprofen 600 to 800 mg tid, indomethacin 50 mg tid) for 1 to 2 wk. Proton pump inhibitor should be provided for gastric protection. NSAIDs should be avoided in patients with recent MI, CHF, acute renal failure, and upper GI bleed.
- Colchicine 0.5 to 0.6 mg once daily (<70 kg) or bid (>70 kg) for 3 mo. Current evidence (COPE, CORE, CORP, ICAP, CORP-2 trials)[6] supports the effectiveness of colchicine in symptomatic relief and prevention of recurrent pericarditis.
- Corticosteroids are prescribed for refractory recurrent pericarditis, or in the setting of established rheumatologic disease, renal failure, or other contraindications to NSAID or colchicine therapies. They can be associated with severe adverse effects, more hospitalizations, and high rate of recurrence.
- In tuberculous pericarditis, adjunctive corticosteroids can prevent development of constriction with tapering dose of 120 mg prednisolone over 6 wk in patients without HIV.

TABLE 3 Diagnostic Pathway and Sequence of Performance in Acute Pericarditis

Diagnostic Measure	Characteristic Findings
Obligatory	
Auscultation	Pericardial rub (monophasic, biphasic, or triphasic)
ECG*	*Stage I:* Anterior and inferior concave ST segment elevation. PR segment deviations opposite to P wave polarity
	Early stage II: All ST junctions return to the baseline. PR segments deviated
	Late stage II: T waves progressively flatten and invert
	Stage III: Generalized T-wave inversions in most or all leads
	Stage IV: ECG returns to prepericarditis state
Echocardiography	Effusion types B to D (Horowitz)
	Signs of tamponade
Blood analyses	Erythrocyte sedimentation rate, C-reactive protein, lactate dehydrogenase, leukocytes (inflammation markers)
	Troponin I,[†] CK-MB (markers of myocardial involvement)
Chest radiograph	Ranging from normal to "water bottle" shape of the heart shadow
	Performed primarily to reveal pulmonary or mediastinal pathology
Mandatory in Tamponade, Optional in Large/Recurrent Effusions or if Previous Tests Inconclusive in Small Effusions	
Pericardiocentesis/drainage	Polymerase chain reaction and histochemistry for etiopathogenetic classification of infection or neoplasia
Optional or if Previous Tests Inconclusive	
CT	Effusions, pericardium, and epicardium
MRI	Effusions, pericardium, and epicardium
Pericardioscopy, pericardial/epicardial biopsy	Establishing the specific etiology

CK-MB, Creatine kinase-MB; *CT,* computed tomography; *ECG,* electrocardiogram; *MRI,* magnetic resonance imaging.

* Typical lead involvement: I, II, aVL, aVF, and V3-V6. The ST segment is always depressed in aVR, frequently in V1, and occasionally in V2. Stage IV may not occur, and there are permanent T-wave inversions and flattenings. If an ECG is first recorded in stage III, pericarditis cannot be differentiated by ECG from diffuse myocardial injury, "biventricular strain," or myocarditis. ECG in early repolarization is very similar to stage I. Unlike stage I, this ECG does not acutely evolve, and J-point elevations are usually accompanied by a slur, oscillation, or notch at the end of the QRS just before and including the J point (best seen with tall R and T waves—large in an early repolarization pattern). Pericarditis is likely if, in lead V6, the J point is greater than 25% of the height of the T-wave apex (using the PR segment as a baseline).

[†]A rise in cardiac muscle troponin I (cTnI) is detected in 32.2% of patients, more frequently in younger, male patients, with ST segment elevation and pericardial effusion at presentation. An increase beyond 1.5 ng/ml is uncommon (7.6%) and associated with CK-MB elevation. cTnI increase and is not a negative prognostic marker for the incidence of recurrences, constrictive pericarditis, cardiac tamponade, or residual left ventricular dysfunction.

From Vincent JL et al: *Textbook of critical care,* ed 7, Philadelphia, 2017, Elsevier.

TABLE 4 Initial Approach to the Patient With Definite or Suspected Acute Pericarditis

1. If the diagnosis is suspected but not certain, listen often for pericardial rub and obtain ECGs frequently to check for diagnostic findings.
2. If the diagnosis is suspected or certain, obtain the following tests to help confirm the diagnosis (if necessary) and determine whether a specific causative diagnosis and/or significant associated conditions and/or complications are present:

   Hemogram hsCRP

   Troponin I

   Chest radiograph

   Echocardiogram

   Consider additional testing on the basis of clinical suspicion of a specific etiology.
3. If the diagnosis is likely or certain, initiate therapy with an NSAID plus colchicine.

From Zipes DP: *Braunwald's heart disease, a textbook of cardiovascular medicine,* ed 11, Philadelphia, 2019, Elsevier.

Because of increased risk of malignancy, corticosteroids should be avoided in persons with combined TB and HIV infection.

- When corticosteroids are indicated, recommended dosing is as follows: Low- to moderate-dose (0.25 to 0.5 mg/kg/day) systemic steroid therapy for 1 mo, followed by a long taper (6 to 12 wk).
- Azathioprine, intravenous immunoglobulins, and anti–interleukin-1 therapies (e.g., anakinra) can be considered for patients with refractory recurrent pericarditis.[7] In addition, a phase 3 trial demonstrated reduction of recurrent pericarditis with interleukin 1-α/1-β inhibition (rilonacept).[8]
- Pericardiectomy and pericardiotomy at specialized centers are a last-resort procedure reserved for recurrent cardiac tamponade, refractory pericarditis, and hemodynamically significant constrictive pericarditis.
- Avoidance of anticoagulants (increased risk of hemopericardium).

TREATMENT OF UNDERLYING CAUSE

- Purulent bacterial pericarditis: Systemic antibiotics and drainage of pericardium
- Collagen vascular disease: Corticosteroid therapy (prednisone)
- Tuberculous pericarditis: Rifampicin, isoniazid, pyrazinamide, and ethambutol for 2 mo, then isoniazid and rifampicin for 6 mo. Isoniazid is the most effective agent in penetrating the pericardial space
- Thyroid-related pericardial effusion: Thyroid replacement therapy
- Uremic: Dialysis
- Malignant pericardial effusion: Fig. 5

POTENTIAL COMPLICATIONS FROM PERICARDITIS

- **Chronic constrictive pericarditis:** Occurs in <1% of patients with acute idiopathic pericarditis. New awareness of subset of patients with "transient constrictive pericarditis" who have an initial hyperacute stage of inflammation that must be identified before progression to fibrosis and calcification of the pericardium.
  1. Physical examination: Signs of right heart failure—hepatomegaly, splenomegaly, ascites, pedal edema, scrotal edema,

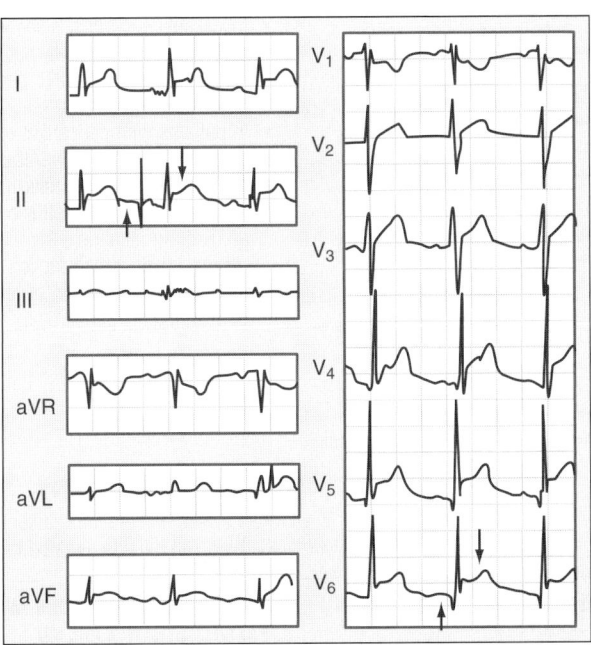

FIG. 1 Typical electrocardiographic changes in acute pericarditis: PR depression *(small arrow)* and concave ST-segment elevation *(large arrow)*. *aVF,* Augmented vector foot; *aVL,* augmented vector left; *aVR,* augmented vector right. (From Vincent JL et al: *Textbook of critical care,* ed 7, Philadelphia, 2017, Elsevier.)

possible anasarca, jugular venous pressure, Kussmaul sign (paradoxical increase in jugular venous pressure during inspiration), pericardial knock (early diastolic filling sound heard 0.06 to 0.1 sec after S2), and clear lungs.
2. ECG: Low QRS voltage, nonspecific ST-segment changes, biatrial enlargement.
3. Chest radiograph: Mild alveolar edema, pleural effusions, biatrial enlargement, pericardial calcification (seen in tuberculous pericarditis).
4. Echocardiography: May show thickened pericardium (>4 mm), >25% mitral and >50% tricuspid valve inflow variation with respiration, interventricular septal bounce; and mitral annulus reversus (medial e' velocity > lateral e' velocity) suggests constrictive pericarditis.
5. Hemodynamics (Fig. E6): Elevation of right-sided filling pressures, equalization of diastolic pressures, as well as prominent "x" and rapid "y" descent in the atrial tracing are seen in constrictive pericarditis. Right ventricular pressure tracing typically shows a "dip and plateau" (square root sign) that is a result of the unimpeded early filling of the RV with an abrupt halt to the late diastolic filling by the stiff pericardium. Discordance of right ventricular and left ventricular systolic pressures during respiration is also suggestive of constrictive pericarditis.
6. Therapy: Complex surgical stripping or removal of both layers of the constricting pericardium improves the functional class in majority of late survivors, but has high operative mortality.

• **Cardiac tamponade:** Occurs in 5% to 15% of patients with idiopathic pericarditis, but in up to 60% of those with neoplastic, tuberculous, or purulent pericarditis.
1. Signs and symptoms: Dyspnea, orthopnea, chest pain, fatigue.
2. Physical examination: Beck triad (distended neck veins, distant heart sounds, hypotension), reduced apical impulse, diaphoresis, tachypnea, tachycardia, narrowed pulse pressure, or pulsus paradoxus (decrease in systolic blood pressure ≥10 mm Hg during inspiration; most specific sign).
3. ECG: Decreased amplitude of the QRS complex, electrical alternans (occurs more frequently with large neoplastic effusions).
4. Chest x-ray: Cardiomegaly ("water-bottle" configuration of the cardiac silhouette may be seen) with clear lungs.
5. Echocardiography (Table 5): Pericardial effusion, >30% mitral and >60% tricuspid valve inflow variation with respiration, paradoxical motion of interventricular septum, diastolic right or left atrium collapse, diastolic right ventricular collapse (pathognomonic).[9]
6. Hemodynamics: Equalization of diastolic pressures within chambers of the heart, elevation of right atrial pressure with a prominent "x" but blunted "y" descent. Table 6 summarizes hemodynamics in cardiac tamponade and constrictive pericarditis.
7. Therapy: Cardiac tamponade is a life-threatening condition usually requiring emergent pericardiocentesis. Avoid drugs (diuretics, nitrates) or therapies (high PEEP) that reduce the preload. Fluid resuscitation can temporize hemodynamics while awaiting pericardiocentesis. In patients with recurrent effusions (e.g., neoplasms), placement of a percutaneous drainage catheter or pericardial window may be necessary.

• **Effusive-constrictive pericarditis:** Uncommon syndrome characterized by concomitant tamponade caused by tense pericardial effusion and constriction caused by the visceral pericardium.
1. Signs and symptoms of both tamponade and/or constriction. Pulsus paradoxus is present, but Kussmaul sign and pericardial knock are typically absent.
2. Echocardiography: Low sensitivity to distinguish effusive-constrictive pericarditis from other types.
3. Cardiac catheterization: Before drainage, "y" descent is usually less prominent than expected, and right atrial "v" wave persists. After drainage, may continue to have elevated right atrial and pulmonary wedge pressures.
4. Therapy: Extensive epicardiectomy (with disruption of the visceral layer of pericardium) is the procedure of choice in symptomatic patients.

• **Myopericarditis:** Defined by an elevated cardiac biomarker. Myocarditis and pericarditis may coexist in 20% to 30% of patients presenting with pericarditis. Hospitalization and cardiac MRI are favored in these patients. Overall, myopericarditis has a good prognosis with appropriate guideline medical therapies and has very low rates of morbidity, mortality, and heart failure.

DISPOSITION

• Complete resolution of pain and other signs and symptoms during the initial 3 wk of therapy occurs in 70% to 90% of cases.
• Admission is highly recommended if any of the following high risk and poor prognostic features exist: Fever >38° C (>100.4° F) during tamponade, failure to respond to 1 wk of outpatient treatment.
• The following are considered moderate risk factors but should also prompt admission: Myopericarditis, trauma, immunosuppression, oral anticoagulant therapy.
• Recurrent pericarditis occurs after a symptom-free interval (4 to 6 wk) following the initial episode of pericarditis. Incidence is reported as 10% to 15% and increases to 50% in patients who are not on colchicine. Standard first line treatment for recurring pericarditis is colchicine plus an NSAID. Colchicine plus low dose prednisone can be used for second-line treatment. Rilonacept, an interleukin-1 antagonist is now FDA approved for treatment of recurrent pericarditis and prevention of further recurrences in patients greater than or equal to 12 yr old. Its use should be reserved for patients with recurrences refractory to colchicine-based regimens.

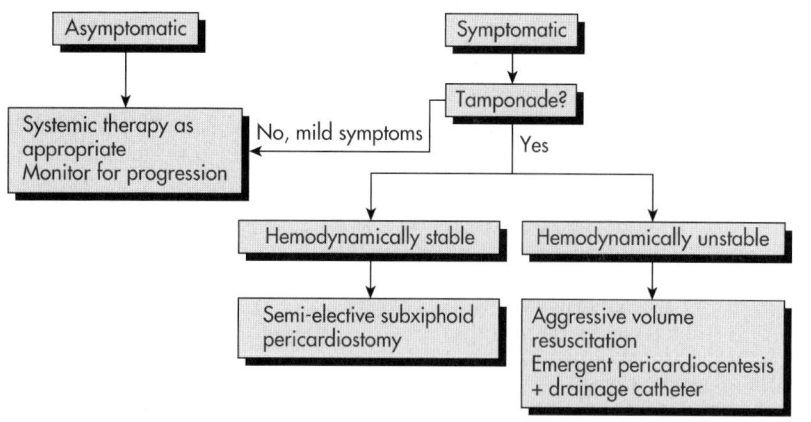

FIG. 5 Treatment approach algorithm to malignant pericardial effusions. (From Niederhuber JE: *Abeloff's clinical oncology*, ed 6, Philadelphia, 2020, Elsevier.)

- Incessant pericarditis is defined as pericarditis lasting for >4 to 6 wk but <3 mo without remission, while chronic pericarditis is pericarditis lasting for >3 mo.
- In patients with pericardial effusion after cardiac surgery, use of NSAIDs are not recommended because they have not been shown to reduce the size of the effusions or prevent late cardiac tamponade. The COPPS trial suggested that prophylactic colchicine may reduce the risk of developing a post-pericardiotomy pericarditis.[10]

REFERENCES
Available at eBooks.Health.Elsevier.com.

RELATED CONTENT
Pericarditis (Patient Information)
Cardiac Tamponade (Related Key Topic)

AUTHORS: **AARON ALI SHAIKH, MD,** and **MAXWELL EYRAM AFARI, MD**

TABLE 5 Hemodynamic and Echocardiographic Features of Constrictive Pericarditis Compared With Restrictive Cardiomyopathy

	Constriction	Restriction
Prominent y descent in venous pressure	Present	Variable
Paradoxical pulse	~1/3 cases	Absent
Pericardial knock	Present	Absent
Equal right- and left-sided filling pressures	Present	Left at least 3-5 mm Hg higher than right
Filling pressures >25 mm Hg	Rare	Common
Pulmonary artery systolic pressure >60 mm Hg	No	Common
"Square root" sign	Present	Variable
Respiratory variation in left-sided and-right-sided pressures/flows	Exaggerated	Normal
Ventricular wall thickness	Normal	Usually increased
Pericardial thickness	Increased	Normal
Atrial size	Possible LA enlargement	Biatrial enlargement
Septal bounce	Present	Absent
Tissue Doppler E' velocity	Increased	Reduced
Speckle tracking	Normal longitudinal, decreased circumferential restoration	Decreased longitudinal, normal circumferential restoration

From Zipes DP: *Braunwald's heart disease, a textbook of cardiovascular medicine*, ed 11, Philadelphia, 2019, Elsevier.

TABLE 6 Hemodynamics in Cardiac Tamponade and Constrictive Pericarditis

	Tamponade	Constriction
Paradoxical pulse	Usually present	Present in ~1/3
Equal left/right-sided filling pressure	Present	Present
Systemic venous wave morphology	Absent y descent	Prominent y descent (M or W shape)
Inspiratory change in systemic venous pressure	Decrease (normal)	Increase or no change (Kussmaul sign)
"Square root" sign in ventricular pressure	Absent	Present

From Mann DL et al: *Braunwald's heart disease*, ed 10, Philadelphia, 2015, Elsevier.

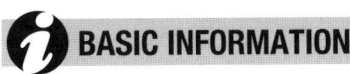
BASIC INFORMATION

DEFINITION

Peripheral artery disease (PAD) refers to atherosclerotic, inflammatory, occlusive, and aneurysmal diseases that lead to acute or chronic obstruction of the arteries involving the noncerebral and noncoronary arteries. (This topic focuses on lower-extremity PAD.)

SYNONYMS

PAD
Peripheral vascular disease (PVD)
Arteriosclerosis obliterans
Atherosclerotic occlusive disease
Atherosclerosis of the extremities
Peripheral arterial stenosis
Vasoocclusive disease of the legs
Chronic critical limb ischemia
Acute limb ischemia
Intermittent claudication

ICD-10CM CODES

I70	Atherosclerosis
I70.2	Atherosclerosis of native arteries of the extremities
I70.21	Atherosclerosis of native arteries of extremities with intermittent claudication
I70.22	Atherosclerosis of native arteries of extremities with rest pain
170.23	Atherosclerosis of native arteries of right leg w/ulceration
170.24	Atherosclerosis of native arteries of left leg w/ulceration
170.25	Atherosclerosis of native arteries of other extremities w/ulceration
170.26	Atherosclerosis of native arteries of extremities with gangrene
170.29	Other atherosclerosis of native arteries of extremities
I73	Other specified peripheral vascular diseases
I70.3	Atherosclerosis of unspecified type of bypass graft(s) of the extremities
170.31	Atherosclerosis of unspec. type of bypass graft(s) of extremities w/intermittent claudication
170.32	Atherosclerosis of unspec. type of bypass graft(s) of extremities w/rest pain
170.33	Atherosclerosis of unspec. type of bypass graft(s) of right leg w/ulceration
170.34	Atherosclerosis of unspec. type of bypass graft(s) of left leg w/ulceration
170.35	Atherosclerosis of unspec. type of bypass graft(s) of other extremity w/ulceration
170.4	Atherosclerosis of autologous vein bypass graft(s) of the extremities
170.5	Atherosclerosis of non-autologous biological bypass graft(s) of the extremities
170.6	Atherosclerosis of non-biological bypass graft(s) of the extremities
170.7	Atherosclerosis of other type of bypass graft(s) of the extremities
I73.8	Other specified peripheral vascular diseases
I73.9	Peripheral vascular disease, unspecified
I79	Disorders of arteries, arterioles, and capillaries in diseases classified elsewhere

EPIDEMIOLOGY & DEMOGRAPHICS

- There are more than 200 million patients afflicted with PAD globally (ankle-brachial index [ABI] $\leq$0.9); it affects approximately 8 to 12 million Americans.[1]
- The prevalence is nearly equal in men and women. It increases with age, from roughly 6% in those aged 40 to 49 yr to 15% to 20% in those aged 70 to 79 yr. However, symptoms of claudication are more likely to be present in males with PAD (50%) vs. in women with PAD (25%).[2]
- Risk factors for PAD include:
  1. Smoking
  2. Diabetes
  3. Hypertension
  4. Hypercholesterolemia
  5. Chronic kidney disease
  6. C-reactive protein
- As per the PARTNERS study, the prevalence of PAD in patients >70 yr or 50 to 69 yr with history of smoking or diabetes was 29%.[3]
- Smoking is three times more likely to lead to PAD than CAD. Conversely, the association of hypertension (HTN) and hyperlipidemia with PAD is lower than that with CAD and cerebrovascular disease.[3]
- Patients at increased risk of PAD include those >65 yr, those aged 50 to 64 yr with risk factors of atherosclerosis, those <50 yr with diabetes and an additional risk factor, as well as those individuals with known atherosclerotic disease in another vascular bed.[2]
- Black race and female sex are particularly sensitive to aggregate effects of multiple risk factors (HTN, diabetes, hypercholesterolemia, smoking, kidney disease). With one of these risk factors, the odds ratio (OR) of developing PAD was found to be 4.9 in Blacks and 2.8 in females. For >3 of these risk factors, the OR was 14.7 in Blacks and 18.6 in females.[4]
- Patients with newly diagnosed PAD are six times more likely to die within the next 10 yr when compared with patients without PAD.[4]
- Patients with heart failure and PAD have increased risk of mortality (hazard ratio [HR] 1.36), increased risk of myocardial infarction (MI), and less improvement in a structural physical exercise program.[4]
- Concomitant renal failure (Cr >2) is associated with worse overall cardiovascular (CV) prognosis in addition to lower rates of amputation-free survival to the point that the *European Journal of Vascular Medicine* guidelines recommend a special attention to be paid to atherosclerosis in lower extremities in these patients.[4]
- The total annual costs associated with the hospitalization of patients with PAD in the U.S. exceed $21 billion and account for ~13% of all Medicare Part A and B expenditures.[5]
- Those with PAD had average annual expenditures of $11,553 compared with only $4219 in matched cohort without PAD.[5]

PHYSICAL FINDINGS & CLINICAL PRESENTATION

- PAD may present in a variety of ways:
  1. 20% to 50%: Asymptomatic (estimated three times more than symptomatic patients)
  2. 10% to 35%: Intermittent claudication (IC), defined as aching pain, cramping, weakness, numbness, or heaviness of the leg induced by exercise, particularly walking, and relieved by rest
  3. 1% to 2%: Critical limb ischemia (CLI), defined as chronic (>2 wk) rest pain, or tissue loss with nonhealing ulceration, necrosis, or gangrene (Fig. E1)
  4. 40% to 50%: Atypical symptoms involving the calf, thigh, or buttock
  5. Acute limb ischemia (ALI) will be present in 14 per 100,000 individuals in the general population. It is defined as acute (<2 wk) onset of symptoms due to severe poor perfusion of the extremities, and further categorized into the following:
     a. Viable: No sensory or muscle weakness with audible Doppler pulses
     b. Threatened: Mild to moderate sensory or motor loss; inaudible arterial Doppler
     c. Irreversible: Severe sensory loss and muscle weakness; inaudible arterial Doppler
        (1) Claudication can be categorized using the Rutherford and Fontaine classification symptoms.
- Physical findings include:
  1. Diminished pulses and/or cool skin temperature of lower extremities
  2. Bruits heard over the distal aorta, iliac, or femoral arteries (femoral bruit is an independent marker for ischemic cardiac events)
  3. Change in skin color:
     a. Dependent rubor in CLI
     b. Livedo reticularis, or a mottled reticulated vascular pattern that appears lacelike
     c. Severe limb ischemia may also have petechiae, persistent cyanosis or pallor, pedal edema, skin fissures, ulceration, or gangrene
  4. Trophic changes of hair loss, thickened and brittle toenails, smooth and shiny skin, and muscle atrophy

ETIOLOGY

- PAD is primarily the result of atherosclerotic narrowing of the arterial lumen that results in impaired blood flow to the lower-extremity tissues and an oxygen supply-demand mismatch. Fig. 2 illustrates the pathophysiology of IC, from which symptoms initially manifest with exercise as metabolic demands increase.
- The mechanism of oxygen supply-demand mismatch is multifactorial, including stenosis-related turbulent flow and loss of kinetic energy with subsequent pressure loss

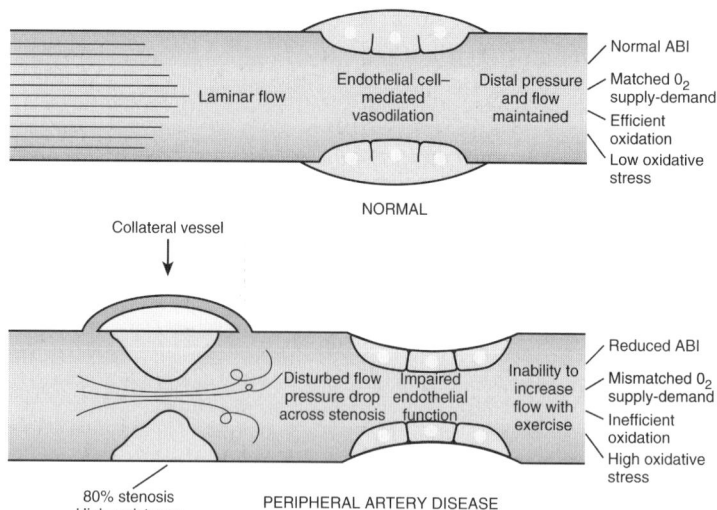

FIG. 2 Pathophysiology of intermittent claudication. In healthy arteries *(top)*, flow is laminar and endothelial function is normal; therefore blood flow and oxygen delivery match muscle metabolic demand at rest and during exercise. Muscle metabolism is efficient and results in low oxidative stress. In contrast, in peripheral artery disease *(PAD)* *(bottom)*, arterial stenosis results in disturbed flow, and the loss of kinetic energy results in a drop in pressure across the stenosis. Collateral vessels have high resistance and only partially compensate for the arterial stenosis. In addition, endothelial function is impaired, thereby resulting in further loss of vascular function. These changes limit the blood flow response to exercise and result in a mismatch of oxygen delivery to muscle metabolic demand. Changes in skeletal muscle metabolism further compromise the efficient generation of high-energy phosphates. Oxidant stress, the result of inefficient oxidation, further impairs endothelial function and muscle metabolism. *ABI,* Ankle-brachial index. (From the text *Anatomie, physiologie, pathologie des vaisseaux lymphatiques* by PC Sappey [1874], courtesy Harvard Medical Library, Francis A. Countway Library of Medicine. In Hiatt WR, Brass EP: Pathophysiology of intermittent claudication. In Creager MA et al [eds]: *Vascular medicine: a companion to Braunwald's heart disease,* ed 2, Philadelphia, 2013, Elsevier.)

across a stenosis, endothelial dysfunction, abnormal skeletal muscle metabolism, and increased oxidant stress.
- CLI may develop gradually from progressive atherosclerosis or in a subacute fashion from multisegmental atherothrombosis or atheroembolization, such that blood supply at rest cannot sufficiently supply the nutritional needs of the affected limb, leading to rest pain and tissue loss.
- ALI is marked by a sudden onset of symptoms (<2 wk) due to arterial occlusion and reduced blow flow to the affected extremity.

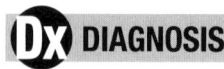 **DIAGNOSIS**

DIFFERENTIAL DIAGNOSIS
- Vascular etiologies
  1. Thrombus or embolism
  2. Vasculitis, such as thromboangiitis obliterans, giant cell arteritis, and Takayasu arteritis
  3. Fibromuscular dysplasia
  4. Aortopathy, including coarctation of the aorta
  5. Raynaud phenomenon
  6. Irradiation-related vascular fibrosis or injury
  7. Extravascular compression, such as compartment syndrome or popliteal artery entrapment
  8. Direct vascular injury
  9. Deep venous thrombosis
- Nonvascular etiologies
  1. Musculoskeletal disorder, such as arthritis or myositis
  2. Spinal stenosis or nerve root compression (neurogenic or pseudoclaudication)

  3. Peripheral neuropathy
  4. Reflex sympathetic dystrophy

WORKUP
- Thorough history, including identifying walking distance, speed, and incline to qualitatively assess for claudication, presence of ischemic rest pain, or presence of nonhealing wounds in patients ≥70 yr or those ≥50 yr with a history of smoking and/or diabetes.
- Careful physical examination includes:
  1. Measurement of blood pressure in both arms; pressure difference of >15 to 20 mm Hg is abnormal and suggestive of subclavian artery stenosis (marker of vascular disease risk and death)
  2. Palpation and recording of carotid pulses, upstroke, amplitude, and presence of bruits
  3. Auscultation and palpation of abdomen for bruits, aortic pulsation, and diameter
  4. Palpation of brachial, radial, ulnar, femoral, popliteal, dorsalis pedis, and posterior tibial pulses. Pulse intensity should be recorded as follows: 0, absent; 1+, diminished; 2+, normal; 3+, bounding
  5. Auscultation of femoral arteries for the presence of bruits
  6. Extremities should be inspected for color, temperature, integrity of the skin, hair loss, and hypertrophic nails
- Categorization of the clinical symptoms helps to identify risk and types of therapeutic intervention. One such classification is the Fontaine staging system (Table 1) for PAD:
  1. I: Asymptomatic
  2. II: Intermittent claudication
  3. IIa: Claudication walking >200 m (mild)
  4. IIb: Claudication walking <200 m (moderate)

  5. III: Nocturnal or rest pain
  6. IV: Evidence of tissue lost with ulceration, gangrene, or necrosis
- Segmental pressure measurement, where pneumatic cuffs are placed on multiple portions of the upper and lower extremity, is a simple tool that can identify the presence and severity of stenosis in the peripheral arteries.
- Resting ABI, a simplified form of segmental pressure measurement, is a first-line noninvasive test to establish a diagnosis of PAD in individuals with symptoms or signs suggestive of disease (individuals with one or more of the following exertional leg symptoms: Nonhealing wounds, age >65 yr, or age >50 yr with smoking or diabetes history).
- ABI of each leg is calculated by dividing the highest dorsalis pedis or posterior tibial systolic blood pressure by the highest systolic brachial pressure obtained from either the right or left arm.
  1. Noncompressible/calcified: >1.40

TABLE 1 Fontaine Classification of Peripheral Artery Disease

Stage	Symptoms
I	Asymptomatic
II	Intermittent claudication
IIa	Pain free, claudication walking >200 m
IIb	Pain free, claudication walking <200 m
III	Rest and nocturnal pain
IV	Necrosis, gangrene

From Bonow RO et al: *Braunwald's heart disease: a textbook of cardiovascular medicine,* ed 9, Philadelphia, 2012, Saunders.

2. Normal: 1.00 to 1.40 at rest
3. Borderline: 0.91 to 0.99 at rest
4. Abnormal: ≤0.90
   a. ABI <0.5 severe PAD
   b. 0.5 <ABI <0.75 moderate PAD
   c. 0.75 <ABI <0.9 mild PADc.
- ABI should be measured in both legs in all new patients (Fig. 3).
- Exercise ABI is recommended if resting ABI is borderline or normal (>0.9) and symptoms of claudication are present; a 25% or greater decrease in ABI after exercise is considered diagnostic.
- Toe-brachial index (TBI) should be used in patients suspected of PAD with an ABI of >1.40. A TBI of <0.70 is abnormal and diagnostic of PAD. TBI may be used to assess perfusion in patients with suspected CLI.
- Routine screening for lower-extremity PAD in the absence of risk factors, history, signs, or symptoms is not recommended.
- PAD is recognized as a risk factor for abdominal aortic aneurysm (AAA), and in observational studies the prevalence of AAA was higher in patients with symptomatic PAD.

LABORATORY TESTS

Laboratory tests can help identify risk factors or other potential causative etiologies. These include lipid profile, hemoglobin A_{1C}, D-dimer, and C-reactive protein/erythrocyte sedimentation rate.

ADDITIONAL PHYSIOLOGIC TESTING & IMAGING STUDIES

- Rest or exercise pulse volume recordings are also useful, depicting the volume of limb flow per pulse in different segments of the limb (e.g., thigh, calf, ankle, metatarsal, and toes). Segmental analysis of the pulse wave may identify the location and severity of a lesion and assess the integrity of blood flow in noncompressible vessels.
- Duplex ultrasound incorporates anatomic and physiologic evaluation by combining 2D ultrasound to visualize arterial segments and pulse wave Doppler to sample blood flow velocities at specific locations in the arterial lumen.

Conventional contrast-enhanced digital subtraction angiography (DSA) remains the gold standard, but duplex ultrasonography, computed tomography angiography, and magnetic resonance angiography have largely replaced catheter-based angiography in anatomic assessment for revascularization. DSA (Fig. E4) is now reserved for patients with PAD who are being considered for endovascular revascularization. It allows assessment of translesional pressure gradients before percutaneous intervention.

℞ TREATMENT

The treatment goal in patients with PAD is to focus on CV risk factor reduction to decrease morbidity and mortality as well as to improve limb-related symptoms. There are also medical and surgical approaches to management of limb-related symptoms to improve blood supply and preserve limb viability. Fig. 5 illustrates an approach to a patient with PAD. 2016 American College of Cardiology Foundation/American Heart Association (ACCF/AHA) guidelines for medical management of patients with PAD are summarized in Table 2.

MEDICAL THERAPY (TABLE 3)
LOWERING CV RISK FACTORS, MORBIDITY, AND MORTALITY:

- Smoking cessation or avoidance of second-hand smoke should be emphasized in patients with PAD at each visit with assistance of behavioral and pharmacologic treatment (Class I).[6]
- E-cigarettes may be considered as an interim activity to reduce habituation and to make smoking cessation possible.
- Control of blood sugar in diabetic patients with PAD is recommended (hemoglobin A_{1C} goal <6.5), although studies have failed to demonstrate a beneficial effect on intensive insulin therapy in lowering risk of PAD.
- In all patients with diabetes and lower-extremity PAD, proper foot care, including use of appropriate footwear, chiropody/podiatric medicine, daily foot inspection, skin cleansing, and use of topical moisturizing creams, should be encouraged, and skin lesions and ulcerations should be addressed urgently (Class I).
- A foot infection should be suspected in patients presenting with local pain, periwound erythema, edema, or discharge; these patients should undergo prompt diagnosis and treatment with an interdisciplinary care team to avoid amputation.
- Antihypertensive therapy also provides reduced CV risk in patients with PAD, and while data regarding specific targets for blood pressure goal and types of agents to be used are mixed, standard therapy per the AHA/ACC guidelines should be utilized (Class I).[7]
- Antiplatelet therapy is indicated to reduce risk of MI, stroke, and vascular death in individuals with symptomatic PAD with either aspirin (75 to 325 mg) or clopidogrel (75 mg) (Class I) and in asymptomatic patients (Class IIa). Uncertain benefit has been observed with combination aspirin and clopidogrel therapy (Class IIb). There are limited data on the use of newer P2Y12 receptor antagonists in PAD. In the EUCLID trial, ticagrelor was not shown to be superior to clopidogrel for the reduction of CV events, with major bleeding being similar in the two groups.[8] There is uncertain benefit with vorapaxar (Class IIb).
- Anticoagulation with low-dose (2.5 mg twice daily) rivaroxaban (Xarelto) plus aspirin 100 mg daily showed significant reductions in both major CV and limb events, including amputations, in patients with PAD in the COMPASS trial. (Class IIa – Level B per 2019 *European Journal of Vascular Medicine* PAD guidelines).[9]
- Similarly, the VOYAGER PAD trial studied patients who had undergone lower-extremity revascularization with therapy with rivaroxaban 2.5 mg twice daily plus aspirin or aspirin alone. The rivaroxaban/aspirin group had significantly lower incidence of the composite outcome of ALI, major amputation for vascular causes, MI, ischemic stroke, or death from CV causes.[10]

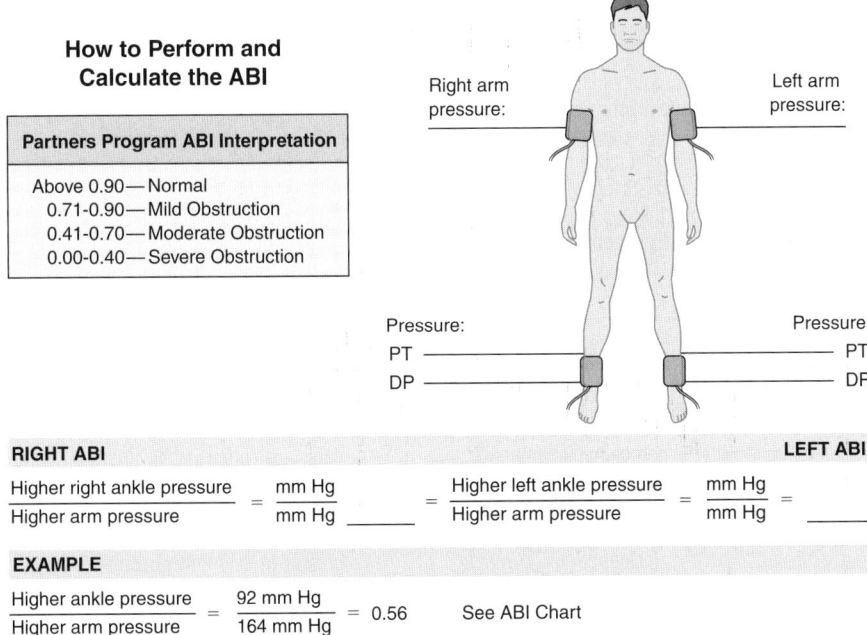

How to Perform and Calculate the ABI

Partners Program ABI Interpretation
Above 0.90— Normal
0.71-0.90 — Mild Obstruction
0.41-0.70 — Moderate Obstruction
0.00-0.40 — Severe Obstruction

Right arm pressure:

Left arm pressure:

Pressure:
PT
DP

Pressure:
PT
DP

RIGHT ABI

$$\frac{\text{Higher right ankle pressure}}{\text{Higher arm pressure}} = \frac{\text{mm Hg}}{\text{mm Hg}} \underline{\quad} =$$

LEFT ABI

$$\frac{\text{Higher left ankle pressure}}{\text{Higher arm pressure}} = \frac{\text{mm Hg}}{\text{mm Hg}} = \underline{\quad}$$

EXAMPLE

$$\frac{\text{Higher ankle pressure}}{\text{Higher arm pressure}} = \frac{92 \text{ mm Hg}}{164 \text{ mm Hg}} = 0.56 \qquad \text{See ABI Chart}$$

FIG. 3 Performing pressure measurements and calculating the ankle-brachial index *(ABI)*. To calculate the ABI, systolic pressures are determined in both arms and both ankles with the use of a handheld Doppler instrument. The highest readings for the dorsalis pedis *(DP)* and posterior tibial *(PT)* arteries are used to calculate the index. (From Goldman L, Schafer AI: *Goldman's Cecil medicine*, ed 24, Philadelphia, 2012, Saunders.)

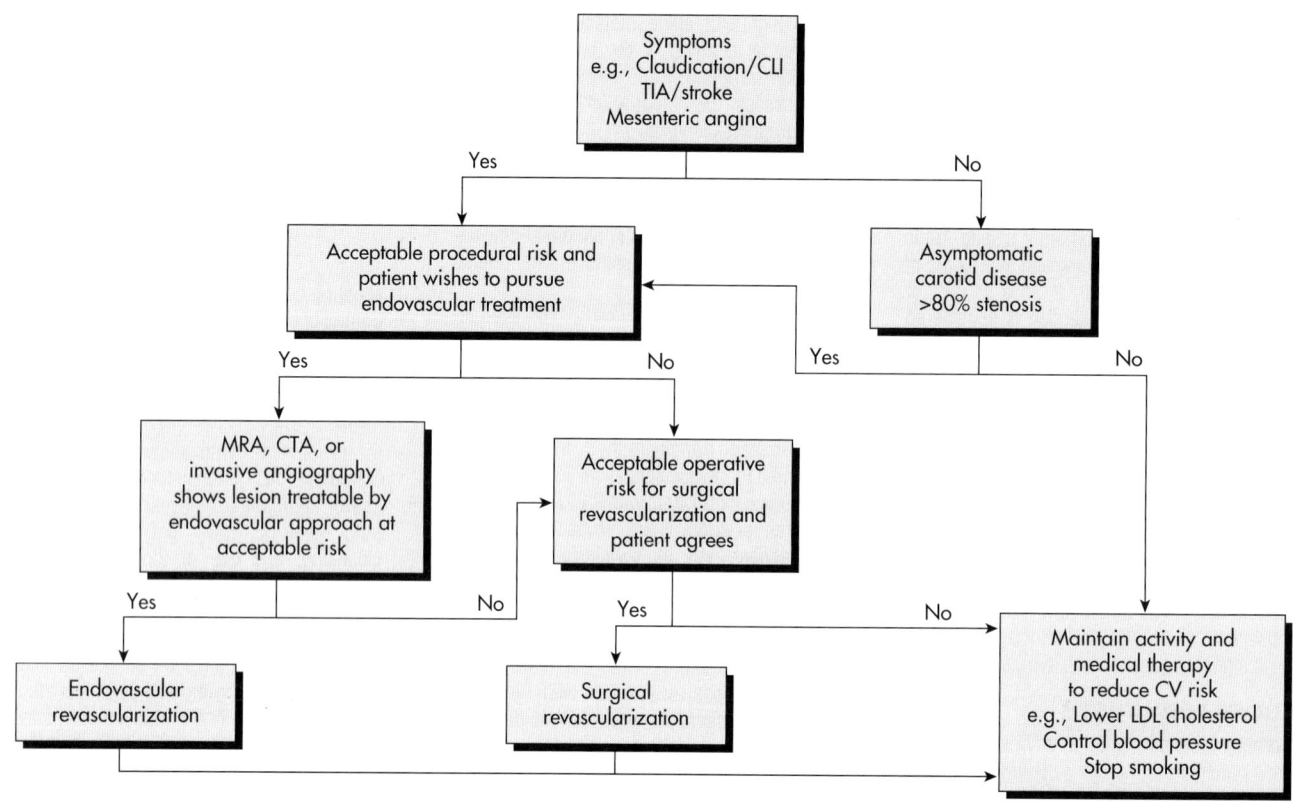

FIG. 5 Approach to a patient with peripheral artery disease. This strategy is based on assessment of the risk for adverse events with and without treatment by taking into consideration procedural or operative risks and the patient's informed decision to proceed with revascularization. *CLI,* Critical limb ischemia; *CTA,* computed tomographic angiography; *CV,* cardiovascular; *LDL,* low-density lipoprotein; *MRA,* magnetic resonance angiography; *TIA,* transient ischemic attack. (From Zipes DP: *Braunwald's heart disease, a textbook of cardiovascular medicine,* ed 11, Philadelphia, 2019, Elsevier.)

- Lipid-lowering therapy in patients with lower limb PAD has been shown to help slow disease progression, alleviate symptoms, and improve walking distance. The 2018 ACC/AHA Guideline on the Treatment of Blood Cholesterol recommends that patients with atherosclerotic PAD receive high-intensity statin therapy to lower risk of CV events regardless of baseline cholesterol values (Class I). In patients who are judged to be at very high risk and considered for PCSK9 inhibitor therapy, maximally tolerated low-density lipoprotein–cholesterol (LDL-C) lowering therapy should include maximally tolerated statin therapy and ezetimibe (Class I). 2019 *European Journal of Vascular Medicine* PAD guidelines also recommends addition of ezetimibe to get better tolerance of the statin medication (with reduced dose) or to achieve target level of LDL <70 mg/dl or >50% decrease.[11,12]

TREATMENT OF CLAUDICATION:

- Exercise therapy: Supervised exercise-training may be as beneficial as stent revascularization in symptomatic improvement. Patients should be prescribed exercise for a minimum of 30 to 45 min, in sessions performed at least three times per week for a minimum of 12 wk (Class I). ACCF/AHA guidelines for exercise therapy in patients with PAD are summarized in Table 4.
- Pharmacologic therapy:
  1. Cilostazol (100 mg PO twice daily) is indicated as effective therapy for enabling pain-free and maximal walking distance (Class 1). It is a phosphodiesterase (PDE-3)

inhibitor that reduces platelet aggregation and causes vasodilatation. It may have an added benefit of reducing restenosis and repeat revascularization following endovascular therapy. Cilostazol is contraindicated in patients with systolic heart failure.
  2. Pentoxifylline, prostanoids, L-arginine, buflomedil, ginkgo biloba, and chelation therapy are no longer considered effective in the treatment of claudication.
  3. No clear evidence exists for effectiveness of hyperbaric oxygen therapy as an adjunctive therapy for wound treatment in severe PAD.

REVASCULARIZATION

In general, there is no difference in clinical outcomes in percutaneous vs. surgical revascularization in iliac and femoropopliteal disease except for the higher morbidity with surgery and greater reinterventions with the percutaneous approach. A recent trial[12a] in patients with chronic limb-threatening ischemia (CLTI) who had adequate great saphenous vein for surgical revascularization revealed that the incidence of a major adverse limb event or death was significantly lower in the surgical group than in the endovascular group. Among patients who lacked an adequate saphenous vein conduit, the outcomes in the two groups were similar.

- The 2016 ACCF/AHA guidelines on PAD (Table 5) have recommended revascularization as a reasonable treatment option for the patient

with lifestyle-limiting claudication with inadequate response to guideline-directed medical therapy. A multidisciplinary approach by vascular specialists in all chronic limb ischemia patients for management of pain, risk factors, and comorbidities is appropriate. ACC/AHA guidelines for wound healing therapies for patients with CLI are summarized in Table 6.
- The following approach is discussed:
  1. Considerations in percutaneous/endovascular treatment:
     a. In patients with a vocational- or lifestyle-limiting disability due to claudication or limb ischemia from either significant aortoiliac or femoropopliteal disease despite optimal medical therapy when clinical features suggest a reasonable likelihood of symptomatic improvement with endovascular intervention.
     b. Endovascular intervention is not indicated as prophylactic therapy in an asymptomatic patient with lower-extremity PAD.
     c. Durability of endovascular intervention is greater in iliac and proximal (including proximal popliteal) artery than in the femoropopliteal segment.
  2. Considerations in surgical revascularization:
     a. Individuals with claudication symptoms who have a significant functional disability that is vocational or lifestyle limiting. These patients need to also be unresponsive to exercise or

TABLE 2 ACCF/AHA Guidelines for Medical Therapy for Patients With Peripheral Artery Disease

COR	Indication	LOE
I	1. Antiplatelet therapy with aspirin alone (range, 75-325 mg/day) or clopidogrel alone (75 mg/day) is recommended to reduce MI, stroke, and vascular death in patients with symptomatic PAD.	A
	2. Treatment with a statin medication is indicated for all patients with PAD.	A
	3. Antihypertensive therapy should be administered to patients with hypertension and PAD to reduce the risk of MI, stroke, heart failure, and cardiovascular (CV) death.	A
	4. Patients with PAD who smoke cigarettes or use other forms of tobacco should be advised at every visit to quit.	A
	5. Patients with PAD who smoke cigarettes should be assisted in developing a plan for quitting that includes pharmacotherapy (varenicline, bupropion, and/or nicotine replacement therapy) and/or referral to a smoking cessation program.	A
	6. Patients with PAD should avoid exposure to environmental tobacco smoke at work, at home, and in public places.	B-NR
	7. Management of diabetes mellitus in the patient with PAD should be coordinated between members of the health care team.	C-EO
	8. Cilostazol is an effective therapy to improve symptoms and increase walking distance in patients with claudication.	A
	9. Patients with PAD should have an annual influenza vaccination.	C-EO
IIa	1. In asymptomatic patients with PAD (ABI ≤0.90), antiplatelet therapy is reasonable to reduce the risk of MI, stroke, or vascular death.	C-EO
	2. The use of angiotensin-converting enzyme inhibitors or angiotensin receptor blockers can be effective to reduce the risk of CV ischemic events in patients with PAD.	A
	3. Glycemic control can be beneficial for patients with CLI to reduce limb-related outcomes.	B-NR
IIb	1. In asymptomatic patients with borderline ABI (0.91-0.99), the usefulness of antiplatelet therapy to reduce the risk of MI, stroke, or vascular death is uncertain.	B-R
	2. The effectiveness of dual-antiplatelet therapy (aspirin and clopidogrel) to reduce the risk of CV ischemic events in patients with symptomatic PAD is not well established.	B-R
	3. Dual-antiplatelet therapy (aspirin and clopidogrel) may be reasonable to reduce the risk of limb-related events in patients with symptomatic PAD after lower extremity revascularization.	C-LD
	4. The overall clinical benefit of vorapaxar added to existing antiplatelet therapy in patients with symptomatic PAD is uncertain.	B-R
	5. The usefulness of anticoagulation to improve patency after lower extremity autogenous vein or prosthetic bypass is uncertain.	B-R
III	1. Anticoagulation should not be used to reduce the risk of CV ischemic events in patients with PAD.	A
	2. Pentoxifylline is not effective for treatment of claudication.	B-R
	3. Chelation therapy (e.g., ethylenediaminetetraacetic acid) is not beneficial for treatment of claudication.	B-R
	4. B-complex vitamin supplementation to lower homocysteine levels for prevention of CV events in patients with PAD is not recommended.	B-R

ABI, Ankle-brachial index; *ACCF,* American College of Cardiology Foundation; *AHA,* American Heart Association; *CLI,* critical limb ischemia; *COR,* class of recommendation; *CV,* cardiovascular; *LOE,* level of evidence; *MI,* myocardial infarction; *PAD,* peripheral artery disease.
From Zipes DP: *Braunwald's heart disease: a textbook of cardiovascular medicine,* ed 11, Philadelphia, 2019, Elsevier.

pharmacotherapy and should have a reasonable likelihood of symptomatic improvement with an acceptable surgical risk and technical factors favoring surgical vs. endovascular approach.
  b. Autogenous vein graft is superior to prosthetic graft if surgical revascularization is performed (Class I).
  c. Iliac or femoropopliteal disease with long segments; multifocal segments; long segment occlusions; and eccentric, calcified stenosis, which are less amenable to percutaneous interventions.
  d. Surgical intervention is not indicated to prevent progression to limb-threatening ischemia in patients with IC as generally claudication does not progress to severe ischemia.
3. Revascularization for ALI (Table 7):
  a. Management approach is dependent on whether affected limb is viable, threatened, or irreversible. Initial management will depend on the absence of sensation and movement. If absent, then urgent surgery should be considered.
  b. Heparin should be given to all patients with ALI; direct thrombin inhibitor is used if patient has history of HIT.

  c. Catheter-based thrombolysis is effective in ALI with salvageable limb.
  d. Amputation should be performed in patients with irreversible damage.
4. Rivaroxaban 2.5 mg PO bid is now FDA approved to reduce the risk of major thrombotic vascular events in patients with PAD, including those who have recently undergone a lower extremity revascularization procedure for symptomatic PAD.

DISPOSITION

Risk factors for atherosclerosis should be assessed, and appropriate modification instituted. Focus should be placed on smoking cessation, dietary adjustment, and pharmacotherapy for dyslipidemia, hyperglycemia, and hypertension. All patients with PAD should receive aspirin therapy unless contraindicated. Revascularization should be considered for refractory lifestyle-limiting symptoms.

More than one in six patients with peripheral arterial disease who undergo peripheral arterial revascularization have unplanned readmission within 30 days with high associated mortality risks and costs. Procedure- and patient-related factors were the primary reasons for readmission.[13]

REFERRAL

Consultation with vascular medicine, vascular surgery, interventional cardiology, or other physicians with expertise in PAD is recommended in patients with rest pain, functional disability from pain, ABI <0.90 at rest, or any physical signs of limb ischemia or gangrene.

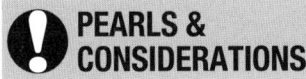

PEARLS & CONSIDERATIONS

COMMENTS
- PAD is a highly prevalent disease process that remains underdiagnosed and undertreated.
- Patients with PAD are at markedly higher risk of future coronary, cerebrovascular, and other vascular events.
- Medical treatment is aimed mainly at cardiovascular risk factor modification, except for cilostazol.
- Studies of the natural history of claudication show the relative safety of initial conservative treatment of PAD in the absence of CLI.
- When PAD limits a patient's ability to walk and exercise, revascularization should be considered.

TABLE 3 Approved Medical Therapies for Patients With Peripheral Artery Disease

Therapy	Mechanism of Action	Key Clinical Trials	INDICATIONS European Medicines Agency	European Society of Cardiology	FDA	ACC/AHA
Statin (Class effect)	Cholesterol-lowering HMG-CoA reductase inhibitor	Heart Protection Study 3% RRR with simvastatin 40 mg/day vs. placebo in all-cause mortality, 18% RRR in coronary heart death Approval for PAD based on subgroup of 6748 patients, 2700 had PAD and no CHD	Reduction in MACE and mortality	Class I for lipid lowering with LDL <2.5 mmol/L, optimally <1.8 mmol/L	Reduction in MACE and mortality	Class I, LOE A
ACEI or ARB (Class effect)	Blood pressure lowering and other vascular effects Renin-angiotensin system inhibition	HOPE 22% RRR with ramipril 10 mg daily vs. placebo for composite of MI, stroke, or CV death Approval for PAD based on subgroup of 4051 patients, 1725 with "clinical PAD"	Reduction in MACE	Class I for blood pressure lowering to ≤40/90 mm Hg	Reduction in MACE	Class I, LOE A for antihypertensive therapy Class IIa, LOE A for ACEI/ARB specifically
Clopidogrel	Antiplatelet P2Y$_{12}$ inhibitor	CAPRIE 8.7% RRR vs. aspirin for composite of ischemic stroke, MI, or vascular death Approval for PAD based on subgroup of 6452 patients	As monotherapy Reduction in MACE	Class I monotherapy for risk reduction Class I added to ASA after lower-extremity stenting	As monotherapy Reduction in MACE	Class I, LOE A for monotherapy Class IIb, LOE B-R, C-LD, when added to aspirin as DAPT
Vorapaxar	Antiplatelet PAR-1 antagonist	TRA2P-TIMI 50 20% RRR vs. placebo for composite of MI, stroke, or CV death Approval for PAD based on subgroup of 3787 patients	Added to aspirin or clopidogrel Reduction in MACE, limb benefits mentioned	Approved after most recent guidelines	Added to aspirin and/or clopidogrel Reduction in MACE	Class IIb, LOE B-R added to aspirin and/or clopidogrel
Pentoxifylline	Decreases blood viscosity Mechanism not fully understood	Meta-analysis of six studies including 788 patients who showed minimal increase in maximal walking distance with (+59 m)	Improve function and symptoms in patients with intermittent claudication	Described but no clear recommendation	Improve function and symptoms in patients with intermittent claudication	Class III, LOE B-R
Cilostazol	Antiplatelet and vasodilator Mechanism not fully understood	50 mg bid ($n = 303$), 100 mg bid ($n = 998$), and placebo ($n = 973$) Improvement in maximal walking distance with 100 mg bid, expressed as the percent mean change from baseline, 28%-100% vs. placebo, which were −10%-41%	Reduction of symptoms of intermittent claudication, as indicated by an increased walking distance	Class I for symptoms	Reduction of symptoms of intermittent claudication, as indicated by an increased walking distance	Class I, LOE A

ACC/AHA, American College of Cardiology/American Heart Association; *ACEI,* angiotensin-converting enzyme inhibitor; *ARB,* angiotensin receptor blocker; *bid,* twice daily; *ASA,* acetylsalicylic acid; *CAPRIE,* Clopidogrel versus Aspirin in Patients at Risk of Ischaemic Events; *CHD,* coronary heart disease; *CV,* cardiovascular; *DAPT,* dual-antiplatelet therapy; *FDA,* U.S. Food and Drug Administration; *HOPE,* Heart Outcomes Prevention Evaluation; *LDL,* low-density lipoprotein; *LOE,* level of evidence *(B-R,* moderate-quality evidence from one or more randomized clinical trials; *C-LD,* randomized or nonrandomized observational/registry studies or a meta-analysis); *MACE,* major adverse cardiovascular events; *MI,* myocardial infarction; *PAR-1,* protease-activated receptor 1; *RRR,* relative risk reduction; *TRA2P-TIMI 50,* Thrombin Receptor Antagonist in Secondary Prevention of Atherothrombotic Ischemic Events–Thrombolysis in Myocardial Infarction.
From Zipes DP: *Braunwald's heart disease: a textbook of cardiovascular medicine,* ed 11, Philadelphia, 2019, Elsevier.

TABLE 4 ACCF/AHA Guidelines for Exercise Therapy in Patients With Peripheral Artery Disease

COR	Indication	LOE
I	1. In patients with claudication, a supervised exercise program is recommended to improve functional status and quality of life and to reduce leg symptoms.	A
	2. A supervised exercise program should be discussed as a treatment option for claudication before possible revascularization.	B-R
IIa	1. In patients with PAD, a structured community- or home-based exercise program with behavioral change techniques can be beneficial to improve walking ability and functional status.	A
	2. In patients with claudication, alternative strategies of exercise therapy, including upper-body ergometry, cycling, and pain-free or low-intensity walking that avoids moderate to maximum claudication while walking, can be beneficial to improve walking ability and functional status.	A

COR, Class of recommendation; *LOE*, level of evidence; *PAD*, peripheral artery disease.
From Zipes DP: *Braunwald's heart disease: a textbook of cardiovascular medicine,* ed 11, Philadelphia, 2019, Elsevier.

TABLE 5 ACCF/AHA Guidelines for Revascularization of Patients With Peripheral Artery Disease

COR	Indication	LOE
I	1. In patients with CLI, revascularization should be performed when possible to minimize tissue loss.	B-NR
	2. An evaluation for revascularization options should be performed by an interdisciplinary care team before amputation in the patient with CLI.	C-EO
	3. Endovascular procedures are recommended to establish in-line blood flow to the foot in patients with nonhealing wounds or gangrene.	B-R
	4. Surgical procedures are recommended to establish in-line blood flow to the foot in patients with nonhealing wounds or gangrene.	C-LD
	5. When surgery is performed for CLI, bypass to the popliteal or infrapopliteal arteries (i.e., tibial, pedal) should be constructed with suitable autogenous vein.	A
	6. Endovascular procedures are effective as a revascularization option for patients with lifestyle-limiting claudication and hemodynamically significant aortoiliac occlusive disease.	A
	7. When surgical revascularization is performed, bypass to the popliteal artery with autogenous vein is recommended in preference to prosthetic graft material.	A
IIa	1. Revascularization is a reasonable treatment option for the patient with lifestyle-limiting claudication with an inadequate response to GDMT.	A
	2. Endovascular procedures are reasonable as a revascularization option for patients with lifestyle-limiting claudication and hemodynamically significant femoropopliteal disease.	B-R
	3. Surgical procedures are reasonable as a revascularization option for patients with lifestyle-limiting claudication with inadequate response to GDMT, acceptable perioperative risk, and technical factors suggesting advantages over endovascular procedures.	B-NR
	4. A staged approach to endovascular procedures is reasonable in patients with ischemic rest pain.	C-LD
	5. Evaluation of lesion characteristics can be useful in selecting the endovascular approach for CLI.	B-R
	6. In patients with CLI for whom endovascular revascularization has failed and a suitable autogenous vein is not available, prosthetic material can be effective for bypass to the below-knee popliteal and tibial arteries.	B-NR
	7. A staged approach to surgical procedures is reasonable in patients with ischemic rest pain.	C-LD
IIb	1. The usefulness of endovascular procedures as a revascularization option for patients with claudication due to isolated infrapopliteal artery disease is unknown.	C-LD
	2. Use of angiosome-directed endovascular therapy may be reasonable for patients with CLI and nonhealing wounds or gangrene.	B-NR
III	1. Endovascular procedures should *not* be performed in patients with PAD solely to prevent progression to CLI.	B-NR
	2. Surgical procedures should not be performed in patients with PAD solely to prevent progression to CLI.	B-NR
	3. Femoral-tibial artery bypasses with prosthetic graft material should not be used for the treatment of claudication.	B-R

CLI, critical limb ischemia; *COR*, Class of recommendation; *GDMT*, guideline-directed medical therapy; *LOE*, level of evidence; *PAD*, peripheral artery disease.
From Zipes DP: *Braunwald's heart disease: a textbook of cardiovascular medicine,* ed 11, Philadelphia, 2019, Elsevier.

- Exercise training is an important and often neglected treatment strategy that has proven beneficial in improving functional status, reducing symptoms, and improving quality of life. Exercise capacity alone is the strongest predictor of mortality in patients with PAD.
- Surgical intervention should be considered in patients who meet the criteria for intervention but have lesions that are not amenable to PTA/stenting or in older patients with a low surgical risk. Advances in endovascular therapy have broadened the range of revascularization options for refractory claudication and critical ischemia and ALI in patients with multiple comorbidities.

PREVENTION

CV disease is the major cause of death in patients with IC. Therefore, the treatment of claudication is directed not only at improving walking distance but also at reducing CV risk.

PATIENT & FAMILY EDUCATION

The following organization offers more information about PAD:

- American College of Cardiology (http://www.acc.org/)

REFERENCES

Available at eBooks.Health.Elsevier.com.

AUTHORS: **MURTAZA BHARMAL, MD,** and **PRANAV M. PATEL, MD, FACC, FAHA, FSCAI**

P

Diseases and Disorders

Peripheral Artery Disease

TABLE 6 ACCF/AHA Guidelines for Wound Healing Therapies for Patients With Critical Limb Ischemia

COR	Indication	LOE
I	1. An interdisciplinary care team should evaluate and provide comprehensive care for patients with CLI and tissue loss to achieve complete wound healing and a functional foot.	B-NR
	2. In patients with CLI, wound care after revascularization should be performed with the goal of complete wound healing.	C-LD
IIb	1. In patients with CLI, intermittent pneumatic compression (arterial pump) devices may be considered to augment wound healing and/or ameliorate severe ischemic rest pain.	B-NR
	2. In patients with CLI, the effectiveness of hyperbaric oxygen therapy for wound healing is unknown.	C-LD
III	Prostanoids are not indicated in patients with CLI.	B-R

CLI, Critical limb ischemia; *COR,* class of recommendation; *LOE,* level of evidence.
From Zipes DP: *Braunwald's heart disease: a textbook of cardiovascular medicine,* ed 11, Philadelphia, 2019, Elsevier.

TABLE 7 ACCF/AHA Guidelines for Management of Patients With Acute Limb Ischemia

COR	Indication	LOE
I	1. Patients with ALI should be emergently evaluated by a clinician with sufficient experience to assess limb viability and implement appropriate therapy.	C-EO
	2. In patients with suspected ALI, initial clinical evaluation should rapidly assess limb viability and potential for salvage and does not require imaging.	C-LD
	3. In patients with ALI, systemic anticoagulation with heparin should be administered unless contraindicated.	C-EO
	4. In patients with ALI, the revascularization strategy should be determined by local resources and patient factors (e.g., etiology, degree of ischemia).	C-LD
	5. Catheter-based thrombolysis is effective for patients with ALI and a salvageable limb.	A
	6. Amputation should be performed as the first procedure in patients with a nonsalvageable limb.	C-LD
	7. Patients with ALI should be monitored and treated (e.g., fasciotomy) for compartment syndrome after revascularization.	C-LD
	8. In the patient with ALI, a comprehensive history should be obtained to determine the cause of thrombosis and/or embolization.	C-EO
IIa	1. In patients with ALI with a salvageable limb, percutaneous mechanical thrombectomy can be useful as adjunctive therapy to thrombolysis.	B-NR
	2. In patients with ALI due to embolism and with a salvageable limb, surgical thromboembolectomy can be effective.	C-LD
	3. In the patient with a history of ALI, testing for a cardiovascular cause of thromboembolism can be useful.	C-EO
IIb	The usefulness of ultrasound-accelerated catheter-based thrombolysis for patients with ALI with a salvageable limb is unknown.	C-LD

ACCF, American College of Cardiology Foundation; *AHA,* American Heart Association; *ALI,* acute limb ischemia; *COR,* class of recommendation; *LOE,* level of evidence.
From Zipes DP: *Braunwald's heart disease: a textbook of cardiovascular medicine,* ed 11, Philadelphia, 2019, Elsevier.

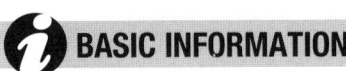
BASIC INFORMATION

DEFINITION

A perirectal abscess is a localized inflammatory process that can be associated with infections of soft tissue and anal glands based on anatomic location. Perianal and perirectal abscesses may be simple or complex, causing suppuration. Infections in these spaces may be classified as superficial perianal or perirectal with involvement in the following anatomic spaces: Ischiorectal, Intersphincteric, perianal, and supralevator. The Parks classification of anorectal abscess is subdivided into intersphincteric, transsphincteric, suprasphincteric, and extrasphincteric abscess (Fig. 1).

SYNONYMS

Rectal abscess
Perianal abscess
Anorectal abscess

ICD-10CM CODES
K61.0   Anal abscess
K61.1   Rectal abscess

EPIDEMIOLOGY & DEMOGRAPHICS

INCIDENCE (IN U.S.): Commonly encountered
PREDOMINANT SEX: Male > female
PREDOMINANT AGE: All ages
PEAK INCIDENCE: Not seasonal; common
GENETICS: None known

PHYSICAL FINDINGS & CLINICAL PRESENTATION

- Localized perirectal or anal pain—often worsened with movement or straining
- Perirectal erythema or cellulitis
- Perirectal mass by inspection or palpation
- Fever and signs of sepsis with deep abscess
- Urinary retention

ETIOLOGY

- Polymicrobial aerobic and anaerobic bacteria involving one of the anatomic spaces (see "Definition"), often associated with localized trauma
- Microbiology: Most infections are polymicrobial, mixed enteric, and skin flora
- Predominant anaerobic bacteria:

1. *Bacteroides fragilis*
2. *Peptostreptococcus* spp.
3. *Prevotella* spp.
4. *Porphyromonas* spp.
5. *Clostridioides* spp.
6. *Fusobacterium* spp.
- Predominant aerobic bacteria:
1. *Staphylococcus aureus*
2. *Streptococcus* spp.
3. *Escherichia coli*
4. *Enterococcus* spp.

DIAGNOSIS

Many patients will have predisposing underlying conditions including:
- Malignancy or leukemia
- Immune deficiency
- Diabetes mellitus
- Recent surgery
- Steroid therapy

DIFFERENTIAL DIAGNOSIS

- Neutropenic enterocolitis
- Crohn disease (inflammatory bowel disease)
- Pilonidal disease
- Hidradenitis suppurativa
- Tuberculosis or actinomycosis; Chagas disease
- Cancerous lesions
- Chronic anal fistula
- Rectovaginal fistula
- Proctitis—often STD-associated, including syphilis, gonococcal, chlamydia, chancroid, condylomata acuminata
- AIDS-associated: Kaposi sarcoma, lymphoma, cytomegalovirus

WORKUP

- Examination of rectal, perirectal/perineal areas
- Rule out necrotic process and crepitance suggesting deep tissue involvement
- Local aerobic and anaerobic culture
- Blood cultures if toxic, febrile, or compromised
- Possible sigmoidoscopy

IMAGING STUDIES

Usually not indicated unless extensive disease is suspected. CT has a sensitivity of 77% and is relatively poor in detecting a perirectal abscess in immunocompromised patients.

TREATMENT

ACUTE GENERAL Rx

- Incision and drainage of abscess
- Debridement of necrotic tissue
- Rule out need for fistulectomy
- Local wound care—packing
- Sitz baths
- Antibiotic treatment: Directed toward coverage for mixed skin and enteric flora

OUTPATIENT—ORAL:
- Trimethoprim/sulfamethoxazole DS bid or ciprofloxacin 500 mg bid or levofloxacin 500 mg q24h plus metronidazole 500 mg q8h × 7 to 10 days
- Amoxicillin/clavulanic acid 875 to 1000 mg 1 tabs bid
- Clindamycin 150 to 300 mg PO q6 to 8h

INPATIENT—INTRAVENOUS:
- Piperacillin/tazobactam 3.375 g IV q6 to 8h
- Ampicillin/sulbactam 1.5 to 3 g IV q6h
- Cefotetan 1 to 2 g IV q8h
- Imipenem or meropenem 500 to 1000 mg IV q8h

DISPOSITION

Follow-up with a general surgeon or infectious disease physician is often warranted.

REFERRAL

- General surgeon or colorectal surgeon for drainage.
- AIDS specialist may be needed for perirectal complications of HIV infection.
- Gastroenterologist follow-up may be warranted in Crohn disease with perirectal fistula and other complications.
- Endoscopic ultrasound–guided perirectal abscess drainage is a recently described promising alternative treatment.

PEARLS & CONSIDERATIONS

Perirectal abscess may be a presenting manifestation of type 2 diabetes mellitus in older adults. Check the blood sugar in patients to exclude the possibility of undiagnosed diabetes mellitus.

SUGGESTED READINGS
Available at eBooks.Health.Elsevier.com.

RELATED CONTENT
Perirectal Abscess (Patient Information)

AUTHOR: **GLENN G. FORT, MD, MPH**

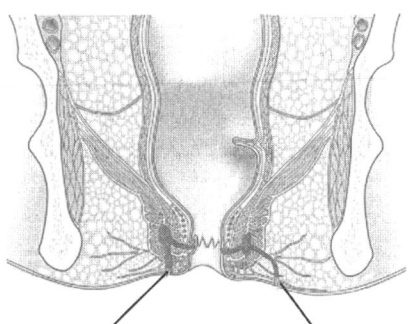
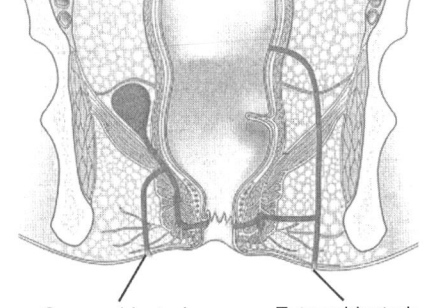

Intersphincteric   Trans-sphincteric   Suprasphincteric   Extrasphincteric

FIG. 1 Parks classification of anorectal abscess. (From Cameron JL, Cameron AM: *Current surgical therapy,* ed 10, Philadelphia, 2011, Saunders.)

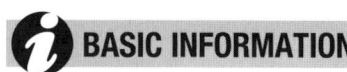

BASIC INFORMATION

DEFINITION

Peritonitis refers to the acute onset of severe abdominal pain caused by peritoneal inflammation.

Secondary peritonitis is peritonitis stemming from another condition; commonly a defect in an abdominal viscus.

SYNONYMS

Acute abdomen
Surgical abdomen

ICD-10CM CODES

K65.0	Generalized (acute) peritonitis
K65.8	Other peritonitis
K65.9	Peritonitis, unspecified
A18.31	Tuberculous peritonitis
A54.85	Gonococcal peritonitis
A74.81	Chlamydial peritonitis
K35.2	Acute appendicitis with generalized peritonitis
K35.3	Acute appendicitis with localized peritonitis
K65.2	Spontaneous bacterial peritonitis
N73.3	Female acute pelvic peritonitis
N73.4	Female chronic pelvic peritonitis
N73.5	Female pelvic peritonitis, unspecified
P78.1	Other neonatal peritonitis

EPIDEMIOLOGY & DEMOGRAPHICS

Common presentation as a result of diverse etiologies; for example, 5% to 10% of the population has acute appendicitis at some point in their lives.

PHYSICAL FINDINGS & CLINICAL PRESENTATION

- Acute abdominal pain
- Abdominal distention and ascites
- Abdominal rigidity, rebound, and guarding
- Altered mental status
- Fever, chills
- Exacerbation with movement
- Anorexia, nausea, and vomiting
- Constipation or diarrhea
- Decreased bowel sounds
- Hypotension and tachycardia
- Tachypnea, dyspnea

ETIOLOGY

- One of the early steps is disturbance in gut flora with overgrowth and extraintestinal organismal overtake. Most common are gram-negative bacteria *(Escherichia coli, Enterobacter, Klebsiella, Proteus)*, gram-positive bacteria (enterococci, streptococci, staphylococci), anaerobic bacteria *(Bacteroides, Clostridioides)*, and fungi.
- It can be acute perforation peritonitis: Gastrointestinal perforation, intestinal ischemia, pelvic peritonitis, and other forms.

- Postoperative peritonitis: Anastomotic leak, accidental perforation, and devascularization.
- Posttraumatic peritonitis: After blunt or penetrating abdominal trauma.

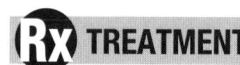

DIAGNOSIS

DIFFERENTIAL DIAGNOSIS

- Postoperative: Abscess, sepsis, bowel obstruction, injury to internal organs
- Gastrointestinal: Perforated viscus, appendicitis, inflammatory bowel disease, infectious colitis, diverticulitis, acute cholecystitis, peptic ulcer perforation, pancreatitis, bowel obstruction
- Gynecologic: Ruptured ectopic pregnancy, pelvic inflammatory disease, ruptured hemorrhagic ovarian cyst, ovarian torsion, degenerating leiomyoma
- Urologic: Nephrolithiasis, interstitial cystitis
- Miscellaneous: Abdominal trauma, penetrating wounds, infections caused by intraperitoneal dialysis

WORKUP

- Acute peritonitis is mainly a clinical diagnosis based on patient history and physical examination.
- Laboratory and imaging studies assist in determining the need for and type of intervention. Typical pretreatment peritoneal fluid and blood culture results in peritonitis are summarized in Table E1.
- If patient is hemodynamically unstable, immediate diagnostic laparotomy should be performed in lieu of adjuvant diagnostic studies.

LABORATORY TESTS

- Ascitic fluid testing
  1. Anaerobic and aerobic cultures
  2. Cell count and differential
  3. Albumin, protein, amylase, bilirubin
  4. Glucose
  5. Lactate dehydrogenase (LDH)
- CBC: Leukocytosis, left shift, anemia
- SMA7: Electrolyte imbalances, kidney dysfunction
- Liver function tests: Indicative of cirrhosis as ascites from liver disease, cholelithiasis
- Amylase: Pancreatitis
- Blood cultures: Bacteremia, sepsis
- Blood gas: Respiratory versus metabolic acidosis
- Urinalysis and culture: Urinary tract infection
- Cervical cultures for gonorrhea and *Chlamydia*
- Urine/serum human chorionic gonadotropin

IMAGING STUDIES

- Abdominal series: Free air from perforation, small or large bowel dilation from obstruction, identification of fecalith

- Chest x-ray examination: Elevated diaphragm, pneumonia
- Pelvic/abdominal ultrasound: Abscess formation, abdominal mass, intrauterine versus ectopic pregnancy, identify free fluid suggestive of hemorrhage or ascites
- Computed tomography (CT): Mass, ascites

TREATMENT

NONPHARMACOLOGIC THERAPY

- Intravenous (IV) hydration to correct dehydration, hypovolemia
- Blood transfusion to correct anemia from hemorrhage
- Nasogastric decompression, especially if obstruction is present
- Oxygen: Intubation if necessary
- Bed rest

ACUTE GENERAL Rx

- Surgery to correct underlying pathology, such as controlling hemorrhage, correcting perforation, and draining abscess
- Broad-spectrum antibiotics to cover both gram-negative aerobic and gram-negative anaerobic bacteria:
  1. Mild-moderate disease: Piperacillin-tazobactam 3.375 g IV q6h or 4.5 g IV q8h *or* ticarcillin-clavulanate 3.1 g IV q6h. Alternative agents are ciprofloxacin 400 mg IV q12h or levofloxacin 750 mg IV q24h *plus* metronidazole 1 g IV q12h.
  2. Severe life-threatening disease: Imipenem 500 mg IV q6h or meropenem 1 g IV q8h. Alternative agents are ampicillin *plus* metronidazole *plus* ciprofloxacin.
  3. Antibiotic therapy should be tailored to culture results and sensitivities.
- Pain control: Morphine or meperidine as needed (hold until diagnosis confirmed)

DISPOSITION

Depends on etiology of peritonitis, age of patient, coexisting medical disease, and duration of process before presentation.

REFERRAL

Surgical consultation is required in all cases of acute peritonitis.

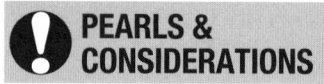

PEARLS & CONSIDERATIONS

CT scan guides therapeutic approach and should be considered as the primary imaging study if available. As with forms of sepsis, early administration of broad-spectrum antibiotics, fluid resuscitation, and rapidly obtaining anatomic source control (when appropriate) will lead to improved outcomes.

AUTHOR: **GHAMAR BITAR, MD**

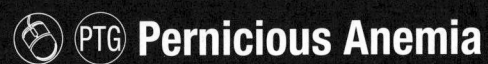

 BASIC INFORMATION

DEFINITION

Pernicious anemia (PA) is an autoimmune disease resulting from antibodies against gastric intrinsic factor and gastric parietal cells that results in vitamin B_{12} deficiency leading to megaloblastic anemia.

SYNONYMS

Megaloblastic anemia resulting from vitamin B_{12} deficiency
Addison-Biermer anemia
Anemia, pernicious

ICD-10CM CODES
D51.0 Vitamin B_{12} deficiency anemia due to intrinsic factor deficiency
D51.8 Other vitamin B_{12} deficiency anemias
D51.9 Vitamin B_{12} deficiency anemia, unspecified
D51.1 Vitamin B_{12} deficiency anemia due to selective vitamin B_{12} malabsorption with proteinuria

EPIDEMIOLOGY & DEMOGRAPHICS

- Increased incidence in females and older adults (40 to 70 yr)
- More frequent in patients of northern European ancestry
- Overall prevalence of undiagnosed PA after age 60 yr is 1.9%
- Prevalence is higher in women (2.7%), particularly in black women (4.3%)
- Associated with other autoimmune diseases (e.g., type 1 diabetes mellitus, Graves disease, Addison disease), along with possible *Helicobacter pylori* association

PHYSICAL FINDINGS & CLINICAL PRESENTATION[1,2]

- Mucosal pallor and/or glossitis ("beefy red tongue")
- Angular cheilosis
- Mild jaundice (representative of intramedullary hemolysis of megaloblastic cells); "lemon yellow" skin due to pallor and jaundice
- Peripheral sensory neuropathy with paresthesias initially and absent reflexes in advanced disease
- Delirium or dementia
- Worsening weakness and possible subacute combined degeneration of spinal cord (Fig. E1)
- Loss of proprioception and an unsteady gait
- Gastrointestinal symptoms including anorexia, pyrosis, nausea, and vomiting
- Possible splenomegaly and mild hepatomegaly

ETIOLOGY[3,4]

- Parietal cell antibodies are present in >70% of patients, while intrinsic factor antibodies are noted in >50% of patients.
- Atrophic gastric mucosa (Fig. E2) with achlorhydria.
- Inborn errors of cobalamin-cofactor synthesis are rare. Fig. E3 illustrates the components and mechanism of cobalamin absorption. An etiopathophysiologic classification of cobalamin deficiency is described in Section II.

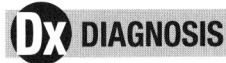 DIAGNOSIS

DIFFERENTIAL DIAGNOSIS

- Nutritional vitamin B_{12} deficiency
- Malabsorption (e.g., celiac disease)
- Chronic alcoholism (multifactorial)
- Chronic gastritis related to *H. pylori* infection
- Folic acid deficiency
- Myelodysplasia
- Thyroid abnormalities
- Atrophic gastritis
- Paraproteinemias
- Gastrectomy or use of H2 blockers
- Insufficient pancreatic enzymes (Zollinger-Ellison syndrome, chronic pancreatitis, post-Whipple procedure)

WORKUP

- The clinical presentation of PA varies with the stage. Initially, patients may be asymptomatic. In advanced stages, patients may have impaired memory, depression, gait disturbances, paresthesias, and generalized weakness.
- Investigation consists primarily of laboratory evaluation. Table 1 describes a step-wise approach to the diagnosis of cobalamin and folate deficiency.
- Endoscopy and biopsy for atrophic gastritis may be performed in selected cases.
- Diagnosis is crucial because failure to treat may result in irreversible neurologic deficits.

LABORATORY TESTS

- Complete blood count generally reveals macrocytic anemia, thrombocytopenia, and mild leukopenia with hypersegmented neutrophils (Fig. E4).
- Mean corpuscular volume (MCV) is significantly elevated in advanced stages.
- Reticulocyte count is low to normal.
- False low serum cobalamin levels can occur in patients who are pregnant or taking oral contraceptives, have multiple myeloma, have transcobalamin I (TCI) deficiency, have severe folic acid deficiency, or are taking large doses of ascorbic acid. False high normal levels in patients with cobalamin deficiency can occur in several conditions including hepatomas, severe liver disease, or monoblastic leukemias (Table 2).

TABLE 1 Stepwise Approach to the Diagnosis of Cobalamin and Folate Deficiency

Megaloblastic Anemia or Neurologic-Psychiatric Manifestations Consistent With Cobalamin Deficiency *Plus* Test Results on Serum Cobalamin and Serum Folate

Cobalamin[a] (pg/ml)	Folate[b] (ng/ml)	Provisional Diagnosis	Proceed with Metabolites?[c]
>300	>4	Cobalamin or folate deficiency is unlikely	No
<200	>4	Consistent with cobalamin deficiency	No
200-300	>4	Rule out cobalamin deficiency	Yes
>300	<2	Consistent with folate deficiency	No
<200	<2	Consistent with (1) combined cobalamin plus folate deficiency or (2) isolated folate deficiency	Yes
>300	2-4	Consistent with (1) folate deficiency or (2) an anemia unrelated to vitamin deficiency	Yes

Test Results on Metabolites: Serum Methylmalonic Acid and Total Homocysteine

Methylmalonic Acid (Normal, 70-270 nM)	Total Homocysteine (Normal, 5-14 μM)	Diagnosis
Increased	Increased	Cobalamin deficiency confirmed; folate deficiency still possible (i.e., combined cobalamin plus folate deficiency possible)
Normal	Increased	Folate deficiency is likely
Normal	Normal	Cobalamin and folate deficiency is excluded

[a]Serum cobalamin levels: Abnormally low, <200 pg/ml; clinically relevant low-normal range, 200-300 pg/ml.
[b]Serum folate levels: Abnormally low, <2 ng/ml; clinically relevant low-normal range, 2-4 ng/ml.
[c]Any frozen-over sample from serum folate/cobalamin determination can be subjected to metabolite tests.
From Hoffman R et al: *Hematology, basic principles and practice*, ed 7, Philadelphia, 2018, Saunders.

TABLE 2 Serum Cobalamin: False-Positive and False-Negative Test Results

Falsely Low Serum Cobalamin in the Absence of True Cobalamin Deficiency

- Folate deficiency (one third of patients)
- Multiple myeloma
- TCI deficiency
- Megadose vitamin C therapy
- Pregnancy
- Oral contraceptives

Falsely Raised Cobalamin Levels in the Presence of a True Deficiency[a]

- Cobalamin binders (TCI and II) increased (e.g., myeloproliferative states, hepatomas, and fibrolamellar hepatic tumors)
- TCII-producing macrophages are activated (e.g., autoimmune diseases, monoblastic leukemias and lymphomas)
- Release of cobalamin from hepatocytes (e.g., active liver disease)
- High serum anti-IF antibody titer

IF, Intrinsic factor; *TC,* transcobalamin.
[a]Although a low serum cobalamin level is not synonymous with cobalamin deficiency, 5% of patients with true cobalamin deficiency have low-normal cobalamin levels, a potentially serious problem because the patient's underlying cobalamin deficiency will progress if uncorrected.
From Hoffman R et al: *Hematology, basic principles and practice,* ed 6, Philadelphia, 2013, Saunders.

- The absence of anemia or macrocytosis does not exclude the diagnosis of cobalamin deficiency. Anemia is absent in 20% of patients with cobalamin deficiency, and macrocytosis is absent in >30% of patients at the time of diagnosis. Macrocytosis can be masked by concurrent iron deficiency, anemia of chronic disease, or thalassemia trait.
- Laboratory tests used for detecting cobalamin deficiency in patients with normal vitamin B_{12} levels include serum and urinary methylmalonic acid (MMA) level (elevated), total homocysteine level (elevated), and intrinsic factor antibody (positive). Cobalamin is a cofactor for the enzymes L-methylmalonyl coenzyme A mutase and methionine synthase. Inadequate levels of cobalamin will thus result in increased MMA and homocysteine levels. Plasma MMA levels can also be used to differentiate cobalamin deficiency from folate deficiency because patients with folate deficiency have normal or mild elevations of MMA levels.
- An increased concentration of plasma MMA does not predict clinical manifestations of vitamin B_{12} deficiency and should not be used as the only marker for diagnosis of B_{12} deficiency.
- Additional laboratory abnormalities can include elevated lactate dehydrogenase, direct hyperbilirubinemia, and decreased

haptoglobin, due to rapid destruction of red blood cells.
- Bone marrow aspirate is not necessary to diagnose cobalamin deficiency. It may show giant C-shaped neutrophil bands and megaloblastic normoblasts (Fig. E5).
- Schilling test: No longer used. It was historically used to identify the locus of cobalamin malabsorption and the cause of cobalamin deficiency.

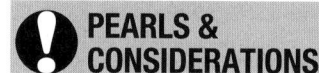

Ⓡ TREATMENT[5-7]

NONPHARMACOLOGIC THERAPY

Avoid folic acid supplementation without proper vitamin B_{12} supplementation. Folic acid supplementation alone may result in hematologic remission in patients with vitamin B_{12} deficiency but will not treat or prevent neurologic manifestations.

ACUTE GENERAL Rx

Traditional therapy of cobalamin deficiency consists of intramuscular (IM) or deep subcutaneous (SC) injections of vitamin B_{12} 1000 mcg/day for 1 wk, followed by 1000 mcg/mo, indefinitely. Monitor response and increase dosing if serum B_{12} levels decline.

CHRONIC Rx

- Parenteral vitamin B_{12} 1000 mcg/mo or intranasal cyanocobalamin 500 mcg/wk for the remainder of life.
- In patients who have no nervous system involvement, intranasal cyanocobalamin may be used in place of parenteral cyanocobalamin after hematologic parameters have returned to normal range. Macrocytosis correction can be noted during the first month of treatment. The initial dose of intranasal cyanocobalamin is 1 spray (500 mcg) in one nostril once per week. Nasal cyanocobalamin is expensive.
- Oral cobalamin (1000 to 2000 mcg/day) is also being effective in mild cases of pernicious anemia because approximately 1% of an oral dose is absorbed by passive diffusion, a pathway that does not require intrinsic factor. Cost for 1 mo of therapy is approximately $5. Consider returning to IM vitamin B_{12} supplementation if decline recurs.

DISPOSITION

Anemia generally resolves with appropriate cobalamin replacement therapy. Neurologic deficits, on the other hand, may be corrected only if treated early on.

REFERRAL

Gastroenterology referral for endoscopy on diagnosis of PA followed by periodic surveillance endoscopies to rule out gastric adenocarcinoma or carcinoid tumors.

TABLE 3 Causes of Megaloblastosis Not Responding to Therapy With Cobalamin or Folate

Wrong Diagnosis

Combined folate and cobalamin deficiencies being treated with only one vitamin

Associated iron deficiency

Associated hemoglobinopathy (e.g., sickle cell disease, thalassemia)

Associated anemia of chronic disease

Associated hypothyroidism

From Hoffman R et al: *Hematology, basic principles and practice,* ed 7, Philadelphia, 2018, Elsevier.

❶ PEARLS & CONSIDERATIONS

COMMENTS

- Early manifestations of negative cobalamin balance are increased serum methylmalonic acid and total homocysteine levels. This occurs when the total cobalamin in serum is still in the low-normal range.
- Vitamin B_{12} deficiency that is allowed to progress for longer than 3 mo may produce permanent degenerative lesions of the spinal cord (e.g., subacute combined degeneration of spinal cord).
- Vitamin B_{12} deficiency may suppress signs of polycythemia vera; treatment of B_{12} deficiency may unmask this disorder.
- Blunted or impeded therapeutic response to vitamin B_{12} may be due to concurrent iron or folic acid deficiency, uremia, infections, or use of drugs with bone marrow suppressant properties. Causes of megaloblastosis not responding to therapy with cobalamin or folate are summarized in Table 3.
- Drugs that interfere with B_{12} absorption include metformin, colchicine, neomycin, and aminosalicylic acid.
- Patients must understand that cobalamin replacement therapy is lifelong.
- Self-injection of vitamin B_{12} may be taught in selected patients. Cost of monthly injections is less than $10.
- Patients who have had bariatric surgery should receive 1 mg of oral vitamin B_{12} per day indefinitely.

REFERENCES
Available at eBooks.Health.Elsevier.com.

RELATED CONTENT
Pernicious Anemia (Patient Information)

AUTHOR: **SHIVA KUMAR R. MUKKAMALLA, MD, MPH, FACP**

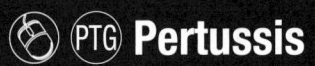

P

BASIC INFORMATION

DEFINITION

Pertussis is a prolonged infection of the upper respiratory tract caused by the bacterium *Bordetella pertussis* and characterized by paroxysms of an intense cough. Humans are the only known host.[1] Infection is spread by respiratory droplets, with an incubation period of 7 to 10 days.[1,2]

SYNONYM

Whooping cough

ICD-10CM CODES

A37.00	Whooping cough due to *Bordetella pertussis* without pneumonia
A37.01	Whooping cough due to *Bordetella pertussis* with pneumonia
A37.10	Whooping cough due to *Bordetella parapertussis* without pneumonia
A37.11	Whooping cough due to *Bordetella parapertussis* with pneumonia
A37.80	Whooping cough due to other *Bordetella* spp. without pneumonia
A37.81	Whooping cough due to other *Bordetella* spp. with pneumonia
A37.90	Whooping cough, unspecified species without pneumonia
A37.91	Whooping cough, unspecified species with pneumonia

EPIDEMIOLOGY & DEMOGRAPHICS

INCIDENCE (IN U.S.):

- Reported pertussis cases to the CDC from 2021 were 1609, for an overall incidence of 0.5/100,000.[3] This is decreased from 2019 when 18,617 cases were reported, for an overall incidence of 5.7/100,000.[4] Seven deaths were reported in 2019 whereas four deaths were reported in 2021.[3,4]
- Primarily a disease of infants, children, and adolescents, although can affect all ages.

PREDOMINANT AGE:

- Infants age <1 yr, usually from underimmunized status[3]
- Children and adults, usually from waning immunity[1,6,7]

PEAK INCIDENCE:

- Children <6 mo (3.6/100,000), 30.8% of whom required hospitalization.[3]
- Children 6 to 11 mo (4.1/100,000), 2.3% of whom required hospitalization.[3]
- Incidence of infection declines with age.
- Pertussis can be transmitted year-round but peak infection rates occur in late summer through fall.[5]

PHYSICAL FINDINGS & CLINICAL PRESENTATION

- Infection is characterized by three phases: Catarrhal, paroxysmal, and convalescent.[1,5,8]
- Catarrhal phase: Usually begins with a 1- to 2-wk prodrome that resembles a common cold. This phase may be mild or absent in adolescents and adults given partial immunity from prior immunization. This is typically the most contagious phase.[5]

- After this initial phase, increased production of mucus occurs. Excessive lacrimation and conjunctival infection should heighten the suspicion for pertussis.
- Paroxysmal phase: Increased mucus production is followed by an intense, paroxysmal cough, typically 5 to 10 coughs during a single expiration, ending with gasps and an inspiratory whoop.[1] Whoop can be absent in infants <6 mo and in immunized patients.[5,8]
- Cough tends to be more frequent at night.[8]
- In some children, apnea and cyanosis are noted; posttussive gagging and vomiting are characteristic of pertussis.[5,8] Fever is typically absent or minimal.
- Cases can be severe and life-threatening in young infants, particularly children <6 mo, and in rare cases has been associated with sudden death. Mortality is usually from prolonged paroxysms leading to frank exhaustion and apnea.
- The paroxysmal phase lasts from 2 wk to 2 mo.[1,8]
- Convalescent phase: Lasts over 2 mo and is characterized by cough of decreasing severity. Other respiratory infections during this stage may lead to worsening of paroxysms.[1]
- Complications include apnea, respiratory failure, secondary bacterial pneumonia (most common), anorexia, rectal prolapse, seizures, encephalopathy, periorbital edema, subconjunctival hemorrhage, petechiae, subcutaneous emphysema, pneumothorax, and pneumomediastinum.[8,9]

ETIOLOGY

Bordetella pertussis, a gram-negative rod that adheres to human cilia and respiratory epithelia[2]

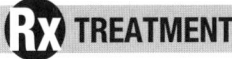 DIAGNOSIS

DIFFERENTIAL DIAGNOSIS

- Croup
- Epiglottitis
- Foreign body aspiration
- Bacterial pneumonia
- Viral pneumonia
- Bronchiolitis
- Asthma exacerbation

WORKUP

- Thorough history and physical exam may provide a clinical diagnosis of pertussis. Providers should screen for specific symptoms in adults/adolescents: Paroxysmal cough, nighttime cough, posttussive vomiting, inspiratory whooping, and absence of fever.
- Culture of bacteria is the gold standard laboratory test and most specific.[9] Culture should be from nasopharyngeal specimen by aspiration or by swabbing the posterior nasopharynx with a polyester-tipped, flocked-rayon, or calcium alginate swab.[9] Highest isolation rate within the first 2 wk of infection. False negatives tend to present after first 2 wk of infection, in previously vaccinated patients, and in patients who have received antibiotics.[9]

- Polymerase chain reaction (PCR) is the most sensitive method for rapid detection of pertussis.[9] PCR testing should be used only to confirm a diagnosis in persons with signs and symptoms consistent with pertussis. PCR testing sensitivity declines and is unlikely to be positive after 4 wk of infection.[9] PCR testing after 5 days of treatment with antibiotics can cause false-negative results and is generally not recommended. PCR testing should be paired with culture for outbreak identification.[1,9]
- Serologic tests for immunoglobulin G (IgG) can be considered 2 to 8 wk after symptom onset if other tests are negative/likely to be negative.[9]
- Chest x-ray if there is concern for concomitant pneumonia.

LABORATORY TESTS

CBC, which usually demonstrates marked leukocytosis (as high as 60,000) and marked lymphocytosis[10]:
Up to 18,000 lymphocytes
- 70% to 80% of total WBCs are lymphocytes

IMAGING STUDIES

Chest x-ray examination is of value if secondary bacterial pneumonia is suspected.

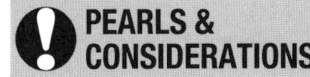 TREATMENT

NONPHARMACOLOGIC THERAPY

- Adequate hydration
- Control of secretions
- Maintenance of airway

ACUTE GENERAL Rx

Antibiotics (Table 1) are indicated:
- Azithromycin, clarithromycin, or erythromycin is recommended for child care workers in close contact with infected children and for all household contacts. Antimicrobial therapy should be given to all persons at high risk of severe disease from pertussis and who were in contact with a pertussis case within 21 days of cough onset: TMP/SMX can be given in two oral doses per day for those who do not tolerate macrolides.

DISPOSITION

- Hospitalization and observation for apnea in infants <4 mo should be considered with younger age, report of color change, and other interventions being predictors of complicated hospital course.[5,11]

REFERRAL

To intensive care setting for life-threatening infections:
- Pulmonologist
- Infectious disease specialist

PEARLS & CONSIDERATIONS

- The diagnosis of pertussis in a young child is easily recognized, but in adolescents and

TABLE 1 Recommended Antimicrobial Treatment and Postexposure Prophylaxis for Pertussis, by Age Group

| Age Group | PRIMARY AGENTS | | ALTERNATIVE AGENT* | |
	Azithromycin	Erythromycin	Clarithromycin	Trimethoprim-Sulfamethoxazole (TMP-SMZ)
<1 mo	Recommended agent. 10 mg/kg/day in a single dose for 5 days (only limited safety data available)	Not preferred. Erythromycin is substantially associated with infantile hypertrophic pyloric stenosis. Use if azithromycin is unavailable; 40 mg/kg/day in 4 divided doses for 14 days	Not recommended (safety data unavailable)	Contraindicated for infants aged <2 mo (risk for kernicterus)
1-5 mo	10 mg/kg/day in a single dose for 5 days	40 mg/kg/day in 4 divided doses for 14 days	15 mg/kg/day in 2 divided doses for 7 days	Contraindicated at age <2 mo. For infants aged ≥2 mo: TMP 8 mg/kg/day plus SMZ 40 mg/kg/day in 2 divided doses for 14 days
Infants aged ≥6 mo and children	10 mg/kg in a single dose on day 1 (maximum 500 mg), then 5 mg/kg/day (maximum 250 mg) on days 2-5	40 mg/kg/day (maximum 2 g/day) in 4 divided doses for 7-14 days	15 mg/kg/day in 2 divided doses (maximum 1 g/day) for 7 days	TMP 8 mg/kg/day plus SMZ 40 mg/kg/day in 2 divided doses (maximum 320 mg TMP/day and 1600 mg SMX/day) for 14 days
Adolescents and adults	500 mg in a single dose on day 1, then 250 mg/day on days 2-5	2 g/day in 4 divided doses for 7-14 days	1 g/day in 2 divided doses for 7 days	TMP 320 mg/day, SMZ 1600 mg/day in 2 divided doses for 14 days

SMZ, Sulfamethoxazole; *TMP,* trimethoprim.

From Centers for Disease Control and Prevention: Recommended antimicrobial agents for treatment and postexposure prophylaxis of pertussis: 2005 CDC guidelines, MMWR Morbid Mortal Wkly Rep 54:1-16, 2005. With Data From Committee on Infectious Diseases AA of P, Kimberlin DW, Barnett ED, Lynfield R, Sawyer MH, eds. Pertussis (Whooping Cough). In: Red Book: 2021 -2024 Report of the Committee on Infectious Diseases. American Academy of Pediatrics; 2021:0. doi:10.1542/9781610025782-S3_102

adults pertussis can be a subtle diagnosis and is often missed. The tip-off is often a persistent, hacking, and productive cough with minor or no fever in a previously healthy person that lasts >2 wk.
- Prevention through vaccination remains the standard in limiting pertussis.
  1. Universal vaccination is advised for all children and adults. Children are recommended to receive the five-dose DTaP series at months 2, 4, 6, and 15 to 18 and at ages 4 to 6 yr.[9]

2. A booster Tdap should be provided to all patients >11 yr of age.[9]
3. Tdap should be administered during each pregnancy regardless of maternal Tdap history.[9]

REFERENCES

Available at eBooks.Health.Elsevier.com.

RELATED CONTENT

Childhood and Adolescent Immunizations (Patient Information)
Pertussis (Patient Information)

AUTHORS: **MATTHEW AUTHEMENT, MD,** and **RUSSELL J. MCCULLOH, MD**

BASIC INFORMATION

DEFINITION

Sore throat may represent pain or soreness in the pharynx or surrounding anatomy. Pharyngitis specifically refers to inflammation of the pharynx. Tonsillitis refers to inflammation of the tonsils, which are situated in the rear of the pharynx. Either pharyngitis or tonsillitis may present with pain, erythema, edema, exudates or enanthems (e.g., ulcers, vesicles).[1]

SYNONYMS

Sore throat
Acute pharyngitis
Pharyngitis
Tonsillitis
Group A *Streptococcus* (GAS)
Group A beta-hemolytic *Streptococcus* (GABHS)

ICD-10CM CODES
J02.0	Streptococcal pharyngitis
J02.8	Acute pharyngitis due to other specified organisms
J02.9	Acute pharyngitis, unspecified
J03.0	Streptococcal tonsillitis
J03.8	Acute tonsillitis due to other specified organisms
J03.9	Acute tonsillitis, unspecified

EPIDEMIOLOGY & DEMOGRAPHICS

Acute pharyngitis accounts for 1% to 2% of all ambulatory care visits and 12 million outpatient visits each year in the U.S.[2]

PREDOMINANT SEX: Females = males
PREDOMINANT AGE:

- All ages are affected (children <3 yr have atypical symptoms and rarely complain of sore throat).
- Incidence peaks in childhood and adolescence, with 50% of cases before age 18 yr.
- Streptococcal pharyngitis is the most common among school-age children (ages 5 to 15 yr). GAS infections are responsible for 5% to 15% of cases of pharyngitis in adults and 35% to 40% of cases in children (ages 5 to 15 yr).

PEAK INCIDENCE:
- Late winter/early spring (GAS infections)[3]

PHYSICAL FINDINGS & CLINICAL PRESENTATION

- Pharynx:
  1. May appear normal to severely erythematous (Fig. E1).
  2. Tonsillar hypertrophy and exudates are commonly seen but do not confirm etiology.
- Common associated viral symptoms:
  1. Coryza
  2. Conjunctivitis
  3. Cough
  4. Cervical lymphadenopathy
     a. Findings associated with specific viral etiology
        (1) Herpes simplex or enterovirus infection: Exudates and vesicles
        (2) Severe acute respiratory syndrome coronavirus 2 (SARS-CoV-2): Fever, cough, diarrhea, and vomiting

     (3) Epstein-Barr virus (EBV): Malaise, cervical node enlargement
  5. Rhinorrhea
- Common candidal symptoms:
  1. Pseudomembranous white plaques on buccal mucosa, palate, tongue
- Common bacterial symptoms, especially for GAS:
  1. High fever >38° C (100.4° F)
  2. Tonsillar exudate
  3. Scarlatiniform rash
  4. Strawberry tongue
  5. Systemic signs of infection
- Rare complications associated with GAS infection:
  1. Scarlet fever
  2. Rheumatic fever
  3. Acute glomerulonephritis
  4. Streptococcal toxic shock syndrome
  5. Pediatric autoimmune neuropsychiatric disorders associated with streptococcal infections (PANDAS) syndrome
- Extension of infection (Fig. E2): Tonsillar, parapharyngeal, or retropharyngeal abscess presenting with severe pain, high fever, trismus, respiratory distress, difficulty swallowing, and drooling.
- Streptococcal tonsillitis is manifested as acute onset of fever, headache, neck pain, dysphagia, odynophagia, sore throat, otalgia, red tongue with enlargement of papillae, sore throat, red swollen uvula, palatal petechiae, and tender anterior cervical adenitis.
- Peritonsillar abscess (accumulation of pus between the tonsil and its capsule) is the most common complication of acute tonsillitis. Clinical signs include dysphagia, odynophagia, drooling, neck stiffness, deformed posterior pharynx, medial displacement of the uvula, trismus, muffled voice (hot-potato voice), and respiratory distress.
- Lingual tonsillitis is a rarely diagnosed cause of pharyngitis that predominantly occurs in patients who have had their palatine tonsils removed. The lingual tonsils are located below the inferior pole of the palatine tonsils and anterior to the vallecula at the base of the tongue. The lymphoid tissue may enlarge after tonsillectomy and repeated infections. Patients have a sore throat that worsens with movement of the tongue. Physical findings often include a normal-appearing pharynx and hyperemia. Lateral soft tissue neck films reveal a normal-appearing epiglottis and a scalloped appearance of the lingual tonsil (Fig. E3).[4]
- Box 1 describes seven danger signs in patients with sore throat.

ETIOLOGY

- Viruses:
  1. Adenovirus
  2. Coronavirus, including SARS-CoV-2
  3. Cytomegalovirus
  4. Enterovirus
  5. Epstein-Barr virus
  6. Herpes simplex virus
  7. Human metapneumovirus
  8. Influenza

  9. Parainfluenza
  10. Respiratory syncytial virus
  11. Rhinovirus
- Bacteria:
  1. GAS: The most common cause of acute tonsillitis
  2. *Fusobacterium necrophorum* (10% of pharyngitis): Highest incidence in patients ages 15 to 30 yr
  3. *Haemophilus influenzae* B
  4. *Neisseria gonorrhoeae*
  5. *Peptostreptococcus*
  6. *Prevotella*
- Other organisms:
  1. *Arcanobacterium haemolyticum*
  2. *Candida albicans*
  3. *Chlamydophila pneumoniae*
  4. *Chlamydia trachomatis*
  5. *Mycoplasma pneumoniae*

DIAGNOSIS

DIFFERENTIAL DIAGNOSIS

- Infectious: Viral, bacterial, fungal, peritonsillar abscess, Lemierre syndrome, epiglottitis, tracheitis, croup, lateral or retropharyngeal abscess, uvulitis. Table 1 summarizes characteristics of viral and bacterial pharyngitis
- Allergic/inflammatory: Allergic rhinitis/sinusitis, gastroesophageal reflux disease, Kawasaki disease, periodic fever with aphthous stomatitis, Stevens-Johnson syndrome, Behçet syndrome, angioedema, anaphylaxis, sore throat associated with granulocytopenia, thyroiditis
- Environmental exposure: Foreign body ingestion, chemical exposure (e.g., smoke), irritative pharyngitis, trauma
- Referred pain: Psychogenic pharyngitis, referred pain from dental abscess, otitis media, cervical adenitis
- Oncologic: Tonsillar hypertrophy associated with lymphoma, lymphangioma, or hemangioma of airway
- Section II describes the differential diagnosis of sore throat

---

BOX 1   Seven Danger Signs in Patients With Sore Throat

1. Persistence of symptoms longer than 1 wk without improvement
2. Respiratory difficulty, particularly stridor
3. Difficulty in handling secretions
4. Difficulty in swallowing
5. Severe pain in the absence of erythema
6. A palpable mass
7. Blood, even in small amounts, in the pharynx or ear

From Andreoli TE et al: *Andreoli and Carpenter's Cecil essentials of medicine*, ed 8, Philadelphia, 2010, Saunders.

TABLE 1 Characteristics of Viral and Bacterial Pharyngitis

	Viral Pharyngitis	Infectious Mononucleosis	Group A Streptococcal Pharyngitis	Diphtheria
Population	Any	Older Children	Peak 5-6 Yr Old	Unimmunized
Onset	Slow	Variable	Rapid	Rapid
Associated symptoms	Rhinorrhea, congestion, hoarseness, oral ulcers	General malaise, headache	Headache, otalgia, nausea, abdominal pain	None
Fever	None or low-grade	High	High	High
Sore throat severity	Mild to moderate	Moderate to severe	Severe	Severe
Dysphagia	Possible	Yes	Yes	Yes
Odynophagia	None	Yes	Yes	Yes
Toxic appearance	No	Sometimes airway obstruction	No	Yes, severe upper airway obstruction
PE findings	Pharyngeal erythema; no exudate; ± tonsil hypertrophy	Palatal petechiae ± tonsil hypertrophy ± exudate; large tender cervical lymphadenopathy; splenomegaly; hepatomegaly	Palatal petechiae, pharyngeal erythema, tonsil hypertrophy ± exudate; large tender cervical lymphadenopathy; scalariform rash; strawberry tongue	Thick exudate, pharyngeal membrane
Diagnostic testing	None	Heterophile or EBV titers	Rapid strep or strep culture	Culture on tellurite media
Treatment	Supportive	Supportive, ibuprofen, steroids, rare airway obstruction	Penicillin or amoxicillin	Antitoxin, penicillin G, amoxicillin

EBV, Epstein-Barr virus; *PE,* Physical examination.
From Flint PW et al: *Cummings otolaryngology, head and neck surgery,* ed 7, Philadelphia, 2021, Elsevier.

BOX 2 Centor Score (Modified/McIsaac) for Determining Group A Beta-Hemolytic Streptococcal Pharyngitis

- Age
- Tonsillar exudate or swelling
- Tender/swollen anterior lymphadenopathy or lymphadenitis
- Absence of cough
- History of fever 38° C (100.4° F) or higher

TABLE 3 Screening for Group A β-Hemolytic *Streptococcus* Carrier State

Screening for GABHS carrier state is not indicated except:
1. In patients with a history or family history of rheumatic fever
2. During a community outbreak of rheumatic fever, poststreptococcal glomerulonephritis, or invasive GABHS infection
3. When tonsillectomy is being considered
4. When symptomatic GABHS spreads among household members

Although both have positive throat culture results, true infections are distinguished from the carrier state by the addition of:
1. A rise in the antistreptolysin-O titer of $\geq 0.2 \log_{10}$ between the acute and convalescent phase (2-4 wk after presentation)
2. Relevant history of symptoms and signs during episode
Documented response to antibiotics

GABHS, Group A β-hemolytic *Streptococcus.*
From Flint PW et al: *Cummings otolaryngology, head and neck surgery,* ed 7, Philadelphia, 2021, Elsevier.

TABLE 2 Centor Criteria (Modified/McIsaac) Scoring for Determining Testing and Treatment for Group A Beta-Hemolytic Streptococcal Pharyngitis

Centor Score	Testing and Treatment
0-1	No further testing or antibiotics
2	Optional rapid strep testing and/or culture
3	Consider rapid strep testing and/or culture
4	Consider rapid strep testing and/or culture. Empiric antibiotics may be appropriate depending on the specific scenario

WORKUP

The Centor criteria identify patients at risk for GAS and consist of (1) fever subjective or measured >38° C (100.5° F), (2) absence of cough, (3) tonsillar exudates, and (4) tender anterior cervical lymphadenopathy. The Mcisaac criteria add 1 point for ages 3 to 14 and subtract 1 point for ages ≥45 yr (Box 2 and Table 2). Patients with ≤1 criteria are at low risk and do not need additional testing. Indications for screening for GABHS carrier state are summarized in Table 3.
- Rapid antigen detection test (RADT) (culture should be performed if RADT negative)
- Gold standard: Throat swab for culture

LABORATORY TESTS
- Testing for bacteria other than GAS is performed infrequently.
- Reserved for patients with persistent signs or symptoms suggestive of a specific non-GAS bacteria.
- For example, gonococcal testing in a sexually active patient. In a patient with suspected EBV, a CBC may show atypical lymphocytes or a mononucleosis slide agglutination test (Monospot) may confirm clinical diagnosis of EBV. When indicated based on population prevalence and supply availability, a nasal swab for a general respiratory viral panel or specifically SARS-CoV-2 will help indicate a viral etiology.

IMAGING STUDIES
- Seldom indicated.
- Imaging is not necessary to make the diagnosis of a peritonsillar abscess.
- If there is concern for parapharyngeal or retropharyngeal space infection, CT or MRI is preferred over plain radiographs.[5]

BOX 3 Indications for Tonsillectomy in Treatment of Recurrent Strep Tonsillitis

1. **Well-documented clinical features for each episode:**
   - Sore throat associated with fever >38.3° C (>100.9° F)
   - Cervical lymphadenopathy, tonsillar exudate, or GABHS positive testing
   - Frequency of seven episodes or more in the preceding year, five or more episodes in each of the preceding 2 yr, or three or more episodes in each of the preceding 3 yr
2. **Other factors that inform decision making about surgical intervention:**
   - How well infections have responded to medical therapy
   - Quality-of-life issues (e.g., days of work/school missed)
   - Children who have multiple antibiotic allergies or intolerance
   - Periodic fever with aphthous stomatitis, pharyngitis, and adenitis
   - History of peritonsillar abscess

From Flint PW et al: *Cummings otolaryngology, head and neck surgery,* ed 7, Philadelphia, 2021, Elsevier.

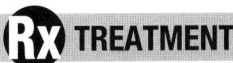 **TREATMENT**

NONPHARMACOLOGIC THERAPY
- Rest
- Soft diet
- Hydration
- Warm saltwater gargles
- Warm beverages with honey or lemon (avoid honey in children <12 mo of age due to risk of infantile botulism)
- Cold beverages/ice chips
- Anesthetic spray/lozenges (Avoid lozenges in children <4 yr due to choking hazard. Avoid benzocaine-containing sprays in children <2 due to risk of methemoglobinemia)

ACUTE GENERAL Rx
- Analgesics: Acetaminophen (adults and children) or ibuprofen (adults and children ≥6 mo of age). Systemic glucocorticoids are not recommended in uncomplicated pharyngitis/tonsillitis because of increased risk of adverse events; analgesics are effective for pain.
- The primary benefit and intent of antibiotic treatment in GAS pharyngitis is the prevention of acute rheumatic fever.[6]
- If streptococcal infection is proven or suspected:
  1. Amoxicillin Immediate Release Tablets: 50 mg/kg/day PO once daily or divided every 12 h for 10 days. Maximum daily dose: 1000 mg/day.
  2. Amoxicillin Extended Release (≥12 yr old): 775 mg PO once daily for 10 days.

3. Penicillin V (≤27 kg) 250 mg PO every 8 to 12 h for 10 days or (>27 kg) 500 mg PO every 8 to 12 h for 10 days.
4. Benzathine penicillin (≤27 kg) 600,000 U IM once or (>27 kg) 1.2 million U IM once.
5. If avoiding penicillin, cephalexin 40 mg/kg/day PO divided every 12 h for 10 days. Maximum 500 mg/dose.
- If uncomplicated gonococcal pharyngitis infection:
  1. <150 kg: Ceftriaxone 500 mg IM once; ≥150 kg: Ceftriaxone 1g IM once.
  2. If chlamydia coinfection is identified: Doxycycline 100 mg PO twice a day for 7 days. If pregnant: Azithromycin 1g PO once.
  3. Consult infectious disease specialist for alternative regimen if anaphylaxis or severe allergic reaction to ceftriaxone.[7]
- Treatment of peritonsillar abscess is drainage through needle or incision.

CHRONIC Rx
- Recurrent streptococcal infections are common and may represent chronic carrier status, reinfection before antibody development, new infection to a different GAS M subtype, poor compliance to antibiotic, or rarely, an immune disorder.
- Recurrence in children is defined as seven or more infections in 1 yr, five or more infections in 2 yr, or three or more infections in 3 yr.
- Chronic carrier: Oral treatment options include clindamycin, amoxicillin-clavulanate, and penicillin plus rifampin.

- In adults, tonsillectomy is rarely indicated for patients with recurrent GAS.
- In children, tonsillectomy may lower the incidence for recurrent pharyngitis.
- In both children and adults, each individual case is reviewed based on patient age, frequency or severity of infections, history of antibiotic use, and patient preferences.[8,9]
- Indications for tonsillectomy in treatment of recurrent streptococcal tonsillitis are summarized in Box 3.

DISPOSITION
- Tonsillopharyngitis is generally managed in an outpatient setting with follow-up arranged in 1 to 2 wk.
- Admission to the hospital is indicated for local suppurative complications (peritonsillar abscess; lateral pharyngeal, posterior, or retropharyngeal abscess; concern for impending airway closure or respiratory distress; or inability to swallow food, medications, or water).

REFERRAL
- To otolaryngologist:
  1. If peritonsillar or other abscess is suspected
  2. If tonsillar hypertrophy persists

PREVENTION
- Hand hygiene.
- Antimicrobial prophylaxis is only recommended in patients with a history of acute rheumatic fever and is based on the risk of recurrence and severity of disease.
- Influenza vaccine for children ≥6 mo. COVID-19 vaccine for children ≥6 mo.[10,11]

REFERENCES
Available at eBooks.Health.Elsevier.com.

RELATED CONTENT
Sore Throat (Patient Information)
Strep Throat (Patient Information)
Tonsillitis (Patient Information)

AUTHORS: **SHIVALI CHOXI, MD,** and **RISA BOCHNER, MD**

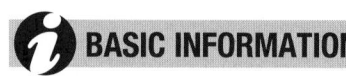
BASIC INFORMATION

DEFINITION

Pheochromocytomas are catecholamine-producing tumors that originate from the chromaffin cells of the adrenergic system. While they generally secrete both norepinephrine and epinephrine, norepinephrine is usually the predominant amine.

SYNONYM

Paraganglioma

ICD-10CM CODES

C74.9 Malignant neoplasm of adrenal gland, unspecified
C75.9 Malignant neoplasm of endocrine gland, unspecified
E27.5 Adrenomedullary hyperfunction

EPIDEMIOLOGY & DEMOGRAPHICS

- Incidence: 0.05% of population; peak incidence in 30s and 40s.
- Approximately 25% of patients with apparently sporadic pheochromocytoma may be carriers of mutations.
- Approximately 25% of pheochromocytomas are familial and associated with genetic disorders (Table 1). Pheochromocytoma is a feature of two disorders with an autosomal dominant pattern of inheritance:
  1. Multiple endocrine neoplasia (MEN) type 2
  2. von Hippel-Lindau disease: Angioma of the retina, hemangioblastoma of the central nervous system, renal cell carcinoma, pancreatic cysts, and epididymal cystoadenoma
- Pheochromocytomas occur in 5% of patients with neurofibromatosis type 1.

PHYSICAL FINDINGS & CLINICAL PRESENTATION

- Hypertension: Can be sustained (55%) or paroxysmal (45%).
- Headache (80%): Usually paroxysmal in nature and described as "pounding" and severe.
- Palpitations (70%): Can be present with or without tachycardia.
- Hyperhidrosis (60%): Most evident during paroxysmal attacks of hypertension.
- Physical examination may be entirely normal if done in a symptom-free interval; during a paroxysm the patient may demonstrate marked increase in both systolic and diastolic pressure, profuse sweating, visual disturbances (caused by hypertensive retinopathy), dilated pupils (from catecholamine excess), paresthesias in the lower extremities (caused by severe vasoconstriction), tremor, and tachycardia.
- Orthostatic hypotension is common among patients with pheochromocytoma due to reduction of blood volume and desensitization of adrenergic receptors by the chronic excess of catecholamines.
- Box E1 summarizes features suggestive of pheochromocytoma.

ETIOLOGY

- Catecholamine-producing tumors that are usually located in the adrenal medulla.
- Specific mutations of the RET protooncogene cause familial predisposition to pheochromocytoma in MEN-2.
- Mutations in the von Hippel-Lindau tumor suppressor gene (VHL gene) cause familial disposition to pheochromocytoma in von Hippel-Lindau disease.
- Recently identified genes for succinate dehydrogenase subunit D (SDHD) and succinate dehydrogenase subunit B (SDHB) predispose carriers to pheochromocytoma and globus tumors.

DIAGNOSIS

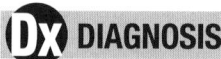

DIFFERENTIAL DIAGNOSIS

- Anxiety disorder
- Thyrotoxicosis
- Amphetamine or cocaine abuse
- Carcinoid
- Essential hypertension
- The differential diagnosis of pheochromocytoma-type spells is summarized in Box 2

WORKUP

Laboratory evaluation and imaging studies to locate the neoplasm (Fig. 1). Anatomic and functional imaging studies that can be used to localize pheochromocytomas are summarized in Table E2. Misdiagnosis of pheochromocytoma is

---

TABLE 1 Autosomal Dominant Syndromes Associated With Pheochromocytoma and Paraganglioma

Syndrome	Gene	Gene Locus	Protein Product	Protein Function	Gene Mechanism	Typical Tumor Location
SDHD (familial paraganglioma type 1)*	SDHD	11q23	SDH D subunit	ATP production	Tumor suppressor	Skull base and neck; occasionally adrenal medulla, mediastinum, abdomen, pelvis
Familial paraganglioma type 2*	SDHAF2	11q13.1	Flavination cofactor	ATP production	Tumor suppressor	Skull base and neck; occasionally abdomen and pelvis
SDHC (familial paraganglioma type 3)	SDHC	1q21	SDH C subunit	ATP production	Tumor suppressor	Skull base and neck
SDHB (familial paraganglioma type 4)	SDHB	1p36.1-35	SDH B subunit	ATP production	Tumor suppressor	Abdomen, pelvis and mediastinum; rarely adrenal medulla, skull base, and neck
MEN-1	MEN-1	11q13	Menin	Transcription regulation	Tumor suppressor	Adrenal medulla
MEN-2A and MEN-2B	RET	10q11.2	RET	Tyrosine kinase receptor	Protooncogene	Adrenal medulla, bilaterally
Neurofibromatosis type 1	NF1	17q11.2	Neurofibromin	GTP hydrolysis	Tumor suppressor	Adrenal-periadrenal
von Hippel-Lindau disease	VHL	3p25-26	VHL	Transcription elongation suppression	Tumor suppressor	Adrenal medulla, bilaterally; occasionally paraganglioma
Familial pheochromocytoma	FP/TMEM127	2q11	Transmembrane protein	Regulation of the mTORC1 signaling complex	Tumor suppressor	Adrenal medulla

ATP, Adenosine triphosphate; *GTP*, guanosine triphosphate; *MEN*, multiple endocrine neoplasia; *mTORC1*, mammalian target of rapamycin complex 1; *RET*, "rearranged during transfection" proto-oncogene; *SDH*, succinate dehydrogenase; *VHL*, von Hippel-Lindau disease.
*Associated with maternal imprinting.
From Melmed S: *Williams textbook of endocrinology*, ed 12, Philadelphia, 2011, Saunders.

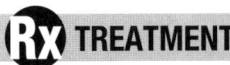

BOX 2 Differential Diagnosis of Pheochromocytoma-Type Spells

Endocrine Causes
Carbohydrate intolerance
Hyperadrenergic spells
Hypoglycemia
Pancreatic tumors (e.g., insulinoma)
Pheochromocytoma
Primary hypogonadism (menopausal syndrome)
Thyrotoxicosis

Cardiovascular Causes
Angina
Cardiovascular deconditioning
Labile essential hypertension
Orthostatic hypotension
Paroxysmal cardiac arrhythmia
Pulmonary edema
Renovascular disease
Syncope (e.g., vasovagal reaction)

Psychologic Causes
Factitious (e.g., drugs, Valsalva maneuver)
Hyperventilation
Severe anxiety and panic disorders
Somatization disorder

Pharmacologic Causes
Chlorpropamide-alcohol flush
Combination of a monoamine oxidase inhibitor and a decongestant
Illegal drug ingestion (cocaine, phencyclidine, lysergic acid diethylamide)
Sympathomimetic drug ingestion
Vancomycin (red man syndrome)
Withdrawal of adrenergic-inhibitor

Neurologic Causes
Autonomic neuropathy
Cerebrovascular insufficiency
Diencephalic epilepsy (autonomic seizures)
Migraine headache
Postural orthostatic tachycardia syndrome
Stroke

Other Causes
Carcinoid syndrome
Mast cell disease
Recurrent idiopathic anaphylaxis
Unexplained flushing spells

From Melmed S et al: *Williams textbook of endocrinology,* ed 14, Philadelphia, 2020, Elsevier.

common. Correct interpretation of biochemical tests and imaging is crucial to a correct diagnosis.

LABORATORY TESTS

- Although there is no consensus on the best test, plasma-free metanephrines have been suggested as the test of first choice for excluding the tumor. Elevated plasma concentrations of normetanephrine or metanephrine have a sensitivity of up to 100%, but the specificity is markedly lower (85%).
- 24-h urine collection will also show increased metanephrines (90% sensitivity, 95% specificity); the accuracy of the 24-h urinary levels for metanephrines can be improved by indexing urinary metanephrine levels by urine creatinine levels.

- Cutoff values for biochemical diagnosis of pheochromocytoma are summarized in Table 3.
- Medications that may increase measured levels of fractionated catecholamines and metanephrines are summarized in Box 3.

IMAGING STUDIES

- Abdominal computed tomography (CT) scan (Fig. E2) with and without contrast (88% sensitivity) is useful in locating pheochromocytomas >0.5 inch in diameter (90% to 95% accurate).
- MRI with contrast: Pheochromocytomas demonstrate a distinctive MRI appearance (up to 100% sensitivity); MRI may become the diagnostic imaging modality of choice.

- Scintigraphy with 131 or 1-123 I-MIBG (up to 100% sensitivity) (see Fig. E2): This norepinephrine analog localizes in adrenergic tissue; it is particularly useful in locating extraadrenal pheochromocytomas.
- 6-[18F]Fluorodopamine positron emission tomography is reserved for cases in which clinical symptoms and signs suggest pheochromocytoma, and results of biochemical tests are positive but conventional imaging studies cannot locate the tumor. It is also used for identification of metastatic disease.

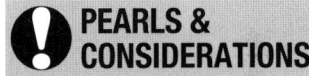 **TREATMENT**

GENERAL Rx

Laparoscopic adrenalectomy (surgical resection for both benign and malignant disease):

- Preoperative stabilization with combination of alpha-adrenergic blocking agents (phenoxybenzamine, prazosin, doxazosin, or terazosin), β-blocker, and liberal fluid and salt intake starting 10 to 14 days before surgery. β-Blockers should be avoided until patients receive adequate alpha-adrenergic blockade for several days to avoid hypertensive crisis due to unopposed alpha stimulation. Amlodipine or verapamil can be added to β-blockers if blood pressure control is still inadequate. Table 4 describes orally administered drugs to treat pheochromocytoma.
- Hypertensive crisis preoperatively and intraoperatively can be controlled with nitroprusside. Table 5 summarizes intravenously administered drugs used to treat pheochromocytoma.

PEARLS & CONSIDERATIONS

COMMENTS

- Obtaining a detailed family history is important because 25% of pheochromocytomas are familial.
- Screening for pheochromocytoma should be considered in patients with any of the following:
  1. Malignant hypertension
  2. Poor response to antihypertensive therapy
  3. Paradoxic hypertensive response
  4. Hypertension during induction of anesthesia, parturition, surgery, or thyrotropin-releasing hormone testing
  5. Hypertension associated with imipramine or desipramine
  6. Neurofibromatosis (increased incidence of pheochromocytoma)
- All patients with pheochromocytoma should be screened for MEN-2 and von Hippel-Lindau disease with the pentagastrin test, serum parathyroid hormone, ophthalmoscopy, MRI of the brain, CT scan of the kidneys and pancreas, and ultrasonography of the testes.

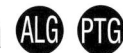

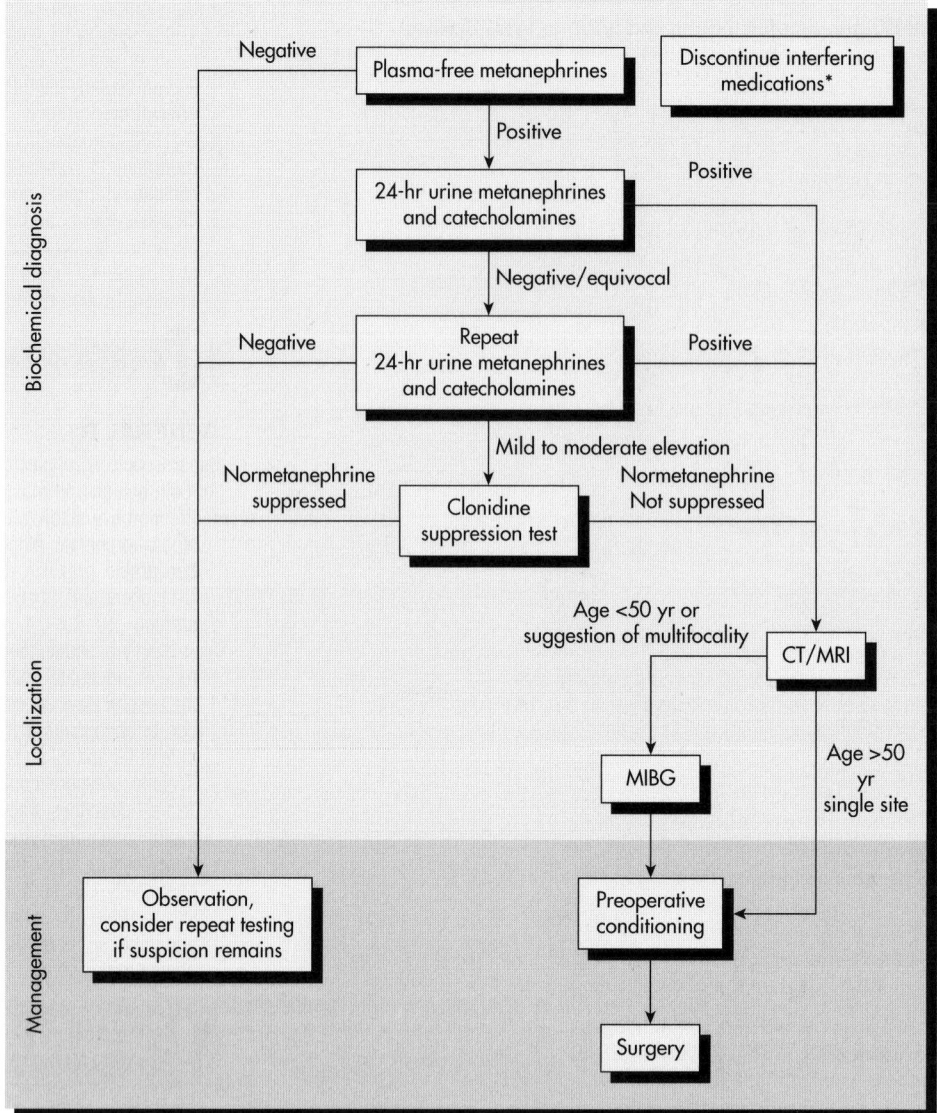

*Including sympathomimetics, phenoxybenzamine, acetaminophen, many psychotropic drugs.

FIG. 1 Algorithm for the diagnosis, localization, and management of pheochromocytoma. Initial plasma-free metanephrine testing can effectively exclude the diagnosis if the result is negative. A 24-h urine collection for catecholamines and their metabolites is generally performed twice, with cutoffs approximately twice the upper limit of normal being criteria for positivity (see Table 3). Clonidine suppression testing can be used for the small fraction of patients in whom the diagnosis remains uncertain after urine testing. Localization with computed tomography *(CT)* or magnetic resonance imaging *(MRI)* follows biochemical confirmation of the diagnosis, with meta-iodobenzylguanidine *(MIBG)* scanning performed for younger patients and those otherwise at risk for multifocal disease. Phenoxybenzamine is given in escalating doses for at least 2 wk before surgery. (From Townsend CM et al: *Sabiston textbook of surgery,* ed 21, St Louis, 2022, Elsevier.)

- In patients with pheochromocytoma, routine analysis for mutations of RET, VHL, SDHD, and SDHB is indicated to identify pheochromocytoma-associated syndromes.

RELATED CONTENT

Pheochromocytoma (Patient Information)
Hypertension (Related Key Topic)

AUTHORS: **BRETT PATRICK, MD, MARK F. BRADY, MD, MPH, MMSc,** and **FRED F. FERRI, MD**

SUGGESTED READINGS
Available at eBooks.Health.Elsevier.com.

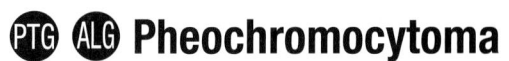

TABLE 3 Cutoff Values for Biochemical Diagnosis of Pheochromocytoma

Test*	CUTOFF VALUE		Definitions	Sensitivity (%)	Specificity (%)
	mol	**g**			
Plasma-free metanephrine	03 nmol/L	59 µg/L	Paired test, positive result if either or both values are elevated	99	85-89
Plasma-free normetanephrine	06 nmol/L	110 µg/L			
Urinary total metanephrines	66 µmol/day	13 mg/day		71	996
Urinary epinephrine	191 nmol/day	35 µg/day		29	996
Urinary norepinephrine	1005 nmol/day	170 µg/day		50	996
Urinary dopamine	4571 nmol/day	700 µg/day		8	100
Urinary total metanephrines and catecholamines	—		Grouped test, positive result if any one of the following three urinary values is elevated: Total metanephrines, epinephrine, norepinephrine, dopamine	88	99
Urinary vanillylmandelic acid	40 µmol/day	79 mg/day		64	95
Clonidine suppression test			Positive result = elevated level after clonidine and fall of <40	96	100
Plasma-free normetanephrine	061 nmol/L	112 µg/L			

*When it is performed twice, 24-h urine testing of urinary total metanephrines and catecholamines (grouped test) is highly sensitive and highly specific.
From Townsend CM et al: *Sabiston textbook of surgery,* ed 21, St Louis, 2022, Elsevier.

BOX 3 Medications That May Increase Measured Levels of Fractionated Catecholamines and Metanephrines

Tricyclic antidepressants (including cyclobenzaprine)
Levodopa
Drugs containing adrenergic receptor agonists (e.g., decongestants)
Amphetamines
Buspirone and antipsychotic agents
Prochlorperazine
Reserpine
Withdrawal from clonidine and other drugs (e.g., illicit drugs)
Illicit drugs (e.g., cocaine, heroin)
Ethanol

From Melmed S et al: *Williams textbook of endocrinology,* ed 14, Philadelphia, 2020, Elsevier.

TABLE 4 Orally Administered Drugs Used to Treat Pheochromocytoma

Drug	Initial Dosage, mg/day* (Maximum)	Side Effects
α-Adrenergic Blocking Agents		
Phenoxybenzamine	10[†] (100)[†]	Postural hypotension, tachycardia, meiosis, nasal congestion, diarrhea, inhibition of ejaculation, fatigue
Prazosin	1 (20)[‡]	First-dose effect, dizziness, drowsiness, headache, fatigue, palpitations, nausea
Terazosin	1 (20)[†]	First-dose effect, asthenia, blurred vision, dizziness, nasal congestion, nausea, peripheral edema, palpitations, somnolence
Doxazosin	1 (20)	First-dose effect, orthostasis, peripheral edema, fatigue, somnolence
Combined α- and β-Adrenergic Blocking Agent		
Labetalol	200[†] (1200)[†]	Dizziness, fatigue, nausea, nasal congestion, impotence
Calcium Channel Blocker		
Nicardipine sustained-release	30[†] (120)[†]	Edema, dizziness, headache, flushing, nausea, dyspepsia
Catecholamine Synthesis Inhibitor		
α-Methyl-ρ-l tyrosine (metyrosine)	1000[‡] (4000)[‡]	Sedation, diarrhea, anxiety, nightmares, crystalluria, galactorrhea, extrapyramidal symptoms

*Given once daily unless otherwise indicated.
[†]Given in two doses daily.
[‡]Given in three or four doses daily.
From Melmed S: *Williams textbook of endocrinology,* ed 12, Philadelphia, 2011, Saunders.

TABLE 5 Intravenously Administered Drugs Used to Treat Pheochromocytoma

Agent	Dosage Range
For Hypertension	
Phentolamine	Administer a 1-mg IV test dose, then 2- to 5-mg IV boluses as needed or continuous infusion.
Nitroprusside	IV infusion rates of 2 μg/kg of body weight per min are suggested as safe. Rates >4 μg/kg/min may lead to cyanide toxicity within 3 h. Doses >10 μg/kg/min are rarely required, and the maximal dose should not exceed 800 μg/min.
Nicardipine	Initiate therapy at 5 mg/h; the IV infusion rate may be increased by 2.5 mg/h q15min up to a maximum of 15 mg/h.
For Cardiac Arrhythmia	
Lidocaine	Initiate therapy with an IV bolus of 1-1.5 mg/kg (75-100 mg); additional boluses of 0.5-0.75 mg/kg (25-50 mg) can be given q5-10min if needed up to a maximum of 3 mg/kg. Loading is followed by maintenance IV infusion of 2-4 mg/min (30-50 μg/kg/min) adjusted for effect and settings of altered metabolism (e.g., heart failure, liver congestion) and as guided by blood level monitoring.
Esmolol	An initial IV loading dose of 0.5 mg/kg is infused over 1 min, followed by a maintenance infusion of 0.05 mg/kg/min for the next 4 min. Depending on the desired ventricular response, the maintenance infusion may then be continued at 0.05 mg/kg/min or increased stepwise (e.g., by 0.1 mg/kg/min increments to a maximum of 0.2 mg/kg/min), with each step being maintained for ≥4 min.

IV, Intravenous.
From Melmed S: *Williams textbook of endocrinology,* ed 12, Philadelphia, 2011, Saunders.

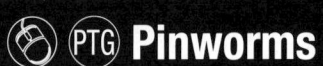

P

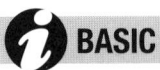 **BASIC INFORMATION**

DEFINITION

Enterobius vermicularis is a small (6-13 mm) helminth of the nematode (roundworm) family that can cause noninvasive infestation of the large intestine.[1] Females have a notably long, pointed tail that is similar in appearance to a pin; therefore *E. vermicularis* is also referred to as pinworms. Other species such as *Enterobius gregorii* and *Syphacia obvelata* have been described to cause pinworms; however, *E. vermicularis* is the most frequent culprit.[2]

SYNONYMS

Pinworms
Enterobiasis
Oxyuriasis
Seatworms
Threadworms

ICD-10CM CODE
B80 Enterobiasis

EPIDEMIOLOGY & DEMOGRAPHICS

- *E. vermicularis* is the most prevalent helminth infection in the U.S., with an estimated prevalence of 20 to 40 million infected individuals.[3,4]
- *E. vermicularis* is found worldwide, although most common in temperate climates.[4]
- Preschool/early grade school age children and their caretakers, as well as institutionalized persons, have the highest risk of infection.[2]
- Close proximity and poor hand hygiene raise the risk of infection.[2]
- Pinworms are easily spread in day care settings, institutions, and within homes.[3]

PHYSICAL FINDINGS & CLINICAL PRESENTATION

- Many individuals (30%-50%) with pinworms are asymptomatic.[3]
- The most common symptom is perianal pruritus, which is often worse at night. Itching can lead to excoriation and secondary bacterial infection.[2]
- Abdominal pain and nausea/vomiting may occur in individuals with high worm burden.[1]
- Symptomatic individuals may display insomnia, enuresis, teeth-grinding, and irritability. Anorexia secondary to pinworms has been described.[4]
- Pinworm infestations are not just limited to the gastrointestinal tract; pinworms can also infest the urethra and vulva and present as urethritis and vaginitis, respectively. Though rare, salpingitis and oophoritis have been reported.[3]
- Rare complications can include appendicitis, resulting from a high worm burden obstructing the lumen of the appendix, and eosinophilic enteritis.[1]

ETIOLOGY & PATHOGENESIS

- Humans are the definitive host for *E. vermicularis*.[2]
- *E. vermicularis* has a fecal-oral transmission pattern. It is spread directly via hand-to-mouth contact, indirectly via fomites, through person-to-person contact, and through ingestion of contaminated food.[4]
- In rare cases, pinworm eggs can become airborne and subsequently inhaled.[3]
- *E. vermicularis* may be transmitted between sexual partners, especially those engaging in oral-anal sex.[5]
- The pinworm species that infect humans and animals are different from each other and do not spread between species.[2]
- Upon ingestion of embryonated eggs, larvae hatch in the small intestine and then migrate to the large intestine after they have matured (1-2 mo). Gravid females tend to occupy the more distal aspects of the large intestine; each gravid female migrates to the perianal region at night to release approximately 10,000 eggs.[2]
- The larvae within the eggs mature and become infectious within 4 to 6 hr of deposition. Eggs may survive and remain infectious for up to 2 to 3 wk in an indoor environment.[2]
- Embryonated eggs are pruritic, and when the host scratches the perianal region, the eggs are retained under the fingernails. This can lead to autoinfection via hand-to-mouth contact or infection of others via the fecal-oral route.[2]
- Retroinfection, when newly hatched larvae migrate from the perianal region into the rectum, can occur but is not thought to be common.[5]
- In the absence of autoinfection, *Enterobius* infestation lasts only 4 to 6 wk.[1]

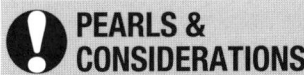 **DIAGNOSIS**

DIFFERENTIAL DIAGNOSIS

- Perianal itching related to poor hygiene. Section II describes the causes of pruritus ani, which include infectious (e.g., group A strep, *Mycoplasma pneumoniae*) and inflammatory (e.g., lichen sclerosis) pathologies
- Perineal yeast/fungal infection
- Sexually transmitted infections
- Hemorrhoids and anal fissures

WORKUP

E. vermicularis ova are 50 by 30 microns with one flattened side and surrounded by a thick, smooth, and colorless shell (Fig. E1).[4] The eggs can be identified via the cellophane (Scotch) tape test in which transparent tape (Fig. E2) is placed on the perianal skin and viewed under the microscope.[6] The test is most effective on awakening prior to bathing.[4] A single examination detects 50% of infections, three examinations detect 90%, and five examinations detect 99%.[4] Examinations should be conducted on different days. Five consecutive negative tests effectively rule out the diagnosis. Pinworm paddles are clear plastic paddles that can be used in place of transparent tape. Ova will not be present in the stool because the eggs are not passed in stool.[3] On rare occasions, adult *E. vermicularis* can be identified in the stool and confirm the diagnosis. No serologic testing for *E. vermicularis* is available. Given that *E. vermicularis* does not cause invasive disease, there is no associated peripheral eosinophilia.[4]

Rx TREATMENT

- It is reasonable to empirically treat patients with anal pruritus.
- Treatment options include either a single dose of mebendazole (100 mg), albendazole (400 mg), or pyrantel pamoate (11 mg/kg up to 1 g) followed by a repeat dose in 2 wk. Mebendazole and albendazole require a prescription whereas pyrantel pamoate is available over the counter.[2,4,5]
- It can be difficult to eradicate the infestation due to reinfection and autoinfection.[5] Retreatment at 2 wk targets newly hatched pinworms before they can lay eggs.[2,5]
- Other infected family members and asymptomatic close contacts and sexual contacts should be treated.[4,5]
- Clothing and bedding should be cleaned to prevent reinfection.[4]

PEARLS & CONSIDERATIONS

- Good hand hygiene is the most effective method of prevention.[2-4]
- Morning bathing to clear the eggs deposited overnight helps to prevent recurrent autoinfection.[2]
- Showering is preferred over taking baths to limit the risk of ingesting pinworms from contaminated bath water.[2]
- Control of *E. vermicularis* infection requires treatment of contacts and family members and decontamination of the environment by frequent changing of clothing and bedding.[2]
- Personal hygiene and cleanliness are crucial. Fingernails should be cut short and scrubbed frequently as pinworm eggs can reside beneath the nails.[2,3]

REFERENCES
Available at eBooks.Health.Elsevier.com.

RELATED CONTENT
Pinworms (Patient Information)

AUTHORS: **LAURA MIYARES, MD,** and **JEREMY MICHEL, MD, MHS**

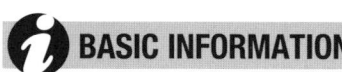
i BASIC INFORMATION

DEFINITION

A pituitary adenoma is a benign neoplasm of the anterior lobe of the pituitary. Pituitary adenomas may cause symptoms, either by excess secretion of hormones or by a local mass effect as the tumor impinges on other nearby structures (e.g., the optic chiasm, hypothalamus, or pituitary stalk). Pituitary adenomas are classified by their size, function, and features that characterize their appearance. Microadenomas are <10 mm in size, macroadenomas are ≥10 mm in size, and giant adenomas are ≥40 mm in size. Depending on the anterior pituitary cell type of origin of the tumor, a pituitary adenoma may be secretory or nonsecretory.

- *Nonsecretory pituitary adenomas* are those in which the neoplasm is a space-occupying lesion whose secretory products do not cause a specific disease state.
- *Secretory pituitary adenomas* (Table 1) can cause endocrine manifestations related to the hormone they are secreting.

Endocrine manifestations of secretory adenomas include:

- *Acromegaly,* a disease state characterized by a pituitary adenoma with somatotroph cell origin that secretes growth hormone (GH); notably, a significant majority of somatotroph adenomas are clinically silent
- Galactorrhea, which is the result of a *prolactinoma* with lactotroph cell origin that secretes prolactin (PRL)
- *Cushing disease,* a disease state of hypersecretion of adrenocorticotropic hormone (ACTH) due to corticotroph cell origin of the tumor
- *Hyperthyroidism* due to a thyrotropin-secreting pituitary adenoma, due to a thyrotroph cell origin which secretes primarily thyroid-stimulating hormone (TSH); notably, thyrotroph adenomas may also present as nonsecretory sellar masses

ICD-10CM CODE
D35.2 Benign neoplasm of pituitary gland

EPIDEMIOLOGY & DEMOGRAPHICS

CLASSIFICATION (BY HORMONE SECRETED):
- No hormone: 30%
- PRL only: 35%
- GH only: 20%
- PRL and GH: 7%
- ACTH: 7%
- Luteinizing hormone (LH), follicle-stimulating hormone (FSH), TSH: 1%

INCIDENCE & PREVALENCE:
- Pituitary adenomas: Up to 15% of all intracranial neoplasms; 3% to 27% at autopsy series. The prevalence of pituitary adenomas has increased to 100 cases/100,000 over the past decades, likely as a result of enhanced awareness and improved diagnostic imaging and hormone assays. True prevalence is likely underestimated due to nonfunctioning pituitary adenomas going undiagnosed until they

are large. There is a higher prevalence in females.
- Prolactinomas: Up to 20% in women with unexplained primary or secondary amenorrhea.
- GH-secreting pituitary adenoma: Prevalence of 3.3 to 13.7 cases/100,000. They account for 8% to 16% of pituitary tumors and are most common in men over age 50.
- Thyrotropin-secreting pituitary adenoma: 1% of pituitary adenomas with a slight female:male predominance of 1.7:1.
- Corticotropin-secreting pituitary adenomas: Female:male predominance of 8:1 but overall uncommon diagnosis, accounting for 2% to 6% of adenomas.

PHYSICAL FINDINGS & CLINICAL PRESENTATION

Most individuals remain asymptomatic.
All sellar masses can cause visual defects by compression of the optic chiasm (bitemporal hemianopsia (Fig. E1) or headaches.

PROLACTINOMAS:
- Females:
  1. Galactorrhea
  2. Amenorrhea
  3. Oligomenorrhea with anovulation
  4. Infertility
  5. Estrogen deficiency and associated osteopenia
  6. Decreased vaginal lubrication
- Males:
  1. Large tumors more common as a result of delayed diagnosis
  2. Possible impotence, decreased libido, or hypogonadism
  3. Galactorrhea rare because males lack the estrogen-dependent breast growth and differentiation

GH-SECRETING PITUITARY ADENOMA—ACROMEGALY:
- Coarse facial features
- Oily skin

- Prognathism
- Carpal tunnel syndrome
- Osteoarthritis
- History of increased hat, glove, or shoe size
- Decreased exercise capacity
- Visual field deficits
- Diabetes mellitus

CORTICOTROPIN-SECRETING PITUITARY ADENOMA—CUSHING DISEASE:
- Usually present when the tumor is small (1 to 2 mm)
- 50% of the tumors are <5 mm
- Other symptoms:
  1. Truncal obesity
  2. Round facies (moon face)
  3. Dorsocervical fat accumulation (buffalo hump)
  4. Hirsutism
  5. Acne
  6. Menstrual disorders
  7. Hypertension
  8. Striae
  9. Bruising
  10. Thin skin
  11. Hyperglycemia

THYROTROPIN-SECRETING PITUITARY ADENOMA:
- In males, larger, more invasive, and more rapidly growing tumors that present later in life
- Other symptoms: Thyrotoxicosis, goiter, visual impairment

NONSECRETORY PITUITARY ADENOMAS (ENDOCRINE INACTIVE PITUITARY ADENOMA):
- Usually large at the time of diagnosis
- Symptoms:
  1. Bitemporal hemianopsia as a result of compression of the optic chiasm
  2. Hypopituitarism from compression of the pituitary gland
  3. Hypogonadism in men and in premenopausal women
  4. Cranial nerve deficits caused by extension into the cavernous sinus

TABLE 1 Types of Pituitary Adenomas Based on Hormones Secreted

Adenoma Type	Hormones	Possible Clinical Manifestations
Somatotroph adenoma	Growth hormone	Gigantism, acromegaly
Mammosomatotroph	Growth hormone + prolactin	Gigantism or acromegaly along with galactorrhea or amenorrhea
Corticotroph adenoma	Adrenocorticotropic hormone	Cushing disease
Lactotroph adenoma*	Prolactin	Women: Reproductive or sexual dysfunction, galactorrhea, amenorrhea, ovulatory disorders Men: Erectile dysfunction, decreased libido
Gonadotroph adenoma	Follicle-stimulating hormone or luteinizing hormone	Most are clinically silent and usually present due to mass effect
Thyrotroph adenoma	Thyroid-stimulating hormone	Hyperthyroidism
Plurihormonal	Growth hormone, prolactin, thyroid-stimulating hormone, various hormonal combinations	Most are clinically silent
Null cell adenoma	No hormones	No symptoms of hormonal excess, usually present due to mass effect

*Most common type of adenoma (~40% of cases).
From Jankovic J et al: *Bradley and Daroff's neurology in clinical practice,* ed 8, Philadelphia, 2022, Elsevier.

5. Hydrocephalus from extension into the third ventricle, compressing the foramen of Monro
6. Diabetes insipidus resulting from compression of the hypothalamus or pituitary stalk (a rare complication)

ETIOLOGY

Benign neoplasms of epithelial origin. Genetic mutations of *MEN1, Gs-Alpha,* and *AIP* are related to the development of pituitary adenomas.

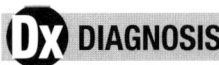 **DIAGNOSIS**

DIFFERENTIAL DIAGNOSIS
PROLACTINOMA:
- Pregnancy
- Postpartum puerperium
- Primary hypothyroidism
- Breast disease
- Breast stimulation
- Drug ingestion (especially phenothiazines, antidepressants, haloperidol, methyldopa, reserpine, opiates, amphetamines, and cimetidine)
- Chronic renal failure
- Liver disease
- Polycystic ovarian disease
- Chest wall disorders
- Spinal cord lesions
- Previous cranial irradiation

ACROMEGALY:
- Ectopic production of GH-releasing hormone from a carcinoid or other neuroendocrine tumor

CUSHING DISEASE:
- Diseases that cause ectopic sources of ACTH overproduction (including small cell carcinoma of the lung, bronchial carcinoid, intestinal carcinoid, pancreatic islet cell tumor, medullary thyroid carcinoma, or pheochromocytoma)
- Adrenal adenomas, adrenal carcinoma
- Nelson syndrome

THYROTROPIN-SECRETING PITUITARY ADENOMAS:
- Primary hypothyroidism

NONSECRETORY PITUITARY ADENOMA:
- Nonneoplastic mass lesions of various etiologies (e.g., infectious, granulomatous, cystic, pituitary hyperplasia)
- Other sellar tumors (e.g., craniopharyngioma, meningioma, pituicytoma)
- Metastases to the hypothalamus or pituitary gland (e.g., breast cancer in females, lung cancer in males)

WORKUP
- Pituitary adenomas should be identified at an early stage so that effective treatment can be implemented.
- Screening tests for functional pituitary adenomas are described in Table 2.

PROLACTINOMA: First step: Measurement of basal PRL levels (practitioners should be aware of discriminatory values in their own institutions).
- Elevated PRL levels are correlated with tumor size.

- Level >200 ng/ml indicates likely prolactinoma, with levels of 100 to 200 ng/ml being equivocal and possibly associated with medications or other sources.
- Basal PRL levels between 20 and 100 suggest a microadenoma but can be due to common medications (estrogen, antidepressants, metoclopramide, Aldomet, and others) or recent breast stimulation.
- Basal level <20 ng/ml is usually considered normal. Each laboratory should develop its own normative values, however, and practitioners should refer to these values.
- Threshold level for obtaining imaging such as MRI should be developed by individual providers depending on the level of specificity and sensitivity desired.

ACROMEGALY:
- First screening tests are the measurement of the serum insulin-like growth factor I level, postprandial serum GH, and thyrotropin-releasing hormone (TRH) stimulation test.
- Follow with an oral glucose tolerance test.
- Failure to suppress serum GH to <2 ng/ml with an oral load of 100 g glucose is considered conclusive.
- A GH-releasing hormone level >300 ng/ml is indicative of an ectopic source of GH.

CUSHING DISEASE:
- Measurement of late-night salivary cortisol level is the best screening test.
- Normal or slightly elevated corticotropin levels ranging from 20 to 200 pg/ml; normal is 10 to 50 pg/ml (normative data should be developed by each institution for its population).
- Level <10 pg/ml usually indicates an autonomously secreting adrenal tumor.
- Level >200 pg/ml suggests an ectopic corticotropin-secreting neoplasm.
- Cushing disease can be assessed by absence of cortisol suppression with the low-dose dexamethasone test but with the presence of cortisol suppression after the high-dose test.

As a method to distinguish Cushing disease from an ectopic source of ACTH, this test is robust.
- 24-h urine collection should demonstrate an increased level of cortisol excretion.

THYROTROPIN-SECRETING PITUITARY ADENOMA:
- Highly sensitive thyrotropin assays, which evaluate the presence of thyrotoxicosis, are one way to detect a thyrotropin-secreting tumor.
- Free alpha subunit is secreted by >80% of tumors, with the ratio of the alpha subunit to thyrotropin <1.
- With central resistance to thyroid hormone, ratio is <1, and the sella is normal.
- Laboratory tests show elevated serum levels of both T_3 and T_4.

NONSECRETORY PITUITARY ADENOMA:
- Visual field testing
- Assessment of the pituitary and organ function to determine if there is hypopituitarism or hypersecretion of hormones (even if the effects of hypersecretion are subclinical)
- TRH to provoke secretion of FSH, LH, and LH-beta-subunit; will not elicit response in normal persons
- Exclusion of Klinefelter syndrome in patient with long-standing primary hypogonadism, elevated gonadotropin levels, and enlargement of the sella

IMAGING STUDIES
Study of choice: MRI of the pituitary and hypothalamus. If an MRI shows the tumor impinging on the optic chiasm, then formal visual field testing is indicated.
- When evaluating Cushing disease, small size at the onset of symptoms noted.
- MRI, in this case, only 60% sensitive at best and may yield false-positive results.
- CT scan only when MRI is unavailable or is otherwise contraindicated.

TABLE 2 Screening Tests for Functional Pituitary Adenomas

Disorder	Test	Comments
Acromegaly	IGF-1 OGTT with GH obtained at 0, 30, and 60 min	Interpret IGF-1 relative to age- and gender-matched controls. Normal subjects should suppress GH to <1 μg/L.
Prolactinoma	Serum PRL level	A level >500 μg/L is pathognomonic for macroprolactinoma. If >200 μg/L, prolactinoma is likely.*
Cushing disease	24-h UFC nighttime salivary cortisol dexamethasone (1 mg) at 11 P.M. and fasting plasma cortisol measured at 8 A.M. ACTH assay	Ensure that urine collection is total and accurate by measuring urinary creatinine. Free salivary cortisol reflects circadian rhythm, and elevated levels may indicate Cushing disease. Normal subjects suppress to <1.8 μg/dl. Distinguishes adrenal adenoma from ectopic ACTH or Cushing disease.
TSH-secreting tumor	TSH measurement free T_4 by dialysis total T_3	If T_4 or T_3 is elevated and TSH is measurable or elevated, a TSH-secreting tumor may be present.

ACTH, Adrenocorticotropic hormone; *GH,* growth hormone; *IGF-1,* insulin-like growth factor type 1; *OGTT,* oral glucose tolerance test; *PRL,* prolactin; T_3, triiodothyronine; T_4, thyroxine; *TSH,* thyroid-stimulating hormone; *UFC,* urinary free cortisol.
*Risperidone may result in prolactin levels >200 μg/L.
From Melmed S et al: *Williams textbook of endocrinology,* ed 12, Philadelphia, 2011, Saunders.

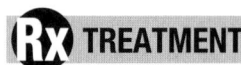

TREATMENT

NONPHARMACOLOGIC THERAPY

SURGERY:

- Selective transsphenoidal resection of the adenoma (Table 3) is the treatment of choice for acromegaly, Cushing disease, and thyrotropin-secreting pituitary adenomas, all

---

TABLE 3 Transsphenoidal Pituitary Surgery

Primary Indications

General

Visual tract or central nervous system compression arising from within sella
Relief of compressive hypopituitarism by presenting, residual, or recurrent tumor tissue
Tumor recurrence after surgery or irradiation
Pituitary hemorrhage
Cerebrospinal fluid leak
Resistance to medical therapy
Intolerance of medical therapy
Personal choice
Desire for immediate pregnancy with macroadenoma
Requirement for diagnostic tissue histology

Specific

Acromegaly
Cushing disease
Clinically nonfunctioning macroadenoma
Prolactinoma
Nelson syndrome
TSH-secreting adenoma

Side Effects

Transient

Diabetes insipidus
Cerebrospinal fluid leak and rhinorrhea
Inappropriate ADH secretion
Arachnoiditis
Meningitis
Postoperative psychosis
Local hematoma
Arterial wall damage
Epistaxis
Local abscess
Pulmonary embolism
Narcolepsy

Permanent (up to 10%)

Diabetes insipidus
Total or partial hypopituitarism
Visual loss
Inappropriate ADH secretion
Vascular occlusion
CNS damage: Oculomotor palsy, hemiparesis, encephalopathy
Nasal septum perforation

Surgery-Related Mortality (up to 1%)

Brain, hypothalamic
Vascular damage
Postoperative meningitis
Cerebrospinal fluid leak
Pneumocephalus
Acute cardiopulmonary disease
Anesthesia-related
Seizure

ADH, Antidiuretic hormone; *CNS*, central nervous system; *TSH*, thyroid-stimulating hormone.
From Melmed S et al: *Williams textbook of endocrinology,* ed 12, Philadelphia, 2011, Saunders.

---

of which tend to be microadenomas at the time of onset of symptoms.
- Macroadenomas, such as the nonsecretory pituitary adenoma, may also be surgically removed, but risk of recurrence is greater with these tumors and adjunctive therapy such as irradiation may also be necessary.
- Bilateral adrenalectomy has been performed in patients with Cushing disease after failure of other therapies; complications that may occur include requiring lifelong hormone replacement or Nelson syndrome (rapid enlargement of pituitary tumor due to adrenal resection).

RADIOTHERAPY:

- Radiotherapy is used primarily as adjuvant treatment. It is reserved for patients who have not responded to surgical treatment and who still have symptoms of the adenoma.
- Used with varying degrees of success in all types of pituitary adenomas.
- Radiotherapy complications include long-term hypopituitarism (40% of patients) and secondary neoplasms (1.5% of patients).

ACUTE GENERAL Rx

PROLACTINOMA:

- For prolactinomas, initial therapy is generally dopamine agonists. Bromocriptine, a dopamine analogue, is generally given orally in divided doses of 1.5 to 10 mg. Cabergoline is given once or twice weekly. It is better tolerated and more effective than bromocriptine for tumor shrinkage but more expensive.
- Side effects of these treatments include orthostatic hypotension, nausea, and dizziness and may be avoided by beginning with low-dose therapy.
- Other compounds include pergolide mesylate, a long-acting ergot derivative with dopaminergic properties, as well as other nonergot derivatives.

ACROMEGALY:

- Somatostatin analogues: Octreotide, lanreotide administered as monthly injections.
- Cabergoline or bromocriptine may also be used. They have modest activity but can be administered orally and are less expensive than somatostatin analogues.
- Pegvisomant may also be used to normalize IGF-1 levels.

CUSHING DISEASE:

- Ketoconazole, which inhibits the cytochrome P-450 enzymes involved in steroid biosynthesis, is effective in managing mild to moderate disease in daily oral doses of 600 to 1200 mg.
- Metyrapone and aminoglutethimide may be used to control hypersecretion of cortisol but are generally used when preparing a patient for surgery or while waiting for a response to radiotherapy.

THYROTROPIN-SECRETING PITUITARY ADENOMA:

- Ablative therapy with either radioactive iodide or surgery is indicated.
- Treatment directed to the thyroid alone may accelerate growth of the pituitary adenoma.
- Octreotide has been shown to be effective in doses similar to those used for acromegaly.

NONSECRETORY PITUITARY ADENOMA:

- There is no role for medical therapy at this time.
- Surgery and radiotherapy may be indicated. An algorithm for the management of nonfunctioning pituitary adenomas is described in Fig. E2.

CHRONIC Rx

For all pituitary adenomas:

- Careful follow-up is necessary. Patients undergoing transsphenoidal microsurgical resection should be seen in 4 to 6 wk to ensure that the adenoma has been completely removed and that any endocrine hypersecretion is resolved.
- If there is good clinical response, patient should be monitored yearly for recurrence and to follow the level of the hypersecreted hormone.
- Patients who have undergone irradiation should experience close follow-up with backup medical therapy, because response to radiotherapy may be delayed; incidence of hypopituitarism also increases with time.
- Surgical resection is not indicated in pituitary incidentalomas that are microadenomas, as only 10% will experience tumor growth.
- Approximately 30% of surgically resected adenomas have persistent or progressive postoperative growth for several decades. Tumors particularly prone to invasive growth and recurrence include those arising from sparsely granulated somatotrophs, silent corticotrophs, corticotroph Crooke cells, and lactotrophs in middle-aged or older men.

SUGGESTED READINGS

Available at eBooks.Health.Elsevier.com.

RELATED CONTENT

Pituitary Adenoma (Patient Information)
Acromegaly (Related Key Topic)
Amenorrhea (Related Key Topic)
Cushing Disease and Syndrome (Related Key Topic)
Galactorrhea (Related Key Topic)
Prolactinoma (Related Key Topic)

AUTHORS: **AMANDA JONES, MD,** and **ANTHONY SCISCIONE, DO**

P

BASIC INFORMATION

DEFINITION
The diagnosis of placenta previa is based on sonography and requires the identification of echogenic homogeneous placental tissue over the internal cervical os. When the placental edge is <2 cm from the internal os, the placenta is called "low-lying." The historic terms "marginal" and "partial" for characterizing a placenta previa are no longer used. A classification of placenta previa in "major" or "minor" is described in Table 1 and illustrated in Fig. 1.

One hypothesis is that the lower uterine cavity contains more vascularized decidua, which promotes implantation of trophoblast toward the cervical os. Another hypothesis is that a particularly large placental surface area increases the probability that the placenta will implant over the cervical os.

ICD-10CM CODES
O44	Placenta previa
O44.0	Complete placenta previa NOS or without hemorrhage
O44.1	Complete placenta previa with hemorrhage
O44.2	Partial placenta previa without hemorrhage
O44.3	Partial placenta previa with hemorrhage
O44.4	Low-lying placenta NOS or without hemorrhage
O44.5	Low-lying placenta with hemorrhage

TABLE 1 Classification of Placenta Previa

Minor	I	Encroaches the lower uterine segment
	II	Reaches internal os of the cervix (marginal)
Major	III	Covers part of internal os (partial)
	IV	Completely covers the internal os (complete)

From Magowan BA: *Clinical obstetrics and gynecology,* ed 4, London, 2019, Elsevier.

EPIDEMIOLOGY & DEMOGRAPHICS
INCIDENCE: The pooled prevalence of major placenta previa was 4.3 cases/1000 pregnancies. Prevalence was highest among Asian studies (12.2/1000) and lower among studies from Europe (3.6/1000), North America (2.9/1000), and sub-Saharan Africa (2.7/1000).
RISK FACTORS:
- Previous placenta previa (recurs in 4% to 8% of subsequent pregnancies)
- Previous cesarean delivery (increases incidence by 47% to 60%)
- Multiparity
- Multiple gestation (increases prevalence by 40%)
- Smoking and cocaine use
- Previous intrauterine surgical procedure or Asherman syndrome
- Abnormal or large placenta

PHYSICAL FINDINGS & CLINICAL PRESENTATION
The classic presentation of placenta previa is painless vaginal bleeding, usually in the second or third trimester. 10% to 20% of women present with uterine contractions, pain, and bleeding. On physical examination, the uterus is soft and pain free. The fetus is often in breech, transverse lie, or high. Fetal distress is usually not present.

DIAGNOSIS

DIFFERENTIAL DIAGNOSIS
- Morbidly adherent placenta (accreta, increta, percreta)
- Vasa previa
- Abruptio placentae
- Vaginal or cervical trauma
- Labor
- Local malignancy

WORKUP
- Do *not* perform a digital vaginal examination.
- Perform a speculum examination in a hospital setting to exclude any local bleeding.
- Perform a transvaginal ultrasonography to assess for placental location.
- Exclude the presence of placenta previa-accreta in patients with a history of cesarean sections. In a prospective study, the frequency of placenta accreta increased with an increasing number of cesarean deliveries: 3% for first cesarean, 11% for second cesarean, 40% for third cesarean, 61% for fourth cesarean, and up to 67% for fifth or more cesarean sections.

LABORATORY TESTS
- A CBC can be used to monitor hemoglobin and hematocrit.
- A Kleihauer-Betke preparation of maternal blood in all Rh-negative women and Rh-immune globulin when indicated.

IMAGING STUDIES
- The simplest and safest method of placental localization is transabdominal sonography with confirmatory imaging by transvaginal ultrasonography (TVUS). Transabdominal ultrasonography alone is inaccurate in the diagnosis of placenta previa and should be used only as a screening tool. TVUS (Fig. 2) has become the gold standard for the diagnosis of placenta previa. It is safe even in the presence of active bleeding.
- MRI has also been effective in detecting placenta previa, although sonography remains the preferred method due to lower cost, widespread availability, and well-established accuracy.

TREATMENT

MANAGEMENT OF ASYMPTOMATIC PLACENTA PREVIA
- Avoid sexual activity, digital exams, and extraneous exercise.
- Review bleeding precautions and anticipatory guidance, including the need for cesarean section and the risk for hysterectomy early in pregnancy.

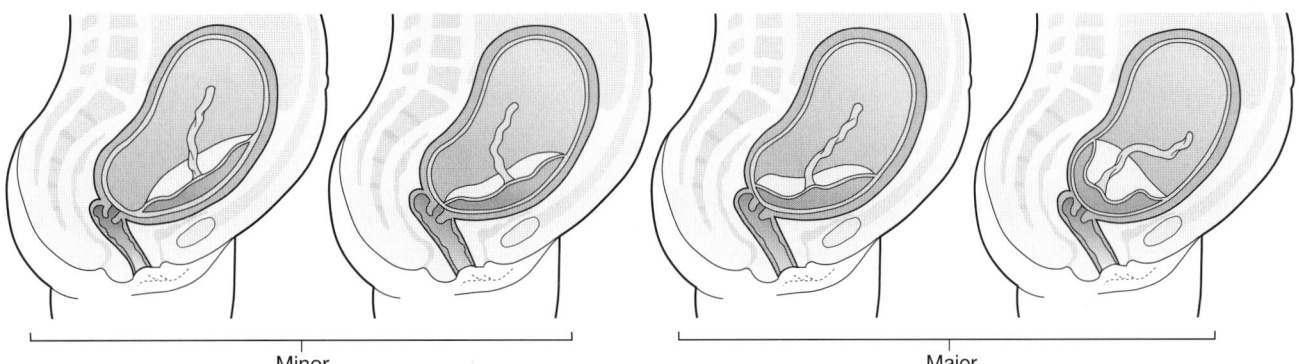

Minor   Major

FIG. 1 Classification into "major" and "minor" placenta previa depends on the distance of the placenta from the internal os of the cervix. In the presence of a cesarean section scar, an anterior placenta previa may result in abnormal invasion (morbidly adherent placenta, placenta accreta). (From Magowan BA: *Clinical obstetrics and gynecology,* ed 4, London, 2019, Elsevier.)

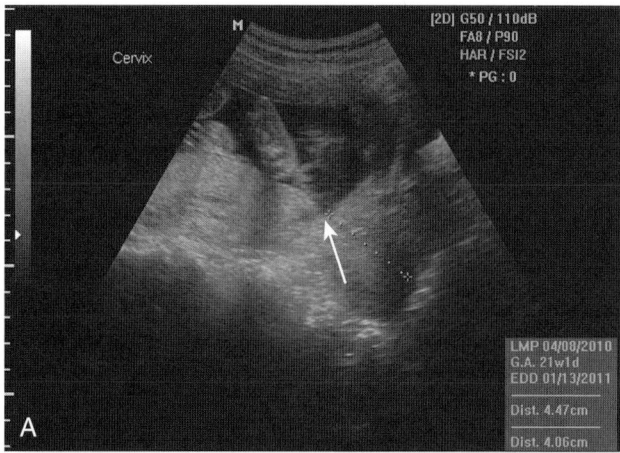
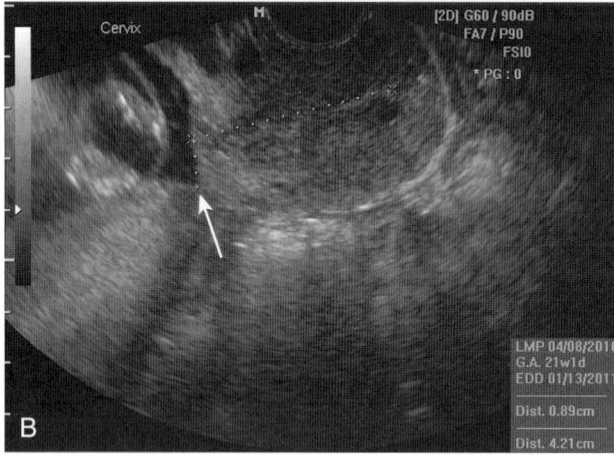

FIG. 2 Transabdominal ultrasonography and transvaginal ultrasonography of marginal placenta previa. *Arrows* identify placental edge. (Courtesy K. Francois. From Gabbe SG: *Obstetrics,* ed 6, Philadelphia, 2012, Saunders.)

Sequential assessment of placental location:
- At 32 wk, follow-up is indicated:
  1. If the placental edge is ≥2 cm from the internal os, placenta previa has resolved, and no further assessment is required.
  2. If the placental edge is over or <2 cm from the internal os, placenta previa persists, and repeat at 36 wk is indicated.
- At 36 wk:
  1. If the placental edge is ≥2 cm, the patient is consented for vaginal delivery.
  2. If the placental edge is over the internal os, cesarean delivery is scheduled.

Timing of delivery:
- Cesarean delivery at 36+0 to 37+6 wk in pregnancies with uncomplicated placenta previa

MANAGEMENT OF SYMPTOMATIC PLACENTA PREVIA
- Initial assessment for signs of maternal hemodynamic compromise or hemorrhagic shock; large-bore IV access with crystalloid fluid resuscitation.
- Assess fetal status and gestational age by sonogram and continuous fetal heart rate monitoring.
- Cross-matched blood should be made available during bleeding episodes.
- Tocolytic therapy should not be administered in an actively bleeding patient.
- Magnesium sulfate therapy for fetal neuroprotection should be considered in those with symptomatic preterm (<32 wk) placenta

previa if the decision has been made to likely deliver the patient within 24 hr. Emergent delivery should not be delayed to administer magnesium.
- Cesarean delivery is indicated for active labor, nonreassuring fetal heart rate tracing, active bleeding with hemodynamic instability, and significant bleeding after 34 wks' gestation.

Expectant management after a resolved bleed:
- Antenatal corticosteroid should be administered to symptomatic women between 23+0 and 36+6 wks' gestation to enhance fetal pulmonary maturity.
- Correct anemia.
- Administer anti-D immune globulin to D-negative women.

DISPOSITION
Inpatient versus outpatient: Consider discharge for women whose bleeding has stopped for 24 h and live in close proximity to the hospital, demonstrate compliance with medical management, can maintain bed rest, understand bleeding precautions, and have an adult companion available for transport 24 h a day.

PEARLS & CONSIDERATIONS

COMMENTS
- Placenta previa is diagnosed by TVUS, with repeat assessment at 32 and 36 wk when indicated.
- Asymptomatic placenta previa can be managed expectantly with a planned cesarean delivery at 36+0 to 37+6 wk.
- Symptomatic placenta previa is managed by assessing hemodynamic stability, considering steroids for fetal lung maturity, magnesium sulfate for fetal neuroprotection when indicated, and cesarean delivery.

SUGGESTED READINGS
Available at eBooks.Health.Elsevier.com.

RELATED CONTENT
Placenta Previa (Patient Information)
Vaginal Bleeding During Pregnancy (Related Key Topic)

AUTHORS: **HELEN B. GOMEZ SLAGLE, MD,** and **ANTHONY SCISCIONE, DO**

BASIC INFORMATION

DEFINITION

A pleural effusion is the pathologic accumulation of fluid in the pleural space, stemming from a wide range of etiologies.

SYNONYMS

Exudates
Transudates
Hydrothorax
Hemothorax
Chylothorax
Empyema

ICD-10CM CODES

J90 Pleural effusion, not elsewhere classified
J91.8 Pleural effusion in other conditions classified elsewhere

PHYSICAL FINDINGS & CLINICAL PRESENTATION

- Subjective symptoms largely depend on the underlying etiology and may include dyspnea, cough, fatigue, fever, chest pain.
- Box 1 summarizes signs and symptoms of pleural effusion.
- Physical examination findings include asymmetric chest wall expansion, dullness to percussion, decreased tactile fremitus, and decreased breath sounds.

ETIOLOGY

A pleural effusion may be caused by a number of factors, including increased capillary permeability, increased vascular hydrostatic pressure, decreased vascular oncotic pressure, inflammation of the pleura, traumatic/iatrogenic causes, and/or obstruction of normal pleural fluid efflux. Box 2 summarizes causes of pleural effusion.[1]

BOX 1 Signs and Symptoms of Effusion

Dyspnea
Cough (dry, nonproductive)
Chest pain (pleuritic or nonpleuritic)
Chest wall discomfort
Decreased breath sounds
Dullness to percussion
Egophony, decreased tactile fremitus
Pleural friction rub
Asymmetric chest wall excursion
Disease-specific signs and symptoms
  may include:
Orthopnea
Paroxysmal nocturnal dyspnea
Fever
Night sweats

From Adams JG et al: *Emergency medicine: clinical essentials*, ed 2, Philadelphia, 2013, Elsevier.

BOX 2 Causes of Pleural Effusions

Transudates
Atelectasis (early)
Congestive heart failure
Central venous occlusion
Glomerulonephritis
Hepatic hydrothorax
Hypoalbuminemia
Myxedema
Nephrotic syndrome
Peritoneal dialysis
Pulmonary embolism
Veno-occlusive disease

Exudates
Infectious
Bacterial infection
Fungal infection
Lung abscess
Parasitic infection
Traumatic hemothorax
Tuberculosis
Viral illness

Malignancies
Lymphoma
Mesothelioma
Primary lung cancer
Pulmonary metastasis

Connective Tissue Disease
Eosinophilic granulomatosis
Granulomatosis with polyangiitis
Rheumatoid arthritis
Systemic lupus erythematosus
Sjögren syndrome

Abdominal/Gastrointestinal
Esophageal rupture
Pancreatic disorders
Subphrenic abscess

Other
Asbestos
Atelectasis (chronic)
Chylothorax
Cerebrospinal fluid leak or ventriculopleural
  shunt
Drug reactions (amiodarone, nitrofurantoin)
Hemothorax
Meigs syndrome
Myxedema
Postpartum state
Postsurgical (abdominal, cardiac bypass)
Pulmonary infarction or embolism
Thoracic endometriosis
Uremia
Superior vena cava syndrome
Yellow nail syndrome

From Adams JG et al: *Emergency medicine: clinical essentials*, ed 2, Philadelphia, 2013, Elsevier.

DIAGNOSIS

DIFFERENTIAL DIAGNOSIS

Differential diagnosis for causes of pleural effusion includes:

- **Transudate**—effusions that stem from hydrostatic and oncotic imbalances; characterized by pleural: serum lactate dehydrogenase (LDH) ratio ≤ 0.6, pleural: serum protein ratio ≤ 0.5, and pleural LDH ratio $\leq \frac{2}{3}$ upper limit of normal serum LDH.[2] Possible causes of transudative pleural effusions include:
  1. Heart failure
  2. Cirrhosis (hepatic hydrothorax)
  3. Chronic renal insufficiency (nephrotic syndrome or peritoneal dialysis)
  4. Hypoalbuminemia
  5. Myxedema
  6. Pericardial disease
  7. Urinothorax
- **Exudate**—effusions that stem from an infiltrative or inflammatory process; characterized by pleural to serum LDH ratio >0.6 or total protein ratio >0.5 or pleural to upper limit of normal for serum LDH ratio $>2:3$. Box 3 describes cellular differential of pleural effusions.

BOX 3 Cellular Differential of Pleural Effusions

Neutrophilia (>50%)
- Bacterial pneumonia (parapneumonic effusion)
- Pulmonary infarction
- Pancreatitis
- Subphrenic abscess
- Early tuberculosis
- Transudates (>10%)

Lymphocytosis (>50%)
- Tuberculosis
- Viral infection
- Malignancy (lymphoma, other neoplasms)
- True chylothorax
- Rheumatoid pleuritis
- Systemic lupus erythematosus
- Uremic effusions
- Transudates ($\approx$30%)

Eosinophilia (>10%)
- Pneumothorax (air in pleural space)
- Trauma
- Pulmonary infarction
- Congestive heart failure
- Infection (especially parasitic, fungal)
- Hypersensitivity syndromes
- Drug reaction
- Rheumatologic diseases
- Hodgkin disease
- Idiopathic
- Iatrogenic (repeat taps introducing blood/air)

From McPherson RA, Pincus MR: *Henry's clinical diagnosis and management by laboratory methods*, ed 23, St Louis, 2017, Elsevier.

Possible causes of exudative pleural effusions include:
1. Malignancy: metastatic cancer or primary (e.g., mesothelioma)
2. Infection
   a. Parapneumonic effusion (simple = pH >7.2, complicated = ≤7.2 or glucose <60)[3]
   b. Empyema (pus in the pleural space, positive pleural fluid cultures or Gram stain from pleural fluid) [See chapter on "Empyema"]
   c. Fungal
   d. Tuberculous effusion
   e. Viral
3. Pulmonary embolism (rarely can present as transudate)
4. Hemothorax
5. Chylothorax
6. Esophageal perforation
7. Pleuropancreatic fistula
8. Biliothorax
9. Collagen vascular disease (e.g., rheumatoid arthritis, systemic lupus erythematosus, eosinophilic granulomatosis, granulomatosis with polyangiitis)
10. Asbestos
11. Meigs syndrome (association of pleural effusion with ascites and ovarian fibroma)

WORKUP

Thoracentesis can help to establish the etiology of a pleural effusion. The Light criteria should be used for classification of the pleural effusion (summarized in Box 4). Fig. 1 illustrates a diagnostic algorithm for pleural effusions. A thorough history and physical examination can avoid unnecessary instrumentation, as it is important to remember that not all pleural effusions need to be immediately sampled (e.g., clear history of heart failure).[1,4] Fig. E2 illustrates an approach to malignant pleural effusions.

LABORATORY TESTS

See Table 1.

IMAGING STUDIES

- **Chest x-ray examination** (Fig. 3)**:** Blunting of the costophrenic angle, ipsilateral atelectasis, contralateral shift of the mediastinum with large effusions, elevated hemidiaphragm with subpulmonic effusions, "spine sign" on lateral chest x-ray examination, may be free-flowing or fixed on lateral decubitus film depending on etiology.
- **Ultrasonography** (Fig. E4): Bedside transthoracic ultrasound can be helpful to identify characteristics of pleural effusions, including:
  1. Size, location, and laterality
  2. Echogenicity of pleural fluid, presence of loculations, pleural adhesions, or pleural implants
  3. Procedure planning (e.g., thoracentesis, chest tube)
  4. Underlying lung parenchymal pathology (e.g., pulmonary edema, consolidation, pneumothorax)
  5. Signs of other pathologies (e.g., ascites, B lines)
  6. Diaphragmatic excursion
- **Computed tomography** (Fig. E5): Useful to identify loculated effusions and to assess underlying lung parenchyma to aid in establishing a diagnosis. In empyema, can demonstrate heterogeneity and gas bubbles. (See chapter on "Empyema.")

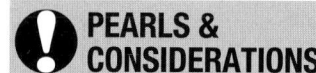 **TREATMENT**

- Table 2 summarizes treatment options for pleural effusions.
- Table 3 summarizes options for control of symptomatic malignant effusions. Fig. 6 describes a treatment approach to malignant pleural effusions.

REFERRAL

Negative diagnostic workup after initial pleural fluid sampling should be followed by referral to a pulmonologist for further evaluation (including consideration for thoracoscopy for pleural biopsy).

❶ PEARLS & CONSIDERATIONS

- One-time drainage of a pleural effusion is seldom a definitive therapy.
- Early identification of the underlying etiology of new effusions should be pursued. Pleural biopsy should be considered when the underlying etiology is uncertain.[4]
- Pleural drainage with a catheter should be considered when the pleural infection is suspected.[4]
- Managing patients with malignant pleural effusion can be challenging and should be tailored to the patient on a case-by-case basis. In patients near the end of life with malignant pleural effusions that are slow to reaccumulate fluid, repeat thoracentesis, as needed, is a reasonable strategy.[4]
- Tunneled indwelling pleural catheters have gained favor for ambulatory management of malignant pleural effusions[5] and are increasingly utilized for the management of refractory noncancerous pleural effusions.[6]
- The LENT score is a validated prognostic score (incorporating LDH in pleural fluid, ECOG score, neutrophil to lymphocyte ratio in serum, and tumor type) that can be used to predict survival in malignant pleural effusions and to help inform treatment decisions in patients.[7]
- Pleurodesis should also be considered when feasible. A recent trial showed that, among patients with malignant pleural effusion, outpatient administration of talc via an indwelling tunneled pleural catheter resulted in a higher rate of pleurodesis and catheter removal than placement of a tunneled catheter alone.[8]

REFERENCES & SUGGESTED READING

Available at eBooks.Health.Elsevier.com.

RELATED CONTENT

Empyema (Related Key Topic)
Heart Failure (Related Key Topic)
Lung Neoplasms, Primary (Related Key Topic)

AUTHORS: **YARON B. GESTHALTER, MD,** and **ILANA KRUMM, MD**

BOX 4 Light Criteria for Classification of Pleural Effusions

In 1972, Light et al. developed the currently accepted benchmark for classifying pleural fluid, as follows:
Pleural fluid protein to serum protein ratio >0.5:1
Pleural fluid lactate dehydrogenase (LDH) to serum LDH ratio >0.6:1
Pleural fluid LDH greater than two thirds the upper limit of normal for serum LDH (a cutoff value of 200 IU/L was used previously)
   Pleural fluid is classified as an exudate if it meets any of the aforementioned criteria. Conversely, if all three characteristics are absent, the fluid is classified as a transudate. These researchers achieved a diagnostic sensitivity of 99% and a specificity of 98% for classification of an exudate.

From Adams JG etal: *Emergency medicine: clinical essentials,* ed 2, Philadelphia, 2013, Elsevier.

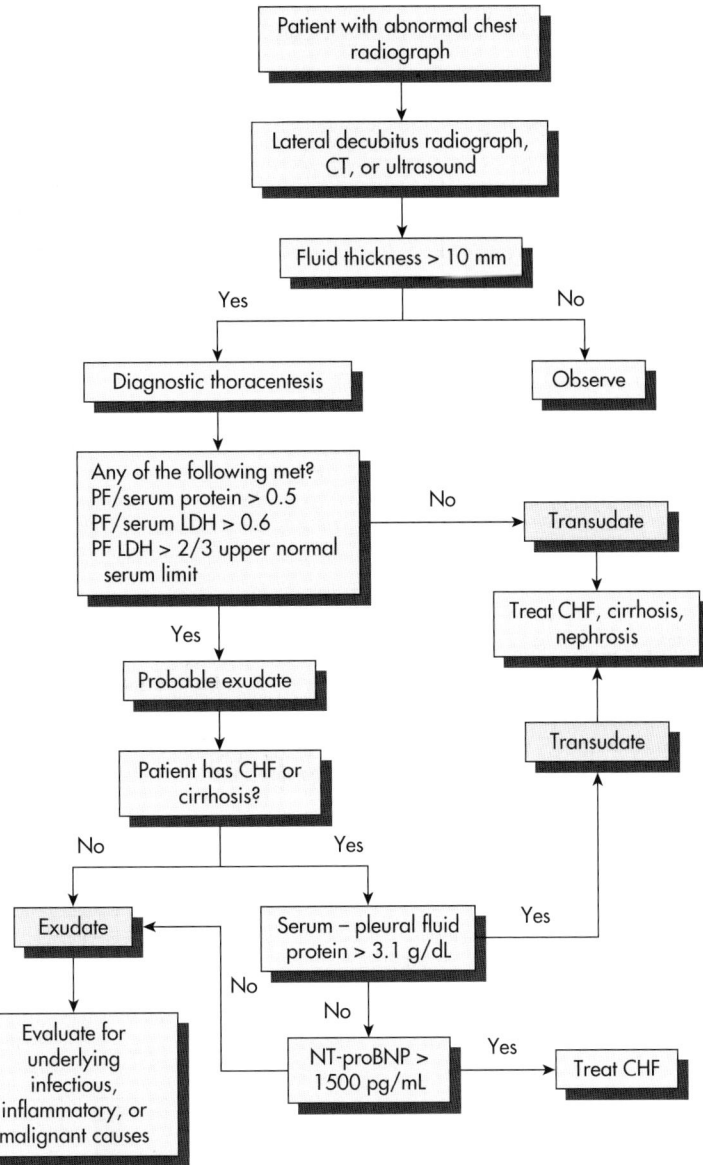

FIG. 1 Algorithm for distinguishing transudative from exudative pleural effusions. With the results of the initial thoracentesis, one can usually determine whether the effusion is an exudate or a transudate. If a transudate, the treatment can be directed to the likely causes—*congestive heart failure* (CHF), liver disease, or kidney disease. If the protein and *lactate dehydrogenase* (LDH) results are borderline exudative and there is also CHF or cirrhosis present, there is a possibility that the effusion is still transudative. To determine this, one can use two additional tests: If the difference between the serum and pleural fluid protein concentrations is greater than 3.1 g/dl, one can assume that the effusion is transudative. If not, one can test the pleural or serum *N-terminal pro–brain natriuretic peptide* (NT-proBNP); if greater than 1500 pg/ml, one can conclude that CHF is at least one of the causes of the effusion. Once the effusion is determined to be exudative, one can focus on further evaluation of the underlying inflammatory, infectious, or malignant cause. *CT*, Computed tomography; *PF*, Pleural fluid. (From Broaddus VC et al: *Murray & Nadel's textbook of respiratory medicine*, ed 7, Philadelphia, 2022, Elsevier.)

TABLE 1   Selected Laboratory Tests Used to Diagnose Pleural Effusion

Test	Diagnostic Utility	Comments
Adenosine deaminase (ADA)	<40 IU/L excludes tuberculous pleurisy	Values >72 IU/L highly specific for tuberculosis, with improved yield with pleural biopsy and PCR, can also be elevated in lymphoma and parapneumonic effusions
Albumin	Pleural: Serum albumin ratio <0.83 more consistent with transudate	Can be used to corroborate mixed findings from LDH and protein ratios
Amylase	Esophageal perforation, pancreatitis, malignancy	
Cell count	**Lymphocyte** predominance suggestive of tuberculosis, lymphoma, malignancy, pulmonary embolism **Neutrophil** predominant effusions seen with bacterial infection, occasionally with malignancy (20%) **Eosinophil** (>10%) predominance is suggestive of air or blood	Helpful in distinguishing causes of exudative effusions
Chylomicrons	Positive finding adds to specificity of triglycerides for establishing chylothorax	Consider thoracic duct defect (due to malignancy, trauma or iatrogenic)
Creatinine	Pleural: Serum creatinine >1 suggests urinothorax	
Culture	Positive findings used to narrow therapy	Should be sent from every suspected parapneumonic effusion to guide antimicrobial selection
Cytology	Sensitivity for malignancy of ~65%	Diagnostic yield increases with two serial samples (~90%)
Glucose	<60 mg/dl suggests complicated parapneumonic effusion, malignancy, tuberculous pleurisy, or rheumatoid effusion	
Hematocrit	Pleural fluid hematocrit >50% peripheral blood hematocrit consistent with hemothorax	Pleural fluid with relatively low hematocrit can appear bloody on gross exam, does not necessarily represent hemothorax
Lactate dehydrogenase (LDH)	Pleural to serum LDH ratio >0.6 or pleural LDH >$^2/_3$ the upper limit of normal serum LDH suggests exudate	
pH	≤7.2 with clinical suspicion highly suggestive of complicated parapneumonic effusion	Can also have low pH with malignant pleural effusions and esophageal perforation
Protein	Pleural to serum protein ratio >0.5 suggests exudate	Very low pleural protein (<0.5g/dl) suggests urinothorax or peritoneal dialysis associated effusion
NT-proBNP	>1500 pg/ml suggests heart failure even if effusion meets criteria for exudate	Chronic pleural effusions related to heart failure in patients on diuretic therapy may appear exudative
Triglycerides	Triglycerides >110 mg/dl seen with chylothorax <50 mg/dl argues against the presence of a chylothorax	Absent triglycerides with high suspicion for chylothorax can be confirmed with pleural chylomicrons

NT-proBNP, N-terminal pro b-type natriuretic peptide; *PCR,* polymerase chain reaction.

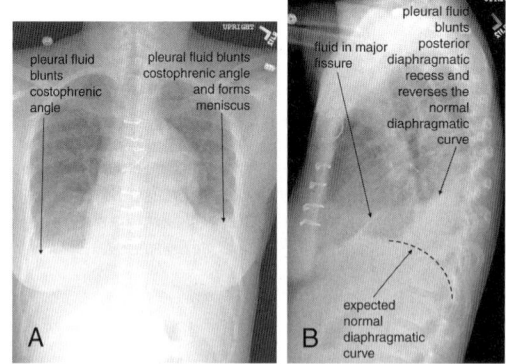

FIG. 3 Pleural effusions. A, Posterior-anterior upright view in which a pleural effusion is most evident on this patient's left side. Both costophrenic angles are blunted. The pleural effusion forms a meniscus against the left lateral chest wall. **B,** Lateral upright view shows two meniscus densities, suggesting bilateral pleural effusions. The posterior diaphragmatic recess is filled with pleural fluid, which forms a meniscus with the posterior chest wall. (From Broder JS: *Diagnostic imaging for the emergency physician,* Philadelphia, 2011, Saunders.)

TABLE 2 Treatment Options for Pleural Effusion

Thoracentesis	Site selection should be guided by ultrasonography whenever possible; evacuation of pleural fluid can be limited when the lung cannot fully re-expand, including central airway obstruction, chronic atelectasis, and the presence of extensive pleural adhesions; aspiration in these circumstances can lead to pneumothorax ex vacuo
Tube thoracostomy	Consider when ongoing drainage will be needed, especially for empyema or hemothorax
Indwelling tunneled pleural catheter	A cuffed pleural drainage catheter tunneled through subcutaneous tissue, drained regularly on an outpatient basis, most commonly used to manage malignant pleural effusions
Pleurodesis	Instillation of a chemical irritant under direct thoracoscopic visualization (e.g., talc poudrage) or via tube thoracostomy to adhere the visceral and parietal pleurae, can also be done with mechanical pleurodesis via video-assisted thoracic surgery
Pharmacotherapy	Based on underlying etiology (e.g., diuretics, antimicrobials, chemotherapy)

TABLE 3 Options for Control of Symptomatic Malignant Effusions

Option	Patient Eligibility and Considerations
Chemotherapy, targeted therapy	Responsive tumor
Therapeutic thoracentesis	Slowly recurring effusion
	Used for patients with very short life expectancy
Pleurodesis	
Via chest tube	Lung able to reinflate
Via thoracoscopy	Can free up lung tacked down by adhesions, obtain biopsies
	Thoracoscopy must be available
Indwelling pleural catheter	Can be used as first line and coupled with talc pleurodesis if suitable
	Good outpatient situation
	Good for trapped lung
Pleuroperitoneal shunt	Patient able to operate pump
	Good for trapped lung
	Good for chylothorax (provided there is no concurrent ascites)
Pleurectomy	
Via thoracoscopy	When other less-invasive options have failed
Via thoracotomy	Good patient status and life expectancy

From Broaddus VC et al: *Murray & Nadel's textbook of respiratory medicine,* ed 7, Philadelphia, 2022, Elsevier.

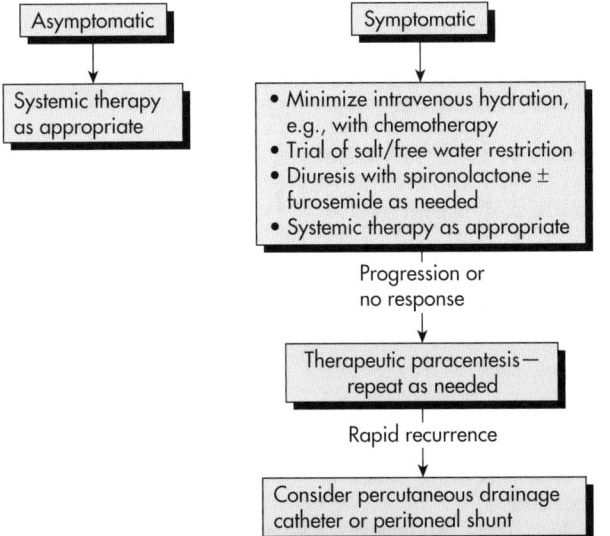

FIG. 6 Treatment approach algorithm to malignant pleural effusions. (From Niederhuber JE: *Abeloff's clinical oncology,* ed 6, Philadelphia, 2020, Elsevier.)

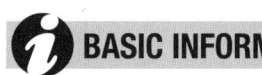
BASIC INFORMATION

DEFINITION

Pneumonia is defined as inflammation of the pulmonary parenchyma caused by an infectious agent (in this case, bacteria). It can be further categorized as community-acquired or health care-associated. The definition of community-acquired pneumonia (CAP), traditionally referred to alveolar infection that develops in the outpatient setting or within 48 hr of admission, now includes patients previously categorized as having health care-associated pneumonia (HCAP) since the microbiology and treatment is similar. Hospital-acquired pneumonia (HAP) is pneumonia occurring ≥48 h after hospital admission and not incubating at the time of admission.[1]

SYNONYMS

Community-acquired pneumonia
CAP
Health care-associated pneumonia
Hospital-acquired pneumonia

ICD-10CM CODES

J15.9	Unspecified bacterial pneumonia
J13	Pneumonia due to *Streptococcus pneumoniae*
J15.1	Pneumonia due to *Pseudomonas*
J15.20	Pneumonia due to staphylococcus, unspecified
J15.0	Pneumonia due to *Klebsiella pneumoniae*
J14	Pneumonia due to *Haemophilus influenzae*
J15.211	Pneumonia due to methicillin-susceptible *Staphylococcus aureus*
J15.212	Pneumonia due to methicillin-resistant *Staphylococcus aureus*
J15.6	Pneumonia due to other aerobic gram-negative bacteria
J15.7	Pneumonia due to *Mycoplasma pneumoniae*

EPIDEMIOLOGY & DEMOGRAPHICS

- The annual incidence of pneumonia in the U.S. is 24.8 cases per 10,000 adults, with the highest rates among adults between 65 to 79 yr of age (63 cases per 10,000 adults) and those >80 yr old (164.3 cases per 10,000 adults). Health care expenditures for CAP exceed $10 billion annually.
- Hospitalization rate for pneumonia is 15% to 20%. Incidence is highest among the oldest adults.
- In 2017, the tenth leading cause of mortality in the U.S. reported by the National Center for Health Statistics was influenza and pneumonia together. Deaths per 100,000 population: 15.1.
- Globally, *Streptococcus pneumoniae* (pneumococcus) is the most common pathogen causing community-acquired pneumonia.

PHYSICAL FINDINGS & CLINICAL PRESENTATION

- Fever, tachypnea, chills, tachycardia, cough, and sometimes pleuritic chest pain (especially if a pleural effusion is present)

- Presentation varies with the cause of pneumonia, the patient's age, and the clinical situation:
  1. Patients with streptococcal pneumonia usually present with high fever, chills, atypical chest pain, cough, and copious production of rusty-appearing purulent sputum. Pleurisy in the setting of parapneumonic effusions can also occur. Potential complications include bacteremia, empyema, and distant infections (e.g., meningitis).
  2. *Mycoplasma pneumoniae:* Insidious onset; headache; dry, paroxysmal cough that is worse at night; myalgias; malaise; sore throat; extrapulmonary manifestations (e.g., erythema multiforme, aseptic meningitis, urticaria, erythema nodosum) may be present. (See chapter on "Mycoplasma Pneumonia.")
  3. *Chlamydia pneumoniae:* Persistent, nonproductive cough, low-grade fever, headache, sore throat.
  4. *Legionella pneumophila:* High fever, mild cough, mental status change, myalgias, diarrhea, respiratory failure. (See chapter on "Legionnaires Disease.")
  5. MRSA pneumonia: Often preceded by influenza, may present with shock and respiratory failure.
  6. Elderly or immunocompromised hosts with pneumonia may initially present with only minimal symptoms (e.g., low-grade fever, confusion); respiratory and nonrespiratory symptoms are less commonly reported by older patients with pneumonia.
- In general, auscultation of lungs in patients with pneumonia reveals crackles/rhonchi and diminished breath sounds. Egophany may also be present.
- Dullness on percussion or decreased fremitus may be an indication that a pleural effusion is present.

ETIOLOGY[2]

- Table 1 summarizes common pathogens causing CAP
- *Streptococcus pneumoniae* (5% to 15% of hospitalized CAP cases): Incidence has been declining due to widespread use of pneumococcal vaccination and reduced rate of cigarette smoking
- *Haemophilus influenzae* (3% to 10% of CAP cases)
- *L. pneumophila* (1% to 5% of adult pneumonias) (2% to 8% of CAP cases)
- *Klebsiella pneumoniae, Pseudomonas aeruginosa, Escherichia coli*
- *Staphylococcus aureus* (3% to 5% of CAP cases)
- Atypical organisms such as *Mycoplasma pneumoniae, Chlamydia pneumoniae,* and *Legionella pneumophila* implicated in up to 40% of cases of CAP
- Gram-negative organisms cause >80% of nosocomial pneumonias
- Predisposing factors (Table 2 and Table 3):
  1. Influenza infection is one of the important predisposing factors to *S. pneumoniae* and *S. aureus* pneumonia

  2. Chronic obstructive pulmonary disease: *H. influenzae, S. pneumoniae, Legionella, Moraxella catarrhalis*
  3. Seizures: Aspiration pneumonia
  4. Compromised hosts: *Legionella,* gram-negative organisms
  5. Alcoholism: *K. pneumoniae, S. pneumoniae, H. influenzae*
  6. HIV: *S. pneumoniae*
  7. IV drug addicts with right-sided bacterial endocarditis: *S. aureus*
  8. Older patient with comorbid diseases: *C. pneumoniae*

DIAGNOSIS

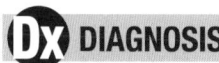

DIFFERENTIAL DIAGNOSIS

- Viral pneumonias (see chapter on "Viral Pneumonia")
- Aspiration pneumonia (see chapter on "Aspiration Pneumonia")
- Exacerbation of chronic bronchitis
- Pulmonary embolism or infarction (see chapter on "Pulmonary Embolism")
- Lung neoplasm
- Bronchiolitis
- Sarcoidosis (see chapter on "Sarcoidosis")
- Hypersensitivity pneumonitis (see chapter on "Hypersensitivity Pneumonitis")
- Pulmonary edema
- Drug-induced lung injury
- Fungal pneumonias
- Parasitic pneumonias
- Atypical pneumonia
- Tuberculosis
- Cryptogenic organizing pneumonia

WORKUP

Diagnostic testing for CAP is summarized in Table 4. Useful tools for assessing severity of illness are the *CURB-65* (see "Disposition") and *Pneumonia Severity Index* (Fig. 1 and Box 1). Poor prognostic indicators are hypotension (SBP <90 or DBP <60), respiratory rate >30/min, fever (>40° C; 104° F), or hypothermia (<35° C; 95° F). None of these indices is as valuable as clinical judgment.[3]

LABORATORY TESTS

- Complete blood count with differential; white blood cell count is elevated, usually with left shift or the presence of bandemia
- Sputum culture should be obtained, ideally prior to initiation of antibiotics, in hospitalized patients or if drug-resistant or unusual pathogen is suspected
- Blood cultures (hospitalized patients only): Positive in approximately 20% of cases of pneumococcal pneumonia
- Pneumococcal urinary antigen test can be used to detect the C-polysaccharide antigen of *S. pneumoniae* (70% sensitivity). It is a useful tool in the treatment of hospitalized adult patients with CAP[4]
- When suspecting *Legionella,* a respiratory specimen culture on special media and/or a urinary antigen should be requested
- Serologic testing for HIV in selected patients

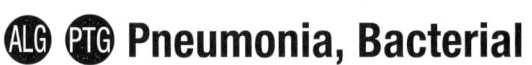

TABLE 1 Common Pathogens Causing Community-Acquired Pneumonia

Inpatient, With No Cardiopulmonary Disease or Modifying Factors

Streptococcus pneumoniae, Haemophilus influenzae, Mycoplasma pneumoniae, Chlamydophila pneumoniae, mixed infection (bacteria plus atypical pathogen), viruses (including influenza), *Legionella* spp., and others *(Mycobacterium tuberculosis,* endemic fungi, *Pneumocystis jirovecii)*

Inpatient, With Cardiopulmonary Disease and/or Modifying Factors

All of the above, but drug-resistant *S. pneumoniae* (DRSP) and enteric gram-negative organisms are more of a concern

Severe Community-Acquired Pneumonia, With No Risks for *Pseudomonas Aeruginosa*

S. pneumoniae (including DRSP), *Legionella* spp., *H. influenzae,* enteric gram-negative bacilli, *Staphylococcus aureus* (including methicillin-resistant *S. aureus*), *M. pneumoniae,* respiratory viruses (including influenza), others *(C. pneumoniae, M. tuberculosis,* endemic fungi)

Severe CAP, With Risks for *P. Aeruginosa*

All of the pathogens above plus *P. aeruginosa*

From Vincent JL et al: *Textbook of critical care,* ed 7, Philadelphia, 2017, Elsevier.

TABLE 2 Risk Factors for Developing Severe Community-Acquired Pneumonia

Advanced age
Comorbid illness (e.g., chronic respiratory illness, cardiovascular disease, diabetes mellitus, neurologic illness, renal insufficiency, malignancy)
Cigarette smoking
Alcohol abuse
Absence of antibiotic therapy before hospitalization
Failure to contain infection to its initial site of entry
Immune suppression
Genetic polymorphisms in the immune response

From Vincent JL et al: *Textbook of critical care,* ed 7, Philadelphia, 2017, Elsevier.

TABLE 3 Clinical Associations With Specific Pathogens

Condition	Commonly Encountered Pathogens
Alcoholism	*Streptococcus pneumoniae* (including penicillin-resistant), anaerobes, gram-negative bacilli (possibly *Klebsiella pneumoniae*), tuberculosis
Chronic obstructive pulmonary disease/current or former smoker	*S. pneumoniae, Haemophilus influenzae, Moraxella catarrhalis*
Residence in nursing home	*S. pneumoniae,* gram-negative bacilli, *H. influenzae, Staphylococcus aureus, Chlamydophila pneumoniae;* consider *M. tuberculosis.* Consider anaerobes, but these are less common
Poor dental hygiene	Anaerobes
Bat exposure	*Histoplasma capsulatum*
Bird exposure	*Chlamydophila psittaci, Cryptococcus neoformans, H. capsulatum*
Rabbit exposure	*Francisella tularensis*
Travel to southwestern United States	*Coccidioidomycosis;* hantavirus in selected areas
Exposure to farm animals or parturient cats	*Coxiella burnetii* (Q fever)
Postinfluenza pneumonia	*S. pneumoniae, S. aureus* (including the community-acquired strain of methicillin-resistant *S. aureus), H. influenzae*
Structural disease of the lung (e.g., bronchiectasis, cystic fibrosis)	*Pseudomonas aeruginosa, Pseudomonas cepacia,* or *S. aureus*
Sickle cell disease, asplenia	Pneumococcus, *H. influenzae*
Suspected bioterrorism	Anthrax, tularemia, plague
Travel to Asia	Severe acute respiratory syndrome, tuberculosis, melioidosis

From Vincent JL et al: *Textbook of critical care,* ed 7, Philadelphia, 2017, Elsevier.

- Serum electrolytes (hyponatremia in suspected *Legionella* pneumonia), BUN, creatinine
- Nasopharyngeal swab for rapid and PCR testing for influenza
- Serum procalcitonin level: Often used to distinguish pneumonia from heart failure in patients presenting to the emergency department with acute dyspnea. The procalcitonin level is significantly higher in patients with pneumonia than in those without. However, serum procalcitonin should not be used to determine initiation or duration of antibiotic therapy in patients with radiographically confirmed CAP unless antibiotic therapy is being extended beyond 5 to 7 days. Recent trials regarding procalcitonin-guided use of antibiotics for lower respiratory tract infections did not result in less use of antibiotics than did usual care among patients with suspected lower respiratory tract infection[5]
- Pulse oximetry or arterial blood gases: Hypoxemia with partial pressure of oxygen <60 mm Hg while the patient is breathing room air, a standard criterion for hospital admission
- Table 5 summarizes recommended microbiologic evaluation in patients with community acquired pneumonia
- Fig. 2 illustrates an algorithm for the diagnosis and treatment of nosocomial pneumonia
- Ventilator-associated pneumonia: Table 6 and Fig. E3 summarizes a proposed strategy for managing antimicrobial therapy in patients with ventilator-associated pneumonia

IMAGING STUDIES

Chest x-ray (PA and lateral) (Fig. 4): Findings vary with the stage and type of pneumonia and the hydration of the patient:

- Classically, pneumococcal pneumonia presents with a segmental lobe infiltrate (Fig. E5).
- Diffuse infiltrates on chest x-ray can be seen with *L. pneumophila* (Fig. 6), *M. pneumoniae,* viral pneumonias, *P. jirovecii (carinii),* miliary tuberculosis, aspiration, aspergillosis.
- An initial chest x-ray is also useful to rule out the presence of complications (pneumothorax, empyema, abscesses).

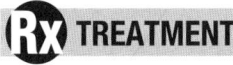 TREATMENT

NONPHARMACOLOGIC THERAPY

- Avoidance of tobacco use
- Oxygen to maintain partial oxygen pressure in arterial blood >60 mm Hg or oxygen saturation >88% in COPD patients and >92% in non-COPD patients
- IV hydration, correction of dehydration
- Assisted ventilation in patients with significant respiratory failure

ACUTE GENERAL Rx

- Antibiotic therapy should be based on clinical, radiographic, and laboratory evaluation.[6-8] Empiric therapy regimens for community-acquired pneumonia are summarized in Tables 7 and 8.

TABLE 4 Diagnostic Testing for Community-Acquired Pneumonia

Test	Sensitivity	Specificity	Comment
Chest radiograph	65%-85%	85%-95%	Computed tomography is more sensitive to infiltrates. Recommended for all patients.
Computed tomography	Gold standard	Not infection specific	Should not be performed routinely but helpful to identify cavitation and loculated pleural fluid. Recommended in the evaluation of nonresponding patients.
Blood cultures	10%-20%	High when positive	Usually shows pneumococcus (in 50%-80% of positive samples) and defines antibiotic susceptibility. Recommended in patients with severe CAP, particularly if not on antibiotic therapy at the time of testing.
Sputum Gram stain	40%-100% depending on criteria	0%-100% depending on criteria	Can correlate with sputum culture to define predominant organism and can be used to identify unsuspected pathogens. Recommended if sputum culture is obtained. May not be able to narrow empiric therapy choices.
Sputum culture			Use if suspect drug-resistant or unusual pathogen, but a positive result cannot differentiate colonization from infection. Obtain via tracheal aspirate in all intubated patients.
Oximetry or arterial blood gas			Define both severity of infection and need for oxygen; if hypercarbia is suspected, a blood gas sample is needed. Recommended in severe community-acquired pneumonia.
Serologic testing for *Legionella*, *Chlamydophila pneumoniae*, *Mycobacterium pneumoniae*, viruses			Accurate, but usually requires acute and convalescent titers collected 4 to 6 wk apart. Not routinely recommended.
Legionella urinary antigen	50%-80%		Specific to serogroup 1, but the best acute diagnostic test for *Legionella*.
Pneumococcal urinary antigen	70%-100%	80%	False positives if recent pneumococcal infection. Can increase sensitivity with concentrated urine.
Serum procalcitonin			Not a routine test, but if performed, should be measured with the highly sensitive Kryptor assay. May help guide duration of therapy and need for ICU admission.

From Vincent JL et al: *Textbook of critical care,* ed 7, Philadelphia, 2017, Elsevier.

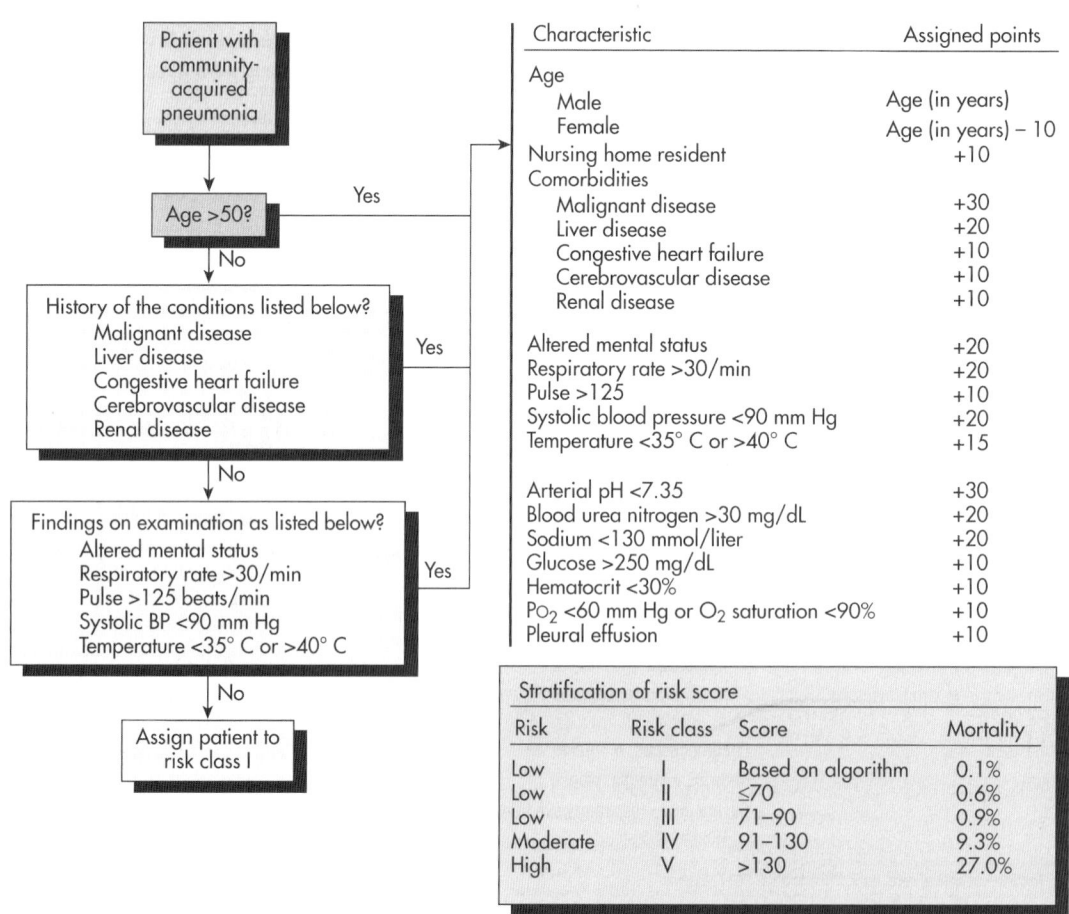

FIG. 1 The pneumonia severity index. *BP,* Blood pressure; *O₂,* oxygen; *Po₂,* partial pressure of oxygen. (From Sellke FW et al: *Sabiston & Spencer surgery of the chest,* ed 9, Philadelphia, 2016, Elsevier.)

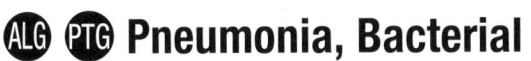
P

Diseases
and Disorders

I

Major Criteria
Invasive mechanical ventilation
Use of vasopressors to maintain blood
  pressure
Minor Criteria
Respiratory rate ≥30 breaths/min
Multilobar infiltrates
New-onset confusion/disorientation
Uremia (BUN >20 mg/dl)
Leukopenia (WBC count <4000 cells/μL)
Pao_2/Fio_2 ratio ≥250
Thrombocytopenia (platelet
  count <100,000 cells/μL)
Hypothermia (core temperature <36° C;
  96.8° F)
Hypotension requiring aggressive fluid
  resuscitation

*According to ATS/IDSA 2007 guidelines.
From Parrillo JE, Dellinger RP: *Critical care medicine:
principles of diagnosis and management in the adult,*
ed 4, Philadelphia, 2014, Saunders.

- Macrolides (azithromycin or clarithromycin) or doxycycline can be used for empiric outpatient treatment of CAP as long as the patient has not received antibiotics within the past 3 mo and does not reside in a community in which the prevalence of macrolide resistance is high.[9] Updated guidelines from the American Thoracic Society and Infectious Diseases Society of America have added amoxicillin as a first-line agent for healthy adult outpatients with CAP.[10] The treatment of choice in suspected *Legionella* pneumonia is either a quinolone (e.g., moxifloxacin) or a macrolide (e.g., azithromycin) antibiotic. A beta-lactam antibiotic is usually added to macrolides.
- In the hospital setting, patients not requiring ICU care can be treated empirically with a second- or third-generation cephalosporin (ceftriaxone, cefotaxime, or cefuroxime) plus a macrolide (azithromycin or clarithromycin) or doxycycline. An antipseudomonal quinolone (levofloxacin or moxifloxacin) can be substituted in place of the macrolide or doxycycline.[11]

- Empiric therapy in ICU patients: IV beta-lactam (ceftriaxone, cefotaxime, ampicillin-sulbactam) plus an IV quinolone (levofloxacin, moxifloxacin) or IV azithromycin.
- In hospitalized patients at risk for *P. aeruginosa* infection, empiric treatment should consist of an antipseudomonal beta-lactam (meropenem, doripenem, imipenem, or piperacillin-tazobactam) with or without a second antipseudomonal agent such as an aminoglycoside or an antipseudomonal quinolone.
- In patients with suspected methicillin-resistant *S. aureus,* vancomycin or linezolid is effective.
- Corticosteroids: Clinical trials evaluating adjunctive use of corticosteroids in severe CAP have produced mixed results. There is no evidence that adjunctive use of corticosteroids improves outcomes in mild to moderate CAP. Guidelines advise against adjunctive treatment of CAP with corticosteroids except in patients with septic shock that is refractory to fluid resuscitation and vasopressor support.[12,13]

TABLE 5 Recommended Microbiologic Evaluation in Patients With Community-Acquired Pneumonia

Patients Who do not Require Hospitalization
None*
Patients Who Require Hospitalization
Two sets of blood cultures (obtained prior to antibiotics) in selected patients

Gram stain and culture of a valid sputum sample in selected patients

Urinary antigen test for detection of *Legionella pneumophila* (in endemic areas or during outbreaks)

Stain for acid-fast bacilli and culture of sputum (if tuberculosis is suggested by clinical history or radiologic findings)

Fungal stain and culture of sputum, and fungal serologies (if infection by an endemic fungus is suggested by the clinical history or radiologic findings)

Sputum examination for *Pneumocystis jirovecii* (if suggested by clinical history, HIV infection, or radiologic findings)

Nucleic acid amplification tests for *Mycoplasma pneumoniae, Chlamydophila pneumoniae, Chlamydophila psittaci, Coxiella burnetii, Legionella* species, respiratory viruses (in endemic areas or during outbreaks) and other agents (e.g., *Streptococcus pneumoniae*) if available

Culture and microscopic evaluation of pleural fluid (if significant fluid is present)
Additional Tests for Patients Who Require Treatment in an ICU
Gram stain and culture of endotracheal aspirate or bronchoscopically obtained specimens using a protected specimen brush or BAL

BAL, Bronchoalveolar lavage; *ICU,* intensive care unit.
*Gram stain and culture should be strongly considered in patients with risk factors for infection by an antimicrobial-resistant organism or unusual pathogen.
From Broaddus VC et al: *Murray & Nadel's textbook of respiratory medicine,* ed 7, Philadelphia, 2022, Elsevier.

TABLE 6 Proposed Strategy for Managing Antimicrobial Therapy in Patients With Ventilator-Associated Pneumonia

Proposed Strategy	Rationale
Step 1: Start therapy using broad-spectrum antibiotics	Due to the emergence of multiresistant GNB, such as *P. aeruginosa* and ESBL-producing GNB, and the increasing role of MRSA, empirical treatment with broad-spectrum antibiotics is justified in most patients with a clinical suspicion of VAP.
Step 2: Stop therapy if the diagnosis of infection becomes unlikely	The goal is to ensure that ICU patients with true bacterial infection receive immediate appropriate treatment. However, this can result in more patients receiving antimicrobial therapy than necessary because clinical signs of infection are nonspecific.
Step 3: Use narrower spectrum antibiotics once the etiologic agent is identified	For many patients with VAP, including those with late-onset infection, therapy can be narrowed once the results of respiratory tract and blood cultures are available, either because an anticipated organism (e.g., *P. aeruginosa* and *Acinetobacter* spp or MRSA) was not recovered, or because the organism isolated is sensitive to a more narrow-spectrum antibiotic than used in the initial regimen.
Step 4: Use pharmacokinetic-pharmacodynamic data to optimize treatment	Clinical and bacteriologic outcomes can be improved by optimizing the therapeutic regimen according to pharmacokinetic and pharmacodynamic properties of the agents selected for treatment.
Step 5: Switch to monotherapy on days 3 to 5	There are no clinical benefits to using a regimen combining two antibiotics for more than days 3 to 5, provided that initial therapy was appropriate, the clinical course appears favorable, and microbiologic data do not point to a very difficult-to-treat microorganism.
Step 6: Shorten the duration of therapy	Reducing duration of therapy in patients with VAP has led to good outcomes with less antibiotic use. Prolonged therapy leads to colonization with antibiotic-resistant bacteria, which may precede a recurrent episode of VAP.

ESBL, Extended-spectrum β-lactamase; *GNB,* gram-negative bacteria; *ICU,* intensive care unit; *MRSA,* methicillin-resistant *Staphylococcus aureus; VAP,* ventilator-associated pneumonia.
From Broaddus VC et al: *Murray & Nadel's textbook of respiratory medicine,* ed 7, Philadelphia, 2022, Elsevier.

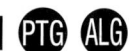

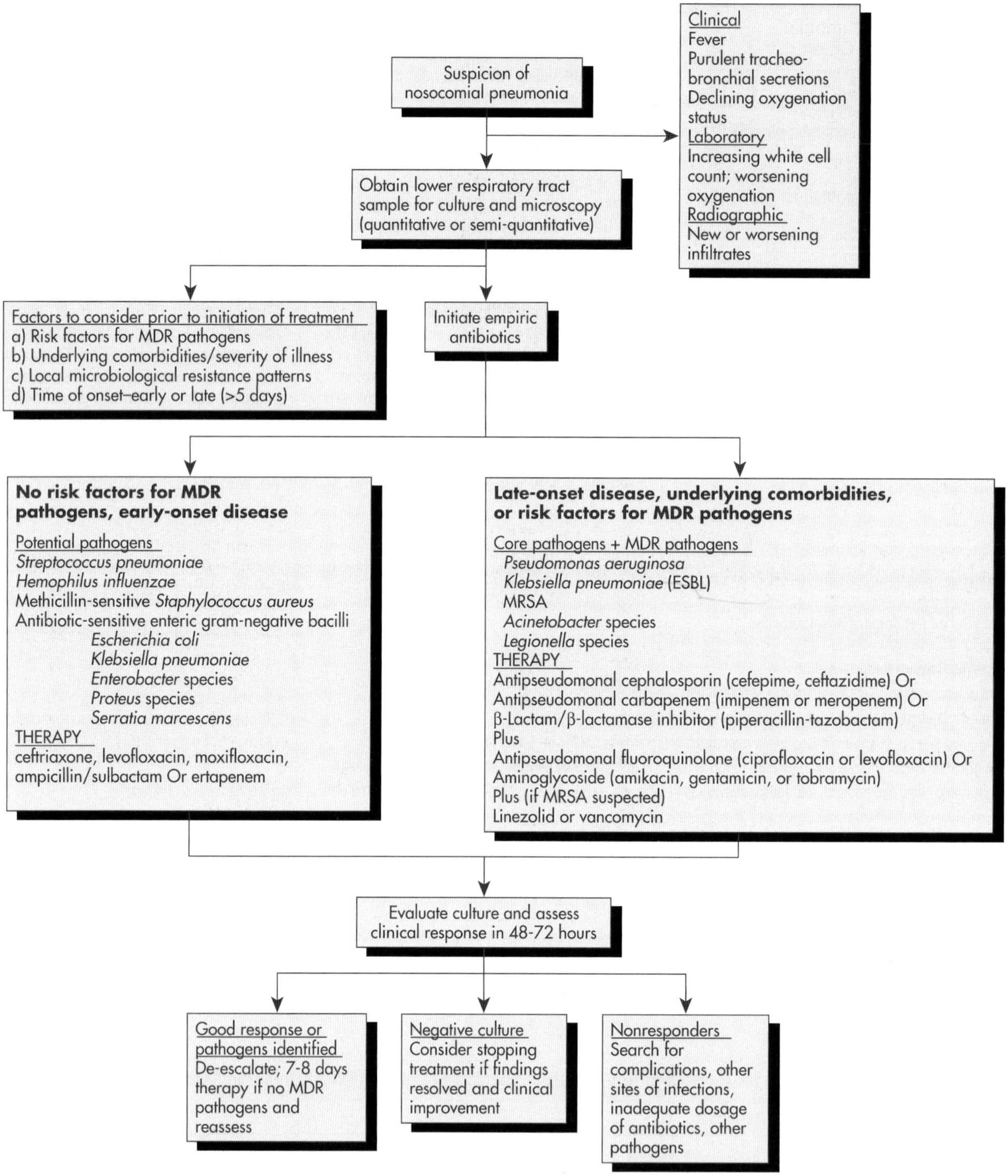

Clinical
Fever
Purulent tracheo-
bronchial secretions
Declining oxygenation
status
Laboratory
Increasing white cell
count; worsening
oxygenation
Radiographic
New or worsening
infiltrates

Suspicion of
nosocomial pneumonia

Obtain lower respiratory tract
sample for culture and microscopy
(quantitative or semi-quantitative)

Factors to consider prior to initiation of treatment
a) Risk factors for MDR pathogens
b) Underlying comorbidities/severity of illness
c) Local microbiological resistance patterns
d) Time of onset–early or late (>5 days)

Initiate empiric
antibiotics

No risk factors for MDR pathogens, early-onset disease

Potential pathogens
Streptococcus pneumoniae
Hemophilus influenzae
Methicillin-sensitive *Staphylococcus aureus*
Antibiotic-sensitive enteric gram-negative bacilli
    Escherichia coli
    Klebsiella pneumoniae
    Enterobacter species
    Proteus species
    Serratia marcescens
THERAPY
ceftriaxone, levofloxacin, moxifloxacin,
ampicillin/sulbactam Or ertapenem

Late-onset disease, underlying comorbidities, or risk factors for MDR pathogens

Core pathogens + MDR pathogens
  Pseudomonas aeruginosa
  Klebsiella pneumoniae (ESBL)
  MRSA
  Acinetobacter species
  Legionella species
THERAPY
Antipseudomonal cephalosporin (cefepime, ceftazidime) Or
Antipseudomonal carbapenem (imipenem or meropenem) Or
β-Lactam/β-lactamase inhibitor (piperacillin-tazobactam)
Plus
Antipseudomonal fluoroquinolone (ciprofloxacin or levofloxacin) Or
Aminoglycoside (amikacin, gentamicin, or tobramycin)
Plus (if MRSA suspected)
Linezolid or vancomycin

Evaluate culture and assess
clinical response in 48-72 hours

Good response or
pathogens identified
De-escalate; 7-8 days
therapy if no MDR
pathogens and
reassess

Negative culture
Consider stopping
treatment if findings
resolved and clinical
improvement

Nonresponders
Search for
complications, other
sites of infections,
inadequate dosage
of antibiotics, other
pathogens

FIG. 2 A suggested algorithm for the diagnosis and treatment of nosocomial pneumonia. (From Parrillo JE, Dellinger RP: *Critical care medicine, principles of diagnosis and management in the adult*, ed 4, Philadelphia, 2014, Elsevier.)

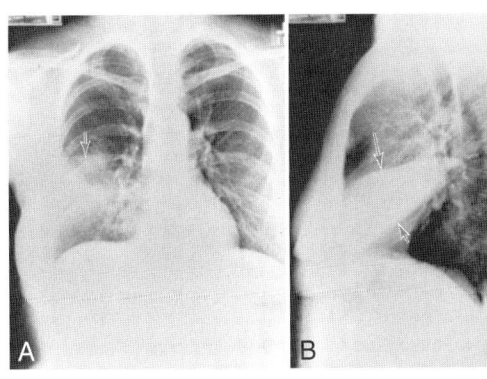

FIG. 4 Posteroanterior (A) and lateral (B) chest radiographs show lobar pneumonia (probably caused by _Streptococcus pneumoniae_) affecting the right middle lobe. In **(A)** the _arrow_ points to a minor fissure, which defines the upper border of the middle lobe. In **(B)** the _long arrow_ points to a minor fissure, and the _short arrow_ points to a major fissure. (From Weinberger SE: _Principles of pulmonary medicine,_ ed 7, Philadelphia, 2019, Elsevier.)

- Duration of antibiotic treatment ranges from 5 to 14 days. Trials have shown that in adults hospitalized with CAP, stopping antibiotic treatment after 5 days in clinically stable patients is reasonable and noninferior to usual care.[8,14] Hematogenous _Staphylococcus_ infection, abscesses, and cavitary lesions might require prolonged antibiotic therapy, sometimes until radiologic resolution is documented.

CHRONIC Rx

Parapneumonic effusion and empyema can be managed with chest tube placement for drainage. (See chapters on "Pleural Effusion" and "Empyema.")

DISPOSITION

Risk factors for a poor outcome from CAP are summarized in Table 9. Indications for hospital admission are:
- Hypoxemia (oxygen saturation <90% while patient is breathing room air)
- Hemodynamic instability
- Inability to tolerate medications
- Active coexisting condition requiring hospitalization. A criterion often used to determine

hospital admission is known as the **"CURB-65": C**onfusion, **B**UN >19.6 mg/dl, **R**espiratory rate >30 breaths/min, systolic **B**P <90 mg Hg, and diastolic BP ≤60 mm Hg, age **≥65.** Patients are generally admitted to the hospital if they fulfill two or more criteria and to the ICU if they have three or more criteria.[15]

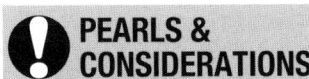

⚠ PEARLS & CONSIDERATIONS

COMMENTS

- "Recurrent pneumonia": Table 10 summarizes the differential diagnosis of recurrent pneumonia.
- Causes of slowly resolving or nonresolving pneumonia:
  1. Difficult to treat infections: Viral pneumonia, _Legionella,_ pneumococci or staphylococci with impaired host response, tuberculosis, atypical mycobacteria, nocardia, or fungi
  2. Neoplasm: Lung, lymphoma, metastasis
  3. Congestive heart failure
  4. Pulmonary embolism

  5. Immunologic or idiopathic: Cryptogenic organizing pneumonia, eosinophilic pneumonia, granulomatosis with polyangiitis
  6. Drug toxicity (e.g., amiodarone, methotrexate)
- Repeat imaging: If patients with pneumonia are not improving, repeat thoracic imaging should be done promptly. In those with complete clinical recovery, it is reasonable to wait 6 to 8 wk before repeating the imaging study to document clearing of the infiltrate. However, the latest guidelines (2019 ATS/IDSA) do not recommend follow-up imaging.[10]

  Patients may be eligible for lung cancer screening, which should be performed as clinically indicated.
- Prevention: Four pneumococcal vaccines are currently available: The 23-valent pneumococcal polysaccharides vaccine (PPSV23), the pneumococcal conjugated vaccine (PCV13), a new 15 valent PVC (PVC-15), and a 20-valent PVC-20 (Prevnar). The Centers for Disease Control and Prevention (CDC) recommends giving the PCV13 to all children. PPSV20 is recommended as a single dose for all adults >65 yr and any other individual with risk factors (including smoking; alcoholism; diabetes mellitus; or chronic heart, lung, or liver disease). It is administered as a single dose. Eligible adults who have received only PPSV23 may receive either PVC-20 or PVC-15 1yr later. Eligible adults who have received PVC-13 alone should receive a chaser dose of PPSV23 at 1 year later. During the influenza season, patients should also receive influenza vaccination.

REFERENCES

Available at eBooks.Health.Elsevier.com.

RELATED CONTENT

Bacterial Pneumonia (Patient Information)
Aspiration Pneumonia (Related Key Topic)
Pneumonia, Mycoplasma (Related Key Topic)

AUTHOR: **JORGE MERCADO, MD**

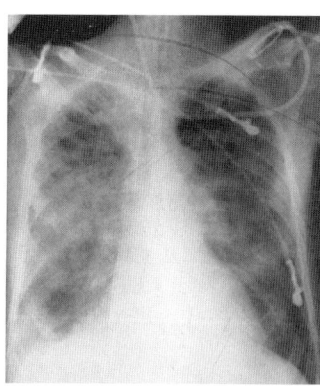

FIG. 6 Chest radiograph of a patient with extensive gram-negative pneumonia. Note the patchy infiltrates throughout both lungs, which are more prominent on the right. (From Weinberger SE: *Principles of pulmonary medicine,* ed 7, Philadelphia, 2019, Elsevier.)

TABLE 7 Guidelines for Empirical Oral Outpatient Treatment of Immunocompetent Adults With Community-Acquired Pneumonia

ATS/IDSA

No modifying factors[a]: Amoxicillin,[b] doxycycline or advanced macrolide if *S. pneumoniae* macrolide resistance <25%[c,d]
Comorbidities[a]: Beta-lactam,[e] macrolide[f] or doxycycline,[d] or fluoroquinolone[g] alone

BTS

Primary: Amoxicillin
Alternatives: Clarithromycin or doxycycline

ERs/ESCMID

Amoxicillin or doxycycline with macrolide as alternative if low levels of resistance

DRSPTWG

Primary: Amoxicillin, amoxicillin-clavulanate, cefuroxime, doxycycline, macrolide (if low rate of resistance)
Alternative: Fluoroquinolone[h]

ATS/IDSA, American Thoracic Society/Infectious Diseases Society of America; *BTS,* British Thoracic Society; *DRSPTWG,* Drug-Resistant *Streptococcus pneumoniae* Therapeutic Working Group; *ERS/ESCMID,* European Respiratory Society and European Society for Clinical Microbiology and Infectious Diseases.
[a]American Thoracic Society/Infectious Disease Society of America comorbidities (modifying factors) include chronic heart, lung, liver or kidney disease; diabetes; asplenia; alcoholism; and malignancy.
[b]Amoxicillin 1 g q8h, doxycycline 100 mg q12h, azithromycin 500 mg on first day then 250 mg/day, clarithromycin 500 mg q8h, or clarithromycin extended release 1000 mg/day.
[c]Advanced macrolides are azithromycin and clarithromycin.
[d]Second-choice agent.
[e]Amoxicillin-clavulanate (500 mg amoxicillin plus 125 mg clavulanate q8h, 875 mg amoxicillin plus 125 mg clavulanate q12h or 2 g amoxicillin plus 125 mg clavulanic acid q12h), cefpodoxime, cefprozil, or cefuroxime.
[f]Because of increasing macrolide resistance, erythromycin cannot be relied upon to ensure coverage of beta-lactamase–producing *Haemophilus influenzae.* A combination of a beta-lactam/beta-lactamase inhibitor is preferred.
[g]Antipneumococcal fluoroquinolones include levofloxacin, and moxifloxacin.
[h]Levofloxacin or moxifloxacin.
From Broaddus VC et al: *Murray & Nadel's textbook of respiratory medicine,* ed 7, Philadelphia, 2022, Elsevier.

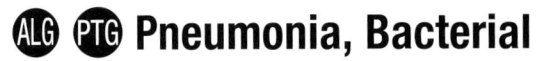
TABLE 8 Guidelines for Empirical Parenteral Inpatient Treatment of Immunocompetent Adults With Community-Acquired Pneumonia

Mild to Moderate Disease

ATS/IDSA
- Primary:[c] Ampicillin and sulbactam, cefotaxime, ceftriaxone, or ceftaroline with azithromycin or clarithromycin
- Alternative: Fluoroquinolone[a] alone or, if history of prior respiratory isolation of MRSA[d] or *Pseudomonas aeruginosa*,[e] treatment to cover these agents

BTS
- Mild: Oral amoxicillin. Alternatives parenteral amoxicillin or benzylpenicillin or clarithromycin
- Moderate: Oral amoxicillin and clarithromycin (can consider clarithromycin monotherapy if prior therapy with amoxicillin)
- Alternative if unable to take oral medication: Parenteral amoxicillin or benzylpenicillin plus clarithromycin (if intolerant of penicillin but able to take a cephalosporin parenteral second- or third-generation cephalosporin plus clarithromycin)
- Alternative: If unable to take penicillin or macrolide,[b] oral doxycycline, or if not able to take any of these, a respiratory fluoroquinolone[a]

ERS/ESCMID
- Aminopenicillin, aminopenicillin with beta-lactamase inhibitor, penicillin, cefotaxime, ceftriaxone with or without macrolide[b]
- Respiratory fluoroquinolone alone[a]

DRSPTWG
- Primary: Cefuroxime, cefotaxime, ceftriaxone, or ampicillin-sulbactam; macrolide[b]
- Alternative: Fluoroquinolone[a]

Severe Disease

ATS/IDSA
- Primary[c]: Ampicillin and sulbactam, cefotaxime, ceftriaxone, or ceftaroline with azithromycin or clarithromycin
- Alternative: Broad-spectrum β-lactam as for primary with fluoroquinolone[a] or, if history of prior respiratory isolation or prior hospitalization with parenteral antimicrobials within 90 days in setting of locally validated risk factors for MRSA[d] or *P. aeruginosa*,[e] treatment to cover these agents

BTS
- Primary: Amoxicillin/clavulanate (or if penicillin intolerant cefuroxime, cefotaxime, or ceftriaxone) plus macrolide[b]

ERS/ESCMID
- Cefotaxime or ceftriaxone plus macrolide or respiratory fluoroquinolone
- Alternative: Respiratory fluoroquinolone alone if no sepsis
- Alternative if risk factors for *P. aeruginosa*: Piperacillin/tazobactam, antipseudomonal cephalosporin (ceftazidime[f] or cefepime) plus ciprofloxacin or plus macrolide[b] and aminoglycoside[g]

DRSPTWG
- Primary: Ceftriaxone or cefotaxime, macrolide;[b] or ceftriaxone or cefotaxime, fluoroquinolone[a]
- Alternative (with caution): Fluoroquinolone[a]

ATS/IDSA, American Thoracic Society/Infectious Diseases Society of America; *BTS*, British Thoracic Society; *DRSPTWG*, Drug-Resistant *Streptococcus pneumoniae* Therapeutic Working Group; *ERS/ESCMID*, European Respiratory Society and European Society for Clinical Microbiology and Infectious Diseases.
[a]Antipneumococcal fluoroquinolones include levofloxacin 750 mg/day and moxifloxacin 400 mg/day.
[b]Advanced macrolides are azithromycin and clarithromycin.
[c]Ampicillin and sulbactam 1.5-3 g q6h, cefotaxime 1-2 g q8h, ceftriaxone 1-2 g/day, or ceftaroline 600 mg q12h and azithromycin 500 mg/day or 500 mg on day 1 and 250 mg once a day thereafter for mild disease or clarithromycin 500 mg bid.
[d]Antistaphylococcal treatments include vancomycin (15 mg/kg q12h, adjust based on levels) or linezolid (600 mg q12h).
[e]Antipseudomonal β-lactams include piperacillin-tazobactam (4.5 g q6h), cefepime (2 g q8h), ceftazidime (2 g q8h), imipenem (500 mg q6h), meropenem (1 g q8h), or aztreonam (2 g q8h).
[f]If ceftazidime used should be combined with penicillin to ensure coverage of pneumococci per ERS/ESCMID guideline.
[g]Recommendation to double cover *P. aeruginosa* with both a β-lactam and either ciprofloxacin or an aminoglycoside per ERS/ESCMID guideline.
From Broaddus VC et al: *Murray & Nadel's textbook of respiratory medicine*, ed 7, Philadelphia, 2022, Elsevier.

TABLE 9 Risk Factors for a Poor Outcome From Community-Acquired Pneumonia

Patient-Related Factors

Male sex
Absence of pleuritic chest pain
Nonclassic clinical presentation
Neoplastic illness
Neurologic illness
Age >65 yr old
Family history of severe pneumonia or death from sepsis

Abnormal Physical Findings

Respiratory rate >30 breaths/min on admission
Systolic (<90 mm Hg) or diastolic (<60 mm Hg) hypotension
Tachycardia (>125 beats/min)
High fever (>40° C; 104° F) or afebrile
Confusion

Laboratory Abnormalities

Blood urea nitrogen >19.6 mg/dl
Leukocytosis or leukopenia (<4000/mm^3)
Multilobar radiographic abnormalities
Rapidly progressive radiographic abnormalities during therapy
Bacteremia
Hyponatremia (<130 mmol/L)
Multiple organ failure
Respiratory failure
Hypoalbuminemia
Thrombocytopenia (<100,000/mm^3) or thrombocytosis (>400,000/mm^3)
Arterial pH <7.35
Pleural effusion

Pathogen-Related Factors

High-risk organisms
Type III pneumococcus, *Staphylococcus aureus,* gram-negative bacilli (including *Pseudomonas aeruginosa*), aspiration organisms, severe acute respiratory syndrome
Possibly high levels of penicillin resistance (minimal inhibitory concentration of at least 4 mg/L) in pneumococcus

Therapy-Related Factors

Delay in initial antibiotic therapy (more than 4 h)
Initial therapy with inappropriate antibiotic therapy
Failure to have a clinical response to empiric therapy within 72 h

From Vincent JL et al: *Textbook of critical care,* ed 7, Philadelphia, 2017, Elsevier.

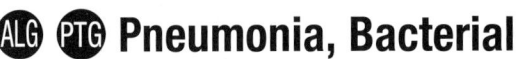

TABLE 10 Differential Diagnosis of Recurrent Pneumonia

Hereditary Disorders

Cystic fibrosis

Sickle cell disease

Disorders of Immunity

Aids

Bruton agammaglobulinemia

Complement deficiency

Selective IgG subclass deficiencies

Common variable immunodeficiency syndrome

Severe combined immunodeficiency syndrome

Disorders of Leukocytes

Chronic granulomatous disease

Hyperimmunoglobulin E syndrome (Job syndrome)

Leukocyte adhesion defect

Disorders of Cilia

Primary ciliary dyskinesia

Kartagener syndrome

Anatomic Disorders

Sequestration

Lobar emphysema

Foreign body

Tracheoesophageal fistula (H type)

Congenital pulmonary airway malformation (cystic adenomatoid malformation)

Gastroesophageal reflux

Bronchiectasis

Aspiration (oropharyngeal incoordination)

Noninfectious Mimics of Pneumonia

Autoimmune diseases (e.g., granulomatosis with polyangiitis)

Hypersensitivity pneumonitis

From Marcdante KJ et al: *Nelson essentials of pediatrics,* ed 9, Philadelphia, 2023, Elsevier.

Diseases and Disorders

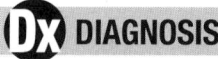

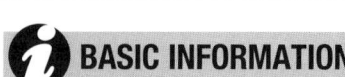

BASIC INFORMATION

DEFINITION

Pneumocystis jirovecii pneumonia (PJP) or *Pneumocystis* pneumonia (PCP) is a respiratory infection caused by the fungal pathogen *P. jirovecii* (formerly known as *P. carinii*).

SYNONYMS

Pneumocystis jirovecii pneumonia
PJP
Pneumocystis pneumonia
PCP

ICD-10CM CODE
B59 Pneumocystosis

EPIDEMIOLOGY & DEMOGRAPHICS

INCIDENCE (IN U.S.):

- In the early days of the HIV epidemic most PCP cases occurred in people with HIV with CD4 counts <200/mm^3. Given improvements in HIV treatment, >70% of cases are now found in HIV-negative individuals.[1]
- Risk factors for infection in people with HIV include CD4 cell count <200/mm^3 or CD4% <14%, elevated HIV RNA levels, and history of PCP.
- Among people with HIV, incidence of PCP remains high in those who are unaware of their HIV-infected status and/or are not on antiretroviral therapy (ART) or PCP prophylaxis.
- PCP also occurs in patients with severe cell-mediated immune deficiency (congenital T-cell deficiency, acute leukemia, lymphoma, bone marrow or solid organ transplant), as well as in patients with hematologic cancers, rheumatologic and chronic lung diseases.[1]
- The major risk factor for infection in HIV-negative individuals is immunosuppression, and it is most commonly seen in patients on chronic high-dose glucocorticoid therapy.[2] PCP also occurs in patients on treatment with antilymphocyte monoclonal antibodies, tumor necrosis factor (TNF) alpha inhibitors, ibrutinib, or idelalisib.[1] In addition to glucocorticoid use, risk factors for mortality among HIV-negative individuals include increased age, solid tumors, CMV coinfection, elevated LDH, lower lymphocyte count, pneumothorax, concurrent pulmonary disease, and need for invasive ventilation.[3]
- Bacterial and viral coinfections with PCP can occur.
- *Pneumocystis* is ubiquitous in the environment and is also frequently found as a colonizer in the airways of infants, children, and adults.

PREDOMINANT SEX: Equal incidence when adjusted for HIV status.
PREDOMINANT AGE: During the AIDS epidemic, age at PCP diagnosis closely correlated with age of HIV infection. Currently the predominant age is 50 to 60 yr of age given the changes in the populations at risk.[1]
PEAK INCIDENCE: Widely variable based on patient's risk profile.

GENETICS:
- Most frequent opportunistic infection among HIV-infected children, with serologic studies suggesting exposure typically occurs in childhood.[4]

PHYSICAL FINDINGS & CLINICAL PRESENTATION

- PCP can present as an acute (3 to 5 days) or subacute (2 to 4 wk) pneumonia with fever, nonproductive cough, and progressive dyspnea. Patients progress to respiratory failure if not treated. Fulminant pneumonia is observed more commonly in immunosuppressed patients without HIV than people with HIV.[2,5]
- Purulent sputum argues against PCP.
- Hemoptysis is unusual.
- Extrapulmonary manifestations are rare but can involve nearly any organ.
- Vital signs: Notable for fever, tachypnea, low oxygen saturation. Oxygen desaturation with ambulation/exertion.
- Pulmonary exam is often normal. Dry rales can be auscultated.
- Spontaneous pneumothorax is possible, so monitor for unilateral decreased or absent breath sounds.

ETIOLOGY

- *P. jirovecii* (formerly *P. carinii*) is a fungal organism (previously classified as a protozoan) (Fig. E1).
- Infection can occur either as a result of activation of latent infection or by new acquisition.
- Infection occurs via airborne transmission.
- No transmission from vertebrate animals (mammals) to humans.
- Increasing number of reports of nosocomial PCP transmission among immunocompromised patients (commonly solid organ transplant recipients).[6]

DIAGNOSIS

DIFFERENTIAL DIAGNOSIS

- Infectious etiologies:
  1. Tuberculosis (especially in low- and middle-income countries)
  2. Bacterial pneumonia
  3. Viral pneumonia, including COVID-19 (SARS CoV-2)
  4. Atypical pneumonia, such as *Mycoplasma* pneumonia
  5. Cryptococcal pneumonia
  6. Histoplasma pneumonia (in endemic areas and advanced AIDS with CD4 cell count <50 cells/mm^3)
  7. *Coccidioides* pneumonia (in endemic areas and advanced AIDS with CD4 cell count <50 cells/mm^3)
  8. CMV pneumonitis (in CD4 cell count <50 cells/mm^3)
  9. *Mycobacterium avium* complex (MAC) (in CD4 cell count <50 cells/mm^3)
  10. Toxoplasmosis
  11. *Legionella* pneumonia
  12. Other fungal pneumonias, such as *Aspergillus* and *Blastomycosis*
  13. Strongyloidiasis
- Noninfectious etiologies:
  1. Kaposi sarcoma
  2. Non-Hodgkin lymphoma
  3. Drug-induced lung injury
  4. Pulmonary edema
  5. Lymphocytic interstitial pneumonia

WORKUP

- Chest x-ray (Fig. 2) or chest computed tomography (CT) (Fig. E3).
- Arterial blood gas for evaluation of severity of hypoxemia and risk stratification.
- Because *Pneumocystis* cannot be cultured, diagnosis must be made through

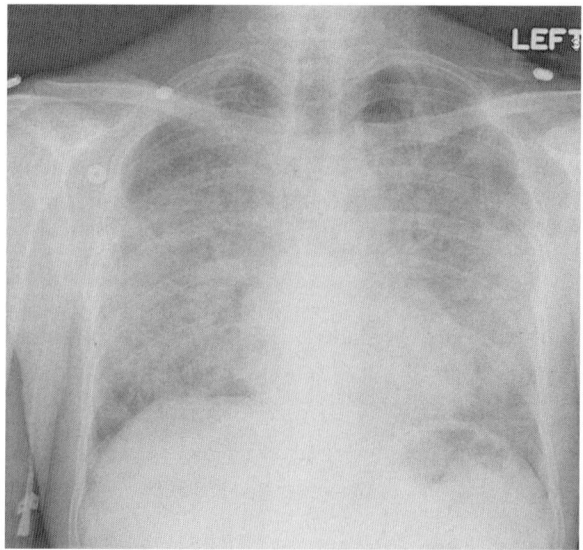

FIG. 2 Chest radiograph showing diffuse interstitial infiltrate in a patient with *Pneumocystis jirovecii* pneumonia. (From Firestein GS et al [eds]: *Kelly's textbook of rheumatology,* ed 9, Philadelphia, 2013, Saunders.)

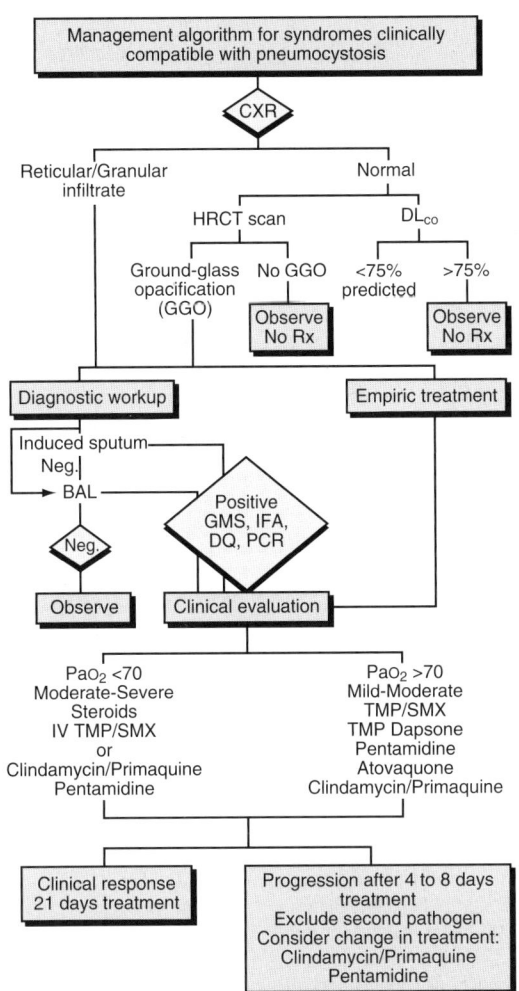

FIG. 5 **Algorithm for the diagnostic evaluation and management of patients with suspected *Pneumocystis* pneumonia.** *BAL,* Bronchoalveolar lavage; *CXR,* chest x-ray; DL_{CO}, single-breath diffusing capacity for carbon monoxide; *DQ,* Diff-Quik (stain); *GGO,* ground-glass opacities; *GMS,* Gomori methenamine silver (stain); *HRCT,* high-resolution computed tomography; *IFA,* immunofluorescent antibody (stain); *IV,* intravenous; *Neg.,* negative; PaO_2, partial pressure of oxygen in arterial blood; *PCR,* polymerase chain reaction; *Rx,* treatment; *TMP/SMX,* trimethoprim-sulfamethoxazole. (From Bennett JE et al: *Mandell, Douglas, and Bennett's principles and practice of infectious diseases,* ed 8, Philadelphia, 2015, Saunders.)

histopathologic or cytopathologic visualization of the organism from induced sputum, bronchoalveolar lavage (BAL) fluid, or tissue. Induced sputum is a common first diagnostic procedure. If negative, bronchoscopy with BAL is performed, which has sensitivity >90% to 97%,[7] and rarely a transbronchial biopsy can be done to augment BAL results and to exclude other pathogens.

- Several stains can be performed (Fig. E4), such as Giemsa, Diff-Quik, and Wright (all stain both the cystic and the trophic forms of the organism but not the cyst wall); Grocott-Gomori methenamine silver, Gram-Weigert, toluidine blue, and cresyl violet stain (stain the cyst wall), as well as immunofluorescent stains, with results depending on the lab experience and the quality of the specimen.
- Polymerase chain reaction (PCR) can be used; however, this cannot distinguish between colonization and active disease.[8]

- Serum 1,3-β-D glucan has a good negative predictive value (very sensitive, less specific); test characteristics are slightly better in people with HIV.[9]
- Lactate dehydrogenase (LDH) is nonspecific; it is often elevated, but a normal LDH does not rule out PCP. Persistently elevated LDH may be predictive of mortality or lack of response to treatment.[3,10]
- Metagenomic next-generation sequencing (mNGS) in blood or BAL fluid has demonstrated good performance for diagnosis of PCP.[11]
- Fig. 5 describes an algorithm for the diagnostic evaluation and management of patients with suspected *Pneumocystis* pneumonia.

LABORATORY TESTS
- HIV antibody test and CD4 cell count (with CD4%) if cause of underlying immune deficiency state is unclear.

- Arterial blood gas and calculation of the alveolar-arterial (A-a) oxygen gradient for determination of disease severity and need for adjunctive corticosteroids:
  1. Mild disease: A-a gradient <35 mm Hg and/or PaO_2 >70 mm Hg
  2. Moderate disease: A-a gradient 35 to 45 mm Hg and PaO_2 >60 mm Hg and <70 mm Hg
  3. Severe disease: A-a gradient >45 mm Hg and PaO_2 <60 mm Hg
- Elevated 1,3-β-D-glucan (>80 pg/ml).
- Elevated lactate dehydrogenase.

IMAGING STUDIES
- Early in the disease course, the chest x-ray can be normal. In these cases, a high-resolution chest CT is recommended. This test is mostly useful in ruling out PCP as a chest CT without ground-glass opacities makes the diagnosis extremely unlikely.
- Classically, PCP presents as bilateral, symmetric interstitial, reticular, or granular infiltrates in the perihilar region ("butterfly pattern") on chest x-ray, and CT chest typically shows ground-glass opacities; however, variable radiographic presentations are possible (unilateral, asymmetric, nodular, miliary, etc.).[8] Pneumatoceles, or cysts, which may cause pneumothorax, are more common in people with HIV.

OTHER STUDIES
If diagnostic uncertainty, PFTs can be used as adjunctive test. Low DLCO is highly sensitive but not specific for PCP infection. A normal DLCO argues against PCP.

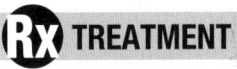 **TREATMENT**

NONPHARMACOLOGIC THERAPY
- Supplemental oxygen
- Noninvasive or invasive ventilatory support if needed
- Prompt chest tube placement if pneumothorax develops

ACUTE GENERAL RX[12]
For confirmed or suspected PCP:
- Preferred therapy: Trimethoprim-sulfamethoxazole (TMP-SMX; 15 to 20 mg/kg trimethoprim and 75 to 100 mg/kg sulfamethoxazole) divided and given q6 to 8h. Recent systematic reviews and meta-analyses have suggested that lower doses of TMP-SMX may be as effective and may be considered in older adults or those with renal dysfunction; however, official guidelines continue to recommend the higher dose of TMP-SMX at this time.[13]
  1. Mild PCP can be treated with PO formulation of TMP-SMX, usually two double-strength (DS) tablets PO tid.
  2. Moderate and severe disease should be treated with intravenous (IV) formulation of TMP-SMX at first but can be switched to PO after clinical improvement.

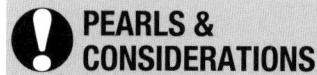
TABLE 1 Causes of Deterioration in an HIV-Infected Person Receiving Treatment for PCP

Etiology	Explanation
Severe Progressive PCP	
Iatrogenic	Pulmonary edema due to IV fluid overload when giving TMP-SMX IRIS following early initiation of ART
Side effects of therapy	Anemia (e.g., caused by TMP-SMX), methemoglobinemia (e.g., caused by dapsone, primaquine)
Inadequate therapy	Incorrect dosage or route of administration Adjuvant glucocorticoids not given for treatment of moderate or severe PCP
Post bronchoscopy	Sedation Pneumothorax
Pneumothorax	Spontaneous Associated with intubation and positive pressure ventilation
Co-pathology in lung	Bacterial infection Pulmonary Kaposi sarcoma Intercurrent pulmonary embolism
Wrong diagnosis	Empiric diagnosis of PCP, and correct diagnosis is another pathology (e.g., bacterial pneumonia)

ART, Antiretroviral therapy; *HIV,* human immunodeficiency virus; *IRIS,* immune reconstitution inflammatory syndrome; *IV,* intravenous; *PCP, Pneumocystis jirovecii* pneumonia; *TMP-SMX,* trimethoprim-sulfamethoxazole.
Bennett JE et al: *Mandell, Douglas, and Bennett's principles and practice of infectious diseases,* ed 8, Philadelphia, 2015, Saunders.

- Alternative therapies: Use only if severe contraindication to TMP-SMX (e.g., Stevens-Johnson syndrome or toxic epidermal necrolysis [TEN]) and after development of treatment-limiting adverse reaction.
  1. Mild-moderate disease:
     a. TMP 15 mg/kg/day split into tid dosing plus dapsone 100 mg PO daily, OR
     b. Clindamycin 600 mg PO q8h plus primaquine 30 mg (base) PO daily, OR
     c. Atovaquone 750 mg PO bid (with food)
  2. Moderate-severe disease:
     a. Clindamycin (600 mg q6h or 900 q8h) IV and primaquine 30 mg (base) PO daily, OR
     b. Pentamidine (4 mg/kg) IV daily. May reduce dose to 3 mg/kg IV daily if toxicity develops. Careful monitoring is required, as IV pentamidine can cause nephrotoxicity, numerous electrolyte disturbances, and cardiac arrhythmias.
- Adjunctive corticosteroids are indicated in moderate to severe PCP (PaO$_2$ <70 mm Hg and A-a gradient >35 mm Hg):
  1. Prednisone 40 mg bid × 5 days, followed by 40 mg/day × 5 days, followed by 20 mg/day × 11 days (for total of 21 days)
  2. Alternative: IV methylprednisolone at 75% of prednisone dose
- Therapy continued for 21 days.
- Antiretroviral therapy in HIV positive individuals should be initiated as soon as possible, ideally within 2 wk of PCP diagnosis. Monitor for immune reconstitution inflammatory syndrome (IRIS).
- Table 1 summarizes causes of deterioration in an HIV-infected patient receiving treatment for PCP.

PROPHYLAXIS
- Primary prophylaxis:
  1. In people with HIV, primary prophylaxis is indicated when CD4 count <200 cells/mm^3 or CD4% <14%. Acceptable regimens include one double-strength tablet PO daily, one single-strength tablet PO daily or one double-strength tablet PO three times a week. Can consider discontinuation of prophylaxis if CD4 cell count between 100 and 200/mm^3 with undetectable HIV viral load for 3 to 6 mo following ART initiation[12]
  2. Commonly also applied to individuals on prolonged courses of steroids (e.g., >4 wk of >20 mg prednisone daily)
  3. Indicated in certain immunosuppressed adults with malignancy[14]
  4. Recommended in patients with rheumatologic, autoimmune, dermatologic diseases on biologic therapy, as well as in patients with solid organ transplant[2,4,15]
- Secondary prophylaxis:
  1. After completion of therapy, secondary prophylaxis should be maintained in people with HIV with TMP-SMX (one single-strength tablet PO daily OR one double-strength tablet PO daily OR [alternative] one double-strength tablet PO three times weekly) until the CD4 cell count is >200 cells/mm^3 and viral load is undetectable for at least 3 mo after ART initiation[12]
  2. If PCP occurs at a CD4 cell count >200 cells/mm^3 while on ART, continue PCP prophylaxis for life, regardless of how high the CD4 cell count rises as a result of ART.
- Patients intolerant of TMP-SMX should be treated with dapsone (100 mg PO daily) or atovaquone (1500 mg PO daily).

- Inhaled pentamidine (300 mg mo by standardized nebulizer) is less effective and is reserved for patients intolerant to other forms of prophylaxis. Inhaled pentamidine or dapsone without pyrimethamine should not be used for PCP prophylaxis in patients with HIV who are also seropositive for *Toxoplasma gondii.*[12]

DISPOSITION
- After completion of therapy, long-term ambulatory follow-up is mandatory to provide secondary prophylaxis of PCP and management of the underlying immunodeficiency syndrome.
- Many patients have chronic respiratory complaints such as exertional dyspnea and may develop chronic obstructive pulmonary disease (COPD). These patients should be referred to a pulmonologist for evaluation and management.

REFERRAL
- To a pulmonologist for bronchoscopy if diagnosis cannot be confirmed by sputum examination
- To an infectious disease specialist if case is severe or difficult to manage and to evaluate for underlying immune deficiency
- To a pulmonologist for evaluation if persistent respiratory complaints such as exertional dyspnea after PCP treatment

PEARLS & CONSIDERATIONS

COMMENTS
- All patients, especially those with severe infection or intolerant of conventional therapy, should be followed by a physician experienced in the management of PCP and, if appropriate, in the long-term management of HIV infection or other underlying disease.
- Patients with suspected PCP should be started on empiric PCP therapy (and adjunctive corticosteroids if indicated) without waiting for diagnostic procedures. *Pneumocystis* can be seen on microscopic examination days to weeks into PCP therapy.
- Before administration of dapsone or primaquine, patients should be tested for G6PD deficiency.
- Clinical and chest x-ray findings in patients with PCP may worsen in the first 5 days after treatment initiation. Wait to declare treatment failure until after at least 7 to 10 days of therapy.[8]
- Mutations associated with resistance to sulfa drugs in other microorganisms have been documented in *P. jirovecii,* but their effect on clinical outcomes is uncertain.
- Monitor for IRIS after ART initiation.
- TMP-SMX can have a range of side effects, including neutropenia (absolute neutrophil count <500 cells/mm^3), fever, hyperkalemia, acute kidney injury, rash. May be able to slowly

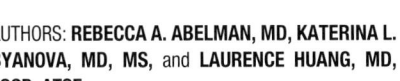
reintroduce medication after resolution of most mild side effects. Most severe and deadly TMP-SMX side effect is Stevens-Johnson syndrome/TEN; avoid all sulfa drugs thereafter.
- Severe and life-threatening hypoglycemia may occur 1 or 2 wk after starting IV pentamidine. Monitor closely and advise the patient of symptoms of hypoglycemia.

- Coinfection with other pathogens can be seen.[8]
- Consider indications for primary PCP prophylaxis in all immunosuppressed patients regardless of HIV status.

REFERENCES
Available at eBooks.Health.Elsevier.com.

RELATED CONTENT
Pneumocystis Pneumonia (Patient Information)
Acquired Immunodeficiency Syndrome (Related Key Topic)

AUTHORS: **REBECCA A. ABELMAN, MD, KATERINA L. BYANOVA, MD, MS,** and **LAURENCE HUANG, MD, FCCP, ATSF**

P

Diseases and Disorders

I

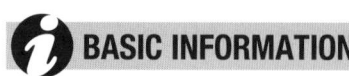

BASIC INFORMATION

DEFINITION
Viral pneumonia is a lung infection caused by any of a large number of viral pathogens. Some of the most important viruses are discussed in this chapter.

SYNONYMS
Viral pneumonia
Nonbacterial pneumonia

ICD-10CM CODES
J12.9   Viral pneumonia, unspecified
J12.89   Other viral pneumonia

EPIDEMIOLOGY & DEMOGRAPHICS
INCIDENCE (IN U.S.):
- COVID-19 (SARS-CoV-2 virus):
  1. The novel coronavirus disease (COVID-19) was first detected in December 2019 and became a worldwide pandemic in 2020. (See "COVID-19 Disease" and "COVID-19 Cardiac Effects" chapters for further information.)
- Influenza virus:
  1. The CDC estimated ~13 million illnesses, ~6.1 million medical visits, 170,000 hospitalizations, and ~14,000 deaths caused by influenza in the 2021 to 2022 influenza season.[1]
  2. Secondary bacterial pneumonia develops in a small percentage of infected persons.
- Incidence of other important viral pathogens can vary widely depending on setting, geography, and testing modalities. With the more widespread use of rapid molecular testing of respiratory secretions, an increase in the detection of viral pathogens has been observed. However, determining causality of the identified virus to the suspected pneumonia remains challenging because respiratory viruses remain detectable for several weeks after initial infection, and the pneumonia may be due to secondary bacterial infection.

PREVALENCE (IN U.S.):
- Often related to immune status of the population or presence of an epidemic/pandemic
- Normal hosts (estimates):
  1. Viral pneumonia requiring children's hospitalization accounts for ~66% cases.
  2. Viruses have been detected in ~23% of adults with clinical pneumonia.

PREDOMINANT SEX:
- Equal predominance.
- Male sex may predispose to more severe respiratory disease in RSV infection.
- Case fatality ratio of COVID-19 is greater among men than among women.

PREDOMINANT AGE:
- COVID-19:
  1. Hospitalizations and deaths increase with age
  2. More prevalent in adults >30 yr

- Influenza:
  1. Overall incidence greatest in children <5 yr
  2. In general, lower incidence with increasing age
  3. Hospitalizations are greatest in infants and children aged <5 yr and adults aged >64 yr
  4. Mortality is greater in adults >64 yr
- RSV and parainfluenza virus:
  1. Young children (as the major cause of pneumonia)
  2. Occurs throughout life
- Human metapneumovirus:
  1. Children: Peak incidence 11 mo
  2. Increasingly detected in adults (bronchitis, chronic obstructive pulmonary disease [COPD] exacerbation, pneumonia)
  3. Frequent cause of lower respiratory tract infection (LRTI) in lung transplant recipients
- Adenoviruses:
  1. Young children
  2. Adults, primarily military recruits
- Varicella:
  1. Approximately 16% of adults (not infected in childhood) who contract varicella develop pneumonia
  2. Acute varicella during pregnancy is more likely to be complicated by severe pneumonia
  3. 90% of reported varicella pneumonia cases are in adults (highest incidence ages 20 to 60 yr)
- Measles:
  1. Young adults and older children who only received a single vaccination (5% failure rate)
  2. Currently most cases are seen in unvaccinated individuals
  3. Measles during pregnancy more likely to be complicated by pneumonia
  4. Underlying cardiopulmonary diseases and immunosuppression predispose to serious pneumonia
  5. Before availability of measles vaccine, 90% of pneumonias in those <10 yr
  6. ~6% of measles cases are complicated by pneumonia
- Cytomegalovirus (CMV):
  1. Neonatal through adult
  2. Immunosuppression is key predisposing factor
  3. Hematopoietic stem cell transplant recipients are at highest risk

PEAK INCIDENCE:
- COVID-19:
  1. Onset in December 2019 without clear seasonal variation
- Influenza:
  1. Winter months for influenza A
  2. Year-round for influenza B
  3. Peak of pneumonia seen weeks into the outbreak of infection
- Respiratory syncytial virus (RSV) and parainfluenza virus: Winter and spring
- Human metapneumovirus: Winter months
- Adenovirus: Endemic (military)
- Varicella: Spring in temperate zones
- Measles: Year-round

- Cytomegalovirus (CMV): Year-round

GENETICS:
Familial disposition:
- Close contact, not genetics, is important in acquisition
- Congenital anomalies and immunosuppression worsen course of RSV pneumonia

Congenital infection:
- CMV is the most common intrauterine infection in the U.S.
- Pneumonia occurs occasionally in infants with symptomatic congenital infection

Neonatal infection:
- Severe RSV pneumonia
- Adenovirus pneumonia
  1. 5% to 20% mortality rate
  2. Can lead to residual restrictive or obstructive functional abnormalities
- "Varicella neonatorum"
  1. Disseminated visceral disease including pneumonia
  2. May develop in neonates whose mothers develop peripartum chickenpox
- CMV pneumonia:
  1. Generally fatal
  2. Associated with severe cerebral damage in this population

PHYSICAL FINDINGS & CLINICAL PRESENTATION
- COVID-19: Wide range, from mild symptoms to severe illness
  1. Fever, chills, fatigue, myalgias, headache
  2. Cough, shortness of breath, sore throat, congestion, rhinorrhea
  3. Loss of taste or smell
  4. Nausea, vomiting, diarrhea
- Influenza:
  1. Fever, cough, or sore throat (referred to as influenza-like illness [ILI])
  2. Uncomfortable or lethargic appearance
  3. Prominent dry cough (rarely hemoptysis)
  4. Flushed skin and erythematous mucous membranes
  5. Rales or rhonchi
- RSV, parainfluenza, and human metapneumovirus:
  1. Fever
  2. Tachypnea
  3. Prolonged expiration
  4. Wheezes and rales
  5. Diarrhea[2]
- Adenoviruses:
  1. Hoarseness, pharyngitis
  2. Conjunctivitis
  3. Tachypnea
  4. Cervical adenitis
- Measles:
  1. Conjunctivitis
  2. Rhinorrhea
  3. Koplik spots (white lesions on the buccal mucosa)
  4. Exanthem (maculopapular rash that starts on the head, then moves down to rest of body)
  5. Pneumonitis (coincident with rash, may also develop after apparent recovery from measles)

6. Fever
7. Dry cough
- Varicella:
  1. Fever
  2. Maculopapular or vesicular rash (all lesions at the same stage) becomes encrusted
  3. Pneumonia typically 1 to 6 days after rash appears. Pneumonia (Fig. E1) may be accompanied by cough and occasionally hemoptysis
  4. Few auscultatory abnormalities noted on examination of the lungs
- CMV:
  1. Fever
  2. Paroxysmal cough
  3. Occasional hemoptysis
  4. Diffuse adenopathy when pneumonia occurs after transfusion
  5. Severe immunosuppression associated with symptomatic CMV pneumonia (may be reactivation of latent infection or in previously seronegative recipients from the donor)

ETIOLOGY

Viral infection can lead to pneumonia in both immunocompetent and immunocompromised hosts.

Dx DIAGNOSIS

DIFFERENTIAL DIAGNOSIS

- Bacterial pneumonia; primary bacterial, secondary bacterial infection, or bacterial coinfection
- Other causes of atypical pneumonia:
  1. *Mycoplasma* spp.
  2. *Chlamydia* spp.
  3. *Coxiella* spp.
  4. Legionnaires disease.
  5. In certain patient populations (e.g., immunocompromised) consider fungal infections, pneumocystis, tuberculosis, or atypical mycobacterium.
- Acute respiratory distress syndrome (ARDS)
- Pulmonary emboli

WORKUP

- Information about the current prevalent strain of influenza virus or local prevalence of COVID-19 can be obtained from local health departments or from the Centers for Disease Control and Prevention.
- Influenza and other viruses may be cultured from respiratory secretions during the initial few days of the illness (special media and techniques necessary).
- Respiratory viral panels that use PCR-based assays from nasopharyngeal or bronchoalveolar lavage samples to test for a variety of viruses are extremely sensitive and are becoming the test of choice.
- Rapid flu tests have a 50% to 70% sensitivity in diagnosing influenza (a negative test does not mean the patient does not have influenza).

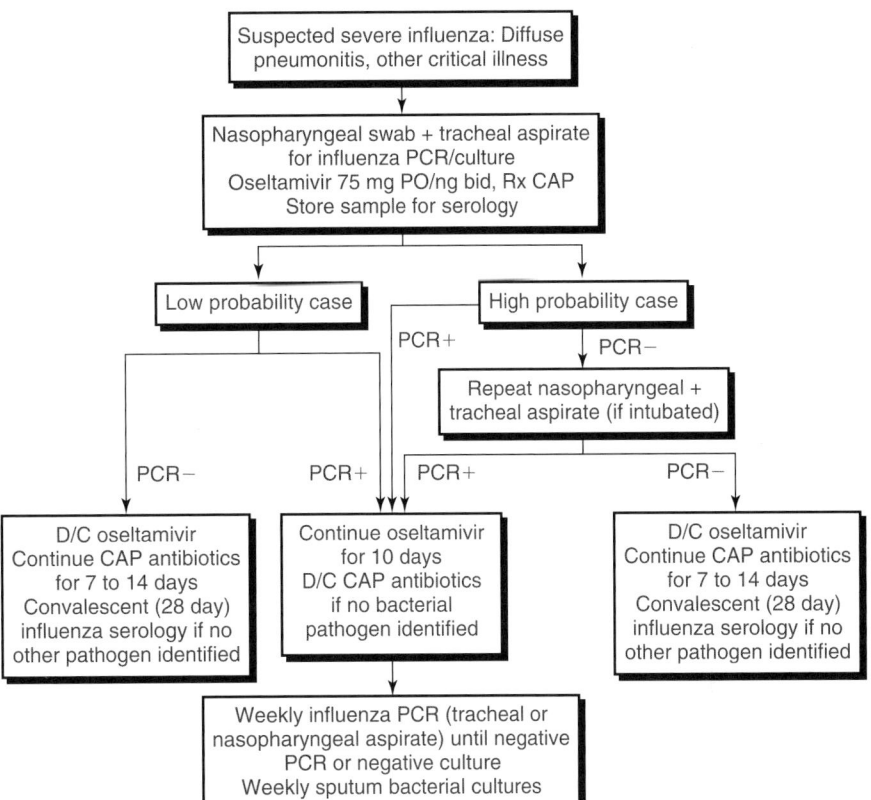

FIG. 2 Suggested algorithm in the workup and management of suspected severe influenza pneumonia in the critical care unit. *CAP,* Community-acquired pneumonia; *D/C,* discontinue; *PCR,* polymerase chain reaction; *PO,* by mouth; *Rx,* prescription. (From Vincent JL et al: *Textbook of critical care,* ed 6, Philadelphia, 2011, Saunders.)

- Measles and adenovirus pneumonia are usually diagnosed clinically and can be confirmed with serology.
- CMV may be grown in culture or PCR amplified from bronchoalveolar lavage samples.
- An algorithm for the workup and management of suspected severe influenza pneumonia in the critical care unit is described in Fig. 2.
- COVID-19 can be assessed by nasopharyngeal or tracheal aspirate PCR tests for diagnostic workup. Rapid antigen tests are also available and provide results more quickly; however, a single negative test does not rule out an infection, especially in those who are asymptomatic. Antibody serology testing is not generally useful for acute diagnosis.

LABORATORY TESTS

- COVID-19, influenza, RSV, and several other respiratory viruses can be assessed by nasopharyngeal or tracheal aspirate PCR tests for diagnostic workup.
- Sputum Gram stain (usually produced in scanty amounts) typically shows few polymorphonuclear leukocytes and few bacteria.
- White blood cell count may vary from leukopenia to modest elevation, usually without a leftward shift. COVID-19 is particularly characterized by leukopenia with predominant lymphopenia.

- Disseminated intravascular coagulation occasionally complicates adenovirus type 7 pneumonia.
- Multinucleated giant cells on Tzanck preparation of an unroofed vesicular lesion are useful in diagnosing varicella (also found in herpes simplex).
- CMV PCR can detect CMV virus but may be negative even with organ involvement in immunosuppressed patients.
- Cultures (blood, sputum, or bronchoalveolar lavage) may be helpful in identifying superinfecting bacterial pathogens.

IMAGING STUDIES

- Chest x-rays may demonstrate a spectrum of findings from ill-defined, patchy, or generalized interstitial opacities (Fig E1), which can be associated with ARDS.
- Chest CT most commonly demonstrates ground glass opacities, which are usually patchy and peripheral in COVID-19.
- A localized dense alveolar opacification suggests a superimposed bacterial pneumonia.
- Small, calcified nodules may develop as a radiographic residual of varicella pneumonia.

Rx TREATMENT

NONPHARMACOLOGIC THERAPY

General:

- Measures to diminish person-to-person transmission.
- Maintenance of adequate hydration.
- Possible ventilation support for severe pneumonia or ARDS.

COVID-19:
- Facial coverings, social distancing, and quarantine are important in limiting spread of disease.
- COVID-19 vaccines became available in the United States in December 2020. The messenger RNA vaccines (Pfizer and Moderna) require two doses and a booster. The Janssen vaccine requires a single dose and can be given as a booster, but the CDC generally recommends Pfizer or Moderna for both primary series and booster.[3] Vaccines have been proven to be effective in reducing severity of illness in COVID-19 pneumonia.

Influenza:
- Yearly prophylactic strain-specific influenza vaccination can be given to prevent infection.

RSV:
- Isolation techniques are important in limiting spread of RSV infections.
- Immunoglobulins with a high RSV-neutralizing antibody titer are beneficial in treatment.

Adenoviruses:
- Intestinal inoculation of respiratory adenoviruses has been used to successfully immunize military recruits.
- Although they produce no disease in recipients, the viruses may be shed chronically and may infect others at a later date.
- These vaccines are not available for civilian populations.

Varicella:
- Live, attenuated varicella vaccine has been successfully used in clinical trials.
- Varicella-zoster immune globulin should be administered within 4 days of exposure to prevent or modify the disease in susceptible persons.
- Nonimmunized persons exposed to varicella are potentially infectious between 10 and 21 days after exposure.

Measles:
- Effective measles vaccine (MMR) is available.
  1. The vaccine should be administered at age 15 mo.
  2. A second dose should be administered at the time of school entry.
- Live, attenuated vaccine or gammaglobulin can prevent measles in unvaccinated persons if administered early after exposure.
- Vitamin A given PO for 2 days reduces morbidity and mortality rates from measles in exposed children.

ACUTE GENERAL Rx

- General: Administer antibiotics for bacterial superinfections when appropriate.

COVID-19:
1. Supportive care is the mainstay of treatment in outpatient and inpatient cases.
2. Remdesivir has been shown to shorten the time to recovery in adults hospitalized with COVID-19 with lower respiratory tract infection.
3. Dexamethasone decreases 28-day mortality in patients requiring respiratory support.
4. Paxlovid has been shown to reduce the risk of hospitalization and death when used in the outpatient setting in patients who are at high risk for progression to severe disease. Individuals considered at high risk include age >50 yr, unvaccinated status, and specific medical conditions (e.g., diabetes, immunocompromised individuals).[4]
5. In situations when Paxlovid and remdesivir are not available or cannot be administered, bebtelovimab and molnupiravir can be used.[4]

- Influenza:
  1. Oseltamivir is recommended in patients of any age suspected or confirmed to have influenza.
  2. Oseltamivir is recommended in outpatients with complicated disease or exacerbation of preexisting conditions with suspected or confirmed influenza.
  3. Baloxavir, oseltamivir, peramivir, or zanamivir may be used in uncomplicated outpatients suspected or confirmed to have influenza.
  4. Amantadine and rimantadine are not recommended for treatment in the United States due to high resistance.

- RSV and parainfluenza:
  1. Ribavirin aerosol may be effective for severe RSV pneumonia.
  2. No approved antiviral therapy for parainfluenza virus pneumonia.

- Human metapneumovirus: No specific antiviral treatment is available.

- Adenoviruses: No approved antiviral therapy for adenovirus; cidofovir has been used in severe cases.

- Varicella:
  1. Patients over age 12 yr who develop chickenpox should be treated with acyclovir or valacyclovir, which may prevent the development of pneumonia.
  2. Varicella pneumonia can be treated with IV acyclovir.

- Measles:
  1. No effective antiviral agent.
  2. Vitamin A should be given to children with measles.

- CMV:
  1. Acyclovir, ganciclovir, and valganciclovir are used to prevent CMV infection in transplant recipients.

2. Ganciclovir and foscarnet, with or without CMV hyperimmune globulin, are used to treat CMV infection, including pneumonia.

DISPOSITION

- Supportive therapy is useful.
- Death is possible during acute illness.
- Residual functional abnormalities may be persistent or develop into or predispose to chronic respiratory diseases later in life.
- Morbidity and mortality rates after most viral pneumonias are increased by bacterial superinfection.

REFERRAL

- To infectious disease specialist and/or pulmonologist if uncertainty about the diagnosis.
- If symptoms or findings are progressive, with severe respiratory compromise, diffuse infiltrates, or the development of ARDS, referral for supportive care on extracorporeal life support could be considered in select patients.

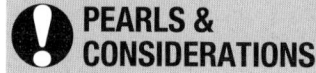

❗ PEARLS & CONSIDERATIONS

COMMENTS

- Facial coverings, social distancing, and quarantine are important in reduction of COVID-19 transmission, which is spread by droplets and aerosols.
- Influenza spreads through close contact and by small droplets transmitted by cough.
- RSV is effectively transmitted by fomites and by direct contact (little by aerosol).
- Varicella is transmitted by direct contact or by aerosol.
- Of the three major forms of parainfluenza viruses (types 1 to 3), type 3 is the most common cause of viral pneumonia; types 1 and 2 primarily cause laryngotracheitis.
- Human metapneumovirus is a common cause of upper respiratory infections and pneumonia.

REFERENCES AND SUGGESTED READINGS

Available at eBooks.Health.Elsevier.com.

RELATED CONTENT

Viral Pneumonia (Patient Information)
Cytomegalovirus Infection (Related Key Topic)
Influenza (Related Key Topic)
Varicella (Related Key Topic)
COVID-19 Disease (Related Key Topic)

AUTHORS: **BETELHEM KIFLE, MD,** and **LEKSHMI SANTHOSH, MD, MAEd**

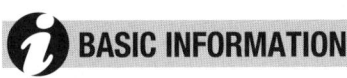

BASIC INFORMATION

DEFINITION

A spontaneous pneumothorax (SP) is defined as air in the pleural space, collapsing the lung without a precipitating event. This can be primary SP (otherwise healthy people without any obvious underlying lung disease) or secondary SP (with underlying lung disease).

SYNONYMS

SP
Primary spontaneous pneumothorax (PSP)
Secondary spontaneous pneumothorax (SSP)
Tension pneumothorax

ICD-10CM CODES

J93.0	Spontaneous tension pneumothorax
J93.11	Primary spontaneous pneumothorax
J93.12	Secondary spontaneous pneumothorax
J93.81	Chronic pneumothorax
J93.83	Other pneumothorax
J93.9	Pneumothorax, unspecified
J95.811	Postprocedural pneumothorax
P25.1	Pneumothorax originating in the perinatal period
S27.0XXA	Traumatic pneumothorax, initial encounter
S27.0XXD	Traumatic pneumothorax, subsequent encounter
S27.0XXS	Traumatic pneumothorax, sequela

EPIDEMIOLOGY & DEMOGRAPHICS

- Approximately 20,000 new cases of SP occur each year in the U.S.
- SP is more common in men than women (6:1).
- Incidence of primary SP is 7.4 per 100,000 in men and 1.2 per 100,000 in women.
- Incidence of secondary SP is 6.3 per 100,000 in men and 2.0 per 100,000 in women.
- SP is commonly seen in tall, thin young men aged 20 to 40 yr.
- Risk factors include smoking, family history, Marfan syndrome, homocystinuria, and thoracic endometriosis.
- Anorexia nervosa is thought to be a risk factor due to pulmonary parenchymal consequences of malnutrition.

PHYSICAL FINDINGS & CLINICAL PRESENTATION

- Sudden onset of pleuritic chest pain (90%), usually at rest and no relationship between the onset of pneumothorax and physical activity, which often becomes dull after a few hours
- Pain is usually unilateral and can be sharp, agonizing, and associated with considerable apprehension
- Dyspnea (80%), which often resolves within 24 h, despite persistence of pneumothorax
- Cough (10%)
- Asymptomatic (5%); may take up to 7 days to come to medical attention
- Tachycardia
- Hypoxemia

- Hypercapnia is rare because the alveolar ventilation is maintained by the contralateral lung
- Decreased chest excursion on the affected side (Fig. 1)
- Diminished breath sounds
- Subcutaneous emphysema may be present
- Hyperresonance on percussion
   Tension pneumothorax (Fig. 2) is a medical emergency and should be suspected when the patient is hemodynamically unstable or experiencing significant respiratory distress. Other signs of tension pneumothorax include jugular venous distention and contralateral tracheal deviation.

ETIOLOGY

- In primary SP, rupture of small blebs and bullae, usually located near the apex of the upper lobes, is a common cause.
- In secondary SP, chronic obstructive pulmonary disease is the most common cause, but it can also be associated with pneumonia, bronchogenic carcinoma, mesothelioma, sarcoidosis, tuberculosis, cystic fibrosis, and many other lung diseases. Causes of secondary SP are summarized in Box 1.
- Catamenial pneumothorax is a rare condition characterized by recurrent SP coinciding with the onset of menses. It usually affects the right lung and is believed to be caused by endometriosis with involvement of the diaphragm and/or pleura. It is believed to be hormonally related, and treatment is aimed at endometrial suppression.

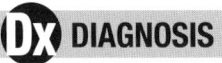

DIAGNOSIS

Established by the chest x-ray examination (CXR) (Fig. 3) or bedside ultrasound

DIFFERENTIAL DIAGNOSIS

- Pleurisy
- Pulmonary embolism
- Myocardial infarction
- Pericarditis
- Asthma
- Pneumonia

WORKUP

CXR

LABORATORY TESTS

Arterial blood gases may show hypoxemia and hypocapnia as a result of hyperventilation.

IMAGING STUDIES

- SP is usually confirmed by upright CXR:
  1. A white visceral pleural line. The absence of vessel markings peripheral to this line helps differentiate from mimicking conditions such as an overlying skin fold. A lateral width of 1 cm corresponds to 27% pneumothorax, and 2 cm occupies 49% of the hemithorax.
  2. The left lateral decubitus position is the most sensitive and the supine position the

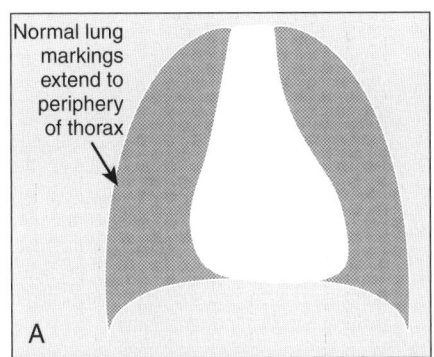
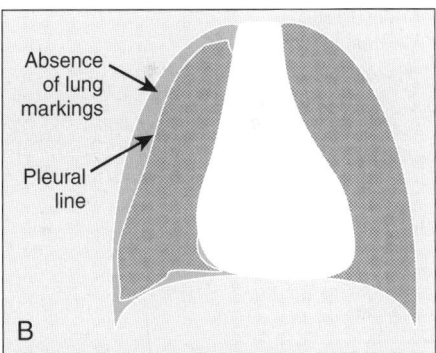

Normal lung markings extend to periphery of thorax

A

Absence of lung markings

Pleural line

B

FIG. 1 Pneumothorax. A, Schematic of normal lung. **B,** Schematic of pneumothorax. Pneumothoraces can range in size from tiny to massive. Because of the variability in their size and location, pneumothoraces can be difficult to detect on chest x-ray examination. For example, a pneumothorax that is anterior or posterior rather than lateral may be hidden on frontal chest x-ray examination, particularly one taken in the supine position. An upright chest x-ray examination should be obtained if possible. An expiratory film is thought to be more sensitive, because the lung and thorax decrease in size during expiration, but air trapped in the pleural space remains the same size and thus appears relatively larger. Subtle pneumothoraces may not be visible on chest x-ray examination. In some cases, subcutaneous air may be the only visible clue to underlying lung injury. Computed tomography (CT) is extremely sensitive for pneumothorax, although controversy remains over the proper management of pneumothoraces seen only on CT. Ultrasound is also thought to be more sensitive than chest x-ray examination for detection of pneumothorax, although, again, the management of pneumothorax seen only on ultrasound is uncertain because this is a relatively newly described method of detection. The chest x-ray examination findings of pneumothorax include a lack of the normal lung markings, which should be visible to the periphery of the chest wall. Sometimes a line marking the boundary of the lung and visceral pleura is visible, although this can be confused with ribs and with the medial margin of the scapula. Depending on the degree of pneumothorax and lung collapse, the lung parenchyma may appear denser than the opposite side. In extreme cases of tension pneumothorax, the pressure exerted by the air in the pleural space may begin to displace other structures, including the diaphragm and mediastinum. In tension pneumothorax, the hyperinflated hemithorax may also have abnormally positioned ribs, with a position more horizontal than usual. (From Broder JS: *Diagnostic imaging for the emergency physician,* Philadelphia, 2011, Saunders.)

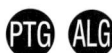

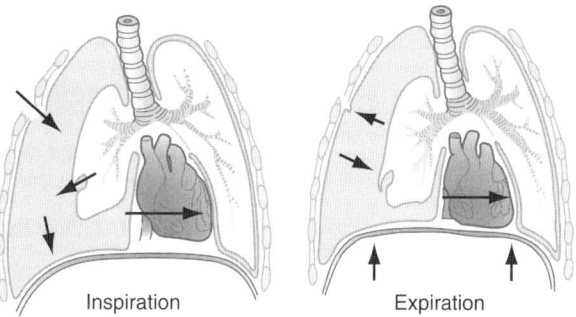

FIG. 2 Tension pneumothorax with total collapse of the right lung and shift of mediastinal structures to the left. Air is forced into the pleural space during inspiration and cannot escape during expiration. (From Marx JA et al: *Rosen's emergency medicine,* ed 8, Philadelphia, 2014, Elsevier.)

BOX 1 Causes of Secondary Spontaneous Pneumothorax

Airway Disease
Chronic obstructive pulmonary disease
Asthma
Cystic fibrosis

Infections
Necrotizing bacterial pneumonia, lung abscess
Pneumocystis jirovecii pneumonia
Tuberculosis

Interstitial Lung Disease
Sarcoidosis
Idiopathic pulmonary fibrosis
Lymphangiomyomatosis
Tuberous sclerosis
Pneumoconioses

Neoplasms
Primary lung cancers
Pulmonary or pleural metastases

Miscellaneous
Connective tissue diseases
Pulmonary infarction
Endometriosis, catamenial pneumothorax

From Marx JA et al: *Rosen's emergency medicine,* ed 8, Philadelphia, 2014, Elsevier.

least sensitive. Inspiratory and expiratory films have equal sensitivities.
3. As little as 50 ml of air can be detected on upright film.
- Tension pneumothorax should be suspected with contralateral tracheal and mediastinal deviation and ipsilateral flattening or inversion of the diaphragm on the CXR (Fig. 4).
- Chest computed tomography scan should be considered for a patient with recurrent pneumothorax or persistent air leak, and for planning surgery.
- Lung ultrasound has emerged as a rapid and accurate screening tool for pneumothorax. Fig. 5 illustrates an algorithm for evaluation of suspected pneumothorax using ultrasound.

- The absence of lung sliding and a positive "stratosphere sign" on M-mode are suggestive of pneumothorax. The lung point sign, a sonographic representation of the point of the chest wall where the pleural layers re-adhere, is 100% specific to confirm the diagnosis.[1]

℞ TREATMENT

INITIAL MANAGEMENT
- When tension pneumothorax is suspected or the patient has severe respiratory distress, emergent needle decompression or tube thoracostomy should be performed. Needle decompression can be done at the bedside using a large bore angiocatheter needle. The needle is introduced in the second intercostal space midclavicular line. The needle is retracted, and the catheter is left in place and attached to a three-way stopcock and a three-chamber system connected to suction. Alternative sites for needle decompression include the fourth or fifth intercostal space in the anterior axillary or mid-axillary line.
- 100% oxygen administration reduces the partial pressure of nitrogen in pleural capillaries, consequently quadrupling the rate of pneumothorax absorption, and should be administered to all patients with pneumothorax.
- When the patient is hemodynamically stable and tension pneumothorax is not suspected, further treatment is based on the size of the pneumothorax and the presence or absence of associated symptoms.
- If the pneumothorax is small (<2 cm between lung and chest wall on CXR) and the patient is asymptomatic, the patient can be treated with observation alone. Repeat imaging should be performed to ensure stability/resorption of the pneumothorax. Some studies have shown that using a cutoff of 35 mm for deciding which patients can be managed with observation is reasonable in selected patients with nonoccult traumatic pneumothoraces after consultation with trauma consultants.
- If the pneumothorax is large (>2 cm), or if the patient is symptomatic with chest pain and dyspnea, initial management should focus on removing air from the pleural space.

- Needle aspiration is the treatment of choice in the clinically stable patient with a large primary SP. Needle aspiration can be done at the bedside using a large bore angiocatheter needle or a commercially available catheter aspiration kit. The needle is introduced in the second intercostal space midclavicular line. The needle is retracted, and the catheter is left in place and attached to a three-way stopcock and a large syringe. Air is aspirated until resistance is met or the patient experiences significant coughing. Repeat CXR is done immediately after aspiration and again in 4 to 24 h to document reexpansion of the lung.
- If there is improvement but not complete resolution of pneumothorax after the aspiration, the catheter can be attached to a Heimlich (one-way) valve or to waterseal to allow further lung expansion. Some stable patients can be discharged home with a Heimlich valve in place if close follow-up monitoring can be obtained.
- Tube thoracostomy is the treatment of choice for patients with a large secondary SP or in patients with large primary SP that did not resolve with needle aspiration. Tube thoracostomy can be performed at the bedside preferably using the Seldinger technique with a small to medium bore chest tube (<14 Fr). The chest tube should be inserted in the second intercostal space in the midclavicular line. Alternate sites for tube thoracostomy include the fourth or fifth intercostal space in the anterior axillary line.
- An algorithmic approach to the treatment of primary SP is outlined in Fig. 6.

PREVENTION
- Approximately 25% to 50% of patients with primary SP will have a recurrence within 5 yr. The recurrence rate is higher in patients with secondary SP.
- Surgical bullectomy and pleurodesis can decrease rate of recurrence. These interventions should be considered in all patients after their first instance of secondary SP, as well as in patients with recurrent primary SP.
- Additional indications for intervention include simultaneous bilateral SP, persistent air leak (>5 to 7 days), failure of lung reexpansion by the chest tube, and professions at risk (e.g., pilots, divers).
- The current recommended surgical approach is the use of video-assisted thoracoscopy (VATS) with bullectomy and/or pleurodesis. Surgical chemical pleurodesis is best achieved with sterile talc. The overall recurrence rate is estimated at <5% after VATS.
- Chemical pleurodesis can also occur via instillation of a sclerosing agent through a chest tube. Talc slurry is the preferred agent; doxycycline, iodine, and minocycline are considered to be acceptable alternatives. The recurrence rates for chemical pleurodesis via a chest tube are higher than for VATS (<25%); therefore, this should be reserved for patients who are poor surgical candidates.

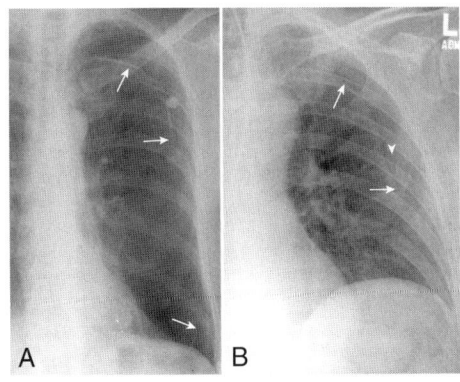

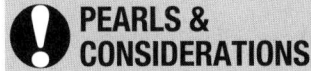

FIG. 3 **A,** Chest x-ray examination of a pneumothorax. The pleural line has lucency on either side, representing air in the pleural space on one side of the line and air in the lung on the other. The line is sharply demarcated and can be traced along its course *(lower arrow)*. No blood vessels can be seen beyond the superior *(upper arrow)* and lateral *(middle arrow)* extent of the line. **B,** Chest x-ray examination of a skinfold *(arrows)* that could be mistaken for a pneumothorax. The border is more of an edge, with lucency on only one side. The edge is poorly defined and cannot be followed continuously *(lower arrow)*. Blood vessels can be traced beyond the border of the fold *(arrowhead)*. (Courtesy Michael B. Gotway, MD, Scottsdale Medical Imaging, and the Department of Radiology, University of California, San Francisco. From Mason RJ et al: *Murray & Nadel's textbook of respiratory medicine*, ed 5, Philadelphia, 2010, Saunders.)

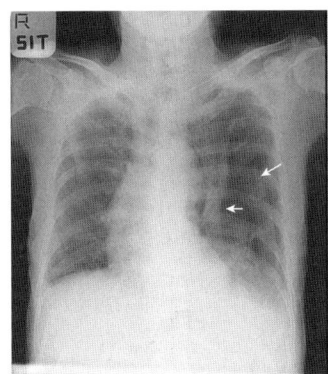

FIG. 4 **Chest x-ray examination showing left pneumothorax with shift of the mediastinum and trachea to the right side *(white arrows).*** The left lung is not completely collapsed, suggesting the presence of a loculated tension pneumothorax. (From Chan SSW: Tension pneumothorax managed without immediate needle decompression, *Am J Emerg Med* 36[3]:242-245, 2009.)

DISPOSITION

- Smoking cessation should be advised.
- Death from primary SP is uncommon.
- In patients with secondary SP and chronic obstructive pulmonary disease, mortality rates range from 1% to 16%.

REFERRAL

Pulmonary and surgical consultations are recommended.

! PEARLS & CONSIDERATIONS

- The rate of pleural air absorption is approximately 1.25% of the volume of the hemithorax per day. This rate can be used to estimate the time interval for complete resolution of pneumothorax with observation.
- Air travel should be avoided until complete resolution of pneumothorax.
- Scuba diving is contraindicated following SP. It may be considered on a case-by-case basis in patients who have had surgical pleurectomy.

COMMENTS

- A recent trial revealed that conservative management of SP is safe and effective and noninferior to interventional management, and it also has a lower risk of serious adverse events.[2]
- Patients with AIDS and *Pneumocystis jirovecii* infection have a high incidence of SP. Treatment typically requires chest tube placement and either thoracoscopy or open thoracotomy.

REFERENCES

Available at eBooks.Health.Elsevier.com.

RELATED CONTENT

Pneumothorax (Patient Information)

AUTHOR: **MIHIR PARIKH, MD**

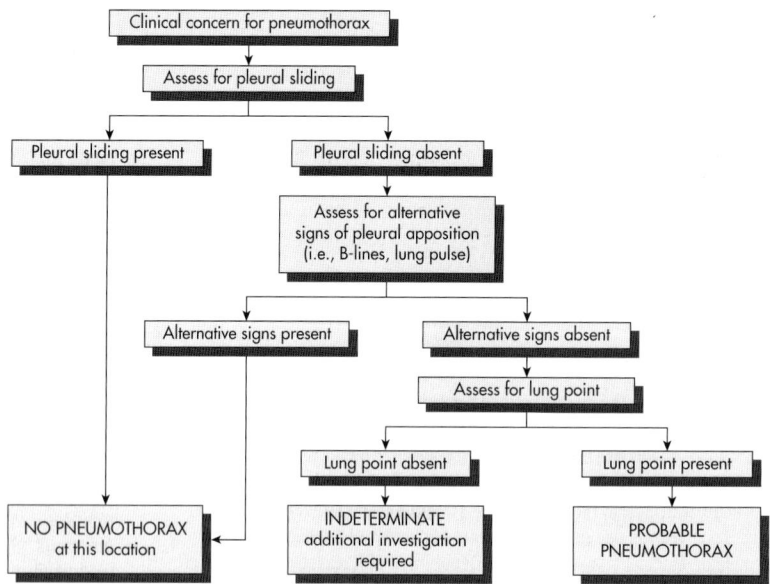

FIG. 5 Sample algorithm for evaluation of suspected pneumothorax using ultrasound. The presence of pleural sliding rules out this diagnosis at the scanned location, but its absence is not confirmatory of that diagnosis. When pleural sliding is absent, one can look for alternative findings to suggest pleural apposition, such as B-lines or a lung pulse. Absent these, finding a lung point is highly suggestive of a pneumothorax; otherwise, the examination is indeterminate at that location. As shown in this algorithm, it is easier to use ultrasound to exclude a pneumothorax than to make the diagnosis. (From Broaddus VC et al: *Murray & Nadel's textbook of respiratory medicine*, ed 7, Philadelphia, 2022, Elsevier.)

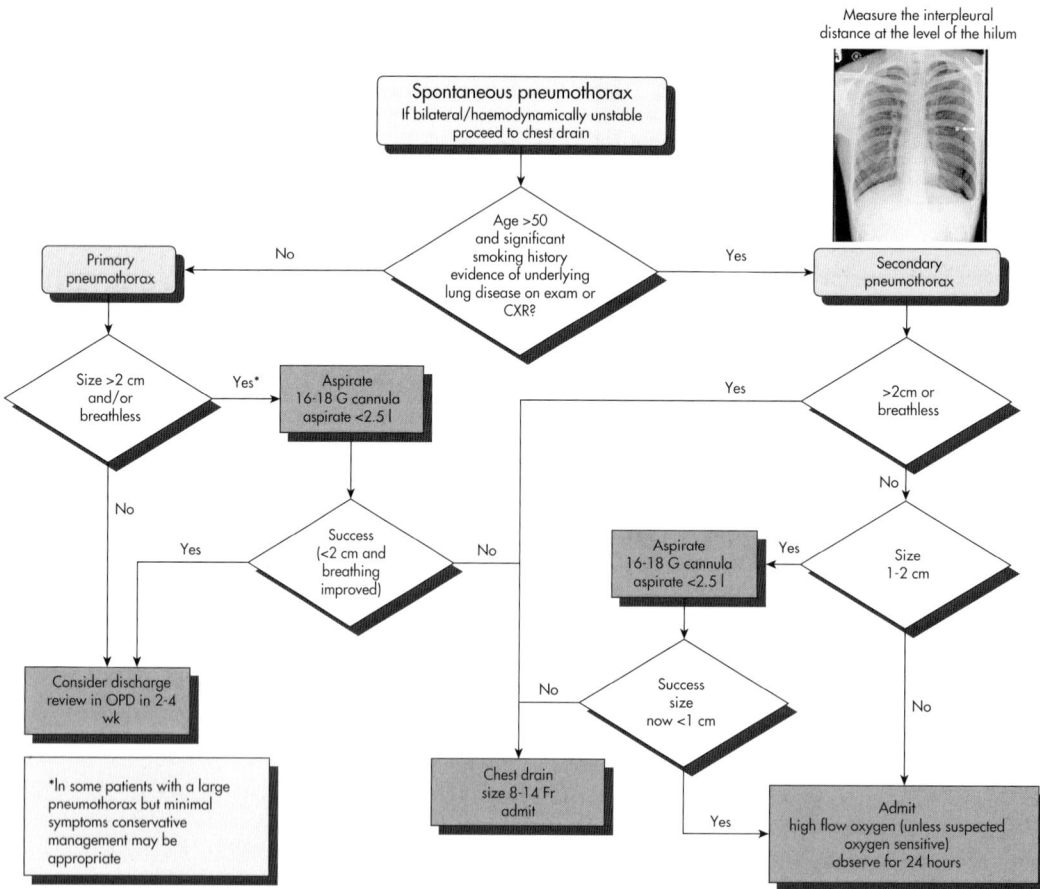

FIG. 6 Management of spontaneous pneumothorax. *CXR,* Chest x-ray examination; *OPD,* outpatient department; *PTX,* pneumothorax. (From Macduff A et al: Management of spontaneous pneumothorax: British Thoracic Society pleural disease guideline 2010, *Thorax* 65:ii18-ii31, 2010.)

BASIC INFORMATION

DEFINITION

Polycystic ovary syndrome (PCOS) is characterized by an accumulation of incompletely developed follicles in the ovaries due to anovulation and associated with ovarian androgen production. In its complete form, it is associated with polycystic ovaries, amenorrhea, hirsutism, and obesity. Table 1 describes criteria for a diagnosis of PCOS.

SYNONYMS

Polycystic ovarian syndrome
Stein-Leventhal syndrome
PCOS

ICD-10CM CODE
E28.2 Polycystic ovarian syndrome

EPIDEMIOLOGY & DEMOGRAPHICS

- 6% to 25% of reproductive-age women (most common endocrine disorder in this population).
- Symptoms usually begin around the time of menarche, and the diagnosis is often made during adolescence or young adulthood.
- Increased risk of endometrial and ovarian cancers.
- PCOS is the most common cause of anovulatory infertility.

PHYSICAL FINDINGS & CLINICAL PRESENTATION

- Oligomenorrhea or amenorrhea
- Dysfunctional uterine bleeding
- Infertility
- Hirsutism
- Acne, alopecia, acanthosis nigricans (Fig. E1)
- Obesity (40% only), predominantly abdominal obesity
- Insulin resistance (type 2 diabetes mellitus)
- Hypertension

ETIOLOGY & PATHOGENESIS

Elevated serum luteinizing hormone (LH) concentrations and an increased serum LH/follicle-stimulating hormone (FSH) ratio result either from an increased gonadotropin-releasing hormone hypothalamic secretion or less likely from a primary pituitary abnormality. This results in dysregulation of androgen secretion and increased intraovarian androgen, the effect of which in the ovary is follicular atresia, maturation arrest, polycystic ovaries, and anovulation. Hyperinsulinemia is a contributing factor to ovarian hyperandrogenism, independent of LH excess. A role for insulin growth factor (IGF) receptors has been postulated for the association of PCOS and diabetes. Fig. E2 illustrates the pathologic mechanisms in PCOS.

DIAGNOSIS

The diagnosis of PCOS excludes secondary causes (androgen-producing neoplasm, hyperprolactinemia, adult-onset congenital adrenal hyperplasia).
Clinical:
- The symptoms, signs, and biochemical features of PCOS vary greatly among women and may change over time.
- PCOS is the most common cause of chronic anovulation with estrogen present. A positive progesterone withdrawal test establishes the presence of estrogen. Medroxyprogesterone (Provera) 10 mg qd is administered for 5 days and bleeding occurs if estrogen is present.
- The presence of oligomenorrhea, hirsutism, obesity, and documented polycystic ovaries establishes the diagnosis.

DIFFERENTIAL DIAGNOSIS

Causes of amenorrhea:
- Primary (unusual in PCOS):
  1. Genetic disorder (Turner syndrome)
  2. Anatomic abnormality (e.g., imperforate hymen)
- Secondary:
  1. Pregnancy
  2. Functional (cause unknown, anorexia nervosa, stress, excessive exercise, hyperthyroidism, less commonly hypothyroidism, adrenal dysfunction, pituitary dysfunction, severe systemic illness, drugs such as oral contraceptives, estrogens, or dopamine agonists)
  3. Abnormalities of the genital tract (uterine tumor, endometrial scarring, ovarian tumor)

LABORATORY TESTS

- Glucose tolerance test at the initial presentation and every 2 yr thereafter (rule out diabetes mellitus). Impaired glucose tolerance is very common, occurring in approximately 30% of women with PCOS
- Fasting lipid panel (rule out dyslipidemia), alanine aminotransferase, aspartate aminotransferase (rule out hepatic steatosis)
- Elevated LH/FSH ratio >2.5
- Prolactin level elevation in 25%
- Elevated androgens (testosterone [free and total levels], DHEA-S) (rule out androgen-secreting tumor)
- Other: Thyroid-stimulating hormone (rule out hypothyroidism), 17-hydroxyprogesterone (rule out congenital adrenal hyperplasia), 24-h urine for cortisol and creatinine (rule out Cushing syndrome)
- TSH
- Table 2 summarizes laboratory testing to exclude other causes of ovulatory dysfunction and hyperandrogenism

IMAGING STUDIES

Pelvic ultrasound (Fig. E3) reveals the presence of twofold to fivefold ovarian enlargement with a thickened tunica albuginea, thecal hyperplasia, and 20 or more subcapsular follicles from 1 to 15 mm in diameter. It is important to note that having polycystic ovaries alone does not make the diagnosis of PCOS because 20% of women with polycystic ovaries have no symptoms.

TREATMENT (TABLE 3)

The goal is to interrupt the self-perpetuating abnormal hormone cycle:
- Reduction of ovarian androgen secretion by laparoscopic ovarian wedge resection. Laparoscopic ovarian surgery (laparoscopic ovarian drilling [LOD]) is a useful alternative that does not trigger ovarian hyperstimulation.

TABLE 1 Criteria for Diagnosis of Polycystic Ovary Syndrome

Study*	Criteria
National Institute of Child Health and Human Development 1990	Menstrual irregularity Hyperandrogenism (clinical or biochemical)
ESHRE-ASRM 2003 Rotterdam criteria	Menstrual irregularity Hyperandrogenism (clinical or biochemical) Polycystic ovaries on ultrasound (two of three required)
AEPCOS Society 2006	Hyperandrogenism (clinical or biochemical) and menstrual irregularity Polycystic ovaries on ultrasound (either or both of the latter two)
NIH Workshop 2012	Endorsement of Rotterdam criteria, acknowledging its limitations, and suggesting the name PCOS should be changed

*All required the exclusion of other underlying hormonal disorders or tumors.
AEPCOS, Androgen Excess and PCOS; *ASRM,* American Society for Reproductive Medicine; *ESHRE,* European Society of Human Reproduction and Embryology; *NIH,* National Institutes of Health; *PCOS,* polycystic ovary syndrome.
From Gershenson DM et al: *Comprehensive gynecology,* ed 8, Philadelphia, 2022, Elsevier.

TABLE 2 Laboratory Testing to Exclude Other Causes of Ovulatory Dysfunction and Hyperandrogenism

Lab	Evaluation for:	Comment
Total and/or bioavailable testosterone	Androgen-secreting tumor	Measure if there are symptoms concerning for an androgen-secreting tumor or if biochemical evidence of hyperandrogenism is needed to make the diagnosis of polycystic ovary syndrome. Rapid progression or a total testosterone >200 ng/dl should prompt a workup for an androgen-secreting tumor.
Dehydroepiandrosterone sulfate	Androgen-secreting tumor	Measure if there are symptoms concerning for an androgen-secreting tumor. Although modest elevations in dehydroepiandrosterone sulfate can be seen in polycystic ovary syndrome, rapid progression or greater elevations should prompt a workup for an adrenal androgen-secreting tumor.
Morning 17-hydroxyprogesterone	Late-onset congenital adrenal hyperplasia	This disorder is caused by a partial adrenal enzyme defect that leads to impaired cortisol production, compensatory elevation in adrenocorticotropic hormone, and subsequent excess androgen production. Symptoms may mimic polycystic ovary syndrome. Normal values <200 ng/dl. If higher than this, adrenocorticotropic hormone stimulation test recommended.
24-h urine for cortisol and creatinine; dexamethasone suppression test; salivary cortisol	Cushing syndrome	Consider ruling out Cushing syndrome in women with an abrupt change in menstrual pattern, later-onset hirsutism, or other evidence of cortisol excess such as hypertension, facial plethora, supraclavicular fullness, hyperpigmented striae, and fragile skin.
Prolactin	Hyperprolactinemia	May be accompanied by galactorrhea. Consider ruling this out in all women with irregular menstrual cycles.
Thyroid function studies	Hyperthyroidism or hypothyroidism	Consider ruling out thyroid dysfunction in all women with irregular menstrual cycles.

From Setji TL, Brown AJ: Polycystic ovary syndrome: update on diagnosis and treatment, *Am J Med* 127:912-919, 2014.

- Reduction of ovarian androgen secretion by using oral contraceptives or LH-releasing hormone (LHRH) analogs.
- Weight reduction for all obese women with PCOS. Loss of abdominal fat seems to be crucial to restore ovulation.
- FSH stimulation with clomiphene HMG or pulsatile LHRH.
- Urofollitropin (pure FSH) administration.
- Metformin improves ovulation, insulin sensitivity, and possibly hyperandrogenemia.

Choice of treatment:
- The management of hirsutism without risking pregnancy includes oral contraceptives, glucocorticoids, LHRH analogs, or spironolactone (an antiandrogen). Finasteride and flutamide may be similarly effective in reducing hirsutism as spironolactone.
- Pregnancy can be achieved with clomiphene (alone or with glucocorticoids, human chorionic gonadotropin, or bromocriptine), HMG, urofollitropin, pulsatile LHRH, or ovarian wedge resection. Metformin may also induce ovulation. Recent trials comparing the aromatase inhibitor letrozole to clomiphene for infertility have shown higher live-birth and ovulation among infertile women with PCOS treated with letrozole. When considering in vitro fertilization (IVF), the transfer of fresh embryos is generally preferred over the transfer of frozen embryos; however, a recent trial among infertile women with PCOS undergoing IVF revealed that frozen-embryo transfer is associated with a higher rate of live birth, a lower risk of the ovarian hyperstimulation syndrome, and a higher risk of preeclampsia after the first transfer than with fresh-embryo transfer.
- Psychologic screening for depression is recommended. Women with PCOS are fourfold more likely to have abnormal depression scores.

DISPOSITION

Table 4 summarizes metabolic complications in PCOS. Cardiovascular risk factors associated with PCOS are described in Table 5.

SUGGESTED READINGS
Available at eBooks.Health.Elsevier.com.

RELATED CONTENT

Polycystic Ovarian Syndrome (Patient Information)
Amenorrhea (Related Key Topic)
Abnormal Uterine Bleeding (Related Key Topic)

AUTHOR: **FRED F. FERRI, MD**

TABLE 3 Treatment for Women With Polycystic Ovary Syndrome

Complaint	Treatment Options
Infertility	Letrozole, clomiphene, with or without metformin, gonadotropins, ovarian cautery ("drilling")
Skin manifestations	Oral contraceptive + antiandrogen (spironolactone, finasteride), GnRH agonists
Abnormal bleeding	Cyclic progestogen, oral contraceptives
Weight, metabolic concerns	Diet/lifestyle management, metformin

From Gershenson DM et al: *Comprehensive gynecology,* ed 8, Philadelphia, 2022, Elsevier.

TABLE 4 Metabolic Complications in Polycystic Ovary Syndrome

Abnormal glucose tolerance (impaired glucose tolerance or type 2 diabetes)	30% of obese polycystic ovary syndrome women have impaired glucose tolerance, and 10% have type 2 diabetes by age 40. In thin women with polycystic ovary syndrome, 10% have impaired glucose tolerance, and 1.5% have type 2 diabetes.
Obesity	Prevalence of obesity varies considerably in women with polycystic ovary syndrome. Previously, prevalence rates of obesity were estimated based on populations of women with polycystic ovary syndrome seeking care. A recent study comparing patients presenting for care in a polycystic ovary syndrome clinic with an unselected population evaluated during a preemployment physical suggests that obesity and overweight may not be more common in polycystic ovary syndrome. In that study, 63.7% of polycystic ovary syndrome clinic patients were obese, compared with 28% of unselected women with polycystic ovary syndrome identified during screening, and 28% of nonpolycystic ovary syndrome controls. Polycystic ovary syndrome symptoms, including hyperandrogenism and oligo-ovulation, are exacerbated by obesity.
Metabolic syndrome	33%-50% of U.S. women with polycystic ovary syndrome have metabolic syndrome compared to only 12% in a similarly aged National Health and Nutrition Examination Survey population. In contrast, only 8.2% of women with polycystic ovary syndrome in Italy met criteria for metabolic syndrome. Thus, metabolic syndrome varies by geographic location, a finding likely related to different body mass index, though other causes including genetics and diet could also be playing a part.
High blood pressure	Data have been conflicting, but a large Kaiser Permanente study demonstrated that hypertension or elevated blood pressure was more than twice as common in women with polycystic ovary syndrome (27% vs. 12%).
Dyslipidemia	Dyslipidemia is more prevalent in women with polycystic ovary syndrome compared to controls (15% vs. 6%). In a meta-analysis, triglyceride values were 26 mg/dl higher (95% CI 17-35), low-density lipoprotein cholesterol was 12 mg/dl higher (95% CI 10-16), and high-density lipoprotein-cholesterol was 6 mg/dl lower (95% CI 4-9) in women with polycystic ovary syndrome compared with controls. Women with polycystic ovary syndrome also have higher concentrations and proportions of small, dense low-density lipoprotein cholesterol.
Nonalcoholic fatty liver disease and nonalcoholic steatohepatitis	Nonalcoholic fatty liver disease and nonalcoholic steatohepatitis have recently been recognized as a potential complication in women with polycystic ovary syndrome. Prevalence of fatty liver disease in polycystic ovary syndrome women has been estimated to be 15%-55%, depending on the diagnostic parameter used (level of serum alanine aminotransferase or ultrasound). Individuals that may be at higher risk of nonalcoholic fatty liver disease including nonalcoholic steatohepatitis include those with metabolic syndrome, insulin resistance, and possibly hyperandrogenemia.
Cardiovascular disease	Many studies demonstrate abnormal surrogate markers of cardiovascular disease in women with polycystic ovary syndrome. However, data regarding cardiovascular disease risk are conflicting with some studies suggesting an increased risk in women with polycystic ovary syndrome, whereas other studies have not found this difference in cardiovascular risk. While it is important to recognize and treat cardiovascular risk factors in this population, further research of cardiovascular risk and complications is still needed to clarify the long-term risk.

CI, Confidence interval.
From Setji TL, Brown AJ: Polycystic ovary syndrome: update on diagnosis and treatment, *Am J Med* 127:912-919, 2014.

TABLE 5 Cardiovascular Risk Factors in Polycystic Ovary Syndrome

Risk Factor	Features
Traditional risk factors	Obesity, insulin resistance, dyslipidemia, abnormal homocysteine, C-reactive protein, plasminogen activator inhibitor-1, increase in inflammatory adipocytokines such as TNF-α, decrease in adiponectin; higher prevalence of diabetes, hypertension
Atherosclerosis	Coronary catheterization studies, increase in carotid intima-media thickness, coronary calcium
Endothelial dysfunction by blood flow studies	All increased in classic PCOS; less of a concern with milder phenotypes using Rotterdam criteria

PCOS, Polycystic ovary syndrome; *TNF-α,* tumor necrosis factor alpha.
From Gershenson DM et al: *Comprehensive gynecology,* ed 8, Philadelphia, 2022, Elsevier.

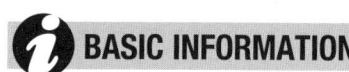
BASIC INFORMATION

DEFINITION

Polycythemia vera is a clonal disorder of abnormal hematopoietic stem/progenitor cells resulting in an increase in blood cell counts (particularly red blood cells), a predisposition to thrombosis (predominantly) and hemorrhage, and a cumulative risk of progression to myelofibrosis (MF) and/or acute myeloid leukemia.[1]

SYNONYMS

PV
Primary polycythemia
Polycythemia rubra vera
P. vera

ICD-10-CM CODE
D45 Polycythemia vera

EPIDEMIOLOGY & DEMOGRAPHICS
INCIDENCE[1]:
- Peak incidence: 2.3 to 2.8 cases per 100,000 persons
- Prevalence: 44 to 57/100,000 (U.S.)[2]
- Median age at diagnosis: 60 yr
- Male/female ratio: 1.2:1
- Genetics: Acquired JAK2 mutation JAK2V617F (97%); JAK2 Exon 12 (3%)
- Risk factors: Nothing definitive

PHYSICAL FINDINGS & CLINICAL PRESENTATION

Signs and symptoms of PV can be insidious and relate to the degree of cytosis and cellular function.[3-5]
- Plethora/ruddy complexion/flushing; retinal/conjunctival vascular engorgement
- Splenomegaly (>75%) and hepatomegaly, early satiety, abdominal discomfort
- Venous or arterial thrombosis (~30% of patients during the course of their disease), myocardial ischemia, stroke
- Mesenteric, portal, or splenic vein thrombosis, Budd-Chiari
- Headache, dizziness, visual changes, paresthesias, hypertension
- Pruritus (particularly after bathing, called aquagenic pruritus), erythromelalgia (erythema/swelling/warmth of the skin of the hands/feet), gout, diaphoresis
- Fatigue, bone pain
- Bleeding: Epistaxis, upper gastrointestinal bleeding (increased incidence of peptic ulcer disease and gastroduodenal erosions[6])

ETIOLOGY

JAK2 V617F mutation leads to constitutive tyrosine kinase phosphorylation, which promotes cytokine hypersensitivity and erythrocytosis (progenitor cells with this mutation grow in the presence and absence of erythropoietin).[7]

DIAGNOSIS

DIFFERENTIAL DIAGNOSIS

Secondary polycythemia[8]:
- Congenital (no splenomegaly)—rare

1. Erythropoietin (Epo) normal/increased
   a. High-affinity hemoglobinopathy (P50 low)
   b. 2,3DPG deficiency (P50 low)
   c. VHL mutation (P50 normal)
   d. PHD2/H1F2alpha (P50 normal)
2. Epo decreased
   a. EPOR mutations
- Acquired (no splenomegaly), Epo typically elevated
  1. Hypoxia associated
     a. Cardiac/pulmonary disease (e.g., congenital cardiac abnormalities with right-to-left shunt, chronic pulmonary disease)
     b. High altitude
     c. Smoking, CO (L shift of oxygen dissociation curve)
     d. OSA, hypoventilation
     e. Renal artery stenosis
  2. O_2 independent
     a. Drugs (EPO, androgens)
     b. Post–renal transplant
     c. Malignant tumors (e.g., renal cell carcinoma, hepatoma)
     d. Other tumors (e.g., hemangioblastoma, uterine fibroids, polycystic kidney)

RELATIVE POLYCYTHEMIA
- Plasma volume depletion

WORKUP

The revised 2016 WHO diagnostic criteria for PV suggest the appropriate workup to include an evaluation of the hemoglobin (Hgb) and hematocrit (Hct) levels, a bone marrow examination, a JAK2 mutation by PCR, and a serum Epo level. The diagnosis of PV requires all 3 major or the first 2 major plus the minor criteria.[3,8,9]
- Major criteria
  1. The Hgb (>16.5g/dl in men; >16g/dl in women) or Hct (>49% in men; >48% in women); increased RBC mass >25% above mean normal predicted value
  2. Bone marrow showing age-adjusted hypercellularity with trilineage growth (panmyelosis) of erythroid/granulocytic/megakaryocytic lines with pleomorphic mature megakaryocytes
  3. Presence of JAK2 V617F (>95% are + for this) or JAK2 exon 12 mutation
- Minor criterion
  1. Subnormal serum erythropoietin level (>85% have this)
- Caveat
  1. Major criterion 2 (bone marrow biopsy) may not be required in patients with sustained absolute erythrocytosis (Hgb >18.6g/dl in men or >16.5g/dl in women; Hct >55.5% in men or >49.5% in women), if major criterion 3 (JAK2+) and the minor criterion are present (subnormal serum erythropoietin).

LABORATORY TESTS[3,6]
- Elevated Hgb (>16.5 g/dl in men, >16 g/dl in women), Hct (>49% in men, >48% in women), or elevated red cell mass (RCM), the latter of which is no longer done routinely

- Increased white blood cell count in 66% (often with basophilia, increased eosinophils, and can have immature myeloid cells)
- Thrombocytosis >50%
- Elevated leukocyte alkaline phosphatase, serum vitamin B_{12}, and uric acid levels (not done routinely), elevated LDH
- Low serum erythropoietin level
- Peripheral blood smear: Anisocytosis, poikilocytosis, hypochromia, microcytosis (consistent with iron deficiency), basophilia, increased eosinophils, immature WBCs, leucoerythroblastic changes (if changing to MF), large platelets
- Bone marrow biopsy: Hypercellularity, panmyelosis (growth of all three cell lines), pleomorphic megakaryocytes, reticulin fibrosis, and absent iron stores

IMAGING STUDIES
- US or CT can be used to evaluate splenomegaly

TREATMENT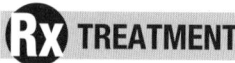

NONPHARMACOLOGIC THERAPY
Phlebotomy to keep Hct <45%[4]

ACUTE GENERAL Rx[4]

Treatments have not proven to modify the natural history of PV, so management has primarily been focused on minimizing the risk of thrombotic/hemorrhagic complications, which are the main causes of morbidity and mortality.[1,5]
- Low-risk patients (age <60 yr and no prior thrombosis): Aspirin (81-100 mg/day) and phlebotomy (maintain Hct <45%)
- High-risk patients (age >60 yr and/or prior thrombosis): Aspirin (81-100 mg/day) and phlebotomy (maintain Hct <45%) and cytoreductive therapy (hydroxyurea [HU]) to reduce thrombotic risk
- Low-dose aspirin is associated with a 60% reduction of combined risk of nonfatal MI, nonfatal stroke, PE, major venous thrombosis, and death from other cardiovascular causes. Twice-daily dosing may be more effective in some cases (resistant to once daily or considered at higher risk of arterial thrombosis).
- Busulfan is an oral alkylating agent not commonly used now.
- Pegylated interferon (IFN)-alpha-2b, used primarily in patients who are refractory or resistant to HU, is very effective, but is associated with significant adverse events. IFN can induce deep and long molecular remissions, even after years of therapy discontinuation, so should perhaps be considered early.
- Ruxolitinib, a JAK 1/2 inhibitor, can be considered for patients who are resistant to or intolerant of HU; it may offer better Hct control, spleen volume reduction, and fewer symptoms.[10]
- Ropeg-IFN-alpha-2b is an interferon, FDA approved 11/21, with good results, regardless of previous treatment, albeit with some significant adverse events. As many as ~60%

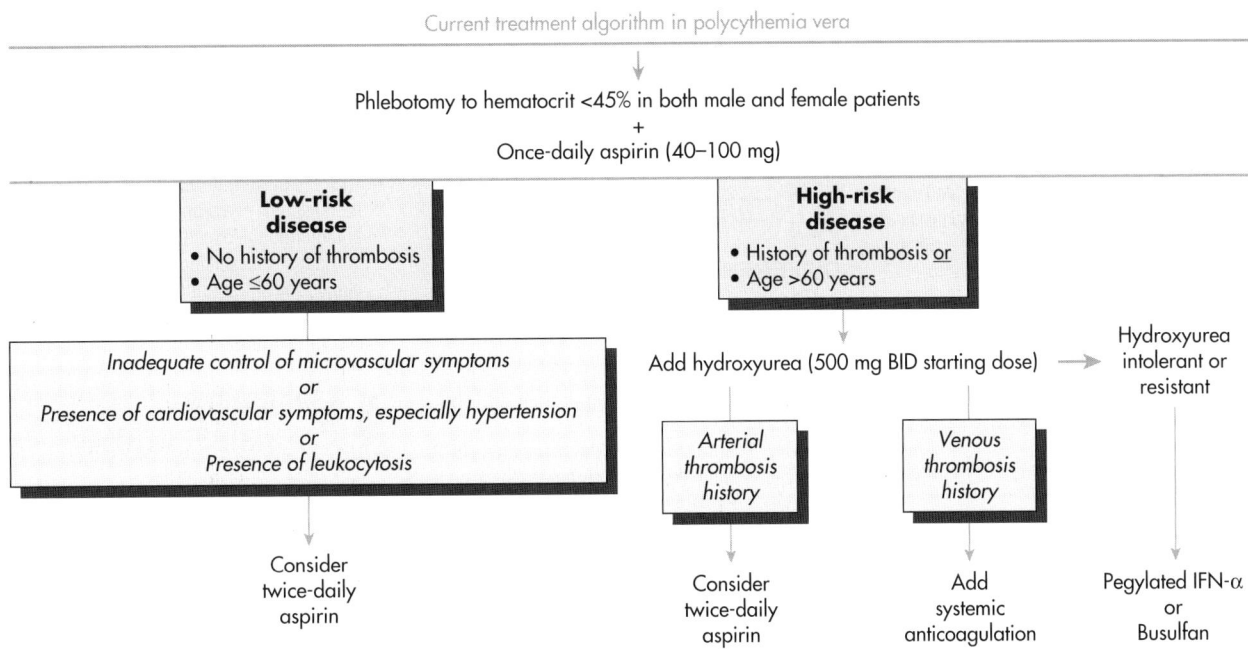

FIG. 1 Current treatment algorithm in polycythemia vera. (From Tefferi A et al: Polycythemia vera treatment algorithm 2018, *Blood Center J* 8:3, 2018.)

may have a complete hematologic response over 5 yr, and discontinuation with a continued response is considered possible.[10]

- Fig. 1 describes an algorithm for management of patients with polycythemia vera.[5]
- There are multiple treatments under investigation with a goal to arrest or delay disease progression. Givinostat, a histone deacetylase inhibitor, and idasanutlin, an MDM2 antagonist, are being evaluated with encouraging early results.[1]

CHRONIC Rx

- Patient education regarding need for lifelong monitoring and treatment

- Adjunctive therapy:
  1. Treatment of pruritus with antihistamines[4]
  2. Control of significant hyperuricemia with allopurinol
  3. Reduction of gastric hyperacidity with antacids or H_2 blockers
  4. Low-dose aspirin to treat vasomotor symptoms in patients without bleeding diathesis

DISPOSITION[5]

- The median survival with standard antiplatelet and cytoreductive therapy is 14 yr.
- The major life-threatening complications are leukemic transformation, fibrotic progression,

and thrombosis (incidence range of 5.5%-18.7%, 6%-14%, and 6%-17%, respectively, over 15, 15, and 3 yr).

- Prognosis (overall survival) is worse in patients >61 yr, WBC >10.5K/mcl, venous thrombosis, and abnormal karyotype.

REFERENCES

Available at eBooks.Health.Elsevier.com.

AUTHOR: **NANCY FREEMAN, MD**

Polymyalgia Rheumatica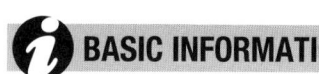

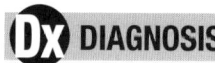 BASIC INFORMATION

DEFINITION

Polymyalgia rheumatica (PMR) is an inflammatory condition characterized by muscle pain and stiffness of the neck, shoulder, and pelvic girdle. PMR primarily affects the elderly and can occur alone or in conjunction with giant cell arteritis (GCA).[1]

SYNONYMS

PMR
Anarthritic rheumatoid syndrome

ICD-10CM CODES

M31.5 Polymyalgia rheumatica with giant cell arteritis
M35.3 Polymyalgia rheumatica

EPIDEMIOLOGY & DEMOGRAPHICS

- PMR almost exclusively occurs above age 50 with peak incidence between ages 70 and 79 with a female:male ratio 2:1.[1]
- In the U.S., incidence is 52.5 cases per 100,000, increasing with advancing age, with a prevalence of 0.5% to 0.7%. A recent literature review showed the global epidemiology of PMR is more limited with a greater variation in prevalence and estimates. Of note, GCA is higher in populations of Northern European ancestry.[1]

PHYSICAL FINDINGS & CLINICAL PRESENTATION

- Patients with PMR often have symptoms for 1 to 3 mo before a diagnosis is made.
- Onset of symmetric muscle pain and stiffness, which is worse in the morning (similar to other inflammatory disorders) and recurs with periods of inactivity.[2]
- Neck, shoulders, lower back, hips, thighs, and occasionally trunk and arms are involved. Shoulders are usually affected first. Pain distribution in PMR is illustrated in Fig. E1.
- Constitutional symptoms of fatigue, malaise, weight loss, loss of appetite, and low-grade fever may accompany pain and stiffness.
- Physical exam may reveal limited range of motion of shoulder (most common), cervical spine, and hips. May have subdeltoid and subacromial bursitis and peripheral joint synovitis. Motor exam is normal, although can be limited by pain.
- High-spiking fevers, night sweats, visual disturbances, headaches, or jaw claudication should raise suspicion of giant cell arteritis and be further evaluated promptly.[3]

ETIOLOGY

The cause is unknown, but both PMR and GCA are associated with HLA-DRB1 haplotype. With both conditions, also see elevated Th17 cells and decreased regulatory T-cells.[2]

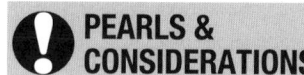 DIAGNOSIS

DIFFERENTIAL DIAGNOSIS

See Box 1.

WORKUP

- Initial laboratory evaluation: ESR, CRP, CBC, CPK.[3]
- ESR >30 mm/h in majority of patients. CRP elevation may be more common than high ESR.
- CBC may show a normocytic anemia and thrombocytosis.
- CPK is normal. Antibodies (ANA, RF, CCP) are typically negative.
- An algorithm for diagnosing polymyalgia rheumatica without giant cell arteritis (GCA) is described in Fig. E2, and Tables 1 and 2 describe various classification criteria for PMR.
- Ultrasonography, MRI, and PET may identify bursitis or tenosynovitis, (features of the 2012 PMR classification of criteria), which increase sensitivity and specificity.[4]

Rx TREATMENT

- Start prednisone 12.5 to 25 mg/day. Dramatic improvement usually occurs within 3 days.
- Dosage should be tailored to patient's weight, symptom severity, and comorbidities (e.g., diabetes, hypertension, or heart failure). If nighttime side effects are experienced, can divide prednisone dose. If symptoms persist after 1 wk, increase dose by 5 mg. Ongoing symptoms require consideration of alternative diagnosis.
- Initial prednisone dose should be maintained for 4 to 8 wk. Steroid dose is then tapered every 2 to 4 wk as tolerated to minimum amount required to remain symptom free. When dose reaches 10 mg/day, taper slowly, usually by 1 mg/mo.
- Flares are typical during tapering, can manage by increasing prednisone 10% to 20%. Most require treatment for 1 to 2 yr with steroids; others are unable to taper off fully.
- Monitor both clinical response and ESR and CRP intermittently.
- Gastroprotection should be considered. Start calcium and vitamin D supplementation for bone health. Start prophylactic bisphosphonates if indicated.

- Although routine use of adjunctive therapy is not recommended, up to one-third of patients have incomplete response to oral prednisone. Consider methotrexate for refractory disease or those at risk of steroid-related side effects. TNFi has not been shown to have benefit.
- A recent systematic literature review found the monoclonal antibody tocilizumab (an antiinterleukin-6 receptor antibody) is effective in cases of isolated PMR while having a glucocorticoid-sparing effect. However, monotherapy with tocilizumab was not recommended.[5a]

(!) PEARLS & CONSIDERATIONS

Patients with PMR should be monitored closely for the development of GCA. Patients who have incomplete response to prednisone or have an evolving pattern of pain and swelling should be reevaluated for the possibility of a different diagnosis such as rheumatoid arthritis.

REFERENCES
Available at eBooks.Health.Elsevier.com.

RELATED CONTENT

Polymyalgia Rheumatica (PMR) (Patient Information)
Giant Cell Arteritis (Related Key Topic)
Vasculitis, Systemic (Related Key Topic)

AUTHORS: **LUCA KATZ, BA,** and **MANUEL F. DASILVA, MD**

BOX 1 Differential Diagnosis of Polymyalgia Rheumatica

- Rheumatoid arthritis
- Rotator cuff syndrome
- Osteoarthritis of shoulder and hip joints
- Fibromyalgia
- Polymyositis/dermatomyositis
- Spondyloarthritis
- Systemic lupus erythematosus
- Vasculitides
- Paraneoplastic myalgias
- Infection-associated myalgias
- RS3PE (remitting seronegative symmetric synovitis and pitting edema)
- Parkinson disease
- Hypothyroidism
- There has been a report of a case of polymyalgia rheumatica being an adverse event after administration of a COVID-19 vaccine, but this is uncommon[6]

TABLE 1 2012 European League Against Rheumatism/American College of
Rheumatology Classification Criteria for Polymyalgia Rheumatica*

Criteria	Points With Ultrasonography	Points Without Ultrasonography
1. Morning stiffness duration >45 min	2	2
2. Hip pain or limited range of movement	1	1
3. Absence of rheumatoid factor or anticitrullinated protein antibody	2	2
4. Absence of other joint involvement	1	1
5. ≥1 shoulder with subdeltoid bursitis and/or biceps tenosynovitis and/or glenohumeral synovitis (either posterior or axillary) and ≥1 hip with synovitis and/or trochanteric bursitis	1	Not applicable
6. Both shoulders with subdeltoid bursitis, biceps tenosynovitis, or glenohumeral synovitis	1	Not applicable

*Score ≥4 without ultrasonography or ≥5 with ultrasonography is categorized as polymyalgia rheumatica.

TABLE 2 Classification Criteria for Polymyalgia Rheumatica

Chuang Criteria

1. Patients aged 50 yr or older
2. Bilateral aching and stiffness persisting for 1 mo or more involving two of the following areas: Neck or torso, shoulders or proximal regions of the arms, and hips or proximal aspects of the thighs
3. ESR >40 mm/h
4. Exclusion of other diagnoses except GCA

The presence of all these criteria defines diagnosis of PMR.

Healey Criteria (22)

1. Persistent pain (for at least 1 mo) involving two of the following areas: Neck, shoulders, and pelvic girdle
2. Morning stiffness lasting >1 h
3. Rapid response to prednisone (≤20 mg/day)
4. Absence of other diseases capable of causing the musculoskeletal symptoms
5. Age >50 yr
6. ESR >40 mm/h

The diagnosis of PMR is made if all the above criteria are satisfied.

Bird Criteria (23)*

1. Bilateral shoulder pain and/or stiffness
2. Onset of illness within 2 wk
3. Initial ESR >40 mm/h
4. Morning stiffness >1 h
5. Age >65 yr
6. Depression or loss of weight
7. Bilateral upper arm tenderness

ESR, Erythrocyte sedimentation rate; GCA, giant cell arteritis.

*A diagnosis of probable polymyalgia rheumatica (PMR) is made if any three or more of these criteria are fulfilled. The presence of any three or more criteria yields a sensitivity of 92% and a specificity of 80%.

From Hochberg MC: Rheumatology, ed 7, Philadelphia, 2019, Elsevier.

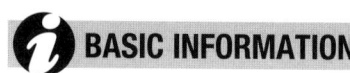

BASIC INFORMATION

DEFINITION

Clinically significant portal hypertension is defined as a portal vein pressure >10 mm Hg, most commonly attributable to liver disease.

ICD-10CM CODE
K76.6 Portal hypertension

EPIDEMIOLOGY & DEMOGRAPHICS

- Incidence of portal hypertension is not known.
- Cirrhosis is the most common cause of portal hypertension in the U.S.
- Portal hypertension is developed by >90% of patients with cirrhosis.
- Alcoholic and viral liver diseases are the most common causes of cirrhosis and portal hypertension in the U.S.
- Schistosomiasis is the main cause of portal hypertension outside the U.S.
- Esophageal varices may appear when portal vein pressure rises to >10 mm Hg.
- Variceal hemorrhage is the most serious complication of portal hypertension and may occur when portal pressures rise >12 mm Hg.

PHYSICAL FINDINGS & CLINICAL PRESENTATION

- Jaundice
- Ascites (Fig. 1)
- Spider angiomata
- Testicular atrophy
- Gynecomastia
- Palmar erythema
- Dupuytren contracture
- Asterixis (with advanced liver failure)
- Irritability, encephalopathy
- Splenomegaly
- Dilated veins in the anterior abdominal wall
- Venous pattern on the flanks

- Caput medusae (tortuous collateral veins around the umbilicus)
- Hemorrhoids
- Hematemesis
- Melena
- Pruritus

ETIOLOGY

Pathophysiologically caused by:
- Conditions resulting in an increased resistance to flow:
  1. **Prehepatic** (e.g., portal vein thrombosis, splenic vein thrombosis, congenital stenosis)
  2. **Hepatic** (e.g., cirrhosis, alcoholic liver disease, primary biliary cirrhosis, schistosomiasis)
  3. **Posthepatic** (e.g., Budd-Chiari syndrome, constrictive pericarditis, inferior vena cava **obstruction**, cor pulmonale, tricuspid regurgitation)
- Conditions leading to increase in portal blood flow:
  1. Splanchnic arterial vasodilation accompanying portal hypertension, mediated by local release of nitric oxide
  2. Arterial-portal venous fistulae

Table 1 describes the pathophysiologic changes in portal hypertension, and Table 2 summarizes the etiologies of portal hypertension.

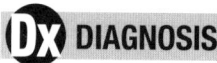 DIAGNOSIS

- The diagnosis of portal hypertension is made on clinical grounds after a comprehensive history and physical examination.
- Noninvasive and invasive procedures confirm diagnosis and determine the severity of portal hypertension.

DIFFERENTIAL DIAGNOSIS

- Ascites from infection, neoplasm, or other inflammatory processes
- Obesity
- Abdominal organomegaly

WORKUP

The workup of portal hypertension includes blood tests and noninvasive imaging studies to determine if the cause of portal hypertension is prehepatic, hepatic, or posthepatic. Ascitic fluid analysis is a key part of the diagnosis.

LABORATORY TESTS

- Complete blood count with platelets
- Liver function tests with serum albumin
- Prothrombin and partial thromboplastin times
- Hepatitis B surface antigen and antibody
- Hepatitis C antibody
- In selected cases: Iron, total iron-binding capacity, and ferritin; antinuclear antibody, anti–smooth muscle antibodies, antimitochondrial antibody, ceruloplasmin, alpha-1 antitrypsin
- Ascitic fluid analysis: A serum-ascites albumin gradient ≥1.1 mg/dl suggests portal hypertension. Polymorphonuclear cells ≥250 cells/ml or positive Gram stain or culture suggest complicating spontaneous bacterial peritonitis (SBP)

IMAGING STUDIES

- Duplex-Doppler ultrasound is effective in screening for portal hypertension.
- Less commonly, CT/MRI/MRA scanning (Figs. E2 and E3) or liver-spleen nuclear medicine scanning can be used if the results from ultrasound are equivocal.
- Upper endoscopy is the most reliable test documenting the presence of esophageal varices.

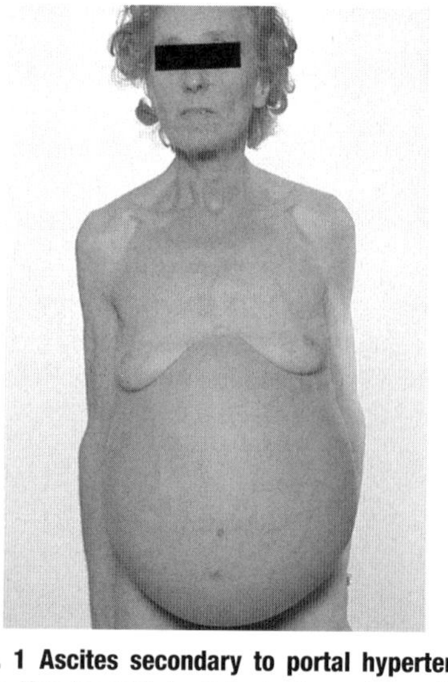

FIG. 1 Ascites secondary to portal hypertension. Note the dilated collateral vein running up the right side of the abdomen. (From Forbes A et al [eds]: *Atlas of clinical gastroenterology*, ed 3, Oxford, 2005, Mosby.)

TABLE 1 Pathophysiologic Changes in Portal Hypertension	
Pathophysiologic Change	**Specifics**
Hepatic resistance	
	Passive, mechanical component: 60%-70%
	Active, dynamic component: 30%-40%
Portal hypertension	
Shunts	
Splanchnic vasodilation	
Increased portal inflow	
Decrease in effective circulating volume; redistribution total blood volume	
Increase in endogenous vasopressors (RAA, SNS, VP)	
	Increase in endothelin-1
	Angiotensin II
	Norepinephrine
	Vasopressin
	PGF-2 alpha
Decrease in NO, CO	

CO, Carbon monoxide; *NO,* nitrogen monoxide; *PGF,* prostaglandin; *RAA,* renin-angiotensin-aldosterone; *SNS,* sympathetic nervous system; *VP,* vasopressin.
From Vincent JL et al: *Textbook of critical care,* ed 7, Philadelphia, 2017, Elsevier.

P

TABLE 2 Etiology of Portal Hypertension Grouped by Location of Insult

Site of Increased Resistance	Condition	FHVP	WHVP	HVGP	SPP
Presinusoidal (extrahepatic)	Extrahepatic portal, splenic, or mesenteric vein thrombosis	Normal	Normal	Normal	Increased
Presinusoidal (intrahepatic)	Early primary biliary cirrhosis	Normal	Normal/raised (?)	Normal/raised (?)	Increased
Presinusoidal (intrahepatic)	PSC	Normal	Normal/raised (?)	Normal/raised (?)	Increased
Presinusoidal (intrahepatic)	Sarcoid	Normal	Normal/raised (?)	Normal/raised (?)	Increased
Presinusoidal (intrahepatic)	Schistosomiasis	Normal	Normal/raised (?)	Normal/raised (?)	Increased
Presinusoidal (intrahepatic)	Congestive heart failure	Normal	Normal/raised (?)	Normal/raised (?)	Increased
Presinusoidal (intrahepatic)	Noncirrhotic portal fibrosis	Normal	Normal/raised (?)	Normal/raised (?)	Increased
Intrahepatic sinusoidal	Cirrhosis (any etiology)	Normal	Increased	Increased	Increased
Intrahepatic sinusoidal	Alcoholic hepatitis	Normal	Increased	Increased	Increased
Intrahepatic sinusoidal	Fulminant liver failure (any etiology)	Normal	Increased	Increased	Increased
Extrahepatic postsinusoidal hypertension	Budd-Chiari syndrome	Increased	Increased	Normal	Increased
Extrahepatic postsinusoidal hypertension	Constrictive pericarditis	Increased	Increased	Normal	Increased
Extrahepatic postsinusoidal hypertension	Inferior vena cava obstruction	Increased	Increased	Normal	Increased
Extrahepatic postsinusoidal hypertension	Congenital inferior vena cava web	Increased	Increased	Normal	Increased
Extrahepatic postsinusoidal hypertension	Right heart failure	Increased	Increased	Normal	Increased

FHVP, Free hepatic venous pressure; *HVPG,* hepatic venous pressure gradient; *PSC,* primary sclerosing cholangitis; *SPP,* systolic pulse pressure; *WHVP,* wedged hepatic venous pressure.
From Vincent JL et al: *Textbook of critical care,* ed 7, Philadelphia, 2017, Elsevier.

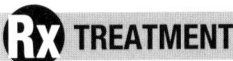 **TREATMENT**

The treatment of portal hypertension is complex and involves measures to reduce the hypertension directly, minimize volume overload, correct underlying disorders, and prevent complications (most notably SBP and variceal bleeding).

NONPHARMACOLOGIC THERAPY

Dietary sodium restriction to generally 2000 mg/day forms the basis of therapy to limit fluid overload.

ACUTE GENERAL Rx

- For tense ascites, serial large-volume paracentesis (LVP) is generally recommended. The use of albumin infusion (8 to 10 g/L of ascites fluid removed) during LVP >5 L has been shown to reduce the incidence of post-paracentesis circulatory dysfunction, although its use remains somewhat controversial.
- IV diuretics, typically furosemide and spironolactone, are used to achieve natriuresis and net negative salt and water balance. Renal function and serum electrolytes are monitored frequently, with transition to an oral regimen for long-term therapy.
- SBP is treated with IV antibiotics directed against enteric bacteria.
- Acute variceal hemorrhage is treated with crystalloid and blood product resuscitation, IV octreotide, terlipressin/vasopressin or somatostatin, and urgent upper endoscopy, often with sclerotherapy or band ligation.

Patients with acute variceal hemorrhage should receive empiric antibiotic therapy for SBP.
- Traditionally, a transjugular intrahepatic portosystemic shunt (TIPS) or surgical shunt placement may be considered in patients not responding to above measures. However, recent data show *early* TIPS placement improved outcomes in acute variceal hemorrhage. Table 3 summarizes indications, contraindications, and complications of the TIPS procedure.
- Table 4 compares treatment modalities for portal hypertension.

CHRONIC Rx

- Dietary sodium restriction in combination with diuretics: The typical ratio of furosemide 40 mg to spironolactone 100 mg retains normal serum potassium levels in most patients.
- Nonselective beta-blockers (propranolol and nadolol) in dosages sufficient to reduce the resting heart rate by 25% have been shown to be effective in primary prophylaxis for first-time variceal bleeding and for preventing recurrent variceal bleeding. Dosages are usually given bid and decreased if heart rate falls to <55 beats/min or systolic blood pressure drops to <90 mm Hg. The addition of a long-acting nitrate (e.g., isosorbide-5-mononitrate) has been shown to improve portal hemodynamics. Findings of a prospective trial of beta-blockers to prevent the formation of varices were negative. The

combination of beta-blockade plus endoscopic esophageal variceal banding is superior to either intervention alone.
- Intermittent LVP may be needed in "diuretic-resistant" patients.
- Patients with prior SBP merit lifelong antibiotics for secondary prevention.
- Abstinence from alcohol or treatment for hepatitis B or hepatitis C. Vaccination for hepatitis A and B as appropriate.
- Hepatic transplantation is an option in selected patients.

DISPOSITION

- The most common complication associated with portal hypertension is variceal bleeding. The risk of bleeding from varices is approximately 15% at 1 yr.
- Development of the hepatorenal syndrome (HRS) is associated with high near-term mortality. In particular, HRS may complicate SBP, which emphasizes the importance of making the diagnosis of SBP and instituting appropriate prophylaxis.

REFERRAL

Consultation with a gastroenterologist is recommended in all patients with portal hypertension to screen for esophageal varices.

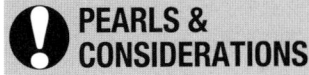 **PEARLS & CONSIDERATIONS**

Splanchnic arterial vasodilation is increasingly recognized as an important component of the

TABLE 3 Indications, Contraindications, and Complications of the TIPS Procedure

Indications	Relative Contraindications	Contraindications	Acute Complications	Chronic Complications
Upper GI bleeding	Pulmonary hypertension	Right-sided heart failure	Neck hematoma	Congestive heart failure
Ascites	Severe liver failure	Biliary tract obstruction	Arrhythmia	Portal vein thrombosis
Hepatic hydrothorax	Portal vein thrombosis	Uncontrolled infection	Stent displacement	Progressive liver failure
	Multiple hepatic cysts	Chronic recurrent disabling hepatic encephalopathy	Hemolysis	Chronic recurrent encephalopathy
		Hepatocellular carcinoma involving hepatic veins	Bilhemia	Stent dysfunction
			Hepatic vein obstruction	TIPSitis
			Shunt thrombosis	
			Hemoperitoneum	
			Hemobilia	
			Liver ischemia	
			Cardiac failure	
			Sepsis	

GI, Gastrointestinal; *TIPS,* transjugular intrahepatic portosystemic shunt.
From Vincent JL et al: *Textbook of critical care,* ed 7, Philadelphia, 2017, Elsevier.

TABLE 4 Comparison of Treatment Modalities

Treatment Modality	No (%), N = 77	Age, Yr (Mean)	Female %	Initial Meld (Mean, Range)	Child-Pugh Score (N = 74)	Ascites Size	Death (No, %) (N = 44)	Days from Presentation Until Death or End of Study
Medical management	64/77 (83%)	52	23/64 (36%)	16 (4-46)	A = 1 B = 31	None: 6 Small: 34 Moderate: 16 Large: 8	40/64 (63%)	321 ± 463
TIPS	8/77 (10%)	56	5/8 (63%)	12 (7-28)	A = 0 B = 5 C = 2	None: 1 Small: 3 Moderate: 3 Large: 1	4/8 (50%)	845 ± 407
Transplant	5/77 (7%)	54	0	21 (10-40)	A = 1 B = 1 C = 1	Large: 1	0	1896 ± 1752

TIPS, Transjugular intrahepatic portosystemic shunt.
From Vincent JL et al: *Textbook of critical care,* ed 7, Philadelphia, 2017, Elsevier.

pathophysiology of portal hypertension and ascites. There may be vasodilation in other capillary beds as well; of note, pulmonary arteriolar vasodilation can create a significant shunt fraction and resultant hypoxemia in the absence of chest radiograph or CT chest evidence of parenchymal disease. The diagnosis is suspected when otherwise unexplained hypoxia arises in a patient with cirrhosis, along with platypnea (dyspnea worse when sitting upright) and orthodeoxia (desaturation with upright posture). The diagnosis is confirmed by echocardiography with agitated saline, in which there is delayed appearance of bubbles in the left heart after injection into a peripheral vein.

COMMENTS

Portal hypertension and its complications carry significant morbidity and mortality rates. Emphasize ethanol abstinence, provide vaccinations and prophylactic therapy where indicated, and consider early referral to a specialist for assistance with management and consideration for hepatic transplantation.

AUTHOR: **FRED F. FERRI, MD**

P

BASIC INFORMATION

DEFINITION

Postconcussion syndrome (PCS) refers to nonspecific neurologic, cognitive, and psychologic symptoms that result from traumatic brain injury (TBI) and persist beyond the expected recovery period. Concussion is an acute trauma-induced alteration of mental function lasting <24 hr, with or without preceding loss of consciousness. Approximately 90% of concussion symptoms resolve within 10 to 14 days, but some may linger.[1] The extent and severity of lingering symptoms are highly dependent on the testing and reporting used. PCS can also follow moderate and severe brain injury, although it is more commonly associated with mild brain injury or concussion often without loss of consciousness.

SYNONYMS

PCS
Postconcussive syndrome
Posttraumatic nervous instability or brain injury
Postcontusion syndrome or encephalopathy
Status post commotio cerebri

ICD-10CM CODE
F07.81 Postconcussional syndrome

EPIDEMIOLOGY & DEMOGRAPHICS

- Incidence is approximately 27 cases per 100,000 persons/yr.
- From 30% to 80% of patients with mild to moderate brain injury will experience some symptoms of PCS though this is variable.[1]
- Risk factors for prolonged symptoms include children, female sex, low socioeconomic status, anxiety sensitivity, previous TBI, severe bodily injury from TBI, headaches, and unsettled litigation.[2]
- Recurrent TBI, especially when symptoms of previous injuries still exist, significantly increases the risk and severity of future postconcussive syndrome.
- Acute postinjury symptoms such as headache, dizziness, photophobia, diplopia, or tinnitus are associated with development of persistent symptoms.[1]

PHYSICAL FINDINGS & CLINICAL PRESENTATION

- Symptoms start within a few days to weeks after the head injury and usually persist after 3 mo; 15% of patients or more will have persistent symptoms 1 yr later.[2]
- At least three of the following symptoms after TBI are required to meet ICD-10 criteria:
  1. Headache (usually of frontooccipital location and showing characteristics of tension or migraine headache)—occurring in 25% to 78% of persons after mild TBI.
  2. Fatigue.
  3. Dizziness and/or vertigo—occurring in approximately 50%. Associated with risk for prolonged recovery.
  4. Impaired memory.
  5. Difficulty in concentrating.
  6. Insomnia—occurring in approximately 33% acutely and 25% more chronically.
  7. Irritability/frustration.
  8. Lowered tolerance of stress, emotion, or alcohol.
- Other associated symptoms: Noise sensitivity, neck pain, nondermatomal paresthesias, interference with social role functioning.
- Detailed neurologic exam focusing on orthostatic intolerance, cognitive function, vestibular function, extraocular movements, gait, balance, and coordination. Abnormalities are often subtle.[3,4]
- May need to test for impaired saccades or vestibulo-ocular reflex abnormalities, cervical motion abnormalities, and impairment on tandem gait forward and backward.[4]

ETIOLOGY

- The inciting TBI may occur as a result of events such as falls, motor vehicle accidents, military injuries, and contact sports.
- The primary injury triggers a slew of pathophysiological changes at the cellular level secondary to the axonal stretching and injury, leading to alterations in membrane and intracellular physiology, thereby affecting neurotransmission. These changes are believed to be a factor in determining whether the outcome will be an apparent normal recovery or persistent postconcussion symptoms.
- Postmortem findings reveal diffuse axonal injury as the primary pathologic finding, along with small petechial hemorrhages and local edema.
- Prior history of anxiety is a strong risk factor for occurrence of PCS.

DIAGNOSIS

A careful history will usually establish the diagnosis and rule out other etiologies.

DIFFERENTIAL DIAGNOSIS

- Headache (dissection of the vertebral artery, occipital neuralgia)
- Epidural hematoma
- Subdural hematoma
- Skull fracture
- Cervical spine disk disease
- Whiplash
- Cerebrovascular accident
- Benign paroxysmal positional vertigo—common after head injury
- Depression
- Anxiety
- Posttraumatic stress disorder

WORKUP

- Neuropsychologic testing, which often reveals difficulties in concentration, memory, language, and executive function
- To exclude other causes of neurologic symptoms after TBI:
  1. Normal results of electroencephalography
  2. Normal evoked potentials

LABORATORY TESTS

Various biomarkers in blood and cerebrospinal fluid and genetic testing have been proposed and studied in patients with TBI, but these tests are not specific and are not routinely used in clinical practice.

Chronically, if not improving, consider growth factor and other neuroendocrine markers.[5]

IMAGING STUDIES

- There is no imaging modality to diagnose PCS. PCS is primarily a clinical diagnosis. The American College of Emergency Physicians' clinical policy regarding neuroimaging in adults with mild traumatic brain injury is summarized in Box 1.
- 10% of computed tomography (CT) scans of the head following mild TBI are abnormal, showing mild subarachnoid hemorrhage, subdural hemorrhage, or contusions.[1,2]
- MRI of the head after a mild traumatic brain injury (mTBI) is abnormal in 30% of patients with normal CT scans and may show irregular brain contours or old cerebral contusions.
- More advanced imaging modalities, including diffuse tensor imaging (DTI) and susceptibility weighted imaging (SWI) in MRI, functional MRI (fMRI), and metabolic imaging such as magnetic resonance spectroscopy (MRS), positron emission tomography (PET), and single-photon emission computed tomography (SPECT) imaging, can show acute and chronic changes even after one mTBI, although they have not found a major role in clinical practice yet.[3]
- None of the imaging modalities have been able to predict the occurrence of PCS in patients with mild TBI.[3]

TREATMENT

PCS must be recognized as a physiologic and psychologic problem and treated accordingly. Treatment should be individualized to target the patient's particular symptoms and is typically completed on an outpatient basis. Some symptoms may be refractory to treatment.

NONPHARMACOLOGIC THERAPY

- Early reassurance and patient education are major components of treatment. Explanation of symptoms and expectations, combined with early follow-up with reassurance, may hasten resolution of symptoms.
- Early and graduated physical activity is preferred over prolonged cognitive and physical rest. Light aerobic activity that avoids risk for reinjury has been shown beneficial in mitigating refractory concussion symptoms. Physical and occupational therapy may be beneficial.[3]
- Cognitive behavioral therapy may be effective in treating symptoms.

BOX 1 American College of Emergency Physicians' Clinical Policy
Regarding Neuroimaging in Adults With Mild Traumatic Brain Injury

A noncontrast head CT is indicated (level one recommendation) in adults with LOC or post-traumatic amnesia only if at least one of the following is present:
- Headache
- Vomiting
- Age older than 60 yr
- Drug or alcohol intoxication
- Deficits in short-term memory
- Physical evidence of trauma above the clavicle
- Posttraumatic seizure
- GCS score below 15
- Focal neurologic deficit
- Coagulopathy

A noncontrast head CT should be considered (level two recommendation) in head trauma patients with no LOC or posttraumatic amnesia if any of the following is present:
- Focal neurologic deficit
- Vomiting
- Severe headache
- Age 65 yr or older
- Physical signs of a basilar skull fracture
- GCS score below 15
- Coagulopathy
- A dangerous mechanism (e.g., ejection from motor vehicle, pedestrian struck, fall of more than 3 feet or 5 stairs)

CT, Computed tomography; *GCS,* Glasgow Coma Scale; *LOC,* level of consciousness.
From Marx J et al: *Rosen's emergency medicine: concepts and clinical practice,* ed 7, Philadelphia, 2010, Mosby.

- Avoidance of alcohol, narcotics, and sleep deprivation.

PHARMACOLOGIC THERAPY

- Supportive symptomatic care may include the use of nonnarcotic analgesics and antiemetics.
- Amitriptyline has been widely used for post-traumatic tension-type headaches as well as for nonspecific symptoms such as irritability, dizziness, insomnia, and depression.[2] Amantadine is also a consideration.
- Posttraumatic migraine-type headaches can be treated with a trial of propranolol or amitriptyline alone or in combination.
- Depression can be treated with selective serotonin reuptake inhibitors but may not respond as well when compared with patients without PCS who have depression.

- If symptoms are not improving, consider testing for hypopituitarism since complete or partial hypopituitarism (most commonly growth factor) can be a sequelae of mild TBI and has overlapping symptoms with post-concussion syndrome.[5]

DISPOSITION

- Most patients improve after mild TBI without any residual deficits within 3 mo, though the cognitive and emotional symptoms resolve more slowly.
- Although good improvement is typically seen within the first 6 mo, patients can continue to show improvement for up to 12 to 18 mo.
- Patients with very severe brain injuries (low Glasgow Coma Scale [GCS] score) and prolonged anterograde amnesia are at increased risk of development of some degree of permanent cognitive and personality disturbance.

- Predictors for the development of persistent PCS include:
  1. Female sex
  2. Ongoing litigation (conflicting studies)
  3. Low socioeconomic status
  4. Prior headaches
  5. Prior TBI
  6. Prior psychiatric illnesses, particularly anxiety

REFERRAL

Early consultations with psychologists, psychiatrists, neurologists, and rehabilitation specialists in an outpatient setting may be beneficial.

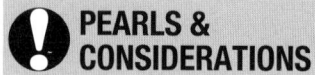

❗ PEARLS & CONSIDERATIONS

- PCS starts within a few days after the injury.
- Recognizing depression and treating pain symptoms early in the course may help prevent the development of persistent PCS (>1 yr).
- The severity of the trauma does not clearly predict the risk of PCS and symptoms do not cluster in a predictable manner.
- The severity of brain injury is usually documented by initial GCS score, duration of loss of consciousness, and duration of amnesia; however, there is a move toward tests of function, such as neuropsychologic testing or fMRI.
- Engaging in physical activity within 2 days after concussion is associated with a lower rate of persistent postconcussive symptoms.

REFERENCES
Available at eBooks.Health.Elsevier.com

RELATED CONTENT
Postconcussion Syndrome (Patient Information)
Concussion (Related Key Topic)
Traumatic Brain Injury (Related Key Topic)

AUTHOR: **COREY ELAM GOLDSMITH, MD, FAAN**

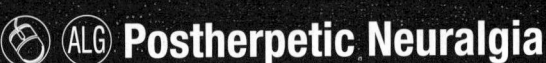

P

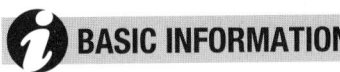 BASIC INFORMATION

DEFINITION

Postherpetic neuralgia (PHN) is a pain syndrome that results as a complication of herpes zoster (HZ). HZ, also known as shingles, is a painful vesicular eruption in a dermatomal distribution. HZ is caused by the reactivation of varicella zoster virus (VZV) in someone with a known history of varicella. PHN is pain and/or dysesthesia that persist for 3 or more mo at the site of resolved HZ.[1]

SYNONYMS

PHN
Shingles neuropathy

ICD-10CM CODE
B02.29 Other postherpetic nervous system involvement

EPIDEMIOLOGY & DEMOGRAPHICS

INCIDENCE: PHN occurs in up to 12.8% of HZ patients. It is the most frequent chronic complication of HZ and the most common neuropathic pain disorder resulting from infection.[2] From 1994 through 2018, the overall incidence of PHN increased across all ages, races/ethnicities, and sexes.[2] The median age of patients with PHN was 65.9 yr old, nearly 10 yr older than the median age of patients with HZ, indicating its predominance in the elderly.[2] In one study, approximately 60% of patients with HZ developed PHN at age 60 yr, and 75% developed PHN at age 70 yr. In another study, the incidence of PHN at 9 yr post-HZ eruption was 21%.[3]

PREDOMINANT SEX & AGE:
- PHN occurs equally in males and females.
- The likelihood of developing PHN significantly increases with advancing age.

PEAK INCIDENCE: Unknown.

RISK FACTORS:
- Advanced age
- Greater severity of HZ prodromal pain
- Greater severity of pain during acute HZ eruption
- Location—specifically ophthalmic (V1) location and brachial plexus
- Severe immunosuppression
- Severe rash[4]

GENETICS: Family history of HZ is considered a risk factor for HZ, with higher risk if multiple family members have had HZ.[5]

PHYSICAL FINDINGS & CLINICAL PRESENTATION

- HZ typically presents as a painful vesicular eruption in a dermatomal distribution. Rarely, HZ can occur subclinically with dermatomal pain in the absence of a rash (zoster sine herpete).[6]
- PHN is pain that continues for 3 mo at the dermatomal site of the resolved HZ. The pain may be described as burning, stabbing, shooting, or shock-like.
- Patients may note an amplified response to stimuli at the site of PHN, with increased pain response (hyperalgesia), pain to typically nonnoxious stimuli (allodynia), or focal changes in autonomic function (e.g., increased sweating).

- Physical examination should include a comparison of sensory function in the affected dermatome with that on the contralateral side.

ETIOLOGY

PHN is associated with damage and scarring to the dorsal root ganglion secondary to inflammation related to active herpes zoster infection.[6]

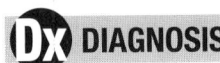 DIAGNOSIS

DIFFERENTIAL DIAGNOSIS

Zoster sine herpete (subclinical HZ without skin eruption)

Rx TREATMENT

ACUTE GENERAL Rx

- Administration of acyclovir or valacyclovir within 72 hr of HZ onset is thought to help reduce the likelihood of developing PNH. However, one Cochrane review paper found no difference with acyclovir administration.[7]
- A single published study supports the use of amitriptyline (25 mg daily) as an adjunct to an antiviral agent in acute HZ to decrease the incidence of PHN and the pain associated with subsequent PHN.[8]
- A suggestive noncontrolled study with co-administration of valacyclovir and gabapentin during acute HZ reduced the incidence of PHN as well.[9]
- Corticosteroids do NOT prevent PHN.[10]

CHRONIC Rx (Table E1)[11-15]

TOPICAL TREATMENTS:
- Lidocaine 5% patches may be used for mild pain.
- Capsaicin 0.075% cream (although little reported efficacy)[16] 5 times per day.
- Capsaicin 8% patch has greater efficacy,[16] but overall analgesia may be minimal at best, with one third of patients unable to tolerate the agent due to burning, stinging, and erythema. However, a single 60-minute treatment with high concentration capsaicin patch was found in one study to reduce PHN for up to 12 wk regardless of concomitant systemic neuropathic pain medication use.[17]

ORAL TREATMENTS:
First line:
- Gabapentinoids (gabapentin, pregabalin) are the only FDA-approved oral therapy for PHN and are some of the most used first-line therapies for chronic PHN pain.[18] Gabapentin may be administered in the immediate-release or extended-release formulation. Dosing includes gabapentin 300 mg 3 times a day (titrating up to max 3600 mg/day) and pregabalin 75 mg nightly (titrating up to 300 mg twice daily).
- Tricyclic antidepressants such as amitriptyline (25 mg/day, increased by 25 mg every night to a maximum of 75 mg/night), desipramine (10-25 mg/day, increased by 25 mg/day every 3 days as needed to a maximum of 150 mg/day), and nortriptyline (10-25 mg/day,

increased by 25 mg/day weekly as needed to maximum of 75 mg day) are other first-line treatments.[19] These medications have a delayed onset of action and may not work as well in patients with certain types of pain, such as burning pain or allodynia. They have a considerable side effect profile. Their use in elderly patients should be carefully considered. A randomized controlled crossover study showed the combination of gabapentin and nortriptyline was more efficacious than either drug as monotherapy for neuropathic pain.[20]

Second line:
- Opiates (e.g., controlled-release oxycodone)[21]: Side effects, the possibility of misuse, and the potential for abuse must be weighed.

Other modalities:
- Dorsal root entry zone (DREZ) lesioning has been used with an improvement rate of up to 45% in long-term studies.[22]
- For recalcitrant cases, epidural corticosteroids[23] and nerve blocks,[24] botulinum toxin,[25,26], cryotherapy,[27] and pulsed radiofrequency.[28]
- Fig. 1 describes a treatment algorithm for HZ and PHN.

COMPLEMENTARY & ALTERNATIVE MEDICINE

Acupuncture: Studies on acupuncture and PHN pain have had varying results. A recent systematic review and meta-analysis of seven randomized, controlled studies showed superior pain reduction in the acupuncture arm compared with pharmacologic therapy, although their effects on improving the global impression or life quality were similar.[29]

REFERRAL

For complicated cases, dermatology, neurology, and/or pain management input can be helpful.

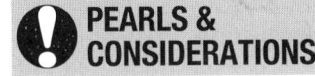 PEARLS & CONSIDERATIONS

COMMENTS

- Careful consideration of treatment side effects and drug interactions is needed.
- The natural history of PHN is slow resolution, and most individuals respond to medical therapy. However, a subtype of patients may develop severe, long-lasting pain that is recalcitrant to medical therapy.
- In a questionnaire study of 385 adults age >65 yr with persistent acute pain, the mean duration of PHN was 3.3 yr.[30]
- Only consider topical capsaicin on intact skin.[31]

PREVENTION

- Vaccination:
  1. A non-live VZV vaccine (Shingrix®) is approved by the FDA for individuals age 50 and older. It is administered as two shots spaced 2 mo apart and is 97% effective against shingles in people ages 50 to 69,[32] and 91% effective against PHN in people 50 and older.[33] It is more effective than the live attenuated VZV vaccine (Zostavax).[34]

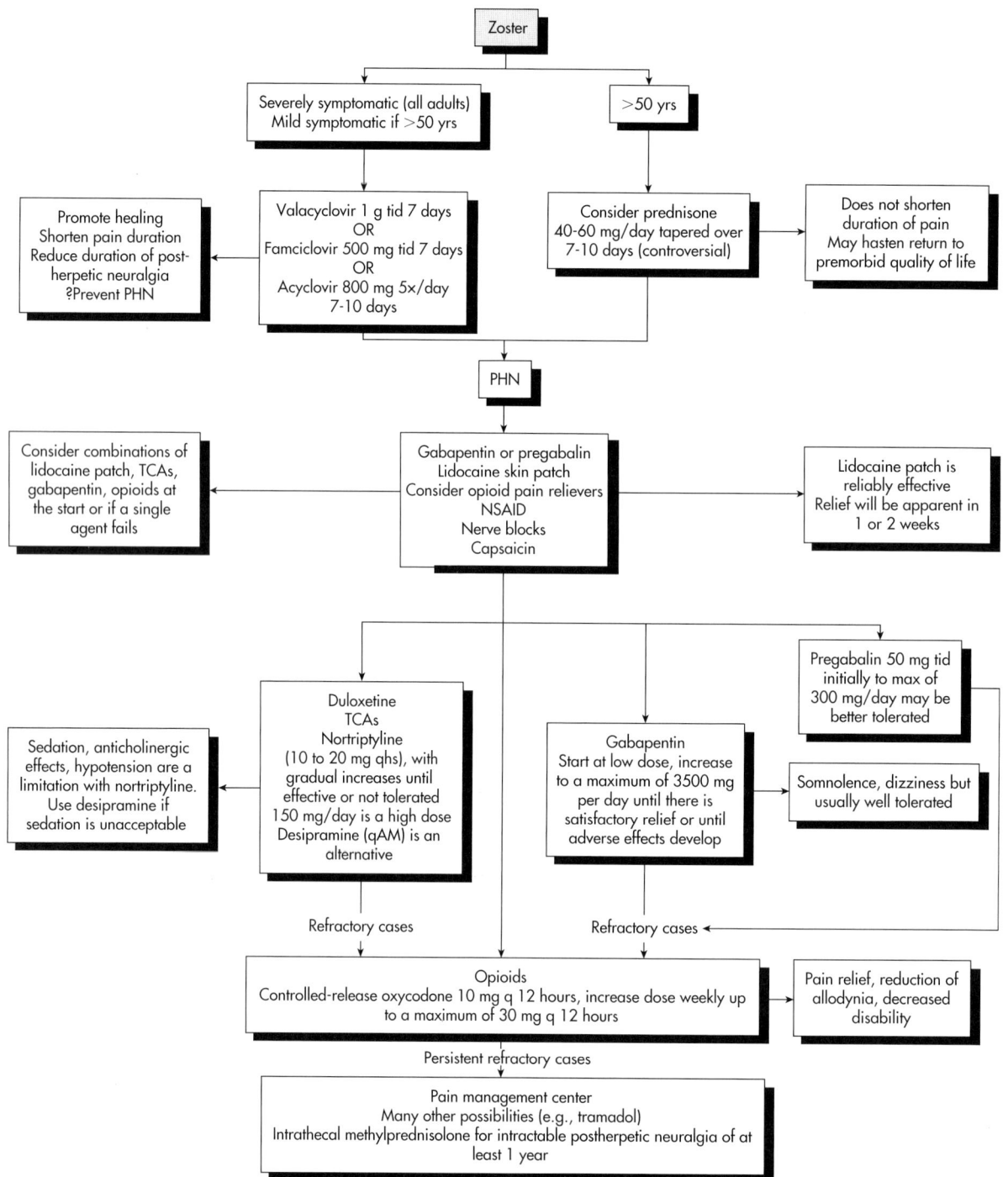

FIG. 1 Treatment of herpes zoster and postherpetic neuralgia. *NSAID,* Nonsteroidal antiinflammatory drug; *PHN,* postherpetic neuralgia; *TCA,* Tricyclic antidepressants. (Modified from Habif TA: *Clinical dermatology,* ed 6, St Louis, 2016, Elsevier.)

2. The Centers for Disease Control and Prevention (CDC) recommends that those who received Zostavax be revaccinated with Shingrix.[35]
3. Those who have had HZ should still receive the vaccine.[36]
4. All immunosuppressed individuals, regardless of age, should receive VZV vaccine.[36]
• Combination therapies can be effective in preventing PHN. Continuous epidural blocks with local anesthetics, antiviral agents with intracutaneous or subcutaneous injection with local anesthetics and steroid, and paravertebral

block combined with antiviral antiepileptic agents have shown efficacy in preventing PHN.[37]

PATIENT & FAMILY EDUCATION
• The only well-documented means of preventing PHN is the prevention of herpes zoster through vaccination.
• Patients should understand both the benefits and the potential adverse effects of treatment.
  1. They should be informed that pain relief will likely not be immediate.

2. Frequent reassessment may be needed, and drug doses should be increased as necessary.

REFERENCES
Available at eBooks.Health.Elsevier.com.

RELATED CONTENT
Herpes Zoster (Related Key Topic)

AUTHORS: **JULIANNE KLEITSCH, BA,** and **LISA PAPPAS-TAFFER, MD**

BASIC INFORMATION

DEFINITION

Postpartum hemorrhage (PPH) is defined, for both vaginal and cesarean deliveries, as an estimated blood loss $\geqq$1000 ml OR blood loss resulting in signs/symptoms of hypovolemia within 24 h following delivery. PPH is further categorized into primary or secondary. Primary PPH occurs within the first 24 h after delivery. Secondary PPH occurs more than 24 h after delivery but within 12 wk following delivery.

SYNONYMS

Obstetric hemorrhage
Maternal hemorrhage
PPH

ICD-10CM CODES

O72.0	Third stage hemorrhage
O72.1	Other immediate postpartum hemorrhage
O72.2	Delayed and secondary postpartum hemorrhage
O72.3	Postpartum coagulation defects

EPIDEMIOLOGY & DEMOGRAPHICS

INCIDENCE: Depending on definitions used and scope considered, anywhere from 1% to 6% of obstetric patients will experience postpartum hemorrhage. Postpartum hemorrhage is the leading cause of maternal mortality worldwide and is implicated in >11% of maternal deaths in the United States and 20% of maternal deaths in developing nations.[1]
PREDOMINANT SEX & AGE: Female of reproductive age
RISK FACTORS:
- Antepartum factors: History of PPH, primiparity or high parity, fetal macrosomia, multiple gestation, polyhydramnios, uterine fibroids, prior uterine surgery, abnormal placentation, bleeding disorder
- Intrapartum factors: Prolonged labor, augmented labor, rapid labor, preeclampsia, chorioamnionitis, operative delivery, episiotomy, lacerations, retained products, placental abruption, fetal demise

PHYSICAL FINDINGS & CLINICAL PRESENTATION (TABLE 1)

- Bleeding is generally brisk at time of delivery.
- Examination findings can include a boggy uterus with continued passage of clot or blood with fundal pressure.
- Objective findings can also include hypotension, tachycardia, and oliguria with substantial blood loss.

ETIOLOGY

- Primary: Uterine atony (70% to 80%), retained placenta, lacerations, and coagulopathies
- Secondary: Subinvolution of placental site, retained products (includes abnormal placentation), infection, and coagulopathies

DIAGNOSIS

WORKUP

- Bimanual examination to evaluate for atony; remove clots; massage if it is present
- Bladder should be emptied
- Examination to verify that placenta is intact
- Ensure adequate IV access
- Consider ultrasonography at bedside to evaluate for retained tissue or clot
- Examination to verify that no lacerations are present, including cervical examination with necessary lighting and retractors (may require examination in OR for adequate exposure)

LABORATORY TESTS

Significant hemorrhage can lead to disseminated intravascular coagulation (DIC). If DIC is suspected, complete blood count and coagulation panels should be ordered. Similarly, if coagulopathy is suspected, evaluation of clotting factors should be ordered. Thromboelastography (TEG) is a useful test to guide product replacement in association with coagulation cascade dysfunction.

IMAGING STUDIES

Ultrasonography can be used to scan for retained products, including clot or placenta. It can be performed to assess the need for more invasive measures, such as instrumentation or a manual sweep.

TREATMENT

The most effective strategy for the prevention of postpartum hemorrhage is active management of the third stage of labor (AMTSL). Medical management with uterotonics is generally the first line of treatment. None of the following medications has been demonstrated to be superior in treating PPH compared with the others.
- Oxytocin (IV, 10 to 40 units diluted into IV solution, or 10 units IM); often given prophylactically immediately after delivery to minimize EBL with delivery of placenta
- Methylergonovine (IM, 0.2 mg)—contraindicated in hypertensive patient
- Carboprost (IM, 0.25 mg)—contraindicated in patient with history of asthma
- Misoprostol (400 to 800 mcg sublingually, buccally, or rectally)

Other medical management:
- Tranexamic acid (IV, 1 g): Trials[2] have shown that among women who undergo cesarean delivery tranexamic acid treatment results in significantly longer incidents of blood loss greater than 1000 ml or red-cell transfusion by day 2 than placebo, but it does not result in lower incidence of hemorrhage-related secondary clinical outcomes (use of additional uterotonic agents, provider-assessed clinically significant postpartum hemorrhage).

NONPHARMACOLOGIC THERAPY

- Active management of third stage of labor: Controlled cord traction (Brandt-Andrews maneuver) and uterine massage after delivery of placenta (in addition to Pitocin)
- Uterine tamponade (Fig. E1): Packing with gauze, Foley catheter, or tamponade balloon (Bakri)
- Intrauterine negative pressure system (Jada system)
- Uterine curettage for suspected retained products
- Uterine artery embolization
- Surgical management with laparotomy:
  1. Hypogastric artery ligation
  2. Bilateral uterine artery ligation (O'Leary sutures)
  3. B-lynch sutures
  4. Hysterectomy

ACUTE GENERAL Rx

- Uterotonics, surgical management, embolization, blood transfusion. Fig. E2 outlines the management of postpartum hemorrhage.
- Table 2 describes therapeutic response to initial fluid resuscitation. Dosing regimen for oxytocic drugs is summarized in Table 3. Blood product replacement is described in Box 1.

CHRONIC Rx

For anemia (Hb <10 g/dl): Ferrous sulfate and ascorbic acid supplementation to support new red blood cell production. Can also consider IV iron replacement.

DISPOSITION

- The patient should be closely watched for at least 24 h after a postpartum hemorrhage. Vital signs should be monitored for evidence of hemodynamic stability and appropriate

---

TABLE 1 Presentation of Symptoms in Postpartum Hemorrhage

% Blood Loss (ml)	Systolic Blood Pressure (mm Hg)	Signs and Symptoms
10-15 (500-1000)	Normal	Tachycardia, palpitations, dizziness
15-25 (1000-1500)	Low-normal	Tachycardia, weakness, diaphoresis
25-35 (1500-2000)	70-80	Restlessness, pallor, oliguria
35-45 (2000-3000)	50-70	Collapse, air hunger, anuria

From Vincent JL et al: *Textbook of critical care,* ed 6, Philadelphia, 2011, Saunders.

TABLE 2 Therapeutic Response to Initial Fluid Resuscitation

Response	Description	Follow-Up Treatment
Rapid response	<20% of blood volume lost	No additional fluids or blood are needed
Transient response	20%-40% of blood volume lost; responds to initial fluid bolus but later has worsening vital signs	Continue fluids and consider blood transfusions
Minimal or no response	Ongoing severe hemorrhage with >40% blood volume lost	Continue aggressive fluid and blood product replacements

From Vincent JL et al: *Textbook of critical care,* ed 6, Philadelphia, 2011, Saunders.

TABLE 3 Dosing Regimens for Oxytocic Drugs

Drugs	Regimens
Oxytocin (Pitocin)	5-unit IV bolus
	Add 20-40 units oxytocin to 1 L of fluids for continuous infusion
	10 units intramyometrially
Methylergonovine (Methergine)	0.2 mg IM every 2-4 h
Ergonovine maleate (Ergotrate)	100-125 μg IM or intramyometrially every 2-4 h
	200-250 μg IM
	Total dose 1.25 mg
Carboprost (Hemabate)	250 μg IM or intramyometrially every 15-90 min
	Total dose 2 mg (8 doses maximum)
Misoprostol	800-1000 μg PR, oral, or sublingual

IM, Intramuscular; *IV,* intravenous; *PR,* per rectum.
From Vincent JL et al: *Textbook of critical care,* ed 7, Philadelphia, 2017, Elsevier.

BOX 1 Blood Product Replacement

Crossmatched blood
  Type-specific or "saline crossmatched" blood
Compatible ABO and Rh blood types
Rh-negative blood is preferable
  Warm the blood, if possible, especially if the rate of infusion is >100 ml/min or if the total volume transfused is high; cold blood is associated with an increased incidence of arrhythmias and paradoxic hypotension
  Administer calcium if blood is transfused rapidly at >100 ml/min because of binding of calcium by anticoagulants in banked blood
  Give 6-10 units fresh frozen plasma (FFP) for every 10 units of packed red blood cell (PRBC) transfusions
Give 10-12 units of platelets if the platelet count decreases to <50 × 10^9/L
Cryoprecipitate can be given to replace fibrinogen in addition to the FFP
Consider 60-120 μg/kg intravenous bolus injection of recombinant activated factor VII (rFVIIa)

From Vincent JL et al: *Textbook of critical care,* ed 7, Philadelphia, 2017, Elsevier.

response to anemia. Serial laboratory tests can be performed in the setting of concern for ongoing bleeding.
- Morbidity can include: Shock, acute respiratory distress syndrome, Sheehan syndrome, thromboembolic disease, and loss of fertility.
- For cases with large blood loss (e.g., >2 L) and hemodynamic instability, surgical intensive care unit admission may be warranted.

REFERRAL

During the course of a postpartum hemorrhage, the anesthesiology department, blood bank, and OR staff should be notified, and adequate nursing should be available. Early considerations should be made to notify obstetricians. If bleeding is brisk or estimated blood loss is considerable, preparation should be made for transfusion of blood products, including notification of the blood bank to facilitate type and crossmatching blood products.

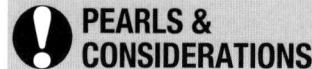

PEARLS & CONSIDERATIONS

PREVENTION
- Active management of third stage of labor

- Implementation of institution-specific PPH risk assessment tools effective for identifying patients at increased risk, though clinical suspicion should be maintained in all patients

REFERENCES & SUGGESTED READINGS

Available at eBooks.Health.Elsevier.com.

AUTHORS: **SCOTT J. MERRILL, MD,** and **MARWAN MA'AYEH, MD**

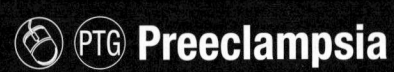
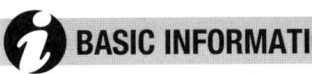 **BASIC INFORMATION**

DEFINITION

Hypertensive disorders of pregnancy represent a spectrum of disease ranging from gestational hypertension to severe preeclampsia. Preeclampsia is defined as new-onset hypertension (systolic blood pressure $\geq$140 or diastolic $\geq$90) after 20 wk gestation or up to 6 wk postpartum in the presence of proteinuria or evidence of end-organ injury.[1] In the absence of proteinuria, other criteria, including thrombocytopenia, acute kidney injury, impaired liver function, pulmonary edema, and new-onset neurologic symptoms, can be used for diagnosis. In 2013, the American College of Obstetrics and Gynecology (ACOG) Task Force on Hypertension in Pregnancy revised the criteria, making the presence of proteinuria unnecessary to make the diagnosis.[2] The task force reinforced the importance of hypertension as a necessary condition and deemphasized proteinuria.

Hypertensive disorders of pregnancy can be categorized as follows:[1]

- Gestational hypertension: Hypertension in pregnancy after 20 wk without proteinuria or evidence of end-organ injury
- Preeclampsia: Hypertension in pregnancy after 20 wk, with proteinuria but without evidence of end-organ injury
- Preeclampsia with severe features (Table 1)
- Chronic hypertension: Hypertension predating pregnancy or present at <20 wk gestation
- Chronic hypertension with superimposed preeclampsia: The presence of chronic hypertension with elevation in blood pressure from baseline often requiring increasing antihypertensives or with development of new onset of signs or symptoms meeting criteria for severe preeclampsia (Table 1)
- Hemolysis, elevated liver enzymes, and low platelet count (HELLP) syndrome: A severe form of preeclampsia defined by LDH greater than 600 IU/L, liver enzymes (AST, ALT) greater than twice the upper limit of normal, and a platelet count less than 100×10^9/L

SYNONYMS

Pregnancy-induced hypertension (PIH)
Hypertensive disorders of pregnancy (HDP)
Severe gestational hypertension

ICD-10CM CODES

011.1	Pre-existing hypertension with pre-eclampsia, first trimester
011.2	Pre-existing hypertension with pre-eclampsia, second trimester
011.3	Pre-existing hypertension with pre-eclampsia, third trimester
011.9	Pre-existing hypertension with pre-eclampsia, unspecified trimester
014.00	Mild to moderate pre-eclampsia, unspecified trimester
014.02	Mild to moderate pre-eclampsia, second trimester
014.03	Mild to moderate pre-eclampsia, third trimester
014.10	Severe pre-eclampsia, unspecified trimester
014.12	Severe pre-eclampsia, second trimester
014.13	Severe pre-eclampsia, third trimester
014.90	Unspecified pre-eclampsia, unspecified trimester
014.92	Unspecified pre-eclampsia, second trimester
014.93	Unspecified pre-eclampsia, third trimester

EPIDEMIOLOGY & DEMOGRAPHICS

INCIDENCE: Hypertensive disorders of pregnancy are recognized as the second leading cause of maternal mortality (after hemorrhage) and are attributed to 18% of maternal mortality globally. The global incidence of preeclampsia is estimated to be 2-4% with significant regional variation.[3,4] The disease burden is borne disproportionately by women in low- and middle-income countries or who are otherwise disadvantaged.[4a]

RISK FACTORS: See Table 2. Recently, SARS-COV-2 infection has been associated with a twofold increased risk of preeclampsia. Vaccination has been shown to be safe in pregnancy and reduce the likelihood of infection.[5,6]

GENETICS: Preeclampsia is a complex genetic disorder that is not yet well understood.[7] However, large studies describing the epigenetics of maternal hypertension have implicated alterations of the fetal FLT1 locus in the development of preeclampsia.[8] There are both fetal and maternal genetic factors influencing the risk of developing preeclampsia. The maternal genetic contribution has been estimated at 30% to 35% and the fetal contribution at 20%.[9]

PATHOGENESIS

The underlying causes of preeclampsia have been studied extensively for over a century; however, many uncertainties remain.[10]

PHYSICAL FINDINGS & CLINICAL PRESENTATION

Headache that persists despite treatment with acetaminophen is one of the classic neurologic symptoms of preeclampsia. **Visual changes** associated with preeclampsia, including scotoma, blurred vision, or aura.[1,11] Classic neurologic exam findings of preeclampsia include hyperreflexia, clonus, or cranial nerve VI palsy.[12]

Endothelial dysfunction and elevated perfusion pressure accompanied by cerebral edema are considered the underlying cause of cerebral injury, including posterior reversible encephalopathy syndrome (PRES), in patients with preeclampsia. PRES is characterized by cerebral edema classically affecting the occipital and parietal lobes. Patients with PRES may manifest headache, visual loss or disturbance, altered sensorium, or altered consciousness.[12] Severe cases of PRES may result in seizure or coma. PRES is also associated with increased risk of hemorrhagic and ischemic CVA. Importantly, patients with hypertensive disorders of pregnancy have a fivefold increased risk for occurrence of hemorrhagic or ischemic stroke.[12]

Patients with persistent neurologic symptoms are at highest risk for developing PRES. Management of PRES includes controlling hypertension, possible antiepileptic therapy, and indicated follow-up care.

Shortness of breath is often an indicator of underlying pulmonary edema from elevated pulmonary perfusion pressure accompanied by endothelial dysfunction. Rales may be auscultated, and a chest x-ray may be useful in confirming the presence of edema. Management includes fluid restriction and use of diuretics as clinically indicated.[1]

Diseases and Disorders

TABLE 1 Criteria for the Diagnosis of Preeclampsia With Severe Features

In patients with preeclampsia, **severe features** can be diagnosed if any one of the following criteria is present:

Blood pressure $\geq$160 mm Hg systolic or $\geq$110 mm Hg diastolic on two separate occasions at least 4 h apart (unless antihypertensive therapy is initiated before this time)

Serum creatinine >1.1 mg/dl or a doubling of the serum creatinine

New onset of visual disturbances

New-onset headache unresponsive to medication and not accounted for by alternative diagnoses

Pulmonary edema

Hepatocellular injury (serum transaminases at least twice the upper limit of normal) or severe persistent right upper quadrant or epigastric pain unresponsive to medications

Thrombocytopenia (platelet count <100 $\times$ 10^9/L)

TABLE 2 Risk Factors for Preeclampsia

Nulliparity
Multifetal gestations
Preeclampsia in a previous pregnancy
Chronic hypertension
Pregestational diabetes
Gestational diabetes
Thrombophilia
Systemic lupus erythematosus
Prepregnancy body mass index greater than 30
Antiphospholipid antibody syndrome
Maternal age 35 yr or older
Kidney disease
Assisted reproductive technology
Obstructive sleep apnea

From American College of Obstetricians and Gynecologists: Gestational hypertension and preeclampsia: ACOG Practice Bulletin No. 222, *Obstet Gynecol* 135:e237-e260, 2020.

Dependent edema, which may affect the lower extremities, vulva, or back, is also frequently seen. It occurs due to increased vascular permeability and sodium retention related to renal injury and abnormal RAAS activation. It can be managed with compression and diuretics. Physiologic edema of pregnancy can sometimes be distinguished from pathologic edema by timing of onset. Rapidly progressing edema >4 to 5 lbs of weight gain per week and facial edema are not typical of healthy pregnancy.[1]

The **right upper quadrant** or **epigastric pain** classically associated with preeclampsia is thought to be the result of periportal and parenchymal necrosis, with hepatocellular edema sometimes resulting in distension of the Glisson capsule. However, no strong correlation between symptoms and laboratory abnormalities exists.[13]

Oliguria in preeclampsia is due to decreased intravascular volume as a result of vascular endothelial dysfunction and RAAS activation.[1,11]

1% of patients with preeclampsia and 3% of patients with severe preeclampsia will develop placental abruption. **Vaginal bleeding** in a preeclamptic patient should prompt a workup for abruption.[1]

It is important to remember that patients can be asymptomatic with elevated blood pressures and high risk. Rarely, HELLP or eclampsia may present in a normotensive patient. It is important to maintain a high level of suspicion for preeclampsia in patients at increased risk.

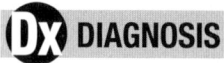 **DIAGNOSIS**

DIFFERENTIAL DIAGNOSIS

- Acute fatty liver of pregnancy
- Appendicitis
- Autoimmune hepatitis
- Chronic hypertension
- Chronic kidney disease
- Diabetic ketoacidosis
- Gallbladder disease
- Gastroenteritis
- Glomerulonephritis
- Hemolytic-uremic syndrome
- Idiopathic thrombocytopenia
- Thrombotic thrombocytopenic purpura
- Pancreatitis
- Peptic ulcer disease
- Secondary hypertension
- Systemic lupus erythematosus
- Viral hepatitis
- Medications or medication withdrawal
- Migraine headache

WORKUP

Hypertension:
- Two blood pressure measurements at least 4 h apart, with a systolic BP of 140 mm Hg or more or a diastolic blood pressure of 90 mm Hg or more.
- Severe hypertension with systolic BP of 160 mm Hg or more or a diastolic blood pressure of 110 mm Hg or more.
- Severe hypertension can be confirmed in a brief period to allow for immediate treatment of severe range blood pressure.

Proteinuria:
- ≥300 mg per 24-h urine collection
- Protein/creatinine ratio ≥0.3
- 2+ on dipstick (only if other methods not available)

Other diagnostic labs:
- See Table 1

LABORATORY TESTS

Generally, the recommended laboratory testing is consistent with labs that can be used to identify end-organ dysfunction.

Complete blood count (CBC) to assess for anemia or thrombocytopenia.

Liver function tests (aspartate aminotransferase, alanine aminotransferase) are useful in determining the presence of hepatic injury and are also useful in excluding HELLP syndrome.

Serum creatinine (and uric acid).

Prothrombin time, partial thromboplastin time, and fibrinogen can be checked to rule out disseminated intravascular coagulation, if clinically appropriate.

IMAGING STUDIES

- CT or MRI scan of head if persistent headache or neurologic symptoms raising concern for PRES or stroke
- Chest x-ray if there is concern for pulmonary edema
- Sonogram of fetus to evaluate for intrauterine growth restriction, amniotic fluid level, placental location
- Sonogram of maternal liver if subcapsular hematoma suspected

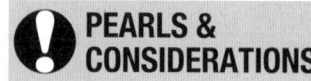 **TREATMENT**

ACUTE GENERAL Rx[1,2,14]

Delivery is the treatment of choice and the only cure for the disease. This must be taken in the context of the gestational age of the fetus and severity of the preeclampsia.
- For preeclampsia with severe features, administer magnesium sulfate 4 to 6 g IV loading dose, with 2 g/h maintenance (adjust dosage for renal insufficiency). If there is a contraindication to magnesium sulfate, such as myasthenia gravis, then use phenytoin at 10 to 15 mg/kg loading dose, then 200 mg IV q8h starting 12 h after loading dose.
- Treat blood pressure (BP) >160 mm Hg systolic or >110 mm Hg diastolic either with hydralazine 5 to 10 mg IV, then 10 mg, every 20 min to a max dose of 20 mg; or with labetalol hydrochloride 20, 40, 60, 80 mg IV, escalating dosage every 10 min to a max dose of 300 mg IV; or with nifedipine 10 to 20 mg orally every 20 min to a max dose of 180 mg/day for acute blood pressure control. If maximum dose of one medication is reached, add an additional medication to reach goal of BP 140 to 150/90 to 100 mm Hg.
- Continuous fetal monitoring.
- Epidural is anesthesia of choice for pain management in labor or cesarean section.
- All patients undergoing induction of labor or cesarean section should receive antiseizure

medications (magnesium sulfate) if disease with severe features, for delivery and 12 to 24 h postpartum.

CHRONIC Rx[1,2,14]

Preeclampsia without severe features: If <37 wk, close observation for worsening maternal or fetal condition with delivery at 37 wk. If 24 to 36 wk, consider antenatal corticosteroids. If severe features develop or there is evidence of fetal compromise, earlier delivery is appropriate.

Preeclampsia with severe features: Delivery in the presence of maternal or fetal compromise, labor, or 34 wk. From 24 to 34 wk consider steroids with close monitoring, and at <24 wk offer termination of pregnancy. Risks of expectant management include severe worsening of disease, eclampsia, abruptio placenta, stillbirth, HELLP syndrome, and ICU admission. Contraindications to expectant management include eclampsia, HELLP syndrome, pulmonary edema, disseminated intravascular coagulation, abruptio placenta, uncontrollable severe hypertension, fetal demise, and nonreassuring fetal status. Labetalol, hydralazine, and nifedipine are the drugs of choice for long-term blood-pressure control during pregnancy.

DISPOSITION

- Preeclampsia is a progressive and unpredictable disease process; a course of expectancy should be managed with caution. Up to 20% of patients who have seizures are normotensive.
- The reoccurrence rate for preeclampsia in a subsequent pregnancy is approximately 20%, and higher in cases with a second trimester presentation or complications. This risk may be decreased with the use of daily low-dose aspirin.
- For high-risk patients, baseline assessment of renal function (24-h urine collection for total protein and creatinine clearance or protein: creatinine ratio), complete blood count, serum creatinine, liver function tests (LFTs), and uric acid should be obtained at the first prenatal visit.

REFERRAL

Obstetric management with input from maternal-fetal subspecialists in severe cases. Transfer of care to facilities with appropriate level of care for all cases <34 wk.

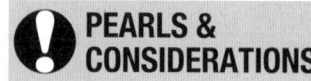 **PEARLS & CONSIDERATIONS**

COMMENTS

- Low-dose aspirin exposure during the early stages of placentation decreases the risk of preeclampsia, preterm birth, and intrauterine growth restriction in women who are at high risk of preeclampsia. The American College of Obstetricians and Gynecologists (ACOG) and the U.S. Preventive Services Task Force (USPSTF) recommend the use of low-dose aspirin as preventive medication starting after 12 wk of gestation (ideally before 16 wk) in

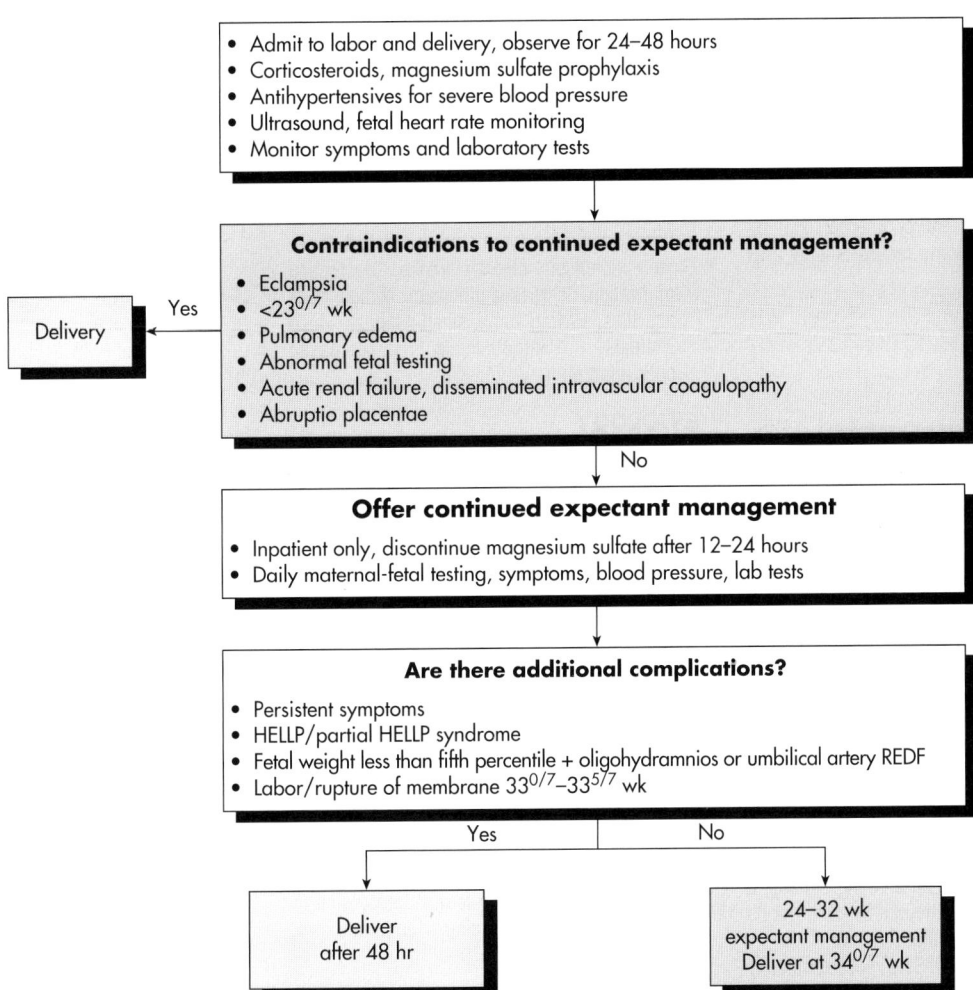

- Admit to labor and delivery, observe for 24–48 hours
- Corticosteroids, magnesium sulfate prophylaxis
- Antihypertensives for severe blood pressure
- Ultrasound, fetal heart rate monitoring
- Monitor symptoms and laboratory tests

Contraindications to continued expectant management?
- Eclampsia
- $<23^{0/7}$ wk
- Pulmonary edema
- Abnormal fetal testing
- Acute renal failure, disseminated intravascular coagulopathy
- Abruptio placentae

Yes → Delivery

No

Offer continued expectant management
- Inpatient only, discontinue magnesium sulfate after 12–24 hours
- Daily maternal-fetal testing, symptoms, blood pressure, lab tests

Are there additional complications?
- Persistent symptoms
- HELLP/partial HELLP syndrome
- Fetal weight less than fifth percentile + oligohydramnios or umbilical artery REDF
- Labor/rupture of membrane $33^{0/7}$–$33^{5/7}$ wk

Yes → Deliver after 48 hr

No → 24–32 wk expectant management Deliver at $34^{0/7}$ wk

FIG. 1 Management plan for patients with preeclampsia with severe features before 34 wks' gestation. *HELLP,* Hemolysis, elevated liver enzymes, and low platelets; *REDF,* reversed end-diastolic flow. (From Gabbe SG et al: *Obstetrics: normal and problem pregnancies,* ed 7, Philadelphia, 2017, Elsevier.)

women who are at high risk for preeclampsia.[15,16]
- The development of preeclampsia may be one of the earliest identifiable risk markers for potential future cardiovascular disease in women. Women with a history of preeclampsia are at increased risk for cardiovascular disease, and appropriate follow-up should be encouraged.

REFERENCES
Available at eBooks.Health.Elsevier.com.

RELATED CONTENT
Preeclampsia (Patient Information)
Eclampsia (Related Key Topic)
Hypertension (Related Key Topic)

AUTHORS: **BETHANY K. SEDERDAHL, MD, MPH,** and **PHILIP A. SHLOSSMAN, MD**

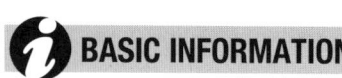
BASIC INFORMATION

DEFINITION

Premenstrual syndrome (PMS) consists of various somatic and physical complaints that develop during the luteal phase of the menstrual cycle and that are of sufficient severity to interfere with daily functioning and/or interpersonal relationships. The symptoms resolve shortly after the onset of menses.[1]

SYNONYM

PMS

ICD-10CM CODE
N94.3 Premenstrual tension syndrome

EPIDEMIOLOGY & DEMOGRAPHICS

- Premenstrual disorders affect about 12% of reproductive-age women, although as many as 80% of women will report at least one somatic or affective symptom during their luteal phase (Table 1).[2]
- Severe cases of premenstrual dysphoric disorder (PMDD), which is more of a psychiatric diagnosis, occur in approximately 3% to 8% of women in the U.S.[3]
- The prevalence of PMS is not associated with age, race, or socioeconomic status.
- Those seeking treatment for PMS are usually in their 30s or 40s.
- Based on some identical twinning studies, a genetic component is thought to exist, but no genes have been identified.[4]
- The natural history of PMS has not been clearly elucidated.

PHYSICAL FINDINGS & CLINICAL PRESENTATION

- Diverse and potentially disabling symptoms. Table 1 summarizes common symptoms of PMS[2]
- Associated with multiple psychologic, physical, and behavioral symptoms
- Most frequent reason for seeking treatment: Emotional symptoms
- Most common emotional symptoms: Depression, irritability, anxiety, labile moods, anger, crying easily, sadness, extreme sensitivity, nervous tension
- Most common physical symptoms: Headache, bloating, cramps, breast tenderness, migraines, fatigue, weight gain, aches and pains, palpitations
- Most common behavior symptom: Food cravings
- Other behavioral symptoms: Increased appetite, increased alcohol intake, decreased motivation, decreased efficiency, avoidance of activities, staying home, sleep changes, libido changes, forgetfulness, decreased concentration

ETIOLOGY

- Etiology is poorly understood and complex. It involves ovarian hormones, central neurotransmitters, and neurosteroids including Serotonin and GABS-A pathways and inflammatory pathways resulting in neuroinflammation.[1,3,5]
- Because of the multifactorial, multiorgan nature of PMS, a single etiologic cause is unlikely.

DIAGNOSIS

DIFFERENTIAL DIAGNOSIS

- A diagnosis of exclusion, so other medical or psychologic disorders should be ruled out (Box 1)
- Common disorders to rule out: Depression or anxiety, anemia, migraines, endometriosis, thyroid disease

WORKUP

- History
- Physical examination
- Laboratory studies to rule out alternative diagnosis
- If no alternative diagnosis, confirm by either history of regular menses, basal body temperature charting, or elevated luteal progesterone that patient is ovulatory
  1. If she is not ovulating, it is not PMS.
  2. A prospective questionnaire given over two menstrual cycles has been found to be the most accurate way to assess the presence of PMS or PMDD.[1] If symptoms are not occurring only in the luteal phase, it is not PMS, and further investigation is needed.
     a. If symptoms occur in the follicular phase, patient has premenstrual exacerbation of another condition.
     b. If symptoms do not occur in the follicular phase, diagnosis of PMS is confirmed.

LABORATORY TESTS

- None available to specifically confirm the diagnosis of PMS
- Thyroid function tests to rule out thyroid disease

TREATMENT

NONPHARMACOLOGIC THERAPY

- Individualization of the treatment plan to maximize therapeutic response
- Psychosocial intervention:
  1. Education
  2. Stress management
  3. Environmental changes
  4. Adequate rest and sleep
  5. Regular exercise
- Nutritional recommendations:
  1. Regularly eaten, well-balanced meals
  2. Adequate amounts of protein, fiber, and complex carbohydrates; low fat
  3. Avoidance of foods that are high in salt and simple sugars; may promote water retention, weight gain, and physical discomfort
  4. Avoidance of alcohol and illicit drugs; may worsen emotional lability
  5. Calcium supplementation (1000 mg/day for women 19 to 50 yr, 1300 mg/day for girls 14 to 18 yr) to reduce the physical and emotional symptoms[2]
  6. The data are mixed regarding the benefits of vitamin D supplementation in reducing

---

BOX 1 Considerations in the Differential Diagnosis of Premenstrual Dysphoric Disorder

Premenstrual syndrome
Endometriosis
Dysmenorrhea
Physical disorders with premenstrual
  exacerbations
Autoimmune disorders
Diabetes mellitus
Anemia
Hypothyroidism
Psychiatric disorders with luteal phase
  exacerbation
Depression
Anxiety
Dysthymic disorder
Bipolar disorder

From Gershenson DM et al: *Comprehensive Gynecology*, ed 8, Philadelphia, 2022, Elsevier.

TABLE 1 Common Symptoms of Cyclic Premenstrual Syndrome

Somatic Symptoms

Abdominal bloating	Constipation or diarrhea
Acne	Headache
Alcohol intolerance	Peripheral edema
Breast engorgement and tenderness	Weight gain
Clumsiness	

Emotional and Mental Symptoms

Anxiety	Insomnia
Change in libido	Irritability
Depression	Lethargy
Fatigue	Mood swings
Food cravings (especially salt and sugar)	Panic attacks
Hostility	Paranoia
Inability to concentrate	Violence toward self and others
Increased appetite	Withdrawal from others

From Goldman L, Schafer AI: *Goldman's Cecil medicine*, ed 24, Philadelphia, 2012, Saunders.

TABLE 2 SSRIs for Premenstrual Dysphoric Disorder

SSRI	Effective Doses
Fluoxetine hydrochloride*	20 mg/day
Sertraline hydrochloride	50-150 mg/day
Paroxetine hydrochloride*	20-30 mg/day
Paroxetine controlled release (CR)	25 mg/day
Citalopram	20-30 mg/day
Escitalopram	10-20 mg/day
SNRI	
Venlafaxine	37.5-112.5 mg/day

PMDD, Premenstrual dysphoric disorder; SNRI, selective norepinephrine reuptake inhibitor; SSRI, selective serotonin reuptake inhibitor.
*Only fluoxetine and paroxetine are approved for PMDD.
From Gershenson DM et al: *Comprehensive Gynecology,* ed 8, Philadelphia, 2022, Elsevier.

PMS symptoms, so more studies are needed
7. Pyridoxine (vitamin B_6) 80 mg qd to improve depression, fatigue, and irritability has been suggested in small studies

ACUTE GENERAL Rx

Suppression of ovulation:
- Oral contraceptives: One pill per day; continuous use of a combinaton pill with drospirenone is associated with better treatment effect[3]
- Progestin-only oral contraceptive: One pill per day
- Oral micronized progesterone: 100 mg every morning and 200 mg every evening on days 17 through 28 of menstrual cycle
- Progestin suppository: 200 to 400 mg bid on days 17 through 28 of menstrual cycle
- Medroxyprogesterone: 150 mg IM q3mo
- Levonorgestrel implants: Surgical insertion every 5 yr
- Transdermal estradiol: One or two 100-μg patches every 3 days
- Danazol: 100 to 200 mg/day (ovulation not suppressed at this dose); has significant side-effect profile and is not commonly utilized
- Gonadotropin-releasing hormone (GnRH) agonists: Daily by intranasal spray or monthly by depot injection; profound hypoestrogenism, concerns for osteoporosis and vasomotor symptoms

Suppression of physical symptoms:
- Spironolactone: 25 to 50 mg bid on days 14 through 28 of menstrual cycle—need a reliable form of birth control
- Mefenamic acid
  1. For fluid retention: 250 mg tid on days 24 through 28 of cycle
  2. For pain: 500 mg tid on days 19 through 28 of cycle
- Bromocriptine: 5 mg/day on days 10 through 26 of cycle
- Naproxen: 550 mg bid on days 17 through 28 of cycle, Naprosyn-500 mg bid on days 17 through 28 of cycle

Suppression of psychologic symptoms (Table 2):
- SSRI, or serotonergic antidepressants, are first-line treatment for PMS/PMDD, treating mostly the psychologic aspects but also some physical aspects[2,4,5]
- Sertraline, paroxetine, fluoxetine, citalopram, escitalopram are most commonly used[4,5]
- In 2013 the *Cochrane Reviews* reported a statistically significant benefit over placebo when taken either continuously or in the luteal phase[4]
- Serotonin-norepinephrine reuptake inhibitors (SNRI) such as venlafaxine; use is off-label, but onset of action is quick and has been found to be helpful[2]
- Seroquel: Smaller studies[2]
- Wellbutrin: Not as effective as the other options
- Ulipristal Acetate is a second-generation Selective Progesterone Receptor Modulator (SPRM) that shows promise at low doses (5 mg/day) in ameliorating symptoms of PMDD[6]
- Off-label use of Dutasteride to increase local allopregnanolone levels and ameliorate physical and psychologic symptoms of PMDD[3]

CHRONIC Rx

- Therapy is largely trial and error, with the goal of providing effective treatment with the safest therapy. Provider should initially attempt to ameliorate the most pronounced symptom(s).
- Limited evidence exists that acupuncture and/ or acupressure may ameliorate some symptoms associated with PMS and improve quality of life.[1,6] More studies are needed to determine if this option is as good as or better than conventional therapies such as treatment with an SSRI.
- Newer pharmacologic therapies that target neurotransmitter systems in the brain through the action of allopregnanolone on the GABA receptor show promise.[3,7]
- For severe intractable PMS bilateral oophorectomy has been considered but should be last resort after a trial of GnRH agonists have been shown to resolve symptoms.[1] This course of action should be exceedingly rare.

DISPOSITION

Improved symptoms in 90% of women over time

REFERENCES

Available at eBooks.Health.Elsevier.com.

RELATED CONTENT

Premenstrual Syndrome (Patient Information)
Dysmenorrhea (Related Key Topic)
Premenstrual Dysphoric Disorder (Related Key Topic)

AUTHOR: **ADRIENNE B. NEITHARDT, MD**

Diseases and Disorders

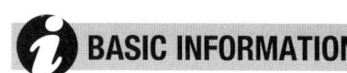
BASIC INFORMATION

DEFINITION

Preterm labor is defined as regular contractions that result in cervical dilation or effacement prior to 37 wk gestation. Preterm birth is one that occurs after 20 wk gestation and before the completion of 37 wk gestational age.

SYNONYM

Premature labor

ICD-10CM CODES

060.0 Preterm labor without delivery
060.1 Preterm spontaneous labor with preterm delivery
060.2 Preterm spontaneous labor with term delivery

EPIDEMIOLOGY & DEMOGRAPHICS

INCIDENCE: The incidence of preterm births in the U.S. increased from 9.5% in 1981 to 12.7% in 2006 before falling gradually to 11.4% by 2013, then to 10% in 2019. The increase since 1981 is attributed to improvements in pregnancy dating by ultrasound, increased use of assisted reproductive technology, and increased preterm induction or preterm operative delivery for maternal or fetal indications. Between 40% and 45% of these births follow spontaneous preterm labor; either the remaining preterm births result from preterm premature rupture of membranes (PPROM), or they occur secondary to intentional delivery for maternal or fetal indications.

PREDOMINANT AGE & RACIAL DIFFERENCES: Pregnant women at the extremes of reproductive age (<17 yr and >35 yr) are at greatest risk. Black race is one of the most significant risk factors with the rate of preterm birth averaging 13.9% between 2016 and 2018 compared to 8.7% among Asian Americans and 9.6% in white women. The disparity between African-American and other ethnic American races persists after adjusting for income, education, and other medical risk factors.

RISK FACTORS: Risk factors for premature labor include a prior preterm delivery, intrauterine infection, systemic or genital tract infections, periodontal disease, short interpregnancy interval (<6 mo), short cervical length (<25 to 30 mm), low prepregnancy body mass index (BMI) (<19.8 kg/m^2), age (<17 yr or >35 yr), a history of elective pregnancy termination, history of prior stillbirth, African-American race, vaginal bleeding, polyhydramnios or oligohydramnios, multiple gestation, structural abnormalities of the uterus, history of cervical cone biopsy or loop electrocautery excision, in vitro fertilization or ovulation induction, tobacco use, heavy alcohol consumption, cocaine use, heroin use, and psychologic or social stress. The strongest historic risk factor for preterm birth is a previous birth between 16 and 36 wk gestation.

GENETICS: A genetic component has been suggested. Women with sisters who have had preterm births and women with grandparents who were born preterm may be at increased risk for having preterm deliveries themselves. Single-nucleotide polymorphisms have also been associated with preterm labor.

PHYSICAL FINDINGS & CLINICAL PRESENTATION

Presenting symptoms include increased pelvic pressure, abdominal cramping or contractions, increased vaginal discharge, vaginal bleeding or spotting, or leakage of fluid.

ETIOLOGY

Causes of premature labor are varied and often difficult to determine. Premature labor may be secondary to infection, systemic illness, trauma, anatomic abnormalities (i.e., uterine anomaly), or a combination of factors. It is thought that cervical ripening is the most common first step to premature labor or delivery. Subsequently, decidual-membrane activation occurs followed by contractions (Box 1).

DIAGNOSIS

DIFFERENTIAL DIAGNOSIS

The differential diagnosis for preterm labor should include preterm rupture of membranes, preterm contractions (contractions before 37 wk gestation that do not result in cervical change), and abdominal pain or cramping secondary to other medical conditions. There are many medical conditions that may cause preterm contractions or premature labor. Treating some of these underlying conditions may improve the prognosis for stopping the preterm labor.
Possible medical conditions include:
- Infection
  1. Chorioamnionitis
  2. Genital tract infections, including bacterial vaginosis, gonorrhea, chlamydia
  3. Urinary tract infections, including pyelonephritis, cystitis, or asymptomatic bacteriuria
  4. Gastroenteritis
- Trauma
- Placental abruption
- Illicit drug use
- Preterm premature rupture of membranes
- Appendicitis
- Nephrolithiasis
- Pancreatitis
- Cholelithiasis
- Uterine fibroids

WORKUP

- History and physical exam to rule out trauma, abuse, other causes of abdominal pain, and infection
- Fetal heart rate monitoring and tocometry to determine fetal status and contraction frequency
- Speculum exam to visually assess the cervix and assess for rupture of membranes, bleeding, infection, or advanced cervical dilation
  1. If the patient is <35 wk gestation, a Fetal Fibronectin (FFN) test should be collected prior to performing a digital exam or transvaginal ultrasound. A FFN test can help predict preterm labor.
- Digital exam in the unruptured patient with normal placentation to determine cervical dilation and effacement, and fetal station

LABORATORY TESTS

- CBC
- Urine analysis and culture
- Urine toxicology screen
- Collect tests for GBS, gonorrhea, and *Chlamydia*
- Perform a wet prep for yeast, bacterial vaginosis, and *Trichomonas*

BOX 1 Factors Linked to Preterm Labor

Demographic and Psychosocial
- Extremes of age (>40 yr, teenagers)
- Lower socioeconomic status
- Tobacco use
- Cocaine abuse
- Prolonged standing (occupation)
- Psychosocial stressors

Reproductive and Gynecologic
- Prior preterm delivery
- Diethylstilbestrol exposure
- Multiple gestations
- Anatomic endometrial cavity anomalies
- Cervical incompetence
- Low pregnancy weight gain
- First-trimester vaginal bleeding
- Placental abruption or previa

Surgical
- Prior reproductive organ surgery
- Prior paraendometrial surgery other than genitourinary (appendectomy)

Infectious
- Urinary tract infections
- Nonuterine infections
- Genital tract infections (bacterial vaginosis)

From Marx JA et al: *Rosen's emergency medicine: concepts and clinical practice,* ed 7, Philadelphia, 2010, Elsevier.

- Fetal fibronectin swab as described earlier
- Consider PT, PTT, INR, CMP, amylase, and lipase
- Amniocentesis may be performed if an intra-amniotic infection is suspected

IMAGING STUDIES

- A formal ultrasound is indicated to determine estimated fetal weight, fetal presentation, amniotic fluid volume, placental location and appearance, and cervical length.

The diagnosis of preterm labor is confirmed in the presence of regular contractions with subsequent cervical change. Suspicion for preterm labor may be heightened if FFN is positive.

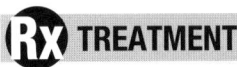 TREATMENT

Patients with premature labor should be delivered promptly when an intraamniotic infection is suspected or when they have advanced cervical dilation >5 cm, a persistently nonreassuring fetal heart rate tracing, or significant vaginal bleeding concerning for placental abruption having maternal or neonatal implications.

NONPHARMACOLOGIC THERAPY

- Bedrest, activity restriction, and pelvic rest are often recommended by clinicians, but there are insufficient data to support this practice, and it is currently not recommended.

ACUTE GENERAL Rx

- Antenatal administration of corticosteroids between 24 wk and 33 6/7 wk gestation is recommended for women at risk of preterm delivery to prevent neonatal respiratory distress syndrome and decrease the incidence of intraventricular hemorrhage and necrotizing enterocolitis. It is also recommended between 34.0 and 36.6 wk gestation if there is no prior steroid exposure.
- Numerous tocolytic agents have been used in an attempt to inhibit contractions (Box 2).

BOX 2   Commonly Used Tocolytic Agents

Magnesium sulfate
- 4-6 g IV bolus over 30 min
- 2-4 g/h IV infusion

Terbutaline
- 5-10 mg PO q4-6h
- 0.25-0.5 mg SC q30 min to 6 h
- 10-80 μg/min IV

Ritodrine*
- 10 mg PO q2-4 h
- 5-10 mg IM q2-4 h
- 50-350 μg/min IV

Isoxsuprine
- 20 mg PO q4-6 h
- 0.05-0.5 mg/min IV

*Ritodrine is currently discontinued in the U.S.
From Marx JA et al: *Rosen's emergency medicine: concepts and clinical practice,* ed 7, Philadelphia, 2010, Elsevier.

Although efficacy is unclear, they can be utilized during an observation period in an effort to prolong gestation for administration and exposure of steroids or to transfer the mother to a facility capable of caring for preterm infants. This, of course, assumes there are no maternal or fetal medical contraindications to use of tocolytic drugs and no indications for rapid delivery. The most commonly used tocolytics are beta-mimetics (terbutaline), intravenous magnesium sulfate, calcium channel blockers (nifedipine), or prostaglandin synthetase inhibitors (indomethacin, ketorolac, sulindac). Table E1 summarizes side effect profiles of tocolytic agents.
- Routine antibiotic use has failed to show benefit in the absence of a known infection. But all mothers in preterm labor (without a documented negative group B strep culture) should be given antibiotics to prevent neonatal GBS infection.

- Intravenous magnesium sulfate has been shown to decrease cerebral palsy in children exposed antenatally with premature labor or premature rupture of the membranes at less than 32 wk gestation.

PROPHYLACTIC OR CHRONIC Rx

- Patients with a history of prior spontaneous preterm birth may be candidates for prophylactic use of 17 alpha-hydroxyprogesterone caproate between 16 wk and 36 wk gestation. These patients may also benefit from transvaginal cervical length screening in pregnancy to monitor for short cervix.
- Patients with a history of preterm birth and short cervix may also be candidates for prophylactic or rescue cerclage.
- Patients with a short cervix may be candidates for vaginal progesterone for prevention and, in some clinical studies, vaginal pessary.
- There is no evidence supporting the use of maintenance tocolytic therapy.

REFERRAL

- Women who present in preterm labor should be referred to an obstetrician and transferred to a facility with a neonatal intensive care unit.
- For women who present for prenatal care with a history of preterm delivery, early referral to an obstetrician is also recommended.

SUGGESTED READINGS

Available at eBooks.Health.Elsevier.com.

RELATED CONTENT

Abruptio Placentae (Related Key Topic)
Breech Birth (Related Key Topic)

AUTHORS: **EMILY E. NUSS, MD,** and **ANTHONY SCISCIONE, DO**

BASIC INFORMATION

DEFINITION

Primary biliary cholangitis (PBC), previously known as primary biliary cirrhosis, is a chronic, variably progressive immune-mediated cholestatic liver disease manifested by fatigue and pruritus. Most often diagnosed in middle-aged women, this condition is characterized by autoimmune destruction of small intralobular bile ducts leading to portal inflammation, hepatic cell necrosis, fibrosis, and, if left untreated, cirrhosis, liver failure, and death.[1]

SYNONYMS

PBC
Primary biliary cirrhosis
Biliary cirrhosis
Nonsuppurative destructive cholangitis
Autoimmune cholangiopathy (AIC)

ICD-10CM CODE
K74.3 Primary biliary cholangitis

EPIDEMIOLOGY & DEMOGRAPHICS

INCIDENCE:
- Most recent annual incidence rate in European countries is 1.87 new cases per 100,000 patients.[1]
- Most recent annual incidence rate in the Asia-Pacific region is 0.86 new cases per 100,000 patients.[2]
- Most recent annual incidence rate in North America is 2.75 new cases per 100,000 patients.[3]
- Pooled global annual incidence is estimated at 1.76 new cases per 100,000 patients.[3]

PREVALENCE: Prevalence is greatest in North America and Northern Europe and varies tremendously by time and geographic areas, but most recent data show an incidence of 22.27 cases per 100,000 patients in European countries, 11.88 cases per 100,000 patients in the Asia-Pacific region, and 21.81 per 100,000 patients in North America.[1,3] Pooled global prevalence is estimated at 14.60 per 100,000 patients. Disease incidence and prevalence appear to be increasing worldwide, particularly in North America.[3,4]

PREDOMINANT SEX: While a female:male ratio of 9:1 is often described, recent studies suggests that PBC may be more common in men than previously understood with a female:male ratio of 4 or 5:1.[5,6] Men with PBC typically present with more advance disease at the time of diagnosis, and those with well-compensated cirrhosis have been reported to have a higher risk of death and liver-related death or transplantation.[6]

PREDOMINANT AGE: Onset typically occurs between the ages of 30 and 65 yr and is uncommon before age 25 yr.

PREDOMINANT RACE: Most often described in Caucasians, but PBC affects all races.

GENETICS:
- Pathogenesis is unknown, but it is thought to be in the setting of environmental influences and genetic predisposition.[7]

- There are no clearly identified genetic factors associated with PBC; however, there is a clear familial occurrence.
- Up to 73% of patients with PBC have at least one other extrahepatic autoimmune disorder such as thyroiditis, Sjögren syndrome, rheumatoid arthritis, cutaneous scleroderma (including CREST syndrome), systemic lupus erythematosus, pernicious anemia, celiac disease, inflammatory bowel disease, autoimmune thrombocytopenia purpura, autoimmune diabetes mellitus, and/or other autoimmune diseases.[8]
- A variant form of PBC exists as an overlap syndrome with autoimmune hepatitis (AIH).
- PBC is closely associated with a greater risk of hepatocellular carcinoma as well as an overall greater risk of cancer.

PHYSICAL FINDINGS & CLINICAL PRESENTATION

Clinical stages:
- Asymptomatic
- Symptomatic
- Cirrhotic
- Hepatic failure

Symptoms:
- 50% to 65% of patients may be asymptomatic at time of diagnosis; between 35% and 89% become symptomatic within 4.5 to 17.8 yr.[9]
- Fatigue (50% to 78% of patients) and pruritus (20% to 70% of patients) are the usual presenting symptoms and are independent of disease severity.[9]
- Fatigue can be chronic and correlate with daytime somnolence and autonomic dysfunction.
- Pruritus is present predominantly on the palm and soles, is worse at night and with constricting garments, and is worse with dry skin and humid weather. The cause is unknown but elevated histamine, bile salt concentration, endogenous opioids, lysophosphatidic acid, and female steroid hormones and their metabolites have been discussed as potential causes. Pruritus may first occur during pregnancy but is distinguished from pruritus of pregnancy because it persists into the postpartum period and beyond.
- Symptoms include jaundice, unexplained right upper quadrant pain, manifestations of portal hypertension, dyslipidemia, xanthomas, and osteoporosis, and may be associated with Sjögren syndrome, rheumatoid arthritis, systemic lupus erythematosus, celiac disease, and thyroid disorders (with the most common being Hashimoto thyroiditis).
- Other symptoms can include steatorrhea, osteopenia, fat-soluble vitamin deficiencies, and anemia.

Physical examination:
- Variable: Findings depend on stage of disease at time of presentation; patients at the early stage may be completely unaffected.
- Excoriations may be present due to extensive scratching from pruritus and can be severe enough to cause bleeding.
- Hepatomegaly and splenomegaly can worsen with disease progression.

- Xanthomas and jaundice generally appear in advanced disease. Kayser-Fleischer rings are rare and result from copper retention. Hyperpigmentation of the skin due to melanin deposition may also occur.
- Late physical findings mirror those of cirrhosis: Spider nevi, caput medusae, temporal and proximal limb wasting, ascites, palmar erythema, digital clubbing, gynecomastia, and edema.

ETIOLOGY

- Although the cause of PBC remains unknown, it is believed to require both a genetic susceptibility as well as an environmental trigger ultimately leading to the modification of mitochondrial proteins triggering a persistent T lymphocyte–mediated attack on intrahepatic biliary epithelial cells.
- PBC is associated most strongly with HLA alleles DRA, DRB1, DPB1, DQB1, BTNL2, and c6orf10. PBC is also associated with ORMDL3, CD80, STAT1/STAT4, IL12A, NF-κB, and RPL3/SYNGR1. However, there is variation across ethnic groups.
- Possible environmental triggers include infectious agents, cigarette smoking, environmental pollutants, radiation, urinary tract infections, reproductive hormone replacement, prior pregnancy, toxic waste sites (particularly exposure to halogenated hydrocarbons), electrophilic drugs, and xenobiotics found in food additives and cosmetics.
- The enzyme complex subunit PDC-E2 is an autoantigen that plays a major role in the early pathogenesis of PBC. Patients with PBC have a tenfold increased concentration of PDC-E2-specific cytotoxic CD8$^+$ lymphocytes in their livers compared to their blood, and antimitochondrial antibodies (AMAs), which are the serologic hallmark of this disease, react to the PDC-E2 subunit leading to a strong inflammatory response. In addition, biliary epithelial cells handle PDC-E2 in a unique way that exposes them to immune-mediated attack. Future therapies may be specific immunomodulation directed at these peptides.
- Damage to bile ducts results in bile leaking into liver parenchyma resulting in hepatocyte necrosis, which can lead to fibrosis and eventual cirrhosis.

DIAGNOSIS

The diagnosis of PBC can be established when two of the following three criteria are met in the absence of extrahepatic biliary obstruction.
- Positive serum AMA (titer >1:40) or PBC-specific antibodies to sp100 or gp210 in AMA-negative patients[9]
- Biochemical evidence of cholestasis (mainly alkaline phosphatase elevation [ALP] ≥1.5 times the upper limit of normal [ULN])
- Characteristic liver histology demonstrating nonsuppurative destruction of small to medium-sized interlobular biliary ducts
- Recent guidelines suggest that the above criteria may lead to a delay in diagnosis, so

clinical judgment and expert referral should be considered[4]

DIFFERENTIAL DIAGNOSIS

- Drug-induced cholestasis (common medications: Phenothiazines, anabolic steroids, some antibiotics as TMP-SMX, oxacillin, and ampicillin)
- PBC-AIH overlap syndrome; reported in 1% to 14.2% of patients initially diagnosed with PBC. Transition from stable PBC to AIH and vice versa also seen
- Other etiologies of chronic liver disease and cirrhosis, such as alcoholic cirrhosis, chronic viral hepatitis, primary sclerosing cholangitis, AIH, sarcoidosis, hepatic amyloidosis, chemical/toxin-induced cirrhosis, other hereditary or familial disorders (e.g., cystic fibrosis, α-1-antitrypsin deficiency)
- Biliary obstruction
- Secondary biliary cirrhosis or secondary sclerosing cholangitis

WORKUP

History, physical examination, laboratory evaluation, liver biopsy

LABORATORY TESTS

- AMAs are found in 90% to 95% of patients with PBC and are 98% specific, although ANA-negative PBC is possible.[9] ANA is also found in about 30% to 50% of patients.[10] Most patients have ANA or AMAs, or both.
- Cholestatic pattern of liver biochemical markers; markedly increased ALP (of hepatic origin). ALP levels below 1.5 times ULN are associated with more favorable prognosis.
- γ-Glutamyl transpeptidase is increased and may be indicative of biliary origin of ALP elevation.
- Serum IgM levels are increased (lower in AMA-negative PBC).
- Bilirubin level is normal early on and increases with disease progression (direct and indirect). Increased serum bilirubin level is generally regarded as a poor prognostic indicator.
- Rising serum hyaluronate levels correlate with the serum bilirubin and histologic worsening of the disease.
- Aminotransferase level may be normal and, if increased, is rarely more than $5\times$ ULN.
- Bile acid levels are strikingly elevated and this accumulation is thought to cause foamy degeneration of hepatocytes due to toxic effects.
- Serum ceruloplasmin may also be elevated.
- Markedly increased serum lipids is largely due to increased lipoprotein X (LpX). Total cholesterol may surpass 1000 mg/dl (with increased xanthomas rather than xanthelasmas). In the early stages of PBC, patients can have relatively higher HDL in comparison to LDL and VLDL. This rise in HDL might explain the lack of increased risk for cardiovascular disease. However, cardiovascular risk may still exist due to other risk factors (e.g., family history and metabolic syndrome).
- Percutaneous liver biopsy is helpful to rule out or confirm PBC in patients with superimposed

NASH or AIH overlap syndrome, but is not always necessary for diagnosis.[11] Biopsy is also helpful for disease staging.

- Histology is not uniform, so histologic stage is based on the most advanced lesion present.
  1. Stage I: Nonsuppurative cholangitis indicated by lymphocytic infiltration of small bile ducts with or without epithelioid granulomas or plasma cells, limited to portal areas
  2. Stage II: Extension of inflammatory cells to periportal parenchyma, ductular proliferation
  3. Stage III: Bridging necrosis or fibrous septa linking portal triads
  4. Stage IV: Frank cirrhosis with regenerative nodules

IMAGING STUDIES

If history, physical examination, blood tests, and liver biopsy are all consistent with PBC, neither imaging nor cholangiography (Fig. E1) is necessary. MRI or transient elastography (TE) is important for determination of degree of cirrhosis if present and may be indicated for monitoring of disease progression. Notably, the cutoffs for transient elastography are different than those established for other diseases, such as hepatitis C.

PROGNOSIS

- There is widespread variation in progression between phases of PBC. Some patients advance rapidly to cirrhosis and require transplant whereas others remain asymptomatic for decades.
- Median time to development of extensive fibrosis in untreated patients is 2 yr.[9]
- Median survival is 7.5 yr in untreated patients and 16 yr in asymptomatic patients; however, this has improved with earlier diagnosis and initiation of treatment.[9] Table 1 summarizes time course of histologic progression to a higher stage in patients with PBC.
- Neither presence nor total titer level of AMAs predicts survival, disease progression, or response to therapy. As such, AMA should not be serially measured.
- Serum bilirubin is the best predictor of survival and the most heavily weighted factor in prognostic models. Box 1 summarizes independent predictors of survival in patients with PBC.[1]

TABLE 1 Time Course of Histologic Progression to a Higher Stage in Patients With PBC

Histologic Progression*	INITIAL HISTOLOGIC STAGE		
	1	2	3
1 yr	41	43	35
2 yr	62	62	50

*Percent of patients in whom the histologic stage increases at 1 yr and 2 yr.

From Feldman M et al: *Sleisenger and Fordtran's gastrointestinal and liver disease*, ed 10, Philadelphia, 2016, Elsevier.

- Serum ALP >1.5 ULN has been shown to be a risk factor for a more progressive course of PBC including cirrhosis.[12]
- Response to ursodeoxycholic acid (UDCA) therapy can be prognostic, with approximately 40% of patients failing to respond. There are multiple biochemical response criteria that, if met after 1 yr of treatment with UDCA, are associated with improved clinical outcomes. Three of these criteria are Barcelona (decrease in ALP level of at least 40% or to the reference range), Paris I (ALP $<3 \times$ ULN, AST $<2 \times$ ULN and bilirubin within normal limits), and Paris II (ALP $<1.5 \times$ ULN, ALT $<1.5 \times$ ULN and bilirubin within normal limits).[13-15]
- Nonresponse to UDCA is also associated with increased HCC risk compared to UDCA-responsive PBC.
- Similarly, the Mayo Risk score, a predictor of short-term survival probability in non-transplanted patients (www.mayoclinic.org/medical-professionals/transplant-medicine/the-updated-natural-histo/the-updated-natural-history-model-for-primary-biliary-cirrhosis/itt-20434724), can also reliably predict life expectancy when calculated after 6 mo of UDCA therapy.[16]
- Several predictive models based upon laboratory and clinical data have been proposed, and two such models (GLOBE score and UK-PBC score) are based on multicenter studies including large cohorts of patients with PBC.
  1. GLOBE score: Includes the following five variables: Serum bilirubin, albumin, serum ALP, platelet count after 1 yr of UDCA treatment, and age at start of therapy. It estimates the duration of transplant-free survival.[17]
  2. UK-PBC score: Includes serum ALP, aminotransferases, and bilirubin after 12 mo of UDCA therapy, in addition to baseline

BOX 1 Independent Predictors of Survival in Patients With PBC in Various Clinical Studies

Clinical
Age
Ascites
Edema
Hepatomegaly
Variceal bleeding

Laboratory
Serum albumin level
Serum alkaline phosphatase level
Serum bilirubin level
Prothrombin time

Liver Histology
Cholestasis
Cirrhosis
Fibrosis
Mallory hyaline

From Feldman M et al: *Sleisenger and Fordtran's gastrointestinal and liver disease*, ed 10, Philadelphia, 2016, Elsevier.

albumin and platelet count. This model estimates the risk of liver transplantation or liver-related death.[18]

- Transient elastography is a valuable noninvasive means of determining prognosis and treatment response. It has been reported to be significantly superior to biochemical markers and risk scores (APRI, FIB-4, Mayo risk score) in predicting fibrosis and cirrhosis in PBC. In a prospective study of PBC patients treated with UDCA, noncirrhotic PBC patients (F0 to F3 stages) were found to have either limited or no significant progression of liver stiffness whereas cirrhotic PBC patients developed significant increases in liver stiffness. Increasing liver stiffness (>2.1 kPa/yr) has been associated with an 8.4-fold increased risk of decompensation, liver transplantation, or death.[19]
- Poorer prognosis is associated with jaundice, advanced histologic stage, elevated bilirubin or ALP, low albumin, hepatocellular carcinoma, nonresponse to UDCA, and esophageal varices.

🆁🆇 TREATMENT

- Treatment is guided by the clinical stage of the disease.
- Asymptomatic stage:
  1. Follow liver function tests every 3 mo.
  2. Once ALP is elevated up to 1.5 × ULN, begin UDCA at 13 to 15 mg/kg/day in two to four divided doses regardless of histologic stage.
     a. Side effects may include headaches, dizziness, diarrhea or constipation, dyspepsia, nausea, weight gain, back pain, and upper respiratory infections.
     b. Watch for interactions with fibric acid derivatives, bile acid sequestrants, estrogen derivatives, and aluminum hydroxide, which may interfere with the therapeutic effect or serum concentration of UDCA.
     c. Efficacy is best if started during stage I or II disease but should be started at any stage of disease. Lifelong therapy is currently recommended.
- Treatment also includes treatment of associated conditions such as fatigue, pruritus, osteoporosis, hypercholesterolemia, malabsorption, fat-soluble vitamin deficiencies, anemia, hypothyroidism, and any complications of cirrhosis.

ACUTE GENERAL Rx

- Symptomatic stage: Goals of treatment are resolution of symptoms such as pruritus, treatment of chronic cholestatic complications, and delay of liver failure.
- Obeticholic acid (OCA), a farnesoid X receptor agonist, has been approved as a second-line treatment for PBC and is indicated in patients who are nonresponders to UDCA as evidenced by persistently elevated ALP, lack of

normalization of bilirubin, high risk on predictive models, and/or evidence of fibrosis by any modality.[4]
  1. It is initially dosed at 5 mg once daily and can be increased to 10 mg once daily after 3 mo if there has been an inadequate decrease in bilirubin and/or ALP.
  2. OCA may be given as adjunctive therapy along with UDCA, or as an alternative in patients intolerant of UDCA.
  3. The most common adverse event noted is pruritus, and therefore this drug may not be ideal for patients with that symptom.
  4. OCA has been associated with severe liver injury and close monitoring of liver function is warranted. OCA use is contraindicated in those with advanced cirrhosis with current or prior decompensation and/or portal hypertension. It should be used with caution and with frequent monitoring in those with cirrhosis that is not advanced.[20]

- Prednisone, azathioprine, colchicine, methotrexate, fibrates, penicillamine, cyclosporine, silymarin, and mycophenolate mofetil are no longer used because of limited efficacy and/or significant toxicity.
- For the pruritus, cholestyramine resin (4 to 16 g/day) reduces pruritus in most patients but must be given at least 4 h before UDCA to avoid reducing the efficacy of that drug. Antihistamines at bedtime help nighttime symptoms. Rifampin (150 to 300 mg bid), oral opiate antagonists such as naltrexone (12.5 to 50 mg daily) and sertraline (75 to 100 mg daily) can be used for pruritus refractory to bile acid sequestrants. Table E2 summarizes treatment recommendations for pruritus in PBC. Intractable pruritus can be an indication for liver transplantation.
- Newer agents that are being investigated for pruritus include ileal bile acid transporter inhibitors and fibrates such as bezafibrate.
- Fibrates may be used in those with inadequate response to UDCA, but should be avoided in those with decompensated liver disease.[20]

CHRONIC Rx

- Liver function tests should be checked every 3 to 6 mo.
- Management of chronic liver disease: Immunization against hepatitis A and B, minimizing ETOH consumption, monitoring for HCC via alpha fetoprotein and ultrasound every 6 mo, and monitoring for varices via EGD every 1 to 3 yr in patients with cirrhosis or Mayo risk score >4.1.
- Management of sicca syndrome: Artificial tears can be used initially for dry eyes. Saliva substitutes can be used for xerostomia and dysphagia; pilocarpine or cevimeline can be used for refractory cases. Moisturizers can be given for vaginal dryness.
- Treatment/prevention of osteopenia/osteoporosis: Patients with PBC should be given 1000 to 1200 mg calcium daily in divided doses and 1000 IU of vitamin D daily in the diet and as

supplements if needed. Weight-bearing exercises are also recommended. Bone densitometry should be done at time of diagnosis, after a fragility fracture, in patients with cirrhosis, prior to transplant, or in patients receiving steroids more than 3 mo. It should then be performed every 2 to 4 yr. Alendronate (70 mg weekly) or other bisphosphonates should be considered if patients have osteopenia in the absence of acid reflux or known varices.
- Hyperlipidemia is common in patients with PBC. However, there is no elevated risk of cardiovascular disease. Statins are safe and effective in patients who may need treatment even if liver chemistry is abnormal.
- Vitamin A, K, and E deficiencies can be clinically important in advanced cases and respond to oral replacement.
- Liver transplantation is the only effective treatment for patients with liver failure, and approximately 25% of PBC patients ultimately need a liver transplant. Indications for transplantation include hepatic decompensation (encephalopathy, recurrent variceal bleeding, intractable ascites and spontaneous bacterial peritonitis), hepatocellular carcinoma fulfilling Milan criteria (see "Hepatocellular Carcinoma"), and intractable pruritus. Liver transplant should also be considered with a Mayo risk score >7.8, MELD score >12, and bilirubin ≥6 mg/dl.
- The outcome of liver transplantation for patients with PBC is more favorable than that of nearly all other liver disease categories. The survival rates at 1 yr are now up to 90% to 95%. Although recurrent disease may develop in about one third of patients after liver transplantation, patient and graft survival is usually not affected.

DISPOSITION

Definitive treatment requires liver transplantation. Patients treated with UDCA have been reported to have transplant-free survival of 90%, 78%, and 66% at 5, 10, and 15 yr, respectively. Among untreated patients, transplant-free survival is 79%, 59%, and 32% at 5, 10, and 15 yr, respectively.[21,22]

REFERRAL

Refer to gastroenterology and/or hepatology for treatment, evaluation for liver transplantation, and management of portal hypertension.

REFERENCES
Available at eBooks.Health.Elsevier.com.

RELATED CONTENT
Primary Biliary Cirrhosis (PBC) (Patient Information)

AUTHORS: **AVERILL GUO, MD,** and **JEANETTE G. SMITH, MD**

Diseases and Disorders

I

BASIC INFORMATION

DEFINITION

Primary ovarian insufficiency is a disorder in women younger than 40 yr of age that is characterized by a decline in ovarian function, loss of oocytes and follicologenesis, and evelevated gonadotropin levels.[1]

SYNONYMS

POI
Hypergonadotropic hypogonadism
Premature ovarian failure
Premature menopause
Gonadal dysgenesis
Early menopause

ICD-10CM CODES
E28.3	Primary ovarian failure
E28.310	Symptomatic premature menopause
E28.39	Other primary ovarian failure
E28.9	Ovarian dysfunction, unspecified

EPIDEMIOLOGY & DEMOGRAPHICS

INCIDENCE: Affects 1% of the female population in the U.S. and 3.7% worldwide. There are significant differences in prevalence among ethnic groups: White 1%, Black 1.4%; Hispanic 1.5%, Chinese 0.5%, and Japanese 0.1%.[1]
PREDOMINANT AGE: 1:250 incident cases by age 35 and 1:100 by age 40

PHYSICAL FINDINGS & CLINICAL PRESENTATION

- The most common presentation is disturbance in menstrual pattern due to intermittent ovarian function.
- Between 5% and 30% of affected women have another affected female relative.
- Between 10% and 30% of affected women already have a concurrent autoimmune condition, the most common of which is hypothyroidism.
- Symptoms of estrogen deficiency include hot flashes, night sweats, poor concentration, drying of the vagina, and infertility.
- Physical exam may reveal stigmata of an autoimmune condition such as vitiligo, thyroid enlargement, or Turner syndrome (webbed neck, short stature, and high-arched palate).

ETIOLOGY (SEE TABLE 1)

Idiopathic in 95% of cases

DIAGNOSIS

DIFFERENTIAL DIAGNOSIS

- Pregnancy.

- Causes of secondary amenorrhea include eating disorder, exercise, drugs, sarcoidosis, polycystic ovarian disease, hypothalamic amenorrhea, hyperprolactinemia/prolactinoma, and Cushing disease.

WORKUP

- After pregnancy is ruled out, the initial evaluation should include the measurement of serum prolactin, FSH, and thyrotropin (TSH) levels.
- If the FSH level is in the menopausal range (>40 μIU/ml by radioimmunoassay), the test should be repeated in 1 mo along with a serum estradiol measurement to confirm the diagnosis of primary ovarian insufficiency.

LABORATORY TESTS

- Once a diagnosis of premature ovarian failure is made, other evaluations include:
- Autoimmune disorders, adrenal insufficiency (seen in 3% of cases): Serum antiadrenal and anti-21 hydroxylase antibodies should be measured.
- Hypothyroidism: Serum TSH, T_4, and anti-TPO antibodies.
- All cases should be screened for osteoporosis by DXA for bone mineral density.
- A karyotype analysis should be performed for all patients to look for chromosomal defects including Turner variant or deletions of the X chromosome.
- Permutations for the fragile X syndrome (FMR1 gene) should be checked for as well.

IMAGING STUDIES

Pelvic ultrasound has no proven benefit in the management of these patients.

TREATMENT

NONPHARMACOLOGIC THERAPY

Counseling or patient support group should be offered to all women with low self-esteem and depression due to the psychological scar left by the diagnosis.

ACUTE GENERAL Rx

- Physiologic estrogen and progestin replacement is reasonable in the cases of young women until they reach the age of natural menopause.
- A dose of 100 mcg of estradiol per day, administered by transdermal patch, achieves average estradiol level observed in normal menstruating women and effectively treats symptoms.
- Cyclic medroxyprogesterone at a dose of 10 mg per day for 12 days each month is the

preferred progestin to provide protection against endometrial cancer.
- Pregnancy may occur while a woman is taking estrogen and progesterone therapy, and the therapy should be stopped immediately if the pregnancy test is found to be positive.

CHRONIC Rx

- Intake of 1200 mg of elemental calcium and 800 units of vitamin D_3 per day should be encouraged to prevent bone loss. A serum 25-hydroxyvitamin D level of 30 ng per ml or higher should be maintained.
- Patients with positive tests for adrenal antibodies should be evaluated annually for adrenal insufficiency by corticotropin stimulation test.
- Patients who wish to avoid pregnancy should use a barrier method or an IUD.
- Options for parenthood include adoption, foster parenthood, egg donation, and embryo donation.

DISPOSITION

Women with the known diagnosis should be encouraged to maintain a lifestyle that optimizes bone and cardiovascular health, including regular weight-bearing exercises, adequate intake of calcium (1200 mg daily) and vitamin D (800 IU daily), healthy diet to prevent obesity, and screening for cardiovascular risk factors.

REFERRAL

Referral to gynecologist and reproductive endocrinologist may be helpful in patients who decide to pursue parenthood.

PEARLS & CONSIDERATIONS

COMMENTS

- Common etiologies should be ruled out, including chromosomal abnormalities, fragile X premutations, and autoimmune causes.
- Management directed at symptom resolution and bone protection primarily, but should include psychosocial support for women facing this devastating diagnosis.

PREVENTION

Early diagnosis of primary ovarian insufficiency important for osteoporosis prevention and possibly prevention of coronary artery disease.

PATIENT & FAMILY EDUCATION

- https://medlineplus.gov/primaryovarianinsufficiency.html.
- www.earlymenopause.com/.
- www.nichd.nih.gov/health/topics/poi/resources/patients.

REFERENCE

Available at eBooks.Health.Elsevier.com.

RELATED CONTENT

Amenorrhea (Related Key Topic)

AUTHOR: **FRED F. FERRI, MD**

TABLE 1 Mechanisms and Causes of Primary Ovarian Insufficiency

Accelerated Follicular Depletion
Genetic: Turner syndrome, fragile X permutations, galactosemia
Toxic: Chemotherapy, radiation, infections such as mumps or cytomegalovirus
Autoimmune: Polyglandular failure, hypothyroidism, Addison disease, vitiligo, myasthenia gravis
Abnormal Follicular Stimulation
Gonadotropin receptor function: Follicle stimulating hormone/luteinizing hormone receptor mutation
Enzyme defects: Aromatase deficiency, luteinized follicles

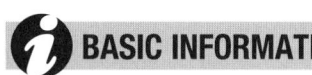

BASIC INFORMATION

DEFINITION
Primary sclerosing cholangitis (PSC) is a chronic, cholestatic, immune-mediated liver disease characterized by progressive inflammation and fibrosis of the intrahepatic and extrahepatic bile ducts. PSC has a strong association with inflammatory bowel disease (IBD) and may be complicated by recurrent cholangitis, colorectal and hepatobiliary malignancies, and cirrhosis.[1]

SYNONYMS
PSC
Chronic obliterative cholangitis
Fibrosing cholangitis
Stenosing cholangitis

ICD-10CM CODES
K83.0   Cholangitis
K83.9   Disease of biliary tract, unspecified

EPIDEMIOLOGY & DEMOGRAPHICS
- The incidence and prevalence of PSC are 1 case/100,000 persons per yr and 6 to 16 cases/100,000 persons, respectively.[2]
- About 60% of patients with PSC are men.
- PSC can present at any age. The median age of diagnosis is 41 yr.[3]
- Over 70% of patients with PSC also have IBD, most commonly with an ulcerative colitis (UC) phenotype. Approximately 5% to 10% of patients with IBD will develop PSC. PSC-IBD may represent a phenotypic entity on its own and typically presents with pancolitis, "backwash" ileitis, and rectal sparing.
- PSC is an independent risk factor for developing colorectal cancer in patients with IBD. PSC-IBD is associated with a fourfold increased risk of colorectal cancer compared to IBD alone.[4]
- Patients with PSC are at increased risk of hepatobiliary cancers, most commonly cholangiocarcinoma (CCA). CCA is present in 1% to 2% of PSC patients at diagnosis. PSC should be considered a premalignant disease with a lifetime risk of developing CCA between 5% and 10%.[5]
- PSC can coexist with other autoimmune liver diseases. PSC–autoimmune hepatitis (AIH) overlap syndrome is more common in young adults and children.[6]
- Box 1 summarizes a classification of diseases associated with sclerosing cholangitis.
- The median survival from time of diagnosis is 10 to 15 yr without liver transplantation.[7]

PHYSICAL FINDINGS & CLINICAL PRESENTATION
- Up to 50% of patients are asymptomatic at the time of diagnosis, with normal physical examination findings. Abnormal liver tests and a known diagnosis of IBD are often the only signs at diagnosis.
- The most common symptoms on presentation include right upper quadrant abdominal pain, pruritus, and fatigue. Additional symptoms include abdominal distention, confusion, jaundice, recurrent cholangitis, or other symptoms related to portal hypertension. On physical exam, patients may have jaundice, skin excoriation and hyperpigmentation from scratching, hepatosplenomegaly, and xanthelasmas.

ETIOLOGY
- The cause of PSC is unknown. Like other autoimmune diseases, the most likely mechanism is immunologic priming in a genetically susceptible patient causing phenotypic expression of the disease.[2]
- Genetic and immunologic factors are supported by reports of familial occurrence of this disorder and increased frequency of human leukocyte antigen (HLA) B8 and DR3. Genome-wide association studies have discovered novel loci associated with PSC, but the functional aspects of these genes are still unknown.
- Portosystemic inflammation caused by translocation of the gut microbiota is an increasing area of research. The close association with UC and PSC may be secondary to gut-activated T lymphocytes in IBD causing portal inflammation because of overlapping adhesion molecules in the gut and liver. Furthermore, intestinal dysbiosis in PSC has also been seen and remains an area of ongoing research.
- Dysregulated inflammatory cytokine production by cholangiocytes is also more recently suggested to be playing a role in the pathogenesis of PSC.

DIAGNOSIS

DIFFERENTIAL DIAGNOSIS
- Immunoglobulin G4 (IgG4)-associated cholangitis (IAC)
- Surgical biliary trauma
- Ischemic cholangitis, recurrent pyogenic cholangitis, recurrent pancreatitis
- Choledocholithiasis, cholangiocarcinoma
- Intraarterial chemotherapy (5-FU/floxuridine)
- Diffuse intrahepatic metastasis, sarcoidosis, or amyloidosis
- AIDS-related, eosinophilic, or mast cell cholangiopathy
- Histiocytosis X, graft-versus-host disease
- Hepatic inflammatory pseudotumor, portal hypertensive biliopathy
- Primary biliary cholangitis (Table 1)

WORKUP
Diagnosis is based on characteristic (1) laboratory findings, (2) cholangiographic findings, and (3) the exclusion of secondary cholangitis. Though liver biopsy is now rarely used to diagnose PSC, it may be indicated in patients with normal cholangiograms and a high suspicion of small-duct PSC, or if PSC-AIH overlap is being considered. Table 2 describes the staging of PSC.

LABORATORY TESTS
- A persistent elevated serum alkaline phosphatase is characteristic of PSC.
- Also, patients frequently have elevated serum aminotransferase levels, and this may suggest an overlap syndrome, such as PSC-AIH.
- However, liver enzymes fluctuate as part of the natural history of PSC, and some patients may have normal liver enzymes.
- Serum bilirubin is usually normal at the time of diagnosis unless the patient has advanced stricturing disease or advanced liver disease. Initial elevation of bilirubin at diagnosis may be related to a worse prognosis.[5]
- A wide range of autoantibodies can be detected in patients with PSC, including antineutrophil cytoplasmic antibodies (ANCAs; 26%-96% of PSC patients), antinuclear antibody (ANA; 8%-77% of PSC patients), and anti–smooth muscle antibody (ASMA; 83% of PSC patients).[8] These antibodies are not specific for PSC and do not reflect prognosis.
  1. Antimitochondrial antibody (AMA), which is characteristic of primary biliary cholangitis (PBC), is *NOT* found in PSC and can be helpful in excluding PSC.
  2. Serum IgG levels are useful in the diagnosis of PSC-AIH overlap syndrome (more common in pediatric patients) and IAC with autoimmune pancreatitis.
  3. In particular, elevated levels of IgG4 are found in 10% to 20% of PSC patients, with a subset of these patients displaying features of autoimmune pancreatitis. PSC patients with elevated IgG4 tend to have worse outcomes and seem to respond to corticosteroid therapy; hence, IgG4 levels should be checked at least once in all patients with PSC.

IMAGING STUDIES
- Cholangiography with magnetic resonance cholangiopancreatography (MRCP), endoscopic retrograde cholangiopancreatography (ERCP), and percutaneous transhepatic cholangiography (PTC) are considered to be the gold standard for the diagnosis of PSC. Characteristic findings reveal segmental fibrosis of bile ducts with saccular dilation of normal intervening areas resulting in a "beads-on-a-string" appearance (Fig. 1).
- MRCP has largely supplanted ERCP and PTC as the diagnostic study of choice because it is noninvasive, less expensive.
- In a meta-analysis of six studies, the sensitivity and specificity of MRCP for diagnosing PSC were 86% and 94%, respectively.[9]
- MRCP, however, does not allow sampling of strictures for brush cytology or biopsy, nor does it allow therapeutic interventions if a mechanical reason for obstruction is found such as stone, stricture, or tumor.[4]
- Noninvasive measurements of liver elastography including MR elastography are promising methods for evaluating for cirrhosis but have not yet been validated in this patient cohort.[10]

BOX 1   Classification of and Diseases Associated With Sclerosing Cholangitis

Primary sclerosing cholangitis
Principal disease associations

Inflammatory bowel disease:
  Crohn colitis or ileocolitis
  Ulcerative colitis

Other disease associations

Systemic diseases with fibrosis:
  Inflammatory pseudotumor
  Mediastinal fibrosis
  Peyronie disease
  Pseudotumor of the orbit
  Retroperitoneal fibrosis
  Riedel thyroiditis
Autoimmune or collagen vascular disorders:
  Autoimmune hemolytic anemia
  Celiac disease
  Chronic sclerosing sialadenitis
  Membranous nephropathy
  Progressive systemic sclerosis
  Rapidly progressive glomerulonephritis
  Rheumatoid arthritis
  Sjögren syndrome
  Systemic lupus erythematosus
  Type 1 diabetes mellitus
Alloimmune diseases:
  Hepatic allograft rejection
  Hepatic graft-versus-host disease after bone marrow transplantation
Infiltrative diseases:
  Hypereosinophilic syndrome
  Histiocytosis X
  Sarcoidosis
  Systemic mastocytosis
Immunodeficiency:
  Congenital immunodeficiency
    Combined immunodeficiency

Dysgammaglobulinemia
X-lined agammaglobulinemia
Acquired immunodeficiency:
  AIDS
  Angioimmunoblastic lymphadenopathy
  Opportunistic infections (e.g., cryptosporidiosis, cytomegalovirus, microsporidiosis)
  Selective IgA deficiency

Secondary sclerosing cholangitis
Obstructive

Autoimmune pancreatitis
Biliary parasites
Caroli disease
Choledocholithiasis
Chronic pancreatitis
Congenital abnormalities:
  Cystic fibrosis
  Choledochal cyst
Fungal infection
Recurrent pyogenic cholangitis
Surgical stricture

Toxic

Intraarterial floxuridine (FUDR)
Intraductal formaldehyde or hypertonic saline (echinococcal cyst treatment)

Ischemic

Hepatic allograft arterial occlusion
Paroxysmal nocturnal hemoglobinuria
Toxic vasculitis (FUDR)
Vascular trauma

Neoplastic

Cholangiocarcinoma
Hepatocellular carcinoma
Lymphoma
Metastatic cancer

From Feldman M et al: *Sleisenger and Fordtran's gastrointestinal and liver disease*, ed 10, Philadelphia, 2016, Elsevier.

(Rx) TREATMENT

- No medical therapy has been established to be effective in treating PSC. Management of PSC patients is aimed at symptom relief and management of complications from PSC (i.e., obstruction/strictures, portal hypertension).[3]
- Ursodeoxycholic acid (UDCA) has shown variable benefit in randomized controlled trials. Although biochemical improvement has been seen with UDCA, there has been no proven benefit on survival. The American Association for Liver Diseases (AASLD) currently recommends against the use of UDCA in PSC.
- Bile acid–based therapy options being tested in clinical trials include 24-norursodeoxycholic acid (norUDCA), steroidal and nonsteroidal bile acid receptor/farnesoid X receptor (FXR) agonists (e.g., obeticholic acid, cilofexor), and the FXR-downstream target fibroblast growth factor-19 (FGF19: nontumorigenic recombinant FGF19/NGM-282 [aldafermin]).[11]

- The use of corticosteroids and other immunosuppressive agents is not recommended in patients with PSC alone; however, it is recommended in patients with PSC-AIH overlap syndrome or elevated IgG4.[2] Randomized control trials are ongoing exploring the use of immune modulators and have shown some promise in reducing ALP levels, especially in patients with worse disease.[12]
- Manipulation of the microbiome is an exciting area being explored as a future treatment for PSC. This is being tried with antibiotics (e.g., vancomycin), fecal microbiota transplantation (FMT), and bacteriophage-based therapy.
  1. Oral vancomycin may show clinical and biochemical response in pediatric patients, but no randomized clinical trial has been performed.[3]
  2. Recent studies have shown that FMT in PSC is safe, improves liver biochemistries, and improves microbiome diversity. This is a rapidly expanding area of gastroenterology that shows promise. However, larger studies are needed to determine if such

treatments can affect mortality or reduce liver transplantation.[13]

ACUTE GENERAL Rx

- For mild pruritus, cooling gels (e.g., menthol gels), skin emollients, and antihistamines are recommended as the first-line treatment.[5]
- For moderate or severe pruritus, bezafibrate and rifampicin are now recommended first-line agents.[11] Alternative agents include cholestyramine, naltrexone, sertraline, and phenobarbital.[14]
- Patients who present with increasing serum bilirubin, worsening pruritus, progressive bile duct dilation on imaging studies, or cholangitis should be evaluated for dominant strictures with imaging. A dominant stricture is a stenosis <1.5 mm in the common bile duct or <1 mm in the hepatic duct.[5]
- ERCP with brushings, cytology, and fluorescent in situ hybridization (FISH) is recommended to evaluate dominant strictures for CCA, which is found in 15% to 20% of cases. Once malignancy is excluded, balloon dilation

TABLE 1 Primary Sclerosing Cholangitis (PSC) Versus Primary Biliary Cholangitis (PBC)

Feature	PSC	PBC
Age	Young	Middle-aged and elderly
Sex	Typically men (70%)	Typically women (90%)
Clinical	Pain Cholangitis Hepatosplenomegaly ALP elevated	Pruritus Xanthomas, xanthelasma Hyperpigmentation Hepatosplenomegaly ALP elevated
Liver function tests	Bilirubin fluctuates	
Antimitochondrial antibody	Negative	Positive in 90% (also elevated in chronic hepatitis, connective tissue disease)
pANCA	Positive (up to 80%)	Negative
MRCP	Irregular and beaded ducts	Pruned ducts
Associated diseases	Ulcerative colitis (70%) Crohn disease (rare) Sjögren syndrome (rare) Thyroiditis (rare) Hypothyroidism (rare) Pancreatitis (rare) Retroorbital and retroperitoneal fibrosis (rare)	CREST syndrome Sjögren syndrome Thyroiditis Renal tubular acidosis
Complications	Portal hypertension Liver failure Bile duct carcinoma	Osteomalacia Steatorrhea (due to bile acid deficiency, associated pancreatic insufficiency or coexisting celiac disease) Portal hypertension, liver failure (late)
Treatment	Ursodeoxycholic acid Liver transplant	Liver transplant

ALP, Serum alkaline phosphatase; *CREST,* calcinosis, Raynaud syndrome, esophageal dysmotility, sclerodactyly, and telangiectasia; *MRCP,* magnetic resonance cholangiopancreatography; *pANCA,* perinuclear antineutrophil cytoplasmic antibody.
From Talley NJ et al: *Essentials of internal medicine,* ed 4, Chatswood, NSW, 2021, Elsevier Australia.

TABLE 2 Staging of Primary Sclerosing Cholangitis

Stage	Description
I—Portal	Portal edema, inflammation, ductal proliferation; abnormalities do not extend beyond the limiting plate
II—Periportal	Periportal fibrosis with or without inflammation extending beyond the limiting plate
III—Septal	Septal fibrosis, bridging necrosis, or both
IV—Cirrhotic	Biliary cirrhosis

From Cameron JL, Cameron AM: *Current surgical therapy,* ed 10, Philadelphia, 2011, Saunders.

with or without stenting is recommended to treat symptomatic patients. Routine stenting is not required, but short-term stenting may be helpful in patients with severe stricture. If ERCP is unsuccessful, percutaneous cholangiopancreatography with stenting should be considered.[5]

- The Role Probe–based confocal laser endomicroscopy (pCLE): Can visualize the gut epithelium at ultra-high magnification (1000×) and resolution (<10 microns) and allows targeted biopsy. pCLE enhances standard imaging by offering in vivo histopathology and visualization of vasculature and architecture using fluorescein dye.
- Recent literature has shown that the combination of ERCP and pCLE was more accurate than ERCP and tissue sampling (90% vs. 73%, $P = .001$).[15,16]
- In noncirrhotic patients with dominant strictures refractory to endoscopic or percutaneous management, surgery should be considered, although this may complicate future liver transplantation surgery.[5]
- Antibiotic usage is recommended in patients with dominant strictures/obstructions both acutely and for long-term prophylaxis in patients with recurrent cholangitis.[5]

CHRONIC Rx

- Avoidance of alcohol and vaccination against hepatitis A and B are advised.
- Patients with PSC are at risk for osteoporosis and osteopenia; therefore DEXA scan should be performed at diagnosis and repeated every 2 to 4 yr. The pathophysiology of osteopathy in PSC is not well understood, but has been hypothesized to be related to decreased absorption of fat-soluble vitamins and impairment of osteoblasts by bilirubin.[5]

- With advanced disease, fat-soluble vitamin deficiencies such as A, E, and D should be assessed and replaced as needed.
- Patients with newly diagnosed PSC should undergo colonoscopy with biopsies to exclude concurrent IBD and for surveillance of colorectal cancer. In patients with PSC and IBD, continued surveillance colonoscopy with biopsies, or chromoendoscopy, at 1- to 2-yr intervals is recommended. In patients without IBD, a 3- to 5-yr surveillance interval has been recommended due to an increased risk of colorectal cancer.[5]
- Screening for CCA and gallbladder cancer should be performed at least yearly with ultrasound and/or MRI/MRCP, with or without serum CA 19-9 regardless of disease stage. CCA screening is not indicated in PSC patients <20 yr of age or in those who have small duct PSC. ERCP with brush cytology or cholangioscopy should be performed in patients who have biochemical or symptomatic deterioration or dominant stricture to rule out CCA.[5]
- Annual transabdominal ultrasound is recommended due to the increased risk of gallbladder malignancy, even in patients who are not cirrhotic. The AASLD recommends cholecystectomy for all gallbladder masses/polyps in PSC patients, whereas the American College of Gastroenterology (ACG) recommends cholecystectomy only for lesions >8 mm.[5]
- Patients with PSC and cirrhosis are recommended to have hepatocellular carcinoma (HCC) surveillance with ultrasound, with or without α-fetoprotein, every 6 months and gastroesophageal variceal surveillance at regular intervals.[17]
- In patients with HCC and CCA, resection versus liver transplantation may be indicated depending on the extent of disease.[5]

DISPOSITION

Liver transplantation is the only effective treatment for patients with decompensated cirrhosis, liver failure, intractable pruritus, and recurrent bacterial cholangitis. Survival is excellent, with 90% and 80% survival rates at 1 and 5 yr, respectively. The recurrence of PSC after transplant is reportedly 5% to 20%, with IBD and younger age at transplant being important risk factors.[2] Transplant referral is warranted in patients with MELD score ≥15, refractory cholangitis, and early-stage HCC/CCA.[4]

REFERRAL

All patients with suspected PSC should be referred to a gastroenterologist or hepatologist for formal diagnosis, management of complications, surveillance of associated malignancies, and evaluation for liver transplantation.

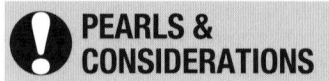 **PEARLS & CONSIDERATIONS**

- Diagnosis of PSC is made by a combination of clinical presentation, cholestatic liver function tests, cholangiographic evidence of multifocal

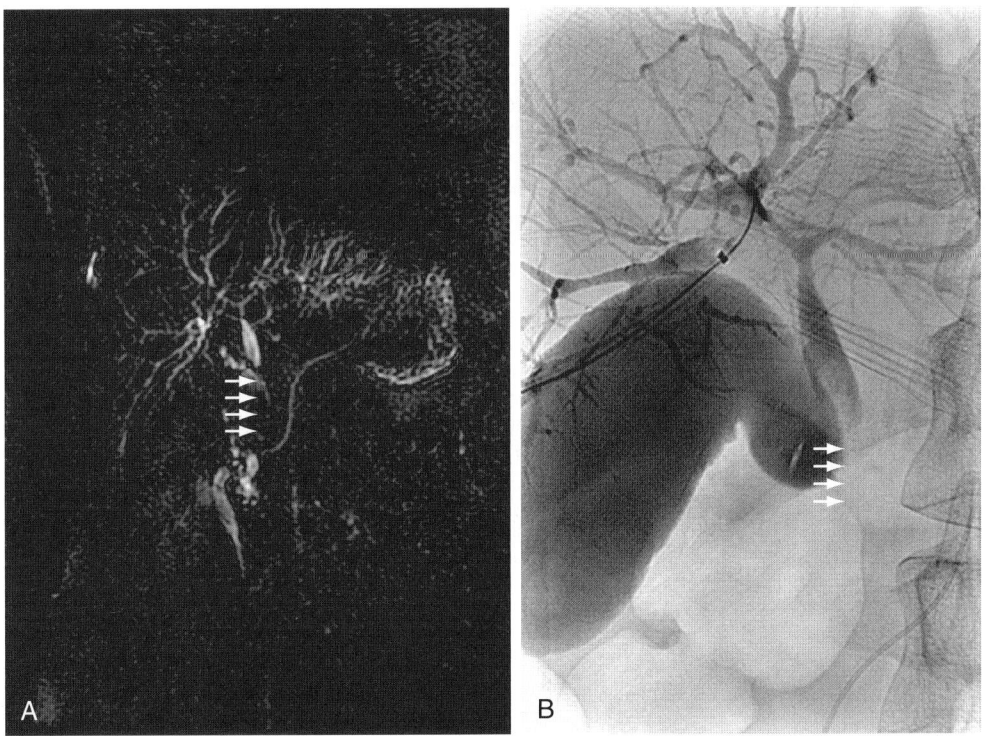

FIG. 1 A, Reconstructed magnetic resonance cholangiopancreatography images in a patient with primary sclerosing cholangitis. The intrahepatic biliary radicles are diffusely abnormal and characterized by pruning and a beaded appearance. There is a dominant stricture at the level of the distal bile duct *(arrows)* indicated by a signal void on magnetic resonance image. **B,** A percutaneous cholangiogram in the same patient. Note the high-grade, dominant, distal bile duct stenosis *(arrows)* with a markedly enlarged gallbladder, suggesting that the stricture involves the insertion of the cystic duct. Similar findings could be seen in a patient with a distal cholangiocarcinoma. (From Feldman M et al: *Sleisenger and Fortran's gastrointestinal and liver disease*, ed 11, Philadelphia, 2021, Elsevier.)

biliary strictures, and the exclusion of secondary cholangitis.
- There is currently no effective medical treatment of PSC. Management of PSC targets symptom relief, complications of PSC, cirrhosis, early hepatobiliary and colorectal cancer detection, and timely referral for liver transplantation. Liver transplant remains the only definitive therapy for complications of PSC.
- Patients are at increased risk for the development of colorectal cancer, gallbladder cancer, and cholangiocarcinoma and need surveillance.
- In patients with cirrhosis, surveillance for gastroesophageal varices and HCC is recommended.

RELATED CONTENT

Ulcerative Colitis (Related Key Topic)

REFERENCES

Available at eBooks.Health.Elsevier.com.

AUTHORS: **MAYA DEEB, MD,** and **TALIA ZENLEA, MD**

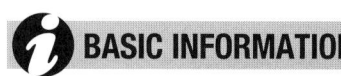

BASIC INFORMATION

DEFINITION

Prolactinomas are monoclonal tumors that secrete prolactin.

ICD-10CM CODES
D35.2 Benign neoplasm of pituitary gland
E22.8 Other hyperfunction of pituitary gland

EPIDEMIOLOGY & DEMOGRAPHICS

INCIDENCE: Most common pituitary tumor; nearly 30% of all pituitary adenomas secrete enough prolactin to cause hyperprolactinemia.
PREDOMINANT SEX: Microadenomas are more common in women; macroadenomas are found more frequently in men.

PHYSICAL FINDINGS & CLINICAL PRESENTATION

- Men: Decreased facial and body hair, infertility, small testicles; may also have decreased libido, erectile dysfunction, and delayed puberty (caused by decreased testosterone as a result of inhibition of gonadotropin secretion).
- Women: Physical examination may be normal; history may reveal amenorrhea, galactorrhea (Fig. E1), oligomenorrhea, and anovulation.
- Both sexes: Visual field defects and headache may occur depending on size of tumor and its expansion.

ETIOLOGY

Prolactin-secreting pituitary adenomas: Microadenomas (<10 mm diameter) or macroadenomas (>10 mm diameter). No risk factors have been identified for sporadic prolactinomas. Rarely prolactinomas can be part of multiple endocrine neoplasia (MEN) type 1 syndrome.

DIAGNOSIS

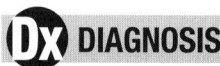

DIFFERENTIAL DIAGNOSIS

Secretion of prolactin is under tonic inhibitory control by hypothalamic dopamine. Hyperprolactinemia may be caused by the following:
- Drugs: Risperidone, phenothiazines, methyldopa, reserpine, monoamine oxidase inhibitors, androgens, progesterone, cimetidine, tricyclic antidepressants, haloperidol, meprobamate, chlordiazepoxide, estrogens, opioids, metoclopramide, verapamil, amoxapine, cocaine, oral contraceptives
- Hepatic cirrhosis, renal failure, primary hypothyroidism
- Ectopic prolactin-secreting tumors (hypernephroma, bronchogenic carcinoma)
- Infiltrating diseases of the pituitary (sarcoidosis, histiocytosis)
- Head trauma, chest wall injury, spinal cord injury
- Polycystic ovary disease, pregnancy, nipple stimulation
- Idiopathic hyperprolactinemia, stress, exercise

WORKUP

- The diagnosis of prolactinoma is established by demonstration of an elevated serum prolactin level (after exclusion of other causes of hyperprolactinemia) and radiographic evidence of a pituitary adenoma.
  1. Normal mean prolactin levels are 8 ng/ml in women and 5 ng/ml in men.
  2. Prolactin levels >100 ng/ml are suspicious for prolactinomas. Most macroprolactinomas raise prolactin levels >250 ng/ml, and levels >500 ng/ml are virtually diagnostic of macroprolactinomas.
  3. Prolactin levels can vary with time of day, stress, sleep cycle, and meals. More accurate measurements can be obtained 2 to 3 hr after awakening, preprandially, and when patient is not distressed.
  4. Serial measurements are recommended in patients with mild prolactin elevations.
- Thyroid-stimulating hormone (TSH), free T_4, blood urea nitrogen (BUN), creatinine, aspartate aminotransferase (ALT), alanine aminotransferase (AST) are useful tests. Pregnancy test in all women of childbearing age.
- All patients with prolactinomas should undergo visual field testing. Serial evaluation is recommended, particularly during pregnancy in patients with macroadenomas.

IMAGING STUDIES

- MRI (Fig. E2) with gadolinium enhancement is the procedure of choice in the radiographic evaluation of pituitary disease.
- In absence of MRI, a radiographic diagnosis is best accomplished with a high-resolution computed tomography (CT) scanner and special coronal cuts through the pituitary region.

TREATMENT

NONPHARMACOLOGIC THERAPY

Pregnancy and breastfeeding should be avoided because they can encourage tumor growth. The management of patients with prolactinoma planning pregnancy is summarized in Table E1.

ACUTE GENERAL Rx

- Management of prolactinomas depends on their size and encroachment on the optic chiasm and other vital structures, the presence or absence of gonadal dysfunction, and the patient's desires regarding fertility. Patients with microprolactinomas without symptoms of hypogonadism do not require treatment. Fig. 3 describes a management algorithm for prolactinomas. Women with hypogonadism related to a microadenoma who do not desire fertility can be treated with a combined oral contraceptive.
- Medical therapy is preferred when fertility is an important consideration. Prolactinomas are treated with the dopamine agonists (DA) bromocriptine and cabergoline.
  1. Bromocriptine: Initial dose is 0.625 mg at bedtime for the first wk. After 1 wk, add

morning dose of 1.25 mg. Gradually increase dose by 1.25 mg/wk until dose of 5 to 10 mg/day is achieved. Bromocriptine decreases size of the tumor and generally lowers the prolactin level into the normal range when the initial serum prolactin is <500 ng/ml. Side effects of bromocriptine are nausea, constipation, dizziness, and nasal stuffiness. Bromocriptine appears to be safe during pregnancy.
  2. Cabergoline is a longer-acting dopamine agonist that is more expensive but may be more effective and better tolerated than bromocriptine; initial dose is 0.25 mg twice weekly.
  3. After therapy is initiated, MRI should be repeated in 1 yr for microprolactinomas if the prolactin level normalizes. For macroprolactinomas, MRI is repeated after 2 mo and every 6 to 12 mo until stable on serial studies.
- Transsphenoidal resection: Option in an infertile patient who cannot tolerate bromocriptine or cabergoline or when medical therapy is ineffective. The success rate depends on the location of the tumor (entirely intrasellar), experience of the neurosurgeon, and size of the tumor (<10 mm in diameter); the recurrence rate may reach 80% within 5 yr. Possible complications of transsphenoidal surgery vary with experience and skill of the neurosurgeon and tumor anatomy and include transient diabetes insipidus, hypopituitarism, cerebrospinal fluid rhinorrhea, and infections (meningitis, wound infection).
- Pituitary irradiation is useful as adjunctive therapy of macroadenomas (>10 mm in diameter) and in patients with persistent hypersecretion after surgery. Potential complications include cranial nerve damage, radionecrosis, and cognitive abnormalities.
- Stereotactic radiosurgery (gamma knife) has become popular as a modality in the treatment of prolactinomas. A high dose of ionizing radiation is delivered to the tumor through multiple ports. Its advantage is minimal irradiation to surrounding tissues. Proximity of the tumor to the optic chiasm limits this therapeutic modality.

CHRONIC Rx

- Patients on medical therapy require periodic measurement of prolactin levels. An attempt to reduce the dose of bromocriptine or cabergoline can be made after the prolactin level has been normal for 2 yr. An MRI scan of the pituitary should be obtained to rule out tumor enlargement within 6 mo of initiation of tapering regimen.
- Evaluation and monitoring of pituitary function are recommended after transsphenoidal surgery.

DISPOSITION

- Transsphenoidal surgery will result in a cure in nearly 50% to 75% of patients with microadenomas and 10% to 20% of patients with macroadenomas.
- Nearly 20% of microprolactinomas resolve during long-term dopamine agonist treatment.

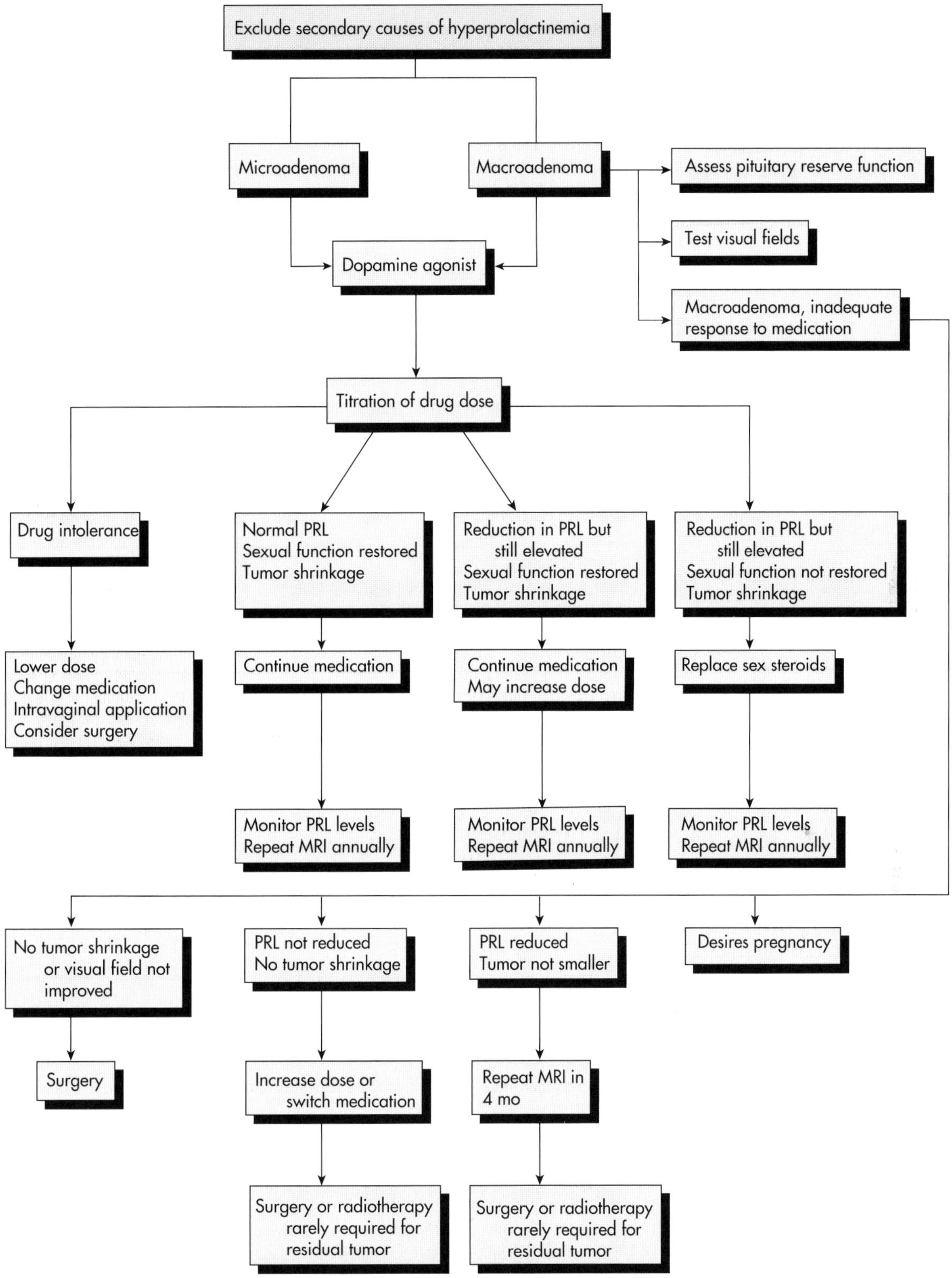

P

```
                    ┌─────────────────────────────────────────────┐
                    │ Exclude secondary causes of hyperprolactinemia │
                    └─────────────────────────────────────────────┘
```

Exclude secondary causes of hyperprolactinemia

Microadenoma | Macroadenoma → Assess pituitary reserve function

→ Test visual fields

→ Macroadenoma, inadequate response to medication

Dopamine agonist

Titration of drug dose

Drug intolerance
- Lower dose
- Change medication
- Intravaginal application
- Consider surgery

Normal PRL / Sexual function restored / Tumor shrinkage
- Continue medication
- Monitor PRL levels / Repeat MRI annually

Reduction in PRL but still elevated / Sexual function restored / Tumor shrinkage
- Continue medication / May increase dose
- Monitor PRL levels / Repeat MRI annually

Reduction in PRL but still elevated / Sexual function not restored / Tumor shrinkage
- Replace sex steroids
- Monitor PRL levels / Repeat MRI annually

No tumor shrinkage or visual field not improved → Surgery

PRL not reduced / No tumor shrinkage → Increase dose or switch medication → Surgery or radiotherapy rarely required for residual tumor

PRL reduced / Tumor not smaller → Repeat MRI in 4 mo → Surgery or radiotherapy rarely required for residual tumor

Desires pregnancy

FIG. 3 Prolactinoma management. After secondary causes of hyperprolactinemia have been excluded, subsequent management decisions are based on clinical imaging and biochemical criteria. *MRI,* Magnetic resonance imaging; *PRL,* prolactin. (From Melmed S et al: *Williams textbook of endocrinology,* ed 14, Philadelphia, 2020, Saunders.)

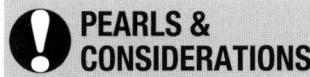

PEARLS & CONSIDERATIONS

COMMENTS
- Patients must be monitored for several years after surgery because up to 50% of microadenomas and nearly 90% of macroadenomas can recur.
- Pituitary microadenomas are found in 10.9% of autopsies, and 44% of these microadenomas are prolactinomas.

RELATED CONTENT
Prolactinoma (Patient Information)
Pituitary Adenoma (Related Key Topic)

AUTHOR: **FRED F. FERRI, MD**

 BASIC INFORMATION

DEFINITION & CLASSIFICATION

Prostate cancer is a neoplasm involving the prostate. Various classifications have been developed to evaluate malignancy potential and prognosis.

- The degree of malignancy varies with the stage:
  1. Stage A: Confined to the prostate, no nodule palpable.
  2. Stage B: Palpable nodule confined to the gland.
  3. Stage C: Local extension.
  4. Stage D: Regional lymph nodes or distant metastases.
- In the Gleason classification (Box 1 and Fig. E1), two histologic patterns are independently assigned numbers 1 to 5 (best to least differentiated). These numbers are added to give a total tumor score between 2 and 10. Prognosis is best for highly differentiated tumors (e.g., Gleason score 2-6) compared with most poorly differentiated tumors (Gleason score 7-10).
- Another commonly used classification is the Tumor-Node-Metastasis (TNM) classification of prostate cancer (Table 1).
- Table 2 summarizes the definition of risk groups and biopsy criteria.

ICD-10CM CODES
C61   Malignant neoplasm of prostate
D07.5 Carcinoma in situ of prostate

EPIDEMIOLOGY & DEMOGRAPHICS

- Prostate cancer has surpassed lung cancer as the most common nonskin cancer in men.
- In the United States, more than 220,000 new cases are diagnosed yearly, and nearly 30,000 males die from prostate cancer each year (second leading cause of death from cancer in U.S. men).
- Incidence of prostate cancer increases with age: Uncommon <50 yr; 80% of new cases are diagnosed in patients aged ≥65 yr. Widespread prostate-specific antigen (PSA) testing has doubled the incidence of prostate cancer and the lifetime risk for prostate cancer to approximately 16%. Prostate cancer is also diagnosed earlier, and the incidence of clinically "silent" T_1 tumors has increased from 17% in 1989 to 48% in 2001 since the advent of PSA screening. Currently, approximately 80% of prostate cancer cases are diagnosed as localized disease and only 4% as metastatic disease. The incidence of metastatic prostate cancer for middle-aged men was stable from 2004 to 2010 and then increased from 12 to 17 cases/100,000 from 2010 to 2018.[1] It is unclear if this increase was due to U.S. Preventive Services Task Force (USPSTF) recommendations against PSA screening in 2008 and 2012 or to more aggressive diagnostic strategies.
- Prostate cancer is found at autopsy in more than half of U.S. men older than 50 yr but is the cause of death in only 3%.
- Average age at time of diagnosis is 72 yr.

- Blacks in the U.S. have the highest incidence of prostate cancer in the world (one in every nine males).
- Incidence is low in Asians.
- Approximately 9% of all prostate cancers may be familial. Obesity is a risk factor for prostate cancer. High-fat, low-fiber diet increases risk. High insulin levels may also increase the risk of prostate cancer. Dietary supplementation with vitamin E has been reported to significantly increase the risk of prostate cancer among healthy men. Linkage studies have implicated chromosome 17p21-22 as a possible location of a prostate-cancer susceptibility gene. Germline mutations in *HOXB13* are associated with a significantly increased risk of hereditary prostate cancer.
- Mortality rates of prostate cancer have declined substantially in the past 15 yr from 34% in 1990 to <20% currently.

PHYSICAL FINDINGS & CLINICAL PRESENTATION

- Generally silent disease until it reaches advanced stages.
- Bone pain and pathologic fractures may be initial symptoms of prostate cancer.
- Local growth can cause symptoms of outflow obstruction.
- Digital rectal examination (DRE) may reveal an area of increased firmness; 10% of patients will have a negative DRE.
- Prostate may be hard, fixed, with extension of tumor to the seminal vesicles in advanced stages.

Dx DIAGNOSIS

DIFFERENTIAL DIAGNOSIS

- Benign prostatic hypertrophy

- Prostatitis
- Prostate stones

LABORATORY TESTS

- Measurement of PSA is controversial in early diagnosis of prostate cancer. PSA screening is associated with psychological harm, and its potential benefits remain uncertain. In asymptomatic men with no history of prostate cancer, screening using PSA does not reduce all-cause mortality or death from prostate cancer. Normal PSA is found in >20% of patients with prostate cancer, whereas only 20% of men with PSA levels between 4 and 10 ng/ml have prostate cancer. Most guidelines encourage a shared decision-making approach between patient and physician regarding PSA testing. Available evidence favors clinician discussion of the pros and cons of PSA screening with average-risk men aged 65 to 69 yr. Only men who express a definite preference for screening should have PSA testing. Rather than widespread annual PSA screening, a reasonable approach may be to focus on high-risk men (those with PSA levels ≥2 ng/ml at age 60). The American Cancer Society recommends offering the PSA test and DRE yearly to men aged ≥50 yr who have a life expectancy of at least 10 yr. Earlier testing, starting at age 40 to 45 yr, is recommended for men at high risk (e.g., blacks, men with family history of prostate cancer). An isolated elevation in PSA level should be confirmed several weeks later before proceeding with further testing, including prostate biopsy. Screening for prostate cancer in men aged ≥75 yr is controversial and generally not recommended. The American College of Physicians (ACP) recommends that clinicians should not screen for prostate cancer using the PSA in average-risk men under age 50, men

---

BOX 1   2005 International Society of Urological Pathology Modified Gleason System

Pattern 1
Circumscribed nodule of closely packed but separate, uniform, rounded to oval, medium-sized acini (larger glands than pattern 3)

Pattern 2
Like pattern 1, fairly circumscribed, yet at the edge of the tumor nodule there may be minimal infiltration
Glands are more loosely arranged and not quite as uniform as Gleason pattern 1

Pattern 3
Discrete glandular units
Typically smaller glands than seen in Gleason pattern 1 or 2
Infiltrates in and among nonneoplastic prostate acini
Marked variation in size and shape

Pattern 4
Fused microacinar glands
Ill-defined glands with poorly formed glandular lumens
Large cribriform glands
Cribriform glands
Hypernephromatoid

Pattern 5
Essentially no glandular differentiation, composed of solid sheets, cords, or single cells
Comedocarcinoma with central necrosis surrounded by papillary, cribriform, or solid masses

From Wein AJ et al: *Campbell-Walsh urology,* ed 11, Philadelphia, 2016, Elsevier.

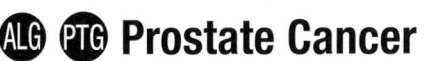

over age 69, or men with a life expectancy of <10 to 15 yr. The U.S. Preventive Services Task Force (USPSTF) recommends against PSA-based screening for prostate cancer in all age groups. According to the USPSTF:

1. The magnitude of harms from screening (e.g., falsely high PSA levels, psychological effects, unnecessary biopsies, over-diagnosis of indolent tumors) is "at least small."
2. The magnitude of treatment-associated harms (i.e., adverse effects of surgery, radiation, and hormonal therapy) is "at least moderate."
3. The 10-yr mortality benefit of PSA-based prostate cancer screening is "small to none."
4. The overall balance of benefits and harms results in "moderate certainty that PSA-based screening has no net benefit."

- The USPSTF currently recommends individualized screening decisions for men between ages 55 and 69 and advises against screening for older men.
- Free PSA: The use of serum free PSA for prostate screening has been proposed by some urologists as a means to decrease unwarranted biopsies without missing a significant number of prostate cancers. This approach is based on the higher free PSA in men with benign prostatic hyperplasia and the higher protein-bound PSA levels in men with prostate cancer. For example, in men with total PSA levels of 4 to 10 ng/ml, the cancer probability is 0.25, but if the percentage of free PSA is ≤17%, the probability of cancer increases to 0.45.
- PSA velocity: The rate of increase of serum PSA over time (PSA velocity) can aid in the diagnosis of prostate cancer. A yearly PSA velocity >0.75 ng/ml increases the likelihood of later malignancy when total PSA is still within normal range. Proper interpretation of PSA velocity requires at least three PSA measurements over an 18-mo period because most PSA variations are physiologic. Recent trials have cast a doubt on the value of PSA velocity by showing that adding PSA velocity as a trigger for biopsy did not improve predictive accuracy beyond that of using PSA threshold values alone. Retrospective studies[2] have also shown that PSA velocity threshold is different in black and non-Hispanic white men treated for low-risk prostate cancer with active surveillance. PSA velocity associated significantly with grade progression was 0.44 mg/ml/yr in black patients and 1.18 mg/ml/yr in non-Hispanic whites. The optimal PSA velocity threshold for development of metastases was 1.77 mg/ml/yr.
- Age-adjusted PSA: There is evidence that the current threshold of 4.0 ng/ml is inadequate for younger men, because in a recent study 22% of men with PSA levels between 2.6 and 4.0 were found to have prostate cancer. The concept of age-related cutoffs remains controversial. Lowering the upper limit of normal for PSA would improve sensitivity but decrease specificity.
- Prostatic acid phosphatase can be used for evaluation of nonlocalized disease.
- Prostate cancer gene 3 (PCA3) is overexpressed in prostate cancer cell, and high levels are suggestive of prostate cancer. Measurement of PCA3 in urine specimens collected after digital exams is helpful to make decisions about prostate biopsy in men with elevated PSA.
- Ultrasound-guided transrectal biopsy and fine-needle aspiration of prostate can confirm the diagnosis. Indications for biopsy include an abnormal PSA level, an abnormal DRE, or a previous biopsy specimen that showed prostatic intraepithelial neoplasia or prostatic atypia. The number of cores taken is patient specific, typically including a minimum of 10 cores. Prostate volume negatively affects cancer detection rate (23% in glands >50 cm^3, 38% in glands <50 cm^3). MRI-targeted biopsy identifies clinically significant prostate cancers more accurately than conventional systematic biopsy in men with suspected localized prostate cancer but misses one in five clinically significant cancers.[2b]

IMAGING STUDIES (FIGS. E2 TO E5)

- MRI can be used to guide decisions on whether to perform biopsies in men with elevated PSA

TABLE 1 Prostate Cancer

T Stage

T_x	Primary tumor is not assessable	
T_0	There is no evidence of primary tumor	
T_1	Tumor is not clinically palpable or detected with imaging	
	T_{1a}	*An incidental histologic finding in ≤5% of resected tissue (e.g., TURP)*
	T_{1b}	*An incidental histologic finding in >5% of resected tissue (e.g., TURP)*
	T_{1c}	*Tumor is identified by needle biopsy*
T_2	Prostate-confined tumor that is clinically palpable or detected with imaging	
	T_{2a}	*Tumor involves ≤1/2 of one prostate lobe*
	T_{2b}	*Tumor involves >1/2 of one prostate lobe (but not both lobes)*
	T_{2c}	*Tumor involves both lobes*
T_3	There is tumor extension through the prostate capsule	
	T_{3a}	*Unilateral or bilateral tumor extension through the prostate capsule*
	T_{3b}	*Seminal vesical involvement*
T_4	Tumor invades structures other than the seminal vesicles (e.g., the bladder neck, rectum, or pelvic wall)	

N Stage

N_x	The lymph nodes are not assessable
N_0	There is no tumor spread
N_1	There is tumor spread to one or more regional pelvic nodes

M Stage

M_0	There is no tumor spread beyond the regional pelvic nodes	
M_1	There is tumor spread beyond the regional pelvic nodes	
	M_{1a}	*Tumor spread to nodes outside of the pelvis*
	M_{1b}	*Tumor spread to bones*
	M_{1c}	*Tumor spread to other organs (e.g., lung, liver and brain) ± bone involvement*

From Grant LA: *Grainger & Allison's diagnostic radiology essentials*, ed 2, Philadelphia, 2019, Elsevier.

TABLE 2 Definition of Risk Groups

Risk Group	Clinical Stage	PSA (ng/ml)	Gleason Score	Biopsy Criteria
Low	T_{1a} or T_{1c}	<10	2-6	Unilateral or <50% of core involved
Intermediate	T_{1b}, T_{1c}, or T_{2a}	<10	3 + 4 = 7	Bilateral
High	T_{1b}, T_{1c}, T_{2b}, or T_3	10-20	4 + 3 = 7	>50% of core involved or perineural invasion or ductal differentiation
Very high	T_4	>20	8-10	Lymphovascular invasion or neuroendocrine differentiation

From Wein AJ et al: *Campbell-Walsh urology*, ed 11, Philadelphia, 2016, Elsevier.

levels on prostate cancer screening. MRI also facilitates targeted biopsy or suspicious areas.[3] However the avoidance of systematic biopsy in favor of MRI-directed targeted biopsy for screening and early detection in persons with elevated PSA levels reduces the risk of over-diagnosis by half at the cost of delaying detection of intermediate-risk tumors in a small proportion of patients.[2b]

- Bone scan is useful to evaluate bone metastasis (present or eventually develops in almost 80% of patients). However, according to the American Urological Association (AUA), the routine use of bone scanning is not required for staging of prostate cancer in asymptomatic men with clinically localized cancer if the PSA level is ≤20 ng/ml.
- CT scan, MRI, and transrectal ultrasonography may be useful in selected patients to assess extent of prostate cancer. High-resolution has been used for the detection of small and otherwise undetectable lymph node metastases in patients with prostate cancer. However, according to the AUA, transrectal ultrasonography adds little to the combination of PSA and DRE. Similarly, CT and MRI imaging are generally not indicated for cancer staging in men with clinically localized cancer and PSA <25 ng/ml. With regard to pelvic lymph node dissection in staging, the AUA states that it may not be required in patients with PSA levels <10 ng/ml and when PSA level is <20 ng/ml and the Gleason score is <6.

(Rx) TREATMENT

NONPHARMACOLOGIC THERAPY
Watchful waiting is reasonable in selected patients with early-stage (T_{1a}) and projected life expectancy <10 yr or in patients with focal and moderately differentiated carcinoma.

ACUTE GENERAL Rx
- Therapeutic approach varies with the following:
  1. Stage of the tumor
  2. Patient's life expectancy
  3. General medical condition
  4. Patient's treatment preference (e.g., patient may be opposed to orchiectomy)

- The optimal treatment of clinically localized prostate cancer is unclear. It is important to remember that all forms of treatment have potential adverse effects. Management requires careful consideration of the potential benefits and harms of intervention and the patient's age, health status, and individual preferences. A treatment algorithm for prostate cancer is described in Fig. 6. Table 3 summarizes recommended treatment based on risk group and life expectancy.
  1. Radical prostatectomy is generally performed in patients with localized prostate cancer and life expectancy >10 yr. Radical prostatectomy reduces disease-specific mortality, overall mortality, and the risks of metastasis and local progression. The absolute reduction in the risk of death after 10 yr is small, but the reductions in the risks of metastasis and local tumor progression are substantial. A 29-yr follow-up comparing radical prostatectomy with watchful waiting showed that men with clinically detected, localized prostate cancer and a long life expectancy benefited from radical prostatectomy with a mean 2.9

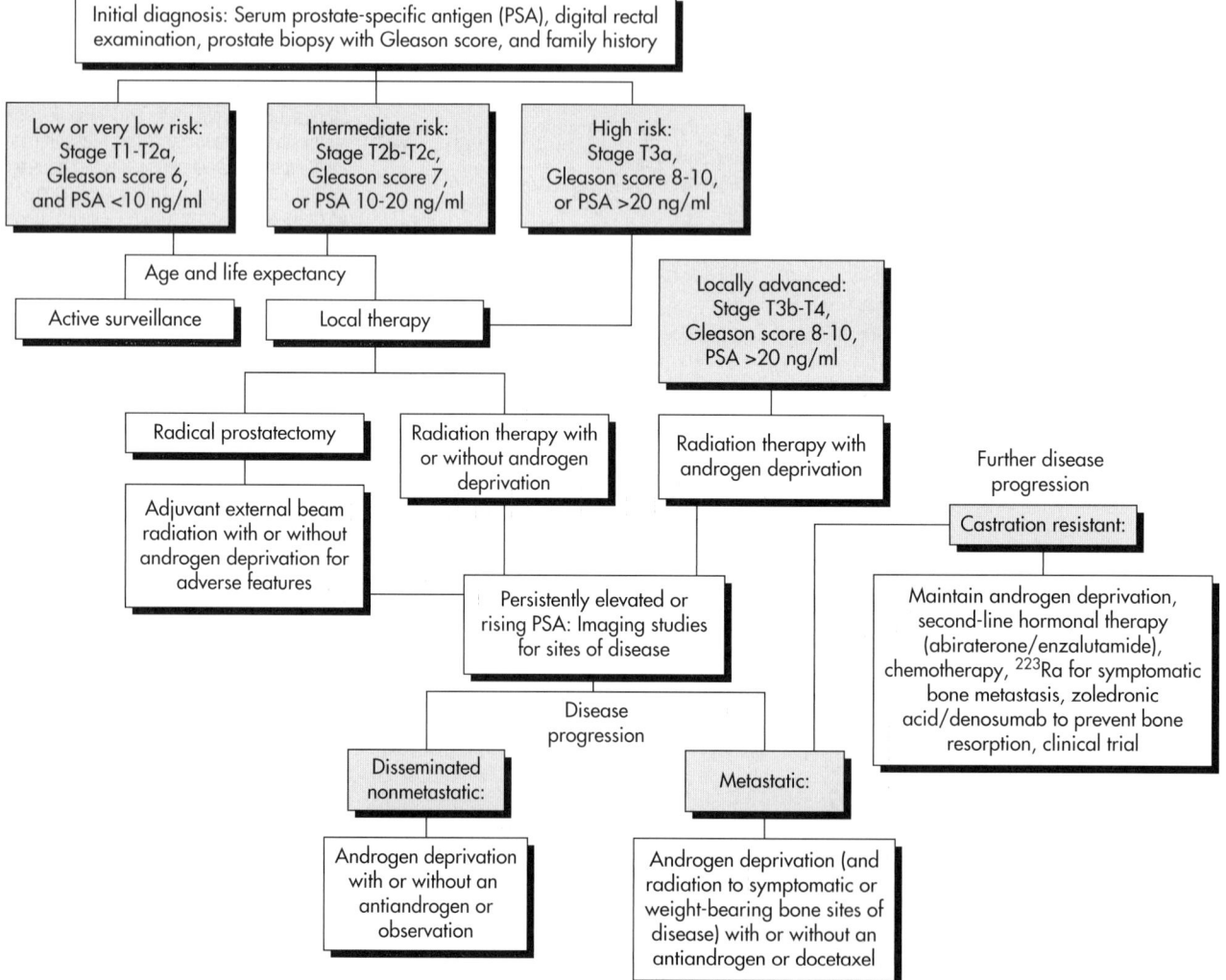

FIG. 6 Treatment algorithm. [223]*Ra*, Radium-223. (From Niederhuber JE: *Abeloff's clinical oncology*, ed 6, Philadelphia, 2020, Elsevier.)

yr of life gained. A trial[4] comparing surgery with radiation therapy for high-risk localized prostate cancer showed that prostate cancer-specific mortality at 5 yr was significantly lower with surgery than with external beam radiation therapy (2.3% vs 4.1% PS 0.001). Postoperative complications of radical prostatectomy include urinary incontinence (10%-20% depending on degree of neurovascular bundle and urethral preservation, patient age, and correct mucosal apposition) and erectile dysfunction (percentage >50% and varies with patient age, preoperative erectile dysfunction, stage of tumor at time of surgery, and preservation of neurovascular bundle). Lower complication rates occur in hospitals that perform a large number of prostatectomies. Fewer men will have postsurgical erectile dysfunction after unilateral or bilateral nerve-sparing surgery. In men undergoing prostatectomy, robotic-assisted laparoscopic surgery represents an alternative to open retropubic radical prostatectomy. Despite advertisements that suggest that there are fewer complications after robotic surgery, data show that sexual dysfunction occurs postoperatively in about 88% of patients who have undergone robotic-assisted or conventional prostatectomy and that incontinence problems are more prevalent (33%) with robotic surgery

than with open retropubic radical prostatectomy (RPP) (27%). Trials have shown that prostatectomy is preferred over "watchful waiting" in patients with localized prostate cancer detected by PSA if the PSA level is >10 ng/ml. In this subgroup, the 10-yr mortality is 48.4% with prostatectomy versus 61.6% with watchful waiting. In men who have low-risk disease (PSA level <10 mcg/L, stage <T_{2a}, Gleason score ≤3 + 3), and <6% risk for prostate cancer–specific death at 15 yr, watchful waiting and active surveillance are reasonable and underutilized options.

2. Radiation therapy (external-beam irradiation or brachytherapy with implantation of radioactive pellets [iodine-125 or palladium-103 seeds] into the prostate gland) represents an alternative in patients with localized prostate cancer, especially poor surgical candidates or patients with a high-grade malignancy. The efficacy of brachytherapy is comparable to external radiation and radical prostatectomy. In patients receiving external-beam radiation, a total dose of 79.2 Gy (high dose) compared with a total dose of 70.2 Gy (conventional dose) has been reported to lower the risk of recurrence without increased risk of morbidity and mortality. Newer radiation treatments such as intensity-modulated radiation therapy (IMRT) and proton

therapy are becoming increasingly popular and replacing the older technique of conformal radiation therapy over the past 10 yr. Trials have shown that among patients with nonmetastatic prostate cancer, the use of IMRT compared with conformal therapy is associated with less GI morbidity and fewer hip fractures but more erectile dysfunction; IMRT compared with proton therapy is associated with less GI morbidity. Patients with localized prostate cancer and high risk for extraprostatic disease and disease recurrence (e.g., Gleason score ≤7 with multiple positive biopsy cores and clinical stage T_{1b}-T_{2b}) may benefit (increased overall survival) with the addition of 6 mo of androgen suppression therapy to radiation therapy. High-intensity focused ultrasound (HIFU) is a newer treatment option for patients with prostate cancer. It ablates localized areas of the prostate with the goal of sparing patients the morbidity of whole-gland therapy. Longer-term studies comparing HIFU with standard therapy are needed. Hemigland cryoablation is another newer treatment modality for intermediate-risk prostate cancer. Longer studies are needed before drawing conclusions.

3. Watchful waiting is reasonable in patients who are too old or too ill to survive longer than 10 yr. If the cancer progresses to the point at which it becomes symptomatic, palliation can be attempted with several methods. Conservative management is also reasonable for patients with Gleason score of 2 to 4 because these patients do not have a shortened life expectancy and treatment is associated with long-term side effects. Watchful waiting also appears to be safe in older men with less-aggressive disease. Individual preferences play a central role in the decision whether to treat or to pursue active surveillance.

- Patients with advanced disease and projected life expectancy <10 yr are candidates for radiation therapy and hormonal therapy (diethylstilbestrol, luteinizing hormone–releasing hormone analogues, antiandrogens, bilateral orchiectomy).
- Recommended treatment of patients with regional metastatic prostate cancer with projected life expectancy ≥10 yr includes radiation therapy and hormonal therapy.
- Prostate cancer is an androgen receptor–dependent disease, and the blocking of androgen-receptor signaling is an effective treatment modality. Table 4 summarizes major

TABLE 3 Recommended Treatment

Risk Group	Life Expectancy (Yr)	Recommended Treatment
Low	0-5	AS, HT
	5-10	AS, RT, HT, O
	>10	RP, RT, AS, O
Intermediate*	0-5	AS, HT, RT, O
	5-10	RT, HT, RP, O
	>10	RP, RT, O, HT
High*	0-5	AS, RT + HT, O
	5-10	RT + HT, HT, RP, O
	>10	RT + HT, RP + RT + HT, HT
Very high*	0-5	AS, RT + HT, O
	5-10	H, RT + HT, ST
	>10	RT + HT, RP + RT + HT, HT, ST, IT

AS, Active surveillance; *HT*, hormone therapy; *IT*, investigational multimodal therapy; *O*, others; *RP*, radical prostatectomy; *RT*, radiation therapy; *ST*, systemic therapy.
*If there is more than a 20% probability of positive lymph nodes, AS, HT, ST + HT.
From Wein AJ et al: *Campbell-Walsh urology*, ed 11, Philadelphia, 2016, Elsevier.

TABLE 4 Major Circulating Androgens

Source	Androgen	Amount Produced/Day (mg)	Relative Potency	Relative Potency/Amount Produced
Testes	Testosterone	6.6	100	15.2
Testes and peripheral tissues	Dihydrotestosterone	0.3	160-190	533-633
Adrenal glands	Androstenedione	1.4	39	27.9
Adrenal glands	Dehydroepiandrosterone	29	15	0.5

From Wein AJ et al: *Campbell-Walsh urology*, ed 11, Philadelphia, 2016, Elsevier.

circulating androgens. Androgen deprivation therapy (ADT) is the mainstay of treatment for metastatic prostate cancer. Adverse effects of ADT include decreased libido, impotence, hot flashes, osteopenia with increased fracture risk, metabolic alterations, and changes in mood and cognition. Adjuvant treatment with luteinizing hormone-releasing hormone (LHRH) agonists (goserelin, leuprolide, or triptorelin) plus antiandrogens (flutamide, bicalutamide, or nilutamide), when started simultaneously with external-beam radiation, improves local control and survival in patients with locally advanced prostate cancer. Pamidronate inhibits osteoclast-mediated bone resorption and prevents bone loss in the hip and lumbar spine in men receiving treatment for prostate cancer. Gonadotropin-releasing hormone (GnRH) receptor antagonists can be used for rapid medical castration of men with advanced prostate cancer. Degarelix is an injectable GnRH agonist useful to suppress testosterone in patients with prostate cancer who are not good candidates for LHRH agonists and refuse surgical castration. Assessment of bone density and treatment with once-weekly oral alendronate can prevent and improve the bone loss that occurs in men receiving ADT for prostate cancer.
- Docetaxel plus prednisone or docetaxel plus estramustine can be used in metastatic hormone–refractory prostate cancer. Newer treatments for hormone–refractory prostate cancer (castration-resistant cancer) include immunotherapy with sipuleucel and cabazitaxel, a microtubule inhibitor that interferes with cell mitosis and replication. Both agents can prolong survival but adverse effects can be severe, and both agents are very expensive. Abiraterone is an oral agent that blocks biosynthesis of androgens by inhibiting CYP17, an enzyme required for androgen biosynthesis. It has been FDA approved for oral treatment, in combination with prednisone, of metastatic castration-resistant prostate cancer in patients previously treated with docetaxel. Darolutamide is an androgen-receptor inhibitor approved for the treatment of nonmetastatic castration-resistant prostate cancer. The addition of darolutamide to androgen-deprivation therapy and docetaxel has also been shown to prolong survival in patients with metastatic, hormone-sensitive prostate cancer.[5]
- Enzalutamide is a newer nonsteroidal antiandrogen. Trials have shown it to be highly effective in extending survival in patients with metastatic castration-resistant prostate cancer. It can be used sequentially with other agents such as docetaxel, abiraterone, cabazitaxel, and immunotherapy.
- Radium-223, an alpha emitter, selectively targets bone metastases and has been found effective in improving survival in men with

castration-resistant prostate cancer and bone metastases.
- The polyadenosine diphosphate [ADP]-ribose) polymerase (PARP) inhibitor olaparib has shown a high response rate in trials in patients whose prostate cancers were no longer responding to standard treatments with enzalutamide or abiraterone and who had defects in DNA-repair genes.

CHRONIC Rx

- Patients should be monitored at 3- to 6-mo intervals with clinical examination and PSA for the first year, then every 6 mo for the second year, then yearly if stable. For patients who have undergone radical prostatectomy, a rising PSA level suggests evidence of residual or recurrent prostate cancer. A recent study revealed that if the PSA level remains undetectable 3 to 5 yr after radical prostatectomy, the probability of biochemical recurrence is extremely low, and it is reasonable to stop PSA monitoring. Salvage radiotherapy may potentially cure patients with disease recurrence after radical prostatectomy. Recent trials have shown that addition of 24 mo of antiandrogen therapy with daily bicalutamide to salvage radiation therapy results in significantly higher rates of long-term overall survival and lower incidences of metastatic prostate cancer and death from prostate cancer than radiation therapy plus placebo.
- Chest radiography and bone scan should be performed yearly or sooner if patient develops symptoms.

DISPOSITION

- Prognosis varies with the stage of the disease and the Gleason classification (see "Definition"). For patients between ages 65 and 69 yr at diagnosis and a Gleason score of 2 to 4, the probability of dying from prostate cancer 15 yr after diagnosis is 0.06 and that of dying from other causes is 0.56. If the Gleason score is 7 to 10, the probability of dying from prostate cancer increases to 0.72 and from other causes varies from 0.25 to 0.36.
- The ploidy of the tumor also has prognostic value; prognosis is better with diploid tumor cells and worse with aneuploid tumor cells.
- For grade 1 tumors, the extended 10-yr, disease-specific survival is similar for patients with prostatectomy (94%), radiotherapy (90%), and conservative management (93%); survival rate is better with surgery than with radiotherapy or conservative management in patients with grade 2 or 3 localized prostate cancer.
- Expression of the gene *EZH2* has been identified as an important factor in the determination of the aggressiveness of prostate cancer. A recent study revealed that expression of the *EZH2* gene may be a better predictor of clinical failure than Gleason score, tumor stage, or surgical margin status. Testing for

EZH2 protein in prostate cancer tissue may be useful to determine prognosis and direct treatment.
- Preoperative PSA level and PSA velocity have prognostic significance. Men whose PSA level increases by >2.0 mcg/ml during the year before the diagnosis of cancer may have a relatively high risk of death from prostate cancer despite undergoing radical prostatectomy.
- Extraprostatic disease is detected at radical prostatectomy in 38% to 52% of patients and is associated with a risk of disease recurrence, progression, and death. In these patients, adjuvant radiotherapy results in significantly reduced risk of PSA relapse and disease recurrence; however, the improvements in metastases-free survival and overall survival are not statistically significant. Table 5 summarizes common pain syndromes in metastatic castration-resistant prostate cancer.
- The Prostate Cancer Prevention trial revealed that the use of 5-alpha-reductase inhibitors lowers the incidence of prostate cancer but also increases the incidence of high-grade tumors (Gleason score >7). It is possible that these agents delay diagnosis of prostate cancer by lowering PSA levels and decreasing prostate size. The trade-off inherent in using 5-alpha-reductase inhibitors for prostate cancer prevention is risk of one additional high-grade cancer in order to avert three or four lower-grade cancers. Based on these results, the FDA's Oncologic Drugs Advisory Committee concluded that finasteride and dutasteride do not have a favorable risk-benefit profile for chemoprevention of prostate cancer in healthy men.
- Patients undergoing prostatectomy are more likely to have urinary incontinence than those undergoing radiotherapy at 2 yr and 5 yr. However, at 15 yr there are no significant relative differences in disease-specific functional outcomes among men undergoing prostatectomy or radiotherapy.
- Bone health is a significant concern in men with prostate cancer. Trials involving bisphosphonates and denosumab reveal that both improve bone mineral density (BMD) in men with nonmetastatic prostate cancer receiving androgen deprivation therapy. Denosumab has also been shown to reduce the risk of vertebral fractures.

REFERENCES & SUGGESTED READINGS
Available at eBooks.Health.Elsevier.com.

RELATED CONTENT
Prostate Cancer (Patient Information)

AUTHOR: **FRED F. FERRI, MD**

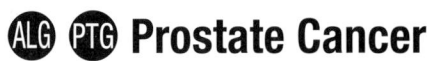

TABLE 5 Common Pain Syndromes in Metastatic Castration-Resistant Prostate Cancer

Pain Syndrome	Initial Management	Other Therapeutic Alternatives
Localized bone pain	Pharmacologic pain management	Surgical stabilization of pathologic fractures or extensive bone erosions
	Localized radiotherapy (special attention to weight-bearing areas, lytic metastasis, and extremities)	Epidural metastasis and cord compression should be evaluated in all patients with focal back pain
		Radiopharmaceuticals should be considered if local radiation therapy falls
Diffuse bone pain	Pharmacologic pain management	Corticosteroids
	"Multispot" or wide-field radiotherapy	Bisphosphonates or RANK ligand inhibitors
	Radiopharmaceuticals	Calcitonin
		Chemotherapy
Epidural metastasis and cord compression	High-dose corticosteroids	Pharmacologic pain management
	Radiation therapy	Physical therapy for recovery of neurologic function
	Surgical decompression and stabilization are indicated in high-grade epidural compressions, extensive bone involvement, or recurrence after irradiation	
Nerve plexopathies caused by direct tumor extension or previous therapy (rare)	Pharmacologic pain management	Tricyclic antidepressants (amitriptyline)
	Radiation therapy (if not previously used)	Anticonvulsants (gabapentin, pregabalin)
	Neurolytic procedures (nerve blocks)	
Miscellaneous neurogenic causes: Postherpetic neuralgia, peripheral neuropathies	Complete neurologic evaluation	Tricyclic antidepressants (amitriptyline)
	Pharmacologic pain management	Anticonvulsants (gabapentin, pregabalin)
	Discontinuation of neurotoxic drugs: Docetaxel, platinum compounds	
Other uncommon pain syndromes: Extensive skull metastasis with cranial nerve/skull base involvement, extensive painful liver metastasis, or pelvic masses	Radiation therapy	Chemotherapy
	Pharmacologic pain management	Intrathecal chemotherapy may ameliorate symptoms of meningeal involvement
	Corticosteroids (cranial nerve involvement)	

RANK, Receptor activator of nuclear factor-κB.
From Wein AJ et al: *Campbell-Walsh urology,* ed 11, Philadelphia, 2016, Elsevier.

BASIC INFORMATION

DEFINITION
A prostate abscess is a rare but severe inflammatory reaction to an infectious process of the prostate gland that usually results as a complication of suboptimally treated acute prostatitis. Infections are typically introduced when infected urine is refluxed into the prostatic ducts or introduced through instrumentation transrectally via prostate biopsy.

SYNONYMS
Prostate Gland Abscess
Prostatic Abscess
Acute Prostatic Abscess
Abscess of Prostate

ICD 10-CM CODE
N41.2 Abscess of Prostate

EPIDEMIOLOGY & DEMOGRAPHICS
INCIDENCE: Rare
PREVALENCE: 0.5% of all urologic disease
PREDOMINANT SEX & AGE: Male, adults and elderly
RISK FACTORS:
- Poorly controlled diabetes mellitus
- Cirrhosis
- CKD
- Immunocompromised
- Preexisting prostatic disease
- Recent Instrumentation of the lower urinary tract (Foleys, biopsy)
- Neurogenic bladder
- HIV positive

PHYSICAL FINDINGS & CLINICAL PRESENTATION
PHYSICAL FINDINGS:
- Fever
- Purulent urethral discharge
- Painful digital rectal examination
- Fluctuance of the prostate (not always present)
CLINICAL PRESENTATION:
- Chills
- Malaise
- Body aches
- Dysuria
- Urinary frequency
- Urinary urgency
- Nocturia
- Hematuria
- Urethritis/urethral burning
- Difficulty urinating or urinary retention
- Pyuria
- Perineal discomfort
- Unresponsive to acute prostatitis treatment within 48 hours

ETIOLOGY
- Historically caused by complication of acute bacterial prostatitis via reflux of infected urine into the prostatic ducts during voiding. However, more recently associated with complications following introduction of instrumentation during prostate biopsy.
- It is more likely to occur in patients with uncontrolled diabetes, compromised immune systems, and suboptimal treatment of acute prostatitis.
- Associated with foreign body instrumentation such as intermittent self-catheterization and bladder outlet obstruction.
- *Escherichia coli* is the most common cause followed by *Klebsiella, Pseudomonas, Proteus, Enterobacter, Serratia,* and *Enterococcus* species.
- In young and/or sexually active patients (age <35 yr) consider *Neisseria gonorrhoeae* and *Chlamydia trachomatis* as the inciting organisms.

DIAGNOSIS

DIFFERENTIAL DIAGNOSIS
- Acute prostatitis
- Chronic prostatitis
- Perirectal abscess
- Perineal abscess
- Chronic pelvic pain syndrome
- Urethritis
- Urinary tract infection

WORKUP
- Largely based on clinical history and physical exam.
- Classical findings include a severely tender prostate with areas of fluctuance on digital rectal examination (DRE).
- DREs could potentially lead to introduction of more bacteria into the bloodstream.
- Other important clinical history is patients who do not improve within 48 hours of treatment for acute prostatitis.

LABORATORY TEST(S)
- Urinalysis with urine culture
- G/C and *Chlamydia* testing by NAAT testing of urine
- CBC and CMP
- Blood cultures

IMAGING STUDIES (FIG. 1)
- Transrectal ultrasound (TRUS) is the preferred imaging modality for diagnosing prostate abscess. Typical findings are irregular hypoechoic areas with ill-defined margins (Fig. 2) usually noted in the transition zone and central zone of the prostate.
- CT with and without contrast can be helpful in delineating extraprostatic collections and extent of spread of the abscess.
- MRI will show an abscess as hypointense on T1 and hyperintense on T2; however, use of this modality has not been standardized.

TREATMENT

NONPHARMACOLOGIC THERAPY
Surgical
Includes ultrasound-guided drainage, transurethral drainage, and open drainage:
- Surgical drainage depends on the size of the abscess; if it is >2 cm, it may benefit from surgical intervention.
- Ultrasound-guided aspiration involves TRUS-guided aspiration or transperineal ultrasound-guided aspiration. TRUS-guided ultrasound aspiration utilizes a needle through the rectal wall into the prostate abscess for drainage.
- Transperineal aspiration involves utilizing a needle to puncture the perineum into the prostate abscess. For recurrent or not completely evacuated abscess, transurethral drainage can be performed.
- Open drainage involves a transperineal incision and drainage for cases where the abscess has penetrated through the levator ani muscle.

ACUTE GENERAL Rx
- Fluid resuscitation with IVF if systemic symptoms present such as sepsis
- Antibiotic therapy depends on the organism isolated but is typically a gram-negative bacteria and usually involves broad spectrum parenteral antibiotics
- Incision and drainage of abscess
- Debridement of necrotic tissue

INPATIENT—INTRAVENOUS
- Levofloxacin 500 mg or moxifloxacin 400 mg IV Q24 x 2 wk
- Ceftriaxone 1 gm IV Q24 x 2 wk
- TMP-SMX 2.5 mg/kg IV q6h x 2 wk or aztreonam 2 gm IV q8h x 2 wk

OUTPATIENT—PO
- Quinolone (levofloxacin/moxifloxacin 500/400 PO q24h x 2 wk)
- Doxycycline 200 mg PO q12h x 3 days followed by 100 mg PO q24h x 11 days
- TMP-SMX 1 SS tablet PO q12h x 2 wk

DISPOSITION
Follow up with surgeon and infectious disease physician is often warranted.

REFERRAL
General surgeon or colorectal surgeon for drainage
Endocrinologist or PCP may be needed if DM is uncontrolled
Infectious disease specialist
TRUS is needed for abscess drainage if conservative measures fail

PEARLS & CONSIDERATIONS

COMMENTS
A prostate abscess may be the first sign of a debilitating or chronic issue such as diabetes. Check the blood glucose to rule out the possibility of undiagnosed diabetes mellitus.

PREVENTION
Ensure optimal management of diabetes mellitus and other chronic conditions.

P

Diseases
and Disorders

I

PATIENT & FAMILY EDUCATION

Advise patients with lower urinary tract infections/prostate infections to be vigilant of warning signs of abscess formation, especially patients who have just received a prostate biopsy or other instrumentation of the lower urinary tract.

SUGGESTED READINGS

Available at eBooks.Health.Elsevier.com

RELATED CONTENT

Prostatitis (Related Key Topic)

AUTHORS: **FRANK A. SANCHEZ, MD, MBA,** and **GLENN G. FORT, MD, MPH**

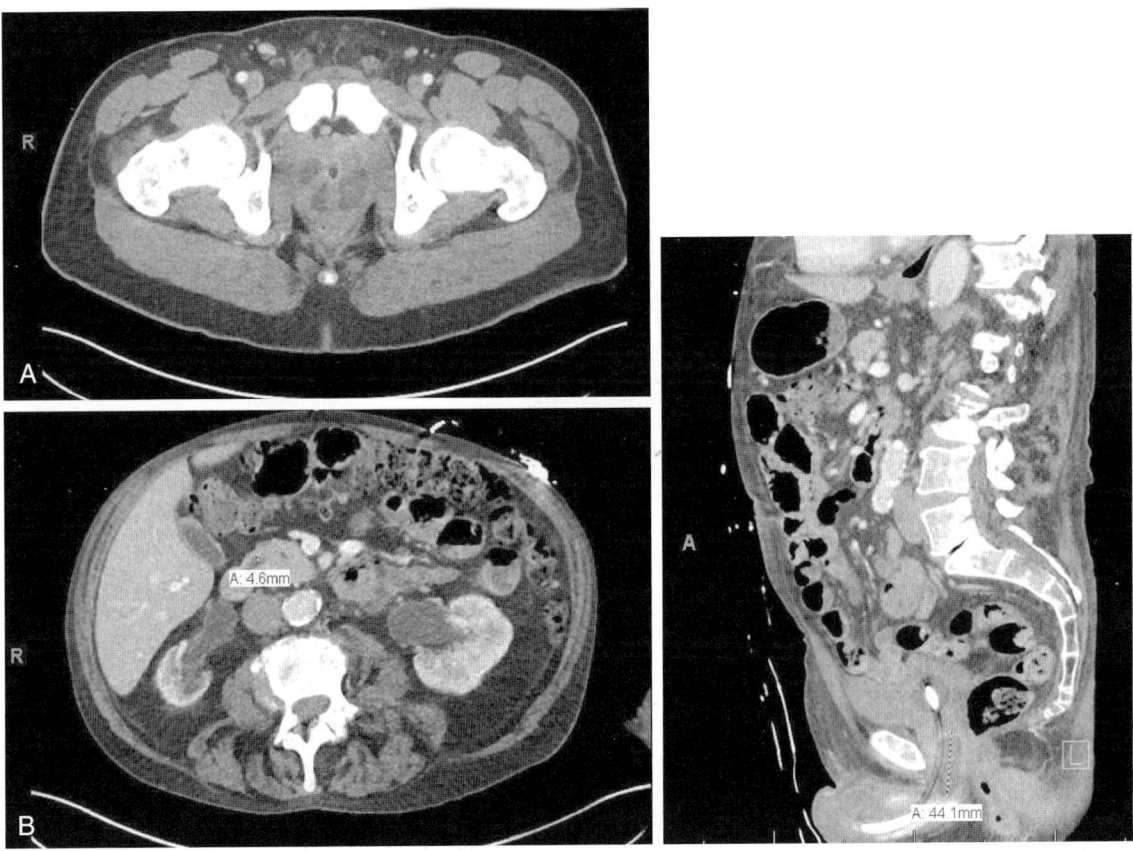

FIG. 1 CT scans from two patients at time of admission with prostatic abscesses. A, A 42-year-old patient with multifocal fluid/purulent attenuation locules measuring up to 3 cm in long axis diameter on CT scan with contrast. **B,** A 64-year-old patient with CT scan with contrast demonstrating an enlarged prostate gland with 4.4 × 2.8 × 2.2 cm rim-enhancing collection extending from mid gland to gland apex. (From Wooster ME et al: Prostatic abscess: clinical features, management, and outcomes of a "stealth" infection: retrospective case series and review of the literature, *Diagnostic microbiology and infectious disease* 99(4), 2021, 115285. https://doi.org/10.1016/j.diagmicrobio.2020.115285.)

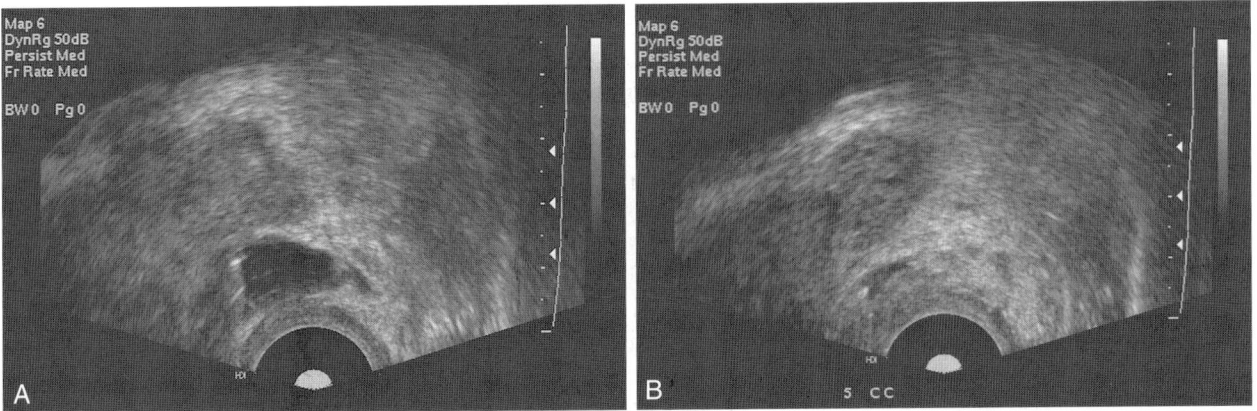

FIG. 2 A, A transrectal sonographic image of a 68-year-old patient with a prostatic abscess that is seen as an irregular hypoechoic collection. **B,** A transrectal sonographic image of the prostate after transrectal drainage of the abscess. The echogenic needle may be seen. (From Soto JA, Lucey BC: *Emergency radiology, the requisites*, ed 2, Philadelphia, 2017, Elsevier.)

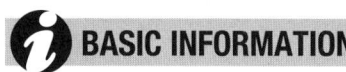
BASIC INFORMATION

DEFINITION

Prostatitis refers to inflammation of the prostate gland. There are four major categories (Table 1):
1. Acute bacterial prostatitis (type I)
2. Chronic bacterial prostatitis (type II)
3. Chronic prostatitis/pelvic pain syndrome (CP/CPPS) (type III): Subdivided into type IIIA (inflammatory) and IIIB (noninflammatory)
4. Asymptomatic inflammatory prostatitis (type IV)

ICD-10CM CODES
N41.0 Acute prostatitis
N41.1 Chronic prostatitis

EPIDEMIOLOGY & DEMOGRAPHICS

- 50% of men will have symptoms of prostatitis in their lifetime.
- Prostatitis accounts for >8% of visits to urologists and 1% of visits to primary care physicians.
- The prevalence of chronic bacterial prostatitis is 5% to 10%.
- CP/CPPS is the most common of the clinically defined prostatitis syndromes, with prevalence ranging from 9% to 12% of men.
- Acute bacterial prostatitis accounts for 10% of all cases of prostatitis.

PHYSICAL FINDINGS & CLINICAL PRESENTATION

- Acute bacterial prostatitis:
  1. Sudden or rapidly progressive onset of:
     a. Dysuria
     b. Frequency
     c. Urgency
     d. Nocturia
     e. Perineal pain that may radiate to the back, rectum, or penis
  2. Hematuria or a purulent urethral discharge may occur.
  3. Occasionally urinary retention complicates the course.
  4. Fever, chills, and signs of sepsis can also be part of the clinical picture.
  5. On rectal examination the prostate is typically tender.
- Chronic bacterial prostatitis:
  1. Characterized by positive culture of expressed prostatic secretions. May cause symptoms such as suprapubic, low back, or perineal pain; mild urgency, frequency, and dysuria with urination; and possibly recurrent urinary tract infections.
  2. May be asymptomatic when the infection is confined to the prostate.
  3. May present as an increase in severity of baseline symptoms of benign prostatic hypertrophy (BPH).
  4. When cystitis is also present, urinary frequency, urgency, and burning may be reported.
  5. Hematuria may be a presenting complaint.
  6. In elderly men, new onset of urinary incontinence may be noted.

- CP/CPPS:
  1. Presents similarly with pain in the pelvic region lasting >3 mo. Symptoms also can include pain in the suprapubic region, low back, penis, testes, or scrotum.
  2. The symptoms can be of variable severity and may include lower urinary tract symptoms, sexual dysfunction, and reduced quality of life.

ETIOLOGY

- Acute bacterial prostatitis:
  1. Acute, usually gram-negative infection of the prostate gland. *Escherichia coli* is the most commonly isolated organism.
     a. Generally associated with cystitis.
     b. Results from the ascent of bacteria into the urethra.
  2. Occasionally the route of infection is hematogenous or a lymphatogenous spread of rectal bacteria.
  3. Consider *Neisseria gonorrhoeae* or *Chlamydia trachomatis* in young patients (age <35 yr) with risk of sexually transmitted disease (STD).
- Chronic bacterial prostatitis:
  1. Often asymptomatic. *E. coli* is the most commonly isolated organism.
  2. Exacerbation of symptoms of BPH caused by the same mechanism as in acute bacterial prostatitis.
- CP/CPPS:
  1. Type IIIA: Refers to symptoms of prostatic inflammation associated with the presence of white blood cells in prostatic secretions with no identifiable bacterial organism.
  2. *Chlamydia* infection may be etiologically implicated in some cases.
  3. Type IIIB: Refers to symptoms of prostatic inflammation with no or few white blood cells in the prostatic secretion. Its cause is multifactorial (Fig. 1).

DIAGNOSIS

DIFFERENTIAL DIAGNOSIS

- BPH with lower urinary tract symptoms
- Prostate cancer
- Interstitial cystitis/bladder pain syndrome
- Pelvic floor dysfunction
- Bladder cancer
- Urolithiasis
- UTI
- Proctitis

WORKUP

- Rectal examination:
  1. Tender prostate most suggestive of acute bacterial prostatitis
  2. Enlarged prostate common in chronic bacterial prostatitis
  3. Normal prostate is consistent with chronic bacterial prostatitis and CP/CPPS
- Expression of prostatic secretions by prostate massage is contraindicated in acute bacterial prostatitis but is appropriate in the other three situations.

LABORATORY TESTS

- Urinalysis
- Urine culture and sensitivity
- Bacterial localization studies can be performed but are cumbersome and impractical in most clinical settings
- Cell count and culture of expressed prostatic secretions
- Prostate-specific antigen (PSA) is not used to diagnose prostatitis and is not recommended unless a nodule is present on digital examination. A rapid rise over baseline should raise the possibility of prostatitis even in the absence of symptoms. In such cases, a follow-up PSA after treatment of prostatitis is appropriate
- CBC and blood cultures if fever, chills, or signs of sepsis exist

TABLE 1 Classification System for the Prostatitis Syndromes

Traditional	National Institutes of Health	Description
Acute bacterial prostatitis	Category I	Acute infection of the prostate gland
Chronic bacterial prostatitis	Category II	Chronic infection of the prostate gland
N/A	Category III Chronic pelvic pain syndrome (CPPS)	Chronic genitourinary pain in the absence of uropathogenic bacteria localized to the prostate gland employing standard methodology
Nonbacterial prostatitis	Category IIIA Inflammatory CPPS	Significant number of white blood cells in expressed prostatic secretions, postprostatic massage urine sediment (VB3), or semen
Prostatodynia	Category IIIB Noninflammatory CPPS	Insignificant number of white blood cells in expressed prostatic secretions, postprostatic massage urine sediment (VB3), or semen
N/A	Category IV Asymptomatic inflammatory prostatitis (AIP)	White blood cells (and/or bacteria) in expressed prostatic secretions, postprostatic massage urine sediment (VB3), semen, or histologic specimens of prostate gland

From Wein AJ et al: *Campbell-Walsh urology*, ed 11, Philadelphia, 2016, Elsevier.

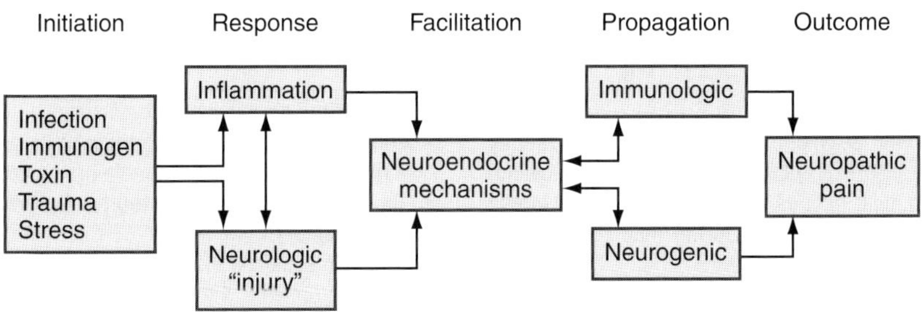

| Initiation | Response | Facilitation | Propagation | Outcome |

FIG. 1 The cause and pathogenesis of chronic prostatitis/chronic pelvic pain syndrome (category III chronic pelvic pain syndrome) appear to involve a pluricausal, multifactorial mechanism. An initiating stimulus, such as infection, reflux of some toxic or immunogenic urine substance, or perineal or pelvic trauma, starts a cascade of events in an anatomically or genetically susceptible man, resulting in a local response of inflammation or neurogenic injury or both. Further interrelated immunologic, neuropathic, endocrinologic, and psychologic mechanisms propagate or sustain the chronicity of the initial (or ongoing) event. The final outcome is the clinical manifestation of chronic perineal or pelvic pain and associated symptoms with local and central neuropathic mechanisms involving areas outside the prostate or pelvic area. (From Wein AJ et al: *Campbell-Walsh urology,* ed 11, Philadelphia, 2016, Elsevier.)

BOX 1 Suggested Therapies for Chronic Prostatitis and Chronic Pelvic Pain Syndrome (National Institutes of Health Category III)

Recommended
1. α-Blocker therapy as part of a multimodal treatment strategy for newly diagnosed, α-blocker–naive patients who have voiding symptoms
2. Antimicrobial therapy trial for selected newly diagnosed, antimicrobial-naive patients
3. Selected phytotherapies: Cernilton and quercetin
4. Multimodal therapy directed by clinical phenotype
5. Directed physiotherapy. Although level 1 evidence is not available, evidence from multiple weak trials and vast clinical experience strongly suggests benefit for selected patients

Not Recommended
1. α-Blocker monotherapy, particularly in patients previously treated with α-blockers
2. Antiinflammatory monotherapy
3. Antimicrobial therapy as primary therapy, particularly for patients in whom treatment with antibiotics has previously failed
4. 5α-Reductase inhibitor monotherapy; can be considered in older patients with coexisting benign prostatic hyperplasia
5. Most minimally invasive therapies such as transurethral needle ablation (TUNA), laser therapies
6. Invasive surgical therapies such as transurethral resection of the prostate (TURP) and radical prostatectomy

Requiring Further Evaluation
1. Low-intensity shock wave treatment
2. Acupuncture
3. Biofeedback
4. Invasive neuromodulation (e.g., pudendal nerve modulation)
5. Electromagnetic stimulation
6. Botulinum toxin A injection
7. Medical therapies including mepartricin, muscle relaxants, neuromodulators, and immunomodulators

Modified from Nickel JC et al: Male chronic pelvic pain syndrome (CPPS). In Chapple C, Abrams P (eds): Male lower urinary tract symptoms (LUTS): an international consultation on male LUTS, Fukuoka, Japan, Sept 30-Oct 4, 2012, Montreal, 2013, Société Internationale d'Urologie. From Wein AJ et al: *Campbell-Walsh urology,* ed 11, Philadelphia, 2016, Elsevier.

Rx TREATMENT

- Acute bacterial prostatitis:
  1. Uncomplicated (with risk of STD, age <35 yr): Ceftriaxone 250 mg IM × 1 dose *or* cefixime 400 mg PO × 1, *then* doxycycline 100 mg bid × 10 days
  2. Uncomplicated with low risk of STD: Levofloxacin 500 mg qid or ciprofloxacin 500 mg bid × 10 to 14 days
- Chronic bacterial prostatitis:
  1. First-line choice is a quinolone (ciprofloxacin or levofloxacin) for 4 wk.
  2. Trimethoprim-sulfamethoxazole (TMP-SMX) is second-line choice for 1 to 3 mo if the organism is sensitive. Tissue penetration for TMP-SMX is not as good as quinolones, and there is evidence of increasing uropathogenic resistance.
- CP/CPPS:
- Suggested therapies for CP/CPPS are summarized in Box 1.

SUGGESTED READINGS
Available at eBooks.Health.Elsevier.com.

RELATED CONTENT
Prostatitis (Patient Information)

AUTHOR: **FRED F. FERRI, MD**

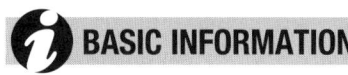

![] BASIC INFORMATION

DEFINITION
Psoriasis is a chronic skin disorder characterized by excessive proliferation of keratinocytes, resulting in the formation of thickened scaly plaques, itching, and inflammatory changes of the epidermis and dermis. Psoriasis is also associated with cardiovascular, metabolic, and neuropsychiatric effects. The various forms of psoriasis include plaque (most common), guttate, erythrodermic, pustular, inverse, and arthritis variants.

ICD-10CM CODES
L40	Psoriasis
L40.0	Psoriasis vulgaris
L40.1	Generalized pustular psoriasis
L40.4	Guttate psoriasis
L40.8	Other psoriasis
L40.9	Psoriasis unspecified
L40.54	Psoriatic juvenile arthropathy

EPIDEMIOLOGY & DEMOGRAPHICS
- Psoriasis affects 2% to 4% of the world's population. Most patients have limited psoriasis involving <5% of their body surface.
- There is a strong association between psoriasis and human leukocyte antigens (HLAs) B13, B17, and B27 (pustular psoriasis).
- Peak age of onset is bimodal (age 30 to 39 yr and at age 60 yr). Mean age at diagnosis is 34 yr.
- Men and women are affected equally. Approximately 20% of patients with psoriasis also have psoriatic arthritis. Median time from development of joint symptoms to diagnosis of psoriatic arthritis is 5 yr. Nail psoriasis affects over 50% of patients with psoriasis and can occur with any of the subtypes.

PHYSICAL FINDINGS & CLINICAL PRESENTATION
- Approximately 67% of patients with psoriasis have mild-to-moderate disease.
- The primary psoriatic lesion is an erythematous papule topped by a loosely adherent scale. Scraping the scale results in several bleeding points *(Auspitz sign)*.
- Chronic plaque psoriasis generally manifests with symmetric, sharply demarcated, erythematous, silver-scaled patches affecting primarily the intergluteal folds, elbows, scalp, fingernails, toenails, and knees (Figs. 1 and 2). This form accounts for 80% of psoriasis cases. Psoriasis may also involve the forehead, particularly contiguous to the scalp (Fig. E3).
- Psoriasis can also develop at the site of any physical trauma (sunburn, scratching). This is known as *Koebner phenomenon.*
- Nail involvement is common (pitting of the nail plate), resulting in hyperkeratosis, onychodystrophy with onycholysis (Fig. E4).
- Pruritus is variable; soreness and bleeding may occur.
- Joint involvement can result in sacroiliitis and spondylitis.

- Guttate psoriasis is generally preceded by streptococcal pharyngitis and manifests with multiple drop-like lesions on the extremities and the trunk.
- Erythrodermic psoriasis is characterized by widespread cutaneous erythema and scaling.
- Pustular psoriasis manifests with widespread pustules. Localized forms may affect palms and soles.
- Inverse psoriasis is characterized by red and sharply demarcated thinner patches involving intertriginous areas (axillae, inguinal areas).
- Adverse effect on psychological and social functioning, with affected persons often feeling stigmatized.

ETIOLOGY
- Unknown, but there is a strong genetic component and high heritability. There are at least nine chromosomal loci with linkage to psoriasis. These loci are called psoriasis susceptibility 1 through 9 (PSORS1-PSORS9). PSORS1 locus in the major histocompatibility complex (MHC) region on chromosome 6 is considered the most important susceptibility locus and is believed to account for 35% to 50% of the heritability of the disease.
- Familial clustering (genetic transmission with a dominant mode with variable penetrants).
- One third of persons affected have a positive family history.
- A high prevalence of celiac disease has been noted in patients with psoriasis.

![] DIAGNOSIS

DIFFERENTIAL DIAGNOSIS
- Contact dermatitis
- Atopic dermatitis
- Stasis dermatitis
- Tinea
- Nummular dermatitis
- Candidiasis
- Mycosis fungoides, Sezary syndrome
- Cutaneous systemic lupus erythematosus
- Secondary and tertiary syphilis

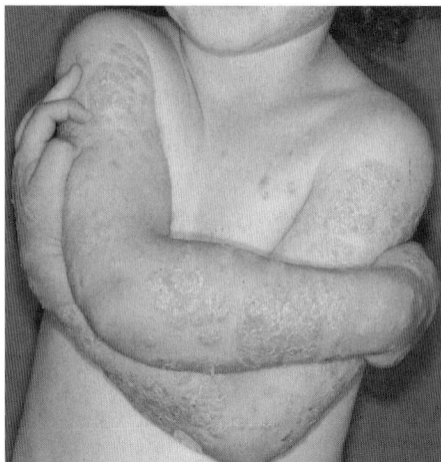

FIG. 1 Psoriasis. Variably sized erythematous plaques with moderately thick overlying scale. (From Paller AS, Mancini AJ: *Hurwitz clinical pediatric dermatology: a textbook of skin disorders of childhood and adolescence*, ed 5, Philadelphia, 2016, Elsevier.)

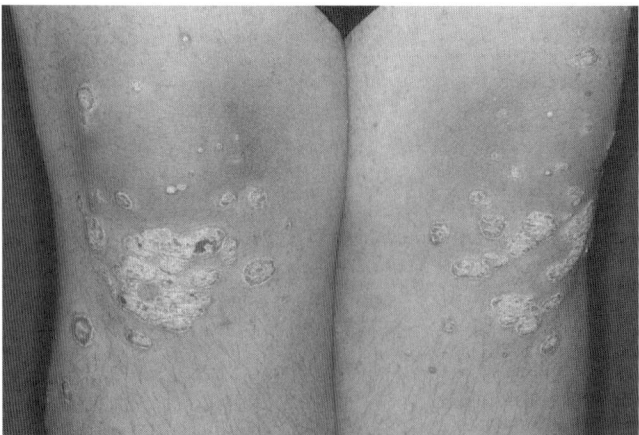

FIG. 2 Typical plaques of psoriasis with thick, micaceous scale overlying erythema. (From Paller AS, Mancini AJ: *Hurwitz clinical pediatric dermatology: a textbook of skin disorders of childhood and adolescence*, ed 5, Philadelphia, 2016, Elsevier.)

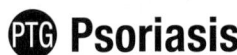

- Drug eruption
- Dermatomyositis (DM)
- Lupus erythematosus (LE)
- Seborrheic dermatitis
- Pityriasis rosea
- Lichen planus
- Pityriasis rubra pilaris

WORKUP

- Diagnosis is clinical. Blood work is rarely needed. A rapid plasma reagin test is useful when ruling out syphilis. Antinuclear antibody (ANA) and anti-Ro and anti-La antibodies are helpful in ruling out subacute cutaneous lupus.
- Skin biopsy is rarely necessary.

LABORATORY TESTS

Generally not necessary for diagnosis.
- Skin biopsy (only if the clinical diagnosis of psoriasis is uncertain)
- Serum electrolytes and calcium for patients with generalized pustular psoriasis (GPP)
- ASO or bacterial cultures for patients with guttate psoriasis
- Appropriate drug-related monitoring for patients on systemic therapies including annual TB testing except for acitretin and apremilast

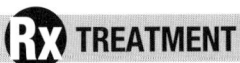 **TREATMENT**

NONPHARMACOLOGIC THERAPY

- Sunbathing generally leads to improvement.
- Eliminate triggering factors (e.g., stress, certain medications [e.g., lithium, β-blockers, antimalarials]). Severe emotional stress tends to aggravate psoriasis.
- Patients with psoriasis benefit from a daily bath in warm water followed by application of a cream or ointment moisturizer. Regular use of an emollient moisturizer limits evaporation of water from the skin and allows the stratum corneum to rehydrate itself.
- Psoralen and ultraviolet A (PUVA) therapy (see "General Rx").
- Local hyperthermia has been used successfully to clear psoriatic plaques, but relapse is common.
- Occlusive treatment with surgical tape or dressings is effective as monotherapy or in combination with topical medications.
- Avoidance of tobacco. Smoking tobacco may worsen psoriasis.

GENERAL Rx

Therapeutic options vary according to the extent of disease and comorbidities. Topical therapies remain the cornerstone for treating mild psoriasis. Approximately 70% to 80% of all patients can be treated adequately with topical therapy.
- Patients with limited disease (<20% of the body) can be treated with the following:
  1. Topical steroids: Disadvantages are brief remissions, expense, and decreased effect with continued use. Salicylic acid can be compounded by pharmacist in concentrations of 2% to 10% and used in combination with a corticosteroid to decrease the amount of scale.

  2. Calcipotriene: A vitamin D analogue effective for moderate plaque psoriasis. Adults should comb the hair, apply solution to the lesions, and rub it in, avoiding uninvolved skin. Disadvantages include its cost and potential burning and skin irritation. It should not be used concurrently with salicylic acid because calcipotriene is inactivated by the acidic nature of salicylic acid. Taclonex ointment and Enstilar aerosol foam formulation are a combination of calcipotriene and the high-potency corticosteroid betamethasone dipropionate. They are well tolerated and more effective than either agent used alone but also much more expensive.
  3. Tar products (Estar, liquor carbonis detergens [LCD], Psorigel) can be used overnight and are most effective when combined with ultraviolet B (UVB) light (Goeckerman regimen).
  4. Anthralin: Useful for chronic plaques; can result in purple-brown staining; best used with UVB light.
  5. Retinoids, such as tazarotene 0.05%, 0.1% cream or gel, are effective in thinning plaques but are expensive and can cause irritation.
  6. Other useful measures include tape or occlusive dressing, UVB and lubricating agents, and interlesional steroids.
- Therapeutic options for persons with generalized disease (affecting >20% of the body) and for those with inadequate response to topical agents:
  1. UVB light exposure three times a wk: This therapy does not require administration of a systemic drug (unlike psoralen plus ultraviolet A [PUVA]), but to be effective, it requires removal of scale with keratolytic agents and emollients.
  2. Oral PUVA administered two to three times weekly is effective for generalized disease. It is often considered in patients for whom narrow-band UVB therapy is ineffective. However, many PUVA treatments are required, necessitating frequent office visits, and it may be associated with phototoxicity, such as erythema and blistering, and increased risk of skin cancer.
- Systemic treatments include methotrexate 25 mg/wk for severe psoriasis. Etretinate (a synthetic retinoid) is most effective for palmarplantar pustular psoriasis. Dose is 0.5 to 1 mg/kg/day. It can cause liver enzyme and lipid abnormalities and is teratogenic.
- Apremilast is a phosphodiesterase type-4 inhibitor used in moderate to severe plaque psoriasis. Side effects include diarrhea, nausea, headache, and worsening depression.
- Cyclosporine is also effective in severe psoriasis; however, relapses are common.
- Chronic plaque psoriasis may be treated with alefacept, a recombinant protein that selectively targets T lymphocytes. Treatment with alefacept for 12 wk (0.025, 0.075, or 0.150 mg/kg of body weight intravenous (IV) weekly) may result in significant improvement. Some patients also demonstrate a sustained

clinical response after the cessation of treatment. This medication is very expensive (a 12-wk course can cost >$8000).
- Tapinarof (Vtama), 1% cream formulation, has been FDA approved for treatment of adults with plaque psoriasis.
- Biologic therapies are now routinely used when traditional systemic agents are ineffective or poorly tolerated. Screening for tuberculosis is necessary before initiating treatment with these agents. Active, serious infection is a contraindication to the use of biologics.
- Tumor necrosis factor (TNF) inhibitors (adalimumab [Humira], etanercept [Enbrel], infliximab [Remicade]): Trials revealed a reduction in severity of plaque psoriasis. Efalizumab, a humanized monoclonal antibody that inhibits the activation of T cells, has also been reported to produce significant improvement in plaque psoriasis treatment period. Adalimumab has been reported to be effective for joint and skin manifestations of psoriasis.
- Newer biologic agents in patients with moderate to severe plaque psoriasis are ustekinumab (Stelara; an interleukin-12 and interleukin-23 blocker), brodalumab (SILIQ), ixekizumab (Taltz), secukinumab (Cosentyx) antiinterleukin-17 receptor antagonists, and guselkumab (Tremfya), risankizumab (Skyrizi), and tildrakizumab (ILUMYA) interleukin-23 blockers. Cost is a limiting factor with all these agents.
- The topical PDE4 inhibitor Roflumilast has been approved for plaque psoriasis.

DISPOSITION

The course of psoriasis is chronic, and the disease may be refractory to treatment.

REFERRAL

- Dermatology referral is recommended in all patients with generalized disease.
- Hospital admission may be necessary for severe diffuse or poorly responsive psoriasis. The Goeckerman regimen combines daily application of tar with UVB exposure and can result in prolonged remissions.

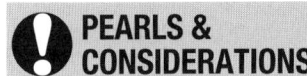 **PEARLS & CONSIDERATIONS**

COMMENTS

Psoriasis is more emotionally than physically disabling for most patients. Counseling may be indicated, particularly when it affects younger patients.

SUGGESTED READINGS

Available at eBooks.Health.Elsevier.com.

RELATED CONTENT

Psoriasis (Patient Information)
Psoriatic Arthritis (Related Key Topic)

AUTHOR: **FRED F. FERRI, MD**

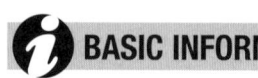
ℹ️ BASIC INFORMATION

DEFINITION

Psoriatic arthritis (PsA) is an inflammatory arthropathy, often included in a class of disorders called the *seronegative spondyloarthropathies (SpA)*, a family of diseases characterized by inflammation of the spine, peripheral joints, and entheses (sites of insertion of tendon into bone).[1] Both the Moll and Wright and CASPAR classification criteria are described in Table 1.

ICD-10CM CODES

L40.5+ Arthropathic psoriasis
L40.54 Psoriatic juvenile arthropathy
L40.52 Psoriatic arthritis mutilans

EPIDEMIOLOGY & DEMOGRAPHICS

INCIDENCE: Three to seven per 100,000 per year[2]
PREVALENCE: One to two per 1000 in the general population.[3] Variable estimates of 4% to 30% of patients with underlying psoriasis[3]
PREDOMINANT SEX: Equal male-to-female distribution[3]
PREDOMINANT AGE: Symptom onset generally between age 30 to 55, although it can begin during childhood[4]

PHYSICAL FINDINGS & CLINICAL PRESENTATION

- Psoriasis precedes arthritis in 67% of cases by an average of 8 to 10 years.[5]
- Arthritis precedes psoriasis or occurs concomitantly in 33% of patients.[5]
  1. There is a weak relationship between the severity of skin disease and arthritic involvement, with only a minority of patients noting a relationship between the activity of the skin and joint manifestations.
- Arthritis, dactylitis, spondylitis, and enthesitis are the main features.[6]

- Arthritis is inflammatory and commonly characterized by prolonged morning stiffness, improvement with activity, joint erythema, warmth, or swelling.[3]
- There are five classically described patterns of joint involvement (Box 1).
- Some patients may present with more than one pattern, which can evolve over time.[3] The distal interphalangeal (DIP) joints (Fig. E1) and spine are each affected in 40% to 50% of cases. It is rare to have spondyloarthritis alone, and it usually occurs with peripheral involvement.[3]
- Dactylitis, also known as "sausage digit," refers to diffuse swelling of a finger or toe (Fig. E2); it is fairly common and occurs in approximately 30% to 40% of patients during the disease course.[7] It is associated with increased risk of radiographic joint damage.[7]
- Enthesitis commonly occurs at the Achilles tendon and plantar fascia (Fig. E3), and swelling and tenderness may be seen upon exam.[6] Subclinical disease may be evident by ultrasonography.[3]
- Dystrophic changes of the nails (pitting, onycholysis, and leukonychia) may occur in association with joint inflammation in involved digits.[6]
- Spondyloarthritis may include sacroiliitis but is generally less likely to cause fusion to the extent seen in ankylosing spondylitis.[3] It is more common to have asymmetric sacroiliac joint involvement (usually bilateral in ankylosing spondylitis).[3]
- Ocular inflammation including conjunctivitis and uveitis can be seen.[7]

ETIOLOGY

Experts theorize the cause of PsA to be an interplay of genetic, immunologic, and environmental factors. Fig. 4 illustrates the pathogenetic pathways in PsA. There is a higher frequency of HLA-B12, HLA-B17, HLA-B57, HLA-Cw*0602 in PsA. Those with PsA versus psoriasis alone have higher frequency of HLA-B27.[6]

Dx DIAGNOSIS
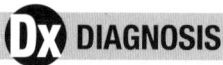

DIFFERENTIAL DIAGNOSIS

- Rheumatoid arthritis (Table 2)
- Erosive osteoarthritis
- Crystalline arthritis, including gout and pseudogout
- Other seronegative spondyloarthropathies, which include reactive arthritis, enteropathic arthritis, and ankylosing spondylitis (also see "Differential Diagnosis of Psoriatic Arthritis" in Section III)

WORKUP

- Diagnosis is generally made on clinical grounds based on history, exam, and radiographic findings given lack of specific lab findings. An algorithm for the diagnosis of PsA is described in Fig. 5.
- Early diagnosis can be difficult to establish when the joint symptoms develop before skin and nail findings.[7]

BOX 1   Subtypes of Psoriatic Arthritis

- Distal interphalangeal joint–predominant arthritis (10%)
- Symmetric polyarthritis–predominant arthritis (5%-20%)
- Asymmetric oligoarthritis or monoarthritis (70%-80%)
- Axial disease predominant (spondylitis, sacroiliitis, or both) (5%-20%)
- Arthritis mutilans (rare)

From Hochberg MC: *Rheumatology*, ed 7, Philadelphia, 2019, Elsevier.

TABLE 1   Classifications of Psoriatic Arthritis

| Moll and Wright | Points | CASPAR* | |
		Category	Description
Presence of PsO and an inflammatory arthritis (peripheral arthritis and/or sacroiliitis or spondylitis)	2	Current PsO	Psoriatic skin or scalp disease confirmed by a dermatologist or rheumatologist; history of PsO from the patient, family physician, dermatologist, rheumatologist, or other qualified practitioner; patient-reported history of PsO in a first- or second-degree relative
The (usual) absence of serologic tests for RF	1	Personal or family history of PsO	
	1	Psoriatic nail dystrophy on current physical examination	Includes onycholysis, pitting, and hyperkeratosis
	1	Negative test for RF	ELISA or nephelometry preferred (no latex) using the local laboratory reference range
	1	Current dactylitis or history of dactylitis documented by a rheumatologist	Swelling of the entire digit
	1	Radiographic evidence of juxtaarticular new bone formation	Ill-defined ossification near joint margins in the hand or foot, excluding osteophyte formation on plain radiographs

CASPAR, Classification Criteria for the Study of Psoriatic Arthritis; *ELISA*, enzyme-linked immunosorbent assay; *PsO*, psoriasis; *RF*, rheumatoid factor.
*Psoriatic arthritis is diagnosed when three or more points are assigned in the presence of inflammatory articular disease (joint, spine, or entheseal).
From Hochberg MC: *Rheumatology*, ed 7, Philadelphia, 2019, Elsevier.

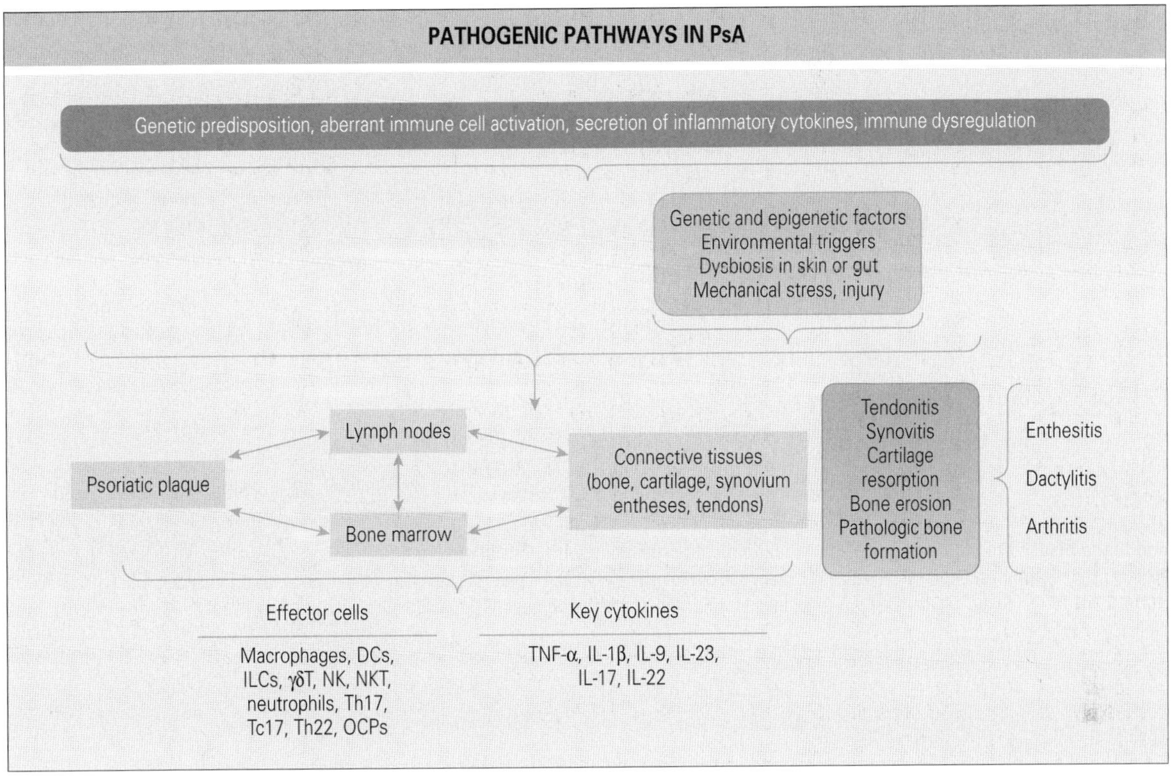

PATHOGENIC PATHWAYS IN PsA

Genetic predisposition, aberrant immune cell activation, secretion of inflammatory cytokines, immune dysregulation

Genetic and epigenetic factors
Environmental triggers
Dysbiosis in skin or gut
Mechanical stress, injury

Lymph nodes

Psoriatic plaque

Bone marrow

Connective tissues
(bone, cartilage, synovium
entheses, tendons)

Tendonitis
Synovitis
Cartilage
resorption
Bone erosion
Pathologic bone
formation

Enthesitis

Dactylitis

Arthritis

Effector cells

Macrophages, DCs,
ILCs, γδT, NK, NKT,
neutrophils, Th17,
Tc17, Th22, OCPs

Key cytokines

TNF-α, IL-1β, IL-9, IL-23,
IL-17, IL-22

FIG. 4 Activation of Th1 and Th17 immune cells in genetically predisposed individuals by an array of poorly defined environmental factors results in psoriatic plaque formation. In a subset of patients with psoriasis, epigenetic and environmental events in patients with specific genetic risk variants result in musculoskeletal inflammation in an array of connective tissues. Effector cells release cytokines that promote inflammation in tendon–ligament–synovial capsule insertion sites, tendons, synovium, and bone. This is accompanied by bone and cartilage damage and pathologic new bone formation. The resulting clinical phenotypes manifest as enthesitis, synovitis, and dactylitis. *DC,* Dendritic cell; *IL,* interleukin; *ILC,* innate lymphocyte; *NK,* natural killer; *OCP,* osteoclast precursors; *PsA,* psoriatic arthritis; *Tc17,* CD8+ IL-17 secreting cell; *Th17,* CD4+ IL-17 secreting cell; *Th22,* IL-22 secreting CD4+ cell; *TNF,* tumor necrosis factor. (From Hochberg MC: *Rheumatology,* ed 7, Philadelphia, 2019, Elsevier.)

TABLE 2 Clinical Features That Distinguish Psoriatic Arthritis From Rheumatoid Arthritis

	Psoriatic Arthritis	Rheumatoid Arthritis
Psoriasis	+	−
Symmetric	+	++
Asymmetric	++	+
Enthesopathy	+	−
Dactylitis	+	−
Nail dystrophy	+	−
HIV association	+	−

From Firestein GS et al: *Firestein & Kelley's textbook of rheumatology,* ed 11, Philadelphia, 2021, Elsevier.

LABORATORY TESTS

- No specific diagnostic lab tests.
- Acute phase reactants such as erythrocyte sedimentation rate (ESR) and C-reactive protein (CRP) may be elevated, although less commonly than in patients with rheumatoid arthritis.[6,8]
- Anemia of chronic disease may be seen.[9]

- Rheumatoid factor (RF) and anti-CCP are generally negative but can be present in up to 10% of patients.[10,11]
- *HLA-B27* is significantly more common in patients with axial inflammation.[6]
- Arthrocentesis generally demonstrates inflammatory synovial fluid without crystals.[7]

IMAGING STUDIES

- Radiographic findings of involved joints may include soft tissue swelling, joint space narrowing, subluxation, erosive changes, and new bone formation (periostitis, fusion). As opposed to rheumatoid arthritis, patients with PsA see more asymmetric joint involvement and DIP joint changes.[8]
- Severe digital erosive change with adjacent heterotopic bone formation may give rise to "pencil in cup" deformity.[7] Whittling of the phalanges may occur.
- With axial involvement, sacroiliac joint changes (sclerosis, erosions, pseudowidening, ankylosis) and bridging vertebral syndesmophytes may be present.[3,6]
- Musculoskeletal ultrasonography can be used in the evaluation of enthesitis or arthritis.[3]
- MRI may be helpful in further evaluation of sacroiliac and spinal involvement.[7]

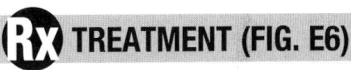

Rx TREATMENT (FIG. E6)

PHARMACOLOGIC THERAPY

The choice of therapeutic agent depends on the type of clinical manifestations, as not all agents are effective for all manifestations. For example, enthesis and spinal involvement are not responsive to traditional oral disease-modifying agents such as methotrexate or leflunomide but are responsive to tumor necrosis factor blocking agents (TNFi).[8]

- NSAIDs may be used for mild or limited disease.[8]
- Intraarticular corticosteroid injections can be used as adjunctive Rx for involved joints.[12]
- Oral glucocorticoids should generally be avoided, given increased risk for development of erythrodermic or pustular psoriasis.[8]
- In patients with active peripheral joint disease, elevated acute phase reactants, or evidence of changes on imaging, traditional DMARDs such as methotrexate, sulfasalazine, and leflunomide should be considered early on. However, data supporting their use is limited.[8]
- Apremilast is an oral phosphodiesterase 4 (PDE 4) inhibitor and is safe to use, especially

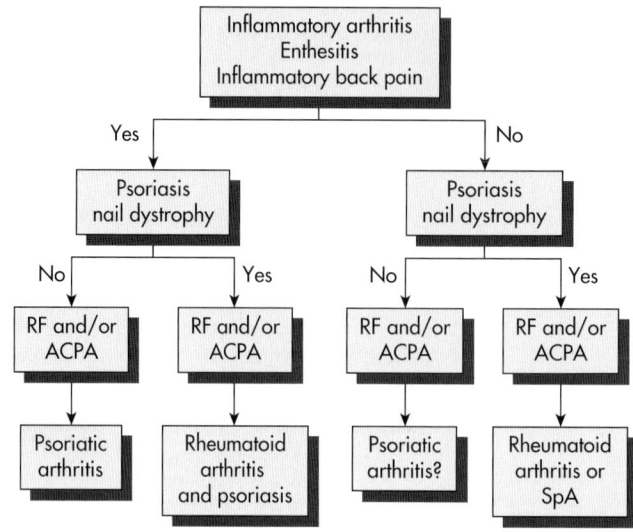

FIG. 5 Algorithm to be used in the diagnosis of individual patients presenting with possible psoriatic arthritis. Some patients may present with typical articular manifestations of psoriatic arthritis, but in the absence of skin or nail disease. They can be diagnosed as having definite psoriatic arthritis only when psoriasis subsequently develops. *ACPA,* Anticitrullinated protein antibody; *RF,* rheumatoid factor; *SpA,* spondyloarthropathy. (From Firestein GS et al: *Firestein & Kelly's textbook of rheumatology,* ed 11, Philadelphia, 2021, Elsevier.)

in those with multiple comorbidities. Apremilast may also be beneficial for enthesitis and dactylitis.[8]

- In patients with peripheral arthritis who fail to respond to nonbiologic DMARDs, escalation of therapy should be considered. All five TNFi's (etanercept, infliximab, adalimumab, golimumab, certolizumab pegol) are FDA-approved to treat PsA. In those resistant to one TNFi, a second TNFi can be considered. If adequate response is still not achieved, a different mechanism of action (interleukin [IL]-17i, IL-12/23 blockade) can be considered.[13,14]

- Secukinumab, an IL-17 inhibitor, is approved to treat psoriasis, PsA, and ankylosing spondylitis (AS). Ixekizumab, an anti-IL-17 monoclonal antibody, can also be used to treat psoriasis, PsA, and AS. Brodalumab, an anti-IL-17RA monoclonal antibody, treats psoriasis alone currently. Guselkumab, an anti-IL-23 antibody, has recently been approved to treat PsA.[12]

- Ustekinumab is a human immunoglobulin G (IgG) monoclonal antibody that binds to the p40 subunit of IL-12 and IL-23 and is approved to treat psoriasis, PsA, and Crohn disease.[12]

- Abatacept (selective T-cell costimulation modulator) was approved to treat PsA but has shown limited efficacy in treatment of psoriasis. It can be used to treat peripheral arthritis. Tofacitinib (oral Janus kinase inhibitor) has also been approved.[8]

- In patients with predominantly axial disease not responsive to NSAIDs, TNFi or IL17i can be considered. For enthesitis and dactylitis, TNFi, IL-17i, IL-12/23, or apremilast can be considered.[8]

REFERRAL

Rheumatology, dermatology

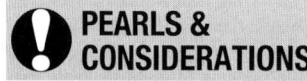 **PEARLS & CONSIDERATIONS**

COMMENTS

- Patients frequently have a positive family history of psoriasis or PsA.

- In addition to pharmacotherapy, patient education regarding the importance of controlling inflammation with lifestyle modifications such as smoking cessation, weight reduction, joint protection, physical activity, exercise, and stress management is vital for treatment.

REFERENCES

Available at eBooks.Health.Elsevier.com

RELATED CONTENT

Psoriatic Arthritis (Patient Information)

AUTHORS: **KENNY CHANG, BS,** and **MANUEL F. DASILVA, MD**

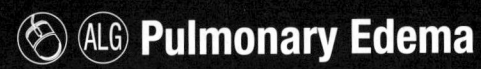
Diseases
and Disorders

I

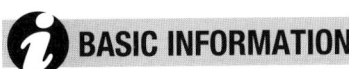 BASIC INFORMATION

DEFINITION

Acute cardiogenic pulmonary edema (ACPE) is a clinically observed consequence of increased capillary leakage of fluid into the interstitial space in the pulmonary vasculature, resulting in the constellation of clinical signs and symptoms of decreased gaseous exchange in the alveoli.[1]

SYNONYMS

ACPE
ADHF
CPE
Cardiogenic pulmonary edema (CPE)
Acute cardiogenic pulmonary edema (ACPE)
Acute decompensated heart failure (ADHF) with pulmonary edema
Acute diastolic heart failure with pulmonary edema
Acute systolic heart failure with pulmonary edema
Acute combined heart failure with pulmonary edema

ICD-10CM CODES
J81.0 Acute pulmonary edema
J81.1 Chronic pulmonary edema
I50.1 Left ventricular failure
J68.1 Pulmonary edema due to chemicals, gases, fumes and vapors

EPIDEMIOLOGY & DEMOGRAPHICS

- The prevalence of heart failure (HF) is estimated around 6.5 million people in the U.S. and about 23 million people globally. In the U.S. this number is expected to increase to 8 million by the year 2030.[2]
- In 2012, 1.7 million HF-related visits to U.S. physician offices, and half a million emergency department visits were reported.
- Approximately 20% of all-cause admissions in the age group older than 65 was related to HF.
- Within 30 days, 25% to 30% of these patients are readmitted with recurrent ADHF.
- In-hospital mortality rate is 10% to 20%, particularly when associated with acute myocardial infarction (MI).

PHYSICAL FINDINGS & CLINICAL PRESENTATION

- Hypertension (in cardiogenic shock could be hypotensive)
- Tachycardia
- Elevated jugular venous pressure with hepatojugular reflex
- Bilateral pulmonary rales/decreased or pleural effusions
- S3 gallop/S4 and/or laterally displaced apex
- Abdominal distention/ascites
- Peripheral edema
- Cold and clammy skin
- Weight gain
- Altered mental status
- Dyspnea (exertional or at rest, paroxysmal nocturnal dyspnea, orthopnea)
- Cough and wheezing (cardiac asthma)
- Diaphoresis
- Perioral and peripheral cyanosis

- Pink, frothy sputum

ETIOLOGY

Common causes of acute pulmonary edema include:
- Acute MI
- Poor dietary compliance or medication nonadherence
- Atrial and ventricular arrhythmias
- Valvular heart disease (mitral, aortic, tricuspid, and pulmonary valve disease)
- Renal and liver disease
- Endocrine (thyrotoxicosis, obesity, metabolic syndrome, diabetes)
- Toxin mediated (cocaine, alcohol, chemotherapy agents, ephedra)
- Peripartum cardiomyopathy/HF of pregnancy
- Infections (myopericarditis, endocarditis, HIV, Chagas)
- Uncontrolled hypertension
- Structural heart disease (ventricular septal defect, infiltrative heart disease, hypertrophic cardiomyopathy)
- Pulmonary embolism
- Postcardioversion syndrome
   Box 1 summarizes common causes of cardiogenic and noncardiogenic pulmonary edema.

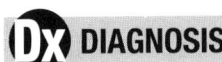 DIAGNOSIS

DIFFERENTIAL DIAGNOSIS

- Noncardiogenic pulmonary edema (Fig. 1 and Table 1)
- Viral pneumonitis including COVID 19[3] and other pulmonary infections

---

BOX 1 Common Causes of Cardiogenic and Noncardiogenic Pulmonary Edema

- Acute exacerbation of heart failure
- Acute valve dysfunction (e.g., mitral valve chordae tendineae rupture)
- Arrhythmia/myocardial infarction
- Hypertensive crisis
- Fluid overload following aggressive volume resuscitation (e.g., postoperative)
- Ventricular septal rupture
- Pericardial tamponade

Noncardiogenic Pulmonary Edema
- Direct lung injury
   1. Pneumonia
   2. Gastric aspiration
   3. Toxic inhalation
   4. Negative pressure related (e.g., strangulation)
- Indirect causes of lung injury
   1. Sepsis
   2. Trauma
   3. Pancreatitis
   4. Multiple blood transfusions
   5. Burn injury
Cardiogenic Pulmonary Edema

From Vincent JL et al: *Textbook of critical care*, ed 7, Philadelphia, 2017, Elsevier.

- Pulmonary embolism
- Exacerbation of asthma/chronic obstructive pulmonary disease
- High-altitude pulmonary edema (HAPE)
- Sarcoidosis
- Pulmonary fibrosis
- Lymphangitic carcinomatosis

LABORATORY TESTS

1. Arterial blood gases (ABGs): Respiratory and metabolic acidosis, decreased PaO_2, increased $PaCO_2$, low pH. (NOTE: The patient may initially show respiratory alkalosis as a result of hyperventilation in attempts to maintain PaO_2.)
2. B-type natriuretic peptide (BNP) and NT-pro BNP add diagnostic value to the history and physical examination as evidenced in the Breathing Not Properly (BNP) study.
3. Cardiac biomarkers: Troponin T or I if suspicion for acute coronary syndrome.
4. Basic metabolic profile: Assess for electrolyte abnormalities and kidney function.
5. Elevated liver function tests (LFTs) are indicative of congestive hepatopathy or shock liver.
6. Serology for suspected inciting agents, including HIV, Chagas, adenovirus, enterovirus, parvovirus, herpes virus, and more recently the novel Coronavirus disease (COVID-19).[3]
7. CBC: Anemia can trigger acute pulmonary edema.
8. Glucose, HgbA1c, fasting lipid profile, thyroid-stimulating hormone (TSH) for risk stratification.
9. Urinalysis and urine toxicology if indicated.
10. Genetic testing for unexplained cardiomyopathies.[4]

IMAGING STUDIES
NONINVASIVE IMAGING:

- ECG: May elucidate the etiology of pulmonary edema. Causes may include ischemia/infarct, arrhythmias, left ventricular (LV) hypertrophy, and atrial enlargement.
- Chest x-ray (Fig. 2):
   1. Bilateral interstitial and alveolar infiltrates
   2. Cephalization of the pulmonary vessels
   3. Kerley B lines; fluffy perihilar infiltrates
   4. Pleural effusions
   5. Enlarged cardiac silhouette
- Echocardiogram:
   1. Assess left and right ventricular systolic/diastolic function.
   2. Structural abnormalities (VSD, LV rupture).
   3. Evaluate valvular abnormalities including endocarditis.
   4. Engorged inferior vena cava (IVC) and IVC plethora, based on bedside ultrasound, suggests elevated filling pressures.
- Computed tomography (CT) of the chest; may differentiate between cardiogenic and noncardiogenic pulmonary edema.
- Lung ultrasound (LUS) has emerged as a tool to diagnose pulmonary edema. It is easy to use, accessible, and noninvasive, and has a high negative predictive value. Positive

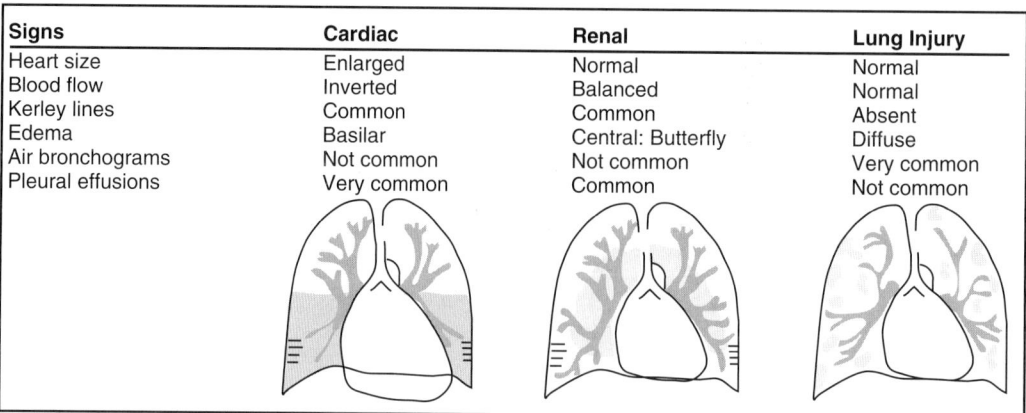

Signs	Cardiac	Renal	Lung Injury
Heart size	Enlarged	Normal	Normal
Blood flow	Inverted	Balanced	Normal
Kerley lines	Common	Common	Absent
Edema	Basilar	Central: Butterfly	Diffuse
Air bronchograms	Not common	Not common	Very common
Pleural effusions	Very common	Common	Not common

FIG. 1 Types of pulmonary edema. (From Weissleder R et al: *Primer of diagnostic imaging,* St Louis, 2007, Mosby.)

TABLE 1 Distinguishing Cardiogenic and Noncardiogenic Pulmonary Edema

	History	Exam	Labs	Imaging	Pulmonary Artery Catheter
Cardiogenic	Heart disease Renal disease Uncontrolled HTN Edema Orthopnea Recent administration of IV fluids or blood products	Heart failure exam findings: Distended neck veins S3 heart sound Dependent edema Elevated blood pressure Cool extremities	↑BNP >1200 pg/ml ↑Creatinine (in setting of volume overload) ↑Troponin	CXR: CMG pleural effusions Kerley B lines TEE: ↓LVEF Diastolic filling defect Severe mitral or aortic valvular disease Pericardial effusion with tamponade VSD	PCWP >18 mm Hg Prominent V-waves (mitral regurgitation) Elevation and equilibration of right atrial pressure, pulmonary artery diastolic and PCWP (tamponade physiology) CVP >12 mm Hg
Noncardiogenic	Sepsis Aspiration event Trauma (long bone fractures) Burn injury Pancreatitis Multiple transfusions	Signs of active infection Extensive burn injury Evidence of trauma (absence of heart failure exam findings)	↑WBC BNP <200 pg/ml	CXR: Diffuse central and peripheral infiltrates Normal heart size No or minimal pleural effusions TEE: Normal LV and valvular function No evidence of volume overload	PCWP <18 mm Hg CVP <12 mm Hg

BNP, Brain natriuretic peptide; *CVP,* central venous pressure; *CXR,* chest x-ray; *HTN,* hypertension; *IV,* intravenous; *LVEF,* left ventricle ejection fraction; *PCWP,* pulmonary capillary wedge pressure; *S3,* third heart sound; *TEE,* transesophageal echocardiogram; *VSD,* ventricular septal defect; *WBC,* white blood count.
From Vincent JL et al: *Textbook of critical care,* ed 7, Philadelphia, 2017, Elsevier.

predictive value for LUS is slightly lower, but LUS remains a versatile, easily accessible and reliable tool at points of triage.[1] Kerley B lines and pleural effusions are highly suggestive of pulmonary edema.[5-7]

INVASIVE IMAGING:
- Right heart catheterization (RHC): Obtain estimated filling pressures, assess cardiac output, differentiate between different shocks, and use to guide tailored inotropic and pressor therapy. Despite the widespread availability of Swan-Ganz catheters the ESCAPE trial failed to demonstrate the utility of pulmonary artery catheters in acute decompensated HF.
- Coronary angiogram: Rule out acute MI/progressive coronary artery disease.
- Left heart catheterization (LHC): Measure left ventricular end-diastolic pressure (LVEDP) to estimate left-sided filling pressure.

- CardioMEMS (St. Jude Medical) is an invasive pulmonary artery pressure monitoring device that can provide remote monitoring capability and aid in reduction of frequency of HF hospitalizations.[2]

ⓇⓍ TREATMENT

ACUTE GENERAL Rx (Fig. 3)
Nonpharmacologic treatment:
- Sodium restriction in American College of Cardiology (ACC)/American Heart Association (AHA) class C and D HF patients has conflicting data.
- Restrict 1.5 to 2 L of free water in the setting of hyponatremia.
- Risk factor modification (blood pressure [BP] and glucose control, dietary modifications).
- Oxygen supplementation if signs of hypoxia are present.

- Noninvasive ventilation (continuous positive airway pressure [CPAP]) or bilevel noninvasive positive-pressure ventilation [NPPV]) reduces dyspnea and may reduce the need for endotracheal intubation. Positive pressure ventilation (invasive or noninvasive) decreases preload and afterload and reduces the work of breathing, while positive end expiratory pressure improves oxygenation.
- HF teaching.

Pharmacologic Treatment:
- Loop diuretics such as furosemide, torsemide, bumetanide, and ethacrynic acid are the cornerstones of the treatment of volume overload. Intravenous treatment might be required in acute pulmonary edema due to coexistent gut edema that is a barrier to effective GI absorption. There is no difference in symptoms or kidney function whether the diuretic is given as a bolus or continuous infusion (DOSE trial;

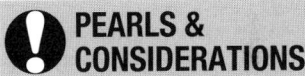

FIG. 2 Pulmonary edema. A, Anterior-posterior chest x-ray. **B,** Close-up from **A.** This 53-yr-old woman with end-stage renal disease missed dialysis and presented to the emergency department. Her examination demonstrated bilateral rales. Her x-ray shows mild cardiomegaly, bilateral interstitial opacities, and cephalization of the pulmonary vascular markings. The minor fissure appears thickened. These findings are consistent with pulmonary edema. In addition, peribronchial cuffing is present. As discussed elsewhere, this is a nonspecific thickening of the bronchial wall that can occur from edema in the setting of heart failure, asthma, viral illness, or even infections such as pertussis. The thickened wall appears white, whereas the air-filled bronchiole appears black and has a circular short-axis cross section. (From Broder JS: *Diagnostic imaging for the emergency physician,* Philadelphia, 2011, Saunders.)

New England Journal of Medicine, March 3, 2011).[8]
- Nitrates: Particularly useful if the patient has concomitant chest pain or is hypertensive.
  1. Nitroglycerin: 0.4 to 0.8 mg sublingual (SL) or nitroglycerin spray may be given immediately on arrival and repeated every 5 min up to three times if the patient remains symptomatic and BP remains stable.
  2. 2% nitroglycerin ointment: 1 to 3 inches out of the tube applied continuously; absorption may be erratic.
  3. IV nitroglycerin for refractory chest pain and hypertension: Start at 0.2 to 0.4 mcg/kg/min.
- Nitroprusside is useful for afterload reduction in severe hypertension, acute mitral regurgitation, or acute aortic regurgitation.
  1. Start at low-dose 0.5 μg/kg/min with an arterial line in place.
  2. Monitor for cyanide toxicity.
- ACE inhibitors, angiotensin II receptor blockers, aldosterone antagonist, and angiotensin receptor–neprilysin inhibitors are vasodilators with long-term mortality benefit in patients with HF with reduced ejection fraction.[4,9,10]
- In patients with HF with reduced ejection fraction, with and without type 2 diabetes, SGLT2 inhibitors decrease frequency of hospitalization for HF, an urgent visit resulting in intravenous therapy for HF, or death from

cardiovascular causes (EMPA-REG OUTCOME, DAPA HF trial). They can be initiated before discharge during acute hospitalizations for ADHF.
- Ultrafiltration/aquapheresis if diuretic resistant.
- Morphine was previously thought to be beneficial in patients with ACPE, but recent data suggested that it can be detrimental with increase in rates of in hospital mortality, increased need for invasive and noninvasive ventilation, and increased need for pressors/inotropes.[11]

Pharmacologic-vasopressors:
- Patients with profound hypotension benefit from vasopressors.
  1. Norepinephrine: Powerful vasoconstrictor with small inotropic effect.[12]
  2. Dopamine: Low doses (0.5 to 3 μg/kg/min) increase blood flow to coronary, renal, and cerebral beds. Intermediate doses (3 to 10 μg/kg/min) increase cardiac contractility while high doses (10 to 20 μg/kg/min) have a pressor effect.

Pharmacologic-inotropes:
- Dobutamine: Potent inotrope, mild chronotropic effects. Dose ranges from 2.5 to 20 mcg/kg/min.
- Phosphodiesterase inhibitors (amrinone, milrinone, and enoximone [not available in U.S.]) may be useful in refractory cases.

Mechanical support:
- Intraaortic balloon pump (IABP): Decreases afterload, increases coronary blood flow.

- Impella: Axial-flow pump on a pigtail catheter that crosses the aortic valve and unloads the left ventricle.
- Tandem heart device: Oxygenated blood is pumped from the left atrium into the femoral artery. It can provide 3.5 to 4.5 L/min of cardiac output.
- Extracorporeal membrane oxygenation (ECMO) as a bridge to heart transplant or recovery.
- Durable mechanical circulatory support such as left ventricular assist device can be considered for those in cardiogenic shock refractory to medical therapy.

DISPOSITION
Admit to intensive care unit (ICU)/critical care unit (CCU) if:
- Need for intubation
- Signs and symptoms of hypoperfusion/shock
- SpO_2 <90% despite supplemental oxygen
- Use of accessory muscles/respiratory rate (RR) >25/min
- Heart rate <40 or >130, systolic BP <90

ⓘ PEARLS & CONSIDERATIONS

- ACPE is the outcome of decompensation of mechanical function of the heart due to variable etiologies
- Accurate identification of etiology and prompt steps in management concurrent to management of pulmonary edema itself can improve outcomes
- Use of bedside LUS or other easily accessible noninvasive and reliable methods to be used in rapid diagnosis to facilitate early initiation of therapy
- Choice of pharmacologic agents on case-by-case basis depending on etiology. Early use of mechanical support in addition if indicated
- Emphasis to be placed on patient education and utilization of quality metrics after discharge as well as continued follow-up in the outpatient setting.

COMMENTS
Accumulated evidence still favors the use of noninvasive ventilation, especially CPAP, in patients with ACPE, especially as this therapy reduces dyspnea and helps correct metabolic abnormalities more rapidly than standard oxygen therapy. The role of morphine in the treatment of ACPE has come into question.

REFERENCES
Available at eBooks.Health.Elsevier.com.

RELATED CONTENT
Heart Failure (Related Key Topic)

AUTHOR: **GEMINI YESODHARAN, MD**

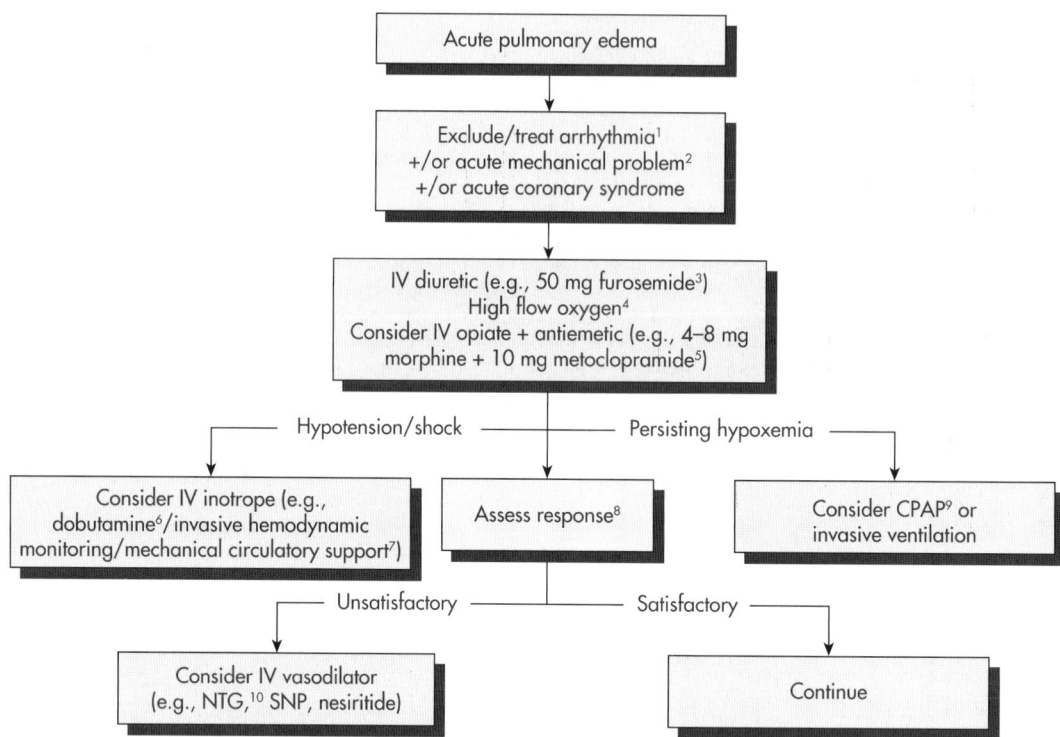

¹ Casual arrhythmia (e.g., ventricular tachycardia). It can be difficult to determine whether atrial fibrillation is a primary cause of acute pulmonary edema or secondary to it. An ECG is an essential investigation.

² Acute mechanical problems include ventricular septal rupture and mitral valve papillary muscle rupture. Mechanical support (e.g., an intraaortic balloon pump) and urgent surgery should be considered. An echocardiogram should be performed as soon as possible, especially in a patient without a prior diagnosis of heart failure/other relevant heart disease (e.g., prior myocardial infarction or valve disease).

³ Dose of diuretic depends on prior diuretic use and renal function—a lower dose may suffice if preserved renal function and no prior diuretic use.

⁴ Oxygen causes an increase in systemic vascular resistance and a reduction in heart rate and cardiac output and should only be administered to patients with hypoxemia.

⁵ Consider if patient is agitated/distressed/in pain; may cause respiratory depression and dose should be reduced in very elderly.

⁶ An intravenous infusion of dobutamine may be started at a dose of 2.5 μg/kg/min, doubling every 15 minutes according to response and tolerability (dose titration usually limited by excessive tachycardia, arrhythmias, or ischemia). A dose above 20 μg/kg/min is rarely needed.

⁷ E.g., an intraaortic balloon pump

⁸ Improvement in symptoms and peripheral perfusion and adequate urine output—patient should be monitored closely, and usually a response will occur within 30 minutes. Bladder catheterization may help in monitoring urine output.

⁹ Continuous positive airways pressure (CPAP) is valuable in severe pulmonary edema, especially if associated with hypoxemia. Endotracheal intubation and invasive mechanical ventilation should be considered in patients with persisting hypoxemia and physical ventilatory exhaustion.

¹⁰ If systolic blood pressure is adequate (>100 mm Hg), an intravenous infusion of nitroglycerin (NTG) can be considered. Start at a dose of 10 μg/min and double every 10 minutes according to response and tolerability (usually dose up-titration is limited by hypotension). A dose of more than 100 μg/min is rarely needed.

FIG. 3 Approach to the patient with acute pulmonary edema. *IV*, Intravenous; *SNP*, sodium nitroprusside. (From Goldman L, Shafer AI: *Goldman-Cecil medicine*, ed 26, Philadelphia, 2019, Elsevier.)

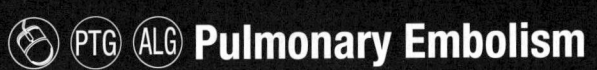
BASIC INFORMATION

DEFINITION
Pulmonary embolism (PE) refers to the lodging of a thrombus or other embolic material from a distant site in the pulmonary circulation. A classification of acute PE is described in Table 1.

SYNONYMS
PE
Pulmonary thromboembolism

ICD-10CM CODES
I26	Pulmonary embolism
I26.01	Septic pulmonary embolism with acute cor pulmonale
I26.09	Other pulmonary embolism with acute cor pulmonale
I26.90	Septic pulmonary embolism without acute cor pulmonale
I26.99	Other pulmonary embolism without acute cor pulmonale
I27.82	Chronic pulmonary embolism
Z86.711	Personal history of pulmonary embolism

EPIDEMIOLOGY & DEMOGRAPHICS
- Approximately 650,000 cases of PE occur in the U.S. each year (increased incidence in women and with advanced age); annually, as many as 100,000 people in the U.S. die from acute PE, and the diagnosis is often not made until after autopsy. The incidence of PE is increasing with the increasing use of spiral CT scans, with a lower severity of illness and lower mortality, suggesting that the increase is the result of earlier diagnosis.

- More than 90% of PEs originate in the deep venous system of the lower extremities. (See chapter "Deep Vein Thrombosis".)
- Pulmonary thromboembolism is associated with >200,000 hospitalizations per year.
- Up to 8% to 10% of victims of PE die within the first hour.
- Although nearly 20% of patients who are treated for PE die within 90 days, PE is not commonly the cause of death because it frequently coexists with other serious conditions, such as cancer, sepsis, or illness leading to hospitalization. The true mortality associated with undiagnosed PE is estimated to be less than 5%.[1a]

PHYSICAL FINDINGS & CLINICAL PRESENTATION
- Most common symptom: Dyspnea (82% to 85%)
- Tachypnea (30% to 60%)
- Cough (30% to 40%)
- Wheezing (20%)
- Chest pain: May be nonpleuritic or pleuritic (infarction) (40% to 49%); angina may reflect right ventricle (RV) ischemia
- Syncope (massive PE) (10% to 14%)
- Fever, diaphoresis, apprehension
- Hemoptysis (2%)
- Evidence of deep vein thrombosis (DVT) may be present (e.g., swelling and tenderness of extremities)
- Cardiac examination may reveal: Tachycardia (23%), increased pulmonic component of S2, murmur of tricuspid insufficiency, right ventricular heave, right-sided S3
- Pulmonary examination: May demonstrate rales, localized wheezing, friction rub

ETIOLOGY
- Thrombus, fat, air, tumor, or other foreign material
- Major transient risk factors for PE:
  1. Postoperative state, major surgery including hip or knee replacement
  2. Trauma to lower extremities, immobilizer, or cast
  3. Prolonged immobilization, reduced mobility
  4. Central venous catheter
  5. Pregnancy and early puerperium
- Minor transient risk factors for PE:
  1. Estrogen-containing birth control pills, hormone replacement therapy, estrogen-modulators (e.g., raloxifene, tamoxifen)
  2. Prolonged air travel
  3. Acute medical illness (e.g., infection, disseminated intravascular coagulation)
- Persistent risk factors for PE:
  1. History of DVT or PE
  2. Heart failure
  3. Visceral cancer (lung, pancreas, alimentary and genitourinary tracts)
  4. Spinal cord injury
  5. Advanced age
  6. Obesity
  7. Hematologic disease (e.g., factor V Leiden mutation, antithrombin III deficiency, protein C deficiency, protein S deficiency, lupus anticoagulant, polycythemia vera, dysfibrinogenemia, paroxysmal nocturnal hemoglobinuria, acquired protein C resistance without factor V Leiden, G20210A prothrombin mutation)
  8. Chronic obstructive pulmonary disease (COPD)
  9. Diabetes mellitus
  Autoimmune diseases (systemic lupus erythematosus, inflammatory bowel disease, rheumatoid arthritis)

DIAGNOSIS

DIFFERENTIAL DIAGNOSIS
- Myocardial infarction
- Pericarditis
- Pneumonia
- Pneumothorax
- Chest wall pain
- GI abnormalities (e.g., peptic ulcer, esophageal rupture, gastritis)
- Heart failure
- Pleuritis
- Anxiety disorder with hyperventilation
- Pericardial tamponade
- Dissection of aorta
- Asthma or COPD exacerbation
- Chronic thromboembolic pulmonary hypertension (CTEPH)

WORKUP
- Guidelines from the Clinical Guidelines Committee of the American College of Physicians for the Evaluation of Patients with Suspected Acute Pulmonary Embolism recommend the following:
  1. Use of validated clinical prediction rules to estimate pretest probability in patients in whom acute PE is being considered.

TABLE 1 Classification of Acute Pulmonary Embolism

Category (Frequency)	Presentation	Therapy
Massive PE (5%-10%)	Systolic blood pressure <90 mm Hg or drop ≥40 mm Hg or poor tissue perfusion or multisystem organ failure plus extensive thrombosis, such as "saddle" PE or right or left main pulmonary artery thrombus	Anticoagulation (usually with high-dose intravenous UFH or LMWH), plus advanced therapy: Systemic thrombolysis, pharmacomechanical catheter-directed therapy, surgical embolectomy, and/or inferior vena cava (IVC) filter.
Submassive PE, high risk (15%)	Hemodynamically stable but moderate or severe RV dysfunction or enlargement, coupled with biomarker elevation indicative of RV microinfarction and/or RV pressure overload	Anticoagulation until decision made regarding implementation of advanced therapy; controversy centers on this group. For systemic thrombolysis, reducing the rate of cardiovascular collapse and death must be balanced against the increased rate of hemorrhagic stroke.
Submassive PE, low risk (5%-10%)	Hemodynamically stable with RV dysfunction or biomarker elevation, but not both	Anticoagulation followed by "watch and wait." Implement advanced therapy if there is clinical deterioration.
Small to moderate PE (70%)	Normal hemodynamics and normal RV size and function	Anticoagulation and consider brief hospital stay or entirely outpatient therapy.

PE, Pulmonary embolism; *RV*, right ventricular; *UFH*, unfractionated heparin.
From Zipes DP: *Braunwald's heart disease: a textbook of cardiovascular medicine*, ed 11, Philadelphia, 2019, Elsevier.

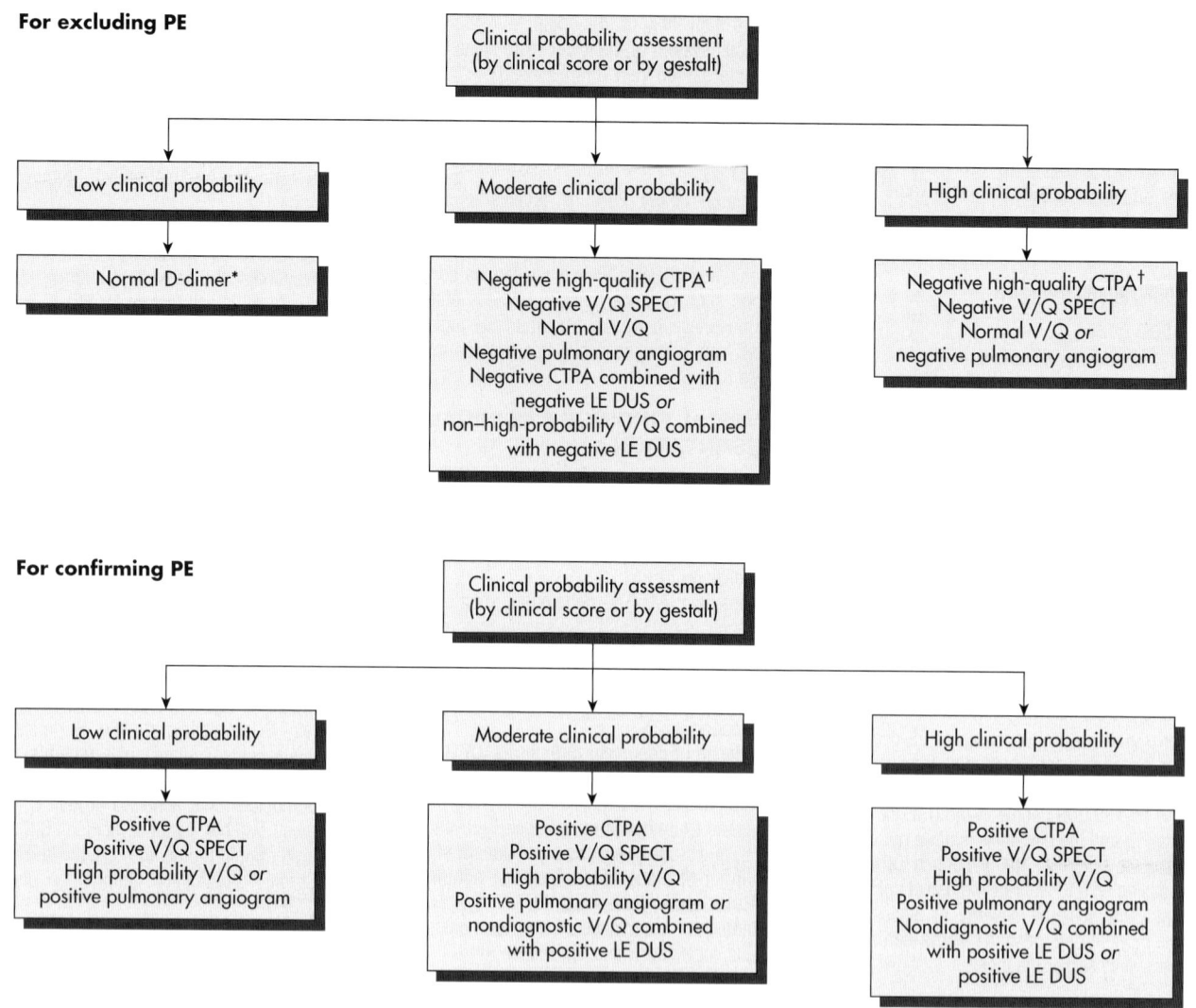

For excluding PE

For confirming PE

FIG. 1 Diagnostic strategies capable of excluding or confirming the diagnosis of pulmonary embolism. Depending on the assessed clinical probability, the tests and their results can be used either to exclude or to confirm a diagnosis of pulmonary embolism. *CTPA,* Computed tomographic pulmonary angiography; *DUS,* Doppler ultrasound; *LE,* lower extremity; *V/Q,* ventilation-perfusion scan; *V/Q SPECT,* ventilation-perfusion scan performed with a SPECT (single-photon emission computerized tomography) protocol. *The limits of normal for D-dimer are best appreciated when the patient's age is taken into account. †Artifacts may interfere with the sensitivity of CTPA, especially in scanners with four or fewer detectors. (From Broaddus VC et al: *Murray & Nadel's textbook of respiratory medicine,* ed 7, Philadelphia, 2022, Elsevier.)

2. Not obtaining a D-dimer measurement or imaging studies in patients with low pretest probability of PE and who meet all PE rule-out criteria.
3. Obtaining a high-sensitivity D-dimer measurement as the initial diagnostic test in patients who have an intermediate pretest probability of PE or in patients with low pretest probability of PE who do not meet all PE rule-out criteria. Clinicians should not use imaging studies as the initial test in patients who have a low or intermediate pretest probability of PE.
4. Use of age-adjusted D-dimer thresholds (age × 10 ng/ml rather than a generic 500 ng/ml) in patients >50 yr to determine whether imaging is warranted.
5. Clinicians should not obtain any imaging studies in patients with a D-dimer level below the age-adjusted cutoff.

6. CT pulmonary angiography (CTPA) should be obtained in patients with high pretest probability of PE. Ventilation-perfusion (V/Q) scans should be reserved for patients who have a contraindication to CTPA or if CTPA is not available.
7. A D-dimer measurement should not be obtained in patients with a high pretest probability of PE.

- Clinical assessment alone is insufficient to diagnose or rule out PE. It is also important to remember that no single noninvasive test has both high sensitivity and high specificity for PE. Consequently, in addition to clinical assessment, most patients require an imaging test to diagnose PE. An integrated diagnostic approach to PE is illustrated in Fig. 1. Prediction models for PE are summarized in Table 2.
- CTPA (Fig. E2) is an excellent diagnostic modality (83% sensitivity and 96% specificity).

- V/Q scan is reserved for patients with clinically significant contrast allergies or renal insufficiency, or when CTPA is not available.
- Pulmonary angiogram (gold standard) can confirm the diagnosis in equivocal cases, but is rarely used.
- Serial compressive duplex ultrasonography of lower extremities can be used in patients with "low-probability" V/Q scans and high clinical suspicion (see "Imaging Studies"). It is useful if positive; negative results do not exclude PE.

LABORATORY TESTS

- ABGs may reveal hypoxemia and respiratory alkalosis (decreased PaO_2 and $PaCO_2$ and increased pH); normal results do not rule out PE.
- Alveolar-arteriolar (A-a) oxygen gradient, a measure of the difference in oxygen concentration between alveoli and arterial blood, may

TABLE 2 Prediction Models for Pulmonary Embolism

Clinical Variable	SCORING MODEL			
	Wells Clinical Model	**Revised Geneva**	**PERC**	**YEARS****
Patient population in which clinical rule was validated	ED patients suspected of having PE	ED patients suspected of having PE	ED patients at low or very low risk of PE	Outpatients and inpatients suspected of having PE
Clinical signs/symptoms of deep venous thrombosis	3	4	1	1
PE is most likely or as likely as alternative diagnosis	3			1
Heart rate:				
75-94 beats/min		3		
≥95 beats/min		5		
≥100 beats/min	1.5		1	
Immobilization, surgery or trauma in the previous 4 wk requiring hospitalization or fracture of the lower limb within 1 mo (Geneva)	1.5	2	1	
Prior DVT or PE	1.5	3	1	
Hemoptysis	1	2	1	1
Malignancy (on treatment, treated in last 6 mo, cured <1 yr or palliative)	1	2		
SaO₂< 95% on room air			1	
Unilateral lower limb pain		3		
Exogenous estrogen use			1	
Age:				
≥50 yr			1	
≥65 yr		1		
Clinical Assessment Probability:				
Low probability	<2 points	0-3 total	0 points*	0 points†
Intermediate probability	2-6 points	4-10 total		
High probability	>6 points	≥11 total		
Dichotomous Wells Score With D-Dimer[446]				
Pulmonary embolism "unlikely"	≤4 points		D-dimer <500 ng/ml: PE excluded; D-dimer >500 ng/ml, consider CTPA	
Pulmonary embolism "likely"	>4 points		PE not excluded, consider additional testing with CTPA	

Age-Adjusted D-Dimer Cutoff for VTE [212]:
Formula for use in patients ≥50 yr of age in whom clinical suspicion for PE is low or intermediate

Units	Age-Adjusted D-Dimer	Interpretation/Recommendation
FEU (fibrinogen equivalent units)‡	Age × 10 μg/L	Above age-adjusted cutoff: VTE *likely*, consider confirmatory testing
DDU (D-dimer units) ‡	Age × 5 μg/L	Below age-adjusted cutoff: VTE *unlikely*, consider alternative diagnosis

CTPA, Computed tomography pulmonary angiography; *DVT,* deep venous thrombosis; *ED,* emergency department; *PE,* pulmonary embolism; *PERC,* Pulmonary Embolism Rule out Criteria; *SaO₂,* arterial saturation of oxygen; *VTE,* venous thromboembolism.
*If no criteria are positive and the clinician's pretest probability of PE <15%, PERC criteria is satisfied, and there is <2% chance of PE.
†In patients with no YEARS items and D-dimer <1000 ng/ml, PE is excluded. In patients with one or more YEARS items, PE is excluded if D-dimer is <500 ng/ml. If PE is not excluded, CTPA is recommended.
‡Must check laboratory closely to ensure correct use of units.
**Years algorithm is a modification of the Wells Clinical Decision Rule. It combines an evaluation of three characteristics (clinical signs of DVT, hemoptysis, and whether PE is the most likely diagnosis) with a differential analysis of D-dimer concentrations.
From Broaddus VC et al: *Murray & Nadel's textbook of Respiratory Medicine*, Ed 7, Philadelphia, 2022, Elsevier.

be elevated. However, a normal A-a gradient does not rule out PE.
- High-sensitivity plasma D-dimer measurement: D-dimer assays by ELISA detect the presence of plasmin-mediated degradation products of fibrin that contain cross-linked D fragments in the whole blood or plasma. A normal plasma D-dimer level is useful to exclude PE in patients with a low pretest probability of PE. However, it cannot be used to "rule in" the diagnosis because it increases with many other disorders (e.g., metastatic cancer, trauma, sepsis, postoperative state). Plasma D-dimer can also be used in conjunction with lower-extremity compression ultrasonography in patients with indeterminate V/Q and spiral CT scans. Absence of DVT and presence of a normal D-dimer level in these settings generally rule out clinically significant PE.
- Elevated cardiac troponin levels also occur in patients with PE because of RV dilation and myocardial injury; therefore, PE should be considered in the differential diagnosis of all patients presenting with chest pain or dyspnea and elevated cardiac troponin levels.

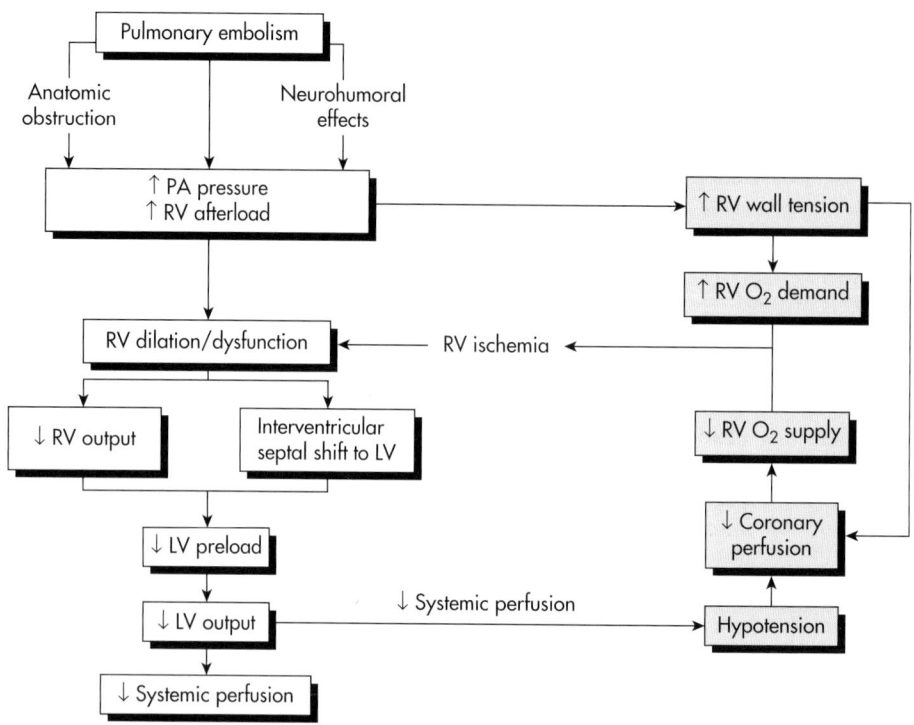

FIG. 3 Pathophysiology of right ventricular dysfunction and its deleterious effects of causing decreased systemic arterial pressure, decreased coronary perfusion, and deteriorating ventricular function. *LV,* Left ventricle/ventricular; *PA,* pulmonary artery; *RV,* right ventricle/ventricular. (From Zipes DP: Braunwald's heart disease: a textbook of cardiovascular medicine, ed 11, Philadelphia, 2019, Elsevier.)

- Elevated serum BNP levels in patients with acute PE may reflect RV overload. The pathophysiology of RV dysfunction in PE is illustrated in Fig. 3.
- ECG is abnormal in 85% of patients with acute PE. Frequent abnormalities are sinus tachycardia; nonspecific ST-segment or T-wave changes; S-1, Q-3, T-3 pattern (10% of patients); S-1, S-2, S-3 pattern; T-wave inversion in V_1 to V_6 acute RBBB; new-onset atrial fibrillation; ST segment depression in lead II; RV strain. An RV strain pattern on ECG in patients with PE and normal blood pressure is associated with adverse short-term outcome and adds incremental prognostic value to echocardiographic evidence of RV function.

IMAGING STUDIES

- Chest x-ray can be normal but is typically abnormal (Fig. E4); suggestive findings include elevated diaphragm, pleural effusion, dilation of pulmonary artery, infiltrate or consolidation, abrupt vessel cut-off, oligemia distal to the PE *(Westermark sign),* or atelectasis. A wedge-shaped consolidation in the middle and lower lobes is suggestive of a pulmonary infarction and is known as a *Hampton hump.*
- CT pulmonary angiography (CTPA) is an accurate, noninvasive tool in the diagnosis of PE (Fig. E5) at the main, lobar, and segmental pulmonary artery levels. A major advantage of CTPA over standard pulmonary angiography is its ability to diagnose intrathoracic disease other than PE that may account for the patient's clinical picture. It is also less invasive,

less costly, and more widely available. Its major shortcoming is its poor sensitivity for subsegmental emboli. It is important to recognize signs of chronic clot on CT scan. These signs include eccentric thrombus, intraluminal webs/bands, mosaic attenuation of lung fields, and presence of bronchial artery collaterals, which may suggest chronic rather than acute PE, warranting a different treatment approach (see Fig. E2).

- V/Q lung scan (in patient with normal chest x-ray examination): This test must be interpreted within the pretest probability of having a PE.
  1. A normal lung scan rules out PE.
  2. A V/Q mismatch is suggestive of PE, and a lung scan interpretation of high probability is confirmatory (Fig. E6).
  3. If the clinical suspicion of PE is high and the V/Q lung scan is interpreted as low probability, moderate probability, or indeterminate, a pulmonary angiogram is diagnostic. A positive angiogram confirms diagnosis. A positive compressive duplex ultrasonography for DVT obviates the need for an angiogram, because treatment with anticoagulants is indicated in these patients. The overall sensitivity of compressive ultrasonography for DVT in patients with PE is 29% with a specificity of 97%. Adding ultrasonography in patients with a nondiagnostic lung scan prevents 9% of angiographies; however, this improvement in efficacy is achieved at the cost of unnecessary anticoagulant therapy in 26% of patients who have false-positive ultrasonography results.

- Pulmonary angiography is the historic gold standard; however, it is invasive, expensive, and not readily available in some clinical settings. False-positive pulmonary angiograms may result from mediastinal disorders such as radiation fibrosis and tumors.
- Echocardiography is useful for identifying patients with PE who are high risk for poor outcomes. Moderate or severe RV hypokinesis, persistent pulmonary hypertension, patent foramen ovale, and free-floating right heart thrombus are markers of increased risk of death or recurrent thrombosis. RV pressure overload may be inferred from a RV:LV ratio ≥ 1.0 and predicts higher rates of in-hospital death or clinical deterioration. McConnell's sign, akinesia of mid-free wall with normal motion at apex, is 77% sensitive and 94% specific for acute PE.
- Gadolinium-enhanced magnetic resonance angiography (MRA/MRV) of the pulmonary arteries has a moderate sensitivity and high specificity for the diagnosis of PE at experienced centers, but obtaining acceptable images is technically challenging and should only be performed if other imaging tests are contraindicated.

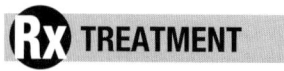
TREATMENT

NONPHARMACOLOGIC THERAPY
Modification of risk factors (see "Etiology") to prevent future PE.

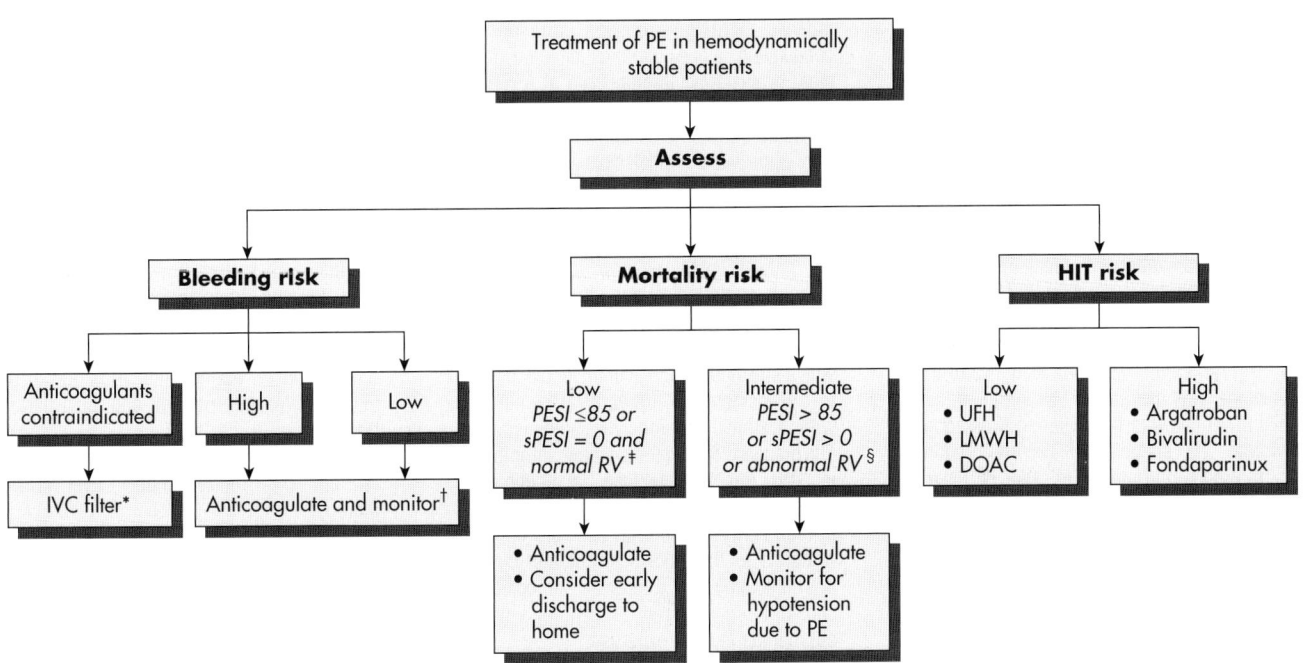

FIG. 7 Treatment of pulmonary embolism (PE) in hemodynamically stable patients. Decisions require assessment of bleeding risk, mortality risk, and risk of *heparin-induced thrombocytopenia* (HIT). *DOAC*, Direct oral anticoagulant; *LMWH*, low-molecular-weight heparin; *PESI*, pulmonary embolism severity index; *sPESI*, simplified PESI; *UFH*, unfractionated heparin.
*Consider echocardiography to rule out pulmonary embolism in transit (if not already done) before *inferior vena cava* (IVC) filter placement.
†See Table 3 for assessment of bleeding risk and recommendations for anticoagulation in patients at high risk for major bleeding.
‡No abnormality of the *right ventricle* (RV) is detected on initial diagnostic testing (e.g., computed tomography pulmonary angiography, echocardiography, troponin).
§Obtain an echocardiogram and biomarker test (e.g., troponin or natriuretic peptides) if not done previously. (From Broaddus VC et al: *Murray & Nadel's textbook of respiratory medicine*, ed 7, Philadelphia, 2022, Elsevier.)

TABLE 3 Anticoagulant Treatments for Acute Pulmonary Embolism

Clinical	Initial*	Long-Term*	Extended*
Unstable	UFH† (5+ days)	DOAC or warfarin‡	DOAC or warfarin‡
High risk for bleed§	UFH† (5+ days)	DOAC or warfarin‡	DOAC or warfarin‡
Stable, cancer	Dalteparin 200 IU/kg/day‖ (1 mo)	Dalteparin 150 IU/kg/day	Dalteparin 150 IU/kg/day
Stable, cancer	Enoxaparin 1 mg/kg/bid‖	Enoxaparin 1 mg/kg/bid	Enoxaparin 1 mg/kg/bid
Stable, cancer	Enoxaparin 1 mg/kg bid (7 days)	Edoxaban 60 mg/day¶	Edoxaban 60 mg/day¶
Stable, no cancer	Apixaban 10 mg bid (7 days)	Apixaban 5 mg bid	Apixaban 2.5 mg bid
Stable, no cancer	Rivaroxaban 15 mg bid (21 days)	Rivaroxaban 20 mg qd	Rivaroxaban 20 mg qd
Stable, no cancer	Enoxaparin 1 mg/kg bid (5-7 days)	Dabigatran 150 mg bid	Dabigatran 150 mg bid

aPTT, Activated partial thromboplastin time; *bid*, twice daily; *DOAC*, direct oral anticoagulant; *HIT*, heparin-induced thrombocytopenia; *INR*, international normalized ratio; *LMWH*, low-molecular-weight heparin; *PE*, pulmonary embolism; *qd*, once daily; *UFH*, unfractionated heparin.
*Initial anticoagulant period from day 1 to day 5 to 7 of treatment, followed by long-term anticoagulation from day 5 to 7 to 3 mo, with anticoagulation extended beyond 3 mo when the risk of recurrent PE exceeds the risk of major bleeding.
†UFH dosed according to a standardized protocol[164]; monitor for HIT.
‡If oral vitamin K antagonist (e.g., warfarin) treatment is planned, begin with 4 to 5 mg once daily and transition entirely to warfarin after all the following criteria are satisfied: (1) at least 5 days of UFH or LMWH; (2) INR >2.0 for two determinations; (3) PE symptoms and PE-related hypoxemia significantly improved, then monitor INR; and (4) adjust dose to maintain INR in range of 2.0 to 3.0.
§High risk for bleeding as defined by Kearon and colleagues. Some experts advise intravenous UFH 400 U/h without a bolus and observe for bleeding/hemostasis. After 6 h with hemostasis, increase to 600 U/h with continued observation. Keep aPTT <50 sec and anti–factor Xa level <0.5 U/ml. If hemostasis is maintained, then slowly increase UFH dose over 24 h to 800 U/h.
‖LMWHs accumulate with renal dysfunction. Titrate doses to produce anti–factor Xa levels of 0.4 to 0.85 U/ml and monitor for HIT.
¶Edoxaban 30 mg once daily for creatinine clearance 15 to 50 ml/min or body weight <60 kg.
From Broaddus VC et al: *Murray & Nadel's textbook of respiratory medicine*, ed 7, Philadelphia, 2022, Elsevier.

ACUTE GENERAL Rx

Patients with acute PE should be initially stratified according to risk (see Table 1) so that higher-risk therapies (e.g., thrombolysis, embolectomy) are offered to patients with the greatest chance of benefit. Many tertiary and quaternary care centers deploy a multidisciplinary Pulmonary Embolism Response Team (PERT) to determine the optimal course of treatment for patients with intermediate- and high-risk PE, given the highly variable mortality risk in the intermediate-risk group.

Anticoagulation is recommended as initial therapy in all patients with small to moderate PE without a contraindication. Fig. 7 illustrates the treatment of PE in hemodynamically stable patients. Anticoagulant treatments for acute PE are summarized in Table 3.

- For patients with low-risk or intermediate-low–risk PE, anticoagulation can be initiated right away with the direct oral anticoagulant (DOAC) rivaroxaban or apixaban; subcutaneous low-molecular-weight heparin (LMWH) or fondaparinux; or IV unfractionated heparin (UFH). When oral anticoagulation is initiated, a DOAC is recommended over a vitamin K antagonist. (See Table 3 in Deep Vein Thrombosis.)
  1. Oral rivaroxaban, a factor Xa inhibitor (15 mg bid for 3 wk, then 20 mg/day), has been studied as a treatment for DVT and PE, without prior parenteral therapy. For both DVT and PE, treatment with rivaroxaban alone was noninferior to treatment with LMWH followed by a vitamin K antagonist with the endpoint of recurrent venous thromboembolism (VTE). Use of rivaroxaban should be avoided in patients with severe renal failure.
  2. Apixaban, a factor Xa inhibitor (10 mg bid for a week, followed by 5 mg bid), is approved for the treatment of acute PE based on the data in the AMPLIFY and AMPLIFY-EXT trials, in which apixaban met its noninferiority mark in terms of efficacy and improved safety compared to warfarin.
  3. Dabigatran, a direct thrombin inhibitor (150 mg bid following 5 to 10 days of parenteral anticoagulation), is approved for treatment of DVT and PE in patients with CrCl >30 ml/min based on data in the RE-COVER and RE-COVER II trials, in which it was noninferior to warfarin.
  4. Edoxaban, a factor Xa inhibitor (60 mg/day, or 30 mg/day if CrCl 15 to 50 ml/min or body weight ≤60 kg or if on certain P-glycoprotein inhibitors, following 5 to 10 days of parenteral anticoagulation) is approved for treatment of DVT and PE based on the Hokusai VTE trial, in which it was noninferior to warfarin.
  5. UFH, subcutaneous LMWH, or subcutaneous fondaparinux can be used for initial treatment for at least 5 days when used with warfarin, dabigatran, or edoxaban. If IV UFH is used, a bolus dose (80 U/kg) followed by a weight-based (18 U/kg/h) continuous infusion to achieve therapeutic anti–factor Xa (or aPTT) levels should be used. LMWH and fondaparinux should be avoided in patients with severe renal failure.
- For patients with intermediate-high risk or high-risk PE, anticoagulation with LMWH or IV UFH (if LMWH is contraindicated due to renal failure or bleeding concerns) is recommended and can be transitioned to an oral agent prior to hospital discharge.
- For patients with contraindications to anticoagulation, consider placement of a *temporary* inferior vena cava (IVC) filter and frequent reassessment of safety for initiation of anticoagulation as soon as possible.
- For patients with intermediate-high risk PE (demonstrating RV strain by imaging and myocardial injury with positive biomarkers), attempts should be made to risk stratify individual patients as this cohort may have multiple therapeutic options including anticoagulation alone, catheter-directed therapies, or systemic thrombolysis at a reduced dose. In high-volume centers, the distinction between treatment strategies in this group may occur via a multidisciplinary PERT team, often consisting of pulmonary and critical care, cardiology, hematology, and interventional radiology specialists.
- For patients with massive or high-risk PE without contraindications to thrombolytics (Box 1), thrombolytic agents (urokinase, tPA, streptokinase) provide rapid resolution of clots with some increased risk of major bleeding (up to 3% incidence of intracranial hemorrhage with systemic thrombolytic administration). The standard dosing for systemic thrombolytic is 100 mg of alteplase (synthetic tPA), administered over 2 h.
- In high-risk patients with absolute contraindications to thrombolytics, catheter-directed thrombectomy or surgical embolectomy should be considered at centers with the appropriate level of expertise.
- For high-risk PE patients in refractory shock or with cardiac arrest, additional mechanical support, such as extracorporeal membrane oxygenation (ECMO), may serve as a bridge to advanced therapies or recovery. Fig. 8 illustrates the approach to a patient with suspected pulmonary embolism and hypotension.
- Long-term treatment for PE not associated with malignancy can be carried out with a DOAC, LMWH, or warfarin.
- For PE associated with malignancy, DOACs or LMWH is recommended for long-term therapy.
- If thrombolytics and anticoagulants are contraindicated (e.g., GI bleeding, recent CNS surgery, recent trauma) or if the patient continues to have recurrent PE despite anticoagulation therapy, an IVC filter is recommended.
- In older adults, IVC filters are associated with higher 30-day and 1-yr mortality (11.6% and 20.5%, respectively, versus 9.3% and 13.4% in those who do not undergo filters); however, these patients tended to be sicker. An IVC filter is not advised for patients with recurrent VTE, unless risk for cardiopulmonary deterioration outweighs risk for IVC filter replacement.
- For PE occurring in the setting of pregnancy, LMWH is the treatment of choice. Dosing is based on early pregnancy weight. Planned delivery should be strongly considered to avoid complications with anticoagulation and spinal anesthesia. For a patient with a recent PE, LMWH should be switched to UFH approximately 36 h prior to planned delivery and the drip should be stopped 4 to 6 h prior to delivery, with a normal partial thromboplastin time (PTT) at the time of spinal anesthesia initiation. LMWH should be restarted as soon as it is deemed safe by the obstetrician. Duration of anticoagulation should be at least 3 mo total with at least 6 wk of anticoagulation after delivery. Breastfeeding mothers can be prescribed either LMWH or warfarin. Thrombolytic therapy should only be used for life-threatening PE during pregnancy due to the high risk of peri-partum and post-partum bleeding.
- For patients with antiphospholipid syndrome, Warfarin is recommended over DOAC therapy.[1]
- For patients with isolated subsegmental PE, rule proximal out. If risk of recurrent venous thromboembolism (VTE) is low, surveillance is recommended over anticoagulation. If risk for recurrent VTE is high, anticoagulation is recommended.[1] However, a recent study revealed that overall, patients with subsegmental PE who did not have proximal DVT had a higher-than-expected rate of recurrent VTE.[2]

CHRONIC Rx

- Elimination of risk factors (see "Etiology").
- Duration of anticoagulation:
  1. Patients with PE attributed to a major transient risk factor that is no longer present should complete at least 3 mo of therapeutic anticoagulation.
  2. Patients with PE occurring in the setting of a minor transient risk factor should complete at least 6 mo of therapeutic anticoagulation. If bleeding risk is low and patient is tolerating therapy well, consider low-dose extended DOAC (apixaban 2.5 mg PO bid or rivaroxaban 10 mg/day) indefinitely.
  3. Patients with PE occurring in the setting of persistent risk factors such as hematologic thrombotic disorders, antiphospholipid syndrome, and ongoing active malignancy, therapeutic anticoagulation should continue during the presence of the persistent risk factor.
  4. For unprovoked PE, lifelong anticoagulation should be considered, as long as bleeding risk is low. If bleeding risk is moderate or high after a single unprovoked PE, stopping

---

BOX 1   Contraindications to Systemic Thrombolysis

Absolute contraindication to systemic thrombolytics tPA:

(Prior intracranial hemorrhage, known structural intracranial cerebrovascular disease, known malignant intracranial neoplasm, ischemic CVA within 3 mo, suspected aortic dissection, active bleeding, recent surgery encroaching on spinal canal or brain, recent significant closed head or facial trauma)

Relative contraindication to systemic thrombolytics

(Age >75, current use of anticoagulation, pregnancy, noncompressible vascular punctures, CPR >10 min, recent internal bleeding, dementia, remote history of CVA [<3 mo], major surgery within 3 wk)

Modified from Parrillo JE, Dellinger RP: *Critical care medicine, principles of diagnosis and management in the adult*, ed 5, Philadelphia, 2019, Elsevier.

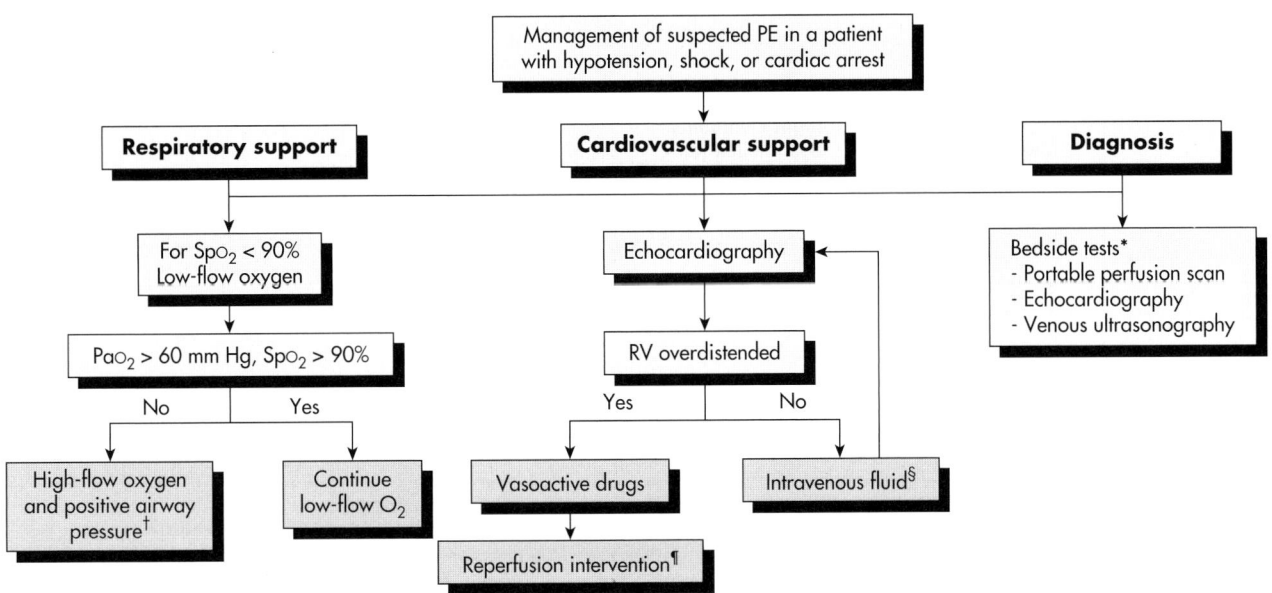

FIG. 8 Management of a patient with suspected pulmonary embolism and hypotension. Hypotension (defined by systolic **blood pressure <90 mm Hg), shock, and cardiac arrest represent a life-threatening spectrum of hemodynamic compromise, and these conditions often limit diagnostic options. At times, thrombolysis must be tried even though the diagnosis of pulmonary embolism (PE) is unproven.** *Pao2,* arterial partial pressure of oxygen; *Spo2,* oxygen saturation as measured by pulse oximetry. *A bedside echocardiogram can support the diagnosis of acute pulmonary embolism (e.g., McConnell's sign) or can provide another diagnosis (e.g., pericardial tamponade), and venous ultrasonography can show deep venous thrombosis. ¶Reperfusion interventions include thrombolysis, surgical embolectomy, and catheter-based treatment. The choice of reperfusion strategy depends on patient-related factors (e.g., bleeding risk and hemodynamic stability) and the institutional resources that can be mobilized (e.g., cardiovascular surgical team). †Suspect right-to-left shunting of venous blood when low-flow oxygen is insufficient. Provide high-flow oxygen. Assess the location of shunting (e.g., atelectasis and/or shunt through the foramen ovale). Provide positive airway pressure with mask ventilation and avoid intubation, if possible, for intrapulmonary shunt, and monitor and manage adverse effects of positive airway pressure on cardiac output. §Intravenous fluids should be titrated carefully to avoid overdistention of the right ventricle (RV). (From Broaddus VC et al: *Murray & Nadel's Textbook of Respiratory Medicine,* ed 7, Philadelphia 2022, Elsevier.)

anticoagulation can be considered. Indefinite long-term anticoagulation should be used in patients with recurrent unprovoked PE.
5. Recurrence risk calculators help inform the risk/benefit discussion with patients interested in avoiding indefinite anticoagulation. Such calculators include the modified Vienna prediction model, the HERDOO-2 score, the DASH model, and the Louzada score.
• Patients with unprovoked DVT/PE have a high rate of recurrent VTE. Longer durations of chronic anticoagulation after unprovoked DVT/PE result in lower rates of recurrent DVT/PE while on anticoagulation, but benefits are lost once anticoagulation is halted. The use of indefinite anticoagulation in select individuals with apparently unprovoked DVT/PE must be weighed against ongoing bleeding risk and other factors.
• Aspirin (100 mg/day) is superior to placebo in preventing recurrence of VTE in patients with a first-ever unprovoked VTE who completed 6 to 18 mo of oral anticoagulation. This suggests that aspirin could be offered as an alternative

to oral anticoagulants for prevention of recurrent VTE in patients who refuse to or cannot continue oral anticoagulant therapy but who have a high risk of recurrent VTE.

DISPOSITION
• Mortality can be reduced to <10% by rapid and effective treatment. Stratification of risk of death associated with PE and severity-adjusted treatment is described in Table 4. Indicators of poor prognosis include hemodynamic instability/hypotension, signs of RV dysfunction, elevated BNP, elevated troponin, thrombus burden, coexisting DVT, and RV thrombus. The Pulmonary Embolism Severity Index (PESI) is summarized in Table 5.
• Risk stratification tools may be used to identify select low-risk patients who may be considered for home treatment.
• Mortality from recurrent PE is 8% with effective treatment and >30% in patients with untreated PE.

OUTPATIENT FOLLOW-UP
• Monitor for recurrent, persistent, or progressive symptoms after PE.

• Determine appropriate plan for type, dosing, duration, and monitoring of anticoagulation.
• Ensure appropriate evaluation of underlying factors contributing to the development of the PE, including hypercoagulable workup and age-appropriate cancer screening.
• Facilitate appropriate and expeditious removal of temporary IVC filters.
• Monitor for sequelae of PE, such as post-PE syndrome (functional and exercise limitation 1 yr post PE), chronic thromboembolic disease (CTED), and chronic thromboembolic pulmonary hypertension (CTEPH). Between 0.1% and 9% of patients who experience PE develop CTEPH, which can be a life-threatening disease if not identified and treated in a timely fashion.

REFERENCES
Available at eBooks.Health.Elsevier.com.

AUTHORS: **ALEXANDER SHERMAN, MD,** and **SONIA JASUJA, MD**

TABLE 4 Stratification of Risk of Death Associated With Pulmonary Embolism and Severity-Adjusted Treatment*

Early Risk of Death	RISK FACTOR			Recommended Treatment
	Shock or Hypotension (on Clinical Examination)	Right Ventricular Dysfunction (on Echocardiography or Multidetector CT)	Myocardial Injury (on Cardiac Troponin Testing)	
High	Present	Present[†]	NA[‡]	LMWH or unfractionated heparin plus thrombolysis or embolectomy
Intermediate-high	Absent	Both present		LMWH, fondaparinux, or UFH; consideration of reperfusion therapy
Intermediate-low	Absent	Only one present		LMWH, fondaparinux, or UFH; avoid early thrombolysis; monitor clinical status and right ventricular function
Low	Absent	Absent	Absent	DOAC, LMWH, fondaparinux, or UFH; consider outpatient treatment

CT, Computed tomography; *RV*, right ventricle; *LMWH*, low-molecular-weight heparin; *UFH*, unfractionated heparin; *DOAC*, direct oral anticoagulant.
*Adapted with modifications from the 2019 Guidelines on the Diagnosis and Management of Acute Pulmonary Embolism of the European Society of Cardiology. NA denotes not applicable.
[†]If RV function is normal on echocardiography, or if a CT scan shows no RV dilation in a patient with hemodynamic compromise and clinically suspected pulmonary embolism, an alternative diagnosis should be sought.
[‡]Troponin test results do not influence risk assessment or treatment in hemodynamically compromised patients with acute pulmonary embolism.
From Konstantinides S: Acute pulmonary embolism, *N Engl J Med* 359:2804-2813, 2008.

TABLE 5 Original and Simplified Pulmonary Embolism Severity Index (PESI)

Variable	Original PESI	Simplified PESI
Age	Age, in yr	1 (if age >80 yr)
Male sex	+10	—
History of cancer	+30	1
History of heart failure	+10	1 for either or both of these items
History of chronic lung disease	+10	
Pulse >110 beats/min	+20	1
Systolic blood pressure <100 mm Hg	+30	1
Respiratory rate >30 breaths/min	+20	—
Temperature <36° C	+20	—
Altered mental status	+60	—
Arterial oxyhemoglobin saturation (Sa O_2) <90%	+20	1

30-DAY MORTALITY RISK STRATA (BASED ON THE SUM OF POINTS)

LOW-RISK PESI

Class I: <65 Points

(event rate 95% CI, 0-1.6)

Class II: 66-85 Points

(event rate 95% CI, 1.7-3.5)

HIGH-RISK PESI

Class III: 86-105 Points

(event rate 95% CI, 3.2-7.1)

Class IV: 106-125 Points

(event rate 95% CI, 4.0-11.4)

Class V: >125 Points

(event rate 95% CI, 10.0-24.5)

LOW-RISK sPESI

0 Points

(event rate 95% CI, 0-2.1)

HIGH-RISK sPESI

≥1 Point

(event rate 95% CI, 8.5-13.2)

CI, Confidence interval; *PESI*, Pulmonary Embolism Severity Index; *sPESI*, simplified P.
From Vincent JL et al: *Textbook of critical care*, ed 7, Philadelphia, 2017, Elsevier.

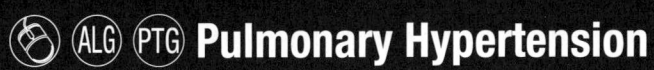 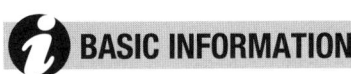
Diseases and Disorders

I

BASIC INFORMATION

DEFINITION

Pulmonary hypertension (PH) is defined as the presence of an elevated mean pulmonary arterial pressure (mPAP) ≥20 mm Hg at rest (previously ≥25 mm Hg), measured by right heart catheterization. However because an mPAP >20 mm Hg does not separate pulmonary vascular disease from increased cardiac output or pulmonary capillary wedge pressures, a pulmonary vascular resistance >3 Woods units (WU) was recently added to the definition of all forms of precapillary PH associated with an mPAP >20 mm Hg. The updated hemodynamic definitions of PH are listed in Table 1.[1]

PH groups:

PH is classified into five major groups based on shared disease histology and pathophysiology, clinical presentation, and therapeutic strategies:

- Group I is caused by pulmonary arterial hypertension (PAH) and is categorized based on etiology.
- Group 2 is caused by left heart disease.
- Group 3 is caused by chronic lung disease and/or hypoxia.
- Group 4 is due to chronic thromboembolic PH (CTEPH).
- Group 5 encompasses PH associated with unclear and/or multifactorial mechanisms.

Table 2 shows most updated classification of various PH groups.[2]

PAH, the primary subtype of PH, is characterized by progressive increases in pulmonary vascular resistance (PVR) primarily due to uncontrolled pulmonary vascular remodeling, sustained vasoconstriction, and thrombosis in situ. The causes of PAH include idiopathic, heritable, drug- and toxin-induced, and associated disorders such as connective tissue disorders, human immunodeficiency virus (HIV) infection, portal hypertension, congenital heart diseases, and schistosomiasis. PAH can also result from pulmonary veno-occlusive disease and/or pulmonary capillary hemangiomatosis and persistent pulmonary hypertension of the newborn. Idiopathic PAH is responsible for more than 50% of all PAH cases. It requires extensive investigation (diagnosis of exclusion), whereas heritable PAH results from gene mutations or familial cases regardless of mutations. The Sixth World Symposium on Pulmonary Hypertension (WSPH) updated the group 1 pulmonary hypertension classification to include new drugs and toxins as known agents associated with PAH. For example, amphetamines, methamphetamines, and dasatinib were added to the definite association category. Leflunomide, bosutinib, and direct-acting antivirals for hepatitis C virus (e.g., sofosbuvir) were added as agents having a possible association.[3] This topic will mostly focus on PAH.

SYNONYMS

PH
Pulmonary arterial hypertension
Idiopathic pulmonary arterial hypertension
IPAH
Associated pulmonary arterial hypertension
PAHA, also known as secondary pulmonary hypertension
Heritable pulmonary arterial hypertension
HPAH
Group I pulmonary hypertension

ICD-10CM CODES
I27.0 Primary pulmonary hypertension
I27.2 Other secondary pulmonary hypertension

EPIDEMIOLOGY & DEMOGRAPHICS

- IPAH is rare, occurring in 1 to 2 cases/1 million people per year, with an overall prevalence estimated at 15 to 50/1 million.
- Idiopathic, heritable, and anorexigen-induced PAH make up 52.6% of all PAH cases. Based on contemporerory registries, PAH is more common in women than men (4.8:1) and usually affects women aged between 30 and 60 yr. However, it can occur in males and is often associated with worse clinical outcomes.[4,5]
- Prevalence of secondary PAH could range from 8% to 12% in cases of scleroderma, 0.5% of HIV, 3% to 4% of mixed connective tissue disorders, and 1% to 5% cases of systemic lupus erythematosus.[6]

PHYSICAL FINDINGS & CLINICAL PRESENTATION

Symptoms:
- Insidious, may go undetected for years
- Exertional dyspnea, the most common presenting symptom (60%)
- Fatigue and weakness
- Anorexia/abdominal pain

- Syncope, classically exertion-related or after a warm shower with peripheral vasodilation
- Chest pain
- Hoarse voice from compression of recurrent laryngeal nerve by an enlarged pulmonary artery (Ortner syndrome)
- Hemoptysis
- Rarely, palpitations due to atrial fibrillation or atrial flutter

Clinical signs:
- Loud P2 component of the second heart sound and paradoxic splitting of second heart sound
- Right-sided S4
- Jugular venous distension
- Abdominal distension and ascites
- Prominent parasternal (right ventricular [RV]) impulse
- Holosystolic tricuspid regurgitation murmur heard best along the left fourth parasternal line that increases in intensity with inspiration
- Peripheral edema
- Features of the physical exam pertinent to the evaluation of PH are summarized in Table 3

ETIOLOGY

- The triggering etiology that initiates the pathogenesis of PAH is likely multifactorial, including inappropriate angiogenesis, metabolic derangements, DNA damage, genetic mutations, and impaired vasoreactivity. Endothelial cell injury along with impaired vascular regeneration, abnormal vascular remodeling, and loss of the small pulmonary arteries are all known to occur as part of the PAH pathogenesis.
- Autoantibodies, proinflammatory cytokines, and inflammatory infiltrates have also been implicated in the pathogenesis of PAH. Individuals with PAH have increased von Willebrand factor levels, plasma fibrinopeptide A, plasminogen activator inhibitor-1, serotonin (5-HT), and thromboxane. In addition, tissue plasminogen activator, thrombomodulin, NO, and PGI2 are decreased, creating an imbalance that favors thrombosis.[3]
- Associated PAH (APAH) has several known risk factors: Connective tissue disorders such as systemic sclerosis, portal hypertension and liver cirrhosis, appetite-suppressant drugs (e.g., fenfluramine), and infections, including schistosomiasis and HIV disease. High altitude, schistosomiasis, and HIV disease are common causes of PH worldwide; however, pulmonary venous hypertension from left ventricular failure and PH related to chronic obstructive pulmonary disease (COPD) are more common causes of PH in developed nations.
- Several genetic abnormalities have been associated with HPAH (heritable PAH), many of which are mutations in the genes that code for members of the tumor growth factor-β family of receptors (BMPR-II, ALK-1, endoglin) on chromosome 2q33.
- The most important gene mutation is in the bone morphogenetic protein receptor-2 (BMPR-II), normally involved with inducing osteogenesis and cell differentiation. Up to

---

TABLE 1 Hemodynamic Definitions of Pulmonary Hypertension Based on Right-Heart Catheterization

	mPAP (mm Hg)	PCWP (mm Hg)	PVR (WU)	Group
Precapillary pulmonary hypertension	mPAP > 20	<15	≥3	1, 3, 4, 5
Isolated postcapillary pulmonary hypertension	mPAP > 20	>15	<3	2, 5
Combined pre- and postcapillary pulmonary hypertension	mPAP > 20	>15	≥3	2, 5

mPAP, Mean pulmonary artery pressure; *PCWP*, pulmonary capillary wedge pressure; *PVR*, pulmonary vascular resistance; *WU*, Woods units.
From Gelzinis TA: Pulmonary hypertension in 2021: part I-definition, classification, pathophysiology, and presentation, *Journal of Cardiothoracic and Vascular Anesthesia* 36(6):1552-1564, 2022. https://doi.org/10.1053/j.jvca.2021.06.036.

TABLE 2 Updated Clinical Classification of Pulmonary Hypertension

1. PAH	**3. PH due to lung disease and/or hypoxia**
a) Idiopathic PAH	a) Obstructive lung disease
b) Heritable PAH	b) Restrictive lung disease
c) Drug- and toxin-induced PAH	c) Other lung disease with mixed restrictive/obstructive pattern
d) PAH associated with:	d) Hypoxia without lung disease
I. Connective tissue disease	e) Developmental lung disorders
II. HIV infection	**4. PH due to pulmonary artery obstructions**
III. Portal hypertension	a) Chronic thromboembolic PH
IV. Congenital heart disease	b) Other pulmonary artery obstructions
V. Schistosomiasis	**5. PH with unclear and/or multifactorial mechanisms**
e) PAH long-term responders to calcium channel blockers	a) Hematologic disorders
f) PAH with overt features of venous/capillaries (PVOD/PCH) involvement	b) Systemic and metabolic disorders
g) Persistent PH of the newborn syndrome	c) Others
2. PH due to left heart disease	d) Complex congenital heart disease
a) PH due to heart failure with preserved LVEF	
b) PH due to heart failure with reduced LVEF	
c) Valvular heart disease	
d) Congenital/acquired cardiovascular conditions leading to postcapillary PH	

HIV, Human immunodeficiency virus; *LVEF,* left ventricular ejection fraction; *PAH,* pulmonary arterial hypertension; *PCH,* pulmonary capillary hemangiomatosis; *PH,* pulmonary hypertension; *PVOD,* pulmonary venoocclusive disease.
From Simonneau G et al: Haemodynamic definitions and updated clinical classification of pulmonary hypertension, *Eur Respir J* 53(1):1801913, 2019, http://doi.org/10.1183/13993003.01913-2018.

25% of patients with IPAH have abnormal BMPR-II structure or function, while up to 80% of hereditary PAH is due to mutations in BMPR-II. Women are more susceptible to PAH, because estrogen inhibits normal BMPR- II.[7]

- Additional mutations that are implicated in PAH development involve ligands of BMPR2 and include GDF2 (encoding BMP9), type I receptor (ACVRL1), and SMAD9 (encoding Smad8). Potassium channel subfamily K member 3 (KCNK3) mutations and caveloin-1 (CAV1) mutations have also been identified along with many others.[8]
- Heritable PAH is an autosomal-dominant disease with variable penetrance, affecting only about 10% to 20% of carriers.

🅓🅧 DIAGNOSIS

- PAH is a hemodynamic diagnosis involving the detection of elevated pressure in the pulmonary arteries and elevated pulmonary vascular resistance in the pulmonary vascular bed, occurring in the absence of significant pulmonary venous hypertension.
- Right-sided heart catheterization must be performed in all patients suspected of having PAH to establish the diagnosis and to assess pulmonary hemodynamics including reactivity response to vasodilators.
- One of the most challenging differential diagnoses of IPAH is heart failure with preserved ejection fraction (EF) (HFpEF). In such patients, the pulmonary capillary wedge pressure (PCWP) may be at the higher limit of normal at rest. Exercise or fluid challenge at the time of right heart catheterization can result in disproportionate rise in PCWP, which favors group 2 PH.
- IPAH is a diagnosis of exclusion; causes that lead to groups 2 to 5 PH must be ruled out.

Transthoracic echocardiogram (TTE), high-resolution computed tomography (HR-CT), pulmonary function tests (PFTs), and ventilation-perfusion (V/Q) scan must be performed before the diagnosis of IPAH is established and treatment started.

DIFFERENTIAL DIAGNOSIS

The differential diagnosis is as listed under "Etiology." Table 4 summarizes distinguishing PAH from heart failure with preserved EF.

EVALUATION

- Consists of establishing the diagnosis and etiology. Fig. E1 illustrates an approach to evaluation of patients with chronic lung disease with possible PH.
- Echocardiography with Doppler technique can provide a noninvasive but limited estimation of systolic PAP. Common findings include tricuspid regurgitation, right heart enlargement, abnormal movement of septum and, rarely, pericardial effusion. However, the diagnosis of PH cannot be established by echocardiography alone, as echocardiography can overestimate or underestimate PAP.
- ECG (Fig. 2) showing RV enlargement, strain pattern, and right axis deviation.
- Chest x-ray examination (Fig. 3) shows enlarged central pulmonary arteries and right heart enlargement. Chest x-ray examination is abnormal in 90% of patients at diagnosis.
- A normal chest x-ray does not rule out the diagnosis. High-resolution CT (Fig. E4) can assist in the evaluation for emphysema or interstitial lung disease. V/Q lung scan has high sensitivity for chronic thromboembolic disease. CT angiography is less sensitive for diagnosing chronic thromboembolic disease. The diagnosis can be confirmed by pulmonary angiography, which has high specificity.

- Cardiac magnetic resonance (CMR) imaging can provide accurate noninvasive evaluation of the right ventricular size, morphology, and function.
- PFTs may show obstructive (airway disease) and/or restrictive disease (parenchymal disease) depending on etiology. Diffusion capacity of carbon monoxide in the lung is reduced due to pulmonary vascular destruction in PAH.
- In asymptomatic patients the severity of PAH disease should be evaluated in a systematic and consistent manner, using a combination of World Health Organization (WHO) functional class (FC), exercise capacity, and echocardiographic, laboratory, and hemodynamic variables to inform therapeutic decisions.
- Right heart catheterization is required to assess pulmonary hemodynamics, exclude shunts and left heart disease, and perform acute vasoreactivity response testing.
- Symptomatic patients with PAH, in the absence of contraindications, should undergo acute vasoreactivity testing using a short-acting agent at a center with experience in the performance and interpretation of vasoreactivity testing.
- Screening for the presence of PAH with Doppler echocardiography is warranted in individuals with a known predisposing genetic mutation or first-degree relative with IPAH, connective tissue diseases (especially scleroderma), congenital heart disease with left-to-right shunt, HIV, sickle cell disease, or portal hypertension undergoing evaluation for orthotopic liver transplantation.
- Determining the degree of functional impairment, as assessed by the WHO functional classification system (classes I-IV) and the 6-min walk test (6MWT), is a useful way to monitor disease progression and assess response to treatment.

TABLE 3 Features of the Physical Examination Pertinent to the Evaluation of Pulmonary Hypertension

Sign	Implication
PHYSICAL SIGNS THAT REFLECT THE SEVERITY OF PULMONARY HYPERTENSION	
Accentuated pulmonary component of S_2 (audible at the apex in >90%)	High pulmonary pressure that increases force of pulmonic valve closure
Early systolic click	Sudden interruption of opening of the pulmonary valve into a high-pressure artery
Midsystolic ejection murmur	Turbulent transvalvular pulmonary outflow
Left parasternal lift	High right ventricular pressure and hypertrophy present
Right ventricular S4 (in 38%)	High right ventricular pressure and hypertrophy present
Increased jugular A wave	Poor right ventricular compliance
PHYSICAL SIGNS THAT SUGGEST MODERATE TO SEVERE PULMONARY HYPERTENSION	
Moderate to severe pulmonary hypertension	
Holosystolic murmur that increases with inspiration	Tricuspid regurgitation
Increased jugular V waves	
Pulsatile liver	
Diastolic murmur	Pulmonary regurgitation
Hepatojugular reflux	High central venous pressure
Advanced pulmonary hypertension with right ventricular failure	
Right ventricular S_3 (in 23%)	Right ventricular dysfunction
Distension of jugular veins	Right ventricular dysfunction or tricuspid regurgitation, or both
Hepatomegaly	Right ventricular dysfunction or tricuspid regurgitation, or both
Peripheral edema (in 32%)	
Ascites	
Low blood pressure, diminished pulse pressure, cool extremities	Reduced cardiac output, peripheral vasoconstriction
PHYSICAL SIGNS THAT SUGGEST A POSSIBLE UNDERLYING CAUSE FOR OR ASSOCIATIONS WITH PULMONARY HYPERTENSION	
Central cyanosis	Abnormal ventilation-perfusion ratio, intrapulmonary shunt, hypoxemia, pulmonary-to-systemic shunt
Clubbing	Congenital heart disease, pulmonary venopathy
Cardiac auscultatory findings, including systolic murmurs, diastolic murmurs, opening snap, and gallop	Congenital or acquired heart or valvular disease
Rales, dullness, or decreased breath sounds	Pulmonary congestion or effusion, or both
Fine rales, accessory muscle use, wheezing, protracted expiration, productive cough	Pulmonary parenchymal disease
Obesity, kyphoscoliosis, enlarged tonsils	Possible substrate for disordered ventilation
Sclerodactyly, arthritis, telangiectasia, Raynaud phenomenon, rash	Connective tissue disorder
Peripheral venous insufficiency or obstruction	Possible venous thrombosis
Venous stasis ulcers	Possible sickle cell disease
Pulmonary vascular bruits	Chronic thromboembolic pulmonary hypertension
Splenomegaly, spider angiomas, palmar erythema, icterus, caput medusae, ascites	Portal hypertension

From McLaughlin VV et al: ACCF/AHA 2009 expert consensus document on pulmonary hypertension: a report of the American College of Cardiology Foundation Task Force on Expert Consensus Documents and the American Heart Association developed in collaboration with the American College of Chest Physicians; American Thoracic Society, Inc., and the Pulmonary Hypertension Association, *J Am Coll Cardiol* 53:1573, 2009; and Mann DL et al: *Braunwald's heart disease*, ed 11, Philadelphia, 2019, Elsevier.

- The longitudinal evaluation of patients with PAH is summarized in Table 5.

LABORATORY AND DIAGNOSTIC TESTS
- CBC is usually normal in PAH but may show secondary polycythemia.
- Other blood tests: antineutrophil antibodies (ANA), antineutrophil cytoplasmic antibodies (ANCA), anti-Scl-70, anticentromere, antitopoisomerase, anti-Ro, anti-La, anti-RNA polymerase III, ribonucleoprotein antibody levels, and rheumatoid factor (RF) to screen for underlying connective tissue disease, HIV serology, liver function tests, and antiphospholipid antibodies.
- Schistosoma stool serologies.

- Brain natriuretic peptide (BNP) level can provide prognostic information, with elevation in BNP level being associated with increased mortality.

Rx TREATMENT (FIG. E5)
- Most of the evidence in management of PAH is limited to IPAH/HPAH. There is some evidence in treatment of APAH associated with connective tissue disease, especially scleroderma, and congenital heart disease. The recommendations for treating PAH associated with other causes are limited to case studies and expert opinions.
- There is some evidence for the use of advanced therapies for sarcoidosis-associated

PH. The heterogeneity of sarcoid-associated PH complicates the interpretation.
- Therapeutic strategies for PH due to chronic lung disease are summarized in Table E6.

GENERAL MEASURES AND TREATMENT:
- Patients should be encouraged to remain active within symptom limits and avoid excessive physical activity.
- Exercise training appears to be beneficial for patients with PH. It is associated with improved exercise capacity, muscular function, quality of life, and possibly RV function and pulmonary hemodynamics.[9]
- PAH is a contraindication to pregnancy as it carries a 30% to 50% mortality risk.
- PAH patients have a higher risk of death from infections and should receive age-appropriate

vaccines as well as be vaccinated against influenza, pneumococcal pneumonia, and SARS-COV-2.

- Although patients with PH were found to have a similar incidence of SAR-COV-2 as the general population, a higher mortality rate (12%) was noted in this patient population.
- Although there are no randomized data to suggest that long-term oxygen therapy is beneficial, O_2 administration has shown to reduce pulmonary vascular resistance (PVR) and improves exercise tolerance in patients with PAH. Ambulatory O_2 may be considered for exercise-induced desaturations to maintain O_2 saturations of >90%.
- Diuretics are recommended if patients develop signs of right-sided heart failure and edema. The three main classes of diuretics—loop diuretics, thiazides, and mineralocorticoid receptor antagonists—are used as monotherapy or in combination, as determined by the patient's clinical need and kidney function.[9] Diuretics improve dyspnea by reducing preload and peripheral edema. Avoid excessive diuresis in patients who are preload dependent.
- Digoxin has been used in patients with IPAH with inconclusive benefits. It can be considered in patients who develop atrial tachyarrhythmia. There is no conclusive data regarding the use of β-blockers, ACE inhibitors, or angiotensin-receptor blockers (ARB) in IPAH unless required by comorbidities such as concurrent hypertension or cardiomyopathy.[9]
- Evidence for the use of oral anticoagulation with warfarin for IPAH is derived mostly from retrospective single-center experience. Data from randomized controlled trials (RCT) and registries remain heterogenous and inconclusive. A large multicenter observational longitudinal registry of patients with IPAH (REVEAL Registry) assessed the effect of warfarin treatment on survival and found no benefit;[10] it also found poorer survival in patients with PAH associated with systemic sclerosis. Generally, patients with IPAH who are undergoing intravenous (IV) prostaglandin therapy are anticoagulated if there are no contraindications to anticoagulation, as they are at high risk for catheter-related thrombosis. There are no data regarding the role of direct oral anticoagulants in IPAH.
- Iron deficiency with or without anemia is common and is associated with reduced exercise capacity, impaired myocardial function, aggravated symptoms, and increased mortality risk; it should be closely monitored and replenished as needed. In patients with severe

TABLE 4 Distinguishing Pulmonary Arterial Hypertension (PAH) From Heart Failure With Preserved Ejection Fraction (HFpEF)

Characteristic	PAH More Likely	HFpEF More Likely
Age	Younger	Older
Comorbid conditions—DM, HTN, CAD, obesity (metabolic syndrome)	Often absent	Often multiple present
Symptoms—PND, orthopnea	Often absent	Often present
Cardiac examination	RV heave, loud P2, TR murmur	Sustained LV impulse, LS4
CXR	Clear lung fields	Pulmonary vascular congestion, pleural effusions, pulmonary edema
Chest CT	Often clear lungs	Mosaic perfusion pattern, ground-glass opacities consistent with chronic interstitial edema
ECG	RAD, RVE	LAE, LVE, atrial fibrillation, no RAD
Natriuretic peptides	Often elevated	Often elevated
Echo—LAE, LVH	Absent	Often present
Echo—diastolic dysfunction	Grade 1 common	Grade 2, 3 common
Echo—right ventricle	Often enlarged, may share the apex	Often normal, mildly enlarged
Echo—pericardial effusion	Sometimes	Rare

CAD, Coronary artery disease; *CT,* computed tomography; *CXR,* chest x-ray; *DM,* diabetes mellitus; *ECG,* electrocardiogram; *Echo,* echocardiography; *HTN,* hypertension; *LAE,* left atrial enlargement; *LS4,* left-sided fourth heart sound; *LV,* left ventricular; *LVE,* left ventricular enlargement; *LVH,* left ventricular hypertrophy; *PND,* paroxysmal nocturnal dyspnea; *RAD,* right-axis deviation; *RV,* right ventricular; *RVE,* right ventricular enlargement; *TR,* tricuspid regurgitation.
From Mann DL et al: *Braunwald's heart disease,* ed 10, Philadelphia, 2015, Elsevier.

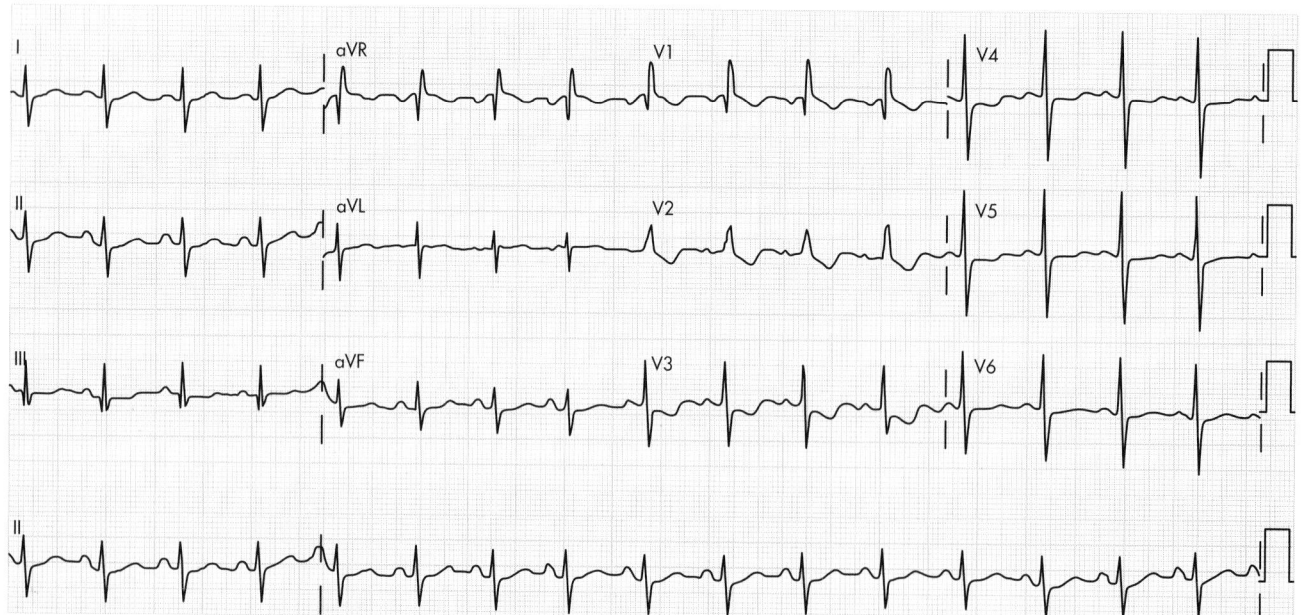

FIG. 2 Electrocardiogram from a patient with pulmonary hypertension. Findings include a prominent "p pulmonale" and increased R wave voltage in the anterior precordial leads suggestive of right atrial and right ventricular abnormalities. (From Broaddus VC et al: *Murray & Nadel's Textbook of Respiratory Medicine,* ed 7, Philadelphia, 2022, Elsevier.)

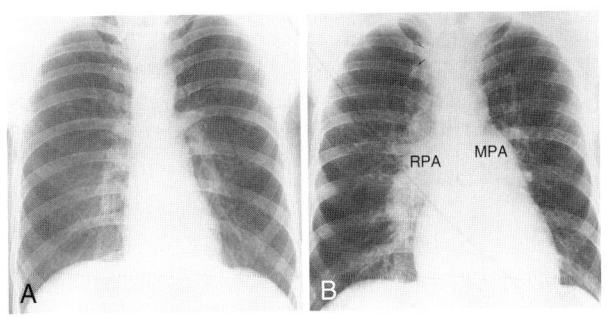

FIG. 3 Progressive pulmonary arterial hypertension. (A) This patient initially presented with a relatively normal chest x-ray film. **(B)** However, several years later, there is increasing heart size and marked dilation of the main pulmonary artery *(MPA)* and right pulmonary artery *(RPA)*. Rapid tapering of the arteries as they proceed peripherally is suggestive of pulmonary hypertension and is sometimes referred to as pruning. (From Mettler FA [ed]: *Primary care radiology,* Philadelphia, 2000, Saunders.)

TABLE 5 Longitudinal Evaluation of Patients With Pulmonary Arterial Hypertension*

	Low Risk	High Risk
Clinical course	Stable; no increase in symptoms and/or decompensation	Unstable; increase in symptoms and/or decompensation
Physical examination	No evidence of right-sided heart failure	Signs of right-sided heart failure
Functional class[†]	I/II	IV
6MWT distance[†]	>400 m	<300 m
Echocardiogram	RV size/function normal	RV enlargement/dysfunction
Hemodynamics	RAP normal/CI normal	RAP high/CI low
BNP	Nearly normal/remaining stable or decreasing	Elevated/increasing
Treatment	Oral therapy	Intravenous prostacyclin and/or combination treatment
Frequency of evaluation	Every 3-6 mo[‡]	Every 1-3 mo
FC assessment	Every clinic visit	Every clinic visit
6MWT distance	Every clinic visit	Every clinic visit
Echocardiogram[§]	Yearly or center dependent	Every 6-12 mo or center dependent
BNP[¶]	Center dependent	Center dependent
RHC	Clinical deterioration and center dependent	Every 6-12 mo or clinical deterioration

BNP, Brain natriuretic peptide; *CI,* cardiac index; *FC,* functional class; *IV,* intravenous; *RAP,* right atrial pressure; *RV,* right ventricle; *6MWT,* 6-min walk.

*For patients in the high-risk category, consider referral to a PAH specialty center for consideration of advanced therapies, clinical trials, and/or lung transplantation.

[†]The frequency of follow-up evaluation for patients in functional class III and/or 6MWT distance between 300 and 400 m would depend on a composite of detailed assessments of the other clinical and objective characteristics listed.

[‡]For patients who remain stable with established therapy, follow-up assessments can be performed by referring physicians or PH specialty centers.

[§]Echocardiographic measurement of pulmonary artery systolic pressure is an estimation only, and it is strongly advised that its evaluation not be relied on as the sole parameter to make therapeutic decisions.

[¶]The usefulness of serial BNP levels to guide management in individual patients has not been established.

From McLaughlin VV et al: ACCF/AHA 2009 expert consensus document on pulmonary hypertension. A report of the American College of Cardiology Foundation Task Force on Expert Consensus Documents and the American Heart Association developed in collaboration with the American College of Chest Physicians; American Thoracic Society, Inc.; and the Pulmonary Hypertension Association, *J Am Coll Cardiol* 53:1573, 2009; and Mann DL et al: *Braunwald's heart disease,* ed 10, Philadelphia, 2015, Elsevier.

iron deficiency anaemia (hemoglobin, 7 to 8 g/dL), IV supplementation is recommended.[11]

CHRONIC Rx

Calcium channel blocker (CCB):
- Acute vasoreactivity response testing should be done in all patients at the time of right heart catheterization. Epoprostenol, adenosine, or nitric oxide is generally used to assess the response. A positive response is a fall in mean PAP of ≥10 mm Hg to a value of <40 mm Hg, with increased or unchanged cardiac output. Fewer than 10% of patients are responders in IPAH, and they are the only patients who can be safely treated with this type of therapy. Acute vasoreactivity study is not recommended for patients in groups 2 to 5.
- The positive responders may benefit from treatment with CCBs (diltiazem, amlodipine, or nifedipine). All patients should be reassessed

in 6 to 8 wk to demonstrate sustained benefit from the CCB.
- CCBs should not be used empirically to treat PAH in the absence of demonstrated acute vasoreactivity because of potential severe side effects.
- If patients do not show an adequate response, additional PAH therapy should be started.

PROSTANOIDS

- These synthetic prostacyclin analogues act as potent vasodilators of pulmonary arteries and inhibitors of platelet aggregation, and also have both cytoprotective and anti-proliferative activities. They all have shown improvement in symptoms, exercise capacity including 6MWD, and hemodynamics. They are ideal for WHO functional class III and IV patients.
  1. Epoprostenol: IV formulation with very short half-life (3 to 5 min). It is the most studied

drug, and it is the only one that has shown to improve mortality. It requires long-term IV access with associated risks of infection and thrombosis. Rapid tachyphylaxis with dose escalation is seen. Common side effects include flushing, headache, jaw pain, abdominal cramping, and diarrhea. Limited evidence exists for use in secondary PAH patients.
  2. Treprostinil: IV and subcutaneous (SQ) formulation with longer half-life. Main disadvantage is pain at SQ pump site (no long-term evidence for IV formulation). Treprostinil is also available as an oral or nebulized inhaled solution.
  3. Iloprost: Aerosolized formulation with short half-life requiring 6 to 8 treatments/day. Oral (PO) and IV forms are also available. Well tolerated, with flushing and jaw pain being the most frequent side effects.

TABLE 7 Pulmonary Arterial Hypertension: Determinants of Prognosis*

Determinants of Risk (estimated 1-yr mortality)	Lower Risk (<5%)	Intermediate Risk (5%-10%)	Higher Risk (>10%)
Clinical evidence of RV failure	No	No	Yes
Progression of symptoms	No	Gradual	Rapid
WHO class[†]	I, II	III	IV
6MWT distance[‡]	>440 m	164-440 m	<165 m
CPET	Peak V_{O_2}>15 ml/kg/min	Peak V_{O_2} 11-15 ml/kg/min	Peak V_{O_2}<11 ml/kg/min
Echocardiography	No pericardial effusion, no RA enlargement, minimal RV dysfunction	No or minimal pericardial effusion, minimal RA enlargement	Pericardial effusion, significant RV enlargement/dysfunction, right atrial enlargement
Hemodynamics	RAP <8 mm Hg, CI >2.5 L/min/m^2	RAP 8-14 mm HgCI 2-2.4 L/min/m^2	RAP >14 mm Hg, CI <2.0 L/min/m^2
BNP[§]	Not elevated	Mildly elevated	Significantly elevated

BNP, Brain natriuretic peptide; *CI*, cardiac index; *CPET*, cardiopulmonary exercise testing; *peak V$_{O_2}$*, average peak oxygen uptake during exercise; *RA*, right arterial; *RAP*, right atrial pressure; *RV*, right ventricular; *WHO*, World Health Organization.

*Most data available pertain to IPAH, with little data available for other forms of PAH. One should not rely on any single factor to make risk predictions.

[†]The WHO class is the functional classification for PAH and is a modification of the NHYA functional class.

[‡]6MWT distance is also influenced by age, sex, and height.

[§]Because data regarding the influence of BNP on prognosis are currently limited and many factors, including renal function, weight, age, and sex, may influence BNP, absolute numbers are not given for this variable.

From McLaughlin VV et al: ACCF/AHA 2009 expert consensus document on pulmonary hypertension. A report of the American College of Cardiology Foundation Task Force on Expert Consensus Documents and the American Heart Association developed in collaboration with the American College of Chest Physicians; American Thoracic Society, Inc.; and the Pulmonary Hypertension Association, *J Am Coll Cardiol* 53:1573, 2009; and Mann DL et al: *Braunwald's heart disease,* ed 10, Philadelphia, 2015, Elsevier.

4. Beraprost: PO formulation. Not approved in the U.S.

PROSTACYCLIN AGONISTS: Selexipag is an oral selective nonprostanoid prostacyclin IP receptor agonist approved for PAH.[12] The IP receptor promotes vasodilation and antiproliferation. Selexipag has been shown to decrease disease progression and hospitalizations without any effect on mortality. Side effects are mild and consist of headache, jaw pain, flushing, and diarrhea.

RIOCIGUAT: GUANYLATE CYCLASE STIMULATORS

Guanylate cyclase stimulators enhance cyclic guanosine monophosphate (cGMP) production and in preclinical studies show antiproliferative and antiremodeling properties in animal models. These oral agents are useful for class II and III patients and have shown favorable results on exercise capacity, hemodynamics (decrease in PVR), WHO functional class, and time to clinical worsening without any mortality benefit. There has also been reported benefit in patients with inoperable and persistent chronic group IV PH with improvement in 6MWD and reduction in PVR. The most serious side effect is syncope.

ENDOTHELIN RECEPTOR ANTAGONISTS (ERAS): Activation of the endothelin system results in vasoconstriction of the pulmonary vascular smooth muscles. Most of these oral pulmonary vasodilators require monthly liver function tests, and often the response is delayed by weeks. Thus it is not an ideal starting therapy for WHO class IV patients. It is effective in class II and III patients and improves symptoms, exercise capacity, and hemodynamics without any improvement in mortality.

- Bosentan is an oral nonselective endothelin A and B receptor blocker, whereas sitaxsentan and pumbrisentan are oral selective endothelin A receptor blockers. Ambrisentan does not require monitoring of liver function tests.

- ERAs have been shown to cause improvement in exercise capacity, WHO functional class, hemodynamic and echocardiographic variables without affecting mortality.

- Macitentan is a nonselective endothelin receptor antagonist that showed significant reduction in composite end point of death in patients with IPAH. It was thought not to cause liver toxicity, but postmarketing analysis suggested it can cause liver toxicity. However, it more frequently can cause anemia and pharyngitis.

PHOSPHODIESTERASE (PDE-5) INHIBITORS:

- These are oral agents that act by inhibiting phosphodiesterase type 5 enzyme (PDE-5), resulting in increased concentration of nitric oxide causing vasodilation through the cGMP/NO pathway. In addition, they exert antiproliferative effects. Highly effective in WHO class II patients, both in IPAH and scleroderma-associated PAH. Improve symptoms, exercise capacity including 6MWD, hemodynamics, and time to clinical worsening. Mortality benefit was not studied. Side effects include headache, flushing, and epistaxis.

- Sildenafil is administered as 20 mg PO tid. Tadalafil dose is 40 mg once daily. They are also used as combination therapy with epoprostenol and endothelin receptor antagonists.

Treatment considerations depending on WHO functional class:

- According to consensus definition, patients with PAH who demonstrate acute vasoreactivity should be considered candidates for therapy with an oral CCB, except in the case of right heart failure or other contraindications.

- CCBs should not be used empirically to treat PAH in the absence of demonstrated acute vasoreactivity, as described previously.

- For treatment-naïve PAH patients with WHO functional class (FC) II or III symptoms who are not candidates for, or who have failed, CCB therapy, monotherapy should be initiated with an approved ERA, phosphodiesterase-5 (PDE5) inhibitor, or the soluble guanylate cyclase stimulator riociguat.

- For treatment-naïve PAH patients with WHO FC IV, prostanoids are first line.

- For treatment-naïve PAH patients with WHO FC III symptoms who have evidence of rapid progression of their disease or other markers of a poor clinical prognosis, consideration of initial treatment with a parenteral prostanoid is recommended.

- For treatment-naïve PAH patients in WHO FC IV who are unable, or do not desire, to manage parenteral prostanoid therapy, treatment with an inhaled prostanoid in combination with an ERA is recommended.

- For WHO FC III or IV PAH patients with unacceptable clinical status despite established PAH-specific monotherapy, addition of a second class of PAH therapy to improve exercise capacity is recommended. Such patients should be evaluated at centers with expertise in the evaluation and treatment of complex patients with PAH.

- Combination therapies: Considered when there is no improvement or deterioration on monotherapy. The FDA has approved the use of ambrisentan and tadalafil together as the first two-drug regimen for PAH because it is associated with a significant reduction in the rate of clinical failure compared with monotherapy with either drug alone (AMBITION trial). Starting dose is 5 mg for ambrisentan and 20 mg for tadalafil once daily.

- Bosentan + inhaled iloprost (STEP trial) showed some benefit over monotherapy.

- IV epoprostenol + PO bosentan (BREATH-2 trial) did not show a statistically significant difference when compared with monotherapy.

- IV epoprostenol + PO sildenafil (PACES trial) showed benefit over monotherapy.

- Inhalation of treprostinil, a stable analogue of prostacyclin, impaired exercise capacity in patients with PH due to interstitial lung disease in a recent trial.

INVASIVE Rx

- Lung transplantation and heart-lung transplantation are other options in patients with end-stage class IV disease.
- Atrial septostomy may be performed as a bridge to transplant. It involves creation of an interatrial communication, resulting in right-to-left shunt, which decreases right-sided pressure and increases LV preload and cardiac output. Atrial septostomy is recommended for individuals with a room air SaO$_2$ >90% who have severe right-sided heart failure (with refractory ascites) despite maximal diuretic therapy, or who have signs of impaired systemic blood flow (such as syncope) from reduced left heart filling.
- Extracorporeal membrane oxygenation (ECMO) is also commonly used as a bridge to transplant.
- Patients should be referred for lung transplant if:
  1. They have WHO FC III or IV during escalating treatment
  2. They have rapidly progressive disease
  3. Parenteral therapy is utilized
  4. Pulmonary venoocclusive disease (PVOD) or pulmonary capillary hemangiomatosis is known or suspected

Lung transplant recipients with IPAH have survival rates of 52% to 75% at 5 yr and 45% to 66% at 10 yr.

TREATMENT OF SECONDARY PAH, APAH:

- Directed toward cause. Some situations merit mention:
  1. PAH with uncorrected congenital heart disease: Eisenmenger syndrome. Medical treatment is generally ineffective. Heart-lung transplantation required in most patients. PH may persist after surgical correction of congenital heart disease, and pulmonary vasodilators can be effective therapies in this patient population.
  2. PAH with scleroderma: Selective pulmonary vasodilators are effective.
  3. PAH with lung disease or hypoxia: O$_2$ therapy for hypoxemia, CPAP for OSA, control of primary disease process.
  4. PAH with chronic thromboembolic disease: Pulmonary endarterectomy is curative; may consider pulmonary vasodilators, notably riociguat, after anticoagulation (for at least 3 mo and if endarterectomy is not an option) if continued symptoms and elevation in PVR and transpulmonary gradient. Fig. 6

illustrates an approach to the diagnosis of chronic thromboembolic PH and determination of operability.
  5. PAH with HIV: Control of viral load by antiretroviral therapy.

DISPOSITION

- The 6MWT is predictive of survival in patients with idiopathic PAH. A baseline 6MWT <250 m is associated with a 50% risk of death at 2 yr. Drop in O$_2$ saturation >10% during the test increases mortality risk 2.9 times over a median follow-up of 26 mo.
- Cardiopulmonary exercise testing (CPET) is also performed, during which gaseous exchange and ventilation are continuously measured during incremental exercise. A peak oxygen uptake (pVO$_2$) of <10 ml/kg/min independently predicts a worse prognosis.
- WHO class II and III patients with PAH have a mean survival of 3.5 yr.
- WHO class IV patients have a mean survival of 6 mo.
- As per the REVEAL 2.0 (Registry to Evaluate Early and Long-term Pulmonary Arterial Hypertension Disease Management) risk score, poor prognostic signs include:
  1. PAH associated with portopulmonary hypertension
  2. WHO functional class IV
  3. Walk a distance of <165 m in 6MWT
  4. Elevated BNP levels >800 pg/ml or NT-proBNP >1100 pg/ml
  5. Presence of pericardial effusion
  6. Right atrial pressure >20 mm Hg within 1 yr on right heart catheterization
  7. Increased heart rate >96 or BP <110 mm Hg
  8. Male gender >60 yr of age
  9. Concomitant renal dysfunction with estimated glomerular filtration rate <60 ml/min/m
  10. Diffusion capacity of lung for carbon monoxide (DLCO) <40%
  11. All-cause hospitalization within the last 6 mo

REFERRAL

If the diagnosis of IPAH/HPAH is suspected, a consultation with a pulmonary specialist is recommended. PHA may require disease-specific consultations. Advanced cases need to be transferred to transplant centers.

❗ PEARLS & CONSIDERATIONS

- The exertional dyspnea of PAH is typically described by patients as being relentlessly

progressive over several months to a year, often out of proportion to, or in the absence of, underlying heart or lung disease.
- Over 20% of patients in the Registry to Evaluate Early and Long-term PAH Disease Management had symptoms for more than 2 yr before PAH was recognized. Consideration of the diagnosis of PAH in the differential diagnosis of unexplained dyspnea, especially in younger individuals, is essential.
- Chest x-ray may reveal evidence of interstitial fluid or fibrosis within the lungs in cases of secondary PH. IPAH is not associated with infiltrates on chest x-ray.

COMMENTS

- RV systolic pressure (RVSP) as estimated by echocardiography is not a good indicator of the presence of PAH because RVSP increases with age and body mass index. Athletically conditioned men also have a higher resting RVSP. Thus these measurements can be misleading.
- Abrupt development of pulmonary edema during acute vasodilator testing suggests pulmonary venoocclusive disease or pulmonary capillary hemangiomatosis and is a contraindication to long-term vasodilator treatment.
- In advanced PAH, heart rate increase is the main compensatory mechanism and reflects increased sympathetic tone. A higher heart rate at rest is an important marker of prognosis and should be assessed at frequent intervals after initiation of treatment for PAH.
- Current therapies significantly improve exercise capacity, quality of life, and pulmonary hemodynamics, but none of these therapies is curative and long-term prognosis remains poor. Many therapies are still under clinical development, and there are some promising results. These therapies include tyrosine kinase inhibitors, rho kinase inhibitors, and pulmonary artery denervation, among others.

REFERENCES
Available at eBooks.Health.Elsevier.com.

RELATED CONTENT
Pulmonary Hypertension (Patient Information)

AUTHORS: **CRAIG L. BASMAN, MD, FACC, FSCAI**, and **ARPANJEET KAUR, MD**

Diseases and Disorders

P

I

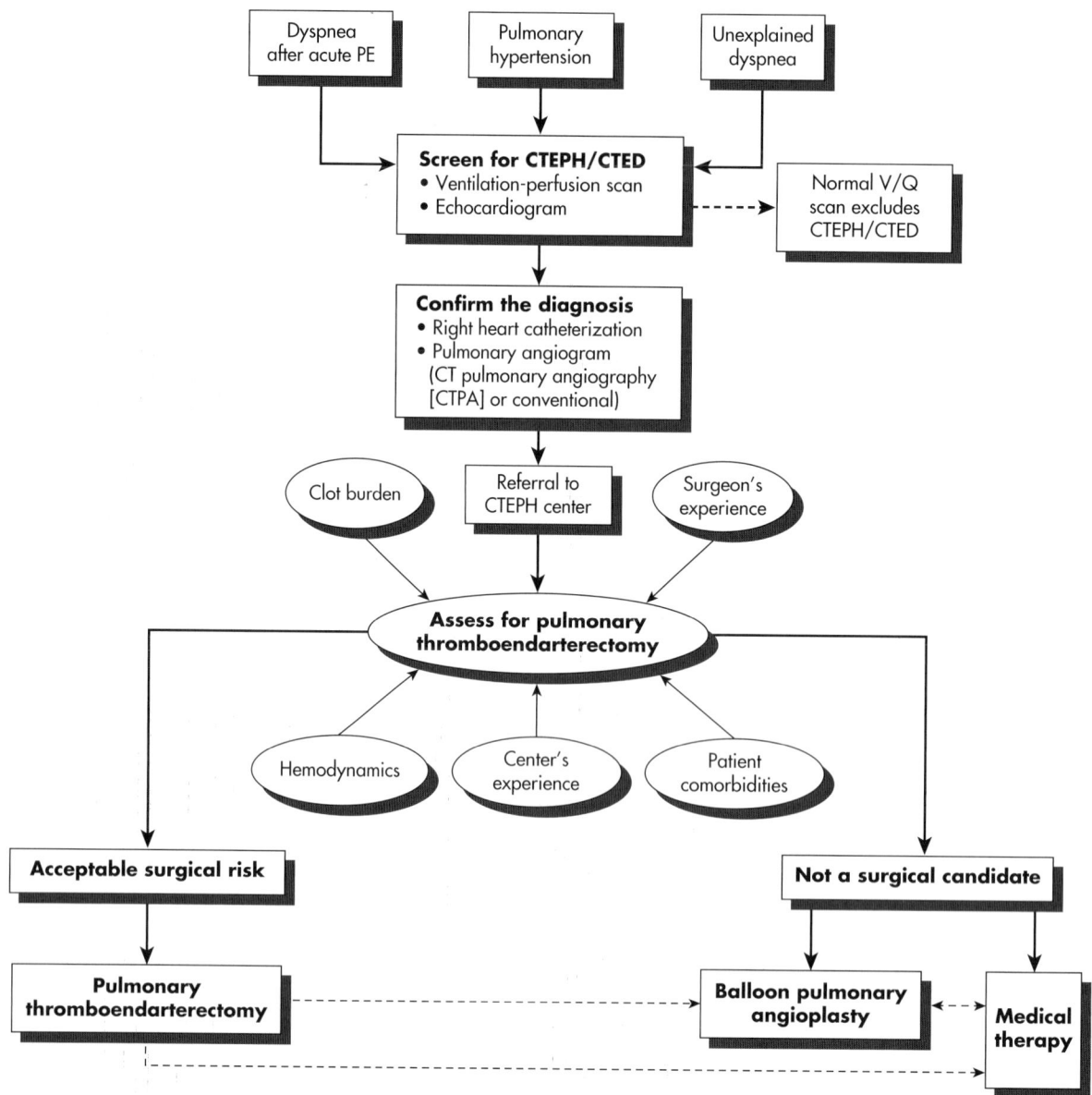

FIG. 6 Approach to the diagnosis of chronic thromboembolic pulmonary hypertension and determination of operability. Patients with residual dyspnea after acute pulmonary embolism *(PE)*, pulmonary hypertension, or unexplained dyspnea should be screened for chronic thromboembolic pulmonary hypertension *(CTEPH)*. Initial screening is done with a ventilation-perfusion *(V/Q)* scan (to look for perfusion defects) and an echocardiogram (to screen for resting pulmonary hypertension). The diagnosis of CTEPH is confirmed with right heart catheterization to assess hemodynamics and pulmonary angiography to determine the amount and proximity of the chronic thrombotic material. Once the diagnosis is established, the key is referral to a CTEPH center where both pulmonary thromboendarterectomy *(PTE)* surgery and balloon pulmonary angioplasty *(BPA)* are offered. The first management decision the CTEPH center makes is determining whether the patient is a surgical candidate. Clot burden, location of disease, hemodynamics, comorbidities, and experience of both the surgeon and the center factor into the decision. PTE surgery is offered to all patients with an acceptable risk/benefit ratio because PTE is curative in the majority of patients. In those with residual pulmonary hypertension following PTE, BPA and/or pulmonary hypertension–targeted therapy can be considered. For those deemed not to be surgical candidates (either due to disease that is too distal or to an unacceptable PTE risk/benefit ratio), therapeutic options include BPA, medical therapy, or a combination of both. All patients with CTEPH require lifelong anticoagulation to prevent recurrent thrombosis. *CTED,* Chronic thromboembolic disease. (From Broaddus VC et al: *Murray & Nadel's textbook of respiratory medicine,* ed 7, Philadelphia, 2022, Elsevier.)

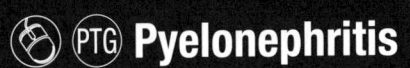
P

I

BASIC INFORMATION

DEFINITION

Pyelonephritis is an ascending infection of a bacterial pathogen that infects the renal pelvis and kidney. It primarily presents as a urinary tract infection (UTI) characterized by painful urination (dysuria) with associated flank pain/tenderness, nausea, vomiting, and/or fever. Older adults may also present with failure-to-thrive, unexplained anorexia, other organ system decompensation, or generalized deterioration.

CONSISTS OF TWO GROUPS:

- *Uncomplicated:* Can be treated as an outpatient with oral (PO) antibiotics.
- *Complicated:* Inpatient treatment with intravenous (IV) antibiotics is required. Hospitalization is indicated for persistent vomiting, progression of uncomplicated UTI, suspected sepsis, immunosuppression, or urinary tract obstruction. This is a potentially life-threatening infection that can lead to renal parenchymal damage. Timely diagnosis and management can significantly impact patient outcomes.

SYNONYMS

Acute pyelonephritis
Pyonephrosis
Renal carbuncle
Lobar nephronia
Acute bacterial nephritis

ICD-10CM CODES
N10	Acute pyelonephritis
N11	Chronic tubulo-interstitial nephritis
N11.0	Nonobstructive reflux-associated chronic pyelonephritis
N11.1	Chronic obstructive pyelonephritis
N11.8	Other chronic tubulo-interstitial nephritis
N11.9	Chronic tubulo-interstitial nephritis, unspecified
N12	Tubulo-interstitial nephritis, not specified as acute or chronic
N20.9	Calculus pyelonephritis

Use additional code (B95-B97) to identify infectious agent.

EPIDEMIOLOGY & DEMOGRAPHICS

INCIDENCE: Pyelonephritis is common in the U.S. with overall rates of 15 to 17 cases/10,000 women and 3 to 4 cases/10,000 men. Pyelonephritis accounts for 9.1% to 31% of severe sepsis cases annually, depending on geographic area. Average annual mortality is 16.1%, ranging from 5% for patients <25 yr to 43% for ages >64 yr.
PREDOMINANT SEX: Women are 5 times more likely to be hospitalized than men until the age of 65 yr. In men beyond the age of 65 yr, the difference in prevalence narrows. Risk factors associated with pyelonephritis in healthy women are sexual intercourse (≥3 times wk over the previous 30 days), a new sex partner in the past year, use of spermicide, UTI during the past 12 mo, mother with a history of UTI, diabetes mellitus, and urinary incontinence. Urinary tract obstruction is the most important risk factor for a complicated UTI.

PREDOMINANT AGE: Trimodal distribution described in female patients:
- Girls, ages 0 to 4 yr
- Women, ages 15 to 35 yr, especially if sexually active
- Gradual increase in frequency after age 50 yr, with peak incidence at 80 yr

Bimodal distribution in male patients:
- Boys, ages 0 to 4 yr
- Gradual increase in prevalence after age 35 yr, with peak incidence at 85 yr

GENETICS: Congenital urologic structural disorders associated with vesicoureteral reflux predispose individuals to infections at an early age (<5 yr) and produce renal scarring in most male and some female patients. Pyelonephritis may produce an Ask-Upmark kidney (segmental renal hypoplasia) that is found more often in young female patients with severe hypertension.

PHYSICAL FINDINGS & CLINICAL PRESENTATION

Diagnosis established by clinical presentation, history, and physical examination.

Pyelonephritis is suspected in cases of lower urinary tract symptoms (e.g., urinary frequency, urgency, and dysuria) and frequently accompanied by any of the following:
- Fever, rigors, chills (fever may not be present in older adults or the immunosuppressed)
- Flank pain
- Hematuria: Gross hematuria occurs rarely in acute pyelonephritis and raises suspicion for acute cystitis, papillary necrosis, or lower genitourinary malignancy
- Toxic appearance
- Nausea and vomiting
- Headache
- Diarrhea

Physical examination may elicit costovertebral angle tenderness with flank pain, a nearly universal finding. Its absence suggests an alternative diagnosis. Patients presenting with nephrolithiasis/ureterolithiasis usually do not present with costovertebral angle tenderness. Usually, abdominal or suprapubic tenderness is present.

ETIOLOGY

Ascending infections from intestinal bacteria that colonize the perineum and vulvae in women account for most infections. Less commonly, bacteria, viruses, or fungal pathogens may produce hematogenously induced pyelonephritis.
- Gram-negative bacilli cause >80% of cases (e.g., *Escherichia coli* and *Klebsiella* species).
- Less common gram-negative bacteria may produce infection, particularly after urinary tract instrumentation (e.g., *Proteus mirabilis, Enterobacter, Serratia,* and *Pseudomonas* species).
- Resistant gram-negative organisms or fungi such as *Candida* may colonize indwelling catheters.
- Gram-positive organisms such as enterococci and rarely, *Staphylococcus saprophyticus.*
- *Staphylococcus aureus* indicates hematogenous spread to the kidneys.
- Viruses generally are limited to the lower urinary tract.

- Urea-splitting organisms generate alkaline urine that fosters production of staghorn calculi. These stones may grow to large size and cause infection, obstruction, or both.

In older adults, *E. coli* is less common (60%). Patients with diabetes develop infections from *Klebsiella* species, Enterobacteriaceae, *Clostridioides* species, or *Candida* species.

During the past decade, community-acquired bacteria (particularly *E. coli*) that produce extended-spectrum beta-lactamases have emerged as a cause of acute pyelonephritis worldwide. The most common risk factors for these uropathogens include frequent visits to health care centers, recent use of antimicrobials (e.g., cephalosporins and fluoroquinolones), older age, immunosuppression, recurrent pyelonephritis, nephrolithiasis, and comorbid conditions such as diabetes mellitus and recurrent UTIs.

DIAGNOSIS

DIFFERENTIAL DIAGNOSIS

Differential diagnosis includes the following:
- Abdominal abscess
- Acute abdomen
- Appendicitis
- Basilar pleural process
- Diverticulitis
- Endometriosis
- Herpes zoster
- Lower rib fracture
- Metastatic disease
- Musculoskeletal disorders
- Nephrolithiasis
- Pancreatitis
- Papillary necrosis
- Pelvic inflammatory disease
- Prostatitis
- Pulmonary infarctions
- Renal corticomedullary necrosis
- Renal vein thrombosis
- Retroperitoneal hemorrhage or abscess
- Splenic abscess or infarct
- Urinary tract obstruction
- Vascular pathology

WORKUP

URINALYSIS: Obtained from and conducted on a clean-catch voided or catheterized specimen, if unable to void or cooperate. Dipstick and microscopic examination must be performed on a fresh specimen for preservation of formed elements (e.g., cells, casts, and microorganisms). Most cases demonstrate pyuria and positive leukocyte esterase in association with a positive blood reaction and microhematuria. Leukocyte casts are generally of kidney origin but may be absent.
URINE CULTURE: Historically, clean, midstream cultures are obtained from all patients suspected of having acute pyelonephritis to guide antibiotic therapy. However, a clean-catch specimen may not be necessary. Recent evidence demonstrates no significant difference in the number of contaminated or unreliable culture results when urine is collected with or without preparatory cleansing. Obtain a catheterized

urine sample if the patient is unable to void, uncooperative, or has an altered mental status. There is no difference in colony counts or organisms between catheterized and midstream voiding samples.

More than 95% of acute pyelonephritis cases exhibit $>10^5$ colony forming units of a single bacterium per milliliter of urine. However, it is important to obtain an accurate history regarding the timing of culture acquisition and prior antibiotic administration. A negative culture with classic clinical and radiologic findings does not rule out acute pyelonephritis, as shown by a prospective study, in which only 23.5% of 196 patients with clinical and radiologic evidence of acute pyelonephritis had demonstrated positive urine cultures. A urine Gram stain may aid in the choice of empiric antimicrobial therapy pending urine culture. If gram-positive cocci are seen, consider *Enterococcus* species or *S. saprophyticus* as causative.

Posttreatment urinalysis and culture are unnecessary if symptomatic improvement occurs, but these studies should be obtained when symptomatic improvement does not occur after 2 or 3 days of antibiotic treatment, or if symptoms recur within 2 wk of treatment. Urinary tract imaging is recommended in such cases.

BLOOD CULTURES: Cultures are obtained from hospitalized patients but may not be routinely required in uncomplicated cases. Approximately 15% to 30% of patients with acute pyelonephritis are bacteremic. Older adults and individuals with complicated acute pyelonephritis are more likely to develop bacteremia and sepsis.

Urine cultures yield a causative organism in nearly all cases of acute pyelonephritis. Therefore, a positive blood culture may be diagnostically redundant. However, in unclear cases, or when an alternative diagnosis to acute pyelonephritis is considered, blood cultures should be obtained.

IMAGING STUDIES: The primary imaging modalities used in patients with pyelonephritis are computed tomography (CT), MRI, and ultrasound. Most uncomplicated cases of acute pyelonephritis do not require imaging studies unless symptoms do not improve, recurrence occurs, or if the patient has prolonged fever (>72 h) or persistent bacteremia. Abdominal radiographs (i.e., kidney, ureter, and bladder x-ray [KUB]) are of limited

utility in acute pyelonephritis, unless staghorn calculi are present. Retrograde or antegrade pyelography may be helpful in severe obstruction that is not evident after noninvasive evaluations. Voiding cystourethrography demonstrates vesicoureteral reflux and generally is conducted routinely only in children.

Recommendations for radiologic tests:

- Healthy patients with uncomplicated pyelonephritis typically do not require radiologic evaluation when therapeutic responses occur within 72 h of antibiotic therapy.
- If no response to therapy occurs within 72 h, abdominal CT is the study of choice.
- Patients with diabetes and immunocompromised patients should undergo precontrast and postcontrast abdominal and pelvic CT scans (Fig. 1) within 24 h of diagnosis when response to therapy is not prompt.
- Ultrasound (Fig. 2) is reserved for patients in whom exposure to contrast or radiation is considered hazardous. There is a high false-negative rate for renal abscess with ultrasound. In a prospective study of acute pyelonephritis that included 213 patients who had a CT/nuclear magnetic resonance (NMR) study done, 50 patients (23.5%) had a renal abscess, yet only 2 were detected by ultrasound.
- All other adults with complicated cases (i.e., history of stones or other urologic conditions, prior urologic surgery, repeated episodes of pyelonephritis) should be evaluated early by CT.
- Helical CT detects calculi with high sensitivity.
- Urologic imaging studies should be conducted in all young men and boys.

Although the risk of contrast-induced nephropathy has declined substantially, exert caution during contrast administration in patients with chronic kidney disease or for those taking metformin. When evaluating kidney function, diagnostic decision-making must include estimated glomerular filtration rate trends, not serum creatinine levels, especially in older adults with reduced muscle mass. Patients with acute pyelonephritis and acutely elevated baseline serum creatinine concentrations may warrant CT imaging to rule out obstruction. If the risk of radiocontrast media administration outweighs its benefits, consider MRI or retrograde or antegrade pyelography.

The purpose of imaging is to identify underlying structural abnormalities such as occult obstruction from a stone or abscess and serious complications such as emphysematous pyelonephritis (EPN). In a prospective study of 213 patients with acute pyelonephritis, there were no differences in frequency of fever, leukocytosis, C-reactive protein, pyuria, urine cultures, and duration of symptoms before hospitalization for positive or negative CT. Accordingly, systematic CT or MRI is not required to exclude an anatomic abnormality. Such abnormalities cannot be predicted based on clinical, biochemical, or culture parameters.

EPN is a necrotizing infection that produces intraparenchymal kidney gas visualized by renal imaging. This disorder is associated with high mortality. Risk factors include diabetes mellitus and/or urinary tract obstruction. Gas-forming bacteria, most commonly *E. coli*, produce gas typically restricted within the Gerota fascia. Studies suggest an overall EPN mortality rate of 19%, reporting significant treatment success rates with percutaneous drainage and antibiotics (66%) and with nephrectomy (90%). EPN must be differentiated from a renal abscess, which can also be associated with a gas collection. With drainage and antibiotic treatment, a renal abscess has a favorable prognosis.

LABORATORY TESTS

A basic metabolic profile and CBC with differential count are required to estimate kidney function in patients with suspected acute pyelonephritis. If the diagnosis is in doubt, other laboratory tests may be appropriate to clarify the differential diagnosis (e.g., lipase, transaminase, and β-hCG levels).

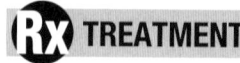 **TREATMENT**

ACUTE GENERAL Rx
UNCOMPLICATED ACUTE PYELONEPHRITIS:
Close outpatient follow-up is possible for patients with minimal GI symptoms and the ability to maintain fluid intake and oral medications. Prompt antibiotic therapy prevents progression of infection and must be initiated following acquisition of appropriate cultures. Begin empiric therapy based on risk of adverse effects, local community bacterial profiles, and

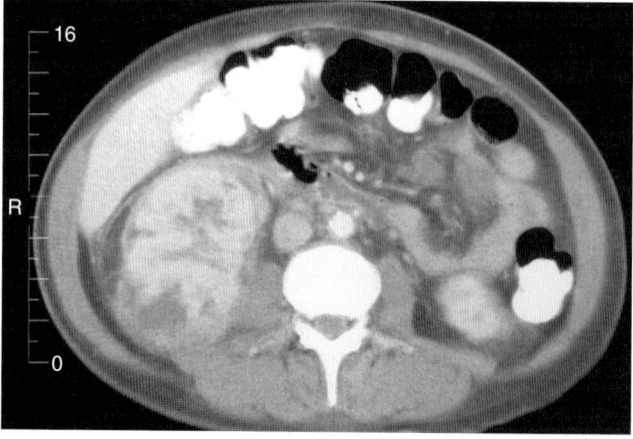

FIG. 1 Acute pyelonephritis: Contrast material–enhanced computed tomography (CT) scan. The heterogeneous CT nephrogram shows the diffuse involvement of the right kidney. Stranding and some fluid are visible in the perinephric space with thickening of Gerota fascia. (From Skorecki K et al: *Brenner & Rector's the kidney,* ed 10, Philadelphia, 2016, Elsevier.)

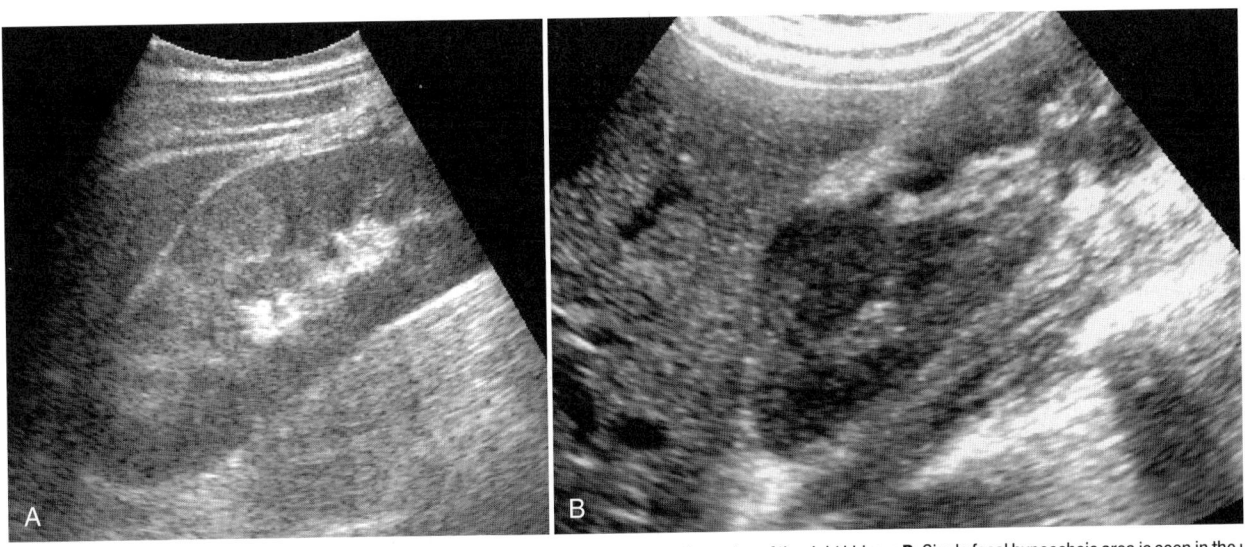

FIG. 2 Acute pyelonephritis. A, Subtle focal increased echogenic areas are seen in the anterior cortex of the right kidney. **B**, Single focal hypoechoic area is seen in the upper pole of the kidney in another patient. (From Rumack CM et al: *Diagnostic ultrasound,* ed 4, Philadelphia, 2011, Elsevier.)

resistance rates. Antibiotics are revised after urine culture results are available.

The concept of requiring long-term treatment for acute pyelonephritis has been questioned. Women with acute pyelonephritis were randomized to PO treatment with ciprofloxacin 500 mg bid for 7 days or 14 days, and 27% of these patients experienced bacteremia from *E. coli.* No differences in the cure rates were found (87% and 96%, respectively).

Outpatient regimens:
- Fluoroquinolones are preferred in communities where the local prevalence of resistant *E. coli* is ≤10%.
- Ciprofloxacin 500 mg PO bid or a single, 1000-mg/day PO dose in the extended-release form for 7 days.
- Levofloxacin 750 mg/day PO for 5 to 7 days.
- The initial dose may be administered intravenously (ciprofloxacin 400 mg or levofloxacin 500 mg).
- When a fluoroquinolone is contraindicated, alternative treatment with trimethoprim-sulfamethoxazole (TMP-SMX) 160/800 mg PO bid for 10 to 14 days may be administered if the pathogen is susceptible.

Because of the high prevalence of resistance to PO beta-lactam antibiotics and TMP-SMX, these agents usually are reserved for cases in which susceptibility results are known. Additional factors (e.g., allergy history, potential drug–drug interactions, drug availability) may require empiric treatment with these agents before susceptibility testing results are known. In this circumstance, a long-acting, broad-spectrum parenteral drug (e.g., ceftriaxone 1 g or gentamicin 5 mg/kg) may be administered as a one-time dose or longer, until sensitivities of the organism are known. If the local prevalence of fluoroquinolone resistance to *E. coli* exceeds 10%, an initial IV dose of ceftriaxone or gentamicin is recommended, followed by an oral fluoroquinolone regimen.

Significant clinical improvement during appropriate empiric antibiotic therapy should occur within 48 to 72 h. If improvement does not occur, a complication of acute pyelonephritis or an alternative diagnosis such as an abscess, EPN, or an obstructing calculus should be considered. Any unexpected change in the clinical picture warrants immediate investigation with a CT scan.

COMPLICATED ACUTE PYELONEPHRITIS:
Hospitalization is indicated for the following reasons:
- Toxic patients
- Complicated infections
- Diabetes or otherwise immunosuppressed
- Suspected bacteremia

Inpatient care includes supportive care, monitoring of culture results, adjustment of antibiotic regimen, and IV volume repletion as required. IV antibiotics are continued until defervescence occurs and clinical improvement occurs. Next, there is conversion to a PO antibiotic regimen for a total duration of 10 to 14 days.
- IV antibiotic options for more toxic patients pending cultures include IV ceftriaxone (once daily), IV ciprofloxacin (400 mg bid), IV levofloxacin (500 mg/day), piperacillin/tazobactam (3.375 g IV qid), or carbapenems such as meropenem (500 mg IV tid).
- Ceftazidime 1 to 2 g IV tid, piperacillin/tazobactam, or carbapenems are optimal choices for *Pseudomonas* because of increasing ciprofloxacin resistance.
- Aminoglycosides are potentially nephrotoxic. These agents should be used only if no better alternative exists.
- Vancomycin 1 g IV bid, linezolid 600 mg IV or PO bid, or daptomycin 4 to 6 mg/kg/day IV for gram-positive cocci (e.g., enterococci, staphylococci).
- Ampicillin 1 to 2 g IV every 4 to 6 h for ampicillin-sensitive enterococci with aminoglycoside for synergy. Urinary obstruction is promptly drained by nephrostomy tube. Surgical drainage of abscess formation(s).

- Pregnant women with acute pyelonephritis are hospitalized and treated initially with a second- or third-generation cephalosporin.

RENAL ABSCESSES (RENAL CARBUNCLES):
Cortical abscesses historically required surgical drainage; however, using current antibiotics is commonly sufficient for cure.
- Semisynthetic penicillin, cephalosporin, fluoroquinolone, or vancomycin with guidance from culture and sensitivity results.
  1. Parenteral therapy for 10 to 14 days followed by PO therapy for 2 to 4 wk.
  2. Fever should resolve in 5 to 6 days and pain within 24 h.
  3. If no clinical response occurs within 48 h, percutaneous (preferred) or open drainage should be considered. More extreme measures are occasionally required, including enucleation or nephrectomy.

CORTICOMEDULLARY ABSCESSES:
- Parenteral therapy for at least 48 h is generally successful.
- May require incision and drainage and possibly, nephrectomy.
- If defervescence occurs, IV antibiotic treatment may be switched to complete a 2-wk course of PO antibiotic therapy.

PERINEPHRIC ABSCESSES:
- Serious complication with mortality in the 25% to 50% range.
- Lesions require early recognition, surgical drainage, and parenteral antibiotics (not adequate alone) to reduce mortality.
- Initial antibiotic therapy may include piperacillin-tazobactam, cefepime, or meropenem.
- Empiric therapy in the setting of *S. aureus* bacteremia includes nafcillin, oxacillin, cefazolin, or vancomycin (when methicillin-resistant *Staphylococcus aureus* is suspected).
- Tuberculosis and fungi are rare reported causes.
- Nephrectomy may be considered with clinical deterioration despite aggressive therapy.

CALCULI-RELATED INFECTIONS: Chronic pyelonephritis may lead to formation of struvite stones (magnesium ammonium phosphate stones). Formation requires infection with a urease-producing organism such as *Proteus* or *Klebsiella*. Symptoms directly attributable to struvite stones are uncommon. Typically, patients will present with symptoms of a UTI, mild flank pain, or hematuria. The stone may grow rapidly over a period of weeks to months if treatment is inadequate. Medical treatment for struvite stones is often ineffective and only indicated when surgery is not an option. The most common surgical intervention is percutaneous nephrolithotomy. Open surgery, once the gold standard, is now rarely used.

Surgical intervention is generally recommended in patients with newly discovered stones or in patients with a solitary kidney or two equally functioning kidneys. Nephrectomy is a reasonable option in patients with a nonfunctional kidney, particularly when chronic infection is present.

RENAL PAPILLARY NECROSIS:
- Admission for parenteral antibiotics:
  1. Initial therapy should cover *E. coli*, *Enterobacter*, *Proteus*, and *Klebsiella* species, pending culture results.
  2. For more serious infections, *Pseudomonas* and *Enterococcus* should also be covered.
  3. Empiric therapy agent options include the following:
     a. Aminoglycosides
     b. Cefotaxime
     c. Ceftriaxone
     d. Ceftazidime
     e. Cefepime
     f. Piperacillin-tazobactam
     g. Imipenem-cilastatin
     h. Meropenem
     i. Ciprofloxacin
  4. Continue parenteral therapy until fever and clinical symptoms improve.

Xanthogranulomatous pyelonephritis (XGP) is a rare variant of chronic pyelonephritis with destruction of renal parenchyma.
- Generally unilateral
- Affects women more than men from newborn to advanced age
- Usually in individuals with obstructing stones
- Presents with flank or abdominal pain, lower urinary tract symptoms, fever, palpable mass, gross hematuria, or weight loss

- Urine cultures commonly demonstrate *E. coli* or *Proteus mirabilis*
- CT is the diagnostic modality of choice and provides staging information
- Can be confused with malignancy
- Treatment is surgical nephrectomy

Chronic nephrolithiasis, especially in high-risk populations such as patients with diabetes or immunosuppressed patients, can predispose individuals and promote complicated infections leading to XGP and ENP. These are very rare disorders that are difficult to diagnose, and an unrecognized renal tumor can be hidden behind a suspected diagnosis of XGP and ENP.

CHRONIC Rx
- Repair underlying structural problems, especially when kidney function is compromised.
  1. Reflux
     a. Obstruction
     b. Suspect nephrolithiasis
- Avoid urinary catheters.

DISPOSITION
- If pyelonephritis is uncomplicated with no significant GI symptoms, treatment may be initiated on an outpatient basis with close monitoring of therapeutic response(s) in 48 to 72 h.
- If pyelonephritis is complicated and symptoms persist for >48 to 72 h, admission is recommended for any of the following: Significant GI symptoms that preclude PO therapy, pregnancy, urinary tract obstruction, suspected renal or perinephric abscess, bacterial sepsis, diabetes or other immunocompromised states, recurrent or refractory pyelonephritis, or infection with unusual or antibiotic-resistant microorganisms.
- If sepsis is present, consider intensive care unit hospitalization.
- Acute pyelonephritis may be fatal when complications develop such as EPN (mortality rate, 20% to 80%), perinephric abscess (mortality rate, 20% to 50%), or sepsis syndrome (>25% overall mortality rate).
- Acute deterioration or nonresponse to conventional therapy may be due to a complication, resistant organism, or unrecognized comorbidity.
- Patients with diabetes and acute pyelonephritis are prone to bacteremia, longer hospital stays, and greater mortality. Those with diabetes should be considered to have complicated status.
- Patients older than 65 yr have greater mortality, septic shock, bedridden status, and immunosuppression. In men, mortality is also increased with the use of antibiotics in the previous month.

REFERRAL
- General surgery or urology for suspected abscess
- Infectious disease for resistant organisms and poor response to routine antibiotic therapy as outlined
- Urology to correct underlying urologic problems (e.g., reflux and hydronephrosis)
- Nephrology consult for renal dysfunction or nephrolithiasis evaluation
- Critical care monitoring, if intensive care unit admission is required

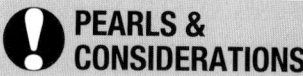 **PEARLS & CONSIDERATIONS**

- Consider acute pyelonephritis in patients with urinary symptoms, flank pain, and fever.
- Obtain a urinalysis and culture before starting empiric antibiotic therapy. Adjust treatment pending antibiotic sensitivity testing.
- Evaluate clinical response in 48 to 72 h during outpatient therapy. If there is no or delayed improvement, continue evaluation to rule out urinary tract obstruction.
- Pursue urology consultation in all cases of urinary tract obstruction or detection of urinary tract gas (e.g., emphysematous pyelonephritis).
- Treat all patients who have diabetes as having complicated acute pyelonephritis.

SUGGESTED READINGS
Available at eBooks.Health.Elsevier.com.

RELATED CONTENT
Pyelonephritis (Patient Information)

AUTHORS: **JAMES P. REICHART, MD,** and **NELSON KOPYT, DO**

BASIC INFORMATION

DEFINITION

Raynaud phenomenon (RP) is a vasospastic disorder that causes an exaggerated response to cold temperatures and/or emotional stress, resulting in episodic digital ischemia. It presents as a cold-induced, symmetric, sharply demarcated white or blue discoloration of the distal fingers or toes, followed by erythema at a variable time after rewarming.

SYNONYMS

Primary Raynaud phenomenon or Raynaud disease
Secondary Raynaud phenomenon
RP

ICD-10CM CODES
I73.0   Raynaud syndrome
I73.00 Raynaud syndrome without gangrene
I73.01 Raynaud syndrome with gangrene

EPIDEMIOLOGY & DEMOGRAPHICS

- RP is classified clinically into primary or secondary forms and affects approximately 3% to 5% of the general population, 15% of children younger than 12 yr, and less than 1% of adults older than 60 yr.
- Occurs more commonly in colder climates.
- Primary RP usually occurs between the ages of 12 and 25 yr.
- It is more likely to affect more women than men (4:1).
- 5% to 15% of patients with primary RP develop a secondary cause later in the course of the disease (mostly a connective tissue disorder).
- Secondary RP tends to begin after age 35 to 40 yr.
- Secondary RP occurs in more than 90% of patients with scleroderma and in approximately 30% of patients with systemic lupus erythematosus or Sjögren syndrome.

PHYSICAL FINDINGS & CLINICAL PRESENTATION

- The typical manifestation of RP is the biphasic color response of the digits to cold exposure and rewarming, which may or may not be accompanied by pain. RP most often affects the hand (Fig. E1).
  1. White (pallor) or blue (cyanotic) discoloration of the digit(s) resulting from vasospasm on cold or vibration exposure.
  2. Red (rubor) with or without pain and paresthesia when vasospasm resolves and blood returns to the digit.
- Color changes can sometimes be induced by placing the hand in an ice bath, although this is not recommended as a diagnostic maneuver because responses may be inconsistent even in patients with definite RP.
- Color changes are well delineated, symmetric, and usually bilateral, involving the fingers and toes. The index, middle, and ring fingers are commonly involved and the thumb

infrequently; however, if the thumb is involved, that suggests secondary causes of RP.
- Fingertips are most often involved, but feet, ears, nose, tongue, and nipples can also be affected.
- Patients with RP may exhibit a violaceous or reticular pattern of skin of arms and legs, sometimes with regular, unbroken circles (livedo reticularis).
- Duration of attacks can range from seconds to hours and averages 15 to 20 min.
- Chronic skin changes resulting from repeated attacks may include skin thickening and brittle nails. Ulcerations and, rarely, gangrene may occur.
- Physical examination should also include examination for symptoms associated with autoimmune disease, such as fever, rash, arthritis, dry eyes, dry mouth, myalgias, or cardiopulmonary abnormalities.

ETIOLOGY

- Primary RP can also be called idiopathic RP, primary Raynaud syndrome, or Raynaud disease. It occurs in the absence of any associated disease.
- With primary RP, the possibility that another first-degree family member is affected is reported as approximately 25%.
- Secondary RP is associated with an underlying pathologic condition or disorder, use of certain drugs, or related occupation. Secondary causes of RP are summarized in Box 1.

DX DIAGNOSIS

Clinical criteria:
- Definite RP: Repeated episodes of biphasic color change on cold exposure
- Possible RP: Uniphasic color changes plus numbness or paresthesia on cold exposure
- No RP: No color change on cold exposure
The suggested criteria for primary RP are:
- Symmetric attacks
- Absence of tissue necrosis, ulceration, gangrene, or peripheral vascular disease
- Absence of a secondary cause on the basis of a patient's history and general physical examination
- Negative nail-fold capillary examination
- Negative test for antinuclear antibody (ANA)
- Normal erythrocyte sedimentation rate (ESR)
Secondary RP is suggested by the following findings:
- Onset of symptoms after age 30 yr
- Male gender
- Episodes that are painful, asymmetric, or associated with ischemic skin lesions
- Clinical features suggestive of a connective-tissue disease
- Elevated specific autoantibody tests and ESR
- Evidence of microvascular disease on microscopy of nail-fold capillaries
- It is critical to differentiate primary and secondary RP since management is significantly different for the two conditions. Table 1

BOX 1   Secondary Causes of Raynaud Phenomenon

Rheumatologic
Systemic sclerosis (CREST syndrome)
Sjögren syndrome
Systemic lupus erythematosus
Ehlers-Danlos syndrome
Rheumatoid arthritis
Dermatomyositis
Polymyositis
Mixed connective tissue disease

Autoimmune
Reiter syndrome
Vasculitis (polyarteritis nodosa, Henoch-Schönlein purpura)
Antiphospholipid syndrome
Primary pulmonary hypertension

Endocrine
Hypothyroidism
Pheochromocytoma
Carcinoid

Infectious
Hepatitis B and C infection
Mycoplasma pneumonia

Medications
Cyclosporine
Ergotamine
Beta-blockers
Cytotoxic (bleomycin, cisplatin, vinblastine)
Bromocriptine
Nicotine
Cocaine
Sulfasalazine
Interferon-alpha and interferon-beta
Clonidine
Sympathomimetics
Estrogen in oral contraceptives
Caffeine

Occlusive Vascular
Arteriosclerosis
Vascular trauma (hypothenar hammer syndrome)
Buerger disease
Thoracic outlet syndrome
Thromboembolism

Hematologic Proliferative
Leukemia
Lymphoma
Polycythemia vera
Multiple myeloma
Disseminated intravascular coagulation
Cryoglobulinemia
Cold agglutinin disease

Neurologic
Migraines
Carpal tunnel syndrome
Polyneuropathy

Environmental
Emotional stress
Frostbite
Repetitive trauma or injuries to hand

Malignancy
Lung, stomach, small bowel
Paraneoplastic syndrome
Neurofibromatosis

From Cameron JL, Cameron AM: *Current surgical therapy,* ed 12, Philadelphia, 2017, Elsevier.

TABLE 1 Characteristics of Primary and Secondary Raynaud Phenomenon

Characteristic	Primary	Secondary
Age	Younger (<30 yr)	Older (>30 yr)
Gender preference	Female	Male (depending on secondary cause)
Incidence	Most common	Less common
Familial predisposition	Yes	Yes
Combination with other disease	No, idiopathic	Associated with systemic disease
Vascular defect	Functional dysregulation of autonomic nervous system	Structural changes in connective tissue or vessels
Associated signs	None	Arthritis, sclerodactyly, cardiopulmonary abnormality, rash
Frequency	Precipitated by stimuli	Periodic and stimuli trigger
Severity of symptoms	Long history of mild attacks	Severe and disabling pain
Distribution	Symmetric	Asymmetric
Duration	Self-limited	Need for additional treatment (pharmacologic, surgery)
Critical complications	None	Ischemia and ulcers
Capillaroscopy	Normal (symmetric, thin, and uniform)	Abnormal (dilated, irregular, elongated, and tortuous vessel)
Vascular examination	Normal pulses	Abnormal pulses
Erythrocyte sedimentation rate	Normal	Elevated
Serologic studies	Negative	Antinuclear antibody, autoantibodies
C-reactive protein	Normal	Elevated

From Cameron JL, Cameron AM: *Current surgical therapy,* ed 12, Philadelphia, 2017, Elsevier.

summarizes characteristics of primary and secondary RP

DIFFERENTIAL DIAGNOSIS

- Neurogenic thoracic outlet syndrome or carpal tunnel syndrome
- Frostbite or cold weather injury
- Medication reaction (ergotamine, chemotherapeutic agents)
- Atherosclerosis, thromboembolic disease
- Buerger disease, embolic disease
- Acrocyanosis
- Livedo reticularis
- Injury from repetitive motion

WORKUP

- An algorithm for the evaluation of RP is illustrated in Fig. 2.
- Once the diagnosis of RP is established, differentiating primary from secondary is helpful in treatment and prognosis.
- Patients who are younger when their symptoms occur, have a normal history and physical examination and normal nail-fold capillaries, and have no history of digital ischemic lesions can be considered as having primary RP. These patients can be monitored clinically without any further testing.
- If a secondary cause of RP is suspected, appropriate laboratory testing is recommended (see "Laboratory Tests"). Secondary RP has associated abnormal nail-fold microscopy.

LABORATORY TESTS

- CBC, serum electrolytes, blood urea nitrogen, creatinine, ESR, ANAs, VDRL antibody test, rheumatoid factor, and urinalysis should be included in the initial evaluation.

- If the history, physical examination, and initial laboratory tests suggest a possible secondary cause, specific serologic testing (e.g., anticentromere antibodies, anti-Scl 70, cryoglobulins, complement testing, and serum protein electrophoresis) may be indicated.
- Noninvasive vascular testing includes finger systolic blood pressures, segmental blood pressure measurements, cold recovery time (measure vasoconstrictor and vasodilator responses of finger to cold), fingertip thermography, and laser Doppler with thermal challenge (measures relative change in skin blood flow with ambient warming).

IMAGING STUDIES

- The diagnosis of RP should not be made on the basis of laboratory tests, and imaging studies should not replace a good history and physical examination.
- Duplex ultrasound can image the palmar arch and digital arteries for patency.
- Magnetic resonance angiography is useful for imaging larger arteries.
- Contrast angiography is the gold standard for arterial imaging.
- Nail-fold capillary microscopy can differentiate primary from secondary RP.
- Videomicroscopy and thermography are also useful for diagnosis of RP.

Ⓡ TREATMENT

NONPHARMACOLOGIC THERAPY

- Avoid drugs that may precipitate RP (see "Etiology").

- Avoid cold exposure and sudden temperature shifts. Use warm gloves, hats, and garments during the winter months or before going into cold environments (e.g., air-conditioned rooms).
- Avoid stressful situations, and use relaxation techniques in preventing RP attacks.

ACUTE GENERAL Rx

- Acute measures to terminate an attack include rotating the arms in a windmill pattern, placing the hands under warm water or in a warm body fold such as the axilla, and the swing-arm maneuver.
- Medications are indicated in the treatment of RP if there are signs of critical ischemia or if the quality of life of the patient is affected to the degree that activities of normal living are no longer possible and preventive techniques do not work. Fig. 3 illustrates an approach to drug treatment of RP. Table E2 summarizes drugs commonly used in RP.

CHRONIC Rx

- Dihydropyridine calcium channel blockers (e.g., nifedipine, amlodipine, felodipine, nisoldipine, isradipine) are the most effective pharmacologic treatment for RP and are the drugs of choice. Amlodipine or nifedipine are commonly used.
- Amlodipine dosage ranges from 2.5 to 10 mg/day. Nifedipine is most often prescribed at a dose of 10 to 20 mg 30 min before cold exposure. If symptoms occur with long duration, nifedipine XL 30 to 180 mg PO qd is often effective.
- When calcium channel blockers do not appropriately control symptoms, phosphodiesterase inhibitors (cilostazol, pentoxifylline, and sildenafil) can be added or substituted. Sildenafil can be started at a dosage of 20 mg/day. Angiotensin 2 receptor antagonists (losartan), and selective serotonin reuptake inhibitors (fluoxetine) have also been used with some limited success.
- Some potential therapeutic options include direct vasodilators such as nitroprusside, hydralazine, papaverine, minoxidil, niacin, and griseofulvin. Topical 1% nitroglycerin or topical l-arginine, ethyl nicotinate, hexyl nicotinate, thurfyl salicylate may also be useful, particularly if low blood pressure is a concern.
- Alpha receptor antagonists such as prazosin and phenoxybenzamine have also shown some effectiveness in treating RP.
- The prostaglandins, including inhaled iloprost, intravenous (IV) epoprostenol, alprostadil, and tadalafil, may be promising in severe RP. However, additional experience and controlled studies are needed.
- Antioxidants like zinc gluconate have been used to decrease tissue damage.
- N-Acetylcysteine and probucol have been shown to lead to improvement in RP.
- Anticoagulation with IV unfractionated heparin or subcutaneous low–molecular-weight heparin and addition of aspirin can be considered during the acute phase of a severe ischemic event. Aspirin (81 mg/day) therapy can be

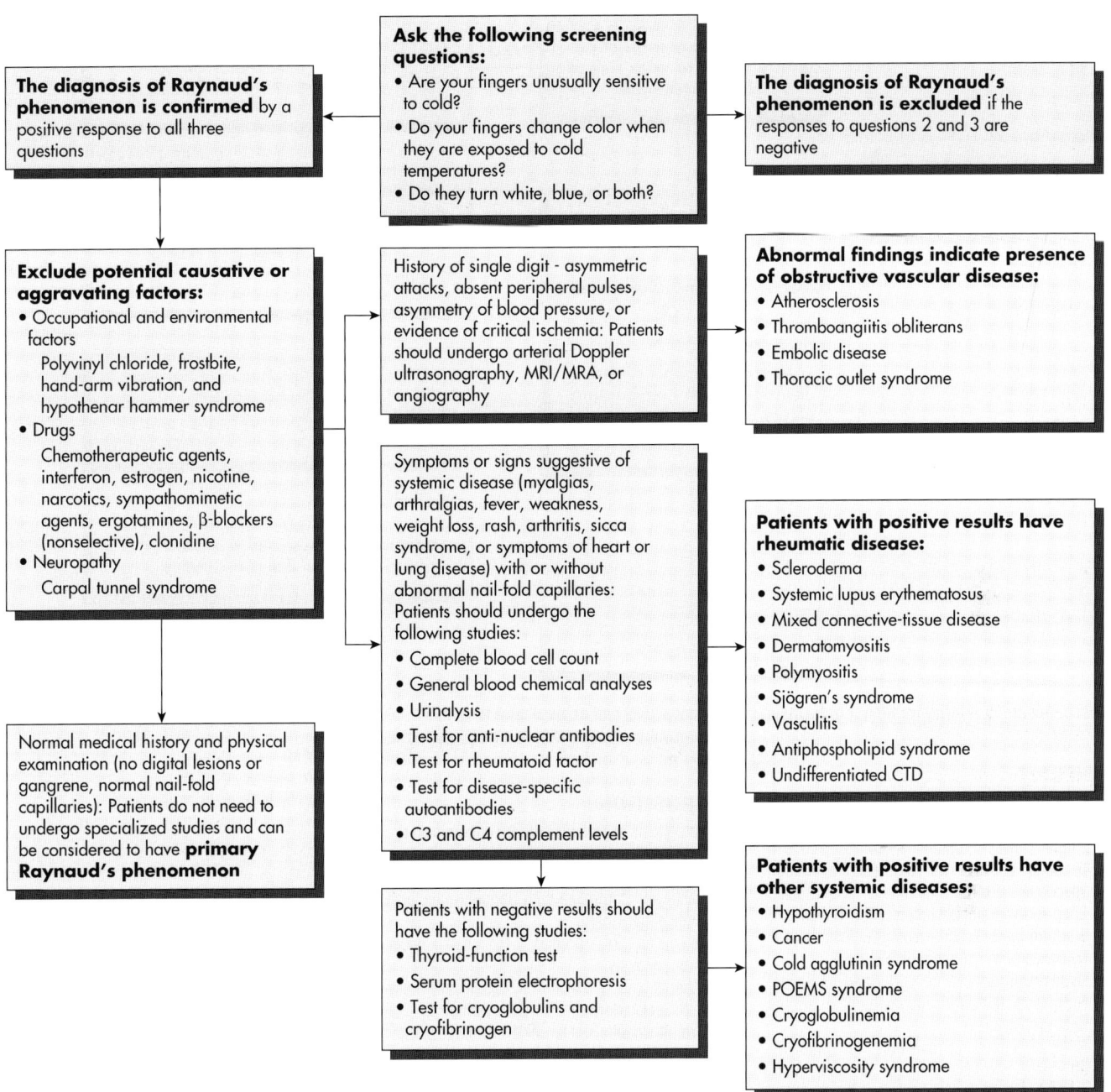

Ask the following screening questions:
- Are your fingers unusually sensitive to cold?
- Do your fingers change color when they are exposed to cold temperatures?
- Do they turn white, blue, or both?

The diagnosis of Raynaud's phenomenon is confirmed by a positive response to all three questions

The diagnosis of Raynaud's phenomenon is excluded if the responses to questions 2 and 3 are negative

Exclude potential causative or aggravating factors:
- Occupational and environmental factors
  Polyvinyl chloride, frostbite, hand-arm vibration, and hypothenar hammer syndrome
- Drugs
  Chemotherapeutic agents, interferon, estrogen, nicotine, narcotics, sympathomimetic agents, ergotamines, β-blockers (nonselective), clonidine
- Neuropathy
  Carpal tunnel syndrome

History of single digit - asymmetric attacks, absent peripheral pulses, asymmetry of blood pressure, or evidence of critical ischemia: Patients should undergo arterial Doppler ultrasonography, MRI/MRA, or angiography

Abnormal findings indicate presence of obstructive vascular disease:
- Atherosclerosis
- Thromboangiitis obliterans
- Embolic disease
- Thoracic outlet syndrome

Symptoms or signs suggestive of systemic disease (myalgias, arthralgias, fever, weakness, weight loss, rash, arthritis, sicca syndrome, or symptoms of heart or lung disease) with or without abnormal nail-fold capillaries: Patients should undergo the following studies:
- Complete blood cell count
- General blood chemical analyses
- Urinalysis
- Test for anti-nuclear antibodies
- Test for rheumatoid factor
- Test for disease-specific autoantibodies
- C3 and C4 complement levels

Patients with positive results have rheumatic disease:
- Scleroderma
- Systemic lupus erythematosus
- Mixed connective-tissue disease
- Dermatomyositis
- Polymyositis
- Sjögren's syndrome
- Vasculitis
- Antiphospholipid syndrome
- Undifferentiated CTD

Normal medical history and physical examination (no digital lesions or gangrene, normal nail-fold capillaries): Patients do not need to undergo specialized studies and can be considered to have **primary Raynaud's phenomenon**

Patients with negative results should have the following studies:
- Thyroid-function test
- Serum protein electrophoresis
- Test for cryoglobulins and cryofibrinogen

Patients with positive results have other systemic diseases:
- Hypothyroidism
- Cancer
- Cold agglutinin syndrome
- POEMS syndrome
- Cryoglobulinemia
- Cryofibrinogenemia
- Hyperviscosity syndrome

FIG. 2 Approach to diagnosis of Raynaud phenomenon. *CTD,* Connective tissue disease; *MRA,* magnetic resonance angiography; *POEMS,* polyneuropathy, organomegaly, endocrinopathy, monoclonal gammopathy, and skin changes. (From Firestein GS et al: *Firestein & Kelley's textbook of rheumatology,* ed 11, Philadelphia, 2021, Elsevier.)

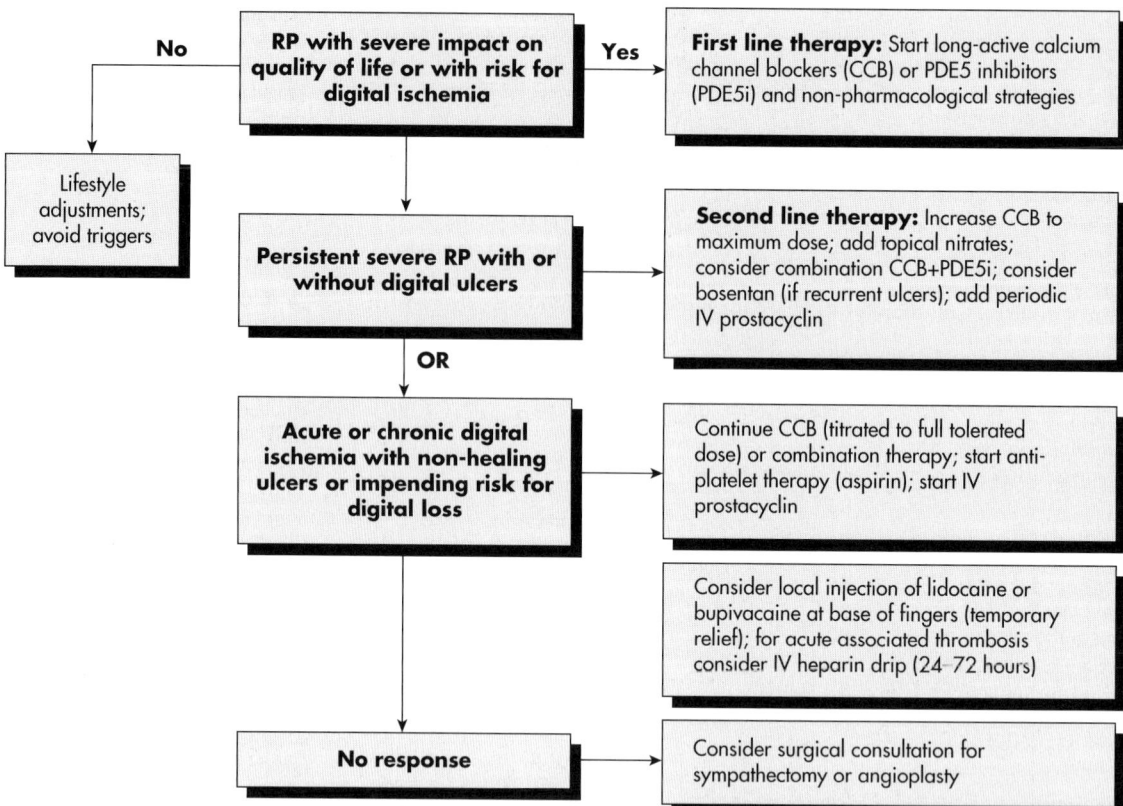

FIG. 3 Approach to drug treatment of Raynaud phenomenon (RP) and acute digital ischemia. *CCB,* Calcium channel blockers; *IV,* intravenous; *PDE-5,* phosphodiesterase-5. (From Firestein GS et al: *Firestein & Kelley's textbook of rheumatology,* ed 11, Philadelphia, 2021, Elsevier.)

considered in all patients with secondary RP with a history of ischemic ulcers or thrombotic events; however, caution should be exercised because aspirin can theoretically worsen vasospasm by the inhibition of prostacyclin. Long-term anticoagulation with heparin or warfarin is not recommended unless there is evidence of a hypercoagulable state.
- Bypass surgery can be performed for severe RP associated with reconstructible arterial occlusive disease.
- Sympathectomy is available for unreconstructible occlusive disease or pure vasospastic disease refractory to medical treatment.
- Microsurgical revascularization of the hand and digital reconstruction may improve digital vascular perfusion and heal digital ulcers when proximal arterial occlusion is associated with digital vasospasm.
- Ischemic digital lesions should be treated with topical antibiotics and daily cleansing with soap and water. Digits that progress to dry gangrene should be permitted to undergo autoamputation. Surgical amputation is limited for intractable pain or deep tissue infection.

DISPOSITION
The prognosis of patients with RP depends on the etiology.
- Primary RP is fairly benign, usually remaining stable and controlled with nonpharmacologic medical treatment.
- Remission of primary RP can occur spontaneously.
- Patients with secondary RP, specifically those with scleroderma, CREST syndrome, or thromboangiitis obliterans, may develop severe ischemic digits with ulceration, gangrene, and autoamputation.
- Box E2 summarizes features suggestive of progression of Raynaud phenomenon.

REFERRAL
- Rheumatology consult is indicated if secondary collagen vascular disease is diagnosed.
- Vascular surgery consult is indicated if ulcers, gangrene, or threatened digit loss is noted.

ⓘ PEARLS & CONSIDERATIONS

- Most patients with RP can be managed by a primary care provider.

- It is important to differentiate primary from secondary forms. Secondary forms may become manifest as far out as 10 yr from the diagnosis of RP. It is important to take immediate action during an attack, and patients are encouraged to:
1. Keep warm
2. Not use tobacco products
3. Avoid aggravating medications
4. Control stress
5. Exercise
6. Follow up with a physician

SUGGESTED READINGS
Available at eBooks.Health.Elsevier.com.

RELATED CONTENT
Raynaud Phenomenon (Patient Information)
Clinical

AUTHOR: **FRED F. FERRI, MD**

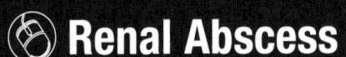

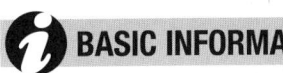 **BASIC INFORMATION**

DEFINITION

Renal abscess and perinephric abscess are purulent complications of an underlying urinary infection of the ascending tract with an obstructed pyelonephritis. Predisposing factors include diabetes and renal stones. There is lobar necrosis with renal abscess and perirenal fat necrosis in perinephric abscess.

SYNONYMS

Intrarenal abscess
Perinephric abscess
Kidney abscess

ICD-10CM CODE
N15.1 Renal and perinephric abscess

EPIDEMIOLOGY & DEMOGRAPHICS

INCIDENCE: Ranges from 1 to 10/10,000 hospital admissions
PREDOMINANT SEX & AGE: In one study, median age was 59.8 yr
RISK FACTORS: Diabetes and renal stones

PHYSICAL FINDINGS & CLINICAL PRESENTATION

- Symptoms include fever, flank pain, abdominal pain, and urinary frequency or dysuria.
- At times, renal abscess can present insidiously in the elderly or persons with diabetes.

ETIOLOGY

These infections may be a complication of a urinary tract infection that ascends to the upper tract, usually due to gram-negative bacteria, or a complication of a bacteremia with hematogenous seeding to the kidney, usually secondary to a *Staphylococcus aureus* infection.

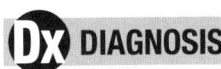 **DIAGNOSIS**

DIFFERENTIAL DIAGNOSIS

- Acute pyelonephritis with papillary necrosis
- Acute lobar nephronia: Acute nonsuppurative renal infection
- Renal cell carcinoma

- Malakoplakia: Rare granulomatous inflammatory disease seen with *Escherichia coli* infection
- Emphysematous pyelonephritis: Gas formation within the renal parenchyma caused by infection by facultative anaerobes or *Candida* spp.

WORKUP

Combination of laboratory tests and imaging

LABORATORY TESTS

- Blood cultures, urine cultures, urinalysis, and CBC are basic tests.
- Elevated erythrocyte sedimentation rate (ESR) or C-reactive protein may be marker for a deep-seated infection.

IMAGING STUDIES

- Ultrasound (US) may show thick-walled fluid-filled cavity in renal parenchyma. A perinephric abscess is confined to the perinephric space by Gerota fascia.
- Computed tomography (CT) with contrast (Fig. E1) is preferred over ultrasound for the diagnosis.
- MRI and nuclear scans are of limited value.

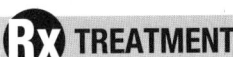 **TREATMENT**

Antibiotic therapy and, when necessary, interventional radiology or surgical drainage procedure

NONPHARMACOLOGIC THERAPY

- Therapy for a renal abscess greater than 5 cm in diameter should be percutaneous drainage by CT- or US-guided therapy along with intravenous (IV) antibiotics.
- A perinephric abscess should be drained percutaneously with CT or US guidance.
- At times a nephrectomy may be required for severe cases, usually in diabetic patients.

ACUTE GENERAL Rx

A renal abscess less than 5 cm in diameter can be treated successfully with targeted IV therapy (92% success rate for abscess 3 to 5 cm in diameter). Antibiotic choices are based on culture results but initially should target gram-negative bacteria unless infection is secondary to staphylococcal

bacteremia. Empiric antibiotic therapy in geographic areas where fluoroquinolone resistance rates are <10% consists of ciprofloxacin 400 mg IV loading dose. In areas with high fluoroquinolone resistance rates, ceftriaxone 1 g IV is appropriate. If perinephric abscess is associated with staphylococcal bacteremia, give IV nafcillin if methicillin-susceptible *Staphylococcus aureus* (MSSA) or vancomycin 1 g IV q12h if methicillin-resistant *S. aureus*.

CHRONIC Rx

Antibiotic therapy generally continues for 2 to 3 wk, some of which can be completed with oral therapy.

DISPOSITION

Antibiotics such as trimethoprim-sulfamethoxazole and quinolone antibiotics penetrate well in the kidney and are ideal oral agents for therapy.

REFERRAL

Interventional radiology, urologic surgeon, and infectious diseases consult

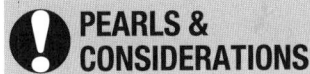 **PEARLS & CONSIDERATIONS**

COMMENTS

This diagnosis should be considered in patients who are being treated for pyelonephritis with appropriate antibiotics and fail to respond clinically after 5 days.

PREVENTION

Early and targeted therapy for urinary tract infections, especially in diabetic patients

SUGGESTED READINGS
Available at eBooks.Health.Elsevier.com.

RELATED CONTENT
Pyelonephritis (Related Key Topic)
Urinary Tract Infection (Related Key Topic)

AUTHOR: **GLENN G. FORT, MD, MPH**

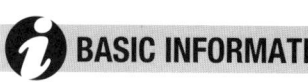
BASIC INFORMATION

DEFINITION
Renal artery stenosis (RAS) is progressive narrowing of the renal artery, which is most commonly due to atherosclerosis or fibromuscular dysplasia (FMD). RAS is an important, potentially reversible cause of hypertension, ischemic nephropathy, and destabilizing cardiac syndromes. RAS increases the risk of renal artery occlusion via progressive stenosis.

SYNONYMS
RAS
Fibromuscular disease
FMD
Renovascular disease

ICD-10CM CODES
Q27.1 Congenital renal artery stenosis
I70.1 Atherosclerosis of renal artery
I15.0 Renovascular hypertension
I77.9 Disorder of arteries and arterioles, unspecified

EPIDEMIOLOGY & DEMOGRAPHICS
- Atherosclerotic renal artery stenosis:
  1. Atherosclerotic renal artery stenosis (ARAS) accounts for ~90% of cases. The true prevalence of ARAS is unknown.[1]
     a. General population autopsy studies: 10% to 27% over 50 yr; hypertensive patients, 0.2% to 5%.
     b. In a general population older than 65 yr, the prevalence is 6.8% by Doppler ultrasound (5.5% of women, 9.1% of men; 6.7% African Americans, and 6.9% White). Bilateral disease was present in 12% of affected individuals.
     c. In patients with malignant hypertension, the prevalence is 43% in White patients and 7% in African American patients. In patients with mild hypertension, the prevalence is <1%.
     d. In patients with peripheral artery disease, the prevalence is 22% to 59%.
  2. Fibromuscular dysplasia:
     a. FMD accounts for ~10% of chronic RAS and is typically encountered in women (90%). FMD was previously thought to be a disease of the young and healthy, with few risk factors. Recent data suggest that the average age of onset of hypertension is 43 yr. Bilateral renal artery involvement is seen in 25% to 35% of cases.[2]

PHYSICAL FINDINGS & CLINICAL PRESENTATION
Progressive RAS:
- RAS should be considered in any White female patients <30 yr with hypertension not attributed to any other cause, any patients >50 yr with new-onset refractory hypertension, or patients with stable hypertension that has abruptly and/or significantly worsened.
- RAS most often presents as a clinically asymptomatic finding. Manifestations can include renovascular hypertension, ischemic nephropathy, or flash pulmonary edema.
- Flash pulmonary edema in the absence of cardiac disease most often indicates severe bilateral RAS.
- Renovascular hypertension should be considered in individuals with resistant hypertension (lack of blood pressure control on a medication regimen that includes 3 maximally dosed medications, one of which is a diuretic).
- Ischemic nephropathy should be considered if kidney function is rapidly deteriorating or kidney sizes are decreasing on serial imaging, particularly with bilateral disease.
- Acute elevations of serum creatinine (>30%) after starting ACE inhibitors or angiotensin receptor blockers (ARBs) may be seen in bilateral disease.
- A bruit heard in either upper quadrant on abdominal auscultation may suggest RAS. Patients with ARAS will often have bruits heard in other vascular beds.

ETIOLOGY
- Atherosclerosis: ARAS has similar risk factors to atherosclerosis in other vascular beds, including family history, smoking, diabetes, hypertension, and hyperlipidemia. ARAS most often involves the ostium and proximal third of the main renal artery.
- FMD (Figs. 1 and 2): Etiology is unknown. Classified into three categories based on the affected layer of arterial wall: Medial (>90%), intimal (<10%), and adventitial (<1%). FMD typically involves the distal main renal artery and intrarenal branches.

PATHOGENESIS
- Pathogenesis of FMD is unknown. FMD involves abnormal constrictions and dilations of the renal artery leading to a typical "string of beads" appearance on angiography.
- The pathogenesis of atherosclerotic RAS is similar to that of atherosclerosis in other vascular beds.

- The pathogenesis of renovascular hypertension is related to the neurohormonal cascade resulting from renal ischemia. Renal hypoperfusion or ischemia secondary to arterial stenosis produces an increase in plasma renin and secondary elevations of angiotensin II, with consequent vasoconstriction, aldosterone elevation, sodium retention, and renal potassium wasting. Hypertension results and can be self-sustaining, even in the case of unilateral RAS due to hypertensive damage of the contralateral kidney[3].
- The pathogenesis of ischemic nephropathy is due to the activation of numerous mechanisms of tissue injury resulting in progressive renal parenchymal loss and fibrosis.
- "Flash" or sudden-onset pulmonary edema, a manifestation usually seen in bilateral ARAS, results from sodium and water retention and upregulation of the sympathetic nervous system[2].

NATURAL HISTORY
- RAS caused by FMD rarely causes renal artery occlusion or ischemic nephropathy.
- ARAS rarely progresses to total occlusion. One study of serial ultrasounds of patients with RAS demonstrated that only 5% of those with >60% stenosis progressed to total occlusion in 1 yr, and an additional 11% progressed to total occlusion by 2 yr.

DIAGNOSIS

SCREENING
American College of Cardiology and American Heart Association (ACC/AHA) guidelines for identification of patients who should be screened for RAS:
- Onset of hypertension at age <30 yr or severe hypertension at age >55 yr
- Clinical findings that suggest secondary hypertension as opposed to essential hypertension in the absence of a more likely cause of

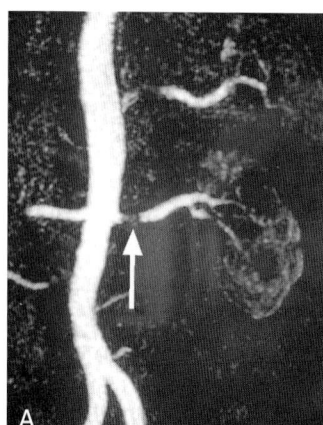
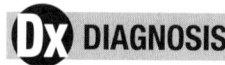

FIG. 1 Magnetic resonance angiogram. A, Coronal maximum intensity projection (MIP) of a patient with significant left renal artery stenosis *(white arrow).* **B,** Axial MIP of the same patient. (From Adam A et al: *Grainger & Allison's diagnostic radiology,* ed 5, 2007, Churchill Livingstone; and Grant LA: *Grainger & Allison's diagnostic radiology essentials,* ed 2, 2019, Philadelphia, Elsevier.)

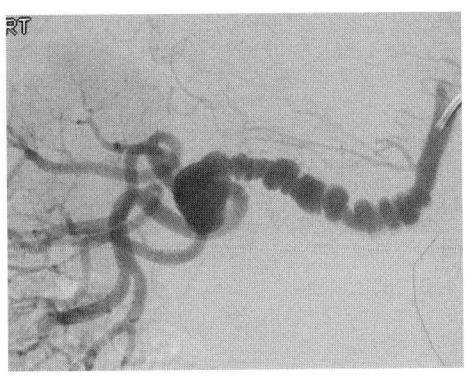

FIG. 2 Fibromuscular dysplasia. On a selective right anterior oblique (RAO) digital subtraction angiogram, the characteristic saccular dilations and weblike stenoses are clearly evident. (From Adam A et al: *Grainger & Allison's diagnostic radiology*, ed 5, 2007, Churchill Livingstone; and Grant LA: Grainger & Allison's diagnostic radiology essentials, ed 2, 2019, Philadelphia, Elsevier.)

secondary hypertension, such as pheochromocytoma
- Malignant hypertension: Hypertension with coexistent evidence of acute end-organ damage (acute renal failure, acute decompensated heart failure, new visual or neurologic disturbance, and/or advanced retinopathy)
- Accelerated hypertension: Sudden and persistent worsening of previously controlled hypertension
- Resistant hypertension: Full doses of a 3-drug regimen that includes a diuretic
- Sudden unexplained pulmonary edema
- New acute kidney injury following initiation of an ACE inhibitor or ARB
- Unexplained atrophic kidney or variation in size of kidneys by >1.5 cm, with smaller kidney affected by RAS

LABORATORY TESTS
- Urinalysis.
- Basic chemistry panel including sodium, potassium, blood urea nitrogen, and serum creatinine.
- Renal vein renin sampling determines whether one or both kidneys are overproducing renin in cases of suspected renovascular hypertension (RVH). A positive result has strong predictive value. However, 50% of patients with no evidence for lateralization can still respond to unilateral intervention.
- Renal vein sampling is typically performed at specialized hypertension centers.

IMAGING STUDIES
Renal duplex Doppler ultrasonography, CT angiography (CTA), and magnetic resonance angiography (MRA) are effective diagnostic screening methods.[1] The choice of imaging modality will depend on the availability of the diagnostic tool, experience and local accuracy of each modality, patient characteristics including body size, renal function, history of contrast media allergy, and presence of prior vascular stents.
RENAL DOPPLER ULTRASOUND:
- Renal Doppler ultrasound is a noninvasive, inexpensive screening study and can determine whether a stenosis of >60% is present.

- Abnormal results in RAS:
  1. Peak systolic velocity (PSV) >250 cm/sec
  2. Peak diastolic velocity >150 cm/sec
  3. Renal-to-aortic ratio (RAR) >3.5
  4. Acceleration time >100 msec
  5. Exact definitions of a positive renal Doppler ultrasound for RAS varies by institution
- Compared to renal angiography, Doppler studies have shown varied performance, with a sensitivity of 84% to 98% and a specificity of 62% to 99%.
- Limitations include high user variability. Valid test performance requires technicians who perform a high volume of these tests to reduce user error. If significant user variability exists at certain institutions, renal Doppler ultrasound may be excluded from the diagnostic algorithm. Patients with a large body habitus may have limited imaging results. It is not as sensitive or specific as MR or CT methods. Detection of RAS is limited to identifying whether stenosis of 60% to 99% is present.
- Duplex Doppler ultrasound is a good modality for monitoring patency following therapeutic, vascular stent insertion.

MAGNETIC RESONANCE ANGIOGRAPHY (MRA):
- MRA provides good visualization of main and accessory renal arteries. The test has high sensitivity (90%-100%) and specificity (76%-94%). MRA is superior to renal Doppler ultrasonography and equivalent to CTA.[3]
- Benefits include the lack of exposure to radiocontrast media or radiation.
- Limitations include claustrophobia, high cost, and inability to image within a previously placed metallic stent.

COMPUTED TOMOGRAPHY ANGIOGRAPHY (CTA):
- CTA is rapid and effective. When compared with angiography, this modality has a sensitivity of 59% to 96% and a specificity of 82% to 99%. It is superior to renal Doppler ultrasonography and equivalent to MRA. Radiocontrast media uptake in kidneys can also be used to estimate the viability of affected kidneys.[3]
- CTA has good spatial resolution and can detect restenosis through metal stents.

- CTA can be used more easily than MRA in obese or claustrophobic patients.
- Limitations include radiation exposure and potentially nephrotoxic, iodinated radiocontrast exposure to patients with chronic kidney disease. Heavily calcified arteries may appear narrower than in actuality.
DIRECT ANGIOGRAPHY:
- IV digital subtraction angiography (DSA) has an 88% sensitivity and 90% specificity. It is the gold standard for anatomic diagnosis of RAS. It is not a first-line screening tool and is recommended after a positive noninvasive test. DSA is used when there is a high clinical suspicion for RAS with inconclusive noninvasive tests and when the decision has already been made that correction of stenosis will produce clinical benefit. DSA allows for angioplasty with stenting during the same procedure. This modality is reserved for patients with a high likelihood of intervention.
- Limitations include its invasive nature, that is, requirement for intraaortic catheterization, which may lead to aortic and/or renal artery trauma and/or aortic dissection, rupture, thrombosis, or embolization.
- Procedure requires a certified interventionalist (radiologist, cardiologist, nephrologist, or vascular surgeon).
- Procedure requires iodinated contrast that must be used cautiously with patients who have chronic kidney disease. Carbon dioxide contrast imaging and limiting image acquisition number reduce kidney injury risk.
NUCLEAR RENOGRAPHY (WITHOUT CAPTOPRIL): A noninvasive test conducted when renal atrophy is present to document differential kidney function. This test is useful when determining whether to revascularize an atrophic kidney or to remove it. Atrophic kidneys with <20% differential renal function are unlikely contributing to overall renal functional decline but may still contribute to renovascular hypertension.

Rx TREATMENT

PHARMACOLOGIC THERAPY
- Because of RAAS activation, ACE inhibitors or ARB are recommended and well-tolerated (92%) as treatment of RVH. Kidney function should be monitored carefully when initiating or titrating these medications, particularly when bilateral RAS (78% tolerability) or unilateral stenosis with a solitary kidney is present to avoid precipitating acute kidney injury.
- Diuretics should be considered in patients with congestive heart failure or flash pulmonary edema.
- Antiplatelet therapy and statin therapy.

NONPHARMACOLOGIC THERAPY
- If blood pressure is not controlled by medications alone, flash pulmonary edema occurs, or kidney function rapidly declines, referral for renal angiography, angioplasty, or stenting may be indicated.
- Angioplasty without stenting is insufficient for atherosclerotic lesions due to a high failure rate or a high rate of restenosis.

- Occasionally, a kidney that has lost function from RAS may cause refractory hypertension. This situation would be discovered only by renal vein renin sampling in a patient with unilateral renal atrophy. In such cases, nephrectomy of the atrophied kidney may be the best method to control blood pressure.
- Renal artery bypass is rarely required.
- If RAS is suspected as the cause of flash pulmonary edema or rapidly declining kidney function, bilateral disease is likely. If confirmed by angiography, both renal arteries should be stented.
- Hypertension is rarely cured with revascularization of RAS due to longstanding hypertension. The goal of intervention is blood pressure control.
- The ACC/AHA guidelines for clinical indications of renal artery revascularization in the presence of significant stenosis include the following:
  1. Accelerated, resistant, or malignant hypertension (class IIa)
  2. Hypertension with unilateral small kidney (class IIa)
  3. Hypertension with intolerance to medication (class IIa)
  4. Treatment of cardiac destabilization syndromes such as unexplained heart failure exacerbations or episodes of flash pulmonary edema (class I) and refractory or unstable angina (class IIa)
  5. Progressive chronic kidney disease with bilateral RAS or RAS associated with a solitary functioning kidney (class IIa)
- Many patients who meet these criteria will not have a beneficial response to renal revascularization. Careful patient selection for angiography and intervention is recommended.
- Multiple randomized controlled trials (e.g., ASTRAL, CORAL, DRASTIC, and STAR) have shown no benefit of revascularization versus medical therapy, with end points of blood pressure control, renal function, and cardiovascular events.[2,4,5] Therefore the decision to refer a patient for revascularization should be made by specialists skilled and practiced in RAS.

FIBROMUSCULAR DYSPLASIA

- Medical therapy should include an ACE inhibitors or ARB to control blood pressure unless severe bilateral disease is present (rare).
- RVH from FMD is often cured by renal artery revascularization because many younger patients do not have background essential hypertension.
- In most cases, patients should be referred for renal artery angioplasty regardless of whether blood pressure can be controlled medically.
- Stenting is not appropriate in patients with FMD because angioplasty alone usually yields a durable result. In addition, recurrence of FMD is common, and the presence of stents may hinder additional interventions.[6]
- Renal artery bypass may be necessary in patients in whom FMD recurs multiple times or in whom angioplasty failed to yield an improvement in blood pressure.

ACUTE GENERAL Rx

The treatment of RAS is targeted to the clinical presentation:

- Asymptomatic disease requires no treatment.
- Patients with chronic hypertension, in the setting of incidentally discovered RAS, require only antihypertensive medical therapy.
- When RVH is suspected, initial therapy is antihypertensive therapy, specifically medications that block the renin-angiotensin-aldosterone system (RAAS). As discussed later, failure to control blood pressure despite an adequate antihypertensive regimen is an indication to consider renal revascularization.
- Patients with ischemic nephropathy should be considered for intervention only if the renal function is declining rapidly or flash pulmonary edema occurs in the setting of bilateral RAS.

DISPOSITION & REFERRAL

- Patients with uncontrolled hypertension on multiple agents should be referred for management by a hypertension specialist.
- Percutaneous intervention for ARAS must be reserved for selected patients until further data are available.

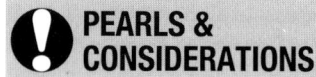 **PEARLS & CONSIDERATIONS**

- RAS is most commonly an incidental finding and clinically silent.
- RAS may present variably as hypertension, renal dysfunction, or both, or flash pulmonary edema.
- Stenting is inappropriate for most patients with RAS. Consideration should be made only in high-risk patients and after consultation with a specialist in the field.
- The modality for the type of imaging should depend on the expertise of the institution.

REFERENCES
Available at eBooks.Health.Elsevier.com.

RELATED CONTENT

Renal Artery Stenosis (Patient Information)
Hypertension (Related Key Topic)

AUTHOR: **KAUSIK UMANATH, MD, MS, FACP FASN**

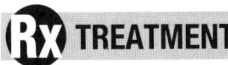

R

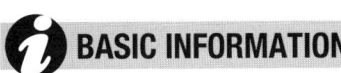 **BASIC INFORMATION**

DEFINITION

Renal cell carcinoma (RCC) is a primary carcinoma originating in the renal parenchyma from the malignant transformation of proximal renal tubular epithelial cells. The majority of renal cell cancers are of clear cell type; papillary tumors comprise 15%, and chromophobe cancers comprise 10%.

SYNONYMS

RCC
Hypernephroma
Renal cell adenocarcinoma

ICD-10CM CODES
C64.9 Malignant neoplasm of kidney, except renal pelvis
C64.1 Malignant neoplasm of right kidney, except renal pelvis
C64.2 Malignant neoplasm of left kidney, except renal pelvis
C64.9 Malignant neoplasm of unspecified kidney, except renal pelvis
C65.9 Malignant neoplasm of renal pelvis

EPIDEMIOLOGY & DEMOGRAPHICS

INCIDENCE: In 2022, there were an estimated 79,000 new cases and 13,920 deaths in the U.S.[1] Two percent of cases of renal cancer are associated with inherited syndromes.
PREDOMINANT SEX: Male:female ratio is approximately 2:1.
PREDOMINANT AGE: Peak incidence is at age 50 to 70 yr.
RISK FACTORS:
- Cigarette smoking
- Obesity
- Phenacetin-containing analgesics
- Asbestos, lead, Thorotrast, and chromium exposure
- Gasoline and other petroleum products
- Role of the *VHL* gene on chromosome 3

PHYSICAL FINDINGS & CLINICAL PRESENTATION

- Patients are often asymptomatic until they have advanced disease.
- Paraneoplastic syndromes such as hypercalcemia, erythrocytosis, anemia, and hepatic dysfunction (Stauffer syndrome) may occur with RCC.
- The classic triad of flank pain, hematuria, and a palpable abdominal mass currently represents an unusual presentation.

- Current presenting findings in RCC include:

Hematuria	50%-60%
Elevated erythrocyte sedimentation rate	50%-60%
Abdominal mass	25%-45%
Anemia	20%-40%
Flank pain	35%-40%
Hypertension	20%-40%
Weight loss	30%-35%
Fever	5%-15%
Hepatic dysfunction	10%-15%
Classic triad (hematuria, abdominal mass, flank pain)	5%-10%
Hypercalcemia	3%-6%
Erythrocytosis	3%-4%
Varicocele	2%-3%

ETIOLOGY

Hereditary forms:
- Familial renal carcinoma
- Renal carcinoma associated with von Hippel-Lindau disease
- Hereditary papillary RCC

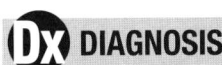 **DIAGNOSIS**

DIFFERENTIAL DIAGNOSIS

- Transitional cell carcinomas of the renal pelvis (8% of all renal cancers)
- Wilms tumor
- Other primary renal carcinomas and sarcomas
- Renal cysts
- Retroperitoneal tumors

WORKUP
LABORATORY TESTS:
- Urinalysis: Hematuria
- CBC: Anemia or erythrocytosis
- Chemistry panel: Renal failure and electrolyte issues, including hypercalcemia
- Liver function tests: Hepatic dysfunction with elevated alkaline phosphatase, prolonged prothrombin time, and hypoalbuminemia

IMAGING STUDIES

Nearly 50% of renal cancers are now detected because a renal mass is incidentally detected on radiographic evaluation.
- Renal ultrasound
- Abdominal computed tomography (CT) scan with contrast (Fig. E1)

- CT-guided biopsy is generally not necessary for diagnosis of solid masses >4 cm (high likelihood of cancer)
- MRI
- Renal arteriogram
- Intravenous pyelography

STAGING
See Table 1.

Rx TREATMENT

NONMETASTATIC CANCERS
- Surgery:
  1. Surgical nephrectomy [open and laparoscopic approaches] is the only effective management for stages I, II, and some stage III tumors. Although radical nephrectomy had long been the standard treatment, retrospective studies have shown that partial rather than radical nephrectomy is associated with improved survival and is appropriate for patients with renal cell neoplasms <4 cm that are not adjacent to the renal pelvis or invading the vena cava.[2]
  2. Laparoscopic robotic-assisted nephrectomy has been adopted in multiple centers, primarily for nephron-sparing surgery in the case of tumors <4 cm. Advantages include less blood loss, minimal effects on renal function, and similar oncologic outcomes. Disadvantages include increased costs and limitations in tumor size and locations eligible for robotic surgery.
  3. Various forms of partial nephrectomy may be available for patients with bilateral cancers or with a solitary kidney.
- Systemic therapy:
  Adjuvant therapy with the tyrosine kinase inhibitor sunitinib has shown modest improved in resected high-risk cases but has not been readily adopted into clinical practice. A randomized trial of adjuvant pembrolizumab after resection in high-risk patients has demonstrated improvement in disease-free survival and overall survival.[3] Adjuvant atezolizumab immunotherapy in patients with increased risk of recurrence though showed no evidence of improved clinical outcomes versus placebo.
Metastatic cancers
- Surgery:
  Cytoreductive nephrectomy in patients with metastatic RCC before immunotherapy improved survival in patients compared with immunotherapy alone based on randomized trials data. However, recent results from the randomized Clinical Trial to Assess the Importance of

TABLE 1 TNM Staging of Renal Cell Carcinomas as per the AJCC Eighth Edition

T Stage	Description
T_x	Tumor cannot be assessed
T_1: Tumor $\leq$7 cm, limited to kidney	T_{1a}: Tumor <4 cm T_{1b}: Tumor $\geq$4 cm to $\leq$7 cm
T_2: Tumor >7 cm, limited to kidney	T_{2a}: Tumor >7 cm but $\leq$10 cm T_{2b}: Tumor >10 cm
T_3: Tumor extending into major veins or perinephric tissue but not into ipsilateral adrenal gland or beyond Gerota fascia	T_{3a}: Tumor extends to renal vein/branches or invades perirenal and/or renal sinus fat T_{3b}: Tumor extends into IVC below diaphragm
	T_{3c}: Tumor extends into IVC above diaphragm or wall of IVC
T_4	Tumor invades beyond Gerota fascia (including contiguous extension into ipsilateral adrenal gland)
N stage	Description
N_x	Regional nodes cannot be assessed
N_1	No regional nodes involved
N_2	Metastasis in regional node(s)
M stage	Description
M_0	No distant metastases
M_1	Distant metastasis present
Stage	TNM grouping
I	$T_1N_0M_0$
II	$T_2N_0M_0$
III	$T_3N_0M_0$ or $T_{1-3}N_1M_0$
IV	$T_4N_{any}M_{any}$ or $T_{any}N_{any}M_1$

AJCC, American Joint Committee on Cancer; *IVC*, intravenous cholangiography; *TNM*, tumor, node, metastases.

Nephrectomy (CARMENA) demonstrated no benefit for intermediate- and poor-risk patients in the setting of modern tyrosine kinase inhibitor (sunitinib) therapy. Additional trials data are awaited to assess the role of nephrectomy in favorable risk patients and with the use of neo-adjuvant tyrosine kinase inhibitor therapy.

- Angioinfarction, cryoablation, or radiotherapy (for palliation).
- Systemic therapy:
  1. Risk stratification using prognostic scoring systems such as the International mRCC Database Consortium Prognostic Model (IMDC score) is the initial step in planning systemic therapy.[4] Absence of any of the following risk factors confers the most favorable risk status (IMDC-Fav), one to two risk factors increase this to intermediate risk (IMDC-Int), and a patient with three or more risk factors has poor-risk disease (IMDC-Poor):
     a. Karnofsky performance status <80%
     b. Time from diagnosis to treatment <1 yr
     c. Hemoglobin concentration < lower limit of normal
     d. Serum calcium > upper limit of normal
     e. Neutrophil count > upper limit of normal
     f. Platelet count > upper limit of normal
  2. Until recently, monotherapy with multi-targeted kinase inhibitors was the initial option for treatment of metastatic cancers followed using mTOR inhibitors as second-line therapy. However, the evolving data with the use of immunotherapy has now moved combinations of dual immu-

notherapy combinations or immuno-therapy/targeted therapy combinations to the frontline as initial therapy in this setting[5]:

a. Checkpoint inhibitors: The checkpoint inhibitors have demonstrated efficacy in both treatment-naïve and previously treated patients. Combination checkpoint inhibition with ipilimumab plus nivolumab has demonstrated superior efficacy for treatment-naïve patients with IMDC intermediate and poor risk status.

b. Combination tyrosine kinase inhibitors and immune checkpoint inhibitors: Regimens combining tyrosine kinase inhibition plus immune checkpoint inhibition (axitinib plus pembrolizumab, axitinib plus avelumab, cabozantinib plus nivolumab, and lenvatinib plus pembrolizumab) all have demonstrated superiority compared to sunitinib monotherapy in upfront therapy.

c. Tyrosine kinase inhibitors: In patients with unresectable disease, therapy with the multitargeted inhibitors axitinib, sunitinib, pazopanib, cabozantinib, lenvatinib, tivozanib, and sorafenib as well as mTOR kinase inhibitors everolimus and temsirolimus can be used as therapy options in sequence. The combination of lenvatinib plus everolimus has also been approved in second-line therapy after demonstrating improved outcomes compared to single-agent

everolimus use. Most responses with these agents are typically partial or stable disease, and relapse is the norm.

d. Immunotherapy: High-dose interleukin-2 therapy may achieve a 15% response rate, which is often durable and associated with long-term survival in highly selected patients with excellent performance status. Severe toxicities associated with this therapy have limited the use of this approach.

PROGNOSIS

The 5-yr overall survival rate among patients with kidney cancer has increased from 57% in 1987 to 76% in 2015. According to a SEER database report, the outcomes of surgically treated patients is shown in the following table though it does not reflect gains made in the immunotherapy era:

Stage	5-Yr Survival (%)
Localized	90-95
Regional	70
Distant	13
Total	76

REFERRAL

- To urologist for staging and surgery
- To medical oncologist if metastatic disease is present

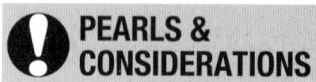 **PEARLS & CONSIDERATIONS**

- Patients should be considered for nephron-sparing surgery in case of smaller tumors (<4 cm).
- Laparoscopic robotic-assisted surgery is utilized for standard nephron-sparing surgery routinely; it is utilized for central tumors and tumors >4 cm in some experienced centers.
- Adjuvant use of tyrosine kinase inhibitors has showed mixed results and is not approved in this setting. An intergroup study showed no survival benefit, whereas a smaller study limited to high-risk patients showed a progression-free survival benefit.
- High-dose interleukin-2 can lead to long-term remissions in 10% to 15% of carefully selected patients with metastatic cancers.

REFERENCES

Available at eBooks.Health.Elsevier.com.

RELATED CONTENT

Kidney Cancer (Patient Information)

AUTHOR: **BHARTI RATHORE, MD**

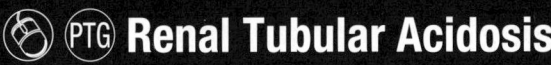

R

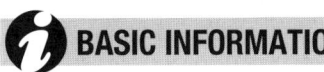 BASIC INFORMATION

DEFINITION

Renal tubular acidosis (RTA) is a group of chronic diseases characterized by hyperchloremic metabolic acidosis (HCMA) produced by the inability of the renal tubules to either excrete hydrogen ions (H^+) or retain bicarbonate ions (HCO_3^-). Factors differentiating the four major types of RTA are described in Table 1.

- Type 1 (classic, distal RTA): Abnormality in distal tubule hydrogen secretion, resulting in hypokalemic HCMA
- Type 2 (proximal RTA): Decreased proximal tubule bicarbonate reabsorption, resulting in hypokalemic HCMA
- Type 3 (mixed RTA): Rare autosomal recessive disorder with features of distal and proximal RTA
- Type 4 (hyporeninemic, hypoaldosteronism RTA): Aldosterone deficiency or a disease of the cortical collecting duct characterized by decreased distal sodium reabsorption and decreased distal tubule acidification hyperkalemic HCMA

SYNONYM

RTA

ICD-10CM CODE

N25.89 Other disorders resulting from impaired renal tubular function

EPIDEMIOLOGY & DEMOGRAPHICS

RTA type 4 primarily affects adults, whereas RTA types 1 and 2 are more frequent in children.

PHYSICAL FINDINGS & CLINICAL PRESENTATION

- Physical examination may be normal.
- Reduced skin turgor may be present from polyuria and dehydration.
- Muscle weakness and aches, paralysis, and cardiac arrhythmias from hypokalemia may occur.
- Low back pain and bone pain may be present in patients with abnormalities of calcium and phosphorus metabolism (RTA type 2).
- Failure to thrive or delayed growth in children.
- Some patients may present with sensorineural deafness in RTA type 1 (H^+–ATPase sequence variants).

ETIOLOGY

- Type 1 RTA: Inherited as a primary disorder with sequence variation of the basolateral chloride-bicarbonate exchanger (*SLC4A1* gene) or apical proton-ATPase (H^+–ATPase). Acquired causes: Autoimmune disorders (systemic lupus erythematosus [SLE], Sjögren syndrome); primary biliary cirrhosis and other liver diseases; medications (amphotericin, nonsteroidal antiinflammatory drugs [NSAID], lithium carbonate, ifosfamide); genetic disorders (Ehlers-Danlos syndrome, Marfan syndrome, hereditary elliptocytosis); toxins (toluene); disorders with nephrocalcinosis (primary hyperparathyroidism, vitamin D intoxication, idiopathic hypercalciuria); and tubulointerstitial disease (renal transplantation, renal medullary cystic disease, obstructive uropathy, chronic urinary tract infections, and analgesic nephropathy).
- Type 2 RTA: Inherited genetic defects of the proximal tubule cell sodium bicarbonate co-transporter (NBCe1 variant) or the carbonic anhydrase type 2 protein, as well as Fanconi syndrome. Genetic etiologies of Fanconi syndrome include cystinosis, Wilson disease, hereditary fructose intolerance, Lowe syndrome, Fanconi-Bickel syndrome, Dent disease, tyrosinemia, and galactosemia. Acquired causes include primary hyperparathyroidism, multiple myeloma, amyloidosis, light chain deposition diseases, heavy metals (copper, lead, mercury, and cadmium), chronic rejection of a transplanted kidney, and medications. Medication-induced RTA may arise from prolonged use of acetazolamide, topiramate, outdated tetracycline, ifosfamide, zidovudine, didanosine, and aminoglycosides.
- Type 3 RTA: Rare inherited recessive disorder with carbonic anhydrase 2 deficiency or drugs (topiramate).
- Type 4 RTA: Inherited disorders such as pseudohypoaldosteronism types 1 or 2 (Gordon syndrome). Acquired causes include diabetes mellitus, HIV/AIDS, sickle cell disease, obstructive uropathy, lupus, amyloidosis, adrenal insufficiency, kidney transplant rejection, drugs (spironolactone, eplerenone, amiloride, angiotensin–converting enzyme [ACE] inhibitors, angiotensin II type 1 receptor blockers [ARBs], trimethoprim, pentamidine, heparin, NSAIDs, and calcineurin inhibitors [cyclosporine, tacrolimus]).

Dx DIAGNOSIS

DIFFERENTIAL DIAGNOSIS: EXTRARENAL ETIOLOGY

- Diarrhea with significant bicarbonate loss
- External loss of biliary and pancreatic secretions (e.g., fistula)
- Bowel-urinary diversion procedures (e.g., ureterosigmoidostomy, ileal conduit)
- Respiratory acidosis
- Drugs: Calcium chloride, magnesium sulfate, cholestyramine

WORKUP

Detection of HCMA by serum electrolyte and arterial blood gas (ABG) analysis followed by evaluation of potential causes (see "Etiology"). Fig 1 describes an approach to the patient with RTA.[1,2]

LABORATORY TESTS[2]

- ABG reveals metabolic acidosis.
- Serum anion gap is normal: i.e., Anion Gap = $[Na^+] - ([Cl^-] + [HCO_3-])$ = 6 to 10 mEq/L.
- Serum potassium is low in RTA types 1 and 2, normal in type 3, and high in type 4 RTA.
- First-morning urine pH is >5.5 in RTA type 1, <5.5 in types 2 and 3, and <5.5 (low mineralocorticoid secretion) or >5.5 (collecting duct abnormality) in type 4 RTA.
- Urinary ammonium is low in renal tubular acidosis. If urinary ammonium test is not available, urine anion gap and urine osmolar gap can be used for calculating urinary ammonium.
- Urine Anion Gap (UAG = Urine $[Na^+ + K^+]$ – Urine $[Cl^-]$) is an indirect evaluation of urinary ammonium excretion and can differentiate renal from extrarenal causes of normal anion

---

TABLE 1 Contrasting Features and Diagnostic Studies in Renal Tubular Acidosis

	TYPES OF RENAL TUBULAR ACIDOSIS		
Finding	Proximal (Type 2)	Classical Distal (Type 1)	Generalized Distal Dysfunction (Type 4)
Plasma potassium	Low	Low	High
Urine pH during metabolic acidosis (ABG pH <7.3)	<5.5	>5.5	<5.5 or >5.5
Urine net charge	Positive	Positive	Positive
Fanconi lesion	Present	Absent	Absent
Fractional bicarbonate excretion	10%-15%	2%-5%	5%-10%
Urine to blood CO_2 pressure difference	Normal	Low	Low
H^+–ATPase defect		Low	
HCO_3^-/Cl^- transporter defect		High	
Amphotericin B		Normal	
Response to therapy	Least responsive	Responsive	Less responsive
Associated features	Fanconi syndrome	Nephrocalcinosis/hypergammaglobulinemia	Chronic kidney disease

ATPase, Adenosine triphosphatase; urine to blood CO_2 pressure difference: <30 mm Hg is low.
Modified from DuBose TD: Disorders of acid-base balance. In *Brenner and Rector's the kidney*, ed 9, Philadelphia, 2011, Saunders.

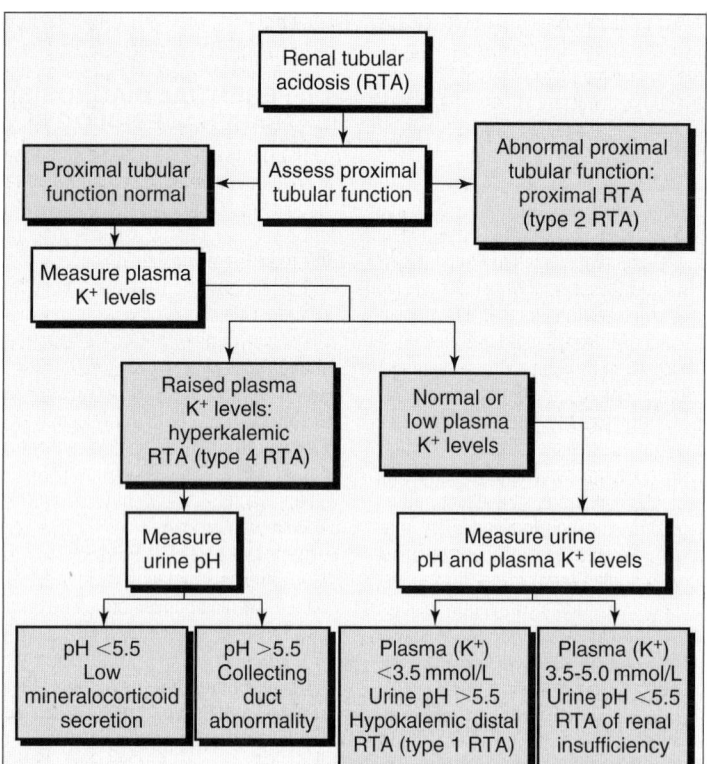

FIG. 1 Approach to the patient with renal tubular acidosis. (From Feehally J et al: *Comprehensive clinical nephrology,* ed 6, Philadelphia, 2019, Elsevier.)

gap metabolic acidosis (e.g., diarrhea). UAG is zero or positive in all types of RTA.

- UAG should be calculated only if U_{Na} >20 mEq/L and urine pH <6.5.
- Urine osmolar gap (UOG) is an independent surrogate of urinary ammonium concentration and is not affected by the presence of other nonreabsorbable anions (e.g., keto-acids, 5-oxoproline/pyroglutamic acid, bicarbonate, or hippurate).
- Calculated urine ammonium (U_{NH4}^{+} (mmol/L) = 0.5 (Measured U_{osm} − Calculated U_{osm} [2 (Na^+ + K^+) + Urine Urea Nitrogen (mg/dL; divided by 2.8) + glucose (mg/dL/18]).
- Calculated urine ammonium ≥75 mEq/L denotes intact renal tubular function and supports an extrarenal origin of HCMA.
- Calculated urine ammonium ≤25 mEq/L denotes inappropriately low concentration.
- UOG cannot be used if there are other neutral substances in the urine (e.g., mannitol, alcohols) or during a urinary tract infection from urease-producing bacteria.

- Additional studies include urine and serum calcium concentrations.
- Intact parathyroid hormone measurement when primary hyperparathyroidism is suspected (type 2 RTA).

IMAGING STUDIES

- Plain abdominal radiographs for evaluation of nephrocalcinosis
- Kidney ultrasound to determine kidney sizes and/or presence of stones
- Noncontrast-enhanced computed tomography (CT) scan in patients with nephrocalcinosis or nephrolithiasis

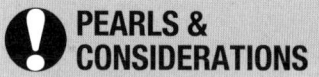 **TREATMENT**

ACUTE GENERAL Rx[3]

- Types 1 and 2 RTA are treated with oral sodium bicarbonate (1 to 2 mEq/kg per day in type 1 RTA, and 2 to 4 mEq/kg per day in type 2

RTA) titrated to correct metabolic acidosis (serum total carbon dioxide >22 mEq/L).
- Potassium supplementation is required for hypokalemic patients.
- Type 4 RTA can be treated with diuretics to lower elevated potassium levels and sodium bicarbonate to correct significant acidosis. Fludrocortisone 0.1 to 0.3 mg/day can be used to correct mineralocorticoid deficiency.

CHRONIC Rx

- Monitor potassium levels in type 4 RTA.
- Monitor for bone disease (osteomalacia) in type 2 RTA.
- Monitor for nephrolithiasis and nephrocalcinosis in type 1 RTA.

DISPOSITION

- Prognosis varies with the associated conditions (see "Etiology").
- Untreated distal RTA may result in hypocalcemia, hypophosphatemia, nephrolithiasis, and nephrocalcinosis.

❗ PEARLS & CONSIDERATIONS

- Nonanion gap metabolic acidosis: Evaluate urine ammonium (urine anion and osmolar gaps) to differentiate nonrenal vs. renal causes of HCMA.
- Examine serum potassium to differentiate between types 1 or 2 RTA vs. type 4 RTA.
- In hyperkalemic type 4 RTA, review medication list and rule out urinary obstruction, especially in older men.

COMMENTS

Patient education materials can be obtained from the National Kidney and Urologic Diseases Information Clearinghouse, Box NKUDIC, Bethesda, MD 20893.

REFERENCES

Available at eBooks.Health.Elsevier.com.

AUTHOR: **JIAN LI, MD, PHD**

ℹ️ BASIC INFORMATION

DEFINITION

Respiratory distress syndrome (RDS) is a clinical condition predominantly seen in preterm infants and is caused by a deficiency of surfactant production and secretion. Due to immaturity, the quantity of surfactant secreted by the lungs may be insufficient to decrease alveolar surface tension and prevent atelectasis.[1,2]

SYNONYMS

Hyaline membrane disease
RDS

ICD-10CM CODE
P22.0   Respiratory distress syndrome of newborn

EPIDEMIOLOGY & DEMOGRAPHICS

INCIDENCE: RDS occurs in 60% to 80% of infants <28 weeks gestation and in 15% to 30% of infants between 32 and 36 weeks gestation. RDS is rare in infants >37 weeks gestation. RDS has a slight male predominance and is more common in males of European descent.[1]

PEAK INCIDENCE: The incidence of RDS is inversely proportional to gestational age, occurring in nearly all infants born at 22 to 24 weeks gestation, and decreasing to less than 1% of infants born at 37 weeks.[2]

PREDOMINANT SEX & AGE: Premature infants: Slight male predominance[1,2]

RISK FACTORS: Risk factors for RDS include prematurity, low birth weight, European descent, elective delivery in the absence of labor, maternal diabetes mellitus, and perinatal hypoxia-ischemia. The risk of RDS is decreased in infants of mothers with chronic or pregnancy-induced hypertension, prolonged rupture of membranes, and exposure to antenatal corticosteroids.[1,2]

GENETICS: RDS is believed to have a genetic contribution, based on twin studies in which the concordance of RDS in monozygotic twins is greater than that in dizygotic twins.[2] In addition, mutations in genes encoding surfactant proteins can be a rare cause of RDS.[1]

PHYSICAL FINDINGS & CLINICAL PRESENTATION

Typically, RDS will present in the first minutes to hours after birth, with signs of respiratory distress that include tachypnea (>60 breaths/min), intercostal and subcostal retractions, nasal flaring, grunting, cyanosis, and increased oxygen requirement.[1,2] Retractions on inspiration are visible as a result of a compliant chest wall, with high negative intrathoracic pressures needed to expand poorly compliant, surfactant-deficient lungs. Grunting occurs on expiration and is believed to be due to the generation of increased functional residual capacity by partial closure of the glottis on exhalation. Cyanosis at birth is due to right-to-left shunting and may be exacerbated by impaired cardiac output due to respiratory compromise. Breath sounds on auscultation may be diminished or coarse. Breath sounds are

uniform, and nonuniform or delayed development of these symptoms may be suggestive of pulmonary air leak. In worsening cases of RDS, hypotension may result, with worsening respiratory distress followed by apnea and respiratory failure.[2]

ETIOLOGY

RDS is caused by a deficiency of surfactant production and secretion. Surfactant's role is to decrease the surface tension within alveoli, increase functional residual capacity, decrease atelectasis, and facilitate adequate gas exchange. Surfactant is produced by type II pneumocytes in adequate quantities by 20 weeks gestation but is not secreted in adequate quantities until 28 to 32 weeks gestation. Mature concentrations of surfactant are present in amniotic fluid after 35 weeks gestation. With RDS, alveolar atelectasis, collection of fibrinous material within the alveoli, and interstitial edema lead to decreased compliance of the lungs, with higher pressures required to achieve adequate functional residual capacity. This results in lung segments that are perfused but not ventilated, leading to hypoxia and hypercapnia. Hypoxia, hypercapnia, and acidosis result in pulmonary vasoconstriction, leading to ischemic injury and release of additional fibrinous material into the alveolar space, further diminishing ventilated segments of lung.[1,2] Causes of RDS are illustrated in Fig. 1.

🅳🆇 DIAGNOSIS

DIFFERENTIAL DIAGNOSIS

The differential diagnosis of RDS is broad. Transient tachypnea of the newborn can be seen in term and preterm newborns and is differentiated by its mild course of illness and the need for minimal or no oxygen supplementation. Early-onset sepsis may not be distinguished from RDS, and in particular pneumonia at the time of birth may present with similar symptoms and chest x-ray findings. Persistent pulmonary hypertension of the newborn may present concurrently in a patient with RDS. In addition, aspiration of meconium, blood, or amniotic fluid may cause surfactant inactivation, leading to a clinical presentation that may resemble RDS. Conditions such as spontaneous pneumothorax, pleural effusions, and congenital anomalies may also present with respiratory distress and may be distinguished from RDS by examination of the chest x-ray.[1]

WORKUP

In addition to physical examination, chest radiography and blood gas sampling are most useful in establishing this diagnosis and may help exclude other causes of acute respiratory distress.

LABORATORY TESTS

Arterial blood gas sampling is preferred to assess the infant's gas exchange in the setting of RDS. Respiratory acidosis noted on blood gas indicates

a need for assisted ventilation, and serial blood gases will guide escalation or titration of support.

Evaluation may also include a complete blood count, blood culture to assess for infectious etiology of respiratory distress, and electrolyte panels to help guide fluid management as the infant experiences increased insensible fluid loss and diuresis in the first few days of life.

IMAGING STUDIES

Typical radiographic findings in infants with RDS include low lung volumes; a diffuse, reticulogranular "ground-glass" appearance of the lung fields bilaterally; and widely distributed air bronchograms. The ground-glass appearance is due to alveolar atelectasis and the air bronchograms are easily visualized due to the contrast of the aerated bronchioles with the collapsed alveoli[2] (Fig. 2).

Echocardiography may also be indicated to assess for patency of the ductus arteriosus, which can complicate management of RDS and have effects on perfusion and hemodynamic stability.[2]

🆁🆇 TREATMENT

NONPHARMACOLOGIC THERAPY

Careful respiratory support is essential for treatment of infants with RDS. Positive pressure ventilation improves gas exchange by increasing airway and alveolar distention and may be achieved via noninvasive as well as invasive strategies. Nasal continuous positive airway pressure (CPAP) and noninvasive positive pressure ventilation (NIPPV) are common initial respiratory support modalities in even the most premature infants, with some studies supporting NIPPV as the most effective primary mode.[3] Although early noninvasive support is associated with improved survival, failure may occur in up to 50% of very preterm patients.[3] Some infants will require conventional or high-frequency mechanical ventilation if oxygenation and ventilation are inadequate or if work of breathing is significant despite noninvasive measures. Continuous monitoring of oxygenation via pulse oximetry and ventilation via end tidal or transcutaneous carbon dioxide monitoring are valuable noninvasive tools to aid in this assessment.

Other supportive care measures such as optimization of enteral nutrition, treatment of anemia with blood transfusion and iron supplementation, caffeine prophylaxis, and medical management of hemodynamically-significant patent ductus arteriosus (PDA) are mainstays of treatment. Fig. 3 illustrates management strategies for RDS.

ACUTE GENERAL Rx

Surfactant therapy is one of the most effective interventions in the management of newborns with RDS. Typically administered endotracheally, exogenous surfactant decreases surface tension in alveoli leading to improved oxygenation, lung compliance, and functional residual capacity. Early surfactant delivery followed by rapid extubation and noninvasive respiratory support (the

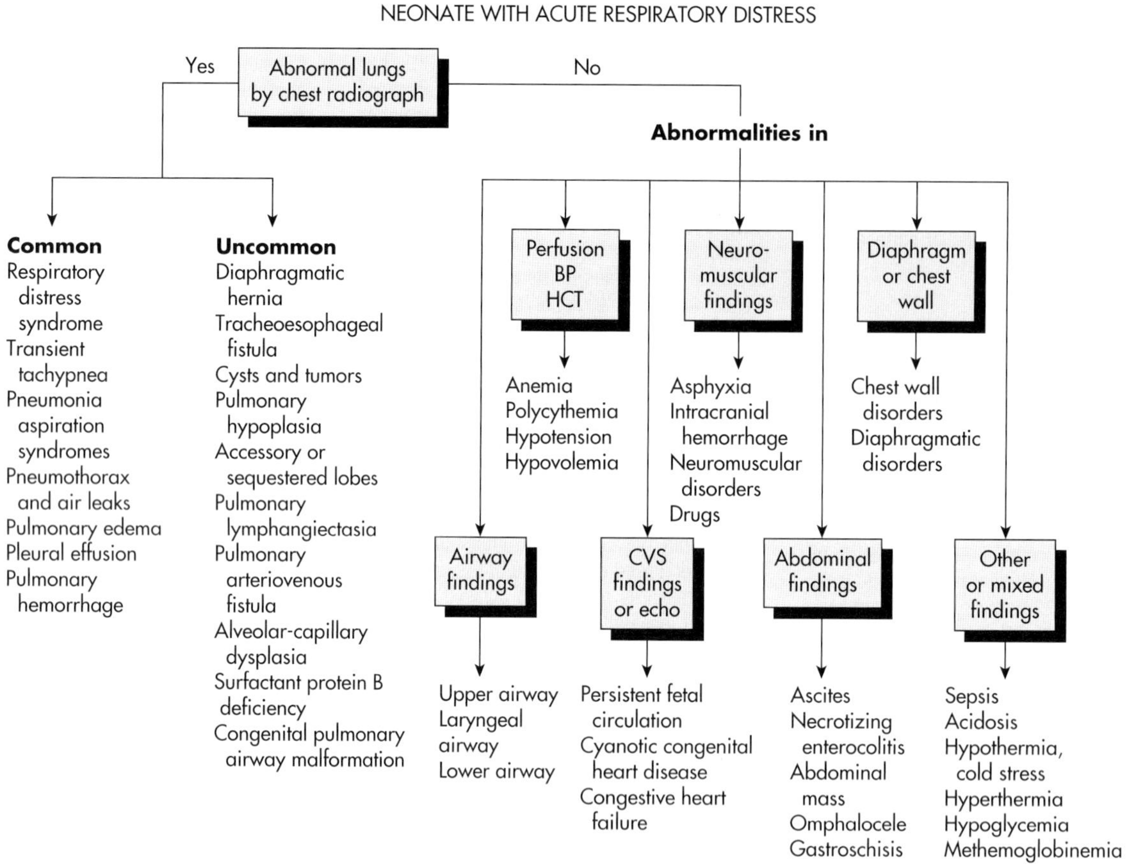

NEONATE WITH ACUTE RESPIRATORY DISTRESS

Yes ← Abnormal lungs by chest radiograph → No

Abnormalities in

Common
Respiratory
 distress
 syndrome
Transient
 tachypnea
Pneumonia
 aspiration
 syndromes
Pneumothorax
 and air leaks
Pulmonary edema
Pleural effusion
Pulmonary
 hemorrhage

Uncommon
Diaphragmatic
 hernia
Tracheoesophageal
 fistula
Cysts and tumors
Pulmonary
 hypoplasia
Accessory or
 sequestered lobes
Pulmonary
 lymphangiectasia
Pulmonary
 arteriovenous
 fistula
Alveolar-capillary
 dysplasia
Surfactant protein B
 deficiency
Congenital pulmonary
 airway malformation

Perfusion
BP
HCT
→
Anemia
Polycythemia
Hypotension
Hypovolemia

Airway
findings
→
Upper airway
Laryngeal
 airway
Lower airway

Neuro-
muscular
findings
→
Asphyxia
Intracranial
 hemorrhage
Neuromuscular
 disorders
Drugs

CVS
findings
or echo
→
Persistent fetal
 circulation
Cyanotic congenital
 heart disease
Congestive heart
 failure

Diaphragm
or chest
wall
→
Chest wall
 disorders
Diaphragmatic
 disorders

Abdominal
findings
→
Ascites
Necrotizing
 enterocolitis
Abdominal
 mass
Omphalocele
Gastroschisis

Other
or mixed
findings
→
Sepsis
Acidosis
Hypothermia,
 cold stress
Hyperthermia
Hypoglycemia
Methemoglobinemia

FIG. 1 **Diagram of causes of respiratory distress in neonates.** *BP*, Blood pressure; *CVS*, cardiovascular system; *echo*, echocardiogram; *HCT*, hematocrit. (Modified from Fanaroff AA, Fanaroff JM: *Klaus & Fanaroff's care of the high-risk neonate*, ed 6, Philadelphia 2013, Elsevier, pg. 271 [Fig. 11-1].)

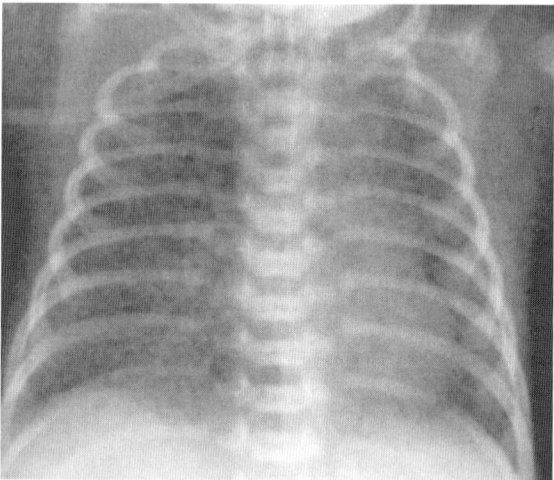

FIG. 2 **Radiographic appearance of respiratory distress syndrome with retriculogranular infiltrates and air bronchograms.** (From Martin RJ et al [eds]: *Fanaroff and Martin's neonatal-perinatal medicine: diseases of the fetus and infant,* ed 11, Philadelphia, 2020, Elsevier.)

INSURE method) is associated with decreased risk of acute injury and chronic lung disease. Surfactant may be administered multiple times every 8 to 12 hr but is most efficacious when given within the first 72 hr of life.[3,5] FiO_2 requirement of greater than 0.3 to 0.4 despite appropriate respiratory support is a common indication for repeat dosing. Surfactant may also be administered via thin tracheal catheter (less invasive surfactant administration [LISA] or minimally invasive surfactant treatment [MIST]). These methods are safe and efficacious with data suggesting a reduced incidence of major complications compared with endotracheal intubation.[4] Complications of surfactant therapy include endotracheal tube occlusion, inadvertent right main stem bronchus instillation, and pulmonary hemorrhage.

CHRONIC Rx

Patients with RDS may develop chronic lung disease of infancy or bronchopulmonary dysplasia, particularly if they require prolonged invasive respiratory support. Systemic dexamethasone regimens have been used to treat infants with evolving chronic lung disease. Although these regimens may facilitate transition to noninvasive support, treatment is associated with increased risk of cerebral palsy and other neurodevelopmental complications.[1] Comparison of these risks with long-term morbidity and mortality associated with prolonged mechanical ventilation should be discussed before initiation of dexamethasone therapy.

DISPOSITION

Patients with RDS continue to be at risk for significant morbidity and mortality, including nonpulmonary complications such as intracranial hemorrhage, sepsis, growth failure, and neurodevelopmental impairment. It is not clear if these complications are sequelae of extreme prematurity or adverse effects associated with management of RDS. Nonetheless, outcomes for this patient population continue to improve.[1,2]

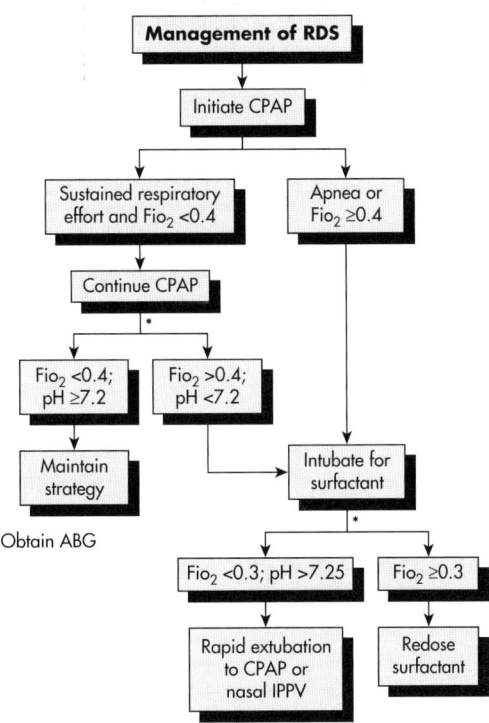

FIG. 3 Algorithm suggesting management strategy of respiratory distress syndrome (RDS). *ABG*, Arterial blood gas; *CPAP*, continuous positive airway pressure; *Fio₂*, fraction of inspired oxygen; *IPPV*, intermittent positive-pressure ventilation. (From Fanaroff AA, Fanaroff JM: *Klaus & Fanaroff's care of the high-risk neonate*, ed 6, Philadelphia, 2013, Elsevier, pg. 253 [Fig. 10-5].)

REFERRAL

Consultation with a multidisciplinary chronic lung disease of infancy team is helpful for the management of patients who develop bronchopulmonary dysplasia and continue to require significant respiratory support beyond 36 weeks corrected gestational age.

PREVENTION

Antenatal corticosteroid administration in pregnant persons at least 24 to 48 hours before delivery significantly reduces severity and improves outcomes for newborns with RDS and should be recommended to obstetrics providers when preterm delivery is likely.[1]

REFERENCES

Available at eBooks.Health.Elsevier.com

AUTHORS: **CRYSTAL T. BASS, MD,** and **JOSEPH A. ASARO, DO**

Diseases and Disorders

I

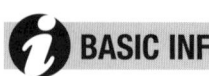

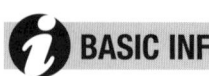 BASIC INFORMATION

DEFINITION

Restless legs syndrome (RLS) is an awake phenomenon consisting of an urge to move legs, usually associated with feeling of discomfort in legs. Symptoms typically are present only at rest and at least partially improve with movement. Additionally, symptoms are usually worse at night. RLS can result in sleep disturbance with associated executive dysfunction and depression.

SYNONYMS

RLS
Wittmaack-Ekbom syndrome

ICD-10CM CODE
G25.81 Restless legs syndrome

EPIDEMIOLOGY & DEMOGRAPHICS

PREVALENCE: Average prevalence rate is 1% to 29%. Prevalence estimates in Europe are around 10%, and 0.1% to 12% in East Asian population.[1-2]
PREDOMINANT SEX: Early-onset RLS is more common in females, with 2:1 female:male ratio.[1-4]
PREDOMINANT AGE: Prevalence of RLS increases with age, and it is more commonly seen in the elderly population but can occur in children.
PEAK PREVALENCE: 10% in persons aged 30 to 79 and 19% in persons aged 80 or above.[1-4]
RISK FACTORS:
- Iron deficiency anemia (IDA): 25% to 35%.
- Pregnancy: Increases in severity and prevalence with each passing trimester.
- End-stage renal disease (ESRD) requiring hemodialysis: Improves with transplant but not dialysis.
- Peripheral neuropathy: 5% to 54% of patients with peripheral neuropathy also have symptoms of RLS.[5]
- Many other neurologic diseases such as Parkinson disease, multiple sclerosis, and myelopathy increase risk as do mood disorders, other inflammatory disease, and cardiovascular disease.
GENETICS: Genetic basis of RLS has been reported, particularly in early-onset RLS.
- Autosomal dominant disorder.
- Common among first-degree relatives.
- RLS associated with certain sequences in chromosomes 6p, 12q, 14q, 9p, 20p, 2p, 16p.
- These include polymorphisms in the genes *BTBD9, MEIS1, PTPRD, MAP2K5, SKOR1,* and *TOX3.*

CLASSIFICATION

- Primary RLS is without any obvious cause, with no associated disorder.
- Secondary RLS results from other medical conditions.

PHYSICAL FINDINGS & CLINICAL PRESENTATION

- Wide spectrum of severity of clinical manifestations has been reported in RLS.[1]

- Most common symptom is unpleasant sensations in legs ("dysesthesias"), reported as discomfort or "creepy-crawling" sensations, mostly bilateral. Arms are occasionally involved.
- There is an extreme urge to move legs, and relief is sustained as long as the movement continues.
- Symptoms are worse at night or evening. Best sleep is usually early in the morning.

ETIOLOGY

The exact etiology remains unknown. Pharmacologic, pathologic, physiologic, and imaging studies have implicated dopaminergic pathways, brain iron metabolism, and endogenous opioid pathways. Drugs that may be associated with RLS are summarized in Table E1.

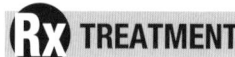 DIAGNOSIS

DIFFERENTIAL DIAGNOSIS

- Periodic limb movement disorder
- Nocturnal leg cramps
- Painful peripheral neuropathy
- Akathisia
- Positional discomfort
- Volitional movements, foot tapping, leg rocking

WORKUP

- Diagnosis of RLS is based on established clinical criteria (Table 2) and normal neurologic examination.
- Testing is done to determine possible cause of secondary RLS. All patients with RLS should be screened for iron deficiency because iron supplementation in patients with iron deficiency may resolve the symptoms.[1]
- Polysomnography with leg activity monitors to determine limb movements during sleep, but they are unable to distinguish periodic limb movements from periodic movements associated with sleep apnea.
- Nerve conduction studies and electromyography for associated peripheral neuropathy given the high prevalence.[5]

LABORATORY TESTS

- Iron status: Serum ferritin, total iron binding capacity, percent saturation
- CBC for anemia in case of iron deficiency
- Metabolic panel: Blood urea nitrogen and serum creatinine for renal insufficiency

IMAGING STUDIES

No imaging studies are required for diagnosis of RLS.

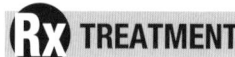 TREATMENT

NONPHARMACOLOGIC THERAPY[5]

- Avoid caffeine, alcohol, and nicotine, which can exacerbate RLS.

- Review and adjust medications that may exacerbate or cause RLS (selective serotonin reuptake inhibitors, dopamine blocking agents, stimulants).
- Physical and mental activity.
- Good sleep hygiene.
- Monitoring for depression as RLS has an elevated suicide risk. Bupropion may be the best agent for depression in RLS due to lack of dopamine effects.
- Mild symptoms are associated with resolution or quick response to treatment.[6]

CHRONIC Rx

Once the diagnosis of RLS is considered based on clinical criteria as mentioned in Table 2 and causes impairment of quality of life, an anticonvulsant (gabapentin, enacarbil, or pregabalin) or dopamine agonist (bromocriptine, pramipexole, or ropinirole) should be started at low dose and then gradually tapered depending on tolerance.
Treatment options (Table 3) for RLS include:
- Anticonvulsants, such as gabapentin, have been shown to be effective in multiple studies. Gabapentin, enacarbil, and pregabalin are now considered first-line agents in the treatment of RLS. These agents do not cause iatrogenic worsening (augmentation) of RLS with long-term treatment. Carbamazepine and valproic acid likely are efficacious.[7]
- Dopaminergic agents such as levodopa and dopamine agonists help to ameliorate RLS symptoms, decrease periodic limb movements, and improve sleep. Dopamine agonists, pramipexole and ropinirole, can be first-line agents in the treatment of RLS but often cause augmentation of RLS with long-term treatment.
- Rotigotine patch (Neupro) is also effective and FDA approved for moderate to severe RLS.[7]
- Opiates, mostly methadone, are generally reserved as last line of treatment.[8]
- Iron replacement with vitamin C should be started concurrently in case of iron deficiency. Iron supplements are indicated even with low-normal ferritin levels (<45 ng/ml).[7-8] Sometimes intravenous iron replacement is used.

REFERRAL

Refer to neurologist if diagnosis is uncertain or an underlying disorder is suspected.

REFERENCES
Available at eBooks.Health.Elsevier.com.

RELATED CONTENT

Restless Legs Syndrome (Patient Information)

AUTHOR: **COREY ELAM GOLDSMITH, MD, FAAN**

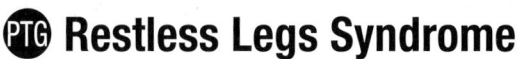 **Restless Legs Syndrome** 1209

R

Diseases and Disorders

I

TABLE 2 Diagnostic Criteria for Restless Legs Syndrome

Minimal Criteria
- Desire to move the legs usually associated with paresthesias
- Motor restlessness, as characterized by floor pacing, leg rubbing, stretching, and flexing
- Worse at rest, with relief by activity
- Worse at night

Additional Criteria
- Sleep disturbances, as difficulty in sleep onset and maintaining sleep, daytime fatigue, or somnolence
- Involuntary movements, as periodic limb or leg movements in sleep and periodic or aperiodic limb movements while awake
- Neurologic examination is normal in idiopathic restless legs syndrome
- Clinical course may begin at any age but most severe in middle and older age
- Family history suggests autosomal dominant mode of inheritance in one third of the cases

From Stiasny K et al: Clinical symptomatology and treatment of restless legs syndrome and periodic limb movement disorder, *Sleep Med Rev* 6(4):253-265, 2002.

TABLE 3 Management of Restless Legs Syndrome

Agent and Daily Dosage	Side Effects	Countermeasures
Step 1: α2δ Agents First-line treatment, particularly if sleep disturbance, pain, or anxiety is present		
Gabapentin enacarbil, 300-600 mg Pregabalin, 50-450 mg* Gabapentin, 100-1800 mg*	Dizziness	Reduce dose and add alternate medication class as needed. If fall risk, then discontinue and change to alternate medication class.
	Somnolence, daytime fatigue	Reduce dose and add alternate medication class as needed. If significant, discontinue and change to alternate medication class.
	Tolerance	Discontinue, take drug holiday with return to medication. Switch to alternate medication class.
	Weight gain	Reduce dose and add alternate medication class as needed. If significant, discontinue and change to alternate medication class.
Step 2: Dopamine Agonists Alternative first-line treatment if depression is present and dose kept low.		
Pramipexole, 0.125-0.5 mg* (0.75 mg in Europe), Ropinirole, 0.5-4.0 mg* Rotigotine, 1-3 mg/24 h	Nausea and orthostatic hypotension	Slowly increase dosage or use domperidone if available (10-30 mg).
	Insomnia	Add or switch to α2δ agent. Use a small dose of benzodiazepines in association with dopamine agonists.
	Daytime fatigue and somnolence	Reduce dosage or discontinue dopamine agonists.
	Compulsive or impulsive behavior	Reduce dose and add alternate medication class as needed. If significant, discontinue and change to alternate medication class.
	Tolerance	Discontinue and switch to longer-acting dopamine agonist or alternate medication class.
	Augmentation	Discontinue and switch to alternate medication class or longer-acting dopamine agonist.
Step 3: Dopamine Precursors Useful for intermittent treatment, such as twice a wk		
Levodopa-benserazide or levodopa-carbidopa (regular or slow release), 100/25 or 200/50 mg†	Same as for dopamine agonists	See "Countermeasures" for dopamine agonists.
	Morning rebound or augmentation of restless legs syndrome in early evening	Use small extra dose of levodopa during daytime or reduce dosage or combine levodopa with dopamine agonists or benzodiazepines or discontinue levodopa (if severe and persistent).
	Augmentation	Do not use daily. Discontinue and switch to dopamine agonists or a nondopamine medication.
Benzodiazepines Useful for sleep promotion		
Clonazepam, 0.5-2.0 mg‡ Temazepam, 15-30 mg‡ Nitrazepam, 5-10 mg*	Daytime somnolence	Reduce dosage.
	Tolerance	Take drug holiday for 2 wk then return to lower dosage.
Opiates Second-line treatment		
Oxycodone-naloxone, 10/5 to 40/20 mg/day Methadone, 2.5-20 mg Oxycodone, 5-40 mg	Constipation	Use for symptom treatment.
	Dependency	Take a drug holiday. Discontinue and switch to alternate medication.
Oral Iron Always consider if serum iron ≤75 mcg/L *or* transferrin saturation ≤17%		
Ferrous sulfate, 650 mg (325 mg with vitamin C, 100 mg twice a day)	Constipation, stomach upset and pain	Reduce dose, discontinue, take with food.
	Diarrhea, nausea, vomiting	Reduce dose, discontinue, take with food.

*One hour before onset of symptoms in the evening or 1-2 h before bedtime if symptoms are not present in the evening.
†Considered most appropriate for PRN dosing not more than 3 times a wk rather than daily use.
‡Before bedtime usually to promote sleep with restless legs syndrome.
From Kryger M et al: *Principles and practice of sleep medicine,* ed 6, Philadelphia, 2017, Elsevier.

BASIC INFORMATION

DEFINITION

- Retinal vein occlusions (RVOs) are defined as retinal vascular disorders caused by complete or partial obstruction of a retinal vein characterized by tortuosity and dilation of the retinal veins with secondary intraretinal hemorrhages, macular edema times, and retinal ischemia (including cotton-wool spots and retinal neovascularization).
- Central retinal vein occlusion (CRVO) is defined by obstruction at or posterior to the optic nerve head.
- Branch retinal vein occlusion (BRVO) is defined by partial or complete obstruction at a tributary or branch of the central retinal vein.

SYNONYMS

RVO
CRVO
BRVO

ICD 10-CM CODES

H34.819	Central retinal vein occlusion, unspecified eye
H34.811	Central retinal vein occlusion, right eye
H34.812	Central retinal vein occlusion, left eye
H34.813	Central retinal vein occlusion, bilateral
H34.8130	Central retinal vein occlusion, bilateral, with macular edema
H34.8131	Central retinal vein occlusion, bilateral, with retinal neovascularization
H34.831	Tributary (branch) retinal vein occlusion, right eye
H34.832	Tributary (branch) retinal vein occlusion, left eye
H34.8190	Central retinal vein occlusion, unspecified eye, with macular edema
H34.8111	Central retinal vein occlusion, right eye, with retinal neovascularization
H34.8121	Central retinal vein occlusion, left eye, with retinal neovascularization
H348191	Central retinal vein occlusion, unspecified eye, with retinal neovascularization
H34.833	Tributary (branch) retinal vein occlusion, bilateral
H34.8311	Tributary (branch) retinal vein occlusion, right eye, with retinal neovascularization
H34.8321	Tributary (branch) retinal vein occlusion, left eye, with retinal neovascularization
H34.8331	Tributary (branch) retinal vein occlusion, bilateral, with retinal neovascularization
H34.8391	Tributary (branch) retinal vein occlusion, unspecified eye, with retinal neovascularization
H34.8330	Tributary (branch) retinal vein occlusion, bilateral, with macular edema
H34.8390	Tributary (branch) retinal vein occlusion, unspecified eye, with macular edema
H34.8392	Tributary (branch) retinal vein occlusion, unspecified eye, stable
H34.9	Unspecified retinal vascular occlusion
H34.8110	Central retinal vein occlusion, right eye, with macular edema
H34.233	Retinal artery branch occlusion, bilateral Bilateral branch retinal artery occlusion; Occlusion of bilateral branch retinal arteries
H34.8310	Tributary (branch) retinal vein occlusion, right eye, with macular edema
H34.8320	Tributary (branch) retinal vein occlusion, left eye, with macular edema

EPIDEMIOLOGY & DEMOGRAPHICS

INCIDENCE:
- BRVO is 6 to 7 times more prevalent than CRVO.

PREDOMINANT SEX & AGE:
- Over 50% of cases occur in patients older than 65.
- Population-based studies report the prevalence of CRVO at <0.1% to 0.4%.

PEAK INCIDENCE:
- 0.7% incidence for patients ages 49 to 60 yr and 4.6% incidence for those older than 80 yr

RISK FACTORS:
- Risk factors for BRVO and CRVO differ.
- A prior RVO is a risk for RVO in the other eye.
- Age: Most important factor for both BRVO and CRVO; majority of cases occur in elderly patients.
- Glaucoma: Open-angle glaucoma is the most common ocular factor predisposing to CRVO.

Systemic conditions that impair vascular health:
- Hypertension: A common finding is recently diagnosed or uncontrolled hypertension. This major risk factor is more prevalent in patients with BRVO than in those with CRVO. More than 64% of RVO patients in the age group over 50 yr are hypertensive, and it is a predominant finding in recurrent RVO (88%).
- Diabetes mellitus: Diabetes mellitus is significantly associated with CRVO.
- Hyperlipidemia: This is the predominant risk factor for RVO in patients under 50 yr old. It is also found in up to 50% of older patients.
- Coagulation defects:
  1. Consider workup only in atypical situations such as patients with family history of clotting at a young age (deep venous thrombosis, pulmonary emboli, or multiple spontaneous abortions), personal history of clotting, or bilateral simultaneous RVO.
  2. Thrombophilia: Factor V Leiden mutation increases the risk of RVO by about 50% to 60%, whereas other prothrombotic defects (i.e., prothrombin G21201A and deficiencies of antithrombin and of protein C or S) are not associated with RVO.
- The role of lupus anticoagulant and anticardiolipin antibodies in RVO is uncertain. The relationship between fibrinolysis and RVO is not strong. Since RVO occurs at arteriovenous crossings, where the blood flow is locally turbulent, changes in platelet reactivity due to polymorphisms in the platelet receptors may be important.
- Hyperhomocysteinemia.
- High body mass index (BMI) and smoking have also been implicated in RVO, but these associations are less consistent.
- High plasma viscosity (e.g., leukemia or multiple myeloma).
- Waldenström macroglobulinemia.
- Myelofibrosis.
- Systemic inflammatory conditions (Behçet disease, polyarteritis nodosa, sarcoidosis, granulomatosis with polyangiitis, Goodpasture syndrome).

PHYSICAL FINDINGS & CLINICAL PRESENTATION

Visual acuity (VA) is reduced compared with unaffected eye, but it varies by occlusion severity and site. Ischemic central retinal vein and branch retinal vein occlusions are associated with worse visual acuity (20/400 or worse) than nonischemic central and branch retinal vein occlusions (better than 20/200). In BRVO, visual function and recovery of vision are correlated with thickness of the central macula, and that is correlated with the integrity of the inner and outer segments of the photoreceptors in the fovea.

Pupillary reflexes may be affected. Patients may or may not show relative afferent pupillary defect (Marcus Gunn pupil), depending on severity.
- Fundoscopic exam may reveal:
  1. Optic disc edema (Fig. E1) in central retinal vein occlusion (may or may not be present in branch retinal vein occlusion) and macular edema
  2. Increased dilation and tortuosity of retinal veins
  3. Central retinal vein occlusion: All retinal veins are dilated and tortuous
  4. Branch retinal vein occlusion: Only affected branch is dilated and tortuous
  5. Widespread deep and superficial hemorrhages (dot-and-blot and flame shaped)
  6. Cotton-wool spots
  7. Neovascularization in advanced cases
- Findings outside fundus may include neovascularization of iris (rubeosis iridis) and/or anterior chamber (iridocorneal) angle (in advanced cases)

Presentation of retinal vein occlusion is variable:
- Clinically ischemic CRVO is generally painless and may present with unilateral loss of vision on awakening.
- Nonischemic central retinal vein occlusion may be asymptomatic and be discovered on routine ophthalmic examination. It most commonly presents with gradual development of central visual blurring that is usually worse on awakening in the morning with a variable degree of improvement after a few hours or in the afternoon. VA is impaired to a variable degree dependent on severity; eyes with

initially good VA tend to have a good prognosis and vice versa; initial VA in the middle range (6/30 to 6/60) is an unreliable predictor of outcome. VA worse than 6/60 commonly indicates that substantial ischemia is present. In cases that do not become ischemic, vision returns to normal or near normal in about 50%.
- In some instances, patients may complain of transient visual blurring before a constant diminution of vision followed by permanent central scotoma.
- Branch retinal vein occlusion usually presents with a sudden painless decrease in visual acuity or a visual field defect. It may also be asymptomatic and discovered on routine ophthalmic examination.

ETIOLOGY
- Compression of retinal vein wall or obstruction by thrombosis.
- In BRVO, arteriolosclerotic thickening of a branch retinal arteriole is associated with compression of a venule at an arteriovenous crossing point, exacerbated by sharing an adventitial sheath. This leads to secondary changes that include endothelial cell loss, turbulent flow, and thrombus formation. Similarly, the central retinal vein and artery possess a common sheath at crossing points posterior to the lamina cribrosa so that atherosclerotic changes of the artery may precipitate CRVO. Hematologic prothrombotic factors are thought to be important in a minority, amplifying an atherosclerotic anatomic predisposition. Once venous occlusion has occurred, elevation of venous and capillary pressure with stagnation of blood flow ensues, resulting in retinal hypoxia, which in turn results in damage to the capillary endothelial cells, extravasation of blood constituents, and liberation of mediators such as vascular endothelial growth factor (VEGF).

Dx DIAGNOSIS

DIFFERENTIAL DIAGNOSIS (IN ORDER OF IMPORTANCE)
- Ocular ischemic syndrome
- Diabetic retinopathy
- Chronic hypertensive retinopathy
- Papilledema

WORKUP
- History and physical examination, including direct funduscopy and measurement of visual acuity by Snellen chart; both eyes are examined
- Slit-lamp biomicroscopy (directed or performed by ophthalmologist): Indicated in all cases when history and physical examination findings lead to suspicion of retinal vein occlusion
- Ophthalmologist-performed assessment
- Evaluation for afferent pupillary defect that corresponds with level of ischemia and risk of neovascular complications

- Measure intraocular pressure before dilated indirect funduscopic examination
- Careful slit-lamp iris examination for neovascularization before dilation
- Dilated binocular funduscopic examination
- Visual field findings may help differentiate vein occlusion findings from ischemic optic neuropathy
- Optical coherence tomography (OCT): Indicated to detect presence and quantify severity of macular edema
- OCT angiography may help in quantifying capillary nonperfusion and foveal ischemia
- Fluorescein angiography (Figs. E2 and E3):
  1. Valuable to help determine location and extent of venous occlusion and to differentiate ischemic from nonischemic retinal vein occlusion, as well as extent of macular edema
  2. Also helps differentiate neovascularization from collateral vessels that form with chronicity
  3. May help guide laser treatment
- Electroretinography: May be used to differentiate ischemic from nonischemic retinal vein occlusion but not used widely

LABORATORY TESTS
In general, there are no clear guidelines for systemic testing in these patients unless the RVO is bilateral, in a person younger than age 40 yr, or there is medical history and/or systemic symptoms to warrant a workup.
- CBC, sedimentation rate, C-reactive protein
- FBS, HBA1c
- Lipid panel
- Evaluation for hypercoagulable state when suspecting thrombotic occlusion: Factor V Leyden, lupus anticoagulant, antithrombin II, INR, aPTT, anticardiolipin antibodies, anti–beta 2-glycoprotein-I antibodies
- Plasma homocysteine level
- ANA

IMAGING STUDIES
- Optical coherence tomography: Provides visualization of central macula to detect edema and to measure macular thickness
- Fluorescein angiography: Indicated for suspected retinal vein occlusion to determine site of occlusion, perfusion status of retina, presence of neovascularization, and presence of macular edema

Rx TREATMENT

NONPHARMACOLOGIC THERAPY
- Control of systemic risk factors: Investigating major systemic risk factors is essential as patients with RVO are at increased risk of cardiovascular disease, cerebrovascular accidents, and all-cause mortality. Addressing these as appropriate is critical, and as well as conferring systemic benefit this may also reduce the risk of the recurrence of retinal vein occlusion.

1. Lifestyle changes to correct hypertension, hyperglycemia, hyperlipidemia, hyperhomocysteinemia
2. Avoidance of tobacco products
3. Reduction of obesity to maintain normal BMI

ACUTE GENERAL Rx
VEGF-A plays a major role in the pathology of retinal vein occlusions and therefore treatment with intravitreal antivascular endothelial growth factor agents is very effective and has become the standard of care for reducing macular edema and ocular neovascularization.
Medications:
- Vascular endothelial growth factor inhibitors
  1. Ranibizumab
  2. Aflibercept
  3. Bevacizumab
  4. Injected monthly but interval may be extended in some patients; over 50% will have persistent macular edema and require ongoing injections more than 5 yr after onset
- Corticosteroids
  1. Typically a second- or third-line treatment after exhaustion of all anti-VEGF drugs
  2. Reduce pro–permeability factors that cause macular edema in RVO
  3. Glaucoma may influence risk-benefit assessment of intravitreal steroids, as corticosteroids can produce a rise in intraocular pressure
  4. Promotes cataract so more commonly used in pseudophakic eyes
- Intravitreal dexamethasone: Dexamethasone intraocular implant; sustained delivery formulation (containing 0.7 mg dexamethasone in a solid polymer delivery system) approved for injection every 6 mo
- Intravitreal triamcinolone: Triamcinolone acetonide suspension for injection; adults: 1 to 4 mg (100 μL of 40 mg/ml suspension) injected into the vitreous cavity

PROCEDURES: LASER PHOTOCOAGULATION:
- Two types of laser treatment may be performed: Focal macular laser photocoagulation to treat macular edema when the edema is noncentral (more common in BRVO) and panretinal photocoagulation to ischemic peripheral retina to manage neovascular complications, particularly iris neovascularization (more common in CRVO).
- Peripheral scatter photocoagulation is indicated for BRVO with retinal or disc neovascularization to lessen the risk of vitreous hemorrhage.
- The 2019 guidelines from the European Society of Retina Specialists suggest that focal laser photocoagulation should be considered only as a second-line treatment of macular edema secondary to BRVO. Intravitreal anti-VEGF injections remain the standard of care for center-involving macular edema for any RVO.

CHRONIC Rx

Monitor monthly during initial therapy using slit-lamp examination to detect neovascularization and to assess iris and anterior chamber (irido-corneal) angle.

- Subsequent follow-up plan depends on degree of ischemia found:
  1. In patients with significant ischemia (i.e., more than 10 disc areas of retinal capillary nonperfusion), evaluate every 3 mo for 1 yr; then continue monitoring for another year, with frequency determined by the treatment given and any complications experienced.
  2. In patients without significant ischemia, evaluate at 3 mo and at 6 mo, and then as determined by the treatment given and any complications experienced.
  3. In patients receiving injection therapy for macular edema, follow up more frequently (e.g., every 4 wk).

DISPOSITION

- In patients with nonischemic (well-perfused) CRVO and good visual acuity on presentation (better than 20/40, corrected), prognosis is favorable; however, 30% of eyes with initially nonischemic CRVO may convert to ischemic subtype.
- According to the Central Vein Occlusion Study:

1. 20% of eyes with visual acuity at presentation of 20/50 to 20/200 improve spontaneously to 20/50
2. 80% of patients with initial visual acuity worse than 20/200 have no improvement or have deterioration

- The ischemic form accounts for 20% of all cases of CRVO. The most concerning complication of CRVO is neovascular glaucoma, occurring in approximately 50% of ischemic cases.
- Prognosis is guarded in cases that have progressed to macular ischemia as demonstrated by fluorescein angiography.
- In BRVO with perfused periphery and normal visual acuity, prognosis is favorable, even with monitoring alone and no therapy.
- Because visual disturbance is often mild to moderate at first but progresses with no treatment, prognosis is generally improved with early diagnosis and treatment.
- CRVO is usually a unilateral disease; however, the annual risk of developing a CRVO in the other eye is approximately 1% per yr, and it is estimated that up to 7% of persons with CRVO may develop CRVO in the other eye within 5 yr of onset in the first eye.

REFERRAL

- Urgent referral to an ophthalmologist (retina specialist if available)

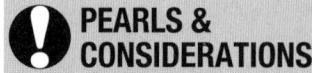

PEARLS & CONSIDERATIONS

PREVENTION

- Appropriate management of chronic systemic diseases associated with the development of vascular disease (e.g., hypertension, diabetes mellitus, hyperlipidemia, coagulation disorders, systemic inflammatory conditions) is important for prevention of RVO.
- Smoking cessation reduces risk of developing RVO.
- Appropriate management of glaucoma may also reduce risk of RVO because open-angle glaucoma is the most common ocular factor predisposing to RVO.

SUGGESTED READINGS

Available at eBooks.Health.Elsevier.com.

RELATED TOPICS

Glaucoma, Open Angle (Related Key Topic)
Diabetes Mellitus (Related Key Topic)
Hypertension (Related Key Topic)

AUTHORS: **ROBERT H. JANIGIAN, JR., MD,** and **FRED F. FERRI, MD**

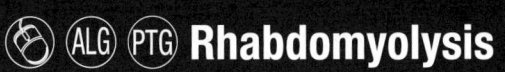

 BASIC INFORMATION

DEFINITION

Rhabdomyolysis is a syndrome characterized by striated muscle lysis with resulting muscle damage and leakage of intracellular contents into the circulation. The presentation may range from an asymptomatic elevation of creatine kinase (CK) to severe muscle injury with irreversible kidney failure. In general, a 5- to 10-fold elevation of CK levels, muscle pain, and myoglobinuria in an appropriate clinical setting (see below) are sufficient criteria for the diagnosis of rhabdomyolysis. Acute kidney injury (AKI), which is not a diagnostic criterion of rhabdomyolysis, typically results from multiple factors, including volume depletion, tubular obstruction, direct heme pigment–induced proximal tubular cell injury, and renal vasoconstriction.

ICD-10CM CODES
M62.82   Rhabdomyolysis (idiopathic)
T79.6   Traumatic ischemia of muscle
M62.89   Other specified disorders of muscle

EPIDEMIOLOGY & DEMOGRAPHICS

PREDOMINANT AGE: Incidence is approximately 1 per 10,000 persons in the U.S.
- Rare in children, increased risk with age, i.e., >80 yr.
- Reported incidence of AKI with rhabdomyolysis is 10% to 55%.
- 7% to 10% of cases of AKI are due to rhabdomyolysis.

MORTALITY RATE: 5% to 8%, with better prognosis when AKI is absent.

ONSET:
- Evidence is limited regarding the onset of physical exertion–induced rhabdomyolysis. Exercise levels that exceed an individual's usual exercise tolerance level commonly induce rhabdomyolysis. Extracellular volume depletion and vasoconstriction are common predisposing features. Patients with risk factors (e.g., metabolic myopathies, advanced age) develop symptoms associated with rhabdomyolysis within 2 to 6 hr after activity. Concurrent electrolyte abnormalities such as hypokalemia, hyponatremia, hypernatremia, hypomagnesemia, hypophosphatemia, and hypocalcemia increase the risk for rhabdomyolysis. Patients without risk factors generally become symptomatic 12 to 36 hr after muscle injury.
- CK levels increase within 2 to 12 hr of the onset of muscle injury, generally peak after 24 to 72 hr, and decline 3 to 5 days after cessation of muscle injury. Peak CK levels may predict development of AKI.
- Rhabdomyolysis from cholesterol-lowering therapy by HMG-CoA reductase inhibitors (statins) requires hospitalization in less than 0.1% of cases. The mechanism of damage is multifactorial: Bioavailability, lipophilicity, efficiency of uptake of transport proteins in hepatocytes, blood level of statins, and level of extrahepatic inhibition of mitochondrial respiration, bioavailability, and lipophilicity. Among the

statins, pravastatin has a lower risk for induction of rhabdomyolysis than other statins, presumably due to lower lipid solubility. The average duration of statin therapy before onset of myopathy is 6 mo. Symptom resolution with normalization of serum CK concentrations occurs in days to weeks following drug discontinuation. The average time for onset of rhabdomyolysis after the addition of a fibrate to statin therapy is 32 days. Rare genetic variants are associated with statin-induced myopathy.

PHYSICAL FINDINGS & CLINICAL PRESENTATION
- Classic triad of muscle pain, weakness, and dark urine from myoglobinuria
- Muscle tenderness is present in half of cases
- Muscle swelling occurs after intravenous fluid repletion
- Muscular rigidity
- Fever
- In rhabdomyolysis secondary to long-term statin administration, fatigue (74%) is nearly as common as muscle pain (88%)
- Oliguria or anuria with AKI

ETIOLOGY
Causes can be divided into three categories:
- Traumatic or muscle compression
  1. High-current electrical injury
  2. Crush injury and compartment syndrome
  3. Tourniquet and limb ischemia
  4. Reperfusion after revascularization procedures for ischemia
  5. Extensive surgical (spinal) dissection, bariatric surgery
- Nontraumatic exertional
  1. Exercise: More than 10 genetically predisposing gene sequence variants are associated with exertional rhabdomyolysis
  2. Sickle cell trait, rarely: Usually additional predisposing factors are involved (e.g., body mass index [BMI] >30 kg/m^2, tobacco use, statin use, antipsychotic use, high altitude)
  3. Heat stroke
  4. Metabolic myopathies
  5. Malignant hyperthermia and neuroleptic malignant syndrome
  6. Seizure activity
- Nontraumatic, nonexertional
  1. Drug-induced (statins alone, combinations of statins with fibrates or erythromycin, simvastatin and amiodarone, amphetamines, haloperidol, levofloxacin, macrolide antibiotics)
  2. Chronic ethanol ingestion
  3. Hypothyroidism
  4. Infectious and inflammatory myositis

Table 1 summarizes various causes of rhabdomyolysis.

DX **DIAGNOSIS**

DIFFERENTIAL DIAGNOSIS
"Creatine Kinase Elevation" in Section IV describes a clinical algorithm for the evaluation of CK elevation.

LABORATORY TESTS
- Creatine kinase: Usually CK is 5 to 10 times the upper limit of the normal range and typically peaks 24 to 72 hr after the initial insult (Fig. 1). Levels >15,000 IU/L are more likely associated with AKI. However, in patients with concomitant risk factors such as hypokalemia or volume depletion, CK levels as low as 5000 U/L may be associated with AKI.
- Myoglobin: Filtration into urine produces a "port wine" color at concentrations of 100 to 300 mg/dl. Myoglobinuria can be suspected by a positive urine dipstick test for blood within urine or by light microscopy detection of red blood cells. Due to its rapid hepatic metabolism, myoglobin lacks sensitivity for detection and diagnosis of rhabdomyolysis. Therefore serum and/or urine myoglobin measurement is not recommended to establish the diagnosis of rhabdomyolysis. Blood urea nitrogen and plasma creatinine concentrations are used to monitor severity of AKI.
- Potassium, calcium, phosphorus, and uric acid are released from damaged muscle, and levels should be monitored. Hyperkalemia is less common in nontraumatic rhabdomyolysis.
- Calcium: Hypocalcemia from deposition of calcium phosphate complexes in damaged muscle tissue. Hypercalcemia may follow resolution of rhabdomyolysis from liberation of calcium from damaged muscle into the

TABLE 1 Causes of Rhabdomyolysis	
Muscle injury/ischemia	Trauma, pressure necrosis, electric shock, burns, acute vascular disease
Myofiber exhaustion	Seizures, excessive exercise, heat exhaustion
Toxins	Alcohol, cocaine, heroin, amphetamines, ecstasy, phencyclidine, snakebite
Drugs	Statins, fibrates, zidovudine, neuroleptic malignant syndrome, azathioprine, theophylline, lithium, diuretics, colchicine
Electrolyte disorders	Hypophosphatemia, hypokalemia, excess water shifts (hyperosmolality)
Infections	Viral (influenza, HIV, coxsackievirus, Epstein-Barr virus), bacterial (*Legionella, Francisella, Streptococcus pneumoniae, Salmonella, Staphylococcus aureus*)
Familial	McArdle disease, carnitine palmitoyl transferase deficiency, malignant hyperthermia
Other	Hypothyroidism, polymyositis, dermatomyositis

From Floege J et al: *Comprehensive clinical nephrology*, ed 4, Philadelphia, 2010, Saunders.

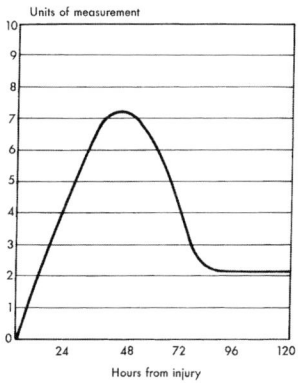

FIG. 1 Typical creatine kinase elimination curve.

circulation and increased gut calcium absorption from enhanced vitamin D production.
- Anion gap metabolic acidosis may occur from release of organic acids and phosphates from damaged muscle. Metabolic acidosis is less common in nontraumatic rhabdomyolysis.
- Urinalysis: Myoglobin is detected as blood on dipstick, but red blood cells are absent on microscopy. Microscopic identification of pigmented tubular casts establishes acute tubular necrosis.
- Rhabdomyolysis-induced acute tubular necrosis may occur with a low fractional excretion of sodium (FE_{Na} <1%).
- Box 1 summarizes laboratory abnormalities observed with rhabdomyolysis.

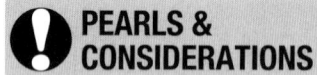 **TREATMENT**

ACUTE GENERAL Rx
- Identify precipitating factor(s) and discontinue potentially contributory drugs or toxins.
- Early, aggressive, high-volume intravenous fluid replacement with normal saline. Extracellular fluid volume-loading and diuresis reduce the risk for renal damage by elimination of urate and phosphate that can precipitate in the kidneys. Fig. 2 describes a treatment algorithm for rhabdomyolysis.
- Fasciotomy is indicated in compartment syndrome for preservation of muscle and nerve function.
- Initiate volume repletion with normal saline at a rate of 200 to 1000 ml/hr, depending on clinical circumstances and severity of muscle damage. Titrate the infusion rate to maintain a urine output of at least 200 ml/hr. Consider treatment with mannitol (up to 200 g per day with cumulative dose up to 800 g) to enhance urine flow rate. Typically, a 20% mannitol

infusion at a dose of 0.5 g/kg is given over a 15-min interval followed by an infusion at 0.1 gram/kg per hr. Discontinue mannitol and volume resuscitation if a diuresis threshold of >20 ml/hr is not established. Maintain volume repletion until myoglobinuria stops (negative urine dipstick blood test) or plasma CK levels decrease to <5000 U/L.
- Correct hypocalcemia if symptomatic or hyperkalemia that produces electrocardiographic changes.
- Treatment of all electrolyte imbalances.
- Urine alkalinization: Maintain urine pH at 6 to 7 and plasma pH at ~7.50. This recommendation is controversial. Early volume resuscitation and expansion are the most important treatments.
- Initiation of renal replacement therapy is determined by severity of kidney injury and/or electrolyte imbalances. Continuous renal replacement therapy and specialized hemodialysis membranes to enhance myoglobin clearance have not been systematically studied or proven superior to intermittent hemodialysis.

DISPOSITION
Early diagnosis and management are required to prevent AKI.

REFERRAL
Renal consultation and surgical consultation if compartment syndrome develops

⚠ PEARLS & CONSIDERATIONS

COMMENTS
- Statin-induced rhabdomyolysis occurs 12 times more frequently when statins are combined with fibrates than when used alone.
- Short-term, high-dose glucocorticoid steroid administration (500 to 1000 mg methylprednisolone) has been used for treatment of alcohol-induced rhabdomyolysis that is refractory to volume repletion. This treatment may be efficacious in cases of severe rhabdomyolysis by reducing secondary leukocyte inflammatory muscle injury.

RELATED CONTENT
Rhabdomyolysis (Patient Information)
Statin-Induced Muscle Syndrome (Related Key Topic)

AUTHORS: **HESHAM SHABAN, MD,** and **JUNIOR UDUMAN, MD**

BOX 1 Laboratory Abnormalities Observed With Rhabdomyolysis

Potassium
Elevated
Risk for acute kidney injury

Bicarbonate
Decreased (20 mEq/L)
Metabolic acidosis

Uric Acid
Elevated (>7 mg/dl)
Marker of acute renal failure

Sodium
Usually normal
Can decrease with mannitol therapy
Use serum osmolality values as a guide

Phosphate
Elevated
Risk for precipitation of calcium phosphate
May need phosphate binders if phosphate >7 mg/dl

Creatine Kinase
Elevated
Associated with creatine kinase level of 15 to 75,000

Blood Urea Nitrogen
Elevated (>20 mg/dl)

Creatinine
Elevated

Calcium
Initially low
Rebound phase may demonstrate hypercalcemia

Liver Function Tests
Occasionally elevated
Serum aspartate transaminase, lactate dehydrogenase, aldolase, muscle enzyme levels elevated

Troponin
Normal
Suspect myocardial damage as a cause (or effect) if elevated
7% false-positive rate for troponin I

Anion Gap
Sometimes elevated
May predict acute kidney injury

Prothrombin Time, Partial Thromboplastin Time, D-Dimer
Disseminated intravascular coagulation in up to 30% of severe cases
Associated with greater mortality

From Adams JG et al: *Emergency medicine, clinical essentials,* ed 2, Philadelphia, 2013, Elsevier.

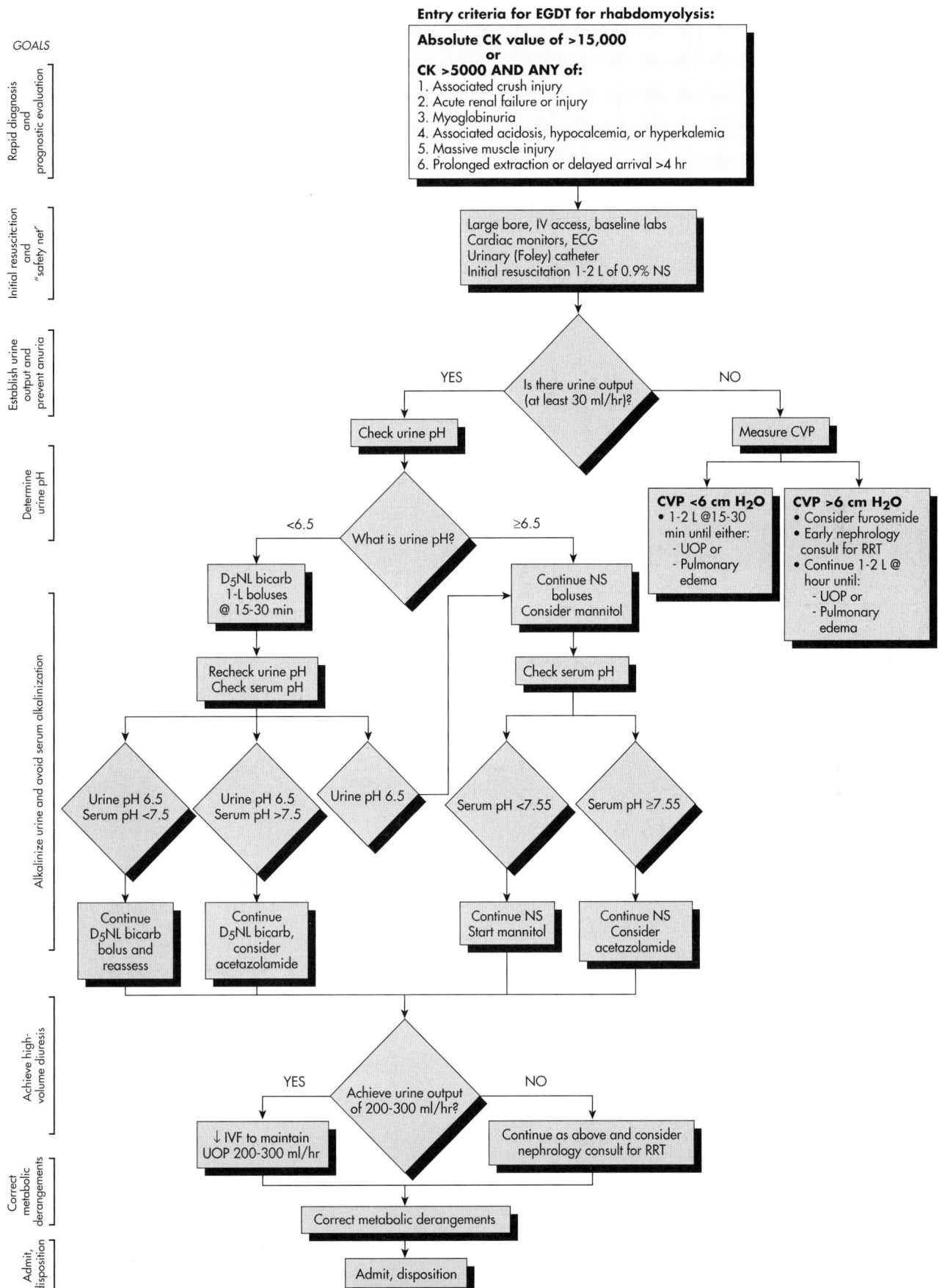

FIG. 2 Early goal-directed therapy for rhabdomyolysis. *CK*, Creatine kinase; *CVP*, central venous pressure; *D5NL bicarb*, 5% dextrose in normal sodium bicarbonate solution; *EGDT*, early goal-directed therapy; *IV*, intravenous; *IVF*, intravenous fluid; *NS*, normal saline; *RRT*, renal replacement therapy; *UOP*, urinary output. (From Adams JG et al: *Emergency medicine, clinical essentials*, ed 2, Philadelphia, 2013, Elsevier.)

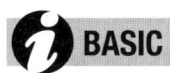

ℹ️ BASIC INFORMATION

DEFINITION

Rheumatoid arthritis (RA) is a systemic autoimmune disease characterized by inflammatory polyarthritis that affects peripheral joints, especially the small joints of the hands and feet.[1] It is a chronic, progressive disease in which untreated inflammation may lead to cartilage and bone erosions and joint destruction resulting in functional impairment.[1]

SYNONYM

RA

ICD-10CM CODES

M06.9	Rheumatoid arthritis, unspecified
M05.10	Rheumatoid lung disease with rheumatoid arthritis of unspecified site
M05.20	Rheumatoid vasculitis with rheumatoid arthritis of unspecified site
M05.39	Rheumatoid heart disease with rheumatoid arthritis of multiple sites
M05.49	Rheumatoid myopathy with rheumatoid arthritis of multiple sites
M05.59	Rheumatoid polyneuropathy with rheumatoid arthritis of multiple sites
M05.69	Rheumatoid arthritis of multiple sites with involvement of other organs and systems
M05.79	Rheumatoid arthritis with rheumatoid factor of multiple sites without organ or systems involvement
M05.80	Other rheumatoid arthritis with rheumatoid factor of unspecified site

EPIDEMIOLOGY & DEMOGRAPHICS

INCIDENCE: Annual incidence of 12 to 1200 per 100,000[2]
PREVALENCE: 0.5% to 1.0% of the worldwide population, with different rates in different ethnic groups[2]
PREDOMINANT SEX: Females are at higher risk of developing RA than males (2 to 3:1)[3]
RISK FACTORS: Female gender, age, tobacco use, silica exposure, and obesity, family history. Smoking has an additive detrimental effect in RA patients (twofold excess mortality risk).[2]
TYPICAL AGE AT DIAGNOSIS: Usually between age 30 and 50.[4] Steadily increases with age until the mid-70s

PHYSICAL FINDINGS & CLINICAL PRESENTATION

Initial presentation:
- Pain, swelling, warmth in one or more peripheral joints, frequently with symmetric small joint involvement, often associated with >1 hour of morning stiffness and constitutional symptoms such as fatigue, malaise, low-grade fevers, and weight loss occurring over a period of weeks to months.[4] A subset of patients can also present with acute-onset polyarthritis instead of insidious symptoms.[2]
- Most common joints involved include metacarpophalangeal (MCP) joints, proximal interphalangeal (PIP) joints (Fig. E1), and metatarsophalangeal (MTP) joints (Fig. E2), as well as wrists.[4]
- Other affected joints involved include elbows, shoulders, hips, knees, and ankles.[4]
- Distal interphalangeal (DIP) joints are spared.[1]
- Sacroiliac and vertebral joints are spared, except for the C1 and C2 articulations.[4]

Chronic longstanding disease:
- "Swan-neck" (DIP flexion and PIP hyperextension) (Fig. E3), "boutonniere" (DIP hyperextension and PIP flexion), and "Z-thumb" (MCP flexion and IP hyperextension) deformities (Fig. 4), ulnar deviation, and subluxation of the MCP joints as well as radial deviation of the wrists.
- C1-C2 (atlantoaxial) inflammation can lead to odontoid erosion and transverse ligament laxity/rupture, resulting in atlantoaxial subluxation (Fig. E5) and cord compression.[5]
- Joint damage of wrists, elbows, shoulders, hips, and knees can lead to severe secondary osteoarthritis, necessitating joint surgery and/or replacement.[4]

Extraarticular manifestations:
- Secondary Sjögren syndrome (~35%): Immune-mediated inflammation of lacrimal and salivary glands, resulting in dry mouth (xerostomia) and eyes (keratoconjunctivitis sicca).[6]
- Rheumatoid nodules (25%): Nontender, firm nodules on extensor surfaces and pressure points, usually in rheumatoid factor positive (RF+) disease.[6] Histopathology demonstrates palisading histiocytes surrounding a central area of fibrinoid necrosis.[7]
- Felty syndrome: RA with splenomegaly and leukopenia.[4] Most patients are positive for HLA-DR4 and RF.

Pulmonary disease:
- Pleural disease (exudative effusions, pleuritis)[4]
- Interstitial lung disease (up to 10% clinically significant)[4]
- Bronchiolitis obliterans[4]
- Cryptogenic organizing pneumonia[4]
- Pulmonary nodules: A combination of RA and pneumoconiosis is called Caplan syndrome[4]

Neuromuscular:
- Entrapment neuropathy (carpal tunnel, tarsal tunnel, and cubital tunnel are most commonly involved)[4,8,9]
- Mononeuritis multiplex[4]
- Peripheral neuropathy[9]
- Cervical myelopathy and cord compression secondary to atlantoaxial subluxation[4]
- Pachymeningitis (rare)[10]
- Vasculitis[4]

Cardiac disease:
- Pericarditis (most common)[4]
- Myocarditis[11]
- Valvular nodules[11]
- There is an increased risk of cardiovascular disease compared to the general population, thought to be secondary to accelerated atherosclerosis from systemic inflammation[11]

Ocular disease:
- Keratoconjunctivitis sicca (dry eye, without dry mouth) (10%)[4]
- Episcleritis, scleritis, scleral thinning, scleromalacia perforans, ulcerative keratitis[4]
  Amyloidosis: Occurs in longstanding, poorly controlled RA. Usually presents as nephrotic syndrome. Organs affected include the heart, kidney, liver, spleen, intestines, and skin[4]
  Osteoporosis[12]

ETIOLOGY

The exact cause of RA remains unknown despite extensive research. It is likely that a combination of genetic, hormonal, and environmental factors leads to aberrant immune activation and inflammatory response in the joint. A common genetic background plays a role in susceptibility to disease, as twins and first-degree relatives of RA patients are at an increased risk of developing the disease compared to the general population.[13] Patients with HLA-DR4, DR1, and DR14 alleles have increased susceptibility to RA; in particular, one amino acid sequence in the DR β chain, known as the shared epitope, is overrepresented in these patients.[13] Other identified genetic associations include polymorphisms in *PTPN22*, *PADI4*, *CTLA4*, *TRAF1-C5*, *STAT4*, *TNFAIP3*.[13] Epigenetic factors are also likely to be involved.[13]

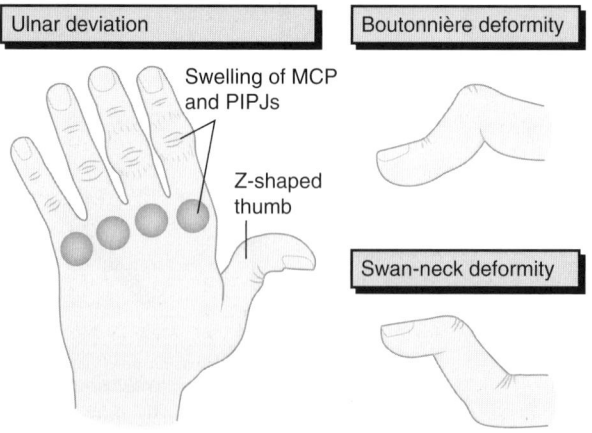

FIG. 4 Characteristic hand deformities in rheumatoid arthritis. *MCP,* Metacarpophalanges; *PIPJs,* proximal interphalangeal joints. (From Ballinger A: *Kumar & Clark's essentials of clinical medicine,* ed 6, Edinburgh, 2012, Saunders.)

Multiple environmental factors have also been implicated as possible etiologic factors, including cigarette smoking, silica exposure, and low socioeconomic class.[13] Infectious agents such as *P. gingivalis*, Epstein-Barr virus, and parvovirus B19 have also been reported as possible triggers.[13]

Stages of disease development presumably include:

- Initiation of the innate immune response through toll-like receptor (TLR) activation by a stimulating signal.[13] The preclinical stages of seropositive rheumatoid arthritis are characterized by disordered immunity, often associated with mucosal surfaces, including the oral cavity, lungs, and gastrointestinal tract, and by local and systemic generation of anti-citrullinated protein antibodies (ACPAs). These autoantibodies can be detected in the blood a median of 4.5 yr before the onset of arthritis.[13a]
- Perpetuation of inflammatory response through activation of the adaptive immune system. There is migration of inflammatory cells (autoreactive B and T cells, monocytes) into the joint space, activation of macrophage-like and fibroblast-like synoviocytes, and development of a "synovial pannus," a thickened synovial membrane.[14]
- The pannus releases proinflammatory cytokines (tumor necrosis factor alpha [TNF-α], interleukin [IL]-1, IL-6, IL-15, IL-17, IL-18) as well as proteases, which erode cartilage and bone.[14] Bone erosions are caused mainly by osteoclasts, which express the receptor activator of NF-κB (RANK).[13] TNF-α, IL-1, IL-6, and IL-17 promote the expression of RANK ligand (RANKL) on T cells and fibroblast-like synoviocytes, thus creating a positive feedback loop.[13] IL-6 and TNF-α act synergistically to increase vascular endothelial growth factor levels, which in turn stimulate angiogenesis, thereby maintaining pannus formation. B-cell differentiation is also promoted by IL-6, leading to the production of autoantibodies.[13]
- Many of the new "biologic" disease-modifying antirheumatic drugs (DMARDs) are engineered to target these cytokines (see "Treatment" section).[15]

DX DIAGNOSIS

The American College of Rheumatology (ACR) and the European League Against Rheumatism (EULAR) developed new classification criteria for RA in 2010 (Table 1). These are based on a point system where patients with score $\geq$6/10 are considered to have "definite RA." Four variables constitute the new criteria:

- The number and size of involved joints (0 to 5 points, with higher scores for a larger number of small joints affected)
- Levels of rheumatoid factor (RF) and anti-cyclic citrullinated peptide (CCP) antibody (0 to 3 points, with a higher score for a high-titer positive RF or anti-CCP)
- Elevated erythrocyte sedimentation rate (ESR) or C-reactive protein (CRP) (1 point)

TABLE 1 The 2010 American College of Rheumatology/European League Against Rheumatism Classification Criteria for Rheumatoid Arthritis[a]

Criteria	Score
Joint involvement	
2-10 large joints	1
1-3 small joints (with or without involvement of large joints)	2
4-10 small joints (with or without involvement of large joints)	3
>10 joints (with at least one small joint)	5
Serology (at least one test result is needed for classification)	
Negative RF and negative ACPA	0
Low-positive RF or low-positive ACPA	2
High-positive RF or high-positive ACPA	3
Acute-phase reactants	
Normal CRP and normal ESR	0
Abnormal CRP or abnormal ESR	1
Duration of symptoms	
<6 wk	0
$\geq$6 wk	1

A score of 6 or greater is needed for classification of a patient as having definite rheumatoid arthritis.

If incontrovertible radiographic evidence of rheumatoid arthritis exists, the diagnosis can be made even if the criteria provided are not fulfilled.

If a patient has previously fulfilled the criteria for rheumatoid arthritis, the diagnosis is maintained even if the criteria are not fulfilled on current reexamination.

ACPA, Anticitrullinated protein antibodies; *CRP*, C-reactive protein; *ESR*, erythrocyte sedimentation rate; *RF*, rheumatoid factor.

[a]Target population (patients who can be evaluated using these criteria): Those who have *at least one joint with definite clinical synovitis* (swelling), with the synovitis not better explained by another disease.

From Firestein GS et al: *Firestein & Kelley's textbook of rheumatology,* ed 11, Philadelphia, 2021, Elsevier.

- Symptom duration $\geq$6 wk (1 point)

DIFFERENTIAL DIAGNOSIS

- Infectious causes: Parvovirus B19, hepatitis B, hepatitis C, poststreptococcal reactive arthritis, acute rheumatic fever[4]
- Connective tissue diseases: Systemic lupus erythematosus, scleroderma, mixed connective tissue disease, Sjögren syndrome[4]
- Seronegative spondyloarthropathies[4]
- Calcium pyrophosphate deposition (CPPD or "pseudo-RA")[4]
- Polyarticular gout[4]
- Polymyalgia rheumatica[4]
- Remitting seronegative symmetric synovitis with pitting edema (RS3PE) can resemble seronegative RA in elderly patients[16]
- Hemochromatosis[17]
- Paraneoplastic syndromes
- Osteoarthritis, a degenerative arthritis that lacks prolonged morning stiffness and that usually lacks synovitis, should not be confused with RA (see Table 2)

LABORATORY TESTS

- RF (sensitivity ~60%; specificity ~80%). False positives are seen with hepatitis C, subacute bacterial endocarditis, primary biliary cirrhosis, sarcoidosis, malignancy, Sjögren syndrome, systemic lupus erythematosus (SLE), and increasing age.[4]
- Anti-CCP antibodies. Sensitivity is similar to RF, but it is more specific for RA than RF (up to 95% to 98%).[18]

- The presence of either RF or anti-CCP ("seropositive RA") is associated with more severe disease, more extraarticular manifestations, and worse prognosis.[18]
- Elevated ESR and/or CRP. These markers decline with treatment; thus they can be used to monitor disease activity along with physical examination and clinical presentation.[18]
- CBC with differential. RA may lead to anemia of chronic disease (through upregulation of the iron-regulating hormone, hepcidin) and thrombocytosis.[18]
- Hypoalbuminemia and hypergammaglobulinemia.
- Antinuclear antibody (ANA) is present in 20% to 30% of patients. However, complement will usually be normal or increased, in contrast to patients with systemic lupus erythematosus. Many patients will have secondary Sjögren syndrome (positive ANA with negative SSA and SSB).[18]
- Inflammatory synovial fluid with >2000 polymorphonuclear neutrophils (PMNs). Of note, patients with RA have an increased risk of developing septic arthritis.[19] Hence, synovial fluid with white blood cells >50,000 cells/mm³ is concerning for an infectious process and must always be ruled out.[19]

IMAGING STUDIES

Recommendations for the use of imaging in the clinical management of rheumatoid arthritis are summarized in Table 3.

Plain radiography (Table E4):

TABLE 2 Factors Useful for Differentiating Early Rheumatoid Arthritis From Osteoarthritis

	Rheumatoid Arthritis	Osteoarthritis
Age at onset	Across age spectrum, peak incidence in 50s	Increases with age
Predisposing factors	Susceptibility epitopes (HLA-DRB1*01, HLA-DRB1*04)	Trauma, overuse
	PTPN22, PADI4 polymorphisms; RF and ACPA positivity	Congenital abnormalities (e.g., shallow acetabulum)
	Smoking	
Early symptoms	Morning stiffness and gelling phenomenon, pain improves with activity	Pain increases through the day and with use
Joints involved	Proximal interphalangeal joints, metacarpophalangeal joints, wrists most often; distal interphalangeal joints almost never	Distal interphalangeal joints (Heberden's nodes), proximal interphalangeal joints (Bouchard's nodes), knees, lumbar spine
Physical findings	Soft tissue swelling, warmth	Bony osteophytes, minimal soft tissue swelling early
Radiographic findings	Periarticular osteopenia, marginal erosions, symmetric joint space narrowing in large joints	Subchondral sclerosis, osteophytes, asymmetric joint space loss in large joints
Laboratory findings	Increased C-reactive protein, positive RF, positive ACPA, anemia, thrombocytosis	Normal

ACPA, Anticitrullinated protein antibody; *HLA,* human leukocyte antigen; *RF,* rheumatoid factor.
From Firestein GS et al: *Firestein & Kelley's textbook of rheumatology,* ed 11, Philadelphia, 2021, Elsevier.

TABLE 3 EULAR Recommendations for the Use of Imaging in the Clinical Management of Rheumatoid Arthritis[a]

When there is diagnostic doubt, conventional radiography, ultrasonography, or MRI can be used to improve the certainty of a diagnosis of RA in addition to clinical criteria alone.[b]

The presence of inflammation seen with ultrasonography or MRI can be used to predict the progression to clinical RA from undifferentiated inflammatory arthritis.

Ultrasonography and MRI are superior to clinical examination in the detection of joint inflammation; these techniques should be considered for more accurate assessment of inflammation. Conventional radiography of the hands and feet should be used as the initial imaging technique to detect damage. However, ultrasonography and/or MRI should be considered if conventional radiographs do not show damage and may be used to detect damage at an earlier time point (especially in early-stage RA).

MRI bone edema is a strong independent predictor of subsequent radiographic progression in early RA, and should be considered as a prognostic indicator. Joint inflammation (synovitis) detected by MRI or ultrasonography as well as joint damage detected by conventional radiographs, MRI, or ultrasonography can also be considered for the prediction of further joint damage.

Inflammation seen on imaging may be more predictive of a therapeutic response than clinical features of disease activity; imaging may be used to predict response to treatment.

Given the superior detection of inflammation by MRI and ultrasonography versus clinical examination, they may be useful in monitoring disease activity.

The periodic evaluation of joint damage, usually by radiographs of the hands and feet, should be considered. MRI (and possibly ultrasonography) is more responsive to change in joint damage and can be used to monitor disease progression.

Monitoring of functional instability of the cervical spine by lateral radiography obtained in flexion and neutral positions should be performed in patients with clinical suspicion of cervical involvement. When radiography is positive or specific neurologic symptoms and signs are present, MRI should be performed.

MRI and ultrasonography can detect inflammation that predicts subsequent joint damage, even when clinical remission is present and can be used to assess persistent inflammation.

EULAR, European League Against Rheumatism; *MRI,* magnetic resonance imaging; *RA,* rheumatoid arthritis.
[a]Recommendations are based on data from imaging studies that have mainly focused on the hands (particularly wrists, metacarpophalangeal, and proximal interphalangeal joints). There are few data with specific guidance on which joints to image.[8]
[b]In patients with at least one joint with definite clinical synovitis, which is not better explained by another disease.
From Firestein GS et al: *Firestein & Kelley's textbook of rheumatology,* ed 11, Philadelphia, 2021, Elsevier.

- Early changes include soft tissue swelling, symmetric joint space narrowing, and periarticular osteopenia.
- Later changes include periarticular erosions and deformities. This reflects cartilage and bone destruction secondary to pannus formation (Fig. E6).
- Radiographs of hands and feet should be obtained at disease onset and repeated to monitor disease progression and to ensure that adequate treatment is achieved.

MRI and musculoskeletal US:
- More sensitive for detecting erosive disease and joint effusions/synovitis.

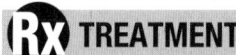 **TREATMENT**

- Early identification and treatment of RA with DMARDs is crucial.[20] More than half of patients have radiographic joint damage within 2 yr of disease onset, but early aggressive treatment with DMARDs and/or biologic agents is associated with decreased progression of synovitis and bone erosions, and with decreased disability.[21]
- There are several tools to measure disease activity (Table 5) and define remission in rheumatoid arthritis, including (but not limited to) the following: Clinical Disease Activity Index (CDAI), Simplified Disease Activity Index (SDAI), Disease Activity Score (DAS) 28, Routine Assessment of Patient Index Data 3 (RAPID3), Stanford Health Assessment Questionnaire (HAQ), and Patient Activity Scale (PAS).

ACUTE GENERAL Rx
- NSAIDs: Can be used initially to relieve pain and mild inflammation or used later in the disease course for additional control of mild pain.[4] NSAIDs are not disease modifying.
- Corticosteroids: Oral or intraarticular, frequently used initially to reduce inflammation rapidly until oral DMARD treatments take effect.[4] They may also be used during acute flares or in low doses for additional control of inflammation.[4] The use of corticosteroids at the lowest dose possible and shortest duration is recommended.[4] Corticosteroids have many side effects, including but not limited to weight gain, increased risk of diabetes, osteoporosis, cataract formation, peptic ulcer disease (especially when used in combination with NSAIDs), and avascular necrosis.

CHRONIC Rx
- DMARDs: Can be classified into "nonbiologic" and "biologic" treatments (Table 6).
  1. Nonbiologic DMARDs: Most commonly used agents are methotrexate (MTX), hydroxychloroquine (HCQ), sulfasalazine (SSZ), and leflunomide (LEF).[4] Most of these are associated with potential toxicity and

require close monitoring. They are also slow-acting drugs that generally require >8 wk to start taking effect.

2. MTX is the most commonly used DMARD worldwide for the treatment of RA.[4] It is effective as monotherapy in about 30% of patients with RA.

3. "Triple therapy"—MTX, HCQ, and SSZ—has been shown to be superior to MTX alone.[20]

- Biologic DMARDs: Newer biologically engineered therapies, which target cytokines and cells involved in the RA inflammatory response.[4] Major side effects include an increased risk of infections, with potential reactivation of tuberculosis.[4] A negative purified protein derivative (PPD) or interferon γ-release assay is a prerequisite to initiate therapy.[4] Biologic DMARDs are most effective when used in combination with a nonbiologic DMARD, usually MTX.[4]
- The five approved tumor necrosis factor α inhibitors (TNFI) include infliximab, etanercept, adalimumab, certolizumab pegol, and golimumab.[4]
- Abatacept (CTLA-4Ig) is a recombinant protein that prevents costimulatory binding of antigen presenting cell to T cell, preventing T-cell activation.[4]
- Tocilizumab (anti–IL-6) is a monoclonal antibody against the IL-6 receptor.[4]
- Sarilumab is another IL-6 inhibitor monoclonal antibody, approved by the FDA in 2017 for treatment of RA, and can be used as monotherapy or in combination with MTX or other conventional DMARDs.[22]
- Tofacitinib (JAK1/2/3 inhibitor) inhibits the JAK-STAT intracellular signaling pathway, thus preventing the production of inflammatory mediators.[13] The first oral biologic DMARD, it can be used as monotherapy or in combination with MTX. Baricitinib, an oral, once-daily Janus kinase (JAK1 and JAK2) inhibitor, was approved by the FDA in May 2018 for treatment of moderate to severe RA in patients who did not respond adequately to one or more TNFIs.[23] A dose of 2 mg was approved, with concerns that higher doses had increased adverse events. Upadacitinib (JAK1 > JAK2/3 inhibitor) was approved in 2019 at 15 mg once daily for moderate to severely active RA resistant or intolerant to MTX, or in combination with MTX with other nonbiologic DMARDs.[23]
- Rituximab (anti-CD20) is a monoclonal antibody against the CD20 antigen on B lymphocytes.[4]
- Biosimilars are beginning to be available.[24] These molecules are highly similar, but not identical, to the original drugs. Legal disputes have delayed the widespread adoption of these drugs in the U.S., but they are likely to be of increasing prevalence in the future.

- Treatment recommendations in RA patient with high-risk comorbidities:
  1. TNFI should be avoided in patients with congestive heart failure, as it can worsen the condition.[25]
  2. In patients with hepatitis B, immunosuppressive therapy can be safely prescribed along with concomitant antiviral therapy.[4]
  3. Treatment of hepatitis C patients with RA should be done following standard guidelines in collaboration with gastroenterology/hepatology.[4] Immunosuppressive therapy can be used safely in conjunction with antiviral therapy; avoidance of DMARDs such as MTX and LEF should be taken into consideration.[15]
  4. In patients with a history of skin cancer, DMARDs are recommended over the use of biologics.[26] For patients with previously treated lymphoproliferative disorders, use of rituximab should be considered first, as well as combination DMARDs and non-TNF biologics.[27] One should avoid TNFI, as there is an increased risk of lymphoma with these agents. Recommendations for treatment of patients with previously treated solid organ malignancy are the same as for patients without the condition.

Rx in pregnancy:[28]

- Patients with active rheumatoid arthritis should be tested for anti-Ro/SSA and anti-La/SSB antibodies once before or early in pregnancy, due to their associated increased in risk for neonatal lupus and congenital heart block.[29]
- Fluorinated glucocorticoids (e.g., betamethasone and dexamethasone) cross the placenta at higher concentrations without significant metabolism and can hasten lung maturity. These should not be used routinely for the management of active RA during pregnancy.[30] Glucocorticoids (e.g., prednisone, prednisolone, and methylprednisolone) should be maintained at the lowest dose possible.[31]
- Hydroxychloroquine (HCQ) has been shown to cross the placenta. However, most studies have not described fetal toxicity with HCQ doses used for the treatment of rheumatic diseases.[32]
- Methotrexate (MTX) should be stopped 1 to 3 mo before conception because of its teratogenic risks. If conception occurs while a woman is taking MTX, the medication should be stopped immediately and folic acid 5 mg/day taken for the remainder of the pregnancy.[33]
- Leflunomide (LEF) should be avoided in pregnancy due to its teratogenic effects. Conception should be delayed until LEF is undetectable in the serum (<0.02 mg/L), typically 2 yr after discontinuation. An enhanced drug elimination procedure using

cholestyramine can be used for faster results.[32]

- TNF-α inhibitors, DMARDs, and other biologics can be continued throughout pregnancy. Most professional societies recommend discontinuing these medications in the third trimester. Noteworthy exception is certolizumab. It is pegylated and does not cross the placenta in significant amounts and can be continued throughout the pregnancy.[34]

Immunization, cardiovascular disease prevention (smoking cessation, blood pressure control, cholesterol control), and osteoporosis prevention (with calcium and vitamin D supplementation and bisphosphonate therapy) should be addressed in all RA patients.

DISPOSITION

- Remissions and exacerbations are common, but condition is chronically progressive in the majority of cases.
- Joint degeneration and deformity often lead to disability. Joint replacement is indicated for patients with severe joint damage whose symptoms are poorly controlled by medical management. The ACR published guidelines in 2017 concerning the perioperative management of antirheumatic medications in patients undergoing elective total hip or total knee arthroplasty.[35]
- Early and aggressive diagnosis and treatment are crucial in preventing or slowing joint destruction.
- Factors associated with poorer prognosis in rheumatoid arthritis are summarized in Table 7.

REFERRAL

- Early referral to rheumatologist
- Orthopedic consultation for corrective surgery

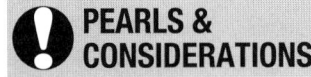

PEARLS & CONSIDERATIONS

RA sometimes develops acutely in the postpartum patient; conversely, as high as 75% of pregnant RA patients will experience remission during pregnancy.

REFERENCES
Available at eBooks.Health.Elsevier.com

RELATED CONTENT
Rheumatoid Arthritis (Patient Information)

AUTHORS: **KENNY CHANG, BS,** and **MANUEL F. DASILVA, MD**

TABLE 5 Instruments Used to Measure Rheumatoid Arthritis Disease Activity

			THRESHOLDS OF DISEASE ACTIVITY		
Instrument	Score Range	Remission	Low	Moderate	High
Disease Activity Score in 28 joints (DAS28)	0-9.4	≤2.6	≤3.2	>3.2 and ≤5.1	>5.1
Simplified Disease Activity Index (SDAI)	0.1-86.0	≤3.3	≤11	>11 and ≤26	>26
Clinical Disease Activity Index (CDAI)	0-76.0	≤2.8	≤10	>10 and ≤22	>22
Rheumatoid Arthritis Disease Activity Index (RADAI)	0-10	≤1.4	<2.2	2.2 and <4.9	>4.9
Patient Activity Scale (PAS or PASII)	0-10	≤1.25	<1.9	≥1.9 and ≤5.3	>5.3
Routine Assessment Patient Index Data (RAPID)	0-30	≤1	<6	≥6 and ≤12	>12

From Firestein GS et al: *Firestein & Kelley's textbook of rheumatology*, ed 11, Philadelphia, 2021, Elsevier.

TABLE 6 Disease-Modifying Drugs and Biologics for Rheumatoid Arthritis

Drugs	Usual Dose	Side Effects and Cautions
DMARDs		
Methotrexate	7.5-25 mg/wk in a single dose orally or SQ. Start low and increase by 5 mg every 1-2 mo until desired effects are achieved	Myelosuppression, hepatotoxicity, hepatic fibrosis, cirrhosis, pulmonary infiltrates or fibrosis, mouth sores (daily folic acid can prevent this), nausea, hair loss
Sulfasalazine (Azulfidine, Azulfidine EC)	500-3000 mg/day in 2-4 divided doses orally	Myelosuppression, hepatotoxicity, nausea
Hydroxychloroquine sulfate (Plaquenil)	200-400 mg per day in 2 divided doses orally Not to exceed 6.5 mg/kg of actual body weight	Retinal toxicity, rash
Leflunomide (Arava)	10-20 mg per day in a single dose orally	Myelosuppression, hepatotoxicity, cirrhosis, diarrhea, hair loss
Azathioprine (Imuran)	50-150 mg per day in 1-3 divided doses orally	Myelosuppression, hepatotoxicity, lymphoproliferative disorders, nausea, hair loss; check TPMT before initiation
BIOLOGICS		Must check T-SPOT and hepatitis B and C serology before starting all biologics; discuss updating vaccinations before initiation
TNF blockers: Adalimumab (Humira) Etanercept (Enbrel) Infliximab (Remicade) Golimumab (Simponi) Certolizumab (Cimzia)	40 mg SQ once a wk or every 2 wk 25 mg SQ twice a wk, or 50 mg SQ once a wk 3-10 mg/kg IV. Given at 0, 2, 6 wk then every 8 wk (usually taken with methotrexate) 50 mg SQ once a mo 400 mg SQ loading at 0, 2, 4 then 200 mg every 2 wk vs. 400 mg q 4 wk	Increased risk of infections, tuberculosis, histoplasmosis, or others Injection site or infusion reaction Congestive heart failure
T-cell costimulation blocker: Abatacept (Orencia)	500-1000 mg IV 0, 2, 4 wk then every 4 wk or 500-1000 mg IV one time, then 125 mg SQ weekly	Increased risk of infections; injection site or infusion reaction; COPD exacerbation
IL-6 blocker: Tocilizumab (Actemra)	4-8 mg/kg IV every 4 wk; 162 mg SQ once every other wk or every wk	Increased risk of infections; myelosuppression; hepatotoxicity; hyperlipidemia
B-cell depletion: Rituximab	1000 mg IV 0, 2 wk and again when arthritis becomes active; on average every 6 mo	Increased risk of infection; progressive multifocal leukoencephalopathy (PML); tumor lysis syndrome
IL-1 blocker: Anakinra	100 mg SQ daily, 100 mg SQ every other day in severe kidney disease	Increased risk of infections; injection site reaction

COPD, Chronic obstructive pulmonary disease; *DMARDs*, disease-modifying antirheumatic drugs; *IL*, interleukin; *SQ*, subcutaneously; *TNF*, tumor necrosis factor; *TPMT*, thiopurine S-methyltransferase.
From Warshaw G et al: *Ham's primary care geriatrics*, ed 7, Philadelphia, 2022, Elsevier.

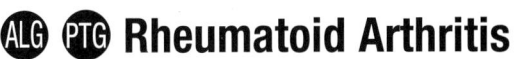

TABLE 7   Factors Associated With Poorer Prognosis in Rheumatoid Arthritis

Presence of rheumatoid factor and titer
Presence of antibodies to CCP and titer
Presence of shared epitope and number of alleles
Presence of erosive disease at presentation
Disease activity at presentation
Magnitude of ESR or CRP elevations
Presence of nodules or extraarticular features
Female sex
Smoking currently and in the past
Obesity

CCP, Cyclic citrullinated peptide; *CRP,* C-reactive protein; *ESR,* erythrocyte sedimentation rate.
From Firestein GS et al: *Firestein & Kelley's textbook of rheumatology,* ed 11, Philadelphia, 2021, Elsevier.

R

Diseases
and Disorders

I

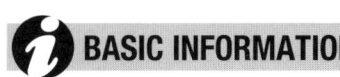

ⓘ BASIC INFORMATION

DEFINITION

Rosacea is a common, chronic, heterogenous, inflammatory skin disease, seen most often in adults of both genders and all skin types. It predominantly involves the central face and is characterized by intermittent flares that present with transient findings (flushing, papules/pustules) and by persistence of some fixed clinical manifestations (telangiectasias, persistent facial erythema).

SYNONYM

Acne rosacea

ICD-10CM CODES
L71	Rosacea
L71.9	Rosacea unspecified
L71.1	Rhinophyma
L71.8	Other rosacea
L71.0	Perioral dermatitis

EPIDEMIOLOGY & DEMOGRAPHICS

- Rosacea occurs in 1 in 20 Americans
- Onset often between ages 30 and 50 yr
- More common in people of Celtic origin; however, this disease may be overlooked in nonwhites because skin pigmentation results in atypical presentation
- Female:male ratio of 3:1

PHYSICAL FINDINGS & CLINICAL PRESENTATION

- Facial erythema, presence of papules, pustules, and telangiectasia (Fig. E1).
- Excessive facial warmth and redness are the predominant presenting symptoms.
- Itching is generally absent.
- Comedones are absent (unlike acne).
- Women are more likely to show symptoms on the chin and cheeks, whereas in men the nose is commonly involved.
- Ocular findings (mild dryness and irritation with blepharitis, conjunctival injection, burning, stinging, tearing, eyelid inflammation, swelling, and redness) are present in 50% of patients.

Rosacea can be classified into four major subtypes (Table E1):
- Erythematotelangiectatic (vascular): Erythema in central part of face, telangiectasia, flushing
- Papulopustular (inflammatory): Presence of dome-shaped erythematous papules and small pustules, in addition to facial erythema, flushing, and telangiectasia
- Phymatosis/glandular rosacea (Fig. E2): Presence of thickened skin with prominent pores that may affect the nose (rhinophyma) (Fig. E3), chin (gnathophyma), forehead (metophyma), eyelids (blepharophyma), and ears (otophyma)
- Ocular: Conjunctival injection, sensation of foreign body in the eye, telangiectasia and erythema of lid margins, scaling

ETIOLOGY

- The pathophysiology of rosacea is incompletely understood but believed to involve the vasculature.
- Hot drinks, alcohol, and sun exposure may accentuate the erythema by causing vasodilation of the skin.
- Flare-ups may also result from reactions to medications (e.g., simvastatin, ACE inhibitors, vasodilators, fluorinated corticosteroids), stress, extreme heat or cold, wind, humidity, strenuous exercise, spicy drinks, menstruation.

Ⓓ DIAGNOSIS

The presence of at least one of the following primary features in a central distribution of the face is generally sufficient to diagnose rosacea: Papules and pustules, telangiectasia, flushing (transient erythema), nontransient erythema.

DIFFERENTIAL DIAGNOSIS

- Drug eruption
- Acne vulgaris (Box 1)
- Contact dermatitis
- Systemic lupus erythematosus
- Carcinoid flush
- Idiopathic facial flushing
- Seborrheic dermatitis
- Facial sarcoidosis
- Photodermatitis
- Mastocytosis
- Perioral dermatitis (Box 1)
- Granulomas of the skin

WORKUP

Diagnosis is based on clinical findings. Distinguishing features between acne and rosacea are the presence of telangiectasia and deep diffuse erythema and absence of comedones in rosacea.

Ⓡ TREATMENT

NONPHARMACOLOGIC THERAPY

- Instruct patients to keep a diary to identify stimuli and triggers that exacerbate rosacea (e.g., spicy foods, drugs, cosmetics) and avoid identified triggers.
- Avoid alcohol, excessive sun exposure, and hot drinks of any type.
- Use of mild, nondrying soap or soap-free cleansers and nonoily moisturizers is recommended; local skin irritants should be avoided. General recommendations for skin care in patients with rosacea are summarized in Table 2.
- Sunscreens are an important component of therapy and should be applied each morning.
- Daily circular massage for several minutes of the central portion of the face is helpful in decreasing lymphedema and inflammation in this area.
- Reassure patient that rosacea is completely unrelated to poor hygiene.

- Vascular laser surgery is effective for telangiectasia.
- Surgical options are available for telangiectasia and rhinophyma and include dermabrasion, laser ablation, heated scalpel, electrocautery, and radiofrequency electrosurgery.

GENERAL Rx

- Several classes of drugs are used in treatment of rosacea, including the metronidazole family, the tetracycline family, ivermectin cream, and azelaic acid.
- Vascular rosacea: Topical therapy with metronidazole aqueous gel is effective as initial therapy for mild cases. Clindamycin lotion (Cleocin), sulfacetamide, or erythromycin 2% solution may also be effective. A 1.5% topical foam formulation of minocycline is also available for treatment of inflammatory lesions of rosacea in adults. Cost is a limiting factor. Brimonidine is a selective alpha$_2$-adrenergic receptor agonist FDA-approved as a gel preparation for topical treatment of adults with persistent facial erythema of rosacea. Oxymetazoline 1% cream is also an FDA-approved selecting alpha1a-adrenergic receptor agonist for topical treatment of persistent facial erythema in adults. Neither brimonidine or oxymetazoline are indicated for the treatment of inflammatory lesions of rosacea.
- Pustular and ocular rosacea: Systemic antibiotics (doxycycline 100 mg daily or tetracycline 250 mg qid until symptoms diminish, then taper off). Minocycline 50 to 100 mg is useful daily in resistant cases. Oral metronidazole (200 mg daily to bid) for 4 to 6 wk is also effective. A 1% cream formulation of the antiparasitic drug ivermectin is effective for papulopustular rosacea with minimal adverse effects. After 3 mo of therapy, it will produce clearing of rosacea lesions in up to 80% of patients with moderate to severe symptoms. Its mechanism of action is unknown, but it may be due to the combination of its antiinflammatory effects and its antiparasitic effects on the *Demodex* mite, which may contribute to the symptoms of rosacea.
- Isotretinoin 0.5 to 1 mg/kg/day in two divided doses for 15 to 20 wk can be used for refractory papular and pustular rosacea; use of retinoids may, however, worsen erythema and telangiectasis.
- Erythema and flushing may respond to low-dose clonidine (0.05 mg bid).
- Treatment of phymatous rosacea: Oral tetracyclines, oral isotretinoin, ablative/pulsed dye laser therapy, electrosurgery.
- Treatment of ocular rosacea: Topical or oral tetracyclines, artificial tears, and/or lid cleansing for eyelid hygiene. Medical and surgical therapies for rosacea are summarized in Table E3.
- A 5% benzoyl peroxide cream (epsolay) has been FDA approved for treatment of inflammatory lesions of rosacea in adults. Cost and formulary are major barriers to its use, less

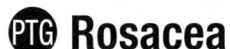

BOX 1 Differentiation of Acne Vulgaris, Periorificial Dermatitis, and Rosacea

Acne vulgaris
- Commences at puberty
- Comedones, pustules, cysts
- Affects face and trunk
- Can be a sign of androgen excess in females; side-effect of steroid use, including corticosteroids

Periorificial dermatitis
- More common 14 yr old to 45 yr old (can occur at any age)
- Female preponderance
- Background erythema with studded erythematous papules and pseudopustules (no comedones)
- Affects one or more of the mouth, nose, and eyelids
- Spares the vermillion border
- No systemic associations
- May have a family history
- Unknown initial trigger but made worse by topical corticosteroids and topical calcineurin inhibitors

Rosacea
- Generally occurs in middle age
- Caucasian skin predominantly
- Female preponderance
- Papules, telangiectasia, pustules (no comedones)
- Centrofacial, often with rhinophyma, and blepharitis
- No systemic disease associations
- Facial flushing, especially with alcohol use

From Talley NJ et al: *Essentials of internal medicine*, ed 4, Chatswood, NSW, 2021, Elsevier Australia.

TABLE 2 General Recommendations for Facial Skin Care and Education in Patients With Rosacea

Facial Skin Care
- Wash with lukewarm water and use soap-free cleansers that are pH balanced.
- Cleansers are applied gently with fingertips.
- Use sunscreens with both UVA and UVB protection and an SPF $\geq$30.
- Sunscreens containing the inorganic filters titanium dioxide and/or zinc oxide are usually well tolerated.
- Use cosmetics and sunscreens that contain protective silicones.
- Water-soluble facial powder containing inert green pigment helps to neutralize the perception of erythema.
- Moisturizers containing humectants (e.g., glycerin) and occlusives (e.g., petrolatum) help to repair the epidermal barrier.
- Avoid astringents, toners, and abrasive exfoliators.
- Avoid cosmetics that contain alcohol, menthols, camphor, witch hazel, fragrance, peppermint, and eucalyptus oil.
- Avoid waterproof cosmetics and heavy foundations that are difficult to remove without irritating solvents or physical scrubbing.
- Avoid procedures such as glycolic peels or dermabrasion.

Patient Education
- Reassure the patient about the benign nature of the disorder and the rarity of rhinophyma, particularly in women.
- Emphasize the chronicity of the disease and the likelihood of exacerbations.
- Direct patients to information websites such as those of the National Rosacea Society (http://www.rosacea.org/) or the American Academy of Dermatology (http://www.aad.org/).
- Advise to avoid recognized triggers.
- Explain the importance of compliance with topical regimens.
- Educate on the importance of sun avoidance.

SPF, Sun protective factor; *UVA,* ultraviolet A; *UVB,* ultraviolet B.
Adapted from Del Rosso JQ, Baum EW: Comprehensive medical management of rosacea: an interim study report and literature review, *J Clin Aesthet Dermatol* 1:20-25, 2008; Powell FC: Rosacea, *N Engl J Med* 352:793-803, 2005; and Pelle MT et al: Rosacea: II. Therapy, *J Am Acad Dermatol* 51:499-512, 2004. In Bolognia J: *Dermatology*, ed 4, Philadelphia, 2018, Elsevier.

expensive generic medications (metronidazole, azelaic acid) are preferred for initial treatment.

DISPOSITION
- Rosacea is often resistant to initial treatment and recurrent. Periods of remission and relapse are common.
- The progression of rosacea is variable. Typical stages include:
  1. Facial flushing
  2. Erythema and/or edema and ocular symptoms
  3. Papules and pustules
  4. Rhinophyma

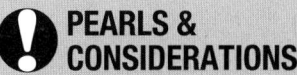 **PEARLS & CONSIDERATIONS**

COMMENTS
- The course of the disease is typically chronic, with remissions and relapses.
- Patients with resistant cases may have *Demodex folliculorum* mite infestation or tinea infection (diagnosis can be confirmed with potassium hydroxide examination); the role of *D. folliculorum* in rosacea is unclear. These mites can sometimes be found in large numbers in the lesions; however, their numbers do not generally decline with treatment.
- Rosacea can result in emotional and social stigmas, especially because many people associate rosacea and rhinophyma with alcohol abuse.
- Early consultation with an ophthalmologist is recommended in patients with suspected ocular involvement.

SUGGESTED READINGS
Available at eBooks.Health.Elsevier.com.

RELATED CONTENT
Rosacea (Patient Information)

AUTHOR: **FRED F. FERRI, MD**

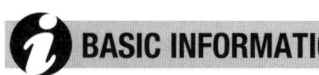
BASIC INFORMATION

DEFINITION

Salmonellosis is an infection caused by one of several serotypes of a gram-negative bacillus of the genus *Salmonella*. Salmonella infection can be typhoidal (serotype Typhi or Paratyphi) or nontyphoidal. Current *Salmonella* nomenclature is described in Box 1.

SYNONYMS

Typhoid fever
Paratyphoid fever
Enteric fever

ICD-10CM CODES
A02.0 *Salmonella* enteritis
A02.1 *Salmonella* sepsis
A02.2 Localized *Salmonella* infections
A02.8 Other specified *Salmonella* infections
A0.9   *Salmonella* infection, unspecified

EPIDEMIOLOGY & DEMOGRAPHICS

INCIDENCE (IN U.S.):
- Epidemiologically, the clinical syndromes are divided into those that cause a typhoidal type of infection (systemic illness with fever and abdominal pain) such as *Salmonella typhi* and those that do not: Nontyphoidal *Salmonella* infections (gastroenteritis) such as *S. enteritidis*, *S. newport*, and *S. typhimurium*.
- Estimated 1 million cases/yr of nontyphoidal salmonellosis in the United States (leading cause of foodborne illness in the U.S.). In 2017 an outbreak occurred linked to live poultry in backyard flocks with over 960 cases in 48 states caused by several different *Salmonella* bacteria. In 2020 an outbreak associated with onions occurred in the U.S.
- Largest outbreak of gastroenteritis syndrome (nontyphoidal): 200,000 who ingested contaminated milk.
- Approximately 500 cases of *Salmonella typhi* infection are reported each year, of which nearly 80% is associated with foreign travel.

PREDOMINANT AGE:
- <20 yr old.
- >70 yr old.
- Highest rates of infection in infants, especially neonates.

PEAK INCIDENCE: Summer and fall.
GENETICS: Neonatal infection.
- Highly susceptible to infection with non-typhoidal *Salmonella*.

PHYSICAL FINDINGS & CLINICAL PRESENTATION (TABLE 1)

- Infections:
  1. Localized to GI tract (gastroenteritis)
  2. Systemic (typhoid fever)
  3. Localized outside of GI tract
- Gastroenteritis:
  1. Incubation period: 12 to 48 h
  2. Nausea, vomiting
  3. Diarrhea, abdominal cramps
  4. Fever

5. Bacteremia: Occurs mostly in the immu-nocompromised host or those with under-lying conditions, including HIV infection
6. Self-limited illness lasting 3 or 4 days
7. Colonization of GI tract persistent for months, especially in those treated with antibiotics
- Typhoid fever:
  1. Incubation period of few days to several wk
  2. Prolonged fever, often with a stepwise-increasing temperature pattern
  3. Myalgias
  4. Headache, cough, sore throat
  5. Malaise, anorexia
  6. Abdominal pain
  7. Hepatosplenomegaly
  8. Diarrhea or constipation early in the course of illness
  9. Rose spots (faint, maculopapular, blanch-ing lesions) sometimes seen on chest or abdomen
- Untreated disease:
  1. Fever lasting 1 to 2 mo
  2. Main complication: GI bleeding caused by perforation from ulceration of Peyer patches in the ileum
  3. Rare complications:
     a. Mental status changes
     b. Shock
  4. Relapse rate of approximately 10%
- Infections outside GI tract:
  1. Can occur in virtually any location
  2. Usually occur in patients with underlying diseases
  3. Endocarditis, endovascular infections are caused by seeding of atherosclerotic pla-ques or aneurysms

---

BOX 1 Nomenclature of *Salmonella* Infections

The multiple microbiologic, serologic, and clinical designations applied to *Salmonella* infections are confusing.[1] Most pathogenic *Salmonella* belong to a single subspecies designated *Salmonella enterica* subspecies enterica. In addition to this species designation, *Salmonella* are classified serologically. The serogroup is assigned based on the O antigen alone, whereas the serotype designation, from which the name is derived, is based on both the O and H antigens.

Salmonella enterica subsp. enterica includes over 1400 serotypes. Although the full name of the cause of typhoid fever is *Salmonella enterica* subsp. enterica serotype Typhi, it is normally shortened to *S.* Typhi. Although serogroup designation is performed routinely in many laboratories, the test lacks clinical utility. Complete serotype identification is often performed in a reference laboratory; however, *S.* Typhi and Paratyphi A can also be identified by biochemical tests in a routine microbiology laboratory. Identification of *S.* Typhi and Paratyphi A are reviewed in detail in the World Health Organization's "The Diagnosis, Treatment and Prevention of Typhoid Fever."[2]

Clinically *Salmonella* are classified as typhoidal or nontyphoidal. The typhoidal serotypes are *S.* Typhi and Paratyphi A, B, and C. All others are classified as nontyphoidal. However, this is also misleading, as many nontyphoidal strains also cause invasive infection, which may mimic typhoid fever.

Examples of Clinical and Serologic Classification of Pathogenic *Salmonella*

Clinical Classification	Serotype	Formal Designation	Serogroup
Typhoidal	Typhi	*S. enterica* subsp. enterica ser. Typhi	D
	Paratyphi A	*S. enterica* subsp. enterica ser. Paratyphi A	A
	Paratyphi B (schottmuelleri)	*S. enterica* subsp. enterica ser. Paratyphi B	B
	Paratyphi C (hirschfeldii)	*S. enterica* subsp. enterica ser. Paratyphi C	C
Nontyphoidal	Typhimurium	*S. enterica* subsp. enterica ser. Typhimurium	B
	Enteritidis	*S. enterica* subsp. enterica ser. Enteritidis	D
	Newport	*S. enterica* subsp. enterica ser. Newport	C

[1]Brenner FW et al: Salmonella nomenclature, *J Clin Microbiol* 38:2465-2467, 2000.
[2]World Health Organization: *Background document: the diagnosis, treatment and prevention of typhoid fever*, Geneva, 2003, WHO.
From Ryan ET et al: *Hunter's tropical medicine and emerging infectious diseases*, ed 10, Philadelphia, 2019, Elsevier.

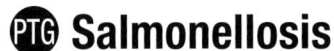
TABLE 1 Clinical Features of Typhoid and Paratyphoid Fever

	Clinical Feature	Approx. Frequency*
Flulike symptoms	Fever	>95%
	Headache	80%
	Chills	40%
	Cough	30%
	Myalgia	20%
	Arthralgia	<5%
Abdominal symptoms	Anorexia	50%
	Abdominal pain	30%
	Diarrhea	20%
	Constipation	20%
Physical findings	Coated tongue	50%
	Hepatomegaly	10%
	Splenomegaly	10%
	Abdominal tenderness	5%
	Rash	<5%
	Generalized adenopathy	<5%

* The proportion of patients demonstrating these clinical features of enteric fever varies depending on the time, region, and type of clinical population (hospitalized or ambulatory) assessed. Estimates are drawn from case series in an endemic area presenting for ambulatory or inpatient care.
From Ryan ET et al: *Hunter's tropical medicine and emerging infectious diseases*, ed 10, Philadelphia, 2019, Elsevier.

TABLE 2 Complications of Typhoid and Paratyphoid Fever

System	Complication	Notes
Gastrointestinal	Hemorrhage	10%-15% hospitalized patients
	Perforation	3% hospitalized patients
Hepatobiliary	Jaundice	1%-3% hospitalized patients
	Hepatitis	Usually subclinical (↑ ALT/AST)
	Acute cholecystitis	Rare, gallbladder may perforate
Neurologic	Mild encephalopathy	Confusion or apathy common
	Severe encephalopathy	Delirium, stupor, or coma
	Seizures	Common in children ≤5 yr
	Meningitis	Rare, primarily infants
	Guillain-Barré syndrome	Reported
Respiratory	Bronchitis	Cough is common
	Pneumonia	May be other concomitant bacterial infection (e.g., *S. pneumoniae*)
Cardiovascular	Myocarditis	Usually subclinical (ECG changes)
	Shock	Uncommon
Hematologic	Anemia	Usually subclinical
	DIC	Usually subclinical (↑ PT/PTT)
Other	Pyogenic infections	Uncommon
	Hemolytic uremic syndrome	Reported
	Miscarriage	Reported

ALT, Alanine aminotransferase; *AST*, aspartate aminotransferase; *DIC*, disseminated intravascular coagulation; *ECG*, echocardiogram; *PT*, prothrombin time; *PTT*, partial thromboplastin time.
From Ryan ET et al: *Hunter's tropical medicine and emerging infectious diseases*, ed 10, Philadelphia, 2019, Elsevier.

4. Hepatic or splenic abscesses in patients with underlying disease in these organs
5. Urinary tract infections in patients with renal tuberculosis (TB) or schistosomiasis
6. *Salmonellae* are a frequent cause of gram-negative meningitis in neonates
7. Osteomyelitis in children with hemoglobinopathies (particularly sickle cell disease)
8. Complications of typhoid and paratyphoid fever are summarized in Table 2

TABLE 3 Host Factors and Conditions Predisposing to the Development of Systemic Disease With Nontyphoidal *Salmonella* Strains

Neonates and young infants (≤3 mo of age)
HIV/AIDS
Other immunodeficiencies and chronic granulomatous disease
Immunosuppressive and corticosteroid therapies
Malignancies, especially leukemia and lymphoma
Hemolytic anemia, including sickle cell disease, malaria, and bartonellosis
Collagen vascular disease
Inflammatory bowel disease
Achlorhydria or use of antacid medications
Impaired intestinal motility
Schistosomiasis, malaria
Malnutrition

AIDS, Acquired immunodeficiency syndrome; *HIV*, human immunodeficiency virus.
From Kliegman RM et al: *Nelson textbook of pediatrics*, ed 19, Philadelphia, 2011, Saunders.

ETIOLOGY

- More than 2000 serotypes of *Salmonella* exist, but only a few cause disease in humans. Host factors and conditions predisposing to the development of systemic disease with nontyphoidal *Salmonella* strains are described in Table 3 and Table 4.
- Raw produce is an increasingly recognized vehicle for salmonellosis. In 2008 there was a large outbreak due to contaminated jalapeno and Serrano peppers with *Salmonella Saintpaul* involving 1500 persons, of whom 21% were hospitalized and two died. In 2009 there was an outbreak associated with contaminated peanut butter and peanuts. In 2017 there was an outbreak associated with papaya.
- Some found only in humans are the cause of enteric fever:
  1. *S. typhi*
  2. *S. paratyphi*
- Some responsible for gastroenteritis and frequently isolated from raw meat and poultry and uncooked or undercooked eggs:
  1. *S. typhimurium*
  2. *S. enteritidis*
- *S. choleraesuis* is a prototype organism that causes extraintestinal nontyphoidal disease.
- Transmission generally via ingestion of contaminated food or drink.
- Outbreaks of gastroenteritis related to contaminated poultry, meat, and dairy products are common.
- Typhoid fever is a systemic illness caused by serotypes exclusive to humans:
  1. Acquisition by ingestion of food or water contaminated by other humans.
  2. Most cases in the United States are:
     a. Acquired during foreign travel: 80% of cases.
     b. Acquired by ingestion of food prepared by chronic carriers, many of whom have acquired the organism outside of the United States.

Diseases and Disorders

TABLE 4 Susceptibility to *Salmonella* spp. Infection

Patient Group at Risk	Mechanism
Newborn	Achlorhydria, rapid gastric emptying
	Poorly developed cell-mediated immunity
	Complement deficiency
	Immunoglobulin deficiency in premature infants
Sickle-cell anemia	Reticuloendothelial system overload owing to hemolysis
	Functional asplenia
	Tissue infarcts
	Defective opsonization
Neutropenia (congenital or acquired)	Polymorphonuclear neutrophils needed for killing
Chronic granulomatous disease	Defective killing by polymorphonuclear neutrophils
Defects of immune system interleukin (IL)-12/interferon-γ axis	Defective signaling resulting in failure to activate macrophages and recurrent/persistent infection by nontyphoid *Salmonella*
Acquired immunodeficiency syndrome	Low CD4
	Effects of malnutrition on cell-mediated immunity
	Survival of organisms in macrophages (owing to *Salmonella* genes *PhoP/PhoQ, spvA-D, R*)
Organ transplantation, immunosuppression	Defective cell-mediated immunity
Gastrectomy	Loss of stomach acid barrier
Malaria	Reticuloendothelial overload during hemolysis
	Abnormal complement levels
	Abnormal macrophage function
Bartonellosis (verruga peruana)	Reticuloendothelial overload during hemolysis
Schistosomiasis	*Salmonella* sequestered in schistosomes protected from host defenses and antibiotics

From Cherry JD et al: *Feigin and Cherry's textbook of pediatric infectious diseases*, ed 8, Philadelphia, 2019, Elsevier.

TABLE 5 Treatment of Salmonella Gastroenteritis in Children

Organism and Indication	Dose and Duration of Treatment
Salmonella infections in infants <3 mo of age or immunocompromised persons (in addition to appropriate treatment for underlying disorder)	Cefotaxime 100-200 mg/kg/day every 6 hr for 5-14 days *or* Ceftriaxone 75 mg/kg/day once daily for 7 days *or* Ampicillin 100 mg/kg/day every 6 hr for 7 days *or* Cefixime 15 mg/kg/day for 7-10 days

From Kliegman RM et al: *Nelson textbook of pediatrics*, ed 19, Philadelphia, 2011, Saunders.

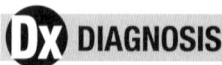 **DIAGNOSIS**

DIFFERENTIAL DIAGNOSIS

- Other causes of prolonged fever:
  1. Malaria
  2. TB
  3. Brucellosis
  4. Amebic liver abscess
- Other causes of gastroenteritis:
  1. Bacterial: *Shigella, Yersinia, Campylobacter* spp.
  2. Viral: Norwalk virus, rotavirus
  3. Parasitic: *Entamoeba histolytica, Giardia lamblia*
  4. Toxic: *Enterotoxigenic E. coli, Clostridium difficile*

WORKUP

- Typhoid fever:
  1. Cultures of blood, stool, urine; repeat if initially negative.
  2. Blood cultures are more likely to be positive early in the course of illness.
  3. Stool and urine cultures are more commonly positive in the second and third wk of illness.
  4. Highest yield with bone marrow biopsy cultures: 90% positive.
  5. Serology using Widal test is helpful in retrospect, showing a fourfold increase in convalescent titers.

- Gastroenteritis: Stool cultures and/or newer polymerase chain reaction (PCR) gastrointestinal panels
- Extraintestinal localized infection:
  1. Blood cultures.
  2. Cultures from the site of infection.

LABORATORY TESTS

- Neutropenia is common.
- Transaminitis is possible.
- Culture to grow organism: Blood, body fluids, biopsy specimens.

IMAGING STUDIES

- Not routinely indicated.
- Radiographs of bone may be suggestive of osteomyelitis (particularly in patients with sickle cell disease and bone infarctions).
- Computed tomography (CT) scan or sonogram of abdomen:
  1. May reveal hepatic or splenic abscesses or pleural involvement
  2. May reveal aortic aneurysm

TREATMENT

NONPHARMACOLOGIC THERAPY

Adequate hydration and electrolyte replacement in people with diarrhea.

ACUTE GENERAL Rx

Treatment decisions must consider the severity of infection and the risk for extraintestinal disease.

- Typhoid fever:
  1. Levofloxacin 750 mg orally (PO)/intravenous (IV) q24h or ciprofloxacin 500 mg PO bid or 400 mg IV bid for 7 to 10 days. Should not be used as first line in patients from South Asia due to resistance unless known to be susceptible
  2. Ceftriaxone 2 g IV qd for 7 to 14 days or cefixime (20-30 mg/kg/day orally divided into q12h dosing for 7 to 14 days)
  3. Another alternative agent: Azithromycin (1 g orally then 500 mg daily for 5 to 7 days)
  4. Children (Table 5): In general, quinolones are avoided in children unless a multidrug-resistant strain is involved due to concerns of possible cartilage damage. Another alternative for children: Azithromycin (10-20 mg/kg to 1 g maximum once daily for 5-7 days)
  5. If tests show susceptibility, can also use amoxicillin or trimethoprim/sulfamethoxazole in adults and children (Table 6)
  6. Dexamethasone 3 mg IV initially, followed by 1 mg IV q6h for eight doses for patients with shock or mental status changes
- Gastroenteritis:
  1. Usually not indicated for gastroenteritis alone because this illness usually self-limited
  2. Treatment may prolong the carrier state and is discouraged for healthy patients <50 yr of age who have relatively mild disease
  3. Prophylactic treatment for patients who are at high risk of developing complications from bacteremia (see Table 5):
     a. Neonates
     b. Patients with hemoglobinopathies
     c. Patients with atherosclerosis
     d. Patients with aneurysms
     e. Patients with prosthetic devices
     f. Immunocompromised patients

TABLE 6 Antibiotics Commonly Used in the Treatment of *Salmonella* Infections

Drug	Dose	Comments
Ciprofloxacin	20-30 mg/kg per day in 2 doses PO or IV	First-line therapy[a]
Ceftriaxone	75-100 mg/kg per day in 1 or 2 doses IM or IV	First-line therapy
Cefotaxime	100-300 mg/kg per day in 3-4 doses IM or IV	First-line therapy
Cefixime	20-30 mg/kg per day in 1 or 2 doses PO	Alternative therapy
Azithromycin	10 mg/kg per day in 1 dose PO	Alternative therapy
Chloramphenicol	50-100 mg/kg per day in 4 doses PO	High frequency of resistance; use only for susceptible strains
Ampicillin	200-400 mg/kg per day in 4 doses PO, IM, or IV	High frequency of resistance; use only for susceptible strains
TMP-SMX	10 mg/kg per day TMP, 50 mg/kg per day SMX in 2 doses PO or IV	High frequency of resistance; use only for susceptible strains

[a]Not approved by the US Food and Drug Administration in children <18 yr; current expert opinion agrees in recommending this agent as an effective therapy for regions with susceptible *Salmonella* strains and especially for severe infections.
IM, Intramuscular; *IV*, intravenous; *PO*, by mouth; *TMP-SMX*, trimethoprim-sulfamethoxazole.
From Cherry JD et al: *Feigin and Cherry's textbook of pediatric infectious diseases*, ed 8, Philadelphia, 2019, Elsevier.

CHRONIC Rx

- Carrier states are possible in those with typhoid fever.
- More common in people >60 yr of age and in people with gallstones.
- Usual site of colonization is the gallbladder.
- Treatment should be considered for those with persistently positive stool cultures and for food handlers.
- Suggested regimens for eradication of carrier state:
  1. Ciprofloxacin 500 mg PO bid for 4 wk.
  2. SMX/TMP 1 to 2 DS tabs PO bid for 6 wk (if susceptible).
  3. Amoxicillin 2 g PO q8h for 6 wk (if susceptible).
- Cholecystectomy may be required in carriers with gallstones who fail medical therapy, but this is rarely indicated for nontyphoidal salmonellosis currently.
- Prolonged course of oral therapy or lifetime suppression for patients with AIDS who have chronic infection.

DISPOSITION

- Typhoid fever:
  1. Treated patients usually respond to therapy; small percentage of chronic carriers.
  2. Untreated patients may have serious complications.
- Gastroenteritis:
  1. Usually self-limited
  2. May be recurrent or persistent in AIDS patients

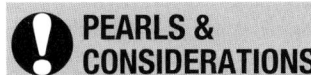 **PEARLS & CONSIDERATIONS**

COMMENTS

- Fluoroquinolones remain the most reliably effective class of antibiotics for empiric therapy despite increasing resistance. They should not be used in children or pregnant women.
- Infections should be reported to local health departments.

- Other recent outbreaks in the U.S. have been traced back to raw tomatoes, peanut butter, pet turtles, frozen pot pies, and onions. In 2022 outbreaks occurred related to backyard poultry and pet turtles less than 4 inches in size.
- Vaccine is available for *Salmonella typhi*. Oral live weakened vaccine (four doses, one every other day) for age >6 yr and lasts for 5 yr or one dose of inactivated injectable vaccine for persons >2 yr old that lasts for 2 yr, but neither vaccine is greater than 75% effective.
- Outbreaks of extensively drug resistant (XDR) typhoid fever have occurred in Pakistan (resistant to ampicillin, sulfa, chloramphenicol, quinolones, and ceftriaxone). Drug of choice for these cases has been azithromycin for milder cases and carbapenems for more severe cases. Some of these cases have been detected in travelers returning from Pakistan.

SUGGESTED READINGS
Available at eBooks.Health.Elsevier.com.

RELATED CONTENT
Salmonellosis (Patient Information)
Typhoid Fever (Related Key Topic)

AUTHOR: **GLENN G. FORT, MD, MPH**

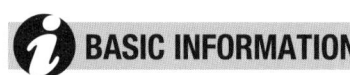
BASIC INFORMATION

DEFINITION

Sarcoidosis is a chronic multisystem granulomatous disease of unknown cause characterized histologically by the presence of noncaseating granulomas and manifesting with a wide range of clinical disturbances.

SYNONYM

Boeck sarcoid

ICD-10CM CODES

D86	Sarcoidosis
D86.0	Sarcoidosis of lung
D86.1	Sarcoidosis of lymph nodes
D86.2	Sarcoidosis of lung with sarcoidosis of lymph nodes
D86.3	Sarcoidosis of skin
D86.8	Sarcoidosis of other and combined sites
D86.9	Sarcoidosis, unspecified

EPIDEMIOLOGY & DEMOGRAPHICS

INCIDENCE (IN U.S.): Incidence is 11 in 100,000 in whites and 35 in 100,000 in blacks; presents most commonly in the winter and early spring. (The adjusted annual incidence among black Americans is roughly 3 times higher than among white Americans [35.5 cases/100,000, as compared with 10.9/100,000] and is likely more chronic and fatal in black Americans.)
PREDOMINANT SEX: Increased incidence in females.
PREDOMINANT AGE: 20 to 50 yr, second peak after 60 yr[1]
GENETICS: Familial clustering has been described. Having a first-degree relative with sarcoidosis increases the risk for disease fivefold.[2] There have been reports of association between sarcoidosis and gene products, specifically human leukocyte antigen (HLA) class II antigens, encoded by HLA-DRB1 and DQB1 alleles.[3]

PHYSICAL FINDINGS & CLINICAL PRESENTATION

- Clinical manifestations often vary with the stage of the disease and degree of organ involvement. Patients may be asymptomatic, but a chest radiograph may demonstrate findings consistent with sarcoidosis (see "Imaging Studies"). Nearly 50% of patients with sarcoidosis are diagnosed by incidental findings on chest radiograph. Lung involvement occurs in >90% of patients with sarcoidosis.
- Frequent manifestations:
  1. Pulmonary manifestations: Dry, nonproductive cough; dyspnea; chest discomfort. Pleural effusion is an uncommon manifestation but can occur in stage II or III of pulmonary involvement.
  2. Constitutional symptoms: Fatigue, weight loss, anorexia, malaise, night sweats.
  3. Visual disturbances: Blurred vision, ocular discomfort, conjunctivitis, iritis, uveitis (65% of patients).

  4. Dermatologic manifestations (30% of patients): Erythema nodosum (10% of patients), macules, papules, subcutaneous nodules, hyperpigmentation, lupus pernio (indurated violaceous lesions on the nose, lips, ears, and cheeks that can erode into underlying cartilage and bone) (Fig. E1).
  5. Myocardial disturbances, arrhythmias, cardiomyopathy, various conduction abnormalities, and pericardial effusion. Cardiac sarcoidosis is much more common than clinically appreciated and is found in up to 25% of patients in the U.S.
  6. Splenomegaly, hepatomegaly, and rarely, can involve the pancreas.
  7. Rheumatologic manifestations: Arthralgias have been reported in up to 40% of patients. It typically affects the ankles but can also involve the knees, wrists, and small joints of the hands and feet.
  8. **Löfgren syndrome,** consisting of the triad of arthritis, erythema nodosum, and bilateral hilar adenopathy, occurs in 9% to 34% of patients. Fever is frequently present.
  9. Neurologic and other manifestations: Cranial nerve palsies, diabetes insipidus, meningeal involvement, parotid enlargement, hypothalamic and pituitary lesions, peripheral adenopathy. Neurosarcoidosis is detected in up to 25% of patients and can occur in the absence of apparent disease elsewhere. Cranial nerve dysfunction is the most common neurologic complication of sarcoidosis. Basilar granulomatous meningitis is the usual cause (Fig. E2), but the facial nerve may also be involved when parotitis is present.
  10. The presence of anterior uveitis, parotiditis, fevers, and facial nerve palsy is known as **Heerfordt syndrome.**
  11. Renal involvement in 7% to 22% in multisystem disease. Epididymis and the testis can be involved in male patients. Initial presentation can be of hydronephrosis due to external compression by retroperitoneal lymph nodes.
  12. Hypercalcemia is seen in about 10% to 13% of patients with multisystem involvement. Abnormal production of 1-alpha-hydroxylase and PTHrp is thought to contribute to the hypercalcemia in some patients with sarcoidosis. Hypercalciuria is also common.

ETIOLOGY & PATHOGENESIS

A cardinal feature of sarcoidosis is the presence of CD4+ T cells that interact with antigen-presenting cells to initiate the formation and maintenance of granulomas (Fig. E3). Multiple lines of evidence suggest that sarcoidosis may result from the interaction of multiple genes with environmental exposures or infection.

GENETIC PREDISPOSITION TO SARCOIDOSIS:
Various HLA antigens have been implicated in diverse patient populations. Familial

predisposition has been reported dating back to 1923, with a wide percentage of variability of affected relatives (0.4% to 21%) and heterogeneity based on genetic background. A more recent study was published by the ACCESS (A Case Controlled Etiologic Survey of Sarcoidosis) study group, which confirmed increased risk for family members with an odds ratio of 4.6 for all relatives. Absolute risk, however, for a family member to be affected was less than 1%. This study also showed a higher risk in white versus black American siblings and parents.
IMMUNOPATHOGENESIS OF SARCOIDOSIS:
Numerous chemokines and cytokines have been implicated in the development and/or resolution of the disease. In sarcoidosis, the alveolitis seen at disease presentation represents an increase in primarily lymphocytic cellularity, predominated by CD4 cells. Presence of increased neutrophils in the bronchoalveolar lavage of patients with sarcoidosis has been associated with persistence of disease, with spontaneous remission noted in 36% of patients with elevated neutrophil counts.

DIAGNOSIS

DIFFERENTIAL DIAGNOSIS

- Infection:
  1. Tuberculosis
  2. Fungal infection (e.g., *Coccidioides*, histoplasmosis, blastomycosis)
  3. Infectious mononucleosis
- Malignancies:
  1. Lymphoma
  2. Metastatic cancer
  3. Lymphangitic carcinomatosis
- Pneumoconioses including berylliosis and silicosis
- Other interstitial lung diseases (e.g., hypersensitivity pneumonitis)
- Vascular abnormalities (e.g., enlarged pulmonary arteries)
- Parasitic infection
- Other diseases such as amyloidosis

WORKUP

- No pathognomonic diagnostic test exists for sarcoidosis, so the diagnosis remains one of exclusion. The presence of noncaseating granulomas does not establish the diagnosis, because conditions such as tuberculosis and malignancies, among others, can cause granulomas.
- Workup is aimed at excluding critical organ involvement, determining extent and severity of disease, and excluding other disease. A complete neurologic and ophthalmologic examination is mandatory.
- A complete occupational and environmental exposure history is recommended.
- In patients with a history of beryllium exposure, beryllium lymphocyte proliferation testing should be obtained to assess for berylliosis.
- Initial laboratory evaluation should include complete blood count, serum chemistries (alanine aminotransferase, aspartate

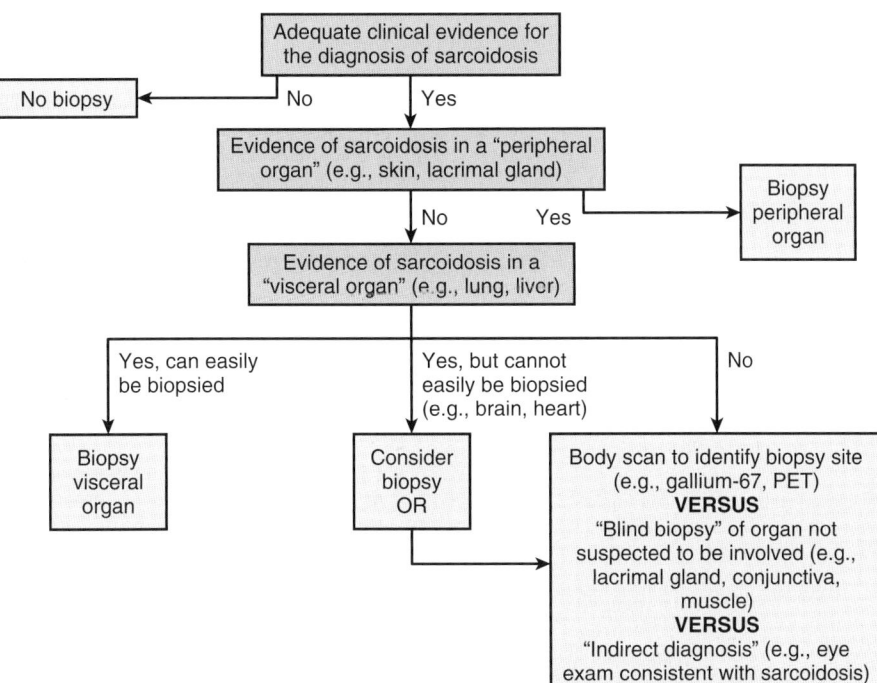

FIG. 4 Diagnostic approach to selecting a biopsy site for pathologic confirmation of granulomatous inflammation consistent with sarcoidosis. This approach emphasizes selection of a relatively noninvasive biopsy site when possible, biopsy of a site suspected to be clinically involved unless the biopsy would be highly invasive, and various approaches when no obvious organ involvement is demonstrated or only organs requiring very invasive biopsies demonstrate potential involvement. *PET,* positron emission tomography. (From Broaddus VC et al: *Murray & Nadel's textbook of respiratory medicine,* ed 7, Philadelphia 2022, Elsevier.)

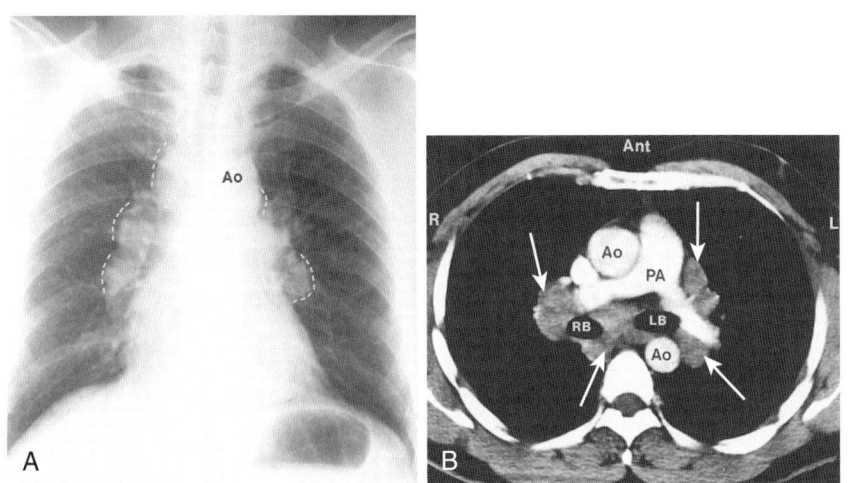

FIG. 5 Sarcoid. Marked lymphadenopathy *(dotted lines)* is seen in the region of both hila in the right paratracheal region **(A).** The transverse contrast-enhanced computed tomography (CT) scan of the upper chest **(B)** clearly shows the ascending and descending aorta *(Ao)* as well as the pulmonary artery *(PA)* and superior vena cava. The right and left mainstem bronchus area is also seen. The *arrows* indicate the extensive lymphadenopathy. *LB,* Left bronchus; *RB,* right bronchus. (From Mettler FA [ed]: *Primary care radiology,* Philadelphia, 2000, Saunders.)

sarcoid involvement (conjunctiva, skin, lymph nodes); bronchoscopy with transbronchial biopsy (85% diagnostic yield) is often performed in patients without any readily accessible site. Among patients with suspected Stage I/II pulmonary sarcoidosis undergoing tissue confirmation, the addition of endobronchial ultrasound (EBUS) transbronchial needle aspiration (TBNA) resulted in greater diagnostic yield. EBUS-TBNA of lymph nodes has a diagnostic yield of approximately 87%. Although in some studies, mediastinoscopy may have a higher diagnostic yield than EBUS-guided lymph node biopsy (98% and 87%, respectively), EBUS-TBNA is less invasive and has become the standard diagnostic modality for patients with mediastinal adenopathy with high clinical suspicion for sarcoidosis.

LABORATORY TESTS
The following laboratory abnormalities are often present in sarcoidosis:
- Hypergammaglobulinemia, anemia, leukopenia may be present.
- Liver function test abnormalities are common, e.g., elevated alkaline phosphatase.
- Hypercalcemia (11% of patients), hypercalciuria (40% of patients; attributable to increased gastrointestinal absorption, abnormal vitamin D metabolism, and increased calcitriol production by sarcoid granuloma).
- Angiotensin-converting enzyme: Elevated in approximately 75% of patients with untreated sarcoidosis; nonspecific and poor sensitivity; generally not useful as a diagnostic tool or in following the course of the disease.
- Serum adenosine deaminase (ADA); serum amyloid A (SAA) elevated but nonspecific.

IMAGING STUDIES
- Chest x-ray (Fig. 5): Pulmonary sarcoidosis is classified based on radiographic pattern. Adenopathy of the hilar and paratracheal nodes is a frequent finding. Parenchymal changes may also be present, depending on the stage of the disease (stage 0, normal radiograph; stage I, bilateral hilar adenopathy; stage II, stage I plus pulmonary infiltrate; stage III, pulmonary infiltrate without adenopathy; stage IV, advanced fibrosis with evidence of "honeycombing," hilar retraction, bullae, cysts, and emphysema).
- Computed tomography (CT) imaging: High-resolution CT may help detect early parenchymal abnormalities. A chest CT scan with contrast can better define mediastinal adenopathy.
- For patients without apparent lung involvement, ^{18}F-fluorodeoxyglucose positron emission tomography (FDG-PET) (Fig. E6) is useful in identifying sites for diagnostic biopsy.
- FDG-PET and MRI with gadolinium are useful in patients with suspected cardiac and neurologic involvement.
- Gallium-67 scan: Represents an older testing modality. It will localize in areas of granulomatous infiltrates; however, it is not specific and not necessary. The "panda" sign

aminotransferase, alkaline phosphatase, electrolytes, blood urea nitrogen, creatinine, serum calcium), urinalysis, 24-hour urinary excretion of calcium, C-reactive protein (CRP), erythrocyte sedimentation rate (ESR), and tuberculin skin test or QuantiFERON gold test for tuberculosis. Routine vitamin D screening is generally not recommended; if done, it should measure both 25-hydroxyvitamin D and 1,25-dihydroxyvitamin

D because sarcoidosis increases conversion of the former to the latter.[4]
- Chest radiograph and ECG should also be obtained in all patients suspected to have sarcoidosis.
- Pulmonary function testing: Spirometry, diffusion capacity of carbon monoxide.
- Biopsy (Fig. 4) in symptomatic patients should be done on accessible tissues suspected of

TABLE 1 Indications for Use of Corticosteroids in Sarcoidosis

Disorder	Treatment
Iridocyclitis	Corticosteroid eye drops; local subconjunctival deposit of cortisone
Posterior uveitis	Oral prednisone
Pulmonary involvement	Steroids rarely recommended for stage I; typically used if infiltrate remains static or worsens over 3-mo period or the patient is symptomatic
Upper airway obstruction	Rare indication for intravenous steroids
Lupus pernio	Oral prednisone shrinks the disfiguring lesions
Hypercalcemia	Responds well to corticosteroids
Cardiac involvement	Corticosteroids usually recommended if patient has arrhythmias or conduction disturbances
Central nervous system involvement	Response is best in patients with acute symptoms
Lacrimal/salivary gland involvement	Corticosteroids recommended for disordered function, not gland swelling
Bone cysts	Corticosteroids recommended if symptomatic

From Andreoli TE (ed): *Cecil essentials of medicine*, ed 8, Philadelphia, 2010, Saunders.

(localization in the lacrimal and salivary glands, giving a "panda" appearance to the face) is suggestive of sarcoidosis.

Additional diagnostic tests:
- Pulmonary function tests (spirometry, lung volumes, and diffusing capacity for carbon monoxide): May be normal; may reveal a restrictive ventilatory defect with reduced forced vital capacity and/or reduced DLCO; may reveal an obstructive pattern; or may reveal a combination.
- Bronchoscopy: Flexible bronchoscopy and bronchoalveolar lavage (BAL) with transbronchial biopsy (showing noncaseating granulomas) are traditional methods for the minimally invasive diagnosis of sarcoidosis. With hilar adenopathy, EBUS-TBNA is the preferred method for lymph node sampling. BAL may show predominantly lymphocytosis, elevated ADA levels, and elevated CD4:CD8 ratio (4:1).
- Mediastinoscopy: Now rarely used for lymph node sampling and diagnosis.
- Routine eye examination is recommended, even for patients without ocular symptoms.
- For patients with extracardiac sarcoidosis or suspected cardiac involvement, cardiac MRI is indicated.
- Echocardiogram is indicated in patients with suspected pulmonary hypertension. If suggested by transthoracic echocardiogram, right heart catheterization should be done.

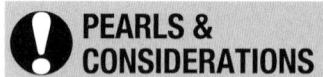 **TREATMENT**

- Many patients with sarcoidosis will not require any treatment, and the disease resolves spontaneously.
- Multisystem sarcoidosis is best treated with a multidisciplinary approach that may include a pulmonologist, rheumatologist, cardiologist, and thoracic radiologist.
- Treatment should be instituted when organ function is threatened.
- Corticosteroids (Table 1) are the mainstay of therapy when treatment is required (e.g., prednisone 40 mg daily for 8 to 12 wk with gradual tapering of the dose to 10 mg every other day over 8 to 12 mo). Corticosteroids should be

considered in patients with severe symptoms (e.g., dyspnea, chest pain); hypercalcemia; ocular, central nervous system, or cardiac involvement; or progressive pulmonary disease. Patients with interstitial lung disease benefit from oral steroid therapy for 6 to 24 mo. A lack of response to steroid therapy may be due to the presence of irreversible fibrotic disease.
- Methotrexate: Patients with progressive disease refractory to corticosteroids or in patients unable to locate corticosteroids may be treated with methotrexate 7.5 to 15 mg once per week or another immunosuppressant such as azathioprine, leflunomide, or mycophenolate mofetil.
- The antimalarial agent hydroxychloroquine is also a corticosteroid sparing agent particularly useful for cutaneous disease, hypercalcemia, and in some cases of neurosarcoidosis.[1]
- Immunomodulators: Represent third line alternatives. Adalimumab and infliximab may be considered. Infliximab has been used with some benefits in cutaneous, pulmonary, and neurologic disease.
- NSAIDs are useful for musculoskeletal symptoms and erythema nodosum.
- Pulmonary rehabilitation is recommended for patients with significant respiratory impairment.
- Lung transplantation should be considered in patients with advanced lung disease, unresponsive to medical therapy.

DISPOSITION
- The majority of patients with sarcoidosis have spontaneous remission within 2 years and do not require treatment. Their course can be followed by periodic clinical evaluation, chest CT scans, and pulmonary function tests.
- Blacks have increased rates of pulmonary involvement, a worse long-term prognosis, and more frequent relapses.
- Up to one third of patients have unrelenting disease, leading to clinically significant organ impairment. Adverse prognostic factors in sarcoidosis include age of onset >40 years, cardiac involvement, neurosarcoidosis, progressive pulmonary fibrosis, chronic hypercalcemia, chronic uveitis, involvement of nasal

mucosa, nephrocalcinosis, and presence of cystic bone lesions and lupus pernio.
- Prognosis for Loeffler syndrome is good with remittance within 16 weeks in most patients. Symptoms can generally be controlled with NSAIDs. Low-dose glucocorticoids, hydroxychloroquine, and colchicine are also effective.
- Pulmonary hypertension is a poor prognostic sign and warrants consideration of referral for lung transplant evaluation. Transplantation for sarcoidosis is performed in 3% to 5% of patients and posttransplant survival rate is approximately 70% at 5 yr. The main factors associated with worse survival are older age and extensive preoperative lung fibrosis.[1]

REFERRAL
- Patients with progressive pulmonary disease or development of pulmonary hypertension despite therapy should be referred for consideration of lung transplant candidacy.
- Ophthalmologic examination is indicated in all patients with suspected sarcoidosis because ocular findings (iridocyclitis, uveitis, conjunctivitis, and keratopathy) are found in ≥25% of documented cases.
- Dermatology consultation for possible biopsy is indicated for patients with possible skin manifestations.
- Patients with suspected cardiac involvement should be referred to cardiology and those with CNS involvement referred to neurology.

! PEARLS & CONSIDERATIONS

COMMENTS
- Serial spirometry and measurement of DLCO can be useful in following response to therapy and disease progression.
- Approximately 15% to 20% of patients with lung involvement advance to irreversible lung impairment (bronchiectasis, cavitation, progressive fibrosis, pneumothorax, and respiratory failure). Death from pulmonary failure occurs in 5% to 7% of patients with sarcoidosis.
- Newer treatment approaches are aimed at targeting mechanisms involving CD4 type 1 helper T cells.
- The diagnosis of sarcoidosis should be reconsidered in the presence of atypical manifestations or persistent/progressive disease despite appropriate therapy.
- Diagnostic biopsy may not be necessary in most patients presenting with asymptomatic bilateral lymphadenopathy (with no other evidence of malignancy), in those with Lofgren syndrome, or in those with Heerfordt syndrome.

REFERENCES
Available at eBooks.Health.Elsevier.com.

RELATED CONTENT
Sarcoidosis (Patient Information)

AUTHOR: **IMRANA QAWI, MD**

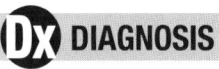
Diseases
and Disorders

I

BASIC INFORMATION

DEFINITION

Scabies is a parasitic skin infestation caused by the mite *Sarcoptes scabiei.*

ICD-10CM CODE
B86   Scabies

EPIDEMIOLOGY & DEMOGRAPHICS

- Scabies is generally acquired by prolonged direct skin-to-skin contact with an infected individual.
- Scabies is endemic in many developing countries; however, it can affect individuals of any age and socioeconomic status.
- Prevalence is 100 to 200 million people worldwide,[1] with more than 200,000 U.S. cases/yr.
- Risk factors include living in crowded conditions (homes, shelters, nursing homes, extended care facilities, and prisons). More common in resource-limited areas and in tropical climates.[1]

PHYSICAL FINDINGS & CLINICAL PRESENTATION

- Primary lesions are caused when the microscopic mite burrows into the upper layer of the skin, laying eggs within the tract she leaves behind; burrows (linear or serpiginous tracts, see Fig. E1) end with a minute papule or vesicle.
- The distribution of primary lesions (Fig. E2) is usually widespread, and lesions are most commonly found in the web spaces of the hands, flexor aspects of wrists, buttocks, genitalia, breasts, axillae, and knees. In

children, they can also involve the head, neck, face, palms of the hands, and soles of the feet.[2] They are often confused with eczema (Fig. E3).
- Secondary lesions result from repeatedly scratching or secondary staphylococcal or streptococcal infections.
- Intense itching, especially at night, is the hallmark of this condition; it is caused by a delayed hypersensitivity to the mite or fecal pellets and is usually noted 2 to 6 wk after the primary infestation.
- Examination of the skin may reveal burrows, tiny vesicles, excoriations, or inflammatory papules.[2]
- Widespread and crusted lesions (Norwegian or crusted scabies) may be seen in the elderly, in immunocompromised patients, or in patients who do not have the ability to scratch (Fig. E4). Pruritus may be mild or absent due to impaired host immune response.
- Table 1 summarizes the different presenting forms of scabies.

ETIOLOGY

- Human scabies is caused by the mite *Sarcoptes scabiei* var. *hominis* (Fig. 5). After impregnation on the skin surface, the gravid female burrows in the stratum corneum and gradually extends the tract along the boundary with the stratum granulosum laying two to three eggs per day for 4 to 6 wk.[3] The eggs hatch in 3 to 4 days, and larvae move to the skin surface and mature in 2 to 3 wk, resuming the cycle.
- Transmission is usually due to prolonged skin-to-skin contact. Transmission can occasionally be due to fomites (especially in crusted scabies) as they can survive off a host for 24 to 36 h.

- Clinical manifestations result from a delayed type IV hypersensitivity reaction to the mite, eggs, saliva, or scybala (fecal pellets).

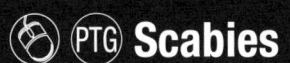 DIAGNOSIS

DIFFERENTIAL DIAGNOSIS

- Pediculosis
- Atopic dermatitis
- Flea bites
- Seborrheic dermatitis
- Dermatitis herpetiformis
- Contact dermatitis
- Nummular eczema
- Infantile acropustulosis
- Langerhans cell histiocytosis
- Arthropod bites

WORKUP

Diagnosis is made based on the clinical appearance of the rash and burrows and should be suspected if the patient presents with intense itching out of proportion to skin findings or there is a history of other family members with similar symptoms. Diagnosis can be confirmed by microscopic detection of mites, eggs, or mite feces.

LABORATORY TESTS

- Microscopic demonstration of the mites, feces, or eggs: A drop of mineral oil may be placed over the suspected lesion before removal (Box 1); the scrapings are transferred directly to a glass slide; a drop of potassium hydroxide is added, and a cover slip is applied.[3]
- Skin biopsy is rarely necessary to make the diagnosis.

TABLE 1   Different Presenting Forms of Scabies

Presenting Forms of Scabies	Specific High-Risk Populations	Clinical Manifestations	Limited Differential Diagnoses
Classic scabies (scabies vulgaris)	Infants and children; sexually active adults; men who have sex with men	Intense generalized pruritus, worse at night; inflammatory pruritic papules localized to finger webs, flexor aspects of wrists, elbows, axillae, buttocks, genitalia, female breasts; lesions and pruritus spare the face, head, and neck; secondary lesions include eczematization, excoriation, impetigo	Dermatitis herpetiformis, drug reactions, eczema, pediculosis corporis, lichen planus, pityriasis rosea
Scalp scabies	Infants and children; institutionalized older adults; AIDS patients; patients with preexisting crusted scabies	Atypical crusted papular lesions of the scalp, face, palms, and soles	Dermatomyositis, ringworm, seborrheic dermatitis
Crusted scabies (Norwegian scabies, scabies norvegica, scabies crustosa)	Institutionalized older adults; institutionalized developmentally disabled (Down syndrome); homeless, especially HIV-positive; all immunocompromised patients, particularly those with AIDS or positive for HIV or HTLV-1; transplant recipients; patients on prolonged systemic corticosteroids and chemotherapy	Psoriasiform hyperkeratotic papular lesions of the scalp, face, neck, hands, feet, with extensive nail involvement; eczematization and impetigo common	Contact dermatitis, drug reactions, eczema, erythroderma, ichthyosis, psoriasis
Nodular scabies	Sexually active adults; men who have sex with men; HIV-positive men > HIV-positive women	Violaceous pruritic nodules localized to male genitalia, groin, axillae, representing hypersensitivity reaction to mite antigens	Acropustulosis, atopic dermatitis, Darier disease, lupus erythematosus, lymphomatoid papulosis, papular urticaria, necrotizing vasculitis, secondary syphilis

AIDS, Acquired immunodeficiency syndrome; *HIV,* human immunodeficiency virus; *HTLV-1,* human T-cell lymphotropic virus type 1.
From Bennett JE et al: *Mandell, Douglas, and Bennett's principles and practice of infectious diseases,* ed 8, Philadelphia, 2015, Saunders.

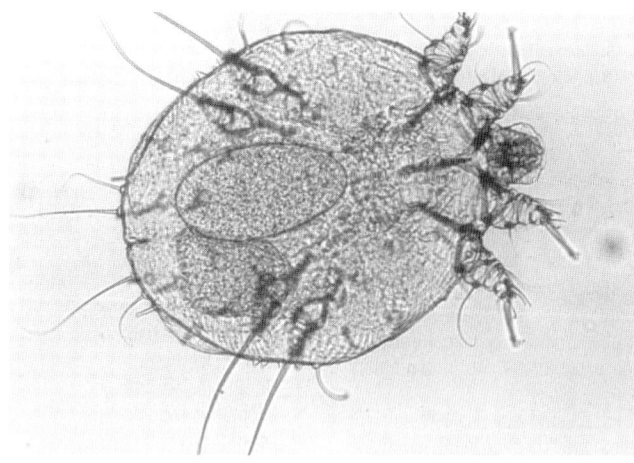

FIG. 5 Scabies mite. Note the eggs within the body of the mite. (Live scabies mite, ×40 magnification.) (From Paller AS, Mancini AJ: *Hurwitz clinical pediatric dermatology: a textbook of skin disorders of childhood and adolescence*, ed 5, Philadelphia, 2016, Elsevier.)

BOX 1   Performing a Mineral-Oil Examination for Scabies

1. Apply a drop of mineral oil to the lesion(s) to be scraped.
2. Scrape through the lesion with a number 15 scalpel blade (a small amount of bleeding is expected with appropriately deep scrapings).
3. Smear contents of scraping on a clean glass slide.
4. Add a few more drops of mineral oil.
5. Place cover slip over oil and examine under microscope at low power.
   Criteria for a positive mineral oil examination:
   Scabies mite.
   or
   Ova (eggs).
   or
   Scybala (feces).

From Paller AS, Mancini AJ: *Hurwitz clinical pediatric dermatology: a textbook of skin disorders of childhood and adolescence*, ed 5, Philadelphia, 2016, Elsevier.

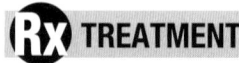 **TREATMENT**

NONPHARMACOLOGIC THERAPY

Clothing, underwear, bedding, and towels used 72 h before treatment must be washed in hot water and put in a dryer or sealed in a plastic bag for at least 72 h. Scabies mites generally do not survive more than 2 to 3 days away from human skin.

ACUTE GENERAL Rx

- Permethrin 5% cream is usually effective with one treatment; it should be massaged into the skin from head to soles of feet and applied under fingernails and toenails. Cream should be applied overnight and then washed off after 8 to 14 h. In children, cream should also be applied to the scalp and face. May need a second application in 1 to 2 wk. Permethrin is safe for children >2 mo old.[4]
- A single dose of ivermectin (200 μg/kg), an antiparasitic agent, can be used as initial therapy or for those who have failed topical treatment. Repeat doses, along with topical therapy, are recommended for Norwegian (crusted) scabies.[4]
- Pruritus generally abates 24 to 48 h after treatment but can last up to 2 wk; oral antihistamines can be effective. Retreatment may be necessary if pruritus is persistent for 2 to 4 wk or if new burrows or rash appears.
- Any sores that become infected should be treated with appropriate antibiotics if needed.
- It is essential that all close contacts and household members are treated at the same time whether symptomatic or not. If the patient is a resident of an extended care facility, it is important to educate the patients, staff, family, and frequent visitors about scabies and the need to have full cooperation with treatment.
- Table 2 summarizes currently recommended treatment for scabies.

DISPOSITION

Treatment failure is often result of poor adherence to treatment regimen or reinfestation. Scabies infection can be complicated by *Streptococcus pyogenes* and *Staphylococcus aureus* impetigo.[3] Refractory cases are usually only seen with immunocompromised hosts or patients with underlying skin diseases. ***Norwegian scabies (crusted scabies)*** refers to a highly contagious, severe variant often found in institutions caring for the elderly or physically and mentally disabled individuals.[5]

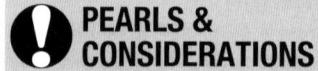 **PEARLS & CONSIDERATIONS**

COMMENTS

- Symptoms can take 4 to 6 wk to develop; however, individuals can still spread scabies before symptoms arise.
- Sexual partners and household members should be notified and treated.
- It is important to decontaminate all bedding, clothing, and towels used by infested persons.
- Lindane is potentially neurotoxic and should not be used on infants or pregnant women (permethrin is safe in pregnancy and infants over 2 mo old).

REFERENCES
Available at eBooks.Health.Elsevier.com.

RELATED CONTENT
Scabies (Patient Information)

AUTHOR: **MARY E. BOVE, MD**

TABLE 2 Currently Recommended Treatment for Scabies

Scabicides	FDA Approved?	Pregnancy Category*	Dosing Schedule	Safety Profile	Contraindications
5% Permethrin cream (Actin, Nix, Elimite)	Yes	B	Apply from neck down; wash off after 8-14 hr; good residual activity, but second application recommended after 1 wk	Excellent; itching and stinging on application	Prior allergic reactions; infants <2 mo of age; breastfeeding
1% Lindane lotion or cream	Yes	B	Apply 30-60 ml from neck down; wash off after 8-12 hr; no residual activity; increasing drug resistance	Potential for central nervous system toxicity from organochloride poisoning, usually manifesting as seizures, with overapplication and ingestions	Preexisting seizure disorder; infants and children <6 mo of age; pregnancy; breastfeeding
10% Crotamiton cream or lotion (Eurax)	Yes	C	Apply from neck down on two consecutive nights; wash off 24 hr after second application	Excellent; not very effective; exacerbates pruritus	None
2%-10% Sulfur in petrolatum ointments	No	C	Apply for 2-3 days, then wash	Excellent; not very effective	Preexisting sulfur allergy
10%-25% Benzoyl benzoate lotion	No	None	Two applications for 24 hr with 1-day to 1-wk interval	Irritant; exacerbates pruritus; can induce contact irritant dermatitis and pruritic cutaneous xerosis	Preexisting eczema
0.5% Malathion lotion (Ovide), 1% malathion shampoo (unavailable in the U.S.)	No	B	95% ovicidal; rapid (5 min) killing; good residual activity; increasing drug resistance	Flammable 78% isopropyl alcohol vehicle stings eyes, skin, mucosa; increasing drug resistance; organophosphate poisoning risk with overapplication and ingestions	Infants and children <6 mo of age; pregnancy; breastfeeding
Ivermectin (Stromectol)	Yes	C	200 µg/kg single PO dose, may be repeated in 14-15 days; not ovicidal, second dose on day 14 or 15 highly recommended; recommended for endemic or epidemic scabies in institutions and refugee camps	Excellent; may cause nausea and vomiting; take on empty stomach with water	Safety in pregnancy uncertain; probably safe during breastfeeding; not recommended for children younger than 5 yr of age or weighing <15 kg

*U.S. Food and Drug Administration (FDA) safety in pregnancy categories: A, safety established; B, presumed safe; C, uncertain safety; D, unsafe; X, highly unsafe.
FDA, U.S. Food and Drug Administration; *PO*, by mouth.
From Bennett JE et al: *Mandell, Douglas, and Bennett's principles and practice of infectious diseases*, ed 8, Philadelphia, 2015, Saunders.

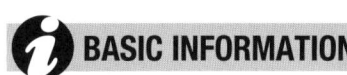
BASIC INFORMATION

DEFINITION
Sciatica is a clinical diagnosis of neuralgia along the sciatic nerve distribution. Sciatica usually occurs unilaterally. Pain is described as sharp or aching and typically radiates from the buttock down the leg posteriorly, laterally, or anteriorly depending on the level of nerve root compression.

SYNONYMS[1-3]
Radicular pain
Lumbosacral radicular syndrome
Deep gluteal syndrome
Ischialgia
Low back pain—sciatica
Lumbago with sciatica
Lumbar nerve root pain
Neuropathy—sciatic nerve
Sciatic nerve dysfunction
Sciatic neuritis

ICD-10CM CODES
G57.00	Lesion of sciatic nerve, unspecified lower limb
G57.01	Lesion of sciatic nerve, right lower limb lesion
G57.02	Lesion of sciatic nerve, left lower limb
M54.30	Sciatica, unspecified side
M54.31	Sciatica, right side
M54.32	Sciatica, left side
M54.40	Lumbago with sciatica, unspecified side
M54.41	Lumbago with sciatica, right side
M54.42	Lumbago with sciatica, left side

EPIDEMIOLOGY & DEMOGRAPHICS[1-3]
INCIDENCE: Very few studies have determined the incidence of sciatica. However, 2% to 11% of patients with low back pain have sciatica
PREVALENCE: Annual prevalence of disc-related sciatica in the general population is estimated at 2.2%
PEAK INCIDENCE: Fourth decade
RISK FACTORS:
- Increasing risk with height in the 50 to 60 age group
- Physical activity in those with prior sciatic symptoms
- Smoking
- Diabetes
- Obesity
- Prolonged sitting and sedentary lifestyle
- Occupational factors:
  1. Strenuous physical activity (e.g., frequent lifting while bending and twisting)
  2. Driving

PHYSICAL FINDINGS & CLINICAL PRESENTATION[4]
- Unilateral leg pain worse than low back pain
- Pain radiating to foot or toes
- Numbness and paresthesia in the same distribution
- Straight leg raise test induces more leg pain
- Localized neuropathy limited to one nerve root

ETIOLOGY[5,6]
- Sciatica is caused by inflammation or compression of the sciatic nerve roots (L4 to S2). L4 root involvement causes pain localized to the frontal and lateral sides of the thigh.
- The most common cause is from disc herniation resulting from age-related degenerative changes.
- Other causes include lumbar spinal stenosis, facet joint osteoarthritis or other arthropathies, sacroiliac joint dysfunction, isthmic spondylolisthesis, soft tissue stenosis, neoplasm, trauma, spinal cord infection, gynecologic conditions, and muscle entrapment (e.g., piriformis syndrome).

DIAGNOSIS

DIFFERENTIAL DIAGNOSIS[5,6]
- Nonspecific low back pain
- Piriformis syndrome
- Muscular problems (e.g., sprain, spasm)
- Vascular problems (e.g., claudication, compartment syndrome)
- Pott disease
- Chronic edema
- Box 1 summarizes the differential diagnosis for low back pain

WORKUP
Sciatica is a clinical diagnosis. Historical clues to the cause of low back pain are summarized in Table 1. Red flags indicating cauda equina or spinal infection mandate emergent workup. Fig. 1 summarizes an algorithm for the management of low back pain.
HISTORY TAKING:
- Onset and duration
- Leg pain more severe than back pain
- Severity of pain
- Complaints of radiating pain in the leg following a dermatomal pattern, generally below the knee, into the foot
- Sensory symptoms (e.g., tingling, numbness)
- Muscle weakness in the legs

BOX 1 Differential Diagnosis for Low Back Pain

Localized and Common	Polymyalgia rheumatica
Uncomplicated musculoskeletal back pain	Reiter syndrome
Intervertebral disk herniation	**Vascular**
Spinal stenosis	Arteriovenous malformation of spinal cord
Spondylolisthesis	Epidural hematoma
Osteoarthritis	Life-threatening referred pain
Fracture	Abdominal aortic aneurysm
Localized and Uncommon	**Gastrointestinal System**
Infection	Biliary pathology
Spondylitis	Pancreatitis
Epidural abscess	Peptic ulcer disease
Discitis	Diverticulitis
Herpes zoster	**Genitourinary System**
Malignancy	Renal colic
Metastatic	Pyelonephritis
Breast	Prostatitis
Lung	Cystitis
Prostate	**Gynecologic System**
Kidney, thyroid, colon (less common)	Menstrual cramps
Primary	Spontaneous abortion
Multiple myeloma	Labor
Lymphoma	Ectopic pregnancy
Leukemia	Pelvic inflammatory disease
Primary cord or extradural tumors	Endometriosis
Osteoid osteoma	Ovarian cyst
Other primary bone tumors	Ovarian torsion
Pediatric	**Hematologic System**
Spondylolisthesis, spondylolysis	Sickle cell vaso-occlusive crisis
Severe scoliosis	**Functional**
Scheuermann disease	Somatization disorder
Rheumatologic	Depression
Ankylosing spondylitis	Fibrositis
Psoriatic arthritis	Malingering

From Marx JA et al: *Rosen's emergency medicine,* ed 8, Philadelphia, 2014, Elsevier.

TABLE 1 Historical Clues to the Cause of Low Back Pain

Questions for Patient	Potential Diagnosis
Does the back pain radiate down past the knees?	Radiculopathy and likely a herniated disk
Is the pain worse with walking and better with bending forward and sitting?	Spinal stenosis
Do you have morning back stiffness that improves with exercise?	Ankylosing spondylitis
Are you older than 50 yr?	Osteoporotic fracture, spinal malignancy
Has there been any recent history of blunt trauma?	Fracture
Do you take long-term corticosteroids?	Fracture, spinal infection
Do you have a history of cancer?	Spinal metastatic malignancy
Does your pain persist at rest?	Spinal malignancy, spinal infection
Has there been persistent pain for longer than 6 wk?	Spinal malignancy
Has there been unexplained weight loss?	Spinal malignancy
Is the pain worse at night?	Spinal malignancy, spinal infection
Are you immunocompromised (e.g., HIV infection, alcoholism, diabetes)?	Spinal infection
Have you had fevers or chills?	Spinal infection
Do you have pain, weakness, or numbness in both legs?	Cauda equina syndrome
Do you have bladder or bowel control problems?	Cauda equina syndrome

HIV, Human immunodeficiency virus.
From Walls RM et al: *Rosen's emergency medicine: concepts and clinical practice*, ed 9, Philadelphia, 2018, Elsevier.

- Influence of coughing, movement, or rest on severity of pain

PHYSICAL EXAMINATION: Neurologic testing
- Myotomes
- Reflexes (patellar - L4, medial hamstring - L5, Achilles - S1)
- Sensations (dermatomes; see Fig. E2)

LUMBAR MOBILITY ASSESSMENT: Neural tension tests
- Straight leg raise test (L5 to S1)
- Reversed straight leg raise test (L2 to L4)
- Bragard test
- Crossed straight leg raise test
- Slump test
- Femoral nerve tension test

Major maneuvers:
- Knee extension (L4)
- Lumbar lateral bending
- Hip flexion
- Lasègue test
- Bechterew test
- Fajersztajn test

Minor maneuvers:
- Ankle dorsal flexion (L5)
- Ankle plantar flexion (S1)
- Cervical flexion
- Spinal flexion
- Hip internal rotation
- Hip adduction
- Great toe dorsiflexion
- Increased intrathecal/intradiscal pressure

LABORATORY TESTS

No laboratory tests specifically identify sciatica.
- Occasionally, laboratory tests such as CBC and erythrocyte sedimentation rate may suggest infection or inflammation, anemia due to certain cancers, or other unusual causes of sciatica.
- Urinalysis may suggest a kidney stone if hematuria is present or infection if bacteria and white blood cells are present.

IMAGING STUDIES

- Routine imaging is not advised in nonspecific low back pain.
- If pain lasts for longer than 12 wk or if neurologic deficits or pain progress, MRI scans of the spine can evaluate for other causes. A repeat MRI is not helpful.
- Computed tomography is not preferred. Plain radiography is not useful.
- If the patient has a history of cancer, HIV infection, or intravenous drug use, or has been taking steroids chronically, imaging is recommended.
- Electromyography.

Rx TREATMENT

Initial treatment for sciatica includes managing pain and maintaining activity and function. Surgery can be considered if there are anatomic abnormalities or pain progresses. If pain is severe and not relieved by previous measures, then narcotic medications may be prescribed for a short period.

NONPHARMACOLOGIC THERAPY[7]

- Exercise minimally reduces intensity of pain. Individual pain and ability to exercise must be considered
- Bed rest is not recommended

- Physical and exercise therapy
- Manual therapy (e.g., spinal mobilization)
- Ice or heat on affected area for 20 min every 2 h
- Reducing pressure on the nerve root

ACUTE GENERAL Rx[8]

- Pain medications should be used sparingly, in minimal doses, and for a short time period due to their uncertain benefit for sciatica and possible adverse effects.
- Acetaminophen for mild pain.
- Corticosteroids may improve symptoms for a short term. However, adverse effects limit usage.
- Benzodiazepines, opioids, and antidepressants are not recommended for sciatica.
- Anticonvulsants or biologic agents have uncertain benefits.
- Gabapentin or pregabalin are frequently prescribed, but trials have failed to show reduced intensity of leg pain or improved outcomes.

PROCEDURES

- Epidural injection of local anesthetic and steroids in the lumbar nerve root area may be considered in acute, severe sciatica. However, evidence is limited and beneficial effect is low.[9]
- Surgery may be recommended if the pain continues for more than 6 to 8 wk despite conservative treatment and if imaging shows an anatomic problem with disc or bone. Surgery is also indicated in serious or progressive neurologic deficits (e.g., motor weakness, bladder dysfunction).
- In a recent trial involving patients with sciatica lasting more than 4 mo and caused by lumbar disk herniation, micro discectomy was superior to nonsurgical care with respect to pain intensity at 6 mo of follow-up.

CHRONIC Rx

If pain is severe and unrelieved by previous measures, then consider a short course of narcotics; however, the medical community is increasingly turning away from long-term opioids due to the associated morbidity and mortality.

DISPOSITION

Outpatient workup and assessment, including:
- Screening for red flags that may indicate malignancies, osteoporotic fractures, trauma, infection, or cauda equina syndrome
- Taking a history to determine localization, severity, loss of strength, sensation, duration, course, influence of coughing, rest or movement
- Physical examination, including straight leg raising test
- Imaging or laboratory diagnostic testing if red flags are present
- Prescribing medication as needed

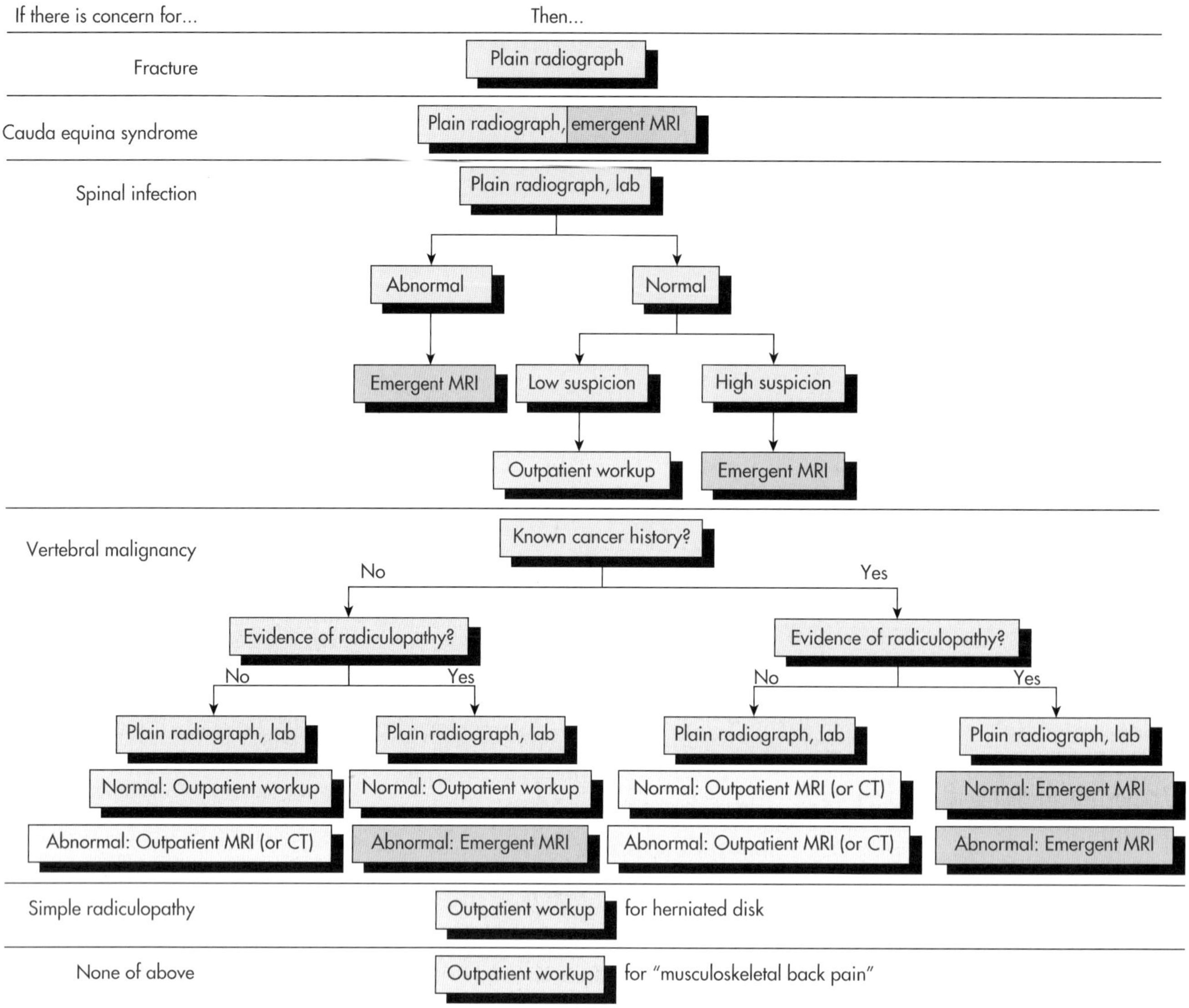

If there is concern for...	Then...

Fracture → Plain radiograph

Cauda equina syndrome → Plain radiograph, emergent MRI

Spinal infection → Plain radiograph, lab

- Abnormal → Emergent MRI
- Normal → Low suspicion → Outpatient workup
- Normal → High suspicion → Emergent MRI

Vertebral malignancy → Known cancer history?

- No → Evidence of radiculopathy?
  - No → Plain radiograph, lab
    - Normal: Outpatient workup
    - Abnormal: Outpatient MRI (or CT)
  - Yes → Plain radiograph, lab
    - Normal: Outpatient workup
    - Abnormal: Emergent MRI
- Yes → Evidence of radiculopathy?
  - No → Plain radiograph, lab
    - Normal: Outpatient MRI (or CT)
    - Abnormal: Outpatient MRI (or CT)
  - Yes → Plain radiograph, lab
    - Normal: Emergent MRI
    - Abnormal: Emergent MRI

Simple radiculopathy → Outpatient workup for herniated disk

None of above → 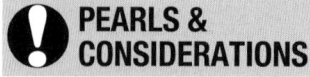 Outpatient workup for "musculoskeletal back pain"

FIG. 1 Algorithm for management of low back pain. The patient's history may be concerning for more than one red flag diagnosis. *CT,* Computed tomography; *MRI,* magnetic resonance imaging. (From Marx JA et al: *Rosen's emergency medicine,* ed 8, Philadelphia, 2014, Elsevier.)

COMPLEMENTARY & ALTERNATIVE MEDICINE

- Acupuncture is not recommended in sciatica.
- Traction and electrotherapy are not recommended in back pain.

REFERRAL

- Physical therapist
- Pain management
- Orthopedic surgeon
- Refer to neurosurgeon immediately in cases of cauda equina syndrome or acute severe paresis or progressive paresis (within a few days)
- Refer to neurosurgeon or orthopedic surgeon for consideration of surgery in cases of intractable radicular pain or if pain does

not diminish after 12 wk of conservative care

❗ PEARLS & CONSIDERATIONS

COMMENTS

- Most patients will recover fully from sciatica and often without treatment, but permanent nerve damage can occur. The following should prompt emergent workup as these symptoms could indicate spinal cord compression: Loss of feeling in affected leg; weakness in affected leg; or loss of bowel or bladder function.
- Sciatica does tend to recur.
- Bed rest is not recommended.

PREVENTION

- Exercise regularly.
- Maintain proper posture when you sit.
- Use good body mechanics.

REFERENCES

Available at eBooks.Health.Elsevier.com.

RELATED CONTENT

Lumbar Disk Syndrome (Related Key Topic)
Piriformis Syndrome (Related Key Topic)

AUTHORS: **EMILY MYLHOUSEN, MD,** and **ANA CASTANEDA-GUARDERAS, MD**

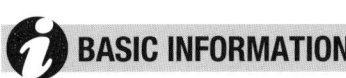
BASIC INFORMATION

DEFINITION

Scleroderma or systemic sclerosis (SSc) is a term used to describe a connective tissue disorder that is characterized by thickening and fibrosis of the skin. Scleroderma is divided into two forms: Localized scleroderma and systemic sclerosis. Localized scleroderma is skin thickening without any organ involvement and includes three subset conditions (Box 1). Systemic sclerosis is a multiorgan disease characterized by fibrosis and vasculopathy. Systemic sclerosis includes skin fibrosis along with variable severe involvement of diverse internal organs. It is further divided into two major subgroups: (1) Limited cutaneous SSc (lcSSc), which involves skin thickening of the face, neck, and distal to the elbows and knees; and (2) diffuse cutaneous SSc (dcSSc), which affects the skin in a more generalized distribution including the proximal and distal extremities, face, neck, and trunk.[1] Clinical features of the major subsets of systemic sclerosis are summarized in Box 2.

SYNONYMS

SSc
Systemic sclerosis
Morphea applies to localized scleroderma that affects only the skin.
Scleredema is a disease of the skin that mimics but is distinct from scleroderma.

ICD-10CM CODES

L94.0	Localized scleroderma (morphea)
L94.1	Linear scleroderma
M34.0	Progressive systemic sclerosis
M34.1	CREST syndrome
M34.2	Systemic sclerosis induced by drug and chemical
M34.81	Systemic sclerosis with lung involvement
M34.82	Systemic sclerosis with myopathy
M34.83	Systemic sclerosis with polyneuropathy
M34.89	Other systemic sclerosis
M34.9	Systemic sclerosis, unspecified

BOX 1 **Classification of Scleroderma**

I. Localized scleroderma
  A. Morphea
  B. Linear scleroderma
  C. Scleroderma en coup de sabre
II. Systemic sclerosis
  A. Limited cutaneous systemic sclerosis
  B. Diffuse cutaneous systemic sclerosis

From Hochberg MC et al: *Rheumatology,* ed 5, St Louis, 2011, Mosby.

EPIDEMIOLOGY & DEMOGRAPHICS

Incidence and prevalence of SSc differs between studies due to variations between geographic regions and time periods.

INCIDENCE: There are an estimated 19 cases per 1 million persons/yr, but many mild cases go unrecognized.
PREVALENCE: 276 cases per 1 million persons per yr.
PREDOMINANT SEX: Female/male ratio of 4:1. However, studies suggest there is greater severity of disease, organ involvement, and relative prevalence of diffuse cutaneous in males vs. females.
PREDOMINANT AGE: 30 to 50 yr.

PHYSICAL FINDINGS & CLINICAL PRESENTATION

PHYSICAL FINDINGS:
- Skin:
  1. Initial presentation of puffy hands and fingers may occur in some patients.
  2. Tightening of the skin begins on the hands and can then progress to the forearms, face, and neck. The skin is shiny, taut, and sometimes red with loss of creases and hair. Skin thickening involving the fingers or toes is known as sclerodactyly (Fig. E1). Skin involvement in scleroderma is classified as lcSSc or dcSSc depending on the distribution of the skin thickening (see previously) (Fig. E2). Fig. E3 illustrates the method used to quantify skin thickness in scleroderma.
  3. Skin tightening may limit movement by causing flexion contractures of the fingers, wrists, and elbows. Perioral skin tightening (Fig. E4) results in decreased oral aperture, furrowing around the lips, and dry membranes.
  4. Pigmentary skin changes (hypo- or hyperpigmentation) may occur (e.g., "salt and pepper").
  5. Telangiectasias (dilated capillaries) may be seen on face, hands, mucous membranes (Fig. E4), and trunk.
  6. Subcutaneous calcinosis, calcinosis cutis.
  7. In dcSSc patients, the skin fibrosis can soften over time (generally occurring at least 2 yr after onset of skin manifestation), with improved joint mobility.
  8. Skin atrophy and thinning can also occur in the late stages of SSc.
- Musculoskeletal:
  1. Arthralgias and swelling
  2. Inflammatory arthritis, tendinitis
  3. Myalgias, myopathy
  4. Joint contractures
  5. Tendon friction rubs (physical exam finding of a palpable rub felt over tendon sheaths—fingers, wrists, elbows, knees, and/or ankles)
- Gastrointestinal involvement:
  1. Esophageal dysmotility with heartburn[2]
  2. Esophageal stricture with dysphagia and odynophagia
  3. Delayed gastric emptying
  4. Gastrointestinal bleeding from mucosal telangiectasias, gastric antral vascular ectasias, or gastritis
  5. Small bowel dysmotility with abdominal cramps, bloating, and diarrhea[2]

BOX 2 **Clinical Features of the Major Subsets of Systemic Sclerosis**

Limited SSc
- Skin sclerosis, distal limbs, and face
- Long preexisting RP symptoms
- Lower frequency of severe lung fibrosis and renal crisis
- High burden of nonlethal morbidity

Diffuse SSc
- Proximal skin sclerosis
- Shorter preexisting RP history
- High frequency of severe lung fibrosis
- Increased risk of scleroderma renal crisis
- Inflammatory skin changes and pruritus common for first 1-3 yr

Sine SSc
- Features of RP with scleroderma-associated ANA reactivity and at least one internal organ manifestation of SSc
- Frequency uncertain because of likely underdiagnosis

Overlap SSc
- Cases that fulfill classification criteria for SSc and that are diagnosed as SSc but also show features of another autoimmune rheumatic disease
- Most often myositis
- Other cases of lupus, arthritis, or vasculitis
- Comprise up to 20% of SSc cohorts

ANA, antinuclear antibody; *RP,* Raynaud phenomenon; *SSc,* systemic sclerosis.
From Hochberg MC: *Rheumatology,* ed 7, Philadelphia, 2019, Elsevier.

6. Colon dysmotility with constipation[2]
7. Intestinal bacterial overgrowth resulting in irregular bowel movements (diarrhea alternating with constipation)[2]
8. Pseudoobstruction (functional ileus)
9. Primary biliary cholangitis
- Pulmonary:
  1. Interstitial lung disease (ILD): Pulmonary fibrosis with symptoms of dyspnea and nonproductive cough as well as fine inspiratory crackles on examination. Seen in both lcSSc and dcSSc, but more common and severe in dcSSc.
  2. Pulmonary arterial hypertension (PAH): Presenting with dyspnea and/or fatigue. Can be identified in both lcSSc and dcSSc, but more commonly seen in lcSSc.
- Cardiac:
  1. Pericarditis or pericardial effusion
  2. Myocardial fibrosis or ischemia that can lead to congestive heart failure or arrhythmias
  3. Left or right systolic or diastolic dysfunction
- Renal:
  1. Rapidly progressive renal failure, also known as scleroderma renal crisis (SRC): New-onset hypertension, anemia with schistocytes on peripheral blood smear, thrombocytopenia and renal insufficiency with active urinary sediment and proteinuria

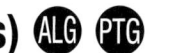
- Vascular:
  1. Raynaud phenomenon (RP): Vasospasm of the fingers with exposure to cold, resulting in color changes of the digits along with numbness/tingling and discomfort[3]
  2. Complications of vascular involvement can include digital pitted scars or ulcers, nonreversible ischemic changes with impending tissue loss, dry gangrene, and auto-amputation
  3. Nailfold capillary abnormalities: Seen with nailfold capillaroscopy, including capillary dilation, avascularity, or "drop out" of capillaries[3]
- Other organ involvement:
  1. Hypothyroidism
  2. Erectile dysfunction
  3. Sjögren syndrome
  4. Entrapment neuropathies
  5. Depression

CLINICAL PRESENTATION

- RP: Initial complaint in 70% of patients (note: The prevalence of RP is 5%-10% in the general population; most cases do not progress to scleroderma)
- Finger or hand swelling that is sometimes associated with carpal tunnel syndrome
- Arthralgias/arthritis
- Internal organ involvement (Table 1, Table E2, Fig. E5, Fig. E6)
- LcSSc (previously known as CREST syndrome): Calcinosis, Raynaud phenomenon, Esophageal dysmotility, Sclerodactyly telangiectasias—skin fibrosis is limited to the distal extremities. This acronym is now considered obsolete by many because it does not accurately reflect the burden of internal organ involvement

ETIOLOGY

The etiology of this condition is unknown, but genetic and environmental factors (infectious agents, occupational exposures, drugs) contribute to the manifestation of the disease.[1] Genetic profiles show clustering of different alleles according to the subtype of SSc.

Pathologically, small- and medium-sized arteries become injured. This leads to fibrin deposition and ultimately luminal occlusion, which causes chronic tissue hypoxia (Fig. E7). There is also an abnormal selection of fibroblasts and aberrant control of connective tissue synthesis by fibroblasts and other cells (Fig. E8). This fibrosis occurs in different organs, causing dysfunction and eventual failure. Although there are characteristic autoantibodies detected, whether they directly participate in the pathogenesis of the disease is not clear.

DIAGNOSIS

The American College of Rheumatology (ACR) and European League Against Rheumatism (EULAR) have created criteria as a guide in diagnosing and classifying SSc (Table 3). These include a scoring system for both clinical and laboratory findings (sclerodactyly, fingertip

TABLE 3 ACR/EULAR 2013 Classification Criteria for Systemic Sclerosis*

Item	Subitem	Weight or Score
Skin thickening of fingers on both hands extending proximal to the MCP joints (sufficient criterion)	—	9
Skin thickening on the fingers (only count the higher score)	Puffy fingers	2
	Sclerodactyly of fingers (distal to MCP joints but proximal to proximal interphalangeal joints)	4
Fingertip lesions (only count higher score)	Digital tip ulcers	2
	Fingertip pitting scars	3
Telangiectasia	—	2
Abnormal nailfold capillaries	—	2
Pulmonary arterial hypertension or ILD (maximum score, 2)	PAH	2
	ILD	2
Raynaud phenomenon	—	3
SSc-related antibodies (anticentromere, antitopoisomerase 1 [anti–SCL-70], anti–RNA polymerase III (max score 3)	Anticentromere Antitopoisomerase I Antipolymerase III	3

*The score is determined by adding the maximum weight or score in each category. Patients with scores ≥9 have definite systemic sclerosis (SSc).

ACR, American College of Rheumatology; *EULAR,* European League Against Rheumatism; *ILD,* interstitial lung disease; *MCP,* metacarpophalangeal; *PAH,* pulmonary arterial hypertension; *SSc,* systemic sclerosis.
From Hochberg MC: *Rheumatology,* ed 7, Philadelphia, 2019, Elsevier.

TABLE 1 Overview of Musculoskeletal Complications of Systemic Sclerosis

Manifestation	Clinical Features	Serologic Associations
Contractures	Typical feature of dcSSc Associated with ARA positivity Palmar fibrosis	ARA, ATA, RF, ACPA
Tendonitis or tendon friction rubs	Overlap arthritis	ARA
Arthritis	May resemble RA in overlap Associated with RF positivity and ACPA positivity More with U1RNP reactivity Contributes to deformity and contractures May have Jaccoud pattern but with fixed deformity	U1RNP, ACPA, RF
Myositis	Minor elevation in CK common, especially in dcSSc Weakness and loss of muscle bulk Severe myositis less frequent Overlap syndromes with myositis most common Serologic associations include anti–PM-Scl, antiU1RNP, antifibrillarin	U1RNP, PM-Scl, U3RNP
Acroosteolysis	More common in environmentally triggered SSc Association with vasculopathy and Raynaud phenomenon Possible association with calcinosis	ACA, ATA

ACA, Anticentromere; *ACPA,* anticyclic citrullinated protein antibody; *ARA,* anti-RNA polymerase III antibody; *ATA,* antitopoisomerase; *CK,* creatine kinase; *dcSSc,* diffuse cutaneous systemic sclerosis; *PM-Scl,* antipolymyositis scleroderma antibody; *RA,* rheumatoid arthritis; *RF,* rheumatoid factor; *SSc,* systemic sclerosis; *U1RNP,* anti–U1-ribonucleoprotein antibody; *U3RNP,* anti–U3-ribonucleoprotein antibody.
From Hochberg MC: *Rheumatology,* ed 7, Philadelphia, 2019, Elsevier.

S

TABLE 4 Distinguishing Features of Scleroderma and Scleroderma-Like Conditions

Condition	Skin Changes and Distribution	Extradermal Involvement	Dermatopathology	Other
Localized scleroderma	Amorphous plaques (morphea) or lines involving the face (linear) and extremities and sparing the fingers	None	Dermal sclerosis, mononuclear inflammation	Linear especially common in children, autoantibodies common
Scleredema	Trunk, back, neck	Rare	Swollen collagen bundles, mucin accumulation	
Scleromyxedema	Induration, sclerodactyly Limited mouth opening	Rare	Excessive dermal mucin deposition	Serum paraprotein (especially IgG λ)
Nephrogenic systemic fibrosis	Extremities, fingers; symmetric	Frequent, mild (muscle, fascia, lungs)	Fibroblast proliferation, mucin deposition, dermal spindle cell proliferation	After gadolinium exposure in end-stage renal disease
Eosinophilic fasciitis	Extremities, trunk; spares fingers	Rare; low-grade myositis	Dermal and hypodermal sclerosis, normal epidermis, muscle inflammation occasionally	Peripheral blood eosinophilia frequent

From Hochberg MC: *Rheumatology,* ed 7, Philadelphia, 2019, Elsevier.

TABLE 5 Autoantigens and Autoantibodies in Scleroderma

Autoantigen	Molecular Structure	Autoantibody Frequency
Scl-70	100-kD native and 70-kD degradation product; DNA topoisomerase I	75% in diffuse scleroderma; 20%-59% in all patients; 13% in CREST
Centromere	Proteins 17, 80, and 140 kD; localized at inner and outer kinetochore plates	57%-82% in CREST; 8% in diffuse form
RNA Pol I	RNA Pol I complex of subunit proteins, 210-211 kD	4%-30% in scleroderma; 13% in diffuse form
RNA Pol II	Transcripts mRNA	4%
RNA Pol III	Transcripts 5S rRNA, tRNA	23% in scleroderma; 45% in diffuse form; 6% in CREST
Fibrillarin	Protein 34 kD, component of U3 RNP particle	6%-8%; 5% in diffuse form; 10% in CREST
U1nRNP	Spliceosome complex	2%-5% in all patients; 24% in PM/scleroderma overlap
PM-Scl	Complex of 11 proteins, 110-120 kD	4%-11%; 24% in PM/scleroderma overlap
Ku	DNA-binding protein	1%-14% in scleroderma; 26%-55% in PM/scleroderma overlap
Th/To	Protein 40 kD, complexes with 7S and 8S RNAs	1%-13% in scleroderma; 1%-11% in diffuse form; 8%-19% in CREST; up to 3% in PM/scleroderma overlap
NOR-90	Protein 90 kD, human upstream binding factor, localized in nucleolus organizer region	Rare

CREST, Calcinosis, Raynaud phenomenon, esophageal dysfunction, sclerodactyly, and telangiectasia; *DNA,* deoxyribonucleic acid; *mRNA,* messenger RNA; *PM,* polymyositis; *RNA,* ribonucleic acid; *RNP,* ribonucleoprotein; *rRNA,* ribosomal RNA; *tRNA,* transfer RNA. From McPherson RA, Pincus MR: *Henry's clinical diagnosis and management by laboratory methods,* ed 23, Philadelphia, 2017, Elsevier.

lesions, telangiectasias, abnormal nailfold capillaries, RP, PAH/ILD, and SSc-related autoantibodies).

DIFFERENTIAL DIAGNOSIS
DERMATOLOGIC:
- Scleroderma
- Amyloidosis
- Porphyria cutanea tarda
- Eosinophilic fasciitis
- Reflex sympathetic dystrophy
- Nephrogenic systemic fibrosis
- Table 4 summarizes distinguishing features of scleroderma and scleroderma-like conditions

SYSTEMIC:
- Idiopathic pulmonary fibrosis
- Primary pulmonary hypertension
- Primary biliary cirrhosis
- Cardiomyopathies
- Gastrointestinal dysmotility problems
- Systemic lupus erythematosus and overlap syndromes

WORKUP
Laboratory tests and imaging studies

LABORATORY TESTS
- Antinuclear antibodies: Nucleolar (more common), homogeneous, or speckled patterns
- Rheumatoid factor positive in 20% of patients
- Routine biochemistry tests may indicate specific organ involvement (e.g., liver, kidney, muscle); should check complete blood count with differential, creatine kinase, comprehensive metabolic panel, urinalysis

The following extractable nuclear antigens are either present or absent in SSc:
- Anticentromere antibodies: Generally positive in one third of patients with lcSSc
- Anti-Scl-70 antibody (antitopoisomerase I): Positive in 40% of patients with dcSSc and has an increased risk of developing ILD
- Anti-RNA polymerase III antibody: Portends a worse prognosis, with rapidly progressive skin fibrosis and increased risk of developing SRC.[4] May also indicate increased cancer risk
- Antiribonucleoprotein (anti-RNP): Positive in 20%, can see with overlap conditions
- Other possible antibodies include U3 RNP, U1 RNP, PM-Scl, Th/To, Anti-Ku
- Table 5 summarizes autoantigens and autoantibodies in scleroderma

IMAGING & OTHER STUDIES
- Arthritis: Joint radiographs
- Gastrointestinal:
  1. Upper endoscopy (diagnostic procedure of choice; may be therapeutic)
  2. Cine-esophagography (in rare circumstances)
  3. Barium swallow (occasionally indicated)
  4. Esophageal manometry
- Pulmonary:
  1. Chest x-ray examination

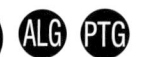
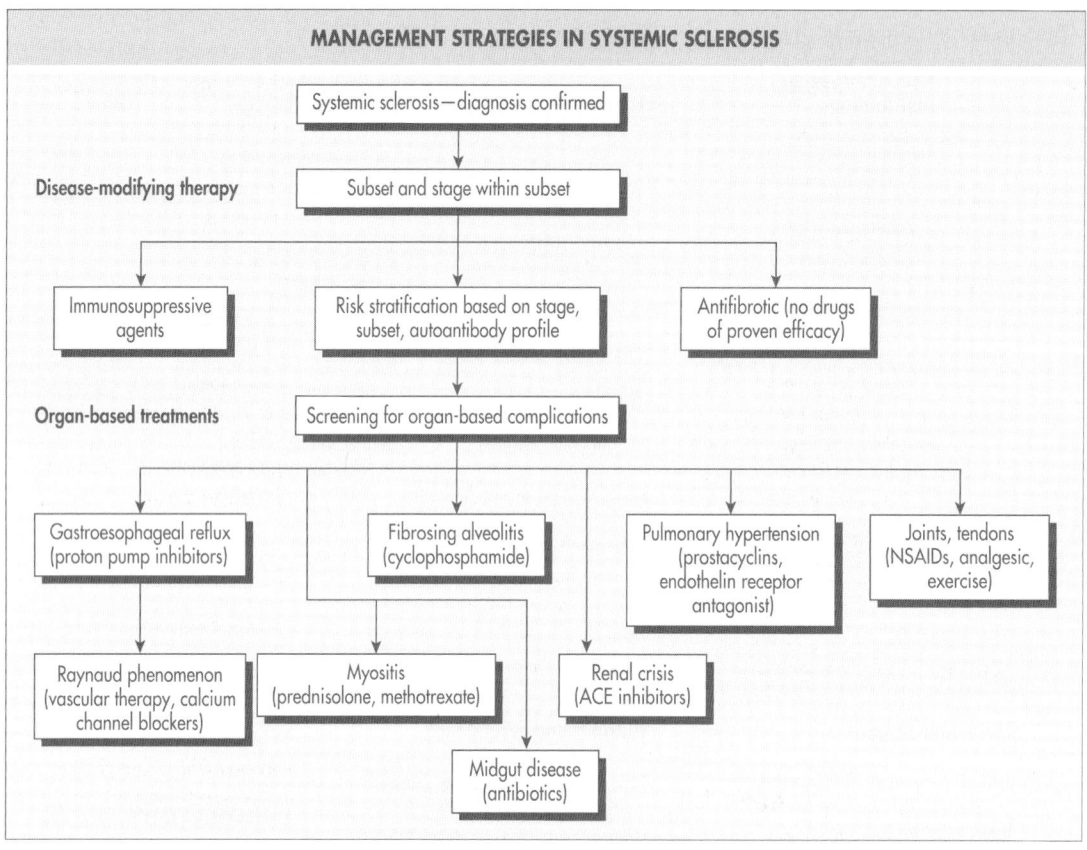

FIG. 9 Management of scleroderma requires multiple strategies depending on the specific problems that are present in individual patients. *ACE,* Angiotensin-converting enzyme; *NSAID,* nonsteroidal antiinflammatory drug. (From Hochberg MC: *Rheumatology,* ed 7, Philadelphia, 2019, Elsevier.)

2. Pulmonary function tests (especially single-breath diffusion capacity for carbon monoxide—DLCO)
3. Thoracic high-resolution computed tomography scan
4. Bronchoscopy with biopsy, bronchoalveolar lavage
- Cardiac:
  1. ECG
  2. Ambulatory (Holter) ECG monitoring
  3. Echocardiography (screen for pulmonary arterial hypertension)
  4. Cardiac catheterization
- Kidney: Renal biopsy
- Skin: Skin biopsy
- Vascular: Nailfold capillaroscopy

TREATMENT

Currently, there is no disease-modifying therapy available for SSc. However, the internal organ involvement of the disease is generally treatable. Fig. 9 and Table 6 illustrate management strategies in SSc. Immunosuppressive agents are used in individual patients. Prednisone should be used with extreme caution, especially in doses >20 mg/day (can precipitate SRC).[4,5]
- RP:
  1. Keep hands and body warm
  2. Avoid smoking and using vasoconstricting drugs

3. Calcium channel blockers (i.e., long-acting dihydropyridines)[5]
4. Peripheral α1-adrenergic blockers
5. Angiotensin II receptor blockers
6. Topical nitrate
7. Phosphodiesterase inhibitors[5]
8. Stellate ganglion blockades
9. Digital sympathectomy
10. Table E7 summarizes vascular therapies for RP
- Arthralgias: NSAIDs or low-dose corticosteroids (5-10 mg of prednisone per day)
- Myositis: Methotrexate or azathioprine with low-dose corticosteroids
- Skin: For skin fibrosis, immunomodulatory drugs have been used, generally started within 3 yr of onset (methotrexate,[5] mycophenolate mofetil[6]). Cyclophosphamide can be used for refractory or rapidly progressive involvement. Table E8 summarizes immunomodulatory and antifibrotic strategies for disease-modifying treatment of systemic sclerosis skin disease
- GI tract: Table E9 summarizes treatment of GI tract complications in systemic sclerosis
- Esophageal reflux:
  1. H2-receptor blockers[2,5]
  2. Proton pump inhibitors[2,5]
- ILD:
  1. Mycophenolate mofetil or cyclophosphamide for symptomatic ILD[5,6]

2. Nintedanib, a small molecule that inhibits several kinases linked to the pathogenesis of ILDs (receptor tyrosine kinases and nonreceptor tyrosine kinases), recently received FDA approval for the treatment of ILD associated with systemic sclerosis.[7]
3. Lung transplantation for patients with advanced pulmonary involvement
- Pulmonary hypertension (Fig. E10):
  1. Oxygen
  2. Diuretics (with caution)
  3. Prostacyclins (epoprostenol,[5] iloprost,[5] reprostinil)
  4. Endothelin-1 receptor inhibitors (bosentan,[5,8] ambrisentan)
  5. Phosphodiesterase 5 inhibitors (sildenafil, tadalafil)[5]
  6. Table E10 summarizes approved therapies for treatment of pulmonary arterial hypertension
- Renal involvement (Fig. E11):
  1. ACE inhibitors[5]
  2. Dialysis
  3. Renal transplantation

REFERRAL

Rheumatology consultation is indicated. Consider pulmonary, cardiology, or gastrointestinal consultations depending on organ involvement.

TABLE 6 Current Recommendations for Treatment of Scleroderma

Manifestation	Primary Therapy	Alternative/Second-Line Therapy
Raynaud phenomenon	Vasodilators (CCB or PDE5 inhibitors) Antiplatelet	PDE5 inhibitors, prostacyclin, ETA
Hypertensive renal disease	ACE inhibitors	ARBs, CCB, prostacyclin, renal transplant (wait at least 12 mo)
GI involvement	**Upper GI** Dental/periodontal care, lifestyle modifications, proton pump inhibitors, prokinetics	EGD to treat stenosis and/or GAVE
	Lower GI Probiotics, rotational antibiotics	Prokinetics Total parenteral nutrition
Skin	Mycophenolate mofetil, cyclophosphamide	IVIG, ATG, HSCT (severe, progressive cases), research trial
Interstitial lung disease	Mycophenolate mofetil, cyclophosphamide	Research trial (novel biologics and antifibrotic drugs)
Pulmonary arterial hypertension	PDE5 inhibitors, ETA, combination (PDE5i+ETA), prostacyclin, PRA, soluble guanylate-cyclase stimulators	Combination therapy, atrioseptostomy, lung transplant, research trial
Cardiac involvement	Heart failure therapy, diuretics, CCB	Immunosuppression, IVIG (myocardial inflammation)
Joints	Prednisone, methotrexate, TNF inhibitors, rituximab, tocilizumab	IVIG (if contractures and rubs are present), PT/OT
Muscles	Prednisone, methotrexate, azathioprine	IVIG
Psychosocial	Antidepressants, pain control, sleep control	Support group

ACE, Angiotensin-converting enzyme; *ARBs,* angiotensin receptor blockers; *ATG,* antithymocyte globulin; *CCB,* calcium channel blockers; *EGD,* esophagogastroduodenoscopy; *ETA,* endothelin receptor antagonist; *GAVE,* gastric antral vascular ectasia; *GI,* gastrointestinal; *HSCT,* hematopoietic stem cell transplantation; *IVIG,* intravenous immunoglobulin; *PDE5,* phosphodiesterase-5 inhibitor; *PRA,* prostacyclin IP receptor agonist; *PT/OT,* physical therapy/occupational therapy.
From Firestein GS et al: *Firestein & Kelley's textbook of rheumatology,* ed 11, Philadelphia, 2021, Elsevier.

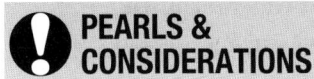

PEARLS & CONSIDERATIONS

COMMENTS
Autologous hematopoietic stem cell therapy (HSCT) has shown some benefit in patients with severe diffuse cutaneous systemic sclerosis, but there was greater treatment-related mortality and morbidity associated with HSCT.[5,9-12]

REFERENCES
Available at eBooks.Health.Elsevier.com.

RELATED CONTENT
Scleroderma (Patient Information)

AUTHORS: **MOHNISH NADELLA, BS,** and **MANUEL F. DASILVA, MD**

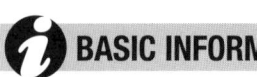

ⓘ BASIC INFORMATION

DEFINITION

Seborrheic dermatitis (SD) is a common inflammatory skin condition characterized by a mild to severe rash with scaling, erythema, and pruritus that occurs in areas of the skin rich in sebaceous glands.

SYNONYMS

SD
Dandruff
Cradle cap (Fig. E1)
Sebopsoriasis
Seborrheic eczema
Pityriasis wapitis
Seborrhea

ICD-10CM CODES
L21.9   Seborrheic dermatitis, unspecified
L21.1   Seborrheic infantile dermatitis
L21.8   Other seborrheic dermatitis

EPIDEMIOLOGY & DEMOGRAPHICS

PREVALENCE: Affects 3% to 5% of otherwise healthy adults; increases to 34% to 83% in immunocompromised patients
PREDOMINANT SEX & AGE: Can occur from infancy through old age, with peak incidence in adolescents and young adults and increasing again after age 50 yr. More common in men than women.
RISK FACTORS: More common in patients with HIV/AIDS, Parkinson disease, other neurologic disorders, mood disorders, chronic alcoholic pancreatitis, hepatitis, cancer, and genetic disorders (e.g., Down syndrome). Recent evidence linking obesity and metabolic syndrome with an increased occurrence of SD. Occurs more often during winter season and during periods of increased stress. Incidence of SD has increased with the use of facial masks during the COVID-19 pandemic.

PHYSICAL FINDINGS & CLINICAL PRESENTATION

- Mild, greasy scaling of the scalp and nasolabial folds (Fig. E2); postauricular skin (Fig. E3), beard area, eyebrows, trunk, and sometimes the central face. Blepharitis, otitis externa, and coexisting acne vulgaris or pityriasis may also be present. Itching and stinging of lesions can occur. Increased occurrence during times of stress or sleep deprivation.
- The scale often has a yellow, greasy appearance.

ETIOLOGY

Newer studies indicate that defects in the immune system may trigger proliferation of the *Malassezia* yeast and the associated skin changes. Patients with SD may show upregulation of interferon (IFN)-α, expressed interleukin-6 (IL-6), expressed IL-1β, and IL-4.

ⒹⓍ DIAGNOSIS

DIFFERENTIAL DIAGNOSIS

- Atopic dermatitis
- Candidiasis
- Dermatophytosis
- Impetigo
- Psoriasis
- Rosacea
- Systemic lupus erythematosus
- Tinea infection
- Contact dermatitis
- Nummular dermatitis

WORKUP

- Diagnosis usually based on clinical identification of lesions (distribution and appearance).
- Skin biopsies can be performed, if warranted, to distinguish SD from similar disorders.

LABORATORY TESTS

- Microscopic examination with special stains can be used to determine whether yeast cells are present in keratinocytes.
- Biopsy can demonstrate parakeratosis in the epidermis, plugged follicular ostia, and spongiosis.
- HIV testing.

ⓡ TREATMENT

NONPHARMACOLOGIC THERAPY

- Patient education that SD is a chronic condition and treatment is aimed at resolving lesions but does not prevent recurrence.
- General recommendations: Wash skin regularly, soften and remove scales, and apply moisturizing emollients after washing.
- Scale removal can be accomplished through the application of mineral or olive oil and removed with a comb or brush after 1 hr.

ACUTE GENERAL Rx

- Antifungals (e.g., Nizoral, selenium sulfide, ketoconazole 2% [the most evidence for effectiveness among antifungals], ciclopirox, terbinafine, miconazole). Considered first-line therapy. Shampoos should be kept on the skin for 5 min before washing off. Antifungal therapy is associated with fewer adverse effects than topical steroids.
- Reserve oral antifungal therapy for patients with widespread SD or SD that is refractory to topical therapy.
- Topical steroids: Can be in the form of shampoos, creams, or ointments. Can be used alone or in more severe SD with antifungals. Low-to-moderate potency steroids are preferred. Desonide and mometasone display the lowest recurrence rates and highest clearance. Avoid prolonged use due to side effects.
- Immunomodulators/calcineurin inhibitors (e.g., tacrolimus ointment, pimecrolimus cream): Good when face and ears are affected. Limit use due to potential side effects. Can be used in combination with topical nonsteroidal

antiinflammatory agents. Excellent modality for patients with skin of color.
- Keratolytics (e.g., coal tar, salicylic acid, zinc pyrithione).
- Other topical modalities for consideration: Nonsteroidal antiinflammatory agents (e.g., Promiseb cream, bisabolol, glycyrrhetinic acid, lactoferrin, selenium sulfide, lithium gluconate/succinate ointment, metronidazole gel).
- Treatment of any secondary bacterial infection with oral antibiotics.

CHRONIC Rx

- Recalcitrant SD: Topical azole combined with desonide regimen (limit use to 2 wk), pimecrolimus cream
- Systemic treatment (moderate to severe SD)
  1. Oral terbinafine (daily for 4 to 6 wk), itraconazole (200 mg daily) and fluconazole (weekly dosing for 4 wk)—mainstay of therapy
  2. Prednisone (0.5 mg/g/day) for 15 days—avoid prolonged or frequent use
  3. Isotretinoin (0.1 mg/kg/day every other day) for 6 mo

COMPLEMENTARY & ALTERNATIVE MEDICINE

- Borage and tea tree oil (melaleuca oil)
- Crude honey
- Aloe vera
- *Quassia amara* (extract from South African tree)

REFERRAL

Consider referral to dermatology for recalcitrant cases or uncertain diagnosis.

ⓘ PEARLS & CONSIDERATIONS

- Use a combination of topical steroids and antifungal cream for severe SD.
- Limit use of steroids to 2-wk course of treatment due to risk of cutaneous atrophy and telangiectasias.
- SD of the scalp can be treated with an antifungal (e.g., 2% ketoconazole) or keratolytic shampoo. Limit use of antifungal shampoos to twice a week to prevent drying of the scalp. Alternate the use of antifungal shampoos with a moisturizing shampoo.
- In patients with widespread SD, consider testing for HIV infection. In patients with HIV/AIDS, the severity of seborrheic dermatitis is inversely correlated with the CDs counts.

SUGGESTED READINGS
Available at eBooks.Health.Elsevier.com.

RELATED CONTENT
Seborrheic Dermatitis (Patient Information)

AUTHOR: **ANNGENE ANTHONY, MD, MPH, FAAFP**

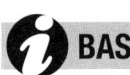
S

Diseases and Disorders

I

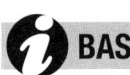 BASIC INFORMATION

DEFINITION

Tonic clonic seizures are characterized by sudden loss of consciousness, muscle contraction (tonic phase), followed by rhythmic jerking activity (clonic phase).

SYNONYMS

Bilateral tonic-clonic seizures
Convulsive seizures
Grand mal seizures
Generalized tonic clonic seizures

ICD-10CM CODES
G40.6   Grand mal seizures, unspecified
G41.0   Grand mal status epilepticus

EPIDEMIOLOGY & DEMOGRAPHICS

INCIDENCE: 40 to 70 cases per 100,000 person-year (epilepsy incidence)[1]
PREVALENCE: 4 to 12 cases/1000 persons (epilepsy prevalence)[1]
PREDOMINANT SEX & AGE: No gender preference
PEAK INCIDENCE: Not applicable

PHYSICAL FINDINGS & CLINICAL PRESENTATION

- Patients with unprovoked tonic clonic seizures usually have normal physical and neurologic examinations.[2]
- A generalized seizure may start without warning and can typically last from 1 to 3 minutes, during which the patient will be unconscious and may have increased rigidity and/or jerking of the whole body, or staring spells. Cyanosis (especially of the lips and face) can result from temporary airway compromise due to muscle spasms. Tonic-clonic seizures can cause injuries, tongue biting, and bladder incontinence.[3] Patients are usually unaware of the seizure afterwards. A post-ictal state characterized by confusion, lethargy, headaches, or drowsiness may result and can last from minutes to hours depending on the severity of the seizure (Fig. 1).
- Tonic clonic seizures are associated with injuries, bladder incontinence, and tongue biting.[3]
- Any warning or aura before onset of the seizure or focal post-ictal weakness (Todd paralysis) may point toward a focal neurologic lesion.[2]

ETIOLOGY

- Seizures are a cardinal sign of cortical neurologic injury. Generalized seizures include both hemispheres of the brain at onset. However, seizures can start focally and then quickly generalize across both hemispheres of the brain and be almost identical to primary generalized seizures. Any warning or aura symptoms before the generalized seizure starts would point to a focal onset.
- Acute symptomatic generalized seizures can be due to systemic causes (e.g., systemic infections, meningitis, encephalitis, electrolyte abnormalities, hypoglycemia, hyperthyroidism, malignant hypertension, eclampsia, drug intoxication or withdrawal).[4]
- Generalized seizures are seen in many epilepsy syndromes with genetic causes.[3]

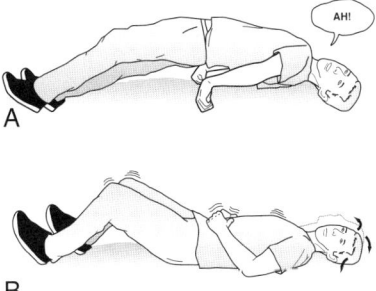

FIG. 1 A, This man in the tonic phase of a tonic-clonic seizure arches his torso and extends his arms and legs. He assumes this position because of the relatively greater strength of the extensor muscles compared to the flexor muscles. Simultaneous diaphragm, chest wall, and laryngeal muscle contractions force air through his tightened larynx to produce the shrill "epileptic cry." During this phase, he may also bite his tongue and lose control of his urine. **B,** In the clonic phase, his head, neck, and legs contract symmetrically and forcefully for about 10 to 20 seconds. Saliva, aerated and often blood-tinged from tongue lacerations, froths from his mouth. His pupils dilate, and he sweats profusely. Finally, his muscular contractions lose strength. The seizure usually ends with stertorous breathing. In the immediate post-ictal period, he remains unresponsive. Before regaining consciousness, he may pass through a state of confusion and agitation. (From Kaufman DM et al: *Kaufman's clinical neurology for psychiatrists,* ed 8, Philadelphia, 2017, Elsevier.)

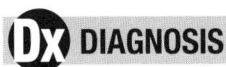 DIAGNOSIS

DIFFERENTIAL DIAGNOSIS

- Convulsive syncope
- Psychogenic nonepileptic spells, conversion disorder, somatic symptom disorder, dissociative disorder
- Focal seizure with secondary generalization
- Transient ischemic attack
- Vertigo
- Factitious disorder
- Malingering
- Myoclonus (from metabolic disturbance)

WORKUP

- Electroencephalogram (EEG) (Fig. 2). An EEG can help confirm the presence of epilepsy but cannot be used to exclude the diagnosis.[5]
- Ambulatory EEG and/or video EEG recommended for patients with diagnostic uncertainty.[5]

LABORATORY TESTS

- Routine blood workup (CBC, comprehensive metabolic panel, glucose, electrolytes)[2]

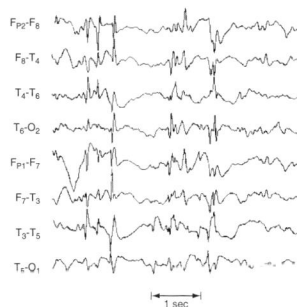

FIG. 2 During a tonic-clonic seizure, the EEG ideally shows paroxysms of spikes, polyspikes, and occasional slow waves in all channels; however, muscle artifact can obscure this pattern. Even during interictal periods, the EEG contains multiple bursts of generalized spikes in the background. In contrast to occasional temporal lobe spikes, this pattern confirms a diagnosis of epilepsy in patients with seizures. (From Kaufman DM et al: *Kaufman's clinical neurology for psychiatrists.* ed 8, Philadelphia, 2017, Elsevier.)

- Urine drug screen[2]
- Lumbar puncture is recommended in patients with suspicion of meningitis

IMAGING STUDIES

- Neurodiagnostic imaging studies such as computed tomography (CT) of the head or, preferably, MRI of the brain should be performed in all patients with first unprovoked seizure.[2]
- CT scans of the head should be avoided in children due to unnecessary exposure to radiation and the low yield of the test.[6] CT scans of the head are reserved for neurologic emergencies and are adjusted for weight in children.

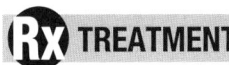 TREATMENT

ACUTE Rx

- The immediate management of a seizure focuses on stabilization of the patient with focus on the airway and vital signs and rapid identification and correction of reversible causes.
- Seizures lasting >5 min or multiple seizures without return to baseline in between should be treated as status epilepticus.[7]
- Treatment is based on the type and etiology of seizures (i.e., metabolic disturbance, infectious, etc.).[2]
- Provoked seizures due to metabolic derangements, infections, fever, alcohol, or drug withdrawal are typically generalized and likely do not need long-term treatment.[2]
- Multiple antiseizure medication choices are available. Choice depends on side effect profile as well as whether the seizure started focally or is secondary to an idiopathic generalized epilepsy syndrome.[2]

NONPHARMACOLOGIC THERAPY

Not applicable

GENERAL Rx

- Patients with a first unprovoked seizure who have a normal EEG, imaging, lab values, and physical exam do not require treatment with antiseizure medications but may be offered therapy because the use of an antiseizure medication after a first unprovoked seizure In an adult reduces the absolute risk of seizure recurrence at 2 yr by 35%. However, there is no difference at 3 yr. This decision should be made in conjunction with the patient and should take into consideration the patient's job, risks of medications, and individual preferences.[2]
- Patients with two or more unprovoked seizures, or those with one seizure and an abnormal workup consistent with epilepsy findings, should be started or continued on antiseizure medications. Patients on antiseizure therapy with negative workup may be considered for weaning off antiseizure medication if seizure-free after 2 yr.[2]
- Primary generalized epilepsies:
  1. Levetiracetam (Keppra): Initial dose 250 to 500 bid, maximum dose 2000 mg bid.
  2. Lamotrigine (Lamictal): Initial dose 25 mg daily and increase slowly to goal dose 200 to 300 mg daily (depends on combination of other medications).
  3. Topiramate (Topamax): Initial dose 25 mg bid and increase to usual dose of 100 to 400 mg bid.
  4. Perampanel (Fycompa): Initial dose of 2 mg once daily at bedtime, increments of 2 mg once daily at weekly intervals to a recommended maintenance dose of 4 to 8 mg (adjunctive treatment in patients with epilepsy 12 yr of age and older).
  5. Valproic acid (Depakote): Initial dose: 10 to 15 mg/kg/day (divided bid), maximum dose 60 mg/kg/day. Valproic acid should be avoided in girls and women with child-bearing potential due to the risk of teratogenicity.[4]
- Focal epilepsies with secondary generalization: Almost all antiseizure medications are approved for focal seizures, either in monotherapy or in adjunct. Carbamazepine, oxcarbazepine, eslicarbazepine, lamotrigine, levetiracetam, or lacosamide are all possibilities, among others.
- Patients who continue to have seizures despite adequate trials on at least two antiseizure medications should be referred to a tertiary care epilepsy center for evaluation of surgical treatment of epilepsy.

DISPOSITION

- Patients should avoid situations that may cause injuries or accidents in the event of a seizure, such as climbing ladders, swimming unsupervised, or taking baths (rather than showers).
- No driving until seizure-free in accordance with local laws and regulations.

REFERRAL

Patients with epilepsy and seizures should be referred for a consultation by a neurologist.

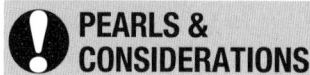

❗ PEARLS & CONSIDERATIONS

COMMENTS

- It is crucial to understand that tonic-clonic seizures can occur in a variety of acute neurologic diseases.
- Successful treatment depends on the correct choice of antiseizure medications based on the type (focal onset vs. generalized onset) and etiology of the seizures.
- All women of childbearing age taking antiseizure medications should take folic acid supplementation (1 to 4 mg/day) for the prevention of neural tube defects.
- Many antiseizure medications also affect vitamin D absorption or metabolism, prompting attention to patients' bone health.

PREVENTION

Sleep deprivation and alcohol consumption should be avoided.

PATIENT & FAMILY EDUCATION

Patients with ongoing seizures are forbidden to drive; check your state regulations and laws regarding driving and epilepsy.

REFERENCES

Available at eBooks.Health.Elsevier.com.

RELATED CONTENT

Generalized Tonic-Clonic Seizures (Patient Information)
Status Epilepticus (Related Key Topic)

AUTHOR: **PEDRO BALAGUERA, MD**

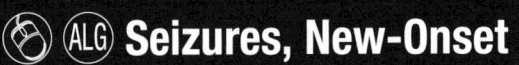

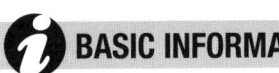 **BASIC INFORMATION**

DEFINITION

An unprovoked seizure is a seizure that occurs without triggers or precipitating factors. In contrast, an acute symptomatic seizure occurs in the setting of an insult to the brain (infectious, toxic, etc.).[1,2] The presentation of a new seizure can vary greatly depending on the type (focal or generalized), progression, and severity.

Epilepsy is a disorder of the brain characterized by an enduring predisposition to generate seizures. For epidemiologic and, commonly, for clinical purposes, epilepsy is considered present when two or more unprovoked seizures occur in a time frame of longer than 24 h or after a single event that occurs in a person who is considered to have a high risk of recurrence (>60% risk in a 10-yr period).[3,4] A classification of seizure descriptions is summarized in Box 1.

SYNONYM

Convulsions

ICD-10CM CODES

G40.001	Localization-related (focal) (partial) idiopathic epilepsy and epileptic syndromes with seizures of localized onset, not intractable, with status epilepticus
G40.009	Localization-related (focal) (partial) idiopathic epilepsy and epileptic syndromes with seizures of localized onset, not intractable, without status epilepticus
G40.10	Localization-related (focal) (partial) symptomatic epilepsy and epileptic syndromes with simple partial seizures, not intractable
G40.101	Localization-related (focal) (partial) symptomatic epilepsy and epileptic syndromes with simple partial seizures, not intractable, with status epilepticus
G40.109	Localization-related (focal) (partial) symptomatic epilepsy and epileptic syndromes with simple partial seizures, not intractable, without status epilepticus
G40.201	Localization-related (focal) (partial) symptomatic epilepsy and epileptic syndromes with complex partial seizures, not intractable, with status epilepticus
G40.209	Localization-related (focal) (partial) symptomatic epilepsy and epileptic syndromes with complex partial seizures, not intractable, without status epilepticus
G40.301	Generalized idiopathic epilepsy and epileptic syndromes, not intractable, with status epilepticus
G40.309	Generalized idiopathic epilepsy and epileptic syndromes, not intractable, without status epilepticus
G40.A01	Absence epileptic syndrome, not intractable, with status epilepticus
G40.A09	Absence epileptic syndrome, not intractable, without status epilepticus
G40.4	Other generalized epilepsy and epileptic syndromes
G40.401	Other generalized epilepsy and epileptic syndromes, not intractable, with status epilepticus
G40.409	Other generalized epilepsy and epileptic syndromes, not intractable, without status epilepticus
G40.501	Epileptic seizures related to external causes, not intractable, with status epilepticus
G40.509	Epileptic seizures related to external causes, not intractable, without status epilepticus
G40.909	Epilepsy, unspecified, not intractable, without status epilepticus

---

BOX 1 Classification of Seizure Descriptions (International League Against Epilepsy, 2017 Revision, Modified)

Focal onset
Aware vs. impaired awareness (formerly called complex partial)
Motor onset vs. nonmotor onset
Focal to bilateral tonic-clonic (formerly called secondarily generalized)
Generalized onset
Motor
Tonic-clonic (formerly called grand mal)
Other motor: Myoclonic, tonic
Nonmotor: Absence
Unknown onset
Motor
Tonic-clonic
Other motor: Myoclonic, tonic
Nonmotor: Absence
Unclassified

EPIDEMIOLOGY & DEMOGRAPHICS

INCIDENCE: 29 to 39 per 100,000 per yr for acute symptomatic seizures. 23 to 61 per 100,000 person-yr for unprovoked seizures.[1] Approximately 8% to 10% of the population will experience a seizure during their lifetime; however, less than 3% go on to develop epilepsy
PREVALENCE: 5 to 8.4 cases per 1000 persons
PREDOMINANT SEX & AGE: Males younger than 12 mo and older than 65 yr[1]
RISK FACTORS[1]:
- Age of onset
- Family history of epilepsy
- Excessive sleep deprivation, use of alcohol, or illicit drugs
- History of head trauma, diseases of the brain, brain surgeries, and strokes
- History of congenital cerebral anomalies or developmental delay
GENETICS: Although some new onset seizures are related to specific genes, most are not

PHYSICAL FINDINGS & CLINICAL PRESENTATION

- Patients with generalized seizures will typically have normal physical exams. Patients with focal seizures due to persistent structural CNS damage may have exam findings consistent with the location of the lesion.
- A generalized seizure may start without warning[5] and can typically last from 30 to 120 sec, during which the patient will be unconscious and may have increased rigidity and/or jerking of the whole body, or staring spells. Cyanosis (especially of the lips and face) can result from temporary airway compromise due to muscle spasms. Tonic-clonic seizures can cause injuries, tongue biting, and bladder incontinence. Patients are usually unaware of the seizure afterwards. A post-ictal state characterized by confusion, lethargy, headaches, or drowsiness may result and can last from minutes to hours depending on the severity of the seizure.
- During a focal seizure, a patient may be aware (focal aware seizure) or have impaired consciousness (focal impaired awareness seizures).[6] A focal impaired awareness seizure may be associated with an aura (itself a focal aware seizure) and lasts between 30 and 120 sec. Motor or nonmotor symptoms may predominate in focal seizures, including jerking of one limb, automatisms, head turning, auditory hallucinations, or feelings of derealization. A focal seizure may progress to a generalized seizure, which usually involves the head and eye turning to one side. Post-ictal weakness may result after focal seizures and can last for hours but usually resolves within 1 day. Patients with associated focal neurologic deficits, fever, persistent headache, cognitive changes, or a recent history of head trauma should be investigated.

ETIOLOGY (TABLE 1)

- New, unprovoked seizures are often idiopathic.
- Acute symptomatic seizures can be due to cerebral abnormalities (e.g., infections/abscesses, subarachnoid hemorrhages, ischemic strokes, tumors, vascular malformations) or systemic causes (e.g., systemic infections, electrolyte abnormalities, hypoglycemia, hyperthyroidism, malignant hypertension, drug intoxication or withdrawal).[2]

DX **DIAGNOSIS**

DIFFERENTIAL DIAGNOSIS[5,7]

- Syncope
- Transient ischemic attacks
- Migraines
- Sleep disorders
- Paroxysmal movement disorders
- Panic attacks, hallucinations, and other psychiatric disorders

WORKUP

- Ambulatory 30-min electroencephalogram (EEG) if patient fully recovers after seizure

S

Diseases and Disorders

I

TABLE 1 Causes of Seizures

Etiology	Examples
Infection and inflammation	Infective (meningo)encephalitis Chronic CNS infection (e.g., neurocysticercosis) Autoimmune limbic encephalitis (may present bizarrely) Cerebral lupus
Neoplasia	Gliomas and other primary CNS neoplasms Metastases Lymphoma
Vascular	Stroke* Subarachnoid hemorrhage* Subdural hematoma Eclampsia Hypertensive encephalopathy
Metabolic	Hyponatremia Hypoglycemia Hypocalcemia Uremia Porphyria
Trauma	Head injury* Neurosurgery*
Drugs and withdrawal	Alcohol Amphetamines, MDMA Pethidine Benzodiazepine or barbiturate withdrawal Many others
Neurodegeneration	Alzheimer disease Creutzfeldt-Jakob disease
Epilepsy	Multiple causes
Psychiatric	Psychogenic nonepileptic seizures

*May occur at the time of the insult or may occur up to years later.
From Talley NJ et al: *Essentials of internal medicine,* ed 4, Chatswood, NSW, 2021, Elsevier Australia.

within 30 to 60 min. May be delayed if treatment does not depend on EEG result.[5]
- Consider inpatient continuous EEG if patient does not fully recover within 60 min or for recurrent seizures.
- ECG.
- Fig. 1 illustrates an algorithm for the approach to the child with a suspected convulsive disorder.

LABORATORY TESTS

Comprehensive metabolic panel and urine drug screen[5]

IMAGING STUDIES

- Acutely, computed tomography (CT) of the head with and without contrast to evaluate for hemorrhage and space-occupying lesions
- Brain MRI with and without contrast with epilepsy protocol in patients with no clear provoking cause of a seizure, in consultation with a neurologist[5]

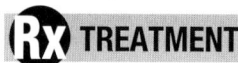 **TREATMENT**

ACUTE Rx

- The immediate management of a seizure focuses on stabilization of the patient with

focus on the airway and vital signs and rapid identification and correction of reversible causes.[8]
- Seizures lasting >5 min or multiple seizures without return to baseline in between should be treated as status epilepticus.[7]
- Treatment is based on the type and etiology of seizures (i.e., metabolic disturbance, infectious, unprovoked, etc.).[5]

CHRONIC Rx

- Provoked seizures do not need long-term treatment.[5]
- Patients with a first unprovoked seizure who have a normal EEG, imaging, lab values, and physical exam do not require treatment with

antiseizure medications but may be offered therapy because the use of an antiseizure medication after a first unprovoked seizure in an adult reduces the absolute risk of seizure recurrence at 2 yr by 35%. However, there is no difference at 3 yr.[8] This decision should be made in conjunction with the patient and should take into consideration the patient's job, risks of medications, and individual preferences.
- Patients with two or more unprovoked seizures, or those with one seizure and an abnormal workup consistent with epilepsy findings, should be started or continued on antiseizure medications. Patients on antiseizure therapy with negative workup may be

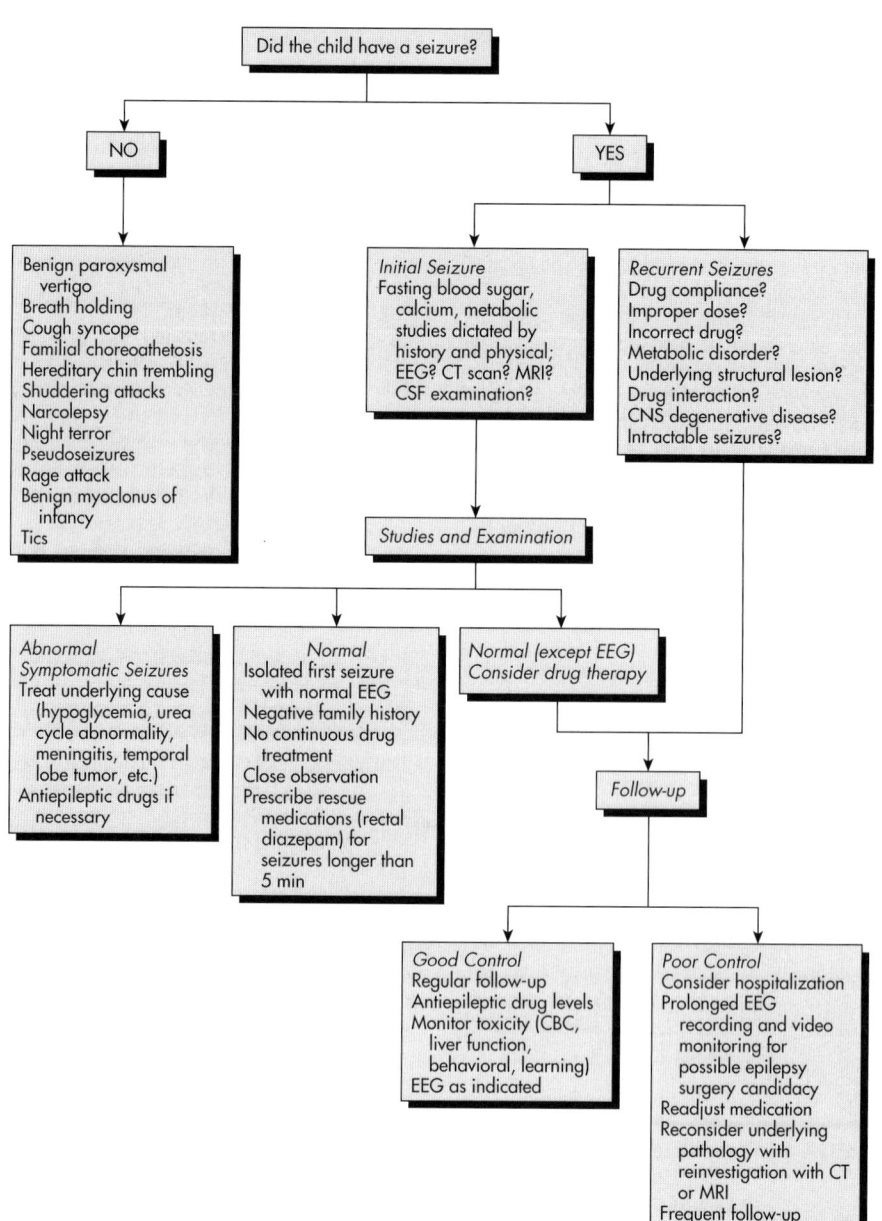

FIG. 1 **Algorithm for the approach to the child with a suspected convulsive disorder.** *CBC,* Complete blood count; *CT,* computed tomography; *CNS,* central nervous system; *CSF,* cerebrospinal fluid; *EEG,* electroencephalogram; *MRI,* magnetic resonance imaging. (From Kliegman RM: *Nelson textbook of pediatrics,* ed 21, Philadelphia, 2020, Elsevier.)

considered for weaning off antiseizure medication if seizure-free after 2 yr.[5]
- The choice of treatment depends largely on seizure type and etiology (Table E2). Antiseizure medications may be thought of as narrow- or wide-spectrum drugs. Treatment with wide-spectrum antiseizure medications is advisable in generalized seizures or those of unknown type, whereas partial seizures are better controlled with narrow-spectrum antiseizure medications.[5]
- Narrow-spectrum drugs include carbamazepine, oxcarbazepine, eslicarbazepine, gabapentin, lacosamide, and phenytoin. Wide-spectrum drugs include valproate, topiramate, zonisamide, lamotrigine, and levetiracetam.[5]
- In patients with significant comorbidities, the use of antiseizure medications with limited drug interactions is advised (lamotrigine, levetiracetam, lacosamide).[5]
- Older patients may benefit from lamotrigine, levetiracetam, or gabapentin due to a lower risk of adverse events.[5]
- Some patients may benefit from having a seizure rescue medication that could be used if they have a prolonged seizure or cluster of seizures.

DISPOSITION
- Patients should avoid swimming unobserved, bathing alone, working at heights, using heavy machinery, or other activities that may be high-risk in the event of a seizure.[5]
- Discontinue driving until seizures are well controlled and in accordance with state laws.[5]

REFERRAL
Patients should be referred to a neurologist, especially if they experience recurrent unprovoked seizures.[5]

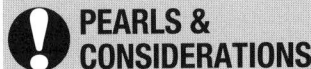

PEARLS & CONSIDERATIONS

COMMENTS
- Driving: Physicians should be aware of the law in their jurisdiction about driving after a seizure. Although a few U.S. states require physicians to notify the state government authority that issues driver's licenses, most do not impose such an obligation on physicians. However, states do require patients to self-report and abstain from driving until seizure-free for a specified period of time, depending on the state.[5]
- Recurrence risk: After a first unprovoked seizure, the overall risk of recurrence may be as high as 60% and is highest within the first 2 years. Greatest recurrence risk in an adult with a first unprovoked seizure is within the first 2 yr and is between 21% and 45%. The recurrence risk is lower in patients treated with an antiseizure medication and higher in patients with a brain MRI abnormality causing the seizure or an EEG showing epileptiform activity.[8]

PREVENTION
Patients with recurrent seizures should be extensively counseled on avoiding seizure triggers such as sleep deprivation, alcohol or drug use, stress, and exposure to excessive flashing lights. Such patients may need dose titration of antiseizure medication and referral to a neurologist.[5]

PATIENT & FAMILY EDUCATION
- Physicians should inform patients with first-time seizures that they are subject to state law restrictions on driving after a seizure.

Physicians should also counsel patients with epilepsy about not swimming unattended, not climbing heights, and taking showers rather than baths (because of the risk of drowning in a bathtub during a generalized seizure).[5] Physicians should counsel women of child-bearing potential about effects of antiseizure medications on both oral contraceptive efficacy and on a developing fetus.[5] They should recommend supplemental folic acid for such women if they are taking antiseizure medications. They should also recommend that women plan pregnancy if they are on antiseizure medications to minimize adverse effects on the pregnancy. All such counseling should be documented in the medical record.
- Patients must be informed of the potential risks of recurrent seizures, including aspiration, status epilepticus, and sudden unexpected death in epilepsy (SUDEP).
- A diagnosis of epilepsy has significant medical, social, and emotional consequences. Patient information on seizures and locating support groups can be found at the Epilepsy Foundation website: https://www.epilepsy.com.

REFERENCES
Available at eBooks.Health.Elsevier.com.

RELATED CONTENT
Absence Seizures (Related Key Topic)
Febrile Seizures (Related Key Topic)
Seizures, Generalized Tonic-Clonic (Related Key Topic)
Focal Seizures (Related Key Topic)
Status Epilepticus (Related Key Topic)

AUTHOR: **PEDRO BALAGUERA, MD**

Sepsis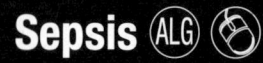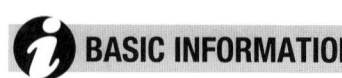

BASIC INFORMATION

DEFINITION

Sepsis is an exaggerated inflammatory response to an infectious stimulus. It is usually caused by generalized bacterial or fungal infection and characterized by evidence of infection, fever or hypothermia, hypotension, and evidence of end-organ compromise. The Sepsis Definitions Task Force in 2016 updated definitions for sepsis and septic shock (Table 1). A major change in the definitions is the elimination of mention of SIRS.* According to the new definitions, sepsis is now defined as evidence of infection plus life-threatening organ dysfunction, clinically codified by an acute change in 2 points or greater in the SOFA score (Table 2). The new clinical criteria for septic shock include sepsis with fluid, unresponsive hypotension, serum lactate level greater than 2 mmol/L, and the need for vasopressors to maintain mean arterial pressure of 65 mm Hg or greater.

SYNONYMS

Septicemia
Sepsis syndrome
Severe sepsis
Systemic inflammatory response syndrome
Septic shock

ICD-10CM CODES

A41.9	Sepsis, unspecified organism
A41.50	Gram-negative sepsis, unspecified
A41.2	Sepsis due to unspecified *Staphylococcus*
A41.4	Sepsis due to anaerobes
A41.51	Sepsis due to *Escherichia coli* [E. Coli]
A41.52	Sepsis due to Pseudomonas
A54.86	Gonococcal sepsis
B37.7	Candidal sepsis
A32.7	Listerial sepsis
A40.0	Sepsis due to streptococcus, group A
A40.1	Sepsis due to streptococcus, group B
A40.3	Sepsis due to Streptococcus pneumoniae
A40.8	Other streptococcal sepsis
A40.9	Streptococcal sepsis, unspecified
A41.01	Sepsis due to Methicillin susceptible *Staphylococcus aureus*
A41.02	Sepsis due to Methicillin resistant *Staphylococcus aureus*

EPIDEMIOLOGY & DEMOGRAPHICS

INCIDENCE (IN U.S.):

- Sepsis occurs in 6% of hospitalized patients; approximately half require intensive care unit (ICU) admission.
- More than 1 million cases of sepsis occur each year in the U.S. 15% of sepsis patients die in the hospital; 6% are discharged to hospice.

PREDOMINANT SEX: Males are slightly more commonly affected than females.

PREDOMINANT AGE:

- Neonatal period.
- Patients >65 yr of age account for 60% of all cases of sepsis.

GENETICS:

- Familial disposition: A great variety of congenital immunodeficiency states and other inherited disorders may predispose to septicemia.
- Neonatal infection: Incidence is high in neonatal period.

PHYSICAL FINDINGS & CLINICAL PRESENTATION

- Fever or hypothermia
- Hypotension
- Tachycardia
- Tachypnea
- Altered mental status
- Bleeding diathesis
- Skin rashes
- Symptoms that reflect primary site of infection: Urinary tract, GI tract, central nervous system (CNS), respiratory tract
- Table 3 describes some clinical signs and symptoms of sepsis

ETIOLOGY

- Disseminated infection with a great variety of bacteria:
  1. Gram-negative bacteria:
     a. *Escherichia coli*
     b. *Klebsiella* spp.
     c. *Pseudomonas aeruginosa*
     d. *Proteus* spp.
     e. *Neisseria meningitides*
  2. Gram-positive bacteria:
     a. *Staphylococcus aureus* (including MRSA)
     b. *Streptococcus* spp.
     c. *Enterococcus* spp.
- Less common infections:

TABLE 1 Proposed New Definitions of Sepsis

Term	Definition	Criteria	Notes
Sepsis[a] (previously severe sepsis)	Life-threatening organ dysfunction caused by a dysregulated host response to infection	Organ dysfunction is identified as an acute change in the SOFA score, ≥ 2 points from the baseline consequent to the infection.	qSOFA (quick Sequential Organ Failure Assessment) Prolonged ICU stay or in-hospital mortality can be identified at the bedside with qSOFA. 1. Respiratory rate ≥ 22 breaths/min 2. Acute mental status change 3. Systolic blood pressure ≤ 100 mm Hg An increase in SOFA of ≥ 2 predicts a 10% mortality in the general hospital population. Presume a baseline SOFA of 0 unless the patient has known (acute or chronic) organ dysfunction before the onset of infection.
Septic shock	It is a subset of sepsis in which the underlying circulatory and cellular/metabolic abnormalities are profound enough to substantially increase mortality.	A clinical construct of sepsis with persisting hypotension requiring vasopressors to maintain MAP ≥ 65 mm Hg and having a serum lactate level ≥ 2 mmol/L despite adequate volume resuscitation	Septic shock portends hospital mortality in excess of 40%.

MAP, Mean arterial pressure.

[a]Note that the proposed new definitions abandon the previous term "severe sepsis" to describe infection-induced organ dysfunction and now use "sepsis" in its place. The previous condition called "sepsis" is now just called "infection," and when infection is not associated with organ dysfunction, there is no differentiation between infection with or without systemic manifestations.
From Parrillo JE, Dellinger RP: *Critical care medicine, principles of diagnosis and management in the adult,* ed 5, Philadelphia, 2019, Elsevier.

---

*SIRS (Systemic Inflammatory Response Syndrome): Variables in SIRS criteria include respiratory rate (breaths/min), white blood cell count (109/L), hands (%), heart rate (beats/min), temperature (°C), and arterial carbon dioxide tension (mm Hg). Score range is 0 to 4.

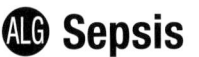

TABLE 2 The Sequential Organ Failure Assessment (SOFA) Score

Score	0	1	2	3	4
Respiration PaO_2/FiO_2, mm Hg	>400	≤400	≤300	≤200 With respiratory support	≤100
Coagulation Platelets × $10^3/mm^3$	>150	≤150	≤100	≤50	≤20
Liver Bilirubin, mg/dl (μmol/L)	<1.2 (<20)	1.2-1.9 (20-32)	2.0-5.9 (33-101)	6.0-11.9 (102-204)	>12.0 (>204)
Cardiovascular Hypotension	No hypotension	MAP <70 mm Hg	Dopamine ≤5 or dobutamine (any dose)*	Dopamine >5 or epinephrine ≤0.1 or norepinephrine ≤0.1*	Dopamine >15 or epinephrine >0.1 or norepinephrine >0.1*
Central Nervous System Glasgow coma score	15	13-14	10-12	6-9	<6
Renal Creatinine, mg/dl (μmol/L) OR urine output	<1.2 (<110)	1.2-1.9 (110- 170)	2.0-3.4 (171-299)	3.5-4.9 (300-440) <500 ml/d	>5.0 (>440) <200 ml/d

*Adrenergic agents administered for at least 1 h (doses given are in mcg/kg per min).
From Ronco C et al: *Critical care nephrology*, ed 3, Philadelphia, 2019, Elsevier.

TABLE 3 Clinical Signs and Symptoms of Sepsis

Infection	General	Inflammatory	Hemodynamic	Tissue Perfusion
Documented or suspected	Temperature >38° C (100.4° F) or <36° C (96.8° F) Heart rate >90 beats/min Respiratory rate ≥20 breaths/min Altered mental status Hyperglycemia Third spacing of fluid	WBC count <4000 or >12,000 cells/μL or ≥10% bands	Hypotension: Systolic blood pressure <90 mm Hg MAP <70 mm Hg SVo_2 >70 CI >3.5 L/min/m²	Hypoxemia: (Pao_2/Fio_2 <300) Acute oliguria (urine output <0.5 ml/kg/h) Coagulopathy Abnormal liver function tests Platelet count <100,000 cells/μL Lactic acidosis Skin mottling

CI, Cardiac index; *MAP*, mean arterial pressure; *SVo₂*, mixed venous oxygen saturation; *WBC*, white blood cell.
From Cameron JL, Cameron AM: *Current surgical therapy*, ed 10, Philadelphia, 2011, Saunders.

1. Fungal
2. Viral
3. Rickettsial
4. Parasitic

- Sepsis is a complex dysregulation of both inflammation and coagulation (Fig. E1). There is activation of coagulation, inflammatory cytokines, complement, and kinin cascades with release of a variety of vasoactive endogenous mediators. The innate immune system recognizes pathogens by means of pattern-recognition receptors (toll-like receptors [TLRs], Table 4). TLRs bind to structures on microorganisms and, based on the composite information gained, generate a tailored response to the invading pathogen.
- Predisposing host factors:
  1. General medical condition
  2. Extremes of age
  3. Immunosuppressive therapy
  4. Recent surgery
  5. Granulocytopenia
  6. Hyposplenism
  7. Diabetes
  8. Instrumentation

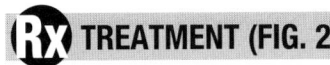 **DIAGNOSIS**

DIFFERENTIAL DIAGNOSIS

- Cardiogenic shock
- Acute pancreatitis
- Pulmonary embolism
- Systemic vasculitis
- Toxic ingestion
- Exposure-induced hypothermia
- Fulminant hepatic failure
- Collagen-vascular diseases

WORKUP

- Evaluation should focus on identifying a specific pathogen and localizing the site of primary infection. Box 1 summarizes a general approach to shock.
- Hemodynamic, metabolic, coagulation disorders should be carefully characterized.
- Intensive monitoring.

LABORATORY TESTS

- Cultures of blood and examination and culture of sputum, urine, wound drainage, stool, and cerebrospinal fluid (CSF), depending on the presenting signs and symptoms for each patient
- CBC with differential, coagulation profile
- Routine chemistries, liver function tests (LFTs)
- Arterial blood gases (ABGs), lactic acid level
- Procalcitonin can be useful as a serum marker of bacterial infection as a cause of the sepsis, and has been shown to improve survival and facilitate earlier discontinuation of antibiotics
- Urinalysis

IMAGING STUDIES

- Chest x-ray
- Other radiographic and radioisotope procedures according to suspected site of primary infection

TREATMENT (FIG. 2)

NONPHARMACOLOGIC THERAPY

- Tissue oxygenation: Mixed venous oxygen saturation maintained >70% if possible; early mechanical ventilation with low tidal

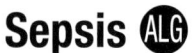

TABLE 4 Toll-Like Receptors

Toll-Like Receptor	Pathogen or Disease State
TLR1	Lyme disease
	Neisseria meningitidis
TLR2	*Mycobacterium tuberculosis*
	Chagas disease
	Leptospirosis
	Fungal sepsis
	CMV viremia
TLR3	Many
TLR4	Gram-negative bacteria
	Septic shock
	Chlamydia trachomatis
	Chlamydia pneumoniae
	Certain viruses
	Mycobacterium tuberculosis
TLR5	Flagellated bacteria (e.g., *Salmonella*)
TLR7	Viral infections
TLR8	Viral infections
TLR9	Bacterial and viral infections
TLR10	Unknown

CMV, Cytomegalovirus; *TLR,* toll-like receptor.
From Parrillo JE, Dellinger RP: *Critical care medicine, principles of diagnosis and management in the adult,* ed 5, Philadelphia, 2019, Elsevier.

BOX 1 General Approach to Shock: Initial Diagnosis and Evaluation

Clinical (primary diagnosis)
 Tachycardia, hypotension (systolic blood pressure <90 mm Hg) tachypnea, oliguria, encephalopathy (confusion), peripheral hypoperfusion (mottled extremities), cyanosis
Laboratory (confirmatory)
 Hemoglobin, WBC, platelets
Prothrombin time/partial thromboplastin time
 Electrolytes, arterial blood gases, Ca, Mg, BUN, creatinine, serum lactate
 ECG
Monitoring (continuous ECG and respiratory monitors)
 Pulse oximetry
 Urinary catheter (urine output)
 Point-of-care ultrasonography (heart, lung, abdominal, and major vessels)
 Arterial pressure catheter
 Central venous pressure monitor (uncomplicated shock)
 Pulmonary artery flotation catheter
  Cardiac output
  Pulmonary artery occlusion pressure
  Central and/or mixed venous oxygen saturation (intermittent or continuous)
 Oximetry*
Imaging
 Chest x-ray
 X-ray views of abdomen
 Computed tomographic scan: Abdomen or chest
 Formal transthoracic and/or transesophageal echocardiogram[a]

BUN, Blood urea nitrogen; *ECG,* electrocardiogram; *WBC,* white blood cell.
*SIRS (Systemic Inflammatory Response Syndrome): Variables in SIRS criteria include respiratory rate (breaths/min), white blood cell count (109/L), hands (%), heart rate (beats/min), temperature (°C), and arterial carbon dioxide tension (mm Hg). Score range is 0 to 4.
From Parrillo JE, Dellinger RP: *Critical care medicine, principles of diagnosis and management in the adult,* ed 5, Philadelphia, 2019, Elsevier.

volume (6 ml/kg predicted body weight) to protect lung parenchyma from overstretching and "volutrauma." Recommended plateau pressure for sepsis-related acute respiratory distress syndrome (ARDS) is ≤30 cm H2O.
- Focal infection should be drained if possible, and potentially infected catheters should be removed.

ACUTE GENERAL Rx

- Blood pressure support, intravenous (IV) fluid resuscitation and vasopressors (Table 5), if needed, with the goal of reestablishing a mean arterial blood pressure >65 mm Hg; reduction in blood lactate and improved mixed venous oxygen saturation >70% within 6 h of recognition of septic shock is associated with improved survival. If possible, measure vena cava oxygen saturation (ScvO2) to assess adequacy of resuscitation. If the ScvO2 is <70%, consider packed red blood cell transfusion to achieve Hct >30%. Start inotropic agents if ScvO2 is <70% despite transfusion and adequate fluid resuscitation.
  1. IV hydration; patients receiving balanced crystalloids as resuscitation fluids appear to have a lower 30-day mortality compared with patients who received saline (26% versus 31%) in a recent trial. Use of the fluid challenge technique to evaluate the effect (and safety) of fluid administration has been downgraded

from a strong recommendation to a weak one in recent guidelines.[1] For sepsis-induced hypoperfusion, give 30 ml/kg of IV crystalloids within 3 h, with additional fluid based on frequent reassessment using dynamic variables (e.g., passive leg raise test or pulse or stroke volume variations induced by mechanical ventilation) rather than previous guidelines using target-specific values of central venous pressure. Fluid administration should be discontinued when the response to fluids is no longer beneficial. Most patients need 4 to 6 L of fluid in the first 6 h. Trials have shown that resuscitation with balanced crystalloids or albumin compared with other fluids seems to be associated with reduced mortality, and that albumin replacement in addition to crystalloids alone does not improve the rate of survival at 28 and 90 days. There is considerable debate about how much fluid is enough fluid before initiating vasopressors. A recent trial comparing a restrictive fluid strategy (prioritizing vasopressors and lower intravenous fluid volumes) with a liberal fluid strategy (prioritizing higher intravenous fluids before vasopressor use) for a 24h period did not result in significantly lower liberal fluid strategy.[2]

2. Therapy with vasopressors if mean arterial blood pressure of >65 mm Hg cannot be maintained by hydration alone. Use norepinephrine as a first-choice vasopressor and target a mean arterial pressure (MAP) of 65 mm Hg. Administration of vasopressors should be initiated via peripheral access, as opposed to waited for placement of central venous access.[1]
- Correction of acidosis by improving the tissue perfusion, not by giving bicarbonate.
- Mechanical ventilation as needed.
- Antibiotics:
  1. Directed at the most likely sources of infection. Table 6 describes initial antibiotic recommendations for septic patients.
  2. Should generally provide broad coverage of gram-positive and gram-negative bacteria (or fungi if clinically indicated).
  3. Antibiotics should be administered within 1 h of the diagnosis of septic shock—this is a medical emergency.
- Updated guidelines[1] recommend that patients with ongoing vasopressor requirements should receive IV corticosteroids. Patients with relative adrenal insufficiency may benefit from low-dose therapy with hydrocortisone (200 mg IV by continuous infusion for 7 days). Current evidence and guidelines support limiting the use of IV hydrocortisone for patients with septic

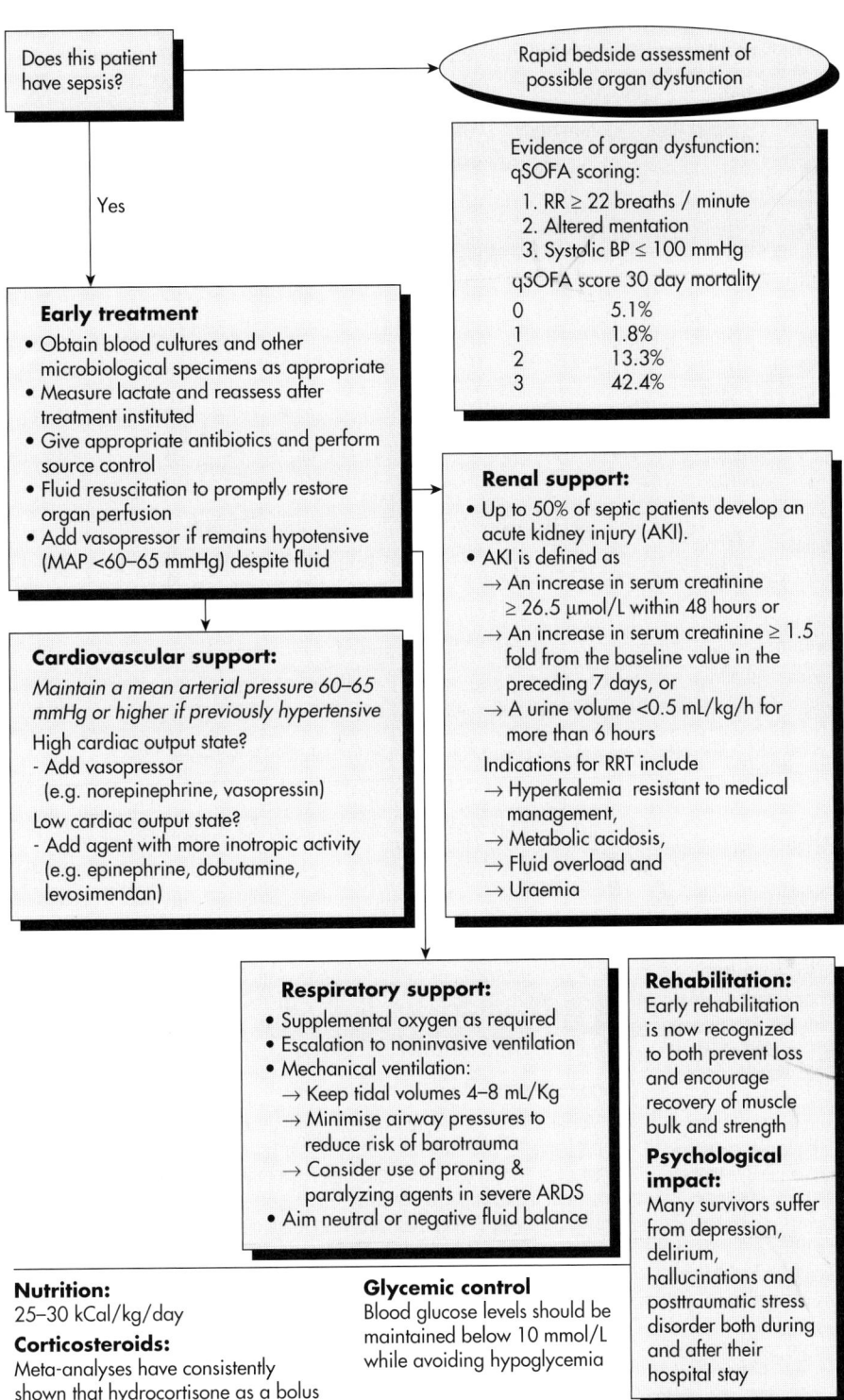

FIG. 2 Flow diagram for the management of sepsis and septic shock. Starting with rapid recognition of the septic patient, early initiation of appropriate antibiotics, and fluid resuscitation with supportive management. *ARDS,* Acute respiratory distress syndrome; *BP,* blood pressure; *MAP,* mean arterial pressure; *RR,* respiratory rate. (From Newman M et al: *Perioperative medicine,* ed 2, Philadelphia, 2022, Elsevier.)

shock to these instances with fluid resuscitation and vasopressor therapy are inadequate to restore hemodynamic stability. The corticotropin (ACTH) stimulation test is not helpful and should not be used to determine the need for corticosteroid in these patients. During the COVID-19 pandemic, the RECOVERY trial provided evidence that treatment with dexamethasone in hospitalized patients at a dose of 6 mg once a day (IV or oral) for up to 10 days reduced 28-day mortality in patients with COVID-19.
• Blood transfusion: A lower hemoglobin threshold is preferred. Trials have shown that among patients with septic shock, mortality at 90 days and rates of ischemic events and use of life support is similar among those assigned to blood transfusion at a higher hemoglobin threshold (hemoglobin level of 9 g/dl or less) and those assigned to blood transfusion at a lower threshold (hemoglobin level of 7 g/dl or less).

TABLE 5 Relative Potency of Intravenously Administered Vasopressors/Inotropes Used in Shock[a]

Drug	Dose	CARDIAC		PERIPHERAL VASCULATURE			
		Heart Rate	Contractility	Vasoconstriction	Vasodilation	Dopaminergic	Typical Clinical Use
Dopamine	1-4 µg/kg/min	1+	1-2+	0	1+	4+	All shock
	5-10 µg/kg/min	2+	2+	1-2+	1+	4+	
	11-20 µg/kg/min	2+	2+	2-3+	1+	4+	
Norepinephrine	0.01-0.3 µg/kg/min	2+	2+	4+	0	0	Refractory shock
Dobutamine	1-20 µg/kg/min	1-2+	3+	1+	2+	0	CHF; cardiogenic, obstructive and septic shock
Dopexamine[b]	0.5-6 µg/kg/min	2+	1+	0	3-4+	4+	CHF; cardiogenic shock
Epinephrine	0.05-0.2 µg/kg/min	4+	4+	4+	3+	0	Refractory or anaphylactic shock
Phenylephrine	0.1-1 µg/kg/min	0	1+	4+	0	0	Neurogenic or septic shock
Isoproterenol	1-8 µg/min	4+	4+	0	4+	0	Cardiogenic shock (bradyarrhythmia), torsades de pointes, ventricular tachycardia
Vasopressin	0.02-0.04 U/min	0	0	4+	0	0	Vasodilatory (e.g., septic) shock
Milrinone	37.5-75 µg/kg bolus over 10 min; 0.375-0.75 µg/ kg/min infusion	1+	3+	0	2+	0	CHF; cardiogenic shock

CHF, Congestive heart failure.
[a]The 1 to 4+ scoring system represents an arbitrary quantitation of the comparative potency of different vasopressors/inotropes.
[b]Not clinically released in the U.S.
From Parrillo JE, Dellinger RP: *Critical care medicine, principles of diagnosis and management in the adult*, ed 5, Philadelphia, 2019, Elsevier.

CHRONIC Rx

- Adjust antibiotic therapy on the basis of culture results.
- In general, continue antibiotic therapy for a minimum of 7 to 10 days.
- Infection source control (e.g., removal of catheter/device suspected to be infected).
- If hyperglycemia develops during treatment, start continuous insulin IV infusion, maintain blood glucose in the 110 to 180 mg/dl level, and avoid insulin-induced hypoglycemia.
- All adult patients who survive to discharge should have follow-up for physical, cognitive, and emotional problems associated with their admission.[1]

DISPOSITION

- All patients with sepsis should be hospitalized and given access to intensive monitoring and nursing care.
- Among adults with suspected infection admitted to an ICU, an increase in SOFA score of 2 or more has greater prognostic accuracy for in-hospital mortality than SIRS criteria or the qSOFA score (quick SOFA). The qSOFA can be done at bedside and consists of increased respiratory rate ≥22/min, altered mentation

and systolic blood pressure (BP) ≤100 mm Hg with each allocated 1 point.

REFERRAL

- To infectious diseases expert
- To physician experienced in critical care

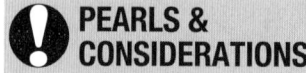 **PEARLS & CONSIDERATIONS**

COMMENTS

- Mortality rises quickly if antibiotic therapy is not instituted promptly (preferably within 1 h of onset of shock) and metabolic derangements are not treated aggressively.
- The Surviving Sepsis Campaign hr-1 bundle 2018 update recommends: Measure lactate level. Remeasure if initial lactate is >2 mmol/ L. [weak recommendation, low quality of evidence] Obtain blood cultures prior to administration of antibiotics. [best practice statement] Administer broad spectrum antibiotics. [strong recommendation, moderate quality of evidence] Rapidly administer 30 ml/ kg crystalloid for hypotension or lactate ≥4 mmol/L [strong recommendation, low quality of evidence] and apply

vasopressors if patient is hypotensive during or after fluid resuscitation to maintain MAP ≥65 mm Hg. [strong recommendation, moderate quality of evidence.]
- Recent trials have shown that early, goal-directed therapy (EGDT) does not result in better outcomes than usual care and is associated with higher hospitalization costs across a broad range of patient and hospital characteristics.
- A recent trial (ACTS Randomized Clinical Trial) in which patients with septic shock were given the combination of ascorbic acid, corticosteroids, and thiamine did not show significant reduction in SOFA score in first 72 h, and thus this combination should not be used in septic shock.
- Use of vitamin C is not recommended for sepsis.[1]

AUTHORS: **GLENN G. FORT, MD, MPH,** and **FRED F. FERRI, MD**

REFERENCES & SUGGESTED READINGS

Available at eBooks.Health.Elsevier.com.

TABLE 6 Empiric Antibiotic Options for Patients With Severe Sepsis or Septic Shock

	SUSPECTED SOURCE				
	Lung	**Abdomen**	**Skin/Soft Tissue**	**Urinary Tract**	**Source Uncertain**
Major Community-Acquired Pathogens	*Streptococcus pneumoniae* *Haemophilus influenzae* *Legionella* *Chlamydia pneumoniae*	*Escherichia coli* *Bacteroides fragilis*	*Streptococcus pyogenes* *Staphylococcus aureus* Polymicrobial	*E. Coli* *Klebsiella* spp. *Enterobacter* spp. *Proteus* spp. Enterococci	
Empirical Antibiotic Therapy	Moxifloxacin *or* levofloxacin *or* azithromycin *plus* cefotaxime *or* ceftazidime *or* cefepime *or* piperacillin-tazobactam	Imipenem *or* meropenem *or* doripenem *or* Piperacillin-tazobactam ± aminoglycosideIf biliary source: Piperacillin-tazobactam, ampicillin-sulbactam, *or* ceftriaxone with metronidazole	Vancomycin *or* daptomycin *plus either* imipenem *or* meropenem *or* piperacillin-tazobactam; ± clindamycin (see text)	Ciprofloxacin *or* levofloxacin (if gram-positive cocci, use ampicillin *or* vancomycin ± gentamicin)	Vancomycin *plus either* doripenem *or* ertapenem *or* imipenem *or* meropenem
Major Commensal or Nosocomial Microorganisms	Aerobic gram-negative bacilli	Aerobic gram-negative rods Anaerobes *Candida* spp.	*Staphylococcus aureus* (? MRSA) Aerobic gram-negative rods	Aerobic gram-negative rods *Enterococci*	Consider MDRO if in area of high prevalence. Consider echinocandin if neutropenic or indwelling intravascular catheter
Empirical Antibiotic Therapy	Imipenem *or* meropenem *or* doripenem *or* cefepime (if *Acinetobacter baumannii* or carbapenem-resistant *Klebsiella* in ICU, add colistin)	Imipenem *or* meropenem ± aminoglycoside (consider echinocandin)	Vancomycin *or* daptomycin *plus* imipenem-cilastatin *or* meropenem *or* cefepime, ± clindamycin	Vancomycin *plus* imipenem *or* meropenem *or* cefepime	Cefepime *plus* vancomycin ± caspofungin

Dosages for intravenous administration (normal renal function):
- Imipenem-cilastatin, 0.5-1.0 g q6-8h
- Meropenem, 1-2 g q8h
- Doripenem, 0.5 g q8h
- Piperacillin-tazobactam, 3.375 g q4h or 4.5 g q6h
- Vancomycin, load 25-30 mg/kg, then 15-20 mg/kg q8-12h
- Cefepime, 1-2 g q8h
- Levofloxacin, 750 mg q24h
- Ciprofloxacin, 400 mg q8-12h
- Moxifloxacin, 400 mg daily
- Ceftriaxone, 2 g q24h
- Caspofungin, 70 mg, followed by 50 mg q24h
- Colistin: Loading dose = 5 mg/kg body weight

ICU, Intensive care unit; *MDRO*, multidrug-resistant organisms; *MRSA*, methicillin-resistant *Staphylococcus aureus*. For MDRO, resistance usually includes carbapenems. Carbapenems are less susceptible to extended-spectrum β-lactamases; base choice on local resistance pattern.
From Bennett JE et al: *Mandell, Douglas, and Bennett's principles and practice of infectious diseases*, ed 8, Philadelphia, 2015, Saunders.

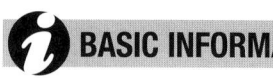

BASIC INFORMATION

DEFINITION

Septic arthritis is a highly destructive form of joint disease most often caused by hematogenous spread of organisms from a distant site of infection. Direct penetration of the joint as a result of trauma or surgery and spread from adjacent osteomyelitis may also cause bacterial arthritis. Any joint in the body may be affected.

SYNONYMS

Infectious arthritis
Bacterial arthritis
Pyogenic arthritis

ICD-10CM CODE

M00.9 Pyogenic arthritis, unspecified

EPIDEMIOLOGY & DEMOGRAPHICS

INCIDENCE (IN U.S.): Between 2 and 6 cases per 100,000 people per year
PREVALENCE (IN U.S.): Unknown
PREDOMINANT SEX: Gonococcal arthritis in females
PREDOMINANT AGE: Gonococcal arthritis in sexually active adults
PEAK INCIDENCE:
- Gonococcal arthritis: Young adults
- Other bacterial causes: All ages

PHYSICAL FINDINGS & CLINICAL PRESENTATION

- Hallmark: Acute onset of monoarticular joint pain, erythema, heat, and immobility
- Limited range of motion of the joint
- Effusion, with varying degrees of erythema and increased warmth around the joint
- Single joint affected in 80% to 90% of cases of nongonococcal arthritis
- Gonococcal dermatitis-arthritis syndrome:
  1. Typical pattern is a migratory polyarthritis or tenosynovitis
  2. Small pustules on the trunk or extremities
- Febrile patient at presentation
- Most commonly affected joints in adult: Knee and hip, but any joint may be involved; in children—hip

ETIOLOGY

- Bacteria spread from another locus of infection.
  1. Highly vascular synovium is invaded by hematogenously spread bacteria.
  2. White blood cell (WBC) enzymes cause necrosis of synovium, cartilage, and bone.
  3. Extensive joint destruction is rapid if infection is not treated with appropriate intravenous (IV) antibiotics and drainage of necrotic material.
- Predisposing factors: Rheumatoid arthritis, prosthetic joints, advanced age, immunodeficiency (HIV, diabetes mellitus [DM], immunosuppressive drugs), gout, sexual activity (gonococcal arthritis), skin infections, cutaneous ulcers (contiguous spread), recent joint surgery, recent intraarticular infection. Risk

factors for development of septic arthritis are summarized in Table 1. Fig. E1 illustrates routes by which bacteria can reach the joint.
- The most common nongonococcal organisms are staphylococci (40%), streptococci (28%), and gram-negative bacilli (19%). Less common are mycobacteria (8%), gram-negative cocci (3%), anaerobes (1%), and gram-positive bacilli (1%).
- Staphylococci (*S. aureus* and coagulase-negative staphylococcal species) account for >50% of prosthetic-hip and prosthetic-knee infections. *S. aureus* is very common in patients with rheumatoid arthritis.

DIAGNOSIS

DIFFERENTIAL DIAGNOSIS

- Gout
- Pseudogout
- Trauma
- Hemarthrosis
- Rheumatic fever
- Adult or juvenile rheumatoid arthritis
- Spondyloarthropathies such as reactive arthritis (Reiter syndrome)
- Osteomyelitis
- Viral arthritides
- Septic bursitis
- Lyme disease caused by *Borrelia burgdorferi*

WORKUP

- Joint aspiration, Gram stain, and culture of the synovial fluid. Fig. 2 describes an algorithm for synovial fluid analysis in septic arthritis.

TABLE 1 Risk Factors for Development of Septic Arthritis

Age >80 yr

Diabetes mellitus

Presence of a prosthetic joint in the knee or the hip

Recent joint surgery

Skin infection

Previous septic arthritis

Recent intra-articular injection

HIV or AIDS

Intravenous drug abuse

End-stage renal disease on hemodialysis

Advanced hepatic disease

Hemophilia with or without AIDS

Sickle cell disease

Underlying malignancy

Hypogammaglobulinemia (susceptible to *Mycoplasma* infections)

Late complement-component deficiency (susceptible to *Neisseria* infections)

Low socioeconomic status with high rate of comorbidities

AIDS, Acquired immunodeficiency virus; *HIV,* human immunodeficiency virus.
From Firestein GS et al: *Firestein & Kelley's textbook of rheumatology,* ed 11, Philadelphia, 2021, Elsevier.

- Immediate arthrocentesis before other studies are undertaken or antibiotics instituted. Synovial fluid should be evaluated at bedside and then sent for lab evaluation.
- Criteria for diagnosis of prosthetic joint infections are summarized in Table 2.

LABORATORY TESTS

- Joint fluid analysis:
  1. Synovial fluid leukocyte count is usually elevated >50,000 cells/mm^3 with >80% polymorphonuclear cells.
  2. Counts are highly variable, with similar findings in gout, pseudogout, or rheumatoid arthritis. Lower WBC counts can occur in joint replacement, disseminated gonococcal disease, and peripheral leukopenia.
  3. Synovial fluid glucose or protein is not helpful because results are not specific for septic arthritis. The differential diagnosis of synovial fluid abnormalities is described in Section IV.
  4. Polymerase chain reaction (PCR) testing: Useful for detection of uncommon organisms (e.g., Lyme disease).
  5. Crystal analysis: Septic arthritis can coexist with crystal arthropathy; therefore the presence of crystals does not preclude a diagnosis of septic arthritis.
- Blood cultures: Positive in 25% to 50% of patients with septic arthritis.
- Culture of possible extraarticular sources of infection.
- Elevated peripheral WBC count, erythrocyte sedimentation rate (ESR) (nonspecific), C-reactive protein (CRP) (nonspecific). When elevated, ESR and CRP may be useful to monitor therapeutic response.
- If gonococcus is suspected, perform nucleic acid amplification tests (NAATs) on synovial fluid.

IMAGING STUDIES

- Radiograph of the affected joint (Fig. 3): Useful to rule out osteomyelitis, fractures, chondrocalcinosis, or inflammatory arthritis
- MRI: Findings that suggest an acute intra-articular infection include the combination of bony erosions with marrow edema
- Computed tomography (CT) scan: Useful for early diagnosis of infections of the spine, hips, and sternoclavicular and sacroiliac joints
- Ultrasound: Can be useful for detecting effusions in joints that are more difficult to examine (e.g., hip)

TREATMENT
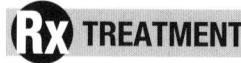

NONPHARMACOLOGIC THERAPY

- Affected joints aspirated daily to remove necrotic material and to follow serial WBC counts and cultures
- If no resolution with IV antibiotics and closed drainage: Open debridement and lavage, particularly in nongonococcal infections
- Prevention of contractures:
  1. After acute stage of inflammation, range-of-motion exercises of the affected joint
  2. Physical therapy helpful

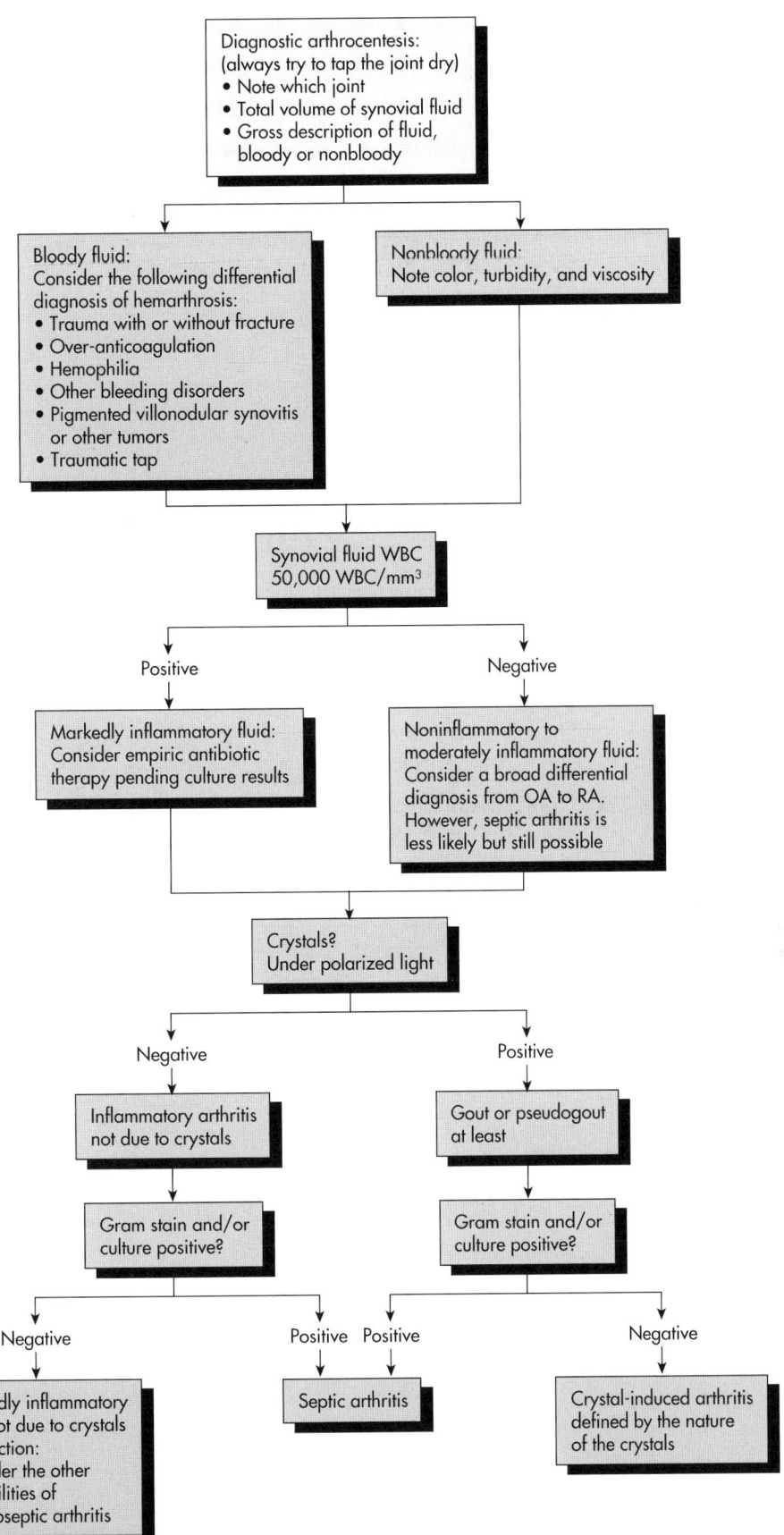

FIG. 2 Algorithm for synovial fluid analysis in septic arthritis. *OA,* Osteoarthritis; *RA,* rheumatoid arthritis; *WBC,* white blood cell count. (From Harris ED et al: *Kelley's textbook of rheumatology,* ed 7, Philadelphia, 2005, Saunders.)

TABLE 2 Criteria for Diagnosis of Prosthetic Joint Infection

Major Criteria (One or More of the Following)	Decision
Two positive cultures of same organism or sinus tract with communication to the joint/ prosthesis	Infected
Minor Criteria	**Score[a]**
Elevated serum CRP or D-dimer	2
Elevated ESR	1
Elevated synovial WBC or leukocyte esterase	3
Positive synovial alpha-defensin	3
Elevated synovial PMN (%)	2
Elevated synovial CRP	1

[a]Score of 6 or more, infected; score of 2-5, possibly infected; score of 0-1, not infected.
CRP, C-reactive protein; *ESR,* erythrocyte sedimentation rate; *PMN,* polymorphonuclear leukocyte; *WBC,* white blood count.
From Firestein GS et al: *Firestein & Kelley's textbook of rheumatology,* ed 11, Philadelphia, 2021, Elsevier.

ACUTE GENERAL Rx

- IV antibiotics immediately after joint aspiration and Gram stain of the synovial fluid. Empiric antibiotic therapy (Table 3) is based on organism found on Gram stain of synovial fluid:
  1. Gram-positive cocci: Vancomycin: 15 to 20 mg/kg IV q8 to 12h. Keep trough levels at 15 to 20 mcg/ml. Alternatives include daptomycin and linezolid
  2. Gram-negative cocci: Ceftriaxone: 1 to 2 g IV daily in adults (children: 50-100 mg/kg IV daily). Alternative includes cefotaxime
  3. Gram-negative rods: Ceftriaxone, cefepime: 1 to 2 g IV q8 to 12h in adults (children: 100-150 mg/kg/day divided in q8h dosing), piperacillin-tazobactam: 3.375 g IV to 4.5 g IV q6h. Aztreonam or fluoroquinolones can be used in patients with allergy to penicillin or cephalosporins
  4. Negative Gram stain: Vancomycin plus either cefepime or a carbapenem such as meropenem: 1 g IV q8h in adults (children: 60 mg/kg/day divided in q8h dosing) or ertapenem
- The optimal duration of antibiotic use in septic arthritis has traditionally been 3 to 6 wk usually following surgical drainage. Recent trials (Gjika et al, *Ann Rheum Dis* Aug 2019, 78: 1114) support a 2-wk course in conjunction with surgery. The duration of antimicrobial therapy in patients with prosthetic joint infections remains unclear however trials have shown that outcomes are better with a 12-wk antibiotic course than with a 6-wk course.[1]

REFERENCE & SUGGESTED READINGS

Available at eBooks.Health.Elsevier.com.

RELATED CONTENT

Septic Arthritis (Patient Information)

AUTHOR: **GLENN G. FORT, MD, MPH**

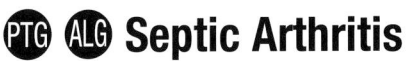

S

TABLE 3 Antibiotic Agents Used in Adults

Synovial Fluid Gram Stain	Organism	Antibiotic	Dose
Gram-positive cocci (clusters)	*Staphylococcus aureus* (methicillin-sensitive)	Nafcillin/oxacillin Or	2 g IV q4h or 12 g daily continuous infusion
		Cefazolin	1-2 g IV q8h
	S. aureus (methicillin-resistant)	Vancomycin or	15 mg/kg IV q12h[a] (serum trough level of 15-20 µg/ml)
		Daptomycin Or	6-8 mg/kg q24h
		Linezolid	600 mg IV or po q12h
Gram-positive cocci (chains)	*Streptococcus*	Penicillin or	2-4 million units IV q4h or 18-24 million units daily continuous infusion
		Cefazolin	1-2 g IV q8h
Gram-negative diplococci	*Neisseria gonorrhoeae*	Ceftriaxone Or	2 g IV q24h
		Cefotaxime Or	1 g IV q8h
		Ciprofloxacin	400 mg IV q12h
Gram-negative bacilli	*Enterobacteriaceae (Escherichia coli, Proteus, Serratia)*	Ceftriaxone or	2 g IV daily
		Ciprofloxacin	750 mg po q12h
		Ertapenem	1 g IV daily
	Pseudomonas	Cefepime Or	2 g IV q8h
		Piperacillin-tazobactam or	3.375 g IV q6h or 3.375 g IV q8h infused over 4 h or 14 g daily continuous infusion
		Ciprofloxacin Meropenem	750 mg po q12h or 400 mg IV q 12h 1-2 g IV q8h
		Plus	
		Gentamicin/tobramycin	7 mg/kg IV daily
Polymicrobial infection	*S. aureus, Streptococcus,* gram-negative bacilli	Nafcillin/oxacillin[a]	2 g IV q4h or 12 g daily continuous infusion
		Plus	
		Ceftriaxone Or	2 g IV q24h
		Cefotaxime Or	2 g IV q8h
		Ciprofloxacin	400 mg IV q12h or 750 mg po q12h

[a]If patient is penicillin allergic, use vancomycin plus third-generation cephalosporin or ciprofloxacin.
IV, Intravenous; *q4h,* every 4 hours; *q6h,* every 6 hours; *q8h,* every 8 hours; *q12h,* every 12 hours; *q24h,* every 24 hours.
From Firestein GS et al: *Firestein & Kelley's textbook of rheumatology,* ed 11, Philadelphia, 2021, Elsevier.

Diseases and Disorders

I

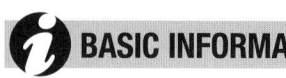
BASIC INFORMATION

DEFINITION

Serotonin syndrome (SS) is an iatrogenic medical condition resulting from excessive serotonergic stimulation of $5-HT_{1A}$ and $5-HT_{2a}$ receptors[1] in the central nervous system (CNS) and peripheral nervous system (PNS). SS is a disorder that is classically characterized by a constellation of various symptoms that are classically defined by the triad of mental status changes, neuromuscular hyperactivity, and autonomic dysfunction.[1,2]

SYNONYMS

SS
Hyperserotonemia
Serotonergic syndrome
Serotonin toxicity

ICD-10CM CODES

Y49	Adverse effects due to psychotropic drugs
Y49.0	Adverse effects due to tricyclic and tetracyclic antidepressants
Y49.1	Adverse effects due to monoamine-oxidase-inhibitor antidepressants
Y49.2	Adverse effects due to other and unspecified antidepressants
Y49.3	Adverse effects due to phenothiazine antipsychotics and neuroleptics
G25.89	Other specified extrapyramidal and movement disorders

EPIDEMIOLOGY & DEMOGRAPHICS

- While the exact incidence of SS is not known, as clinical manifestations may go unnoticed or be attributed to another condition, the overall incidence is known to be rising in the face of increased use of serotonergic medications.[1]
- SS is seen in all age groups.
- SS classically occurs in patients receiving two or more serotonergic drugs, but it can also occur occasionally with monotherapy.
- Selective serotonin reuptake inhibitor (SSRI) is the most commonly implicated medication associated with SS.
- Concomitant use of an SSRI with a monoamine oxidase inhibitor (MAOI) poses the greatest risk of developing severe SS.
- Combination of SSRIs with other serotonergic drugs (e.g., tryptophan, illicit drugs like cocaine and MDMA, "Ecstasy") or drugs with serotonergic properties (e.g., methylene blue, lithium, meperidine, triptans, linezolid) may also lead to SS.

PHYSICAL FINDINGS & CLINICAL PRESENTATION[1-3]

- Findings of clonus and tremor with hyperreflexia in the setting of recent use of serotonergic agents strongly suggest the diagnosis of SS.
- Symptoms can manifest within minutes to hours after starting a new psychopharmacologic treatment, increasing the dose of a serotonergic drug, or administering a second serotonergic drug. Nearly all patients develop symptoms within 24 h of exposure.
- Clonus (inducible, spontaneous, and ocular) is the key finding in establishing a diagnosis of SS.
- Classic triad of clinical features:
  1. Neuromuscular excitation: Hyperreflexia, myoclonus, muscle rigidity, tremor, ocular clonus, bilateral Babinski signs
  2. Autonomic nervous system excitation: Nausea/vomiting, diarrhea, hypertension, tachycardia, diaphoresis, fever >38° C (100° F) to severe hyperthermia, dilated pupils, dry mucous membranes, flushed skin
  3. Altered mental status: Anxiety, agitation, confusion, coma

ETIOLOGY

- Hyperstimulation of the brain stem and spinal cord serotonin receptors leading to the neuromuscular and autonomic symptoms.[1,2]
- Psychopharmacologic drugs—in particular, fluoxetine and sertraline taken with MAOI (e.g., tranylcypromine and phenelzine)—have been cited as a common cause of SS. Triptans (serotonin-receptor agonists used in the treatment of migraines) may also precipitate the SS when used in combination with SSRIs and serotonin-norepinephrine reuptake inhibitors. Box 1 describes classes of medications that produce SS.

DIAGNOSIS

- SS is a clinical diagnosis. There are no specific laboratory tests for SS. A high index of suspicion along with a detailed medication history is the mainstay of diagnosis.[4]
- Diagnostic criteria: Most accurate is Hunter Serotonin Toxicity Criteria (sensitivity 84%, specificity 97%, confirmation by toxicologist). Sternbach diagnostic criteria (Table E1) are also commonly used with statistics of sensitivity 75% and specificity 96%.[4]

DIFFERENTIAL DIAGNOSIS

- Medical: Neuroleptic malignant syndrome, malignant hyperthermia, infection (e.g., meningitis, encephalitis), hyperthyroidism, tetanus.[1,2]
- Toxins: Anticholinergic, amphetamines, cocaine, lithium, LSD, PCP, salicylates.
- Classic features in differentiation of NMS from SS are that SS develops over 24 h, involves neuromuscular hyperactivity (hyperreflexia, myoclonus), and begins to resolve within 24 h with appropriate therapy, whereas NMS develops gradually over days to weeks, involves sluggish neuromuscular response, and resolves over an average period of 1 wk to 10 days.[5]

WORKUP

- Because SS is a clinical diagnosis, there is no laboratory test that confirms the diagnosis, and serum serotonin concentration does not correlate with the clinical picture.[3]
- However, patients with SS may develop leukocytosis, elevated creatinine phosphokinase, and decreased sodium bicarbonate levels.
- Patients with severe SS may develop complications including disseminated intravascular coagulation, rhabdomyolysis, metabolic acidosis, renal failure, myoglobinuria, and acute respiratory distress syndrome.
- All patients should receive more extensive workup to evaluate for other life-threatening illnesses.[1,2,5]

LABORATORY TESTS (USED TO NARROW DIFFERENTIAL DIAGNOSIS)[1,3]

- CBC with differential when considering sepsis
- Urine and blood cultures
- Electrolytes, blood urea nitrogen, and creatinine to rule out acidosis and renal failure
- Coagulation studies to rule out disseminated intravascular coagulation
- Blood and urine toxicology screen, including acetaminophen and salicylate levels if overdose was intentional to rule out complicating co-ingestions
- It should be noted that urine drug screening is of limited utility due to its lack of sensitivity for many drugs
- Thyroid function tests
- Creatine-phosphokinase (CPK) with isoenzymes
- ECG because ventricular rhythm disturbance is a potentially fatal complication
- Cerebrospinal fluid studies to rule out meningitis

IMAGING STUDIES (USED TO NARROW DIFFERENTIAL DIAGNOSIS)

- Plain chest x-ray examination
- Head computed tomography

BOX 1 Classes of Medications That Produce Serotonin Syndrome in Psychiatric Patients

Selective serotonin reuptake inhibitors
Monoamine oxidase inhibitors
Atypical antipsychotics
Heterocyclic antidepressants
Trazodone
Dual-uptake inhibitors
Psychostimulants
Buspirone
Mood stabilizers
Analgesics
Antiemetics
Cough suppressants
Dietary supplements
Linezolid

From Goldman L, Schafer AI: *Goldman-Cecil medicine*, ed 24, Philadelphia, 2012, Saunders.

(Rx) TREATMENT[1-3]

- Once a diagnosis of SS is established, consultation with a medical toxicologist, clinical pharmacologist, and/or poison control center should be considered.
- Management includes:
  1. Discontinue use of all potential precipitating drugs.
  2. Provide supportive management.
  3. Control agitation.
  4. Administer serotonin antagonists.
  5. Control autonomic instability.
  6. Control hyperthermia.
  7. Reassess the need to resume the use of the serotonergic agent once the symptoms have resolved.

NONPHARMACOLOGIC THERAPY

- Discontinuation of the drug is the mainstay of therapy.[1]
- Supportive treatment aimed at normalizing vital signs.
- Patients who are severely hyperthermic with temperatures >41° C (106° F) should be given intravenous (IV) sedation, paralyzed, and intubated. Cooling blankets can be used for patients with mild to moderate hyperthermia. There is no role for acetaminophen. (This lack of utility is due to the etiology of the hyperthermia; Tylenol focuses the thermoregulatory nature of the hypothalamus whereas SS hyperthermia is entirely derived from muscle activity.)[3,4]
- Intubation is recommended for patients who are unable to protect their airways as a result of mental status changes or seizures.[3]

ACUTE GENERAL Rx

- Benzodiazepines for control of agitation are preferred to physical restraints.[1]
  1. Lorazepam 2 to 4 mg IV every 30 min has been used effectively in treating agitation, muscle rigidity, myoclonus, and seizure complications, but while that is a good starting point, effective treatment often requires escalating to much higher doses.
  2. Diazepam 5 to 10 mg is an alternative choice.
- Patients may have rapid changes in blood pressure and heart rate. Hypertensive patients

should be treated with short-acting titratable agents (e.g., esmolol or nitroprusside). Hypotensive patients may require both IV fluids and vasopressor therapy.
- Serotonin antagonists should be titrated to clinical effectiveness in patients for whom nonpharmacologic therapy and benzodiazepines are not achieving adequate response. Although, limited evidence is available for these treatments.
  1. Cyproheptadine (4 mg tablet or 2 mg/5 ml syrup available)–widely accepted as standard of care
     a. Adults: 12 mg initially followed by 2 mg every 2 h until therapeutic response (up to 32 mg/day)
     b. Children (ages 7 to 14): 4 mg every 6 h (up to 16 mg/day)
     c. Children (ages 2 to 6): 2 mg every 6 h (up to 12 mg/day)
     d. Children (younger than 2 yr): 0.06 mg/kg every 6 h (up to 0.25 mg/kg/day)
  2. Atypical antipsychotic agents with serotonin antagonist properties (e.g., olanzapine 10 mg sublingual [SL]) have been tried with some success, but efficacy is unproven. It also has been reported in some instances to cause SS.[3]
  3. Chlorpromazine 50 to 100 mg intramuscularly may be considered in severe cases, but intravenous fluid loading is essential to prevent hypotension. This may also increase the likelihood of the patient seizing.
  4. Dantrolene and Bromocriptine which is used in treating NMS have no role in treating SS.[3,5]

CHRONIC Rx

For patients not requiring hospital admission, lorazepam can be given in an oral dose on a prn basis with close follow-up.

DISPOSITION[2,3]

- SS is a potentially life-threatening condition if not recognized early, although it does exist on a spectrum.
- Prompt diagnosis and withdrawal of the medication results in improvement of symptoms within 24 h.
- Seizures, rhabdomyolysis, hyperthermia, ventricular arrhythmia, respiratory arrest, and coma are all complicating features of SS.

REFERRAL

All cases of SS secondary to psychotropic medications should be referred to a psychiatrist.

PREVENTION

Modify prescription practices by avoiding multidrug regimens.

Detailed pharmacy review before starting high risk drugs (see Box 1).

(!) PEARLS & CONSIDERATIONS

The combined use of SSRIs and MAOIs is contraindicated.

- Despite serotonin syndrome being relatively rare, it is worth consideration in a differential even if common supporting elements to the diagnosis are absent such as meeting Hunter criteria, MAOI involvement, rapid onset, and hyperthermia.[4]
- Studies have suggested that genetic polymorphisms at the sites of CYP2D6 and T102C may contribute to individuals developing serotonin syndrome.[3]

COMMENTS

- The use of SSRIs and other serotonergic agents is not an absolute contraindication; however, prompt withdrawal of the medication is recommended if any symptoms suggesting SS occur.
- SS is usually found in patients being treated for depression, bipolar disorders, obsessive-compulsive disorder, attention deficit disorder, and Parkinson disease.
- SS can occur without an elevation of body temperature.
- Absence of MOAI does not exclude SS from one's differential; any other combinations of SSRIs or serotoninergic modulating drugs can precipitate SS.

REFERENCES

Available at eBooks.Health.Elsevier.com.

AUTHORS: **NATHAN STANFORD, MD,** and **ALAN TAYLOR, MD**

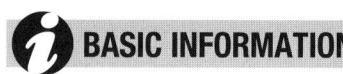

BASIC INFORMATION

DEFINITION

Sialolithiasis is the existence of hardened intra-luminal deposits in the ductal system of a salivary gland.

SYNONYMS

Salivary gland stone
Salivary calculus

ICD-10CM CODE
K11.5 Sialolithiasis

EPIDEMIOLOGY & DEMOGRAPHICS

Affects patients mostly in the fifth to eighth decades and occurs most commonly in the submandibular gland (85%); 15% of occurrences are located in a parotid gland (Table E1).

PHYSICAL FINDINGS & CLINICAL PRESENTATION

- Symptoms: Colicky postprandial pain and swelling of a salivary gland. Tends to have a remitting/relapsing course.
- Signs: Swelling and tenderness of a salivary gland. The stone may be felt with bimanual palpation of the floor of the mouth or inner cheek.

ETIOLOGY

- The cause is unknown. Contributing factors include saliva stagnation, sialadenitis (inflammation of a salivary gland), ductal inflammation, or injury (Fig. 1).
- Gout is a known cause of salivary gland calculi.
- Salivary calculus composition is mainly calcium phosphate and carbonate, often combined with small proportions of magnesium, zinc, ammonium salts, and organic materials or debris.

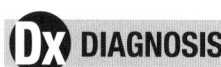

DIAGNOSIS

DIFFERENTIAL DIAGNOSIS

- Lymphadenitis
- Salivary gland tumor
- Salivary gland bacterial (*Staphylococcus* or *Streptococcus*), viral (mumps), or fungal infection (sialadenitis)
- Noninfectious salivary gland inflammation (e.g., Sjögren syndrome, sarcoidosis, lymphoma)
- Salivary duct stricture
- Dental abscess

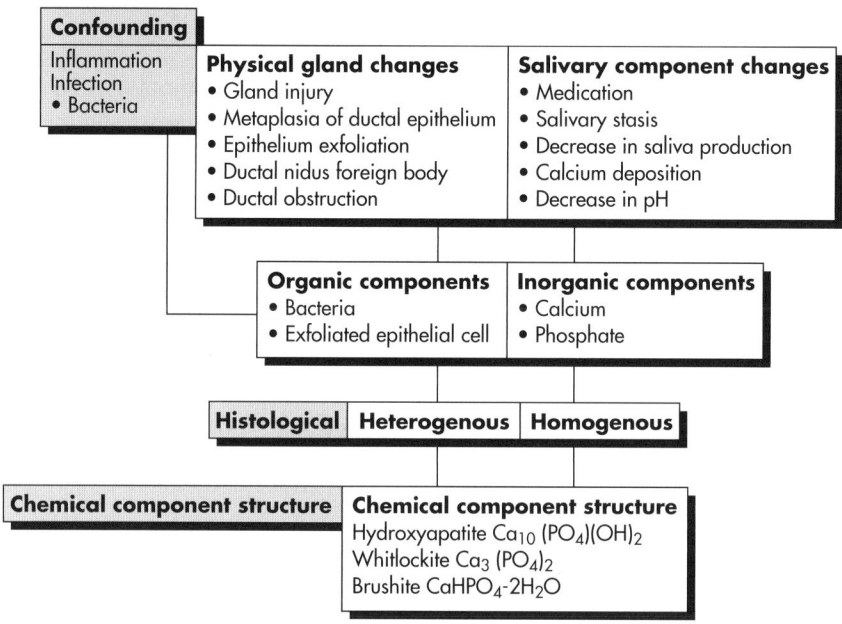

FIG. 1 Algorithm of clinical findings and pathogenesis of sialolithiasis. (From Lee LT, Wong YK: Sialolithiasis in minor salivary glands, *J Oral Maxillofac Surg*, 2010.)

IMAGING STUDIES

- X-ray: 90% of submandibular stones are radiopaque and will show up on x-ray. 90% of parotid stones are radiolucent and will not show up on x-ray.
- Noncontrast-enhanced computed tomography is very useful in detecting nearly all salivary stones.
- Ultrasound can detect 90% of salivary stones >2 mm.
- Sialography has a 95% to 100% sensitivity in detecting stones (Figs. E2 and E3), although it is more invasive than the above options and requires contrast injection into the affected duct.

TREATMENT

- Nonsurgical management is usually the first-line treatment.
  1. Warm compresses, gland massages, sialogogues (lemon wedges, sour candies), IV or oral hydration.
  2. Antibiotics if associated bacterial sialadenitis is present.
- Surgical treatment:

1. The surgical approach depends on the location of the stone. Submandibular stones in the distal aspect of the duct that are palpable may be excised transorally under local anesthesia. More proximal stones may require removal of the submandibular gland. Sialoendoscopy is a newer technique where a rigid endoscope and specialized instruments and/or lasers are used to visualize and remove the stones. Stones in the parotid duct also may be accessible via the transoral approach or may require parotidectomy. Sialoendoscopy is also an option for parotid stones.
2. Extracorporeal shock wave lithotripsy is an alternative technique that breaks up the stones into smaller fragments that can be secreted naturally through the duct.

REFERRAL

To otorhinolaryngologist

RELATED CONTENT

Salivary Gland Stones (Patient Information)
Sialadenitis (Related Key Topic)

AUTHOR: **LOUIS F. INSALACO, MD**

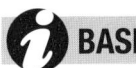

BASIC INFORMATION

DEFINITION

Sinus node dysfunction is a group of cardiac rhythm disturbances characterized by abnormalities of the sinus node leading to the inability of the SA node to react to heart rate changes to meet physiologic demands. This entity includes (1) sinus bradycardia (sinus rate <50 beats per minutes [BPM]); (2) ectopic atrial bradycardia; (3) sinus pauses or arrest; (4) sinoatrial exit block; (5) chronotropic incompetence; (6) alternating sinus bradycardia with paroxysmal supraventricular tachyarrhythmias (frequently atrial fibrillation), known as tachycardia-bradycardia syndrome; and (7) isorhythmic dissociation. When sinus node dysfunction is associated with symptoms, it is called sick sinus syndrome (SSS). The term *chronotropic incompetence* represents the inability to augment heart rates appropriately in response to exercise or activities of daily living.

SYNONYMS

Sinus pause
Sinus arrest
Inappropriate persistent sinus bradycardia
Tachycardia-bradycardia syndrome
Sinoatrial exit block
SSS
Bradycardia-tachycardia syndrome

ICD-10CM CODE
I49.5 Sick sinus syndrome

EPIDEMIOLOGY & DEMOGRAPHICS

- In children: Associated with genetic, congenital, and acquired heart disease, particularly after cardiac surgery.
- In adults: It is primarily a disease of the elderly secondary to progressive idiopathic degenerative disease. A modern population study has suggested that White race, increased body mass index, prolonged baseline QRS or right bundle branch block, elevated N-terminal pro-B-type natriuretic peptide, hypertension, or other cardiovascular diseases are associated with increased incidence of sick sinus syndrome. With an aging population, the annual incidence of SSS is projected to increase significantly.

PHYSICAL FINDINGS & CLINICAL PRESENTATION

- Fatigue, light-headedness, syncope, presyncope, palpitations. Other manifestations include dyspnea on exertion and chest pain. Usually symptoms are progressive; however, abrupt symptoms can occur (i.e., syncope).
- Physical examination may be normal or reveal abnormalities (e.g., irregular heart rhythm, signs of congestive heart failure, heart murmurs or gallop sounds) associated with the underlying heart disease.

TABLE 1 Indications for Permanent Pacing in Chronic Sinus Node Dysfunction

Class	Indications
I	• In patients who are symptomatic due to sinus node dysfunction, permanent pacing is indicated to increase heart rate and improve symptoms. • In patients with symptomatic sinus bradycardia as a consequence of necessary therapy for which there is no alternative treatment, permanent pacing is recommended to increase heart rate and improve symptoms.
IIa	• For patients with tachy-brady syndrome and symptomatic bradycardia, permanent pacing is reasonable to increase heart rate and reduce symptoms attributable to hypoperfusion. • In patients with symptomatic chronotropic incompetence, permanent pacing with rate-responsiveness is reasonable to improve symptoms and increase exertional heart rates.
IIb	• In patients with symptoms that are likely attributable to SND, a trial of oral theophylline may be considered to increase heart rate, improve symptoms, and help determine the potential benefits of permanent pacing.
III	• In asymptomatic patients with sinus bradycardia or sinus pauses that are secondary to physiologically elevated parasympathetic tone, permanent pacing should not be performed. • In patients with sleep-related sinus bradycardia or transient sinus pauses occurring during sleep, permanent pacing should not be performed in the absence of other indications for pacing. • In patients with asymptomatic SND, or in those in whom the symptoms have been documented to occur in the absence of bradycardia or chronotropic incompetence, permanent pacing is not indicated.

ACC, American College of Cardiology; *AHA*, American Heart Association; *HRS*, Heart Rhythm Society.
Adapted from Kusumoto FM et al: 2018 ACC/AHA/HRS guideline on the evaluation and management of patients with bradycardia and cardiac conduction delay, *J Am Coll Cardiol* 74(7): 932-987, 2019. doi:10.1016/j.jacc.2018.10.044.

ETIOLOGY

- Sinus node fibrosis is the primary etiology, which may also affect the atrioventricular node, the His bundle, or its branches. Polypharmacy should be considered and obtaining an accurate medicine list is essential. Common medications include β-blockers, non-dihydropyridine calcium channel blockers, digoxin, and antiarrhythmic medications.
- Additional etiologies include acute coronary syndromes, diseases of the SA nodal artery, inflammatory and infiltrative diseases (hemochromatosis, amyloidosis, sarcoidosis), collagen vascular diseases (systemic lupus erythematosus and scleroderma), epicardial and pericardial diseases, trauma following cardiac surgery, hypothyroidism, hypothermia, hypoxia, sepsis, muscular dystrophies (e.g., myotonic dystrophy, Friedreich ataxia), infectious etiologies such as Lyme disease and increased intracranial pressure.
- Note that the sinus node artery arises from right coronary artery in 60% of people and the left circumflex artery in 40%.

DIAGNOSIS

DIFFERENTIAL DIAGNOSIS

- Atrioventricular block
- Medication toxicity
- Carotid sinus hypersensitivity
- Metabolic abnormality (e.g., hyperkalemia in acute kidney injury)

WORKUP

- ECG (Fig. E1)

- Ambulatory cardiac rhythm monitoring with diary to correlate symptoms to findings. Event recorders, wearable ECG devices, or an implantable loop recorder if symptoms are less frequent. Note that establishment of diagnosis is more effective with longer-term recording (at least 2 to 4 wk) compared with 24-hr ambulatory ECG.
- Exercise stress testing to evaluate the severity of chronotropic incompetence.
- Electrophysiologic testing, including sinus node recovery time and sinoatrial conduction time.

TREATMENT

- Permanent pacemaker placement is primarily indicated if bradycardia is symptomatic and a reversible etiology is not identified. Indications for permanent pacemaker in sinus node dysfunction are described in Table 1.
- In tachycardia-bradycardia syndrome, drug treatment or ablation is often indicated for tachycardia after placement of a permanent pacemaker for bradycardia.

AUTHORS: **MICHAEL LAWRENZ CO, MD, MSC,** and **DANIEL R. FRISCH, MD**

Sickle Cell Disease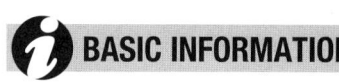

BASIC INFORMATION

DEFINITION

- Sickle cell disease (SCD) is a hemoglobin synthesis disorder in which the substitution of valine for glutamic acid at position six of the beta-globin chain yields a variant molecule, hemoglobin S. In its deoxygenated form, hemoglobin S (deoxy HgbS) polymerizes into long strands, deforming red blood cells (RBCs) into a characteristic sickle shape. Chronic RBC membrane damage from this process locks cells into an abnormal sickle shape; along with abnormal adherence to vascular endothelium, this leads to obstruction in the microcirculation and causes painful crises—the hallmark of sickle cell disease.
SCD patients include those who are homozygous sickle cell hemoglobin (HbS) and those with one sickle hemoglobin gene inherited with other hemoglobin abnormalities, notably beta thalassemia (Hgb S/β^0 or Hgb S/β^+ thalassemia) and hemoglobin C (HbSC). A comparison of sickle cell syndromes is summarized in Table 1.

SYNONYMS

Sickle cell anemia
SCD
Hemoglobin S disease

ICD-10CM CODES

D57.1	Sickle-cell disease without crisis
D57.20	Sickle-cell/Hb-C disease without crisis
D57.211	Sickle-cell/Hb-C disease with acute chest syndrome
D57.212	Sickle-cell/Hb-C disease with splenic sequestration
D57.219	Sickle-cell/Hb-C disease with crisis, unspecified
D57.3	Sickle-cell trait
D57.40	Sickle-cell thalassemia without crisis
D57.411	Sickle-cell thalassemia with acute chest syndrome
D57.412	Sickle-cell thalassemia with splenic sequestration
D57.419	Sickle-cell thalassemia with crisis, unspecified
D57.80	Other sickle-cell disorders without crisis
D57.811	Other sickle-cell disorders with acute chest syndrome
D57.812	Other sickle-cell disorders with splenic sequestration
D57.819	Other sickle-cell disorders with crisis, unspecified

EPIDEMIOLOGY & DEMOGRAPHICS

- SCD is an autosomal-recessive disorder. Sickle cell disease affects approximately 100,000 Americans. One in 13 children born to African Americans has sickle cell trait, and approximately 1 in 365 black children born in the U.S. has sickle cell anemia. Among children born to Hispanic Americans, the incidence of SCD is 1 in 16,300 live births.
- Sickle cell trait occurs in approximately 300 million people worldwide, with the highest prevalence of approximately 30% to 40% in sub-Saharan Africa, but also in the southern Mediterranean region (usually as Hgb S/β^0 or Hgb S/β^+), parts of the Middle East, and India. In the U.S., it is found in nearly 10% of African Americans.
- An estimated 2000 babies are born with sickle cell disease in the U.S. each year, and worldwide 275,000 infants are born with the disease annually.
- There is no predominant sex.

PHYSICAL FINDINGS & CLINICAL PRESENTATION

- Physical examination is variable depending on the degree of anemia and presence of acute vasoocclusive syndromes, as well as acute pulmonary, neurologic, cardiovascular, genitourinary, and musculoskeletal complications. Clinical manifestations of sickle cell disease are described in Table 2. Table 3 summarizes organ damage seen in sickle cell disease. Table 4 summarizes acute problems in sickle cell disease.
- A study of the prevalence of pain in sickle cell patients found that they complained of pain on 55% of days surveyed; another study showed 40% to 80% complained. Chronic pain may be due to avascular necrosis of joints and is sometimes poorly explained.
- There is no clinical laboratory finding that is pathognomonic of an episode of painful SCD crisis. The diagnosis is made solely on the basis of the medical history and physical examination. Elevated total bilirubin, reticulocytosis, and lactate dehydrogenase (LDH) are sometimes seen with crisis due to increased hemolysis. However, hemolytic anemia is typical for sickle cell disease at baseline. "Aplastic crisis" refers to crisis presenting with severe anemia and low reticulocyte count, usually caused by B19 parvovirus infection.
- Bones are the most common site of pain. Dactylitis, or hand-foot syndrome (acute, painful swelling of the hands and feet), is the first manifestation of sickle cell disease in many infants. Irritability and refusal to walk are other common symptoms. After infancy, musculoskeletal pain can be symmetric, asymmetric, or migratory, and it may or may not be associated with swelling, low-grade fever, redness, or warmth.
- In both children and adults, sickle vasoocclusive episodes are difficult to distinguish from osteomyelitis, septic arthritis, synovitis, rheumatic fever, or gout.
- Cholecystitis presents with abdominal pain commonly in patients with chronic hemolysis. In general, localizing symptoms for infections should be evaluated because these can trigger sickle crisis. Adult patients with severe SCD have splenic atrophy, whereas patients with milder disease (e.g., Hgb S/C) may have splenic infarct-related pain.
- Acute chest syndrome is a potentially life-threatening complication that manifests with chest pain, fever, wheezing, tachypnea, and cough and pulmonary infiltrates on imaging. Causes include infection (*Mycoplasma, Chlamydia,* viruses), infarction, and fat embolism; Fig. E1 illustrates the pathogenesis of the acute chest syndrome.

TABLE 1 Comparison of Sickle Cell Syndromes

GENOTYPE	CLINICAL CONDITION	PERCENT HEMOGLOBIN					OTHER FINDING(S)
		HB A	HB S	HB A$_2$	HB F	HB C	
SA	Sickle cell trait	55-60	40-45	2-3	–	–	Usually asymptomatic
SS	Sickle cell anemia	0	85-95	2-3	5-15	–	Clinically severe anemia; Hb F heterogeneous in distribution
S-β^0 thalassemia	Sickle cell β^0-thalassemia	0	70-80	3-5	10-20	–	Moderately severe anemia; splenomegaly in 50%; smear: hypochromic, microcytic anemia
S-β^+ thalassemia	Sickle cell β^+-thalassemia	10-20	60-75	3-5	10-20	–	Hb F distributed heterogeneously; mild microcytic anemia
SC	Hb SC disease	0	45-50	–	–	45-50	Moderately severe anemia; splenomegaly; retinopathy; target cells
S-HPFH	Sickle-hereditary persistence of Hb F	0	70-80	1-2	20-30	–	Often asymptomatic; Hb F is uniformly distributed

From Andreoli T et al: Cecil essentials of medicine, ed 7, Philadelphia, 2007, Saunders. In Marcdante KJ et al: *Nelson essentials of pediatrics,* ed 9, Philadelphia, 2023, Elsevier.

TABLE 2   Clinical Manifestations of Sickle Cell Disease*

MANIFESTATION	COMMENTS
Anemia	Chronic, onset 3-4 mo of age; hemoglobin usually 6-10 g/dl
Aplastic crisis	Parvovirus infection, reticulocytopenia; acute and reversible; may need transfusion
Sequestration crisis	Massive splenomegaly (may involve liver), shock; treat with transfusion
Hemolytic crisis	May be associated with G6PD deficiency
Dactylitis	Hand foot swelling in early infancy
Pain	Microvascular painful vasoocclusive infarcts of muscle, bone, bone marrow, lung, intestines; chronic pain (nervous system sensitization)
Cerebrovascular accidents (overt and silent)	Large and small vessel occlusion → thrombosis/bleeding (stroke); requires chronic transfusion; neurocognitive deficits
Acute chest syndrome	Infection, asthma, atelectasis, infarction, fat emboli, severe hypoxemia, infiltrate, dyspnea, absent breath sounds; treated with transfusions, antibiotics, oxygen, bronchodilators
Chronic lung disease	Pulmonary fibrosis, restrictive lung disease, cor pulmonale, pulmonary hypertension
Priapism	Causes eventual impotence; treated with transfusion, oxygen, or corpora cavernosa-to-spongiosa shunt
Ocular	Retinopathy
Gallbladder disease	Bilirubin stones; cholecystitis
Renal	Hematuria, papillary necrosis, renal concentrating defect; nephropathy
Cardiomyopathy	Heart failure
Skeletal	Osteonecrosis (avascular) of femoral or humeral head
Leg ulceration	Seen in older patients
Infections	Functional asplenia, defects in properdin system; pneumococcal bacteremia, meningitis, and arthritis; deafness from meningitis; *Salmonella* and *Staphylococcus aureus* osteomyelitis; severe *Mycoplasma* pneumonia
Growth failure, delayed puberty	May respond to nutritional supplements
Psychosocial issues	Depression, anxiety, attention deficit hyperactivity disorder (ADHD)

G6PD, Glucose-6-phosphate dehydrogenase.

*Clinical manifestations with sickle cell trait are unusual but include renal papillary necrosis (hematuria), sudden death on exertion, intraocular hyphema extension, and sickling in unpressurized airplanes.

From Marcdante KJ et al: *Nelson essentials of pediatrics,* ed 9, Philadelphia, 2023, Elsevier.

TABLE 3   Organ Damage Seen in Sickle Cell Disease

Organ or System	Injury
Skin	Stasis ulcer
Central nervous system	Cerebrovascular accident
Eye	Retinal hemorrhage, retinopathy
Cardiac	Congestive heart failure
Pulmonary	Intrapulmonary shunting, embolism, infarct, infection
Vascular	Occlusive phenomenon at any site
Liver	Hepatic infarct, hepatitis resulting from transfusion, hepatic sequestration, intrahepatic cholestasis
Gallbladder	Increased incidence of bilirubin gallstones caused by hemolysis
Spleen	Acute sequestration
Urinary	Hyposthenuria, hematuria
Genital	Decreased fertility, impotence, priapism
Skeletal	Bone infarcts, osteomyelitis, aseptic necrosis
Placenta	Insufficiency with fetal wastage
Leukocytes	Relative immunodeficiency
Erythrocytes	Chronic hemolysis

From Marx J et al: *Rosen's emergency medicine: concepts and clinical practice,* ed 7, Philadelphia, 2010, Mosby.

- Musculoskeletal and skin abnormalities include leg ulcers (particularly on the malleoli) and limb-girdle deformities caused by avascular necrosis of the femoral and humeral heads. Osteonecrosis of the heads of the femur and humerus is found in nearly 50% of adults with Hgb S/S disease.
- Endocrine abnormalities include delayed sexual maturation and late physical maturation, especially evident in boys.
- Neurologic abnormalities on examination may include seizures and altered mental status. Strokes occur in about 10% of children and adults with sickle cell anemia and approximately 35% of children with sickle cell anemia have cerebrovascular disease.
- Infections, particularly involving *Salmonella, Staphylococcus aureus, Mycoplasma,* and *Streptococcus,* are relatively common. Catheter-associated bacteremia should be considered if a vascular access device is present; these may present without fever.
- Severe splenomegaly as a result of sequestration often occurs in children before splenic atrophy.

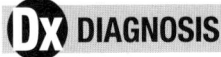 **DIAGNOSIS**

DIFFERENTIAL DIAGNOSIS
- Thalassemia
- Other hemolytic anemias
- The differential diagnosis of patients presenting with a painful crisis is discussed in "Physical Findings"

WORKUP (TABLE 5)
- Screening of all newborns regardless of racial background is performed in the U.S. Screening can be performed with sodium metabisulfite reduction test (Sickledex test).
- Hemoglobin electrophoresis will also confirm the diagnosis and is useful to identify hemoglobin variants such as fetal hemoglobin and hemoglobin C.
- Patients will have evidence of hemolysis (elevated reticulocyte count, low haptoglobin, variable elevation of LDH and total bilirubin).
- Chest x-ray often reveals typical vertebral body changes ("fish mouth" vertebrae) caused by chronic vasoocclusive injury to vertebral bodies.
- For prenatal diagnosis, initial step is identification of parenteral globin gene mutation by DNA-based testing. If positive, then DNA-based testing of chorionic villus sampling or amniotic fluid cells is performed.

LABORATORY TESTS
- Anemia (from chronic hemolysis), reticulocytosis, leukocytosis, and thrombocytosis are common. Hgb S/β^0 and Hgb S/β^+ thalassemia will have microcytosis; Hgb S/C is also typically microcytic. Hgb S/C may have normal or near-normal hematocrit but will have characteristic changes on peripheral smear (target cells).
- Elevations of bilirubin, lactate dehydrogenase, and low haptoglobin are consistent with chronic hemolysis.
- Peripheral blood smear may reveal sickle cells, target cells, poikilocytosis, and hypochromia (Fig. 2).

TABLE 4 Acute Problems in Sickle Cell Disease

Dactylitis. Typically the bones of the hands and feet are affected, with fever and leukocytosis. It is often the first event in young children and can occur multiple times until the age 3 yr.

Painful crises. Typically occurs after the first few years in bones or occasionally abdominal viscera. Pain is caused by ischemia and can be very severe. Crises are associated with low-grade fever and mild leukocytosis compared with osteomyelitis, in which fever and leukocytosis are more pronounced. Pain relief with paracetamol, nonsteroidal antiinflammatory drugs, or opioids, as appropriate, should be instigated immediately. Supportive measures such as hydration, intravenously if necessary, and oxygen also help to reduce the duration of the pain crisis. Any precipitating cause such as infection should be treated.

Central nervous system events. Strokes occur in up to 17% of children and young adults. The pathogenesis is unclear, but angiography often shows occlusions or stenosis. Recurrence is likely unless a long-term transfusion program is initiated.

Acute chest syndrome. This is a common cause of death presenting with fever, tachypnea, chest pain, and leukocytosis, often with a sudden drop in hemoglobin. It can be difficult to differentiate among infection, infarction, and embolism. Common precipitating causes are pulmonary fat embolism and infections. Treatment is with transfusion (simple or exchange), antibiotics, and aggressive treatment of hypoxia.

Splenic sequestration. This occurs in children between ages 6 mo and 2 yr. It is caused by sudden trapping of red cells within the spleen, producing a sudden drop in hemoglobin and rapidly enlarging spleen, eventually leading to hypovolemic shock and death. Management includes early detection of the rapidly enlarging spleen and blood transfusion.

Priapism. Engorgement of the penis can be short-lived and self-terminating, or it can last in excess of 24 hr and may lead to impotence. Initial management is with fluids and analgesia, but persistent priapism (>12 hr) may need partial exchange transfusion and corporal aspiration.

Infections. Overwhelming infection with *Streptococcus pneumoniae* is the most common cause of death in children. Other common causes of infections in sickle cell disease include *Haemophilus influenzae* and *Salmonella*. A significant reduction in the number of deaths from sepsis has resulted from the routine use of vaccinations against these organisms and antibiotic prophylaxis. Malaria prophylaxis should be considered in endemic areas.

From Ryan ET et al: *Hunter's tropical medicine and emerging infectious diseases*, ed 10, Philadelphia, 2019, Elsevier.

TABLE 5 Baseline Evaluations to Consider

	Tests
Blood tests	CBC with differential
	Reticulocyte count
	Hemoglobin HPLC or electrophoresis
	LDH
	Renal function tests
	Liver function tests
	Mineral panel
	Serum iron, ferritin, TIBC
	Vitamin D level
	Hepatitis B sAg
	Hepatitis C antibody
	RBC alloantibody screen
	RBC typing
	D-dimer[a]
	C-reactive protein[a]
	Brain natriuretic peptide
Urine and kidney tests	Urinalysis
	Renal ultrasonography[b]
Radiology	MRI or MRA brain (adults)[c] or transcranial Doppler ultrasonography starting at age 2 yr (children)
	Chest radiography[d]
	Hip or shoulder radiograph or MRI (or both)[c]
	Bone density in teenagers and adults
Cardiology and pulmonary	Echocardiogram
Neurocognitive	Neurocognitive testing[d]

CBC, Complete blood count; *HPLC*, high-performance liquid chromatography; *LDH*, lactate dehydrogenase; *MRA*, magnetic resonance angiography; *MRI*, magnetic resonance imaging; *RBC*, red blood cell; *sAg*, surface antigen; *TIBC*, total iron-binding capacity.
[a]Consider following as surrogate markers after initiation of disease-modifying intervention.
[b]If hematuria with red blood cells in urine.
[c]As clinically indicated.
[d]If the patient has poor school performance, an abnormal memory, or abnormal MRI findings.
From Hoffman R et al: *Hematology: basic principles and practice*, ed 7, Philadelphia, 2018, Elsevier.

- Elevated blood urea nitrogen and creatinine may be present in patients presenting acutely with dehydration or chronically with progressive renal insufficiency.
- Urinalysis may reveal hematuria and proteinuria. Patients with SCD should be screened for microalbuminuria and proteinuria with spot urine testing by 10 yr of age.

IMAGING STUDIES (FIGS. E3 AND E4)

- Chest x-ray or noncontrast chest CT scan to evaluate acute and chronic lung changes is helpful.
- Routine skeletal imaging is rarely helpful in acute crisis and should usually be reserved for pain that is not consistent with transient acute crisis.
- MRI or bone scan is useful to address chronic avascular necrosis or, in the acute setting, osteomyelitis.
- CT or MRI scan of brain is not indicated in asymptomatic adults and children with SCD but is often needed in patients with neurologic complications, such as transient ischemic attack, cerebrovascular accident, seizures, or altered mental status.
- Transcranial Doppler ultrasonography (TCD) is used to identify children with sickle cell anemia who are at risk for stroke. There should be an annual screening starting at age 2 until age 16. Patients determined to be at risk (transcranial Doppler velocity ≥200 cm/s) should be enrolled in long-term transfusion programs. These transfusions are effective in reducing risk of stroke by >90%. In adults, magnetic resonance angiography (MRA) can be used instead of TCD to identify those at risk for stroke.
- Doppler echocardiography should be performed in patients with unexplained respiratory symptoms to evaluate for pulmonary hypertension (Fig. E5), with right heart catheterization performed if abnormal. Screening for vasculopathy is done by estimating the tricuspid regurgitant jet velocity (TRV). Elevated values are predictive of early mortality. The prevalence of pulmonary hypertension when right heart catheterization is performed is approximately 6% in adults with sickle cell disease.

🆁🆇 TREATMENT

NONPHARMACOLOGIC THERAPY

- Patients should be instructed to avoid conditions that may precipitate sickling crisis, such as extremes of cold and heat and dehydration.
- Maintain adequate hydration (PO or IV).
- Correct hypoxia when present.

ACUTE GENERAL Rx

- Initiate aggressive IV and oral hydration; most patients in crisis have evidence of dehydration. Use hypo-osmolar fluids, such as LR or 0.45 normal saline, for intravenous hydration during acute crisis in the hospitalized patient. Normal

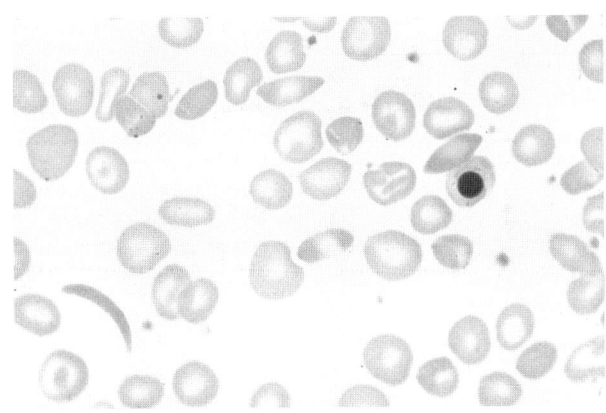

FIG. 2 Photomicrograph of a blood film. Sickle cell anemia (homozygosity for hemoglobin S). Shown are a sickle cell, boat-shaped cells, a nucleated red cell, and target cells. (From Bain BJ et al: *Dacie and Lewis practical haematology,* ed 12, Philadelphia, 2017, Elsevier.)

TABLE 6 Bacteria and Viruses That Most Frequently Cause Serious Infection in Patients With Sickle Cell Disease

Microorganism	Type of Infection	Comments
Streptococcus pneumoniae	Septicemia	Common despite prophylactic penicillin and pneumococcal vaccine
	Meningitis	Less frequent than in years past
	Pneumonia	Rarely documented except in infants and young children
	Septic arthritis	Uncommon
Haemophilus influenzae type b	Septicemia	
Meningitis		
Pneumonia	Much less common in recent years because of immunization with conjugate vaccine	
Salmonella species	Osteomyelitis	
Septicemia	Most common cause of bone and joint infection	
Escherichia coli and other gram-negative enteric pathogens	Septicemia	
Urinary tract infection		
Osteomyelitis	Focus sometimes not apparent	
Staphylococcus aureus	Osteomyelitis	Uncommon
Mycoplasma pneumoniae	Pneumonia	Pleural effusions; multilobe involvement
Chlamydia pneumoniae	Pneumonia	
Parvovirus B19	Bone marrow suppression (aplastic crisis)	High fever common; rash and other organ involvement infrequent
Hepatitis viruses (A, B, and C)	Hepatitis	Marked hyperbilirubinemia

Data from Buchanan GR, Glader BE: Benign course of extreme hyperbilirubinemia in sickle cell anemia: analysis of six cases, *J Pediatr* 91:21, 1977. From Hoffman R et al: *Hematology: basic principles and practice,* ed 7, Philadelphia, 2018, Elsevier.

saline has adverse biochemical effects on sickled cells and may lead to increase pain.

- L-arginine 1000 mg/kg TID, decreases narcotic use by approximately 54% in the hospitalized patient during a vaso-occlusive crisis.
- Aggressively diagnose and treat suspected infections such as urinary infection, respiratory infections, or catheter-associated line infections. Table 6 summarizes bacteria and viruses that most frequently cause serious infection in patients with sickle cell disease.

- Provide pain relief during the vaso-occlusive crisis (Table 7). Most patients will have a treatment history that can guide dosing. Opiate management is complicated by high levels of tolerance in patients often treated over many years. Patient-controlled analgesic pumps are often helpful; caution should be used when employing continuous infusions, which are usually not necessary or helpful. Morphine and hydromorphone are most commonly used. Meperidine is rarely used now and generally discouraged because of neurologic side effects, although some patients state a preference for it.

- Oral diphenhydramine is used to control pruritus, which is commonly associated with opiate analgesics; preferred to IV therapy in guidelines.
- Tables 8 and 9 summarize overall strategies for the management of acute chest syndrome.
- Follow oxygenation in patients presenting with chest pain or respiratory symptoms; assess for evolving acute chest syndrome if oxygenation deteriorates.
- Urology evaluation for priapism.

CHRONIC Rx

- Hydroxyurea increases hemoglobin F levels, reduces the incidence of vasoocclusive complications, and improves survival. It is helpful in patients with Hgb S/S and S/β[o] thalassemia; its value in other variants is less certain. There is strong evidence to support use of hydroxyurea therapy in children ages 9 mo and older to decrease the frequency of vasoocclusive crises and acute chest syndrome. Hydroxyurea is also strongly recommended for adults with three or more crises during any 12-mo period, with SCD pain or chronic anemia interfering with daily activities, or with severe or recurrent episodes of acute chest syndrome. It should be stopped in pregnancy, and contraception counseling should be given to all patients.
- Recommended starting doses for hydroxyurea are 15 mg/kg/day in adults and 5 to 10 mg/kg/day in patients with renal disease. A recent randomized study has shown markedly superior efficacy with a dose escalation strategy of up to 30 mg/kg/day compared with traditional dosing of 20 mg/kg/day.
- Pharmaceutical grade L-glutamine is approved for use to decrease crisis symptoms in patients with Hgb S/S and Hgb S/β[o] thalassemia; benefits include decrease in acute crisis episodes, reduced hospitalization, and decrease in episodes of acute chest syndrome. Dosing is 5 to 15 g tid, taken with food or 8 oz of cold or room-temperature fluid. Constipation, nausea, headache, and abdominal discomfort were common side effects, occurring in approximately 15% to 20% of patients. It may work with or without concomitant use of hydroxyurea. Caution may be warranted in prescribing L-glutamine to patients with clinically significant renal or hepatic dysfunction.
- Replace folic acid (1 mg PO daily) to replace increased utilization of folic acid stores from chronic hemolysis. Patients also have mineral and vitamin deficiencies (calcium; zinc; and vitamins A, C, D, and E) and may need oral supplementation.
- Chronic pain management represents an enduring challenge, made more difficult by the current opiate addiction and overdose epidemic. In one study, patients reported pain in 55% of days. Review of guidelines for safe opiate prescribing is strongly recommended

TABLE 7 Recommended Dose and Interval of Analgesics Necessary to Obtain Adequate Pain Control in Patients With Sickle Cell Disease

	Dose/Rate	Comments
Severe to Moderate Pain		
Morphine	Parenteral: 0.1-0.15 mg/kg every 3-4 h Recommended maximum single dose, 10 mg PO: 0.3-0.6 mg/kg every 4 h	Drug of choice for pain; lower doses in elderly adults and infants and in patients with liver failure or impaired ventilation
Meperidine	Parenteral: 0.75-1.5 mg/kg every 2-4 h Recommended maximum dose, 100 mg PO: 1.5 mg/kg every 4 h	Increased incidence of seizures; avoid in patients with renal or neurologic disease and those who receive MAOIs
Hydromorphone	Parenteral: 0.01-0.02 mg/kg every 3-4 h PO: 0.04-0.06 mg/kg every 4 h	
Oxycodone	PO: 0.15 mg/kg/dose every 4 h	
Ketorolac	IM: Adults: 30 or 60 mg initial dose followed by 15-30 mg; children: 1 mg/kg load followed by 0.5 mg/kg every 6 h	Equal efficacy to 6 mg MS; helps narcotic-sparing effect; not to exceed 5 days; maximum, 150 mg first day, 120 mg maximum on subsequent days; may cause gastric irritation
Butorphanol	Parenteral: Adults: 2 mg every 3-4 h	Agonist–antagonist; can precipitate withdrawal if given to patients who are being treated with agonists
Mild Pain		
Codeine	PO: 0.5-1 mg/kg every 4 h Maximum dose, 60 mg	Mild to moderate pain not relieved by aspirin or acetaminophen; can cause nausea and vomiting
Aspirin	PO: Adults: 0.3-6 mg every 4-6 h; children: 10 mg/kg every 4 h	Often given with a narcotic to enhance analgesia; can cause gastric irritation; avoid in febrile children
Acetaminophen	PO: Adults: 0.3-0.6 g every 4 h; children: 10 mg/kg	Often given with a narcotic to enhance analgesia
Ibuprofen	PO: Adults: 300-400 mg every 4 h; children: 5-10 mg/kg every 6-8 h	Can cause gastric irritation
Naproxen	PO: Adults: 500 mg/dose initially and then 250 every 8-12 h; children: 10 mg/kg/day (5 mg/kg every 12 h)	Long duration of action; can cause gastric irritation
Indomethacin	PO: Adults: 25 mg every 8 h; children: 1-3 mg/kg/day given 3 or 4 times	Contraindicated in psychiatric, neurologic, renal diseases; high incidence of gastric irritation; useful in gout

IM, Intramuscular; *MAOI*, monoamine oxidase inhibitor; *MS*, morphine sulphate; *PO*, oral.

Adapted from Charache S et al: Effect of hydroxyurea on the frequency of painful crises in sickle cell anemia: investigators of the multicenter study of hydroxyurea in sickle cell anemia, *N Engl J Med* 332:1317, 1995. In Hoffman R et al: *Hematology: basic principles and practice,* ed 7, Philadelphia, 2018, Elsevier.

TABLE 8 Overall Strategies for the Management of Acute Chest Syndrome

Prevention

Incentive spirometry and periodic ambulation in patients admitted for sickle cell pain, surgery, or febrile episodes

Watchful waiting in any hospitalized child or adult with sickle cell disease (pulse oximetry monitoring and frequent respiratory assessments)

Cautious use of intravenous fluids

Intense education and optimum care of patients who have sickle cell anemia and asthma

Diagnostic Testing and Laboratory Monitoring

Blood cultures, if febrile

Nasopharyngeal samples for viral culture (respiratory syncytial virus, influenza), depending on clinical setting

Complete blood counts every day and appropriate chemistries

Continuous pulse oximetry

Chest radiographs for persistent or progressive illness

Treatment

Blood transfusion (simple or exchange) depending on clinical features; consider maintaining an active type and crossmatch

Supplemental O_2 for drop in pulse oximetry by 4% over baseline, or values <90%

Empirical antibiotics (third-generation cephalosporin and macrolide)

Continued respiratory therapy (incentive spirometry and chest physiotherapy as necessary)

Bronchodilators and corticosteroids for patients with asthma

Optimum pain control and fluid management

From Kliegman RM: *Nelson textbook of pediatrics,* ed 21, Philadelphia, 2020, Elsevier.

and management with pain management specialists is also strongly recommended.

- Indications for PRBC transfusion in SCD are described in Table 10. Urgent exchange transfusion for acute chest syndrome with progressive hypoxia (arterial oxygen saturation <90%) or multiorgan failure may be lifesaving. Simple transfusion may be adequate in milder cases with a target Hgb of 10 g/dl. Transfusion therapy is appropriate for patients with stroke or at high risk by transcranial Doppler study (see earlier) if possible.

Transfusion has shown to be beneficial in children with silent infarcts by MRI in preventing progression. Transfusion to Hgb 10 g/dl is recommended in anemic patients undergoing general anesthesia to reduce crisis and respiratory complications after surgery. Patients on chronic transfusion therapy should receive RBC matched at C, E, and K antigens to avoid alloimmunization. Transfusion is not recommended for asymptomatic anemia. Serum ferritin level should be monitored quarterly. Iron overload due to blood transfusions (transfusional hemosiderosis) can be treated with chelating agents (deferoxamine [SC infusion], deferasirox [PO], and deferiprone [PO]).

- Annual screening for proteinuria is recommended. ACE inhibitor therapy should be started for microalbuminuria in adults with SCD to prevent progression of renal injury. Progressive renal injury may cause worsening anemia and responds to erythropoietin.
- Annual retinopathy screening should be performed beginning at age 10, especially for patients with Hgb S/C variant, in whom proliferative retinopathy occurs in about 30% to 50%. It is less common in Hgb S/S and other variants.
- Gene therapy for SCD patients represents a novel approach. Clinical trials with lentiviral vector-mediated addition of an antisickling

TABLE 9 Treatment of the Acute Chest Syndrome

Oxygen therapy to maintain arterial hemoglobin oxygen saturation >92%

Pain control and incentive spirometry to reduce chest wall splinting and pulmonary atelectasis

Close clinical observation
- Monitor Po2/Fio2 ratio
- Particular attention to worsening respiratory function

Asthma therapy if indicated

Empirical antibiotics
- Cover typical and atypical respiratory pathogens
- Consider regional and seasonal risk of methicillin-resistant *Staphylococcus aureus*
- Anticipate influenza A or B infections and treat/prevent accordingly

Transfusion therapy
- Main indication for transfusion therapy in ACS is worsening respiratory function
- Simple transfusion is as effective as erythrocytapheresis in the usual patient
- Patients with high initial hemoglobin concentrations (≥9 g/dl) or patients with more severe disease should receive erythrocytapheresis
- Transfused blood should be matched to Rh, C, E, and Kell antigens, and transfusion records documenting history of prior alloantibodies should be obtained

ACS, Acute chest syndrome; *Fio2,* fractional concentration of oxygen in inspired gas; *Po2,* partial pressure of oxygen.
From Broaddus VC et al: *Murray & Nadel's textbook of respiratory medicine*, ed 7, Philadelphia, 2022, Elsevier.

TABLE 10 Indications for Transfusion in Sickle Cell Disease

	Duration	Consensus	Method	Goal*
Stroke, acute	Single	+	Ex	HbS <30%
Stroke, ongoing care	Chronic	+	Either	HbS <30%
High-velocity transcranial Doppler	Chronic	+	Either	HbS <30%
ACS, initial episode	Single	+	Dir > Ex	Hgb 10
ACS, recurrent	6-12 mo	+	Either	
Pulmonary hypertension	Chronic	+	Either	
Multiorgan failure	Single	+	Ex	
Major surgery	Single	+	Dir	Hgb 10
Acute anemia	Single	+	Dir	
Recurrent spleen sequestration	Chronic	+		
Sepsis/meningitis	Single	+	Dir	
Severe chronic pain	6-12 mo	+		
Congestive heart failure	Chronic	+		
Silent infarct with abnormal neuropsychology	Chronic	−		
Pregnancy		−		
Anemia/renal failure	Chronic	−		
Leg ulcers	6-12 mo	−		
Severe growth delay		−		
Severe eye disease		−		
Priapism		−		

ACS, Acute chest syndrome; *Dir,* direct; *Ex,* exchange; *Hb,* hemoglobin type; *Hgb,* hemoglobin concentration; +, consensus reached; −, consensus not reached.
*Goal of transfusion if a consensus has been reached.
From Fuhrman BP et al: *Pediatric critical care*, ed 4, Philadelphia, 2011, Saunders.

β-globin gene into autologous hematopoietic stem cells are ongoing with encouraging early results in terms of reduction of sickle cell crises and correction of the biologic hallmarks of the disease. A level of erythrocyte fetal hemoglobin (HbF) comprising alpha and gamma globins may ameliorate the hemolytic anemia of sickle cell disease by mitigating sickle hemoglobin polymerization and erythrocyte sickling. BCL11A is a repressor of gamma-globin expression and HbF production in adult erythrocytes. Its down-regulation is a promising therapeutic strategy for induction of HbF. Gene therapy trials with the use of LentiGlobin have shown sustained production of HbA^T87Q in most red cells, leading to reduced hemolysis and complete resolution of severe vaso-occlusive events.[1]

- Allogeneic stem cell transplantation can be curative in young patients with symptomatic SCD.
- Crizanlizumab, an antibody against the adhesion molecule p-selectin, revealed a significantly lower rate of sickle cell–related pain crisis than placebo and was associated with a low incidence of adverse events in a recent study. It has been approved for the prevention of vasoocclusive crises in adults and pediatric patients ages 16 yr and older.
- Voxelotor, an inhibitor of sickle hemoglobin (HbS) polymerization, significantly increases hemoglobin levels and reduces markers of hemolysis and is approved for the therapy of adults and children over age 12 yr.
- Penicillin V 125 mg PO bid should be administered by age 2 mo and increased to 250 mg bid by age 3 yr. Penicillin prophylaxis can be discontinued after age 5 yr, except in children who have had splenectomy.
- Table 11 summarizes disease-modifying treatments to consider.

REFERRAL

- Hospitalization for pain crisis unresponsive to oral analgesics, or involving fever, respiratory symptoms, or vomiting and diarrhea.
- Optimal management requires coordination with hematology, blood banking, pain management, and psychosocial counseling and support.
- Referral for patients with organ-specific complications, notably pulmonary hypertension, acute/chronic kidney disease, and ophthalmologic complications.
- Referral to an ophthalmologist for an annual dilated retinal examination beginning at 10 yr of age.

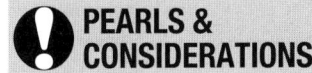

PEARLS & CONSIDERATIONS

COMMENTS

- The average life span of individuals with sickle cell trait is similar to that of the general population. It may be associated with hematuria, often painless, and rhabdomyolysis under extreme conditions. Chronic pain and acute pain are not typical of sickle cell trait. It is also associated with a higher incidence of renal medullary cancer. Chronic problems in sickle cell disease are summarized in Table 12.
- Regular immunizations, especially pneumococcal vaccination, are recommended. The prophylactic administration of penicillin soon after birth and the timely administration of pneumococcal and *Haemophilus influenzae* type b vaccines have resulted in a significant decline in the incidence of these infections. The heptavalent conjugated pneumococcal vaccine (Prevnar) should be administered from 2 mo of age. The 23-valent unconjugated pneumococcal vaccine (Pneumovax) is given from age 2 yr and can be boosted once 3 yr

TABLE 11 Disease-Modifying Treatments to Consider[a]

Robust clinical data	Penicillin prophylaxis
	Streptococcus pneumoniae vaccination
	Hydroxyurea
	Chronic exchange transfusion
	Iron chelation for chronic iron overload[b]
Limited clinical data	Daily multivitamin without iron or folate supplementation *and* vitamin D replacement[c]
	Haemophilus influenzae vaccination
	Influenza vaccination
	Erythropoietin
	Phlebotomy
Experimental	Hb F reactivation with decitabine, histone deacetylase inhibitors, or imids
	Erythropoietin for chronic relative reticulocytopenia
	Nutritional supplements and antioxidants (e.g., glutamine, zinc, multivitamins)
	N-acetylcysteine

Hb F, Fetal hemoglobin.
[a]See text for specific indications and limitations.
[b]Best data from thalassemia patient experience.
[c]Risks minimal; therefore it is generally done.
From Hoffman R et al: *Hematology: basic principles and practice,* ed 7, Philadelphia, 2018, Elsevier.

TABLE 12 Chronic Problems in Sickle Cell Disease

Growth and development	Reduced height and weight
	Pubertal delay
	Cognitive impairment (recurrent small strokes)
Locomotor	Osteonecrosis of humeral and femoral heads
	Chronic leg ulcers
Cardiovascular	Myocardial infarction
	Left and right ventricular dilatation
Pulmonary	Pulmonary fibrosis
	Pulmonary hypertension
	Cor pulmonale
Genitourinary	Renal papillary necrosis—hematuria and tubular defects
	Chronic renal failure
	Frequent urinary tract infections in women
	Impotence (secondary to priapism)
Ocular	Proliferative retinopathy (30% of patients)
	Blindness (especially in SC disease)
	Retinal detachment

SC, Sickle cell.
From Ryan ET et al: *Hunter's tropical medicine and emerging infectious diseases,* ed 10, Philadelphia, 2019, Elsevier.

later. Influenza vaccination can be given after 6 mo of age.

- In patients with SCD presenting with acute crisis, intravenous hydration with hypotonic saline is favored over normal saline. Normal saline can have adverse biochemical effects on sickle cell and possibly lead to increased pain.
- Pulmonary hypertension is a complication of chronic hemolysis and is associated with a high risk of death. It can be detected by Doppler echocardiography in more than 30% of adult patients with sickle cell disease. Cardiac catheterization will confirm the diagnosis. It is resistant to hydroxyurea therapy.
- Malnutrition can lead to poor clinical outcomes in patients with SCD. Identifying patients at risk might improve outcomes.
- Vitamin D deficiency is common and should be treated to prevent adverse skeletal outcomes.
- Metformin increases fetal hemoglobin (HbF) levels in patients with SCD. A recent study revealed that metformin use in SCD patients with diabetes is associated with fewer episodes of consequential SCD complications and with lower health care utilization.
- Exposure to systemic corticosteroids is associated with a fourfold excess risk for hospitalization for a vaso-occlusive episode (VOE).[2]

REFERENCES & SUGGESTED READINGS
Available at eBooks.Health.Elsevier.com.

RELATED CONTENT
Sickle Cell Anemia (Patient Information)

AUTHOR: **RELINDIS AZENWI FRU, MD**

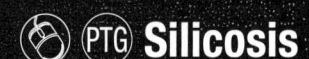

S

 BASIC INFORMATION

DEFINITION

Silicosis is a spectrum of chronic fibrotic lung disease caused by inhalation of crystalline silica.

SYNONYMS

Pneumoconiosis caused by silica
Silicoproteinosis
Progressive massive fibrosis

ICD-10CM CODE

J62.8 Pneumoconiosis due to other dust containing silica

EPIDEMIOLOGY & DEMOGRAPHICS

- Occupational lung disease impacting workers exposed to respirable crystalline silica across a number of professions. Jobs associated with an increased risk of silicosis are described in Box 1.
- According to the Occupational Safety and Health Administration (OSHA), approximately 2.3 million Americans are exposed to respirable crystalline silica at work.[1]
- Within the U.S., age-adjusted death rates due to silicosis have decreased over time.[2] However, the quality of mortality data is limited. New outbreaks of silicosis have been described worldwide in the past 5 yrs among engineered stone fabricators.[3]

PHYSICAL FINDINGS & CLINICAL PRESENTATION

There are three patterns of silicosis: Acute silicoproteinosis, simple chronic silicosis, and progressive massive fibrosis.[4]
- Acute silicosis is also known as silicoproteinosis. Develops within days to weeks of a high level respirable crystalline silica exposure. Presents with rapid onset acute hypoxic respiratory failure, cough, and fatigue.
- Chronic silicosis is the most common clinical presentation, and onset occurs after decades of repeated exposure. It has two types:
  1. Simple silicosis, which may be asymptomatic, with the only manifestation being an abnormal chest x-ray. Latency period is 10 to 20 yrs. Over time, patients may develop increasing dyspnea and cough.
  2. Progressive massive fibrosis characterized by x-ray progression and resulting fibrosis. Patients report dyspnea, cough, and pleuritic chest pain, and may be hypoxic on examination.
- Patients with chronic silicosis may develop an accelerated form of disease, with rapid progression to progressive massive fibrosis (less than 10 yrs after first exposure). Patients with recurrent, high-level exposures have a greater risk of developing accelerated disease.

ETIOLOGY

- Inhaled respirable crystalline silica becomes lodged in the terminal bronchioles
- Engulfed by alveolar macrophages, which release interleukin-1 (IL-1) and tumor necrosis factor alpha (TNF-alpha) triggering the inflammatory cascade
- Persistent inflammatory cytokine release recruits type 2 pneumocytes and fibroblasts
- Collagen deposition in the interstitium, leading to fibrosis (Fig. E1)

DIAGNOSIS

DIFFERENTIAL DIAGNOSIS

- Other pneumoconiosis (coal workers' pneumoconiosis, siderosis, talcosis)
- Sarcoidosis
- Fungal infection (blastomycosis, coccidioidomycosis, histoplasmosis)
- Tuberculosis
- Interstitial lung disease
- Lung cancer
- Amyloidosis

WORKUP

- Occupational and exposure history
- Chest x-ray (Fig. E2)
- High resolution computed tomography (CT) imaging (Fig. E3)
- Pulmonary function testing
- Lung biopsy (not required if history and imaging are suggestive)

Acute silicosis:
- Chest x-ray examination demonstrates typical pattern of perihilar or basilar opacities.
- Chest CT demonstrates diffuse nodular and ground glass opacities with enlargement of hilar lymph nodes.
- Bronchoscopy: Milky and lipoproteinaceous effluent is seen on bronchoalveolar lavage (BAL).
- Lung biopsy is not necessary in the setting of a definite exposure history.
- Exclusion of other causes like pulmonary edema, alveolar hemorrhage, and pulmonary alveolar proteinosis is necessary.

Chronic silicosis:
- Chest x-ray demonstrates multiple small, rounded opacities (<1 cm in diameter) distributed in the upper lung zones. Eggshell calcification of the hilar lymph nodes may be noted.
- Conglomerate masses >1 cm in diameter with an upper lobe predominance are characteristic of primary myelofibrosis (PMF) (Fig. E4).
- Pulmonary function tests (PFT) show mixed obstructive and restrictive defect.
- Bronchoscopy and lung biopsies have limited diagnostic role unless atypical x-ray features are noted.[4]

Accelerated silicosis:
- Chest x-ray pattern initially suggestive of simple silicosis, with rapid (less than 10 yr) progression to changes characteristic of PMF.

TREATMENT

- Treatment is symptomatic (supplemental O_2 for hypoxemia, bronchodilators, antibiotics for infections)
- Prevention (industrial hygiene)
- Smoking cessation
- Pulmonary rehabilitation
- Vaccination against influenza and pneumococcus
- Treatment of associated tuberculosis if present
- Consider lung transplant for patients who develop chronic respiratory failure

ASSOCIATED COMPLICATIONS

Silica exposure/silicosis is associated with an increased risk of the following:
- Lung and renal cancer[5]
- Acute kidney injury[6]
- Mycobacterial and chronic fungal infections[5]
- Rheumatologic disease, particularly rheumatoid arthritis and scleroderma[5]

REFERENCES

Available at eBooks.Health.Elsevier.com.

RELATED CONTENT

Interstitial Lung Disease (Related Key Topic)
Silicosis (Patient Information)

AUTHOR: **MAEVE G. MACMURDO, MBChB, MPH**

BOX 1   Occupational Exposures Associated With Silicosis

Mining: Surface or underground mining (tunneling)
Milling: Ground silica for abrasives and filler
Quarrying
Sandblasting (e.g., of buildings, preparing steel for painting)
Pottery; ceramic or clay work
Grinding, polishing using silica wheels
Engineered stone fabrication: Cutting, grinding engineered stone products
Foundry work: Grinding, molding, chipping
Refractory brick work
Glass making: To polish and as an abrasive
Boiler work: Cleaning boilers
Manufacture of abrasives
Hydraulic fracturing

Adapted from Goldman L, Schafer AI: *Goldman's Cecil medicine*, ed 24, Philadelphia, 2012, Saunders.

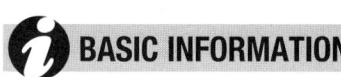
BASIC INFORMATION

DEFINITION
Sinus venous thrombosis (SVT) is an uncommon form of stroke due to thrombosis of one of the intracranial veins or sinuses resulting in increased intracranial pressure and possibly venous infarction or hemorrhage.

SYNONYMS
SVT
Intracranial venous sinus thrombosis or thrombophlebitis
Dural sinus thrombosis
Cerebral venous thrombosis
Venous sinus thrombosis

ICD-10CM CODES
I67.6 Nonpyogenic thrombosis of intracranial venous system
O87.3 Cerebral venous thrombosis in the puerperium

EPIDEMIOLOGY & DEMOGRAPHICS
INCIDENCE:
- 5 to 12 per million people annually[1-2]
- SVT represents 0.5% to 1% of all strokes
- 78% in people <50 yr old[1-3]
- 3:1 female-to-male ratio mainly due to the higher incidence during pregnancy and the postpartum period

RISK FACTORS[3-4]:
- Prior prothrombotic medical conditions including thrombophilias, inflammatory bowel disease, nephrotic syndrome, iron deficiency anemia, polycythemia, antiphospholipid syndrome, antithrombin III deficiency, protein C deficiency, protein S deficiency, factor V Leiden gene mutation, Coronavirus (COVID-19) vaccines[4a] hyperhomocysteinemia, and cancers
- Transient conditions causing a prothrombotic state including pregnancy and the postpartum period, dehydration
- Infections (usually parameningeal—ear, sinus, mouth, face, neck)
- Medications including oral contraceptives and cytotoxic medications
- Mechanical factors such as head trauma, lumbar puncture, and neurosurgery

PHYSICAL FINDINGS & CLINICAL PRESENTATION
- Symptom onset occurs acutely within 48 hr in 37% and chronically over more than 30 days in up to 10%.[3]
- Headache, although not specific, is the most common presenting symptom in up to 90% of patients. It is often diffuse and progressive over days and weeks, although it may present more acutely. Up to 25% present with only headache without other focal neurological symptoms or papilledema.[2-3]
- Papilledema and/or isolated cranial VI nerve palsies as a manifestation of increased cerebral pressure.
- Seizures occur in ~40%.[2-3]

- Bilateral involvement and symptoms are frequent.
- The physical findings and presentation depend on the venous sinus involved.[1]
  1. Superior sagittal sinus (62%)—headache, papilledema, focal motor weakness
  2. Lateral sinus thrombosis (41%-45%)—hemianopia, contralateral weakness, aphasia
  3. Cavernous sinus—ptosis, vision loss, ophthalmoplegia, hypoesthesia or hyperesthesia of V1 and V2, chemosis, periorbital edema, and proptosis due to involvement of cranial nerves III to VI, as well as impaired venous drainage from the orbit and eye
  4. Deep cerebral veins (internal cerebral vein, vein of Galen, straight sinus)—alteration in consciousness due to bilateral thalamic or basal ganglia infarction

ETIOLOGY
- 34% had an inherited or acquired prothrombotic condition.[2-4]
- 25% of patients had more than one risk factor.
- Infective sinus venous thrombosis, usually in the cavernous sinus, most commonly results from contiguous spread of an infection from either the sinuses (sphenoid, ethmoid, or frontal) or the medial third of the face (areas around the eyes and nose that drain to the ophthalmic vein). Hematogenous spread can also occur.

DIAGNOSIS

- The diagnosis of VST is made by clinical suspicion and confirmed by appropriate imaging studies.

DIFFERENTIAL DIAGNOSIS
- Idiopathic intracranial hypertension
- Arterial ischemic infarction
- Primary intracerebral hemorrhage
- Migraine headache
- Meningitis
- Epidural and subdural infections
- Epidural and subdural hematoma
- Subarachnoid hemorrhage
- Trauma

WORKUP
CST is a clinical diagnosis, with laboratory tests and imaging studies confirming the clinical impression.

LABORATORY TESTS
- CBC, CMP, PT/PTT.
- Screening of potential prothrombotic conditions included infections, underlying inflammatory disease, or inherited/acquired prothrombotic conditions.
- A normal D-dimer assay may make the diagnosis of SVT very unlikely except in the setting of isolated headache.[1]
- Lumbar puncture (LP) is not often necessary except in cases of infection where it may help distinguish from more localized processes (e.g., sinusitis, orbital cellulitis). Elevated opening pressure is a common finding and may be a clue to consider SVT in patients

presenting with isolated headache.[2] Elevated cell counts and protein are often but not always present. In the setting of an infection, the cerebrospinal fluid profile is typical for a parameningeal focus (high white blood cells with polymorphonuclear and/or mononuclear cells, normal glucose, normal protein, culture negative), and in one third may be similar to that of bacterial meningitis.

IMAGING STUDIES
- CT head without contrast—30% to 40% present with ICH. Bilateral ICH or lobar ICH of unclear etiology should raise a strong suspicion for SVT. However CT head without contrast by itself is often normal, with only one third of cases showing a hyperdense sinus. CT head with contrast may sometimes show enhancement of the dural lining of the sinus with an associated filling defect like the "empty delta sign."
- MRI with gadolinium, including magnetic resonance angiography and magnetic resonance venogram (Fig. 1), is more sensitive than computed tomography (CT) scan and is the imaging study of choice to diagnose SVT. Findings may include an obvious signal hyperintensity within thrombosed vascular sinuses, focal edema, and/or hemorrhage in a nonarterial or bilateral distribution or associated with a venous sinus.[2]
- If high level of suspicion or not visualized, CT or MR venogram may demonstrate the thrombosis.

TREATMENT

ACUTE GENERAL Rx
- Acute treatment with anticoagulation, even in the setting of already present intracerebral hemorrhage, is necessary to prevent thrombus growth, facilitate recanalization, and prevent DVT or PE.[2]
  1. Cerebral hemorrhage on presentation is associated with adverse outcomes, but anticoagulation does not result in further worsening outcomes.
- LMWH is preferred to unfractionated heparin when medically indicated.[5]
- Anticoagulation alone is sometimes not sufficient to dissolve a large and extensive thrombus. In the setting of clinical deterioration, direct catheter thrombolysis, mechanical thrombectomy, or surgical thrombectomy could be considered.[2]
- If concern for infection due to local invasion (from otitis, mastoiditis) or systemic (meningitis), broad-spectrum intravenous antibiotics are used as empiric therapy until a definite pathogen is found, considering the source.
- Treatment of intracranial pressure, seizures, and hydrocephalus if and when required may be necessary.[2] Acetazolamide treatment can be helpful.

CHRONIC Rx
- Overall 6.5% annual risk of any type of recurrent thrombosis; however, VTE is more common than recurrent SVT.[2]

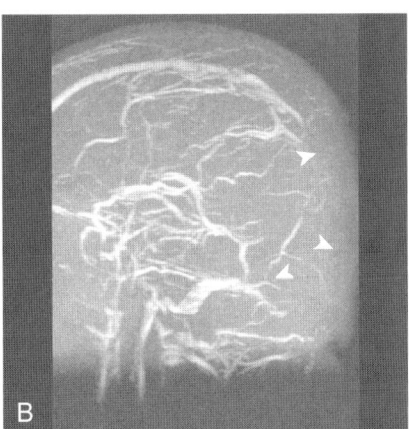

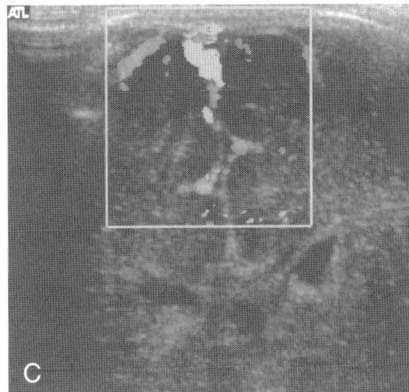

FIG. 1 Superior sagittal sinus (SSS) thrombosis on magnetic resonance venogram (MRV). Sagittal T1 magnetic resonance imaging **(A)** shows intermediate signal intensity in sagittal and straight sinuses *(arrowheads)*. No flow is seen on MRV **(B)** in these vessels *(arrowheads)*, which is consistent with thrombosis. Color Doppler evacuation **(C)** of the SSS in another 6-mo-old patient with suspected thrombosis demonstrated a patent SSS with normal draining cortical veins. (From Fuhrman BP, et al: *Pediatric critical care,* ed 4, Philadelphia, 2011, Saunders.)

- In patients with provoked SVT associated with a transient risk factor, treatment with warfarin or a DOAC for 3 to 6 mo is recommended. If the SVT occurred in the setting of pregnancy, LMWH should be continued for at least 6 wk postpartum.
- In patients with an unprovoked SVT, warfarin or a DOAC should be continued for 6 to 12 mo.[2,6]
- Testing for prothrombotic conditions, including protein C, protein S, antithrombin deficiency, antiphospholipid syndrome, prothrombin G20210A mutation, and factor V Leiden is recommended 2 to 4 wk after completion of anticoagulation. If positive, indefinite anticoagulation should be considered.[2]
- In women with a history of SVT, prophylaxis with LMWH during future pregnancies and the postpartum period is recommended.[2]
- Patients with infected VST are usually treated with prolonged courses (3 to 4 wk) of IV antibiotics. If there is evidence of complications, such as intracranial suppuration, 6 to 8 wk of total therapy may be warranted.
- Headache is common chronically and often is not related to recurrent VST, although this may need to be investigated.[2]

- SVT of the cavernous, lateral, or sagittal sinus can induce dural arteriovenous fistula formation.[2]

DISPOSITION
- SVT can be a life-threatening, rapidly progressive, or more indolent disease with high morbidity and mortality rates. Mortality ranges from 8% to 10% with complete recovery in 79% of patients.
- Risk factors for long-term poor outcome include central nervous system infection, malignancy, thrombosis of deep venous system, intracranial hemorrhage on admission, Glasgow Coma Scale <9, mental status disturbance, age >37, and male sex.[3]
- Complications of untreated SVT include extension of thrombus to other dural sinuses, carotid thrombosis with concomitant strokes, subdural empyema, brain abscess, or meningitis. Septic embolization may also occur.

REFERRAL
If suspected, VST should be considered a medical emergency.

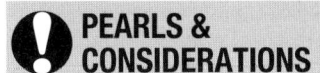

PEARLS & CONSIDERATIONS

COMMENTS
Venous sinus thrombosis can present with isolated headache and papilledema mimicking idiopathic intracranial hypertension. In a patient with possible intracranial hypertension, evaluation of the cerebral venous sinuses is required to rule out a secondary cause.

Delays in diagnosis of CVT are common, and a high level of suspicion is necessary.

REFERENCES
Available at eBooks.Health.Elsevier.com.

RELATED CONTENT
Idiopathic Intracranial Hypertension (Related Key Topic)

AUTHOR: **COREY E. GOLDSMITH, MD, FAAN**

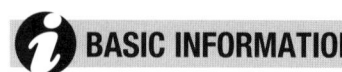

BASIC INFORMATION

DEFINITION

Sinusitis is inflammation of the mucous membranes lining one or more of the paranasal sinuses. The various presentations are:
- Acute sinusitis: Infection lasting <4 wk, with complete resolution of symptoms.
- Subacute infection: Lasts from 4 to 12 wk, with complete resolution of symptoms.
- Recurrent acute infection: Episodes of acute infection lasting <30 days, with resolution of symptoms, which recur at intervals at least 10 days apart.
- Chronic sinusitis: Inflammation of the paranasal sinuses and nasal cavities lasting >12 wk, with persistent upper respiratory symptoms. It accounts for 1% to 2% of total physician encounters.
- Acute bacterial sinusitis superimposed on chronic sinusitis: New symptoms that occur in patients with residual symptoms from prior infection(s). With treatment, the new symptoms resolve, but the residual ones do not.

SYNONYM

Rhinosinusitis: Sinusitis is almost always accompanied by inflammation of the nasal mucosa; thus it is now the preferred term.

ICD-10CM CODES
J32.9	Chronic sinusitis, unspecified
J01.90	Acute sinusitis, unspecified
J01.00	Acute maxillary sinusitis, unspecified
J01.01	Acute recurrent maxillary sinusitis
J01.10	Acute frontal sinusitis, unspecified
J01.11	Acute recurrent frontal sinusitis
J01.20	Acute ethmoidal sinusitis, unspecified
J01.21	Acute recurrent ethmoidal sinusitis
J01.30	Acute sphenoidal sinusitis, unspecified
J01.31	Acute recurrent sphenoidal sinusitis
J01.80	Other acute sinusitis
J01.81	Other acute recurrent sinusitis
J01.91	Acute recurrent sinusitis, unspecified
J32.0	Chronic maxillary sinusitis
J32.1	Chronic frontal sinusitis
J32.2	Chronic ethmoidal sinusitis
J32.3	Chronic sphenoidal sinusitis
J32.8	Other chronic sinusitis

EPIDEMIOLOGY & DEMOGRAPHICS

INCIDENCE (IN U.S.): Seems to correlate with the incidence of upper respiratory tract infections and higher in women than men; 30 million cases per yr in the U.S.
PEAK INCIDENCE:
- Fall, winter, spring: September through March
- In adults: Greatest incidence between 45 and 74 yr of age
- Approximately 6% to 7% of children presenting with respiratory symptoms have acute sinusitis

PHYSICAL FINDINGS & CLINICAL PRESENTATION

- Patients often give a history of a recent upper respiratory illness with some improvement, then a relapse.
- Mucopurulent secretions in the nasal passage:
  1. Purulent nasal and postnasal discharge lasting 7 to 10 days
  2. Facial tightness, pressure, or pain
  3. Nasal obstruction
  4. Headache
  5. Decreased sense of smell
  6. Purulent pharyngeal secretions, brought up with cough, often worse at night
- Erythema, swelling, and tenderness over the infected sinus in a small proportion of patients:
  1. Diagnosis cannot be excluded by the absence of such findings.
  2. These findings are not common, and do not correlate with number of positive sinus aspirates.
- Intermittent low-grade fever in about half of adults with acute bacterial sinusitis.
- Toothache is a common complaint when the maxillary sinus is involved.
- Periorbital cellulitis and excessive tearing with ethmoid sinusitis:
  1. Orbital extension of infection: Chemosis, proptosis, impaired extraocular movements
- Characteristics of acute sinusitis in children with upper respiratory tract infections:
  1. Persistence of symptoms
  2. Cough
  3. Bad breath
- Symptoms of chronic sinusitis (may or may not be present):
  1. Nasal or postnasal discharge
  2. Fever
  3. Facial pain or pressure
  4. Headache
- Nosocomial sinusitis is typically seen in patients with nasogastric tubes or nasotracheal intubation.

ETIOLOGY

- Each of the four paranasal sinuses is connected to the nasal cavity by narrow tubes (ostia), 1 to 3 mm in diameter; these drain directly into the nose through the turbinates. The sinuses are lined with a ciliated mucous membrane (mucoperiosteum).
- Acute viral infection:
  1. Infection with the common cold or influenza
  2. Mucosal edema and sinus inflammation
  3. Decreased drainage of thick secretions/obstruction of the sinus ostia
  4. Subsequent entrapment of bacteria
    a. Multiplication of bacteria
    b. Secondary bacterial infection
- Other predisposing factors:
  1. Tumors
  2. Polyps
  3. Foreign bodies
  4. Congenital choanal atresia
  5. Other entities that cause obstruction of sinus drainage
  6. Allergies
  7. Asthma
- Dental infections lead to maxillary sinusitis.
- Viruses recovered alone or in combination with bacteria (in 16% of cases):
  1. Rhinovirus
  2. Coronavirus
  3. Adenovirus
  4. Parainfluenza virus
  5. Respiratory syncytial virus
- The principal bacterial pathogens in sinusitis are *Streptococcus pneumoniae*, nontypable *Haemophilus influenzae*, and *Moraxella catarrhalis* (Table 1).
- In the remainder of cases *Streptococcus pyogenes*, *Staphylococcus aureus*, beta-hemolytic streptococci, and mixed anaerobic infections (*Peptostreptococcus*, *Fusobacterium*, *Bacteroides*, and *Prevotella* spp.) are found.
- Infection is polymicrobial in about one third of cases.
- Anaerobic infections are seen more often in cases of chronic sinusitis and in cases associated with dental infection; anaerobes are unlikely pathogens in sinusitis in children.
- Fungal pathogens are isolated with increasing frequency in immunocompromised patients but remain uncommon pathogens in the paranasal sinuses. Fungal pathogens include *Phaeohyphomycosis*, *Aspergillus*, *Pseudallescheria*, *Sporothrix*, and *Zygomycetes spp.*
- Nosocomial infections: Occur in patients with nasogastric tubes, nasotracheal intubation, cystic fibrosis, and immunocompromised state.
  1. *S. aureus* (including MRSA)
  2. *Pseudomonas aeruginosa*
  3. *Klebsiella pneumoniae*
  4. *Enterobacter* spp.
  5. *Proteus mirabilis*
- Organisms typically isolated in chronic sinusitis:

TABLE 1 Microbiology of Acute Bacterial Rhinosinusitis in Adults

Organism	Range of Prevalence (%)
Streptococcus pneumoniae	20–43
Haemophilus influenzae	22–35
Streptococcus spp	3–9
Anaerobes	0–9
Moraxella catarrhalis	2–10
Staphylococcus aureus	0–8
Other	4

From Broaddus VC et al: *Murray & Nadel's textbook of respiratory medicine*, ed 7, Philadelphia, 2022, Elsevier.

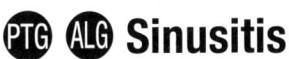

1. *S. aureus*
2. *S. pneumoniae*
3. *H. influenzae*
4. *P. aeruginosa*
5. *Anaerobes*

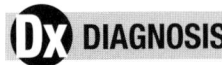 **DIAGNOSIS**

DIFFERENTIAL DIAGNOSIS

- Temporomandibular joint disease
- Migraine headache
- Cluster headache
- Dental infection
- Trigeminal neuralgia
- Allergic rhinitis
- Drugs (cocaine, decongestant overuse)
- Gastroesophageal reflux disease
- Wegener granulomatosis
- Cystic fibrosis

WORKUP

- The diagnosis is generally based on clinical signs and symptoms (purulent rhinorrhea and facial pain). Radiologic tests and cultures are not recommended initially and should be considered only when treatment is ineffective, and sinusitis persists.
- In the normal healthy host, the paranasal sinuses should be sterile. Although the contiguous structures are colonized with bacteria and likely contaminate the sinuses, the mucociliary lining functions to remove these bacteria.
- Gold standard for diagnosis: Recovery of bacteria in high-density $\geq 10^4$ colony-forming units/ml from a paranasal sinus, in the setting of a patient with history of upper respiratory infection and symptoms persisting for 7 to 10 days. Sinus aspiration is the best method for obtaining cultures; however, it must be performed by an otorhinolaryngologist and is not practical for the primary care practitioner. Therefore, most diagnoses are based on the clinical history and presentation, possibly supported by radiologic evaluations.
  1. Overall, standard radiographs are of limited use in diagnosis, although negative films are strong evidence against the diagnosis
  2. Computed tomography (CT) scans (Figs. E1 and E2):
     a. Much more sensitive than plain x-rays in detecting acute changes and disease in the sinuses
     b. Recommended for patients requiring surgical intervention, including sinus aspiration; it is a useful adjunct to guide therapy
  3. Transillumination:
     a. Used for diagnosis of frontal and maxillary sinusitis
     b. Absence of light transmission indicates that sinus is filled with fluid
     c. Dullness (decreased light transmission) is less helpful in diagnosing infection
  4. Endoscopy:
     a. Used to visualize secretions coming from the ostia of infected sinuses
     b. Culture collection via endoscopy often contaminated by nasal flora; not nearly as good as sinus puncture
  5. Sinus puncture:
     a. Gold standard for collecting sinus cultures
     b. Generally reserved for treatment failures, suspected intracranial extension, and nosocomial sinusitis

TREATMENT

NONPHARMACOLOGIC THERAPY

To help promote sinus drainage:
- Air humidification with vaporizers (for steam) or humidifiers (for a cool mist)
- Application of hot, wet towel over the face
- Sipping hot beverages
- Hydration

ACUTE GENERAL Rx

- Sinus drainage:
  1. Nasal vasoconstrictors, such as phenylephrine nose drops, 0.25% or 0.5%.
  2. Topical decongestants should not be used for more than a few days because of the risk of rebound congestion.
  3. Systemic decongestants.
  4. Corticosteroids: Nasal or systemic corticosteroids, such as nasal beclomethasone. Oral corticosteroids combined with antibiotics may be associated with modest benefit for short-term relief of symptoms in adults with severe symptoms of acute sinusitis compared with antibiotics alone. Oral corticosteroids as monotherapy are not associated with improved clinical outcomes in adults with clinically diagnosed acute sinusitis.
  5. Nasal irrigation, with hypertonic or normal saline (saline may act as a mild vasoconstrictor of nasal blood flow).
  6. Use of antihistamines has no proven benefit, and the drying effect on the mucous membranes may cause crusting, which blocks the ostia, thus interfering with sinus drainage.
- Analgesics, antipyretics

Antimicrobial therapy:
- Most cases of acute sinusitis have a viral cause and will resolve within 2 wk without antibiotics.
- Current treatment recommendations favor symptomatic treatment for those with mild symptoms. 85% of persons have a reduction or resolution of symptoms within 7 to 15 days without antibiotic therapy. Physicians grossly overprescribe antibiotics for presumed bacterial sinusitis despite a much higher prevalence of viral infections.
- Antibiotics should not be prescribed for mild to moderate sinusitis within the first wk of illness. They should be reserved for those with persistent symptoms for more than 10 days, high fever and purulent nasal discharge or facial pain lasting for at least 3 consecutive days, or worsening symptoms after a typical viral illness lasting >5 days that had initially improved ("double sickening").
- Antibiotic therapy is usually empiric, targeting the common pathogens:
  1. First-line antibiotics in children include amoxicillin or amoxicillin/clavulanate. For adults, amoxicillin/clavulanate or doxycycline is first-line agent, with quinolones (levofloxacin or moxifloxacin) reserved as second-line agents unless patient is penicillin allergic.
  2. Second-line antibiotics include the newer macrolides: Clarithromycin and oral cephalosporins: Cefuroxime axetil, cefprozil, cefaclor, loracarbef, but high rate of resistance of *S. pneumoniae* is a concern with these agents as is *H. influenzae* resistance with TMP-SMX and azithromycin such that they should no longer be used as first-line agents.
  3. For patients with uncomplicated acute sinusitis, the less expensive first-line agents appear to be as effective as the costlier second-line agents.
- Hospitalization and intravenous (IV) antibiotics may be required for more severe infection and those with suspected intracranial complications. Broader-spectrum antibiotic coverage may be indicated in severe cases, to cover for MRSA, *Pseudomonas*, and fungal pathogens.
- Duration of therapy generally 5 to 7 days in adults rather than 10 to 14 days as recommended in the past.
  1. Optimal duration of treatment in children varies from 10 to 28 days.

Surgery:
- Surgical drainage indicated
  1. If intracranial or orbital complications suspected
  2. Many cases of frontal and sphenoid sinusitis
  3. Chronic sinusitis recalcitrant to medical therapy
- Surgical debridement imperative in the treatment of fungal sinusitis

Complications:
- Untreated, sinusitis may lead to a number of serious, life-threatening complications.
- Intracranial complications include meningitis, brain abscess, and epidural and subdural empyema.
- Intracranial sequelae are more common with frontal and ethmoid infections.
- Extracranial complications include orbital cellulitis, blindness, orbital abscess, osteomyelitis.
- Extracranial sequelae are more commonly seen with ethmoid sinusitis.

CHRONIC Rx

- Chronic sinusitis: Evidence supports daily high-volume saline irrigation with topical corticosteroid therapy as a first-line therapy for chronic sinusitis. A short course of systemic corticosteroids (1 to 3 wk), short course of doxycycline (3 wk), or a leukotriene antagonist may be considered in patients with nasal polyps. A prolonged course (3 mo) of macrolide antibiotic may be considered for patients without polyps. A clinical algorithm for the

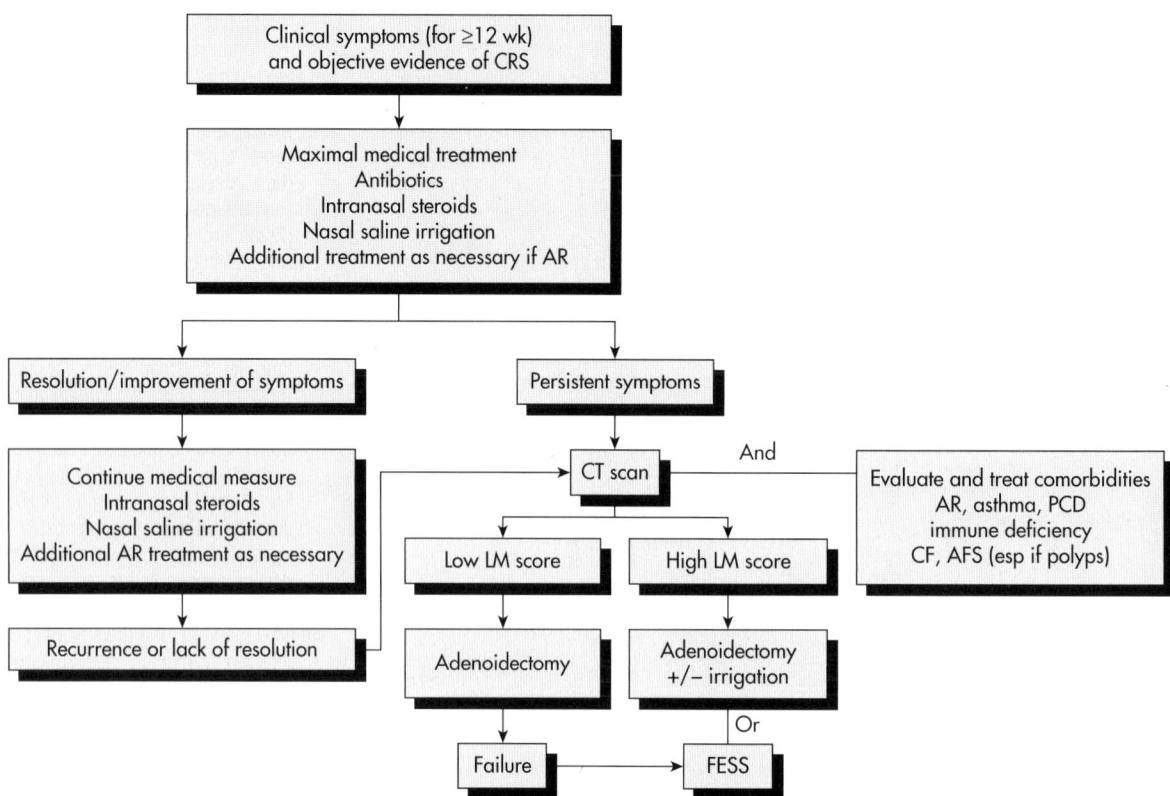

FIG. 3 General clinical algorithm for the management of chronic rhinosinusitis (CRS) in children. If symptoms improve or resolve after maximal medical therapy, one can continue conservative medical management with intranasal steroids and nasal saline irrigation as necessary. If a child has persistent symptoms after maximal medical management, then one should obtain a computed tomography *(CT)* scan at the end of the course of treatment to evaluate for extent of disease. One would also initiate investigations into possible coexisting comorbidities such as allergic rhinitis, immune deficiencies, and primary ciliary dyskinesia. Surgical management would be informed by the severity of disease on CT scan. If the severity is low, as evidenced by a Lund MacKay score <5, then one can move forward with an adenoidectomy. If the score is greater than 5, then most would choose adenoidectomy with maxillary sinus irrigation. Clearly, factors such as age, the presence of asthma and the severity of disease on the CT scan might mandate concomitant adenoidectomy and limited FESS. Finally, in patients with significant disease such as nasal polyps, mucoceles associated with cystic fibrosis, or expansile disease such as with allergic fungal sinusitis, one would go directly to FESS. *AFS,* Allergic fungal sinusitis; *AR,* allergic rhinitis; *CF,* cystic fibrosis; *FESS,* functional endoscopic sinus surgery; *LM,* Lund MacKay; *PCD,* primary ciliary dyskinesia. (From Flint PW et al: *Cummings otolaryngology, head and neck surgery,* ed 7, Philadelphia, 2021, Elsevier.)

management of chronic rhinosinusitis in children is illustrated in Fig. 3.

- Dupilumab (Dupixent), a monoclonal antibody that targets interleukin -4 and -13 was recently FDA approved for chronic rhinosinusitis with nasal polyps (CRSwNP). Cost is a limiting factor.
- Surgical intervention may be necessary in nonresponders.

REFERRAL

- To infectious disease specialist if failure to respond to initial therapy
- To otorhinolaryngologist for:
  1. Failure to respond to therapy
  2. Suspected fungal infection
  3. Suspected intracranial or orbital complications

SUGGESTED READINGS

Available at eBook.Health.Elsevier.com.

RELATED CONTENT

Sinusitis (Patient Information)

AUTHOR: **GLENN G. FORT, MD, MPH**

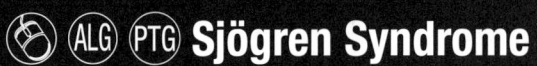

S

 BASIC INFORMATION

DEFINITION

Sjögren Syndrome (SS) is a chronic autoimmune disorder that targets exocrine glands. It is characterized by lymphocytic and plasma cell infiltration and destruction of salivary, lacrimal, and parotid glands, resulting predominantly in dry eyes and dry mouth. Clinical presentation varies from mild symptoms to severe systemic symptoms involving multiple organ systems. There are multiple classification criteria but no universally accepted classification criterion for the diagnosis of Sjögren syndrome.

Primary and secondary forms have been described:

- Primary: Dry mouth (xerostomia) and dry eyes (xerophthalmia) develop as isolated entities. It is immunogenetically associated with HLA-DRB1*0301 and DRB1*1501 and serologically associated with antibodies to Ro/SS-A and La/SS-B.
- Secondary: Associated with other autoimmune connective tissue diseases, including rheumatoid arthritis (RA), systemic lupus erythematosus (SLE), scleroderma, and polymyositis. The immunogenetic and serologic findings are usually those of the accompanying disease (e.g., HLA-DR4 if associated with RA).

SYNONYMS

- SS
- pSS (primary Sjögren syndrome)
- sSS (secondary Sjögren syndrome)
- Sicca syndrome
- Keratoconjunctivitis sicca
- Sicca complex
- Dry eye syndrome/dysfunctional tear syndrome

ICD-10CM CODES

M35.00	Sicca syndrome, unspecified
M35.01	Sicca syndrome with keratoconjunctivitis
M35.02	Sicca syndrome with lung involvement
M35.03	Sicca syndrome with myopathy
M35.04	Sicca syndrome with tubulo-interstitial nephropathy
M35.09	Sicca syndrome with other organ involvement

EPIDEMIOLOGY & DEMOGRAPHICS

INCIDENCE: 4 per 100,000; of these cases, 70% had primary SS.[1]

PREVALENCE: Prevalence is 0.2% to 2.7% of the population; secondary SS is also common and can affect up to 19% of patients with SLE and 26% to 31% of RA and scleroderma patients.[1]

PREDOMINANT SEX: Female:male ratio is approximately 10:1.[1]

PREDOMINANT AGE: Peak incidence is the fourth and fifth decade but can occur in all ages. Rarely reported in children.

RISK FACTOR: Seen in all races/ethnicities, but more common in Caucasians.

PHYSICAL FINDINGS & CLINICAL PRESENTATION

SS is one of the most common autoimmune diseases and should be considered in any patient with unexplained symptoms and a positive antinuclear antibody.

- 2016 American College of Rheumatology/European League Against Rheumatism classification criteria for primary SS is described in Table 1.

MANIFESTATIONS (TABLE 2):

- Dry mouth, dry lips (cheilosis), erythema, and hyperlobulated tongue (Fig. E1) and other mucosal surfaces, carious teeth. Dry throat, hoarseness, and dysphonia can also occur.
- Dry eyes (conjunctival injection, corneal ulceration, blurred vision, decreased luster, enlargement of lacrimal glands, and irregularity of the corneal light reflex).
- Salivary gland enlargement (Fig. E2) and dysfunction, with subsequent difficulty in chewing and swallowing food and in speaking without frequent water intake, thickened saliva, and burning sensation in mouth.
- Extraglandular involvement occurs in 50% of patients. There are multiple systemic manifestations associated with SS, which include the following:
  1. Fever/fatigue.
  2. Cutaneous vasculitis may be present, usually of lower extremities.
  3. Skin ulceration, photosensitivity, Raynaud phenomenon.
  4. Dyspareunia and pruritus can occur secondary to vaginal dryness.
  5. Pulmonary involvement includes interstitial lung disease (nonspecific interstitial pneumonitis (NSIP), usual interstitial pneumonia (UIP)); lymphocytic interstitial pneumonitis (LIP) and cryptogenic organizing pneumonia (COP); chronic obstructive pulmonary disease; fibrosis; and xerotrachea.
  6. Gastrointestinal: Celiac disease, esophageal dysmotility, type I autoimmune hepatitis, primary biliary cirrhosis, and pancreatitis can occur.
  7. Renal manifestations: Type 1 renal tubular acidosis, Fanconi syndrome, glomerulonephritis, and interstitial nephritis.
  8. Neurologic involvement: Peripheral, cranial, or autonomic neuropathy; central nervous system (CNS) involvement also possible, cognitive dysfunction ("brain fog").
  9. Musculoskeletal: Arthralgias and myopathy.
  10. Hematologic: Cytopenias, hyper-gammaglobulinemia, cryoglobulins. Increased lymphoma risk, with 5% to 10% developing non-Hodgkin lymphoma.
  11. RA and other connective tissue diseases are seen commonly with secondary SS.
  12. Autoimmune thyroiditis may be observed in patients with SS.
  13. Pregnancy: Patients with anti-SSA antibodies have an increased risk of delivering a baby with neonatal lupus, with cutaneous manifestations or congenital heart block.

ETIOLOGY

Sjögren syndrome is an autoimmune disorder of unclear etiology. It is associated with certain HLA-DQ and HLA-DR alleles. It has been postulated that viral agents (e.g., hepatitis C and Epstein-

---

TABLE 1 2016 American College of Rheumatology/European League Against Rheumatism Classification Criteria for Sjögren Syndrome

Item	Score
Histopathology showing focal lymphocytic sialadenitis with a focus score $\geq$ 1 per 4 mm^2	3
The presence of anti-Ro/SS-A antibodies	3
SICCA ocular staining score $\geq$5 using lissamine green and fluorescein dye (or Rose Bengal score $\geq$4 by the van Bijsterveld scoring system)	1
Schirmer's test $\leq$5 mm per 5 minutes in at least one eye	1
Unstimulated whole salivary flow of less than 0.1 mL per minute	1

Rules for Classification

Patients may be classified as primary Sjögren's syndrome if they display at least one symptom of ocular or oral dryness and a total score of 4 or greater when the weights from the five criteria items above are summed.

Exclusion Criteria

History of head and neck radiation treatment
Active hepatitis C infection (with confirmation by PCR)
AIDS
Sarcoidosis
Amyloidosis
Graft vs. host disease (GVHD)
IgG4-related disease (IgG4-RD)

AIDS, Acquired immunodeficiency syndrome; *SICCA*, Sjogren's International Collaborative Clinical Alliance.
From Firestein GS et al: *Firestein & Kelley's textbook of rheumatology*, ed 11, Philadelphia, 2021, Elsevier.

TABLE 2   Clinical Manifestations of Sjögren Syndrome

Dry eyes	Keratoconjunctivitis sicca
	Corneal ulcers, keratitis
Dry mouth	Increased caries
Major salivary gland swelling	Parotid
	Submandibular
Extraglandular manifestations	Fatigue
	Arthritis
	Arthralgia/myalgia
	Raynaud phenomenon
Pulmonary involvement	Chronic cough
	Interstitial lung disease: nonspecific interstitial pneumonia, Lymphocytic interstitial pneumonia, usual interstitial pneumonia
	Small airways disease
Renal involvement	Tubulointerstitial nephritis
	Renal tubular acidosis (distal more common)
Neurological involvement	Peripheral neuropathy
	Central nervous system disease: demyelinating disease, neuromyelitis optica

From Petty RE et al: *Textbook of Pediatric Rheumatology*, ed 8, Philadelphia, 2021, Elsevier.

Barr virus) may trigger the clinical manifestations. The pathogenesis involves a complex interplay of several factors, including genetic and epigenetic controls of immune homeostasis and gene expression, age, gender, and environmental insults.

Over 90% of the infiltrating cells are CD4+ T lymphocytes with memory phenotype (70%) and B lymphocytes (20%). The remaining 10% are an admixture of plasma cells, CD8+ T lymphocytes, T regulatory cells, natural killer cells, and dendritic cells. Predominantly Th1- and Th17-driven response.

🅓🅧 DIAGNOSIS

DIFFERENTIAL DIAGNOSIS (TABLE E1)

- Medication-related dryness (e.g., anticholinergics, antihistamines, diuretics, benzodiazepines, antidepressants)
- Age-related exocrine gland dysfunction
- Mouth breathing, anxiety
- Infections such as viruses, HIV, hepatitis C
- Diabetes mellitus, acromegaly, type V hyperlipidemia
- Chronic sialadenitis
- Graft-versus-host disease
- IgG4-related disease
- Ocular herpetic lesions, blepharitis, corneal abrasions, contact lens irritation
- Vitamin A deficiency
- Other: Sarcoidosis, primary salivary hypofunction, radiation injury, amyloidosis

WORKUP

Workup involves ocular and oral examination and laboratory and radiographic testing to demonstrate the criteria for diagnosis of primary and secondary. An algorithm for diagnosis of SS is provided in Fig. 3.

- Symptoms and objective signs of ocular dryness:
  1. Schirmer test (Fig. E4): <5 mm wetting per 5 min. (Normal wetting is >15 mm in 5 min). There is a 15% false-positive and false-negative rate.
  2. Zone-quick diagnostic threads: A sterile cotton thread with pH indicator, phenol red. Yellow turns to red in contact with tears.
  3. Positive Rose Bengal stains dead/dying cells.
  4. Tear breakup time and tear osmolality measured after instillation of fluorescein.
- Symptoms and objective signs of dry mouth:
  1. Decreased parotid flow using Lashley cups or other methods.
  2. Abnormal biopsy result of minor salivary gland (focus score >1 based on average of four assessable lobules).
  3. Sialometry (sensitivity 56%, specificity 81%): Assessment of rate of saliva production in which collection of ≤1.5 ml after two expectorations 15 min apart is considered positive.
- Evidence of systemic autoimmune disorder:
  1. Elevated rheumatoid factor (70% to 90% of patients).
  2. Elevated titer of antinuclear antibodies (ANA)>1:320 (80% of patients).
  3. Presence of anti-SS-A (Ro) (>60% of patients) or anti-SS-B (La) antibodies (40% of patients).

SECONDARY:

- Characteristic signs and symptoms of SS.
- Clinical features sufficient to allow a diagnosis of RA, SLE, polymyositis, or scleroderma.

LABORATORY TESTS

- Positive ANA (80% of patients) with autoantibodies anti-SS-A and anti-SS-B may be present.

- Additional laboratory abnormalities may include elevated erythrocyte sedimentation rate, anemia, leukopenia, thrombocytopenia, abnormal liver function studies, elevated serum beta$_2$ microglobulin levels, rheumatoid factor (50% to 60%), hypergammaglobulinemia, antibodies to double-stranded DNA (in cases with proteinuria), depressed C3 and C4, and the presence of cryoglobulins (30% of patients).[2]
- A definite diagnosis of SS can be made with a salivary gland biopsy (gold standard) showing focal lymphocytic sialadenitis with focus score of 1 per 4 mm^2 of glandular tissue.[3]
- Salivary gland ultrasound can be done to characterize changes in salivary gland parenchyma (sensitivity 75%, specificity 78%). Diseased gland shows hypoechoic areas with convex borders.
- MRI of the gland shows inhomogeneous parenchyma. Finding generally correlates with biopsy of the gland.

🅡🅧 TREATMENT

NONPHARMACOLOGIC THERAPY

- Adequate fluid replacement: Ameliorate skin dryness by gently blotting dry after bathing, leaving a small amount of moisture, and then applying a moisturizer.
- Increased environmental moisture by using humidifiers.
- Proper oral hygiene (daily topical fluoride use, antimicrobial mouth rinses, and stabilization of oral cavity pH) to reduce the incidence of caries.
- Sugar-free chewing gum and sour lemon lozenges to stimulate salivary secretion.
- Periodic dental and ophthalmologic evaluations to screen for complications.
- Exercise: Education about self-care measures to reduce fatigue, participation in regular low-impact aerobic exercise.
- Reduce caffeine intake and smoking.

GENERAL Rx

- Use artificial tears frequently.
- Muscarinic agonists: Pilocarpine (5 mg PO qid) or cevimeline (30 mg PO tid) can be useful to improve oral dryness, but should only be considered for patients with significant symptoms, and/or experiencing salivary flow rate of <0.3mL/min.[4]
- Ophthalmic cyclosporine and lifitegrast drops may be useful for dry eyes.
- While some studies suggest hydroxychloroquine (HCQ) alone or in conjunction with methotrexate may be useful for arthralgias and cutaneous manifestations, the JOQUER randomized control trial showed no improvement in pSS when taking HCQ for 24 wk.[5]
- Oral cyclosporine only improves the symptoms of subjective dryness.
- Tumor necrosis factor antagonists have not shown benefit in short-duration placebo-controlled trials.[6]

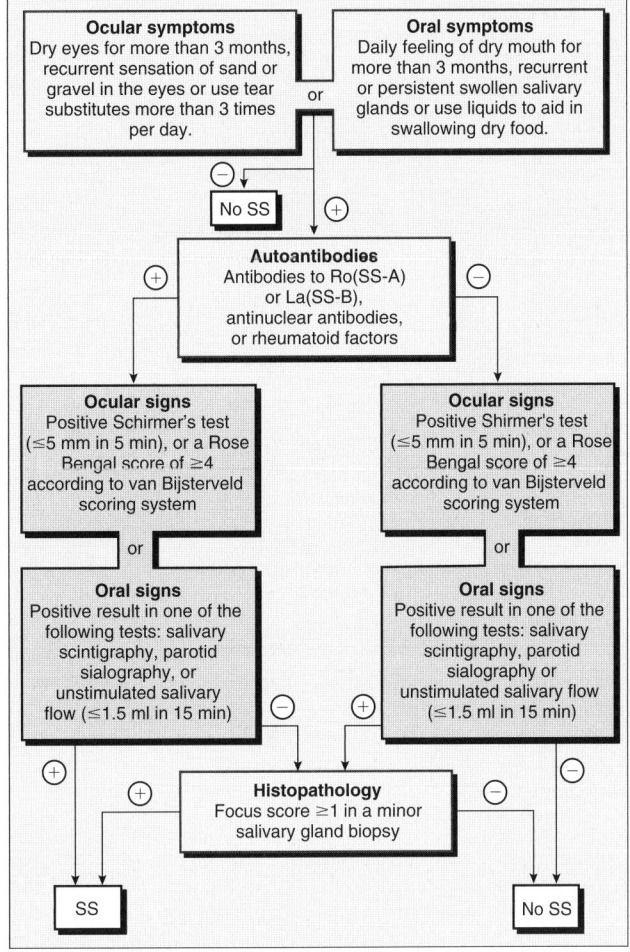

FIG. 3 Suggested algorithm for the diagnosis of Sjögren syndrome. Exclusion criteria include hepatitis C or HIV, sarcoidosis, graft-versus-host disease, preexisting lymphoma, previous head or neck irradiation, and use of anticholinergic drugs. (From Hochberg MC et al: *Rheumatology,* ed 5, St Louis, 2011, Mosby.)

- Dehydroepiandrosterone is not recommended for treatment of fatigue.
- Rituximab (RTX) has been shown to improve oral dry mouth symptoms, relieving marked salivary and lacrimal gland swelling in a retrospective review. A randomized control trial in 2010 also demonstrated RTX to be a safe and effective treatment for the management of pSS.[7]
- Propionic acid gel can be used for vaginal dryness.
- Systemic manifestations are treated according to symptoms and complications.
- Cyclophosphamide, azathioprine, and mycophenolate mofetil are generally reserved for life-threatening extraglandular manifestations.
- Fig. 5 describes a treatment algorithm for Sjögren syndrome.

REFERRAL

- Rheumatology referral is generally indicated.
- Referral should be made to an oncologist when lymphoma is suspected.
- During pregnancy, if the patient tests positive for SSA/SSB antibody, they should seek consultation with a perinatologist.

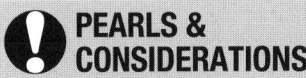 **PEARLS & CONSIDERATIONS**

COMMENTS

- Unusual presentations of SS may occur in association with polymyalgia rheumatica, chronic fatigue syndrome, fever of unknown origin, and inflammatory myositis.
- The most serious complication of primary SS is the development of non-Hodgkin lymphoma and other lymphoproliferative disorders, which occur at a 10-fold to 44-fold increased rate as compared to age-matched controls.[8]
- The presence of parotid gland enlargement, rheumatoid factor, low C4, cryoglobulinemia, lymphopenia, and higher levels of disease activity as measured by EULAR Sjögren Syndrome Disease Activity Index (ESSDAI) predicts a higher lymphoma risk.[9]

REFERENCES
Available at eBooks.Health.Elsevier.com.

RELATED CONTENT
Sjögren Syndrome (Patient Information)

AUTHORS: **OMAR KARIM, BS,** and **MANUEL F. DASILVA, MD**

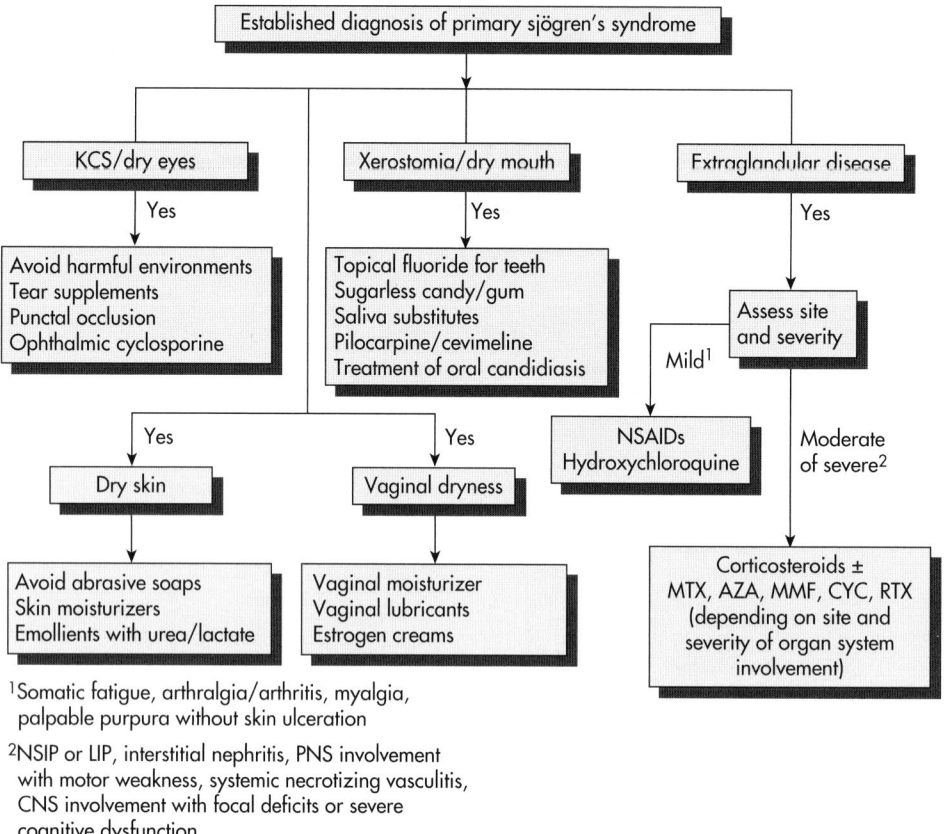

FIG. 5 Treatment algorithm for Sjögren syndrome. The treatment of Sjögren syndrome usually requires a multidisciplinary approach involving rheumatologists, ophthalmologists, dentists/oral surgeons, otolaryngologists, and other subspecialists, depending on the extent of extraglandular disease. In all cases, it is prudent to minimize the use of medications that can exacerbate the symptoms of dryness, such as antihistamines, antidepressants, muscle relaxers, and other drugs with anticholinergic properties. The treatment of extraglandular disease is individualized according to the site and severity of organ system involvement. The approaches indicated in the algorithm for the treatment of extraglandular disease are not supported by evidence from randomized controlled trials, but rather from expert opinion based on retrospective case series and clinical experience. *AZA,* Azathioprine; *CYC,* cyclophosphamide; *KCS,* keratoconjunctivitis sicca; *LIP,* lymphocytic interstitial pneumonitis; *MMF,* mycophenolate mofetil; *MTX,* methotrexate; *NSAIDs,* nonsteroidal antiinflammatory drugs; *NSIP,* nonspecific interstitial pneumonitis; *PNS,* peripheral nervous system; *RTX,* rituximab. (From Firestein GS et al: *Firestein & Kelley's textbook of rheumatology,* ed 11, Philadelphia, 2021, Elsevier.)

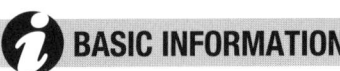 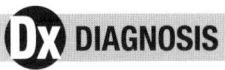

S

BASIC INFORMATION

DEFINITION

Small bowel bacterial overgrowth (SIBO) is the presence of excessive native and/or nonnative bacteria in the small intestine (bacterial count $>10^5$/ml per jejunal aspirate) causing chronic diarrhea and malabsorption.

SYNONYMS

Bacterial overgrowth syndrome
SIBO

ICD-10CM CODES
K90.4 Malabsorption due to intolerance, NEC
K90.89 Other intestinal malabsorption

EPIDEMIOLOGY & DEMOGRAPHICS

PREVALENCE: The prevalence of SIBO is varied based on the population studied and the diagnostic tests used. It has shown to be prevalent in up to 12.5% to 20% of the healthy population using glucose and lactulose breath test.
PREDOMINANT SEX & AGE: SIBO affects predominantly the elderly population or those with recent upper GI (UGI) surgery, including bariatric surgery. The elderly population has decreased gastric secretion and hypomotility due to age-associated decline as well as increased use of motility-altering medications.
RISK FACTORS:
- Advanced age is a known risk factor as there is thought to be an age-associated decline in GI motility.
- Patients with irritable bowel syndrome have a higher prevalence of SIBO compared to the general population. Initial studies have shown up to 65% to 80% of irritable bowel syndrome (IBS) patients with confirmed SIBO with an abnormal lactulose breath test.
- Other risk factors include UGI tract surgery, inflammatory bowel disease, chronic pancreatitis, immunodeficiency, liver disease, and obesity.

PHYSICAL FINDINGS & CLINICAL PRESENTATION

- Patients will present with nonspecific findings, which include abdominal distention, bloating, and/or pain. Other common symptoms include diarrhea and subsequent weight loss and weakness. Pathophysiology of symptoms and clinical consequences of SIBO are summarized in Table 1.
- The severity of symptoms reflects the extent of bacterial overgrowth.
- Severe malabsorption can present as symptoms secondary to vitamin deficiencies. Fat-soluble vitamin deficiencies can present as night blindness (vitamin A), osteomalacia and hypocalcemia (vitamin D), or prolonged bleeding (vitamin K). Bacterial overgrowth can affect vitamin B_{12} absorption in the ileum, leading to neuropathies with sensory ataxia.

ETIOLOGY

Disorders that disrupt protective mechanisms against bacterial burden predispose patients to SIBO. Box 1 summarizes diseases and disorders linked to SIBO based on pathophysiology.
- Patients with structural or anatomic abnormalities are at greater risk. These include patients with small bowel diverticula, small intestinal strictures, surgical blind loops, ileocecal resections, or gastric resections (increasing common cause of SIBO).
- Motility disorders predispose to SIBO because of the ineffective clearance of bacteria from the proximal bowel into the colon. Examples of this include gastroparesis and small bowel dysmotility, both suggestive of poorly controlled diabetes. Long-standing celiac disease can also interfere with small bowel motility.
- It is thought that recent antibiotic use as well as antacid medication can alter the normal bacterial flora in the small intestine, contributing to SIBO.

DIAGNOSIS

DIFFERENTIAL DIAGNOSIS

- Celiac disease
- Chronic pancreatitis
- Inflammatory bowel disease
- Irritable bowel syndrome
- Tropical sprue
- Whipple disease
- Lactose intolerance

WORKUP

Diagnostic testing should include workup for diarrhea, anemia, and malabsorption. Although endoscopy with jejunal aspirate and culture was a diagnostic tool of choice, its role is limited because of low specificity. Hydrogen breath tests have their limitations as well, but they are noninvasive and easy to perform.

LABORATORY TESTS

- Breath tests have become more commonplace in diagnosing SIBO. Typically fermenting bacteria reside in the colon. In SIBO, fermenting bacteria is present in the small intestine as well. A carbohydrate test dose (typically lactulose or glucose) is given, and its byproduct (hydrogen) is measured as it is excreted in the breath. In SIBO, exhaled hydrogen concentrations rise early.
- Standard anemia workup is essential. CBC may suggest macrocytic anemia secondary to B_{12} deficiency.
- Nutritional status should be evaluated with albumin levels.
- Stool evaluation can aid in the diagnosis as well. An increase in fecal fat may be suggestive of SIBO. Stool WBC, culture, ova, and

Diseases and Disorders

TABLE 1 Pathophysiology of Symptoms and Clinical Consequences in Small Bowel Bacterial Overgrowth

Process	Mechanisms of Action	Clinical Consequences
Mucosal injury induced by bacteria and/or their toxins or products	Loss of brush-border enzymes	Carbohydrate maldigestion
	Injury to epithelial barrier leading to enhanced intestinal permeability	Protein-losing enteropathy; bacterial translocation and portal and systemic endotoxemia
	Inflammatory response generating inflammatory cytokines	Liver injury and inflammation, systemic inflammatory responses
Luminal competition with the host for nutrients	Consumption of dietary protein	Hypoproteinemia, edema
	Consumption of vitamin B_{12}	B_{12} deficiency, megaloblastic anemia, neurologic symptoms
	Consumption of thiamine	Thiamine deficiency
	Consumption of nicotinamide	Nicotinamide deficiency
Bacterial metabolism	Fermentation of unabsorbed carbohydrates	Bloating, distension, flatulence
	Deconjugation of primary bile acids	Diarrhea due to the effects of deconjugated bile acids in the colon; depletion of the bile acid pool leading to fat and fat-soluble vitamin malabsorption
	Synthesis of vitamin K	Interference with dosing of vitamin K antagonists (e.g., warfarin)
	Synthesis of folate	High serum folate levels
	Synthesis of D-lactic acid	D-lactic acidosis
	Synthesis of alcohol	Liver injury
	Synthesis of acetaldehyde	Liver injury

From Feldman M et al: *Sleisenger and Fordtran's gastrointestinal and liver disease*, ed 10, Philadelphia, 2016, Elsevier.

BOX 1 Diseases and Disorders Linked to Small Bowel Bacterial Overgrowth (SIBO) Based on Pathophysiology

Dysmotility
Acromegaly:
  Amyloidosis
  Chronic opiate use
  Diabetic autonomic neuropathy
  Gastroparesis
  Hypothyroidism
  Idiopathic intestinal pseudo-obstruction
  Long-standing use of motility-suppressing drugs
  Myotonic muscular dystrophy
  Systemic sclerosis/scleroderma

Altered Anatomy
Blind loops:
  Gastrocolic or jejunocolic fistula
  Ileocecal valve resection
  Small intestinal diverticulosis
  Strictures (Crohn disease, radiation, surgery)
  Surgically induced alterations in anatomy (Billroth II gastrectomy, end-to-side anastomosis)

Hypochlorhydria
Long-term acid suppression (?)
  Postsurgical

Immune Deficiency
Acquired immune deficiency syndrome (e.g., AIDS, severe malnutrition)
  Inherited immune deficiencies

Multifactorial Causes
Advanced age:
  Celiac disease
  Chronic pancreatitis
  Crohn disease
  Cystic fibrosis
  End-stage kidney disease
  Intestinal failure
  Liver disease
  Radiation enteropathy
  Tropical sprue

Unclear or Undefined Relationship to SIBO
Erosive esophagitis:
  Interstitial cystitis
  Irritable bowel syndrome
  Parkinson disease
  Restless legs syndrome
  Rosacea
  Severe obesity

From Feldman M et al: *Sleisenger and Fordtran's gastrointestinal and liver disease,* ed 10, Philadelphia, 2016, Elsevier.

parasites should be ordered as well to rule out other infectious etiology.

IMAGING STUDIES
- Endoscopic evaluation of the small intestine can be useful in finding structural and motility causes of bacterial overgrowth such as diverticula and strictures. Small bowel biopsy may aid in the diagnosis of celiac disease as well.
- Jejunal aspirate cultures via endoscopy are considered a standard of diagnosis. Aspirate cultures that exceed 10^5 organisms/ml suggest the presence of SIBO.

- There are several limitations to jejunal aspirate cultures. Bacterial overgrowth is not uniform and may be in inaccessible areas to endoscopist and can easily be missed. Contamination from oropharyngeal flora can lead to false-positive tests. Also, endoscopy is an invasive test, and other methods of testing such as a breath test may be a more practical initial approach.

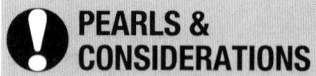 **TREATMENT**

The goal is to treat the underlying cause and treat the bacterial overgrowth with antibiotic therapy.

NONPHARMACOLOGIC THERAPY
Structural disorders such as strictures, fistula, and diverticula may require surgical intervention.

ACUTE GENERAL Rx
- 7- to 10-day course of antibiotic therapy with rifaximin, amoxicillin-clavulanate, or metronidazole and ciprofloxacin has been shown to be beneficial.
- Nutritional support with vitamin replacement and dietary modification (lactose-free diet).

CHRONIC Rx
- Recurrence is common after antibiotic therapy. These patients may require subsequent courses of antibiotic therapy.
- Avoid using antacid medication.
- Avoid drugs that reduce GI motility (opioids).
- Consider lactose-free diet if the response to antimicrobial agents is incomplete.

DISPOSITION
Prognosis is dependent on underlying cause of SIBO. Although recurrence rate is high, antibiotic therapy remains the mainstay of therapy often requiring repeated courses if the underlying condition cannot be resolved.

REFERRAL
- Gastroenterology consultation for small bowel evaluation
- Surgical consultation with an underlying structural disorder

🛈 **PEARLS & CONSIDERATIONS**

COMMENTS
- SIBO is due to a disruption of protective mechanisms against bacterial burden.
- Look for risk factors including UGI tract surgery, structural disorders, inflammatory bowel disease (IBD), IBS, and disorders decreasing GI motility.
- Diagnosis can be made with hydrogen breath test or endoscopic jejunal aspirate culture.
- Treatment is with antibiotics.
- The combination of vitamin B_{12} deficiency (due to bacterial consumption) and an elevated serum folate level (due to bacterial production) is suggestive of SIBO.
- SIBO can contribute to symptoms of IBS or IBD.

RELATED CONTENT
Small Intestinal Bacterial Overgrowth (Patient Information)
Irritable Bowel Syndrome (Related Key Topic)
Malabsorption (Related Key Topic)

AUTHOR: **FRED F. FERRI, MD**

S

BASIC INFORMATION

DEFINITION

- Small bowel obstruction can be **functional** (as a result of intrinsic abnormal intestinal pathology; dysfunction peristalsis, also called "ileus") or **mechanical** (which may occur acutely or may be chronic).
- Small bowel obstruction is due to intraluminal or extraluminal mechanical compression.
- Mechanical obstruction means the blockage of the intestinal lumen, preventing the passage of luminal contents through the gut tube. Intraabdominal adhesion disease is the most common cause of mechanical small bowel obstruction in developed countries.
- Mechanical obstruction may be either:
  1. **Simple obstruction:** In which the lumen may be *partially* or *completely blocked* but with intact intestinal blood flow OR
  2. **Strangulated obstruction:**
     a. This is a surgical emergency.
     b. Usually the obstruction is complete; blood flow to the obstructed segment is cut off; and tissue necrosis, gangrene, and perforation may occur.

ICD-10CM CODES
K56	Paralytic ileus and intestinal obstruction
K56.1	Intussusception
K56.2	Volvulus
K56.3	Gallstone ileus
K56.4	Other impaction of intestine
K56.5	Intestinal adhesions (bands) with obstruction
K56.6	Other and unspecified intestinal obstruction
K56.9	Ileus, unspecified

EPIDEMIOLOGY & DEMOGRAPHICS

- An estimated 300,000 laparotomies are performed yearly in the U.S. for small bowel obstruction.
- The most frequently encountered surgical disorder of the small intestines is mechanical small bowel obstruction (SBO). This is a common surgical emergency accounting for 2% to 4% of emergency room visits and 15% of hospital admissions.
- 75% of all cases of small bowel obstruction result from intraabdominal adhesion related to prior abdominal surgery, such as appendectomy, colorectal surgery, and gynecologic procedures.

PREDOMINANT SEX & AGE: Incidence is similar for males and females.

RISK FACTORS:
- Previous abdominal or pelvic surgery—most important risk factor for mechanical SBO in the U.S.
- Hernia (abdominal wall or groin)
- Prior abdominal irradiation
- Bowel neoplasm
- Foreign-body ingestion
- Parasitic infestation
- Gallstones
- Inflammatory/ischemic stricture

PHYSICAL FINDINGS & CLINICAL PRESENTATION

PHYSICAL FINDINGS: These may include:
- Dehydration (manifested by tachycardia, decreased urine output, orthostatic hypotension, dry mucous membrane)
- Abdominal distention may suggest an abnormal accumulation of air or fluid
- Hyperactive bowel sounds (an early occurrence)
- Tympany to abdominal percussion over a distended abdomen may indicate the presence of air
- Percussion dullness over a distended abdomen may indicate fluid
- High-pitched "tinkling" sound on auscultation of the abdomen
- Hypoactive bowel sounds (late finding)
- Hernia
- Rectal examination may reveal:
  1. Blood (suggestive of neoplasm or strangulation or mucosal ischemia)
  2. Masses (may suggest obturator hernia)
  3. Fecal impaction

CLINICAL PRESENTATION: There are four key symptoms: Abdominal pain, vomiting, distention, and constipation
- Abdominal pain (abrupt onset):
  1. Intermittent, crampy, or colicky
  2. Constant pain (that is, change in pain's character) signifies serious complication
- Abdominal distention: Indicates abnormal accumulation of air or fluid
- Nausea
- Vomiting (bilious vomiting seen in proximal obstructions)
- Diarrhea (early finding)
- Constipation (a late finding)
- Obstipation (inability to pass gas or stool)
- Hypotension, fever, tachycardia, leukocytosis, and peritoneal signs (these late findings may be seen with strangulation or intestinal ischemia) should compel urgency toward operative management
- It is important to perform serial abdominal examinations to detect changes early

ETIOLOGY

- Postoperative adhesions, especially prior abdominopelvic operations (may cause acute obstruction usually within 1 mo of surgery; or chronic obstructions can occur years later)
- Incarcerated inguinal hernia
- Malignant tumor
- Inflammatory bowel disease
- Gallstone ileus
- Stool impaction
- Stricture
- Cystic fibrosis
- Volvulus
- In children consider pyloric stenosis, intussusception, congenital atresia

Dx DIAGNOSIS

DIFFERENTIAL DIAGNOSIS

- Paralytic ileus
- Pseudoobstruction
- Acute cholangitis
- Cholecystitis
- Gastroenteritis
- Inflammatory bowel disease
- Diverticulitis
- Endometriosis
- Mesenteric ischemia
- Pancreatitis
- Dysmenorrhea
- Ovarian torsion

WORKUP

All patients diagnosed with acute small bowel obstruction should be admitted to the hospital, as they need immediate surgical evaluation. During the initial evaluation, the primary objectives are to gauge the degree of metabolic derangement and volume depletion, and to assess the need for gastrointestinal decompression with nasogastric (NG) tube and expediency of surgery. It is also important to exclude sepsis, perforation, and bowel ischemia. As with many surgical conditions, determining the correct diagnosis and management strategy hinges on a focused, yet thorough history and physical examination.

LABORATORY TESTS

- Laboratory abnormalities are not diagnostic of bowel obstruction but instead may indicate complications of obstruction. Essential laboratory tests include:
  1. Basic metabolic panel (hyponatremia, hypokalemia)
  2. CBC: Hemoconcentration, leukocytosis
  3. Urinalysis
  4. Serum amylase: May be elevated
  5. Lactate dehydrogenase
  6. Hepatic panel
  7. Check serum lactate, blood cultures, arterial blood gas in patients with signs such as fever, hypotension, or change in mental status
  8. Type and cross-match (in anticipation of possible surgical intervention)

IMAGING STUDIES

- Image to confirm diagnosis, identify the location of the obstruction, and access the type of obstruction.
- Imaging also helps identify complications (perforation, necrosis, etc.) and possible cause of the obstruction.
- Initial radiographic evaluation begins with plain x-ray films of the abdomen (supine and upright) and an upright chest radiograph. An upright chest radiograph is of paramount importance to inspect for pneumoperitoneum and also for evidence of aspiration in a patient with a history of vomiting. A supine and upright plain abdominal x-ray in patients with suspected small bowel obstruction may show:
  1. Ladderlike pattern of dilated small bowel loops with air-fluid levels (Fig. 1) indicating small bowel obstruction
  2. Accumulation of air and fluid proximal and clearance of fluid and air distal to the point of obstruction

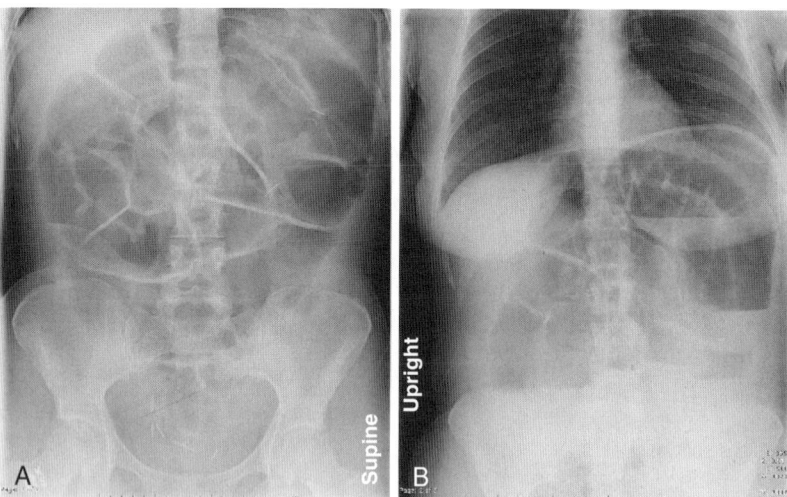
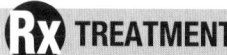

FIG. 1 A, Supine film showing dilated loops of small bowel in a patient with small bowel obstruction. **B,** Upright abdominal film revealing multiple air-fluid levels and small bowel dilation, consistent with a diagnosis of small bowel obstruction. (From Marx J: *Rosen's emergency medicine: concepts and clinical practice,* ed 6, Philadelphia, 2006, Saunders.)

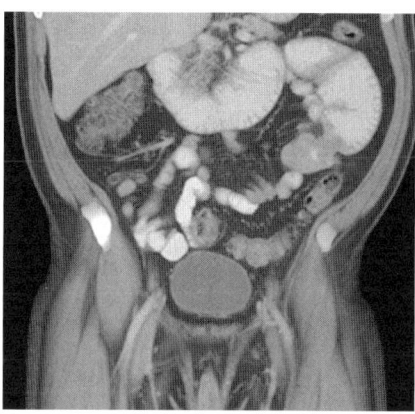

FIG. 4 Coronal image of computed tomographic scan showing mass in proximal small bowel with decompressed loops of small bowel distal to obstruction. (From Cameron JL, Cameron AM: *Current surgical therapy,* ed 10, Philadelphia, 2011, Saunders.)

3. Proximal small bowel dilation with distal loop collapse
- Enteroclysis (a fluoroscopic x-ray of the small intestine) is useful in detecting obstruction and can distinguish partial from complete blockage and adhesions from metastases.
- Computed tomography (CT) scan of the abdomen and pelvis with contrast is the gold standard imaging modality.
- CT scan is the study of choice if the patient has fever, tachycardia, abdominal pain, and leukocytosis. It can reveal the etiology of the obstruction: Abscess, inflammatory process, extra-luminal pathology, and/or metastases.
- CT can elucidate the cause, such as the presence of a mass (Fig. E2) or a hernia with subsequent obstruction (Fig. E3). In addition, CT has high sensitivity for detecting strangulation and pneumoperitoneum indicative of a perforation and is particularly useful in the early postoperative setting to rule out ischemia, intraabdominal abscess, or morbidity as the underlying cause. It is also useful in patients with a history of malignancy to differentiate potentially recurrent disease from adhesions (Fig. 4).
- CT enterography, in which intraluminal distention is achieved with administration of large volumes of oral contrast such as water-methylcellulose solution, can be useful. This modality is most often used to diagnose patients with Crohn disease–related strictures, and its benefit is high-resolution imaging of the bowel wall; however, it is impractical in the patient with GI distress who is nauseated and vomiting.

TREATMENT

- Immediate admission to the hospital if acute small bowel obstruction is suspected.
- Prompt surgical consultation to determine if surgical intervention is needed.

EMERGENCY ROOM CARE

- Vigorous fluid resuscitation and correction of electrolyte disorders underpin the initial therapeutic goals of both nonoperative and preoperative management strategies. Placing a Foley catheter to measure urinary output, establishing adequate intravenous access, and reassessing hemodynamic and electrolyte status are all essential in the initial management.
- Initial treatment:
  1. Designate the patient nothing by mouth; *nil per os* ("NPO")
  2. Fluid resuscitation (with isotonic Ringer or normal saline solution)
  3. Bowel decompression (via NG tube placement): A standard NG tube provides symptomatic relief, prevents added gas and fluid accumulation proximally, and enables the serial assessment of antegrade fluid movement
  4. Correction of metabolic and electrolyte abnormalities
  5. Pain management
  6. Antiemetic administration
  7. Surgical consultation: Must be done early
  8. Antibiotic administration

NONSURGICAL INPATIENT CARE

General principles:

- Bowel rest
- Continue NG suction for decompression
- Serial abdominal examination (q4 to 6h)
- Check labs, for example, CBC, basic metabolic panel, lactic acid q6h
- Provide adequate fluid

Patients with low-grade partial SBOs are prone to spontaneous resolution with conservative interventions such as bowel rest, NG decompression, and appropriate fluid resuscitation. For partial or simple obstructions resolution usually occurs within 72 h.

SURGICAL CARE

More than 25% of inpatients admitted because of SBO will require an operation. Patients with complete or high-grade partial SBO are most likely to need surgery, with less than 20% successfully managed nonoperatively. Surgery is indicated in:

- Strangulated obstruction (which is a surgical emergency)
- Patients with clinical signs including fever, tachycardia, and peritonitis
- Patients with radiologic signs of ischemia/necrosis or perforation (require prompt surgery)
- Simple complete obstruction: After failed nonoperative care

SUGGESTED READINGS

Available at eBooks.Health.Elsevier.com.

AUTHOR: **DANIEL K. ASIEDU, MD, PhD, FACP**

ⓘ BASIC INFORMATION

DEFINITION

A spinal epidural abscess (SEA) is a focal suppurative infection occurring in the spinal epidural space.

SYNONYM

SEA
Intraspinal abscess

ICD-10CM CODE
G06.1 Intraspinal abscess and granuloma

EPIDEMIOLOGY & DEMOGRAPHICS

INCIDENCE (IN U.S.):
- 2 to 25 cases/100,000 hospitalized patients/yr
- May be increasing over the past 3 decades

PREDOMINANT AGE:
- Median age of onset approximately 50 yr (35 yr in intravenous drug users)
- Peak incidence in seventh and eighth decades of life

PHYSICAL FINDINGS & CLINICAL PRESENTATION

- The presentation of SEA can be nonspecific.
- Fever, malaise, and back pain are the most consistent early symptoms.
- Pain is often focal. It may initially be mild but can progress to become severe.
- As the disease progresses, root pain can occur, followed by motor weakness, sensory changes, bladder and bowel dysfunction, and paralysis.
- Physical findings may be limited to fever or spinal tenderness.
- The evolution to neurologic deficits can occur as quickly as a few hours, or over weeks to months.
- Once paralysis occurs, it may quickly become irreversible without the appropriate intervention.

ETIOLOGY

- SEA most commonly results from hematogenous dissemination.
- Pyogenic bacteria account for the majority of cases in the U.S. Immigrants from tuberculosis (TB)-endemic areas may present with tuberculous SEAs. Fungi and parasites can also cause this condition. The most common causative organism is *Staphylococcus aureus*. Gram-negative bacilli and anaerobes may be seen if the infection has a urinary or GI source.
- Most posterior SEAs are thought to originate from distant focus (e.g., skin and soft tissue infections), whereas anterior SEAs are commonly associated with diskitis or vertebral osteomyelitis. No source was found in approximately one third of cases.
- Associated predisposing conditions include diabetes mellitus, alcoholism, cancer, AIDS, and chronic renal failure, or following epidural anesthesia, spinal surgery or trauma, prolonged epidural catheter placement, paraspinal glucocorticoid or analgesic injections,

acupuncture, or intravenous (IV) drug use. No predisposing condition is found in approximately 20% of patients.
- Damage to the spinal cord can be caused by direct compression of the spinal cord, vascular compromise, bacterial toxins, and inflammation.

Ⓓ DIAGNOSIS

DIFFERENTIAL DIAGNOSIS
- Herniated disk
- Vertebral osteomyelitis and diskitis
- Metastatic tumors
- Meningitis

LABORATORY TESTS

- White blood count (WBC) may be normal or elevated.
- Erythrocyte sedimentation rate (ESR) and C-reactive proteins are usually elevated.
- Blood cultures are positive in approximately 60% of patients with SEA and should be obtained before starting antibiotics.
- CSF cultures are positive in 19%, but lumbar puncture is unnecessary, and may be contraindicated.
- Once imaging is done, computed tomography (CT)-guided aspiration or open biopsy should be done to determine causative organism.

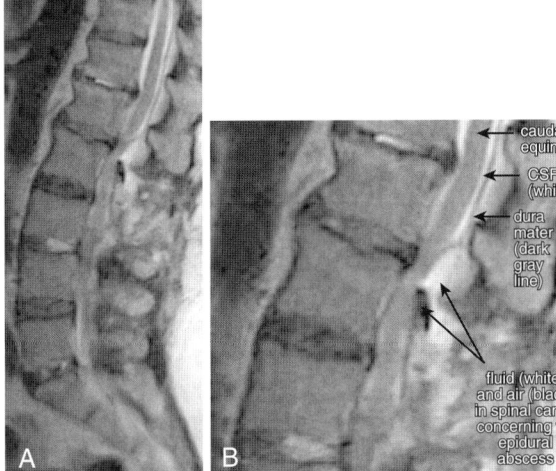

FIG. 1 Same patient as in Fig. 2, in whom noncontrast computed tomography showed air in the spinal canal, concerning for epidural abscess. Magnetic resonance imaging (MRI) of the lumbar spine without contrast was performed, as the patient was in acute renal failure. **A,** This T2-weighted sagittal MRI provides useful information even without gadolinium contrast. **B,** Close-up. On T_2-weighted MRI sequences, fluid including cerebrospinal fluid *(CSF)* appears white. Fat-containing tissues such as bone marrow and the spinal cord or cauda equina appear dark gray. Calcified bone appears nearly black due to an absence of resonating protons. Air appears completely black for the same reason. The midline sagittal image shows the cauda equina to be impinged upon by an epidural fluid collection containing air—an epidural abscess. The dura mater is visible as a thin, dark-gray line parallel to the spinal cord. It is indented in the region of the epidural abscess. (From Broder JS: *Diagnostic imaging for the emergency physician,* Philadelphia, 2011, Saunders.)

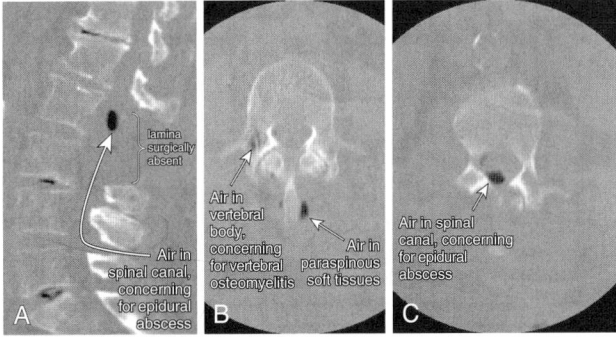

FIG. 2 This 67-yr-old female presented with delirium and fever. She had undergone lumbar laminectomy 3 mo prior, and her wound had been treated with a wound VAC dressing. Magnetic resonance imaging was not initially available, so noncontrast computed tomography (CT) was performed. Noncontrast CT is excellent at delineating air, which appears black on bone windows. **A,** The midsagittal view demonstrates air *(black)* in the spinal canal at the L2 and L3 levels. On the axial views **(B, C),** air is visible in the spinal canal, in paraspinal soft tissues, and within the vertebral body. These findings are concerning for a paraspinal infection that has developed into an epidural abscess with vertebral osteomyelitis. (From Broder JS: *Diagnostic imaging for the emergency physician,* Philadelphia, 2011, Saunders.)

Abscess content culture is positive in 90% of patients.

IMAGING STUDIES

- MRI with gadolinium is the imaging modality of choice (Fig. 1); CT scan with contrast may show the abscess (Fig. 2) but is less sensitive than MRI.
- CT with myelography is more sensitive for cord compression.

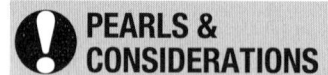 **TREATMENT**

NONPHARMACOLOGIC THERAPY

- Surgical decompression is the mainstay of treatment. Decompression within the first 24 h has been related to an improved prognosis.
- Nonsurgical treatment is effective in some patients, but failure rate may be excessive. This approach should not be considered and should only be attempted in the absence of signs of compressive myelopathy and with very careful follow-up.

ACUTE GENERAL Rx

- In addition to surgery, antibiotics directed at the most likely organism should be initiated. Fig. 3 describes an algorithm for the management of patients with SEA.
- If the organism is unknown, broad coverage against staphylococci, streptococci, and gram-negative bacilli should be initiated. Empiric antimicrobial intravenous therapy typically includes vancomycin (loading dose: 25 to 30 mg/kg, then 15 to 20 mg/kg q8 to 12h, aiming for trough levels of 15 to 20) plus an antipseudomonal cephalosporin such as piperacillin/tazobactam at high dose (4.5 g IV q6h) or carbapenem such as meropenem (1 to 2 g IV q8h) or imipenem. The regimen can be adjusted according to culture results. Therapy should continue for at least 4 to 6 wk.

CHRONIC Rx

Neurologic deficits may remain despite aggressive treatment.

DISPOSITION

Irreversible paralysis and death can occur in up to 25% of patients.

REFERRAL

All cases should be referred to a neurosurgeon and an infectious disease specialist.

❗ PEARLS & CONSIDERATIONS

- Follow-up imaging with MRI is not necessary unless patient develops new neurologic signs or symptoms, has poor clinical response, or has persistent elevation of inflammatory markers.
- It is critically important to recognize this process early; the prognosis is generally excellent if treatment is initiated while symptoms are localized and before evidence of myelopathy develops.
- The likelihood of success postsurgery is low in patients who have developed complete paralysis for longer than 36 h.

SUGGESTED READINGS
Available at eBooks.Health.Elsevier.com.

AUTHOR: **GLENN G. FORT, MD, MPH**

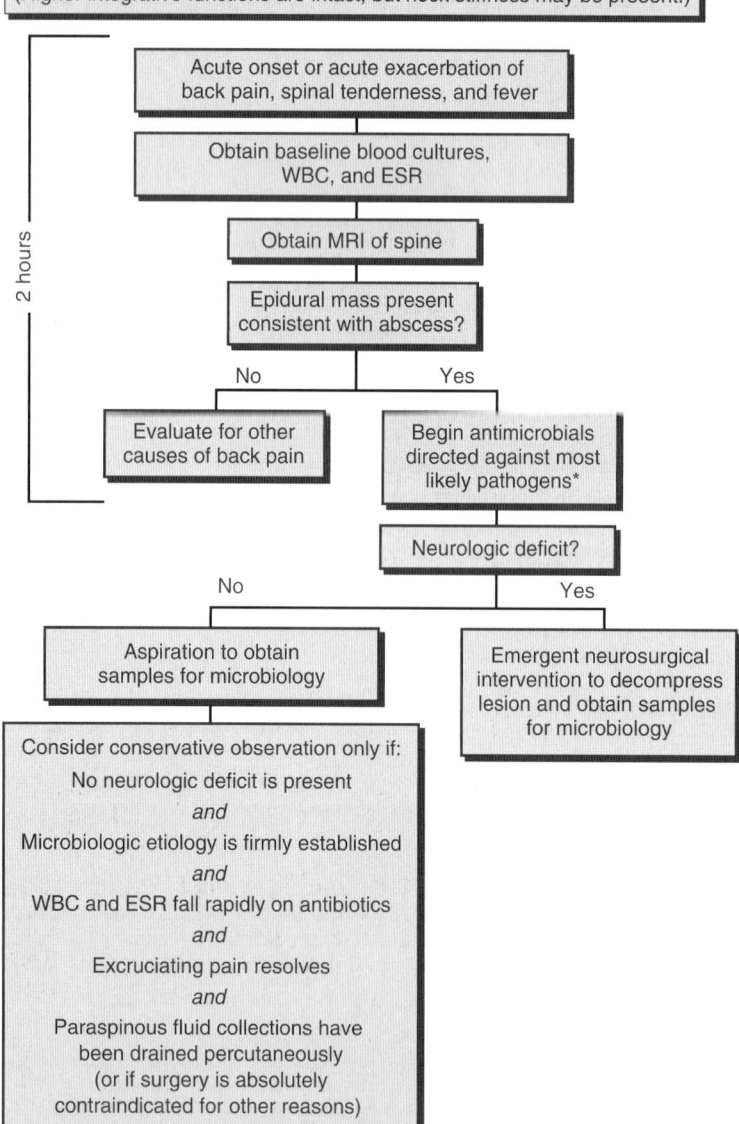

FIG. 3 Algorithm for the management of patients with spinal epidural abscess syndrome. If MRI cannot be performed, myelography, high-contrast computed tomography (CT), or CT-myelography may be an acceptable alternative to localize an epidural abscess. If abscess drainage can be performed promptly, antimicrobial drugs may be withheld until specimens for microbial analysis are obtained. *ESR,* Erythrocyte sedimentation rate; *MRI,* magnetic resonance imaging; *WBC,* white blood cell. (From Vincent JL et al: *Textbook of critical care,* ed 6, Philadelphia, 2011, Saunders.)

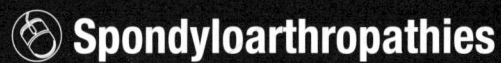
 BASIC INFORMATION

DEFINITION

Spondyloarthropathies (SpAs) are a group of diverse interrelated systemic autoinflammatory conditions that are serologically negative for rheumatoid factor, connected by an underlying genetic risk (HLA-B27) with similar patterns of inflammation. This group encompasses ankylosing spondylitis, psoriatic arthritis, reactive arthritis, enteropathic arthritis, undifferentiated spondyloarthritis, and juvenile-onset spondyloarthritis (Table 1). SpAs are broadly classified by axial vs. peripheral joint involvement, and with or without radiographic progression.

SYNONYMS

Spondyloarthritides
Spondylopathy
Spondylitis

ICD-10CM CODES
M46.80	Other specified inflammatory spondylopathies, unspecified site	
M46.82	Other specified inflammatory spondylopathies, cervical region	
M46.83	Other specified inflammatory spondylopathies, cervicothoracic region	
M46.86	Other specified inflammatory spondylopathies, lumbar region	
M46.87	Other specified inflammatory spondylopathies, lumbosacral region	
M46.89	Other specified inflammatory spondylopathies, multiple sites	
M46.81	Other specified inflammatory spondylopathies, occipito-atlanto-axial region	
M46.88	Other specified inflammatory spondylopathies, sacrococcygeal region	
M46.84	Other specified inflammatory spondylopathies, thoracic region	
M46.85	Other specified inflammatory spondylopathies, thoracolumbar region	

EPIDEMIOLOGY & DEMOGRAPHICS

PREVALENCE: Worldwide prevalence of SpA is 0.2% to 1.6%, with approximately 1% of the U.S. population affected. Varies regionally with prevalence of HLA-B27. The most prevalent subtype is ankylosing spondylitis followed by psoriatic arthritis.
PREDOMINANT SEX & AGE: Males younger than age 45 yr are predominantly affected. Previously, the male:female ratio was thought to be 10:1; more recently, approximately 3:1.

Patients >45 yr may present with chronic, severe disease due to diagnostic delays.
RISK FACTORS: HLA-B27 allele,* male sex,* smoking,* ethnic background, family history of SpA, and certain infections. (*Associated with more severe disease.)
GENETICS: Association with the HLA-B27 allele is the strongest known genetic risk factor; approximately 95% of patients with ankylosing spondylitis have the HLA-B27 allele.

PHYSICAL FINDINGS & CLINICAL PRESENTATION

- History:
  1. Inflammatory low back pain may be the primary presenting symptom:
     a. Pain and stiffness in the low back or buttocks that is worse in the morning, may awaken the patient from sleep, and improves with exercise
     b. Morning stiffness generally lasting longer than 1 h
     c. Improvement with NSAIDs
     d. Sensitivity up to 90% and positive likelihood ratio up to 2.2 for axial SpA
  2. Symptoms of systemic and peripheral inflammation are additional clues that can be elicited in a comprehensive review of systems:
     a. Uveitis: Painful ocular inflammation
     b. Psoriasis: Chronic skin inflammation with red patches and silvery scales
     c. Inflammatory bowel disease: Crohn disease and ulcerative colitis
     d. Synovitis: Inflammation of the synovial membrane of joints
     e. Enthesitis: Inflammation at the site of tendon or ligament insertion onto bone
     f. Dactylitis: Tenosynovitis of the digits causing classic sausage-like appearance
- Physical exam:
  1. Axial joints: Spine and sacroiliac (SI) joints.
  2. Inspect curvature, palpate for tenderness, and evaluate range of motion for cervical, thoracic, and lumbar spine. Measure degree of axial involvement with occiput wall, thoracic expansion. Patients with SpA may have an abnormal Schober test result (Fig. E1). This test is performed by having the patient stand erect and marking the distance between the midpoint of the posterior superior iliac spines ("dimples of Venus") and 10 cm above that point. The patient is then asked to maximally flex forward while the more caudal spot is kept stationary. The more cephalad point on the tape measure should demonstrate at least 5 cm of excursion. This abnormality also can be seen with lumbar degenerative disk disease. Test for sacroiliitis with Patrick and Gaenslen tests.
  3. Peripheral joints: Lower extremity predominance.
  4. Inspect for signs of inflammation, including dactylitis, synovitis, and enthesitis.
  5. Evaluate for systemic involvement manifesting as anterior uveitis and psoriasis:
     a. Slit lamp is necessary to diagnose anterior uveitis.
     b. Full skin exam is critical to detect occult psoriasis; look for nail changes.
- Musculoskeletal manifestations commonly affect weight-bearing joints with high mechanical stress; thus it is particularly important to examine the lumbar spine, SI joints, and lower extremities.
- Degree of axial involvement can be measured via specialized exam techniques, which are used to track disease activity and response to treatment over time.

ETIOLOGY

The exact etiology of SpAs is still unknown; however, evidence indicates a combination of genetics and environmental factors play an important role in susceptibility and pathogenesis.
- Genetic:
  1. The HLA-B27 allele has a strong association with SpA, through mechanisms that are not fully understood. The subset of HLA-B27 patients with SpAs are at an increased risk for axial skeleton involvement and earlier age of onset.
- Environmental:
  1. Microbial infections, disruptions in barrier defense mechanisms (skin and intestinal mucosa), and mechanical articular stressors may trigger an inflammatory response, which then develops into signs and symptoms specific to each type of SpA.
- Autoinflammatory:
  1. Key components of the inflammatory cascade involved in the pathogenesis of SpA are tumor necrosis factor (TNF), interleukin (IL)-12, IL-17, IL-23, and

TABLE 1 Comparison of Ankylosing Spondylitis and Related Disorders

Feature	Ankylosing Spondylitis	Psoriatic Arthritis	Reactive Arthritis	Enteropathic Arthropathy
Sex (male:female)	2-3:1	1:1	1:1	1:1
Age of onset	<40 yr	35-55 yr	20-40 yr	Any age
Sacroiliitis or spondylitis (%)	100	~20	~40	<20
Symmetry of sacroiliitis	Symmetrical	Asymmetrical	Asymmetrical	Symmetrical
Peripheral arthritis (%)	~25	95	90	5-20
Distribution	Axial and lower limbs	Variable	Lower limbs	Variable
HLA-B27 positivity (%)	85-95	25-60*	30-70	7-70†
Uveitis	0-40	~20	~50	<15

*60% when spondylitis is present.
†70% when spondylitis is present.
From Hochberg MC: *Rheumatology*, ed 7, Philadelphia, 2019, Elsevier.

prostaglandins. Success in treatment with targeted therapies to each of these molecules has helped us understand their role in the etiology of SpA.

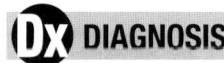 **DIAGNOSIS**

Several classification criteria now exist for the SpAs. In 1991, the European Spondyloarthropathy Study Group (ESSG) criteria were developed to establish criteria for the SpAs (Fig. 2). These criteria have been demonstrated to be 87% sensitive and specific for the diagnosis of SpA. They are somewhat less well suited for diagnosis of early disease but extremely useful for established disease.

Table 2 summarizes current diagnostic criteria for SpA.

DIFFERENTIAL DIAGNOSIS

- Seronegative rheumatoid arthritis (peripheral presentation)
- Degenerative disc disease (axial presentation) or DISH
- Inflammatory osteoarthritis (axial or peripheral presentation)
- Hypertrophic osteoarthropathy (peripheral presentation)

WORKUP

- Young patients, particularly men <45 yr, with chronic inflammatory low back pain responsive to NSAIDs should be screened.
- Patients with psoriasis, inflammatory bowel disease, or recent gastrointestinal or genitourinary infections presenting with new-onset low back or peripheral joint pain should also be screened.
- Screening begins with a comprehensive history and physical exam.
- HLA-B27 testing and imaging of SI joints and/or lumbar spine are indicated based on clinical suspicion.

LABORATORY TESTS

- HLA-B27:
  1. Negative test does not rule out SpA.
  2. Sensitivity: 95% for ankylosing spondylitis, 80% for reactive arthritis, 70% for psoriatic arthritis, and 50% for enteropathic arthritis.
- Elevated erythrocyte sedimentation rate (ESR) and C-reactive protein (CRP), anemia of chronic disease, leukocytosis, and thrombocytosis may reflect active inflammation. A normal CRP or ESR does not rule out spondyloarthropathies.
- Testing for rheumatoid arthritis antibodies is generally negative (rheumatoid factor, cyclic citrullinated peptide).
- Synovial fluid is inflammatory and nonspecific, with white blood cell>2,000/mm^2.

IMAGING STUDIES

- **X-Ray:** SI joints and lumbar spine:
  1. May not detect early inflammation
  2. 20% to 80% have nonradiographic disease at time of presentation

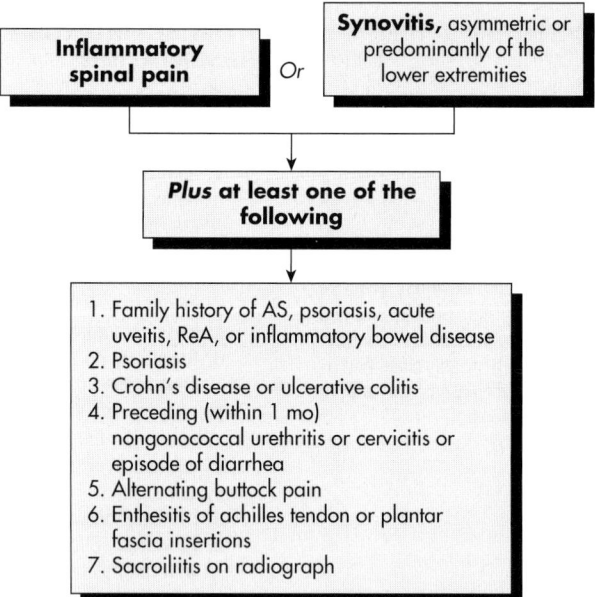

FIG. 2 European Spondyloarthropathy Study Group (ESSG) criteria for spondyloarthritis. *AS,* Ankylosing spondylitis/axial spondyloarthritis; *ReA,* reactive arthritis. (From https://omicsgroup.org. Accessed September 29, 2014. In Firestein GS et al: *Firestein & Kelley's Textbook of Rheumatology,* ed 11, Philadelphia, 2021, Elsevier.)

TABLE 2 Criteria for Spondyloarthritis (SpA)*

Amor Criteria	ESSG Criteria
Past or current clinical manifestations:	Inflammatory back pain *or* synovitis:
1. Back pain at night and/or back stiffness in the morning (1 point)	- Asymmetric synovitis or
2. Asymmetric oligoarthritis (2 points)	- Predominantly lower limb synovitis
3. Gluteal pain without other details (1 point) or alternating gluteal pain (2 points)	AND
	One or more of the following:
4. Sausage-like digit or toe (2 points)	- Positive family history
5. Heel pain or other enthesopathy (2 points)	- Psoriasis
	- Inflammatory bowel disease
6. Iritis (2 points)	- Urethritis, cervicitis, or acute diarrhea within 1 mo before arthritis
7. Nongonococcal urethritis within 1 mo before the onset of arthritis (1 point)	- Buttock pain alternating between right and left gluteal areas
8. Acute diarrhea within 1 mo before the onset of arthritis (1 point)	- Enthesopathy
9. Past or current psoriasis and/or balanitis and/or inflammatory bowel disease (2 points)	- Sacroiliitis (radiography)
Radiographic changes:	
1. Sacroiliitis grade 2 or more if bilateral, grade 3 or more if unilateral (3 points)	
Predisposing genetic factors:	
1. Presence of HLA-B27 antigen and/or family history of ankylosing spondylitis, Reiter syndrome, psoriasis, uveitis, or chronic bowel disease (2 points)	
Responsiveness to treatment:	
1. Improvement within 48 hr after initiation of an NSAID and/or recurrence within 48 hr after discontinuation of an NSAID (2 points)	

*Definite SpA if ≥6 points; probable SpA if 5 points.
ESSG, European Spondyloarthropathy Study Group; *NSAID,* nonsteroidal antiinflammatory drug.
From Hochberg MC: *Rheumatology,* ed 7, Philadelphia, 2019, Elsevier.

3. May show signs of structural damage such as erosions, syndesmophytes, sclerosis, and ankylosis in chronic axial disease
- **MRI:** SI joints and lumbar spine:
  1. Subchondral bone marrow edema in early disease
  2. Useful when x-ray and clinical findings are nondiagnostic but clinician's suspicion for axial SpA remains high

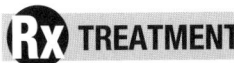 ## TREATMENT

Improvement in symptoms, preservation of function, and prevention of structural damage can be achieved through a multidisciplinary approach.

NONPHARMACOLOGIC THERAPY
- Physical and occupational therapies improve functional outcomes.
- Surgery:
  1. Joint replacements (high-impact joints such as hips)
  2. Spinal wedge osteotomy (advanced axial disease)
  3. Colectomy (advanced enteropathic arthritis)

ACUTE GENERAL Rx
- NSAIDs are first line.
- Avoid steroids in psoriatic arthritis due to risk of life-threatening pustular psoriasis and erythroderma.

CHRONIC Rx
- **NSAIDs:**
  1. Up to 35% of patients may achieve remission.
  2. Best response in early disease.
  3. Continuous dosing may prevent radiographic progression of axial disease.
- **Disease-modifying antirheumatic drugs (DMARDs):** Effective for peripheral involvement only, not effective in axial disease
  1. Methotrexate, leflunomide, sulfasalazine
- **TNF inhibitors:** NSAID or DMARD failure

1. Infliximab, adalimumab, golimumab, etanercept, certolizumab pegol
- **IL-17 and IL-12/23 inhibitors:** 2nd TNF inhibitor failure
  1. Recent studies show similar efficacy compared to TNF inhibitors.
  2. Ixekizumab (IL-17 inhibitor) recently approved for ankylosing spondylitis.
  3. Ustekinumab (IL-12/23 inhibitor) and secukinumab (IL-17 inhibitor) are effective in psoriatic arthritis. Secukinumab also is approved for ankylosing spondylitis.
  4. Ustekinumab is also effective in Crohn-enteropathic arthritis.
- **Janus kinase inhibitors:** Phase II clinical trial Tofacitinib (JAK 1, 2, 3 inhibitor) was shown to improve clinical and imaging outcomes in axial SpA, with phase III trial data pending.

Tofacitinib is approved to treat both UC and psoriatic arthritis.

DISPOSITION
- Function and mobility may be limited in advanced axial disease.
- Psoriatic arthritis is an independent risk factor for cardiovascular disease.

COMPLEMENTARY & ALTERNATIVE MEDICINE
- Strong clinical trials are lacking.
- Small studies have shown Pilates, t'ai chi, deep tissue massage, and hydroelectric therapy can be beneficial in axial SpA.

REFERRAL
Rheumatology, dermatology, ophthalmology, gastroenterology, infectious disease

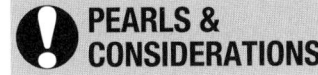 ## PEARLS & CONSIDERATIONS

COMMENTS
Young patients with chronic inflammatory low back pain deserve referral to a rheumatologist.

HLA-B27 positivity is not required for diagnosis if strong clinical features are present. MRI may be needed to detect early axial disease. Repeated spinal x-rays at scheduled intervals (e.g., every 2 yr) are not recommended in patients with active or stable nonradiographic axial SpA. Track axial disease activity with clinical scoring systems and physical exam measurements. Traditional DMARDs are not effective in axial disease.

PREVENTION
High index of suspicion and prompt referral allows for early diagnosis. Early treatment with treat-to-target approach may prevent symptomatic and radiographic progression.

PATIENT & FAMILY EDUCATION
Smoking cessation is key. Discuss with family the implications of strong genetic component. Educate patients with psoriasis and inflammatory bowel disease about symptoms of inflammatory low back or peripheral joint pain to monitor for development of SpA in these high-risk individuals.

SUGGESTED READINGS
Available at eBooks.Health.Elsevier.com.

RELATED CONTENT
Ankylosing Spondylitis (Related Key Topic)
Psoriatic Arthritis (Related Key Topic)
Reactive Arthritis (Reiter Syndrome) (Related Key Topic)
Enteropathic Arthritis (Related Key Topic)

AUTHORS: **OZAIR K. MEGHANI, BA,** and **MANUEL F. DASILVA, MD**

S

Diseases and Disorders

I

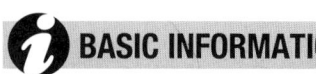
BASIC INFORMATION

DEFINITION

Spontaneous abortion is fetal loss before wk 20 of pregnancy, calculated from the patient's last menstrual period, or the delivery of a fetus weighing <500 g. Early loss is before gestational age 12 6/7 wk, whereas late loss refers to losses from wk 13 to 20.[1]

Spontaneous abortion can also be classified as incomplete (partial passage of fetal tissue through partially dilated cervix), complete (spontaneous passage of all fetal tissue), threatened (uterine bleeding without cervical dilation or passage of tissue), inevitable (bleeding with cervical dilation without passage of fetal tissue), or missed abortion (intrauterine fetal demise without passage of tissue).

Recurrent spontaneous abortion involves three or more spontaneous pregnancy losses before wk 20. It affects approximately 1% of couples attempting to conceive. However, in actual practice, most reproductive experts consider two spontaneous pregnancy losses sufficient to initiate an evaluation for habitual or recurrent spontaneous abortion, since the risk of another loss is similar at this point, and the emotional stress is high. As many as 5% of couples and probably even a higher proportion of couples in which the woman is over age 35 are affected by two or more consecutive spontaneous abortions.[2]

SYNONYMS

Spontaneous miscarriage
Miscarriage
Spontaneous pregnancy loss

ICD-10CM CODES
003.89 Complete or unspecified spontaneous abortion with other complications
003.9 Complete or unspecified spontaneous abortion without complication

EPIDEMIOLOGY & DEMOGRAPHICS

INCIDENCE: 10% to 20% of clinically recognized pregnancies; 80% of miscarriages occur in the first trimester.[1] Recurrent miscarriage occurs in <1% of couples attempting to have children.[2]

RISK FACTORS:
- Vaginal bleeding, which may have as high as a 50% chance of spontaneous abortion[3]
- Advancing maternal age
- Two or more prior miscarriages
- Significant underlying maternal health issues such as uncontrolled diabetes, thyroid disease, or other endocrine disturbances[4]
- Illicit substance use
- Obesity
- Alcohol, smoking, and excessive caffeine intake
- Use of fluconazole in pregnancy is associated with a statistically significant increased risk of spontaneous miscarriage[5]

GENETICS:
- Fetal chromosomal aneuploidy and polyploidy account for the overwhelming majority of first-trimester losses.[1,2,6]

- Autosomal trisomy accounts for the majority of abnormalities, followed by monosomy X, tetraploidy, and, lastly, structural chromosomal abnormalities.[6]
- The incidence of trisomy increases as maternal age increases.[1,6]

MATERNAL CAUSES:
- Uterine anomalies: Müllerian abnormalities such as unicornuate, bicornuate, or septated uterus are associated with increased miscarriage risk, although rates vary in different studies. A septated uterus is most highly associated with recurrent loss and can be surgically corrected and thus is important to diagnose.[7] Other intrauterine pathologies such as synechiae, leiomyomas, or prior DES exposure are important to rule out also.
- Incompetent cervix (iatrogenic or congenital, associated with 20% of midtrimester losses).
- Antiphospholipid antibody syndrome.
- Uncontrolled diabetes mellitus.[4]
- Rare or controversial causes include HLA associations between mother and father; infections such as tuberculosis, *Chlamydia,* and *Ureaplasma;* smoking and alcohol use; irradiation; progesterone deficiency; and environmental toxins. Most of the literature is observational in nature, which may skew risk factor data.[2,4,5]
- With two or more spontaneous miscarriages, a karyotype can be performed on the products of conception to evaluate for aneuploidy, which may be associated with a balanced translocation in one of the parents, and which has a substantially increased risk for abortion (depending on the actual type of translocation); if the pregnancy is carried to term, it has a 3% to 5% risk for an unbalanced karyotype.[6] In patients with recurrent miscarriages, evaluation for anatomic defects such as uterine septum and for antiphospholipid syndrome (lupus anticoagulant, beta 2 glycoprotein IgG/IgM, and anticardiolipin antibody IgG/IgM) should also be obtained.[2,4]

PHYSICAL FINDINGS & CLINICAL PRESENTATION

- Profuse bleeding and cramping have a higher association with miscarriage than bleeding without cramping, which is more consistent with a threatened miscarriage.
- Cervical dilation with history or finding of fetal tissue at cervical os may be present.
- In cases of missed abortion, uterine size may be smaller than menstrual dating, in contrast to molar gestation, where size may be greater than dates.
- The presence of nausea and vomiting in early pregnancy is associated with a reduced risk for pregnancy loss.[8]

ETIOLOGY

In a general overview the etiology can be classified in terms of maternal (environmental) and fetal (genetic) factors, with the majority of miscarriages being related to genetic or chromosomal causes.

DIAGNOSIS

DIFFERENTIAL DIAGNOSIS

- Normal pregnancy
- Hydatidiform molar gestation
- Ectopic pregnancy
- Dysfunctional uterine bleeding
- Pathologic endometrial or cervical lesions

WORKUP

- All patients with bleeding in the first trimester should have an evaluation for possible ectopic pregnancy.
- If there are three early, prior pregnancy losses, a workup and treatment for recurrent miscarriage should begin before next conception. If there is a strong history for second-trimester loss, consideration for cerclage should be given if the history is consistent with incompetent cervix (e.g., painless cervical dilation).
- Most providers will initiate an evaluation for couples who have had two previous losses.
- One unexplained fetal loss beyond 10 wk or 1 birth before 34 wk because of preeclampsia should prompt an evaluation for antiphospholipid antibody syndrome.

LABORATORY TESTS

- Type and antibody screen are used to evaluate the need for Rh immune globulin.
- Recurrent pregnancy loss: During the preconception period in patients with recurrent pregnancy loss, hemoglobin A_{1c}, TSH, prolactin, anticardiolipin antibody, lupus anticoagulant, 20210A beta 2 glycoprotein antibodies, karyotyping, and anatomic evaluation with hysterosalpingography, or saline ultrasonography (2D/3D) to assess for uterine septum. With increasing age, oocyte quality is a factor, and some practitioners will perform day 3 of the menstrual cycle FSH and anti-müllerian hormone to assess for diminished ovarian reserve. Progesterone level <5 mg/dl suggests nonviable gestation vs. >25 mg/dl, which suggests a good prognosis.[2,6]

IMAGING STUDIES

Transvaginal sonogram (preferred) (Figs. 1, 2, and E3) can be used with menstrual dating and serum quantitative human chorionic gonadotropin to document pregnancy location, fetal heart presence, gestational sac size, and adnexal pathology.

TREATMENT

NONPHARMACOLOGIC THERAPY

Depending on the patient's clinical status, desire to continue the pregnancy, and certainty of the diagnosis, expectant management can be considered. In pregnancies <8 weeks, complete expulsion of fetal tissue usually occurs, and surgical intervention such as D&C may be avoided especially if the women is symptomatic.[1] However, expectant management is generally

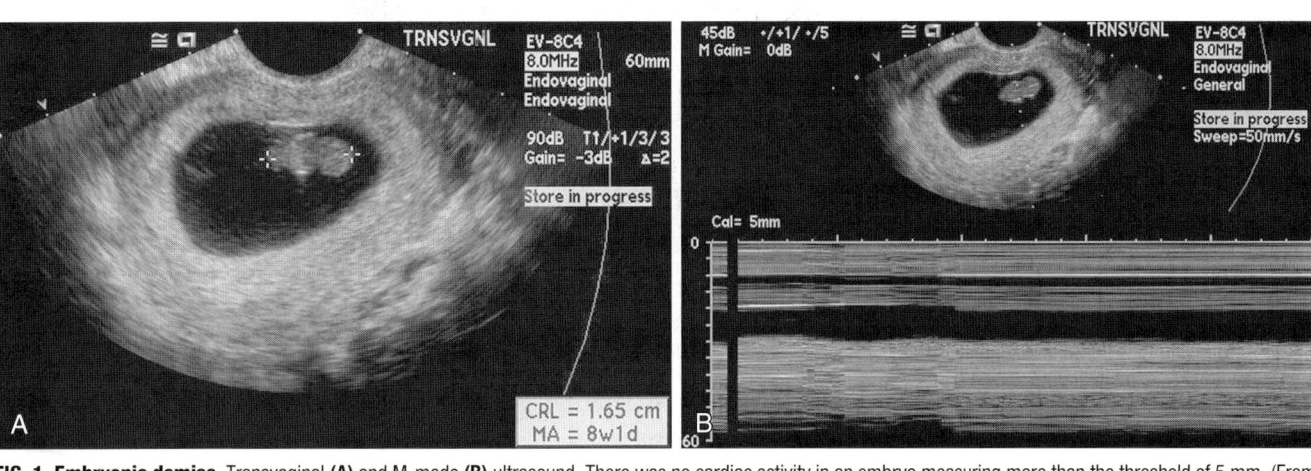

FIG. 1 Embryonic demise. Transvaginal **(A)** and M-mode **(B)** ultrasound. There was no cardiac activity in an embryo measuring more than the threshold of 5 mm. (From Fielding JR et al: *Gynecologic imaging*, Philadelphia, 2011, Saunders.)

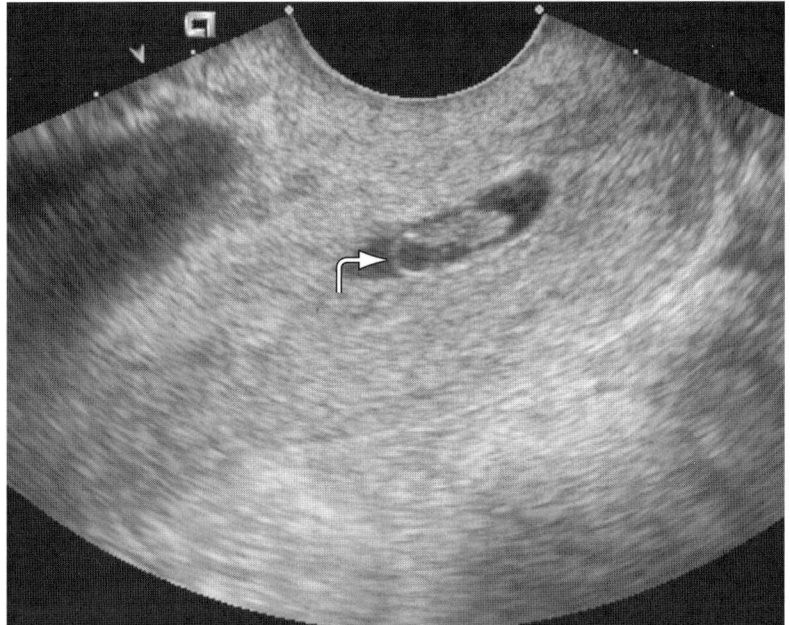

FIG. 2 Inevitable abortion. Transvaginal ultrasonography shows a sac in the cervical canal, past the internal os. The embryo *(curved arrow)* was nonviable. (From Fielding JR et al: *Gynecologic imaging*, Philadelphia, 2011, Saunders.)

associated with longer time to resolution of pregnancy event and potentially higher risk of extensive blood loss and/or infection compared to surgical and/or medical management of a missed abortion.[1]

ACUTE GENERAL Rx

- Incomplete miscarriage greater than 8 wk and especially in the second trimester can be associated with great blood loss; consideration should be given to D&C versus limited expectant or medical management based on the clinical presentation and patient's wishes.
- In cases of missed abortion, if fetal demise has occurred >6 wk before or gestational age is >14 wk, there is an increased risk of hypofibrinogenemia with disseminated intravascular coagulation. Thus D&C or manual vacuum aspiration should be performed early in the disease course. Consider use of misoprostol (Cytotec) in appropriate cases with or without pretreatment with mifepristone (200 mg orally) where the patient wishes to avoid surgery.[1,9]
- There is evidence that a surgical approach leads to quicker resolution of the pregnancy event with fewer visits being required.[1,8,10]
- Rh-negative patients should be given RhoGAM 50 mcg IM to prevent Rh isoimmunization.

ⓘ PEARLS & CONSIDERATIONS

Spontaneous pregnancy loss is recommended as a replacement for the term *abortion* and to acknowledge the emotional aspects of losing a pregnancy.

REFERENCES

Available at eBooks.Health.Elsevier.com.

RELATED CONTENT

Miscarriage (Patient Information)

AUTHOR: **ADRIENNE B. NEITHARDT, MD**

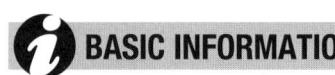

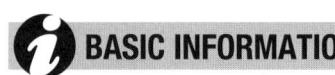 BASIC INFORMATION

DEFINITION

Spontaneous bacterial peritonitis (SBP) is an inflammatory reaction of the peritoneum secondary to the presence of bacteria or other microorganisms. More specifically, SBP is defined as an ascitic fluid infection without an evident intraabdominal surgically treatable source occurring primarily in patients with advanced cirrhosis of the liver.

SYNONYMS

Primary peritonitis
SBP
Peritonitis, spontaneous bacterial

ICD-10CM CODE
K65.2 Spontaneous bacterial peritonitis

EPIDEMIOLOGY & DEMOGRAPHICS

PREVALENCE: The prevalence of SBP in cirrhotic patients admitted to the hospital has been estimated at 10% to 30%.
PREDOMINANT SEX: Males are affected more often than females.

PHYSICAL FINDINGS & CLINICAL PRESENTATION

- Acute fever with accompanying abdominal pain/ascites, nausea, vomiting, diarrhea.
- In cirrhotic patients, presentation may be subtle with a low-grade temperature (100° F [37.8° C]) with or without abdominal abnormalities.
- In patients with ascites, a heightened degree of awareness is necessary for detection.
- Jaundice and encephalopathy.
- Deterioration of mental status and/or renal function.
- Table E1 summarizes symptoms and signs of ascetic fluid infection.

ETIOLOGY

- *Escherichia coli*
- *Klebsiella pneumoniae*
- *Streptococcus pneumoniae*
- *Streptococcus* and *Enterococcus* spp.
- *Staphylococcus aureus*
- Anaerobic pathogens: *Bacteroides, Clostridium* organisms
- Other: Fungal, mycobacterial, viral

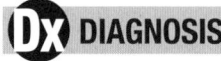 DIAGNOSIS

The diagnosis of SBP is established by a positive ascitic fluid bacterial culture and an elevated ascitic fluid absolute polymorphonuclear leukocyte count ($\geq$250 cells/mm^3).

DIFFERENTIAL DIAGNOSIS

- Appendicitis (in children)

- Perforated peptic ulcer
- Secondary bacterial peritonitis
- Peritoneal abscess
- Splenic, hepatic, or pancreatic abscess
- Cholecystitis
- Cholangitis

WORKUP

Paracentesis and ascitic fluid analysis will confirm diagnosis (see "Laboratory Tests").

LABORATORY TESTS

Ascitic fluid analysis reveals the following:
- Cell count with an absolute polymorphonuclear cell count $>250/mm^3$
- Presence of bacteria on Gram stain
- pH <7.31
- Lactic acid >32 mg/dl
- Protein <1 g/dl
- Glucose >50 mg/dl
- Lactate dehydrogenase <225 µU/ml
- Positive culture of peritoneal fluid
- Measurement of the serum/ascites/albumin gradient: The serum/ascites/albumin gradient indirectly measures portal pressure. The albumin concentration of ascitic fluid and serum must be obtained on the same day. The ascitic fluid value is subtracted from the serum value to obtain the gradient. If the difference (not a ratio) is >1.1 g/dl, the patient has portal hypertension, with 97% accuracy. If the difference is <1.1 g/dl, portal hypertension is not present. The majority of patients with SBP have portal hypertension as a result of cirrhosis

IMAGING STUDIES

- Abdominal ultrasound: If there is clinical difficulty in performing paracentesis
- CT scan: To rule out secondary peritonitis (if indicated) and to exclude abscess, mass

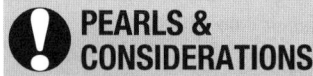 TREATMENT

ACUTE GENERAL Rx

- Cefotaxime (2 g IV q8h) or ceftriaxone (2 g IV q24h). Alternative agents include ticarcillin-clavulanate, piperacillin-tazobactam, cefoxitin, and meropenem (for multidrug resistant gram-negative rods). Continue therapy for 5 to 7 days. Repeat diagnostic paracentesis can be done at day 2. Repeat paracentesis at 48 hr will demonstrate a significant decrease in polymorphonuclear count in patients with SBP. If ascites PMN count decreases by at least 25% at day 2, IV therapy can be switched to PO (levofloxacin 500 to 750 mg qd) to complete 7 days of therapy if organisms are susceptible.
- IV albumin (1.5 g/kg of body weight upon initial diagnosis and 1 g/kg of albumin on day 3) if BUN >30 mg/dl, serum creatinine >1 mg/dl, bilirubin >4 mg/dl.

PROPHYLAXIS

- Ciprofloxacin 500 mg PO qd or levofloxacin 250 mg PO qd.
- Alternative therapy: TMP-SMX one double-strength tablet PO qd.
- Rifaximin 1200 mg a day was shown in a recent study to be superior to norfloxacin.
- Prophylaxis should be continued until disappearance of ascites or until liver transplantation.

DISPOSITION

The overall mortality rate from an episode of SBP is 20%, and following an episode, the 1-yr mortality rate approaches 70%. Patients that develop SBP should be considered for liver transplantation.

! PEARLS & CONSIDERATIONS

COMMENTS

- Renal failure is a major cause of morbidity in cirrhotic patients with SBP. The use of IV albumin (1.5 g/kg at the time of diagnosis and 1 g/kg on day 3) may lower the rate of renal failure and mortality in patients with SBP.
- The criteria for the diagnosis of SBP require that abdominal paracentesis be performed and ascitic fluid be analyzed before a diagnosis of SBP can be made.
- Culturing ascitic fluid as if it were blood (with bedside inoculation of at least 10 ml of ascitic fluid directly into blood culture bottles at the bedside) has been shown to significantly increase the culture positivity of the ascitic fluid in the 80% to 100% range.
- Avoid therapeutic paracenteses during active infection.
- Positive blood cultures in an individual with ascites require exclusion of a peritoneal source by paracentesis.
- Follow-up paracentesis is indicated only in selected cases (worsening clinical status, nosocomial SBP, infection with atypical organism, recent β-lactam exposure).
- All patients with ascites and upper gastrointestinal hemorrhage should receive prophylaxis for SBP with IV ceftriaxone for as long as 7 days.[1]

REFERENCE & SUGGESTED READINGS
Available at eBooks.Health.Elsevier.com.

AUTHOR: **GLENN G. FORT, MD, MPH**

BASIC INFORMATION

DEFINITION

Squamous cell carcinoma (SCC) is a malignant neoplasm of keratinocytes. It originates from keratinizing cells of the epidermis or its appendages.

SYNONYMS

SCC
Skin cancer

ICD-10CM CODES
C44.5	Malignant neoplasm of skin of trunk
C44.4	Malignant neoplasm of skin of scalp and neck
D04	Carcinoma in situ of skin
C44.9	Malignant neoplasm of skin, unspecified
C44.0	Malignant neoplasm of skin of lip
C44.2	Malignant neoplasm of skin of ear and external auricular canal
C44.3	Malignant neoplasm of skin of other and unspecified parts of skin
C44.02	Squamous cell carcinoma of skin of lip
C44.121	Squamous cell carcinoma of skin of unspecified eyelid, including canthus
C44.122	Squamous cell carcinoma of skin of right eyelid, including canthus
C44.129	Squamous cell carcinoma of skin of left eyelid, including canthus
C44.221	Squamous cell carcinoma of skin of unspecified ear and external auricular canal
C44.222	Squamous cell carcinoma of skin of right ear and external auricular canal
C44.229	Squamous cell carcinoma of skin of left ear and external auricular canal
C44.320	Squamous cell carcinoma of skin of unspecified parts of face
C44.321	Squamous cell carcinoma of skin of nose
C44.329	Squamous cell carcinoma of skin of other parts of face
C44.42	Squamous cell carcinoma of skin of scalp and neck
C44.520	Squamous cell carcinoma of anal skin
C44.521	Squamous cell carcinoma of skin of breast
C44.529	Squamous cell carcinoma of skin of other part of trunk
C44.621	Squamous cell carcinoma of skin of unspecified upper limb, including shoulder
C44.622	Squamous cell carcinoma of skin of right upper limb, including shoulder
C44.629	Squamous cell carcinoma of skin of left upper limb, including shoulder
C44.721	Squamous cell carcinoma of skin of unspecified lower limb, including hip
C44.722	Squamous cell carcinoma of skin of right lower limb, including hip
C44.729	Squamous cell carcinoma of skin of left lower limb, including hip
C44.82	Squamous cell carcinoma of overlapping sites of skin

EPIDEMIOLOGY & DEMOGRAPHICS

- SCC is the second most common cutaneous malignancy, comprising 20% of all cases of nonmelanoma skin cancer.
- Incidence is highest in lower latitudes (e.g., southern U.S., Australia).
- Male:female ratio is 2:1.
- Incidence increases with age and sun exposure.
- In Black patients, SCC are 20% more common than basal cell carcinomas (BCC).
- Average age at diagnosis is 66 yr.
- The lifetime risk for SCC is increasing worldwide, escalating 50% to 300% in the last three decades.

PHYSICAL FINDINGS & CLINICAL PRESENTATION

- SCC frequently begins at the site of actinic keratosis and commonly affects the scalp, neck region, back of hands (Fig. E1), superior surface of the pinna, and the lip (Fig. E2). On the lower lip, SCC often develops on actinic cheilitis. A history of smoking is a significant predisposing factor.
- Bowen disease refers to SCC in situ.
- SCC lesions may have a scaly, erythematous macule or plaque.
- Telangiectasia, central ulceration may also be present. The ulcer may be superficial and hidden by a crust. Removal of the crust may reveal a well-defined papillary base.
- Most SCCs present as exophytic lesions that grow over a period of mo.
- Although most SCCs are relatively slow growing and nonaggressive, some (2% to 5%) can exhibit rapid growth and metastases. Aggressive tumors are more common in immunocompromised patients and when arising from scars, burns, or prior injury (Marjolin ulcer). Presence of SCC on ears, lips, or size >2 cm are high-risk features of SCC.

ETIOLOGY

Risk factors include ultraviolet B radiation, immunosuppression (kidney transplant recipients have a significantly increased risk), arsenic exposure, human papillomavirus (HPV) infection, medications (azathioprine, sorafenib, tumor necrosis factor [TNF] inhibitors), discoid lupus erythematosus (LE), erosive lichen planus, chronic ulcers, prior radiation exposure, and tobacco abuse.

DIAGNOSIS

DIFFERENTIAL DIAGNOSIS

- Keratoacanthomas
- Actinic keratosis
- Amelanotic melanoma
- Basal cell carcinoma
- Benign tumors
- Healing traumatic wounds
- Spindle cell tumors
- Warts

WORKUP

Diagnosis is made by full-thickness skin biopsy (incisional or excisional).
- Biopsy
- Staging
- Radiologic examination (PET, MRI, computed tomography [CT], ultrasound) if high-risk tumor
- Sentinel lymph node biopsy (controversial) may be considered for very high-risk tumors

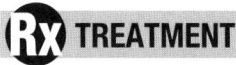

TREATMENT

ACUTE GENERAL Rx

- The goals of treatment of primary cutaneous SCC are to completely remove the tumor, to minimize the risk of metastasis and recurrence, to restore normal function after treatment, and to provide the best possible cosmetic outcome.
- Electrodesiccation and curettage for small SCCs (<2 mm in diameter), superficial tumors, and lesions located in extremity and trunk.
- Tumors thinner than 4 mm can be managed by simple local removal.
- Lesions 4 to 8 mm thick or those with deep dermal invasion should be excised.
- Tumors penetrating the dermis can be treated with several modalities, including excision and Mohs surgery, radiation therapy, and chemotherapy. Mohs surgery is commonly used for lesions on the face.
- Metastatic SCC can be treated with cryotherapy and combination of chemotherapy using 13-*cis*-retinoic acid and interferon-alpha 2A.
- A treatment algorithm for squamous cell carcinoma is illustrated in Fig. 3.
- In a recent phase 1 study of PD-1 blockade with cemiplimab among patients with advanced cutaneous squamous cell carcinoma, cemiplimab induced a response in approximately half the patients.

DISPOSITION

- Survival is related to size, location, degree of differentiation, immunologic status of the patient, depth of invasion, and presence of metastases. Risk factors for metastasis include lesions on the lip or ear, increasing lesion depth, and poor cell differentiation.
- Patients whose tumors penetrate through the dermis or exceed 8 mm in thickness are at risk of tumor recurrence.
- Risk factors for local recurrence or metastases in squamous cell carcinoma of the skin are summarized in Table E1.
- The most common metastatic locations are regional lymph nodes, liver, and lung.
- Tumors on the scalp, forehead, ears, nose, and lips also carry a higher risk.

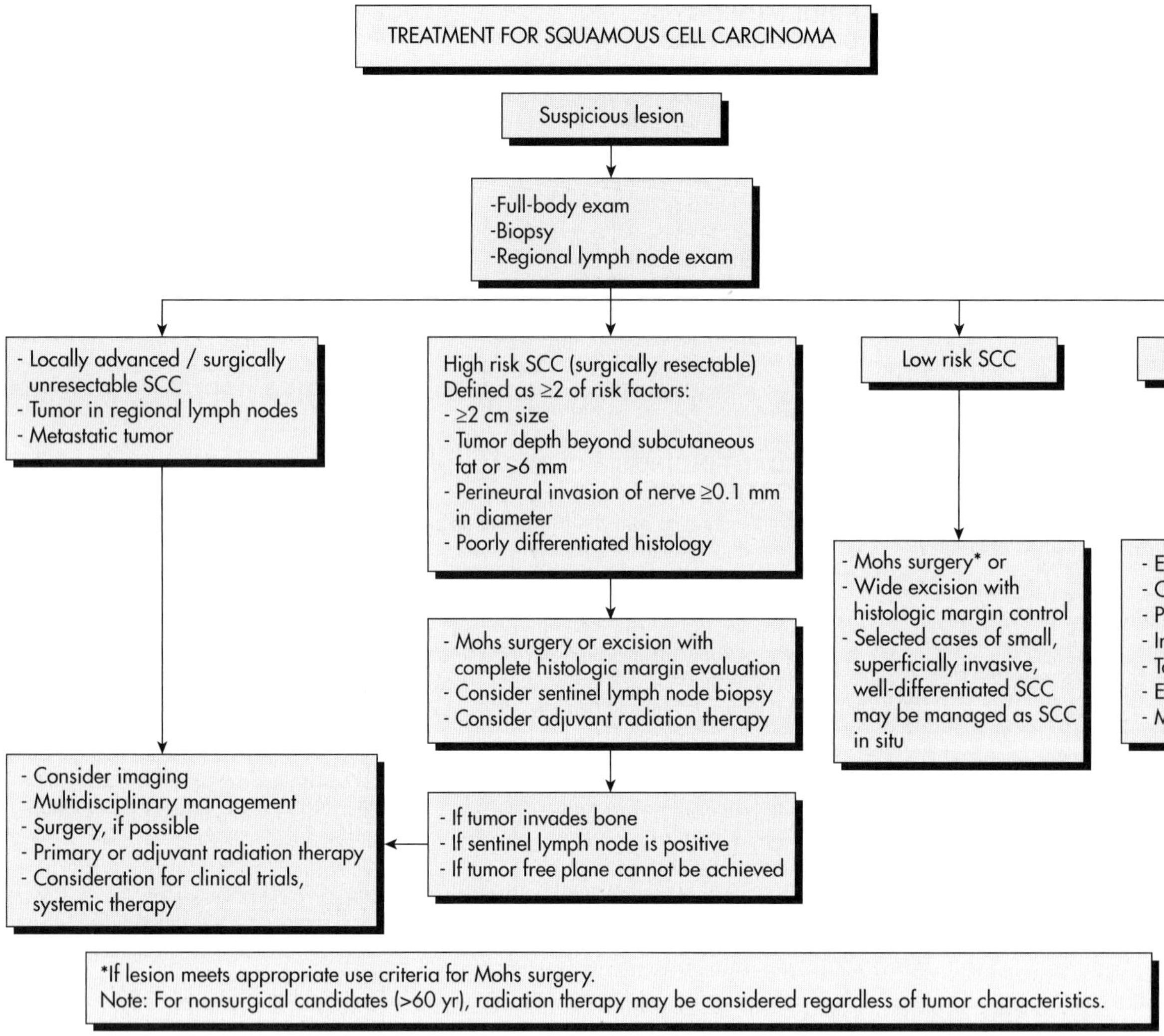

TREATMENT FOR SQUAMOUS CELL CARCINOMA

Suspicious lesion

- Full-body exam
- Biopsy
- Regional lymph node exam

- Locally advanced / surgically unresectable SCC
- Tumor in regional lymph nodes
- Metastatic tumor

High risk SCC (surgically resectable)
Defined as ≥2 of risk factors:
- ≥2 cm size
- Tumor depth beyond subcutaneous fat or >6 mm
- Perineural invasion of nerve ≥0.1 mm in diameter
- Poorly differentiated histology

Low risk SCC

SCC in situ

- Mohs surgery or excision with complete histologic margin evaluation
- Consider sentinel lymph node biopsy
- Consider adjuvant radiation therapy

- Mohs surgery* or
- Wide excision with histologic margin control
- Selected cases of small, superficially invasive, well-differentiated SCC may be managed as SCC in situ

- EDC
- Cryosurgery
- PDT
- Imiquimod
- Topical 5-FU
- Excision
- Mohs surgery*

- Consider imaging
- Multidisciplinary management
- Surgery, if possible
- Primary or adjuvant radiation therapy
- Consideration for clinical trials, systemic therapy

- If tumor invades bone
- If sentinel lymph node is positive
- If tumor free plane cannot be achieved

---

*If lesion meets appropriate use criteria for Mohs surgery.
Note: For nonsurgical candidates (>60 yr), radiation therapy may be considered regardless of tumor characteristics.

FIG. 3 Treatment algorithm for squamous cell carcinoma (SCC). *EDC*, Electrodesiccation and curettage; *5-FU*, 5-fluorouracil; *PDT*, photodynamic therapy. (From Niederhuber JE: *Abeloff's clinical oncology*, ed 6, Philadelphia, 2020, Elsevier.)

- The rate of SCC metastasis from all skin sites ranges from 0.5% to 5.2%.
- SCCs originating in the lip and pinna metastasize in 10% to 20% of cases.
- 5-yr survival for metastatic SCC is 34%.

REFERRAL
Oncology referral for metastatic SCC

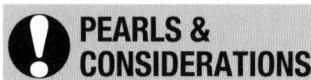 **PEARLS & CONSIDERATIONS**

COMMENTS
- SCC arising in areas of prior radiation, thermal injury, and areas of chronic ulcers or chronic draining sinuses are more aggressive and have a higher frequency of metastasis than those originating in actinic damaged skin.
- Oral retinoids may be useful as a preventive strategy in patients with immunosuppression.
- Nicotinamide (500 mg bid, available over the counter) mitigates some of the deleterious effects of ultraviolet (UV) radiation and has been reported to lower the incidence of non-melanoma skin cancer (NMSCO) by 23%.

SUGGESTED READINGS
Available at eBooks.Health.Elsevier.com.

RELATED CONTENT
Squamous Cell Carcinoma (Patient Information)

AUTHOR: **FRED F. FERRI, MD**

BASIC INFORMATION

DEFINITION

Statin-induced muscle syndromes (SIMS) include myopathy, myalgia, myositis, and rhabdomyolysis. Definitions for these syndromes are inconsistent in the medical literature.

- Myopathy: A general term defined as any disease of muscles
- Myalgia: Muscle weakness or pain without serum creatinine kinase elevation
- Myositis: Muscle weakness or pain with an increased serum creatinine kinase level
- Rhabdomyolysis: Muscle weakness or pain and a marked serum creatinine kinase level usually greater than 10× the upper limit of normal and serum creatinine elevation as well as signs of brown urine and elevated urine myoglobin. A rare **immune-mediated necrotizing myopathy (IMNM)**, also known as **statin-associated autoimmune myopathy**, has also been associated with the use of statins with symptoms persisting after discontinuation of the drug. This condition presents with symmetric proximal arm and leg weakness and severe elevations of muscle enzymes

SYNONYMS

SIMS
Statin-induced myopathies
Statin-induced myositis
Statin-induced myalgias
Statin-induced rhabdomyolysis
Statin-associated autoimmune myopathy

ICD-10CM CODES

M60.9	Myositis, unspecified
M62.82	Rhabdomyolysis
G72.2	Myopathy due to other toxic agents
G72.9	Myopathy, unspecified
G72.81	Critical illness myopathy
G72.89	Other specified myopathies
M60.89	Other myositis, multiple sites

EPIDEMIOLOGY & DEMOGRAPHICS

INCIDENCE: Risk of statin-induced rhabdomyolysis is 1.2 per 10,000 persons/yr. Rhabdomyolysis risk of death is 0.15 deaths per 1 million prescriptions. SIMS most commonly occur in people aged 51 to 75, which may reflect the pattern of statin use. Statin-associated autoimmune myopathy occurs in an estimated 2 or 3 of every 100,000 patients treated with statins.
PREVALENCE: The prevalence of statin-induced myalgias is about 1% to 5%, similar to placebo in clinical trials, although observational studies have suggested a prevalence of 10% or higher. Statins may cause elevated transaminases (ALT, AST) at a prevalence of 0.5% to 2.0% and rhabdomyolysis ~0.08%.
PREDOMINANT SEX & AGE: The mean age of hospitalized patients with statin-induced myopathy or rhabdomyolysis was 64 yr old and was slightly more common in women (56%).

PEAK INCIDENCE: Patients on high-dose statins have a 0.9% incidence of statin-induced rhabdomyolysis.
RISK FACTORS: Small body frame; age over 80 yr; women, particularly frail elderly women; patients taking multiple drugs, especially gemfibrozil, niacin, cyclosporine, itraconazole, ketoconazole, erythromycin, clarithromycin, verapamil, amiodarone; renal or liver impairment; pharmacogenetic variability; hypothyroidism; excessive alcohol intake; vigorous exercise; severe infections; excessive grapefruit juice ingestion; low vitamin D levels; inherited defects of muscle metabolism such as carnitine palmityl transferase II deficiency, McArdle disease, and myoadenylate deaminase deficiency; acquired myopathies such as postpoliomyelitis syndrome; lipophilic statins (simvastatin, atorvastatin, lovastatin); multiple conditions such as diabetes; renal impairment, and prior elevated CK; and drugs of abuse (amphetamines, heroin, cocaine, phencyclidine).
GENETICS: Interpatient variability exists in the activity of the *CYP3A4* gene for the metabolism of simvastatin, atorvastatin, and lovastatin. Homozygous carriers of *CYP2D6* (poor metabolizers) had a higher rate of discontinuation of simvastatin due to muscle syndromes compared with the *CYP2D6* wild-type genotype; patients taking atorvastatin and having a muscle event were more likely to have the CYP2D6*4 allele. *SLCO1B1* polymorphisms encode for the organic anion transport of statins into the liver cells. The variant C allele may increase the risk of the *SLCO1B1* statin–induced myopathy in patients taking simvastatin and atorvastatin. Simvastatin-induced myopathy is more likely to be associated with *SLO1B1* genotype and not *ABCB1* genotype. However, a statin-associated autoimmune myopathy has shown a link to class II HLA allele DRB1*11:01 in the development of anti-HMG CoA reductase antibodies, leading to an increase in expression of the antibodies in the muscles of patients exposed to statins. Deficiencies in ubiquinone (coenzyme Q10) may exist in patients with a mutation in the *COQ2* gene. The *EYS* gene can affect neuromuscular tissue and may have a role. In addition, *RYR1* and *CACNA1S* genetic variants may be associated with statin-induced muscle syndromes and elevated CK levels.

PHYSICAL FINDINGS & CLINICAL PRESENTATION

- Myopathy can occur at any time, although it is more common within the first 4 wk of therapy; statin-associated necrotizing myopathy may occur after months of using statins
- Proximal generalized muscle aches, body aches, and pains, and may be mild or severe
- Dark-colored urine
- Muscle cramps, spasms, tenderness, or stiffness
- Unusually tired or weak
- Nocturnal cramping
- Tendon pain

ETIOLOGY

- History of current statin use.

- May be explained by one of three deficiencies of end products of the 3-hydroxy-3-methyl-glutaryl-coA reductase pathway: Cell signaling and apoptosis, mitochondrial function and ubiquinone concentrations, and cholesterol concentrations and cell membrane integrity.
- The risk may be enhanced by drug interactions that interfere with hepatic metabolism and gut wall transport of interacting medications and by pharmacodynamic effects.
- Underlying metabolic muscle disorder may predispose a patient to develop myopathy.
- Patients with statin-associated autoimmune myopathy have been found to have anti–HMG-CoA reductase antibodies even prior to exposure to statin therapy.

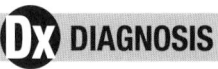 DIAGNOSIS

DIFFERENTIAL DIAGNOSIS

Bursitis, tendinitis, radiculopathy, osteoarthritis, muscle strain, myofascial pain, hypothyroidism, proton pump inhibitor–induced polymyositis, viral illness, polymyositis, idiopathic inflammatory myositis, and polymyalgia rheumatica

WORKUP

Workup consists of a thorough history, including exercise history, urine color, medication history, and physical exam to palpate tenderness and obtain blood tests to evaluate muscle and kidney damage.

LABORATORY TESTS

If severe myopathy or rhabdomyolysis is suspected:
- Elevated CPK, positive serum myoglobin, elevated BUN, serum creatinine, AST, ALT, LDH, and potassium
- Urine creatinine, positive casts, and hemoglobin in urine with absence of red blood cells
- Anti-3-hydroxy-3-methylglutaryl-coenzyme A (anti–HMG-CoA) antibody
- Consider electrocardiogram and assessment of calcium, phosphate, and uric acid

If mild to moderate myopathy is suspected:
- Monitor TSH and CPK levels; CPK may only be elevated when sudden severe myopathy occurs.
- If the patient has brown or dark urine or elevated CPK, monitor BUN and serum creatinine.
- In statin-associated autoimmune myopathy, the creatine kinase level is usually ≥10 times the upper limit of normal. In these patients, muscle biopsy specimens will be positive for autoantibodies against HMG-CoA reductase and may have necrosis.

IMAGING STUDIES

- Not recommended.
- In statin-associated autoimmune myopathy, electromyography shows small-amplitude motor-unit potentials with increased spontaneous activity characteristic of an active myopathic process. Muscle edema is evident on MRI.
- Statin Intolerance Tool:

1. The American College of Cardiology has created a tool to assess statin muscle symptoms and to guide clinicians that can be of value: http://tools.acc.org/statinintolerance/#!/

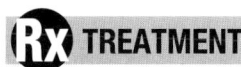 **TREATMENT**

NONPHARMACOLOGIC THERAPY
Treatment of rhabdomyolysis is generally supportive in nature (see "Rhabdomyolysis" topic).

ACUTE GENERAL Rx
- Stop statin therapy immediately if muscle symptoms occur. Check history, potential drug-drug interactions, CPK, TSH, renal function, hepatic function, and urinalysis.
- If patients have suspected rhabdomyolysis, they should be hospitalized and treated with supportive therapy and monitoring of complications.
- If CPK <10× the upper limit of normal without symptoms, continue statin therapy at the same or lower dosage.
- If CPK <10× the upper limit of normal with intolerable symptoms, discontinue statin.
- If CPK >10× the upper limit of normal, discontinue statin.

Box E1 describes recommendations of the National Lipid Association Statin Safety Assessment Task Force regarding statin and muscle safety.

CHRONIC Rx
- After stopping the statin and symptom or CPK resolution, which may take up to 4 mo, consider the same statin at a lower dosage or a different statin at an equivalent or lower dosage.
- When restarting therapy, consider statins such as low-dose rosuvastatin; pravastatin; and alternate-day dosing of rosuvastatin or atorvastatin.
- If patient had rhabdomyolysis secondary to statin therapy, consider nonstatin treatments.
- If the patient develops myopathy after a second trial of therapy, statin treatment should be permanently discontinued and nonstatin cholesterol-lowering therapy initiated.
- A nocebo effect of statin-induced myopathy has been demonstrated in some patients.
- Bempedoic acid may offer a safe and effective lipid-lowering therapeutic option for patients unable to tolerate statins.
- For IMNM (statin-associated autoimmune myopathy and idiopathic inflammatory myositis), immunosuppressive therapy with prednisone (1 mg per kg of body weight per day) and at least one agent (methotrexate, azathioprine, or mycophenolate mofetil) have been used. In resistant cases, IV immune globulin or another agent such as rituximab may be added.

INTEGRATIVE MEDICINE
- The effect of coenzyme Q10 on reducing or preventing SIMS remains controversial; although it may be effective in reducing muscle pain, weakness, cramps, and tiredness, it has no effect on lowering CK levels. Given its safety, coenzyme Q10 can be recommended if the actions listed under "Chronic Rx" are insufficient to continue the use of the statin and if the muscle symptoms have been limited to myalgias. Use coenzyme Q10 with caution in patients taking warfarin, as its anticoagulant effect may be decreased.
- A 2015 meta-analysis of observational studies reported that vitamin D levels were lower in patients with statin-induced myalgias than in individuals who did not have these symptoms.
- A more recent trial[1] comparing statin users who took vitamin D supplements to those who took placebo revealed that both had the same incidence of muscle symptoms. The mean 25 hydroxyvitamin D level at baseline was 30 mg/mL. Vitamin D did not prevent symptoms in subgroups with baseline levels less than 30 mg/mL or <20 mg/mL.

DISPOSITION
- Usually resolves within 1 wk up to 4 mo after discontinuing statin therapy.
- Once the patient has a full recovery, an alternative statin can be tried.
- Statins should not be restarted in IMNM or idiopathic inflammatory myositis.

REFERRAL
If rhabdomyolysis is suspected, immediate referral for hospitalization is suggested.

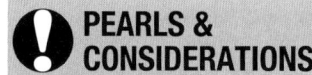 **PEARLS & CONSIDERATIONS**

COMMENTS
- SIMS are usually mild and will resolve within a few wk after discontinuing statin therapy. However, such syndromes may progress to rhabdomyolysis.
- A recent meta-analysis[2] revealed that among participants taking statins 27.1% reported muscle symptoms compared with 26.6% in the placebo group for a 3% small increase during a median of 4 yr which is considered barely significant. All excess risk occurred in the first year of therapy.

PREVENTION
- Follow the 2013 AHA/ACC treatment guidelines and the 2017 ACC focused update on nonstatin therapies for LDL cholesterol and limit the concomitant use of fibrates with statins.
- Discontinue statin therapy prior to and during surgical procedures.
- If patient requires a short-term therapy with an interacting medication such as an azole antifungal, temporarily discontinue statin until interacting therapy is completed.
- If statin–fibric acid therapy is warranted, fenofibrate is preferred over gemfibrozil to decrease risk of myopathy.
- Baseline liver function testing before initiation of statin therapy and only if clinically indicated thereafter.

PATIENT & FAMILY EDUCATION
- Inform patients to promptly report muscle weakness, unexpected muscle pain, or brownish urine.
- Providers should be cautious of the impact of media coverage of statin-induced side effects, which may include the nocebo effect.
- Ensure that the pharmacist and/or primary care physician checks for drug-drug interactions with every new prescription, including those from dentists and physicians from other specialties.
- Coenzyme Q10 may lessen milder muscle symptoms from statins, but patients should inform their physician and pharmacist if they decide to use this supplement.
- A recent clinical trial comparing lipid-lowering efficacy for two nonstatin therapies, ezetimibe and evolocumab, among patients with statin intolerance revealed that evolocumab resulted in a significantly greater reduction in LDL-C levels after 24 wk. Further studies are needed to assess long-term efficacy and safety.

SUGGESTED READINGS & REFERENCES
Available at eBooks.Health.Elsevier.com.

RELATED CONTENT
Rhabdomyolysis (Related Key Topic)

AUTHORS: **LISA COHEN, PHARMD,** and **ANNE L. HUME, PHARMD**

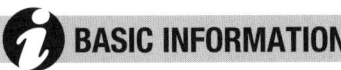
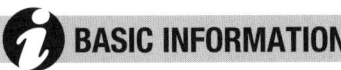 BASIC INFORMATION

DEFINITIONS

Status epilepticus is a medical neurologic emergency. It is historically defined as 30 min of continuous seizure activity or two or more seizures without full recovery of consciousness between seizures. However, in practice, a continuous seizure that lasts >5 min is treated as status epilepticus.[1]

Refractory status epilepticus: Status epilepticus persisting despite administration of at least two appropriately selected and dosed parenteral medications including a benzodiazepine. No specific seizure duration is required.[2]

Super-refractory status epilepticus exists if status epilepticus continues for 24 h or longer after anesthesia is administered.[2]

SYNONYMS

Convulsive status epilepticus
Nonconvulsive status epilepticus

ICD-10CM CODES
G41   Status epilepticus
G40.301 Generalized idiopathic epilepsy and epileptic syndromes, not intractable, with status epilepticus

EPIDEMIOLOGY & DEMOGRAPHICS

INCIDENCE: 18.3 to 41 per 100,000 people per year in the U.S.[3]
PREDOMINANT SEX & AGE: From population-based studies, it seems that status epilepticus is more common in Black males and in either young children or older adults.[4]
PEAK INCIDENCE: The highest incidences occur in young children and in those aged 60 and above. The incidence in the elderly is about 3 to 10 times that of younger adults.[4]

PHYSICAL FINDINGS & CLINICAL MANIFESTATIONS

- Patients can present with repetitive tonic-clonic movements of the body (convulsive status epilepticus); other patients are comatose and nonresponsive (nonconvulsive status epilepticus).[5]
- Patients may also present with lethargy, intermittent confusion, and involuntary movements.

ETIOLOGY

- Status epilepticus can be the result of an acute neurologic injury, such as stroke, meningitis, brain tumor.[6] Table 1 summarizes causes of status epilepticus in adults presenting in the community.
- In patients with epilepsy, low antiseizure medication levels can result in status.[2]

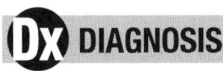 DIAGNOSIS

DIFFERENTIAL DIAGNOSIS

- Encephalopathies: Metabolic, infectious, toxic, cerebral hypoperfusion, etc.
- Nonepileptic psychogenic events

WORKUP

- ABCs
- ICU admission
- Emergent electroencephalogram (EEG), especially if the patient does not start returning to baseline[2]
- Continuous EEG in refractory cases[2]

TABLE 1 Causes of Status Epilepticus in Adults Presenting From the Community

Previous Seizures	No Previous Seizures
Common	
Subtherapeutic anticonvulsant	Ethanol-related
Ethanol-related	Drug toxicity
Intractable epilepsy	CNS infection
	Head trauma
	CNS tumor
Less Common	
CNS infection	Metabolic aberration
Metabolic aberration	Stroke
Drug toxicity	
Stroke	
CNS tumor	
Head trauma	

CNS, Central nervous system.
From Vincent JL et al: *Textbook of critical care,* ed 7, Philadelphia, 2017, Elsevier.

- Table 2 describes a suggested timetable for emergency diagnosis and treatment of status epilepticus. A treatment approach is summarized in Table 3 and Fig. 1

LABORATORY TESTS

- Routine blood workup (CBC, CMP, glucose, electrolytes)
- Urine drug screen
- Lumbar puncture and CSF analysis in patients with suspected infectious meningitis or encephalitis or suspected autoimmune or paraneoplastic encephalitis

IMAGING STUDIES

- Immediate CT scan of the head.
- MRI of the brain with and without contrast should be performed once the patient is in a stable condition.[2,6]

(Rx) TREATMENT

- The longer a patient is in status epilepticus, the harder it is to treat and the more likely permanent damage is done.[2]
- Patients with continuous seizure activity over 5 min should be given intravenous lorazepam 0.1 mg/kg/dose, max: 4 mg/dose, may repeat dose once (or diazepam 0.15 to 0.2 mg/kg/dose, max 10 mg/dose, may repeat dose once only when lorazepam is not available).[2,7]
- In the absence of intravenous access, intramuscular administration of midazolam 10 mg in an adult is a superior alternative.[2,7]

TABLE 2 Suggested Timetable for Emergency Diagnosis and Treatment of Status Epilepticus

Time	Exam/Intervention	Testing
Initial presentation: 0 min	Airway, breathing, circulation, IV access, monitoring	Glucose, oxygenation via pulse oximetry ± blood gas analysis
Primary survey: 5 min	Neurologic exam Administer antiseizure medications Lorazepam, 0.1 mg/kg IV Phenobarbital, 20 mg/kg IV Normal saline maintenance IV Reduce fever	Electrolytes, renal and liver function, ammonia, anticonvulsant levels, toxicology, complete blood cell count, urinalysis
Secondary survey: 15-30 min	Evaluate treatment results Second-line antiseizure medication if seizure persists Fosphenytoin, 20 mg/kg IV; or phenytoin, 20 mg/kg IV	Patient-specific: Cranial imaging (CT vs. MRI), lumbar puncture, EEG, ECG
Status epilepticus: >30 min	Intubation and mechanical ventilation	
Refractory status epilepticus: >60 min	Titrate antiseizure medications to burst suppression Pentobarbital, 10 mg/kg IV given over 30 min, then 5 mg/kg every h for 3 doses, then 1 mg/kg/h; titrate to effect Midazolam, 0.15 mg/kg IV, then 1-2 μg/kg/min, titrate to effect Phenobarbital, 5-10 mg/kg IV every 20 min to achieve burst suppression, then every 12 h Evaluate need for vasopressors	Continuous EEG Neurologic consultation Consider anesthesia consultation for treatment with inhaled anesthetic

CT, Computed tomography; *ECG,* electrocardiogram; *EEG,* electroencephalogram; *IV,* intravenous; *MRI,* magnetic resonance imaging.
From Vincent JL et al: *Textbook of critical care,* ed 7, Philadelphia, 2017, Elsevier.

Diseases and Disorders

I

TABLE 3   Treatment Approach to Status Epilepticus

1. Appropriate critical care treatment should be provided as soon as possible and simultaneously with emergent initial therapy for seizures. Treatment should be escalated quickly until seizures are controlled.

2. Critical care treatment (dictated by clinical circumstances):
   a. Intubation for airway protection and mechanical ventilation
   b. Vital sign monitoring
   c. Peripheral IV access
   d. Treatment of hypotension with vasopressors
   e. Finger stick blood glucose
   f. Nutrient resuscitation (thiamine before dextrose)
   g. Hypertension may be related to ongoing seizure activity, and termination of status epilepticus often substantially corrects it. Additionally, many agents used to terminate status epilepticus can produce hypotension

3. Emergent initial therapy with benzodiazepines:
   a. Lorazepam 0.1 mg/kg up to 4 mg per dose, may repeat after 5-10 min
   b. Midazolam 0.2 mg/kg IM/IV up to 10 mg
   c. Diazepam 0.15 mg/kg up to 10 mg per dose, may repeat after 5 min

4. Urgent control therapy—antiseizure drugs available in IV formulations:
   a. Fosphenytoin/phenytoin 20 mg PE/kg IV, may repeat bolus of 5 mg/kg IV
   b. Valproic acid 20-40 mg/kg IV, may repeat bolus of 20 mg/kg IV
   c. Levetiracetam 1000-3000 mg IV
   d. Phenobarbital 20 mg/kg IV, may repeat bolus of 5-10 mg/kg
   e. Lacosamide 200-400 mg IV
   f. Midazolam bolus 0.2 mg/kg IV, followed by 0.05-2 mg/kg/h continuous infusion

5. Refractory therapy–continuous infusion of antiseizure drugs, titrated to either seizure cessation, suppression-burst, or complete suppression on EEG:
   a. Midazolam bolus 0.2 mg/kg IV, followed by 0.05-2 mg/kg/h continuous infusion
   b. Propofol bolus 1-2 mg/kg, followed by 20 mcg/kg/min continuous infusion, titrate up to 30-200 mcg/kg/min
   c. Pentobarbital 5-15 mg/kg, may repeat bolus of 5-10 mg/kg, followed by 0.5-5 mg/kg/h continuous infusion

6. Treat complications

7. Complications of status epilepticus are numerous and can involve multiple organ systems. In particular, convulsive status epilepticus is associated with cardiac complications such as hypertension and tachycardia, as well as rhabdomyolysis and hyperthermia. Respiratory complications, including respiratory failure, hypoxia, and neurogenic pulmonary edema, may be seen. Status epilepticus is associated with neuronal damage and cerebral edema with increased intracranial pressure, which may require intracranial pressure monitoring and aggressive treatment with hypertonic agents

From Vincent JL et al: *Textbook of critical care,* ed 7, Philadelphia, 2017, Elsevier.

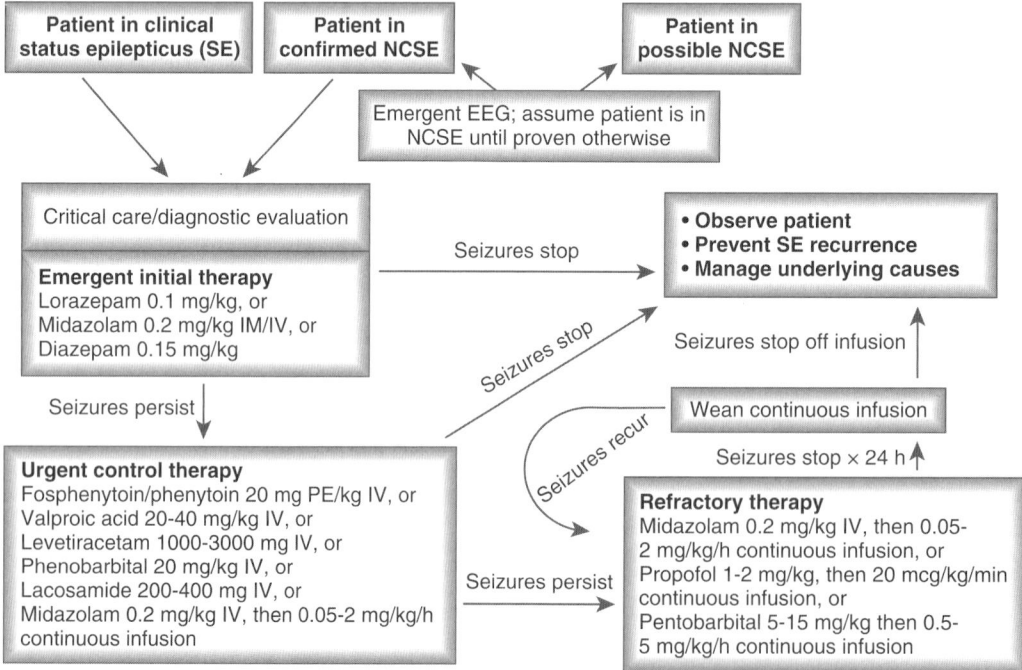

FIG. 1 Management algorithm for status epilepticus. *EEG,* Electroencephalogram; *IM,* intramuscular; *IV,* intravenous; *NCSE,* nonconvulsive status epilepticus; *SE,* status epilepticus. (From Vincent JL et al: *Textbook of critical care,* ed 7, Philadelphia, 2017, Elsevier.)

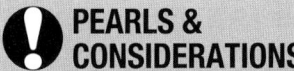

TABLE 4 Treatment Alternatives for Refractory and Super-Refractory Status Epilepticus

	Comments	Adverse Events
Thiopental	Metabolized to pentobarbital	Hypotension Respiratory depression Cardiac depression
Ketamine	Mechanism of action particularly well-suited to treat refractory and super-refractory SE (NMDA receptor antagonist)	High intracranial pressure Hypotension Hallucinations
Inhaled anesthetics	High rate of complications Needs closed system (gas recovery)	Hypotension Infection Paralytic ileus
Ketogenic diet	Relatively safe (no respiratory and cardiocirculatory instability) Slow onset of action Requires skilled dietitian	Gastroesophageal reflux Constipation Acidosis Hypertriglyceridemia
Lidocaine	Minor respiratory depression compared with other drugs	Cardiocirculatory instability Possible induction of seizures
Hypothermia	Only transitory control (cannot be a prolonged therapy)	Hypotension Cardiovascular instability Impaired coagulation (bleeding risks)
Resective surgery	Long-term treatment of seizures Not all patients are eligible	Surgical risks

NMDA, N-methyl-ᴅ-aspartate; *SE,* status epilepticus.
From Swaiman KF et al: *Swaiman's pediatric neurology, principles and practice,* ed 6, Philadelphia, 2017, Elsevier. See original table for references.

- It is not uncommon for patients in convulsive status epilepticus to transition to non-convulsive status epilepticus with time or with benzodiazepine treatment. If a patient does not start improving or has any subtle signs of ongoing seizures, consider nonconvulsive status epilepticus.
- Failure of response to lorazepam or midazolam is referred to as established status epilepticus and should be followed by second-line therapy of intravenous fosphenytoin 20 mg/kg (PE) at a rate not greater than 150 mg/min, phenytoin 20 mg/kg IV at up to 50 mg/min as tolerated, intravenous valproic acid 40 mg/kg IV (max: 300 mg/dose), or intravenous levetiracetam 60 mg/kg IV (max: 4500 mg/dose). Vital signs should be monitored during the infusion.[2,7]
- If seizures continue, an additional infusion of intravenous valproate; levetiracetam; lacosamide; or continuous infusions of pentobarbital, midazolam, and propofol are alternatives. Superiority of any one agent is not established.[2,6] Treatment alternatives for refractory and super-refractory status epilepticus are summarized in Table 4.

GENERAL Rx

It is important to find out the etiology of the status epilepticus (e.g., metabolic disturbance, infection). The appropriate treatment/understanding of the underlying cause of the status epilepticus will impact successful treatment.

CHRONIC Rx

- Chronic treatment of status epilepticus depends on underlying etiology.
- Patient with status epilepticus due to epilepsy will need chronic treatment.

DISPOSITION

- Response to treatment depends on the etiology of the status epilepticus.
- When there is no CNS injury as a cause or result of the status epilepticus, the prognosis is good.
- No driving until seizure freedom in accordance with local laws and regulations.

REFERRAL

Status epilepticus is a neurologic emergency; therefore immediate inpatient neurologic consultation is warranted.

ⓘ PEARLS & CONSIDERATIONS

COMMENTS

- Status epilepticus is a medical emergency that carries a high risk of mortality. Mortality among patients who present in status epilepticus approaches 20%. Among those who survive, functional ability will decline in 25% of cases.[5]
- Continuous video EEG is crucial in the treatment of these patients because some of them may not be clinically seizing (convulsing) but electrographically they may still have subclinical repetitive seizures or subclinical status epilepticus.[2]
- In the context of benzodiazepine-refractory convulsive status epilepticus, the anticonvulsant drugs levetiracetam, fosphenytoin, and valproate each led to seizure cessation and improved alertness by 60 min in approximately half the patients, and the three drugs were associated with similar incidences of adverse events.[8]

PREVENTION

Medication compliance is crucial in patients with epilepsy.

PATIENT & FAMILY EDUCATION

- Patients with epilepsy have normal lives.
- The goal of treatment is no seizures and no side effects to medications.
- Patient education and information can be obtained at the Epilepsy Foundation: www.epilepsyfoundation.org.
- Pregnant women with epilepsy should visit the Antiepileptic Drug Pregnancy Registry website for information and assistance: www.aedpregnancyregistry.org.
- Patients with ongoing seizures are forbidden from driving; check state regulations and laws regarding driving and epilepsy.

REFERENCES

Available at eBooks.Health.Elsevier.com.

AUTHOR: **PEDRO BALAGUERA, MD**

S

Diseases and Disorders

I

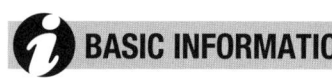
BASIC INFORMATION

DEFINITION

Ischemic stroke is the sudden onset of a focal neurologic deficit as a result of cerebral ischemia resulting in cell death.[1] The purpose of this chapter is to help the provider make decisions about the management of the acute stroke patient within the first several hours of symptoms—this is the crucial time for definitive treatment interventions.

SYNONYMS

Stroke
Brain attack
Cerebrovascular accident (this is a nonspecific term and should not be used)

ICD-10CM CODES

I63	Cerebral infarction
I63.3	Cerebral infarction due to thrombosis of cerebral arteries
I63.4	Cerebral infarction due to embolism of cerebral arteries
I63.5	Cerebral infarction due to unspecified occlusion or stenosis of cerebral arteries
I63.6	Cerebral infarction due to cerebral venous thrombosis, nonpyogenic
I63.8	Other cerebral infarction
I63.9	Cerebral infarction, unspecified
I67.89	Other cerebrovascular disease

EPIDEMIOLOGY & DEMOGRAPHICS

INCIDENCE:

- ~795,000 new or recurrent strokes occur each year in the U.S.[2]
- Stroke is the fifth leading cause of death (150,000 deaths every year) and the leading cause of long-term disability in the U.S.[2]

PREVALENCE: There are ~7 million stroke survivors in the U.S., two thirds of which are currently disabled.[2]

RISK FACTORS: Hypertension, dyslipidemia, diabetes mellitus, and smoking are the four major modifiable risk factors. Other risk factors include age, gender, atrial fibrillation (most common cause of cardioembolic stroke), mechanical heart valve, patent foramen ovale, recent myocardial infarction, metabolic syndrome, carotid artery stenosis, vertebral artery stenosis, intracranial artery stenosis, hypercoagulable states, subclinical atrial tachyarrhythmias without clinical atrial fibrillation, sickle cell disease, and obesity.[3] Inherited and miscellaneous disorders causing cerebral infarction are summarized in Box 1.

GENETICS: Multifactorial

PHYSICAL FINDINGS & CLINICAL PRESENTATION

When a patient presents with an acute ischemic stroke acutely, the most important considerations are determination of the time the patient was last known normal, the etiology (ischemic or hemorrhagic), and the severity, because these aspects will determine acute treatment. The time last known normal was when the patient was last seen normal (by themselves or by someone else).

If they awoke with the deficits, the time last seen normal was when they went to bed.[4]

Clinical presentation varies with the artery and region of CNS affected. Clinical presentation cannot reliably distinguish between hemorrhagic and ischemic causes, and so imaging must be done. Following is a noncomprehensive list of common stroke syndrome presentations based on the cerebral vascular territory affected. Please note that this list is not comprehensive and that all findings for a particular syndrome may not be listed here.[4]

- Large- to medium-sized arteries:
  1. Dominant middle cerebral artery (MCA) (left in 90% of people): Right face and arm > leg weakness and sensory loss with aphasia (expressive, receptive, or both); possible hemianopia
  2. Nondominant MCA: Contralateral face and arm > leg weakness and sensory loss with hemineglect; possible hemianopia
  3. Anterior cerebral artery (ACA): Contralateral leg weakness and sensory loss
  4. Internal carotid artery: Combination of contralateral MCA and ACA
  5. Basilar artery: Typically an acute loss of consciousness preceded by vertigo, nausea, vomiting, and diplopia; quadriparesis or quadriplegia may be seen, including "locked-in" syndrome
  6. Posterior cerebral artery: Unilateral hemianopia; blindness with anosognosia if bilateral (Anton syndrome)
  7. Posterior inferior cerebellar artery: Lateral medullary (Wallenberg) syndrome—ipsilesional loss of pinprick and temperature on the face and contralateral loss of pinprick and temperature on the body; ipsilesional Horner syndrome and ipsilesional palatal weakness with resulting dysphagia, dysarthria. Also with vertigo, nystagmus, ataxia.
- **Small arteries: Lacunar syndromes;** no cortical signs are present in lacunar syndromes.[5]

1. Pure motor hemiparesis: Typically due to an ischemic lesion in either the internal capsule or pons
2. Pure hemisensory loss: Typically due to an ischemic lesion of the thalamus
3. Ataxic hemiparesis: Ataxia out of proportion to the hemiparesis; typically due to an ischemic lesion of either the internal capsule or pons
4. Sensorimotor stroke: Typically due to ischemic lesion involving both the thalamus and internal capsule
5. Dysarthria–clumsy hand syndrome: Multiple localizations possible but typically the pons; facial weakness, dysarthria, and mild clumsiness and weakness of the hand

ETIOLOGY

Etiologies include atherosclerosis, cardioembolism, artery-to-artery embolism, small-vessel lipohyalinosis, arterial dissection, and vasospasm.[6]

DIAGNOSIS

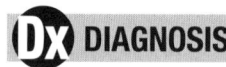

DIFFERENTIAL DIAGNOSIS

The differential diagnosis of acute ischemic stroke includes hemorrhagic stroke (intracerebral hemorrhage), subarachnoid or subdural hemorrhage, seizure with postictal paralysis, migraine with hemiparesis or other aura, syncope, hypoglycemia, hypertensive encephalopathy, and conversion disorder.[7]

LABORATORY TESTS

- Immediate (Box 2): Complete blood count, metabolic panel that includes blood glucose and renal function, PT/INR, aPTT, troponin I, and urinalysis. Blood glucose is the only test required before initiation of IV thrombolysis (t-PA or tissue Plasminogen Activator). Although it is desirable to know the results of CBC and PT/INR/aPTT before giving a patient tPA, thrombolytic therapy should not be delayed while awaiting the results unless (1) there is

---

BOX 1 Inherited and Miscellaneous Disorders Causing Cerebral Infarction

- Homocystinuria
- Fabry disease
- Marfan syndrome
- Ehlers-Danlos syndrome
- Pseudoxanthoma elasticum
- Sneddon syndrome
- Hereditary hemorrhagic telangiectasia
- Neoplastic angioendotheliomatosis
- Susac syndrome
- Eales disease
- Reversible cerebral segmental vasoconstriction syndrome
- Hypereosinophilic syndrome
- Cerebral amyloid angiopathy
- Coils and kinks
- Arterial dolichoectasia
- Complications of coarctation of the aorta
- Air, fat, amniotic fluid, bone marrow, and foreign particle embolism

From Jankovic J et al: *Bradley and Daroff's neurology in clinical practice,* ed 8, Philadelphia, 2022, Elsevier.

BOX 2 Immediate Diagnostic Studies: Evaluation of a Patient With Suspected Acute Ischemic Stroke

All Patients
Noncontrast brain computed tomographic scan (magnetic resonance imaging, if immediately available, preferred at the institution, and only DWI/ADC sequence)
Blood glucose level
Serum electrolyte and renal function tests
Electrocardiography
Markers of cardiac ischemia
Complete blood count, including platelet count
Prothrombin time/international normalized ratio
Activated partial thromboplastin time
Oxygen saturation

Selected Patients
CT angiogram head and neck or MR angiogram head and neck
CT or MR perfusion
Hepatic function tests
Toxicology screen
Blood alcohol level
Pregnancy test
Arterial blood gas tests (if hypoxia is suspected)
Chest radiography (if lung disease is suspected)
Lumbar puncture (if subarachnoid hemorrhage is suspected and computed tomography scan is negative for blood)
Electroencephalogram (if seizures are suspected)

From Christensen H et al: Abnormalities on ECG and telemetry predict stroke outcome at 3 months, *J Neurol Sci* 234:99-103, 2005.

BOX 3 Specialized Laboratory Tests for Thrombophilia

- Antithrombin activity
- Protein C
- Protein S (total and free antigen levels)
- Activated protein C resistance
- Factor V Leiden
- Prothrombin gene (G20210 A) mutation
- Cardiolipin (IgG, IgM) antibodies
- β_2-Glycoprotein 1 (IgG, IgM) antibodies
- Lupus anticoagulant
- Fibrinogen
- Plasminogen
- Plasminogen activator inhibitor
- Plasmin functional activity
- Factors V, VII, VIII, IX, X, XI, and XIII levels
- Hemoglobin electrophoresis
- Plasma homocysteine

From Jankovic J et al: *Bradley and Daroff's neurology in clinical practice*, ed 8, Philadelphia, 2022, Elsevier.

---

clinical suspicion of a bleeding abnormality or thrombocytopenia; (2) the patient has received heparin or warfarin; or (3) the patient's use of anticoagulants is not known.[8]
- Specialized laboratory tests for thrombophilia are summarized in Box 3.
- National Institutes of Health Stroke Scale (Table 1): A brief, focused neurologic examination aimed at providing a numeric estimate of the severity of stroke; can be performed by any health care provider trained in its use.[8]
- ECG and telemetry monitoring.
- Echocardiogram to look for potential cardiogenic source of embolism, infective endocarditis, and intracardiac shunts.[9]

IMAGING STUDIES
- Immediate (Fig. 1): Computed tomography (CT) of the head without contrast to rule out hemorrhage, required before initiation of IV thrombolysis (t-PA).[10]
- CT angiogram of the head and neck is necessary acutely in selected patients if deficits are severe to assess whether there is a thrombus that is amenable to intervention as well as CT head perfusion to assess for the degree of salvageable tissue (Table 2).[10]
- MRI of the brain with stroke protocol to assess the extent of stroke (because CT typically will not show an ischemic stroke for several hours), but it is rarely needed in the hyperacute

setting to determine appropriateness of reperfusion strategy.[10]
Cross reference: See "Transient Ischemic Attack" for general workup, which is identical to that for ischemic stroke.

RX TREATMENT

NONPHARMACOLOGIC THERAPY
GENERAL CONSIDERATIONS:
- Airway and breathing should be maintained.
- Supplemental oxygen should be provided to keep the oxygen saturation $\geq$92%.
- Pneumatic compression devices or pharmacologic means should be applied to help prevent deep venous thrombosis.
- Avoid any and all oral intake until swallowing is evaluated and found to be unimpaired; this helps to avoid aspiration pneumonia.
- Early mobilization for rehabilitation is desirable.
- Consider neurosurgical intervention for craniectomy in select cases. Typical cases in which craniectomy may be performed include cerebellar ischemia with compression of the brain stem and/or the fourth ventricle as well as large middle cerebral artery ischemia. Available evidence suggests that it may be better to perform early hemicraniectomy (<48 h) to achieve better outcomes in malignant hemispheric strokes. Decompressive hemicraniectomy has shown good benefit in terms of mortality and morbidity.[11]

ACUTE GENERAL RX (TABLE 3)
INTRAVENOUS THROMBOLYSIS:
- IV t-PA, or alteplase, is currently the only medical therapy approved by the U.S.[12-15] FDA for the treatment of acute ischemic stroke. Tenecteplase has been shown to be noninferior and is used as an alternative to alteplase in some centers but is not discussed here.[16]
- The time window for administration of alteplase is generally accepted to be within 4.5 h of symptom onset, although the FDA indication is still within 3 h. The American Heart Association/American Stroke Association recommends a t-PA administration window of up to 4.5 h with certain additional exclusion criteria when compared to the 3-h administration.[12] Time goals for evaluation and treatment of patients with acute ischemic stroke are summarized in Table 4.[17]
- There are strict criteria for the administration of IV t-PA[12,18] (Tables 5 and 6).
- The protocol is weight based, with 90 mg being the maximum allowable dose.
- The risk of brain hemorrhage with IV t-PA is about 6% in stroke patients. The management of suspected intracranial hemorrhage after use of t-PA is summarized in Box 4.[19]
- Endovascular intervention is useful only for large, accessible thrombi. Therefore, if a stroke patient is a candidate for IV t-PA, treatment with IV t-PA should be started and then the patient should be assessed for possible endovascular therapy.[12] Table 7

TABLE 1 National Institutes of Health Stroke Scale

1A. Level of Consciousness (LOC)

0 = Alert
1 = Not alert, but arousable
2 = Not alert, obtunded
3 = Coma

1B. LOC Questions

Ask the month and his/her age.
0 = Answers both correctly
1 = Answers one correctly
2 = Answers neither correctly

1C. LOC Commands

Open and close the eyes.
Open and close the nonparetic hand.
0 = Performs both tasks correctly
1 = Performs one task correctly
2 = Performs neither task correctly

2. Best Gaze (Horizontal)

0 = Normal
1 = Partial gaze palsy
2 = Forced deviation or total gaze paresis

3. Visual Fields

0 = No visual loss
1 = Partial hemianopia
2 = Complete hemianopia
3 = Bilateral hemianopia

4. Facial Palsy

0 = Normal
1 = Minor paralysis
2 = Partial paralysis (total or near total paralysis of lower face)
3 = Complete paralysis of upper and lower face

5. Motor Arm

Right

Arm extended with palms down 90 degrees (if sitting) or 45 degrees (if supine) for 10 sec
0 = No drift
1 = Drift; limb drifts down from position and does not hit bed or support in 10 sec
2 = Some effort against gravity
3 = No effort against gravity
4 = No movement
Left

6. Motor Leg

Right

Leg extended at 30 degrees, always tested supine for 5 sec
0 = No drift
1 = Drift; limb drifts down from position and does not hit bed or support in 5 sec
2 = Some effort against gravity
3 = No effort against gravity
4 = No movement
Left

7. Limb Ataxia

The finger-nose-finger and heel-shin tests
0 = Absent
1 = Present in one limb
2 = Present in two limbs

8. Sensory

To Pinprick or Noxious Stimuli

0 = Normal
1 = Mild to moderate sensory loss
2 = Severe to total sensory loss

9. Best Language

0 = No aphasia, normal
1 = Mild-to-moderate aphasia
2 = Severe aphasia
3 = Mute, global aphasia, coma

10. Dysarthria

0 = Normal
1 = Mild-to-moderate
2 = Severe (including mute/ anarthric due to aphasia)
Do not score if intubated.

11. Extinction and Inattention

0 = No abnormality
1 = Present
2 = Profound (two modalities)

Total Score:

From Vincent JL et al: *Textbook of critical care*, ed 7, Philadelphia, 2017, Elsevier.

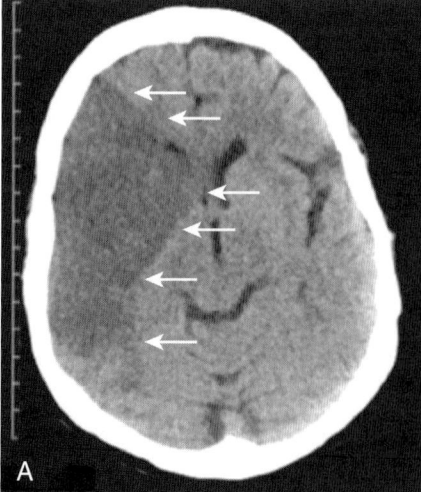 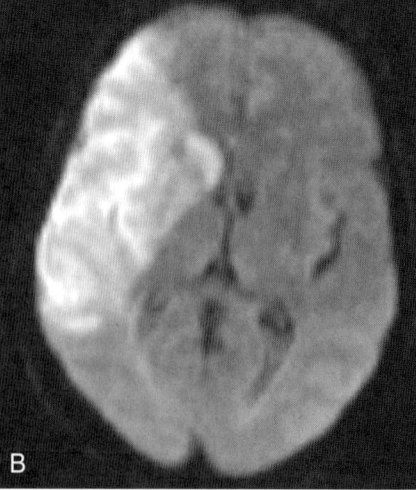

FIG. 1 Large right middle cerebral artery infarct on an unenhanced computed tomographic scan **(A)** and a diffusion-weighted magnetic resonance image **(B)**. There is a mass effect, and this patient is at risk for cerebral herniation syndromes.

summarizes AHA recommendations for endovascular therapy in patients with acute ischemic stroke.

IMMEDIATE CATHETER CEREBRAL ANGIOGRAPHY FOR ENDOVASCULAR INTERVENTION

(Figs. 2 and 3): Methods available:

- The American Heart Association/American Stroke Association 2018 guidelines with an update in 2019 recommend mechanical thrombectomy with a stent-retriever device for highly selected patients who present with large vessel occlusion (LVO) up to 16 h after last known normal and suggest that it is reasonable up to 24 h.[12,20,21]
  1. IV t-PA should be administered in this group if eligible.
  2. All patients should be assessed with CT angiogram head and neck or MRA head and neck for possible LVO if they have an NIHSS of ≥6 or suspicion of a large vessel stroke.
  3. In selected patients with acute ischemic stroke within 6 to 24 h of last known normal who have LVO on noninvasive angiogram, obtaining a CT perfusion, DW-MRI, or perfusion is recommended to aid in patient selection for mechanical thrombectomy.[20,21]
- Adult patients should receive mechanical thrombectomy with a stent retriever if they present within 6 h of last known normal with a causative LVO (especially of the internal carotid artery or MCA segment 1 [M1] but reasonable in the setting of a causative MCA segment 2 or 3 [M2/3] or other large vessel cerebral artery) if they were relatively independent before the stroke and have an NIHSS score of ≥6 and an ASPECTS score of ≥6.[22-27]
- Patients should receive mechanical thrombectomy with a stent retriever if treatment can be initiated within 16 h (and up to 24 h) of last known normal with a large anterior circulation LVO and they meet the DAWN[21] or DEFUSE-3[20] criteria (a defined mismatch between clinical severity and/or infarct volume compared to the penumbra [tissue at risk]). The number needed to treat to improve functional outcomes is only 2.8, and so patients should be aggressively evaluated for possible treatment.
- Complications can ensue from the endovascular procedure itself, including an intracerebral hemorrhage rate that is similar to that associated with IV t-PA. A recent meta-analysis revealed that among patients with acute ischemic stroke, endovascular therapy with mechanical thrombectomy versus standard medical care with t-PA was associated with improved functional outcomes and higher rates of angiographic revascularization, but no significant difference in symptomatic intracranial hemorrhage or all-cause mortality at 90 days.[28]
- Endovascular intervention is typically available only at comprehensive stroke centers.

HYPERTENSION: Elevated blood pressure is common during acute stroke, and it often subsides without specific therapy. In general,

TABLE 2 Imaging Modalities for Stroke

Imaging Modality	Advantage	Disadvantage
Cerebral catheter angiography	• Allows for the definitive assessment of cerebral circulation (gold standard) • Allows for the deployment of intraarterial thrombolysis and thrombectomy devices if a thrombus is found • Allows for the assessment of collateral circulation	• Invasive (significant risks) • High cost • Not available at all facilities
Doppler studies	• Noninvasive • May be performed at the patient's bedside	• Can be limited by the patient's body habitus • Operator dependent
Magnetic resonance angiography	• Excellent view of the large arteries of the neck and brain • No contrast material needed	• Cannot be performed in patients who are critically ill, who are unable to tolerate supine positioning, who have a pacemaker or other ferromagnetic hardware, or who are claustrophobic
Magnetic resonance perfusion	• Assesses cerebral hemodynamics • May show ischemic penumbra (i.e., the area of the brain that may be saved by timely intervention)	• Not commonly available • Not well standardized
CT angiography	• Excellent view of the large arteries of the neck and brain • Similar to magnetic resonance angiography with regard to resolution	• Requires intravenous contrast
CT perfusion	• Assesses cerebral hemodynamics • May show ischemic penumbra (i.e., the area of the brain that may be saved by timely intervention)	• Challenging to interpret in some cases • Not routinely available at many facilities • Requires intravenous contrast

CT, Computed tomography.

TABLE 3 Treatment Options for Acute Ischemic Stroke

Time Window	Treatment Options
0-3 h	IV thrombolysis with alteplase Mechanical thrombectomy (terminal ICA or M1 occlusion)
3-4.5 h	IV thrombolysis with alteplase (relative contraindications) Mechanical thrombectomy (terminal ICA or M1 occlusion)
4.5-6 h	Mechanical thrombectomy (terminal ICA or M1 occlusion)

6-24 h	a. Mechanical thrombectomy (large vessel occlusion + favorable perfusion imaging) 6-16 h (DEFUSE 3 Criteria):
	  i. Occlusion of terminal ICA or MCA - M1
	  ii. Clinical imaging mismatch
	b. Infarct core volume <70 ml
	c. Mismatch volume >15 ml
	d. Mismatch ratio (penumbra/core) >1.8
	e. 16-24 h (DAWN Criteria):
	  i. Occlusion of terminal ICA or MCA - M1
	  ii. Clinical imaging mismatch:
	f. ≥80 yr, NIHSS ≥10 + core <21 ml
	g. <80 yr, NIHSS ≥10 + core <31 ml
	h. <80 yr, NIHSS ≥20 + core <51 ml

Wake-up stroke	• Age 18-80 yr old • Stroke symptoms at awakening or could not report symptom onset • MRI brain including DWI, FLAIR, a sequence sensitive to hemorrhage, and time-of-flight magnetic resonance angiography of circle of Willis • Patients are eligible for thrombolysis if: 1. Abnormal signal in DWI + no signal change in FLAIR

DWI, Diffusion-weighted imaging; *FLAIR,* fluid-attenuated inversion recovery; *ICA,* internal carotid artery; *MCA,* middle cerebral artery; *MRI,* magnetic resonance imaging; *NIHSS,* National Institutes of Health stroke scale.
From Warshaw G et al: *Ham's primary care geriatrics,* ed 7, Philadelphia, 2022, Elsevier.

TABLE 4 Time Goals for Evaluation and Treatment of Patients With Acute Ischemic Stroke

Time After Emergency Department Arrival	Goals
10 min	Assess ABCs, vital signs
	Provide oxygen if hypoxemic
	Obtain intravenous access
	Obtain laboratory studies
	CBC, coagulation, electrolytes
	Check glucose level, treat if indicated
	Perform screening neurologic assessment
	Activate stroke team
	Order "stroke code" brain CT or MRI
	Obtain 12-lead ECG
25 min	Review history
	Establish time at onset or last known normal
	Perform neurologic examination
	NIH Stroke Scale
45 min	Review laboratory studies
	Review brain CT or MRI results
	Evaluate inclusion and exclusion criteria (see Table 4)
60 min	Review risks and benefits
	Obtain consent
	Begin infusion

ABCs, Airway, breathing, circulation; *CBC*, complete blood count; *CT*, computed tomography; *ECG*, electrocardiogram; *MRI*, magnetic resonance imaging; *NIH*, National Institutes of Health.
From Goldman L, Schafer AI: *Goldman-Cecil medicine,* ed 26, Philadelphia, 2019, Elsevier.

TABLE 5 Eligibility Criteria for Acute Thrombolysis in Acute Ischemic Stroke

Eligibility Criteria
- Diagnosis of ischemic stroke causing measurable and "disabling" neurologic deficit
- The neurologic signs should not be minor and isolated. Caution should be exercised in treating a patient with major deficits
- Onset of symptoms <4.5 h before beginning treatment
- The neurologic signs should not be clearing spontaneously
- The symptoms of stroke should not be suggestive of subarachnoid hemorrhage
- The patient or family members should understand the potential risks and benefits from treatment

Contraindications for Thrombolysis
- Evidence of intracranial hemorrhage on CT
- Head trauma or prior stroke in previous 3 mo
- Myocardial infarction in the previous 3 mo
- Gastrointestinal or urinary tract hemorrhage in previous 21 days
- Arterial puncture at a noncompressible site in the previous 7 days
- Major surgery in the previous 14 days
- History of previous intracranial hemorrhage
- Elevated blood pressure (systolic >185 mm Hg and diastolic >110 mm Hg)
- Evidence of active bleeding or acute trauma (fracture) on examination
- Taking an oral anticoagulant or, if taking anticoagulant, INR ≥1.7 is a contraindication
- If receiving heparin in previous 48 h, aPTT must be in normal range
- Platelet count ≤100,000 mm^3
- Blood glucose concentration ≥50 mg/dl (2.7 mmol/L)
- Seizure with postictal residual neurologic impairments
- CT shows a multilobar infarction (hypodensity >1/3 cerebral hemisphere)

aPTT, Activated partial thromboplastin time; *CT*, computed tomography; *INR*, international normalized ratio.
From Hoffman R et al: *Hematology: basic principles and practice,* ed 7, Philadelphia, 2018, Elsevier.

hypertension is not treated acutely unless it is extremely high (e.g., >220 mm Hg systolic blood pressure), there is evidence of hypertension-induced organ damage, or thrombolysis is being considered, in which case the blood pressure needs to be reduced (if it can be safely accomplished) to <185/110 mm Hg. It is risky to decrease blood pressure dramatically and quickly in the presence of acute ischemic stroke as it can cause an extension of the infarction into the ischemic penumbra. A gradual 15% to 25% decrease over the first 24 h is recommended when more acute lowering is not required. Blood pressure goals and treatment options in acute ischemic stroke are summarized in Box 5.[29]

HYPOTENSION: The presence of systemic hypotension in acute ischemic stroke portends a poor outcome. The cause should be sought, and volume depletion should be corrected with normal saline. Cardiac arrhythmias should be treated. Induced hypertension with vasopressor agents may be useful for select cases with an ischemic penumbra that is at risk, but caution is strongly advised.[12]

HYPOGLYCEMIA: Hypoglycemia can mimic stroke. Prompt assessment of serum glucose level and replacement as necessary are important.[12]

HYPERGLYCEMIA: Hyperglycemia should be treated with sliding scale insulin, taking into consideration the patient's oral intake. The presence of hyperglycemia worsens ischemic stroke outcomes, but recent evidence has not shown that aggressive treatment with an insulin pump improves outcomes and in-hospital goals of <180 are considered adequate.[30]

FEVER: Fever is harmful during acute stroke. Ascertaining and addressing the cause while lowering an elevated temperature is strongly advised.

ELEVATED INTRACRANIAL PRESSURE: Traditional treatment of increased intracranial pressure associated with acute ischemic stroke is shown in Box 6.

ANTIPLATELET THERAPY: Oral, rectal, or feeding tube administration of aspirin (81 to 325 mg/day) within 48 h of stroke onset is advised to decrease the likelihood of a repeat ischemic stroke. Other oral antiplatelet regimens including dual antiplatelet therapy may be indicated.[31] Please see further discussion in Stroke, Secondary Prevention. Patients who have received t-PA should not be given antithrombotic or anticoagulant agents within the first 24 h after administration.

ANTICOAGULATION THERAPY: In patients with acute ischemic stroke presumed secondary to embolism and atrial fibrillation, full-dose anticoagulation with heparin infusion or low-molecular-weight heparin is seldom indicated in the acute setting due to the relatively high risk of hemorrhagic conversion and little evidence to suggest any benefit except in very select

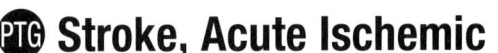

TABLE 6 Administration of rtPA for Acute Ischemic Stroke

Infuse 0.9 mg/kg (maximum dose 90 mg) over 60 min, with 10% of the dose given as a bolus over 1 min.

Admit the patient to an intensive care or stroke unit for monitoring.

If the patient develops severe headache, acute hypertension, nausea, or vomiting or has a worsening neurologic examination, discontinue the infusion (if IV rtPA is being administered) and obtain emergent CT scan.

Measure blood pressure and perform neurologic assessments every 15 min during and after IV rtPA infusion for 2 h, then every 30 min for 6 h, then hourly until 24 h after IV rtPA treatment.

Increase the frequency of blood pressure measurements if systolic blood pressure is >180 mm Hg or if diastolic blood pressure is >105 mm Hg; administer antihypertensive medications to maintain blood pressure at or below these levels.

Delay placement of nasogastric tubes, indwelling bladder catheters, or intraarterial pressure catheters if the patient can be safely managed without them.

Obtain a follow-up CT or MRI scan at 24 h after IV rtPA before starting anticoagulants or antiplatelet agents.

CT, Computed tomography; *IV*, intravenous; *MRI*, magnetic resonance imaging; *rtPA*, recombinant tissue plasminogen activator.
From Powers WJ et al: Guidelines for the early management of patients with acute ischemic stroke: 2019 update to the 2018 guidelines for the early management of acute ischemic stroke: a guideline for healthcare professionals from the American Heart Association/American Stroke Association, *Stroke* 50:e344-e418, 2019.

BOX 4 Management of Suspected Intracerebral Hemorrhage After Use of Tissue Plasminogen Activator

Discontinue the t-PA infusion if it remains in progress.
Obtain noncontrast CT scan of the head stat.
Order PT, PTT, platelet count, fibrinogen level, type and cross-match stat.
In event of hemorrhage, consult hematology and neurosurgery.
Give 6 to 8 units of cryoprecipitate, then 6 to 8 units of platelets.
Administer aminocaproic acid 4 to 5 g IV over 1 h, followed by 1 g PO or IV per h.
Check fibrinogen every 4 h and give cryoprecipitate to keep fibrinogen >150 mg/dl.
Monitor blood pressure every 15 min.
Periodically repeat CBC, PT, PTT.
Consider repeat head CT.

From Parrillo JE, Dellinger RP: *Critical care medicine: principles of diagnosis and management in the adult,* ed 5, Philadelphia, 2019, Elsevier.

TABLE 7 AHA Recommendations for Endovascular Therapy in Patients With Acute Ischemic Stroke

Patients should receive endovascular therapy with a stent retriever if they meet all of the following criteria (class I; level of evidence, A):
1. Prestroke modified Rankin score 0 to 1 (functionally independent)
2. Acute ischemic stroke receiving intravenous recombinant tissue plasminogen activator within 4.5 h of onset according to guidelines from professional medical societies
3. Causative occlusion of the internal carotid artery or proximal middle cerebral artery
4. Age 18 yr or older
5. National Institutes of Health Stroke Scale (NIHSS) score of 6 or greater
6. Alberta Stroke Program Early CT Score (ASPECTS) of 6 or greater
7. Treatment can be initiated (groin puncture) within 6 h of symptom onset

CT, Computed tomography.
From Zipes DP: *Braunwald's heart disease: a textbook of cardiovascular medicine,* ed 11, Philadelphia, 2019, Elsevier.

circumstances. However, chronic anticoagulation is indicated after the acute period has passed.[31]

DISPOSITION
Patients with acute ischemic stroke should be cared for in a stroke unit or an intensive care unit. Nurses with skills in stroke care and telemetry monitoring should be routine. Once the patient is stable and the workup is complete, rehabilitation should be arranged.[5-33]

REFERRAL
Patients with acute ischemic stroke should be transported to a hospital in which providers are skilled in stroke care. Depending on the severity and duration of symptoms, the patient may qualify for immediate endovascular intervention at a comprehensive stroke center, even if he or she is not a candidate for IV t-PA. If complications from brain edema develop, further evaluation by a neurosurgeon may be helpful during the acute phase.[12]

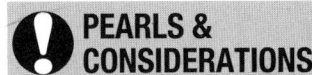 **PEARLS & CONSIDERATIONS**

PREVENTION
- The prevention of acute ischemic stroke depends on the aggressive management of risk factors in individual patients.
- Cross reference: Stroke, secondary prevention.
- Paroxysmal atrial fibrillation is common in patients with cryptogenic stroke. Ambulatory ECG monitoring with a loop recorder or other device for 30 days or more significantly improved the detection of atrial fibrillation by a factor of >5 and nearly doubled the rate of anticoagulant treatment compared to the standard practice of short-duration ECG monitoring.

PATIENT & FAMILY EDUCATION
Patients and families need to be taught about ways to reduce the risk for recurrent stroke, including lifestyle modifications. Education about rehabilitation goals, when appropriate, should also be accomplished.

REFERENCES & SUGGESTED READINGS
Available at eBooks.Health.Elsevier.com.

RELATED CONTENT
Stroke (Patient Information)
Stroke, Secondary Prevention (Related Key Topic)
Transient Ischemic Attack (Related Key Topic)
Atrial Fibrillation (Related Key Topic)

AUTHORS: **CÉSAR E. ESCAMILLA-OCAÑAS, MD,** and **COREY ELAM GOLDSMITH, MD, FAAN**

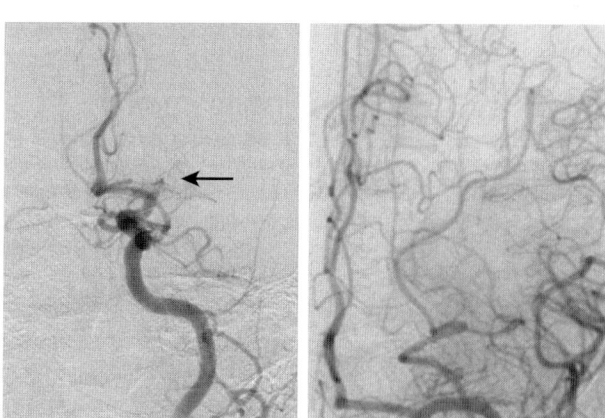

FIG. 2 A, A catheter angiogram showing left middle cerebral artery occlusion, which caused severe stroke symptoms for several hours. **B,** The artery was opened with the Merci clot retrieval system, and this resulted in normal flow.

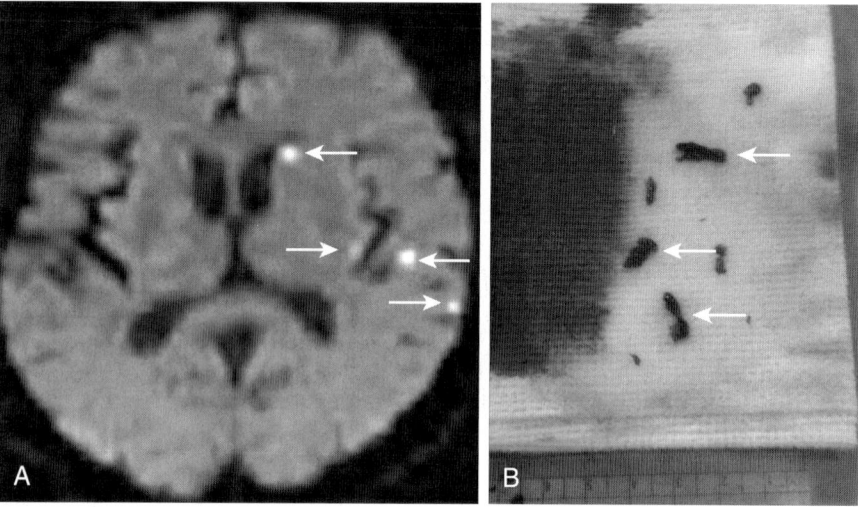

FIG. 3 A, A diffusion-weighted magnetic resonance image of the same patient as shown in previous figure, this time showing only mild left cerebral ischemia after intervention. The patient was clinically normal. **B,** Thrombi removed from the middle cerebral artery using the Merci clot retrieval system.

BOX 6 Medical Management Guidelines for Elevated Intracranial Pressure in Patients with Acute Ischemic Stroke

---

Correction of Factors Exacerbating Increased Intracranial Pressure
- Hypercarbia
- Hypoxia
- Hyperthermia
- Acidosis
- Hypotension
- Hypovolemia

Positional
- Avoidance of head and neck positions compressing jugular veins
- Avoidance of flat supine position; elevation of head of bed 15 degrees

Medical Therapy
- Endotracheal intubation and mechanical ventilation if Glasgow Coma Scale score ≤ 8
- Hyperventilation to a P_{CO_2} of 35 ± 3 mm Hg (if herniating)
- Hyperosmolar therapy with mannitol or hypertonic saline

Fluid Management
- Maintenance of euvolemia with isotonic solutions using normal saline; avoidance of glucose-containing solutions because hyperglycemia is associated with worse prognosis for stroke; replacement of urinary losses with normal saline in patients receiving mannitol

From Jankovic J et al: Bradley and Daroff's neurology in clinical practice, ed 8, Philadelphia, 2022, Elsevier.

BOX 5 Blood Pressure Goals in Acute Ischemic Stroke

- If not a candidate for thrombolysis: <220/120 mm Hg
- If candidate for thrombolysis: <185/110 mm Hg
- After thrombolysis: <180/105 mm Hg
- After revascularization: <140/80 mm Hg

From Warshaw G et al: *Ham's primary care geriatrics,* ed 7, Philadelphia, 2022, Elsevier.

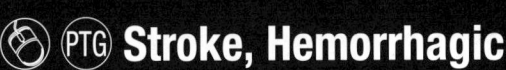
 BASIC INFORMATION

DEFINITION

Hemorrhagic stroke is the sudden onset of a focal neurologic deficit caused by hemorrhage into (intracerebral hemorrhage) or around (subarachnoid hemorrhage) the brain.

Subarachnoid hemorrhage commonly occurs as a result of a ruptured aneurysm. Please see "Subarachnoid Hemorrhage" for additional information.

This section will discuss intracerebral hemorrhage only.

Intracerebral hemorrhage (ICH) can have associated intraventricular extension/hemorrhage (IVH).

SYNONYMS

Intracerebral hemorrhage
Intracranial hemorrhage
Cerebrovascular attack (this is a nonspecific term and should not be used)

ICD-10CM CODES

I61	Intracerebral hemorrhage
I61.0	Intracerebral hemorrhage in hemisphere, subcortical
I61.1	Intracerebral hemorrhage in hemisphere, cortical
I61.2	Intracerebral hemorrhage in hemisphere, unspecified
I61.3	Intracerebral hemorrhage in brainstem
I61.4	Intracerebral hemorrhage in cerebellum
I61.5	Intracerebral hemorrhage, intraventricular
I61.6	Intracerebral hemorrhage, multiple localized
I61.9	Nontraumatic intracerebral hemorrhage, unspecified

EPIDEMIOLOGY & DEMOGRAPHICS

INCIDENCE: There are approximately 795,000 new or recurrent strokes per year in the U.S., of which approximately 10% are hemorrhagic.[1,2] Risk increases sharply with age. Intracerebral hemorrhage has a mortality rate of 30% to 40%.[3]

RISK FACTORS:
- Increased age
- Hypertension
- Cerebral amyloid angiopathy
- Anticoagulant use
- Antithrombotic medication
- Sympathomimetic drugs (e.g., cocaine, heroin, amphetamine, ephedrine)
- Alcoholism
- African American race
- Low cholesterol, low-density lipoprotein, and triglycerides
- Minuscule increase in absolute risk from antiplatelet therapy

GENETICS: Multifactorial

PHYSICAL FINDINGS & CLINICAL PRESENTATION

Patients with intracerebral hemorrhage present with focal neurologic signs that are abrupt in onset but not instantaneous, as occurs with embolic stroke. The evolution is typically over minutes and may be associated with headache, nausea, or vomiting and, in many cases, a depressed level of consciousness.[3a] The presentation varies with the region of the brain that is affected. Table 1 summarizes clinical features of anatomic forms of intracerebral hemorrhage. There is no exact clinical way to distinguish between a primary cerebral hemorrhage and an ischemic stroke; therefore imaging is required. Imaging can also help determine if the diagnosis is ischemic stroke with hemorrhagic conversion versus primary hemorrhage.[3,4]

The following are common locations for hypertensive hemorrhage:
- Basal ganglia
- Cerebellum
- Pons

Lobar hemorrhage in an older adult is likely due to amyloid angiopathy.

A systematic, detailed examination is necessary when approaching a comatose patient (Box 1). The ICH score is a widely used grading scale to estimate mortality based on computed tomography (CT) scan results. Parameters used to calculate the ICH score include Glasgow Coma Scale (GCS) (0 to 2 points) at presentation, patient age ≥80 (1 point), ICH volume ≥30 ml (1 point), presence of intraventricular blood (1 point), and infratentorial origin of blood (1 point). Scores range from 0 to 6, with a score of 0 conferring 0% mortality and a score of 6 with estimated 100% mortality.[5] This score, however, should not be used as the sole prognostic indicator or decision maker for discontinuing aggressive care. Accuracy of prognosis, especially early after ICH onset, is difficult, and aggressive treatment is recommended for at least the first 48 h before discussing prognosis.[3]

ETIOLOGY

- Arteriolosclerosis
- Amyloid angiopathy
- Aneurysm
- Arteriovenous malformation
- Brain tumor

Nonhypertensive causes of intracerebral hemorrhage are summarized in Box 2.

DX DIAGNOSIS

DIFFERENTIAL DIAGNOSIS

- Ischemic stroke, possibly with hemorrhagic conversion
- Seizure with postictal paralysis
- Syncope
- Migraine with hemiparesis
- Conversion disorder

LABORATORY TESTS

- CBC, metabolic panel including blood glucose, renal and liver function, prothrombin time/international normalized ratio, activated partial thromboplastin time, urinalysis, cardiac troponin, and toxicology screens[3]
- ECG and telemetry monitoring

IMAGING STUDIES

- Immediate: CT scan of the head without contrast is highly sensitive for hemorrhage (Fig. E1).
- Intraventricular extension of ICH occurs in 30% to 50% of patients with ICH and predisposes to the development of hydrocephalus in approximately half of patients. IVH predicts a worse prognosis.
- CT or MR angiogram to rule out an underlying vascular malformation. CT spot sign on the CT angiography has been shown to be a reliable early predictor of hematoma expansion.[6]
- MRI of the brain with a gradient echo sequence is also highly sensitive for hemorrhage, including intracerebral microhemorrhages that may not be visible with computed tomography scanning. While CT and MRI are equivalent for detecting acute ICH, MRI is more accurate to detect chronic ICH.[3] MRI may also help to identify underlying brain tumors or vascular malformations, especially if the bleeding occurs at atypical sites. In the acute setting the MRI may show only the hematoma, but repeat MRI approximately 6 wk after initial hemorrhage may help exclude these other etiologies.

Rx TREATMENT

NONPHARMACOLOGIC THERAPY

- Urgent neurosurgical evaluation is needed in many cases either for evacuation of the hematoma or for relieving raised intracranial pressure by procedures such as external ventricular drain (EVD) placement or decompressive surgeries.
- Surgery should be performed promptly for cases of cerebellar hemorrhage of >3 cm when the patient is deteriorating clinically, showing brain stem edema or hydrocephalus.[4]
- Surgery for evacuation of lobar or deep brain clots may be considered for select cases, although the level of evidence for efficacy is not high. Surgery is often considered in lobar hemorrhages close to the surface and/or when the patient is neurologically deteriorating.[3]
- Minimally invasive surgery for hematoma evacuation in ICH >20 to 30 ml can be effective in improving mortality.[3]
- In patients with ICH <30 ml and IVH, the addition of thrombolytic irrigation with alteplase or urokinase with the EVD placement hastens intraventricular clot removal and results in further mortality reduction.[3]

ACUTE GENERAL Rx

The cornerstones of medical management of acute intracerebral hemorrhage (Table 2) include:
- Control of hypertension
- Correction of coagulopathy
- Management of elevated intracranial pressure
- Treatment of seizures

HYPERTENSION (BOX 3): Blood pressure should be quickly lowered by 15% and then gradually and safely brought to the individual patient's target range. In theory, this may diminish the expansion of the hematoma. More aggressive

TABLE 1 Clinical Features of Anatomic Forms of Intracerebral Hemorrhage

Type of Intracerebral Hemorrhage	Hemiplegia	Hemisensory Syndrome	Aphasia	Homonymous Visual Defects	GAZE PALSY		Brainstem Signs
					Horizontal	Vertical	
Putaminal	Generally dense	Frequent	Global > motor > conduction	In large hematomas	Contralateral	No	No (only present with herniation)
Caudate	Absent or mild, transient	Absent	Transcortical motor (in dominant hemisphere hematomas)	No	Generally absent	No	No
Thalamic	Generally dense	Frequent, prominent	Occasional, thalamic variety	In large hematomas	Contralateral, occasionally ipsilateral	Yes, upward	Skew deviation, Horner syndrome, Parinaud syndrome
Lobar	Prominent in frontoparietal location	Prominent in frontoparietal location	In dominant temporoparietal location	In occipital hematomas	Contralateral in frontal hematomas	No	No (only present with herniation)
Cerebellar	Absent	Absent	No	No	Ipsilateral	No	Ipsilateral fifth through seventh nerve palsy, Horner syndrome
Pontine	Variable, usually bilateral	Variable, usually bilateral	No	No	Bilateral	No	Pinpoint reactive pupils, ocular "bobbing," decerebrate rigidity, respiratory rhythm abnormalities
Mesencephalic	Variable, usually present	Rare	No	No	No	Occasional, upward	Unilateral or bilateral third nerve palsy
Medullary	Generally absent	Occasional	No	No	No	No	Nystagmus, ataxia, hiccups, facial hypesthesia, dysarthria, dysphagia, 12th nerve palsy, Horner syndrome
Intraventricular	Generally absent	Rare	No	No	Occasional	Occasional	Rare (decerebrate rigidity)

From Jankovic J et al: *Bradley and Daroff's neurology in clinical practice,* ed 8, Philadelphia, 2022, Elsevier.

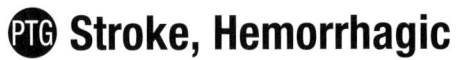

BOX 1 Neurologic Profile: A Modified Glasgow Coma Scale

Verbal Response
Oriented speech
Confused conversation
Inappropriate speech
Incomprehensible speech
No speech

Eye Opening
Spontaneous
Response to verbal stimuli
Response to noxious stimuli
None

Motor Response
Obeys
Localizes
Withdraws (flexion)
Abnormal flexion
None

Pupillary Reaction
Present
Absent

Spontaneous Eye Movement
Orienting
Roving conjugate
Roving disconjugate
Miscellaneous abnormal movements
None

Oculocephalic Response
Normal (unpredictable)
Full
Minimal
None

Oculovestibular Response
Normal (nystagmus)
Tonic conjugate
Minimal or disconjugate
None

Deep Tendon Reflexes
Normal
Increased
Absent

From Parrillo JE, Dellinger RP: *Critical care medicine: principles of diagnosis and management in the adult,* ed 4, Philadelphia, 2014, Elsevier.

BOX 2 Nonhypertensive Causes of Intracerebral Hemorrhage

- Vascular malformations (saccular or mycotic aneurysms, arteriovenous malformations, cavernous angiomas)
- Intracranial tumors
- Bleeding disorders, anticoagulant and fibrinolytic treatment
- Cerebral amyloid angiopathy
- Granulomatous angiitis of the central nervous system and other vasculitides, such as polyarteritis nodosa
- Sympathomimetic agents (including amphetamine and cocaine)
- Hemorrhagic infarction
- Head trauma
- Miscellaneous: Other vasculopathies (e.g., moyamoya disease, reversible cerebral vasoconstriction syndrome, cerebral autosomal dominant arteriopathy with subcortical infarcts and leukoencephalopathy [rarely]), and septic emboli/arteritis in the setting of infective endocarditis (all discussed elsewhere)

From Jankovic J et al: *Bradley and Daroff's neurology in clinical practice,* ed 8, Philadelphia, 2022, Elsevier.

control of systolic blood pressure (SBP) to 140 or less in the acute setting has been shown to be safe in clinical trials (INTERACT2 trial) with nonsignificant improvement in outcomes compared to less aggressive BP control (target SBP <180 mm Hg).[7] ATACH 2 studied aggressive blood pressure lowering in patients randomized within 4.5 h of symptom onset. Patients were randomized to aggressive blood pressure lowering to a target SBP of 110 to 139 mm Hg compared to standard blood pressure lowering to target SBP of 179 to 140 mm Hg. The trial was stopped early because there was no difference in neurologic outcome or death, but patients in the aggressive blood pressure lowering arm suffered more kidney injury.[8] More recent analysis has failed to demonstrate functional outcome improvement but found it to be safe.[9]

The most recent guidelines state that for ICH patients presenting with SBP between 150 and 220 mm Hg and without contraindication to acute BP treatment, acute lowering of SBP to a target range of 140 to 130 mm Hg is safe and can be effective for improving functional outcome. For ICH patients presenting with SBP >220 mm Hg, it may be reasonable to consider aggressive reduction of BP with a continuous intravenous infusion and frequent BP monitoring.[3]

CORRECTION OF COAGULOPATHY:
- Anticoagulation-associated ICH accounts for about 20% of all cases. Early hematoma expansion has been associated with poor outcome. Rapid reversal of coagulopathy should be performed as soon as possible after diagnosis of ICH to improve outcome.[3]

- Protamine sulfate is used to treat cases of heparin-induced intracerebral hemorrhage. Protamine dosage is 1 mg intravenous (IV) for every 100 units of heparin administered in the previous 2 to 3 h (maximum dose is 50 mg).
- Prothrombin concentrate complex (PCC) is recommended for reversal of warfarin-associated ICH in INR >2 and may be reasonable in INR 1.9 to 1.3 at a lower dose. FFP may be used instead if PCC not available but showed slower reversal of coagulopathy and was associated with more hematoma expansion compared to PCC. Vitamin K should be administered IV along with PCC for sustained effects. Routine use of recombinant factor VII concentrates is not recommended due to insufficient evidence and concern for increased risk of thromboembolic events.[3,10]
- Idarucizumab (Praxbind) is a humanized monoclonal antibody fragment that can be used for urgent reversal of the anticoagulant effect of the direct thrombin inhibitor dabigatran (Pradaxa). PCC infusion is also recommended if idarucizumab is not available.[3,10]
- Andexanet alfa, a recombinant modified human factor X2 decoy protein, has been effective for reversion of the anticoagulant effect of apixaban (Eliquis), rivaroxaban (Xarelto), and edoxaban (Savaysa), though it requires continuous infusion. PCC infusion is also recommended if andexanet alfa is not available.[3,10]
- Recommendations for thrombolytic-associated intracerebral hemorrhage treatment include the consideration of the infusion of platelets and cryoprecipitate.
- Platelet transfusion for patients experiencing ICH while on aspirin appears to result in worse outcomes than no platelet transfusion according to the PATCH trial is not recommended unless the patient requires emergency neurosurgery.[3,11]

ELEVATED INTRACRANIAL PRESSURE: This condition should be treated with a graded approach, which may include the elevation of the head of the bed, analgesia/sedation, hyperventilation, and osmotic therapy. In patients clinically suspected to have elevated ICP or with GCS <8, invasive monitoring of the ICP may be required. If conservative treatment fails to control ICP, EVD placement or other decompressive procedures like craniotomy should be pursued.[3]

SEIZURES: If seizures occur, they should be treated aggressively, including with intravenous medications, if needed. Although widely practiced, routine use of prophylactic antiepileptic medications is not recommended and, if used, should be stopped after 7 days if no evidence of seizures. Continuous EEG monitoring should be employed in patients with suspected seizures or unexplained low levels of consciousness.[3]

SUPPORTIVE TREATMENT[3]:
- Hyperglycemia: A high blood glucose level predicts a worse outcome. Markedly elevated glucose levels should be lowered to <180 mg/dl.

TABLE 2   Medical Management Protocol for Acute Intracranial Hemorrhage

Blood pressure	• Maintain mean arterial pressure <140 mm Hg with continuous infusion labetalol (2-10 mg/min), nicardipine (5-15 mg/h), or clevidipine (2-6 mg/h) • If stuporous or comatose, measure ICP and maintain CPP >70 mm Hg.

Reversal of anticoagulation	• For elevated INR: Vitamin K 10 mg IV push and 4F-PCC
	  1. INR 1.3-1.9: consider 10-20 units/kg
	  2. INR 2 to <4: 25 units/kg; not to exceed 2500 units
	  3. INR 4-6: 35 units/kg; not to exceed 3500 units
	  4. INR >6: 50 units/kg; not to exceed 5000 units
	• For heparin: Protamine sulfate 10 to 50 mg slow IV push (1 mg reverses approximately 100 units of heparin)
	• For dabigatran: Idarucizumab 5g IV (Praxbind)
	• For the factor Xa inhibitors (rivaroxaban, apixaban, and edoxaban): Andexanet-alpha IV. Low dose (≤10 mg rivaroxaban or ≤5 mg apixaban per dose): 400 mg IV bolus, followed by 4 mg/kg for 2 h. High dose (higher doses given within 8 h): 800 mg bolus, followed by 8 mg/kg for 2 h.
	• For thrombocytopenia or platelet dysfunction: Desmopressin 0.3 µg/kg intravenous push. Platelet transfusion is reasonable in the setting of thrombocytopenia but is not effective and may be harmful when given to patients on NSAIDs or other antiplatelet agents.
	• Expedited INR reversal for life-saving neurosurgical intervention: Recombinant activated factor VII 40-80 µg/kg (approximately 3.0-6.0 mg) intravenous push

Intracranial hypertension	• Elevate head of bed to 30 degrees • Hyperventilate to pCO$_2$ of 30 mm Hg • EVD placement • Mannitol 1.0-1.5 g IV prn to surgery
Fluids and nutrition	• Normal (0.9%) saline at 1.0 ml/kg/h • Begin enteral feeding via nasoduodenal tube within 24 h
Seizure	• For coma, start continuous EEG monitoring. • If clinical or electrographic seizures, treat with phenytoin or levetiracetam
Physiologic homeostasis	• Cooling blankets to maintain temperature ≤37.5° C • Insulin as needed to maintain glucose 120-180 mg/dl

CPP, Cerebral perfusion pressure; *FEIBA,* factor VIII inhibitor bypass activity; *4F-PCC,* four factor prothrombin complex concentrate, containing factors II, VII, IX, and X; *INR,* international normalization ratio; *IV,* intravenous; *NSAIDs,* nonsteroidal antiinflammatory drugs.
From Goldman L, Schafer AI: *Goldman-Cecil medicine,* ed 26, Philadelphia, 2019, Elsevier.

BOX 3   Suggested Recommended Guidelines for the Treatment of Elevated Blood Pressure in Patients With Spontaneous Intracerebral Hemorrhage

1. SBP of >200 mm Hg or MAP of >150 mm Hg: Consider the aggressive reduction of BP with continuous intravenous infusion, with BP monitoring every 5 min.
2. SBP of >180 mm Hg or MAP of >130 mm Hg with evidence or suspicion of elevated ICP: Consider ICP monitor and reducing BP with intermittent or continuous intravenous medications to keep cerebral perfusion pressure >60 to 80 mm Hg.
3. SBP of >180 mm Hg or MAP of >130 mm Hg without evidence or suspicion of elevated ICP: Consider a modest reduction of BP (e.g., MAP of 110 mm Hg or target blood pressure of 160/90 mm Hg) with intermittent or continuous intravenous medications, and clinically reexamine the patient every 15 min.

BP, Blood pressure; *ICP,* intracranial pressure; *MAP,* mean arterial pressure; *SBP,* systolic blood pressure.
Modified from Broderick J et al: Guidelines for the management of spontaneous intracerebral hemorrhage in adults: 2007 update, *Stroke* 38:2001-2023, 2007.

• Antipyretics should be administered for fever in addition to searching for a cause of the fever.
• Care should be taken to avoid hypoxia. Airway and ventilatory management should happen early and concurrently with the primary management of ICH.

• Pneumatic compression devices should be applied from the start of hospitalization to help prevent deep venous thrombosis. Chemical deep venous thrombosis prophylaxis can be started after 24 to 48 h in most situations once the bleed has been determined to be stable.

• Early mobilization for rehabilitation is desirable in the first 24 to 48 h.

DISPOSITION
For large hemorrhages or unstable patients, immediate referral to a stroke center

REFERRAL
Patients with hemorrhagic stroke should be transported to a hospital where providers are skilled in the treatment of stroke and cerebrovascular diseases including the availability of neurosurgery services and neurocritical care. Depending on the severity and duration of symptoms, the patient may require neurosurgical intervention.

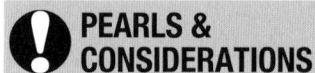 **PEARLS & CONSIDERATIONS**

• Outcomes are inversely correlated with hemorrhage size. However, specific reversal agents may be useful for warfarin-, heparin-, direct oral anticoagulant- (DOAC), or thrombolysis-associated hemorrhage.
• No procoagulant medications have yet been shown to be safe and effective for the mitigation of spontaneous intracerebral hemorrhage in placebo-controlled trials.

PREVENTION
• Prevention depends on the aggressive management of risk factors in individual patients, including hypertension, smoking, alcohol use, and cocaine use.
• Uncontrolled hypertension accounts for more than 70% of the attributable risk for ICH. Patients with prior ICH attributable to hypertension should have a blood pressure goal of <130/80 mm Hg.[3] DOACs dabigatran, apixaban, rivaroxaban, and edoxaban are uniformly associated with an overall reduced risk of iatrogenic ICH when used for stroke prevention in atrial fibrillation when compared to warfarin. Any of the currently available DOACs can be considered first line for patients at high risk for ICH.

PATIENT & FAMILY EDUCATION
Patients and families need to understand that most patients will not soon achieve functional independence and that rehabilitation will be a long process. Education about avoiding antithrombotic agents should be stressed as appropriate for individual circumstances.

REFERENCES
Available at eBooks.Health.Elsevier.com.

RELATED CONTENT
Stroke (Patient Information)
Stroke, Secondary Prevention (Related Key Topic)

AUTHOR: **COREY ELAM GOLDSMITH, MD, FAAN**

Diseases and Disorders

I

i BASIC INFORMATION

DEFINITION

Subarachnoid hemorrhage (SAH) is defined as hemorrhage into the subarachnoid space surrounding the brain. This can be either non-traumatic or traumatic in nature. Cerebral aneurysms are the most common cause of nontraumatic SAH (up to 85%) and have the most devastating consequences. Other causes include venous bleed, which have less severe sequelae. Here we will focus on aneurysmal nontraumatic subarachnoid hemorrhage.

SYNONYMS

Subarachnoid bleed
SAH

ICD-10CM CODES

I60	Subarachnoid hemorrhage
I60.1	Subarachnoid hemorrhage from middle cerebral artery
I60.2	Subarachnoid hemorrhage from anterior communicating artery
I60.3	Subarachnoid hemorrhage from posterior communicating artery
I60.4	Subarachnoid hemorrhage from basilar artery
I60.5	Subarachnoid hemorrhage from vertebral artery
I60.7	Subarachnoid hemorrhage from intracranial artery, unspecified

EPIDEMIOLOGY & DEMOGRAPHICS

INCIDENCE: Aneurysmal SAH: 6.67/100,000 persons worldwide and varies from 0.71 to 12.38 per 100,000 persons depending on geography. Annual incidence estimated at 500,000 cases worldwide.[1]
PREDOMINANT SEX & AGE: Women in the fifth and sixth decades of life.[2]
PEAK INCIDENCE: Most aneurysmal SAH occurs in people who are between the ages of 55 and 60 yr.

RISK FACTORS: Although genetics seem to play a factor in aneurysm formation, lifestyle factors are more important for determining overall risk of rupture. These risk factors include smoking, hypertension, oral contraception, pregnancy, and sympathomimetic use.
GENETICS:
- Several genes and medical conditions such as collagen vascular disease and autosomal dominant polycystic kidney disease have been associated with aneurysm formation, but their association with SAH remains controversial.[3,4]
- Current guidelines recommend screening for aneurysms only if 2 or more first-degree relatives have a history of SAH or cerebral aneurysms.
- Genetic screening is not recommended for patients with SAH.[4]

PHYSICAL FINDINGS & CLINICAL PRESENTATION

- The primary symptom is a sudden, severe headache in >90% of cases. About 50% have a headache that is classically described as the "worst headache of my life" and reaches maximal intensity within 1 min—the so-called thunderclap headache. This headache may be associated with nausea/vomiting, neck pain, seizure, or complete loss of consciousness.
- Most patients report a history of headaches during the weeks preceding the actual hemorrhage event. These are most likely sentinel bleeds that represent microhemorrhages.
- A posterior communicating artery aneurysm may present as oculomotor (cranial nerve III) palsy, typically involving the pupillary fibers, even in a nonruptured setting.
- The World Federation of Neurosurgeons (WFNS) score and the Hunt and Hess score are clinical scores that correlate with mortality (higher numbers indicating higher mortality) (Table 1).

ETIOLOGY
- Trauma.

- About 85% of nontraumatic SAHs are caused by a ruptured berry aneurysm, whereas 10% do not reveal a bleeding source despite modern imaging techniques. About 5% are due to other causes, which include arteriovenous malformations (AVMs), tumors, vasculitis, reversible cerebrovascular vasoconstriction syndrome, cerebral sinus venous thrombosis, and coagulopathies.
- Table 2 summarizes nonaneurysmal causes of subarachnoid hemorrhage.

Dx DIAGNOSIS

DIFFERENTIAL DIAGNOSIS
- Other headache syndromes: Thunderclap headaches due to reversible cerebral vasoconstriction syndrome (often with recurrent thunderclap headaches), migraine headache, sexual headache, cough headache, exertional headache, secondary causes including, but not limited to, pituitary apoplexy or acute hydrocephalus.

WORKUP
IMAGING STUDIES:
- The Ottawa SAH Rule can assist in selecting patients who require further neuroimaging and workup (Fig. 1).
- Computed tomography (CT) of the brain without contrast (Fig. 2) shows hemorrhage in around 95% of cases, especially during the acute phase (i.e., 24 to 48 hr) after the onset of bleeding. Box 1 describes a CT scan classification of subarachnoid hemorrhage. About 3% to 5% of SAH may be missed on initial CT of the head. MRI brain, specifically FLAIR sequence, is helpful in detecting subarachnoid blood if clinically suspected.
- Lumbar puncture should be performed in all cases of suspected SAH with "normal CT of the head," especially when clinical suspicion is high. The following suggest SAH:
  1. An RBC count of more than $100,000/m^3$ in tubes 1 AND 4. This is to differentiate from a traumatic tap in which there will be a drop in RBC count from tube 1 to 4.

TABLE 1 Most Commonly Used Clinical Grading Scales for Subarachnoid Hemorrhage

Hunt and Hess Scale

- Grade 0: Asymptomatic
- Grade 1: Mild headache and mild nuchal rigidity, no neurologic deficit
- Grade 2: Moderate to severe headache but no neurologic deficit other than cranial nerve palsy
- Grade 3: Drowsy, confused, or mild focal deficit
- Grade 4: Stupor, moderate to severe hemiparesis, and early decerebrate posturing
- Grade 5: Deep comatose, decerebrate posturing

WORLD FEDERATION OF NEUROLOGICAL SURGEONS SCALE

	Glasgow Coma Scale	Motor Deficit
Grade 0	15	Absent
Grade 1	15	Absent
Grade 2	13-14	Absent
Grade 3	13-14	Present
Grade 4	7-12	Present or absent
Grade 5	3-6	Present or absent

From Jankovic J et al: *Bradley and Daroff's neurology in clinical practice,* ed 8, Philadelphia, 2022, Elsevier.

BOX 1 Computed Tomography Scan Classification of Subarachnoid Hemorrhage (Fisher Scale)

Group 1: No blood detected
Group 2: Diffuse deposition or thin layer of blood, with all vertical layers of blood (interhemispheric fissure, insular cistern, ambient cistern) <1 mm thick
Group 3: Localized clots or vertical layers of blood 1 mm or greater in thickness
Group 4: Diffuse or no subarachnoid hemorrhage but with intraparenchymal or intraventricular clots

From Jankovic J et al: *Bradley and Daroff's neurology in clinical practice,* ed 8, Philadelphia, 2022, Elsevier.

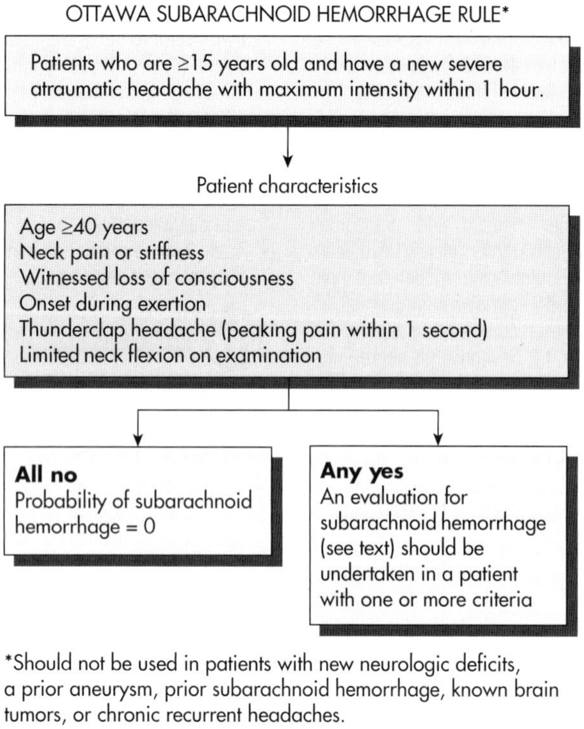

OTTAWA SUBARACHNOID HEMORRHAGE RULE*

Patients who are ≥15 years old and have a new severe
atraumatic headache with maximum intensity within 1 hour.

↓

Patient characteristics

Age ≥40 years
Neck pain or stiffness
Witnessed loss of consciousness
Onset during exertion
Thunderclap headache (peaking pain within 1 second)
Limited neck flexion on examination

All no
Probability of subarachnoid
hemorrhage = 0

Any yes
An evaluation for
subarachnoid hemorrhage
(see text) should be
undertaken in a patient
with one or more criteria

*Should not be used in patients with new neurologic deficits,
a prior aneurysm, prior subarachnoid hemorrhage, known brain
tumors, or chronic recurrent headaches.

FIG. 1 The Ottawa Subarachnoid Hemorrhage Rule. (From Goldman L, Shafer AI: *Goldman-Cecil medicine*, ed 26, 2019, Elsevier.)

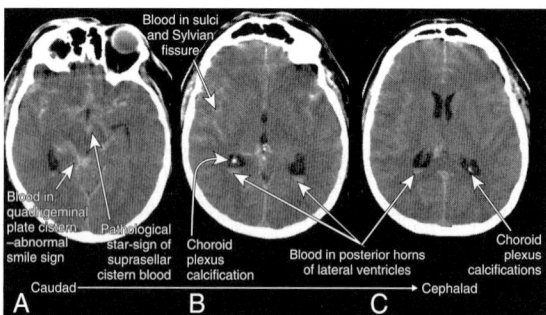

FIG. 2 Subarachnoid hemorrhage (SAH), noncontrast computed tomography (CT), brain windows.
Acute SAH appears white on noncontrast CT brain windows. **A** through **C,** Nonconsecutive axial slices, progressing
from caudad to cephalad. In this case of diffuse SAH, note the presence of subarachnoid blood filling the sulci, as
well as extending into the cisterns, Sylvian fissures, and even lateral ventricles. In **A,** blood *(white)* fills the
suprasellar cistern. This star-shaped structure is normally filled with cerebrospinal fluid (CSF) *(black)*. The
quadrigeminal plate cistern is normally a smile-shaped black crescent, filled with CSF, but in this case it is filled
with blood. Extremely bright calcifications in the choroid plexus of the posterior horns of the lateral ventricles are
common, normal findings—do not mistake these for hemorrhage. Note their similarity in density to bone of the
calvarium. (From Broder JS: *Diagnostic imaging for the emergency physician,* Philadelphia, 2011, Saunders.)

2. Presence of xanthochromia or bilirubin in
the cerebrospinal fluid.
3. SAH can also be excluded by the following
two criteria: CSF RBC count $<2000 \times 10^6$/L
and no xanthochromia.
- CT angiogram of the brain (Fig. E3 and Fig. E4).
- Digital subtraction angiography with 3D processing when indicated is the gold standard
for diagnosis of etiology in subarachnoid
hemorrhage.
- ECG may reveal diffuse repolarization abnormalities in precordial leads (Fig. E5).[5]

LABORATORY TESTS
- Basic laboratory values, including CBC,
chemistry panel, prothrombin time, partial
thromboplastin time, and platelet count.
- Serum troponin to evaluate for severe cardiac
stress; elevated troponins indicate cardiac
damage secondary to a catecholamine surge
and can be associated with poor outcomes.
- Patients with SAH are prone to developing
cerebral salt wasting, resulting in hyponatremia. Sodium levels should be monitored
frequently.

**TABLE 2 Nonaneurysmal Causes
of Subarachnoid Hemorrhage**

Trauma
Idiopathic perimesencephalic subarachnoid
  hemorrhage
Arteriovenous malformation
Intracranial arterial dissection
Cocaine and amphetamine use
Mycotic aneurysm
Pituitary apoplexy
Moyamoya disease
Central nervous system vasculitis
Sickle cell disease
Coagulation disorders
Primary or metastatic neoplasm

Causes are listed in approximate order of frequency.
From Goldman L, Shafer AI: *Goldman-Cecil medicine*, ed 26,
  2019, Elsevier.

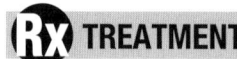 **TREATMENT**

NONPHARMACOLOGIC THERAPY
- Airway, breathing, and circulation
- Once stabilized, good neurologic exam
- Cerebrospinal fluid (CSF) drainage may be
required for patients who develop hydro-
cephalus and increased intracranial pressure.
It is also recommended for patients with Hunt
and Hess grade 3 or higher

ACUTE GENERAL Rx
- Critical care management: Initial management
strategies are geared toward stabilizing the
patient and preventing re-hemorrhage and
hydrocephalus. Re-hemorrhage occurs within
72 hr in up to 23% and is associated with very
high mortality rates.
- Blood pressure control: Tight blood pressure
control is paramount before securing the
aneurysm to protect against re-rupture. Blood
pressure control can be achieved with the use
of antihypertensive infusions such as intravenous nicardipine. A systolic blood pressure of
less than 140 mm Hg is recommended.
Placement of arterial line is recommended.
After securing of the aneurysm, liberalization
of blood pressure parameters is the standard.
- Intracranial pressure control: Raised intracranial pressure occurs in more than 50% of
patients with subarachnoid hemorrhage secondary to hydrocephalus, cerebral edema,
cerebral infarction or other causes. Insertion of
a ventricular catheter to treat acute hydrocephalus and maintain intracranial
pressure <20 mm Hg can be lifesaving. Patients who are unable to be weaned may
require permanent CSF diversion.
- In cases of aneurysmal SAH, treatment focuses on occlusion/exclusion of the aneurysm
to prevent rebleeding. Most aneurysms
currently are treated endovascularly. The most
common treatment methods are:

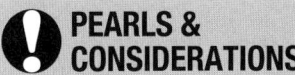

1. Microsurgical clipping: Performed through a craniotomy by placing a clip around the neck of the aneurysm
2. Endovascular coiling (Fig. E6): Performed via digital subtraction angiography; it consists of deploying platinum coils inside the aneurysm (Fig. E7) or stents in the parent artery to cause thrombosis of the aneurysmal sac.
3. Flow diverters and the Woven EndoBridge (WEB) device are also treatment options.

- Vasospasm: Cerebral vasospasm is a morbid complication leading to cerebral ischemia, disability, and death after SAH. It typically develops between day 4 and 14 (but may occur up to day 21) after the hemorrhage, and it reaches a peak on day 6 to 8. Treatment strategies include:
  1. Induced hypertension with typical mean arterial pressure goals of 90 to 100 (after aneurysm is secured) and with euvolemia instead of hypervolemia, as the latter was found to lead to significant cardiopulmonary and hemodynamic complications. "Triple H" therapy—*H*ypertension, *H*ypervolemia, and *H*emodilution—was originally employed to maintain cerebral perfusion, but it has fallen out of favor due to its many complications.
  2. Nimodipine (60 mg q4h or 30 mg q2h if blood pressure is low) has been shown to improve outcomes if it is administered between days 4 and 21 after the hemorrhage. Nimodipine has not been shown to reduce the incidence of vasospasm but does have a mortality benefit, likely acting as a neuroprotective agent.
  3. Intraarterial therapies such as intraarterial calcium channel blockers and balloon angioplasty may be employed as needed for symptomatic vasospasm.
- Seizures occur in about 3% of patients during the acute phase. Use of prophylactic antiepileptics is controversial and not recommended, but patients presenting with seizures should be treated appropriately with anticonvulsants.
- Pain control: Use short-acting and less-sedating medications (e.g., codeine, low-dose morphine).
- Monitor and treat for cerebral salt wasting and any other electrolyte abnormalities or anemia.
- Maintain normothermia.
- Avoid hyperglycemia or hypoglycemia.
- Management of SAH is complex and requires a multidisciplinary approach that includes expertise from neurology, critical care, neurosurgery, neuro-interventionalists, cardiologists, and endocrinologists, to name a few. A brief summary of the management is outlined above, but a detailed discussion is outside the scope of this text. The authors recommend supplementing this material with society guidelines such as those laid out by the Neurocritical Care Society.[6]

CHRONIC Rx

- Management of reversible risk factors mentioned earlier (smoking, hypertension, drug use)
- Management of neurologic disability through physical therapy and rehabilitation

DISPOSITION

- Outcomes after SAH have been improving over the years, with a 17% to 50% decrease in case fatality. The prehospital and 30-day mortality rates are still reported at around 15% to 33%.
- Almost half of those who survive hospitalization have cognitive impairments or disability that affect their lifestyles.[7]

REFERRAL

All patients should be managed at high-volume SAH centers, which are defined as having a case volume of more than 35 SAHs a year. Patients who present to alternative facilities should be transferred to a high-volume SAH center as soon as possible.

PEARLS & CONSIDERATIONS

COMMENTS

- "Thunderclap" headaches should be considered SAH until proven otherwise and evaluated by CT of the head with/without LP. MRI FLAIR sequence is also a helpful modality.
- All SAH should be managed in a critical care setting (preferably neurocritical care unit) with neurosurgical care available.
- Measures to prevent rebleeding include adequate control of blood pressure and aneurysm treatment with the use of coiling or clipping.

PREVENTION

Controlling some of the modifiable risk factors, especially smoking and blood pressure, may help to decrease the risk of aneurysmal rupture.

PATIENT & FAMILY EDUCATION

- SAH is a devastating condition, with most survivors developing significant neurologic or cognitive deficits. A good support system and an adequate physical and cognitive rehabilitation program may prove useful to survivors.
- Screening may be useful for patients with two or more first-degree relatives with SAH.

REFERENCES

Available at eBooks.Health.Elsevier.com.

RELATED CONTENT

Subarachnoid Hemorrhage (Patient Information)

AUTHOR: **KHAWJA A. SIDDIQUI, MD**

Diseases and Disorders

BASIC INFORMATION

DEFINITION

Subclavian steal syndrome is an occlusion or severe stenosis of the proximal subclavian artery leading to decreased antegrade flow or retrograde flow in the ipsilateral vertebral artery and neurologic symptoms referable to the posterior circulation.

SYNONYM

Proximal subclavian (or innominate) artery stenosis or occlusion

ICD-10CM CODE

G45.8   Other transient cerebral ischemic attacks and related syndromes

EPIDEMIOLOGY & DEMOGRAPHICS

- Similar to that of other manifestations of atherosclerosis (coronary artery disease, cerebrovascular disease, or peripheral vascular disease)
- Affects middle-aged persons (men somewhat younger than women on average) with arteriosclerotic risk factors, including family history, smoking, diabetes mellitus, hyperlipidemia, hypertension, and sedentary lifestyle

PHYSICAL FINDINGS & CLINICAL PRESENTATION

SYMPTOMS:

- Many patients are asymptomatic.
- Upper-extremity ischemic symptoms: Fatigue, exercise-related aching, coolness, numbness of the involved upper extremity.

- Neurologic symptoms are reported by 25% of patients with known unilateral subclavian steal. These include brief spells of:
  1. Vertigo
  2. Diplopia
  3. Decreased vision
  4. Oscillopsia
  5. Gait unsteadiness
  These spells are only occasionally provoked by exercising the ischemic upper extremity (classic subclavian steal). Left subclavian steal is more common than right, but the latter is more serious.
- Posterior circulation stroke related to subclavian steal is rare.
- Innominate artery stenosis can cause decreased right carotid artery flow and cerebrovascular symptoms of the anterior cerebral circulation, but this is uncommon.

Physical findings:
- Delayed and smaller volume pulse (wrist or antecubital) in the affected upper extremity
- Lower blood pressure in the affected upper extremity
- Supraclavicular bruit

NOTE: Inflating a blood pressure cuff will increase the bruit if it originates from a vertebral artery stenosis and decrease the bruit if it originates from a subclavian artery stenosis.

ETIOLOGY & PATHOGENESIS

ETIOLOGY:

- Atherosclerosis
- Arteritis (Takayasu disease and temporal arteritis)
- Embolism to the subclavian or innominate artery
- Cervical rib
- Long-term use of a crutch

- Occupational (baseball pitchers and cricket bowlers)

Pathogenesis: The vertebral artery originates from the subclavian artery. For subclavian steal to occur, the occlusion must be proximal to the takeoff of the vertebral artery. On the right side, only a small distance separates the bifurcation of the innominate artery and the takeoff of the vertebral artery, explaining why the condition occurs less commonly on the right side. Occlusion of the innominate artery must affect right carotid artery flow.

DIAGNOSIS

The carotid arteries should be evaluated at least noninvasively in all cases.

DIFFERENTIAL DIAGNOSIS

- Posterior circulation transient ischemic attack or stroke
- Upper-extremity ischemia:
  1. Distal subclavian artery stenosis or occlusion
  2. Raynaud phenomenon
  3. Thoracic outlet syndrome

WORKUP

- Noninvasive upper-extremity arterial flow studies
- Doppler sonography of the vertebral, subclavian, and innominate arteries
- Arteriography, magnetic resonance arteriogram (Fig. 1)

TREATMENT

- In most patients the disease is benign and requires no treatment other than atherosclerosis risk factor modification and aspirin. Symptoms tend to improve over time as collateral circulation develops.
- Vascular surgical reconstruction requires a thoracotomy; it may be indicated in innominate artery stenosis or when upper-extremity ischemia is incapacitating.

AUTHOR: **FRED F. FERRI, MD**

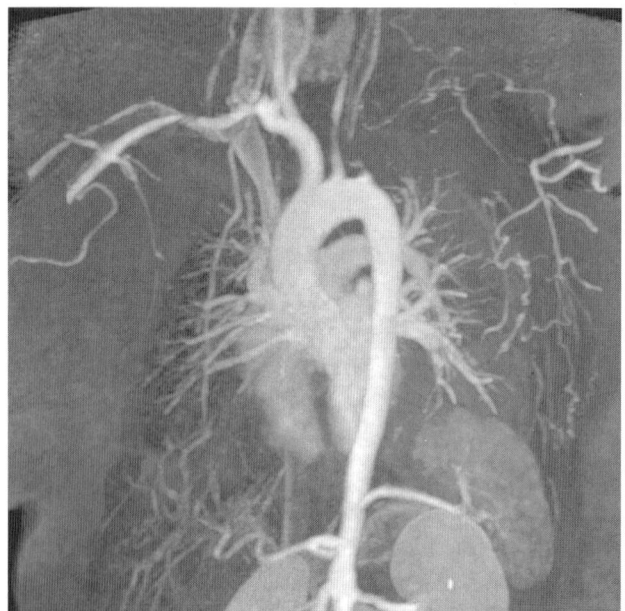

FIG. 1   Magnetic resonance arteriogram demonstrating diffuse moderate stenosis of the proximal left common carotid and proximal occlusion of the left subclavian artery coming off the aortic arch with development of an extensive collateral network. (From Hochberg MC et al: *Rheumatology*, ed 5, St Louis, 2011, Mosby.)

BASIC INFORMATION

DEFINITION

A subdural hematoma (SDH) is a collection of blood or blood products between the brain and dura mater. Subdural hematomas can be acute (ASDH) or chronic (CSDH) and vary significantly in presentation and treatment.

SYNONYMS

Acute subdural hematoma
ASDH
Chronic subdural hematoma
CSDH
Subdural hemorrhage

ICD-10CM CODES

I62.01   Acute subdural hematoma
I62.03   Chronic subdural hematoma
S06.5   Traumatic subdural hemorrhage

EPIDEMIOLOGY & DEMOGRAPHICS

INCIDENCE:

- The exact incidence of ASDH is unknown, but it is commonly seen in patients with head injury.
- CSDH is most common in the elderly with an estimated incidence of 1.72 to 20.6 per 100,000.[1]
- Between 10% and 20% of cases will experience reaccumulation of CSDH after evacuation.[1]

PREVALENCE: Unknown

PREDOMINANT SEX & AGE:

- Peak incidence of CSDH is in the eighth decade and is notably higher in males.
- ASDHs usually present with trauma and can happen in all age groups. In particular, shaken baby syndrome can be associated with SDH in the infant population.[1]

RISK FACTORS:

- Factors such as antithrombotic therapy, coagulopathy, thrombocytopenia, early childhood, advanced age, brain atrophy, and chronic alcoholism can increase the risk of bleeding.[2,3] Intracranial hypotension associated with CSF shunts or leaks is uncommon but can result in acute or chronic SDH.[2,4]

PHYSICAL FINDINGS & CLINICAL PRESENTATION

- Symptoms vary on the basis of acuity, size, and location. Acute traumatic SDHs are often seen in traumatic brain injury patients, and their Glasgow Coma Scale may vary according to the extent of brain injury, size of hematoma, and associated compression. When associated with a midline shift (i.e., >5 mm), they can cause signs of cerebral herniation (e.g., ipsilateral pupil dilation, contralateral weakness) requiring prompt surgical evacuation.[5]
- Patients with CSDH may present with diverse nonspecific symptoms such as headaches, confusion, gait disturbance, incontinence, aphasia, hemiparesis, transient ischemic attack-like symptoms, and seizures.

ETIOLOGY

ASDH is usually the result of shearing and tearing of bridging veins between the brain parenchyma and the dura mater. Other causes of bleeding into the subdural space include contusion and extension of parenchymal hemorrhage. In the setting of spontaneous SDH, vascular abnormalities, such as arteriovenous (AV) malformation, aneurysm, and dural AV fistula, should be considered.[5] For CSDH, it has been proposed that initial minor trauma splits the inner dural cell layer, leading to a self-perpetuating inflammatory cascade that causes membrane formation and neovascularization in the subdural space through the release of procollagen, fibrinolytic, and angiogenic factors. The resulting weak and rigid blood vessels and ongoing fibrinolysis lead to recurrent accumulation of blood in the subdural space.[1]

DIAGNOSIS

DIFFERENTIAL DIAGNOSIS

Cerebrospinal fluid (CSF) hygromas, abscesses, and tumor infiltrations

WORKUP

- Clinical assessment: Patient history screening for provoking factors, including medications, specifically anticoagulants/antiplatelets; alcohol abuse; recent trauma; cancer; and recent bacterial infections
- Neurologic examination: Glasgow Coma Scale, cranial nerves, motor/sensory exam CT head

LABORATORY TESTS

Assessment of the patient's coagulation status including CBC with platelet count, prothrombin time, partial thromboplastin time, and liver function test (especially with a history of alcoholism or liver failure)

IMAGING STUDIES

CT head (Fig. 1): Demonstrates the classic crescentic collection between the brain and inner table. For comatose and trauma patients, include

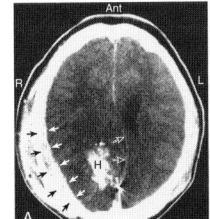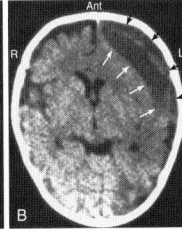

FIG. 1 A, Noncontrast computed tomography scan of an acute subdural hematoma shows a crescentic area of increased density in the right posterior parietal region between the brain and the skull *(black and white arrows)*. An area of intraparenchymal hemorrhage *(H)* is also seen. **B,** A chronic subdural hematoma for a different patient is shown. There is an area of decreased density in the left frontoparietal region *(arrows)* that effaces the sulci, compresses the anterior horn of the left lateral ventricle, and shifts the midline somewhat to the right. (From Mettler FA [ed]: *Primary care radiology,* Philadelphia, 2000, Saunders.)

a cervical spine CT scan. ASDH is usually hyperdense, whereas a CSDH is usually hypodense on noncontrast CT. Contrast is only needed if there are concerns about tumor or infection.

TREATMENT

- Admission for monitoring in the setting of ASDH.
- Correction of underlying coagulopathy, if present (e.g., warfarin/DOAC/ASA/clopidogrel reversal).
- The majority of SDH can be managed without surgery in awake patients with normal neurologic examinations.
- Atorvastatin and tranexamic acid have shown promising results in reducing the reaccumulation of CSDH, although results from larger randomized controlled trials are still awaited, and these drugs are not used in routine clinical practice.[6-8]
- Steroids have not demonstrated any clinical benefit and may be associated with more adverse events in two randomized controlled trials.[9,10]
- The irritative effects of blood products on the brain can contribute to seizures, in both acute and chronic subdural hematomas. If seizures occur, aggressive treatment with antiepileptic drugs should be undertaken. Nonclinical seizures should be considered in cases with depressed or fluctuating mental status, and video EEG monitoring should be instituted in such cases. In traumatic ASDH, seizure prophylaxis with phenytoin or levetiracetam for 7 days can be considered as there is underlying injury to the brain parenchyma.[11,12]

NONPHARMACOLOGIC THERAPY

Surgical treatment is indicated in:
- ASDHs measuring >10 mm in thickness with a midline shift >5 mm on CT scan and a compromised neurologic status (Glasgow Coma Scale <9, pupillary asymmetry or fixation) should be immediately evacuated.[5]
- In CSDH with a mass effect, a clear change in the neurologic examination from baseline, and/or enlargement of the hematoma size, evacuation (Fig. 2) via craniotomy or burr hole should be considered.
- In cases of recurrent CSDHs or otherwise high-risk patients who need antithrombotics, middle meningeal artery embolization has emerged as an effective treatment option.[13]

DISPOSITION

Depending on the size and location of the SDH and the examination of the patient, disposition can range from the ICU to outpatient management. When observation of the patient is considered, clinical examinations should be serially performed. Patient baseline and follow-up clinical examinations are more important than CT scan findings.

REFERRAL

Neurosurgical and operative consultation should be made available.

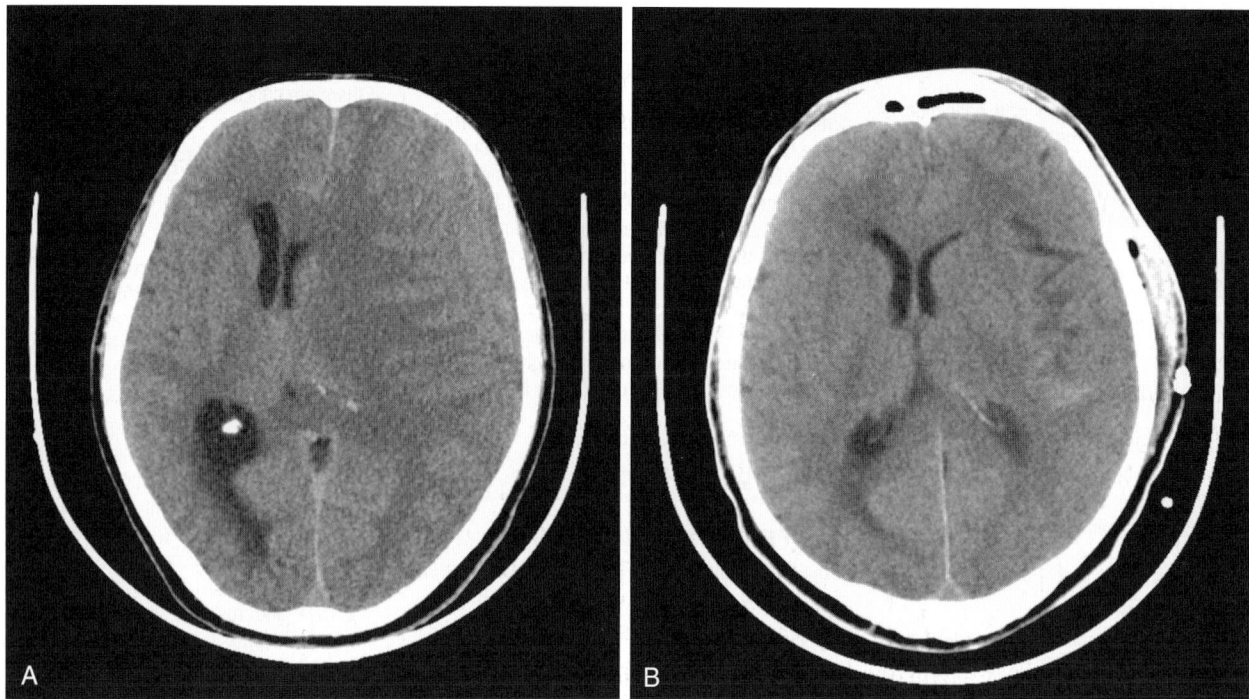

FIG. 2 An isodense subdural hematoma. A, Sulcal effacement and a midline shift to the right are clues to the presence of a left-sided subdural hematoma. **B,** Reexpansion of the left Sylvian fissure and a reduction in midline shift after evacuation. (From Soto JA, Lucey BC: *Emergency radiology, the requisites*, ed 2, Philadelphia, 2017, Elsevier.)

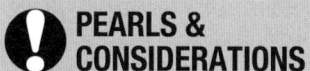

PEARLS & CONSIDERATIONS

COMMENTS
- Many elderly patients have small CSDHs or hygromas. Unless these are associated with seizures or clinical or radiographic progression, they are usually not emergent and usually do not require neurosurgical intervention.

- SDHs in elderly patients can have a mixed hyperdense and hypodense appearance on noncontrast CT scan; this finding is suggestive of subdural membranes and chronic components.

PATIENT & FAMILY EDUCATION
Individuals with SDHs are at higher risk for seizure, so surveillance is important.

REFERENCES
Available at eBooks.Health.Elsevier.com.

RELATED CONTENT
Subdural Hematoma (Patient Information)

AUTHOR: **MUHAMMAD UBAID HAFEEZ, MD**

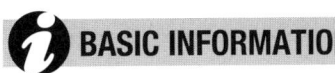

ⓘ BASIC INFORMATION

DEFINITION

Superior vena cava (SVC) syndrome is a set of symptoms that results when blood flow from the head, neck, upper torso, or extremities to the right atrium is partially or completely obstructed. Most commonly, this results from a mediastinal mass that compresses the SVC or the veins that drain into it.

SYNONYM

SVC syndrome

ICD-10CM CODES
I87.1	Compression of vein
S25.20XA	Unspecified injury of superior vena cava, initial encounter
S25.29XA	Other specified injury of superior vena cava, initial encounter

EPIDEMIOLOGY & DEMOGRAPHICS

- SVC syndrome occurs in 15,000 persons in the U.S. every year.
- More than 60% of patients presenting with SVC syndrome have a previously undiagnosed malignancy.[1]
- SVC syndrome mirrors lung cancer (especially small cell carcinoma) and lymphoma.

PREDOMINANT SEX & AGE:
- SVC syndrome secondary to malignancy is more common in men than women due to a higher incidence of lung cancer in men.
- Incidence increases with age, and the median age of diagnosis is 40 to 60 yr.

RISK FACTORS:
- Intrathoracic malignancy
- Thrombosis
- Postradiation fibrosis
- Mediastinitis

PHYSICAL FINDINGS & CLINICAL PRESENTATION[2]

The pathophysiology of SVC syndrome involves increased pressure in the venous system draining into the SVC producing edema of the head, neck, and upper extremities. Symptoms develop over a period of 2 wk in one third of patients and include:
- Shortness of breath
- Chest pain
- Cough
- Dysphagia, hoarseness, stridor
- Headache
- Syncope
- Visual disturbances

Signs:
- Chest wall vein distention (Fig. E1)
- Neck vein distention
- Facial edema, facial plethora
- Upper extremity swelling
- Cyanosis

ETIOLOGY
- Lung cancer (65% of all cases, of which half are small cell lung cancer)
- Lymphoma (15%)
- Thymoma

- Tuberculosis
- Goiter
- Aortic aneurysm (arteriosclerotic or syphilitic)
- SVC thrombosis:
  1. Primary: Associated with a central venous catheter, endocardial defibrillator, or pacemaker leads
  2. Secondary: Complication of SVC syndrome associated with one of the abovementioned causes
- Inflammatory process, fibrosing mediastinitis
- Fig. E2 illustrates the anatomy of superior vena cava syndrome. Table 1 summarizes common malignancies associated with SVC syndrome in adults

ⒹⓍ DIAGNOSIS

Diagnostic imaging (Fig. E3 and E4): Computed tomography (CT) scan of the chest with contrast is the most useful diagnostic study. Magnetic resonance imaging (MRI) is usually adequate to establish the diagnosis of SVC obstruction and to assist in the differential diagnosis of probable cause.[3]

DIFFERENTIAL DIAGNOSIS

SVC syndrome is characteristic enough to exclude other diagnoses. The differential diagnosis concerns the underlying etiologies listed previously.

WORKUP

Percutaneous needle biopsy, endobronchial ultrasound-guided needle biopsy (EBUS), and mediastinoscopy are the most common initial diagnostic modalities used to establish a histologic diagnosis.

IMAGING STUDIES[3]
- Chest x-ray can demonstrate mediastinal widening and pleural effusion.
- Chest CT with contrast or MRI (for contrast-intolerant patients) usually confirms the diagnosis.

- Venography is rarely needed and is warranted only when an intervention (e.g., stent or surgery) is planned.
- Box 1 summarizes an approach to patients with superior vena cava obstruction.

ⓇⓍ TREATMENT[2]

Tissue diagnosis is usually needed before commencing therapy. EBUS is now considered the first step in evaluation. Mediastinoscopy can be considered if EBUS is nondiagnostic or there is high clinical suspicion for lymphoma. Management is guided by the severity of the symptoms and the underlying etiology. Table E2 compares treatment modalities for malignancy-related SVC obstruction.

NONPHARMACOLOGIC TREATMENT
- Most patients with SVC syndrome do not require emergency intervention. Emergency empiric radiation is indicated in critical situations such as respiratory failure or central nervous system signs associated with increased intracranial pressure.
- Treatment of the underlying malignancy:
  1. Radiotherapy: Most tumors causing SVC syndrome are sensitive to radiotherapy
  2. Systemic chemotherapy
- For SVC syndrome secondary to benign disease, upright positioning and fluid restriction allow collateral channels to develop and promotes clinical regression.
- Percutaneous self-expandable stents that can be placed under local anesthesia with radiologic manipulation to bypass the obstruction are useful in the treatment of SVC syndrome, especially in cases associated with malignant tumors.
- Surgical bypass grafting is infrequently used to treat SVC syndrome.

CHRONIC Rx
- Anticoagulant or fibrinolytic therapies are employed for patients who do not respond to

TABLE 1 Malignancies Associated With Superior Vena Cava (SVC) Syndrome in Adults*

Neoplastic Diagnosis	Percentage of SVC Syndrome	Percentage of Disease-Associated SVC Syndrome
Lung cancer, stage 3B or 4:	48-81	
Small cell lung cancer		15-45
Squamous cell cancer		20-25
Adenocarcinoma		5-25
Large cell carcinoma		4-30
Lymphoma:	2-21	
Diffuse large cell lymphoma		64
Lymphoblastic lymphoma		33
Breast cancer	11	

*Includes lung cancer, lymphomas, and metastases from other solid tumors. 75% to 85% of patients with SVC have neoplastic disease.
From Zipes DP et al (eds): *Braunwald's heart disease*, ed 7, Philadelphia, 2005, Saunders.

BOX 1 Approach to Patients With Superior Vena Cava Obstruction

The diagnosis is established by physical examination and clinical presentation.
- Respiratory status should be assessed promptly. Only patients in extremis should be treated urgently with radiation therapy or stent placement without a histologic diagnosis. Emergency therapy is necessary in fewer than 5% of all SVC obstruction cases.
- Diagnostic evaluation should proceed with the least invasive procedures performed initially, followed by more invasive procedures as needed to obtain histologic diagnosis:
  1. Chest radiography
  2. Sputum cytology
  3. Thoracentesis with cytologic evaluation of fluid
  4. Node biopsy if a palpable node is present; avoid fine-needle aspiration if lymphoma is suspected
  5. Fiber-optic bronchoscopy with endobronchial ultrasound
  6. Mediastinoscopy with video-assisted imaging
  7. Thoracostomy with video-assisted imaging
- Evaluation may vary depending on the age and sex of the patient:
  1. In older adults (i.e., ≥50 yr), the most common cause of SVC obstruction is lung cancer; lymphoma and metastatic cancer are less common, and benign processes are uncommon.
  2. In young adults (<50 yr old), the most common cause of SVC obstruction is lymphoma (usually large cell or lymphoblastic lymphoma; rarely Hodgkin disease). Lung cancer and thoracic malignancy are less common. Germ cell cancer (almost never in female patients) and benign causes are uncommon. The preceding evaluation should be modified to include the following studies before more invasive procedures are performed:
     a. Serum tumor markers (e.g., β-human chorionic gonadotropin, α-fetoprotein, and lactate dehydrogenase)
     b. Bone marrow aspiration and biopsy

From Niederhuber JE: *Abeloff's clinical oncology,* ed 6, Philadelphia, 2020, Elsevier.

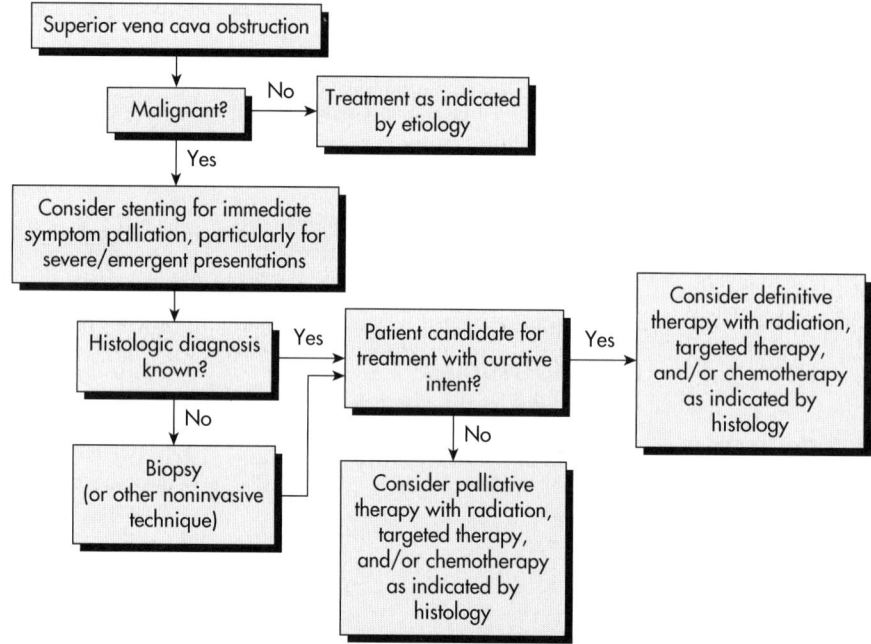

FIG. 5 A management algorithm for superior vena cava obstruction. (From Niederhuber JE: *Abeloff's clinical oncology,* ed 6, Philadelphia, 2020, Elsevier.)

cancer treatment within 1 week or if an obstructing thrombus has been documented.
- Loop diuretics are often used, but their effect is limited.
- Steroids (e.g., dexamethasone 4 mg q6h) may be useful in reducing the tumor burden in lymphoma and thymoma after definitive diagnosis is made.

- Fig. 5 illustrates a management algorithm for superior vena cava obstruction.

REFERRAL
- To a thoracic surgeon, pulmonary specialist, and/or oncologist

REFERENCES

Available at eBooks.Health.Elsevier.com.

AUTHORS: **CHELSIE ANDERSON, MD, MS,** and **LORRIANA E. LEARD, MD**

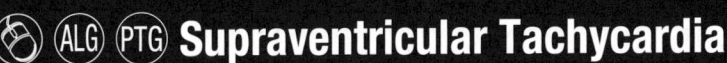

S

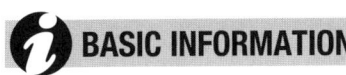 **BASIC INFORMATION**

DEFINITION

Supraventricular tachycardia (SVT) refers to a group of rapid regular tachyarrhythmia. There are three major categories of SVT:

1. Atrial tachycardia (AT): An arrhythmia that originates from the atrium and does not involve the AV node. This is usually a focal arrhythmia. In some cases, the underlying mechanism may be a reentry circuit, either a small circuit (micro-reentry) or a large circuit (macro-reentry)
2. AV nodal reentrant tachycardia (AVNRT)
3. AV reentrant tachycardia (AVRT) (Fig. 1)

The latter two are reentrant arrhythmia that always involve the AV node as part of the circuit (see Fig. 1).

Other forms of arrhythmia that involve the atria, such as atrial fibrillation and atrial flutter, have distinct electrocardiographic features and are covered in separate chapters. Rare forms of SVT such as inappropriate sinus tachycardia, sinus mode reentry tachycardia, and junctional tachycardia are beyond the scope of this chapter.

SYNONYMS

SVT
Paroxysmal supraventricular tachycardia
PSVT

ICD-10CM CODE
I47.1 Supraventricular tachycardia

EPIDEMIOLOGY & DEMOGRAPHICS

The exact epidemiology of SVT is difficult to estimate because there is poor differentiation between SVT and atrial fibrillation/flutter in the literature. According to older reports from the U.S., the estimated prevalence of SVT was 225/100,000 persons and estimated incidence was 35/100,000 persons/yr.[1] Yet, most contemporary data suggest a remarkable rise in the prevalence and incidence of SVT in the U.S., which were estimated at 332.9/100,000 people and 57.8/100,000 people/yr, respectively.[2] SVT is most commonly diagnosed between the second and fourth decades of life and mostly in patients without prior cardiac conditions.[3] AVNRT is the most common type of SVT in both genders and in all ages, but is most common among young women.[4] AVRT is the second most common SVT, and it is typically diagnosed in younger patients as compared to the age of patients with AVNRT.[4] AT is more commonly associated with structural heart disease.[4]

PHYSICAL FINDINGS & CLINICAL PRESENTATION

- Patients may be either symptomatic or asymptomatic.
- Patient may be aware of "fast" regular heartbeat (but sometimes complain of irregular heartbeat, palpitations); may complain of weakness, dyspnea, dizziness, chest pain, presyncope or, rarely, syncope.[5]

- Patients with AVNRT may complain of neck pounding during the episode due to simultaneous contraction of the atria and ventricles with closed AV valves causing a sharp increase in atrial and jugular venous pressure.[6]
- In some cases the episodes can be triggered by physical activity or psychological stress, but in others there may not be an obvious trigger.[5] In patients with AVNRT, sometimes the arrhythmia is reproducibly initiated when bending forward to pick up an item from the floor.[7]
- Hemodynamic status during the arrhythmia may vary and depend on the patient's comorbidities and presence of underlying structural heart disease. Usually, patients are hemodynamically stable.[7]
- Physical examination is most commonly normal and unrevealing, except rapid regular heart rate and occasionally hypotension. In patients with AVNRT sharp tall jugular vein A waves may be seen when the right atrium contracts against a closed tricuspid valve.[6]

ETIOLOGY (SEE FIG. 1)

- AVNRT: Dual electrical pathways within the AV node. In typical AVNRT the anterograde limb conducts slowly (slow pathway), and the retrograde limb has fast conduction properties (fast pathway), and vice versa in atypical AVNRT.[3]
- AVRT is accessory pathway mediated, either orthodromic (antegrade through the AV node and retrograde through the accessory pathway) or, much less commonly, antidromic (antegrade through the accessory pathway and retrograde through the AV node). In the case of antidromic tachycardia, the QRS will be wide and fully preexcited. In some patients, the presence of accessory pathway is not

evident on the baseline ECG (concealed accessory pathway), while in others it is manifest in the baseline ECG, presenting the typical features of the Wolff-Parkinson-White (WPW) syndrome.
- Paroxysmal atrial tachycardia and multifocal atrial tachycardia: Abnormal automaticity of atrial tissue or triggered activity. In some cases (especially in patients who underwent previous cardiac surgery such as valve replacement or atrial septal defect [ASD] closure), the underlying mechanism is macroreentrant AT.[3]

Dx DIAGNOSIS

The diagnosis of SVT relies principally on the 12-lead ECG. Every patient suspected of having an episode of SVT should have a 12-lead ECG done immediately. Typically, patients with SVT will present with a narrow complex QRS tachycardia with a ventricular rate faster than 100 beats per minute (bpm) and typically faster than 130 to 150 bpm.[8]

P wave morphology can be useful in discriminating rhythms. P waves with a similar axis to the sinus node can be atrial tachycardias and sinus tachycardias. P waves with retrograde depolarization of the atria (seen as inverted in the inferior leads) can be seen in AVNRT, AVRT, and atrial tachycardia. Sawtooth P waves are indicative of atrial flutter, and an absence of P waves with irregular R-R intervals points to atrial fibrillation. Variable (>3) morphologies of P wave are suggestive of multifocal atrial tachycardia. Wide QRS complex (>0.12 sec) with initial slurring (delta wave) during sinus rhythm and short PR (<0.12 sec) is characteristic of Wolff-Parkinson-White syndrome.

In typical AVNRT, due to the small size of the circuit within the AV node and the fast retrograde

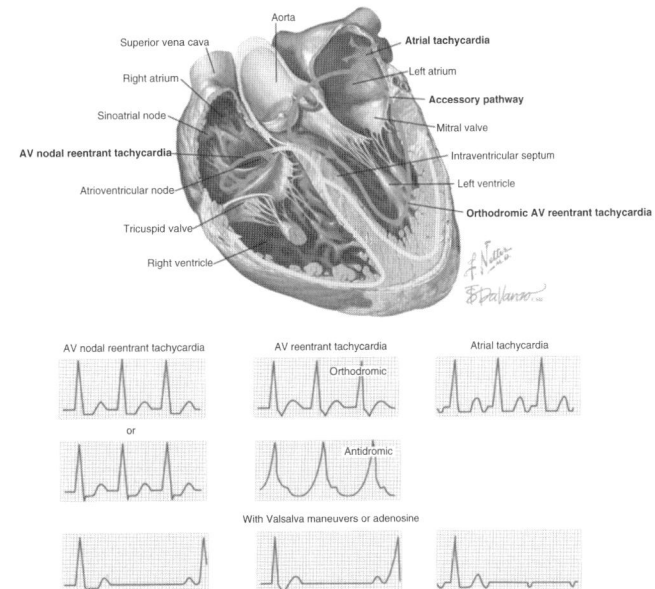

FIG. 1 Typical electrocardiographic recordings and anatomic representation of the common supraventricular tachycardias. (From Runge MS et al [eds]: *Netter's cardiology,* ed 2, Philadelphia, 2010, Saunders. Adapted from Delacretaz E: Clinical practice: supraventricular tachycardia, *N Engl J Med* 354:1039-1051, 2006.)

conduction, there is simultaneous depolarization of the ventricles and atria, thus making the P wave "buried" in the QRS and therefore not visible or inscribed very close to the QRS at the final part of the QRS complex, and sometimes creating a "pseudo terminal S wave" usually seen in leads II, III, and aVF and "pseudo terminal R waves" at the end of the QRS in V1 and avR[3,8] (see Fig. 1).

In orthodromic AVRT, the P wave is usually visible close after the QRS due to the rapid conduction properties of the accessory pathway (short RP tachycardia). In AT, the P wave is usually noticed farther away after the QRS (long RP tachycardia)[3,8] (see Fig. 1). A unique form of orthodromic AVRT termed *paroxysmal junctional reentrant tachycardia* (PJRT) involves a concealed accessory pathway, usually located in the posteroseptal region, and typically presents with deeply inverted retrograde P waves in leads II, III, and aVF, with a long RP interval.[9]

Other diagnostic maneuvers that may assist in the differential diagnosis are vagal maneuvers (such as carotid sinus massage) or giving intravenous AV nodal blocking agents (such as adenosine or verapamil) to produce AV nodal conduction block. This will terminate reentrant arrhythmia dependent on the AV node—AVNRT and AVRT—but not AT, which will continue, albeit with nonconducted P waves.[10,11]

Other arrhythmias that present with narrow complex tachycardia like PSVT are:
- Fascicular VT
- Junctional tachycardias
- Artifact such as with Parkinson disease

SVT can conduct with bundle branch block (BBB) and wide QRS either due to preexisting BBB on the baseline ECG or due to aberrant conduction (rapid rate–dependent BBB). When a patient presents with wide QRS tachycardia, VT must be excluded first.[12] Features to distinguish SVT from ventricular tachycardia are outlined in Table 1.

WORKUP

- Electrocardiography
- Echocardiography to exclude structural heart disease
- Thyroid function tests
- Complete blood count to exclude anemia or infection as an underlying trigger for the event
- In most cases the workup will be negative, with no underlying cardiac or systemic pathology and no clear triggers for an acute episode
- Holter or event monitor to document the arrhythmias if they are paroxysmal and not documented yet

🆁🆇 TREATMENT (FIG. 2)

NONPHARMACOLOGIC THERAPY

Acute termination: If the patient is hemodynamically unstable, prompt synchronized cardioversion with an external deflbrillator using 50 to 100 J should be performed.[10,11]

If the patient is stable, Valsalva maneuver in the supine position is the most effective way to terminate most types of SVT; carotid sinus massage (after excluding occlusive carotid disease and murmurs over the carotid arteries) is also commonly used to elicit vagal efferent impulses. These are effective in terminating AVRT, AVNRT, and may occasionally terminate some types of atrial tachycardia, but in the case of sinus

TABLE 1 Features That May Differentiate Ventricular Tachycardia From Supraventricular Tachycardia With Aberrancy

Helpful Features	Implications
Positive QRS concordance	Diagnostic of VT
Presence of AV dissociation, capture beats, or fusion beats	Diagnostic of VT
R to S interval >100 ms in any one precordial lead	Suggests VT
Atypical RBBB (monophasic R, QR, RS, or triphasic QRS in V_1; R:S ratio <1, QS or QR, monophasic R in V_6)	Suggests VT
Atypical LBBB (R >30 min or R to S [nadir or notch] >60 min in V_1 or V_2; R:S ratio <1, QS or QR in V_6)	Suggests VT
Shift of axis from baseline	Suggests VT
History of CAD	Suggests VT
QRS during tachycardia identical to QRS during sinus rhythm	Suggests SVT
Termination with adenosine	Suggests SVT

AV, Atrioventricular; *CAD*, coronary artery disease; *LBBB*, left bundle branch block; *RBBB*, right bundle branch block; *SVT*, supraventricular tachycardia; *VT*, ventricular tachycardia.
From Stambler BS et al: Etripamil nasal spray for rapid conversion of supraventricular tachycardia to sinus rhythm, *J Am Coll Cardiol* 72:489-497, 2018.

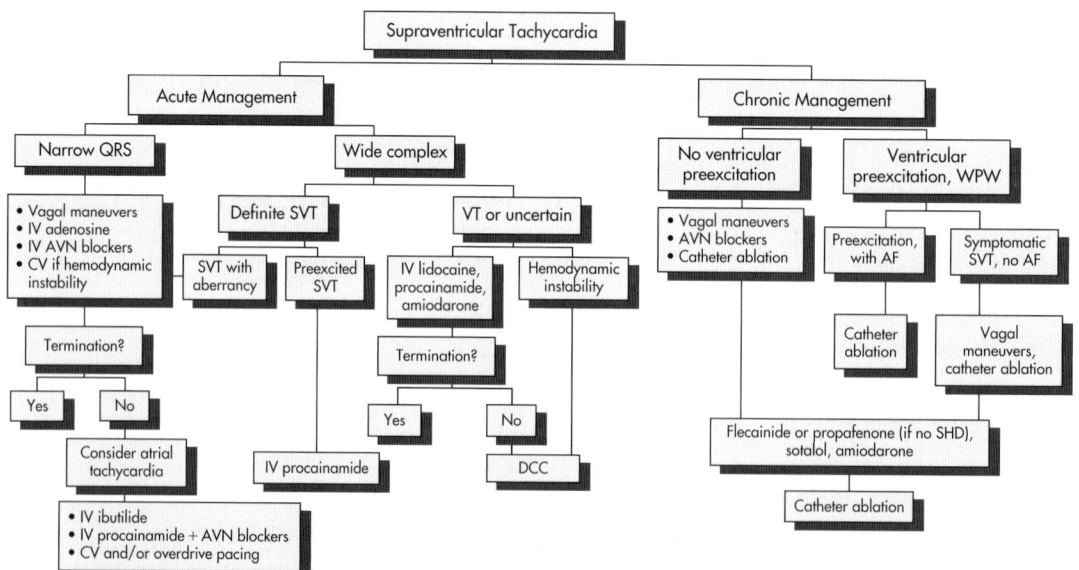

FIG. 2 Supraventricular tachycardia. *AF,* Atrial fibrillation; *AVN,* atrioventricular node; *DCC,* direct current cardioversion; *CV,* cardioversion; *IV,* intravenous; *SHD,* structural heart disease (no overt evidence of myocardial, valvular, congenital, or coronary heart disease); *SVT,* supraventricular tachycardia; *VT,* ventricular tachycardia; *WPW,* Wolff-Parkinson-White. (From Olshansky B et al: *Arrhythmia essentials,* ed 2, Philadelphia, 2017, Elsevier.)

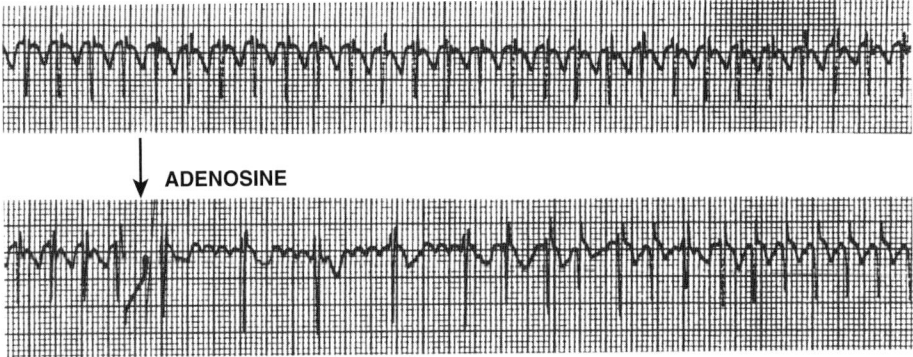

FIG. 3 Adenosine can uncover the mechanism of supraventricular tachycardia. A 3-month-old infant developed an extremely fast, narrow QRS complex tachycardia and a heart rate of 220 beats/min after insertion of a central line through a jugular vein. Adenosine produced a transient atrioventricular block and unmasked very rapid atrial fibrillation waves (570 beats/min). (From Park MK: *Park's pediatric cardiology for practitioners,* ed 6, Philadelphia, 2014, Elsevier.)

tachycardia, atrial flutter, and atrial fibrillation, they only transiently slow down AV conduction without terminating the actual tachycardia.[10,11]

ACUTE TREATMENT

- Adenosine is useful to terminate acutely orthodromic AVRT and AVNRT and can uncover the underlying rhythm in paroxysmal atrial tachycardia (Fig. 3); it is the first choice of therapy for treatment of almost all episodes of SVT unresponsive to vagal maneuvers. The dose is 6 mg given as a rapid IV bolus; tachycardia is usually terminated within a few seconds. If this fails, one may repeat with 12 mg IV bolus for up to two times. Contraindications are second- or third-degree atrioventricular block; WPW with atrial fibrillation; sick sinus syndrome; and chronic use of drugs such as dipyridamole, theophylline, or aminophylline; and heart transplant. Adenosine may cause bronchospasm in asthmatics as well as chest discomfort, flushing, and shortness of breath, but these usually last for a very short time and serious adverse effects are extremely rare due to the drug's very short half-life.[10,11]
- Verapamil 5 to 10 mg IV is given over 5 min; if no effect, may repeat in 30 min.
  1. Verapamil should be used cautiously in patients with SVT associated with hypotension and should not be used in patients with heart failure with reduced ejection fraction or those who are under regular beta-blocker treatment.
  2. Slow injection of calcium chloride (10 ml of a 10% solution given over 5 to 8 min before verapamil administration) decreases the hypotensive effect without compromising its antiarrhythmic effect.[10,11]

- Metoprolol (IV 5 mg/2 min up to 15 mg) or esmolol (500 μg/kg IV bolus, then 50 μg/kg/min) may be effective in the treatment of SVT.[10,11]
  1. IV digoxin (0.75 to 1 mg slow IV loading in increments of 0.25 mg over several hours) is rarely used in SVT but may tried if other agents are not effective.
  2. Digoxin, beta-blockers, and calcium channel blockers should be avoided in patients with preexcitation syndrome and antidromic AVRT or preexcited atrial fibrillation to avoid increased conduction through the accessory pathway.
- Etripamil, a novel fast-acting intranasal calcium channel blocker, has been suggested to be effective in rapid conversion of SVT to sinus rhythm.[13] The efficacy and safety of this new drug in treating SVT are currently examined in several randomized clinical trials. This drug may prove in the future to be an important treatment modality but is not yet approved for routine clinical use.

ONGOING MANAGEMENT

The main goal of treatment is the prevention of recurrent episodes and eliminating symptoms. Current guidelines recommend referring patients with recurrent, symptomatic SVT to catheter ablation, which is a highly effective mode of treatment with a low risk of complications.[10,11] Recent studies show that ablation therapy is highly effective, safe, and associated with a very low recurrence rate.[14] If catheter ablation therapy is not desirable or feasible, regular treatment with beta blockers or nondihydropyridine calcium channel blockers can be tried; if these fail, class Ic antiarrhythmics are optional.[10,11] Rarely, when all other treatments fail or are contraindicated, class

III antiarrhythmics, such as amiodarone or sotalol, may be tried.[10,11] In patients with infrequent and minimally symptomatic episodes without preexcitation, it is optional to provide treatment only during acute episodes with a "pill-in-the-pocket" strategy with either beta-blockers or other antiarrhythmics.[10,11]

DISPOSITION

Most patients respond well with resolution of the SVT upon treatment (see "Acute General Rx"). Some patients may need chronic AV blocking agents for recurrence.

Radiofrequency ablation (RFA) is the procedure of choice in symptomatic patients with SVT and particularly in AVRT, AVNRT, and atrial flutter.[10,11] RFA has high efficacy rates (single procedure success is 93.2%), low all-cause mortality (0.1%), and low adverse events (2.9%). Recent technologic developments provided the ability to perform RFA with no to minimal radiation using advanced electroanatomic mapping systems and intracardiac echocardiography.[15] Despite high reported success rates and high safety profile, RFA appears to be underused in clinical practice.

REFERENCES & SUGGESTED READINGS

Available at eBooks.Health.Elsevier.com.

RELATED CONTENT

Supraventricular Tachycardia (Patient Information)

AUTHORS: **GAL TSABAN, MD, MPH,** and **YUVAL KONSTANTINO, MD**

Syncope 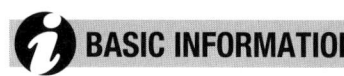 ⒜ ⒢ ⓢ

ⓘ BASIC INFORMATION

DEFINITION

Syncope is a symptom that presents with an abrupt, transient, complete loss of consciousness, associated with inability to maintain postural tone, with rapid and spontaneous recovery. The presumed mechanism is cerebral hypoperfusion. There are three major types: Neurocardiogenic, orthostatic, and cardiac. Syncope is a symptom, and the goal is to distinguish lethal causes from benign causes of transient loss of consciousness.

ICD-10CM CODE
R55 Syncope and collapse

EPIDEMIOLOGY & DEMOGRAPHICS[1-3]

- Syncope accounts for 1% to 3% of emergency department visits and 6% of hospital admissions.
- 40% of the adult population will experience at least one syncopal episode during their lifetimes.
- Incidence of syncope is highest in elderly men and young women.
- 15% of children and adolescents experience syncope; fewer than 5% have cardiac causes.
- Older age (>60 yr), males, known ischemic or structural heart disease, previous arrhythmias, brief or absent prodrome, syncope during exertion or in the supine position, abnormal cardiac examination, family history of inheritable conditions or premature sudden cardiac death, and presence of known congenital heart disease are all associated with increased risk for cardiac etiology of syncope.

PHYSICAL FINDINGS & CLINICAL PRESENTATION

- Blood pressure: If low, consider orthostatic hypotension; if unequal in both arms (difference >20 mm Hg), consider subclavian steal or dissecting aneurysm. (NOTE: Blood pressure [BP] and heart rate [HR] should be recorded in the supine and standing positions, waiting at least 5 min between each position.) If there is a drop in BP but no change in HR, the patient may be taking a β-blocker or may have an autonomic neuropathy.
- Pulse: If patient has tachycardia, bradycardia, or irregular rhythm, consider arrhythmia.
- Heart: If there are murmurs present, consider syncope attributable to left ventricular outflow obstruction (aortic stenosis or idiopathic hypertrophic subaortic stenosis); if there are jugular venous distention and distal heart sounds, consider cardiac tamponade.
- Carotid sinus pressure: Can be diagnostic if it reproduces symptoms and other causes are excluded; a pause >3 sec or a systolic BP drop >50 mm Hg without symptoms or <30 mm Hg with symptoms when sinus pressure is applied separately on each side for <5 sec is considered abnormal. This test should be avoided in patients with carotid bruits or cerebrovascular disease. ECG monitoring,

intravenous (IV) access, and bedside atropine should be available when carotid sinus pressure is applied.

ETIOLOGY

- Consider blood pressure equation: MAP – RAP = CO × resistance
  1. Where MAP = mean arterial pressure, RAP = right atrial pressure or central venous pressure, CO = cardiac output = heart rate × stroke volume
  2. Transient drop in heart rate, stroke volume, and/or resistance causes syncope
- Neurocardiogenic or neurally mediated syncope: Most common type, accounting for two thirds of cases. It includes vasovagal, situational, carotid hypersensitivity, and postexertional syncope (Box 1).
  1. Psychophysiologic (emotional upset, panic disorders, hysteria, hyperventilation)
  2. Visceral reflex (micturition, defecation, food ingestion, coughing, ventricular contraction, glossopharyngeal neuralgia)
  3. Carotid sinus pressure
  4. Reduction of venous return caused by Valsalva maneuver
  5. Postural tachycardia syndrome (POTS)
- Orthostatic hypotension (10% of cases):
  1. Hypovolemia
  2. Vasodilator medications
  3. Neurogenic orthostatic hypotension (primary autonomic failure, Parkinson disease, multiple system atrophy)
  4. Autonomic neuropathy (diabetes, amyloid)
  5. Pheochromocytoma
  6. Carcinoid syndrome
- Cardiac (10% to 20%):
  1. Reduced cardiac output – which should be transient, quickly reversible or compensated by increased resistance:
     a. Left ventricular obstruction (aortic stenosis, hypertrophic cardiomyopathy)
     b. Obstruction to pulmonary flow (pulmonary embolism, pulmonic stenosis, primary pulmonary hypertension); prevalence of pulmonary embolism in patients hospitalized for first episode of syncope up to 17% (mean age 76 yr)[4]
     c. Myocardial infarct with pump failure
     d. Cardiac tamponade
     e. Mitral stenosis
     f. Reduction of venous return (atrial myxoma, valve thrombus)
     g. Aortic dissection
     h. β-blocker therapy

BOX 1 Causes of Syncope

Reflex Syncopal Syndromes
- Vasovagal faint (common faint)
- Carotid sinus syncope
- Situational faint:
  1. Acute hemorrhage
  2. Cough, sneeze
  3. Gastrointestinal stimulation (swallow, defecation, visceral pain)
  4. Micturition (postmicturition)
  5. Postexercise
  6. Pain, anxiety
- Glossopharyngeal and trigeminal neuralgia

Orthostatic
- Aging
- Antihypertensives
- Autonomic failure:
  1. Primary autonomic failure syndromes (e.g., pure autonomic failure, multiple system atrophy, Parkinson disease with autonomic failure)
  2. Secondary autonomic failure syndromes (e.g., diabetic neuropathy, amyloid neuropathy)
- Medications
- Volume depletion:
  1. Hemorrhage, diarrhea, Addison disease, diuretics, febrile illness, hot weather

Cardiac Arrhythmias
- Sinus node dysfunction (including bradycardia-tachycardia syndrome)
- Atrioventricular conduction system disease
- Paroxysmal supraventricular and ventricular tachycardias
- Implanted device (pacemaker, implantable cardioverter defibrillator) malfunction
- Drug-induced proarrhythmias

Structural Cardiac or Cardiopulmonary Disease
- Cardiac valvular disease:
  1. Acute myocardial infarction, ischemia
  2. Obstructive cardiomyopathy
  3. Atrial myxoma
  4. Acute aortic dissection
  5. Pericardial disease, tamponade
  6. Pulmonary embolus, pulmonary hypertension

Cerebrovascular
- Vascular steal syndromes

Multifactorial

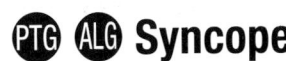
TABLE 1 Drugs That Can Cause or Contribute to Syncope

Drug	Mechanism
Diuretics	Volume depletion
Vasodilators:	Reduction in systemic vascular resistance and venodilation
• Angiotensin-converting enzyme inhibitors	
• Calcium channel blockers	
• Hydralazine	
• Nitrates	
• α-Adrenergic blockers	
• Prazosin	
Other antihypertensive drugs:	Centrally acting antihypertensives
• α-Methyldopa	
• Clonidine	
• Guanethidine	
• Hexamethonium	
• Labetalol	
• Mecamylamine	
• Phenoxybenzamine	
Drugs associated with torsades de pointes:	Ventricular tachycardia associated with a prolonged QT interval
• Amiodarone	
• Disopyramide	
• Encainide	
• Flecainide	
• Quinidine	
• Procainamide	
• Sotalol	
Digoxin	Cardiac arrhythmias
Psychoactive drugs:	Central nervous system effects causing hypotension; cardiac arrhythmias
• Tricyclic antidepressants	
• Phenothiazines	
• Monoamine oxidase inhibitors	
• Barbiturates	
Alcohol	Central nervous system effects causing hypotension; cardiac arrhythmias

From Fillit HM: *Brocklehurst's textbook of geriatric medicine and gerontology*, ed 8, Philadelphia, 2017, Elsevier.

2. Arrhythmias or asystole:
   a. Extreme tachycardia (>160 to 180 beats/min)
   b. Severe bradycardia (<30 to 40 beats/min)
   c. Sick sinus syndrome
   d. Atrioventricular block (second or third degree)
   e. Ventricular tachycardia or fibrillation
   f. Long QT syndrome, with R-on-T leading to polymorphic ventricular tachycardia
   g. Pacemaker malfunction, leading to bradycardia
   h. Psychotropic medications and beta-blockers (Table 1)

DX DIAGNOSIS

DIFFERENTIAL DIAGNOSIS

- Seizure (Table 2)
- Vertebrobasilar transient ischemic attack (TIA) usually manifests as diplopia, vertigo, or ataxia but not loss of consciousness. Isolated episodes of transient loss of consciousness (TLOC, Fig. E1) without accompanying neurologic symptoms are unlikely to be TIAs
- Recreational drugs or alcohol
- Functional causes such as somatoform disorders
- Sleep disorders, such as sleep attacks and narcolepsy, are also in the differential for TLOC
- Head trauma

WORKUP

The history is crucial to diagnosing the cause of syncope and may suggest a diagnosis that can be evaluated with directed testing. History is also important to determine other etiologies for TLOC, such as seizure.

- Sudden loss of consciousness (LOC): Consider cardiac arrhythmias.
- Gradual LOC: Consider orthostatic hypotension, vasodepressor syncope, hypoglycemia.
- History of aura before LOC or prolonged confusion (>1 min), amnesia, or lethargy after LOC suggests seizure rather than syncope.
- Patient's activity at the time of syncope:
  1. Micturition, coughing, defecation: Consider syncope caused by decreased venous return.
  2. Turning head or while shaving: Consider carotid sinus syndrome.
  3. Physical exertion in a patient with murmur: Consider aortic stenosis or hypertrophic obstructive cardiomyopathy.
  4. Arm exercise: Consider subclavian steal syndrome.
  5. Assuming an upright position: Consider orthostatic hypotension.
- Associated events:
  1. Chest pain: Consider myocardial infarction, pulmonary embolism.
  2. Palpitations: Consider arrhythmias or POTS.
  3. Incontinence (urine or fecal) and tongue biting are associated with seizure or syncope.
  4. Brief, transient shaking after LOC may represent myoclonus from global cerebral hypoperfusion and not seizures. However, sustained tonic/clonic muscle action is more suggestive of seizure.
  5. Focal neurologic symptoms or signs point to a neurologic event such as a seizure with residual deficits (e.g., Todd paralysis) or cerebral ischemic injury.
  6. Psychologic stress: Syncope may be vasovagal.
  7. Multiple nonspecific symptoms (fatigue, diffuse weakness, headache, "brain fog," exercise intolerance, "coat hanger sign") can be seen in POTS and neurogenic orthostatic hypotension.
- Review current medications, particularly anti-hypertensive and psychotropic drugs.
- Table 3 differentiates syncope caused by neutrally mediated hypotension, arrhythmias, seizures, and psychogenic causes.
- Fig. 2 illustrates an approach to the evaluation of syncope.

LABORATORY TESTS

Routine blood tests rarely yield diagnostically useful information and should be done only if they are specifically suggested by the results of the history and physical examination. The following are commonly ordered tests:

- Pregnancy test in women of childbearing age
- CBC to look for anemia and signs of infection
- Electrolytes, blood urea nitrogen, creatinine, magnesium, and calcium to look for electrolyte abnormalities and evaluate fluid status
- Serum glucose level
- Cardiac troponins, especially if the patient gives a history of chest pain before the syncopal episode
- Drug and alcohol levels with suspected toxicity

IMAGING STUDIES

- ECG to rule out arrhythmias in all patients; may be diagnostic in 5% to 10% of patients.
- Echocardiography: Indicated in patients where initial evaluation suggests structural heart disease (based on physical exam and/or ECG) or have known heart disease.
- Exercise stress testing can be useful to establish the cause of syncope in selected patients who experience syncope or pre-syncope during exertion.

TABLE 2 Clinical Features That Help Distinguish a Generalized Tonic-Clonic Seizure From Syncope

	Seizure	Syncope
Clinical context and circumstances	Neurologic or systemic conditions that predispose to seizures, family history of seizures. Mental fatigue, sleep deprivation, alcohol use or withdrawal, systemic illness	Cardiovascular disorders, dehydration, anemia. Family history of syncope
Triggers	Usually none (unless reflex epilepsy)	Orthostatic hypotension, venipuncture, painful and noxious stimuli, emotional stress, micturition, Valsalva maneuver
Clinical features		
• Onset	No warning unless there is a warning symptom. Abrupt loss of consciousness, generalized stiffening, and fall. Occurs in any position	Tiredness, nausea, diaphoresis, tunneling of vision. Loss of consciousness over few seconds and fall. Occurs usually standing
• Course	Prominent tonic phase then clonic movements lasting about 1 min, cyanosis, labored breathing, may bite tongue or cheeks, sometimes urinary incontinence	Usually loss of tone, pallor, multifocal myoclonic jerks lasting <15 sec, sometimes urinary incontinence, usually no tongue or cheek biting
• Offset	Postictal sleepiness and confusion lasting up to hours, headache, myalgia	Rapid recovery over seconds to less than few minutes, no confusion, headache, or myalgia. May have fatigue

From Goldman L, Schafer AI: *Goldman-Cecil medicine*, ed 26, Philadelphia, 2019, Elsevier.

TABLE 3 Differentiation of Syncope Caused by Neurally Mediated Hypotension, Arrhythmias, Seizures, and Psychogenic Factors

	Neurally Mediated Hypotension	Arrhythmias	Seizures	Psychogenic
Demographics and clinical setting	Female > male sex Younger age (<55 yr) More episodes (>2) Standing, warm room, emotional upset	Male > female sex Older age (>54 yr) Fewer episodes (<3) During exertion or when supine Family history of sudden death	Younger age (<45 yr) Any setting	Female > male sex Occurs in presence of others Younger age (<40 yr) Many episodes (often many episodes in a day) No identifiable trigger
Premonitory symptoms	Longer duration (>5 sec) Palpitations Blurred vision Nausea Warmth Diaphoresis Lightheadedness	Shorter duration (<6 sec) Palpitations less common	Sudden onset or brief aura (déjà vu, olfactory, gustatory, visual)	Usually absent
Observations during the event	Pallor Diaphoresis Dilated pupils Slow pulse, low BP Incontinence may occur Brief clonic movements may occur	Blue, not pale Incontinence may occur Brief clonic movements may occur	Blue face, no pallor Frothing at the mouth Prolonged syncope (duration >5 min) Tongue biting Horizontal eye deviation Elevated pulse and BP Incontinence more likely* Tonic-clonic movements if grand mal	Normal color Not diaphoretic Eyes closed Normal pulse and BP No incontinence Prolonged duration (minutes) common
Residual symptoms	Residual symptoms common Prolonged fatigue common (>90%) Oriented	Residual symptoms uncommon (unless prolonged unconsciousness) Oriented	Residual symptoms common Aching muscles Disorientation Fatigue Headache Slow recovery	Residual symptoms uncommon Oriented

BP, Blood pressure.

*May be observed with any of these causes of syncope but more common with seizures.

From Zipes DP: *Braunwald's heart disease: a textbook of cardiovascular medicine*, ed 11, Philadelphia, 2019, Elsevier.

- If seizure is suspected, MRI of the brain and electroencephalogram may be useful.
- If head trauma or neurologic signs on examination, computed tomography (CT) or MRI may be helpful.

- If arrhythmias are suspected, a 24-h Holter monitor or admission to a telemetry unit in high risk patients is appropriate. In general, Holter monitoring is rarely useful, revealing a cause for syncope in <3% of cases. Loop recorders

that can be activated after syncopal episode to retrieve information about the cardiac rhythm during the preceding 4 min add considerable diagnostic yield in patients with unexplained syncope.

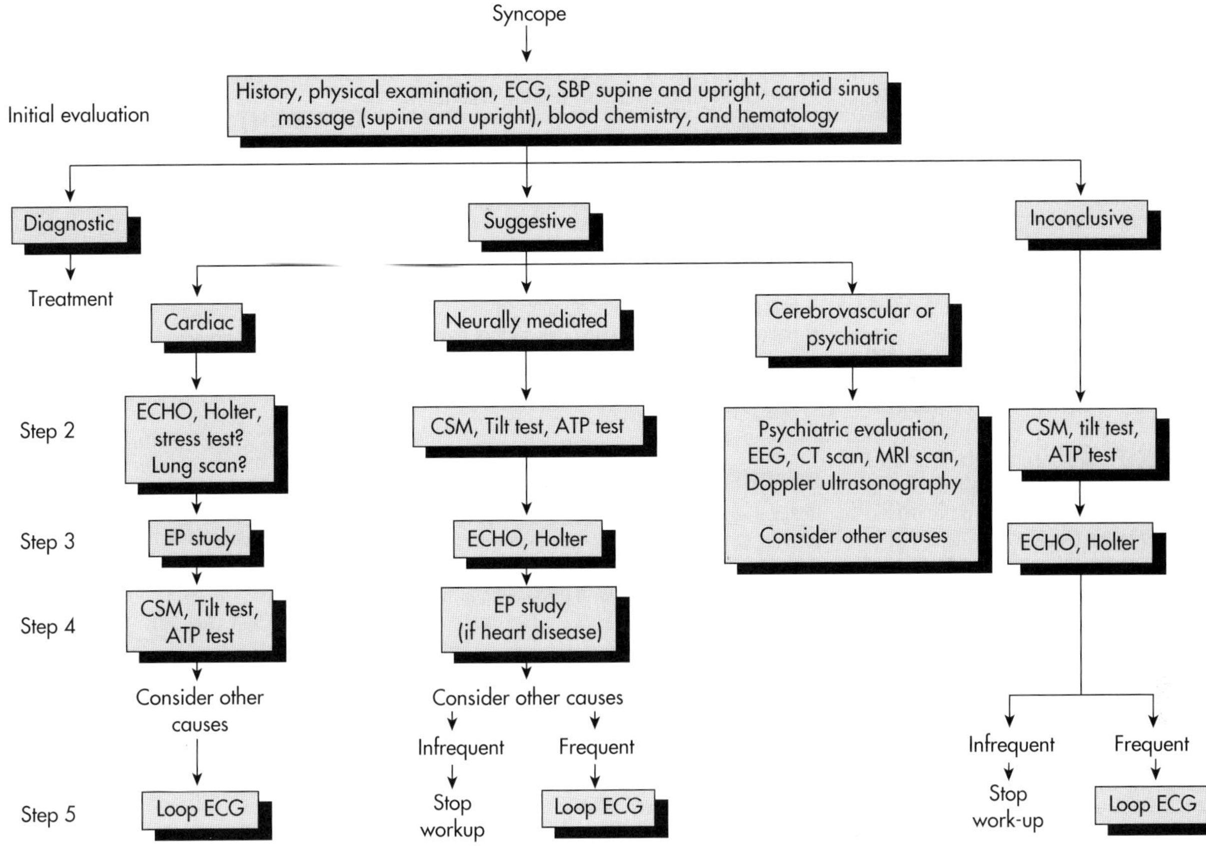

Syncope

History, physical examination, ECG, SBP supine and upright, carotid sinus massage (supine and upright), blood chemistry, and hematology

Initial evaluation

Diagnostic   Suggestive   Inconclusive

Treatment

Cardiac   Neurally mediated   Cerebrovascular or psychiatric

Step 2   ECHO, Holter, stress test? Lung scan?   CSM, Tilt test, ATP test   Psychiatric evaluation, EEG, CT scan, MRI scan, Doppler ultrasonography   CSM, tilt test, ATP test

                                                                              Consider other causes

Step 3   EP study   ECHO, Holter   ECHO, Holter

Step 4   CSM, Tilt test, ATP test   EP study (if heart disease)

         Consider other causes   Consider other causes

                                    Infrequent   Frequent   Infrequent   Frequent

Step 5   Loop ECG   Stop workup   Loop ECG   Stop work-up   Loop ECG

FIG. 2 An approach to the evaluation of syncope for all age groups. *ATP test,* Adenosine provocation test; *CSM,* carotid sinus massage; *CT,* computed tomography; *ECG,* electrocardiogram; *ECHO,* echocardiogram; *EEG,* electroencephalography; *EP study,* electrophysiologic study; *MRI,* magnetic resonance imaging; *SBP,* systolic blood pressure. (From Fillit HM: *Brocklehurst's textbook of geriatric medicine and gerontology,* ed 8, Philadelphia, 2017, Elsevier.)

- Implantable cardiac monitors that function as permanent loop recorders or implantable cardioverter-defibrillators, which are placed subcutaneously in the pectoral region with the patient under local anesthesia, are useful in patients with cardiac syncope.
- Electrophysiologic studies may be indicated in patients with structural heart disease and/or recurrent syncope. The diagnostic yield of EPS was approximately 50% and 10% in patients with and without structural heart disease, respectively.

TILT-TABLE TESTING

- Useful to support a diagnosis of neuro-cardiogenic syncope. Patients age >50 yr should have stress testing before tilt-table testing. Positive results would preclude tilt-table testing.
- Indicated in patients with recurrent episodes of unexplained syncope as well as patients in high-risk occupations (e.g., pilots, bus drivers). The test is also useful for identifying patients with prominent bradycardic response who may benefit from implantation of a permanent pacemaker. The test is contraindicated in patients with recent stroke, MI, and severe coronary or carotid disease.
- It is performed by keeping the patient strapped in an upright posture on a tilt table with

footboard support. The angle of the tilt table varies from 60 to 80 degrees. The duration of upright posture during tilt-table testing varies from 25 to 45 min.
- The hallmark of neurocardiogenic syncope is severe hypotension associated with a paradoxical bradycardia triggered by a specific stimulus. The diagnosis of neurocardiogenic syncope is likely if upright tilt testing reproduces these hemodynamic changes in <15 min and causes presyncope or syncope.
- Postural orthostatic tachycardia syndrome is diagnosed if there is a sustained heart rate increase of not less than 30 beats/min (40 beats/min if age <18 yr old) and above 120 beats/min within 10 min of active standing or head-up tilt without associated orthostatic hypotension and with reproduction of symptoms.

PSYCHIATRIC EVALUATION

- May be indicated in young patients without heart disease who have frequently recurring transient loss of consciousness and other somatic symptoms.
- Generalized anxiety disorder, pain disorder, and major depression predispose patients to neurally mediated reactions and may result in syncope.

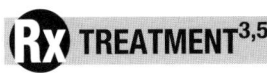 **TREATMENT**[3,5]

NONPHARMACOLOGIC THERAPY

- Education about condition, avoidance of triggers, reassurance of benign nature of neuro-cardiogenic syncope.
- Ensure proper hydration; consider compression stockings and salt tablets in appropriate patients.
- Perform physical counter-pressure maneuvers if sufficient prodrome.
- Eliminate medications that may induce hypotension.
- Elevate the head of the bed by 10 to 30 degrees while sleeping.
- There is uncertainty in orthostatic training/exercise for sustained benefit.

ACUTE GENERAL Rx

- Varies with the underlying etiology of syncope (e.g., pacemaker in patients with syncope resulting from bradycardia or prolonged pauses). Clinical variables for identification of high-risk syncope patients who may benefit from hospitalization or an accelerated outpatient evaluation are summarized in Table E4.
- Syncope caused by orthostatic hypotension is treated with volume replacement in patients with intravascular volume depletion. Also

consider midodrine to promote venous return by adrenergic-mediated vasoconstriction and fludrocortisone for its mineralocorticoid effects to increase intravascular volume, although these medications can cause supine hypertension. Droxidopa is approved for neurogenic orthostatic hypotension in pure autonomic failure or multiple system atrophy.

- The alpha-1 agonist midodrine (starting dose 2.5 mg bid and titrated as tolerated) is effective for the prevention of vasovagal syncope in young healthy patients with frequent vasovagal syncope.[6]
- Beta-blockers in older patients (>42 yr) and selective-serotonin reuptake inhibitors may be considered for recurrent neurocardiogenic syncope.
- Catheter-based cardioneural ablation may have a role in targeting atrial ganglionic plexi to treat refractory cases of neurocardiogenic syncope. The largest multicenter registry (n = 71, 13 sites) in the U.S. showed 82% free of syncope at 8.5-mo median follow-up after single ablation.

DISPOSITION

Prognosis varies with the age of the patient and the etiology of the syncope. In general:

- Benign prognosis (very low 1-yr morbidity rate) in patients:
  1. Age <30 yr and having noncardiac syncope
  2. Age <70 yr and having vasovagal or psychogenic syncope or syncope of unknown cause
- Poor prognosis (high mortality and morbidity rates) in patients with cardiac syncope, with presenting systolic BP <90 mm Hg.
- Patients with the following risk factors have a higher 1-yr mortality rate: Abnormal ECG, history of ventricular arrhythmia, history of congestive heart failure.

REFERRAL

Hospital admission in elderly patients without prior history of syncope or unknown etiology of their syncope and in any patients suspected of having cardiac syncope, with presenting systolic BP <90 mm Hg

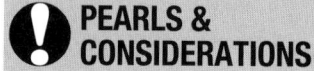

PEARLS & CONSIDERATIONS

COMMENTS

- The etiology of syncope is identified in <50% of cases during the initial evaluation.
- A thorough history and physical examination are the most productive means of establishing a diagnosis in patients with syncope.
- Driving restrictions vary based on state but consider restricting driving if syncope is frequent or unpredictable.

REFERENCES

Available at eBooks.Health.Elsevier.com.

RELATED CONTENT

Syncope (Patient Information)
Orthostatic Hypotension (Related Key Topic)

AUTHOR: **WILSON LAM, MD**

Diseases and Disorders

I

BASIC INFORMATION

DEFINITION

In healthy individuals, the expected physiologic response to serum hypotonicity is inhibition of the hypothalamic synthesis and posterior pituitary gland release of antidiuretic hormone/arginine vasopressin (ADH/AVP). Decreased binding to renal medullary collecting duct vasopressin receptors results in the increased excretion of urine that is dilute (low osmolality) and hypotonic (low sodium and potassium concentrations). The syndrome of inappropriate antidiuresis (SIAD) is defined by inappropriately concentrated urine in patients with hypotonic hyponatremia and normal extracellular fluid (ECF) volume. In the absence of an elevated serum glucose or exogenous osmole such as mannitol, the serum sodium concentration (S_{Na}) is essentially determined by the ratio of total body exchangeable sodium and potassium ($Na_e + K_e$) (mmol) to total body water (TBW) (L).[1]

Hyponatremia results from a reduction in total body exchangeable sodium and potassium ($Na_e + K_e$), increase in TBW, or both. To correct hyponatremia, the normal, appropriate renal response is excretion of urine with (Na + K) concentrations significantly less than serum sodium (S_{Na}). In SIAD, TBW is increased primarily by expansion of the volume of electrolyte-free water (EFW), which is water essentially devoid of Na and K. The severity of hyponatremia in SIAD is determined by the magnitude of electrolyte-free fluid intake and of the urinary dilution defect (the patient's minimum urine osmolality). The definition of SIAD excludes hemodynamic stimuli that stimulate ADH, including reduced ECF volume (decreased total body sodium content), hypotension, and disorders characterized by decreased effective arterial blood volume. The latter group is characterized by increased ECF volume (edema or ascites) from increased total body sodium content. This group includes cardiac disease (e.g., congestive heart failure or chronic pericardial disease), nephrotic syndrome, and cirrhosis.

The term *syndrome of inappropriate antidiuretic hormone* (SIADH) has fallen into disfavor because 10% to 15% of so-called SIADH patients manifest suppressed or undetectable serum ADH concentrations. The group with suppressed ADH may have renal collecting duct cells with increased sensitivity to ADH, secretion of other ADH-like peptides, or altered renal hemodynamics that reduce sodium and water delivery to distal diluting sites, thereby preventing maximal urinary dilution. Establishing a diagnosis of SIAD does not require the measurement of ADH levels. Patients with adrenal insufficiency are excluded from the definition of SIAD. Hypothyroidism has been considered a cause of SIADH previously but is no longer because bioscientific evidence of thyroid hormone influencing water metabolism is lacking. Instead, hyponatremia may result from impaired cardiac output (heart failure) in severe cases of hypothyroidism (i.e., myxedema). SIAD should not be diagnosed in acute or chronic kidney disease.

SYNONYMS

SIADH
SIAD
Syndrome of inappropriate antidiuretic hormone secretion
Syndrome of inappropriate ADH release
Inappropriate secretion of antidiuretic hormone

ICD-10CM CODE
E22.2 Syndrome of inappropriate secretion of antidiuretic hormone

EPIDEMIOLOGY & DEMOGRAPHICS

INCIDENCE: Hyponatremia occurs in nearly 14% of hospitalized patients and represents an acquired disorder in the majority of cases. Nearly half of these patients have SIAD. The adjusted odds ratio for in-hospital mortality in patients with hyponatremia at hospital admission is 1.47 (95% confidence interval, 1.33 to 1.62).

PHYSICAL FINDINGS & CLINICAL PRESENTATION

- SIAD is defined as an S_{Na} <130 mmol/L persisting for more than 48 hr with normal ECF volume with concentrated urine (Uosm >50 to 100) and in the absence of the exclusion criteria noted earlier. Patients are hemodynamically stable with no evidence of edema, ascites, pleural effusion, or pulmonary congestion.
- Manifestations: Weakness, dizziness, headache, nausea, vomiting, muscle cramps in mild exercise-associated hyponatremia (EAH)[2]; confusion, vomiting, seizure, coma, ataxia, collapse, and dyspnea (severe EAH); fever and delirium after 3,4-methylenedioxymethamphetamine (MDMA, ecstasy) administration; stigmata of alcoholism or malnutrition, fever and/or localizing symptoms related to pneumonia or other pulmonary disease, or headaches and visual field defects from an intracranial mass.
- If hyponatremia occurs rapidly, namely, in less than 24 hr, delirium, lethargy, or seizures may occur. Diminished reflexes and extensor plantar responses may occur with severe hyponatremia or an S_{Na} <120 mmol/L.
- Neurologic abnormalities, including ataxia, mood changes, and proximal muscle weakness, are frequent in chronic hyponatremia. Abnormalities may be subtle despite severe hyponatremia.

ETIOLOGY

- Drugs: Thiazide diuretics[3] and selective serotonin reuptake inhibitor (SSRI) antidepressants are the two most common causes of drug-related hyponatremia. Narcotic analgesics, carbamazepine, phenothiazines, tricyclic antidepressants, MDMA (ecstasy), nicotine, clofibrate, haloperidol, nonsteroidal antiinflammatory drugs (NSAIDs), monoamine oxidase inhibitors, chlorpropamide, vasopressin, desmopressin, oxytocin, and chemotherapeutic agents (vincristine,

cyclophosphamide), proton pump inhibitors[4] represent additional etiologies
- Neoplasms: Lung, oropharynx, stomach, duodenum, pancreas, brain, thymus, bladder, prostate, endometrium, mesothelioma, lymphoma, and Ewing sarcoma
- Pulmonary disorders: Coronavirus disease (SARS-CoV-2, COVID-19),[5] pneumonia, aspergillosis, pulmonary abscess, tuberculosis, bronchiectasis, emphysema, cystic fibrosis, status asthmaticus, and respiratory failure associated with positive-pressure breathing
- Intracranial pathology: Trauma, neoplasms, infections (meningitis, encephalitis, brain abscess), hemorrhage, hydrocephalus, multiple sclerosis, and Guillain-Barré syndrome
- Postoperative period: Surgical stress, positive pressure ventilation, anesthetic agents, and pain
- Other: Acute intermittent porphyria, psychosis, delirium tremens, general anesthesia, and EAH (associated with extreme endurance exercise such as marathon running)
- Table 1 summarizes common etiologies of SIAD

DIFFERENTIAL DIAGNOSIS[6]

- Hyponatremia associated with subclinical hypovolemia
- Solute-limited water excretion (e.g., "tea-and-toast" diet, beer-drinker's potomania); an acquired disorder in which the renal capacity to excrete sufficient EFW is impaired from an insufficient osmolar intake (sodium and potassium) and/or metabolism (generation of urea from protein metabolism)
- Primary polydipsia or water intake that exceeds renal dilutional capability and is frequently accompanied by solute-limited water excretion
- Endocrine disorders, including hypothyroidism and adrenal insufficiency
- Severe hypokalemia produces hyponatremia because the exchangeable potassium pool is twice the size of the exchangeable sodium pool. When intracellular potassium is in severe deficit, the resulting intracellular osmolality shifts water from the intracellular to extracellular space. Additionally, sodium ions exit the plasma, enter cells, and cause hyponatremia
- Hypertonic hyponatremia (hyperglycemia, iatrogenic administration of mannitol, sorbitol, glycine)
- Hyponatremia from subclinical heart or liver disease
- Pseudohyponatremia caused by extreme hyperglobulinemia or hyperlipidemia
- Reset osmostat: ADH regulation occurs at a lower-than-normal osmotic threshold, with intact urinary dilution and concentration
- Cerebral salt wasting syndrome (CSWS) in critically ill neurologic patients (Table E2)

WORKUP

- Normal ECF volume by history and physical examination. No history of large-volume fluid

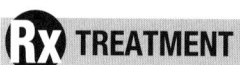

TABLE 1 Common Etiologies of the Syndrome of Inappropriate Antidiuretic Hormone Secretion (SIADH)

Tumors

Pulmonary/mediastinal (bronchogenic carcinoma, mesothelioma, thymoma)

Extrapulmonary (duodenal carcinoma, pancreatic carcinoma, ureteral/prostate carcinoma, uterine carcinoma, nasopharyngeal carcinoma, leukemia)

Central Nervous System Disorders

Mass lesions (tumors, brain abscesses, subdural hematoma)

Inflammatory diseases (encephalitis, meningitis, systemic lupus erythematosus, acute intermittent porphyria, multiple sclerosis)

Degenerative/demyelinating diseases (Guillain-Barré syndrome, spinal cord lesions)

Miscellaneous (subarachnoid hemorrhage, head trauma, acute psychosis, delirium tremens, pituitary stalk section, transsphenoidal adenomectomy, hydrocephalus)

Drug-Related

Stimulated release of AVP (nicotine, phenothiazines, tricyclics)

Direct renal effects and/or potentiation of AVP antidiuretic effects (desmopressin, oxytocin, prostaglandin synthesis inhibitors)

Mixed or uncertain actions (ACE inhibitors, carbamazepine and oxcarbazepine, chlorpropamide, clofibrate, clozapine, cyclophosphamide, 3,4-methylenedioxy-methamphetamine [ecstasy], omeprazole; serotonin reuptake inhibitors [SSRIs], vincristine)

Pulmonary

Infections (tuberculosis, acute bacterial and viral pneumonia, aspergillosis, empyema)

Mechanical/ventilatory causes (acute respiratory failure, COPD, positive-pressure ventilation)

Other Causes

Acquired immunodeficiency syndrome (AIDS) and AIDS-related complex

Prolonged strenuous exercise (marathon, triathlon, ultramarathon, hot-weather hiking)

Senile atrophy

Idiopathic

ACE, Angiotensin-converting enzyme; *AVP,* arginine vasopressin; *COPD,* chronic obstructive pulmonary disease.
From Melmed S: *Williams textbook of endocrinology,* ed 12, Philadelphia, 2011, Saunders.

TABLE 3 Diagnostic Criteria for the Syndrome of Inappropriate Antidiuretic Hormone Release

Essential Diagnostic Criteria

Decreased extracellular fluid effective osmolality ($<$270 mOsm/kg H_2O)Inappropriate urinary concentration ($>$100 mOsm/kg H_2O)

Clinical normovolemia

Elevated urinary sodium concentration under conditions of normal salt and water intake

Absence of adrenal, thyroid, or pituitary insufficiency

Absence of chronic kidney disease

Absence of diuretic use

Supplemental Criteria

Abnormal water loading test (inability to excrete at least 90% of a 20 ml/kg H_2O load in 4 hours and/or failure to dilute urine osmolality to $<$100 mOsm/kg H_2O). Plasma vasopressin level inappropriately elevated relative to the plasma osmolality

No significant correction of S_{Na} with volume expansion, but improvement after fluid restriction

---

S_{Na}, Serum sodium.
From Floege J et al: *Comprehensive clinical nephrology,* ed 4, Philadelphia, 2010, Saunders.

losses. No generalized edema, ascites, pulmonary congestion, or large pleural effusions

- Laboratory evaluation (see "Laboratory Tests") is consistent with excessive ADH secretion or sensitivity in the absence of osmotic or hemodynamic stimuli for ADH secretion
- Normal thyroid, adrenal, and cardiac function
- No recent or concurrent use of loop diuretics
- Failure to correct hyponatremia after ECF volume repletion by isotonic 0.9% saline solution
- Correction of hyponatremia solely by fluid restriction is generally unsuccessful
- Diagnostic criteria for SIADH are described in Table 3

LABORATORY TESTS

- Normal or low blood urea nitrogen (BUN) and/or serum creatinine
- S_{Na} lower than the limit of the normal range
- Decreased serum osmolality ($<$270 mOsm/kg H_2O) corrected for serum glucose, BUN, and exogenous osmoles
- Decreased serum uric acid concentration
- Urine osmolality $>$100 mOsm/kg H_2O with simultaneous plasma hypoosmolality; that is, plasma osmolality $<$270 mOsm/kg H_2O
- Urine Na concentration is generally $>$40 mmol/L with normal dietary salt intake

IMAGING STUDIES

Imaging is not routinely required for diagnosis. Imaging may facilitate the diagnosis of an associated underlying pulmonary or central nervous system (CNS) disease or rule out intracranial pathology.

Rx TREATMENT

NONPHARMACOLOGIC THERAPY

With mild SIAD, fluid restriction (10 to 15 ml/kg per day) combined with increased solute loads (diets high in protein, urea powder, sodium chloride, and potassium chloride) may normalize S_{Na}. The enhanced solute load produces an osmotic diuresis that increases EFW loss. Urea administration should be undertaken with a consulting nephrologist; it has been proven safe for decades[7] and is sold in the U.S. as a "medical food supplement."

ACUTE GENERAL Rx
PHARMACOLOGIC THERAPY:
Rate of Correction: In chronic hyponatremia, it is critical to avoid overly rapid correction of S_{Na} correction to prevent brain injury from osmotic demyelination syndrome.[8] Patients with moderate-to-severe hyponatremia should undergo serial monitoring of S_{Na} and serum potassium concentration (S_K), urine volumes, and urine chemistries (osmolality, K, and Na). Most SIAD patients have chronic hyponatremia (developing over more than 24 to 48 hr) and mild symptoms. Target S_{Na} correction rates are

6 to 8 mmol/L per day in chronic hyponatremia. The S_{Na} should be actively lowered in patients who experience increases of $>$10 mmol/L during a 24-hr period. The rate of S_{Na} change during conservative therapy or 0.9% infusion is often slow or flat because sodium is excreted while water is mostly retained. In cases of hyponatremia from undiagnosed ECF volume depletion or a limitation of EFW excretion due to inadequate urinary solute (tea and toast diet or beer potomania), administration of saline may produce rapid excretion of large volumes of hypotonic urine with overly rapid S_{Na} correction. Therefore close monitoring of serum and urine electrolytes, osmolality, and volume is always recommended.

Acute Hyponatremia: In patients with acute hyponatremia (duration $<$24 hr), the goal of therapy is to increase S_{Na} sufficiently to prevent or reduce the severity of cerebral edema. S_{Na} should be increased by up to 4 to 6 mmol/L within the first 3 hr if symptoms are mild to moderate and within the initial hour with severe symptoms (seizures, coma, obtundation).

Rapid correction of S_{Na} in acute hyponatremia may involve hypertonic saline therapy (3% saline, 513 mmol/L). As a general rule, 1 ml/kg body weight of 3% saline is expected to increase S_{Na} by 1 mmol/L. S_{Na} correction rates may be greater than anticipated when unrecognized ECF volume depletion is concurrently corrected. The simultaneous delivery of the synthetic ADH analog desmopressin can mitigate S_{Na} overcorrection. Intravenous furosemide therapy may augment urinary EFW loss and prevent unintended ECF volume expansion during hypertonic saline therapy, which is contraindicated in individuals with heart failure.

Chronic Hyponatremia: The therapeutic goals of chronic hyponatremia from SIAD are normalization of TBW and restoration of Na and K stores to their respective normal levels. These goals may be achieved as follows.

- Choose a 24-hr target S_{Na}, based on current S_{Na} and safe rates of correction (see "Rate of Correction").
- Estimate TBW and total body cation content. Estimation of current TBW should consider the patient's baseline TBW, volume of additional retained water, and changes in total body content of sodium and potassium (see example that follows).
- Account for all sources of EFW intake and loss (including insensible losses). Add/subtract this total volume to/from net target EFW to determine total EFW volume loss required to attain the target S_{Na}.
- Select a strategy that achieves target EFW volume loss: Collecting duct arginine vasopressin receptor-2 antagonist (e.g., tolvaptan), oral urea therapy, or loop diuretic combined with electrolyte replacement such as sodium chloride (salt) tablets with 17 mmol sodium per 1 g of NaCl.

The following example demonstrates the method to determine the target TBW and EFW loss required to reach an appropriate S_{Na} target after 24 hr of therapy in a patient with chronic hyponatremia.

- S_{Na} is 115 mmol/L in 75 kg, minimally symptomatic older woman who chronically takes an SSRI and hydrochlorothiazide.
  1. *Step 1: Establish target S_{Na}:*
     a. Target S_{Na} after 24 hr = Current S_{Na} + 6 = 121 mmol/L
  2. *Step 2: Estimate current TBW and total body cations:*
     a. Current weight = 75 kg
     b. Estimated TBW fraction = 0.55 (55%)
     c. Current TBW = 0.55 × 75 = 41.2 L
     d. Current total body cation quantity = Current TBW × S_{Na} = 41.2 × 115 = 4743 mmol
  3. *Step 3: Calculate target TBW:*
     a. Target TBW (L) = Current [TBNa$_e$ + TBK$_e$]/Target S_{Na} = 4743 mmol/ 121 mmol/L = 39.2 L
  4. Step 4: Calculation of net EFW loss:
     a. Target net EFW loss after 24 hr = Current TBW − Target TBW = 41.2 L − 39.2 L = 2 L
  5. *Step 5: Calculate total urine EFW volume:*
     a. Target total urine EFW excretion (estimate: 1 L oral fluid intake and 0.5 L net insensible loss) Urine EFW volume = 2 + (1 − 0.5) = 2.5 L
  6. *Step 6: Choose therapeutic strategy*

  7. *Step 7: Implement strategy and monitor results frequently*

Loop Diuretic Plus Saline Strategy: Before the advent of specific arginine vasopressin receptor-2 antagonists, SIAD was typically treated by increasing urine volume and EFW loss with a loop diuretic. In the earlier example a 24-hr net EFW loss of 2.5 L is required. With loop diuretic administration, roughly a 5 L urine output is required to reduce TBW appropriately. The urine can be functionally considered half-normal saline (0.45% saline). The urine may be considered as two proportions: An electrolyte-free fraction, representing 2.5 L of pure water, and 2.5 L of isotonic saline, with the urine cation concentrations of Na and K equaling a concentration of sodium in 0.9% saline. Cation losses can be repaired with 0.9% saline or 3% saline. Administration of the latter requires 70% less volume than 0.9% saline and elevates S_{Na} more rapidly. Alternatively, cation replacement may be carried out by oral administration of NaCl and KCl tablets. Periodic monitoring of S_{Na}, S_K, urine volume, and urine chemistries (osmolality, sodium, and potassium) is recommended to prevent overly rapid correction of S_{Na}.

The use of hypertonic saline solutions should be guided by an expert. Urine potassium loss cannot be ignored, and these losses are corrected separately.

Arginine Vasopressin Receptor Antagonists: Selective arginine vasopressin receptor antagonist therapy is straightforward and convenient for patients and medical personnel. Currently, two agents are available in the U.S: Intravenous (IV) conivaptan (20 mg IV once followed by continuous IV infusion of 20 to 40 mg/day for 2 to 4 days) and oral tolvaptan (15 to 90 mg/day, as needed). Tolvaptan must be initiated in-hospital. Urinary electrolyte losses are minimal, meaning that administration produces virtually electrolyte-free urines. In the earlier example, the dose would be titrated to produce a daily urine output of 2.5 L. Urine output in excess of this amount would require quantitative replacement with oral water or intravenously as D_5W until the effects of the AVP agonist wore off (in approximately 12 to 24 hr in the case of tolvaptan).

CHRONIC Rx

- When SIAD is chronic, fluid restriction (<15 ml/kg per day) may be required indefinitely and combined with high dietary electrolyte and protein.

- NaCl tablets, electrolyte supplements, protein powders to generate urea production, and pharmaceutical-grade urea may be used to correct hyponatremia. Periodic monitoring of electrolytes is recommended in patients with chronic SIAD.
- Tolvaptan has been administered successfully in clinical trials. FDA labeling states that initial therapy must take place in-hospital. Tolvaptan use is restricted to 30 days due to concerns regarding hepatotoxicity, which was detected during clinical trials for polycystic kidney disease. Additional contraindications include volume contraction and concomitant use of strong cytochrome P3A inhibitors. Patients undergoing tolvaptan therapy are not fluid-restricted.
- Demeclocycline variably increases urine EFW losses. This agent is contraindicated in hepatic disease and rarely used today.

DISPOSITION

- Mortality exceeding 40% has been reported in patients with S_{Na} <110 mmol/L.
- Hospital readmission rates are common in chronic SIAD when an underlying cause cannot be eliminated, especially if patients are unwilling or unable to restrict their fluid intake and follow dietary recommendations.
- Chronic, mild-to-moderate hyponatremia is associated with bone loss, falls, and increased fracture risk, particularly in older patients.

REFERRAL

Emergency department evaluation and hospital admission are appropriate for moderate-to-severe hyponatremia due to SIAD, especially when acute or symptomatic. Due to a high complication risk from overly aggressive or ineffective treatment, consultation by a nephrologist, endocrinologist, or critical care physician is recommended.

REFERENCES & SUGGESTED READINGS
Available at eBooks.Health.Elsevier.com.

RELATED CONTENT

Syndrome of Inappropriate Secretion of Antidiuretic Hormone (Patient Information)
Salt-Losing Nephropathy (Related Key Topic)

AUTHOR: **MARK D. FABER, MD, MACM**

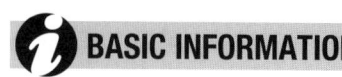
BASIC INFORMATION

DEFINITION

Syphilis is a systemic sexually transmitted disease caused by the spirochete *Treponema pallidum,* with acute and chronic manifestations, characterized by primary skin lesions; secondary eruption involving skin and mucous membranes; long periods of latency; and late lesions of the skin, bone, viscera, central nervous system, and cardiovascular system.[1]

ICD-10CM CODES

A50	Congenital syphilis
A51.0	Primary genital syphilis
A51.1	Primary anal syphilis
A51.2	Primary syphilis of other sites
A51.3	Secondary syphilis of skin and mucous membranes
A51.4	Other secondary syphilis
A51.5	Early syphilis, latent
A51.9	Early syphilis, unspecified
A52	Late syphilis
A52.0	Cardiovascular and cerebrovascular syphilis
A52.1	Symptomatic neurosyphilis
A52.2	Asymptomatic neurosyphilis
A52.3	Neurosyphilis, unspecified
A52.8	Late syphilis, latent
A52.9	Late syphilis, unspecified
A53.9	Syphilis, unspecified

EPIDEMIOLOGY & DEMOGRAPHICS

- Most diagnosed in people 20 to 30 yr old in urban areas and among people of lower socioeconomic status.
- Rates reached historic lows in the U.S. in 2000 but began increasing in 2001 with a continued increase observed. The number of cases reported to the U.S. Centers for Disease Control and Prevention (CDC) increased by 71% from 2014 to 2018, with men accounting for 85% of all cases. Additionally, rates are disproportionately higher among African American and Hispanic men and women, along with men who have sex with men (MSM). Rates of primary and secondary syphilis among women more than doubled between 2014 and 2018, and congenital syphilis rates are also increasing secondary to this.[2,3]

PHYSICAL FINDINGS & CLINICAL PRESENTATION

PRIMARY SYPHILIS[1]:

- Characteristic lesion is a painless chancre on genitalia, most commonly on the penis, cervix, or vagina (Figs. E1 and E2); mouth; or anus.
- May appear 3 days to 12 wk with median around 3 wk postexposure. May resolve without treatment within 6 wk.

SECONDARY SYPHILIS[1]:

- Bacteremia, also called spirochetemia, is associated with generalized lymphadenopathy and a characteristic maculopapular rash, including the palms, soles, trunk, and mucous membranes. Constitutional, flulike symptoms

may also occur, as well as mild disturbances of multiple organ systems. Typically occurs 4 to 6 wk after appearance of chancre and can resolve within 1 wk to 12 mo even without treatment. Of note, there can be relapsing episodes up to 5 yr after the initial episode.
- 60% to 80% have maculopapular lesions on palms and soles (Fig. E3).
- 21% to 58% have mucocutaneous or mucosal lesions (pharyngitis, tonsillitis, "mucous patch" lesion on oral and genital mucosa).
- Condylomata lata intertriginous papules (raised, gray-white lesions) form at areas of friction and moisture, such as the vulva (Fig. E4).

LATENT SYPHILIS—EARLY VS. LATE LATENT[1]:

- Generally asymptomatic, can occur between 1 and 30 yr after a primary infection. Early latent applies to relapses that occur within 1 yr, whereas late latent occurs more than 1 yr after acquisition.
- Seroreactivity is seen without other evidence of primary or secondary disease. Without treatment, one third will progress to tertiary syphilis.

TERTIARY SYPHILIS[1]:

- One half of patients with tertiary syphilis have late benign syphilis characterized by gummas (nodular, ulcerative lesions) that can involve the skin, mucous membranes, skeletal system, and viscera.
- One fourth of patients with tertiary syphilis will have manifestations of cardiovascular syphilis, including aortitis, aneurysm, or aortic regurgitation.
- Manifestations of the central nervous system (CNS); "neurosyphilis," which may be asymptomatic or symptomatic; tabes dorsalis; meningovascular syphilis; general paralysis; or insanity may occur.
- Manifestations of the eye, "ocular syphilis," which can affect any part of the eye, with posterior uveitis being the most common, iritis, choroidoretinitis, and leukoplakia may also occur. The Argyll Robertson pupil, a pupil that does not react to light but accommodates, is pathognomonic of tertiary syphilis.

ETIOLOGY

- *Treponema pallidum,* a spirochete
- Spread by sexual intercourse or by intrauterine transfer

DIAGNOSIS

DIFFERENTIAL DIAGNOSIS

- Other genitoulcerative diseases such as herpes or chancroid (Table 1)

WORKUP

Essentials of a proper sexual history are summarized in Table 2.
- Confirmation is primarily through laboratory diagnosis. Culture of lesions
- Serologic testing (see the following lab tests)

- Cerebrospinal fluid (CSF) testing

LABORATORY TESTS

- Dark-field microscopy of fluid from lesion to look for treponeme is the definitive method for diagnosis of early syphilis. Typically done if a chancre is cultured. It is then sent to the lab for dark-field microscopy.
- Serologic testing:
  1. Nontreponemal tests are sensitive to disease: Venereal Disease Research Laboratory (VDRL) or rapid plasma reagin (RPR).
  2. Treponemal tests are specific to disease: Fluorescent treponemal antibody absorbed (FTA-ABS) tests, the *T. pallidum* passive particle agglutination (TP-PA) assay, various enzyme immunoassays (EIAs), chemiluminescence immunoassays, immunoblots, or rapid treponemal assays.
  3. Antibody titers are used to assess for response to treatment and for reinfection in previously treated patients.
- Screening methods:
  1. Most traditional and most used include screening with nontreponemal tests (sensitive: VDRL, RPR), with confirmation using the treponemal tests (specific: FTA-ABS, TP-PA).
- Lumbar puncture (LP) is used for cerebrospinal fluid VDRL (CSF-VDRL) in patients with evidence of latent syphilis (good specificity, poor sensitivity). If negative with high suspicion, can also perform a CSF FTA-ABS (good sensitivity, less specificity). When reactive in the absence of substantial contamination of CSF with blood, it is considered diagnostic of neurosyphilis. The CDC indications for LP are not commonly used, but are needed in cases of neurologic symptoms, treatment failure, any eye or ear involvement, or evidence of active syphilis (aortitis, gumma, iritis).
- HIV testing in all patients.

TREATMENT[1,4] (BOX E1)

ACUTE GENERAL Rx

- Primary, secondary, early latent:
  1. Penicillin G benzathine 2.4 million U intramuscularly (IM) once.
  2. Infants and children: Benzathine penicillin G 50,000 units/kg IM, up to the adult dose of 2.4 million units in a single dose.
  3. Nonpregnant penicillin-allergic patients: Doxycycline 100 mg bid × 14 days. For pregnancy, patients are admitted as an inpatient and desensitized from penicillin allergy and then are treated with penicillin G once.
  4. Alternative regimens (contraindicated in MSM, persons with HIV, or pregnant women):
     a. Azithromycin 2 g by mouth (PO) × 1 dose
     b. Ceftriaxone 1 to 2 g IM or intravenous (IV) for 10 to 14 days
     c. Tetracycline 500 mg PO qid for 14 days

TABLE 1 Genital Ulcer Disease

Disease	Lesions	Lymphadenopathy	Systemic Symptoms
Primary syphilis	**Painless,** indurated, with a clean base, usually singular	Nontender, rubbery, nonsuppurative bilateral lymphadenopathy	None
Genital herpes	**Painful** vesicles, shallow, usually multiple	Tender, bilateral inguinal adenopathy	Present during primary infection
Chancroid	Tender papule, then **painful,** undermined purulent ulcer, single or multiple	Tender, regional, painful, suppurative nodes	None
Lymphogranuloma	Small, **painless** vesicle or papule progresses to an ulcer	Painful, matted, large nodes with fistulous tracts	Present after genital lesion heals

From Wein AJ et al: *Campbell-Walsh urology,* ed 11, Philadelphia, 2016, Elsevier.

TABLE 2 Essentials of the Sexual History

The Five Ps of the Sexual History	Essential Points to Cover
Partners	Last 3 mo who, how many, where from, risk factors in partners?
Practices	Is sexual contact vaginal, oral, anal and with whom? Are condoms used sometimes, always, never?
Protection	How is risk reduced (e.g., monogamy, condoms)?
Pregnancy	Plans around becoming or preventing pregnancy and details of contraception used
Past STIs	In patient and partners—what infections, when and how were they treated, how were they followed up? Screening since?

STIs, Sexually transmitted infections.
From Cameron P et al: *Textbook of Adult Emergency Medicine,* ed 5, 2019, Elsevier Edinburgh, Australia.

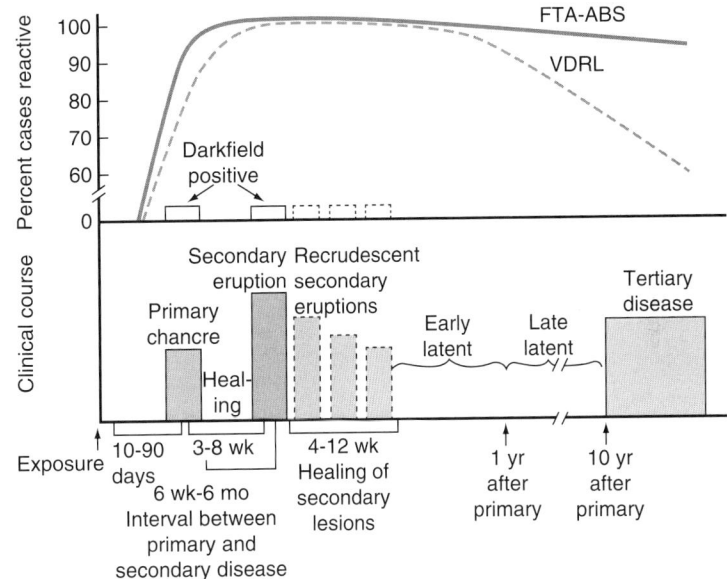

FIG. 6 The course of untreated syphilis. *FTA-ABS,* Fluorescent treponemal antibody absorption; *VDRL,* Venereal Disease Research Laboratory. (From Cherry JD et al: *Feigin and Cherry's textbook of pediatric infectious diseases,* ed 8, Philadelphia, 2019, Elsevier.)

d. Amoxicillin 3 g PO bid + probenecid 500 mg PO bid for 14 days
• Late latent syphilis, tertiary syphilis (not neurosyphilis):
1. Penicillin G benzathine 2.4 million U IM weekly × 3 wk
2. Infants and children: Benzathine penicillin G 50,000 units/kg IM, up to the adult dose of 2.4 million units in a single dose
3. Nonpregnant penicillin-allergic patients: Doxycycline 100 mg PO bid × 4 wk
• Neurosyphilis:
1. Aqueous crystalline penicillin G 18 to 24 million U/day, administered as 3 to 4 million U IV q4h or continuous infusion for 10 to 14 days
2. Alternative regimen: Procaine penicillin 2.4 million U IM/day plus probenecid 500 mg PO qid, both for 10 to 14 days
• Congenital syphilis:
1. Aqueous crystalline penicillin G 50,000 U/kg/dose IV q12h × first 7 days of life and q8h after that for a total of 10 days OR procaine penicillin G 50,000 U/kg/dose IM/day × 10 days
2. An algorithm for evaluation and treatment of infants born to mothers with reactive serologic tests for syphilis is illustrated in Fig. E5

DISPOSITION

Repeat quantitative nontreponemal tests at 6 and 12 mo to ensure adequate treatment. For HIV-infected patients, repeat testing at 3, 6, 9, 12, and 24 mo. Pregnancy requires monthly tests until delivery.
• Findings indicating need for retreatment of syphilis and additional testing for HIV:
1. If a fourfold increase in titer occurs and is sustained over testing performed >2 wk apart
2. If initial high titer fails to drop by fourfold within a year for early syphilis or 24 mo for late syphilis
3. If signs persist or patient develops new signs of infection
• Because treatment failure may be the result of unrecognized CNS infection, CSF examination can be considered in such situations. For retreatment, weekly infusions of benzathine penicillin G 2.4 million units IM for 3 wk is recommended, unless CSF examination indicates that neurosyphilis is present.
• Pregnant women without a fourfold drop in titer by 6 mo compared to pretreatment titer need to be retreated. Inadequate treatment is likely if patient delivers fewer than 30 days

after treatment or if titers are fourfold higher than pretreatment at delivery. Titers should be repeated monthly during pregnancy for those infected.
• Cases should be reported to local or state health department for referral, follow-up, and partner notification.

REFERRAL

Pregnant and possible congenital syphilis
• Pregnant and allergic to penicillin who need to be desensitized for treatment
• Late latent syphilis with serious central nervous system, cardiovascular, or other organ system compromise

⊘ PEARLS & CONSIDERATIONS

• Jarisch-Herxheimer reaction (fever, myalgia, tachycardia, hypotension) may occur within 24 h of treatment.
• Fig. 6 illustrates the course of untreated syphilis. One third of untreated patients develop CNS and/or cardiovascular sequelae.
• Up to 80% of those treated during late stages remain seropositive indefinitely.

- Treponemal tests remain positive even after adequate therapy.
- Male circumcision does not decrease the incidence of syphilis (unlike HIV, herpes simplex virus 2 [HSV-2], and human papillomavirus [HPV] infection).
- Partner notification and treatment:
  1. Persons who are exposed within 90 days preceding the diagnosis of primary, secondary, or early latent syphilis in a sex partner might be infected even if seronegative; therefore, such persons should be treated presumptively.
  2. Persons who were exposed ≥90 days before the diagnosis of syphilis in a sex partner should be treated presumptively if serologic test results are not available immediately and the opportunity for follow-up is uncertain.

REFERENCES

Available at eBooks.Health.Elsevier.com.

RELATED CONTENT

Syphilis (Patient Information)
Tabes Dorsalis (Related Key Topic)

AUTHORS: **LEAH SAYLOR, DO,** and **STEVEN D. JOHNSON, MD**

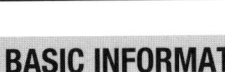

S

Diseases
and Disorders

I

BASIC INFORMATION

DEFINITION

Systemic lupus erythematosus (SLE) is a chronic inflammatory disorder characterized by auto-antibody production responsible for antibody-mediated and immune complex deposition tissue damage. SLE involves multiple organ systems and has heterogeneous disease patterns. Relapses and remissions are a common feature.

SYNONYMS

SLE
Lupus

ICD-10CM CODES

M32	Systemic lupus erythematosus
M32.0	Drug-induced systemic lupus erythematosus
M32.8	Other forms of systemic lupus erythematosus
M32.9	Systemic lupus erythematosus, unspecified
M32.10	Systemic lupus erythematosus, organ or system involvement unspecified
M32.11	Endocarditis in systemic lupus erythematosus
M32.12	Pericarditis in systemic lupus erythematosus
M32.13	Lung involvement in systemic lupus erythematosus
M32.14	Glomerular disease in systemic lupus erythematosus
M32.15	Tubulo-interstitial nephropathy in systemic lupus erythematosus
M32.19	Other organ or system involvement in systemic lupus erythematosus

EPIDEMIOLOGY & DEMOGRAPHICS

INCIDENCE: Varies across gender, racial/ethnic groups, and geography, with a prevalence of 24 to 207 cases per 100,000 persons per year. Prevalence is higher among African Americans, Asian Americans, and Hispanics. There are an estimated 350,000 people diagnosed with SLE in the U.S.[1,2]

PREDOMINANT SEX: Female:male ratio is 9:1. The ratio is highest in reproductive age group, and about half of that in patients younger than 16 and older than 55.[3]

PREDOMINANT AGE: Mean age at diagnosis is 31.

PHYSICAL FINDINGS & CLINICAL PRESENTATION

- Constitutional: Unexplained fever, fatigue (80% to 100% patients), malaise (Table 1)
- Mucocutaneous lesions (more than 80% of patients):
  1. Acute (associated with + Ro antibody): Malar rash (Fig. E1) sparing nasolabial folds (acute cutaneous lupus); annular or papulosquamous rash (subacute cutaneous lupus)
  2. Chronic: Raised erythematous patches with subsequent edematous plaques and adherent scales (discoid cutaneous lupus), lupus profundus, lupus tumidus; alopecia, photosensitivity, nasal, or oropharyngeal ulcerations (classically painless, but discoid lesions [Fig. E2] may be painful); Raynaud phenomenon; leukocytoclastic vasculitis, chilblains; livedo reticularis or livedo racemosa (secondary to antiphospholipid antibody syndrome)
  3. Skin biopsy hallmark: Interface dermatitis
- Musculoskeletal (about 90% of lupus patients): Arthralgias are more common than true arthritis, but nonerosive deforming arthritis is not rare; myositis
- Cardiac: Pericardial rub (pericarditis) is most common; valvular heart disease (e.g., valve sclerosis, Libman-Sacks endocarditis); congestive heart failure, myocarditis, premature atherosclerotic heart disease
- Pulmonary: Pleuritis (most common), acute or chronic pneumonitis, diffuse alveolar hemorrhage, pulmonary hypertension
- Gastrointestinal: Dysphagia, mesenteric vasculitis, peritonitis, pancreatitis, hepatitis
- Neuropsychiatric: Headache, psychosis, seizure, acute confusion states, peripheral or cranial neuropathy, transverse myelitis, stroke (may be associated with antiphospholipid syndrome), cognitive dysfunction
- Hematologic (about 50% of lupus patients): Anemia (hemolytic, anemia of chronic disease, aplastic anemia), thrombocytopenia, leukopenia, lymphadenopathy, secondary antiphospholipid antibody syndrome
- Renal: Acute renal failure, proteinuria, nephritic syndrome, nephrotic syndrome

ETIOLOGY

Lupus may develop in genetically susceptible individuals, triggered by endogenous and exogenous factors. SLE susceptibility involves major histocompatibility complex (MHC) class II polymorphism with commonly observed association with *HLA-DR-2, DR3, DR4,* and *DR8.* SLE is also associated with inherited deficiencies of C1q, C2, C4a, others. There is predilection for familial clustering of SLE with risk in monozygotic twins —about 25% to 50%—and 5% in dizygotic twins. Environmental factors such as ultraviolet (UV) light, Epstein-Barr virus infection, and tobacco smoking may have a triggering role. Autoantibody production is the hallmark of disease development and diagnosis of SLE. Evidence supports the improper processing of nuclear proteins and nucleic acid from cell death. Impairments in neutrophil cell death via a process termed NET-osis (nuclear extracellular trap) contribute to the accumulation of nuclear debris. This, in turn, can lead to the presentation of self-nuclear material to plasmacytoid dendritic cells. Plasmacytoid dendritic cells propagate antibody and immune complex production via a type I interferon-dependent mechanism (Fig. E3).[4]

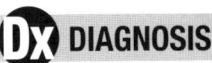 DIAGNOSIS

DIFFERENTIAL DIAGNOSIS

- Rheumatoid arthritis, mixed connective tissue disease, systemic vasculitis
- Neoplastic disorder
- Hematologic malignancy, paraneoplastic syndrome
- Systemic infection
- Other: Thrombotic thrombocytopenic purpura/hemolytic uremic syndrome, primary antiphospholipid antibody syndrome

EVALUATION

The diagnosis of SLE is clinical. The 2019 European League Against Rheumatism/American College of Rheumatology (ACR) classification criteria for SLE (Table 2) includes positive antinuclear antibody (ANA) at least once as obligatory entry criterion, followed by additive weighted criteria grouped in seven clinical (constitutional, hematologic, neuropsychiatric, mucocutaneous, serosal, musculoskeletal, renal), and three immunologic (antiphospholipid antibodies,

---

TABLE 1 Potential Clinical Manifestations of Systemic Lupus Erythematosus

Target Organ	Potential Clinical Manifestations
Constitutional	Fatigue, anorexia, weight loss, fever, lymphadenopathy
Musculoskeletal	Arthritis, myositis, arthralgias, myalgias, avascular necrosis, osteoporosis
Skin	Malar rash, discoid rash, photosensitive rash, cutaneous vasculitis, livedo reticularis, periungual capillary abnormalities, Raynaud phenomenon, alopecia, oral and nasal ulcers
Renal	Hypertension, proteinuria, hematuria, edema, nephrotic syndrome, renal failure
Cardiovascular	Pericarditis, myocarditis, conduction system abnormalities, Libman-Sacks endocarditis
Neurologic	Seizures, psychosis, cerebritis, stroke, transverse myelitis, depression, cognitive impairment, headaches, pseudotumor, peripheral neuropathy, chorea, optic neuritis, cranial nerve palsies
Pulmonary	Pleuritis, interstitial lung disease, pulmonary hemorrhage, pulmonary hypertension, pulmonary embolism
Hematologic	Immune-mediated cytopenias (hemolytic anemia, thrombocytopenia or leukopenia), anemia of chronic inflammation, hypercoagulability, thrombocytopenic thrombotic microangiopathy
Gastroenterology	Hepatosplenomegaly, pancreatitis, vasculitis affecting bowel, protein-losing enteropathy
Ocular	Retinal vasculitis, scleritis, episcleritis, papilledema

TABLE 2 The American College of Rheumatology/European League Against Rheumatism Classification Criteria for Systemic Lupus Erythematosus

Clinical			Immunologic		
Constitutional	Fever	2	aPL	aCL IgG or B2GP1 or LA	2
Cutaneous	Nonscarring alopecia	2	Complement	Low C3 or C4	3
	Oral ulcers	2		Low C3 + C4	4
	SCLE or discoid	4			
	ACLE	6			
Arthritis	Arthritis (synovitis in ≥2 joints or TTP and a.m. stiffness)	6	Antibodies	Anti-DNA	6
				Anti-Sm	6
Neurologic	Delirium	2			
	Psychosis	3			
	Seizure	5			
Serositis	Pleural/pericardial effusion	5			
	Acute pericarditis	6			
Hematologic	Leukopenia	3			
	Thrombocytopenia	4			
	AIHA	4			
Renal	UPCR >0.5	4			
	Class II or V	8			
	Class III or IV	10			

aCL, Anticardiolipin antibodies; *ACLE,* acute cutaneous lupus erythematosus; *AIHA,* autoimmune hemolytic anemia; *aPL,* antiphospholipid antibodies; *IgG,* immunoglobulin G; *SCLE,* subacute cutaneous lupus erythematosus; *Sm,* Smith; *TTP,* thrombotic thrombocytopenic purpura; *UPCR,* urine protein/creatinine ratio.
From Firestein GS et al: *Firestein & Kelley's textbook of rheumatology,* ed 11, Philadelphia, 2021, Elsevier.

complement proteins, SLE-specific antibodies) domains, and weighted from 2 to 10. Patients accumulating ≥10 points are classified as having systemic lupus. The new criteria had a sensitivity of 96.1% and specificity of 93.4%, compared with 82.8% sensitivity and 93.4% specificity of the ACR 1997 (see later) and 96.7% sensitivity and 83.7% specificity of the Systemic Lupus International Collaborating Clinics 2012 criteria.[5]

1997 ACR Criteria:
- Malar rash
- Discoid rash
- Photosensitivity (recurrence of unusual skin rash in sun-exposed areas)
- Oral or nasopharyngeal painless ulceration, observed by physician
- Arthritis (nonerosive)
- Serositis (pleuritis, pericarditis)
- Renal disorder (persistent proteinuria >0.5 g/day, or ≥3+ on dipstick if quantification not performed; cellular casts)
- Neurologic disorder (seizures, psychosis [in absence of offending drugs or metabolic derangement])
- Hematologic disorder:
  1. Hemolytic anemia with reticulocytosis
  2. Leukopenia (<4000/mm³ total on two or more occasions)
  3. Lymphopenia (<1500/mm³ on two or more occasions)
  4. Thrombocytopenia (<100,000/mm³ in the absence of offending drugs)
- Immunologic disorder:
  1. Anti–double-stranded DNA antibody (anti-dsDNA)
  2. Anti-Smith antibody (anti-Sm)
  3. Antiphospholipid antibodies (anticardiolipin immunoglobulin M [IgM] or IgG, lupus anticoagulant, antibeta-2 glycoprotein IgM

or IgG, or false-positive fluorescent treponemal antibody absorption test or *Treponema pallidum* immobilization for 6 mo)
- ANA: An abnormal titer of ANA by immunofluorescence or equivalent assay at any time in the absence of drugs known to be associated with drug-induced lupus syndrome

2012 SLICC Criteria: SLE can be diagnosed if[6]:
- Biopsy-proven nephritis with either ANA or anti-dsDNA antibodies *or*
- Patient satisfies four clinical criteria, requiring at least one clinical and at least one immunologic criterion
- Clinical criteria:
  1. Acute cutaneous lupus (malar rash, bullous lupus, toxic epidermal necrolysis, photosensitive lupus rash, maculopapular lupus, subacute cutaneous lupus)
  2. Chronic cutaneous lupus (discoid, hypertrophic verrucous, panniculitis, mucosal lupus, lupus tumidus, chilblains lupus, lichen planus)
  3. Oral ulcers or nasal ulcers
  4. Nonscarring alopecia
  5. Synovitis (more than two joints or inflammatory arthralgias of more than two joints)
  6. Serositis (pleurisy for more than 1 day, pericardial pain for more than 1 day)
  7. Renal (>500 mg proteinuria/24 h or RBC casts)
  8. Neurologic (seizures, psychosis, mononeuritis multiplex, myelitis, peripheral or cranial neuropathy, acute confusion state)
  9. Hemolytic anemia
  10. Lymphopenia (<1000/mm³ at least once)
  11. Thrombocytopenia (<100,000/mm³ at least once)

- Immunologic criteria:
  1. ANA
  2. Anti-dsDNA (>2× laboratory reference range)
  3. Anti-Smith
  4. Antiphospholipid antibodies (lupus anticoagulant, rapid plasma reagin [RPR], anticardiolipin IgA, IgG, IgM, anti-β2 glycoprotein IgA, IgG, IgM)
  5. Low complement
  6. Direct Coombs test in the absence of hemolytic anemia

Definitions of SLE classification criteria are included in Table 3.

LABORATORY TESTS
Suggested initial laboratory evaluation of suspected SLE:
- ANA by immunofluorescence or similar high-quality method
  1. CBC with differential, blood urea nitrogen and serum creatinine, urinalysis, erythrocyte sedimentation rate (ESR), partial thromboplastin time (PTT), complements (C3, C4)

Consider additional laboratory testing in a patient with strong suspicion for systemic lupus:
- Anti-dsDNA, anti-Smith, anti-SSA, anti-SSB, anti-RNP antibodies. Table 4 summarizes autoantibodies and clinical significance in SLE
- Lupus anticoagulant, RPR, anticardiolipin antibodies, anti-beta-2 glycoprotein antibodies especially in patients with thrombotic events or recurrent miscarriages
- Urinalysis for red blood cell (RBC), cellular casts
- Random spot urine protein: Urine creatinine ratio, 24-h urine protein collection if proteinuria; >0.5 or >500 mg/24 h is abnormal, respectively. Evaluation of renal biopsy specimens in lupus nephritis (LN) is summarized in Table E5

Direct Coombs test

IMAGING STUDIES
- Chest x-ray examination for evaluation of pulmonary involvement (pleural effusion, infiltrates)
- Electrocardiogram for chest pain
- Echocardiogram if murmur, evidence of new or unexplained congestive heart failure, or suspected pericarditis

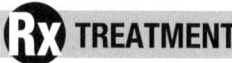 **TREATMENT**

NONPHARMACOLOGIC THERAPY
- Avoidance of sunlight and use of high-SPF sunscreen (>35).
- Screening and counseling for modifiable cardiovascular risk factors such as cigarette smoking, diet, exercise, cholesterol, and uncontrolled hypertension (HTN).
- Counseling for pregnancy planning for patients of childbearing age.
- Calcium and vitamin D supplementation for prevention of early osteoporosis (see "Osteoporosis").[7]

Diseases and Disorders

I

TABLE 3 Definitions of SLE Classification Criteria 2019

Criteria	Definition
Antinuclear antibodies (ANA)	ANA at a titer of ≥1:80 on HEp-2 cells or an equivalent positive test at least once. Testing by immunofluorescence on HEp-2 cells or a solid-phase ANA screening immunoassay with at least equivalent performance is highly recommended.
Fever	Temperature >38.3° C (100.9° F)
Leukopenia	White blood cell count <4000/mm^3
Thrombocytopenia	Platelet count <100,000/mm^3
Autoimmune hemolysis	Evidence of hemolysis, such as reticulocytosis, low haptoglobin, elevated indirect bilirubin, elevated LDH, *AND* positive Coombs (direct antiglobulin) test
Delirium	Characterized by 1) change in consciousness or level of arousal with reduced ability to focus, 2) symptom development over hours to <2 days, 3) symptom fluctuation throughout the day, 4) either 4a) acute/subacute change in cognition (e.g., memory deficit or disorientation) or 4b) change in behavior, mood, or affect (e.g., restlessness, reversal of sleep/wake cycle)
Psychosis	Characterized by 1) delusions and/or hallucinations without insight and 2) absence of delirium
Seizure	Primary generalized seizure or partial/focal seizure
Nonscarring alopecia	Nonscarring alopecia observed by a clinician†
Oral ulcers	Oral ulcers observed by a clinician†
Subacute cutaneous OR discoid lupus	Subacute cutaneous lupus erythematosus observed by a clinician: †Annular or papulosquamous (psoriasiform) cutaneous eruption, usually photodistributed If skin biopsy is performed, typical changes must be present (interface vacuolar dermatitis consisting of a perivascular lymphohistiocytic infiltrate, often with dermal mucin noted) OR Discoid lupus erythematosus observed by a clinician:† Erythematous-violaceous cutaneous lesions with secondary changes of atrophic scarring, dyspigmentation, often follicular hyperkeratosis/plugging (scalp), leading to scarring alopecia on the scalp If skin biopsy is performed, typical changes must be present (interface vacuolar dermatitis consisting of a perivascular and/or lymphohistiocytic infiltrate of the appendages. In the scalp, follicular keratin plugs may be seen. In longstanding lesions, mucin deposition may be noted)
Acute cutaneous lupus	Malar rash or generalized maculopapular rash observed by a clinician.† If skin biopsy is performed, typical changes must be present (interface vacuolar dermatitis consisting of a perivascular lymphohistiocytic infiltrate, often with dermal mucin noted. Perivascular neutrophilic infiltrate may be present early in the course)
Pleural or pericardial effusion	Imaging evidence (such as ultrasound, x-ray, CT scan, MRI) of pleural or pericardial effusion, or both
Acute pericarditis	≥2 of 1) pericardial chest pain (typically sharp, worse with inspiration, improved by leaning forward), 2) pericardial rub, 3) EKG with new widespread ST elevation or PR depression, 4) new or worsened pericardial effusion on imaging (such as ultrasound, x-ray, CT scan, MRI)
Joint involvement	Either 1) synovitis involving two or more joints characterized by swelling or effusion, or 2) tenderness in two or more joints and at least 30 min of morning stiffness
Proteinuria >0.5 g/24 h	Proteinuria >0.5 g/24 h by 24-h urine or equivalent spot urine protein-to-creatinine ratio
Class II or V lupus nephritis on renal biopsy according to ISN/RPS 2003 classification	Class II: Mesangial proliferative lupus nephritis: Purely mesangial hypercellularity of any degree or mesangial matrix expansion by light microscopy, with mesangial immune deposit. A few isolated subepithelial or subendothelial deposits may be visible by immunofluorescence or electron microscopy, but not by light microscopy. Class V: Membranous lupus nephritis: Global or segmental subepithelial immune deposits or their morphologic sequelae by light microscopy and by immunofluorescence or electron microscopy, with or without mesangial alterations
Class III or IV lupus nephritis on renal biopsy according to ISN/RPS 2003 classification	Class III: Focal lupus nephritis: Active or inactive focal, segmental, or global endocapillary or extracapillary glomerulonephritis involving <50% of all glomeruli, typically with focal subendothelial immune deposits, with or without mesangial alterations Class IV: Diffuse lupus nephritis: Active or inactive diffuse, segmental, or global endocapillary or extracapillary glomerulonephritis involving ≥50% of all glomeruli, typically with diffuse subendothelial immune deposits, with or without mesangial alterations. This class includes cases with diffuse wire loop deposits but with little or no glomerular proliferation.
Positive antiphospholipid antibodies	Anticardiolipin antibodies (IgA, IgG, or IgM) at medium or high titer (>40 APL, GPL, or MPL, or >the 99th percentile) or positive anti-β$_2$GPI antibodies (IgA, IgG, or IgM) or positive lupus anticoagulant
Low C3 OR low C4	C3 OR C4 below the lower limit of normal
Low C3 AND low C4	Both C3 AND C4 below their lower limits of normal
Anti-dsDNA antibodies OR anti-Sm antibodies	Anti-dsDNA antibodies in an immunoassay with demonstrated ≥90% specificity for SLE against relevant disease controls OR anti-Sm antibodies

anti-β$_2$GPI, Anti–β$_2$-glycoprotein I; *anti-dsDNA*, anti-double-stranded DNA; *anti-Sm*, anti-Smith *CT*, computed tomography; *EKG*, electrocardiography; *Ig*, immunoglobulin; *ISN*, International Society of Nephrology; *LDH*, lactate dehydrogenase; *MRI*, magnetic resonance imaging; *RPS*, Renal Pathology Society; *SLE*, systemic lupus erythematosus.

†This may include physical examination or review of a photograph.

GENERAL Rx

- There are only four FDA-approved SLE medications: Aspirin, corticosteroids, hydroxychloroquine (1955), and belimumab (2011).
- Treatment should be targeted toward the involved organ(s). Recommended drugs for the treatment of SLE according to stratification of disease severity are described in Fig. 4. Indications for immunosuppressive therapy in SLE are summarized in Table 6.
- Limited and defined courses of corticosteroids are useful for a variety of SLE symptoms. Steroid therapy should be restricted to acute or subacute control of symptoms, due to the increased cardiovascular risk and increased organ damage associated with chronic steroid use. Recommended drug monitoring in SLE is summarized in Table 7.
- Consider checking G6PD in certain ethnic groups more predisposed to antimalarial-induced hemolytic anemia.
- Hydroxychloroquine has best evidence for reducing flares, organ damage, lipids,

TABLE 4 Autoantibodies and Clinical Significance in Systemic Lupus Erythematosus

Autoantibody	Prevalence in SLE (%)	Clinical Associations
Antinuclear Antibody		
Anti-dsDNA	60	95% specificity for SLE; fluctuates with disease activity; associated with glomerulonephritis
Anti-Smith	20-30	99% specificity for SLE; associated with anti-U1RNP antibodies
Anti-U1RNP	30	Antibody associated with mixed connective tissue disease and lower frequency of glomerulonephritis
Anti-Ro/SS-A	30	Associated with Sjögren syndrome, photosensitivity, SCLE, neonatal lupus, congenital heart block
Anti-La/SS-B	20	Associated with Sjögren syndrome, SCLE, neonatal lupus, congenital heart block, anti-Ro/SS-A
Antihistone	70	Also associated with drug-induced lupus
Antiphospholipid	30	Associated with arterial and venous thrombosis, pregnancy morbidity

SCLE, Subacute cutaneous lupus erythematosus; SLE, systemic lupus erythematosus.
From Firestein GS et al: *Firestein & Kelley's textbook of rheumatology*, ed 11, Philadelphia, 2021, Elsevier.

thrombosis; improving survival; augmenting action of mycophenolate mofetil (MMF) in LN; and preventing seizures. Currently recommend not to exceed an oral dose of 5 mg/kg/day to decrease risk of retinal toxicity.[1]

- Methotrexate and azathioprine are used as steroid-sparing agents. Indications include cutaneous and joint involvement.[1]
- Joint pain and mild serositis are generally well controlled with NSAIDs or low-dose corticosteroids. Hydroxychloroquine and methotrexate are also effective for arthritis. Belimumab does well for joint and cutaneous manifestations. Leflunomide and rituximab may be considered for refractory arthritis. Treatment approach for musculoskeletal features of SLE is summarized in Table 8.
- Cutaneous manifestations:
  1. Topical or intradermal corticosteroids are helpful for individual discoid lesions, especially in the scalp.
  2. Hydroxychloroquine alone or in combination with quinacrine and/or chloroquine can be considered for refractory skin disease.
  3. Refractory cases may be treated with belimumab, MMF, dapsone, or combination treatment.[1,8]
  4. Fig. E5 and Table E9 summarize general management of cutaneous lesions in SLE.
- Hematologic manifestations:
  1. Corticosteroids are first-line therapy. Table E10 summarizes the treatment and main hematologic features of SLE.
  2. Azathioprine can be used for thrombocytopenia or hemolytic anemia. Check for TPMT genetic mutation before the first use.
  3. Intravenous immunoglobulin (IVIG) or rituximab may be considered for severe leukopenia, autoimmune hemolytic anemia, or autoimmune thrombocytopenia (Fig. E6).
  4. Central nervous system manifestations:
  5. Headaches are treated symptomatically. Most headaches will not be SLE-related and should be treated according to the underlying cause.

  6. Anticonvulsants and antipsychotics may be indicated.
  7. Standard therapy for other neuropsychiatric SLE symptoms is not established.
- Renal disease: The histologic classification of LN according to the International Society of Nephrology/Renal Pathology Society is summarized in Table E11. Severity of LN is described in Table E12. Treatment recommendations for LN are summarized in Table E13. (Class III, IV, or IV/V with cellular crescents LN; see Table E14.) INDUCTION: 6-mo treatment.
  1. The typical treatment induction period is 6 mo. The use of intravenous cyclophosphamide (CYC) with corticosteroids given at monthly intervals is more effective in preserving renal function than is treatment with glucocorticoids alone. Low-dose "Euro-Lupus" protocol may be equally efficacious and less toxic for certain populations (e.g., Caucasians, Blacks) than high-dose regimen. MMF is considered equivalent to CYC based on high-quality studies, with better tolerability and fertility profile. MMF may be preferred in African Americans and Hispanics. MMF and azathioprine are good options for maintenance treatment.
  2. There is interest in and positive data for use of calcineurin inhibitors, such as tacrolimus, for treatment of LN. Newer and possibly less toxic voclosporin has entered phase III trial and when added to MMF showed better results in renal responses compared with MMF alone.[9]
- Severe nonrenal organ disease:
  1. Evidence from systematic randomized controlled trials for non-renal lupus treatment is comparatively limited.
  2. High-dose intravenous CYC is used as an induction treatment. Azathioprine or MMF may be used as maintenance.
  3. IVIG may be considered in severe disease especially when concomitant infection is present.

  4. Plasmapheresis or plasma exchange may be considered in critical situations: First-line therapy in Guillain-Barré syndrome, thrombotic thrombocytopenic purpura (TTP); second-line for SLE-related hemolytic anemia, cerebritis, and diffuse alveolar hemorrhage (DAH). Infectious complications are common.
- Fever/infection post-immunosuppressive therapy
  1. Immunosuppressive therapy can result in neutropenia and increased susceptibility to infection
  2. Fig. E7 illustrates an approach to SLE patients with fever and other signs of infection post-immunosuppressive therapy
- Therapy targeting B cells:
  1. Rituximab: Anti-CD20 monoclonal antibody. Randomized controlled trials for rituximab as an adjunct induction agent were negative in terms of both renal and nonrenal outcomes but were felt to be limited by study design. Some observational studies have shown efficacy in those who have failed other regimens.[1,10]
  2. Epratuzumab: An anti-CD22 agent. Studies initially showed positive data, but in July 2015 both phase III trials for SLE failed to meet their primary endpoint, and this medication is no longer studied.
  3. Belimumab: Decreases activation of B cells. When used in addition to standard therapy, patients on belimumab showed improvement in cutaneous and musculoskeletal disease. Belimumab-treated patients had decreased SLE activity, a reduced time to disease flare, and lower glucocorticoid exposure. Patients with central nervous system or serious kidney disease were excluded. There is interest in adding belimumab to standard LN regimen, but data from BLISS-LN are not yet available.[8,11]
  4. Abatacept: Downregulates T-cell activation. Data are limited regarding improvement in arthritis, fatigue, sleep if added to routine therapy. Negative data as adjunct agent for lupus arthritis when added to MMF or CYC. Shows limited positive efficacy in patients refractory to other treatments.[1]
  5. Interferon therapy: Interferon α (INFα) has been linked to increased disease activity in SLE. INFα blocking therapies are in phase II clinical trials. Sifalimumab, a monoclonal antibody against INFα, reduced moderate to severe mucocutaneous involvement in SLE and decreased active joint count and fatigue scores in preliminary data analysis. Development of sifalimumab has been terminated in favor of anifrolumab, a similar INFα blocking agent. The TULIP-1 study of that molecule did not meet response criteria based on score used in the BLISS trial. TULIP-2 used BICLA as a response measure and showed statistically significant improvement compared to placebo. The phase III trial is ongoing.[12,13]
  6. There is continuous interest in studying B-cell and interferon-based treatment,

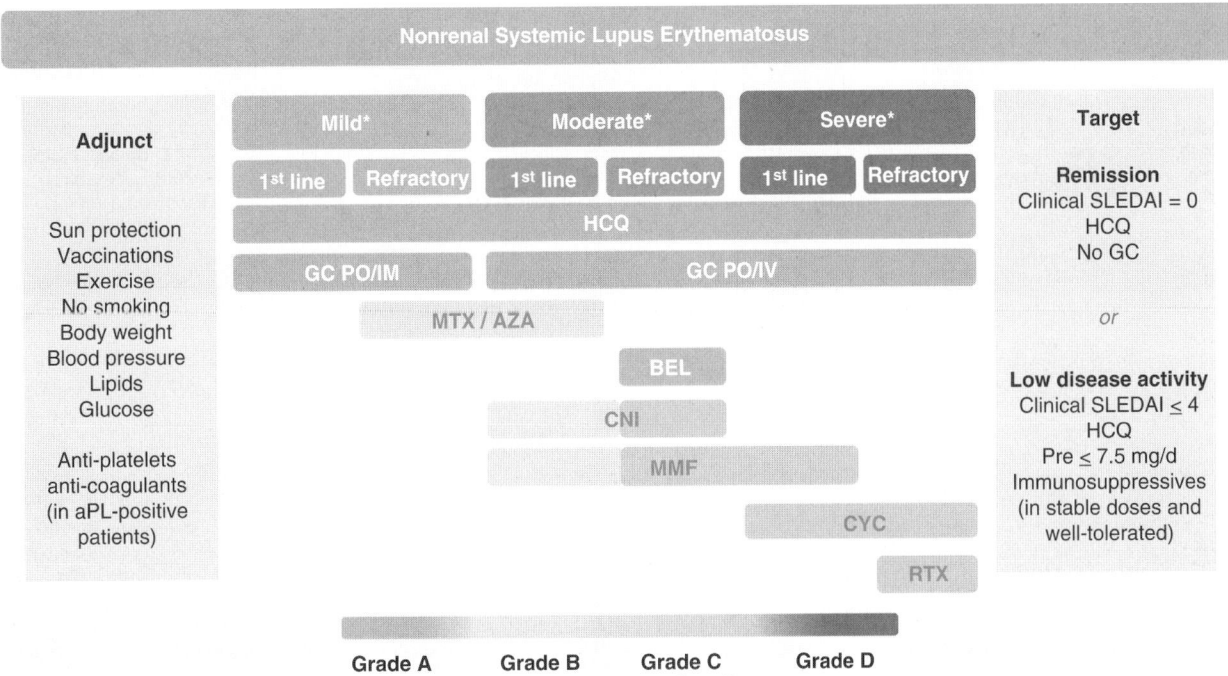

Mild: Constitutional symptoms/mild arthritis/rash ≤ 9% BSA/PLTs 50-100 × 10³/mm³; SLEDAI≤6; BILAG C or ≤ BILAG B manifestation
Moderate: RA-like arthritis/rash 9-18% BSA/cutaneous vasculitis ≤ 18% BSA; PLTs 20-50×10³/mm³/serositis; SLEDAI 7-12; ≥2 BILAG manifestations
Severe: major organ threatening disease (cerebritis, myelitis, pneumonitis, mesenteric vasculitis; thrombocytopenia with platelets <20×10³/mm³; TTP-like disease or acute hemophagocytic syndrome; SLEDAI>12; ≥1 BILAG A manifestations)

FIG. 4 Recommended drugs for the treatment of SLE according to stratification of disease severity. The grading of recommendation/level of evidence refers to extrarenal manifestations. *aPL,* Antiphospholipid antibodies; *AZA,* azathioprine; *BEL,* belimumab; *CNI,* calcineurin inhibitors; *CYC,* cyclophosphamide; *GC,* glucocorticoids; *HCQ,* hydroxychloroquine; *IM,* intramuscular; *IV,* intravenous; *MMF,* mycophenolate mofetil; *MTX,* methotrexate; *PO,* per os; *Pre,* prednisone; *RTX,* rituximab; *SLEDAI,* Systemic Lupus Erythematosus Disease Activity Index. (From Firestein GS et al: *Firestein & Kelley's textbook of rheumatology,* ed 11, Philadelphia, 2021, Elsevier.)

TABLE 6   Indications for Immunosuppressive Therapy in Systemic Lupus Erythematosus

General Indications
Involvement of major organs or extensive involvement of non-major organs (skin) refractory to other agents, or both
Failure to respond to or inability to taper glucocorticoids to acceptable doses (<7.5 mg/day) for long-term use

Specific Organ Involvement

Renal
Proliferative or membranous nephritis, or mixed

Hematologic
Severe thrombocytopenia (platelets <20-30,000/mm³)
Thrombotic thrombocytopenic purpura-like syndrome
Severe autoimmune hemolytic or aplastic anemia (hemoglobin <8 g/dl) not responding to glucocorticoids

Pulmonary
Lupus pneumonitis and/or alveolar hemorrhage

Cardiac
Myocarditis with depressed left ventricular function, pericarditis with impending tamponade

Gastrointestinal
Abdominal vasculitis, peritonitis

Nervous System
Transverse myelitis, optic neuritis, psychosis refractory to glucocorticoids, mononeuritis multiplex, severe peripheral neuropathy, acute confusional state

From Firestein GS et al: *Firestein & Kelley's textbook of rheumatology,* ed 11, Philadelphia, 2021, Elsevier.

but no FDA approved treatment, other than noted earlier, is currently used clinically.
7. Novel potential targeted treatment approaches may include blocking interleukin-17 (IL-17), IL-12/23, and JAK inhibitors (early data for 4-mg baricitinib showed positive results). Research remains very active and ongoing to find new therapeutic targets.[14,15]
- Recommended assessment and monitoring of patients with SLE with nonrenal, noncentral nervous system manifestations are summarized in Box 1.
- SLE in pregnancy (Table E15): Pregnancy in the setting of SLE is associated with a higher risk of complications compared with healthy women (preterm labor, unplanned cesarean delivery, fetal growth restriction, preeclampsia, and eclampsia). Ideally, conception should be attempted in a state of disease remission or stability. If pregnancy occurs during a period of disease relapse, medications need to be adjusted for maternal and fetal safety. Mothers with active SLE should be tested for anti-Ro/SSA and anti-La/SSB antibodies once before or

TABLE 7 Recommended Drug Monitoring in Systemic Lupus Erythematosus

Drug	Dosage	Dose Adjustment	Toxicities Requiring Monitoring	Baseline Evaluation	Laboratory Monitoring
Azathioprine	50-200 mg/day in 1-3 doses with food	↓ 25% if eGFR 10-30 ml/min; ↓ 50% if eGFR <10 ml/min	Myelosuppression, hepatotoxicity, lymphoproliferative diseases	CBC, platelets, Cr, AST or ALT	CBC and platelets every 2 wk, with changes in dosage; during monitoring every 1-3 mo
Mycophenolate mofetil	1-3 g/day in 2 divided doses with food	Maximum 1 g/day if eGFR <25 ml/min	Myelosuppression, hematotoxicity, infection	CBC, platelet, Cr, AST or ALT	CBCs and platelets every 1-2 wk with changes in dosage; during monitoring every 1-3 mo
Cyclophosphamide	50-150 mg/day in a single dose with breakfast. Increase fluid intake (at least 3 L water/day), empty bladder before bedtime	↓ 25% if eGFR 25-50 ml/min; ↓ 30%-50% if eGFR <25 ml/min; ↓ 25% if serum Bil 3.1-5 mg/dl or transaminases >3 times ULN	Myelosuppression, hemorrhagic cystitis, myeloproliferative disease, malignancies	CBC, platelet, Cr, AST or ALT, urinalysis	CBC with differential every 1-2 wk, with changes in dosage and then every 1-3 mo; keep WBC >4000/mm^3 with dose adjustment; urinalysis for hematuria, AST or ALT every 3 mo; urinalysis for hematuria every 6-12 mo following cessation
Methotrexate	7.5-25 mg/wk in 1-3 doses with food or milk/water	↓ 50% if eGFR 10-50 ml/min; avoid use if eGFR <10 ml/min; avoid use in hepatic dysfunction (serum Bil 3.1-5 mg/dl or transaminases >3 times ULN)	Myelosuppression, hepatic fibrosis, pneumonitis	Chest radiograph, hepatitis B/C serology in high-risk patients, AST or ALT, Alb, ALP, Cr	CBC with platelet, AST, Alb, Cr every 1-3 mo
Cyclosporin A	100-400 mg/day in 2 doses at the same time every day with meal or between meals	Avoid in impaired renal function	Renal insufficiency, anemia, hypertension	CBC, Cr, uric acid, AST or ALT, Alb, ALP, blood pressure	Cr every 2 wk until dose is stable, then monthly; CBC, potassium, AST or ALT, Alb, and ALP every 1-3 mo; drug levels only with doses >3 mg/kg/day
Tacrolimus	1-4 mg/day in 2 doses at the same time every day	Cautious use in liver or renal insufficiency	Renal insufficiency, neurotoxicity, malignancy, infections, hyperkalemia	Cr, potassium, AST or ALT, glucose, blood pressure	Once a week for the first 3-4 wk, then every 1-3 mo; monitor drug trough levels
Rituximab	1000 mg on day 1 and 15	None	HBV reactivation (rare)	CBC, Cr, AST or ALT, HBV serology (high-risk patients), TST	CBC and platelets

Note that placebo-controlled studies have failed to demonstrate efficacy in controlled clinical trials.

Alb, Serum albumin; *ALP,* alkaline phosphatase; *ALT,* alanine transaminase; *AST,* aspartate transaminase; *Bil,* bilirubin; *CBC,* complete blood cell count; *Cr,* serum creatinine; *eGFR,* estimated glomerular filtration rate; *HBV,* hepatitis B; *LFTs,* liver function tests; *MTX,* methotrexate; *TST,* tuberculin skin testing; *ULN,* upper limit of normal; *WBC,* white blood cell count.

From Firestein GS et al: *Firestein & Kelley's textbook of rheumatology,* ed 11, Philadelphia, 2021, Elsevier.

TABLE 8 Treatment Approach for Musculoskeletal Features of Systemic Lupus Erythematosus

	First-Line Therapy	Second-Line Therapy	Third-Line Therapy	Experimental Therapy
Arthritis	HCQ or CQ	MTX	Belimumab	Abatacept
	Low doses of glucocorticoids	Leflunomide	RTX	Sifalimumab
			Anti-TNF	
AVN	Avoid high doses of corticosteroid	Antiaggregation in aPL positivity	Core decompression	
			Percutaneous drilling	
			Arthroplasty	
Myositis	High-dose corticosteroid	MTX	IVIG	
		Azathioprine	RTX	

aPL, Antiphospholipid; *AVN,* avascular necrosis; *CQ,* chloroquine; *HCQ,* hydroxychloroquine; *IVIG,* intravenous immunoglobulin; *MTX,* methotrexate; *RTX,* rituximab; *TNF,* tumor necrosis factor.

From Hochberg MC: *Rheumatology,* ed 7, Philadelphia, 2019, Elsevier.

early in pregnancy, due to their associated increase in risk for neonatal lupus and congenital heart block.[16]

1. Recommended during pregnancy: Hydroxychloroquine, low-dose aspirin, antihypertensives (methyldopa, labetalol, nifedipine)
2. Selective use allowed during pregnancy: NSAIDs, glucocorticoids, azathioprine, cyclosporine, tacrolimus, biologics
3. Contraindicated: Cyclophosphamide, mycophenolate mofetil, methotrexate, leflunomide

DISPOSITION

- Most patients with SLE experience remissions and exacerbations.
- 5-yr survival rate has improved to more than 90% in patients with newly diagnosed SLE since the advent of potent immunosuppressive therapy. The 15-yr survival rate is now 85%.[3]

BOX 1 Recommended Assessment and Monitoring of Patients With Systemic Lupus Erythematosus With Nonrenal, Noncentral Nervous System Manifestations

Patient General Assessment
In addition to the standard care of patients without lupus of the same age and sex, the assessment of patients with SLE must include the evaluation of:
- Disease activity by a validated index at each visit
- Organ damage annually
- General quality of life by patient history and/or by a 0-10 VAS (patient global score) at each visit
- Comorbidities
- Drug toxicity

Cardiovascular Risk Factors
At baseline and during follow-up at least once a year:
- Assess smoking, vascular events (cerebral and cardiovascular), physical activity, oral contraceptives, hormonal therapies, and family history of cardiovascular disease
- Perform blood tests: Blood cholesterol, glucose
- Examine for blood pressure and BMI (and/or waist circumference)
- NB: Some patients may need more frequent follow-up (e.g., those taking glucocorticoids).

Osteoporosis Risk
All patients with SLE:
- Should be assessed for adequate calcium and vitamin D intake, regular exercise, and smoking habits
- Should be screened and followed for osteoporosis according to existing guidelines (1) for postmenopausal women and (2) for patients taking glucocorticoids or on any other medication that may reduce BMD

Cancer Risk
Cancer screening is recommended according to the guidelines for the general population, including cervical smear tests.

Infection Risk
Screening: Patients with SLE should be screened for:
- HIV based on the patient's risk factors
- HCV and HBV based on the patient's risk factors, particularly before IS drugs including high-dose glucocorticoids are given
- Tuberculosis, according to local guidelines, especially before IS drugs including high-dose glucocorticoids are given
- CMV testing should be considered during treatment in selected patients.
  Vaccination: Patients with SLE are at high risk of infections, and prevention should be recommended. The administration of inactivated vaccines (especially flu and pneumococcus), following CDC guidelines for patients who are immunosuppressed, should be encouraged strongly in patients with SLE who take IS drugs, preferably administered when the SLE is inactive. For other vaccinations, an individual risk–benefit analysis is recommended.
  Monitoring: At follow-up visits, continuous assessment of the risk of infection by taking into consideration the presence of:

- Severe neutropenia (<500 cells/mm^3)
- Severe lymphopenia (<500 cells/mm^3)
- Low IgG (<500 mg/dl)

Frequency of Assessments
In patients with no activity, no damage, and no comorbidity, assessments are recommended every 6-12 mo. During these visits, preventive measures should be emphasized.

Laboratory Assessment
It is recommended to monitor the following autoantibodies and complement:
- At baseline: ANA, anti-dsDNA, anti-Ro, anti-La, anti-RNP, anti-Sm, antiphospholipid, C3, C4
- Reevaluation of aPLs in previously negative patients before pregnancy, surgery, transplant, and use of estrogen-containing treatments or in the presence of a new neurologic or vascular event; anti-Ro and anti-La antibodies before pregnancy; anti-dsDNA/C3 C4 may support evidence of disease activity or remission
  Other laboratory assessments. At 6- to 12-mo intervals, patients with inactive disease should have:
- CBC
- ESR
- CRP
- Serum albumin
- Serum creatinine (or eGFR)
- Urinalysis and urine protein-to-creatinine ratio
  NB: If a patient is on a specific drug treatment, monitoring for that drug is required as well.

Mucocutaneous Involvement
Mucocutaneous lesions should be characterized, according to existing classification systems, as to whether they may be:
- LE specific
- LE nonspecific
- LE mimickers
- Drug-related
  Lesions should be assessed for activity and damage using validated indices (e.g., CLASI).

Eye Assessment
In patients treated with glucocorticoids or antimalarials, a baseline eye examination is recommended according to standard guidelines. An eye examination during follow-up is recommended:
- In selected patients taking glucocorticoids (high risk of glaucoma or cataracts)
- In patients on antimalarial drugs. (Low risk: HCQ: No further testing is required until after 5 yr of baseline, and after the first 5 yr of treatment, eye assessment is recommended yearly; High risk: Eye assessment is recommended yearly, especially when using CQ.)

ANA, Antinuclear antibodies; anti-RNP, anti-ribonucleoprotein; anti-Sm, anti-Smith; aPLs, antiphospholipid antibodies; BMD, bone mineral density; BMI, body mass index; CBC, complete blood count; CDC, Centers for Disease Control and Prevention; CLASI, cutaneous lupus erythematosus disease area and severity index; CMV, cytomegalovirus; CQ, chloroquine; CRP, C-reactive protein; eGFR, estimated glomerular filtration rate; ESR, erythrocyte sedimentation rate; HBV, hepatitis B virus; HCV, hepatitis C virus; HCQ, hydroxychloroquine; HIV, human immunodeficiency virus; IgG, immunoglobulin G; IS, immunosuppressive; LE, lupus erythematosus; NB, nota bene; SLE, systemic lupus erythematosus; VAS, visual analog scale.
From Hochberg MC: *Rheumatology,* ed 7, Philadelphia, 2019, Elsevier.

- Early death related to SLE activity and infections; late death due to cardiovascular disease.
- LN progression rate to ESRD in 10% to 30% within 15 yr.
- African Americans, Asian Americans, and Hispanic Americans in general have a worse prognosis. The leading cause of death in SLE patients in developed countries is premature atherosclerosis. The quality of life for many

SLE patients is poor due to fatigue, chronic pain, and cognitive impairment.[2]

REFERRAL
- Rheumatology consultation for all patients with SLE
- Hematology consultation for patients with significant hematologic abnormalities (e.g., severe hemolytic anemia or thrombocytopenia)

- Nephrology consultation in patients with proteinuria and/or suspected renal involvement
- Dermatology consultation for patients with unexplained or unusual skin rash
- Cardiology consultation for patients with lupus carditis, arrhythmias
- Ophthalmology referral for all patients on hydroxychloroquine and chloroquine

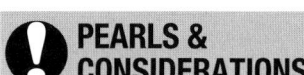
! PEARLS & CONSIDERATIONS

- Arthritis in SLE often has no prolonged morning stiffness and is not erosive on x-rays; reversible joint deformities in lupus are termed Jaccoud arthropathy.
- Myocardial infarction is 50 times more common in young female patients than in age-matched control groups.

- Prevent adverse effects of medications: Consider prophylaxis for infections and appropriate vaccinations, ensure yearly Pap and other cancer screening as clinically indicated; for patients taking CYC, intervention to preserve bladder and fertility should be considered; manage bone health.
- Based on small clinical data, a vitamin D level >40 may have modest reduction in disease activity; in addition, vitamin D may reduce risk of thrombosis, based on oncology research.[7]

RELATED CONTENT

Systemic Lupus Erythematosus (Patient Information)
Discoid Lupus (Related Key Topic)
Renal Lupus (Related Key Topic)

REFERENCES

Available at eBooks.Health.Elsevier.com.

AUTHORS: **OMAR KARIM, BS,** and **MANUEL F. DASILVA, MD**

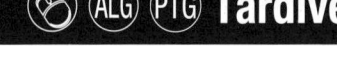
Diseases and Disorders

I

BASIC INFORMATION

DEFINITION

Tardive dyskinesia (TD) is a neurologic disorder of involuntary movements associated with the long-term use of antipsychotic medication, particularly first-generation antipsychotics. Patients exhibit rapid, repetitive, stereotypic movements that mostly involve the oral, lingual, trunk, and limb areas.

SYNONYMS

Orofacial dyskinesia
Tardive syndrome
TD

ICD-10CM CODE
G24.01   Drug induced subacute dyskinesia
DSM-5 CODE
335.85

EPIDEMIOLOGY & DEMOGRAPHICS

- The disorder is caused by dopamine-blocking antipsychotics (e.g., haloperidol) and antiemetics (e.g., metoclopramide, prochlorperazine, and promethazine).
- The reported prevalence of TD can be variable; however, this is a serious clinical concern.[1]
- With first-generation antipsychotics, about 32% of patients are affected with TD, and ~5% are expected to develop TD with each year of antipsychotic treatment.[1,2]
- The incidence of TD with second-generation antipsychotics is about 13% or more. With the increasing use of these medications, TD remains a serious problem.[1,2]
- Risk increases with the duration of antipsychotic treatment, in female and in elderly patients, in patients with brain damage or dementia, with concurrent anticholinergic use, and in patients without schizophrenia spectrum diagnoses.[2]

PHYSICAL FINDINGS & CLINICAL PRESENTATION

- TD is classically described as a chronic condition of insidious onset, but symptoms are variable over time and may even improve despite continued antipsychotic therapy.
- The condition typically appears with the reduction or withdrawal of the antipsychotic medications.
- TD classically involves stereotypic movements of the mouth and tongue, including lip smacking and puckering, tongue twisting and protrusion, and facial grimacing (Fig. 1).
- TD may also involve slow, writhing movements of the trunk or choreoathetoid movements of the fingers and toes.
- The involuntary mouth movements associated with TD may be suppressed by voluntary actions (e.g., putting food in the mouth, talking).
- Many patients may be unaware of or unbothered by the movements, but some find them disfiguring.
- Variants of TD with similar treatment include tardive dystonia (e.g., torticollis,

blepharospasm), tardive myoclonus, tardive akathisia, and tardive tics.

ETIOLOGY

TD is caused by chronic exposure to dopamine receptor antagonists that is thought to result in the upregulation of dopamine receptors in the basal ganglia as well as damage to striatal cholinergic neurons. Dysfunction of striatal GABAergic interneurons has also been implicated. It has been proposed that dopamine receptor hypersensitivity and neurodegenerative changes might cause altered synaptic plasticity of excitatory synapses onto striatal interneurons, resulting in an imbalance between the direct and indirect basal ganglia pathways.

DIAGNOSIS

DIFFERENTIAL DIAGNOSIS

- Acute extrapyramidal symptoms (e.g., short-term withdrawal dyskinesias, Parkinsonism, akathisia)
- Basal ganglia movement disorders (e.g., Huntington chorea, Tourette syndrome, levodopa-induced dyskinesia in Parkinson disease, Wilson disease)
- Autoimmune diseases (Sydenham chorea, multiple sclerosis)
- Other causes of neurologic damage (e.g., lead or mercury toxicity, HIV, neurosyphilis, head injury, neurodegeneration from illicit substances)
- Mannerisms associated with catatonia
- Hyperthyroidism-induced choreoathetosis
- Edentulous dyskinesias and improperly fitted dentures
- Rabbit syndrome (a rare variant of extrapyramidal symptoms with rapid vertical orofacial movements without tongue involvement); may respond to anticholinergic agents

WORKUP

TD is a diagnosis of exclusion, with emphasis on a complete neuropsychiatric and medication history and a thorough physical examination. Abnormal Involuntary Movement Scale (AIMS) can be used to evaluate and monitor the severity of TD.

IMAGING STUDIES

Standard brain imaging is normal in patients with TD.

TREATMENT

ACUTE GENERAL Rx

- Treatment is predicated on prevention (Fig. 2): Limit the indications for antipsychotics; use the lowest effective dose; discontinue the drugs, when feasible; and monitor patients frequently. Anticholinergic medications may worsen symptoms.
- Switch to second-generation antipsychotics, if possible.

CHRONIC Rx

- If continued antipsychotic treatment is needed, switching to clozapine or quetiapine remains the preferred initial treatment if feasible, though evidence is insufficient.[3,4]
- Valbenazine and deutetrabenazine, inhibitors of the vesicular monoamine transporter 2 (VMAT2), are centrally acting synaptic dopamine depleters that are the first FDA-approved treatments for TD and are recommended as first-line treatment options when discontinuation of antipsychotic not indicated. The older version, tetrabenazine, may also improve TD and might be considered.[3-7]

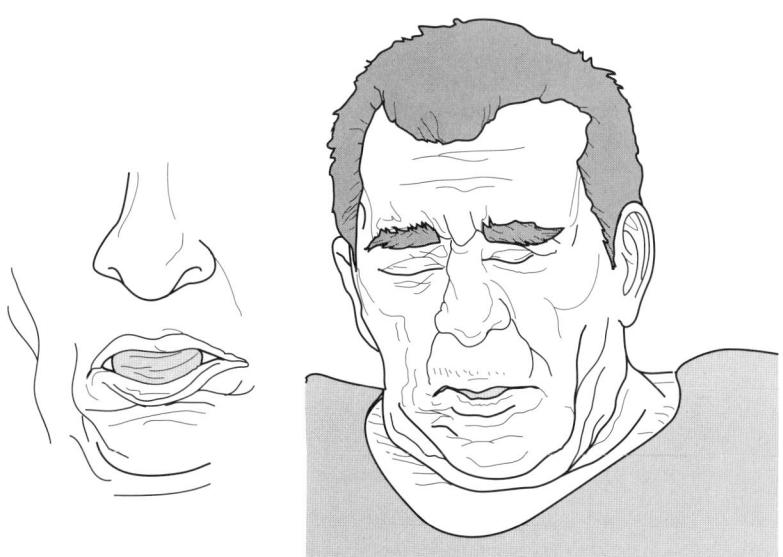

FIG. 1 The oral-buccal-lingual type of tardive dyskinesia consists of repetitive tongue darting, lip smacking, kissing, lip puckering, and chewing. Sometimes blepharospasm also is present. Tongue movements are not only prominent, but they may lead to tongue enlargement *(macroglossia)*. (From Kaufman DM et al: *Kaufman's clinical neurology for psychiatrists,* ed 9, Philadelphia, 2023, Elsevier.)

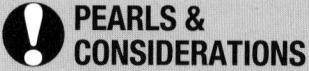

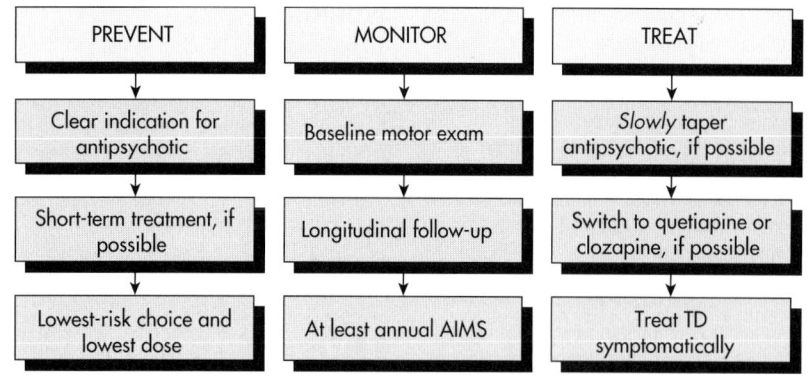

FIG. 2 Prevention and treatment of tardive dyskinesia *(TD)*. (From Stern TA: *Massachusetts General Hospital handbook of general hospital psychiatry*, ed 7, Philadelphia, 2018, Elsevier.)

- Clonazepam, botulinum toxin, amantadine, and ginkgo have limited evidence to improve TD.[3,4]
- For treatment-resistant, disabling TD, deep brain stimulation of internal globus pallidus seems to provide significant symptom reduction without exacerbation of psychiatric symptoms.[3]
- Limited evidence suggests that vitamin E might help prevent progression of TD; however, there is no evidence that this can be a treatment strategy for the condition.[8]
- Using a higher dose of antipsychotic medication to mask TD is not considered a safe practice, as the risks might outweigh the benefits.[9]
- TD is potentially irreversible in nearly two thirds of patients; thus patients undergoing long-term treatment with dopamine receptor blocking agents require frequent monitoring and aggressive management at the onset of TD symptoms.

REFERRAL

Movement disorder specialist consultation if symptoms are severe

PEARLS & CONSIDERATIONS

- After removal of the causative medication, symptoms of tardive dyskinesia can take months to resolve or may become permanent (higher risk in elderly, female sex, prolonged use, and higher dose of causative medication).
- First-generation antipsychotics should be resumed to treat TD in the absence of active psychosis only as a last resort for persistent, disabling, and treatment-resistant TD.
- Avoid anticholinergic medications (e.g., benztropine), which may exacerbate TD symptoms.
- Recent evidence suggests increased overall mortality among patients with TD, which highlights the need for referral for more aggressive specialized interventions.

REFERENCES
Available at eBooks.Health.Elsevier.com.

RELATED CONTENT
Tardive Dyskinesia (Patient Information)

AUTHORS: **SHREEDHAR PAUDEL, MD, MPH,** and **CAROL LIM, MD, MPH**

BASIC INFORMATION

DEFINITION

Temporomandibular joint (TMJ) syndrome refers to a group of disorders leading to symptoms of the TMJ. Box 1 describes a classification of temporomandibular joint disorder (TMD), which also can be classified as intraarticular (within the joint) or extraarticular (involving the surrounding musculature). The TMJ is a diarthrotic joint, meaning neither joint can move independently of the other because each is hinged at both ends. The joint is a true synovial joint capable of two actions of movement: Translational and rotational. The articulating surfaces are the glenoid fossa of the temporal bone and the condylar process of the mandible, with the articular disk interposed between the two.

SYNONYMS

Temporomandibular dysfunction
Painful temporomandibular joint
TMJ
Temporomandibular disorders (TMD)

ICD-10CM CODE
N26.60 Temporomandibular joint disorder, unspecified

EPIDEMIOLOGY & DEMOGRAPHICS

- 15% to 25% of the population have symptoms of TMJ disorders at some point in their lives.
- Females are affected more often than males (up to 4:1 ratio).
- Occurs between the second and fourth decades of life.
- Usually unilateral, affecting either side with equal frequency.

PHYSICAL FINDINGS & CLINICAL PRESENTATION

- Symptoms may appear or be worse during stressful life events.

1. Often unilateral pain in the muscles of mastication, usually described as a "dull" ache
2. Otalgia
3. Odontalgia
4. Headaches (frontal, temporal, retroorbital)
5. Tinnitus
6. Dizziness
7. Clicking or popping sounds with movement of the TMJ
8. Joint locking
- Fig. E1 illustrates the clinical examination of the temporomandibular joint, range of mandibular motion, and muscle palpation.
- Physical exam findings:
  1. Tender to palpation over TMJ in external auditory meatus or preauricular region anterior to tragus
  2. Limited jaw opening or trismus
  3. Clicking or popping of TMJs with joint mobility
  4. Lateral deviation of mandible
  5. TMJ crepitus

ETIOLOGY

- Myofascial pain-dysfunction syndrome: The most common cause of TMJ syndrome and results from teeth grinding and clenching the jaw (bruxism)
- Internal TMJ derangement: Abnormal connection of the articular disk to the mandibular condyle as a result of disk displacement or chronic dislocations
- Degenerative joint disease
- Rheumatoid arthritis
- Gouty arthritis
- Pseudogout
- Ankylosing spondylitis
- Trauma (i.e., fractures)
- Congenital defects (i.e., aplasia, hypoplasia)
- Prior surgery (orthodontic, intraarticular steroid injection)
- Tumors

DIAGNOSIS

Can be made based on history and physical examination in most cases.

DIFFERENTIAL DIAGNOSIS

Includes the list provided earlier. Myofascial pain-dysfunction syndrome, internal TMJ derangement, and degenerative joint disease represent >90% of all causes of TMJ syndrome. Others not mentioned include dental problems such as dental caries, loss of posterior teeth support, and Eagle syndrome (stylohyoid syndrome, carotidynia, and trigeminal neuralgia). Alternative diagnoses such as otitis, mastoiditis, salivary gland disorders, migraine headache, sinusitis, postherpetic neuralgia, trigeminal neuralgia, glossopharyngeal neuralgia, and giant cell arteritis should always be excluded.

WORKUP

The diagnosis is based largely on history and physical examination findings. Radiographic imaging evaluation is used to exclude anatomic or systemic causes of disease when conservative management has failed.

LABORATORY TESTS

Laboratory examination is often not needed but may be helpful in ruling out certain conditions. CBC if infection is suspected. Rheumatoid factor if rheumatoid arthritis is suspected.

IMAGING STUDIES

- Plain radiographs: The most common views are the panoramic, transorbital, and transpharyngeal in both opened and closed positions.
- CT scan is highly accurate in diagnosing osseous derangements of the TMJ.
- MRI is the procedure of choice and has replaced arthrography in cases of disabling pain or if locking occurs. It is used to determine disk position and morphology along with degenerative bony changes.
- Arthrography is helpful in looking for meniscus involvement but is seldom performed anymore, as it is more invasive and less accurate than MRI for TMJ imaging.

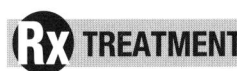 TREATMENT

NONPHARMACOLOGIC THERAPY

- Soft diet to rest the muscles of mastication
- Heat 15 to 20 min 4 to 6 times per day
- Massage of the masseter and temporalis muscles
- Formed splints or bite appliances to reduce compression of retrodiscal tissue (Fig. 2)
- Range-of-motion exercises
- Cognitive-behavioral therapy and biofeedback have been shown to reduce pain
- Acupuncture

ACUTE GENERAL Rx

- NSAIDs: Ibuprofen 800 PO mg tid prn or naproxen 500 mg PO bid prn, titrated to relieve symptoms

---

BOX 1 Classification of Temporomandibular Joint Disorder

Myofascial Pain Disorder and Dysfunction
Most common; primarily of muscular origin
Characterized by myogenous pain and limited mandibular function
May be associated with parafunctional habits, stress, anxiety, depression, or trauma

Temporomandibular Joint Internal Displacement (Disk Displacement)
Reducing or nonreducing (closed lock) with joint sounds and deviation with opening
Most common is anteromedial displacement of the disk
Results in a mechanical interference, leading to moderate to severe restriction in range of motion

Systemic Diseases (Arthritides, e.g., Rheumatoid Arthritis, Psoriatic Arthritis, Osteoarthritis)
Affect the joint through inflammation or degenerative processes
May result in condylar remodeling and degenerative joint disease
Also may be related to infectious processes triggering joint inflammation

Congenital and Developmental Diseases (Including Trauma and Neoplasms)
Hemifacial microsomia or condylar hyperplasia
Idiopathic condylar resorption
Ankylosis
Tumors (e.g., osteochondroma)

From Hochberg MC: *Rheumatology*, ed 7, Philadelphia, 2019, Elsevier.

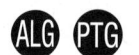
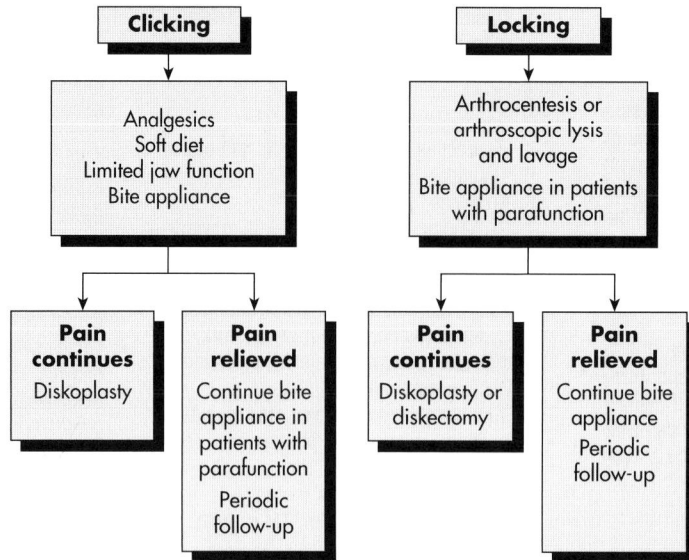

FIG. 2 Management of internal derangements of the temporomandibular joint. Patients with painful clicking or locking are treated medically initially, whereas patients with locking require surgical intervention. (From Firestein GS et al: *Firestein & Kelley's textbook of rheumatology,* ed 11, Philadelphia, 2021, Elsevier.)

- Muscle relaxants or benzodiazepines at bedtime: Diazepam 2.5 to 5 mg PO tid prn or amitriptyline 5 to 100 mg PO daily prn
- In degenerative joint disease of the TMJ, intraarticular steroid injection can be tried
- Botulism toxin injections into the masticatory muscles
- Arthrocentesis with joint lavage and lysis of adhesions (Fig. E3)
- In patients with pain and clicking in the TMJ that is unresponsive to nonsurgical treatment, the disk should be repositioned arthroscopically or by open surgery (discoplasty) (see "Chronic Rx")

CHRONIC Rx

- Most of the above treatments are used for myofascial pain-dysfunction syndrome; however, they can be applied to other causes of TMJ syndrome. Surgery is usually a measure of last resort in patients who do not respond to nonpharmacologic and acute general treatment. Absolute indications for surgical therapy include neoplasms, growth abnormalities, and joint ankylosis.
- Surgical procedures include:
  1. Meniscoplasty
  2. Meniscectomy
  3. Subcondylar osteotomy
  4. TMJ reconstruction

DISPOSITION

The course depends on the underlying etiology; however, less than 5% of adults with temporomandibular symptoms develop chronic symptoms.

REFERRAL

All patients with TMJ syndrome refractory to conservative nonpharmacologic and acute therapy should be referred to a periodontist, oral maxillofacial surgeon, or ear-nose-throat surgeon.

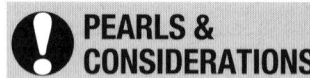

PEARLS & CONSIDERATIONS

Patients with rheumatoid arthritis involving the TMJ usually have bilateral involvement.

COMMENTS

Frequently, emotional stress initiates the myofascial pain-dysfunction, which accounts for 85% of all cases of TMJ syndrome.

SUGGESTED READING

Available at eBooks.Health.Elsevier.com.

RELATED CONTENT

Temporomandibular Joint (TMJ) Syndrome (Patient Information)

AUTHOR: **LOUIS F. INSALACO, MD**

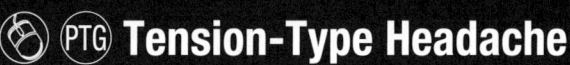

 BASIC INFORMATION

DEFINITION

Tension-type headache (TTH) is a highly prevalent primary headache disorder. In contrast to migraine, it is not typically associated with nausea, vomiting, photophobia, or phonophobia.[1] Although previously thought to be caused by psychological factors and muscle contraction, current thinking implicates neurobiological mechanisms.

ICD-10CM CODES
G44.201 Tension-type headache, unspecified, intractable
G44.209 Tension-type headache, unspecified, not intractable

EPIDEMIOLOGY & DEMOGRAPHICS

Most common type of neurologic dysfunction and type of headache, representing 70% of all headaches presenting to primary care physicians. Yearly prevalence rates in the U.S. are more than 34,000 per 100,000 people. Women are slightly more affected than men.[2]

PHYSICAL FINDINGS & CLINICAL PRESENTATION

Headaches have an insidious progression, ranging from infrequent (<1 day per mo) to chronic (at least 180 days per yr).[1] Although considered a "featureless" headache disorder, either photophobia or phonophobia may still be present, but are typically more mild. Concurrent problems, such as anxiety, depression, and analgesic overuse, may aggravate the headaches. Patients may have pericranial tenderness to palpation on exam. The rest of the examination should be normal.

PATHOPHYSIOLOGY

- TTH is no longer thought to be due to either a psychological problem or abnormal muscle contraction. Similar to migraine, TTH is likely a heterogeneous disorder with several possible pathophysiologic mechanisms.
- In episodic TTH, peripheral mechanisms may predominate, whereas in chronic TTH, central mechanisms are involved.

Dx DIAGNOSIS

The International Headache Society criteria[1] for tension-type headache are as follows:
- At least 10 headaches
- Lasting from 30 min to 7 days
- Having at least two of the following features:
  1. Bilateral
  2. Pressure or tightening (nonpulsating) quality
  3. Mild or moderate intensity
  4. Not aggravated by routine physical activity such as walking or climbing stairs
- Both of the following:
  1. No nausea or vomiting

2. No more than one of either photophobia or phonophobia
- Not better accounted for by another diagnosis

DIFFERENTIAL DIAGNOSIS

- Migraine (would expect associated symptoms [i.e., nausea]; see Table 1 and "Migraine Headache" chapter)
- Cervical spine disease
- Intracranial mass (may present with focal neurologic signs, seizures)
- Idiopathic intracranial hypertension (found more often in obese women of childbearing age)
- Medication overuse headache
- Secondary headache (e.g., obstructive sleep apnea, temporomandibular joint syndrome, hypo- or hyperthyroidism, drug side effects)
- Section II describes the differential diagnosis of headaches

WORKUP

- Routine testing is not needed; the diagnosis may be established clinically.
- Thorough history to identify any red flag features (see topic "Migraine Headache," SSNOOP5 mnemonic in Differential Diagnosis) and physical examination (looking for papilledema) for all patients being evaluated for headache.
- Neuroimaging, preferably with contrast-enhanced MRI, should be performed only when red flag features are identified by history or unexplained neurologic findings are present on examination.
- Erythrocyte sedimentation rate and C-reactive protein in patients 50 yr of age and older to screen for giant cell arteritis.

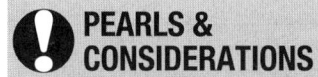 **TREATMENT**

Current evidence supports synergistic benefits of combined nonpharmacologic and pharmacologic interventions. Nonpharmacologic therapy may include behavioral sleep modification, acupuncture, cognitive-behavioral therapy, relaxation training, and biofeedback.[3,4]

ACUTE Rx

- Simple analgesics (i.e., NSAID, acetaminophen).
- Combination analgesics containing caffeine may be used as second-line treatment, although use on more than 10 days per month may lead to medication overuse headache.
- As with migraine headaches, narcotic- and barbiturate-containing analgesics should be avoided in tension-type headaches.

PREVENTIVE Rx

- Tricyclic antidepressants (e.g., amitriptyline 10 to 70 mg qhs) (first choice)
- Other options: Mirtazapine, venlafaxine, and tizanidine
- Muscle relaxers have not been known to show any benefit.[3]

DISPOSITION

For those with episodic or infrequent TTH, prognosis is generally favorable. Chronic TTH can be more difficult to treat as it is generally less responsive to therapeutic agents.[5]

REFERRAL

If red flags are present on history or exam or if the patient is not improving with treatment

⨀ PEARLS & CONSIDERATIONS

It is imperative to avoid overuse of caffeine as well as narcotic- and barbiturate-containing medications because of the risk of rebound headaches.

REFERENCES
Available at eBooks.Health.Elsevier.com.

RELATED CONTENT
Tension Headache (Patient Information)

AUTHOR: **ANJALI SUNDARAMOORTHY, DO**

TABLE 1 Comparison of Tension-Type and Migraine Headaches

	Tension-type	Migraine
Location	Bilateral	Hemicranial*
Nature	Dull ache	Throbbing*
Severity	Slight–moderate	Moderate–severe
Associated symptoms	None	Nausea, hyperacusis, photophobia
Behavior	Continues working	Seeks seclusion
Effect of alcohol	Reduces headache	Worsens headache

*In approximately half of patients, at least at onset.
From Kaufman DM et al: *Kaufman's clinical neurology for psychiatrists*, ed 9, Philadelphia, 2023, Elsevier.

Diseases and Disorders

T

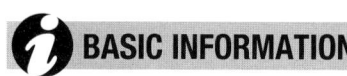

BASIC INFORMATION

DEFINITION

Testicular cancers (TCs) are primary germ cell cancers originating in the testis. They are the most common cancers in men between the ages of 15 and 44 yr.

SYNONYMS

TC
Testis tumor
Testicular neoplasms

ICD-10CM CODES

C62.00	Malignant neoplasm of unspecified undescended testis
C62.01	Malignant neoplasm of undescended right testis
C62.02	Malignant neoplasm of undescended left testis
C62.10	Malignant neoplasm of unspecified descended testis
C62.11	Malignant neoplasm of descended right testis
C62.12	Malignant neoplasm of descended left testis
D40.10	Neoplasm of uncertain behavior of unspecified testis
D40.11	Neoplasm of uncertain behavior of right testis
D40.12	Neoplasm of uncertain behavior of left testis

EPIDEMIOLOGY & DEMOGRAPHICS

INCIDENCE:
- There were an estimated 9910 new cases and 460 deaths associated with testicular cancer in the U.S. in 2022.[1]
- Globally, there were an estimated 74,400 new cases and 7300 deaths from testicular cancer in 2020.[2]
- White men have the highest incidence, whereas Black men have the lowest incidence.

PREVALENCE:
- TC accounts for 0.5% of all cancers in males and is the most common malignancy between the ages of 15 and 35 yr.

PHYSICAL FINDINGS & CLINICAL PRESENTATION

- TC typically presents as a painless testicular mass. Any mass within the testicle should be considered cancer until proven otherwise. It may be found by the patient, who brings it to the attention of a physician, or it may be found by a physician on a routine examination.
- Symptoms other than scrotal or testicular swelling are typically absent unless the cancer has metastasized (10% of patients at diagnosis).[3,4] Occasionally a patient may report scrotal fullness or heaviness. About 10% of patients present with acute pain. Back pain secondary to enlarged retroperitoneal lymph nodes can occur. Gynecomastia from

tumors that secrete beta-human chorionic gonadotropin (hCG) is found in 5% of men with testicular cancer.
- Testicular palpation should be performed with two hands. Transillumination may distinguish a solid mass (e.g., cancer) and a fluid-filled lesion (e.g., hydrocele or spermatocele). The mass is nontender; indeed, it is less sensitive than a normal testicle.

ETIOLOGY, CLASSIFICATION, & PATHOLOGY

- Cryptorchidism (undescended testes) is a major risk factor even if corrected by orchiopexy; however, treatment of undescended testis before puberty decreases the risk of testicular cancer from fivefold to twofold.
- Family history is an important risk factor (risk is four to eight times as high in a brother of a person with testicular cancer and four to six times higher in sons of a father with testicular cancer).
- Other risk factors include genetic disorders (Down syndrome, testicular dysgenesis syndrome), Klinefelter syndrome, infertility, tobacco use, and White race (risk is highest among Whites and lowest among Blacks).
- Classification: TC can be classified as pure seminomas or nonseminomatous germ cell tumors (embryonal carcinoma, choriocarcinoma, yolk sac carcinoma, teratoma, or mixed germ cell tumors).
- Germ-cell neoplasia in situ (GCNIS) is a precursor lesion developing from gonocytes that have failed to mature. Approximately 90% of germ-cell tumors are associated with adjacent GCNIS, which carries a 50% risk of testicular cancer within 5 yr.[4] Table 1 summarizes germ cell tumors and serum markers. More than 80% of TC harbor an isochromosome of the short arm of chromosome 12, while the rest have amplification of 12p genetic material. Genes localized to the 12p region are associated with pluripotency, germ cell proliferation, and survival. After the development of GCNIS, subsequent steps occur that lead to malignant transformation, with a gain of 12p sequences possibly playing a major role.

- The incidence of various subtypes of TC is as below:

Cell Type	Frequency (%)
Seminoma	42
Embryonal cell carcinoma	26
Teratocarcinoma	26
Teratoma	5
Choriocarcinoma	1

- Other rare types:
  1. Yolk sac carcinoma
  2. Mixed germ cell tumors
  3. Carcinoid tumor
  4. Sertoli cell tumors
  5. Leydig cell tumors
  6. Lymphoma
  7. Metastatic cancer to the testes

STAGING

- The TNM staging system for TC is described in Table 2 and Table 3.
- The clinical stages consist of stage I, with tumor confined to the testis; stage II, with positive regional lymph nodes; and stage III, with metastases. Fig. 1 shows the clinical staging of TC.

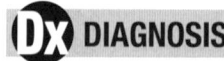 DIAGNOSIS

DIFFERENTIAL DIAGNOSIS

- Spermatocele
- Varicocele
- Hydrocele
- Epididymitis/orchitis
- Epidermoid cyst of the testicle
- Epididymis tumors
- Inguinal hernia
- Hematocele or testicular rupture
- Torsion of testicular appendage

TABLE 1 Germ Cell Tumors and Serum Markers

Histology	Marker Negative (%)	Elevated hCG Alone (%)	Elevated AFP Alone (%)
Seminoma	90	10 (usually <100 IU/ml)	0 (if +, by definition, NSGCT)
All NSGCTs	15	50-60	40
Embryonal		0	10-40
Yolk sac tumors		Rare	80-90 (alone or with elevated hCG)
Choriocarcinoma (or syncytiotrophoblast elements)		>90 (level can be very high)	0

AFP, α-Fetoprotein; *hCG*, human chorionic gonadotropin; *NSGCT*, nonseminoma germ cell tumor.
From Niederhuber JE: *Abeloff's clinical oncology*, ed 6, Philadelphia, 2020, Elsevier.

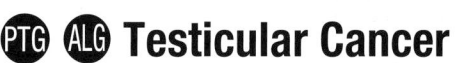

TABLE 2 TNM Staging for Testicular Cancer *(AJCC 8th Edition Staging Cancer Manual)*

pT Stage	Primary Tumor
pT_X	Primary tumor cannot be assessed
pT_0	No evidence of primary tumor
pT_{is}	Germ cell neoplasia in situ
pT_1	Tumor limited to testis (including rete testis invasion) without lymphovascular invasion pT_{1a}: Tumor smaller than 3 cm in size (seminoma only) pT_{1b}: Tumor 3 cm or larger in size (seminoma only)
pT_2	Tumor limited to testis (including rete testis invasion) with lymphovascular invasion OR tumor invading hilar soft tissue or epididymis or penetrating visceral mesothelial layer covering the external surface of tunica albuginea with or without lymphovascular invasion
pT_3	Tumor directly invades spermatic cord soft tissue with or without lymphovascular invasion
pT_4	Tumor invades scrotum with or without lymphovascular invasion
N Stage	**Regional Lymph Nodes**
N_x	Regional lymph nodes cannot be assessed
N_0	No regional lymph node metastasis
N_1	Metastasis with a lymph node mass 2 cm or smaller in greatest dimension OR multiple lymph nodes, none larger than 2 cm in greatest dimension
N_2	Metastasis with a lymph node mass larger than 2 cm but not larger than 5 cm in greatest dimension OR multiple lymph nodes, any one mass larger than 2 cm but not larger than 5 cm in greatest dimension
N_3	Metastasis with a lymph node mass larger than 5 cm in greatest dimension
M Stage	**Distant Metastasis**
M_0	No distant metastasis
M_1	Distant metastasis present M_{1a}: Nonretroperitoneal nodal or pulmonary metastases M_{1b}: Nonpulmonary visceral metastases
S	**Serum Tumor Markers**
S_x	Not available
S_0	Markers within normal levels
S_1	LDH $<1.5 \times$ N *and* hCG (mIU/ml) <5000 *and* AFP (ng/ml) <1000
S_2	LDH $1.5\text{-}10 \times$ N *or* hCG (mIU/ml) 5000-50,000 *or* AFP (ng/ml) 1000-10,000
S_3	LDH $>10 \times$ N *or* hCG (mIU/ml) $>50,000$ *or* AFP (ng/ml) $>10,000$

AJCC, American Joint Committee on Cancer; *TNM,* tumor, necrosis, metastases.

TABLE 3 AJCC Prognostic Stage Groupings

Stage	T	N	M	S
0	pT_{is}	N_0	M_0	S_0
I	$pT_{1\text{-}4}$	N_0	M_0	S_X
I_A	pT_1	N_0	M_0	S_0
I_B	$pT_{2\text{-}4}$	N_0	M_0	S_0
I_S	Any T	N_0	M_0	$S_{1\text{-}3}$
II	Any T	$N_{1\text{-}3}$	M_0	S_X
II_A	Any T	N_1	M_0	$S_0\text{-}S_1$
II_B	Any T	N_2	M_0	$S_0\text{-}S_1$
II_C	Any T	N_3	M_0	$S_0\text{-}S_1$
III	Any T	Any N	M_1	S_X
III_A	Any T	Any N	M_{1a}	$S_0\text{-}S_1$
III_B	Any T	Any N	$M_0\text{-}M_{1a}$	S_2
III_C	Any T	Any N	$M_0\text{-}M_{1a}$	S_3
	Any T	Any N	M_{1b}	Any S

AJCC, American Joint Committee on Cancer.

WORKUP

Physical examination, laboratory tests, and imaging studies (Fig. 2). Immunohistochemical analysis of the testicular specimen is used to determine the histologic composition of the tumor. Staging involves computed tomography (CT) of chest, abdomen, and pelvis and measurement of beta subunit of human chorionic gonadotropins (β-hCG), alpha-fetoprotein (AFP), and lactate dehydrogenase (LDH).

LABORATORY TESTS

- Serum β-hCG is elevated in approximately 20% of patients with pure seminomas.
- Serum AFP is elevated in nonseminoma tumors, never elevated in patients with pure seminomas.
- One or both tumor markers will be elevated in 70% of cases of testicular cancer.
- Serum lactate LDH level is elevated with rapid turnover of malignant cells.
- Testicular biopsy is contraindicated.

IMAGING STUDIES

- Testicular ultrasound
- CT scan of chest, pelvis, and abdomen
- MRI of the brain in patients with neurologic symptoms
- PET scan is not recommended (frequent false positives)

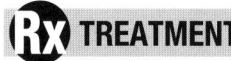 **TREATMENT**

- Fertility preservation is an important but underutilized consideration in the management of these patients. Serum cryopreservation is the most cost-effective procedure for fertility preservation and should be offered to all patients before the start of therapy.
- The initial diagnostic procedure involves usually a radical inguinal orchiectomy, which is both diagnostic and therapeutic. Treatment recommendations are dependent on pathology (seminoma vs. nonseminoma), stage (I vs. II vs. III), and risk (good, intermediate, poor).
- Box E1 summarizes a treatment algorithm for TC.
- Seminoma:
  1. Stage I: Most patients (80% to 85%) are cured with orchiectomy. The addition of adjuvant chemotherapy (one cycle of single-agent carboplatin) or radiation therapy (to the paraaortic lymph nodes) is a standard treatment option that increases cure rates to >95%. In most instances, though, active postorchiectomy surveillance is the routine approach in clinical practice. Recent randomized trials have shown that less intensive surveillance CT imaging strategies are noninferior to aggressive imaging strategies in this stage group. Long-term survival is the norm irrespective of the initial option chosen.
  2. Stage II_A or II_B: Radiotherapy or combination chemotherapy (e.g., bleomycin, etoposide, and cisplatin [BEP] regimen).
- Nonseminoma:
  1. Stage I_A: Radical orchiectomy plus nerve-sparing retroperitoneal lymph node dissection (RPLND)
  2. Stage I_B: Same as stage I_A plus two cycles of chemotherapy (bleomycin, etoposide, and cisplatin [BEP])
  3. Stages II-III: Multiagent cisplatin-based chemotherapy regimens for three or four cycles depending on risk stratification (low/

T

Diseases and Disorders

I

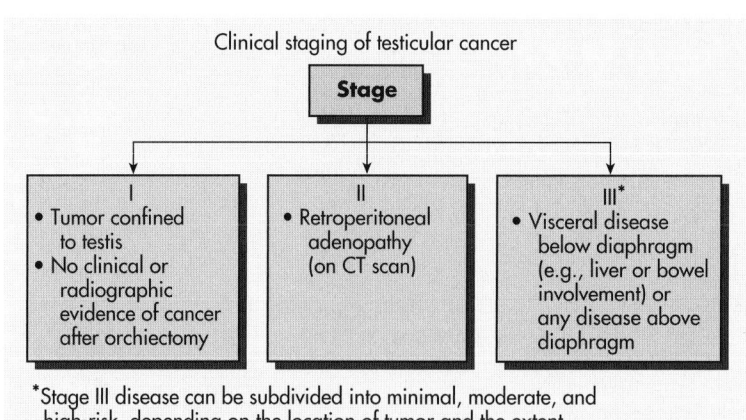

FIG. 1 Clinical staging of testicular cancer. The American Joint Committee on Cancer TNM staging system is less commonly used, because it is based upon histologic evaluation of the orchidectomy specimen and retroperitoneal periaortic lymph node dissection. Because the latter may not be performed in every patient, the clinical staging system is generally more practical. *CT*, Computed tomography; *TNM*, tumor, necrosis, metastases. (From Skarin AT: *Atlas of diagnostic oncology,* ed 4, St Louis, 2010, Mosby.)

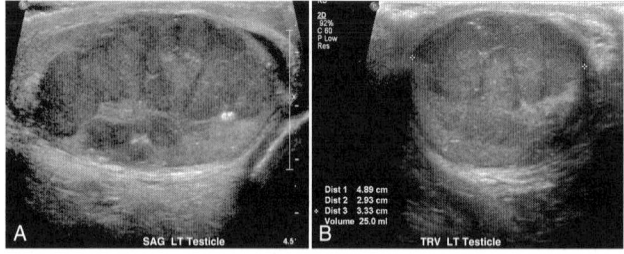

FIG. 2 Seminoma in an 18-yr-old patient with painless left scrotal mass. A and **B,** Sagittal and transverse sonograms of the left testis demonstrate a testicular volume of 25 ml, with a lobulated, heterogeneous, relatively hypoechoic mass occupying most of the testis with a thin rim of normal testis and a few tiny clusters of calcification, as well as multiple, tiny, brightly echoic speckles both inside and outside the mass. The tiny speckles represent microlithiasis. (From Rumack CM et al: *Diagnostic ultrasound,* ed 4, Philadelphia, 2011, Elsevier.)

intermediate or high). RPLND is offered for residual lymph nodal disease after chemotherapy
- Relapsed disease:
  1. Salvage chemotherapy using multiagent regimens is offered. Active chemotherapy regimens include TIP (paclitaxel, ifosfamide, cisplatin) and VIP (vinblastine, ifosfamide, cisplatin) regimens.
  2. Chemotherapy-sensitive patients can be successfully treated with high-dose chemotherapy followed by autologous stem cell transplantation (ASCT).
- Posttreatment surveillance for testicular cancer survivors (annually):
  1. Fertility assessment
  2. Physical examination and skin examination (increased risk of dysplastic nevi)
  3. Testicular examination (3% to 4% risk of second testicular cancer)
  4. Serum tumor markers (hCG, AFP)
  5. Abdominal and pelvic CT every 3 to 4 mo for 2 yr, every 6 to 12 mo in third and fourth yr, and annually thereafter

DISPOSITION

- The overall cure for TC is >95% (80% for metastatic disease). Patients with pure seminomas have a better prognosis. Prognosis can be determined by criteria established by the International Germ Cell Consensus Criteria (Table E4). Given these favorable outcomes, the U.S. Preventive Services Task Force recommends against screening asymptomatic men for testicular cancer.
- There is an increased risk for metabolic syndrome (insulin resistance, hypertension, dyslipidemia, abdominal obesity) after radiation or chemotherapy. Additionally, effects on long-term reproductive health, lower fertility, hearing impairment, neuropathy, and Raynaud phenomenon are long-term toxicities seen with chemotherapy use.[5]
- Therapeutic radiation and chemotherapy are both risk factors for the development of solid and hematologic second malignant neoplasms (SMNs) in survivors. In a recent SEER analysis

of 29,400 patients, the 30-yr cumulative incidences of solid-SMN after radiotherapy, chemotherapy, and surgery alone were 16.9%, 10.1%, and 8.8%, respectively.[6] Increased sevenfold excesses of acute myeloid leukemia were seen 1 to 10 yr after testicular cancer diagnosis. Risks for lymphoma and plasma cell dyscrasias were not elevated. Common reported cancers include those of the thyroid, kidney, pancreas, and stomach, as well as leukemia.

REFERENCES
Available at eBooks.Health.Elsevier.com.

RELATED CONTENT
Testicular Cancer (Patient Information)

AUTHOR: **BHARTI RATHMORE, MD**

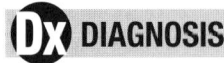

Diseases
and Disorders

I

BASIC INFORMATION

DEFINITION[1-3]

Thoracic outlet syndrome (TOS) describes a condition producing upper extremity symptoms believed to result from neurovascular compression at the thoracic outlet (Fig. E1, Table 1). Three types are described on the basis of point of compression: (1) cervical rib and scalenus syndrome, in which abnormal scalene muscles or the presence of a cervical rib may cause compression; (2) costoclavicular syndrome, in which compression may occur under the clavicle; and (3) subcoracoid pectoralis minor syndrome, in which compression may occur in the subcoracoid area or retropectoralis minor area. The compression occurs in three anatomic structures: Arteries, veins, and nerves, and specific terminology is used to describe TOS depending on the predominantly affected structure: Arterial TOS, venous TOS, and neurogenic TOS.[1] TOS usually is caused by a combination of two factors: (1) having abnormal anatomy that creates compression in the thoracic outlet and (2) having some environmental factor such as injury at the thoracic outlet or excessive repetitive motion that predisposes to compression.
- Neurogenic TOS (nTOS): Caused by compression of brachial nerve plexus
- Arterial TOS (aTOS): Caused by subclavian artery compression and almost always associated with complete cervical rib or anomalous first rib
- Venous TOS (vTOS): Caused by compression of subclavian vein and may also occur in patients with chronic indwelling intravenous catheters

SYNONYM

TOS

ICD-10CM CODE
G54.0 Brachial plexus disorders

EPIDEMIOLOGY & DEMOGRAPHICS[2]

PREVALENCE: TOS is an uncommon disorder. Its prevalence varies from source to source, likely due to a lack of agreement on diagnostic criteria.

Presence of cervical ribs occurs in 0.5% to 1% of the population (50% bilateral), but most are asymptomatic. Approximately 90% to 95% of all TOS disorders are neurogenic, and the remaining 5% to 10% are arterial or venous.

PREDOMINANT SEX: Females affected more often than males (ratio of 3.5:1).

PREDOMINANT AGE: TOS usually occurs in the third to fifth decades of life, although certain types occur in younger individuals.

PHYSICAL FINDINGS & CLINICAL PRESENTATION[2,4]

- Symptoms and signs are related to the degree of involvement of each of the various structures at the level of the first rib.
- True venous or arterial involvement is not common.
- Diagnosis is most often used in the consideration of neural pain affecting the arm, which suggests involvement of the brachial plexus.
  1. Arterial compression: Pallor, pain, paresthesias, diminished pulses, coolness, Raynaud phenomenon, digital gangrene, digital ischemia, supraclavicular bruit or mass, and stroke
  2. Venous compression: Edema, cyanosis and pain, thrombosis causing superficial venous dilation in the shoulder area
  3. Neurologic compression: Pain and/or paresthesia of neck, shoulder region, arm or hand, depending on the root involved; intrinsic weakness and diminished sensation on examination; occipital headache
  4. Possible supraclavicular tenderness
  5. Provocative tests[5]: Adson (Fig. E2), Wright (hyperabduction test where the strength of the radial pulse weakens as the arm is passively abducted and externally rotated), elevated arm stress test or EAST (Roos), upper limb tension test or ULTT (Elvey). May reproduce pain but are of disputed usefulness

ETIOLOGY[2,3]

- Congenital cervical rib or fibrous extension of cervical rib
- Abnormal scalene muscle insertion
- Drooping of shoulder girdle from generalized hypotonia or trauma

- Narrowed costoclavicular interval as a result of downward and backward pressure on shoulder (sometimes seen in individuals who carry heavy backpacks), poor posturing, pregnancy
- Acute venous thrombosis with exercise (effort thrombosis or Paget-Schroetter syndrome)
- Bony abnormalities of first rib
- Abnormal fibromuscular bands
- Malunion of clavicle fracture

DIAGNOSIS

DIFFERENTIAL DIAGNOSIS[5]

- Carpal tunnel syndrome
- Cervical radiculopathy
- Brachial neuritis
- Ulnar nerve compression (cubital tunnel syndrome)
- Complex regional pain syndrome
- Superior sulcus tumor
- Intrinsic shoulder dysfunction

WORKUP

Fig. E3 describes a diagnostic algorithm for thoracic outlet syndrome. Preliminary criteria for the clinical diagnosis of neurogenic thoracic outlet syndrome are summarized in Table 2. Except for venous or arterial pathology, no ancillary diagnostic tests are reliable for diagnostic confirmation.

IMAGING STUDIES[6]

- Electromyography and nerve conduction velocity studies to rule out carpal tunnel syndrome, cervical radiculopathy
- Doppler ultrasound for initial evaluation for arterial or venous thoracic outlet syndrome with provocative maneuvers
- Cervical spine radiographs to rule out cervical disk disease
- Chest x-ray examination to rule out lung tumor
- Computed tomography with intravenous (IV) contrast for detailed anatomic relationship of vascular structure to surrounding muscles and bones
- Computed tomography angiography or contrast-enhanced magnetic resonance angiography can be very useful in assessing

TABLE 1 Sites and Structures Compressed in Thoracic Outlet Syndrome

Site	Description	Abnormalities	Structures Compressed
Sternal-costovertebral circle	This aperture can be narrowed by bony variations	• Cervical first rib • First rib • Long transverse process	• Subclavian artery • Subclavian vein • Brachial plexus
Scalene muscle triangle	The scalenus anterior and middle muscle insert on the first rib, creating a tunnel	Scalenus anterior and middle	• Subclavian artery • Brachial plexus
First rib, clavicular space	The neurovascular structures lie above the rib and below the clavicle	• Costoclavicular ligament • Clavicle • First rib	• Subclavian vein • Subclavian artery • Brachial plexus
Behind the pectoralis minor muscle	The neurovascular structures travel to and from the arm behind this muscle	• Pectoralis minor • Costocoracoid ligament	• Subclavian vein • Subclavian artery • Brachial plexus

From Sellke FW et al: *Sabiston & Spencer surgery of the chest*, ed 9, Philadelphia, 2016, Elsevier.

TABLE 2 Preliminary Criteria for the Clinical Diagnosis of Neurogenic Thoracic Outlet Syndrome

Unilateral or bilateral upper extremity symptoms that:

(1) Extend beyond the distribution of a single cervical nerve root or peripheral nerve

(2) Have been present for at least 12 wk

(3) Have not been explained satisfactorily by another condition

(4) Meet at least one criterion in at least four of the following five categories:

1. Principal symptoms	1A. Pain in the neck, upper back, shoulder, arm, or hand
	1B. Numbness; paresthesias; or weakness in the arm, hand, or digits
2. Symptom characteristics	2A. Pain, paresthesias, or weakness exacerbated with elevated arm positions
	2B. Pain, paresthesias, or weakness exacerbated by prolonged or repetitive arm or hand use or by prolonged work on a keyboard or other repetitive strain
	2C. Pain or paresthesias radiate down the arm from the supraclavicular or infraclavicular space
3. Clinical history	3A. Symptoms began after occupational, recreational, or accidental injury of the head, neck, or upper extremity, including repetitive upper extremity strain or overuse activity
	3B. Previous clavicle or first rib fracture or known cervical rib(s)
	3C. Previous cervical spine or peripheral nerve surgery without sustained improvement
	3D. Previous conservative or surgical treatment for thoracic outlet syndrome
4. Physical examination	4A. Local tenderness on palpation over scalene triangle or subcoracoid space
	4B. Arm, hand, or digit paresthesias on palpation over scalene triangle or subcoracoid space
	4C. Weak handgrip, intrinsic muscles, or digit 5 or thenar or hypothenar atrophy
5. Provocative maneuvers	5A. Positive upper limb tension test (ULTT)
	5B. Positive 1- or 3-min elevated arm stress test (EAST)
	5C. Positive Adson test
	5D. Positive Wright test (or hyperabduction)

From Cameron JL, Cameron AM: *Current surgical therapy*, ed 12, Philadelphia, 2017, Elsevier.

vessel imaging while using provocative arm positions
- MRI with and without IV contrast for evaluation of neurogenic thoracic outlet syndrome
- Arteriography or venography (Fig. E4) can be used for dynamic studies while performing upper extremity maneuvers and also performing thrombolysis, if needed

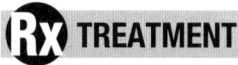 **TREATMENT**

ACUTE GENERAL RX[2,3]
- Avoid weight gain
- Sling for pain relief
- Physical therapy modalities plus shoulder girdle–strengthening exercises

- Postural reeducation
- NSAIDs and other analgesics
- Muscle relaxants
- Muscle block with injection of local anesthetic agent or botulinum toxin A in anterior scalene (for diagnostic and therapeutic reasons, e.g., predicting response to surgical intervention)[7]

CHRONIC RX[2,3]
Surgical treatment is indicated in the presence of the following:
- Symptomatic after failure of physical therapy
- With complications such as thrombosis, aneurysms
- With neurologic compressions
- With sympathetic cervical rib

Surgical options:
- Thoracic outlet decompression including cervical rib resection and anterior scalenectomy
- Thoracic sympathectomy
- Vascular reconstruction
- Catheter-directed thrombolysis or aspiration mechanical thrombectomy, followed by thoracic outlet decompression and anticoagulation for deep vein thrombosis due to venous TOS

DISPOSITION[2,3]
- Nonsurgical treatment is often successful for patients with pain as the primary symptom.
- Nonsurgical management is initially recommended in neurogenic TOS. Operative management is often required in arterial TOS and venous TOS.
- Complications of surgical treatment include transient dysesthesia, hematoma, pneumothorax, hemothorax, venous injury, arterial injuries, or brachial plexus injuries.

REFERRAL
For vascular surgery consultation when venous or arterial impairment is present

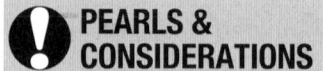 **PEARLS & CONSIDERATIONS**

COMMENTS
- True thoracic outlet syndrome is probably an uncommon condition with considerable disagreement regarding its frequency.
- Diagnosis is often used to describe a wide variety of clinical symptoms and should be modified by the affected structure such as nTOS, aTOS, and vTOS.

REFERENCES
Available at eBooks.Health.Elsevier.com.

RELATED CONTENT
Thoracic Outlet Syndrome (Patient Information)

AUTHOR: **PHILIPPE MONTGRAIN, MD**

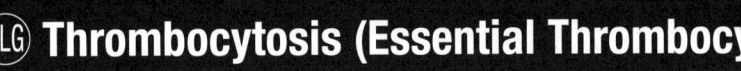
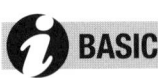 **BASIC INFORMATION**

DEFINITION

Thrombocytosis is defined by an elevated platelet count (>450,000/ml) in peripheral blood. It is caused by overproduction of platelets (reactive thrombocytosis) or clonal expansion of megakaryocytes (clonal thrombocytosis). Reactive thrombocytosis is driven by excessive cytokines induced by various stimuli, such as trauma or inflammation. Clonal thrombocytosis is defined as chronic myeloproliferative neoplasms (MPNs), of which four subgroups are well characterized: Chronic myelogenous leukemia (CML), polycythemia vera (PV), primary myelofibrosis (PMF), and essential thrombocythemia (ET). In addition, platelet count can be spuriously elevated in some conditions (see "Differential Diagnosis"). Extreme thrombocytosis is defined as platelet count >1 million/ml. This chapter deals primarily with essential thrombocythemia.

SYNONYMS

Thrombocythemia
Essential thrombocythemia
ET

ICD-10CM CODES	
D47.3	Essential (hemorrhagic) thrombocythemia
D75.89	Other specified diseases of blood and blood-forming organs
D75.9	Disease of blood and blood-forming organs, unspecified
D77	Other disorders of blood and blood-forming organs in diseases classified elsewhere

EPIDEMIOLOGY & DEMOGRAPHICS

It has been estimated that about 88% to 97% of the cases of thrombocytosis are reactive rather than clonal proliferation.[1]

Epidemiology for essential thrombocythemia:
INCIDENCE: 1 to 2 per 100,000 population/yr.[2]
PREVALENCE: Estimated at 38 to 57 cases/ 100,000 population.[3]
PREDOMINANT SEX & AGE: The median age at diagnosis is 65 to 70 yr. Female:male ratio is 2:1.[4]

PHYSICAL FINDINGS & CLINICAL PRESENTATION

- Regardless of the cause, a high platelet count may be associated with vasomotor symptoms such as headache, visual disturbances, dizziness, atypical chest pain, acral dysesthesia, and erythromelalgia.[1,4]
- Thrombotic and bleeding complications can occur. Thrombosis at unusual sites (hepatic vein, IVC, portal vein, splenic vein) are especially concerning.[1,4]
- Symptoms and complications are much more likely to occur in association with clonal thrombocytosis than reactive thrombocytosis.
- The degree of thrombocytosis does not predict the likelihood of clonal thrombocytosis and does not generally correlate to the risk of thrombosis.[1]

- Splenomegaly is common with MPNs.[5]
- Coexistent leukocytosis and erythrocytosis are common with CML and PV.[5]
- Disease transformation from ET to PV, PMF, and acute myeloid leukemia (AML) is uncommon. In patients with ET, the 15-yr rate of leukemic transformation is estimated at 2% to 5%.[6]

ETIOLOGY

- Essential thrombocytosis, a myeloproliferative neoplasm, is a clonal disorder of a multipotent hematopoietic progenitor cell.[1]
- Abnormality in JAK2-STAT pathway (including *JAK2, CALR,* and *MPL* gene mutations) may play a role in pathogenesis of MPN.[1]

DX DIAGNOSIS

DIFFERENTIAL DIAGNOSIS

- Spurious thrombocytosis:
  1. Mixed cryoglobulinemia—precipitated cryoglobulin particles are counted as platelets by automatic counters; generally occurs at low temperatures
  2. Circulating cytoplasmic fragments miscounted as platelets—seen mainly in patients with leukemia, lymphoma, severe hemolysis, or burns
- Reactive thrombocytosis:
  1. Benign hematologic disorders
  2. Acute hemorrhage, iron deficiency anemia, hemolytic anemia
  3. Chronic infection, such as tuberculosis
  4. Acute and chronic inflammatory disorders
  5. Rheumatologic disorders
  6. Inflammatory bowel disease
  7. Celiac disease
  8. Functional and surgical asplenia
  9. Tissue damage
  10. Trauma, thermal burn
  11. Myocardial infarction
  12. Acute pancreatitis
  13. Recent surgery
  14. Renal failure, nephrotic syndrome
  15. Exercise
  16. Medications, such as vincristine, epinephrine
- Clonal thrombocytosis:
  1. CML
  2. PV
  3. PMF
  4. Myelodysplastic syndrome (5q-syndrome)
  5. AML with inv(3), t(3;3)
  6. Essential thrombocytosis (Box 1)

WORKUP

- Comprehensive history and physical examination to exclude many of the common causes of reactive thrombocytosis: History and physical examination suggestive of acute blood loss, iron deficiency, acute or chronic infection/inflammation, medication use, asplenia, malignancy, and trauma should be evaluated. Fig. E1 describes a diagnostic algorithm for thrombocytosis. The diagnosis of ET requires platelet counts >450 × 10^3/ml on two separate occasions >4 wk apart, absence of BCR-ABL, and exclusion of secondary causes of thrombocytosis.
- Repeat CBC with peripheral blood smear and bone marrow biopsy (Figs. E2 and E3) to exclude spurious thrombocytosis.

LABORATORY TESTS

- CBC with peripheral blood smear: Howell-Jolly bodies and target cells are present in patients with asplenia; nucleated red blood cell (RBC), teardrop RBC and white blood cell (WBC) precursors in patients with PMF.
- Serum ferritin level: Low ferritin level suggests iron deficiency.
- Serum C-reactive protein, erythrocyte sedimentation rate, and plasma fibrinogen: Nonspecific markers of infection or inflammation.

> **BOX 1** World Health Organization Diagnostic Criteria for Essential Thrombocythemia
>
> Diagnosis requires that all of the following criteria be met:
> - Sustained platelet count ≥450 × 10^9/L*
> - Bone marrow biopsy specimen showing proliferation mainly of the megakaryocytic lineage, with increased numbers of enlarged, mature megakaryocytes; no significant increase or left shift of neutrophil granulopoiesis or erythropoiesis
> - Failure to meet the WHO criteria for polycythemia vera,[††] primary myelofibrosis,[‡] BCR-ABL1–positive chronic myelogenous leukemia,[§] myelodysplastic syndrome,[¶] or other myeloid neoplasms
> - Demonstration of *JAK2 V617F* or other clonal marker; or, in the absence of *JAK2 V617F*, no evidence of reactive thrombocytosis[¶]
>
> *Sustained during the workup process.
> ‡Requires the absence of relevant reticulin fibrosis, collagen fibrosis, peripheral blood leukoerythroblastosis, or markedly hypercellular marrow accompanied by megakaryocyte morphology typical for primary myelofibrosis—small to large megakaryocytes with an aberrant nuclear-to-cytoplasmic ratio and hyperchromatic, bulbous, or irregularly folded nuclei and dense clustering.
> †Requires the failure of iron replacement therapy to increase the hemoglobin level to the polycythemia vera range in the presence of decreased serum ferritin. Exclusion of polycythemia vera is based on hemoglobin and hematocrit levels; red cell mass measurement is not required.
> §Requires the absence of BCR-ABL1.
> ¶Causes of reactive thrombocytosis include iron deficiency, splenectomy, surgery, infection, inflammation, connective tissue disease, metastatic cancer, and lymphoproliferative disorders. Requires the absence of dyserythropoiesis and dysgranulopoiesis.
> From Swerdlow SH et al (eds): *WHO classification of tumours of haematopoietic and lymphoid tissues,* Lyon, France, 2008, IARC Press.

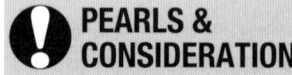
TABLE 1 Choice of Drugs for Treatment of Patients With High-Risk Essential Thrombocythemia

Age (yr)	Treatment of Choice	Second Line
<50	Interferon	Anagrelide
		Hydroxyurea
50-75	Hydroxyurea	Interferon
		Anagrelide
>75	Hydroxyurea	Anagrelide

From Hoffman R et al: *Hematology: basic principles and practice,* ed 7, Philadelphia, 2018, Elsevier.

- Philadelphia chromosome or BCR-ABL rearrangement: Positive in CML.
- Serum erythropoietin assay: Low to normal in PV and ET.
- *JAK2* mutation analysis: PV and ET; *JAK2* mutation is found in 95% of patients with PV and in 50% to 60% of patients with ET and PMF.[7]
- In ET, frequency of *MPL* and *CALR* mutations are estimated to be 5% and 27%, respectively.[8]
  1. These mutations are associated with differences in prognosis and risk of thrombosis.[8]
  2. *JAK2, CALR,* and *MPL* mutations are mutually exclusive. They are not confined to a particular myeloproliferative neoplasm, and their absence does not exclude any of the MPNs.[8]
  3. About 13% of patients with ET will be negative for *JAK2, CALR,* and *MPL* mutations.[8]
- Bone marrow chromosome analysis: 5q-syndrome and other myelodysplastic syndrome, CML.
- Bone marrow exam in ET may show clusters of abnormal megakaryocytes and increased reticulin fibrosis (see Fig. E3).

Rx TREATMENT

No therapies are known to alter survival or leukemic transformation in ET. Reactive thrombocytosis has been rarely associated with thrombosis or bleeding and generally does not require specific therapy.

ACUTE GENERAL Rx

- Vasomotor symptoms easily manageable with low-dose aspirin (<100 mg/day).[5]
- Bleeding:
  1. Discontinue any platelet antiaggregating agent, such as aspirin or nonsteroidal antiinflammatory agents.
  2. Evaluate for disseminated intravascular coagulopathy and coagulation factor deficiency. Acquired factor V deficiency is occasionally present in association with clonal thrombocytosis. In that case, treat with fresh frozen plasma infusion.

3. In case of extreme thrombocytosis (platelet count generally >1,000,000/uL [1000×10⁹/L]), acquired von Willebrand disease may occur. Immediate definitive therapy with a platelet-lowering agent is essential in this instance. Platelet pheresis should be reserved for cases of acute thrombosis or bleeding.
- Thrombosis:
  1. Arterial or venous thrombosis occurs in 10% to 20% of patients.[8]
  2. If the platelet count is >800,000/ml, platelet apheresis coupled with a platelet-lowering agent should be considered with the goal of platelet count <400,000/mm³.
  3. Anticoagulant therapy for 3 mo to indefinite based on the presence or absence of additional thrombophilic defects.

CHRONIC Rx

Treatment strategies for ET are based on the presence or absence of risk factors for thrombosis. Objective risk stratification is done by calculating IPSET-thrombosis score with age, history of thrombosis, cardiac risk factor, and presence of JAK2 mutation. Smoking cessation and obesity management should be discussed with all patients with ET. In low-risk patients (age <60 yr, no history of thrombosis or hemorrhage, platelet count <1 million/ml), observation may be adequate. Treatment with low-dose aspirin is indicated in low-risk patients with vasomotor symptoms or with other indications for aspirin use. The cytoreductive therapy along with low-dose aspirin therapy is indicated in high-risk patients (age >60 yr and/or with previous history of thrombosis) regardless of vasomotor symptoms. Exception is if a high-risk patient has no history of arterial thrombosis but has history of venous thrombosis, in which case systemic anticoagulation instead of low-dose aspirin is recommended.[8]
- Low-dose aspirin (81 mg/day) may be safe and effective in preventing vascular events. It is also effective in preventing recurrent vascular events in high-risk patients and in treating the vasomotor symptoms.
- Cytoreductive therapy (Table 1):
  1. First-line therapy is hydroxyurea in majority of cases. Anagrelide and interferon (if not used previously) generally are considered second line.
  2. Hydroxyurea (HU) vs. anagrelide: A randomized trial comparing HU with aspirin and anagrelide with aspirin in patients with ET found that patients in the anagrelide group had increased rates of arterial thrombosis, serious hemorrhage, and transformation to myelofibrosis, but decreased rate of venous thrombosis.[9] However, another randomized trial found no difference between HU and anagrelide in terms of arterial and venous thrombosis and bleeding complications.[10] Current recommendation is to consider anagrelide after failure of other drug options, including HU, interferon, and busulfan.[8] Monitor liver

function tests and the degree of neutropenia or anemia with HU therapy.
3. The incidence of leukemic conversion in patients with ET treated with HU alone is reported as <1%. Interferon alpha may be effective for controlling platelet count in patients failing treatment with HU. A randomized control trial comparing HU with pegylated interferon (PEG) found no difference in complete response between the two treatments at 12 mo. However, PEG was associated with more Grade 3/4 adverse events compared to HU (46% vs. 28%).[11]
4. To date there is no proven benefit to JAK2 inhibition with ruxolitinib compared to best available therapy in essential thrombocytosis with regard to platelet counts, thrombosis, hemorrhage, or transformation to AML.

DISPOSITION

- Although long survival is expected in patients with ET, it is inferior to the sex- and age-matched U.S. population.
- An International Prognostic Score for Essential Thrombocythemia (IPSET) was proposed by International Working Group on Myelofibrosis Research and Treatment based on age, WBC count, and history of thromboembolism at diagnosis.

REFERRAL

Refer to hematologist/oncologist when platelet count is consistently elevated >450,000/mm³ without causes for reactive thrombocytosis.

! PEARLS & CONSIDERATION

COMMENTS

- Some patients with clinically apparent ET have BCR-ABL rearrangement, even in the absence of other features of CML. It is suggested that it should be tested in all ET patients due to its potential therapeutic implications.
- The risk of bleeding with aspirin use in patients with ET paradoxically increases when the platelet count is >1 million/ml, likely due to acquired von Willebrand disease.

PATIENT & FAMILY EDUCATION

Smoking cessation is encouraged in both patients with ET and reactive thrombocytosis.

REFERENCES

Available at eBooks.Health.Elsevier.com.

AUTHORS: **NIRAV HARIBHAKTI, MD, PHARMD,** and **JOHN L. REAGAN, MD**

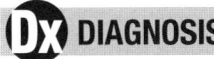

T

Diseases and Disorders

I

BASIC INFORMATION

DEFINITION

Superficial venous thrombophlebitis (SVT) is an inflammation of a vein with subsequent secondary thrombus formation. SVT most frequently involves superficial veins of the leg, but any superficial vein can be affected. SVT has been reported to occur in 125,000 people in the U.S. per year; however, the actual incidence is likely far greater. SVT is not always a benign condition. SVT should be regarded as the superficial venous manifestation of a systemic process known as venous thromboembolism (DVT, PE).

SYNONYMS

SVT
Superficial phlebitis
Superficial suppurative thrombophlebitis
Suppurative thrombophlebitis

ICD-10CM CODES
I80.00	Phlebitis and thrombophlebitis of superficial vessels of unspecified lower extremity
I80.8	Phlebitis and thrombophlebitis of other sites
I80.9	Phlebitis and thrombophlebitis of unspecified site

EPIDEMIOLOGY & DEMOGRAPHICS

- Approximately 30% to 45% of patients diagnosed with SVT are men with an average age of 54 yr.
- Approximately 55% to 70% of patients diagnosed with SVT are women with an average age of 58 yr.
- The overall recurrence of SVT is 18% over an average observation period of 15 mo, equally involving varicose and nonvaricose veins.
- The lifetime incidence of SVT in those with untreated varicose veins has been estimated at 25% to 50%.

PHYSICAL FINDINGS & CLINICAL PRESENTATION

- Subcutaneous vein is palpable as a tender cord or "worm-like" mass with increased warmth and erythema.
- Induration, redness, and tenderness are localized along the course of the vein. This linear appearance (Fig. E1) rather than circular appearance is useful to distinguish thrombophlebitis from other conditions (cellulitis, erythema nodosum).
- There is some swelling of the overlying skin and subcutaneous tissue but without generalized edema of the limb.
- Low-grade fever may be present.

ETIOLOGY

- In the lower extremity, 70% of SVT occurs in patients with varicose veins, with the great saphenous vein being most commonly involved (60% to 80%)
- Intravenous catheters and infusion of caustic drugs are the most common cause of upper-extremity SVT

- Malignancy
- Pregnancy/puerperium
- Hypercoagulable states
- Previous DVT/SVT
- OCP (oral contraceptive pill)/HRT (hormone replacement therapy)

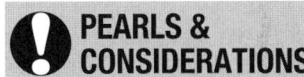 DIAGNOSIS

DIFFERENTIAL DIAGNOSIS

- Lymphangitis
- Cellulitis
- Erythema nodosum
- Panniculitis
- Acute lipodermatosclerosis

WORKUP

The clinical investigation includes not only the local findings but also the presence of varicose veins with or without the stigmata of chronic venous insufficiency. Today, duplex ultrasound is the most important additional diagnostic tool.

IMAGING STUDIES

- Duplex ultrasound offers the advantage of being inexpensive, noninvasive, and repeatable for follow-up examination.
- Ultrasonography confirms the diagnosis, shows the location of the thrombus and its location regarding the saphenofemoral and/or saphenopopliteal junctions.
- Ultrasound examination of patients with SVT has revealed that a concomitant DVT can exist in 15% to 20%.
- In up to 25% of these patients, the DVT may not be contiguous with the SVT and may be found in the contralateral leg.
- Therefore bilateral duplex exam is recommended in all cases of SVT that involve the main trunk of the great saphenous vein (GSV) or small saphenous vein (SSV).

TREATMENT

NONPHARMACOLOGIC THERAPY

- Warm, moist compresses
- Do not restrict activity. Immediate mobilization with walking exercises

ACUTE GENERAL Rx

- Treatment guidelines for SVT are not well established because of the lack of controlled clinical trials. In general, the primary goal of management should be to prevent thrombus extension and the risk of venous thromboembolism. All other therapy is directed at patient comfort with analgesics and NSAIDs (in patients not receiving anticoagulants).
- In patients with migratory SVT (Fig. E2), recurrent SVT, or SVT without varicose veins, the underlying condition should be investigated, and treatment directed accordingly.
- The most common cause of upper-extremity SVT is an intravenous catheter. Treatment starts with removal of the cannula and application of warm compresses. The resultant

lump may persist for months. No anticoagulant therapy is required.
- In patients with lower-extremity SVT in a varicose vein branch, control of pain with analgesics and the use of gradient compression stockings are usually sufficient. Patients are encouraged to continue their usual daily activities.
- Many investigators favor systemic anticoagulation when there is superficial thrombosis of 5 cm or more in length, the thrombus is within 1 cm of the saphenous junctions, or more than 5 cm of the saphenous trunk is involved, as shown by duplex ultrasonography. Anticoagulation is also reasonable for patients with SVT and cancer or previous DVT.
- The American College of Chest Physicians guidelines recommend anticoagulation for 45 days over no anticoagulation in patients with lower-extremity SVT within 1 cm of the saphenofemoral or saphenopopliteal junction.
- In the case of patients with varicose veins secondary to saphenous vein reflux, a catheter vein ablation procedure should be performed only after the acute SVT episode is over in order to avoid the thromboembolic complications induced by such procedures.

! PEARLS & CONSIDERATIONS

SUPERFICIAL SUPPURATIVE THROMBOPHLEBITIS

- Superficial suppurative thrombophlebitis is associated with an intravenous catheter or multiple puncture sites secondary to IV drug abuse and is located primarily in the upper extremity.
- Clinical presentation is similar to that of nonsuppurative SVT but with associated fever, leukocytosis, and/or septicemia.
- Most cases of intravenous catheter sepsis are not complicated by suppurative thrombophlebitis; local IV catheter site infections occur in about 7% of cases and septicemia is found in only 1 of every 400 IV catheterizations.
- The incidence of peripheral vein suppurative thrombophlebitis is highest in patients with specific risk factors such as burns, steroids, and IV drug abuse.
- Treatment consists of antibiotics with adequate coverage of gram-negative rods and *Staphylococcus aureus,* including MRSA. Initial empirical treatment is with IV vancomycin 1 g q12h *plus* ceftriaxone 1 g IV q24h. Alternative regimen consists of daptomycin 6 mg/kg IV q12h *plus* ceftriaxone 1 g IV q24h.

SUGGESTED READING
Available at eBooks.Health.Elsevier.com.

RELATED CONTENT
Thrombophlebitis (Patient Information)
Deep Vein Thrombosis (Related Key Topic)

AUTHOR: **FRANK G. FORT, MD, FACS, RPHS**

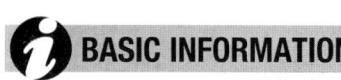

BASIC INFORMATION

DEFINITION

Thrombotic thrombocytopenic purpura (TTP) is a rare autoimmune disorder characterized primarily by thrombocytopenia and microangiopathic hemolytic anemia and can be associated commonly with other hallmarks such as neurologic impairment, renal dysfunction, and fever. The laboratory hallmark of TTP is a severe deficiency of the *ADAMTS13* factor (activity <10%).

SYNONYMS

Immune mediated thrombocytopenic purpura
iTTP
TTP
Upshaw-Schulman syndrome

ICD-10CM CODE
M31.1 Thrombotic microangiopathy

EPIDEMIOLOGY & DEMOGRAPHICS

- About 90% of new TTP cases are seen in adults (mostly females between 18 and 50 yr).
- The incidence of new TTP is 3 to 11 cases per million population per year. The prevalence is ~10 cases per million population.
- There is increased incidence in HIV/AIDS and during pregnancy.

PHYSICAL FINDINGS & CLINICAL PRESENTATION

- The disease often begins as a flulike illness ultimately followed by development of characteristic clinical and laboratory abnormalities.
- Most patients present with nonspecific constitutional symptoms (weakness, nausea, abdominal pain, vomiting).
- Purpura (Fig. E1 and Fig. E2).
- Jaundice and pallor (from hemolysis).
- Mucosal bleeding.
- Fever.
- Fluctuating levels of consciousness (caused by thrombotic occlusion of the cerebral vessels). However, one third of patients have no neurologic abnormalities.
- Renal failure and neurologic events are usually end-stage features.

ETIOLOGY

- Acquired TTP is an autoimmune disorder caused by autoantibody inhibition of *ADAMTS13* activity.[1]
- Hereditary TTP (also called Upshaw-Schulman syndrome) is caused by homozygous or compound heterozygous *ADAMTS13* mutations[2] (Table 1).
- Many drugs, including clopidogrel, ticlopidine, penicillin, antineoplastic agents (gemcitabine, mitomycin C), calcineurin inhibitors (cyclosporine), oral contraceptives, and quinine, have been associated with TTP.
- Other precipitating causes include infectious agents, pregnancy, malignancies, allogeneic stem cell transplantation, and neurologic disorders.
- Acquired TTP has been reported in the setting of COVID-19 infection as well as after vaccination with traditional and mRNA COVID-19 vaccines.

DIAGNOSIS

DIFFERENTIAL DIAGNOSIS

It is challenging to differentiate TTP from other thrombotic microangiopathies given the significant overlap in clinical presentation, but this distinction is critical in selecting an appropriate therapy for patients.

- Disseminated intravascular coagulation (DIC)
- Malignant hypertension
- Vasculitis
- Eclampsia or preeclampsia
- Hemolytic-uremic syndrome (HUS) and atypical HUS
- Gastroenteritis associated with serotoxin-producing serotype of *Escherichia coli*

WORKUP

A comprehensive history, physical examination, and laboratory evaluation usually confirm the diagnosis (Fig. 3).

LABORATORY TESTS

- Severe anemia and thrombocytopenia (platelet count <50,000 or >50% reduction from previous counts)

- Peripheral blood smear (Fig. E4, Fig. E5) with numerous red blood cell (RBC) fragments (schistocytes)
- Elevated blood urea nitrogen and creatinine
- Hemolysis demonstrated by elevated reticulocyte count, indirect bilirubin, lactate dehydrogenase and decreased haptoglobin
- Urinalysis: Hematuria (RBCs and RBC casts in urine sediment) and proteinuria
- No laboratory evidence of DIC (normal fibrin degradation product, fibrinogen)
- Hereditary TTP is diagnosed in cases of *ADAMTS13* deficiency with concurrent absence of *ADAMTS13* autoantibody inhibitor; the confirmation requires documentation of *ADAMTS13* mutations[2]
- Acquired TTP is diagnosed in cases with microangiopathic hemolytic anemia and thrombocytopenia without another apparent cause. An *ADAMTS13* level <10% of normal activity is seen in acquired TTP, while levels >20% suggest other diagnoses

TREATMENT

ACUTE GENERAL Rx

- Discontinue any potential offending agents.
- Initiate *ADAMTS13* replacement by plasma infusion in patients with hereditary TTP.
- TTP therapy consists of complementary approaches:
  1. Therapeutic plasma exchange (TPE)
  2. Immunosuppression
  3. Newer paradigms also include targeting von Willebrand factor-platelet interactions[3]
- TPE reduces mortality rates from >90% to <20%. Daily TPE with replacement of 1.0 to 1.5 times the predicted patient plasma volume is the standard approach. TPE should be continued for a minimum of 2 days after the platelet count returns to normal (>150,000 cells/m³). There is no benefit to a tapering approach with TPE.
- High-dose plasma infusion (25 ml/kg/day) may be useful when TPE cannot be promptly started and in patients with very severe or refractory disease between plasma exchange sessions. This approach can cause volume overload in patients with renal insufficiency.

TABLE 1 Etiology, Epidemiology, and Pathogenesis of TTP, HUS, and *ADAMTS13*–Related Parameters

	Congenital TTP	Acquired TTP	HUS
Etiology	*ADAMTS13* mutation	Antibody to *ADAMTS13*, endothelial cell activation	*Escherichia coli* or other microorganisms
Epidemiology	5-10 cases per year per million	≤1 case per year per million	1-5 cases per year per million, mainly in children
Pathogenesis	Defective cleavage of vWF multimers, massive secretion of ultra-large vWF multimers, increased platelet deposition under shear condition, occlusion of blood vessels in microcirculation		Intoxication with Shiga-like toxin, damage of endothelial cells, enterohemorrhagic colitis, renal disorder
ADAMTS13 antigen	Very low or absent	Low or variable	Normal or moderately decreased
ADAMTS13 activity	≤5%-10%	≤5%-10% or variable	30%-100%
Inhibitor against *ADAMTS13*	No	Mostly yes	No

ADAMTS13, A disintegrin and metalloproteinase with a thrombospondin type 1 motif, member 13; *HUS,* hemolytic uremic syndrome; *TTS,* thrombotic thrombocytopenic purpura; *vWF,* von Willebrand factor.
From McPherson RA, Pincus MR: *Henry's clinical diagnosis and management by laboratory methods,* ed 23, Philadelphia, 2017, Elsevier.

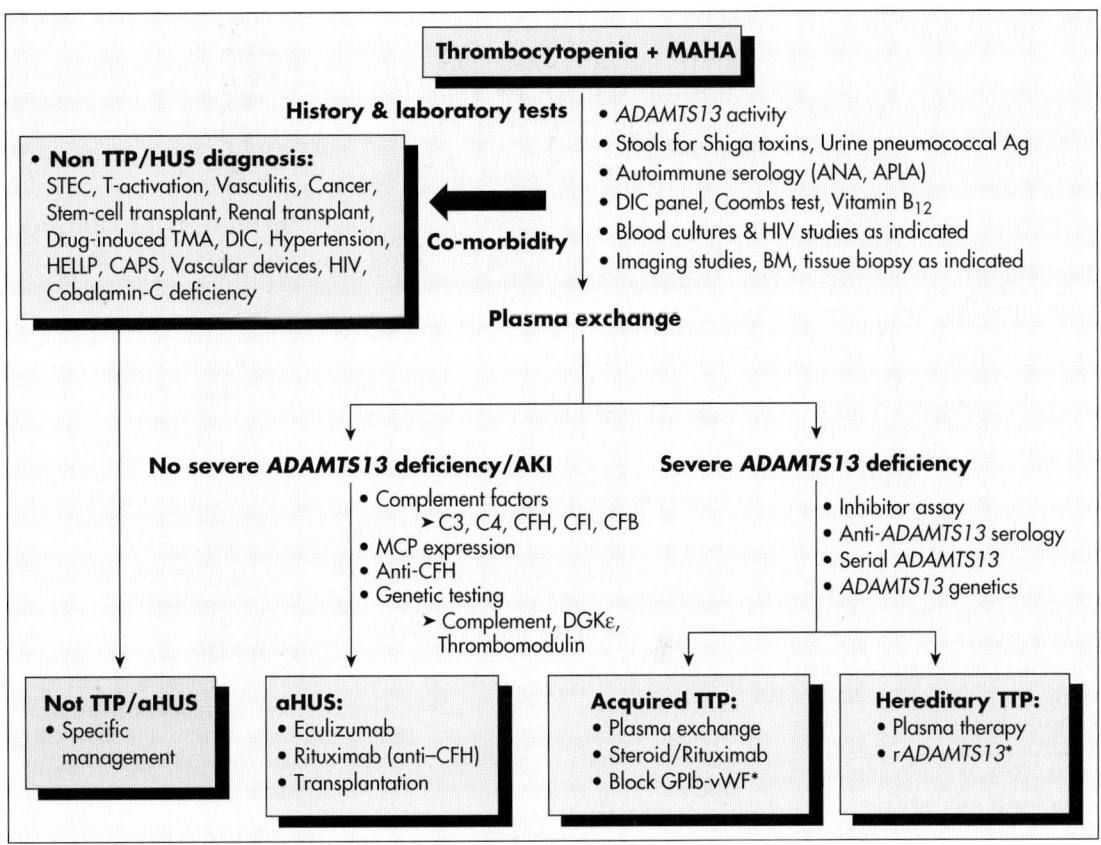

FIG. 3 An approach to diagnosis and management of thrombotic microangiopathies. *ADAMTS13,* A disintegrin and metalloproteinase with thrombospondin type 1 motifs, member 13; *Ag,* antigen; *aHUS,* atypical hemolytic uremic syndrome; *AKI,* acute kidney injury; *ANA,* antinuclear antibody; *APLA,* antiphospholipid antibodies; *BM,* bone marrow; *CAPS,* catastrophic antiphospholipid syndrome; *CFB,* complement factor B; *CFH,* complement factor H; *CFI,* complement factor I; *DGKE,* diacyl glycerol kinase ε; *DIC,* disseminated intravascular coagulation; *GP,* glycoprotein; *HELLP,* hemolysis, elevated liver enzymes, and low platelet count; *HIV,* human immunodeficiency virus; *HUS,* hemolytic uremic syndrome; *MAHA,* macroangiopathic hemolytic anemia; *MCP,* membrane cofactor protein; *rADAMTS13,* recombinant *ADAMTS13; STEC,* Shiga toxin-producing *E. coli; TMA,* thrombotic microangiopathy; *TTP,* thrombotic thrombocytopenic purpura; *vWF,* von Willebrand factor. *Bullet points* are diagnoses or therapies. *Indicates therapies under investigation. (From Hoffman R et al: *Hematology: basic principles and practice,* ed 7, Philadelphia, 2018, Elsevier.)

- Patients with hereditary TTP who experience severe plasma allergic reactions have been effectively treated with plasma-derived factor VIII concentrate that contains *ADAMTS13.*
- Immunosuppression with the concurrent use of corticosteroids (prednisone 1 to 2 mg/kg/day) typically is initiated and tapered over a period of 3 to 4 wk after stable platelet counts are achieved.
- Immunosuppression with the monoclonal anti-CD20 antibody rituximab is used in cases of suboptimally responsive TTP (inadequate platelet recovery after 3 to 5 days of TPE) and results in remissions in most patients.[4] Frontline use of rituximab results in shorter hospitalization with fewer relapses but results in overtreatment in many cases.
- Caplacizumab, an anti–von Willebrand factor humanized, bivalent, variable-domain-only immunoglobulin fragment, inhibits interaction between von Willebrand factor multimers and platelets. In a randomized trial, treatment with caplacizumab and TPE was associated with faster normalization of the platelet count and lower incidence of a composite of TTP-related death, recurrence of TTP, or a thromboembolic event during the treatment period than placebo.[5] It has been FDA approved for use in

combination with plasma exchange and immunosuppressive therapy for treatment of immune-mediated TTP.
- Recombinant *ADAMTS13* is being evaluated, and early data have demonstrated its efficacy in increasing *ADAMTS13* activity in congenital TTP[6] and potential efficacy as an adjunct to TPE.
- Platelet transfusions are contraindicated except in severely thrombocytopenic patients with documented bleeding or those who are facing surgery or other invasive procedures in the setting of severe thrombocytopenia.
- Use of antiplatelet agents (acetylsalicylic acid, dipyridamole) is controversial.
- Splenectomy is performed in refractory cases.
- Dialysis is rarely required.

CHRONIC Rx

- Relapsing TTP may be initially retreated with TPE.
- TTP unresponsive to standard therapy is usually effectively treated with rituximab and occasionally with chemotherapy agents (vincristine, cyclophosphamide, bortezomib).
- Splenectomy done while patients are in remission has been used historically to decrease the frequency of relapses.

DISPOSITION

- Survival of patients with TTP currently exceeds 80% with TPE.
- Relapse occurs in 20% to 40% of patients who have achieved initial remission.

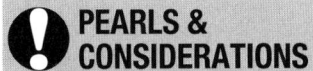

PEARLS & CONSIDERATIONS

COMMENTS

- TTP should be considered in pregnant women with vague neurologic, gastrointestinal, or renal symptoms in either the obstetric triage or emergency department areas.
- TTP is fatal in 90% of patients without therapy.

REFERENCES

Available at eBooks.Health.Elsevier.com.

RELATED CONTENT

Hemolytic-Uremic Syndrome (Related Key Topic)

AUTHOR: **BHARTI RATHORE, MD**

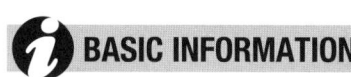

(i) BASIC INFORMATION

DEFINITION[1]

- Thymoma is a rare tumor originating from the thymic epithelial cells. It is the most frequent tumor arising from the thymus gland and the most frequent among the anterior mediastinal neoplasms, despite its unusual Incidence.[1,2]
- Thymoma was once considered to be either benign or malignant. Even though thymoma may be benign by nature, it can infiltrate beyond the thymus capsule (invasive thymoma) or become malignant if it progresses (thymic carcinoma). A benign tumor restricted to the thymus is the most prevalent kind of tumor, followed by locally invasive tumors and carcinomas. However, it is currently regarded as having a high possibility of being malignant. The best approach to tell if the condition will return following therapy is to assess whether the tumors have spread to other locations.[1]
- Thymoma is a slow-growing tumor that spreads primarily through local extension. Extrathoracic metastases are infrequent. In fact, metastases are often restricted to the pleura, pericardium, or diaphragm. Thymomas are frequently associated with neuromuscular conditions such as myasthenia gravis; 10% to 20% of individuals with myasthenia gravis have a thymoma.[1]

ICD-10CM CODES
C37	Malignant neoplasm of thymus
D150	Benign neoplasm of thymus
D384	Neoplasm of uncertain or unknown behavior of thymus
E320	Persistent hyperplasia of thymus
E328	Other diseases of thymus
E329	Disease of thymus, unspecified

EPIDEMIOLOGY & DEMOGRAPHICS

- Thymoma primarily affects adults between the ages of 40 and 70; it is relatively rare in children and adolescents.
- The risk of developing thymoma is comparable for both men and women.[1]

INCIDENCE:
- The incidence of thymomas is remarkably low, at just 1.5 cases per million individuals.
- Thymomas are more prevalent among African Americans, Asians, and Pacific Islanders.[3]

RISK FACTORS:
- It is not well understood what causes thymomas.
- Alcohol consumption, smoking cigarettes, and exposure to ionizing radiation do not appear to be risk factors for developing thymomas.

PHYSICAL FINDINGS & CLINICAL PRESENTATION

- Regarding the clinical presentation, approximately one third of patients are asymptomatic. Those with symptoms typically exhibit chest discomfort, dysphagia, weight loss, appetite loss, cough, or dyspnea.[4]
- There is a strong correlation between thymoma and autoimmune paraneoplastic diseases, the most prevalent of which is myasthenia gravis (30% to 50%), followed by thymoma-associated hypogammaglobulinemia (Good syndrome) and thymoma-associated autoimmune pure red cell aplasia. Myasthenia gravis is characterized by eyelid drooping, double vision, drooling, difficulty ascending stairs, hoarseness, and/or dyspnea.[5]
- Thymomas can invade the local tissue (such as the pleura or the lung), but they seldom extend to nearby lymph nodes or extrathoracic locations. It is possible to develop superior vena cava (SVC) syndrome if the tumor is damaging the primary blood vessel, the superior vena cava, that runs between the brain and the heart. The most typical signs and symptoms of SVC syndrome are face/neck edema, dilated neck veins, cough, dyspnea, orthopnea, proptosis, swelling of the upper extremities, and dilated chest vein collaterals.[2,4]

(Dx) DIAGNOSIS

- Patients who have thymoma in its early stages are usually asymptomatic, and the tumor is frequently discovered inadvertently on a chest

x-ray examination or computed tomography (CT) scan.
- Due to the substantial correlation between myasthenia gravis and thymoma, regular chest CT scans are performed on myasthenia gravis patients as part of their diagnostic evaluation.[4]

DIFFERENTIAL DIAGNOSIS

The thymoma is the most prevalent type of tumor that can be seen in the anterior mediastinum region.[2,6,7]
- Primary anterior mediastinal mass following by thymoma in adults
  1. Substernal goiter
  2. Lymphoma
  3. Germ cell tumor (teratoma)
  4. Carcinoma
- Primary anterior mediastinal mass following by thymoma in children
  1. Lymphoma
  2. Germ cell tumor (teratoma)
  3. Thymic cyst

WORKUP

In patients presenting with anterior mediastinal mass, workup is aimed at differentiating between thymic tumors (the most common type) and nonthymic tumors for further management planning.

LABORATORY TESTS

In cases when myasthenia gravis is suspected, investigations may involve showing antibodies (such as antiacetylcholine receptors or muscle-specific kinase.[5]

IMAGING STUDIES

Contrast-enhanced CT (Fig. 1) is the imaging modality of choice for imaging thymic tumors because of its excellent spatial and temporal resolution, ease of access, and convenience; nonetheless, chest radiographs are the most often performed imaging examination and may be the first modality to suggest a thymic mass. Typical characteristics are a well-defined anterior mediastinal mass in the thymic bed, the absence of tumor markers, the absence of additional

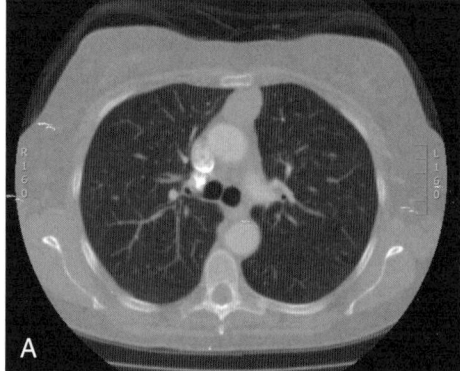 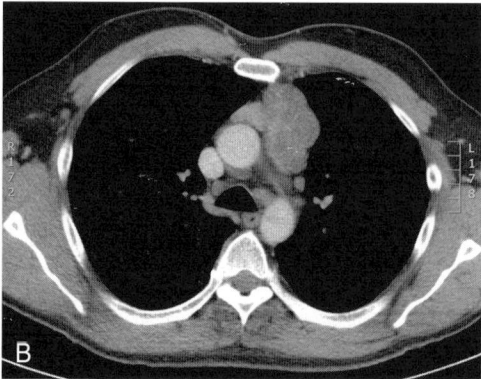

FIG. 1 A, Computed tomography (CT) scan of the chest in a patient with myasthenia gravis and thymoma. The thymoma is small with a plane of separation between the tumor and the pericardium. **B,** Chest CT scan in a patient with a larger mediastinal mass. The location, character, and size are noted. Transthoracic core needle biopsy was performed. Germ cell tumor markers were normal. Pathology demonstrated thymoma. A 6.5-cm thymoma was subsequently resected. There was no invasion of the pericardium. A complete resection (R0) was accomplished. (From Townsend CM et al: *Sabiston textbook of surgery*, ed 21, Philadelphia, 2022, Elsevier.)

adenopathy, and the absence of continuity with the thyroid.[6-8]

MRI is not frequently utilized in the examination of thymic tumors, although it is beneficial in specific situations, such as evaluating for regions of modest local invasion such as in mediastinal organs.[7]

- The importance of PET/CT is particularly evident in aggressive tumors, such as thymic carcinoma, due to a greater total tumor metabolism demonstrated by a much higher absorption of fluorodcoxyglucosc in thymic carcinomas compared to thymomas.[9]

BIOPSY

- If a resectable thymoma is firmly suspected based on clinical and radiologic symptoms (e.g., patients with myasthenia gravis and a distinctive mass on CT), surgical biopsy is not required due to the possibility of tumor seeding when the tumor capsule is breached. In fact, using a transpleural approach to get a thymoma biopsy should be avoided due to the high risk of spreading the tumor within the pleural space, which could result in a stage I thymoma evolving into a stage IV thymoma.[4]
- Small biopsies (fine-needle or core needle biopsies) may not necessarily reveal the presence of invasion. However, if the lesion is sampled using a CT-guided needle biopsy, biopsies are accompanied by a low risk of pneumomediastinum or mediastinitis and an even lower risk of heart or large blood vessel injury.
- Histologically, thymic tumors can be classified according to the World Health Organization (WHO) categories (Table 1). These classifications are based on the appearance of tumor cells under a microscope as follows[10]:
  A: Spindle cell thymoma or medullary thymoma.
  AB: Mixed thymoma, with lymphocytes in the tumor.
  B1: Lymphocytic thymoma, with many lymphocytes in the tumor, but the cells of the thymus appear healthy.
  B2: Cortical thymoma, with many lymphocytes, like type B1 thymoma. However, the thymus cells do not appear healthy.
  B3: Epithelial thymoma, atypical thymoma, squamoid thymoma, and well-differentiated thymic carcinoma. This type of thymoma has few lymphocytes, and the thymus cells look abnormal.

STAGING

Essentially, the tumor, node, metastasis (TNM) staging approach is not useful for thymomas since the majority of patients do not have nodal disease or metastases, and only the extent of the primary tumor is typically imperative. The widely recognized staging system developed by Masaoka et al.[11,12] is provided in Table 2.

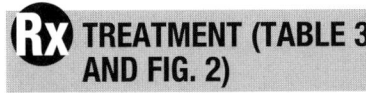 **TREATMENT (TABLE 3 AND FIG. 2)**

- Surgery, including total thymectomy and complete tumor removal, is suggested for all

TABLE 1 World Health Organization (WHO) Classification of Thymoma and Thymic Carcinoma[20]

WHO Type	Histologic Terminology
A	Spindle cell, medullary
AB	Mixed
B1	• Lymphocyte-rich, lymphocytic • Predominantly cortical • Organoid
B2	Cortical
B3	• Epithelial, atypical • Squamoid • Well-differentiated thymic carcinoma
Thymic carcinomas	• Epidermoid keratinizing (squamous cell) carcinoma • Epidermoid nonkeratinizing carcinoma • Lymphoepithelioma-like carcinoma • Sarcomatoid carcinoma (carcinosarcoma) • Clear cell carcinoma • Basaloid carcinoma • Mucoepidermoid carcinoma • Papillary carcinoma • Undifferentiated carcinoma

resectable thymomas in surgically appropriate patients.
- The term "resectability" refers to a complete resection (R0). Indeed, resection completeness is the most significant outcome predictor.[13,14]
- The pericardium, phrenic nerve, pleura, lung, and even significant vascular structures may need to be excised in order to perform a complete resection. The pleural surfaces should be evaluated for pleural metastases during thymectomy. If feasible, pleural metastases should be eradicated to accomplish complete gross resection. However, bilateral phrenic nerve resection should be avoided due to severe respiratory morbidity.[15]
- Adjuvant therapy is not indicated for stage I thymomas that have been totally resected (R0); however, postoperative radiation therapy is recommended for incompletely resected thymomas and patients with thymomas that have capsular invasion after an R0 resection.[14]
- Postoperative radiation is recommended for patients with stage II and stage III thymoma (with macroscopic invasion into adjacent organs) due to the increased risk of disease recurrence. Since thymomas frequently do not disseminate to local lymph nodes, intensive nodal irradiation is rarely a viable option. Postoperative chemotherapy is also not helpful in this situation. The presence of encapsulation has very little impact on the prognosis since all thymomas are classified as malignant when the tumor disrupts the capsule.[16-18]

TABLE 2 Masaoka Clinical Staging of Thymoma[21]

Stage	Description
I	Macroscopically and microscopically completely encapsulated (tumor can invade into but not through the capsule)
IIA	Microscopic invasion through capsule
IIB	Macroscopic invasion into surrounding fatty tissue or mediastinal pleura
IIIA	Macroscopic invasion into neighboring organs (e.g., pericardium or lung)
IIIB	Macroscopic invasion of great vessels
IVA	Pleural or pericardial dissemination
IVB	Lymphogenous or hematogenous metastases

TABLE 3 Masaoka Staging of Thymoma and Treatment Guide Related to Masaoka Staging

Masaoka Stage	Treatment
Stage I	Complete surgical resection
Stage II	Complete surgical resection with consider postoperative RT
Stage III	Complete surgical resection with consider postoperative RT
Stage IV	Complete surgical resection with consider postoperative RT
Any R1 resection	Postoperative Rt
Any R2 resection	Definitive RT +/- chemotherapy

PROGNOSIS

Significance prognostic factors related to shorter overall survival include incomplete tumor resection (R1, R2), increased age, and high staging.[14]

SURVEILLANCE

- Following the primary treatment for resectable thymomas, surveillance for recurrence should comprise chest CT scans every 6 mo for the first 2 yr, followed by yearly screenings for the next 10 yr for thymoma.
- MRI may be utilized for surveillance, including (1) when patients cannot tolerate contrast and (2) when patients are young and will be evaluated for many years to reduce radiation exposure.[19]

REFERENCES & SUGGESTED READING
Available at eBooks.Health.Elsevier.com.

AUTHORS: **VARUT SUPANAKORN, MD,** and **PATAN GULTAWATVICHAI, MD**

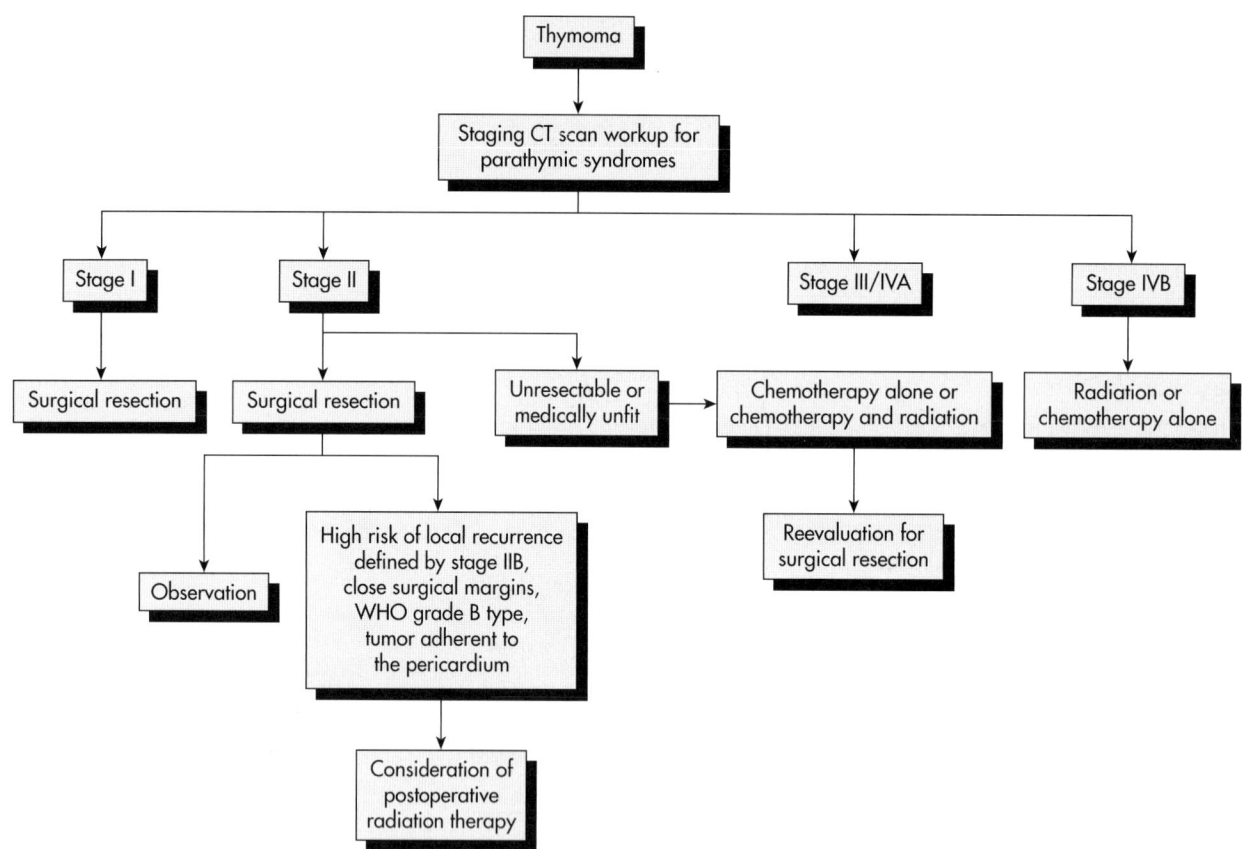

FIG. 2 Algorithm of clinical approach to a patient with thymoma. *CT,* Computed tomography; *WHO,* World Health Organization. (From Niederhuber JE: *Abeloff's clinical oncology,* ed 6, Philadelphia, 2020, Elsevier.)

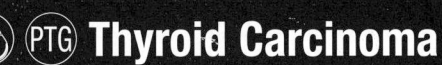

T

 BASIC INFORMATION

DEFINITION

Thyroid carcinoma is a primary neoplasm of the thyroid and consists of four major subtypes: Papillary, follicular, anaplastic, and medullary. A classification of thyroid neoplasms is described in Table E1.

SYNONYMS

Papillary carcinoma of thyroid
Follicular carcinoma of thyroid
Anaplastic carcinoma of thyroid
Medullary carcinoma of thyroid

ICD-10CM CODES
C73	Malignant neoplasm of thyroid gland
D09.3	Carcinoma in situ of thyroid and other endocrine glands
D34	Benign neoplasm of thyroid gland
D44.0	Neoplasm of uncertain behavior of thyroid gland

EPIDEMIOLOGY & DEMOGRAPHICS

- Thyroid cancer is the most common endocrine cancer, with an estimated 43,800 new cases and 2230 deaths occurring in 2022 in the U.S.
- Incidence is 13.9 per 100,000 people in the U.S. and increasing over last 4 decades.
- Female:male ratio is 3:1.
- Median age at diagnosis: 45 to 50 yr.
- Occult thyroid cancer is identified in 20% of autopsy specimens.

PHYSICAL FINDINGS & CLINICAL PRESENTATION

- Thyroid cancer is often identified incidentally.
- Physical exam may reveal:
  1. Presence of thyroid nodule
  2. Hoarseness and cervical lymphadenopathy
  3. Painless swelling in the region of the thyroid

ETIOLOGY

- Risk factors: Prior neck irradiation.
- Multiple endocrine neoplasia II (medullary carcinoma).
- Inherited syndromes associated with thyroid cancer are described in Table 2.
- GLP-1 receptor agonists for the treatment of type 2 DM (e.g., exenatide, albiglutide) can increase the risk of medullary thyroid carcinoma (MTC).

TABLE 2 Inherited Syndromes Associated With Thyroid Cancer

Multiple endocrine neoplasia (MEN) 2A and 2B

Isolated familial medullary thyroid cancer

Gardner syndrome

Familial adenomatous polyposis

Carney complex

Cowden syndrome

Familial nonmedullary thyroid cancer

From Cameron JL, Cameron AM: *Current surgical therapy,* ed 10, Philadelphia, 2011, Saunders.

- Papillary thyroid carcinoma is the commonest type of thyroid carcinoma of follicular origin and encompasses several tumor types that have mutually exclusive mutations that activate thyroid cell abnormal proliferation. BRAF V600E mutation accounts for 60% of these mutations; other mutations include *RAS* or *RET/PTC* rearrangements.[1,2]
- In follicular thyroid carcinoma, oncogenic drivers are primarily *RAS* alterations (40% to 50% of cases) and *PAX8/PPAR*γ rearrangements (30% to 40% of cases). Molecular alterations of the PI3K/Akt pathway and PTEN silencing by inactivating mutations or epigenetic changes also occur in some cases.
- Poorly differentiated thyroid carcinomas are aggressive cancers with a high mutation rate. *RAS* and *BRAF* mutations are found in 20% to 50% and up to 35% of cases, respectively. Genetic alterations that characterize PDTC and are associated with tumor aggressiveness are *TERT* promoter (20% to 50%) mutations and *TP53* mutations (10% to 35%) that cooccur with *RAS* and *BRAF* mutations.[1,2]
- In anaplastic thyroid cancer, as many as 25% to 50% of cases harbor BRAFV600 mutations, which can be targeted with available BRAF/MEK inhibitor combination therapy. Other frequent mutations include *TERT* (75%), *TP53* (63%), and *RAS* (24%). Other actionable molecular drivers with available targeted therapies include *RET* rearrangements, *ALK* rearrangements, *NTRK* fusions, and *TSC2* mutations, suggesting the need for broad molecular profiling.
- Pathways in the development of thyroid cancer are depicted in Fig. E1.

Dx DIAGNOSIS

DIFFERENTIAL DIAGNOSIS

- Multinodular goiter
- Lymphocytic thyroiditis
- Ectopic thyroid

WORKUP

The workup of thyroid carcinoma includes laboratory evaluation and diagnostic imaging. Key features of thyroid malignancies are summarized in Table 3. Diagnosis is confirmed with fine-needle aspiration or surgical biopsy. At diagnosis, the vast majority of thyroid cancers are well differentiated, with excellent prognosis. The characteristics of thyroid carcinoma vary with the type:

- Papillary carcinoma (80%):
  1. Most frequently occurs in women during second or third decades
  2. Histologically, psammoma bodies (calcific bodies present in papillary projections) are pathognomonic; found in 35% to 45% of papillary thyroid carcinomas
  3. Majority are not papillary lesions but mixed papillary follicular carcinomas
  4. Spread is by lymphatics and by local invasion

- Follicular carcinoma (10%):
  1. More aggressive than papillary carcinoma
  2. Incidence increases with age
  3. Tends to metastasize hematogenously to bone, producing pathologic fractures
  4. Tends to concentrate iodine (useful for radiation therapy)
- Poorly differentiated thyroid carcinoma (5% to 6%):
  1. Aggressive cancers with pathology characterized by high mitotic activity and tumor necrosis.
  2. Patients often develop vascular invasion, lymph node metastasis, extrathyroidal extension, and distant metastases.
  3. Associated with a mean survival of 3.2 yr.
  4. Radioiodine therapy is of limited benefit and most patients require systemic therapies.
- Anaplastic carcinoma (1%):
  1. Very aggressive neoplasm
  2. Two major histologic types: Small cell (less aggressive, 5-yr survival approximately 20%) and giant cell (death usually within 6 mo of diagnosis)
- MTC (4%):
  1. Unifocal lesion: Found sporadically in elderly patients
  2. Bilateral lesions: Associated with pheochromocytoma and hyperparathyroidism; this combination is known as MEN-II and is inherited as an autosomal-dominant disorder

LABORATORY TESTS

- Thyroid function studies are generally normal. Thyroid-stimulating hormone (TSH), T4, and serum thyroglobulin levels should be obtained before thyroidectomy in patients with confirmed thyroid carcinoma. Serum thyroglobulin levels can be useful postoperatively to monitor recurrence of thyroid carcinoma (Fig. E2).
- Increased plasma calcitonin assay in patients with medullary carcinoma (tumors produce thyrocalcitonin). RET proto-oncogene sequencing and measurement of plasma free metanephrine and normetanephrine levels to rule out coexistent pheochromocytoma are recommended in all patients with medullary thyroid cancer.
- Fine-needle aspiration biopsy is the best method to assess a thyroid nodule (see "Thyroid Nodule" in Section I). Table 4 describes the Bethesda system for thyroid cytopathology.

IMAGING STUDIES (FIG. E3)

- Thyroid ultrasound can detect solitary solid nodules that have a high risk of malignancy. However, a negative ultrasound does not exclude diagnosis of thyroid carcinoma.
- Thyroid scanning with iodine-123 or technetium-99m can identify hypofunctioning (cold) nodules, which are more likely to be malignant. However, warm nodules can also be malignant.

TABLE 3 Thyroid Malignancies—Key Features

	Description	Pattern of Spread
Papillary carcinoma (70%-80%)	Low-grade tumors with a good prognosis (histologically multicentric) ▶ Tumors concentrate radio-iodine	Early lymph node spread (metastatic lymph nodes may be normal in size, cystic, calcified, hemorrhagic, or contain colloid) ▶ Distant metastases are rare (and usually to the lungs)
Follicular carcinoma (10%-20%)	Slow growing ▶ Tumors concentrate radio-iodine	It rarely metastasizes to the regional lymph nodes ▶ The tendency is to spread via the bloodstream and disseminate to the lungs, bones, or liver
Anaplastic carcinoma (1%-2%)	Undifferentiated malignant tumors that do not concentrate radio-iodine ▶ There is a poor prognosis ▶ They tend to occur in older patients ▶ Punctate calcification and necrosis frequently are present	Lymphatic metastases occur in the majority of patients
Medullary carcinoma (5%-10%)	This originates from the parafollicular C cells ▶ It does not concentrate radio-iodine ▶ It may be sporadic or familial (and associated with the MEN type II syndrome or other endocrine neoplasms) ▶ It is usually a unilateral, solitary lesion ▶ Calcification is seen in 10% ▶ ^{123}I-MIBG and somatostatin analogs (e.g., octreotide) can be used for evaluation ▶ Circulating calcitonin levels are usually elevated	It may invade locally, spread to the regional nodes, or demonstrate hematogenous spread to the lungs, bones, or liver
Lymphoma (10%)	It is usually a non-Hodgkin lymphoma ▶ It occurs in one third of patients with Hashimoto thyroiditis (a MALT-type lymphoma) ▶ It presents as a rapidly enlarging, solitary nodule (80%) or as multiple nodules (imaging cannot distinguish between a lymphoma and thyroiditis) ▶ Necrosis and calcification are uncommon	It can involve the nodes with spread to the GI tract
Metastases (<1%)	The most common primary is renal cell carcinoma	

From Grant LA: *Grainger & Allison's diagnostic radiology essentials*, ed 2, Philadelphia, 2019, Elsevier.

TABLE 4 The Bethesda System for Thyroid Cytopathology

Category	Risk of Malignancy (%)	Recommended Management
Nondiagnostic or unsatisfactory	1-4	Repeat FNA with ultrasound guidance
Benign	0-3	Clinical follow-up
Atypia of undetermined significance (AUS) or follicular lesion of undetermined significance (FLUS)	5-15	Repeat FNA*
Follicular neoplasm or suspicious for follicular neoplasm	15-30	Lobectomy
Suspicious for malignancy	60-75	Lobectomy with or without frozen section or total thyroidectomy
Malignant	97-99	Total thyroidectomy

FNA, Fine-needle aspiration.
*Lobectomy also can be considered depending on clinical or sonographic characteristics.
From Niederhuber JE: *Abeloff's clinical oncology*, ed 6, Philadelphia, 2020, Elsevier.

STAGING (TABLE E5)

- Stage I: Thyroid cancer of any size without distal spread in patient <55 yr. In patients >55 yr, tumor size ≤4 cm without local invasion or positive cervical lymph nodes
- Stage II: Distal spread in patient <55 yr. In patients >55 yr, tumors >2 cm but <4 cm, spread to nearby lymph nodes, not spread to distant sites
- Stage III: Tumors >4 cm in patient >55 yr of age, not spread to distant sites
- Stage IV: Distal spread in patient >55 yr of age

℞ TREATMENT

ACUTE GENERAL Rx

- Papillary carcinoma:
  1. Total thyroidectomy is indicated if the patient has:
     a. Extrathyroid extension
     b. History of radiation exposure
     c. Poorly differentiated
     d. Cervical lymph node involvement
     e. Tumor >4 cm
     f. Known distant metastasis
  2. Lobectomy with isthmectomy may be considered in patients with intrathyroid papillary carcinoma <4 cm and no history of neck or head irradiation; surgery should be followed with suppressive therapy with thyroid hormone because these tumors are TSH responsive. The accepted practice is to suppress serum TSH concentrations to <0.1 microunit/ml in patients with persistent disease, suppression to 0.1 to 0.5 microunit/ml in patients who are disease free but are at high risk of recurrence, and a goal TSH level of 0.3 to 2.0 microunits/ml in patients who are disease free and have a low risk of recurrence.
  3. Radioiodine ablation reduces rates of death and recurrence (Table 6). Radioiodine is administered for stages III and IV disease.[3]
  4. In cases that have progressed after radioiodine therapy, oral targeted inhibitors (lenvatinib, sorafenib) have significant survival benefit.[4-6]
  5. Of note, larotrectinib and entrectinib are both FDA approved for patients with NTRK gene fusion–positive advanced solid tumors.
  6. If a patient is found to have a *BRAF* mutation, one can consider giving vemurafenib or dabrafenib, although these two drugs are not FDA approved for *BRAF*-mutated, metastatic papillary thyroid cancer.
- Follicular carcinoma:
  1. Total thyroidectomy followed by TSH suppression, as previously noted.
  2. Radiotherapy with iodine-131 followed by thyroid suppression therapy with triiodothyronine is useful in patients with metastasis (see Table 6).
  3. In cases that have progressed after radioiodine therapy, oral targeted inhibitors (lenvatinib, sorafenib) have significant survival benefit.
- Anaplastic carcinoma:
  1. At diagnosis, this neoplasm is rarely operable; palliative surgery is indicated for extremely large tumor compressing the trachea.

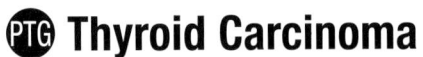
TABLE 6 Indications for Iodine-131 Treatment in Patients With Papillary, Follicular, or Hürthle Cell Thyroid Carcinoma After Initial Definitive Near-Total Thyroidectomy

No Indication

Adult patients at very low risk for cause-specific mortality or relapse: Complete surgical resection, favorable histology, and limited extent of disease (e.g., PTC patients with MACIS scores <6; patients with tumor size <1 cm, N0, and M0).

Definite Indications

Distant metastasis at diagnosis

Incomplete tumor resection

Complete tumor resection but high risk for mortality or recurrence (e.g., PTC patients with MACIS scores >6 and pTNM stage II/III FTC or HCC)

Probable Indications

Incomplete surgery (less than near-total thyroidectomy, no lymph node dissection)

PTC or FTC in a child younger than 16 yr

If PTC, tall cell or columnar cell variant and diffuse sclerosing variant

If FTC, widely invasive or poorly differentiated tumor

Bulky nodal metastases

FTC, Follicular thyroid carcinoma; *HCC,* Hürthle cell carcinoma; *MACIS,* scoring system based on metastasis, age, completeness of resection, invasion, and size; *PTC,* papillary thyroid carcinoma; *pTNM,* pathologic tumor-node-metastasis classification.
From Melmed S et al (eds): *Williams textbook of endocrinology,* ed 12, Philadelphia, 2011, Saunders.

TABLE 7 Characteristics of Thyroid Cancers

Type of Cancer	Percentage of Thyroid Cancers	Age of Onset (yr)	Treatment	Prognosis
Papillary	88	40-80	Thyroidectomy, followed by radioactive iodine ablation and TSH suppression	Good
Follicular	10	45-80	Thyroidectomy, followed by radioactive iodine ablation and TSH suppression	Fair to good
Medullary	3-4	20-50	Thyroidectomy and central compartment lymph node dissection and TSH suppression	Fair
Anaplastic	1	50-80	Isthmusectomy followed by palliative x-ray treatment	Poor
Lymphoma	<1	25-70	X-ray therapy and/or chemotherapy	Fair

From Andreoli TE et al: *Andreoli and Carpenter's Cecil essentials of medicine,* ed 8, Philadelphia, 2010, Saunders.

TABLE 8 Factors Used in Prognostic Classification Systems

	TNM	AMES	AGES	MACIS
Patient Factors				
Age	×	×	×	×
Gender	×	×		
Tumor Factors				
Size	×	×	×	×
Histologic grade		×		
Histologic type	×	×	*	*
Extrathyroid spread	×	×	×	×
Lymph node metastasis	×			
Distant metastasis	×	×	×	×
Incomplete resection				×

AGES, Age at diagnosis, histologic tumor grade, extent of disease at presentation, and tumor size; *AMES,* patient age, metastases, extent of invasion, and tumor size; *MACIS,* metastasis, age at diagnosis, completeness of surgical resection, extrathyroid invasion, and tumor size; *TNM,* tumor/node/metastasis.
*AGES/MACIS classifications for papillary carcinomas only.
From Flint PW et al: *Cummings otolaryngology, head and neck surgery,* ed 7, Philadelphia, 2021, Elsevier.

2. Management is usually restricted to radiation therapy or chemotherapy (combination of doxorubicin, cisplatin, and other antineoplastic agents) (see Table 6); these measures rarely provide significant palliation.

3. Patients with anaplastic thyroid cancer should have their tumors tested for *BRAF V600E* mutation and *NTRK* gene fusion. The FDA has approved dabrafenib 150 mg PO bid and trametinib 2 mg PO daily for patients who harbor the *BRAF* mutation.

4. Larotrectinib or entrectinib can be offered to patients who have an *NTRK* gene mutation.
- Medullary carcinoma:
  1. Thyroidectomy should be performed, followed by TSH suppression.
  2. Vandetanib and cabozantinib are oral tyrosine kinase inhibitors that are FDA-approved for treatment of symptomatic or progressive, unresectable, locally advanced or metastatic medullary thyroid cancer.
  3. Patients and their families should be screened for pheochromocytoma and hyperparathyroidism.

DISPOSITION
- Overall 5-yr survival rate is 98.17, but prognosis varies with the type of thyroid carcinoma: 5-yr survival is over 80% for follicular carcinoma and is approximately 5% with anaplastic carcinoma (Table 7).
- Factors used in prognostic classification systems are summarized in Table 8.
- Risk factors for aggressive behavior of well-differentiated thyroid carcinomas are described in Box 1.
- Box 2 summarizes risk stratification for thyroid cancer recurrence.

BOX 1 Risk Factors for Aggressive Behavior of Well-Differentiated Thyroid Carcinomas

Demographics
Age <20 yr
Men >55 yr
Women >55 yr
Male > female
History of radiation exposure/therapy
Family history of thyroid carcinoma
Physical Examination
Hard, fixed lesion
Rapid growth of mass
Pain
Lymphadenopathy
Vocal cord paralysis
Aerodigestive tract compromise
    Dysphagia
    Stridor
Histopathologic Factors (at Initial Presentation)
Size >4 cm
Extrathyroid spread
Vascular invasion
Lymph node metastasis
Distant metastasis
Histologic type
    Tall cell variant of papillary carcinoma
    Follicular carcinoma
    Hürthle cell carcinoma

From Flint PW et al: *Cummings otolaryngology, head and neck surgery*, ed 7, Philadelphia, 2021, Elsevier.

BOX 2 Risk Stratification for Thyroid Cancer Recurrence

High Risk
Gross extrathyroidal extension, incomplete tumor resection, distant metastases, or lymph node >3 cm

Intermediate Risk
Aggressive histology, minor extrathyroidal extension, vascular invasion, or >5 involved lymph nodes (0.2-3 cm)

Low Risk
Intrathyroidal DTC ≤5 LN micrometastases (<0.2 cm)

FTC, extensive vascular invasion (≈ 30%-55%)
pT4a gross ETE (≈ 30%-40%)
pN1 with extranodal extension, >3 LN involved (≈ 40%) PTC, >1 cm, TERT mutated ± BRAF mutated (≈ 40%) pN1, any LN >3 cm (≈ 30%)
PTC, extrathyroidal, BRAF mutated (≈ 10%-40%)
PTC, vascular invasion (≈ 15%-30%)
Clinical N1 (≈ 20%)
pNI, >5 LN involved (≈ 20%)
Intrathyroidal PTC, <4 cm, BRAF mutated (≈ 10%) pT3 minor ETE (≈ 3%-8%)
pN1, all LN <0.2 cm (≈ 5%)
pN1 ≤5 LN involved (≈ 5%)
Intrathyroidal PTC, 2-4 cm (≈ 5%)
Multifocal PTMC (≈ 4%-6%)
pN1 without extranodal extension, ≤3 LN involved (2%) Minimally invasive FTC (≈ 2%-3%)
Intrathyroidal, <4 cm, BRAF wild type (≈ 1%-2%) Intrathyroidal unifocal PTMC, BRAF mutated, (≈ 1%-2%) Intrathyroidal, encapsulated, FV-PTC (≈ 1%-2%)
Unifocal PTMC (≈ 1%-2%)

From Flint PW et al: *Cummings otolaryngology, head and neck surgery*, ed 7, Philadelphia, 2021, Elsevier.

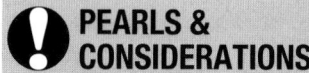

PEARLS & CONSIDERATIONS

COMMENTS

- Follow-up surveillance (Table E9) involves neck ultrasound 6 to 12 mo after initial treatment and periodically and lab evaluation with TSH, serum thyroglobulin (T8), and thyroglobulin antibody (T8 Ab).
- Family members of patients with medullary carcinoma should be screened; DNA analysis for the detection of mutations in the *RET* gene structure permits the identification of *MEN IIA* gene carriers.
- While there is little controversy regarding the benefit of radioactive iodine in iodine-avid advanced-stage well-differentiated thyroid cancer, the indications for radioactive iodine following total thyroidectomy in patients with very low risk disease is controversial. Proponents argue that its use may destroy microscopic metastases, while opponents counter that the risk of secondary cancer due to radioactive iodine is not warranted in patients whose prognosis is typically excellent.[7]
- Metastatic thyroid cancers that are refractory to radioiodine (iodine-131) are associated with a poor prognosis.
- Small-molecule tyrosine kinase inhibitors, including vandetanib, cabozantinib, sorafenib, and lenvatinib, are now FDA-approved and have shown clinical benefit with improved survival in advanced differentiated and medullary thyroid cancer.
- Targeted therapy with a combined regimen of BRAF/MEK inhibitors (dabrafenib plus trametinib) is efficacious and approved in patients with metastatic BRAFV600E-mutated anaplastic thyroid cancer.
- In a subset of patients with anaplastic thyroid cancer, the immune checkpoint inhibitor pembrolizumab may be an effective salvage therapy when added to kinase inhibitors at the time of progression on these drugs. In patients with advanced, differentiated thyroid cancer, pembrolizumab has a manageable safety profile and demonstrates evidence of anti-tumor activity in a minority of treated patients.
- Selpercatinib is approved for thyroid cancers with *RET* gene mutations.

REFERENCES
Available at eBooks.Health.Elsevier.com.

RELATED CONTENT
Thyroid Cancer (Patient Information)
Thyroid Nodule (Related Key Topic)
Multiple Endocrine Neoplasia (Related Key Topic)

AUTHOR: **BHARTI RATHORE, MD**

ⓘ BASIC INFORMATION

DEFINITION
An abnormal growth of thyroid tissue detected on either physical examination or radiographic imaging, and ultimately confirmed by thyroid ultrasound.

ICD-10CM CODES
E04.1	Nontoxic single thyroid nodule or cyst
E04.9	Nontoxic goiter
E05.1	Thyrotoxicosis with toxic single thyroid nodule
E05.2	Thyrotoxicosis with toxic multinodular goiter
E05.11	Thyrotoxicosis with toxic single thyroid nodule with thyrotoxic crisis or storm

EPIDEMIOLOGY & DEMOGRAPHICS
- Thyroid nodules are present in up to 50% of the population.
- Only 5% of the population has a palpable nodule.
- Incidence of thyroid nodules increases after 45 yr. They are more common in women by a ratio of 4:1.
- The vast majority of nodules (approximately 95%), regardless of size, are benign.

PHYSICAL FINDINGS & CLINICAL PRESENTATION
- Anatomic: Characteristics of the nodule include size, firmness (ranges from soft to rock hard), mobility, presence of single or multiple nodules, and presence of enlarged cervical lymph nodes. Additional physical findings to look for include exophthalmos, which would suggest Graves disease, tracheal deviation, and hoarseness suggestive of recurrent laryngeal nerve dysfunction usually associated with advanced malignancy.
- Physiologic: Symptoms of thyrotoxicosis that can be seen with a toxic nodule or toxic multinodular goiter include palpitations, anxiety, insomnia, weight loss, and heat intolerance. The signs of thyrotoxicosis include tremor, lid lag, tachycardia, pressured speech, and restlessness.

ETIOLOGY
- Most nodules are benign. They can be solitary or multiple. Positive family history is common. Iodine deficiency is rarely a cause of nodule formation in developed countries, where salt is iodized.
- Malignancy risks include family history of thyroid cancer and prior head and neck irradiation. Indicators of malignancy: Nodule significantly increasing in size, regional lymphadenopathy, fixation to adjacent tissues, very young or very old age at onset, symptoms of local invasion (dysphagia, hoarseness, neck pain), male sex.
- Inherited syndromes: MEN II predisposes to medullary thyroid cancer, and Cowden syndrome predisposes to follicular neoplasms. Other syndromic causes include Carney complex, Gardner syndrome, and familial adenomatous polyposis.

ⒹⓍ DIAGNOSIS

DIFFERENTIAL DIAGNOSIS
- Benign functioning or nonfunctioning thyroid adenoma
- Benign thyroid cyst
- Thyroid carcinoma
- Multinodular goiter
- Thyroglossal duct cyst (midline neck mass at level of hyoid)
- Epidermoid cyst (subcutaneous firm mobile mass)
- Laryngocele (superior lateral neck mass)
- Nonthyroid neck neoplasm (lymphoma or lymph node metastases)
- Branchial cleft cyst (lateral neck mass, often with a draining fistula tract)

WORKUP (FIG. 1)
Physical exam is helpful if there are overt signs of hyperthyroidism or malignancy, but these are uncommon. Diagnosis usually relies on laboratory tests, radiographic studies, and cytology.[1]

LABORATORY TESTS
- Serum thyroid-stimulating hormone (TSH) required in all patients. If suppressed, obtain free T4 and free T3 and thyroid scan to screen for a "hot nodule," indicative of a hyperfunctioning adenoma. If the TSH is normal or elevated, consider biopsy based on ultrasonographic characteristics.
- Serum calcitonin is only recommended when suspecting medullary carcinoma (MTC), such as a patient with a family history of MEN II or familial MTC, or history of pheochromocytoma or hyperparathyroidism.
- If the patient may have Hashimoto thyroiditis, check an antimicrosomal or antithyroid peroxidase antibody level to confirm (see "Thyroiditis" in Section I). These patients often have marked heterogeneity of the thyroid parenchyma on ultrasound, which can be mistaken for nodular disease.
- Molecular analysis of thyroid tissue is now commercially available, and it may be useful when fine needle aspiration (FNA) biopsy results are indeterminate.[2] Several companies offer the testing, and in general they are beneficial as rule-out tests. They can be used to identify a subpopulation of patients with a low likelihood of cancer, thereby avoiding unnecessary thyroid lobectomy in patients with indeterminate FNA. These tests have a high negative predictive value for cytologically indeterminate nodules (95% for an atypia or follicular lesion of undetermined significance, 94% for a follicular neoplasm). It is less common to find a gene that is highly predictive of cancer, such as BRAF, RET/PTC, and PAX8-PPAR gamma. The presence of RAS mutations is not as helpful, as it is commonly found in benign follicular adenomas, noninvasive follicular thyroid neoplasms with papillary-like nuclear features, and follicular cancers.

BIOPSY
- FNA biopsy is the best means of distinguishing benign from malignant nodules, but it requires the availability of an expert cytopathologist.
- Decision to perform ultrasound-guided biopsy is based on size and ultrasound features. The American Thyroid Association guidelines for thyroid nodules tallies the number of benign or suspicious ultrasound features and then recommends biopsy or observation based on nodule size. The American College of Radiology has published a thyroid nodule scoring system called TI-RADS (thyroid imaging reporting and data system [Table 1]), which is used in a similar way. If the likelihood of malignancy is low, a 1-yr follow-up ultrasound should be performed.
- FNA is discouraged for thyroid nodules <1 cm in diameter unless there are highly concerning features, such as concern for tracheal or nerve involvement, or suspicion of metastatic disease.
- FNA biopsy is very low yield for thyroid cystic lesions because of a paucity of cellular material. Most asymptomatic simple cysts can be observed. Large compressive cysts, or those with a significant solid component, should be considered for resection.
- Previous endocrine, surgery, and radiology algorithms recommended biopsy of all solid thyroid nodules over 1 cm. Over the last 5 yr, there has been a marked shift toward risk stratifying nodules by their ultrasound characteristics using the TI-RADS scoring system or the American Thyroid Association risk assessment. Lower-risk nodules can be followed with ultrasound unless they cross certain size thresholds. Higher-risk nodules still follow the 1-cm cutoff for FNA biopsy.
- FNA biopsy results at most tertiary care institutions are now reported using the Bethesda classification system. The Bethesda Classification system (Table 2) estimates the probability of malignancy at histology based on FNA biopsy cytology and treatment recommendation.[3]

IMAGING STUDIES
- Iodine uptake scanning (Fig. 2) is only indicated in patients with suppressed TSH levels to determine if the nodule is toxic or not. If it is hot, biopsy is not indicated.
- Ultrasonography is an inexpensive and effective modality to stratify malignancy risk. The American College of Radiology (ACR) Thyroid Imaging, Reporting and Data System (TI-RADS) is illustrated in Fig. 3.[4]
- Ultrasound (Fig. E4) is useful to evaluate the size and number of nodules, as well as their characteristics. These include whether it is solid or cystic, echogenicity relative to normal thyroid tissue, irregular vs. smooth borders, presence of calcifications, shape, and vascularity. Table 3 summarizes ultrasound features of benign and malignant thyroid nodules. The three ultrasound characteristics most predictive of malignancy in solid thyroid nodules are shape taller than wide, microcalcifications,

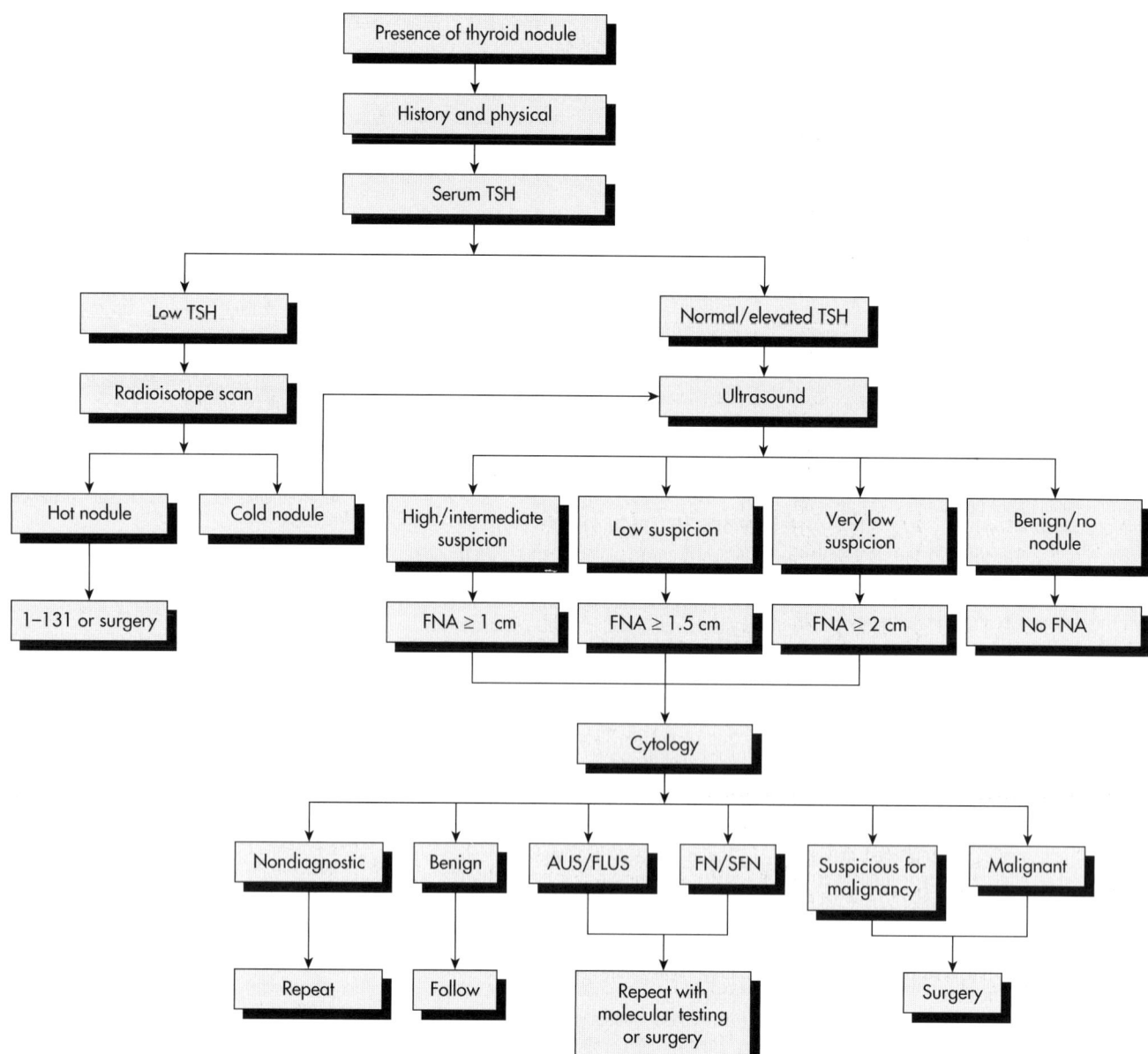

FIG. 1 Workup of a thyroid nodule. *AUS,* Atypia of undetermined significance; *FLUS,* follicular lesion of undetermined significance; *FN,* follicular neoplasm; *FNA,* fine-needle aspiration biopsy; *SFN,* suspicious for follicular neoplasm; *TSH,* thyroid-stimulating hormone. (Modified from Townsend CM et al: *Sabiston textbook of surgery,* ed 21, St Louis, 2022, Elsevier.)

TABLE 1 American College of Radiology Thyroid Nodule Scoring System: TI-RADS

Scoring and Classification	Recommendations
TR1: 0 points	TR1: No FNA required (0.3% risk)
TR2: 2 points	TR2: No FNA required (1.5% risk)
TR3: 3 points	TR3: ≥1.5 cm follow-up at 1, 3, 5 yr, ≥2.5 cm FNA (4.8% risk)
TR4: 4-6 points	TR4: ≥1.0 cm follow-up at 1, 2, 3, 5 yr ≥1.5 cm FNA (9.1% risk)
TR5: ≥7 points	TR5: ≥0.5 cm follow-up each year, ≥1.0 cm FNA (35% risk)

ACR TI-RADS is a reporting system for thyroid nodules on ultrasound proposed by the American College of Radiology (ACR) and is based on composition, echogenicity, shape, margin, and echogenic foci.
From Tessler FN et al: ACR Thyroid Imaging, Reporting and Data System (TI-RADS): white paper of the ACR TI-RADS committee, *J Am Coll Radiol* 14:587-595, 2017.

and hypoechogenicity, in that order. The positive predictive value for malignancy steadily rises as the number of suspicious ultrasound findings mounts. However, FNA biopsy remains necessary for a definitive diagnosis. Very low risk ultrasound features include simple cystic lesions and spongiform nodules (sponge-like in appearance with layers of solid and cystic contents). Ultrasound follow-up is reasonable in such cases without biopsy, although it is acceptable to biopsy spongiform nodules over 2 cm based on practitioner and patient preference.

TABLE 2 Bethesda Classification System for Thyroid Nodules

Diagnostic Category Bethesda Classification	Risk of Malignancy	Action
I Nondiagnostic	1-4	Repeat biopsy after 4 wk; if very low risk, follow with ultrasound
II Benign	1-3	1-yr follow-up ultrasound
III Atypia (follicular lesion) of undetermined significance (AUS/FLUS)	5-15	Repeat biopsy in 3 mo; consider genetic testing
IV Follicular neoplasm	15-30	Thyroid lobectomy; consider genetic testing if nodule appears low risk or patient wishes to avoid surgery
V Suspicious	60-75	Thyroid lobectomy or total thyroidectomy
VI Malignant	97-99	Thyroid lobectomy or total thyroidectomy

Adapted from Cibas ES, Ali SZ: The Bethesda system for reporting thyroid cytopathology, *Am J Clin Pathol* 132:658-665, 2009.

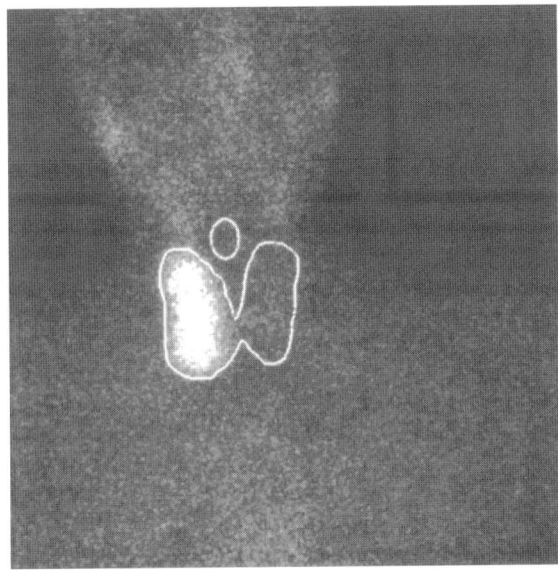

FIG. 2 ^{131}I scan demonstrating an area of increased uptake in the right lobe of a 32-yr-old woman with increased thyroid function test values and a palpable nodule. This scan is consistent with a toxic or hyperfunctioning nodule. (From Townsend CM et al: *Sabiston textbook of surgery*, ed 21, St Louis, 2022, Elsevier.)

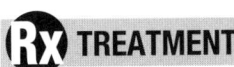 **TREATMENT**

GENERAL Rx

- Evaluation of results of FNA:
  1. Regardless of biopsy result, symptomatic compressive nodules, substernal nodules, and those causing tracheal deviation are all indications for thyroidectomy.
  2. Table 2 contains the guidelines for management of each of the possible results after FNA biopsy. Nondiagnostic biopsies contain insufficient cells and require repeat, unless they are obviously benign cystic lesions.
  3. Benign nodules carry a 5% false-negative biopsy rate and should be reassessed at 1 yr for growth. If they have grown more than 3 mm, repeat biopsy should be considered.
  4. AUS/FLUS carries a 15% risk of malignancy. Usually a repeat biopsy is performed at 3 mo in hopes of obtaining a definitive result. Genetic testing is a consideration.
  5. Follicular neoplasms are higher risk and warrant lobectomy or genetic testing. Ultrasound features should aid in the decision to perform genetic testing.
  6. Suspected malignancy and papillary thyroid cancer are treated similarly with lobectomy or total thyroidectomy.

DISPOSITION

Variable with results of FNA biopsy. Once patients have had a benign biopsy and a 1-yr follow-up ultrasound shows no significant growth, they do *not* require annual thyroid ultrasound exams. They can be followed with an annual neck exam. If growth is detected or symptoms develop, repeat ultrasound is indicated.

REFERRAL

Surgery or radiology referral for possible FNA biopsy if nodule is solid and over 1 cm

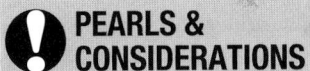 **PEARLS & CONSIDERATIONS**

COMMENTS

- Many solid, benign nodules grow; therefore, an increase in nodule volume alone is not a reliable predictor of malignancy.
- Thyroid nodules incidentally identified as FDG avid on fluorodeoxyglucose-PET (FDG-PET) scan done for other disorders have a higher malignancy rate (25%).
- Highly suspicious nodules should be referred for surgical evaluation even if result of FNA is "benign."
- Most follicular neoplasms are benign, and patients should not be told they have a malignancy based on this cytology result.

REFERENCES

Available at eBooks.Health.Elsevier.com.

RELATED CONTENT

Thyroid Nodule (Patient Information)
Thyroiditis (Related Key Topic)
Thyroid Carcinoma (Related Key Topic)

AUTHOR: **PETER J. MAZZAGLIA, MD**

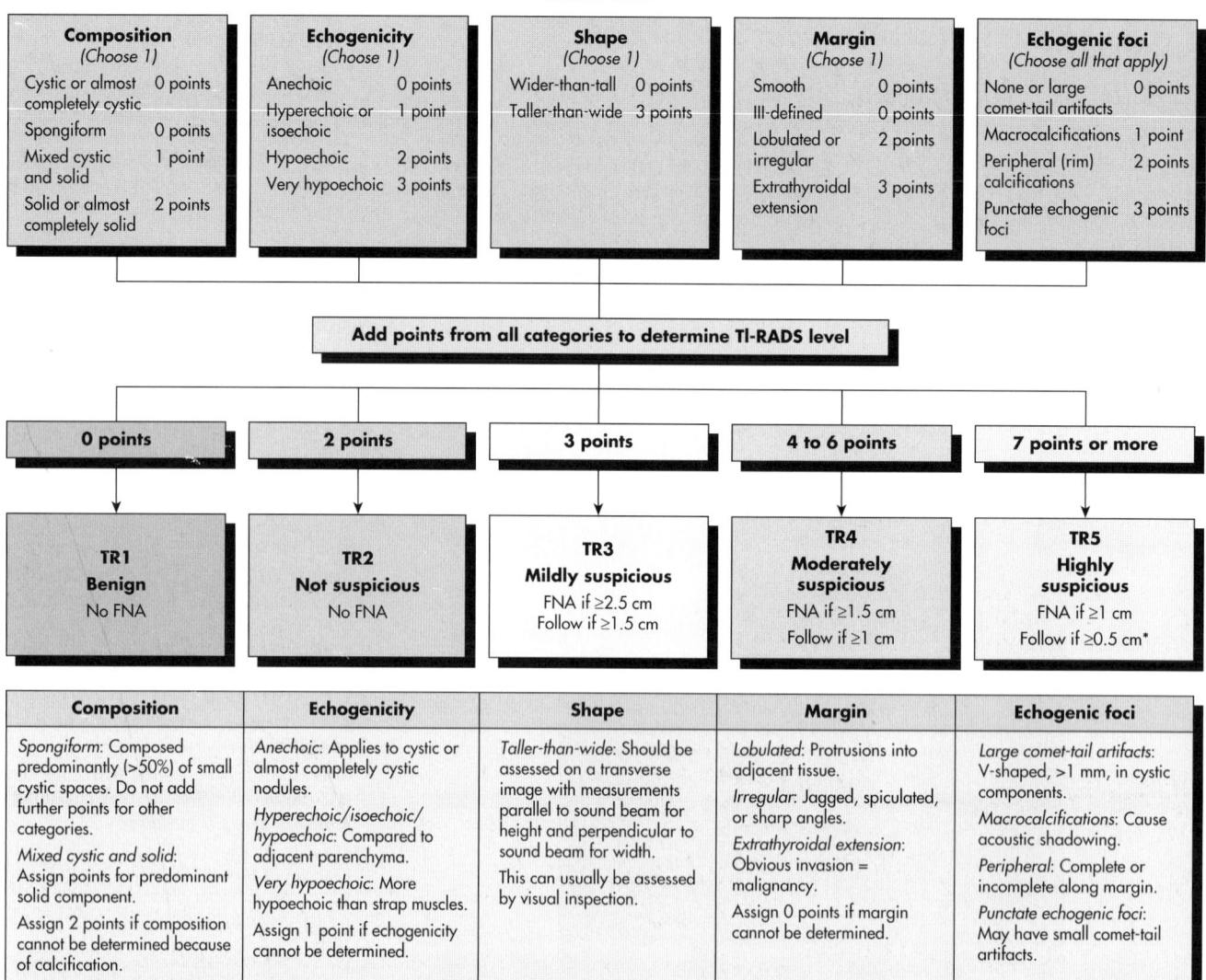

FIG. 3 **The American College of Radiology (ACR) Thyroid Imaging, Reporting and Data System (TI-RADS) lexicon, TR levels, and criteria for fine-needle aspiration biopsy.** (From Tessler FN et al: ACR Thyroid Imaging, Reporting and Data System [TI-RADS]: white paper of the ACR TI-RADS Committee, *J Am Coll Radiol* 14:587-595, 2017.)

TABLE 3 Ultrasound Features Suggestive of Benign and Malignant Thyroid Nodules		
	Benign	**Suspicious for Malignancy**
Nodule characteristics	• Cystic • Spongiform • Hyperechoic • "Comet tail" artefact (seen in colloid nodules; do not confuse with microcalcifications)	• Hypoechoic • Very hypoechoic Shape taller than wide
Nodule margin	• Smooth, regular • Presence of halo	• Irregular, lobulated, or poorly defined • Protrusion outside of thyroid capsule
Calcification	• Absent • Coarse • Eggshell	• Microcalcification • Broken eggshell
Metastatic spread		• Invasion of the adjacent tissues • Enlarged ipsilateral or bilateral cervical lymph nodes; metastatic nodes are round, hyperechoic, and can contain microcalcifications

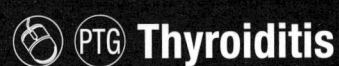

 BASIC INFORMATION

DEFINITION

Thyroiditis is an inflammatory disease of the thyroid. It is a multifaceted disease with various etiologies, different clinical characteristics (depending on the stage), and distinct histopathology. Thyroiditis can be subdivided into three common types (Hashimoto, painful, and painless) and two rare forms (suppurative and Riedel). To add to the confusion, there are various synonyms for each form, and there is no internationally accepted classification of autoimmune thyroid disease.

SYNONYMS

Hashimoto thyroiditis: Chronic lymphocytic thyroiditis, chronic autoimmune thyroiditis, lymphadenoid goiter

Painful subacute thyroiditis: Subacute thyroiditis, giant cell thyroiditis, de Quervain thyroiditis, subacute granulomatous thyroiditis, pseudogranulomatous thyroiditis

Painless postpartum thyroiditis: Subacute lymphocytic thyroiditis, postpartum thyroiditis

Painless sporadic thyroiditis: Silent sporadic thyroiditis, subacute lymphocytic thyroiditis

Infectious thyroiditis: Acute suppurative thyroiditis, bacterial thyroiditis, microbial inflammatory thyroiditis, pyogenic thyroiditis

Riedel thyroiditis: Fibrous thyroiditis

ICD-10CM CODES
E06.3 Autoimmune thyroiditis
E06.1 Subacute thyroiditis
E06.9 Thyroiditis, unspecified
E06.0 Acute thyroiditis
E06.5 Other chronic thyroiditis

PHYSICAL FINDINGS & CLINICAL PRESENTATION

- Thyroiditis typically has three phases: Thyrotoxic and hypothyroid (each lasting approximately 3 mo) and return to euthyroidism.
- Hashimoto: Patients may have signs of hyperthyroidism (tachycardia, diaphoresis, palpitations, weight loss) or hypothyroidism (fatigue, weight gain, delayed reflexes) depending on the stage of the disease. Usually there is diffuse, firm enlargement of the thyroid gland; the gland may also be of normal size (atrophic form with clinically manifested hypothyroidism).
- Painful subacute: Exquisitely tender, enlarged thyroid, fever; signs of hyperthyroidism are initially present; signs of hypothyroidism can subsequently develop.
- Painless thyroiditis: Clinical features are similar to subacute thyroiditis except for the absence of tenderness of the thyroid gland.
- Suppurative: Patient is febrile with severe neck pain, focal tenderness of the involved portion of the thyroid, erythema of the overlying skin.
- Riedel: Slowly enlarging hard mass in the anterior neck; often mistaken for thyroid cancer; signs of hypothyroidism occur in advanced stages.

ETIOLOGY

- Hashimoto: Autoimmune disorder that begins with the activation of CD4 T-helper lymphocytes specific for thyroid antigens. The etiologic factor for the activation of these cells is unknown
- Painful subacute: Possibly postviral; usually follows a respiratory illness not considered to be a form of autoimmune thyroiditis
- Painless thyroiditis: Frequently occurs postpartum
- Infectious (suppurative): Infectious etiology, generally bacterial, although fungi and parasites have also been implicated; often occurs in immunocompromised hosts or after a penetrating neck injury
- Riedel: Fibrous infiltration of the thyroid; etiology unknown
- Drug induced: Typically painless due to lithium, interferon-alfa, amiodarone, interleukin-2
- Radiation thyroiditis: Occurs 5 to 10 days after treatment with radioactive iodine; it is painful and may result in transient exacerbation of hyperthyroidism

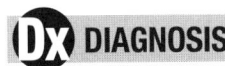 **DIAGNOSIS**

DIFFERENTIAL DIAGNOSIS

- The hyperthyroid phase of Hashimoto, subacute, and silent thyroiditis can be mistaken for Graves disease.
- Riedel thyroiditis can be mistaken for carcinoma of the thyroid.
- Painful subacute thyroiditis can be mistaken for infections of the oropharynx and trachea or for suppurative thyroiditis.
- Factitious hyperthyroidism can mimic silent sporadic thyroiditis.

WORKUP

- The diagnostic workup includes laboratory and x-ray evaluation to rule out other conditions that may mimic thyroiditis (see previously) and differentiate the various forms of thyroiditis.
- The patient's medical history may be helpful in differentiating the various types of thyroiditis (e.g., presentation after childbirth is suggestive of silent [postpartum, painless] thyroiditis; occurrence after a viral respiratory infection suggests subacute thyroiditis; history of penetrating injury to the neck indicates suppurative thyroiditis).

LABORATORY TESTS

- Thyroid-stimulating hormone, free T4: May be normal or indicative of hypothyroidism or hyperthyroidism depending on the stage of the thyroiditis.
- White blood cell (WBC) with differential: Increased WBC with left shift occurs with subacute and suppurative thyroiditis.
- Antimicrosomal antibodies: Detected in >90% of patients with Hashimoto thyroiditis and 50% to 80% of patients with silent thyroiditis.
- Serum thyroglobulin levels are elevated in patients with subacute and silent thyroiditis; this test is nonspecific but may be useful in monitoring the course of subacute thyroiditis

and distinguishing silent thyroiditis from factitious hyperthyroidism (low or absent serum thyroglobulin level).

IMAGING STUDIES (FIGS. E1 AND E2)

24-h radioactive iodine uptake (RAIU) is useful to distinguish Graves disease (increased RAIU) from thyroiditis (normal or low RAIU). Table E1 summarizes factors that influence 24-h thyroid iodide uptake.

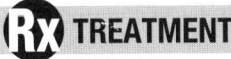 **TREATMENT**

ACUTE GENERAL Rx

- The duration of the thyrotoxic phase of thyroiditis is usually 10 to 12 wk. This phase is followed by a hypothyroid phase typically lasting up to 12 wk.
- Treat hypothyroid phase in symptomatic patients somatic with levothyroxine 25 to 50 mcg/day initially and monitor serum thyroid-stimulating hormone initially every 6 to 8 wk.
- Control symptoms of hyperthyroidism with β-blockers (e.g., propranolol 20 to 40 mg PO q6h or atenolol).
- Control pain in patients with subacute thyroiditis with NSAIDs. Prednisone 20 to 40 mg daily may be used if nonsteroidals are insufficient, but it should be gradually tapered off over several weeks.
- Use intravenous (IV) antibiotics and drain abscess (if present) in patients with suppurative thyroiditis.

DISPOSITION

- Hashimoto thyroiditis: Long-term prognosis is favorable; most patients recover their thyroid function.
- Painful subacute thyroiditis: Permanent hypothyroidism occurs in 10% of patients.
- Painless thyroiditis: 6% of patients have permanent hypothyroidism.
- Infectious thyroiditis: There is usually full recovery after treatment.
- Riedel thyroiditis: Hypothyroidism occurs when fibrous infiltration involves the entire thyroid.

REFERRAL

- Surgical referral in patients with compression of adjacent neck structures and in some patients with infectious (suppurative) thyroiditis.
- Total thyroidectomy has been shown to improve symptoms in patients with Hashimoto thyroiditis who still have symptoms despite having normal thyroid gland function while receiving medical therapy.

SUGGESTED READING
Available at eBooks.Health.Elsevier.com.

RELATED CONTENT
Thyroiditis (Patient Information)
Hyperthyroidism (Related Key Topic)
Hypothyroidism (Related Key Topic)

AUTHOR: **FRED F. FERRI, MD**

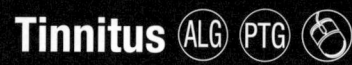 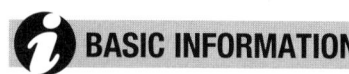

ⓘ BASIC INFORMATION

DEFINITION

Tinnitus is a perceived sound in the absence of acoustic stimulus external to the head. It may be unilateral, bilateral, or lateral dominant. It is commonly described as a ringing, buzzing, roaring, hissing, whistling, humming, cricket-like, or pulsing sound. It is frequently a symptom associated with hearing loss, Ménière disease, acoustic neuroma, drug toxicity, depression, or an autoimmune inner ear disease. The sound may be internal and perceived only by the patient, called subjective or tonal tinnitus, or it may be heard by both the patient and the examiner, called objective or nontonal tinnitus. Tinnitus can be subdivided into three key distinctions: Subjective versus objective, pulsatile versus nonpulsatile, and primary versus secondary. This early classification guides the history, physical examination, and subsequent diagnostic studies, thereby facilitating a simple and efficient approach to tinnitus management. Subjective tinnitus can only be heard by the patient, while objective tinnitus is also appreciated by the examiner. Objective tinnitus is rare: Even at an otolaryngology tertiary referral center, it represents only 1.5% of all tinnitus complaints. By definition, objective tinnitus implies an identifiable source for the acoustic stimulus, including joints, muscles, turbulent blood flow, or rarely, otoacoustic emissions. Objective tinnitus is usually pulsatile or rhythmic and can be auscultated in the periauricular region, ear canal, neck, or chest. Patient confirmation that the sound identified is identical to their perceived tinnitus is required for classifying the symptom as objective tinnitus.

Subjective nonpulsatile tinnitus is by far the most common type of tinnitus, representing an estimated 90% of all tinnitus referrals seen in an otolaryngology practice. Typically described as a "ringing," "hissing," "buzzing," or "roaring," nonpulsatile tinnitus is almost exclusively subjective. Conversely, pulsatile tinnitus, often described as rhythmic or pulse-like, can be either subjective or objective and may be altered by changes in position.

ICD-10CM CODES
H93.1	Tinnitus
H93.2	Other abnormal auditory perceptions
H93.11	Tinnitus, right ear
H93.12	Tinnitus, left ear
H93.13	Tinnitus, bilateral
H93.19	Tinnitus, unspecified ear

EPIDEMIOLOGY & DEMOGRAPHICS

PREVALENCE:
- The American Tinnitus Association reports 50 to 60 million Americans have tinnitus for >6 mo.
- Prevalence increases steadily with age, peaking for persons aged 60 to 69 yr.
- Prevalence in the U.S. based on National Health Interview Survey (NHIS) in 1996:
  1. 2.98% all ages
  2. 0.26% for persons <18 yr old
  3. 1.6% for persons aged 18 to 44 yr
  4. 5.96% for persons aged 45 to 64 yr: 7.7% males, 4.3% females
  5. 9.6% for persons aged 65 to 74 yr: 12% males, 7.7% females
  6. 7.6% for persons >75 yr: 11.4% males, 5.3% females
  7. 2:1 South/Northeast regions
- Up to 18% of people in industrialized societies are mildly affected by chronic tinnitus, and 0.5% report tinnitus having a severe effect on their daily life.
- Only 20% of patients with persistent tinnitus ever seek medical evaluation.

PREDOMINANT SEX & AGE: Persons most affected are male, Caucasian, elderly, persons with hearing impairment, persons living in southern U.S. For military veterans, tinnitus is the third most common service-related disability.

RISK FACTORS: Any condition causing hearing loss or damage to the auditory system can produce tinnitus. Cochlear damage from exposure to noise is the most common cause. Exposure to ototoxic drugs is also important.

PHYSICAL FINDINGS & CLINICAL PRESENTATION
- History should focus on exposure to loud noises, evidence of hearing loss, and ototoxic drugs.
- Patient should be screened for depression.
- Patient who complains of sound in ear may also complain of ear pain or fullness.
- Objective tinnitus is pulsatile and coincides with patient's pulse.
- Physical examination should focus on HEENT, neck, and neurologic exam.
- There may be no significant physical findings.

ETIOLOGY
- The mechanism behind tinnitus is poorly understood. It may originate at any point along the auditory pathway. Causes of tinnitus include injured cochlear hair cells, spontaneous activity in auditory nerve fibers, hyperactivity in the auditory nuclei in the brain stem, or a reduction in the suppressive activity of the central auditory cortex.
- Medications implicated in causing tinnitus include salicylates, NSAIDs, aminoglycosides, loop diuretics, valproate, quinine, chemotherapeutic agents, cisplatin, vincristine, and heavy metals such as lead.

Ⓓ DIAGNOSIS

DIFFERENTIAL DIAGNOSIS (TABLE 1, FIG.1)
- Subjective/tonal tinnitus:
  1. Otologic: Tympanic membrane disorder, inner ear disorder (hair cells, organ of Corti), Ménière disease. Sigmoid sinus diverticula (Fig. E2) may manifest as pulsatile venous tinnitus and account for approximately 20% of cases of pulsatile tinnitus.
  2. Ototoxic medications
  3. Neurologic: Multiple sclerosis, head trauma, cochlear nerve lesion, acoustic schwannoma, neurofibroma, meningioma
  4. Metabolic: Thyroid disorder, hyperlipidemia (leading to plaque formation), vitamin B_{12} deficiency
  5. Psychogenic: Depression, anxiety, fibromyalgia
  6. Infectious: Otitis media, Lyme disease, meningitis, syphilis
- Objective/nontonal tinnitus:
  1. Vascular: Arterial bruit, venous hum, arteriovenous malformation, vascular tumors
  2. Neurologic: Contraction of muscles of the eustachian tube, contraction of the stapedius muscle, contraction of the tensor tympani muscles, or a palatal myoclonus, glomus jugulare tumor
  3. Conductive: Patulous (wide-open) eustachian tube

WORKUP
- Audiometry.
- Tympanometry.
- Electronystagmography is used to evaluate for Ménière disease.
- An algorithm for tinnitus evaluation is described in Fig. 3.
- Targeted history in tinnitus and clinical significance are summarized in Table E2.

LABORATORY TESTS
Evaluate for metabolic abnormalities: TSH, CBC, B_{12}, and lipid panel.

IMAGING STUDIES (FIG. 4)
- CT/MRI: To evaluate for subjective tinnitus.
- MRI/MRA: To evaluate objective tinnitus.
- Imaging should not be part of routine management. Clinicians must distinguish patients with bothersome tinnitus from patients with nonbothersome tinnitus. For patients without persistent and bothersome tinnitus, audiometric testing is optional.

℞ TREATMENT

NONPHARMACOLOGIC THERAPY
- It is best to avoid exposure to excessive noise, ototoxic agents, and to wear protective equipment in noisy environments, or mask the tinnitus through amplification of normal sounds with a hearing aid. Habituation techniques such as tinnitus retraining therapy may help. Cognitive-behavioral therapy helps patients cope with tinnitus distress through biofeedback.
- Recent trials involving brain stimulation in the form of repetitive transcranial magnetic stimulation (rTMS) have shown reduction in the perception or severity of tinnitus.

ACUTE GENERAL Rx
- If the tinnitus is severe enough to cause suicidal symptoms, immediate referral to a psychiatrist and an otolaryngologist is recommended to minimize the time to diagnosis and optimize treatment.

TABLE 1 Differential Diagnosis and Associated Conditions of Subjective Nonpulsatile Tinnitus

	Etiology or Associated Condition
Inner ear	Sensorineural hearing loss, Ménière disease, presbycusis, noise-induced hearing loss
Middle ear	Otosclerosis, ossicular or tympanic membrane abnormalities, cholesteatoma
External ear	Canal occlusion, cerumen impaction
Otologic infections	Otitis externa, otitis media, labyrinthitis, mastoiditis, herpes zoster oticus
Ototoxic medications	Antibiotics, antineoplastic drugs, corticosteroids, nonsteroidal antiinflammatory drugs, diuretics
Social habits	Alcohol, nicotine, and caffeine intake
Neurologic	Multiple sclerosis, Charcot-Marie-Tooth, epilepsy, migraine
Psychologic	Anxiety, depression
Autoimmune	Systemic lupus erythematous, systemic sclerosis, rheumatoid arthritis
Musculoskeletal	Temporomandibular joint disorder
Endocrine	Diabetes mellitus, hyperinsulinemia, hypothyroidism, pregnancy

From Flint PW et al: *Cummings otolaryngology, head and neck surgery,* ed 7, Philadelphia, 2021, Elsevier.

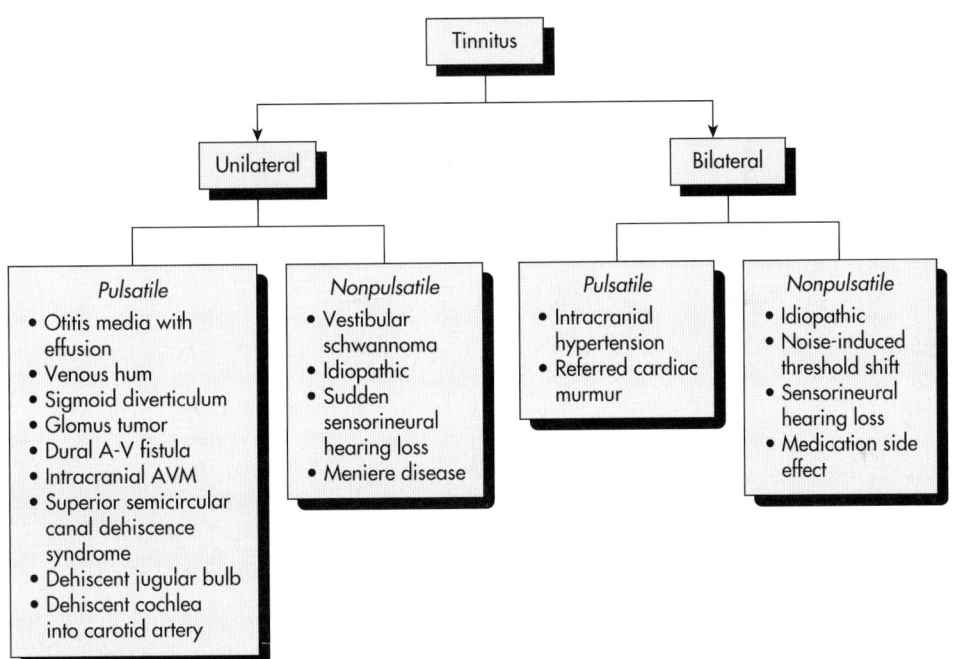

FIG. 1 Establishing a differential diagnosis with a chief complaint of hearing loss. This algorithm encourages the clinician to consider the patient complaint in categorical differential diagnosis families. It is not exhaustive. *SNHL,* Sensorineural hearing loss. (From Flint PW et al: *Cummings otolaryngology, head and neck surgery,* ed 7, Philadelphia, 2021, Elsevier.)

- Patients with persistent symptoms or tinnitus accompanied by visual changes or headache should be evaluated for tumors such as acoustic neuroma.
- Clinicians should not routinely recommend anxiolytics, anticonvulsants, or intratympanic medications.

CHRONIC Rx

There is insufficient evidence to support the use of any medication, vitamin, or nutritional supplement to treat tinnitus. Empirical use of over-the-counter supplements or prescription medications should be discouraged.

DISPOSITION

Clinical course is variable. About 20% to 25% of patients with chronic tinnitus consider it a significant problem. Individualized tinnitus management programs can be beneficial in most patients.

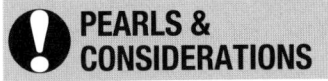 **PEARLS & CONSIDERATIONS**

PREVENTION

- Avoid loud, chronic noise and ototoxic drugs.

- Higher caffeine intake is associated with a lower risk of incidence of tinnitus in women.

SUGGESTED READING
Available at eBooks.Health.Elsevier.com.

RELATED CONTENT
Tinnitus (Patient Information)

AUTHORS: **VICKY H. BHAGAT, MD, MPH,** and **DAWN HOGAN, MD**

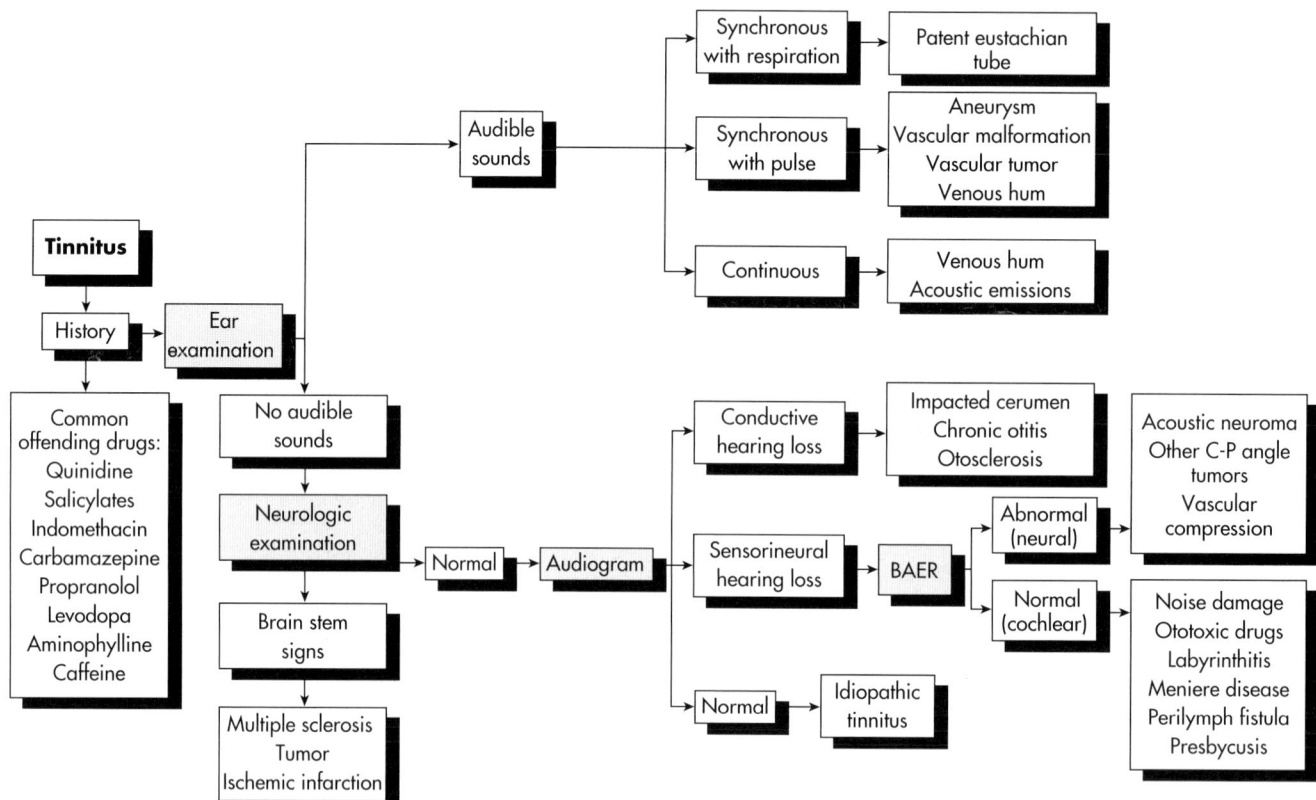

FIG. 3 Evaluation of tinnitus. *BAER,* Brain stem auditory evoked response; *C-P,* cerebellopontine. (From Goldman L, Schafer AI: *Goldman's Cecil medicine,* ed 24, Philadelphia, 2012, Saunders.)

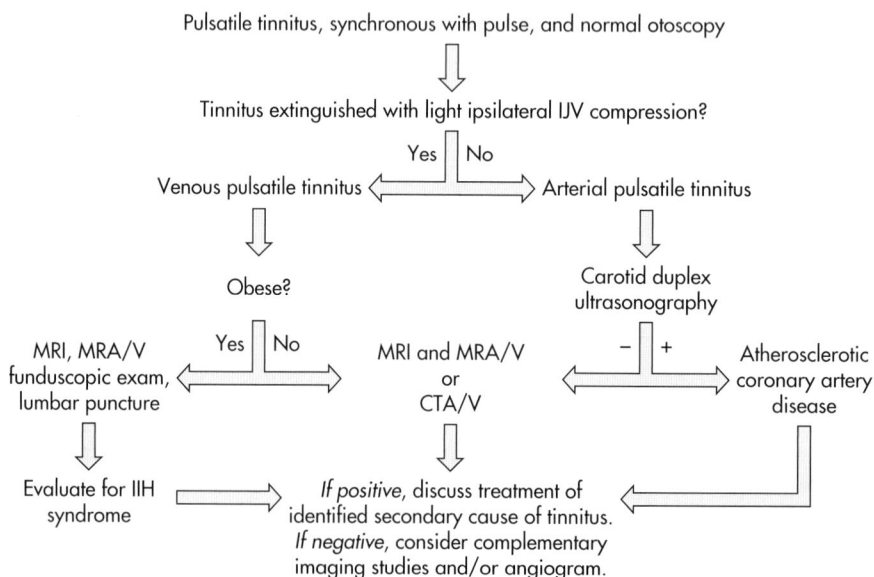

FIG. 4 Diagnostic imaging algorithm for pulsatile tinnitus. *CTA/V,* Computed tomography angiography/venography; *IIH,* idiopathic intracranial hypertension; *IJV,* internal jugular vein; *LP,* lumbar puncture; *MRA/V,* magnetic resonance angiography/venography; *MRI,* magnetic resonance imaging. (From Flint PW et al: *Cummings otolaryngology, head and neck surgery,* ed 7, Philadelphia, 2021, Elsevier.)

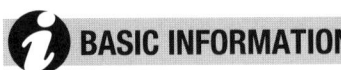

BASIC INFORMATION

DEFINITION

The term *Torsade de Pointes* (TdP) refers to a polymorphic ventricular tachycardia (VT) associated with a prolonged QT interval and electrocardiographically characterized by QRS complexes of changing amplitude that appear to twist around the isoelectric line, hence the name *torsade de pointes,* or "twisting of the points" (Fig. 1).

Torsade is typically initiated by a short-long-short sequence of ventricular beats but can also be initiated by a short-coupled variant. Typically, TdP occurs in the setting of a markedly prolonged QT interval (>500 msec); the QTc prolongs even further during the long diastolic interval of a compensatory pause after an early beat, followed by an early PVC on the T wave, leading to a polymorphic VT with a ventricular rate of 160 to 250 beats per min, irregular RR intervals, and a cycling of the QRS axis through 180 degrees every 5 to 20 beats. It may be repetitive, non-sustained, or sustained and may degenerate into ventricular fibrillation. In some cases, the result is sudden cardiac death.

SYNONYMS

Torsades
TdP

ICD-10CM CODE
I47.2 Ventricular tachycardia

EPIDEMIOLOGY & DEMOGRAPHICS

INCIDENCE: The precise incidence of TdP is unclear but accounts for fewer than 5% of all sudden cardiac arrests. In congenital long QT syndromes (LQTS), TdP may occur in up to 6% of cases at rest and 9% of cases during an exercise test. Among drug-induced causes of TdP, the incidence may vary between <1% in cases of antibiotics and antipsychotics to 2% to 4% when caused by class III antiarrhythmics such as sotalol, ibutilide, and dofetilide.

PREDOMINANT SEX & AGE: Because testosterone shortens the QT interval, women have a longer baseline QT interval, which is believed to be the reason for a two- to threefold increased incidence of TdP in women.

RISK FACTORS:
- TdP in patients with congenital LQTS is often initiated by an external trigger (Table 1). Triggers can include exercise, noise, emotion, sudden waking from sleep by an alarm clock, telephone ringing, thunder, swimming, or diving. TdP in LQT1 patients is classically triggered by vigorous exercise or swimming; in LQT2 by emotion, pregnancy, or noise; and in LQT3 when at rest or asleep. Risk factors for drug-induced TdP are outlined in Table 2.
- The risk factors for developing TdP in patients with acquired long QT are extensive and are outlined in Table 3.

GENETICS:
- Of the congenital LQTS channelopathies, long QT syndromes 1, 2, and 3 account for >70% of all cases. In general, the risk of TdP increases as the QT lengthens; however, there are also genotype-phenotype relationships that help define risk; for example, LQTS3 carries a higher risk of TdP than LQTS1. Similarly, the Jervell and Lange-Nielsen syndrome and Romano-Ward syndrome may lead to TdP.
- It is also likely that genetic factors are at play in acquired LQT and in the development of TdP. For example, in large populations, the QT interval prolongs very little with the administration of QT-prolonging drugs such as fluoroquinolones; however, certain individuals will have markedly exaggerated QT prolongation that leads to TdP; this is likely due to some underlying genetic factor.

PATHOPHYSIOLOGY:
- Changes in the balance of transmembrane ionic currents lead to lengthening of the QT interval and to abnormal action potentials called early afterdepolarizations (EADs). An EAD, in the setting of electrical instability induced by the prolonged QT, initiates the torsades. Perpetuation may be caused by transmural entry, triggered activity, or abnormal automaticity. A distinct group of cells called the M cells, located in the mid-myocardium, has a less rapid delayed rectifier potassium current (IKr), and these cells are central to the genesis of TdP.
- Drugs with the potential to cause TdP most frequently inhibit the rapid potassium channels and result in prolongation of the action potential duration, producing a prolonged QT on ECG.

PHYSICAL FINDINGS & CLINICAL PRESENTATION

- Clinical features depend on whether the TdP is caused by acquired or congenital long QT syndrome. Congenital LQTS patients may have certain specific triggers, such as noise, exercise, and emotions (see "Risk Factors").
- Symptoms of the tachycardia itself include palpitations, presyncope, syncope (sometimes with jerking movements from myoclonus, often misinterpreted as seizures), and sudden cardiac death (SCD).
- Patients resuscitated from SCD have an especially ominous prognosis, with a relative risk of 12.9% of experiencing another cardiac arrest.

ETIOLOGY

The etiology or triggers of TdP may be congenital or acquired causes of QT prolongation (see Table 1). For a comprehensive list of drugs that can cause or have the potential to cause TdP, see "Patient/Family Education."

DIAGNOSIS

DIFFERENTIAL DIAGNOSIS

Other causes of syncope:
- Other causes of broad complex tachycardia such as:
  1. Polymorphic VT
  2. Wolff-Parkinson-White (WPW) syndrome with rapid atrial fibrillation
  3. ECG artifact

WORKUP

- ECG (Fig. 2) and telemetry are the mainstays of diagnosing TdP as they detect the arrhythmia, the preceding prolonged QT interval, and the long-short cycles that trigger it.
- Determination and treatment of the etiology of TdP (see Table 1) is key.

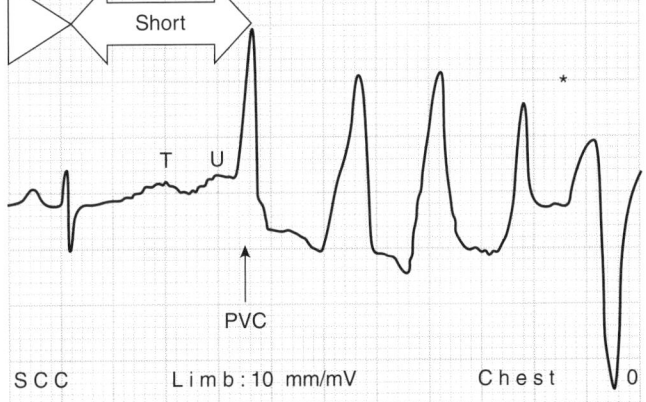

FIG. 1 Onset of Torsade de Pointes during the recording of a standard 12-lead electrocardiogram (ECG) in a young male with a history of drug addiction treated with chronic methadone therapy who presented to a hospital emergency department after ingesting an overdose of prescription and over-the-counter drugs from his parent's drug cabinet. Classic ECG features evident in this rhythm strip include a prolonged QT interval with distorted T-U complex, initiation of the arrhythmia after a short-long-short cycle sequence by a PVC that falls near the peak of the distorted T-U complex, "warm-up" phenomenon with initial R-R cycles longer than subsequent cycles, and abrupt switching of QRS morphology from predominantly positive to predominantly negative complexes *(asterisk).* (From Drew BJ et al: Prevention of torsade de pointes in hospital settings: a scientific statement from the American Heart Association and the American College of Cardiology Foundation, *J Am Coll Cardiol* 55:934-947, 2010.)

TABLE 1   Causes and Triggers of Torsade de Pointes

Congenital	• Romano-Ward syndrome (autosomal dominant) • Jervell and Lange-Nielsen syndrome (autosomal recessive) • LQTS channelopathies
Acquired	
Metabolic syndromes	• Hypokalemia • Hypocalcemia • Hypomagnesemia • Starvation • Anorexia nervosa • Liquid protein diets • Hypothyroidism
Bradyarrhythmias	• Sinus node dysfunction • Second- or third-degree AV block
Antiarrhythmic drugs	• Quinidine • Procainamide • Disopyramide • Amiodarone and dronedarone • Sotalol • Dofetilide, ibutilide, azimilide
Antimicrobial drugs	• Erythromycin, clarithromycin, azithromycin • Pentamidine • Azole antifungals like voriconazole • Fluoroquinolones such as levofloxacin and moxifloxacin • Chloroquine
Antihistaminics	• Terfenadine • Astemizole
Psychiatric drugs	• Phenothiazines • Thioridazine • Tricyclic antidepressants • Haloperidol • Risperidone • Selective serotonin reuptake inhibitors
Antineoplastic agents	• Tyrosine kinase inhibitors such as sunitinib, dasatinib • Vorinostat • Arsenic
Gastric motility agents	• Cisapride, domperidone
Opioid dependence drugs	• Methadone
Other factors	• Myocardial ischemia • Hypothermia • Intracranial disease • HIV infection • Connective tissue disease with anti-Ro/SSA antibodies • Periodic paralysis (Andersen syndrome) • Cocaine

TABLE 2   Risk Factors for Drug-Induced Torsade de Pointes

- Congenital long QT
- Female gender
- Electrolyte abnormalities (hypokalemia, hypomagnesemia, hypocalcemia)
- Diuretic use
- Bradycardia
- Cardiac hypertrophy
- Myocardial fibrosis
- Congestive heart failure
- Renal and liver insufficiency
- Coadministration of drugs blocking P450 isoenzyme CYP3A4
- High doses or rapid intravenous infusion of the drug
- Baseline electrocardiographic abnormalities (prolonged QT, T-wave lability)

From Gowda RM et al: Torsade de pointes: the clinical considerations, *Int J Cardiol* 96(1):1-6, 2004.

TABLE 3   Risk Factors for Torsade de Pointes in Hospitalized Patients

- Clinically recognizable risk factors
- QTc >500 msec
- LQT2-type repolarization: Notched or "bifid" T-wave
- Use of QT-prolonging drugs
- Concurrent use of more than one QT-prolonging drug
- Rapid infusion by intravenous route
- Structural heart disease
- Congestive heart failure
- Myocardial infarction
- Advanced age
- Female sex
- Hypokalemia
- Hypomagnesemia
- Hypocalcemia
- Treatment with diuretics
- Impaired hepatic drug metabolism
- Bradycardia
- Sinus bradycardia, heart block, incomplete heart block with pauses
- Premature QRS complexes leading to short-long-short cycles
- Multiple clinically recognizable risk factors
- Occult (latent) congenital LQTS
- Genetic polymorphisms

From Drew BJ et al: Prevention of torsade de pointes in hospital settings: a scientific statement from the American Heart Association and the American College of Cardiology Foundation, *Circulation* 121(8):1047, 2010.

LABORATORY TESTS

- Electrolytes: Assess for hypokalemia, hypocalcemia, and hypomagnesemia
- Thyroid function tests
- Genetic studies if suspicion of congenital LQT syndrome

IMAGING STUDIES

- Echocardiography to rule out structural heart disease as a cause of VT
- Stress test to rule out myocardial ischemia. Stress ECG with dynamic assessment of the QT interval during varying heart rates may be diagnostic of long QT syndromes and related TdP

- Computed tomography scan of the head if intracranial disease is suspected

Rx TREATMENT

The cornerstone of treatment comprises intravenous magnesium and acceleration of the heart rate, either by mechanical overdrive pacing or by infusion of isoproterenol. Withdrawal of causative drugs and correction of underlying causes such as electrolyte imbalances, hypothermia, and ischemia are also important. The 2017 American Heart Association and the American College of Cardiology (AHA/ACC) guidelines for management of patients with ventricular arrhythmias provide an overview and recommendations for treatment of TdP.[1]

NONPHARMACOLOGIC THERAPY

- Withdrawal of any offending drugs and correction of electrolyte abnormalities are recommended in patients presenting with TdP (Class I recommendation).

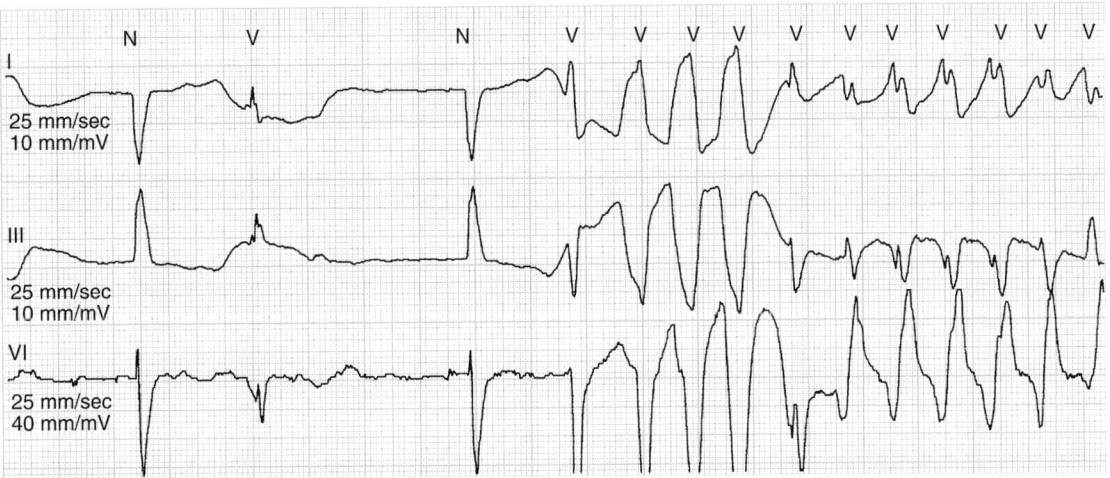

FIG. 2 Torsade de Pointes. This lead I, III, and V₁ rhythm strip shows sinus bradycardia with left bundle branch block and marked QT prolongation with premature ventricular contractions (R-on-T) that initiates a very rapid polymorphic ventricular tachycardia with the characteristic twisting of the QRS complex around the isoelectric baseline. Torsade de Pointes literally means "twisting of the points." (From Olshansky B et al: *Arrhythmia essentials*, ed 2, Philadelphia, 2017, Elsevier.)

- Temporary atrial or ventricular overdrive pacing is a Class I recommendation for all causes of TdP if intravenous magnesium fails.
- Acute and long-term pacing is recommended for patients presenting with TdP due to heart block and symptomatic bradycardia (Class 1) or those with recurrent pause-dependent torsades (Class IIa).
- Active internal and external rewarming if hypothermia is the etiology.
- If TdP degenerates into ventricular fibrillation, defibrillation and advanced cardiac life support protocol should be followed.

ACUTE GENERAL Rx

- Intravenous magnesium sulfate 1 to 2 g given over 1 to 2 min is first-line therapy for patients who present with LQTS and few episodes of TdP (Class IIa). Magnesium is not likely to be effective in patients with a normal QT interval.
- Isoproterenol is reasonable as temporary treatment in patients with acute disease who present with recurrent pause-dependent TdP and who do not have congenital LQTS (Class IIa).
- Beta-blockade combined with pacing is reasonable acute therapy for patients who present with TdP and sinus bradycardia (Class IIa).
- Potassium repletion to 4.5 to 5 mmol/L may be considered for patients who present with TdP and hypokalemia (Class IIb).
- Intravenous lidocaine, oral mexiletine, or phenytoin may be considered in patients who present with LQT3 and TdP (Class IIb).
- TdP is usually self-limited, and cardioversion should be performed only as a last resort in the setting of pulseless VF because of the high likelihood of immediate recurrence of the TdP after cardioversion.

CHRONIC Rx

- TdP resulting from congenital LQTS is treated with beta-blockade (propranolol or nadolol are preferred), pacing, and implantable cardioverter-defibrillator in high-risk cases.

For patients who continue to have syncope despite maximal drug therapy, cervical-thoracic sympathectomy may be considered.
- Long-term pacing is recommended for patients presenting with TdP due to heart block and symptomatic bradycardia.
- Avoid use of QT-prolonging drugs.
- Lifestyle modification in case of congenital LQTS.
- In patients with eating disorders, nutritional rehabilitation will correct the QT prolongation over the long term (3 to 18 mo).
- Psychiatric evaluation of patients with drug overdose and eating disorders.

DISPOSITION

Patients with TdP should be monitored in an intensive care setting.

REFERRAL

Patients should have an urgent cardiology consultation.

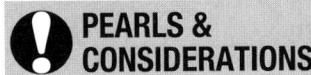

PEARLS & CONSIDERATIONS

COMMENTS

- Identification of the etiology for TdP is key in diagnosis, management, and prognosis of this condition.
- Drugs associated with TdP vary greatly in their risk for arrhythmia; an updated list can be found at https://crediblemeds.org/. The risk-benefit ratio should be assessed for each individual to determine whether the potential therapeutic benefit of a drug outweighs the risk for TdP.
- Risk factors for drug-induced TdP include older age, female sex, heart disease, electrolyte disorders (especially hypokalemia and hypomagnesemia), renal or hepatic dysfunction, bradycardia or rhythms with long pauses, treatment with more than one QT-prolonging drug, and genetic predisposition.
- After initiation of a drug associated with TdP, ECG signs indicative of risk for arrhythmia

include an increase in QTc from predrug baseline of >60 msec, marked QTc interval prolongation >500 msec, T-U wave distortion that becomes more exaggerated in the beat after a pause, visible T-wave alternans, new-onset ventricular ectopy, and couplets and nonsustained polymorphic ventricular tachycardia initiated in the beat after a pause.

PREVENTION

The 2011 AHA/ACC scientific statement on prevention of TdP suggests a strategy of documenting the QTc interval before and at least every 8 to 12 h after the initiation, increased dose, or overdose of QT-prolonging drugs. If QTc prolongation is observed, documentation of more frequent measurements is recommended. The duration of QTc monitoring depends upon the duration of treatment with the QT-prolonging drug and the drug half-life.[2]

PATIENT & FAMILY EDUCATION

- Patients should be educated about avoiding use of QT-prolonging drugs. A complete list of these drugs can be found at https://crediblemeds.org/.
- First-degree relatives of all patients with congenital LQTS should undergo genetic testing.
- Congenital LQTS patients should avoid certain specific triggers (e.g., swimming and exercise in LQTS 1 and LQTS 2 and acoustic stimuli in LQTS 2).
- It is recommended that all patients affected by LQTS avoid competitive sports activity.

RELATED CONTENT

Long QT Syndrome (Related Key Topic)

REFERENCES

Available at eBooks.Health.Elsevier.com.

AUTHOR: **JOHN WYLIE, MD, FACC**

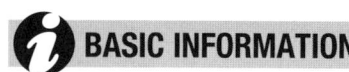
ℹ️ BASIC INFORMATION

DEFINITION

Tourette syndrome (TS) is an inherited neuropsychiatric disorder characterized by motor and phonic tics that wax and wane and change over time. Diagnosis requires onset of symptoms prior to age 18; however, symptom onset typically occurs in early childhood.

Tics are sudden, brief, patterned, repetitive, intermittent, movements (motor tics) or sounds (phonic tics) that may abruptly interrupt otherwise normal motor activity or speech.[1]

SYNONYMS

Gilles de la Tourette syndrome
TS
Tourette disorder

ICD-10CM CODE

F95.2 Combined vocal and multiple motor tic disorder [de la Tourette]

EPIDEMIOLOGY & DEMOGRAPHICS

PREVALENCE (IN U.S.): Estimates range from 0.3% to 3% in children.[2]
PREDOMINANT SEX: Approximate male:female ratio of 4:1.[2]
PREDOMINANT AGE: Typical age of onset is between 2 and 12 yr of age (most frequently between 3 and 8 yr).[3]

PHYSICAL FINDINGS & CLINICAL PRESENTATION

- Neurologic examination is normal.
- Phonic tics are characterized by simple meaningless sounds or noises (e.g., clearing of throat, sniffing, grunting, forceful exhales or inhales) or complex, which are semantically meaningful utterances (e.g., repetition of words or short phrases, swearing [coprolalia]).[3]
- Motor tics can be simple (e.g., blinking, grimacing, head jerking [Fig. E1]) or complex (e.g., gesturing [Fig. E2]). Tics wax, wane, change over time, and are often suppressible. Commonly, they are preceded by a premonitory urge that builds until the tic is performed, during which the urge is resolved and then later builds again.[4]
- TS is often associated with a variety of psychiatric conditions, most commonly attention-deficit/hyperactivity disorder (ADHD) and obsessive-compulsive disorder (OCD).[5]
- Diagnostic criteria of TS according to the *Diagnostic and Statistical Manual of Mental Disorders,* fifth edition, are as follows:
  1. Multiple motor tics and one or more phonic tics must be present for greater than 1 yr, although not necessarily concurrently.
  2. The tics may wax and wane in frequency but have persisted for more than 1 yr since onset.
  3. Age at onset is less than 18 yr.
  4. Disturbance is not attributable to the direct physiologic effects of a substance (e.g., cocaine) or another medical condition (e.g., Huntington disease or post-viral encephalitis).

ETIOLOGY

The exact pathogenesis is unknown; however, current models describe network dysfunction between the cortex, thalamus, and basal ganglia.[6] Genetic predisposition is likely, as there is a strong family history of OCD or TS in patients with tics, and twin studies provide evidence for the importance of genetic factors with a concordance rate of 77%.[7] Multiple genes have been explored as possible links to TS, but no causative gene has yet been identified.

🅳🆇 DIAGNOSIS

DIFFERENTIAL DIAGNOSIS

- Autism spectrum disorder.
- Carbon monoxide poisoning.
- Sydenham chorea.
- Brain tumor.
- Drug intoxication: Many drugs are known to induce or exacerbate tic disorders, including cocaine and supratherapeutic levels of stimulants.
- Postinfectious encephalitis.
- Inherited disorders: Huntington disease, neurodegeneration with brain iron accumulation, and neuroacanthocytosis. These conditions should have other observed abnormalities on neurologic examination.
- Functional neurologic symptom disorder.

WORKUP

Clinical examination and history to confirm diagnosis

LABORATORY TESTS

No laboratory tests are required for the diagnosis

IMAGING STUDIES

Computed tomography scan and MRI of brain are unremarkable in TS and unnecessary when the neurologic examination is within normal limits.

🆁🆇 TREATMENT (FIG. 3)

NONPHARMACOLOGIC THERAPY

- Multidisciplinary: Education of patients, parents, teachers, psychologists, and school nurses is essential.
- Patients with tics require treatment only when movements and sounds are bothersome, impairing, or painful to the patient. If none of these characteristics are present, patient and caregiver education on the natural history of tics is appropriate. However, forceful motor tics involving the neck should be treated more aggressively (these often are bothersome and painful to the child), as these may pose a risk of causing traumatic cervical myelopathy with associated spasticity, weakness, and eventual loss of mobility.[8]
- Cognitive-behavioral therapy, termed habit-reversal treatment or Comprehensive Behavioral Intervention for Tics (CBIT), is often recommended as first-line treatment.[9]
- Screening for comorbid psychiatric disorders such as ADHD, OCD, anxiety, and depression must be performed, as these symptoms often become more impairing than the tics.

ACUTE GENERAL Rx

In general, acute treatment of tics is not necessary unless tics are clearly self-injurious. In this case, one could consider short-term treatment with benzodiazepines until adequate doses of chronic anti-tic medications are achieved.[10]

CHRONIC Rx

Tics require treatment when movements and sounds are painful, bothersome, or impairing to the patient or if lack of treatment would cause imminent self-harm (e.g., forceful motor tics of the neck).[3]

Oral medications include alpha-2 agonists (clonidine, guanfacine), anticonvulsants (topiramate, clonazepam), dopamine-receptor blocking agents (haloperidol, pimozide, aripiprazole, fluphenazine), and vesicular monoamine transporter type 2 (VAMT2) inhibitors (tetrabenazine, valbenazine, deutetrabenazine).
TICS:
- Alpha-2 agonists (clonidine and guanfacine) can be used for treatment of motor and phonic tics; however, they may be limited by adverse effects.[11] They may also be beneficial for management of comorbid psychiatric conditions such as impulsivity.
- Haloperidol, aripiprazole, and pimozide are the only U.S. FDA–approved medications for the treatment of tics in TS; however, other dopamine receptor blocking agents may also be used such as fluphenazine or ziprasidone.[10,11] Dopamine receptor blocking medications carry a small but significant risk of tardive dyskinesia, especially in adults.
- Tetrabenazine, deutetrabenazine, and valbenazine are presynaptic dopamine-depleting agents that inhibit VMAT2 and have been found to provide meaningful benefit in treatment of tics and do not carry a risk of tardive dyskinesia.[12] However, large-scale randomized placebo-controlled trials have not shown the same benefit.[11]
- An antiepileptic (topiramate) has also been found to be helpful in reducing tics.[10,11]
- Botulinum neurotoxin injections are effective for simple motor tics and are particularly useful in forceful neck tics. Injections must be repeated every 3 mo.[13]
- In the case of tics that are refractory to treatments and are impairing, surgical treatment with deep brain stimulation can be considered.[14]

ADHD: Stimulants are the most common medications for the treatment of ADHD. Previous studies have reported exacerbations of tics in

Treatment algorithm for Tourette syndrome

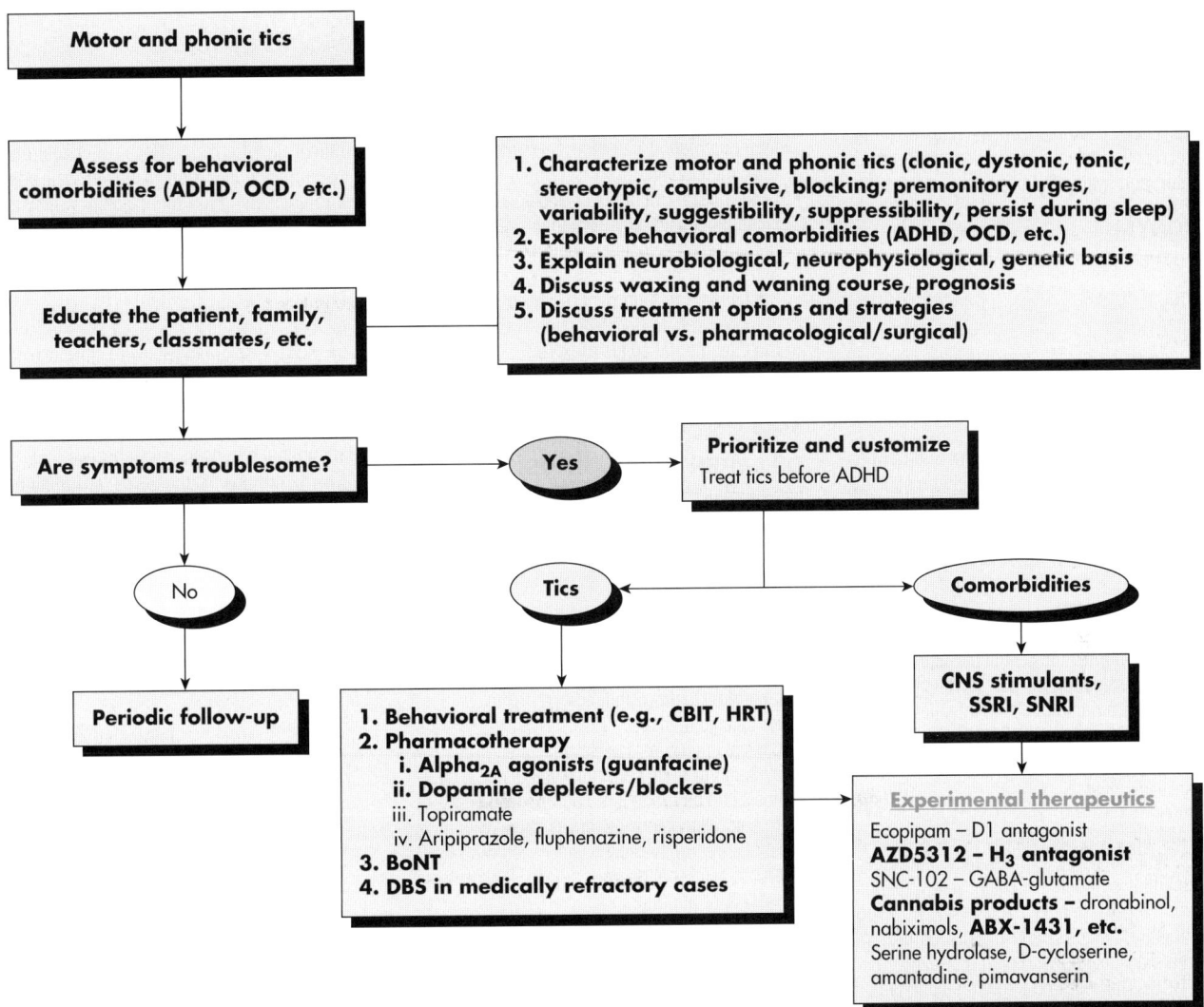

FIG. 3 Treatment algorithm for Tourette syndrome. *ADHD*, Attention-deficit/hyperactivity disorder; *CBIT*, comprehensive behavioral intervention for tics; *CNS*, Central nervous system; *DBS*, deep brain stimulation; *GABA*, γ-aminobutyric acid; *HRT*, habit reversal training; *OCD*, obsessive compulsive disorder; *SNc*, substantia nigra pars compacta; *SNRI*, selective noradrenergic reuptake inhibitor; *SSRI*, selective serotonin reuptake inhibitor. (From Jankovic J et al: *Bradley and Daroff's neurology in clinical practice*, ed 8, Philadelphia, 2022, Elsevier.)

some patients; however, a meta-analysis concluded that there was no concrete evidence that stimulants consistently worsened tic severity.[15] These medications should be used if troublesome ADHD is present.

OCD: Selective serotonin reuptake inhibitors, such as fluoxetine, citalopram, escitalopram, or fluvoxamine, are the most effective medications for OCD.

DISPOSITION

- The intensity and frequency of tics often decrease in late adolescence and early adulthood.
- Approximately 75% of patients will have reduced severity of tics in adulthood; however, 90% will still have mild tics that are often not impairing as adults.[3]

REFERRAL

When tics do not require treatment, no referrals are necessary. The provider should educate the

patient and caregivers on the diagnosis and natural history of tics. However, referrals should be made to neurologists or subspecialty movement disorder neurologists if (1) the diagnosis is unclear, (2) treatment is required or has been refractory, or (3) there is risk of imminent self-harm when untreated. The latter should be expedited whenever possible.

If comorbid psychiatric disorders are bothersome or impairing, referral to a psychiatrist should also be made.

⚠ PEARLS & CONSIDERATIONS

- Tics require treatment when they are bothersome, impairing, or painful.
- An important part of treatment is appropriate evaluation and therapy of coexisting conditions (e.g., ADHD, OCD), as these conditions often cause more disability than the tics themselves.

- Treatment of tics includes comprehensive behavioral intervention for tics, medications, botulinum neurotoxin injections, and deep brain stimulation.

COMMENTS

Patient education may be obtained from the Tourette Syndrome Association, 4240 Bell Blvd., Bayside, NY 11361-2864; 800-237-0717 or 718-224-2999; http://www.tsa-usa.org/.

REFERENCES

Available at eBooks.Health.Elsevier.com.

RELATED CONTENT

Tourette Syndrome (Patient Information)

AUTHOR: **MARIAM HULL, MD**

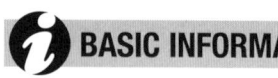

BASIC INFORMATION

DEFINITION

Toxic megacolon (TM) is a rare but severe complication of colonic inflammation, most commonly associated with inflammatory bowel disease (IBD), characterized by total or partial nonobstructive colonic distention (>6 cm in diameter) and systemic toxicity.

SYNONYM

Toxic dilation of the colon

ICD-10CM CODES
A04.7   Megacolon due to *Clostridium difficile*
K59.3   Megacolon, not elsewhere classified

EPIDEMIOLOGY & DEMOGRAPHICS

INCIDENCE: The exact prevalence of TM is underreported and varies depending on etiology. Incidence in patients with ulcerative colitis (UC) is approximately 10% and nearly 5% in patients with Crohn disease. *Clostridium difficile* infections may be complicated by toxic megacolon in up to 3% of cases.

PREDOMINANT SEX & AGE: With increasing rates of *C. diff* infections, patients ages 65 and older are at higher risk for developing toxic megacolon as a result of *C. diff* infection.

RISK FACTORS: Major risk factors include inflammatory, infectious, and ischemic conditions of the colon, especially in individuals who are immunocompromised. Other risk factors include hypokalemia, use of narcotics, antidiarrheal agents, anticholinergics, pregnancy, and recent instrumentation (such as colonoscopy, barium enema). Female gender, age >40 yr, hypoalbuminemia, acidosis, and high blood urea nitrogen are associated with high mortality.

GENETICS: There are no known genetic factors that predispose patients to developing toxic megacolon associated with an inflammatory or infectious etiology.

PHYSICAL FINDINGS & CLINICAL PRESENTATION

- Patients with toxic megacolon usually appear severely ill. Clinical symptoms are similar to those of IBD and acute colitis and may include abdominal pain, diarrhea (usually severe and bloody), and vomiting.
- Physical exam findings may include a distended, tender, and tympanic abdomen with reduced or absent bowel sounds. The patient may also present with signs of shock such as fever, tachycardia, mental status changes, and hypovolemia. Older patients and those on steroid therapy are less likely to demonstrate a peritoneal abdominal examination.
- Laboratory findings may include leukocytosis, lactic acidosis, anemia, increased inflammatory markers, and electrolyte abnormalities. Patients who present with severe volume losses can present with hypokalemia and hypoalbuminemia.

ETIOLOGY

- The mechanism of the development of TM is unclear; however, defective smooth muscle contraction and lowered pressure of the colonic lumen play an important role in its development.
- Most common etiologies are inflammatory conditions such as UC, Crohn disease, and Behçet disease. Infections such as *C. diff, Salmonella, Shigella, E. Coli,* cytomegalovirus, and *Entamoeba* can also be complicated by toxic megacolon.
- Other less common etiologies include ischemic colitis, hypokalemia, medications, barium enema, colonoscopy, bowel preparations, malignancy such as lymphoma, and Kaposi sarcoma. In general, toxic megacolon is more likely to be associated with pancolitis than segmental colitis (Box 1).

DIAGNOSIS

DIFFERENTIAL DIAGNOSIS

Ischemic colitis, Crohn disease, ulcerative colitis, Hirschsprung disease, colonic pseudoobstruction (Ogilvie syndrome), diffuse dysmotility, large/small bowel obstruction, volvulus

WORKUP

- General principles of workup include physical examination to evaluate for an acute abdomen, laboratory testing, and radiography to evaluate for colonic dilation.
- Clinical criteria for toxic megacolon, proposed by Jalan et al in 1969, are still used. A diagnosis can be made if radiographic evidence of colonic distension >6 cm is present with at least three of the following: Fever >38.6° C (101.5° F), heart rate >120, leukocytosis >10.5, or anemia. In addition, at least one of the following must also be present: Hypovolemia, altered level of consciousness, electrolyte abnormalities, or hypotension.
- Patients with suspected toxic megacolon should be triaged emergently to an emergent care setting to facilitate rapid diagnosis and treatment.

LABORATORY TESTS

Initial testing should include a CBC, full chemistry panel, liver function panel, erythrocyte sedimentation rate, C-reactive protein, lactic acid,

---

BOX 1   Disorders Associated With Toxic Megacolon

- Inflammatory bowel disease
  1. Ulcerative colitis
  2. Crohn disease
- Infectious colitis
  1. *Salmonella, Shigella,* amoebic colitis
  2. *Clostridium* difficile
  3. Cytomegalovirus colitis
  4. Human immunodeficiency virus (HIV) infection
- Cancer chemotherapy
- Ischemia

From Vincent JL et al: *Textbook of critical care,* ed 6, Philadelphia, 2011, WB Saunders.

---

blood cultures, coagulation panel, type and screen, and stool studies including *C. diff.*

IMAGING STUDIES

- All patients should initially receive a plain abdominal x-ray examination (Fig. 1) to assess for colonic dilation. Common findings include mucosal irregularity, loss of haustrations, "thumb printing" due to bowel wall edema, and thickening of the colonic wall with a continuous segment of air-filled colon >6 cm in diameter. The transverse or right colon is usually the most dilated segment seen.
- Computed tomography (CT) has been increasingly used to assess disease extent and for surgical planning (Fig. 2). It can also be helpful when differentiating between the various etiologies of toxic megacolon and to assess for complications such as intraabdominal hemorrhage or abscess.
- CT features include colonic distention, abnormal haustra, pericolonic fat stranding, colonic wall thickening, ascites, pleural effusion, and small bowel or gastric distension.
- An abdominal ultrasound provides nonspecific findings.

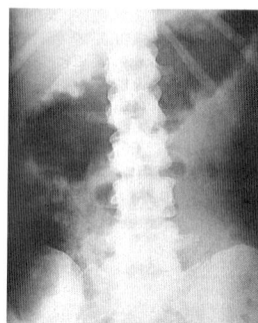

FIG. 1 Toxic megacolon secondary to ulcerative colitis. The smooth indentations seen along the margin of the colon represent pseudopolyps. (From Marx JA et al [eds]: *Rosen's emergency medicine: concepts and clinical practice,* ed 7, Philadelphia, 2010, Elsevier.)

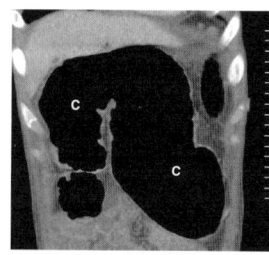

FIG. 2 Toxic megacolon. In a young patient with severe ulcerative colitis, coronal computed tomography demonstrates marked dilation of the colon *(c)* with thinning of its walls. The diameter of the lumen of the colon exceeds 7 cm. This finding places the patient at high risk of colon perforation. (From Webb WR et al: *Fundamentals of body CT,* ed 4, Philadelphia, 2015, Saunders.)

Rx TREATMENT

Treatment includes both medical and surgical options. Principles of initial management include treating the underlying cause, managing shock, analgesia, and early surgical and gastroenterology consultation.

NONPHARMACOLOGIC THERAPY

- Surgery may be required in up to 50% of patients with toxic megacolon who do not show clinical improvement within 24 to 48 h. The preferred first-line surgical treatment is subtotal colectomy with an end ileostomy. Other options include total proctocolectomy or colon decompression via the Turnbull method.
- Timing of surgical treatment is still controversial, with many advocating for aggressive medical treatment and observation before surgical intervention. Some studies conclude that early surgical intervention is favorable, whereas others conclude an increase in mortality, especially in patients older than 65.
- Definitive indications for early surgical treatment include perforation, persistent colonic hemorrhage, full-thickness ischemia, necrosis, abdominal compartment syndrome, or rapid clinical deterioration.

ACUTE GENERAL Rx

- Patients should be on bowel rest. Maneuvers to decrease abdominal distension by passing of colonic gas via walking or rotating patients should be employed.
- Medications that impact colonic motility such as anticholinergics, opioids, and antidiarrheal agents should be discontinued and avoided.
- Electrolyte abnormalities, dehydration, and anemia are common clinical findings and should be addressed early. Fluid resuscitation with an isotonic solution and correction of electrolyte disturbances (especially hypokalemia) can help prevent worsening atony of the colonic wall. Patients with anemia from colonic hemorrhage should receive blood transfusion(s).
- Patients with toxic megacolon should receive broad-spectrum antibiotics as soon as possible as mortality due to TM correlates with the development of sepsis. Infections due to *C. diff* should be treated with vancomycin (oral or rectal) or metronidazole (oral or intravenous [IV]). Toxic megacolon due to cytomegalovirus should be treated with ganciclovir IV.
- Patients with inflammatory etiologies such as UC or Crohn should receive high-dose IV steroids, either hydrocortisone 100 mg IV or methylprednisolone 60 mg IV every 6 to 8 h. Steroids should not be used in patients with a confirmed infectious etiology.
- There are currently no data to support empiric treatment of toxic megacolon due to IBD with cyclosporine or infliximab. These treatment options should be reserved for patients who are not steroid responsive and should be limited to one attempt at clinical improvement so as not to delay surgical intervention.
- A management algorithm for toxic megacolon is outlined in Fig. 3.

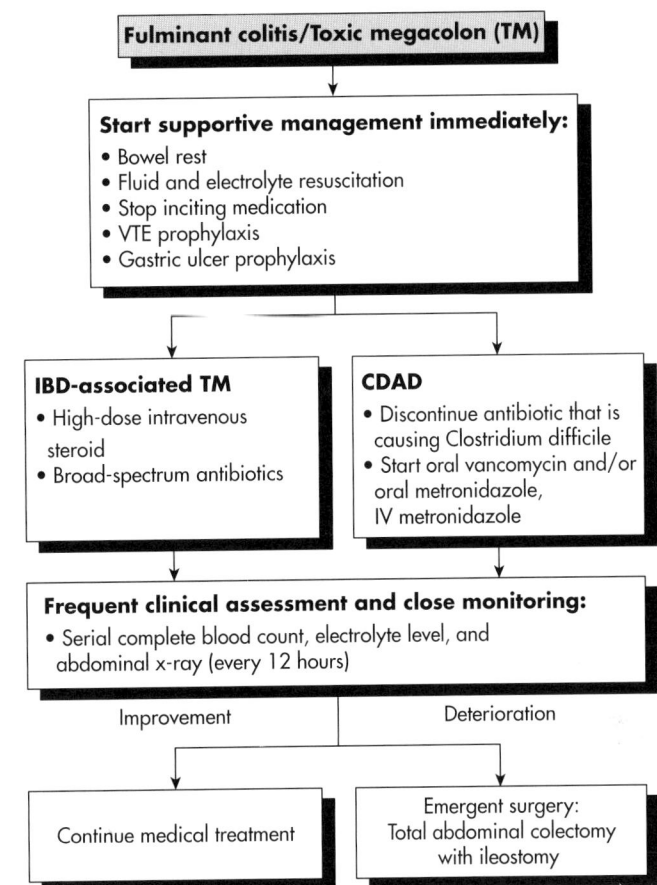

FIG. 3 Management algorithm for toxic megacolon. *CDAD, C. difficile*-associated disease; *IBD,* inflammatory bowel disease; *VTE,* venous thromboembolism. (From Cameron JL, Cameron AM: *Current surgical therapy,* ed 12, Philadelphia, 2017, Elsevier.)

CHRONIC Rx

Patients with IBD will need continued treatment for the underlying disease process once the acute processes associated with toxic megacolon have resolved.

DISPOSITION

All patients with toxic megacolon will require admission, possibly to the intensive care unit, depending on their clinical presentation.

REFERRAL

- Patients with suspected toxic megacolon presenting outside an emergency department should be referred there immediately.
- Surgical consultation should be obtained in all cases.
- All patients with toxic megacolon due to newly diagnosed IBD who are discharged from the hospital should be referred to a gastroenterologist for continued treatment.

ⓘ PEARLS & CONSIDERATIONS

COMMENTS

- Early recognition and treatment of toxic megacolon is critical given the associated high morbidity and mortality.

- Anticholinergic medications, antidiarrheal agents, and opioids can precipitate or worsen toxic megacolon and should be discontinued immediately if TM is suspected.
- Management includes medical and surgical treatment with inpatient hospitalization and treatment of the underlying cause.

PREVENTION

Prevention focuses on treatment of underlying causes of colitis to prevent complications such as toxic megacolon.

SUGGESTED READINGS

Available at eBooks.Health.Elsevier.com.

RELATED CONTENT

Clostridium difficile Infection (Related Key Topic)
Crohn Disease (Related Key Topic)
Small Bowel Obstruction (Related Key Topic)
Ulcerative Colitis (Related Key Topic)

AUTHORS: **RORY MERRITT, MD, MEHP,** and **ERIC EBERT, MD**

Toxoplasmosis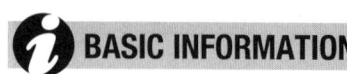

BASIC INFORMATION

DEFINITION

Toxoplasmosis is an infection caused by the protozoal parasite *Toxoplasma gondii* transmitted through ingestion of undercooked meat, undercooked shellfish, or cat feces.

ICD-10CM CODES
B58.9	Toxoplasmosis, unspecified
B58.3	Pulmonary toxoplasmosis
B58.89	Toxoplasmosis with other organ involvement
P37.1	Congenital toxoplasmosis

EPIDEMIOLOGY & DEMOGRAPHICS
INCIDENCE (IN U.S.):
- Seroprevalence varies widely across different geographic locations, increasing with age, prevalence of cats in the area, and certain activities such as working in slaughterhouses or owning cats.
- Seroprevalence among women of childbearing age was 9.1% between 2009 and 2010.
- 0.23 cases of congenital toxoplasmosis per 10,000 live births between 2006 and 2014.
- Among patients with HIV, seroprevalence is approximately 11% in the U.S.

PREDOMINANT SEX: Equal gender distribution.
PREDOMINANT AGE:
- Infancy (congenital infection).
- Prevalence increases with age. Primary infection is usually asymptomatic, but latent infection can reactivate later in life.

PEAK INCIDENCE: Seroprevalence is higher in Latin America, Africa, and other temperate climates than in the U.S.
GENETICS: Congenital infection:
- Incidence and severity vary with the trimester of gestation during which the mother acquired infection.
  1. 10% to 25% (first trimester)
  2. 30% to 54% (second trimester)
  3. 60% to 65% (third trimester)
- Congenital infection occurring in the first trimester is the most severe.
- 89% to 100% of infections in the third trimester are asymptomatic.
- Risk to the fetus is not correlated with symptoms in the mother.

PHYSICAL FINDINGS & CLINICAL PRESENTATION
- Acquired (immunocompetent host): Usually subclinical, though may develop adenopathy, fatigue, and other constitutional symptoms that, although generally mild, can take weeks to resolve.
- Acquired (in patients with AIDS, especially with CD4 count <100, hematopoietic stem cell transplant recipients): Most common presentation is encephalitis with headache, confusion, and fever. May have motor weakness or other focal neurologic abnormalities and seizures. Can also present as pneumonitis, chorioretinitis, or other end-organ involvement.
- Acquired (immunocompromised patients):
  1. Encephalitis
  2. Myocarditis (especially in heart transplant patients)
  3. Pneumonitis
- Ocular infection in the immunocompetent host: If not congenital, then presents in second or third decade of life as a focal necrotizing retinitis with photophobia, blurred vision, pain, and potentially loss of central vision if the macula is involved.
- Congenital: Results from acute infection acquired by the mother within 6 to 8 wk before conception or during gestation and is usually asymptomatic in the mother. In the infant, symptomatic disease is estimated at 40%. Ocular disease can include chorioretinitis and blindness, while central nervous system (CNS) manifestations can include intracranial calcifications resulting in epilepsy, hydrocephalus, microcephaly, psychomotor or developmental delay, and encephalitis.

ETIOLOGY
- *T. gondii:*
  1. Ubiquitous intracellular protozoan
  2. Present worldwide
  3. Cat is the definitive host (Fig. E1)
  4. Oocysts can remain viable up to a year in moist soil, despite freezing temperatures
- Human infection:
  1. Ingestion of oocysts shed by cats in soil, litter boxes, vegetables
  2. Ingestion of inadequately cooked meat or shellfish containing tissue cysts
  3. Vertical transmission

DIAGNOSIS

DIFFERENTIAL DIAGNOSIS
- Lymphadenopathy:
  1. Infectious mononucleosis
  2. Cytomegalovirus (CMV) mononucleosis
  3. Cat-scratch disease
  4. Sarcoidosis
  5. Tuberculosis
  6. Lymphoma
  7. Metastatic cancer
- Cerebral mass lesions in immunocompromised host:
  1. Lymphoma
  2. Tuberculosis
  3. Bacterial abscess
- Pneumonitis in immunocompromised host:
  1. *Pneumocystis jiroveci (carinii)* pneumonia
  2. Tuberculosis
  3. Fungal infection
- Chorioretinitis:
  1. Syphilis
  2. Tuberculosis
  3. Histoplasmosis (competent host)
  4. CMV
  5. Herpes simplex
  6. Fungal infection
  7. Tuberculosis
- Myocarditis:
  1. Organ rejection in heart transplant recipients
- Congenital infection:
  1. Rubella
  2. CMV
  3. Herpes simplex
  4. Syphilis
  5. Listeriosis
  6. Erythroblastosis fetalis
  7. Sepsis

WORKUP
- Acute infection, immunocompetent host:
  1. CBC
  2. *Toxoplasma* serology (immunoglobulin [Ig] G, IgM) in serial blood specimens 3 wk apart
  3. Lymph node biopsy if diagnosis uncertain
  4. Bone marrow exam (Fig. E2) in suspected bone marrow involvement
- Immunocompromised host:
  1. CNS symptoms:
     a. Cerebral computed tomography (CT) scan or MRI if CNS symptoms present
     b. Spinal tap, if safe
     c. Brain biopsy (Fig. E3) if no response to empiric therapy
  2. Ocular symptoms:
     a. Funduscopic examination (Fig. E4)
     b. Serologic studies
     c. Rarely, vitreous tap
  3. Pulmonary symptoms:
     a. Chest x-ray examination
     b. Bronchoalveolar lavage
     c. Transbronchial or open-lung biopsy
  4. Myocarditis:
     a. Cardiac enzymes
     b. Electrocardiogram
     c. Endomyocardial biopsy for definitive diagnosis
- Toxoplasmosis in pregnancy (Fig. E5):
  1. Initial maternal screening with IgM and IgG
     a. If negative, mother at risk of acute infection and should be retested monthly
     b. If both IgG and IgM positive, obtain IgA and IgE enzyme-linked immunoassay (ELISA), differential agglutination (AC/HS) test
     c. IgA and IgE ELISA, AC/HS test elevated in acute infection
     d. Ig high for 1 yr or more
     e. IgG repeated 3 to 4 wk later to determine if titer is stable
  2. Acute maternal infection not excluded or documented:
     a. Fetal blood sampling (for culture, Ig, IgA, IgE)
     b. Amniotic fluid polymerase chain reaction (PCR)
  3. Fetal ultrasound every other week if maternal infection documented to look for ventriculomegaly, calcifications in the brain, and enlarged liver and spleen
- Congenital toxoplasmosis (Fig. E6):
  1. Placental histology
  2. Specific IgM or IgA in infant's blood

LABORATORY TESTS
- Antibody studies:
  1. More than one test necessary to establish diagnosis of acute toxoplasmosis (look for seroconversion or 4× increase)
  2. IgM antibody:

TABLE 1 Guidelines for Interpretation of Serologic Tests for Toxoplasmosis

IgG	IgM	IgG Avidity	Interpretation
Positive	Negative	—	Remote infection, immune. IgG avidity testing is best used when both IgG and IgM are positive and timing of infection is crucial, as in pregnancy (see below).
			False-negative IgM results occur in approximately 25% of cases when evaluating infection in the newborn. If infection is suspected in this setting, further testing (dye test, IgM EIA, IgA EIA, IgE EIA/ISAGA, PCRs, ideally with paired maternal serology tests—see text) is necessary in a reference laboratory (*Toxoplasma* Serology Laboratory, PAMF Research Institute, 795 El Camino Real, Ames Building Palo Alto, CA, 94301; 650-853-4828).
Positive	Positive or equivocal	High	Infection within the past 18 mo but likely >12 wk ago. If pregnant and beyond first trimester, consider sending specimen to reference laboratory for dye test, repeat IgG avidity and IgM EIA, IgA EIA, IgE EIA/ISAGA, and AC/HS testing (see above).
Positive	Positive or equivocal	Low	Infection within the past 12 wk. Consider sending specimen to a reference laboratory (see above) to time infection more accurately (dye test, repeat IgG avidity and IgM EIA, IgA EIA, IgE EIA/ISAGA, and AC/HS) in the setting of pregnancy.
Equivocal	Negative	—	Indeterminate. Test a new specimen or consider a different assay (IFA or ELISA).
Equivocal	Equivocal	—	Indeterminate. Test a new specimen or consider a different assay (IFA or ELISA).
Equivocal	Positive	—	Acute infection or false-positive IgM result. Test a second specimen; if IgG becomes positive or remains equivocal, consider sending specimen to a reference laboratory to time infection more accurately (dye test, IgG avidity, IgM EIA, IgA EIA, IgE EIA/ISAGA, AC/HS—see text) in the setting of pregnancy.
Negative	Negative	—	No evidence of *Toxoplasma* infection; not immune.
Negative	Equivocal	—	Either false-positive IgM result or possible recent infection. Obtain a new specimen and retest. If infection is recent, IgM and IgG should become positive, with low IgG avidity. If repeated testing is still IgG negative and IgM equivocal, patient is likely uninfected. Consider IgM ISAGA.
Negative	Positive	—	Acute infection or false-positive IgM result. Repeat testing on new specimen. If the result is the same, it is likely a false-positive IgM result. Consider IgM ISAGA.

AC/HS, Differential agglutination test; *EIA,* enzyme immunoassay; *ELISA,* enzyme-linked immunosorbent assay; *IFA,* immunofluorescence assay; *Ig,* immunoglobulin; *ISAGA,* immunosorbent agglutination assay; *PCR,* polymerase chain reaction.
From Cherry JD et al: *Feigin and Cherry's pediatric infectious diseases,* ed 8, Philadelphia, 2019, Elsevier.

a. Appears 5 days into infection
b. Peaks at 2 wk
c. Falls to low level or disappears within 2 mo
d. May persist at low levels for 1 yr or more
3. Antibody not measurable:
  a. Ocular toxoplasmosis
  b. Reactivation
  c. Immunocompromised hosts
4. IgG antibody:
  a. Appears 1 to 2 wk after infection
  b. Peaks at 6 to 8 wk
  c. Gradually declines over months to years
5. Guidelines for interpretation of serologic tests for toxoplasmosis are summarized in Table 1

IMAGING STUDIES
- Chest x-ray examination if pulmonary involvement suspected
- Cerebral CT scan (Fig. E7) or MRI (Fig. E8) if encephalitis suspected

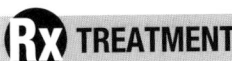 **TREATMENT**

NONPHARMACOLOGIC THERAPY
- Selected cases of ocular infection:
  1. Photocoagulation
  2. Vitrectomy
  3. Lensectomy
- Selected cases of congenital cerebral infection:
  1. Ventricular shunting

ACUTE GENERAL Rx
- Acute infection, immunocompetent, nonpregnant host:
  1. Usually requires no treatment, unless severe and persistent symptoms or vital organ damage
- Acute infection, immunocompromised host, non-AIDS:
  1. Treat even if asymptomatic
  2. Duration:
    a. Until 4 to 6 wk after resolution of all signs and symptoms
    b. Usually 6 mo or longer
- Reactivated infection, immunocompromised host, non-AIDS:
  1. Treat if symptomatic
- Acute or reactivated infection, AIDS:
  1. Treat in all cases
  2. Induction course:
    a. 3 to 6 wk
    b. Maintenance therapy continued for life; consider discontinuation of suppressive therapy if the patient has a good response to antiretroviral therapy and if the CD4 count remains >200 cells/mm^3 for more than 3 mo
  3. Empiric therapy:
    a. AIDS with positive IgG
    b. Multiple ring-enhancing lesions on cerebral CT scan or MRI
    c. Response seen by day 7 in 71% and day 14 in 91%
- Ocular infection:
  1. Treat in all cases

2. Therapy continued for 1 mo or longer if needed
3. Response seen in 70% within 10 days
4. Retreat as needed
5. Steroids may be indicated in patients with signs or symptoms of increased intracranial pressure
6. Surgical treatment in selected cases
- Treatment regimens (Table 2):
  1. Pyrimethamine 200 mg loading dose once PO, then 50 mg (<60 kg) to 75 mg (>60 kg) daily; *plus*
  2. Leucovorin 10 to 25 mg PO daily; *plus*
  3. Sulfadiazine 1 (<60 kg) to 1.5 g (>60 kg) PO q6h
Other treatment options (if sulfa hypersensitivity or allergy is present): Pyrimethamine 50 to 75 mg/day PO with leucovorin 10 to 25 mg/day PO and either (1) clindamycin 600 mg q6h PO or IV q6h, or (2) atovaquone 1500 mg PO q12h, or (3) azithromycin 900 to 1200 mg PO daily.
- Acute infection in pregnancy:
  1. Treat immediately
  2. Risk of fetal infection reduced by 60% with treatment
    a. Seroconversion in the first trimester
      (1) Spiramycin 1 g q8h
    b. Seroconversion beyond the first trimester or positive amniotic fluid PCR/ultrasound findings consistent with congenital toxoplasmosis:
      (1) Sulfadiazine 75 mg/kg daily in two divided doses ×2 days, then 50 mg/kg bid, *plus*

TABLE 2 Treatment of Toxoplasmosis

Disease	Medication	Dosage	Length of Therapy
Acute acquired—generally not treated unless severe or persistent symptoms, vital organ damage, or host immunosuppression[a]	Pyrimethamine *plus*	2 mg/kg daily for 2 days, then 1 mg/kg daily	4-6 wk or 2 wk after symptoms resolve for normal host; 4-6 wk beyond resolution for immunosuppressed hosts. In AIDS patients, treat until CD4+ count >200
	Sulfadiazine *plus*	75-100 mg/kg daily divided twice daily (maximum 4 g/day); consider the lower dose in children >20 kg (see text)	
	Folinic acid	5-20 mg 3 times wkly; use higher doses if marrow suppression	
Ocular, older child	Pyrimethamine *plus*	2 mg/kg daily for 2 days, then 1 mg/kg daily (maximum 50 mg/day)	4-6 wk or 2 wk after symptoms resolve
	Sulfadiazine *plus*	75-100 mg/kg daily divided twice daily (maximum 4 g/day); consider the lower dose in children >20 kg (see text)	Prednisone should be continued until resolution of sight-threatening active chorioretinitis
	Folinic acid *plus*	5-20 mg 3 times wkly	
	Prednisone	1 mg/kg daily divided twice daily	
Congenital	Pyrimethamine *plus*	2 mg/kg daily for 2 days, then 1 mg/kg daily for 6 mo, then 3 times wkly (M-W-F) for 6 mo	1 yr
	Sulfadiazine *plus*	100 mg/kg daily divided twice daily	
	Folinic acid *plus*	5-10 mg 3 times wkly	
	Prednisone	1 mg/kg daily divided twice daily	Until resolution of elevated CSF protein level or sight-threatening active chorioretinitis
Pregnant women—acute infection first 21 wk of gestation	Spiramycin	3 g/day divided twice daily without food	Until fetal infection documented or excluded at 21 wk of gestation; if fetus infected, change to pyrimethamine plus sulfadiazine plus folinic acid until delivery
Pregnant women—fetal infection confirmed (amniotic fluid PCR positive)	Pyrimethamine *plus*	100 mg/day divided twice daily for 2 days, then 50 mg/day	Until delivery
	Sulfadiazine *plus*	3 g/day divided twice daily	
	Folinic acid	5-20 mg/day	

[a]For more detailed recommendations for patients with human immunodeficiency virus infection/AIDS, see http://aidsinfo.nih.gov/guidelines.
AIDS, Acquired immunodeficiency syndrome; *CSF,* cerebrospinal fluid; *PCR,* polymerase chain reaction.
From Cherry JD et al: *Feigin and Cherry's pediatric infectious diseases,* ed 8, Philadelphia, 2019, Elsevier.

    (2) Pyrimethamine 50 mg bid ×2 days, then 50 mg/day PO, *plus*
    (3) Leucovorin 10 to 20 mg/day PO
- Postnatal treatment of congenital infection:
  1. Sulfadiazine 50 mg/kg PO bid, *plus*
  2. Pyrimethamine 2 mg/kg PO for 2 days, then 1 mg/kg PO daily for the first 2 to 6 mo, then 3× wkly, *plus*
  3. Leucovorin 5 to 20 mg PO 3×s wkly
  4. Minimum duration of treatment: 12 mo

CHRONIC Rx

Maintenance therapy in AIDS patients because of the high risk (80%) of relapse:
- Pyrimethamine 25 mg PO qid
- Sulfadiazine 500 mg PO qid
- Leucovorin 10 to 20 mg PO qid

DISPOSITION

- Prognosis:
  1. Excellent in the immunocompetent host
  2. Good in ocular infection (although relapses are common)
- Treatment of acute infection in pregnancy:
  1. Reduces incidence and severity of congenital toxoplasmosis
- Treatment of congenital infection:
  1. Improvement in intellectual function

  2. Regression of retinal lesions
- AIDS:
  1. 70% to 95% response to therapy

REFERRAL

- To infectious disease expert:
  1. Immunocompromised hosts
  2. Pregnant women
  3. Difficulty in making a diagnosis or deciding on treatment
- To pediatric infectious disease expert:
  1. Congenital infection
- To obstetrician:
  1. Pregnant seronegative mother
  2. Acute seroconversion
- To ophthalmologist:
  1. Congenital infection
  2. Any case of ocular infection

❗ PEARLS & CONSIDERATIONS

COMMENTS

- Prevention of toxoplasmosis is most important in seronegative pregnant women and immunocompromised hosts.

- Patient instructions:
  1. Cook meat to 66° C (150.8° F).
  2. Cook eggs.
  3. Do not drink unpasteurized milk.
  4. Wash hands thoroughly after handling raw meat.
  5. Wash kitchen surfaces that come in contact with raw meat.
  6. Wash fruits and vegetables.
  7. Avoid contact with materials potentially contaminated with cat feces.

SUGGESTED READING

Available at eBooks.Health.Elsevier.com.

RELATED CONTENT

Toxoplasmosis (Patient Information)

AUTHORS: **TARA C. BOUTON, MD, MPH, TM, PHILIP A. CHAN, MD, MS,** and **GLENN G. FORT, MD, MPH**

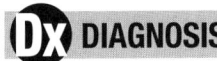

BASIC INFORMATION

DEFINITION

Transient ischemic attack (TIA) is a transient episode of neurologic dysfunction caused by focal brain, spinal cord, or retinal ischemia without acute infarction on MRI.[1] TIA symptoms typically resolve within 60 min and by definition within 24 h. Despite complete symptom resolution, one third (20% to 50%) of patients clinically suspected to have suffered a TIA have evidence of acute tissue infarction on MRI.[1-3]

SYNONYMS

TIA
Amaurosis fugax
Ophthalmologic TIA
"Mini-stroke"
Prestroke

ICD-10CM CODES
G45.9   Transient cerebral ischemic attack, unspecified
G45.8   Other transient cerebral ischemic attacks and related syndromes
Z86.73 Personal history of transient ischemic attack (TIA), and cerebral infarction without residual deficits

EPIDEMIOLOGY & DEMOGRAPHICS

INCIDENCE: 70 to 101 cases/100,000 persons annually[4]
PREVALENCE: 7.6 million persons in the U.S.
Annual risk of stroke after either a TIA or minor stroke is approximately 3% to 4%[3,4]
PREDOMINANT SEX & RACE: Males > females; African American > Caucasian
PEAK INCIDENCE: After age 60 yr[4]
RISK FACTORS: Same as for ischemic stroke (diabetes, hypertension, age, smoking, obesity, alcoholism, unhealthy diet, psychosocial stress, and lack of regular physical activity)

PHYSICAL FINDINGS & CLINICAL PRESENTATION

- TIAs often present with transient neurologic symptoms including ipsilateral transient monocular blindness (amaurosis fugax), contralateral numbness or weakness, contralateral homonymous hemianopsia, and/or aphasia.[1]
- Anatomy of carotid artery is illustrated in Fig. E1. Box 1 summarizes carotid artery TIAs.[5]
- Anatomy of vertebral arteries is illustrated in Fig. E2. Vertebrobasilar artery TIAs are described in Box 2.[5]

ETIOLOGY

Embolic (cardioembolism in 10% to 15%), large vessel atherothrombotic disease (20% to 25%), lacunar disease, hypoperfusion, hypercoagulable state, arteritis[6]

DIAGNOSIS

DIFFERENTIAL DIAGNOSIS

Seizures, hypoglycemia, hemiplegic migraine, intracranial hemorrhage, mass lesion, vestibular disease, Bell palsy, meningitis, multiple sclerosis, subdural hematoma, brain abscess, cervical or lumbar spine disease, conversion disorder.[7]

WORKUP

Given the high risk of stroke within the first 48 h after TIA (up to 10%), hospital admission for workup is advised.[8] Most of the immediate risk of stroke is secondary to carotid disease.

The American Heart Association recommends that the ABCD2 score be used in the evaluation of TIA.[8] It consists of 1 point for age $\geq$60 yr, 1 point for BP $\geq$140 mm Hg systolic or $\geq$90 mm Hg diastolic, clinical features (2 points for unilateral weakness, 1 point for speech impairment), duration of TIA (2 points for duration $\geq$60 min, 1 point for duration 10 to 59 min), presence of diabetes mellitus (1 point).[9,10] According to the guidelines, it is reasonable to hospitalize patients with TIA if they present within 72 h and have an ABCD2 score $\geq$3.[8,11] There is some debate about the usefulness of this scale because it fails to account for changes seen on echocardiogram, carotid Dopplers, or ECG that may place the patient at more imminent risk of stroke (carotid stenosis, atrial fibrillation, cardiac thrombus, etc.). If patient cannot have outpatient evaluation within the next few days, admission is also indicated. Alternatives to this scoring system are being investigated.[12]

LABORATORY TESTS

CBC, basic metabolic panel, prothrombin time, activated partial thromboplastin time, sedimentation rate, fasting lipid panel, serum glucose and hemoglobin A_{1c} (to detect latent diabetes mellitus), and thyroid-stimulating hormone.[8]

BOX 1   Carotid Artery Transient Ischemic Attacks

Symptoms
   Contralateral hemiparesis, hemianopsia, hemisensory loss
   Aphasia, if dominant hemisphere
   Neglect and hemi-inattention, if nondominant hemisphere
   Ipsilateral amaurosis fugax
Associated findings
   Carotid bruit
   Retinal artery emboli
Tests
   Ultrasonography (carotid Doppler studies)
   Magnetic resonance imaging angiography (MRA)
   Cerebral arteriography
Therapy
   Medical: Platelet inhibitors (e.g., aspirin)
   Risk-reduction measures (e.g., control blood pressure, glucose levels, cholesterol)
   Surgical: Carotid endarterectomy, if stenosis >70% and symptomatic
   Endovascular: Placement of stent

From Kaufman DM et al: *Kaufman's clinical neurology for psychiatrists,* ed 8, Philadelphia, 2017, Elsevier.

BOX 2   Vertebrobasilar Artery Transient Ischemic Attacks

Symptoms
   Vertigo, vomiting, tinnitus
   Circumoral paresthesias or numbness
   Dysarthria, dysphasia
   Drop attacks
Associated findings
   Nystagmus
   Ataxia
   Cranial nerve abnormalities
Tests
   Ultrasonography (transcranial Doppler studies)
   Magnetic resonance imaging angiography (MRA)
   Cerebral arteriography
Therapy
   Medical: Platelet inhibitors (see Box 1)
   Risk-reduction measures
   Surgical: None

From Kaufman DM et al: *Kaufman's clinical neurology for psychiatrists,* ed 8, Philadelphia, 2017, Elsevier.

IMAGING STUDIES

- Computed tomography (CT) scan should be obtained to exclude hemorrhage; MRI with diffusion-weighted images if immediately available to determine whether infarction occurred.[8]
- Imaging of the vessels should be obtained via magnetic resonance angiography (MRA) head and neck, computed tomography angiography (CTA) head and neck, or carotid Doppler/transcranial Doppler (CD/TCD). If symptoms are localizable to the posterior circulation, MRA or CTA should be obtained in lieu of CD/TCD.[13,14]
- Transthoracic echocardiogram should be obtained in all patients. A bubble study should be obtained in all patients younger than 50 yr with TIA symptoms.[15]
- ECG should be obtained to exclude the presence of arrhythmias, namely atrial fibrillation.[16,17]
- At least 24 h of heart rhythm monitoring should be accomplished to screen for arrhythmia. Paroxysmal atrial fibrillation is common in patients with TIA and longer monitoring is encouraged.
  Noninvasive ambulatory ECG monitoring for 30 days significantly improved the detection of atrial fibrillation by a factor of more than five and nearly doubled the rate of anticoagulant treatment as compared with the standard practice of short-duration ECG monitoring.[18]
  Furthermore, a randomized study of insertable cardiac monitor vs. conventional follow-up in patients with cryptogenic stroke or TIA found that by 6 mo atrial fibrillation had been detected in 8.9% in the insertable cardiac monitor group vs. 1.4% in the control group.[19]

(RX) TREATMENT

NONPHARMACOLOGIC THERAPY

- Carotid endarterectomy or carotid stenting should be considered for patients found to have carotid stenosis of ≥50% as the cause for TIA. Efficacy is greatest in the 2 wk immediately following a TIA or ischemic stroke.[20] Please refer to the "Carotid Artery Stenosis" chapter for more information.
- Intracranial angioplasty and stenting is only used in select patients who fail maximal medical management with aggressive platelet inhibition, strict risk factor control such as hyperlipidemia, hypertension, diabetes mellitus, weight loss, treatment of sleep apnea, and smoking cessation, among others.[21-23]

ACUTE GENERAL Rx

- In the absence of contraindications, patients with atrial fibrillation should be considered for anticoagulation. Choices for anticoagulants include the direct oral anticoagulants (such as dabigatran, rivaroxaban, apixaban, edoxaban, betrixaban) and/or warfarin. In patients with TIA and atrial fibrillation or a cardiac thrombus, therapeutic anticoagulation should be achieved rapidly. Those who are not candidates for a direct oral anticoagulation and who will need chronic warfarin should first be started on either intravenous (IV) heparin or therapeutic anticoagulant doses of Lovenox, along with warfarin, until target international normalization ratio (INR) between 2.0 and 3.0 is achieved, at which point warfarin should be continued as monotherapy.[8]
- Although no compelling evidence exists for the use of heparin in the acute treatment of TIAs without cardioembolic source, patients who develop recurrent symptoms within the same vascular territory that increase in duration, severity, and/or frequency (crescendo TIA/stuttering TIA) may benefit from its use pending cardiac and vascular imaging and identification of a possible source.
- Patients with high-risk TIA (ABCD2 score >3) or minor stroke may be started on dual antiplatelet therapy of clopidogrel 300 to 600 mg on day 1 followed by 75 mg/day and aspirin for 21 to 30 days based on the CHANCE and POINT trials.[24,25]

CHRONIC Rx

- Please refer to the "Secondary Stroke Prevention" chapter for more complete discussion.
- Chronic therapy includes single antiplatelet (after 21 to 30 days) or anticoagulation therapy and modifying the four major risk factors: Hypertension, dyslipidemia, diabetes mellitus, and smoking cessation.
- If no evidence of atrial fibrillation, antiplatelet therapy alone should be used to reduce the risk of recurrent TIAs or subsequent stroke.[26,27] Antiplatelet agents commonly used in stroke prevention include aspirin, aspirin/dipyridamole, clopidogrel, and ticagrelor. All are reasonable choices, but practitioners should consider their individual patient's comorbidities when selecting an antiplatelet agent. Chronic long-term dual antiplatelet therapy is not recommended as this increases the risk of hemorrhagic complications.
- Warfarin (INR 2.0-3.0) or use of direct oral anticoagulants instead of an antiplatelet is indicated for prevention of future strokes in patients with atrial fibrillation.[8]

(!) PEARLS & CONSIDERATIONS

- All-cause mortality in 1 yr is 25% in patients diagnosed TIA.

- Approximately 20% to 30% of ischemic strokes are heralded by transient ischemic symptoms.
- Patients with nonclassic TIA symptoms (e.g., isolated symptoms of vertigo, ataxia, diplopia, dysarthria, bilateral decreased vision, numbness in one body segment) tent to wait longer before seeking medical attention (♦3 days) and are more likely to have has a recurrent stroke before seeking attention (8% vs 5%). Both classic and nonclassic symptoms of TIA confer similar 90-day stroke risk.[28]
- Previous studies conducted between 1987 and 2003 estimated the risk of stroke or an acute coronary syndrome was 12% to 20% during the first 3 mo after a TIA. New data estimate the 1-yr risk to be 6.2%. Multiple infarctions on brain imaging, large-artery atherosclerosis, and an ABCD score of 6 or 7 were each associated with more than a doubling of the risk of stroke.

PREVENTION

- A healthy lifestyle and management of cardiovascular risk factors should be encouraged.
- Antiplatelet therapy has not been proven efficacious in primary prevention of TIA or stroke but is very beneficial in secondary prevention.

PATIENT & FAMILY EDUCATION

Patients should be counseled on the early signs of stroke symptoms and instructed to promptly seek medical attention if they develop symptoms concerning for stroke. Patients should be encouraged to pursue a healthy lifestyle to include exercise and smoking cessation. In addition, patients should take an active role in controlling blood pressure and blood glucose. Further educational materials can be found online at https://www.strokecenter.org/.

REFERENCES & SUGGESTED READING

Available at eBooks.Health.Elsevier.com.

RELATED CONTENT

- Transient Ischemic Attack (TIA) (Patient Information)
- Carotid Artery Stenosis (Related Key Topic)
- Atrial Fibrillation (Related Key Topic)
- Stroke, Acute Ischemic (Related Key Topic)
- Stroke, Secondary Prevention (Related Key Topic)

AUTHORS: **CÉSAR E. ESCAMILLA-OCAÑAS, MD,** and **COREY ELAM GOLDSMITH, MD, FAAN**

BASIC INFORMATION

DEFINITION

Demyelination in a transverse region of the spinal cord due to an inflammatory process that leads to sensory and motor changes below the lesion and autonomic dysfunction. The term "transverse myelitis" (TM) of late refers to any cause of inflammatory myelopathy, irrespective of severity or degree of structural or functional interruption of pathways through a transverse spinal cord section. TM that extends across three or more segments of the cord is referred to as longitudinally extensive TM. The pathologic hallmark of TM is the presence of focal collections of lymphocytes and monocytes with varying degrees of demyelination, axonal injury, and astroglial and microglial activation within the spinal cord.

SYNONYMS

TM
Idiopathic transverse myelitis (ITM)

ICD-10CM CODES
G37.3   Acute transverse myelitis in demyelinating disease of central nervous system
G04.89 Other myelitis

EPIDEMIOLOGY & DEMOGRAPHICS

INCIDENCE: Annual incidence ranges from 1.3 to 8 cases per million. The incidence increases to 24.6 cases per million annually if causes of acquired demyelination such as multiple sclerosis (MS) or neuromyelitis optic spectrum disorder are included.[1,2]
PREVALENCE: Unknown.
PREDOMINANT SEX: None, but female preponderance seen in cases associated with MS and neuromyelitis optica spectrum disorder (NMOSD).
PEAK INCIDENCE: Can occur at any age. Bimodal peak in the incidence between 10 and 19 yr and 30 and 39 yr. 20% of cases occur in children with a bimodal peak of incidence between 0 to 2 yr and 5 to 17 yr.[1,2]
RISK FACTORS: Infection, vaccination.
GENETICS: No genetic predisposition has been shown.

PHYSICAL FINDINGS & CLINICAL PRESENTATION

- Rapid onset of symmetric or asymmetric paraparesis or paraplegia of the lower extremities over a few days, ascending paresthesia, sensory level at the trunk, back pain, sphincter dysfunction, and positive Babinski, which can be bilateral. The arms may also be involved if the cervical cord is involved, but cervical involvement is less common than thoracic involvement. In the acute phase the weakness is flaccid, with diminished deep tendon reflexes mimicking a peripheral neuropathy such as Guillain-Barré syndrome.
- One third to half of patients present with localizing back pain or a bandlike area of altered sensation, usually at the dermatomal level corresponding to the lesion within the cord.
- There is progression to nadir of clinical deficits between 4 h and 21 days after symptom onset.
- Urinary incontinence or retention, GI disturbances (incontinence or constipation), and sexual dysfunction are common.
- Acute flaccid myelitis is a subtype of myelitis in which patients present with acute limb weakness and have primarily involvement of gray matter on spinal cord imaging.

ETIOLOGY

- The clinical signs are caused by an interruption in ascending and descending sensory, motor, and autonomic pathways in the transverse plane of the spinal cord, resulting in sensory-level weakness and autonomic dysfunction at and below the level of the lesion due to demyelination or inflammation of the spinal cord.
- Can be idiopathic demyelination (15% to 30%) that is a monophasic one-time event or demyelination secondary to neurologic or systemic conditions (Box 1).
- Secondary causes include postinfection, postvaccination, acute demyelinating encephalomyelitis (where TM tends to be monophasic), and others such as MS, NMOSD, connective tissue disorders such as systemic lupus, Sjögren syndrome, antiphospholipid antibody syndrome, sarcoidosis, and paraneoplastic conditions, which can be progressive or relapsing.[1-4]
- Infectious causes of myelitis include HIV, syphilis, varicella zoster (associated with shingles), human T-cell leukemia virus type 1, Lyme disease, COVID-19, arboviruses such as West Nile virus (typically causing a poliomyelitis-type acute flaccid paralysis), or enteroviruses (typically causing acute flaccid paralysis mainly in children).[4]
- About 50% of patients have had a recent upper respiratory infection.

DIAGNOSIS

DIFFERENTIAL DIAGNOSIS

- MS (Table 1)
- Neuromyelitis optica spectrum disorder (NMOSD)[4,5]
- Metastatic disease
- Spinal cord tumors
- Herniated or slipped disks
- Spinal stenosis

BOX 1   Central Nervous System and Systemic Autoimmune Disorders Associated With Acute Transverse Myelitis

Central Nervous System Disorders
Acute disseminated encephalomyelitis
Multiple sclerosis
Neuromyelitis optica

Systemic Autoimmune Disorders
Antiphospholipid antibody syndrome
Behçet disease
Mixed connective tissue disorder
Neurosarcoidosis
Sjögren syndrome
Systemic lupus erythematosus

From Cherry JD et al: *Feigin and Cherry's textbook of pediatric infectious diseases*, ed 8, Philadelphia, 2019, Elsevier.

TABLE 1   Distinguishing Acute Transverse Myelitis From Other Central Nervous System Demyelinating Disorders

Finding	ATM	ADEM	MS	NMO
Myelitis	+	+/−	+/− (partial)	+
Acute mental status changes	−	+	−	+/−
Optic neuritis	−	+/−	+/−	+/−
Abnormal brain MRI	−	+	+	+/−
CSF oligoclonal bands	−	+/−	+	+/−
Serum AQP4-IgG	−	−	−	+/−
Recurrences	+/−	+/−	+	+

+, Always present; +/−, variably present; −, usually absent; *ADEM*, acute disseminated encephalomyelitis; *AQP*, aquaporin 4; *ATM*, acute transverse myelitis; *CSF*, cerebrospinal fluid; *MRI*, magnetic resonance imaging; *MS*, multiple sclerosis; *NMO*, neuromyelitis optica.
From Cherry JD et al: *Feigin and Cherry's textbook of pediatric infectious diseases*, ed 8, Philadelphia, 2019, Elsevier.

TABLE 2 Suggested Diagnostic Workup for Recurrent Central Nervous System Demyelinating Disorders and Systemic Autoimmune Disorders Associated With Acute Transverse Myelitis

All Patients	Suggestive of Neuromyelitis Optica	Also Consider
Brain MRI with gadolinium	Ophthalmology consultation	Angiotensin-converting enzyme (serum, CSF)
CSF oligoclonal bands	Visual evoked potentials	Other autoantibodies
Antinuclear antibodies	Formal visual field testing	Anti-dsDNA
Antiphospholipid antibodies		Anti-La
Serum AQP4-IgG		Anti-Ro
		Anti-Smith

CSF, Cerebrospinal fluid; MRI, magnetic resonance imaging; NMO, neuromyelitis optica.
From Cherry JD et al: Feigin and Cherry's textbook of pediatric infectious diseases, ed 8, Philadelphia, 2019, Elsevier.

TABLE 3 Suggested Diagnostic Workup for Infections Associated With Acute Transverse Myelitis

Blood	Cerebrospinal Fluid	Other
• Blood cultures • Acute and convalescent titers to Borrelia burgdorferi, EBV, Mycoplasma pneumoniae	• Bacterial culture • Viral culture • PCR testing for CMV, EBV, Enterovirus, HSV, M. pneumoniae, VZV	• Viral culture of stool and respiratory secretions • Consider stool ova and parasite testing and serum titers if parasitic infection is suspected

CMV, Cytomegalovirus; EBV, Epstein-Barr virus; HSV, herpes simplex virus; PCR, polymerase chain reaction; VZV, varicella zoster virus.
From Cherry JD et al: Feigin and Cherry's textbook of pediatric infectious diseases, ed 8, Philadelphia, 2019, Elsevier.

- Spinal epidural abscess
- Vascular malformation
  1. Spinal dural arteriovenous fistula (most common)[6]
  2. Arteriovenous malformation of the spinal cord
- Spinal cord infarction due to either anterior spinal artery or posterior spinal artery occlusion

WORKUP

TM should be suspected in patients with a history of rapid (hours to days) onset of motor weakness and sensory abnormalities with bladder or bowel dysfunction that is referable to the spinal cord. The dysfunction is bilateral (not necessarily symmetric), and there is often a clearly defined sensory (dermatomal) level. It is important to distinguish idiopathic TM from TM due to MS or NMOSD because idiopathic TM does not relapse and does not require long-term immunomodulatory therapy.[1-3] A suggested diagnostic workup for recurrent CNS demyelinating disorders and systemic autoimmune disorders associated with acute TM is summarized in Table 2.

LABORATORY TESTS

- Lumbar puncture looking for cerebrospinal fluid pleocytosis, oligoclonal bands for MS, or serology and polymerase chain reaction (PCR) looking for infection (Table 3) such as varicella zoster virus and enterovirus PCR.
- Antinuclear antibody, hepatitis B serology, Lyme disease serology, VDRL, SSA, SSB, anticardiolipin antibody, lupus anticoagulant, copper, ceruloplasmin, vitamin B_{12}, RPR.
- Serum NMO-IgG and myelin oligodendrocyte glycoprotein (MOG) antibodies to evaluate for NMOSD.
- If a paraneoplastic etiology is suspected, then appropriate antibodies should be ordered and appropriate cancer screening undertaken.

IMAGING STUDIES

- Gadolinium-enhanced MRI of brain and MRI of the entire spine (Fig. E1, Fig. E2). This will show demyelinating lesion on T_2 with contrast enhancement. In MS there is usually a short segment lesion (less than three vertebral segments) that is dorsally located. Longitudinally extensive TM that spans more than three or more segments of the cord is more typical of NMOSD, postinfectious, vascular, or other inflammatory causes.[4,5]
- Spinal dural arteriovenous (AV) fistulas are often missed initially on MRI and will worsen with steroid treatment. If suspected, may need a computed tomography (CT) spinal angiogram.[6]
- CT of the spine with and without contrast should be obtained if MRI is unavailable, but CT does not allow for visualization of the spinal cord itself.
- CT myelogram may also be obtained if MRI is unavailable to evaluate for compression; however, this does not image the parenchyma of the cord directly.
- Chest CT with and without contrast if sarcoidosis is suspected.

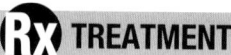 **TREATMENT**

Corticosteroids (intravenous [IV] methylprednisolone 1 g/day for 3 to 7 days) are the first-line treatment for TM.

NONPHARMACOLOGIC THERAPY

- Physical therapy
- Respiratory and oropharyngeal support

ACUTE GENERAL Rx

- High-dose IV corticosteroid (e.g., methylprednisolone 1000 mg/day for 3 to 7 days).
- Rescue therapy with plasma exchange may be helpful in patients who do not respond to corticosteroids.
- Combination therapy with plasmapheresis and corticosteroids or other immunosuppressive agents (e.g., rituximab or cyclophosphamide) may also be effective.
- Analgesia for pain.

CHRONIC Rx

- Baclofen or tizanidine for muscle spasms and spasticity
- Gabapentin or pregabalin for neuropathic pain
- Low-molecular-weight heparin for deep vein thrombosis prophylaxis in patients with immobility
- Need for chronic immunosuppression will depend on underlying etiology

DISPOSITION

- One third of patients with TM will have complete recovery, one third will have fair recovery, and one third have permanent disability and do not recover. Recurrence or relapse is possible, especially if the patient has MS, NMOSD, or sarcoidosis.[4,5]
- If a patient worsens with steroid treatment, strongly consider spinal dural AV fistula.[6]
- Patients who need further care, including those with urinary retention, may need home nursing assistance. Some patients may benefit from rehabilitation, either inpatient or outpatient.

REFERRAL

- Referral to a neurologist to evaluate need for long-term therapy
- Referral for physical and occupational therapy
- Consider psychiatric consultation (high incidence of long-term mood and anxiety disorders)

REFERENCES

Available at eBooks.Health.Elsevier.com.

RELATED CONTENT

Multiple Sclerosis (Related Key Topic)
Neuromyelitis Optica Spectrum Disorder (Related Key Topic)

AUTHOR: **COREY ELAM GOLDSMITH, MD, FAAN**

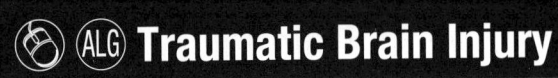

 BASIC INFORMATION

DEFINITION

- Traumatic brain injury (TBI) is a broad term that encompasses multiple intracranial processes (including cerebral contusion, epidural hemorrhages, subdural hemorrhages, subarachnoid hemorrhages, skull fractures, diffuse axonal injury, and cerebral edema) that occur secondary to trauma to the head or if the head experiences a sudden deceleration injury without external trauma that results in injury to the brain.[1] An overview of classification of TBI is summarized in Table 1. These injuries result in varying levels of cellular and macroscopic changes, detected with clinical examination and supplemented by neuroimaging.
- Mild TBI is defined as loss of consciousness <30 minutes, a Glasgow Coma Scale (GCS) of 13 to 15, and normal imaging.
- Moderate TBI is defined as loss of consciousness for 30 minutes to 24 hr with even longer alteration in consciousness, a GCS of 9 to 12, and may or may not have abnormal imaging.
- Severe TBI is defined as >24 hr of loss of consciousness with a GCS of 3 to 8 and prolonged posttraumatic amnesia with normal or abnormal imaging.[1,2]

SYNONYMS

TBI
Head injury
Concussion
Intracranial contusion

ICD-10CM CODES

S06.9X0A   Intracranial injury
S06.1X7A   Traumatic cerebral edema with loss of consciousness of any duration with death due to brain injury prior to regaining consciousness, initial encounter
S06.2X9A   Diffuse traumatic brain injury with loss of consciousness of unspecified duration, initial encounter
S06.300A   Unspecified focal traumatic brain injury without loss of consciousness, initial encounter
S06.305A   Unspecified focal traumatic brain injury with loss of consciousness greater than 24 hours with return to preexisting conscious level, initial encounter
S06.309A   Unspecified focal traumatic brain injury with loss of consciousness of unspecified duration, initial encounter
S09.90   Unspecified injury of the head

EPIDEMIOLOGY & DEMOGRAPHICS

Traumatic brain injury (TBI) is a worldwide leading cause of mortality in the young and elderly. In the 2017 CDC surveillance report, unintentional falls have surpassed motor vehicle crashes as number one cause of TBI.[3]

INCIDENCE: Globally, more than 69 million people suffer from TBI each year, with North America and Europe showing highest incidence and Southeast Asian and Western Pacific countries experiencing the greatest burden of disease. According to one estimate, up to 4.6 million individuals suffer from TBI in United States and Canada each year.[4] In 2014, about 2.87 million emergency department visits, including deaths and hospitalizations, were associated with TBI. The financial burden of TBI has been estimated to be greater than $80 billion per yr in the United States alone and approaching $400 billion dollar worldwide in direct and indirect costs.[5]

PREVALENCE: In 2016, the global prevalence of TBI was estimated at 55.5 million. Between 1990 to 2016, the age-standardized prevalence of TBI increased by 8.4%.[6] According to the CDC, there were 224,000 TBI-related hospitalization in 2017, decreased from 261,000 in 2016, while the number of deaths increased from 59,000 to 61,000.[3]

PEAK INCIDENCE: In the U.S. 792/100,000 individuals, including nonspecific head injury, removing which brings the number to 264/100,000.[3]

PREDOMINANT SEX & AGE: TBI occurs more commonly in males and hospitalizations/deaths are the highest in older adults >75 yr of age.[3]

RISK FACTORS:
- Falls
- Motor vehicle accidents
- Physical violence
- Sport injuries
- Ballistic injuries (gunshot wounds, blast injuries)

GENETICS: TBI and Apo E ε4 synergistically are associated with a tenfold increased risk for Alzheimer disease. Apo E ε4 is also associated with larger intracerebral hematomas and greater ischemia after TBI.[7]

PHYSICAL FINDINGS & CLINICAL PRESENTATION

TBI patients can present with a spectrum of clinical symptoms including nausea, vomiting, headache, seizures, altered mental status, and/or coma. Stigmata of trauma, including bruises, scalp lacerations, and periorbital or mastoid ecchymosis suggesting skull base fractures, are telltale signs of possible underlying traumatic brain injury. Box 1 describes risk stratification in patients with minor head trauma. The spectrum of TBI is most commonly assessed using the GCS, which ranges from 3 to 15 and utilizes eye, motor, and verbal exams (Table 2).

ETIOLOGY

- Mechanical falls (49.1%), motor vehicle accidents (24.5%), and assaults resulting in direct or indirect trauma to the head are the most common etiologies (Fig. E1, Fig. E2).
- Gunshot wounds are the most prevalent **penetrating injuries** (Fig. E3), accounting for 35% of deaths from TBI under the age of 45 yr in the United States. Self-inflicted injuries—for example, with nail guns—can also lead to penetrating injuries (Fig. E4). Gunshot wounds are the most lethal type of brain injury, 90% resulting in death.
- The most common mechanisms of pediatric TBI vary according to age. Falls are the leading cause of TBI in children younger than 14 yr of age. Children younger than 4 yr of age are injured mainly by falls but are also affected by abusive injuries and motor vehicle accidents. Children 4 to 8 yr of age are injured in falls and motor vehicle accidents but also become more at risk for other transportation-related injuries such as bicycle-related incidents. Abusive head trauma (AHT) is particularly common in young infants aged less than 2 yr; approximately 30 of every 100,000 infants aged less than 1 yr were hospitalized for AHT.[8]
- Sports-related TBIs account for roughly one third of all causes of TBI, with males, adolescents, and young adults with higher incidence. Some common sports associated with TBI are football, horse riding, cycling,

TABLE 1 Overview of Classification of Traumatic Brain Injury

Mechanism	Blunt		High velocity (MVC)
			Low velocity (fall, assault)
	Penetrating		GSW
			Other (stab wounds, etc.)
	Blast		Explosive devices
Severity	Mild		GCS 14–15
	Moderate		GCS 9–13
	Severe		GCS 3–8
Morphology	Skull fracture	Vault	Linear versus stellate
			Depressed/nondepressed
			Open/closed
		Basilar	With/without CSF
			With/without CN palsy
	Intracranial lesions	Focal	Epidural
			Subdural
			Intracerebral
		Diffuse	Mild concussion
			Classic concussion
			Diffuse axonal injury

CN, Cranial nerve; *CSF,* cerebrospinal fluid; *GCS,* Glasgow Coma Scale; *GSW,* gunshot wound; *MVC,* motor vehicle collision.
From Jankovic J et al: *Bradley and Daroff's neurology in clinical practice,* ed 8, Philadelphia, 2022, Elsevier.

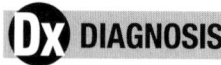
skateboarding, hockey, water sports, and snow sports.[9]

DIAGNOSIS

DIFFERENTIAL DIAGNOSIS

Differential diagnosis of TBI is quite limited; however, there are several considerations and diagnoses considered as a possibility within the realm of TBI. These are enumerated in the imaging section.

WORKUP

TBI workup is always a part of the advanced trauma life support (ATLS) protocol. Primary and secondary survey followed by imaging studies constitutes the standardized approach to TBI. Focused TBI workup includes:

- History: Including timing of injury, duration of loss of consciousness if applicable, seizures (if any), comorbidities, use of anticoagulants and antiplatelet agents (requires reversal in the event of intracranial blood on imaging).

BOX 1 Risk Stratification in Patients With Minor Head Trauma

High Risk
- Focal neurologic findings
- Asymmetrical pupils
- Skull fracture on clinical examination
- Multiple trauma
- Serious, painful, distracting injuries
- External signs of trauma above the clavicles
- Initial Glasgow Coma Scale score of 14 or 15
- Loss of consciousness
- Posttraumatic confusion or amnesia
- Progressively worsening headache
- Vomiting
- Posttraumatic seizure
- History of bleeding disorder or anticoagulation
- Recent ingestion of intoxicants
- Unreliable or unknown history of injury
- Previous neurologic diagnosis
- Previous epilepsy
- Suspected child abuse
- Age above 60 yr or below 2 yr

Medium Risk
- Initial Glasgow Coma Scale score of 15
- Brief loss of consciousness
- Posttraumatic amnesia
- Vomiting
- Headache
- Intoxication

Low Risk
- Currently asymptomatic
- No other injuries
- No focality on examination
- Normal pupils
- No change in consciousness
- Intact orientation and memory
- Initial Glasgow Coma Scale score of 15
- Accurate history
- Trivial mechanism
- Injury less than 24 hr ago
- No or mild headache
- No vomiting
- No preexisting high-risk factors

- Neurologic examination: Glasgow Coma Scale, cranial nerves, motor/sensory exam. Assess for scalp lacerations, specifically overlying a skull fracture as well as cerebrospinal fluid (CSF) otorrhea or rhinorrhea.
- CT imaging of the head if there is a significant history of impact to the head, polytrauma, positive loss of consciousness, or stigmata of trauma to the head. Factors to consider regarding the need for CT imaging in head-injured patients are described in Table 3. The American College of Emergency Physicians Clinical Policy Regarding Neuroimaging in adults with mild TBI is summarized in Box 2.

LABORATORY TESTS

- Basic labs including CBC, basic metabolic panel, prothrombin time, activated partial thromboplastin time, urine drug screen, and ethanol blood level.
- Consider tests for platelet function analysis for unknown antiplatelet use.
- No blood biomarker currently exists (Figs. E5 and E6).

IMAGING STUDIES (TABLE 4)

CT imaging forms the current cornerstone of imaging modalities for head trauma; however, it is not always necessary. Patients over the age of 16 with minimal head injury (i.e., no history of loss of consciousness, amnesia, and confusion), not on blood thinners, and without associated seizure generally do not need a CT scan. Canadian CT head rules for patients with GCS 13 to 15 who do have history of loss of consciousness, amnesia, and/or confusion are a useful guide in determining utility of obtaining a CT scan. If any of these risk factors are present, it is recommended that a CT scan of the head be considered.

HIGH RISK:
- Failure to reach GCS of 15 within 2 hr
- Suspected open or depressed skull fracture
- Any signs of basal skull fracture (hemotympanum, "raccoon" eyes, CSF otorrhea/rhinorrhea, Battle's sign)
- Two or more episodes of vomiting
- Age older than 65

MEDIUM RISK:
- Dangerous mechanism of injury or polytrauma
- Retrograde amnesia to the event >30 minutes

Usually, in addition to a plain CT of the head (Fig. E7), computed tomography angiography (CTA) head/neck or CT of the spine is helpful if arterial or C-spine injury is suspected, respectively. Other imaging modalities such as MRI can be helpful in certain situations but are typically adjuncts in the acute setting to CT-guided management.

Pathologies that can be identified with imaging are noted in the following:
- Primary extraaxial: Epidural, subdural, subarachnoid hemorrhage
- Primary intraaxial: Axonal injury, cortical contusion, intracerebral or intraventricular hemorrhage, encephalomalacia (from prior TBI or vascular insult)
- Skull fracture: Linear, depressed, open, involving frontal sinus or skull base
- Penetrating brain injury: Gunshot wounds, sharp objects resulting in parenchymal and vascular injury
- Vascular injury: Dissection, traumatic carotid-cavernous fistula (CCF), dural arteriovenous fistula (dAVF), pseudoaneurysm formation
- Secondary acute injury: Diffuse cerebral swelling/dysautoregulation (seen more commonly in children from posttraumatic hyperemia), infarction, infection from

---

TABLE 2 Useful Criteria to Assess the Severity of Head Injury[a]

Quantifying the Degree of Head Injury	Glasgow Coma Scale (GCS)	Score
• Moderate TBI (GCS 9-13)	**Eye Opening**	
• Severe TBI (GCS <8)	Spontaneous	4
• Significant head CT:	To speech	3
• Cerebral edema	To pain	2
• Midline shift	None	1
• Subdural/epidural bleeding	**Verbal Response**	
• Open head injury with intracranial air	Oriented	5
	Confused conversation	4
	Inappropriate words	3
	Incomprehensible sounds	2
	None	1
	Best Motor Response	
	Obeys commands	6
	Localizes pain	5
	Flexion withdrawal to pain	4
	Abnormal flexion (decorticate)	3
	Extension (decerebrate)	2
	None (flaccid)	1

TBI, Traumatic brain injury.

[a]Consultation with other specialists (i.e., neurosurgeon) may be valuable for the orthopedic surgeon unfamiliar with the process of "clearing" the patient's head injury for ischemic monomelic neuropathy (IMN) fixation.

From Browner B et al: *Skeletal trauma: basic science, management, and reconstruction,* ed 6, Philadelphia, 2019, Elsevier.

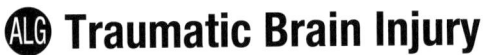

T

Diseases and Disorders

I

TABLE 3 Factors to Consider Regarding the Need for Computed Tomography in Head-Injured Patients

Indications for urgent CT include the following:

- Evidence of skull fracture—basal, depressed, or open
- Abnormal results of neurologic examination
- Seizure
- Vomiting more than once
- High-risk mechanism (e.g., ejection from vehicle; injury to pedestrian or cyclist vs. car occupant)
- Decreasing GCS score or persistently decreased GCS score below 15
- Indications for lower threshold for CT scan include the following:
  - Age >60 yr
  - Persistent anterograde amnesia
  - Retrograde amnesia >30 min
  - Coagulopathy
  - Fall >5 stairs or >3 ft
  - Intoxication (examination unreliable)
  - LOC >30 min
  - Mechanism and location of injury
  - Social factors (e.g., abusive situation at home, language barriers precluding an accurate history)

CT, Computed tomography; *GCS,* Glasgow Coma Scale; *LOC,* loss of consciousness.
From Jankovic J et al: *Bradley and Daroff's neurology in clinical practice,* ed 8, Philadelphia, 2022, Elsevier.

BOX 2 American College of Emergency Physicians Clinical Policy Regarding Neuroimaging in Adults With Mild Traumatic Brain Injury

A noncontrast head computed tomography (CT) is indicated (level-1 recommendation) in adults with level of consciousness (LOC) or posttraumatic amnesia only if one or more of the following is present:
- Headache
- Vomiting
- Age >60 yr
- Drug or alcohol intoxication
- Deficits in short-term memory
- Physical evidence of trauma above the clavicle
- Posttraumatic seizure
- Glasgow Coma Scale (GCS) score <15
- Focal neurologic deficit
- Coagulopathy

A noncontrast head CT should be considered (level-2 recommendation) in head trauma patients with no LOC or posttraumatic amnesia if there is:
- Focal neurologic deficit
- Vomiting
- Severe headache
- Age ≥ 65 yr
- Physical signs of a basilar skull fracture
- GCS score <15
- Coagulopathy
- A dangerous mechanism (e.g., ejection from motor vehicle, pedestrian struck, fall of more than 3 feet or 5 stairs)

From Marx JA et al: *Rosen's emergency medicine,* ed 8, Philadelphia, 2014, Elsevier.

---

penetrating trauma, brain herniation from mass lesion or cerebral edema
- Secondary chronic injury: Hydrocephalus (posttraumatic due to disruption of normal CSF absorption pathways), encephalomalacia, CSF leak (from skull base fractures, manifests as otorrhea or rhinorrhea, leptomeningeal cyst (seen most commonly in infants, skull fracture resulting in underlying dural injury)

(Rx) TREATMENT (FIG. 8)

Prevention of secondary injury is the primary goal of prehospital and early in-hospital management. Most common mechanisms of secondary injury are either intracranial (increased intracranial pressure [ICP], hematoma) or systemic (hypoxia, hypovolemia, hypotension). Early categorization of head trauma patients according to the severity (based on GCS) and transport to facilities equipped with personnel and technology to deal with issues pertaining to head trauma has improved the overall management of head injury patients and prevention of secondary injury.[10] Assessment and treatment recommendations for mild TBI are summarized in Table 5. Airway, breathing, and circulation, however, still remain the most

important parameters to be stabilized, and both directly and indirectly affect GCS and overall outcome. Trauma guidelines suggest intubation should be performed in any patient with a GCS of 8 or less to prevent hypoxemia and hypercapnia. Previously, patients were hyperventilated to decrease pCO_2 in an effort to reduce ICP. Recent evidence suggests normo-ventilation for patients with severe TBI, with hyperventilation only being used as a temporary measure until other methods of reducing ICP are employed.[11] Intravenous fluid resuscitation should also be started early to prevent hypovolemia resulting in hypotension, shown to double mortality. Transfer to and care in a Level 1 trauma center are associated with better outcomes. Monitoring and treatment recommendations for severe TBI are summarized in Table 6.

Details of in-hospital management including critical care and surgical intervention is beyond the scope of this text. Some important points are summarized below.
- Advanced trauma life support (ATLS) protocol (airway, breathing, circulation, disability, exposure).
- Ventilatory support.
- Optimization of oxygenation, ventilation, and fluid status.
- CT head (Fig. E9) to evaluate for mass lesion (hematoma) or cerebral edema. These findings may necessitate either surgical intervention or ICP monitor placement. ATLS guidelines recommend maximum 30 minutes between initial assessment and CT head.
- In case of either a severe TBI (GCS 8 or less) or a moderate TBI (GCS 8 to 13) with an unreliable neurologic exam, patients should be admitted to the intensive care unit for frequent neurologic checks. TBI guidelines suggest ICP monitor placement for GCS 8 or less to monitor intracranial pressure closely.[11] ICP monitors are of various kinds, and the most commonly used include external ventricular drain, intraparenchymal pressure monitor, and a bolt device with brain tissue oxygen pressure monitoring with fiberoptic pressure monitor. Recent research has also supported the use of brain tissue oxygen monitoring for severe TBI patients.[11]
- Surgical decompression may involve evacuation of hematoma (epidural, subdural, intraparenchymal, contusion) through craniotomy alone (replacement of bone after completion of operation) versus decompressive craniectomy (complete removal of bone without replacement). Skull fractures are treated depending on the morphology of the fracture. Open, depressed fractures require surgical debridement and elevation in most cases, in addition to broad-spectrum antibiotics.
- Avoid electrolyte imbalance, especially hyponatremia and hyperglycemia, which may contribute to cerebral edema and increase intracranial pressure. A recent randomized controlled trial studied use of a continuous 20% hypertonic saline infusion vs standard therapy in patients with moderate to severe TBI (COBI trial) and did not improve neurologic status at 6 mo.[12]

TABLE 4 Comparison of Head Imaging Modalities

	Computed Tomography Scans	Magnetic Resonance Imaging	Angiography	Skull Radiography
Advantages	Fast Patient accessible for monitoring Defines acute hemorrhages, mass effects, bone injuries, hydrocephalus, intraventricular blood, edema	Defines contusions and pericontusion edema, posttraumatic ischemic infarction, brainstem injuries	Helps localize acute traumatic lesions Defines vascular injuries, injuries to venous sinuses Detects mass effects	Readily available May help screen some patients for further imaging studies
Disadvantages	Artifacts arise from patient's movement, foreign bodies Streak artifacts may obscure brainstem or posterior fossa	Slow Patients not easily accessible for monitoring Does not define most acute hemorrhagic lesions Not useful for bone injuries	Does not define nature of acute lesion Does not detect infratentorial masses	Does not indicate presence or absence of intracranial injury
Indications	Acute severe head trauma Acute moderate head trauma Suspected depressed skull fracture High-risk minor head trauma Suspected child abuse in minor head trauma Deteriorating neurologic status	Persistent symptoms with postconcussive syndrome Suspected posttraumatic ischemic infarction Suspected contusions not seen on CT scan	Suspected vascular injury CT scan not available	CT scan may not be done Penetrating head trauma

CT, Computed tomography.
From Marx JA et al: *Rosen's emergency medicine: concepts and clinical practice,* ed 7, 2010, Elsevier.

- Elevation of head of bed to allow better venous drainage to reduce intracranial pressure.
- ICP management (Table 7), which may include the following: Drainage of cerebrospinal fluid via external ventricular drain, surgical hematoma evacuation, administration of hyperosmotic fluids to reduce edema, pharmacologic sedation and paralysis, pentobarbital-induced coma, and surgical decompression of the brain.[11]
- Decompressive craniectomy in patients with TBI and refractory intracranial hypertension may reduce ICU stay but does not clearly improve outcomes. DECRA[13] and RESCUE-icp[14] are two randomized controlled trials that assessed decompressive craniectomy (DC) for reduction in ICP vs. medical management. Both trials were unable to provide definite evidence for or against DC, indicating that the decision to proceed with DC should be made on case-by-case basis, after assessment of individual risks and benefits.[11]
- Normothermia: In patients with TBI, hypothermia can reduce intracranial hypertension, but recent trials in patients with an intracranial pressure of more than 20 mm Hg after TBI, therapeutic hypothermia, plus standard care to reduce intracranial pressure did not result in outcomes better than those with standard care alone. The most recent TBI guidelines do not recommend hypothermia.[11]
- Prevention of seizures in the acute setting. Seizure prophylaxis can be considered for the first 7 days. Indications for acute seizure prophylaxis in severe head trauma are described in Box 3. Usually phenytoin or levetiracetam is used.[15] Seizure prophylaxis, however, has not shown to prevent long-term development of traumatic epilepsy.
- Deep vein thrombosis (DVT) prophylaxis is recommended in almost all patients on hospital day 1 in addition to sequential compression devices (SCDs) for immobile or bedbound patients to prevent DVTs.[11]

- Early initiation of parenteral nutrition.
- Early tracheostomy for ventilator-dependent patients is recommended to reduce mechanical ventilation days.[11]

CHRONIC Rx

- TBI can lead to short- or long-term emotional, physiologic, and cognitive sequelae. Patients suffering from TBI are shown to benefit from neurocognitive, occupational, and physical therapy. The Glasgow Outcome Scale is a comprehensive measure of severity and eventual outcome of brain injury. Posttraumatic amnesia, age, length of coma, GCS score within the first 24 hr, and imaging study scales are some of the factors affecting outcome and dictating long-term prognosis.
- Chronic treatment addresses several sequelae of TBI, including, but not limited to, the following: Dysautonomia, agitation, sleep disturbance, posttraumatic epilepsy, spasticity, dysphagia, syndrome of the trephined, posttraumatic hydrocephalus, apathy, fecal/urinary incontinence, headache, and neuropathic pain syndromes.
- Neurostimulants such as amantadine, zolpidem, bromocriptine, amphetamine, and methylphenidate are used in the rehabilitation phase with anecdotal data, but good randomized controlled trials (RCTs) are lacking in this area.

DISPOSITION

- Depending on severity of head injury, patients may require admission to a rehabilitation facility or discharge to home with outpatient neurocognitive therapy.
- Despite individual clinical variability, several common neurobehavioral sequelae of moderate to severe TBI can be identified (Table 8). Cognitive recovery is protracted for moderate to severe TBIs, with most improvements occurring in the first year but measurable

recovery of cognitive functioning still occurring several years after the injury. However, even after a prolonged length of time, individuals do not necessarily return to preinjury levels.

REFERRAL

Early transfer to a Level 1 Trauma Center with neurosurgical personnel if high-risk findings are noted on clinical exam or CT head, and is associated with better outcomes.[10]

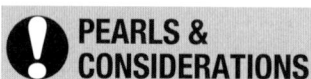 **PEARLS & CONSIDERATIONS**

TBI is major healthcare issue. Guidelines (Table 9) have been developed to address TBI in a timely and effective fashion.[11] Clinical acumen and judgment, however, is irreplaceable and should be exercised for better patient care and outcomes. Early recognition of high-risk patients and early imaging and early evaluation at a Level 1 Trauma Center by a specialist are associated with improved outcomes. The goal of healthcare providers in the field or in the community is to identify patients who need this attention.

PATIENT & FAMILY EDUCATION

- Brain Injury Association of America www.biausa.org/
- Brain Injury Resource Center www.headinjury.com/linktbisup.htm

REFERENCES
Available at eBooks.Health.Elsevier.com.

RELATED CONTENT

Concussion (Related Key Topic)
Postconcussion Syndrome (Related Key Topic)

AUTHOR: **ALI AHMAD, MD**

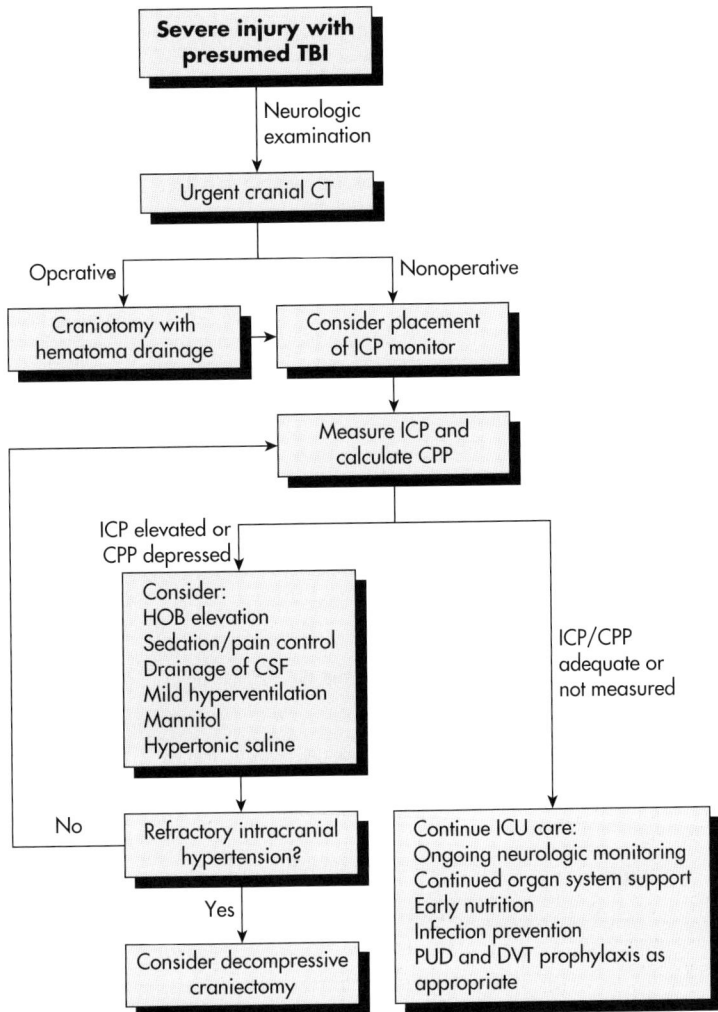

FIG. 8 Algorithm for the management of traumatic brain injury (TBI). *CPP,* Cerebral perfusion pressure; *CSF,* cerebrospinal fluid; *CT,* computed tomography; *DVT,* deep venous thrombosis; *HOB,* head of bed; *ICP,* intracranial pressure; *ICU,* intensive care unit; *PUD,* peptic ulcer disease. (From Townsend CM et al: *Sabiston textbook of surgery,* ed 21, St Louis, 2022, Elsevier.)

TABLE 5 Assessment and Treatment Recommendations for Mild Traumatic Brain Injury

Function	Assessment	Treatment
Overall recovery	Standardized symptom checklist	Physical rest 1-2 days[1] followed by subsymptomatic aerobic exercise[2]
Headache	Determine the type	HA persisting more than 3-4 days may require abortive treatment tailored to phenotype (migraine, tension-type, occipital neuralgia, etc.)
Vertigo	Romberg test, dynamic standing, tandem gait	If Hallpike Dix is normal, or if Epley maneuver does not relieve symptoms, consider physical therapy for vestibular rehabilitation
Eye movements	Examine cranial nerves 3, 4, 6 for tracking, saccades, diplopia, nystagmus	Physical therapy evaluation for vestibular rehabilitation
Near vision	Near-point accommodation and binocular convergence	Ophthalmologic evaluation for vision therapy
Cognitive function	Symptoms, cognitive testing, neuropsychologist evaluation	Sleep hygiene, neuropsychology evaluation for cognitive rehabilitation[3]

HA, Headache.

[1]Thomas DG et al: Benefits of strict rest after acute concussion: a randomized controlled trial, *Pediatrics* 135:213-223, 2015.
[2]Kurowski BG et al: Aerobic exercise for adolescents with prolonged symptoms after mild traumatic brain injury: an exploratory randomized clinical trial, *J Head Trauma Rehabil* 32:79-89, 2017.
[3]Cooper DB et al: Cognitive rehabilitation for military service members with mild traumatic brain injury: a randomized clinical trial, *J Head Trauma Rehabil* 32:E1-E15, 2017.
From Goldman L, Schafer AI: *Goldman-Cecil medicine,* ed 26, Philadelphia, 2019, Elsevier.

TABLE 6 Guidelines for the Management of Severe Traumatic Brain Injury

Topic	Level 1	Level 2	Level 3
Blood pressure and oxygenation	Insufficient data	Avoid systolic blood pressure <90 mm Hg	Avoid hypoxia (Pao₂ <60 mm Hg or O₂ saturation <90%)
Hyperosmolar therapy	Insufficient data	Mannitol is effective for control of raised ICP at doses of 0.25 g/kg to 1 g/kg body weight	Restrict mannitol use prior to ICP monitoring in patients with signs of transtentorial herniation
Prophylactic hypothermia	Insufficient data	Insufficient data	Pooled data indicate that prophylactic hypothermia is not significantly associated with decreased mortality as compared with normothermic controls
Infection prophylaxis	Insufficient data	Periprocedural antibiotics for intubation should be administered to reduce the incidence of pneumonia. Early tracheostomy should be performed to reduce days on mechanical ventilation with pneumonia	To reduce infection, routine ventricular catheter exchange or prophylactic antibiotic use for ventricular catheter placement is not recommended
Deep venous thrombosis prophylaxis	Insufficient data	Insufficient data	Intermittent pneumatic compression stockings are recommended. Low-molecular-weight heparin or low-dose unfractionated heparin should be used in combination with mechanical prophylaxis
Indications for ICP monitoring	Insufficient data	ICP should be monitored in all salvageable patients with a GCS score of 3-8 after resuscitation and an abnormal CT scan	ICP monitoring is indicated in patients with severe TBI with a normal CT scan if >40 yr of age with blood pressure <90 mm Hg
ICP pressure-monitoring technology	N/A	N/A	N/A
ICP thresholds	Insufficient data	Treatment should be initiated with ICP >20 mm Hg	A combination of ICP values and clinical and brain CT findings should be used to determine the need for treatment
Cerebral perfusion thresholds	Insufficient data	Aggressive attempts to maintain CPP above 70 mm Hg with fluids and pressors should be avoided because of the risk of adult respiratory distress syndrome	CPP of <50 mm Hg should be avoided. The CPP value to target lies within the range of 50-70 mm Hg. Patients with intact pressure autoregulation tolerate higher CPP values. Ancillary monitoring of cerebral parameters that include blood flow, oxygenation, or metabolism facilitates CPP management
Brain oxygen monitoring and thresholds	Insufficient data	Insufficient data	Jugular venous saturation (<50%) or brain tissue oxygen tension (<15 mm Hg) are treatment thresholds
Anesthetics, analgesics, sedatives	Insufficient data	Prophylactic administration of barbiturates to induce burst suppression electroencephalogram is not recommended. High-dose barbiturate administration is recommended to control elevated ICP refractory to maximum standard medical and surgical treatment. Hemodynamic stability is essential before and during barbiturate therapy. Propofol is recommended for the control of ICP but not for improvement in mortality or 6-mo outcome	N/A
Nutrition	Insufficient data	Patients should be fed to attain full caloric replacement by day 7 postinjury	N/A
Antiseizure prophylaxis	Insufficient data	Anticonvulsants are indicated to decrease the incidence of early PTS (within 7 days of injury)	N/A
Hyperventilation	Insufficient data	Prophylactic hyperventilation (Paco₂ of 25 mm Hg or less) is not recommended	Hyperventilation is recommended as a temporizing measure for the reduction of ICP. Hyperventilation should be avoided during the first 24 hr after injury, when cerebral blood flow is often critically reduced. If hyperventilation is used, jugular venous oxygen saturation (SjO₂) or brain-tissue oxygen tension (PbtO₂) measurements are recommended to monitor oxygen delivery
Steroids	The use of high-dose methylprednisolone is associated with increased mortality and is contraindicated	N/A	N/A

CT, Computed tomography; *CPP,* cerebral perfusion pressure; *ICP,* intracranial pressure; *GCS,* Glasgow Coma Scale; *PTS,* posttraumatic seizures; *TBI,* traumatic brain injury.
From Jankovic J et al: *Bradley and Daroff's neurology in clinical practice,* ed 8, Philadelphia, 2022, Elsevier.

TABLE 7 Elevated ICP Management

- Verify ICP
  1. Check if EVD is still patent
  2. Check to see if EVD waveform is present and adequate
  3. Check to see if EVD ICP correlates with intraparenchymal monitor if present
- Check for 30-degree head elevation
- Loosen cervical collar if in place
- Open EVD for ICP >20 mm Hg for 10 min and then close and transduce ICP
  1. Repeat once
  2. If ICP >20 mm Hg, keep open at 15 mm Hg above midbrain and proceed with ICP module
- Treat temperature >37.5°C with 650 mg of acetaminophen once
- Sedation
  1. Titrate propofol to a Ramsay score of 4
     a. Do not exceed 5 mg/kg/h for more than 24 h
  2. Check potassium, triglycerides, creatine kinase, and urinalysis for myoglobinuria q 8 h for 24 h
  3. If maximal dose of propofol is reached and ICP >20 mm Hg
  4. Start fentanyl drip at 0.8 μg/kg/h
  5. Apply bispectral index (BIS) monitor
  6. Titrate fentanyl drip to a bispectral index of 30 or to a maximum of 5 μg/kg/h
  7. Start chlorhexidine gluconate (Peridex) with a loading infusion of 1 μg/kg over 10 min
     a. Continue maintenance infusion of 0.2 to 0.7 μg/kg/h
- Hyperosmolar therapy
  1. 3% hypertonic saline bolus of 250 mL
  2. Before administering 3% hypertonic saline bolus, check if Na <130 mEq/L
  3. In emergency, administer mannitol 1-0.5 mg/kg bolus once
  4. Check sodium and serum osmolality q 4 h × 2 after every bolus
  5. Start 3% hypertonic saline drip at 0.5 mL/h if ≥ three 3% hypertonic saline boluses within 6 h
  6. Check sodium and serum osmolality q 2 h while on drip
  7. If sodium >160 mEq/L or serum osmolality >320 sOsm/L, call physician
  8. If serum sodium has increased to >10 mEq/L within the last 24 h, call physician
  9. If CBF > 35 mL/min/100 g white matter or >80 mL/min/100 g gray matter refer to CBF module high flow
- If core body temperature ≥37.5°C, start normothermia protocol
- Hyperventilation
  1. Do not hyperventilate in the first 24 hr (goal of Paco$_2$ of 35-40 mm Hg)
  2. If PbtO$_2$ is <20 mmHg, go to hypoxia module
  3. If CBF <18 mL/min/100 g white matter or <67 mL/min/100 g gray matter, go to CBF module
  4. If PbtO$_2$ and CBF are optimized, hyperventilate to 33-35 mm Hg
- Radiology
  1. Refractory ICP > 20 mm Hg despite intervention, obtain portable head CT without contrast immediately if no head CT since ICP is elevated despite maximal therapy
- Consider surgery
- Induce pentobarbital coma
  1. Only for diffuse nonoperative injuries
  2. Only with attending approval
  3. Order continuous EEG monitoring if not already in place
  4. Have norepinephrine drip ready at the bedside for MAP < 80 mm Hg/CPP < 60 mm Hg
  5. Pentobarbital bolus/loading: 10 mg/kg once over 60 min, then 5 mg/kg qh × 4 or until burst suppression
  6. Pentobarbital maintenance dose: 1 mg/kg/h titrated to burst suppression

CBF, Cerebral blood flow; *CPP*, cerebral perfusion pressure; *EEG*, electroencephalography; *EVD*, external ventricular drain; *ICP*, intracranial pressure; *MAP*, mean arterial pressure; *PbtO$_2$*, Brain tissue oxygen.
From Jankovic J et al: *Bradley and Daroff's neurology in clinical practice,* ed 8, Philadelphia, 2022, Elsevier.

BOX 3 Indications for Acute Seizure Prophylaxis in Severe Head Trauma

- Depressed skull fracture
- Paralyzed and intubated patient
- Seizure at the time of injury
- Seizure at emergency department presentation
- Penetrating brain injury
- Severe head injury (Glasgow Coma Scale score ≤8)
- Acute subdural hematoma
- Acute epidural hematoma
- Acute intracranial hemorrhage
- Prior history of seizures

TABLE 8 Common Neurocognitive Sequelae of Moderate to Severe Traumatic Brain Injury

Cognitive Domain	Clinical Manifestation of Impairment
Attention	Difficulty with sustained attention
	Poor concentration
	Psychomotor impersistence
Memory	Problems with acquiring and retaining new verbal or nonverbal information
	Problems in retrieving verbal and nonverbal memories
Speed of information processing	Slowed sensorimotor skills and information processing
Executive functioning	Problems in convergent and divergent reasoning
	Poor judgment
	Difficulty planning
	Problems in self-monitoring and self-correcting behavior
Awareness of symptoms	Difficulty recognizing deficits
	Unrealistic expectations concerning the recovery of functions
	Problems related to poor treatment compliance
Language and communication	Problems in word comprehension
	Impaired reading, spelling, and writing ability
	Tendency to become fragmented in free speech
Integrative functions	Problems in adequate or time-efficient execution of various perceptual-motor-spatial-sequential tasks

From Jankovic J et al: *Bradley and Daroff's neurology in clinical practice,* ed 8, Philadelphia, 2022, Elsevier.

TABLE 9 Brain Trauma Foundation Recommendations for Traumatic Brain Injury

Parameter	Guideline
Hyperosmolar therapy	Mannitol effective for control of raised ICP (0.25-1 g/kg)
Prophylactic hypothermia	Early (within 2.5 hr), short term (48 hr postinjury) hypothermia not recommended to improve outcomes in patients with diffuse injury
Infection prophylaxis	Routine external ventricular catheter exchange not recommended; oral care is not recommended to reduce ventilator-associated pneumonia; antimicrobial ventricular EVD catheters decrease infection
ICP monitoring	Indicated if GCS score = 3-8 on admission and abnormal CT. In severe traumatic brain injury and normal CT, indicated with two or more of the following: Age >40 yr, unilateral posturing, hypotension with SBP <90 mm Hg
CPP threshold	CPP <50 mm Hg should be avoided; aggressive interventions to maintain it above 70 mm Hg have a considerable risk of acute respiratory distress syndrome
Brain oxygen monitoring and thresholds	Jugular venous saturation (50%) or above
Blood pressure and oxygenation	Maintain SBP >100 mm Hg in patients 50-69 yr of age, >110 mm Hg in patients 15-49 and > 70 yr of age; hypoxia (saturation <90% or Po_2 <60 mm Hg) should be avoided
Nutrition	Should be initiated within at least by day 5 and at most day 7 postinjury
Sedatives	High-dose barbiturates recommended to control refractory ICP in the hemodynamically stable patient; propofol recommended for ICP control but does not improve mortality
Seizure prophylaxis	Decreases early posttraumatic seizures (<7 days after injury); insufficient evidence to recommend levetiracetam over phenytoin
Hyperventilation	Recommended as temporizing measure; Pco_2 below 25 mm Hg not recommended; avoid in first 24 hr after injury
Steroids	Not recommended, contraindicated

CPP, Cerebral perfusion pressure; *CT,* computed tomography; *EVD,* external ventricular drain; *GCS,* Glasgow Coma Scale; *ICP,* intracranial pressure; *SBP,* systolic blood pressure.
From Townsend CM et al: *Sabiston textbook of surgery,* ed 21, St Louis, 2022, Elsevier.

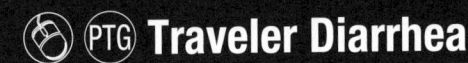
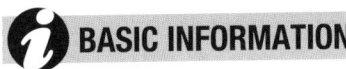 **BASIC INFORMATION**

DEFINITION

Traveler diarrhea (TD) is defined as three or more loose-to-watery stools, with or without associated fever, abdominal cramps, and vomiting, within a 24-hr period. It develops during or within 10 days of traveling to developing areas of the world.

SYNONYMS

TD
Enterotoxigenic *Escherichia coli*
Enteroaggregative *E. coli*
Infectious diarrhea
Postinfectious irritable bowel syndrome

ICD-10CM CODE
A09 Infectious diarrhea

EPIDEMIOLOGY & DEMOGRAPHICS

- TD is mostly caused by bacteria and other pathogens in food and water.
- At least one episode of diarrhea occurs in 40% to 50% of travelers during their stay abroad. Table 1 describes pathogens and epidemiologic features associated with TD.

INCIDENCE:
- **High risk (>20%):** South and Southeast Asia, Africa (except South Africa), South and Central America, and Mexico
- **Moderate risk (10% to 20%):** Caribbean Islands, South Africa, Central and East Asia (including Russia and China), Eastern Europe, and the Middle East, including Israel
- **Low risk (<10%):** Northern and Western Europe, Australia, New Zealand, United States, Canada, Singapore, Japan

PREVALENCE: Acute and chronic diarrhea account for a third of medical visits by returned travelers as per the GeoSentinel database.

PREDOMINANT SEX & AGE:
- Travelers in their 30s are at highest risk, possibly secondary to more adventurous travel.
- Sex does not seem to influence the risk for TD.
- Infants and toddlers are more likely to have a more severe form of TD and are more likely to need hospitalization.

PEAK INCIDENCE:
- Peak incidence occurs during the first week of travel and progressively declines after that.
- Seasonal variation does exist for TD, with lower rates in the winter months.

RISK FACTORS:
- Gastric acid protects against enteropathogens, so medications that reduce gastric acid secretion (i.e., proton pump inhibitor [PPI] or histamine-2 [H_2]-receptor blockers) are known to increase risk for TD by a factor of 12.
- Immunocompromised travelers such as those with HIV/AIDS are at higher risk for parasitic infections.
- Backpackers are at higher risk than those staying at a resort.
- Food bought from street vendors or prepared by persons not wearing gloves carries a higher risk.

GENETICS: Travelers with the O blood group are at higher risk for diarrhea caused by norovirus and *Shigella*.

PHYSICAL FINDINGS & CLINICAL PRESENTATION

- The clinical presentation does not allow determination of infectious cause.
- 90% of cases occur within 2 wk of stay.
- Acute watery diarrhea predominates in 90% of patients.
- Signs of invasive infection, including fever and bloody/mucoid diarrhea, occur in 3% to 30%.

- Most patients report three to five bowel movements a day, but in 20% a higher frequency of up to 20 daily bowel movements occurs.
- Nausea (10% to 70%), vomiting (4% to 36%), abdominal cramps/tenesmus (80%), urgency (90%).
- Other: Myalgia, arthralgia, headache.
- Average episode resolves in 3 to 5 days.
- Prolonged symptoms lasting more than 1 wk: 8% to 15%; chronic diarrhea >30 days: 1% to 3%.
- Severe episodes may result in electrolyte imbalance (K^+ loss).
- 50% of all travelers are incapacitated for at least 24 hr, but up to 20% are ill in bed for 1 to 2 days.

ETIOLOGY

- *E. coli* (Table E2): Accounts for up to 60% of all cases of TD and is most prevalent in Central and South America, South Asia, and Africa. Table E3 summarizes etiology of TD in Latin America, Africa, and Asia.
  1. Enterotoxigenic *E. coli* (ETEC): Produce heat labile and heat stable toxin and are the most common cause, accounting for 10% to 45% of cases. Frequently seen in Latin America, Africa, and South Asia.
  2. Enteroaggregative *E. coli* (EAEC): More commonly seen in Latin America.
  3. Other *E. coli* (enteropathogenic [EPEC], enteroinvasive [EIEC], enterohemorrhagic [EHEC]): Shiga toxin–producing or diffuse adhering *E. coli* are much less common.
- *Campylobacter:* 2% to 32% of cases. More common in Southeast Asia, where it is more frequent than ETEC.
- *Shigella:* 2% to 9%. More common in Africa.
- *Salmonella:* <5% of cases except in Asia, where it is seen in up to 10% of cases.

TABLE 1 Pathogens and Epidemiologic Features Associated With Traveler Diarrhea

Organism	Approximate Percentage of Cases (%)	Epidemiologic Features
Enterotoxigenic *Escherichia coli*	15-50	Most important causative agent of traveler diarrhea overall; not diagnosed by routine microbiologic methods
Enteroaggregative *E. coli*	20-35	Not diagnosed by routine microbiologic methods
Shigella spp. and enteroinvasive *E. coli*	10-25	Most important causes of dysentery; enteroinvasive *E. coli* not diagnosed by routine microbiologic methods
Nontyphoidal *Salmonella* spp.	5-10	
Campylobacter jejuni	3-15	More common in Asia; antimicrobial resistance a concern
Aeromonas	5	
Plesiomonas	5	
Giardia lamblia	<2	Affects hikers and campers who drink from contaminated freshwater streams
Cryptosporidium hominis/parvum	<2	Occasional large-scale waterborne outbreaks
Cyclospora cayetanensis	<2	
Vibrio cholerae		Ongoing outbreaks in Haiti and Zimbabwe, and endemic in many countries in Asia; rare cause of disease in travelers
Norovirus		Outbreaks on cruise ships
Entamoeba histolytica		May cause liver abscess

From Bennett JE et al: *Mandell, Douglas, and Bennett's principles and practice of infectious diseases*, ed 8, Philadelphia, 2015, Saunders.

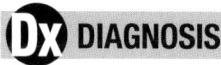
- Other bacteria: *Aeromonas, Arcobacter, Plesiomonas,* enterotoxigenic *Bacteroides fragilis, Vibrio cholera,* noncholera vibrios.
- Viral pathogens:
  1. Norovirus: Up to 17% of cases from Caribbean and Africa
  2. Rotavirus: 4% to 7% of cases
- Protozoans:
  1. *Entamoeba histolytica:* More common in South and Southeast Asia
  2. *Giardia lamblia:* More common in South and Southeast Asia, especially Nepal
  3. *Cryptosporidium, Cyclospora, Isospora*

DIAGNOSIS

DIFFERENTIAL DIAGNOSIS

- Malaria
- Dengue fever
- Influenza
- Rocky Mountain spotted fever
- Irritable bowel syndrome
- Inflammatory bowel disease
- Shellfish poisoning
- Mushroom poisoning

WORKUP

- Most cases of TD are self-limiting, do not require workup, and are treated symptomatically without regard to etiologic agent.
- In patients with diarrhea, fever, and colitic symptoms (bloody stools, cramping), a stool culture should be obtained to look for specific bacterial pathogens.

LABORATORY TESTS

- Stool culture ×3 for bacterial pathogens.
- Stool for ova and parasites to help identify protozoans. Special stains such as modified acid-fast or trichrome stain may be necessary for *Cryptosporidium, Cyclospora,* and *Isospora*. There are PCR gastrointestinal panels that can detect bacteria, viruses, and parasites, all from one stool sample.
- Blood cultures in patients with systemic illness to rule out *Salmonella* spp.

TREATMENT

NONPHARMACOLOGIC THERAPY

- Fluid replacement to treat volume depletion of diarrhea is important.
- Mild cases: Alternate fluids that contain salts and fluids that contain sugars, such as broths or fruit juices. Pedialyte is effective as an over-the-counter product.
- Severe cases: Oral rehydration solution (ORS) packets are available in most pharmacies. They should be mixed with clean water to replace lost electrolytes and are used until patient is urinating regularly. An alternative home-based solution can be made with: $\frac{1}{2}$ teaspoon of salt, $\frac{1}{2}$ teaspoon of baking soda, and 4 tablespoons of sugar in 1 liter of clean water.

ACUTE GENERAL Rx

- Antisecretory agents may reduce symptoms but do not treat underlying cause:
  1. Bismuth subsalicylate: 1 dose of 525 mg (2 tablets of Pepto-Bismol) PO every 30 min up to 8 doses a day. Can reduce number of bowel movements by 50%. Dosages are available for children based on weight, and the product is available in liquid or chewable tablet form.
  2. Loperamide: 4 mg PO, then 2 mg after each loose bowel movement, not to exceed 16 mg/day. Use for up to 48 hr. Has antisecretory and antimotility effect. Antimotility drugs should not be used in cases of bloody diarrhea or dysentery (increased risk of colitis and colonic perforation). When used, they should be given only in conjunction with antimicrobial therapy.
- Antibiotics are warranted only for moderate to severe diarrhea (i.e., more than four bowel movements a day; fever; or blood, pus, or mucus in stool. Antibiotics can reduce duration of diarrhea by 1 to 2 days.
  1. Azithromycin: The preferred antibiotic for empiric treatment of moderate to severe TD. It is also the preferred agent for children and pregnant women. Dose of 1 g PO is the single dose for women. Children: 10 mg/kg daily single dose or for 3 days. Particularly effective against quinolone-resistant *Campylobacter* infections in Southeast Asia. Another option for children: Ceftriaxone 50 mg/kg IV once daily ×3 days.
     a. Ciprofloxacin: 500 mg bid for 1 to 3 days
     b. Levaquin: 500 mg/day for 1 to 3 days
  2. Fluoroquinolones are also effective agents for bacterial causes of TD, but resistance to fluoroquinolones is increasing. Cannot be used in children under 15 and in pregnant women.
  3. Rifaximin: 200 mg PO tid for 3 days for children age >12 and adults is effective for afebrile, noncolitic diarrhea such as ETEC. Does not treat *Salmonella, Shigella,* or *Campylobacter*.
  4. Rifamycin is now FDA approved for TD caused by noninvasive strains of *E. coli*. It is not recommended for TD complicated by fever and/or bloody stools. Dosage is 388 mg (2 tablets) bid ×3 days.
- Concerns of use of antibiotics:
  1. Widespread use of antibiotics has led to resistance. Tetracycline and sulfa agents such as trimethoprim-sulfamethoxazole (TMP-SMX; Bactrim) are no longer used due to widespread resistance.
  2. Antibiotic treatment may lead to prolonged colonization in infections with *Salmonella* and nontyphoid *Salmonella*.
  3. In cases of EHEC (Shiga toxin production) treatment with quinolones, but not rifaximin, may increase risk of complications such as hemolytic uremic syndrome.
  4. *Clostridium difficile* infection can occur with use of antibiotics.

PREVENTION BY ANTIBIOTICS AND NONANTIBIOTIC AGENTS

- Antibiotic prophylaxis can be considered for certain groups, such as persons with underlying illness, athletes, and politicians for up to 2 to 3 wk. Ciprofloxacin 250 to 500 mg/day is effective in preventing 90% of TD. Rifaximin dosed daily has been shown to help prevent TD for U.S. travelers to Mexico, but not as effectively as ciprofloxacin.
- Bismuth subsalicylate can be used. It must be given 4× daily and can cause black tongue and stools. As it contains salicylates, it can interact with anticoagulants and lead to toxicity in patients on long-term salicylate therapy.
- Probiotics are being studied for their potential use but evidence of their effectiveness is limited.

REFERRAL

Infectious diseases physician for more difficult cases lasting more than 72 hr

PEARLS & CONSIDERATIONS

- Travelers on cruises have lower incidence of TD than land-based trips, but cruise ship passengers and staff are at higher risk of large outbreaks of norovirus that are difficult to contain. Norovirus infection needs only a low inoculum of virus to cause illness, and the virus is relatively resistant to cleaning.
- In up to 40% of cases of TD, no pathogen is identified.
- *Giardia* is the most frequent cause of long-lasting TD.

PREVENTION

- There are oral and injectable vaccines against *Salmonella typhi* available in the U.S.
- Dukoral is an oral vaccine available in some countries such as Canada and Australia and in Europe to help prevent cholera and ETEC.

PATIENT & FAMILY EDUCATION

Food hygiene education: Wash hands often, especially after going to bathroom and before eating. Avoid raw fruits and vegetables (unless peeled and washed in clean water). Avoid undercooked meats, fish, and seafood. Avoid tap water and ice. Choose beverages in factory-sealed containers (such as bottled water and carbonated soft drinks). Try to avoid buffet-style foods.

SUGGESTED READINGS

Available at eBooks.Health.Elsevier.com.

RELATED CONTENT

Traveler Diarrhea (Patient Information)

AUTHOR: **GLENN G. FORT, MD, MPH**

BASIC INFORMATION

DEFINITION

Pulmonary tuberculosis (TB) is an infection of the lung and, occasionally, surrounding structures, caused by the bacterium *Mycobacterium tuberculosis* (Mtb). Two states of M. tuberculosis infection are recognized: Latent tuberculosis infection (LTBI) and acute tuberculosis disease, although infection and immunologic control exist across a spectrum. LTBI is a state of persistent immune response to stimulation by *M. tuberculosis* antigens without evidence of clinically manifested active TB and with bacillary replication absent or below some undefined threshold as a result of immunologic control. Most persons with LTBI never become sick with TB; however, 5% to 15% have progression to tuberculosis disease.[1] Multidrug-resistant (MDR) TB is defined as disease caused by strains of Mtb that are at least resistant to treatment with isoniazid (INH) and rifampin (RIF) (two of the most effective first-line drugs); extensively drug-resistant (XDR) TB refers to disease caused by MDR strains that are also resistant to treatment with any fluoroquinolone and bedaquiline or linezolid.

SYNONYM

TB

ICD-10CM CODES
A15.0 Tuberculosis of lung
A15.7 Primary respiratory tuberculosis

EPIDEMIOLOGY & DEMOGRAPHICS

INCIDENCE (WORLDWIDE):
- One fourth of the world's population is infected with TB, and it is one of the world's leading infectious disease killers.
- In 2017, there were an estimated 10 million new cases of active TB; 9% involved coinfection with HIV; 1.3 million deaths from TB, including 300,000 among HIV-infected patients; 457,560 incident cases of multidrug-resistant TB worldwide.

INCIDENCE (IN U.S.):
- In 2018, a total of 9029 new TB cases were reported in the U.S., representing a 0.7% decrease from 2017. The U.S. TB incidence in 2018 was 2.8/100,000 persons.
- The rate among non–U.S.-born persons was >14 times that in the U.S.-born persons. Since 1993, TB case counts and rates have declined in the U.S. As the number of cases decreases overall, an increasing percentage of cases occurs among non–U.S.-born persons.
- More than 90% of new cases each year from reactivated prior infections, and 9% represent new infections.
- Only 10% of patients with purified protein derivative (PPD) conversions will develop TB, most within 1 to 2 yr, though this is higher in HIV-positive patients (8%/yr).
- Two thirds of new TB cases in 2018 occurred in non–U.S.-born persons, for whom the top five countries of birth were Mexico, the Philippines, India, Vietnam, and China.

- In 2017 in the U.S., 1.9% of cases were MDR TB, which is a decline from 8.2% in 2008. There were three cases of XDR TB in the U.S. in 2017.

PREVALENCE (IN U.S.):
- Between 3.1% and 5.0% of the U.S. population is estimated to be infected with latent TB infection (LTBI)
- Varies widely among population groups

PREDOMINANT SEX:
- Globally, in 2017, 6 million men contracted TB compared to 3.2 million women

PREDOMINANT AGE:
- Ages 24 to 45

PEAK INCIDENCE:
- Infancy
- Teenage years
- Pregnancy
- Elderly
- HIV-positive patients at highest risk regardless of age

GENETICS:
- Populations with widespread low native resistance have been intensely infected when initially exposed to TB.
- Following elimination of those with least native resistance, incidence and prevalence of TB tends to decline.

PHYSICAL FINDINGS & CLINICAL PRESENTATION

- See "Etiology"
- Primary pulmonary TB infection generally asymptomatic
- Reactivation pulmonary TB:
  1. Fever
  2. Night sweats
  3. Cough
  4. Hemoptysis
  5. Scanty nonpurulent sputum
  6. Weight loss
  7. Chest pain
- Progressive primary pulmonary TB disease: Same as reactivation pulmonary TB
- TB pleurisy:
  1. Pleuritic chest pain
  2. Fever
  3. Shortness of breath
- Rare massive, suffocating, fatal hemoptysis secondary to erosion of pulmonary artery within a cavity (Rasmussen aneurysm)
- Chest examination:
  1. Not specific
  2. Usually underestimates extent of disease
  3. Rales accentuated after a cough (posttussive rales)

ETIOLOGY

- Mtb, a slow-growing, aerobic, nonspore-forming, nonmotile bacillus, with a lipid-rich cell wall:
  1. Lacks pigment
  2. Produces niacin
  3. Reduces nitrate
  4. Produces heat-labile catalase
  5. Mtb staining, acid-fast and acid-alcohol fast by Ziehl-Neelsen method, appearing as red, slightly bent, beaded rods 2 to 4

microns long (acid-fast bacilli [AFB]), against a blue background
6. Polymerase chain reaction (PCR) to detect <10 organisms/ml in sputum (compared with the requisite 10,000 organisms/ml for AFB smear detection)
7. Culture:
   a. Growth on solid media (Löwenstein-Jensen; Middlebrook 7H11) in 2 to 6 wk
   b. Growth in liquid media (BACTEC, using a radioactive carbon source for early growth detection) often in 9 to 16 days
   c. Enhanced in a 5% to 10% carbon dioxide atmosphere
8. Genome sequencing:
   a. Facilitates immediate identification of Mtb strains and resistance in early growing cultures
   b. False negatives possible if growth suboptimal
9. Humans are the only reservoir for Mtb
10. Transmission:
    a. Aerosolized droplets containing AFB generated through cough, speaking, singing, bronchoscopy, or autopsy are inhaled directly into alveoli
    b. Facilitated by close exposure to high-velocity cough (unprotected by proper mask or respirators) from patients with AFB-positive sputum and cavitary lesions
    c. Locations of increased TB transmission risk include hospitals, homeless shelters, correctional facilities, nursing homes, and residential homes for those with HIV
- Pathogenesis:
  1. Mtb are ingested by macrophages in alveoli, then transported to regional lymph nodes, where spread is contained
  2. Some Mtb may reach bloodstream and disseminate widely
  3. Primary TB (often asymptomatic, minimal pneumonitis in lower or midlung fields, with hilar lymphadenopathy) is essentially an intracellular infection, with multiplication of organisms continuing 2 to 12 wk after primary exposure, until cell-mediated hypersensitivity (detected by positive skin test reaction to tuberculin PPD) matures, and results in subsequent containment of infection
  4. Local and disseminated Mtb are thus contained by the following T-cell–mediated immune responses:
     a. Recruitment of monocytes
     b. Transformation of lymphocytes with secretion of lymphokines
     c. Activation of macrophages and histiocytes
     d. Organization into granulomas, where Mtb may survive within macrophages (Langhans giant cells), but within which multiplication essentially ceases (95%) and from which spread is prohibited
  5. Progressive primary pulmonary disease:

a. May immediately follow the asymptomatic phase
b. Necrotizing pulmonary infiltrates
c. Tuberculous bronchopneumonia
d. Endobronchial TB
e. Interstitial TB
f. Widespread miliary lung lesions

6. Postprimary TB pleurisy with pleural effusion:
   a. Develops after early primary infection, although often before conversion to positive PPD
   b. Results from pleural seeding from a peripheral lung lesion or rupture of lymph node into pleural space
   c. May produce a large (sometimes hemorrhagic) exudative effusion (with polymorphonuclear cells early, rapidly replaced by lymphocytes), frequently without pulmonary infiltrates
   d. Generally resolves without treatment
   e. Portends a high risk of subsequent clinical disease, and therefore must be diagnosed and treated early (pleural biopsy and culture) to prevent future catastrophic TB illness
   f. May result in disseminated extrapulmonary infection

7. Reactivation pulmonary TB:
   a. Occurs months to years after primary TB
   b. Preferentially involves the apical posterior segments of the upper lobes and superior segments of the lower lobes
   c. Associated with necrosis and cavitation of involved lung, hemoptysis, chronic fever, night sweats, weight loss
   d. Spread within lung occurs via cough and inhalation

8. Reinfection TB:
   a. May mimic reactivation TB
   b. Ruptured caseous foci and cavities, which may produce endobronchial spread

9. Mtb in both progressive primary and reactivation pulmonary TB:
   a. Intracellular (macrophage) lesions (undergoing slow multiplication)
   b. Closed caseous lesions (undergoing slow multiplication)
   c. Extracellular, open cavities (undergoing rapid multiplication)
   d. INH and RIF are bactericidal in all three sites
   e. Pyrazinamide (PZA) especially active within acidic macrophage environment
   f. Extrapulmonary reactivation disease also possible

10. Rapid local progression and dissemination in infants with devastating illness before PPD conversion occurs
11. Most symptoms (fever, weight loss, anorexia) and tissue destruction (caseous necrosis) from cytokines and cell-mediated immune responses
12. Mtb has no important endotoxins or exotoxins
13. Granuloma formation related to tumor necrosis factor (TNF) secreted by activated macrophages

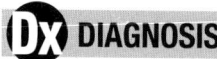

DIAGNOSIS

DIFFERENTIAL DIAGNOSIS

- Necrotizing pneumonia (anaerobic, gram-negative)
- Histoplasmosis
- Coccidioidomycosis
- Melioidosis
- Interstitial lung diseases (rarely)
- Cancer
- Sarcoidosis
- Silicosis
- Rare pneumonias:
  1. *Rhodococcus equi* (cavitation)
  2. *Bacillus cereus* (50% hemoptysis)
  3. *Eikenella corrodens* (cavitation)

WORKUP

- Sputum for AFB stains and Mtb culture.
- Chest x-ray examination (Fig. E1).
- Target groups for LTBI screening are summarized in Table 1. PPD (tuberculin skin test) or interferon gamma release assays (IGRA) can be used for screening of LTBI (Fig. 2):
  1. Recent conversion from negative to positive within 3 mo of exposure is highly suggestive of recent infection.
  2. Negative PPD never rules out acute TB.
  3. Prior positive PPD may become negative after several years and return to positive only after second repeated PPD; repeat second PPD within 1 wk, which thus may mimic skin test conversion.
  4. Positive PPD reaction is determined as follows:
     a. Induration after 72 h of intradermal injection of 0.1 ml of 5 TU-PPD.
     b. 5-mm induration if HIV-positive (or other severe immunosuppressed state affecting cellular immune function), close contact of active TB, fibrotic chest lesions.
     c. 10-mm induration if in high–medical risk groups (immunosuppressive disease or therapy, renal failure, gastrectomy, silicosis, diabetes), foreign-born high-risk group (Southeast Asia, Latin America, Africa, India), low socioeconomic groups, intravenous (IV) drug addict, prisoner, health care worker.
     d. 15-mm induration if low risk.
  5. PPD cannot distinguish between TB disease and TB infection.
- IGRAs: Diagnostic test for LTBI, known as the QuantiFERON TB Gold test (QFT-G) and T-SPOT.TB Assay. These blood tests measure interferon response to specific Mtb antigens. The test may assist in distinguishing true positive reactions from individuals with latent TB from PPD reactions related to non-tuberculous mycobacteria, prior bacillus Calmette-Guérin vaccination, or difficult-to-interpret skin-test results from people with dermatologic conditions or immediate allergic reactions to PPD. IGRAs have a specificity >95% for diagnosis of latent TB. The sensitivity of the T-SPOT assay (90%) appears to be

---

TABLE 1 Target Groups for Latent Tuberculosis Infection Screening

Individuals with Increased Risk of Infection

Contacts of individuals with untreated infectious active tuberculosis

Individuals who have immigrated to the United States within the past 5 yr from tuberculosis endemic areas

Individuals who work and/or reside in high-risk congregate settings (e.g., hospitals, homeless shelters, prisons, nursing homes)

Individuals with Conditions Associated with Increased Risk for Reactivation

High Risk for Reactivation (Risk of Reactivation Is at Least Six Times Higher Than for Healthy Individuals)

Human immunodeficiency virus infection

Severe immunosuppression (e.g., individuals receiving medication for solid-organ transplantation, chemotherapy, tumor necrosis factor-α inhibitors)

Certain malignancies (e.g., hematologic malignancies, head and neck cancers)

Silicosis

End-stage renal disease

Radiographic evidence of prior granulomatous disease (e.g., fibrotic lesions on chest imaging)

Children <5 yr with a positive tuberculin skin test reaction

Moderate Risk for Reactivation (Risk of Reactivation Is Less Than Six Times Higher Than for Healthy Individuals)

Corticosteroid use ($\geq$15 mg daily for $\geq$1 mo)

Diabetes mellitus

Underweight or malnourished individuals (includes malabsorptive conditions, such as gastrectomy, jejunoileal bypass surgeries)

Substance abuse (e.g., smoking, alcohol abuse, injection drug use)

Radiographic evidence of solitary or small granulomas

From Broaddus VC et al: *Murray & Nadel's textbook of respiratory medicine*, ed 7, Philadelphia 2022, Elsevier.

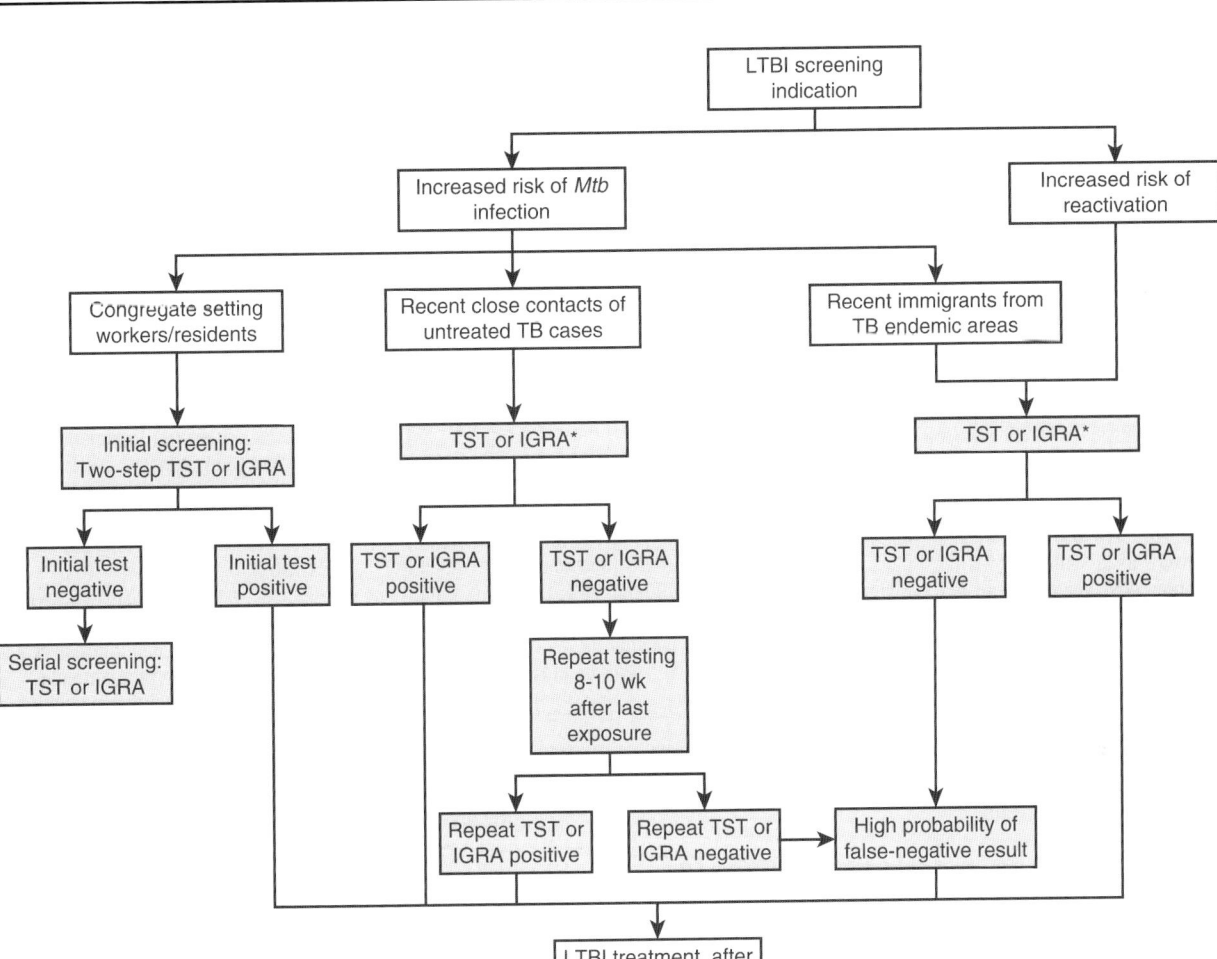

FIG 2 Latent tuberculosis infection screening algorithm. Individuals at high likelihood of having LTBI, due to demographic or specific exposure history or an untreated previously positive TST or IGRA, and a high probability of a presently false-negative result, due to immunodeficiency or immunosuppression, should be considered for treatment. *IGRA preferred for individuals with prior bacillus Calmette-Guérin and individuals at high risk for becoming lost to follow-up. TST preferred for children younger than 5 yr. Dual testing (not shown) may be considered for certain situations. *IGRA,* Interferon gamma release assay; *LTBI,* latent tuberculosis infection; *Mtb, Mycobacterium tuberculosis; TB,* tuberculosis; *TST,* tuberculin skin test. (From Broaddus VC et al: *Murray & Nadel's textbook of respiratory medicine,* ed 7, Philadelphia, 2022, Elsevier.)

higher than the QFT-G test (80%). It should be noted that IGRA sensitivity is diminished by HIV infection. As with PPD, negative tests do not rule out active TB disease, and positive tests cannot distinguish between TB infection and disease.

- The Xpert `MTB/RIF is an automated molecular test for Mtb and resistance to RIF that provides sensitive detection of TB and RIF resistance directly from untreated sputum in less than 2 h with minimal hands-on time.

LABORATORY TESTS

- Sputum for AFB stains and culture:
  1. Induced sputum if patient not coughing productively
- Sputum from bronchoscopy if high suspicion of TB in patients unable to produce expectorated induced sputum for AFB:
  1. Positive AFB smear is essential before or shortly after treatment to ensure subsequent growth for definitive diagnosis and sensitivity testing

  2. Consider lung biopsy if sputum negative, especially if infiltrates are predominantly interstitial
- AFB stain–negative sputum may grow Mtb subsequently (especially in HIV)
- Gastric aspirates may be helpful, especially in children
- CBC:
  1. Variable values:
     a. White blood cells (WBCs): Low, normal, or elevated (including leukemoid reaction: >50,000)
     b. Normocytic, normochromic anemia often
- Rarely helpful diagnostically
- Erythrocyte sedimentation rate usually elevated
- Thoracentesis:
  1. Exudative effusion:
     a. Elevated protein and adenosine deaminase
     b. Decreased glucose
     c. Elevated WBCs (polymorphonuclear leukocytes early, replaced later by lymphocytes)

     d. May be hemorrhagic
  2. Pleural fluid usually AFB-negative
  3. Pleural biopsy often diagnostic—may need to be repeated for diagnosis
  4. Culture pleural biopsy tissue for AFB
- Bone marrow biopsy is often diagnostic in difficult-to-diagnose cases, especially miliary TB

IMAGING STUDIES

- Chest x-ray examination:
  1. Primary infection reflected by calcified peripheral lung nodule with calcified hilar lymph node
  2. Reactivation pulmonary TB:
     a. Necrosis
     b. Cavitation (especially on apical lordotic views)
     c. Fibrosis and hilar retraction
     d. Bronchopneumonia
     e. Interstitial infiltrates
     f. Miliary pattern
     g. Many of the previous findings may also accompany progressive primary TB

3. TB pleurisy:
   a. Pleural effusion, often rapidly accumulating and massive
4. TB activity not established by single chest x-ray examination
5. Serial chest x-ray examinations are excellent indicators of progression or regression

🆁🆇 TREATMENT

NONPHARMACOLOGIC THERAPY

- Increased rest during acute phase of treatment
- High-calorie, high-protein diet to reverse malnutrition and enhance immune response to TB
- Isolation in negative-pressure rooms with high-volume air replacement and circulation, with health care provider wearing proper protective 0.5- to 1-micron filter respirators, until three consecutive sputum AFB smears are negative during workup (taken in 8- to 24-h intervals, with at least one being an early morning specimen) or a diagnosed patient has been on standard multidrug treatment for at least 2 wk and is clinically improving

ACUTE GENERAL Rx

- Generally, treatment of active TB consists of two phases: An intensive phase, followed by a continuation phase
- Compliance (rigid adherence to treatment regimen) chief determinant of success:
  1. Supervised directly observed therapy (DOT) recommended for all patients and mandatory for patients with high likelihood of loss to follow-up
- Adult initial regimen:
  1. INH 5 mg/kg (INH; max 300 mg) PO, RIF 10 mg/kg (RIF; max 600 mg) PO, ethambutol (EMB) by weight increments (EMB: 40 to 55 kg, 800 mg; 56 to 75 kg,1200 mg; 76 to 90 kg, 1600 mg) PO, and PZA by weight increments (PZA: 40 to 55 kg, 1000 mg; 56 to 75 kg, 1500 mg; 76 to 90 kg, 2000 mg) PO dosed daily
  2. Pyridoxine (vitamin B_6, 25 mg/day) should be given with INH to prevent peripheral neuropathy

  3. Usually decreased to INH and RIF after 8 wk depending on susceptibilities, with ultimate duration of therapy dependent on HIV treatment status, extent of disease, regimen used, and treatment response, but generally at least 6 mo
  4. Alternative, more complicated DOT regimens
  5. In patients with rifampin-susceptible TB, a strategy involving initial treatment with an 8-week bedaquiline-linezolid regimen was shown to be noninferior to standard treatment for TB with respect to clinical outcomes. This strategy was associated with a shorter duration of treatment and with no evident safety concerns.[2]
- Monitor for clinical toxicity (especially hepatitis). Pharmacology and adverse effects of antituberculosis medications are summarized in Table 2.
  1. Patient and physician awareness that anorexia, nausea, right upper quadrant pain, and unexplained malaise require immediate cessation of treatment
  2. Evaluation of liver function testing:

TABLE 2 Pharmacology and Adverse Effects of Antituberculosis Medications

Drug	Pharmacology	Adverse Effects
INH	Prodrug, activated by bacterial catalase/peroxidase, KatG Peak plasma concentration: 1-2 hr after ingestion C_{max}: 3-5 µg/ml Half-life: 2-5 hr (slow acetylators), 0.5-2 hr (fast acetylators) Metabolism: Hepatic acetylation (NAT2 enzyme) and excreted in urine	Liver injury Peripheral neuropathy due to pyridoxine deficiency; give pyridoxine (25-50 mg) with each INH dose if at risk (patients with diabetes, HIV, renal disease, alcohol abuse, malnutrition, pregnancy) or if neuropathy develops CNS toxicity: Headache, poor concentration, depression, seizures, optic neuritis Rash Hematologic abnormalities INH inhibition of cytochrome P-450 causes increases in serum concentrations of certain medications, including phenytoin, carbamazepine, valproic acid, clopidogrel, warfarin, theophylline, ketoconazole
RIF	Peak plasma concentration: 1-4 hr after ingestion C_{max}: 8-24 µg/ml Half-life: 2-3 hr; prolonged with liver disease Metabolism: Hepatic deacetylation to enterohepatically recirculated active metabolite	Liver injury: Usually cholestatic pattern of injury GI upset Hypersensitivity (flulike syndrome); symptoms include fever, headache, malaise, myalgias that start 1-2 hr postadministration; may resolve with change from intermittent to daily RIF therapy Rash Hematologic abnormalities Discoloration of body fluids (e.g., urine, feces, tears) Cytochrome P-450 induction causes decrease in serum concentrations of many medications, including antiretrovirals, anticonvulsants, anticoagulation, immunosuppressants, chemotherapy, methadone, oral contraceptives, levothyroxine, and antihypertensives
PZA	Prodrug, activated by bacterial pyrazinamidase enzymes Peak plasma concentration: 1-4 hr after ingestion C_{max}: 20-40 µg/mlHalf-life: 10 hr Metabolism: Hydrolyzed by liver, excreted in urine	Liver injury Arthralgias, gout: Consider avoiding in patients with gout GI upset Rash Photosensitivity
EMB	Peak plasma concentration: 2-4 hr after ingestion C_{max}: 2-6 µg/ml Half-life: 3-4 hr Primarily excreted through kidneys in unchanged form Reduce dose in patients with impaired renal function	Optic neuritis: Perform patient education, baseline and monthly assessment of visual acuity, and color discrimination while receiving EMB Rash GI upset
Levofloxacin	Peak plasma concentration: 1-2 hr postingestion C_{max}: 8-12 µg/ml Half-life: 6-8 hr Primarily excreted through kidneys in unchanged form; if CrCl <30 ml/min, administer tiw (not daily)	GI: Nausea, vomiting, diarrhea, abdominal pain CNS toxicity: Headache, insomnia, dizziness, tremulousness QT prolongation Tendon effects: Tendonitis, tendon rupture (more common in elderly) Arthralgias Peripheral neuropathy Rash

TABLE 2 Pharmacology and Adverse Effects of Antituberculosis Medications—cont'd

Drug	Pharmacology	Adverse Effects
Moxifloxacin	Peak plasma concentration: 1-3 hr postingestion C_{max}: 3-5 µg/ml Half-life: 11-13 hr Hepatic metabolism via glucuronide and sulfate conjugation; approximately 45% excreted unchanged in urine and feces	GI: Nausea, vomiting, diarrhea, abdominal pain CNS toxicity: Dizziness, headache, insomnia, tremulousness, confusion QT prolongation Tendon effects: Tendonitis, tendon rupture (more common in elderly) Arthralgias Peripheral neuropathy Rash Liver injury (rare)
Bedaquiline	Peak plasma concentration: 5 hr after ingestion (should be taken with food, which increases bioavailability) C_{max}: 2.7 µg/ml (200-mg dose) Half-life: ~5.5 mo Hepatic metabolism via CYP3A4, excreted in feces	Nausea QT prolongation Headache Rash Arthralgia Transaminitis
Linezolid	Peak plasma concentration: 1-2 hr after ingestion C_{max}: 12-24 µg/ml Half-life: 5 hr Hepatic metabolism, urinary excretion	Peripheral neuropathy Hematologic: Thrombocytopenia, leukopenia, anemia GI: Diarrhea, nausea Optic neuropathy Serotonin syndrome: Risk increased in presence of other serotonergic medications
Clofazimine	Peak plasma concentration: 4-8 hr if taken with food (take with food to improve absorption and tolerability) C_{max}: 0.5-2.0 µg/ml Half-life: 70 days Hepatic metabolism, excretion unknown	Skin discoloration (reversible) in 75%-100% of patients Photosensitivity GI: Abdominal pain, nausea, splenic infarction Dry skin QT prolongation
Cycloserine	Peak plasma concentration: 2-4 hr after ingestion, C_{max}: 20-35 µg/ml Half-life: 12 hr Hepatic metabolism; approximately 65% excreted unchanged in urine	CNS toxicity: Lethargy, difficulty with concentration, depression, confusion, psychosis, seizures; pyridoxine may prevent/treat symptoms Peripheral neuropathy Rash
Delamanid	Prodrug, activated by bacterial nitroreductase Peak plasma concentration: 4 hr after ingestion (take with food, which increases bioavailability threefold) C_{max}: 0.37 µg/ml Half-life: 30-38 hr Metabolized by plasma albumin, excreted in feces	GI: Nausea, vomiting, abdominal pain Headache, insomnia, dizziness, tinnitus QT prolongation Palpitations
Pretomanid	Prodrug, activated by bacterial nitroreductase Peak plasma concentration: 4-5 hr after ingestion (take with food, which increases bioavailability 75%) C_{max}: 2 µg/ml Half-life: 16-20 hr No single major metabolic pathway identified, although CYP3A4 contributes ~20% to metabolism; excreted in urine and feces	Adverse effects reported based on combination treatment with bedaquiline and linezolid: Peripheral and optic neuropathy, QT prolongation Myelosuppression: Hematologic: Thrombocytopenia, leukopenia, anemia Transaminitis, hepatic toxicity Lactic acidosis GI: Diarrhea, nausea Rash Headache

C_{max}, Maximum concentration; *CNS*, central nervous system; *CrCl*, creatinine clearance; *CYP3A4*, cytochrome P-450 enzyme; *EMB*, ethambutol; *GI*, gastrointestinal; *HIV*, human immunodeficiency virus; *INH*, isoniazid; *NAT2*, N-acetyltransferase 2; *RIF*, rifampin; *PZA*, pyrazinamide; *tiw*, three times weekly.
From Broaddus VC et al: *Murray & Nadel's textbook of respiratory medicine*, ed 7, Philadelphia 2022, Elsevier.

a. Minimal aspartate aminotransferase/alanine transaminase elevations without symptoms generally transient and not clinically significant
- Drug resistance (often multiple drug resistance TB [MDRTB]) increased by:
  1. Prior treatment
  2. Acquisition of TB in countries with high TB burden
  3. Known contact with MDR TB
  4. Other factors associated with increased risk: Homelessness, incarceration, AIDS, IV drug use
- Other medications used in MDR or XDR TB include levofloxacin, moxifloxacin, cycloserine, aminoglycosides such as amikacin or kanamycin, PAS, clofazimine, bedaquiline, delamanid, pretomanid, linezolid, and ethionamide. A recent trial with the combination of bedaquiline, pretomanid, and

linezolid revealed a favorable outcome at 6 mo after the end of therapy in a high percentage of patients with highly drug-resistant forms of TB. Other trials[3] have shown that a 6-month bedaquiline pretomanid-moxifloxacin regimen that included linezolid at a dose of 600 mg daily may be used in place of longer regimens in persons older than 14 yr of age who have multidrug-resistant or rifampin-resistant TB, regardless of their HIV status
- Drug-resistant TB should be treated in consultation with a TB expert
- Preventive treatment for PPD conversion only (infection without disease)
  1. Must be certain that chest x-ray examination is negative and patient has no symptoms of TB
  2. Most important groups:
     a. HIV-positive and other severely immunocompromised patients

b. Close contact with active TB
c. Recent converter
d. Old TB on chest x-ray examination
e. IV drug addict
f. Medical risk factor
g. High-risk foreign country
h. Homeless
i. Box 1 summarizes persons in whom preventive therapy should be initiated to prevent progression to TB
3. Treatment of latent *M. tuberculosis* (Tables 3 and 4)
- Infants generally given prophylaxis immediately if recent contact with active TB (even if infant PPD negative), then retested with PPD in 3 mo (continuing INH if PPD becomes positive and stopping preventive treatment if PPD remains negative)

BOX 1 Persons in Whom Treatment Should Be Initiated to Prevent Progression to Tuberculosis

Household members and other close associates of persons with potentially infectious tuberculosis
    Contacts of any age with a Mantoux tuberculin skin test reading of 5 mm or greater and no documented history of reaction in the past, or with a positive interferon gamma release assay (IGRA), should be considered recently infected and receive therapy if they have not been treated previously
Newly infected people, regardless of age, who have had a tuberculin skin test or IGRA conversion within the past 2 yr
People with HIV infection who have a reaction of 5 mm or greater to a Mantoux test or positive IGRA
People of any age with past tuberculosis infection who received inadequate treatment
People of any age with a positive tuberculin skin test or positive IGRA and an abnormal but stable chest radiograph
People with significant tuberculin reactions or positive IGRAs who have special clinical situations, including silicosis, diabetes mellitus, prolonged corticosteroid therapy, immunosuppressive therapy, hematologic malignant disease, or end-stage renal disease
All children and adolescents with a positive tuberculin skin test reaction or interferon release assay result

Adapted from Cherry JD et al: *Feigin and Cherry's textbook of pediatric infectious diseases,* ed 8, Philadelphia, 2019, Elsevier.

TABLE 3 Recommendations for Regimens to Treat Latent Tuberculosis Infection

Priority Rank*	Regimen	Recommendation (strong or conditional)	Evidence (high, moderate, low, or very low)
Preferred	3 mo INH plus rifapentine given once weekly	Strong	Moderate
Preferred	4 mo RIF given daily	Strong	Moderate (HIV negative)[†]
Preferred	3 mo INH plus RIF given daily	Conditional	Very low (HIV negative)
		Conditional	Low (HIV positive)
Alternative	6 mo INH given daily	Strong[§]	Moderate (HIV negative)
		Conditional	Moderate (HIV positive)
Alternative	9 mo isoniazid given daily	Conditional	Moderate

*Preferred: Excellent tolerability and efficacy, shorter treatment duration, higher completion rates than longer regimens and therefore higher effectiveness. *Alternative:* Excellent efficacy but concerns regarding longer treatment duration, lower completion rates, and therefore lower effectiveness.
[†]No evidence reported in HIV-positive persons.
[§]Strong recommendation for those persons unable to take a preferred regimen (e.g., due to drug intolerability or drug-drug interactions).
HIV, Human immunodeficiency virus; *INH,* isoniazid; *RIF,* rifampin.
From Sterling TR et al: Guidelines for the treatment of latent tuberculosis infection: recommendations from the National Tuberculosis Controllers Association and CDC, 2020, *MMWR Morb Mortal Wkly Rep* 69(1):1-11, 2020, Table 3.

CHRONIC Rx

Generally not indicated beyond treatment described previously

DISPOSITION

- Monthly follow-up by physician experienced in TB treatment.
- Confirm sensitivity testing and alter treatment appropriately.
- Frequent sputum samples until culture is negative.
- Confirm regression on chest x-ray examination at 2 to 3 mo.
- Approximately 5% of patients with drug-susceptible TB have a relapse after 6 mo of first-line therapy. Higher minimum inhibitory concentration values of INH or RIF in predominant isolates of *M. tuberculosis* are associated with a greater risk of relapse.

REFERRAL

- To infectious disease expert for:
  1. HIV-positive patient
  2. Patient with suspected drug-resistant TB
  3. Patients previously treated for TB
  4. Patients whose fever has not decreased and sputum has not converted to negative in 2 to 4 wk

5. Patients with overwhelming pulmonary or extrapulmonary TB
- To pulmonologist for bronchoscopy or pleural biopsy, if necessary for diagnosis

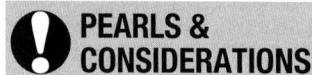 **PEARLS & CONSIDERATIONS**

COMMENTS

- All contacts (especially close household contacts and infants) should be properly tested for PPD or IGRA conversions during 3 mo after exposure.
- Those with positive PPD or IGRA should be evaluated for active TB and properly treated or given prophylaxis.
- Previous treatment is a common risk factor for XDR and MDR TB.
- In treatment of LTBIs, evidence exists for the efficacy and safety of INH monotherapy, rifampicin monotherapy, and combination therapies.
- Left untreated, 5% to 10% of patients with latent TB develop active TB. Updated guidelines from the CDC and the National Tuberculosis Controllers Association for latent TB

treatment include any of the following regimens:
1. Once-weekly INH plus rifapentine for 3 mo administered under direct observation. The guideline recommends this regimen for adults and children (age <2 yr), including patients who are HIV-positive.
2. Daily RIF for 4 mo is also strongly recommended, especially for HIV-negative people, and perhaps has the lowest toxicity.
3. Daily RIF plus INH for 3 mo is another alternative.
4. A recent 4 mo trial of rifapentine regimens with or without moxifloxacin for tuberculosis revealed that the efficacy of a 4-mo rifapentine-based regimen containing moxifloxacin was noninferior to the standard 6-mo regimen in the treatment of tuberculosis.[1]

AUTHORS: **TARA C. BOUTON, MD, MPH, TM,** and **GLENN G. FORT, MD, MPH**

REFERENCES & SUGGESTED READINGS

Available at eBooks.Health.Elsevier.com.

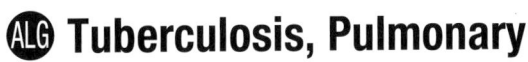
TABLE 4 Dosages for Recommended Latent Tuberculosis Infection Treatment Regimens

Drug	Duration	Dose and Age Group	Frequency	Total Doses
INH* and rifapentine†	3 mo	Adults and children aged ≥12 yr INH: 15 mg/kg rounded up to the nearest 50 or 100 mg; 900 mg maximum Rifapentine: 10-14 kg, 300 mg 14.1-25 kg, 450 mg 25.1-32 kg, 600 mg 32.1-49.9 kg, 750 mg ≥50 kg, 900 mg maximum **Children aged 2-11 yr** INH*: 25 mg/kg; 900 mg maximum Rifapentine†: See earlier	Once weekly	12
RIF¶	4 mo	**Adults:** 10 mg/kg **Children:** 15-20 mg/kg** **Maximum dose:** 600 mg	Daily	120
INH* and RIF¶	3 mo	**Adults** INH*: 5 mg/kg; 300 mg maximum RIF¶: 10 mg/kg; 600 mg maximum **Children** INH*: 10-20 mg/kg††; 300 mg maximum RIF¶: 15-20 mg/kg; 600 mg maximum	Daily	90
INH*	6 mo	**Adults:** 5 mg/kg **Children:** 10-20 mg/kg†† **Maximum dose:** 300 mg	Daily	180
		Adults: 15 mg/kg **Children:** 20-40 mg/kg†† **Maximum dose:** 900 mg	Twice weekly§	52
	9 mo	**Adults:** 5 mg/kg **Children:** 10-20 mg/kg†† **Maximum dose:** 300 mg	Daily	270
		Adults: 15 mg/kg **Children:** 20-40 mg/kg†† **Maximum dose:** 900 mg	Twice weekly§	76

*Isoniazid is formulated as 100- and 300-mg tablets.
†Rifapentine is formulated as 150-mg tablets in blister packs that should be kept sealed until use.
§Intermittent regimens must be provided via directly observed therapy (i.e., a health care worker observes the ingestion of medication).
¶RIF (rifampicin) is formulated as 150- and 300-mg capsules.
**The American Academy of Pediatrics acknowledges that some experts use rifampin at 20-30 mg/kg for the daily regimen when prescribing for infants and toddlers. (From American Academy of Pediatrics: Tuberculosis. In Kimberlin DW et al [eds]: *Red book: 2018 report of the Committee on Infectious Diseases,* ed 31, Itasca, IL: 2018, American Academy of Pediatrics, pp. 829-853.)
††The American Academy of Pediatrics recommends an isoniazid dosage of 10-15 mg/kg for the daily regimen and 20-30 mg/kg for the twice-weekly regimen.
INH, Isoniazid; *RIF,* rifampin.
From Sterling TR et al: Guidelines for the treatment of latent tuberculosis infection: recommendations from the National Tuberculosis Controllers Association and CDC, 2020, *MMWR Morb Mortal Wkly Rep* 69(1):1-11, 2020, Table 4.

Diseases and Disorders

I

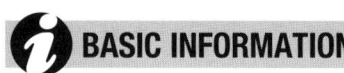

BASIC INFORMATION

DEFINITION
Ulcerative colitis (UC) is an idiopathic, remitting and relapsing, chronic inflammatory bowel disease (IBD) that starts in the rectum and extends proximally.

SYNONYMS
UC
Inflammatory bowel disease (IBD)
Idiopathic proctocolitis
Pancolitis

ICD-10CM CODES
K51.0	Ulcerative pancolitis
K51.2	Ulcerative proctitis
K51.3	Ulcerative rectosigmoiditis
K51.5	Left-sided colitis
K51.90	Ulcerative colitis, unspecified, without complications
K51.80	Other ulcerative colitis without complications
K51.811	Other ulcerative colitis with rectal bleeding
K51.812	Other ulcerative colitis with intestinal obstruction
K51.813	Other ulcerative colitis with fistula
K51.814	Other ulcerative colitis with abscess
K51.818	Other ulcerative colitis with other complication
K51.819	Other ulcerative colitis with unspecified complications
K51.911	Ulcerative colitis, unspecified with rectal bleeding
K51.912	Ulcerative colitis, unspecified with intestinal obstruction
K51.913	Ulcerative colitis, unspecified with fistula
K51.914	Ulcerative colitis, unspecified with abscess
K51.918	Ulcerative colitis, unspecified with other complication
K51.919	Ulcerative colitis, unspecified with unspecified complications

EPIDEMIOLOGY & DEMOGRAPHICS
INCIDENCE: The incidence of UC is 9 to 12 cases/100,000 persons per yr in the U.S.; worldwide, the estimated incidence ranges from 1.2 to 20.3 cases/100,000 person-yr, and its prevalence ranges from 7.6 to 246.0/100,000 persons. It is most common between ages 15 and 40 yr, with a second peak between 50 and 80 yr. The disease affects men and women at similar rates. Infection with nontyphoid *Salmonella* or *Campylobacter* is associated with an 8 to 10 times higher risk of developing UC in the following year. Worldwide, UC is more common than Crohn disease.
PREVALENCE: The prevalence of UC is 7.6 to 246.0 cases/100,000 per yr. Higher prevalence in Ashkenazi Jewish descendants.
GENETICS:
- Both specific and nonspecific gene variants are associated with UC.

- There are 47 loci associated with UC, of which 19 are specific for UC and 28 are shared with Crohn disease.
- Abnormalities in humoral and cellular adaptive immunity are also found in UC.

GEOGRAPHIC DISTRIBUTION: The highest incidence and prevalence of IBD are seen in northern Europe and North America, and the lowest in continental Asia.

PHYSICAL FINDINGS & CLINICAL PRESENTATION
- Patients with UC often present with acute onset of bloody diarrhea accompanied by tenesmus, fever, and dehydration. At presentation 40% of adults have proctitis, 40% have left-sided colitis, and 20% have pancolitis. Diarrhea is not always present in UC patients with proctosigmoiditis and proctitis, and patients may have constipation.
- Abdominal pain is not usually a prominent symptom. Abdominal distention and tenderness may indicate the presence of complications such as toxic megacolon.
- The onset of symptoms is typically acute and is generally followed by periods of spontaneous remission and frequent relapses.
- Fever, evidence of dehydration may be present during the acute flare-up.
- Evidence of extraintestinal manifestations may be present in nearly 25% of patients: Liver disease, sclerosing cholangitis, iritis, uveitis, episcleritis, arthritis, erythema nodosum, pyoderma gangrenosum, aphthous stomatitis. Box 1 summarizes common extraintestinal manifestations of UC.

ETIOLOGY & PATHOGENESIS
Accumulating evidence suggests that it may result from an inappropriate inflammatory response to environmental triggers and immune dysregulation involving CD4+ T-cell Th2 response in a genetically susceptible host.

DIAGNOSIS

DIFFERENTIAL DIAGNOSIS (TABLE 1, BOX 2)
- Crohn disease
- Bacterial infections:
  1. Acute: *Campylobacter, Yersinia, Salmonella, Shigella, Chlamydia, Escherichia coli, Clostridioides difficile,* gonococcal proctitis
  2. Chronic: Whipple disease, tuberculosis, enterocolitis
- Irritable bowel syndrome
- Protozoal and parasitic infections (amebiasis, giardiasis, cryptosporidiosis)
- Neoplasm (intestinal lymphoma, carcinoma of colon)
- Ischemic bowel disease
- Diverticulitis
- Celiac sprue, lymphocytic or collagenous colitis, radiation enteritis, endometriosis
- Solitary rectal ulcer
- Acute self-limited colitis
- Medication (NSAIDs, chemotherapy)

WORKUP
An accurate diagnosis of UC should define the extent and severity of inflammation. Diagnostic workup includes:
- Comprehensive history, physical examination
- Laboratory tests (see "Laboratory Tests")
- Colonoscopy to establish the presence of mucosal inflammation; typical endoscopic findings in UC are areas of continuous friable mucosa; diffuse, uniform erythema replacing the usual mucosal vascular pattern (Table 2); and pseudopolyps. The transition from abnormal to normal tissue tends to be abrupt. Rectal involvement is invariably present if the disease is active. Pathologic findings suggestive of UC include crypt abscesses and atrophy, mucin depletion, basal plasmacytosis, basal lymphoid aggregates, increased lamina propria cellularity, and Paneth cell metaplasia

LABORATORY TESTS
- Anemia and high erythrocyte sedimentation rate (in severe colitis) are common, but normal levels do not rule out the disorder.

BOX 1   Common Extraintestinal Manifestations of Ulcerative Colitis

Cutaneous/Oral
Angular stomatitis
Aphthous stomatitis
Erythema nodosum
Oral ulcerations
Psoriasis
Pyoderma gangrenosum
Pyostomatitis vegetans
Sweet syndrome (acute febrile neutrophilic dermatosis)

Ophthalmologic
Conjunctivitis
Episcleritis
Retinal vascular disease
Scleritis
Uveitis, iritis

Musculoskeletal
Ankylosing spondylitis
Osteomalacia
Osteonecrosis
Osteopenia
Osteoporosis
Peripheral arthropathy
Sacroiliitis

Hepatobiliary
Autoimmune hepatitis
Cholangiocarcinoma
Pericholangitis
Primary sclerosing cholangitis
Hepatic steatosis

Hematologic
Anemia of chronic disease
Autoimmune hemolytic anemia
Hypercoagulable state
Iron deficiency anemia
Leukocytosis or thrombocytosis
Leukopenia or thrombocytopenia

From Feldman M et al: Sleisenger and Fordtran's gastrointestinal and liver disease, ed 10, Philadelphia, 2016, Elsevier.

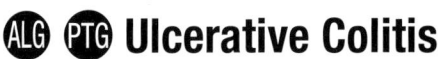
TABLE 1 Features That Distinguish Ulcerative Colitis From Other Diagnoses

Diagnosis	Clinical Features	Radiologic and Colonoscopic Features	Histologic Features
UC	Bloody diarrhea	Extends proximally from rectum; fine mucosal ulceration	Distortion of crypts; acute and chronic diffuse inflammatory cell infiltrate; goblet cell depletion; crypt abscesses; lymphoid aggregates
Crohn colitis	Perianal lesions are common; may be associated with ileitis; frank bleeding is less common than in UC	Segmental disease; rectal sparing; strictures, fissures, ulcers, fistulas; small bowel involvement	Focal inflammation; submucosal involvement; granulomas; goblet cell preservation; transmural inflammation, fissuring
Ischemic colitis	Occurs in older adults; sudden onset, often painful; usually resolves spontaneously in several days	Segmental splenic flexure and sigmoid involvement are most common, with thumbprinting early and ulceration after 24-72 hr; rectal involvement is rare	Mucosal necrosis with ghost cells; congestion with red blood cells; hemosiderin-laden macrophages and fibrosis (when disease is chronic)
Microscopic colitis	Watery diarrhea; normal-appearing mucosa at colonoscopy	Usually normal	Chronic inflammatory infiltrate; increased intraepithelial lymphocytes (lymphocytic colitis) and/or subepithelial collagen band (collagenous colitis)
Infectious colitis	Sudden onset; identifiable source in some cases (e.g., *Salmonella* spp.); pain may predominate (e.g., *Campylobacter* spp.); pathogens are present in stool	Nonspecific findings	Crypt architecture is usually normal; edema, superficial neutrophilic infiltrate, crypt abscesses
Amebic colitis	History of travel to endemic area; amebae may be detected in a fresh stool specimen, but ELISA for amebic lectin antigen is the preferable diagnostic test	Discrete ulcers; ameboma or strictures	Similar to UC; amebae present in lamina propria or in flask-shaped ulcers, identified by periodic acid–Schiff stain
Gonococcal proctitis	Rectal pain; pus	Granular changes in rectum	Intense polymorphonuclear neutrophil infiltration; purulent exudate; gram-negative diplococci
Pseudomembranous colitis	Often a history of antibiotic use; characteristic pseudomembranes may be seen on sigmoidoscopy; *Clostridioides difficile* toxin is detectable in stools	Edematous; shaggy outline of colon; pseudomembranes may be identified radiologically or seen at colonoscopy	May resemble acute ischemic colitis; summit lesions of fibrinopurulent exudate

ELISA, Enzyme-linked immunosorbent assay; *UC,* ulcerative colitis.
From Feldman M et al: *Sleisenger and Fordtran's gastrointestinal and liver disease,* ed 10, Philadelphia, 2016, Elsevier.

Diseases and Disorders

- Potassium, magnesium, calcium, and albumin may be decreased.
- Antineutrophil cytoplasmic antibodies (ANCA) with a perinuclear staining pattern (pANCA) can be found in >45% of patients; there is an increased frequency in treatment-resistant left-sided colitis, suggesting a possible association between these antibodies and a relative resistance to medical therapy in patients with UC.
- Calprotectin is a protein that is measured in feces as a marker of intestinal mucosa leukocyte activity that may be useful for screening of patients with suspected IBD. Trials have shown that based on a pretest probability of IBD of 32% in adults, an abnormal fecal calprotectin test would increase the posttest probability to 91% and a normal result would reduce the probability to 3%.
- Fecal lactoferrin is also a sensitive marker of intestinal inflammation.
- Stool examinations for ova and parasites, stool culture, and testing for *C. difficile* toxin and *E. coli* O157:H7 may be useful to eliminate other causes of diarrhea in selected patients with risk factors.

IMAGING STUDIES

Image studies (plain radiography, CT scan [Fig. E1]) are generally reserved for suspected complications such as perforation of bowel or toxic megacolon.

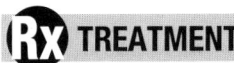 **TREATMENT**

NONPHARMACOLOGIC THERAPY

- Correct nutritional deficiencies; total parenteral nutrition with bowel rest may be necessary in severe cases. Folate supplementation may reduce the incidence of dysplasia and cancer in chronic UC.
- Avoid oral feedings during acute exacerbation to decrease colonic activity; a low-roughage diet may be helpful in early relapse.
- Psychotherapy is useful in most patients. Referral to self-help groups is also important because of the chronicity of the disease and the young age of the patients.

ACUTE GENERAL Rx

The therapeutic options (Table 3) vary with the degree of disease (mild, severe, fulminant) and areas of involvement (distal, extensive).

- Mild disease can be treated with 5-aminosalicylate agents (mesalamine, olsalazine, balsalazide, sulfasalazine). It can be administered as an enema (40 mg once daily at bedtime for 3 to 6 wk) or suppository (500 mg bid) for patients with distal colonic disease. Oral forms in which the 5-acetyl salicylic acid is in a slow-release or pH-dependent matrix (Pentasa 1 g qid, Asacol 800 mg PO tid) can deliver therapeutic concentrations to the more proximal small bowel or distal ileum. Olsalazine can be useful for maintenance of remission of UC in patients intolerant to sulfasalazine. Usual dose is 500 mg bid taken with food. Balsalazide is indicated for mild to moderately active UC. Usual dose is three 750-mg capsules tid. Probiotics may also be helpful in inducing remission in mild-to-moderate UC.
- Mild-to-moderate UC is often treated with a combination of rectal and oral 5-aminosalicylate. Refractory patients are candidates for oral glucocorticoids or immunosuppressive agents (e.g., cyclosporine).
- Severe disease usually responds to oral corticosteroids (e.g., prednisone 40 to 60 mg/

Infectious Causes
Aeromonas hydrophila
Campylobacter jejuni
Chlamydia spp.
Clostridioides difficile
Cytomegalovirus
Entamoeba histolytica
Escherichia coli O157:H7, other EHEC
Herpes simplex virus (HSV)
Listeria monocytogenes
Neisseria gonorrhoeae
Salmonella spp.
Schistosomiasis
Shigella spp.
Yersinia enterocolitica

Noninfectious Causes
Acute self-limited colitis
Behçet disease
Crohn disease
Diversion colitis
Diverticulitis
Drugs and toxins
  Chemotherapy
  Gold
  Penicillamine
Eosinophilic colitis
Graft-versus-host disease
Ischemic colitis
Microscopic colitis
  Collagenous
  Lymphocytic
Neutropenic colitis (typhlitis)
NSAIDs
Radiation colitis
Segmental colitis associated with diverticulosis
Solitary rectal ulcer syndrome

From Feldman M et al: *Sleisenger and Fordtran's gastrointestinal and liver disease,* ed 10, Philadelphia, 2016, Elsevier.

TABLE 2 Endoscopic Differentiation of Ulcerative Colitis and Crohn Disease

Feature	Ulcerative Colitis	Crohn Disease
Distribution	Diffuse inflammation that extends proximally from the anorectal junction	Rectal sparing, frequent skip lesions
Inflammation	Diffuse erythema, early loss of vascular markings with mucosal granularity or friability	Focal and asymmetric, cobblestoning; granularity and friability less commonly seen
Ulceration	Small ulcers in a diffusely inflamed mucosa; deep, ragged ulcers in severe disease	Aphthoid ulcers, linear or serpiginous ulceration; intervening mucosa is often normal
Colonic lumen	Often narrowed in long-standing chronic disease; tubular colon; strictures are rare	Strictures are common

From Feldman M et al: *Sleisenger and Fordtran's gastrointestinal and liver disease,* ed 10, Philadelphia, 2016, Elsevier.

maintenance of remission. In patients with moderately to severely active ulcerative colitis who cannot tolerate or respond poorly to TNF inhibitors oral Janus kinase inhibitors (tofacitinib or upadacitinib) may be effective. The FDA has also approved ozanimod, an oral sphingosine 1-phosphate (S1P) receptor modulator for treatment of adults with moderately to severe active ulcerative colitis who had an inadequate response to or would not tolerate other drugs.

- Fulminant disease generally requires hospital admission and parenteral corticosteroids (e.g., IV hydrocortisone 100 mg q6h). When bowel movements have returned to normal and the patient is able to eat normally, PO prednisone is resumed. IV cyclosporine can also be used in severe refractory cases; renal toxicity is a potential complication.
- Surgery is indicated in patients who do not respond to intensive medical therapy. Fig. 2 illustrates the surgical management of chronic UC.
- Proctocolectomy is usually curative in these patients and also eliminates the high risk of developing adenocarcinoma of the colon (10% to 20% of patients develop it after 10 yr with the disease). Total proctocolectomy with ileal pouch–anal anastomosis (IPAA) is the procedure of choice for most patients who require elective surgery, since it preserves anal sphincter function. Continent ileostomy is an alternative procedure.

CHRONIC Rx

- Colonoscopic surveillance and multiple biopsies should be instituted approximately 10 yr after diagnosis because of the increased risk of colon carcinoma.

- Erythropoietin is useful in patients with anemia refractory to treatment with iron and vitamins.
- In patients on long-term steroid therapy, periodic bone density scans are recommended to screen for glucocorticoid-induced osteoporosis.

DISPOSITION

- The natural history of the disease is one of remission and episodic flares.
- The clinical course is variable. ~66% of patients will achieve clinical remission with medical therapy, and nearly 80% of treatment-compliant patients maintain remission. 15% to 20% of patients eventually require colectomy. Pouchitis is the most common long-term complication of IPAA (up to 40% of patients). >75% of patients treated medically will experience relapse.

REFERRAL

- GI consultation for initial diagnostic sigmoidoscopy/colonoscopy in suspected cases.
- Surgical referral for patients with severe disease unresponsive to medical therapy. Indications for surgery in patients with UC are summarized in Box 3.

SUGGESTED READINGS
Available at eBooks.Health.Elsevier.com.

RELATED CONTENT
Ulcerative Colitis (Patient Information)

AUTHOR: **FRED F. FERRI, MD**

day); the FDA has recently approved an extended-release formulation of the corticosteroid budesonide for induction of remission in mild to moderate UC. Corticosteroid suppositories or enemas are also useful for distal colitis. The immunosuppressant azathioprine or mercaptopurine also provides effective long-term treatment for Crohn disease. In patients with moderately to severely active disease, a tumor necrosis factor (TNF) inhibitor (infliximab, adalimumab, golimumab), an integrin receptor antagonist (vedolizumab), or an interleukin (IL) 12-23 antagonist (ustekinumab) are useful for both induction and

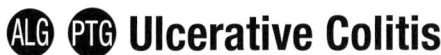

TABLE 3 Medical Therapy Used in Ulcerative Colitis

Drug	Release Site	Treatment of UC	Side Effects
Oral 5-aminosalicylates			
Sulfasalazine	Colon	Induce and maintain remission in mild-to-moderate UC	Sulfasalazine: Idiosyncratic (rash, hepatitis, aplastic anemia), dose-related (nausea, hemolytic anemia, inhibits folic acid transport), oligospermia (reversible)
Mesalamine (mesalazine)	Distal ileum, colon	Use in combination with topical mesalamine for distal colitis	
Mesalamine (mesalazine) (controlled-release)	Duodenum, jejunum, ileum, colon		
Olsalazine	Colon		
Balsalazide	Colon		
Topical 5-aminosalicylates			
Mesalamine (mesalazine) enema	Rectum, sigmoid	Induce and maintain remission in mild-to-moderate distal disease	
Mesalamine (mesalazine) suppository	Rectum	Combination therapy with oral aminosalicylates are superior to monotherapy	
Antibiotics			
Ciprofloxacin	Systemic	Antibiotics are not used for the treatment of UC but are used for pouchitis	Ciprofloxacin: Tendonitis and rupture
Metronidazole			Metronidazole: Neuropathy
Amoxicillin/clavulanic acid			Amoxicillin/clavulanic acid: Hepatitis
Rifaximin			
Corticosteroids			
Budesonide extended-release	Colon	Induce remission in mild-to-moderate UC Should not be used for maintenance	High first-pass metabolism More favorable side-effect profile than prednisone
Prednisone	Systemic	Induce remission in mild-to-moderate and some moderate-to-severe UC flares Not used for maintenance therapy	Infection, diabetes mellitus, osteoporosis, osteonecrosis, cataracts, glaucoma, and myopathy. Increase risk of mortality
Methylprednisolone	Systemic	Induce remission in severe UC	As for prednisone
Immunomodulators			
6-Mercaptopurine	Systemic	Maintain remission in steroid-dependent, steroid-refractory, or steroid-induced-remission UC	Allergic reactions, pancreatitis, myelosuppression, nausea, infections, hepatotoxicity, and malignancy, in particular lymphoma
Azathioprine	Systemic	Not used to induce remission	
Cyclosporine	Systemic	Rescue therapy to induce remission in severe UC not responding to IV methylprednisolone	Infections, hypertension, renal insufficiency, tremor, headache, hepatotoxicity
Biologicals			
Infliximab	Systemic	Can be used to induce and maintain moderate-to-severe UC and are steroid-sparing	Infections (tuberculosis, fungal infections), autoantibody formation, psoriasis, drug-induced lupus
Adalimumab	Systemic	Infliximab is also used as a rescue therapy to induce remission in severe UC not responding to IV methylprednisolone	Infusion reactions (infliximab), injection-site reaction (adalimumab and golimumab), delayed hypersensitivity reaction (infliximab)
Golimumab	Systemic		Lymphoma (higher in combination therapy)
Vedolizumab	Systemic	Effective in the induction and maintenance of remission in moderate-to-severe UC	Headache, infections, abdominal pain, infusion reactions
Tofacitinib (small molecules)	Systemic	Effective in induction and maintenance	Infections (especially herpes zoster), lymphoma

UC, Ulcerative colitis.
From Talley NJ et al: *Essentials of internal medicine,* ed 4, Chatswood, NSW, 2021, Elsevier Australia.

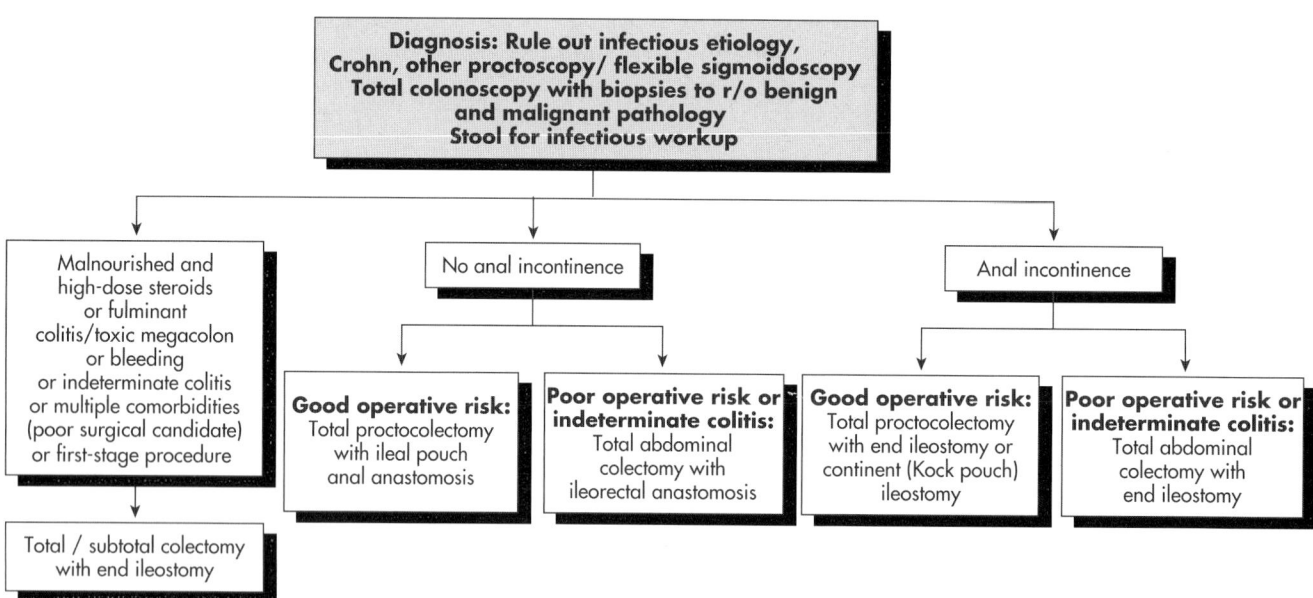

FIG. 2 Surgical management of chronic ulcerative colitis. (From Cameron JL, Cameron AM: *Current surgical therapy,* ed 12, Philadelphia, 2017, Elsevier.)

BOX 3 Indications for Surgery in Patients With Ulcerative Colitis

Colonic dysplasia or carcinoma
Colonic perforation
Growth retardation
Intolerable or unacceptable side effects of medical therapy
Medically refractory disease
Systemic complications that are recurrent or unmanageable
Toxic megacolon
Uncontrollable colonic hemorrhage

From Feldman M et al: *Sleisenger and Fordtran's gastrointestinal and liver disease,* ed 10, Philadelphia, 2016, Elsevier.

BASIC INFORMATION

DEFINITION

Urethritis is a well-defined clinical syndrome manifested by dysuria, a urethral discharge, or both.

SYNONYMS

Gonococcal urethritis
GCU

ICD-10CM CODE

A54.00 Gonococcal infection of lower genitourinary tract, unspecified

EPIDEMIOLOGY & DEMOGRAPHICS

- Urethritis commonly is divided into two major categories based on etiology: Gonococcal urethritis (GCU, *Neisseria gonorrhoeae* spp.) and nongonococcal urethritis (NGU, all other pathogens, most commonly *Chlamydia trachomatis*).
- This differentiation is based historically on *N. gonorrhoeae*'s easy visualization on Gram stain as gram-negative, kidney-shaped diplococci.
- In the U.S., rates of gonorrheal urethritis are rising; however, the incidence varies greatly based on race and geography; the prevalence of GCU is disproportionately higher in the South and among Black, non-Hispanic men. The urethra is the most common site of infection in all men.

PHYSICAL FINDINGS & CLINICAL PRESENTATION

- Symptoms of GCU: Dysuria is the most common chief complaint in patients with GCU, which is often accompanied by discharge and pruritus. Acute-onset purulent discharge is a hallmark of this infection. Additionally, meatal edema and urethral tenderness to palpation may occur. Approximately 5% to 10% of patients with GCU remain asymptomatic.

- GCU may spread to other parts of the genitourinary system. Prostatic involvement can cause urinary frequency, urgency, and nocturia and may present with mucopurulent discharge. Epididymal involvement can result in unilateral testicular pain and edema.
- Time frame: The incubation period of GCU is variable but is commonly 4 to 7 days. Without treatment, urethritis will persist for 3 to 7 wk, with 95% of men becoming asymptomatic after 3 mo.
- Complications: Periurethritis leading to urethral stenosis can occur. Additionally, disseminated infection can lead to tenosynovitis and arthritis. Rarely, hepatitis, myocarditis, endocarditis, and meningitis can occur.

DIAGNOSIS

DIFFERENTIAL DIAGNOSIS (TABLE 1)

- NGU
- Herpes simplex virus

LABORATORY TESTS

- Urethritis is diagnosed when a symptomatic male has any of the following characteristics:
  1. Mucopurulent/purulent discharge on examination
  2. Urethral swab showing:
     a. $\geq$2 WBCs per field in high-prevalence settings or $\geq$5 WBCs per field in lower prevalence settings
     b. Gram-negative diplococci seen within WBCs
- Urethritis can be diagnosed by culture or by NAATs.[1] The performance of NAATs with respect to overall sensitivity, specificity, and ease of specimen transport is better than that of any of the other tests available for the diagnosis of chlamydial and gonococcal infections. NAATs should be used as first line to detect chlamydia and gonorrhea, except in cases of child sexual assault, rectal and

oropharyngeal infections in prepubescent girls, and when evaluating a potential gonorrhea treatment failure, in which case culture and susceptibility testing might be required.
- Of note, a presumptive diagnosis can be made without the earlier diagnostic criteria for males who are at high risk for sexually transmitted infections (i.e., more than one partner and >25 yr) and who are unlikely to return for follow-up. In these patients, empirical treatment to cover both gonococcal and nongonococcal infections can be given before the results of a nucleic acid amplification test (NAAT).
- Similarly, when in-person testing is not feasible in situations such as the COVID-19 pandemic, sexually active patients with symptoms consistent with urethritis should be treated with a regimen active against gonorrhea. (Dear Colleague Letter: Providing effective care and prevention when facility-based services and in-person patient-clinician contact is limited, 2020).
- If Gram staining is available, it is indicated and should be performed with modified Thayer-Martin media, as this helps differentiate GCU from NGU.
- NAATs have largely replaced culture in many health care settings. They are not more sensitive than culture for detecting *N. gonorrhoeae* in cervical or urethral specimens; however, they have specificities of >99% and retain sensitivity when used to test first-catch urine.
- For culture and susceptibility testing: Rayon, Dacron, or calcium alginate tips with plastic or wire shafts should be used (not cotton-tipped swabs, which are bactericidal). A swab of the urethra should be performed within 2 to 4 hr after voiding to prevent bacterial washout with urination. Collect cultures of the pharynx and rectum when indicated for concomitant *Chlamydia* testing on all patients.
- Concomitant serologic testing for syphilis and HIV infections should be offered to all patients.

TREATMENT

Regimen for adults and adolescents weighing >45 kg with GCU :
- Ceftriaxone 500 mg IM as a single dose for persons weighing <150 kg (300 lbs)
- For persons weighing $\geq$150 kg (300 lbs), 1 g of IM ceftriaxone should be administered.
- If chlamydial infection has not been excluded, providers should treat for chlamydia with doxycycline 100 mg PO twice daily for 7 days.
Alternative regimen for GCU if cephalosporin allergy:
- Gentamicin 240 mg IM as a single dose plus azithromycin 2 g PO as a single dose.
Alternative regimen for GCU if ceftriaxone not available or administration is not feasible:
- Cefixime 800 mg PO once. If chlamydial infection has not been excluded, providers should treat for chlamydia with doxycycline 100 mg PO twice daily for 7 days.
Regimen for infants and children weighing $\leq$45 kg

TABLE 1 Etiology of Urethritis

Infectious	Noninfectious
Sexually Transmitted Infections	**Vasculitides**
Neisseria gonorrhoeae	Reiter syndrome
Chlamydia trachomatis	Erythema multiforme
Trichomonas vaginalis	Kawasaki disease
Herpes simplex virus type 2	
Mycoplasma spp.	
Nonsexually Transmitted Infections	**Mechanical**
Staphylococcus saprophyticus	Masturbation
Enterobacteriaceae	Foreign body
Gardnerella vaginalis	Trauma
Streptococcus spp.	Dysfunctional elimination
Enterobius vermicularis	**Chemical**
	Soaps
	Detergents
	Drugs

From Cherry JD: *Feigin and Cherry's pediatric infectious diseases*, ed 8, Philadelphia, 2019, Elsevier.

- Ceftriaxone 25 to 50 mg/kg body weight IV or IM as a single dose, but not exceeding 250 mg IM[2]

FOLLOW UP

It is imperative to appropriately counsel patients on the avoidance of intercourse or use of barrier protection until a cure has been obtained and sexual partners have been evaluated. Once treated, patients should be advised to abstain from sex for 7 days.

In cases of suspected cephalosporin treatment failure, clinicians should obtain relevant clinical specimens for culture and antimicrobial susceptibility testing, consult an infectious disease specialist or STD clinical expert (www.stdccn.org/) for guidance in clinical management, and report the case to the Centers for Disease Control and Prevention (CDC) through state and local public health authorities within 24 hr. Health departments should prioritize notification and culture evaluation for the patient's sex partner(s) from the preceding 60 days for those with suspected cephalosporin treatment failure or persons whose gonococcal isolates demonstrate reduced susceptibility to cephalosporins.

A test of cure (repeat testing 1 to 3 wk after initial treatment) is unnecessary for persons with uncomplicated GCU treated with any of the recommended or alternative regimens. However, for persons with pharyngeal gonorrhea, a test of cure is recommended, using culture or NAATs 7 to 14 days after initial treatment, regardless of the treatment regimen.

Alternatively, repeat testing 3 mo after treatment is recommended for all persons diagnosed with GCU, regardless of treatment, because reinfections rates are so high: Reinfection within 12 mo ranges from 7% to 12% among persons previously treated for gonorrhea. If retesting at 3 mo is not possible, clinicians should retest within 12 mo after initial treatment.

CHRONIC INFECTION

- Reinfection is the most common cause of recurrence.
- Repeat swab and culture of the urethra, pharynx, and rectum (where applicable) are mandatory.
- Persistence of *N. gonorrhoeae* by smear or culture requires treatment for *N. gonorrhoeae.*
- Postgonococcal urethritis (PGU): Persistence of polymorphonuclear cells (PMNs) in the absence of gram-negative intracellular diplococci. This occurs when GCU is treated with a regimen that is ineffective against coincident nongonococcal infection; it represents NGU after GCU and should be treated as such.

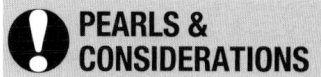

❗ PEARLS & CONSIDERATIONS

COMMENTS

- Partner notification: The names and contact information of sexual partners should be gathered at the time of diagnosis and referred to the health department, or the patient can notify the contact directly.
- Expedited partner treatment is recommended by the CDC and is approved in most states. This consists of giving prescriptions to the infected patient for their partner(s) who has not been evaluated by a physician and for whom health department partner-management strategies are impractical or unavailable.[2]
- On examination of the urethral smear, the presence of small numbers of PMNs provides objective evidence of urethritis. The complete absence of PMNs on a urethral smear argues against urethritis. If in addition to the PMNs there are gram-negative, intracellular diplococci, the diagnosis of gonorrhea is established.

REFERENCES & SUGGESTED READINGS

Available at eBooks.Health.Elsevier.com.

RELATED CONTENT

Gonococcal Urethritis (Patient Information)
Gonorrhea (Related Key Topic)

AUTHORS: **LAUREN ROBY, MD,** and **ANTHONY C. SCISCIONE, DO**

BASIC INFORMATION

DEFINITION

Nongonococcal urethritis (NGU) is urethral inflammation caused by any of several organisms (see "Etiology").

SYNONYMS

NGU
Nongonococcal urethritis

ICD-10CM CODES

A56.0 Chlamydial infection of lower genitourinary tract
N34.1 Nonspecific urethritis

EPIDEMIOLOGY & DEMOGRAPHICS

- The occurrence is 50% in sexually transmitted disease clinics. *Chlamydia trachomatis* is the most common notifiable disease in the U.S., with >1.5 million infections reported to the Centers for Disease Control and Prevention (CDC) in 2016.
- NGU most commonly affects men in a higher socioeconomic class, affecting heterosexual men more frequently than men who have sex with men.
- NGU carries a greater morbidity rate than gonococcal urethritis (GCU).

PHYSICAL FINDINGS & CLINICAL PRESENTATION

- Incubation period: 2 to 35 days.
- Symptoms: Dysuria, whitish-clear urethral discharge, and urethral itching. The onset of symptoms in NGU is less acute than in GCU. The majority of persons with *C. trachomatis* infection are not aware of their infection because they do not have symptoms that would prompt them to seek medical care.
- Signs: Whitish-clear urethral discharge, meatal edema, and erythema. Infected women manifest pyuria, and the disease can present as acute urethral syndrome.

COMPLICATIONS

- Epididymitis in men may be linked to nonbacterial prostatitis, proctitis in men who have sex with men, or Reiter syndrome.
- Urethritis complications are more common in women and can be associated with ectopic pregnancy, pelvic inflammatory disease, or infertility.

ETIOLOGY

- Most common agent is *Chlamydia* spp., an obligate intracellular parasite possessing both DNA and RNA, which replicates by binary fission. It causes 20% to 50% of NGU cases. Two species exist:
  1. *Chlamydia psittaci*
  2. *Chlamydia trachomatis* with its 15 serotypes:
     a. Serotypes A through C cause hyperendemic-blinding trachoma.
     b. Serotypes D through K cause genital tract infection.
     c. Serotypes L1 through L3 cause lymphogranuloma venereum.
- Other causes of NGU: *Mycoplasma genitalium* (found in 44% of treatment failures with double infection with *C. trachomatis* in up to 15% of cases); *Ureaplasma urealyticum,* causing 15% to 30% of the cases of NGU; *Trichomonas vaginalis;* herpes simplex virus; and *Adenovirus*. However, the cause of up to 50% of the cases of NGU may not be identified.
- Asymptomatic infection occurs in 28% of the contacts of women with chlamydial cervical infection.

DIAGNOSIS

DIFFERENTIAL DIAGNOSIS

- Gonococcal urethritis
- Herpes simplex virus
- Trichomoniasis

LABORATORY TESTS

- Requires demonstration of urethritis and exclusion of infection with *N. gonorrhoeae.*
- Nucleic acid amplification tests (NAATs) have replaced culture where persons are screened for asymptomatic genital infection, and yields more sensitivity, specificity, and ease of specimen transport than any other tests available for the diagnosis of chlamydial and gonococcal infections. NAATs should be used to detect chlamydia and gonorrhea except in cases of child sexual assault, rectal and oropharyngeal infections in prepubescent girls, and when evaluating a potential gonorrhea treatment failure, in which case culture and susceptibility testing might be required.
- *Chlamydia* culture: The appearance of polymorphonuclear cells on urethral smear confirms the diagnosis of urethritis. Because *Chlamydia* is an intracellular parasite of the columnar epithelium, the best specimen for culture is an endourethral swab taken from an area 2 to 4 cm inside the urethra. For culture, a Dacron-tipped swab is used; avoid calcium alginate or cotton swabs. The organism can only be grown in tissue culture, which is expensive.

TREATMENT

- Because it is impossible to differentiate among the common causes of NGU, the condition is treated syndromically, including in the initial treatment regimen those drugs effective against the common causative agents.
- In patients with isolated uncomplicated NGU, the recommended regimen is doxycycline 100 mg bid for 7 days. An alternative regimen is azithromycin 1 g PO single dose or 500 mg PO in a single dose followed by 250 mg PO daily for 4 days.

- Recommended treatment for isolated uncomplicated NGU in pregnancy is azithromycin, 1 g PO as a single dose or amoxicillin 500 mg tid for 7 days.
- In patients with confirmed urethritis and unclear etiology, concurrent treatment for gonorrhea and *Chlamydia* is recommended. In these patients, uncomplicated infections of the urethra can be treated with combination of a single 1-g dose of oral azithromycin or 100 mg doxycycline bid for 7 days *plus* ceftriaxone 250 mg × 1 dose.
- In areas where *T. vaginitis* is prevalent, men who have sex with women and have persistent or recurrent urethritis should be presumably treated with metronidazole 2 g PO or a single dose of tinidazole 2 g PO.
- Patients with recurrent NGU should initially be assessed for compliance with treatment or reexposure; retreatment of initial therapy should be considered. Alternative retreatment regimens should take into consideration the original treatment. For patients initially treated with doxycycline, consider retreatment with a single dose of azithromycin 1 g. If azithromycin was used for initial treatment, consider retreatment with moxifloxacin 400 mg/day for 6 days.

PEARLS & CONSIDERATIONS

COMMENTS

- Partner notification: The names and contact information of all sexual partners within preceding 60 days should be gathered at the time of the visit and referred to the health department, or the patient notifies the contacts directly. Expedited partner treatment is recommended by the CDC and approved in several states. This consists of giving prescriptions to the infected patient for their partner(s) who have not been evaluated by a physician and are unlikely to seek medical care.
- Patients should abstain from intercourse for 7 days after therapy completion.
- Test of cure for NGU in pregnancy should be performed 4 wk after therapy completion and patients should be rescreened 3 mo after treatment.

SUGGESTED READING

Available at eBooks.Health.Elsevier.com.

RELATED CONTENT

Nongonococcal Urethritis (Patient Information)
Cervicitis (Related Key Topic)
Chlamydia Genital Infections (Related Key Topic)

AUTHORS: **RACHEL WRIGHT HEINLE, MD, FACOG,** and **CHRISTINE BURKE, MD**

Diseases and Disorders

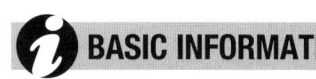

BASIC INFORMATION

DEFINITION

Urinary tract infection (UTI) is a term that encompasses a broad range of clinical entities that have in common a positive urine culture. Most cases are caused by bacteria ascending from the urethra into the bladder. A conventional threshold is growth of >100,000 colony-forming units (CFUs)/ml from a midstream-catch urine sample with no more than two species of organisms and at least one sign or symptom of UTI (urgency, frequency, dysuria, suprapubic tenderness, fever >38.0° C [100.4° F]). In symptomatic patients, using a lower threshold of between 100 and 10,000 CFUs/ml increases diagnostic sensitivity without significantly compromising specificity.

SYNONYM

UTI

ICD-10CM CODES

N39.0	Urinary tract infection, site not specified
N99.521	Infection of other external stoma of urinary tract
N99.531	Infection of other stoma of urinary tract
N30.00	Acute cystitis without hematuria
N30.30	Trigonitis without hematuria
N30.20	Other chronic cystitis without hematuria

CLASSIFICATION

- Uncomplicated UTI: Occurs in a normal urinary tract and resolves rapidly with conventional antimicrobials. These patients have a low risk of upper UTI.
- Complicated UTI: Occurs in patients with coexisting pathology (strictures, stones, comorbidities [diabetes mellitus, multiple sclerosis, spinal cord injuries]). These patients are considered at high risk for upper UTI.
- First infection: The first documented UTI; tends to be uncomplicated and is easily treated.
- Unresolved bacteriuria: UTI in which the urinary tract is not sterilized during therapy. Main causes are bacterial resistance, patient noncompliance with treatment, mixed bacterial infection, rapid reinfection, azotemia, infected stones, Munchausen syndrome, and papillary necrosis.
- Bacterial persistence: UTI in which the urine cultures become sterile during therapy, but a persistent source of infection gives rise to reinfection by the same organism. Causes include chronic bacterial prostatitis, atrophic infected kidney, vesicovaginal or enterovesical fistulas, obstructive uropathy, infected pyelocaliceal diverticula, infected ureteral stump after nephrectomy, infected necrotic papillae from papillary necrosis, infected urachal cysts, infected medullary sponge kidney, urethral diverticula, and foreign bodies.
- Reinfection: UTI in which a new infection occurs with new pathogens at variable intervals after a previous infection has been eradicated.
- Relapse: A less common form of recurrent infection; occurs within 2 wk of treatment when the same organism reappears in the same site as the previous infection. Relapsing infections of the urinary tract most commonly occur in pyelonephritis, kidney obstruction from a stone, foreign body, and prostatitis.

EPIDEMIOLOGY & DEMOGRAPHICS

INCIDENCE:

- UTI is the most common bacterial infection encountered in the ambulatory care setting in the U.S. The self-reported annual incidence of UTI in women is 12%, and half of all women report having had at least one UTI by 32 yr of age.
- UTIs account for 8 million health care visits per year and 15% of all outpatient prescriptions.
- Incidence by age group:
  1. In neonates: More common in boys as a result of anatomic abnormalities such as the posterior urethral valves.
  2. In preschool children: More common in girls than in boys (4.5% vs. 0.5%).
  3. In adulthood: More common in women, with a 1% to 3% prevalence in nonpregnant women. Table 1 describes risk factors for acute uncomplicated UTIs in women.
  4. In pregnancy: At 12 wk gestation, the incidence of asymptomatic bacteriuria is similar to that in nonpregnant women (2% to 10%). However, 25% to 30% of pregnant women with untreated asymptomatic bacteriuria develop acute pyelonephritis, especially in the second and third trimesters, and pregnant women have a pyelonephritic recurrence rate of 10%; therefore treatment of asymptomatic bacteriuria in pregnancy is recommended.
  5. In adults aged ≥65: At least 10% of men and 20% of women have bacteriuria.

PHYSICAL FINDINGS & CLINICAL PRESENTATION

- Typical symptoms of UTI include:
  1. Urinary frequency and/or urgency
  2. Dysuria
  3. Suprapubic pain
  4. Gross or microscopic hematuria
- The probability of cystitis is greater than 50% in women with any symptom of UTI and greater than 90% in women who have dysuria and frequency without vaginal symptoms.

- Clinical symptoms alone can be used to make the diagnosis of uncomplicated UTI in women without a urine culture.
- When negative cultures are associated with significant pyuria, vaginal discharge, or hematuria, infections with *Chlamydia trachomatis*, *Neisseria gonorrhoeae*, and *Trichomonas vaginalis* should be considered.
- Acute pyelonephritis presents with fever, flank or abdominal pain, chills, malaise, and vomiting. It is these systemic symptoms that distinguish pyelonephritis from cystitis. Complications of acute pyelonephritis are renal abscess, perinephric abscess, emphysematous pyelonephritis, and pyonephrosis.

ETIOLOGY & PATHOGENESIS

- Most UTIs are caused by fecal flora, which can colonize the vaginal and periurethral tissues and ascend into the bladder.
- Other risk factors include incomplete bladder emptying due to neurologic disease, bladder outlet obstruction or urethral stricture, renal failure, diabetes, vesicoureteral reflux, fistula, urinary diversion, advanced age, pregnancy, recent sexual activity, and instrumentation.
- Catheters: Patients who require a long-term Foley catheter will eventually develop significant levels of bacteriuria. Treatment is reserved for individuals who become symptomatic (fever, chills, malaise, loss of appetite, pain, etc.). Using prophylactic antibiotics to treat patients who have chronic catheters is not indicated because of the risk of acquiring bacteria resistant to antibiotic therapy.
- Once bacteria reach the urinary tract, three factors determine whether symptomatic infection occurs (Box 1). These factors also determine the anatomic level of the UTI:
  1. Virulence of the microorganism
  2. Inoculum size
  3. Adequacy of the host defense mechanisms
- Urinary pathogens: In 90% of UTIs the infecting organism is gram-negative bacilli. *Escherichia coli* is the most common pathogen, causing 85% of UTI cases (predominantly O, K, and H antigen serotypes). *Staphylococcus saprophyticus* causes 10% of infections, especially in young, sexually active women. Other less

---

TABLE 1 Factors Modulating Risk for Acute Uncomplicated Urinary Tract Infections in Women

Host Determinants	Uropathogen Determinants
Behavioral: Sexual intercourse, use of spermicidal products, recent antimicrobial use, suboptimal voiding habits	*Escherichia coli* virulence determinants: P, S, Dr, and type I fimbriae; hemolysin; aerobactin; serum resistance
Genetic: Innate and adaptive immune response, enhanced epithelial cell adherence, antibacterial factors in urine and bladder mucosa, nonsecretor of ABO blood group antigens, P_1 blood group phenotype, reduced *CXCR1* expression, previous history of recurrent cystitis	
Biologic: Estrogen deficiency in postmenopausal women, micturition	

From Floege J et al: *Comprehensive clinical nephrology,* ed 4, Philadelphia, 2010, Saunders.

BOX 1 Bacterial Factors

- The size of the inoculum
- The virulence of the infecting organism
  1. Virulence factors
     a. P-fimbriae facilitate the adherence of bacteria to biologic surfaces.
     b. K-antigens facilitate adherence and protect the organisms from the host-immune response.
     c. O-antigens are an important source of systemic reactions such as fever and shock that occur with bacterial infections.
     d. H-antigens are associated with flagella and are related to bacterial locomotion.
     e. Hemolysin may potentiate tissue damage and facilitate local bacterial growth.
     f. Urease alkalinizes the urine and facilitates stone formation, thus potentiating infection.
  2. Biofilms harbor bacteria on prosthetic devices and may be a source of recurrent infections.
  3. The presence of sialosyl galactosyl globoside on the surface of kidney cells. This compound is a highly powerful receptor for *Escherichia coli* bacteria.
  4. Women with a deficiency in human beta-defensin-1 are at greater risk for urinary tract infection.

common urinary pathogens include *Klebsiella, Enterobacter, Serratia, Proteus,* and *Pseudomonas.*

- In contrast, the organisms that commonly colonize the distal urethra and skin of both men and women and the vagina of women are *Staphylococcus epidermidis,* diphtheroids, lactobacilli, *Gardnerella vaginalis,* and a variety of anaerobes that rarely cause UTIs. In general, the isolation of two or more bacterial species from a urine culture signifies a contaminated specimen unless the patient is being managed with an indwelling catheter or urinary diversion, or has a chronic complicated infection.
- Innate defense mechanisms against cystitis include low urine pH and high urine osmolarity, mucopolysaccharide glycosaminoglycan (GAG) protective layer, complete bladder emptying, and low vaginal pH due to the

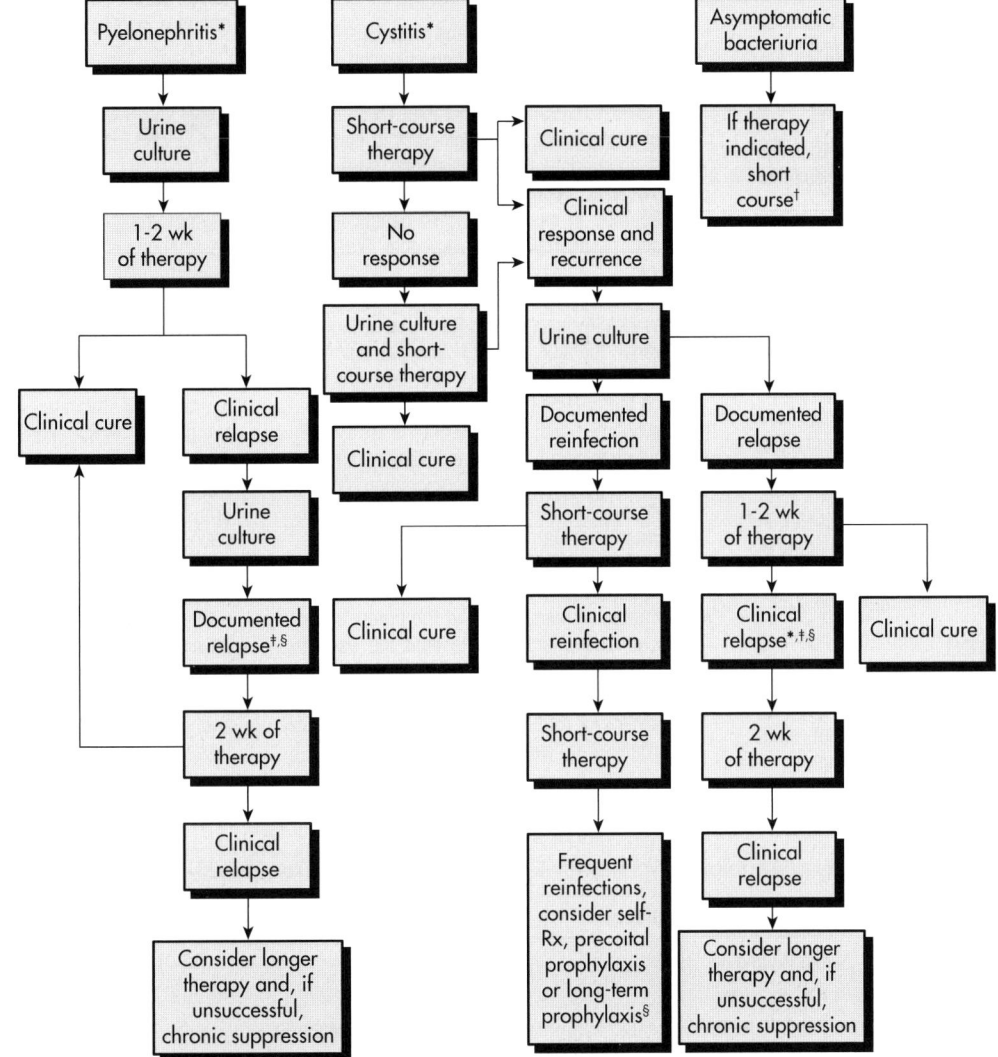

*Consider imaging studies in all men and in women with complicated urinary tract infection.
†No therapy except for renal transplant patients or prior to urologic procedures. Follow-up culture only in transplant patients.
‡Evaluate men for chronic bacterial prostatitis.
§Consider imaging studies in women.

FIG. 1 Approach to the management of urinary tract infection in nonpregnant adults. (From Bennett JE et al: *Mandell, Douglas, and Bennett's principles and practice of infectious diseases,* ed 8, Philadelphia, 2015, Saunders.)

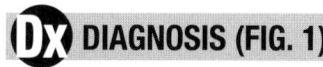

presence of estrogen and resulting colonization of the genital tract by lactobacillus. At the level of the kidney, uromodulin (also known as Tamm-Horsfall protein) is secreted by renal tubular epithelial cells to inhibit adherence of bacteria to urothelial cells.

• In uncomplicated, nonpregnant patients, cystitis rarely progresses to pyelonephritis or other serious infections such as bacteremia.

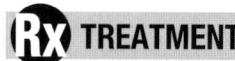 DIAGNOSIS (FIG. 1)

DIFFERENTIAL DIAGNOSIS
• Vaginitis
• Urethritis (gonococcal, nongonococcal, *Trichomonas*)
• Interstitial cystitis (painful bladder syndrome)
• Pelvic inflammatory disease
• Nephrolithiasis
• Structural urethral abnormalities such as diverticulum or stricture

LABORATORY TESTS
• Microscopic urinalysis of clean-catch urine for bacteria and pyuria. The presence of ≥10 leukocytes/µl of unspun urine from a midstream catch indicates possible UTI. The absence of pyuria should call into question the diagnosis of UTI.
• Dipstick urinalysis with the presence of nitrites or leukocyte esterase is indicative of UTI. However, dipstick urinalysis may not be useful in symptomatic patients, as a negative dipstick urinalysis does not exclude the diagnosis of UTI. Additionally, dipsticks may be falsely positive when the urine is contaminated. Overall, a dipstick positive for nitrites and leukocyte esterase has a sensitivity of 75% and specificity of 82% in patients with >100,000 CFU/ml.
• Urine culture and sensitivity are useful in complicated UTIs and to help guide therapy in patients who fail initial therapy. They are generally not needed in uncomplicated UTIs.

IMAGING STUDIES
• Warranted only if renal infection or genitourinary abnormality is suspected
• CT urogram, voiding cystourethrogram, renal ultrasound, and intravenous pyelogram

• Specialty examination: Cystoscopy and retrograde pyelography to rule out obstructive uropathy, urethral diverticulum, mesh obstruction, or malignancy

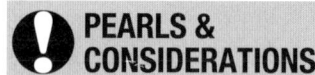 TREATMENT

SUPPORTIVE THERAPY
Urinary analgesics such as phenazopyridine and aggressive hydration

ACUTE GENERAL Rx
• First-line antimicrobials for uncomplicated UTI recommended by the Infectious Disease Society of North America, the American Urologic Society, and the American College of Obstetricians and Gynecologists include nitrofurantoin twice daily for 5 days, trimethoprim plus sulfamethoxazole (TMP-SMX) twice daily for 3 days, or fosfomycin 3-g sachet in a single dose.
• Antimicrobial stewardship and drug resistance needs to be considered when choosing antibiotic therapy. Nitrofurantoin continues to have the lowest rates of antimicrobial resistance. Empiric treatment with TMP-SMX is considered appropriate when resistance rates are below 20%. Beta-lactam antibiotics may be appropriate in cases of known patient intolerance or allergy to conventional first-line agents.
• Nitrofurantoin may have lower rates of bioavailability in patients >65 yr due to decline in renal function. If CrCl is <30 ml/min, nitrofurantoin should be avoided, as it may not reach therapeutic concentration in the urine.
• Many women with a history of UTIs are aware of symptom onset. Patient-initiated therapy, in which a patient is given a prescription for the treatment of an uncomplicated UTI and instructed to start therapy when symptoms develop, has been found to be safe, effective, and less costly.
• High rates of resistance and the potential for serious side effects should limit the use of fluoroquinolone antimicrobials. The U.S. FDA has warned against the use of fluoroquinolone antibiotics for routine infections when suitable alternatives are available.

• Pyelonephritis may be treated as an outpatient in stable, well-hydrated patients with close follow-up. Antimicrobial selection is ideally based on urine culture results. Empiric treatment with fluoroquinolone antimicrobials or TMP-SMX is acceptable. Initiation of treatment in the emergency room setting with a single parenteral dose of a long-acting beta-lactam or aminoglycoside antibiotic followed by oral treatment with fluoroquinolones or TMP-SMX is an acceptable regimen. Patients should be assessed for a proper response to treatment within 48 hr. Nitrofurantoin and fosfomycin are not indicated for the treatment of pyelonephritis due to inadequate renal tissue levels.
• Inpatient management of pyelonephritis should begin with parenteral antimicrobials followed by transition to oral agents based on clinical response and culture results.
• Pyelonephritis may require a total duration of 10 to 14 days of therapy, although evidence exists that 7 to 10 days may be equally effective in low-risk patients (Table 2).

! PEARLS & CONSIDERATIONS

COMMENTS
• Asymptomatic bacteriuria occurs commonly in postmenopausal women. Treatment of asymptomatic bacteriuria with antimicrobials is discouraged because it seldom resolves and can result in the development of drug-resistant organisms. Patients with cloudy or foul-smelling urine should be encouraged to aggressively hydrate to eliminate these symptoms. Postmenopausal women with vaginal atrophy can be treated with vaginal estrogen to reduce the incidence of bacteriuria. Exceptions include immunocompromised patients, patients with structural urinary tract abnormalities, and pregnant patients.
• Pregnancy: 25% to 30% of pregnant women with untreated asymptomatic bacteriuria develop pyelonephritis. All pregnant women should be screened for asymptomatic bacteriuria and treated. Nitrofurantoin, TMP-SMX, and beta-lactam antibiotics are appropriate first-line choices in pregnancy.

TABLE 2 Dosage and Toxicity of Antibiotics Commonly Used to Treat Urinary Tract Infections

Drug	Oral Dose and Frequency	Minor Toxicity	Major Toxicity
Trimethoprim-sulfamethoxazole	160 mg/800 mg, q12h	Allergic	Serious skin reactions, blood dyscrasia
Nitrofurantoin macrocrystals	100 mg, q12h	GI upset	Peripheral neuropathy, pneumonitis
Ampicillin	250-500 mg, q6h	Allergic, candidal overgrowth	Allergic reactions, pseudomembranous colitis
Tetracycline	250-500 mg, q6h	GI upset, skin rash, candidal overgrowth	Hepatic dysfunction, nephrotoxicity
Cephalexin	250-500 mg, q6h	Allergic	Hepatic dysfunction
Ciprofloxacin	250 mg, q12h	Nausea, vomiting, diarrhea, abdominal pain, headache, skin rash	Arrhythmias, angina, convulsions, GI bleeding, nephritis

GI, Gastrointestinal.
From Walters M, Karram M: *Urogynecology and reconstructive pelvic surgery*, ed 4, Philadelphia, 2015, Elsevier.

TABLE 3 Spectrum of Antimicrobial Activity Against Common Lower Urinary Tract Pathogens

Organism	Nitrofurantoin	TMP-SMX	Ciprofloxacin	Levofloxacin	Cephalexin	Ampicillin	Fosfomycin
Escherichia coli	+	±	+	+	+	±	+
Pseudomonas	−	−	+	±	−	−	+
Klebsiella	−	±	+	+	+	−	+
Proteus	±	±	+	+	±	+	±
Enterobacter	±	±	+	+	−	−	±
Enterococcus	+	−	−	±	−	+	±
Staphylococcus	+	+	±	±	±	+	+
Serratia marcescens	−	±	+	+	−	−	±

From Walters M, Karram M: *Urogynecology and reconstructive pelvic surgery,* ed 4, Philadelphia, 2015, Elsevier.

- Recurrent UTI: Two or more symptomatic UTIs over a 6-mo period or three or more episodes over a 12-mo period. Causes include unresolved infection, abnormal vaginal colonization by the originally infecting organism, or reinfection with a new strain. Management of recurrent UTI includes antibiotic prophylaxis for 6 mo or longer, intermittent self-treatment, and postcoital prophylaxis depending on the circumstances. Patients with recurrent UTIs can be considered for an anatomic evaluation including office cystoscopy and upper urinary tract imaging (renal ultrasound or CT urography).
- Nonantimicrobial strategies to prevent UTI have shown mixed results. Nonantimicrobial agents with antiseptic effects on the lower urinary tract include cranberry supplements with vitamin C, D-mannose, and methenamine. Studies demonstrating clinical effectiveness of these agents show modest effects with few side effects. Topical estrogen has been shown to normalize the vaginal flora and may increase the thickness of the urothelium over time and should be used as an adjunct in postmenopausal women with recurrent UTI. Oral probiotics may also be beneficial by decreasing the vaginal pH.

ANTIMICROBIAL RESISTANCE:
- Because of the overuse of antibiotics, organisms once sensitive to a number of antimicrobial agents are now increasingly resistant, making effective treatment of UTI and pyelonephritis more challenging. Most important has been the increasing resistance to TMP-SMX, the current primary care provider drug of choice for acute uncomplicated UTI in women.
- Fluoroquinolone use for the treatment of acute cystitis in women should be avoided when suitable alternatives exist. The U.S. FDA has changed the labeling of quinolone antibiotics to reflect this recommendation.
- When choosing a treatment regimen, physicians should consider such factors as:
  1. In vitro susceptibility
  2. Adverse effects on individual patients
  3. Adverse effects on the population (stewardship)
  4. Cost-effectiveness
  5. Resistance rates in their respective communities
- Meropenem (1 g IV q8h) or IV plazomicin (15 mg/kg body weight once daily) are effective for the treatment of complicated UTIs and acute pyelonephritis caused by *Enterobacteriaceae,* including multidrug-resistant strains (Table 3).

SUGGESTED READINGS
Available at eBooks.Health.Elsevier.com.

RELATED CONTENT
Urinary Tract Infection (Patient Information)
Urinary Tract Infection (Child) (Patient Information)
Pyelonephritis (Related Key Topic)

AUTHORS: **SYDNEY FORD, MD, MPH,** and **ANTHONY SCISCIONE, DO**

Diseases and Disorders

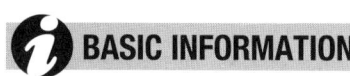

BASIC INFORMATION

DEFINITION
Urolithiasis is the presence of calculi (urinary stones) within the urinary tract. The five major types of urinary stones are calcium oxalate (60% to 70%), calcium phosphate (20%), uric acid (7%), struvite (7%), and cystine (1%) (Table 1).[1]

SYNONYMS
Kidney stones
Kidney calculi
Renal stones
Renal calculi
Ureteral stones
Ureteral calculi
Nephrolithiasis
Ureterolithiasis

ICD-10CM CODES
N20.0 Calculus of kidney
N20.1 Calculus of ureter
N20.2 Calculus of kidney with calculus of ureter
N20.9 Urinary calculus, unspecified
N21.0 Calculus in bladder
N21.1 Calculus in urethra
N21.8 Other lower urinary tract calculus
N21.9 Calculus of lower urinary tract, unspecified

EPIDEMIOLOGY & DEMOGRAPHICS
INCIDENCE: Urinary stones affect approximately 1 in 11 persons in the United States.[2]
PREVALENCE: Approximately 10% and 7% in men and women, respectively.[2]
PREDOMINANT SEX & AGE: Most common in men in their 30 to 50s.[2]
PEAK INCIDENCE: Fourth to sixth decade of life.[2]
RISK FACTORS: Dehydration, warm weather, prior stone episodes, metabolic syndrome

PHYSICAL FINDINGS & CLINICAL PRESENTATION
Obstructing ureter stones, although asymptomatic at times, cause the following signs and symptoms:
- Renal colic: Acute, often severe flank pain
- Referred pain: Pain radiating from the flank downward to the lower back and abdomen and anteriorly to the groin and genitalia
- Inability to find a comfortable position
- Nausea and vomiting
- Hematuria, gross or microscopic
- Urinary urgency and frequency with distal ureteral stones mimicking a urinary tract infection
- Fever and chills accompanying acute renal colic from superimposed infection
- Older adult patients; children; and patients with diabetes mellitus, neurologic deficits, or kidney transplant may present with nonspecific and vague abdominal discomfort and pain

ETIOLOGY
- Low urine output
- Low or high urine pH, hypercalciuria, hypocitraturia, hyperoxaluria, and/or hyperuricosuria predispose patients to urinary stone formation.[3]
- Diets high in sodium and animal protein, excessive oxalate content, and heavy intake of phosphoric acid can all increase the risk of urinary stone formation.[2]
- Anatomic factors predisposing patients to urinary stasis: Malrotated, horseshoe, or ectopic kidney; ureteropelvic junction obstruction, bladder outlet obstruction, and urinary strictures affecting the urinary tract.[4,5]

DIAGNOSIS

DIFFERENTIAL DIAGNOSIS
- Gastrointestinal: Appendicitis, constipation, diverticulitis, small bowel obstruction
- Genitourinary: Testicular torsion, ureteropelvic junction obstruction, urinary tract infection
- Obstetric-gynecologic: Dysmenorrhea, ectopic pregnancy, pelvic inflammatory disease, ovarian torsion
- Other: Malignancy (primary) urinary tract or retroperitoneal lymphadenopathy causing ureteral/kidney obstruction, musculoskeletal back pain, malingering or factitious disorder

WORKUP
- Imaging studies should be performed to determine the location of obstructing urinary stones. Urine and blood studies are obtained to assess the acuity of stone presentation and elucidate possible etiologies.

LABORATORY TESTS
- Bloodwork should include the following:
  1. A CBC should be obtained in anticipation of possible intervention associated with a significant bleeding risk or in those with bleeding disorders. Additionally, the presence of leukocytosis in the acute setting may influence the management approach.[4]
  2. A basic metabolic panel is appropriate in the acute setting. Patients undergoing a formal metabolic evaluation should have a comprehensive metabolic panel in addition to assessing levels of uric acid and parathyroid home.[2-5]
- Urine studies:
  1. A urinalysis (UA) should always be part of the workup for urolithiasis. Hematuria is often present, but the absence of hematuria does not exclude stones. Urine pH may help identify stone type, where pH >7.5 is associated with struvite stones, pH <5.5 is generally associated with uric acid stones, and low serum bicarbonate concentration with urine pH $\geq$6 is consistent with a renal tubular acidosis.[4,5]
  2. Urine culture and sensitivity should be obtained in patients suspected to have an underlying urinary tract infection or when surgery is planned.[4,5]
- A 24-h urine collection evaluates for urine chemistries. It is generally reserved for patients with recurrent stones, bilateral stones, large stone burden, young, and/or motivated first-time stone formers who are interested in preventive measures.[2,3,5]

IMAGING STUDIES
- Noncontrast computed tomography (CT) is the standard for diagnosing urolithiasis. It is rapid and accurate, has the greatest sensitivity (nearly 100%) and specificity (94% to 96%), and can identify almost all stone types in essentially all locations. CT scan is the best test upon which to base stone treatment recommendations, evaluate stone persistence or passage, and plan for surgery.[4,6]
- Renal-bladder ultrasonography (RBUS) may be an adequate initial study to detect stone presence (i.e., hydronephrosis, absent ureteral jet), especially in patients known to have a history of stones and in patients where radiation should be avoided (e.g., pregnancy and children). RBUS is 50% to 70% sensitive in detecting stones within the kidneys and approximately 90% sensitive in detecting hydronephrosis. Initial RBUS may be associated with lower cumulative radiation exposure than initial CT, without significant differences in missing, serious, or alternative diagnoses; adverse events; pain scores; return emergency department visits; or hospitalizations.[4,6]

TABLE 1 Types of Urinary Tract Stones and Their Etiology

Composition	Etiological Factors	Percentage of All Stones
Calcium oxalate/calcium oxalate mixed with calcium phosphate	An underlying metabolic disorder (e.g., idiopathic hypercalciuria or hyperoxaluria) ▶ in 25% no metabolic abnormality is identified	75
Struvite or matrix calculi (composed of magnesium ammonium phosphate)	Renal infection	10-15
Uric acid	Hyperuricemia or hyperuricosuria ▶ it is idiopathic in 50%	6
Cysteine	A renal tubular defect	1-2

Other stones (e.g., xanthine stones, which may be related to a metabolic abnormality, or indinavir stones, which are drug related) are uncommon and account for <5% of all renal stones.
From Grant LA: *Grainger & Allison's diagnostic radiology essentials*, ed 2, Philadelphia, 2019, Elsevier.

- A kidney-ureter-bladder x-ray (KUB) can identify radioopaque stones (e.g., calcium-containing) but not radiolucent stones (uric acid stones). However, the KUB has much lower detection rates than CT, with an estimated sensitivity of 44% and specificity of 77%.[5]

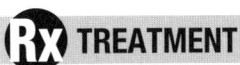

TREATMENT

ACUTE GENERAL Rx

- NSAIDs are excellent for managing renal colic and are preferred first-line agents (e.g., ketorolac, ibuprofen). Opiates may be required for severe pain. Initial pain control with NSAIDs can reduce overall opiate dosing for renal colic.
- For patients who have a stone with a high probability of passage (i.e., small stone, especially in the distal ureter), medical expulsive therapy with alpha-blockers or calcium channel blockers (used less often due to side effects) may be helpful, particularly for stones in the distal ureter >5 mm in size.[5]
- Intravenous fluids and antiemetics may be required.
- Antibiotics are indicated if a urinary tract infection is present or suspected.

PREVENTION

Preventive measures for urolithiasis center around dietary measures, hydration, and lifestyle modifications.[2,5] Diets high in sodium and animal protein should be avoided in favor of those rich in vegetables and fiber and normal amounts of calcium. Fluid intake near 3 liters per day is advocated, with the goal of having a urine output of 2 liters or more on a daily basis. Furthermore, an active lifestyle with adequate physical activity is advocated in addition to maintaining a body mass index in the normal range. Pharmaceutical therapy may be necessary in those with recurrent urolithiasis despite following the aforementioned preventive measures.

- Thiazide diuretic agents are widely used for "prevention of recurrence of kidney stones," but a recent trial among patients with recurrent kidney stones revealed that the incidence of recurrence did not differ substantially among patients receiving hydrochlorothiazide once daily at a dose of 12.5 mg, 25 mg, or 50 mg or placebo daily.[6a]

CHRONIC Rx

- Pharmaceutical therapy may be indicated in patients with certain stone composition, specific metabolic abnormalities, and/or those with stone recurrence or stone growth despite preventive measures.[2,3] This includes allopurinol (normalcalciuria with hyperuricosuria), potassium citrate (normalcalciuria with hypocitraturia; normalcemia with hypercalciuria; uric acid stone formers, cystinuria), thiazides (normalcemia with hypercalciuria), calcium citrate (normalcalciuria with hyperoxaluria), and tiopronin (cystine stone formers).[3]

DISPOSITION

- Patients with uncomplicated obstructing ureter stones may safely be observed. A 4- to 6-wk monitoring period is preferred, which may be paired with medical expulsion therapy.[4,5]
- Stone passage is influence by size and location of stone. Smaller and more distal stones are more likely to pass spontaneously.[4,5]
- For high-risk patients, stone recurrence rates are estimated to be 50% at 10 yr compared to 10% to 20% in those with lower risk profile.[7]
- A formal metabolic evaluation should be considered in those with stone recurrence, motivated first-time stone formers, and children after their first stone episode.

REFERRAL

- Urology referral is appropriate for any patient with urinary stones when a patient cannot be discharged from the emergency department; when a patient has an obstructing kidney stone and presumed or associated urinary tract infection; when there are large or recurrent stones; when patients have solitary kidneys or complex anatomy that may predispose them to stones; and when spontaneous passage is unlikely or does not occur despite an appropriate monitoring period.

PEARLS & CONSIDERATIONS

COMMENTS

- Uncomplicated obstructing ureteral stones can safely be monitored for 4 to 6 wk.
- Medical expulsion therapy includes improved hydration, analgesics, and medications that may help with stone passage such as alpha-blockers or calcium channel blockers.
- Consider NSAIDs as first-line therapy for pain control with kidney stones, unless there are contraindications (e.g., allergy or acute kidney injury).
- Imaging is key to diagnosing urolithiases. Ultrasound or KUB is a suitable screening test, while CT scan is most accurate and often determines treatment recommendations.
- Escalation of care is indicated if (1) spontaneous passage does not occur, (2) the patient is persistently symptomatic, (3) an underlying urinary tract infection is suspected, (4) significant acute kidney injury is present despite adequate hydration, and (5) concerns for systemic inflammatory response syndrome are present. Urology consultation is appropriate at this point to determine the need for prompt urinary tract drainage via insertion of a ureteral stent or percutaneous nephrostomy.
- The removal of small, asymptomatic kidney stones during surgery to remove ureteral or contralateral kidney stones is up to the urologist and the patient. Trials have shown that removal of small asymptomatic stones results in a lower incidence of relapse than nonremoval and in a similar number of emergency department visits related to the surgery.[8]

REFERENCES

Available at eBooks.Health.Elsevier.com.

AUTHORS: **ISAAC PALMA-ZAMORA, MD,** and **DAVID A. LEAVITT, MD**

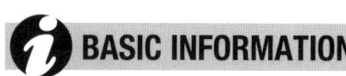
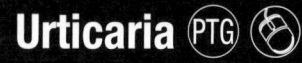 **BASIC INFORMATION**

DEFINITION

Urticaria is a pruritic rash involving the epidermis and the upper portions of the dermis caused by localized capillary vasodilation and the release of histamine and other vasoactive mediators. It is followed by transudation of protein-rich fluid in the surrounding tissue and manifests clinically with the presence of raised erythematous, circumscribed lesions with central pallor. Urticaria is classified according to its chronicity into acute (<6-wk duration) and chronic (≥6-wk duration). Chronic urticaria has been categorized on the basis of consensus criteria and guidelines as spontaneous urticaria (previously designated as chronic idiopathic urticarias) in which urticaria, angioedema, or both occur in unprompted fashion, or as inducible urticaria (previously designated as physical urticaria) in which urticaria, angioedema, or both are elicited by factors such as cold, heat, or pressure.[1a]

SYNONYMS

Hives
Wheals

ICD-10CM CODES
L50.0	Allergic urticaria
L50.1	Idiopathic urticaria
L50.2	Urticaria due to cold and heat
L50.3	Dermatographic urticaria
L50.4	Vibratory urticaria
L50.5	Cholinergic urticaria
L50.6	Contact urticaria
L50.8	Other urticaria
L50.9	Urticaria, unspecified

EPIDEMIOLOGY & DEMOGRAPHICS

- Between 15% and 25% of the population will have at least one episode of urticaria during their lifetime.[1]
- The incidence of chronic urticaria (CU) is thought to be around 1.4% annually. It is more common in adults, with the average age of occurrence between the third and fifth decades of life. Females are twice as likely to be affected as males.[1,2]
- Incidence is increased in atopic patients.[1]

PHYSICAL FINDINGS & CLINICAL PRESENTATION

- Presence of elevated, erythematous, or white circumscribed lesions that change in size and shape over time (Fig. E1) in no specific distribution; they are characterized by extreme pruritus and are evanescent, with individual lesions generally lasting <24 h in duration and disappearing without scarring. If the patient has persistent symptoms, new lesions typically have a novel distribution.
- Stroking of the skin can lead to urticarial reaction (dermatographism) (Fig. E2).
- Angioedema occurs in approximately 40% of cases of urticaria and is caused by mast cell

mediator release in the subcutaneous tissue and deep dermis.[2]
- Although not yet well understood, patients with CU may have a range of concurrent systemic symptoms such as fatigue, rhinorrhea, dyspnea, gastritis, joint pain, and hypertension. These patients also have higher rates of depression and anxiety.[2]

PATHOGENESIS

- Cellular mechanisms of acute and chronic urticaria are heterogenous and incompletely understood, but are known to involve pathologic activation of mast cells and basophils, which leads to the release of proinflammatory mediators, such as histamine, leukotrienes, and prostaglandins.[1]
- Autoimmunity plays a central role specifically in the pathogenesis of chronic spontaneous urticaria (CSU), with contributions from immunoglobulin G (IgG)- and IgE-specific autoantibodies (against interleukin-24 [IL-24] and FcεR1, the latter being found on the surface of dermal mast cells and basophils). CSU patients also tend to have higher levels of proinflammatory cytokines: IL-17, IL-31, and IL-33. The clinical significance of these antibodies and inflammatory markers is currently being studied and reviewed for potential therapeutic targets.[1,3]

ETIOLOGY

Acute urticaria (Table 1):
- Food allergies (e.g., shellfish [Fig. E3], tree nuts, legumes, milk, eggs)
- Medication allergies (e.g., penicillin, aspirin, sulfonamides, hormone therapy)
- Insect sting allergies (e.g., honey bee, *Hymenoptera,* fire ant)
- Systemic diseases (e.g., systemic lupus erythematosus, serum sickness, autoimmune thyroid disease, cutaneous mastocytosis, cryoglobulinemia)
- Infections (e.g., viral upper respiratory infections, hepatitis B and C, fungal infections, chronic bacterial infections, helminthic)
- Nonimmunologic contact urticaria (e.g., caterpillars, plants)
- Immunologic contact urticaria (e.g., natural rubber latex, nickel, parabens, benzoic acid, salicylic acid)
- Other: Pregnancy, hair bleaches, saliva, pemphigoid, emotional stress, malignancy (lymphomas, endocrine tumors)
- Idiopathic urticaria is diagnosed in ~50% of patients with acute urticaria
Chronic urticaria:
- CU is classified as either CSU or chronic inducible urticaria, depending on whether the skin lesions appear spontaneously or can be induced.
- Physical stimuli (e.g., pressure, cholinergic, solar, cold/heat, aquagenic, or vibration) are found in ~20% of patients.[2]
- Autoimmune component in up to 50% of cases.[1]

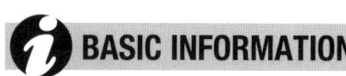 **DIAGNOSIS**

DIFFERENTIAL DIAGNOSIS

- Erythema multiforme
- Erythema marginatum
- Erythema infectiosum
- Urticarial vasculitis
- Herpes gestationis
- Drug eruption
- Multiple insect bites
- Bullous pemphigoid
- Mastocytosis or other mast cell disease
- Viral exanthema
- Pityriasis rosea
- Atopic dermatitis
- Contact dermatitis
- Henoch-Schönlein purpura

WORKUP

- It is useful to determine whether hives are acute or chronic; a medical history focused on various etiologic factors is necessary before embarking on additional laboratory testing.
- Most cases of acute urticaria resolve spontaneously and diagnostic testing is not required. However, in patients with acute urticaria, it is crucial to consider anaphylaxis before further workup of urticaria because this may require urgent management.
- The cause of CU is often never determined, and diagnostic testing may be unnecessary based on a detailed history and physical examination. Targeted laboratory testing based on clinical findings is appropriate.[2]

LABORATORY TESTS

- If the history is consistent with allergen-induced contact urticaria, skin testing with allergen extracts and screening for dermatographism (i.e., by attempting to elicit a wheal after application of linear skin pressure) should be performed only after withholding antihistamines for 36 to 72 h to prevent false-negative results.[2]
- CBC with differential, erythrocyte sedimentation rate (ESR), thyroid-stimulating hormone (TSH), and liver function tests should be considered only in patients with a history or physical exam concerning for an underlying systemic condition. Routine laboratory testing is not indicated. Even with extensive testing, the cause of CU is rarely established.[2]
- Measurement of C4, C1 inhibitor antigenic level and function, and C1q may be helpful in patients who present with angioedema alone. In these patients, C1-inhibitor deficiency should be considered.[2]
- Skin biopsy is helpful in patients with fever, arthralgias, and elevated ESR. Histologic evidence of leukocytoclasia (neutrophilic infiltration with fragmentation of nuclei) is indicative of urticarial vasculitis.[2]
- When food or contact allergy is suspected in acute urticaria, testing can be performed using

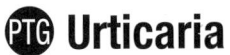

TABLE 1 Some Causes of Urticaria*

Infections	Eggs†
Bacterial infections	Cheese
Dental abscess	Inhalants
Sinusitis	Animal dander
Otitis	Pollen
Pneumonitis	Contactants
Gastritis	Wool
Hepatitis	Silk
Cholecystitis	Occupational exposure
Cystitis	Potatoes
Vaginitis	Antibiotics
Fungal infections	Cosmetics
Dermatophytes	Dyes
Candida	Hairspray
Other Infections/Infestations	Nail polish
Scabies	Mouthwash
Helminth	Toothpaste
Protozoa	Perfumes
Trichomonas	Hand cream
Drugs and Chemicals	Soap
Salicylates	Insect repellent
Indomethacin and other, newer nonsteroidal antiinflammatory agents†	Physical stimuli
Opiates†	Light
Radiocontrast material†	Pressure
Penicillin (medication, milk, blue cheese)	Heat
Sulfonamides	Cold
Sodium benzoate	Water
Douches	Vibration
Ear drops or eye drops	Endocrinopathies
Insulin	Thyroid disease
Menthol (cigarettes, toothpaste, iced tea, hand cream, lozenges, candy)	Diabetes mellitus
Tartrazine (vitamins, birth control pills, antibiotics, FDC yellow #5)	Pregnancy
	Menstruation
Foods	Menopause
Nuts	Systemic diseases
Berries†	Rheumatic fever
Fish	Connective tissue diseases (lupus erythematosus, Sjögren syndrome, rheumatoid arthritis, Still disease, dermatomyositis, polymyositis, other)
Seafood	
Shellfish†	Leukemia
Bananas	Lymphoma
Grapes	Acquired immunodeficiency disease
Tomatoes	Ovarian tumors

*Partial list of most frequently described causes in each category.
†May be mediated by nonimmunologic mechanisms independent of immunoglobulin E.
From Callen JP et al: *Dermatological signs of systemic disease*, ed 5, Philadelphia, 2017, Elsevier.

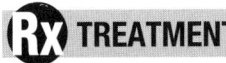 TREATMENT

NONPHARMACOLOGIC THERAPY

Remove all suspected etiologic agents (e.g., stop all nonessential drugs) and avoid any triggers that may have been observed to precipitate an attack.

ACUTE URTICARIA Rx

- Oral antihistamines: Use of second-generation H_1 antihistamines (e.g., cetirizine 10 mg/day, levocetirizine 5 mg/day, loratadine 10 mg/day, fexofenadine 180 mg/day) is preferred over first-generation sedating antihistamines (e.g., hydroxyzine, diphenhydramine). Higher doses of second-generation antihistamines up to four times the FDA-approved dose may be required to achieve adequate control of symptoms.[5]
- Leukotriene receptor antagonists (e.g., montelukast) can be added to H_1 antagonists in refractory cases, although the utility of this has not been consistently shown.[5]
- Oral corticosteroids should be reserved for refractory cases of acute urticaria and prescribed for a very limited course (e.g., prednisone 20 mg/day or 20 mg bid for 5 days).[5,6]

CHRONIC URTICARIA Rx

Stepwise approach for management of CU is described in Fig. E4.
- Step 1: Monotherapy with second-generation H_1 antihistamines. Avoidance of triggers if known (e.g., NSAIDs, alcohol, opiates, physical triggers).[5]
- Step 2: Dose advancement of second-generation antihistamine (up to 4× the daily recommended dose). Consider addition of leukotriene receptor antagonist (e.g., montelukast) or first-generation H_1 antihistamine (hydroxyzine or doxepin) to be taken at bedtime.[5]
- Step 3: Referral to an allergy specialist for evaluation and management. Consider addition of omalizumab (monoclonal anti-IgE antibody that downregulates surface IgE receptors) to antihistamine therapy.[5]
- Step 4: If adequate control is not reached by 18 wk, alternative agents should be considered, including antiinflammatory (dapsone, hydroxychloroquine, sulfasalazine, methotrexate) or immunosuppressive agents (cyclosporine A, mycophenolate, tacrolimus, sirolimus).[5]
- Step 5: Consider addition of immunomodulatory biologic agents (tumor necrosis factor-α [TNF-α] inhibitor, IL-1) or alternative therapies such as ultraviolet light therapy, intravenous immunoglobulin, or plasmapheresis.[5]
- Patients should be evaluated at each visit and, if symptoms are well managed, should be considered for step down in treatment.

skin prick or serum testing for allergen-specific IgE.[2]
- Recent studies have demonstrated a possible link between vitamin D deficiency and CU and suggested that vitamin D supplementation may reduce symptom severity in patients who are deficient, although additional studies are needed.[4]

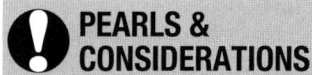
DISPOSITION

- Most cases of urticaria resolve within 6 wk.[7]
- >50% of patients may not achieve satisfactory control of CU with antihistamines alone and may require additional therapies. The median duration of CU is between 3 and 5 yr, but it can often be present for much longer durations.

❗ PEARLS & CONSIDERATIONS

COMMENTS

- Topical treatment (e.g., starch baths or oatmeal baths) may be temporarily soothing in selected patients; however, they are not recommended for long-term control of CU.
- If individual urticarial lesions leave residual ecchymoses, pigmentation, and/or lesions that typically last >24 h at a single location, consider skin biopsy to evaluate for urticarial vasculitis.
- Be judicious when prescribing NSAIDs in CU patients, as up to 30% of these patients will experience an exacerbation of urticaria and/or angioedema.

REFERENCES

Available at eBooks.Health.Elsevier.com.

RELATED CONTENT

Hives (Patient Information)
Chronic Urticaria (Related Key Topic)

AUTHORS: **TIMOTHY KADDIS, MD,** and **SHYAM JOSHI, MD**

ⓘ BASIC INFORMATION

DEFINITION

Uterine fibroids, also called leiomyomas or uterine myomas, are benign myometrial tumors of muscle and connective tissue. The incidence of malignancy is <1/770 to 10,000.[1] They are typically discrete nodular tumors that vary in size and number.

Fibroids are classified by location in the uterus relative to the myometrium

- Subserosal: Located underneath the uterine serosa
- Intramural: Located in the myometrium proper
- Submucosal: Also known as intracavitary as they are located adjacent to the endometrium and protrude into the uterine cavity
- Pedunculated: Located on a pedicle or stalk, either from the serosa or in the cavity
- The above classifications are further detailed by the FIGO classification system (types 0 to 8)

Fibroids can occur singly but are often multiple. They can be located infrequently within the cervix, broad ligament, adnexa, vagina, vulva, or other unexpected structures. Parasitic fibroids attach to nearby pelvic structures and acquire a blood supply from a nonuterine source with potential detachment from the parent myometrium (Fig. 1). After uncontained morcellation, disseminated peritoneal leiomyomatosis can occur.[1]

SYNONYMS

Uterine leiomyomas
Uterine myomas
Fibroids

ICD-10CM CODES
D25.0 Submucous leiomyoma of uterus
D25.1 Intramural leiomyoma of uterus
D25.2 Subserosal leiomyoma of uterus
D25.9 Leiomyoma of uterus, unspecified

EPIDEMIOLOGY & DEMOGRAPHICS

- Estimated cumulative incidence of >70% in women by age 50
- 50% of fibroids are asymptomatic, but symptomatic uterine fibroids affect 25% to 50% of all women and 30% to 40% of perimenopausal women with possible effect on daily activities
- Most common benign solid pelvic tumor diagnosed in women and most common reason for benign hysterectomy
- Risk factors include age, family history, African American race, early menarche, exposure to diethylstilbestrol, obesity, hypertension, polycystic ovary syndrome, vitamin D deficiency, and nulliparity
- Black women typically develop fibroids and clinically significant symptoms at a younger age[2]
- Frequently diagnosed incidentally on pelvic examination
- Potential to enlarge during pregnancy as well as regress after menopause

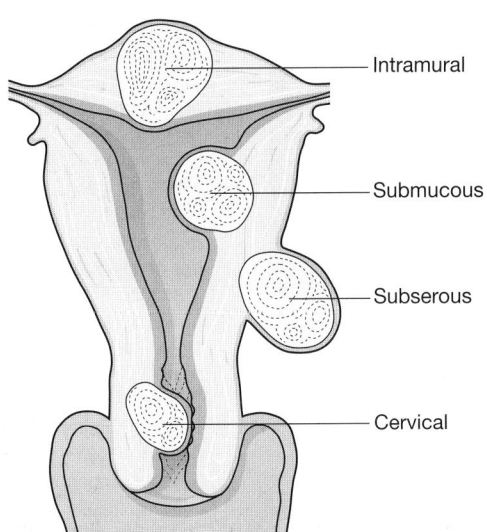

FIG. 1 Sites of fibroids throughout the uterus. (From Magowan BA: *Clinical obstetrics & gynecology*, ed 4, London, 2019, Elsevier.)

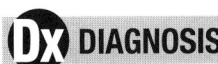

- Approximately 200,000 hysterectomies, 30,000 myomectomies, thousands of selective uterine-artery embolizations and high-intensity focused MRI/ultrasound procedures, and a growing number of radiofrequency ablations are performed annually in the U.S. to remove or destroy uterine fibroids.

PHYSICAL FINDINGS & CLINICAL PRESENTATION

- Presenting symptoms:
  1. Abnormal uterine bleeding (most common, AUB-L) due to dilated endometrial vessels
  2. Chronic pelvic pain (dysmenorrhea, dyspareunia, pelvic pressure)
  3. Bulk symptoms (bloating, increase in abdominal girth)
  4. Anemia from menorrhagia
  5. Acute pain (torsion of pedunculated fibroid, infarction, degeneration)
  6. Urinary symptoms (frequency from bladder pressure, ureteral obstruction, urinary retention, incontinence in setting of prolapse)
  7. GI symptoms (rectosigmoid compression with constipation or intestinal obstruction, pain with defecation)
  8. Prolapse through cervix of pedunculated submucosal fibroid
  9. Infertility (sole etiology in 1%-3%, more likely subfertility with submucosal fibroid)[3]
  10. Pregnancy complications including preterm birth, small fetus for gestational age, malpresentation
  11. Enlarged, irregular uterus on pelvic examination

ETIOLOGY

Fibroids arise from a single progenitor smooth muscle cell in the myometrium and are monoclonal. They are sensitive to endogenous but not exogenous estrogen and progesterone hormones, thus develop during the reproductive years. Malignant transformation of preexisting leiomyoma is extremely uncommon (<0.5%). There is a racial disparity in the prevalence, suggesting a genetic component, with most fibroids having a normal chromosomal makeup. A small group of individuals have an autosomal dominant disorder, hereditary leiomyomatosis and renal cell carcinoma syndrome (HLRCC), in which there is a genetic mutation in the fumarate hydratase gene, causing diminished suppressor function in fibroid formation.[3]

ⓓⓧ DIAGNOSIS

DIFFERENTIAL DIAGNOSIS

- Ovarian mass (neoplastic, nonneoplastic, endometrioma)
- Adenomyosis/adenomyoma
- Endometriosis
- Endometrial polyp
- Endometrial carcinoma or hyperplasia
- Leiomyosarcoma/uterine carcinosarcoma
- Inflammatory mass (reproductive organ or GI origin)
- Pregnancy

WORKUP

- Complete pelvic examination, including speculum exam and bimanual exam
- Estimation of size of uterus/mass and location of fibroids via imaging
- Endometrial sampling may be indicated (biopsy or dilation and curettage) when abnormal bleeding and pelvic mass are present to evaluate for endometrial carcinoma; may identify but cannot rule out leiomyosarcoma, which has no reliable nonsurgical test available
- Fibroid biopsy not recommended[1]
- If significant urinary symptoms are prominent, intravenous pyelogram to rule out impingement on urinary system

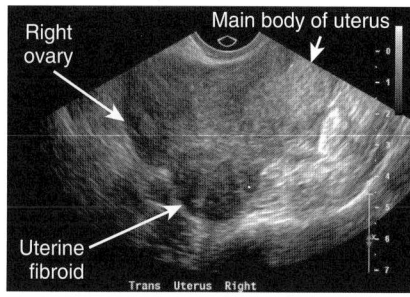

FIG. 2 Fibroid uterus: Endovaginal ultrasound.
Ultrasound is the primary modality used for evaluation of uterine fibroids (leiomyomas). Typical features include a well-circumscribed appearance. Fibroids may be hypoechoic or hyperechoic relative to the uterus. They may be exophytic or intramural, or they may project into the uterine cavity. Whereas malignant uterine tumors may invade adjacent structures, a fibroid is contained within the uterine serosa. Uterine tumors, both benign and malignant, can show central necrosis, which usually appears hypoechoic with ultrasound. In this 38-yr-old woman, the fibroid is exophytic. The right ovary lies adjacent and is difficult to distinguish in this case. (From Broder JS: *Diagnostic imaging for the emergency physician,* Philadelphia, 2011, Saunders.)

LABORATORY TESTS

- Pregnancy test
- CBC
- Blood urea nitrogen/creatinine
- Thyroid-stimulating hormone

IMAGING STUDIES

- Pelvic ultrasound (Fig. 2) is the primary diagnostic modality, with higher diagnostic accuracy via transvaginal ultrasound.
- MRI with contrast (Fig. E3) is helpful in planning treatment or if malignancy is strongly suspected. Also relevant to localize fibroid size, number, and location, especially if myomectomy or uterine artery embolism is contemplated.
- Saline infusion sonography can be helpful in determining location and protrusion into uterine cavity of submucosal fibroids.
- Diagnostic hysteroscopy can be performed in the office and may provide direct evidence of intrauterine pathology or submucosal fibroid that distorts uterine cavity.

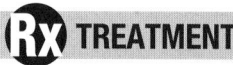 **TREATMENT**

Management (Fig. 4) should be based on primary symptoms and patient goals; this may include observation with close follow-up, medical management, temporizing surgical therapies, embolization (Fig. E5), or definitive surgical procedures. Treatment is indicated if bleeding requires blood transfusions, renal function is affected by size of the enlarged fibroid uterus, or when symptoms are present and are severe enough to be unacceptable to the patient.

NONSURGICAL Rx

- Patient observation and follow-up with periodic repeat pelvic exams to ensure that tumors are not growing rapidly, which could suggest malignancy.
- Hormonal therapies reduce bleeding symptoms and many have the added benefit of contraception. There is no evidence that exogenous estrogen or progestin increases risk of myomas.
  1. Combined hormonal methods with estrogen and progestin, including oral contraceptives, contraceptive patch, contraceptive vaginal ring
  2. Progestin-only agents including oral progestins, intramuscular progestin injection, levonorgestrel intrauterine device (IUD)
  3. Progesterone IUD significantly improves menorrhagia, but expulsion rate with myomas is 10% to 15%, and intracavitary fibroids are a contraindication. Enormous uteri may lead to migrated strings precluding simple retrieval
  Gonadotropin-releasing hormone (GnRH) agonist, leuprolide, results in 25% to 50% reduction in uterine volume and cessation of menses within 3 mo of initiating treatment. Hypoestrogenism, reversible bone loss, and hot flushes are side effects. Consider low-dose progesterone replacement (add-back therapy) to minimize hypoestrogenic effects. GnRH agonist therapy is not recommended for longer than 6 mo without add-back or 12 mo with add-back due to these effects, so goal is to bridge to other treatment.
- Regrowth and return of bleeding symptoms occurs in 50% of treated patients within 3 mo after cessation.
- Indications for GnRH agonist:
  1. Anemia treatment to normalize hemoglobin before surgery
  2. Avoiding surgery in patients approaching menopause
  3. Preoperatively for large myomas to make hysterectomy, hysteroscopic resection/ablation more feasible
  4. Medical contraindication for surgery
- Use of GnRH agonists alters the consistency of the fibroid, making myomectomy more challenging.
- GnRH antagonists (FDA approved 2020 and 2021)—elagolix and relugolix. Both treatment options contain hormonal add-back (estradiol and norethindrone acetate) and can be prescribed for max of 2 yr. May still have light menses. Possible adverse effects include high blood pressure, worsening of lipids and liver enzymes, and loss of bone mineral density. Patients with history of venous thromboembolism or those who are over the age of 35 and smoke should not take these medications.
- Nonhormonal medical therapies:
- Nonsteroidal antiinflammatory drugs for pain; data do not support use as monotherapy for AUB-L menorrhagia.[3]
- Tranexamic acid, an oral antifibrinolytic, can decrease menorrhagia by 40% to 65%. Side effects include abdominal cramps,

headaches, fatigue, and increased risk of venous thromboembolism.
- Other drugs used and under investigation:
- Danazol: Androgen and inhibitor of steroidogenesis, side effect of hirsutism.
- Mifepristone: Antiprogesterone reduces fibroid volume 40% to 50% with amenorrhea.
- Raloxifene: Selective estrogen receptor modulator, either alone or with GnRH agonist, reduces fibroid volume 70% up to 1 yr but only in postmenopausal patients.

SURGICAL Rx

- Indications:
  1. Abnormal uterine bleeding with anemia refractory to hormonal therapy
  2. Chronic pain with severe dysmenorrhea, dyspareunia, or lower abdominal pressure/pain
  3. Acute pain, torsion, or prolapsing submucosal fibroid
  4. Urinary symptoms or signs such as hydronephrosis
  5. Infertility or recurrent pregnancy loss with endometrial cavity-distorting fibroid as only finding[4]
  6. Enlarged uterus with compression symptoms or discomfort
  7. Rapid uterine enlargement premenopausal or any growth after menopause—this indication should involve gynecologic oncologist
- Procedures:
  1. Hysterectomy (definitive procedure): Vaginal, laparoscopic, robotic, or abdominal approach, dependent on surgical preference/expertise and uterine size.
  2. Myomectomy (preserves fertility): May be performed via abdominal, laparoscopic, or robotic approach; 60% recurrence at 5 yr postop[5]; significant hemorrhage risk, so control anemia preop
  3. Vaginal myomectomy for prolapsed pedunculated submucosal fibroid
  4. Hysteroscopic resection: Typically at least 50% of the fibroid must be intracavitary for a hysteroscopic approach to be successful. May need to be done in stages.
  5. Radiofrequency volumetric thermal ablation: FDA-approved uterine-sparing procedure in which laparoscopic or transcervical ultrasound-guided ablation of fibroids induces myolysis (necrosis) resulting in fibroid shrinking. Preliminary data on subsequent pregnancy are limited, but encouraging.[3, 6]
  6. Magnetic resonance–guided focused ultrasound: ultrasound energy focused to cause fibroid coagulative necrosis. Enables fertility preservation, but due to numerous contraindications, many patients are ineligible.[3]
  7. Uterine artery embolization (UAE): Alternative to surgery performed by interventional radiologist, but its less invasive nature should be balanced against a higher rate for treatment failure or complications at 5 yr. Age 40 or less at time of embolization and

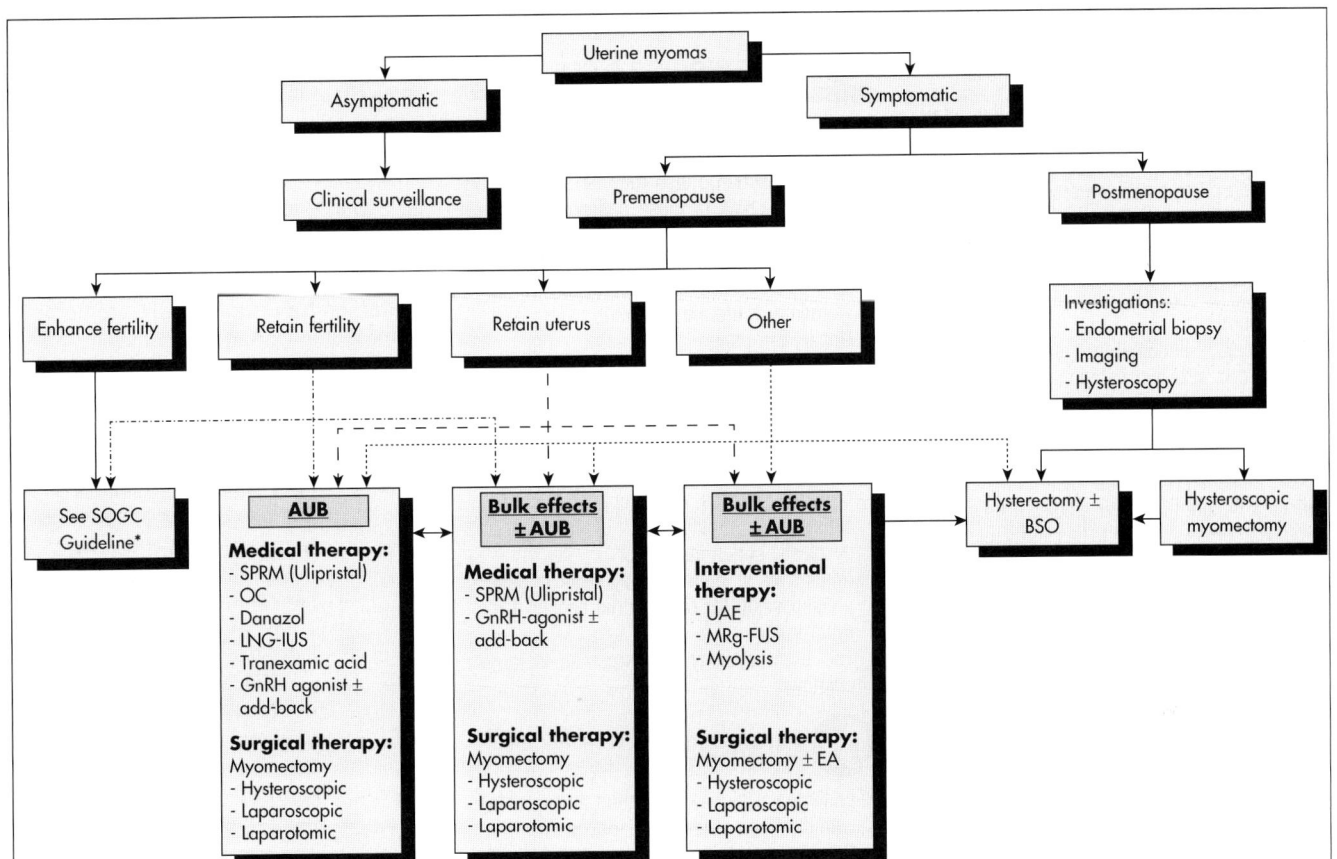

FIG. 4 Algorithm for the management of uterine fibroids. *AUB, Abnormal uterine bleeding; BSO,* Bilateral salpingo-oophorectomy; *GnRH,* Gonadotropin-releasing hormone; *LNG-IUS, levonorgestrel-releasing intrauterine system; MRg-FUS,* magnetic resonance-guided focused ultrasound; *OC,* oral contraceptives; SPRM, selective progesterone-receptor modulator; UAE, uterine artery embolization. (From Vilos GA et al: The management of uterine leiomyomas, *J Obstet Gynaecol Can* 37[2]:163, 2015; and Carranza-Mamane B et al; Society of Obstetrics and Gynaecology Canada Reproductive Endocrinology and Infertility Committee: the management of uterine fibroids in women with otherwise unexplained infertility, SOGC Clinical Practice Guidelines, *J Obstet Gynaecol Can* 37[3]:277-285, 2015.)

history of previous myomectomy are predictors of UAE failure. If the patient wishes to preserve future fertility, UAE should not be performed. Contraindicated if history of GnRH agonist use or salpingectomy.[3]

8. Endometrial ablation: Decreases menorrhagia, has limitations based on uterine cavity distortion.

9. Patients who receive procedures other than definitive management are more likely to result in a second surgery if younger age/less proximity to menopause.

COMPLICATIONS

- Degeneration occurs when the fibroid outgrows its blood supply. During pregnancy, rare but typically seen in the second trimester. May see fever and leukocytosis, but symptoms improve within 48 h.[3]

- Leiomyosarcoma (<0.1%). The U.S. FDA voiced concern regarding the use of power morcellation in the peritoneal cavity during minimally invasive laparoscopy if a tissue containment system is not used due to the possibility of spreading occult malignancy. In 2020, FDA recommended against power morcellation if age >50 yr or postmenopausal.[1]

DISPOSITION

Fibroids continue to grow during reproductive years, but symptoms improve after menopause.

COMPLEMENTARY & ALTERNATIVE THERAPY

Lack of evidence to support acupuncture or herbal therapy.[2] There is some research supporting use of vitamin D.[7]

REFERRAL

Consultation with gynecologist for management and with gynecologic oncologist if suspicious of malignancy

REFERENCES

Available at eBooks.Health.Elsevier.com.

RELATED CONTENT

Uterine Fibroids (Patient Information)
Dysfunctional Uterine Bleeding (Related Key Topic)

AUTHORS: **LISA BIRD, MD,** and **NIMA R. PATEL, MD**

Diseases and Disorders

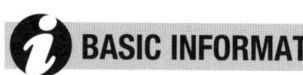

BASIC INFORMATION

DEFINITION

Cancers of the uterus include tumors that originate from epithelial or mesenchymal tissue. Tumors that arise from the epithelium are referred to as adenocarcinomas, whereas tumors that arise from mesenchymal tissue (i.e., connective, muscular, vascular) are referred to as sarcomas. These tumors may be found in various locations of the uterus including the endometrium or myometrium.

Historically, endometrial adenocarcinomas were divided into two categories: Type 1 and Type 2. Type 1 endometrial carcinomas refer to endometrioid subtypes, whereas Type 2 endometrial carcinomas refer to serous, clear cell, and mixed Mullerian subtypes (see "Endometrial Cancer"). Recent molecular studies have shown carcinosarcomas (MMMT) to be closely related to epithelial tumors compared to sarcomas.

This chapter will focus on sarcomas of the uterus arising from the endometrial stroma or myometrium.

SARCOMAS OF THE UTERUS

Leiomyosarcomas
Endometrial stromal sarcoma
Adenosarcomas
Undifferentiated sarcoma

ICD-10CM CODES
C54.1 Malignant neoplasm of endometrium
C54.2 Malignant neoplasm of the myometrium
C54.0 Malignant neoplasm of isthmus uteri
C54.8 Malignant neoplasm of overlapping sites of corpus uteri

EPIDEMIOLOGY & DEMOGRAPHICS

INCIDENCE & PREVALENCE: Incidence of all uterine cancer is 28.1 per 100,000 women per yr with 4.9 deaths per 100,000 women as of 2018. In the most recent update from SEER Annual Report to the Nation, uterine cancer showed the highest increase frequency in death of all cancers among U.S. women. Endometrial cancer remains the most common uterine malignancy in the U.S; however, sarcomas of the uterus are rare. Sarcomas account for approximately 3% to 8% of all cancers of the uterine corpus. Sarcomas are associated with a poor prognosis compared to endometrial cancer.
RISK FACTORS: Box 1 describes risk factors for uterine sarcoma.

BOX 1 Risk Factors for Uterine Sarcoma

- Nulliparity
- Obesity
- History of pelvic radiation
- Exposure to tamoxifen

From Fielding JR et al: *Gynecologic imaging,* Philadelphia, 2011, Saunders.

MEAN AGE AT DIAGNOSIS: 50 yr old.

PHYSICAL FINDINGS & CLINICAL PRESENTATION

- Abnormal vaginal bleeding is the most common symptom (90% of women with diagnosis)
- Vaginal discharge also may be a presenting symptom (10% of these patients have non-bloody discharge)
- May also present as pelvic pain or pressure and pelvic mass on examination (10% of women with uterine sarcoma)
- Urinary symptoms
- Abdominal pain or distention
- Weight loss

ETIOLOGY

- Endometrial cancers are thought to derive from an excess of unopposed estrogen causing a proliferation of disorganized dysplastic endometrium.
- A minority of patients may have a genetic predisposition for endometrial cancer (Lynch syndrome).
- The exact etiology for sarcomas is largely unknown.

DIAGNOSIS

- Endometrial biopsy or dilation and curettage with histologic evidence of malignancy
OR
- Postsurgical histologic examination of uterine tissue

DIFFERENTIAL DIAGNOSIS

- Endometrial hyperplasia
- Endometrial polyp
- Leiomyoma

WORKUP

Diagnosis can be made histologically by biopsy for abnormal bleeding. Workup includes biopsy (in the office or operating room, in conjunction with hysteroscopy) and imaging (see "Imaging Studies" below). Surgical removal of the uterus is the most common way to diagnose a uterine sarcoma. Histologic criteria include mitotic index, cellular atypia, loss of polarity, and necrosis.

LABORATORY TESTS

- CBC
- Comprehensive metabolic panel (CMP)
- CA-125 (high levels can be a sign of metastasis, not diagnostic, not always elevated)

IMAGING STUDIES

- Pelvic ultrasound is a lower-cost method of detecting uterine corpus mass or thickened endometrial lining. Features concerning for uterine sarcoma: Heterogeneous texture, central necrosis, irregular vessel distribution, and rapid growth of the uterus.
- Chest x-ray examination should be considered for preoperative testing with suspicion of uterine sarcoma.
- Computed tomography (CT) scans (Fig. 1), MRI, and PET may be useful for assessing

tumor spread once diagnosis is made or characterizing a uterine mass.

STAGING

Staging of endometrial carcinoma and uterine adenosarcoma is summarized in Tables 1 and 2.

TABLE 1 International Federation of Gynecology and Obstetrics 2009 Staging for Endometrial Carcinoma (Including Carcinosarcoma)

Stage	
I	Tumor confined to uterine corpus including endocervical glands
I_A	Tumor confined to endometrium or invades <50% of the myometrium
I_B	Tumor invades 50% or more the myometrium
II	Tumor invades cervical stroma but confined to uterus
III	Tumor involving the serosa, adnexa, vagina, or parametria
III_A	Tumor invades uterine serosa or adnexa
III_B	Involvement of vagina or parametrium
III_{C1}	Metastasis to pelvic lymph nodes
III_{C2}	Metastasis to paraaortic lymph nodes
IV	Tumor involves bladder and/or bowel mucosa or distant metastasis
IV_A	Invasion of bladder or bowel mucosa
IV_B	Distant metastases including intraabdominal metastasis, inguinal lymph nodes, or both

From Niederhuber JE: *Abeloff's clinical oncology,* ed 6, Philadelphia, 2020, Elsevier.

TABLE 2 International Federation of Gynecology and Obstetrics 2009 Staging for Uterine Sarcoma (Including Leiomyosarcoma and Endometrial Stromal Sarcoma)

Stage	
I	Tumor limited to the uterus
I_A	Tumor 5 cm or less in greatest dimension
I_B	Tumor more than 5 cm
II	Tumor extends beyond the uterus, within the pelvis
II_A	Adnexal involvement
II_B	Extrauterine pelvic tissue involvement
III	Involvement of abdominal tissues
III_A	1 site
III_B	>1 site
III_C	Regional lymph node metastasis
IV	
IV_A	Tumor invades bladder or rectum
IV_B	Distant metastases

From Niederhuber JE: *Abeloff's clinical oncology,* ed 6, Philadelphia, 2020, Elsevier.

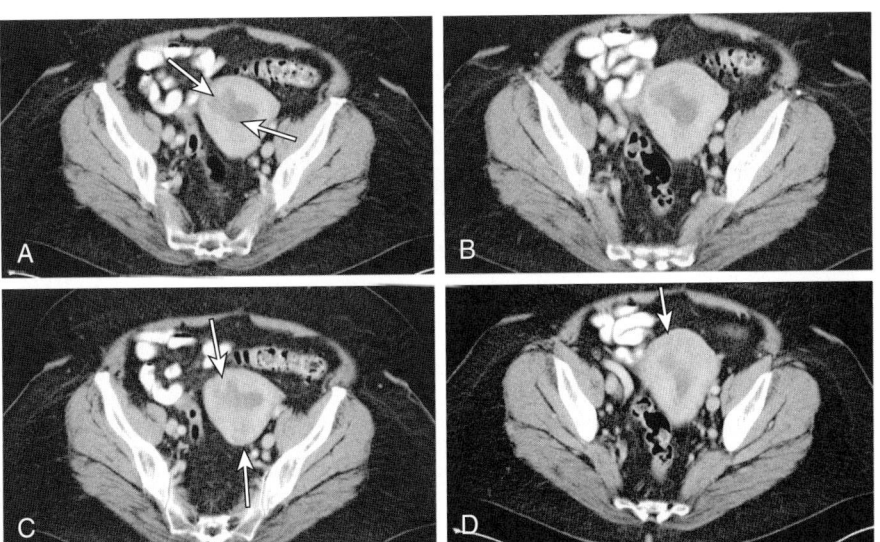

FIG. 1 A 50-yr-old patient with uterine sarcoma. A, Axial contrast-enhanced computed tomographic (CT) image. Low-attenuation lobulated and infiltrating soft tissue fills the endometrial canal *(arrows)*, extending into the myometrium. **B,** Axial contrast-enhanced CT image showing same as **A.** Low-attenuation, lobulated, and infiltrating soft tissue fills the endometrial canal, extending into the myometrium. **C,** Axial contrast-enhanced CT image. Low-attenuation lobulated and infiltrating soft tissue fills the endometrial canal. Subtle myometrial invasion is seen anterior and posterior *(arrows)*. **D,** Axial contrast-enhanced CT image. Low-attenuation lobulated and infiltrating soft tissue fills the endometrial canal *(arrow)*, showing same. Subtle myometrial invasion is seen fundally. (From Fielding JR et al: *Gynecologic imaging,* Philadelphia, 2011, Saunders.)

BOX 2	Uterine Sarcoma Prognostic Factors

- Tumor stage
- Tumor grade
- Tumor size
- Patient age
- Vascular space involvement
- Mitotic count
- Residual disease at surgery or uterine morcellation
- Adjuvant chemotherapy

From Fielding JR et al: *Gynecologic imaging,* Philadelphia, 2011, Saunders.

RX TREATMENT

- Treatment for sarcomas is based on the method in which diagnosis was made. If diagnosed after a hysterectomy, surgical resection for residual tumor or tube/ovary may be performed. If diagnosis made by biopsy, surgical resection is based on the symptoms and extent of the disease.
- Further treatment depends on the type of cancer, histologic grade, and stage.
  1. Low-grade endometrial stromal sarcoma: Stage 1 disease is usually followed up by

---

BOX 3	Uterine Sarcoma: Key Points

- The disease mainly affects women aged 40-60 yr old depending on the type of sarcoma.
- Patients may present with abnormal uterine bleeding, abdominal distention, enlarging pelvic mass, pelvic pain/pressure, or may be asymptomatic.
- The primary treatment is hysterectomy and bilateral salpingo-oophorectomy.
- Adjuvant radiotherapy to the pelvis and/or systemic chemotherapy may be considered if > stage 1 sarcoma.

From Greer IA et al: *Mosby's color atlas and text of obstetrics and gynecology,* London, 2001, Harcourt.

surveillance after surgery. A higher staged disease may be offered external beam radiation therapy and/or antiestrogen hormone therapy.
  2. High-grade endometrial stromal sarcoma, undifferentiated uterine sarcoma, and uterine leiomyosarcoma: Stage 1 disease can be followed with surveillance. Chemotherapeutic agents and external beam radiation therapy can be considered for stage 2 or higher.

DISPOSITION

- Survival varies with each type of sarcoma but is generally very poor. Box 2 describes uterine prognostic factors.
- 5-yr survival for grade I endometrial stromal sarcoma is 91% and drops to 42% for grade III.
- 5-yr survival for leiomyosarcoma ranges from 76% for stage 1 to 29% for stage 4.
- 5-yr survival for undifferentiated sarcoma ranges from 70% for stage 1 to 23% for stage 4.

REFERRAL

A gynecologic oncologist should manage uterine sarcoma.
Key points in the management of uterine sarcoma are described in Box 3.

SUGGESTED READINGS

Available at eBooks.Health.Elsevier.com.

RELATED CONTENT

Uterine Cancer (Patient Information)
Endometrial Cancer (Related Key Topic)

AUTHORS: **CHRISTINA NESTLERODE, DO,** and **ROBERT NEFF, MD**

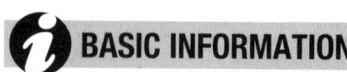
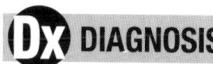 BASIC INFORMATION

DEFINITION

Prepubescent vulvovaginitis is an inflammatory condition of the vulva and vagina.

SYNONYM

Prepubertal vulvovaginitis

ICD-10CM CODES	
N76.0	Acute vaginitis
N76.1	Subacute and chronic vaginitis
N76.2	Acute vulvitis
N76.3	Subacute and chronic vulvitis
N76.89	Other specified inflammation of vagina and vulva

EPIDEMIOLOGY & DEMOGRAPHICS

- Most common gynecologic problem of pre-menarchal girls.[1,2]
- Prepubertal girls are susceptible to irritation and trauma because of the absence of protective hair and labial fat pads, as well as the presence of a more alkaline environment and unestrogenized atrophic mucosa, poor hygiene, obesity, and choice of apparel.[1]
- Symptoms of vulvovaginitis and introital irritation and discharge account for 80% to 90% of gynecologic visits.[2]
- Nonspecific etiology in up to 75% of children with vulvovaginitis.
- Majority of vulvovaginitis in girls involves a primary irritation of the vulva with secondary involvement of the lower third of the vagina.[1]

PHYSICAL FINDINGS & CLINICAL PRESENTATION

- Erythema, rash.
- Vulvar pain, dysuria, pruritus.
- Discharge can also be present.
- If present, vaginal discharge may be foul smelling or bloody.

ETIOLOGY

- Most commonly attributed to poor hygiene or nonspecific irritants. Etiologic factors in pre-menarcheal vulvovaginitis are summarized in Box 1.[1,2]
- Hypoestrogenic state increases risk of infection or irritation due to:
  1. Atrophic, friable vaginal mucosa
  2. Higher vaginal pH (more hospitable to infectious agents)
  3. Underdeveloped labia minora and lack of significant adipose and hair of labia majora (less intrinsic protection of the vagina from trauma, irritants, infectious agents)
- Infections:
  1. Bacterial: Often respiratory or enteric organisms[2]
  2. Protozoal/parasitic
  3. Mycotic
  4. Viral[3,4]
- Endocrine disorders
- Labial adhesions[5]
- Skin disorders
- Sexual abuse[3,4]

- Allergic substance
- Trauma
- Foreign body
- Masturbation
- Constipation

DX DIAGNOSIS

DIFFERENTIAL DIAGNOSIS

- Physiologic leukorrhea
- Foreign body
- Bacterial vaginosis
- Fungal vulvovaginitis
- Precocious puberty
- Sexual abuse or trauma and possibly an associated sexually transmitted infection such as gonorrhea, *Chlamydia,* or *Trichomonas*[3,4]
- Pinworms
- Cutaneous vulvar disease

WORKUP

- History regarding symptoms, hygiene practices, exposures to known irritants, types of clothing.[1,2]
- Examination, including Tanner staging, pelvic/genital examination; possibly speculum examination.[1,2]
- Knee-chest position for examination may be easier for the child to tolerate. May need to consider exam under anesthesia for more thorough evaluation or for intolerance of exam, if necessary.[1,2]
- May need rectal examination.
- KOH and normal saline preparation of discharge.[6]
- Vaginoscopy if considering a foreign body.[2]
- Sexual abuse/assault screening if indicated.[1-4]

LABORATORY TESTS

- Urinalysis to rule out urinary tract infection and diabetes
- Cultures including sexually transmitted diseases[3,4]
- Wet mount[6]

Rx TREATMENT

NONPHARMACOLOGIC THERAPY

- Avoid tight clothing. Counsel on loose-fitting pants and underwear to allow air circulation[1,2]
- Avoid staying in wet swimsuits after swimming
- Appropriate hygiene education
- Avoid chemical irritants
- If foreign body, removal via irrigation or exam under anesthesia
- If vulva is irritated, can use a topical over-the-counter emollient
- Reassurance

ACUTE GENERAL Rx

- *Streptococcal* and *staphylococcal* spp., *Haemophilus influenzae:* Adolescents: Ampicillin 50 to 100 mg/kg/day divided q6h (max daily dose 2 g/day)
- *Chlamydia trachomatis:* Children <45 kg: Erythromycin 50 mg/kg/day orally (PO) divided q6h ×14 days (max dose 2 g/day).

Children ≥45 kg but younger than 8 yr: Erythromycin 500 mg qid ×7 days. Children ≥8 yr: Doxycycline 2.2 mg/kg/dose twice daily ×7 days (max dose 100 mg/dose). Adolescents: Doxycycline 100 mg bid ×7 days[4]
- *Neisseria gonorrhoeae:* Children ≤45 kg: Ceftriaxone 25 to 50 mg/kg intravenous (IV) or intramuscular (IM) in a single dose, not to exceed 125 mg/dose. Children >45 kg: Ceftriaxone 500 mg IM once; 1000 mg recommended for patients ≥150 kg. If chlamydia has not been excluded in adolescents, add Doxycycline 100 mg PO bid ×7 days[3,4]
- *Trichomonas:* Children <45 kg: Metronidazole 45 mg/kg/day PO in divided doses 3×/day for 7 days (max daily dose 2g/day). Children >45 kg: 500 mg PO bid for 7 days or 2 g once as a single dose[4]
- *Bacterial vaginosis:* Children and adolescents >45 kg: Metronidazole 500 mg PO bid ×7 days[6]
- *Candida:* Fluconazole 150 mg PO once
- *Recurrent candida:* Fluconazole 100 to 200 mg PO q72 h for 3 doses; maintenance 100 to 200 mg weekly for 6 mo
- *Pinworms:* Mebendazole 100-mg chewable tablet once, repeat in 2 wk; Pyrantel pamoate 11 mg/kg (max 1 g) PO repeat in 2 wk (available over the counter)
- *Labial agglutination:* Spontaneous resolution if asymptomatic or topical estrogen cream twice daily if symptomatic until resolution then A&D Ointment for 6 to 12 mo[5]
- Condyloma acuminatum: Treatment is optional as most spontaneously resolve in a few years. If symptomatic, cryotherapy ablative laser therapy, or Imiquimod 5% cream 3×per wk for up to 16 wk

DISPOSITION

Further education:
- Discuss appropriate hygiene.[1]
- If sexually active, discuss pregnancy prevention and safe sexual practices. Have a high suspicion of sexual abuse and report to child protective services with any concerns for abuse.[1,3,4]

REFERRAL

- To Obstetrician/Gynecologist, preferably a physician with specialized training in Pediatric and Adolescent Gynecology if available
- To pediatrician
- To dermatologist

REFERENCES

Available at eBooks.Health.Elsevier.com

RELATED CONTENT

Chlamydia Genital Infections (Related Key Topic)
Pruritus Vulvae (Related Key Topic)
Vaginitis, Fungal (Related Key Topic)
Vaginitis, *Trichomonas* (Related Key Topic)
Vaginosis, Bacterial (Related Key Topic)

AUTHORS: **MORGAN WILHOITE, DO,** and **NIMA R. PATEL, MD, MS**

BOX 1 Etiologic Factors in Premenarcheal Vulvovaginitis

Bacterial Infections
Nonspecific mixed infections secondary to:
  Poor perineal hygiene
  Foreign body in vagina
  Respiratory tract infections
  Skin infections (impetigo)
  Urinary tract infection
Specific nonvenereal infection:
  Hemolytic streptococci (groups A, B, F)
  Escherichia coli
  Shigella flexneri, Shigella sonnei
  Neisseria meningitidis, Neisseria sicca
  Haemophilus influenzae type b, nontypeable strains
  Streptococcus pneumoniae
  Corynebacterium diphtheriae
  Yersinia enterocolitica
  Mycobacterium tuberculosis
  Moraxella (Branhamella) catarrhalis
  Staphylococcus aureus
Specific venereal infections:
  Neisseria gonorrhoeae
  Treponema pallidum
  Chlamydia trachomatis
  Chancroid *(Haemophilus ducreyi)*
  Granuloma inguinale
Bacterial vaginosis:
  Gardnerella vaginalis
  Mobiluncus species
Fungal Infections
  Candida albicans
  Other yeasts
  Dermatophytes

Protozoan and Parasitic Infections
  Trichomoniasis
  Amebiasis
  Enterobius vermicularis
  Hirudiniasis
  Schistosomiasis
  Other parasitic infections (ascariasis, trichuriasis)

Viral Infections
Venereal:
  Herpes simplex
  Condyloma acuminatum (papillomavirus)
  Molluscum contagiosum
Involvement as part of systemic infection:
  Measles
  Varicella
  Mononucleosis (Epstein-Barr virus)
  Coxsackievirus
  Smallpox

Infestations
Pediculosis
Scabies

Contact Irritation or Allergic Reactions
Bubble bath preparations
Hair shampoos
Vulvar deodorant sprays
Soaps, laundry detergents
Other medications

Vulvar or Perineal Skin Diseases
Local:
  Seborrhea
  Lichen sclerosus et atrophicus
  Lichen planus
  Lichen simplex chronicus
  Premalignant leukoplakia
  Erythrasma *(Corynebacterium minutissimum)*
  Bartholinitis
  Skenitis
Involvement as part of a systemic disorder:
  Psoriasis
  Bullous pemphigoid
  Atopic dermatitis
  Drug eruption
  Generalized pruritus with excoriation
  Chronic liver disease
  Chronic renal disease
  Metabolic errors
  Psychosomatic
  Crohn disease
  Sjögren syndrome
  Henoch-Schönlein purpura
  Histiocytosis
  Kawasaki disease
  Stevens-Johnson syndrome
  Typhoid
  Zinc deficiency

Physical Factors
Sand (sandbox)
Chemical or thermal trauma
Physical trauma (accidents, abuse, masturbation)
Nylon, rayon underclothing
Tight garments (maceration in warm climates)
Anatomic abnormalities:
  Neoplasms (sarcoma botryoides)
  Polyps
  Labial agglutination, adhesion
  Prolapsed urethra
  Ectopic ureter
  Rectal fistula
  Draining pelvic abscess via fistula

From Cherry JD et al: *Feigin and Cherry's textbook of pediatric infectious diseases,* ed 8, Philadelphia, 2019, Elsevier.

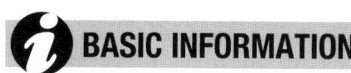
BASIC INFORMATION

DEFINITION

Trichomonas vulvovaginitis is inflammation of the vulva and vagina caused by the protozoan *Trichomonas vaginalis*.[1]

SYNONYMS

Trichomonas vaginalis
T. vaginalis
Trichomoniasis
Trich
TV

ICD-10CM CODE

A59.01 Trichomonal vulvovaginitis

EPIDEMIOLOGY & DEMOGRAPHICS

- Most common nonviral sexually transmitted infection in the U.S., caused by a parasitic protozoan[2]
- Acquired through sexual contact
  1. Commonly transmitted male to female, female to male, and female to female
  2. Rarely transmitted male to male
- Overall prevalence is 2% in women 18 to 59; incidence increases with age
- Diagnosed in:[3]

1. 9.6% Black women, 1.4% Hispanic women, 0.8% non-Hispanic white women
2. 14.6% to 27% women presenting to STI clinics
3. 9% to 32% incarcerated women
4. Up to 70% of male partners of women with trichomonas

RISK FACTORS[5]:

- African descent
- Multiple sexual partners
- HIV infection
- IV drug use
- History of previous STIs
- History of incarceration
- Concurrent bacterial vaginosis (BV) infection
- Others: Less than a high school education, living below the national poverty level

PHYSICAL FINDINGS & CLINICAL PRESENTATION

These symptoms and physical findings may or may not be present depending on the case:[3,4]
- Yellow-green, malodorous vaginal discharge
- Vaginal and/or vulvar pruritus
- Dysuria
- Dyspareunia
- Intense erythema of the vaginal mucosa
- Cervical petechiae ("strawberry cervix")
- Infected men may have symptoms of urethritis, epididymitis, or prostatitis

- Asymptomatic in approximately 85% of women and 75% of men

ETIOLOGY

Single-cell protozoan *Trichomonas vaginalis*

DIAGNOSIS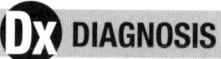

DIFFERENTIAL DIAGNOSIS[4] (TABLE 1)

- Bacterial vaginosis
- Candida vulvovaginitis
- STI (gonorrhea or chlamydia)
- Others: Atrophic vulvovaginitis, contact dermatitis

WORKUP

- Pelvic examination
- Speculum examination
- Wet mount: Look for motile trichomonads on normal saline preparation (Fig. 1)
  1. 40% to 70% sensitivity[3]
  2. Evaluate within 10 min; sensitivity decreases over time
- Assess vaginal pH: Trichomonas is associated with elevated pH ($>$4.5)
- Laboratory testing (see later)
  1. Note: If wet mount negative, should evaluate with lab test if possible

---

TABLE 1 Features of Sexually Transmitted Infections Characterized by Vaginal Discharge

FEATURE	PHYSIOLOGIC LEUKORRHEA (NORMAL)	TRICHOMONIASIS	BACTERIAL VAGINOSIS
Agent	Normal flora	*Trichomonas vaginalis*	Reduction in *Lactobacillus* and overgrowth organisms including *Gardnerella vaginalis*, *Bacteroides*, *Mobiluncus*, and *Peptostreptococcus*
Incubation	—	5-28 days	Not necessarily sexually transmitted
Predominant Symptoms			
Pruritus	None	Mild to moderate	None to mild
Discharge	Minimal	Moderate to severe	Mild to moderate
Pain	None	Mild	Uncommon
Vulvar inflammation	None	Common	Uncommon
Characteristics of Discharge			
Amount	Small	Profuse	Moderate
Color	Clear, milky	Yellow-green or gray	Gray
Consistency	Flocculent	Frothy	Homogeneous
Viscosity	Thin	Thin	Thin
Foul odor	None	Possible	Yes
Odor with KOH	None	Possible	Characteristic fishy odor (amine)
pH	$<$4.5	$>$5.0	$>$4.5
Diagnosis			
Saline drop	Squamous and few WBCs	WBC; motile flagellates, slightly larger than WBCs	Squamous cells studded with bacteria ("clue cells") and WBCs
Gram stain	Gram-positive and gram-negative rods and cocci	*Trichomonas*	Predominance of gram-negative rods and cocci with paucity of gram-positive rods
Culture	Mixed flora with *Lactobacillus* predominant	Culture generally not indicated; antibody and nucleic acid tests available	Culture not useful
Treatment	Reassurance	Metronidazole or tinidazole	Metronidazole or clindamycin

KOH, Potassium hydroxide; *WBCs*, white blood cells.
From Marcdante KJ et al: *Nelson essentials of pediatrics*, ed 9, Philadelphia, 2023, Elsevier.

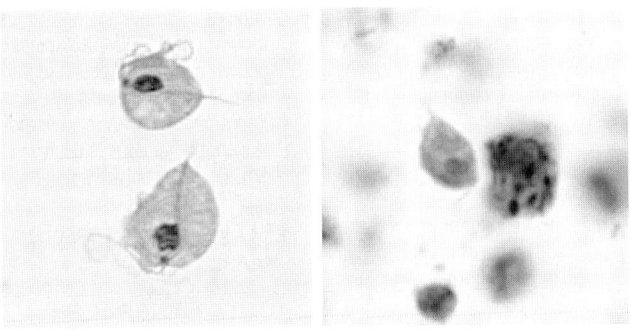

FIG. 1 *Trichomonas vaginalis* **trophozoites stained with Giemsa** *(right and left).* ((From Centers for Disease Control and Prevention: Laboratory identification of parasites of public health concern, Trichomoniasis. (https://www.cdc.gov/dpdx/trichomoniasis/index.html.))

- Recommend also screening for gonorrhea and chlamydia

LABORATORY TESTS

- Nucleic acid amplification tests (NAATs): Most sensitive and specific test (gold standard)[3]
  1. Can be collected as endocervical swab, vaginal swab, or urine
  2. Pros: More rapid turnaround time compared with culture
  3. Cons: More expensive, test results take 24 to 72 hr
  4. Brands: Aptima, Amplicor, BD Max
- Rapid tests: Useful in areas with high prevalence of trichomonas[3]
  1. Pros: Sensitivity 80% to 95%, specificity 97% to 100%; more accurate than wet mount
  2. Cons: More expensive
  3. Brands: OSOM Trichomonas Rapid Test (10 min), Affirm VP III (45 min)
- Culture: Was gold standard before PCR[3]
  1. Useful if negative wet mount or NAAT not available
  2. Pros: Sensitivity up to 93%, specificity up to 100%; can be used for antimicrobial susceptibility
  3. Cons: Not widely available, can take 3 to 7 days to get results
  4. Brands: InPouch
- PAP smear: Incidental finding of trichomonads is sometimes reported on PAP smear[4]
  1. Liquid-based cytology: High specificity, reasonable to treat if presence reported
  2. Conventional PAP smear: Lower specificity, recommend evaluating with diagnostic test, although still reasonable to treat if patient reports symptoms

Rx TREATMENT

NONPHARMACOLOGIC THERAPY

- Barrier methods: Recommend using condoms, internal condoms, dental dams, or other barrier methods during all oral, anal, or vaginal intercourse.
- Hygiene: Recommend not sharing sex toys and cleaning after each use with a dedicated cleaner.
- Screening: Recommend regular STI screening if concern for a new partner or new exposure.

ACUTE GENERAL Rx

- Preferred initial treatment for women:[6] Metronidazole 500 mg PO bid × 7 days
  1. Second-line treatment for women:[6] Metronidazole, secnidazole, or tinidazole 2 g PO × 1 dose
- Preferred initial treatment for men:[3] Metronidazole 2 g PO × 1 dose
  1. Second-line treatment for men:[3] Tinidazole or secnidazole 2 g PO × 1 dose
- Special populations:
  1. Pregnancy:[3] Metronidazole only (either 500 mg PO bid × 7d or 2 g PO × 1 dose)
     a. Avoid tinidazole and secnidazole, minimal research has been done
     b. Trichomonas is associated with premature rupture of membranes, preterm delivery, and small-for-gestational-age infants; unclear if treatment improves outcomes
  2. Breastfeeding:[3] Consider deferring breastfeeding for 12 to 24 hr after taking traditional dose of metronidazole
     a. Lowest concentration in breast milk: Metronidazole 400 mg PO tid × 7 days
  3. HIV:[3] Metronidazole 500 mg PO bid × 7 days
     a. Higher treatment failure with single-dose regimen
- Expedited partner therapy (EPT): Recommend sending Rx for sex partners and abstaining from sex for 7 days or until both partners are treated and symptoms resolved.[4]
- CDC recommends retesting sexually active women between 3 wk and 3 mo after completing treatment.[3]

- NOTE: Consider recommending avoidance of alcohol consumption during treatment with metronidazole (at least 24 hr after completion of therapy) and tinidazole (at least 72 hr after completion of therapy) to reduce the possibility of disulfiram-like reaction, although is likely unnecessary.[5]

CHRONIC Rx

- For persistent infections:[3] Repeat metronidazole 500 mg PO bid × 7 days
- If treatment is still unsuccessful:[3] Metronidazole or tinidazole 2 g PO daily × 7 days
- If still unsuccessful:[3]
  1. Option 1: Tinidazole 2 g PO daily PLUS intravaginal tinidazole 500 mg bid × 14 days
  2. Option 2: Tinidazole 1 g PO tid PLUS intravaginal paromomycin 4 g nightly (6.25% cream) × 14 days
  3. Option 3: Culture and susceptibility testing per the CDC (404-718-4141)
- Allergy, intolerance, or adverse reactions: Alternatives to metronidazole or tinidazole are not recommended. Patients who are allergic to nitroimidazoles can be managed by desensitization.[3,4]

DISPOSITION

- Trichomonas is considered an STI and treatment of sex partners is recommended.
- If diagnosed with trichomonas, testing for other STIs is recommended, including HIV, syphilis, and gonorrhea/chlamydia.
- Trichomonas is associated with 1.5- to 2-fold increased risk for HIV acquisition.
- Trichomonas in pregnancy is associated with premature rupture of membranes, preterm birth, and delivery of low-birth-weight infants.

REFERRAL

- To obstetrician/gynecologist for recurrent infection or pregnancy

REFERENCES
Available at eBooks.Health.Elsevier.com.

RELATED CONTENT
Trichomoniasis (Patient Information)
Pruritus Vulvae (Related Key Topic)

AUTHORS: **ALEXANDRA H. SMICK, MD,** and **STEVEN D. JOHNSON, MD**

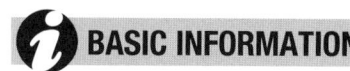

BASIC INFORMATION

DEFINITION

Bacterial vaginosis (BV) is a polymicrobial infection in which anaerobic bacteria overgrow and replace the normal hydrogen peroxide-producing lactobacilli, resulting in thin, gray, and malodorous vaginal discharge.

SYNONYMS

Bacterial vaginosis
BV
Nonspecific vaginitis
Gardnerella vaginalis vaginitis

ICD-10CM CODES
N76.0 Acute vaginitis
N77.1 Vaginitis, vulvitis and vulvovaginitis in diseases classified elsewhere

EPIDEMIOLOGY & DEMOGRAPHICS

- Most common cause of vaginal discharge in women of reproductive age.
- Most common organisms include *Gardnerella vaginalis*, *Porphyromonas* species, *Mycoplasma hominis*, *Bacteroides* species, *Peptostreptococcus* species, *Ureaplasma urealyticum*, *Fusobacterium* species, *Prevotella* species, and *Atopobium vaginae*, and other facultative anaerobes.
- Women with BV are at increased risk for acquiring other sexually transmitted diseases (STDs) such as human immunodeficiency virus (HIV), *N. gonorrhoeae*, *C. trachomatis*, and herpes simplex virus type 2 (HSV-2). BV may also contribute to persistent human papillomavirus (HPV) infection.
- May be associated with pelvic inflammatory disease (PID) and complications after gynecologic surgery. Preoperative evaluation and treatment before planned hysterectomy or abortion decreases the infection complication rate.
- May be associated with low birth weight, premature rupture of membranes (PROM), and prematurity in the obstetric setting.
- BV may recur in 30% of cases within the first 3 mo after treatment, which may be due to:
  1. Persistence of pathogenic bacteria
  2. Reinfection from exogenous sources including sexual partners
  3. Failure of the normal lactobacillus-dominant flora to reestablish
- Risk factors: Multiple female or male sexual partners, sexually transmitted infections, douching, tobacco use, lack of condom use, and lack of vaginal lactobacilli.

PHYSICAL FINDINGS & CLINICAL PRESENTATION

- 50% to 75% of patients are asymptomatic
- A thin, dull, and gray homogeneous discharge (Fig. 1)
- Characterized by a "fishy" odor from the vagina
- Vaginal pH >4.5

- BV alone does not typically cause dysuria or dyspareunia, and presence may suggest concomitant infection with another pathogen
- Clue cells on microscopic examination (Fig. 2)

ETIOLOGY

- *Gardnerella vaginalis* is detected in 40% to 50% of vaginal secretions.
- Increase in vaginal pH secondary to decrease in hydrogen peroxide producing lactobacilli allows predominance of anaerobes that produce amines.
- It is unclear how the vaginal floral imbalance occurs and the role sexual activity plays in the pathogenesis of BV.
- *G. vaginalis* may be important in epithelial biofilm formation.
- Ethnicity and age may contribute to the vaginal microbial environment.

DIAGNOSIS

WORKUP

- At least three of the Amsel clinical diagnostic criteria must be present for diagnosis (sensitivity of 92% and specificity of 77%):
  1. Thin, gray, and homogeneous, malodorous discharge that adheres to the vaginal walls
  2. Vaginal pH >4.5
  3. Positive whiff-amine test
     a. Conducted by placing wet mount specimen and adding 10% potassium hydroxide, which creates a fishy odor.
  4. More than 20% of the epithelial cells on microscopy are clue cells
- Gram staining: Considered the gold-standard laboratory method to determine the concentration of lactobacilli and gram-negative and gram-positive bacteria.
- If microscopy is unavailable, other diagnostic tests include Affirm VPIII (Becton Dickinson, Sparks, MD), a DNA-hybridization probe test for high concentrations of *G. vaginalis*, and the OSOM BV Blue test (Sekisui Diagnostics, Framingham, MA), which detects vaginal fluid sialidase activity. A molecular test for the

vaginal microbiome for BV, candidiasis, and trichomonas (BD MAX Vaginal Panel) has also shown promising results in early studies.
- Cultures are unnecessary.
- Pap smear is not a reliable test for BV.
- Rule out other causes such as vulvar diseases, STDs, and atrophic vaginitis.

TREATMENT

ACUTE GENERAL Rx

- Recommended regimens (similar efficacy):
  1. Metronidazole 500 mg PO bid for 7 days *or*
  2. Metronidazole 0.75% gel, one full applicator (5 g) intravaginally daily for 5 days *or*
  3. Clindamycin 2% cream, one full applicator (5 g) intravaginally at bedtime for 7 days
- Alternative regimens:
  1. Clindamycin 300 mg PO bid for 7 days or clindamycin 100 mg ovules intravaginally once at bedtime for 3 days.
- May be associated with antimicrobial resistance
  1. Tinidazole 1g PO once daily for 5 days
- Longer half-life than metronidazole (~12 to 14 hr vs. ~6 to 7 hr)
  1. Secnidazole 2 g PO once
- Longer half-life than metronidazole (~17 hr vs. ~8 hr). Shown to be superior to placebo in phase 3 trial and at least as effective as metronidazole 500 mg PO bid in noninferiority trial. Single 1-g oral dose appears to be effective also. Single dose improves compliance but is more expensive than multidose metronidazole therapy.
- Disulfiram-type reactions may occur while taking oral or topical metronidazole, and patients should be advised to avoid alcohol while undergoing treatment.
- Sexual partners: It is not necessary to treat male partners of affected females; however, females who partner with females need to be aware of the signs and symptoms of BV, and treatment is indicated in this population if symptoms occur.

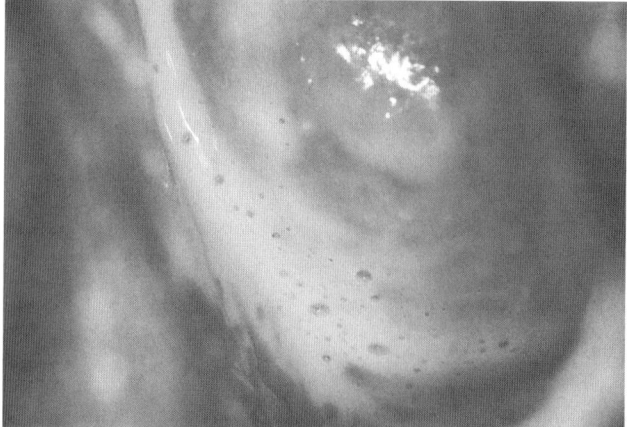

FIG. 1 Bacterial vaginosis. The gray, homogeneous discharge that coats the tissues is characteristic. (From Bennett JE et al: *Mandell, Douglas, and Bennett's principles and practice of infectious diseases*, ed 8, Philadelphia, 2015, Saunders.)

V

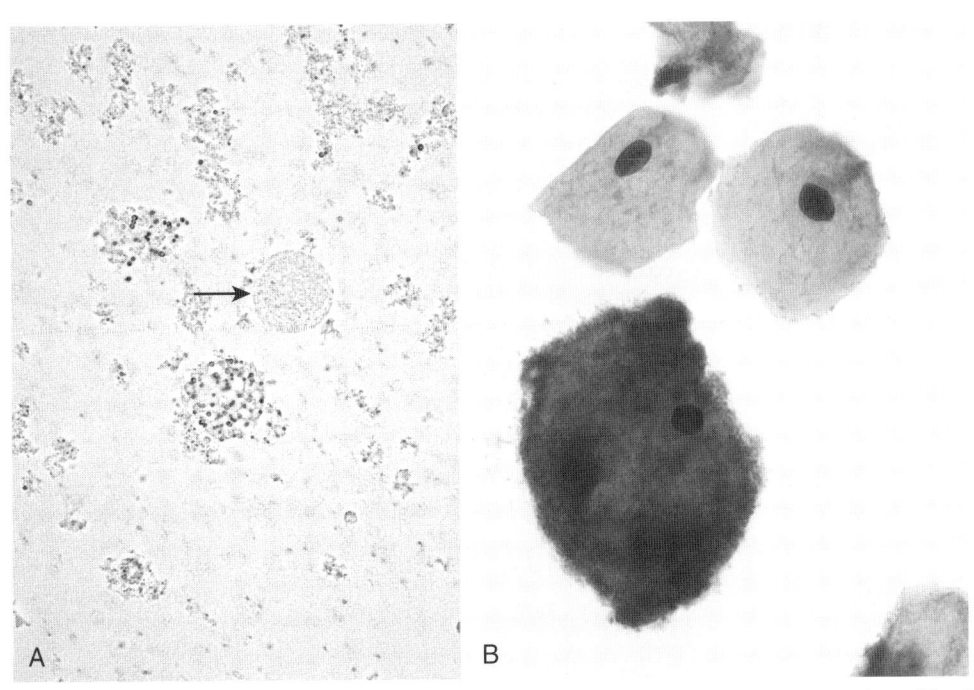

FIG. 2 Bacterial vaginosis, seen as dense, evenly distributed collections of rod-like bacteria forms in squamous cells as seen on a wet prep **(A)** or Papanicolaou stain (clue cells; **B**). (From Crum CP et al: *Diagnostic gynecologic and obstetric pathology,* ed 3, Philadelphia, 2018, Elsevier.)

- Follow-up visits after treatment and resolution of symptoms are unnecessary, but patients are advised to return if symptoms recur.
- Not enough evidence for or against probiotic use for treatment and prevention.
- Clindamycin cream may weaken latex condoms if used together. Avoid treatment of asymptomatic patients.
- Treatment in pregnancy:
  1. Symptomatic pregnant patients with BV should be treated to relieve bothersome symptoms.
  2. Insufficient evidence to recommend routine screening for BV in asymptomatic pregnant women at high or low risk of preterm delivery.
  3. Can use oral or topical therapy for symptomatic pregnant women with same regimen as nonpregnant women.

4. There is no evidence that metronidazole or clindamycin have any teratogenic effect during pregnancy. Tinidazole should be avoided in pregnancy.
- Recurrent BV:
  1. Condom use may help reduce the risk of recurrence.
  2. Chronic suppressive therapy has been proven to reduce the development or recurrence of BV.

PEARLS & CONSIDERATIONS

- BV is the most common cause of vaginitis in reproductive women.
- BV has been associated with pelvic inflammatory disease (PID), postprocedural gynecologic complications, and other STDs. It is reasonable to treat asymptomatic women who are to undergo gynecologic surgery and screen for other STDs.
- American College of Obstetricians and Gynecologists, U.S. Preventive Services Task Force (USPSFT), and CDC all agree to not routinely screen and treat all pregnant women with asymptomatic BV to prevent preterm birth.

SUGGESTED READINGS
Available at eBooks.Health.Elsevier.com.

RELATED CONTENT
Bacterial Vaginal Infections (Patient Information)

AUTHORS: **DEVON SMITH, DO,** and **EMILY SAKS, MD, MSCE**

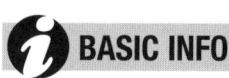
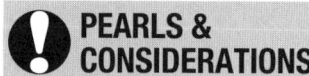 BASIC INFORMATION

DEFINITION

Enterococci are gram-positive, facultative anaerobic organisms usually oval in shape and can be seen as single cells, pairs, or chains. Vancomycin-resistant *Enterococcus* (VRE) are enterococci that have become resistant to vancomycin and several antibiotics normally used to treat enterococcal infections.

SYNONYM

VRE

ICD-10CM CODE

Z16.39 Resistance to other specified antimicrobial drug

EPIDEMIOLOGY & DEMOGRAPHICS

INCIDENCE:
- VRE may be associated with the use or overuse of specific classes of antibiotics.
- VRE can spread within hospital units, causing widespread colonization or clinical outbreaks, and is generally considered hospital acquired or nursing home acquired.

PEAK INCIDENCE: VRE was first reported in Europe in 1986, and there has been a steady rise in the incidence of enterococcal strains resistant to vancomycin. In 2007, 80% of *E. faecium* isolates and 7% of *E. faecalis* isolates were resistant to vancomycin.

RISK FACTORS:
- Prior antimicrobial therapy, especially vancomycin
- Prolonged hospitalization
- Chronic medical conditions, renal failure
- Invasive devices
- ICU stay
- Colonization: VRE colonize the gastrointestinal tract; can be found on skin or perirectal swab culture or stool culture

OUTCOMES: VRE infections are associated with adverse outcomes, with mortality rates significantly higher in patients with VRE infections versus vancomycin-susceptible enterococcal infections.

PHYSICAL FINDINGS & CLINICAL PRESENTATION

Patients may be asymptomatic and have gastrointestinal colonization; it can be associated with diarrhea. In hospitalized patients, infection is associated with colonization and can cause wound infections, bacteremia, abscesses (intra-abdominal), and, rarely, pneumonia, urinary tract infections, and endocarditis.

ETIOLOGY

- The Clinical and Laboratory Standards Institute uses the following MIC definitions for vancomycin susceptibility and resistance in enterococci:
  1. Vancomycin susceptible: $\leq$4 mcg/ml
  2. Vancomycin resistant: $\geq$32 mcg/ml
  3. Vancomycin intermediate: 8 to 16 mcg/ml (vancomycin not recommended)
- Enterococci are primarily found in the human digestive tract and female genital tract, where they make up a significant portion of the normal bacterial population in healthy people. Enterococci can cause urinary tract, wound, bloodstream, heart valve, and brain infections. In the great majority of cases, VRE infections occur in hospitalized patients who have compromised immune systems. Most cases of VRE are caused by the *E. faecium* strains that have acquired resistance when they came in contact with other bacteria and shared genetic information.
- VRE is most commonly transmitted from one patient to another by health care workers whose hands have become contaminated inadvertently with feces or fluids of a person carrying the organism. VRE are not airborne but can survive on surfaces for several weeks.

DX DIAGNOSIS

DIFFERENTIAL DIAGNOSIS

- Other bacterial pathogens in blood, wounds, or urine
- Once colonized, increased incidence to become infected

LABORATORY TESTS

- VRE rectal swab culture
- VRE stool culture
- Blood, urine, and wound cultures

RX TREATMENT

- For rectal or stool colonization, therapy is not recommended.
- Therapy is complicated by the fact that strains exhibit inherent resistance to many commonly used antibiotics.
- More than 80% of vancomycin-resistant *E. faecium* strains are also resistant to ampicillin.
- In symptomatic patients, if VRE strains are known to be susceptible, potential therapeutic agents include:
  1. Linezolid: 600 mg IV or PO q12h
  2. Daptomycin: 4 mg/kg/day IV for non-bacteremia infections and 6 mg/kg/day IV for bacteremias
  3. Tigecycline: 100 mg IV load dose, then 50 mg IV q12h. Although not specifically FDA approved for VRE strains, it offers an option for patients intolerant to other agents
  4. Quinupristin-dalfopristin (Synercid) only effective for *E. faecium* strains with no activity for *E. faecalis* strains: 7.5 mg/kg q8 to 12h. Can cause severe myalgias and arthralgias and venous irritation that often requires use of a central line, which has limited the use of this antibiotic
  5. Salvage regimens for severe VRE infections include:
     a. Daptomycin plus gentamicin and/or ampicillin or ceftaroline
     b. Daptomycin plus tigecycline
  6. The Healthcare Infection Control Practices Advisory Committee recommends that between one and three negative stool/rectal cultures be obtained at weekly intervals to remove a patient from contact precautions

REFERRAL

To infectious disease specialist

! PEARLS & CONSIDERATIONS

COMMENTS

- Patients who are colonized with VRE have about an 8% rate of developing a true VRE infection in hospital or after discharge. The rate is higher in immunocompromised and severely ill patients.
- Incidence increases with comorbidity and hospitalization.
- The number of patients already colonized with VRE in a defined geographic area (colonization pressure) is the most significant factor for predicting new acquisition of VRE.
- An association between VRE colonization and *Clostridium difficile* infection has been reported in patients with hematologic malignancies.

PREVENTION

- Hand hygiene: Most important and practical method of preventing spread in hospital environment. Soap and water (used as a 30-sec wash) and alcohol-based hand rubs are effective, as is chlorhexidine.
- Cohorting and isolation (contact precautions) techniques: Use of private rooms and use of gowns and gloves have been shown to decrease the risk of spread of multidrug-resistant bacteria. In 2018 the Society of Healthcare Epidemiology of America (SHEA) published guidelines that suggested isolation could be discontinued after between one and three negative stool swabs except for immunocompromised patients, patients in burn units, or patients in units with high VRE colonization rates.
- Cleaning contaminated objects or surfaces with standard hospital disinfectants, antibiotic management (prudent vancomycin use and antibiotic stewardship), and surveillance also help prevent spread.

SUGGESTED READINGS

Available at eBooks.Health.Elsevier.com.

RELATED CONTENT

Health Care-Related Infections (Related Key Topic)

AUTHOR: **GLENN G. FORT, MD, MPH**

BASIC INFORMATION

DEFINITION

Vasculitis refers generically to inflammation occurring within the walls of blood vessels. Blood vessel inflammation can result in either perforation of affected vessels with hemorrhage into adjacent structures or thrombosis with subsequent ischemia and infarction of supplied tissues. Vasculitis can occur as a primary process or secondary to another connective tissue disease, infection, or drug exposure. The systemic vasculitides are a heterogeneous group of disorders (Table 1) characterized by blood vessel inflammation affecting vessels of varying size and location resulting in a wide range of clinical manifestations dictated largely by which vessels are affected (Fig. 1 and Fig. E2). Vasculitis is traditionally classified according to the size of the blood vessels predominantly affected (Table 2). Antineutrophilic cytoplasmic autoantibody (ANCA)–associated vasculitis (AAV) includes granulomatosis with polyangiitis (GPA); microscopic polyangiitis (MPA), including renal-limited vasculitis (RLV); and eosinophilic granulomatosis with polyangiitis (EGPA). All are associated with ANCA and have similar features on renal histology (e.g., a focal necrotizing, and often crescentic, pauciimmune glomerulonephritis). Several of these are covered in individual topics, including topics on ANCA-associated vasculitis, giant cell arteritis (GCA), Takayasu arteritis, and Henoch-Schönlein purpura (HSP). Severity varies between and within specific vasculitides from a relatively benign, self-limited process to severe, life-threatening multisystem organ involvement with significant morbidity and mortality.

ICD-10CM CODES
M30.0	Polyarteritis nodosa
M30.3	Mucocutaneous lymph node syndrome [Kawasaki]
M31.30 31	Wegener granulomatosis without renal involvement
M31.5	Giant cell arteritis with polymyalgia rheumatica
M31.6	Other giant cell arteritis
M31.4	Aortic arch syndrome [Takayasu]
D 69.0	Allergic purpura
L95.9	Vasculitis limited to the skin, unspecified

EPIDEMIOLOGY & DEMOGRAPHICS

- The epidemiology and demographics of the various vasculitides vary by the individual disease and, where applicable, are covered under the relevant vasculitis disease chapters.
- The most common form of systemic vasculitis in the U.S. is giant cell arteritis, with an approximate incidence of 170 cases/1 million per year in individuals older than 50 yr.
- ANCA-associated vasculitis is significantly less common with aggregate incidence estimated at ~20 per million in the U.S.
- Polyarteritis nodosa (PAN) has an annual incidence of 1/100,000 persons but has a higher incidence in patients with existing hepatitis B or C infections.

TABLE 1 Comparing the Vasculitides

Disease	Pathophysiology	Classic Features	Testing	Treatment
Giant cell arteritis	Mononuclear cell infiltration and giant cell formation	Headache, scalp tenderness, visual disturbance	ESR, CRP biopsy	Prednisone and aspirin, may need tocilizumab or sarilumab
Takayasu arteritis	Mononuclear cell infiltration and giant cell formation	Visual disturbance, chest pain, abdominal pain, differences in extremity blood pressure and pulses	Angiography	Prednisone Surgical or angiographic intervention
Polyarteritis nodosa	Polymorphonuclear infiltration	Fever, hypertension, myalgias, abdominal pain, hematuria, CHF, GI bleeding, orchitis	ESR, CRP biopsy Angiography	Prednisone (mild disease) plus cyclophosphamide (moderate-severe disease) Antiviral therapy if concurrent hepatitis B or C Azathioprine or methotrexate for maintenance of remission
Kawasaki disease	Polymorphonuclear infiltration	5-day fever, conjunctivitis, oral lesions, rash, red palms and soles, edema, cervical lymphadenopathy	ESR, CRP leukocytosis Thrombocytosis Echocardiography	Aspirin plus IV gamma globulin
Granulomatosis with polyangiitis (Wegener granulomatosis)	Granuloma formation secondary to aggregating neutrophils	Upper and lower respiratory symptoms, renal insufficiency, skin lesions, visual disturbance	ESR, CRP c-ANCA/PR3	Prednisone and methotrexate (mild disease) Cyclophosphamide or rituximab plus prednisone (moderate to severe disease)
Eosinophilic granulomatosis with polyangiitis (Churg-Strauss syndrome)	Eosinophilic infiltration Allergic granulomas	Allergic rhinitis, nasal polyps, asthma	Leukocytosis Eosinophilia ESR, CRP biopsy	Prednisone with or without cyclophosphamide, mepolizumab
Henoch-Schönlein purpura	IgA complex deposition	Palpable purpura, arthralgias, GI disturbances, glomerulonephritis	Leukocytosis Eosinophilia Ig A elevation, skin biopsy	Usually self-limited NSAIDs Prednisone if necessary Rituximab (refractory cases)
Cryoglobulinemic vasculitis	Cold precipitable monoclonal or polyclonal immunoglobulins	Palpable purpura, glomerulonephritis, myalgias, weakness, peripheral neuropathy	Low complement levels, hepatitis C Renal biopsy	Rituximab with or without prednisone Peg interferon plus ribavirin (HCV infection)
Cutaneous leukocytoclastic vasculitis	Neutrophilic infiltration Mononuclear and eosinophilic infiltration	Palpable purpura, macules, vesicles, bullae, urticaria	Skin biopsy	Prednisone Colchicine Dapsone
Behçet syndrome	Polymorphonuclear infiltration	Recurrent oral aphthous ulcers, genital ulcers, skin lesions, visual disturbance	ESR, CRP leukocytosis Oral mucosa autoantibodies	Topical corticosteroids Prednisone with azathioprine (end-organ disease) Colchicine (aphthous ulcer and arthritis) Apremilast Infliximab (refractory disease)

c-ANCA, Cytoplasmic antineutrophil cytoplasmic antibody; *CHF,* congestive heart failure; *CRP,* C-reactive protein; *ESR,* erythrocyte sedimentation rate; *GI,* gastrointestinal; *IgA,* immunoglobulin A; *IV,* intravenous.
From Adams JG et al: *Emergency medicine: clinical essentials,* ed 2, Philadelphia, 2013, Elsevier.

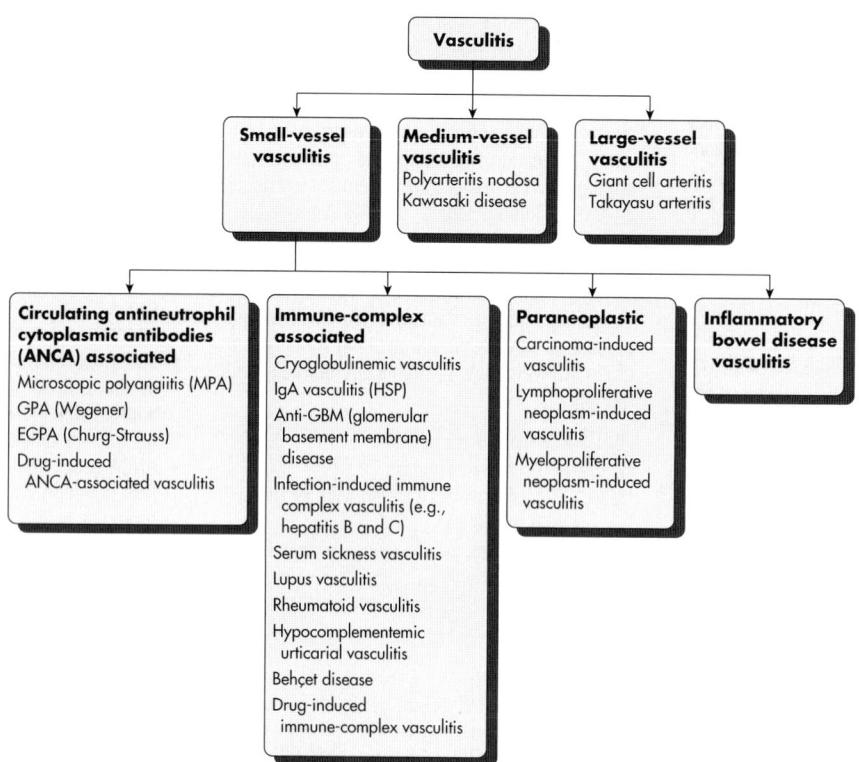

FIG. 1 Major categories of noninfectious vasculitis. Not included are vasculitides that are known to be caused by direct invasion of vessel walls by infectious pathogens, such as rickettsial vasculitis and neisserial vasculitis. *EGPA,* Eosinophilic granulomatous polyangiitis; *GPA,* granulomatous polyangiitis; *HSP,* Henoch-Schönlein purpura. (From Freehally J et al: *Comprehensive clinical nephrology,* ed 6, Philadelphia, 2019, Saunders.)

TABLE 2 Names and Definitions of Small Vessel Vasculitides as Presented by the 2012 Chapel Hill Consensus Conference

Name	Definition and Comments
Small-vessel vasculitis	Vasculitis predominantly affecting small vessels, defined as small intraparenchymal arteries, arterioles, capillaries, and venules. Medium-sized arteries and veins may be affected.
ANCA-associated vasculitis	Necrotizing vasculitis with few or no immune deposits predominantly affecting small vessels (i.e., capillaries, venules, arterioles, and small arteries), associated with MPO ANCA or PR3 ANCA. Not all patients have ANCA. Add a prefix indicating ANCA reactivity (e.g., MPO-ANCA, PR3-ANCA, ANCA-negative).
Granulomatosis with polyangiitis	Necrotizing granulomatous inflammation usually involving the upper and lower respiratory tract, and necrotizing vasculitis affecting predominantly small- to medium-sized vessels (e.g., capillaries, venules, arterioles, arteries, and veins). Necrotizing glomerulonephritis is common.
Microscopic polyangiitis	Necrotizing vasculitis with few or no immune deposits predominantly affecting small vessels (i.e., capillaries, venules, or arterioles). Necrotizing arteritis involving small- and medium-sized arteries may be present. Necrotizing glomerulonephritis is very common. Pulmonary capillaritis often occurs. Granulomatous inflammation is absent.
Eosinophilic granulomatosis with polyangiitis (Churg-Strauss syndrome)	Eosinophil-rich and necrotizing granulomatous inflammation often involving the respiratory tract, and necrotizing vasculitis predominantly affecting small- to medium-sized vessels, and associated with asthma and eosinophilia. ANCA is more frequent when glomerulonephritis is present.
Immune complex vasculitis	Vasculitis with moderate to marked vessel wall deposits of Ig and/or complement components predominantly affecting small vessels (i.e., capillaries, venules, arterioles, and small arteries). Glomerulonephritis is frequent.
Anti–glomerular basement membrane disease	Vasculitis affecting glomerular capillaries, pulmonary capillaries, or both, with GBM deposition of anti-GBM autoantibodies. Lung involvement causes pulmonary hemorrhage, and renal involvement causes glomerulonephritis with necrosis and crescents.
Cryoglobulinemic vasculitis	Vasculitis with cryoglobulin immune deposits affecting small vessels (predominantly capillaries, venules, or arterioles) and associated with serum cryoglobulins. Skin, glomeruli, and peripheral nerves are often involved.
IgA vasculitis (Henoch-Schönlein purpura)	Vasculitis, with IgA1-dominant immune deposits, affecting small vessels (predominantly capillaries, venules, or arterioles). Often involves skin and GI tract, and frequently causes arthritis. Glomerulonephritis indistinguishable from IgA nephropathy may occur.
Hypocomplementemic urticarial vasculitis (anti-C1q vasculitis)	Vasculitis accompanied by urticaria and hypocomplementemia affecting small vessels (i.e., capillaries, venules, or arterioles), and associated with anti-C1q antibodies. Glomerulonephritis, arthritis, obstructive pulmonary disease, and ocular inflammation are common.

ANCA, Anti-neutrophil cytoplasmic antibody; *GBM,* glomerular basement membrane; *GI,* gastrointestinal; *MPO,* myeloperoxidase; *PR3,* proteinase 3.
From Firestein GS et al: *Firestein & Kelley's textbook of rheumatology,* ed 11, Philadelphia, 2021, Elsevier.

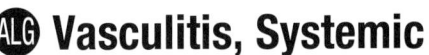

V

I

- Age distribution can demonstrate significant variability between the vasculitides as shown by the fact that GCA generally does not occur before age 50, whereas 90% of cases of HSP occur in the pediatric population, and 80% of patients with Kawasaki disease are under age 5.
- Although genetic factors clearly play a role in disease susceptibility, familial cases of vasculitis are rare.

PHYSICAL FINDINGS & CLINICAL PRESENTATION

- Clinical presentation often includes nonspecific constitutional symptoms including fever, malaise, headache, and weight loss.
- Signs and symptoms are generally dictated by the tropism of involved vessels.
- Skin manifestations of vasculitis include petechiae, palpable purpura (Fig. E3), subcutaneous nodules, livedo reticularis, ulcerations, and digital ischemia.
- Kidney involvement of medium-sized and large vessel vasculitis is often in the form of renovascular hypertension. Glomerulonephritis may be seen in small vessel vasculitis.
- Pulmonary small vessel involvement can cause alveolar hemorrhage, which can present with cough, dyspnea, and alveolar hemorrhage.
- Organ involvement in polyarteritis nodosa is summarized in Table 3.
- Mononeuritis multiplex is the characteristic finding of vasculitis affecting the vasa nervorum of the peripheral nervous system.
- GI involvement of the mesenteric vasculature can cause postprandial pain, bleeding, and perforation.
- Testicular pain or tenderness can be seen with hepatitis B infection in PAN.
- Cardiac involvement can include chest pain secondary to ischemic infarcts in the coronary arteries, pericarditis, cardiomyopathy, and arrhythmias.
- Arthritis, while nonspecific, can be present.
- Significant clinical variability exists between the various vasculitides, although overlapping symptoms may be seen.

ETIOLOGY

Most forms of systemic vasculitis are of unknown etiology. Cryoglobulinemia vasculitis is often secondary to hepatitis C infection, and cutaneous leukocytoclastic vasculitis is often related to a drug exposure.

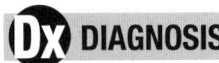 DIAGNOSIS

DIFFERENTIAL DIAGNOSIS

- Infective endocarditis
- Atrial myxoma
- Cholesterol emboli
- Malignancy
- Hypercoagulopathy
- Congenital collagen vascular disorder

WORKUP

- The diagnosis of most forms of systemic vasculitis relies on the history and physical

TABLE 3 Organ Involvement in Polyarteritis Nodosa

System	Comment	Frequency
Constitutional	Fever and weight loss (current and previous)	>90%
Musculoskeletal	Arthritis, arthralgia, myalgia, or weakness; when muscle is involved, it provides a useful site for biopsy	24%-80%
Skin	Purpura, nodules, livedo reticularis, ulcers, bullous or vesicular eruptions, and segmental skin edema	44%-50%
Cardiovascular	Cardiac ischemia, cardiomyopathy, hypertension	35%
Ear, nose, and throat	No involvement; nasal crusting, sinusitis, and hearing loss suggest an alternative diagnosis such as granulomatosis with polyangiitis	None
Respiratory	Lung involvement not seen in PAN; abnormal respiratory findings suggest an alternative diagnosis	None
Abdominal	Pain is an early feature of mesenteric artery involvement; progressive involvement may cause bowel, liver, or splenic infarction, bowel perforation, or bleeding from a ruptured arterial aneurysm; less common presentations include appendicitis, pancreatitis, or cholecystitis as a result of ischemia or infarction; the presence of abdominal tenderness or peritonitis and blood loss on rectal examination should be assessed	33%-36%
Renal	Vasculitis involving the renal arteries is present in many cases but does not commonly give rise to clinical features; it can present with renal impairment, renal infarcts, or rupture of renal arterial aneurysms; glomerular ischemia may result in mild proteinuria or hematuria, but red cell casts are absent because glomerular inflammation is not a feature; if evidence of glomerular inflammation exists, then an alternative diagnosis such as microscopic polyangiitis or granulomatosis with polyangiitis must be considered; hypertension is a manifestation of renal ischemia causing activation of the renin-angiotensin system	11%-66%
Nervous system	Mononeuritis multiplex, with sensory symptoms preceding motor deficits; CNS involvement is a less frequent finding and can present with encephalopathy, seizures, and stroke	55%-79%
Ocular	Visual impairment, retinal hemorrhage, and optic ischemia	Rare
Other	Breast or uterine involvement is rare; testicular pain from ischemic orchitis is a characteristic feature, albeit an uncommon presentation	Rare

PAN, Polyarteritis nodosa.
From Firestein GS et al: *Firestein & Kelley's textbook of rheumatology,* ed 11, Philadelphia, 2021, Elsevier.

examination as well as supportive laboratory testing. Table 4 describes differential diagnostic features of selected forms of small vessel vasculitis.
- Tissue biopsy is important in establishing an accurate diagnosis; biopsy sites should target affected tissues.
- Electromyography and nerve conduction studies can evaluate for site of nerve or muscle involvement before biopsy in patients with neuropathy or myopathy.
- Imaging such as mesenteric angiography can be supportive and may obviate the need for tissue biopsy.

LABORATORY TESTS

- Laboratory markers of systemic inflammation include elevated erythrocyte sedimentation rate (ESR), C-reactive protein (CRP), and anemia of chronic disease.
- ANCA targeting myeloperoxidase (MPO) and proteinase 3 (PR3) are frequently found in several small vessel vasculitides, including GPA (Wegener), microscopic polyangiitis (MPA), and EGPA (Churg-Strauss).
- Hepatitis C antibodies and rheumatoid factor are often present in cryoglobulinemic vasculitis.
- Positive hepatitis B serologies are commonly found in PAN.

- Urinalysis in patients with glomerulonephritis due to small vessel ANCA-associated vasculitis will generally demonstrate hematuria with active urinary sediment, with red blood cell casts and proteinuria.

IMAGING STUDIES

- CT angiography, magnetic resonance angiography, and angiography can demonstrate vascular narrowing and aneurysm formation in suspected medium-size and large-vessel vasculitis.
- Pulmonary and sinus CT scans can demonstrate active pulmonary and upper airway disease in ANCA-associated vasculitis.

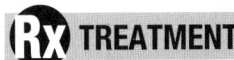 TREATMENT

Treatment of vasculitis depends on the specific type of vasculitis and is tailored to the severity of disease activity. Novel treatments are covered under the relevant vasculitis disease chapters.

ACUTE GENERAL Rx

- Systemic corticosteroids are generally required to gain initial control of active vasculitis, although mild cases of drug-induced cutaneous leukocytoclastic vasculitis

TABLE 4 Differential Diagnostic Features of Selected Forms of Small Vessel Vasculitis

Features	Microscopic Polyangiitis (MPA)	Granulomatosis With Polyangiitis (GPA)	Eosinophilic Granulomatosis With Polyangiitis	Henoch-Schönlein Purpura (HSP)	Cryoglobulinemic Vasculitis
Vasculitic signs and symptoms	+	+	+	+	+
Immunoglobulin A–dominant immune deposits	−	−	−	+	−
Cryoglobulins in blood and vessels	−	−	−	−	+
Antineutrophil cytoplasmic antibodies in blood	+	+	+	−	−
Necrotizing granulomas	−	+	+	−	−
Asthma and eosinophils	−	−	+	−	−

From Freehally J et al: *Comprehensive clinical nephrology,* ed 6, Philadelphia, 2019, Saunders.

often require cessation of the offending medication and at times, low-dose corticosteroid use.

- HSP and vasculitis limited to the skin, including cutaneous PAN, can often be managed without further immunosuppression.
- Major organ-threatening disease in systemic vasculitis has traditionally required pulse steroids and oral or intravenous cyclophosphamide for induction of remission.
- Studies have demonstrated noninferiority of rituximab compared to cyclophosphamide in ANCA-associated vasculitis with major organ involvement, and it is approved for this use.
- Rituximab with prednisone has also been shown to be effective in the treatment of relapsing flares of disease activity in ANCA-associated vasculitis.
- Less severe disease such as GPA limited to the upper airways can be managed with methotrexate rather than cyclophosphamide.
- Trimethoprim-sulfamethoxazole should be used to prevent *Pneumocystis jiroveci* infection with concurrent immunosuppressive therapy.
- The goal of acute therapy is to induce remission of disease activity and is generally continued for 1 to 2 mo once this is achieved, at which point chronic therapy is used.

CHRONIC Rx

- The goal of chronic therapy is to prevent disease relapse and minimize medication side effects.
- Steroids are gradually tapered as allowed by disease activity.
- Immunomodulatory agents such as methotrexate or azathioprine are commonly used for maintenance therapy in place of cyclophosphamide to reduce side effects.
- Cryoglobulinemic vasculitis due to chronic hepatitis C virus infection will often improve with treatment of the underlying viral infection.
- In PAN with concurrent hepatitis B infection, appropriate antiviral treatment (interferon alpha-2b or lamivudine with or without plasma exchange) is indicated.
- Rituximab may also be an appropriate remission maintenance agent in ANCA-associated vasculitis. For GPA or MPA, scheduled redosing of rituximab every 4 to 6 mo is conditionally recommended over redosing based on ANCA titers or CD19 B-cell counts.

DISPOSITION

Varies widely among the various vasculitides

REFERRAL

Systemic vasculitis care is generally coordinated by a rheumatologist. Renal, pulmonary, neurology, and GI consultations are often needed when vasculitis involves these organ systems. Isolated cutaneous leukocytoclastic vasculitis is often managed by dermatology.

SUGGESTED READINGS

Available at eBooks.Health.Elsevier.com.

RELATED CONTENT

Cogan Syndrome (Related Key Topic)
Cryoglobulinemia (Related Key Topic)
Giant Cell Arteritis (Related Key Topic)
ANCA-Associated Vasculitis (Related Key Topic)
IgA Vasculitis (Related Key Topic)
Kawasaki Disease (Related Key Topic)
Takayasu Arteritis (Related Key Topic)

AUTHOR: **NICHOLAS J. LEMME, MD**

V

I

BASIC INFORMATION

DEFINITION

The spectrum of chronic venous disease (CVD) ranges from varicose veins to leg edema and skin manifestations consisting of hyperpigmentation, eczema, lipodermatosclerosis, and venous ulcer. These latter venous-specific skin changes constitute an advanced form of CVD known as chronic venous insufficiency (CVI).

SYNONYMS

Stasis dermatitis
Postthrombotic syndrome (PTS)
Chronic venous disease

ICD-10CM CODES

I87.2	Venous insufficiency (chronic) (peripheral)
I87.8	Other specified disorders of veins
I87.9	Disorder of vein, unspecified
I83.10	Varicose veins of unspecified lower extremity with inflammation

EPIDEMIOLOGY & DEMOGRAPHICS

- From 10% to 35% of adults in the U.S. have some form of CVI.
- Venous ulcers are the complication of CVI that results in the greatest morbidity and affects 4% of people over the age of 65.
- The population-based costs to the U.S. government for CVI treatment and venous ulcer care have been estimated at >$1 billion/yr.
- In addition, 4.6 million workdays/yr are lost to chronic venous-related diseases.

PHYSICAL FINDINGS & CLINICAL PRESENTATION

The manifestations of CVI can be viewed using the internationally accepted classification system, CEAP (clinical, etiology, anatomy, and pathophysiology) (Table E1). The spectrum of cutaneous changes of CVI in the affected leg include:

- Varicose eczema: The most common and earliest sign, this involves the skin above the medial ankle and consists of pruritic, red, and scaly eczematous patches and plaques.
- Hyperpigmentation: Caused by the breakdown of red blood cells and leads to hemosiderin deposition and dark staining of the skin (Fig. 1).
- Atrophie blanche: Usually presents as hypopigmented white patches with focal red punctate dots or telangiectasia surrounded by hyperpigmentation. Skin in this condition is avascular and prone to ulceration (Fig. 2).
- Lipodermatosclerosis: A chronic, brawny induration of the skin and underlying fat that usually involves the skin from medial malleolus up to the lower border of the calf. Progression of the disease leads to an "inverted champagne bottle" appearance. The induration and lack of perfusion of the skin in this area make it susceptible to ulcer formation.

ETIOLOGY

- CVI occurs as a result of sustained venous hypertension in the leg, which can be caused by the following:
  1. Primary: Vein valve failure with reflux in the superficial venous system or perforating veins (most common cause of CVI)
  2. Secondary: Postthrombotic syndrome in which a deep vein thrombosis causes outflow obstruction *or*
  3. Combination of the two previous processes
- This sustained elevation in venous pressure or venous hypertension results in pathologic effects in the skin and subcutaneous tissues such as edema, eczema, hyperpigmentation, fibrosis, and ultimately venous ulceration.

DIAGNOSIS

The diagnosis and evaluation of CVI are directed primarily by a detailed history and physical examination.

DIFFERENTIAL DIAGNOSIS

- Contact dermatitis
- Atopic dermatitis
- Cellulitis
- Dermatophyte infection
- Pretibial myxedema
- Nummular eczema
- Xerosis
- Asteatotic eczema

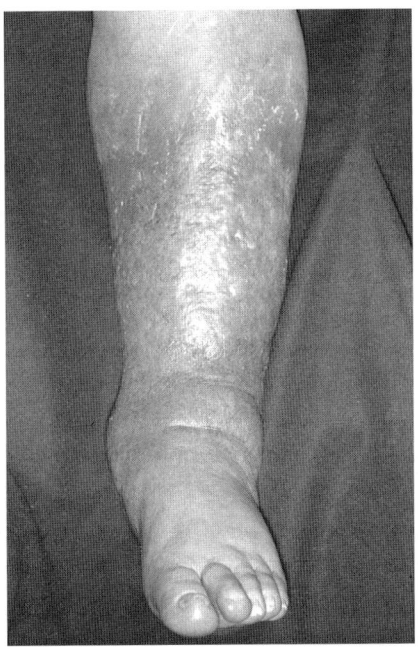

FIG. 1 Stasis dermatitis, venous insufficiency. (From James WD et al: *Andrews' diseases of the skin,* ed 12, Philadelphia, 2016, Elsevier.)

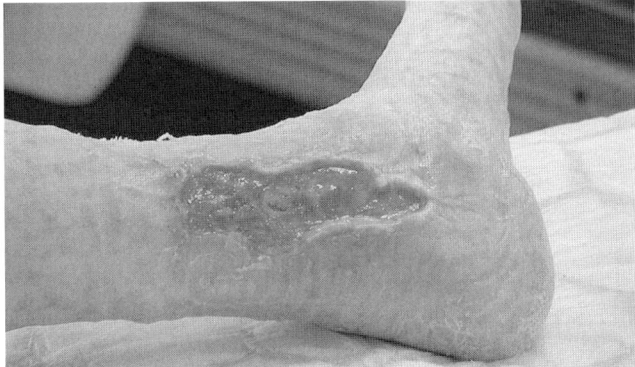

FIG. 2 Chronic venous ulcer likely to be resistant to treatment as it involves the space behind the medial malleolus, which is difficult to compress. (From Fillit HM: *Brocklehurst's textbook of geriatric medicine and gerontology,* ed 8, London, 2017, Elsevier.)

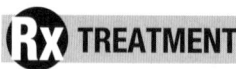

WORKUP

The primary goal is to identify the cause of sustained venous hypertension.

LABORATORY TESTS

Generally not indicated

IMAGING STUDIES

- Evaluation of the patient is performed in the standing position with duplex ultrasonography to identify reflux in the superficial, deep, and perforating veins as well as obstruction of the deep veins.
- No exam of a leg with CVI is complete without palpation of pulses and/or determination of ankle-brachial index (ABI).

Rx TREATMENT

NONPHARMACOLOGIC THERAPY

- Leg elevation above heart level for 30 min three to four times a day
- Weight reduction because obesity is a risk factor for deep vein thrombosis and CVI
- Walking exercises to improve calf function
- Physical therapy to improve ankle joint mobility
- For weeping skin lesions, wet-to-dry dressing changes

ACUTE GENERAL Rx

- The fundamental role of compression in the treatment of CVI is well recognized and has been validated by randomized controlled trials.
- The beneficial effects of gradient compression stockings (decrease in edema and control of discomfort) are due to their effect on microvascular hemodynamics and Starling forces.
- Below-knee compression stocking with a gradient of at least 20 to 30 mm Hg will control edema, alleviate pain, and improve the quality of life in CVI patients.

- Compression stockings are contraindicated in patients with an ABI of <0.6.
- Some patients (acute lipodermatosclerosis) may benefit from nonelastic compression with the unna gel paste gauze boot to alleviate their symptoms and acute increase in their swelling. The Unna boot is changed once a week.
- Topical corticosteroid creams or ointments (e.g., triamcinolone 0.12% bid) may be used to help reduce inflammation and itching. Steroids should never be applied to ulcer.
- Antibiotics should only be used when treating a clinically apparent, culture-proved infection. Most secondary infections are the result of *Staphylococcus* or *Streptococcus* organisms.
- Diuretics have no role in the treatment of CVI-related edema.

CHRONIC Rx

- Although conservative care is fundamental, patients with CVI should be considered for correction of their underlying venous hypertension.
- The majority of patients with CVI have superficial vein or perforator vein reflux as their underlying pathology and would benefit from the newer vein ablation procedures listed below.
  1. Endovenous ablation of superficial (saphenous) or perforator vein reflux.
  2. Radiofrequency ablation with VNUS closure.
  3. Endovenous laser therapy (EVLT).
  4. Ultrasound-guided foam sclerotherapy.

COMPLEMENTARY & ALTERNATIVE MEDICINE

Several groups of drugs have been evaluated in the treatment of CVI, including coumarins, flavonoids, and saponosides (horse chestnut extracts). These drugs have venoactive properties

and are widely used in Europe but are not approved for use in the U.S. The precise mechanism of action is not known. Horse chestnut seed extract has been found, in the short term, to be as effective as compression stockings in reducing pain and edema, but long-term efficacy has not been established.

REFERRAL

- Phlebology
- Vascular surgery
- Indications for referral:
  1. Skin and subcutaneous changes consistent with CVI
  2. Associated peripheral arterial insufficiency (peripheral artery disease)
  3. Long-standing varicose vein disease
  4. Consideration for vein ablation procedure

❗ PEARLS & CONSIDERATIONS

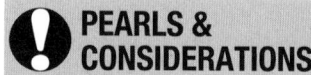

COMMENTS

- Inflammatory skin changes from CVI are irreversible. The goal of therapy is to eliminate venous hypertension and prevent progression.
- Venous ulcers are often an end-stage manifestation of CVI. Refer to "Venous Ulcers" for more information.

SUGGESTED READINGS

Available at eBooks.Health.Elsevier.com.

RELATED CONTENT

Stasis Dermatitis (Patient Information)
Varicose Veins (Related Key Topic)
Venous Ulcers (Related Key Topic)

AUTHOR: **FRANK G. FORT, MD, FACS, RPHS**

BASIC INFORMATION

DEFINITION

Venous ulcers are defined as chronic defects of the skin that fail to heal spontaneously and persist for longer than 4 wk. Venous ulcers account for about 70% of all lower-extremity ulcerations. They are usually located in the "gaiter" region and can be accompanied by varicose veins, edema, hyperpigmentation, and lipodermatosclerosis. Venous ulceration develops in patients as a result of sustained venous hypertension.

SYNONYM

Stasis ulcers

ICD-10CM CODES
I87.2   Venous insufficiency (chronic) (peripheral)
L97.909 Non-pressure chronic ulcer of unspecified part of unspecified lower leg with unspecified severity

EPIDEMIOLOGY & DEMOGRAPHICS

In industrialized nations, up to 1.5% of the population will suffer from venous ulcers. In patients ≥65 yr, the incidence increases to 4%. In the U.S., >500,000 people suffer from stasis ulcers.

RISK FACTORS:
- Obesity
- Increasing age
- Family history of chronic venous insufficiency
- History of deep venous thromboembolism

PHYSICAL FINDINGS & CLINICAL PRESENTATION

Venous ulcers are most commonly located in the lower leg just above the ankle (gaiter region). They are a partial-thickness, irregularly shaped wound with well-defined borders with granulation tissue and fibrin present in the ulcer base (Figs. E1 and E2). Venous ulcers are relatively painless and are surrounded by brown-stained skin and/or dry, itchy, and reddened skin. In about 50% of patients, there are visible varicose veins in an aching, swollen leg.

ETIOLOGY

The exact mechanism of the role of venous hypertension in the etiology of venous ulcers is not certain. Hemodynamic forces such as venous hypertension, circulatory stasis, and modified conditions of shear stress appear to play an important role in an inflammatory reaction accompanied by leukocyte activation that clinically leads to fibrosclerotic remodeling of the skin and then to ulceration.

DIAGNOSIS

DIFFERENTIAL DIAGNOSIS
- Arterial ulcer
- Neurotrophic ulcers (located predominantly in the foot)
- Vasculitis
- Pyoderma gangrenosum
- Ulcerated skin tumors like basal cell or squamous cell carcinoma (Marjolin ulcer)
- Rheumatoid arthritis

WORKUP
- The history and clinical signs and symptoms of leg ulcers are often misleading and may not differentiate venous ulcers from other leg ulcers; about 30% of leg ulcers are not of venous origin.
- Measurement of the ankle-brachial index (ABI) is essential in excluding peripheral arterial disease, which can be present in 20% of patients and is required before starting compression therapy. Arterial insufficiency is suggested by an ABI <0.9.
- Patients with lower-extremity ulcers should also be evaluated for diabetes.
- Coagulation defects have been found in 40% of patients with leg ulcers. This finding suggests that many patients with leg ulcers have a known or suspected history of deep venous thrombosis and a thrombophilia workup is indicated.
- If vasculitis is suspected, a biopsy of the edge of the ulcer can confirm the diagnosis.
- Any wound that has failed to improve after therapy of 4 wk should have a biopsy to rule out malignancy.

IMAGING STUDIES
- Evaluation of patients with venous leg ulcer should include duplex sonography to identify reflux in the superficial, deep, and perforating veins as well as possible obstruction of the deep veins.
- If the ulcer appears to be infected, consider tissue for culture, plain x-ray films, and bone scan to evaluate for osteomyelitis.

TREATMENT

NONPHARMACOLOGIC THERAPY
- Fig. 3 describes an algorithm for the treatment of venous ulcers.
- Surgical debridement to remove all nonviable material can be accomplished in the office setting with the use of a topical xylocaine gel. Debridement produces the release of growth factors that allow the development of healthy granulation tissue and the initiation of the healing process.
- The first-line treatment of ulcers includes below-knee compression stockings to improve venous return to the heart, thereby decreasing edema, inflammation, and tissue ischemia (used only if the ABI is between 0.6 and 0.85 because compression can cause limb ischemia).
- There is Level A evidence that graduated compression stockings alone can lead to healing of a venous ulcer. The stockings should be worn during the day and removed at night.
- Regular, brisk walking 30 min a day, five times a wk is recommended.
- Elevate leg above heart level and raise the foot of bed with 3-in blocks to reduce edema.
- Role of surgery: In a randomized controlled trial, endovenous catheter ablation of superficial reflux showed no improvement in the healing rate of ulcers but did demonstrate a reduction of ulcer recurrence from 28% to 12% at 12 mo. Longer term follow-up (median 3 to 5 yr) also confirmed that abrasive procedures lowered incidence of recurrent ulcers.

ACUTE GENERAL Rx
- Dressings are used under compression stockings to provide a clean, moist environment to promote healing.
- Modern, more complex dressings have been developed and include occlusive and semi-occlusive dressings, classified according to their physical composition and ability to control wound drainage.
- Semiocclusive dressings have varying ability to absorb wound drainage. Some examples of this type are hydrocolloids (DuoDERM), hydrogels (DuoDERM hydrogel), foam dressings (Allevyn), and alginates.
- Biologic wound dressings (Apligraf) and tissue-engineered products (Oasis) have been developed, and these products can either directly provide growth factors or indirectly stimulate growth factors in the ulcer bed.
- Pentoxifylline (800 mg PO tid) has been shown to be an effective adjuvant to compression therapy as reported in a meta-analysis of nine clinical trials.
- Skin grafting should be considered for large or refractory ulcers as long as the wound is clean and there is healthy granulation tissue.
- Published randomized clinical trials on the value of the different types of dressings in the management of leg ulcers have not shown effects on ulcer healing. Despite the lack of evidence to support their use, modern dressings remain a part of the standard of care. Decisions regarding their use should be based on local cost of the dressings and the physician's clinical experience.
- Trials have shown that endovenous ablation of superficial veins lowers the probability of long-term recurrent venous ulcers.[1]
- Trials involving the use of weekly, low-dose, high-frequency ultrasound for hard-to-heal venous leg ulcers do not support adding therapeutic ultrasound to standard care for venous leg ulcers.

DISPOSITION

The overall prognosis for this condition is poor; the healing rate depends on the initial size of the ulcer. Although 65% to 70% of venous ulcers are healed within 6 mo, the 5-yr recurrence rate of healed venous ulcers can be as high as 40%. Maintenance of lifelong compression therapy is recommended.

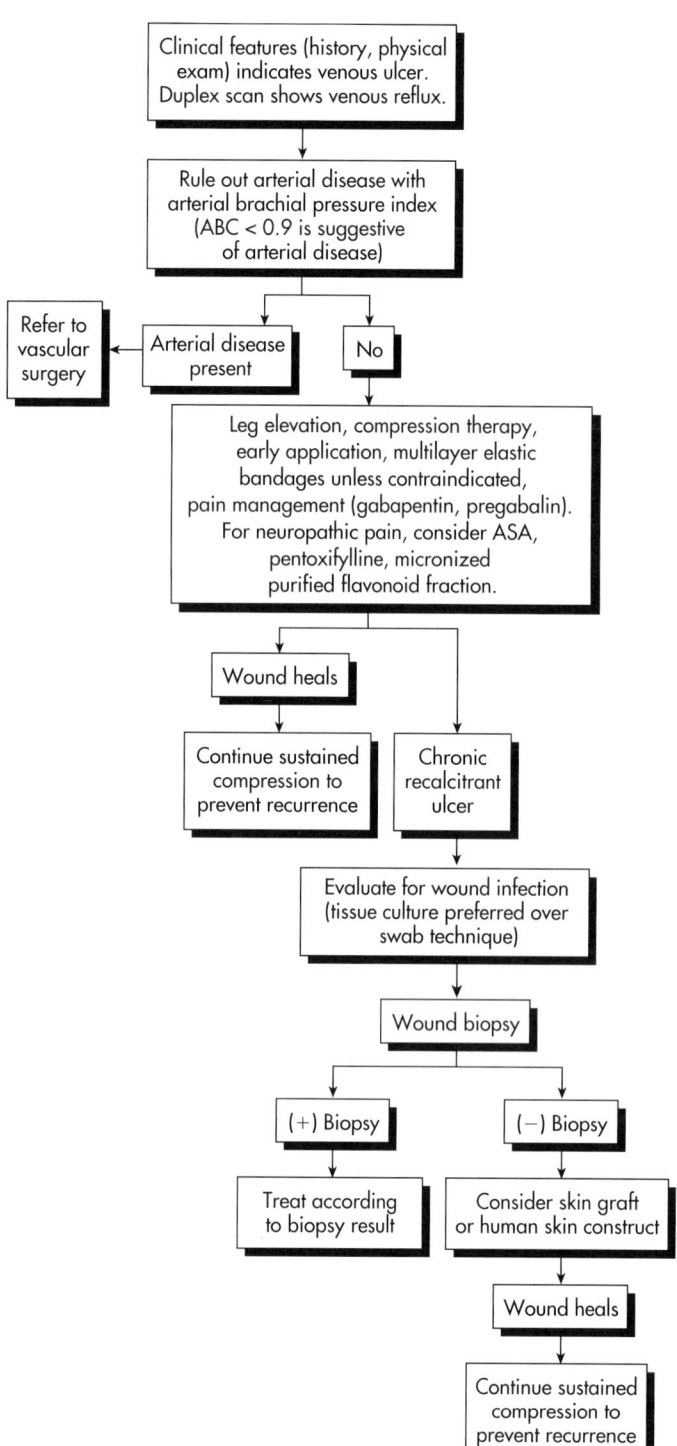

FIG. 3 Algorithm for the care of a patient with a venous leg ulcer.

REFERRAL

All patients should be evaluated weekly during the first month of therapy. Nonhealing ulcers with little to no improvement should also be referred to a wound care clinic.

REFERENCE & SUGGESTED READINGS

Available at eBooks.Health.Elsevier.com.

AUTHOR: **FRANK G. FORT, MD, FACS, RPHS**

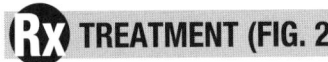

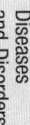

BASIC INFORMATION

DEFINITION

Vertebral compression fractures (VCFs) are defined as fractures of spinal vertebrae in which a bony surface is driven toward another bony surface. These fractures are classified as radiographic reductions in vertebral body height of more than 15%.

SYNONYMS

Thoracolumbar vertebral compression fractures
Osteoporotic fractures
VCF

ICD-10CM CODES

M80.0	Post-menopausal osteoporosis with pathologic fracture
M80.4	Drug-induced osteoporosis with pathological fracture
M80.5	Idiopathic osteoporosis with pathological fracture
M80.8	Other osteoporosis with pathological fracture
M80.9	Unspecified osteoporosis with pathological fracture
S32.009A	Unspecified fracture of unspecified lumbar vertebra, initial encounter for closed fracture
S22.009A	Unspecified fracture of unspecified thoracic vertebra, initial encounter for closed fracture

EPIDEMIOLOGY & DEMOGRAPHICS

Approximately 700,000 VCFs occur in the United States each year, and they affect up to 25% of postmenopausal women. They are the most common complication of osteoporosis. The prevalence increases with age, reaching a peak of 40% to 50% among women aged >80 yr. Compression fractures are also a major concern among men, although their rates of VCF are lower.

RISK FACTORS:

- Modifiable: Tobacco or alcohol use, osteoporosis, estrogen deficiency (i.e., early menopause, bilateral oophorectomy, premenopausal amenorrhea for >1 yr), frailty, impaired vision, abusive situations, inadequate physical activity, low body mass index, and deficiency of vitamin D or calcium.
- Nonmodifiable: Advanced age, female gender, dementia, Caucasian descent, history of fractures in adulthood and among first-degree relatives, and falls.

PHYSICAL FINDINGS & CONSIDERATIONS

- Asymptomatic: Most VCFs are asymptomatic, except for height loss or kyphosis (i.e., dowager's hump [Fig. E1]), which is often a sign of multiple VCFs and height loss of >6 cm has a sensitivity/specificity of 94% and 30%, respectively, for VCF.
- Symptomatic: When symptomatic, VCFs usually present as acute back pain after activity (e.g., bending, lifting) or coughing; neck strain and radicular rib pain may also be present.

ETIOLOGY

- VCFs take place when the combination of bending and the axial load on the spine exceed the strength of the vertebral body.
- The primary etiology of VCF is osteoporosis, though a pathologic fracture from an underlying malignancy, typically metastatic disease, must be ruled out.

DIAGNOSIS

DIFFERENTIAL DIAGNOSIS

- Osteoporosis
- Malignancy, most often metastases
- Hyperparathyroidism
- Osteomalacia
- Granulomatous diseases (e.g., tuberculosis)
- Hematologic/oncologic diseases (e.g., multiple myeloma, primary bone malignancy)

WORKUP

- Only one third of VCFs are diagnosed. Guidelines for patient selection for vertebral fractural assessment are described in Box E1.
- VCFs can be clinically suspected from the history and physical alone, though they are often diagnosed incidentally by imaging performed for another indication.
- There may or may not be a specific injury or a remembered event that led to the VCF.

LABORATORY TESTS

Tests to rule out infection or cancer may be helpful, such as a CBC, an erythrocyte sedimentation rate, an alkaline phosphatase level, and a C-reactive protein level; these tests can be reserved for individuals for whom there is clinical suspicion.

IMAGING STUDIES

- Plain frontal and lateral radiographs (x-rays) are the initial imaging method and may be sufficient, particularly when no neurologic abnormalities are present. MRI and computed tomography (CT) scans may be uncomfortable or painful for the patient, especially during the acute phase.
- Although CT scans are not routinely necessary for the diagnosis, they can be helpful for visualizing fractures that are not seen on plain films, for evaluating the integrity of the posterior vertebral wall, for ruling out other causes of back pain, for detecting spinal canal narrowing, and for assessing instability.
- MRI may be useful when spinal cord compression is suspected, if neurologic symptoms are present, or to distinguish malignancy from osteoporosis (e.g., in patients <55 yr with VCF after minimal or no trauma).
- Bone density studies may be helpful to determine the severity of osteoporosis, which is a key risk factor for future fractures.

TREATMENT (FIG. 2)

NONPHARMACOLOGIC THERAPY

- Physical therapy.
- External back braces: Frequently recommended to relieve pain and improve mobility, however, controlled trials have not shown any effect in patients with vertebral compression fractures.
- Exercise programs: Getting active as soon as possible is extremely important for both short- and long-term recovery.

ACUTE GENERAL Rx

- Analgesics are first line for pain control, including acetaminophen and opioids (oral or parenteral), and pain can be expected to diminish over 4 to 6 wk.
- NSAIDs are helpful but must be used with caution among elderly patients or when contraindicated.
- Muscle relaxants should be used judiciously because they have significant side effects, particularly in the elderly.
- Intranasal calcitonin (200 units once daily, alternating nostrils) has been shown in some small trials to hasten relief from pain when used as an adjunct to oral analgesics, and a 2- to 4-wk course may be useful for patients who do not achieve adequate control with oral analgesics alone.
- Early mobilization with physical therapy is important for recovery and prevention of subsequent fractures.
- The efficacy of vertebroplasty vs. kyphoplasty vs. conservative treatment remains controversial.
- Percutaneous vertebroplasty (Fig. E3) involves the injection of acrylic bone cement into the affected vertebral body in an effort to stabilize the fracture and reduce pain, whereas in kyphoplasty, a high-pressure inflatable bone tamp or balloon is expanded within the body of the affected vertebra to restore prefracture vertebral height before the injection of bone cement. These two procedures were thought to be helpful in patients who did not respond to conservative therapy; however, further studies showed them to be no more effective than sham procedures. Nonetheless, Klazen et al (2010)[1] demonstrated in an open-label prospective randomized trial that for the subgroup of patients with acute osteoporotic VCFs and persistent pain, percutaneous vertebroplasty may provide immediate pain relief, sustained for at least a year, which may be significantly greater than that achieved with conservative treatment. Zampini (2010)[2] showed in a nonrandomized cohort study that elderly patients who underwent kyphoplasty were more likely to be discharged home. Analysis of Medicare claims of patients with VCF treated with kyphoplasty or vertebroplasty compared with medical management revealed no difference in mortality or major medical outcomes but decreased health care utilization in the

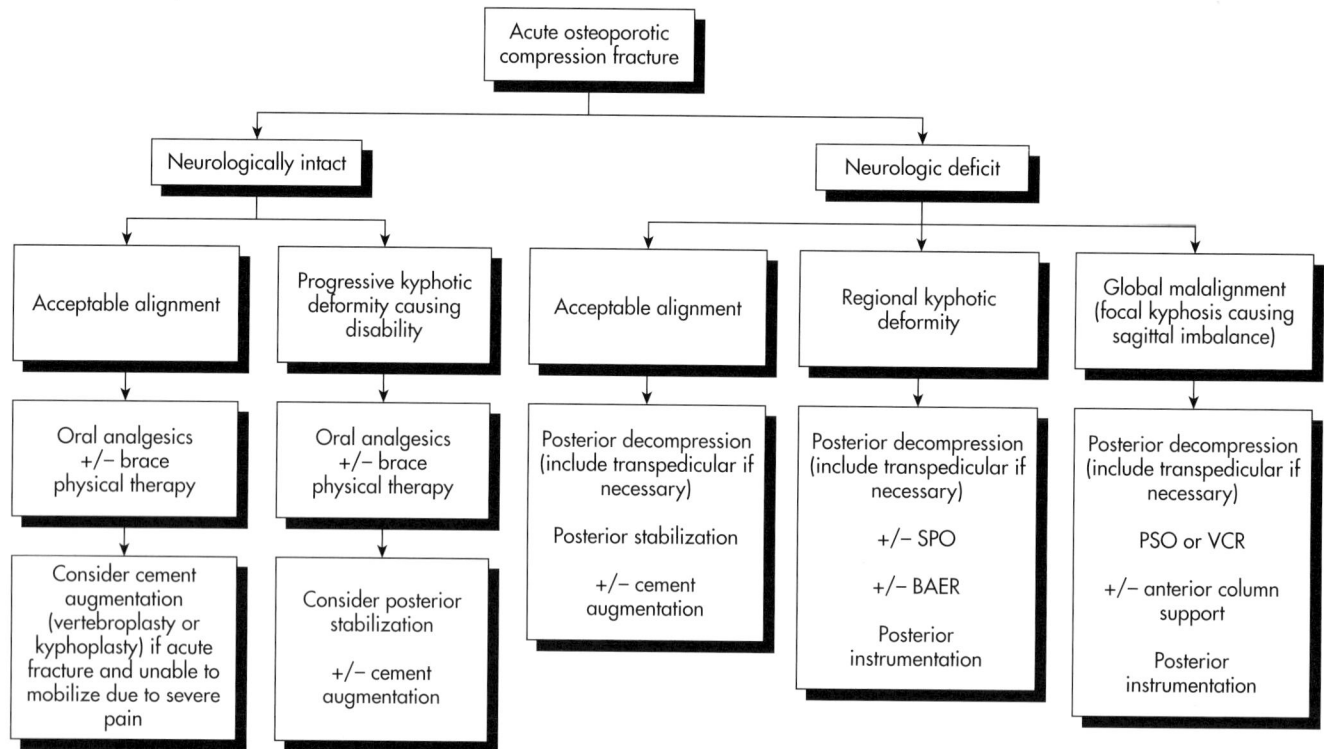

FIG. 2 A generalized treatment algorithm for osteoporotic spine fractures. *BAER,* Balloon-assisted endplate reduction; *PSO,* pedicle subtraction osteotomy; *SPO,* Smith–Petersen osteotomy; *VCR,* vertebral column resection. (From Browner BD et al: *Skeletal trauma: basic science, management, and reconstruction,* ed 6, Philadelphia, 2020, Elsevier.)

conservatively managed group. These procedures are still in their infancy, and more answers should be forthcoming as to their efficacy, as well as questions regarding the amount of time that conservative therapy alone should be pursued and which procedure, if any, should be advised. Most current guidelines recommend 4 to 6 wk of medical therapy before pursuing surgical intervention in neurologically intact VCF.

CHRONIC Rx

Osteoporosis should be treated with the reduction of risk factors (e.g., smoking, alcohol), diet, exercise, calcium and vitamin D supplements, and with medications used to treat osteoporosis (e.g., bisphosphonates).

REFERRAL

Referral is indicated for neurologic abnormalities, unremitting pain, instability, continued disability, or when the investigation of the cause of the fracture reveals serious underlying pathology.

⚠ PEARLS & CONSIDERATIONS

Prevention of osteoporosis and conservative therapy remain the mainstay of treatment.

COMMENTS

- VCFs should be suspected in anyone aged >50 yr with the acute onset of low back pain. There are many opportunities for diagnosis and treatment that are easy to miss, especially for males.
- Solitary vertebral fractures higher than T7 are unusual and should raise suspicion for other pathologic causes.
- Diagnosing and treating osteoporosis reduce the incidence of VCFs.
- Getting people with VCF physically active as soon as possible will be efficacious both acutely and in the long term.
- In general, VCF will be best managed through a partnership of the patient, the primary care

physician, an orthopedist, a physical therapist, a dietitian, and a social worker.
- Concerns that vertebroplasty and kyphoplasty increased risk for a new "secondary" fracture in adjacent vertebrae have not been confirmed in retrospective studies.[3]

PREVENTION

Reducing the effects of modifiable risk factors is key.

REFERENCES & SUGGESTED READINGS

Available at eBooks.Health.Elsevier.com.

AUTHOR: **FRED F. FERRI, MD**

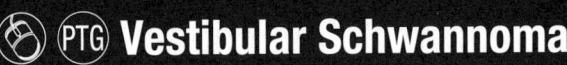
V

I

BASIC INFORMATION

DEFINITION

Acoustic neuroma is a benign proliferation of the Schwann cells that cover the vestibular branch of the eighth cranial nerve (CN VIII). Symptoms are commonly a result of compression of the acoustic branch of CN VIII, the facial nerve (CN VII), and the trigeminal nerve (CN V). The glossopharyngeal nerve (CN IX) and vagus nerve (CN X) are less commonly involved. In extreme cases, compression of the brain stem may lead to obstruction of cerebrospinal fluid (CSF) outflow and elevated intracranial pressure (ICP).[1]

SYNONYMS

Acoustic neuroma
Acoustic schwannoma

ICD-10CM CODE
D33.3 Benign neoplasm of cranial nerves

EPIDEMIOLOGY & DEMOGRAPHICS

- Vestibular schwannomas account for 8% of all intracranial tumors and are the most common neoplasm of the cerebellopontine angle in adults.[1a]
- Overall incidence is approximately 1 in 100,000 person-years in the U.S., with a higher incidence in patients with neurofibromatosis type 2 (NF2). About 3000 new cases of acoustic neuroma are diagnosed each year. The tumor most commonly presents in the fifth and sixth decades.[2]

PHYSICAL FINDINGS & CLINICAL PRESENTATION

- Most frequently unilateral hearing loss and/or tinnitus. Also balance problems, vertigo, facial pain (trigeminal neuralgia) and weakness, difficulty swallowing, fullness or pain of the involved ear. Headache may occur.[3]
- With elevated ICP, patients may also have vomiting, fever, and visual changes.
- Hearing loss is the most common presenting complaint and is usually high frequency.

ETIOLOGY

The etiology is incompletely understood, but long-term exposure to acoustic trauma has been implicated.[4] Bilateral acoustic neuromas may be inherited in an autosomal-dominant manner as part of NF2. This disease is associated with a defect on chromosome 22q1.[5] Childhood exposure to low-dose radiation for benign head and neck conditions may increase risk for acoustic neuromas.[6] There is inconclusive evidence to link chronic exposure to radiofrequency radiation from cellular telephone use and the risk for developing brain tumors.[7]

DIAGNOSIS

DIFFERENTIAL DIAGNOSIS

- Benign positional vertigo
- Ménière disease
- Trigeminal neuralgia
- Cerebellar disease
- Normal-pressure hydrocephalus
- Presbycusis
- Glomus tumors
- Vertebrobasilar insufficiency
- Ototoxicity from medications
- Other tumors:
  1. Meningioma, glioma
  2. Facial nerve schwannoma
  3. Cavernous hemangioma
  4. Metastatic tumors

WORKUP

- A detailed neurologic examination with special attention to the cranial nerves is crucial.
- Rinne and Weber tests help determine conductive or sensorineural hearing loss.
- Common office balance tests (i.e., Romberg, Dix-Hallpike) are typically normal.
- Otoscopic evaluation may help rule out other causes of hearing loss.[8,9]

LABORATORY TESTS

- Audiometry is useful, often showing asymmetric, sensorineural, high-frequency hearing loss.
- CSF protein may be elevated.

IMAGING STUDIES

- MRI with gadolinium (Fig. 1, Fig. 2, Fig. 3) is the preferred test. It can detect tumors as small as 2 mm in diameter.[8]
- High-resolution computed tomography scan with and without contrast can detect tumors 1 cm in diameter or larger.
- Treatment decisions should be based on the size of the tumor, rate of growth (older patients tend to have slower-growing tumors), degree of neurologic deficit, desire to preserve hearing, life expectancy, age of the patient, and surgical risk. A combination of treatments can also be used.[9]

TREATMENT

NONPHARMACOLOGIC THERAPY

- Surgery is the definitive treatment. Choice of approach (middle cranial fossa, translabyrinthine, or retromastoid suboccipital) may vary depending on the size of the tumor, amount of residual hearing desired, and degree of surgical risk that can be tolerated. Partial resection is sometimes undertaken to minimize the risk of injury to nearby structures. Intraoperative facial nerve monitoring is recommended.[9]
- Radiation therapy (stereotactic radiotherapy, stereotactic radiosurgery, or proton beam radiotherapy) is useful for tumors <3 cm in diameter or for those in whom surgery is not an option. Radiotherapy after partial resection has also been used to minimize complications.[10,11]
- Age alone is not a contraindication to surgery.

GENERAL Rx

- Bevacizumab, an antivascular endothelial growth factor monoclonal antibody, has been

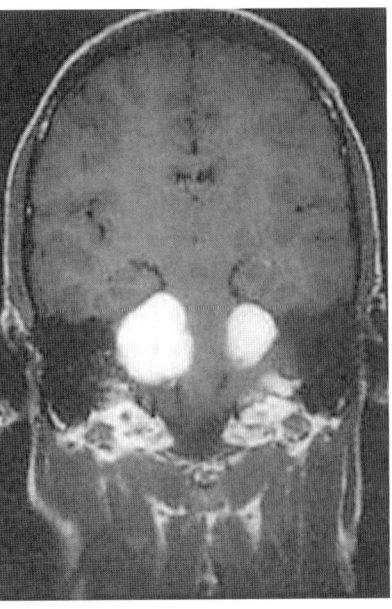

FIG. 1 Magnetic resonance imaging with enhancement shows bilateral acoustic neuromas. Coronal view. (From Kanski JJ, Bowling B: *Clinical ophthalmology, a systematic approach*, ed 7, Philadelphia, 2011, Saunders.)

shown to improve hearing and reduce the volume of growing acoustic neuromas in some neurofibromatosis type 2 patients.[8]
- New therapeutic strategies being investigated include gene therapy and molecular targeted therapy.[12]
- Observation with MRI every 6 to 12 mo may be appropriate for frail patients with small tumors, but risk of unrecoverable hearing loss may increase if surgery is delayed. Also, progressive hearing loss may occur despite absence of growth on subsequent imaging.[8,9]

DISPOSITION

Hearing can be preserved at near-preoperative levels in more than two thirds of patients with small- to medium-sized tumors. Occurrence of secondary radiation-related tumors following radiosurgery is rare. There are no standard posttreatment follow-up recommendations. Therefore an individualized approach to follow-up imaging and audiometry is recommended.[2,8,9]

REFERRAL

Prompt referral to an otolaryngologist or neurosurgeon who is facile with all three surgical approaches is recommended.

PEARLS & CONSIDERATIONS

COMMENTS

- Presents most commonly as unilateral, sensorineural hearing loss.

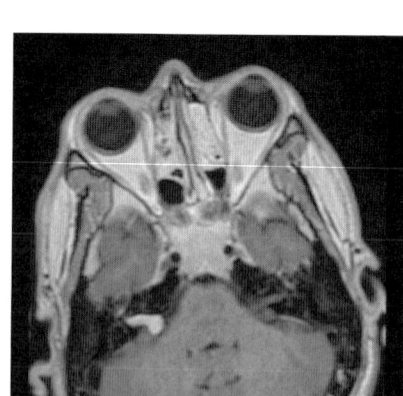 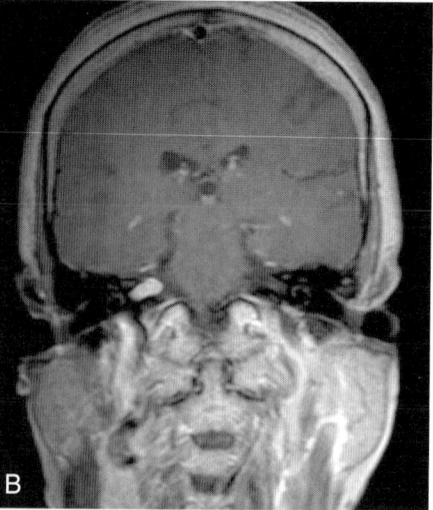

FIG. 2 T1-weighted postgadolinium contrast magnetic resonance image demonstrating a unilateral right enhancing mass within the internal auditory canal and cerebellopontine angle consistent on axial **(A)** and coronal **(B)** images consistent with a vestibular schwannoma. (From Flint PW et al: *Cummings otolaryngology, head and neck surgery,* ed 7, Philadelphia, 2021, Elsevier.)

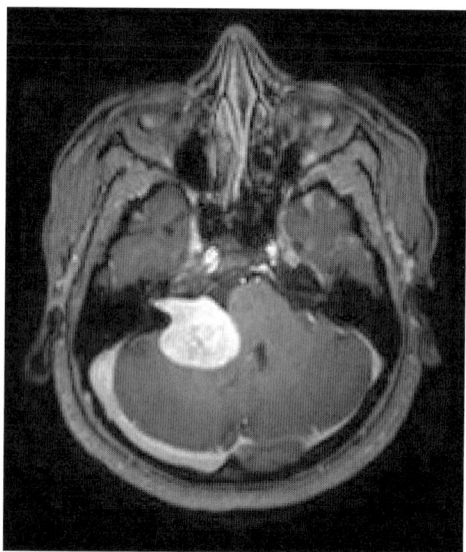

- Treatment outcomes are excellent, with surgical cure rates greater than 95%.
- Of those who are managed with observation only, approximately half have continued enlargement, and approximately one fifth eventually have a surgical intervention.

PATIENT & FAMILY EDUCATION

Acoustic Neuroma Association: www.anausa.org/

REFERENCES

Available at eBooks.Health.Elsevier.com.

RELATED CONTENT

Acoustic Neuroma (Patient Information)
Tinnitus (Related Key Topic)

AUTHOR: **COURTNEY CLARK BILODEAU, MD, FACP**

FIG. 3 **A large acoustic neuroma, originating from the right cerebellopontine angle, compresses the pons and shifts the fourth ventricle.** Patients with neurofibromatosis type 2, because they tend to develop bilateral acoustic neuromas, routinely undergo MRI with views of the internal auditory canals. (From Kaufman DM et al: *Kaufman's clinical neurology for psychiatrists, clinical atlas,* ed 9, Philadelphia, 2023, Elsevier.)

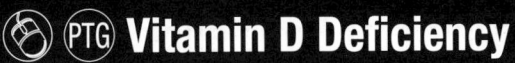

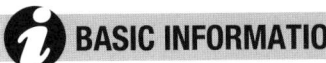 **BASIC INFORMATION**

- Vitamin D is a hormone and a steroid and, by definition, not a vitamin. There are two forms of vitamin D: Vitamin D_2 and vitamin D_3.
- Vitamin D_2 (ergocalciferol) is mainly found in some plant foods.
- Vitamin D_3 (cholecalciferol) is produced in skin exposed to ultraviolet (UV) B radiation from sunlight (Fig. E1). Gloson, Whistler, and DeBoot independently described rickets in the mid-seventeenth century. Sniadecki first reported the association of rickets with inadequate exposure to sunlight in 1822.
- The major functions of vitamin D include:
  1. Increasing calcium, magnesium, and phosphorus absorption from the small intestines
  2. Promoting the maturation of osteoclast to resorb calcium from bones

DEFINITION

Vitamin D deficiency is characterized by hypocalcemia and/or hypophosphatemia leading to impaired bone mineralization. It is classified as a serum 25-hydroxyvitamin D (25[OH]D) level of <20 ng/ml (50 nmol/L). This standard definition of vitamin D deficiency has been recently challenged, and some endocrinologists recommend a cutoff of 12 mg/ml for vitamin D deficiency. Vitamin D insufficiency is defined as a 25(OH)D between 12 and 20 ng/ml.

The consequences of vitamin D deficiency include:
- Bone disease (rickets, osteoporosis, low bone mass)
- May impair reproductive success
- Decrease the ability to combat infection (especially tuberculosis, influenza, viral infection)
- May induce or worsen autoimmune disorders
- May increase the incidence of death due to heart disease, inflammatory bowel disease, fracture, and cancer of the breast, colon, and prostate
- Subclinical vitamin D deficiency may occur in developed countries and be associated with increased fall risk and osteoporosis

SYNONYMS

The sunshine vitamin
The antirachitic factor
Cholecalciferol

ICD-10CM CODE
E55.9 Vitamin D deficiency, unspecified

EPIDEMIOLOGY & DEMOGRAPHICS

INCIDENCE:
- Vitamin D insufficiency is very high among older adults and hospitalized and institutionalized people.
- Worldwide deficiency and insufficiency affect about 1 billion people.
- Children and young adults: 40% to 50% of preadolescent Caucasian girls, and Hispanic and African American adolescents, are vitamin D deficient.

PREVALENCE: 41.6% of adults (at least 20 yr old) have 25(OH)D levels <20 ng/dl.

PREDOMINANT SEX & AGE:
- Decreased skin production of vitamin D with age
- Increased prevalence among darker-skinned individuals

PEAK INCIDENCE: In the U.S., 40% to 100% of the elderly are vitamin D deficient.

Sixty percent of nursing home residents may be vitamin D deficient.

RISK FACTORS:
- Age (due to decreased ability to produce D_3)
- Sunshine-deficient areas (geographic location, living in higher latitudes)
- Dark-skinned individuals (melanin competes with vitamin D_3 precursors for UV photons and thus decreases pre-D_3 formation)
- Obese individuals
- Institutionalized individuals
- Pregnant and lactating women
- Use of sunscreen (sun radiation that causes skin cancer also produces pre-vitamin D_3 in skin)
- Patients on certain medications that antagonize vitamin D action (phenobarbital, phenytoin)
- Intestinal resection
- Severe chronic liver diseases (such as cirrhosis)
- Kidney disease (e.g., nephritic syndrome)
- Sarcoidosis and lymphomas (increased catabolism of 25[OH]D to 1,25[OH]2D)
- Intestinal malabsorption disease (caused by celiac sprue, cystic fibrosis, Whipple disease)

PHYSICAL FINDINGS & CLINICAL PRESENTATION

- Clinical presentation of vitamin D deficiency is dependent on the duration and severity of deficiency
- Most patients with mild to moderate vitamin D deficiency are asymptomatic
- Severe deficiency may lead to rickets (in children), osteomalacia (in adults), bone demineralization, hypokalemia, and phosphaturia
- Mild deficiency can lead to hypocalcemia and hyperparathyroidism
- Rickets: Seen in children; caused by defective mineralization in the skeleton (Fig. E2)
  1. Bowing of the legs
  2. Leg bone pain
  3. Delayed growth
  4. Seizure due to hypocalcemia
- Osteomalacia: Seen in adults with severe and prolonged vitamin D deficiency
  1. Periosteal bone pain (best detected by putting firm pressure on tibia or sternal bones)
  2. Proximal muscle weakness
  3. Chronic muscle aches/pain
- Fracture with very minimal trauma (brittle and easily broken bones)
- Severe hypocalcemia: Especially in late vitamin D deficiency leading to seizure tetany
- Hypophosphatemia
- Paresthesia
- Tetany
- Muscle cramps

ETIOLOGY

- Inadequate exposure to sunlight, such as:
  1. During winter
  2. In nursing home and health care institution residents
  3. With excessive use of sunscreen
- Medications: Individuals on certain medications, such as phenobarbital, phenytoin, and rifampin (antagonize vitamin D action/increase vitamin D catabolism)
- Diseases and disease states:
  1. Diseases causing vitamin D malabsorption:
     a. Cystic fibrosis
     b. Whipple disease
     c. Celiac sprue
  2. Diseases increasing vitamin D catabolism:
     a. Lymphoma
     b. Sarcoidosis
  3. Intestinal resection
  4. Decreased 25(OH)D production:
     a. Kidney disease
     b. Liver cirrhosis

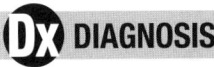 **DIAGNOSIS**

DIFFERENTIAL DIAGNOSIS

- Arthritis
- Fibromyalgia

WORKUP

- Population-wide screening for vitamin D deficiency is not recommended because evidence to support this practice is lacking. Appropriate to screen high-risk individuals.
- Screening is needed for individuals at risk (osteoporosis, history of falls, obese persons, pregnant and lactating women, diseases causing vitamin D malabsorption, African Americans). Workup involves blood and urine tests as well as radiography, as outlined in the next section.

LABORATORY TESTS (TABLE 1)

- Serum 25(OH)D: This is the best test to determine vitamin D status.
- Parathyroid hormone (PTH): Increased levels in vitamin D insufficiency. It is a marker of vitamin D insufficiency.
- Increased (serum or bone) alkaline phosphatase.
- Decreased 24-h urine calcium (patient should not be on a thiazide).
- In patients at risk for osteomalacia [s-25(OH)D is less than 10 ng/ml], check calcium, Ph, alkaline phosphatase, PTH, basic metabolic panel, and tissue transglutaminase antibodies.

IMAGING STUDIES

- Radiographs may show:
  1. Pseudofractures of the pelvis, femur, metatarsals
  2. Nontraumatic fractures
- Bone density:
  1. Decreased bone mineral density (osteopenia or osteoporosis). Note that bone mineral density is not routinely performed in patients whose only risk factor is decreased Vitamin D levels.

TABLE 1 Laboratory Tests

	SERUM			URINE
	Calcium	Phosphorus	Alkaline phosphatase	Calcium
Osteoporosis	N	N	N	N
Hyperparathyroidism				
Primary	↑		N or ↑	N or ↑
Secondary	N or ↑	↑	↑	↓
Tertiary	↑	N or ↓	N or ↑	N or ↑
Hypoparathyroidism	↓	↑	N	↓
Pseudohypoparathyroidism	↓	↑	N	↓
Rickets/osteomalacia				
Vit D deficient	↓	↓	↑	
Vit D refractory	N	↓	↑	↓
Hypophosphatasia	N or ↑	N	↓	N or ↑

Vit, Vitamin.
From Grant LA: *Grainger & Allison's diagnostic radiology essentials,* ed 2, Philadelphia, 2019, Elsevier.

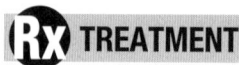 **TREATMENT**

NONPHARMACOLOGIC THERAPY
- Natural sources of vitamin D. These include:
  1. Exposure to sunlight. A mild sunburn is equivalent to consuming 10,000 to 25,000 IU of dietary vitamin D.
  2. Dietary sources are not enough to meet daily requirements. Oily fish such as salmon, cod, and mackerel are rich sources of vitamin D_3.
- Foods fortified with vitamin D
  1. Mainly fortified dairy products
  2. Fortified orange juice

ACUTE GENERAL Rx
- Treating deficiency (general population): Cholecalciferol (vitamin D_3), when available, is preferred for vitamin D supplementation
  1. 50,000 IU of vitamin D every week for 8 wk, *or*
  2. 6000 IU daily to achieve a serum level of 25(OH)D of at least 30 ng/ml
- Maintenance measures after treatment (general population): 1500 to 2000 IU daily
- Treating deficiency (obese patients, patients with malabsorption syndromes, or those taking certain medications, as indicated earlier)
  1. 10,000 IU daily maintenance dose is recommended once s-25(OH)D level exceeds 30 ng/ml.
  2. After treating deficiency, recheck 25(OH)D in 12 to 16 wk.
  3. Maintenance measures after treatment (obese patients, patients with malabsorption syndromes, or those taking certain medications, as indicated earlier): 3000 to 6000 IU daily.

If deficiency persists after several attempts at treatment, try UV B light therapy.

REFERRAL
Referral to an endocrinologist is recommended if there is no response to treatment.

PREVENTION
- Food fortification with vitamin D_2 or vitamin D_3.
- Adequate sun exposure, for example, exposure in the middle of the day (between 10:00 A.M. and 3:00 P.M.).
- Use vitamin D_3 for supplementation when available.
- Vitamin D supplementation (per the Endocrine Society):
  1. Infants (age range 1 to 12 mo) require at least 400 IU/day of vitamin D
  2. Children (age range 1 to 18 yr) require 600 IU/day of vitamin D
  3. Adult supplementation (adults 19 to 70 yr): 600 IU of vitamin D daily
  4. Adult supplementation (persons ≥70 yr): 800 IU of vitamin D daily
  5. Exceptions: Pregnant or lactating women, obese persons, and patients on antiseizure medications, steroids, antifungals, and AIDS medications should be given 2× to 3× more vitamin D
  6. To reduce the risk of fracture and falls, the American Geriatric Society recommends a daily intake of at least 1000 IU and the National Osteoporosis Foundation 800 to 1000 IU in adults 65 yr or older

SCREENING: Routine screening for low-risk adults is not recommended. Screening is recommended only for individuals at high risk for vitamin D deficiency such as Blacks and Hispanics, obese individuals (body mass index >30 kg/m²), patients with osteoporosis, the elderly, and patients with certain chronic diseases (see "Risk Factors"). According to the U.S. Preventive Services Task Force, current evidence is insufficient to assess the balance of benefits and harms of screening for vitamin D deficiency in asymptomatic adults.

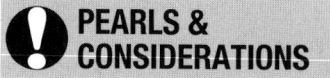 **PEARLS & CONSIDERATIONS**

- In the U.S., vitamin D supplements are available by prescription as vitamin D_2 (ergocalciferol) or over the counter as vitamin D_3 (cholecalciferol, usually in 400- to 1000-IU doses). Both vitamin D_2 and vitamin D_3 are acceptable as supplements. On average, oral vitamin D_3 raises blood levels more than does vitamin D_2.
- Upper limit of maintenance tolerability in healthy adults is 4000 IU a day. More than 4000 IU of vitamin D daily in nondeficient individuals increases the risk of harm. High-level supplements (>10,000 IU daily) are associated with kidney and tissue damage.
- Vitamin D supplementation is recommended for fall prevention. A recent study showed that vitamin D supplementation did not result in a significant lower risk of fractures. Trials have revealed that Vitamin D supplementation at doses of 1000 IU daily or higher did not prevent falls in older adults, and fall risk increased with higher doses.[1]
- Prescribing more than the recommended daily amount to improve quality of life or prevent cardiovascular disease or death is not advised.
- Trials have shown that low vitamin D levels are associated with depressive symptoms, especially in persons with a history of depression. These findings suggest that measuring vitamin D levels may be useful in patients with a history of depression.
- Recent data suggest that vitamin D deficiency is associated with the risk of developing certain cancers (including breast, colon, and prostate).
- A randomized trial has shown that 5 yr of routing vitamin D supplementation does not lower 6 yr mortality in older adults.[2]
- Vitamin D deficiency is associated with some autoimmune diseases (types 1 and 2 diabetes, metabolic syndrome, multiple sclerosis). Daily vitamin D supplementation was found to be beneficial in preventing some new autoimmune diseases in older adults.[3]

REFERENCES & SUGGESTED READINGS
Available at eBooks.Health.Elsevier.com.

RELATED CONTENT
Vitamin D Deficiency (Patient Information)
Osteomalacia and Rickets (Related Key Topic)
Vitamin Deficiency (Related Key Topic)

AUTHOR: **DANIEL K. ASIEDU, MD, PHD, FACP**

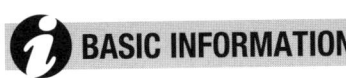
BASIC INFORMATION

DEFINITION

Vitamins are organic compounds that cannot be synthesized by humans but are required as nutrients in minute amounts for normal metabolism. Vitamins have several different functions: They may regulate cell growth and differentiation, as catalysts, as antioxidants, and as coenzymes. Vitamins are classified as either fat soluble (vitamins A, D, E, K) or water soluble (B group of vitamins and C). Deficiency of most vitamins is rare in Western countries. Certain groups may be prone to vitamin deficiency, and these are discussed here. Vitamin D deficiency is discussed in a separate topic.

SYNONYMS

Hypovitaminosis
Vitamin A: Retinol
Vitamin E: Alpha tocopherol
Vitamin K: Phytonadione or menadiol
Vitamin B_1: Thiamine
Vitamin B_2: Riboflavin
Niacin: Vitamin B_3; nicotinic acid
Vitamin B_5: Pantothenic acid
Vitamin B_6: Pyridoxine; pyridoxal phosphate
Folic acid: Vitamin B_9; folate
Vitamin B_{12}: Cyanocobalamin
Vitamin C: Ascorbic acid

ICD-10CM CODES
E50 Vitamin A deficiency
E51 Thiamine deficiency
E53 Deficiency of other B group vitamins
E55 Vitamin D deficiency
E56 Other vitamin deficiencies
E56.0 Deficiency of vitamin E
E56.1 Deficiency of vitamin K
E53.0 Riboflavin deficiency
E52 Niacin deficiency [pellagra]
E53.1 Pyridoxine deficiency
E53.8 Deficiency of other specified B group vitamins
E54 Ascorbic acid deficiency

EPIDEMIOLOGY & DEMOGRAPHICS

Deficiency can occur in all age groups but is most common in the elderly.
- Vitamin A deficiency: Affects 250 million preschool children worldwide.
- Vitamin E deficiency: Deficiency is rare in humans. Usually occurs in individuals with severe protein-energy malnutrition.
- Vitamin K deficiency: Varies by geographic regions; no race predilection; affects both sexes equally. Encountered often in infants. In normal healthy adults, 8% to 31% have vitamin K deficiency, but it rarely leads to significant bleeding.
- Vitamin B_1 (thiamine) deficiency: Incidence is unknown; no sex, race, or age predilection. Deficiency is usually due to inadequate intake, especially if consuming diet made up of polished rice and grains.
- Vitamin B_2 (riboflavin): More common than previously appreciated. Deficiency is referred to as ariboflavinosis.
- Vitamin B_5 (pantothenic acid) deficiency: Rare, as it is present in all foods.
- Vitamin B_{12} (cobalamin) deficiency: Relatively common. Of patients with anemia, about 1% to 2% is due to B_{12} deficiency. Among patients with macrocytosis (mean corpuscular volume [MCV] > 100) 18% to 20% is due to B_{12} deficiency. Occurs in all age groups but more common in the elderly. B_{12} deficiency due to pernicious anemia is common in Northern Europe.
- Vitamin B_9 (folic acid) deficiency: Mandatory fortification started in 1998. Prevalence before fortification 16% and after 0.5%. Neural tube defect associated with low maternal folate status during pregnancy. Pregnant women and the elderly are at greatest risk of folic acid deficiency.
- Vitamin C (ascorbic acid) deficiency: Smokers and low-income persons are at increased risk. Vitamin C deficiency is associated with access to food and/or socioeconomic status. Prevalence vary worldwide, but the rate is about 7.1% in the U.S.

Fig. 1 shows environmental and nutritional factors in disease.

PHYSICAL FINDINGS & CLINICAL PRESENTATION

- Vitamin A: Xerophthalmia, xerosis of the cornea, keratomalacia, Bitot spots (abnormal squamous cell proliferation and keratinization of the conjunctiva), nyctalopia (poor adaptation to darkness)/night blindness, poor bone growth, dry skin and hair, follicular hyperkeratosis (caused by blockage of hair follicles by keratin), pruritus, broken fingernails
- Vitamin K: Clinical manifestation usually occurs if hypoprothrombinemia is present. Major symptom is bleeding to minor trauma. Also can show easy bruisability, epistaxis, hematoma, gum bleeding, melena, hematuria, or splinter hemorrhage
- Vitamin E: Neuromuscular disorders (ataxia; hyporeflexia, peripheral neuropathy); bone weakness, hemolysis

Vitamin	Function	Consequences of deficiency
A	Retinal function, epithelial growth control	Night blindness, keratomalacia, xerophthalmia
B_1 (thiamine)	Coenzyme	Beriberi, Wernicke's encephalopathy
B_2 (riboflavin)	Coenzyme	Dermatitis, glossitis, keratitis, neuropathy, confusion
B_6 (pyridoxine)	Coenzyme	Neuropathy
B_{12} (cobalamin)	Nucleic acid synthesis	Megaloblastic anemia / Subacute combined degeneration of spinal cord
Niacin	Coenzyme NAD, NADP	Pellagra (diarrhea, dermatitis, and dementia)
Folate	Coenzyme in nucleic acid synthesis	Megaloblastic anemia, villous atrophy of gut
Vitamin C	Cofactor in hydroxylation	Scurvy
Vitamin D	Calcium and phosphate absorption	Rickets (childhood) / Osteomalacia (adults)
Vitamin E	Antioxidant	Spinocerebellar degeneration
Vitamin K	Cofactor for coagulation factor synthesis	Bleeding due to coagulation defects

FIG. 1 Environmental and nutritional factors in disease. (From Stevens A: *Core pathology,* St Louis, 2009, Elsevier.)

- Vitamin B_1 (thiamine): Beriberi, which has two subtypes (infantile and adult). Adult type is described below:
  1. Dry beriberi (affecting the nervous system): Symmetrical peripheral neuropathy (with sensory and motor impairments), Wernicke encephalopathy (nystagmus, ataxia, ophthalmoplegia, and confusion), Korsakoff syndrome (impaired short-term memory loss and confabulation but normal cognition)
  2. Wet beriberi (affecting the cardiovascular system): Cardiomegaly, cardiomyopathy, heart failure, tachycardia, hypotension, chest pain, peripheral edema
  3. Gastrointestinal (GI): Anorexia; constipation
- Vitamin B_2 (riboflavin):
  1. Cheilosis (chapping and fissure of the lip)
  2. Glossitis (sore red tongue)
  3. Oily, scaly rashes on nasolabial folds, eyelids, scrotum, labia majora
  4. Red itchy eyes
  5. Normocytic or normochromic anemia
  6. Peripheral neuropathy
- Vitamin B_3 (niacin):
  1. Pellagra (4 *D*s—diarrhea, dermatitis, dementia, and ultimately death)
  2. Hyperpigmentation of sun-exposed skin
  3. "Raw beef" swollen and painful tongue
  4. Deficiency can be seen in prolonged use of Isoniazid, in carcinoid syndrome, and in Hartnup syndrome
- Vitamin B_5 (pantothenic acid):
  1. Deficiency is rare
  2. Deficiency leads to "burning feet syndrome" (distal paresthesia and dysesthesia)
  3. Anemia
  4. GI symptoms
- Vitamin B_6 (Pyridoxine): Rare to see overt deficiency
  1. Mild deficiency—glossitis, cheilosis, impaired proprioception; sensory ataxia, confusion, depression
  2. Severe deficiency—seborrheic dermatitis, seizure, microcytic
- Vitamin B_{12} (cyanocobalamin):
  1. Megaloblastic anemia (pernicious anemia)
  2. Neurologic symptoms including peripheral neuropathy, ataxia (shuffling gait), paresthesia; subacute degeneration of the spinal cord (demyelination of the dorsal column), visual disturbances due to optic atrophy
  3. Glossitis and GI symptoms such as nausea, vomiting, and anorexia are also common
  4. Patients may also have dementia/mental sluggishness, depression, and weakness
- Vitamin B_9 (folic acid):
  1. Patchy hyperpigmentation of skin (especially between fingers and toes) and mucous membranes
  2. Moderate fever (temp $<102°$ F; $38.9°$ C) despite the absence of infection
  3. Neural tube defect
  4. Angular stomatitis
  5. Red, beefy, smooth, and shiny tongue
  6. Megaloblastic anemia
- Vitamin C: Scurvy (bruising, petechiae, follicular hyperkeratosis, perifollicular hemorrhage,

corkscrew hairs), poor wound healing, fatigue, gingivitis/bleeding gums, weight loss, bone abnormalities (Fig. E2). Also, loss of teeth, abnormal nail (koilonychia and splint hemorrhages). Vitamin C deficiency may be associated with nonalcoholic fatty liver

ETIOLOGY

- Fat-soluble vitamins (vitamins A, D, E, K):
  1. Decreased ingestion, malnutrition, eating disorders
  2. Diseases that affect fat absorption decrease the absorption of fat-soluble vitamins—for example, cystic fibrosis, celiac sprue, inflammatory bowel disease, cholestasis, hepatobiliary disease, small bowel surgery
  3. Change in vitamin metabolism:
     a. Alcoholism
     b. Drugs such as cholestyramine, warfarin, anticonvulsants, antibiotics (e.g., cephalosporins)
     c. Chronic kidney disease
- Increased risk in:
  1. Vegans
  2. Recent immigrants
  3. Refugees
  4. Toddlers/preschoolers living below the poverty line
- Water-soluble vitamins (the B group of vitamins and vitamin C)—there are several etiologic factors, including:
  1. Inadequate intake
  2. Decreased absorption
  3. Alcoholism
  4. Pregnancy/lactation
  5. Peritoneal dialysis
  6. Medications (e.g., isoniazid, phenothiazines, tricyclic antidepressants, metformin [vit B_{12}])
  7. Malabsorption
  8. Low income
  9. Advanced age
- Vitamin B_{12} deficiency—caused by:
  1. Insufficient dietary intake, as in strict vegans
  2. Decreased absorption secondary to intrinsic factor deficiency, decreased intrinsic factor secretion, gastric atrophy, gastrectomy/gastric bypass
  3. Terminal ileum disease such as celiac disease, enteritis, tropical sprue
- Folic acid deficiency:
  1. Increased needs can lead to deficiency (e.g., pregnancy, lactation, malignancy)
  2. Derangement of folate metabolism by:
     a. Medication (e.g., methotrexate)
     b. Disease (e.g., hypothyroidism)
     c. Increased excretion: As seen in alcoholics

Dx DIAGNOSIS

WORKUP

Table 1 summarizes clinical clues in identifying vitamin deficiency.

LABORATORY TESTS

General initial laboratory tests include:

- CBC
- Liver function tests
- Basic metabolic panel
- Albumin
- Measurement of serum levels of the specific vitamin in question

Specific tests may be considered in the following cases:

- Vitamin A:
  1. Serum retinol level (best test, a direct measure, expensive)
  2. Retinol binding protein (easier to perform, less expensive)
  3. Dark-adaptation threshold test
- Vitamin K:
  1. Protein induced by vitamin K absence or antagonism is the current best test available to determine vitamin K status. The level is increased in vitamin K deficiency
  2. Prothrombin time/partial thromboplastin time
  3. Prothrombin
  4. Des-gamma-carboxyprothrombin (most sensitive test)
  5. Niacin: Urine-*N*-methylnicotinamide (level <0.8 mg/day indicates niacin deficiency)
- Vitamin B_1 (thiamine):
  1. Blood thiamine levels
  2. Thiamine pyrophosphate levels in blood
  3. Erythrocyte thiamine transketolase activity
  4. Urinary thiamine excretion
- Vitamin B_3 (niacin): Check urinary N-methylnicotinamide or erythrocyte NAD/NADP ratio (tests are not readily available)
- Vitamin B_2: Check plasma riboflavin concentration
- Vitamin B_{12}:
  1. Serum vitamin B_{12} <190 pg/ml is diagnostic of vitamin B_{12} deficiency
  2. Serum methylmalonic acid, which is elevated in B_{12} deficiency
  3. Antiparietal antibody
  4. Intrinsic factor antibody is decreased
  5. CBC shows increased MCV, anemia with low hemoglobin, and low hematocrit
  6. Blood smear shows macrocytosis and hypersegmentation of megaloblasts
  7. Megaloblastic anemia
- Folic acid:
  1. Check serum folate level.
  2. Additional testing includes checking for serum homocysteine level, which will be elevated.
  3. Red cell folate level shows chronic folate status.

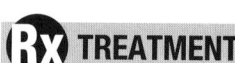 TREATMENT

Most of the vitamins are available over the counter individually or in different multivitamin formulations.

- Vitamin A deficiency: Treat with oral supplementation 10,000 IU daily.
  1. Consume vitamin A–rich foods such as liver, beef, carrots, oranges, mangoes.
  2. Five servings of fruit and vegetables give enough carotenoids for a day.

TABLE 1 Clinical Clues in Identifying Vitamin Deficiency

Clinical Features	Causes and Diagnosis	Treatment and Notes
Vitamin A deficiency		
Can take years to cause symptoms Xerophthalmia causing night blindness and Bitot's spots (conjunctival squamous cell proliferation and keratinization) is the earliest sign Poor bone growth Follicular hyperkeratosis Impaired immune system Conjunctival xerosis Keratomalacia	Low dietary intake (preformed vitamin A is from animals; provitamin A is found in plants) Diagnosis is made by measuring serum retinol levels	Vitamin A supplementation Daily requirement (RDA) for adult males is 3000 IU and for females is 2300 IU Vitamin A toxicity is related to chronic ingestion ($\geq$25,000 IU/d); serum retinol levels are not helpful as vitamin A is stored in the liver
Vitamin B$_{12}$ deficiency		
Can take several years to show symptoms Macrocytic anemia Smooth tongue In severe deficiency—subacute combined degeneration of the spinal cord Peripheral sensory neuropathy affecting large and small fibers Dementia	Low dietary intake Pernicious anemia Terminal ileum disease	Vitamin B$_{12}$ supplementation If both folate and vitamin B$_{12}$ deficiency are present, you must replace vitamin B$_{12}$ first to avoid subacute combined degeneration of the spinal cord
Vitamin B$_6$ (pyridoxine) deficiency		
Can take weeks to become symptomatic Glossitis Cheilosis Vomiting Seizures Scrotal dermatitis	Mainly secondary to drugs, e.g., isoniazid, cycloserine, penicillamine, phenobarbital Can measure serum levels of pyridoxal-phosphate	Vitamin supplementation Large doses can cause both impaired position and vibratory sense
Vitamin B$_2$ (riboflavin) deficiency		
Can take weeks to become symptomatic Normochromic normocytic anemia Sore throat and magenta tongue Glossitis Cheilosis Seborrheic dermatitis in perianal area, nose	Associated with phenothiazine and tricyclic antidepressants	Vitamin supplementation
Vitamin B$_1$ (thiamine) deficiency		
Can take weeks to become symptomatic Wet beriberi—heart failure secondary to cardiomyopathy Dry beriberi (neuropathy)— Wernicke encephalopathy (WE)—nystagmus, ophthalmoplegia, and ataxia Peripheral neuropathy Korsakoff syndrome	Low dietary intake Alcoholic patients, chronic dialysis patients IV glucose can precipitate WE: Give thiamine before glucose Can directly measure thiamine levels in serum	Thiamine supplementation
Vitamin C deficiency (scurvy)		
First symptoms are petechial hemorrhage and ecchymoses Bleeding, swollen gums Hyperkeratotic papules Hemorrhagia into joints, nail beds Loosening of teeth Periosteal hemorrhages Coiled hairs Impaired wound healing Weak bones Sjögren's syndrome	Low dietary intake	Vitamin C supplementation Large doses can cause oxalate renal stones and impaired absorption of vitamin B$_{12}$
Iodine deficiency		
Hypothyroidism	Low dietary intake Drug and alcohol abusers	Improve dietary intake
Niacin deficiency (pellagra)		
The 3 'D's: —Dermatizis (sun-exposed areas) —Diarrhea — Depression to dementia to psychosis (altered mental state)Hyperpigmentation Glossitis Stomatitis	Low dietary intake; tryptophan is used in the body to make niacin Carcinoid syndrome (tryptophan is used up) Isoniazid (increased excretion of tryptophan—pyroxidine supplement must be used concurrently to prevent this) Hartnup disease (autosomal recessive, cerebellar ataxia)	Replacement treatment

Continued

TABLE 1 Clinical Clues in Identifying Vitamin Deficiency—cont'd

Clinical Features	Causes and Diagnosis	Treatment and Notes
Zinc deficiency		
Rash (face, body: Pustular, bullous, vesicular, seborrheic, acneiform), skin ulcers, alopecia, dysgeusia Impaired immunity Night blindness Decreased spermatogenesis Diarrhea	Low dietary intake	Zinc supplementation
Vitamin E deficiency		
Peripheral sensory and motor neuropathy Hemolytic anemia Retinal degeneration Dry skin		Vitamin E supplementation Large doses can potentiate the effects of oral anticoagulation
Vitamin K deficiency		
Bleeding tendency Easy bruisability	Low dietary intake Systemic diseases that cause fat-soluble vitamin malabsorption Can detect by checking coagulation profile (INR and PT)	Vitamin K supplementation
Clinical Features	Causes and Diagnosis	Treatment and Notes
Vitamin D deficiency		
The major source of vitamin D is from sun exposure. Secondary sources are from diet or supplementation and intestinal absorption In the liver, vitamin D undergoes hydroxylation by 25-hydroxylase to 25-hydroxyvitamin D, 25 (OH)D. Further hydroxylation takes place in the kidneys to activated vitamin D (1,25-dihydroxyvitamin D). Activated vitamin D is important in bone mineralization Vitamin D deficiency leads to: —Rickets in children —Osteomalacia in adults —Hypocalcemia — Secondary hyperparathyroidism which leads to phosphaturia	Decreased exposure to the sun Decreased intestinal absorption from the intestine Renal disease Systemic diseases that cause fat malabsorption Can be directly measured by checking for serum 25(OH)D	Increase casual exposure to sunlight Vitamin D supplementation: —25(OH)D (Ostelin 1000) —Activated vitamin D (calcitriol; this form should be used in renal disease) The RDA for vitamin D is 600 IU for adults Avoid excessive doses, as toxicity can cause hypercalcemia, confusion, polyuria, polydipsia, anorexia, vomiting, and muscle weakness Long-term toxicity results in bone demineralization and pain

INR, International normalized ratio; *RDA*, recommended dietary allowance; *PT*, prothrombin time.
From Talley NJ et al: *Essentials of internal medicine*, ed 4, Chatswood, NSW, 2021, Elsevier Australia.

- Vitamin K deficiency: Treatment depends on the severity of bleeding, administered subcutaneously or intramuscularly (IM).
- Vitamin B_1 (thiamine) deficiency: Give IM thiamine 50 mg for several days.
  1. If B_1 deficiency is suspected and patient needs intravenous glucose, give thiamine first before intravenous glucose. This prevents the development of Korsakoff psychosis.
- Vitamin B_{12} deficiency: Give 1000 mcg IM daily for 7 days, then once a wk for 1 mo, then once a month indefinitely.
  1. A potential option is oral supplementation.
- Folic acid deficiency: Daily requirement is 400 to 1000 mcg (1 mg) daily.

1. Centers for Disease Control and Prevention recommend that women of childbearing age take 400 mcg of folic acid daily.
- The U.S. Preventive Services Task Force (USPSTF) found no benefit and likely harm from use of β-carotene and lack of either benefit or harm from use of vitamin E, leading to a recommendation against use of either one for preventing cardiovascular disease or cancer.[1]

REFERENCE & SUGGESTED READINGS
Available at eBooks.Health.Elsevier.com.

RELATED CONTENT
Anemia, Pernicious (Related Key Topic)
Osteomalacia and Rickets (Related Key Topic)
Vitamin D Deficiency (Related Key Topic)
Wernicke Syndrome (Related Key Topic)
Vitamins and Their Functions (Appendix IIb) (Related Key Topic)

AUTHOR: **DANIEL K. ASIEDU, MD, PHD, FACP**

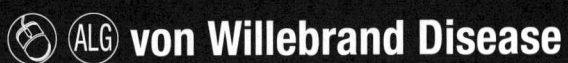

V

I

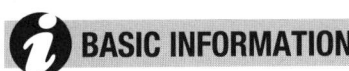 **BASIC INFORMATION**

DEFINITION

von Willebrand disease (vWD) is an inherited disorder of hemostasis characterized by a quantitative or qualitative deficiency in von Willebrand factor (vWF), which results in defective platelet adhesion and aggregation.

SYNONYMS

vWD
Pseudohemophilia

ICD-10CM CODE
D68.0   von Willebrand disease

EPIDEMIOLOGY & DEMOGRAPHICS

- Most common inherited bleeding disorder.
- Prevalence is 0.6% to 1.3% according to population studies and is consistent across all races and ethnicities.
- Estimates based on referral for symptoms of bleeding suggest a prevalence of 1 case/10,000 persons.[1]

PHYSICAL FINDINGS & CLINICAL PRESENTATION

- Generally normal physical examination.
- Mucosal bleeding (gingival bleeding, epistaxis) and easy bruising occurs.
- GI bleeding may occur because of angiodysplasia in type 2 or type 3 vWD.
- Bleeding after surgery or dental extraction.
- Most women have menorrhagia.
- Rarely, muscle or joint bleeding occurs in type 3 vWD.

ETIOLOGY

- vWD is usually an autosomal-dominant disorder but is rarely recessive or double-heterozygotic.
- vWF is a protein product of a gene located on the short arm of chromosome 12. vWD results from a failure to synthesize or secrete vWF or an accelerated clearance of vWF.
- Binding of vWF multimers to denuded subendothelial collagen or glycosaminoglycans causes platelet adhesion by acting as a ligand for glycoprotein IB on the platelet surface.[2] This latter activity can be measured by the ristocetin cofactor (RCo) assay. In vWD, the RCo level is <30% of normal. Low vWF (mild vWD) exists when the RCo level is between 30% and 60%, with such patients potentially exhibiting a bleeding phenotype.
- There are three broad clinically defined types of vWD:
  1. Type 1 is the most common (80% cases), in which levels of vWF, FVIII:C, and RCo are reduced but concordant. Within type 1, there is type 1 mild, which is common; type 1 severe (T1S), which is rare; and type 1C, in which the low vWF is due to accelerated clearance.
  2. Type 2 has four subtypes: Type 2A, type 2B, type 2N, and type 2M. All of these variants have a qualitative defect in vWF, low levels of RCo, and show a discordancy between levels of RCo and FVIII:C.
  3. Type 3 is rare and either an autosomal recessive disorder or double heterozygote and has a near-complete quantitative deficiency of vWF and very low FVIII:C.
- Acquired vWD disease presents with mucocutaneous bleeding abnormalities but no family history. It is seen often in association with hematoproliferative or autoimmune

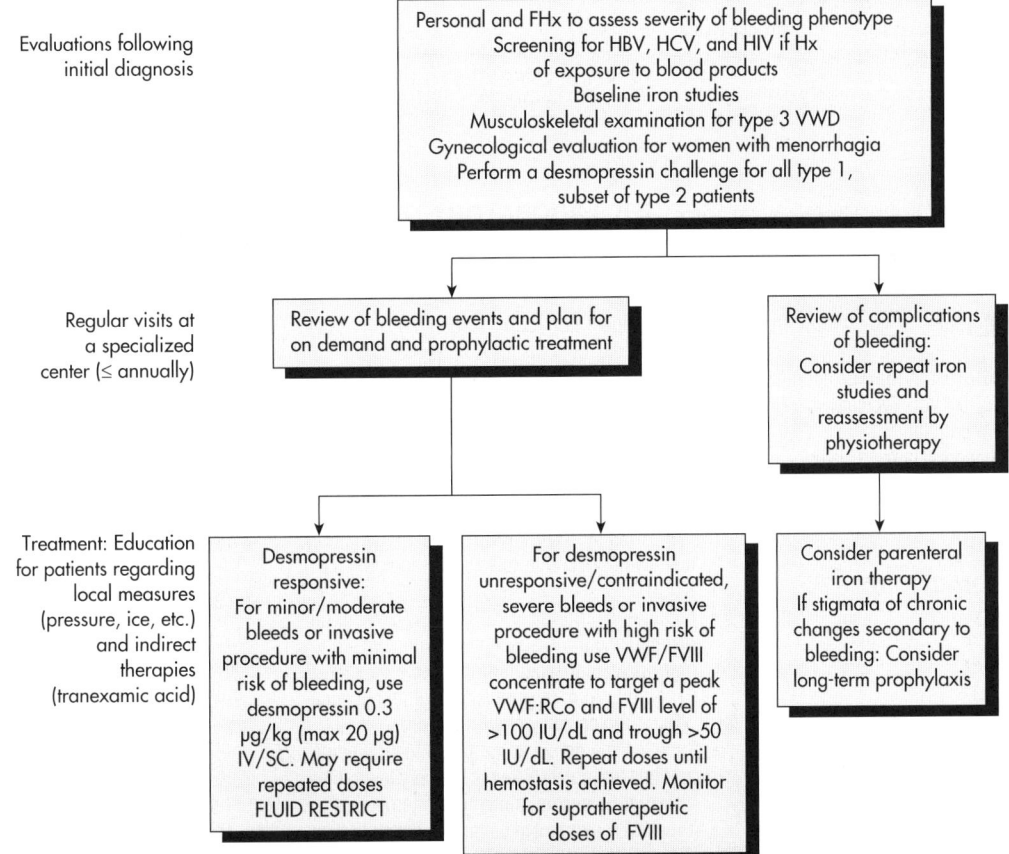

Evaluations following initial diagnosis

> Personal and FHx to assess severity of bleeding phenotype
> Screening for HBV, HCV, and HIV if Hx of exposure to blood products
> Baseline iron studies
> Musculoskeletal examination for type 3 VWD
> Gynecological evaluation for women with menorrhagia
> Perform a desmopressin challenge for all type 1, subset of type 2 patients

Regular visits at a specialized center (≤ annually)

> Review of bleeding events and plan for on demand and prophylactic treatment

> Review of complications of bleeding: Consider repeat iron studies and reassessment by physiotherapy

Treatment: Education for patients regarding local measures (pressure, ice, etc.) and indirect therapies (tranexamic acid)

> Desmopressin responsive: For minor/moderate bleeds or invasive procedure with minimal risk of bleeding, use desmopressin 0.3 μg/kg (max 20 μg) IV/SC. May require repeated doses FLUID RESTRICT

> For desmopressin unresponsive/contraindicated, severe bleeds or invasive procedure with high risk of bleeding use VWF/FVIII concentrate to target a peak VWF:RCo and FVIII level of >100 IU/dL and trough >50 IU/dL. Repeat doses until hemostasis achieved. Monitor for supratherapeutic doses of FVIII

> Consider parenteral iron therapy If stigmata of chronic changes secondary to bleeding: Consider long-term prophylaxis

FIG. 1 Approach to the management of von Willebrand disease. *FHx,* Family history; *FVIII,* factor VIII; *HBV,* hepatitis B virus; *HCV,* hepatitis C virus; *HIV,* human immunodeficiency virus; *Hx,* history; *IV,* intravenous; *RCo,* ristocetin cofactor; *SC,* subcutaneous; *vWD,* von Willebrand disease; *vWF,* von Willebrand factor. (From Hoffman R: *Hematology: basic principles and practice,* ed 7, Philadelphia, 2018, Elsevier.)

TABLE 1 Table of Investigations

vWD Type	vWF:RCo IU/dl[a]	vWF:Ag IU/dl[a]	RCo/Ag IU/dl[a]	FVIII:C IU/dl[a]	Multimer Pattern[b]	Other
1	Low	Low	Equivalent	~1.5× vWF:Ag	Normal	
2A	Low	Low	vWF:RCo <vWF:Ag	Low or normal	Abnormal↓ HMWM	
2B	Low	Low	vWF:RCo <vWF:Ag	Low or normal	Abnormal↓ HMWM	↑ RIPA[c] (↓ platelet count)
2M	Low	Low	vWF:RCo <vWF:Ag	Low or normal	Normal	
2N	Normal/low	Normal/low	Equivalent	<30	Normal	↓ vWF:FVIIIB[d]
3	Absent	Absent	NA	<10	Absent	

[a]Relative to the reference range (approximate values); vWF:RCo (50-200 IU/dl); vWF:Ag (50-200 IU/dl); FVIII:C (50-150 IU/dl).
[b]HMWM, High-molecular-weight multimers.
[c]Increased agglutination at low concentrations of ristocetin.
[d]The ability of vWF to bind and protect FVIII is reduced. vWF and FVIII levels can look exactly like those in males with mild hemophilia A or in symptomatic hemophilia A carrier females.
Ag, Antigen; *FVIII:C,* FVIII level; *NA,* not applicable; *RCo,* ristocetin cofactor; *RIPA,* ristocetin-induced platelet aggregation; *vWD,* von Willebrand disease; *vWF:FVIIIB,* FVIII-binding assay.
From Hoffman R: *Hematology: basic principles and practice,* ed 7, Philadelphia, 2018, Elsevier.

TABLE 2 Desmopressin Responsiveness in the Various Subtypes of von Willebrand Disease

vWD Type	vWF:RCo	vWF:Ag	RCo/Ag	FVIII:C IU/dl	vWF:CB	vWF:CB/vWF:Ag
1	Increase	Increase	Remains >0.7	Increase	Increase	Remains >0.7
2A	No/little change	Increase	Remains <0.7	Increase	No/little change	Remains <0.7
2M (GP1B-binding dysfunction)	No/little change	Increase	Remains <0.7	Increase	Increase	Remains >0.7
3	No/little change	No/little change		No/little change	No/little change	

Ag, Antigen; *FVIII:C,* factor VIII level; *GP1B,* glycoprotein 1B; *RCo,* ristocetin cofactor; *vWD,* von Willebrand disease; *vWF,* von Willebrand factor; *CB,* collagen assays–binding.
Modified from Favaloro EJ: Rethinking the diagnosis of von Willebrand disease, *Thromb Res* 127(Suppl 2):17, 2011; and Hoffman R: *Hematology, basic principles and practice,* ed 7, Philadelphia, 2018, Elsevier.

disorders or may occur in hypothyroidism. Successful treatment of the underlying illness can reverse the clinical course.

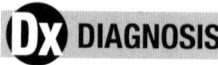 **DIAGNOSIS**

A definitive diagnosis of vWD may be made if vWF:RCo levels are <30 IU/dl. Typically, a vWD diagnosis requires two criteria:

(1) A personal history, family history, or physical evidence of mucocutaneous bleeding and (2) a qualitative or quantitative decrease in functional activity of vWD.

DIFFERENTIAL DIAGNOSIS

Platelet function disorders, clotting factor deficiencies

WORKUP (FIG. 1)

Screening Laboratory Tests:
- Laboratory evaluation (Table 1).
- Initial testing includes prothrombin time (normal), partial thromboplastin time (normal or slightly increased), platelet count (normal), and PFA-100 (abnormal or may show high normal values in type 1 vWD).

SPECIFIC LABORATORY TESTS

- Factor VIII coagulant activity (FVIII:C, typically decreased but normal in some type 2 cases).
- vWF antigen, RCo, and collagen binding assay are typically decreased.
- Normal platelet number and morphology.
- Prolonged bleeding time or prolonged PFA-100 closure times.
- von Willebrand propeptide.[3] This measures the N-terminal propeptide of vWF. This vWFpp is secreted in equimolar amounts to the mature vWF. The ratio of vWFpp to vWF assists in identifying vWD due to rapid clearance, as in type 1C.
- Multimeric analysis: Type 2A vWD can be distinguished by absence of medium- and high-molecular-weight multimers.
- Type 2B vWD is distinguished by the absence of high-molecular-weight multimers.
- Type 2N is a defect in the factor VIII:C binding and has normal vWF levels but very low factor VIII:C with a normal multimer pattern.
- Type 2M is a defect in binding to platelets (low RCo, low collagen-binding activity) but normal multimers.

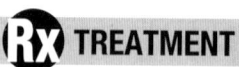 **TREATMENT**

NONPHARMACOLOGIC THERAPY

- Avoidance of aspirin and other NSAIDs
- Antifibrinolytics such as tranexamic acid (1g PO TID-QID), especially for menorrhagia or oral bleeding

ACUTE GENERAL Rx

- Treatment of vWD is based on normalizing factor VIII land vWF levels on spontaneous bleeding or before a planned intervention.
- Desmopressin (DDAVP) (Table 2): This binds to receptors on endothelial cells and causes vWF release and is suitable in milder forms of vWD. DDAVP is administered at a dose of 0.3 mcg/kg in 50 to 100 ml of intravenous normal saline solution infused over 20 to 30 min. It is also available as a nasal spray (150 mcg spray to each nostril) before minor surgery and for the management of minor bleeding episodes.
- The use of therapeutic products to replete vWF levels is required in cases unresponsive to DDAVP or those with severe vWD. Currently

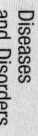

available vWF products can be grouped into the following categories: (1) vWF/factor VIII plasma-derived concentrates, (2) plasma-derived vWF-only concentrate, and (3) recombinant-derived vWF-only concentrate.[4]

- Recombinant-derived vWF is a treatment approach that overcomes the limitations associated with plasma-derived vWF concentrates such as variable vWD levels and risk

of pathogen transmission.[5] In severe vWD, the prophylactic use of recombinant-derived vWF-only concentrate is superior to on-demand use by reducing rate of bleeding and reduction in bleeding risk.

- In patients with severe vWD undergoing surgery or those who receive repeated therapeutic doses of concentrates, use of a plasma-derived vWF-only concentrate or

recombinant-derived vWF-only concentrate need to be administered.

REFERENCES
Available at eBooks.Health.Elsevier.com.

AUTHOR: **RITESH RATHORE, MD**

V

Diseases and Disorders

I

Waldenström Macroglobulinemia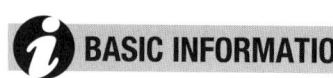

BASIC INFORMATION

DEFINITION

Waldenström macroglobulinemia (WM) is an indolent B-cell lymphoplasmacytic lymphoma (LPL) characterized by lymphoplasmacytic infiltration in the bone marrow (BM) and other organs, a monoclonal immunoglobulin M (IgM) paraprotein in the serum, and presence of the *MYD88 L265P* mutation.[1] Less than 5% of LPLs secrete IgG, IgA, or light chains, or they can be nonsecretory.

SYNONYMS

WM
Monoclonal macroglobulinemia
Lymphoplasmacytic lymphoma

ICD-10CM CODE
C88.0 Waldenström macroglobulinemia

EPIDEMIOLOGY & DEMOGRAPHICS

- Accounts for 1% of all non-Hodgkin lymphoma cases
- A reported 1500 to 2000 new cases diagnosed every year in the U.S.
- Overall incidence: 3.4 per million person-year in men, 1.7 per million person-year in women
- Median age at diagnosis: 69 yr
- More common among men than women and among whites than blacks

PHYSICAL FINDINGS & CLINICAL PRESENTATION

- 25% to 30% of patients can be asymptomatic at presentation
- Weakness, fatigue, and pallor, usually associated with anemia (50%)
- Fever, night sweats, and weight loss (30%)
- Demyelinating peripheral sensory neuropathy, slowly progressive and usually affecting the feet symmetrically, associated with anti-MAG antibodies in half of the cases (20%)
- Lymphadenopathy (15%)
- Hepatosplenomegaly (15%)
- Hyperviscosity syndrome (10%), characterized by headaches, recurrent nosebleeds, blurry vision due to retinal hemorrhages (Fig. E1); retinal vein link: Sausage shaped
- Acquired von Willebrand disease (5% to 10%)
- Acrocyanosis, livedo reticularis, purpura, and/or peripheral ulcerations usually associated with symptomatic cryoglobulinemia (5% to 10%)
- Hemolytic anemia caused by cold agglutinin disease (5%)
- Amyloidosis causing renal dysfunction, neuropathy, and/or cardiac dysfunction (<5%)
- Kidney dysfunction (2% to 3%)
- Meningeal signs caused by CNS involvement by WM (Bing Neel syndrome, 1%)
- Pleural effusion (<1%)

ETIOLOGY

- The main risk factor for development of WM is having IgM monoclonal gammopathy of unknown significance (MGUS).

- Other risk factors are older age and male sex.
- Multiple reports suggest familial clustering in about 20% of the patients, which may indicate a genetic predisposition to WM and other blood cancers.
- Approximately 20% of the patients have an Ashkenazi Jewish ancestry.
- There is an increased risk of WM in people with a personal history of autoimmune diseases.

DIAGNOSIS

The diagnosis of WM is usually established by laboratory blood tests and by BM biopsy.[2] Diagnosis requires demonstration of LPL involving the BM space and the presence of an IgM monoclonal paraprotein (Table 1). *MYD88 L265P* is a commonly recurring mutation in WM seen in >90% of the patients with WM and 50% to 60% of patients with IgM MGUS and can be useful in differentiating WM from other IgM-secreting B-cell disorders such as marginal zone lymphoma, IgM multiple myeloma, and atypical forms of chronic lymphocytic leukemia.[3] Non–L265P *MYD88* mutations rarely have been described (<5%) and should be excluded in patients who test negative for *MYD88 L265P* by polymerase chain reaction–based assays. Mutations in the *CXCR4* gene have been described in 30% to 40% of patients and may affect clinical presentation and response to treatment with Bruton tyrosine kinase (BTK) inhibitors.[4,5]

DIFFERENTIAL DIAGNOSIS

- IgM MGUS
- IgM multiple myeloma

- Marginal zone lymphoma
- Atypical chronic lymphocytic leukemia

WORKUP

In any patient suspected of having WM, specific blood tests (CBC, serum or urine protein electrophoresis [SPEP or UPEP, respectively], serum IgM level, beta 2-microglobulin, serum viscosity) should be ordered. BM biopsy confirms the diagnosis. *MYD88 L265P* mutation testing can be helpful in supporting the diagnosis of WM.

LABORATORY TESTS

- CBC with differential:
  1. Anemia is a common finding, with a median hemoglobin value of approximately 10 g/dl. WBC count is usually normal; thrombocytopenia can occur.
  2. Peripheral smear may reveal "stacked coin" rouleaux formations and malignant lymphoid cells in some patients.
- SPEP: Homogeneous M spike (monoclonal gammopathy).
- Immunoelectrophoresis: Confirms IgM responsible for the M spike.
- Serum IgM levels are elevated.
- Serum viscosity. Hyperviscosity usually occurs when the serum viscosity is four times the viscosity of normal serum; classic feature although present in only 10% of cases.
- Cryoglobulins or cold agglutinins may be present.
- BM biopsy: BM reveals infiltration by a lymphoplasmacytic cell population constituted by small lymphocytes with evidence of plasmacytoid and plasma cell differentiation. The BM

TABLE 1 Physicochemical and Immunologic Properties of the Monoclonal Immunoglobulin M Protein in Waldenström Macroglobulinemia

Properties of IgM Monoclonal Protein	Diagnostic Condition	Clinical Manifestations
Pentameric structure	Hyperviscosity	Headaches, blurred vision, epistaxis, retinal hemorrhages, leg cramps, impaired mentation, intracranial hemorrhage
Precipitation on cooling	Cryoglobulinemia (type I)	Raynaud phenomenon, acrocyanosis, ulcers, purpura, cold urticaria
Autoantibody activity to myelin-associated glycoprotein, ganglioside M_1, sulfatide moieties on peripheral nerve sheaths	Peripheral neuropathies	Sensorimotor neuropathies, painful neuropathies, ataxic gait, bilateral foot drop
Autoantibody activity to IgG	Cryoglobulinemia (type II)	Purpura, arthralgia, renal failure, sensorimotor neuropathies
Autoantibody activity to red blood cell antigens	Cold agglutinins	Hemolytic anemia, Raynaud phenomenon, acrocyanosis, livedo reticularis
Tissue deposition as amorphous aggregates	Organ dysfunction	Skin: Bullous skin disease, papules, Schnitzler syndrome Gastrointestinal: Diarrhea, malabsorption, bleeding Kidney: Proteinuria, renal failure (light-chain component)
Tissue deposition as amyloid fibrils (light-chain component most commonly)	Organ dysfunction	Fatigue, weight loss, edema, hepatomegaly, macroglossia, organ dysfunction of involved organs (heart, kidney, liver, peripheral sensory and autonomic nerves)

IgM, Immunoglobulin M.
From Hoffman R: *Hematology: basic principles and practice*, ed 7, Philadelphia, 2018, Elsevier.

TABLE 2 Summary of Consensus Response Criteria for Waldenström Macroglobulinemia

Response Type	Abbreviation	Criteria
Complete response	CR	Absence of serum monoclonal IgM protein by immunofixation Normal serum IgM level Complete resolution of extramedullary disease (i.e., lymphadenopathy/splenomegaly if present at baseline) Morphologically normal bone marrow aspirate and trephine biopsy
Very good partial response	VGPR	Monoclonal IgM protein is detectable 90% reduction in serum IgM level from baseline or normalization of serum IgM level Complete resolution of extramedullary disease (i.e., lymphadenopathy/splenomegaly if present at baseline) No new signs or symptoms of active disease
Partial response	PR	Monoclonal IgM protein is detectable ≥50% but <90% reduction in serum IgM level from baseline Reduction in extramedullary disease (i.e., lymphadenopathy/splenomegaly if present at baseline) No new signs or symptoms of active disease
Minor response	MR	Monoclonal IgM protein is detectable ≥25% but <50% reduction in serum IgM level from baseline No new signs or symptoms of active disease
Stable disease	SD	Monoclonal IgM protein is detectable <25% reduction and <25% increase in serum IgM level from baseline No progression in extramedullary disease (i.e., lymphadenopathy/splenomegaly) No new signs or symptoms of active disease
Progressive disease	PD	>25% increase in serum IgM level from lowest nadir (requires confirmation) and/or progression in clinical features attributable to the disease

IgM, Immunoglobulin M.
From Owen RG et al: Response assessment in Waldenström macroglobulinemia. *Br J Haematol* 160:171, 2013; and Hoffman R et al: *Hematology: basic principles and practice,* ed 7, Philadelphia, 2018, Elsevier.

infiltration should be confirmed by immunophenotypic studies (flow cytometry and immunohistochemistry) showing the following profile: sIgM+ CD19+ CD20+ CD22+ CD79+ CD5– CD10–.

IMAGING STUDIES

CT of the chest, abdomen, and pelvis may show lymphadenopathy, hepatosplenomegaly, and rarely, extralymphatic/extramedullary areas of disease.

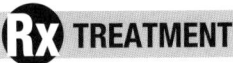 **TREATMENT**

- Because of the incurable nature of WM, the aim of treatment is to relieve symptoms and reduce the risk of organ damage. Initiation of therapy should not be based on the IgM levels alone because this may not correlate with either disease burden or symptomatic status. Patients with smoldering or asymptomatic WM and preserved hematologic function should be observed without therapy.
- Considerations for the initiation of treatment include the following: Significant adenopathy or organomegaly, symptomatic hyperviscosity, moderate to severe neuropathy, amyloidosis, symptomatic cryoglobulinemia or cold agglutinin disease, symptomatic anemia, constitutional symptoms, or evidence of disease transformation.[6]

NONPHARMACOLOGIC THERAPY

Asymptomatic patients do not require treatment, and these patients should be monitored periodically for the onset of symptoms or changes in blood tests (e.g., worsening anemia, thrombocytopenia, rising IgM levels, and serum viscosity). Plasmapheresis should be the initial treatment in patients with symptoms of hyperviscosity or cryoglobulinemia followed immediately by more definitive therapy. Serum IgM level, percentage of

BM involvement, serum albumin level, and serum beta 2-microglobulin level can be used to estimate the risk of requiring therapy (https://awmrisk.com/).[7]

INITIAL Rx

- Treatment of the lymphoproliferative disorder includes single or combination therapy. There is no universally agreed upon standard of care:
  1. Combination regimens include alkylating agents (cyclophosphamide and bendamustine) or proteasome inhibitors (bortezomib, carfilzomib, and ixazomib) in combination with rituximab.[8-11] Response rates are 80% to 90% with any of these regimens.
  2. Rituximab, a monoclonal anti-CD20 antibody, can be used in symptomatic patients who are not candidates for combination therapy.[12,13] Response rates are 40% to 50%.
  3. In April 2015, the FDA granted approval for the oral Bruton tyrosine kinase (BTK) inhibitor ibrutinib to be used in patients with symptomatic WM. The response rate to ibrutinib is 90%, with a median time to response of 4 wk.[14-17] Major responses were absent in patients who do not carry the *MYD88* mutation. The response was delayed in patients who carry a *CXCR4* mutation.
  4. In August 2018, the FDA approved the combination of ibrutinib and rituximab for the treatment of symptomatic WM patients. The combination was associated with higher response rate and longer median progression-free survival than rituximab and placebo.[18,19]
  5. Acalabrutinib and zanubrutinib are new BTK inhibitors that have been shown to be safe and effective in WM patients.[20,21] These agents have higher affinity for BTK, have

fewer off-target effects, and might be associated with lower rates of atrial fibrillation than ibrutinib.
  6. Zanubrutinib was approved by the FDA for the treatment of WM in November 2021.
  7. Treatment with BTK inhibitors should continue until disease progression or unacceptable toxicity.

Rx ON RELAPSED/REFRACTORY DISEASE

- Previously treated patients can be retried on original therapy if the disease was not refractory to the prior therapy and the length of response from initial therapy was substantial. If the response from the initial therapy was short, alternative first-line agents can be used.
- Other treatment options include venetoclax,[22] fludarabine,[23] thalidomide,[24] everolimus,[25] and clinical trials. Autologous stem cell transplantation should be considered in heavily pretreated patients.[26]

DISPOSITION

- The progression of WM is slow and insidious, with median survival from time of diagnosis of about 10 yr.[27] About 10% to 20% of patients die from progression of the disease.
- Table 2 summarizes consensus response criteria for WM.[28]
- Younger patients tend to have more prolonged survival.[29]
- Some patients develop myelodysplasia or acute myelogenous leukemia, usually secondary to exposure to chemotherapy,[30] and some patients can develop more aggressive lymphomas.[31]
- The risk of thyroid cancer, kidney cancer, and melanoma is increased in patients with WM.[32]
- A staging system using age, serum beta 2-microglobulin level, hemoglobin level, platelet count, and serum IgM concentration

TABLE 3 Prognostic Scoring Systems in Waldenström Macroglobulinemia

Study	Adverse Prognostic Factors	Number of Groups	Survival
Gobbi et al[1]	Hgb <9 g/dl Age >70 yr Weight loss Cryoglobulinemia	0-1 prognostic factors 2-4 prognostic factors	Median: 48 mo Median: 80 mo
Morel et al[2]	Age ≥65 yr Albumin <4 g/dl Number of cytopenias: Hgb <12 g/dl Platelets <150 × 10⁹/L WBC <4 × 10⁹/L	0-1 prognostic factors 2 prognostic factors 3-4 prognostic factors	5-yr: 87% of patients 5-yr: 62% 5-yr: 25%
Dhodapkar et al[3]	β_2M ≥3 g/dl Hgb <12 g/dl IgM <4 g/dl	β_2M <3 mg/dl + Hgb ≥12 g/dl β_2M <3 mg/dl + Hgb <12 g/dl β_2M ≥3 mg/dl + IgM ≥4 g/dl β_2M ≥3 mg/dl + IgM <4 g/dl	5-yr: 87% of patients 5-yr: 63% 5-yr: 53% 5-yr: 21%
Dimopoulos et al[4]	Albumin ≤3.5 g/dl β_2M ≥3.5 mg/L	Albumin ≥3.5 g/dl + β_2M <3.5 mg/dl Albumin ≤3.5 g/dl + β_2M <3.5 or β_2M 3.5-5.5 mg/dl β_2M >5.5 mg/dl	Median: NR Median: 116 mo Median: 54 mo
Morel et al[5]	Age >65 yr Hgb <11.5 g/dl Platelets <100 × 10⁹/L β_2M >3 mg/L IgM >7 g/dl	0-1 prognostic factors (excluding age) 2 prognostic factors (or age >65 yr) 3-5 prognostic factors	5 yr: 87% of patients 5 yr: 68% 5 yr: 36%

β_2M, β_2-Microglobulin; *Hgb,* hemoglobulin; *IgM,* immunoglobulin M; *NR,* not reported; *WBC,* white blood cell count.

[1]Gobbi PG et al: Study of prognosis in Waldenström's macroglobulinemia: a proposal for a simple binary classification with clinical and investigational utility, *Blood* 83:2939, 1994.

[2]Morel P et al: Prognostic factors in Waldenström macroglobulinemia: a report on 232 patients with the description of a new scoring system and its validation on 253 other patients, *Blood* 96:852, 2000.

[3]Dhodapkar MV et al: Prognostic factors and response to fludarabine therapy in patients with Waldenström macroglobulinemia: results of United States intergroup trial (Southwest Oncology Group S9003), *Blood* 98:41, 2001.

[4]Dimopoulos M et al: The international staging system for multiple myeloma is applicable in symptomatic Waldenström's macroglobulinemia, *Leuk Lymphoma* 45:1809, 2004.

[5]Morel P et al: International prognostic scoring system for Waldenström macroglobulinemia, *Blood* 113:4163, 2009.

From Hoffman R et al: *Hematology, basic principles and practice,* ed 7, Philadelphia, 2018, Elsevier.

before treatment provide insight into prognosis and survival in patients treated with chemotherapy.[33] Prognostic scoring systems in WM are summarized in Table 3.

REFERRAL

A hematology consultation is helpful in guiding future workup, treatment, and monitoring. Participation in clinical trials is highly encouraged in patients with WM.

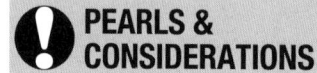 **PEARLS & CONSIDERATIONS**

COMMENTS

WM was first described in 1944 by the Swedish physician Jan Gösta Waldenström, who also described the X-linked Bruton agammaglobulinemia.

REFERENCES & SUGGESTED READINGS

Available at eBooks.Health.Elsevier.com.

AUTHOR: **JORGE J. CASTILLO, MD**

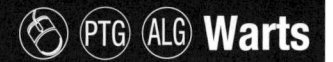
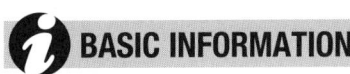 **BASIC INFORMATION**

DEFINITION

Warts are benign epidermal lesions caused by human papillomavirus (HPV).

SYNONYMS

Verruca vulgaris (common warts)
Verruca plana (flat warts)
Condyloma acuminatum (venereal warts)
Verruca plantaris (plantar warts)
Mosaic warts (cluster of many warts)
HPV infection

ICD-10CM CODES
B07.9 Viral wart, unspecified
B07.8 Other viral warts
A63.0 Anogenital (venereal) warts
B07.0 Plantar wart

EPIDEMIOLOGY & DEMOGRAPHICS

- HPV infection causes up to 4.5% of all new cancer cases worldwide and represents 29.5% of all infection-related cancers.[1]
- Risk factors include use of communal showers, occupational handling of meat, and immunosuppression. Common warts occur most frequently in children and young adults.
- Anogenital warts are most common in young, sexually active patients. Genital warts are the most common viral sexually transmitted disease in the U.S., with up to 79 million Americans carrying the causative virus and 14 million persons are newly infected each year in the U.S.
- Persistent infection with oncogenic HPV types can cause cervical cancer in women as well as other anogenital and oropharyngeal cancers in women and men. 66% of cervical cancers, 55% of vaginal cancers, 79% of anal cancers, and 62% of oropharyngeal cancers are attributable to HPV types 16 or 18.
- Common warts are longer lasting and more frequent in immunocompromised patients (e.g., lymphoma, AIDS, immunosuppressive drugs).
- Plantar warts occur most frequently at points of maximal pressure (over the heads of the metatarsal bones or on the heels).

PHYSICAL FINDINGS & CLINICAL PRESENTATION (TABLE E1)

- Common warts (Fig. E1) have an initial appearance of a flesh-colored papule with a rough surface; they subsequently develop a hyperkeratotic appearance with black dots on the surface (thrombosed capillaries). They may be single or multiple and are most common on the hands.
- Warts obscure normal skin lines (important diagnostic feature). Cylindrical projections from the wart may become fused, forming a mosaic pattern.
- Flat warts (Fig. E2) generally are pink or light yellow, slightly elevated, and often found on the forehead, back of hands, mouth, and beard area. They often occur in lines corresponding

to trauma (e.g., a scratch), are often misdiagnosed (particularly when present on the face), and are inappropriately treated with topical corticosteroids.
- Filiform warts have a fingerlike appearance with various projections; they are generally found near the mouth, beard, or periorbital and paranasal regions.
- Plantar warts (Fig. E3) are slightly raised and have a roughened surface; they may cause pain when walking; as they involute, small hemorrhages (caused by thrombosed capillaries) may be noted.
- Genital warts (Fig. E4) are generally pale pink with several projections and a broad base. They may coalesce in the perineal area to form masses with a cauliflower-like appearance. Intraanal warts occur predominantly in patients who have had receptive anal intercourse, in contrast with perianal warts, which may occur in men and women without a history of anal sex.
- Genital warts on the cervical epithelium can produce subclinical changes that may be noted on Pap smear or colposcopy.

ETIOLOGY

- HPV infection: >150 types of viral DNA have been identified. Transmission of warts is by direct contact. ~40 different types of HPV are transmitted through sexual contact.
- Genital warts: 90% are caused by HPV types 6 or 11. HPV types 16, 18, 31, 33, and 35 are found occasionally in visible genital warts (usually as coinfections with HPV 6 or 11) and can be associated with foci of high-grade, intraepithelial neoplasia, particularly in persons who are infected with HIV infection. In addition to warts on genital areas, HPV types 6 and 11 have been associated with conjunctival, nasal, oral, and laryngeal warts.

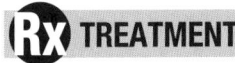 **DIAGNOSIS**

DIFFERENTIAL DIAGNOSIS

- Molluscum contagiosum
- Condyloma latum
- Acrochordon (skin tags) or seborrheic keratosis
- Epidermal nevi
- Hypertrophic actinic keratosis
- Squamous cell carcinomas
- Acquired digital fibrokeratoma
- Varicella-zoster virus in patients with AIDS
- Recurrent infantile digital fibroma
- Plantar corns (may be mistaken for plantar warts)

WORKUP

- Diagnosis is generally based on clinical findings.
- Suspect lesions should be biopsied.
- The application of 3% to 5% acetic acid, which causes skin color to turn white, has been used by some providers to detect HPV-infected genital mucosa. However, acetic acid application is not a specific test for HPV infection. Therefore, the routine use of this procedure for

screening to detect mucosal changes attributed to HPV infection is not recommended.

LABORATORY TESTS

- Screening for cervical cancer with cytology, which is performed by either Pap smear or liquid-based cytology. Screening guidelines recommend starting screening at age 21. Annual cytology is recommended until at least three normal cytology results are obtained.
- Colposcopy with biopsy is recommended in patients with cervical squamous cell changes.

Rx TREATMENT

NONPHARMACOLOGIC THERAPY

- Importance of use of condoms to reduce transmission of genital warts should be emphasized.
- Watchful waiting is an acceptable option in the treatment of nongenital cutaneous warts because many warts will disappear without intervention over time. However, many patients often request treatment because of social stigma or discomfort.
- Plantar warts that are not painful do not need treatment.
- Factors that influence selection of treatment include wart size, wart number, anatomic site of the wart, wart morphology, patient preference, cost of treatment, convenience, adverse effects, and provider experience. Factors that might affect response to therapy include the presence of immunosuppression and compliance with therapy.

GENERAL Rx

- Common warts:
  1. Application of topical salicylic acid 17%. Soak area for 5 min in warm water and dry. Apply thin layer once or twice daily for up to 12 wk, avoiding normal skin. Bandage.
  2. Liquid nitrogen and electrocautery are also common methods of removal. Cure rates for cryotherapy are 50% to 70% after three or four treatments.
  3. Blunt dissection can be used in large lesions or resistant lesions.
  4. Duct tape occlusion is also effective for treating common warts. It is cut to cover warts and left in place for 6 days. It is removed after 6 days, and the warts are soaked in water and then filed with pumice stones. New tape is applied 12 h later. This treatment can be repeated until warts resolve.
  5. Recalcitrant warts can be treated with injection of *Candida* or mumps skin antigen into the wart every 3 to 4 wk for up to three treatments, photodynamic therapy with aminolevulinic acid, pulsed dye laser, and intralesional bleomycin.
- Filiform warts: Surgical removal is necessary.
- Flat warts: Generally more difficult to treat.
  1. Tretinoin cream applied at bedtime over the involved area for several weeks may be effective.
  2. Application of liquid nitrogen.

3. Electrocautery.
4. 5-Fluorouracil cream applied once or twice a day for 3 to 5 wk is also effective. Persistent hyperpigmentation may occur after Efudex use.

- Plantar warts:
1. Salicylic acid therapy (e.g., Occlusal-HP). Soak wart in warm water for 5 min, remove loose tissue, dry. Apply to area, allow to dry, reapply. Use once or twice daily; maximum 12 wk. Use of 40% salicylic acid plasters (Mediplast) is also a safe, nonscarring treatment; it is particularly useful in treating mosaic warts covering a large area.
2. Blunt dissection is also a fast and effective treatment modality.
3. Laser therapy can be used for plantar warts and recurrent warts; however, it leaves open wounds that require 4 to 6 wk to fill with granulation tissue.
4. Interlesional bleomycin is also effective but generally used when all other treatments fail.

- Genital warts:
1. Can be effectively treated with 20% podophyllin resin in compound tincture of benzoin applied with a cotton tip applicator by the treating physician and allowed to air dry. The treatment can be repeated weekly if necessary.
2. Podofilox (Condylox 0.5% gel) is available for application by the patient. Local adverse effects include pain, burning, and inflammation at the site.
3. Cryosurgery with liquid nitrogen delivered with a probe or as a spray is effective for treating smaller genital warts.
4. Carbon dioxide laser can also be used for treating primary or recurrent genital warts (cure rate >90%).
5. Imiquimod cream, 5%, is a patient-applied immune response modifier effective in the treatment of external genital and perianal warts (complete clearing of genital warts in >70% of females and >30% of males in 4 to 16 wk). Sexual contact should be avoided while the cream is on the skin. It is applied three times weekly before normal sleeping hours and is left on the skin for 6 to 10 h.

6. Sinecatechins (Veregen), a botanical drug product, is also effective for treatment of external genital and perianal warts. Formulation is a 15% ointment applied to affected area three times daily for up to 16 wk.
- Application of trichloroacetic acid or bichloroacetic acid 80% to 90% is also effective for external genital warts. A small amount should be applied only to warts and allowed to dry, at which time a white "frosting" develops. This treatment can be repeated weekly if necessary.

DISPOSITION

- Warts can be effectively treated with the previous modalities with complete resolution in the majority of patients; however, the recurrence rate is high.
- Cervical carcinomas and precancerous lesions in women are associated with genital papillomavirus infection.
- Squamous cell anal cancer is also associated with a history of genital warts.

REFERRAL

- Dermatology referral for warts resistant to conservative therapy
- Surgical referral in selected cases
- Sexually transmitted disease counseling for patients with anogenital warts

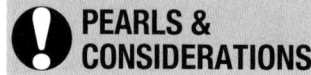

❗ PEARLS & CONSIDERATIONS

COMMENTS

- Subungual and periungual warts are generally more resistant to treatment. Dermatology referral for cryosurgery is recommended in resistant cases.
- Examination of sex partners is not necessary for the management of genital warts because no data indicate that reinfection plays a role.

PREVENTION

- The HPV vaccines (Gardasil, Gardasil-9, Cervarix) have been licensed in the U.S. Advisory Committee on Immunization Practices (ACIP) recommends routine vaccination with HPV4 or HPV2 for females aged 11 to 12 yr and HPV4 for males aged 11 to 12 yr. Vaccination is also recommended for females aged 13 to 26 yr and for males aged 13 through 21 yr who were not vaccinated previously. Delaying vaccination until after first sexual activity is associated with higher prevalence of vaginal human papillomavirus.[2] Males aged 22 through 26 may be vaccinated. ACIP recommends vaccination of men who have sex with men and immunocompromised persons (including those with infection) through age 26 yr if not previously vaccinated. The 9-valent HPV vaccine (Gardasil-9) is approved for use in girls and women 9 to 26 yr old and boys 9 to 15 yr old. It is indicated to prevent diseases associated with HPV infection with types 6, 11, 16, 18, 31, 33, 45, 52, and 58. It appears to be more effective than the other two currently available vaccines. It consists of two doses. The first dose is administered at 11 to 12 yr of age, and the second dose 6 to 12 mo later. However, if the second dose is given <5 mo apart, a third dose will be needed at age 9 to 14. Patients with a weak immune system and in those starting vaccination at age 15 to 26 yr will need three doses. ACIP does not recommend catch-up HPV vaccination for all adults over 26 yr old. Shared decision-making regarding HPV vaccination is recommended for some adults ages 27 through 65 who are unvaccinated.
- Male circumcision decreases heterosexual transmission of HPV.

REFERENCES & SUGGESTED READINGS

Available at eBooks.Health.Elsevier.com.

RELATED CONTENT

Human Papillomavirus Infection (Patient Information)
Warts (Patient Information)
Condyloma Acuminatum (Related Key Topic)

AUTHOR: **FRED F. FERRI, MD**

BASIC INFORMATION

DEFINITION

Wolff-Parkinson-White (WPW) syndrome is a congenital heart condition in which, in addition to the normal electrical conduction through the atrioventricular (AV) node, there is an accessory pathway (AP) that connects the atria to the ventricles. Consequently, a portion of the ventricular myocardium is depolarized via the AP earlier than the normal AV nodal conduction, resulting in ventricular preexcitation. The terms "WPW syndrome" and "WPW pattern" often are used in describing patients with ventricular preexcitation. Patients with WPW syndrome have ECG findings of preexcitation, including short PR and slurring of the initial segment of the QRS complex known as the delta wave together with symptoms suggestive of arrhythmia or documented arrhythmia, which may be AV reentrant tachycardia, atrial fibrillation (AF), or both. Patients with the WPW pattern have characteristic ECG findings of preexcitation without evidence of symptoms or arrhythmia.

SYNONYMS

WPW
Preexcitation syndrome

ICD-10CM CODE
I45.6 Preexcitation syndrome

EPIDEMIOLOGY & DEMOGRAPHICS[1-5]

- The prevalence of a WPW pattern on the surface ECG is 0.1% to 0.3% in the general population. The prevalence is increased to 0.55% in first-degree relatives of affected patients. It is estimated that ~65% of adolescents and 40% of individuals older than 30 yr with WPW pattern on a resting ECG are asymptomatic.
- The prevalence of WPW is higher among males and decreases with age.
- Most patients with WPW have structurally normal hearts, but it may also occur in patients with congenital heart disease, most notably in patients with Ebstein anomaly, which is associated with right-side AP and often multiple and slowly conducting APs.

PHYSICAL FINDINGS & CLINICAL PRESENTATION

- The physical examination is usually unremarkable.
- Symptoms are typically related to tachyarrhythmias, including the following:
  1. Palpitations, light-headedness, anxiety, dyspnea, or chest pain
  2. Syncope or near syncope
  3. Sudden cardiac death
- The common arrhythmias in WPW syndrome are:
  1. Supraventricular tachycardia (SVT): AV reciprocating tachycardia (AVRT). This is the most common arrhythmia, further classified as orthodromic AVRT (narrow complex tachycardia, with antegrade

conduction through the AV node and retrograde conduction via the AP that occurs in 70% of symptomatic patients) or antidromic AVRT (wide complex tachycardia with antegrade conduction via the AP and retrogradely through the AV node, which occurs in 4% to 5% of patients).
  2. AF (~10% to 38%), the second most common tachycardia, can be complicated by a very rapid ventricular response due to conduction over the AP, which can lead to ventricular fibrillation (VF) and sudden death. This risk is dependent on the antegrade refractory period of AP during AF.
  3. The risk of sudden death in symptomatic patients with WPW syndrome is estimated to be ~0.25%/yr or 3% to 4% over a lifetime.
- In a meta-analysis including ~2000 subjects with asymptomatic WPW, children had a sudden death rate of 1.9 compared with 0.9 in adults per 1000 patient-years of follow-up. This incidence is comparable with the estimated 0.1%/yr risk of death in the general population in Europe, Japan, and the U.S.

ETIOLOGY & PATHOGENESIS[6]

- APs are thought to be an embryologic remnant, as substantiated by reports of SVT in uterus and by a greater prevalence of WPW in newborns and infants.
- Left free wall APs are most common followed by posteroseptal, right free wall, and anteroseptal locations.
- Some patients with WPW syndrome (~5% to 10%) have multiple APs.
- In subjects with WPW, two parallel routes of AV conduction are present: One is subject to delay through the AV node, and the other occurs without delay through the AP and results in preexcitation of the ventricles. The resulting QRS complex is a fusion beat, as a portion of the ventricle is preexcited and activated via the AP giving rise to the delta wave, and the remainder of the ventricle is activated by the normal activation pathway (Fig. 1).
- Reciprocating tachycardias occur when conduction is anterograde in one pathway (usually the AV node, i.e., orthodromic AVRT) and retrograde in the other (usually the AP) as a result of different refractory periods. This is usually initiated by a premature atrial or ventricular depolarization.

DIAGNOSIS

- Three basic features characterize the ECG abnormalities associated with WPW pattern:
  1. PR interval <120 ms.
  2. QRS complex can be >120 ms with a slurred, slowly rising onset of QRS in some leads (delta wave) and a normal terminal QRS portion. The width of the QRS complex depends on the amount of preexcited ventricular tissue.

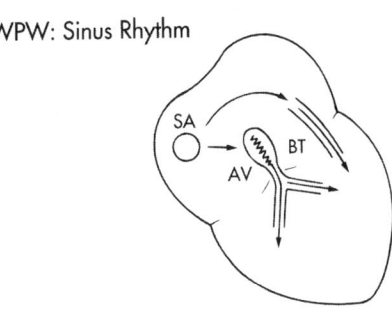

WPW: Sinus Rhythm

FIG. 1 With Wolff-Parkinson-White (WPW) syndrome, an abnormal accessory pathway called a bypass tract connects the atria and the ventricles.

  3. Secondary ST-T wave changes directed in an opposite direction to the major delta and QRS vectors may be present.
- ECG patterns with abnormal QRS complexes and ST and T changes can mask or mimic myocardial infarction (in particular posteroseptal AP with negative delta waves in the inferior wall, which mimics old inferior wall myocardial infarction), bundle branch block (Fig. 2), or ventricular hypertrophy.
- Most commonly seen tachycardia (orthodromic AVRT) is characterized by a normal QRS with a regular rate of 150 to 250 bpm. Onset and termination are abrupt.
- Variants of preexcitation:
  1. Lown-Ganong-Levine syndrome is characterized by a short PR interval, a narrow QRS complex without a delta wave, and a clinical syndrome of paroxysmal SVTs. Postulated mechanisms to the short PR interval include a variant of the normal, enhanced sympathetic tone or specialized intranodal fibers with enhanced AV nodal conduction.
  2. Atriofascicular AP: A slowly conducting AP with AV-nodal like properties that conducts only in antegrade direction and connects the right atrium with the right bundle branch or the apical myocardium. In the baseline state, minimal or no preexcitation may be present. During preexcitation the QRS appears like a typical left bundle branch (LBBB) pattern. The typical arrhythmia in patients with atriofascicular AP is antidromic tachycardia with LBBB morphology.
  3. Nodoventricular or nodofascicular APs (Mahaim fiber): Rare variants that connect the AV node and the ventricle or the bundle branch appropriately.
- An electrophysiology study is the gold standard to confirm the diagnosis, determine the location, and assess the conduction properties of the AP.

RISK STRATIFICATION[7,8]

- Intermittent and abrupt loss of preexcitation on a beat-to-beat basis is usually indicative of

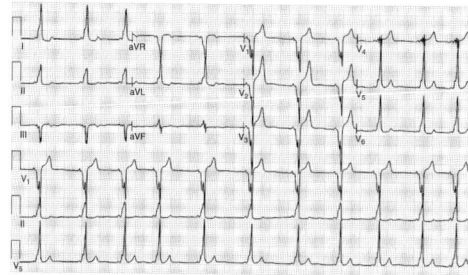

FIG. 2 Wolff-Parkinson-White (WPW) syndrome. This 12-lead electrocardiogram with rhythm strips shows preexcitation with an accessory pathway connecting the right atrium to the right ventricle. This gives rise to a pattern like left bundle branch block because the ventricles are activated over the right-sided accessory pathway. The tracing shows the typical characteristics of WPW syndrome, including a short PR interval, a wide QRS complex, and a delta wave. (From Olshansky B et al: *Arrhythmia essentials,* ed 2, Philadelphia, 2017, Elsevier.)

BOX 1   Goals of Electrophysiologic Evaluation in Patients With Wolff-Parkinson-White Syndrome

- Confirmation of the presence of an accessory pathway (AP)
- Evaluation for the presence of multiple APs
- Localization of the AP(s)
- Evaluation of the refractory period of the AP and its implications for life-threatening arrhythmias
- Induction and evaluation of tachycardias
- Demonstration of the AP role in the tachycardia
- Evaluation of other tachycardias not dependent on the presence of the AP
- Ablation of the AP, when indicated.

From Issa Z et al: *Clinical arrhythmology and electrophysiology,* ed 2, Philadelphia, 2012, Saunders.

---

lower risk, assessed with Holter monitoring or with an exercise stress test. The loss of preexcitation after administration of the antiarrhythmic drug procainamide has also been used to indicate a low-risk subgroup. More recent evidence, however, has begun to demonstrate that intermittent preexcitation is not 100% specific for identification of a "low-risk" AP. In a study of 295 children at a single institution, "high-risk" intracardiac electrophysiology study (EPS) characteristics were identified in 5% of patients with intermittent preexcitation and 31% with abrupt loss of preexcitation on exercise test.

- In patients with a persistent preexcitation pattern, electrophysiology study is the procedure of choice for risk stratification.

🆁🆇 TREATMENT[9]

Goals of electrophysiologic evaluation in patients with WPW syndrome are described in Box 1.

ACUTE MANAGEMENT

- Urgent cardioversion for an acute tachycardia episode with hemodynamic instability.
- Narrow QRS tachycardia (consistent with orthodromic AVRT):
  1. Vagal maneuvers and/or IV adenosine.
  2. IV β-blockers, diltiazem, or verapamil can be administered for regular and **narrow**

QRS tachycardia, implying antegrade conduction via the AV node, when the patient is hemodynamically stable and IV adenosine is ineffective.

- Wide QRS complex tachycardias (WCTs):
  1. Most commonly caused by AF with antegrade conduction via the AP and the AV node. AV nodal blocking therapies (i.e., β-blockers, calcium channel blockers, digoxin, and adenosine) are potentially dangerous and should be avoided in these cases because of the risk of causing VF by enhancement of the ventricular response through the AP when the AV node is blocked and the blood pressure is lowered.
  2. Stable patients with preexcited AF can be managed with IV procainamide. Procainamide can decrease ventricular rate by slowing conduction over the AP and have the additional benefit of possibly terminating AF. Electrical cardioversion should be performed if the patient is hemodynamically unstable.
  3. In a patient with WCT due to antidromic tachycardia, drug treatment may be directed at the AP (IV procainamide) or at the AV node because both are critical components of the tachycardia circuit.

LONG-TERM MANAGEMENT

- Asymptomatic:

  1. In low-risk patients with AP effective refractory period (APERP) >250 ms, or shortest preexcited RR interval (SPERRI) >250 ms, no therapy is required. An electrophysiology study may be considered in asymptomatic patients with intermittent loss of preexcitation for further risk stratification in order to assess the APERP and SPERRI.
  2. In high-risk patients with APERP <250 ms or SPERRI <250 ms, competitive athletes, or high-risk occupation (i.e., pilots), ablation should be considered.
- Symptomatic:
  1. Patients who presented with aborted sudden cardiac death, preexcited tachycardia (i.e., AF, flutter, atrial tachycardia), or syncope suggestive of cardiac origin should undergo an electrophysiology study for further characterization and ablation of the AP accordingly. Patients with symptomatic palpitations or documented AVRT should be offered an electrophysiology study and ablation of the AP to prevent recurrence and to allow the patient to avoid long-term medical therapy. Ongoing management for stable patients with history of orthodromic AVRT who are not candidates for, or prefer not to undergo, catheter ablation:
     a. Class IC antiarrhythmics (flecainide, propafenone), in the absence of structural heart disease.
     b. Class III antiarrhythmics (amiodarone, sotalol or dofetilide).
     c. Oral β-blockers, diltiazem, or verapamil.

REFERENCES

Available at eBooks.Health.Elsevier.com.

RELATED CONTENT

Wolff-Parkinson-White Syndrome (Patient Information)

AUTHORS: **ROI WESTREICH, MD, PHD,** and **YUVAL KONSTANTINO, MD**

SECTION II

Differential Diagnosis

ABDOMINAL DISTENTION

ICD-10CM # R14.0 Abdominal distension (gaseous)

NONMECHANICAL OBSTRUCTION

Excessive intraluminal gas.
Intraabdominal infection.
Trauma.
Retroperitoneal irritation (renal colic, neoplasms, infections, hemorrhage).
Vascular insufficiency (thrombosis, embolism).
Mechanical ventilation.
Extraabdominal infection (sepsis, pneumonia, empyema, osteomyelitis of spine).
Metabolic/toxic abnormalities (hypokalemia, uremia, lead poisoning).
Chemical irritation (perforated ulcer, bile, pancreatitis).
Peritoneal inflammation.
Severe pain, pain medications.

MECHANICAL OBSTRUCTION

Neoplasm (intraluminal, extraluminal).
Adhesions, endometriosis.
Infection (intraabdominal abscess, diverticulitis).
Gallstones.
Foreign body, bezoars.
Pregnancy.
Hernias.
Volvulus.
Stenosis at surgical anastomosis, radiation stenosis.
Fecaliths.
Inflammatory bowel disease.
Gastric outlet obstruction.
Hematoma.
Other: parasites, superior mesenteric artery (SMA) syndrome, pneumatosis intestinalis, annular pancreas, Hirschsprung disease, intussusception, meconium.

ABDOMINAL PAIN, ADOLESCENCE[1]

ICD-10CM # R10.817 Generalized abdominal tenderness
R10.827 Generalized rebound abdominal tenderness

Acute gastroenteritis.
Irritable bowel syndrome (IBS).
Anxiety.
Mittelschmerz.
Appendicitis.
Inflammatory bowel disease.
Peptic ulcer disease (PUD).
Cholecystitis.
Neoplasm.
Diabetic ketoacidosis.
Functional abdominal pain.
Pelvic inflammatory disease (PID).
Pregnancy.

Pyelonephritis.
Renal stone.
Trauma.

ABDOMINAL PAIN, CHILDHOOD[1]

ICD-10CM # R10.817 Generalized abdominal tenderness
R10.827 Generalized rebound abdominal tenderness

Acute gastroenteritis.
Appendicitis.
Constipation.
Cholecystitis, acute.
Intestinal obstruction.
Pancreatitis.
Neoplasm.
Inflammatory bowel disease.
Other:
Functional abdominal pain.
Pyelonephritis.
Pneumonia.
Diabetic ketoacidosis.
Heavy metal poisoning.
Sickle cell crisis.
Trauma.
Anxiety.
Sexual abuse.

ABDOMINAL PAIN, CHRONIC LOWER[2]

ICD-10CM # R10.814 Left lower quadrant abdominal tenderness
R10.824 Left lower quadrant rebound abdominal tenderness
R10.813 Right lower quadrant abdominal tenderness
R10.823 Right lower quadrant rebound abdominal tenderness
R10.30 Lower abdominal pain, unspecified

ORGANIC DISORDERS

Common
Gynecologic disease.
Lactase deficiency.
Diverticulitis/diverticulosis.
Crohn disease.
Intestinal obstruction.
Uncommon
Chronic intestinal pseudoobstruction.
Mesenteric ischemia.
Malignancy (e.g., ovarian carcinoma).
Abdominal wall pain.
Spinal disease.
Testicular disease.
Metabolic diseases (e.g., diabetes mellitus, familial Mediterranean fever, C1 esterase deficiency [angioneurotic edema], porphyria, lead poisoning, tabes dorsalis, renal failure).

FUNCTIONAL DISORDERS

Common
Irritable bowel syndrome.
Functional abdominal bloating.
Uncommon
Functional abdominal pain.

ABDOMINAL PAIN, DIFFUSE

ICD-10CM # R10.817 Generalized abdominal tenderness
R10.827 Generalized rebound abdominal tenderness

Early appendicitis.
Aortic aneurysm.
Gastroenteritis.
Intestinal obstruction.
Diverticulitis.
Peritonitis.
Mesenteric insufficiency or infarction.
Pancreatitis.
Inflammatory bowel disease.
Irritable bowel.
Mesenteric adenitis.
Metabolic: toxins, lead poisoning, uremia, drug overdose, diabetic ketoacidosis (DKA), heavy metal poisoning.
Sickle cell crisis.
Pneumonia (rare).
Trauma.
Urinary tract infection, PID.
Other: anxiety, acute intermittent porphyria, tabes dorsalis, periarteritis nodosa, Henoch-Schönlein purpura, adrenal insufficiency.

ABDOMINAL PAIN, EPIGASTRIC

ICD-10CM # R10.816 Epigastric abdominal tenderness
R10.826 Epigastric rebound abdominal tenderness

Gastric: PUD, gastric outlet obstruction, gastric ulcer.
Duodenal: PUD, duodenitis.
Biliary: cholecystitis, cholangitis, biliary dyskinesia.
Hepatic: hepatitis.
Pancreatic: pancreatitis.
Intestinal: high small bowel obstruction, early appendicitis.
Cardiac: angina, MI, pericarditis.
Pulmonary: pneumonia, pleurisy, pneumothorax.
Subphrenic abscess.
Vascular: dissecting aneurysm, mesenteric ischemia.
Psychiatric: anxiety.

ABDOMINAL PAIN, EXTRAABDOMINAL AND SYSTEMIC CAUSES[3]

ICD-10CM # R10.817 Generalized abdominal tenderness

Differential Diagnosis

II

EXTRAABDOMINAL AND SYSTEMIC CAUSES OF ACUTE ABDOMINAL PAIN

Cardiac
Endocarditis.
Heart failure.
Myocardial ischemia and infarction.
Myocarditis.

Thoracic
Empyema.
Esophageal rupture (Boerhaave syndrome).
Esophageal spasm.
Esophagitis.
Pleurodynia (Bornholm disease).
Pneumonitis.
Pneumothorax.
Pulmonary embolism and infarction.

Hematologic
Acute leukemia.
Hemolytic anemia.
Henoch-Schönlein purpura.
Sickle cell disease.

Metabolic
Acute adrenal insufficiency (Addison disease).
Diabetes mellitus (especially with ketoacidosis).
Hyperlipidemia.
Hyperparathyroidism.
Hypersensitivity reactions (e.g., to insect bites, reptile venoms).
Lead poisoning.
Porphyria.
Toxins.
Uremia.

Infections
Herpes zoster.
Osteomyelitis.
Typhoid fever.

Neurologic
Abdominal epilepsy.
Radiculopathy, spinal cord or peripheral nerve tumors, degenerative arthritis of spine, herniated vertebral disk.
Tabes dorsalis.

Miscellaneous
Angioedema.
Familial Mediterranean fever.
Heat stroke.
Muscle contusion, hematoma, tumor.
Narcotic withdrawal.
Psychiatric disorders.

ABDOMINAL PAIN, INFANCY[1]

| ICD-10CM # | R10.817 | Generalized abdominal tenderness |
| | R10.827 | Generalized rebound abdominal tenderness |

Acute gastroenteritis.
Appendicitis.
Intussusception.
Volvulus.
Meckel diverticulum.
Other: colic, trauma.

ABDOMINAL PAIN, LEFT LOWER QUADRANT

| ICD-10CM # | R10.814 | Left lower quadrant abdominal tenderness |
| | R10.824 | Left lower quadrant rebound abdominal tenderness |

Intestinal: diverticulitis, diverticulosis, intestinal obstruction, perforated ulcer, inflammatory bowel disease, perforated descending colon, inguinal hernia, neoplasm, appendicitis.
Reproductive: ectopic pregnancy, ovarian cyst, torsion of ovarian cyst, tuboovarian abscess, mittelschmerz, endometriosis, seminal vesiculitis.
Renal: renal or ureteral calculi, pyelonephritis, neoplasm.
Vascular: leaking aortic aneurysm.
Psoas abscess.
Trauma.

ABDOMINAL PAIN, LEFT UPPER QUADRANT

| ICD-10CM # | R19.02 | Left upper quadrant abdominal swelling, mass, and lump |

Gastric: PUD, gastritis, pyloric stenosis, hiatal hernia.
Pancreatic: pancreatitis, neoplasm, stone in pancreatic duct or ampulla.
Cardiac: MI, angina pectoris.
Splenic: splenomegaly, ruptured spleen, splenic abscess, splenic infarction.
Renal: calculi, pyelonephritis, neoplasm.
Pulmonary: pneumonia, empyema, pulmonary infarction.
Vascular: ruptured aortic aneurysm.
Cutaneous: herpes zoster.
Trauma.
Intestinal: high fecal impaction, perforated colon, diverticulitis.

ABDOMINAL PAIN, NONSURGICAL CAUSES

| ICD-10CM # | R19.8 | Other specified symptoms and signs involving the digestive system and abdomen |
| | R10.817 | Generalized abdominal tenderness |

Irritable bowel syndrome.
Urinary tract infection, pyelonephritis, salpingitis, PID.
Gastroenteritis, gastritis, peptic ulcer.
Diverticular spasm.
Hepatitis, mononucleosis.
Pancreatitis.
Inferior wall myocardial infarction.
Basilar pneumonia, pulmonary embolism.
Diabetic ketoacidosis.

Strain or hematoma of rectus muscle.
Ruptured Graafian follicle.
Herpes zoster.
Nerve root compression.
Sickle cell crisis.
Acute adrenal insufficiency.
Other: acute porphyria, familial Mediterranean fever, tabes dorsalis, anxiety, sexual abuse.

ABDOMINAL PAIN, PERIUMBILICAL

| ICD-10CM # | R10.815 | Periumbilic abdominal tenderness |
| | R10.825 | Periumbilic rebound abdominal tenderness |

Intestinal: small bowel obstruction or gangrene, early appendicitis.
Vascular: mesenteric thrombosis, dissecting aortic aneurysm.
Pancreatic: pancreatitis.
Metabolic: uremia, DKA.
Trauma.

ABDOMINAL PAIN, POORLY LOCALIZED[1]

| ICD-10CM # | R10.819 | Abdominal tenderness, unspecified site |

EXTRAABDOMINAL

Metabolic
DKA, acute intermittent porphyria, hyperthyroidism, hypothyroidism, hypercalcemia, hypokalemia, uremia, hyperlipidemia, hyperparathyroidism.

Hematologic
Sickle cell crisis, leukemia or lymphoma, Henoch-Schönlein purpura.

Infectious
Infectious mononucleosis, Rocky Mountain spotted fever, acquired immunodeficiency syndrome (AIDS), streptococcal pharyngitis (in children), herpes zoster.

Drugs and Toxins
Heavy metal poisoning, black widow spider bites, withdrawal syndromes, mushroom ingestion.

Referred Pain
Pulmonary: pneumonia, pulmonary embolism, pneumothorax.
Cardiac: angina, MI, pericarditis, myocarditis.
Genitourinary: prostatitis, epididymitis, orchitis, testicular torsion.
Musculoskeletal: rectus sheath hematoma.

Functional
Somatization disorder, malingering, hypochondriasis, Munchausen syndrome.

INTRAABDOMINAL
Early appendicitis, gastroenteritis, peritonitis, pancreatitis, abdominal aortic aneurysm, mesenteric insufficiency or infarction, intestinal obstruction, volvulus, ulcerative colitis.

ABDOMINAL PAIN, POST-CHOLECYSTECTOMY[3]

ICD-10CM # R10.817 Generalized abdominal tenderness

CAUSES OF ABDOMINAL PAIN AFTER CHOLECYSTECTOMY

Biliary Causes
Biliary stricture.
Biliary tract malignancy.
Choledocholithiasis.
Choledochocele.
Cystic duct remnant.
SOD.
Pancreatic Causes
Pancreatitis.
Pseudocyst.
Malignancy.
Other GI Disorders
Esophageal motor disorders.
GERD.
Intestinal malignancy.
Intraabdominal adhesions.
IBS.
Mesenteric ischemia.
PUD.
Extraintestinal Disorders
Coronary artery disease.
Intercostal neuritis.
Neurologic disorders.
Psychiatric disorders.
Wound neuroma.

ABDOMINAL PAIN, PREGNANT PATIENT[4]

ICD-10CM # R10.817 Generalized abdominal tenderness

COMMON CAUSES OF ABDOMINAL PAIN IN PREGNANT PATIENTS

Right Upper Quadrant
Gastroesophageal reflux.
Peptic ulcer disease.
Acute cholecystitis.
Biliary colic.
Acute pancreatitis.
Hepatitis.
Acute fatty liver of pregnancy.
HELLP syndrome.
Preeclampsia.
Pneumothorax.
Pneumonia.
Acute appendicitis.
Hepatic adenoma.
Hemangioma.
Right Lower Quadrant
Acute appendicitis.
Ectopic pregnancy.
Renal or ureteral colic.
Pelvic inflammatory disease.
Tuboovarian abscess.
Endometriosis.
Adnexal torsion.

Ruptured ovarian cyst.
Ruptured corpus luteum.
Lower Abdomen
Threatened, incomplete, or complete abortion.
Abruptio placentae.
Preterm labor.
Pelvic inflammatory disease.
Tuboovarian abscess.
Inflammatory bowel disease.
Irritable bowel syndrome.
Pycloncphritis.
Flank
Pyelonephritis.
Hydronephrosis of pregnancy.
Acute appendicitis (retrocecal appendix).
Diffuse Abdominal Pain
Early acute appendicitis.
Small bowel obstruction.
Acute intermittent porphyria.
Sickle cell crisis.

HELLP, Hemolysis, elevated liver enzymes, low platelets.

ABDOMINAL PAIN, RIGHT LOWER QUADRANT

ICD-10CM # R10.813 Right lower quadrant abdominal tenderness
R10.823 Right lower quadrant rebound abdominal tenderness

Intestinal: acute appendicitis, regional enteritis, incarcerated hernia, cecal diverticulitis, intestinal obstruction, perforated ulcer, perforated cecum, Meckel diverticulitis.
Reproductive: ectopic pregnancy, ovarian cyst, torsion of ovarian cyst, salpingitis, tuboovarian abscess, mittelschmerz, endometriosis, seminal vesiculitis.
Renal: renal and ureteral calculi, neoplasms, pyelonephritis.
Vascular: leaking aortic aneurysm.
Cutaneous: herpes zoster.
Psoas abscess.
Trauma.
Cholecystitis.

ABDOMINAL PAIN, RIGHT UPPER QUADRANT

ICD-10CM # R10.811 Right upper quadrant abdominal tenderness
R10.821 Right upper quadrant rebound abdominal tenderness

Biliary: calculi, infection, inflammation, neoplasm.
Hepatic: hepatitis, abscess, hepatic congestion, neoplasm, trauma.
Gastric: PUD, pyloric stenosis, neoplasm, alcoholic gastritis, hiatal hernia.
Pancreatic: pancreatitis, neoplasm, stone in pancreatic duct or ampulla.
Renal: calculi, infection, inflammation, neoplasm, rupture of kidney.
Pulmonary: pneumonia, pulmonary infarction, right-sided pleurisy.

Intestinal: retrocecal appendicitis, intestinal obstruction, high fecal impaction, diverticulitis.
Cardiac: myocardial ischemia (particularly involving the inferior wall), pericarditis.
Cutaneous: herpes zoster.
Trauma.
Fitz-Hugh-Curtis syndrome (perihepatitis).

ABDOMINAL PAIN, SUPRAPUBIC

ICD-10CM # R10.30 Lower abdominal pain, unspecified

Intestinal: colon obstruction or gangrene, diverticulitis, appendicitis.
Reproductive system: ectopic pregnancy, mittelschmerz, torsion of ovarian cyst, PID, salpingitis, endometriosis, rupture of endometrioma.
Cystitis, rupture of urinary bladder.

ABDOMINAL WALL MASSES[2]

ICD-10CM # R19.00 Intraabdominal and pelvic swelling, mass and lump, unspecified site

LUMPS ARISING IN THE SKIN AND SUBCUTANEOUS FAT (THAT COULD OCCUR ANYWHERE ON THE BODY)

Lipoma.
Sebaceous cyst.

LUMPS ARISING IN THE SKIN AND SUBCUTANEOUS FAT (SPECIFIC TO THE ANTERIOR ABDOMINAL WALL)

Tumor nodule of the umbilicus (secondary to the intraperitoneal malignancy, also called *Sister Mary Joseph nodule*).

LUMPS ARISING IN THE FASCIA AND MUSCLE

Rectus sheath hematoma (usually painful).
Desmoid tumor (associated with Gardner syndrome).

HERNIA

Incisional:	It has an overlying scar. The sac may be very much larger than the neck of the hernia.
Umbilical:	The hernia is through the umbilical scar. Those presenting at birth commonly resolve in the first years of life.
Paraumbilical:	The neck is just lateral to the umbilical scar. Patients usually present later in life.
Epigastric:	It occurs in the midline between the xiphoid process and the umbilicus. They are usually small (<2 cm). They result when a knuckle of extraperitoneal fat extrudes

Differential Diagnosis

II

Spigelian: through a small defect in the linea alba. Commonly irreducible and without an expansile cough impulse.
Spigelian: A rare hernia found along the linea semilunaris at the lateral edge of the rectus sheath, most commonly a third of the way between the umbilicus and the pubis.

DIVARICATION OF THE RECTI
Supraumbilical elliptical swelling of the attenuated linea alba (no cough impulse).

ABORTION, RECURRENT
ICD-10CM # P01.8 Newborn (suspected to be) affected by other maternal complications of pregnancy

Congenital anatomic abnormalities.
Adhesions (uterine synechiae).
Uterine fibroids.
Endometriosis.
Endocrine abnormalities (luteal phase insufficiency, hypothyroidism, uncontrolled diabetes mellitus [DM]).
Parenteral chromosome abnormalities.
Maternal infections (cervical *Mycoplasma, Ureaplasma, Chlamydia*).
DES exposure, heavy metal exposure.
Thrombocytosis.
Allogenic immunity, autoimmunity, lupus anticoagulant.

ACALCULOUS GALLBLADDER DISEASE[5]
ICD-10CM # K82.9 Other diseases of gallbladder

Biliary tract anomaly (e.g., choledochal cyst).
Bone marrow transplant.
Burns.
Chemotherapy in oncology patients.
Critical illness in intensive care unit patients.
Crohn disease, Henoch-Schönlein purpura, Kawasaki disease, systemic lupus erythematosus.
Infectious agents (atypical microbes).
Microlithiasis.
Postoperative state (e.g., cardiac surgery).
Sepsis.
Sludge.
Systemic inflammatory states.
Total parenteral nutrition.
Traumatic spinal cord injury.

ACHES AND PAINS, DIFFUSE[6]
ICD-10CM # M25.50 Pain in unspecified joint

Postviral arthralgias/myalgias.
Bilateral soft tissue rheumatism.
Overuse syndromes.
Fibrositis.
Hypothyroidism.
Metabolic bone disease.
Paraneoplastic syndrome.
Myopathy (polymyositis, dermatomyositis).
Rheumatoid arthritis (RA).
Sjögren syndrome.
Polymyalgia rheumatica.
Hypermobility.
Benign arthralgias/myalgias.
Chronic fatigue syndrome.
Hypophosphatemia.

ACIDOSIS, HYPERCHLORIC METABOLIC[7]
ICD-10CM # E87.2 Acidosis

GASTROINTESTINAL BICARBONATE LOSS
Diarrhea.
External pancreatic or small bowel drainage.
Ureterosigmoidostomy, jejunal loop.
Drugs:
Calcium chloride (acidifying agent).
Magnesium sulfate (diarrhea).
Cholestyramine (bile acid diarrhea).

RENAL ACIDOSIS
Hypokalemic:
Proximal RTA (type 2).
Distal (classic) RTA (type 1).
Drug-induced hypokalemia:
Acetazolamide (proximal RTA).
Amphotericin B (distal RTA).
Hyperkalemic:
Generalized distal nephron dysfunction (type 4 RTA).
Mineralocorticoid deficiency or resistance (pseudohypoaldosteronism type 1) PHA-I, PHA-II.
↓ Na^+ delivery to distal nephron.
Tubulointerstitial disease.
Ammonium excretion defect.
Drug-induced hyperkalemia:
Potassium-sparing diuretics (amiloride, triamterene, spironolactone).
Trimethoprim.
Pentamidine.
Angiotensin-converting enzyme inhibitors and angiotensin II receptor blockers.
Nonsteroidal antiinflammatory drugs.
Cyclosporine, tacrolimus.
Normokalemic:
Early renal insufficiency.

OTHER
Acid loads (ammonium chloride, hyperalimentation).

Loss of potential bicarbonate: ketosis with ketone excretion.
Dilution acidosis (rapid saline administration).
Hippurate.
Cation-exchange resins.

ACIDOSIS, LACTIC[7]
ICD-10CM # E87.2 Acidosis

CAUSES OF LACTIC ACIDOSIS
L-Lactic Acidosis
Conditions associated with type A lactic acidosis:
Poor tissue perfusion.
Shock:
Cardiogenic.
Hemorrhagic.
Septic.
Profound hypoxemia:
Severe asthma.
Carbon monoxide poisoning.
Conditions associated with type B lactic acidosis:
Liver disease.
Metformin.
Inborn errors of metabolism.
Pyroglutamic acidosis.
Kombucha tea.
d-Lactic Acidosis
Short bowel syndrome.
Ischemic bowel.
Small bowel obstruction.

ACIDOSIS, METABOLIC
ICD-10CM # E87.2 Acidosis

METABOLIC ACIDOSIS WITH INCREASED ANION GAP (AG ACIDOSIS)
Lactic acidosis.
Ketoacidosis (DM, alcoholic ketoacidosis).
Uremia (chronic renal failure).
Ingestion of toxins (paraldehyde, methanol, salicylate, ethylene glycol).
High-fat diet (mild acidosis).

METABOLIC ACIDOSIS WITH NORMAL AG (HYPERCHLOREMIC ACIDOSIS)
Renal tubular acidosis (including acidosis of aldosterone deficiency).
Intestinal loss of HCO_3- (diarrhea, pancreatic fistula).
Carbonic anhydrase inhibitors (e.g., acetazolamide).
Dilutional acidosis (as a result of rapid infusion of bicarbonate-free isotonic saline).
Ingestion of exogenous acids (ammonium chloride, methionine, cystine, calcium chloride).
Ileostomy.
Ureterosigmoidostomy.
Drugs: amiloride, triamterene, spironolactone, β-blockers.

ACIDOSIS, RESPIRATORY

ICD-10CM # E87.2 Acidosis

Pulmonary disease (COPD, severe pneumonia, pulmonary edema, interstitial fibrosis).

Airway obstruction (foreign body, severe bronchospasm, laryngospasm).

Thoracic cage disorders (pneumothorax, flail chest, kyphoscoliosis).

Defects in muscles of respiration (myasthenia gravis, hypokalemia, muscular dystrophy).

Defects in peripheral nervous system (amyotrophic lateral sclerosis, poliomyelitis, Guillain-Barré syndrome, botulism, tetanus, organophosphate poisoning, spinal cord injury).

Depression of respiratory center (anesthesia, narcotics, sedatives, vertebral artery embolism or thrombosis, increased intracranial pressure).

Failure of mechanical ventilator.

ACUTE KIDNEY INJURY AND LIVER DISEASE, CAUSES[8,9]

| ICD-10CM # | S37.009A | Unspecified injury of unspecified kidney, initial encounter |
| | K76.89 | Other specified diseases of liver |

Prerenal uremia:	Diuretic use, GI loss, peritoneal aspiration, hypoalbuminemia.
Hepatorenal syndrome.	
Acute tubular necrosis:	Hyperbilirubinemia, sepsis, toxic shock syndrome.
Drugs:	Acetaminophen (paracetamol), NSAIDs, tetracycline, rifampicin, isoniazid, anesthetic agents, sulfonamides, allopurinol, methotrexate.
Infections:	Hepatitis C and cryoglobulinemia, hepatitis B and polyarteritis nodosa, leptospirosis, hantavirus, Epstein-Barr virus, gram-negative sepsis, spontaneous bacterial peritonitis.
Other:	Papillary necrosis and obstruction, inhalation of chlorinated hydrocarbons, mushroom poisoning (*Amanita phalloides*).

ACUTE KIDNEY INJURY DUE TO INTRINSIC RENAL DISEASES[10]

ICD-10CM # Varies with specific diagnosis

INTRINSIC RENAL DISEASES THAT CAUSE ACUTE KIDNEY INJURY

Vascular Diseases

Large-Vessel Diseases

Renal artery thrombosis or stenosis.

Renal vein thrombosis.

Atheroembolic disease.

Small- and Medium-Vessel Diseases

Scleroderma.

Malignant hypertension.

Hemolytic uremic syndrome.

Thrombotic thrombocytopenic purpura.

HIV-associated microangiopathy.

Glomerular Diseases

Systemic Diseases

Systemic lupus erythematosus.

Infective endocarditis.

Systemic vasculitis (e.g., periarteritis nodosa, granulomatosis with polyangiitis).

Henoch-Schönlein purpura.

HIV-associated nephropathy.

Essential mixed cryoglobulinemia.

Goodpasture syndrome.

Primary Renal Diseases

Poststreptococcal glomerulonephritis.

Other postinfectious glomerulonephritis.

Rapidly progressive glomerulonephritis.

Tubulointerstitial Diseases and Conditions

Drugs (many).

Toxins (e.g., heavy metals, ethylene glycol).

Infections.

Multiple myeloma.

Acute Tubular Necrosis

Ischemia

Shock.

Sepsis.

Severe prerenal azotemia.

Nephrotoxins

Antibiotics.

Radiographic contrast agents.

Myoglobinuria.

Hemoglobinuria.

Other Diseases and Conditions

Severe liver disease.

Allergic reactions.

NSAIDs.

ACUTE KIDNEY INJURY, HIV PATIENT, CAUSES[8,9]

| ICD-10CM # | S37.009A | Unspecified injury of unspecified kidney, initial encounter with B20 human immunodeficiency virus (HIV) disease |

Prerenal:	Diarrhea, nausea and vomiting, cirrhosis and hepatorenal syndrome, sepsis.
Vascular:	Thrombotic microangiopathy.
Glomerular:	Immune complex glomerulonephritis

(MPGN secondary to hepatitis C virus, postinfectious glomerulonephritis), HIVAN.

Acute tubular necrosis:	Sepsis, hypotension, nephrotoxins (aminoglycosides, amphotericin, acyclovir, cidofovir, tenofovir, pentamidine).
Acute interstitial nephritis:	Drug-induced (co-trimoxazole), rifampicin, foscarnet, nevirapine), CMV infection, DILS.
Drug-induced intratubular obstruction:	Sulfadiazine, indinavir, foscarnet, acyclovir.
Postrenal obstruction:	Stones, tuberculosis, fungal ball, tumor.
Associated with IV drug use:	Sepsis, endocarditis, heroin-associated nephropathy (FSGS), rhabdomyolysis.

CMV, Cytomegalovirus; *DILS*, diffusive infiltrative lymphocytosis syndrome; *FSGS*, focal segmental glomerulosclerosis; *HIVAN*, HIV-associated nephropathy; *MPGN*, membranoproliferative glomerulonephritis.

ACUTE KIDNEY INJURY IN SPECIFIC CLINICAL SETTINGS[11]

| ICD-10CM # | N17.9 | Acute kidney failure, unspecified |

MAJOR CAUSES OF ACUTE KIDNEY INJURY IN SPECIFIC CLINICAL SETTINGS

AKI in the Cancer Patient

Prerenal azotemia:

Hypovolemia (e.g., poor intake, vomiting, diarrhea).

Intrinsic AKI:

Exogenous nephrotoxins: chemotherapy, antibiotics, contrast media.

Endogenous toxins: hyperuricemia, hypercalcemia, tumor lysis, paraproteins.

Other: radiation, HUS/TTP, glomerulonephritis, amyloid, malignant infiltration.

Postrenal AKI:

Ureteric or bladder neck obstruction.

AKI After Cardiac Surgery

Prerenal azotemia:

Hypovolemia (surgical losses, diuretics), cardiac failure, vasodilators.

Intrinsic AKI:

Ischemic ATN (even in absence of hypotension).

Atheroembolic disease after aortic manipulation/intraaortic balloon pump.

Preoperative or perioperative administration of contrast medium.

Allergic interstitial nephritis induced by perioperative antibiotics.

Postrenal AKI:

Obstructed urinary catheter, exacerbation of voiding dysfunction.

AKI in Pregnancy

Prerenal azotemia:

Acute fatty liver of pregnancy with fulminant hepatic failure.

Intrinsic AKI:

Preeclampsia or eclampsia.

Postpartum HUS/TTP.

HELLP syndrome.

Ischemia: postpartum hemorrhage, abruptio placentae, amniotic fluid embolus.

Direct toxicity of illegal abortifacients.

Postrenal AKI:

Obstruction with pyelonephritis.

AKI After Solid Organ or Bone Marrow Transplantation

Prerenal azotemia:

Intravascular volume depletion (e.g., diuretic therapy).

Vasoactive drugs (e.g., calcineurin inhibitors, amphotericin B).

Hepatorenal syndrome, venoocclusive disease of liver (BMT).

Intrinsic AKI:

Postoperative ischemic ATN (even in absence of hypotension).

Sepsis.

Exogenous nephrotoxins: aminoglycosides, amphotericin B, radiocontrast media.

HUS/TTP (e.g., cyclosporine or myeloablative radiotherapy related).

Allergic tubulointerstitial nephritis.

Postrenal AKI:

Obstructed urinary catheter.

AKI and Pulmonary Disease (Pulmonary Renal Syndrome)

Prerenal azotemia:

Diminished cardiac output complicating pulmonary embolism, severe pulmonary hypertension, or positive-pressure mechanical ventilation.

Intrinsic AKI:

Vasculitis.

Goodpasture syndrome, ANCA-associated vasculitis, SLE, eosinophilic granulomatosis with polyangiitis, polyarteritis nodosa, cryoglobulinemia, right-sided endocarditis, lymphomatoid granulomatosis, sarcoidosis, scleroderma.

Toxins:

Ingestion of paraquat or diquat.

Infections:

Legionnaires disease, *Mycoplasma* infection, tuberculosis, disseminated viral or fungal infection.

AKI from any cause with hypervolemia and pulmonary edema.

Lung cancer with hypercalcemia, tumor lysis, or glomerulonephritis.

AKI and Liver Disease

Prerenal azotemia:

Reduced true (GI hemorrhage, GI losses from lactulose, diuretics, large-volume paracentesis) circulatory volume or effective (hypoalbuminemia, splanchnic vasodilation).

Hepatorenal syndrome type 1 or 2.

Tense ascites with abdominal compartment syndrome.

Intrinsic AKI:

Ischemic (severe hypoperfusion—see earlier) or direct nephrotoxicity and hepatotoxicity of drugs or toxins (e.g., carbon tetrachloride, acetaminophen, tetracyclines, methoxyflurane).

Tubulointerstitial nephritis plus hepatitis caused by drugs (e.g., sulfonamides, rifampin, phenytoin, allopurinol, phenindione), infections (leptospirosis, brucellosis, Epstein-Barr virus infection, cytomegalovirus infection), malignant infiltration (leukemia, lymphoma), or sarcoidosis.

Glomerulonephritis or vasculitis (e.g., polyarteritis nodosa, ANCA-associated glomerulonephritis, cryoglobulinemia, SLE, postinfectious hepatitis or liver abscess).

AKI and Nephrotic Syndrome

Prerenal azotemia:

Intravascular volume depletion (diuretic therapy, hypoalbuminemia).

Intrinsic AKI:

Manifestation of primary glomerular disease.

Collapsing glomerulopathy (e.g., HIV, pamidronate).

Associated ATN (older hypertensive males).

Associated interstitial nephritis (NSAIDs, rifampin, interferon alfa).

Other: amyloid or light-chain deposition disease, renal vein thrombosis, severe interstitial edema.

AKI, Acute kidney injury; *ANCA,* antineutrophil cytoplasmic antibody; *ATN,* acute tubular necrosis; *BMT,* bone marrow transplantation; *GI,* gastrointestinal; *HELLP,* hemolysis, elevated liver enzymes, low platelets; *HIV,* human immunodeficiency virus; *HUS,* hemolytic uremic syndrome; *NSAID,* nonsteroidal antiinflammatory drug; *SLE,* systemic lupus erythematosus; *TTP,* thrombotic thrombocytopenic purpura.

ACUTE KIDNEY INJURY, PIGMENT INDUCED[10]

ICD-10CM # Varies with specific diagnosis

CAUSES OF PIGMENT-INDUCED ACUTE KIDNEY INJURY

Rhabdomyolysis and myoglobinuria.

Vigorous exercise.

Arterial embolization.

Status epilepticus.

Status asthmaticus.

Coma-induced and pressure-induced myonecrosis.

Heat stress.

Diabetic ketoacidosis.

Myopathy.

Alcoholism.

Hypokalemia.

Hypophosphatemia.

Hemoglobinuria.

Transfusion reactions.

Snake envenomation.

Malaria.

Mechanical destruction of RBCs by prosthetic valves.

G6PD deficiency.

G6PD, Glucose-6-phosphate dehydrogenase.

ACUTE LIVER FAILURE[12]

ICD-10CM # K71.01 Toxic liver disease with hepatic necrosis

DIFFERENTIAL DIAGNOSIS OF ACUTE LIVER FAILURE

Viruses	Hepatitis A and B viruses (typical viruses causing viral hepatitis).
	Hepatitis C virus (rare).
	Hepatitis D virus.
	Hepatitis E virus (often in pregnant women in endemic areas).
	Cytomegalovirus.
	Hemorrhagic fever viruses.
	Herpes simplex virus.
	Paramyxovirus.
	Epstein-Barr virus.
Drugs	Paracetamol hepatotoxicity.
	Idiosyncratic hypersensitivity reactions (e.g., isoniazid, statins, halothane).
	Illicit drugs (e.g., Ecstasy, cocaine).
	Alternative medicines (e.g., chaparral and *Teucrium polium*), traditional Chinese medicine.
Toxins	Mushroom poisoning (usually *Amanita phalloides*).
	Bacillus cereus toxin.
	Cyanobacteria toxin.
	Organic solvents (e.g., carbon tetrachloride).
	Yellow phosphorus.
Vasculopathy	Ischemic hepatitis.
	Hepatic vein thrombosis (Budd-Chiari syndrome).
	Hepatic venoocclusive disease.
	Portal vein thrombosis.
	Hepatic arterial thrombosis.
Metabolic	Acute fatty liver of pregnancy/hemolysis, elevated liver enzymes, low platelet count (HELLP) syndrome.
	α_1-antitrypsin deficiency.
	Fructose intolerance.
	Galactosemia.
	Lecithin-cholesterol acyltransferase deficiency.
	Reye syndrome.
	Tyrosinemia.
	Wilson disease.
Autoimmune	Autoimmune hepatitis.

Malignancy   Primary liver malignancy (hepatocellular carcinoma or cholangiocarcinoma).
     Secondary (e.g., extensive hepatic metastases or infiltration of adenocarcinoma).

Miscellaneous   Adult-onset Still disease.
     Heat stroke.
     Primary graft nonfunction (in liver transplant recipients).
     Indeterminate etiology (approximately 20% of acute liver failure cases).

ACUTE LUNG INJURY, DISEASE AND DISORDER ASSOCIATIONS[13]

ICD-10CM #   S27.3   Injury, lung

CLINICAL DISORDERS ASSOCIATED WITH ACUTE LUNG INJURY

Infectious Causes
Gram-negative or gram-positive sepsis.
Bacterial pneumonia.
Viral pneumonia.
Fungal pneumonia
Parasitic infections.
Mycobacterial disease.

Aspiration
Gastric acid.
Food and other particulate matter.
Fresh or sea water (near drowning).
Hydrocarbon fluids.

Trauma
Lung contusion.
Fat emboli.
Nonthoracic trauma.
Thermal injury (burns).
Blast injury (explosion, lightning).
Overdistention (mechanical ventilation).
Inhaled gases (phosgene, ammonia).

Hemodynamic Disturbances
Shock of any etiology.
Anaphylaxis.
High-altitude pulmonary edema.
Reperfusion.
Air embolism.
Amniotic fluid embolism.

Drugs
Heroin.
Methadone.
Propoxyphene.
Naloxone.
Cocaine.
Barbiturates.
Colchicine.
Salicylates.
Ethchlorvynol.
Interleukin-2.
Protamine.

Hydrochlorothiazide.

Hematologic Disorders
Disseminated intravascular coagulation.
Incompatible blood transfusion.
Rh incompatibility.
Antileukocyte antibodies.
Leucoagglutinin reactions.
Postcardiopulmonary bypass, pump oxygenator.

Metabolic Disorders
Pancreatitis.
Diabetic ketoacidosis.

Neurologic Disorders
Head trauma.
Grand mal seizures.
Increased intracranial pressure (any cause).
Subarachnoid or intracerebral hemorrhage.

Miscellaneous Disorders
Lung reexpansion.
Upper airway obstruction.

ACUTE RESPIRATORY DISTRESS IN PREGNANCY[14]

ICD-10CM #   J96.00   Acute respiratory failure

Disorder	Distinguishing Features
Pregnancy-Specific	
Amniotic fluid embolism:	Cardiorespiratory collapse, seizures, DIC.
Pulmonary edema secondary to preeclampsia:	Hypertension, proteinuria.
ARDS secondary to obstetric sepsis:	Evidence of obstetric sepsis, shock.
Tocolytic pulmonary edema:	Tocolytic administration, rapid improvement.
Peripartum cardiomyopathy:	Gradual onset, cardiac gallop, cardiomegaly.
Trophoblastic embolism:	Nodular infiltrate, molar pregnancy.
Risk Increased by Pregnancy	
Aspiration pneumonitis:	Vomiting, aspiration.
Venous thromboembolism:	Evidence of DVT, positive V̇/Q̇ scan, leg Doppler, CT angiogram.
Pneumomediastinum:	Occurs during delivery, subcutaneous emphysema.
Valvular heart disease:	Pulmonary edema, cardiac murmur, cardiomegaly.
ARDS secondary to sepsis:	Evidence of sepsis (e.g., pyelonephritis).
Unrelated to Pregnancy	
Asthma:	Features similar to nonpregnant patient.
Pneumonia:	Features similar to nonpregnant patient.

ARDS, Acute respiratory distress syndrome; *CT*, computed tomography; *DIC*, disseminated intravascular coagulopathy; *DVT*, deep venous thrombosis; V̇/Q̇, ventilation-perfusion.

ACUTE SCROTUM

ICD-10CM #   R10.2   Pelvic and perineal pain

Testicular torsion.
Epididymitis.
Testicular neoplasm.
Orchitis.
Trauma.

ADNEXAL MASS[1]

ICD-10CM #   R19.00   Intraabdominal and pelvic swelling, mass and lump, unspecified site

Ovary (neoplasm, endometriosis, functional cyst).
Fallopian tube (ectopic pregnancy, neoplasm, tuboovarian abscess, hydrosalpinx, paratubal cyst).
Uterus (fibroid, neoplasm).
Retroperitoneum (neoplasm, abdominal wall hematoma or abscess).
Urinary tract (pelvic kidney, distended bladder, urachal cyst).
Inflammatory bowel disease.
GI tract neoplasm.
Diverticular disease.
Appendicitis.
Bowel loop with feces.

ADRENAL CALCIFICATIONS[15]

ICD-10CM #   E27.8   Other specified disorder of adrenal gland

CAUSES OF ADRENAL CALCIFICATION

Infection:
   Tuberculosis.
   Histoplasmosis.
   Echinococcus.
Prior hemorrhage.
Neoplasm:
   Adrenocortical carcinoma.
   Myelolipoma.
   Pheochromocytoma.
Hemangioma (rare).

ADRENAL CYSTIC LESIONS[15]

ICD-10CM #   E27.8   Other specified disorder of adrenal gland

CYSTIC ADRENAL LESIONS

Pseudocyst.
Endothelial cyst.
Epithelial cyst.
Infection (*Echinococcus*, abscess).
Necrotic neoplasm.
Cystic pheochromocytoma.
Lymphangioma.

ADRENAL INSUFFICIENCY, CRITICALLY ILL PATIENT[16]

ICD-10CM #	E27.40	Unspecified adrenocortical insufficiency

CAUSES OF ADRENAL INSUFFICIENCY IN CRITICALLY ILL PATIENTS
Reversible Dysfunction of the HPA Axis
Sepsis/septic shock.
Acute lung injury.
Burns.
Pancreatitis.
Liver failure.
Hypothermia.
Drugs:
    Etomidate (primary AI).
    Corticosteroids (secondary AI).
    Ketoconazole (primary AI).
    Megestrol acetate (secondary AI).
    Rifampin (increased cortisol metabolism).
    Phenytoin (increased cortisol metabolism).
    Metyrapone (primary AI).
    Mitotane (primary AI).
Primary Adrenal Insufficiency (Adrenal Failure)
Autoimmune adrenalitis.
HIV infection:
    HART therapy.
    HIV virus.
    CMV.
Metastatic carcinoma:
    Lung.
    Breast.
    Kidney.
Systemic fungal infection:
    Histoplasmosis.
    Cryptococcus.
    Blastomycosis.
Tuberculosis.
Adrenal hemorrhage/infarction:
    DIC.
    Meningococcemia.
    Anticoagulation.
    Antiphospholipid syndrome.
    HIT.
    Trauma.

AI, Adrenal insufficiency; *CMV*, cytomegalovirus; *DIC*, disseminated intravascular coagulation; *HIT*, heparin-induced thrombocytopenia; *HPA*, hypothalamic-pituitary axis.

ADRENAL MASSES[17]

ICD-10CM #	C74.90	Malignant neoplasm of unspecified part of unspecified adrenal gland
	E27.8	Other specified disorders of adrenal gland

UNILATERAL ADRENAL MASSES
Functional Lesions
Adrenal adenoma.
Adrenal carcinoma.
Pheochromocytoma.
Primary aldosteronism, adenomatous type.
Nonfunctional Lesions
Incidentaloma of adrenal.
Ganglioneuroma.
Myelolipoma.
Hematoma.
Adenolipoma.
Metastasis.

BILATERAL ADRENAL MASSES
Functional Lesions
ACTH-dependent Cushing syndrome.
Congenital adrenal hyperplasia.
Pheochromocytoma.
Conn syndrome, hyperplastic variety.
Micronodular adrenal disease.
Idiopathic bilateral adrenal hypertrophy.
Nonfunctional Lesions
Infection (tuberculosis, fungi).
Infiltration (leukemia, lymphoma).
Replacement (amyloidosis).
Hemorrhage.
Bilateral metastases.

ADRENAL PSEUDOMASSES[15]

ICD-10CM #	E27.8	Other specified disorder of adrenal gland

Thickened diaphragmatic crus.
Accessory spleen.
Gastric fundus.
Gastric diverticulum.
Renal vein.
Retrocrural and retroperitoneal adenopathy.
Upper-pole renal cysts and tumors.
Pancreatic tumors.
Hypertrophied caudate lobe of liver.
Fluid-filled colon interposed between stomach and kidney.

ADRENERGIC TOXIDROME[16]

ICD-10CM #	T44.8X1S	Poisoning by centrally acting and adrenergic-neuron-blocking agents, accidental (unintentional), sequela

COMMON CAUSES OF THE ADRENERGIC TOXIDROME
Recreational drugs:
Cocaine.
Amphetamines and other "designer drugs"; "Ecstasy" (3,4-methylenedioxymethamphetamine [MDMA]); 3,4-methylenedioxyamphetamine (MDA); 3,4-methylenedioxyethylamphetamine (MDEA); paramethoxyamphetamine (PMA); methamphetamine.
β_1-Adrenergic agents:
    Salbutamol.
Theophylline.
Inotropic agents:
    Norepinephrine.
    Epinephrine.
    Isoproterenol.
Over-the-counter cough and cold preparations and nasal decongestants:
    Phenylpropanolamine.
    Pseudoephedrine.
Amphetamine-like agents prescribed for ADD or weight loss:
    Methylphenidate.
    Dextroamphetamine.
Psychostimulants.

ADD, Attention deficit disorder.

ADRENOCORTICAL HYPERFUNCTION[18]

ICD-10CM #	E26.9	Hyperaldosteronism, unspecified

SYNDROMES OF ADRENOCORTICAL HYPERFUNCTION
States of Glucocorticoid Excess
Physiologic States
Stress.
Strenuous exercise.
Last trimester of pregnancy.

Pathologic States
Psychiatric conditions (pseudo-Cushing disorders):
    Depression.
    Alcoholism.
    Anorexia nervosa.
    Panic disorders.
    Alcohol and drug withdrawal.
ACTH-dependent states:
    Pituitary adenoma (Cushing disease).
    Ectopic ACTH syndrome.
    Bronchial carcinoid.
    Thymic carcinoid.
    Islet cell tumor.
    Small cell lung carcinoma.
    Ectopic CRH secretion.
ACTH-independent states:
    Adrenal adenoma.
    Adrenal carcinoma.
    Micronodular adrenal disease.

Exogenous Sources
Glucocorticoid intake.
ACTH intake.
States of Mineralocorticoid Excess
Primary Aldosteronism
Aldosterone-secreting adenoma.
Bilateral adrenal hyperplasia.
Aldosterone-secreting carcinoma.
Glucocorticoid-suppressible hyperaldosteronism.
Adrenal Enzyme Deficiencies
11b-Hydroxylase deficiency.

17a-Hydroxylase deficiency.
11b-Hydroxysteroid dehydrogenase, type II.
Exogenous Mineralocorticoids
Licorice.
Carbenoxolone.
Fludrocortisone.
Secondary Hyperaldosteronism
Associated with hypertension:
　Accelerated hypertension.
　Renovascular hypertension.
　Estrogen administration.
　Renin-secreting tumors.
Without hypertension:
　Bartter syndrome.
　Sodium-wasting nephropathy.
　Renal tubular acidosis.
　Diuretic and laxative abuse.
　Edematous states (cirrhosis, nephrosis, congestive heart failure).

ACTH, Adrenocorticotropin hormone; _CRH_, corticotropin-releasing hormone.

ADRENOCORTICAL HYPOFUNCTION

ICD-10CM # E27.49 Other adrenocortical insufficiency

SYNDROMES OF ADRENOCORTICAL HYPOFUNCTION
Primary Adrenal Disorders
Combined Glucocorticoid and Mineralocorticoid Deficiency
Autoimmune:
　Isolated autoimmune disease (Addison disease).
　Polyglandular autoimmune syndrome, type I.
　Polyglandular autoimmune syndrome, type II.
Infectious:
　Tuberculosis.
　Fungal.
　Cytomegalovirus.
　Human immunodeficiency virus.
Vascular:
　Bilateral adrenal hemorrhage.
　Sepsis.
　Coagulopathy.
　Thrombosis; embolism.
　Adrenal infarction.
Infiltration:
　Metastatic carcinoma and lymphoma.
　Sarcoidosis.
　Amyloidosis.
　Hemochromatosis.
Congenital:
　Congenital adrenal hyperplasia.
　　21-Hydroxylase deficiency.
　　3b-ol Dehydrogenase deficiency.
　　20,22-Desmolase deficiency.
Adrenal unresponsiveness to ACTH.
Congenital adrenal hypoplasia.

Adrenoleukodystrophy.
Adrenomyeloneuropathy.
Iatrogenic
Bilateral adrenalectomy.
Drugs:
　Metyrapone, aminoglutethimide, trilostane, ketoconazole, o,p'-DDD, mifepristone.
Mineralocorticoid Deficiency without Glucocorticoid Deficiency
Corticosterone methyl oxidase deficiency.
Isolated zona glomerulosa defect.
Heparin therapy.
Critical illness.
Converting-enzyme inhibitors.
Secondary Adrenal Disorders
Secondary Adrenal Insufficiency
Hypothalamic-pituitary dysfunction.
Exogenous glucocorticoids.
After removal of an ACTH-secreting tumor.
Hyporeninemic Hypoaldosteronism
Diabetic nephropathy.
Tubulointerstitial diseases.
Obstructive uropathy.
Autonomic neuropathy.
Nonsteroidal antiinflammatory drugs.
β-Adrenergic drugs.

ACTH, Adrenocorticotropic hormone.

ADVERSE FOOD REACTIONS, DIFFERENTIAL DIAGNOSIS[19]

ICD-10CM # T78.1XXA Other adverse food reactions, not elsewhere classified, initial encounter

GASTROINTESTINAL DISORDERS (WITH VOMITING AND/OR DIARRHEA)
Structural abnormalities (pyloric stenosis, Hirschsprung disease).
Enzyme deficiencies (primary or secondary):
　Disaccharidase deficiency: lactase, fructose, sucrase-isomaltase.
　Galactosemia.
Other: pancreatic insufficiency (cystic fibrosis), peptic disease.

CONTAMINANTS AND ADDITIVES
Flavorings and preservatives—rarely cause symptoms: sodium metabisulfite, monosodium glutamate, nitrites.
Dyes and colorings—very rarely cause symptoms (urticaria, eczema): tartrazine.
Toxins: bacterial, fungal (aflatoxin), fish-related (scombroid, ciguatera).
Infectious organisms:
　Bacteria (_Salmonella, Escherichia coli, Shigella_).
　Virus (rotavirus, enterovirus).
　Parasites (_Giardia,_ Anisakis simplex [in fish]).
Accidental contaminants: heavy metals, pesticides.

Pharmacologic agents: caffeine, glycosidal alkaloid solanine (potato spuds), histamine (fish), serotonin (banana, tomato), tryptamine (tomato), tyramine (cheese).

PSYCHOLOGIC REACTIONS
Food phobias.

ADYNAMIC ILEUS[1]

ICD-10CM # K56.0 Paralytic ileus
　　　　　　 K56.7 Ileus, unspecified

Abdominal trauma.
Infection (retroperitoneal, pelvic, intrathoracic).
Laparotomy.
Metabolic disease (hypokalemia).
Renal colic.
Skeletal injury (rib fracture, vertebral fracture).
Medications (e.g., narcotics).

AEROPHAGIA (BELCHING, ERUCTATION)

ICD-10CM # R14.0 Abdominal distention (gaseous)
　　　　　　 R14.1 Gas pain
　　　　　　 R14.2 Eructation
　　　　　　 R14.3 Flatulence

Anxiety disorders.
Rapid food ingestion.
Carbonated beverages.
Nursing infants (especially when nursing in horizontal position).
Eating or drinking in supine position.
Gum chewing.
Poorly fitting dentures, orthodontic appliances.
Hiatal hernia, gastritis, nonnuclear dyspepsia.
Cholelithiasis, cholecystitis.
Ingestion of legumes, onions, peppers.

AGITATION AND CONFUSION[20]

ICD-10CM # Varies with specific diagnosis.

Causes
Epileptic
Absence status.[a]
Complex partial seizure.[a]
Epileptic encephalopathies.[a]
Infectious Disorders
Bacterial infections.
　Cat-scratch disease.[a]
　Meningitis.[a]
Rickettsial infections.
　Lyme disease.[a]
　Rocky Mountain spotted fever.[a]
Viral infections.
　Arboviruses.
　Aseptic meningitis.
　Herpes simplex encephalitis.[a]
　Measles encephalitis.
　Postinfectious encephalomyelitis.
　Reye syndrome.

Metabolic and Systemic Disorders
Disorders of osmolality.
  Hypoglycemia.[a]
  Hyponatremia.[a]
Endocrine disorders.
  Adrenal insufficiency.[a]
  Hypoparathyroidism.[a]
  Thyroid disorders.[a]
Hepatic encephalopathy.
Inborn errors of metabolism.
  Disorders of pyruvate metabolism.
  Medium-chain acyl-CoA dehydrogenase (MCAD) deficiency.
  Respiratory chain disorders.
  Urea cycle disorder, heterozygote.
Renal disease.
  Hypertensive encephalopathy.[a]
  Uremic encephalopathy.[a]

Migraine
Acute confusional.[a]
Aphasic.[a]
Transient global amnesia.[a]

Psychological
Panic disorder.[a]
Schizophrenia.

Toxic
Immunosuppressive drugs.[a]
Prescription drugs.[a]
Substance abuse.[a]
Toxins.[a]

Vascular
Congestive heart failure.[a]
Embolism.[a]
Hypertensive encephalopathy.[a]
Lupus erythematosus.[a]
Anti-NMDA antibody encephalitis.
Subarachnoid hemorrhage.[a]
  Vasculitis.[a]

---

[a]Denotes the most common conditions and the ones with disease-modifying treatments.
NMDA, N-methyl-D-aspartate.

AIR-SPACE OPACIFICATION ON X-RAY[21]

ICD-10CM #   R91.8   Other nonspecific abnormal finding of lung field

CAUSES OF AIR-SPACE OPACIFICATION
Edema
Cardiogenic.
Noncardiogenic.
Inflammation/Infection
Granulomatosis with polyangiitis.
Cryptogenic organizing pneumonia.
Blood
Idiopathic pulmonary hemosiderosis.
Antibasement membrane antibody disease.
Systemic lupus erythematosus.
Miscellaneous Causes
Eosinophilic pneumonia.
Alveolar proteinosis.
Alveolar cell carcinoma.
Alveolar microlithiasis.

Lymphoma (MALToma).
Sarcoidosis.

AIRWAY OBSTRUCTION, CENTRAL[22]

ICD-10CM #   Varies with specific diagnosis

ETIOLOGY OF CENTRAL AIRWAY OBSTRUCTION

Nonmalignant	Malignant
Vascular sling.	Primary airway tumors.
	Bronchogenic.
	Mucoepidermoid.
	Adenoid cystic.
	Carcinoid.
Lymphadenopathy.	Lymphadenopathy due
Infection (histoplasmosis and tuberculosis).	to malignancy.
Sarcoidosis.	
Relapsing polychondritis.	Metastatic tumor to airway.
	Bronchogenic.
	Renal cell.
	Esophageal carcinoma.
	Breast.
	Thyroid.
	Colon.
	Melanoma.
Granulation tissue associated with:	Mediastinal tumors
Artificial airways.	Lymphoma.
Airway stents.	Thymus.
Aspirated foreign bodies.	Thyroid.
Surgical anastomosis.	
Inflammatory lesions.	
Amyloidosis.	
Papillomatosis.	
Granulomatosis with polyangiitis.	

AIRWAY OBSTRUCTION, PEDIATRIC AGE[23]

ICD-10CM #		
	J44.9	Chronic obstructive pulmonary disease, unspecified
	T17.900A	Unspecified foreign body in respiratory tract, part unspecified causing asphyxiation, initial encounter
	T17.908A	Unspecified foreign body in respiratory tract, part unspecified causing other injury, initial encounter
	T17.910A	Gastric contents in respiratory tract, part unspecified causing asphyxiation, initial encounter
	T17.918A	Gastric contents in respiratory tract, part unspecified causing other injury, initial encounter
	T17.920A	Food in respiratory tract, part unspecified causing asphyxiation, initial encounter
	T17.928A	Food in respiratory tract, part unspecified causing other injury, initial encounter
	T17.990A	Other foreign object in respiratory tract, part unspecified in causing asphyxiation, initial encounter
	T17.998A	Other foreign object in respiratory tract, part unspecified causing other injury, initial encounter
	J38.5	Laryngeal spasm
	J68.9	Unspecified respiratory condition due to chemicals, gases, fumes, and vapors

CONGENITAL CAUSES
Craniofacial dysmorphism.
Hemangioma.
Laryngeal cleft/web.
Laryngoceles, cysts.
Laryngomalacia.
Macroglossia.
Tracheal stenosis.
Vascular ring.
Vocal cord paralysis.

ACQUIRED INFECTIOUS CAUSES
Acute laryngotracheobronchitis.
Epiglottitis.
Laryngeal papillomatosis.
Membranous croup (bacterial tracheitis).
Mononucleosis.
Retropharyngeal abscess.
Spasmodic croup.
Diphtheria.

ACQUIRED NONINFECTIOUS CAUSES
Anaphylaxis.
Foreign body aspiration.
Supraglottic hypotonia.
Thermal/chemical burn.
Trauma.
Vocal cord paralysis.
Angioneurotic edema.

AKINETIC/RIGID SYNDROME[18]

ICD-10CM #   R29.8   Akinesis

Parkinsonism (idiopathic, drug-induced).
Catatonia (psychosis).
Progressive supranuclear palsy.
Multisystem atrophy (Shy-Drager syndrome, olivopontocerebellar atrophy).
Diffuse Lewy-body disease.
Toxins (MPTP, manganese, carbon monoxide).
Huntington disease and other hereditary neurodegenerative disorders.

ALCOHOL-RELATED SEIZURES[10]

ICD-10CM #	F10.232 Alcohol dependence with withdrawal with perceptual disturbance

DIFFERENTIAL DIAGNOSIS OF ALCOHOL-RELATED SEIZURES

Withdrawal (alcohol or drugs).
Exacerbation of idiopathic or posttraumatic seizures.
Acute intoxication (amphetamines, anticholinergics, cocaine, isoniazid, organophosphates, phenothiazines, tricyclic antidepressants, salicylates, lithium).
Metabolic (hypoglycemia, hyponatremia, hypernatremia, hypocalcemia, hepatic failure).
Infectious (meningitis, encephalitis, brain abscess).
Trauma (intracranial hemorrhage).
Cerebrovascular accident.
Sleep deprivation.
Noncompliance with anticonvulsants.

ALKALOSIS, METABOLIC

ICD-10CM #	E87.3 Alkalosis

CAUSES OF METABOLIC ALKALOSIS

Exogenous HCO_3- loads.
Acute alkali administration.
Milk-alkali syndrome.
Effective Extracellular Volume Contraction, Normotension, Hypokalemia, and Secondary Hyperreninemic Hyperaldosteronism
GI origin:
  Vomiting.
  Gastric aspiration.
  Congenital chloridorrhea.
  Villous adenoma.
  Combined administration of sodium polystyrene sulfonate (Kayexalate and aluminum hydroxide).
Renal origin:
  Diuretics (especially thiazides and loop diuretics).
  Acute.
  Chronic.
  Edematous states.
  Posthypercapnic state.
  Hypercalcemia-hypoparathyroidism.
  Recovery from lactic acidosis or ketoacidosis.

Nonreabsorbable anions such as penicillin, carbenicillin.
Mg^{++} deficiency.
K^+ depletion.
Bartter syndrome (loss-of-function mutation of Cl^- transport in thick ascending limb of Henle loop).
Gitelman syndrome (loss-of-function mutation in Na^+/Cl^- cotransporter).
Carbohydrate refeeding after starvation.
Extracellular Volume Expansion, Hypertension, K^+ Deficiency, and Hypermineralocorticoidism
Associated with high renin:
  Renal artery stenosis.
  Accelerated hypertension.
  Renin-secreting tumor.
  Estrogen therapy.
Associated with low renin:
  Primary aldosteronism.
  Adenoma.
  Hyperplasia.
  Carcinoma.
  Glucocorticoid suppressible.
Adrenal enzymatic defects:
  11β-Hydroxylase deficiency.
  17α-Hydroxylase deficiency.
Cushing syndrome or disease:
  Ectopic corticotropin.
  Adrenal carcinoma.
  Adrenal adenoma.
  Primary pituitary.
Other:
  Licorice.
  Carbenoxolone.
  Chewer's tobacco.
  Lydia Pinkham tablets.
Gain-of-Function Mutation of ENaC with Extracellular Fluid Volume Expansion, Hypertension, K^+ Deficiency, and Hyporeninemic Hypoaldosteronism
Liddle syndrome.

ALKALOSIS, RESPIRATORY

ICD-10CM #	E87.3 Alkalosis

Hypoxemia (pneumonia, pulmonary embolism, atelectasis, high-altitude living).
Drugs (salicylates, xanthenes, progesterone, epinephrine, thyroxine, nicotine).
Central nervous system (CNS) disorders (tumor, cerebrovascular accident [CVA], trauma, infections).
Psychogenic hyperventilation (anxiety, hysteria).
Hepatic encephalopathy.
Gram-negative sepsis.
Hyponatremia.
Sudden recovery from metabolic acidosis.
Assisted ventilation.

ALOPECIA[13,24]

ICD-10CM #	L65.9 Nonscarring hair loss, unspecified

	L63.2	Ophiasis
	L63.8	Other alopecia areata
	Q84.0	Congenital alopecia
	Q84.1	Congenital morphological disturbances of hair, not elsewhere classified
	Q84.2	Other congenital malformations of hair
	F54	Psychological and behavioral factors associated with disorders or diseases classified elsewhere

SCARRING ALOPECIA

Congenital (aplasia cutis).
Tinea capitis with inflammation (kerion).
Bacterial folliculitis.
Discoid lupus erythematosus.
Lichen planopilaris.
Folliculitis decalvans.
Neoplasm.
Trauma.

NONSCARRING ALOPECIA

Cosmetic treatment.
Tinea capitis.
Structural hair shaft disease.
Trichotillomania (hair pulling).
Anagen arrest.
Telogen arrest.
Alopecia areata.
Androgenetic alopecia.

ALOPECIA AND HYPOTRICHOSIS, IN CHILDREN AND ADOLESCENTS

ICD-10CM #	L65.9	Nonscarring hair loss, unspecified
	L63.2	Ophiasis
	L63.8	Other alopecia areata
	Q84.0	Congenital alopecia
	Q84.1	Congenital morphological disturbances of hair, not elsewhere classified
	Q84.2	Other congenital malformations of hair

Congenital total alopecia: atrichia with papules, Moynahan alopecia syndrome.
Congenital localized alopecia: aplasia cutis, triangular alopecia, sebaceous nevus.
Hereditary hypotrichosis: Marie-Unna syndrome, hypotrichosis with juvenile macular dystrophy, hypotrichosis–Mari type, ichthyosis with hypotrichosis, cartilage-hair hypoplasia, Hallermann-Streiff syndrome, trichorhinophalangeal syndrome, ectodermal dysplasia ("pure" hair and nail and other ectodermal dysplasias).

Differential Diagnosis

II

Diffuse alopecia of endocrine origin: hypopituitarism, hypothyroidism, hypoparathyroidism, hyperthyroidism.

Alopecia of nutritional origin: marasmus, kwashiorkor, iron deficiency, zinc deficiency (acrodermatitis enteropathica), gluten-sensitive enteropathy, essential fatty acid deficiency, biotinidase deficiency.

Disturbances of the hair cycle: telogen effluvium.

Toxic alopecia: anagen effluvium.

Autoimmune alopecia: alopecia areata.

Traumatic alopecia: traction alopecia, trichotillomania.

Cicatricial alopecia: lupus erythematosus, lichen planopilaris, pseudopelade, morphea (en coup de saber), dermatomyositis, infection (kerion, favus, tuberculosis, syphilis, folliculitis, leishmaniasis, herpes zoster, varicella), acne keloidalis, follicular mucinosis, sarcoidosis.

Hair shaft abnormalities: monilethrix, pili annulati, pili torti, trichorrhexis invaginata, trichorrhexis nodosa, woolly hair syndrome, Menkes disease, trichothiodystrophy, trichodento-osseous syndrome, uncombable hair syndrome (spun-glass hair, pili trianguli et canaliculi).

ALOPECIA, DRUG-INDUCED

ICD-10CM # L65.9 Nonscarring hair loss, unspecified
L63.8 Alopecia areata

DRUGS REPORTED TO INDUCE HAIR LOSS

ACE inhibitors (captopril, enalapril, moexipril, ramipril).
Allopurinol.
Amiodarone.
Amphetamines.*,[†]
Analgesics, antiinflammatories (ibuprofen, indomethacin, naproxen).
Androgens.[‡]
Anticoagulants (coumarin, dextran, heparin/heparinoids).
Antiepileptics (carbamazepine, hydantoins, lamotrigine, troxidone, valproic acid, vigabatrin).
Antipsychotics (flupentixol decanoate, fluphenazine decanoate).
Antithyroid drugs (carbimazole, iodine, thiouracil).
Appetite suppressants.
Aromatase inhibitors (fadrozole, 4-OHA, vorozole).
Benzimidazoles (albendazole, mebendazole)
β-Blockers (levobunolol, metoprolol, nadolol, propranolol, timolol).
Bromocriptine.
Buspirone.
Butyrophenones.

Cantharidin.
Chloramphenicol.
Cholestyramine.
Cidofovir.
Cimetidine.
Clonazepam.
Clotrimazole.
Colchicine.
Contraceptive (oral).[§]
Danazol.
Diazoxide.
Diclofenac.
Dixyrazine.
Ethambutol.
Ethionamide.
Fibrates (clofibrate, fenofibrate).
G-CSF (granulocyte-colony stimulating factor)
Gefitinib.[¶]
Gentamicin.
Glatiramer acetate.
Glibenclamide.
Gold salts.
Haloperidol.
Immunoglobulins.
Indanediones.
Indinavir.
Interferons.
Isonicotinic acid hydrazide.**
Leflunomide.
Levodopa.
Lithium.
Maprotiline.
Mesalazine.
Methyldopa.
Methysergide.
Metyrapone.
Minoxidil.
Nicotinic acid.
Nitrofurantoin.
Octreotide.
Olanzapine.
Pentosan polysulfate.
Phenindione.
Potassium thiocyanate.
Pyridostigmine.
Radiation (<700 Gy).
Retinoids (acitretin, etretinate, isotretinoin).
Retinol (vitamin A).
Risperidone.
Salicylates.
Serotonin reuptake inhibitors (fluoxetine, fluvoxamine, paroxetine, sertraline).
Sorafenib.
Spironolactone.
Strontium ranelate.
Sulfasalazine.

Tamoxifen.
Terbinafine.
Terfenadine.
Thiamphenicol.
Thyroxine.
Tocopherol (vitamin E).
Trazodone.
Triazoles (fluconazole, itraconazole).
Tricyclic antidepressants (amitriptyline, desipramine, doxepin, imipramine, maprotiline).
Trimethadione.
Triparanol.
Vasopressin.[††]

[††]Hair loss usually severe.

ALVEOLAR CONSOLIDATION

ICD-10CM # J18.2 Hypostatic pneumonia, unspecified organism
J81.1 Hypostatic pneumonia, unspecified organism

Infection.
Neoplasm (bronchoalveolar carcinoma, lymphoma).
Aspiration.
Trauma.
Hemorrhage (granulomatosis with polyangiitis, Goodpasture, bleeding diathesis).
ARDS.
CHF.
Renal failure.
Eosinophilic pneumonia.
Bronchiolitis obliterans.
Pulmonary alveolar proteinosis.

ALVEOLAR HEMORRHAGE[25]

ICD-10CM # P26.1 Massive pulmonary hemorrhage originating in the perinatal period
K08.8 Alveolar hemorrhage
P26.8 Other pulmonary hemorrhages originating in the perinatal period

Hematologic disorders (coagulopathies, thrombocytopenia).
Goodpasture syndrome (antibasement membrane antibody disease).
Granulomatosis with polyangiitis.
Immune complex-mediated vasculitis.
Idiopathic pulmonary hemosiderosis.
Drugs (penicillamine).
Lymphangiogram contrast.
Mitral stenosis.

AMENORRHEA

ICD-10CM # N91.2 Amenorrhea, unspecified

PREGNANCY
Early Menopause
Hypothalamic Dysfunction
Defective synthesis or release of LHRH, anorexia nervosa, stress, exercise.

---

[*]Haidar G, Singh N: Fever of unknown origin, *N Engl J Med* 386(5):463-477, 2022.
[†]More frequent cause.
[‡]More frequent cause.

[§]Genetic transmission.
[¶]Not listed as a syndrome by ILAE but instead recognized under absence seizures with special features.
**Includes schizophrenia, schizophreniform disorder, brief reactive psychosis.

Pituitary Dysfunction
Neoplasm, postpartum hemorrhage, surgery, radiotherapy.
Ovarian Dysfunction
Gonadal dysgenesis, 17a-hydroxylase deficiency, premature ovarian failure, polycystic ovarian disease, gonadal stromal tumors.

UTEROVAGINAL ABNORMALITIES
Congenital: imperforate hymen, imperforate cervix, imperforate or absent vagina, Müllerian agenesis.
   Acquired: destruction of endometrium with curettage (Asherman syndrome), closure of cervix or vagina caused by traumatic injury, hysterectomy.

OTHER
Metabolic diseases (liver, kidney), malnutrition, rapid weight loss, exogenous obesity, endocrine abnormalities (Cushing syndrome, Graves disease, hypothyroidism).

AMNESIA

ICD-10CM # F19.96 Other psychoactive substance use, unspecified with psychoactive substance-induced persisting amnestic disorder
F44.0 Dissociative amnesia
R41.2 Retrograde amnesia
G45.4 Transient global amnesia

Degenerative diseases (e.g., Alzheimer, Huntington disease).
CVA (especially when involving thalamus, basal forebrain, and hippocampus).
Head trauma.
Postsurgical (e.g., mammillary body surgery, bilateral temporal lobectomy).
Infections (herpes simplex encephalitis, meningitis).
Wernicke-Korsakoff syndrome.
Cerebral hypoxia.
Hypoglycemia.
CNS neoplasms.
Creutzfeldt-Jakob disease.
Medications (e.g., midazolam and other benzodiazepines).
Psychosis.
Malingering.

AMNIOTIC FLUID α-FETOPROTEIN ELEVATION[21]

ICD-10CM # Z36 Encounter for antenatal screening of mother

CAUSES OF ELEVATED AMNIOTIC FLUID α-FETOPROTEIN
Craniospinal defect (open neural tube defect).
Omphalocele.
Gastroschisis.
Duodenal atresia.

Congenital nephrosis.
Cystic hygroma.
Unbalanced D/G dislocation.
Down, Tay-Sachs, Klinefelter, Turner syndromes.
Fetal tumors.
Epidermolysis bullosa.
Pilonidal sinus.
Rhesus disease.
Fetal demise.
Incorrect dates.
Multiple pregnancies.

ANAL ABSCESS AND FISTULA[2]

ICD-10CM # K61.0 Anal abscess
K61.1 Rectal abscess
K61.3 Ischiorectal abscess
K60.3 Anal fistula

Primary anal gland infection.
Secondary abscess:
   Inflammatory bowel disease:
      Crohn disease.
      Ulcerative colitis.
Infection:
   Tuberculosis.
   Actinomycosis.
   Threadworm.
Trauma.
Leukopenia.
Immunosuppression:
   HIV.
   Drugs.
Rectal cancer.
Diabetes mellitus.

ANAL INCONTINENCE[1]

ICD-10CM # R15.9 Full incontinence of feces

TRAUMATIC
Nerve injured in surgery.
Spinal cord injury.
Obstetric trauma.
Sphincter injury.

NEUROLOGIC
Spinal cord lesions.
Dementia.
Autonomic neuropathy (e.g., DM).
Obstetrics: pudendal nerve stretched during surgery.
Hirschsprung disease.

MASS EFFECT
Carcinoma of anal canal.
Carcinoma of rectum.
Foreign body.
Fecal impaction.
Hemorrhoids.

MEDICAL
Procidentia.
Inflammatory disease.

Diarrhea.
Laxative abuse.

PEDIATRIC
Congenital.
Meningocele.
Myelomeningocele.
Spina bifida.
After corrective surgery for imperforate anus.
Sexual abuse.
Encopresis.

ANAPHYLAXIS[26]

ICD-10CM # T78.2 Anaphylactic shock, unspecified, initial encounter

PULMONARY
Laryngeal edema.
Epiglottitis.
Foreign body aspiration.
Pulmonary embolus.
Asphyxiation.
Hyperventilation.

CARDIOVASCULAR
Myocardial infarction.
Arrhythmia.
Hypovolemic shock.
Cardiac arrest.

CNS
Vasovagal reaction.
CVA.
Seizure disorder.
Drug overdose.

ENDOCRINE
Hypoglycemia.
Pheochromocytoma.
Carcinoid syndrome.
Catamenial (progesterone-induced anaphylaxis).

PSYCHIATRIC
Vocal cord dysfunction syndrome.
Munchausen syndrome.
Panic attack/globus hystericus.

OTHER
Hereditary angioedema.
Cord urticaria.
Idiopathic urticaria.
Mastocytosis.
Serum sickness.
Idiopathic capillary leak syndrome.
Sulfite exposure.
Scombroid poisoning (tuna, blue fish, mackerel).

ANAPHYLAXIS MIMICS[27]

ICD-10CM # Varies with specific diagnosis

CONDITIONS THAT MIMIC ANAPHYLAXIS
Vasovagal episodes.
Acute pulmonary events:

Acute asthmatic attacks.
Acute pulmonary edema.
Pulmonary embolus.
Spontaneous pneumothorax.
Foreign body aspiration.
Acute cardiac events:
  Supraventricular tachycardias.
  Acute myocardial infarction/ischemia.
Drug overdoses.
Insulin shock.
Carcinoid attacks.

ANAPHYLAXIS, PATHOPHYSIOLOGIC CLASSIFICATION[28]

ICD-10CM # T78.2 Anaphylactic shock, unspecified, initial encounter

PATHOPHYSIOLOGIC CLASSIFICATION OF ANAPHYLAXIS

IgE Dependent, Immunologic
Foods.
Drugs.
Insect stings and bites.
Exercise (food dependent).
Other causes.
IgE Independent, Immunologic
Immune aggregates.
IgG anti-IgA.
Cytotoxic.
Disturbance of arachidonic acid metabolism:
  Aspirin.
  Other nonsteroidal antiinflammatory drugs.
Activation of kallikrein-kinin contact system:
  Dialysis membranes.
  Radiocontrast media.
Multimediator recruitment:
  Complement.
  Clotting.
  Clot lysis.
  Kallikrein-kinin contact system.
Other causes.
Nonimmunologic
Direct mediator release from mast cells and basophils:
  Drugs, e.g., opiates.
  Physical factors, e.g., cold and sunlight.
Exercise.
c-kit Mutation (D816V).
Other causes.
Idiopathic.

ANAPHYLACTOID SYNDROME OF PREGNANCY[29]

ICD-10CM # O88.113

CARDIOVASCULAR COLLAPSE, HYPOTENSION

Acute coronary syndromes, myocardial infarction.
Cardiomyopathy.
Pulmonary embolism.
Anesthesia complications, transfusion reaction.
Sepsis, systemic inflammatory response syndrome.

RESPIRATORY ARREST

Pulmonary embolism, air embolism.
Anesthesia complications, transfusion reaction.
Aspiration.

ALTERED MENTAL STATUS, SEIZURE

Eclampsia.
Cerebrovascular accident.
Hypoglycemia.

COAGULOPATHY

Disseminated intravascular coagulation.
Consumptive coagulopathy from hemorrhage.

ANDROGEN EXCESS, REPRODUCTIVE-AGE WOMAN

ICD-10CM # E28.1 Androgen excess

Polycystic ovary syndrome.
Idiopathic.
Medications (e.g., anabolizing agents, testosterone, danazol).
Pregnancy (luteoma, hyperreaction luteinalis).
Sertoli-Leydig ovarian neoplasm.
Adrenal adenoma or hyperplasia.
Cushing syndrome.
Glucocorticoid resistance.
Hypothyroidism.
Hyperprolactinemia.

ANDROGEN RESISTANCE[30]

ICD-10CM # E34.5 Androgen resistance syndrome

CONGENITAL OR DEVELOPMENTAL DISORDERS

Uncommon causes:
  Kennedy disease (spinal and bulbar muscular atrophy).
  Partial androgen insensitivity syndrome (AR mutations).
  5α-reductase type 2 deficiency.
  Complete androgen insensitivity syndrome (female phenotype).

ACQUIRED DISORDERS

Common causes:
  AR antagonists (bicalutamide, nilutamide).

Drugs (spironolactone, cyproterone acetate, marijuana, histamine 2 receptor antagonists).
Uncommon causes:
  Celiac disease.

ANEMIA, APLASTIC[31]

ICD-10CM # D61.09 Other constitutional aplastic anemia

ACQUIRED APLASTIC ANEMIA

Secondary aplastic anemia.
Irradiation.
Drugs and chemicals.
Regular effects.
Cytotoxic agents.
Benzene.
Idiosyncratic reactions.
Chloramphenicol.
Nonsteroidal antiinflammatory drugs.
Antiepileptics.
Gold.
Other drugs and chemicals.
Viruses.
Epstein-Barr virus (infectious mononucleosis).
Hepatitis virus (non-A, non-B, non-C, non-G hepatitis).
Parvovirus (transient aplastic crisis, some pure red cell aplasia).
Human immunodeficiency virus (acquired immunodeficiency syndrome).
Immune diseases.
Eosinophilic fasciitis.
Hyperimmunoglobulinemia.
Thymoma and thymic carcinoma.
Graft-versus-host disease in immunodeficiency.
Paroxysmal nocturnal hemoglobinuria.
Pregnancy.
Idiopathic aplastic anemia.

INHERITED APLASTIC ANEMIA

Fanconi anemia.
Dyskeratosis congenita.
Shwachman-Diamond syndrome.
Reticular dysgenesis.
Amegakaryocytic thrombocytopenia.
Familial aplastic anemias.
Preleukemia (e.g., monosomy 7).
Nonhematologic syndromes (e.g., Down, Dubowitz, Seckel).

ANEMIA, APLASTIC, DUE TO DRUGS AND CHEMICALS[29]

ICD-10CM # D61.1 Drug-induced aplastic anemia
             D61.2 Aplastic anemia due to other external agents

	D61.89	Other specified aplastic anemias and other bone marrow failure syndromes

Agents that regularly produce marrow depression as a major toxic effect when used in commonly employed doses or normal exposures:

Cytotoxic drugs used in cancer chemotherapy.
Alkylating agents (busulfan, melphalan, cyclophosphamide).
Antimetabolites (antifolic compounds, nucleotide analogs), antimitotics (vincristine, vinblastine, colchicine).
Some antibiotics (daunorubicin, doxorubicin [Adriamycin]).
Benzene (and less often benzene-containing chemicals; kerosene, carbon tetrachloride, Stoddard solvent, chlorophenols).

Agents probably associated with aplastic anemia but with a relatively low probability relative to their use:

Chloramphenicol.
Insecticides.
Antiprotozoals (quinacrine and chloroquine).
NSAIDs (including phenylbutazone, indomethacin, ibuprofen, sulindac, diclofenac, naproxen, piroxicam, fenoprofen, fenbufen, aspirin).
Anticonvulsants (hydantoins, carbamazepine, phenacemide, ethosuximide).
Gold, arsenic, and other heavy metals such as bismuth and mercury.
Sulfonamides as a class.
Antithyroid medications (methimazole, methylthiouracil, propylthiouracil).
Antidiabetes drugs (tolbutamide, carbutamide, chlorpropamide).
Carbonic anhydrase inhibitors (acetazolamide, methazolamide, mesalazine).
D-Penicillamine.
2-Chlorodeoxyadenosine.

Agents more rarely associated with aplastic anemia:

Antibiotics (streptomycin, tetracycline, methicillin, ampicillin, mebendazole and albendazole, sulfonamides, flucytosine, mefloquine, dapsone).
Antihistamines (cimetidine, ranitidine, chlorpheniramine).
Sedatives and tranquilizers (chlorpromazine, prochlorperazine, piperacetazine, chlordiazepoxide, meprobamate, methyprylon, remoxipride).
Antiarrhythmics (tocainide, amiodarone).
Allopurinol (can potentiate marrow suppression by cytotoxic drugs).
Ticlopidine.
Methyldopa.
Quinidine.
Lithium.
Guanidine.

Canthaxanthin.
Thiocyanate.
Carbimazole.
Cyanamide.
Deferoxamine.
Amphetamines.

ANEMIA, CAUSES IN PREGNANCY[32]

ICD-10CM #	D50.8	Other iron deficiency anemias
	D50.9	Iron deficiency anemia, unspecified
	D51.0	Vitamin B_{12} deficiency anemia due to intrinsic factor deficiency
	D51.1	Vitamin B_{12} deficiency anemia due to selective vitamin B_{12} malabsorption with proteinuria
	D51.3	Other dietary vitamin B_{12} deficiency anemia
	D51.8	Other vitamin B_{12} deficiency anemias
	D52.0	Dietary folate deficiency anemia
	D52.1	Drug-induced folate deficiency anemia
	D52.8	Other folate deficiency anemias
	D52.9	Folate deficiency anemia, unspecified
	D53.1	Other megaloblastic anemias, not elsewhere classified
	D53.0	Protein deficiency anemia
	D53.2	Scorbutic anemia
	D53.8	Other specified nutritional anemias
	D53.9	Nutritional anemia, unspecified
	D64.0	Hereditary sideroblastic anemia
	D64.1	Secondary sideroblastic anemia due to disease
	D64.2	Secondary sideroblastic anemia due to drugs and toxins
	D64.3	Other sideroblastic anemias

CAUSES OF ANEMIA DURING PREGNANCY

Common causes—85% of anemia:
  Physiologic anemia.
  Iron deficiency.
Uncommon causes:
  Folic acid deficiency.
  Vitamin B_{12} deficiency (due to the rapid increase in bariatric surgery).
  Hemoglobinopathies:
    Sickle cell disease.
    Hemoglobin SC.
    β-Thalassemia minor.
  Bariatric surgery.

GI bleeding.
Rare causes:
  Hemoglobinopathies.
  β-Thalassemia major.
  α-Thalassemia.
Syndromes of chronic hemolysis:
  Hereditary spherocytosis.
  Paroxysmal nocturnal hemoglobinuria.
Hematologic malignancy.

ANEMIA, DRUG-INDUCED[33]

ICD-10CM #	D61.1	Drug-induced aplastic anemia

DRUGS THAT MAY INTERFERE WITH RED CELL PRODUCTION BY INDUCING MARROW SUPPRESSION OR APLASIA

Alcohol.
Antineoplastic drugs.
Antithyroid drugs.
Antibiotics.
Oral hypoglycemic agents.
Phenylbutazone.
Azidothymidine (AZT).

DRUGS THAT INTERFERE WITH VITAMIN B_{12}, FOLATE, OR IRON ABSORPTION OR UTILIZATION

Nitrous oxide.
Anticonvulsant drugs.
Antineoplastic drugs.
Isoniazid.
Cycloserine A.

DRUGS CAPABLE OF PROMOTING HEMOLYSIS

Immune Mediated
Penicillins.
Quinine.
α-methyldopa.
Procainamide.
Mitomycin C.
Oxidative Stress
Antimalarials.
Sulfonamide drugs.
Nalidixic acid.

DRUGS THAT MAY PRODUCE OR PROMOTE BLOOD LOSS

Aspirin.
Alcohol.
Nonsteroidal antiinflammatory agents.
Corticosteroids.
Anticoagulants.

ANEMIA, HYPOCHROMIC[31]

ICD-10CM #	D50.8	Other Iron deficiency anemias
	D50.9	Iron deficiency anemia, unspecified
	D64.0	Hereditary sideroblastic anemia

D64.1	Secondary sideroblastic anemia due to disease
D64.2	Secondary sideroblastic anemia due to drugs and toxins
D64.3	Other sideroblastic anemias

DECREASED BODY IRON STORES

Iron deficiency anemia.

NORMAL OR INCREASED BODY IRON STORES

Impaired iron metabolism.

Anemia of chronic disease.

Defective absorption, transport, or use of iron.

Disorders of globin synthesis:

Thalassemia.

Other microcytic hemoglobinopathies.

Disorders of heme synthesis: sideroblastic anemias:

Hereditary.

Acquired.

ANEMIA, LOW RETICULOCYTE COUNT[18]

ICD-10CM # D64.9 Anemia, unspecified

MICROCYTIC ANEMIA (MCV <80)

Iron deficiency.

Thalassemia minor.

Sideroblastic anemia.

Lead poisoning.

MACROCYTIC ANEMIA (MCV >100)

Megaloblastic anemias.

Folate deficiency.

Vitamin B_{12} deficiency.

Drug-induced megaloblastic anemia.

Nonmegaloblastic macrocytosis.

Liver disease.

Hypothyroidism.

NORMOCYTIC ANEMIA (MCV 80-100)

Early iron deficiency.

Aplastic anemia.

Myelophthisic disorders.

Endocrinopathies.

Anemia of chronic disease.

Uremia.

Mixed nutritional deficiency.

ANEMIA, MEGALOBLASTIC[17]

ICD-10CM #	D51.0	Vitamin B_{12} deficiency anemia due to intrinsic factor deficiency
	D51.1	Vitamin B_{12} deficiency anemia due to selective vitamin B_{12} malabsorption with proteinuria

D51.3	Other dietary vitamin B_{12} deficiency anemia
D51.8	Other vitamin B_{12} deficiency anemias
D52.0	Dietary folate deficiency anemia
D52.1	Drug-induced folate deficiency anemia
D52.8	Other folate deficiency anemias
D52.9	Folate deficiency anemia, unspecified
D53.1	Other megaloblastic anemias, not elsewhere classified
D53.0	Protein deficiency anemia
D53.2	Scorbutic anemia
D53.8	Other specified nutritional anemias
D53.9	Nutritional anemia, unspecified

COBALAMIN (CBL) DEFICIENCY

Nutritional CBL Deficiency (Insufficient CBL Intake)

Vegetarians, vegans, breastfed infants of mothers with pernicious anemia.

Abnormal Intragastric Events (Inadequate Proteolysis of Food CBL)

Atrophic gastritis, partial gastrectomy with hypochlorhydria.

Loss/Atrophy of Gastric Oxyntic Mucosa (Deficient Intrinsic Factor [IF] Molecules)

Total or partial gastrectomy, pernicious anemia (PA), caustic destruction (lye).

Abnormal Events in Small Bowel Lumen

Inadequate pancreatic protease (R-CBL not degraded, CBL not transferred to IF).

Insufficiency of pancreatic protease—pancreatic insufficiency.

Inactivation of pancreatic protease—Zollinger-Ellison syndrome.

Usurping of luminal CBL (inadequate CBL binding to IF).

By bacteria—stasis syndromes (blind loops, pouches of diverticulosis, strictures, fistulas, anastomoses); impaired bowel motility (scleroderma, pseudoobstruction), hypogammaglobulinemia.

By *Diphyllobothrium latum.*

Disorders of Ileal Mucosa/IF Receptors (IF-CBL not Bound to IF Receptors)

Diminished or absent IF receptors—ileal bypass/resection/fistula.

Abnormal mucosal architecture/function—tropical/nontropical sprue, Crohn disease, TB ileitis, infiltration by lymphomas, amyloidosis.

IF-/post IF-receptor defects—Imerslund-Gräsbeck syndrome, TC II deficiency.

Drug-induced effects (slow K, biguanides, cholestyramine, colchicine, neomycin, PAS).

DISORDERS OF PLASMA CBL TRANSPORT (TC II-CBL NOT DELIVERED TO TC II RECEPTORS)

Congenital TC II deficiency, defective binding of TC II-CBL to TC II receptors (rare).

METABOLIC DISORDERS (CBL NOT UTILIZED BY CELL)

Inborn enzyme errors (rare).

Acquired disorders: (CBL oxidized to cob[III]alamin)—N_2O inhalation.

FOLATE DEFICIENCY

Nutritional Causes

Decreased dietary intake—poverty and famine (associated with kwashiorkor, marasmus), institutionalized individuals (psychiatric/nursing homes), chronic debilitating disease/goats' milk (low in folate), special diets (slimming), cultural/ethnic cooking techniques (food folate destroyed) or habits (folate-rich foods not consumed).

Decreased diet and increased requirements:

Physiologic: pregnancy and lactation, prematurity, infancy.

Pathologic: intrinsic hematologic disease (autoimmune hemolytic disease), drugs, malaria; hemoglobinopathies (SS, thalassemia), RBC membrane defects (hereditary spherocytosis, paroxysmal nocturnal hemoglobinopathy); abnormal hematopoiesis (leukemia/lymphoma, myelodysplastic syndrome, agnogenic myeloid metaplasia with myelofibrosis); infiltration with malignant disease; dermatologic (psoriasis).

Folate Malabsorption

With normal intestinal mucosa:

Some drugs (controversial).

Congenital folate malabsorption (rare).

With mucosal abnormalities—tropical and nontropical sprue, regional enteritis.

Defective Cellular Folate Uptake—Familial Aplastic Anemia (Rare), Inadequate Cellular Utilization

Folate antagonists (methotrexate).

Hereditary enzyme deficiencies involving folate.

Drugs (Multiple Effects on Folate Metabolism)

Alcohol, sulfasalazine, triamterene, pyrimethamine, trimethoprim-sulfamethoxazole, diphenylhydantoin, barbiturates.

MISCELLANEOUS MEGALOBLASTIC ANEMIAS (NOT CAUSED BY CBL OR FOLATE DEFICIENCY)

Congenital Disorders of DNA Synthesis (Rare)

Orotic aciduria, Lesch-Nyhan syndrome, congenital dyserythropoietic anemia.

Acquired Disorders of DNA Synthesis

Thiamine-responsive megaloblastosis (rare).

Malignancy—erythroleukemia—refractory sideroblastic anemias—all antineoplastic drugs that inhibit DNA synthesis.

Toxins: alcohol.

ANEMIA, MICROCYTIC, HYPOCHROMIC, DIFFERENTIAL DIAGNOSIS[34]

ICD-10CM #	D50.8	Other iron deficiency anemias
	D50.9	Iron deficiency anemia, unspecified
	D64.0	Hereditary sideroblastic anemia
	D64.1	Secondary sideroblastic anemia due to disease
	D64.2	Secondary sideroblastic anemia due to drugs and toxins
	D64.3	Other sideroblastic anemias

DIFFERENTIAL DIAGNOSIS OF MICROCYTIC HYPOCHROMIC ANEMIA

Decreased Body Iron Stores
Iron deficiency anemia.
Normal or Increased Body Iron Stores
Anemia of chronic disease.
Defective absorption, transport, or use of iron.
Iron-refractory, iron deficiency anemia after parenteral iron.
Atransferrinemia.
Aceruloplasminemia.
Divalent metal transporter 1 (DMT1 or SLC11A2) deficiency.
Ferroportin-associated hemochromatosis with impaired iron export (type 4A).
Heme oxygenase 1 deficiency.
Disorders of globin synthesis.

Decreased Body Iron Stores
Thalassemia.
  Other microcytic hemoglobinopathies.
  Disorders of heme synthesis.
Sideroblastic anemias.
  Hereditary.
  Acquired.

ANERGY, CUTANEOUS[17]

ICD-10CM #	D89.9	Disorder involving the immune mechanism, unspecified

IMMUNOLOGIC

Acquired (AIDS, acute leukemia, carcinoma, CLL, Hodgkin lymphoma, NHL).
Congenital (ataxia-telangiectasia, Di George syndrome, severe combined immunodeficiency, Wiskott-Aldrich syndrome).

INFECTIONS

Bacterial (bacterial pneumonia, brucellosis).
Disseminated mycotic infections.
Mycobacterial (lepromatous leprosy, TB).
Viral (varicella, hepatitis, influenza, mononucleosis, measles, mumps).

IMMUNOSUPPRESSIVE MEDICATIONS

Systemic corticosteroids.
Methotrexate, cyclophosphamide.
Rifampin.

OTHER

Alcoholic cirrhosis, biliary cirrhosis, sarcoidosis, rheumatic disease.
Diabetes, Crohn disease, uremia.
Anemia, pyridoxine deficiency, sickle cell anemia.
Burns, malnutrition, pregnancy, old age, surgery.

ANEURYSMS, THORACIC AORTA

ICD-10CM #	I71.2	Thoracic aortic aneurysm, without rupture

Trauma.
Infection.
Inflammatory (syphilis, Takayasu disease).
Collagen vascular disease (RA, ankylosing spondylitis).
Annuloaortic ectasia (Marfan syndrome, Ehlers-Danlos syndrome).
Congenital.
Coarctation.
Cystic medial necrosis.

ANHIDROSIS

ICD-10CM #	L74.0	Miliaria rubra
	L74.1	Miliaria crystallina
	L74.2	Miliaria profunda

Drugs (anticholinergics).
Dehydration.
Hysteria.
Obstruction of sweat ducts (e.g., inflammation, miliaria).
Local radiant heat or pressure.
CNS lesions (medulla, hypothalamus, pons).
Spinal cord lesions.
Lesions of sympathetic nerves.
Congenital sweat gland disturbances.

ANION GAP ACIDOSIS[7]

ICD-10CM #	E87.2	Acidosis

CLINICAL CAUSES OF HIGH ANION GAP AND NORMAL ANION GAP ACIDOSIS

High Anion Gap
Ketoacidosis:
  Diabetic ketoacidosis (acetoacetate).
  Alcoholic (β-hydroxybutyrate).
  Starvation.
Lactic acid acidosis:
  L-Lactic acid acidosis (types A and B).
  D-Lactic acid acidosis.
Renal failure: sulfate, phosphate, urate, hippurate.
Ingestions (toxins and their metabolites):

Ethylene glycol → glycolate, oxalate.
Methyl alcohol → formate.
Salicylate → ketones, lactate, salicylate.
Paraldehyde → organic anions.
Toluene → hippurate (commonly presents with normal anion gap).
Propylene glycol → lactate.
Pyroglutamic acidosis (acetaminophen use) → 5-oxoproline.
Normal Anion Gap
GI loss of HCO_3- (negative urine anion gap):
  Diarrhea.
  Fistula, external.
Renal loss of HCO_3- or failure to excrete NH_4^+ (positive urine anion gap):
  Proximal renal tubular acidosis (RTA type 2).
  Acetazolamide.
  Classic distal renal tubular acidosis (low serum K^+) RTA type 1.
  Generalized distal renal tubular defect (high serum K^+) RTA type 4.
Miscellaneous:
  NH_4Cl ingestion.
  Sulfur ingestion.
  Dilutional acidosis.
  Late stages in treatment of diabetic ketoacidosis.

ANION GAP INCREASE

ICD-10CM #	E87.8	Other disorders of electrolyte and fluid balance, not elsewhere classified

Uremia.
Ketoacidosis (diabetic, starvation, alcoholic).
Lactic acidosis.
Ethylene glycol poisoning.
Salicylate overdose.
Methanol poisoning.

ANISOCORIA

ICD-10CM #	H57.02	Anisocoria

Mydriatic or miotic drugs.
Prosthetic eye.
Inflammation (keratitis, iridocyclitis).
Infections (herpes zoster, syphilis, meningitis, encephalitis, TB, diphtheria, botulism).
Subdural hemorrhage.
Cavernous sinus thrombosis.
Intracranial neoplasm.
Cerebral aneurysm.
Glaucoma.
CNS degenerative diseases.
Internal carotid ischemia.
Toxic polyneuritis (alcohol, lead).
Adie syndrome.
Horner syndrome.
DM.
Trauma.
Congenital.

ANKLE AND FOOT PAIN[35]

ICD-10CM # M25.579 Pain in unspecified ankle and joint pain in unspecified foot

Anterior ankle:	Anterior impingement.
	Ankle arthritis or synovitis.
	Osteochondral defect or lesion (cartilage injury).
	Loose body within the joint.
	Talar avascular necrosis.
	Talar stress fracture.
	Tenosynovitis of the extensor hallucis longus, extensor digitorum longus.
	Deep (central) or superficial (anterolateral) peroneal nerve injury.
	Saphenous (anteromedial) nerve injury.
Posterior ankle:	Os trigonum (accessory ossicle involving the posterior lateral tubercle of the talus).
	Posterior impingement.
	Retrocalcaneal bursitis.
	Achilles tendinopathy.
	Flexor hallucis longus tendinopathy or stenosis.
Posterolateral ankle:	Peroneal tendinopathy.
	Subfibular impingement caused by flatfoot and impingement.
	Fibular stress fracture.
	Sural nerve injury.
	Lateral ligament injury (sprain).
Posteromedial ankle:	Posterior tibial tendinopathy.
	Flexor digitorum longus or flexor hallucis longus tendinopathy.
	Tibial stress fracture.
	Medial malleolar stress fracture.
	Tarsal tunnel syndrome.
	Tibial nerve injury.
	Deltoid ligament injury.
Heel:	Achilles insertional tendinopathy.
	Inflammatory enthesitis.
	Plantar fasciitis.
	Haglund disease (pump bump).
	Calcaneal stress fracture.
Hindfoot:	Subtalar, talonavicular, or calcaneocuboid arthritis or synovitis.
	Posterior tibial tendon dysfunction or tendinopathy (medial) or peroneal tendon dysfunction (lateral).
	Occult fracture of the talus, calcaneus cuboid, or navicular.
	Accessory navicular.
Midfoot:	Insertional tendinopathy (peroneal, posterior tibial, tibialis anterior).
	Arthritis or synovitis (navicular–cuneiform, cuneiform–metatarsal, cuboid–metatarsal).
	Navicular stress fracture.
	Spring ligament strain.
Forefoot	
First ray, first MTP joint, hallux:	Arthritis or synovitis MTP (hallux limitus/rigidus) and IP joints.
	Hallux valgus.
	Hallux varus.
	Sesamoiditis.
	Gouty monoarthritis.
Second to fifth rays, MTP joints, lesser toes:	Arthritis or synovitis (MTP, proximal and distal IP joints).
	Lesser toe deformities (hammer and claw toes).
	Metatarsalgia.
	MTP instability.
	MTP dislocations.
	Morton neuroma (interdigital neuralgia).
	Stress fracture of the metatarsals.
	Bunionette (fifth metatarsal phalangeal deviation).
	Rheumatoid nodules.
	Bursitis (intermetatarsal or adventitious).
	Ulcer.
	Infection.

IP, Interphalangeal; *MTP*, metatarsophalangeal.

ANORECTAL ABSCESS[4]

ICD-10CM # K61.2 Anorectal abscess

ETIOLOGY OF ANORECTAL ABSCESS

Nonspecific Etiology
Cryptoglandular.
Specific Etiology
Inflammatory condition.
Crohn disease.
Tuberculosis.
Actinomycosis.
Lymphogranuloma venereum.
Traumatic Etiology
Impalement.
Foreign body.
Anal fissure.
Iatrogenic.
Episiotomy.
Hemorrhoidectomy.
Prostatectomy.
Radiation.
Malignancy
Rectal or anal carcinoma.
Leukemia.
Lymphoma.

ANORECTAL DISEASE, AIDS PATIENT[3]

ICD-10CM # Varies with specific diagnosis

DIFFERENTIAL DIAGNOSIS OF ANORECTAL DISEASE IN PATIENTS WITH AIDS
Infections
Bacteria
*Chlamydia trachomatis.**
Lymphogranuloma venereum.
*Neisseria gonorrhoeae.**
Shigella flexneri.
Mycobacterium tuberculosis.
Protozoa
Entamoeba histolytica.
   Leishmania donovani.
Viruses
HSV.*
Cytomegalovirus.*
Fungi
Candida albicans.
Histoplasma capsulatum.
Neoplasms
Lymphoma.*
   Kaposi sarcoma.
   Squamous cell carcinoma.
   Cloacogenic carcinoma.
   Condyloma acuminatum.
Other
Idiopathic ulcers.*
Perirectal abscess, fistula.*

*More frequent diagnosis.

ANOREXIA[2]

ICD-10CM # R63.0 Anorexia

SELECTED CAUSES OF ANOREXIA
Gastrointestinal Tract/Liver
Gastric outlet obstruction or small bowel obstruction.
Gastric cancer.
Hepatic metastases.
Acute viral hepatitis.
Metabolic
Addison disease.
Hypopituitarism.
Hyperparathyroidism.
Functional
Extremely unpleasant sight/smell.
Systemic
Chronic pain.
Renal failure.
Severe congestive heart failure.
Respiratory failure.
Psychiatric
Depression.
Anorexia nervosa.
Medications
Digoxin.
Narcotic analgesics.

Diuretics.
Antihypertensives.
Chemotherapeutic agents.
Amphetamines.
Miscellaneous
Excessive smoking.
Excessive alcohol intake.
Oral cavity disease.
Thiamine deficiency.
Early pregnancy.
Hypogeusia or dysgeusia.

ANOVULATION

ICD-10CM # N97.0 Female infertility associated with anovulation

Anorexia and bulimia.
Strenuous exercise.
Weight loss/malnutrition.
Empty sella syndrome.
Pituitary disorders (infarction, infection, trauma, irradiation, surgery, microadenomas, macroadenomas).
Idiopathic hypopituitarism.
Drug induced.
Thyroid dysfunction (hypothyroidism, hyperthyroidism).
Systemic diseases (e.g., liver disease).
Adrenal hyperfunction (Cushing syndrome, congenital adrenal hyperplasia).
Polycystic ovarian syndrome.
Isolated gonadotropin deficiency.

ANOVULATION, HYPOTHALAMIC PITUITARY CAUSES[36]

ICD-10CM # N97.0 Female infertility associated with anovulation

CLASSIFICATION OF ANOVULATION CAUSED BY DISORDERS OF THE HYPOTHALAMIC-PITUITARY UNIT

Functional hypothalamic anovulation (amenorrhea):
Stress (psychogenic or physical).
Dieting.
Vigorous exercise.
Chronic illness (e.g., chronic liver or renal insufficiency, AIDS).
Psychiatric-medical emergencies:
Anorexia nervosa.
Medications:
Antipsychotics (e.g., olanzapine, risperidone, amisulpride, clozapine).
Opiates.
Hypothyroidism.

ANATOMICALLY OR GENETICALLY DEFINED PATHOLOGIC CONDITIONS OF THE HYPOTHALAMIC-PITUITARY UNIT

Pituitary tumors.
Prolactinoma.
Clinically nonfunctioning adenoma.
GH-secreting adenoma (acromegaly).
ACTH-secreting adenoma (Cushing disease).
Other pituitary tumors (e.g., metastasis, meningioma).
Pituitary stalk section.
Hemorrhagic pituitary destruction, including pituitary apoplexy and Sheehan syndrome.
Pituitary aneurysm.
Infiltrative disease of the pituitary (e.g., lymphocytic hypophysitis, sarcoidosis, histiocytosis X, tuberculosis).
Empty sella syndrome.
Tumors that affect hypothalamic function (e.g., metastasis, craniopharyngioma).
Infiltrative granulomatous disease of the hypothalamus (e.g., sarcoidosis, histiocytosis X, tuberculosis).
Head trauma.
Irradiation to the head.
CNS infection.
Isolated gonadotropin deficiency (including Kallmann syndrome).
Other.

ACTH, Adrenocorticotropic hormone; *AIDS,* acquired immunodeficiency syndrome; *CNS,* central nervous system; *GH,* growth hormone.

AORTIC ARCH SEGMENT ABNORMALITIES[37]

ICD-10CM # Q25.49 Other congenital malformations of aorta

DIFFERENTIAL DIAGNOSIS OF AORTIC ARCH SEGMENT ABNORMALITIES

Dilated aortic arch:
Aortic aneurysm.
Aortic dissection.
Aortic pseudoaneurysm.
Mass silhouetting aortic arch.
Small or inapparent arch:
Right-sided aortic arch.
Coarctation of the aorta.
Interruption of the aortic arch.
Double aortic arch.

APPENDICITIS, DIFFERENTIAL DIAGNOSIS IN PREGNANCY[32]

ICD-10CM # Varies with specific diagnosis

DIFFERENTIAL DIAGNOSIS OF APPENDICITIS DURING PREGNANCY

Gynecologic Conditions
Ruptured ovarian cyst.
Adnexal torsion.
Pelvic inflammatory disease or salpingitis.
Endometriosis.
Ovarian cancer.
Obstetrical Causes
Abruptio placentae.
Chorioamnionitis.
Endometritis.
Uterine fibroid degeneration.
Labor (preterm or term).
Viscus perforation after abortion.
Ruptured ectopic pregnancy.
Gastrointestinal Causes
Crohn disease.
Colonic diverticulitis (right side).
Cholecystitis.
Pancreatitis.
Mesenteric lymphadenitis.
Gastroenteritis.
Colon cancer.
Intestinal obstruction.
Hernia (incarcerated inguinal or internal).
Colonic intussusception.
Ruptured Meckel diverticulum.
Colonic perforation.
Acute mesenteric ischemia.
Other Causes
Pyelonephritis.
Urolithiasis.

APPETITE LOSS IN INFANTS AND CHILDREN[23]

ICD-10CM # R63.0 Anorexia
F50.8 Other eating disorders
F98.29 Other feeding disorders of infancy and early childhood

ORGANIC DISEASE

Infection (Acute or Chronic) Neurologic
Congenital degenerative disease.
Hypothalamic lesion.
Increased intracranial pressure (including a brain tumor).
Swallowing disorders (neuromuscular).
Gastrointestinal
Oral lesions (e.g., thrush or herpes simplex).
Gastroesophageal reflux.
Obstruction (especially with gastric or intestinal distention).
Inflammatory bowel disease.
Celiac disease.
Constipation.

Cardiac
Congestive heart failure (especially associated with cyanotic lesions).
Metabolic
Renal failure and/or renal tubule acidosis.
Liver failure.
Congenital metabolic disease.
Lead poisoning.
Nutritional
Marasmus.
Iron deficiency.
Zinc deficiency.
Fever
RA.
Rheumatic fever.
Drugs
Morphine.
Digitalis.
Antimetabolites.
Methylphenidate.
Amphetamines.
Miscellaneous
Prolonged restriction of oral feedings, beginning in the neonatal period.
Systemic lupus erythematosus (SLE).
Tumor.

PSYCHOLOGIC FACTORS

Anxiety, fear, depression, mania (limbic influence on the hypothalamus).
Avoidance of symptoms associated with meals (abdominal pain, diarrhea, bloating, urgency, dumping syndrome).
Anorexia nervosa.
Excessive weight loss and food aversion in athletes, simulating anorexia nervosa.

AQUEDUCTAL STENOSIS, CONGENITAL[38]

ICD-10CM #　Varies with specific diagnosis

CAUSES OF CONGENITAL AQUEDUCTAL STENOSIS

Genetic or Presumed Genetic Causes
Holoprosencephaly.
Chiari II malformation.
X-linked hydrocephalus with aqueductal stenosis and pachygyria.
Autosomal recessive hydrocephalus with aqueductal stenosis.
Mutation of dorsalizing gene in vertical axis of neural tube.
Agenesis of mesencephalic and metencephalic neuromeres.
Primary defective ependymal and choroid plexus epithelia.
Acquired Causes in Utero
Intraventricular hemorrhage with thrombus in aqueduct.
Congenital infections (e.g., cytomegalovirus infection, mumps).

Ependymitis/ventriculitis with gliosis around and within aqueduct.
Chronic arachnoiditis.
Hydranencephaly.
Aqueductal membrane across lumen.
Amnion rupture sequence.
Aneurysms, venous angiomas, and other vascular malformations.
Cystic dilation of perivascular Virchow-Robin spaces in midbrain.
Tumors of aqueduct (e.g., ependymoma, astrocytoma, glioneuronal hamartoma, neuroepithelial tumor of subcommissural organ).
Tumors that compress the midbrain tectum from above (e.g., pineal tumors and cysts, arachnoidal cysts, lipomas).

ARTERIAL OCCLUSION[39]

ICD-10CM #　I74.3　Embolism and thrombosis of arteries of the lower extremities
　　　　　　　I74.2　Embolism and thrombosis of arteries of the upper extremities

Thromboembolism (post-MI, mitral stenosis, rheumatic valve disease, atrial fibrillation, atrial myxoma, marantic endocarditis, bacterial endocarditis, Libman-Sacks endocarditis).
Atheroembolism (microemboli composed of cholesterol, calcium, and platelets from proximal atherosclerotic plaques).
Arterial thrombosis (endothelial injury, altered arterial blood flow, trauma, severe atherosclerosis, acute vasculitis).
Vasospasm.
Trauma.
Hypercoagulable states.
Miscellaneous (irradiation, drugs, infections, necrotizing).

ARTHRITIS AND ABDOMINAL PAIN

ICD-10CM #　M00.9　Pyogenic arthritis, unspecified
　　　　　　　R10.817　Generalized abdominal tenderness
　　　　　　　M02.9　Reactive arthropathy

Viral syndrome.
Inflammatory bowel disease.
Celiac disease.
Vasculitis.
SLE.
RA.
Scleroderma.
Amyloidosis.
Chronic hepatitis C.
Whipple disease.
Polyarteritis nodosa.
Behçet disease.

Familial Mediterranean fever.
Blind loop syndrome.
Babesiosis.
Lyme disease.
Ehrlichiosis.

ARTHRITIS AND DIARRHEA

ICD-10CM #　M00.9　Pyogenic arthritis, unspecified
　　　　　　　R19.7　Diarrhea, unspecified

Viral syndrome.
Inflammatory bowel disease.
Celiac disease.
Whipple disease.
Enterogenic (bacterial) reactive arthritis.
Collagenous colitis.
Behçet disease.
Hyperthyroidism.
Spondyloarthropathy.
Blind loop syndrome.

ARTHRITIS AND EYE LESIONS[40]

ICD-10CM #　M00.9　Pyogenic arthritis, unspecified
　　　　　　　M02.3　Reiter disease
　　　　　　　M02.9　Reactive arthropathy

SLE.
Sjögren syndrome.
Behçet syndrome.
Sarcoidosis.
Subacute bacterial endocarditis (SBE).
Lyme disease.
Granulomatosis with polyangiitis.
Giant cell arteritis.
Takayasu arteritis.
RA, JRA.
Scleroderma.
Inflammatory bowel disease.
Whipple disease.
Ankylosing spondylitis.
Reactive arthritis.
Psoriatic arthritis.

ARTHRITIS AND HEART MURMUR[40]

ICD-10CM #　M00.9　Pyogenic arthritis, unspecified
　　　　　　　I01.8　Other acute rheumatic heart disease
　　　　　　　M02.9　Reactive arthropathy

SBE.
Cardiac myxoma.
Ankylosing spondylitis.
Reactive arthritis.
Acute rheumatic fever.
RA.
SLE with Libman-Sacks endocarditis.
Relapsing polychondritis.

ARTHRITIS AND MUSCLE WEAKNESS[41]

ICD-10CM #	M00.9	Pyogenic arthritis, unspecified
	M62.9	Disorder of muscle, unspecified
	M02.9	Reactive arthropathy

RA.
Ankylosing spondylitis.
Polymyositis.
Dermatomyositis.
SLE, scleroderma, mixed connective tissue disease.
Sarcoidosis.
HIV-associated arthritis.
Whipple disease.

ARTHRITIS AND RASH[40]

ICD-10CM #	M00.9	Pyogenic arthritis, unspecified
	R21	Rash and other nonspecific skin eruption
	M02.9	Reactive arthropathy

Chronic urticaria.
Vasculitic urticaria.
SLE.
Dermatomyositis.
Polymyositis.
Psoriatic arthritis.
Reactive arthritis.
Chronic sarcoidosis.
Serum sickness.
Sweet syndrome.
Leprosy.

ARTHRITIS AND SUBCUTANEOUS NODULES[40]

ICD-10CM #	M00.9	Pyogenic arthritis, unspecified
	A18.4	Tuberculosis of skin and subcutaneous tissue
	M02.9	Reactive arthropathy

RA.
Gout.
Pseudogout (rare).
Sarcoidosis.
Light chain (LA) amyloidosis (primary, multiple myeloma).
Acute rheumatic fever (ARF).
Hemochromatosis.
Whipple disease.
Multicentric reticulohistiocytosis.

ARTHRITIS AND WEIGHT LOSS[40]

ICD-10CM #	M00.9	Pyogenic arthritis, unspecified
	R63.4	Abnormal weight loss
	M02.9	Reactive arthropathy

Severe RA.
RA with vasculitis.
Reactive arthritis.
RA or psoriatic arthritis or ankylosing spondylitis with amyloidosis.
Cancer.
Enteropathic arthritis (Crohn, ulcerative colitis).
HIV infection.
Whipple disease.
Blind loop syndrome.
Scleroderma with intestinal bacterial overgrowth.

ARTHRITIS OR EXTREMITY PAIN, IN CHILDREN AND ADOLESCENTS[19]

| ICD-10CM # | M02.9 | Reactive arthropathy |

CAUSES OF ARTHRITIS OR EXTREMITY PAIN IN CHILDREN AND ADOLESCENTS

Rheumatic and Inflammatory Diseases
Juvenile idiopathic arthritis.
Systemic lupus erythematosus.
Juvenile dermatomyositis.
Polyarteritis.
Vasculitis.
Scleroderma.
Sjögren syndrome.
Behçet disease.
Overlap syndromes.
Granulomatosis with polyangiitis (Wegener granulomatosis).
Sarcoidosis.
Kawasaki syndrome.
Henoch-Schönlein purpura.
Chronic recurrent multifocal osteomyelitis.
Seronegative Spondyloarthropathies
Juvenile ankylosing spondylitis.
Inflammatory bowel disease.
Psoriatic arthritis.
Reactive arthritis associated with urethritis, iridocyclitis, and mucocutaneous lesions.
Infectious Illnesses
Bacterial arthritis (septic arthritis, *Staphylococcus aureus*, pneumococcus, gonococcus, *Haemophilus influenzae*).
Lyme disease.
Viral illness (parvovirus, rubella, mumps, Epstein-Barr virus, hepatitis B).
Fungal arthritis.
Mycobacterial infection.
Spirochetal infection.
Endocarditis.
Reactive Arthritis
Acute rheumatic fever.
Reactive arthritis (postinfectious due to *Shigella*, *Salmonella*, *Yersinia*, *Chlamydia*, or meningococcus).
Serum sickness.
Toxic synovitis of the hip.
Postimmunization.
Immunodeficiencies
Hypogammaglobulinemia.

Immunoglobulin A deficiency.
Human immunodeficiency virus.
Congenital and Metabolic Disorders
Gout.
Pseudogout.
Mucopolysaccharidoses.
Thyroid disease (hypothyroidism, hyperthyroidism).
Hyperparathyroidism.
Vitamin C deficiency (scurvy).
Hereditary connective tissue disease (Marfan syndrome, Ehlers-Danlos syndrome).
Fabry disease.
Farber disease.
Amyloidosis (familial Mediterranean fever).
Bone and Cartilage Disorders
Trauma.
Patellofemoral syndrome.
Hypermobility syndrome.
Osteochondritis dissecans.
Avascular necrosis (including Legg-Calvé-Perthes disease).
Hypertrophic osteoarthropathy.
Slipped capital femoral epiphysis.
Osteolysis.
Benign bone tumors (including osteoid osteoma).
Histiocytosis.
Rickets.
Neuropathic Disorders
Peripheral neuropathies.
Carpal tunnel syndrome.
Charcot joints.
Neoplastic Disorders
Leukemia.
Neuroblastoma.
Lymphoma.
Bone tumors (osteosarcoma, Ewing sarcoma).
Histiocytic syndromes.
Synovial tumors.
Hematologic Disorders
Hemophilia.
Hemoglobinopathies (including sickle cell disease).
Miscellaneous Disorders
Pigmented villonodular synovitis.
Plant-thorn synovitis (foreign body arthritis).
Myositis ossificans.
Eosinophilic fasciitis.
Tendinitis (overuse injury).
Raynaud phenomenon.
Pain Syndromes
Fibromyalgia.
Growing pains.
Depression (with somatization).
Reflex sympathetic dystrophy.
Regional myofascial pain syndromes.

ARTHRITIS, AXIAL SKELETON

| ICD-10CM # | M45.9 | Ankylosing spondylitis of unspecified sites in spine |
| | L40.54 | Psoriatic juvenile arthropathy |

Differential Diagnosis

II

	L40.59	Other psoriatic arthropathy
	M15.9	Polyosteoarthritis, unspecified
	M45.9	Ankylosing spondylitis of unspecified sites in spine

RA.

Psoriatic arthritis.

Reiter syndrome (reactive arthritis).

Ankylosing spondylitis.

Juvenile RA.

Degenerative disease of the nucleus pulposus.

Spondylosis deformans.

Diffuse idiopathic skeletal hyperostosis (DISH).

Alkaptonuria.

Infection.

ARTHRITIS, CHRONIC, MONOARTICULAR OR OLIGOARTICULAR, INFECTIOUS CAUSES[42]

ICD-10CM # Varies with specific diagnosis

INFECTIOUS CAUSES OF CHRONIC MONOARTICULAR OR OLIGOARTICULAR ARTHRITIS

Bacterial

Borrelia burgdorferi.

Tropheryma whipplei.

Treponema pallidum.

Nocardia spp.

Fungi

Candida spp.

Cryptococcus neoformans.

Blastomyces dermatitidis.

Coccidioides spp.

Paracoccidioides brasiliensis.

Sporothrix schenckii.

Aspergillus spp. and other molds, including *Rhizopus, Scedosporium,* and *Fusarium.*

Mycobacteria

Mycobacterium tuberculosis.

M. kansasii.

M. marinum.

M. avium-intracellulare complex.

M. terrae.

M. fortuitum, M. chelonae, M. abscessus.

M. haemophilum.

M. leprae.

Parasites

Helminths.

Filariae.

ARTHRITIS, FEVER, AND RASH[40]

ICD-10CM #	M00.9	Pyogenic arthritis, unspecified
	M02.9	Reactive arthropathy

	R21	Rash and other nonspecific skin eruption
	R50.9	Fever, unspecified

Rubella, parvovirus B19.

Gonococcemia, meningococcemia.

Secondary syphilis, Lyme borreliosis.

Adult acute rheumatic fever, adult Still disease, adult Kawasaki disease.

Vasculitic urticaria.

Acute sarcoidosis.

Familial Mediterranean fever.

Hyperimmunoglobulinemia D and periodic fever syndrome.

ARTHRITIS, MONOARTICULAR AND OLIGOARTICULAR[43]

ICD-10CM #	M19.90	Unspecified osteoarthritis, unspecified site
	M01.X0	Direct infection of unspecified joint in infectious and parasitic diseases classified elsewhere
	M13.10	Monoarthritis, not elsewhere classified, unspecified site

Septic arthritis (*S. aureus, Neisseria gonor- rhoeae,* meningococci, streptococci, *Strepto- coccus pneumoniae,* enteric gram-negative bacilli).

Crystalline-induced arthritis (gout, pseudogout, calcium oxalate, hydroxyapatite and other basic calcium/phosphate crystals).

Traumatic joint injury.

Hemarthrosis.

Monoarticular or oligoarticular flare of an in- flammatory polyarticular rheumatic disease (RA, psoriatic arthritis, Reiter syndrome [reactive arthritis], SLE).

ARTHRITIS, PEDIATRIC AGE[23]

ICD-10CM #	M01.X0	Direct infection of unspecified joint in infectious and parasitic diseases classified elsewhere
	M08.00	Unspecified juvenile rheumatoid arthritis of unspecified site
	M08.3	Juvenile rheumatoid polyarthritis (seronegative)
	M08.40	Pauciarticular juvenile rheumatoid arthritis, unspecified site

RHEUMATIC DISEASES OF CHILDHOOD

Acute rheumatic fever.

SLE.

Juvenile ankylosing spondylitis.

Polymyositis and dermatomyositis.

Vasculitis.

Scleroderma.

Psoriatic arthritis.

Mixed connective tissue disease and overlap syndromes.

Kawasaki disease.

Behçet syndrome.

Familial Mediterranean fever.

Reiter syndrome (reactive arthritis).

Reflex sympathetic dystrophy.

Fibromyalgia (fibrositis).

INFECTIOUS DISEASES

Bacterial arthritis.

Viral or postviral arthritis.

Fungal arthritis.

Osteomyelitis.

Reactive arthritis.

NEOPLASTIC DISEASES

Leukemia.

Lymphoma.

Neuroblastoma.

Primary bone tumors.

NONINFLAMMATORY DISORDERS

Trauma.

Avascular necrosis syndromes.

Osteochondroses.

Slipped capital femoral epiphysis.

Diskitis.

Patellofemoral dysfunction (chondromalacia patellae).

Toxic synovitis of the hip.

Overuse syndromes.

GENETIC OR CONGENITAL SYNDROMES

Hematologic Disorders

Sickle cell disease.

Hemophilia.

INFLAMMATORY BOWEL DISEASE

Miscellaneous

Growing pains.

Psychogenic arthralgias (conversion reactions).

Hypermobility syndrome.

Villonodular synovitis.

Foreign body arthritis.

ARTHRITIS, POLYARTICULAR

ICD-10CM #	M15.0	Primary generalized (osteo)arthritis
	M12.89	Other specific arthropathies, not elsewhere classified, multiple sites
	M08.3	Juvenile rheumatoid polyarthritis (seronegative)

RA, juvenile (rheumatoid) polyarthritis.

SLE, other connective tissue diseases, erythema nodosum, palindromic rheumatism, relapsing polychondritis.

Psoriatic arthritis, ankylosing spondylitis.

Sarcoidosis.

Lyme arthritis, bacterial endocarditis, *Neisseria gonorrhoeae* infection, rheumatic fever, Reiter disease (reactive arthritis).

Crystal deposition disease.

Hypersensitivity to serum or drugs.

Hepatitis B, HIV, rubella, mumps.

Other: serum sickness, leukemias, lymphomas, enteropathic arthropathy, Whipple disease, Behçet syndrome, Henoch-Schönlein purpura, familial Mediterranean fever, hypertrophic pulmonary osteoarthropathy.

ASCENDING AORTA, ABNORMAL SEGMENT[44]

ICD-10CM # Q25.49 Other congenital malformations of aorta

DIFFERENTIAL DIAGNOSIS OF AN ABNORMAL ASCENDING AORTA SEGMENT

Aortic aneurysm.

Aortic dissection.

Poststenotic dilation in aortic stenosis.

Aortic dilation in aortic insufficiency.

ASCITES

ICD-10CM # R18.0 Malignant ascites
| | C78.6 | Secondary malignant neoplasm of retroperitoneum and peritoneum |
| | I89.8 | Other specified noninfective disorders of lymphatic vessels and lymph nodes |

Hypoalbuminemia: nephrotic syndrome, protein-losing gastroenteropathy, starvation.

Cirrhosis.

Hepatic congestion: CHF, constrictive pericarditis, tricuspid insufficiency, hepatic vein obstruction (Budd-Chiari syndrome), inferior vena cava or portal vein obstruction.

Peritoneal infections: TB and other bacterial infections, fungal diseases, parasites.

Neoplasms: primary hepatic neoplasms, metastases to liver or peritoneum, lymphomas, leukemias, myeloid metaplasia.

Lymphatic obstruction: mediastinal tumors, trauma to the thoracic duct, filariasis.

Ovarian disease: Meigs syndrome, struma ovarii.

Chronic pancreatitis or pseudocyst: pancreatic ascites.

Leakage of bile: bile ascites.

Urinary obstruction or trauma: urine ascites.

Myxedema.

Chylous ascites.

ASPIRATION, CHRONIC[22]

ICD-10CM # Varies with specific diagnosis

CAUSES OF CHRONIC ASPIRATION

Cerebrovascular accidents.

Atherosclerotic thrombosis.

Embolism.

Intracranial hemorrhage.

DEGENERATIVE NEUROLOGIC DISEASES

Parkinson disease.

Amyotrophic lateral sclerosis.

Progressive supranuclear palsy.

Multiple sclerosis.

NEUROMUSCULAR AND MUSCULAR DISORDERS

Poliomyelitis.

Myasthenia gravis.

Muscular dystrophy.

Myopathies.

PERIPHERAL NERVE DISORDERS

Cranial nerves.

Guillain-Barré syndrome.

Intracranial neoplasms.

Primary dysfunction related to neoplasm.

Postsurgical dysfunction.

Trauma.

Closed head injury.

Hematoma.

Anoxic brain injury.

Intracranial infection.

PHARYNGEAL DISORDERS

Neoplasms.

Postsurgical dysfunction.

Postirradiation dysfunction.

Zenker diverticulum.

Cricopharyngeal dysfunction.

Stricture.

ESOPHAGEAL DISORDERS

Reflux.

Achalasia.

Caustic injury.

MISCELLANEOUS

Severe illness.

Multisystem disease.

Drug intoxication.

ASPIRATION LUNG INJURY, CHILDREN[19]

ICD-10CM # P24.8 Neonatal aspiration syndromes

CONDITIONS PREDISPOSING TO ASPIRATION LUNG INJURY IN CHILDREN

Anatomic and Mechanical

Tracheoesophageal fistula.

Laryngeal cleft.

Vascular ring.

Cleft palate.

Micrognathia.

Macroglossia.

Achalasia.

Esophageal foreign body.

Tracheostomy.

Endotracheal tube.

Nasoenteric tube.

Collagen vascular disease (scleroderma, dermatomyositis).

Gastroesophageal reflux disease.

Obesity.

Neuromuscular

Altered consciousness.

Immaturity of swallowing/prematurity.

Dysautonomia.

Increased intracranial pressure.

Hydrocephalus.

Vocal cord paralysis.

Cerebral palsy.

Muscular dystrophy.

Myasthenia gravis.

Guillain-Barré syndrome.

Werdnig-Hoffmann disease.

Ataxia-telangiectasia.

Cerebral vascular accident.

Miscellaneous

Poor oral hygiene.

Gingivitis.

Prolonged hospitalization.

Gastric outlet or intestinal obstruction.

Poor feeding techniques (bottle propping, over-feeding, inappropriate foods for toddlers).

Bronchopulmonary dysplasia.

Viral infection.

ASTHENIA

ICD-10CM # G93.3 Postviral fatigue syndrome
	R53.1	Weakness
	R53.81	Other malaise
	R53.83	Other fatigue

Depression.

Chronic fatigue syndrome.

Sleep disorders.

Anemia.

Hypothyroidism.

Sedentary lifestyle.

Medications (e.g., narcotics, sedatives).

Infections.

Dehydration/electrolyte disorders.

COPD and other pulmonary disorders.

Renal failure.

CHF.

Diabetes.

Addison disease.

Paraneoplastic syndrome.

ASTHMA, CHILDHOOD[45]

ICD-10CM # J45.20 Mild intermittent asthma, uncomplicated
| | J45.22 | Mild intermittent asthma with status asthmaticus |

Differential Diagnosis

II

INFECTIONS
Bronchiolitis (RSV).
Pneumonia.
Croup.
Tuberculosis, histoplasmosis.
Bronchiectasis.
Bronchiolitis obliterans.
Bronchitis.
Sinusitis.

ANATOMIC, CONGENITAL
Cystic fibrosis.
Vascular rings.
Ciliary dyskinesia.
B-lymphocyte immune defect.
Congestive heart failure.
Laryngotracheomalacia.
Tumor, lymphoma.
H-type tracheoesophageal fistula.
Repaired tracheoesophageal fistula.
Gastroesophageal reflux.

VASCULITIS, HYPERSENSITIVITY
Allergic bronchopulmonary aspergillosis.
Allergic alveolitis, hypersensitivity pneumonitis.
Churg-Strauss syndrome.
Periarteritis nodosa.

OTHER
Foreign body aspiration.
Pulmonary thromboembolism.
Psychogenic cough.
Sarcoidosis.
Bronchopulmonary dysplasia.
Vocal cord dysfunction.

ATAXIA

ICD-10CM #		
	R27.0	Ataxia, unspecified
	R27.8	Other lack of coordination
	R27.9	Unspecified lack of coordination
	F10.229	Alcohol dependence with intoxication, unspecified
	F10.20	Alcohol dependence, uncomplicated
	G11.1	Early-onset cerebellar ataxia
	G31.89	Other specified degenerative diseases of nervous system
	F44.4	Conversion disorder with motor symptom or deficit
	F44.6	Conversion disorder with sensory symptom or deficit

Vertebral-basilar artery ischemia.
Diabetic neuropathy.
Tabes dorsalis.

Vitamin B_{12} deficiency.
Multiple sclerosis and other demyelinating diseases.
Meningomyelopathy.
Cerebellar neoplasms, hemorrhage, abscess, infarct.
Nutritional (Wernicke encephalopathy).
Paraneoplastic syndromes.
Parainfectious: Guillain-Barré syndrome, acute ataxia of childhood and young adults.
Toxins: phenytoin, alcohol, sedatives, organophosphates.
Wilson disease (hepatolenticular degeneration).
Hypothyroidism.
Myopathy.
Cerebellar and spinocerebellar degeneration: ataxia/telangiectasia, Friedreich ataxia.
Frontal lobe lesions: tumors, thrombosis of anterior cerebral artery, hydrocephalus.
Labyrinthine destruction: neoplasm, injury, inflammation, compression.
Hysteria.
AIDS.

ATAXIA, ACUTE OR RECURRENT[46]

ICD-10CM #		
	R27.0	Ataxia, unspecified
	R27.8	Other lack of coordination
	R27.9	Unspecified lack of coordination
	F10.229	Alcohol dependence with intoxication, unspecified
	F10.20	Alcohol dependence, uncomplicated
	G11.1	Early-onset cerebellar ataxia
	G31.89	Other specified degenerative diseases of nervous system
	F44.4	Conversion disorder motor symptom or deficit
	F44.6	Conversion disorder with sensory symptom or deficit

Drug ingestion (e.g., phenytoin, carbamazepine, sedatives, hypnotics, and phencyclidine) or intoxication (e.g., alcohol, ethylene glycol, hydrocarbon fumes, lead, mercury, or thallium).
Postinfectious (cerebellitis [e.g., varicella], acute disseminated encephalomyelitis).
Head trauma.
Basilar migraine.
Benign paroxysmal vertigo (migraine equivalent).
Brain tumor or neuroblastoma (if accompanied by opsoclonus or myoclonus [i.e., "dancing eyes, dancing feet"]).
Hydrocephalus.
Infection (e.g., labyrinthitis, abscess).

Seizure (ictal or postictal).
Vascular events (e.g., cerebellar hemorrhage or stroke).
Miller-Fisher variant of Guillain-Barré syndrome (ataxia, ophthalmoplegia, and areflexia). Warning: if bulbar signs present, disease is likely progressive; patient may lose ability to protect airway and/or ability to breathe.
Inherited ataxias.
Inborn errors of metabolism (e.g., mitochondrial disorders, amino-acidopathies, urea cycle defects).
Conversion reaction.
Multiple sclerosis.

ATAXIA, CEREBELLAR, ADULT ONSET[47]

ICD-10CM #		
	G11.0	Congenital nonprogressive ataxia
	G11.2	Late-onset cerebellar ataxia

CAUSES OF ADULT ONSET CEREBELLAR ATAXIA
Inherited
Later onset SCA syndromes.
Rarely Friedreich ataxia.
Congenital
Arnold–Chiari malformation (cerebellar ectopia).
Inflammatory
Multiple sclerosis.
Sarcoidosis.
Infections (TB, viral).
Neoplastic
Often metastatic in adults.
Meningioma, neurofibroma.
Hemangioblastoma.
Paraneoplastic
Usually with small cell bronchial carcinoma.
Vascular
Infarction, hemorrhage.
Arteriovenous malformations.
Trauma
Head injury.
Postsurgical.
Toxic
Alcohol, phenytoin, solvent abuse.
Endocrine
Hypothyroidism (very rare).
Degenerative
Multiple system atrophy (MSA).

ATAXIA, CEREBELLAR, CHILDREN[47]

ICD-10CM #		
	G11.0	Congenital nonprogressive ataxia
	G11.2	Late-onset cerebellar ataxia

CAUSES OF CEREBELLAR ATAXIA IN CHILDREN
Congenital Malformations
Cerebellar agenesis/hypoplasia.

Dandy–Walker syndrome.
Arnold–Chiari malformation.
Hereditary Ataxias
Friedreich ataxia.
Trauma
Birth trauma.
Head injury in childhood.
Infectious
Secondary to bacterial meningitis.
Secondary to encephalitis.
Hydrocephalus
Tumors
Medulloblastoma.
Astrocytoma.
Hemangioblastoma.

ATAXIA, CHRONIC OR PROGRESSIVE[46]

ICD-10CM #	R27.0	Ataxia, unspecified
	R27.8	Other lack of coordination
	R27.9	Unspecified lack of coordination
	G11.1	Early-onset cerebellar ataxia
	G11.0	Congenital nonprogressive ataxia
	G11.2	Late-onset cerebellar ataxia
	G11.3	Cerebellar ataxia with defective DNA repair
	G11.8	Other hereditary ataxia

Hydrocephalus.
Hypothyroidism.
Tumor or paraneoplastic syndrome.
Low vitamin E levels (e.g., cystic fibrosis).
Wilson disease.
Inborn errors of metabolism.
Inherited ataxias (e.g., ataxia-telangiectasia, Friedreich ataxia).

ATAXIA IN CHILDHOOD[48]

ICD-10CM #	G11.1	Early-onset cerebellar ataxia

SELECTED CAUSES OF ATAXIA IN CHILDHOOD

Congenital:
  Agenesis of vermis of the cerebellum.
  Aplasia or dysplasia of the cerebellum.
  Basilar impression.
  Cerebellar dysplasia with microgyria, macrogyria, or agyria.
  Cervical spinal bifida with herniation of the cerebellum (Chiari malformation, type 3).
  Chiari malformation.
  Dandy-Walker syndrome.
  Encephalocele.
  Hydrocephalus (progressive).
  Hypoplasia of the cerebellum.
Degenerative and/or genetic:

Acute intermittent cerebellar ataxia.
  Ataxia, retinitis pigmentosa, deafness, vestibular abnormality, and intellectual deterioration.
  Ataxia-telangiectasia.
  Biemond posterior column ataxia.
  Cerebellar ataxia with deafness, anosmia, absent caloric responses, nonreactive pupils, and hyporeflexia.
  Cockayne syndrome.
  Dentate cerebellar ataxia (dyssynergia cerebellaris progressiva).
  Familial ataxia with macular degeneration.
  Friedreich ataxia.
  Hereditary cerebellar ataxia, intellectual retardation, choreoathetosis, and eunuchoidism.
  Hereditary cerebellar ataxia with myotonia and cataracts.
  Hypertrophic interstitial neuritis.
  Marie ataxia.
  Marinesco-Sjögren syndrome.
  Pelizaeus-Merzbacher disease.
  Periodic attacks of vertigo, diplopia, and ataxia —autosomal dominant inheritance.
  Posterior and lateral column difficulties, nystagmus, and muscle atrophy.
  Progressive cerebellar ataxia and epilepsy.
  Ramsay Hunt syndrome (myoclonic seizures and ataxia).
  Roussy-Lévy syndrome.
  Spinocerebellar ataxia (SCAs); olivopontocerebellar ataxias.
Endocrinologic:
  Cretinism.
  Hypothyroidism.
Infectious or postinfectious:
  Acute cerebellar ataxia.
  Acute disseminated encephalomyelitis.
  Cerebellar abscess.
  Coxsackievirus.
  Diphtheria.
  Echovirus.
  Fisher syndrome.
  Infectious mononucleosis (Epstein-Barr virus infection).
  Infectious polyneuropathy.
  Japanese B encephalitis.
  Mumps encephalitis.
  Mycoplasma pneumoniae.
  Pertussis.
  Polio.
  Postbacterial meningitis.
  Rubeola.
  Tuberculosis.
  Typhoid.
  Varicella.
Metabolic:
  Abetalipoproteinemia.
  Argininosuccinic aciduria.

Ataxia with vitamin E deficiency (AVED).
  GM2 gangliosidosis (late).
  Hartnup disease.
  Hyperalaninemia.
  Hyperammonemia I and II.
  Hypoglycemia.
  Kearns-Sayre syndrome.
  Leigh disease.
  Maple syrup urine disease (intermittent).
  MERRF (myoclonic epilepsy with ragged red fibers).
  Metachromatic leukodystrophy.
  Mitochondrial complex defects (I, III, IV).
  Multiple carboxylase deficiency (biotinidase deficiency).
  Neuronal ceroid-lipofuscinosis.
  Neuropathy, ataxia, retinitis pigmentosa (NARP).
  Niemann-Pick disease (late infantile).
  5-Oxoprolinuria.
  Pyruvate decarboxylase deficiency.
  Refsum disease.
  Sialidosis.
  Triose-phosphate isomerase deficiency.
  Tryptophanuria.
  Wernicke encephalopathy (thiamine or B_1 deficiency).
Neoplastic:
  Frontal lobe tumors.
  Hemispheric cerebellar tumors.
  Midline cerebellar tumors.
  Neuroblastoma.
  Pontine tumors (primarily gliomas).
  Spinal cord tumors.
Primary psychogenic:
  Conversion reaction.
Toxic:
  Alcohol.
  Benzodiazepines.
  Carbamazepine.
  Clonazepam.
  Lead encephalopathy.
  Phenobarbital.
  Phenytoin.
  Primidone.
  Tick paralysis poisoning.
Traumatic:
  Acute cerebellar edema.
  Acute frontal lobe edema.
Vascular:
  Angioblastoma of cerebellum.
  Basilar migraine.
  Cerebellar embolism.
  Cerebellar hemorrhage.
  Cerebellar thrombosis.
  Posterior cerebellar artery disease.
  Vasculitis.
  von Hippel-Lindau disease.

ATAXIA, TOXIC CAUSES[49]

ICD-10CM #   R27.0   Early-onset cerebellar ataxia

SELECTED TOXIC CAUSES OF ATAXIA

Medications:
  Acetohexamide.
  Amiodarone.
  Anticholinergic agents.
  Antidepressants, including selective serotonin reuptake inhibitors.
  Antiepileptic drugs.
  Antihistamines.
  Antimicrobials, antifungals.
  Antineoplastics.
  Antiparasitics.
  Baclofen.
  Buspirone.
  Dextromethorphan.
  Disulfiram.
  Ethanol.
  Fenfluramine.
  Lithium.
  Lysergic acid diethylamide (LSD), phencyclidine palmitate (PCP).
  Mexiletine.
  Sedatives, narcotics.
Industrial toxins:
  Aluminum compounds.
  Butyl alcohol.
  Carbon monoxide.
  Carbon tetrachloride.
  Ethylene glycol.
  Formaldehyde.
  Gasoline.
  Manganese.
  Metaldehyde (snail bait, fire starters).
  Paradichlorobenzene (moth repellent, diaper pail deodorant).
  Rodenticides: aluminum phosphide, sodium monofluoroacetate.
  Solvents.
Biologic toxins:
  Belladonna, hyoscyamine.
  Buckeye (*Aesculus* spp.).
  Mayapple (*Podophyllum peltatum*).
  Mescaline, peyote.
  Podophyllum (ingested).
  Poison hemlock (*Conium maculatum*).

ATELECTASIS

ICD-10CM #   J98.11   Atelectasis

Lung neoplasm (primary or metastatic).
Infection (pneumonia, TB, fungal, histoplasmosis).
Postoperative (lower lobes).
Sarcoidosis.
Mucoid impaction.
Foreign body.
Postinflammatory (middle lobe syndrome).
Pneumothorax.
Pleural effusion.
Pneumoconiosis.
Interstitial fibrosis.
Bulla.
Mediastinal or adjacent mass.

ATRIAL ENLARGEMENT, LEFT ATRIUM[21]

ICD-10CM #   I51.7   Cardiomegaly

CAUSES OF LARGE LEFT ATRIUM
Causes Due to Volume Overload
Mitral regurgitation (often with left ventricular failure).
Ventricular septal defect.
Patent ductus arteriosus.
Atrial septal defect with shunt reversal (i.e., pulmonary hypertension).
ASD with tricuspid atresia (obligatory shunt reversal).
Aortopulmonary window.
Causes Due to Pressure Overload
Mitral stenosis.
Noncompliant left ventricle: hypertension, hypertrophic cardiomyopathy, aortic stenosis.
Left ventricular failure (often with secondary mitral regurgitation).
Left atrial myxoma.
Other Causes (Both Rare)
Atrial fibrillation.
Isolated/idiopathic.

ATRIAL ENLARGEMENT, RIGHT ATRIUM

ICD-10CM #   I51.7   Cardiomegaly

Right ventricular failure.
Atrial septal defect.
Tricuspid regurgitation.
Tricuspid stenosis.
Pulmonary hypertension.
Restrictive cardiomyopathy.
Right atrial myxoma.
Ebstein anomaly.
Anomalous pulmonary venous drainage to the right atrium.
Endomyocardial fibrosis.
Sinus of Valsalva fistula.
Arrhythmogenic right ventricular dysplasia.

ATYPICAL LYMPHOCYTOSIS, HETEROPHIL NEGATIVE, INFECTIOUS CAUSES[18]

ICD-10CM #   D72.820   Lymphocytosis (symptomatic)

MOST COMMON INFECTIOUS CAUSES OF HETEROPHIL-NEGATIVE ATYPICAL LYMPHOCYTOSIS

Babesiosis.
Cytomegalovirus.
Epstein-Barr virus (particularly in children).
Human herpesvirus 6.
Human immunodeficiency virus (especially during acute seroconversion).
Infectious mononucleosis.
Malaria.
Measles.
Toxoplasmosis.
Varicella.
Infectious hepatitis.

AV NODAL BLOCK[39]

ICD-10CM #   I44.30   Unspecified atrioventricular block
                I44.2   Atrioventricular block, complete

Idiopathic fibrosis (Lenègre disease).
Sclerodegenerative processes (e.g., Lev disease with calcification of the mitral and aortic annuli).
AV node radiofrequency ablation procedure.
Medications (e.g., digoxin, β-blockers, calcium channel blockers, class III antiarrhythmics).
Acute inferior wall MI.
Myocarditis.
Infections (endocarditis, Lyme disease).
Infiltrative diseases (e.g., hemochromatosis, sarcoidosis, amyloidosis).
Trauma (including cardiac surgical procedures).
Collagen vascular diseases.
Aortic root diseases (e.g., spondylitis).
Electrolyte abnormalities (e.g., hyperkalemia).

BACK PAIN

ICD-10CM #		
	M54.89	Other dorsalgia
	M54.9	Dorsalgia, unspecified
	M54.5	Low back pain
	F45.42	Pain disorder with related psychological factors
	M54.08	Panniculitis affecting regions of neck and back, sacral and sacrococcygeal region
	S23.9XXA	Sprain of unspecified parts of thorax, initial encounter
	M43.27	Fusion of spine, lumbosacral region
	M43.28	Fusion of spine, sacral and sacrococcygeal region
	M53.2X7	Spinal instabilities, lumbosacral region
	M53.3	Sacrococcygeal disorders, not elsewhere classified

Trauma: injury to bone, joint, or ligament.
Mechanical: pregnancy, obesity, fatigue, scoliosis.
Degenerative: osteoarthritis.
Infections: osteomyelitis, subarachnoid or spinal abscess, TB, meningitis, basilar pneumonia.

Metabolic: osteoporosis, osteomalacia.

Vascular: leaking aortic aneurysm, subarachnoid or spinal hemorrhage/infarction.

Neoplastic: myeloma, Hodgkin disease, carcinoma of pancreas, metastatic neoplasm from breast, prostate, lung.

GI: penetrating ulcer, pancreatitis, cholelithiasis, inflammatory bowel disease.

Renal: hydronephrosis, calculus, neoplasm, renal infarction, pyelonephritis.

Hematologic: sickle cell crisis, acute hemolysis.

Gynecologic: neoplasm of uterus or ovary, dysmenorrhea, salpingitis, uterine prolapse.

Inflammatory: ankylosing spondylitis, psoriatic arthritis, Reiter syndrome (reactive arthritis).

Lumbosacral strain.

Psychogenic: malingering, hysteria, anxiety.

Endocrine: adrenal hemorrhage or infarction.

BACK PAIN, CHILDREN AND ADOLESCENTS[19]

| ICD-10CM # | M54.5 | Low back pain |
| | M54.9 | Dorsalgia |

INFLAMMATORY OR INFECTIOUS

Diskitis.
Vertebral osteomyelitis (pyogenic, tuberculous).
Spinal epidural abscess.
Pyelonephritis.
Pancreatitis.

RHEUMATOLOGIC

Pauciarticular juvenile rheumatoid arthritis.
Reiter syndrome (reactive arthritis).
Ankylosing spondylitis.
Psoriatic arthritis.

DEVELOPMENTAL

Spondylolysis.
Spondylolisthesis.
Scheuermann disease.
Scoliosis.

TRAUMATIC (ACUTE VERSUS REPETITIVE)

Hip-pelvis anomalies.
Herniated disk.
Overuse syndromes.
Vertebral stress fractures.
Upper cervical spine instability.

NEOPLASTIC

Vertebral Tumors
Benign
Eosinophilic granuloma.
Aneurysmal bone cyst.
Osteoid osteoma.
Osteoblastoma.
Malignant
Osteogenic sarcoma.
Leukemia.
Lymphoma.

Metastatic tumors.

Spinal Cord, Ganglia, and Nerve Roots
Intramedullary spinal cord tumor.
Sympathetic chain.
Ganglioneuroma.
Ganglioneuroblastoma.
Neuroblastoma.

OTHER

Intraabdominal or pelvic pathology.
Following lumbar puncture.
Conversion reaction.
Juvenile osteoporosis.

BACK PAIN, LOW, ACUTE[43]

| ICD-10CM # | M54.5 | Low back pain |

DIFFERENTIAL CONSIDERATIONS IN ACUTE LOW BACK PAIN

Emergent
Aortic dissection.
Cauda equina syndrome.
Epidural abscess or hematoma.
Meningitis.
Ruptured/expanding aortic aneurysm.
Spinal fracture or subluxation with cord or root impingement.
Urgent
Back pain with neurologic deficits.
Disk herniation causing neurologic compromise.
Malignancy.
Sciatica with motor nerve root compression.
Spinal fractures without cord impingement.
Spinal stenosis.
Transverse myelitis.
Vertebral osteomyelitis.
Common or Stable
Acute ligamentous injury.
Acute muscle strain.
Ankylosing spondylitis.
Degenerative joint disease.
Intervertebral disk disease without impingement.
Pathologic fracture without impingement.
Seropositive arthritis.
Spondylolisthesis.
Referred or Visceral
Cholecystitis.
Esophageal disease.
Nephrolithiasis.
Ovarian torsion, mass, or tumor.
Pancreatitis.
Peptic ulcer disease.
Pleural effusion.
Pneumonia.
Pulmonary embolism.
Pyelonephritis.
Retroperitoneal hemorrhage or mass.

BACK PAIN, VISCEROGENIC ORIGIN

ICD-10CM #	F45.41	Pain disorder exclusively related to psychological factors
	M54	Dorsalgia
	M54.5	Low back pain

Urolithiasis.
Aortic aneurysm.
Colorectal carcinoma.
Endometriosis.
Tubal pregnancy.
Prostatitis.
Peptic ulcer.
Pancreatitis.
Diverticular spasm.
Metastatic neoplasm (e.g., bladder, uterus, ovary, kidney).

BACTERIAL OVERGROWTH, SMALL INTESTINE[2]

| ICD-10CM # | A04.9 | Bacterial Intestinal Infection, Unspecified |

Gastric surgery—Billroth II.
Small bowel diverticula.
Small bowel stricture:
  Crohn disease.
  Radiation enteritis.
Impaired small intestinal motility:
  Scleroderma.
  Diabetes mellitus.
  Chronic intestinal pseudoobstruction.
Miscellaneous/multifactorial:
  Elderly.
  Immune deficiency syndromes.
  Chronic pancreatitis.
  Cirrhosis.

BALLISM[43]

| ICD-10CM # | G25.4 | Drug-induced chorea |
| | G25.5 | Other chorea |

Cerebral infarction or hemorrhage.
Medications (e.g., dopamine agonists, phenytoin).
CNS neoplasm (primary or metastatic).
Nonketotic hyperosmolar state.

BENIGN SLEEP MYOCLONUS OF INFANCY (BSMI)[50]

| ICD-10CM # | Varies with specific diagnosis |

Common Mimics of BSMI

Mimics	Distinguishing Features
Myoclonic seizures.	BSMI occurs only during sleep and stops abruptly and consistently when infants are aroused,

Differential
Diagnosis

II

whereas seizures can occur during wakefulness. Epileptiform activity on electroencephalogram (EEG) is present during epileptic myoclonus but not with BSMI.

BSMI is seen typically in neurologically and developmentally normal infants, whereas myoclonic seizures may be associated with perinatal disorders (i.e., hypoxic-ischemic encephalopathy, infection, or metabolic abnormalities).

Infantile spasms (West syndrome).	Often seen after the first month of life. Manifested by sudden head flexion with arm extension and lower extremity flexion. Epileptiform activity on EEG is present; usually associated with an abnormal EEG pattern known as hypsarrhythmia.
Pyridoxine-dependency seizures.	Can occur while infants are awake, whereas BSMI will stop abruptly and consistently when infants are aroused. EEG slowing is supportive of encephalopathy versus BSMI. Responsive to vitamin B_6 (pyridoxine).
Hyperekplexia (startle disease).	Generalized stiffness while awake. Exaggerated startle reflex. Typical movements occur as an excessive response to stimulation, such as touch or loud noise.
Jitteriness.	Occurs during wakefulness in response to tactile or auditory stimuli, whereas BSMI occurs during sleep.

BSMI, Benign sleep myoclonus of infancy.

BILE DUCT, DILATED[2]

ICD-10CM # K83.1 Obstruction of bile duct

Normal variant.
Postcholecystectomy.
Unsuspected bile duct stone.
Sphincter of Oddi stenosis.
Occult bile duct stricture.
Previous bile duct injury.
Early carcinoma of the pancreas, carcinoma of the bile duct, or carcinoma of the ampulla.

Extrinsic compression of the bile duct by a primary or secondary neoplasm.

BILIARY OBSTRUCTION[15]

ICD-10CM # Varies with specific diagnosis

CAUSES OF BILIARY OBSTRUCTION
Benign Miscellaneous
Choledocholithiasis.
Hemobilia.
Congenital biliary diseases.
Caroli disease.
Choledochal cysts.
Cholangitis.
Infectious.
Acute pyogenic cholangitis.
Biliary parasites.
Recurrent pyogenic cholangitis.
HIV cholangiopathy.
Sclerosing cholangitis.
Neoplasms
Cholangiocarcinoma.
Gallbladder carcinoma.
Locally invasive tumors (esp. pancreatic adenocarcinoma).
Ampullary tumors.
Metastases.
Extrinsic Compression
Mirizzi syndrome.
Pancreatitis.
Adenopathy.

BILIARY TREE, REFLUX OF GAS OR BOWEL[48]

ICD-10CM # Varies with specific diagnosis

CAUSES OF REFLUX OF GAS OR BOWEL CONTRAST INTO THE BILIARY TREE
Iatrogenic.
Sphincterotomy.
Choledochojejunostomy.
Gallstone fistula.
Cholecystoduodenal fistula.
Perforated ulcer.
Choledochoduodenal fistula.
Carcinoma.
Choledochoenteric fistula.

BLADDER (URINARY) WALL THICKENING[15]

ICD-10CM # Varies with specific diagnosis

CAUSES OF BLADDER WALL THICKENING
Focal
Neoplasm
Transitional cell carcinoma.
Squamous cell carcinoma.

Adenocarcinoma.
Lymphoma.
Metastases.
Infectious/inflammatory.
Tuberculosis (acute).
Schistosomiasis (acute).
Cystitis.
Malakoplakia.
Cystitis cystica.
Cystitis glandularis.
Fistula.
Medical Diseases
Endometriosis.
Amyloidosis.
Trauma
Hematoma.
Diffuse
Neoplasm
Transitional cell carcinoma.
Squamous cell carcinoma.
Adenocarcinoma.
Infectious/Inflammatory
Cystitis.
Tuberculosis (chronic).
Schistosomiasis (chronic).
Medical Diseases
Interstitial cystitis.
Amyloidosis.
Neurogenic Bladder
Detrusor hyperreflexia.
Bladder Outlet Obstruction
With muscular hypertrophy.

BLEEDING, GI IN PATIENTS WITH AIDS[3]

ICD-10CM # K92.2 Gastrointestinal bleeding, unspecified

(EXCLUDING NON-AIDS-SPECIFIC DIAGNOSES)
Esophagus
Candida spp.
Cytomegalovirus.
HSV.
Idiopathic ulcer.
Stomach
Cytomegalovirus.*
Kaposi sarcoma.*
Cryptosporidiosis.
Lymphoma.
Small Intestine
Kaposi sarcoma.
Lymphoma.
Cytomegalovirus.
Salmonella spp.
Cryptosporidium.

---
*More frequent diagnosis.

Colon
Cytomegalovirus.*
Kaposi sarcoma.*
Entamoeba histolytica.
Campylobacter jejuni.
Clostridium difficile.
Shigella spp.
Idiopathic ulcerations.
Lymphoma.

---

*More frequent diagnosis.

BLEEDING, LOWER GI

ICD-10CM # K92.2 Gastrointestinal hemorrhage, unspecified

(ORIGINATING BELOW THE LIGAMENT OF TREITZ)
Small Intestine
Ischemic bowel disease (mesenteric thrombosis, embolism, vasculitis, trauma).
Small bowel neoplasm: leiomyomas, carcinoids.
Hereditary hemorrhagic telangiectasia (Rendu-Osler-Weber syndrome).
Meckel diverticulum and other small intestine diverticula.
Aortoenteric fistula.
Intestinal hemangiomas: blue rubber-bleb nevi, intestinal hemangiomas, cutaneous vascular nevi.
Hamartomatous polyps: Peutz-Jeghers syndrome (intestinal polyps, mucocutaneous pigmentation).
Infections of small bowel: tuberculous enteritis, enteritis necroticans.
Volvulus.
Intussusception.
Lymphoma of small bowel, sarcoma, Kaposi sarcoma.
Irradiation ileitis.
AV malformation of small intestine.
Inflammatory bowel disease.
Polyarteritis nodosa.
Other: pancreatoenteric fistulas, Henoch-Schönlein purpura, Ehlers-Danlos syndrome, SLE, amyloidosis, metastatic melanoma.
Colon
Carcinoma (particularly left colon).
Diverticular disease.
Inflammatory bowel disease.
Ischemic colitis.
Colonic polyps.
Vascular abnormalities: angiodysplasia, vascular ectasia.
Radiation colitis.
Infectious colitis.
Uremic colitis.
Aortoenteric fistula.
Lymphoma of large bowel.
Hemorrhoids.
Anal fissure.

Trauma, foreign body.
Solitary rectal/cecal ulcers.
Long-distance running.

BLEEDING, LOWER GI, PEDIATRIC[43]

ICD-10CM # K92.2 Gastrointestinal hemorrhage, unspecified

<3 MO
Swallowed maternal blood.
Infectious colitis.
Milk allergy.
Bleeding diathesis.
Intussusception.
Midgut volvulus.
Meckel diverticulum.
Necrotizing enterocolitis.

<2 YR
Anal fissure.
Infectious colitis.
Milk allergy.
Colitis.
Intussusception.
Meckel diverticulum.
Polyp.
Duplication.
Hemolytic-uremic syndrome.
Inflammatory bowel disease.
Pseudomembranous enterocolitis.

<5 YR
Infectious colitis.
Anal fissure.
Polyp.
Intussusception.
Meckel diverticulum.
Henoch-Schönlein purpura.
Hemolytic-uremic syndrome.
Inflammatory bowel disease.
Pseudomembranous enterocolitis.

5 TO 18 YR
Infectious colitis.
Inflammatory bowel disease.
Pseudomembranous enterocolitis.
Polyp.
Hemolytic-uremic syndrome.
Hemorrhoids.

BLEEDING, RECTAL[2]

ICD-10CM # K92.2 Gastrointestinal hemorrhage, unspecified

IN PATIENTS <40 YR
Very Common
Hemorrhoids.
Anal fissure.
Inflammatory bowel disease (mainly proctitis).

Less Common
Polyps (hamartomatous or adenomatous).
Infective colitis.
Meckel diverticulum.
Intussusception.
Rare
Colorectal cancer.

IN PATIENTS >40 YR
Hemorrhoids.
Anal fissure.
Colorectal cancer.
Colorectal polyps (mostly adenomas).
Angiodysplasia.
Diverticular disease.
Inflammatory bowel disease.
Ischemic colitis.
Infective colitis.

BLEEDING, THIRD TRIMESTER[29]

ICD-10CM # N93.9 Abnormal uterine and vaginal bleeding, unspecified

Placental abruption.
Placenta previa.
Bloody show (extrusion of cervical mucus).
Vasa previa.
Disseminated intravascular coagulopathy.
Uterine rupture.
Cervicitis, cervical cancer, or other cervical abnormality.
Vaginal laceration.

BLEEDING, UPPER GI

ICD-10CM # K92.2 Gastrointestinal hemorrhage, unspecified

(ORIGINATING ABOVE THE LIGAMENT OF TREITZ)
Swallowed Hemoptysis
Oral or pharyngeal lesions: swallowed blood from nose or oropharynx.
Esophageal: varices, ulceration, esophagitis, Mallory-Weiss tear, carcinoma, trauma.
Gastric: peptic ulcer (including Cushing and Curling ulcers), gastritis, angiodysplasia, gastric neoplasms, hiatal hernia, gastric diverticulum, pseudoxanthoma elasticum, Rendu-Osler-Weber syndrome.
Duodenal: peptic ulcer, duodenitis, angiodysplasia, aortoduodenal fistula, duodenal diverticulum, duodenal tumors, carcinoma of ampulla of Vater, parasites (e.g., hookworm), Crohn disease.
Biliary: hematobilia (e.g., penetrating injury to liver, hepatobiliary malignancy, endoscopic papillotomy).

Differential Diagnosis

II

BLEEDING, UPPER GI, PEDIATRIC[43]

ICD-10CM # K92.2 Gastrointestinal hemorrhage, unspecified

<3 MO
Swallowed maternal blood.
Gastritis.
Ulcer, stress.
Bleeding diathesis.
Foreign body (NG tube).
Vascular malformation.
　Duplication.

<2 YR
Esophagitis.
Gastritis.
Ulcer.
Pyloric stenosis.
Mallory-Weiss syndrome.
Vascular malformation.
Duplication.

<5 YR
Esophagitis.
Gastritis.
Ulcer.
Esophageal varices.
Foreign body.
Mallory-Weiss syndrome.
Hemophilia.
Vascular malformations.

5 TO 18 YR
Esophagitis.
Gastritis.
Ulcer.
Esophageal varices.
Mallory-Weiss syndrome.
Inflammatory bowel disease.
Hemophilia.
Vascular malformation.

BLEEDING, VAGINAL, NONPREGNANT FEMALE[29]

ICD-10CM # N93.9 Abnormal uterine and vaginal bleeding, unspecified

TRAUMA
Blunt force.
Penetrating force.
Foreign bodies.

INFECTIOUS
Vaginitis.
Cervicitis.
Endometritis.

DYSFUNCTIONAL UTERINE BLEEDING
Ovulatory.
Anovulatory.
Adenomyosis.

BENIGN GROWTHS
Uterine leiomyomas.
Cervical polyps.

MALIGNANCY
Vulvar.
Cervical.
Uterine.
Ovarian.

SYSTEMIC DISEASE
Medications
Anticoagulation (warfarin [Coumadin], low-molecular-weight heparin, clopidogrel [Plavix]).
Antipsychotics.
Corticosteroids.
Tamoxifen.
Selective serotonin reuptake inhibitors.
Contraceptives (oral, intrauterine devices, intramuscular).

BLINDNESS, GERIATRIC AGE

ICD-10CM # H54.8 Legal blindness, as defined in USA

Cataracts.
Glaucoma.
Diabetic retinopathy.
Macular degeneration.
Trauma.
CVA.
Corneal scarring.
Giant cell arteritis.
Ocular herpes zoster.

BLINDNESS, MONOCULAR, TRANSIENT

ICD-10CM # H54.41 Blindness, right eye, normal vision left eye
H54.42 Blindness, left eye, normal vision right eye

Migraine (vasospasm).
Embolic cerebrovascular disease.
Intermittent angle-closure glaucoma.
Partial retinal vein occlusion.
Hyphema.
Optic disc edema.
Giant cell arteritis.
Psychogenic.
Hypotension.
Hypercoagulopathy disorders.
Multiple sclerosis.

BLINDNESS, PEDIATRIC AGE[51]

ICD-10CM # H54.41 Blindness, right eye, normal vision left eye
H54.42 Blindness, left eye, normal vision right eye

CONGENITAL
Optic nerve hypoplasia or aplasia.
Optic coloboma.
Congenital hydrocephalus.
Hydranencephaly.
Porencephaly.
Microencephaly.
Encephalocele, particularly occipital type.
Morning glory disc.
Aniridia.
Anterior microphthalmia.
Peter anomaly.
Persistent pupillary membrane.
Glaucoma.
Cataracts.
Persistent hyperplastic primary vitreous.

PHAKOMATOSES
Tuberous sclerosis.
Neurofibromatosis (special association with optic glioma).
Sturge-Weber syndrome.
von Hippel–Lindau disease.

TUMORS
Retinoblastoma.
Optic glioma.
Perioptic meningioma.
Craniopharyngioma.
Cerebral glioma.
Posterior and intraventricular tumors when complicated by hydrocephalus.
Pseudotumor cerebri.

NEURODEGENERATIVE DISEASES
Cerebral storage disease.
Gangliosidoses, particularly Tay-Sachs disease (infantile amaurotic familial idiocy), Sandhoff variant, generalized gangliosidosis.
Other lipidoses and ceroid lipofuscinoses, particularly the late-onset amaurotic familial idiocies such as those of Jansky-Bielschowsky and of Batten-Mayou-Spielmeyer-Vogt.
Mucopolysaccharidoses, particularly Hurler syndrome and Hunter syndrome.
Leukodystrophies (dysmyelination disorders), particularly metachromatic leukodystrophy and Canavan disease.
Demyelinating sclerosis (myelinoclastic diseases), especially Schilder disease and Devic neuromyelitis optica.
Special types: Dawson disease, Leigh disease, Bassen-Kornzweig syndrome, Refsum disease.
Retinal degenerations: retinitis pigmentosa and its variants, Leber congenital type.
Optic atrophies: congenital autosomal recessive type, infantile and congenital autosomal dominant types, Leber disease, and atrophies associated with hereditary ataxias—the types of Behr, of Marie, and of Sanger-Brown.

INFECTIOUS PROCESSES

Encephalitis, especially in the prenatal infection syndromes caused by *Toxoplasma gondii,* cytomegalovirus, rubella virus, *Treponema pallidum,* herpes simplex.
Meningitis, arachnoiditis.
Chorioretinitis.
Endophthalmitis.
Keratitis.

HEMATOLOGIC DISORDERS

Leukemia with CNS involvement.

VASCULAR AND CIRCULATORY DISORDERS

Collagen vascular diseases.
Arteriovenous malformations: intracerebral hemorrhage, subarachnoid hemorrhage.
Central retinal occlusion.

TRAUMA

Contusion or avulsion of optic nerves, chiasm, globe, cornea.
Cerebral contusion or laceration.
Intracerebral, subarachnoid, or subdural hemorrhage.

DRUGS AND TOXINS OTHER

Retinopathy of prematurity.
Sclerocornea.
Conversion reaction.
Optic neuritis.
Osteopetrosis.

BLISTERS, SUBEPIDERMAL

ICD-10CM # T07 Unspecified multiple injuries

Burns.
Porphyria cutanea tarda.
Bullous pemphigoid.
Bullous drug reaction.
Arthropod bite reaction.
Toxic epidermal necrosis.
Dermatitis herpetiformis.
Polymorphous light eruption.
Variegate porphyria.
SLE.
Epidermolysis bullosa.
Pseudoporphyria.
Acute graft-versus-host reaction.
Linear IgA disease.
Leukocytoclastic vasculitis.
Pressure necrosis.
Urticaria pigmentosa.
Amyloidosis.

BONE AND/OR SOFT TISSUE HYPERTROPHY[52]

ICD-10CM # M85.80 Other specified disorders of bone density and structure, unspecified site

DISORDERS ASSOCIATED WITH BONE AND/OR SOFT TISSUE HYPERTROPHY

Conditions Associated with Generalized Overgrowth

Pituitary gigantism and acromegaly.
Other endocrine disorders.
Cerebral gigantism (Sotos).

Conditions Associated with Limb Hemihypertrophy

Lipomatosis.
Idiopathic congenital hemihypertrophy (associated with tumors, e.g., Wilms tumor, adrenocortical tumors, hepatoblastoma).
Proteus syndrome (capillary port-wine hemangiomas, lymphangiomas, lipomas, epidermal nevi, hypertrophy hands and feet, macrocephaly).
Maffucci syndrome (enchondromas, exostosis, lymphangiomas, venous angiomas).
Klippel-Trenaunay syndrome (capillary port-wine hemangiomas, varicosities, lymphangiomas).
Parkes Weber syndrome (capillary port-wine hemangiomas, varicosities, arteriovenous fistula).
Blue rubber bleb nevus syndrome (cavernous hemangiomas of skin, GI tract).
Other angiodysplasias (e.g., Servelle-Martorell syndrome; venous arterial malformations with limb hypertrophy and bony hypoplasia).
Beckwith-Wiedemann syndrome (macroglossia, visceromegaly, omphaloceles, hemihypertrophy, etc.).

Conditions Associated with Macrodactyly

Neurofibromatosis.
Macrodystrophia lipomatosa.
Proteus syndrome.
Bannayan-Zonana syndrome (lipomatosis, angiomatosis, macrocephaly).
Hemangiomatosis and other vascular malformations (Klippel-Trenaunay and Parkes Weber).
Lymphangiomatosis.
Arteriovenous malformation.
Maffucci syndrome, Ollier disease.
Epidermal nevus syndrome.

BONE DENSITY, DECREASED, GENERALIZED[21]

ICD-10CM # M85.80 Other specified disorders of bone density and structure, unspecified site

DISORDERS ASSOCIATED WITH GENERALIZED LOSS OF BONE DENSITY

Disorders of Multiple or Uncertain Cause

Senile osteoporosis.*

---

*Patients who cannot synthesize Lewis blood group antigens (∼5% of the population) do not produce CA–19–9 antigen.

Juvenile osteoporosis.
Osteoporosis imperfecta.[†]

Secondary Bone Disorders
Endocrine
Adrenal cortex:
  Cushing disease.
  Addison disease.
Gonadal disorders:
  Postmenopausal osteoporosis.
  Hypogonadism.
Pituitary:
  Acromegaly.
  Hypopituitarism.
Pancreas:
  Diabetes mellitus.
Thyroid:
  Hyperthyroidism.
  Hypothyroidism.
Parathyroid:
  Hyperparathyroidism.

Marrow Replacement and Expansion
Myeloma.
Leukemia.
Lymphoma.
Metastatic disease.
Gaucher disease.
Anemias (sickle cell, thalassemia, hemophilia).

Drugs and Other Substances
Steroids.
Heparin (osteoporosis).
Anticonvulsants (osteomalacia).
Immunosuppressants.
Alcohol.

Chronic Disease
Chronic renal disease.
Hepatic insufficiency.
GI malabsorption syndromes.
Chronic inflammatory polyarthropathies.
Chronic debility or immobilization.

[†]Common cause of decrease in bone density in children.

BONE DENSITY, DECREASED, LOCALIZED[21]

ICD-10CM # Z82.62 Family history of osteoporosis
          M85.80 Other specified disorders of bone density and structure, unspecified site

DISORDERS ASSOCIATED WITH LOCALIZED LOSS OF BONE DENSITY

Disuse osteoporosis.[‡]
Reflex sympathetic dystrophy (Sudeck).
Osteolytic syndromes:
  Acroosteolysis, primary and secondary.
  Massive osteolysis of Gorham.
  Carpotarsal osteolysis.

[‡]Common causes.

Transient regional osteoporosis.
Neuromuscular disorders.
Infection.
Arthropathies.
Tumors, primary and secondary, myelomatosis.

BONE DISEASE, PROLIFERATIVE[53]

ICD-10CM # Varies with specific diagnosis

CLASSIFICATION CRITERIA FOR SYSTEMIC LUPUS ERYTHEMATOSUS
American College of Rheumatology (ACR) 1997 Revised Classification Criteria*
Malar rash.
Discoid rash.
Photosensitivity.
Arthritis (nonerosive, affecting two or more joints).
Serositis (pleuritis, pericarditis, or peritonitis).
Seizure or psychosis.
Hematologic manifestations (hemolytic anemia, leukopenia [<4000 leukocytes/mm^3], lymphopenia [<1500 lymphocytes/mm^3], thrombocytopenia [<100,000 platelets /mm^3]).
Immunologic abnormalities (positive anti–double-stranded DNA or anti-Smith antibody).
False-positive rapid plasma reagin (RPR), positive lupus anticoagulant test result in elevated anticardiolipin immunoglobulin (Ig)G or IgM anticardiolipin antibody.
Antinuclear antibody.
Systemic Lupus International Collaborating Clinics (SLICC) Classification Criteria[†]

Clinical Criteria
Acute cutaneous lupus.
Chronic cutaneous lupus.
Oral or nasal ulcers.
Nonscarring alopecia.
Synovitis (two or more joints).
Serositis.
Glomerulonephritis.
Neurologic disorder (seizures, psychosis, mononeuritis multiplex, myelitis, peripheral or cranial neuropathy, acute confusional state).
Hemolytic anemia.
Leukopenia (<4000 leukocytes/mm^3) or lymphopenia (<1000 lymphocytes/mm^3).
Thrombocytopenia (<100,000 platelets/mm^3).
Immunologic Criteria
Antinuclear antibody (ANA).
Anti–double-stranded DNA antibody.
Anti-Smith antibody.
Antiphospholipid antibody (false-positive RPR; medium- or high-titer IgA, IgG, or IgM anticardiolipin antibody; IgG, IgA, or IgM anti–β2 glycoprotein I antibody).
Low complement (C3, C4, CH50).
Positive direct Coombs test in the absence of hemolytic anemia.

*For ACR criteria, the presence of 4 or more of 11 criteria is needed.
†For SLICC criteria, the presence of four or more criteria (at least one clinical and one laboratory criterion) is needed or a biopsy demonstrating lupus nephritis with a positive ANA or anti–double-stranded DNA is needed.

BONE LESIONS, PREFERENTIAL SITE OF ORIGIN[54]

ICD-10CM #		
C41.0	Malignant neoplasm of bones of skull and face
C41.1	Malignant neoplasm of mandible
C41.2	Malignant neoplasm of vertebral column
C41.3	Malignant neoplasm of ribs, sternum and clavicle
C40.00	Malignant neoplasm of scapula and long bones of unspecified upper limb
C40.10	Malignant neoplasm of short bones of unspecified upper limb
C41.4	Malignant neoplasm of pelvic bones, sacrum and coccyx
C40.20	Malignant neoplasm of long bones of unspecified lower limb
C40.30	Malignant neoplasm of short bones of unspecified lower limb
C41.9	Malignant neoplasm of bone and articular cartilage, unspecified
C79.51	Secondary malignant neoplasm of bone
C79.52	Secondary malignant neoplasm of bone marrow

EPIPHYSIS
Chondroblastoma.
Giant cell tumor—after fusion of growth plate.
Langerhans cell histiocytosis.
Clear cell chondrosarcoma.
Osteosarcoma.

METAPHYSIS
Parosteal sarcoma.
Chondrosarcoma.
Fibrosarcoma.
Nonossifying fibroma.
Giant cell tumor—before fusion of growth plate.
Unicameral bone cyst.
Aneurysmal bone cyst.

DIAPHYSIS
Myeloma.
Ewing tumor.
Reticulum cell sarcoma.

METADIAPHYSEAL
Fibrosarcoma.
Fibrous dysplasia.
Enchondroma.
Osteoid osteoma.
Chondromyofibroma.

BONE MARROW FAILURE SYNDROMES, INHERITED[31]

ICD-10CM # D61.89 Other specified aplastic anemias and other bone marrow failure syndromes

BI-LINEAGE AND TRI-LINEAGE CYTOPENIAS
Fanconi anemia.
Shwachman-Diamond syndrome.
Dyskeratosis congenita.
Amegakaryocytic thrombocytopenia:
    Other inherited thrombocytopenia disorders.
Other genetic syndromes:
    Down syndrome.
    Dubowitz syndrome.
    Seckel syndrome.
    Reticular dysgenesis.
    Schimke immunoosseous dysplasia.
    Noonan syndrome.
    Cartilage-hair hypoplasia.
    Familial marrow failure (non-Fanconi).

UNI-LINEAGE CYTOPENIA
Diamond-Blackfan anemia.
Kostmann syndrome/congenital neutropenia:
    ELA2 mutations.
    HAX1 mutations.
    GFI1 mutations.
    WASP mutations.
    Constitutive cell surface G-CSF-R mutations.
Other inherited neutropenia syndromes:
    Barth syndrome.
    Glycogen storage disease 1b.
    Miscellaneous.
Thrombocytopenia with absent radii.
Congenital dyserythropoietic anemias (CDAs):
    Types I, II, III, IV.
    Variants.
    Nonclassifiable CDAs.
    Groups IV, V, VI, VII.

BONE MARROW FIBROSIS[24]

ICD-10CM # D75.9 Disease of blood and blood-forming organs, unspecified

MYELOID DISORDERS
Myelofibrosis with myeloid metaplasia.
Metastatic cancer.
Chronic myeloid leukemia.
Myelodysplastic syndrome.
Atypical myeloid disorder.
Acute megakaryocytic leukemia.
Other acute myeloid leukemias.
Gray platelet syndrome.

LYMPHOID DISORDERS
Hairy cell leukemia.
Multiple myeloma.
Lymphoma.

NONHEMATOLOGIC DISORDERS
Connective tissue disorder.
Infections (tuberculosis, kala-azar).
Vitamin D deficiency (rickets).
Renal osteodystrophy.

BONE MASS, LOW[18]

| ICD-10CM # | M85.80 | Other specified disorders of bone density and structure, unspecified site |

SECONDARY CAUSES OF LOW BONE MASS
Endocrine Diseases
Female hypogonadism.
Hyperprolactinemia.
Hypothalamic amenorrhea.
Anorexia nervosa.
Premature and primary ovarian failure.
Female athlete triad.
Male hypogonadism.
Primary gonadal failure (e.g., Klinefelter syndrome).
Secondary gonadal failure (e.g., idiopathic hypogonadotropic hypogonadism, androgen deprivation therapy for prostate cancer).
Hyperthyroidism.
Hyperparathyroidism.
Hypercortisolism.
Vitamin D insufficiency or deficiency.
Gastrointestinal Diseases
Subtotal gastrectomy.
Gastric bypass surgery.
Malabsorption syndromes.
Chronic obstructive jaundice.
Primary biliary cirrhosis and other cirrhoses.
Bone Marrow Disorders
Multiple myeloma.
Monoclonal gammopathy of unknown significance (MGUS).
Lymphoma.
Leukemia.
Hemolytic anemias.
Systemic mastocytosis.
Disseminated carcinoma.
Connective Tissue Diseases
Osteogenesis imperfecta.
Ehlers-Danlos syndrome.
Marfan syndrome.
Homocystinuria.
Drugs
Alcohol.
Antiseizure medications.
Aromatase inhibitors.
Chemotherapy.
Cyclosporine.
Depo-medroxyprogesterone.
Excess thyroid hormone.
Glucocorticoids.
Gonadotropin-releasing hormone agonists.
Heparin.

Miscellaneous Causes
Immobilization.
Rheumatoid arthritis.
Chronic obstructive pulmonary disease.
Weight loss.

BONE MINERAL DENSITY, INCREASED

ICD-10CM #	M89.30	Hypertrophy of bone, unspecified site
	M89.8X9	Other specified disorders of bone, unspecified site
	M94.8X9	Other specified disorders of cartilage, unspecified sites

Paget disease of bone.
Skeletal metastases.
DISH.
Osteonecrosis.
Sarcoidosis.
Hypoparathyroidism, pseudohypoparathyroidism.
Milk-alkali syndrome.
Osteopetrosis.
Hypervitaminosis A or D.
Dysplasias (craniodiaphyseal, craniometaphyseal, frontometaphyseal).
Endosteal hyperostosis.
Fluorosis.
Heavy metal poisoning.
Ionizing radiation.
Other: lymphoma, leukemia, mastocytosis, multiple myeloma, polycythemia vera.

BONE PAIN

| ICD-10CM # | M89.8 | Pain, bone |

Trauma.
Neoplasm (primary or metastatic).
Osteoporosis with compression fracture.
Paget disease of bone.
Infection (osteomyelitis, septic arthritis).
Osteomalacia.
Viral syndrome.
Sickle cell disease.
Anxiety.

BONE RESORPTION[54]

| ICD-10CM # | M89.9 | Disorder of bone, unspecified |
| | M94.9 | Disorder of cartilage, unspecified |

DISTAL CLAVICLE
Hyperparathyroidism.
RA.
Scleroderma.
Posttraumatic osteolysis.
Progeria.
Pycnodysostosis.
Cleidocranial dysplasia.

INFERIOR ASPECT OF RIBS
Vascular impression associated with but not limited to coarctation of the aorta.
Hyperparathyroidism.
Neurofibromatosis.

TERMINAL PHALANGEAL TUFTS
Scleroderma.
Raynaud phenomenon.
Vascular disease.
Frostbite, electrical burns.
Psoriasis.
Tabes dorsalis.
Hyperparathyroidism.

GENERALIZED RESORPTION
Paraplegia.
Myositis ossificans.
Osteoporosis.

BOWEL WALL THICKENING[48]

| ICD-10CM # | Varies with specific diagnosis |

BENIGN VERSUS MALIGNANT BOWEL WALL THICKENING
Benign
Homogeneous attenuation.
Symmetrical.
Circumferential.
Thickening <1 cm.
Segmental or diffuse involvement.
Double halo sign.
Dark inner ring.
Bright outer ring.
Target sign.
Bright inner ring.
Dark middle ring.
Bright outer ring.
Malignant
Heterogeneous attenuation.
Asymmetrical.
Eccentric.
Thickening >1 to 2 cm.
Focal mass.
Abrupt transition.
Lobulated contour.
Spiculated contour.
Narrowed bowel lumen.
Enlarged lymph nodes.
Liver metastases.

BOW LEGS (GENU VARUM), CLASSIFICATION[19]

| ICD-10CM # | E64.3 | Genu varum, acquired |
| | Q74.1 | Congenital malformation of knee |

PHYSIOLOGIC
Asymmetric Growth
Tibia vara (Blount disease):
Infantile.
Juvenile.

Differential Diagnosis

II

Adolescent.
Focal fibrocartilaginous dysplasia.
Physeal injury.
Trauma.
Infection.
Tumor.

METABOLIC DISORDERS

Vitamin D deficiency (nutritional rickets).
Vitamin D–resistant rickets.
Hypophosphatasia.

SKELETAL DYSPLASIA

Metaphyseal dysplasia.
Achondroplasia.
Enchondromatosis.

BRACHYCARDIA, ICU PATIENT[7]

ICD-10CM #   R00.1   Bradycardia, unspecified

COMMON CAUSES OF BRADYCARDIA IN THE ICU

Medications: antiarrhythmics, β-blockers, calcium channel blockers, clonidine, dexmedetomidine, digoxin, lithium, opioids, phenytoin, and propofol.
Age-related degeneration.
Cardiac ischemia.
Electrolyte abnormalities.
Elevated intracranial pressure.
Elevated vagal tone.
Endotracheal intubation.
Hypertension.
Hypothermia.
Hypothyroidism.
Hypoxia.
Inflammatory disease.
Obstructive sleep apnea.
Postcardiac surgery.

BRADYCARDIA, SINUS[39]

ICD-10CM #   I49.8   Other specified cardiac arrhythmias
               R00.1   Bradycardia, unspecified

Idiopathic.
Degenerative processes (e.g., Lev disease, Lenègre disease).
Medications
  β-Blockers.
  Some calcium channel blockers (diltiazem, verapamil).
  Digoxin (when vagal tone is high).
  Class I antiarrhythmic agents (e.g., procainamide).
  Class III antiarrhythmic agents (amiodarone, sotalol).
  Clonidine.
  Lithium carbonate.

ACUTE MYOCARDIAL ISCHEMIA AND INFARCTION

Right or left circumflex coronary artery occlusion or spasm.
High vagal tone (e.g., athletes).

BRAIN MASS[29]

ICD-10CM #   C71   Malignant neoplasm of brain
               D33   Benign neoplasm of brain
               I61.9   Intracranial hemorrhage, unspecified

METASTATIC BRAIN TUMOR
Primary Brain Tumor
Meningioma.
Glioma.
Pituitary adenoma.
Vestibular schwannoma.
Primary or secondary CNS lymphoma.
Infections
Abscess.
Toxoplasmosis.
Neurocysticercosis.
Tuberculoma.
Progressive multifocal leukoencephalopathy.

VASCULAR DISEASE
Hemorrhage
Anomalies (arteriovenous malformation).
Intratumoral.
Hypertensive.
Infarct
Embolism.
Thrombosis (sinus venous).
Inflammatory
Multiple sclerosis.
Encephalomyelitis.

BRAIN TUMORS, CHILDREN[20]

ICD-10CM #   C71   Malignant neoplasm of brain
               D33   Benign neoplasm of brain

Brain Tumors in Children
Hemispheric Tumors

Choroid plexus papilloma
Glial tumors.
  Astrocytoma.
  Ependymoma.
  Oligodendroglioma.
  Ganglioglioma.
  Primitive neuroectodermal tumors.
Pineal region tumors.
  Pineal parenchymal tumors.
    Pineoblastoma.
    Pineocytoma.
Germ cell tumors.
  Embryonal cell carcinoma.
  Germinoma.
  Teratoma.
Other tumors.
  Angiomas.

Dysplasia.
Meningioma.
Metastatic tumors.
Middle Fossa Tumors
Optic glioma.
Sellar and parasellar tumors.
Posterior Fossa Tumors
Astrocytoma.
Brain stem glioma.
Ependymoma.
Hemangioblastoma.
Medulloblastoma.

BREAST INFLAMMATORY LESION[55]

ICD-10CM #   N61   Inflammatory disorders of breast
               N60.19   Diffuse cystic mastopathy of unspecified breast
               P39.0   Neonatal infective mastitis
               P83.4   Breast engorgement of newborn

Mastitis (*S. aureus*, β-hemolytic *Streptococcus*).
Trauma.
Foreign body (sutures, breast implants).
Granuloma (TB, fungal).
Fat necrosis post biopsy.
Necrosis or infarction (anticoagulant therapy, pregnancy).
Breast malignancy.

BREAST MASS

ICD-10CM #   N63   Unspecified lump in breast

Fibrocystic breasts.
Benign tumors (fibroadenoma, papilloma).
Mastitis (acute bacterial mastitis, chronic mastitis).
Malignant neoplasm.
Fat necrosis.
Hematoma.
Duct ectasia.
Mammary adenosis.

BREAST MASS, ADOLESCENTS[56]

ICD-10CM #   N63   Unspecified lump in breast

ETIOLOGY OF BREAST MASSES IN ADOLESCENTS

Classic or juvenile fibroadenoma (70%).
Fibrocystic disease.
Breast cyst.
Abscess/mastitis.
Intraductal papilloma.
Fat necrosis/lipoma.
Cystosarcoma phyllodes (low-grade malignancy).
Adenomatous hyperplasia.
Hemangioma, lymphangioma, lymphoma (rare).
Carcinoma ($<$1%).

BREATH ODOR[57]

ICD-10CM # R19.6 Halitosis

Sweet, fruity: DKA, starvation ketosis.
Fishy, stale: uremia (trimethylamines).
Ammonia-like: uremia (ammonia).
Musty fish, clover: fetor hepaticus (hepatic failure).
Foul, feculent: intestinal obstruction/diverticulum.
Foul, putrid: nasal/sinus pathology (infection, foreign body, cancer), respiratory infections (empyema, lung abscess, bronchiectasis).
Halitosis: tonsillitis, gingivitis, respiratory infections, Vincent angina, gastroesophageal reflux, achalasia, certain foods (garlic, onions, protein drinks, etc.).
Cinnamon: pulmonary TB.

BREATHING DISORDERS, SLEEP RELATED[22]

ICD-10CM # Varies with specific diagnosis

SLEEP-RELATED BREATHING DISORDERS

Central Sleep Apnea Syndromes
Central sleep apnea with Cheyne-Stokes breathing.
Central sleep apnea due to high-altitude periodic breathing.
Central sleep apnea due to a medical disorder without Cheyne-Stokes breathing.
Central sleep apnea due to a medication or substance.
Primary central sleep apnea.
Primary sleep apnea of infancy.
Primary central sleep apnea of prematurity.
Treatment-emergent central sleep apnea.

OBSTRUCTIVE SLEEP APNEA DISORDERS

Obstructive sleep apnea, adult.
Obstructive sleep apnea, pediatric.

SLEEP-RELATED HYPOVENTILATION/HYPOXEMIC DISORDERS

Obesity hypoventilation syndrome.
Idiopathic central alveolar hypoventilation.

LATE-ONSET CENTRAL HYPOVENTILATION WITH HYPOTHALAMIC DYSFUNCTION

Congenital central alveolar hypoventilation syndrome.
Sleep-related hypoventilation due to a medical disorder.
Sleep-related hypoventilation due to a medication or substance.
Sleep-related hypoxemia.

BREATHING, NOISY[57]

ICD-10CM #		
R06.00	Dyspnea, unspecified
R06.09	Other forms of dyspnea
R06.3	Periodic breathing
R06.83	Snoring
R06.89	Other abnormalities of breathing
R06.1	Stridor

Infection: upper respiratory infection, peritonsillar abscess, retropharyngeal abscess, epiglottitis, laryngitis, tracheitis, bronchitis, bronchiolitis.
Irritants and allergens: hyperactive airway, asthma (reactive airway disease), rhinitis, angioneurotic edema.
Compression from outside of the airway: esophageal cysts or foreign body, neoplasms, lymphadenopathy.
Congenital malformation and abnormality: vascular rings, laryngeal webs, laryngomalacia, tracheomalacia, hemangiomas within the upper airway, stenoses within the upper airway, cystic fibrosis.
Acquired abnormality (at every level of the airway): nasal polyps, hypertrophied adenoids and/or tonsils, foreign body, intraluminal tumors, bronchiectasis.
Neurogenic disorder: vocal cord paralysis.

BRONCHIAL OBSTRUCTION[21]

ICD-10CM # J98.0 Tracheobronchial collapse

CAUSES OF BRONCHIAL OBSTRUCTION

Outside the Bronchus
Lymph nodes and other masses.
In the Wall of the Bronchus
Tumors
Lung carcinoma (commonly squamous cell).
Bronchial carcinoid.
Metastasis.
Hamartoma.
Inflammation
Tuberculosis.
Sarcoidosis.
Granulomatosis with polyangiitis.
Inflammatory bowel disease.
Bronchomalacia
Broncholith.
Inside the Bronchus
Mucus plug.
Inhaled foreign body.

BRONCHOPLEURAL FISTULA[21]

ICD-10CM # J86.0 Bronchopleural fistula

CAUSES OF BRONCHOPLEURAL FISTULA

Trauma
Penetrating.

Iatrogenic (especially postpneumonectomy, postlobectomy, postbiopsy).
Infection
Necrotizing pneumonia.
Empyema.
Tuberculosis.
Septic embolus.
Infected pulmonary infarct.

BROWN URINE

ICD-10CM # R82 Other abnormal findings in urine

Bile pigments.
Myoglobin.
Concentrated urine.
Use of multivitamin supplements.
Medications (antimalarials, metronidazole, nitrofurantoin, levodopa, methyldopa, phenazopyridine).
Diet rich in fava beans.
Urinary tract infection.

BRUISING

ICD-10CM # I99.8 Other disorder of circulatory system

Medication-induced (warfarin, aspirin, NSAIDs, prednisone).
Alcohol abuse.
Senile purpura.
Purpura simplex.
Physical abuse.
Vasculitis.
Platelet disorders.
Coagulation factor deficiencies.
Cushing disease.
Vitamin C deficiency.
Marfan syndrome.
Ehlers-Danlos syndrome.
Disseminated intravascular coagulation.
Leukemia.
Hereditary hemorrhagic telangiectasia.

BULLOUS DISEASES

ICD-10CM #		
L13.9	Bullous disorder, unspecified
L12.0	Bullous pemphigoid
L12.8	Other pemphigoid
L10.0	Pemphigus vulgaris
L10.1	Pemphigus vegetans
L10.2	Pemphigus foliaceous
L10.4	Pemphigus erythematosus
L10.9	Pemphigus, unspecified

Bullous pemphigoid.
Pemphigus vulgaris.
Pemphigus foliaceus.
Paraneoplastic pemphigus.
Cicatricial pemphigoid.
Erythema multiforme.
Dermatitis herpetiformis.
Herpes gestationis.
Impetigo.

Erosive lichen planus.
Linear IgA bullous dermatosis.
Epidermolysis bullosa acquisita.

CAFÉ-AU-LAIT SPOTS[19]

| ICD-10CM # | L81.3 Cafe au lait spots |

Neurofibromatosis types 1 and 2.
McCune-Albright syndrome.
Russell-Silver syndrome.
Ataxia-telangiectasia.
Fanconi anemia.
Tuberous sclerosis.
Bloom syndrome.
Basal cell nevus syndrome.
Gaucher disease.
Chédiak-Higashi syndrome.
Hunter syndrome.
Maffucci syndrome.
Multiple mucosal neuroma syndrome.
Watson syndrome.
Proteus syndrome.
Turner syndrome.
Ring chromosome syndrome.
Jaffe-Campanacci syndrome.

CALCIFICATION ON CHEST X-RAY

ICD-10CM #	J98.4	Calcification of lung
	M51.84	Other intervertebral disc disorders, thoracic region
	M51.85	Other intervertebral disc disorders, thoracolumbar region

Lung neoplasm (primary or metastatic).
Silicosis.
Idiopathic pulmonary fibrosis.
Tuberculosis.
Histoplasmosis.
Disseminated varicella infection.
Mitral stenosis (end-stage).
Secondary hyperparathyroidism.

CALCIFICATIONS, ABDOMINAL, NONVISCERAL ON X-RAY[21]

| ICD-10CM # | M61.9 | Calcification and ossification of muscle, unspecified |

NONVISCERAL ABDOMINAL CALCIFICATION
Common
Atherosclerosis.
Mesenteric lymph nodes.
Phleboliths.
Aneurysm.
Dermoid cyst.
Differentiate
Rib cartilage.
Injections in the buttocks.

Uncommon
Infestations:
  Armillifer armillatus.
  Cysticercosis.
  Guinea worm.
  Hydatid.
Tumors:
  Lipoma.
  Hemangioma.
  Neuroblastoma.
  Osteo/chondrosarcoma of soft tissues.
  Retroperitoneal sarcoma of soft tissues.
  Peritoneal metastases.
  Pheochromocytoma.
Tuberculosis:
  Peritonitis.
  Psoas abscess.
Meconium peritonitis.
Pseudomyxoma Peritonei
Mesenteric cyst.
Pancreatitis with saponification.
Lithopedion.
Appendices Epiploicae
Ligaments.
Foreign bodies.
Posttraumatic buttock cysts.

CALCIFICATIONS, ADRENAL GLAND ON X-RAY[21]

| ICD-10CM # | E27.4 Calcification, adrenal gland |

ADRENAL GLAND CALCIFICATION
Common
Idiopathic.
Hemorrhage.
Tuberculosis.
Neuroblastoma/ganglioneuroma.
Pheochromocytoma.
Uncommon
Other tumors:
  Adenoma.
  Carcinoma.
  Dermoid.
Addison disease.
Cyst.
Histoplasmosis.

CALCIFICATIONS, CARDIAC ON X-RAY[21]

| ICD-10CM # | I51.5 | Calcification, myocardium |
| | I25.1 | Calcification, arteriosclerotic |

CAUSES OF VISIBLE CALCIFICATION WITHIN THE HEART
Coronary Artery
Atherosclerosis.
Aortic Root
Atherosclerotic aorta.
Thrombus.
Syphilis.
Ankylosing spondylitis.

Homograft calcification.
Pericardium
Chronic pericarditis, tuberculosis, hemopericardium, pyogenic or viral pericarditis.
Posttraumatic.
Postoperative.
Uremic pericarditis.
Asbestosis (may be pleural calcification applied to pericardium).
Myocardium
Ventricular aneurysm (may mimic pericardial calcification).
Calcified myocardial infarction.
Postmyocarditis.
Endocardium
Endomyocardial fibrosis.
Thrombus.
Valve Cusps
Calcified valves (particularly mitral and aortic valves).
Mitral annulus calcification.
Homograft calcification.
Old vegetation.
Valve Annulus
Submitral.
Mitral.
Aortic.
Left Atrium
Wall.
Thrombus.
Atrial myxoma.
Pulmonary Artery
Pulmonary hypertension.
Postoperative:
  Postoperative serumoma calcified hydatid cyst.

CALCIFICATIONS, CUTANEOUS

| ICD-10CM # | L94.2 | Calcinosis cutis |
| | L98.8 | Other specified disorders of the skin and subcutaneous tissue |

Calcification, Raynaud phenomenon, esophageal dysmotility, sclerodactyly, and telangiectasia (CREST) syndrome.
Trauma.
Pancreatitis or pancreatic cancer.
Chronic renal failure.
Sarcoidosis.
Hyperparathyroidism.
Milk-alkali syndrome.
Hypervitaminosis D.
Panniculitis.
Idiopathic.
Iatrogenic (e.g., application of calcium alginate dressing to skin).
Multiple myeloma.
Dermatomyositis.
Parasitic infections.
Leukemia.
Lymphoma.

CALCIFICATIONS, GENITAL TRACT, FEMALE ON X-RAY[21]

ICD-10CM # E83.59 Other disorders of calcium metabolism

FEMALE GENITAL TRACT CALCIFICATION

Uterus
Leiomyomas.
Squamous cell carcinoma.
Adenocarcinoma of endometrium.
Leiomyosarcoma.
Lithopedion.
Fallopian Tubes
Ovary.
Dermoid cyst.
Serous cystadenoma/carcinoma.
Tuberculosis.
Cysts.
Autoamputation.

CALCIFICATIONS, LIVER ON X-RAY[21]

ICD-10CM # K76.89 Other specified diseases of liver
NEC K75.3 Granuloma, hepatic

LIVER CALCIFICATION

Common
Granuloma (tuberculosis, histoplasmosis, brucellosis).
Multiple scattered round densities.
Hydatid cyst:
Fine curvilinear in wall, or dense and irregular if contracted.
Primary liver tumor (hemangioma, hepatoblastoma, hepatoma, cholangiocarcinoma).
Irregular patterns or multiple nodules.
Metastases (mucinous primary of colon or breast, cystadenocarcinoma of ovary).
Finely stippled, may be extensive.
Uncommon
Hepatic artery aneurysm.
Armillifer armillatus infestation.
Chronic granulomatous disease of childhood.
Cyst (congenital or acquired).
Hematoma.
Intrahepatic gallstones.
Old liver abscess.
Portal vein thrombosis.
Differentiate
Hemochromatosis.
Thorotrast, thallium, iron.

CALCIFICATIONS, PANCREAS ON X-RAY[21]

ICD-10CM # K86.8 Calcification, pancreas

PANCREATIC CALCIFICATION

Common
Chronic pancreatitis.

Uncommon
Acute pancreatitis (saponification).
Tumors:
Cystadenoma.
Cystadenocarcinoma.
Islet cell tumor.
Metastases.
Hereditary pancreatitis (large clumps).
Hemorrhage.
Hyperparathyroidism.
Pseudocyst.
Cavernous lymphangioma.
Mucoviscidosis.
Kwashiorkor.

CALCIFICATIONS, SPLEEN ON X-RAY[21]

ICD-10CM # D73.8 Calcification, spleen

SPLENIC CALCIFICATION

Larger than 10 mm
Splenic artery aneurysm.
Splenic artery atheroma.
Cyst:
Posttraumatic.
Dermoid.
Epidermoid.
Hydatid.
Hematoma.
Infarct.
Abscess.
Tuberculosis.
Smaller than 10 mm
Histoplasmosis.
Tuberculosis.
Phleboliths.
Armillifer armillatus infestation.
Brucellosis.
Infarcts.

CALCIFICATIONS, VALVULAR ON X-RAY[21]

ICD-10CM # I51.5 Calcification, heart

CAUSES OF RADIOGRAPHICALLY VISIBLE VALVE CALCIFICATION

Aortic Valve
Rheumatic aortic valve disease.
Bicuspid aortic valve.
Age/degenerate aortic valve.
Syphilis.
Ankylosing spondylitis.
Homograft calcification.
Mitral Valve
Rheumatic mitral valve disease.
Mitral annulus calcification.
Old vegetation (may only be visible on CT).
Homograft calcification.
Pulmonary Valve
Congenital pulmonary valve stenosis.
Rheumatic pulmonary valve disease (rare).
Fallot tetralogy (usually after repair).

Pulmonary hypertension.
Homograft calcification.
Tricuspid Valve
Rheumatic tricuspid valve disease.
Old vegetation (may only be visible on ultrafast CT).

CALCIUM STONES

ICD-10CM # N20.9 Urinary calculus, unspecified

Medications (e.g., antacids, loop diuretics, vitamin D, acetazolamide, glucocorticoids).
Primary hyperparathyroidism.
Hypercalcemia from malignancy.
Sarcoidosis.
Prolonged immobilization.
Hyperoxaluria (e.g., Crohn disease, celiac disease, chronic pancreatitis).
Hyperuricosuria (e.g., hyperuricemia, excessive dietary purine, allopurinol, probenecid).
Renal tubular acidosis.
Milk-alkali syndrome.
Thyrotoxicosis.
Hypocitraturia (e.g., metabolic acidosis, hypomagnesemia, hypokalemia).

CARDIAC ARREST, NONTRAUMATIC[1]

ICD-10CM # I46.9 Cardiac arrest, cause unspecified

Cardiac (coronary artery disease, cardiomyopathies, structural abnormalities, valve dysfunction, arrhythmias).
Respiratory (upper airway obstruction, hypoventilation, pulmonary embolism, asthma, COPD exacerbation, pulmonary edema).
Circulatory (tension pneumothorax, pericardial tamponade, PE, hemorrhage, sepsis).
Electrolyte abnormalities (hypokalemia or hyperkalemia, hypomagnesemia or hypermagnesemia, hypocalcemia).
Medications (tricyclic antidepressants, digoxin, theophylline, calcium channel blockers).
Drug abuse (cocaine, heroin, amphetamines).
Toxins (carbon monoxide, cyanide).
Environmental (drowning/near-drowning, electrocution, lightning, hypothermia or hyperthermia, venomous snakes).

CARDIAC DEATH, SUDDEN[18]

ICD-10CM # Z86.74 Personal history of sudden cardiac arrest

Ventricular tachycardia.
Bradyarrhythmia, sick sinus syndrome.
Aortic stenosis.
Tetralogy of Fallot.
Pericardial tamponade.
Cardiac tumors.
Complications of infective endocarditis.

Differential
Diagnosis

II

Hypertrophic cardiomyopathy (arrhythmia or obstruction).
Myocardial ischemia.
Atherosclerosis.
Prinzmetal angina.
Kawasaki arteritis.

CARDIAC ENLARGEMENT[39]

ICD-10CM #	I51.7	Cardiomegaly
	Q23.8	Other congenital malformations of aortic and mitral valves
	Q24.8	Other specified congenital malformations of heart
	I11.9	Hypertensive heart disease without heart failure

CHAMBER ENLARGEMENT
Chronic Volume Overload
Mitral or aortic regurgitation.
Left-to-right shunt (PDA, VSD, AV fistula).
Cardiomyopathy
Ischemic.
Nonischemic.
Decompensated Pressure Overload
Aortic stenosis.
Hypertension.
High-Output States
Severe anemia.
Thyrotoxicosis.
Bradycardia
Severe sinus bradycardia.
Complete heart block.

LEFT ATRIUM
LV failure of any cause.
Mitral valve disease.
Myxoma.

RIGHT VENTRICLE
Chronic volume overload.
Tricuspid or pulmonic regurgitation.
Left-to-right shunt (ASD).
Decompensated pressure overload:
    Pulmonic stenosis.
    Pulmonary artery hypertension:
        Primary.
        Secondary (PE, COPD).
        Pulmonary venoocclusive disease.

RIGHT ATRIUM
RV failure of any cause.
Tricuspid valve disease.
Myxoma.
Ebstein anomaly.

MULTICHAMBER ENLARGEMENT
Hypertrophic cardiomyopathy.
Acromegaly.
Severe obesity.

PERICARDIAL DISEASE
Pericardial effusion with or without tamponade.
Effusive constrictive disease.

Pericardial cyst, loculated effusion.

PSEUDOCARDIOMEGALY
Epicardial fat.
Chest wall deformity (pectus excavatum, straight back syndrome).
Low lung volumes.
AP chest x-ray.
Mediastinal tumor, cyst.

CARDIAC MASSES[58]

ICD-10CM #	C38.0	Malignant neoplasm of heart
	D15.1	Benign neoplasm of heart

Intracardiac thrombus.
Focal myocardial hypertrophy.
Left ventricular noncompaction.
Infectious disease (abscess).
Primary cardiac tumor.
Secondary cardiac tumor (metastasis).
Lipomatous hypertrophy of septum.
Cyst.
Imaging artifact.

CARDIAC MURMURS

ICD-10CM #	R01.0	Benign and innocent cardiac murmurs
	R01.1	Cardiac murmur, unspecified

SYSTOLIC
Mitral regurgitation (MR).
Tricuspid regurgitation (TR).
Ventricular septal defect (VSD).
Aortic stenosis (AS).
Idiopathic hypertrophic subaortic stenosis (IHSS).
Pulmonic stenosis (PS).
Innocent murmur of childhood.
Coarctation of aorta.
Mitral valve prolapse (MVP).

DIASTOLIC
Aortic regurgitation (AR).
Atrial myxoma.
Mitral stenosis (MS).
Pulmonary artery branch stenosis.
Tricuspid stenosis (TS).
Graham Steell murmur (diastolic decrescendo murmur heard in severe pulmonary hypertension).
Pulmonic regurgitation (PR).
Severe mitral regurgitation (MR).
Austin Flint murmur (diastolic rumble heard in severe AR).
Severe VSD and patent ductus arteriosus.

CONTINUOUS
Patent ductus arteriosus.
Pulmonary AV fistula.

CARDIAC TUMORS[59]

ICD-10CM #	C38.0	Malignant neoplasm of heart
	D15.1	Benign neoplasm of heart

PRIMARY
Benign:
    Myxoma.
    Lipoma.
    Fibroma.
    Rhabdomyoma.
    Fibroelastoma.
Malignant:
    Sarcoma.
    Mesothelioma.
    Lymphoma.

SECONDARY
Direct Extension
Lung cancer.
Breast cancer.
Mediastinal tumors.
Metastatic Tumors
Malignant melanoma.
Leukemia.
Lymphoma.
Venous Extension
Renal cell cancer.
Adrenal cancer.
Liver cancer.

CARDIOEMBOLISM

ICD-10CM #	I21.3 ST	Elevation (STEMI) myocardial infarction of unspecified site
	I21.9	Acute myocardial infarction, unspecified

Acute MI.
Atrial fibrillation.
Left ventricular aneurysm.
Valvular heart disease (e.g., rheumatic mitral valve disease, mitral valve prolapse).
Dilated cardiomyopathy.
Atrial septal defect.
Patent foramen ovale.
Cardioversion for atrial fibrillation.
Infective endocarditis.
Atrial septal aneurysm.
Sick sinus syndrome and cardiac arrhythmias.
Nonbacterial thrombotic endocarditis.
Prosthetic heart valves.
Atrial myxoma and other intracardiac tumors.
Cyanotic heart disease.
Balloon angioplasty.
Coronary artery bypass grafting.
Aneurysms of sinus of Valsalva.
Other: VVI pacing, ventricular support devices, heart transplantation, intracardiac defects with paradoxical embolism.

CARDIOGENIC SHOCK

ICD-10CM #   R57.0   Cardiogenic shock

Myocardial infarction.
Arrhythmias.
Pericardial effusion/tamponade.
Chest trauma.
Valvular heart disease.
Myocarditis.
Cardiomyopathy.
CHF, end-stage.

CATAPLEXY[38]

ICD-10CM #   G47.4   Narcolepsy and cataplexy

DIFFERENTIAL DIAGNOSIS OF CATAPLEXY

Partial complex seizure.
Absence spell.
Atonic seizure.
Drop attack.
Syncope.
Vertebrobasilar insufficiency.
Basilar migraines.
Pseudocataplexy.

CATARACTS, PEDIATRIC AGE

ICD-10CM #   H26.0   Infantile, juvenile, and presenile cataracts

DEVELOPMENTAL VARIANTS

Prematurity (Y-suture vacuoles) with or without retinopathy of prematurity.

GENETIC DISORDERS

Simple Mendelian Inheritance
Autosomal dominant (most common).
Autosomal recessive.
X-linked.
Major Chromosomal Defects
Trisomy disorders (13, 18, 21).
Turner syndrome (45X).
Deletion syndromes (11p13, 18p, 18q).
Duplication syndromes (3q, 20p, 10q).
Multisystem Genetic Disorders
Alport syndrome (hearing loss, renal disease).
Alström syndrome (nerve deafness, diabetes mellitus).
Apert disease (craniosynostosis, syndactyly).
Cockayne syndrome (premature senility, skin photosensitivity).
Conradi disease (chondrodysplasia punctata).
Crouzon disease (dysostosis craniofacialis).
Hallermann-Streiff syndrome (microphthalmia, small pinched nose, skin atrophy, hypotrichosis).
Hypohidrotic ectodermal dysplasia (anomalous dentition, hypohidrosis, hypotrichosis).
Ichthyosis (keratinizing disorder with thick, scaly skin).

Incontinentia pigmenti (dental anomalies, mental retardation, cutaneous lesions).
Lowe syndrome (oculocerebrorenal syndrome: hypotonia, renal disease).
Marfan syndrome.
Marinesco-Sjögren syndrome (cerebellar ataxia, hypotonia).
Meckel-Gruber syndrome (renal dysplasia, encephalocele).
Myotonic dystrophy.
Nail-patella syndrome (renal dysfunction, dysplastic nails, hypoplastic patella).
Nevoid basal cell carcinoma syndrome (autosomal dominant, basal cell carcinoma erupts in childhood).
Peters anomaly (corneal opacifications with iris-corneal dysgenesis).
Reiger syndrome (iris dysplasia, myotonic dystrophy).
Rothmund-Thomson syndrome (poikiloderma: skin atrophy).
Rubinstein-Taybi syndrome (broad great toe, mental retardation).
Smith-Lemli-Opitz syndrome (toe syndactyly, hypospadias, mental retardation).
Sotos syndrome (cerebral gigantism).
Spondyloepiphyseal dysplasia (dwarfism, short trunk).
Werner syndrome (premature aging in second decade of life).
Inborn Errors of Metabolism
Abetalipoproteinemia (absent chylomicrons, retinal degeneration).
Fabry disease (α-galactosidase A deficiency).
Galactokinase deficiency.
Galactosemia (galactose-1-phosphate uridyl transferase deficiency).
Homocystinemia (subluxation of lens, mental retardation).
Mannosidosis (acid α-mannosidase deficiency).
Niemann-Pick disease (sphingomyelinase deficiency).
Refsum disease (phytanic acid α-hydrolase deficiency).
Wilson disease (accumulation of copper leads to cirrhosis and neurologic symptoms).

ENDOCRINOPATHIES

Hypocalcemia (hypoparathyroidism).
Hypoglycemia.
Diabetes mellitus.

CONGENITAL INFECTIONS

Toxoplasmosis.
Cytomegalovirus infection.
Syphilis.
Rubella.
Perinatal herpes simplex infection.
Measles (rubeola).
Poliomyelitis.
Influenza.
Varicella-zoster.

OCULAR ANOMALIES

Microphthalmia.
Coloboma.
Aniridia.
Mesodermal dysgenesis.
Persistent papillary membrane.
Posterior lenticonus.
Persistent hyperplastic primary vitreous.
Primitive hyaloid vascular system.

MISCELLANEOUS DISORDERS

Atopic dermatitis.
Drugs (corticosteroids).
Radiation.
Trauma.
Idiopathic

CAVITARY LESION ON CHEST X-RAY[60]

ICD-10CM #   R91.8   Other nonspecific abnormal finding of lung field

NECROTIZING INFECTIONS

Bacteria: anaerobes, *Staphylococcus aureus,* enteric gram-negative bacteria, *Pseudomonas aeruginosa, Legionella* spp., *Haemophilus influenzae, Streptococcus pyogenes, Streptococcus pneumoniae, Rhodococcus, Actinomyces.*
Mycobacteria: *Mycobacterium tuberculosis, Mycobacterium kansasii,* MAI.
Bacteria-like: *Nocardia* spp.
Fungi: *Coccidioides immitis, Histoplasma capsulatum, Blastomyces hominis, Aspergillus* spp., *Mucor* spp.
Parasitic: *Entamoeba histolytica, Echinococcus, Paragonimus westermani.*

CAVITARY INFARCTION

Bland infarction (with or without superimposed infection).
Lung contusion.

SEPTIC EMBOLISM

S. aureus, anaerobes, others.

VASCULITIS

Granulomatosis with polyangiitis, periarteritis.

NEOPLASMS

Bronchogenic carcinoma, metastatic carcinoma, lymphoma.

MISCELLANEOUS LESIONS

Cysts, blebs, bullae, or pneumatocele with or without fluid collections.
Sequestration.
Empyema with air-fluid level.
Bronchiectasis.

Differential Diagnosis

II

CEREBRAL INFARCTION SECONDARY TO INHERITED DISORDERS

ICD-10CM # I63.50 Cerebral infarction due to unspecified occlusion or stenosis of unspecified cerebral artery

Homocystinuria.
Marfan syndrome.
Ehlers-Danlos syndrome.
Rendu-Osler-Weber syndrome.
Pseudoxanthoma elasticum.
Fabry disease.

CEREBRAL VASCULITIS, CAUSES[61]

ICD-10CM # Varies with specific diagnosis

PRIMARY CEREBRAL VASCULITIDES
Takayasu arteritis.
Primary cerebral vasculitis.
Polyarteritis nodosa.

SECONDARY VASCULITIDES
Immune Disorders
Systemic lupus erythematosus.
Wegner granulomatosis.
Kawasaki syndrome.
Sarcoidosis.
Henoch-Schönlein purpura.
Primary Intracranial Infections
Bacterial meningitis (especially *Diplococcus pneumoniae*).
Tuberculous meningitis.
Mycotic infections.
Cat-scratch disease.
Human immunodeficiency virus/acquired immunodeficiency syndrome.
Malaria.
Lyme disease.
Rickettsial infections.
Brucellosis.

CEREBROVASCULAR DISEASE, ISCHEMIC[62]

ICD-10CM # I67.9 Cerebrovascular disease, unspecified

VASCULAR DISORDERS
Large-vessel atherothrombotic disease.
Lacunar disease.
Arterial-to-arterial embolization.
Carotid or vertebral artery dissection.
Fibromuscular dysplasia.
Migraine.
Venous thrombosis.
Radiation.
Complications of arteriography.
Multiple, progressive intracranial arterial occlusions.

INFLAMMATORY DISORDERS
Giant cell arteritis.
Polyarteritis nodosa.
SLE.
Granulomatous angiitis.
Takayasu disease.
Arteritis associated with amphetamine, cocaine, or phenylpropanolamine.
Syphilis, mucormycosis.
Sjögren syndrome.
Behçet syndrome.

CARDIAC DISORDERS
Rheumatic heart disease.
Mural thrombus.
Arrhythmias.
Mitral valve prolapse.
Prosthetic heart valve.
Endocarditis.
Myxoma.
Paradoxical embolus.

HEMATOLOGIC DISORDERS
Thrombotic thrombocytopenic purpura.
Sickle cell disease.
Hypercoagulable states.
Polycythemia.
Thrombocytosis.
Leukocytosis.
Lupus anticoagulant.

CERVICAL INSTABILITY, PEDIATRIC

ICD-10CM # M50 Cervical disc disorders

CONGENITAL
Vertebral (Bony Anomalies)
Craniooccipital defects (occipital vertebrae, basilar impression, occipital dysplasias, condylar hypoplasia, occipitalized atlas).
Atlantoaxial defects (aplasia of atlas arch, aplasia of odontoid process).
Subaxial anomalies (failure of segmentation and/or fusion, spina bifida, spondylolisthesis).
Ligamentous or Combined Anomalies
Found at birth as an element of somatogenic aberration.
Syndromic Disorders
Down syndrome.
Klippel-Feil syndrome.
22q11.2 deletion syndrome.
Larsen syndrome.
Marfan syndrome.
Ehlers-Danlos syndrome.

ACQUIRED
Trauma.
Infection (pyogenic, granulomatous).
Tumor (including neurofibromatosis).
Inflammatory conditions (e.g., juvenile rheumatoid arthritis).
Osteochondrodysplasias (e.g., achondroplasia, diastrophic dysplasia, metatropic dysplasia, spondyloepiphyseal dysplasia).

Storage disorders (e.g., mucopolysaccharidoses).
Metabolic disorders (rickets).
Miscellaneous (including osteogenesis imperfecta, sequela of surgery).

CHEST PAIN, CHILDREN[45]

ICD-10CM # R07.9 Chest pain, unspecified
R07.82 Intercostal pain
R07.89 Other chest pain
R07.1 Chest pain on breathing
R07.81 Pleurodynia

MUSCULOSKELETAL (COMMON)
Trauma (accidental, abuse).
Exercise, overuse injury (strain, bursitis).
Costochondritis (Tietze syndrome).
Herpes zoster (cutaneous).
Pleurodynia.
Fibrositis.
Slipping rib.
Sickle cell anemia vasoocclusive crisis.
Osteomyelitis (rare).
Primary or metastatic tumor (rare).

PULMONARY (COMMON)
Pneumonia.
Pleurisy.
Asthma.
Chronic cough.
Pneumothorax.
Infarction (sickle cell anemia).
Foreign body.
Embolism (rare).
Pulmonary hypertension (rare).
Tumor (rare).

GASTROINTESTINAL (LESS COMMON)
Esophagitis (gastroesophageal reflux).
Esophageal foreign body.
Esophageal spasm.
Cholecystitis.
Subdiaphragmatic abscess.
Perihepatitis (Fitz-Hugh-Curtis syndrome).
Peptic ulcer disease.

CARDIAC (LESS COMMON)
Pericarditis.
Postpericardiotomy syndrome.
Endocarditis.
Mitral valve prolapse.
Aortic or subaortic stenosis.
Arrhythmias.
Marfan syndrome (dissecting aortic aneurysm).
Anomalous coronary artery.
Kawasaki disease.
Cocaine, sympathomimetic ingestion.
Angina (familial hypercholesterolemia).

IDIOPATHIC (COMMON)
Anxiety, hyperventilation.
Panic disorder.

OTHER (LESS COMMON)

Spinal cord or nerve root compression.
Breast-related pathologic condition.
Castleman disease (lymph node neoplasm).

CHEST PAIN, NONPLEURITIC[63]

ICD-10CM #	R07.9	Chest pain, unspecified
	R07.82	Intercostal pain
	R07.89	Other chest pain

Cardiac: myocardial ischemia/infarction, myocarditis.

Esophageal: spasm, esophagitis, ulceration, neoplasm, achalasia, diverticula, foreign body.

Referred pain from subdiaphragmatic GI structures.

Gastric and duodenal: hiatal hernia, neoplasm, PUD.

Gallbladder and biliary: cholecystitis, cholelithiasis, impacted stone, neoplasm.

Pancreatic: pancreatitis, neoplasm.

Dissecting aortic aneurysm.

Pain originating from skin, breasts, and musculoskeletal structures: herpes zoster, mastitis, cervical spondylosis.

Mediastinal tumors: lymphoma, thymoma.

Pulmonary: neoplasm, pneumonia, pulmonary embolism/infarction.

Psychoneurosis.

Chest pain associated with mitral valve prolapse.

CHEST PAIN, PLEURITIC

| ICD-10CM # | R07.1 | Chest pain on breathing |
| | R07.81 | Pleurodynia |

Cardiac: pericarditis, postpericardiotomy/Dressler syndrome.

Pulmonary: pneumothorax, hemothorax, embolism/infarction, pneumonia, empyema, neoplasm, bronchiectasis, pneumomediastinum, TB, carcinomatous effusion.

GI: liver abscess, pancreatitis, esophageal rupture, Whipple disease with associated pericarditis or pleuritis.

Subdiaphragmatic abscess.

Pain originating from skin and musculoskeletal tissues: costochondritis, chest wall trauma, fractured rib, interstitial fibrosis, myositis, strain of pectoralis muscle, herpes zoster, soft tissue and bone tumors.

Collagen vascular diseases with pleuritis.

Psychoneurosis.

Familial Mediterranean fever.

CHEST WALL TUMORS, PRIMARY[64]

| ICD-10CM # | Varies with specific diagnosis |

SOFT TISSUE

Benign

Lipoma.

Hemangioma.
Lymphangioma.
Fibroma.
Rhabdomyoma.
Neurofibroma.
Desmoid tumor.

Malignant

Malignant fibrous histiocytoma.
Rhabdosarcoma.
Liposarcoma.
Neurofibrosarcoma.
Leiomyosarcoma.

BONY AND CARTILAGINOUS

Benign

Fibrous dysplasia.
Osteochondroma.
Chondroma.
Askin tumor.
Plasmacytoma.

Malignant

Chondrosarcoma.
Osteogenic sarcoma.
Ewing sarcoma.

CHIASMAL DISEASE[44]

| ICD-10CM # | Varies with specific diagnosis |

CAUSES OF CHIASMAL DISEASE

Tumors

Pituitary adenomas.
Craniopharyngioma.
Meningioma.
Glioma.
Chordoma.
Dysgerminoma.
Nasopharyngeal tumors.
Metastases.

Nonneoplastic Masses

Aneurysm.
Rathke pouch cysts.
Fibrous dysplasia.
Sphenoidal sinus mucocele.
Arachnoid cysts.

Miscellaneous

Demyelination.
Inflammation (e.g., sarcoidosis).
Trauma.
Radiation-induced necrosis.
Toxicity (e.g., ethambutol).
Vasculitis.

CHILDHOOD EOSINOPHILIA

| ICD-10CM # | D72.1 | Eosinophilia |

PHYSIOLOGIC

Prematurity.
Infants receiving hyperalimentation.
Familial.

INFECTIOUS

Parasitic (with tissue-invasive helminths, e.g., trichinosis, strongyloidiasis, pneumocystosis, filariasis, cysticercosis, cutaneous and visceral larva migrans, echinococcosis).

Bacterial (brucellosis, tularemia, cat-scratch disease, *Chlamydia*).

Fungal (histoplasmosis, blastomycosis, coccidioidomycosis, allergic bronchopulmonary aspergillosis).

Mycobacterial (tuberculosis, leprosy).

Viral (hepatitis A, hepatitis B, hepatitis C, Epstein-Barr virus).

PULMONARY

Allergic (rhinitis, asthma).
Loeffler syndrome.
Hypersensitivity pneumonitis.
Eosinophilic pneumonia.
Pulmonary interstitial eosinophilia.

DERMATOLOGIC

Atopic dermatitis.
Pemphigus.
Dermatitis herpetiformis.
Infantile eosinophilic pustular folliculitis.
Episodic angioedema and urticaria.
Eosinophilic fasciitis (Shulman syndrome).
Eosinophilic cellulitis (Wells syndrome).
Kimura disease.

ONCOLOGIC

Neoplasm (lung, GI, uterine).
Hodgkin disease.
Leukemia.
Myelofibrosis.

IMMUNOLOGIC

T-cell immunodeficiencies.
Hyperimmunoglobulin E (Job) syndrome.
Wiskott-Aldrich syndrome.
Graft-versus-host disease.
Drug hypersensitivity.
Postirradiation.
Postsplenectomy.

ENDOCRINE

Postadrenalectomy.
Addison disease.
Panhypopituitarism.

CARDIOVASCULAR

Loeffler disease (fibroplastic endocarditis).
Congenital heart disease.
Hypersensitivity vasculitis.

GASTROINTESTINAL

Milk protein allergy.
Inflammatory bowel disease.
Eosinophilic esophagitis.
Eosinophilic gastroenteritis.

CHOLANGITIS, ACUTE[64]

| ICD-10CM # | K83.0 | Cholangitis |

NONIATROGENIC

Benign Conditions

Choledocholithiasis.
  Primary.
  Secondary.
Pancreatitis (chronic/acute), including pancreatic pseudocyst.
Papillary stenosis.
Mirizzi syndrome.
Choledochal cysts (type V, Caroli disease).
Primary sclerosing cholangitis.

Malignancies

Pancreatic cancer.
Cholangiocarcinoma.
Porta hepatis tumor/metastasis.

IATROGENIC

Obstructed biliary endoprosthesis.
Iatrogenic biliary stricture.
Direct surgical trauma.
Ischemia-induced stricture.
Anastomotic stricture (biliobiliary/bilioenteric anastomosis).

CHOLESTASIS[24]

ICD-10CM #	K80.65	Calculus of gallbladder and bile duct with chronic cholecystitis with obstruction

EXTRAHEPATIC

Choledocholithiasis.
Bile duct stricture.
Cholangiocarcinoma.
Pancreatic carcinoma.
Chronic pancreatitis.
Papillary stenosis.
Ampullary cancer.
Primary sclerosing cholangitis.
Choledochal cysts.
Parasites (e.g., ascaris, clonorchis).
AIDS.
Cholangiography.
Biliary atresia.
Portal lymphadenopathy.
Mirizzi syndrome.

INTRAHEPATIC

Viral hepatitis.
Alcoholic hepatitis.
Drug induced.
Ductopenia syndromes.
Primary biliary cirrhosis.
Benign recurrent intrahepatic cholestasis.
Byler disease.
Primary sclerosing cholangitis.
Alagille syndrome.
Sarcoid.
Lymphoma.
Postoperative.
Total parenteral nutrition.
α-1-antitrypsin deficiency.

CHOLESTASIS, NEONATAL AND INFANTILE, DIFFERENTIAL DIAGNOSIS[19]

ICD-10CM #	026.6	Liver disorders in pregnancy, childbirth and the puerperium

INFECTIOUS

Generalized bacterial sepsis.
Viral hepatitis:
  Hepatitis A, B, C, D.
  Cytomegalovirus.
  Rubella virus.
  Herpesvirus: herpes simplex, human herpesvirus 6 and 7.
  Varicella virus.
  Coxsackievirus.
  Echovirus.
  Reovirus type 3.
  Parvovirus B19.
  HIV.
  Adenovirus.
Others:
  Toxoplasmosis.
  Syphilis.
  Tuberculosis.
  Listeriosis.
  Urinary tract infection.

TOXIC

Sepsis.
Parenteral nutrition related.
Drug related.

METABOLIC

Disorders of amino acid metabolism:
  Tyrosinemia.
Disorders of lipid metabolism:
  Wolman disease.
  Niemann-Pick disease (type C).
  Gaucher disease.
Cholesterol ester storage disease.
Disorders of carbohydrate metabolism:
  Galactosemia.
  Fructosemia.
  Glycogenosis IV.
Disorders of bile acid biosynthesis.
Other metabolic defects:
  α1-Antitrypsin deficiency.
  Cystic fibrosis.
  Hypopituitarism.
  Hypothyroidism.
  Zellweger (cerebrohepatorenal) syndrome.
  Neonatal iron storage disease.
  Indian childhood cirrhosis/infantile copper overload.
  Congenital disorders of glycosylation.
  Mitochondrial hepatopathies.
  Citrin deficiency.

GENETIC OR CHROMOSOMAL

Trisomy 17, 18, 21.
Donahue syndrome.

INTRAHEPATIC CHOLESTASIS SYNDROMES

"Idiopathic" neonatal hepatitis.
Alagille syndrome (arteriohepatic dysplasia).
Nonsyndromic bile duct paucity syndrome.
Intrahepatic cholestasis (PFIC):
  FIC-1 deficiency.
  BSEP deficiency.
  MDR3 deficiency.
Familial benign recurrent cholestasis associated with lymphedema (Aagenaes).
Congenital hepatic fibrosis.
Caroli disease (cystic dilation of intrahepatic ducts).

EXTRAHEPATIC DISEASES

Biliary atresia.
Sclerosing cholangitis.
Bile duct stricture/stenosis.
Choledochal-pancreaticoductal junction anomaly.
Spontaneous perforation of the bile duct.
Choledochal cyst.
Mass (neoplasia, stone).
Bile/mucous plug ("inspissated bile").

MISCELLANEOUS

Shock and hypoperfusion.
Associated with enteritis.
Associated with intestinal obstruction.
Neonatal lupus erythematosus.
Myeloproliferative disease (trisomy 21).
Hemophagocytic lymphohistiocytosis.
Arthrogryposis cholestatic pigmentary syndrome.

CHOLESTATIC LIVER ENZYME ELEVATION, EXTRAHEPATIC CAUSES[3]

ICD-10CM #	Varies with specific diagnosis

EXTRAHEPATIC CAUSES OF CHOLESTATIC LIVER ENZYMES IN ADULTS

Intrinsic

Choledocholithiasis.
Immune-mediated duct injury:
  Autoimmune pancreatitis.
  PSC.
Malignancy:
  Ampullary cancer.
  Cholangiocarcinoma.
Infections:
  AIDS cholangiopathy:
    Cytomegalovirus.
    Cryptosporidiosis.
    Microsporidiosis.
  Parasitic infections:
    Ascariasis.

Extrinsic

Malignancy:

Gallbladder cancer.

Metastases, including portal adenopathy from metastases.

Pancreatic cancer.

Mirizzi syndrome.

Pancreatitis.

Pancreatic pseudocyst.

CHOLESTATIC LIVER ENZYME ELEVATION, INTRAHEPATIC CAUSES[3]

ICD-10CM #   Varies with specific causes

INTRAHEPATIC CAUSES OF CHOLESTATIC LIVER ENZYME ELEVATIONS IN ADULTS

Drugs*

Bland cholestasis:[††]

Anabolic steroids.

Estrogens.

Cholestatic hepatitis:

Angiotensin-converting enzyme inhibitors: captopril, enalapril.

Antimicrobials: amoxicillin-clavulanic acid, ketoconazole.

Azathioprine.

Chlorpromazine.

NSAIDs: sulindac, piroxicam.

Granulomatous hepatitis:

Allopurinol.

Antibiotics: sulfonamides.

Antiepileptics: carbamazepine, phenytoin.

Cardiovascular agents: hydralazine, procainamide, quinidine.

Phenylbutazone.

Vanishing bile duct syndrome:

Amoxicillin-clavulanic acid.

Chlorpromazine.

Dicloxacillin.

Flucloxacillin.

Macrolides.

PBC

PSC

Granulomatous Liver Disease

Infections:

Brucellosis.

Fungal: histoplasmosis, coccidioidomycosis.

Leprosy.

Q fever.

Schistosomiasis.

TB, *Mycobacterium avium* complex, bacillus Calmette-Guérin.

Sarcoidosis.

Idiopathic granulomatous hepatitis.

Other:

Crohn disease.

Heavy metal exposure: beryllium, copper.

Hodgkin disease.

Viral Hepatitis

HAV and HEV.

HBV and HCV, including fibrosing cholestatic hepatitis.

EBV.

Cytomegalovirus.

Idiopathic Adulthood Ductopenia

Genetic Conditions

Progressive familial intrahepatic cholestasis:

Type 1 (formerly Byler disease).

Type 2.

Type 3.

Benign recurrent intrahepatic cholestasis:

Type 1.

Type 2.

CF.

Malignancy

Hepatocellular carcinoma.

Metastatic disease.

Paraneoplastic syndrome:

Non-Hodgkin lymphoma.

Prostate cancer.

Renal cell cancer.

Infiltrative Liver Disease

Amyloidosis.

Lymphoma.

Intrahepatic Cholestasis of Pregnancy

TPN:

Graft-versus-host disease.

Sepsis.

CHOREA

ICD-10CM #   G25.4   Drug-induced chorea

G25.5   Other chorea

Medications (e.g., neuroleptics, tricyclics, antiparkinsonian drugs).

Cerebral palsy.

Huntington disease.

Benign hereditary chorea.

Thyroid disorder (hyperthyroidism, hypothyroidism).

Friedreich ataxia.

Ataxia-telangiectasia.

Hypoglycemia, hyperglycemia.

Electrolyte abnormalities (hyponatremia, hypocalcemia, hypomagnesemia, hypernatremia).

Vitamin B_{12} deficiency.

SLE.

Wilson disease.

Alcohol.

Cocaine.

Carbon monoxide poisoning.

Mercury poisoning.

CHOREA, PEDIATRIC PATIENT[49]

ICD-10CM #   G25.5   Other chorea

CAUSES OF CHOREA IN CHILDHOOD

Static Injury/Structural Disorders

Cerebral palsy.

Stroke.

Trauma.

Moyamoya disease.

Vasculitis.

Tumors.

Congenital malformations.

Joubert syndrome.

Hereditary/Degenerative Disorders

Ataxia-telangiectasia (A-T) and ataxia-telangiectasia-like disorder (ATLD).

Ataxia oculomotor apraxia (AOA) (includes AOA-1, AOA-2, and early onset cerebellar ataxia and hypoalbuminemia [EOCA-HA]).

Fahr disease.

Pantothenate kinase-associated neurodegeneration (PKAN, associated with mutations in the pantothenate kinase-2 [*PANK-2*] gene), and other causes of neuronal brain iron accumulation (NBIA).

Metabolic Disorders

Acyl-CoA dehydrogenase deficiencies.

Mitochondrial disorders, including Leigh syndrome.

GM_1 gangliosidosis.

Lesch-Nyhan disease.

Niemann-Pick type C.

Methylmalonic aciduria.

Nonketotic hyperglycemia.

Kernicterus.

Hypoparathyroidism.

Propionic acidemia.

Hypernatremia.

Hypomagnesemia.

Hypocalcemia.

Hypo- or hyperglycemia.

Vitamin E deficiency or malabsorption.

Bassen-Kornzweig disease.

Complications of cardiac bypass.

Infectious/Parainfectious Disease

Encephalitis/postencephalitis.

Immune-Mediated/Demyelinating Disorders

Sydenham chorea.

Lupus erythematosus.

Henoch-Schönlein purpura.

Anticardiolipin or antiphospholipid antibody syndrome.

Anti-NMDA antibody syndrome.

Drugs/Toxins

Neuroleptic medications, and neuroleptic-like antiemetics (haloperidol, chlorpromazine, pimozide, prochlorperazine, metoclopramide).

Calcium channel blockers (flunarizine, cinnarizine).

Antiseizure medications (phenytoin, carbamazepine, valproate, phenobarbital).

Anticholinergic medications (trihexyphenidyl, benztropine).

Antihistamines.

Tricyclic antidepressants.

Differential Diagnosis

II

[††]Diffuse, uniform loss, but many hairs left randomly distributed in area of loss.

Clomipramine.
Stimulants (including methylphenidate, dex-amphetamine, pemoline, and bronchodilators).
Clonidine.
L-dopa.
Cocaine.
Bismuth.
Lithium.
Manganese.
Ethanol.
Carbon monoxide.
Oral contraceptives.
General anesthesia (including propofol)—during induction or emergence.
Paroxysmal Disorders
Complex migraine.
Alternating hemiplegia of childhood.
Paroxysmal kinesigenic dyskinesia (PKD).
Paroxysmal nonkinesigenic dyskinesia (PNKD).
Paroxysmal exercise-induced dyskinesia (PED).
Endocrine Disorders
Hyperthyroidism.
Pheochromocytoma.

CHOREOATHETOSIS[25]

ICD-10CM # G25.5 Choreoathetosis

SYSTEMIC DISEASES
SLE.
Polycythemia.
Thyrotoxicosis.
Rheumatic fever.
Cirrhosis of the liver (acquired hepatocerebral degeneration).
DM.
Wilson disease.

PRIMARY DEGENERATIVE BRAIN DISEASES
Huntington chorea.
Olivopontocerebellar atrophies.
Neuroacanthocytosis.

FOCAL BRAIN DISEASES
Hemichorea.
Stroke.
Tumor.
Arteriovenous malformation.

DRUG-INDUCED CHOREOATHETOSIS
Parkinson Disease Drugs
Levodopa.

EPILEPSY DRUGS
Phenytoin.
Carbamazepine.
Phenobarbital.
Gabapentin.
Valproate.
Psychostimulant Drugs
Cocaine.
Amphetamine.
Methamphetamine.

Dextroamphetamine.
Methylphenidate.
Pemoline.
Psychotropic Drugs
Lithium.
Tricyclic antidepressant drugs.
Oral Contraceptive Drugs
Cimetidine

CHRONIC PNEUMONIA[65]

ICD-10CM # J17 Pneumonia in diseases classified elsewhere

CAUSES OF CHRONIC PNEUMONIA
Infectious
Bacteria
Mixed aerobic and anaerobic bacteria.
Actinomyces spp.
Burkholderia pseudomallei.
Nocardia spp.
Rhodococcus equi.
Mycobacteria
Mycobacterium abscessus.
Mycobacterium avium complex.
Mycobacterium kansasii.
Mycobacterium tuberculosis.
Parasites
Dirofilaria.
Echinococcus granulosus.
Filaria.
Paragonimus westermani.
Fungi
Aspergillus spp.
Blastomyces dermatitidis.
Coccidioides spp.
Cryptococcus spp.
Histoplasma capsulatum.
Scedosporium spp.
Sporothrix schenckii.
Noninfectious
Neoplasia.
Cystic fibrosis.
Sarcoidosis.
Amyloidosis.
Vasculitis.
Drugs.
Radiation.
Recurrent pulmonary emboli.
Bronchial obstruction.
Pulmonary infiltration with eosinophilia syndrome.
Pneumoconiosis.

CHYLOTHORAX[4]

ICD-10CM # I89.8 Other specified noninfective disorders of lymphatic vessels and lymph nodes

Traumatic (Chest and Neck)
  Blunt.
  Penetrating.
Iatrogenic
  Catheterization, particularly subclavian vein.
  Postsurgical.

Excision of cervical/supraclavicular lymph nodes.
Radical lymph node dissections of the neck or chest.
Lung, esophageal, or mediastinal resection.
Thoracic aneurysm repair.
Sympathectomy.
Congenital cardiovascular surgery.
Neoplasms
  Lymphoma, lung, esophageal, or mediastinal neoplasms.
  Metastatic carcinoma.
Infectious
  Tuberculous lymphadenosis.
  Mediastinitis.
  Ascending lymphangitis.
Other
  Lymphangioleiomyomatosis.
  Venous thrombosis.
  Congenital.

CLOUDY URINE

ICD-10CM # R82 Other abnormal findings in urine

Concentrated urine.
Use of multivitamin supplements.
Diet high in purine-rich foods.
Pyuria.
Phosphaturia.
Urinary tract infection.
Lipiduria.
Chyluria.
Hyperoxaluria.

CLUBBING

ICD-10CM # R68.3 Clubbing of fingers

Pulmonary neoplasm (lung, pleura).
Other neoplasm (GI, liver, Hodgkin, thymus, osteogenic sarcoma).
Pulmonary infectious process (empyema, abscess, bronchiectasis, TB, chronic pneumonitis).
Extrapulmonary infectious process (subacute bacterial endocarditis, intestinal TB, bacterial or amebic dysentery, arterial graft sepsis).
Pneumoconiosis.
Cystic fibrosis.
Sarcoidosis.
Cyanotic congenital heart disease.
Endocrine (Graves disease, hyperparathyroidism).
Inflammatory bowel disease.
Celiac disease.
Chronic liver disease, cirrhosis (particularly biliary and juvenile).
Pulmonary AV malformations.
Idiopathic.
Thyroid acropachy.
Hereditary (pachydermoperiostosis).
Chronic trauma (jackhammer operators, machine workers).

COBALAMIN DEFICIENCY[31]

ICD-10CM # E53.8 Deficiency of other specified B group vitamins

ETIOPATHOPHYSIOLOGIC CLASSIFICATION OF COBALAMIN DEFICIENCY

Nutritional cobalamin deficiency (i.e., insufficient cobalamin intake):

Vegetarians, poverty-imposed near-vegetarians, breastfed infants of mothers with pernicious anemia.

Abnormal intragastric events (i.e., inadequate proteolysis of food cobalamin):

Atrophic gastritis, partial gastritis with hypochlorhydria, proton-pump inhibitors, H_2 blockers.

Loss or atrophy of gastric oxyntic mucosa (i.e., deficient intrinsic factor [IF] molecules):

Total or partial gastrectomy, pernicious anemia, caustic destruction (lye).

Abnormal events in small bowel lumen:

Inadequate pancreatic protease (e.g., R-cobalamin not degraded, cobalamin not transferred to IF):

Insufficient pancreatic protease (i.e., pancreatic insufficiency).

Inactivation of pancreatic protease (i.e., Zollinger-Ellison syndrome).

Usurping of luminal cobalamin (i.e., inadequate cobalamin binding to IF):

By bacteria, during stasis syndromes (e.g., blind loops, pouches of diverticulosis, strictures, fistulas, anastomosis), impaired bowel motility (e.g., scleroderma), hypogammaglobulinemia.

By *Diphyllobothrium latum* (fish tapeworm).

Disorders of ileal mucosa/IF–cobalamin receptors (i.e., IF–cobalamin not bound to IF–cobalamin receptors):

Diminished or absent IF–cobalamin receptors (e.g., ileal bypass, resection, fistula).

Abnormal mucosal architecture/function (e.g., tropical or nontropical sprue, Crohn disease, tuberculosis ileitis, infiltration by lymphomas, amyloidosis).

IF-/post-IF–cobalamin receptor defects (e.g., Imerslund-Gräsbeck syndrome, transcobalamin II [TC II] deficiency).

Drug effects (e.g., slow K, metformin, cholestyramine, colchicine, neomycin).

Disorders of plasma cobalamin transport (i.e., TC II–cobalamin not delivered to TC II receptors):

Congenital TC II deficiency, defective binding of TC II–cobalamin to TC II receptors (rare).

Metabolic disorders (i.e., cobalamin not used by cells):

Inborn enzyme errors (rare).

Acquired disorders (e.g., cobalamin functionally inactivated by irreversible oxidation, N_2O inhalation).

COGNITIVE IMPAIRMENT[66]

ICD-10CM # G31.84 Mild cognitive impairment, so stated

CAUSES OF COGNITIVE IMPAIRMENT: DIAGNOSES BY CATEGORIES WITH REPRESENTATIVE EXAMPLES

Degenerative
Alzheimer disease.
Frontotemporal dementias.
Dementia with Lewy bodies.
Corticobasal degeneration.
Huntington disease.
Wilson disease.
Parkinson disease.
Multiple system atrophy.
Progressive supranuclear palsy.

Psychiatric
Depression.
Schizophrenia.

Vascular
Vascular dementia.
Binswanger encephalopathy.
Amyloid dementia.
Diffuse hypoxic/ischemic injury.

Obstructive
Normal-pressure hydrocephalus.
Obstructive hydrocephalus.

Traumatic
Chronic subdural hematoma.
Chronic traumatic encephalopathy.
Post Aagenaes concussion syndrome.

Neoplastic
Tumor: malignant, primary and secondary.
Tumor: benign (e.g., frontal meningioma).
Paraneoplastic limbic encephalitis.

Infections
Chronic meningitis.
Postherpes encephalitis.
Focal cerebritis/abscesses.
HIV dementia.
HIV-associated infection.
Syphilis.
Lyme encephalopathy.
Subacute sclerosing panencephalitis.
Creutzfeldt–Jakob disease.
Progressive multifocal leukoencephalopathy.
Parenchymal sarcoidosis.
Chronic systemic infection.

Demyelinating
Multiple sclerosis.
Adrenoleukodystrophy.
Metachromatic leukodystrophy.

Autoimmune
Systemic lupus erythematosus.
Polyarteritis nodosa.

Drugs/Toxins
Medications:
Anticholinergics.
Antihistamines.
Anticonvulsants.
β-blockers.
Sedative–hypnotics.

Substance abuse
Alcohol.
Inhalants.
Phencyclidine (PCP).
Toxins
Arsenic.
Bromide.
Carbon monoxide.
Lead.
Mercury.
Organophosphates.

COLIC, ACUTE ABDOMINAL[2]

ICD-10CM # R10.0 Acute abdomen

Acute gastroenteritis.
Food poisoning.
Nonspecific causes.
Constipation.
Gastric outlet obstruction:
Chronic peptic ulceration.
Gastric cancer.
Small bowel obstruction:
Adhesions:
Postsurgical.
Inflammatory (e.g., diverticular).
Radiation.
Meckel diverticulum.
Metastatic.
Stricture:
Ischemic.
Radiation.
Inflammatory (e.g., Crohn disease).
Volvulus intussusception:
Tumor (e.g., Peutz-Jeghers syndrome).
Superior mesenteric artery syndrome.
Intraluminal bolus:
Gallstone.
Bezoar.
Hernia:
Abdominal wall.
Internal.
Neoplasm:
Benign (e.g., leiomyoma).
Malignant (e.g., carcinoid tumor, adenocarcinoma).
Large bowel obstruction:
Colon cancer.
Diverticular disease.
Volvulus.
Uterine:
Missed abortion.
Parturition.
Period pain.

COLON ISCHEMIA[3]

ICD-10CM # Varies with specific diagnosis

CAUSES OF COLON ISCHEMIA

Acute pancreatitis.
Allergy.
Amyloidosis.

Heart failure or cardiac arrhythmias.
Hematologic disorders and coagulopathies:
    Activated protein C resistance.
    Antithrombin deficiency.
    Factor V Leiden mutation.
    Paroxysmal nocturnal hemoglobinuria.
    Polycythemia vera.
    Protein C and S deficiencies.
    Prothrombin G20210A mutation.
    Sickle cell disease.
Infection:
    Bacteria (*Escherichia coli* O157:H7).
    Parasites (*Angiostrongylus costaricensis*).
    Viruses (HBV, HCV, cytomegalovirus).
Inferior mesenteric artery thrombosis.
Long-distance running.
Medications and toxins:
    Alosetron.
    Cocaine.
    Danazol.
    Digitalis compounds.
    Ergots.
    Estrogens.
    Flutamide.
    Glycerin enema.
    Gold salts.
    Immunosuppressive agents.
    Interferon-α.
    Methamphetamine.
    NSAIDs.
    Penicillin.
    Phenylephrine.
    Polyethylene glycol 3350 colon lavage solutions.
    Pit viper toxin.
    Progestins.
    Pseudoephedrine.
    Psychotropic drugs.
    Saline laxatives.
    Sumatriptan.
    Tegaserod.
    Vasopressin.
Pheochromocytoma.
Ruptured ectopic pregnancy.
Shock.
Strangulated hernia.
Surgery/procedures:
    Aortic aneurysmectomy.
    Aortoiliac reconstruction.
    Barium enema.
    Colectomy with inferior mesenteric artery ligation.
    Colon bypass.
    Colonoscopy.
    Exchange transfusions.
    Gynecologic operations.
    Lumbar aortography.
Thromboembolism:
    Cholesterol (atheroembolism).
    Myxoma (left atrial).
Trauma (blunt or penetrating).
Vasculitis and vasculopathy:

Buerger disease.
Eosinophilic granulomatosis with angiitis.
Fibromuscular dysplasia.
Kawasaki disease.
Polyarteritis nodosa.
Rheumatoid vasculitis.
SLE.
Takayasu arteritis.
Volvulus.

COLOR CHANGES, CUTANEOUS[57]

ICD-10CM # L81.9 Disorder of pigmentation, unspecified

BROWN
Generalized: pituitary, adrenal, liver disease, ACTH-producing tumor (e.g., oat cell lung carcinoma).
Localized: nevi, neurofibromatosis.

WHITE
Generalized: albinism.
Localized: vitiligo, Raynaud phenomenon.

RED (ERYTHEMA)
Generalized: fever, polycythemia, urticaria, viral exanthems.
Localized: inflammation, infection, Raynaud phenomenon.

YELLOW
Generalized: liver disease, chronic renal disease, anemia.
Generalized (except sclera): hypothyroidism, increased intake of vegetables containing carotene.
Localized: resolving hematoma, infection, peripheral vascular insufficiency.

BLUE
Lips, mouth, nail beds: cardiovascular and pulmonary diseases, Raynaud phenomenon.

COMA

ICD-10CM # R40.20 Unspecified coma

Vascular: hemorrhage, thrombosis, embolism.
CNS infections: meningitis, encephalitis, cerebral abscess.
Cerebral neoplasms with herniation.
Head injury: subdural hematoma, cerebral concussion, cerebral contusion.
Drugs: narcotics, sedatives, hypnotics.
Ingestion or inhalation of toxins: CO, alcohol, lead.
Metabolic disturbances.
Hypoxia.
Acid-base disorders.
Hypoglycemia, hyperglycemia.
Hepatic failure.
Electrolyte disorders.
Uremia.
Hypothyroidism.

Hypothermia, hyperthermia.
Hypotension, malignant hypertension.
Postictal.

COMA, NORMAL COMPUTED TOMOGRAPHY[18]

ICD-10CM # R40.20 Unspecified coma

MENINGEAL DISORDERS
Subarachnoid hemorrhage (uncommon).
Bacterial meningitis.
Encephalitis.
Subdural empyema.

EXOGENOUS TOXINS
Sedative drugs and barbiturates.
Anesthetics and γ hydroxybutyrate.*
Alcohols.
Stimulants:
    phencyclidines.[†]
    Cocaine and amphetamines.[‡]
Psychotropic drugs:
    Cyclic antidepressants.
    Phenothiazines.
    Lithium.
Anticonvulsants.
Opioids.
Clonidine.[§]
Penicillins.
Salicylates.
Anticholinergics.
Carbon monoxide, cyanide, and methemoglobinemia.

ENDOGENOUS TOXINS/ DEFICIENCIES/DERANGEMENTS
Hypoxia and ischemia.
Hypoglycemia.
Hypercalcemia.
Osmolar:
    Hyperglycemia.
    Hyponatremia.
    Hypernatremia.
Organ system failure:
    Hepatic encephalopathy.
    Uremic encephalopathy.
    Pulmonary insufficiency (carbon dioxide narcosis).

SEIZURES
Prolonged postictal state.
Spike-wave stupor.

---

*Involvement principally of cancellous bone.
[†]Involvement of cancellous and cortical bone.
[‡]Coma after seizures or status (i.e., a prolonged post-ictal state).
[§]An antihypertensive agent active through the opiate receptor system; frequent overdose when used to treat narcotic withdrawal.

HYPOTHERMIA OR HYPERTHERMIA

Brain stem ischemia.
Basilar artery stroke.
Brain stem or cerebellar hemorrhage.
Conversion or malingering.

COMA, PEDIATRIC POPULATION[67]

ICD-10CM #   R40.20   Unspecified coma

ANOXIA

Birth asphyxia.
Carbon monoxide poisoning.
Croup/epiglottitis.
Meconium aspiration.

INFECTION

Hemolysis.
Blood loss.
Hydrops fetalis.
Infection.
Meningoencephalitis.
Sepsis.
Postimmunization encephalitis.

INCREASED INTRACRANIAL PRESSURE

Anoxia.
Inborn metabolic errors.
Toxic encephalopathy.
Reye syndrome.
Head trauma/intracranial bleed.
Hydrocephalus.
Posterior fossa tumors.

HYPERTENSIVE ENCEPHALOPATHY

Coarctation of aorta.
Nephritis.
Vasculitis.
Pheochromocytoma.

ISCHEMIA

Hypoplastic left heart.
Shunting lesions.
Aortic stenosis.
Cardiovascular collapse (any cause).

PURPURIC CAUSES

Disseminated intravascular coagulation.
Hemolytic-uremic syndrome.
Leukemia.
Thrombotic purpura.

HYPERCAPNIA

Cystic fibrosis.
Bronchopulmonary dysplasia.
Congenital lung anomalies.

NEOPLASM

Medulloblastoma.
Glioma of brain stem.
Posterior fossa tumors.

DRUGS/TOXINS

Maternal sedation.
Alcohol.
Any drug.
Lead.
Salicylism.
Arsenic.
Pesticides.

ELECTROLYTE ABNORMALITIES

Hypernatremia (diarrhea, dehydration, salt poisoning).
Hyponatremia (SIADH, androgenital syndrome, gastroenteritis).
Hyperkalemia (renal failure, salicylism, androgenitalism).
Hypokalemia (diarrhea, hyperaldosteronism, salicylism, DKA).
Hypocalcemia (vitamin D deficiency, hyperparathyroidism).
Severe acidosis (sepsis, cold injury, salicylism, DKA).

HYPOGLYCEMIA

Birth injury or stress.
Diabetes.
Alcohol.
Salicylism.
Hyperinsulinemia.
Iatrogenic.

POSTSEIZURE

Renal Causes
Nephritis.
Hypoplastic kidneys.
Hepatic Causes
Acute hepatitis.
Fulminant hepatic failure.
Inborn metabolic errors.
Bile duct atresia.

COMPRESSION SYNDROMES, NEUROVASCULAR CAUSES[27]

ICD-10CM #	M47.016	Anterior spinal artery compression syndromes, lumbar region
	M47.019	Anterior spinal artery compression syndromes, site unspecified
	M47.013	Anterior spinal artery compression syndromes, cervicothoracic region
	M47.021	Vertebral artery compression syndromes, occipito-atlanto-axial region
	M47.022	Vertebral artery compression syndromes, cervical region

Anatomic

Potential sites of neurovascular compression:
    Interscalene triangle.
    Costoclavicular space.
    Subcoracoid area.

Congenital

Cervical rib and its fascial remnants.
Rudimentary first thoracic rib.
Scalene muscles:
    Anterior.
    Middle.
    Minimus.
Adventitious fibrous bands.
Bifid clavicle or first rib.
Exostosis of first thoracic rib.
Enlarged transverse process of C7.
Omohyoid muscle.
Anomalous course of transverse cervical artery.
Abnormal lateral insertion of costoclavicular ligament.
Flat clavicle.

Traumatic

Fracture of clavicle.
Dislocation of head of humerus.
Crushing injury to upper thorax.
Sudden, unaccustomed muscular efforts involving shoulder girdle muscles.
Cervical spondylosis and injuries to cervical spine.
Atherosclerosis.

CONGESTIVE HEART FAILURE AND CARDIOMYOPATHY[18]

ICD-10CM #	I50.9	Heart failure, unspecified
	I42.7	Cardiomyopathy due to drug and external agent

CAUSES OF CONGESTIVE HEART FAILURE AND CARDIOMYOPATHY

Coronary Artery Disease
Acute ischemia.
Myocardial infarction.
Ischemic cardiomyopathy with hibernating myocardium.

Idiopathic
Idiopathic dilated cardiomyopathy.
Idiopathic restrictive cardiomyopathy.
Peripartum.

Pressure Overload
Hypertension.
Aortic stenosis.

Volume Overload
Mitral regurgitation.
Aortic insufficiency.
Anemia.
Atrioventricular fistula.

Toxins
Ethanol.
Cocaine.
Doxorubicin (Adriamycin).
Methamphetamine.

Metabolic-Endocrine
Thiamine deficiency.
Diabetes.
Hemochromatosis.
Thyrotoxicosis.
Obesity.
Infiltrative
Amyloidosis.
Inflammatory
Viral myocarditis.
Hereditary
Hypertrophic.
Dilated.

Genetic bases for these cardiomyopathies have been identified in a large number of individual patients and families. Most of the mutations have been found in cardiac contractile or structural proteins.

CONGESTIVE HEART FAILURE, INFANT[29]

ICD-10CM # 105.9 Heart failure, unspecified

Critical coarctation of the aorta.
Interrupted aortic arch.
Congenital aortic stenosis.
Hypoplastic left heart syndrome.
Large ventricular septal defect.
Truncus arteriosus.
Unrecognized supraventricular tachycardia.
Cardiac tamponade.
Myocarditis.

CONJUNCTIVAL NEOPLASM

ICD-10CM # Varies with specific diagnosis

MALIGNANT
Squamous cell carcinoma.
Melanoma.
Sebaceous carcinoma.
Kaposi sarcoma.
Metastatic neoplasms.

BENIGN
Melanocytic nevus.
Squamous papilloma.
Hemangioma.
Lymphangioma.
Myxoma.

CONNECTIVE TISSUE DISORDERS, HEREDITARY[38]

ICD-10CM # Varies with specific diagnosis

CLASSIFICATION OF HEREDITARY DISORDERS OF CONNECTIVE TISSUE
Skeletal (Primarily Type I Collagen)
Osteogenesis imperfecta.
Dermis, Tendons, and Ligaments (Primarily Type I Collagen)
Hypermobile Ehlers-Danlos syndrome (type III).
Classic Ehlers-Danlos syndrome (type I).

Vascular Ehlers-Danlos syndrome.
Cartilage (Primarily Fibrils of Type II Collagen, Proteoglycans)
Chondrodysplasias.
Achondroplasia.
Pseudoachondroplasia.
Stickler syndrome.
Craniosynostosis (syndromic).
Skeletal, Cardiovascular, and Eye (Type I and Type III Collagen, Fibrillin, Elastin)
Marfan syndrome.
MASS phenotype (mitral valve prolapse, aortic dilation, skin, and skeletal features).
Loeys-Dietz syndrome.
Beals syndrome (congenital contractual arachnodactyly).
Dermal/epidermal (keratin, laminin, type VII collagen, plectin, integrin).
Epidermolysis bullosa.
Basal lamina (type IV collagen, laminin, nidogen).
Alport syndrome.

CONSCIOUSNESS IMPAIRMENT, ACUTE, IN CRITICALLY ILL PATIENT

ICD-10CM # F05.9 Delirium, unspecified

GENERAL CAUSES OF ACUTELY IMPAIRED CONSCIOUSNESS IN THE CRITICALLY ILL
Infection
Sepsis encephalopathy.
CNS infection.
Drugs
Narcotics.
Benzodiazepines.
Anticholinergics.
Anticonvulsants.
Tricyclic antidepressants.
Selective serotonin uptake inhibitors.
Phenothiazines.
Steroids.
Immunosuppressants (cyclosporine, FK-506, OKT3).
Anesthetics.
Electrolyte and Acid-Base Disturbances
Hyponatremia.
Hypernatremia.
Hypercalcemia.
Hypermagnesemia.
Severe acidemia and alkalemia.
Organ System Failure
Shock.
Renal failure.
Hepatic failure.
Pancreatitis.
Respiratory failure (hypoxia, hypercapnia).
Endocrine Disorders
Hypoglycemia.
Hyperglycemia.
Hypothyroidism.
Hyperthyroidism.
Pituitary apoplexy.

Drug Withdrawal
Alcohol.
Opiates.
Barbiturates.
Benzodiazepines.
Vascular Causes
Shock.
Hypotension.
Hypertensive encephalopathy.
CNS vasculitis.
Cerebral venous sinus thrombosis.
Central Nervous System Disorders
Hemorrhage.
Stroke.
Brain edema.
Hydrocephalus.
Increased intracranial pressure.
Meningitis.
Ventriculitis.
Brain abscess.
Subdural empyema.
Seizures.
Vasculitis.
Seizures
Convulsive and nonconvulsive status epilepticus.
Miscellaneous
Fat embolism syndrome.
Neuroleptic malignant syndrome.
Thiamine deficiency (Wernicke encephalopathy).
Psychogenic unresponsiveness.

CONSTIPATION

ICD-10CM # K59.00 Constipation, unspecified

Intestinal obstruction.
Fecal impaction.
Diverticular disease.
GI neoplasm.
Strangulated femoral hernia.
Gallstone ileus.
Tuberculous stricture.
Adhesions.
Ameboma.
Volvulus.
Intussusception.
Inflammatory bowel disease.
Hematoma of bowel wall, secondary to trauma or anticoagulants.
Poor dietary habits: insufficient bulk in diet, inadequate fluid intake.
Change from daily routine: travel, hospital admission, physical inactivity.
Acute abdominal conditions: renal colic, salpingitis, biliary colic, appendicitis, ischemia.
Hypercalcemia or hypokalemia, uremia.
Irritable bowel syndrome, pregnancy, anorexia nervosa, depression.
Painful anal conditions: hemorrhoids, fissure, stricture.
Decreased intestinal peristalsis: old age, spinal cord injuries, myxedema, diabetes, multiple sclerosis, parkinsonism and other neurologic diseases.

Drugs: codeine, morphine, antacids with aluminum, verapamil, anticonvulsants, anticholinergics, disopyramide, cholestyramine, alosetron, iron supplements.

Hirschsprung disease, meconium ileus, congenital atresia in infants.

CONSTIPATION, ADULT PATIENT[2]

ICD-10CM # K59.00 Constipation, unspecified

NO GROSS STRUCTURAL ABNORMALITY

Inadequate fiber intake.

Irritable bowel syndrome (associated with abdominal pain) or functional constipation.

Idiopathic slow-transit constipation.

"Obstructed defecation" pelvic floor dysfunction (or dyssynergia).

STRUCTURAL DISORDERS

Anal fissure, infection, or stenosis.

Colon cancer or stricture.

Aganglionosis and/or abnormal myenteric plexus:

Hirschsprung disease.

Chagas disease.

Neuropathic pseudoobstruction.

Abnormal colonic muscle:

Myopathy.

Dystrophia myotonica.

Systemic sclerosis.

Idiopathic megarectum and/or megacolon.

Proximal megacolon.

NEUROLOGIC CAUSES

Diabetic autonomic neuropathy.

Damage to the sacral parasympathetic outflow.

Spinal cord damage or disease (e.g., multiple sclerosis).

Parkinson disease.

Blunting of consciousness, mental retardation, psychosis.

Pain induced by straining (e.g., sciatic nerve compression).

ENDOCRINE OR METABOLIC CAUSES

Hypothyroidism.

Hypercalcemia.

Porphyria.

Pregnancy.

PSYCHOLOGIC DISORDERS

Depression.

Anorexia nervosa.

Denied bowel habit.

Drug side effects.

CONSTIPATION, PEDIATRIC PATIENT[68]

ICD-10CM # K59.00 Constipation

Nonorganic (Functional)—Retentive

Anatomic

Anal stenosis, atresia with fistula.

Imperforate anus.

Anteriorly displaced anus.

Intestinal stricture (postnecrotizing enterocolitis).

Anal stricture.

Abnormal Musculature

Prune-belly syndrome.

Gastroschisis.

Down syndrome.

Muscular dystrophy.

Intestinal Nerve or Muscle Abnormalities

Hirschsprung disease.

Pseudoobstruction (visceral myopathy or neuropathy).

Intestinal neuronal dysplasia.

Spinal cord lesions.

Tethered cord.

Autonomic neuropathy.

Spinal cord trauma.

Spina bifida.

Chagas disease.

Drugs

Anticholinergics.

Narcotics.

Methylphenidate.

Phenytoin.

Antidepressants.

Chemotherapeutic agents (vincristine).

Pancreatic enzymes (fibrosing colonopathy).

Lead, arsenic, mercury.

Vitamin D intoxication.

Calcium channel blocking agents.

Metabolic Disorders

Hypokalemia.

Hypercalcemia.

Hypothyroidism.

Diabetes mellitus, diabetes insipidus.

Porphyria.

Intestinal Disorders

Celiac disease.

Cow's milk protein intolerance.

Cystic fibrosis (meconium ileus equivalent).

Inflammatory bowel disease (stricture).

Tumor.

Connective tissue disorders.

Systemic lupus erythematosus.

Scleroderma.

Psychiatric Diagnosis

Anorexia nervosa.

COPD DECOMPENSATION[10]

ICD-10CM # J44.1 Chronic obstructive pulmonary distress with acute exacerbation

CAUSES OF ACUTE DECOMPENSATION IN THE PATIENT WITH CHRONIC OBSTRUCTIVE PULMONARY DISEASE

Acute Exacerbations

Infectious

Viral.

Rhinovirus, respiratory syncytial virus, coronavirus, influenza virus.

Bacterial.

Haemophilus influenzae, Streptococcus pneumoniae, Moraxella (Branhamella) catarrhalis, Pseudomonas aeruginosa.

Atypical bacteria.

Chlamydia pneumoniae, Legionella.

Air Pollution

Nitrogen dioxide.

Ozone.

Particulates, dust.

Other Critical Events

Pneumothorax.

Pulmonary embolism.

Lobar atelectasis.

Congestive heart failure.

Pneumonia.

Pulmonary compression (e.g., obesity, ascites, gastric distention, pleural effusion).

Trauma (e.g., rib fractures, pulmonary contusion).

Neuromuscular and metabolic disorders.

Unrelated treatable chronic pulmonary disease (bronchiectasis, tuberculosis, sarcoidosis).

Noncompliance with prescribed treatment regimens.

Iatrogenic:

Inadequate therapy.

Inappropriate therapy (e.g., deleterious drugs).

CORNEAL CLOUDING, PEDIATRIC AGE[20]

ICD-10CM # Varies with specific diagnosis

Cerebrohepatorenal syndrome (Zellweger syndrome).

Congenital syphilis.[a]

Fabry disease (ceramide trihexosidosis).

Familial high-density lipoprotein deficiency (Tangier island disease).

Fetal alcohol syndrome.

Glaucoma.[a]

Infantile GM1 gangliosidosis.

Juvenile metachromatic dystrophy.

Marinesco-Sjögren disease.

Mucolipidosis.

Mucopolysaccharidoses.

Multiple sulfatase deficiency.

Pelizaeus-Merzbacher disease.

Trauma (forceps at birth).

[a] Denotes the most common conditions and the ones with disease-modifying treatments.

CORNEAL SENSATION, DECREASED

ICD-10CM # H18.899 Other specified disorders of cornea, unspecified eye

Herpes (simplex, zoster).

Differential Diagnosis

II

Contact lens wear.

Topical agents (NSAIDs, anesthetics, β-blockers).

Diabetes.

Eye trauma.

Postsurgery.

COUGH

ICD-10CM # R05 Cough

Infectious process (viral, bacterial).

Postinfectious.

"Smoker's cough."

Rhinitis (allergic, vasomotor, postinfectious).

Asthma.

Exposure to irritants (noxious fumes, smoke, cold air).

Drug-induced (especially ACE inhibitors, β-blockers).

GERD.

Interstitial lung disease.

Lung neoplasms.

Lymphomas, mediastinal neoplasms.

Bronchiectasis.

Cardiac (CHF, pulmonary edema, mitral stenosis, pericardial inflammation).

Recurrent aspiration.

Inflammation of larynx, pleura, diaphragm, mediastinum.

Cystic fibrosis.

Anxiety.

Other: pulmonary embolism, foreign body inhalation, aortic aneurysm, Zenker diverticulum, osteophytes, substernal thyroid, thyroiditis, PMR.

COUGH, CHRONIC, ADULT PATIENT[28]

ICD-10CM # R05 Cough

CAUSES OF CHRONIC COUGH IN ADULTS

Intrathoracic Causes

Lungs and Airways

Asthma.

Nonasthmatic eosinophilic bronchitis.

Chronic bronchitis.

Bronchiectasis.

ACEIs.

Inhaled medications.

Chronic exposure to environmental and occupational irritants.

Bronchogenic and metastatic carcinoma.

Bronchial carcinoid.

Foreign body or endobronchial suture.

Broncholith.

Infectious and noninfectious bronchiolitis.

Chronic infectious pneumonias (e.g., bacterial, tuberculous, fungal, parasitic).

Chronic infectious tracheobronchitis (as in tuberculosis or aspergillosis).

Chronic interstitial lung disease (e.g., sarcoidosis, HSP, IPF, asbestosis).

Pulmonary vasculitis (as in granulomatosis with polyangiitis).

Sjögren syndrome with xerotrachea.

Relapsing polychondritis.

Pleura

Chronic effusion.

Diaphragm

Transvenous pacemaker stimulation.

Mediastinum

Neural tumors.

Thymoma.

Teratoma.

Lymphoma.

Metastatic lymphadenopathy.

Intrathoracic goiter.

Bronchogenic cyst.

Cardiovascular

Mitral stenosis.

Left ventricular failure.

Pulmonary thromboembolism.

Enlarged left atrium.

Vascular ring.

Aberrant innominate artery.

Aortic aneurysm.

Pericardial stimulation by transvenous pacemaker.

Extrathoracic Causes

Head and Neck

Rhinitis and sinusitis.

Nasal polyps.

Rhinolith.

Oropharyngeal dysphagia.

Laryngeal disorders (e.g., vocal fold dysfunction, laryngomalacia).

Postviral vagal neuropathy.

Recurrent aspiration.

Elongated uvula.

Chronically infected tonsils.

Neurilemmoma of vagus nerve.

Neuroma of internal laryngeal nerve.

Ascending palatine artery aneurysm.

Osteophytes of cervical spine.

Mammomanogamus (Syngamus) laryngeus infection.

Thyroiditis.

Upper Gastrointestinal

Gastroesophageal reflux disease.

Esophageal cyst or diverticulum.

Tracheoesophageal fistula.

Central Nervous System

Psychogenic or habit cough.

Tic disorders.

Gilles de la Tourette syndrome.

ACEI, Angiotensin-converting enzyme inhibitor; *HSP*, hypersensitivity pneumonitis; *IPF*, idiopathic pulmonary fibrosis.

COUGH, CHRONIC, PEDIATRIC PATIENT[68]

ICD-10CM # R05 Cough

DIFFERENTIAL DIAGNOSIS OF RECURRENT AND PERSISTENT COUGH IN CHILDREN

Recurrent Cough

Reactive airway disease (asthma).

Drainage from upper airways.

Aspiration.

Frequently recurring respiratory tract infections in immunocompetent or immunodeficient patients.

Symptomatic Chiari malformation.

Idiopathic pulmonary hemosiderosis.

Hypersensitivity (allergic) pneumonitis.

Persistent Cough

Hypersensitivity of cough receptors after infection.

Reactive airway disease (asthma).

Chronic sinusitis.

Chronic rhinitis (allergic or nonallergic).

Bronchitis or tracheitis caused by infection or smoke exposure.

Bronchiectasis, including cystic fibrosis, primary ciliary dyskinesia, immunodeficiency.

Habit cough.

Foreign-body aspiration.

Recurrent aspiration owing to pharyngeal incompetence, tracheolaryngoesophageal cleft or tracheoesophageal fistula.

Gastroesophageal reflux, with or without aspiration.

Pertussis.

Extrinsic compression of the tracheobronchial tract (vascular ring, neoplasm, lymph node, lung cyst).

Tracheomalacia, bronchomalacia.

Endobronchial or endotracheal tumors.

Endobronchial tuberculosis.

Hypersensitivity pneumonitis.

Fungal infections.

Inhaled irritants, including tobacco smoke.

Irritation of external auditory canal.

Angiotensin-converting enzyme inhibitors.

CRAMPS[38]

ICD-10CM # R25.2 Cramps and spasm

Cramp Syndromes

Ordinary:

Common in normal individuals, especially gastrocnemius muscle, older age.

Pregnancy.

Systemic disorders:

Dehydration: hidrosis, diuretics, hemodialysis.

Metabolic: low Na^+, $Mg2^+$, $Ca2^+$, glucose, uremia, cirrhosis, Gitelman syndrome.

Endocrine: thyroid (hyper- or hypothyroid), hypoadrenal, hyperparathyroid.

Ischemia.

Drug-induced.

Denervation, partial: motor neuron disease, spinal stenosis, radiculopathy, neuropathy (including small-fiber neuropathy).

Syndromes: cramp-fasciculation, Satoyoshi syndrome.

Other Contraction Syndromes

Central disorders: stiff person syndrome, spasticity, tetanus, dystonia.

Peripheral nerve disorders: neuromyotonia, tetany, myokymia, partial denervation.

Muscle: contractures, myotonia, myoedema.

Genetic Muscle Contraction Syndromes

Muscular dystrophy: Becker; LGMD 1C.

Myotonia: myotonia congenita, myotonia fluctuans, acetazolamide-responsive myotonia, myotonic dystrophy.

Contractures:

Brody syndrome: *ATP2A1*.

Glycogen storage disorders: deficiency of myophosphorylase; phosphorylase kinase regulatory subunit α1; phosphoglycerate mutase; phosphofructokinase, muscle.

Rippling muscle syndrome: caveolin-3.

Hereditary angiopathy with nephropathy, aneurysms, and muscle cramps (HANAC): *COL4A1*.

Neuropathic.

Cramps: autosomal dominant:

Schwartz-Jampel: perlecan, *LIFR*.

Neuromyotonia and myokymia: *KCNQ2*; *KCNA1*.

Geniospasm.

Crisponi: *CRLF1*.

Myofibrillar myopathy.

Cramps: autosomal recessive:

Autosomal recessive axonal neuropathy with neuromyotonia *HINT1*.

Possible Treatments for Cramps and Other Muscle Spasms

Normalize metabolic abnormalities.

Quinine sulfate.

Carbamazepine.

Phenytoin.

Gabapentin.

Tocainide.

Verapamil.

Amitriptyline.

Vitamin E.

Riboflavin.

Mexiletine.

---

*Usual features: sudden involuntary, painful muscle contractions (usually involve single muscles, especially gastrocnemius); local cramps in other muscles often associated with neuromuscular disease. Precipitants: muscle contraction, occasionally during sleep. Relief: passive muscle stretch, local massage.

CREEPING ERUPTION, TRAVELERS[69]

ICD-10CM # Varies with specific diagnosis

CAUSES OF CREEPING ERUPTION IN TRAVELERS

Nematode Larvae

Animal hookworms (HrCLM)*, *Pelodera strongyloides*, zoonotic *Strongyloides* spp.

Gnathostomiasis (*Gnathostoma* spp.).

Larva currens (*Strongyloides stercoralis*).

Adult Nematodes

Loiasis (*Loa loa*).

Dracunculiasis (*Dracunculus medinensis*).

Dirofilariasis (*Dirofilaria immitis*).

Trematode Larvae

Fascioliasis (*Fasciola gigantica*).

Fly Maggots

Migratory myiasis (*Gasterophilus* spp.).

Mites

Scabies (*Sarcoptes scabiei*).*

Pyemotes dermatitis (*Pyemotes ventricosus*).

HrCLM, Hookworm-related cutaneous larva migrans.*

---

*Common cause.

CUTANEOUS CALCIFICATIONS[70]

ICD-10CM # Varies with specific diagnosis

Disorders of Cutaneous Calcification

Dystrophic

Autoimmune connective tissue diseases, especially dermatomyositis, CREST.

Cutaneous tumors or cysts (e.g., pilomatricomas, pilar cysts).

Infections, especially parasitic.

Trauma, including "heel sticks" in neonates, injection sites, surgical scars.

Panniculitis.

Genetic disorders (e.g., pseudoxanthoma elasticum, Ehlers–Danlos syndrome).

Metastatic

Advanced chronic kidney disease.

Calciphylaxis.*

Benign nodular calcification of renal disease.

Hypervitaminosis D.

Milk-alkali syndrome.

Sarcoidosis.

Tumoral calcinosis (familial).

Hyperparathyroidism.

Neoplasms (e.g., multiple myeloma, adult T-cell leukemia/lymphoma, SCC of the lung or head and neck).

Idiopathic

Idiopathic calcified nodules of the scrotum.

Subepidermal calcified nodule.

Tumoral calcinosis (sporadic).

Milia-like calcinosis.

Iatrogenic

Extravasation of intravenous solutions containing calcium or phosphate

Application of calcium-containing electrode paste for EMGs and EEGs

Application of calcium alginate dressings to denuded skin

Organ transplantation, especially liver

Gadolinium (nephrogenic systemic fibrosis).

CREST, Calcification, Raynaud phenomenon, esophageal dysmotility, sclerodactyly and telangiectasia; EEG, electroencephalogram; EMG, electromyography; SCC, squamous cell carcinoma.

CUTANEOUS INFECTIONS, ATHLETES

ICD-10CM # L08.9 Local infection of the skin and subcutaneous tissue, unspecified

Tinea pedis.

Tinea cruris.

Molluscum contagiosum.

Herpes simplex.

Verruca vulgaris.

Folliculitis.

Impetigo.

Furuncles.

Otitis externa.

Erythrasma.

CUTANEOUS ULCERS, TRAVELERS[69]

ICD-10CM # Varies with specific diagnosis

CAUSES OF CUTANEOUS ULCER IN TRAVELERS

Noninfectious Causes

Spider bite.

Cupping.

Bacterial Infection

Ecthyma.*

Tick eschar* (rickettsiosis).

Anthrax.

Mycobacterial infection (*M. ulcerans*).

Melioidosis.

Glanders.

Tularemia.

Cutaneous diphtheria.

Plague.

Parasitic Infection

Leishmaniasis.*

Trypanosomal chancre (African trypanosomiasis).

Chagoma (American trypanosomiasis).

Cutaneous amebiasis.

Fungal Infection

Sporotrichosis.

Mycetomas.

West African histoplasmosis.

North American blastomycosis.

Paracoccidioidomycosis.

Chromomycosis.

Viral Infection

Herpes simplex infection.

---

*Common cause.

CYANOSIS[43]

ICD-10CM # R23.0 Cyanosis

DIFFERENTIAL DIAGNOSIS OF CYANOSIS

Peripheral Cyanosis

Low Cardiac Output States

Shock.

Left ventricular failure.

Hypovolemia.

Environmental Exposure (Cold)

Air or water.

Arterial Occlusion

Thrombosis.

Embolism.

Vasospasm (Raynaud phenomenon).

Peripheral vascular disease.

Venous Obstruction
Redistribution of blood flow from extremities
Central Cyanosis
Decreased arterial oxygen saturation
High altitude (>8000 ft).
Impaired pulmonary function:
　Hypoventilation.
　Impaired oxygen diffusion.
　Ventilation-perfusion mismatching:
　　Pulmonary embolism.
　　Acute respiratory distress syndrome.
　　Pulmonary hypertension.
　Respiratory compromise:
　　Upper airway obstruction.
　　Pneumonia.
　　Diaphragmatic hernia.
　　Tension pneumothorax.
　　Polycythemia.
Anatomic Shunts
Pulmonary arteriovenous fistulae and intra-pulmonary shunts.
Cerebral, hepatic, peripheral arteriovenous fistulae.
Cyanotic congenital heart disease:
　Endocardial cushion defects.
　Ventricular septal defects.
　Coarctation of aorta.
　Tetralogy of Fallot.
　Total anomalous pulmonary venous drainage.
　Hypoplastic left ventricle.
　Pulmonary vein stenosis.
　Tricuspid atresia and anomalies.
　Premature closure of foramen ovale.
　Dextrocardia.
　Pulmonary stenosis of atrial septal defect.
　Patent ductus arteriosus with reversed shunt.
Abnormal Hemoglobin
Methemoglobinemia:
　Hereditary.
　Acquired.
Sulfhemoglobinemia.
Mutant hemoglobin with low oxygen affinity (e.g., hemoglobin Kansas).

CYANOSIS, CENTRAL, SECONDARY TO CARDIAC DEFECT[58]

ICD-10CM # R23.0　Cyanosis

Transposition of the great arteries.
Tetralogy of Fallot.
Tricuspid atresia.
Truncus arteriosus.
Total anomalous pulmonary venous return.

Ebstein anomaly.
Eisenmenger physiology.
Critical pulmonary stenosis or atresia.
Functionally single ventricle.

Note 5 Ts and 2 Es.

CYANOSIS, NEONATAL[29]

ICD-10CM # R23.0　Cyanosis

RESPIRATORY
Upper Airway
Choanal atresia.
Macroglossia.
Glossoptosis (secondary to micrognathia).
Laryngomalacia.
Laryngeal web or cyst.
Vascular anomalies (e.g., cystic hygromas, rings).
Subglottic stenosis (commonly secondary to intubation).
Foreign body.
Lower Airway
Pneumonia.
Bronchiolitis.
Pulmonary edema.
Atelectasis.
Bronchopulmonary dysplasia.

SYSTEMIC
Sepsis.
Trauma.
Poisons.

CARDIAC
Cyanotic congenital heart diseases.
Transposition of the great vessels (most common neonatal).
Tetralogy of Fallot.
Truncus arteriosus.
Tricuspid atresia.
Total anomalous pulmonary venous return.
Ebstein anomaly.
GI.
Gastroesophageal reflux.

NEUROLOGIC
Seizures.
Central hypoventilation syndrome (Ondine curse).
Spinal muscular atrophy type I (Werdnig-Hoffmann).
Botulism.
Congenital myopathies.

HEMATOLOGIC
Methemoglobinemia.

CYTOPENIAS, OLDER ADULTS[71]

ICD-10CM # D46.A　Refractory cytopenia with multilineage dysplasia

Cytopenia of one or more lineages.
Hematologic neoplasm.
Vitamin B_{12} deficiency.
Autoimmune disorder.
Consumptive coagulopathy.
Systemic inflammation.
Alcohol.
Splenomegaly.
Thyroid dysfunction.

Human immunodeficiency virus.

DAYTIME SLEEPINESS

ICD-10CM # R53.82　Chronic fatigue, unspecified

Sleep deprivation.
Medication induced (e.g., benzodiazepines, β-blockers, narcotics, sedative antidepressants, gabapentin).
Depression.
Obstructive sleep apnea.
Medical illness (e.g., severe anemia, hypothyroidism, COPD, hepatic failure, renal insufficiency, CHF, electrolyte disturbances).
Circadian rhythm abnormalities (e.g., jet lag, shift work sleep disorder).
Restless legs syndrome.
Posttrauma.
Narcolepsy.
Neurologic disorders (e.g., neurodegenerative disorders; parkinsonism; multiple sclerosis; lesions affecting thalamus, hypothalamus, or brain stem).

DEAFNESS, ACQUIRED

ICD-10CM #		
	H91.93	Unspecified hearing loss, bilateral
	H91.92	Unspecified hearing loss, left ear
	H91.91	Unspecified hearing loss, right ear
	H91.90	Unspecified hearing loss, unspecified ear
	H91.9	Unspecified hearing loss
	H91	Other and unspecified hearing loss
	H90.5	Unspecified sensorineural hearing loss
	H91.09	Ototoxic hearing loss, unspecified ear
	H90.2	Conductive hearing loss, unspecified
	H91.8X9	Other specified hearing loss, unspecified ear

COMMON CAUSES OF ACQUIRED DEAFNESS
Conductive Hearing Loss
Acute otitis media, otitis media with effusion, chronic otitis media.
Sensorineural Hearing Loss
Severe hypoxia.
Lassa fever.
Sepsis neonatorum.
Bacterial meningitis.
Viral infections (e.g., mumps).
Hyperbilirubinemia.
Noise-induced damage.
Autoimmune sensorineural hearing loss.
Presbycusis.
Head trauma.
Ménière's disease.
Scrub typhus.

Sudden idiopathic sensorineural hearing loss.
HIV/AIDS, tuberculosis.
Ototoxicity.
Tumors, hydatid cyst in the cerebellopontine angle.

DELAYED PASSAGE OF MECONIUM[21]

ICD-10CM # P76.0 Meconium plug syndrome

Ileal atresia.
Meconium ileus.
Functional immaturity of the colon.
Colon atresia.
Anorectal malformations.
Hirschsprung disease.
Megacystis-microcolon-intestinal hypoperistalsis syndrome.
Extrinsic compression of the distal bowel by a mass lesion.
  Mesenteric cyst.
  Enteric duplication cyst.
Paralytic ileus, sepsis, drugs, and metabolic upset.

DELIRIUM[1]

ICD-10CM # R40.0 Somnolence
R40.1 Stupor
F05 Delirium due to known physiological condition

PHARMACOLOGIC AGENTS

Anxiolytics (benzodiazepines).
Antidepressants (e.g., amitriptyline, doxepin, imipramine).
Cardiovascular agents (e.g., methyldopa, digitalis, reserpine, propranolol, procainamide, captopril, disopyramide).
Antihistamine.
Cimetidine.
Corticosteroids.
Antineoplastics.
Drugs of abuse (alcohol, cannabis, amphetamines, cocaine, hallucinogens, opioids, sedative-hypnotics, phencyclidine).

METABOLIC DISORDERS

Hypercalcemia.
Hypercarbia.
Hypoglycemia.
Hyponatremia.
Hypoxia.

INFLAMMATORY DISORDERS

Sarcoidosis.
SLE.
Giant cell arteritis.

ORGAN FAILURE

Hepatic encephalopathy.
Uremia.

NEUROLOGIC DISORDERS

Alzheimer disease.
CVA.
Encephalitis (including HIV).
Encephalopathies.
Epilepsy.
Huntington disease.
Multiple sclerosis.
Neoplasms.
Normal-pressure hydrocephalus.
Parkinson disease.
Pick disease.
Wilson disease.

ENDOCRINE DISORDERS

Addison disease.
Cushing syndrome.
Panhypopituitarism.
Parathyroid disease.
Postpartum psychosis.
Recurrent menstrual psychosis.
Sydenham chorea.
Thyroid disease.

DEFICIENCY STATES

Niacin.
Thiamine, vitamin B_{12}, and folate.

DELIRIUM AND AGITATION, DRUG-INDUCED

ICD-10CM # F05.9 Delirium, unspecified

COMMONLY USED DRUGS ASSOCIATED WITH DELIRIUM AND AGITATION

Benzodiazepines.
Opiates (especially meperidine).
Anticholinergics.
Antihistamines.
H_2 blockers.
Antibiotics.
Corticosteroids.
Metoclopramide.

DELIRIUM, AGITATED[43]

ICD-10CM # F05 Delirium due to known physiological condition

Metabolic causes:
  Electrolyte abnormalities.
  Hypoglycemia.
  Hypoxia.
  Uremia/hyperammonemia.
Structural lesions of the CNS:
  Trauma.
  Stroke.
  Hemorrhage.
  Mass.
Endocrine disease:
  Thyrotoxicosis.
Infections:

Bacterial/viral meningitis/encephalitis.
Toxicologic causes:
  Sympathomimetic/stimulants.
  Cocaine.
  Amphetamines and derivatives.
  Caffeine.
  Phencyclidine/ketamine.
  Anticholinergics.
  Serotonin syndrome.
  Sedative-hypnotic withdrawal.
Heatstroke.
Postictal state.

CNS, Central nervous system.

DELIRIUM, DIALYSIS PATIENT[1]

ICD-10CM # F05 Delirium due to known physiological condition
F06.8 Other specified mental disorders due to known physiological condition

STRUCTURAL

Cerebrovascular accident (particularly hemorrhage).
Subdural hematoma.
Intracerebral abscess.
Brain tumor.

METABOLIC

Disequilibrium syndrome.
Uremia.
Drug effects.
Meningitis.
Hypertensive encephalopathy.
Hypotension.
Postictal state.
Hypernatremia or hyponatremia.
Hypercalcemia.
Hypermagnesemia.
Hypoglycemia.
Severe hyperglycemia.
Hypoxemia.
Dialysis dementia.

DEMENTIA, ADOLESCENT PATIENT[72]

ICD-10CM # F03 Unspecified dementia
F03.90 Unspecified dementia without behavioral disturbance

CAUSES OF DEMENTIA IN ADOLESCENTS

Autoimmune or inflammatory diseases:
  Paraneoplastic syndromes, including NMDA antibody encephalitis.
  Vasculitis.
Cerebral and noncerebral neoplasms:
  Chemotherapy (intrathecal).

Differential Diagnosis

II

Radiotherapy treatment.

Drug, inhalant, and alcohol abuse, including overdose.

Head trauma, including child abuse.

Infections:

HIV-associated dementia.

Variant Creutzfeldt–Jakob disease (vCJD).

Subacute sclerosing panencephalitis (SSPE).

Metabolic abnormalities:

Adrenoleukodystrophy.

Wilson disease.

Neurodegenerative illnesses:

Huntington disease.

Metachromatic leukodystrophy.

Other rare, usually genetically transmitted, illnesses.

DEMENTIAS, NONDEGENERATIVE[38]

ICD-10CM # F03 Unspecified Dementia

PARTIAL LIST OF NONDEGENERATIVE DEMENTIAS

Vascular
Vasculitis (primary or secondary).
Chronic subdural hematoma.

Infectious Causes
Syphilis.
Chronic meningitis.
CJD and other prion diseases.
Whipple.
PML.
Sequelae of herpes encephalitis.
HIV/AIDS-associated dementia.
Neurobrucellosis.
CNS tuberculosis.
Parasitic infections (e.g., cysticercosis).
Lyme disease.
Subacute sclerosing panencephalitis.

Toxic/Metabolic Causes
Hypothyroidism.
Liver disease.
Kidney disease.
Vitamin B_{12} deficiency.
Thiamine deficiency.
Vitamin E deficiency.
Marchiafava-Bignami disease.
Deficiency of nicotinic acid (pellagra).
Heavy metal toxicity.
Parathyroid hormone dysfunction.
Adrenal and pituitary disorders.
Carbon monoxide poisoning.
Drugs (see prior table for list of drugs that can affect cognition).

Structural Causes
Primary or metastatic neoplasm.
Hydrocephalus.

Immune/Inflammatory
Autoimmune dementia.
Multiple sclerosis.
Sarcoidosis.
Collagen vascular diseases (e.g., systemic lupus erythematosus, Sjögren syndrome).
Behçet.

Neoplastic
Slow-growing neoplasm (e.g., meningioma, pituitary tumors).
Gliomatosis cerebri.
Radiation effect.
Paraneoplastic syndromes.
Lymphoma.

Psychiatric
Depression.

Inherited Disorders
Leukodystrophies (e.g., metachromatic leukodystrophy, adrenoleukodystrophy).
Krabbe disease.
Storage disorders: Gaucher disease, Niemann-Pick disease, cerebrotendinous xanthomatosis, and polysaccharidoses, neuronal ceroid lipofuscinoses.
Wilson disease.

AIDS, acquired immunodeficiency syndrome; *CJD*, Creutzfeldt-Jakob disease; *CNS*, central nervous system; *HIV*, human immunodeficiency virus; *PML*, progressive multifocal leukoencephalopathy.

DEMYELINATING DISEASES[62]

ICD-10CM # G37.9 Demyelinating disease of central nervous system, unspecified

MULTIPLE SCLEROSIS
Relapsing and chronic progressive forms.
Acute multiple sclerosis.
Neuromyelitis optica (Devic disease).

DIFFUSE CEREBRAL SCLEROSIS
Schilder encephalitis periaxialis diffusa.
Baló concentric sclerosis.

ACUTE DISSEMINATED ENCEPHALOMYELITIS
After measles, chickenpox, rubella, influenza, mumps.
After rabies or smallpox vaccination.

NECROTIZING HEMORRHAGIC ENCEPHALITIS
Hemorrhagic leukoencephalitis.

LEUKODYSTROPHIES
Krabbe globoid leukodystrophy.
Metachromatic leukodystrophy.
Adrenoleukodystrophy.
Adrenomyeloneuropathy.
Pelizaeus-Merzbacher leukodystrophy.
Canavan disease.
Alexander disease.

DEVELOPMENTAL DELAY, NO REGRESSION[20]

ICD-10CM # Varies with specific diagnosis

Predominant Speech Delay
Bilateral hippocampal sclerosis.
Congenital bilateral perisylvian syndrome.
Hearing impairment.[§]
Autism.

Predominant Motor Delay
Ataxia.
Hemiplegia.
Hypotonia.
Neuromuscular disorders.[a]
Paraplegia.

Global Developmental Delay
Cerebral malformations.
Chromosomal disturbances.
Intrauterine infection.
Perinatal disorders.
Progressive encephalopathies.

---

[a]Denotes the most common conditions and the ones with disease-modifying treatments.

DEXTROCARDIA[37]

ICD-10CM # Q24.0 Dextrocardia

TYPES OF DEXTROCARDIA

Primary Dextrocardia
Dextroversion: the left ventricle is to the left of the right ventricle, as it is in the normal heart.
Mirror-image dextrocardia: the left ventricle is to the right of the right ventricle.

Secondary Dextrocardia
Skeletal causes:
Scoliosis.
Sternal or rib deformity.
Lung causes:
Pneumonectomy.
Collapse.
Pneumothorax.
Unilateral airtrapping.
Pleural causes:
Diaphragmatic hernia with displacement of the gut into left thorax.

DIAPER DERMATITIS[73]

ICD-10CM # L22 Diaper dermatitis

DIFFERENTIAL DIAGNOSIS OF DIAPER DERMATITIS

Chafing dermatitis.
Irritant contact dermatitis.
Diaper candidiasis.
Seborrheic dermatitis.
Psoriasis.
Intertrigo.
Jacquet dermatitis.
Perianal pseudoverrucous papules and nodules.
Miliaria.
Folliculitis.
Impetigo.
Scabies.
Nutritional deficiency (i.e., acrodermatitis enteropathica, cystic fibrosis, biotin deficiency).
Allergic contact dermatitis.
Atopic dermatitis.
Granuloma gluteale infantum.
Langerhans cell histiocytosis.
Burns.
Child abuse.

Epidermolysis bullosa.
Congenital syphilis.
Varicella/herpes.
Tinea cruris.
Chronic bullous dermatosis of childhood.
Bullous mastocytosis.

DIAPHRAGM ELEVATION, BILATERAL, SYMMETRICAL[21]

ICD-10CM # J98.6 Disorders of diaphragm

CAUSES OF BILATERAL SYMMETRICAL ELEVATION OF THE DIAPHRAGM

Supine position.
Poor inspiration.
Obesity.
Pregnancy.
Abdominal distention (ascites, intestinal obstruction, abdominal mass).
Diffuse pulmonary fibrosis.
Lymphangitis carcinomatosa.
Disseminated lupus erythematosus.
Bilateral basal pulmonary emboli.
Painful conditions (after abdominal surgery).
Bilateral diaphragmatic paralysis.

DIAPHRAGM ELEVATION, UNILATERAL[21]

ICD-10CM # J98.6 Disorders of diaphragm

CAUSES OF UNILATERAL ELEVATION OF THE DIAPHRAGM

Posture—lateral decubitus position (dependent side).
Gaseous distention of stomach or colon.
Dorsal scoliosis.
Pulmonary hypoplasia.
Pulmonary collapse.
Phrenic nerve palsy.
Eventration.
Pneumonia or pleurisy.
Pulmonary thromboembolism.
Rib fracture and other painful conditions.
Subphrenic infection.
Subphrenic mass.

DIAPHRAGM WEAKNESS AND PARALYSIS[74]

ICD-10CM # J98.6 Paralysis of diaphragm

NEUROPATHIC CAUSES

Trauma
Cardiac surgery with cold.
Cardioplegia.
Blunt trauma.
Spinal cord injury.
Radiation injury.
Cervical manipulation.

Scalene and brachial nerve block.
Tumor compression.
Lung cancer.
Metastatic mediastinal tumor.
Metabolic
Diabetes.
Vitamin deficiency (B_6, B_{12}, folate).
Hypothyroidism.
Inflammatory Neuritis
Idiopathic (neuralgic amyotrophy, Parsonage-Turner).
Mononeuritis multiplex.
Vasculitis.
Paraneoplastic.
Miscellaneous
Cervical spondylosis.
Poliomyelitis.
Amyotrophic lateral sclerosis.

MYOPATHIC CAUSES

Muscular Dystrophies
Limb-girdle.
Duchenne and Becker.
Metabolic Myopathies
Hyper- or hypothyroidism.
Acid maltase deficiency.
Rheumatologic
Systemic lupus erythematosus.
Dermatomyositis.
Mixed connective disease.
Miscellaneous
Amyloidosis.
Malnutrition.
Idiopathic.

DIARRHEA, ACUTE WATERY AND BLOODY[2]

ICD-10CM #		
	K52.2	Allergic and dietetic gastroenteritis and colitis
	K52.89	Other specified noninfective gastroenteritis and colitis
	R19.7	Diarrhea, unspecified

ACUTE WATERY DIARRHEA

GI infections:
  Protozoal (e.g., *Giardia*).
  Bacterial (e.g., enterotoxigenic *Escherichia coli*, cholera).
  Viral (e.g., rotavirus, Norwalk virus).
Drugs.
Toxins.
Dietary constituents (e.g., lactose intolerance).
Onset of chronic diarrheal illness.

ACUTE BLOODY DIARRHEA

Infectious colitis:
  Confluent proctocolitis (e.g., *Shigella*, *Campylobacter*, *Salmonella*, *Entamoeba histolytica*).
  Segmental colitis (e.g., *Campylobacter*, *Salmonella*, enteroinvasive *E. coli*, *Aeromonas*, *E. histolytica*).

Drug-induced colitis (e.g., NSAIDs).
Inflammatory bowel disease.
Ischemic colitis (usually elderly patient with underlying heart disease or arrhythmias).
Antibiotic-associated colitis.

DIARRHEA, CRITICALLY ILL PATIENT[11]

ICD-10CM # R19.7 Diarrhea, unspecified

COMMON CAUSES OF DIARRHEA IN CRITICALLY ILL PATIENTS

Medication
Antibiotics.
H_2-receptor antagonists, antacids.
Drugs: significant amounts of sorbitol, magnesium, or hypertonic medications.
Laxative use (unintended).
Gastrointestinal Dysfunction
Gastric or small bowel resection.
Inflammatory bowel disease.
Pancreatic insufficiency.
Radiation enteritis.
Sprue.
Protein-losing gastroenteropathies.
Bowel impaction (paradoxic).
Malnutrition
Hypoproteinemia.
Micronutrient deficiencies.
Enteral Nutrition–Associated
Excessive feeding rate, concentration, volume, or osmolality.
Adaptation in malnourished patients or those whose GI tract has not been used recently.
Intolerance or allergy to feeding formula.
Infection
Clostridium difficile enterocolitis.
Opportunistic GI infection.
Significant amounts of contaminated feeding formula.
Altered GI flora.
Endocrine Dysfunction
Diabetes mellitus.
Hyperthyroidism.
Hypocortisolism.

DIARRHEA, INFECTIOUS[43]

ICD-10CM # A09 Infectious gastroenteritis and colitis, unspecified

ETIOLOGIC AGENTS OF INFECTIOUS DIARRHEA

Viral (60% of Cases)
Astrovirus.
Calicivirus.
Coronavirus.
Cytomegalovirus.*
Enteric adenovirus.
Hepatitis A through G.

---

*All of these disorders may cause localized low back pain.

II

Herpes simplex virus.
HIV enteropathy.
Norwalk-like agents.
Pararotavirus.
Norwalk virus.
Picornavirus.
Rotavirus.
Small round viruses.
Bacterial (20% of Cases)
Invasive
Aeromonas spp.
Campylobacter spp.
Clostridium difficile.
Enteroinvasive *E. coli.*
Mycobacterium spp.
Plesiomonas shigelloides.
Salmonella spp.
Shigella spp.
Vibrio fluvialis.
Vibrio parahaemolyticus.
Vibrio vulnificus.
Yersinia enterocolitica.
Yersinia pseudotuberculosis.
Toxigenic
Food poisoning with preformed toxins:
  Bacillus cereus.
  Clostridium botulinum.
  Staphylococcus aureus.
Toxin formation after colonization:
  Aeromonas hydrophila.
  Clostridium perfringens.
  Enterohemorrhagic *E. coli* 0157:H7.
  Enterotoxigenic *E. coli.*
  Klebsiella pneumoniae.
  Shigella spp.
  Vibrio cholerae.
  Other bacteria
Parasitic (5% of Cases)
Protozoa
Balantidium coli.
Blastocystis hominis.
Cryptosporidium.
Cyclospora.
Dientamoeba fragilis.
Entamoeba histolytica.
Entamoeba polecki.
Enteromonas hominis.
Giardia lamblia.
Isospora belli.
Microsporidia.
Sarcocystis hominis.
Helminths
Angiostrongylus costarricense.
Anisakiasis.
Ascaris lumbricoides.
Diphyllobothrium latum.
Enterobius vermicularis.
Hookworms.
Schistosoma spp.
Strongyloides stercoralis.
Taenia spp.
Trichinella spiralis.
Trichuris trichiura.

DIARRHEA, NONINFECTIOUS[43]

ICD-10CM # K59.1 Functional diarrhea

CAUSES OF NONINFECTIOUS DIARRHEA
Toxins
Drugs
ACE inhibitors.
Alprazolam.
Antacids (Mg).
Antibiotics.
Antidepressants.
Antiepileptic drugs.
Antihypertensives.
Antiparkinson drugs.
β-blockers.
Caffeine.
Cardiac antiarrhythmics.
Chemotherapy agents.
Cholesterol-lowering drugs.
Cholinergic agents.
Cholinesterase inhibitors.
Colchicine.
Digitalis.
Diuretics.
Fluorouracil.
Fluoxetine.
Histamine H_2-receptor antagonists.
Hydralazine.
Lactulose.
Laxatives/cathartics.
Levodopa.
Lithium.
NSAIDs.
Neomycin.
Podophyllin.
Procainamide.
Prostaglandins.
Quinidine.
Ricinoleic acid.
Theophylline.
Thyroid hormone.
Valproic acid.
Dietetic Foods
Mannitol.
Sorbitol.
Xylitol.
Fish-Associated Toxins
Amnestic shellfish poisoning.
Ciguatera.
Echinoderms.
Neurotoxic shellfish poisoning.
Paralytic shellfish poisoning.
Scombroid.
Tetroton.
Plant-Associated Toxins
Herbal preparations.
Horse chestnut.
Mushrooms—*Amanita* spp.
Nicotine.

Other plant toxins:
  Pesticides—organophosphates.
  Pokeweed.
  Rhubarb.
Miscellaneous:
  Allergic reactions.
  Carbon monoxide poisoning.
  Ethanol.
  Heavy metals.
  Monosodium glutamate (MSG).
  Opiate withdrawal.
Gastrointestinal Pathology
Appendicitis.
Autonomic dysfunction.
Bile acid malabsorption.
Blind loop.
Bowel obstruction.
Celiac disease.
Cirrhosis.
Defects in amino acid transport.
Diverticular disease.
Familial dysautonomia.
Fecal impaction.
Fecal incontinence.
GI bleed.
GI cancer.
Hirschsprung disease.
Inflammatory bowel disease (ulcerative colitis, Crohn disease).
Intussusception.
Irritable bowel syndrome.
Ischemic bowel.
Lactose/fructose intolerance.
Malabsorption syndromes.
Malrotation.
Postsurgical.
Postvagotomy.
Radiation therapy.
Short gut syndrome.
Small bowel resection.
Strictures.
Toxic megacolon.
Tropical sprue.
Volvulus.
Whipple disease.
Endocrine Related
Carcinoid syndrome (serotonin).
Hormonal hypersecretion.
Hyperthyroidism (thyroid hormone).
Medullary carcinoma of the thyroid (calcitonin).
Pancreatic cholera (VIP).
Somatostatinoma (somatostatin).
Systemic mastocytosis (histamine).
Zollinger-Ellison syndrome (gastrin).
Endocrine Pathology
Adrenal insufficiency.
Diabetes enteropathy.
Hypoparathyroidism.
Pancreatic insufficiency.
Systemic Illness/Other
Alcoholism.
Amyloidosis.

Connective tissue disease.
Cystic fibrosis.
Ectopic pregnancy.
Hemolytic-uremic syndrome.
Henoch-Schönlein purpura.
Lymphoma.
Otitis media—infants.
Pelvic inflammatory disease.
Pneumonia/sepsis.
Pyelonephritis.
Scleroderma/SLE.
Severe malnutrition.
Stevens-Johnson syndrome.
Toxic shock syndrome.
Wilson disease.
Miscellaneous:
Factitious diarrhea.
Runner's diarrhea.

ACE, Angiotensin-converting enzyme; *GI,* gastrointestinal; *NSAIDs,* nonsteroidal antiinflammatory drugs; *SLE,* systemic lupus erythematosus; *VIP,* vasoactive intestinal polypeptide.

DIARRHEA IN PATIENTS WITH AIDS[3]

ICD-10CM # R19.7 Diarrhea, unspecified

PROTOZOA

Microsporidium.*
Cryptosporidium spp.*
Isospora belli.
Toxoplasma spp.
Giardia lamblia.
Entamoeba histolytica.
Leishmania donovani.
Blastocystis hominis.
Cyclospora spp.
Pneumocystis jiroveci.

BACTERIA

Clostridium difficile.
Salmonella spp.
Shigella spp.
Campylobacter jejuni
Mycobacterium avium complex.
Mycobacterium tuberculosis.
SIBO.
Vibrio spp.

VIRUSES

CMV.
HSV.
Adenoviruses.
Rotavirus spp.
Norovirus.
HIV.

FUNGI

Histoplasmosis.
Coccidioidomycosis.
Cryptococcosis.
Candidiasis.
Penicillium marneffei.

NEOPLASMS

Lymphoma.
Kaposi sarcoma.

IDIOPATHIC

"AIDS enteropathy."

DRUG INDUCED

HIV protease inhibitors.

PANCREATIC DISEASE

Pancreatic insufficiency.
Chronic pancreatitis.
Infectious pancreatitis (CMV, MAC).
Drug-induced pancreatitis (e.g., pentamidine).

CMV, Cytomegalovirus.

DIARRHEA, PEDIATRIC PATIENT[68]

ICD-10CM # R19.7 Diarrhea, unspecified

Acute
Common
Gastroenteritis (viral > bacterial > protozoal).
Systemic infection.
Antibiotic associated.
Overfeeding.
Rare
Primary disaccharidase deficiency.
Hirschsprung toxic colitis.
Adrenogenital syndrome.
Neonatal opiate withdrawal.
Chronic
Common
Postinfectious secondary lactase deficiency.
Cow's milk or soy protein intolerance (allergy).
Chronic nonspecific diarrhea of infancy.
Excessive fruit juice (sorbitol) ingestion.
Celiac disease.
Cystic fibrosis.
AIDS enteropathy.
Rare
Primary immune defects.
Autoimmune enteropathy.
IPEX and IPEX-like syndromes.
Glucose-galactose malabsorption.
Microvillus inclusion disease (microvillus atrophy).
Congenital transport defects (chloride, sodium).
Primary bile acid malabsorption.
Factitious syndrome by proxy.
Hirschsprung disease.
Shwachman syndrome.
Secretory tumors.

Acrodermatitis enteropathica.
Lymphangiectasia.
Abetalipoproteinemia.
Eosinophilic gastroenteritis.
Short bowel syndrome.

CHILD
Acute
Common
Gastroenteritis (viral > bacterial > protozoal).
Food poisoning.
Systemic infection.
Antibiotic associated.
Rare
Toxic ingestion.
Hemolytic uremic syndrome.
Intussusception.
Chronic
Common
Postinfectious secondary.
Lactase deficiency.
Irritable bowel syndrome.
Celiac disease.
Cystic fibrosis.
Lactose intolerance.
Excessive fruit juice (sorbitol) ingestion.
Giardiasis.
Inflammatory bowel disease.
AIDS enteropathy.
Rare
Primary and acquired immune defects.
Secretory tumors.
Pseudoobstruction.
Sucrase-isomaltase deficiency.
Eosinophilic gastroenteritis.
Secretory tumors.

ADOLESCENT
Acute
Common
Gastroenteritis (viral > bacterial > protozoal).
Food poisoning.
Antibiotic associated.
Rare
Hyperthyroidism.
Appendicitis.
Chronic
Common
Irritable bowel syndrome.
Inflammatory bowel disease.
Lactose intolerance.
Giardiasis.
Laxative abuse (anorexia nervosa).
Constipation with encopresis.
Rare
Secretory tumor.
Primary bowel tumor.
Parasitic infections and venereal diseases.
Appendiceal abscess.
Addison disease.

IPEX, Immunodysregulation polyendocrinopathy enteropathy X-linked.

Differential Diagnosis

II

DIARRHEA, TUBE-FED PATIENT[24]

ICD-10CM # K91.89 Other postprocedural complications and disorders of digestive system

COMMON CAUSES UNRELATED TO TUBE FEEDING

Elixir medications containing sorbitol.
Magnesium-containing antacids.
Antibiotic-induced sterile gut.
Pseudomembranous colitis.

POSSIBLE CAUSES RELATED TO TUBE FEEDING

Inadequate fiber to form stool bulk.
High fat content of formula (in the presence of fat malabsorption syndrome).
Bacterial contamination of enteral products and delivery systems (causal association with diarrhea not documented).
Rapid advancement in rate (after the GI tract is unused for prolonged periods).

UNLIKELY CAUSES RELATED TO TUBE FEEDING

Formula hyperosmolality (proven not to be the cause of diarrhea).
Lactose (absent from nearly all enteral feeding formulas).

DIFFUSE PARENCHYMAL LUNG DISEASE, DRUG-INDUCED[75]

ICD-10CM # J84.89 Other specified interstitial pulmonary diseases

CYTOTOXIC CHEMOTHERAPY

Bleomycin.
Busulfan.
Cyclophosphamide.
Gemcitabine.
Nitrosoureas.
Taxanes (e.g., paclitaxel, docetaxel).

ANTIMETABOLITES

Methotrexate.

TARGETED BIOLOGIC AGENTS

Tumor necrosis factor (TNF)-α inhibitors or soluble receptors:
Infliximab.
Adalimumab.
Certolizumab pegol.
Etanercept.
Tyrosine kinase inhibitors:
Afatinib.
Erlotinib.
Gefitinib.
Idelalisib.
Imatinib.
Osimertinib.
Trametinib.

Checkpoint inhibitors (antibodies against PD-1, PD-1 ligand, or CTLA-4):
Ipilimumab.
Nivolumab.
Pembrolizumab.
Inhibitors of anaplastic lymphoma kinase (ALK):
Alectinib.
Ceritinib.
Crizotinib.

MISCELLANEOUS

Trastuzumab (monoclonal antibody against HER2).
Rituximab (monoclonal antibody against CD20).
Inhibitors of mechanistic target of rapamycin (mTOR, e.g., everolimus).

MISCELLANEOUS OTHER DRUGS

Nitrofurantoin.
Amiodarone.

DRUG-INDUCED SYNDROMES

Drug-induced lupus (e.g., procainamide, hydralazine).
Drug-induced pulmonary infiltrates with eosinophilia (e.g., sulfa-containing drugs).

DIPLOPIA, BINOCULAR

ICD-10CM # H53.2 Diplopia

Cranial nerve palsy (third, fourth, sixth).
Thyroid eye disease.
Myasthenia gravis.
Decompensated strabismus.
Orbital trauma with blowout fracture.
Orbital pseudotumor.
Cavernous sinus thrombosis.

DIPLOPIA, MONOCULAR

ICD-10CM # H53.2 Diplopia

Postoperative corrected long-standing tropia.
Defective contact lenses.
Poorly fitting bifocals.
Trauma to iris.
Corneal disorder (e.g., dry eye, astigmatism).
Cataracts.
Lens subluxation.
Nystagmus.
Eyelid twitching.
Foreign body in aqueous or vitreous media.
Migraine.
Lesions of occipital cortex.
Psychogenic.

DIPLOPIA, VERTICAL[38]

ICD-10CM # H53.2 Diplopia

COMMON CAUSES

Superior oblique palsy.
Thyroid eye disease (muscle infiltration).
Myasthenia gravis.
Skew deviation (brain stem, cerebellar, hydrocephalus).

LESS COMMON CAUSES

Orbital inflammation (myositis, idiopathic orbital inflammatory syndrome [previously designated "orbital pseudotumor"]).
Orbital infiltration (lymphoma, metastases, amyloid, IgG-4–related disease).
Primary orbital tumor.
Entrapment of the inferior rectus (blowout fracture).
Third nerve palsy with or without aberrant innervation.
Superior division third nerve palsy.
Partial third nuclear lesion (very rare).
Brown syndrome (congenital, acquired).
Congenital extraocular muscle fibrosis or muscle absence.
Double elevator palsy (monocular elevator deficiency); controversial in origin.
Sagging eye syndrome (see discussion in section on sixth nerve mimics).

OTHER CAUSES

Chronic progressive external ophthalmoplegia.
Miller Fisher syndrome.
Botulism.
Monocular supranuclear gaze palsy.
Stiff person syndrome.
Superior oblique myokymia.
Dissociated vertical deviation (divergence).
Wernicke encephalopathy.
Vertical one-and-a-half syndrome.

DIZZINESS

ICD-10CM # R42 Dizziness and giddiness

Viral syndrome.
Anxiety, hyperventilation.
Benign positional paroxysmal vertigo.
Medications (e.g., sedatives, antihypertensives, analgesics).
Withdrawal from medications (e.g., benzodiazepines, SSRIs).
Alcohol or drug abuse.
Postural hypotension.
Hypoglycemia, hyperglycemia.
Hematologic disorders (e.g., anemia, polycythemia, leukemia).
Head trauma.
Menière disease.
Vertebrobasilar ischemia.
Cervical osteoarthritis.
Cardiac abnormalities (arrhythmias, cardiomyopathy, CHF, pericarditis).
Multiple sclerosis.
Peripheral vestibulopathy.
Air or sea travel.
Electrolyte abnormalities.
Eye problems (cornea, lens, retina).
Migraine.
Brain stem infarct.
Autonomic neuropathy.
Chronic otomastoiditis.

Complex partial seizures.
Ramsey Hunt syndrome.
Arteritis.
Syncope and presyncope.
Perilymph fistula.
Cerebellopontine tumor.
Hepatic or renal disease.

DORSAL MIDBRAIN SYNDROME[38]

ICD-10CM #   Code varies with specific diagnosis

Pineal and other tumors.
Stroke.
Trauma (including iatrogenic from surgery).
Hydrocephalus and shunt malfunction.
Multiple sclerosis.
Transtentorial herniation.
Congenital aqueductal stenosis.
Infections:
  Encephalitis.
  Cysticercosis.
  Midbrain arteriovenous malformation.
Metabolic disorders:
  Lipid storage disease.
  Wilson disease.
  Kernicterus.
Wernicke encephalopathy.

DRUG-INDUCED LUPUS[35]

ICD-10CM #   M32.0   Drug-induced lupus

DRY EYE

ICD-10CM #   H04.129   Dry eye syndrome of unspecified lacrimal gland

Contacts.
Medications (antihistamines, clonidine, β-blockers, ibuprofen, scopolamine).
Keratoconjunctivitis sicca.
Trauma.
Environmental causes (air conditioning in patient with contacts).

DYSENTERY AND INFLAMMATORY ENTEROCOLITIS[42]

ICD-10CM #   Varies with specific diagnosis

DIFFERENTIAL DIAGNOSIS OF ACUTE BACTERIAL DYSENTERY AND INFLAMMATORY ENTEROCOLITIS

Specific Infectious Processes
Bacillary dysentery (*Shigella dysenteriae, Shigella flexneri, Shigella sonnei, Shigella boydii; invasive Escherichia coli*).
Campylobacteriosis (*Campylobacter jejuni*).
Amebic dysentery (*Entamoeba histolytica*).
Ciliary dysentery (*Balantidium coli*).
Vibriosis (*Vibrio parahaemolyticus*).

Salmonellosis (*Salmonella typhimurium*).
Typhoid fever (*Salmonella typhi*).
Enteric fever (*Salmonella choleraesuis, Salmonella paratyphi*).
Yersiniosis (*Yersinia enterocolitica*).
Proctitis
Gonococcal (*Neisseria gonorrhoeae*).
Herpetic (herpes simplex virus).
Chlamydial (*Chlamydia trachomatis*).
Syphilitic (*Treponema pallidum*).
Other Syndromes
Necrotizing enterocolitis of the newborn.
Enteritis necroticans.
Pseudomembranous enterocolitis or *Clostridium difficile* colitis without overt pseudomembranes (*C. difficile*).
Diverticulitis.
Typhlitis.
Chronic Inflammatory Processes
Enteropathogenic and enteroaggregative *E. coli.*
Syphilis.
GI tuberculosis.
GI mycosis (including *Basidiobolus ranarum*).
Parasitic enteritis.
Syndromes without Known Infectious Cause
Idiopathic ulcerative colitis.
Crohn disease.
Radiation enteritis.
Ischemic colitis.
Allergic enteritis.
Brainerd diarrhea.

DYSLIPOPROTEINEMIAS, SECONDARY CAUSES[58]

ICD-10CM #   E78.4   Other hyperlipidemia

Cause	Disorder
Metabolic	Diabetes.
	Lipodystrophy.
	Glycogen storage disorders.
Renal	Chronic renal failure.
	Glomerulonephritis with nephritic syndrome.
Hepatic	Cirrhosis.
	Biliary obstruction.
	Porphyria.
	Primary biliary cirrhosis (with secondary LCAT deficiency).
Hormonal	Estrogens.
	Progesterones.
	Growth hormone.
	Thyroid disorders (hypothyroidism).
	Corticosteroids.
Lifestyle	Physical inactivity.
	Obesity.
	Diet rich in fats, saturated fats.
	Alcohol intake.
	Smoking.
Medications	Retinoic acid derivatives.
	Glucocorticoids.
	Exogenous estrogens.
	Thiazide diuretics.
	β-adrenergic blockers (selective).
	Testosterone and other anabolizing steroids.

Immunosuppressive medications (cyclosporine).
Antiviral medications (HIV protease inhibitors).
Antischizophrenic medications.

HIV, Human immunodeficiency virus; *LCAT,* lecithin-cholesterol acyltransferase.

DYSPAREUNIA[55]

ICD-10CM #	N94.1	Dyspareunia
	N44.8	Other noninflammatory disorders of the testis
	N50.8	Other specified disorders of male genital organs
	N53.12	Painful ejaculation
	F52.6	Dyspareunia not due to a substance or known physiological condition

INTROITAL
Vaginismus.
Intact or rigid hymen.
Clitoral problems.
Vulvovaginitis.
Vaginal atrophy: hypoestrogen.
Vulvar dystrophy.
Bartholin or Skene gland infection.
Inadequate lubrication.
Operative scarring.

MIDVAGINAL
Urethritis.
Trigonitis.
Cystitis.
Short vagina.
Operative scarring.
Inadequate lubrication.

DEEP
Endometriosis.
Pelvic infection.
Uterine retroversion.
Ovarian pathology.
GI.
Orthopedic.
Abnormal penile size or shape.

DYSPEPSIA AND PYROSIS, DIFFERENTIAL DIAGNOSIS DURING PREGNANCY[32]

ICD-10CM #	K30	Dyspepsia, atonic
	F45.3	Dyspepsia, psychogenic

DIFFERENTIAL DIAGNOSIS OF DYSPEPSIA OR PYROSIS DURING PREGNANCY

Gastroesophageal reflux disease.
Peptic ulcer disease.
Nausea and vomiting of pregnancy.
Hyperemesis gravidarum.
Pancreatitis.
Biliary colic.
Acute cholecystitis.

Differential Diagnosis

II

Viral hepatitis.
Appendicitis.
Acute fatty liver of pregnancy (in late pregnancy).
Irritable bowel syndrome/nonulcer dyspepsia.

DYSPHAGIA

ICD-10CM # R13.10 Dysphagia, unspecified

Esophageal obstruction: neoplasm, foreign body, achalasia, stricture, spasm, esophageal web, diverticulum, Schatzki ring.
Peptic esophagitis with stricture, Barrett stricture.
External esophageal compression: neoplasms (thyroid neoplasm, lymphoma, mediastinal tumors), thyroid enlargement, aortic aneurysm, vertebral spurs, aberrant right subclavian artery (dysphagia lusoria).
Hiatal hernia, GERD.
Oropharyngeal lesions: pharyngitis, glossitis, stomatitis, neoplasms.
Hysteria: globus hystericus.
Neurologic and/or neuromuscular disturbances: bulbar paralysis, myasthenia gravis, ALS, multiple sclerosis, parkinsonism, CVA, diabetic neuropathy.
Toxins: poisoning, botulism, tetanus, post-diphtheritic dysphagia.
Systemic diseases: scleroderma, amyloidosis, dermatomyositis.
Candida and herpes esophagitis.
Presbyesophagus.

DYSPHAGIA, ESOPHAGEAL[3]

ICD-10CM # R13-14 Dysphagia, pharyngoesophageal phase

COMMON CAUSES OF ESOPHAGEAL DYSPHAGIA
Motility (Neuromuscular) Disorders
Primary
Achalasia.
Distal esophageal spasm.
Hypercontractile (jackhammer) esophagus.
Hypertensive LES.
Nutcracker (high-pressure) esophagus.
Other peristaltic abnormalities.*
Secondary
Chagas disease.
Reflux-related dysmotility.
Scleroderma and other rheumatologic disorders.
Structural (Mechanical) Disorders
Intrinsic
Carcinoma and benign tumors.
Diverticula.
Eosinophilic esophagitis.
Esophageal rings and webs (other than Schatzki ring).
Foreign body.

Lower esophageal (Schatzki) ring.
Medication-induced stricture.
Peptic stricture.
Extrinsic
Mediastinal mass.
Spinal osteophytes.
Vascular compression.
LES, Lower esophageal sphincter.

DYSPHAGIA, OROPHARYNGEAL[2]

ICD-10CM # R13.12 Dysphagia, oropharyngeal phase

FUNCTIONAL DISORDERS
Central Nervous System
Stroke.
Head injury.
Parkinson disease.
Motor neuron disease.
Multiple sclerosis.
Tumor.
Drugs (e.g., phenothiazines).
Malformations (e.g., syrinx, Arnold-Chiari).
Neural
Motor neuron disease.
Myasthenia gravis.
Radiotherapy.
Poliomyelitis.
Familial dysautonomia.
Muscle
Autoimmune myopathy (polymyositis, dermatomyositis, systemic lupus erythematosus).
Thyrotoxic myopathy.
Guillain-Barré motor neuropathy.
Muscular dystrophies.

STRUCTURAL DISORDERS
Head/neck surgery.
Stricture.
Radiotherapy.
Tumor.
Pharyngeal pouch.
Web.
Extrinsic (e.g., osteophytes).

MISCELLANEOUS
Xerostomia.

DYSPNEA

ICD-10CM # R06.9 Unspecified abnormalities of breathing

Upper airway obstruction: trauma, neoplasm, epiglottitis, laryngeal edema, tongue retraction, laryngospasm, abductor paralysis of vocal cords, aspiration of foreign body.
Lower airway obstruction: neoplasm, COPD, asthma, aspiration of foreign body.
Pulmonary infection: pneumonia, abscess, empyema, TB, bronchiectasis.
Pulmonary hypertension.
Pulmonary embolism/infarction.
Parenchymal lung disease.

Pulmonary vascular congestion.
Cardiac disease: ASHD, valvular lesions, cardiac dysrhythmias, cardiomyopathy, pericardial effusion, cardiac shunts.
Space-occupying lesions: neoplasm, large hiatal hernia, pleural effusions.
Disease of chest wall: severe kyphoscoliosis, fractured ribs, sternal compression, morbid obesity.
Neurologic dysfunction: Guillain-Barré syndrome, botulism, polio, spinal cord injury.
Interstitial pulmonary disease: sarcoidosis, collagen vascular diseases, DIP, Hamman-Rich pneumonitis, etc.
Pneumoconioses: silicosis, berylliosis, etc.
Mesothelioma.
Pneumothorax, hemothorax, pleural effusion.
Inhalation of toxins.
Cholinergic drug intoxication.
Carcinoid syndrome.
Hematologic: anemia, polycythemia, hemoglobinopathies.
Thyrotoxicosis, myxedema.
Diaphragmatic compression caused by abdominal distention, subphrenic abscess, ascites.
Lung resection.
Metabolic abnormalities: uremia, hepatic coma, DKA.
Sepsis.
Atelectasis.
Psychoneurosis.
Diaphragmatic paralysis.
Pregnancy.

DYSTONIA, PEDIATRIC PATIENT[49]

ICD-10CM # G24.9 Dystonia, unspecified
G24.2 Idiopathic nonfamilial dystonia
G24.1 Genetic torsion dystonia

CAUSES OF DYSTONIA IN CHILDHOOD
Static Injury/Structural Disorders
Cerebral palsy.
Hypoxic-ischemic injury.
Kernicterus.
Head trauma.
Encephalitis.
Tumors.
Stroke in the basal ganglia (which may be due to vascular abnormalities or varicella).
Congenital malformations affecting basal ganglia.
Hereditary/Degenerative Disorders
DYT1 (autosomal dominant, Torsin A).
DYT2 (autosomal-recessive, hippocalcin).
DYT4 (autosomal dominant, β-tubulin 4a).
DYT5 (autosomal dominant, GTP cyclohydrolase 1).
DYT6 (autosomal dominant, THAP1).
DYT8 (autosomal dominant, myofibrillogenesis regulator 1).
DYT9 (autosomal dominant, GLUT1).

---

*Peristaltic abnormalities include absent peristalsis and weak peristalsis, as well as hypertensive peristalsis (nutcracker esophagus).

DYT10 (autosomal dominant, PRRT2).

DYT11 (autosomal dominant [maternal imprinting], ε-Sarcoglycan).

DYT12 (autosomal dominant, Na$^+$/K$^+$ATPase α3 subunit).

DYT15 (autosomal dominant, unknown).

DYT16 (autosomal recessive, protein kinase activator PRKRA).

Pantothenate kinase-associated neuro-degeneration (PKAN; neuronal brain iron accumulation type 1, due to mutations in *PANK2*).

PLA2G6-associated neurodegeneration (PLAN).

Huntington disease (Westphal variant, IT15–4p16.3).

Spinocerebellar ataxias (SCAs, particularly SCA3/Machado-Joseph disease).

Striatal necrosis.

Leigh syndrome.

Neuroacanthocytosis.

HARP syndrome (hypoprebetalipoproteinemia, acanthocytosis, retinitis pigmentosa, and pallidal degeneration).

Tay-Sachs disease.

Sandhoff disease.

Niemann-Pick type C.

Metabolic Disease

Glutaric aciduria types 1 and 2.

Acyl-CoA dehydrogenase deficiencies.

Neurotransmitter disorders.

Mitochondrial disorders.

GM$_1$ gangliosidosis.

Lesch-Nyhan disease.

Wilson disease.

Vitamin E deficiency.

Methylmalonic aciduria.

Tyrosinemia.

Drugs/Toxins

Neuroleptic and neuroleptic-like antiemetic medications (haloperidol, chlorpromazine, olanzapine, risperidone, prochlorperazine).

Calcium channel blockers.

Stimulants (amphetamine, cocaine, ergot alkaloids).

Anticonvulsants (carbamazepine, phenytoin).

Thallium.

Manganese.

Carbon monoxide.

Ethylene glycol.

Cyanide.

Methanol.

Paroxysmal Disorders

Paroxysmal kinesigenic dyskinesia (PKD).

Paroxysmal nonkinesigenic dyskinesia (PNKD).

Exercise-induced dyskinesia (PED).

DYSURIA

ICD-10CM #   R30.0   Dysuria
            R30.9   Painful micturition, unspecified

Urinary tract infection.

Estrogen deficiency (in postmenopausal female).

Vaginitis.

Genital infection (e.g., herpes, condyloma).

Interstitial cystitis.

Chemical irritation (e.g., deodorant aerosols, douches).

Meatal stenosis or stricture.

Reiter syndrome.

Bladder neoplasm.

GI etiology (diverticulitis, Crohn disease).

Impaired bladder or sphincter action.

Urethral carbuncle.

Chronic fibrosis posttrauma.

Radiation therapy.

Prostatitis.

Urethritis (gonococcal, *Chlamydia*).

Behçet syndrome.

Stevens-Johnson syndrome.

EARACHE[76]

ICD-10CM #   H92.09   Otalgia, unspecified ear

Otitis media.

Serous otitis media.

Eustachitis.

Otitis externa.

Otitic barotrauma.

Mastoiditis.

Foreign body.

Impacted cerumen.

Referred otalgia, as with TMJ dysfunction, dental problems, and tumors.

ECTOPIC ACTH SECRETION[24]

ICD-10CM #   E34.2   Ectopic hormone secretion, not elsewhere classified

Small cell carcinoma of lung.

Endocrine tumors of foregut origin.

    Thymic carcinoid.

    Islet cell tumor.

    Medullary carcinoid, thyroid.

    Bronchial carcinoid.

Pheochromocytoma.

Ovarian tumors.

EDEMA, CHILDREN[23]

ICD-10CM #   R60.0   Localized edema
            R60.1   Generalized edema
            R60.9   Edema, unspecified

CARDIOVASCULAR

Congestive heart failure.

Acute thrombi or emboli.

Vasculitis of many types.

RENAL

Nephrotic syndrome.

Glomerulonephritis of many types.

End-stage renal failure.

ENDOCRINE OR METABOLIC

Thyroid disease.

Starvation.

Hereditary angioedema.

IATROGENIC

Drugs (diuretics and steroids).

Water or salt overload.

HEMATOLOGIC

Hemolytic disease of the newborn.

GASTROINTESTINAL

Hepatic cirrhosis.

Protein-losing enteritis.

Lymphangiectasis.

Cystic fibrosis.

Celiac disease.

Enteritis of many types.

LYMPHATIC ABNORMALITIES

Congenital (gonadal dysgenesis).

Acquired.

EDEMA, GENERALIZED

ICD-10CM #   R60.0   Localized edema
            R60.1   Generalized edema
            R60.9   Edema, unspecified

Congestive heart failure (CHF).

Cirrhosis.

Nephrotic syndrome.

Pregnancy.

Idiopathic.

Acute nephritic syndrome.

Myxedema.

Medications (NSAIDs, estrogens, vasodilators).

EDEMA, LEG, UNILATERAL[1]

ICD-10CM #   R60.0   Localized edema
            R60.9   Edema, unspecified

WITH PAIN

DVT.

Postphlebitic syndrome.

Popliteal cyst rupture.

Gastrocnemius rupture.

Cellulitis.

Psoas or other abscess.

WITHOUT PAIN

DVT.

Postphlebitic syndrome.

Other venous insufficiency (after saphenous vein harvest, varicosities).

Lymphatic obstruction/lymphedema (carcinoma, lymphoma, sarcoidosis, filariasis, retroperitoneal fibrosis).

EDEMA OF LOWER EXTREMITIES

ICD-10CM #   R60.0   Localized edema
            R60.9   Edema, unspecified

CHF (right-sided).

Hepatic cirrhosis.

Differential Diagnosis

II

Nephrosis.
Myxedema.
Lymphedema.
Pregnancy.
Abdominal mass: neoplasm, cyst.
Venous compression from abdominal aneurysm.
Varicose veins.
Bilateral cellulitis.
Bilateral thrombophlebitis.
Vena cava thrombosis, venous thrombosis.
Retroperitoneal fibrosis.

EJECTION SOUND OR CLICK

ICD-10CM # R01.2 Other cardiac sounds

Aortic regurgitation.
Aortic root dilation.
Systemic hypertension.
Chronic pulmonary hypertension.
Tetralogy of Fallot.
Atrial septal defect.
Pulmonary valve stenosis.
Aortic aneurysm.

ELBOW PAIN

ICD-10CM # M25.529 Pain in unspecified elbow

Trauma.
Infection.
Inflammatory arthritis.
Lateral or medial epicondylitis.
Entrapment neuropathy.
Olecranon bursitis.
Osteoarthritis.
Gout.
Cervical disease (referred pain).
Shoulder disease (referred pain).
Partial subluxation.
Synovial osteochondromatosis.
Loose body.

ELEVATED HEMIDIAPHRAGM

ICD-10CM # J98.6 Disorders of diaphragm
Q79.0 Congenital diaphragmatic hernia
Q79.1 Other congenital malformations of diaphragm

Neoplasm (bronchogenic carcinoma, mediastinal neoplasm, intrahepatic lesion).
Substernal thyroid.
Infectious process (pneumonia, empyema, TB, subphrenic abscess, hepatic abscess).
Atelectasis.
Idiopathic.
Eventration.
Phrenic nerve dysfunction (myelitis, myotonia, herpes zoster).
Trauma to phrenic nerve or diaphragm (e.g., surgery).
Aortic aneurysm.
Intraabdominal mass.

Pulmonary infarction.
Pleurisy.
Radiation therapy.
Rib fracture.

EMBOLI, ARTERIAL[1]

ICD-10CM # I74.3 Embolism and thrombosis of arteries of the lower extremities
I74.2 Embolism and thrombosis of arteries of the upper extremities

Myocardial infarction with mural thrombi.
Atrial fibrillation.
Cardiomyopathies.
Prosthetic heart valves.
CHF.
Endocarditis.
Left ventricular aneurysm.
Left atrial myxoma.
Sick sinus syndrome.
Paradoxical embolus from venous thrombosis.
Aneurysms of large blood vessels.
Atheromatous ulcers of large blood vessels.

EMESIS, PEDIATRIC AGE[23]

ICD-10CM # R11.10 Vomiting, unspecified
R11.11 Vomiting without nausea
R11.12 Projectile vomiting

INFANCY
Gastrointestinal Tract
Congenital
Regurgitation: chalasia, gastroesophageal reflux.
Atresia: stenosis (tracheoesophageal fistula, prepyloric diaphragm, intestinal atresia).
Duplication.
Volvulus (errors in rotation and fixation, Meckel diverticulum).
Congenital bands.
Hirschsprung disease.
Meconium ileus (cystic fibrosis), meconium plug.

Acquired
Acute infectious gastroenteritis, food poisoning (staphylococcal, clostridial).
Pyloric stenosis.
Gastritis, duodenitis.
Intussusception.
Incarcerated hernia—inguinal, internal secondary to old adhesions.
Cow's milk protein intolerance, food allergy, eosinophilic gastroenteritis.
Disaccharidase deficiency.
Celiac disease—presents after introduction of gluten in diet; inherited risk.
Adynamic ileus—the mediator for many non-gastrointestinal causes.
Neonatal necrotizing enterocolitis.
Chronic granulomatous disease with gastric outlet obstruction.

Nongastrointestinal Tract
Infectious: otitis, urinary tract infection, pneumonia, upper respiratory tract infection, sepsis, meningitis.
Metabolic: aminoaciduria and organic aciduria, galactosemia, fructosemia, adrenogenital syndrome, renal tubular acidosis, diabetic ketoacidosis, Reye syndrome.
CNS: trauma, tumor, infection, diencephalic syndrome, rumination, autonomic responses (pain, shock).
Medications: anticholinergics, aspirin, alcohol, idiosyncratic reaction (e.g., codeine).

CHILDHOOD
Gastrointestinal Tract
Peptic ulcer—vomiting is a common presentation in children younger than 6 yr old.
Trauma: duodenal hematoma, traumatic pancreatitis, perforated bowel.
Pancreatitis: mumps, trauma, cystic fibrosis, hyperparathyroidism, hyperlipidemia, organic acidemias.
Crohn disease.
Idiopathic intestinal pseudoobstruction.
Superior mesenteric artery syndrome.
Nongastrointestinal Tract
CNS: cyclic vomiting, migraine, anorexia nervosa, bulimia.

ENCEPHALOMYELITIS, NONVIRAL CAUSES[1]

ICD-10CM # G04.81 Other encephalitis and encephalomyelitis

Subacute bacterial endocarditis.
Rocky Mountain spotted fever.
Typhus.
Ehrlichia.
Q fever.
Chlamydia.
Mycoplasma.
Legionella.
Brucellosis.
Listeria.
Whipple disease.
Cat-scratch disease.
Syphilis (meningovascular).
Relapsing fever.
Lyme disease.
Leptospirosis.
Nocardia.
Actinomycosis.
Tuberculosis.
Cryptococcus.
Histoplasma.
Toxoplasma.
Plasmodium falciparum.
Trypanosomiasis.
Behçet disease.
Vasculitis.
Carcinoma.
Drug reactions.

ENCEPHALOPATHY, HYPERTENSIVE[7]

ICD-10CM # Varies with specific diagnosis

Cerebral infarction.
Subarachnoid hemorrhage.
Intracerebral hemorrhage.
Subdural or epidural hematoma.
Brain tumor or other mass lesion.
Seizure disorder.
CNS vasculitis.
Encephalitis/meningitis.
Drug ingestion.
Drug withdrawal.

ENCEPHALOPATHY, METABOLIC[17]

ICD-10CM #		
	F10.27	Alcohol dependence with alcohol-induced persisting dementia
	K72.90	Hepatic failure, unspecified without coma
	K72.91	Hepatic failure, unspecified with coma
	G92	Toxic encephalopathy
	T56.0X1A	Toxic effect of lead and its compounds, accidental (unintentional), initial encounter
	T56.0X2A	Toxic effect of lead and its compounds, intentional self-harm, initial encounter

Substrate deficiency: hypoxia/ischemia, carbon monoxide poisoning, hypoglycemia.
Cofactor deficiency: thiamine, vitamin B_{12}, pyridoxine (INH administration).
Electrolyte disorders: hyponatremia, hypercalcemia, carbon dioxide narcosis, dialysis, hypermagnesemia, disequilibrium syndrome.
Endocrinopathies: DKA, hyperosmolar coma, hypothyroidism, hyperadrenocorticism, hyperparathyroidism.
Endogenous toxins: liver disease, uremia, porphyria.
Exogenous toxins: drug overdose (sedative/hypnotics, ethanol, narcotics, salicylates, tricyclic antidepressants), drug withdrawal, toxicity of therapeutic medications, industrial toxins (e.g., organophosphates, heavy metals), sepsis.
Heat stroke.
Epilepsy (postictal).

ENCEPHALOPATHY, PROGRESSIVE, ONSET AFTER AGE 2[20]

ICD-10CM # Varies with specific diagnosis

DISORDERS OF LYSOSOMAL ENZYMES

Gaucher disease type III (glucosylceramide lipidosis).
Globoid cell leukodystrophy (late-onset Krabbe disease).
Glycoprotein degradation disorders.
Aspartylglycosaminuria.
Mannosidosis type II.
GM2 gangliosidosis (juvenile Tay-Sachs disease).
Metachromatic leukodystrophy (late-onset sulfatide lipidosis).
Mucopolysaccharidoses types II and VII.
Niemann-Pick type C (sphingomyelin lipidosis).

INFECTIOUS DISEASE

Acquired immunodeficiency syndrome encephalopathy.[a]
Congenital syphilis.[a]
Subacute sclerosing panencephalitis.

OTHER DISORDERS OF GRAY MATTER

Ceroid lipofuscinosis.
  Juvenile.
  Late infantile (Bielschowsky-Jansky disease).
Huntington disease.
Mitochondrial disorders.
  Late-onset poliodystrophy.
  Myoclonic epilepsy and ragged-red fibers.
Progressive neuronal degeneration with liver disease.
Xeroderma pigmentosum.

OTHER DISORDERS OF WHITE MATTER

Adrenoleukodystrophy.
Alexander disease.
Cerebrotendinous xanthomatosis.
Progressive cavitating leukoencephalopathy.

---

[a] Denotes the most common conditions and the ones with disease-modifying treatments.

ENCEPHALOPATHY, PROGRESSIVE, ONSET BEFORE AGE 2[20]

ICD-10CM # Varies with specific diagnosis

ACQUIRED IMMUNODEFICIENCY SYNDROME ENCEPHALOPATHY.[a]

DISORDERS OF AMINO ACID METABOLISM.

Guanidinoacetate methyltransferase deficiency.[a]
Homocystinuria (21q22).[a]
Maple syrup urine disease (intermediate and thiamine-response forms).[a]
Phenylketonuria.

DISORDERS OF LYSOSOMAL ENZYMES.

Ganglioside storage disorders.

GM1 gangliosidosis.
GM2 gangliosidosis (Tay-Sachs disease, Sandhoff disease).
Gaucher disease type II (glucosylceramide lipidosis).[a]
Globoid cell leukodystrophy (Krabbe disease).
Glycoprotein degradation disorders.
I-cell disease.
  Mucopolysaccharidoses.[a]
  Type I (Hurler syndrome).[a]
  Type III (Sanfilippo disease).
Niemann-Pick disease type A (sphingomyelin lipidosis).
Sulfatase deficiency disorders.
  Metachromatic leukodystrophy (sulfatide lipidosis).
  Multiple sulfatase deficiency.
Carbohydrate-deficient glycoprotein syndromes.
Hypothyroidism.[a]

MITOCHONDRIAL DISORDERS.

Alexander disease.
Mitochondrial myopathy, encephalopathy, lactic acidosis, stroke.
Progressive infantile poliodystrophy (Alpers disease).
Subacute necrotizing encephalomyelopathy (Leigh disease).
Trichopoliodystrophy (Menkes disease).

NEUROCUTANEOUS SYNDROMES.

Chediak-Higashi syndrome.
Neurofibromatosis.[a]
Tuberous sclerosis.[a]

OTHER DISORDERS OF GRAY MATTER.

Infantile ceroid lipofuscinosis (Santavuori-Haltia disease).
Infantile neuroaxonal dystrophy.
Lesch-Nyhan disease.[a]
Progressive neuronal degeneration with liver disease.
Rett syndrome.

OTHER DISORDERS OF WHITE MATTER.

Aspartoacylase deficiency (Canavan disease).
Galactosemia: transferase deficiency.[a]
Neonatal adrenoleukodystrophy.[a]
Pelizaeus-Merzbacher disease.
Progressive cavitating leukoencephalopathy.

PROGRESSIVE HYDROCEPHALUS.[a]

---

[a] Denotes the most common conditions and the ones with disease-modifying treatments.

ENDOMETRIAL THICKENING[15]

ICD-10CM # Varies with specific diagnosis

CAUSES OF ENDOMETRIAL THICKENING

Early intrauterine pregnancy.
Incomplete abortion.
Ectopic pregnancy.

Retained products of conception.
Trophoblastic disease.
Endometritis.
Adhesions.
Hyperplasia.
Polyps.
Carcinoma.

ENTERIC FEVER[5]

ICD-10CM #	A01.00	Typhoid fever, unspecified
	A01.3	Paratyphoid fever
	R50.9	Fever, unspecified

Epstein-Barr infection.
Dengue.
Tuberculosis.
Brucellosis.
Bartonella henselae.
Leptospirosis.
Tularemia.
Ehrlichiosis.
Plague.
Typhus.
Malaria.
Disseminated histoplasmosis.

ENTHESOPATHY

ICD-10CM #	M46.00	Spinal enthesopathy, site unspecified

Viremia or bacteremia.
Ankylosing spondylitis.
Psoriatic arthritis.
Drug-induced (quinolones, etretinate).
Reactive arthritis.
DISH.
Reiter syndrome.

EOSINOPHILIA, DISEASE ASSOCIATIONS[77]

ICD-10CM #	D72.1	Eosinophilia
	NEC J82	Eosinophilia, pulmonary

DISEASES, SYNDROMES, AND CONDITIONS COMMONLY ASSOCIATED WITH PERIPHERAL BLOOD EOSINOPHILIA AND/OR TISSUE EOSINOPHILIA

Infectious Agents
Parasitic Infections
Tropical eosinophilia.
Visceral larval migrans (VLM, toxocariasis).
Helminth infections.
Filariasis (*Wuchereria bancrofti, Brugia malayi*).
Onchocerciasis.
Schistosomiasis.
Fascioliasis.
Paragonimiasis.
Strongyloidiasis.
Trichinosis.
Hookworm.
Ascariasis.

Echinococcosis/hydatid disease.
Fungal Infections
Coccidioidomycosis.
Cryptococcosis (CSF eosinophilia) in HIV.
Allergic Diseases
Asthma (atopic and intrinsic, nasal polyps, aspirin intolerance syndromes).
Bronchopulmonary aspergillosis.
Allergic rhinitis.
Urticarias (acute allergic and chronic idiopathic).
Atopic dermatitis.
Acute drug (hypersensitivity) reactions (interstitial nephritis, cholestatic hepatitis, exfoliative dermatitis).
Respiratory Tract Disorders
Hypersensitivity pneumonitis (rare).
Allergic bronchopulmonary aspergillosis.
Eosinophilic pneumonia.
Transient pulmonary infiltrates (Löeffler syndrome).
Prolonged pulmonary infiltrates with eosinophilia (PIE syndrome).
Tropical pulmonary eosinophilia (TPE).
Bronchiectasis.
Cystic fibrosis.
Endocrinologic Disorders
Addison disease.
Gastrointestinal Diseases
Inflammatory bowel disease (IBD).
Eosinophilic gastroenteritis, eosinophilic esophagitis (EE).
Allergic gastroenteritis (young children).
Celiac disease (when associated with EE).
Toxic Reactions to Ingested Agents
Eosinophil myalgia syndrome (L-tryptophan).
Toxic oil syndrome.
Reactions to Cytokine Therapies
IL-2 and IL-2 plus lymphokine activated killer (LAK) cells.
GM-CSF therapy.
Cutaneous Disorders
Atopic dermatitis.
Immunologic skin diseases.
Scabies.
Myiasis.
Chlamydial pneumonia of infancy.
Scarlet fever and pneumococcal pneumonia (convalescent phase).
Cat-scratch disease.
Eosinophilic cellulitis (Wells syndrome).
Episodic angioedema with eosinophilia.
Chronic idiopathic urticaria.
Bullous pemphigoid.
Herpes gestationis.
Angioblastic lymphoid hyperplasia (Kimura disease).
Immunodeficiency Syndromes
Wiskott-Aldrich syndrome.
Selective IgA deficiency with atopy.
Hyper-IgE recurrent infection syndrome (Job syndrome).
Swiss-type and sex-linked combined immunodeficiency.
Nezelof syndrome.

Graft-versus-host-disease (GVHD).
Connective Tissue Diseases
Vasculitis/Collagen Vascular Disorders
  Hypersensitivity vasculitis.
  Allergic granulomatosis with angiitis (Churg-Strauss syndrome).
  Serum sickness.
  Eosinophilic fasciitis.
  Sjögren syndrome.
  Rheumatoid arthritis (severe).
Neoplastic, Myeloproliferative, and Lymphoproliferative Neoplasms and Syndromes
Neoplastic
  Ovarian carcinoma.
  Solid tumors (mucin-secreting, epithelial cell origin).
Chronic eosinophil leukemia.
Idiopathic hypereosinophilic syndromes (HES).
Systemic mastocytosis.
Myeloproliferative
  Chronic myelogenous leukemia (CML), acute myelogenous leukemia (AML), and myelodysplastic syndrome (MDS).
  Myelomonocytic leukemia with bone marrow eosinophilia (M4Eo, inversion 16).
Lymphoproliferative
  T-cell lymphocytic leukemia.
  Lymphomas (T cell, Hodgkin disease).
  Angioimmunoblastic lymphadenopathy.
Rare Causes
Chronic active hepatitis.
Chronic dialysis.
Acute pancreatitis.
Postirradiation.
Hypopituitarism.

EOSINOPHILIA, GI[3]

ICD-10CM #	D72.1	Eosinophilia

CAUSES OF GI EOSINOPHILIA

GERD
Eosinophilic GI disorders:
  Eosinophilic esophagitis:
    Connective tissue disease-associated eosinophilic esophagitis.
    Familial eosinophilic esophagitis.
  Eosinophilic gastritis.
  Eosinophilic enteritis.
  Eosinophilic gastroenteritis.
Infections:
  Schistosomiasis.
  Anisakiasis.
  GI basidiobolomycosis.
  Toxocariasis.
Celiac disease.
Hypereosinophilic syndrome.
Drug hypersensitivity response.
IBD.
Transplant-associated eosinophilic enteritis.
Eosinophilic granulomatosis with polyangiitis.
Toxic injury.
Graft-versus-host disease.

EOSINOPHILIC LUNG DISEASE[21]

ICD-10CM # NEC J82 Eosinophilia, pulmonary

IDIOPATHIC
Simple pulmonary eosinophilia (Löffler syndrome).
Acute eosinophilic pneumonia.
Chronic eosinophilic pneumonia.
Hypereosinophilic syndrome.

DRUG-INDUCED
Aminosalicylic acid.
Para-aminosalicylic acid.
NSAIDs.
Captopril.
Cocaine.
Minocycline.
Nitrofurantoin.
Phenytoin.

INFECTION
Parasitic (ascariasis, paragonimiasis. tropical eosinophilia).
Fungal (Aspergillus).
Bacterial (TB, atypical mycobacterial infection, brucella).
Viral (respiratory syncytial virus).

IMMUNOLOGIC DISEASES
Granulomatosis with polyangiitis.
Churg-Strauss syndrome.
Rheumatoid disease.
Sarcoidosis.

NEOPLASMS
Bronchogenic carcinoma.
Bronchial carcinoid.
Lymphoma (Hodgkin, non-Hodgkin).

EOSINOPHILIA, PARASITIC CAUSES[42]

ICD-10CM # Varies with specific diagnosis

PARASITIC CAUSES OF EOSINOPHILIA
Widespread Geographic Distribution
Ascariasis (migratory phase).
Hookworm.[†]
Strongyloidiasis.[*,‡]
Tropical pulmonary eosinophilia.
Lymphatic filariasis.
Schistosomiasis.
Toxocariasis.
Cysticercosis (Taenia solium).

[†]Although these are most common neoplastic lesions of the lumbosacral spine, most occur infrequently.
[*]Most frequent parasitic causes of massive eosinophilia (>5000/mm³).
[‡]Absent in disseminated infection in compromised hosts.

Echinococcosis (cyst rupture).
Trichinosis.
Trichuriasis.
Aberrant helminthiasis from animals.
Limited Geographic Distribution
Clonorchiasis.
Paragonimiasis.
Fascioliasis.
Angiostrongyliasis.
Opisthorchiasis.
Onchocerciasis, loiasis, and other nonlymphatic filariases.
Gnathostomiasis.
Capillariasis.
Trichostrongyliasis.

EPIGASTRIC PAIN[2]

ICD-10CM #		
	R10.816	Epigastric abdominal tenderness
	R10.826	Epigastric rebound abdominal tenderness

Peptic ulceration (uncomplicated).*
Peptic ulceration (perforated).
Biliary colic.
Acute pancreatitis.
Abdominal aortic aneurysm.
Anxiety.
Inferior wall MI.

---

*Conditions that also cause right upper quadrant pain

EPILEPSY

ICD-10CM #	G40.909	Epilepsy, unspecified, not intractable, without status epilepticus

Psychogenic spells.
Transient ischemic attack.
Hypoglycemia.
Syncope.
Narcolepsy.
Migraine.
Paroxysmal vertigo.
Arrhythmias.
Drug reaction.

EPILEPSY MIMICS, PEDIATRIC PATIENT[49]

ICD-10CM # Varies with specific diagnosis

DISORDERS THAT MAY MIMIC CHILDHOOD EPILEPSY
Confused with Generalized Tonic-Clonic Seizures
Pallid syncope (reflex anoxic seizure).
Vasodepressor syncope (reflex anoxic seizure).
Cyanotic breath-holding attacks.
Collapsing attacks with cardiac dysrhythmias.
Cataplexy.
Confused with Generalized Absence Seizures
Behavioral staring attacks.
Complex partial (dyscognitive) seizures.

Tic disorder.
Confused with Complex Partial (Dyscognitive) Seizures
Self-stimulatory behavior, especially in children with autistic spectrum disorders.
Sleep walking.
Night terrors.
Temper tantrums with amnesia for the rage event.
Benign paroxysmal vertigo.
Migraine-related disorders.
Confused with Epileptic Myoclonus
Physiologic hypnagogic myoclonus.
Benign infantile sleep myoclonus.
Startle disease.

EPILEPSY SYNDROMES, AGE SPECIFIC[5]

ICD-10CM #	G40.90	Epilepsy, unspecified, not intractable
	G40.301	Generalized idiopathic epilepsy and epileptic syndromes, not intractable, with status epilepticus
	G40.40	Other generalized epilepsy and epileptic syndromes, not intractable

EPILEPSY SYNDROMES BY AGE OF ONSET
Neonatal
Benign familial neonatal epilepsy.
Early myoclonic encephalopathy.
Ohtahara syndrome.
Infancy
Epilepsy of infancy with migrating focal seizures.
West syndrome (infantile spasms, hypsarrhythmia; to be distinguished from benign myoclonus of early infancy, a nonepilepsy).
Myoclonic epilepsy in infancy (benign Dravet variant).
Benign infantile epilepsy.
Benign familial infantile epilepsy.
Severe myoclonic epilepsy of infancy (classic Dravet syndrome).
Myoclonic encephalopathy in nonprogressive disorders.
Childhood
Genetic epilepsy with febrile seizures plus (GEFS+; can begin in infancy).
Panayiotopoulos syndrome.
Epilepsy with myoclonic atonic (previously astatic) seizures (Doose syndrome).
Benign epilepsy with centrotemporal spikes (BECTS, or benign rolandic epilepsy).
Autosomal-dominant nocturnal frontal lobe epilepsy (ADNFLE).
Late-onset childhood occipital epilepsy (Gastaut syndrome).
Epilepsy with myoclonic absences (Tassinari syndrome).
Lennox-Gastaut syndrome.

Epileptic encephalopathy with continuous spike-and-wave during sleep (CSWS).

Landau-Kleffner syndrome (LKS).

Childhood absence epilepsy (pyknolepsy).

Generalized epilepsy with eyelid myoclonia (Jeavons syndrome).*

Adolescence–Adult

Juvenile absence epilepsy (JAE).

Juvenile myoclonic epilepsy (JME).

Epilepsy with generalized tonic-clonic seizures alone.

Progressive myoclonus epilepsies (PME).

Autosomal-dominant epilepsy with auditory features.

Other familial temporal lobe epilepsies.

Less Specific Age Relationship

Familial focal epilepsy with variable foci (childhood to adult).

Reflex epilepsies (e.g., photosensitive, audiogenic, or reading-induced seizures; may or may not coexist with spontaneous seizures).

---

*Not listed as a syndrome by ILAE but instead recognized under absence seizures with special features.

EPISTAXIS

ICD-10CM #   R04.0   Epistaxis

Trauma.

Medications (nasal sprays, NSAIDs, anticoagulants, antiplatelets).

Nasal polyps.

Cocaine use.

Coagulopathy (hemophilia, liver disease, DIC, thrombocytopenia).

Systemic disorders (hypertension, uremia).

Infections.

Anatomic malformations.

Rhinitis.

Nasal polyps.

Local neoplasms (benign and malignant).

Desiccation.

Foreign body.

ERECTILE DYSFUNCTION, ORGANIC[67]

ICD-10CM #   N52.9   Male erectile dysfunction, unspecified

Neurogenic abnormalities: somatic nerve neuropathy, CNS abnormalities.

Psychogenic causes: depression, performance anxiety, marital conflict.

Endocrine causes: hyperprolactinemia, hypogonadotropic hypogonadism, testicular failure, estrogen excess.

Trauma: pelvic fracture, prostate surgery, penile fracture.

Systemic disease: DM, renal failure, hepatic cirrhosis.

Medications: diuretics, antidepressants, H_2 blockers, exogenous hormones, alcohol, antihypertensives, nicotine abuse, finasteride, etc.

Structural abnormalities: Peyronie disease.

EROSIONS, GENITALIA

ICD-10CM #   N36.8   Other specified disorders of urethra

Candidiasis.

Intraepithelial neoplasia.

Squamous cell carcinoma.

Lichen planus.

Pemphigus vulgaris.

Erythema multiforme.

Lichen sclerosus.

Bullous pemphigoid.

Extramammary Paget disease.

Impetigo.

ERYTHEMATOUS ANNULAR SKIN LESIONS

ICD-10CM #   L53.8   Other specified erythematous conditions

Tinea corporis.

Warfarin plaques.

Erythema multiforme.

Erythema annulare.

Cutaneous lupus.

Cutaneous sarcoidosis.

Trauma.

Acute febrile neutrophilic dermatosis (Sweet syndrome).

ERYTHROCYTOSIS[31]

ICD-10CM #   D75.0   Familial erythrocytosis

CAUSES OF ERYTHROCYTOSIS

Relative or Spurious Erythrocytosis (Normal Red Cell Mass)

Hemoconcentration secondary to dehydration (diarrhea, diaphoresis, diuretics, water deprivation, emesis, ethanol, hypertension, preeclampsia, pheochromocytoma, carbon monoxide intoxication).

True or Absolute Erythrocytosis

Polycythemia vera.

Primary congenital polycythemia.

Secondary erythrocytosis caused by:

Congenital causes (e.g., activating mutation of erythropoietin receptor).

Hypoxia caused by carbon monoxide poisoning, high oxygen affinity hemoglobin, high-altitude residence, chronic pulmonary disease, hypoventilation syndromes such as sleep apnea, right to left cardiac shunt, neurologic defects involving the respiratory center.

Nonhypoxic causes with pathologic erythropoietin production.

Renal disease (cysts, hydronephrosis, renal artery stenosis, focal glomerulonephritis, renal transplantation).

Tumors (renal cell cancer, hepatocellular carcinoma, cerebellar hemangioblastoma, uterine

fibromyoma, adrenal tumors, meningioma, pheochromocytoma).

Drug-associated causes:

Androgen therapy.

Exogenous erythropoietin growth factor therapy.

ERYTHRODERMA

ICD-10CM #   L53.9   Erythematous condition, unspecified

Drug reaction (e.g., allopurinol, ampicillin, phenytoin, vancomycin, dapsone, omeprazole, carbamazepine).

Atopic dermatitis.

Psoriasis.

Contact dermatitis.

Idiopathic.

Pityriasis rubra.

Chronic actinic dermatitis.

Bullous pemphigoid.

Paraneoplastic.

Cutaneous T-cell lymphoma.

Connective tissue disease.

Hypereosinophilia syndrome.

ESOPHAGEAL PERFORATION[1]

ICD-10CM #   K22.3   Perforation of esophagus
             S27.819A Unspecified injury of esophagus (thoracic part), initial encounter

Trauma.

Caustic burns.

Iatrogenic.

Foreign bodies.

Spontaneous rupture (Boerhaave syndrome).

Postoperative breakdown of anastomosis.

ESOPHAGEAL STRICTURES[78]

ICD-10CM #   Varies with specific diagnosis

BENIGN

Congenital

Esophageal atresia.

Tracheoesophageal fistula.

Web.

ACQUIRED

Peptic:

Gastroesophageal reflux.

Scleroderma.

Schatzki ring.

Caustic ingestion.

Drug-induced:

Anticholinergic medications.

Aspirin.

Ferrous sulfate.

Fosamax.

Nonsteroidal antiinflammatory.

Quinidine.

Potassium supplements.
Tetracycline.
Vitamin C.
Eosinophilic esophagitis.
Iatrogenic:
  Variceal ligation/injection.
  Endoscopic mucosal resection.
  Ablation therapy (cryotherapy/radiofrequency).
  Postoperative (anastomotic).
  Radiation.
  Instrumentation.
  Nasogastric tube.
Infections:
  Fungal: moniliasis.
  Bacterial: syphilis.
  Mycobacterial: tuberculosis.
Granulomatous:
  Crohn disease.
Dermatosis:
  Epidermolysis bullosa dystrophica.
  Pemphigoid.
  Behçet syndrome.

MALIGNANT

Primary.
Secondary.

ESOPHAGEAL TUMORS, BENIGN[78]

ICD-10CM # Varies with specific diagnosis

CLASSIFICATION OF BENIGN ESOPHAGEAL TUMORS

Mucosa (First and Second Esophageal Ultrasound [EUS] Layers)
Squamous papilloma.
Fibrovascular polyp.
Retention cyst.
Submucosa (Third EUS Layer)
Lipoma.
Fibroma.
Neurofibroma.
Granular cell tumor.
Hemangiomas.
Salivary gland–type tumor.
Muscularis Propria (Fourth EUS Layer)
Leiomyoma.
Duplication cyst.
Periesophageal Tissue (Fifth EUS Layer)
Foregut cyst.

ESOPHAGITIS[1]

ICD-10CM # K20.9 Esophagitis, unspecified

INFECTIOUS

Candidiasis.
Cytomegalovirus.
Herpes simplex virus.
HIV infection, acute.

NONINFECTIOUS

Gastroesophageal reflux.
Mucositis from cancer chemotherapy.
Mucositis from radiation therapy.
Aphthous ulcers.

ESOPHAGUS, SYSTEMIC DISEASES[78]

ICD-10CM # Varies with specific diagnosis

SYSTEMIC DISEASES OF THE ESOPHAGUS

Connective Tissue Disorders
Scleroderma.
Systemic lupus erythematosus.
Polymyositis.
Dermatomyositis.
Mixed connective tissue disorder.
Raynaud phenomenon.
Allergic Disease
Eosinophilic esophagitis.
Metabolic Diseases
Amyloidosis.
Diabetes mellitus.
Hypothyroidism.
Hyperthyroidism.
Dermatologic Diseases
Epidermolysis bullosa.
Pemphigus vulgaris.
Pemphigoid.
Erythema multiforme.
Lichen planus.
Behçet disease.
Infectious Diseases
Histoplasmosis.
Tuberculosis.
Actinomycosis.
Immunocompromised host:
  Fungal: *Candida* spp.
  Viral: herpes simplex, cytomegalovirus.
  Mycobacterial.
  Bacterial: *Streptococcus viridans, Staphylococcus,* bacilli, *Treponema pallidum.*
  Protozoal.
Miscellaneous Disorders
Sarcoidosis.
Crohn disease.

ESOTROPIA

ICD-10CM # H50.00 Unspecified esotropia
           H50.43 Accommodative component in esotropia
           H50.05 Alternating esotropia

Congenital.
Accommodative esotropia.
Myasthenia gravis.
Abducens palsy.
Pseudo-sixth nerve palsy.
Medial rectus entrapment (e.g., blowout fracture).
Posterior internuclear ophthalmoplegia.
Wernicke encephalopathy.
Thyroid myopathy.
Chiari malformation.

EXANTHEMS[25]

ICD-10CM # R21 Rash and other nonspecific skin eruption

Measles.
Rubella.
Erythema infectiosum (fifth disease).
Roseola exanthema.
Varicella.
Enterovirus.
Adenovirus.
Epstein-Barr virus.
Kawasaki disease.
Staphylococcal scalded skin.
Scarlet fever.
Meningococcemia.
Rocky Mountain spotted fever.

EYELID NEOPLASM

ICD-10CM # C44.101 Unspecified malignant neoplasm of skin of unspecified eyelid, including canthus

MALIGNANT

Melanoma.
Basal cell carcinoma.
Squamous cell carcinoma.
Bowen disease.
Sebaceous cell carcinoma.
Metastatic lymphoma/leukemia.

BENIGN

Melanocytic nevus.
Pilar, eccrine, or apocrine tumor.
Neurofibroma.
Keratosis.
Squamous papilloma.
Keratoacanthoma.

EYELID RETRACTION

ICD-10CM # H02.89 Other specified disorders of eyelid

Congenital.
Graves ophthalmopathy.
Myasthenia gravis.
Postsurgical.
Guillain-Barré syndrome.
Cerebellar disease.
Horizontal gaze palsy.
Partial palsy of superior rectus muscle.
Encephalitis.
Closed head injury.
Disseminated sclerosis.
Eye trauma.
Contact lens wear.
Proptosis.
Eyelid neoplasm.
Atopic dermatitis.
Herpes zoster ophthalmicus.
Botulinum toxin injection.
Cyclic oculomotor paralysis.

Differential Diagnosis

II

Spheroid wing meningioma.
Hepatic cirrhosis.
Down syndrome.
Essential hypertension.
Meningitis.
Paget disease of bone.

EYE PAIN

ICD-10CM # H57.13 Ocular pain, bilateral

Foreign body.
Herpes zoster.
Trauma.
Conjunctivitis.
Iritis.
Iridocyclitis.
Uveitis.
Blepharitis.
Ingrown lashes.
Orbital or periorbital cellulitis/abscess.
Sinusitis.
Headache.
Glaucoma.
Inflammation of lacrimal gland.
Tic douloureux.
Cerebral aneurysm.
Cerebral neoplasm.
Entropion.
Retrobulbar neuritis.
UV light.
Dry eyes.
Irritation or inflammation from eye drops, dust, cosmetics, etc.

FACIAL PAIN

ICD-10CM # G50.1 Atypical facial pain

Infection, abscess.
Postherpetic neuralgia.
Trauma, posttraumatic neuralgia.
Tic douloureux.
Cluster headache, "lower-half headache."
Geniculate neuralgia.
Anxiety, somatization syndrome.
Glossopharyngeal neuralgia.
Carotidynia.

FACIAL PARALYSIS[25]

ICD-10CM # G51.0 Bell palsy

INFECTION

Bacterial: otitis media, mastoiditis, meningitis, Lyme disease.
Viral: herpes zoster, mononucleosis, varicella, rubella, mumps, Bell palsy.
Mycobacterial: TB, meningitis, leprosy.
Miscellaneous: syphilis, malaria.

TRAUMA

Temporal bone fracture, facial laceration.
Surgery.

NEOPLASM

Malignant: squamous cell carcinoma, basal cell and adenocystic tumors, leukemia, parotid neoplasms, metastatic tumors.
Benign: facial nerve neuroma, vestibular schwannoma, congenital cholesteatoma.

IMMUNOLOGIC

Guillain-Barré syndrome, periarteritis nodosa.
Reaction to tetanus antiserum.

METABOLIC

Pregnancy.
Hypothyroidism.
DM.

FACIAL WEAKNESS, CONGENITAL[20]

ICD-10CM # Varies with specific diagnosis

CAUSES

Aplasia of facial muscles.
Birth injury.
Congenital myotonic dystrophy.
Congenital bilateral perisylvian syndrome.
Fiber-type disproportion myopathies.
    Myasthenic syndromes.*
    Congenital myasthenia.
    Familial infantile myasthenia.
    Transitory neonatal myasthenia.

*Denotes the most common conditions and the ones with disease-modifying treatments.

FACIAL WEAKNESS, POSTNATAL[20]

ICD-10CM # Varies with specific diagnosis

CAUSES

Autoimmune and postinfectious.
    Bell palsy.[a]
    Idiopathic cranial polyneuropathy.
    Miller Fisher syndrome.[a]
    Myasthenia gravis.[a]
Genetic.
    Juvenile progressive bulbar palsy (Fazio-Londe disease).
    Muscular disorders.
    Facioscapulohumeral syndrome.
    Facioscapulohumeral syndrome, infantile form.
    Fiber-type disproportion myopathies.
    Melkersson syndrome.
    Myotonic dystrophy.
    Oculopharyngeal dystrophy.
    Myasthenic syndromes.[a]
    Congenital myasthenia.[a]
    Familial infantile myasthenia.[a]

[a]Denotes the most common conditions and the ones with disease-modifying treatments.

Osteopetrosis (Albers-Schönberg disease).
Recurrent facial palsy.
Hypertension.
Infectious.
    Diphtheria.
    Herpes zoster oticus.[a]
    Infectious mononucleosis.
    Lyme disease.[a]
    Otitis media.[a]
    Sarcoidosis.[a]
    Tuberculosis.[a]
Metabolic disorders.
    Hyperparathyroidism.[a]
    Hypothyroidism.[a]
Multiple sclerosis.
Syringobulbia.[a]
Toxins.
Trauma.
    Delayed.
    Immediate.
Tumor.
    Glioma of brain stem.
    Histiocytosis X.
    Leukemia.
    Meningeal carcinoma.
    Neurofibromatosis.

FAILURE TO THRIVE

ICD-10CM # R62.50 Unspecified lack of expected normal physiological development in childhood

PSYCHOSOCIAL/BEHAVIORAL

Inadequate diet because of poverty/food insufficiency, errors in food preparation.
Poor parenting skills (lack of knowledge of sufficient diet).
Child/parent interaction problems (autonomy struggles, coercive feeding, maternal depression).
Food refusal.
Rumination.
Parental cognitive or mental health problems.
Child abuse or neglect; emotional deprivation.

NEUROLOGIC

Cerebral palsy.
Hypothalamic and other CNS tumors (diencephalic syndrome).
Neuromuscular disorders.
Neurodegenerative disorders.

RENAL

Recurrent urinary tract infection.
Renal tubular acidosis.
Renal failure.

ENDOCRINE

Diabetes mellitus.
Diabetes insipidus.
Hypothyroidism/hyperthyroidism.
Growth hormone deficiency.
Adrenal insufficiency.

GENETIC/METABOLIC/CONGENITAL

Sickle cell disease.
Inborn errors of metabolism (organic acidosis, hyperammonemia, storage disease).
Fetal alcohol syndrome.
Skeletal dysplasias.
Chromosomal disorders.
Multiple congenital anomaly syndromes (VATER [vertebral defects, imperforate anus, tracheoesophageal fistula, radial and renal dysplasia], CHARGE [coloboma, heart disease, atresia choanae, retarded growth and retarded development and/or CNS anomalies, genital hypoplasia, ear anomalies and/or deafness]).

GASTROINTESTINAL

Pyloric stenosis.
Gastroesophageal reflux.
Repair of tracheoesophageal fistula.
Malrotation.
Malabsorption syndromes.
Celiac disease.
Milk intolerance: lactose, protein.
Pancreatic insufficiency syndromes (cystic fibrosis).
Chronic cholestasis.
Inflammatory bowel disease.
Chronic congenital diarrhea states.
Short bowel syndrome.
Pseudoobstruction.
Hirschsprung disease.
Food allergy.

CARDIAC

Cyanotic heart lesions.
Congestive heart failure.
Vascular rings.

PULMONARY/RESPIRATORY

Severe asthma.
Cystic fibrosis; bronchiectasis.
Chronic respiratory failure.
Bronchopulmonary dysplasia.
Adenoid/tonsillar hypertrophy.
Obstructive sleep apnea.

MISCELLANEOUS

Collagen vascular disease.
Malignancy.
Primary immunodeficiency.
Transplantation.

INFECTIONS

Perinatal infection (TORCHES [toxoplasma, other, rubella, cytomegalovirus, herpes simplex]).
Occult/chronic infections.
Parasitic infestation.
Tuberculosis.
HIV.

FATIGUE

| ICD-10CM # | R53.83 | Other fatigue |
| | F48.0 | Neurasthenia |

Depression.
Anxiety, emotional stress.
Inadequate sleep.
Chronic fatigue syndrome.
Prolonged physical activity.
Pregnancy and postpartum period.
Anemia.
Hypothyroidism.
Medications (β-blockers, anxiolytics, antidepressants, sedating antihistamines, clonidine, methyldopa).
Viral or bacterial infections.
Sleep apnea syndrome.
Dieting.
Renal failure, CHF, COPD, liver disease.

FATIGUE, CHRONIC

| ICD-10CM # | R53.83 | Other fatigue |
| | F48.0 | Neurasthenia |

CHRONIC INFECTIONS

Hepatitis C.
Lyme disease.
Parasitic and fungal infections.
Tuberculosis.
Human immunodeficiency virus.
Xenotropic murine leukemia retrovirus.

SLEEP DISORDERS

Obstructive sleep apnea.
Restless leg syndrome.
Circadian rhythm disorder.
Upper airway resistance syndrome.
Narcolepsy/parasomnias.
Alpha-delta sleep disorder.

ENDOCRINE/METABOLIC DISORDERS

Addison disease.
Cushing syndrome.
Poorly controlled diabetes.
Thyroid disorders.
Hemochromatosis.
Hypopituitarism.
Diabetes insipidus.

GENERAL MEDICAL DISORDERS

Anemia (any cause).
Chronic renal/hepatic failure.
Malnutrition.
Medication side effects.
Chronic pain disorders.

PSYCHOLOGICAL

Mood disorders (depression, anxiety, bipolar).
Schizophrenia.
Posttraumatic stress disorder.
Anorexia nervosa/bulimia.
Childhood abuse and/or neglect.

CHRONIC INFLAMMATION

Rheumatoid arthritis.
Systemic lupus erythematosus.
Sjögren syndrome.
Polymyositis/dermatomyositis.
Vasculitis.
Sarcoidosis.

CARDIOPULMONARY

Congestive heart failure.
Neurally mediated hypotension.
Postural orthostatic tachycardia syndrome.
Pulmonary hypertension.
Chronic obstructive pulmonary disease.
Mitral valve prolapse.

GASTROINTESTINAL

Celiac disease.
Inflammatory bowel disease.
Autoimmune hepatitis.
Hepatic cirrhosis.

MALIGNANCY

Lymphoma and occult malignancies.
Postchemotherapy syndrome.

NEUROLOGIC DISORDERS

Multiple sclerosis.
Myasthenia gravis.
Muscular dystrophies.
Parkinson disease.
Early dementia.

LIFESTYLE FACTORS

Chronic overwork.
Persistent unresolved stress.
Inadequate exercise.
Morbid obesity (body mass index >40).
Alcoholism/drug abuse.

FATTY LIVER

| ICD-10CM # | K76.0 | Fatty (change of) liver, not elsewhere classified |
| | K76.89 | Other specified diseases of liver |

Obesity.
Alcohol abuse.
DM.
Acute fatty liver of pregnancy.
Medications (tetracycline, valproic acid, glucocorticoids, amiodarone, estrogen, methotrexate).
Reye syndrome.
Wilson disease.
Nonalcoholic steatosis.

FEVER, ABDOMINAL PAIN, JAUNDICE IN PEDIATRIC PATIENT[5]

| ICD-10CM # | R50.9 | Fever, unspecified |

Cholangitis.
Cholecystitis.

Cholelithiasis.
Sepsis.
Hepatitis.
Choledochal cyst.
Pancreatitis.
Urinary tract infection.
Leptospirosis and other systemic infections with hepatic involvement.
Spontaneous perforation of common bile duct.
Biliary cyst.
Appendicitis.

FEVER AND CARDIOPULMONARY FAILURE[79]

ICD-10CM # R50.9 Fever, unspecified

DIFFERENTIAL DIAGNOSIS OF FEVER AND RAPIDLY PROGRESSIVE CARDIOPULMONARY FAILURE

Bacterial Infection
Severe community-acquired pneumonia.
Meningitis, endocarditis.
Rickettsial disease (babesiosis, ehrlichiosis, Rocky Mountain spotted fever, scrub typhus, Mediterranean spotted fever).
Q-Fever (*Coxiella burnetii*).
Brucellosis.
Plague (*Yersinia pestis*).
Tularemia (*Francisella tularensis*).
Typhoid fever/salmonellosis.
Leptospirosis (*Leptospira interrogans*).
Anthrax.
Mycobacterial infections.

Viral Infections
Viral pneumonia (influenza, CMV, EBV, VZV, SARS).
Hantavirus.
Dengue fever and yellow fever.
Hemorrhagic fever (Lassa, Marburg, or Ebola viruses).

Fungal Infections
Coccidiomycosis.
Cryptococcus.
Histoplasmosis.
Blastomycosis.

Parasitic Infections
Malaria.
Leishmaniasis.
Schistosomiasis.
Strongyloides.

Noninfectious Causes
Inflammatory:
Rapid-onset interstitial pneumonia (acute interstitial pneumonia, acute hypersensitivity pneumonitis).
Acute eosinophilic pneumonia.
ARDS due to other causes (inhalation injury, drug overdose, trauma).
Rheumatologic disorders:

Wegener granulomatosis, Churg-Strauss disease, Goodpasture syndrome.
Systemic lupus erythematosus, antiphospholipid syndrome.
Other:
Malignancy, lymphoma, lymphoproliferative disease, leukemia.
Pulmonary embolism, aortic dissection, acute myocardial infarction.
Adrenal insufficiency, thyroid storm.

ARDS, Acute respiratory distress syndrome; *CMV*, cytomegalovirus; *EBV*, Epstein-Barr virus; *SARS*, severe acute respiratory syndrome; *VZV*, varicella zoster virus.

FEVER AND JAUNDICE

ICD-10CM # R50.9 Fever, unspecified
R17 Unspecified jaundice

Bacterial sepsis.
Cholangitis.
Hepatic abscess.
Leptospirosis.
Malaria.
Viral hepatitis.
Yellow fever.

FEVER AND LYMPHADENOPATHY

ICD-10CM # R59.9 Enlarged lymph nodes, unspecified
R50.9 Fever, unspecified

REGIONAL
Cervical
Streptococci.
Tuberculosis.
Viral upper respiratory infection.
Peripheral
Bartonella henselae.
Herpesviruses.
Lymphoma.
Metastatic cancer.
Sporotrichosis.
Streptococci.
Inguinal
Chancroid.
Herpes.
Lymphogranuloma venereum.
Syphilis (primary).

GENERALIZED
Cytomegalovirus.
Epstein-Barr virus.
HIV.
Lymphoma.
Sarcoidosis.
Syphilis (secondary).
Toxoplasmosis.
Viral hepatitis.

FEVER AND RASH

ICD-10CM # R21 Rash and other nonspecific skin eruption
R21 Rash and other nonspecific skin eruption
R50.9 Fever, unspecified

Drug hypersensitivity: penicillin, sulfonamides, thiazides, anticonvulsants, allopurinol.
Viral infection: measles, rubella, varicella, erythema infectiosum, roseola, enterovirus infection, viral hepatitis, infectious mononucleosis, acute HIV.
Other infections: meningococcemia, staphylococcemia, scarlet fever, typhoid fever, *Pseudomonas* bacteremia, Rocky Mountain spotted fever, Lyme disease, secondary syphilis, bacterial endocarditis, babesiosis, brucellosis, listeriosis.
Serum sickness.
Erythema multiforme.
Erythema marginatum.
Erythema nodosum.
SLE.
Dermatomyositis.
Allergic vasculitis.
Pityriasis rosea.
Herpes zoster.

FEVER AND RASH IN ICU[2]

ICD-10CM # R21 Rash and other nonspecific skin eruption
R50.9 Fever, unspecified

DIFFERENTIAL DIAGNOSTIC CLINICAL FEATURES OF FEVER AND RASH IN THE ICU
Rash with Shock
Infectious causes: toxic shock syndrome, meningococcemia, postsplenectomy sepsis, overwhelming *Staphylococcus aureus* bacteremia/acute bacterial endocarditis, arboviral hemorrhagic fevers, hemorrhagic smallpox, *Vibrio vulnificus*, gas gangrene, dengue fever.
Noninfectious cause: systemic lupus erythematosus (on steroids).

RASH WITH MENTAL CHANGES
Infectious causes: Rocky Mountain spotted fever, meningococcemia (with meningitis), *S. aureus* acute bacterial endocarditis, Chikungunya fever, typhus.
Noninfectious cause: systemic lupus erythematosus.

RASH WITH CONJUNCTIVAL SUFFUSION
Infectious causes: Rocky Mountain spotted fever, dengue fever, arboviral hemorrhagic fevers, toxic shock syndrome.

Noninfectious cause: adult Kawasaki disease.

RASH WITH RELATIVE BRADYCARDIA

Infectious causes: Rocky Mountain spotted fever, typhus, dengue fever, typhoid, arboviral hemorrhagic fevers.
Noninfectious cause: drug rash.

RASH WITH ABDOMINAL PAIN

Infectious causes: V. vulnificus, gas gangrene, Clostridium sordelli, scarlet fever.
Noninfectious causes: cholesterol emboli syndrome, systemic lupus erythematosus.

RASH ON PALMS AND SOLES

Infectious causes: Rocky Mountain spotted fever, toxic shock syndrome, chickenpox, smallpox, monkeypox, scarlet fever.
Noninfectious cause: drug rash.

RASH WITH DIARRHEA

Infectious causes: V. vulnificus, gas gangrene, toxic shock syndrome, dengue fever, arboviral hemorrhagic fevers.
Noninfectious cause: none.

RASH WITH EDEMA OF DORSUM OF HANDS/FEET

Infectious causes: Rocky Mountain spotted fever, toxic shock syndrome.
Noninfectious cause: adult Kawasaki disease.

RASH WITH BULLAE

Infectious causes: V. vulnificus, S. aureus complicated skin/skin structure infection, gas gangrene.
Noninfectious cause: none.

RASH WITH HEART MURMUR

Infectious cause: acute bacterial endocarditis.
Noninfectious cause: systemic lupus erythematosus.
Rash with gangrene of nose tip
Infectious cause: S. aureus acute bacterial endocarditis.
Noninfectious causes: systemic lupus erythematosus, vasculitis.

RASH WITH CEREBROVASCULAR ACCIDENT

Infectious causes: cholesterol emboli syndrome, S. aureus acute bacterial endocarditis.
Noninfectious cause: none.

RASH WITH SPLENOMEGALY

Infectious causes: Rocky Mountain spotted fever, typhus.
Noninfectious causes: systemic lupus erythematosus, adult Kawasaki disease.

RASH WITH DEAFNESS

Infectious causes: Rocky Mountain spotted fever, typhus, meningococcal meningitis.
Noninfectious cause: none.

RASH WITH HEPATOSPLENOMEGALY

Infectious causes: Rocky Mountain spotted fever, typhus.
Noninfectious cause: atypical measles.

RASH WITH HEPATOMEGALY

Infectious cause: typhus.
Noninfectious cause: none.

FEVER, AFTER TRAVEL TO THE TROPICS[18]

ICD-10CM # R50.81 Fever presenting with conditions classified elsewhere

CAUSES OF FEVER AFTER TRAVEL TO THE TROPICS

80% of Specific Infections Causing Fever (Includes Respiratory and Urinary Tract Infection)
Malaria.
Viral hepatitis.
Febrile illness unrelated to foreign travel.
Dengue fever.
Enteric fever (typhoid and paratyphoid fevers).
Other Causes
Gastroenteritis.
Rickettsia.
Leptospirosis.
Schistosomiasis.
Amebic liver abscess.
Tuberculosis.
Acute HIV infection.
Others.

FEVER, COMMON INFECTIOUS CAUSES[7]

ICD-10CM # R50.9 Fever, unspecified

CENTRAL NERVOUS SYSTEM

Meningitis:
Encephalitis.
Brain abscess.
Epidural abscess.

HEAD AND NECK

Acute suppurative parotitis:
Acute sinusitis.
Parapharyngeal and retropharyngeal space infections.
Acute suppurative otitis media.

CARDIOVASCULAR

Catheter-related infection:
Endocarditis.

PULMONARY AND MEDIASTINAL

Pneumonia:
Empyema.
Mediastinitis.

HEPATOBILIARY AND GASTROINTESTINAL

Diverticulitis:
Appendicitis.
Peritonitis (spontaneous or secondary).
Intraperitoneal abscess.
Perirectal abscess.
Infected pancreatitis.
Acute cholecystitis.
Cholangitis.
Hepatic abscess.
Acute viral hepatitis.

GENITOURINARY

Bacterial or fungal cystitis:
Pyelonephritis.
Perinephric abscess.
Tuboovarian abscess.
Endometritis.
Prostatitis.

BREAST

Mastitis:
Breast abscess.

CUTANEOUS AND MUSCULAR

Cellulitis:
Suppurative wound infection.
Necrotizing fasciitis.
Bacterial myositis or myonecrosis.
Herpes zoster.

OSSEOUS

Osteomyelitis.

FEVER, DRUG-INDUCED[59]

ICD-10CM # R50.2 Drug induced fever

SELECTED AGENTS ASSOCIATED WITH DRUG-INDUCED FEVER

Common
Antimicrobial:
Amphotericin B.
β-Lactams.
Sulfonamides.
Cardiovascular:
Procainamide.
Quinidine.
CNS:
Carbamazepine.
Phenytoin.
Miscellaneous:
Bleomycin.
Interferon-α.
Interleukin-2.
Less Common
Antimicrobial:
Clindamycin.
Fluoroquinolones.
Rifampin.
Cardiovascular:
Diltiazem.
Hydralazine.

1216 of 1712

CNS:
Haloperidol.
Serotonin reuptake inhibitors.
Miscellaneous:
Allopurinol.
Cimetidine.
Tacrolimus.

FEVER, HOSPITAL ASSOCIATED[59]

ICD-10CM # R50.2 Drug induced fever
R50.9 Fever, unspecified

SELECTED CAUSES OF HOSPITAL-ASSOCIATED FEVER

Common
Infectious:
Clostridium difficile enterocolitis.
Pneumonia.
Surgical wound.
Urinary tract.
Vascular catheter.
Noninfectious:
Drug-induced fever.
Hematoma.
Immediate postoperative state.
Transfusion reaction.
Venous thromboembolism.

Less Common
Infectious:
Biliary tract disease.
Endometritis.
Intraabdominal abscess.
Mediastinitis.
Sinusitis.
Noninfectious:
Adrenal insufficiency.
Gout.
Myocardial infarction.
Organ infarction.
Pancreatitis.

FEVER IN RETURNING TRAVELERS AND IMMIGRANTS[25]

ICD-10CM # R50.81 Fever presenting with conditions classified elsewhere

COMMON*
Acute respiratory tract infection (worldwide).*
Gastroenteritis (worldwide) [foodborne, waterborne, fecal-oral].
Enteric fever, including typhoid (worldwide) [food, water].

Urinary tract infection (worldwide) [sexual contact].
Drug reactions [antibiotics, prophylactic agents, other] {rash frequent}.
Malaria (tropics, limited areas of temperate zones) [mosquitoes].
Arboviruses (Africa; tropics) [mosquitoes, ticks, mites].
Dengue (Asia, Caribbean, Africa) [mosquitoes].
Viral hepatitis (worldwide).
Hepatitis A (worldwide) [food, fecal-oral].
Hepatitis B (worldwide, especially Asia, sub-Saharan Africa) [sexual contact] {long incubation period}.
Hepatitis C (worldwide) [blood or sexual contact].
Hepatitis E (Asia, North Africa, Mexico, others) [food, water].
Tuberculosis (worldwide) [airborne, milk] {long period to symptomatic infection}.
Sexually transmitted diseases (worldwide) [sexual contact].

LESS COMMON*
Filariasis (Asia, Africa, South America) [biting insects] {long incubation period, eosinophilia}.*
Measles (developing world) [airborne] {in susceptible individual}.
Amebic abscess (worldwide) [food].
Brucellosis (worldwide) [milk, cheese, food, animal contact].
Listeriosis (worldwide) [foodborne] {meningitis}.
Leptospirosis (worldwide) [animal contact, open fresh water] {jaundice, meningitis}.
Strongyloidiasis (warm and tropical areas) [soil contact] {eosinophilia}.
Toxoplasmosis (worldwide) [undercooked meat].

RARE
Relapsing fever (western Americas, Asia, northern Africa) [ticks, lice].
Hemorrhagic fevers (worldwide) [arthropod and nonarthropod transmitted].
Yellow fever (tropics) [mosquitoes] {hepatitis}.
Hemorrhagic fever with renal syndrome (Europe, Asia, North America) [rodent urine] {renal impairment}.
Hantavirus pulmonary syndrome (western North America, other) [rodent urine] {respiratory distress syndrome}.
Lassa fever (Africa) [rodent excreta, person to person] {high mortality rate}.
Other: chikungunya, Rift Valley, Ebola-Marburg, etc. (various) [insect bites, rodent excreta, aerosols, person to person] {often severe}.

Rickettsial infections {rashes and eschars}.
Leishmaniasis, visceral (Middle East, Mediterranean, Africa, Asia, South America) [biting flies] {long incubation period}.
Acute schistosomiasis (Africa, Asia, South America, Caribbean) [fresh water].
Chagas disease (South and Central America) [reduviid bug bites] {often asymptomatic}.
African trypanosomiasis (Africa) [tsetse fly bite] {neurologic syndromes, sleeping sickness}.
Bartonellosis (South America) [sandfly bite] {skin nodules}.
HIV infection/AIDS (worldwide) [sexual and blood contact].
Trichinosis (worldwide) [undercooked meat] {eosinophilia}.
Plague (temperate and tropical plains) [animal exposures and fleas].
Tularemia (worldwide) [animal contact, fleas, aerosols] {ulcers, lymph nodes}.
Anthrax (worldwide) [animal, animal product contact] {ulcers}.
Lyme disease (North America, Europe) [tick bites] {arthritis, meningitis, cardiac abnormalities}.

FEVER, NONINFECTIOUS CAUSES[43]

ICD-10CM # R50.9 Fever, unspecified

DIFFERENTIAL DIAGNOSIS—NONINFECTIOUS CAUSES OF FEVER

Critical Diagnoses
Acute myocardial infarction.
Pulmonary embolism/infarction.
Intracranial hemorrhage.
Cerebrovascular accident.
Neuroleptic-malignant syndrome.
Thyroid storm.
Acute adrenal insufficiency.
Transfusion reaction.
Pulmonary edema.

Emergent Diagnoses
Congestive heart failure.
Dehydration.
Recent seizure.
Sickle cell disease.
Transplant rejection.
Pancreatitis.
Deep vein thrombosis.

Nonemergent Diagnoses
Drug fever.
Malignancy.
Gout.
Sarcoidosis.
Crohn disease.
Postmyocardiotomy syndrome.

FEVER OF UNKNOWN ORIGIN, PEDIATRIC PATIENT[5]

ICD-10CM # R50.9 Fever, unspecified

---

*A vegetative state may not necessarily begin with coma but can also develop as the end stage of neurodegenerative diseases (e.g., Alzheimer disease) of adults or children and can accompany severe congenital developmental abnormalities of the brain such as anencephaly.

*Diagnoses for which particular symptoms are indicative are in *italics*. Exposure to regions of the world that are most likely to be significant to the diagnosis are presented in (parentheses). Vectors, risk behaviors, and sources associated with acquisition are presented in [brackets]. Special clinical characteristics are listed within {braces}.

INFECTIOUS DISEASES

Bacterial
Bacterial endocarditis.
Brucellosis.
Cat-scratch disease.
Leptospirosis.
Liver abscess.
Mastoiditis (chronic).
Osteomyelitis.
Pelvic abscess.
Perinephric abscess.
Pyelonephritis.
Salmonellosis.
Sinusitis.
Subdiaphragmatic abscess.
Tuberculosis.
Tularemia.
Viral
Adenovirus.
Arboviruses.
Cytomegalovirus.
Epstein-Barr virus (infectious mononucleosis).
Hepatitis viruses.
Chlamydial
Lymphogranuloma venereum.
Psittacosis.
Rickettsial
Q fever.
Rocky Mountain spotted fever.
Fungal
Blastomycosis (nonpulmonary).
Histoplasmosis (disseminated).
Parasitic
Malaria.
Toxoplasmosis.
Visceral larva migrans.
Unclassified
Sarcoidosis.
Collagen Vascular Diseases
Juvenile rheumatoid arthritis.
Polyarteritis nodosa.
Systemic lupus erythematosus.
Malignancies
Hodgkin disease.
Leukemia and lymphoma.
Neuroblastoma.
Miscellaneous
Central diabetes insipidus.
Drug fever.
Ectodermal dysplasia.
Factitious fever.
Familial dysautonomia.
Granulomatous colitis.
Hemophagocytic lymphohistiocytosis.
Infantile cortical hyperostosis.
Kikuchi-Fujimoto disease.
Nephrogenic diabetes insipidus.
Pancreatitis.
Periodic fever.
Serum sickness.
Thyrotoxicosis.
Ulcerative colitis.

FEVER, PEDIATRIC, ACUTE[29]

ICD-10CM # R50.9 Fever, unspecified

COMMON VIRAL INFECTIONS

Central Nervous System
Meningitis.
Encephalitis.
Tumor.
Brain abscess.
Head, Ears, Eyes, Nose, and Throat
Otitis media.
Pharyngitis.
Retropharyngeal abscess.
Peritonsillar abscess.
Lateral pharyngeal wall abscess.
Stomatitis.
Influenza.
Sinusitis.
Parotitis.
Cervical adenitis.
Periorbital cellulitis.
Orbital cellulitis or abscess.
Respiratory System
Bronchiolitis.
Croup.
Epiglottitis.
Pneumonia.
Upper respiratory infection.
Cardiovascular System
Myocarditis.
Pericarditis.
Endocarditis.
Genitourinary System
Urinary tract infection.
Tuboovarian abscess.
Gastrointestinal Tract
Acute viral gastroenteritis.
Bacterial enteritis.
Appendicitis.
Focal Soft Tissue Infections
Cellulitis.
Musculoskeletal System
Osteomyelitis.
Septic arthritis.
Rheumatologic Disorders
Acute rheumatic fever.
Juvenile rheumatoid arthritis.
Henoch-Schönlein purpura.
Vasculitis
Behçet syndrome.
Malignancy
Leukemia.
Lymphoma.
Sarcoma.
Systemic Illness
Bacteremia.
Viremia.
Sepsis.
Kawasaki disease.
Toxic shock syndrome.
Rocky Mountain spotted fever.
Meningococcemia.

MISCELLANEOUS DISORDERS

Toxicologic
Anticholinergic toxidromes.
Salicylate overdose.
Amphetamine.
Cocaine.
Endocrine
Thyrotoxicosis.

FEVER, PERIODIC[53]

ICD-10CM # R50.9 Fever, unspecified

DIFFERENTIAL DIAGNOSIS OF PERIODIC FEVER

Hereditary.
Nonhereditary.
   Infectious.
      Hidden infectious focus (e.g., aortoenteric fistula, Caroli disease).
      Recurrent reinfection (e.g., chronic meningococcemia, host defense defect).
      Specific infection (e.g., Whipple disease, malaria).
   Noninfectious inflammatory disorder, e.g.:
      Adult-onset Still disease.
      Juvenile chronic rheumatoid arthritis.
      Periodic fever, aphthous stomatitis, pharyngitis, and adenitis.
      Schnitzler syndrome.
      Behçet disease.
      Crohn disease.
      Sarcoidosis.
      Extrinsic alveolitis.
      Humidifier lung, polymer fume fever.
   Neoplastic
Lymphoma (e.g., Hodgkin disease, angioimmunoblastic lymphoma).
   Solid tumor (e.g., pheochromocytoma, myxoma, colon carcinoma).
Vascular (e.g., recurrent pulmonary embolism).
Hypothalamic.
Psychogenic periodic fever.
Factitious or fraudulent.

FEVER, POSTOPERATIVE[4]

ICD-10CM # R50.9 Fever, unspecified

Infectious
Abscess.
Acalculous cholecystitis.
Bacteremia.
Decubitus ulcers.
Device-related infections.
Empyema.
Endocarditis.
Fungal sepsis.
Hepatitis.
Meningitis.
Osteomyelitis.
Pseudomembranous colitis.

Differential Diagnosis

II

Parotitis.
Perineal infections.
Peritonitis.
Pharyngitis.
Pneumonia.
Retained foreign body.
Sinusitis.
Soft tissue infection.
Tracheobronchitis.
Urinary tract infection.
Noninfectious
Acute hepatic necrosis.
Adrenal insufficiency.
Allergic reaction.
Atelectasis.
Dehydration.
Drug reaction.
Head injury.
Hepatoma.
Hyperthyroidism.
Lymphoma.
Myocardial infarction.
Pancreatitis.
Pheochromocytoma.
Pulmonary embolus.
Retroperitoneal hematoma.
Solid organ hematoma.
Subarachnoid hemorrhage.
Systemic inflammatory response syndrome.
Thrombophlebitis.
Transfusion reaction.
Withdrawal syndromes.
Wound infection.

FEVER, POSTPARTUM[29]

ICD-10CM # R50.9 Fever, unspecified

MOST COMMON
Metritis.
Urinary tract infection.
Pneumonia.
Wound infection.
Mastitis.
Superficial or deep vein thrombosis.

MOST THREATENING
Toxic shock syndrome.
Necrotizing fasciitis.
Pelvic phlegmon.
Pelvic abscess.
Peritonitis.
Septic pelvic thrombosis.
Breast abscess.

FEVER, RECURRENT OR PERIODIC, IN CHILDREN[19]

ICD-10CM # R50.2 Drug induced fever
R50.9 Fever, unspecified

INFECTIOUS DISEASES
Brucellosis.
Rat-bite fever.

Relapsing fever.

RHEUMATIC DISEASES
Juvenile idiopathic arthritis (systemic onset).
Behçet disease.
Systemic lupus erythematosus.
Relapsing polychondritis.
Crohn disease.

HEREDITARY AUTOINFLAMMATORY SYNDROMES
Familial Mediterranean fever (FMF).
Cryopyrinopathies:
　Familial cold autoinflammatory syndrome (FCAS).
　Muckle-Wells syndrome (MWS).
　Chronic infantile neurologic cutaneous and articular (CINCA) syndrome, also called neonatal-onset multisystem inflammatory disease (NOMID).
Tumor necrosis factor receptor–associated periodic syndrome (TRAPS).
Hyperimmunoglobulinemia D with periodic fever syndrome (HIDS).

CYCLIC HEMATOPOIESIS
Hereditary form.
Acquired form.

IDIOPATHIC CONDITIONS
Periodic fever with aphthous stomatitis, pharyngitis, and adenitis (PFAPA).

FEVER WITH MACULOPAPULAR OR PETECHIAL RASH[27]

ICD-10CM # R21 Rash and nonspecific skin eruption
ICD-10CM # R50.9 Fever, unspecified

DIFFERENTIAL DIAGNOSIS OF FEVER WITH MACULOPAPULAR OR PETECHIAL RASH
Rocky Mountain spotted fever.
Meningococcal disease.
Enteroviral infection (echovirus and coxsackievirus).
Human herpesvirus 6 infection (roseola).
Human parvovirus B19 infection (fifth disease).
Epstein-Barr virus infection.
Disseminated gonococcal infection.
Murine typhus.
Ehrlichiosis.
Group A streptococcal pharyngitis.
Mycoplasma pneumoniae infection.
Leptospirosis.
Secondary syphilis.
Kawasaki disease.
Thrombotic thrombocytopenic purpura (TTP).
Drug reactions.
Immune complex–mediated illness.
Toxic shock syndrome.

Erythema multiforme.
Stevens-Johnson syndrome.

FEVERS PRONE TO RELAPSE[35]

ICD-10CM # R50.9 Fever, unspecified

Infectious Causes
Relapsing fever (*Borrelia recurrentis*).
Q fever (*Coxiella burnetii*).
Typhoid fever (*Salmonella typhi*).
Syphilis (*Treponema pallidum*).
Tuberculosis.
Histoplasmosis.
Coccidioidomycosis.
Blastomycosis.
Melioidosis (*Pseudomonas pseudomallei*).
Lymphocytic choriomeningitis (LCM) infection.
Dengue fever.
Yellow fever.
Chronic meningococcemia.
Colorado tick fever.
Leptospirosis.
Brucellosis.
Oroya fever (*Bartonella bacilliformis*).
Acute rheumatic fever.
Rat-bite fever (*Spirillum minus*).
Visceral leishmaniasis.
Lyme disease (*Borrelia burgdorferi*).
Malaria.
Babesiosis.
Noninfluenza respiratory viral infection.
Epstein-Barr virus infection.
Noninfectious Causes
Behçet disease.
Crohn disease.
Weber-Christian disease (panniculitis).
Leukoclastic angiitis syndromes.
Sweet syndrome.
Systemic lupus erythematosus and other autoimmune disorders.
Periodic Fever Syndromes
Familial Mediterranean fever.
Cyclic neutropenia.
Periodic fever, aphthous stomatitis, pharyngitis, and adenopathy (PFAPA).
Hyper–immunoglobulin D syndrome.
Hibernian fever (tumor necrosis factor superfamily immunoglobulin A–associated syndrome [TRAPS]).
Muckle-Wells syndrome.
Others.

FINGER LESIONS, INFLAMMATORY

ICD-10CM # B08.8 Other specified viral infections characterized by skin and mucous membrane lesions
L03.0 Cellulitis of finger 6

Paronychia.
Herpes simplex type 1 (herpetic whitlow).
Dyshidrotic eczema (pompholyx).
Herpes zoster.
Bacterial endocarditis (Osler nodes).
Psoriatic arthritis.

FLACCID PARALYSIS, ACUTE, DIFFERENTIAL DIAGNOSIS[19]

ICD-10CM # G83.9 Paralytic syndrome, unspecified

Brain stem stroke.
Brain stem encephalitis.
Acute anterior poliomyelitis.
   Caused by poliovirus.
   Caused by other neurotropic viruses.
Acute myelopathy.
   Space-occupying lesions.
   Acute transverse myelitis.
Peripheral neuropathy.
   Guillain-Barré syndrome.
   Post-rabies vaccine neuropathy.
   Diphtheritic neuropathy.
   Heavy metals, biologic toxins, or drug intoxication.
   Acute intermittent porphyria.
   Vasculitic neuropathy.
   Critical illness neuropathy.
   Lymphomatous neuropathy.
Disorders of neuromuscular transmission.
   Myasthenia gravis.
   Biologic or industrial toxins.
   Tic paralysis.
Disorders of muscle.
   Hypokalemia.
   Hypophosphatemia.
   Inflammatory myopathy.
   Acute rhabdomyolysis.
   Trichinosis.
   Periodic paralyses.

FLATULENCE AND BLOATING[76]

ICD-10CM # R14.0 Abdominal distension (gaseous)
           R14.1 Gas pain
           R14.2 Eructation
           R14.3 Flatulence

Ingestion of nonabsorbable carbohydrates.
Ingestion of carbonated beverages.
Malabsorption: pancreatic insufficiency, biliary disease, celiac disease, bacterial overgrowth in small intestine.
Lactase deficiency.
Irritable bowel syndrome.
Anxiety disorders.
Food poisoning, giardiasis.

FLOPPY INFANT[38]

ICD-10CM # P94.2 Congenital hypotonia

DIFFERENTIAL DIAGNOSIS OF THE FLOPPY INFANT

Cerebral hypotonia.
Chromosomal Disorders
Prader-Willi syndrome.

Chronic nonprogressive encephalopathy.
Chronic progressive encephalopathy.
Benign congenital hypotonia.
Combined Cerebral and Motor Unit Disorders
Acid maltase deficiency.
Congenital myotonic dystrophy.
Syndromic congenital muscular dystrophies.
Congenital disorders of glycosylation.
Lysosomal disorders.
Infantile neuroaxonal dystrophy.
Spinal Cord Disorders
Acquired spinal cord lesions.
Spinal muscular atrophy.
Infantile spinal muscular atrophy with respiratory distress.
X-linked spinal muscular atrophy.
Peripheral Nerve Disorders
Congenital hypomyelinating neuropathy/Dejerine-Sottas disease.
Neuromuscular Junction Disorders
Juvenile myasthenia gravis.
Neonatal myasthenia gravis.
Congenital myasthenic syndromes.
Infant botulism.
Muscle Disorders
Congenital myopathies:
   Centronuclear myopathy.
   Nemaline myopathy.
   Central core disease.
Nonsyndromic congenital muscular dystrophies:
   Merosin-deficient congenital muscular dystrophy.
   Ullrich congenital muscular dystrophy.
Other muscular dystrophies:
   Infantile facioscapulohumeral dystrophy.

FLUSHING[80]

ICD-10CM # R23.2 Flushing

Physiologic flushing: menopause, ingestion of monosodium glutamate (Chinese restaurant syndrome), ingestion of hot drinks.
Drugs: alcohol (with or without disulfiram, metronidazole, or chlorpropamide), nicotinic acid, diltiazem, nifedipine, levodopa, bromocriptine, vancomycin, amyl nitrate.
Neoplastic disorders: carcinoid syndrome, VIPoma syndrome, medullary carcinoma of thyroid, systemic mastocytosis, basophilic chronic myelocytic leukemia, renal cell carcinoma.
Anxiety.
Agnogenic flushing.

FOLATE DEFICIENCY[31]

ICD-10CM # D52.0 Dietary folate deficiency anemia
           D52.1 Drug-induced folate deficiency anemia
           D52.8 Other folate deficiency anemias
           D52.9 Folate deficiency anemia, unspecified

ETIOPATHOPHYSIOLOGIC CLASSIFICATION OF FOLATE DEFICIENCY

Nutritional causes:
   Decreased dietary intake:
      Poverty and famine.
      Institutionalized individuals (e.g., psychiatric, nursing homes), chronic debilitating disease.
      Prolonged feeding of infants with goat's milk, special slimming diets or food fads (i.e., folate-rich foods not consumed), cultural or ethnic cooking techniques (i.e., food folate destroyed).
Decreased diet and increased requirements:
   Physiologic (e.g., pregnancy and lactation, prematurity, hyperemesis gravidarum, infancy).
   Pathologic (e.g., intrinsic hematologic diseases involving hemolysis with compensatory erythropoiesis, abnormal hematopoiesis, or bone marrow infiltration with malignant disease and dermatologic disease such as psoriasis).
Folate malabsorption:
   With normal intestinal mucosa:
      Some drugs (controversial).
      Congenital folate malabsorption (rare).
   With mucosal abnormalities (e.g., tropical and nontropical sprue, regional enteritis).
Defective cellular folate uptake:
   Familial aplastic anemia (rare).
   Acute cerebral folate deficiency.
Inadequate cellular use:
   Folate antagonists (e.g., methotrexate).
   Hereditary enzyme deficiencies involving folate.
Drugs:
   Multiple effects on folate metabolism (e.g., alcohol, sulfasalazine, triamterene, pyrimethamine, trimethoprim-sulfamethoxazole, diphenylhydantoin, barbiturates).
Acute folate deficiency:
   Intensive care unit setting.
   Uncertain origin.

FOOT AND ANKLE PAIN[8]

ICD-10CM # M25.5 Pain in joint
           M25.9 Joint disorder, unspecified

TENDON, LIGAMENT, AND MUSCLE

Gastrocnemius-soleus strain.
Plantaris rupture.
Anterior talofibular ligament tear.
Calcaneofibular ligament tear.
Deltoid ligament tear.
Anterolateral impingement due to complete tear of anterior talofibular ligament and anterior inferior tibiofibular ligament.

Syndesmotic impingement due to tear of syndesmosis.

Sinus tarsi syndrome (lateral hindfoot pain and instability due to injury of contents of the sinus and tarsal tunnel).

Achilles tendinitis.

Achilles rupture.

Plantar fasciitis.

Posterior tibial tendon dysfunction.

Flexor hallucis longus dysfunction.

Tibialis anterior tendon tear.

Peroneus brevis tendon tear.

BONE

Fracture of talus.

Calcaneal fracture.

Navicular fractures.

Lisfranc fracture-dislocation (fracture of the first metatarsal base with dislocation of medial cuneiform).

Metatarsal stress fracture.

Freiberg infraction (sclerosis and flattening of the second metatarsal head due to trauma or microtrauma).

Avascular necrosis of the talus.

Fracture of the phalanges.

Fracture of the sesamoids.

Sesamoiditis.

Metatarsalgia.

JOINT

Osteoarthritis.

Gout.

Rheumatoid arthritis.

Other inflammatory arthritides.

Charcot joint.

Osteochondral lesion of the talus.

PERIARTICULAR STRUCTURES

Shin splint (periosteal avulsion and periostitis at the insertion of the medial soleus due to repetitive overuse, such as in running and hiking).

Hallux rigidus.

Hallux valgus.

Ingrown toenail.

Toe deformities.

Turf toe (sprain of the first metatarsophalangeal joint due to hyperextension forces).

Plantar fasciitis.

Plantar fibromatosis.

NERVES

Anterior tarsal tunnel syndrome (involvement of deep peroneal nerve under the superficial fascia of the ankle).

Morton neuroma.

VESSELS

Atherosclerosis.

Compartment syndrome.

REFERRED PAIN

Complex regional pain syndrome.

FOOT AND ANKLE PAIN, IN DIFFERENT AGE GROUPS[41]

ICD-10CM #	M25.579	Pain in unspecified ankle and joints of unspecified foot

COMMON CAUSES OF FOOT AND ANKLE PAIN IN DIFFERENT AGE GROUPS

Childhood (2 to 10 yr)
Intraarticular

Club foot.

Congenital midfoot and forefoot deformities.

Septic arthritis.

Periarticular

Osteomyelitis.

Adolescence (10 to 18 yr)
Intraarticular

Arch disorders (pes cavus, pes planus).

Periarticular

Osteomyelitis.

Tumors.

Early Adulthood (18 to 30 yr)
Intraarticular

Metatarsalgia.

Hallux valgus.

Hallux rigidus.

Osteochondritis.

Accessory ossicles.

Periarticular

Achilles tendonitis.

Achilles tendon rupture.

Fasciitis.

Referred

Lumbar spine.

Knee.

Adulthood (30 to 50 yr)
Intraarticular

Osteoarthritis.

Inflammatory arthritis.

Gout.

Metatarsalgia.

Hallux valgus.

Hallux rigidus.

Osteochondritis.

Accessory ossicles.

Periarticular

Ischemic foot pain.

Diabetes.

Bursitis.

Tendonitis.

Plantar fasciitis.

Corns.

Referred

Lumbar spine.

Knee.

Old Age (>50 yr)
Intraarticular

Osteoarthritis.

Inflammatory arthritis.

Gout.

Metatarsalgia.

Hallux valgus.

Hallux rigidus.

Periarticular

Ischemic foot pain.

Diabetes.

Bursitis.

Tendonitis.

Plantar fasciitis.

Corns.

Referred

Lumbar spine.

Knee.

FOOT DERMATITIS

ICD-10CM #	B35.3	Tinea pedis
	K25	Unspecified contact dermatitis

Tinea pedis.

Dyshidrotic eczema.

Tylosis (mechanically induced hyperkeratosis, fissuring, and dryness).

Allergic contact dermatitis.

Psoriasis.

Peripheral vascular insufficiency.

Neuropathic foot ulcers (DM, poorly fitting shoes).

Acquired plantar keratoderma.

Sézary syndrome.

FOOTDROP

ICD-10CM #	M21.379	Foot drop, unspecified foot

Peripheral neuropathy.

L5 radiculopathy.

Peroneal nerve compression.

Sciatic nerve palsy.

Scapuloperoneal syndromes.

Spasticity.

Peroneal nerve compression.

Myopathy.

Dystonia.

FOOT LESION, ULCERATING

ICD-10CM #	S90.929A	Unspecified superficial injury of unspecified foot, initial encounter
	S90.933A	Unspecified superficial injury of unspecified great toe, initial encounter
	S90.936A	Unspecified superficial injury of unspecified lesser toe(s), initial encounter
	L08.89	Other specified local infections of the skin and subcutaneous tissue

Cellulitis.

Plantar wart.

Squamous cell carcinoma.
Actinomycosis (Madura foot).
Plantar fibromatosis.
Pseudoepitheliomatous hyperplasia.

FOOT PAIN

ICD-10CM #   M25.579   Pain in unspecified ankle and joints of unspecified foot

Trauma (fractures, musculoskeletal and ligamentous strain).
Inflammation (plantar fasciitis, Achilles tendonitis or bursitis, calcaneal apophysitis).
Arterial insufficiency, Raynaud phenomenon, thromboangiitis obliterans.
Gout, pseudogout.
Calcaneal spur.
Infection (cellulitis, abscess, lymphangitis, gangrene).
Decubitus ulcer.
Paronychia, ingrown toenail.
Thrombophlebitis, postphlebitic syndrome.

FOOT PAIN BY AGE[19]

ICD-10CM #   M25.579   Pain in unspecified ankle and joints of unspecified foot

0 TO 6 YEARS
Poorly fitting shoes.
Foreign body.
Fracture.
Osteomyelitis.
Leukemia.
Puncture wound.
Drawing of blood.
Dactylitis.
Juvenile rheumatoid arthritis (JRA).

6 TO 12 YEARS
Poorly fitting shoes.
Sever disease.
Enthesopathy (JRA).
Foreign body.
Accessory navicular.
Tarsal coalition.
Ewing sarcoma.
Hypermobile flatfoot.
Trauma (sprains, fractures).
Puncture wound.

12 TO 20 YEARS
Poorly fitting shoes.
Stress fracture.
Foreign body.
Ingrown toenail.
Metatarsalgia.
Plantar fasciitis.
Osteochondroses (avascular necrosis).
Freiberg infarction.
Köhler disease.
Achilles tendinitis.

Trauma (sprains).
Plantar warts.
Tarsal coalition.

FOREARM AND HAND PAIN

ICD-10CM #   S59.809A   Other specified injuries of unspecified elbow, initial encounter
     S59.919A   Unspecified injury of unspecified forearm, initial encounter
     S69.80XA   Other specified injuries of unspecified wrist, hand and finger(s), initial encounter
     S69.90XA   Unspecified injury of unspecified wrist, hand and finger(s), initial encounter

Epicondylitis.
Tenosynovitis.
Osteoarthritis.
Cubital tunnel syndrome.
Carpal tunnel syndrome.
Trauma.
Herpes zoster.
Peripheral vascular insufficiency.
Infection (cellulitis, abscess).

FOREARM FRACTURES[18]

ICD-10CM #   S52   Fracture of forearm

TRAUMATIC
Wrist sprain, elbow sprain.
Ligamentous injuries, forearm contusions, hematomas.
Dislocations of the elbow or wrist (including nursemaid's elbow).

INFECTIOUS
Cellulitis of the forearm, abscesses.
Necrotizing fasciitis.

VASCULAR
Acute arterial occlusion.
Venous thrombosis.

NEUROLOGIC
Neurapraxias, carpal tunnel syndrome.
Systemic neurologic syndromes involving the nerves of the upper extremities.

ARTHRITIS
Septic joint, gonococcal arthritis, rheumatoid arthritis, osteoarthritis.
Pseudogout, gout.
Systemic lupus erythematosus, rheumatic fever, viral syndrome.
Reiter syndrome, Lyme disease, serum sickness.

OTHER
Olecranon bursitis, soft tissue masses.
Normal growth plates, nutrient vessels.

GAIT ABNORMALITY

ICD-10CM #   R26.0   Ataxic gait
     R26.1   Paralytic gait
     R26.89   Other abnormalities of gait and mobility
     R26.9   Unspecified abnormalities of gait and mobility

Parkinsonism.
Degenerative joint disease (hips, back, knees).
Multiple sclerosis.
Trauma, foot pain.
CVA.
Cerebellar lesions.
Infections (tabes, encephalitis, meningitis).
Sensory ataxia.
Dystonia, cerebral palsy, neuromuscular disorders.
Metabolic abnormalities.

GALACTORRHEA[25]

ICD-10CM #   N64.3   Galactorrhea not associated with childbirth

Prolonged suckling.
Drugs (INH, phenothiazines, reserpine derivatives, amphetamines, spironolactone and tricyclic antidepressants).
Major stressors (surgery, trauma).
Hypothyroidism.
Pituitary tumors.

GALLBLADDER SONOGRAPHIC NONVISUALIZATION[15]

ICD-10CM #   Varies with specific diagnosis

CAUSES OF SONOGRAPHIC NONVISUALIZATION OF GALLBLADDER
Previous cholecystectomy.
Physiologic contraction.
Fibrosed gallbladder duct—chronic cholecystitis.
Air-filled gallbladder or emphysematous cholecystitis.
Tumefactive sludge.
Agenesis of gallbladder.
Ectopic location.

GALLBLADDER WALL THICKENING[15]

ICD-10CM #   Varies with specific diagnosis

CAUSES OF GALLBLADDER WALL THICKENING
Generalized Edematous States
Congestive heart failure.
Renal failure.
End-stage cirrhosis.
Hypoalbuminemia.

Inflammatory Conditions
Primary:
    Acute cholecystitis.
    Cholangitis.
    Chronic cholecystitis.
Secondary:
    Acute hepatitis.
    Perforated duodenal ulcer.
    Pancreatitis.
    Diverticulitis/colitis.
Neoplastic Conditions
Gallbladder adenocarcinoma.
Metastases.
Miscellaneous
Adenomyomatosis.
Mural varicosities.

GALLSTONE DISEASE, PEDIATRIC PATIENT[5]

ICD-10CM #   K80.20   Calculus of gallbladder without cholecystitis without obstruction

Biliary tract anomaly (e.g., choledochal cyst).
Cephalosporin use.
Crohn disease.
Cystic fibrosis.
Genetic predisposition (e.g., ABCB4, UGT1A1 mutations).
Hemolytic disorders (e.g., sickle-cell anemia, hereditary spherocytosis).
Hispanic or Latino ancestry.
Malabsorption.
Metabolic syndrome.
Obesity.
Parasitic disease (*Ascaris lumbricoides*).
Pregnancy.
Rapid weight loss.
Solid organ and hematologic transplant (e.g., liver, kidney, heart, bone marrow).
Total parenteral nutrition.

GASTRIC DILATION[21]

ICD-10CM #   K31.0   Acute dilation of stomach

CAUSES OF A MASSIVELY DILATED STOMACH
Mechanical Gastric Outlet Obstruction
Duodenal or pyloric canal ulceration.
Carcinoma of pyloric antrum.
Extrinsic compression.
Paralytic Ileus
Surgery.
Trauma.
Peritonitis.
Pancreatitis.
Cholecystitis.
Diabetes mellitus.
Hepatic coma.
Drugs.
Gastric Volvulus
Intubation.
Air swallowing.

GASTRIC EMPTYING, DELAYED[18]

ICD-10CM #   K30   Functional dyspepsia

CAUSES OF DELAYED GASTRIC EMPTYING
Mechanical Causes
Peptic ulcer disease, scarred pylorus.
Malignancy: gastric cancer, gastric lymphoma, pancreatic cancer.
Gastric surgery: vagotomy, gastric resection, Roux-en-Y anastomosis.
Crohn disease.
Endocrine and Metabolic Causes
Diabetes mellitus.
Hypothyroidism.
Hypoadrenal states.
Electrolyte abnormalities.
Chronic renal failure.
Medications.
Anticholinergics.
Opiates.
Dopamine agonists.
Tricyclic antidepressants.
Abnormalities of Gastric Smooth Muscle
Scleroderma.
Polymyositis, dermatomyositis.
Amyloidosis.
Pseudoobstruction.
Myotonic dystrophy.
Neuropathy.
Scleroderma.
Amyloidosis.
Autonomic neuropathy.
Central Nervous System or Psychiatric Disorders
Brain stem tumors.
Spinal cord injury.
Anorexia nervosa.
Stress.
Miscellaneous
Idiopathic gastroparesis.
Gastroesophageal reflux disease.
Nonulcer (functional) dyspepsia.
Cancer cachexia or anorexia.

GASTRIC EMPTYING, RAPID

ICD-10CM #   K30   Functional dyspepsia

Pancreatic insufficiency.
Dumping syndrome.
Peptic ulcer.
Celiac disease.
Promotility agents.
Zollinger-Ellison disease.

GASTROINTESTINAL BLEEDING, PEDIATRIC PATIENT[68]

ICD-10CM #   K92.2   Gastrointestinal hemorrhage, unspecified

INFANT
Common
Bacterial enteritis.
Milk protein allergy intolerance.
Intussusception.
Swallowed maternal blood.
Anal fissure.
Lymphonodular hyperplasia
Rare
Volvulus.
Necrotizing enterocolitis.
Meckel diverticulum.
Stress ulcer, gastritis.
Coagulation disorder (hemorrhagic disease of newborn).
Esophagitis.

CHILD
Common
Bacterial enteritis.
Anal fissure.
Colonic polyps.
Intussusception.
Peptic ulcer/gastritis.
Swallowed epistaxis.
Prolapse (traumatic) gastropathy secondary to emesis.
Mallory-Weiss syndrome.
Rare
Esophageal varices.
Esophagitis.
Meckel diverticulum.
Lymphonodular hyperplasia.
Henoch-Schönlein purpura.
Foreign body.
Hemangioma, arteriovenous malformation.
Sexual abuse.
Hemolytic-uremic syndrome.
Inflammatory bowel disease.
Coagulopathy.
    Duplication cyst:
    Angiodysplasia.
    Angiodysplasia with von Willebrand disease.
    Blue rubber bleb nevus syndrome.

ADOLESCENT
Common
Bacterial enteritis.
Inflammatory bowel disease.
Peptic ulcer/gastritis.
Prolapse (traumatic) gastropathy secondary to emesis.
Mallory-Weiss syndrome.
Colonic polyps.
Anal fissure.
Rare
Hemorrhoids.
Esophageal varices.
Esophagitis.
Pill ulcer.
Telangiectasia-angiodysplasia.
Graft-versus-host disease.
    Duplication cyst:
    Angiodysplasia.

Angiodysplasia with von Willebrand disease.
Blue rubber bleb nevus syndrome.

GASTROINTESTINAL OBSTRUCTION, PEDIATRIC PATIENT[68]

ICD-10CM #	K56.2K5.	VolvulusIntus
	1K56.9	susceptionIleus
	K56.6	unspecified
		Other and unspecified intestinal obstruction

Esophagus
Congenital
Esophageal atresia.
Vascular rings.
Schatzki ring.
Tracheobronchial remnant.
Acquired
Esophageal stricture.
Foreign body.
Achalasia.
Chagas disease.
Collagen vascular disease.
Stomach
Congenital
Antral webs.
Pyloric stenosis.
Acquired
Bezoar, foreign body.
Pyloric stricture (ulcer).
Chronic granulomatous disease of childhood.
Eosinophilic gastroenteritis.
Crohn disease.
Epidermolysis bullosa.
Small Intestine
Congenital
Duodenal atresia.
Annular pancreas.
Malrotation/volvulus.
Malrotation/Ladd bands.
Ileal atresia.
Meconium ileus.
Meckel diverticulum with volvulus or intussusception.
Inguinal hernia.
Internal hernia.
Intestinal duplication.
Pseudoobstruction.
Acquired
Postsurgical adhesions.
Crohn disease.
Intussusception.
Distal ileal obstruction syndrome (cystic fibrosis).
Duodenal hematoma.
Superior mesenteric artery syndrome.
Colon
Congenital
Meconium plug.
Hirschsprung disease.
Colonic atresia, stenosis.
Imperforate anus.
Rectal stenosis.

Pseudoobstruction.
Volvulus.
Colonic duplication.
Acquired
Ulcerative colitis (toxic megacolon).
Chagas disease.
Crohn disease.
Fibrosing colonopathy (cystic fibrosis).

GASTROINTESTINAL SYMPTOMS IN CHILDREN, NONDIGESTIVE CAUSES[68]

| ICD-10CM # | Varies with specific diagnosis |

Anorexia
Systemic disease: inflammatory, neoplastic.
Cardiorespiratory compromise.
Iatrogenic: drug therapy, unpalatable therapeutic diets.
Depression.
Anorexia nervosa.
Vomiting
Inborn errors of metabolism.
Medications: erythromycin, chemotherapy, nonsteroidal antiinflammatory drugs, marijuana.
Increased intracranial pressure.
Brain tumor.
Infection of the urinary tract.
Labyrinthitis.
Adrenal insufficiency.
Pregnancy.
Psychogenic.
Abdominal migraine.
Poisoning/toxins.
Renal disease.
Diarrhea
Infection: otitis media, urinary tract infection.
Uremia.
Medications: antibiotics, cisapride.
Tumors: neuroblastoma.
Pericarditis.
Adrenal insufficiency.
Constipation
Hypothyroidism.
Spina bifida.
Developmental delay.
Dehydration: diabetes insipidus, renal tubular lesions.
Medications: narcotics.
Lead poisoning.
Infant botulism.
Abdominal Pain
Pyelonephritis, hydronephrosis, renal colic.
Pneumonia (lower lobe).
Pelvic inflammatory disease.
Porphyria.
Fabry disease.
Angioedema.
Endocarditis.
Abdominal migraine.
Familial Mediterranean fever.
Sexual or physical abuse.
Systemic lupus erythematosus.
School phobia.

Sickle cell crisis.
Vertebral disk inflammation.
Psoas abscess.
Pelvic osteomyelitis or myositis.
Medications.
Abdominal Distention or Mass
Ascites: nephrotic syndrome, neoplasm, heart failure.
Discrete mass: Wilms tumor, hydronephrosis, neuroblastoma, mesenteric cyst, hepatoblastoma, lymphoma.
Pregnancy.
Jaundice
Hemolytic disease.
Urinary tract infection.
Sepsis.
Hypothyroidism.
Panhypopituitarism.

GAZE PALSIES[20]

| ICD-10CM # | Varies with specific diagnosis |

APRAXIA OF HORIZONTAL GAZE
Ataxia-telangiectasia.
Ataxia-ocular motor apraxia.
Brain stem glioma.
Congenital ocular motor apraxia.
Huntington disease.

INTERNUCLEAR OPHTHALMOPLEGIA
Brain stem stroke.
Brain stem tumor.
Exotropia (pseudo-internuclear ophthalmoplegia [INO]).
Multiple sclerosis.
Myasthenia gravis (pseudo-INO).
Toxic-metabolic.

VERTICAL GAZE PALSY
Aqueductal stenosis.
Congenital vertical ocular motor apraxia.
Gaucher disease.
Hydrocephalus.
Miller Fisher syndrome.
Niemann-Pick disease type C.
Tumor:
    Midbrain.
    Pineal region.
    Third ventricle.

HORIZONTAL GAZE PALSY
Adversive seizures.
Brain stem tumors.
Destructive lesions of the frontal lobe.
Familial horizontal gaze palsy.

CONVERGENCE PARALYSIS
Head trauma.
Idiopathic.
Multiple sclerosis.
Pineal region tumors.

Differential Diagnosis

II

GENITAL DISCHARGE, FEMALE[55]

ICD-10CM # N94.9 Unspecified condition associated with female genital organs and menstrual cycle

Physiologic discharge: cervical mucus, vaginal transudation, bacteria, squamous epithelial cells.
Individual variation.
Pregnancy.
Sexual response.
Menstrual cycle variation.
Infection.
Foreign body: tampon, cervical cap, other.
Neoplasm.
Fistula.
IUD.
Cervical ectropion.
Spermicide.
Nongenital causes: urinary incontinence, urinary tract fistula, Crohn disease, rectovaginal fistula.

GENITAL LESIONS, INFECTIOUS CAUSES[42]

ICD-10CM # Varies with specific diagnosis

INFECTIOUS CAUSES OF GENITAL LESIONS
Sexually Transmitted Infections
Syphilis:
    Primary (chancre).
    Secondary (condyloma latum).
Herpes simplex virus types 1 and 2.
Chancroid *(Haemophilus ducreyi)*.
Lymphogranuloma venereum.
Granuloma inguinale (donovanosis).
Human papillomavirus.
Sarcoptes scabiei.
Molluscum contagiosum.
Nonsexually Transmitted Infections
Folliculitis.
Tuberculosis.
Tularemia.
Histoplasmosis.
Candida (balanitis or vaginitis).
Amebiasis.

GENITAL LESIONS, NONINFECTIOUS CAUSES[42]

ICD-10CM # Varies with specific diagnosis

NONVENEREAL CAUSES OF GENITAL LESIONS
Trauma.
Malignancies (e.g., squamous cell carcinoma).
Behçet syndrome.
Lipschütz vulvar ulcers.
Peyronie disease.
Fixed-drug eruption.
Eczema.

Psoriasis.
Inflammatory bowel disease.
Contact dermatitis.
Lichen planus.
Hidradenitis suppurativa.
Postinflammatory hypopigmentation.
Aphthous ulcers (associated with human immunodeficiency virus).

GENITAL SORES[18]

ICD-10CM #	A60.9	Anogenital herpesviral infection, unspecified
	A51.0	Primary genital syphilis
	A63.0	Anogenital (venereal) warts
	A57	Chancroid
	A58	Granuloma inguinale
	A55	Chlamydial lymphogranuloma (venereum)
	N94.89	Other specified conditions associated with female genital organs and menstrual cycle
	N50.8	Other specified disorders of male genital organs

Herpes genitalis.
Syphilis.
Chancroid.
Lymphogranuloma venereum.
Granuloma inguinale.
Condyloma acuminatum.
Neoplastic lesion.
Trauma.

GLOMERULONEPHRITIS ASSOCIATED WITH MALIGNANCY[11]

ICD-10CM # N00.9 Acute nephritic syndrome with unspecified morphologic changes

Membranous glomerulonephritis:
Breast cancer.
Lung cancer.
Colon cancer.
Prostate cancer.
Graft-versus-host disease.
Minimal change disease:
Hodgkin lymphoma.
Non-Hodgkin lymphoma.
Graft-versus-host disease.
Case reports.
Immunoglobulin A nephritis.
Antineutrophil cytoplasmic antibody vasculitis.
Focal segmental glomerulosclerosis.

GLOMERULONEPHRITIS, RAPIDLY PROGRESSIVE[18]

ICD-10CM # N05.9 Unspecified nephritic syndrome with unspecified morphologic changes

DIFFERENTIAL DIAGNOSIS OF RAPIDLY PROGRESSIVE GLOMERULONEPHRITIS
Linear Immune Staining
Anti-GBM disease.
Goodpasture syndrome.
Rarely membranous glomerulonephritis.
Granular Immune Staining
Subacute bacterial endocarditis (past infectious).
Lupus nephritis.
Cryoglobulinemia.
Membranoproliferative glomerulonephritis (type II more than type I).
Immunoglobulin A nephropathy, Henoch-Schönlein purpura.
Idiopathic.
No Immune Staining (Pauci-immune)
Antineutrophil cytoplasmic antibody-associated vasculitis (Wegener granulomatosis, microscopic polyangiitis, Churg-Strauss syndrome).
Idiopathic.

GLOMERULOPATHIES, THROMBOTIC, MICROANGIOPATHIC[18]

ICD-10CM # M31.1 Thrombotic microangiopathy

THROMBOTIC MICROANGIOPATHIC GLOMERULOPATHIES
Thrombotic thrombocytopenic purpura.
Hemolytic-uremic syndrome.
Malignant hypertension.
Scleroderma renal crisis.
Preeclampsia, eclampsia.
HELLP syndrome (hemolysis, elevated liver enzymes, low platelets).
Antiphospholipid antibody syndrome.
Drugs: oral contraceptives, quinine, cyclosporine, tacrolimus, ticlopidine, clopidogrel.

GLOMERULOSCLEROSIS, FOCAL SEGMENTAL[18]

ICD-10CM # N03.3 Chronic nephritic syndrome with diffuse mesangial proliferative glomerulonephritis

ETIOLOGY OF FOCAL SEGMENTAL GLOMERULOSCLEROSIS (FSGS)
Primary idiopathic FSGS.
Secondary FSGS.
HIV (usually collapsing variant).
Reflux nephropathy.
Heroin abuse.
Sickle cell disease.
Oligomeganephronia.
Renal dysgenesis or agenesis (low nephron mass).
Radiation nephritis.
Familial podocytopathies.

NPHS1 (nephrin) mutation.
NPHS2 (podocin) mutation.
TRPC6 (cation channel) mutation.
ACTN4 (a-actinin 4 mutation).

GLOSSODYNIA[2]

ICD-10CM #	K14.6	Glossodynia

DENTURE-RELATED

Dentures (ill-fitting, monomer from denture base).
Dental plaque.
Oral parafunction.

INFECTIVE/DERMATOLOGIC

Candidiasis.
Lichen planus.

DEFICIENCY STATES

Iron, vitamin B_{12}, folate, B_2 (riboflavin), B_6 (pyridoxine), zinc.

ENDOCRINE

Diabetes.
Myxedema.
Hormonal changes occurring during menopause.

NEUROLOGICALLY MEDIATED

Referred from tonsils, teeth.
Lingual nerve neuropathy.
Glossopharyngeal neuralgia.
Esophageal reflux.

IATROGENIC

Mouthwash.
Xerostomia

GLUCOCORTICOID DEFICIENCY[24]

ICD-10CM #	E27.1	Primary adrenocortical insufficiency
	E27.3	Drug-induced adrenocortical insufficiency

ACTH-independent causes.
TB.
Autoimmune (idiopathic).
Other rare causes:
  Fungal infection.
  Adrenal hemorrhage.
  Metastases.
  Sarcoidosis.
  Amyloidosis.
  Adrenoleukodystrophy.
  Adrenomyeloneuropathy.
  HIV infection.
  Congenital adrenal hyperplasia.
  Medications (e.g., ketoconazole).
ACTH-dependent causes:
  Hypothalamic-pituitary-adrenal suppression.
  Exogenous.
  Glucocorticoid.

ACTH.
  Endogenous—cure of Cushing syndrome.
Hypothalamic-pituitary lesions.
  Neoplasm:
    Primary pituitary tumor.
    Metastatic tumor.
    Craniopharyngioma.
  Infection:
    Tuberculosis.
    Actinomycosis.
    Nocardiosis.
  Sarcoid.
  Head trauma.
  Isolated ACTH deficiency.

GOITER

ICD-10CM #	E01.2	Iodine-deficiency related (endemic) goiter, unspecified
	E04.9	Nontoxic goiter, unspecified
	E04.9	Nontoxic goiter, unspecified
	E07.1	Dyshormonogenetic goiter
	E01.2	Iodine-deficiency related (endemic) goiter, unspecified
	E04.9	Nontoxic goiter, unspecified
	E04.2	Nontoxic multinodular goiter
	E04.0	Nontoxic diffuse goiter
	E05.10	Thyrotoxicosis with toxic single thyroid nodule without thyrotoxic crisis or storm

Thyroiditis.
Toxic multinodular goiter.
Graves disease.
Medications (PTU, methimazole, sulfonamides, sulfonylureas, ethionamide, amiodarone, lithium, etc.).
Iodine deficiency.
Sarcoidosis, amyloidosis.
Defective thyroid hormone synthesis.
Resistance to thyroid hormone.

GRANULOMATOUS DERMATITIDES

ICD-10CM #	L92.9	Granulomatous disorder of the skin and subcutaneous tissue, unspecified

Granuloma annulare.
Sarcoidosis.
Necrobiosis lipoidica diabeticorum.
Cutaneous Crohn disease.
Rheumatoid nodules.
Annular elastolytic giant cell granuloma (actinic granuloma).
Foreign body granuloma.

GRANULOMATOUS DISORDERS[81]

ICD-10CM #	M31.30	Granulomatosis with polyangiitis without renal involvement
	K75.3	Granulomatous hepatitis
	L92.9	Granulomatous disorder of skin and subcutaneous tissue, unspecified

INFECTIONS

Fungi
Histoplasma.
Coccidioides.
Blastomyces.
Sporothrix.
Aspergillus.
Cryptococcus.
Protozoa
Toxoplasma.
Leishmania.
Metazoa
Toxocara.
Schistosoma.
Spirochetes
Treponema pallidum.
T. pertenue.
T. carateum.
Mycobacteria
M. tuberculosis.
M. leprae.
M. kansasii.
M. marinum.
M. avian.
Bacille Calmette-Guérin (BCG) vaccine.
Bacteria
Brucella.
Yersinia.
Other Infections
Cat-scratch disease.
Lymphogranuloma.

NEOPLASIA

Carcinoma.
Reticulosis.
Pinealoma.
Dysgerminoma.
Seminoma.
Reticulum cell sarcoma.
Malignant nasal granuloma.

CHEMICALS

Beryllium.
Zirconium.
Silica.
Starch.

IMMUNOLOGIC ABERRATIONS

Sarcoidosis.
Crohn disease.
Primary biliary cirrhosis.
Granulomatosis with polyangiitis.

Differential Diagnosis

II

Giant cell arteritis.
Peyronie disease.
Hypogammaglobulinemia.
SLE.
Lymphomatoid granulomatosis.
Histiocytosis X.
Hepatic granulomatous disease.
Immune complex disease.
Rosenthal-Melkersson syndrome.
Churg-Strauss allergic granulomatosis.

LEUKOCYTE OXIDASE DEFECT
Chronic granulomatous disease of childhood.

EXTRINSIC ALLERGIC ALVEOLITIS
Farmer's lung.
Bird fancier's.
Mushroom worker's.
Suberosis (cork dust).
Bagassosis.
Maple bark stripper's.
Paprika splitter's.
Coffee bean.
Spatlese lung.

OTHER DISORDERS
Whipple disease.
Pyrexia of unknown origin.
Radiotherapy.
Cancer chemotherapy.
Panniculitis.
Chalazion.
Sebaceous cyst.
Dermoid.
Sea urchin spine injury.

GRANULOMATOUS LIVER DISEASE

ICD-10CM #   K75.3   Granulomatous hepatitis

Sarcoidosis.
Granulomatosis with polyangiitis.
Vasculitis.
Inflammatory bowel disease.
Allergic granulomatosis.
Erythema nodosum.
Infections (fungal, viral, parasitic).
Primary biliary cirrhosis.
Lymphoma.
Hodgkin disease.
Drugs (e.g., allopurinol, hydralazine, sulfon-
   amides, penicillins).
Toxins (copper sulfate, beryllium).

GREEN OR BLUE URINE

ICD-10CM #   R82   Other abnormal findings in
                         urine

Pseudomonal urinary tract infection
Medications: triamterene, amitriptyline, IV
   cimetidine, IV promethazine.
Biliverdin.
Dyes (methylene blue, indigo carmine).

GROIN AND SCROTAL MASSES[4]

ICD-10CM #   Code varies with specific diagnosis

DIFFERENTIAL DIAGNOSIS OF GROIN AND SCROTAL MASSES
Inguinal hernia.
Hydrocele.
Varicocele.
Ectopic testis.
Epididymitis.
Testicular torsion.
Lipoma.
Hematoma.
Sebaceous cyst.
Hidradenitis of inguinal apocrine glands.
Inguinal lymphadenopathy.
Lymphoma.
Metastatic neoplasm.
Femoral hernia.
Femoral lymphadenopathy.
Femoral artery aneurysm or pseudoaneurysm.

GROIN LUMP[2]

| **ICD-10CM #** | R19.09 | Other intraabdominal and pelvic swelling, mass and lump |
| | R22.9 | Localized swelling, mass and lump, unspecified |

COMMON CAUSES
Inguinal hernia.
Femoral hernia.
Lymph node.

OTHER CAUSES
Saphena varix.
Femoral artery aneurysm/pseudoaneurysm.
Psoas abscess.
Lipoma of the cord.
Encysted hydrocele of the cord (male).
Testicular maldescent (male).
Hydrocele of canal of Nuck (female).

GROIN MASSES

| **ICD-10CM #** | R22.9 | Localized swelling, mass and lump, unspecified |
| | S39.848A | Other specified injuries of external genitals, initial encounter |

Hernia (inguinal, femoral).
Hydrocele.
Varicocele.
Sebaceous cyst.
Hidradenitis of inguinal apocrine glands.
Neoplasm: lymphoma, metastases.
Lipoma.
Hematoma.
Reactive inguinal adenopathy, femoral adenitis.
Folliculitis, psoas abscess.

Epididymitis, testicular torsion, ectopic testes.
Aneurysm or pseudoaneurysm of femoral artery.

GROIN PAIN[64]

ICD-10CM #   R52   Pain, unspecified

DIFFERENTIAL DIAGNOSIS OF GROIN PAIN
Surgery
Workers' compensation.
Hernia.
Recurrent hernia.
Posthernia.
Orthopedic
Hip disorders:
   Acetabular labral tears.
   Avascular necrosis.
   Chondritis dissecans.
   Legg-Calvé-Perthes disease.
   Osteoarthritis.
   Pelvic stress fractures.
   Slipped femoral capital epiphysis.
   Synovitis.
Urology
Cystitis.
Epididymitis.
Nephrolithiasis.
Prostate cancer.
Prostatitis.
Torsion of testes.
Urethral extravasation.
Urinary tract infection.
Vas granuloma/fibrosis.
Dermatology
Lymphadenitis.
Psoriasis/burn.
Sebaceous cyst/hidradenitis.
Thrombophlebitis/cellulitis.
Neurosurgery
Disk disease.
Spinal injuries, inflammation, tumors.
Spondylolisthesis.
Spondylolysis.
Rheumatology
Connective tissue disorders.
Iliopsoas bursitis.
Osteitis pubis.
Systemic lupus erythematosus.
Neurology
Lumbosacral disorders.
Neurofibromatosis.
Infectious Disease
Herpes zoster.
HIV/tuberculosis.
Lyme disease.
Psoas abscess.
Sports Medicine
"Sports hernia" (adductor strains).
Gilmore groin.
Vascular
Abscess hematoma.
Postvein stripping.
Pseudoaneurysm.
Vascular graft.

Gastroenterology
Appendicitis/adhesions.
Diverticulitis.
Inflammatory retroperitoneal phlegmon (pancreatitis).
Meckel diverticulum.
Granulomatous colitis.
Gynecology
Cesarean section.
Cervical cancer.
Endometriosis.
Tubal/ovarian disorders.

GROIN PAIN, ACTIVE PATIENT[82]

| ICD-10CM # | S39.848A | Other specified injuries of external genitals, initial encounter |
| | R52 | Pain, unspecified |

MUSCULOSKELETAL
Avascular necrosis of the femoral head.
Avulsion fracture (lesser trochanter, anterior superior iliac spine, anterior inferior iliac spine).
Bursitis (iliopectineal, trochanteric).
Entrapment of the ilioinguinal or iliofemoral nerve.
Gracilis syndrome.
Muscle tear (adductors, iliopsoas, rectus abdominis, gracilis, sartorius, rectus femoris).
Myositis ossificans of the hip muscles.
Osteitis pubis.
Osteoarthritis of the femoral head.
Slipped capital femoral epiphysis.
Stress fracture of the femoral head or neck and pubis.
Synovitis.

HERNIA-RELATED
Avulsion of the internal oblique muscle in the conjoined tendon.
Defect at the insertion of the rectus abdominis muscle.
Direct inguinal hernia.
Femoral ring hernia.
Indirect inguinal hernia.
Inguinal canal weakness.

UROLOGIC
Epididymitis.
Fracture of the testis.
Hydrocele.
Kidney stone.
Posterior urethritis.
Prostatitis.
Testicular cancer.
Torsion of the testis.
Urinary tract infection.
Varicocele.

GYNECOLOGIC
Ectopic pregnancy.
Ovarian cyst.

Pelvic inflammatory disease.
Torsion of the ovary.
Vaginitis.
Lymphatic enlargement in groin.

GROIN PAIN, ATHLETES[83]

| ICD-10CM # | R52 | Pain, unspecified |

DIFFERENTIAL DIAGNOSIS OF GROIN PAIN IN ATHLETES
Hip-Associated Causes
Acetabular labral tear and femoroacetabular impingement.
Osteoarthritis.
Snapping hip syndrome and iliopsoas tendonitis.
Avascular necrosis.
Iliotibial band syndrome.
Visceral Causes
Inguinal hernia.
Other abdominal hernias.
Testicular torsion.
Infectious Causes
Septic arthritis.
Osteomyelitis.
Pelvic inflammatory disease.
Prostatitis.
Epididymitis and orchitis.
Herpes infection.
Inflammatory Causes
Endometriosis.
Inflammatory bowel disease.
Pelvic inflammatory disease.
Primary osteitis pubis.
Traumatic Causes
Stress fracture.
Tendon avulsion.
Muscle contusion.
Baseball pitcher–hockey goalie syndrome.
Developmental Causes
Apophysitis.
Growth plate stress injury or fracture.
Legg-Calvé-Perthes disease.
Developmental dysplasia.
Slipped capital femoral epiphysis.
Neurologic Causes
Nerve entrapment syndromes.
Referred pain.
Sacroiliitis.
Sciatic entrapment (piriformis syndrome).
Hamstring strain.
Knee pain.
Neoplastic Causes
Testicular carcinoma.
Osteoid osteoma.

GYNECOMASTIA

| ICD-10CM # | N62 | Hypertrophy of breast |

Physiologic (puberty, newborns, aging).
Drugs (estrogen and estrogen precursors, 5-a reductase inhibitors, digitalis, testosterone and exogenous androgens, clomiphene, cimetidine, spironolactone, ketoconazole,

amiodarone, ACE inhibitors, isoniazid, phenytoin, methyldopa, metoclopramide, phenothiazine).
Increased prolactin level (prolactinoma).
Liver disease.
Adrenal disease.
Thyrotoxicosis.
Increased estrogen production (hCG-producing tumor, testicular tumor, bronchogenic carcinoma).
Secondary hypogonadism.
Primary gonadal failure (trauma, castration, viral orchitis, granulomatous disease).
Defects in androgen synthesis.
Testosterone deficiency.
Klinefelter syndrome.

HAIR LOSS[84]

ICD-10CM #	L63.8	Other alopecia areata
	L63.9	Alopecia areata, unspecified
	L64.0	Drug-induced androgenic alopecia
	L64.8	Other androgenic alopecia

GENERALIZED
Acute blood loss.*
Childbirth.
Crash diets (inadequate protein).
Drugs:
    Coumarin.
    Heparin.
    Propranolol.
    Vitamin A.
    High fever.
Hypothyroidism and hyperthyroidisms.
Physical stress (e.g., surgery).
Physiologic stress (e.g., neonate).
Psychologic stress.
Severe illness (e.g., systemic lupus erythematosus).
Cancer chemotherapeutic agents.
Poisoning:
    Thallium (rat poison).
    Arsenic.
Radiation therapy.
Secondary syphilis: "moth eaten" alopecia.

LOCALIZED
Androgenetic alopecia.†
    Male pattern.
    Female pattern.
Hirsutism.
Alopecia areata.
Trichotillomania.
Traction alopecia.
Scarring alopecia:
    Developmental defects: aplasia cutis.

*Diffuse, uniform loss, but many hairs left randomly distributed in area of loss.
†Most or all hair missing from involved area.

Physical injury: burns, pressure.
Infection:
   Fungal: kerion.
   Bacterial: folliculitis, furuncle.
   Viral: herpes zoster.
Neoplasms:
   Metastatic carcinoma.
   Sclerosing basal cell carcinoma.
Lupus erythematosus.
Lichen planus.
Cicatricial pemphigoid.
Scleroderma.

HALITOSIS

ICD-10CM # R19.6 Halitosis

Tobacco use.
Alcohol use.
Dry mouth (mouth breathing, inadequate fluid intake).
Foods (onion, garlic, meats, nuts, protein drinks).
Disease of mouth or nose (infections, cancer, inflammation).
Medications (antihistamines, antidepressants).
Systemic disorders (diabetes, uremia).
GI disorders (esophageal diverticula, hiatal hernia, GERD, achalasia).
Sinusitis.
Pulmonary disorders (bronchiectasis, pneumonia, neoplasms, TB).

HALLUCINATIONS, VISUAL, NEUROLOGIC CAUSES[72]

ICD-10CM # R44.1 Visual hallucinations

Blindness/sensory deprivation—Charles Bonnet syndrome.
Palinopsia.
Dementia-producing diseases:
   Alzheimer.
   Dementia with Lewy bodies.*
   Parkinson.†
Intoxications:
   Alcoholic hallucinosis.
      Delirium tremens (DTs).
Hallucinogens:
   Amphetamines.
   Cocaine.
   Lysergic acid diethylamide (LSD).
   Phencyclidine (PCP).
Medicines:
   Atropine, scopolamine.
   Levodopa and dopamine agonists.
   Steroids.
Migraine with aura (classic migraine).

---

*Although visual hallucinations are likely to complicate almost any form of dementia, they are characteristic of dementia with Lewy bodies disease.
†Dopaminergic medications such as levodopa-carbidopa (Sinemet) are more likely than Parkinson disease itself to produce hallucinations.

Narcolepsy: hypnopompic (awakening) and hypnagogic (falling asleep) hallucinations.
Seizures.
Peduncular hallucinations.

HAND PAIN AND SWELLING[40]

ICD-10CM # 729.5 Pain in limb

Trauma.
Gout.
Pseudogout.
Cellulitis.
Lymphangitis.
DVT of upper extremity.
Thrombophlebitis.
RA.
Remitting seronegative symmetrical synovitis with pitting edema (RS3PE).
Polymyalgia rheumatica.
Mixed connective tissue disease.
Scleroderma.
Rupture of the olecranon bursa.
Metzger syndrome (neoplasia).
The puffy hand of drug addiction.
Reflex sympathetic dystrophy.
Eosinophilic fasciitis.
Sickle cell (hand-foot syndrome).
Leprosy.
Factitial (the rubber band syndrome).

HEADACHE[85]

ICD-10CM #		
	G44.1	Vascular headache, not elsewhere classified
	R51	Headache
	G44.209	Tension-type headache, unspecified, not intractable
	G44.009	Cluster headache syndrome, unspecified, not intractable
	G43.909	Migraine, unspecified, not intractable, without status migrainosus
	G44.1	Vascular headache, not elsewhere classified

Vascular: migraine, cluster headaches, temporal arteritis, hypertension, cavernous sinus thrombosis.
Musculoskeletal: neck and shoulder muscle contraction, strain of extraocular and/or intraocular muscles, cervical spondylosis, temporomandibular arthritis.
Infections: meningitis, encephalitis, brain abscess, sepsis, sinusitis, osteomyelitis, parotitis, mastoiditis.
Cerebral neoplasm.
Subdural hematoma.
Cerebral hemorrhage/infarct.
Pseudotumor cerebri.

Normal-pressure hydrocephalus (NPH).
Postlumbar puncture.
Cerebral aneurysm, arteriovenous malformations.
Posttrauma.
Dental problems: abscess, periodontitis, poorly fitting dentures.
Trigeminal neuralgia, glossopharyngeal neuralgia.
Otitis and other ear diseases.
Glaucoma and other eye diseases.
Metabolic: uremia, carbon monoxide inhalation, hypoxia.
Pheochromocytoma, hypoglycemia, hypothyroidism.
Effort induced: benign exertional headache, cough, headache, coital cephalalgia.
Drugs: alcohol, nitrates, histamine antagonists.
Paget disease of the skull.
Emotional, psychiatric.

HEADACHE, ACUTE[46]

ICD-10CM # R51 Headache

DIFFERENTIAL DIAGNOSIS OF ACUTE HEADACHE

Evaluation of the first acute headache should exclude pathologic causes listed here before consideration of more common etiologies.
Increased intracranial pressure (ICP): trauma, hemorrhage, tumor, hydrocephalus, pseudotumor cerebri, abscess, arachnoid cyst, cerebral edema.
Decreased ICP: after ventriculoperitoneal shunt, lumbar puncture, cerebrospinal fluid leak from basilar skull fracture.
Meningeal inflammation: meningitis, leukemia, subarachnoid or subdural hemorrhage.
Vascular: vasculitis, arteriovenous malformation, hypertension, cerebrovascular accident.
Bone, soft tissue: referred pain from scalp, eyes, ears, sinuses, nose, teeth, pharynx, cervical spine, temporomandibular joint.
Infection: systemic infection, encephalitis, sinusitis, etc.
First migraine.

HEADACHE AND FACIAL PAIN[17]

ICD-10CM #	R51	Headache
	G44.1	Vascular headache, not elsewhere classified

VASCULAR HEADACHES
Migraine
Migraine with headaches and inconspicuous neurologic features:
   Migraine without aura ("common migraine").

Migraine with headaches and conspicuous neurologic features:
With transient neurologic symptoms:
Migraine with typical aura ("classic migraine").
Sensory, basilar, and hemiplegic migraine.
With prolonged or permanent neurologic features ("complicated migraine"):
Ophthalmoplegic migraine.
Migrainous infarction.
Migraine without headaches but with conspicuous neurologic features ("migraine equivalents"):
Abdominal migraine.
Benign paroxysmal vertigo of childhood.
Migraine aura without headache ("isolated auras," transient migrainous accompaniments).
Cluster Headaches
Episodic cluster headache ("cyclic cluster headaches").
Chronic cluster headaches.
Chronic paroxysmal hemicrania.
Other Vascular Headaches
Headaches of reactive vasodilation (fever, drug-induced, postictal, hypoglycemia, hypoxia, hypercarbia, hyperthyroidism).
Headaches associated with arterial hypertension:
Chronic severe hypertension (diastolic 120 mm Hg).
Paroxysmal severe hypertension (pheochromocytoma, some coital headaches).
Headaches caused by cranial arteritis:
Giant cell arteritis ("temporal arteritis").
Other vasculitides.

HEADACHES ASSOCIATED WITH DEMONSTRABLE MUSCLE SPASM

Headache caused by posturally induced or perilesional muscle spasm:
Headaches of sustained or impaired posture (e.g., prolonged close work, driving).
Headaches associated with cervical spondylosis and other diseases of cervical spine.
Myofascial pain dysfunction syndrome (headache or facial pain associated with disorders of teeth, jaws, and related structures, or "TMJ syndrome").
Headaches caused by psychophysiologic muscular contraction ("muscle contraction headaches," or tension-type headache associated with disorder of pericranial muscles).

HEADACHES AND FACIAL PAIN WITHOUT DEMONSTRABLE PHYSICAL SUBSTRATE

Headaches of uncertain etiology:
"Tension headaches" (tension-type headache unassociated with disorder of pericranial muscles).
Some forms of posttraumatic headache.
Psychogenic headaches (e.g., hypochondriacal, conversional, malingered).

Facial pain of uncertain etiology ("atypical facial pain").

COMBINED TENSION-MIGRAINE HEADACHES

Episodic migraine superimposed on chronic tension headaches.
Chronic daily headaches:
Associated with analgesic and/or ergotamine overuse ("rebound headaches").
Not associated with drug overuse.

HEADACHES AND HEAD PAINS CAUSED BY DISEASES OF EYES, EARS, NOSE, SINUSES, TEETH, OR SKULL
Headaches Caused by Meningeal Inflammation
Subarachnoid hemorrhage.
Meningitis and meningoencephalitis.
Others (e.g., meningeal carcinomatosis).

HEADACHES ASSOCIATED WITH ALTERED INTRACRANIAL PRESSURE ("TRACTION HEADACHES")
Increased Intracranial Pressure
Intracranial mass lesions (neoplasm, hematoma, abscess, etc.).
Hydrocephalus.
Benign intracranial hypertension.
Venous sinus thrombosis.
Decreased Intracranial Pressure
Postlumbar puncture headaches.
Spontaneous hypoliquorrheic headaches.

HEADACHES AND HEAD PAINS CAUSED BY CRANIAL NEURALGIAS
Presumed Irritation of Superficial Nerves
Occipital neuralgia.
Supraorbital neuralgia.
Presumed Irritation of Intracranial Nerves
Trigeminal neuralgia ("tic douloureux").
Glossopharyngeal neuralgia.

HEADACHE, CHRONIC[46]

ICD-10CM #   R51   Headache

DIFFERENTIAL DIAGNOSIS OF RECURRENT OR CHRONIC HEADACHES

Migraine (with or without aura).
Tension.
Analgesic rebound.
Caffeine withdrawal.
Sleep deprivation (e.g., in children with sleep apnea) or chronic hypoxia.
Tumor.
Psychogenic: conversion disorder, malingering.
Cluster headache.

HEAD AND NECK, SOFT TISSUE MASSES

ICD-10CM #   R22.0   Localized swelling, mass and lump, head
               R22.1   Localized swelling, mass and lump, neck

Lipoma.
Pilar cyst.
Epidermal inclusion cyst.
Dermoid cyst.
Bone cyst.
Hemangioma.
Eosinophilic granuloma.
Other: facial nerve neuroma, teratoma, rhabdomyoma, rhabdomyosarcoma, branchial cleft cyst.

HEARING IMPAIRMENT AND DEAFNESS[20]

ICD-10CM #   Varies with specific diagnosis

Congenital.
Aplasia of inner ear.
Michel defect.
Mondini defect.
Scheibe defect.
Chromosome disorders.
Trisomy 13.
Trisomy 18.
18q syndrome.
Genetic disorders.
Isolated deafness.
Pendred syndrome.
Usher syndrome.
Waardenburg syndrome.
Intrauterine viral infection.
Maternal drug use.
Drugs.
Antibiotics.
β-Blockers.
Chemotherapy.
Genetic neurologic disorders.
Familial spastic paraplegia.
Hereditary motor sensory neuropathies.
Hereditary sensory autonomic neuropathies.
Infantile Refsum disease.
Neurofibromatosis type 2.
Pontobulbar palsy with deafness.
Mitochondrial disorders.
Spinocerebellar degenerations.
Wolfram syndrome.
Xeroderma pigmentosum.
Infectious diseases.
Bacterial meningitis.[a]
Otitis media.[a]
Sarcoidosis.[a]
Viral encephalitis.
Viral exanthemas.

[a]Denotes the most common conditions and the ones with disease-modifying treatments.

Differential Diagnosis

II

Metabolic disorders.
 Hypothyroidism.*
 Ménière disease.
Skeletal disorders.
 Apert acrocephalosyndactyly.
 Cleidocranial dysostosis.
 Craniofacial dysostosis (Crouzon disease).
 Craniometaphyseal dysplasia (Pyle disease).
 Klippel-Feil syndrome.
 Mandibulofacial dysostosis (Treacher-Collins
  syndrome).
 Osteogenesis imperfecta.
 Osteopetrosis (Albers-Schönberg disease).
Susac syndrome.
Trauma.
Tumor.
 Acoustic neuroma.*
 Cholesteatoma.*

HEARING LOSS, ACUTE[1]

ICD-10CM # H91.23 Sudden idiopathic
        hearing loss, bilateral

Infectious: mumps, measles, influenza, herpes
 simplex, herpes zoster, CMV, mononucleosis,
 syphilis.
Vascular: macroglobulinemia, sickle cell disease,
 Berger disease, leukemia, polycythemia, fat
 emboli, hypercoagulable states.
Metabolic: diabetes, pregnancy,
 hyperlipoproteinemia.
Conductive: cerumen impaction, foreign bodies,
 otitis media, otitis externa, barotrauma,
 trauma.
Medications: aminoglycosides, loop diuretics,
 antineoplastics, salicylates, vancomycin.
Neoplasm: acoustic neuroma, metastatic
 neoplasm.

HEARTBURN AND INDIGESTION[76]

ICD-10CM # R12 Heartburn
        K30 Functional dyspepsia

Reflux esophagitis.
Gastritis.
Nonulcer dyspepsia.
Functional GI disorder (anxiety disorder, social/
 environmental stresses).
Excessive intestinal gas (ingestion of flatulogenic
 foods, GI stasis, constipation).
Gas entrapment (hepatitis or splenic flexure
 syndrome).
Neoplasm (adenocarcinoma of stomach or
 esophagus, lymphoma).
Gallbladder disease.

HEART DISEASE, TRAUMATIC CAUSES[86]

ICD-10CM # S26.020 Mild laceration of heart
         with hemopericardium

S26.021	Moderate laceration of heart with hemopericardium
S26.022	Major laceration of heart with hemopericardium

Penetrating:
 Stab wounds: knives, swords, ice picks, fence
  posts, wire, sports.
 Projectile wounds: handguns, rifles, nail guns,
  lawnmower projectiles.
 Shotgun wounds: pellets, close-range versus
  distant.
Nonpenetrating (blunt):
 Motor vehicle accident:
  Seat belt.
  Air bag.
  Dashboard/steering wheel.
Vehicular-pedestrian accident.
Falls from a height.
Crushing: industrial accident.
Blasts: improvised explosive devices, grenades,
 fragments (combined blunt/penetrating).
Assault.
Sternal or rib fractures.
Recreational: sporting events (e.g., rodeo,
 baseball).

HEART FAILURE WITH PRESERVED LEFT VENTRICULAR EJECTION FRACTION[59]

ICD-10CM # I50.9 Heart failure, unspecified

CAUSES OF (AND ALTERNATIVE EXPLANATIONS FOR) HEART FAILURE WITH PRESERVED LEFT VENTRICULAR EJECTION FRACTION (>45% TO 50%)

Inaccurate diagnosis of heart failure (e.g., pul-
 monary disease, obesity).
Inaccurate measurements of ejection fraction.
Systolic function overestimated by ejection frac-
 tion (e.g., mitral regurgitation).
Episodic, unrecognized systolic dysfunction.
Intermittent ischemia.
Arrhythmia.
Severe hypertension.
Alcohol abuse.
Diastolic dysfunction.
Abnormalities of myocardial relaxation:
 Ischemia.
 Hypertrophy.
Abnormalities of myocardial compliance:
 Hypertrophy.
 Aging.
 Fibrosis.
 Diabetes mellitus.
 Infiltrative disease (amyloidosis, sarcoidosis).
 Storage disease (hemochromatosis).
 Endomyocardial disease (endomyocardial
  fibrosis, radiation, anthracyclines).

Pericardial disease (constriction, tamponade).

HEART FAILURE, ACUTE[43]

ICD-10CM # I50.9 Heart failure, unspecified

COMMON PRECIPITATING CAUSES OF ACUTE HF

Systemic hypertension.
Myocardial infarction or ischemia.
Dysrhythmia.
Systemic infection.
Anemia.
Dietary, physical, environmental, and emotional
 excesses.
Pregnancy.
Thyrotoxicosis or hypothyroidism.
Acute myocarditis.
Acute valvular dysfunction.
Pulmonary embolus.
Pharmacologic complications.

HEART FAILURE, CHRONIC[87]

ICD-10CM # I50.9 Heart failure, unspecified

Myocardial disease.
Coronary artery disease:
 Myocardial infarction.*
 Myocardial ischemia.
Chronic pressure overload:
 Hypertension.
 Obstructive valvular disease.
Chronic volume overload:
 Regurgitant valvular disease.
 Intracardiac (left-to-right) shunting.
 Extracardiac shunting.
Nonischemic dilated cardiomyopathy:
 Familial or genetic disorders.
 Infiltrative disorders.
 Toxic or drug-induced damage.
 Metabolic disorder.
 Viral or other infectious agents.
Disorders of rate and rhythm:
 Chronic bradyarrhythmias.
 Chronic tachyarrhythmias.
 Pulmonary heart disease
 Cor pulmonale.
 Pulmonary vascular disorders.
High-output states.
Metabolic disorders:
 Thyrotoxicosis.
 Nutritional disorders (beriberi).
Excessive blood flow requirements:
 Systemic arteriovenous shunting.
 Chronic anemia.

---

*Indicates conditions that can also lead to HF with a
 preserved EF.

HEART FAILURE, CONGENITAL HEART DISEASE CAUSES[88]

ICD-10CM # I50.9   Heart failure, unspecified

CAUSES OF CONGESTIVE HEART FAILURE RESULTING FROM CONGENITAL HEART DISEASE

Age of Onset	Cause

At birth:	HLHS.
	Volume overload lesions:
	  severe tricuspid or pulmonary insufficiency.
	  Large systemic arteriovenous fistula.

First week:	TGA. PDA in small premature infants. HLHS (with more favorable anatomy). TAPVR, particularly those with pulmonary venous obstruction. Others. Systemic arteriovenous fistula. Critical AS or PS.
1 to 4 wk:	COA with associated anomalies. Critical AS. Large left-to-right shunt lesions (VSD, PDA) in premature infants. All other lesions previously listed.
4 to 6 wk:	Some left-to-right shunt lesions such as ECD.
6 wk to 4 mo:	Large VSD. Large PDA. Others, such as anomalous left coronary artery from the PA.

AS, Aortic stenosis; *COA*, coarctation of the aorta; *ECD*, endocardial cushion defect; *HLHS*, hypoplastic left heart syndrome; *PA*, pulmonary artery; *PDA*, patent ductus arteriosus; *PS*, pulmonary stenosis; *TAPVR*, total anomalous pulmonary venous return; *TGA*, transposition of the great arteries; *VSD*, ventricular septal defect.

HEART FAILURE, PATHOGENIC CAUSES[59]

ICD-10CM # I50.9   Heart failure, unspecified

IMPAIRED SYSTOLIC (CONTRACTILE) FUNCTION

Ischemic damage or dysfunction:
  Myocardial infarction.
  Persistent or intermittent myocardial ischemia.
  Hypoperfusion (shock).
Chronic pressure overloading:
  Hypertension.
  Obstructive valvular disease.
Chronic volume overload:
  Regurgitant valvular disease.

Intracardiac left-to-right shunting.
Extracardiac shunting.
Nonischemic dilated cardiomyopathy:
  Familial/genetic disorders.
  Toxic/drug-induced damage
  Immunologically mediated necrosis.
  Infectious agents.
  Metabolic disorders.
  Infiltrative processes.
  Idiopathic conditions.

IMPAIRED DIASTOLIC FUNCTION (RESTRICTED FILLING, INCREASED STIFFNESS)

Pathologic myocardial hypertrophy:
  Primary (hypertrophic cardiomyopathies).
  Secondary (hypertension).
  Aging.
  Ischemic fibrosis.
  Restrictive cardiomyopathy:
    Infiltrative disorders (amyloidosis, sarcoidosis).
    Storage diseases (hemochromatosis, genetic abnormalities).
Endomyocardial disorders.

MECHANICAL ABNORMALITIES

Intracardiac:
  Obstructive valvular disease.
  Regurgitant valvular disease.
  Intracardiac shunts.
  Other congenital abnormalities.
Extracardiac:
  Obstructive (coarctation, supravalvular aortic stenosis).
  Left-to-right shunting (patent ductus arteriosus).

DISORDERS OF RATE AND RHYTHM

Bradyarrhythmias (sinus node dysfunction, conduction abnormalities).
Tachyarrhythmias (ineffective rhythms, chronic tachycardia).

PULMONARY HEART DISEASE

Cor pulmonale.
Pulmonary vascular disorders.

HIGH-OUTPUT STATES

Metabolic disorders:
  Thyrotoxicosis.
  Nutritional disorders (beriberi).
  Excessive blood flow requirements:
    Chronic anemia.
    Systemic arteriovenous shunting.

HEART FAILURE, PREGNANCY

ICD-10CM # I50.9   Heart failure, unspecified

Congenital valvular heart disease exacerbated by pregnancy.
Peripartum cardiomyopathy.

Untreated thyrotoxicosis.
Hypothyroidism.
Pulmonary hypertension.
Myocardial infarction.

HEAT STROKE[29]

ICD-10CM # T67.0   Heatstroke and sunstroke

Sepsis.
Encephalitis.
Meningitis.
Brain abscess.
Malaria (cerebral falciparum).
Typhoid fever.
Tetanus.
Alcohol withdrawal syndrome.
Neuroleptic malignant syndrome.
Anticholinergic toxicity.
Salicylate toxicity.
Phencyclidine hydrochloride (PCP), cocaine, or amphetamine toxicity.
Status epilepticus.
Cerebral hemorrhage.
Diabetic ketoacidosis.
Thyroid storm.

HEEL PAIN

ICD-10CM # M25.50   Pain in unspecified joint

Achilles tendonitis/tendinopathy (insertional, noninsertional).
Retrocalcaneal bursitis (superficial, deep).
Plantar fasciopathy.
Neuropathy (tarsal tunnel, posterior tibial nerve [medial calcaneal branch], abductor digiti quinti).
Calcaneal stress fracture.
Puncture wound, foreign body.
Cellulitis.
Spondyloarthropathy.
Fat pad atrophy.
Soft tissue tumor.
S1 radiculopathy.
Paget disease of bone.
Haglund deformity.
Primary or metastatic bone tumor.

HEEL PAIN, PLANTAR

ICD-10CM # M79.609   Pain in unspecified limb

SKIN

Keratoses.
Verruca.
Ulcer.
Fissure.

CONNECTIVE TISSUE

Fat
Atrophy.
Panniculitis.
Dense Connective Tissue
Inflammatory fasciitis.
Fibromatosis.

Enthesopathy.
Bursitis.
Bone (Calcaneus)
Stress fracture.
Paget disease.
Benign bone cyst/tumor.
Malignant bone tumor.
Metabolic bone disease (osteopenia).
Nerve
Tarsal tunnel.
Plantar nerve entrapment.
S1 nerve root radiculopathy.
Painful peripheral neuropathy.

INFECTION
Dermatomycoses.
Acute osteomyelitis.
Plantar abscess.

MISCELLANEOUS
Foreign body.
Nonunion calcaneus fracture.
Psychogenic.
Idiopathic.

HEMARTHROSIS
ICD-10CM # T14.90 Injury, unspecified

Trauma.
Anticoagulant therapy.
Thrombocytopenia, thrombocytosis.
Bleeding disorders (e.g., von Willebrand disease).
Charcot joint.
Idiopathic.
Other: pigmented villonodular synovitis, hemangioma, synovioma, AV fistula, ruptured aneurysm.

HEMATEMESIS[2]
ICD-10CM # K92.0 Hematemesis

CAUSES OF HEMATEMESIS
Very Common
Gastric or duodenal ulcer or erosions.
Common
Mallory-Weiss tear (a laceration at the gastro-esophageal junction).
Ulcerative esophagitis.
Esophageal varices.
Uncommon
Vascular malformations.
Ulcerated GI stromal tumor.
Carcinoma of esophagus or stomach.
Aortoenteric fistula.

HEMATURIA
ICD-10CM # R31.9 Hematuria, unspecified

Use the mnemonic TICS:
T (Trauma): blow to kidney, insertion of Foley catheter or foreign body in urethra, prolonged and severe exercise, very rapid emptying of overdistended bladder. (Tumor): hypernephroma, Wilms tumor, papillary carcinoma of the bladder, prostatic and urethral neoplasms. (Toxins): turpentine, phenols, sulfonamides and other antibiotics, cyclophosphamide, NSAIDs.
I (Infections): glomerulonephritis, TB, cystitis, prostatitis, urethritis, *Schistosoma haematobium,* yellow fever, blackwater fever. (Inflammatory processes): Goodpasture syndrome, periarteritis, postirradiation.
C (Calculi): renal, ureteral, bladder, urethra. (Cysts): simple cysts, polycystic disease. (Congenital anomalies): hemangiomas, aneurysms, AVM.
S (Surgery): invasive procedures, prostatic resection, cystoscopy. (Sickle cell disease and other hematologic disturbances): hemophilia, thrombocytopenia, anticoagulants. (Somewhere else): bleeding genitals, factitious (drug addicts).

HEMATURIA, DIFFERENTIAL BASED ON AGE AND SEX
ICD-10CM # R31.9 Hematuria, unspecified

0 TO 20 YR
Acute urinary tract infections.
Acute glomerulonephritis.
Congenital urinary tract anomalies with obstruction.
Trauma to genitals.

20 TO 40 YR
Acute urinary tract infection.
Trauma to genitals.
Urolithiasis.
Bladder cancer.

40 TO 60 YR (WOMEN)
Acute urinary tract infection.
Bladder cancer.
Urolithiasis.

40 TO 60 YR (MEN)
Acute urinary tract infection.
Bladder cancer.
Urolithiasis.

60 YR AND OLDER (WOMEN)
Acute urinary tract infection.
Bladder cancer.
Vaginal trauma or irritation.
Urolithiasis.

60 YR AND OLDER (MEN)
Acute urinary tract infection.
Benign prostatic hyperplasia.
Bladder cancer.
Urolithiasis.
Trauma.

HEMATURIA, IN CHILDREN[43]
ICD-10CM # R31.9 Hematuria, unspecified

EXTRARENAL
Trauma.
Meatal stenosis or posterior urethral valves.
Exercise.
Menstruation or rectal bleeding.
Foreign bodies.
Cystitis, urethritis, or epididymitis.

INTRARENAL
Pyelonephritis.
Renal or bladder stones or tumors.
Poststreptococcal or idiopathic glomerulonephritis.
Acute interstitial nephritis.
Acute tubular necrosis.
Basement membrane glomerular disease.
Renal vein or arterial thrombosis.
Recurrent familial hematuria.
Polycystic kidney disease.

SYSTEMIC
Henoch-Schönlein purpura.
Systemic lupus erythematosus.
Hemolytic-uremic syndrome.
Infectious mononucleosis.
Sickle cell disease or other hemoglobinopathies.
Bacterial endocarditis or artificial cardiac valves.
Bleeding disorders, warfarin, or aspirin.
Medications such as amitriptyline or chlorpromazine, radiocontrast dyes.
Munchausen syndrome or factitious.

HEMIBALLISM[38]
ICD-10CM # G25.5 Other chorea

ETIOLOGY
Structural Lesions
Cerebrovascular Disease
Infarction.
Transient ischemic attack.
Hemorrhage.
Arteriovenous malformation.
Subarachnoid hemorrhage.
Subclavian steal syndrome.
Infection
Syphilis.
Tuberculoma.
Toxoplasmosis.
Acquired immunodeficiency syndrome.
Influenza A.
Tumor
Pituitary microadenoma.
Metastasis.
Immune-Mediated
Systemic lupus erythematosus.
Sydenham chorea.
Behçet disease.
Scleroderma.

Other
Static encephalopathy.
Head injury.
Demyelinating disease.
Thalamotomy.
Heredodegenerative disease.
Metabolic
Nonketotic hyperosmolar hyperglycemia.
Drug-Induced
Phenytoin and other anticonvulsants.
Oral contraceptives.
Neuroleptics (tardive).

HEMIPLEGIA, ACUTE[20]

ICD-10CM # Varies with specific diagnosis

Alternating hemiplegia.
Asthmatic amyotrophy.
Cerebrovascular disease.[a]
Diabetes mellitus.
Epilepsy.
Hypoglycemia.
Kawasaki disease.
Migraine.[a]
Trauma.
Tumor.[a]

[a]Denotes the most common conditions and the ones with disease-modifying treatments.

HEMIPLEGIA, PROGRESSIVE[20]

ICD-10CM # Varies with specific diagnosis

Adrenoleukodystrophy.
Arteriovenous malformation.
Brain abscess.
Cerebral hemisphere tumor.
Demyelinating diseases.
Late-onset globoid leukodystrophy.
Multiple sclerosis.
Sturge-Weber syndrome.

HEMIPARESIS/HEMIPLEGIA

| ICD-10CM # | G81.00 | Flaccid hemiplegia affecting unspecified side |
| | G81.10 | Spastic hemiplegia affecting unspecified side |

CVA.
Transient ischemic attack.
Cerebral neoplasm.
Multiple sclerosis or other demyelinating disorder.
CNS infection.
Migraine.
Hypoglycemia
Subdural hematoma.
Vasculitis.
Todd paralysis.
Epidural hematoma.
Metabolic (hyperosmolar state, electrolyte imbalance).

Psychiatric disorders.
Congenital disorders.
Leukodystrophies.

HEMOLYSIS AND HEMOGLOBINURIA

ICD-10CM #	P55.8	Other hemolytic diseases of newborn
	P55.9	Hemolytic disease of newborn, unspecified
	R82.3	Hemoglobinuria

Erythrocyte trauma (prosthetic cardiac valves, marching and severe trauma, extensive burns).
Infections (malaria, Bartonella, Clostridium welchii).
Brown recluse spider bite.
Incompatible blood transfusions.
Hemolytic-uremic syndrome.
Thrombotic thrombocytopenic purpura (TTP).
Paroxysmal nocturnal hemoglobinuria (PNH).
Drugs (penicillins, quinidine, methyldopa, sulfonamides, nitrofurantoin).
Erythrocyte enzyme deficiencies (e.g., exposure to fava beans in patients with glucose-6-phosphate dehydrogenase deficiency).

HEMOLYSIS, INTRAVASCULAR

| ICD-10CM # | D59.6 | Hemoglobinuria due to hemolysis from other external causes |
| | D59.8 | Other acquired hemolytic anemias |

Infections.
Exertional hemolysis (e.g., prolonged march).
Valve hemolysis.
Microangiopathic hemolytic anemia.
Osmotic and chemical agents.
Thermal injury.
Cold agglutinins.
Venoms (snakes, spiders).
Paroxysmal nocturnal hemoglobinuria (PNH).

HEMOLYSIS, MECHANICAL

| ICD-10CM # | D59.4 | Other nonautoimmune hemolytic anemias |

Prosthetic heart valves.
Aortic stenosis.
Malignant hypertension.
Metastatic adenocarcinoma.
Traumatic exercise.
Renal transplants.
Renal cortical necrosis.
Glomerulonephritis.
Thrombotic thrombocytopenic purpura (TTP), hemolytic-uremic syndrome (HUS).
Renal vasculitis.
Scleroderma.
Diabetes mellitus.

HEMOLYSIS, OXIDATIVE, DRUG-INDUCED[71]

| ICD-10CM # | D59 | Acquired hemolytic anemia |
| | D59.1 | Other autoimmune hemolytic anemias |

AGENTS THAT CAUSE OXIDATIVE HEMOLYSIS
Therapeutic Agents
Nitrofurantoin (Furadantin).
Sulfasalazine (Azulfidine).
p-Aminosalicylic acid.
Phenazopyridine (Pyridium).
Cotrimoxazole.
Quinolones.
Phenacetin.
Rasburicase.
Dapsone and other sulfones.
Primaquine.
Recreational Drugs
Isobutyl nitrate.
Amyl nitrite.
Miscellaneous Agents
Naphthalene mothballs.
Methylene blue.
Paraquat.
Hydrogen peroxide.

HEMOPERITONEUM

| ICD-10CM # | K66.1 | Hemoperitoneum |

Ruptured Graafian follicle.
Ruptured spleen.
Ectopic pregnancy.
Traumatic laceration of liver.
Ruptured aneurysm.
Ruptured bladder.
Traumatic laceration of bowel, pancreas, uterus.

HEMOPTYSIS

| ICD-10CM # | R04.2 | Hemoptysis |

CARDIOVASCULAR
Pulmonary embolism/infarction.
Left ventricular failure.
Mitral stenosis.
AV fistula.
Severe hypertension.
Erosion of aortic aneurysm.

PULMONARY
Neoplasm (primary or metastatic).
Infection.
Pneumonia: Streptococcus pneumoniae, Klebsiella pneumoniae, Staphylococcus aureus, Legionella pneumophila.
Bronchiectasis.
Abscess.
TB.
Bronchitis.

Differential Diagnosis

II

Fungal infections (aspergillosis, coccidioidomycosis).

Parasitic infections (amebiasis, ascariasis, paragonimiasis).

Vasculitis: granulomatosis with polyangiitis, Churg-Strauss syndrome, Henoch-Schönlein purpura.

Goodpasture syndrome.

Trauma (needle biopsy, foreign body, right-sided heart catheterization, prolonged and severe cough).

Cystic fibrosis, bullous emphysema.

Pulmonary sequestration.

Pulmonary AV fistula.

SLE.

Idiopathic pulmonary hemosiderosis.

Drugs: aspirin, anticoagulants, penicillamine.

Pulmonary hypertension.

Mediastinal fibrosis.

OTHER

Epistaxis, trauma.

Laryngeal bleeding (laryngitis, laryngeal neoplasm).

Hematologic disorders (clotting abnormalities, DIC, thrombocytopenia).

HEMOPTYSIS/PULMONARY HEMORRHAGE[20]

ICD-10CM # R04.2 Hemoptysis

CARDIOVASCULAR DISORDERS

Heart failure with pulmonary edema.

Pulmonary hypertension with Eisenmenger syndrome.

Mitral stenosis.

Venoocclusive disease.

Arteriovenous malformation (Osler-Weber-Rendu syndrome).

Pulmonary embolism.

Portal vein obstruction.

PULMONARY DISORDERS

Bronchogenic cyst.

Bronchopulmonary sequestration.

Pneumonia (bacterial, mycobacterial, fungal, parasitic, or viral).

Bronchiectasis (cystic fibrosis, primary ciliary dyskinesia, immunodeficiency, retained foreign body).

Tracheobronchitis.

Lung abscess.

Tumor (adenoma, carcinoid, hemangioma, metastasis).

Trauma (contusion, laceration).

IMMUNE DISORDERS

Henoch-Schönlein purpura.

Pulmonary capillaritis.

Idiopathic pulmonary hemosiderosis.

Anti–glomerular basement membrane disease (Goodpasture disease).

Granulomatosis with polyangiitis (formerly known as Wegener granulomatosis).

Systemic lupus erythematosus.

Polyarteritis nodosa.

OTHER CONDITIONS/FACTORS

Coagulopathy (Von Willebrand factor).

Toxic inhalation (nitrogen dioxide, pesticides, crack cocaine).

Post–bone marrow transplantation.

Catamenial hemoptysis (females).

HEMORRHAGIC CYSTITIS[89]

ICD-10CM # N39.0 Urinary tract infection

DIFFERENTIAL DIAGNOSIS FOR HEMORRHAGIC CYSTITIS[27]

Infectious.*

Bacterial.

Viral (especially BK virus, adenovirus).

Fungal.

Parasitic.

Trauma:

External.

Postsurgical (e.g., transurethral resection of the bladder).

Malignancy:

Bladder primary.

Bladder invasion from local/distant primary.

Vascular malformation.

Chemical exposure:

Cyclophosphamide.

Ifosfamide.

Busulfan.

Thiotepa.

Temozolomide.

Aniline dye.

Ether.

Nonoxynol-9 (accidental urethral insertion of vaginal contraceptive).

Radiation therapy history (e.g., prostate cancer, cervical cancer).

Medication induced:

Penicillin and derivatives (via immune reaction).

Bleomycin.

Danazol.

Tiaprofenic.

Allopurinol.

Phensuximide.

Methenamine mandelate.

Acetic acid.

Manifestation of systemic disease:

Amyloidosis.

Rheumatoid arthritis.

Crohn disease.

---

*Bleeding localized to bladder after diagnostic workup for gross hematuria with cystoscopy, urine cytology, and upper tract imaging is without clear cause of alternative bleeding source.

HEPATIC CYSTS[17]

ICD-10CM # Q44.6 Cystic disease of liver
B67.8 Echinococcosis, unspecified, of liver

CONGENITAL HEPATIC CYSTS

Parenchymal: solitary cyst, polycystic disease.

Ductal: localized dilation, multiple cystic dilatations of intrahepatic ducts (Caroli disease).

ACQUIRED HEPATIC CYSTS

Inflammatory cysts: retention cysts, echinococcal cyst, amebic cyst.

Neoplastic cyst.

Peliosis hepatis.

HEPATIC DYSFUNCTION, POSTOPERATIVE[3]

ICD-10CM # K91.82 Postprocedural hepatic failure

CAUSES OF POSTOPERATIVE HEPATIC DYSFUNCTION

Hepatocellular Injury (predominant serum ALT elevation, with or without hyperbilirubinemia)

Acute transfusion-associated viral hepatitis.

Hepatic allograft rejection.

Hepatic artery thrombosis.

Inhalational anesthetics: halothane, others.

Ischemic hepatitis (shock liver).

Other drugs: antihypertensives (e.g., labetalol), heparin.

Unrecognized chronic liver disease: NASH, hepatitis C, other disorders.

Cholestatic Jaundice (elevated serum alkaline phosphatase ± ALT; direct hyperbilirubinemia)

Acalculous cholecystitis.

Benign postoperative cholestasis.

Bile duct injury: after cholecystectomy or liver transplantation.

Bile duct obstruction: gallstones, pancreatitis.

Cardiac bypass of prolonged duration.

Cholangitis.

Drugs: amoxicillin-clavulanic acid, chlorpromazine, erythromycin, telithromycin, trimethoprim/sulfamethoxazole, warfarin, others.

Hemobilia.

Microlithiasis (biliary sludge).

Prolonged TPN.

Sepsis.

Indirect Hyperbilirubinemia (serum alkaline phosphatase and ALT often normal)

Gilbert syndrome.

Hemolytic anemia (G6PD deficiency, other causes).

Multiple transfusions.

Resorbing hematoma.

G6PD, Glucose-6-phosphate dehydrogenase; *NASH,* nonalcoholic steatohepatitis.

HEPATIC GRANULOMAS[18]

ICD-10CM # K75.3 Granulomatous hepatitis

INFECTIONS

Bacterial, spirochetal: TB and atypical mycobacterial infections, tularemia, brucellosis, leprosy, syphilis, Whipple disease, listeriosis.

Viral: mononucleosis, CMV.

Rickettsial: Q fever.

Fungal: coccidioidomycosis, histoplasmosis, cryptococcal infections, actinomycosis, aspergillosis, nocardiosis.

Parasitic: schistosomiasis, clonorchiasis, toxocariasis, ascariasis, toxoplasmosis, amebiasis.

HEPATOBILIARY DISORDERS

Primary biliary cirrhosis, granulomatous hepatitis, jejunoileal bypass.

SYSTEMIC DISORDERS

Sarcoidosis, granulomatosis with polyangiitis, inflammatory bowel disease, Hodgkin disease, lymphoma.

DRUGS/TOXINS

Beryllium, parenteral foreign material (starch, talc, silicone, etc.), phenylbutazone, α-methyldopa, procainamide, allopurinol, phenytoin, nitrofurantoin, hydralazine.

HEPATITIS, ACUTE[1]

ICD-10CM #	B17.8	Acute viral hepatitis, unspecified
	B15	Acute hepatitis A
	B16	Acute hepatitis B
	B17.1	Acute hepatitis C
	B17.2	Acute hepatitis E

Infectious:
  Hepatitis A, B, C, D, E.
  Epstein-Barr virus.
  Cytomegalovirus.
  Herpes simplex virus.
  Yellow fever.
  Leptospirosis.
  Q fever.
  HIV.
  Brucellosis.
  Lyme disease.
  Syphilis.
Noninfectious:
  Drug induced.
  Autoimmune.
  Ischemic.
  Acute fatty liver of pregnancy.
  Acute Budd-Chiari syndrome.
  Wilson disease.

HEPATITIS, CHRONIC[1]

ICD-10CM #	K73.9	Chronic hepatitis, unspecified
	B18.0	Chronic viral hepatitis B with δ-agent
	B18.2	Chronic viral hepatitis C

Chronic viral hepatitis:
  Hepatitis B.
  Hepatitis C.
  Hepatitis D.
Autoimmune hepatitis and variant syndromes.
Hereditary hemochromatosis.

Wilson disease.
α_1-Antitrypsin deficiency.
Fatty liver and nonalcoholic steatohepatitis.
Alcoholic liver disease.
Drug-induced liver disease.
Hepatic granulomas:
  Infectious.
  Drug induced.
  Neoplastic.
  Idiopathic.

HEPATITIS, IN CHILDREN[19]

ICD-10CM #	B17.9	Acute viral hepatitis, unspecified
	K73.9	Chronic hepatitis, unspecified

CAUSES AND DIFFERENTIAL DIAGNOSIS OF HEPATITIS IN CHILDREN

Infectious
Hepatotropic viruses:
  HAV.
  HBV.
  HCV.
  HDV.
  HEV.
  Hepatitis non–A-E viruses.
Systemic infection that can include hepatitis:
  Adenovirus.
  Arbovirus.
  Coxsackievirus.
  Cytomegalovirus.
  Enterovirus.
  Epstein-Barr virus.
  "Exotic" viruses (e.g., yellow fever).
  Herpes simplex virus.
  Human immunodeficiency virus.
  Paramyxovirus.
  Rubella.
  Varicella zoster.
Other.

Nonviral Liver Infections
Abscess.
Amebiasis.
Bacterial sepsis.
Brucellosis.
Fitz-Hugh-Curtis syndrome.
Histoplasmosis.
Leptospirosis.
Tuberculosis.
Other.

Autoimmune
Autoimmune hepatitis.
Sclerosing cholangitis.
Other (e.g., systemic lupus erythematosus, juvenile rheumatoid arthritis).

Metabolic
α_1-Antitrypsin deficiency.
Tyrosinemia.
Wilson disease.

Other.

Toxic
Iatrogenic or drug induced (e.g., acetaminophen).
Environmental (e.g., pesticides).

Anatomic
Choledochal cyst.
Biliary atresia.
Other.

Hemodynamic
Shock.
Congestive heart failure.
Budd-Chiari syndrome.
Other.

Nonalcoholic Fatty Liver Disease
Idiopathic.
Reye syndrome.
Other.

HEPATOMEGALY

ICD-10CM #	R16.0	Hepatomegaly, not elsewhere classified

FREQUENT JAUNDICE

Infectious hepatitis.
Toxic hepatitis.
Carcinoma: liver, pancreas, bile ducts, metastatic neoplasm to liver.
Cirrhosis.
Obstruction of common bile duct.
Alcoholic hepatitis.
Biliary cirrhosis.
Cholangitis.
Hemochromatosis with cirrhosis.

INFREQUENT JAUNDICE

CHF.
Amyloidosis.
Liver abscess.
Sarcoidosis.
Infectious mononucleosis.
Alcoholic fatty infiltration.
Nonalcoholic steatohepatitis.
Lymphoma.
Leukemia.
Budd-Chiari syndrome.
Myelofibrosis with myeloid metaplasia.
Familial hyperlipoproteinemia type 1.
Other: amebiasis, hydatid disease of liver, schistosomiasis, kala-azar (Leishmania donovani), Hurler syndrome, Gaucher disease, kwashiorkor.

HEPATOMEGALY, BY SHAPE OF LIVER[2]

ICD-10CM #	R16.0	Hepatomegaly, not elsewhere classified

DIFFUSELY ENLARGED AND SMOOTH

Massive
Metastatic disease.

Alcoholic liver disease with fatty infiltration.
Myeloproliferative diseases (e.g., polycythemia rubra vera, myelofibrosis).
Moderate
The above causes.
Hemochromatosis.
Hematologic disease (e.g., chronic myeloid leukemia, lymphoma).
Fatty liver (e.g., diabetes mellitus, obesity).
Infiltrative disorders (e.g., amyloid).
Mild
The above causes.
Hepatitis (viral, drugs).
Cirrhosis.
Biliary obstruction.
Granulomatous disorders (e.g., sarcoid).
HIV infection.

DIFFUSELY ENLARGED AND IRREGULAR

Metastatic disease.
Cirrhosis.
Hydatid disease.
Polycystic liver disease.

LOCALIZED SWELLINGS

Riedel lobe (a normal variant—the lobe may be palpable in the right lumbar region).
Metastasis.
Large simple hepatic cyst.
Hydatid cyst.
Hepatoma.
Liver abscess (e.g., amebic abscess).

HERMAPHRODITISM[45]

| ICD-10CM # | Q56.3 | Pseudohermaphroditism, unspecified |
| | Q56.4 | Indeterminate sex, unspecified |

Female Pseudohermaphroditism
  Androgen exposure:
    Fetal source:
    21-Hydroxylase (P450 c21) deficiency.
    11β-Hydroxylase (P450 c11) deficiency.
    3β-Hydroxysteroid dehydrogenase II (3β-HSD II) deficiency.
    Aromatase (P450arom) deficiency.
    Maternal source.
    Virilizing ovarian tumor.
    Virilizing adrenal tumor.
    Androgenic drugs.
  Undetermined origin:
    Associated with genitourinary and GI tract defects.

MALE PSEUDOHERMAPHRODITISM

Defects in testicular differentiation:
  Denys-Drash syndrome (mutation in WT1 gene).
  WAGR syndrome (Wilms tumor, aniridia, genitourinary malformation, retardation).
  Deletion of 11p13.

Camptomelic syndrome (autosomal gene at 17q24.3-q25.1) and SOX 9 mutation.
XY pure gonadal dysgenesis (Swyer syndrome).
Mutation in SRY gene.
Unknown cause.
XY gonadal agenesis.
Deficiency of testicular hormones:
  Leydig cell aplasia.
  Mutation in LH receptor.
  Lipoid adrenal hyperplasia (P450 scc) deficiency; mutation in StAR (steroidogenic acute regulatory protein).
  3α-HSD II deficiency.
  17-Hydroxylase/17, 20-lyase (P450 c17) deficiency.
  Persistent Müllerian duct syndrome.
  Gene mutations, Müllerian-inhibiting substance (MIS).
  Receptor defects for MIS.
Defect in androgen action:
  5α-Reductase II mutations.
  Androgen receptor defects:
    Complete androgen insensitivity syndrome.
    Partial androgen insensitivity syndrome.
    Reifenstein and other syndromes.
    Smith-Lemli-Opitz syndrome.
Defect in conversion of 7-dehydrocholesterol to cholesterol.

TRUE HERMAPHRODITISM

XX.
XY.
XX/XY chimeras.

HERNIATION SYNDROMES[20]

| ICD-10CM # | Varies with specific diagnosis |

UNILATERAL (UNCAL) TRANSTENTORIAL HERNIATION

Declining consciousness.
Increased blood pressure, slow pulse.
Dilated and fixed pupils.
Homonymous hemianopia.
Respiratory irregularity.
Decerebrate rigidity.

BILATERAL (CENTRAL) TRANSTENTORIAL HERNIATION

Decerebrate or decorticate rigidity.
Declining consciousness.
Impaired upward gaze.
Irregular respiration.
Pupillary constriction or dilation.

CEREBELLAR (DOWNWARD) HERNIATION

Declining consciousness.
Impaired upward gaze.
Irregular respirations.
Lower cranial nerve palsies.
Neck stiffness or head tilt.

HICCUPS[26]

| ICD-10CM # | R06.6 | Hiccough |

TRANSIENT HICCUPS

Sudden excitement, emotion.
Gastric distention.
Esophageal obstruction.
Alcohol ingestion.
Sudden change in temperature.

PERSISTENT OR CHRONIC HICCUPS

Toxic/metabolic: uremia, DM, hyperventilation, hypocalcemia, hypokalemia, hyponatremia, gout, fever.
Drugs: benzodiazepines, steroids, α-methyldopa, barbiturates.
Surgery/general anesthesia.
Thoracic/diaphragmatic disorders: pneumonia, lung cancer, asthma, pleuritis, pericarditis, myocardial infarction, aortic aneurysm, esophagitis, esophageal obstruction, diaphragmatic hernia or irritation.
Abdominal disorders: gastric ulcer or cancer, hepatobiliary or pancreatic disease, IBD, bowel obstruction, intraabdominal or subphrenic abscess, prostatic infection or cancer.
CNS disorders: traumatic, infectious, vascular, structural.
Ear, nose, and throat disorders: pharyngitis, laryngitis, tumor, irritation of auditory canal.
Psychogenic disorders.
Idiopathic disorders.

HILAR AND MEDIASTINAL LYMPH NODE ENLARGEMENT[59]

| ICD-10CM # | R59.0 | Mediastinal adenopathy |

DISORDERS ASSOCIATED WITH HILAR AND MEDIASTINAL LYMPH NODE ENLARGEMENT

Sarcoidosis.
Lymphoma.
Fungal disease.
Tuberculosis.
Metastatic cancer.
Silicosis, coal worker's pneumoconiosis, beryllium lung.

HIP PAIN, CHILDREN[1]

ICD-10CM #	S79.819A	Other specified injuries of unspecified hip, initial encounter
	S79.829A	Other specified injuries of unspecified thigh, initial encounter
	S79.919A	Unspecified injury of unspecified hip, initial encounter

TRAUMA
Hip or pelvis fractures.
Overuse injuries.

INFECTION
Septic arthritis.
Osteomyelitis.

INFLAMMATION
Transient synovitis.
Juvenile RA.
Rheumatic fever.

NEOPLASM
Leukemia.
Osteogenic or Ewing sarcoma.
Metastatic disease.

HEMATOLOGIC DISORDERS
Hemophilia.
Sickle cell anemia.

MISCELLANEOUS
Legg-Calvé-Perthes disease.
Slipped capital femoral epiphysis.

HIP PAIN, DIFFERENTIAL DIAGNOSIS[90]

ICD-10CM #   M25.559   Pain in unspecified hip

ARTICULAR

Inflammatory Joint Disease
Rheumatoid arthritis.
Spondyloarthropathies.
Polymyalgia rheumatica.

Degenerative Joint Disease
Primary osteoarthritis.
Secondary osteoarthritis.

Metabolic Joint Diseases
Gout.
Pseudogout.
Ochronosis.
Hemochromatosis.
Wilson disease.
Acromegaly.

Femoroacetabular Impingement
Acetabular Labral Tear
   Infections.
   Tumors.
Benign:
   Pigmented villonodular sclerosis.
   Osteochondromatosis.
Malignant:
   Synovial sarcoma.
   Synovial metastasis.

Hemarthrosis in children
Toxic synovitis.
Juvenile chronic arthritis.

REFERRED PAIN
Thoracolumbar spine:
   Intraabdominal structures.

Retroperitoneal structures.

PERIARTICULAR
Bursitis:
   Trochanteric.
   Iliopsoas.
   Ischiogluteal.
Tendinitis:
   Trochanteric.
   Adductor.
Acute calciflc periarthritis.
Heterotropic ossification.

OSSEOUS
Bone lesions.
Fractures.
Neoplasms.
Infection.
Osteonecrosis of the femoral head.
Paget disease.
Metabolic bone disease.
Stress fracture.
Transient osteoporosis.
In children:
   Congenital dislocation of the hip.
   Acetabular dysplasia.
   Coxa vara.
   Slipped capital femoral epiphysis.
   Legg-Calvé-Perthes disease.
   Rickets.

NEUROLOGIC
Entrapment neuropathies.
Lateral femoral cutaneous nerve (meralgia paresthetica).
Lumbar nerve root compression.
L2, L3, and L4.

VASCULAR
Atherosclerosis of aorta, iliac vessels.

HIP PAIN, IN DIFFERENT AGE GROUPS[41]

ICD-10CM #   M25.559   Pain in unspecified hip

COMMON CAUSES OF HIP PAIN IN DIFFERENT AGE GROUPS
Childhood (2 to 10 yr)
Intraarticular
Developmental dislocation of the hip.
Perthes disease.
Irritable hip.
Rickets.

Periarticular
Osteomyelitis.

Referred
Abdominal.
Adolescence (10 to 18 yr)
Intraarticular
Slipped upper femoral epiphysis.
Torn labrum.

Periarticular
Trochanteric bursitis.
Snapping hip.
Osteomyelitis.
Tumors.

Referred
Abdominal.
Lumbar spine.
Early Adulthood (18 to 30 yr)
Intraarticular
Inflammatory arthritis.
Torn labrum.

Periarticular
Bursitis.

Referred
Abdominal.
Lumbar spine.
Adulthood (30 to 50 yr)
Intraarticular
Osteoarthritis.
Inflammatory arthritis.
Osteonecrosis.
Transient osteoporosis.

Periarticular
Bursitis.

Referred
Abdominal.
Lumbar spine.
Old Age (50 yr)
Intraarticular
Osteoarthritis.
Inflammatory arthritis.

Referred
Abdominal.
Lumbar spine.

HIP PAIN WITHOUT OBVIOUS FRACTURE[43]

ICD-10CM #   R52   Pain, unspecified
            M25.559   Pain in unspecified hip

DIFFERENTIAL DIAGNOSIS OF A PAINFUL HIP WITHOUT OBVIOUS FRACTURE

Referred pain (lumbar spine, hip, or knee).
Avascular necrosis of the femoral head.
Degenerative joint disease or osteoarthritis.
Herniation of a lumbar disk.
Diskitis.
Toxic synovitis of the hip.
Septic arthritis.
Bursitis.
Tendonitis.
Ligamentous injuries of the knee or hip.
Occult fracture.
Slipped capital femoral epiphysis.
Perthes disease.
Tumor (lymphoma).
Deep venous thrombosis.
Arterial insufficiency.

Osteomyelitis.
Iliopsoas abscess.
Retroperitoneal hematoma.
Inguinal hernia.
Inguinal lymphadenopathy.
Genitourinary complaints.
Sports-related hernia.

HIRSUTISM

ICD-10CM # L68.0 Hirsutism

Idiopathic: familial, possibly increased sensitivity to androgens.
Menopause.
Polycystic ovarian syndrome.
Drugs: androgens, anabolic steroids, methyl-testosterone, minoxidil, diazoxide, phenytoin, glucocorticoids, cyclosporine.
Congenital adrenal hyperplasia.
Adrenal virilizing tumor.
Ovarian virilizing tumor: arrhenoblastoma, hilus cell tumor.
Pituitary adenoma.
Cushing syndrome.
Hypothyroidism (congenital and juvenile).
Acromegaly.
Testicular feminization.

HIV INFECTION, ANORECTAL LESIONS[1]

ICD-10CM # B20 Human immunodeficiency virus [HIV] disease
Z21 Asymptomatic human immunodeficiency virus [HIV] infection status

COMMON CONDITIONS
Anal fissure.
Abscess and fistula.
Hemorrhoids.
Pruritus ani.
Pilonidal disease.

COMMON STDS
Gonorrhea.
Chlamydia.
Herpes.
Chancroid.
Syphilis.
Condylomata acuminata.

ATYPICAL CONDITIONS
Infectious: TB, CMV, actinomycosis, *Cryptococcus.*
Neoplastic: lymphoma, Kaposi sarcoma, squamous cell carcinoma.
Other: idiopathic and ulcer.

HIV INFECTION, CHEST RADIOGRAPHIC ABNORMALITIES[1]

ICD-10CM # B20 Human immunodeficiency virus [HIV] disease

Z21 Asymptomatic human immunodeficiency virus [HIV] infection status

DIFFUSE INTERSTITIAL INFILTRATION
Pneumocystis jiroveci.
Cytomegalovirus.
Mycobacterium tuberculosis.
Mycobacterium avium complex.
Histoplasmosis.
Coccidioidomycosis.
Lymphoid interstitial pneumonitis.

FOCAL CONSOLIDATION
Bacterial pneumonia.
Mycoplasma pneumoniae.
Pneumocystis jiroveci.
Mycobacterium tuberculosis.
Mycobacterium avium complex.

NODULAR LESIONS
Kaposi sarcoma.
Mycobacterium tuberculosis.
Mycobacterium avium complex.
Fungal lesions.
Toxoplasmosis.

CAVITARY LESIONS
Pneumocystis jiroveci.
Mycobacterium tuberculosis.
Bacterial infection.

PLEURAL EFFUSION
Kaposi sarcoma.
(Small effusion may be associated with any infection).

ADENOPATHY
Kaposi sarcoma.
Lymphoma.
Mycobacterium tuberculosis.
Cryptococcus.

PNEUMOTHORAX
Kaposi sarcoma.

HIV INFECTION, COGNITIVE IMPAIRMENT[1]

ICD-10CM # B20 Human immunodeficiency virus [HIV] disease

EARLY TO MID-STAGE HIV DISEASE
Depression.
Alcohol and substance abuse.
Medication-induced cognitive impairment.
Metabolic encephalopathies.
HIV-related cognitive impairment.

ADVANCED HIV DISEASE (CD4+ <100/MM^3)
Opportunistic infection of CNS.
Neurosyphilis.
CNS lymphoma.
Progressive multifocal leukoencephalopathy.

Depression.
Metabolic encephalopathies.
Medication-induced cognitive impairment.
Stroke.
HIV dementia.

HIV INFECTION, CUTANEOUS MANIFESTATIONS[26]

ICD-10CM # B20 Human immunodeficiency virus [HIV] disease
Z21 Asymptomatic human immunodeficiency virus [HIV] infection status

BACTERIAL INFECTION
Bacillary angiomatosis: numerous angiomatous nodules associated with fever, chills, weight loss.
Staphylococcus aureus: folliculitis, ecthyma, impetigo, bullous impetigo, furuncles, carbuncles.
Syphilis: may occur in different forms (primary, secondary, tertiary); chancre may become painful because of secondary infection.

FUNGAL INFECTION
Candidiasis: mucous membranes (oral, vulvovaginal), less commonly candida intertrigo or paronychia.
Cryptococcoses: papules or nodules that strongly resemble molluscum contagiosum; other forms include pustules, purpuric papules, and vegetating plaques.
Seborrheic dermatitis: scaling and erythema in the hair-bearing areas (eyebrows, scalp, chest, and pubic area).

ARTHROPOD INFESTATIONS
Scabies: pruritus with or without rash, usually generalized but can be limited to a single digit.

VIRAL INFECTION
Herpes simplex: vesicular lesion in clusters; perianal, genital, orofacial, or digital; can be disseminated.
Herpes zoster: painful dermatomal vesicles that may ulcerate or disseminate.
HIV: discrete erythematous macules and papules on the upper trunk, palms, and soles are the most characteristic cutaneous finding of acute HIV infection.
Human papillomavirus: genital warts (may become unusually extensive).
Kaposi sarcoma (herpesvirus): erythematous macules or papules; enlarge at varying rates; violaceous nodules or plaques; occasionally painful.
Molluscum contagiosum: discrete umbilicated papules commonly on the face, neck, and intertriginous sites (axilla, groin, or buttocks).

NONINFECTIOUS
Drug reactions: more frequent and severe in HIV patients.

Nutritional deficiencies: mainly seen in children and patients with chronic diarrhea; diffuse skin manifestations, depending upon the deficiency.

Psoriasis: scaly lesions; diffuse or localized; can be associated with arthritis.

Vasculitis: palpable purpuric eruption (can resemble septic emboli).

HIV INFECTION, ESOPHAGEAL DISEASE

ICD-10CM #	B20	Human immunodeficiency virus [HIV] disease
	K21.9	Gastro-esophageal reflux disease without esophagitis

Candida infection.
Cytomegalovirus infection.
Aphthous ulcer.
Herpes simplex.

HIV INFECTION, HEPATIC DISEASE[1]

ICD-10CM #	B20	Human immunodeficiency virus [HIV] disease

VIRUSES
Hepatitis A.
Hepatitis B.
Hepatitis C.
Hepatitis D (with HBV).
Epstein-Barr virus.
Cytomegalovirus.
Herpes simplex virus.
Adenovirus.
Varicella-zoster virus.

MYCOBACTERIA
Mycobacterium avium complex.
Mycobacterium tuberculosis.

FUNGI
Histoplasma capsulatum.
Cryptococcus neoformans.
Coccidioides immitis.
Candida albicans.
Pneumocystis jiroveci.
Penicillium marneffei.

PROTOZOA
Toxoplasma gondii.
Cryptosporidium parvum.
Microsporida.
Schistosoma.

BACTERIA
Bartonella henselae (peliosis hepatis).

MALIGNANCY
Kaposi sarcoma (HHV-8).
Non-Hodgkin lymphoma.
Hepatocellular carcinoma.

MEDICATIONS
Zidovudine.
Didanosine.
Ritonavir.
Other HIV-1 protease inhibitors.
Fluconazole.
Macrolide antibiotics.
Isoniazid.
Rifampin.
Trimethoprim-sulfamethoxazole.

HIV INFECTION, LOWER GI TRACT DISEASE[1]

ICD-10CM #	B20	Human immunodeficiency virus [HIV] disease

CAUSES OF ENTEROCOLITIS
Bacteria
Campylobacter jejuni and other spp.
Salmonella spp.
Shigella flexneri.
Aeromonas hydrophila.
Plesiomonas shigelloides.
Yersinia enterocolitica.
Vibrio spp.
Mycobacterium avium complex.
Mycobacterium tuberculosis.
Escherichia coli (enterotoxigenic, enteroadherent).
Bacterial overgrowth.
Clostridium difficile (toxin).
Parasites
Cryptosporidium parvum.
Microsporidia (*Enterocytozoon bieneusi, Septata intestinalis*).
Isospora belli.
Entamoeba histolytica.
Giardia lamblia.
Cyclospora cayetanensis.
Viruses
Cytomegalovirus.
Adenovirus.
Calicivirus.
Astrovirus.
Picobirnavirus.
Human immunodeficiency virus.
Fungi
Histoplasma capsulatum.

CAUSES OF PROCTITIS
Bacteria
Chlamydia trachomatis.
Neisseria gonorrhoeae.
Treponema pallidum.
Viruses
Herpes simplex.
Cytomegalovirus.

HIV INFECTION, MUSCULOSKELETAL DISORDERS[52]

ICD-10CM #	B20	Human immunodeficiency virus [HIV] disease

MUSCULOSKELETAL DISORDERS ASSOCIATED WITH HIV INFECTION
Joints, Ligaments, and Soft Tissues
Painful articular syndrome.
HIV-associated arthritis.
Reactive arthritis.
Septic arthritis.
Psoriatic arthritis.
Diffuse infiltrative lymphocytosis syndrome.
Systemic lupus erythematosus.
Rheumatoid arthritis.
Vasculitis (polyarteritis nodosa, drug induced).
Immune reconstitution inflammatory syndrome.
Cellulitis and soft tissue abscesses.
Fasciitis (including necrotizing fasciitis).
Bursitis and tenosynovitis.
Muscles
HIV myopathy.
Nucleoside reverse transcriptase inhibitor (NRTI) myopathy.
Muscle infections (pyomyositis, toxoplasmosis).
Other (rhabdomyolysis, non-Hodgkin lymphoma, myasthenia gravis, nemaline [rod] myopathy, and inclusion body myositis).
Bones
Osteomyelitis.
Osteopenia and osteoporosis.
Osteonecrosis.
Hypertrophic osteoarthropathy.
Opportunistic Infections, HIV/AIDS-Defining Neoplastic Disorders, and Other Disorders Affecting Any Part of the Musculoskeletal System in HIV Infection
Neoplasia:
   Kaposi sarcoma.
   Non-Hodgkin lymphoma.
   Hodgkin lymphoma.
   Leiomyosarcoma.
   Ewing sarcoma.
Infection:
   Tuberculosis.
   Disseminated *Mycobacterium avium* complex infection.
   Coccidioidomycosis.
   Toxoplasmosis.
   Bacillary angiomatosis.
Other:
   HIV-related lipodystrophy.
   HIV wasting syndrome.

HIV INFECTION, OCULAR MANIFESTATIONS[17]

ICD-10CM #	B20	Human immunodeficiency virus [HIV] disease
	Z21	Asymptomatic human immunodeficiency virus [HIV] infection status

EYELIDS
Molluscum contagiosum.
Kaposi sarcoma.

CORNEA/CONJUNCTIVA
Keratoconjunctivitis sicca.

Bacterial/fungal ulcerative keratitis.
Herpes simplex.
Herpes zoster ophthalmicus.
Conjunctival microvasculopathy.
Kaposi sarcoma.

RETINA, CHOROID, AND VITREOUS

Microvasculopathy.
Endophthalmitis.
Cytomegalovirus retinitis.
Acute retinal necrosis.
Syphilis.
Toxoplasmosis.
Pneumocystis choroidopathy.
Cryptococcosis.
Mycobacterial infection.
Intraocular lymphoma.
Candidiasis.
Histoplasmosis.

DRUGS ASSOCIATED WITH OCULAR TOXICITY

Rifabutin.
Didanosine.

NEUROOPHTHALMIC

Disc edema.
Primary or secondary optic neuropathy.
Cranial nerve palsies.

ORBITAL

Lymphoma.
Infection.
Pseudotumor.

HIV INFECTION, PULMONARY DISEASE[1,42]

| ICD-10CM # | B20 | Human immunodeficiency virus [HIV] disease |
| | I28.8 | Other diseases of pulmonary vessels |

RADIOGRAPHIC APPEARANCE

Diffuse Interstitial Infiltrates
Pneumocystis jiroveci.
Mycobacterium tuberculosis, especially with advanced human immunodeficiency virus disease.
Histoplasma capsulatum.
Coccidioides spp.
Cryptococcus neoformans.
Toxoplasma gondii.
Cytomegalovirus.
Influenza.
Lymphocytic interstitial pneumonitis.
Abacavir hypersensitivity.

Focal Consolidation
Pyogenic bacterial pneumonia from Streptococcus pneumoniae, Haemophilus influenzae.
M. tuberculosis.
Legionella spp.
Rhodococcus equi.

Hilar Adenopathy
M. tuberculosis.

H. capsulatum.
Coccidioides spp.
Non-Hodgkin or Hodgkin lymphoma.
Mycobacterium avium complex.

Cavitary Disease
Pyogenic bacterial pneumonia from Pseudomonas aeruginosa, Staphylococcus aureus, Enterobacteriaceae.
M. tuberculosis.
C. neoformans.
R. equi.
Aspergillus spp.
Nocardia spp.
Mycobacterium avium complex.
P. jiroveci.

Nodules or Masses
M. tuberculosis.
C. neoformans.
Aspergillus spp.
H. capsulatum.
Nocardia spp.
Non-Hodgkin lymphoma.
Kaposi sarcoma.
Lung cancer.

Normal Radiograph
P. jiroveci.
M. tuberculosis.

CAUSES

Mycobacterial
M. tuberculosis.
M. kansasii.
M. avium complex.
Other nontuberculous mycobacteria.

Other Bacterial
Streptococcus pneumoniae.
Staphylococcus aureus.
Haemophilus influenzae.
Enterobacteriaceae.
Pseudomonas aeruginosa.
Moraxella catarrhalis.
Group A Streptococcus.
Nocardia spp.
Rhodococcus equi.
Chlamydia pneumoniae.

Fungal
Pneumocystis carinii.
Cryptococcus neoformans.
Histoplasma capsulatum.
Coccidioides immitis.
Aspergillus spp.
Blastomyces dermatitidis.
Penicillium marneffei.

Viral
Cytomegalovirus.
Herpes simplex virus.
Adenovirus.
Respiratory syncytial virus.
Influenza viruses.
Parainfluenza virus.

Other
Toxoplasma gondii.
Strongyloides stercoralis.
Kaposi sarcoma.

Lymphoma.
Lung cancer.
Lymphocytic interstitial pneumonitis.
Nonspecific interstitial pneumonitis.
Bronchiolitis obliterans with organizing pneumonia.
Pulmonary hypertension.
Emphysema-like or bullous disease.
Pneumothorax.
Congestive heart failure.
Diffuse alveolar damage.
Pulmonary embolus.

HOARSENESS

| ICD-10CM # | R49.8 | Other voice and resonance disorders |

Allergic rhinitis.
Infections (laryngitis, epiglottitis, tracheitis, croup).
Vocal cord polyps.
Voice strain.
Irritants (tobacco smoke).
Vocal cord trauma (intubation, surgery).
Neoplastic involvement of vocal cord (primary or metastatic).
Neurologic abnormalities (multiple sclerosis, ALS, parkinsonism).
Endocrine abnormalities (puberty, menopause, hypothyroidism).
Other (laryngeal webs or cysts, psychogenic, muscle tension abnormalities).

HYDROCEPHALUS[20]

| ICD-10CM # | Varies with specific diagnosis |

Head trauma.
Brain neoplasm (primary or metastatic).
Spinal cord tumor.
Cerebellar infarction.
Exudative or granulomatous meningitis.
Cerebellar hemorrhage.
Subarachnoid hemorrhage.
Aqueductal stenosis.
Third ventricle colloid cyst.
Hindbrain malformation.
Viral encephalitis.
Metastases to leptomeninges.
Causes in pediatric age

COMMUNICATING
Achondroplasia.
Basilar impression.
Choroid plexus papilloma.[a]
Meningeal malignancy.
Meningitis.[a]
Posthemorrhagic.

NONCOMMUNICATING
Abscess.[a]
Aqueductal stenosis.[a]
Chiari malformation.

[a]Denotes the most common conditions and the ones with disease-modifying treatments.

Dandy-Walker malformation.
Hematoma.[a]
Infectious.[a]
Klippel-Feil syndrome.
Mass lesions.[a]
Tumors and neurocutaneous disorders.
Vein of Galen malformation.[a]
Walker-Warburg syndrome.
X-linked.

OTHER CAUSES OF INCREASED INTRACRANIAL CEREBROSPINAL FLUID

Benign enlargement of subarachnoid space.
Holoprosencephaly.
Hydranencephaly.
Porencephaly.

---

[a]Denotes the most common conditions and the ones with disease-modifying treatments

HYPERCALCEMIA

ICD-10CM #   E83.52   Hypercalcemia

Malignancy: increased bone resorption via osteoclast-activating factors, secretion of PTH-like substances, prostaglandin E2, direct erosion by tumor cells, transforming growth factors, colony-stimulating activity. Hypercalcemia is common in the following neoplasms:
  Solid tumors: breast, lung, pancreas, kidneys, ovary.
  Hematologic cancers: myeloma, lymphosarcoma, adult T-cell lymphoma, Burkitt lymphoma.
Hyperparathyroidism: increased bone resorption, GI absorption, and renal absorption; etiology: Parathyroid hyperplasia, adenoma.
  Hyperparathyroidism or renal failure with secondary hyperparathyroidism.
Granulomatous disorders: increased GI absorption (e.g., sarcoidosis).
Paget disease: increased bone resorption, seen only during periods of immobilization.
Vitamin D intoxication, milk-alkali syndrome; increased GI absorption.
Thiazides: increased renal absorption.
Other causes: familial hypocalciuric hypercalcemia, thyrotoxicosis, adrenal insufficiency, prolonged immobilization, vitamin A intoxication, recovery from acute renal failure, lithium administration, pheochromocytoma, disseminated SLE.

HYPERCALCEMIA, MALIGNANCY-INDUCED

ICD-10CM #   E83.52   Hypercalcemia

Lung carcinoma:	(6% frequency, 35% of hypercalcemic cases)
Breast carcinoma:	(10% frequency, 25% of hypercalcemic cases)
Multiple myeloma:	(33% frequency, 10% of hypercalcemic cases)
Lymphoma:	(4% of hypercalcemic cases)

Genitourinary cancer:	(6% of hypercalcemic cases)

HYPERCAPNIA, PERSISTENT[17]

ICD-10CM #   R06.00   Dyspnea, unspecified
                R06.09   Other forms of dyspnea
                R06.89   Other abnormalities of breathing

Hypercapnia with normal lungs: CNS disturbances (CVA, parkinsonism, encephalitis), metabolic alkalosis, myxedema, primary alveolar hypoventilation, spinal cord lesions.
Diseases of the chest wall (e.g., kyphoscoliosis, ankylosing spondylitis).
Neuromuscular disorders (e.g., myasthenia gravis, Guillain-Barré syndrome, amyotrophic lateral sclerosis, muscular dystrophy, poliomyelitis).
COPD.

HYPERCOAGULABLE STATE, ASSOCIATED DISORDERS[31]

ICD-10CM #   D68.69   Other thrombophilia

Systemic lupus erythematosus in association with the presence of a lupus anticoagulant or antiphospholipid antibodies.

MALIGNANCY

Disease-related: includes migratory superficial thrombophlebitis (Trousseau syndrome), nonbacterial thrombotic endocarditis, thrombosis associated with chronic DIC, thrombotic microangiopathy.
Treatment-related: associated with the administration of various chemotherapeutic agents (L-asparaginase, mitomycin, some adjuvant chemotherapeutic agents for treatment of breast cancer, thalidomide or lenalidomide in conjunction with high doses of dexamethasone).
Infusion of prothrombin complex concentrates.
Nephrotic syndrome.
Heparin-induced thrombocytopenia.
Myeloproliferative disorders.
Paroxysmal nocturnal hemoglobinuria.
DIC, Disseminated intravascular coagulopathy.

HYPERGASTRINEMIA

ICD-10CM #   E16.4   Abnormal secretion of gastrin

Decreased gastrin release inhibition from medications (proton pump inhibitors [PPIs], H_2 receptor antagonists), vagotomy.
Chronic renal failure.
Hypochlorhydria due to atrophic gastritis, gastric carcinoma, pernicious anemia.
Gastrinoma (Zollinger-Ellison syndrome).
Pyloric obstruction.
Hyperplasia of antral G cells.
RA.

HYPERHIDROSIS[45]

ICD-10CM #   R61   Generalized hyperhidrosis

CORTICAL

Emotional.
Familial dysautonomia.
Congenital ichthyosiform erythroderma.
Epidermolysis bullosa.
Nail-patella syndrome.
Jadassohn-Lewandowsky syndrome.
Pachyonychia congenita.
Palmoplantar keratoderma.

HYPOTHALAMIC

Drugs
Antipyretics.
Emetics.
Insulin.
Meperidine.
Exercise Infection
Defervescence.
Chronic illness.
Metabolic
Debility.
DM.
Hyperpituitarism.
Hyperthyroidism.
Hypoglycemia.
Obesity.
Porphyria.
Pregnancy.
Rickets.
Infantile scurvy.
Cardiovascular
Heart failure.
Shock.
Vasomotor
Cold injury.
Raynaud phenomenon.
RA.
Neurologic
Abscess.
Familial dysautonomia.
Postencephalitic.
Tumor.
Miscellaneous
Chédiak-Higashi syndrome.
Compensatory.
Phenylketonuria.
Pheochromocytoma.
Vitiligo.
Medullary
Physiologic gustatory sweating.
Encephalitis.
Granulosis rubra nasi.
Syringomyelia.
Thoracic sympathetic trunk injury.
Spinal
Cord transection.
Syringomyelia.
Changes in Blood Flow
Mallucci syndrome.
Arteriovenous fistula.
Klippel-Trenaunay syndrome.
Glomus tumor.

Blue rubber bleb nevus syndrome.

HYPERKALEMIA

ICD-10CM # E87.5 Hyperkalemia

Pseudohyperkalemia.
Hemolyzed specimen.
Severe thrombocytosis (platelet count 0.106 ml).
Severe leukocytosis (white blood cell count 0.105 ml).
Fist clenching during phlebotomy.
Excessive potassium intake (often in setting of impaired excretion).
Potassium replacement therapy.
High-potassium diet.
Salt substitutes with potassium.
Potassium salts of antibiotics.
Decreased renal excretion.
Potassium-sparing diuretics (e.g., spironolactone, triamterene, amiloride).
Renal insufficiency.
Mineralocorticoid deficiency.
Hyporeninemic hypoaldosteronism.
Tubular unresponsiveness to aldosterone (e.g., SLE, multiple myeloma, sickle cell disease).
Type 4 RTA.
ACE inhibitors.
Heparin administration.
NSAIDs.
Trimethoprim-sulfamethoxazole.
β-blockers.
Pentamidine.
Redistribution (excessive cellular release):
Acidemia (each 0.1 decrease in pH increases the serum potassium by 0.4 to 0.6 mEq/L). Lactic acidosis and ketoacidosis cause minimal redistribution.
Insulin deficiency.
Drugs (e.g., succinylcholine, markedly increased digitalis level, arginine, β-adrenergic blockers).
Hypertonicity.
Hemolysis.
Tissue necrosis, rhabdomyolysis, burns.
Hyperkalemic periodic paralysis.

HYPERKALEMIA, DRUG-INDUCED[7]

ICD-10CM # E87.5 Hyperkalemia

IMPAIRED RENIN-ALDOSTERONE ELABORATION/FUNCTION

Cyclooxygenase inhibitors (NSAIDs).
β-Adrenergic antagonists.
Spironolactone.
Angiotensin-converting enzyme inhibitors and angiotensin II receptor blockers.
Heparin.

INHIBITORS OF RENAL POTASSIUM SECRETION

Potassium-sparing diuretics (amiloride, triamterene).
Trimethoprim.
Pentamidine.
Cyclosporine.
Digitalis overdose.
Lithium.

ALTERED POTASSIUM DISTRIBUTION

Insulin antagonists (somatostatin, diazoxide).
β-Adrenergic antagonists.
α-Adrenergic agonists.
Hypertonic solutions.
Digitalis.
Succinylcholine.
Arginine hydrochloride, lysine hydrochloride.

HYPERKALEMIA IN CHILDREN[11]

ICD-10CM # E87.5 Hyperkalemia

MOST RELEVANT CAUSES OF HYPERKALEMIA IN PEDIATRIC PATIENTS

Pseudohyperkalemia
Improper collection of blood.
Hematologic disorders: leukocytosis, thrombocytosis, spherocytosis.
Transcellular Shift of Potassium
Acidosis.
Insulin deficiency.
Hyperosmolality.
Exercise with nonselective β-blockers.
Familial hyperkalemic periodic paralysis.
Increased Potassium Load
From exogenous origin: pharmacologic supplements.
From endogenous origin (cellular lysis): burns, trauma, intravascular hemolysis, rhabdomyolysis, tumor mass destruction.
Decreased Urinary Excretion
Renal failure.
Mineralocorticoid deficiency.
Addison disease.
Hypoaldosteronism.
Mineralocorticoid resistance.
Type 1 and type 2 pseudohypoaldosteronism.
Renal tubular acidosis: type 4 and hyperkalemic form of type 1.
"Hyperkalemic" drugs: potassium-sparing diuretics, trimethoprim, calcineurin inhibitors, blockers of the renin angiotensin aldosterone system.

HYPERKINETIC MOVEMENT DISORDERS[91]

ICD-10CM # F90.8 Attention-deficit hyperactivity disorder, other type

E83.00	Disorder of copper metabolism, unspecified
E83.01	Wilson disease
E83.09	Other disorders of copper metabolism
G24.02	Drug induced acute dystonia
G24.1	Genetic torsion dystonia

Chorea, choreoathetosis: drug-induced, Huntington chorea, Sydenham chorea.
Tardive dyskinesia (e.g., phenothiazines).
Hemiballismus (lacunar CVA near subthalamic nuclei in basal ganglia, metastatic lesions, toxoplasmosis [in AIDS]).
Dystonia (idiopathic, familial, drug-induced [prochlorperazine, metoclopramide]), Wilson disease.
Liver failure.
Thyrotoxicosis.
SLE, polycythemia.

HYPERMAGNESEMIA

ICD-10CM # E83.40	Disorders of magnesium metabolism, unspecified
E83.41	Hypermagnesemia

Renal failure (decreased GFR).
Decreased renal excretion secondary to salt depletion.
Abuse of antacids and laxatives containing magnesium in patients with renal insufficiency.
Endocrinopathies (deficiency of mineralocorticoid or thyroid hormone).
Increased tissue breakdown (rhabdomyolysis).
Redistribution: acute DKA, pheochromocytoma.
Other: lithium, volume depletion, familial hypocalciuric hypercalcemia.

HYPEROSTOSIS, CORTICAL BONE[21]

ICD-10CM # M48.19 Ankylosing hyperostosis [Forestier], multiple sites in spine

DISORDERS ASSOCIATED WITH HYPEROSTOSIS OF CORTICAL BONE

Progressive diaphyseal dysplasia.
Endosteal hyperostosis.
Pachydermoperiostosis.
Hypertrophic osteoarthropathy.
Thyroid acropachy.
Hypervitaminosis A.
Paget disease.
Infantile cortical hyperostosis.

HYPERPHOSPHATEMIA

ICD-10CM # E83.30 Disorder of phosphorus metabolism, unspecified

Excessive phosphate administration.
Excessive oral intake or IV administration.

Laxatives containing phosphate (phosphate tablets, phosphate enemas).

Decreased renal phosphate excretion.

Acute or chronic renal failure.

Hypoparathyroidism or pseudohypoparathyroidism.

Acromegaly, thyrotoxicosis.

Bisphosphonate therapy.

Tumor calcinosis.

Sickle cell anemia.

Transcellular shift out of cells.

Chemotherapy of lymphoma or leukemia, tumor lysis syndrome, hemolysis.

Acidosis.

Rhabdomyolysis, malignant hyperthermia.

Artifact: in vitro hemolysis.

Pseudohyperphosphatemia: hyperlipidemia, paraproteinemia, hyperbilirubinemia.

HYPERPHOSPHATEMIA IN CHILDREN[11]

ICD-10CM # E83.30 Disorder of phosphorus metabolism, unspecified

CAUSES OF HYPERPHOSPHATEMIA

Impaired Renal Excretion of Phosphate

Renal insufficiency.

Hypoparathyroidism, pseudohypoparathyroidism.

Transient parathyroid resistance of infancy.

Acromegaly.

Tumoral calcinosis.

Hyperthyroidism.

Juvenile hypogonadism.

High ambient temperature.

Heparin.

Bisphosphonate etidronate.

Increased Phosphate Intake

Exogenous Loads

Phosphate salts: laxatives and enemas.

Vitamin D intoxication.

Blood transfusion.

White phosphorus burns.

Liposomal amphotericin B.

Fosphenytoin.

Parenteral phosphate.

Endogenous Loads

Crush injury.

Rhabdomyolysis.

Cytotoxic therapy of neoplasms: tumor lysis.

Hemolysis.

Malignant hyperthermia.

Catabolic states.

Lactic acidosis.

Fulminant hepatitis.

Transcellular Shift of Phosphate

Cellular shift in diabetes ketoacidosis.

Metabolic acidosis.

Respiratory acidosis.

Miscellaneous

Hyperostosis.

HYPERPIGMENTATION[92]

ICD-10CM # L81.4 Other melanin hyperpigmentation

Addison disease.*

Arsenic ingestion.

ACTH- or MSH-producing tumors (e.g., oat cell carcinoma of the lung).

Drug induced (e.g., antimalarials, some cytotoxic agents).

Hemochromatosis ("bronze" diabetes).

Malabsorption syndrome (Whipple disease and celiac sprue).

Melanoma.

Melanotropic hormone injection.

Pheochromocytoma.

Porphyrias (porphyria cutanea tarda and variegate porphyria).

Pregnancy.

Progressive systemic sclerosis and related conditions.

PUVA therapy (psoralen administration) for psoriasis and vitiligo.

ACTH, Adrenocorticotropic hormone; *MSH*, melanocyte-stimulating hormone; *PUVA*, psoralen plus ultraviolet A.

*Accentuation on sun-exposed surfaces.

HYPERPROLACTINEMIA[30]

ICD-10CM # E22.1 Hyperprolactinemia

PHYSIOLOGIC

Pregnancy.

Lactation.

Stress.

Sleep.

Coitus.

Exercise.

PATHOLOGIC

Hypothalamic-Pituitary Stalk Damage

Tumors: craniopharyngioma, suprasellar pituitary mass extension, meningioma, dysgerminoma, hypothalamic metastases.

Granulomas.

Infiltrations.

Rathke cyst.

Irradiation.

Trauma: pituitary stalk section, sellar surgery, head trauma.

Pituitary

Prolactinoma.

Acromegaly.

Macroadenoma (compressive).

Idiopathic.

Plurihormonal adenoma.

Lymphocytic hypophysitis or parasellar mass.

Macroprolactinemia.

Systemic Disorders

Chronic renal failure.

Polycystic ovary syndrome.

Cirrhosis.

Pseudocyesis.

Epileptic seizures.

Cranial irradiation.

Chest: neurogenic chest wall trauma, surgery, herpes zoster.

PHARMACOLOGIC

Neuropeptide

Thyrotropin-releasing hormone.

Drug-Induced Hypersecretion

Dopamine receptor blockers:

    Phenothiazines: chlorpromazine, perphenazine.

    Butyrophenones: haloperidol.

    Thioxanthenes.

    Metoclopramide.

Dopamine synthesis inhibitors:

    α-Methyldopa.

Catecholamine depleters:

    Reserpine.

Cholinergic Agonist

Physostigmine.

Antihypertensives

Labetalol.

Reserpine.

Verapamil.

H2 Antihistamines

Cimetidine.

Ranitidine.

Estrogens

Oral contraceptives.

Oral contraceptive withdrawal.

Anticonvulsant

Phenytoin.

Anesthetics

Neuroleptics

Chlorpromazine.

Risperidone.

Promazine.

Promethazine.

Trifluoperazine.

Fluphenazine.

Butaperazine.

Perphenazine.

Thiethylperazine.

Thioridazine.

Haloperidol.

Pimozide.

Thiothixene.

Molindone.

Opiates and Opiate Antagonists

Heroin.

Methadone.

Apomorphine.

Morphine.

Antidepressants

Tricyclic antidepressants: clomipramine, amitriptyline.

Selective serotonin reuptake inhibitors: fluoxetine.

HYPERSPLENISM, ASSOCIATED CONDITIONS

ICD-10CM # D73.1 Hypersplenism

Cirrhosis.
Portal vein thrombosis.
Myeloproliferative diseases.
Lymphomas.
Leukemias.
Splenic vein thrombosis.
Autoimmune disease.
Sickle cell disease.
Thalassemias.
Gaucher disease.
Niemann-Pick disease.

HYPERTENSION, ADRENOCORTICAL CAUSES[30]

ICD-10CM # I15.8 Other secondary hypertension

LOW RENIN AND HIGH ALDOSTERONE

Primary Aldosteronism

Aldosterone-producing adenoma (APA)	35% of cases
Bilateral idiopathic hyperplasia (IHA)	60% of cases
Primary (unilateral) adrenal hyperplasia	2% of cases
Aldosterone-producing adrenocortical carcinoma	<1% of cases

Familial Hyperaldosteronism (FH)

Glucocorticoid-remediable aldosteronism (FH type I)	<1% of cases
FH type II (APA or IHA)	<2% of cases
Ectopic aldosterone-producing adenoma or carcinoma	<0.1% of cases

LOW RENIN AND LOW ALDOSTERONE

Hyperdeoxycorticosteronism
Congenital adrenal hyperplasia:
  11β-Hydroxylase deficiency.
  17α-Hydroxylase deficiency.
Deoxycorticosterone-producing tumor.
Primary cortisol resistance.
Apparent mineralocorticoid excess (AME)/11β-HSD* deficiency.
  Genetic: Type 1 AME.
Acquired: licorice or carbenoxolone ingestion (type 1 AME), Cushing syndrome (type 2 AME).
Cushing Syndrome
Exogenous glucocorticoid administration—most common cause.
Endogenous:

ACTH[†]-department-85% of cases: pituitary, ectopic.
ACTH-independent—15% of cases: unilateral adrenal disease (adenoma or carcinoma), bilateral adrenal disease (massive macronodular hyperplasia [rare], primary pigmented nodular adrenal disease [rare]).

[†]ACTH, corticotropin.

HYPERTENSION, ENDOCRINE CAUSES[30]

ICD-10CM # I15.8 Other secondary hypertension

ADRENAL-DEPENDENT CAUSES

Pheochromocytoma.
Primary aldosteronism.
Hyperdeoxycorticosteronism:
  Congenital adrenal hyperplasia: 11β-hydroxylase deficiency, 17α-hydroxylase deficiency.
  Deoxycorticosterone-producing tumor.
  Primary cortisol resistance.
Cushing syndrome.

AME/11β-HSD (HYDROXYSTEROID DEHYDROGENASE) DEFICIENCY

Genetic:
  Type 1 apparent mineralocorticoid excess (AME).
Acquired:
  Licorice or carbenoxolone ingestion (type 1 AME).
  Cushing syndrome (type 2 AME).

THYROID-DEPENDENT CAUSES

Hypothyroidism.
Hyperthyroidism.

PARATHYROID-DEPENDENT CAUSES

Hyperparathyroidism.

PITUITARY-DEPENDENT CAUSES

Acromegaly.
Cushing syndrome.

HYPERTENSION, IN CHILDREN[43]

ICD-10CM # I10 Essential (primary) hypertension

PRIMARY

Essential hypertension.

SECONDARY

Renal
Glomerulonephritis.
Henoch-Schönlein purpura.
Pyelonephritis.
Obstruction of reflux.
Polycystic kidney disease.
Diabetic nephropathy.

Trauma.
Renal transplant or hemodialysis.
Tuberous sclerosis.
Systemic lupus nephritis.
Endocrine
Pheochromocytoma.
Cushing syndrome.
Congenital adrenal hyperplasia.
Corticosteroid treatment.
Hyperthyroidism.
Neuroblastoma.
Ovarian tumor.
Cardiac
Congestive heart failure.
Coarctation of the aorta.
Vascular
Hemolytic-uremic syndrome.
Kawasaki syndrome.
Renal artery thrombosis or stenosis.
Neurologic
CNS tumor or infection.
CNS trauma or abuse.
Increased intracranial pressure.
Guillain-Barré syndrome.
Neoplastic
Neuroblastoma.
Wilms tumor.
Pheochromocytoma.
Adrenal carcinoma.
Drugs
Corticosteroids.
Cocaine.
Sympathomimetics.
Oral contraceptives.
Phencyclidine.
β-blocker or clonidine withdrawal.
Lead, mercury.
Others
Iatrogenic fluid overload.
Volume overload from end-stage renal disease.

HYPERTENSION, RESISTANT[11]

ICD-10CM # I10 Essential (primary) hypertension
ICD-10CM # I15 Secondary hypertension

CAUSES OF RESISTANT HYPERTENSION

Pseudoresistance:
  White coat hypertension or office elevations.
  Pseudohypertension in older patients.
  Use of small cuff on very obese arm.
Nonadherence to therapeutic regimen.
Volume overload.
Drug-related causes:
  Antihypertensive drug dosage too low.
  Wrong type of diuretic.
  Inappropriate combinations of antihypertensive drugs.
Drug actions and interactions:
  Sympathomimetics.
  Nasal decongestants.

*Includes alcohol, barbiturates, benzodiazepines.

Appetite suppressants.
Cocaine.
Caffeine.
Oral contraceptives.
Adrenal steroids.
Licorice (may be found in chewing tobacco).
Cyclosporine, tacrolimus.
Erythropoiesis-stimulating agents (ESAs) and erythropoietin.
Antidepressants.
Nonsteroidal antiinflammatory drugs.
Concomitant conditions:
Obesity.
Sleep apnea.
Ethanol intake >1 oz (30 ml)/day.
Anxiety, hyperventilation.
Secondary causes of hypertension:
Renovascular hypertension.
Primary aldosteronism.
Pheochromocytoma.
Hypothyroidism.
Hyperthyroidism.
Hyperparathyroidism.
Aortic coarctation.
Renal disease.

HYPERTENSIVE CRISIS SYNDROMES[7]

ICD-10CM # I13 Hypertensive heart and renal disease
I15 Secondary hypertension

Malignant hypertension.
Nonmalignant hypertension with target organ disorders:
Patient requiring emergency surgery with poorly controlled hypertension.
Hyperviscosity syndrome.
Postoperative patient.
Renal transplant patient: acute rejection, transplant renal artery stenosis.
Quadriplegic patient with autonomic hyperreflexia.
Severe burns.
Acute aortic dissection.
Intracranial hemorrhage, ischemic stroke, or subarachnoid hemorrhage.
Hypertensive encephalopathy.
Myocardial ischemia/acute left ventricular failure.
Preeclampsia/eclampsia.
Antiphospholipid antibody syndrome.
Acute renal failure:
Scleroderma renal crisis.
Chronic glomerulonephritis.
Reflux nephropathy.
Analgesic nephropathy.
Acute glomerulonephritis.
Radiation nephritis.
Ask-Upmark kidney.
Chronic lead intoxication.
Renovascular hypertension:
Fibromuscular dysplasia.

Atherosclerosis.
Endocrine hypertension:
Congenital adrenal hyperplasia.
Pheochromocytoma.
Oral contraceptives.
Aldosteronism.
Cushing disease.
Systemic vasculitis.
Atheroembolic renal crisis.
Drugs:
Oral contraceptives.
Nonsteroidal antiinflammatory agents.
Atropine.
Corticosteroids.
Sympathomimetics.
Cyclosporine.
Erythropoietin.
Lead intoxication.
Catecholamine excess states:
Pheochromocytoma.
MAO/tyramine interaction.
Antihypertensive withdrawal.
Cocaine intoxication, sympathomimetic overdose.

HYPERTENSIVE ENCEPHALOPATHY[14]

ICD-10CM # I67.4 Hypertensive encephalopathy

Ischemic stroke.
Intracerebral hemorrhage.
Subarachnoid hemorrhage.
Subdural hematoma.
Epidural hematoma.
Central nervous vasculitis.
Brain mass.
Seizure disorder.
Central nervous system infection.
Drug toxicity.
Withdrawal syndrome.

HYPERTRICHOSIS[93]

ICD-10CM # L68.0 Hirsutism
L68.1 Acquired hypertrichosis lanuginosa
L68.3 Polytrichia
L68.9 Hypertrichosis, unspecified
Q84.1 Congenital morphological disturbances of hair, not elsewhere classified

DRUGS

Dilantin.
Streptomycin.
Hexachlorobenzene.
Penicillamine.
Diazoxide.
Minoxidil.
Cyclosporine.

SYSTEMIC ILLNESS

Hypothyroidism.
Anorexia nervosa.
Malnutrition.
Porphyria.
Dermatomyositis.
Idiopathic

HYPERTRICHOSIS, CONGENITAL, GENERALIZED[73]

ICD-10CM # L68.9 Hypertrichosis, unspecified

Congenital Syndromes Associated with Generalized Hypertrichosis

Barber-Say syndrome.
Cantú syndrome (hypertrichosis with osteochondrodysplasia).
Coffin-Siris syndrome.
Cornelia de Lange (Brachmann–de Lange) syndrome.
Craniofacial dysostosis.
Hemimaxillofacial dysplasia.
Lipodystrophies:
Berardinelli-Seip syndrome.
Donohue syndrome (leprechaunism).
Mitochondrial encephalopathy, lactic acidosis, and strokelike episodes (MELAS) syndrome.
Mucopolysaccharidoses:
Hunter syndrome.
Hurler syndrome.
Sanfilippo syndrome.
Rubinstein-Taybi syndrome.
Schinzel-Giedion syndrome.
Porphyrias:
Erythropoietic porphyria (Gunther disease).
Familial porphyria cutanea tarda.
Hepatoerythropoietic porphyria.
Stiff skin syndrome.
Toxin exposure:
Fetal alcohol syndrome.
Fetal hydantoin syndrome.
Winchester syndrome.

HYPERTROPHIC OSTEOARTHROPATHY

ICD-10CM # M89.40 Other hypertrophic osteoarthropathy, unspecified site

Idiopathic.
Pulmonary disease (e.g., pulmonary fibrosis, cystic fibrosis, sarcoidosis).
Bronchogenic carcinoma.
AIDS.
GI neoplasm (e.g., esophagus, colon).
Hepatic neoplasm, cirrhosis.
Cardiovascular diseases, aortic aneurysm, aortic prosthesis.
Congenital cyanotic heart disease, patent ductus arteriosus.
Pulmonary infections, bacterial endocarditis, amebic dysentery.

Inflammatory bowel disease.
Connective tissue diseases.
Lymphomas.
Thyroid acropachy.

HYPERVENTILATION, PERSISTENT[17]

ICD-10CM # R06.4 Hyperventilation

Fibrotic lung disease.
Metabolic acidosis (e.g., diabetes, uremia).
CNS disorders (midbrain and pontine lesions).
Hepatic coma.
Salicylate intoxication.
Fever.
Sepsis.
Psychogenic (e.g., anxiety).

HYPOCALCEMIA

ICD-10CM # E83.51 Hypocalcemia

Renal insufficiency: hypocalcemia caused by:
  Increased calcium deposits in bone and soft tissue secondary to increased serum phosphate level.
  Decreased production of 1,25-dihydroxyvitamin D.
  Excessive loss of 25-OHD (nephrotic syndrome).
Hypoalbuminemia: each decrease in serum albumin (g/L) will decrease serum calcium by 0.8 mg/dl but will not change free (ionized) calcium.
Vitamin D deficiency:
  Malabsorption (most common cause).
  Inadequate intake.
  Decreased production of 1,25-dihydroxyvitamin D (vitamin D–dependent rickets, renal failure).
  Decreased production of 25-OHD (parenchymal liver disease).
  Accelerated 25-OHD catabolism (phenytoin, phenobarbital).
  End-organ resistance to 1,25-dihydroxyvitamin D.
Hypomagnesemia: hypocalcemia caused by:
  Decreased PTH secretion.
  Inhibition of PTH effect on bone.
Pancreatitis, hyperphosphatemia, osteoblastic metastases: hypocalcemia is secondary to increased calcium deposits (bone, abdomen).
Pseudohypoparathyroidism (PHP): autosomal recessive disorder characterized by short stature, shortening of metacarpal bones, obesity, and mental retardation; the hypocalcemia is secondary to congenital end-organ resistance to PTH.
Idiopathic hypoparathyroidism, surgical removal of parathyroids (e.g., neck surgery).

"Hungry bones syndrome": rapid transfer of calcium from plasma into bones after removal of a parathyroid tumor.
Sepsis.
Massive blood transfusion (as a result of EDTA in blood).

HYPOCALCEMIA IN PEDIATRIC PATIENTS[11]

ICD-10CM # E83.51 Hypocalcemia

CAUSES OF HYPOCALCEMIA
Neonatal Hypocalcemia
Early neonatal hypocalcemia (first few days of life)
Maternal hyperparathyroidism.
Maternal diabetes mellitus.
Toxemia of pregnancy.
Sepsis.
SGA, IUGR, prematurity.
Asphyxia.
Transfusion (citrated blood products).
Congenital rubella.
Hypomagnesemia.
Respiratory or metabolic alkalosis.
Late neonatal hypocalcemia (fourth to tenth day of life)
Vitamin D deficiency: nutritional deficiency; VDR loss-of-function mutation; deficient 1α-hydroxylase activity.
Phosphate overload: excessive intake of evaporated/whole milk.
Nutritional calcium deficiency.
Hypomagnesemia.
Hypoalbuminemia (nephrotic syndrome).
Transfusion (citrated blood products).
Acute/chronic kidney insufficiency.
Diuretics (furosemide).
Organic acidemia.
Primary hypoparathyroidism: DiGeorge syndrome; familial hypoparathyroidism; pseudohypoparathyroidism; Kenny-Caffey syndrome; partial deletion of GCMB; retardation dysmorphism syndrome; Pearson mitochondriopathy; Kerns-Sayre mitochondriopathy; PTH gene defects; CaSR-activating gene mutation.
Hypocalcemia in Childhood
Parathyroid-related hypocalcemia
Primary hypoparathyroidism: DiGeorge syndrome; familial hypoparathyroidism; pseudohypoparathyroidism; Kenny-Caffey syndrome; Sanjad-Sakati syndrome; partial deletion of GCMB; retardation dysmorphism syndrome; Pearson mitochondriopathy; Kerns-Sayre mitochondropathy; PTH gene defects; CaSR-activating gene mutation; Bartter syndrome type 5.
Secondary hypoparathyroidism: radiation; surgery; infiltration (hemochromatosis, thalassemia, Wilson disease).
Autoimmune polyglandular syndrome type 1.

Vitamin D–related hypocalcemia
Nutritional vitamin D deficiency.
Defective 1α-hydroxylase activity.
VDR loss-of-function mutation.
Nutritional calcium deficiency
Hypomagnesemia
Hyperphosphatemia: kidney failure, rhabdomyolysis, tumor lysis
Hypoalbuminemia (nephrotic syndrome)
Medications: diuretics, chemotherapy, transfusion (citrated blood)
Organic acidemia (IVA, MMA, PPA)

CaSR, Calcium-sensing receptor; *GCMB*, glial cell missing homolog B (a parathyroid-specific transcription factor); *IUGR*, intrauterine growth retardation; *IVA*, isovaleric acidemia; *MMA*, methylmalonic acidemia; *PPA*, propionic acidemia; *PTH*, parathyroid hormone; *SGA*, small for gestational age; *VDR*, vitamin D receptor.

HYPOCAPNIA

ICD-10CM # R06.8 Hypoventilation

Hyperventilation.
Pneumonia, pneumonitis.
Fever, sepsis.
Medications (salicylates, β-adrenergic agonists, progesterone, methylxanthines).
Pulmonary disease (asthma, interstitial fibrosis).
Pulmonary embolism.
Hepatic failure.
Metabolic acidosis.
High altitude.
CHF.
Pregnancy.
Pain.
CNS lesions.

HYPOGLYCEMIA

ICD-10CM #		
	E16.2	Hypoglycemia, unspecified
	E10.65	Type 1 diabetes mellitus with hyperglycemia
	E15	Nondiabetic hypoglycemic coma
	K91.2	Postsurgical malabsorption, not elsewhere classified
	E16.2	Hypoglycemia, unspecified

Oral hypoglycemics (therapeutic, factitious).
Exogenous insulin (therapeutic, factitious).
Postoperative gastric emptying (alimentary hyperinsulinism).
Severe malnutrition.
Liver disease.
Hypermetabolic state (sepsis).
Ketotic hypoglycemia.
Insulinoma.
Antibodies to endogenous insulin.

Hormone deficiencies (glucagon, growth hormone, hypoadrenalism).

Enzyme disorders in metabolism of glycogen, hexose, glycolysis, and Krebs cycle.

Idiopathic.

HYPOGLYCEMIA, IN INFANTS AND CHILDREN[19]

ICD-10CM # E16.2 Hypoglycemia, unspecified

CLASSIFICATION OF HYPOGLYCEMIA IN INFANTS AND CHILDREN

Neonatal Transient Hypoglycemia Associated with Inadequate Substrate or Immature Enzyme Function in Otherwise Normal Neonates

Prematurity.

Small for gestational age.

Normal newborn.

Transient Neonatal Hyperinsulinism Also Present in

Infant of diabetic mother.

Discordant twin.

Birth asphyxia.

Infant of toxemic mother.

NEONATAL, INFANTILE, OR CHILDHOOD PERSISTENT HYPOGLYCEMIAS

Hormonal Disorders

Hyperinsulinism.

Recessive KATP channel HI.

Recessive HADH (hydroxyl acyl CoA dehydrogenase) mutation HI.

Recessive UCP2 (mitochondrial uncoupling protein 2) mutation HI.

Focal KATP channel HI.

Dominant KATP channel HI.

Dominant glucokinase HI.

Dominant glutamate dehydrogenase HI (hyperinsulinism/hyperammonemia syndrome).

Dominant mutation in HNF4A (hepatic nuclear factor 4 alpha) HI with MODY later in life.

Dominant mutation in SLC16A1 (the pyruvate transporter)-exercise-induced hypoglycemia.

Acquired islet adenoma.

Beckwith-Wiedemann syndrome.

Insulin administration (Munchausen syndrome by proxy).

Oral sulfonylurea drugs.

Congenital disorders of glycosylation.

Counter-Regulatory Hormone Deficiency

Panhypopituitarism.

Isolated growth hormone deficiency.

Addison disease.

Epinephrine deficiency.

Glycogenolysis and Gluconeogenesis Disorders

Glucose-6-phosphatase deficiency (GSD 1a).

Glucose-6-phosphate translocase deficiency (GSD 1b).

Amylo-1,6-glucosidase (debranching enzyme) deficiency (GSD 3).

Liver phosphorylase deficiency (GSD 6).

Phosphorylase kinase deficiency (GSD 9).

Glycogen synthetase deficiency (GSD 0).

Fructose-1,6-diphosphatase deficiency.

Pyruvate carboxylase deficiency.

Galactosemia.

Hereditary fructose intolerance.

Lipolysis Disorders

Fatty Acid Oxidation Disorders

Carnitine transporter deficiency (primary carnitine deficiency).

Carnitine palmitoyltransferase-1 deficiency.

Carnitine translocase deficiency.

Carnitine palmitoyltransferase-2 deficiency.

Secondary carnitine deficiencies.

Very long-, long-, medium-, short-chain acyl-CoA dehydrogenase deficiency.

OTHER ETIOLOGIES

Substrate-Limited

Ketotic hypoglycemia.

Poisoning: drugs.

Salicylates.

Alcohol.

Oral hypoglycemic agents.

Insulin.

Propranolol.

Pentamidine.

Quinine.

Disopyramide.

Ackee fruit (unripe): hypoglycin.

Vacor (rat poison).

Trimethoprim-sulfamethoxazole (with renal failure).

Liver Disease

Reye syndrome.

Hepatitis.

Cirrhosis.

Hepatoma.

Amino Acid and Organic Acid Disorders

Maple syrup urine disease.

Propionic acidemia.

Methylmalonic acidemia.

Tyrosinosis.

Glutaric aciduria.

3-Hydroxy-3-methylglutaric aciduria.

Systemic Disorders

Sepsis.

Carcinoma/sarcoma (secreting—insulin-like growth factor II).

Heart failure.

Malnutrition.

Malabsorption.

Antiinsulin receptor antibodies.

Antiinsulin antibodies.

Neonatal hyperviscosity.

Renal failure.

Diarrhea.

Burns.

Shock.

Postsurgical.

Pseudohypoglycemia (leukocytosis, polycythemia).

Excessive insulin therapy of insulin-dependent diabetes mellitus.

Factitious.

Nissen fundoplication (dumping syndrome).

Falciparum malaria.

GSD, Glycogen storage disease; *HI*, hyperinsulinemia; *KATP*, regulated potassium channel.

HYPOGONADISM

ICD-10CM #		
	E28.310	Symptomatic premature menopause
	E29.1	Testicular hypofunction
	E28.39	Other primary ovarian failure
	E23.6	Other disorders of pituitary gland

HYPERGONADOTROPIC HYPOGONADISM

Hormone resistance (androgen, LH insensitivity).

Gonadal defects (e.g., Klinefelter syndrome, myotonic dystrophy).

Drug-induced (e.g., spironolactone, cytotoxins).

Alcoholism, radiation-induced.

Mumps orchitis.

Anatomic defects, castration.

HYPOGONADOTROPIC HYPOGONADISM

Pituitary lesions (neoplasms, granulomas, infarction, hemochromatosis, vasculitis).

Drug-induced (e.g., glucocorticoids).

Hyperprolactinemia.

Genetic disorders (Laurence-Moon-Biedl syndrome, Prader-Willi).

Delayed puberty.

Other: chronic disease, nutritional deficiency, Kallmann syndrome, idiopathic isolated LH or FSH deficiency.

HYPOKALEMIA

ICD-10CM # E87.6 Hypokalemia

Cellular shift (redistribution) and undetermined mechanisms.

Alkalosis (each 0.1 increase in pH decreases serum potassium by 0.4 to 0.6 mEq/L).

Insulin administration.

Vitamin B_{12} therapy for megaloblastic anemias, acute leukemias.

Hypokalemic periodic paralysis: rare familial disorder manifested by recurrent attacks of flaccid paralysis and hypokalemia.

β-adrenergic agonists (e.g., terbutaline), decongestants, bronchodilators, theophylline, caffeine.

Barium poisoning, toluene intoxication, verapamil intoxication, chloroquine intoxication.

Correction of digoxin intoxication with digoxin antibody fragments (Digibind).
Increased renal excretion.
Drugs:
   Diuretics, including carbonic anhydrase inhibitors (e.g., acetazolamide).
   Amphotericin B.
   High-dose sodium penicillin, nafcillin, ampicillin, or carbenicillin.
   Cisplatin.
   Aminoglycosides.
   Corticosteroids, mineralocorticoids.
   Foscarnet sodium.
RTA: distal (type 1) or proximal (type 2).
Diabetic ketoacidosis (DKA), ureteroenterostomy.
Magnesium deficiency.
Postobstruction diuresis, diuretic phase of ATN.
Osmotic diuresis (e.g., mannitol).
Bartter syndrome: hyperplasia of juxtaglomerular cells leading to increased renin and aldosterone, metabolic alkalosis, hypokalemia, muscle weakness, and tetany (seen in young adults).
Increased mineralocorticoid activity (primary or secondary aldosteronism), Cushing syndrome.
Chronic metabolic alkalosis from loss of gastric fluid (increased renal potassium secretion).
GI loss:
   Vomiting, nasogastric suction.
   Diarrhea.
   Laxative abuse.
   Villous adenoma.
   Fistulas.
   Inadequate dietary intake (e.g., anorexia nervosa).
   Cutaneous loss (excessive sweating).
   High dietary sodium intake, excessive use of licorice.

HYPOKALEMIA IN PEDIATRIC PATIENTS[11]

ICD-10CM # E87.6 Hypokalemia

MOST RELEVANT CAUSES OF HYPOKALEMIA IN PEDIATRIC PATIENTS
Acute Redistribution of Potassium to the Intracellular Compartment
Metabolic alkalosis.
Insulin administration.
Hypokalemic periodic paralysis.
Prolonged Lack of Intake
Increased Renal Loss
Drugs: diuretics, antibiotics, aminoglycosides, penicillin, amphotericin B, capreomycin.
Metabolic acidosis and diabetic ketoacidosis.
Increased mineralocorticoid activity.
Cushing syndrome.
Congenital adrenal hyperplasia.
Primary or secondary hyperaldosteronism.

Primary tubulopathies.
Bartter syndrome.
Gitelman syndrome.
Liddle syndrome.
Types 1 and 2 renal tubular acidosis.
Epilepsy, ataxia, sensorineural deafness, and tubulopathy (EAST) syndrome.
Fanconi syndrome.
Increased Gastrointestinal Loss
Vomiting (hypertrophic pyloric stenosis).
Diarrhea.

HYPOMAGNESEMIA

ICD-10CM # E83.40 Disorders of magnesium metabolism, unspecified
E83.42 Hypomagnesemia

GASTROINTESTINAL AND NUTRITIONAL
Defective GI absorption (malabsorption).
Inadequate dietary intake (e.g., alcoholics).
Parenteral therapy without magnesium.
Chronic diarrhea, villous adenoma, prolonged nasogastric suction, fistulas (small bowel, biliary).

EXCESSIVE RENAL LOSSES
Diuretics.
RTA.
Diuretic phase of ATN.
Endocrine disturbances (DKA, hyperaldosteronism, hyperthyroidism, hyperparathyroidism), SIADH, Bartter syndrome, hypercalciuria, hypokalemia.
Cisplatin, alcohol, cyclosporine, digoxin, pentamidine, mannitol, amphotericin B, foscarnet, methotrexate.
Antibiotics (gentamicin, ticarcillin, carbenicillin).
Redistribution: hypoalbuminemia, cirrhosis, administration of insulin and glucose, theophylline, epinephrine, acute pancreatitis, cardiopulmonary bypass.
Miscellaneous: sweating, burns, prolonged exercise, lactation, "hungry-bones" syndrome.

HYPOMAGNESEMIA IN PEDIATRIC PATIENTS[11]

ICD-10CM # E83.42 Hypomagnesemia

MAIN CAUSES OF HYPOMAGNESEMIA IN CHILDREN
Primary Inherited Disorders
Familial hypomagnesemia with hypercalciuria and nephrocalcinosis.
Hypomagnesemia with secondary hypocalcemia.
Autosomal dominant hypomagnesemia.
Isolated autosomal recessive hypomagnesemia with normocalciuria.

Activating mutations of calcium-sensing receptor.
Gitelman syndrome.
Bartter syndrome.
Secondary Disorders
Decreased GI absorption:
   Malabsorptive syndromes.
   Vomiting and diarrhea.
Increased urinary excretion:
   Extracellular volume expansion.
   Polyuric states: obstructive uropathy, kidney transplant.
Drugs:
   Diuretics.
   Calcineurin antagonists.
   Others: cisplatinum, aminoglycosides, amphotericin B.
   Metabolic acidosis.
Miscellaneous: "hungry bone," low-birth-weight newborn, infant of diabetic mother.

HYPONATREMIA

ICD-10CM # E87.1 Hypo-osmolality and hyponatremia

Renal loss from renal disease, diuretics.
GI loss (diarrhea, vomiting, suction).
Hypertonic hyponatremia (e.g., increased serum osmolality from hyperglycemia).
Transcutaneous loss (extensive burns, excessive sweating).
Fluid sequestration (e.g., ascites).
Osmotic diuresis (e.g., mannitol, glucose).
Dilutional (psychogenic polydipsia, iatrogenic).
Syndrome of inappropriate antidiuretic hormone secretion.
Edema with water and sodium retention.
Artifact (e.g., severe hyperlipidemia).
Laboratory error.
Adrenal insufficiency.

HYPOPHOSPHATEMIA

ICD-10CM # E83.30 Disorder of phosphorus metabolism, unspecified
E83.31 Familial hypophosphatemia

Decreased intake (prolonged starvation [alcoholics], hyperalimentation, or IV infusion without phosphate).
Malabsorption.
Phosphate-binding antacids.
Renal loss:
   RTA.
   Fanconi syndrome, vitamin D–resistant rickets.
   ATN (diuretic phase).
   Hyperparathyroidism (primary or secondary).
   Familial hypophosphatemia.
   Hypokalemia, hypomagnesemia.
   Acute volume expansion.

Glycosuria, idiopathic hypercalciuria.
Acetazolamide.
Transcellular shift into cells:
Alcohol withdrawal.
DKA (recovery phase).
Glucose-insulin or catecholamine infusion.
Anabolic steroids.
Total parenteral nutrition.
Theophylline overdose.
Severe hyperthermia; recovery from hypothermia.
"Hungry bones" syndrome.

HYPOPHOSPHATEMIA IN PEDIATRIC PATIENTS[11]

ICD-10CM # E83.30 Disorder of phosphorus metabolism, unspecified

CAUSES OF HYPOPHOSPHATEMIA
Decreased Phosphate Intake
Starvation, inadequate phosphate intake, chronic diarrhea, chronic alcoholism.
Total parenteral nutrition with insufficient phosphate content.
Increased Loss of Phosphate
Increased renal phosphate excretion:
Primary hyperparathyroidism.
Secondary hyperparathyroidism: vitamin D deficiency or resistance (including 1α-hydroxylase deficiency, VDR mutations, VDDR); imatinib.
Excess FGF-23 or phosphatonins: X-linked hypophosphatemia, AD hypophosphatemic rickets, tumor-induced osteomalacia, epidermal nevus, McCune-Albright syndrome.
Fanconi syndrome, cystinosis, Wilson disease Dent disease, Lowe syndrome, multiple myeloma, amyloidosis, heavy-metal toxicity, rewarming of hyperthermia, Na/Pi-IIa and Na/Pi-IIc mutation (HHRH).
PTHrP-dependent hypercalcemia of malignancy.
Hypomagnesemia.
Decreased intestinal absorption:
Vitamin D deficiency or resistance (VDDR I and II).
Malabsorption.
Increased intestinal loss:
Phosphate binding antacids used in treating peptic ulcers.
Increased loss from other routes:
Skin: severe burns.
Vomiting.
Phosphate Shifting from Extracellular Compartment to Cells and Bones
Diabetic ketoacidosis.
Alcohol intoxication.
Acute respiratory alkalosis, salicylate intoxication, gram-negative sepsis, toxic shock syndrome, acute gout.

Refeeding syndromes from starvation, anorexia nervosa, hepatic failure: acute intravenous glucose, fructose, glycerol.
Rapid cellular proliferation: intensive erythropoietin therapy, GM-CSF therapy, leukemic blast crisis.
Recovery from hypothermia.
Heat stroke.
Post parathyroidectomy; "hungry bone" disease: osteoblastic metastases, antiresorptive treatment of severe Paget disease.
Catecholamine (albuterol, dopamine, terbutaline, epinephrine).
Thyrotoxic periodic paralysis.
Hypocalcemic periodic paralysis.
Miscellaneous
Hyperaldosteronism.
Oncogenic hypophosphatemia.
Post kidney transplantation.
Post partial hepatectomy.
High-dose corticosteroids, estrogens.
Medications: ifosfamide, toluene, calcitonin, bisphosphonate, tenofovir, paraquat, cisplatin, acetazolamide, and other diuretics.
Post obstructive diuresis.

AD, Autosomal dominant; *FGF-23,* fibroblast growth factor 23; *GM-CSF,* granulocyte-macrophage colony-stimulating factor; *HHRH,* hereditary hypophosphatemic rickets with hypercalciuria; *Na/Pi-II,* type II sodium-dependent phosphate cotransporter; *PTHrP,* parathyroid hormone–related peptide; *VDR,* vitamin D receptor; *VDDR,* vitamin D–dependent rickets.

HYPOPIGMENTATION

ICD-10CM # L81.9 Disorder of pigmentation, unspecified

Vitiligo.
Tinea versicolor.
Atopic dermatitis.
Chemical leukoderma.
Idiopathic hypomelanosis.
Sarcoidosis.
SLE.
Scleroderma.
Oculocutaneous albinism.
Phenylketonuria.
Nevoid hypopigmentation.

HYPOTENSION, POSTURAL

ICD-10CM # I95.89 Other hypotension

Antihypertensive medications (especially α-blockers, diuretics, ACE inhibitors).
Volume depletion (hemorrhage, dehydration).
Impaired cardiac output (constrictive pericarditis, aortic stenosis).
Peripheral autonomic dysfunction (DM, Guillain-Barré).
Idiopathic orthostatic hypotension.

Central autonomic dysfunction (Shy-Drager syndrome).
Peripheral venous disease.
Adrenal insufficiency.

HYPOTHYROIDISM, CONGENITAL[19]

ICD-10CM # E03.0 Congenital hypothyroidism with diffuse goiter
E03.1 Congenital hypothyroidism without goiter

ETIOLOGIC CLASSIFICATION OF CONGENITAL HYPOTHYROIDISM
Primary Hypothyroidism
Defect of fetal thyroid development (dysgenesis):
Aplasia.
Hypoplasia.
Ectopia.
Defect in thyroid hormone synthesis (dyshormonogenesis):
Iodide transport defect: mutation in thyroglobulin gene.
Thyroid organification, or coupling defect: mutation in thyroid peroxidase gene.
Defects in H_2O_2 generation: mutations in DUOXA2 maturation factor or DUOX2 gene.
Thyroglobulin synthesis defect: mutation in thyroglobulin gene.
Deiodination defect: mutation in *DEHAL1* gene.
TSH unresponsiveness:
$G_s\alpha$ mutation (e.g., type 1A pseudohypothyroidism).
Mutation in TSH receptor.
Defect in thyroid hormone transport: mutation in monocarboxylate transporter 8 (MCT8) gene.
Iodine deficiency (endemic goiter).
Maternal antibodies: thyrotropin receptor–blocking antibody (TRBAb, also termed thyrotropin-binding inhibitor immunoglobulin).
Maternal medications:
Iodides, amiodarone.
Propylthiouracil, methimazole.
Radioiodine.

CENTRAL (HYPOPITUITARY) HYPOTHYROIDISM
PIT-1 mutations:
Deficiency of thyroid-stimulating hormone (TSH).
Deficiency of growth hormone.
Deficiency of prolactin.
PROP-1 mutations:
Deficiency of TSH.
Deficiency of growth hormone.
Deficiency of prolactin.
Deficiency of luteinizing hormone.
Deficiency of follicle-stimulating hormone.
±Deficiency of adrenocorticotropic hormone.
TSH deficiency: mutation in TSH β subunit gene (manifests as primary hypothyroidism with elevated TSH level).

Differential Diagnosis

II

Multiple pituitary deficiencies (e.g., craniopharyngioma).
Thyroid-releasing hormone (TRH) deficiency: Isolated.
Multiple hypothalamic deficiencies (e.g., septooptic dysplasia).
TRH unresponsiveness.
Mutations in TRH receptor.

HYPOTONIA, INFANTILE, DIFFERENTIAL DIAGNOSIS[19]

ICD-10CM #   H44.40   Unspecified hypotony of eye

Cerebral hypotonia:
Benign congenital hypotonia.
Chromosome disorders.
Prader-Willi syndrome.
Trisomy.
Chronic nonprogressive encephalopathy.
Cerebral malformation.
Perinatal distress.
Postnatal disorders.
Peroxisomal disorders.
Cerebrohepatorenal syndrome (Zellweger syndrome).
Neonatal adrenoleukodystrophy.
Other genetic defects.
Familial dysautonomia.
Oculocerebrorenal syndrome (Lowe syndrome).
Other metabolic defects.
Acid maltase deficiency (see "Metabolic Myopathies").
Infantile GM, gangliosidosis.
Spinal cord disorders.
Spinal muscular atrophies:
Acute infantile.
Autosomal dominant.
Autosomal recessive.
Cytochrome-c oxidase deficiency.
X-linked.
Chronic infantile:
Autosomal dominant.
Autosomal recessive.
Congenital cervical spinal muscular atrophy.
Infantile neuronal degeneration.
Neurogenic arthrogryposis.
Polyneuropathies:
Congenital hypomyelinating neuropathy.
Giant axonal neuropathy.
Hereditary motor-sensory neuropathies.
Disorders of neuromuscular transmission:
Familial infantile myasthenia.
Infantile botulism.
Transitory myasthenia gravis.
Fiber-type disproportion myopathies.
Central core disease.
Congenital fiber-type disproportion myopathy.
Myotubular (centronuclear) myopathy.
Acute.
Chronic.
Nemaline (rod) myopathy.

Autosomal dominant.
Autosomal recessive.
Metabolic myopathies:
Acid maltase deficiency.
Cytochrome-c oxidase deficiency.
Muscular dystrophies:
Bethlem myopathy.
Congenital dystrophinopathy.
Congenital muscular dystrophy.
Merosin deficiency, primary.
Merosin deficiency, secondary.
Merosin positive.
Congenital myotonic dystrophy.

HYPOTONIC POLYURIA[11]

ICD-10CM #   Varies with specific diagnosis

CAUSES OF HYPOTONIC POLYURIA

Central (Neurogenic) Diabetes Insipidus
Congenital (congenital malformations, autosomal dominant, arginine vasopressin [AVP] neurophysin gene mutations).
Drug- or toxin-induced (ethanol, diphenylhydantoin, snake venom).
Granulomatous (histiocytosis, sarcoidosis).
Neoplastic (craniopharyngioma, germinoma, lymphoma, leukemia, meningioma, pituitary tumor; metastases).
Infectious (meningitis, tuberculosis, encephalitis).
Inflammatory, autoimmune (lymphocytic infundibuloneurohypophysitis).
Trauma (neurosurgery, deceleration injury).
Vascular (cerebral hemorrhage or infarction, brain death).
Idiopathic.
Osmoreceptor Dysfunction
Granulomatous (histiocytosis, sarcoidosis).
Neoplastic (craniopharyngioma, pinealoma, meningioma, metastases).
Vascular (anterior communicating artery aneurysm or ligation, intrahypothalamic hemorrhage).
Other (hydrocephalus, ventricular or suprasellar cyst, trauma, degenerative diseases).
Idiopathic.
Increased AVP Metabolism
Pregnancy
Nephrogenic Diabetes Insipidus
Congenital (X-linked recessive, AVP V2 receptor gene mutations, autosomal recessive or dominant, aquaporin-2 water channel gene mutations).
Drug-induced (demeclocycline, lithium, cisplatin, methoxyflurane).
Hypercalcemia.
Hypokalemia.
Infiltrating lesions (sarcoidosis, amyloidosis).
Vascular (sickle cell anemia).
Mechanical (polycystic kidney disease, bilateral ureteral obstruction).
Solute diuresis (glucose, mannitol, sodium, radiocontrast dyes).

Idiopathic.
Primary Polydipsia
Psychogenic (schizophrenia, obsessive-compulsive behaviors).
Dipsogenic (downward resetting of thirst threshold, idiopathic or similar lesions, as with central DI).

HYPOVOLEMIA[11]

ICD-10CM #   Varies with specific diagnosis

CAUSES OF ABSOLUTE AND RELATIVE HYPOVOLEMIA

Absolute
Extrarenal
GI fluid loss.
Bleeding.
Skin fluid loss.
Respiratory fluid loss.
Extracorporeal ultrafiltration.
Renal
Diuretics.
Obstructive uropathy/postobstructive diuresis.
Hormone deficiency.
Hypoaldosteronism.
Adrenal insufficiency.
Na+ wasting tubulopathies.
Genetic.
Acquired tubulointerstitial disease.
Relative
Extrarenal
Edematous states.
Heart failure.
Cirrhosis.
Generalized vasodilation.
Sepsis.
Drugs.
Pregnancy.
Third-space loss.
Renal
Severe nephrotic syndrome.

HYPOVOLEMIC SHOCK, PEDIATRIC POPULATION[61]

ICD-10CM #   R57.1   Hypovolemic shock
              R57.8   Other shock

ETIOLOGIES OF HYPOVOLEMIC SHOCK

Whole blood loss.
Absolute loss: hemorrhage.
External bleeding.
Internal bleeding:
GI.
Intraabdominal (spleen, liver).
Major vessel injury.
Intracranial (in infants).
Fractures.
Relative loss:
Pharmacologic (barbiturates, vasodilators).
Positive pressure ventilation.
Spinal cord injury.

Sepsis.
Anaphylaxis.
Plasma loss.
Burns.
Capillary leak syndromes:
Inflammation, sepsis.
Anaphylaxis.
Protein-losing syndromes.
Fluid and electrolyte loss.
Vomiting and diarrhea.
Excessive diuretic use.
Endocrine:
Adrenal insufficiency.
Diabetes insipidus.
Diabetes mellitus.

HYPOXEMIA AND HYPERCAPNIC RESPIRATORY FAILURE[27]

ICD-10CM # Varies with specific diagnosis

COMMON CAUSES OF HYPOXEMIC AND HYPERCAPNIC RESPIRATORY FAILURE

Brain
Bulbar poliomyelitis.
Central alveolar hypoventilation.
Cerebrovascular accident.
Cerebral malignancy.
Drug overdose (e.g., narcotic, sedative/hypnotic).
Elevated intracranial pressure.
Encephalitis and meningitis.
Pontine herniation.
Postoperative anesthetic depression.
Spinal Cord
Amyotrophic lateral sclerosis.
Cervical cordotomy.
Guillain-Barré syndrome.
Poliomyelitis.
Spinal cord trauma.
Neuromuscular System
Acute intermittent porphyria.
Botulism.
Cholinergic crisis.
Curariform drugs.
Electrolyte disorders (e.g., hypophosphatemia, hypomagnesemia).
Hypokalemic periodic paralysis.
Multiple sclerosis.
Myasthenia gravis.
Myxedema.
Neuromuscular blocking antibiotics (e.g., polymyxin, streptomycin).
Organophosphate insecticides.
Peripheral neuritis.
Polymyositis.
Respiratory muscle fatigue—critical illness polyneuropathy/polymyopathy.
Tetanus.
Upper Airway
Epiglottitis and laryngotracheitis.

Large tonsils and adenoids.
Obstructive sleep apnea.
Postintubation laryngeal edema.
Tracheal obstruction.
Vocal cord paralysis.
Thorax and Pleura
Chest wall burn with eschar formation.
Chest wall trauma—flail chest.
Kyphoscoliosis.
Massive abdominal distention.
Massive obesity.
Muscular dystrophy.
Large pleural effusion/pleural fibrosis.
Pneumothorax.
Rheumatoid spondylitis.
Thoracoplasty.
Cardiovascular System
Cardiogenic pulmonary edema.
Left ventricular failure.
Mitral stenosis.
Biventricular failure.
Fat embolism.
Snake bite.
Uremia.
Volume overload.
Pulmonary venoocclusive disease.
Lower Airway and Alveoli
Acute respiratory distress syndrome (ARDS).
Aspiration.
Asthma.
Atelectasis.
Bronchiectasis.
Bronchiolitis.
Chronic obstructive pulmonary disease.
Cystic fibrosis.
Interstitial lung disease.
Massive bilateral pneumonia.
Near-drowning.
Pancreatitis.
Pulmonary contusion.
Radiation lung injury.
Sepsis.
Smoke inhalation.
Surgical resection of lung parenchyma.

ILIAC FOSSA PAIN, LEFT SIDED[2]

ICD-10CM # M25.5 Pain in joint

GASTROINTESTINAL CAUSES OF ACUTE LEFT ILIAC FOSSA PAIN

Nonspecific left iliac fossa pain including constipation.
Acute gastroenteritis.
Acute diverticulitis.
Colonic carcinoma.
Colonic ischemia.
Localized small bowel perforation.

ILIAC FOSSA PAIN, RIGHT SIDED[2]

ICD-10CM # M25.5 Pain in joint

DIFFERENTIAL DIAGNOSIS OF RIGHT ILIAC FOSSA PAIN

Gastrointestinal Causes
Nonspecific right iliac fossa pain.
Acute appendicitis.
Mesenteric adenitis.
Terminal ileitis.
Acute inflammation of Meckel diverticulum.
Crohn disease of the terminal ileum.
Cecal carcinoma.
Inflammatory cecal lesion (e.g., diverticulitis in a solitary cecal diverticulum).
Inflammatory lesion of the terminal ileum (e.g., foreign body perforation).
Nongastrointestinal Causes
Ruptured ovarian follicle (mittelschmerz).
Acute salpingitis (pelvic inflammatory disease).
Rupture/torsion or hemorrhage of an ovarian cyst.
Endometriosis.
Ectopic pregnancy.
Urinary tract infection.

IMMUNODEFICIENCY, CONGENITAL (PRIMARY)

ICD-10CM #	D80.0	Hereditary hypogammaglobulinemia
	D80.1	Nonfamilial hypogammaglobulinemia
	D80.2	Selective deficiency of IgA
	D80.3	Selective deficiency of IgG
	D80.4	Selective deficiency of IgM

CONGENITAL (PRIMARY) CAUSES OF IMMUNODEFICIENCY

T-lymphocyte Deficiencies
DiGeorge syndrome (thymic aplasia with reduced CD4 and CD3 cells).
Purine nucleoside phosphorylase deficiency (marked T-cell depletion).
B-lymphocyte Deficiencies
Bruton X-linked agammaglobulinemia (absence of B cells, plasma cells, and antibody).
Selective immunoglobulin G (IgG) subclass deficiencies.
Selective IgA deficiency.
Hyper-IgM immunodeficiency (elevated IgM but reduced IgG and IgA).
Mixed T- and B-lymphocyte Deficiencies
Common variable immunodeficiency (leads to various B-cell activation or differentiation defects and gradual deterioration of T-cell number and function).
Severe combined immunodeficiency (severe reduction in IgG and absence of T cells).
Wiskott-Aldrich syndrome (decreased T-cell number and function, low IgM, occasionally low IgG).

Ataxia-telangiectasia (decreased T-cell number and function; IgA, IgE, IgG$_2$, and IgG$_4$ deficiency).

Disorders of Complement
C3 deficiency (congenital absence of C3 or consumption of C3 due to deficiency of C3b inactivator).

Phagocyte Defects
Chronic granulomatous disease (defect in nicotinamide adenine dinucleotide phosphate oxidase in phagocytic cells).

Chédiak-Higashi syndrome (impaired microbicidal activity of phagocytes).

Kostmann syndrome, Shwachman-Diamond syndrome, cyclic neutropenia (low neutrophil count).

IMPAIRED CONSCIOUSNESS AND COMA[49]

ICD-10CM # R40.20 Unspecified coma

INFECTIOUS OR INFLAMMATORY
Infectious
Bacterial meningitis.
Viral encephalitis.
Rickettsial infection.
Protozoan infection.
Helminth infestation.
Inflammatory
Sepsis-associated encephalopathy.
Vasculitis, collagen vascular disorders.
Demyelination.
Acute disseminated encephalomyelitis.
Multiple sclerosis.

STRUCTURAL
Traumatic
Concussion.
Cerebral contusion.
Epidural hematoma or effusion.
Intracerebral hematoma.
Diffuse axonal injury.
Abusive head trauma.
Neoplasms
Vascular Disease
Cerebral infarction:
Thrombosis.
Embolism.
Venous sinus thrombosis.
Cerebral hemorrhage:
Subarachnoid hemorrhage.
Arteriovenous malformation.
Aneurysm.
Congenital abnormality or dysplasia of vascular supply
Trauma to carotid or vertebral arteries in the neck
Focal Infection
Abscess.
Cerebritis.
Hydrocephalus

METABOLIC, NUTRITIONAL, OR TOXIC
Hypoxic-Ischemic Encephalopathy
Shock.
Cardiac or pulmonary failure.
Near-drowning.
Carbon monoxide poisoning.
Cyanide poisoning.
Strangulation.
Metabolic Disorders
Sarcoidosis.
Hypoglycemia.
Fluid and electrolyte imbalance.
Endocrine disorders:
  With acidosis:
  Diabetic ketoacidosis.
  Aminoacidemias.
  Organic acidemias.
With hyperammonemia:
  Hepatic encephalopathy.
  Urea cycle disorders.
  Disorders of fatty acid metabolism.
  Reye syndrome.
  Valproic acid encephalopathy.
Uremia.
Porphyria.
Mitochondrial disorders.
Leigh syndrome.
Nutritional
Thiamine deficiency.
Niacin or nicotinic acid deficiency.
Pyridoxine dependency.
Folate and vitamin B$_{12}$ deficiency.
Exogenous Toxins and Poisons
Alcohol intoxication.
Over-the-counter medications.
Prescription medications (oral and ophthalmic).
Herbal treatments.
Heavy-metal poisoning.
Mushroom and plant intoxication.
Illegal drugs.
Industrial agents.
Hypertensive Encephalopathy
Burn Encephalopathy

IMPOTENCE[80]

ICD-10CM #	F52.21	Male erectile disorder
	F52.8	Other sexual dysfunction not due to a substance or known physiological condition
	N52.9	Male erectile dysfunction, unspecified

Psychogenic.
Endocrine: hyperprolactinemia, DM, Cushing syndrome, hypothyroidism or hyperthyroidism, abnormality of hypothalamic-pituitary-testicular axis.
Vascular: arterial insufficiency, venous leakage, AV malformation, local trauma.
Medications.

Neurogenic: autonomic or sensory neuropathy, spinal cord trauma or tumor, CVA, multiple sclerosis, temporal lobe epilepsy.
Systemic illness: renal failure, COPD, cirrhosis of liver, myotonic dystrophy.
Peyronie disease.
Prostatectomy.

INCONTINENCE, FECAL[2]

ICD-10CM # R15.9 Full incontinence of feces

NORMAL SPHINCTER
Diarrhea.
Anorectal conditions:
  Rectal carcinoma.
  Inflammatory bowel disease.
  Hemorrhoids.
  Mucosal prolapse.
  Fissure-in-ano.
  Abnormal rectal sensation.

ABNORMAL SPHINCTER
Congenital abnormalities.
Anal sepsis.
Neurologic conditions.
Rectal prolapse.
Sphincter trauma.
Neurogenic (idiopathic) incontinence.

INFECTIOUS DIARRHEA IN TROPICS[3]

ICD-10CM # R19.7 Diarrhea, unspecified

CAUSES OF INFECTIOUS DIARRHEA IN THE TROPICS
Bacteria
Aeromonas hydrophila.
Arcobacter butzleri.
Bacteroides fragilis, enterotoxigenic.
Campylobacter jejuni.
Escherichia coli: enterotoxigenic, enteroaggregative, enteroinvasive, enterohemorrhagic.
Laribacter hongkongensis.
Plesiomonas shigelloides.
Salmonella, nontyphoidal.
Shigella spp: S. dysenteriae, S. flexneri, S. sonnei, S. boydii.
Vibrio cholerae O1, 0139, non-O1 non-0139.
Vibrio parahaemolyticus.
Yersinia enterocolitica.
Helminths
Paracapillaria philippinensis.
Fasciolopsis buski.
Heterophyiasis (Metagonimus yokogawai, Haplorchis taichui).
Schistosoma mansoni.
Strongyloides stercoralis.
Protozoa
Blastocystis hominis.
Cryptosporidium parvum.
Cyclospora cayetanensis.
Encephalitozoon intestinalis.

Enterocytozoon bieneusi.
Giardia lamblia.
Isospora belli.
Leishmania donovani.
Viruses
Astroviruses.
Caliciviruses: norovirus and sapovirus.
Enteric adenoviruses.
HIV.
Picornaviruses.
Rotavirus.

INFERTILITY, FEMALE[24]

ICD-10CM #	N97.9	Female infertility, unspecified

FALLOPIAN TUBE PATHOLOGY

PID or puerperal infection.
Congenital anomalies.
Endometriosis.
Secondary to past peritonitis of nongenital origin.
Amenorrhea and anovulation.
Minor anovulatory disturbances.

CERVICAL AND UTERINE FACTORS

Leiomyomas and polyps.
Uterine anomalies.
Intrauterine synechiae (Asherman syndrome).
Destroyed endocervical glands (postsurgery or postinfection).

VAGINAL FACTORS

Congenital absence of vagina.
Imperforate hymen.
Vaginismus.
Vaginitis.

IMMUNOLOGIC FACTORS

Sperm-immobilizing antibodies.
Sperm-agglutinating antibodies.

NUTRITIONAL AND METABOLIC FACTORS

Thyroid disorders.
DM.
Severe nutritional disturbances.

INFERTILITY, MALE[24]

ICD-10CM #	N46.9	Male infertility, unspecified

DECREASED PRODUCTION OF SPERMATOZOA

Varicocele.
Testicular failure.
Endocrine disorders.
Cryptorchidism.
Stress, smoking, caffeine, nicotine, recreational drugs.

DUCTAL OBSTRUCTION

Epididymal (postinfection).
Congenital absence of vas deferens.
Ejaculatory duct (postinfection).

Postvasectomy.

INABILITY TO DELIVER SPERM INTO VAGINA

Ejaculatory disturbances.
Hypospadias.
Sexual problems (i.e., impotence), medical or psychological.

ABNORMAL SEMEN

Infection.
Abnormal volume.
Abnormal viscosity.
Abnormal sperm motion.

IMMUNOLOGIC FACTORS

Sperm-immobilizing antibodies.
Sperm-agglutinating antibodies.

INSOMNIA[76]

ICD-10CM #	780.51	Insomnia with sleep apnea
	G47.00	Insomnia, unspecified
	F51.01	Primary insomnia
	F51.03	Paradoxical insomnia
	F51.09	Other insomnia not due to a substance or known physiological condition

Anxiety disorder, psychophysiologic insomnia.
Depression.
Drugs (e.g., caffeine, amphetamines, cocaine), hypnotic-dependent sleep disorder.
Pain, fibromyalgia.
Inadequate sleep hygiene.
Restless leg syndrome.
Obstructive sleep apnea.
Sleep bruxism.
Medical illness (e.g., GERD, sleep-related asthma, parkinsonism and movement disorders).
Narcolepsy.
Other: periodic leg movement of sleep, central sleep apnea, REM behavioral disorder.

INTESTINAL PSEUDOOBSTRUCTION[17,68]

ICD-10CM #	K56.0	Paralytic ileus
	K56.9	Ileus, unspecified
	K59.9	Functional intestinal disorder, unspecified

"PRIMARY" (IDIOPATHIC INTESTINAL PSEUDOOBSTRUCTION)

Hollow visceral myopathy:
   Familial.
   Sporadic.
Neuropathic:
   Abnormal myenteric plexus.
   Normal myenteric plexus.

SECONDARY

Scleroderma.
Myxedema.

Amyloidosis.
Muscular dystrophy.
Hypokalemia.
Chronic renal failure.
DM.
Drug toxicity caused by:
   Anticholinergics.
   Opiate narcotics.
Ogilvie syndrome.

CAUSES OF SECONDARY CHRONIC INTESTINAL PSEUDOOBSTRUCTION IN CHILDREN

Autoimmune
Autoimmune myositis.
Autoimmune ganglionitis.
Scleroderma.
Endocrine
Diabetes mellitus.
Hypoparathyroidism.
Hypothyroidism.
Gastrointestinal
Celiac disease.
Eosinophilic gastroenteritis.
Inflammatory bowel disease.
Hematology/Oncology
Multiple myeloma.
Paraneoplastic syndromes.
Pheochromocytoma.
Sickle cell disease.
Infection
Chagas disease.
Cytomegalovirus.
Epstein-Barr virus.
Herpes zoster.
JC virus.
Kawasaki disease.
Postviral neuropathy.
Medications and Toxins
Chemotherapy.
Cyclopentolate and phenylephrine eye drops.
Diltiazem and nifedipine.
Fetal alcohol syndrome.
Jellyfish envenomation.
Opioid medications.
Postanesthesia.
Radiation injury.
Mitochondrial Disorders
Mitochondrial neurogastrointestinal encephalomyopathy.
Musculoskeletal Disorders
Ehlers-Danlos syndrome.
Myotonic dystrophy.
Duchenne muscular dystrophy.
Rheumatology
Amyloidosis.
Dermatomyositis.
Polymyositis.
Systemic lupus erythematous.

From Wyllie R, Hyams JS, Kay M (eds): *Pediatric gastrointestinal and liver disease,* ed 5, Philadelphia, 2016, Elsevier, Box. 44.3, p. 548.

Differential Diagnosis

II

INTRAABDOMINAL MASS LESION, NEONATAL[21]

ICD-10CM # R19.00 Intraabdominal and pelvic swelling, mass and lump, unspecified site

CAUSES OF A NEONATAL INTRA-ABDOMINAL MASS LESION

Complicated meconium ileus.
Dilated bowel proximal to an obstruction.
Mesenteric or duplication cyst.
Abscess.
GU causes:
  Hydronephrosis.
  Renal cystic disease.
  Mesoblastic nephroma.
  Wilms tumor.
  Adrenal hemorrhage.
  Neuroblastoma.
  Retroperitoneal teratoma.
  Ovarian cyst.
  Hydrometrocolpos.
Hemangioendothelioma.
Hepatoblastoma.
Choledochal, hepatic, or splenic cysts.

INTRACEREBRAL HEMORRHAGE, NONHYPERTENSIVE CAUSES

ICD-10CM # I61.9 Nontraumatic intracerebral hemorrhage, unspecified

Trauma.
Anticoagulation.
Intracranial tumors.
Vascular malformations.
Bleeding disorders.
Vasculitides (e.g., polyarteritis nodosa, granulomatous angiitis).
Cocaine and other sympathomimetic agents.
Cerebral amyloid angiopathy.

INTRACRANIAL LESION

ICD-10CM # G93.89 Other specified disorders of brain

Tumor (primary or metastatic).
Abscess.
Stroke.
Intracranial hemorrhage.
Angioma.
Multiple sclerosis (initial single lesion).
Granuloma.
Herpes encephalitis.
Artifact.

INTRACRANIAL PRESSURE INCREASE[56]

ICD-10CM # Varies with specific diagnosis

MASS EFFECT
Hydrocephalus.

Hemorrhage.
Tumor.
Abscess.
Cyst.
Inflammatory mass.
Arterial ischemic stroke with edema.
Cerebral sinovenous thrombosis.

DIFFUSE EDEMA
Hypoxic-ischemic injury.
Trauma.
Infection.
Meningitis.
Encephalitis.
Hypertension.
Metabolic derangement or toxin.
Hyponatremia.
Diabetic ketoacidosis.
Dialysis disequilibrium syndrome.
Reye syndrome.
Fulminant hepatic encephalopathy.
Pulmonary insufficiency with hypercarbia.
Lead intoxication.
Idiopathic intracranial hypertension (pseudotumor cerebri).
Drugs.
Withdrawal of long-term steroid administration.
Endocrinologic disturbance.
Obesity.

INTRACRANIAL TUMORS[94]

ICD-10CM # D33.2 Benign neoplasm of brain, unspecified
              C71.9 Malignant neoplasm of brain, unspecified

Differential Diagnosis of Intracranial Tumors
Infection.
Brain abscess.
Bacterial.
Fungal.
Parasitic (e.g., cysticercosis).
Herpes encephalitis.
Vascular disease.
Stroke.
Intracranial hemorrhage.
Inflammatory conditions.
Granuloma (sarcoid).
Multiple sclerosis: tumefactive single large lesion.
Vascular malformations.
Cavernous angiomas.
Venous angiomas.
Congenital abnormalities.
Cortical dysplasia.
Heterotopia.

INTRAOCULAR NEOPLASM

ICD-10CM # C69.9 Malignant disorder of eye, unspecified

MALIGNANT
Retinoblastoma.
Melanoma.
Reticulum cell sarcoma.
Metastatic tumor.

BENIGN
Melanocytic nevus.
Hemangioma.
Reactive lymphoid hyperplasia.

IRON METABOLISM DISORDERS[95]

ICD-10CM # E83.10 Disorder of iron metabolism, unspecified

IRON DEFICIENCY
Deficient Iron Intake
Diet of low bioavailability.
Increased physiological requirements due to rapid growth in early childhood and in adolescence.
Blood loss.
Physiological (e.g., menstruation).
Pathological (e.g., GI).
Malabsorption of Iron
Reduced or absent gastric acid secretion (e.g., after partial or total gastrectomy or with atrophic gastritis).
Reduced duodenal absorption (e.g., in coeliac disease).
Bypass of stomach and duodenum (bariatric surgery).
Rare, inherited iron-refractory iron deficiency anemia (e.g., deficiency of TMPRSS6 [transmembrane protease, serine 6], also known as matriptase-2).
Redistribution of Iron
Macrophage iron accumulation in reticuloendothelial system in inflammatory, infectious, or malignant diseases (anemia of chronic disease, also known as anemia of inflammation).
Macrophage iron accumulation within the lungs in idiopathic pulmonary hemosiderosis.

IRON OVERLOAD
Due to Increased Iron Absorption
Hereditary hemochromatosis—commonly (among Northern Europeans) homozygosity for *HFE* C282Y but sometimes involving non-C282Y *HFE* or other genes (*HAMP, HFE2* [encoding hemojuvelin], *TFR2, SLC40A1*).
Substantial ineffective erythropoiesis (e.g., β thalassemia intermedia and major, some types of sideroblastic anemia, congenital dyserythropoietic anemia).
Sub-Saharan iron overload ("Bantu siderosis")—only in combination with increased dietary iron.
Other rare inherited disorders (e.g., congenital atransferrinemia, DMT1 deficiency, aceruloplasminemia).
Inappropriate iron therapy (rare).

DUE TO MULTIPLE BLOOD TRANSFUSIONS FOR REFRACTORY ANEMIAS OR FOR OTHER REASONS
Thalassemia major.
Aplastic anemia.

Myelodysplastic syndromes.
Sickle cell disease (when regularly transfused).

IRON OVERLOAD[31]

| ICD-10CM # | E83.10 | Disorder of iron metabolism, unspecified |

HEREDITARY IRON OVERLOAD

Hereditary hemochromatosis:
  HFE-associated (type 1).
  Non–HFE-associated:
    Transferrin receptor 2–associated (type 3).
Juvenile hemochromatosis (type 2):
  Hemojuvelin-associated (type 2A).
  Hepcidin-associated (type 2B).
Autosomal dominant hemochromatosis:
  Ferroportin-associated (type 4).
  DMT1-associated hemochromatosis.
  Atransferrinemia.
  Aceruloplasminemia.

ACQUIRED IRON OVERLOAD

Iron-loading anemias (refractory anemias with hypercellular erythroid marrow).
Chronic liver disease.
Porphyria cutanea tarda.
Insulin resistance–associated hepatic iron overload.
African dietary iron overload.*
Medical iron ingestion.
Parenteral iron overload:
  Transfusional iron overload.
  Inadvertent iron overload from therapeutic injections.

PERINATAL IRON OVERLOAD

Neonatal hemochromatosis.
Trichohepatoenteric syndrome.
Cerebrohepatorenal syndrome.
GRACILE (Fellman) syndrome.[†]

FOCAL SEQUESTRATION OF IRON

Idiopathic pulmonary hemosiderosis.
Renal hemosiderosis.
Associated with neurologic abnormalities:
Pantothenate kinase–associated neuro-degeneration (formerly called Hallervorden-Spatz syndrome).
Neuroferritinopathy.
Friedreich ataxia.

*May have a genetic component.
[†]GRACILE, Growth retardation, aminoaciduria, cholestasis, iron overload, lactic acidosis, and early death.

ISCHEMIA, UPPER EXTREMITY, CAUSES[60]

| ICD-10CM # | S45.809A | Unspecified injury of other specified blood vessels at shoulder and upper arm level, |

unspecified arm, initial encounter

VASOSPASM

Raynaud disease.
Medication induced: vasopressors, β-blockers.
Ergot poisoning.

INTRINSIC ARTERIAL DISEASE

Atherosclerosis.
Radiation arteritis.
Azotemic arteriopathy.
Spontaneous dissection.
Fibromuscular dysplasia.

INFLAMMATORY DISEASES

Connective tissue disorders.
Buerger disease.
Takayasu arteritis.
Temporal (giant cell) arteritis.
Hypersensitivity angiitis.

NONINFLAMMATORY MEDICAL DISEASE

Thrombophilic states.
Myeloproliferative disorders.
Cold injury.
Hepatitis-associated vasculitis.
Cryoglobulinemia.
Vinyl chloride exposure.

EMBOLISM

Cardiac (most common).
Proximal aneurysm.
Arterial thoracic outlet syndrome.
Atheroembolism.
Paradoxic embolus (with accompanying septal defect).

TRAUMA

Iatrogenic.
Blunt arterial injury.
Penetrating arterial injury.
Hypothenar hammer syndrome.
Vibration.

ISCHEMIC BOWEL DISEASE[29]

| ICD-10CM # | K55.1 | Vascular disorder of intestine |
| | I99 | Other and unspecified disorders of circulatory system |

Abdominal aortic aneurysm: rupture or expansion.
Perforated ulcer or viscus.
Ruptured ectopic pregnancy (woman of child-bearing age).
Incarcerated or strangulated hernia.
Septic shock.
Intussusception.
Volvulus.
Salpingitis or tuboovarian abscess.

Torsion of the ovary or testicle.
Appendicitis.
Pelvic mass or torsion.
Pancreatitis.
Diverticulitis.
Ruptured ovarian cyst.
Renal colic.
Biliary colic.
Also consider atypical manifestations of:
  Inferior wall myocardial infarction.
  Pulmonary embolism.
  Pneumonia.
  Diabetic ketoacidosis.
  Acute glaucoma.
Differential diagnoses are listed in order of urgency.

ISCHEMIC COLITIS, NONOCCLUSIVE[26]

| ICD-10CM # | K55.1 | Chronic vascular disorders of intestine |

ACUTE DIMINUTION OF COLONIC INTRAMURAL BLOOD FLOW

Small Vessel Obstruction
Collagen-vascular disease.
Vasculitis, diabetes.
Oral contraceptives.
Nonocclusive Hypoperfusion
Hemorrhage.
CHF, MI, arrhythmias.
Sepsis.
Vasoconstricting agents: vasopressin, ergot.
Increased viscosity: polycythemia, sickle cell disease, thrombocytosis.

INCREASED DEMAND ON MARGINAL BLOOD FLOW

Increased Motility
Mass lesion, stricture.
Constipation.
Increased Intraluminal Pressure
Bowel obstruction.
Colonoscopy.
Barium enema.

ISCHEMIC NECROSIS OF CARTILAGE AND BONE[24]

| ICD-10CM # | M89.9 | Disorder of bone, unspecified |
| | M94.9 | Disorder of cartilage, unspecified |

ENDOCRINE/METABOLIC

Ethanol abuse.
Glucocorticoid therapy.
Cushing disease.
DM.
Hyperuricemia.
Osteomalacia.
Hyperlipidemia.

Differential Diagnosis

II

STORAGE DISEASES (E.G., GAUCHER DISEASE)

Hemoglobinopathies (e.g., sickle cell disease).
Trauma (e.g., dislocation, fracture).
HIV infection.
Dysbaric conditions (e.g., caisson disease).
Collagen-vascular disorders.
Irradiation.
Pancreatitis.
Organ transplantation.
Hemodialysis.
Burns.
Intravascular coagulation.
Idiopathic, familial.

JAUNDICE

ICD-10CM #	R17	Unspecified jaundice
	K83.8	Other specified diseases of biliary tract
	E80.7	Disorder of bilirubin metabolism, unspecified

PREDOMINANCE OF DIRECT (CONJUGATED) BILIRUBIN

Extrahepatic obstruction.
Common duct abnormalities: calculi, neoplasm, stricture, cyst, sclerosing cholangitis.
Metastatic carcinoma.
Pancreatic carcinoma, pseudocyst.
Ampullary carcinoma.
Hepatocellular disease: hepatitis, cirrhosis.
Drugs: estrogens, phenothiazines, captopril, methyltestosterone, labetalol.
Cholestatic jaundice of pregnancy.
Hereditary disorders: Dubin-Johnson syndrome, Rotor syndrome.
Recurrent benign intrahepatic cholestasis.

PREDOMINANCE OF INDIRECT (UNCONJUGATED) BILIRUBIN

Hemolysis: hereditary and acquired hemolytic anemias.
Inefficient marrow production.
Impaired hepatic conjugation: chloramphenicol.
Neonatal jaundice.
Hereditary disorders: Gilbert syndrome, Crigler-Najjar syndrome.

JAUNDICE, CLASSIFICATION[18]

ICD-10CM #	R17	Unspecified jaundice

PREHEPATIC (PREDOMINANTLY UNCONJUGATED HYPERBILIRUBINEMIA)

Overproduction

Hemolysis (e.g., spherocytosis, sickle cell disease, hemolysis of the newborn, autoimmune disorders).
Ineffective erythropoiesis (e.g., megaloblastic anemias).
Hematomas.

Pulmonary emboli.

HEPATIC (UNCONJUGATED HYPERBILIRUBINEMIA)

Decreased Hepatic Uptake

Gilbert syndrome.
Drugs (e.g., rifampin, radiographic contrast agents).
Neonatal jaundice.
Posthepatitis.
Decreased systolic binding proteins (e.g., newborn or premature infants).
Portacaval shunt.
Prolonged fasting.

Decreased Conjugation Due to Limited Glucuronyl Transferase Activity

Gilbert disease.
Crigler-Najjar syndrome, types I and II.
Neonatal jaundice.
Breast-milk jaundice.
Chronic persistent hepatitis.
Wilson disease.
Noncirrhotic portal fibrosis.
Drug inhibition (e.g., chloramphenicol).

PREDOMINANTLY CONJUGATED HYPERBILIRUBINEMIA

Impaired Hepatic Excretion

Familial disorders (Dubin-Johnson syndrome, Rotor syndrome, benign recurrent cholestasis, cholestasis of pregnancy).
Hepatocellular infiltrative disorders.
Liver metastasis.
Liver cirrhosis.
Hepatitis (viral, bacterial, parasitic, autoimmune, ethanol, and drug-induced).
Drug-induced cholestasis (especially chlorpromazine, erythromycin estolate, isoniazid, halothane).
Primary biliary cirrhosis.
Primary sclerosing cholangitis.
Pericholangitis.
Congestive heart failure.
Shock.
Toxemia of pregnancy.
Sarcoidosis.
Hepatic trauma.
Amyloidosis.
Autoimmune cholangiopathy.
Vanishing bile duct syndrome.
Sepsis.
Postoperative complications.

EXTRAHEPATIC

Extrahepatic Biliary Obstruction

Gallstones, choledocholithiasis.
Cholecystitis.
Tumors of the head of the pancreas (adenocarcinoma, mucinous duct ectasia, neuroendocrine tumors, metastasis).
Tumors of bile ducts (cholangiocarcinoma, Klatskin tumor: cholangiocarcinoma at the bifurcation).
Gallbladder cancer.

Tumors of the ampulla of Vater (adenoma, adenocarcinoma).
Tumors of the duodenum (adenocarcinoma, lymphoma).
Hemobilia (blood in the biliary tree).
Biliary strictures (postcholecystectomy, post-liver transplantation, primary sclerosing cholangitis).
Congenital disorders (biliary atresia, idiopathic dilation of common bile duct, cystic fibrosis).
Metastasis to the hepatic hilum.
Primary bile duct lymphoma.
Cholangiopathy of acquired immunodeficiency syndrome.
Choledochal cysts.
Infectious cholangiopathy (*Clonorchis sinensis, Ascaris lumbricoides, Fasciola hepatica*).
Chronic pancreatitis (fibrosis of the head of the pancreas).

JAUNDICE IN PREGNANCY[96]

ICD-10CM #	R17	Unspecified jaundice

DIFFERENTIAL DIAGNOSIS

Drug hepatotoxicity (can be seen with α-methyldopa).
Viral hepatitis.
Autoimmune hepatitis (screen for anti-mitochondrial antibodies).
Hyperemesis gravidarum (severe).
Cholelithiasis.
Cholangiocarcinoma (extremely rare).
Overlap syndromes:
   Preeclampsia (HELLP syndrome) (liver rupture, and infarction in rare cases).
   Acute fatty liver of pregnancy.

JAUNDICE, NEONATAL[18]

ICD-10CM #	P59.9	Neonatal jaundice, unspecified

PREHEPATIC

Hereditary spherocytosis.
Nonspherocytic hemolytic anemia (glucose-6-phosphate dehydrogenase deficiency, α-thalassemia, vitamin K_3–induced hemolysis, pyruvate kinase deficiency).

HEPATIC

Crigler-Najjar syndrome, types I and II.
α_1-Antitrypsin deficiency.
Sepsis.
Drug-induced.
Hypothyroidism.
Breast-milk jaundice.
Fetomaternal blood group incompatibility (Rhesus, Landsteiner groups ABO).

POSTHEPATIC

Extrahepatic biliary obstruction.
Biliary atresia.
Bile duct paucity.

Alagille syndrome.

JOINT AND PERIARTICULAR PAIN, ACUTE[8]

ICD-10CM #   M25.50   Joint pain

COMMON ACUTE MONOARTHRITIS

Septic arthritis (nongonococcal, gonococcal).
Crystal arthritis (gout, pseudogout).
Reactive arthritides.
Lyme disease.
Plant thorn synovitis.
Other infections (mycobacterial, viral, soft tissue).

TRAUMA OR INTERNAL DERANGEMENT

Loose bodies.
Stress fractures.
Ischemic necrosis.
Hemarthrosis.

ACUTE MONOARTHRITIS OR POLYARTHRITIS

Psoriatic arthritis.
Enteropathic arthritis.
Rheumatoid arthritis/palindromic rheumatism.
Juvenile inflammatory arthritides.

MONOARTHROPATHIES FROM NONINFLAMMATORY DISEASE

Osteoarthritis.
Charcot joints.
Storage diseases (hemochromatosis, ochronosis).

SYNOVIAL DISEASES

Pigmented villonodular synovitis.
Lipoma arborescens.
Synovial osteochondromatosis.
Reflex sympathetic dystrophy.
Sarcoidosis.
Amyloid.

ACUTE MONOARTHRITIS OF SYSTEMIC DISEASE

Systemic lupus erythematosus.
Vasculitides (antineutrophil cytoplasmic antibody positive and negative).
Henoch-Schönlein purpura.
Behçet disease.
Bacterial endocarditis.
Familial Mediterranean fever.
Relapsing polychondritis.

SOFT TISSUE LESIONS

Bone Diseases
Paget disease.
Osteomyelitis (Brodie abscess).
Osteogenic/osteoid tumors.
Metastatic disease.
Pulmonary hypertrophic osteoarthropathy.

JOINT PAIN, ANTERIOR HIP, MEDIAL THIGH, KNEE[25]

ICD-10CM #	M25.50	Pain in unspecified joint
	M25.559	Pain in unspecified hip
	M25.569	Pain in unspecified knee

ACUTE

Acute rheumatic fever.
Adductor muscle strain.
Avascular necrosis.
Crystal arthritis.
Femoral artery (pseudo) aneurysm.
Fracture (femoral neck or intertrochanteric).
Hemarthrosis.
Hernia.
Herpes zoster.
Iliopectineal bursitis.
Iliopsoas tendinitis.
Inguinal lymphadenitis.
Osteomalacia.
Painful transient osteoporosis of hip.
Septic arthritis.

SUBACUTE AND CHRONIC

Adductory muscle strain.
Amyloidosis.
Acute rheumatic fever.
Femoral artery aneurysm.
Hernia (inguinal or femoral).
Iliopectineal bursitis.
Iliopsoas tendinitis.
Inguinal lymphadenopathy.
Osteochondromatosis.
Osteomyelitis.
Osteitis deformans (Paget disease).
Osteomalacia (pseudofracture).
Postherpetic neuralgia.
Sterile synovitis (e.g., RA, psoriatic, SLE).

JOINT PAIN, HIP, LATERAL THIGH[25]

ICD-10CM #	S79.919A	Unspecified injury of unspecified hip, initial encounter
	S79.929A	Unspecified injury of unspecified thigh, initial encounter
	M25.9	Joint disorder, unspecified

ACUTE

Herpes zoster.
Iliotibial tendinitis.
Impacted fracture of femoral neck.
Lateral femoral cutaneous neuropathy (meralgia paresthetica).
Radiculopathy: L4-5.
Trochanteric avulsion fracture (greater trochanter).
Trochanteric bursitis.

Trochanteric fracture.

SUBACUTE AND CHRONIC

Lateral femoral cutaneous neuropathy (meralgia paresthetica).
Osteomyelitis.
Postherpetic neuralgia.
Radiculopathy: L4-5.
Tumors.

JOINT PAIN, POLYARTICULAR

ICD-10CM #   M25.50   Pain in unspecified joint

Osteoarthritis.
RA.
Fibromyalgia.
Viral syndrome (e.g., human parvovirus B19 infection).
SLE.
Psoriatic arthritis.
Ankylosing spondylitis.

JOINT PAIN, POSTERIOR HIPS, THIGH, BUTTOCKS[25]

ICD-10CM #	M25.50	Pain in unspecified joint
	M25.559	Pain in unspecified hip
	M25.569	Pain in unspecified knee

ACUTE

Gluteal muscle strain.
Herpes zoster.
Ischial bursitis.
Ischial or sacral fracture.
Osteomalacia (pseudofracture).
Sciatic neuropathy.
Radiculopathy: L5-S1.

SUBACUTE AND CHRONIC

Gluteal muscle strain.
Ischial bursitis.
Lumbar spinal stenosis.
Osteoarthritis of hip.
Osteitis deformans (Paget disease).
Osteomyelitis.
Osteochondromatosis.
Osteomalacia (pseudofracture).
Postherpetic neuralgia.
Radiculopathy: L5-S1.
Tumors.

JOINT SWELLING

| ICD-10CM # | M25.40 | Effusion, unspecified joint |

Trauma.
Osteoarthritis.
Gout.
Pyogenic arthritis.
Pseudogout.
RA.
Viral syndrome.

JUGULAR VENOUS DISTENTION

ICD-10CM #   I99.8   Other disorder of circulatory system

Right-sided heart failure.
Cardiac tamponade.
Constrictive pericarditis.
Goiter.
Tension pneumothorax.
Pulmonary hypertension.
Cardiomyopathy (restrictive).
Superior vena cava syndrome.
Valsalva maneuver.
Right atrial myxoma.
COPD.

JUVENILE ARTHRITIS[56]

ICD-10CM #   Varies with specific diagnosis

Connective Tissue Diseases
Juvenile idiopathic arthritis.
Systemic lupus erythematosus.
Juvenile dermatomyositis.
Scleroderma with arthritis.
Infectious Arthritis
Bacterial arthritis.
Viral arthritis.
Fungal arthritis.
Lyme disease.
Reactive Arthritis
Poststreptococcal arthritis.
Rheumatic fever.
Toxic synovitis.
Henoch-Schönlein purpura.
Postinfectious arthritis (formerly Reiter).
Orthopedic Disorders
Traumatic arthritis.
Legg-Calve-Perthes disease.
Slipped capital femoral epiphysis.
Osteochondritis dissecans.
Chondromalacia patellae.
Musculoskeletal Pain Syndromes
Growing pains.
Hypermobility syndromes.
Myofascial pain syndromes/fibromyalgia.
Complex regional pain syndrome.
Hematologic/Oncologic Disorders
Leukemia.
Lymphoma.
Sickle cell disease.
Thalassemia.
Malignant and benign tumors of bone, cartilage, or synovium.
Metastatic bone disease.
Hemophilia.
Miscellaneous
Rickets/metabolic bone disease.
Lysosomal storage diseases.
Heritable disorders of collagen.

KERATITIS, NONINFECTIOUS

ICD-10CM #   H16.9   Unspecified keratitis

Collagen vascular disease.
Atopic keratoconjunctivitis.
Chemical injury.
Thermal injury.
Ectropion/entropion.
Lid defects.
Exophthalmos.
Keratoconjunctivitis sicca.
Erythema multiforme.
Mucous membrane pemphigoid.
DM (delayed epithelial healing).
Neuroparalytic (cranial nerve VII).
Neurotrophic (diabetes, cranial nerve V).

KIDNEY CYSTIC DISEASE[89]

ICD-10CM #   Varies with specific diagnosis

CYSTIC DISEASES OF THE KIDNEY
Inheritable
Autosomal recessive (infantile) polycystic kidney disease.
Autosomal dominant (adult) polycystic kidney disease.
    Juvenile nephronophthisis and medullary cystic disease complex.
    Juvenile nephronophthisis (autosomal recessive).
Medullary cystic disease (autosomal dominant).
Congenital nephrosis (familial nephrotic syndrome) (autosomal recessive).
Familial hypoplastic glomerulocystic disease (autosomal dominant).
Multiple malformation syndromes with renal cysts (e.g., tuberous sclerosis, von Hippel-Lindau disease).
Nonheritable
Multicystic kidney (multicystic dysplastic kidney).
Benign multilocular cyst (cystic nephroma).
Simple cysts.
Medullary sponge kidney.
Sporadic glomerulocystic kidney disease.
Acquired renal cystic disease.
Calyceal diverticulum (pyelogenic cyst).

KIDNEY ENLARGEMENT, UNILATERAL[2]

ICD-10CM #   N13.30   Unspecified hydronephrosis

Hydronephrosis (may be bilateral).
Polycystic kidney (may be bilateral).
Simple cyst of kidney.
Renal cell carcinoma.
Pyonephrosis (may be bilateral).
Acute renal vein thrombosis.

KIDNEY INJURY, CANCER PATIENTS[11]

ICD-10CM #   Varies with specific diagnosis

CAUSES OF ACUTE KIDNEY INJURY IN CANCER PATIENTS
Prerenal
Sepsis
Volume depletion (vomiting, diarrhea, mucositis).
Hepatorenal syndrome (venoocclusive disease of the liver).
Capillary leak syndrome (interleukin-2 administration).
Hypercalcemia.
Intrinsic
Acute tubular necrosis
Ischemia (sepsis/shock).
Nephrotoxic (aminoglycosides, amphotericin B, chemotherapy).

Tubulointerstitial nephritis
Tumor lysis syndrome (urate and phosphate nephropathy).
Allergic reaction.
Pyelonephritis.
Opportunistic infections.
Infiltration (lymphoma/leukemia).

Vascular
Thrombotic microangiopathy.
Cancer treated.
Drug induced.
Bone marrow transplantation.
Radiation injury.

Amyloidosis
Light-chain deposition disease
Paraneoplastic syndromes (membranous, antineutrophil cytoplasmic antibody associated, focal segmental glomerulosclerosis)
Postrenal
Intrarenal (urate, acyclovir, methotrexate)
Extrarenal (retroperitoneal fibrosis, lymphadenopathy, direct invasion)

KNEE PAIN[25]

ICD-10CM #		
	S83.419A	Sprain of medial collateral ligament of unspecified knee, initial encounter
	S83.509A	Sprain of unspecified cruciate ligament of unspecified knee, initial encounter
	M23.50	Chronic instability of knee, unspecified knee
	M23.8X9	Other internal derangements of unspecified knee

S83.289A	Other tear of lateral meniscus, current injury, unspecified knee, initial encounter
S83.249A	Other tear of medial meniscus, current injury, unspecified knee, initial encounter
M25.669	Stiffness of unspecified knee, not elsewhere classified

DIFFUSE
Articular.
Anterior.
Prepatellar bursitis.
Patellar tendon enthesopathy.
Chondromalacia patellae.
Patellofemoral osteoarthritis.
Cruciate ligament injury.
Medial plica syndrome.

MEDIAL
Anserine bursitis.
Spontaneous osteonecrosis.
Osteoarthritis.
Medial meniscal tear.
Medial collateral ligament bursitis.
Referred pain from hip and L3.
Fibromyalgia.

LATERAL
Iliotibial band syndrome.
Meniscal cyst.
Lateral meniscal tear.
Collateral ligament.
Peroneal tenosynovitis.

POSTERIOR
Popliteal cyst (Baker cyst).
Tendinitis.
Aneurysms, ganglions, sarcoma.

KNEE PAIN, IN DIFFERENT AGE GROUPS[41]
ICD-10CM # M25.569 Pain in unspecified knee

COMMON CAUSES OF KNEE PAIN IN DIFFERENT AGE GROUPS
Childhood (2 to 10 yr)
Intraarticular
Juvenile arthritis.
Osteochondritis dissecans.
Infection.
Torn discoid meniscus.
Periarticular
Osteomyelitis.
Referred
Perthes disease.
Irritable hip.
Adolescence (10 to 18 yr)
Intraarticular
Osteochondritis dissecans.

Torn meniscus.
Anterior knee pain syndrome.
Patellar instability.
Periarticular
Osgood-Schlatter disease.
Sinding-Larsen-Johansson syndrome.
Osteomyelitis.
Bone tumors.
Referred
Slipped upper femoral epiphysis.
Early Adulthood (18 to 30 yr)
Intraarticular
Torn meniscus.
Patellar instability.
Anterior knee pain syndrome.
Inflammatory arthritis.
Periarticular
Ligament injuries.
Bursitis.
Adulthood (30 to 50 yr)
Intraarticular
Degenerate meniscal tears.
Osteoarthritis.
Inflammatory arthritis.
Periarticular
Bursitis.
Referred
Osteoarthritis of hip.
Spinal disorders.
Old Age (>50 yr)
Intraarticular
Osteoarthritis.
Inflammatory arthritis.
Periarticular
Bursitis.
Referred
Osteoarthritis of hip.
Spinal disorders.

LARGE BOWEL STRICTURE[21]
ICD-10CM # S36.5 Injury of colon

CAUSES OF LARGE BOWEL STRICTURES
Physiologic:
    Spasm.
    Distended bladder.
Malignant:
    Annular carcinoma.
    Scirrhous carcinoma.
    Lymphoma.
Diverticular disease:
    Muscle thickening.
    Pericolic abscess.
    Superimposed malignancy.
Ischemia.
Radiation colitis.
Inflammatory bowel disease:
    Ulcerative colitis.
    Crohn disease.
    Tuberculosis.
    Lymphogranuloma venereum.

Amebiasis.
Extrinsic disease:
    Intraabdominal masses.
    Metastatic carcinoma.
    Endometriosis.
    Pelvic lipomatosis.
    Cholecystitis.
    Pancreatitis.
Miscellaneous:
    Postoperative anastomosis.
    Trauma.
    Hirschsprung disease.

LEFT AXIS DEVIATION[97]
ICD-10CM #	I44.7	Left bundle-branch block, unspecified
	I44.4	Left anterior fascicular block
	I44.5	Left posterior fascicular block
	I44.60	Unspecified fascicular block
	I44.69	Other fascicular block

Normal variation.
Left anterior fascicular block (hemiblock).
Left bundle branch block.
Left ventricular hypertrophy.
Mechanical shifts causing a horizontal heart, high diaphragm, pregnancy, ascites.
Some forms of ventricular tachycardia.
Endocardial cushion defects and other congenital heart disease.

LEFT BUNDLE BRANCH BLOCK
ICD-10CM # I44.7 Left bundle-branch block, unspecified

Ischemic heart disease.
Electrolyte abnormalities (e.g., hyperkalemia).
Cardiomyopathy.
Idiopathic.
LVH.
Pulmonary embolism.
Cardiac trauma.
Bacterial endocarditis.

LEG CRAMPS, NOCTURNAL
ICD-10CM # R25.2 Cramp and spasm

Diabetic neuropathy.
Medications.
Electrolyte abnormalities (hypokalemia, hyponatremia, hypocalcemia, hyperkalemia, hypophosphatemia).
Respiratory alkalosis.
Uremia.
Hemodialysis.
Peripheral nerve injury.
ALS.
Alcohol use.
Heat cramps.
Vitamin B_{12} deficiency.

Hyperthyroidism.
Contractures.
DVT.
Hypoglycemia.
Peripheral vascular insufficiency.
Baker cyst.

LEG LENGTH DISCREPANCIES[51]

ICD-10CM #	M21.759	Unequal limb length (acquired), unspecified femur
	M21.769	Unequal limb length (acquired), unspecified tibia and fibula
	Q72.899	Other reduction defects of unspecified lower limb

CONGENITAL
Proximal femoral local deficiency.
Coxa vara.
Hematrophy-hemihypertrophy (anisomelia).
Developmental dysplasia of the hip.

DEVELOPMENTAL
Legg-Calvé-Perthes disease.

NEUROMUSCULAR
Polio.
Cerebral palsy (hemiplegia).

INFECTIOUS
Pyogenic osteomyelitis with physeal damage.

TRAUMA
Physeal injury with premature closure.
Overgrowth.
Malunion (shortening).

TUMOR
Physeal destruction.
Radiation-induced physeal injury.
Overgrowth.

LEG MOVEMENT WHEN STANDING, INVOLUNTARY

| ICD-10CM # | R25.8 | Other abnormal involuntary movements |

Benign essential tremor.
Orthostatic tremor.
Spastic ataxia.
Cerebellar truncal tremor.
Postanoxic myoclonus.

LEG PAIN, EXERTIONAL[58]

| ICD-10CM # | R25.2 | Cramp and spasm |

Vascular Causes
Atherosclerosis.
Thrombosis.
Embolism.

Vasculitis:
  Thromboangiitis obliterans.
  Takayasu arteritis.
  Giant cell arteritis.
Aortic coarctation.
Fibromuscular dysplasia.
Irradiation.
Endofibrosis of the external iliac artery.
Extravascular compression:
  Arterial entrapment (e.g., popliteal artery entrapment, thoracic outlet syndrome).
Adventitial cysts.
Nonvascular Causes
Lumbosacral radiculopathy:
Degenerative arthritis.
Spinal stenosis.
Herniated disc.
Arthritis:
Hips, knees.
Venous insufficiency.
Myositis.
Glycogen storage disease type V (McArdle syndrome).

LEG PAIN WITH EXERCISE

| ICD-10CM # | R25.2 | Cramp and spasm |

Shin splints.
Arteriosclerosis obliterans.
Neurogenic (spinal cord compression or ischemia).
Venous claudication.
Popliteal cyst.
DVT.
Thromboangiitis obliterans.
Adventitial cysts.
Popliteal artery entrapment syndrome.
McArdle syndrome.

LEG SWELLING[29]

| ICD-10CM # | R60.0 | Localized edema |

Deep vein thrombosis.
Cellulitis.
Baker cyst rupture or inflammation.
Congestive heart failure.
Renal failure.
Liver failure.
Inferior vena cava compression.
Musculoskeletal trauma.
Polyarteritis nodosa.
Erythema nodosum.
Myositis.
Tendinitis.
Lymphedema.
Superficial thrombophlebitis.
Compartment syndrome.

LEG ULCERS[25]

| ICD-10CM # | I70.25 | Atherosclerosis of native arteries of other extremities with ulceration |
| | L97.909 | Non-pressure chronic ulcer of unspecified part |

of unspecified lower leg with unspecified severity

VASCULAR
Arterial: arteriosclerosis, thromboangiitis obliterans, AV malformation, cholesterol emboli.
Venous: superficial varicosities, incompetent perforators, DVT, lymphatic abnormalities.

VASCULITIS HEMATOLOGIC
Sickle cell anemia, thalassemia, polycythemia vera, leukemia, cold agglutinin disease.
Macroglobulinemia, protein C and protein S deficiency, cryoglobulinemia, lupus anticoagulant, antiphospholipid syndrome.

INFECTIOUS
Fungal: blastomycosis, coccidioidomycosis, histoplasmosis, sporotrichosis.
Bacterial: furuncle, ecthyma, septic emboli.
Protozoal: leishmaniasis.

METABOLIC
Necrobiosis lipoidica diabeticorum.
Localized bullous pemphigoid.
Gout, calcinosis cutis, Gaucher disease.

TUMORS
Basal cell carcinoma, squamous cell carcinoma, melanoma.
Mycosis fungoides, Kaposi sarcoma, metastatic neoplasms.

TRAUMA
Burns, cold injury, radiation dermatitis.
Insect bites.
Factitial, excessive pressure.

NEUROPATHIC
Diabetic trophic ulcers.
Tabes dorsalis, syringomyelia.

DRUGS
Warfarin, IV colchicine extravasation, methotrexate, halogens, ergotism, hydroxyurea.

PANNICULITIS
Weber-Christian disease.
Pancreatic fat necrosis, α-antitrypsinase deficiency.

LEPTOMENINGEAL METASTASES[38]

| ICD-10CM # | Code varies with specific diagnosis |

DIFFERENTIAL DIAGNOSISNEOPLASTIC
Parenchymal metastases.
Dural metastases.
Castleman disease.

INFECTIONS
Bacterial/viral meningitis.
Fungal infections, including *Cryptococcus*.

Lyme disease.
Neurocysticercosis.
Tuberculosis.

GRANULOMATOUS DISORDERS

Histiocytosis.
Sarcoidosis.
Granulomatosis with polyangiitis.

INFLAMMATORY DISORDERS

Multiple sclerosis.
Paraneoplastic encephalomyelitis.
Relapsing polychondritis.
Rheumatoid nodules.
Vasculitis (including granulomatous angiitis).

MISCELLANEOUS

Enhancing meningeal blood vessels.
Post–lumbar puncture changes (intracranial hypotension).

LETHARGY AND COMA[20]

ICD-10CM # Varies with specific diagnosis

Epilepsy
Epileptic encephalopathies.
Postictal state.
Status epilepticus.
Hypoxia-Ischemia
Cardiac arrest.
Cardiac arrhythmia.
Congestive heart failure.
Hypotension.
  Autonomic dysfunction.
  Dehydration.
  Hemorrhage.
  Pulmonary embolism.
Near-drowning.
Neonatal.
Increased Intracranial Pressure
Cerebral abscess.
Cerebral edema.
Cerebral tumor.
Herniation syndromes.
Hydrocephalus.
Intracranial hemorrhage.
  Spontaneous.
  Traumatic.
Infectious Disorders
Bacterial infections.
  Cat-scratch disease.*
  Gram-negative sepsis.*
  Hemorrhagic shock and encephalopathy syndrome.*
  Meningitis.*
  Toxic shock syndrome.
Postimmunization encephalopathy.
Rickettsial infections.
  Lyme disease.*
  Rocky Mountain spotted fever.*
Viral infections.
  Arboviruses.
  Aseptic meningitis.

Herpes simplex encephalitis.
Measles encephalitis.
Postinfectious encephalomyelitis.
Reye syndrome.
Metabolic and Systemic Disorders
Disorders of osmolality.
  Diabetic ketoacidosis (hyperglycemia).
  Hypoglycemia.
  Hypernatremia.
  Hyponatremia.
Endocrine disorders.
  Adrenal insufficiency.
  Hypoparathyroidism.
  Thyroid disorders.
Hepatic encephalopathy.
Inborn errors of metabolism.
  Disorders of pyruvate metabolism.
  Glycogen storage disorders.
  Medium-chain acyl-CoA dehydrogenase (MCAD) deficiency.
  Respiratory chain disorders.
  Urea cycle disorder, heterozygote.
Renal disorders.
  Acute uremic encephalopathy.
  Chronic uremic encephalopathy.
  Dialysis encephalopathy.
  Hypertensive encephalopathy.
Other metabolic disorders.
  Burn encephalopathy.
  Hypomagnesemia.
  Parenteral hyperalimentation.
  Vitamin B complex deficiency.
Migraine coma.
Toxic.
  Immunosuppressive drugs.*
  Prescription drugs.*
  Substance abuse.*
  Toxins.*
Trauma.
Concussion.
  Contusion.
  Intracranial hemorrhage.
    Epidural hematoma.
    Subdural hematoma.
    Intracerebral hemorrhage.
  Neonatal.
Vascular.
  Hypertensive encephalopathy.*
  Intracranial hemorrhage, nontraumatic.*
  Lupus erythematosus.*
  Neonatal idiopathic cerebral venous thrombosis.
  Vasculitis.*

*Denotes the most common conditions and the ones with disease-modifying treatments.

LEUKOCORIA

ICD-10CM # H57.9 Unspecified disorder of eye and adnexa

Cataract.
Retinal detachment.

Retinoblastoma.
Retinal telangiectasia.
Retrolenticular vascularized membrane.
Familial exudative vitreoretinopathy.

LID RETRACTION, CAUSES[98]

ICD-10CM # H02.539 Eyelid retraction unspecified eye, unspecified lid

Thyroid eye disease.
Neurogenic:
  Contralateral unilateral ptosis.
  Unopposed levator action due to facial palsy.
  3rd nerve misdirection.
  Marcus Gunn jaw-winking syndrome.
  Collier sign of the dorsal midbrain (Parinaud syndrome).
  Infantile hydrocephalus (setting sun sign).
  Parkinsonism.
  Sympathomimetic drops.
Mechanical:
  Surgical overcorrection of ptosis.
  Scarring of upper lid skin.
Congenital:
  Isolated.
  Duane retraction syndrome.
  Down syndrome.
  Transient "eye popping" reflex in normal infants.
Miscellaneous:
  Prominent globe (pseudo-lid retraction).
  Uremia (Summerskill sign).
  Idiopathic.

LIGHT-NEAR DISSOCIATION[44]

ICD-10CM # Varies with specific diagnosis

CAUSES OF LIGHT-NEAR DISSOCIATION

Unilateral
Afferent conduction defect.
Adie pupil.
Herpes zoster ophthalmicus.
Aberrant regeneration of the third cranial nerve.
Bilateral
Neurosyphilis.
Type 1 diabetes mellitus.
Myotonic dystrophy.
Parinaud (dorsal midbrain) syndrome.
Familial amyloidosis.
Encephalitis.
Chronic alcoholism.

LIMB ISCHEMIA, ACUTE, NONTRAUMATIC[64]

ICD-10CM # I70.2 Atherosclerosis of arteries of extremities

CAUSES OF NONTRAUMATIC ACUTE LIMB ISCHEMIA

Atherosclerotic
In situ thrombosis.

Atheroembolism from thoracic aortic aneurysm/abdominal aortic aneurysm.

Femoral/popliteal aneurysm with or without compression.

Dissection.

Nonatherosclerotic
Embolism from cardiac thrombosis (atrial fibrillation, post–myocardial infarction akinesis).

Graft thrombosis, graft aneurysm.

Mycotic emboli.

Raynaud phenomenon.

Arteritis with thrombosis.

Inherited and acquired hypercoagulable states.

Drug-induced vasospasm.

External compression (Baker cyst, popliteal entrapment).

Mimics
Phlegmasia cerulea dolens.

Acute neuropathy.

Hypovolemia.

Systemic shock.

LIMP

ICD-10CM #		
	R26.0	Ataxic gait
	R26.1	Paralytic gait
	R26.89	Other abnormalities of gait and mobility
	R26.9	Unspecified abnormalities of gait and mobility
	M25.80	Other specified joint disorders, unspecified joint
	F44.4	Conversion disorder with motor symptom or deficit
	F44.6	Conversion disorder with sensory symptom or deficit

Degenerative joint disease, osteochondritis dissecans, chondromalacia patellae.

Trauma to extremities, vertebral disk, hips.

Poorly fitting shoes, foreign body in shoe, unequal leg length.

Splinter in foot.

Joint infection (septic arthritis, osteomyelitis), viral arthritis.

Abdominal pain (e.g., appendicitis, incarcerated hernia), testicular torsion.

Polio, neuromuscular disorders, Guillain-Barré syndrome, multiple sclerosis.

Osgood-Schlatter disease.

Legg-Calvé-Perthes disease.

Factitious, somatization syndrome.

Neoplasm (local or metastatic).

Other: diskitis, periostitis, sickle cell disease, hemophilia.

LIMPING, PEDIATRIC AGE[51]

ICD-10CM #		
	R26.0	Ataxic gait
	R26.1	Paralytic gait
	R26.89	Other abnormalities of gait and mobility
	R26.9	Unspecified abnormalities of gait and mobility

TODDLER (1 TO 3 YR)
Infection:
  Septic arthritis:
    Hip.
    Knee.
    Osteomyelitis.
    Diskitis.
Occult trauma:
  Toddler's fracture.
Neoplasia.

CHILDHOOD (4 TO 10 YR)
Infection:
  Septic arthritis:
    Hip.
    Knee.
    Osteomyelitis.
    Diskitis.
    Transient synovitis, hip.
LCPD.
Tarsal coalition.
Rheumatologic disorder:
  JRA.
Trauma.
Neoplasia.

ADOLESCENCE (11+ YR)
SCFE.
Rheumatologic disorder:
  JRA.
  Trauma.
  Tarsal coalition.
  Hip dislocation (DDH).
  Neoplasia.

DDH, Developmental dysplasia of the hip; *JRA,* juvenile RA; *LCPD,* Legg-Calvé-Perthes disease; *SCFE,* slipped capital femoral epiphysis.

LIVEDO RETICULARIS

ICD-10CM #	L95.0	Livedoid vasculitis

Emboli (SBE, left atrial myxoma, cholesterol emboli).

Thrombocythemia or polycythemia.

Antiphospholipid antibody syndrome.

Cryoglobulinemia, cryofibrinogenemia.

Leukocytoclastic vasculitis.

SLE, RA, dermatomyositis.

Pancreatitis.

Drugs (quinine, quinidine, amantadine, catecholamines).

Physiologic (cutis marmorata).

Congenital.

LIVER DISEASE, PREGNANCY[2]

ICD-10CM #	K75.89	Other specified inflammatory liver diseases

INCIDENTAL TO PREGNANCY
Viral hepatitis.
Alcohol related.
Autoimmune chronic active hepatitis.

RELATED TO PREGNANCY (POSSIBLY INFLUENCED BY HORMONES PRESENT IN PREGNANCY)
Complicated gallstone disease.
Hepatic adenoma.
Focal nodular hyperplasia.
Budd-Chiari syndrome.

SPECIFIC TO PREGNANCY
Severe hyperemesis gravidarum.
Benign intrahepatic cholestasis.
Acute fatty liver of pregnancy.
Preeclampsia (HELLP).

LIVER LESIONS, BENIGN, OFTEN CONFUSED WITH MALIGNANCY

ICD-10CM #	K76.1	Chronic passive congestion of liver
	K76.89	Other specified diseases of liver

Fatty infiltration.
Adenoma.
Hemangioma.
Cysts.
Flow artifacts.
Focal nodular hyperplasia.
Nonenhanced vessels.

LOWER GI ULCERATIVE LESIONS[99]

ICD-10CM #	Varies with specific diagnosis

INFECTIOUS
Epstein-Barr virus.
Human immunodeficiency virus.
Cytomegalovirus.
Herpes simplex.
Herpes zoster.
Syphilis.
Erosive candidiasis.
Mycobacterial infection.
Chancroid.
Lymphogranuloma venereum.

NOT INFECTIOUS
Behçet disease.
Excoriation.
Aphthous (idiopathic) ulcer.

Erythema multiforme.
Carcinoma.

LOW-VOLTAGE ECG

ICD-10CM #   R94.31   Abnormal electrocardiogram [ECG] [EKG]

Hypothyroidism.
Obesity.
Pericardial effusion.
Anasarca.
Pleural effusion.
Pneumothorax.
Amyloidosis.
Aortic stenosis.

LUMBAR SPINE, VISCEROGENIC PAIN REFERRED TO LUMBAR SPINE[351]*

ICD-10CM #   M54.5   Low back pain

Vascular
Expanding aortic aneurysm.
Genitourinary
Endometriosis.
Tubal pregnancy.
Kidney stone.
Prostatitis.
Gastrointestinal
Pancreatitis.
Peptic ulcers.
Colon cancer.

*All of these disorders may cause localized low back pain.

LUNG CANCER, OCCUPATIONAL CAUSES[21]

ICD-10CM #   C34.90   Malignant neoplasm of unspecified part of unspecified bronchus or lung

CAUSES OF OCCUPATIONAL LUNG CANCER

Asbestos	Lagging, insulation
Arsenic	Metal smelting, pesticide manufacture
Beryllium	Electronics, dental prosthetic manufacture
Chromium	Coloring pigment production, electroplating
Nickel	Electroplating
Silica	Grinding, quarrying, sandblasting
Radon	Mining
Uranium	Mining

LUNG DISEASE AND GASTROINTESTINAL AND LIVER INVOLVEMENT[13]

ICD-10CM #   Varies with specific diagnosis

ESOPHAGEAL REFLUX

Aspiration pneumonia.
Asthma.
Scleroderma.
Bronchitis.
Bronchiectasis.
Cough.
Pulmonary fibrosis.
Mycobacterial disease.

INFLAMMATORY BOWEL DISEASE

Bronchitis.
Bronchiectasis.
Bronchiolitis.
Colobronchial fistula.
Desquamative interstitial lung disease.
Drug reactions for agents that treat inflammatory bowel disease.
Eosinophilic lung disease.
Interstitial lung disease.
Necrobiotic nodules.
Obstructive lung disease.
Organizing pneumonia.
Reduced diffusing capacity.
Sarcoidosis.
Serositis affecting pleura or pericarditis.
Tracheal stenosis.

LIVER

α1-antitrypsin deficiency.
Chronic active hepatitis.
Hepatopulmonary syndrome.
Portopulmonary hypertension.
Primary biliary cirrhosis.
Hepatosplenomegaly.
  Amyloidosis.
  Collagen vascular disease.
  Eosinophilic granulomatosis.
  Lymphatic interstitial pneumonia.
  Sarcoidosis.

LUNG DISEASE AND RENAL INVOLVEMENT[13]

ICD-10CM #   Varies with specific diagnosis

LUNG DISEASE WITH RENAL INVOLVEMENT

Glomerulonephritis
Systemic vasculitis.
Collagen vascular disease.
Antibasement membrane.
Sarcoidosis.
Nephrotic Syndrome
Amyloidosis.
Disseminated Langerhans cell histiocytosis.
Drug-induced lung disease.
Paraneoplastic syndrome.
Posttransplantation.
Pulmonary hydatid disease.
Systemic lupus erythematosus.
Vasculitis.
Venous thrombosis.
Renal mass

Lymphangioleiomyomatosis.
Metastasis neoplasm.
Renal carcinoid.
Tuberous sclerosis.
Granulomatosis with polyangiitis.
Nephrolithiasis
Alveolar proteinosis.
Cystic fibrosis.
Hypercalcemic syndromes.
Osteolysis from mycobacteria or fungi.
Sarcoidosis.
Systemic Hypertension
Collagen vascular disease.
Diffuse alveolar hemorrhage.
Pulmonary renal syndromes.
Neurofibromatosis.
Sleep apnea.

LUNG DISEASE AND SKIN AND SUBCUTANEOUS LESIONS[13]

ICD-10CM #   Varies with specific diagnosis

SKIN AND SUBCUTANEOUS LESIONS ASSOCIATED WITH LUNG DISEASE

Skin Lesions
Diffuse pigment change:
  Acanthosis nigricans—lung neoplasm.
  Albinism—Hermansky-Pudlak syndrome.
  Bronze pigmentation—hemosiderosis.
  Gray-brown—Whipple disease.
Cutaneous draining sinus:
  Fungal infections (especially histoplasmosis).
  Mycobacterial infections (especially tuberculosis).
  Neoplasms (especially mesothelial tumors).
  Necrotizing vasculitis.
  Other bacterial infections (especially actinomycosis).
Cutaneous ulcers:
  Beryllium disease.
  Chronic venous insufficiency.
  Fungal infections (especially histoplasmosis).
  Mycobacterial disease.
  Necrotizing vasculitis.
  Parasitic disease.
  Polycythemia.
  Sickle cell disease.
  Tularemia.
Cutaneous vasculitis:
  Behçet syndrome.
  Churg-Strauss syndrome.
  Collagen vascular disease.
  Sarcoidosis.
  Granulomatosis with polyangiitis.
Erythema multiforme:
  Drug reactions.
  Fungi (especially coccidimycosis).
  Mycoplasma and other infectious agents.
  Neoplasms.
  Exfoliative dermatitis.

Adverse drug reactions.
Chemotherapy.
Disseminated malignancy.
Graft-versus-host disease.
Radiation therapy.
Flushing:
Bronchial carcinoid, pheochromocytoma, other neoplasms.
Carbon dioxide, cyanide, and other toxins.
Drugs.
Foods and vasodilatory substances.
Hormones.
Mastocytosis.
Metabolic states (e.g., hyperthyroidism, fever).
Macular rash:
Antibasement membrane disease.
Café-au-lait spots (neurofibromatosis).
Coal miner's scars.
Collagen vascular disease.
Idiopathic pulmonary fibrosis.
Rose spots (psittacosis).
Sarcoidosis.
Syphilis.
Viral pneumonia.
Maculopapular rash:
Amyloidosis.
Drug-induced lung disease.
Collagen vascular disease.
Gaucher disease.
Kaposi sarcoma.
Lung neoplasm.
Lymphomatoid granulomatosis.
Lymphoma.
Parasites.
Sarcoidosis.
Syphilis.
Vasculitis.
Viral pneumonia
Telangiectasia:
Arteriovenous malformation.
Ataxia-telangiectasia.
Carcinoid syndrome.
Cushing disease.
Hepatopulmonary syndrome and other chronic liver diseases.
Hereditary hemorrhagic telangiectasia (Osler-Weber-Rendu).
Mastocytosis.
Systemic sclerosis and other collagen vascular diseases.
Urticaria:
Asthma.
Drug reactions.
Cystic fibrosis.
Exercise-induced urticaria.
Food allergy.
Hereditary angioneurotic edema.
Inhaled antigens.
Insect bites and stings.
Infectious agents, such as *Mycoplasma* and *Helicobacter*.

Mastocytosis.
Occupational sensitization.
Parasites.
Vasculitis.
Nail Changes with Lung Disease
Color changes:
Cigarette smoking discoloration.
Splinter hemorrhages.
Yellow nail syndrome.
Beau lines (any severe illness):
Dermatomyositis.
Sarcoidosis.
Seronegative arthropathies.
Systemic sclerosis.
Lung Disease with Subcutaneous Involvement
Adenopathy:
Environmental mycobacteria.
Fungal infections.
Human immunodeficiency virus infections.
Metastatic neoplasm.
Leukemia.
Lymphoma.
Sarcoidosis.
Tuberculosis.
Calcinosis:
Dermatomyositis.
Metastatic osteosarcoma.
Mixed connective tissue disease.
Scleroderma.
Tuberculosis.
Uremic metastatic calcification.
Erythema induratum (Bazin disease):
Aortic stenosis.
Cryoglobulinemia.
Nodular vasculitis.
Panniculitis.
Peripheral neuropathy.
Takayasu disease.
Streptococcus infection.
Tuberculosis and other mycobacterial disease.
Weber-Christian disease.
Erythema nodosa:
Neoplasm.
Other infectious and inflammatory diseases.
Primary coccidiomycosis, histoplasmosis.
Primary tuberculosis.
Psittacosis.
Sarcoidosis.
Subcutaneous nodules:
Amyloidosis.
Neoplasm.
Neurofibromatosis.
Rheumatoid arthritis.
Tuberous sclerosis (angiofibromas).
von Recklinghausen.
Weber-Christian disease.
Lung Disease with Salivary Gland Enlargement
Bulimia and aspiration.
Gaucher disease.
Lymphoid interstitial pneumonitis.

Lymphatic carcinoma.
Lymphoma.
Other causes of lymphadenopathy.
Sarcoidosis.
Sjögren disease.

LUNG DISEASE WITH BONE, JOINT, NERVE, AND MUSCLE INVOLVEMENT[13]
ICD-10CM # Varies with specific diagnosis

ARTHRITIS
Ankylosing spondylitis.
Collagen vascular diseases.
Reactive arthritis.
Sarcoidosis.
Systemic vasculitis.
Tuberculosis.

BONE LESIONS
Ankylosing spondylitis.
Blastomycosis and other fungal disease.
Collagen vascular diseases.
Eosinophilic granulomatosis.
Fibrous histiocytoma.
Gaucher disease.
Neoplasm.
Sarcoidosis.
Tuberculosis.

MUSCLE DISEASE
Collagen vascular disease.
l-Tryptophan.
Diabetes insipidus.
Eosinophilic granulomatosis.
Polymyositis.
Sarcoidosis.

NEUROLOGIC DISEASE
Acute inflammatory polyneuropathy.
Amyotrophic lateral sclerosis.
Aspiration.
Botulism.
Lambert-Eaton syndrome.
Myasthenia gravis.
Organophosphate poisoning.
Polio and postpolio syndrome.
Sarcoidosis.
Churg-Strauss syndrome.
Granulomatosis with polyangiitis.

LUNG TUMORS, BENIGN[78]
ICD-10CM # Varies with specific disorder

COMMON BENIGN TUMORS OF THE LUNG BASED ON CELLS OF ORIGIN
Tumors of Epithelial Origin
Mucous gland adenoma.
Clara cell adenoma.
Mucous cystadenoma.

Pleomorphic adenoma.

Tumors of Mesenchymal Origin

Hamartoma.

Inflammatory pseudotumor.

Chondroma.

Fibroma.

Benign endobronchial fibrous histiocytoma.

Leiomyoma.

Lipoma.

Lymphatic lesions.

Tumors of Miscellaneous Origin

Nodular pulmonary amyloidosis.

Clear cell tumor (sugar tumor).

Thymoma.

Granular cell tumor.

Teratoma.

Pulmonary paraganglioma.

LUNG VOLUMES IN DIFFUSE LUNG DISEASE[59]

ICD-10CM #   Varies with specific disorder

LARGE LUNG VOLUMES

Emphysema.

Chronic asthma.

Diffuse bronchiolitis obliterans.

Highly trained athletes.

Lymphangioleiomyomatosis.

SMALL LUNG VOLUMES

End-stage lung fibrosis.

Bilateral diaphragmatic paralysis.

Massive ascites.

NORMAL LUNG VOLUMES

Sarcoidosis.

Langerhans cell histiocytosis.

Neurofibromatosis.

Emphysema with pulmonary fibrosis.

LYMPHADENOPATHY[24]

ICD-10CM #   R59.9   Enlarged lymph nodes, unspecified

GENERALIZED

AIDS.

Lymphoma: Hodgkin disease, non-Hodgkin lymphoma.

Leukemias, reticuloendotheliosis.

Infectious mononucleosis, CMV, and other viral infections.

Diffuse skin infection: generalized furunculosis, multiple tick bites.

Parasitic infections: toxoplasmosis, filariasis, leishmaniasis, Chagas disease.

Serum sickness.

Collagen vascular diseases (RA, SLE).

Dengue (arbovirus infection).

Sarcoidosis and other granulomatous diseases.

Drugs: INH, hydantoin derivatives, antithyroid and antileprosy drugs.

Secondary syphilis.

Hyperthyroidism, lipid-storage diseases.

LOCALIZED

Cervical Nodes

Infections of the head, neck, ears, sinuses, scalp, pharynx.

Mononucleosis.

Lymphoma.

TB.

Malignancy of head and neck.

Rubella.

Scalene/Supraclavicular Nodes

Lymphoma.

Lung neoplasm.

Bacterial or fungal infection of thorax or retroperitoneum.

GI malignancy.

Axillary Nodes

Infections of hands and arms.

Cat-scratch disease.

Neoplasm (lymphoma, melanoma, breast carcinoma).

Brucellosis.

Epitrochlear Nodes

Infections of the hand.

Lymphoma.

Tularemia.

Sarcoidosis, secondary syphilis (usually bilateral).

Inguinal Nodes

Infections of leg or foot, folliculitis (pubic hair).

LGV, syphilis.

Lymphoma.

Pelvic malignancy.

Pasteurella pestis.

Hilar Nodes

Sarcoidosis.

TB.

Lung carcinoma.

Fungal infections, systemic.

Mediastinal Nodes

Sarcoidosis.

Lymphoma.

Lung neoplasm.

TB.

Mononucleosis.

Histoplasmosis.

Abdominal/Retroperitoneal Nodes

Lymphoma.

TB.

Neoplasm (ovary, testes, prostate, and other malignancies).

LYMPHANGITIS[1]

ICD-10CM #   I89.1   Lymphangitis

Acute:

Group A streptococci.

Staphylococcus aureus.

Pasteurella multocida.

Chronic:

Sporothrix schenckii (sporotrichosis).

Mycobacterium marinum (swimming pool granuloma).

Mycobacterium kansasii.

Nocardia brasiliensis.

Wuchereria bancrofti.

LYMPHEDEMA[100]

ICD-10CM #	i89.0	Lymphedema, not elsewhere classified
	I97.2	Postmastectomy lymphedema syndrome
	Q82.0	Hereditary lymphedema

CLASSIFICATION OF LYMPHEDEMA

Primary Lymphedema

Congenital lymphedema (Milroy disease).

Lymphedema praecox.

Lymphedema tarda.

Syndromes Associated with Primary Lymphedema

Yellow nail syndrome.

Turner syndrome.

Noonan syndrome.

Pes cavus.

Phakomatosis pigmentovascularis.

Distichiasis-lymphedema.

Emberger syndrome.

WILD syndrome.

Hypotrichosis-telangiectasia-lymphedema syndrome.

Cutaneous Disorders Sometimes Associated with Primary Lymphedema

Yellow nails.

Hemangiomas.

Xanthomatosis and chylous lymphedema.

Congenital absence of nails.

Secondary Lymphedema

Postmastectomy lymphedema.

Melphalan isolated limb perfusion.

Malignant occlusion with obstruction.

Extrinsic pressure.

Factitial lymphedema.

Postradiation therapy.

Following recurrent lymphangitis/cellulitis.

Lymphedema of upper limb in recurrent eczema.

Granulomatous disease.

Rosaceous lymphedema.

Primary amyloidosis.

Complications of Lymphedema

Cellulitis of lymphedema.

Elephantiasis nostras verrucosa.

Ulceration.

Lymphangiosarcoma.

LYMPHOCYTOSIS, ATYPICAL[1]

ICD-10CM #   D72.89   Other specified disorders of white blood cells

Epstein-Barr virus primary infection (infectious mononucleosis).

Cytomegalovirus primary infection (heterophile-negative mono).

Human herpesvirus 6 primary infection (roseola).

Primary HIV infection.

Toxoplasmosis.
Acute viral hepatitis.
Rubella, mumps.
Drug reactions (e.g., phenytoin, sulfa).

MACROCEPHALY[101]

ICD-10CM #　Varies with specific diagnosis

CAUSES
Hydrocephalus.
Obstructive hydrocephalus from aqueductal stenosis.
Communicating hydrocephalus from meningitis.
Mass lesions.
Subdural hematoma.
Tumors.
Neurocutaneous disorders.
Neurofibromatosis (NF1).
Tuberous sclerosis.
Metabolic storage diseases.
Hurler syndrome.
Leukodystrophies.
Tay-Sachs disease.
Genetic mutations.
47,XYY.
PTEN mutation.
Trisomy 13.
Trisomy 18.
Abnormal skull growth.
Achondroplasia.
Benign familial trait.

MACROTHROMBOCYTOPENIA, INHERITED[31]

ICD-10CM #　Varies with specific disorder

Bernard-Soulier syndrome.
MHY9-related disorders:
　May-Hegglin anomaly.
　Sebastian syndrome.
　Fechtner syndrome.
　Epstein syndrome.
Gray platelet syndrome.
Montreal platelet syndrome.
Mediterranean macrothrombocytopenia.
Mediterranean stomatocytosis/macrothrombocytemia.
GATA1 mutations.
Sialyl-Lewis-S antigen deficiency.
Paris-Trousseau syndrome.
Platelet-type von Willebrand disease.

MACULAR CRYSTALS[44]

ICD-10CM #　Varies with specific diagnosis

OTHER CAUSES OF MACULAR CRYSTALS
Primary hyperoxaluria.
Bietti corneoretinal crystalline dystrophy.
Cystinosis.
Sjögren–Larsson syndrome.

Gyrate atrophy.
Acquired parafoveal telangiectasis.
Talc-corn starch emboli.
West African crystalline maculopathy.

MADAROSIS[44]

ICD-10CM #　H02.729　Madarosis of unspecified eye, unspecified eyelid and periocular area

CAUSES OF MADAROSIS
Local
Chronic anterior lid margin disease.
Infiltrating lid tumors.
Burns.
Radiotherapy or cryotherapy of lid tumors.
Skin Disorders
Generalized alopecia.
Psoriasis.
Systemic diseases.
Myxedema.
Systemic lupus erythematosus.
Acquired syphilis.
Lepromatous leprosy.
Following Removal
Procedures for trichiasis.
Trichotillomania (psychiatric disorder of hair removal).

MALABSORPTION[2]

ICD-10CM #　K90.89　Other intestinal malabsorption

CAUSES OF MALABSORPTION
More Common
Celiac disease.
Chronic pancreatitis.
Post gastrectomy.
Crohn disease.
Small bowel resection.
Small intestinal bacterial overgrowth.
Lactase deficiency.
Less Common
AIDS (*Mycobacterium avium intracellulare*, AIDS enteropathy).
Whipple disease.
Intestinal lymphoma.
Immunoproliferative small intestinal disease (alpha heavy chain disease).
Radiation enteritis.
Collagenous sprue.
Tropical sprue.
Nongranulomatous ulcerative jejunoileitis.
Eosinophilic gastroenteritis.
Amyloidosis.
Zollinger-Ellison syndrome.
Intestinal lymphangiectasia.
Systemic mastocytosis.
Chronic mesenteric ischemia.
Abetalipoproteinemia (autosomal recessive).

MALABSORPTION SYNDROME IN TROPICS[3]

ICD-10CM #　K90.89　Other intestinal malabsorption

CAUSES OF MALABSORPTION SYNDROME IN THE TROPICS
SIBO
Following ulcer surgery.
Secondary to intestinal TB and Crohn disease.
Infections
Bacteria
Mycobacterium avium intracellulare complex.
Mycobacterium tuberculosis.
Helminths
Paracapillaria philippinensis.
Strongyloides stercoralis.
Protozoa
Cryptosporidium parvum.
Cyclospora cayetanensis.
Encephalitozoon intestinalis.
Enterocytozoon bieneusi.
Giardia lamblia.
Isospora belli.
Leishmania donovani.
Lymphatic Obstruction
Intestinal lymphangiectasia.
Mucosal Diseases
Autoimmune enteropathy.
Celiac disease.
Eosinophilic gastroenteritis.
HIV enteropathy.
Immunoproliferative small intestinal disease.
Intestinal lymphoma.
Primary immunodeficiencies.
Tropical sprue.
Neonatal Diseases
Microvillus inclusion disease.
Tufting enteropathy.
Pancreatic Insufficiency
Alcoholic pancreatitis.
CF.
Tropical pancreatitis.
Specific Transport Disorders
Abetalipoproteinemia.
Fructose malabsorption.
Glucose-galactose malabsorption.
Hypolactasia.
Sucrose intolerance.

MALNUTRITION, CAUSES IN EARLY LIFE[19]

ICD-10CM #　E46　Unspecified protein-energy malnutrition

0 TO 6 MO
Breastfeeding difficulties.
Improper formula preparation.
Impaired parent/child interaction.
Congenital syndromes.
Prenatal infections or teratogenic exposures.
Poor feeding (sucking, swallowing) or feeding refusal (aversion).

Maternal psychological disorder (depression or attachment disorder).
Congenital heart disease.
Cystic fibrosis.
Neurologic abnormalities.
Child neglect.
Recurrent infections.

6 TO 12 MO
Celiac disease.
Food intolerance.
Child neglect.
Delayed introduction of age-appropriate foods or poor transition to food.
Recurrent infections.
Food allergy.

AFTER INFANCY
Acquired chronic diseases.
Highly distractible child.
Inappropriate mealtime environment.
Inappropriate diet (e.g., excessive juice consumption, avoidance of high-calorie foods).
Recurrent infections.

MASTALGIA, MEDICATION INDUCED[102]
ICD-10CM # N64.4 Mastodynia

Medications Associated with Mastalgia
Antihypertensives.
Atenolol and other beta-blockers.
Hydrochlorothiazide.
Methyldopa.
Minoxidil.
Spironolactone.
Antidepressants and antipsychotic agents.
Amitriptyline and other tricyclic antid\\ressants.
Chlorpromazine/promethazine.
Fluoxetine.
Haloperidol.
Hormonal agents.
Estrogens.
Progestins.
Androgens.
Ginseng.
Clomiphene citrate.
Digoxin.
Chlorpropamide.

MEDIASTINAL COMPARTMENTS, ANATOMY AND PATHOLOGY[103]
ICD-10CM # Varies with specific disorder

ANTERIOR
Normal Structures
Lymph nodes.
Connective tissue.
Thymus (remnant in adults).
Masses
Thymoma.
Germ cell neoplasm.
Lymphoma.
Thyroid enlargement (intrathoracic goiter).
Other tumors.

MIDDLE
Normal Structures
Pericardium.
Heart.
Vessels: ascending aorta, venae cavae, main pulmonary arteries.
Trachea.
Lymph nodes.
Nerves: phrenic, upper vagus.
Masses
Carcinoma.
Lymphoma.
Pericardial cyst.
Bronchogenic cyst.
Benign lymph node enlargement (granulomatous disease).

POSTERIOR
Normal Structures
Vessels: descending aorta.
Esophagus.
Vertebral column.
Nerves: sympathetic chain, lower vagus.
Lymph nodes.
Connective tissue.
Masses
Neurogenic tumor.
Diaphragmatic hernia.

MEDIASTINAL MASSES OR WIDENING ON CHEST X-RAY
ICD-10CM # R59.9 Enlarged lymph nodes, unspecified
J98.5 Diseases of mediastinum, not elsewhere classified

Lymphoma: Hodgkin disease and non-Hodgkin lymphoma.
Sarcoidosis.
Vascular: aortic aneurysm, ectasia, or tortuosity of aorta or bronchocephalic vessels.
Carcinoma: lungs, esophagus.
Esophageal diverticula.
Hiatal hernia.
Achalasia.
Prominent pulmonary outflow tract: pulmonary hypertension, pulmonary embolism, right-to-left shunts.
Trauma: mediastinal hemorrhage.
Pneumomediastinum.

Lymphadenopathy caused by silicosis and other pneumoconioses.
Leukemias.
Infections: TB, viral (rare), *Mycoplasma* (rare), fungal, tularemia.
Substernal thyroid.
Thymoma.
Teratoma.
Bronchogenic cyst.
Pericardial cyst.
Neurofibroma, neurosarcoma, ganglioneuroma.

MEDIASTINAL MASSES, SITES OF ORIGIN[48]
ICD-10CM # Varies with specific diagnosis

DIFFERENTIAL DIAGNOSIS OF MEDIASTINAL MASSES BASED ON COMMON SITES OF ORIGIN
Prevascular Space (Anterior Mediastinum)
Thymic masses.
Thymoma.
Thymic carcinoma.
Thymic neuroendocrine tumor.
Thymolipoma.
Thymic cyst.
Thymic hyperplasia.
Thymic lymphoma.
Germ cell tumors.
Teratoma and dermoid cyst.
Seminoma.
Nonseminomatous germ cell tumors.
Thyroid abnormalities (goiter and neoplasm).
Parathyroid tumor or hyperplasia.
Lymph node masses (particularly Hodgkin lymphoma).
Vascular abnormalities (aorta and great vessels).
Mesenchymal abnormalities (e.g., lipomatosis, lipoma).
Foregut cyst.
Lymphangioma.
Hemangioma.
Retrosternal Space (Anterior Mediastinum)
Lymph node masses.
Pretracheal Space (Middle Mediastinum)
Lymph node masses.
Lung carcinoma.
Sarcoidosis.
Lymphoma (particularly Hodgkin disease).
Metastases.
Infections (e.g., tuberculosis).
Foregut cyst.
Tracheal tumor.
Mesenchymal masses (e.g., lipomatosis, lipoma).
Thyroid abnormalities.
Vascular abnormalities (aorta and great vessels).
Lymphangioma and hemangioma.
Aortopulmonary Window (Middle Mediastinum)
Lymph node masses.
Lung carcinoma.

Sarcoidosis.
Lymphoma.
Metastases.
Infections (e.g., tuberculosis).
Mesenchymal masses (e.g., lipomatosis, lipoma).
Vascular abnormalities (aorta or pulmonary artery).
Chemodectoma.
Foregut cyst.
Subcarinal Space and Azygoesophageal Recess (Middle Mediastinum)
Lymph node masses.
Lung carcinoma.
Sarcoidosis.
Lymphoma.
Metastases.
Infections (e.g., tuberculosis).
Foregut cyst.
Dilated azygos vein.
Esophageal masses.
Varices.
Hernia.
Paravertebral Masses (Posterior Mediastinum)
Neurogenic tumor.
Nerve sheath tumors.
Sympathetic ganglia tumors.
Paraganglioma.
Meningocele.
Foregut cyst.
Neurenteric cyst.
Thoracic spine abnormalities.
Extramedullary hematopoiesis.
Fluid collections and pseudocyst.
Vascular abnormalities.
Hernias.
Esophageal masses.
Varices.
Mesenchymal masses (e.g., lipomatosis, lipoma).
Lymph node masses.
Lymphoma (particularly non-Hodgkin).
Metastases.
Dilated azygos or hemiazygos vein.
Hernia.
Lymphangioma and hemangioma.
Thymic mass or germ cell tumor.
Anterior cardiophrenic angle masses.
Lymph node masses (particularly lymphoma and metastases).
Pericardial cyst.
Fat pad.
Morgagni hernia.
Thymic masses.
Germ cell tumors.

MEDIASTINITIS, ACUTE[1]

ICD-10CM # J98.5 Diseases of mediastinum, not elsewhere classified

Esophageal perforation.
Iatrogenic.
EGD, esophageal dilation, esophageal variceal sclerotherapy, nasogastric tube, Sengstaken-

Blackmore tube, endotracheal intubation, esophageal surgery, paraesophageal surgery, transesophageal echocardiography, anterior stabilization of cervical vertebral bodies.
Swallowed foreign bodies.
Trauma.
Spontaneous perforation (e.g., emesis, carcinoma).
Head and neck infections (e.g., tonsillitis, pharyngitis, parotitis, epiglottitis, odontogenic).
Infections originating at another site (e.g., TB, pneumonia, pancreatitis, osteomyelitis of sternum, clavicle, ribs).
Cardiothoracic surgery (median sternotomy) (e.g., CABG, valve replacement, other types of cardiothoracic surgery).

MELANONYCHIA

ICD-10CM # NEC   Melanin
         L81.4   hyperpigmentation

Pregnancy.
Trauma.
Medications (e.g., AZT, 5-fluorouracil, doxorubicin, psoralens).
Nail matrix nevus.
HIV infection.
Onychomycosis.
Melanocyte hyperplasia.
Verrucae.
Pustular psoriasis.
Lichen planus.
Basal cell carcinoma.
Nail matrix melanoma.
Subungual keratosis.
Addison disease.
Bowen disease.

MEMORY LOSS SYMPTOMS, ELDERLY PATIENTS

ICD-10CM # R41.2 Retrograde amnesia

Age-related mild cognitive impairment.
Depression (pseudodementia).
Medications (e.g., anticholinergics, sedatives).
Hypothyroidism.
Chronic hypoxia.
Cerebrovascular infarcts.
Alzheimer disease.
Hepatic disease.
Chronic renal failure.
Hyperthyroidism.
Frontotemporal dementia.
Lewy body dementia.

MENINGITIS, CHRONIC[1]

ICD-10CM # G03.1 Chronic meningitis

TB.
Fungal CNS infection.
Tertiary syphilis.
CNS neoplasm.
Metabolic encephalopathies.

Multiple sclerosis.
Chronic subdural hematoma.
SLE cerebritis.
Encephalitides.
Sarcoidosis.
NSAIDs.
Behçet syndrome.
Anatomic defects (traumatic, congenital, postoperative).
Granulomatous angiitis.

MENINGITIS, RECURRENT[1]

ICD-10CM # G03.2 Benign recurrent meningitis [Mollaret]

Drug induced (with rechallenge).
Parameningeal focus.
    Infection (sinusitis, mastoiditis, osteomyelitis, brain abscess).
    Tumor (epidermoid cyst, craniopharyngioma).
Posttraumatic (bacterial).
Mollaret meningitis.
SLE.
Herpes simplex virus.

MENTAL STATUS CHANGES AND COMA[43]

ICD-10CM # R41.82 Altered mental status, unspecified

METABOLIC/SYSTEMIC ETIOLOGY OF ALTERED MENTAL STATUS AND COMA
Hypoxia
Severe pulmonary disease (hypoventilation).
Severe anemia.
Environmental/toxin:
Methemoglobinemia:
    Cyanide.
    Carbon monoxide.
    Decreased atmospheric oxygen (high altitude).
    Near-drowning.
Disorders of Glucose
Hypoglycemia:
    Chronic alcohol abuse and liver disease.
    Excessive use of insulin or other hypoglycemic agents.
    Insulinoma.
Hyperglycemia:
    Diabetic ketoacidosis.
    Nonketotic hyperosmolar coma.
Decreased Cerebral Blood Flow
Hypovolemic shock.
Cardiac:
    Vasovagal syncope.
    Arrhythmias.
    Myocardial infarction.
    Valvular disorders.
    Congestive heart failure.
    Pericardial effusion/tamponade.
    Myocarditis.
Infectious:
    Septic shock.

Bacterial meningitis.

Vascular/hematologic:

Hypertensive encephalopathy.

Pseudotumor cerebri.

Hyperviscosity (sickle cell, polycythemia).

Hyperventilation.

Cerebral lupus vasculitis.

Thrombotic thrombocytopenic purpura.

Disseminated intravascular coagulation.

Metabolic Cofactor Deficiency

Thiamine (Wernicke-Korsakoff syndrome).

Pyridoxine (isoniazid overdose).

Folic acid (chronic alcohol abuse).

Cyanocobalamin.

Niacin.

Electrolyte/pH Disturbances

Acidosis/alkalosis.

Hypernatremia/hyponatremia.*

Hypercalcemia/hypocalcemia.

Hypophosphatemia.

Hypermagnesemia/hypomagnesemia.

Endocrine Disorders

Myxedema coma, thyrotoxicosis.

Hypopituitarism.

Addison disease (primary or secondary).

Cushing disease.

Pheochromocytoma.

Hyperparathyroidism/hypoparathyroidism.

Endogenous Toxins

Hyperammonemia (liver failure).

Uremia (renal disease).

Carbon dioxide narcosis (pulmonary disease).

Porphyria.

Exogenous Toxins

Alcohols:

Ethanol, isopropyl alcohol, methanol, ethylene glycol.

Acid poisons:

Salicylates.

Paraldehyde.

Ammonium chloride.

Antidepressant medications:

Lithium.

Tricyclic antidepressants (TCAs).

Selective serotonin reuptake inhibitors (SSRIs).

Monoamine oxidase inhibitors (MAOIs).

Stimulants:

Amphetamines/methamphetamines.

Cocaine.

Over-the-counter sympathomimetics.

Narcotics/opiates:

Morphine.

Heroin.

Codeine, oxycodone, meperidine, hydrocodone.

Methadone.

Fentanyl.

Propoxyphene.

Sedative-hypnotics:

Benzodiazepines.

*Can be associated with dilution of formula in infant feeding.

Barbiturates.

Rohypnol.

Bromide.

Hallucinogens:

Lysergic acid diethylamide (LSD).

Marijuana.

Mescaline, peyote.

Mushrooms.

Phencyclidine (PCP).

Herbs/plants:

Aconite.

Jimson weed.

Morning glory.

Volatile substances:

Hydrocarbons (gasoline, butane, toluene, benzene, chloroform).

Nitrites.

Anesthetic agents (nitrous oxide, ether).

Other:

γ-Hydroxybutyrate (GHB).

Ketamine.

Penicillin.

Cardiac glycosides.

Anticonvulsants.

Steroids.

Heavy metals.

Cimetidine.

Organophosphates.

Disorders of Temperature Regulation/Environmental

Hypothermia.

Heat stroke.

Malignant hyperthermia.

Neuroleptic malignant syndrome.

High-altitude cerebral edema (HACE).

Dysbarism.

Primary Glial or Neuronal Disorders

Adrenoleukodystrophy.

Creutzfeldt-Jakob disease.

Progressive multifocal leukoencephalopathy.

Marchiafava-Bignami disease.

Gliomatosis cerebri.

Central pontine myelinolysis.

Other Disorders of Unknown Etiology

Seizures.

Postictal states.

Reye syndrome.[†]

Intussusception.

[†]Prominent in the pediatric population.

MENTAL STATUS CHANGES AND COMA, STRUCTURAL CAUSES[29]

ICD-10CM # R40.1 Stupor

COMMON AGE-RELATED CAUSES OF ALTERED MENTAL STATUS AND COMA

Infant

Infection.

Trauma, abuse.

Metabolic.

Child

Toxic ingestion.

Adolescent, Young Adult

Toxic ingestion.

Recreational drug use.

Trauma.

Elderly

Medication changes.

Over-the-counter medications.

Infection.

Alterations in living environment.

Stroke.

Trauma.

MENTAL STATUS CHANGES AND COMA, METABOLIC AND SYSTEMIC CAUSES

ICD-10CM # F05.9 Delirium, unspecified

METABOLIC AND SYSTEMIC CAUSES OF ALTERED MENTAL STATUS AND COMA

Hypoxia, Hypercapnia

Severe pulmonary disease (hypoventilation).

Severe anemia.

Environmental, toxic.

Methemoglobinemia.

Cyanide.

Carbon monoxide.

Decreased atmospheric oxygen (high altitude).

Near-drowning.

Glucose Disorders

Hypoglycemia:

Chronic alcohol abuse and liver disease.

Excessive dosage of insulin or other hypoglycemic agents.

Insulinoma.

Hyperglycemia:

Diabetic ketoacidosis.

Nonketotic hyperosmolar coma.

Decreased Cerebral Blood Flow

Hypovolemic shock.

Cardiac:

Vasovagal syncope.

Arrhythmias.

Myocardial infarction.

Valvular disorders.

Congestive heart failure.

Pericardial effusion, tamponade.

Myocarditis.

Infectious:

Septic shock.

Bacterial meningitis.

Vascular, hematologic

Hypertensive encephalopathy.

Pseudotumor cerebri.

Hyperviscosity (sickle cell, polycythemia).

Hyperventilation.

Cerebral vasculitis as a manifestation of systemic lupus erythematosus.

Thrombotic thrombocytopenic purpura.

Disseminated intravascular coagulation.

Differential Diagnosis

II

Metabolic Cofactor Deficiency
Thiamine (Wernicke-Korsakoff syndrome).
Pyridoxine (isoniazid overdose).
Folic acid (chronic alcohol abuse).
Cyanocobalamin.
Niacin.
Electrolyte, pH Disturbances
Acidosis, alkalosis.
Hypernatremia, hyponatremia.*
Hypercalcemia, hypocalcemia.
Hypophosphatemia.
Hypermagnesemia, hypomagnesemia.
Endocrine Disorders
Myxedema coma, thyrotoxicosis.
Hypopituitarism.
Addison disease (primary or secondary).
Cushing disease.
Pheochromocytoma.
Hyperparathyroidism, hypoparathyroidism.
Endogenous Toxins
Hyperammonemia (liver failure).
Uremia (renal disease).
Carbon dioxide narcosis (pulmonary disease).
Porphyria.
Exogenous Toxins
Alcohols:
   Ethanol, isopropyl alcohol, methanol, ethylene
      glycol.
Acid poisons:
   Salicylates.
   Paraldehyde.
   Ammonium chloride.
Antidepressant medications:
   Lithium.
   Tricyclic antidepressants.
   Selective serotonin reuptake inhibitors.
   Monoamine oxidase inhibitors.
Stimulants:
   Amphetamines, methamphetamines.
   Cocaine.
   Over-the-counter sympathomimetics.
Narcotics, opiates:
   Morphine.
   Heroin.
   Codeine,   oxycodone,   meperidine,
      hydrocodone.
   Methadone.
   Fentanyl.
   Propoxyphene.
Sedative-hypnotics:
   Benzodiazepines.
   Barbiturates.
   Rohypnol.
   Bromide.
Hallucinogens:
   Lysergic acid diethylamide.
   Marijuana.
   Mescaline, peyote.
   Mushrooms.
   Phencyclidine.

Herbs, plants:
   Aconite.
   Jimsonweed.
   Morning glory.
Volatile substances:
   Hydrocarbons (gasoline, butane, toluene,
      benzene, chloroform).
   Nitrites.
   Anesthetic agents (nitrous oxide, ether).
Other:
   γ-Hydroxybutyrate.
   Ketamine.
   Penicillin.
   Cardiac glycosides.
   Anticonvulsants.
   Steroids.
   Heavy metals.
   Cimetidine.
   Organophosphates.
*Disorders of Temperature Regulation,
Environmental*
Hypothermia.
Heat stroke.
Malignant hyperthermia.
Neuroleptic malignant syndrome.
High-altitude cerebral edema.
Dysbarism.
Primary Glial or Neuronal Disorders
Adrenoleukodystrophy.
Creutzfeldt-Jakob disease.
Progressive multifocal leukoencephalopathy.
Marchiafava-Bignami disease.
Gliomatosis cerebri.
Central pontine myelinolysis.
Other Disorders with Unknown Etiology
Seizures.
Postictal states.
Reye syndrome.
Intussusception.

MESENTERIC ARTERIAL EMBOLISM, ASSOCIATED FACTORS[43]

ICD-10CM #	I74.09	Other arterial embolism and thrombosis of abdominal aorta

FACTORS ASSOCIATED WITH MESENTERIC ARTERIAL EMBOLISM

Coronary artery disease:
   Postmyocardial infarction mural thrombi.
   Congestive heart failure.
Valvular heart disease:
   Rheumatic mitral valve disease.
   Nonbacterial endocarditis.
Arrhythmias:
   Chronic atrial fibrillation.
Aortic aneurysms or dissections.
Coronary angiography.

MESENTERIC ISCHEMIA, NONOCCLUSIVE[1]

ICD-10CM #	K55.0	Acute vascular disorders of intestine
	K55.1	Chronic vascular disorders of intestine
	S35.8X9A	Unspecified injury of other blood vessels at abdomen, lower back and pelvis level, initial encounter

Cardiovascular disease resulting in low-flow states (CHF, cardiogenic shock, post cardio-pulmonary bypass, dysrhythmias).
Septic shock.
Drug induced (cocaine, vasopressors, ergot alkaloid poisoning).

MESENTERIC VENOUS THROMBOSIS[1]

ICD-10CM #	I82.91	Chronic embolism and thrombosis of unspecified vein

Hypercoagulable states (protein C or S deficiency, antithrombin III deficiency, Factor V Leyden, malignancy, polycythemia vera, sickle cell disease, homocystinemia, lupus anticoagulant, cardiolipin antibody).
Trauma (operative venous injury, abdominal trauma, postsplenectomy).
Inflammatory conditions (pancreatitis, diverticulitis, appendicitis, cholangitis).
Other: CHF, renal failure, portal hypertension, decompression sickness.

METASTATIC NEOPLASMS

ICD-10CM #	C79.51	Secondary malignant neoplasm of bone
	C79.52	Secondary malignant neoplasm of bone marrow
	C79.31	Secondary malignant neoplasm of brain
	C78.7	Secondary malignant neoplasm of liver and intrahepatic bile duct
	C78.00	Secondary malignant neoplasm of unspecified lung

To Bone	To Brain
Breast.	Lung.
Lung.	Breast.
Prostate.	Melanoma.
Thyroid.	GU tract.
Kidney.	Colon.
Bladder.	Sinuses.
Endometrium.	Sarcoma.
Cervix.	Skin.
Melanoma.	Thyroid.
To Liver	**To Lung**
Colon.	Breast.
Stomach.	Colon.

---

*Can be associated with dilution of formula in infant feeding.

Pancreas.
Breast.
Lymphomas.
Bronchus.
Lung.
Sarcoma.
Choriocarcinoma.
Kidney.
Kidney.
Testis.
Stomach.
Thyroid.
Melanoma.

METHEMOGLOBINEMIA, DRUG-INDUCED[34]

ICD-10CM # D74 Methemoglobinemia

SUBSTANCES ASSOCIATED WITH METHEMOGLOBINEMIA

Acetaminophen (nitrobenzene derivative).
Acetanilide.
Local anesthetics:
  Benzocaine.
  Lidocaine.
  Prilocaine.
Aniline dyes.
Celecoxib.
Dapsone.
Flutamide.
Ifosfamide.
Metoclopramide.
Nitric oxide.
Nitrites:
  Amyl nitrite.
  Isobutyl nitrite.
  Sodium nitrite.
  Nitrates (bacterial conversion to nitrites).
Nitrobenzenes/nitrobenzoates.
Nitroethane (nail polish remover).
Nitrofurans.
Nitroglycerin.
Paraquat/monolinuron.
Phenacetin.
Phenazopyridine (pyridium).
Primaquine.
Rasburicase.
Sulfamethoxazole.

MICROCEPHALY[45,101]

ICD-10CM # Varies with specific diagnosis

PRIMARY (GENETIC)

Familial (autosomal recessive).
Autosomal dominant.
Syndromes:
  Down (21-trisomy).
  Edward (18-trisomy).
  Cri-du-chat (5 p-).
  Cornelia de Lange.
  Rubinstein-Taybi.
  Smith-Lemli-Opitz.

SECONDARY (NONGENETIC)

Radiation.
Congenital infections:
  Cytomegalovirus.
  Rubella.

Toxoplasmosis.
Drugs:
  Fetal alcohol.
  Fetal hydantoin.
  Meningitis/encephalitis.
  Malnutrition.
  Metabolic.
  Hyperthermia.
  Hypoxic ischemic encephalopathy.

Commonly Cited Causes

In utero infections.
  Zika, human immunodeficiency virus (HIV), toxoplasmosis, rubella, cytomegalovirus, herpes.[a]
In utero and neonatal cerebral insults.
  Hypoxia, stroke.
Congenital malformations.
  Neural tube defects, anencephaly.
Genetic mutation syndromes.
  Angelman, Rett, velocardiofacial (VCF).
Toxic exposures.
  Fetal alcohol syndrome.
  Cocaine exposure.

[a] Often neurologists apply the mnemonic "TORCHES" to Toxoplasmosis, Rubella, Cytomegalovirus, Herpes.

MICROPENIS[80]

ICD-10CM # N48.89 Other specified disorders of penis
Q55.62 Hypoplasia of penis

HYPOGONADOTROPIC HYPOGONADISM (HYPOTHALAMIC OR PITUITARY DEFICIENCIES)

Kallmann syndrome: autosomal dominant; associated with hyposmia.
Prader-Willi syndrome: hypotonia, mental retardation, obesity, small hands and feet.
Rud syndrome: hyposomia, ichthyosis, mental retardation.
De Morsier syndrome (septooptic dysplasia): hypopituitarism, hypoplastic optic discs, absent septum pellucidum.

HYPERGONADOTROPIC HYPOGONADISM

Primary testicular defect: disorders of testicular differentiation or inborn errors of testosterone synthesis.
Klinefelter syndrome.
Other X polysomies (i.e., XXXXY, XXXY).
Robinow syndrome: brachymesomelic dwarfism, dysmorphic facies.

PARTIAL ANDROGEN INSENSITIVITY

Idiopathic
Defective morphogenesis of the penis.

MIOSIS

ICD-10CM # H57.03 Miosis

Medications (e.g., morphine, pilocarpine).
Neurosyphilis.
Congenital.
Iritis.
CNS pontine lesion.
CNS infections.
Cavernous sinus thrombosis.
Inflammation/irritation of cornea or conjunctiva.

MONOARTHRITIS, ACUTE

ICD-10CM # M13.10 Monoarthritis, not elsewhere classified, unspecified site

Overuse.
Trauma.
Gout.
Pseudogout.
Osteoarthritis.
Infectious arthritis (e.g., gonococcal, Lyme disease, viral, mycobacteria, fungi).
Osteomyelitis.
Avascular necrosis of bone.
Hemarthrosis.
Bowel disease–associated arthritis.
Bone malignancy.
Psoriatic arthritis.
Juvenile RA.
Sarcoidosis.
Hemoglobinopathies.
Vasculitic syndromes.
Behçet syndrome.
Foreign body synovitis.
Hypertrophic pulmonary osteoarthropathy.
Amyloidosis, familial Mediterranean fever.

MONOCYTOSIS[31]

ICD-10CM # D72.821 Monocytosis (symptomatic)

Inflammatory diseases:
  Autoimmune/granulomatous.
  Systemic lupus erythematosus.
  Rheumatoid arthritis.
  Giant cell arteritis.
  Myositis.
  Polyarteritis.
  Ulcerative colitis.
  Regional enteritis.
  Sarcoidosis.
Infectious diseases:
  Tuberculosis.
  Syphilis.
  Subacute bacterial endocarditis.
Malignant disorders:
  Preleukemia.
  Nonlymphocytic leukemia.

Differential Diagnosis

II

Histiocytoses.
Hodgkin disease.
Non-Hodgkin lymphoma.
Carcinomas.
Miscellaneous:
　Chronic neutropenia.
　Post splenectomy.

MONONEUROPATHY

ICD-10CM #　G58.9　Mononeuropathy, unspecified

Herpes zoster.
Herpes simplex.
Vasculitis.
Trauma, compression.
Diabetes.
Postinfectious or inflammatory.

MONONEUROPATHY, ISOLATED[43]

ICD-10CM #　G56.90　Unspecified mononeuropathy of unspecified upper limb

UPPER EXTREMITY

Radial nerve:
　Axilla.
　Humerus.
　Elbow (posterior interosseous neuropathy).
　Wrist (superficial cutaneous radial neuropathy).
Ulnar nerve:
　Axilla.
　Humerus.
　Elbow.
　Condylar groove.
　Cubital tunnel.
Wrist (Guyon canal):
Hand:
　Superficial terminal ulnar neuropathy.
　Deep terminal ulnar neuropathy:
　　Proximal hypothenar.
　　Distal hypothenar.
Median nerve.
Axilla.
Humerus (musculocutaneous mononeuropathy).
Forearm:
　Anterior interosseus.
　Pronator syndrome.
Wrist (carpal tunnel).
Hand (recurrent motor branch).
Suprascapular mononeuropathy:
　Axillary mononeuropathy.

LOWER EXTREMITY

Sciatic nerve.
Femoral nerve:
　Iliacus compartment (proximal).
　Saphenous mononeuropathy (distal).
Lateral femoral cutaneous (meralgia paresthetica).
Peroneal nerve:

Common peroneal mononeuropathy (fibular head, popliteal fossa).
Deep peroneal mononeuropathy (anterior compartment).
Tibial nerve:
　Popliteal fossa (proximal).
　Tarsal tunnel (distal).
Sural nerve:
　Popliteal fossa, calf (proximal).
　Fifth metatarsal base (distal).
Plantar nerve:
　Distal to tarsal tunnel.
　Interdigital neuropathies (Morton neuroma).
Obturator mononeuropathy.

MONONEUROPATHY MULTIPLEX[10]

ICD-10CM #　G58.9　Mononeuropathy, unspecified

MONONEUROPATHY MULTIPLEX

Vasculitis
Systemic vasculitis:
　Polyarteritis nodosa.
　Rheumatoid arthritis.
　Systemic lupus erythematosus.
　Sjögren syndrome (keratoconjunctivitis sicca).
Nonsystemic vasculitis
Diabetes Mellitus
Neoplastic
Paraneoplastic.
Direct infiltration.
Infectious
Lyme disease.
HIV infection.
Sarcoid
Toxic (lead)
Transient (polycythemia vera)
Cryoglobulinemia (hepatitis C)

MONONUCLEOSIS, MONOSPOT NEGATIVE[18]

ICD-10CM #　B27.90　Infectious mononucleosis, unspecified without complication

DIFFERENTIAL DIAGNOSIS OF MONOSPOT-NEGATIVE MONONUCLEOSIS

Acute HIV infection.
EBV mononucleosis (particularly in children).
Cytomegalovirus.
Acute toxoplasmosis.
Streptococcal pharyngitis.
Acute hepatitis B infection.

EBV, Epstein-Barr virus; HIV, human immunodeficiency virus.

MONOPLEGIA, ACUTE[20]

ICD-10CM #　Varies with specific diagnosis

Complicated migraine.[a]
Dislocation of the radial head.
Hemiparetic seizures.[a]
Monomelic spinal muscular atrophy.
Plexopathy and neuropathy.
　Acute neuritis.
　　Asthmatic plexitis.
　　Idiopathic plexitis.[a]
　　Osteomyelitis plexitis.
　　Poliomyelitis.
　　Tetanus toxoid plexitis.
　Hereditary.
　　Hereditary brachial neuritis.
　　Hereditary neuropathy with liability to pressure palsy.
　Injury.
　　Lacerations.
　　Pressure injuries.
　　Traction injuries.[a]
Stroke.

---

[a] Denotes the most common conditions and the ones with disease-modifying treatments.

MOVEMENT DISORDER, HYPERKINETIC[94]

ICD-10CM #　G25.9　Extrapyramidal and movement disorder, unspecified

Hyperkinetic Movement Disorders
Tremor.
Chorea.
Ballism.
Dystonia.
Athetosis.
Tics.
Myoclonus.
Startle.
Stereotypies.
Miscellaneous.

MOVEMENT DISORDER, PEDIATRIC PATIENT[72]

ICD-10CM #　G25.9　Extrapyramidal and movement disorder, unspecified

COMMONLY CITED MOVEMENT DISORDERS THAT MAY BEGIN IN CHILDHOOD OR ADOLESCENCE

Early Childhood
Athetosis or choreoathetosis.
Lesch-Nyhan syndrome.
Childhood
Dopa-responsive dystonia.
Dystonia associated with *DYT1* gene.
Myoclonus from subacute sclerosing panencephalitis (SSPE).
Parkinson disease.
Sydenham chorea.
Tourette disorder.
Withdrawal-emergent dyskinesia.

Adolescence
Essential tremor.*
Huntington disease (juvenile Huntington disease).*
Medication- and drug-induced movements.
Tardive dyskinesias.
Wilson disease.*

---

*Despite incapacitating movements, many choreoathetosis patients have no mental retardation.

MOVEMENT DISORDERS AND COGNITIVE IMPAIRMENT[72]

| ICD-10CM # | G25.9 | Extrapyramidal and movement disorder, unspecified |

MOVEMENT DISORDERS ASSOCIATED WITH COGNITIVE IMPAIRMENT

Young Children
Athetosis or choreoathetosis.*
Lesch-Nyhan syndrome.
Rett syndrome.
Older Children and Adolescents
Huntington disease.
Subacute sclerosing panencephalitis.
Wilson disease.
Adults
Creutzfeldt-Jakob disease.†
Huntington disease.
Parkinson disease.

---

*Genetic transmission.
†Myoclonus.

MOVEMENT DISORDERS, NEUROLEPTIC-INDUCED[72]

| ICD-10CM # | G25.70 | Drug-induced movement disorder, unspecified |

Acute dyskinesias:
  Akathisia.
  Neuroleptic-malignant syndrome.
  Oculogyric crisis and other dystonias.
Tardive dyskinesias:
  Akathisia.
  Dystonia.
  Oral-buccal-lingual dyskinesia.*
  Tics.
  Tremor.
  Stereotypies.
Dose-dependent dyskinesia:
  Parkinsonism.
Withdrawal-emergent dyskinesias.

---

*Commonly referred to as "tardive dyskinesia."

MULTIVALVULAR HEART DISEASE[58]

| ICD-10CM # | Varies with specific diagnosis |

Acquired
Systemic diseases:
Infective endocarditis.
Carcinoid heart disease.
Systemic lupus erythematosus.
Cardiac diseases:
Infective endocarditis.
Rheumatic heart disease.
Degenerative:
Calcific diseases, increased with age, prior radiation, chronic kidney disease.
Iatrogenic:
Adverse drug effects: ergot-related antagonists.
Radiation therapy.
Functional (annulus dilation), caused by:
Ischemic heart disease.
Hypertensive heart disease.
Chronic arrhythmia.
Pulmonary hypertension.
Cardiomyopathy.
Congenital
Connective tissue disorders:
Marfan syndrome.
Ehlers-Danlos syndrome.
Other:
Trisomy 18, 13, and 15.
Shone syndrome.
Ochronosis.
Mixed
Multiple conditions may contribute to valve dysfunction, such as: Degenerative diseases may lead to associated functional disease. Congenital heart disease may predispose to infective endocarditis or degenerative disease.

MUSCLE DISCOMFORT DUE TO DRUGS AND TOXINS[38]

| ICD-10CM # | Varies with specific diagnosis |

Inflammatory Myopathy
Definite:
  Hydralazine.
  Penicillamine.
  Procainamide.
  1,1'-Ethylidenebis (tryptophan).
  Immune checkpoint inhibitors (ipilimumab, nivolumab, more so anti-PD-1 agents).
  Statin (HMG-CoA reductase antibody myopathy).
  Toxic oil syndrome.
Possible:
  Cimetidine.
  Imatinib mesylate.
  Interferon-α.
  Ipecac.
  Lansoprazole.
  Leuprolide.
  Levodopa.
  Penicillin.
  Phenytoin.
  Propylthiouracil.
  Proton pump inhibitors.
  Sulfonamide.
Rhabdomyolysis ± Chronic Myopathy
Alcohol.

ε-Amino caproic acid.
Amphetamines.
Cocaine.
Cyclosporine.
Daptomycin.
Hypokalemia.
Isoniazid.
Lipid-lowering agents:*
  Bezafibrate.
  Clofibrate.
  Fenofibrate.
  Gemfibrozil.
  Lovastatin.
  Simvastatin.
  Pravastatin.
  Fluvastatin.
  Atorvastatin.
  Cerivastatin.
  Nicotinic acid.
  Red yeast rice.
Labetalol.
Lithium.
Organophosphates.
Propofol.
Snake venom.
Tacrolimus.
Zidovudine.
Painful Myopathy ± Rhabdomyolysis
Colchicine.
Emetine.
Fenoverine.
Germanium.
Hypervitaminosis E.
Taxenes.
Zidovudine.
Myalgia ± Myopathy
Amiodarone.
Amphotericin.
Aromatase inhibitors.
Azathioprine.
Beta-blockers (rare).
Bevacizumab.
Bisphosphonates.
Bortezomib.
Brentuximab.
Bumetanide.
Calcium channel blockers.
Cholesterol-lowering agents.
Corticosteroid withdrawal.
Danazol.
Denosumab.
Eculizumab.
Estrogen.
Evolocumab.
Fluoroquinolones.
HER2 antibodies (trastuzumab, pertuzumab).
Inotersen.
Interferon-α: 2a and 2b.
Ivosidenib.

---

*Especially with concurrent cyclosporine A, danazol, erythromycin, gemfibrozil, niacin, or colchicine.

Differential Diagnosis

II

Lanadelumab (anti-kallikrein monoclonal antibody).

Mercury (organic).

Methotrexate.[†]

Metolazone.

Mushrooms (orellanine/*Psilocybe*).

Opioids.

Oral contraceptives.

Paclitaxel.

Retinoids (all-*trans*-retinoic acid, isotretinoin).

Rifampin.

Serotonin reuptake inhibitor treatment and withdrawal.[‡]

Succinylcholine.

Tyrosine kinase inhibitors (alectinib, acalabrutinib, dasatinib, imatinib, larotrectinib, lenvatinib, lorlatinib, nilotinib, pazopanib, sunitinib, trametinib, as well as BRAF inhibitors [dabrafenib, vemurafenib]).

Vaccines.

Vinca alkaloids.

Cramps

Albuterol.

Anticholinesterase.

Bergamot (bergapten).

Caffeine.

Clofibrate.

Cyclosporine.

Diuretics (chronic, excessive use).

Lithium.

Nifedipine.

Terbutaline.

Tetanus.

Theophylline.

Vitamin A.

[†]With concurrent pantoprazole.
[‡]Especially with withdrawal of medications with a short half-life (paroxetine, venlafaxine).

MUSCLE DISEASE[47]

ICD-10CM # M60.009 Infective myositis, unspecified site

CLASSIFICATION OF MUSCLE DISEASE

Muscular Dystrophies

Duchenne.

Becker.

Limb girdle.

Childhood.

Facioscapulohumeral.

Myotonic Disorders

Dystrophia myotonica.

Myotonica congenita.

Inflammatory

Infective: bacterial, viral, parasitic.

Unknown cause: polymyositis, dermatomyositis, sarcoidosis.

Endocrine

Thyroid disease—hyper- and hypothyroidism.

Cushing disease.

Addison disease.

Hyperparathyroidism.

Metabolic

Glycogen storage diseases.

Periodic paralyses.

Mitochondrial diseases.

Drug-induced

Corticosteroids.

Chloroquine.

Amiodarone.

Penicillamine.

Alcohol.

Zidovudine.

Clofibrate.

Other

Inclusion body myositis.

MUSCLE WEAKNESS

ICD-10CM # M62.9 Disorder of muscle, unspecified

Physical deconditioning.

Impaired cardiac output (e.g., mitral stenosis, mitral regurgitation).

Uremia, liver failure.

Electrolyte abnormalities (hypokalemia, hyperkalemia, hypophosphatemia, hypercalcemia), hypoglycemia.

Drug induced (e.g., statin myopathy).

Muscular dystrophies.

Steroid myopathy.

Alcoholic myopathy.

Myasthenia gravis, Lambert-Eaton syndrome.

Infections (polio, botulism, HIV, hepatitis, diphtheria, tick paralysis, neurosyphilis, brucellosis, TB, trichinosis).

Pernicious anemia, other anemias, beriberi.

Psychiatric illness (depression, somatization syndrome).

Organophosphate or arsenic poisoning.

Inflammatory myopathies (e.g., collagen vascular disease, RA, sarcoidosis).

Endocrinopathies (e.g., adrenal insufficiency, hypothyroidism), diabetic neuropathy.

Other: motor neuron disease, mitochondrial myopathy, L-tryptophan (eosinophilia-myalgia), rhabdomyolysis, glycogen storage disease, lipid storage disease.

MUSCLE WEAKNESS, LOWER MOTOR NEURON VERSUS UPPER MOTOR NEURON

ICD-10CM # M62.9 Disorder of muscle, unspecified

LOWER MOTOR NEURON

Weakness, usually severe.

Marked muscle atrophy.

Fasciculations.

Decreased muscle stretch reflexes.

Clonus not present.

Flaccidity.

No Babinski sign.

Asymmetric and may involve one limb only in the beginning to become generalized as the disease progresses.

UPPER MOTOR NEURON

Weakness, usually less severe.

Minimal disuse muscle atrophy.

No fasciculations.

Increased muscle stretch reflexes.

Clonus may be present.

Spasticity.

Babinski sign.

Often initial impairment of only skilled movements.

In the limbs the following muscles may be the only ones weak or weaker than the others: triceps; wrist and finger extensors; interossei; iliopsoas; hamstrings; and foot dorsiflexors, inverters, and extroverters.

MUSCULOSKELETAL BENIGN TUMORS AND TUMORLIKE LESIONS[52]

ICD-10CM # Varies with specific diagnosis

Fibrous dysplasia.

Enchondromatosis.

Osteochondromatosis.

Synovial cysts.

Brown tumors in hyperparathyroidism.

Langerhans cell histiocytosis (eosinophilic granuloma).

Hemangiomatosis.

Bone islands, osteoma (Gardner syndrome).

Fibrous cortical defect, nonossifying fibroma.

Giant cell tumor.

Neurofibromatosis.

Amyloidosis.

Mastocytosis.

SAPHO, chronic multifocal osteomyelitis.

SAPHO, Synovitis, acne, pustulosis, hyperostosis, osteitis.

MUSCULOSKELETAL MALIGNANT TUMORS AND TUMORLIKE LESIONS[52]

ICD-10CM # Varies with specific diagnosis

Metastases.

Myeloma.

Angiosarcoma.

Leukemia.

Neuroblastoma.

Ewing sarcoma.

Osteosarcomatosis.

Lymphoma.

MYDRIASIS

ICD-10CM # H57.04 Mydriasis

Coma.

Medications (cocaine, atropine, epinephrine, etc.).

Glaucoma.
Cerebral aneurysm.
Ocular trauma.
Head trauma.
Optic atrophy.
Cerebral neoplasm.
Iridocyclitis.

MYELIN DISEASES[38]

ICD-10CM # Varies with specific diagnosis

AUTOIMMUNE

Acute disseminated encephalomyelitis.
Acute hemorrhagic leukoencephalopathy.
Multiple sclerosis.

INFECTIOUS

Progressive multifocal leukoencephalopathy.

TOXIC/METABOLIC

Carbon monoxide poisoning.
Vitamin B_{12} deficiency.
Mercury intoxication (Minamata disease).
Alcohol/tobacco amblyopia.
Central pontine myelinolysis.
Marchiafava-Bignami syndrome.
Hypoxia.
Radiation.

VASCULAR

Binswanger disease.

HEREDITARY DISORDERS OF MYELIN METABOLISM

Adrenoleukodystrophy.
Metachromatic leukodystrophy.
Krabbe disease.
Alexander disease.
Canavan-van Bogaert-Bertrand disease.
Pelizaeus-Merzbacher disease.
Phenylketonuria.

MYELITIS[7]

| ICD-10CM # | G04.91 | Myelitis, unspecified |
| | G04.89 | Other myelitis |

Viral
HIV.
HSV-1 and HSV-2.
VZV.
CMV.
EBV.
WNV.
HTLV.
Bacterial
Mycoplasma pneumoniae.
Borrelia burgdorferi.
Treponema pallidum.
Pyogenic bacteria.
Mycobacterium tuberculosis.
Fungal
Coccidioides immitis.
Actinomyces.

Aspergillus.
Blastomyces dermatitidis.
Histoplasmosis.
Immune-Mediated
Multiple sclerosis.
Neuromyelitis optica.
Connective tissue disorders (neuro-lupus, neuro-Sjögren).
Neurosarcoidosis.
Paraneoplastic.
Noninflammatory Myelopathies
Vitamin B_{12} deficiency.
Folic acid deficiency.
Copper deficiency.
Vitamin E deficiency.
Nitrous oxide toxicity.
Heroin.
Radiation myelopathy.
Traumatic/compressive myelopathy.
Vascular myelopathy.

MYELOPATHY AND MYELITIS[17]

| ICD-10CM # | M51.9 | Unspecified thoracic, thoracolumbar and lumbosacral intervertebral disc disorder |
| | G95.9 | Disease of spinal cord, unspecified |

INFLAMMATORY

Infectious: spirochetal TB, zoster, rabies, HIV, polio, rickettsial, fungal, parasitic.
Noninfectious: idiopathic transverse myelitis, multiple sclerosis.

TOXIC/METABOLIC

DM, pernicious anemia, chronic liver disease, pellagra, arsenic.

TRAUMA COMPRESSION

Spinal neoplasm, cervical spondylosis, epidural abscess, epidural hematoma.

VASCULAR

AV malformation, SLE, periarteritis nodosa, dissecting aortic aneurysm.
Physical Agents
Electrical injury, irradiation.
Neoplastic
Spinal cord tumors, paraneoplastic myelopathy.

MYOCARDIAL ISCHEMIA[17]

ICD-10CM #	I25.5	Ischemic cardiomyopathy
	I25.89	Other forms of chronic ischemic heart disease
	I25.9	Chronic ischemic heart disease, unspecified
	I24.8	Other forms of acute ischemic heart disease

Atherosclerotic obstructive coronary artery disease.
Nonatherosclerotic coronary artery disease:

Coronary artery spasm.
Congenital coronary artery anomalies:
    Anomalous origin of coronary artery from pulmonary artery.
    Aberrant origin of coronary artery from aorta or another coronary artery.
    Coronary arteriovenous fistula.
    Coronary artery aneurysm.
Acquired disorders of coronary arteries:
    Coronary artery embolism.
    Dissection:
        Surgical.
        During percutaneous coronary angioplasty.
        Aortic dissection.
        Spontaneous (e.g., during pregnancy).
Extrinsic compression:
    Tumors.
    Granulomas.
    Amyloidosis.
Collagen-vascular disease:
    Polyarteritis nodosa.
    Temporal arteritis.
    RA.
    SLE.
    Scleroderma.
Miscellaneous disorders:
    Irradiation.
    Trauma.
    Kawasaki disease.
Syphilis.
Hereditary disorders:
    Pseudoxanthoma elasticum.
    Gargoylism.
    Progeria.
    Homocystinuria.
    Primary oxaluria.
"Functional" causes of myocardial ischemia in absence of anatomic coronary artery disease:
    Syndrome X.
    Hypertrophic cardiomyopathy.
    Dilated cardiomyopathy.
    Muscle bridge.
    Hypertensive heart disease.
    Pulmonary hypertension.
    Valvular heart disease; aortic stenosis, aortic regurgitation.

MYOCLONUS

ICD-10CM # G25.3 Myoclonus

Physiologic (e.g., exercise or anxiety induced).
Renal failure.
Hepatic failure.
Hyponatremia.
Hypoglycemia or severe hyperglycemia.
Postdialysis.
Epileptic myoclonus.
Postencephalitis.
CNS lesion (stroke, neoplasm).
CNS trauma.
Parkinson disease.
Medications (e.g., tricyclics, L-dopa).

Friedreich ataxia.
Ataxia-telangiectasia.
Wilson disease.
Huntington disease.
Progressive supranuclear palsy.
Heavy metal poisoning.
Benign familial.

MYOCLONUS, DRUG-INDUCED[49]

ICD-10CM #   G25.79   Other drug-induced
movement disorders

SELECTED AGENTS ASSOCIATED WITH MYOCLONUS

Medications
Antibiotics (β-lactams).
Antidepressants.
Antineoplastics: busulfan, chlorambucil.
Carbamazepine, vigabatrin.
Clozapine.
L-dopa.
Lidocaine.
Lithium.
Lorazepam (preterm infants).
Methaqualone.
Morphine.
Nitroprusside.
Piperazine.
Industrial Toxins
Camphor.
Chlorophenoxy herbicides.
Gasoline.
Biological Toxins
Buckeye (*Aesculus* spp.).
Lupine.
Shellfish (domoic acid poisoning).

MYOCLONUS, PEDIATRIC PATIENT[68]

ICD-10CM #   G25.3   Myoclonus

SELECTED CAUSES OF MYOCLONUS IN CHILDREN

Physiologic Causes
Hiccups.
Hypnic jerks (sleep starts).
Nocturnal (sleep) myoclonus.
Developmental Causes
Benign neonatal sleep myoclonus.
Benign myoclonus of early infancy.
Myoclonus with fever.
Storage Diseases
Juvenile Gaucher disease (type III).
Sialidosis type 1 (cherry-red spot–myoclonus).
GM$_1$ gangliosidosis.
Neuronal ceroid-lipofuscinosis (late infantile).
Inherited Degenerative Diseases
Dentatorubral-pallidoluysian atrophy (DRPLA).
Huntington disease.
Progressive myoclonus ataxia.

Ramsay Hunt syndrome.
Early myoclonic encephalopathy.
Rasmussen encephalitis.
Infectious and Postinfectious Diseases
Meningitis (viral or bacterial).
Encephalitis.
Epstein-Barr virus (EBV).
Coxsackievirus.
Influenza.
Human immunodeficiency virus (HIV).
Acute disseminated encephalomyelitis (ADEM).
Metabolic Causes
Uremia.
Hepatic failure.
Electrolyte disturbances.
Hypoglycemia or hyperglycemia.
Aminoacidurias.
Organic acidurias.
Urea cycle disorders.
POLG1 mutations.
Myoclonic epilepsy with ragged red fibers (MERRF).
Mitochondrial encephalomyopathy, lactic acidosis, and stroke-like episodes (MELAS).
Biotinidase deficiency (usually epileptic).
Cobalamin deficiency (infantile).
Leigh syndrome.
Toxic Causes
Psychotropic medications (tricyclic antidepressants, lithium, selective serotonin reuptake inhibitors, monoamine oxidase inhibitors, neuroleptics).
Antibiotics (penicillin, cephalosporins, quinolones).
Antiepileptics (phenytoin, carbamazepine, lamotrigine, gabapentin, benzodiazepines [in infants], vigabatrin).
Opioids.
General anesthetics.
Antineoplastic drugs.
Strychnine, toluene, lead, carbon monoxide, mercury.
Hypoxia
Lance-Adams syndrome.
Functional (Psychogenic) Causes

MYOPATHIC PAIN SYNDROMES[38]

ICD-10CM #   Code varies with specific diagnosis

INFLAMMATORY

Inflammatory and immune myopathies:
    Systemic connective tissue disease.
    Perimysial pathology: tRNA synthetase antibodies.
    Fasciitis.
    Childhood dermatomyositis.
Muscle infections:
Viral myositis (including hepatitis C [possibly], enterovirus, dengue virus).
Pyomyositis.
Toxoplasmosis.
Trichinosis.

Spirochete (*Borrelia burgdorferi*/Lyme disease).

RHABDOMYOLYSIS ± METABOLIC DISORDER

Glycogen storage disease type V (myophosphorylase deficiency): McArdle disease.
Glycogen storage disease type VII (phosphofructokinase deficiency).
Carnitine palmitoyltransferase II.
Mitochondrial myopathies.
Malignant hyperthermia syndromes.
Familial recurrent rhabdomyolysis (myoglobinuria) in childhood (LPIN1 mutations).

OTHER MYOPATHIES WITH PAIN OR DISCOMFORT

Myopathy with tubular aggregates ± cylindrical spirals.
Adult-onset nemaline rod myopathy.
Multicore disease.
Fiber-type disproportion myopathy.
Myopathy with deficiency of iron-sulfur clusters.
Myopathy with tubulin-reactive crystalline inclusions.
Myopathy with hexagonally cross-linked crystalloid inclusions.
Myoadenylate deaminase deficiency.
Neuromyopathy with internalized capillaries.
Myotonias: myotonic dystrophy 2; dominant myotonia congenita (occasional).
Muscular dystrophies (occasional): Duchenne, Becker, limb-girdle dystrophy types 1A, 1C, 2C, 2D, 2E, 2H, 2I, 2L; ANO5-deficient myopathy.
Selenium deficiency.
Vitamin D deficiency.
Toxic myopathy: eosinophilia myalgia, rhabdomyolysis.
Hypothyroid myopathy.
Mitochondrial disorders (fatigue or myalgias with exercise).
Camurati-Engelmann syndrome (bone pain).
Drugs and Toxins

MYOPATHIC SYNDROMES, DRUG-INDUCED[90]

ICD-10CM #   G72.9   Myopathy, unspecified

TYPE OF MYOPATHY

Necrotizing myopathy.
Inflammatory myopathy.
Mitochondrial myopathy.
Hypokalemic myopathy.
Antimicrotubular myopathy.
Lysosomal storage myopathy.
Corticosteroid myopathy.
Others.

DRUGS

HMG-CoA reductase inhibitors (statins), fibrates, alcohol.

Penicillamine, interferon-a, procainamide.

Zidovudine.

Diuretics, laxatives, licorice, amphotericin B, alcohol.

Colchicine, vincristine.

Chloroquine, hydroxychloroquine, quinacrine, amiodarone, perhexiline.

Corticosteroids, especially fluorinated.

Ipecac syrup, emetine.

MYOPATHIES ASSOCIATED WITH REST PAIN[90]

ICD-10CM # G72.9 Myopathy, unspecified

Childhood dermatomyositis.

Hypothyroid myopathy.

Acute alcoholic myopathy.

Drug-induced myopathies.

Infectious myopathies.

Myopathies associated with metabolic bone disease.

Carnitine palmitoyl transferase deficiency.

Rhabdomyolysis from any cause.

MYOPATHIES, HIV ASSOCIATED[8]

ICD-10CM # G72.9 Myopathy, unspecified

HIV-Associated Myopathies	Myopathies Secondary to Antiretrovirals	Others
HIV polymyositis.	Zidovudine myopathy.	Opportunistic infections involving muscle (toxoplasmosis).
Inclusion body myositis.	Toxic Mitochondrial myopathies related to other NRTIs.	
Nemaline myopathy.		Tumor infiltrations of skeletal muscle.
Diffuse infiltrative lymphocytosis syndrome.	HIV-associated lipodystrophy syndrome.	Rhabdomyolysis.
HIV wasting syndrome.	Immune Reconstitution syndrome related to ART.	
Vasculitic processes.		
Myasthenia gravis and other myasthenic syndromes.		
Chronic fatigue and fibromyalgia.		

ART, Antiretroviral therapy; NRTIs, nucleoside reverse transcriptase inhibitors.

MYOPATHIES, INFECTIOUS

ICD-10CM # G72.9 Myopathy, unspecified

HIV.

Viral myositis.

Trichinosis.

Toxoplasmosis.

Cysticercosis.

MYOPATHIES, INFLAMMATORY

ICD-10CM # G72.9 Myopathy, unspecified

SLE, RA.

Sarcoidosis.

Paraneoplastic syndrome.

Polymyositis, dermatomyositis.

Polyarteritis nodosa.

Mixed connective tissue disease.

Scleroderma.

Inclusion body myositis.

Sjögren syndrome.

Cimetidine, d-penicillamine.

MYOPATHIES, METABOLIC[90]

ICD-10CM # G72.9 Myopathy, unspecified

DISORDERED GLYCOGEN METABOLISM

Myophosphorylase deficiency (McArdle disease).

Phosphorylase b kinase deficiency.

Phosphofructokinase deficiency.

Debrancher enzyme deficiency.

Brancher enzyme deficiency.

Phosphoglycerate kinase deficiency.

Phosphoglycerate mutase deficiency.

Lactate dehydrogenase deficiency.

Acid maltase deficiency.

Aldolase deficiency.

β-Enolase deficiency.

DISORDERED LIPID METABOLISM

Carnitine deficiencies.

Carnitine palmitoyltransferase deficiency.

Fatty acid acyl-CoA dehydrogenase deficiencies.

MITOCHONDRIAL MYOPATHIES

Coenzyme Q10 deficiency.

Respiratory chain complex deficiencies.

ENDOCRINE

Acromegaly.

Hypothyroidism.

Hyperthyroidism.

Hyperparathyroidism.

Cushing disease.

Addison disease.

Hyperaldosteronism.

METABOLIC-NUTRITIONAL

Uremia.

Hepatic failure.

Malabsorption.

Periodic paralysis.

Vitamin D deficiency.

Vitamin E deficiency.

ELECTROLYTE DISORDERS

Sodium: hypernatremia and hyponatremia.

Potassium: hyperkalemia and hypokalemia.

Calcium: hypercalcemia and hypocalcemia.

Phosphate: hypophosphatemia.

Magnesium: hypomagnesemia.

MYOPATHIES, TOXIC[18]

ICD-10CM # G72.2 Myopathy due to other toxic agents

Inflammatory: cimetidine, d-penicillamine.

Noninflammatory necrotizing or vacuolar: cholesterol-lowering agents, chloroquine, colchicine.

Acute muscle necrosis and myoglobinuria: cholesterol-lowering drugs, alcohol, cocaine.

Malignant hyperthermia: halothane, ethylene, others; succinylcholine.

Mitochondrial: zidovudine.

Myosin loss: nondepolarizing neuromuscular blocking agents; glucocorticoids.

MYOPATHY, DRUG-INDUCED[35]

ICD-10CM # G72.9 Myopathy, unspecified

DRUGS AND TOXINS THAT MAY INDUCE MYOPATHY

Example	Comments
Cimetidine.	
Chloroquine.	Vacuolar myopathy.
Colchicine.	Vacuolar myopathy.
Emetine.	
Ethanol.	Acute rhabdomyolysis and chronic myopathy.
Glucocorticoids.	Type II fiber atrophy.
Heroin.	
IFN-α.	Dermatomyositis and polymyositis reported.
Penicillamine.	Typical polymyositis. Mitochondrial myopathy.
Statins and fibrates.	Cases of autoimmune necrotizing myopathy, polymyositis, rhabdomyolysis, and noninflammatory myopathies reported.
Anti-TNF.	In RA patients existing reports of polymyositis, dermatomyositis and anti–Jo-1–positive myositis

Differential Diagnosis

II

during TNF blockade.

Zidovudine (AZT).
(Many others reported at the case level.)

AZT, Zidovudine; *IFN,* interferon; *RA,* rheumatoid arthritis; *TNF,* tumor necrosis factor.

MYOSITIS, INFECTIOUS CAUSES[90]

ICD-10CM #   M60.009   Infective myositis, unspecified site

VIRAL

Influenza A and B viruses.
Enteroviruses (coxsackieviruses, echoviruses).
Human immunodeficiency virus.
Human T-cell lymphotrophic virus type 1.
Hepatitis B and C viruses.
Cytomegalovirus.
Epstein-Barr virus.
Adenovirus.
Varicella-zoster virus.
Parainfluenza.

PARASITIC

Trichinella spp.
Echinococcus spp.
Schistosoma spp.
Toxoplasma gondii.
Trypanosoma cruzi.
Sarcocystis spp.

BACTERIAL

Staphylococcus aureus.
Streptococcus, groups A and B.
Aeromonas hydrophila.
Borrelia burgdorferi.
Clostridium perfringens.
Anaerobic streptococci.
Mycobacterium spp.
Rickettsia spp.

FUNGAL

Candida spp.
Cryptococcus neoformans.
Microsporida.

MYOSITIS, INFLAMMATORY[18]

ICD-10CM #   M60.009   Infective myositis, unspecified site
            M60.9   Myositis, unspecified
            M60.10   Interstitial myositis of unspecified site

INFECTIOUS

Viral myositis:
    Retroviruses (HIV, HTLV-I).
    Enteroviruses (echovirus, coxsackievirus).

Other viruses (influenza, hepatitis A and B, Epstein-Barr virus).
Bacterial: pyomyositis.
    Parasites: trichinosis, cysticercosis.
    Fungi: candidiasis.

IDIOPATHIC

Granulomatous myositis (sarcoid, giant cell).
Eosinophilic myositis.
Eosinophilia-myalgia syndrome.

ENDOCRINE/METABOLIC DISORDERS

Hypothyroidism.
Hyperthyroidism.
Hypercortisolism.
Hyperparathyroidism.
Hypoparathyroidism.
Hypocalcemia.
Hypokalemia.

METABOLIC MYOPATHIES

Myophosphorylase deficiency (McArdle disease).
Phosphofructokinase deficiency.
Myoadenylate deaminase deficiency.
Acid maltase deficiency.
Lipid storage diseases.
Acute rhabdomyolysis.

DRUG-INDUCED MYOPATHIES

Alcohol.
d-Penicillamine.
Zidovudine.
Colchicine.
Chloroquine, hydroxychloroquine.
Lipid-lowering agents.
Cyclosporine.
Cocaine, heroin, barbiturates.
Corticosteroids.

NEUROLOGIC DISORDERS

Muscular dystrophies.
Congenital myopathies.
Motor neuron disease.
Guillain-Barré syndrome.
Myasthenia gravis.

NAIL CLUBBING

ICD-10CM #   R68.3   Clubbing of nails

COPD.
Pulmonary malignancy.
Cirrhosis.
Inflammatory bowel disease.
Chronic bronchitis.
Congenital heart disease.
Endocarditis.
AV malformations.
Asbestosis.
Trauma.
Idiopathic.

NAIL, HORIZONTAL WHITE LINES (BEAU LINES)

ICD-10CM #   L60.4   Beau lines

Malnutrition.
Idiopathic.
Trauma.
Prolonged systemic illnesses.
Pemphigus.
Raynaud phenomenon.

NAIL KOILONYCHIA

ICD-10CM #   L60.8   Other nail disorders

Trauma.
Iron deficiency.
SLE.
Hemochromatosis.
Raynaud phenomenon.
Nail-patella syndrome.
Idiopathic.

NAIL ONYCHOLYSIS

ICD-10CM #   L60.1   Onycholysis

Infection.
Trauma.
Psoriasis.
Connective tissue disorders.
Sarcoidosis.
Hyperthyroidism.
Amyloidosis.
Nutritional deficiencies.

NAIL PITTING

ICD-10CM #   L60.8   Other nail disorders

Psoriasis.
Alopecia areata.
Reiter syndrome.
Trauma.
Idiopathic.

NAIL SPLINTER HEMORRHAGE

ICD-10CM #   L60.8   Other nail disorders

SBE.
Trauma.
Malignancies.
Oral contraceptives.
Pregnancy.
SLE.
Antiphospholipid syndrome.
Psoriasis.
RA.
Peptic ulcer disease.

NAIL STRIATIONS

ICD-10CM #   L60.8   Other nail disorders

Psoriasis.
Alopecia areata.
Trauma.
Atopic dermatitis.
Vitiligo.

NAIL TELANGIECTASIA

ICD-10CM # L60.8 Other nail disorders

RA.
Scleroderma.
Trauma.
SLE.
Dermatomyositis.

NAIL WHITENING (TERRY NAILS)

ICD-10CM # L60.8 Other nail disorders

Malnutrition.
Trauma.
Liver disease (cirrhosis, hepatic failure).
DM.
Hyperthyroidism.
Idiopathic.

NAIL YELLOWING

ICD-10CM # L60.8 Other nail disorders

Tobacco abuse.
Nephrotic syndrome.
Chronic infections (TB, sinusitis).
Bronchiectasis.
Lymphedema.
Raynaud phenomenon.
RA.
Pleural effusions.
Thyroiditis.
Immunodeficiency.

NASAL AND PARANASAL SINUS TUMORS[21]

ICD-10CM # C30.0 Malignant neoplasm of nasal cavity

BENIGN AND MALIGNANT NASAL AND PARANASAL SINUS TUMORS EPITHELIAL TUMORS

BENIGN
Papilloma.
Adenoma.
Inverting papilloma.

MALIGNANT
Squamous carcinoma.
Adenocarcinoma.
Melanoma.
Adenoid cystic carcinoma.
Malignant salivary tumors.

MESENCHYMAL TUMORS
Benign
Osteoma.
Ossifying fibroma complex.
Angiofibroma.
Chondroma.
Malignant
Osteogenic sarcoma.
Fibrosarcoma.
Angiosarcoma.
Chondrosarcoma.
Lymphoma.
Rhabdomyosarcoma.

NASAL BLOCKAGE[96]

ICD-10CM # Code varies with specific diagnosis

CAUSES
Nasal mucosal conditions:
  Allergic rhinitis.
  Nonallergic rhinitis.
  Infective rhinitis.
  Chronic rhinosinusitis (with or without nasal polyps).
Adenoidal hypertrophy.
Vasculitic conditions:
  ANCA-positive vasculitis.
Granulomatous disorders:
  Sarcoidosis.
Mass lesions:
  Tumors of the nasal cavity, paranasal sinuses, or nasopharynx.
Anatomical obstruction:
  Nasal septal deviation.
  Trauma.
  Foreign bodies.

NASAL MASSES, CONGENITAL[21]

ICD-10CM # J34.1 Cyst and mucocele of nose and nasal sinus
ICD-10CM # J34.89 Other specified disorders of nose and nasal sinuses

Dermoid.
Nasal cerebral heterotopia (glioma).
Frontal meningoencephalocele.
Nasolacrimal duct mucocele.
Nasal hamartoma.
Nasal hemangioma.

NASOPHARYNGEAL TUMORS[22]

ICD-10CM # C10.6 Benign neoplasm of nasopharynx
ICD-10CM # C11.3 Malignant neoplasm of nasopharynx

BENIGN TUMORS
Developmental
Thornwaldt cyst.

Hairy polyp.
Teratomas (varied origin).

ECTODERMAL
Papilloma.
Adenomatous polyps.

MESODERMAL
Juvenile angiofibroma.
Fibromyxomatous polyps.
Choanal polyps.
Osteomas.
Fibrous dysplasia.
Craniopharyngioma.
Solitary fibrous tumor.
Desmoid fibromatosis.
Schwannoma.

BENIGN SALIVARY GLAND TUMORS
Pleomorphic adenoma.
Monomorphic adenoma.

MALIGNANT TUMORS
Epithelial
Nasopharyngeal cancer.
Undifferentiated carcinoma.
Squamous cell carcinoma.

EMBRYONAL
Chordoma.

LYMPHOID
Lymphoma.

MESODERMAL
Hemangiopericytoma.
Malignant fibrous histiocytoma.
Rhabdomyosarcoma.

MALIGNANT SALIVARY GLAND TUMORS
Adenoid cystic carcinoma.
Mucoepidermoid carcinoma.
Acinic cell carcinoma.
Adenocarcinoma.

METASTATIC TUMORS
Adenocarcinoma.
Papillary carcinoma.

NAUSEA AND VOMITING

ICD-10CM # R11.2 Nausea with vomiting, unspecified

Infections (viral, bacterial).
Intestinal obstruction.
Metabolic (uremia, electrolyte abnormalities, DKA, acidosis, etc.).
Severe pain.
Anxiety, fear.
Psychiatric disorders (bulimia, anorexia nervosa).
Pregnancy.

Medications (NSAIDs, erythromycin, morphine, codeine, aminophylline, chemotherapeutic agents, etc.).

Withdrawal from substance abuse (drugs, alcohol).

Head trauma.

Vestibular or middle ear disease.

Migraine headache.

CNS neoplasms.

Radiation sickness.

PUD.

Carcinoma of GI tract.

Reye syndrome.

Eye disorders.

Abdominal trauma.

NAUSEA AND VOMITING, CAUSES DURING PREGNANCY[32]

ICD-10CM # R11.2 Nausea with vomiting, unspecified

DIFFERENTIAL DIAGNOSIS OF NAUSEA AND VOMITING DURING PREGNANCY

Nausea and vomiting of pregnancy.

Hyperemesis gravidarum.

Pancreatitis.

Symptomatic cholelithiasis.

Viral hepatitis.

Peptic ulcer disease.

Gastric cancer.

Intestinal obstruction.

Intestinal pseudoobstruction.

Gastroparesis diabeticorum.

Gastritis.

Gastroesophageal reflux disease.

Acute pyelonephritis.

Drug toxicity.

Vagotomy.

Preeclampsia/eclampsia.

Acute fatty liver of pregnancy.

Hemolysis, elevated liver enzymes, and low platelets (HELLP) syndrome.

Anorexia nervosa/bulimia.

Other neuropsychiatric disorders.

NAUSEA AND VOMITING, CHRONIC[3]

ICD-10CM # R11.2 Nausea with vomiting, unspecified

DIFFERENTIAL DIAGNOSIS OF CHRONIC NAUSEA AND VOMITING

Mechanical GI tract obstruction (pylorus, bile duct, small intestine, colon).

Mucosal inflammation.

Peritoneal irritation.

Carcinomas (e.g., gastric, ovarian, renal, bronchogenic).

Metabolic/endocrine disorders (diabetic mellitus, hypothyroidism, hyperthyroidism, adrenal insufficiency, uremia).

Medications (anticholinergics, narcotics, L-dopa, progesterone, calcium channel blockers, digitalis, NSAIDs, antidysrhythmic agents, lubiprostone, cannabis, metformin, amylin analogs).

Gastroparesis.

Gastric dysrhythmias (tachygastria, bradygastria, mixed).

CNS disorders (tumors, migraine, seizures, stroke, orthostatic intolerance).

Psychogenic disorders (anorexia nervosa, bulimia nervosa).

NECK AND ARM PAIN

ICD-10CM #	M54.2	Cervicalgia
	S46.919A	Strain of unspecified muscle, fascia and tendon at shoulder and upper arm level, unspecified arm, initial encounter

Cervical disk syndrome.

Trauma, musculoskeletal strain.

Rotator cuff syndrome.

Bicipital tendonitis.

Glenohumeral arthritis.

Acromioclavicular arthritis.

Thoracic outlet syndrome.

Pancoast tumor.

Infection (cellulitis, abscess).

Angina pectoris.

NECK MASS[25]

ICD-10CM # R22.1 Localized swelling, mass and lump, neck

CONGENITAL ANOMALIES

Thyroglossal duct cyst.

Bronchial apparatus anomalies.

Teratomas.

Ranula.

Dermoid cysts.

Hemangioma.

Laryngoceles.

Cystic hygroma.

NONNEOPLASTIC INFLAMMATORY ETIOLOGIES

Folliculitis.

Adenopathy secondary to peritonsillar abscess.

Retropharyngeal or parapharyngeal abscess.

Salivary gland infections.

Viral infections (mononucleosis, HIV, CMV).

TB.

Cat-scratch disease.

Toxoplasmosis.

Actinomyces.

Atypical *Mycobacterium.*

Jugular vein thrombus.

NEOPLASM (PRIMARY OR METASTATIC)

Lipoma

NECK PAIN[25]

ICD-10CM # M54.2 Cervicalgia

INFLAMMATORY DISEASES

RA.

Spondyloarthropathies.

Juvenile RA.

NONINFLAMMATORY DISEASE

Cervical osteoarthritis.

Diskogenic neck pain.

Diffuse idiopathic skeletal hyperostosis.

Fibromyalgia or myofascial pain.

INFECTIOUS CAUSES

Meningitis.

Osteomyelitis.

Infectious diskitis.

NEOPLASMS

Primary.

Metastatic.

REFERRED PAIN

Temporomandibular joint pain.

Cardiac pain.

Diaphragmatic irritation.

GI sources (gastric ulcer, gallbladder, pancreas).

NECK PAIN FROM RHEUMATOLOGIC DISORDERS[8]

ICD-10CM # M54.2 Cervicalgia

Rheumatoid arthritis:

Without disease of the C1-C2 joint.

With structural cervical abnormalities: C1-C2 subluxation, C1-C2 facet involvement.

Spondyloarthropathies.

Reactive arthritis.

Psoriatic arthritis.

Enteropathic arthritis.

Polymyalgia rheumatica.

Osteoarthritis.

Fibromyalgia.

Nonspecific musculoskeletal pain.

Miscellaneous spondyloarthropathies.

Whipple disease.

Behçet disease.

Paget disease.

Acromegaly.

Ossification of the posterior longitudinal ligament.

Diffuse idiopathic skeletal hyperostosis.

NECK PAIN, NONMUSCULAR CAUSES[35]

ICD-10CM # M54.2 Cervicalgia

Structure	Condition
Pharynx.	Pharyngitis.
Larynx.	Laryngitis.
	Carcinoma.
Trachea.	Tracheitis.
Thyroid.	Thyroiditis.
Lymph nodes.	Lymphadenitis.
Carotid arteries.	Carotidynia.
	Dissection.
	Inflammation.
Aorta.	Aneurysm.
	Dissection.
Heart.	Angina.
	Infarction.
Pericardium.	Pericarditis.
Diaphragm.	Inflammation by blood, infection.

NECROTIZING PNEUMONIAS[18]

ICD-10CM # J15.8 Pneumonia due to other specified bacteria

COMMON
Tuberculosis.
Staphylococcus.
Gram-negative bacilli.
Anaerobes.
Fungi.
Pneumocystis jirovecii.

RARE
Streptococcus pneumoniae.
Legionella.
Viruses.
Mycoplasma pneumoniae.

NEONATAL SEIZURES MIMICS[20]

ICD-10CM # Varies with specific diagnosis

Benign nocturnal myoclonus.[a]
Jitteriness.*
Nonconvulsive apnea.
Normal movement.
Opisthotonos.
Pathologic myoclonus.

[a]Denotes the most common conditions and the ones with disease-modifying treatments.

NEOPLASTIC LESIONS, LUMBOSACRAL SPINE[35]

ICD-10CM # M54.5 Low back pain

BENIGN
Osteoid osteoma.
Osteoblastoma.
Osteochondroma.
Giant cell tumor.
Aneurysmal bone cyst.
Hemangioma.
Eosinophilic granuloma.
Sacroiliac lipoma.

MALIGNANT
Multiple myeloma.
Chondrosarcoma.
Chordoma.
Lymphoma.
Skeletal metastases.

SPINAL CORD TUMORS
Extradural metastases.
Intradural–extramedullary:
 Neurofibroma.
 Meningioma.
Intramedullary:
 Ependymoma.
 Astrocytoma.

NEPHRITIC SYNDROME, ACUTE[18]

ICD-10CM # N00.8 Acute nephritic syndrome with other morphologic changes

LOW SERUM COMPLEMENT LEVEL
Acute postinfectious glomerulonephritis.
Membranoproliferative glomerulonephritis.
SLE.
Subacute bacterial endocarditis.
Visceral abscess "shunt" nephritis.
Cryoglobulinemia.

NORMAL SERUM COMPLEMENT LEVEL
IgA nephropathy.
Antiglomerular basement membrane disease.
Polyarteritis nodosa.
Granulomatosis with polyangiitis.
Henoch-Schönlein purpura.
Goodpasture syndrome.

NEPHROCALCINOSIS

ICD-10CM # E83.59 Other disorders of calcium metabolism

Sarcoidosis.
Hyperparathyroidism.
Chronic glomerulonephritis.
Milk-alkali syndrome.
Distal renal tubular acidosis.
Medullary sponge kidney.
Bartter syndrome.
Hypervitaminosis D.

Idiopathic hypercalciuria.
Hyperoxaluria.
Cortical necrosis.
Tuberculosis.
Idiopathic hypercalciuria.
Rapidly progressive osteoporosis.

NEPHROPATHY, OBSTRUCTIVE[89]

ICD-10CM # Varies with specific diagnosis

POSSIBLE CAUSES OF OBSTRUCTIVE NEPHROPATHY
Renal
Congenital
Polycystic kidney.
Renal cyst.
Peripelvic cyst.
Ureteropelvic junction obstruction.
Neoplastic
Wilms tumor.
Renal cell carcinoma.
Transitional cell carcinoma of the collecting system.
Multiple myeloma.
Inflammatory
Tuberculosis.
Echinococcus infection.
Metabolic
Calculi.
Miscellaneous
Sloughed papillae.
Trauma.
Renal artery aneurysm.
Ureter
Congenital
Stricture.
Ureterocele.
Obstructing megaureter.
Retrocaval ureter.
Prune belly syndrome.
Neoplastic
Primary carcinoma of ureter.
Metastatic carcinoma.
Inflammatory
Tuberculosis.
Amyloidosis.
Schistosomiasis.
Abscess.
Ureteritis cystica.
Endometriosis.
Miscellaneous
Retroperitoneal fibrosis.
Pelvic lipomatosis.
Aortic aneurysm.
Radiation therapy.
Lymphocele.
Trauma.
Urinoma.
Pregnancy.
Radiofrequency ablation.

Differential Diagnosis

II

Bladder and Urethra
Congenital
Posterior urethral valve.
Phimosis.
Hydrocolpos.
Neoplastic
Bladder carcinoma.
Prostate carcinoma.
Carcinoma of urethra.
Carcinoma of penis.
Inflammatory
Prostatitis.
Paraurethral abscess.
Miscellaneous
Benign prostatic hypertrophy.
Neurogenic bladder.
Urethral stricture.

NEUROGENIC BLADDER[104]

ICD-10CM #	N31.9	Neuromuscular dysfunction of bladder, unspecified

SUPRATENTORIAL
CVA.
Parkinson disease.
Alzheimer disease.
Cerebral palsy.

SPINAL CORD
Spinal cord injury.
Spinal stenosis.
Central cord syndrome.
ALS.
Multiple sclerosis.
Myelodysplasia.

PERIPHERAL NEUROPATHY
Diabetes.
Alcohol.
Shingles.
Syphilis.

NEUROLOGIC DEFICIT, FOCAL[1]

ICD-10CM #	G45.9	Transient cerebral ischemic attack, unspecified
	I67.848	Other cerebrovascular vasospasm and vasoconstriction

TRAUMATIC: INTRACRANIAL, INTRASPINAL
Subdural hematoma.
Intraparenchymal hemorrhage.
Epidural hematoma.
Traumatic hemorrhagic necrosis.

INFECTIOUS
Brain abscess.

Epidural and subdural abscesses.
Meningitis.

NEOPLASTIC
Primary CNS tumors.
Metastatic tumors.
Syringomyelia.
Vascular.
Thrombosis.
Embolism.
Spontaneous hemorrhage: arteriovenous malformation, aneurysm, hypertensive.

METABOLIC
Hypoglycemia.
Vitamin B_{12} deficiency.
Postseizure.
Hyperosmolar nonketotic.

OTHER
Migraine.
Bell palsy.
Psychogenic.

NEUROLOGIC DEFICIT, MULTIFOCAL[1]

ICD-10CM #	I67.89	Other cerebrovascular disease
	G45.9	Transient cerebral ischemic attack, unspecified
	I67.848	Other cerebrovascular vasospasm and vasoconstriction

Acute disseminated encephalomyelitis: postviral or postimmunization.
Infectious encephalomyelitis: poliovirus, enteroviruses, arbovirus, herpes zoster, Epstein-Barr virus.
Granulomatous encephalomyelitis: sarcoid.
Autoimmune: SLE.
Other: familial spinocerebellar degenerations.

NEUROMUSCULAR JUNCTION DYSFUNCTION[18]

ICD-10CM #	N31.9	Neuromuscular dysfunction of bladder, unspecified

DISORDERS OF THE NEUROMUSCULAR JUNCTION
Autoimmune
Myasthenia gravis.
Lambert-Eaton myasthenic syndrome.
Congenital
Presynaptic defects in ACh resynthesis, packaging, or release.
Synaptic defect: congenital end plate AChE deficiency.
Postsynaptic defects: slow-channel syndromes.

Postsynaptic defects: decreased response to ACh.
   Fast-channel syndromes.
   AChR deficiency without kinetic abnormality.
Familial limb-girdle myasthenia.
Toxic
Botulism.
Drug-induced disorders.
Organophosphate intoxication.

Ach, Acetylcholine; *AChE,* acetylcholinesterase; *AChR,* acetylcholine receptor.

NEURONOPATHIES, SENSORY (GANGLIONOPATHIES)[43]

ICD-10CM #	G60.0	Hereditary motor and sensory neuropathy

Herpes:
   Herpes simplex I and II.
   Varicella zoster (shingles).
Inflammatory sensory polyganglionopathy (ISP).
Paraneoplastic.
Primary biliary cirrhosis.
Sjögren syndrome (keratoconjunctivitis sicca).
Toxin-induced:
   Pyridoxine (vitamin B_6) overdose.
   Metals:
      Platinum (cisplatin).
      Methyl mercury.
Vitamin E deficiency.

NEUROPATHIC BLADDER (HEAD) NEUROPATHIES, AUTONOMIC[19]

ICD-10CM #	G63	Polyneuropathy in diseases classified elsewhere

GUILLAIN-BARRÉ SYNDROME
Non–Guillain-Barré syndrome autoimmunity.
Paraneoplastic (type I antineuronal nuclear antibody).
Lambert-Eaton syndrome.
Antibodies to neuronal nicotinic acetylcholine receptors.
Antibodies to P/Q type calcium channels.
Other autoantibodies.
Systemic lupus erythematosus.

HEREDITARY
Type I autosomal dominant.
Type II autosomal recessive (Morvan disease).
Type III autosomal recessive (Riley-Day).
Type IV autosomal recessive (congenital insensitivity to pain with anhidrosis).
Type V absence of pain.

METABOLIC
Fabry disease.
Diabetes mellitus.

Tangier disease.
Porphyria.

INFECTIOUS

HIV.
Chagas disease.
Botulism.
Leprosy.
Diphtheria.
TOXINS

OTHER

Triple A (Allgrove) syndrome.
Navajo Indian neuropathy.
Multiple endocrine neoplasia type 2b.

NEUROPATHIES, AUTONOMIC, PERIPHERAL, CAUSES[59]

ICD-10CM #	G90.09	Other idiopathic peripheral autonomic neuropathy

METABOLIC

Diabetes mellitus.
Alcohol.
Acute intermittent porphyria.
Uremia.

AUTOIMMUNE

Autoimmune autonomic ganglionopathy.
Guillain-Barré syndrome.
Morvan syndrome.
Lambert-Eaton myasthenic syndrome.
Chronic inflammatory demyelinating polyradiculoneuropathy.
Sjögren syndrome.
Systemic lupus erythematosus.
Mixed connective tissue diseases.

PARAPROTEINEMIC

Amyloidosis.

NUTRITIONAL

Cyanocobalamin deficiency.
Thiamine deficiency.
Gluten-sensitive neuropathy.

TOXIC

Heavy metals.
Organic solvents.
Organophosphates.
Vacor.
Acrylamide.

DRUG INDUCED

Cisplatin.
Vincristine.
Amiodarone.
Metronidazole.
Perhexiline.
Paclitaxel.

INFECTIOUS

HIV.
Leprosy.
Chagas disease.
Botulism.
Diphtheria.
Lyme disease.

GENETIC

Hereditary sensory and autonomic neuropathies:
   Types I and II.
   Type III (familial dysautonomia).
   Type IV (congenital insensitivity to pain).
   Type V.
Fabry disease.

IDIOPATHIC

Adie syndrome.
Ross syndrome.
Acute cholinergic neuropathy.
Chronic idiopathic anhidrosis.
Amyotrophic lateral sclerosis.

NEUROPATHIES, PAINFUL[62]

ICD-10CM #	G58.9	Mononeuropathy, unspecified
	G62.1	Alcoholic polyneuropathy
	G61.89	Other inflammatory polyneuropathies
	G60.0	Hereditary motor and sensory neuropathy
	G60.0	Hereditary motor and sensory neuropathy
	E11.42	Type 2 diabetes mellitus with diabetic polyneuropathy
	E10.42	Type 1 diabetes mellitus with diabetic polyneuropathy

MONONEUROPATHIES

Compressive neuropathy (carpal tunnel, meralgia paresthetica).
Trigeminal neuralgia.
Ischemic neuropathy.
Polyarteritis nodosa.
Diabetic mononeuropathy.
Herpes zoster.
Idiopathic and familial brachial plexopathy.

POLYNEUROPATHIES

DM.
Paraneoplastic sensory neuropathy.
Nutritional neuropathy.
Multiple myeloma.
Amyloid.
Dominantly inherited sensory neuropathy.
Toxic (arsenic, thallium, metronidazole).
AIDS-associated neuropathy.
Tangier disease.
Fabry disease.

NEUROPATHIES, PERIPHERAL, ASYMMETRICAL PROXIMAL/ DISTAL[43]

ICD-10CM #	G99.0	Autonomic neuropathy in diseases classified elsewhere

BRACHIAL PLEXOPATHY

Open

Direct plexus injury (knife or gunshot wound).
Neurovascular (plexus ischemia).
Iatrogenic (central line insertion).
Closed
Traction injuries:
   "Stingers."
   Traction neurapraxia.
   Partial or complete nerve root avulsion.
Radiation.
Neoplastic.
Idiopathic brachial plexitis.
Thoracic outlet.

LUMBOSACRAL PLEXOPATHIES

Open
Closed
Traction injuries:
   Pelvic double vertical shearing fracture.
   Posterior hip dislocation.
   Retroperitoneal hemorrhage.
Vasospastic (deep buttock injection).
Neoplastic.
Radiation.
Idiopathic lumbosacral plexitis.
Infectious:
   Herpesvirus (sacrococcygeal).
   Herpes simplex II.
   Herpes zoster.
Cytomegalovirus (CMV) polyradiculopathy (HIV).

NEUROPATHIES, SENSORY ATAXIC[38]

ICD-10CM #	Code varies with specific diagnosis

Sensory neuronopathies (polyganglionopathies):
   Paraneoplastic sensory neuronopathy (malignant inflammatory sensory polyganglionopathy):
   Sjögren syndrome.
   Idiopathic.
   Toxic (cisplatin and analogs, vitamin B_6 excess).
Chronic immune sensory polyradiculopathy.
Demyelinating polyradiculoneuropathies:
   Guillain-Barré syndrome (Miller-Fisher variant).
   Immunoglobulin M monoclonal gammopathy MAG** antibody.
Canomad.*
Tabes dorsalis.

**Myelin-associated glycoprotein.
*Chronic ataxic neuropathy with ophthalmoplegia, IgM paraprotein, cold agglutinins, and anti-GD1b disialosyl antibodies.

Differential Diagnosis

II

NEUROPATHIES, SMALL FIBER[38]

ICD-10CM # Code varies with specific diagnosis

Diabetes mellitus and impaired glucose tolerance.
Sjögren (sicca) syndrome.
Celiac disease.
Amyloid neuropathy (early familial and primary).
Human immunodeficiency virus–associated sensory neuropathy.
Hereditary sensory and autonomic neuropathies.
Fabry disease.
Tangier disease.
Cryptogenic small-fiber neuropathy.

NEUROPATHIES, TOXIC AND METABOLIC[19]

ICD-10CM # NEC G62.2 Toxic neuropathy

METALS

Arsenic (insecticide, herbicide).
Lead (paint, batteries, pottery).
Mercury (metallic, vapor).
Thallium (rodenticides).
Gold.

OCCUPATIONAL OR INDUSTRIAL CHEMICALS

Acrylamide (grouting, flocculation).
Carbon disulfide (solvent).
Cyanide.
Dichlorophenoxyacetate.
Dimethylaminopropionitrile.
Ethylene oxide (gas sterilization).
Hexacarbons (glue, solvents).
Organophosphates (insecticides, petroleum additive).
Polychlorinated biphenyls.
Tetrachlorbiphenyl.
Trichloroethylene.

DRUGS

Amiodarone.
Chloramphenicol.
Chloroquine.
Cisplatin.
Colchicine.
Dapsone.
Ethambutol.
Ethanol.
Gold.
Hydralazine.
Isoniazid.
Metronidazole.
Nitrofurantoin.
Nitrous oxide.
Nucleosides (antiretroviral agents ddC, ddI, d4T, others).
Penicillamine.
Pentamidine.
Phenytoin.
Pyridoxine (excessive).
Statins.
Stilbamidine.
Suramin.
Taxanes (paclitaxel, docetaxel).
Thalidomide.
Tryptophan (eosinophilia-myalgia syndrome).
Vincristine.

METABOLIC DISORDER

Fabry disease.
Krabbe disease.
Leukodystrophies.
Porphyria.
Tangier disease.
Tyrosinemia.
Uremia.

NEUROPATHIES WITH AUTONOMIC NERVOUS SYSTEM INVOLVEMENT[38]

ICD-10CM # Code varies with specific diagnosis

ACUTE

Acute pandysautonomic neuropathy (autoimmune, paraneoplastic).
Guillain-Barré syndrome.
Porphyria.
Toxic: vincristine, Vacor (rodenticide).

CHRONIC

Diabetes mellitus.
Amyloid neuropathy (familial and primary).
Paraneoplastic sensory neuronopathy (malignant inflammatory sensory polyganglionopathy).
Human immunodeficiency virus–related autonomic neuropathy.
Hereditary sensory and autonomic neuropathy.

NEUROPATHIES WITH FACIAL NERVE INVOLVEMENT

ICD-10CM # G51.8 Other disorders of facial nerve

Sarcoidosis.
HIV.
Lyme disease.
Guillain-Barré.
Others: chronic inflammatory polyneuropathy, Tangier disease, amyloidosis.

NEUROPENIA, DRUG-INDUCED[34]

ICD-10CM # D70.9 Other neutropenia

DRUGS COMMONLY ASSOCIATED WITH NEUTROPENIA

Antibiotics:
  Vancomycin.
  Semisynthetic penicillins.
  Chloramphenicol.
  Sulfa.
Linezolid.
Antithyroid drugs:
  Methimazole.
  Propylthiouracil.
Cardiovascular:
  Ticlopidine.
  Procainamide.
Antipsychotics:
  Clozapine.
  Olanzapine.
  Chlorpromazine.
Anticonvulsants:
  Phenytoin.
  Carbamazepine
  Valproic acid.
Antiinflammatory agents:
  Indomethacin.
  Sulfasalazine.
  Phenylbutazone.
H_2 blockers:
  Cimetidine.
  Ranitidine.
Analgesics:
  Dipyrone.
Antineoplastic:
  Rituximab.
Anthelminthic:
  Levamisole.

NEUTROPENIA WITH DECREASED MARROW RESERVE[31]

ICD-10CM # D70.8 Other neutropenia

PRIMARY

Severe congenital neutropenia.
Shwachman-Diamond syndrome.
Cyclic neutropenia.

SECONDARY

Lymphoproliferative disorder of granular lymphocytes.
Chemotherapy.
Drug induced (nonimmune).
Nutritional.
Viral infection (varicella, EBV, measles, CMV, hepatitis, HIV).

NEUTROPENIA WITH NORMAL MARROW RESERVE[31]

ICD-10CM # D70.9 Neutropenia, unspecified

Chronic benign neutropenia of infancy and childhood.
Ethnic or benign familial neutropenia.
Autoimmune neutropenia.
Alloimmune neutropenia.
Drug-induced neutropenia.
Infection-related neutropenia.
Hypersplenism.

NEUTROPENIA, IN CHILDHOOD[105]

ICD-10CM #   D70.8   Other neutropenia
           D70.9   Neutropenia unspecified

ACQUIRED

Infection.
Immune mediated.
Hypersplenism.
Vitamin B_{12}, folate, copper deficiency.
Drugs or toxic substances.
Aplastic anemia.
Malignancies or preleukemic disorders.
Ionizing radiation.

CONGENITAL

Cyclic neutropenia.
Severe congenital neutropenia (Kostmann syndrome).
Chronic benign neutropenia of childhood.
Shwachman-Diamond syndrome.
Fanconi anemia.
Metabolic disorders (amino acidopathies, Barth syndrome, glycogen storage disorders).
Osteopetrosis.
Neutropenia with pigmentation abnormalities, e.g., Chédiak-Higashi.

NEUTROPHILIA[31]

ICD-10CM #   D72.0   Neutrophilia, hereditary giant
           D71   Functional disorders of polymorphonuclear neutrophils

CLASSIFICATION OF NEUTROPHILIA

Primary (No Other Evident Associated Disease)
Hereditary neutrophilia.
Chronic idiopathic neutrophilia.
Chronic myelogenous leukemia (CML) and other myeloproliferative diseases.
Familial myeloproliferative disease.
Congenital anomalies and leukemoid reaction.
Leukocyte adhesion factor deficiency (LAD).
Familial cold urticaria and leukocytosis.
Secondary
Infection.
Stress neutrophilia.
Chronic inflammation.
Drug induced.
Nonhematologic malignancy.
Generalized marrow stimulation as in hemolysis.
Asplenia and hyposplenism.

NIPPLE DISCHARGE[68]

ICD-10CM #   Varies with specific diagnosis

Pregnancy.
Hormones (oral contraceptives, estrogen, progesterone).
Blood pressure drugs (methyldopa, verapamil).
Tricyclic antidepressants.
Tranquilizers (antipsychotics).
Antinausea drugs (metoclopramide).
Herbs (nettle, fennel, blessed thistle, anise, fenugreek seed).
Illicit drugs (marijuana, opiates).
Stimulation of the breast (sexual or from exercise).
Thyroid abnormalities.
Chronic emotional stress.
Hypothalamic tumors.
Chest wall conditions.
Herpes zoster.
Trauma.
Burns.
Tumors.
Breast conditions:
Mammary duct ectasia.
Chronic cystic mastitis.
Intraductal cysts.
Intraductal papillomas.

NIPPLE LESIONS

ICD-10CM #   Varies with specific diagnosis

Contact dermatitis.
Trauma.
Paget disease.
Sebaceous hyperplasia.
Neurofibroma.
Accessory nipple.
Papillary adenoma.
Nevoid hyperkeratosis.
Cellulitis.

NODULAR LESIONS, SKIN

ICD-10CM #   R22.9   Localized swelling, mass and lump, unspecified

Lipoma.
Cherry angioma.
Angiokeratoma.
Hemangioma.
Classic Kaposi sarcoma.
Nodular melanoma.
Pyogenic granuloma.
Angiosarcoma.
Eccrine poroma.

NODULES, PAINFUL

ICD-10CM #   R22.9   Localized swelling, mass and lump, unspecified

Arthropod bite or sting.
Erythema nodosum.
Glomus tumor.
Neuroma.
Leiomyoma.
Angiolipoma.
Dermatofibroma.
Osler node.
Blue rubber bleb nevus.
Vasculitis.
Sweet syndrome.

NYSTAGMUS

ICD-10CM #   H55.00   Unspecified nystagmus
           H55.89   Other irregular eye movements

Medications (meperidine, barbiturates, phenytoin, phenothiazines, etc.).
Multiple sclerosis.
Congenital.
Neoplasm (cerebellar, brain stem, cerebral).
Labyrinthine or vestibular lesions.
CNS infections.
Optic atrophy.
Other: Arnold-Chiari malformation, syringobulbia, chorioretinitis, meningeal cysts.

NYSTAGMUS, DOWNBEAT[38]

ICD-10CM #   H55.09   Other forms of nystagmus

CAUSES

Congenital (rare).
Transiently in normal neonates.
Idiopathic (common).
Craniocervical junction abnormalities:
    Basilar invagination (e.g., Paget disease).
    Chiari malformations.
    Dolichoectasia of the vertebrobasilar arterial system.
    Foramen magnum tumors.
    Syringobulbia.
Cerebellar disorders:
    Alcoholic cerebellar degeneration (chronic usage).
    Anoxic cerebellar degeneration.
    Antiglutamic acid decarboxylase antibodies (anti-GAD65 antibodies).
    Cerebellar degeneration following human T-lymphotropic virus types I and II.
    Episodic ataxia.
    Familial spinocerebellar degeneration, particularly SCA-6, and with multiple system atrophy.
    Heat stroke–induced cerebellar degeneration.
    Paraneoplastic cerebellar degeneration.
Metabolic disorders (drugs, toxins, and deficiencies):

Differential Diagnosis

II

Alcohol intoxication.
Amiodarone.
Anticonvulsants.
Lithium.
Magnesium depletion.
Opioids.
Toluene abuse.
Vitamin B_{12} deficiency.
Wernicke encephalopathy (as a chronic, persistent late-stage finding).
Other:
Benign paroxysmal positional vertigo: positional downbeat nystagmus with an anterior canal lesion.
Brain stem encephalitis.
Cardiogenic vertigo.
Cephalic tetanus.
Finger extensor weakness and downbeat nystagmus motor neuron disease (FEW-DON-MND).
Hydrocephalus.
Leukodystrophy.
Multiple sclerosis.
Small-amplitude downbeat nystagmus in carriers of blue-cone monochromatism.
Syncope.
Vertebrobasilar ischemia.

NYSTAGMUS, MONOCULAR

ICD-10CM # H55.09 Other forms of nystagmus
H55.00 Unspecified nystagmus

Amblyopia.
Strabismus.
Multiple sclerosis.
Monocular blindness.
Internuclear ophthalmoplegia.
Lid fasciculations.
Brain stem infarct.

OCULAR MOTOR APRAXIA, ASSOCIATED DISORDERS[38]

ICD-10CM # Varies with specific diagnosis

ASSOCIATED DISORDERS

Aicardi syndrome.
Aplasia or hypoplasia of the corpus callosum.
Aplasia or hypoplasia of the cerebellar vermis (up to 53% of patients).
Ataxia with "ocular motor" apraxia type I syndrome.
Ataxia telangiectasia.
Autosomal recessive AOA associated with axonal peripheral neuropathy, areflexia, and pes cavus (may be the same as EOAH).
Bardet-Biedl syndrome.
Bilateral cerebral cortical lesions.
Birth injuries (see perinatal/postnatal disorders).
Carbohydrate-deficient glycoprotein syndrome type Ia.
Carotid fibromuscular hypoplasia.
Cockayne syndrome.
COMA (occasionally may be familial).

Congenital vertical ocular motor apraxia (rare).
Cornelia de Lange syndrome.
Dandy-Walker malformation.
EOAH (may be the same disorder as AOA).
GM1 gangliosidosis.
Hydrocephalus.
Infantile Gaucher disease.
Infantile Refsum disease.
Joubert syndrome.
Krabbe leukodystrophy.
Leber congenital amaurosis.
Megalocephaly.
Microcephaly.
Microphthalmos.
Neurovisceral lipidosis (e.g., Niemann-Pick type C).
Occipital porencephalic cysts.
Pelizaeus-Merzbacher disease.
Perinatal and postnatal disorders (hypoxia, meningitis, PV leukomalacia, athetoid cerebral palsy, perinatal septicemia and anemia, herpes encephalitis, epilepsy).
Propionic acidemia.
Succinic semialdehyde dehydrogenase deficiency.
Wieacker syndrome.

ODYNOPHAGIA[2]

ICD-10CM # Varies with specific diagnosis

CAUSES OF ODYNOPHAGIA

Infections
Herpes simplex virus.
Cytomegalovirus.
Candidiasis.
Chemical, Inflammatory
Gastroesophageal reflux.
Drug induced (slow-K, tetracyclines, quinidine).
Radiation.
Graft-versus-host disease.
Crohn disease.
Dermatologic diseases (pemphigus and pemphigoid).

OLFACTORY FUNCTION IMPAIRMENT[38]

ICD-10CM # G52.0 Disorders of olfactory nerve

ASSOCIATED DISORDERS AND CONDITIONS, AS MEASURED BY OLFACTORY TESTING

22q11 deletion syndrome.
AIDS/HIV infection.
Adenoid hypertrophy.
Adrenal cortical insufficiency.
Age.
Alcoholism.
Allergies.
Alzheimer disease.
Amyotrophic lateral sclerosis.
Anorexia nervosa.
Asperger syndrome.
Ataxias.

Attention deficit hyperactivity disorder.
Bardet-Biedl syndrome.
Chemical exposure.
Chronic obstructive pulmonary disease.
Congenital.COVID-19 infection.
Creutzfeldt-Jakob disease.
Cushing syndrome.
Cystic fibrosis.
Degenerative ataxias.
Diabetes.
Down syndrome.
Epilepsy.
Facial paralysis.
Frontotemporal lobe degeneration.
Gonadal dysgenesis (Turner syndrome).
Guamanian ALS/PD/dementia syndrome.
Head trauma.
Herpes simplex encephalitis.
Hypothyroidism.
Huntington disease.
Iatrogenesis.
Kallmann syndrome.
Korsakoff psychosis.
Leprosy.
Liver disease.
Lubag.
Medications.
Migraine.
Multiple sclerosis.
Multiple system atrophy.
Multiinfarct dementia.
Narcolepsy with cataplexy.
Neoplasms, cranial/nasal.
Nutritional deficiencies.
Obesity.
Obsessive compulsive disorder.
Obstructive pulmonary disease.
Orthostatic tremor.
Panic disorder.
Parkinson dementia complex of Guam.
Parkinson disease.
Pick disease.
Posttraumatic stress disorder.
Pregnancy.
Pseudohypoparathyroidism.
Psychopathy.
Radiation (therapeutic, cranial).
REM behavior disorder.
Refsum disease.
Renal failure/end-stage kidney disease.
Restless leg syndrome.
Rhinosinusitis/polyposis.
Schizophrenia.
Seasonal affective disorder.
Sjögren syndrome.
Stroke.
Tobacco smoking.
Toxic chemical exposure.
Upper respiratory infections.
Usher syndrome.
Vascular disorders (e.g., aneurysms, hemorrhages).
Vitamin B_{12} deficiency.

AIDS, Acquired immunodeficiency syndrome; *ALS,* advanced life support; *HIV,* human immunodeficiency virus; *PD,* Parkinson disease; *REM,* rapid eye movement.

OPACIFICATION OF HEMIDIAPHRAGM ON X-RAY[21]

ICD-10CM # Varies with specific diagnosis

CAUSES OF OPACIFICATION OF A HEMITHORAX

Pleural effusion.
Consolidation.
Collapse.
Massive tumor.
Fibrothorax.
Combination of above lesions.
Pneumonectomy.
Lung agenesis.

OPHTHALMOPLEGIA[18]

| ICD-10CM # | H51.9 | Unspecified disorder of binocular movement |
| | H49.00 | Third [oculomotor] nerve palsy, unspecified eye |

BILATERAL

Botulism.
Myasthenia gravis.
Wernicke encephalopathy.
Acute cranial polyneuropathy.
Brain stem stroke.

UNILATERAL

Carotid-posterior (third cranial nerve, pupil involved communicating aneurysm).
Diabetic-idiopathic (third or sixth cranial nerve, pupil spared).
Myasthenia gravis.
Brain stem stroke.[‡]

[‡]Spontaneous, multivector, chaotic eye movement.

OPHTHALMOPLEGIA, ACUTE, BILATERAL[38]

ICD-10CM # Varies with specific diagnosis

Basilar meningitis, hypertrophic cranial pachy-meningitis, or neoplastic infiltration.[†]
Botulism.
Brain stem encephalitis.[†]
Brain stem stroke.[†]
Carotid-cavernous or dural shunt fistula.[†]
Cavernous sinus thrombosis (febrile, ill patient).[†]
Central herniation syndrome.
Ciguatera poisoning.
Diphtheria.
Fisher syndrome (Miller Fisher syndrome) with or without ataxia.

Intoxication (sedatives, tricyclics, organophosphates, anticonvulsants—consciousness impaired).
Leigh disease (subacute necrotizing encephalomyelitis).
Multiple sclerosis.
Myasthenia.
Neuroleptic malignant syndrome (personal observation).
Orbital pseudotumor.[†]
Paraneoplastic encephalomyelitis.
Pituitary apoplexy.[†]
Progressive encephalomyelitis with rigidity and myoclonus, a variant of stiff person syndrome.
Psychogenic.
Stiff person syndrome.
Thallium poisoning.
Tick paralysis.
Tolosa-Hunt syndrome.[†]
Trauma (impaired consciousness, signs of injury).[†]
Wernicke encephalopathy.
*All may be unilateral.

[†]Pain may be present.

OPHTHALMOPLEGIA, ACUTE, UNILATERAL[20]

ICD-10CM # Varies with specific diagnosis

Aneurysm.[a,b]
Brain tumors.
Brain stem glioma.
Parasellar tumors.
Tumors of pineal region.
Brain stem stroke.[a]
Cavernous sinus fistula.
Cavernous sinus thrombosis.
Gradenigo syndrome.
Idiopathic ocular motor nerve palsy.[a]
Increased intracranial pressure.
Multiple sclerosis.[a]
Myasthenia gravis.[a]
Ophthalmoplegic migraine.[a,b]
Orbital inflammatory disease.[a,b]
Orbital tumor.[b]
Recurrent familial.[a]
Trauma.
Head.
Orbital.

---

[a] May be recurrent.
[b] May be associated with pain.

OPHTHALMOPLEGIA AND GAZE PALSIES[38]

ICD-10CM # Varies with specific diagnosis

CAUSES OF OPHTHALMOPLEGIA AND GAZE PALSIES

Site	Disorder
Muscle:	Ocular myopathies:

Congenital myopathies:
Central core.
Centronuclear (myotubular).
Fiber-type disproportion.
Multicore (ptosis, spares EOM).
Nemaline.
Neurocristopathy (EOM fibrosis).
Oculopharyngodistal myopathy (Satoyoshi myopathy).
Autosomal dominant.
Autosomal recessive.
Reducing body myopathy (ptosis, spares EOM).
Dystrophies:
Myotonic dystrophy (ptosis, usually spares EOM).
Oculopharyngeal dystrophy.
Inflammatory myopathies:
Dermatomyositis.
Giant cell arteritis (typically by muscle ischemia).
Idiopathic orbital inflammatory syndrome (orbital pseudotumor).
Metabolic and toxic myopathies (act at multiple sites, e.g., anticonvulsants).
Mitochondrial cytopathy:
Chronic progressive external ophthalmoplegia (CPEO).
CPEO-like syndrome: mitochondrial toxicity in long-standing AIDS and long exposure to HAART.
Kearns-Sayre syndrome.
Pearson syndrome.
POLIP syndrome (polyneuropathy, ophthalmoplegia, leukoencephalopathy, intestinal pseudoobstruction).
Infiltrative disorders (thyroid, amyloid, metastases, congenital familial fibrosis, cystinosis).
High myopia (large globes cause mechanical restriction).

Differential Diagnosis

II

Trauma (orbital entrapment).

Neuromuscular junction: Myasthenia gravis.
Toxins (e.g., botulism, cosmetic botulinum toxin, organophosphates).
Lambert-Eaton syndrome (rarely affects EOM, mainly causes ptosis).

Ocular motor nerves:
Gaze palsies: Nuclear and paranuclear:
Brain stem injury (vascular, multiple sclerosis, neuromyelitis optica, encephalitis, paraneoplastic, toxins, tumor).
Familial congenital gaze palsy.
Glycine encephalopathy (nonketotic hyperglycinemia: hiccups, seizures, apneic spells).
Internuclear ophthalmoplegia.
Leigh disease.
Machado-Joseph disease (SCA3).
Maple syrup urine disease.
Möbius and Duane syndromes (agenesis of cranial nerve nuclei).
One-and-a-half syndrome.
Progressive encephalitis with rigidity and myoclonus (PERM), a variant of the stiff person syndrome.
Spinocerebellar degeneration.
Tangier disease.
Vitamin E deficiency.
Prenuclear:
Monocular "supranuclear" elevator palsy.
Ocular tilt reaction.
Skew deviation.
Vertical one-and-a-half syndrome.
Supranuclear (predominantly horizontal).
Acutely, after hemispheric stroke:
Congenital ocular motor apraxia or congenital saccadic palsy.
Ipsiversive or contraversive (wrong-way eyes).
Gaucher disease (types 2 and 3).

Ictal (transient, adversive).
Juvenile-onset GM2 gangliosidosis (mimics juvenile SMA).
Postictal (transient, ipsiversive).
Paraneoplastic disorders.
Supranuclear (predominantly vertical):
Adult-onset GM2 gangliosidosis (mimics multisystem atrophy or spinocerebellar degeneration) (V > H).
Amyotrophic lateral sclerosis (rare, V > H).
Autosomal dominant parkinsonian-dementia complex with pallidopontonigral degeneration (dementia, dystonia, frontal and pyramidal signs, urinary incontinence).
Cerebral amyloid angiopathy with leukoencephalopathy.
Congenital vertical ocular motor apraxia (rare).
Dentatorubral-pallidoluysian atrophy (autosomal dominant, dementia, ataxia, myoclonus, choreoathetosis).
Diffuse Lewy body disease (ophthalmoplegia may be global).
Dorsal midbrain syndrome.
Familial Creutzfeldt-Jakob disease (U > D).
Familial paralysis of vertical gaze.
Gerstmann-Sträussler-Scheinker disease (U > D, dysmetria, nystagmus).
Guamanian Parkinson disease-dementia complex (Lytico-Bodig disease).
HARP syndrome (hypoprebetali-poproteinemia, acanthocytosis, retinitis pigmentosa, pallidal degeneration).
Hydrocephalus (untreated, decompensated shunt).
Joseph disease.
Kernicterus (U > D).

Late-onset cerebelloponto-mesencephalic degeneration (D > U).
Neurovisceral lipidosis; synonyms: DAF syndrome (downgaze palsy-ataxia-foamy macrophages); dystonic lipidosis; Niemann-Pick disease type C (initially loss of downgaze, which may become global, and be associated with ataxia, cognitive changes, sensory neuropathy, and pyramidal findings).
Pallidoluysian atrophy (dysarthria, dystonia, bradykinesia).
Paraneoplastic disorders.
Progressive supranuclear palsy (PSP).
Stiff person syndrome.
Subcortical gliosis (U > D).
Variant Creutzfeldt-Jakob disease (U > D).
Vitamin B$_{12}$ deficiency (U > D).
AIDS encephalopathy.
Alzheimer disease (pursuit).
Cerebral adrenoleukodystrophy.
Corticobasal ganglionic degeneration.
Fahr disease (idiopathic striatopallidodentate calcification).
Gaucher disease.
Hexosaminidase A deficiency.
Huntington disease.
Joubert syndrome.
Leigh disease (infantile striatonigral degeneration).
Malignant neuroleptic syndrome (personal observation).
Methylmalo-nomocystinuria.
Neurosyphilis.
Opportunistic infections.
Paraneoplastic disorders.
Pelizaeus-Merzbacher disease (H > V).
Pick disease (impaired saccades).
Progressive multifocal leukoencephalopathy.
Pseudo-PSP, a selective saccadic palsy, associated with progressive ataxia,

dysarthria, and dysphagia over several months following aortic/cardiac surgery under hypothermic circulatory arrest.

Stiff person syndrome—late.

Tay-Sachs disease (infantile GM2 gangliosidosis) (V > H).

Wernicke encephalopathy.

Whipple disease (V > H).

X-linked dystonia-parkinsonism (Lubag disease).

AIDS, Acquired immunodeficiency syndrome; *D*, loss of downgaze; *EOM*, extraocular muscles; *global*, loss of horizontal and vertical gaze; *H*, loss of horizontal gaze; *HAART*, highly active antiretroviral therapy; *SMA*, spinal muscular atrophy; *U*, loss of upgaze; *V*, loss of vertical gaze.

OPHTHALMOPLEGIA, CHRONIC[38]

ICD-10CM # Varies with specific diagnosis

Brain stem neoplasm.

Chronic ataxic neuropathy, ophthalmoplegia, monoclonal protein, cold agglutinins, and disialosyl antibodies (CANOMAD).

Chronic basal meningitis (infection, sarcoid, or carcinoma).

Chronic ophthalmoplegia with anti-GQ1b antibody.

Congenital extraocular muscle fibrosis.

Dysthyroidism.

Leigh disease.

Multiple sclerosis.

Myasthenia gravis.

Myopathies (e.g., mitochondrial, fiber-type disproportion).

Nuclear, paranuclear, and supranuclear gaze palsies.

OPHTHALMOPLEGIA, COMBINED VERTICAL GAZE[38]

ICD-10CM # Varies with specific diagnosis

DIFFERENTIAL DIAGNOSIS

Stroke.

Progressive supranuclear palsy.

Cortical-basal ganglionic degeneration.

Arteriovenous malformation.

Multiple sclerosis.

Tumor (thalamic, mesencephalic, pineal).

Hydrocephalus.

Whipple disease.

Syphilis.

Metabolic disorders:

Lipid and lysosomal storage diseases (e.g., Niemann-Pick type C).

Wilson disease.

Kernicterus.

Wernicke encephalopathy.

Bulbar-onset amyotrophic lateral sclerosis (associated with TDP-43–positive inclusions).

Paraneoplastic brain stem encephalitis (e.g., with Ma-2 antibodies).

Creutzfeldt-Jakob disease.

OPHTHALMOPLEGIA, INTERNUCLEAR[38]

ICD-10CM # Varies with specific diagnosis

Brain stem (pontine) stroke—unilateral.

Multiple sclerosis—unilateral or bilateral.

Intrinsic tumor—primary or metastatic.

Meningitis (especially tuberculosis, also acquired immunodeficiency syndrome, brucellosis, cysticercosis, syphilis).

Brain stem encephalitis (infective, inflammatory, lupus, paraneoplastic, sarcoid).

Chemotherapy with radiation therapy.

Drug intoxication:

Comatose—anticonvulsants, phenothiazines, tricyclics.

Awake—lithium.

Spinocerebellar degeneration.

Fabry disease (vascular).

Herniation (epidural and acute and chronic subdural hemorrhage, cerebral hematoma).

Vascular malformations.

Vasculitis.

Wernicke encephalopathy.

Progressive supranuclear palsy.

Syringobulbia associated with a Chiari malformation.

Trauma (closed head injury, neck/vertebral artery injury).

Hexosaminidase A deficiency.

Kennedy disease (X-linked recessive progressive spinomuscular atrophy).

Maple syrup urine disease.

Cerebral air embolism.

Vitamin B_{12} deficiency.

Pseudointernuclear ophthalmoplegia.

Long-standing exotropia.

Myasthenia.

Myotonic dystrophy.

Neuromyotonia of the lateral rectus muscle.

Partial palsy of cranial nerve III.

Previous extraocular muscle surgery.

Thyroid orbitopathy (lateral rectus restriction).

Orbital pseudotumor.

Other infiltrative disorders of extraocular muscle (neoplasm, amyloid, etc.).

Miller Fisher syndrome (sometimes may be a true internuclear ophthalmoplegia).

OPHTHALMOPLEGIA, TOTAL[38]

ICD-10CM # Varies with specific diagnosis

Acute

Miller Fisher syndrome.

Guillain-Barré syndrome.

Bilateral pontine or midbrain-thalamic stroke.

Myasthenia gravis.

Pituitary apoplexy.

Botulism.

Anticonvulsant intoxication.

Multiple cranial neuropathies from infection or neoplasm.

Wernicke encephalopathy.

Chronic/Progressive

Chronic progressive external ophthalmoplegia syndromes.

Oculopharyngeal muscular dystrophy.

Myotonic dystrophy and other congenital myopathies.

Congenital cranial dysinnervation syndromes.

Neurodegenerative diseases (e.g., progressive supranuclear palsy, late spinocerebellar ataxia type 2).

Myasthenia gravis.

Thyroid eye disease (especially in combination with myasthenia gravis).

OPSOCLONUS[61]

ICD-10CM # H55.89 Other irregular eye movements

Multiple sclerosis.

Encephalitis.

CNS lymphoma.

Hydrocephalus.

Pontine hemorrhage.

Thalamic disorder (glioma, hemorrhage).

Hyperosmolar coma.

Carcinoma, paraneoplastic.

Cocaine.

Medications (e.g., phenytoin, haloperidol, amitriptyline, diazepam, vidarabine).

OPTIC ATROPHY[47]

ICD-10CM # H47.20 Unspecified optic atrophy

CAUSES OF OPTIC ATROPHY

Optic Nerve Compression

Pituitary tumor.

Carotid aneurysm.

Glaucoma.

Optic nerve tumor.

Sphenoid meningioma.

Olfactory groove meningioma.

Optic Neuritis Following Long-Standing Papilledema Central Retinal Artery Occlusion Toxic/Metabolic

Diabetes.

Methyl alcohol.

Tobacco.

Quinine.
Ethambutol.
Lead and arsenic.
Anemia.
Secondary to Retinal Disease
Senile macular degeneration.
Retinitis pigmentosa.
Severe chorioretinitis.
Secondary to Trauma
Orbital fracture.
Hereditary
Leber optic atrophy.
Hereditary ataxias.
Spinocerebellar degeneration.

OPTIC DISC ELEVATION[44]

ICD-10CM #　Varies with specific diagnosis

CAUSES OF OPTIC DISC ELEVATION
Papilledema.
Accelerated hypertension.
Anterior optic neuropathy.
Ischemic.
Inflammatory.
Infiltrative.
Compressive, including orbital disease.
Pseudopapilledema.
Disc drusen.
Tilted optic disc.
Peripapillary myelinated nerve fibers.
Crowded disc in hypermetropia.
Mitochondrial optic neuropathies.
Leber hereditary optic neuropathy.
Methanol poisoning.
Intraocular disease.
Central retinal vein occlusion.
Uveitis.
Posterior scleritis.
Hypotony.

OPTIC DISC SWELLING[20]

ICD-10CM #　Varies with specific diagnosis

Congenital disk elevation.
Increased intracranial pressure.
Ischemic neuropathy.
Optic glioma.
Optic nerve drusen.
Papillitis.
Retrobulbar mass.

ORAL MUCOSA, ERYTHEMATOUS LESIONS[63]

ICD-10CM #	K12.2	Cellulitis and abscess of mouth
	K13.70	Unspecified lesions of oral mucosa
	K13.79	Other lesions of oral mucosa

Allergy.
Erythroplakia.

Candidiasis.
Geographic tongue.
Stomatitis areata migrans.
Plasma cell gingivitis.
Pemphigus vulgaris.

ORAL MUCOSA, PIGMENTED LESIONS[63]

ICD-10CM #	K12.2	Cellulitis and abscess of mouth
	K13.70	Unspecified lesions of oral mucosa
	K13.79	Other lesions of oral mucosa
	K13.5	Oral submucous fibrosis

Racial pigmentation.
Oral melanotic macule.
Peutz-Jeghers syndrome.
Neurofibromatosis.
Albright syndrome.
Addison disease.
Chloasma.
Drug reaction: quinacrine, Minocin, chlorpromazine, Myleran.
Amalgam tattoo.
Lead line.
Smoker's melanosis.
Nevi.
Melanoma.

ORAL MUCOSA, PUNCTATE EROSIVE LESIONS[63]

ICD-10CM #	K12.2	Cellulitis and abscess of mouth
	K13.70	Unspecified lesions of oral mucosa
	K13.79	Other lesions of oral mucosa

Viral lesion: herpes simplex, coxsackievirus (A, B, A16), herpes zoster.
Aphthous stomatitis.
Sutton disease (giant aphthae).
Behçet syndrome.
Reiter syndrome.
Neutropenia.
Acute necrotizing ulcerative gingivostomatitis (ANUG).
Drug reaction.
Inflammatory bowel disease.
Contact allergy.

ORAL MUCOSA, WHITE LESIONS[63]

ICD-10CM #	K12.2	Cellulitis and abscess of mouth
	K13.70	Unspecified lesions of oral mucosa
	K13.79	Other lesions of oral mucosa
	K13.5	Oral submucous fibrosis

Leukoplakia.

White, hairy leukoplakia.
Squamous cell carcinoma.
Lichen planus.
Stomatitis nicotinica.
Benign intraepithelial dyskeratosis.
White spongy nevus.
Leukoedema.
Darier-White disease.
Pachyonychia congenital.
Candidiasis.
Allergy.
SLE.

ORAL SOFT TISSUE TUMORS[94]

ICD-10CM #　Varies with specific diagnosis

Connective Tissue Hyperplasia (Normal-Appearing Overlying Mucosa)
Irritation fibroma.
Denture-associated hyperplasia.
Palatal papillomatosis (papillary hyperplasia).
Generalized gingival hyperplasias.
Drug-induced (phenytoin, nifedipine, cyclosporine).
Hereditary.
Reactive Hyperplasia (Erythematous Overlying Mucosa)
Pyogenic granuloma/pregnancy tumor.
Peripheral giant cell granuloma.
Inflammatory gingival hyperplasia.
Hyperplastic lingual tonsil.
Epithelial Masses (Usually Irregular White Surface)
Papilloma/oral wart.
Squamous cell carcinoma.
Verrucous carcinoma.
Focal epithelial hyperplasia (Heck disease).
Condyloma acuminatum (venereal wart).
Keratoacanthoma (on lips).
Salivary Duct Obstruction (Minor Salivary Glands)
Mucocele/ranula (usually fluctuant).
Salivary stone (sialolith).
Subepithelial Neoplasms
Primary connective tissue or salivary gland tumors.
Metastatic Lesions (Especially in the Mandible).
Lymphoma (especially in the palate or posterior mandible).
Focal or generalized leukemic infiltrates in the gingiva (especially with acute monocytic leukemia).

ORAL ULCERS, ACUTE

| ICD-10CM # | K13.70 | Unspecified lesions of oral mucosa |
| | K13.79 | Other lesions of oral mucosa |

Trauma (including thermal trauma).
Aphthous stomatitis.
Syphilis.
Herpes simplex infection.
Herpes zoster.

ORAL VESICLES AND ULCERS[18]

| ICD-10CM # | K13.70 | Unspecified lesions of oral mucosa |
| | K13.79 | Other lesions of oral mucosa |

Aphthous stomatitis.
Primary herpes simplex infection.
Vincent stomatitis.
Syphilis.
Coxsackievirus A (herpangina).
Fungi (histoplasmosis).
Behçet syndrome.
SLE.
Reiter syndrome.
Crohn disease.
Erythema multiforme.
Pemphigus.
Pemphigoid.

ORBITAL INFLAMMATION[44]

ICD-10CM #	H05.019	Cellulitis of unspecified orbit
	C69.10	Malignant neoplasm of unspecified orbit
	D31.60	Benign neoplasm of unspecified orbit
	H05.029	Osteomyelitis of unspecified orbit
	H05.049	Tendonitis of unspecified orbit
	H05.229	Edema of unspecified orbit
	H05.239	Hemorrhage of unspecified orbit

DIFFERENTIAL DIAGNOSIS OF AN ACUTELY INFLAMED ORBIT

Infection
Bacterial orbital cellulitis.
Fungal orbital infection.
Dacryocystitis.
Infective dacryoadenitis.
Vascular lesions
Acute orbital hemorrhage,
Cavernous sinus thrombosis.
Carotid–cavernous fistula.
Neoplasia
Rapidly progressive retinoblastoma.
Lacrimal gland tumor.
Other neoplasms (e.g., metastatic lesion with inflammation, lymphoma, Waldenström macroglobulinemia).
Rhabdomyosarcoma, leukemia, lymphangioma, or neuroblastoma in children
Endocrine
Thyroid eye disease of rapid onset.
Nonneoplastic inflammation
Idiopathic orbital inflammatory disease.
Tolosa-Hunt syndrome.
Orbital myositis.
Acute allergic conjunctivitis with lid swelling.
Herpes zoster ophthalmicus.

Herpes simplex skin rash.
Sarcoidosis.
Vasculitides: Wegener granulomatosis, polyarteritis nodosa.
Scleritis, including posterior scleritis.
Ruptured dermoid cyst.

ORBITAL LESIONS, CALCIFIED

| ICD-10CM # | H05.89 | Other disorders of orbit |

Chronic inflammation.
Phlebolith.
Dermoid cyst.
Mucocele walls.
Tumors (lacrimal gland, fibroosseous).
Meningioma (optic sheath).
Lymphangioma.
Orbital varix.

ORBITAL LESIONS, CYSTIC

| ICD-10CM # | H05.9 | Unspecified disorder of orbit |

Sweat gland cyst.
Dermoid cyst.
Lacrimal gland cyst.
Abscess.
Conjunctival cyst.
Lymphangioma.
Schwannoma.

ORBITAL NEOPLASMS, MALIGNANT[106]

| ICD-10CM # | C69.10 | Malignant neoplasm of unspecified orbit |

LESIONS WITH CLINICALLY MALIGNANT BEHAVIOR

Langerhans cell tumors.*
Non-Langerhans cell tumors.
Atypical lymphoid hyperplasia.
Meningioma of optic nerve.

PRIMARY MALIGNANT TUMORS OF ORBIT

Lymphoma.
Lacrimal gland carcinomas.
Rhabdomyosarcoma.
Primitive neuroectodermal tumors.
Malignant peripheral nerve sheath tumor.
Alveolar soft part sarcoma.
Melanoma.
Osteosarcoma.
Fibrosarcoma.
Leiomyosarcoma.
Chondrosarcoma.
Liposarcoma.
Glioma of optic nerve.

---

*Relatively common tumor.

SECONDARY MALIGNANT TUMORS OF ORBIT

Eyelid malignancies.
Conjunctival malignancies.
Uveal melanoma.
Retinoblastoma.
Lacrimal drainage system malignancies.
Paranasal sinus and nasal carcinoma.
Brain tumors.

METASTATIC TUMORS OF ORBIT

Distant carcinomas (e.g., breast, lung, gastrointestinal tract).
Neuroblastoma.
Leukemia (granulocytic sarcoma).
Carcinoid tumor.
Metastatic melanoma.

ORGASM DYSFUNCTION[55]

| ICD-10CM # | F52.31 | Female orgasmic disorder |
| | F52.32 | Male orgasmic disorder |

Anorgasmia: inadequate stimulation or learning.
Spinal cord lesion or injury.
Multiple sclerosis.
Alcoholic neuropathy.
Amyotrophic lateral sclerosis.
Spinal cord accident.
Spinal cord trauma.
Peripheral nerve damage.
Radical pelvic surgery.
Herniated lumbar disk.
Hypothyroidism.
Addison disease.
Cushing disease.
Acromegaly.
Hypopituitarism.
Pharmacologic agents (e.g., SSRIs, β-blockers).
Psychogenic.

OROFACIAL PAIN

| ICD-10CM # | R51 | Facial pain |

Dental abscess.
Sinusitis.
Otitis media.
Otitis externa.
Wisdom tooth eruption.
Sialoadenitis.
Herpes zoster.
Trigeminal neuralgia.
Parotitis.
Anxiety disorder.
Malingering.

OSTEOLYTIC BENIGN BONE LESIONS, MULTIPLE[52]

| ICD-10CM # | Varies with specific diagnosis |

COMMON MULTIPLE OSTEOLYTIC BENIGN LESIONS

Cystic lesions in joint disease.

Amyloidosis.
Brown tumors in hyperparathyroidism.
Enchondromatosis.
Fibrous dysplasia.
Osteomyelitis (including tuberculosis, hydatid, sarcoid, etc.).
Massive osteolysis (Gorham disease).
Mastocytosis.
Neurofibromatosis.
Langerhans cell histiocytosis (histiocytosis X).

OSTEOMYELITIS, PEDIATRIC PATIENT[5]

ICD-10CM # M86 Osteomyelitis

Fractures.
Thrombophlebitis.
Scurvy.
Septicemia.
Cellulitis.
Septic bursitis.
Myositis.
Pyomyositis.
Rheumatic fever.
Toxic synovitis.
Reactive arthritis.
Complex regional pain syndrome.
Chronic recurrent multifocal osteomyelitis.
Osteoid osteoma.
Langerhans cell histiocytosis.
Leukemia.
Ewing sarcoma.
Malignant primary bone tumors.
Bone infarction (sickle-cell or Gaucher disease).

OSTEOPOROSIS IN CHILDREN[52]

ICD-10CM # M81.8 Other osteoporosis without current pathological fracture

CAUSES OF OSTEOPOROSIS IN CHILDREN
Systemic long-term oral glucocorticoid therapy.
Chronic inflammatory disease (e.g., juvenile inflammatory arthritis).
Hypogonadism—primary or secondary.
Prolonged immobilization.
Osteogenesis imperfecta.
Idiopathic juvenile osteoporosis.

OSTEOPOROSIS, SECONDARY CAUSES

ICD-10CM # M81.0 Age-related osteoporosis without current pathological fracture

Medication induced (e.g., glucocorticoids, anticonvulsants, heparin, LHRH agonists or antagonists).
Hyperparathyroidism.
Hyperthyroidism.

Prolonged immobilization.
Chronic renal failure.
Sickle cell disease.
Multiple myeloma.
Myeloproliferative diseases.
Leukemias and lymphomas.
Acromegaly.
Prolactinoma.
DM.
Total parenteral nutrition.
Malabsorption.
Chronic hypophosphatemia.
Connective tissue disorders (e.g., osteogenesis imperfecta, Marfan syndrome, Ehlers-Danlos).
Hepatobiliary disease.
Postgastrectomy.
Aluminum-containing antacids.
Systemic mastocytosis.
Homocystinuria.*

---

*Involvement principally of cancellous bone.

OSTEOSCLEROSIS, DIFFUSE[21]

ICD-10CM # Q77.4 Congenital osteosclerosis

DISORDERS ASSOCIATED WITH DIFFUSE OSTEOSCLEROSIS
*Neoplastic Causes**
Prostate carcinoma, breast carcinoma, GI adenocarcinoma, carcinoid tumors, transitional cell carcinoma of the bladder, myeloma, lymphoma, leukemia.
Hematologic Causes
Sickle cell disorders, mastocytosis, myelofibrosis, polycythemia vera.
Metabolic Causes
Renal osteodystrophy, primary hyperparathyoidism, familial hypophosphatemic osteomalacia, hypervitaminosis D, fluorosis, hypoparathyroidism, pseudohypoparathyroidism.[†]
Primary Osseous Disorders[†]
Osteoporosis.
Pyknodysostosis.
Paget disease.

[†]Involvement of cancellous and cortical bone.

OSTEOSCLEROTIC BENIGN BONE LESIONS, MULTIPLE[52]

ICD-10CM # Q78.2 Osteosclerosis

COMMON MULTIPLE OSTEOSCLEROTIC BENIGN LESIONS
Bone infarcts.
Bone islands.
Callus.
Osteomyelitis (chronic, multifocal).
Paget disease.
Fibrous dysplasia.

Enchondromatosis.
Mastocytosis.
Matured benign lesions (e.g., nonossifying fibromas).
Osteomas (Gardner syndrome).
Osteopathia striata.
Osteopoikilosis.

OVARIAN ENLARGEMENT, NONNEOPLASTIC[99]

ICD-10CM #		
	N83.209	Unspecified ovarian cyst, unspecified side
	N83.29	Other ovarian cysts
	N80.1	Endometriosis of ovary
	O00.209	Unspecified ovarian pregnancy without intrauterine pregnancy

NONNEOPLASTIC CAUSES OF OVARIAN ENLARGEMENT IN THE NONPREGNANT PATIENT
Functional
Hemorrhagic corpus luteum.
Follicle cyst.
Cortical stromal hyperplasia (hyperthecosis).
Polycystic ovarian syndrome (PCOS).
Mesothelial/müllerian.
Endometriotic cyst.
Xanthomatous pseudotumor.
Cystic adhesions/cystic mesothelioma.
Simple cyst.
Vascular
Ovarian torsion/infarction.
Massive ovarian edema.

OVULATORY DYSFUNCTION[26]

ICD-10CM #		
	N97.0	Female infertility associated with anovulation
	N92.3	Ovulation bleeding

HYPERANDROGENIC ANOVULATION
Polycystic ovarian syndrome.
Late-onset congenital adrenal hyperplasias.
Ovarian hyperthecosis.
Androgen-producing ovarian tumors.
Androgen-producing adrenal tumors.
Cushing syndrome.

HYPOESTROGENIC ANOVULATION (HYPOTHALAMIC OR PITUITARY ETIOLOGY)
Hypogonadotropic Hypoestrogenic States
Reversible:
    Functional hypothalamic amenorrheas:
        Eating disorders (anorexia nervosa, excessive weight loss).
        Excessive athletic training.
Neoplastic:
    Craniopharyngioma.
    Pituitary stalk compression.

Infiltrative diseases:
  Histiocytosis-X.
  Sarcoidosis.
Hypophysitis.
Pituitary adenomas:
  Hyperprolactinemia.
  Euprolactinemic galactorrhea.
Endocrinopathies:
  Hypothyroidism/hyperthyroidism.
  Cushing disease.
Irreversible:
  Kallmann syndrome.
  Isolated gonadotropin deficiency (hypothalamic or pituitary origin).
  Panhypopituitarism/pituitary insufficiency:
    Sheehan syndrome, pituitary apoplexy.
    Pituitary irradiation or ablation.

Hypergonadotropic Hypoestrogenic States
Physiologic states:
  Menopause.
  Perimenopause.
Premature ovarian failure.
Immune-related:
  Radiation/chemotherapy-induced.
Ovarian dysgenesis.
Turner syndrome.
46XX with mutations of X.
Androgen insensitivity syndrome.

MISCELLANEOUS
Endometriosis.
Luteal phase defect.

PAIN, MIDFOOT

ICD-10CM # M25.579 Pain in unspecified ankle and joints of unspecified foot

MEDIAL ASPECT
Tendonitis of posterior tibialis.
Tendonitis of flexor digitorum longus.
Tendonitis of flexor hallucis longus.
Infection (osteomyelitis, septic arthritis, cellulitis) of foot.
Peripheral vascular insufficiency.
Fracture.
Osteoarthritis.
Gout, pseudogout.
Neuropathy.
Tumor.

LATERAL ASPECT
Peroneus longus tendonitis.
Peroneus brevis tendonitis.
Infection (osteomyelitis, septic arthritis, cellulitis) of foot.
Peripheral vascular insufficiency.
Fracture.
Osteoarthritis.
Gout, pseudogout.
Neuropathy.
Tumor.

PAIN, PLANTAR ASPECT, HEEL

ICD-10CM # M25.579 Pain in unspecified ankle and joints of unspecified foot

Plantar fasciitis.
Tarsal tunnel syndrome.
Neuroma.
Infection (osteomyelitis, septic arthritis, cellulitis) of foot.
Peripheral vascular insufficiency.
Fracture.
Bone cyst.
Osteoarthritis.
Gout, pseudogout.
Neuropathy.
Tumor.
Heel pad atrophy.
Plantar fascia rupture.

PAIN, POSTERIOR HEEL

ICD-10CM # M79.609 Pain in unspecified limb

Achilles tendonitis.
Retrocalcaneal bursitis.
Retroachilles bursitis.
Infection (osteomyelitis, septic arthritis, cellulitis) of foot.
Peripheral vascular insufficiency.
Fracture.
Osteoarthritis.
Gout, pseudogout.
Neuropathy.
Tumor.

PAIN SYNDROMES WITHOUT CHRONIC MYOPATHY[38]

ICD-10CM # Code varies with specific diagnosis

PAIN OF UNCERTAIN ORIGIN
Polymyalgia rheumatica.
Infections:
  Viral and postviral syndromes.
  Brucellosis.

ENDOCRINE:
Thyroid: decreased (mainly) or increased.
Parathyroid: increased or decreased.
Adrenal insufficiency.
  Familial Mediterranean fever.

PAIN WITH DEFINED ORIGIN
Connective tissue disorders:
  Systemic.
  Fasciitis.
Joint disease.
Bone: osteomalacia, fracture, neoplasm.
Vascular: ischemia, thrombophlebitis.
Polyneuropathy:
  Small-fiber polyneuropathies.
  Guillain-Barré syndrome.

Radiculoneuropathy.
Central nervous system: restless legs syndrome, dystonias (focal).

PAIN OF MUSCLE FROM CENTRAL SENSITIZATION
Fibromyalgia.
Chronic fatigue syndrome/systemic exertion intolerance disease.
Myofascial pain syndrome.
Joint hypermobility syndrome/Ehlers-Danlos syndrome.

PAIN OF MUSCLE ORIGIN WITHOUT CHRONIC MYOPATHY
Muscle ischemia: atherosclerosis, calciphylaxis.
Muscle overuse syndromes:
  Delayed-onset muscle soreness (DOMS).
  Cramps.
Drugs, toxins.
Muscle injury (strain).
Usual features: muscle pain; may interfere with effort but no true weakness; present at rest, may increase with movement; muscle morphology and serum creatine kinase normal.

PALINDROMIC RHEUMATISM[40]

ICD-10CM #
	M12.30	Palindromic rheumatism, unspecified site
	M12.319	Palindromic rheumatism, unspecified shoulder
	M12.329	Palindromic rheumatism, unspecified elbow
	M12.339	Palindromic rheumatism, unspecified wrist
	M12.349	Palindromic rheumatism, unspecified hand
	M12.359	Palindromic rheumatism, unspecified hip
	M12.369	Palindromic rheumatism, unspecified knee
	M12.379	Palindromic rheumatism, unspecified ankle and foot
	M12.38	Palindromic rheumatism, vertebrae
	M12.39	Palindromic rheumatism, multiple sites

Palindromic RA.
Essential palindromic rheumatism.
Crystal synovitis (gout, CPPD, pseudogout, calcific periarthritis).
Lyme borreliosis, stages 2 and 3.
Sarcoidosis.

Whipple disease.
Acute rheumatic fever.
Reactive arthritis (rare).

PALMOPLANTAR HYPERKERATOSIS

ICD-10CM #	L85.1	Acquired keratosis [keratoderma] palmaris et plantaris
	L85.2	Keratosis punctata (palmaris et plantaris)
	L87.0	Keratosis follicularis et parafollicularis in cutem penetrans

Superficial skin infection.
Chronic eczema.
Repeated trauma.
Psoriasis.
Reiter syndrome.
Paraneoplastic acrokeratosis.

PALPABLE GALLBLADDER[96]

ICD-10CM #	Varies with specific diagnosis

CAUSES
With Jaundice
Carcinoma of the head of the pancreas.
Carcinoma of the ampulla of Vater.
Mucocele of the gallbladder due to a stone in Hartmann pouch and a stone in the common bile duct (rare).
Without Jaundice
Mucocele of the gallbladder.
Carcinoma of the gallbladder.

PALPITATIONS[76]

ICD-10CM #	R00.2	Palpitations

Anxiety.
Electrolyte abnormalities (hypokalemia, hypomagnesemia).
Exercise.
Hyperthyroidism.
Ischemic heart disease.
Ingestion of stimulant drugs (cocaine, amphetamines, caffeine).
Medications (digoxin, β-blockers, calcium channel antagonists, hydralazines, diuretics, minoxidil).
Hypoglycemia in type 1 DM.
Mitral valve prolapse.
Wolff-Parkinson-White (WPW) syndrome.
Sick sinus syndrome.

PANCOAST SYNDROME[14]

ICD-10CM #	Varies with specific diagnosis

CAUSES OF PANCOAST SYNDROME
Neoplasms
Primary bronchogenic carcinomas.

Other primary thoracic neoplasms: adenoid cystic carcinomas.
Hemangiopericytoma.
Mesothelioma.
Metastatic neoplasms: carcinoma of the larynx, cervix, urinary bladder, and thyroid gland.
Hematologic neoplasms: plasmacytoma, lymphoid granulomatosis, lymphoma.
Infectious Processes
Bacterial: staphylococcal and pseudomonal pneumonia, thoracic actinomycosis.
Fungal: aspergillosis, allescheriasis, cryptococcosis.
Tuberculosis.
Parasitic: echinococcosis (hydatid cyst).

PANCREATIC CALCIFICATIONS

ICD-10CM #	K86.1	Other chronic pancreatitis
	K86.8	Other specified diseases of pancreas

Chronic pancreatitis.
Hyperparathyroidism.
Metastatic neoplasm.
Pseudocyst.
Hereditary pancreatitis.
Cystoadenoma.
Cystoadenocarcinoma.
Cavernous lymphangioma.
Hemorrhage.
Acute pancreatitis (saponification).

PANCREATIC CYSTIC LESIONS[48]

ICD-10CM #	K86.2	Cyst of pancreas
	K86.3	Pseudocyst of pancreas

Pseudocyst.
Serous cystadenoma.
Mucinous cystic neoplasm.
Intraductal papillary mucinous neoplasm.
Solid and papillary epithelial neoplasm.
True epithelial cyst.
Duodenal diverticulum.
Cystic neuroendocrine tumors.
Ductal adenocarcinoma with cystic degeneration.
Cystic metastases.
Cystic degeneration in sarcoma, hemangioma, and paraganglioma.

PANCREATIC SOLID LESIONS[48]

ICD-10CM #	C25.9	Malignant neoplasm of pancreas, unspecified
	D13.6	Benign neoplasm of pancreas

Neoplastic solid tumors.
Ductal adenocarcinoma.
Pancreatic neuroendocrine tumor.
Pancreatic lymphoma.
Metastases to the pancreas.

Solid pseudopapillary tumor.
Pancreaticoblastoma.
Acinar cell carcinoma.
Mesenchymal tumors (sarcoma, fibrous histiocytoma, etc.).
Nonneoplastic solid lesions.
Focal chronic pancreatitis.
Autoimmune pancreatitis.
Groove pancreatitis.
Focal sparing of diffuse pancreatic fatty infiltration.
Intrapancreatic accessory spleen.
Developmental pancreas lobulation.
Sarcoidosis of the pancreas.

PANCREATITIS, ACUTE, IN CHILDREN[19]

ICD-10CM #	K85	Acute pancreatitis

CAUSES OF ACUTE PANCREATITIS IN CHILDREN
Drugs and Toxins
Acetaminophen overdose.
Alcohol.
L-Asparaginase.
Azathioprine.
Carbamazepine.
Cimetidine.
Corticosteroids.
Enalapril.
Erythromycin.
Estrogen.
Furosemide.
Isoniazid.
Lisinopril.
6-Mercaptopurine.
Methyldopa.
Metronidazole.
Organophosphate poisoning.
Pentamidine.
Retrovirals: DDC, DDI, tenofovir.
Sulfonamides: mesalamine, 5-aminosalicylates, sulfasalazine, trimethoprim/sulfamethoxazole.
Sulindac.
Tetracycline.
Thiazides.
Valproic acid.
Venom (spider, scorpion, Gila monster lizard).
Vincristine.
Genetic
Cationic trypsinogen gene *(PRSS1)*.
Chymotrypsin C gene *(CTRC)*.
Cystic fibrosis gene *(CFTR)*.
Trypsin inhibitor gene *(SPINK1)*.
Infectious
Ascariasis.
Coxsackie B virus.
Epstein-Barr virus.
Hepatitis A, B.
Influenza A, B.
Leptospirosis.
Malaria.

Measles.
Mumps.
Mycoplasma.
Reye syndrome: varicella, influenza B.
Rubella.
Rubeola.
Septic shock.

Obstructive
Ampullary disease.
Ascariasis.
Biliary tract malformations.
Choledochal cyst.
Choledochocele.
Cholelithiasis, microlithiasis, and choledocholithiasis (stones or sludge).
Duplication cyst.
Endoscopic retrograde cholangiopancreatography (ERCP) complication.
Pancreas divisum.
Pancreatic ductal abnormalities.
Postoperative.
Sphincter of Oddi dysfunction.
Tumor.

Systemic Disease
Autoimmune pancreatitis.
Brain tumor.
Collagen vascular diseases.
Crohn disease.
Diabetes mellitus.
Head trauma.
Hemochromatosis.
Hemolytic-uremic syndrome.
Hyperlipidemia: type I, IV, V.
Hyperparathyroidism/hypercalcemia.
Kawasaki disease.
Malnutrition.
Organic acidemia.
Peptic ulcer.
Periarteritis nodosa.
Renal failure.
Systemic lupus erythematosus.
Transplantation: bone marrow, heart, liver, kidney, pancreas.
Vasculitis.

Traumatic
Blunt injury.
Burns.
Child abuse.
Hypothermia.
Surgical trauma.
Total body cast.

PANCREATITIS, DRUG-INDUCED[43]

ICD-10CM # K85.3 Drug induced acute pancreatitis

DEFINITE
Acetaminophen.
Azathioprine.
Cimetidine.
Cisplatin.
Corticosteroids.
Didanosine.

Erythromycin.
Estrogens.
Ethyl alcohol.
Furosemide.
L-Asparaginase.
Mercaptopurine.
Metronidazole.
Methyldopa.
Nitrofurantoin.
Octreotide.
Organophosphates.
Pentamidine.
Ranitidine.
Tetracycline.
Salicylates.
Sulfonamides, trimethoprim-sulfamethoxazole, sulfasalazine.
Sulindac.
Valproic acid.

POSSIBLE
Bumetanide.
Carbamazepine.
Chlorthalidone.
Clonidine.
Colchicine.
Cyclosporine.
Cytarabine.
Diazoxide.
Enalapril.
Ergotamine.
Ethacrynic acid.
Indomethacin.
Isoniazid.
Isotretinoin.
Mefenamic acid.
Opiates.
Phenformin.
Piroxicam.
Procainamide.
Rifampin.
Thiazides.

PANCYTOPENIA[31]

ICD-10CM # D61.818 Other pancytopenia

PANCYTOPENIA WITH HYPOCELLULAR BONE MARROW
Acquired aplastic anemia.
Inherited aplastic anemia (Fanconi anemia and others).
Some myelodysplasia syndromes.
Rare aleukemic leukemia (acute myelogenous leukemia).
Some acute lymphoblastic leukemias.
Some lymphomas of bone marrow.

PANCYTOPENIA WITH CELLULAR BONE MARROW
Primary bone marrow diseases.
Myelodysplasia syndromes.
Paroxysmal nocturnal hemoglobinuria.
Myelofibrosis.
Some aleukemic leukemias.

Myelophthisis.
Bone marrow lymphoma.
Hairy cell leukemia.
Secondary to systemic diseases.
Systemic lupus erythematosus, Sjögren syndrome.
Hypersplenism.
Vitamin B_{12}, folate deficiency (familial defect).
Overwhelming infection.
Alcohol.
Brucellosis.
Ehrlichiosis.
Sarcoidosis.
Tuberculosis and atypical mycobacteria.

HYPOCELLULAR BONE MARROW ± CYTOPENIA
Q fever.
Legionnaires disease.
Mycobacteria.
Tuberculosis.*
Anorexia nervosa, starvation.
Hypothyroidism.

---

*Pancytopenia in tuberculosis only rarely is associated with a hypocellular bone marrow at biopsy or autopsy. Marrow failure in the setting of tuberculosis is almost always fatal; exceptional patients probably had underlying myelodysplasia or acute leukemia.

PANCYTOPENIA SYNDROME, INHERITED[19]

ICD-10CM # D61.818 Other pancytopenia

Fanconi anemia.
Shwachman-Diamond syndrome.
Dyskeratosis congenita.
Congenital amegakaryocytic thrombocytopenia.
Unclassified inherited bone marrow failure syndromes.
Other genetic syndromes:
    Down syndrome.
    Dubowitz syndrome.
    Seckel syndrome.
    Reticular dysgenesis.
    Schimke immunoosseous dysplasia.
    Familial aplastic anemia (non-Fanconi).
    Cartilage-hair hypoplasia.
    Noonan syndrome.

PAPILLEDEMA

ICD-10CM # H47.10 Unspecified papilledema

CNS infections (viral, bacterial, fungal).
Medications (lithium, cisplatin, corticosteroids, tetracycline, etc.).
Head trauma.
CNS neoplasm (primary or metastatic).
Pseudotumor cerebri.
Cavernous sinus thrombosis.
SLE.
Sarcoidosis.
Subarachnoid hemorrhage.
Carbon dioxide retention.
Arnold-Chiari malformation and other developmental or congenital malformations.

Differential Diagnosis

II

Orbital lesions.
Central retinal vein occlusion.
Hypertensive encephalopathy.
Metabolic abnormalities.

PAPULOSQUAMOUS DISEASES[24]

ICD-10CM # L98.8   Other specified disorders of the skin and subcutaneous tissue

Psoriasis.
Pityriasis rubra pilaris.
Pityriasis rosea.
Lichen planus.
Lichen nitidus.
Secondary syphilis.
Pityriasis lichenoides.
Parapsoriasis.
Mycosis fungoides.
Dermatophytosis.
Tinea versicolor.

PARALYSIS AND MUSCULAR RIGIDITY, DRUG-INDUCED[49]

ICD-10CM # G83   Other paralytic syndromes
R29.818   Other symptoms and signs involving the nervous system

SELECTED AGENTS ASSOCIATED WITH PARALYSIS AND MUSCULAR RIGIDITY
Paralysis
Medications and Industrial Toxins
Aminoglycoside antibiotics.
β-blockers.
Chloroquine (with color vision shift).
Cholinesterase inhibitors: neostigmine, pyridostigmine.
d-Penicillamine.
Pesticides: organophosphates, carbamates.
Pyrithioxine.
Trimethadione.
Biologic Toxins
Cobra venom.
Poison hemlock (*Conium maculatum*).
Scorpion fish (*Scorpaenidae*).
Snake venom, ticks, botulinum toxin.
Star of Bethlehem (*Hippobroma longiflora*).
Sweet pea (*Lathyrus odoratus*).
Tetrodotoxin (puffer fish, blue-ringed octopus, others).
Muscular Rigidity
Black widow spider venom (*Latrodectus mactans*).
Strychnine (*Strychnos nux vomica*, "slang nut").
Tetanus toxin.

PARALYTIC ILEUS[107]

ICD-10CM # K56   Paralytic ileus and intestinal obstruction

CAUSES OF A PARALYTIC ILEUS

Peritonitis.
Surgery.
Trauma:
  Spine.
  Ribs.
  Hip.
  Retroperitoneum.
Inflammation:
  Appendicitis
  Pancreatitis.
  Cholecystitis.
  Salpingitis.
Congestive heart failure.
Pneumonia.
Renal colic.
Renal failure.
Leaking abdominal aortic aneurysm.
Low serum potassium.
Drugs (e.g., morphine).
Spinal lesions.
General debility or infection.
Vascular occlusion.

PARANASAL SINUS MALIGNANCIES[22]

ICD-10CM #   Code varies with specific diagnosis

EPITHELIAL MALIGNANCIES
Squamous cell carcinoma:
Verrucous carcinoma.
Papillary squamous cell carcinoma.
Basaloid squamous cell carcinoma.
Spindle cell carcinoma.
Adenosquamous carcinoma.
Acantholytic squamous cell carcinoma.
Lymphoepithelial carcinoma.
Sinonasal undifferentiated carcinoma.
Adenocarcinoma:
Intestinal-type adenocarcinoma.
Nonintestinal-type adenocarcinoma.
Salivary gland–type carcinomas:
Adenoid cystic carcinoma.
Acinic cell carcinoma.
Mucoepidermoid carcinoma.
Epithelial-myoepithelial carcinoma.
Clear cell carcinoma not otherwise specified.
Myoepithelial carcinoma.
Carcinoma ex pleomorphic adenoma.
Polymorphous low-grade adenocarcinoma.
Neuroendocrine tumors:
Typical carcinoid.
Atypical carcinoid.
Small cell carcinoma, neuroendocrine type.

SOFT TISSUE MALIGNANCIES
Fibrosarcoma.
Malignant fibrous histiocytoma.
Leiomyosarcoma.
Rhabdomyosarcoma.
Angiosarcoma.
Malignant peripheral nerve sheath tumor.

BONE AND CARTILAGE MALIGNANCIES
Chondrosarcoma.
Mesenchymal chondrosarcoma.
Osteosarcoma.
Chordoma.

HEMATOLYMPHOID MALIGNANCIES
Extranodal natural killer/T-cell lymphoma.
Diffuse large B-cell lymphoma.

Extramedullary plasmacytoma.
Extramedullary myeloid sarcoma.
Histiocytic sarcoma.
Langerhans cell histiocytosis.

NEUROECTODERMAL MALIGNANCIES
Ewing sarcoma.
Primitive neuroectodermal tumor.
Olfactory neuroblastoma.
Melanotic neuroectodermal tumor of infancy.
Mucosal malignant melanoma.

GERM CELL MALIGNANCIES
Teratoma with malignant transformation.
Sinonasal teratocarcinosarcoma.

PARANEOPLASTIC NEUROLOGIC SYNDROMES

ICD-10CM # G13.0   Paraneoplastic neuromyopathy and neuropathy

Lambert-Eaton myasthenic syndrome.
Myasthenia gravis.
Guillain-Barré syndrome.
Amyotrophic lateral sclerosis.
Dermatomyositis.
Carcinoid myopathy.
Cerebellar degeneration.
Encephalomyelitis.
Optic neuritis, uveitis, retinopathy.
Stiff-man syndrome.
Autonomic neuropathy.
Brachial neuritis.
Sensory neuropathy.
Progressive multifocal leukoencephalopathy.

PARANEOPLASTIC SYNDROMES, ENDOCRINE[17]

ICD-10CM # G13.0   Paraneoplastic neuromyopathy and neuropathy

Hypercalcemia.
Syndrome of inappropriate secretion of antidiuretic hormone.
Hypoglycemia.
Zollinger-Ellison syndrome.
Ectopic secretion of human chorionic gonadotropin.
Cushing syndrome.

PARANEOPLASTIC SYNDROMES, NONENDOCRINE[17]

ICD-10CM # G13.0   Paraneoplastic neuromyopathy and neuropathy

CUTANEOUS
Dermatomyositis.
Acanthosis nigricans.
Sweet syndrome.

Erythema gyratum repens.
Systemic nodular panniculitis (Weber-Christian disease).

RENAL

Nephrotic syndrome.
Nephrogenic diabetes insipidus.

NEUROLOGIC

Subacute cerebellar degeneration.
Progressive multifocal leukoencephalopathy.
Subacute motor neuropathy.
Sensory neuropathy.
Ascending acute polyneuropathy (Guillain-Barré syndrome).
Myasthenic syndrome (Eaton-Lambert syndrome).

HEMATOLOGIC

Microangiopathic hemolytic anemia.
Migratory thrombophlebitis (Trousseau syndrome).
Anemia of chronic disease.

RHEUMATOLOGIC

Polymyalgia rheumatica.
Hypertrophic pulmonary osteoarthropathy.

PARAPARESIS[101]

ICD-10CM #   Varies with specific diagnosis

Causes

Inflammatory central nervous system (CNS) diseases.
Multiple sclerosis (MS).
Neuromyelitis optica (NMO).
Genetic disorders.
Spinal cerebellar ataxias (SCAs).
Hereditary spastic paraparesis (HSP).
Infectious illnesses.
Human T-lymphotropic virus type 1 (HTLV-1) myelopathy.
Compressive lesions.
Cervical spondylosis.
Spinal meningiomas.
Metastatic tumors.
Neurodegenerative illnesses.
Amyotrophic lateral sclerosis (ALS).
Nutritional deficiencies.
Copper deficiency.
Vitamin B_{12} deficiency (combined system disease).

PARAPARESIS, ACUTE OR SUBACUTE[47]

ICD-10CM #   G82.2   Paraparesis

CAUSES OF ACUTE OR SUBACUTE PARAPARESIS

Trauma to a Previously Normal Spine
Vertebral Disease
Metastatic carcinoma.
Cervical spondylosis.

Dorsal disk prolapse.
Paget disease.
Rheumatoid arthritis.
Pott disease of spine.

Tumors

Extradural or intradural carcinoma, lymphoma, myeloma, leukemia.
Dorsal meningioma.
Neurofibroma.

Hematologic Disease

Any cause of thrombocytopenia.
Other clotting disorders.
Leukemia.
Anticoagulant treatment.
Epidural or intramedullary hemorrhage.

Infection

Epidural abscess.
TB abscess.
Syphilitic myelitis.
HIV infection.
Vascular myelopathy.

Vascular

Anterior spinal artery occlusion.
Infarction secondary to hypotension.
Embolic infarction.
Infarction secondary to aortic dissection.
Arteriovenous malformation: infarction or hemorrhage.
Primary intramedullary hemorrhage.
Vasculitis—polyarteritis nodosa (PAN).

Inflammatory

Myelitis of unknown cause.
Multiple sclerosis.
Systemic lupus erythematosus.
Sarcoidosis.

Metabolic

Subacute degeneration of the cord.

PARAPARESIS, CHRONIC PROGRESSIVE[47]

ICD-10CM #   G82.2   Paraparesis

CAUSES OF CHRONIC PROGRESSIVE PARAPARESIS

Vertebral Disease
Cervical spondylosis.
Dorsal disk prolapse.
Rheumatoid arthritis.
Pott disease of spine.
Ankylosing spondylitis.
Tumors
Meningioma.
Neurofibroma.
Glioma.
Ependymoma.
Chordoma.
Lipoma.

Syringomyelia
With Arnold-Chiari malformation.
With tumor.
Posttraumatic.
Infection
Tropical spastic paraparesis (HTLV-1 infection).
Syphilitic myelitis.
Vascular
Arteriovenous malformation.
Inflammatory
Multiple sclerosis.
Sarcoidosis.
Radiation myelopathy.
Arachnoiditis.
Metabolic
Subacute combined degeneration of the cord.
Paget disease.
Degenerative
Motor neuron disease.
Hereditary
Hereditary spastic paraplegia.

PARAPARESIS, PAINLESS[72]

ICD-10CM #   G82   Paraplegia (paraparesis) and quadriplegia (quadriparesis)

FREQUENTLY OCCURRING CAUSES OF PAINLESS PARAPARESIS

Inflammatory CNS diseases:
Multiple sclerosis (MS).
Neuromyelitis optica (NMO).
Genetic disorders:
Spinal cerebellar ataxias (SCAs).
Hereditary spastic paraparesis (HSP).
Infectious illnesses:
Human T-lymphotropic virus type 1 (HTLV-1) myelopathy.
Compressive lesions:*
Cervical spondylosis.
Spinal meningiomas.
Metastatic tumors.
Neurodegenerative illnesses:
ALS.
Nutritional deficiencies:
Copper deficiency.
Vitamin B_{12} deficiency (combined system disease).

*Frequently presents with wrist drop.

PARAPLEGIA

ICD-10CM #	G82.20	Paraplegia, unspecified
	G80.1	Spastic diplegic cerebral palsy
	I69.969	Other paralytic syndrome following unspecified cerebrovascular disease affecting unspecified side

Trauma: penetrating wounds to motor cortex, fracture-dislocation of vertebral column with compression of spinal cord or cauda equina, prolapsed disk, electrical injuries.

Neoplasm: parasagittal region, vertebrae, meninges, spinal cord, cauda equina, Hodgkin disease, NHL, leukemic deposits, pelvic neoplasms.

Multiple sclerosis and other demyelinating disorders.

Mechanical compression of spinal cord, cauda equina, or lumbosacral plexus: Paget disease, kyphoscoliosis, herniation of intervertebral disk, spondylosis, ankylosing spondylitis, RA, aortic aneurysm.

Infections: spinal abscess, syphilis, TB, poliomyelitis, leprosy.

Thrombosis of superior sagittal sinus.

Polyneuritis: Guillain-Barré syndrome, diabetes, alcohol, beriberi, heavy metals.

Heredofamilial muscular dystrophies.

ALS.

Congenital and familial conditions: syringomyelia, myelomeningocele, myelodysplasia.

Hysteria.

PARASELLAR MASSES[30]

ICD-10CM #   Varies with specific diagnosis

GENETIC
Transcription factor mutations (e.g., PROP1*).

CYSTS
Rathke.
Arachnoid.
Epidermoid.
Dermoid.

TUMORS
Hormone-secreting or nonfunctional pituitary adenoma.
Granular cell tumor.
Craniopharyngioma (cystic components).
Chordoma.
Meningioma.
Sarcoma.
Glioma.
Schwannoma.
Germ cell tumor.
Vascular tumor.
Solid or hematological metastasis.

MALFORMATION AND HAMARTOMAS
Ectopic pituitary, neurohypophyseal, or salivary tissue.
Hypothalamic hamartoma.
Gangliocytoma.

MISCELLANEOUS LESIONS
Aneurysms.
Hypophysitis.
Infections.
Sarcoidosis.
Giant cell granuloma.
Histiocytosis X.

*PROP1, prophet of Pit1 (pairedlike homeodomain transcription factor).

PARESTHESIAS

ICD-10CM #   R20.2   Paresthesia of skin
             G54.8   Other nerve root and plexus disorders

Multiple sclerosis.
Nutritional deficiencies (thiamin, vitamin B_{12}, folic acid).
Compression of spinal cord or peripheral nerves.
Medications (e.g., INH, lithium, nitrofurantoin, gold, cisplatin, hydralazine, amitriptyline, sulfonamides, amiodarone, metronidazole, dapsone, disulfiram, chloramphenicol).
Toxic chemicals (e.g., lead, arsenic, cyanide, mercury, organophosphates).
DM.
Myxedema.
Alcohol.
Sarcoidosis.
Neoplasms.
Infections (HIV, Lyme disease, herpes zoster, leprosy, diphtheria).
Charcot-Marie-Tooth syndrome and other hereditary neuropathies.
Guillain-Barré neuropathy.

PARKINSONISM[49]

ICD-10CM #   G20   Parkinson disease
             G21   Secondary parkinsonism
             G21.9   Secondary parkinsonism, unspecified
             G21.19 Other drug-induced Secondary parkinsonism
             G21.4   Vascular parkinsonism
             G21.2   Secondary parkinsonism due to other external agents

CAUSES OF PARKINSONISM
Static Injury/Structural Disorders
Basal ganglia infarcts.
Brain tumor.
Hydrocephalus.
Hereditary/Degenerative Disorders
Juvenile Parkinson disease.
Spinocerebellar ataxia.
Huntington disease (Westphal variant).
Pallidal-pyramidal disorder.
Neurodegeneration with brain iron accumulation (NBIA).
Pantothenate kinase-associated neurodegeneration (PKAN).
Rett syndrome.
Pelizaeus-Merzbacher disease.
Machado-Joseph disease (spinocerebellar ataxia type 3).
Neuronal ceroid lipofuscinoses.
Neuronal intranuclear inclusion body disease.
Metabolic Disorders
Dopa-responsive dystonia.
Tyrosine hydroxylase deficiency and other abnormalities of bioamine metabolism.
Abnormalities of folate metabolism.
Wilson disease.

Basal ganglia calcification (Fahr syndrome, hypoparathyroidism).
Infectious/Parainfectious Disorders
Encephalitis lethargica (Von Economo disease).
Autoimmune encephalitides, including anti-NMDA receptor associated encephalitis.
Viral encephalitis.
Acute demyelinating encephalomyelitis.
Drugs/Toxins
1-methyl-4-phenyl-1,2,3,6-tetrahydropyridine (MPTP) poisoning.
Rotenone.
Tetrabenazine.
Reserpine.
Methyldopa.
Sedatives.
Neuroleptics.
Antiemetics.
Calcium channel blockers.
Isoniazid.
Serotonin reuptake inhibitors (sertraline, fluoxetine).
Meperidine.
Disorders That Mimic Parkinsonism
Catatonia.
Spasticity.
Hypothyroidism.
Depression (with psychomotor retardation).

PARKINSONISM AND OTHER ACUTE EXTRAPYRAMIDAL REACTIONS, DRUG-INDUCED[49]

ICD-10CM #   G21.19   Other drug-induced secondary parkinsonism

SELECTED AGENTS ASSOCIATED WITH PARKINSONISM AND OTHER ACUTE EXTRAPYRAMIDAL REACTIONS
Medications
Amiodarone.
Anticholinergic agents: benztropine.
Antidepressants (including selective serotonin reuptake inhibitors).
Antiepileptic drugs.
Antifungal agents.
Antihistamines.
Antipsychotics and related drugs (including "novel" agents).
Bethanechol.
Bupropion (acute).
Buspirone.
Captopril (acute).
Clonazepam.
Diazoxide.
Digoxin (chorea).
Estrogen (chorea).
Heroin.
Ketamine.
L-dopa.
Lithium (chorea).
l-Methyl-4-phenyl-1,2,3,6,-tetrahydropyridine (MPTP).

Metronidazole (oculogyric crisis).
Ofloxacin (Tourette-like syndrome).
Opiates/opioids.
Reserpine.
Stimulants.
Sulfasalazine (chorea).
Vinblastine.
Industrial Toxins
Carbon monoxide.
Metals: manganese, thallium, aluminum.
Methanol.
Trichloroethylene.
Biologic Toxins
Arthrinium mycotoxin.

PARKINSONISM-PLUS SYNDROMES

ICD-10CM #	G21.8	Other secondary parkinsonism

Parkinson disease.
Shy-Drager syndrome.
Corticobasal degeneration.
Olivo-ponto-cerebellar atrophy.
Dementia with Lewy bodies.
Progressive supranuclear palsy.
Striatonigral degeneration.

PAROTID SWELLING[108]

ICD-10CM #	K11.20	Sialoadenitis, unspecified
	B26.9	Mumps without complication
	K11.8	Other diseases of salivary glands
	K11.5	Sialolithiasis
	K11.3	Abscess of salivary gland

INFECTIOUS
Mumps.
Parainfluenza.
Influenza.
Cytomegalovirus infection.
Coxsackievirus infection.
Lymphocytic choriomeningitis.
Echovirus infection.
Suppuration (bacterial).
Actinomyces infection.
Mycobacterial infection.
Cat-scratch disease.

NONINFECTIOUS
Drug hypersensitivity (thiouracil, phenothiazines, thiocyanate, iodides, copper, isoprenaline, lead, mercury, phenylbutazone).
Sarcoidosis.
Tumors, mixed.
Hemangioma, lymphangioma.
Sialectasis.
Sjögren syndrome.
Mikulicz syndrome (scleroderma, mixed connective tissue disease, SLE).
Recurrent idiopathic parotitis.
Pneumoparotitis.
Trauma.
Sialolithiasis.

Foreign body.
Cystic fibrosis.
Malnutrition (marasmus, alcohol cirrhosis).
Dehydration.
DM.
Waldenström macroglobulinemia.
Reiter syndrome (reactive arthritis).
Amyloidosis.

NONPAROTID SWELLING
Hypertrophy of masseter muscle.
Lymphadenopathy.
Rheumatoid mandibular joint swelling.
Tumors of jaw.
Infantile cortical hyperostosis.

PELVIC AVULSION FRACTURES[52]

ICD-10CM #	M84.350A	Stress fracture pelvis, initial encounter
	M84.454A	Pathological fracture pelvis, initial encounter

ACUTE AVULSION FRACTURE
Nontraumatic avulsion fracture: Bone metastasis, prior graft harvesting.
Soft tissue injury: Tendon tear, muscle strain.
Aggressive-looking appearance: Osteomyelitis, tumor.
Incidental normal variant: Accessory bone.

CHRONIC AVULSION FRACTURE
Apophyseal avulsion injury: Apophysitis, traction periostitis.
Soft tissue injury: Bursitis, degenerative tendinopathy, calcific tendinitis.

PELVIC MASS

ICD-10CM #	R19.09	Other intraabdominal and pelvic swelling, mass and lump

Hemorrhagic ovarian cyst.
Simple ovarian cyst (follicle or corpus luteum).
Ovarian carcinoma, carcinoma of fallopian tube, colorectal carcinoma, metastatic carcinoma, prostate carcinoma, bladder carcinoma, lymphoma, Hodgkin disease.
Cystadenoma, teratoma, endometrioma.
Leiomyoma.
Leiomyosarcoma.
Diverticulitis, diverticular abscess.
Appendiceal abscess, tuboovarian abscess.
Ectopic pregnancy, intrauterine pregnancy.
Paraovarian cyst.
Hydrosalpinx.

PELVIC PAIN, CAUSES IN WOMEN[43]

ICD-10CM #	N94	Pain and other conditions associated with female

genital organs and menstrual cycle

	G10.2	Pelvic and perineal pain
	G89.4	Chronic pain syndrome

POTENTIAL CAUSES OF PELVIC PAIN IN WOMEN
Reproductive Tract
Ovarian torsion.
Ovarian cyst.
Salpingitis/tuboovarian abscess.
Septic pelvic thrombophlebitis.
Endometritis.
Endometriosis.
Uterine perforation.
Uterine fibroids.
Dysmenorrhea.
Pregnancy-related
First Trimester
Ectopic pregnancy.
Threatened abortion.
Nonviable pregnancy.
Ovarian hyperstimulation syndrome.
Second and Third Trimesters
Placenta previa.
Placental abruption.
Round ligament pain.
Intestinal Tract
Appendicitis.
Diverticulitis.
Ischemic bowel.
Perforated viscus.
Bowel obstruction.
Incarcerated/strangulated hernia.
Inflammatory bowel disease.
Gastroenteritis.
Urinary Tract
Pyelonephritis.
Cystitis.
Ureteral stone.

PELVIC PAIN, CHRONIC[93]

ICD-10CM #	N94.89	Other specified conditions associated with female genital organs and menstrual cycle
	R10.2	Pelvic and perineal pain
	R10.10	Upper abdominal pain, unspecified
	R10.2	Pelvic and perineal pain
	R10.30	Lower abdominal pain, unspecified

GYNECOLOGIC DISORDERS
Primary dysmenorrhea.
Endometriosis.
Adenomyosis.
Adhesions.
Fibroids.
Retained ovary syndrome after hysterectomy.
Previous tubal ligation.
Chronic pelvic infection.

II

Differential Diagnosis

MUSCULOSKELETAL DISORDERS
Myofascial pain syndrome.

GASTROINTESTINAL DISORDERS
Irritable bowel syndrome.
Inflammatory bowel disease.

URINARY TRACT DISORDERS
Interstitial cystitis.
Nonbacterial urethritis.

PELVIC PAIN, CYCLIC AND ACYCLIC[12]

ICD-10CM #   R10.10   Abdominal and pelvic pain

CAUSES OF CYCLIC AND ACYCLIC PELVIC PAIN
Cyclic
Mittelschmerz.
Endometriosis.*
Adenomyosis.
Cervical stenosis.*
Leiomyoma (fibroid).
Primary dysmenorrhea.
Acyclic
Chronic PID.
Pelvic adhesions.
Uterine prolapse.
Chronic urethritis.
Diverticulitis.
Irritable bowel syndrome.
Levator syndrome.
Detrusor instability.
Interstitial cystitis.
Abdominal hernia.
Abdominal wall myofascial pain.
Abuse syndromes: physical and sexual.
Depression.

PID, Pelvic inflammatory disease.

*May become acyclic.

PELVIC PAIN, GENITAL ORIGIN[1]

ICD-10CM #   N94.89   Other specified conditions associated with female genital organs and menstrual cycle
      R10.2   Pelvic and perineal pain
      R10.10   Upper abdominal pain, unspecified
      R10.2   Pelvic and perineal pain
      R10.30   Lower abdominal pain, unspecified

PERITONEAL IRRITATION
Ruptured ectopic pregnancy.
Ovarian cyst rupture.
Ruptured tuboovarian abscess.
Uterine perforation.

TORSION
Ovarian cyst or tumor.
Pedunculated fibroid.

INTRATUMOR HEMORRHAGE OR INFARCTION
Ovarian cyst.
Solid ovarian tumor.
Uterine leiomyoma.

INFECTION
Endometritis.
Pelvic inflammatory disease.
Trichomonas cervicitis or vaginitis.
Tuboovarian abscess.

PREGNANCY-RELATED
First Trimester
Ectopic pregnancy.
Abortion.
Corpus luteum hematoma.
Late Pregnancy
Placental problems.
Preeclampsia.
Premature labor.

MISCELLANEOUS
Endometriosis.
Foreign objects.
Pelvic adhesions.
Pelvic neoplasm.
Primary dysmenorrhea.

PELVIC PAIN, NONPREGNANT FEMALE[29]

ICD-10CM #   N94.89   Other specified conditions associated with female genital organs and menstrual cycle
      R10.2   Pelvic and perineal pain
      R10.10   Upper abdominal pain, unspecified
      R10.30   Lower abdominal pain, unspecified

DIFFERENTIAL DIAGNOSIS OF PELVIC PAIN IN NONPREGNANT FEMALES
Gynecologic Diagnoses
Infectious:
    Vaginitis.
    Cervicitis.
    Endometritis.
    Tuboovarian abscess.
    Pelvic inflammatory disease.
Ovarian:
    Ovarian torsion.
    Ruptured ovarian cyst.
    Ovarian tumor.
    Degenerating ovarian tumor.
    Mittelschmerz.
Cervical:
    Cervical polyps.

    Cervical stenosis.
    Cervical cancer.
Uterine:
    Uterine fibroids.
    Degenerating uterine fibroids.
    Adenomyosis.
    Endometrial carcinoma.
Extrauterine:
    Endometriosis.
    Adhesions.
    Residual accessory ovary.
Nongynecologic Diagnoses
GI:
    Acute appendicitis.
    Mesenteric lymphadenitis.
    Diverticulitis.
    Inflammatory bowel disease.
    Irritable bowel syndrome.
    Bowel obstruction.
    Intraabdominal abscess.
    Colorectal carcinoma.
Urinary:
    Cystitis.
    Renal colic.
    Bladder cancer.
Musculoskeletal:
    Abdominal wall pain.
    Lumbar back pain.
    Fibromyalgia.
    Muscular strain.
    Piriformis syndrome.
Neurologic:
    Lumbar radiculopathy.
    Shingles.
    Spondylosis.
Psychologic:
    Personality disorders.
    Major depressive disorder.

PENILE RASH

ICD-10CM #   R21   Rash and other nonspecific skin eruption

Herpes simplex 2.
Balanitis (*Candida*).
Condyloma acuminatum.
Molluscum contagiosum.
Scabies.
Pediculosis pubis.
Pearly penile papules.
Lichen nitidus.
Fox-Fordyce disease (follicular papules).
Trauma.

PERIANAL PAIN[2]

ICD-10CM #   K62.89   Other specified diseases of anus and rectum

Fissure-in-ano.
Anal sepsis:
    Anal abscess.
    Anal fistula.

Hemorrhoids:
Internal hemorrhoids.
External hemorrhoids.
Pruritus ani.
Proctalgia fugax.
Chronic perianal pain syndromes:
Coccygodynia.
Descending perineum syndrome.
Levator ani syndrome.
Idiopathic perineal pain.

PERICARDIAL EFFUSION

| ICD-10CM # | I30.9 | Acute pericarditis, unspecified |
| | I31.3 | Pericardial effusion |

Pericarditis.
Uremia.
Myxedema.
Neoplasm (leukemia, lymphoma, metastatic).
Hemorrhage (trauma, leakage of thoracic aneurysm).
SLE, rheumatoid disease.
Myocardial infarction.

PERIPHERAL ARTERIAL DISEASE, NONATHEROSCLEROTIC CAUSES[71]

ICD-10CM #	I73.9	Peripheral vascular disease, unspecified
	I73.8	Other specified peripheral vascular diseases
	I79.8	Other disorders of arteries, arterioles, and capillaries in diseases classified elsewhere

NONATHEROSCLEROTIC CAUSES OF PERIPHERAL ARTERY DISEASE

Thromboembolism.
Atheroembolism.
Vasculitides:
Large vessel vasculitides, such as giant cell arteritis and Takayasu arteritis.
Small vessel vasculitides, such as thromboangiitis obliterans (Buerger disease).
Trauma.
Popliteal artery entrapment.
Cystic adventitial disease.
Fibromuscular dysplasia.
Iliac artery endofibrosis.

PERIPHERAL INFLAMMATORY ARTHRITIS[53]

| ICD-10CM # | Code varies with specific diagnosis |

DIFFERENTIAL DIAGNOSIS FOR PATIENTS WITH A NEW ONSET OF PERIPHERAL INFLAMMATORY ARTHRITIS

Crystal arthritis (e.g., gout, pseudogout).
Inflammatory osteoarthritis.
Rheumatoid arthritis.
Psoriatic arthritis.
Other spondyloarthropathy.
Systemic lupus erythematosus.
Other connective tissue diseases/vasculitis.
Postinfective arthritis (e.g., reactive arthritis, postviral arthritis).
Sarcoidosis.
Malignancy-associated arthritis.
RS3PE.
Septic arthritis.
Other.
RS3PE, Remitting seronegative symmetrical synovitis with pitting edema.

PERIODIC PARALYSIS, HYPERKALEMIC

| ICD-10CM # | G83.9 | Paralytic syndrome, unspecified |

Chronic renal failure.
Renal insufficiency with excessive potassium supplementation.
Potassium-sparing diuretics.
Endocrinopathies (hypoaldosteronism, adrenal insufficiency).

PERIODIC PARALYSIS, HYPOKALEMIC

| ICD-10CM # | G83.9 | Paralytic syndrome, unspecified |

Chronic diarrhea (laxative abuse, sprue, villous adenoma).
Potassium-depleting diuretics.
Medications (amphotericin B, corticosteroids).
Chronic licorice ingestion.
Thyrotoxicosis.
Renal tubular acidosis.
Conn syndrome.
Bartter syndrome.
Barium intoxication.

PERITONEAL CARCINOMATOSIS[24]

| ICD-10CM # | C78.6 | Secondary malignant neoplasm of retroperitoneum and peritoneum |

PRIMARY DISORDERS OF THE PERITONEUM: MESOTHELIOMA

Metastatic spread from:
Stomach.
Colon.
Pancreas.
Carcinoid.
Other Intraabdominal Organs
Ovary.
Pseudomyxoma peritonei.
Extraabdominal Primary Tumors
Breast.
Lung.
Hematologic Malignancy
Lymphoma.

PERITONEAL EFFUSION[109]

ICD-10CM #	R18	Ascites
	R85.9	Unspecified abnormal finding in specimens from digestive organs and abdominal cavity
	R88.8	Abnormal findings in other body fluids and substances

TRANSUDATES

Increased hydrostatic pressure or decreased plasma oncotic pressure.
Congestive heart failure.
Hepatic cirrhosis.
Hypoproteinemia.

EXUDATES

Increased capillary permeability or decreased lymphatic resorption.
Infections (TB, spontaneous bacterial peritonitis, secondary bacterial peritonitis).
Neoplasms (hepatoma, metastatic carcinoma, lymphoma, mesothelioma).
Trauma.
Pancreatitis.
Bile peritonitis (e.g., ruptured gallbladder).

CHYLOUS EFFUSION

Damage or obstruction to thoracic duct.
Trauma.
Lymphoma.
Carcinoma.
Tuberculosis.
Parasitic infection.

PERIUMBILICAL SWELLING

| ICD-10CM # | R19.00 | Intraabdominal and pelvic swelling, mass and lump, unspecified site |

Umbilical hernia.
Lipoma.
Epigastric hernia.
Umbilical granuloma.
Omphalocele.
Gastroschisis.
Caput medusae.

PHARYNGEAL OBSTRUCTION, CAUSES[13]

| ICD-10CM # | Varies with specific diagnosis |

CAUSES OF PHARYNGEAL OBSTRUCTION

Malignant or benign tumors (e.g., papillomas, polyps).

Infection (e.g., croup, epiglottitis, tonsillar abscess).

Edema or hypertrophy (e.g., angioneurotic edema, anaphylactic reactions, postradiation therapy, obstructive sleep apnea).

Trauma (e.g., cricoid fracture, cervical subluxation, precervical hematoma).

Burn injury.

Extrinsic compression (e.g., goiter or pregnancy-related thyroid enlargement).

Foreign body.

Congenital web (infants).

Sarcoidosis and other granulomatous diseases.

Amyloid.

PHEOCHROMOCYTOMA-TYPE SPELLS[30]

ICD-10CM #   I15.2   Hypertension due to pheochromocytoma

DIFFERENTIAL DIAGNOSIS OF PHEOCHROMOCYTOMA-TYPE SPELLS

Endocrine Causes

Carbohydrate intolerance.

Hyperadrenergic spells.

Hypoglycemia.

Pancreatic tumors (e.g., insulinoma).

Pheochromocytoma.

Primary hypogonadism (menopausal syndrome).

Thyrotoxicosis.

Cardiovascular Causes

Angina.

Cardiovascular deconditioning.

Labile essential hypertension.

Orthostatic hypotension.

Paroxysmal cardiac arrhythmia.

Pulmonary edema.

Renovascular disease.

Syncope (e.g., vasovagal reaction).

Psychologic Causes

Factitious (e.g., drugs, Valsalva).

Hyperventilation.

Severe anxiety and panic disorders.

Somatization disorder.

Pharmacologic Causes

Chlorpropamide-alcohol flush.

Combination of a monoamine oxidase inhibitor and a decongestant.

Illegal drug ingestion (cocaine, phencyclidine, lysergic acid diethylamide).

Sympathomimetic drug ingestion.

Vancomycin ("red man syndrome").

Withdrawal of adrenergic-inhibitor.

Neurologic Causes

Autonomic neuropathy.

Cerebrovascular insufficiency.

Diencephalic epilepsy (autonomic seizures).

Migraine headache.

Postural orthostatic tachycardia syndrome.

Stroke.

Other Causes

Carcinoid syndrome:

   Mast cell disease.

   Recurrent idiopathic anaphylaxis.

   Unexplained flushing spells.

PHOTODERMATOSES[24]

ICD-10CM #   L56.0   Drug phototoxic response
             L56.1   Drug photoallergic response
             L56.2   Photocontact dermatitis [berloque dermatitis]

Polymorphous light eruption.

Chronic actinic dermatitis.

Solar urticaria.

Phototoxicity and photoallergy.

Porphyrias.

PHOTOSENSITIVITY

ICD-10CM #   L56.0   Drug phototoxic response
             L56.1   Drug photoallergic response
             L56.2   Photocontact dermatitis [berloque dermatitis]

Solar urticaria.

Photoallergic reaction.

Phototoxic reaction.

Polymorphous light eruption.

Porphyria cutanea tarda.

SLE.

Drug induced (e.g., tetracyclines).

PIGMENTURIA[43]

ICD-10CM #   R82   Other abnormal findings in urine

HEMOGLOBINURIA

Hemolysis.

HEMATURIA

Renal causes.

Trauma.

ACUTE INTERMITTENT PORPHYRIA

Bilirubinuria

Food

Beets.

Drugs

Vitamin B_{12}.

Rifampin.

Phenytoin.

Laxatives.

PITUITARY INSUFFICIENCY, ACQUIRED[36]

ICD-10CM #   E23.0   Hypopituitarism

E89.3   Postprocedural hypopituitarism
E23.1   Drug-induced hypopituitarism

CAUSES OF ACQUIRED PITUITARY INSUFFICIENCY

Traumatic

Surgical resection.

Radiation damage.

Traumatic brain injury.

Infiltrative/Inflammatory

Primary Hypophysitis

Lymphocytic.

Granulomatous.

Xanthomatous.

Secondary Hypophysitis

Sarcoidosis.

Histiocytosis X.

Infections.

Wegener granulomatosis.

Takayasu disease.

Hemochromatosis.

Infections

Tuberculosis.

Pneumocystis jirovecii infection.

Fungal (histoplasmosis, aspergillosis).

Parasites (toxoplasmosis).

Viral (cytomegalovirus).

Vascular

Pregnancy related.

Aneurysm.

Apoplexy.

Diabetes.

Hypotension.

Arteritis.

Sickle cell disease.

Neoplastic

Pituitary adenoma.

Parasellar mass:

Rathke cyst.

Dermoid cyst.

Meningioma.

Germinoma.

Ependymoma.

Glioma.

Craniopharyngioma.

Hypothalamic hamartoma, gangliocytoma.

Pituitary metastatic deposits.

Hematologic malignancy:

Leukemia.

Lymphoma.

PITUITARY REGION TUMORS[21]

ICD-10CM #   Varies with specific diagnosis

PRIMARY TUMORS IN THE SELLAR AND PARASELLAR REGION

Pituitary macroadenoma.

Meningioma.

Schwannoma (e.g., of fifth nerve).

Chordoma.

Chondrosarcoma.

Craniopharyngioma.
Rathke cleft cyst.
Dermoid.
Epidermoid.
Tuber cinereum hamartoma.
Optic glioma.
Germ cell tumors.

PLATELET DYSFUNCTION, DRUG-INDUCED[71]

ICD-10CM # D69.1 Qualitative platelet defects

Antiplatelet Drugs
COX inhibitors: aspirin.
ADP receptor antagonists:
Thienopyridines: clopidogrel, ticlopidine, prasugrel.
Nonthienopyridines: ticagrelor, cangrelor.
$\alpha_{IIb}\beta_3$ inhibitors: abciximab, eptifibatide, tirofiban.
PDE inhibitors:
Nonselective PDE inhibitors: pentoxifylline, caffeine, theophylline.
PDE3 inhibitors: cilostazol, milrinone, anagrelide.
PDE5 inhibitors: dipyridamole, sildenafil.
Adenyl cyclase stimulators: epoprostenol, iloprost, beraprost.
Drugs that adversely affect platelet function.
NSAIDs: ibuprofen, naproxen, indomethacin.
Cardiovascular agents:
Calcium channel blockers: nifedipine, diltiazem, verapamil.
β-Blockers: propranolol.
Vasodilators: nitrates, nitroprusside.
Diuretics: furosemide.
Angiotensin II receptor antagonist: losartan, valsartan, and olmesartan.
Antibiotics: β-lactams, amphotericin, hydroxychloroquine, nitrofurantoin.
Antifungal drugs: Miconazole, amphotericin B.
Psychiatric drugs: TCAs, fluoxetine, chlorpromazine, promethazine, trifluoperazine.
Oncologic drugs: mithramycin, daunorubicin, BCNU, asparaginase, vincristine, dasatinib, ibrutinib.
Anesthetics: dibucaine, procaine, halothane, sevoflurane, propofol.
Plasma expanders: dextran, hydroxyl ethyl starch.
Heparins and thrombolytic agents.
Miscellaneous: clofibrate, statins, cocaine, ketanserin, radiographic contrast agents, antihistamines, immunosuppressive drugs.

ADP, Adenosine diphosphate; *BCNU,* carmustine; *COX,* cyclooxygenase; *NSAID,* nonsteroidal antiinflammatory drug; *PDE,* phosphodiesterase; *TCA,* tricyclic antidepressant.

PLEURAL EFFUSIONS

ICD-10CM # J91.8 Pleural effusion in other conditions classified elsewhere

EXUDATIVE
Neoplasm: bronchogenic carcinoma, breast carcinoma, mesothelioma, lymphoma, ovarian carcinoma, multiple myeloma, leukemia, Meigs syndrome.
Infections: viral pneumonia, bacterial pneumonia, *Mycoplasma,* TB, fungal and parasitic diseases, extension from subphrenic abscess.
Trauma.
Collagen vascular diseases: SLE, RA, scleroderma, polyarteritis, granulomatosis with polyangiitis.
Pulmonary infarction.
Pancreatitis.
Postcardiotomy/Dressler syndrome.
Drug-induced SLE (hydralazine, procainamide).
Postabdominal surgery.
Ruptured esophagus.
Chronic effusion secondary to congestive failure.

TRANSUDATIVE
CHF.
Hepatic cirrhosis.
Nephrotic syndrome.
Hypoproteinemia from any cause.
Meigs syndrome.

PLEURAL EFFUSIONS, MALIGNANCY-ASSOCIATED

ICD-10CM # C78.2 Secondary malignant neoplasm of pleura

Lung cancer	(30% to 40%)
Breast cancer	(20% to 25%)
Lymphoma	(10% to 15%)
Leukemia	(5% to 10%)
GI tract	(5%)
GU tract	(5%)
Reproductive	(3%)

PLEURAL HYPERPLASIA[78]

ICD-10CM # Varies with specific diagnosis

BENIGN CAUSES OF PLEURAL HYPERPLASIA
Pleural infections.
Radiation.
Surgery.
Trauma.
Intracavitary treatments (chemotherapy or sclerosing agents).
Collagen vascular diseases.
Systemic immune diseases (systemic lupus erythematosus, rheumatoid arthritis, Sjögren syndrome, Wegener granulomatosis).
Subpleural pulmonary abnormalities (infarction, infection, neoplasia).
Pneumothorax.
Drug reactions (nitrofurantoin, bromocriptine, methysergide, procarbazine).
Pancreatitis, uremia.
Pneumoconiosis (asbestosis).

PLEURAL MASSES[78]

ICD-10CM # Varies with specific diagnosis

CAUSES OF PLEURAL MASSES
Inflammatory pleural reactions:
Reactive mesothelial hyperplasia or organizing pleuritis versus atypical mesothelial hyperplasia.
Nodular pleural plaques.
Pulmonary tumors that may resemble pleural tumors:
Inflammatory pseudotumor of the lung.
Benign pleural tumors:
Solitary fibrous tumor.
Lipomas and lipoblastomas.
Adenomatous tumors.
Calcifying fibrous tumors.
Mesothelial cysts.
Multicystic mesothelioma.
Schwannoma.
Pleural tumors with low malignant potential:
Desmoid tumors.
Well-differentiated papillary mesothelioma.
Pleural thymoma.
Primary malignant pleural tumors that may look like benign tumors:
Malignant solitary fibrous tumor.
Pleuropulmonary blastoma.
Localized malignant mesothelioma.
Vascular sarcoma.
Liposarcoma.
Pleuropulmonary synovial sarcoma.
Askin tumor or primitive neuroectodermal tumor (PNET).
Desmoplastic small round cell tumor.
Malignant pleural tumors:
Metastatic malignancies to the pleura.
Malignant mesothelioma.

PNEUMATOSIS INTESTINALIS IN NEONATE AND OLDER CHILD[21]

ICD-10CM # Varies with specific diagnosis

CAUSES OF PNEUMATOSIS INTESTINALIS IN THE NEONATE AND THE OLDER CHILD
Necrotizing enterocolitis.
Bowel ischemia, inflammation, and obstruction.
Cyanotic congenital heart disease.
Hirschsprung disease.
Gastroschisis.
Anorectal atresia.
Inflammatory bowel disease.
Lymphoma.
Leukemia.
CMV and rotavirus gastroenteritis.
Colonoscopy.
Caustic ingestion.
Short bowel syndrome.
Congenital immune deficiency states.

Clostridium infection.
Chronic steroid use.
Posthepatic, renal, or bone marrow transplant.
Collagen vascular disease.
Graft-versus-host disease.
AIDS.

PNEUMONIA, CHRONIC[42]

ICD-10CM #	J15.9	Unspecified bacterial pneumonia
	J12.9	Viral pneumonia, unspecified
	B25.0	Cytomegaloviral pneumonitis
	J18.0	Bronchopneumonia, unspecified organism

INFECTIOUS AGENTS THAT TYPICALLY CAUSE CHRONIC PNEUMONIA
Bacteria
Mixed aerobic and anaerobic bacteria.
Actinomyces spp.
Nocardia spp.
Rhodococcus equi.
Burkholderia pseudomallei.
Mycobacteria
Mycobacterium tuberculosis.
Mycobacterium kansasii.
Mycobacterium avium complex.
Mycobacterium abscessus.
Mycobacterium terrae.
Fungi
Aspergillus spp.
Blastomyces dermatitidis.
Coccidioides spp.
Cryptococcus neoformans.
Cryptococcus gattii.
Dark-walled molds.
Emmonsia parvum var. crescens.
Histoplasma capsulatum.
Sporothrix schenckii complex.
Paracoccidioides brasiliensis.
Penicillium marneffei.
Scedosporium apiospermum.
Parasites
Dirofilaria:
   Echinococcus granulosus.
   Filaria (tropical pulmonary eosinophilia).
   Paragonimus westermani.

NONINFECTIOUS CAUSES OF CHRONIC PNEUMONIA
Neoplasia
Carcinoma (primary or metastatic).
Hodgkin disease and non-Hodgkin lymphoma.
Other lymphoproliferative disorders.
Cystic Fibrosis
Sarcoidosis
Amyloidosis
Vasculitis (autoimmune diseases)
Systemic lupus erythematosus.
Polyarteritis nodosa.
Granulomatosis with polyangiitis.

Allergic angiitis and granulomatosis (Churg-Strauss syndrome).
Goodpasture syndrome.
Microscopic polyangiitis.
Lymphomatoid granulomatosis.
Progressive systemic sclerosis.
Rheumatoid arthritis.
Mixed connective tissue syndrome (overlap syndrome).
Chemicals, Drugs
Radiation
Recurrent pulmonary emboli
Bronchial obstruction with atelectasis (e.g., tumor, foreign body)
Pulmonary sequestration
Pulmonary infiltration with eosinophilia syndrome (Löffler syndrome—usually transient.)
Pneumonia plus asthma (e.g., allergic bronchopulmonary aspergillosis).
Bronchocentric granulomatosis.
Chronic eosinophilic pneumonia.
Pneumoconiosis
Asbestosis.
Berylliosis.
Silicosis.
Anthracosilicosis.

OTHER LUNG DISEASES: CAUSE UNKNOWN
Chronic Organizing Pneumonia
Chronic Interstitial Pneumonia (Fibrosing Alveolitis, Idiopathic Pulmonary Fibrosis)
Usual interstitial pneumonia (UIP).
Desquamative interstitial pneumonia (DIP).
Lymphocytic interstitial pneumonia (LIP).
Giant cell interstitial pneumonia (GIP).
Eosinophilic granuloma (histiocytosis X).
Lymphangioleiomyomatosis.
Pulmonary alveolar proteinosis.
Pulmonary alveolar microlithiasis.
Idiopathic pulmonary hemosiderosis.
Angiocentric immunoproliferative lesions.

PNEUMONIA MIMICS[110]

| ICD-10CM # | Varies with specific diagnosis |

NONINFECTIOUS CAUSES THAT MAY PRESENT AS PNEUMONIA
Radiologic Technique
Inadequate inspiration.
Breast shadow.
Thymus.
Uneven grid on film.
Underpenetrated film.
Primary Pulmonary
Asthma.
Bronchiectasis.
Atelectasis.
Bronchopulmonary dysplasia.
Cystic fibrosis.
Pulmonary sequestration.
Congenital cystic adenomatoid malformation.
α_1-Antitrypsin deficiency.

Aspiration
Foreign body.
Chemical.
Recurrent caused by anatomic or physiologic disorders.
Primary Cardiac
Congenital heart disease.
CHF
Pulmonary Infarction
Sickle cell vasoocclusive crisis.
Pulmonary embolism.
Collagen Vascular Disorders
Acute Respiratory Distress Syndrome
Pleural effusion
Neoplasm.

PNEUMONIA, NONRESPONDING, CAUSES[13]

ICD-10CM #	J15.9	Unspecified bacterial pneumonia
	J12.9	Viral pneumonia, unspecified
	B25.0	Cytomegaloviral pneumonitis
	J18.0	Bronchopneumonia, unspecified organism

CAUSES OF NONRESPONDING PNEUMONIA
Infectious Pneumonia
Resistant microorganisms:
   Community-acquired pneumonia (e.g., *Streptococcus pneumoniae, Staphylococcus aureus*).
   Nosocomial pneumonia (e.g., *Acinetobacter,* methicillin-resistant *Staphylococcus aureus* (MRSA), Pseudomonas aeruginosa).
Uncommon microorganisms (e.g., *Mycobacterium tuberculosis, Nocardia* spp., fungi, *Pneumocystis jirovecii*).
Complications of pneumonia:
Empyema.
Abscess or necrotizing pneumonia.
Metastatic infection.
Noninfectious Pneumonia
Neoplasms.
Pulmonary hemorrhage.
Pulmonary embolism.
Sarcoidosis.
Eosinophilic pneumonia.
Pulmonary edema.
Acute respiratory distress syndrome.
Bronchiolitis obliterans with organizing pneumonia.
Drug-induced pulmonary disease.
Pulmonary vasculitis.

PNEUMONIA, RECURRENT

| ICD-10CM # | J15.9 | Unspecified bacterial pneumonia |
| | J12.9 | Viral pneumonia, unspecified |

B25.0	Cytomegaloviral pneumonitis	
J18.0	Bronchopneumonia, unspecified organism	

Mechanical obstruction from neoplasm.

Chronic aspiration (tube feeding, alcoholism, CVA, neuromuscular disorders, seizure disorder, inability to cough).

Bronchiectasis.

Kyphoscoliosis.

COPD, CHF, asthma, silicosis, pulmonary fibrosis, cystic fibrosis.

Pulmonary TB, chronic sinusitis.

Immunosuppression (HIV, corticosteroids, leukemia, chemotherapy, splenectomy).

PNEUMOPERITONEUM, NEONATAL[21]

ICD-10CM #   Varies with specific diagnosis

CAUSES OF NEONATAL PNEUMOPERITONEUM

Necrotizing enterocolitis.

Spontaneous perforation of a hollow viscus:
    Stomach.
    Duodenum.
    Ileum.
    Colon.

Malrotation and volvulus.

Distal obstruction.

Perforation of Meckel diverticulum.

Anterior abdominal wall defects:
    Pentalogy of Cantrell.
    Omphalocele.
    Gastroschisis.
    Cloacal exstrophy.

Stress and peptic ulcers.

Mechanical ventilation (air leak) or resuscitation ("bagging").

Postlaparotomy.

Iatrogenic gastric perforation with an orogastric tube.

Iatrogenic colon perforation:
    Thermometer.
    During an enema.

Indomethacin.

Dexamethasone treatment.

PNEUMOTHORAX, IN CHILDREN[19]

ICD-10CM #	J93.0	Spontaneous tension pneumothorax
	J93	Pneumothorax
	J93.9	Pneumothorax unspecified

SPONTANEOUS

Primary idiopathic—usually resulting from ruptured subpleural blebs.

Secondary blebs.

Congenital lung disease:
    Congenital cystic adenomatoid malformation.
    Bronchogenic cysts.
    Pulmonary hypoplasia.

Conditions associated with increased intrathoracic pressure:
    Asthma.
    Bronchiolitis.
    Air-block syndrome in neonates.
    Cystic fibrosis.
    Airway foreign body.

Infection:
    Pneumatocele.
    Lung abscess.
    Bronchopleural fistula.

Diffuse lung disease:
    Langerhans cell histiocytosis.
    Tuberous sclerosis.
    Marfan syndrome.
    Ehlers-Danlos syndrome.

Metastatic neoplasm—usually osteosarcoma (rare).

TRAUMATIC

Noniatrogenic:
    Penetrating trauma.
    Blunt trauma.
    Loud music (air pressure).

Iatrogenic:
    Thoracotomy.
    Thoracoscopy, thoracentesis.
    Tracheostomy.
    Tube or needle puncture.

Mechanical ventilation.

POLIOSIS[44]

ICD-10CM #   Varies with specific diagnosis

CAUSES OF POLIOSIS

Ocular

Chronic anterior blepharitis.

Sympathetic ophthalmitis.

Idiopathic uveitis.

Systemic

Vogt-Koyanagi-Harada syndrome.

Waardenburg syndrome.

Vitiligo.

Marfan syndrome.

Tuberous sclerosis.

POLYCYTHEMIA

ICD-10CM #	D45	Polycythemia primary
	D75.1	Polycythemia secondary

Tobacco abuse.

Chronic lung disease.

High altitude.

Sleep apnea.

Right-to-left cardiac shunts.

Erythropoietin administration.

Androgens/anabolic steroids.

Polycystic kidney disease.

Renal cell carcinoma.

Hepatocellular carcinoma.

Polycythemia vera.

Carbon monoxide exposure.

Primary familial and congenital polycythemia.

High-oxygen–affinity hemoglobins.

Uterine leiomyoma, meningioma, pheochromocytoma, parathyroid carcinoma.

Cobalt exposure.

POLYCYTHEMIAS, DIFFERENTIAL DIAGNOSIS[34]

ICD-10CM #	D45	Polycythemia primary
	D75.1	Polycythemia secondary

DIFFERENTIAL DIAGNOSIS OF THE POLYCYTHEMIAS

Relative or Spurious Polycythemia

Decreased plasma volume—reduced fluid intake, marked loss of body fluids (diaphoresis, vomiting, diarrhea, "third spacing").

Gaisböck syndrome.

Overfilling of blood in collection vacuum tubes.

Absolute polycythemia

Secondary polycythemia.

Acquired.

Hypoxia:
    Pulmonary disease.
    Cyanotic congenital heart disease.
    Hypoventilation syndromes:
        Sleep apnea.
        Pickwickian syndrome.
        High altitude.
        Smokers' polycythemia, hookah polycythemia, carbon monoxide intoxication caused by industrial exposure.

Postrenal transplantation erythrocytosis.

Aberrant erythropoietin production.

Tumors:
    Renal cell carcinoma.
    Wilms tumor.
    Hepatic carcinoma.
    Uterine leiomyomata.

Virilizing ovarian tumors.

Vascular cerebellar tumors.

Miscellaneous renal and hepatic disorders:
    Solitary renal cysts.
    Polycystic kidney disease.
    Renal artery stenosis hydronephrosis.
    Viral hepatitis.

Endocrine disorders:
    Cushing syndrome.
    Primary aldosteronism.
    Androgen use.
    Erythropoietin use.

Congenital polycythemias:
    Abnormal high-affinity hemoglobin variants.
    Bisphosphoglycerate deficiency.

Congenital methemoglobinemia.
Chuvash polycythemia (von Hippel Lindau mutations).
Prolyl hydroxylase mutations.
Hypoxia-inducible factor gene mutations.
Primary polycythemias:
  Primary congenital and familial polycythemia.
  Polycythemia vera.

POLYCYTHEMIA, RELATIVE VERSUS ABSOLUTE[31]

ICD-10CM # D75.1 Secondary polycythemia

RELATIVE OR SPURIOUS POLYCYTHEMIA

Decreased plasma volume—reduced fluid intake, marked loss of body fluids (diaphoresis, vomiting, diarrhea, "third-spacing").
Gaisböck syndrome.
Overfilling of blood in collection vacuum tubes.

ABSOLUTE POLYCYTHEMIA

Primary Congenital and Familial Polycythemia
Secondary Polycythemia Acquired
Hypoxia:
  Pulmonary disease.
  Cyanotic congenital heart disease.
  Hypoventilation syndromes: sleep apnea, Pickwickian syndrome.
High altitude.
Smokers' polycythemia, carbon monoxide intoxication due to industrial exposure.
Postrenal transplantation erythrocytosis.
Aberrant erythropoietin production.
Tumors: renal cell carcinoma, Wilms tumor, hepatic carcinoma, uterine leiomyomata, virilizing ovarian tumors, vascular cerebellar tumors.
Miscellaneous renal and hepatic disorders: solitary renal cysts, polycystic kidney disease, renal artery stenosis, hydronephrosis, viral hepatitis.
Endocrine disorders: Cushing syndrome, primary aldosteronism.
Androgen use.
Erythropoietin use.
Congenital:
  Abnormal high-affinity hemoglobin variants.
  Bisphosphoglycerate deficiency.
  Congenital methemoglobinemia.
  Chuvash polycythemia (von Hippel-Lindau mutations).
  Prolyl hydroxylase mutations.
  Polycythemia vera.

POLYMYALGIAS[90]

ICD-10CM # M35.3 Polymyalgia rheumatica

DISEASE ENTITIES WITH POLYMYALGIAS

Rheumatoid arthritis.
Rotator cuff syndrome.

Osteoarthritis of shoulder and hip joints.
Fibromyalgia.
Polymyositis/dermatomyositis.
Spondyloarthritis.
Systemic lupus erythematosus.
Vasculitides.
Paraneoplastic myalgias.
Infection-associated myalgias.
Statin therapy.
RS3PE (remitting seronegative symmetric synovitis and pitting edema).
Parkinson disease.
Hypothyroidism.

POLYNEUROPATHIES WITH PREDOMINANTLY UPPER LIMB MOTOR INVOLVEMENT[38]

ICD-10CM # Code varies with specific diagnosis

Multifocal motor neuropathy.
Multifocal acquired demyelinating sensory and motor neuropathy (MADSAM, Lewis-Sumner syndrome).
Lead neuropathy.*
Porphyria.
Tangier disease.
Familial amyloid neuropathy type 2.
Hereditary motor neuropathy (uncommon forms).

*May be associated with spine pain.

POLYNEUROPATHY[62]

ICD-10CM # G61.9 Inflammatory polyneuropathy, unspecified

PREDOMINANTLY MOTOR

Guillain-Barré syndrome.
Porphyria.
Diphtheria.
Lead.
Hereditary sensorimotor neuropathy, types I and II.
Paraneoplastic neuropathy.

PREDOMINANTLY SENSORY

Diabetes.
Amyloidosis.
Leprosy.
Lyme disease.
Paraneoplastic neuropathy.
Vitamin B_{12} deficiency.
Hereditary sensory neuropathy, types I-IV.

PREDOMINANTLY AUTONOMIC

Diabetes.
Amyloidosis.
Alcoholic neuropathy.
Familial dysautonomias.

MIXED SENSORIMOTOR

Systemic diseases: renal failure, hypothyroidism, acromegaly, RA, periarteritis nodosa, SLE, multiple myeloma, macroglobulinemia, remote effect of malignancy.
Medications: isoniazid, nitrofurantoin, ethambutol, chloramphenicol, chloroquine, vincristine, vinblastine, dapsone, disulfiram, diphenylhydantoin, cisplatin, 1-tryptophan.
Environmental toxins: *N*-hexane, methyl *N*-butyl ketone, acrylamide, carbon disulfide, carbon monoxide, hexachlorophene, organophosphates.
Deficiency disorders: malabsorption, alcoholism, vitamin B_1 deficiency, Refsum disease, metachromatic leukodystrophy.

POLYNEUROPATHY, DEMYELINATING[43]

ICD-10CM # G37.9 Demyelinating disease of central nervous system, unspecified

Guillain-Barré syndrome:
  Acute inflammatory demyelinating polyradiculoneuropathy (AIDP).
  Acute motor axonal neuropathy (AMAN).
  Acute motor and sensory axonal neuropathy (AMSAN).
  Miller Fisher syndrome.
Chronic inflammatory demyelinating polyradiculoplexo-neuropathy.
Malignancy.
HIV.
Hepatitis B.
Buckthorn.
Diphtheria.

POLYNEUROPATHY, DISTAL SENSORIMOTOR[43]

ICD-10CM # G63 Polyneuropathy in diseases classified elsewhere

Diabetes mellitus.
Alcoholism.
Neoplastic or paraneoplastic.
Hereditary motor and sensory neuropathies (Charcot-Marie-Tooth).
Cryptogenic sensorimotor polyneuropathies (CSPN).
HIV.
Toxins:
  Organic or industrial agents:
    Acrylamide.
    Allyl chloride.
    Carbon disulfide.
    Ethylene oxide.
    Hexacarbons.
    Methyl bromide.
    Organophosphate-induced delayed polyneuropathy (OPIDP).
    Polychlorinated biphenyls (PCBs).
    Trichloroethylene.
    Vacor.

Metals:
- Arsenic.
- Gold.
- Mercury (inorganic).
- Thallium.

Therapeutic agents:
- Amiodarone.
- Antiretrovirals.
- Dapsone.
- Disulfiram.
- Isoniazid.
- Metronidazole.
- Nitrofurantoin.
- Paclitaxel (Taxol).
- Phenytoin.
- Statins (HMG-CoA reductase inhibitors).
- Thalidomide.
- Vinca alkaloids (vincristine, vinblastine).

Nutritional:
- Beriberi (thiamine or vitamin B_1).
- Pellagra (niacin, B vitamins).
- Pernicious anemia (vitamin B_{12}).
- Pyridoxine deficiency (vitamin B_6).

End-organ dysfunction
- Acromegaly.
- Chronic pulmonary disease.
- Hypothyroidism.
- Renal failure (uremic neuropathy).

Paraproteinemias:
- Amyloidosis.
- Monoclonal gammopathy of unknown significance (MGUS).
- Multiple myeloma.
- Waldenström macroglobulinemia.

Porphyria

HMG-CoA, Hydroxymethylglutaryl coenzyme A.

POLYNEUROPATHY, DRUG-INDUCED[62]

ICD-10CM # G62.0 Drug-induced polyneuropathy

DRUGS IN ONCOLOGY

Vincristine.
Procarbazine.
Cisplatin.
Misonidazole.
Metronidazole
Taxol.

DRUGS IN INFECTIOUS DISEASES

Isoniazid.
Nitrofurantoin.
Dapsone.
ddC (dideoxycytidine).
ddI (dideoxyinosine).

DRUGS IN CARDIOLOGY

Hydralazine.
Perhexiline maleate.
Procainamide.
Disopyramide.

DRUGS IN RHEUMATOLOGY

Gold salts.
Chloroquine.

DRUGS IN NEUROLOGY AND PSYCHIATRY

Diphenylhydantoin.
Glutethimide.
Methaqualone.

MISCELLANEOUS

Disulfiram (Antabuse).
Vitamin: (pyridoxine in megadoses).

POLYNEUROPATHY, SYMMETRIC[62]

ICD-10CM # G61.9 Inflammatory polyneuropathy, unspecified

ACQUIRED NEUROPATHIES

Toxic:
- Drugs.
- Industrial toxins.
- Heavy metals.
- Abused substances.

Metabolic/endocrine:
- Diabetes.
- Chronic renal failure.
- Hypothyroidism.
- Polyneuropathy of critical illness.

Nutritional deficiency:
- Vitamin B_{12} deficiency.
- Alcoholism.
- Vitamin E deficiency.

Paraneoplastic:
- Carcinoma.
- Lymphoma.

Plasma cell dyscrasia:
- Myeloma, typical, atypical, and solitary forms.
- Primary systemic amyloidosis.

Idiopathic chronic inflammatory demyelinating polyneuropathies.
Polyneuropathies associated with peripheral nerve autoantibodies.
AIDS.

INHERITED NEUROPATHIES

Neuropathies with Biochemical Markers
Refsum disease.
Bassen-Kornzweig disease.
Tangier disease.
Metachromatic leukodystrophy.
Krabbe disease.
Adrenomyeloneuropathy.
Fabry disease.
Neuropathies without Biochemical Markers or Systemic Involvement
Hereditary motor neuropathy.
Hereditary sensory neuropathy.
Hereditary sensorimotor neuropathy.

POLYURIA

ICD-10CM # R35.8 Other polyuria

DM.
Diabetes insipidus.
Primary polydipsia (compulsive water drinking).
Hypercalcemia.
Hypokalemia.
Postobstructive uropathy.
Diuretic phase of renal failure.
Drugs: diuretics, caffeine, alcohol, lithium.
Sickle cell trait or disease, chronic pyelonephritis (failure to concentrate urine).
Anxiety, cold weather.

POPLITEAL SWELLING

ICD-10CM #	I87.1	Compression of vein
	I72.4	Aneurysm of artery of lower extremity
	S85.009A	Unspecified injury of popliteal artery, unspecified leg, initial encounter
	I77.3	Arterial fibromuscular dysplasia
	M71.20	Synovial cyst of popliteal space [Baker], unspecified knee
	I80.3	Phlebitis and thrombophlebitis of lower extremities, unspecified
	M66.369	Spontaneous rupture of flexor tendons, unspecified lower leg

Phlebitis (superficial).
Lymphadenitis.
Trauma: fractured tibia or fibula, contusion, traumatic neuroma.
DVT.
Ruptured varicose vein.
Baker cyst.
Popliteal abscess.
Osteomyelitis.
Ruptured tendon.
Aneurysm of popliteal artery.
Neoplasm: lipoma, osteogenic sarcoma, neurofibroma, fibrosarcoma.

PORTAL HYPERTENSION[18]

ICD-10CM # K76.6 Portal hypertension

INCREASED RESISTANCE TO FLOW

Presinusoidal
Portal or splenic vein occlusion (thrombosis, tumor).
Schistosomiasis.
Congenital hepatic fibrosis.
Sarcoidosis.
Sinusoidal
Cirrhosis (all causes).
Alcoholic hepatitis.

Postsinusoidal
Venoocclusive disease.
Budd-Chiari syndrome.
Constrictive pericarditis.

INCREASED PORTAL BLOOD FLOW
Splenomegaly not caused by liver disease.
Arterioportal fistula.

POSTMENOPAUSAL BLEEDING
ICD-10CM #   N95.0   Postmenopausal bleeding

Hormone replacement therapy.
Neoplasm (uterine, ovarian, cervical, vaginal, vulvar).
Atrophic vaginitis.
Vaginal infection.
Polyp.
Extragenital (GI, urinary).
Tamoxifen.
Trauma.

POSTURAL HYPOTENSION, NONNEUROLOGIC CAUSES
ICD-10CM #   I95.1   Orthostatic hypotension

Diuretics and hypertensive agents.
GI hemorrhage.
Alcohol.
Excessive heat.
Rapid volume loss from diarrhea, vomiting.
Hemodialysis.
Extensive burns.
Pyrexia.
Aortic stenosis (impaired output).
Constrictive pericarditis, atrial myxoma (impaired cardiac filling).
Adrenal insufficiency.
Diabetes insipidus.
Vasodilatory agents (e.g., nitrates).

POSTURING ABNORMALITY[20]
ICD-10CM #   Varies with specific diagnosis

Dystonia.[a]
Conversion disorder.
Muscular dystrophy.
Myotonia.
Neuromyotonia.
Rigidity.
Spasticity.[a]
Stiff person syndrome (Stiff man syndrome).

[a] Denotes the most common conditions and the ones with disease-modifying treatments.

PREMATURE GRAYING, SCALP HAIR
ICD-10CM #   Varies with specific diagnosis

Chemical exposure (e.g., phenol/catechol derivatives, sulfhydryls, arsenic).
Physical agents (e.g., ionizing radiation, lasers).
Hyperthyroidism.

Vitamin B_{12} deficiency.
Down syndrome.
Chronic and severe protein deficiency.
Vitiligo.
Idiopathic.
Myotonic dystrophy.
Ataxia-telangiectasia.
Progeria.
Werner syndrome.

PREMATURE VENTRICULAR CONTRACTIONS AND VENTRICULAR TACHYCARDIA[43]
ICD-10CM #   I49.40   Unspecified premature depolarization
I47.2   Ventricular tachycardia

CAUSES OF PREMATURE VENTRICULAR CONTRACTIONS AND VENTRICULAR TACHYCARDIA
Acute or previous myocardial infarction/ischemia.
Hypokalemia.
Hypoxemia.
Ischemic heart disease.
Valvular disease.
Catecholamine excess.*
Other drug intoxications (especially cyclic antidepressants).
Idiopathic causes.[†]
Digitalis toxicity.
Hypomagnesemia.
Hypercapnia.
Class I antidysrhythmic agents.
Ethanol.
Myocardial contusion.
Cardiomyopathy.
Acidosis.
Alkalosis.
Methylxanthine toxicity.

*Relative increase in sympathetic tone from drugs (direct or indirect) or conditions that augment catecholamine release or decrease parasympathetic tone.
[†]Isolated premature ventricular contractions (PVCs) can occur in up to 50% of young subjects without obvious cardiac or noncardiac disease; however, multiform and repetitive PVCs and ventricular tachycardia are rarely seen in this population.

PREPUBERTAL BLEEDING WITHOUT BREAST DEVELOPMENT[102]
ICD-10CM #   Varies with specific diagnosis

Foreign object.
Genital trauma.
Sexual abuse.
Lichen sclerosus.
Infectious vaginitis (especially from *Shigella*).
Urethral prolapse.
Breakdown of labial adhesions.
Friable genital warts or vulvar lesions.
Vaginal tumor.

Rare presentation of McCune-Albright syndrome (typically have breast development).
Isolated menarche (controversial).
Dermatologic conditions with secondary excoriation.
Nongenital bleeding; mistaken as genital: rectal and urinary.

PRESACRAL MASSES IN CHILDREN[15]
ICD-10CM #   Varies with specific diagnosis

PRESACRAL MASSES IN CHILDREN
Solid
Sacrococcygeal teratoma.
Neuroblastoma.
Rhabdomyosarcoma.
Fibroma.
Lipoma.
Leiomyoma.
Lymphoma.
Hemangioendothelioma.
Sacral bone tumors.
Cystic
Abscess.
Rectal duplication.
Hematoma.
Lymphocele.
Neurenteric cyst.
Sacral osteomyelitis.
Ulcerative colitis.
Anterior meningocele.

PRIMARY ANGIITIS OF CNS[111]
ICD-10CM #   Varies with specific diagnosis

Differential Diagnosis of Primary Angiitis of the CNS
Secondary Cerebral Vasculitis
Primary Systemic Vasculitides
Granulomatosis with polyangiitis
Microscopic polyangiitis
Eosinophilic granulomatosis with polyangiitis
Polyarteritis nodosa
Behçet's disease
Systemic Autoimmune Disease
Systemic lupus erythematosus
Sjögren's syndrome
Inflammatory myositis
Rheumatoid arthritis
Mixed connective tissue disease
Other Multisystem Inflammatory Disorders
Sarcoidosis
Susac's syndrome
Infection
Bacterial
Mycobacterial
Fungal
Viral
Protozoal
Malignancy
CNS lymphoma
Glioma

Angiocentric lymphoma
Lymphomatoid granulomatosis
Metastatic malignancy
Vasospastic Disorders
Reversible cerebral vasoconstrictive syndrome
Drug exposures
Other Arterial Diseases
Atherosclerosis
Fibromuscular dysplasia
Moyamoya disease
Dissection
Hypercoagulable States
Antiphospholipid antibody syndrome
Thrombotic thrombocytopenic purpura
Stroke-like Syndromes
CADASIL
Mitochondrial diseases
Sickle cell disease
Fabry's disease
Sneddon's syndrome
Leukoencephalopathies
Progressive multifocal leukoencephalopathy
Reversible posterior leukoencephalopathy
    syndrome
Cerebral Hemorrhage
Hypertensive
Aneurysmal
Amyloid angiopathy
Arteriovenous malformation
Embolic Disease
Thrombus
Cholesterol emboli
Myxoma
Endocarditis
Air emboli

CADASIL, Cerebral autosomal dominant arteriopathy
    with subcortical infarcts and leukoencephalopathy.-
From *Firestein & Kelley's Textbook of Rheumatology,* Ed 11,
Philadelphia, 2021, Elsevier.

PROLONGED QT SYNDROMES[10]

ICD-10CM #	I45.81	Long QT syndrome

CLASSIFICATION AND CAUSES OF PROLONGED QT SYNDROMES THAT PRODUCE TORSADES DE POINTES

Pause Dependent (Acquired)
Drug induced: class IA and IC antidysrhythmics; many phenothiazines and butyrophenones (notably haloperidol and droperidol), cyclic antidepressants, antibiotics (especially macrolides), organophosphates, antihistamines, antifungals, antiseizure and antiemetic agents.
Electrolyte abnormalities: hypokalemia, hypomagnesemia, hypocalcemia (rarely).
Diet related: starvation, low protein.
Severe bradycardia or atrioventricular block.
Hypothyroidism.
Contrast injection.
Cerebrovascular accident (especially intraparenchymal).
Myocardial ischemia.
Adrenergic Dependent (Tachycardia Prompted)
Congenital:

Jervell and Lange-Nielsen syndrome (deafness, autosomal recessive).
Romano-Ward syndrome (normal hearing, autosomal dominant).
Sporadic (normal hearing, no familial tendency).
Mitral valve prolapse.
Acquired (rare):
Cerebrovascular disease (especially subarachnoid hemorrhage).
Autonomic surgery: radical neck dissection, carotid endarterectomy, truncal vagotomy.

PROPTOSIS[22]

ICD-10CM #	H05.2	Ocular proptosis

Endocrine:
    Graves ophthalmopathy.
    Cushing syndrome.
Orbital neoplasms:
    Primary neoplasms.
    Hemangioma.
    Lymphoma (may be systemic).
    Optic nerve glioma.
    Choroidal melanoma.
    Lacrimal gland tumors.
    Meningioma.
    Rhabdomyosarcoma.
Extension of paranasal sinus tumors.
Metastatic disease:
    Malignant melanoma.
    Breast carcinoma.
    Lung carcinoma.
    Kidney.
    Prostate.
Inflammatory:
    Orbital pseudotumor.
    Orbital myositis.
Granulomatous:
    Sarcoidosis.
    Wegener granulomatosis.
Infectious:
    Orbital cellulitis.
    Syphilis.
    Mucormycosis.
    Parasitic (trypanosomiasis, schistosomiasis, cysticercosis, echinococcal disease).
Vascular/miscellaneous:
    Carotid-cavernous fistula.
    Lithium therapy.
    Cirrhosis.
    Obesity.
    Amyloidosis.
    Dermoid and epidermoid cysts.
Foreign body.

PROPTOSIS AND PALATAL NECROTIC ULCERS

ICD-10CM #	K13.70	Unspecified lesions of oral mucosa
	K13.79	Other lesions of oral mucosa
	H05.20	Unspecified exophthalmos

Cavernous sinus thrombosis.
Bacterial orbital cellulitis.
Metastatic neoplasm.
Rhinocerebral mucormycosis.
Ecthyma gangrenosum.
CNS aspergillosis.

PROTEIN-LOSING ENTEROPATHY, PEDIATRIC AGE[19]

ICD-10CM #	E44.0	Moderate protein-energy malnutrition

CAUSES OF PROTEIN-LOSING ENTEROPATHY

Mucosal inflammation:
Infection:
    Cytomegalovirus.
    Bacterial overgrowth.
    Invasive bacterial infection.
Gastric inflammation:
    Ménétrier disease.
    Eosinophilic gastroenteropathy.
Intestinal inflammation:
    Celiac disease.
    Crohn disease.
Eosinophilic gastroenteropathy:
    Tropical sprue.
    Radiation enteritis.
Primary intestinal lymphangiectasia.
Secondary intestinal lymphangiectasia:
Constrictive pericarditis.
Congestive heart failure.
Post–Fontan procedure.
Malrotation.
Lymphoma.
Sarcoidosis.
Radiation therapy.
Colonic inflammation:
    Inflammatory bowel diseases.
    Necrotizing enterocolitis.
Congenital disorders of glycosylation.

PROTEINURIA

ICD-10CM #	R80.9	Proteinuria, unspecified

Nephrotic syndrome as a result of primary renal diseases.
Malignant hypertension.
Malignancies: multiple myeloma, leukemias, Hodgkin disease.
CHF.
DM.
SLE, RA.
Sickle cell disease.
Goodpasture syndrome.
Malaria.
Amyloidosis, sarcoidosis.
Tubular lesions: cystinosis.
Functional (after heavy exercise).
Pyelonephritis.
Pregnancy.
Constrictive pericarditis.

Differential Diagnosis

II

Renal vein thrombosis.
Toxic nephropathies: heavy metals, drugs.
Radiation nephritis.
Orthostatic (postural) proteinuria.
Benign proteinuria: fever, heat, or cold exposure.

PRURITUS

ICD-10CM #	L29.9	Pruritus, unspecified
	L29.3	Anogenital pruritus, unspecified

Dry skin.
Drug-induced eruption, fiberglass exposure.
Scabies.
Skin diseases.
Myeloproliferative disorders: mycosis fungoides, Hodgkin lymphoma, multiple myeloma, polycythemia vera.
Cholestatic liver disease.
Endocrine disorders: DM, thyroid disease, carcinoid, pregnancy.
Carcinoma: breast, lung, gastric.
Chronic renal failure.
Iron deficiency.
AIDS.
Neurosis.
Sjögren syndrome.

PRURITUS ANI[10]

ICD-10CM #	L29.0	Pruritus ani

FECAL IRRITATION
Poor hygiene.
Anorectal conditions (fissure, fistula, hemorrhoids, skin tags, perianal clefts).
Spicy foods, citrus foods, caffeine, colchicine, quinidine.

CONTACT DERMATITIS
Anesthetic agents, topical corticosteroids, perfumed soap.

DERMATOLOGIC DISORDERS
Psoriasis, seborrhea, lichen simplex, or sclerosus.

SYSTEMIC DISORDERS
Chronic renal failure, myxedema, DM, thyrotoxicosis, polycythemia vera, Hodgkin disease.

SEXUALLY TRANSMITTED DISEASES
Syphilis, herpes simplex virus, human papillomavirus.

OTHER INFECTIOUS AGENTS
Pinworms.
Scabies.
Bacterial infection, viral infection.

PRURITUS VULVAE[47]

ICD-10CM #	L29.3	Anogenital pruritus, unspecified

CAUSES OF PRURITUS VULVAE
Diseases Special to Vulval Skin
Lichen sclerosus et atrophicus.
Leukoplakia.
Carcinoma.
Skin Disease
Psoriasis.
Atopic dermatitis.
Irritant and allergic contact dermatitis (especially medicaments).
Infection
Candidiasis.
Trichomonas.
Infestation
Pediculosis.
Psychogenic
Anxiety.
Depression.
Unknown.

PSEUDOCELLULITIS[70]

ICD-10CM #	Varies with specific diagnosis

CAUSES OF PSEUDOCELLULITIS
Infections and Bites
Arthropod bite reactions (e.g., insect, spider).
Erythema migrans.
Herpes zoster.
Toxin-mediated erythema (e.g., recurrent toxin-mediated perineal erythema).
Neutrophilic Dermatoses
Sweet syndrome, neutrophilic panniculitis.
Familial Mediterranean fever, other auto-inflammatory syndromes.
Drug Reactions
Fixed drug eruptions (especially nonpigmenting).
Vaccine/injection site reactions.
Toxic erythema of chemotherapy (e.g., due to gemcitabine), neutrophilic eccrine hidradenitis.*
Other Inflammatory Disorders
Allergic contact dermatitis (including airborne and dermal), stasis dermatitis.
Phytophotodermatitis.
Well syndrome.
Panniculitis (e.g., lipodermatosclerosis, erythema nodosum).
Thrombophlebitis.
Angioedema.
Interstitial granulomatous dermatitis, patch type granuloma annulare.
Inflammatory morphea.
Acute inflammatory edema of the ICU.
Metabolic Disorders
Gout.
Malignancy
Erysipeloid skin metastases (especially breast carcinoma).

ICU, Intensive care unit.
*Occasionally develops before onset of leukemia or due to infection.

PSEUDOCYANOSIS, ETIOLOGY

ICD-10CM #	Varies with etiology

Medications: amiodarone, minocycline, chlorpromazine.
Heavy metals:
Gold (systemic absorption).
Silver (systemic absorption).
Local contact with color dyes, gold, silver.

PSEUDOHERMAPHRODITISM, FEMALE

ICD-10CM #	E25.0	Congenital adrenogenital disorders associated with enzyme deficiency
	E25.8	Other adrenogenital disorders
	E25.9	Adrenogenital disorder, unspecified
	Q56.3	Pseudohermaphroditism, unspecified
	Q56.4	Indeterminate sex, unspecified

Congenital adrenal hyperplasia.
Maternal use of testosterone or related steroids.
Virilizing ovarian or adrenal tumor.
Virilizing luteoma of pregnancy.
Disturbances in differentiation of urogenital structures, nonandrogen related.
Maternal virilizing adrenal hyperplasia.
Fetal P450 aromatase deficiency.

PSEUDOHERMAPHRODITISM, MALE

ICD-10CM#	E25.0	Congenital adrenogenital disorders associated with enzyme deficiency
	E25.8	Other adrenogenital disorders
	E25.9	Adrenogenital disorder, unspecified
	Q56.3	Pseudohermaphroditism, unspecified
	Q56.4	Indeterminate sex, unspecified

Maternal ingestion of progestogens.
End-organ resistance to androgenic hormones.
5-α-reductase-2 deficiency.
XY gonadal dysgenesis.
Testicular regression syndrome.
Defects in testosterone metabolism by peripheral tissues.
Testosterone biosynthesis defects.

PSEUDOINFARCTION[97]

ICD-10CM #	Varies with specific diagnosis

Cardiac tumors, primary and secondary.
Cardiomyopathy (particularly hypertrophic and dilated).
Chagas disease.
Chest deformity.
COPD (particularly emphysema).
HIV infection.
Hyperkalemia.
Left anterior fascicular block.
Left bundle branch block.
Left ventricular hypertrophy.
Myocarditis and pericarditis.
Normal variant.
Pneumothorax.

Poor R wave progression, rotational changes, and lead placement.
Pulmonary embolism.
Trauma to chest (nonpenetrating).
Wolff-Parkinson-White syndrome.
Rare causes: pancreatitis, amyloidosis, sarcoidosis, scleroderma.

PSYCHOSIS[25]

ICD-10CM #	F29	Unspecified psychosis not due to a substance or known physiological condition
	F29	Unspecified psychosis not due to a substance or known physiological condition
	F10.231	Alcohol dependence with withdrawal delirium
	F01.51	Vascular dementia with behavioral disturbance

PRIMARY
Schizophrenia-related.*
Major depression.
Dementia.
Bipolar disorder.

SECONDARY
Drug use.[†]
Drug withdrawal. [‡]
Drug toxicity.[§]
Charles Bonnet syndrome.
Infections (pneumonia).
Electrolyte imbalance.
Syphilis.
Congestive heart failure.
Parkinson disease.
Trauma to temporal lobe.
Postpartum psychosis.
Hypothyroidism/hyperthyroidism.
Hypomagnesemia.
Epilepsy.
Meningitis.
Encephalitis.
Brain abscess.
Herpes encephalopathy.
Hypoxia.
Hypercarbia.
Hypoglycemia.
Thiamine deficiency.
Postoperative states.

PSYCHOSIS, MEDICAL DISORDERS-INDUCED[10]

ICD-10CM #	F29	Unspecified psychosis not due to a substance or known physiological condition
	F53	Puerperal psychosis

MEDICAL DISORDERS THAT MAY CAUSE ACUTE PSYCHOSIS
Metabolic Disorders
Hypercalcemia.
Hypercarbia.
Hypoglycemia.
Hyponatremia.
Hypoxia.
Inflammatory Disorders
Sarcoidosis.
Systemic lupus erythematosus.
Temporal (giant cell) arteritis.
Organ Failure
Hepatic encephalopathy.
Uremia.
Neurologic Disorders
Alzheimer disease.
Cerebrovascular disease.
Encephalitis (including HIV infection).
Encephalopathies.
Epilepsy.
Huntington disease.
Multiple sclerosis.
Neoplasms.
Normal-pressure hydrocephalus.
Parkinson disease.
Pick disease.
Wilson disease.
Endocrine Disorders
Addison disease.
Cushing disease.
Panhypopituitarism.
Parathyroid disease.
Postpartum psychosis.
Recurrent menstrual psychosis.
Sydenham chorea.
Thyroid disease.
Deficiency States
Niacin.
Thiamine.
Vitamin B_{12} and folate.

PSYCHOSIS, MEDICATION-INDUCED[10]

ICD-10CM #	F10.5	Psychotic disorder due to psychoactive substance use

PHARMACOLOGIC AGENTS THAT MAY CAUSE ACUTE PSYCHOSIS
Antianxiety Agents
Alprazolam.
Chlordiazepoxide.
Clonazepam.
Clorazepate.
Diazepam.

Ethchlorvynol.
Antibiotics
Isoniazid.
Rifampin.
Anticonvulsants
Ethosuximide.
Phenobarbital.
Phenytoin.
Primidone.
Antidepressants
Amitriptyline.
Doxepin.
Imipramine.
Protriptyline.
Trimipramine.
Cardiovascular Drugs
Captopril.
Digitalis.
Disopyramide.
Methyldopa.
Procainamide.
Propranolol.
Reserpine.
Drugs of Abuse
Alcohol.
Amphetamines.
Cannabis.
Cocaine.
Hallucinogens.
Opioids.
Phencyclidine.
Sedative-hypnotics.
Miscellaneous Drugs
Antihistamines.
Antineoplastics.
Bromides.
Cimetidine.
Corticosteroids.
Disulfiram.
Heavy metals.

PTOSIS[20]

ICD-10CM #	Varies with specific diagnosis

Congenital
Congenital fibrosis of extraocular muscles.
Horner syndrome.[a]
Myasthenia.[a]
Oculomotor nerve palsy.[a]

Acquired
Horner syndrome.[a]
Lid inflammation.
Mitochondrial myopathies.
Myasthenia gravis.[a]
Oculomotor nerve palsy.[a]
Oculopharyngeal dystrophy.
Ophthalmoplegic migraine.
Orbital cellulitis.
Trauma.

[a]Denotes the most common conditions and the ones with disease-modifying treatments.

---

*Includes schizophrenia, schizophreniform disorder, brief reactive psychosis.
[†]Includes hypnotics, glucocorticoids, marijuana, phencyclidine, atropine, dopaminergic agents (e.g., amantadine, bromocriptine, L-dopa), immunosuppressants.
[‡]Includes alcohol, barbiturates, benzodiazepines.
[§]Includes digitalis, theophylline, cimetidine, anticholinergics, glucocorticoids, catecholaminergic agents.

PUBERTY, DELAYED[80]

ICD-10CM # E30.0 Delayed puberty

NORMAL OR LOW SERUM GONADOTROPIN LEVELS

Constitutional delay in growth and development.
Hypothalamic and/or pituitary disorders:
  Isolated deficiency of growth hormone.
  Isolated deficiency of GnRH.
  Isolated deficiency of LH and/or FSH.
  Multiple anterior pituitary hormone deficiencies.
  Associated with congenital anomalies: Kallmann syndrome; Prader-Willi syndrome; Laurence-Moon-Biedl syndrome; Friedreich ataxia.
  Trauma.
  Postinfection.
  Hyperprolactinemia.
  Postirradiation.
  Infiltrative disease (histiocytosis).
  Tumor.
  Autoimmune hypophysitis.
  Idiopathic.
Functional:
  Chronic endocrinologic or systemic disorders.
  Emotional disorders.
  Drugs: cannabis.

INCREASED SERUM GONADOTROPIN LEVELS

Gonadal abnormalities:
  Congenital:
    Gonadal dysgenesis.
    Klinefelter syndrome.
    Bilateral anorchism.
    Resistant ovary syndrome.
    Myotonic dystrophy in males.
    17-Hydroxylase deficiency in females.
    Galactosemia.
  Acquired:
    Bilateral gonadal failure resulting from trauma or infection or after surgery, irradiation, or chemotherapy.
    Oophoritis: isolated or with other autoimmune disorders.
Uterine or vaginal disorders:
  Absence of uterus and/or vagina.
  Testicular feminization: complete or incomplete androgen insensitivity.

PUBERTY, PRECOCIOUS

ICD-10CM # E25.0 Congenital adrenogenital disorders associated with enzyme deficiency
           E25.8 Other adrenogenital disorders
           E25.9 Adrenogenital disorder, unspecified

Idiopathic.
Congenital virilizing adrenal hyperplasia.
Hypothalamic tumors.
Head trauma.
Hydrocephalus.
Degenerative CNS disease.

Arachnoid cyst.
Sex chromosome abnormalities (e.g., 47, XXY, 48, XXXY).
Perinatal asphyxia.
CNS infection (e.g., meningitis, encephalitis).

PULMONARY ARTERY SEGMENT ABNORMALITIES[37]

ICD-10CM # Q25.72 Congenital pulmonary arteriovenous malformation

Differential Diagnosis of the Main Pulmonary Artery Segment

DILATED MPA SEGMENT

Increased pulmonary artery volume (shunt):
  VSD.
  ASD.
  PDA.
Increased pulmonary artery pressure (pulmonary hypertension):
  Mitral stenosis.
  COPD/emphysema.
  Interstitial pulmonary fibrosis.
  Cystic fibrosis.
  Chronic thromboembolism.
  Primary PH.
Increased pulmonary artery volume and pressure:
  ASD with PH.
Normal pulmonary artery pressure and flow:
  Valvular pulmonic stenosis.

FLAT OR CONCAVE MPA SEGMENT

Tetralogy of Fallot.
Tetralogy variants.
Tetralogy with pulmonary atresia.
Pulmonary atresia with VSD.
Double-chamber RV.
Double-outlet RV.
Tricuspid atresia.
Ebstein malformation.

NO MPA SEGMENT PRESENT

Persistent truncus arteriosus.
D-transposition of the great arteries.

ASD, Atrial septal defect; *COPD*, chronic obstructive pulmonary disease; *MPA*, main pulmonary artery; *PDA*, patent ductus arteriosus; *PH*, pulmonary hypertension; *RV*, right ventricle; *VSD*, ventricular septal defect.

PULMONARY CRACKLES

ICD-10CM # R09.8 Friction sounds, chest

Pneumonia.
Left ventricular failure.
Asbestosis, silicosis, interstitial lung disease.
Chronic bronchitis.
Alveolitis (allergic, fibrosing).
Neoplasm.

PULMONARY CYSTS ON X-RAY[21]

ICD-10CM # Q33.0 Polycystic lungs, congenital
           J98.4 Pulmonary manifestations

CAUSES OF CYSTS IN THE LUNG ON CHEST RADIOGRAPH

Cystic fibrosis.
Cystic bronchiectasis.
Bronchopulmonary dysplasia (neonate and older).
Tuberculosis (apical thick walled).
Pulmonary abscess (thick wall, fluid level).
Empyema.
Streptococcal pneumatocele (thin wall, postinfective).
Cavitating pneumonia.
Mycetoma (apical cyst with contents).
Cystic congenital adenomatoid malformation (basal cysts of varying size).
Diaphragmatic hernia (cysts of similar size).
Hiatal hernia (posterior).
Morgagni hernia (midline anterior).
Bronchopulmonary sequestration (basal).
Congenital lobar emphysema.
Hydatid disease (in endemic areas).
Kerosene inhalation (pneumatocele).
Histiocytosis and other causes of interstitial disease.

PULMONARY EDEMA, NONCARDIOGENIC[21]

ICD-10CM # J81.0 Acute pulmonary edema

CAUSES OF NONCARDIOGENIC PULMONARY EDEMA

Adult respiratory distress syndrome.
Drowning.
Asphyxia.
Upper airway obstruction (usually with cardiomegaly).
High altitude.
Increased intracranial pressure.
Postictal.
Noxious gases:
  Smoke.
  Nitrous dioxide (silo filler's disease).
  Sulfur dioxide.
  Nitrogen mustard.
Drugs:
  Aspirin.
  Diazepam, chlordiazepoxide, barbiturates.
  Narcotics (heroin, methadone, morphine).
  β-adrenergic drugs (terbutaline).
  Contrast media.
  Colchicine.
  Fluorescein.
  Hydrochlorothiazide.
  Nitrofurantoin.
  Propoxyphene.
Poisons:
  Parathion.

Transfusion reactions.
Renal failure: transplantation.
Bone marrow transplantation.
Fat embolism.
Pancreatitis.

PULMONARY EOSINOPHILIA[28]

ICD-10CM #   NEC J82   Eosinophilia, pulmonary

TYPES AND CAUSES OF PULMONARY EOSINOPHILIA

Drug- and toxin-induced eosinophilic lung diseases.
Helminth and fungal infection-related eosinophilic lung diseases:
  Transpulmonary passage of larvae (i.e., Löffler syndrome): *Ascaris,* hookworm, *Strongyloides.*
  Pulmonary parenchymal invasion: mostly helminths, paragonimiasis.
  Heavy hematogenous seeding with helminths: trichinellosis, disseminated strongyloidiasis, cutaneous and visceral larva migrans, schistosomiasis.
  Tropical pulmonary eosinophilia: filaria.
  Allergic bronchopulmonary aspergillosis.
Chronic eosinophilic pneumonia.
Acute eosinophilic pneumonia.
Churg-Strauss syndrome (vasculitis).
Other: neoplasia, idiopathic hypereosinophilic syndrome, bronchocentric granulomatosis.

PULMONARY HEMORRHAGE, DIFFUSE, ALVEOLAR[14]

ICD-10CM #   R04.8   Pulmonary hemorrhage

IMMUNOLOGIC DISEASES

Antiglomerular basement membrane antibody disease (Goodpasture syndrome).
Vasculitides associated with circulating or in situ immune complexes:
  Systemic lupus erythematosus.
  Mixed connective tissue disease.
  Schönlein-Henoch purpura.
  Essential mixed cryoglobulinemia.
  Tumor-related vasculitis.
  Endocarditis-related vasculitis.
  Polyarteritis nodosa.
  Systemic necrotizing vasculitis.
Vasculitides associated with antineutrophil cytoplasmic antibodies:
  Wegener granulomatosis.
  Microscopic polyangiitis.
  Idiopathic necrotizing crescentic glomerulonephritis.
Rapidly progressive glomerulonephritis.
Associated with other connective tissue diseases, pathophysiology unknown:
  Rheumatoid arthritis.
  Progressive systemic sclerosis.
  Behçet disease.
Associated with other renal diseases.

Immunoglobulin A nephropathy.
Diabetic nephropathy.
Associated with precipitating antibodies to milk (Heiner syndrome).
Idiopathic pulmonary hemosiderosis.
Primary antiphospholipid antibody syndrome.

CHEMICAL OR DRUG-RELATED CAUSES

Amiodarone.
D-Penicillamine.
Isocyanates.
Nitrofurantoin.
Retinoic acid.
Trimellitic anhydride.
"Crack" cocaine.
Sirolimus.
Everolimus.
Propylthiouracil-induced vasculitis.
Erlotinib.
Bevacizumab.
Gemcitabine.
Infliximab.

TRANSPLANT-RELATED CAUSES

Bone marrow transplant.
Renal transplant.
Lung transplant.

BLEEDING DIATHESIS

Thrombocytopenia.
Leukemia with diffuse alveolar damage.
Viral pneumonia.
Bacterial or fungal sepsis.
Radiation.
Chemotherapy toxic to lung.
Blast counts >80,000/μL.
Extrinsic anticoagulants/thrombolytics.
Warfarin overdose.
Tissue plasminogen activator.
Platelet glycoprotein IIb/IIIa inhibitors.
Coagulopathies.
Cirrhosis.
Disseminated intravascular coagulation.

INFECTIONS

Adenovirus.
Aspergillosis (invasive).
Cytomegalovirus.
Dengue.
Hantavirus.
Influenza.
Legionella.
Leptospirosis.
Malaria.
Mycoplasma.
Staphylococcus aureus.

PULMONARY VENOUS HYPERTENSION

Mitral stenosis.
Mitral regurgitation.
Pulmonary capillary hemangiomatosis.
Pulmonary venoocclusive disease.
Fibrosing mediastinitis.

Congenital heart disease.

DIFFUSE LUNG INJURY

Negative-pressure pulmonary hemorrhage.
Breath-hold diving.
Postictal neurogenic pulmonary edema.

PULMONARY HEMORRHAGE, FOCAL[27]

ICD-10CM #   R04.8   Pulmonary hemorrhage

CAUSES OF FOCAL PULMONARY HEMORRHAGE

Iatrogenic Disorders
Bronchoscopy.
Lung biopsy.
Pulmonary artery catheterization.
Transtracheal aspiration.
Radiofrequency ablation.
Brachytherapy.
Infectious Disorders
Lung abscess.
Mycetoma.
Necrotizing pneumonia (*Staphylococcus aureus,* gram-negative aerobes, *Legionella, Actinomyces* spp., *Stenotrophomonas, Kytococcus sedentarius, Leptospira* spp., *Yersinia pestis, Francisella tularensis*).
Parasitic infection (paragonimiasis, amebiasis, ascariasis, clonorchiasis, echinococcosis, hookworm infestation, strongyloidiasis, trichinosis, schistosomiasis).
Parenchymal fungal infection (aspergillosis, mucormycosis, coccidioidomycosis, histoplasmosis, maduromycosis, botryomycosis).
Tuberculosis (active or inactive).
Viral tracheitis.
Herpetic tracheobronchitis.
Interstitial Lung Diseases
Lymphangioleiomyomatosis.
Sarcoidosis.
Tuberous sclerosis.
Pneumoconiosis.
Langerhans cell granulomatosis.
Miscellaneous Disorders
Amyloidosis.
Bronchogenic cyst.
Broncholithiasis.
Bronchopleural fistula.
Thoracic endometriosis.
Foreign body.
Tracheopathia osteoplastica.
Lipoid pneumonia.
Organophosphate aspiration.
Chronic pancreatitis.
Neoplastic Disorders
Bronchial adenoma.
Lung cancer.
Tracheal tumors (mucoepidermoid, squamous cell, adenoid cystic, glomus).
Pulmonary blastoma.
Pleuropulmonary angiosarcoma.
Sarcoma (synovial, myofibroblastic).
Clear cell tumor.

Metastatic disease (prostate, renal, breast, ovarian).

Tracheobronchial schwannoma.

Pulmonary Airway Diseases

Bronchiectasis.

Bronchitis.

Granulomatous tracheobronchitis (ulcerative colitis, Crohn disease, granulomatosis with polyangiitis).

Cystic fibrosis.

Bullous emphysema.

Traumatic Injury

Blunt chest trauma.

Penetrating injury.

Ruptured bronchus.

Lightning injury.

Thoracic splenosis.

Vascular Disorders

Pulmonary embolism, infarction.

Systemic cholesterol emboli.

Intralobar sequestration.

Pulmonary artery aneurysms.

Behçet disease, Hughes-Stovin syndrome, traumatic pseudoaneurysms.

Acquired arteriovenous malformations.

Osler-Weber-Rendu syndrome (hereditary hemorrhagic telangiectasia).

Takayasu arteritis.

Aortic aneurysms.

Trachea–innominate artery fistulas.

Scimitar syndrome.

Vena cava-bronchial.

Dieulafoy disease of bronchus.

Ventriculopulmonary fistulas.

Hemangioma (sclerosing, cavernous, tracheal).

PULMONARY HEMORRHAGE, PEDIATRIC AGE

ICD-10CM #	P26.9	Pulmonary hemorrhage newborn

CAUSES OF PULMONARY HEMORRHAGE (HEMOPTYSIS)

Focal Hemorrhage

Bronchitis and bronchiectasis (especially cystic fibrosis related).

Infection (acute or chronic), pneumonia, abscess.

Tuberculosis.

Trauma.

Pulmonary arteriovenous malformation.

Foreign body (chronic).

Neoplasm including hemangioma.

Pulmonary embolus with or without infarction.

Bronchogenic cysts.

Diffuse hemorrhage

Idiopathic of infancy.

Congenital heart disease (including pulmonary hypertension, venoocclusive disease, congestive heart failure).

Prematurity.

Cow's milk hyperreactivity (Heiner syndrome).

Goodpasture syndrome.

Collagen vascular diseases (systemic lupus erythematosus, rheumatoid arthritis).

Henoch-Schönlein purpura and vasculitic disorders.

Granulomatous disease (Wegener granulomatosis).

Celiac disease.

Coagulopathy (congenital or acquired).

Malignancy.

Immunodeficiency.

Exogenous toxins.

Hyperammonemia.

Pulmonary hypertension.

Pulmonary alveolar hemosiderosis.

Tuberous sclerosis.

Lymphangiomyomatosis or lymphangioleiomyomatosis.

Physical injury or abuse.

PULMONARY HEMORRHAGIC SYNDROMES, DIFFUSE[21]

ICD-10CM #	P26.1	Massive pulmonary hemorrhage originating in the perinatal period
	R04.8	Pulmonary hemorrhage

CLASSIFICATION OF DIFFUSE PULMONARY HEMORRHAGE SYNDROMES

Nonimmunocompromised Patients

Antibasement membrane antibody disease/Goodpasture syndrome.

Diseases of presumed immune etiology, with or without nephropathy:

Systemic lupus erythematosus.

Rheumatoid arthritis.

Systemic sclerosis.

Systemic necrotizing vasculitis.

Granulomatosis with polyangiitis.

Microscopic polyarteritis.

Diseases with no known immune etiology:

Idiopathic pulmonary hemosiderosis.

Rapidly progressive glomerulonephritis without immune complexes.

Fibrillary glomerulonephritis.

Drug-induced (anticoagulants, trimellitic anhydride, cocaine, lymphangiography).

Valvular heart disease.

Disseminated intravascular coagulation.

Acute lung injury.

Tumors.

Immunocompromised Patients

Blood dyscrasias.

Infection.

Tumors.

PULMONARY INFILTRATES ASSOCIATIONS[106]

ICD-10CM #	Varies with specific diagnosis

PULMONARY INFILTRATES AND THEIR ASSOCIATION WITH SPECIFIC INFECTIOUS AND NONINFECTIOUS DISORDERS

Radiologic Sign	Potential Etiologic Disorder(s)
Interstitial infiltrates:	Pulmonary edema.
Diffuse alveolar damage:	Idiopathic pneumonia syndrome. Respiratory virus infection: RSV, parainfluenza virus, influenza virus, adenovirus, enterovirus. Herpesvirus infection: CMV, HSV, VZV, HHV-6. Pneumocystis pneumonia.
Focal airspace disease:	Bacterial pneumonia. Fungal pneumonia.
Nodules:	Fungal pneumonia (aspergillosis). Nocardia infection. Legionella infection. Septic bacterial emboli. Mycobacterial infection (with cavitation). EBV lymphoproliferative disorder. Relapsed malignancy. Pulmonary embolism (pleura based).
Halo sign or air-crescent sign:	Aspergillosis.

CMV, Cytomegalovirus; *EBV*, Epstein-Barr virus; *HHV*, human herpesvirus; *HSV*, herpes simplex virus; *RSV*, respiratory syncytial virus; *VZV*, varicella-zoster virus.

PULMONARY INFILTRATES, IMMUNOCOMPROMISED HOST[103]

ICD-10CM #	J82	Pulmonary eosinophilia, not elsewhere classified
	J98.4	Other disorders of lung

CAUSES OF PULMONARY INFILTRATES IN THE IMMUNOCOMPROMISED HOST

Infections:

Bacteria:

Gram-positive cocci, especially Staphylococcus.

Gram-negative bacilli.

Mycobacterium tuberculosis.

Nontuberculous mycobacteria.

Nocardia.

Viruses:

Cytomegalovirus.

Herpesvirus.

Fungi:

Aspergillus.

Cryptococcus.

Candida.

Mucor.

Pneumocystis jiroveci.
Protozoa:
  Toxoplasma gondii (rare).
Pulmonary effects of therapy:
  Chemotherapeutic agents.
  Radiation therapy.
  Pulmonary hemorrhage.
  Congestive heart failure.
  Disseminated malignancy.
  Nonspecified interstitial pneumonitis (no defined etiology).

PULMONARY LESIONS

ICD-10CM#	J98.4	Other disorders of lung
	J70.9	Respiratory conditions due to unspecified external agent
	S27.309A	Unspecified injury of lung, unspecified, initial encounter

TB.
Legionella pneumonia.
Mycoplasma pneumonia.
Viral pneumonia.
Pneumocystis carinii.
Hypersensitivity pneumonitis.
Aspiration pneumonia.
Fungal disease (aspergillosis, histoplasmosis).
ARDS associated with pneumonia.
Psittacosis.
Sarcoidosis.
Septic emboli.
Metastatic cancer.
Multiple pulmonary emboli.
Rheumatoid nodules.

PULMONARY MASS, SOLITARY, CAUSES[21]

ICD-10CM #	R91.1	Solitary pulmonary nodule

CAUSES OF A SOLITARY PULMONARY MASS

Bronchial carcinoma.
Bronchial carcinoid.
Granuloma.
Hamartoma.
Metastasis.
Chronic pneumonia or abscess.
Hydatid cyst.
Pulmonary hematoma.
Bronchocele.
Fungus ball.
Massive fibrosis in coal workers.
Bronchogenic cyst.
Sequestration.
Arteriovenous malformation.
Pulmonary infarct.
Round atelectasis.

PULMONARY MASS, SOLITARY, MIMICS[21]

ICD-10CM #	Varies with specific diagnosis

SIMULANTS OF A SOLITARY PULMONARY MASS

Extrathoracic artifacts.
Cutaneous masses.
Bony lesions.
Pleural tumors or plaques.
Encysted pleural fluid.
Pulmonary vessels.

PULMONARY NODULE, SOLITARY

ICD-10CM #	J98.4	Other disorders of lung

Bronchogenic carcinoma.
Granuloma from histoplasmosis.
TB granuloma.
Granuloma from coccidioidomycosis.
Metastatic carcinoma.
Bronchial adenoma.
Bronchogenic cyst.
Hamartoma.
AV malformation.
Other: fibroma, intrapulmonary lymph node, sclerosing hemangioma, bronchopulmonary sequestration.

PULMONARY NODULES, MULTIPLE IN PATIENT WITH PRIOR CANCER[74]

ICD-10CM #	Varies with specific diagnosis

Malignant.
Metastasis.
Primary lung cancer.
Benign.
Infectious
Fungal infection.
Mycobacterial infection.
Nocardiosis.
Septic emboli.
Noninfectious
Rheumatoid nodules.
Hamartoma.
Carcinoid.
Sarcoidosis.
Cryptogenic organizing pneumonia.
Vasculitis (granulomatosis with polyangiitis).

PULMONARY OPACITIES[94]

ICD-10CM #	Varies with specific diagnosis

CLASSIFICATION OF LARGE PULMONARY OPACITIES

Diffuse homogeneous.
Multifocal patchy.
Lobar without atelectasis.
Lobar with atelectasis.
Perihilar.
Peripheral.

PULMONARY–RENAL SYNDROMES, CAUSES[9]

ICD-10CM #	Varies with specific diagnosis

Systemic vasculitis: ANCA associated:	Anti-GBM disease (Goodpasture).Granulomatosis with polyangiitis. Microscopic polyarteritis. Churg-Strauss syndrome. Drugs (penicillamine, hydralazine, propylthiouracil). Immune complex disease. Lupus erythematosus. Henoch-Schönlein purpura. Mixed cryoglobulinemia. Rheumatoid vasculitis.
Infection:	Severe bacterial pneumonia, postinfectious glomerulonephritis, *Legionella*, hantavirus, opportunistic infection in immunocompromised patients, infective endocarditis.
Pulmonary edema and AKI:	Volume overload, severe left ventricular failure.
Multiorgan failure:	Acute respiratory distress syndrome and AKI.
Other:	Paraquat poisoning, renal vein or IVC thrombosis with pulmonary emboli.

AKI, Acute kidney injury; *ANCA,* antineutrophil cytoplasmic antibody; *GBM,* glomerular basement membrane; *IVC,* inferior vena cava.

PULSATILE TINNITUS[22]

ICD-10CM #	H93.A9	Pulsatile tinnitus, unspecified ear
	H93.A1	Pulsatile tinnitus right ear
	H93.A2	Pulsatile tinnitus left ear
	H93.A3	Pulsatile tinnitus bilateral

Synchronous With Pulse
Arterial Etiologies

Cardiovascular:	Hypertension. Valvular heart disease.
Intraosseous:	Paget disease, otosclerosis.
Neoplasm:	Paraganglioma (glomus tympanicum or jugulare). Vestibular schwannoma, endolymphatic sac tumor, hemangiopericytoma, temporal bone hemangioma, meningioma, and vascular metastases to the skull base.
Vascular stenosis:	Carotid artery atherosclerosis and subsequent stenosis. Other atherosclerotic disease (subclavian, external carotid).

Differential Diagnosis

II

Fibromuscular dysplasia of the carotid artery.

Skull base variant:
Persistent stapedial artery.
Aberrant or dehiscent internal carotid artery (intratympanic).
Arteriovenous fistula or malformation, aneurysm.
Arterial dissection (carotid, vertebral).
Vascular compression of cranial nerve VIII.
Hyperdynamic states with increased cardiac output (anemia, thyrotoxicosis, pregnancy).

Venous etiologies:
Sigmoid sinus and jugular bulb anomalies.
Idiopathic intracranial hypertension.
Dilated mastoid or condylar emissary veins.
Dural sinus stenosis (transverse or sigmoid sinus).
Idiopathic tinnitus, essential tinnitus, or venous hum.*

Asynchronous with Pulse

Muscular myoclonus:
Palatal, tensor tympani, or stapedial muscle myoclonus.

Otologic—middle ear:
Patulous eustachian tube.
Ossicular or tympanic membrane abnormality.
Otosclerosis.
Semicircular canal dehiscence.
Middle ear effusion.

Joints:
Temporomandibular joint disease.

*Venous hum, also known as idiopathic or essential tinnitus, is a subtype of pulsatile tinnitus whose existence is controversial. Historical cases of venous hum are thought to be secondary to undiagnosed idiopathic intracranial hypertension.

PULSELESS ELECTRICAL ACTIVITY

ICD-10CM # I46.9 Cardiac arrest, cause unspecified

Hypovolemia.
Hypoxia.
Hyperkalemia.
Acidosis.
Cardiac tamponade.
Tension pneumothorax.
Pulmonary embolus.
Drug overdose.
Hypothermia.

PUPILLARY DILATATION, POOR RESPONSE TO DARKNESS

ICD-10CM # H21.569 Pupillary abnormality, unspecified eye

Drugs (narcotics, general anesthetics, cholinergics).

Acute trauma (spasm from prostaglandin release).
Inflammation, infection (interruption of inhibitory fibers to the Edinger-Westphal nucleus).
Old age (loss of inhibition at midbrain from reticular activating formation).
Horner syndrome (sympathetic neuron interruption).
Adie syndrome tonic pupil.
Lymphoma.
Congenital miosis.

PURPURA

ICD-10CM # D69.2 Other nonthrombocytopenic purpura
D69.0 Allergic purpura
D69.49 Other primary thrombocytopenia
M31.1 Thrombotic microangiopathy

THROMBOTIC

Trauma.
Septic emboli, atheromatous emboli.
DIC.
Thrombocytopenia.
Meningococcemia.
Rocky Mountain spotted fever.
Hemolytic-uremic syndrome.
Viral infection: echo, coxsackie.
Scurvy.
Other: left atrial myxoma, cryoglobulinemia, vasculitis, hyperglobulinemic purpura.

PURPURA, NONPALPABLE[31]

ICD-10CM # D69.2 Other nonthrombocytopenic purpura

INCREASED TRANSMURAL PRESSURE GRADIENT

Acute (Valsalva, coughing, vomiting, high altitude, weight lifting).
Chronic—venous stasis.

DECREASED MECHANICAL INTEGRITY OF MICROCIRCULATION AND SUPPORTING TISSUES

Age related (infancy and actinic purpura).
Glucocorticoid excess—Cushing syndrome and glucocorticoid therapy.
Vitamin C deficiency (scurvy).
Abnormal connective tissue—Ehlers-Danlos syndrome.
Amyloid infiltration of blood vessels.
Colloid milium.
Hormonal—female easy bruising syndrome (purpura simplex).
Lorenzo oil.
MELAS syndrome.

TRAUMA TO BLOOD VESSELS

Physical:
Injuries.
Child abuse.
Factitial purpura.
Ultraviolet purpura:
Purpuric sunburn.
Solar purpura.
Infectious:
Bacterial.
Rickettsial.
Fungal.
Viral.
Parasitic.
Embolic:
Infectious organisms.
Atheroemboli (cholesterol crystal emboli).
Fat emboli.
Allergic and/or inflammatory:
Serum sickness.
Pigmented purpuric eruptions.
Pyoderma gangrenosum.
Contact dermatitis.
Familial Mediterranean fever.
Neoplastic.
Metabolic:
Erythropoietic porphyria.
Calciphylaxis.
Immunoglobulin related (hyperglobulinemic purpura of Waldenström and light-chain vasculitis).
Drug related.
Thrombotic:
Disseminated intravascular coagulation.
Warfarin (Coumadin)-induced skin necrosis.
Protein C or protein S deficiency, factor V Leiden, prothrombin G20201A.
Purpura fulminans.
Paroxysmal nocturnal hemoglobinuria.
Antiphospholipid antibody syndrome.
Hemangioma with thrombocytopenia and consumptive coagulopathy (Kasabach-Merritt syndrome).
Unknown Cause-Psychogenic Purpura

PURPURA, NONPURPURIC DISORDERS SIMULATING PURPURA[18]

ICD-10CM # Varies with specific diagnosis

Disorders with telangiectasias:
Cherry angiomas.
Hereditary hemorrhagic telangiectasia.
Chronic actinic telangiectasia.
Scleroderma.
CREST syndrome.
Ataxia-telangiectasia.
Chronic liver disease.
Pregnancy-related telangiectasia.
Kaposi sarcoma and other vascular sarcomas.
Fabry disease.

Neonatal extramedullary hematopoiesis.
Angioma serpiginosum.

PURPURA, PALPABLE[31]

ICD-10CM #	D69.2	Other nonthrombocytopenic purpura

Cutaneous vasculitis:
   Systemic vasculitides.
   Paraneoplastic vasculitis.
   Henoch-Schönlein purpura.
   Acute hemorrhagic edema of infancy.
   Livedoid vasculitis.
   Idiopathic.
   Urticarial.
   Cryoglobulinemia.
   Cryofibrinogenemia.
   Primary cutaneous diseases

QT INTERVAL PROLONGATION[97]

ICD-10CM #	R94.31	Abnormal electrocardiogram [ECG] [EKG]
	I45.81	Long QT syndrome

Drugs:
   Class I antiarrhythmics (e.g., disopyramide, procainamide, quinidine).
   Class III antiarrhythmics.
   Tricyclic antidepressants.
   Phenothiazines.
   Astemizole.
   Terfenadine.
   Adenosine.
   Antibiotics (e.g., erythromycin and other macrolides):
      Antifungal agents.
      Pentamidine, chloroquine.
Ischemic heart disease.
Cerebrovascular disease.
Rheumatic fever.
Myocarditis.
Mitral valve prolapse.
Electrolyte abnormalities.
Hypocalcemia.
Hypothyroidism.
Liquid protein diets.
Organophosphate insecticides.
Congenital prolonged QT syndrome.

RADIATION-INDUCED NEOPLASMS[54]

ICD-10CM #	Varies with specific diagnosis

RADIATION-INDUCED NEOPLASMS
Osteochondroma
Benign.
Exclusively with childhood irradiation.

Histologically identical to spontaneous osteochondroma.
Sarcoma
Malignant.
Latent period of 4 years or more.
Histologically identical to spontaneous sarcoma.
Commonly malignant fibrous histiocytoma or osteosarcoma.
Occurs in either bone or soft tissue.
Tumors in Other Organ Systems
Squamous cell cancer of the skin.
Breast cancer.
Leukemia, with shorter latent period than sarcoma.

RECTAL MASS, PALPABLE[2]

ICD-10CM #	R22.9	Localized swelling, mass and lump, unspecified

Rectal carcinoma.
Rectal polyp.
Hypertrophied anal papilla.
Diverticular phlegmon (prolapsing into the pouch of Douglas).
Sigmoid colon carcinoma (prolapsing into the pouch of Douglas).
Metastatic deposits at the pelvic reflection (Blumer shelf).
Primary pelvic malignancy (uterine, ovarian, prostatic, or cervical).
Mesorectal lymph nodes.
Endometriosis.
Solitary rectal ulcer syndrome.
Foreign body.
Feces.
Presacral cyst.
Amebic granuloma.
Vaginal tampon and even the pubic bone may be mistaken for a rectal mass.

RECTAL PAIN

ICD-10CM #	K62.89	Other specified diseases of anus and rectum

Anal fissure.
Thrombosed hemorrhoid.
Anorectal abscess.
Foreign bodies.
Fecal impaction.
Endometriosis.
Neoplasms (primary or metastatic).
Pelvic inflammatory disease.
Inflammation of sacral nerves.
Compression of sacral nerves.
Prostatitis.
Other: proctalgia fugax, uterine abnormalities, myopathies, coccygodynia.

RED BLOOD CELL APLASIA, ACQUIRED, ETIOLOGY

ICD-10CM #	D61.01	Constitutional (pure) red blood cell aplasia

Idiopathic (>50% of cases).
Medications (most frequent with phenytoin).
Non-Hodgkin lymphoma.
Viral infections (parvovirus B19, EB virus, mumps, hepatitis).
Myelodysplastic syndromes.
Thymoma.
Autoimmune diseases.
Allogenic bone marrow transplant from ABO incompatible donor.
Pregnancy.

RED BLOOD CELL FRAGMENTATION HEMOLYSIS, CAUSES[34]

ICD-10CM #	Varies with specific disorder

CAUSES OF RED BLOOD CELL FRAGMENTATION HEMOLYSIS
Damaged microvasculature.
Thrombotic thrombocytopenic purpura–hemolytic uremic syndrome (TTP–HUS).
Associated with pregnancy: preeclampsia or eclampsia; hemolysis plus elevated liver enzymes plus low platelets (HELLP syndrome).
Associated with malignancy, with or without mitomycin C treatment.
Vasculitis: polyarteritis, Wegener granulomatosis, acute glomerulonephritis, or *Rickettsia*-like infections.
Systemic lupus erythematosus.
Abnormalities of renal vasculature: malignant hypertension, acute glomerulonephritis, scleroderma, or allograft rejection with or without cyclosporine treatment.
Disseminated intravascular coagulation.
Malignant hypertension.
Catastrophic antiphospholipid antibody syndrome.
Atrioventricular malformations.
Kasabach-Merritt syndrome.
Hemangioendotheliomas.
Atrioventricular shunts for congenital and acquired conditions (e.g., stents, coils, trans-jugular intrahepatic portosystemic shunt, Levine shunts).
Cardiac abnormalities:
   Replaced valve, prosthesis, graft, or patch.
   Aortic stenosis or regurgitant jets (e.g., in ruptured sinus of Valsalva).
Drugs:
   Cyclosporine.
   Mitomycin.
   Ticlopidine.
   Clopidogrel.
   Tacrolimus.
   Cocaine.
Systemic infection:
   Bacterial endocarditis.
   Brucellosis.

Differential Diagnosis

II

Cytomegalovirus.
Human immunodeficiency virus.
Ehrlichiosis.
Rocky Mountain spotted fever

RED EYE

ICD-10CM # H57.8 Other specified disorders of eye and adnexa

Infectious conjunctivitis (bacterial, viral).
Allergic conjunctivitis.
Acute glaucoma.
Keratitis (bacterial, viral).
Iritis.
Trauma.

RED EYE, ACUTE[112]

ICD-10CM # H57.8 Other specified disorders of eye and adnexa

Obvious open globe.
Corneal abrasion.
Corneal ulcer.
Subconjunctival hemorrhage.
Hyphema.
Occult open globe.
Herpes simplex virus glaucoma.
Iritis, traumatic iritis.
Scleritis.
Conjunctivitis.
Blepharitis.
Ultraviolet keratitis.
Episcleritis.
Conjunctival foreign body.
Dry eye.
Contact lens overwear syndrome.

RED HOT JOINT

ICD-10CM # Varies with specific diagnosis

Trauma.
Gout.
Infection (septic joint).
Pseudogout (calcium pyrophosphate dehydrate crystal deposition).
Psoriatic arthropathy.
Reactive arthritis.
Palindromic rheumatism.

RED URINE

ICD-10CM # R39.19 Other difficulties with micturition

Hematuria.
Porphyrins.
Hemoglobinuria.
Myoglobinuria.
Medications (phenazopyridine, aminosalicylic acid, deferoxamine, phenazopyridine, phenolphthalein, NSAIDs, rifampin, phenytoin, methyldopa, doxorubicin, phenacetin).
Foods (beets, berries, maize).
Urate crystalluria.

RENAL ALLOGRAFT DYSFUNCTION[59]

ICD-10CM # T86.1 Complications of renal allograft

IMMEDIATE/DELAYED GRAFT FUNCTION (1 TO 3 DAYS)

Acute tubular necrosis.
Hyperacute humoral rejection.
Urinary leak or obstruction.
Renal artery or vein thrombosis.
Recurrence of disease (e.g., focal segmental glomerulosclerosis).

EARLY POSTTRANSPLANTATION PERIOD (FIRST MONTH)

Acute cellular rejection.
Acute humoral rejection.
Calcineurin inhibitor toxicity.
Urinary tract obstruction.
Volume depletion.
Recurrence of disease.

Late Acute Dysfunction
Acute rejection.
Cyclosporine or tacrolimus toxicity.
Recurrence of primary disease.
Tubulointerstitial nephritis, drug-induced.
Renal artery stenosis.
Infection (bacterial urinary tract infection [UTI], cytomegalovirus, BK virus).
Hemodynamic (volume; use of angiotensin-converting enzyme inhibitor, angiotensin II receptor blocker).

Chronic Dysfunction
Chronic rejection.
Cyclosporine or tacrolimus toxicity.
Recurrent renal disease.
De novo renal disease.
Urinary tract obstruction.
Bacterial UTI.
Hypertensive nephrosclerosis.

RENAL ARTERY OCCLUSION, CAUSES

ICD-10CM # N28.0 Ischemia and infarction of kidney

Atrial fibrillation.
Angiography or stent placement.
Abdominal aortic surgery.
Trauma.
Renal artery aneurysm/dissection.
Vasculitis.
Thrombosis in patient with fibromuscular dysplasia.
Atherosclerosis.
Septic embolism.
Mural thrombus thromboembolism.
Atrial myxoma thromboembolism.
Mitral stenosis thromboembolism.
Prosthetic valve thromboembolism.
Renal cell carcinoma.

RENAL COLIC[112]

ICD-10CM # N23 Unspecified renal colic

Vascular:
    Abdominal aortic aneurysm.
    Aortic dissection.
    Renal artery dissection.
    Renal artery stenosis.
    Renal vein thrombosis.
    Renal infarct.
    Mesenteric ischemia.
    Retroperitoneal hemorrhage.
GI:
    Incarcerated hernia.
    Appendicitis.
    Cholecystitis.
    Biliary colic.
    Pancreatitis.
    Bowel obstruction.
    Diverticulitis.
Gynecologic:
    Ectopic pregnancy.
    Ovarian torsion.
    Tuboovarian abscess.
    Pelvic inflammatory disease.
    Endometriosis.
Genitourinary:
    Testicular torsion.
    Pyelonephritis.
    Perinephric abscess.
    Urinary tract tumor.
    Renal papillary necrosis.
    Upper urinary tract hemorrhage.
Musculoskeletal:
    Lumbar strain.
    Radiculopathy.
    Disk herniation.
    Vertebral compression fracture.
Dermatologic:
    Herpes zoster.
Miscellaneous:
    Factitious.

RENAL CYSTIC DISORDERS

ICD-10CM # Q61.01 Congenital single renal cyst

Simple cysts.
Acquired cystic kidney disease.
Autosomal dominant polycystic kidney disease.
Autosomal recessive polycystic kidney disease.
Medullary cystic disease.
Medullary sponge kidney.

RENAL DISEASE, SKIN MANIFESTATIONS[11]

ICD-10CM # Varies with specific diagnosis

SKIN MANIFESTATIONS SECONDARY TO RENAL DISEASE
Nonspecific
Pruritus.

Xerosis.

Acquired ichthyosis.

Pigmentary alteration:

    Pallor (secondary to anemia).

    Hyperpigmentation.

    Dyspigmentation (yellow tint).

Infections (fungal, bacterial, viral).

Purpura.

Somewhat Specific

Acquired perforating dermatosis.

Calciphylaxis.

Metastatic calcification.

Blistering disorders:

    Porphyria cutanea tarda.

    Pseudoporphyria.

Eruptive xanthomas.

Pseudo–Kaposi sarcoma.

Specific

Nephrogenic systemic fibrosis.

Dialysis-associated steal syndrome.

Metastatic renal cell carcinoma.

Dialysis-related amyloidosis.

Arteriovenous shunt dermatitis.

Uremic frost.

RENAL FAILURE, ACUTE, PIGMENT-INDUCED[43]

ICD-10CM #   N19   Unspecified kidney failure

CAUSES OF PIGMENT-INDUCED ACUTE RENAL FAILURE

Rhabdomyolysis and myoglobinuria.

Vigorous exercise.

Arterial embolization.

Status epilepticus.

Status asthmaticus.

Coma-induced and pressure-induced myonecrosis.

Heat stress.

Diabetic ketoacidosis.

Myopathy.

Alcoholism.

Hypokalemia.

Hypophosphatemia.

Hemoglobinuria.

Transfusion reactions.

Snake envenomation.

Malaria.

Mechanical destruction of RBCs by prosthetic valves.

G6PD deficiency.

_G6PD,_ Glucose-6-phosphate dehydrogenase; _RBCs,_ red blood cells.

RENAL FAILURE, CHRONIC[59]

ICD-10CM #   N18.9   Chronic kidney disease, unspecified

CAUSES OF CHRONIC RENAL FAILURE

Diabetic glomerulosclerosis (systemic disease involving the kidney).

Hypertensive nephrosclerosis.

Glomerular disease:

    Glomerulonephritis.

    Amyloidosis, light chain disease (systemic disease involving the kidney).

    Systemic lupus erythematosus, Wegener granulomatosis (systemic disease involving the kidney).

Tubulointerstitial disease:

    Reflux nephropathy (chronic pyelonephritis).

    Analgesic nephropathy.

    Obstructive nephropathy (stones, benign prostatic hypertrophy).

    Myeloma kidney (systemic disease involving the kidney).

Vascular disease:

    Scleroderma (systemic disease involving the kidney).

    Vasculitis (systemic disease involving the kidney).

    Renovascular renal failure (ischemic nephropathy).

    Atheroembolic renal disease (systemic disease involving the kidney).

Cystic disease:

    Autosomal dominant polycystic kidney disease.

    Medullary cystic kidney disease.

RENAL FAILURE, INTRINSIC OR PARENCHYMAL CAUSES[17]

ICD-10CM #	N17.0	Acute kidney failure with tubular necrosis
	N17.1	Acute kidney failure with acute cortical necrosis
	N17.2	Acute kidney failure with medullary necrosis
	N17.8	Other acute kidney failure
	N17.9	Acute kidney failure, unspecified
	N18.9	Chronic kidney disease, unspecified

ABNORMALITIES OF THE VASCULATURE

Renal arteries: atherosclerosis, thromboembolism, arteritis.

Renal veins: thrombosis.

Microvasculature: vasculitis, thrombotic microangiopathy.

ABNORMALITIES OF GLOMERULI (ACUTE GLOMERULONEPHRITIS)

Antiglomerular membrane disease (Goodpasture syndrome).

Immune complex glomerulonephritis: SLE, postinfectious, idiopathic, membranoproliferative.

ABNORMALITIES OF INTERSTITIUM (ACUTE INTERSTITIAL NEPHRITIS)

Drugs (e.g., antibiotics, NSAIDs, diuretics, anticonvulsants, allopurinol).

Infectious pyelonephritis.

Infiltrative: lymphoma, leukemia, sarcoidosis.

ABNORMALITIES OF TUBULES

Physical obstruction (uric acid, oxalate, light chains).

Acute tubular necrosis:

    Ischemic.

    Toxic (antibiotics, chemotherapy, immunosuppressives, radiocontrast dyes, heavy metals, myoglobin, hemolyzed RBCs).

RENAL FAILURE, POSTRENAL CAUSES[17]

ICD-10CM #	N17.0	Acute kidney failure with tubular necrosis
	N17.1	Acute kidney failure with acute cortical necrosis
	N17.2	Acute kidney failure with medullary necrosis
	N17.8	Other acute kidney failure
	N17.9	Acute kidney failure, unspecified
	N18.9	Chronic kidney disease, unspecified

URETER AND RENAL PELVIS

Intrinsic obstruction:

    Blood clots.

    Stones.

    Sloughed papillae: diabetes, sickle cell disease, analgesic nephropathy.

    Inflammatory: fungus ball.

Extrinsic obstruction:

    Malignancy.

    Retroperitoneal fibrosis.

    Iatrogenic: inadvertent ligation of ureters.

BLADDER

Prostatic hypertrophy or malignancy.

Neuropathic bladder.

Blood clots.

Bladder cancer.

Stones.

URETHRAL

Strictures.

Congenital valves.

RENAL FAILURE, PRERENAL CAUSES[17]

ICD-10CM #	N17.0	Acute kidney failure with tubular necrosis
	N17.1	Acute kidney failure with acute cortical necrosis
	N17.2	Acute kidney failure with medullary necrosis

Differential Diagnosis

II

N17.8	Other acute kidney failure
N17.9	Acute kidney failure, unspecified
N18.9	Chronic kidney disease, unspecified

DECREASED CARDIAC OUTPUT
CHF.
Arrhythmias.
Pericardial constriction or tamponade.
Pulmonary embolism.

HYPOVOLEMIA
GI tract loss (vomiting, diarrhea, nasogastric suction).
Blood losses (trauma, GI tract surgery).
Renal losses (diuretics, mineralocorticoid deficiency, postobstructive diuresis).
Skin losses (burns).

VOLUME REDISTRIBUTION (DECREASE IN EFFECTIVE BLOOD VOLUME)
Hypoalbuminemic states (cirrhosis, nephrosis).
Sequestration of fluid in "third" space (ischemic bowel, peritonitis, pancreatitis).
Peripheral vasodilation (sepsis, vasodilators, anaphylaxis).

ALTERED RENAL VASCULAR RESISTANCE
Increase in afferent vascular resistance (NSAIDs, liver disease, sepsis, hypercalcemia, cyclosporine).
Decrease in efferent arteriolar tone (ACE inhibitors).

RENAL INFARCTION[9]

ICD-10CM #	N28.0	Ischemia and infarction of kidney

CAUSES OF RENAL INFARCTION
Thrombosis: Spontaneous
Atherosclerotic disease of aorta and renal artery.
Fibromuscular dysplasia of renal artery.
Aneurysms of aorta or renal artery.
Dissection of aorta or renal artery:
    Marfan syndrome.
    Ehlers-Danlos syndrome.
Vasculitis involving renal artery:
    Polyarteritis nodosa.
    Takayasu arteritis.
    Kawasaki disease.
    Thromboangiitis obliterans.
    Other necrotizing vasculitides.
Inflammatory disease of the aorta or renal artery:
    Syphilis.
    Tuberculosis.
    Mycoses.
Hypercoagulable states:
    Nephrotic syndrome.
    Antiphospholipid syndrome.

Antithrombin III deficiency.
    Homocystinuria.
Thrombotic microangiopathies:
    Hemolytic-uremic syndrome.
    Thrombotic thrombocytopenic purpura.
    Antiphospholipid syndrome.
    Malignant hypertension.
    Scleroderma.
    Sickle cell nephropathy.
    Polycythemia vera.
    Postpartum hemolytic-uremic syndrome.
    Hyperacute vascular allograft rejection.
Thrombosis: Induced
Traumatic.
Following endovascular intervention.
Postrenal transplantation.
Embolism
Cardiac source:
    Atrial fibrillation or other arrhythmias.
    Native and prosthetic valvular heart disease.
    Infective endocarditis.
    Marantic endocarditis.
Myocardial infarction with mural thrombi.
Left atrial myxoma or other tumor.
Noncardiac sources:
    Atheromatous embolic disease.
    Paradoxical emboli.
    Fat emboli.
    Tumor emboli.
Therapeutic renal embolization.
Segmental renal infarction of childhood.
Cisplatinum and gemcitabine.
Sickle cell disease or sickle cell trait.

RENAL PARENCHYMAL DISEASE, CHRONIC[21]

ICD-10CM #	N28.9	Disorder of kidney and ureter, unspecified

DIFFERENTIAL DIAGNOSIS OF CHRONIC RENAL PARENCHYMAL DISEASE
No Papillary/Caliceal Abnormality
Diffuse Parenchymal Loss
Bilateral:
    Chronic glomerulonephritis.
    Diffuse small-vessel disease.
    Hereditary nephropathies.
Unilateral:
    Renal artery stenosis.
    Postirradiation.
    Rare:
        Hypoplastic kidney.
        Postobstructive atrophy.

FOCAL PARENCHYMAL LOSS
Infarct.
Previous trauma.
Papillary/Caliceal Abnormality
Diffuse Parenchymal Loss
Obstructive nephropathy.
Generalized reflux nephropathy.

No Parenchymal Loss
Papillary necrosis.
TB.
Medullary sponge kidney.
Megacalices.
Pelvicaliceal cyst.
Focal Parenchymal Loss
Focal reflux nephropathy (chronic atrophic pyelonephritis).
TB.
Calculus disease.

RENAL VEIN THROMBOSIS, CAUSES

ICD-10CM #	I82.3	Embolism and thrombosis of renal vein

Nephrotic syndrome.
Renal cell carcinoma.
Aortic aneurysm causing compression.
Lymphadenopathy.
Retroperitoneal fibrosis.
Estrogen therapy.
Pregnancy.
Renal cell carcinoma with vein invasion.
Severe dehydration.

RESPIRATORY DISTRESS IN THE NEWBORN, CAUSES[32]

ICD-10CM #	J96.00	Acute respiratory failure

RESPIRATORY DISTRESS IN THE NEWBORN
Noncardiopulmonary
Hypothermia or hyperthermia.
Hypoglycemia.
Metabolic acidosis.
Drug intoxications; withdrawal.
Polycythemia.
CNS insult.
Asphyxia.
Hemorrhage.
Neuromuscular disease.
Werdnig-Hoffman disease.
Myopathies.
Phrenic nerve injury.
Skeletal abnormalities.
Asphyxiating thoracic dystrophy.
Cardiovascular
Left-sided outflow obstruction.
Hypoplastic left heart.
Aortic stenosis.
Coarctation of the aorta.
Cyanotic lesions.
Transposition of the great vessels.
Total anomalous pulmonary venous return.
Tricuspid atresia.
Right-sided outflow obstruction.
Pulmonary
Upper airway obstruction.
Choanal atresia.
Vocal cord paralysis.

Meconium aspiration.
Clear fluid aspiration.
Transient tachypnea.
Pneumonia.
Pulmonary hypoplasia.
Primary.
Secondary.
Hyaline membrane disease.
Pneumothorax.
Pleural effusions.
Mass lesions.
Lobar emphysema.
Cystic adenomatoid malformation.

RESPIRATORY DYSFUNCTION ASSOCIATED WITH CENTRAL NERVOUS SYSTEM[74]

ICD-10CM # Code varies with specific diagnosis

CEREBRAL CORTEX
Stroke.
Neoplasm.
Cerebral degeneration.
Seizures.

BRAIN STEM/BASAL GANGLIA
Stroke.
Neoplasm.
Poliomyelitis.
Central alveolar hypoventilation.
Progressive bulbar palsy.
Multiple system atrophy.
Anoxic encephalopathy.
Encephalitis.
Multiple sclerosis.
Parkinson disease.
Chorea.
Dyskinesias.

SPINAL CORD
Trauma.
Infarction or hemorrhage.
Demyelinating disease.
Disc compression.
Syringomyelia.
Tumor.
Epidural abscess.

RESPIRATORY DYSFUNCTION ASSOCIATED WITH PERIPHERAL NERVOUS SYSTEM[74]

ICD-10CM # Code varies with specific diagnosis

MOTOR NERVES/ANTERIOR HORN CELL
Acute idiopathic polyneuropathy (Guillain-Barré syndrome).
Motor neuron disease.
Amyotrophic lateral sclerosis.

Spinal muscular atrophy.
Primary lateral sclerosis.
Critical illness neuropathy.
Vasculitides.
Toxins (e.g., lithium, arsenic, gold).
Metabolic.
Diabetes.
Porphyria.
Uremia.
Diphtheria.

NEUROMUSCULAR JUNCTION
Myasthenia gravis.
Lambert-Eaton myasthenic syndrome.
Toxins.
Botulism.
Snake venoms.
Scorpion bites.
Shellfish.
Crab poisoning.
Drugs.
Antibiotics.
Neuromuscular junction blockers.
Anticholinesterase inhibitors.
Corticosteroids.
Lidocaine.
Quinidine.
Lithium.
Antirheumatics.

MYOPATHIES
Muscular dystrophies.
Myotonic dystrophy.
Dermatomyositis.
Polymyositis.
Inclusion body myositis.
Glycogen storage diseases.
Pompe disease.
Forbes-Cori disease.
Thick filament myopathy.
Mitochondrial myopathy.
Nemaline body myopathy.
Severe hypokalemia.
Hypophosphatemia.

RESPIRATORY FAILURE, HYPOVENTILATORY[25]

ICD-10CM #   J96.00   Acute respiratory failure, unspecified whether with hypoxia or hypercapnia
       J96.90   Respiratory failure, unspecified, unspecified whether with hypoxia or hypercapnia

ABNORMAL RESPIRATORY CAPACITY (NORMAL RESPIRATORY WORKLOADS)
Acute depression of CNS:
    Various causes.
Chronic central hypoventilation syndromes:
    Obesity-hypoventilation syndrome.
    Sleep apnea syndrome.

Hypothyroidism.
Shy-Drager syndrome (multisystem atrophy syndrome).
Acute toxic paralysis syndromes:
    Botulism.
    Tetanus.
    Toxic ingestion or bites.
    Organophosphate poisoning.
Neuromuscular disorders (acute and chronic):
    Myasthenia gravis.
    Guillain-Barré syndrome.
    Drugs.
    Amyotrophic lateral sclerosis.
    Muscular dystrophies.
    Polymyositis.
    Spinal cord injury.
    Traumatic phrenic nerve paralysis.

ABNORMAL PULMONARY WORKLOADS
Chronic obstructive pulmonary disease:
    Chronic bronchitis.
    Asthmatic bronchitis.
    Emphysema.
Asthma and acute bronchial hyperreactivity syndromes.
Upper airway obstruction.
Interstitial lung diseases.

ABNORMAL EXTRAPULMONARY WORKLOADS
Chronic thoracic cage disorders:
    Severe kyphoscoliosis.
    After thoracoplasty.
    After thoracic cage injury.
Acute thoracic cage trauma and burns.
Pneumothorax.
Pleural fibrosis and effusions.
Abdominal processes.

RESPIRATORY MUSCLE WEAKNESS[27]

ICD-10CM #   Varies with specific diagnosis

CAUSES OF DECREASED RESPIRATORY MUSCLE STRENGTH OR ENDURANCE
Disorders of the phrenic nerve:
    Guillain-Barré syndrome.
    Poliomyelitis.
Respiratory muscle atrophy.
Disorders of neuromuscular transmission:
    Myasthenia gravis.
    Ventilator dependence.
    Malnutrition.
    Myopathy.
    Critical illness polyneuropathy/myopathy.
Altered diaphragmatic force-length relationship:
    Dynamic hyperinflation and diaphragmatic flattening.

RETINOPATHY, HYPERTENSIVE

ICD-10CM # H35.039 Hypertensive retinopathy, unspecified eye

Retinal venous obstruction.
Diabetic retinopathy.
Ocular ischemic syndrome.
Hyperviscosity.
Tortuosity of retinal artery.

RHINITIS

ICD-10CM # J31.0   Chronic rhinitis
J30.0   Vasomotor rhinitis
J30.1   Allergic rhinitis due to pollen
J30.2   Other seasonal allergic rhinitis
J30.5   Allergic rhinitis due to food
J30.89   Other allergic rhinitis
J30.9   Allergic rhinitis, unspecified

Allergic rhinitis.
Infectious rhinitis.
Vasomotor rhinitis.
Exercise-induced rhinitis.
Emotional rhinitis.
Rhinitis medicamentosa.
Hormone-mediated rhinitis (menses, pregnancy, oral contraceptives, hypothyroidism).
GERD.
Chemical- or irritant-induced rhinitis.
Rhinitis mimics:
  Deviated septum.
  Enlarged adenoids.
  Nasal polyps/tumors.
  Foreign bodies.
  CSF rhinorrhea.
  Sarcoidosis.
  Midline granuloma.
  Granulomatosis with polyangiitis.
  SLE.
  Sjögren syndrome.

RHINITIS, CHRONIC[28]

ICD-10CM # J31.0 Chronic rhinitis

CLASSIFICATION OF CHRONIC RHINITIS
Allergic
Systemic.
Local (entopy).
Work-Related
Irritant.
Corrosive.
Immunologic.
Infectious (Rhinosinusitis)
Allergic.
Nonallergic.

Nonallergic
Idiopathic.
Nonallergic with eosinophilia.
Atrophic.
Primary.
Secondary.
Medication-related.
Topical vasoconstrictors (rhinitis medicamentosa).
Oral medications.
Exercise-induced.
Cold air-induced.
Gustatory.
Hormonal.
Aging.
Systemic diseases.

RHINOSINUSITIS, DIFFERENTIAL DIAGNOSIS[13]

ICD-10CM # Varies with specific diagnosis

DIFFERENTIAL DIAGNOSIS OF RHINOSINUSITIS
Allergic Rhinitis
Seasonal.
Perennial.
Combined seasonal and perennial.
Allergic fungal rhinosinusitis.
Nonallergic Rhinitis
Nonallergic, noninflammatory idiopathic rhinopathy (vasomotor rhinitis).
Nonallergic rhinitis with eosinophilia syndrome (NARES).
Cold dry air-induced rhinitis.
Gustatory rhinitis.
Infectious Rhinosinusitis
Bacterial.
Viral.
Fungal.
Granulomatous.
Drug-Induced Rhinitis
Oral contraceptives.
Various antihypertensives and ocular β-blockers.
Topical decongestants (rhinitis medicamentosa).
Phosphodiesterase-5 antagonists.
Mechanical Causes of Rhinosinusitis
Septal deviation.
Nasal foreign body.
Choanal atresia or stenosis.
Adenoid hypertrophy.
Encephalocele.
Glioma.
Dermoid.
Innate and Acquired Immunity Disorders
Congenital or acquired immunodeficiencies.
Cystic fibrosis.
Immotile cilia syndrome.
Systemic Inflammatory Disorders
Sarcoidosis.
Granulomatosis with polyangiitis.
Vasculitis.

Neoplastic Causes
Benign:
  Polyps.
  Nasopharyngeal angiofibroma.
  Inverting papilloma.
Malignant:
  Adenocarcinoma.
  Squamous cell carcinoma.
  Esthesioneuroblastoma.
  Lymphoma.
  Rhabdomyosarcoma.

RIB DEFECTS ON X-RAY[21]

ICD-10CM # Varies with specific diagnosis

CAUSES OF SUPERIOR MARGINAL RIB DEFECTS
Normal
Isolated defects.
Projectional artifacts (due to lordosis).
Neurologic
Paralytic poliomyelitis.
Quadriparesis.
Collagen Vascular Disease
Rheumatoid arthritis.
SLE.
Systemic sclerosis.
Local Pressure
Chest drainage tube.
Osteochondroma.
Neural tumor.
Coarctation of aorta.
Hyperparathyroidism Miscellaneous
Osteogenesis imperfecta.
Marfan syndrome.

RIB NOTCHING ON X-RAY[21]

ICD-10CM # Varies with specific diagnosis

CAUSES OF INFERIOR RIB NOTCHING
Arterial.

AORTIC OBSTRUCTION
Aortic coarctation.
Aortic thrombosis.
Aortitis.

SUBCLAVIAN ARTERY OBSTRUCTION
Blalock-Taussig operation.
Arteritis.
Atherosclerotic occlusion.

PULMONARY OLIGEMIA
Pulmonary atresia.
Tetralogy of Fallot.
Multiple pulmonary arterial stenoses.
  Venous

CHRONIC SUPERIOR VENA CAVAL OBSTRUCTION

Arteriovenous
Arteriovenous Malformation
Pulmonary.
Chest wall.
Neural
    Neurofibromas.

RIGHT AXIS DEVIATION[97]

ICD-10CM #   Varies with specific diagnosis

Normal variation.
Right ventricular hypertrophy.
Left posterior fascicular block.
Lateral myocardial infarction.
Pulmonary embolism.
Dextrocardia.
Mechanical shifts or emphysema causing a vertical heart.

SACCADIC INTRUSIONS AND OSCILLATIONS[38]

ICD-10CM #   H55.81   Deficient saccadic eye movements

Square-wave jerks and square-wave oscillations.
Flutter (voluntary, involuntary).
Flutter dysmetria.
Microsaccadic flutter (variant of voluntary flutter?).
Opsoclonus.
Macro–square wave jerks (now designated square-wave pulses).
Ocular bobbing, reverse and inverse bobbing, dipping, and reverse dipping.
Superior oblique myokymia.
Convergence-retraction nystagmus.
Abduction nystagmus with internuclear ophthalmoplegia.
Ticlike ocular myoclonic jerks (eye tics).

SALIVARY GLAND ENLARGEMENT

ICD-10CM #   K11.1   Hypertrophy of salivary gland

Neoplasm.
Sialolithiasis.
Infection (mumps, bacterial infection, HIV, TB).
Sarcoidosis.
Idiopathic.
Acromegaly.
Anorexia/bulimia.
Chronic pancreatitis.
Medications (e.g., phenylbutazone).
Cirrhosis.
DM.

SALIVARY GLAND SECRETION, DECREASED

ICD-10CM #   K11.7   Disturbances of salivary secretion
             R68.2   Dry mouth, unspecified

Medications (antihistamines, antidepressants, neuroleptics, antihypertensives).
Dehydration.
Anxiety.
Sjögren syndrome.
Sarcoidosis.
Mumps.
Amyloidosis.
CNS disorders.
Head and neck radiation.

SCLERODERMA-LIKE SYNDROMES[18]

ICD-10CM #   Varies with specific diagnosis

OTHER DISEASES

Morphea.
Eosinophilic fasciitis.
Scleredema (of Buschke).
Scleromyxedema.
Graft-versus-host disease.
Nephrogenic-fibrosing dermopathy.

ENVIRONMENTAL AGENTS AND DRUGS

Bleomycin.
l-Tryptophan.
Organic solvents.
Pentazocine.
Toxic oil syndrome.
Vinyl chloride disease.
Gadolinium.

SCLERODERMA-LIKE SYNDROMES, DRUG-INDUCED[53]

ICD-10CM #   M34.2   Systemic sclerosis induced by drug or chemical

CHEMICALS

Silica.
Heavy metals.
Mercury.

ORGANIC CHEMICALS

Vinyl chloride.
Benzene.
Toluene.
Trichloroethylene.

DRUGS

Bleomycin.
Pentazocine.
Taxol.
Cocaine.

DIETARY SUPPLEMENT/APPETITE SUPPRESSANTS

L-tryptophan (or contaminant).
Mazindol.
Fenfluramine.
Diethylpropion.

SCROTAL CALCIFICATIONS[15]

ICD-10CM #   Varies with specific diagnosis

SCROTAL CALCIFICATIONS

Testicular
Solitary, postinflammatory granulomatous, vascular.
Microlithiasis.
"Burned-out" germ cell tumor.
Large-cell calcifying Sertoli cell tumor.
Teratoma.
Mixed germ cell tumor.
Sarcoid.
TB.
Chronic infarct.
Extratesticular
Tunica vaginalis "scrotal pearls."
Chronic epididymitis.
Schistosomiasis.

SCROTAL MASSES, BOYS AND ADOLESCENTS[19]

ICD-10CM #   R22.9   Localized swelling, mass and lump, unspecified

PAINFUL

Testicular torsion.
Torsion of appendix testis.
Epididymitis.
Trauma: ruptured testis, hematocele.
Inguinal hernia (incarcerated).
Mumps orchitis.

PAINLESS

Hydrocele.
Inguinal hernia.*
Varicocele.
Spermatocele.
Testicular tumor.
Henoch-Schönlein purpura.
Idiopathic scrotal edema.

*May be associated with discomfort.

SCROTAL PAIN[25]

ICD-10CM#   S31.30XA   Unspecified open wound of scrotum and testes, initial encounter

Differential Diagnosis

II

	N50.9	Disorder of male genital organs, unspecified
	R10.2	Pelvic and perineal pain
	N49.9	Inflammatory disorder of unspecified male genital organ
	N50.1	Vascular disorders of male genital organs
	N49.9	Inflammatory disorder of unspecified male genital organ

Torsion:
  Appendages.
  Spermatic cord.
Infection:
  Orchitis.
  Abscess.
  Epididymitis.
Neoplasia:
  Benign.
  Malignant.
  Incarcerated hernia.
  Trauma.
  Hydrocele.
  Spermatocele.
  Varicocele.

SCROTAL PAIN, ADOLESCENT OR PEDIATRIC PATIENT[89]

ICD-10CM # Varies with specific diagnosis

DIFFERENTIAL DIAGNOSIS OF PEDIATRIC ADOLESCENT ACUTE SCROTAL PAIN

Appendage torsion:
  Appendix testis.
  Other appendage (epididymis, paradidymis, vas aberrans).
Spermatic cord torsion:
  Intravaginal, acute or intermittent.
  Extravaginal.
Epididymitis:
  Infectious:
    Urinary tract infection.
    Sexually transmitted disease.
    Viral.
  Sterile or traumatic.
Scrotal edema or erythema:
  Diaper dermatitis, insect bite, or other skin lesions.
  Idiopathic scrotal edema.
Orchitis:
  Associated with epididymitis with or without abscess.
  Vasculitis (e.g., Henoch-Schönlein purpura).
  Viral illness (mumps).
Trauma:
  Hematocele or scrotal contusion or testis rupture.

Hernia or hydrocele:
  Inguinal hernia with or without incarceration.
  Communicating hydrocele.
  Encysted hydrocele with or without torsion.
  Associated with acute abdominal pathology (e.g., appendicitis, peritonitis).
Varicocele.
Intrascrotal mass:
  Cystic dysplasia or tumor of testis.
  Epididymal cyst, spermatocele or tumor.
  Other paratesticular tumors.
Musculoskeletal pain from inguinal tendonitis or muscle strain.
Referred pain (e.g., ureteral calculus or anomaly).

SCROTAL SWELLING

ICD-10CM # N50.8 Other specified disorders of male genital organs

Hydrocele.
Varicocele.
Neoplasm.
Acute epididymitis.
Orchitis.
Trauma.
Hernia.
Torsion of spermatic cord.
Torsion of epididymis.
Torsion of testis.
Insect bite.
Folliculitis.
Sebaceous cyst.
Thrombosis of spermatic vein.
Other: lymphedema, dermatitis, fat necrosis, Henoch-Schönlein purpura, idiopathic scrotal edema.

SEIZURE

ICD-10CM # R56.9 Unspecified convulsions

Syncope.
Alcohol abuse/withdrawal.
TIA.
Hemiparetic migraine.
Psychiatric disorders.
Carotid sinus hypersensitivity.
Hyperventilation, prolonged breath holding.
Hypoglycemia.
Narcolepsy.
Movement disorders (tics, hemiballismus).
Hyponatremia.
Brain tumor (primary or metastatic).
Tetanus.
Strychnine, phencyclidine poisoning.

SEIZURE, PEDIATRIC[43]

ICD-10CM # R56.9 Unspecified convulsions
            P90   Convulsions of newborn

FIRST MONTH OF LIFE
First Day
Hypoxia.

Drugs.
Trauma.
Infection.
Hyperglycemia.
Hypoglycemia.
Pyridoxine deficiency.
Day 2 to 3
Infection.
Drug withdrawal.
Hypoglycemia.
Hypocalcemia.
Developmental malformation.
Intracranial hemorrhage.
Inborn error of metabolism.
Hyponatremia or hypernatremia.
Day >4
Infection.
Hypocalcemia.
Hyperphosphatemia.
Hyponatremia.
Developmental malformation.
Drug withdrawal.
Inborn error of metabolism.

1 TO 6 MO
As above.

6 MO TO 3 YR
Febrile seizures.
Birth injury.
Infection.
Toxin.
Trauma.
Metabolic disorder.
Cerebral degenerative disease.

>3 YR
Idiopathic.
Infection.
Trauma.
Cerebral degenerative disease.

SEIZURE MIMICS[18]

ICD-10CM # Varies with specific diagnosis

NONEPILEPTIC EPISODIC DISORDERS THAT MAY RESEMBLE SEIZURES

Movement disorders: myoclonus, paroxysmal choreoathetosis, episodic ataxias, hyperexplexia (startle disease).
Migraine: confusional, vertebrobasilar, visual auras.
Syncope.
Behavioral and psychiatric: psychogenic non-epileptic attacks (pseudoseizures), hyperventilation syndrome, panic or anxiety disorder, dissociative states.
Cataplexy (usually associated with narcolepsy).
Transient ischemic attack.
Alcoholic blackouts.
Hypoglycemia.

SEIZURES, NEONATAL, DUE TO NEUROCUTANEOUS DISORDERS[20]

ICD-10CM # Varies with specific diagnosis

INCONTINENTIA PIGMENTI

Seizure type.
  Neonatal seizures.
Generalized tonic-clonic.
Cutaneous manifestations.
Erythematous bullae (newborn).
Pigmentary whorls (infancy).
Depigmented areas (childhood).

LINEAR NEVUS SEBACEOUS SYNDROME

Seizure type.
  Infantile spasms.
  Lennox-Gastaut syndrome.
  Generalized tonic-clonic.
Cutaneous manifestation.
  Linear facial sebaceous nevus.

NEUROFIBROMATOSIS

Seizure type.
  Generalized tonic-clonic.
  Partial complex.
  Partial simple motor.
Cutaneous manifestations.
  Cafe au lait spots.
  Axillary freckles.
  Neural tumors.

STURGE-WEBER SYNDROME

Seizure type.
  Epilepsia partialis continua.
  Partial simple motor.
  Status epilepticus.
Cutaneous manifestation.
  Hemifacial hemangioma.

TUBEROUS SCLEROSIS

Seizure type.
  Neonatal seizures.
  Infantile spasms.
  Lennox-Gastaut syndrome.
  Generalized tonic-clonic.
  Partial simple motor.
  Partial complex.

CUTANEOUS MANIFESTATIONS

Abnormal hair pigmentation.
Adenoma sebaceum.
Café-au-lait spots.
Depigmented areas.
Shagreen patch.

SEIZURES, NEONATAL PEAK TIME OF ONSET[20]

ICD-10CM # Varies with specific diagnosis

24 HOURS

Bacterial meningitis and sepsis.[a]
Direct drug effect.
Hypoxic-ischemic encephalopathy.[a]
Intrauterine infection.
Intraventricular hemorrhage at term.[a]
Laceration of tentorium or falx.
Pyridoxine dependency.[a]
Subarachnoid hemorrhage.*

24 TO 72 HOURS

Bacterial meningitis and sepsis.[a]
Cerebral contusion with subdural hemorrhage.
Cerebral dysgenesis.[a]
Cerebral infarction.[a]
Drug withdrawal.
Glycine encephalopathy.
Glycogen synthase deficiency.
Hypoparathyroidism-hypocalcemia.
Idiopathic cerebral venous thrombosis.
Incontinentia pigmenti.
Intracerebral hemorrhage.
Intraventricular hemorrhage in premature newborns.[a]
Pyridoxine dependency.[a]
Subarachnoid hemorrhage.
Tuberous sclerosis.
Urea cycle disturbances.

72 HOURS TO 1 WEEK

Cerebral dysgenesis.
Cerebral infarction.[a]
Familial neonatal seizures.
Hypoparathyroidism.
Idiopathic cerebral venous thrombosis.[a]
Intracerebral hemorrhage.
Kernicterus.
Methylmalonic acidemia.
Nutritional hypocalcemia.[a]
Propionic acidemia.
Tuberous sclerosis.
Urea cycle disturbances.

1 TO 4 WEEKS

Adrenoleukodystrophy, neonatal.
Cerebral dysgenesis.
Fructose dysmetabolism.
Gaucher disease type 2.
GM1 gangliosidosis type 1.
Herpes simplex encephalitis.[a]
Idiopathic cerebral venous thrombosis.[a]
Ketotic hyperglycinemias.
Maple syrup urine disease, neonatal.[a]
Tuberous sclerosis.
Urea cycle disturbances.

---

[a]Denotes the most common conditions and the ones with disease-modifying treatments.

SEXUAL DIFFERENTIATION ABNORMALITIES[89]

ICD-10CM # Varies with specific diagnosis

ABNORMAL SEXUAL DIFFERENTIATION

Disorders of gonadal differentiation.
  Seminiferous tubule dysgenesis.
  Klinefelter syndrome.
  46,XX male.
  Syndromes of gonadal dysgenesis:
    Turner syndrome.
    Pure gonadal dysgenesis.
    Mixed gonadal dysgenesis.
    Partial gonadal dysgenesis (dysgenetic male pseudohermaphroditism).
    Bilateral vanishing testis, testicular regression syndromes.
Ovotesticular DSD (true hermaphroditism).
46,XX DSD (masculinized female):
  Congenital adrenal hyperplasia (21-hydroxylase, 11β-hydroxylase, 3β-hydroxysteroid dehydrogenase deficiencies).
Maternal androgens.
46,XY DSD (undermasculinized male).
  Leydig cell agenesis, unresponsiveness.
  Disorders of testosterone biosynthesis.
  Variants of congenital adrenal hyperplasia affecting corticosteroid and testosterone synthesis:
    StAR deficiency (congenital lipoid adrenal hyperplasia).
    Cytochrome P450 oxidoreductase (POR) deficiency.
    3β-Hydroxysteroid dehydrogenase deficiency.
    17β-Hydroxylase deficiency.
Disorders of testosterone biosynthesis:
  17, 20-Lyase deficiency.
  17β-Hydroxysteroid oxidoreductase deficiency.
Disorders of androgen-dependent target tissue:
  Androgen receptor and postreceptor defects.
  Syndrome of complete (severe) androgen insensitivity.
  Syndrome of partial androgen insensitivity.
  Mild androgen insensitivity syndrome (MAIS).
Disorders of testosterone metabolism by peripheral tissues:
  5α-Reductase deficiency.
  Disorders of synthesis, secretion, or response to müllerian-inhibiting substance.
Persistent müllerian duct syndrome.
Unclassified forms:
  In females: Mayer-Rokitansky-Küster-Hauser syndrome.
  Disorder of sex development (DSD).

SEXUAL DYSFUNCTION, FEMALE[18]

ICD-10CM # R37 Sexual dysfunction, unspecified

FACTORS THAT MAY INFLUENCE SEXUAL FUNCTIONING IN WOMEN
Biological
Medications (e.g., antidepressants, antihypertensives).
Vaginal atrophy, pain with intercourse.
Low testosterone levels (e.g., bilateral oophorectomy).
Illness (e.g., diabetes, hypothyroidism, cerebrovascular accident).
Sleep disturbances, fatigue.
Disability or pain from illness (e.g., arthritis).
Incontinence.
Psychological
Depression.
Body image.
Interpersonal
Marital issues.
Poor communication.
Partner's sexual problems (e.g., erectile dysfunction).
Partner's health problems (e.g., myocardial infarction).
Sociocultural
Ageism ("too old" to want sex).
Multiple other obligations and commitments.
Lack of partner.

SEXUALLY TRANSMITTED DISEASES, ANORECTAL REGION[10]

ICD-10CM #	K62.89	Other specified diseases of anus and rectum

ULCERATIVE
Lymphogranuloma venereum.
Herpes simplex virus.
Early (primary) syphilis.
Chancroid (*Haemophilus ducreyi*).
Cytomegalovirus.
Idiopathic (usually HIV positive).

NONULCERATIVE
Condyloma acuminatum.
Gonorrhea.
Chlamydia (*Chlamydia trachomatis*).
Syphilis.

SEXUAL PRECOCITY[113]

ICD-10CM #	E30.1	Precocious puberty
	E30.8	Other disorders of puberty

TRUE PRECOCIOUS PUBERTY
Premature reactivation of LHRH pulse generator.

INCOMPLETE SEXUAL PRECOCITY
(Pituitary gonadotropin independent).
Males
Chorionic gonadotropin-secreting tumor.
Leydig cell tumor.
Familial testotoxicosis.
Virilizing congenital adrenal hyperplasia.
Virilizing adrenal tumor.

Premature adrenarche.
Females
Granulosa cell tumor (follicular cysts may be manifested similarly).
Follicular cyst.
Feminizing adrenal tumor.
Premature thelarche.
Premature adrenarche.
Late-onset virilizing congenital adrenal hyperplasia.
In Both Sexes
McCune-Albright syndrome.
Primary hypothyroidism.

SHOULDER PAIN

ICD-10CM #	M24.819	Other specific joint derangements of unspecified shoulder, not elsewhere classified
	M75.80	Other shoulder lesions, unspecified shoulder
	S43.409A	Unspecified sprain of unspecified shoulder joint, initial encounter
	S46.919A	Strain of unspecified muscle, fascia and tendon at shoulder and upper arm level, unspecified arm, initial encounter

WITH LOCAL FINDINGS IN SHOULDER
Trauma: contusion, fracture, muscle strain, trauma to spinal cord.
Arthrosis, arthritis, RA, ankylosing spondylitis.
Bursitis, synovitis, tendinitis, tenosynovitis.
Aseptic (avascular) necrosis.
Local infection: septic arthritis, osteomyelitis, abscess, herpes zoster, TB.

WITHOUT LOCAL FINDINGS IN SHOULDER
Cardiovascular disorders: ischemic heart disease, pericarditis, aortic aneurysm.
Subdiaphragmatic abscess, liver abscess.
Cholelithiasis, cholecystitis.
Pulmonary lesions: apical bronchial carcinoma, pleurisy, pneumothorax, pneumonia.
GI lesions: PUD, gastric neoplasm, peptic esophagitis.
Pancreatic lesions: carcinoma, calculi, pancreatitis.
CNS abnormalities: neoplasm, vascular abnormalities.
Multiple sclerosis.
Syringomyelia.
Polymyositis/dermatomyositis.
Psychogenic.
Polymyalgia rheumatica.
Ectopic pregnancy.

SHOULDER PAIN BY LOCATION

ICD-10CM #	M75.80	Other shoulder lesions, unspecified shoulder
	S43.499A	Other sprain of unspecified shoulder joint, initial encounter
	S46.019A	Strain of muscle(s) and tendon(s) of the rotator cuff of unspecified shoulder, initial encounter
	S46.819A	Strain of other muscles, fascia and tendons at shoulder and upper arm level, unspecified arm, initial encounter

TOP OF SHOULDER (C4)
Cervical source.
Acromioclavicular.
Sternoclavicular.
Diaphragmatic.

SUPEROLATERAL (C5)
Rotator cuff tendinitis.
Impingement.
Adhesive capsulitis.
Glenohumeral arthritis.

ANTERIOR
Bicipital tendinitis and rupture.
Glenoid labral tear.
Adhesive capsulitis.
Glenohumeral arthritis.
Osteonecrosis.

AXILLARY
Neoplasm (Pancoast, mediastinal).
Herpes zoster.

SHOULDER PAIN, IN DIFFERENT AGE GROUPS[41]

ICD-10CM #	M25.519	Pain in unspecified shoulder

COMMON CAUSES OF SHOULDER PAIN IN DIFFERENT AGE GROUPS
Childhood (2 to 10 yr)
Intraarticular
Instability.
Periarticular
Osteochondromas.
Adolescence (10 to 18 yr)
Intraarticular
Instability.
Early Adulthood (18 to 30 yr)
Intraarticular
Instability.
Acromioclavicular joint sprain.
Periarticular
Calcific tendonitis.
Impingement.

Shoulder Pain (continued)

Referred
Cervical.
Adulthood (30 to 60 yr)
Intraarticular
Osteochondritis.
Osteoarthritis.
Frozen shoulder.
Inflammatory arthritis.
Periarticular
Calcific tendonitis.
Impingement.
Rotator cuff tear.
Bicipital tendonitis.
Referred
Cervical.
Old Age (>60 yr)
Intraarticular
Osteochondritis.
Osteoarthritis.
Frozen shoulder.
Inflammatory arthritis.
Periarticular
Impingement.
Rotator cuff tear.
Referred
Cervical.

SINOVENOUS OCCLUSIVE DISEASE, INTRACRANIAL[38]

ICD-10CM # Varies with specific diagnosis

Facial/orbital/paranasal sinuses/middle ear infections.
Trichinosis.
Syphilis.
Varicella-zoster virus infections.
Human immunodeficiency virus infections.
Sepsis.
Pregnancy and puerperium.
Carcinoma.
Dehydration.
Marasmus.
L-Asparaginase therapy.
Androgen therapy.
Cisplatin and etoposide therapy.
Epsilon-aminocaproic acid therapy.
Medroxyprogesterone therapy.
Cis-diamminedichloroplatinum (CDDP) and etoposide (VP-16) therapy.
IV catheters, cardiac pacemakers.
Polyarteritis nodosa.
Systemic lupus erythematosus.
Granulomatosis with polyangiitis.
Behçet disease.
Kohlmeier-Degos disease (malignant atrophic papulosis).
Osteopetrosis.
Inflammatory bowel disease.
Sarcoidosis.
Osteoporosis.
Congestive heart failure.
Nephrotic syndrome.
Budd-Chiari syndrome.
Chronic lung disease.
Diabetes mellitus.
Cerebral arterial occlusions.
Homocystinuria.
Head injury.
Paroxysmal nocturnal hemoglobinuria.
Sickle cell disease and trait.
Polycythemla vera.
Essential thrombocythemia.
Iron-deficiency anemia.
Hypoplasminogenemia.
Afibrinogenemia.
Cryofibrinogenemia.
Antiphospholipid antibody syndrome (APAS).
Disseminated intravascular coagulation.
Antithrombin deficiency.
Protein S deficiency.
Protein C deficiency.
Combined deficiencies (protein C, protein S, and antithrombin III).
Activated protein C resistance.
Factor V Leiden mutation.
Prothrombin G20210 mutation.
Elevated factor VIII plasma levels.
Heparin-induced thrombocytopenia.
Maternal coagulopathy (twin transfusion reaction).
Familial histidine-rich glycoprotein deficiency.
Arteriovenous malformations.
Sturge-Weber syndrome.
Neoplasm (meningioma, metastasis, glomus tumors).
Idiopathic.

SINUS NODE DYSFUNCTION[59]

ICD-10CM # Varies with specific diagnosis

CAUSES OF SINUS NODE DYSFUNCTION
Intrinsic
Hypothyroidism.
Fibrocalcific degeneration.
Increased vagal tone, especially in sleep apnea.
Congenital mutations.
Scleroderma.
Amyloidosis.
Chagas disease.
Extrinsic
Trauma, including cardiac surgery.
Drugs:
Calcium-channel blockers.
β-Blockers.
Digoxin.
Antiarrhythmic medications (amiodarone, dronedarone, sotalol, flecainide, propafenone).
Lithium.

SINUS OF VALSALVA ANEURYSMS[37]

ICD-10CM # Varies with specific diagnosis

Congenital: single cusp involved with normal aorta.
Localized deficiency of the tissue in the aortic annulus.
Retraction of a cusp into a closing ventricular septal defect.
Inherited: all cusps involved with annuloaortic ectasia.
Marfan syndrome.
Ehlers-Danlos syndrome.
Acquired: saccular false aneurysms.
Aortic root abscess with endocarditis.
Luetic aortitis.
Aortic dissection.

SINUS OSTIAL OBSTRUCTION[42]

ICD-10CM # Varies with specific diagnosis

FACTORS THAT PREDISPOSE TO SINUS OSTIAL OBSTRUCTION
Mucosal Swelling
Systemic factors:
Viral upper respiratory infection.
Allergic inflammation.
Cystic fibrosis.
Immune disorders.
Ciliary dyskinesia.
Tobacco smoke.
Local insult:
Facial trauma.
Swimming, diving.
Rhinitis medicamentosa.
Nasal intubation.
Mechanical Obstruction
Choanal atresia.
Deviated septum.
Nasal polyps.
Foreign body.
Tumor.
Ethmoid bullae.

SINUS TACHYCARDIA[27]

ICD-10CM # R00.0 Tachycardia, unspecified

DIFFERENTIAL DIAGNOSIS OF SINUS TACHYCARDIA
Etiologic Category
Specific Disorders
Hemodynamic:
Heart failure: systolic and diastolic heart failure caused by ischemic, valvular, or non-ischemic myopathy.

Differential Diagnosis

II

Loss of circulating blood volume: GI bleeding, anemia, shifts of intravascular fluid due to changes in colloidal osmotic pressure or inflammation.

Septic shock: dehydration.

Vascular shunts: intracardiac as well as aortovenous malformations, fistulas.

Pulmonary embolism.

Metabolic and neurohumoral:

Sepsis: infections and inflammatory conditions.

Hyperthyroidism.

Paget disease of the bone.

Pheochromocytoma.

Carcinoid syndrome.

Beriberi heart disease.

Carcinoma.

Hyperpyrexia.

Acidosis.

Exercise.

Pharmacologic:

Sympathomimetic agents: isoproterenol, epinephrine, or dopamine.

Vagolytic agents, atropine, scopolamine.

Vasodilators: nitrates, angiotensin-converting enzyme inhibitors, angiotensin receptor blockers, hydrazine, as well as centrally acting vasodilators.

Thyroid preparations, caffeine and nicotine.

Bronchodilators, including theophylline and terbutaline.

Anesthetic agents, including spinal anesthetics, causing peripheral vasodilation.

Drugs of abuse: amphetamines, cocaine, "ecstasy," cannabis.

Neurologic/psychological:

Pain.

Fear, anxiety, and hysteria.

Hyper-β adrenergic phase of neurocardiogenic syncope.

Autonomic dysfunction such as with diabetes.

SKIN AND RENAL[11]

ICD-10CM #   Varies with specific diagnosis

SELECTED CONDITIONS WITH CONCURRENT SKIN AND RENAL INVOLVEMENT

More Common

Lupus erythematosus.

Leukocytoclastic vasculitis.

Henoch-Schönlein purpura.

Mixed cryoglobulinemia.

Diabetes mellitus.

Systemic vasculitis.

Less Common

Nail-patella syndrome.

Hemolytic-uremic syndrome.

Toxic shock syndrome.

Mixed connective tissue disease.

Dermatomyositis.

Rheumatoid arthritis.

Sjögren syndrome.

Dermatitis herpetiformis.

Sarcoidosis.

Systemic sclerosis.

Ulcerative colitis.

Amyloidosis.

Toxic epidermolysis.

Hypothyroidism.

Graves disease.

Fabry disease.

Neurofibromatosis.

Hurler syndrome.

Castleman disease.

Infectious endocarditis.

Staphylococcal scalded skin syndrome (in adults).

SKIN INDURATION, CHRONIC[90]

ICD-10CM #   Varies with specific diagnosis

CONDITIONS ASSOCIATED WITH CHRONIC SKIN INDURATION

Systemic sclerosis.

Localized scleroderma.

Scleroderma variants.

Scleredema:

Scleredema adultorum of Buschke.

Scleredema diabeticorum.

Scleredema neonatorum.

Scleromyxedema.

Nephrogenic fibrosing dermopathy.

Eosinophilic syndromes:

Eosinophilic fasciitis (diffuse fasciitis with eosinophilia, Shulman disease).

Eosinophilia-myalgia syndrome.

Toxic oil syndrome.

Chronic graft-versus-host disease.

Pseudoscleroderma (local injection of vitamin K, bleomycin, pentazocine).

Metabolic diseases:

Porphyria cutanea tarda.

Phenylketonuria.

Werner syndrome.

Acromegaly.

Pachydermoperiostosis.

Polyneuropathy, organomegaly, endocrinopathy, monoclonal gammopathy (POEMS).

Stiff skin syndrome.

Reflex sympathetic dystrophy.

Hemiplegia.

SKIN, THICKENED AND TETHERED[96]

ICD-10CM #   Varies with specific diagnosis

CREST syndrome, scleroderma, or mixed connective tissue disease.

Eosinophilic fasciitis.

Localized morphea—small areas of sclerosis.

Chemicals—vinyl chloride, pentazocine, bleomycin, toxic oil syndrome.

Pseudoscleroderma—secondary to porphyria cutanea tarda, acromegaly, carcinoid syndrome.

Scleredema—people with diabetes develop thick skin over the shoulders and upper back.

Graft-versus-host disease.

Silicosis.

SLEEP-RELATED HALLUCINATIONS[50]

ICD-10CM #   Varies with specific diagnosis

HYPNAGOGIC AND HYPNOPOMPIC HALLUCINATIONS

Sleep deprivation.[‡]

Narcolepsy.[§,¶]

COMPLEX NOCTURNAL VISUAL HALLUCINATIONS

Parkinson disease.[§,**, ††, ‡‡, §§]

Dementia with Lewy bodies.[¶¶,***]

Peduncular hallucinosis.[**, †††, ‡‡‡, §§§]

Charles Bonnet syndrome.[**,¶¶¶]

Schizophrenia.[**]

Metabolic encephalopathy.[**]

Posterior cerebral artery infarction.[**]

Delirium tremens.[**]

Migraine.[**]

Focal epilepsy.[**]

[‡]American Academy of Sleep Medicine: *International classification of sleep disorders*, ed 3. Darien, 2014, American Academy of Sleep Medicine.

[§]Leu-Semenescu S et al: Hallucinations in narcolepsy with and without cataplexy: contrasts with Parkinson disease, *Sleep Med* 12:497-504, 2011.

[¶]Szucs A et al: Misleading hallucinations in unrecognized narcolepsy, *Acta Psychiatr Scand* 108:314-317, 2003.

[**]Manford M, Andermann F: Complex visual hallucinations, *Brain* 121:1819-1840, 1998.

[††]Kulisevsky J, Roldan E: Hallucinations and sleep disturbances in Parkinson's disease, *Neurology* 63(Suppl 3):S28-S30, 2004.

[‡‡]Arnulf I et al: Hallucinations, REM sleep, Parkinson's disease, *Neurology* 55:281-288, 2000.

[§§]Arnulf I et al: Parkinson's disease and sleepiness. An integral part of PD, *Neurology* 58:1019-1024, 2002.

[¶¶]McKeith IG et al: Diagnosis and management of dementia with Lewy bodies: fourth consensus report of the DLB Consortium, *Neurology* 89:88-100, 2017.

[***]Tiraboschi P et al: Absence of rapid eye movement sleep with hypnopompic visual hallucinations; a possible harbinger of dementia with Lewy bodies, *Sleep Med* 14:377-379, 2013.

[†††]Benke T: Peduncular hallucinosis, *J Neurol* 253:1561-1571, 2006.

[‡‡‡]Cervera A et al: Sleep studies in two patients with pontine haematomas and "peduncular" hallucinosis, *J Neurol* 246(Suppl 1):139, 1999.

[§§§]Vetrugno R et al: Peduncullar hallucinosis: a polysomnographic and SPECT study of a patient and efficacy of serotonergic therapy, *Sleep Med* 10:1158-1160, 2009.

[¶¶¶]Lerario A et al: Charles Bonnet syndrome: two case reports and review of the literature, *J Neurol* 260:1180-1186, 2013.

Guillain-Barré syndrome.[****]
Sleepwalking.[‡,††††,‡‡‡‡]
Night terrors.[‡,††††]
Idiopathic hypersomnia.[§§§§]
Anxiety disorder.[§§§§]
Acute alcohol withdrawal.[¶¶¶¶]
Acute barbiturate withdrawal.[§§§§]
Acute benzodiazepine withdrawal.[§§§§]
Lipophilic beta blockers.[‡,††††]
Dopaminergic agents.[‡,††††]

Substances with hallucinogenic properties, such as mescaline, LSD, amphetamine, and cocaine.[‡,††††]

[****]De Cock VC et al: Vivid dreams, hallucinations, psychosis and REM sleep in Guillain-Barré syndrome, *Brain* 128:2535-2545, 2005.

[††††]Rao SC, Silber MH: Sleep-related hallucinations and exploding head syndrome. In Thorpy MJ, Plazzi G (eds.): *The parasomnias and other related sleep-related movement disorders*, 2010, Cambridge University Press,194-201, Cambridge, United Kingdom.

[‡‡‡‡]Mantoan L et al: Adult-onset NREM parasomnia with hypnopompic hallucinatory pain: a case report, *Sleep* 36:287-290, 2013.

[§§§§]Silber MH et al: Complex nocturnal visual hallucinations, *Sleep Med* 6:363-366, 2005.

[¶¶¶¶]The US Xyrem Multicenter Study Group: A randomized, double blind, placebo-controlled multicenter trial comparing the effects of three doses of orally administrated sodium oxybate with placebo for the treatment of narcolepsy, *Sleep* 25:42-49, 2002.

SLEEPTALKING[50]

ICD-10CM #   Varies with specific diagnosis

Confusional arousals.[*****]
Night terrors.[*****]
Sleepwalking.[*****]
Sleep-related eating syndrome.[†††††]
Sexsomnia.[‡‡‡‡‡]
REM   sleep   behavior disorder.[§§§§§,¶¶¶¶,******,††††††]
Status dissociatus.[‡‡‡‡‡‡]

[*****]Oudiette D et al: Dreamlike mentations during sleepwalking and sleep terrors in adults, *Sleep* 32:1621-1627, 2009.

[†††††]Vinai P et al: Defining the borders between sleep-related eating disorder and night eating syndrome, *Sleep Med* 13:686-690, 2012.

[‡‡‡‡‡]Schenck CH et al: Sleep and sex: what can go wrong? A review of the literature on sleep related disorders and abnormal sexual behaviors and experiences, *Sleep* 30:683-702, 2007.

[§§§§§]Iranzo A et al: The clinical and pathophysiological relevance of REM sleep behavior disorder in neurodegenerative diseases, *Sleep Med Rev* 13:385-401, 2009.

[¶¶¶¶¶]Santamaria J et al: Relation between dream content and movement intensity in REM behavior disorder, *Sleep* 27(Suppl):A289, 2003.

[******]De Cock VC et al: Restoration of normal control in Parkinson's disease during REM sleep, *Brain* 130:450-456, 2007.

[††††††]De Cock VC et al: The improvement of movement and speech during rapid eye movement sleep behavior disorder in multiple system atrophy, *Brain* 134:856-862, 2011.

[‡‡‡‡‡‡]Mahowald MW, Schenck CH: Dissociated states of wakefulness and sleep, *Neurology* 42(Suppl 6):44-52, 1992.

Parasomnia overlap disorder.[§§§§§§]
Agrypnia excitata.[¶¶¶¶¶¶]
Anti-IgLON5 disease.[*******]
Sleep-related hypermotor epilepsy.[†††††††]
Periodic limb movement disorder.[‡‡‡‡‡‡‡]
Obstructive sleep apnea.[§§§§§§§]
Nocturnal panic attacks.[†††††††]
Sleep-related dissociative disorder.[†††††††]

[§§§§§§]Schenck CH et al: A parasomnia overlap disorder involving sleepwalking, sleep terrors, and REM sleep behavior disorder in 33 polysomnographic confirmed cases, *Sleep* 20:972-981, 1997.

[¶¶¶¶¶¶]Provini F: Agrypnia excitata, *Curr Neurol Neurosci Rep* 13:341, 2013.

[*******]Sabater L et al: A novel non-rapid-eye movement and rapid-eye-movement parasomnia with sleep breathing disorder associated with antibodies to IgLON5: an observational study: a case series, characterisation of the antigen, and postmortem study, *Lancet Neurol* 13:575-586, 2014.

[†††††††]American Academy of Sleep Medicine: *International classification of sleep disorders*, ed 3, Darien, 2014, American Academy of Sleep Medicine.

[‡‡‡‡‡‡‡]Gaig C et al: Periodic limb movements during sleep mimicking REM sleep behavior disorder: a new form of periodic limb movement disorder, *Sleep* 40(3), 2017, http://dx.doi.org/10.1093/sleep/zsw063.

[§§§§§§§]Iranzo A, Santamaria J: Severe obstructive sleep apnea/hypopnea syndrome mimicking REM sleep behavior disorder, *Sleep* 28:203-206, 2005.

SMALL BOWEL MASSES[2]

ICD-10CM #   Varies with specific diagnosis

Cyst:
  Mesenteric cyst.
Tumor:
  Benign.
  Malignant.
Intussusception.
Inflammation:
  Crohn disease.

SMALL BOWEL OBSTRUCTION[10]

ICD-10CM #	K56.5	Intestinal adhesions [bands] with obstruction (postprocedural) (postinfection)
	Q41.9	Congenital absence, atresia and stenosis of small intestine, part unspecified

INTRINSIC

Congenital (atresia, stenosis).
Inflammatory (Crohn, radiation enteritis).
Neoplasms (metastatic or primary).
Intussusception.
Traumatic (hematoma).

EXTRINSIC

Hernias (internal and external).
Adhesions.
Volvulus.

Compressing masses (tumors, abscesses, hematomas).

INTRALUMINAL

Foreign body.
Gallstones.
Bezoars.
Barium.
Ascaris infestation.

SMALL INTESTINE ULCERATION

ICD-10CM #   K63.3   Ulcer of intestine

Inflammatory bowel disease.
Celiac disease.
Vasculitis, SLE, Behçet syndrome.
Uremia.
Infections (*Campylobacter*, TB, *Yersinia*, parasites, typhoid, cytomegalovirus [CMV], *Clostridium*).
Mesenteric insufficiency.
Neoplasms.
Radiation.
Drugs (salicylates, potassium, indomethacin, antimetabolites).
Meckel diverticulum.
Zollinger-Ellison syndrome.
Lymphocytic enterocolitis.
Stomal ulceration.

SMELL DISTURBANCE

ICD-10CM #   R43.8   Other disturbances of smell and taste

Upper respiratory tract infection.
Nasal or paranasal sinus disease.
Exposure to noxious vapors.
Head trauma.
Idiopathic.
Dental caries, periodontal disease.
Medications.

SODIUM RETENTION, RENAL CAUSES[11]

ICD-10CM #   Varies with specific diagnosis

CAUSES OF RENAL SODIUM RETENTION

Primary
Oliguric acute kidney injury.
Chronic kidney disease.
Glomerular disease.
Severe bilateral renal artery stenosis.
Na+-retaining tubulopathies (genetic).
Mineralocorticoid excess.
Secondary
Heart failure.
Cirrhosis.
Idiopathic edema.

SOFT TISSUE MASS MIMICKING MALIGNANCY[52]

ICD-10CM #   Varies with specific diagnosis

Differential Diagnosis

II

OVERVIEW OF DISEASES THAT CAN PRESENT AS A SOFT TISSUE MASS MIMICKING MALIGNANCY

Etiology	Disease Entity
Trauma:	Muscle contusion.
	Hematoma.
	Muscle herniation.
	Calcific myonecrosis.
	Hypothenar hammer syndrome.
	Myositis ossificans.
Metabolic:	Diabetic myopathy.
	Gout.
	Pseudogout.
	Calcific tendinosis.
Congenital:	Accessory muscle.
Infectious:	Necrotizing fasciitis.
	Abscess.
	Pyomyositis.
	Hydatid cystic disease.
	Cat-scratch disease.
	Actinomycosis.
Inflammation:	Bursitis.
	Sarcoidosis.
	Foreign body reaction.
	Injection granuloma.
	Granuloma annulare.
	Epidermal inclusion cyst.
Vascular:	Adventitial cystic disease.
	Pseudoaneurysm.
	Thrombosed vein.
	Arteriovenous vascular malformation.
Miscellane -ous:	Focal myositis.
	Amyloid tumor of soft tissue.

SOFT TISSUE TUMORS, PEDIATRIC PATIENTS[52]

ICD-10CM # Varies with specific diagnosis

PEDIATRIC SOFT TISSUE TUMORS

Vascular lesions:
  Hemangioma of infancy.*
  Congenital hemangioma.
  Hemangioendothelioma (Kasabach-Merritt syndrome).
  Arteriovenous malformation.
  Venous malformations.
  Lymphatic malformation (lymphangioma, cystic hygroma).
  Capillary malformation.
Adipocytic tumors:
  Lipoma.
  Lipoblastoma.
  Liposarcoma.
Fibrohistiocytic tumors:
  Pigmented villonodular synovitis.
  Giant cell tumor of tendon sheath.
Fibroblastic and myofibroblastic tumors:
  Nodular fasciitis.
  Fibrous hamartoma of infancy.

*Lesions with MR-specific features.

Myofibroma, myofibromatosis.
Infantile fibrosarcoma.
Fibromatosis colli.
Neurogenic tumors:
  Schwannoma.
  Neurofibroma.
  Malignant nerve sheath tumor.
Leiomyoma
Rhabdomyosarcoma
Tumors of uncertain differentiation
  Synovial cell sarcoma.
  Primitive neuroectodermal tumor (Ewing sarcoma).
Pilomatricoma

SORE THROAT[43]

ICD-10CM # J02 Acute pharyngitis

DIFFERENTIAL DIAGNOSIS FOR SORE THROAT

Infectious Causes
Aerobes
Common:
  Streptococcus pyogenes (GABHS).
  Peptostreptococcus spp.
  Nongroup A *Streptococcus*.
  Neisseria gonorrhoeae.
  Neisseria meningitides.
  Mycoplasma pneumoniae.
  Arcanobacterium hemolyticum.
  Chlamydia trachomatis.
  Staphylococcus aureus.
Uncommon:
  Haemophilus influenzae.
  Haemophilus parainfluenzae.
  Coccidioides spp.
  Corynebacterium diphtheriae.
  Streptococcus pneumoniae.
  Yersinia enterocolitica.
  Treponema pallidum.
  Francisella tularensis.
  Legionella pneumophila.
  Mycobacterium spp.

ANAEROBES
Bacteroides spp.
Peptococcus spp.
Clostridium spp.
Fusobacterium spp.
Prevotella spp.

OTHER
Candida spp.

VIRAL
Rhinovirus.
Adenovirus.
Coronavirus.
Herpes simplex 1, 2.
Influenza A, B.
Parainfluenza.

Cytomegalovirus.
Epstein-Barr.
Varicella-zoster.
Hepatitis virus.
Noninfectious Causes

SYSTEMIC
Kawasaki disease.
Stevens-Johnson syndrome.
Cyclic neutropenia.
Thyroiditis.
Connective tissue disease.

TRAUMA, MISCELLANEOUS
Penetrating injury.
Angioneurotic edema.
Retained foreign body.
Anomalous aortic arch.
Laryngeal fracture.
Calcific retropharyngeal tendinitis.
Retropharyngeal hematoma.
Caustic exposure.

TUMOR
Tongue.
Larynx.
Thyroid.
Leukemia.

SPASTIC PARAPLEGIAS

ICD-10CM # G82.20 Paraplegia, unspecified

Cervical spondylosis.
Friedreich ataxia.
Multiple sclerosis.
Spinal cord tumor.
HIV.
Tertiary syphilis.
Vitamin B_{12} deficiency.
Spinocerebellar ataxias.
Syringomyelia.
Spinal cord AV malformations.
Adrenoleukodystrophy.

SPINAL CORD COMPRESSION, EPIDURAL

ICD-10CM # Varies with specific diagnosis

Osteoarthritis.
Meningioma.
Spinal epidural abscess.
Spinal epidural hematoma.
Spinal epidural vascular malformations.
RA.
Metastatic cancer (vertebral, intramedullary, leptomeninges).
Radiation myelopathy.
Neurofibroma.
Sarcoidosis.
Paraneoplastic myelopathy.
Histiocytosis.

SPINAL CORD DYSFUNCTION

ICD-10CM #	G95.9	Disease of spinal cord, unspecified
	Q07.9	Congenital malformation of nervous system, unspecified
	D51.1	Vitamin B_{12} deficiency anemia due to selective vitamin B_{12} malabsorption with proteinuria
	D51.3	Other dietary vitamin B_{12} deficiency anemia
	D51.8	Other vitamin B_{12} deficiency anemias
	G95.89	Other specified diseases of spinal cord
	G95.19	Other vascular myelopathies

Trauma.
Multiple sclerosis.
Transverse myelitis.
Neoplasm (primary, metastatic).
Syringomyelia.
Spinal epidural abscess.
HIV myelopathy.
Diskitis.
Spinal epidural hematoma.
Spinal cord infarction.
Spinal AV malformation.
Subarachnoid hemorrhage.

SPINAL CORD DYSFUNCTION, NONTRAUMATIC[43]

ICD-10CM #	Q07.9	Congenital malformation of nervous system, unspecified

NONTRAUMATIC ETIOLOGIES OF SPINAL CORD DYSFUNCTION
Processes Affecting the Spinal Cord or Blood Supply Directly
Multiple sclerosis.
Transverse myelitis.
Spinal arteriovenous malformation/subarachnoid hemorrhage.
Syringomyelia.
HIV myelopathy.
Other myelopathies.
Spinal cord infarction.
Compressive Lesions Affecting the Spinal Cord
Spinal epidural abscess.
Spinal epidural hematoma.
Diskitis.
Neoplasm.
Metastatic.
Primary CNS.

CNS, Central nervous system; *HIV*, human immunodeficiency virus.

SPINAL CORD ISCHEMIC SYNDROMES[38]

ICD-10CM #	G95.9	Acute infarction of spinal cord

Local mechanical vascular compression.
Regional hemodynamic compromise.
Systemic hypotension.
Occlusive vascular disease.
Thromboembolism.
Endovascular procedures.
Fibrocartilaginous (intervertebral disk) embolism.
Vasculitis.
Arterial dissection.
Thrombosis.
Venous occlusion.

SPINAL TUMORS[24]

ICD-10CM #	Varies with specific diagnosis

EXTRADURAL
Metastases.
Primary bone tumors arising in spine.

INTRADURAL EXTRAMEDULLARY
Meningiomas.
Neurofibromas.
Schwannomas.
Lipomas.
Arachnoid cysts.
Epidermoid cysts.
Metastasis.

INTRAMEDULLARY
Ependymoma.
Glioma.
Hemangioblastoma.
Lipoma.
Metastases.

SPINAL PARAPLEGIA[20]

ICD-10CM #	Varies with specific diagnosis

Congenital malformations.
Arachnoid cyst.
Arteriovenous malformations.
Atlantoaxial dislocation.
Caudal regression syndrome.
Dysraphic states.
Chiari malformation.
Myelomeningocele.
Tethered spinal cord.
Syringomyelia.
Familial spastic paraplegia.
Autosomal dominant.
Autosomal recessive.
X-linked recessive.
Infections.
Asthmatic amyotrophy.
Diskitis.

Epidural abscess.
Herpes zoster myelitis.
Polyradiculoneuropathy.
Tuberculous osteomyelitis.
Lupus myelopathy.
Metabolic disorders.
Adrenomyeloneuropathy (adrenoleukodystrophy).
Argininemia.
Krabbe disease.
Neonatal cord infarction.
Transverse myelitis.
Devic disease.
Encephalomyelitis.
Idiopathic.
Trauma.
Concussion.
Epidural hematoma.
Fracture dislocation.
Neonatal cord trauma.
Tumors.
Astrocytoma.
Ependymoma.
Ewing sarcoma.
Neuroblastoma.

SPLENIC CYSTS, CLASSIFICATION[64]

ICD-10CM #	D73.4	Cyst of spleen

Primary (true).
Parasitic.
Nonparasitic.
Congenital.
Epidermoid.
Dermoid.
Mesothelial (serous).
Transitional.
Neoplastic.
Secondary (false): pseudocysts.
Traumatic.
Degenerative.
Inflammatory.
Hemorrhagic.

SPLENIC MASSES, FOCAL SOLID[15]

ICD-10CM #	Varies with specific diagnosis

FOCAL SOLID SPLENIC MASSES
Benign
Hemangioma.
Hamartoma.
Littoral cell angioma.
Lymphangioma.
Sclerosing angiomatoid nodular transformation (SANT).
Inflammatory pseudotumor.
Malignant
Lymphoma.

Metastases.
Angiosarcoma.
Hemangiopericytoma.
Other
Infarct.

SPLENIC NODULES[15]

ICD-10CM # Varies with specific diagnosis

CAUSES OF SPLENIC NODULES
Infectious
Tuberculosis/*Mycobacterium avium-intra-cellulare* complex.
Pyogenic abscesses.
Histoplasmosis.
Candida abscesses.
Cat-scratch disease.
Pneumocystis jirovecii (formerly *P. carinii* pneumonia).
Inflammatory
Sarcoidosis.
Malignant
Lymphoma.
Metastases.
Other
Gamna-Gandy bodies.
Gaucher disease.

SPLENIC TUMORS, CLASSIFICATION[64]

ICD-10CM # C26.1 Malignant neoplasm of spleen

Malignant.
Lymphoproliferative disease.
Non-Hodgkin lymphoma.
Hodgkin disease.
Hairy cell leukemia.
Chronic lymphocytic leukemia.
Myeloproliferative disease.
Chronic myelogenous leukemia.
Myelofibrosis.
Primary tumors.
Angiosarcoma.
Metastatic tumors.
Benign.
Hemangiomas.
Hamartomas.
Lymphangiomas.
Sclerosing angiomatoid nodular transformation (SANT).

SPLENOMEGALY

ICD-10CM #	R16.1	Splenomegaly, not elsewhere classified
	D73.2	Chronic congestive splenomegaly
	R16.1	Splenomegaly, not elsewhere classified

Hepatic cirrhosis.
Neoplastic involvement: CML, CLL, lymphoma, multiple myeloma.

Bacterial infections: TB, infectious endocarditis, typhoid fever, splenic abscess.
Viral infections: infectious mononucleosis, viral hepatitis, HIV.
Gaucher disease and other lipid storage diseases.
Sarcoidosis.
Parasitic infections (malaria, kala-azar, histoplasmosis).
Hereditary and acquired hemolytic anemias.
Idiopathic thrombocytopenic purpura (ITP).
Collagen vascular disorders: SLE, RA (Felty syndrome), polyarteritis nodosa.
Serum sickness, drug hypersensitivity reaction.
Splenic cysts and benign tumors: hemangioma, lymphangioma.
Thrombosis of splenic or portal vein.
Polycythemia vera, myeloid metaplasia.

SPLENOMEGALY AND HEPATOMEGALY[2]

| ICD-10CM # | R16.1 | Splenomegaly, not elsewhere classified |
| | R16.0 | Hepatomegaly, not elsewhere classified |

CAUSES OF SPLENOMEGALY AND HEPATOSPLENOMEGALY
Massive Splenomegaly
Hematologic disease (e.g., chronic myeloid leukemia, myelofibrosis).
Moderate Splenomegaly
The above causes.
Portal hypertension.
Hematologic disease (e.g., lymphoma, leukemia, thalassemia).
Storage disease (e.g., Gaucher disease).
Small Splenomegaly
The above causes.
Infective (hepatitis, leptospirosis, malaria, bacterial endocarditis).
Hematologic disease (e.g., hemolytic anemias, essential thrombocythemia, polycythemia rubra vera).
Connective tissue diseases or vasculitis (e.g., rheumatoid arthritis, systemic lupus erythematosus, polyarteritis nodosa).
Solitary cyst, polycystic syndrome, hydatid cyst.
Infiltration (amyloid, sarcoid).
Hepatosplenomegaly
Chronic liver disease with portal hypertension.
Hematologic disease (e.g., myeloproliferative disease, lymphoma).
Infection (e.g., amyloid, sarcoid).
Connective tissue disease (e.g., systemic lupus erythematosus).

SPLENOMEGALY AND HYPERSPLENISM[71]

ICD-10CM #	R16.1	Splenomegaly, not elsewhere classified
	D73.1	Hypersplenism
	D73.81	Neutropenic splenomegaly

DIFFERENTIAL DIAGNOSIS OF SPLENOMEGALY AND HYPERSPLENISM
Infections
Acute
Viral (viral hepatitis, infectious mononucleosis, CMV infection).
Bacterial (septicemia, salmonellosis, brucellosis, splenic abscess).
Parasite (toxoplasmosis).
Subacute and Chronic
Subacute bacterial endocarditis.
Tuberculosis.
Malaria.
Kala-azar.
Fungal disease.
Inflammation
Felty syndrome.
SLE.
Serum sickness.
Rheumatic fever.
Sarcoidosis.
ALPS.
Congestive Splenomegaly
Intrahepatic
Cirrhosis.
Extrahepatic
Portal vein obstruction.
Splenic vein obstruction.
Hepatic vein occlusion (Budd-Chiari syndrome).
Chronic Passive Congestion
Heart failure.
Hematologic Disorders
RBC disorders: hemolytic anemias, thalassemia, sickle cell disorders.
Neoplasia
Malignant
MPDs.
Myeloid metaplasia.
Polycythemia rubra vera.
Essential thrombocythemia.
Chronic leukemia.
Chronic myeloid leukemia.
Chronic lymphocytic leukemia.
Hairy cell leukemia.
Lymphoma.
Acute leukemia.
Malignant histiocytosis.
Benign
Hamartoma.
Hemangioma.
Lymphangioma.
Fibroma.
Storage Diseases
Gaucher disease.
Niemann-Pick disease.
Miscellaneous
Amyloidosis.
Cysts.

ALPS, Autoimmune lymphoproliferative syndrome; *CMV*, cytomegalovirus; *MPD*, myeloproliferative disorder; *RBC*, red blood cell; *SLE*, systemic lupus erythematosus.

SPLENOMEGALY, CHILDREN[31]

ICD-10CM # R16.1 Splenomegaly, not elsewhere classified

DISORDERS OF THE BLOOD

Hemolytic anemia: congenital/acquired.
Thalassemia.
Sickle cell disease.
Leukemia.
Osteopetrosis.
Myelofibrosis/myeloid metaplasia/thrombocythemia.

INFECTIONS: ACUTE AND CHRONIC

Viral:
  Congenital (e.g., TORCH association).
  Mononucleosis (e.g., EBV, CMV infection).
  Virus-associated hemophagocytic syndrome.
  HIV.
Bacterial:
  Sepsis/abscess.
  Brucellosis.
  Salmonellosis.
  Tularemia.
  Tuberculosis.
  Subacute bacterial endocarditis.
  Syphilis.
  Lyme disease.
Fungal:
  Histoplasmosis (disseminated).
Rickettsial:
  Rocky Mountain spotted fever.
  Cat-scratch disease.
Parasitic:
  Toxoplasmosis.
  Malaria.
  Leishmaniasis (kala-azar).
  Schistosomiasis.
  Echinococcosis.

HEPATIC/PORTAL SYSTEM DISORDERS

Acute/chronic active hepatitis.
Cirrhosis/hepatic fibrosis/biliary atresia.
Portal or splenic venous obstruction (Banti syndrome).

AUTOIMMUNE DISEASE

Juvenile rheumatoid arthritis.
Systemic lupus erythematosus.
Autoimmune lymphoproliferative syndrome (Canale-Smith syndrome).

NEOPLASMS/CYSTS

Lymphomas (Hodgkin and non-Hodgkin).
Hemangiomas/lymphangiomas.
Hamartomas.
Congenital or acquired (posttraumatic) cysts.

STORAGE DISEASES/INBORN ERRORS OF METABOLISM

Lipidoses: Gaucher disease, Niemann–Pick disease, others.
Mucopolysaccharidoses.
Defects in carbohydrate metabolism: galactosemia, fructose intolerance.
Sea-blue histiocyte syndrome.

MISCELLANEOUS DISORDERS

Histiocytoses:
  Reactive.
  Langerhans cell.
  Malignant.
Sarcoidosis.
Congestive heart failure.
Familial Mediterranean fever.

CMV, Cytomegalovirus; *EBV*, Epstein-Barr virus; *TORCH*, toxoplasmosis, other infections, rubella, cytomegalovirus infection, herpes simplex.

SPONTANEOUS PNEUMOTHORAX[10]

ICD-10CM #	J93.0	Spontaneous tension pneumothorax
	J93.11	Primary spontaneous pneumothorax
	J93.12	Secondary spontaneous pneumothorax

CAUSES OF SECONDARY SPONTANEOUS PNEUMOTHORAX

Airway Disease
Chronic obstructive pulmonary disease.
Asthma.
Cystic fibrosis.
Infections
Necrotizing bacterial pneumonia, lung abscess.
Pneumocystis jiroveci pneumonia.
Tuberculosis.
Interstitial Lung Disease
Sarcoidosis.
Idiopathic pulmonary fibrosis.
Lymphangiomyomatosis.
Tuberous sclerosis.
Pneumoconioses.
Neoplasms
Primary lung cancers.
Pulmonary or pleural metastases.
Miscellaneous
Connective tissue diseases.
Pulmonary infarction.
Endometriosis, catamenial pneumothorax.

STATURAL OVERGROWTH[30]

ICD-10CM # E34.4 Constitutional tall stature

FETAL OVERGROWTH

Maternal diabetes mellitus.

Cerebral gigantism (Sotos syndrome).
Weaver syndrome.
Beckwith-Wiedemann syndrome.
Other insulin-like growth factor 2 (IGF2) excess syndromes.

POSTNATAL OVERGROWTH LEADING TO CHILDHOOD TALL STATURE

Familial (constitutional) tall stature.
Cerebral gigantism.
Beckwith-Wiedemann syndrome.
Exogenous obesity.
Excess growth hormone (GH) secretion (pituitary gigantism).
McCune-Albright syndrome or multiple endocrine neoplasia (MEN) associated with excess GH secretion.
Precocious puberty.
Marfan syndrome.
Klinefelter syndrome (XXY).
Weaver syndrome.
Fragile X syndrome.
Homocystinuria.
XYY.
Hyperthyroidism.

POSTNATAL OVERGROWTH LEADING TO ADULT TALL STATURE

Familial (constitutional) tall stature.
Androgen or estrogen deficiency/estrogen resistance (in males).
Testicular feminization.
Excess GH secretion.
Marfan syndrome.
Klinefelter syndrome (XXY).
XYY.

STEATOHEPATITIS

| ICD-10CM # | K76.0 | Fatty (change of) liver, not elsewhere classified |
| | K76.89 | Other specified diseases of liver |

Alcohol abuse.
Obesity.
DM.
Parenteral nutrition.
Medications (high-dose estrogen, amiodarone, corticosteroids, methotrexate, nifedipine).
Jejunoileal bypass.
Abetalipoproteinemia.
Wilson disease, Weber-Christian disease.

STEATOSIS, MACROVESICULAR AND MICROVESICULAR[94]

| ICD-10CM # | K75.81 | Nonalcoholic steatohepatitis (NASH) |
| | K70.9 | Alcoholic liver disease, unspecified |

Common Causes of Macrovesicular and Microvesicular Steatosis

Macrovesicular Steatosis	Microvesicular Steatosis
Obesity, type 2 diabetes, metabolic syndrome, and dyslipidemia (nonalcoholic fatty liver disease).	Reye syndrome. Medications (valproate, antiretroviral medicines, intravenous tetracycline).
Excessive alcohol consumption.	Heat stroke.
Hepatitis C (genotype 3).	Acute fatty liver of pregnancy.
Wilson disease.	HELLP syndrome.
Lipodystrophy starvation.	Inborn errors of metabolism (lecithin–cholesterol acyltransferase deficiency, cholesterol ester storage disease, Wolman disease).
Jejunoileal bypass.	
Parenteral nutrition.	
Medications (amiodarone, methotrexate, tamoxifen, corticosteroids, antipsychotics).	

HELLP =Hemolysis, elevated liver enzymes, and low platelets.

STERILE PYURIA[12]

ICD-10CM #   R82.998   Other abnormal findings in urine

Common causes of sterile pyuria:
Nonspecific urethritis in males.
Prostatitis.
Renal tract neoplasm.
Renal calculi.
Catheterization.
Renal tuberculosis.
Previous antibiotic treatment.

STOMATITIS, BULLOUS

ICD-10CM #   K12.30   Oral mucositis (ulcerative), unspecified

Erythema multiforme.
Erosive lichen planus.
Bullous pemphigoid.
SLE.
Pemphigus vulgaris.
Mucous membrane pemphigoid.

STRIDOR IN NEONATES[29]

ICD-10CM #   R06.1   Stridor

INTRINSIC LESIONS
Larynx
Laryngomalacia.
Infection (laryngitis).
Vocal cord paralysis.
Laryngeal web.
Laryngocele or laryngeal cyst.
Laryngotracheal esophageal cleft.
Foreign body.
Trachea
Tracheomalacia.
Tracheal stenosis.
Tracheoesophageal fistula.
Subglottic hemangioma.
Tracheal web.
Extrinsic Compression
Vascular ring.
Anomalous innominate artery.
Mediastinal mass.
Esophageal foreign body.
Other
Macroglossia.
Gastroesophageal reflux.

STRIDOR, PEDIATRIC AGE[45]

ICD-10CM #   R06.1   Stridor

RECURRENT
Allergic (spasmodic) croup.
Respiratory infections in a child with otherwise asymptomatic anatomic narrowing of the large airways.
Laryngomalacia.

PERSISTENT
Laryngeal obstruction:
   Laryngomalacia.
   Papillomas, other tumors.
   Cysts and laryngoceles.
   Laryngeal webs.
   Bilateral abductor paralysis of the cords.
   Foreign body.
Tracheobronchial disease:
   Tracheomalacia.
   Subglottic tracheal webs.
Endotracheal, endobronchial tumors.
Subglottic tracheal stenosis.
Congenital.
Acquired.
Extrinsic masses.
Mediastinal masses.
Vascular ring.
Lobar emphysema.
Bronchogenic cysts.
Thyroid enlargement.
Esophageal foreign body.
Tracheoesophageal fistulas.
Other.
Gastroesophageal reflux.
Macroglossia, Pierre Robin syndrome.
Cri-du-chat syndrome.
Hysterical stridor.
Hypocalcemia.

STROKE[17]

ICD-10CM #   Varies with specific diagnosis

STROKE "MIMICS"
Hypoglycemia.
Drug overdose or intoxication.
Hysterical conversion reaction.
Hyperventilation.
Metabolic encephalopathy.
Migraine.
Syncope.
Transient global amnesia.
Seizures.
Vestibular vertigo.

STROKE, PEDIATRIC AGE[97]

ICD-10CM #   I67.89   Other cerebrovascular disease

CARDIAC DISEASE
Congenital:
   Aortic stenosis.
   Mitral stenosis; mitral prolapse.
   Ventricular septal defects.
   Patent ductus arteriosus.
   Cyanotic congenital heart disease involving right-to-left shunt.
Acquired:
   Endocarditis (bacterial, SLE).
   Kawasaki disease.
   Cardiomyopathy.
   Atrial myxoma.
   Arrhythmia.
   Paradoxical emboli through patent foramen ovale.
   Rheumatic fever.
   Prosthetic heart valve.

HEMATOLOGIC ABNORMALITIES
Hemoglobinopathies:
   Sickle cell (SS) disease.
   Sickle (SC) disease.
Polycythemia.
Leukemia/lymphoma.
Thrombocytopenia.
Thrombocytosis.
Disorders of coagulation:
   Protein C deficiency.
   Protein S deficiency.
   Factor V Leiden.
   Antithrombin III deficiency.
   Lupus anticoagulant.
Oral contraceptive pill use.
Pregnancy and the postpartum state.
Disseminated intravascular coagulation.
Paroxysmal nocturnal hemoglobinuria.
Inflammatory bowel disease (thrombosis).

INFLAMMATORY DISORDERS

Meningitis:
  Viral.
  Bacterial.
  Tuberculosis.
Systemic infection:
  Viremia.
  Bacteremia.
  Local head and neck infections.
Drug-induced inflammation:
  Amphetamine.
  Cocaine.
Autoimmune disease:
  SLE.
  Juvenile RA.
  Takayasu arteritis.
  Mixed connective tissue disease.
  Polyarteritis nodosum.
  Primary CNS vasculitis.
  Sarcoidosis.
  Behçet syndrome.
  Granulomatosis with polyangiitis.

METABOLIC DISEASE ASSOCIATED WITH STROKE

Homocystinuria.
Pseudoxanthoma elasticum.
Fabry disease.
Sulfite oxidase deficiency.
Mitochondrial disorders:
  MELAS.
  Leigh syndrome.
Ornithine transcarbamylase deficiency.

INTRACEREBRAL VASCULAR PROCESSES

Ruptured aneurysm.
Arteriovenous malformation.
Fibromuscular dysplasia.
Moyamoya disease.
Migraine headache.
Postsubarachnoid hemorrhage vasospasm.
Hereditary hemorrhagic telangiectasia.
Sturge-Weber syndrome.
Carotid artery dissection.
Postvaricella.

TRAUMA AND OTHER EXTERNAL CAUSES

Child abuse.
Head trauma/neck trauma.
Oral trauma.
Placental embolism.
ECMO therapy.

CNS, Central nervous system; *ECMO*, extracorporeal membrane oxygenation; *MELAS*, mitochondrial encephalomyopathy, lactic acidosis, and stroke.

STROKE, YOUNG ADULT, CAUSES[18]

ICD-10CM #	I64	Stroke
	I67.89	Other cerebrovascular disease

Cardiac factors (ASD, MVP, patent foramen ovale).
Inflammatory factors (SLE, polyarteritis nodosa).
Infections (endocarditis, neurosyphilis).
Drugs (cocaine, heroin, oral contraceptives, decongestants).
Arterial dissection.
Hematologic factors (DIC, TTP, deficiency of protein S, protein C, antithrombin III).
Migraine.
Postpartum angiopathy.
Other: premature atherosclerosis, fibromuscular dysplasia.

ST-SEGMENT DEPRESSION, NONCORONARY CAUSES[87]

ICD-10CM #	R94.31	Abnormal electrocardiogram

NONCORONARY CAUSES OF ST-SEGMENT DEPRESSION

Anemia.
Cardiomyopathy.
Digitalis use.
Glucose load.
Hyperventilation.
Hypokalemia.
Intraventricular conduction disturbance.
Left ventricular hypertrophy.
Mitral valve prolapse.
Preexcitation syndrome.
Severe aortic stenosis.
Severe hypertension.
Severe hypoxia.
Severe volume overload (aortic, mitral regurgitation).
Sudden excessive exercise.
Supraventricular tachyarrhythmias.

ST-SEGMENT ELEVATION[29]

ICD-10CM #	R94.31	Abnormal electrocardiogram [ECG] [EKG]

DIFFERENTIAL DIAGNOSIS OF ST-SEGMENT ELEVATION ON ELECTROCARDIOGRAPHY

ST-segment elevation myocardial infarction.
Pericarditis.
Benign early repolarization.
Left bundle branch block.
Left ventricular hypertrophy.
Left ventricular aneurysm.
Paced ventricular rhythms.
Prinzmetal angina.

Hyperkalemia.
Hypothermia with Osborne waves.
Intracranial hemorrhage.
Brugada syndrome.
Normal variant.

ST SEGMENT ELEVATIONS, NONISCHEMIC

ICD-10CM #	R94.31	Abnormal electrocardiogram [ECG] [EKG]

Early repolarization.
Acute pericarditis.
LVH.
Normal pattern variant.
LBBB.
Pulmonary embolism.
Hyperkalemia.
Postcardioversion.

SUDDEN CARDIAC DEATH[86]

ICD-10CM #	Z86.74	Personal history of sudden cardiac arrest
	Z82.41	Family history of sudden cardiac death

CAUSES OF AND CONTRIBUTING FACTORS IN SUDDEN CARDIAC DEATH

Coronary Artery Abnormalities
Coronary atherosclerosis:
  Chronic coronary atherosclerosis with acute or transient myocardial ischemia—thrombosis, spasm, physical stress.
  Acute myocardial infarction, onset and early phase.
  Chronic atherosclerosis with a change in myocardial substrate, including previous myocardial infarction.
Congenital abnormalities of coronary arteries:
  Anomalous origin from the pulmonary artery.
  Other coronary arteriovenous fistula.
  Origin of a left coronary branch from the right or noncoronary sinus of Valsalva.
  Origin of the right coronary artery from the left sinus of Valsalva.
  Hypoplastic or aplastic coronary arteries.
  Coronary-intracardiac shunt.
Coronary artery embolism:
  Aortic or mitral endocarditis.
  Prosthetic aortic or mitral valves.
  Abnormal native valves or left ventricular mural thrombus.
  Platelet embolism.
Coronary arteritis:
  Polyarteritis nodosa, progressive systemic sclerosis, giant cell arteritis.
  Mucocutaneous lymph node syndrome (Kawasaki disease).
  Syphilitic coronary ostial stenosis.
Miscellaneous mechanical obstruction of the coronary arteries:

Differential Diagnosis

Coronary artery dissection in Marfan syndrome.

Coronary artery dissection in pregnancy.

Prolapse of aortic valve myxomatous polyps into the coronary ostia.

Dissection or rupture of the sinus of Valsalva.

Functional obstruction of the coronary arteries:

Coronary artery spasm with or without atherosclerosis.

Myocardial bridges.

Hypertrophy of the Ventricular Myocardium

Left ventricular hypertrophy associated with coronary heart disease.

Hypertensive heart disease without significant coronary atherosclerosis.

Hypertrophic myocardium secondary to valvular heart disease.

Hypertrophic cardiomyopathy:

Obstructive.

Nonobstructive.

Primary or secondary pulmonary hypertension:

Advanced chronic right ventricular overload.

Pulmonary hypertension in pregnancy (highest risk peripartum).

Myocardial Diseases and Dysfunction, with or without Heart Failure

Chronic congestive heart failure:

Ischemic cardiomyopathy.

Idiopathic dilated cardiomyopathy, acquired.

Hereditary dilated cardiomyopathy.

Alcoholic cardiomyopathy.

Hypertensive cardiomyopathy.

Postmyocarditis cardiomyopathy.

Peripartum cardiomyopathy.

Idiopathic fibrosis.

Acute and subacute cardiac failure:

Massive acute myocardial infarction.

Myocarditis, acute or fulminant.

Acute alcoholic cardiac dysfunction.

Takotsubo syndrome (uncertain risk for sudden death).

Ball valve embolism in aortic stenosis or prosthesis.

Mechanical disruptions of cardiac structures:

Rupture of the ventricular free wall.

Disruption of the mitral apparatus:

Papillary muscle.

Chordae tendineae.

Leaflet.

Rupture of the interventricular septum.

Acute pulmonary edema in noncompliant ventricles.

Inflammatory, Infiltrative, Neoplastic, and Degenerative Processes

Viral myocarditis, with or without ventricular dysfunction:

Acute phase.

Postmyocarditis interstitial fibrosis.

Myocarditis associated with the vasculitides.

Sarcoidosis.

Progressive systemic sclerosis.

Amyloidosis.

Hemochromatosis.

Idiopathic giant cell myocarditis.

Chagas disease.

Cardiac ganglionitis.

Arrhythmogenic right ventricular dysplasia, right ventricular cardiomyopathy.

Neuromuscular diseases (e.g., muscular dystrophy, Friedreich ataxia, myotonic dystrophy).

Intramural tumors:

Primary.

Metastatic.

Obstructive intracavitary tumors:

Neoplastic.

Thrombotic.

Diseases of the Cardiac Valves

Valvular aortic stenosis/insufficiency.

Mitral valve disruption.

Mitral valve prolapse.

Endocarditis.

Prosthetic valve dysfunction.

Congenital Heart Disease

Congenital aortic (potentially high risk) or pulmonic (low risk) valve stenosis.

Congenital septal defects with Eisenmenger physiology:

Advanced disease.

During labor and delivery.

Late after surgical repair of congenital lesions (e.g., tetralogy of Fallot).

Electrophysiologic Abnormalities

Abnormalities of the conducting system:

Fibrosis of the His-Purkinje system:

Primary degeneration (Lenègre disease).

Secondary to fibrosis and calcification of the "cardiac skeleton" (Lev disease).

Postviral conducting system fibrosis.

Hereditary conducting system disease.

Anomalous pathways of conduction (Wolff-Parkinson-White syndrome, short refractory period bypass).

Abnormalities of repolarization:

Congenital abnormalities in duration of the QT interval:

Congenital long–QT interval syndromes:

Romano-Ward syndrome (without deafness).

Jervell and Lange-Nielsen syndrome (with deafness).

Congenital short–QT interval syndrome.

Acquired (or provoked) long–QT interval syndromes:

Drug effect (with genetic predisposition?):

Cardiac, antiarrhythmic.

Noncardiac.

Drug interactions.

Electrolyte abnormality (response modified by genetic predisposition?).

Toxic substances.

Hypothermia.

CNS injury, subarachnoid hemorrhage.

Brugada syndrome—right bundle branch block and ST-segment elevations in the absence of ischemia:

Early repolarization syndrome.

Ventricular fibrillation of unknown or uncertain cause:

Absence of identifiable structural or functional causes:

"Idiopathic" ventricular fibrillation.

Short-coupled torsades de pointes, polymorphic ventricular tachycardia.

Nonspecific fibrofatty infiltration in a previously healthy victim (variation of right ventricular dysplasia?).

Sleep-death in Southeast Asians (see VIIB3, Brugada syndrome):

Bangungut.

Pokkuri.

Lai-tai.

Electrical Instability Related to Neurohumoral and Central Nervous System Influences

Catecholaminergic polymorphic ventricular tachycardia.

Other catecholamine-dependent arrhythmias.

CNS related:

Psychic stress, emotional extremes (Takotsubo syndrome).

Auditory related:

"Voodoo death" in primitive cultures.

Diseases of the cardiac nerves.

Arrhythmia expression in congenital long–QT interval syndrome.

Sudden Infant Death Syndrome and Sudden Death in Children

Sudden infant death syndrome:

Immature respiratory control function.

Long–QT interval syndrome.

Congenital heart disease.

Myocarditis.

Sudden death in children:

Eisenmenger syndrome, aortic stenosis, hypertrophic cardiomyopathy, pulmonary atresia.

After corrective surgery for congenital heart disease.

Myocarditis.

Genetic disorders of electrical function (e.g., long–QT interval syndrome).

No identified structural or functional cause.

Miscellaneous

Sudden death during extreme physical activity (seek predisposing causes).

Commotio cordis—blunt chest trauma.

Mechanical interference with venous return:

Acute cardiac tamponade.

Massive pulmonary embolism.

Acute intracardiac thrombosis.

Dissecting aneurysm of the aorta.

Toxic and metabolic disturbances (other than the QT interval effects listed above):

Electrolyte disturbances.

Metabolic disturbances.

Proarrhythmic effects of antiarrhythmic drugs.

Proarrhythmic effects of noncardiac drugs.

Mimics sudden cardiac death:

"Café coronary."

Acute alcoholic states ("holiday heart").

Acute asthmatic attacks.
Air or amniotic fluid embolism.

SUDDEN DEATH, PEDIATRIC AGE[45]

ICD-10CM # R99 Ill-defined and unknown cause of mortality

SIDS AND SIDS "MIMICS"

SIDS.
Long QT syndromes.
Inborn errors of metabolism.
Child abuse.
Myocarditis.
Duct-dependent congenital heart disease.

CORRECTED OR UNOPERATED CONGENITAL HEART DISEASE

Aortic stenosis.
Tetralogy of Fallot.
Transposition of great vessels (postoperative atrial switch).
Mitral valve prolapse.
Hematologic left heart syndrome.
Eisenmenger syndrome.

CORONARY ARTERIAL DISEASE

Anomalous origin.
Anomalous tract.
Kawasaki disease.
Periarteritis.
Arterial dissection.
Marfan syndrome.
Myocardial infarction.

MYOCARDIAL DISEASE

Myocarditis.
Hypertrophic cardiomyopathy.
Dilated cardiomyopathy.
Arrhythmogenic right ventricular dysplasia.

CONDUCTION SYSTEM ABNORMALITY/ARRHYTHMIA

Long QT syndromes.
Proarrhythmic drugs.
Preexcitation syndromes.
Heart block.
Commotio cordis.
Idiopathic ventricular fibrillation.
Heart tumor.

MISCELLANEOUS

Pulmonary hypertension.
Pulmonary embolism.
Heat stroke.
Cocaine.
Anorexia nervosa.
Electrolyte disturbances.

SIDS, Sudden infant death syndrome.

SUDDEN DEATH, YOUNG ATHLETE

ICD-10CM # R99 Ill-defined and unknown cause of mortality

Hypertrophic cardiomyopathy.
Coronary artery anomalies.
Myocarditis.
Ruptured aortic aneurysm (Marfan syndrome).
Arrhythmias.
Aortic valve stenosis.
Asthma.
Trauma (cerebral, cardiac).
Drug and alcohol abuse.
Heat stroke.
Cardiac sarcoidosis.
Atherosclerotic coronary artery disease.
Dilated cardiomyopathy.

SUPERIOR VENA CAVA SEGMENT ABNORMALITIES[37]

ICD-10CM # Q26.8 Other congenital malformations of great veins

Differential Diagnosis of an Abnormal Superior Vena Cava Segment
Increased SVC Pressure
SVC obstruction:
　Lung cancer.
　Stricture resulting from long-term cannulation.
　Right-sided heart failure.
Increased SVC Volume
　Vein of Galen aneurysm.
　Upper extremity AVM.
　Partial anomalous pulmonary venous connection.
　Interruption of the IVC with azygos continuation.

AVM, Arteriovenous malformation; *IVC,* inferior vena cava; *SVC,* superior vena cava.

SWOLLEN LIMB

ICD-10CM # M79.89 Other specified soft tissue disorders

Trauma.
Insect bite.
Abscess.
Lymphedema.
Thrombophlebitis.
Lipoma.
Neurofibroma.
Postphlebitic syndrome.
Myositis ossificans.
Nephrosis, cirrhosis, CHF.
Hypoalbuminemia.
Varicose veins.

SYMPATHOMIMETIC TOXICITY[12]

ICD-10CM # Varies with specific diagnosis

Substances That Can Cause Sympathomimetic Toxicity
　Methamphetamines (ice [crystals]); speed (powder), pills, base (oily powder).
　3, 4-methylenedioxymethamphetamine (MDMA or Ecstasy).
　Phenylethylamines (bath salts).
　Cocaine.
　Ma huang (herbal ecstasy).
　Paramethoxyamphetamine (PMA or "death").
　Mephedrone (4-MMC).
　Pseudoephedrine.
　Methylphenidate.
　Imidazolines: decongestants (naphazoline, oxymetazoline, tetrahydrozoline).
　Clonidine withdrawal.*
　Dexamphetamine.
　Caffeine.
　Yohimbe-containing supplements (used in combinations with stimulants).

---

*Clonidine is a central α_2 agonist; it does not cause acute sympathomimetic syndrome except in abrupt withdrawals.

TALL STATURE[80]

ICD-10CM # E22.0 Acromegaly and pituitary gigantism

CONSTITUTIONAL (FAMILIAL OR GENETIC)—MOST COMMON CAUSE

Endocrine Causes
Growth hormone excess—gigantism.
Sexual precocity (tall as children, short as adults):
　True sexual precocity.
　Pseudosexual precocity.
Androgen deficiency:
　Klinefelter syndrome.
　Bilateral anorchism.

GENETIC CAUSES

Klinefelter syndrome.
Syndromes of XYY, XXYY.

MISCELLANEOUS SYNDROMES AND DISORDERS

Cerebral gigantism or Sotos syndrome: prominent forehead, hypertelorism, high arched palate, dolichocephaly, mental retardation, large hands and feet, and premature eruption of teeth. Large at birth, with most rapid growth in first 4 yr of life.
Marfan syndrome: disorder of mesodermal tissues, subluxation of the lenses, arachnodactyly, and aortic aneurysm.
Homocystinuria: same phenotype as Marfan syndrome.

Obesity: tall as infants, children, and adolescents.

Total lipodystrophy: large hands and feet, generalized loss of subcutaneous fat, insulin-resistant DM, and hepatomegaly.

Beckwith-Wiedemann syndrome: neonatal tallness, omphalocele, macroglossia, and neonatal hypoglycemia.

Weaver-Smith syndrome: excessive intrauterine growth, mental retardation, megalocephaly, widened bifrontal diameter, hypertelorism, large ears, micrognathia, camptodactyly, broad thumbs, and limited extension of elbows and knees.

Marshall-Smith syndrome: excessive intrauterine growth, mental retardation, blue sclerae, failure to thrive, and early death.

TARDIVE DYSKINESIA[85]

ICD-10CM #	R27.9	Unspecified lack of coordination
	F44.4	Conversion disorder with motor symptom or deficit
	F44.6	Conversion disorder with sensory symptom or deficit
	G24.4	Idiopathic orofacial dystonia

DIFFERENTIAL DIAGNOSIS

Medications (antidepressants, anticholinergics, amphetamines, lithium, L-dopa, phenytoin).

Brain neoplasms.

Ill-fitting dentures.

Huntington disease.

Idiopathic dystonias (tics, blepharospasm, aging).

Wilson disease.

Extrapyramidal syndrome (postanoxic or postencephalitic).

Torsion dystonia.

TASTE AND SMELL LOSS[18]

ICD-10CM #	R43.0	Anosmia
	R43.1	Parosmia
	R43.2	Parageusia

TASTE

Local: radiation therapy.

Systemic: cancer, renal failure, hepatic failure, nutritional deficiency (vitamin B_{12}, zinc), Cushing syndrome, hypothyroidism, DM, infection (influenza), drugs (antirheumatic and antiproliferative).

Neurologic: Bell palsy, familial dysautonomia, multiple sclerosis.

SMELL

Local: allergic rhinitis, sinusitis, nasal polyposis, bronchial asthma.

Systemic: renal failure, hepatic failure, nutritional deficiency (vitamin B_{12}), Cushing syndrome, hypothyroidism, DM, infection (viral hepatitis, influenza), drugs (nasal sprays, antibiotics).

Neurologic: head trauma, multiple sclerosis, Parkinson disease, frontal brain tumor.

TELANGIECTASIA

| ICD-10CM # | I78.8 | Other diseases of capillaries |
| | I78.9 | Disease of capillaries, unspecified |

Oral contraceptive agents.

Pregnancy.

Rosacea.

Varicose veins.

Trauma.

Drug induced (corticosteroids, systemic or topical).

Spider telangiectases.

Hepatic cirrhosis.

Mastocytosis.

SLE, dermatomyositis, systemic sclerosis.

TENDINOPATHY[10]

| ICD-10CM # | M67.90 | Unspecified disorder of synovium and tendon, unspecified site |
| | M71.9 | Bursopathy, unspecified |

INTRINSIC FACTORS

Anatomic Factors

Malalignment.

Muscle weakness or imbalance.

Muscle inflexibility.

Decreased vascularity.

Systemic Factors

Inflammatory conditions (e.g., SLE).

Pregnancy.

Quinolone-induced tendinopathy.

Age-Related Factors

Tendon degeneration.

Increased tendon stiffness.

Tendon calcification.

Decreased vascularity.

EXTRINSIC FACTORS

Repetitive Mechanical Load

Excessive duration.

Excessive frequency.

Excessive intensity.

Poor technique.

Workplace factors.

Equipment Problems

Footwear.

Athletic field surface.

Equipment factors (e.g., racquet size).

Protective gear.

TESTICULAR CYSTIC LESIONS[15]

| ICD-10CM # | Varies with specific diagnosis |

Benign

Tunica albuginea cysts.

Tunica vaginalis cysts.

Intratesticular cysts.

Tubular ectasia of rete testis.

Cystic dysplasia.

Epidermoid cysts.

Abscess.

Malignant

Nonseminomatous germ cell tumor.

Necrosis or hemorrhage in tumor.

Tubular obstruction by tumor.

Lymphoma.

TESTICULAR FAILURE[114]

| ICD-10CM # | E29 | Testicular dysfunction |

PRIMARY

Klinefelter syndrome (XXY).

XYY.

Vanishing testes syndrome (in utero or early postnatal torsion).

Noonan syndrome.

Varicocele.

Myotonic dystrophy.

Orchitis (mumps, gonorrhea).

Cryptorchidism.

Chemical exposure.

Irradiation to testes.

Spinal cord injury.

Polyglandular failure.

Idiopathic oligospermia or azoospermia.

Germinal cell aplasia (Sertoli cell-only syndrome).

Idiopathic testicular failure.

Testicular torsion.

Testicular trauma.

Diethylstilbestrol (maternal use during pregnancy leading to in utero estrogen exposure).

Testicular tumor with subsequent irradiation therapy, chemotherapy, or surgery (retroperitoneal lymph node dissection or orchiectomy).

SECONDARY

Delayed puberty.

Kallmann syndrome.

Isolated gonadotropin deficiency.

Prader-Labhart-Willi syndrome.

Lawrence-Moon-Biedl syndrome.

CNS irradiation.

Prepubertal panhypopituitarism.

Postpubertal panhypopituitarism.

Hypogonadism secondary to hyperprolactinemia.

Adrenogenital syndrome.

Chronic liver disease.

Chronic renal failure/uremia.

Hemochromatosis.

Cushing syndrome.

Malnutrition.

Massive obesity.

Sickle cell anemia.

Hyper/hypothyroidism.

Anabolic steroid use.

TESTICULAR PAIN

| ICD-10CM # | N50.9 | Disorder of male genital organs, unspecified |
| | R10.2 | Pelvic and perineal pain |

Testicular torsion.
Trauma.
Epididymitis.
Orchitis.
Neoplasm.
Urolithiasis.
Inguinal hernia.
Infection (cellulitis, abscess, folliculitis).
Anxiety.

TESTICULAR SIZE VARIATIONS[114]

ICD-10CM #	N50.0	Atrophy of testis
	N44.2	Benign cyst of testis
	N44.8	Other noninflammatory disorders of the testis
	N50.3	Cyst of epididymis
	N50.8	Other specified disorders of male genital organs
	N53.12	Painful ejaculation
	E29.1	Testicular hypofunction

SMALL TESTES

Hypothalamic-pituitary dysfunction.
Gonadotropin deficiency.
Growth hormone deficiency.
Normal variant.
Primary hypogonadism.
Autoimmune destruction.
Chemotherapy.
Cryptorchidism.
Irradiation.
Klinefelter syndrome.
Orchiditis.
Testicular regression syndrome.
Torsion.
Trauma.

LARGE TESTES

Adrenal rest tissue.
Compensatory.
Fragile X syndrome.
Idiopathic.
Tumor.

TETANUS[10]

ICD-10CM #	A35	Other tetanus

TETANUS "MIMICS"

Acute abdomen.
Black widow spider bite.
Dental abscess.
Dislocated mandible.
Dystonic reaction.
Encephalitis.
Head trauma.
Hyperventilation syndrome.
Hypocalcemia.
Meningitis.
Peritonsillar abscess.

Progressive fluctuating muscular rigidity (stiff-man syndrome).
Psychogenic.
Rabies.
Sepsis.
Subarachnoid hemorrhage.
Status epilepticus.
Strychnine poisoning.
Temporomandibular joint syndrome.

THORACIC AORTIC ANEURYSMS[37]

ICD-10CM #	I71.2	Thoracic aortic aneurysm, without rupture

ANEURYSMS OF THE THORACIC AORTA

By Location
Sinuses of Valsalva:
  Infected.
  Congenital.
  Trauma.
  Annuloaortic ectasia.
Ascending aorta:
  Aortitis.
  Takayasu disease.
  Syphilis.
  Trauma.
  Annuloaortic ectasia.
  Marfan syndrome.
  Ehlers-Danlos syndrome.
Aortic arch:
  Trauma.
  Infected.
  Syphilis.
  Of patent ductus arteriosus.
  Coarctation.
  Takayasu disease.
  Duct of Kommerell from aberrant right subclavian artery.
Descending aorta:
  Atherosclerosis.
  Infected.
  Inflammatory.
  Syphilis.
  Takayasu disease.

By Shape
Saccular:
  Trauma.
  Infected.
  Of ductus arteriosus.
  Syphilis.
  Penetrating ulcer.
Fusiform:
  Cystic medial necrosis.
  Atherosclerosis.

By Integrity of the Aortic Wall
True:
  Cystic medial necrosis.
  Atherosclerosis.
  Collagen vascular disease.

Rheumatoid arthritis.
Ankylosing spondylitis.
Aortitis.
False:
  Trauma.
  Infected.
  Penetrating ulcer.
  Rupture.
  After aortotomy.

THROMBOCYTOPENIA

ICD-10CM #	D47.3	Essential (hemorrhagic) thrombocythemia
	D69.59	Other secondary thrombocytopenia
	D69.6	Thrombocytopenia, unspecified

INCREASED DESTRUCTION

Immunologic
Drugs: quinine, quinidine, digitalis, procainamide, thiazide diuretics, sulfonamides, phenytoin, aspirin, penicillin, heparin, gold, meprobamate, sulfa drugs, phenylbutazone, NSAIDs, methyldopa, cimetidine, furosemide, INH, cephalosporins, chlorpropamide, organic arsenicals, chloroquine, platelet glycoprotein IIb/IIIa receptor inhibitors, ranitidine, indomethacin, carboplatin, ticlopidine, clopidogrel.
Idiopathic thrombocytopenic purpura (ITP).
Transfusion reaction: transfusion of platelets with plasminogen activator (PLA) in recipients without PLA-1.
Fetal/maternal incompatibility.
Collagen vascular diseases (e.g., SLE).
Autoimmune hemolytic anemia.
Lymphoreticular disorders (e.g., CLL).

Nonimmunologic
Prosthetic heart valves.
Thrombotic thrombocytopenic purpura (TTP).
Sepsis.
DIC.
Hemolytic-uremic syndrome (HUS).
Giant cavernous hemangioma.

DECREASED PRODUCTION

Abnormal marrow.
Marrow infiltration (e.g., leukemia, lymphoma, fibrosis).
Marrow suppression (e.g., chemotherapy, alcohol, radiation).
Hereditary disorders.
Wiskott-Aldrich syndrome: X-linked disorder characterized by thrombocytopenia, eczema, and repeated infections.
May-Hegglin anomaly: increased megakaryocytes but ineffective thrombopoiesis.
Vitamin deficiencies (e.g., vitamin B_{12}, folic acid).

SPLENIC SEQUESTRATION, HYPERSPLENISM

Dilutional, as a result of massive transfusion.

Differential Diagnosis

II

THROMBOCYTOPENIA, IN PREGNANCY[31]

ICD-10CM # D69.59 Other secondary thrombocytopenia

Incidental thrombocytopenia of pregnancy (gestational thrombocytopenia).
Preeclampsia/eclampsia.
  Peripartum/postpartum thrombotic microangiopathy.
Disseminated intravascular coagulation (DIC) secondary to:
  Abruptio placentae.
  Endometritis.
  Amniotic fluid embolism.
  Retained fetus.
Thrombotic thrombocytopenic purpura.
Hemolytic-uremic syndrome.

THROMBOCYTOPENIA, INHERITED DISORDERS[18]

ICD-10CM # D47.3 Essential (hemorrhagic) thrombocythemia

Amegakaryocytic thrombocytopenia.
Thrombocytopenia–absent radii.
MYH9-related thrombocytopenia:
May-Hegglin anomaly.
Fechtner syndrome.
Epstein syndrome.
Sebastian syndrome.
X-linked macrothrombocytopenia.
Wiskott-Aldrich syndrome.
X-linked thrombocytopenia.
Thrombocytopenia and radioulnar synostosis.
Familial platelet disorder—AML.
Familial dominant thrombocytopenia.
Paris-Trousseau thrombocytopenia.
Bernard-Soulier syndrome.
Bernard-Soulier carrier/Mediterranean macrothrombocytopenia.

THROMBOCYTOPENIA IN NEWBORNS, DIFFERENTIAL DIAGNOSIS[34]

ICD-10CM # D47.3 Essential (hemorrhagic) thrombocythemia
              D69.59 Other secondary thrombocytopenia
              D69.6 Thrombocytopenia, unspecified

DIFFERENTIAL DIAGNOSIS OF THROMBOCYTOPENIA IN NEWBORNS
Perinatal hypoxemia.
Placental insufficiency.
Congenital infection.
  Sepsis.
  Toxoplasmosis.
  Rubella.
  Cytomegalovirus.

Autoimmune:
  Maternal immune thrombocytopenia.
  Maternal systemic lupus erythematosus.
Disseminated intravascular coagulation.
Maternal drug exposure.
Congenital heart disease.
Hereditary thrombocytopenia.
  MYH9 macrothrombocytopenia (including May-Hegglin anomaly).
  Thrombocytopenia absent radii syndrome.
  Amegakaryocytic thrombocytopenia.
  Wiskott-Aldrich syndrome.
  Fanconi anemia.
Hemangioma with thrombocytopenia.
  Kasabach-Merritt syndrome.
Bone marrow infiltration.
  Congenital leukemia.

THROMBOCYTOSIS

ICD-10CM # D75.9 Disease of blood and blood-forming organs, unspecified

Iron deficiency.
Posthemorrhage.
Neoplasms (GI tract).
CML.
Polycythemia vera.
Myelofibrosis with myeloid metaplasia.
Infections.
After splenectomy.
Postpartum.
Hemophilia.
Pancreatitis.
Cirrhosis.
Idiopathic.

THROMBOSIS OR THROMBOTIC DIATHESIS[18]

ICD-10CM # I74.09 Other arterial embolism and thrombosis of abdominal aorta

DIFFERENTIAL DIAGNOSIS OF THE PATIENT PRESENTING WITH THROMBOSIS OR THROMBOTIC DIATHESIS
Inherited (Primary) Hypercoagulable States
Activated protein C resistance caused by factor V Leiden mutation.
Prothrombin gene mutation (G to A transition at position 20210 in the 3-untranslated region).
Antithrombin III deficiency.
Protein C deficiency.
Protein S deficiency.
Dysfibrinogenemias (rare).
Acquired (Secondary) Hypercoagulable States
In association physiologic or thrombogenic stimuli:
  Pregnancy (especially the postpartum period).
  Estrogen use (oral contraceptives, hormone replacement therapy).

  Immobilization.
  Trauma.
  Postoperative state.
Advancing age.
Obesity.
Prolonged air travel.
Lupus anticoagulant or antiphospholipid antibody syndrome.
In association with other clinical disorders.
Mixed/Unknown
Activated protein C resistance in the absence of factor V Leiden.
Elevated factor VIII level.
Elevated factor XI level.
Elevated factor IX level.
Elevated thrombin activatable fibrinolysis inhibitor (TAFI) level.
Decreased free tissue factor pathway inhibitor (TFPI) level.
Decreased plasma fibrinolytic activity.

THYMIC MASSES[78]

ICD-10CM # Varies with specific diagnosis

THYMIC MASSES
Thymic hyperplasia.
Thymoma.
Thymic carcinoma.
Thymic neuroendocrine tumors.
  Carcinoid.
  Small-cell carcinoma.
Thymic cysts (not rhizomatous).
Thymolipoma.
Metastases to the thymus.

THYMOMA, DISEASES ASSOCIATIONS[78]

ICD-10CM # Varies with specific diagnosis

SYSTEMIC DISEASES MOST COMMONLY ASSOCIATED WITH THYMOMA
Myasthenia gravis.
Cytopenias (most commonly red cell hypoplasia).
Nonthymic malignancies.
Hypogammaglobulinemia.
Systemic lupus erythematosus.
Polymyositis.
Rheumatoid arthritis.
Thyroiditis.
Sjögren syndrome.
Ulcerative colitis.

THYROMEGALY

ICD-10CM # Varies with specific diagnosis

Goiter.
Graves disease.
Thyroiditis (lymphocytic, granulomatous, suppurative).
Toxic adenoma.
Neoplasm (primary, metastatic).

THYROTOXICOSIS[30]

ICD-10CM # E05.80

CAUSES OF THYROTOXICOSIS
Sustained Hormone Overproduction (Hyperthyroidism)
Low TSH, high RAIU:
Graves disease (von Basedow disease).
Toxic multinodular goiter.
Toxic adenoma.
Chorionic gonadotropin-induced:
Gestational hyperthyroidism: physiologic hyperthyroidism of pregnancy, familial gestational hyperthyroidism due to TSH receptor mutations.
Trophoblastic tumors.
Inherited nonimmune hyperthyroidism associated with TSH receptor or G protein mutations.
Low TSH, low RAIU:
Iodide-induced hyperthyroidism (Jod-Basedow effect).
Amiodarone-associated hyperthyroidism due to iodide release.
Struma ovarii:
Metastatic functioning thyroid carcinoma.
Normal or elevated TSH:
TSH-secreting pituitary tumors.
Thyroid hormone resistance with pituitary predominance.

TRANSIENT HORMONE EXCESS (THYROTOXICOSIS)
Low TSH, low RAIU
Thyroiditis:
Autoimmune: lymphocytic thyroiditis (silent thyroiditis, painless thyroiditis, postpartum thyroiditis), acute exacerbation of Hashimoto disease.
Viral or postviral:
Subacute (granulomatous, painful, postviral) thyroiditis.
Drug-induced or associated thyroiditis:
Amiodarone.
Lithium, interferon-α, interleukin-2, GM-CSF.
Infectious thyroiditis.
Exogenous thyroid hormone:
Iatrogenic overreplacement.
Thyrotoxicosis factitia.
Ingestion of natural products containing thyroid hormone:
"Hamburger" thyrotoxicosis.
Natural foodstuffs.
Thyromimetic compounds (e.g., tiratricol PLB).
Occupational exposure to thyroid hormone (e.g., pill manufacturing, veterinary occupations).

GM-CSF, granulocyte-macrophage colony-stimulating factor; *RAIU,* radioactive iodine uptake; *TSH,* thyroid-stimulating hormone.

TICK-RELATED INFECTIONS

ICD-10CM #		
	A77.0	Spotted fever due to *Rickettsia rickettsii*
	A93.2	Colorado tick fever
	B60.0	Babesiosis
	A77.8	Other spotted fevers
	A69.20	Lyme disease, unspecified

Lyme disease.
Rocky Mountain spotted fever.
Babesiosis.
Tularemia.
Q fever.
Colorado tick fever.
Ehrlichiosis.
Relapsing fever.

TICS

ICD-10CM # F95.9 Tic disorder, unspecified

Tourette syndrome.
Physiologic tic.
Anxiety disorder.
Huntington disease.
Medications (e.g., antipsychotics, carbamazepine, phenytoin, phenobarbital).
Encephalitis.
Head trauma.
Schizophrenia.
Carbon monoxide poisoning.
Stroke.
Sydenham chorea.
Creutzfeldt-Jakob disease.

TORSADES DE POINTES[97]

ICD-10CM # I47.2 Ventricular tachycardia

Antiarrhythmics known to increase the QT interval (e.g., quinidine, procainamide, amiodarone, disopyramide, sotalol).
Tricyclic antidepressants and phenothiazines.
Histamine (H_1) antagonists (e.g., astemizole, terfenadine).
Antiviral and antifungal agents and antibiotics.
Hypokinemia.
Hypomagnesemia.
Insecticide poisoning.
Bradyarrhythmias.
Congenital long QT syndrome.
Subarachnoid hemorrhage.
Chloroquine, pentamidine.
Cocaine abuse.

TOXIC MEGACOLON, CAUSES[64]

ICD-10CM # K59.3 Megacolon, not elsewhere classified

INFLAMMATORY
Ulcerative colitis.
Crohn disease.

INFECTIOUS
Bacterial:
Clostridium difficile pseudomembranous colitis.
Salmonella (typhoid and nontyphoid).
Shigella.
Campylobacter.
Yersinia.
Parasitic:
Entamoeba histolytica.
Cryptosporidium.
Viral:
Cytomegalovirus colitis.

OTHER
Ischemia.
Kaposi sarcoma.

TRACHEOBRONCHIAL NARROWING ON X-RAY[21]

ICD-10CM # Varies with specific diagnosis

CAUSES OF TRACHEOBRONCHIAL NARROWING
Long-Segment/Diffuse Narrowing
Sarcoidosis.
Amyloidosis.
Granulomatosis with polyangiitis.
Relapsing polychondritis.
Tracheobronchopathia osteochondroplastica.
Pemphigoid.
Short-Segment Narrowing
Previous intubation or tracheostomy.
Congenital stenosis or web.
Extrinsic compression (from thyroid).
Adenoid cystic carcinoma.
Squamous carcinoma.

TRANSIENT AMNESIA[101]

ICD-10CM # Varies with specific diagnosis

Alcohol abuse.
WernickeaKorsakoff syndrome.
Alcoholic blackouts.
Electroconvulsive therapy (ECT).
Head trauma.
Medications.
Benzodiazepines.
Fentanyl.
Gamma hydroxybutyrate (GHB).[a]
Scopolamine, other anticholinergic medications.
Sildenafil (Viagra), tadalafil (Cialis).
Zolpidem (Ambien).

---

[a] When used illicitly, people call GHB the "date-rape drug." Under carefully controlled conditions, neurologists prescribe GHB as oxybate (Xyrem) to treat cataplexy.

TREMOR

ICD-10CM #	R25.0	Abnormal head movements
	R25.1	Tremor, unspecified
	R25.2	Cramp and spasm
	R25.3	Fasciculation
	R25.9	Unspecified abnormal involuntary movements
	G25.0	Essential tremor
	G25.1	Drug-induced tremor
	G25.2	Other specified forms of tremor

REST TREMORS

Parkinson disease.

Other parkinsonian syndromes (less commonly).

Midbrain (rubral) tremor: rest <postural <kinetic.

Wilson disease (also acquired hepatocerebral degeneration).

Essential tremor—only if severe: rest <postural and action.

POSTURAL AND ACTION (TERMINAL) TREMORS

Physiologic tremor.

Exaggerated physiologic tremor (these factors can also aggravate other forms of tremor).

Stress, fatigue, anxiety, emotion.

Endocrine: hypoglycemia, thyrotoxicosis, pheochromocytoma, adrenocorticosteroids.

Drugs and toxins: β-agonists, dopamine agonists, amphetamines, lithium, tricyclic antidepressants, neuroleptics, theophylline, caffeine, valproic acid, alcohol withdrawal, mercury (Hatter shakes), lead, arsenic, others.

Essential tremor (familial or sporadic):

Primary writing tremor.

With other CNS disorders:

Parkinson disease.

Other akinetic-rigid syndromes.

Idiopathic dystonia, including focal dystonias.

With peripheral neuropathy:

Charcot-Marie-Tooth syndrome (controversial whether to call this the Roussy-Levy syndrome).

Variety of other peripheral neuropathies (especially dysgammaglobulinemia).

Cerebellar tremor.

KINETIC (INTENTION) TREMOR

Disease of cerebellar outflow (dentate nucleus and superior cerebellar peduncle): multiple sclerosis, trauma, tumor, vascular disease, Wilson acquired hepatocerebral degeneration, drugs, toxins (e.g., mercury), others.

MISCELLANEOUS RHYTHMICAL MOVEMENT DISORDERS

Psychogenic tremor.

Orthostatic tremor.

Rhythmical movements in dystonia (dystonic tremor).

Rhythmical myoclonus (segmental myoclonus—e.g., palatal or branchial myoclonus, spinal myoclonus, limb myorhythmia).

Oscillatory myoclonus.

Asterixis.

Clonus.

Epilepsia partialis continua.

Hereditary chin quivering.

Spasmus nutans.

Head bobbing with third ventricular cysts.

Nystagmus.

TREMOR, IN CHILDREN, CAUSES[19]

ICD-10CM #	R25.0	Abnormal head movements
	R25.1	Tremor, unspecified
	R25.2	Cramp and spasm
	R25.3	Fasciculation
	R25.9	Unspecified abnormal involuntary movements

BENIGN

Enhanced physiologic tremor.

Shuddering attacks.

Jitteriness.

Spasmus nutans.

STATIC INJURY/STRUCTURAL

Cerebellar malformation.

Stroke (particularly in the midbrain or cerebellum).

Multiple sclerosis.

HEREDITARY/DEGENERATIVE

Familial essential tremor.

Fragile X premutation.

Wilson disease.

Huntington disease.

Juvenile parkinsonism (tremor is rare).

Pallidonigral degeneration.

METABOLIC

Hyperthyroidism.

Hyperadrenergic state (including pheochromocytoma and neuroblastoma).

Hypomagnesemia.

Hypocalcemia.

Hypoglycemia.

Hepatic encephalopathy.

Vitamin B_{12} deficiency.

Inborn errors of metabolism.

Mitochondrial disorders.

DRUGS/TOXINS

Valproate, phenytoin, carbamazepine, lamotrigine, gabapentin, lithium, tricyclic antidepressants, stimulants (cocaine, amphetamine, caffeine, thyroxine, bronchodilators), neuroleptics, cyclosporin, toluene, mercury, thallium, amiodarone, nicotine, lead, manganese, arsenic, cyanide, naphthalene, ethanol, lindane, serotonin reuptake inhibitors.

PERIPHERAL NEUROPATHIES

Psychogenic.

TRICHOMEGALY[44]

ICD-10CM #	Not available

CAUSES OF TRICHOMEGALY

Drug-induced: topical prostaglandin analogues, phenytoin and cyclosporine.

Malnutrition.

AIDS.

Porphyria.

Hypothyroidism.

Familial.

Congenital: Oliver-McFarlane, Cornelia de Lange, Goldstein-Hutt, Hermansky-Pudlak syndromes.

TUBULOINTERSTITIAL DISEASE, ACUTE[24]

ICD-10CM #	N17.0	Acute kidney failure with tubular necrosis

DRUGS

Antibiotics, penicillins, cephalosporins, rifampin.

Sulfonamides: cotrimoxazole, sulfamethoxazole.

NSAIDs: propionic acid derivatives.

Miscellaneous: phenytoin, thiazides, allopurinol, cimetidine, ifosfamide.

INFECTIONS

Invasion of renal parenchyma.

Reaction to systemic infections: streptococcal, diphtheria, hantavirus.

SYSTEMIC DISEASES

Immune mediated: SLE, transplanted kidney, cryoglobulinemias.

Metabolic: urate, oxalate.

Neoplastic: lymphoproliferative diseases.

IDIOPATHIC

TUBULOINTERSTITIAL KIDNEY DISEASE[24]

ICD-10CM #	N17.0	Acute kidney failure with tubular necrosis

Ischemic and toxic acute tubular necrosis.

Allergic interstitial nephritis.

Interstitial nephritis secondary to immune complex-related collagen vascular disease (e.g., SLE, Sjögren).

Granulomatous diseases (sarcoidosis, uveitis).

Pigment-related tubular injury (myoglobinuria, hemoglobinuria).

Hypercalcemia with nephrocalcinosis.

Tubular obstruction (drugs such as indinavir, uric acid in tumor lysis syndrome).

Myeloma kidney or cast nephropathy.

Infection-related interstitial nephritis: *Legionella, Leptospira.*

Infiltrative diseases (e.g., lymphoma).

TUMOR MARKERS ELEVATION[2]

ICD-10CM #   R97.8   Other abnormal tumor markers

CAUSES OF ELEVATED LEVELS OF TUMOR MARKERS

Carcinoembryonic Antigen (CEA)

Colonic cancer (higher levels if the tumor is more differentiated or is extensive or has spread to the liver).

Lung or breast cancer; seminoma.

Cigarette smokers.

Cirrhosis, inflammatory bowel disease, rectal polyps, pancreatitis.

Advanced age.

α-Fetoprotein

Hepatocellular cancer: very high titers or a rising titer is strongly suggestive, but >10% of patients do not have an elevated level.

Hepatic regeneration (e.g., cirrhosis, alcoholic or viral hepatitis).

Cancer of the stomach, colon, pancreas, or lung.

Teratocarcinoma or embryonal cell carcinoma (testis, ovary, extragonadal).

Pregnancy.

Ataxia-telangiectasia.

Normal variant.

Prostate-Specific Antigen

Prostate carcinoma (localized disease).

Prostatic hyperplasia.

Prostatitis.

Prostatic infarction.

Cancer-Associated Antigen (CA-19-9)

Pancreatic carcinoma (80% with advanced, well-differentiated cancer have an elevated level).

Other GI cancers: colon, stomach, bile duct.

Acute or chronic pancreatitis.

Chronic liver disease.

Biliary tract disease.

UPPER AIRWAY OBSTRUCTION[12]

ICD-10CM #   Varies with specific diagnosis

CAUSES OF UPPER AIRWAY OBSTRUCTION

Altered conscious state:

Head injury.

Cerebrovascular accident.

Drugs and toxins.

Metabolic—hypoglycemia, hyponatremia.

Foreign bodies.

Infections:

Tonsillitis.

Peritonsillar abscess (quinsy).

Epiglottitis.

Ludwig angina.

Other abscesses and infections.

Trauma:

Blunt or penetrating trauma resulting in edema or hematoma formation.

Uncontrolled hemorrhage.

Thermal injuries.

Inhalation burns.

Neoplasms:

Larynx, trachea, thyroid.

Allergic reactions:

Anaphylaxis.

Angioedema.

Anatomic:

Tracheomalacia—congenital or acquired (secondary to prolonged intubation).

Other congenital malformations.

Functional upper airway obstruction syndrome.

Acute-on-chronic causes.

Patients with chronic narrowing of the airway (e.g., due to tracheomalacia) may present with worsening obstruction from an acute upper respiratory tract illness or injury.

UREMIC ENCEPHALOPATHY, DIFFERENTIAL DIAGNOSIS[9]

ICD-10CM #   G93.40   Encephalopathy, unspecified

Differential Diagnosis	Comment
Hypertensive encephalopathy	
Systemic inflammatory response syndrome (SIRS):	Observed in septic patients.
Systemic vasculitis:	Vasculitis or lupus with cerebral involvement.
Drug-induced neurotoxicity	
Analgesics:	Meperidine, codeine, morphine, gabapentin.
Antibiotics:	High-dose penicillins (may cause seizures), acyclovir, ethambutol (optic nerve damage), erythromycin and aminoglycosides (may cause ototoxicity), nitrofurantoin and isoniazid (peripheral neuropathy).
Psychotropics:	Lithium, haloperidol, clonazepam, diazepam, chlorpromazine.
Immunosuppressants:	Cyclosporine, tacrolimus.
Chemotherapeutics:	Cisplatinum, ifosfamide.
Others:	High doses of loop diuretics (ototoxic), ephedrine, methyldopa, aluminum.
Cerebral atheroembolic disease:	Follows recent aortic or cardiac angiography; associated with peripheral manifestations, including lower extremity cyanosis, livedo reticularis, and eosinophilia.
Subdural hematoma	
Posterior leukoence-phalopathy:	Observed particularly following renal transplantation due to reversible, abnormal permeability of the blood-brain barrier. Often manifests as headache followed by mental depression, visual loss, and seizures in the context of volume expansion, acute hypertension, and often treatment with corticosteroids or calcineurin inhibitors. Lesions in the parietal, temporal, and occipital lobes may be seen on imaging studies.

URETERAL COLIC[115]

ICD-10CM #   R33.8   Other retention of urine
              N13.8   Other obstructive and reflux uropathy

DIAGNOSTIC DIFFERENTIALS OF RENAL OR URETERAL COLIC

Acute cholecystitis, acute cholelithiasis.

Acute appendicitis.

Pelvic inflammatory disease.

Diverticulosis and/or diverticulitis.

Intestinal obstruction.

Leaking abdominal aortic aneurysm.

Musculoskeletal sprains.

Herniated disk.

Herpes zoster (shingles).

GI dysfunction with ileus and/or toxic colonic dilatation.

URETERAL STRICTURE[89]

ICD-10CM #   Varies with specific diagnosis

ETIOLOGY OF URETERAL STRICTURE

Malignancy (e.g., transitional cell carcinoma, cervical cancer).

Ureteral calculus.

Radiation.

Ischemia or trauma caused by surgical dissection.

Periureteral fibrosis caused by abdominal aortic aneurysm or endometriosis.

Endoscopic instrumentation.
Renal ablation injury.
Infection (tuberculosis).
Idiopathic condition.

URETERIC OBSTRUCTION, CONGENITAL[21]

ICD-10CM #	N13.8	Other obstructive and reflux uropathy
	N20.9	Urolithiasis

CONGENITAL CAUSES OF URETERIC OBSTRUCTION

Primary megaureter.
Ureterocele (ectopic and orthotopic).
Ureteric valve.
Distal ureteric stenosis.
Ureteric atresia.
Circumcaval ureter and variants.
Bladder diverticulum.

URETHRAL BLEEDING[89]

ICD-10CM #	Varies with specific diagnosis

DIFFERENTIAL DIAGNOSIS FOR URETHRAL BLEEDING

Male
Trauma:
  Blunt (straddle injury, kick to perineum).
  Penetrating (foreign body insertion, failed urethral catheterization).
  Intercourse related (penile fracture, masturbation).
Urethritis:
  Bacterial (gonococcal, nongonococcal).
  Viral.
  Chemical.
  Autoimmune (Reiter syndrome).
Malignancy:
  Urothelial carcinoma.
  Squamous cell carcinoma (meatus/glans).
Condyloma.
Calculus disease.
Female
Trauma:
  Blunt (pelvic fracture).
  Penetrating (foreign body).
Urethral diverticulum.
Urethral caruncle.
Urethritis.
Malignancy.
Calculus disease.

URETHRAL DISCHARGE AND DYSURIA

ICD-10CM #	R36.0	Urethral discharge without blood
	R36.9	Urethral discharge, unspecified
	N36.9	Urethral disorder, unspecified
	N39.9	Disorder of urinary system, unspecified
	R30.0	Dysuria
	R30.9	Painful micturition, unspecified

Urethritis (gonococcal, chlamydial, trichomonal).
Cystitis.
Prostatitis.
Vaginitis (candidiasis, chemical).
Meatal stenosis.
Interstitial cystitis.
Trauma (foreign body, masturbation, horseback or bike riding).

URETHRAL OBSTRUCTION, CHILDREN[21]

ICD-10CM #	N13.8	Other obstructive and reflux uropathy

CAUSES OF URETHRAL OBSTRUCTION IN CHILDREN

Intrinsic Lesions
Valve (posterior, anterior, saccular diverticulum).
Stenosis, atresia.
Inflammatory stricture.
Traumatic stricture:
  External trauma (saddle injury, and so on).
  Iatrogenic trauma (catheter, cystoscopy, surgery).
Urethral "tumors":
  Girls: leiomyoma.
  Boys: polyp, rhabdomyosarcoma.
Miscellaneous (epidermolysis bullosa).
Extrinsic Lesions
Presacral mass dissecting inferiorly (tumor, cyst).
Fecal impaction (Hirschsprung, postrepair anal atresia, habitual constipation, neuropathy).
Mass originating in genital organs:
  Boys: utricle cyst, prostate rhabdomyosarcoma, seminal vesicle cyst, Cowper duct cyst.
  Girls: hydrometrocolpos, hydrocolpos, fused labia.

URETHRITIS, PEDIATRIC PATIENT[5]

ICD-10CM #	N34.1	Nonspecific urethritis
	N34.2	Other urethritis

ETIOLOGY OF URETHRITIS

Infectious	Noninfectious
Sexually Transmitted Infections	**Vasculitides**
Neisseria gonorrhoeae.	Reiter syndrome.
Chlamydia trachomatis.	Erythema multiforme.
Trichomonas vaginalis.	Kawasaki disease.
Herpes simplex virus type 2.	Mechanical.
Mycoplasma spp.	Masturbation.
	Foreign body.
Nonsexually Transmitted Infections	Trauma.
Staphylococcus saprophyticus.	Dysfunctional elimination.
Enterobacteriaceae.	Chemical.
Gardnerellavaginalis.	Soaps.
Streptococcus spp.	Detergents.
Enterobius vermicularis.	Drugs.

URIC ACID STONES

ICD-10CM #	N20.9	Urolithiasis

Hyperuricemia.
Excessive dietary purine.
Medications (salicylates, allopurinol, probenecid).
Urine pH <5.5 (e.g., diarrhea, high animal protein diet).
Decreased urine output (dehydration, malabsorption, diarrhea, inadequate fluid intake).
Tumor lysis.
Hemolytic anemia.
Myeloproliferative disorders.

URINARY INCONTINENCE, CHILDREN[19]

ICD-10CM #	R32	Unspecified urinary incontinence

CAUSES OF URINARY INCONTINENCE IN CHILDHOOD

Overactive bladder.
Infrequent voiding.
Detrusor-sphincter dyssynergia.
Nonneurogenic neurogenic bladder (Hinman syndrome).
Vaginal voiding.
Giggle incontinence.
Cystitis.
Bladder outlet obstruction (posterior urethral valves).
Ectopic ureter and fistula.
Sphincter abnormality (epispadias, exstrophy; urogenital sinus abnormality).
Neuropathic.
Overflow incontinence.
Traumatic.
Iatrogenic.
Behavioral.
Combination.

URINARY RETENTION[115]

ICD-10CM #	R33.9	Retention of urine, unspecified

COMMON CAUSES OF URINARY RETENTION

Obstructive Cause
Urethral stricture.
Enlarged prostate.
Lower genitourinary tract malignancy.

Pelvic malignancy.
Bladder stones.
Foreign body.
Blood clot.
Posterior urethral valves.
Ureterocele.
Primary Detrusor Insufficiency
Detrusor areflexia.
Multiple sclerosis.
Iatrogenic injury during abdominal or back surgery.
Spinal cord injury.
Myelomeningocele.

URINARY RETENTION, ACUTE

ICD-10CM #   R33.9   Retention of urine, unspecified

Mechanical obstruction: urethral stone, foreign body, urethral stricture, BPH, prostate carcinoma, prostatitis, trauma with hematoma formation.
Neurogenic bladder.
Neurologic disease (MS, parkinsonism, tabes dorsalis, CVA).
Spinal cord injury.
CNS neoplasm (primary or metastatic).
Spinal anesthesia.
Lower urinary tract instrumentation.
Medications (antihistamines, antidepressants, narcotics, anticholinergics).
Abdominal or pelvic surgery.
Alcohol toxicity.
Pregnancy.
Anxiety.
Encephalitis.
Postoperative pain.
Spina bifida occulta.

URINARY TRACT BLEEDING, UPPER[89]

ICD-10CM #   *Varies with specific diagnosis*

DIFFERENTIAL DIAGNOSIS FOR UPPER URINARY TRACT BLEEDING

Renal glomerular diseases:
    IgA nephropathy (Berger disease).
    Thin basement membrane disease.
    Acute glomerulonephritis (e.g., poststreptococcal).
    Lupus nephritis.
    Hereditary nephritis (e.g., Alport syndrome).
Renal tubulointerstitial diseases:
    Papillary necrosis.
    Sickle cell nephropathy.
    Analgesic nephropathy.
    Polycystic kidney disease.
    Medullary sponge kidney.

Vasculitis:
    Henoch-Schönlein purpura.
    Wegener granulomatosis.
Infection:
    Pyelonephritis.
    Xanthogranulomatous pyelonephritis.
    Renal tuberculosis.
    Fungal infection.
Obstruction:
    Ureteropelvic junction obstruction.
    Ureteral stricture.
Nephrolithiasis.
Malignancy:
    Renal cortical tumors (renal cell carcinoma, benign tumors).
    Upper tract urothelial carcinoma.
Fibroepithelial polyp.
Vascular diseases:
    Renal arteriovenous malformations (congenital, acquired).
    Iliac arterio-ureteral fistula.
    Renal artery aneurysm (especially ruptured).
    Renal artery pseudoaneurysm.
    Renal artery and/or vein thrombosis.
    Hemangioma.
    Atheroembolic disease.
    Nutcracker syndrome.
    Loin-pain hematuria syndrome.
Trauma:
    Blunt.
    Penetrating.
Lateralizing essential hematuria.

URINARY TRACT OBSTRUCTION[59]

ICD-10CM #   N21.8   Other lower urinary tract calculus
              N20.9   Urolithiasis

INTRARENAL

Uric acid nephropathy.
Sulfonamide precipitates.
Acyclovir, indinavir precipitates.
Multiple myeloma.

URETERAL

Intrinsic
Intraluminal:
    Nephrolithiasis.
    Papillary necrosis.
    Blood clots.
    Fungus balls.
Intramural:
    Ureteropelvic junction dysfunction.
    Ureterovesical junction dysfunction.
    Ureteral valve, polyp, or tumor.
    Ureteral stricture.
    Schistosomiasis.
    Tuberculosis.
    Scarring from instrumentation.

Drugs (e.g., NSAIDs).
Extrinsic
Vascular system:
    Aneurysm: abdominal aorta or iliac vessels.
    Aberrant vessels: ureteropelvic junction.
    Venous: retrocaval ureter.
GI tract:
    Crohn disease.
    Diverticulitis.
    Appendiceal abscess.
    Colon cancer.
    Pancreatic tumor, abscess, or cyst.
Reproductive system:
    Uterus: pregnancy, prolapse, tumor, endometriosis.
    Ovary: abscess, tumor, ovarian remnants.
    Gartner duct cyst, tuboovarian abscess.
Retroperitoneal disease:
    Retroperitoneal fibrosis: radiation, drugs, idiopathic.
    Inflammatory: tuberculosis, sarcoidosis.
    Hematoma.
    Primary tumor (e.g., lymphoma, sarcoma).
    Metastatic tumor (e.g., cervix, ovarian, bladder, colon).
    Lymphocele.
    Pelvic lipomatosis.

BLADDER

Neurogenic bladder:
    Diabetes mellitus.
    Spinal cord defect.
    Trauma.
    Multiple sclerosis.
    Stroke.
    Parkinson disease.
    Spinal anesthesia.
    Anticholinergics.
Bladder neck dysfunction.
Bladder calculus.
Bladder cancer.

URETHRA

Urethral stricture.
Prostate hypertrophy or cancer.
Obstruction from instrumentation.

URINARY TRACT OBSTRUCTION, CONGENITAL CAUSES[11]

ICD-10CM #   *Varies with specific diagnosis*

CONGENITAL CAUSES OF URINARY TRACT OBSTRUCTION

Ureteropelvic Junction
Ureteropelvic junction obstruction.
Proximal and Middle Ureter
Ureteral folds.
Ureteral valves.
Strictures.
Benign fibroepithelial polyps.

Differential Diagnosis

II

Retrocaval ureter.
Distal Ureter
Ureterovesical junction obstruction.
Vesicoureteral reflux.
Prune-belly syndrome.
Ureteroceles.
Bladder
Bladder diverticula.
Neurologic conditions (e.g., spina bifida).
Urethra
Posterior urethral valves.
Urethral diverticula.
Anterior urethral valves.
Urethral atresia.
Labial fusion.

URINE CASTS

ICD-10CM #	R82.99	Other abnormal findings in urine

Normal finding.
Pyelonephritis.
Chronic renal disease.
Nephrotic syndrome.
Acute tubular necrosis.
Interstitial nephritis.
Nephritic syndrome.
Glomerulonephritis.
Eclampsia.
Heavy metal ingestion.
Allograft rejection.
Hypothyroidism.

URINE COLOR ABNORMALITIES[115]

ICD-10CM #	R82.5	Elevated urine levels of drugs, medicaments and biological substances
	R82.99	Other abnormal findings in urine

COMMON CAUSES OF ABNORMAL URINE COLOR
Colorless.

DISEASE
Diabetes mellitus.
Diabetes insipidus.

DRUG
Ethyl alcohol.
Diuretics.

MISCELLANEOUS
Overhydration.
Yellow-orange

DRUG
Tetracycline.
Flutamide.
Pyridium.
Azo Gantrisin (Roche Labs, Nutley, NJ).
Sulfasalazine.

Vitamin B.

MISCELLANEOUS
Dehydration.
Milky White

DISEASE
Urinary tract infection/pyuria.
Blue-green

DISEASE
Pseudomonas urinary tract infection.

DRUG
Methylene blue.
Urised (Polymedica Pharmaceuticals, Woburn, MA).
Indigo carmine.
Doan's pills (Novartis Consumer Health, Parsippany, NJ).
Clorets (Cadbury Adams, Parsippany, NJ).
Amitriptyline.
Red-brown

DISEASE
Hematuria.
Hemolytic anemia.
Hemoglobinuria.
Lead poisoning.
Mercury poisoning.
Porphyria.

DRUG
Rifampin.
Ex-Lax (Novartis Consumer Health, Parsippany, NJ).
Phenolphthalein.
Phenothiazines.
Nitrofurantoin.
Doxorubicin.

MISCELLANEOUS
Beets.
Blackberries.
Rhubarb.
Brown-black

DISEASE
Fecaluria.
Methemoglobinuria.
Melaninuria.

DRUG
Metronidazole.
Methyldopa.
Methocarbamol.

MISCELLANEOUS
Fava beans.
Aloe.

URINE, RED[104]

ICD-10CM #	Varies with specific diagnosis

WITH A POSITIVE DIPSTICK
Hematuria.
Hemoglobinuria: negative urinalysis.
Myoglobinuria: negative urinalysis.

WITH A NEGATIVE DIPSTICK
Drugs
Aminosalicylic acid.
Deferoxamine mesylate.
Ibuprofen.
Phenacetin.
Phenolphthalein.
Phensuximide.
Rifampin.
Anthraquinone laxatives.
Doxorubicin.
Methyldopa.
Phenazopyridine.
Phenothiazine.
Phenytoin.
Dyes
Azo dyes.
Eosin.
Foods
Beets, berries, maize.
Rhodamine B.
Metabolic
Porphyrins.
Serratia marcescens (red diaper syndrome).
Urate crystalluria.

UROLITHIASIS-LIKE PAIN[11]

ICD-10CM #	Varies with specific diagnosis

DIFFERENTIAL DIAGNOSIS OF UROLITHIASIS-LIKE PAIN
Category
Disorders
Renal:
  Pyelonephritis.
  Blood clot.
  Renal infarction.
  Tumor (kidney or pelvis).
  Papillary necrosis.
Ureteral:
  Tumor.
  Blood clot.
  Stricture.
Bladder:
  Tumor.
  Blood clot.
  Urinary retention.
Intraabdominal:
  Peritonitis.
  Appendicitis.
  Biliary disease.
  Bowel obstruction.
  Vascular disorder.
  Aortic aneurysm.
  Mesenteric insufficiency.
Retroperitoneal:
  Lymphadenopathy.

Fibrosis.
Tumor.
Gynecologic:
    Ectopic or tubal pregnancy.
    Ovarian torsion, cyst rupture.
    Pelvic inflammatory disease.
    Cervical cancer.
    Endometriosis.
    Ovarian vein syndrome.
Neuromuscular:
    Muscle pain.
    Rib fracture.
    Radiculitis.
Infectious:
    Herpes zoster.
    Pleuritis, pneumonia.
    Fungal bezoar.

UROPATHY, OBSTRUCTIVE[17]

ICD-10CM #   N13.9   Obstructive and reflux
                        uropathy, unspecified
                 N20.9   Urolithiasis

INTRINSIC CAUSES
Intraluminal
Intratubular deposition of crystals (uric acid,
    sulfas).
Stones.
Papillary tissue.
Blood clots.
Intramural
Functional.
Ureter (ureteropelvic or ureterovesical
    dysfunction).
Bladder (neurogenic): spinal cord defect or
    trauma, diabetes, multiple sclerosis, Parkin-
    son disease, cerebrovascular accidents.
Bladder neck dysfunction.
Anatomic
Tumors.
Infection, granuloma.
Strictures.

EXTRINSIC CAUSES
Originating in the Reproductive System
Prostate: benign hypertrophy or cancer.
Uterus: pregnancy, tumors, prolapse,
    endometriosis.
Ovary: abscess, tumor, cysts.
Originating in the Vascular System
Aneurysms (aorta, iliac vessels).
Aberrant arteries (ureteropelvic junction).
Venous (ovarian veins, retrocaval ureter).
Originating in the Gastrointestinal Tract
Crohn disease.
Pancreatitis.
Appendicitis.
Tumors.
Originating in the Retroperitoneal Space
Inflammations.
Fibrosis.
Tumor, hematomas.

UROSEPSIS[115]

ICD-10CM #   A41.9   Sepsis, unspecified
                        organism

COMMON CAUSES OF UROSEPSIS
Obstructing ureteral stone with pyonephrosis.
Staghorn calculus with urinary tract infection.
Ureteral obstruction with proximal urinary tract
    infection.
Urinary retention with urinary tract infection.
Acute prostatitis with prostatic abscess.
Perinephric abscess or renal carbuncle.
Urethral stricture with periurethral abscess.
Fournier gangrene.
Foreign body within urinary tract (e.g., Foley
    catheter).

URTICARIA IN TRAVELERS[69]

ICD-10CM #   L50.9   Urticaria, unspecified

CAUSES OF URTICARIA IN TRAVELERS
Noninfectious causes: adverse drug reaction.*
Viral infection: hepatitis A infection.
Parasitic infection: invasive phase of helminthic
    diseases (ascariasis, hookworm, strongyloi-
    diasis, anisakiasis, gnathostomiasis, schisto-
    somiasis,* fascioliasis), chronic helminthic
    infections where humans are dead-end host
    (trichinellosis, toxocariasis), and rupture of
    cyst during hydatid disease.

---

*Common cause.

UTERINE BLEEDING, ABNORMAL[55]

ICD-10CM #   N92.6   Irregular menstruation,
                        unspecified
                 N93.9   Abnormal uterine and
                        vaginal bleeding,
                        unspecified

PREGNANCY
Threatened abortion.
Incomplete abortion.
Complete abortion.
Molar pregnancy.
Ectopic pregnancy.
Retained products of conception.

OVULATORY
Vulva: infection, laceration, tumor.
Vagina: infection, laceration, tumor, foreign body.
Cervix: polyps, cervical erosion, cervicitis,
    carcinoma.
Uterus: fibroids (submucous fibroids most likely
    to cause abnormal bleeding), polyps, adeno-
    myosis, endometritis, intrauterine device,
    atrophic endometrium.

Pregnancy complications: ectopic pregnancy;
    threatened, incomplete, complete abortion;
    retained products of conception.
Abnormality of clotting system.
Midcycle bleeding.
Halban disease (persistent corpus luteum).
Menorrhagia.
Pelvic inflammatory disease.

ANOVULATORY
Physiologic causes:
Puberty.
Perimenopausal.
    Pathologic causes:
    Ovarian failure (FSH over 40 IU/ml).
    Hyperandrogenism.
    Hyperprolactinemia.
    Obesity.
    Hypothalamic dysfunction (polycystic ovaries);
        LH/FSH ratio greater than 2:1.
    Hyperplasia.
    Endometrial carcinoma.
    Estrogen-producing tumors.
    Hypothyroidism.

UVEITIS, PEDIATRIC AGE

ICD-10CM #   H20.9   Anterior uveitis

ANTERIOR UVEITIS
Juvenile rheumatoid arthritis (pauciarticular).
Sarcoidosis.
Trauma.
Tuberculosis.
Kawasaki disease.
Ulcerative colitis.
Postinfectious (enteric or genital) with arthritis
    and rash.
Spirochetal (syphilis, leptospiral).
Heterochromic iridocyclitis (Fuchs).
Viral (herpes simplex, herpes zoster).
Ankylosing spondylitis.
Stevens-Johnson syndrome.
Idiopathic.
Drugs.

POSTERIOR UVEITIS (CHOROIDITIS—MAY INVOLVE RETINA)
Toxoplasmosis.
Parasites (toxocariasis).
Sarcoidosis.
Tuberculosis.
Viral (rubella, herpes simplex, HIV,
    cytomegalovirus).
Subacute sclerosing panencephalitis.
Idiopathic.

ANTERIOR AND/OR POSTERIOR UVEITIS
Sympathetic ophthalmia (trauma to other eye).

Differential
Diagnosis

II

Vogt-Koyanagi-Harada syndrome (uveo-otocuta-neous syndrome: poliosis, vitiligo, deafness, tinnitus, uveitis, aseptic meningitis, retinitis).

Behçet syndrome.

Lyme disease.

V – Differential Diagnosis

VAGINAL BLEEDING, ABNORMAL

ICD-10CM # N93.9 Abnormal uterine and vaginal bleeding, unspecified

DIFFERENTIAL DIAGNOSIS OF ABNORMAL VAGINAL BLEEDING
Ovulatory Bleeding—Menorrhagia
Anovulatory bleeding—sometimes known as dysfunctional uterine bleeding (DUB).
Uterine and Ovarian Pathology
Uterine fibroids (pelvic pain, dysmenorrhea).
Endometriosis; adenomyosis (dysmenorrhea, dyspareunia, pelvic pain, infertility).
Pelvic inflammatory disease and pelvic infection (fever, vaginal discharge, pelvic pain, inter-menstrual and postcoital bleeding).
Endometrial polyps (intermenstrual bleeding).
Endometrial hyperplasia; endometrial carcinoma (pelvic pain, abnormal bleeding, postcoital bleeding).
Polycystic ovary syndrome (irregular bleeding, infertility, and hirsutism)
Systemic Disease
Coagulation disorder; bleeding diathesis such as von Willebrand disease.
Liver or renal disease.
Hypothyroidism (fatigue, constipation, coarse features, alopecia).

IATROGENIC CAUSE
Anticoagulation.
Intrauterine device.
Chemotherapy.
Sex steroids.

VAGINAL BLEEDING, PREGNANCY[93]

ICD-10CM # N93.9 Abnormal uterine and vaginal bleeding, unspecified

FIRST TRIMESTER
Implantation bleeding.
Abortion:
  Threatened.
  Complete.
  Incomplete.
  Missed.
Ectopic pregnancy.
Neoplasia.
Hydatidiform mole.
Cervix.

THIRD TRIMESTER
Placenta previa.
Placental abruption.
Premature labor.
Choriocarcinoma.

VAGINAL DISCHARGE, PREPUBERTAL GIRLS[23]

ICD-10CM # N89.8 Other specified noninflammatory disorders of vagina

Irritative (bubble baths, sand):
  Poor perineal hygiene.
  Foreign body.
  Associated systemic illness (group A strepto-cocci, chickenpox).
  Infections.
  Escherichia coli with foreign body.
  Shigella organisms.
  Yersinia organisms.
  Infections (consider sexual abuse):
    Chlamydia trachomatis.
    Neisseria gonorrhoeae.
    Trichomonas vaginalis.
Tumor (rare).

VALVULAR HEART DISEASE[18]

ICD-10CM # Varies with specific diagnosis

MAJOR CAUSES OF VALVULAR HEART DISEASE IN ADULTS
Aortic Stenosis
Bicuspid aortic valve.
Rheumatic fever.
Degenerative stenosis.
Aortic Regurgitation
Bicuspid aortic valve.
Aortic dissection.
Endocarditis.
Rheumatic fever.
Aortic root dilation.
Mitral Stenosis
Rheumatic fever.
Mitral Regurgitation

CHRONIC
Mitral valve prolapse.
Left ventricular dilation.
Posterior wall myocardial infarction.
Rheumatic fever.
Endocarditis.

ACUTE
Posterior wall or papillary muscle ischemia.
Papillary muscle or chordal rupture.
Endocarditis.
Prosthetic valve dysfunction.
Systolic anterior motion of mitral valve.

TRICUSPID REGURGITATION
Functional (annular) dilation.

Tricuspid valve prolapse.
Endocarditis.
Carcinoid heart disease.

VASCULAR LESIONS OF GI TRACT[3]

ICD-10CM # Varies with specific diagnosis

Primary Vascular Lesions
Aneurysms of the aorta and its branches.
Angioectasia (angiodysplasia, vascular ectasia).
Arteriovenous malformation.
Blue rubber bleb nevus.
Capillary phlebectasia.
Dieulafoy lesion.
Glomus tumor.
Hemangioma.
Hemangiomatosis.
Hemangioendothelioma.
Hemangiopericytoma.
Hemangiosarcoma.
Hemorrhoids.
Kaposi sarcoma.
Diseases and Syndromes with Vascular Lesions
Blue rubber bleb nevus syndrome.
Ehlers-Danlos syndrome.
Hereditary hemorrhagic telangiectasia (Osler-Weber-Rendu disease).
Klippel-Trenaunay or Parkes Weber syndrome.
Kohlmeier-Degos syndrome.
Marfan syndrome.
Pseudoxanthoma elasticum.
PSS (scleroderma, CREST).
Scurvy.
Turner syndrome.
von Willebrand disease.
Systemic Disorders Associated with Vascular Lesions
Portal hypertension:
  Congestive gastropathy and colopathy.
  GAVE (watermelon stomach).
  Spider telangiectasias.
  Varices.
Renal failure:
  GI telangiectasias.
  GAVE (watermelon stomach).
Vasculitis (e.g., polyarteritis nodosa).
Iatrogenic lesions:
  Radiation telangiectasia.

CREST, Calcinosis, Raynaud phenomenon, esophageal dysmotility, sclerodactyly, telangiectasia; *GAVE*, gastric antral vascular ectasia

VASCULITIS, CLASSIFICATION

ICD-10CM # I77.6 Arteritis, unspecified

LARGE VESSEL DISEASE
Arteritis
Giant cell arteritis.
Takayasu arteritis.

Arteritis associated with Reiter syndrome (reactive arthritis), ankylosing spondylitis.

MEDIUM AND SMALL VESSEL DISEASE
Polyarteritis Nodosa
Primary (idiopathic).
Associated with viruses (hepatitis B or C, CMV, HIV, herpes zoster).
Associated with malignancy (hairy cell leukemia).
Familial Mediterranean fever.
Granulomatous Vasculitis
Granulomatosis with polyangiitis.
Lymphomatoid granulomatosis.
Behçet Disease
Kawasaki Disease (Mucocutaneous Lymph Node Syndrome)

PREDOMINANTLY SMALL VESSEL DISEASE
Hypersensitivity Vasculitis (Leukocytoclastic Vasculitis)
Henoch-Schönlein purpura.
Mixed cryoglobulinemia.
Serum sickness.
Vasculitis associated with connective tissue diseases (SLE, Sjögren syndrome).
Vasculitis associated with specific syndromes:
 Primary biliary cirrhosis.
 Lyme disease.
 Chronic active hepatitis.
 Drug-induced vasculitis.
Churg-Strauss Syndrome
 Goodpasture Syndrome
 Erythema Nodosum
 Panniculitis. Buerger Disease
 (Thrombophlebitis Obliterans)

VASCULITIS (DISEASES THAT MIMIC VASCULITIS)[25]
ICD-10CM # Varies with specific diagnosis

EMBOLIC DISEASE
Infectious or marantic endocarditis.
Cardiac mural thrombus.
Atrial myxoma.
Cholesterol embolization syndrome.

NONINFLAMMATORY VESSEL WALL DISRUPTION
Atherosclerosis.
Arterial fibromuscular dysplasia.
Drug effects (vasoconstrictors, anticoagulants).
Radiation.
Genetic disease (neurofibromatosis, Ehlers-Danlos syndrome).
Amyloidosis.
Intravascular malignant lymphoma.

DIFFUSE COAGULATION
Disseminated intravascular coagulation.
Thrombotic thrombocytopenic purpura.
Hemolytic-uremic syndrome.

Protein C and S deficiencies, factor V/Leiden mutation.
Antiphospholipid syndrome.

VEGETATIVE STATE, PERSISTENT[18]
ICD-10CM # R40.3 Persistent vegetative state

PERSISTENT VEGETATIVE STATE: COMMON CAUSES*
Trauma (diffuse axonal injury).
Cardiac arrest and hypoperfusion (laminar necrosis of cortical mantle and/or thalamic necrosis).
Bihemispheric infarctions.
Purulent meningitis or encephalitis (cortical injury).
Carbon monoxide.
Prolonged hypoglycemic coma.

---

*A vegetative state may not necessarily begin with coma but can also develop as the end stage of neurodegenerative diseases (e.g., Alzheimer disease) of adults or children and can accompany severe congenital developmental abnormalities of the brain such as anencephaly.

VENTILATION DISORDERS[96]
ICD-10CM # Varies with specific diagnosis

UPPER AIRWAY PATHOLOGY
Obstructive sleep apnea.
Upper airway mechanical dysfunction (e.g., tracheal stenosis, vocal cord dysfunction).
Foreign body inhalation.
Oropharyngeal disorders (e.g., tonsillar hypertrophy, epiglottitis, malignancies).

LOWER AIRWAY OBSTRUCTIVE PATHOLOGY
Reversible airway disease: asthma.
Chronic obstructive pulmonary disease: emphysema, chronic bronchitis.
Bronchiectasis.
Lobar collapse (foreign body, neoplasm, mucus plug).

LOWER AIRWAY PARENCHYMAL PATHOLOGY
Infection: pneumonia.
Interstitial disease: idiopathic, pneumoconiosis, autoimmune, granulomatous, drug-induced, hypersensitivity.
Neoplasm.

CHEST WALL AND PLEURAL ABNORMALITIES
Pleural effusion.
Empyema.
Skeletal deformity (e.g., kyphoscoliosis, fractured ribs).
Malignancy—mesothelioma.

Pneumothorax.
Primary or secondary muscle disease (e.g., polymyositis, muscular dystrophy, drug-induced myopathy).

CENTRAL CONTROL PROBLEMS
Central sleep apnea.
Sedation (e.g., due to drugs, primary cerebral disease).

VENTILATION–PERFUSION MISMATCH ON LUNG SCAN
ICD-10CM # Varies with specific diagnosis

Pulmonary embolism.
Emphysema.
Irradiation.
Pulmonary hypertension.
AV malformations.
Pulmonary thrombosis.
External compression of pulmonary artery (neoplasm, cysts, fibrosing mediastinitis).
Vasculitis.
Tuberculosis.
Pulmonary thrombosis.
Congenital (pulmonary artery hypoplasia, congenital heart disease with upper lobe diversion).
Sequestered segment.
Parasitic lung disease.
Intraluminal obstruction from catheter fragments.

VENTRICULAR FAILURE
ICD-10CM # I51.9 Heart disease, unspecified

LEFT VENTRICULAR FAILURE
Systemic hypertension.
Valvular heart disease (AS, AR, MR).
Cardiomyopathy, myocarditis.
Bacterial endocarditis.
Myocardial infarction.
Idiopathic hypertrophic subaortic stenosis.

RIGHT VENTRICULAR FAILURE
Valvular heart disease (mitral stenosis).
Pulmonary hypertension.
Bacterial endocarditis (right-sided).
Right ventricular infarction.

BIVENTRICULAR FAILURE
Left ventricular failure.
Cardiomyopathy.
Myocarditis
Arrhythmias.
Anemia.
Thyrotoxicosis.
Arteriovenous fistula.
Paget disease.
Beriberi.

VERRUCOUS LESIONS
ICD-10CM # Varies with specific diagnosis

Differential Diagnosis

II

Warts.
Seborrheic keratosis.
Lichen simplex.
Acanthosis nigricans.
Scabies (Norwegian, crusted).
Verrucous carcinoma.
Nevus sebaceous.
Deep fungal infection.

VERTEBRAL LESIONS[106]

ICD-10CM #	Varies with specific diagnosis

Anatomic Distribution of Vertebral Lesions

Anterior Elements of the Spine	Posterior Elements of the Spine	Both Anterior and Posterior Elements of the Spine
Multiple myeloma.	Osteoid osteoma.	Metastasis (spares disc end plates).
Hemangioma.	Osteoblastoma.	Infection (involves disc end plates).
Paget disease of bone.	Aneurysmal bone cyst.	Classic osteosarcoma.
Histiocytosis X (vertebra plana).		Postradiation sarcoma.
Giant cell tumor of bone.		Malignant histiocytoid variety.
Reparative granuloma.		Osteosarcoma.
Ewing sarcoma (primitive neuroectodermal tumor).		Osteochondroma.
Lymphoma of bone.		Primary chondrosarcoma.
Malignant fibrous histiocytoma.		Secondary chondrosarcoma.
Chordoma.		

VERTIGO

ICD-10CM #	R42	Dizziness and giddiness
	H81.13	Benign paroxysmal vertigo, bilateral
	H81.49	Vertigo of central origin, unspecified ear
	H81.399	Other peripheral vertigo, unspecified ear
	H81.23	Vestibular neuronitis, bilateral

PERIPHERAL
Otitis media.
Acute labyrinthitis.
Vestibular neuronitis.
Benign positional vertigo.
Ménière disease.

Ototoxic drugs: streptomycin, gentamicin.
Lesions of the eighth nerve: acoustic neuroma, meningioma, mononeuropathy, metastatic carcinoma.
Mastoiditis.

CNS OR SYSTEMIC
Vertebrobasilar artery insufficiency.
Posterior fossa tumor or other brain tumors.
Infarction/hemorrhage of cerebral cortex, cerebellum, or brain stem.
Basilar migraine.
Metabolic: drugs, hypoxia, anemia, fever.
Hypotension/severe hypertension.
Multiple sclerosis.
CNS infections: viral, bacterial.
Temporal lobe epilepsy.
Arnold-Chiari malformation, syringobulbia.
Psychogenic: ventilation, hysteria.

VERTIGO, CENTRAL[29]

ICD-10CM #	R42

MAJOR CAUSES OF CENTRAL VERTIGO
Demyelination:
  Acquired.
  Leukodystrophies.
  Multiple sclerosis.
Familial disorders:
  Friedreich ataxia.
  Spinocerebellar ataxia.
  Familial episodic ataxia (type 1 and type 2).
  Olivopontocerebellar atrophy.
CNS infections:
  Lyme neuroborreliosis.
  Meningitis.
  Tuberculosis.
Intrinsic brain stem lesion:
  Tumor.
  Arteriovenous malformation.
  Trauma.
Migraine:
  Basilar.
  Benign paroxysmal positional vertigo of childhood.
Toxins:
  Drugs, alcohol.
  Analgesics.
  Anticonvulsants.
  Antihypertensives.
  Hypnotics.
  Tranquilizers.
Metabolic and endocrine disorders:
  Hyperinsulinism.
  Impaired glucose tolerance.
  Diabetes mellitus.
  Hypertriglyceridemia.
  Hypothyroidism.
Systemic conditions:
  Paget disease.
Stroke/ischemia:

Vertebrobasilar.
Cerebellar.
Posterior inferior cerebellar artery syndrome.
Lateral medullary syndrome.
Medial medullary infarct.
Basilar artery syndrome.
Anterior inferior cerebellar artery.
Other causes of posterior ischemia:
  Subclavian steal syndrome.
  Rotational vertebral artery occlusion syndrome.
  Vertebral artery dissection.
  Vertebral or basilar artery dolichoectasia.
  Neoplasm of the fourth ventricle.
  Chiari malformation.
  Superficial siderosis of the CNS.
  Vestibular epilepsy.

VESICULAR OR BULLOUS SKIN RASH[12]

ICD-10CM #	R21	Rash and other nonspecific skin eruption

CAUSES OF A VESICULAR OR BULLOUS SKIN RASH
Most Common
Viral:
  Herpes zoster.
  Herpes simplex.
Impetigo.
Scabies.
Insect bites and papular urticaria.
Bullous eczema and pompholyx.
Drugs:
  Sulfonamides.
  Penicillin.
  Barbiturates.
Less Common
Erythema multiforme major ("target lesions" rash, plus one mucous membrane involved) or erythema multiforme minor (1 to 2 cm "target lesions" only):
  Mycoplasma pneumonia.
  Herpes simplex.
  Drugs such as sulfur, penicillins.
  Idiopathic (50%).
SJS and TEN with epidermal detachment and mucosal erosions:
  Drugs such as anticonvulsants, sulfonamides, NSAIDs, and penicillins.
Staphylococcal scalded-skin syndrome (children).
Dermatitis herpetiformis (gluten sensitivity).
Pemphigus and pemphigoid.
Rare
Porphyria cutanea tarda.
Epidermolysis bullosa.

NSAIDs, Nonsteroidal antiinflammatory drugs; *SJS,* Stevens-Johnson syndrome; *TEN,* toxic epidermal necrolysis.

VESICULOBULLOUS DISEASES[24]

ICD-10CM #		
	L94.2	Calcinosis cutis
	L98.8	Other specified disorders of the skin and subcutaneous tissue

IMMUNOLOGICALLY MEDIATED DISEASES

Bullous pemphigoid.
Herpes gestationis.
Mucous membrane pemphigoid.
Epidermolysis bullosa acquisita.
Dermatitis herpetiformis.
Pemphigus (vulgaris, foliaceus, paraneoplastic).

HYPERSENSITIVITY DISEASES

Erythema multiforme minor.
Erythema multiforme major (Stevens-Johnson syndrome).
Toxic epidermal necrolysis.

METABOLIC DISEASES

Porphyria cutanea tarda.
Pseudoporphyria.
Diabetic blisters.

INHERITED GENETIC DISORDERS

Epidermolysis bullosa:
Simplex.
Junctional.
Dystrophic.

INFECTIOUS DISEASES

Impetigo.
Staphylococcal scalded skin syndrome.
Herpes simplex.
Varicella.
Herpes zoster.

VIRAL ENCEPHALITIS, COMMON CAUSES[94]

ICD-10CM #		
	A86	Unspecified viral encephalitis
	A85.2	Arthropod-borne viral encephalitis, unspecified
	A84.9	Tick-borne viral encephalitis, unspecified
	A83.9	Mosquito-borne viral encephalitis, unspecified
	A85.8	Other specified viral encephalitis
	A85	Other viral encephalitis, not elsewhere classified

COMMON CAUSES OF VIRAL ENCEPHALITIS

Causes of Viral Encephalitis

Nonseasonal:
Herpes simplex virus type 1 (herpes simplex encephalitis).
Herpes simplex virus type 2 (neonatal encephalitis or adult meningoencephalitis).

Seasonal—summer and fall—arboviruses (arthropod borne):
West Nile virus.
St. Louis encephalitis virus.
Eastern equine encephalitis virus.
Western equine encephalitis virus.
La Crosse/California encephalitis virus.
Powassan encephalitis virus.
Chikungunya virus.

Seasonal—nonarthropod borne:
Summer and fall: enteroviruses (including coxsackieviruses, echoviruses, polioviruses, and enterovirus 71).
Winter: influenza virus.

Immunosuppressed patients:
Human immunodeficiency virus (chronic HIV encephalitis).
Varicella-zoster virus (subacute encephalitis).
JC virus (progressive multifocal leukoencephalopathy).
Cytomegalovirus (ventriculitis or encephalitis).
Human herpesvirus 6 (subacute encephalitis).
Epstein-Barr virus (subacute encephalitis).

Uncommon Causes in the U.S.

Powassan encephalitis virus.
Zika virus.
Chikungunya virus.
Variegated squirrel bornavirus.
Lymphotropic choriomeningitis virus.
Rabies.
Measles (subacute sclerosing panencephalitis).
Mumps.
Adenovirus.
Herpes B virus (of monkeys).
Rubella (progressive rubella panencephalitis).

Causes Outside the United States

Zika virus (Africa, Asia, Caribbean, Central America, Pacific Islands, South America).
Chikungunya virus (Africa, Asia, Central America, Pacific Islands, South America, Western Europe).
Tick-borne encephalitis virus (Russia, Asia).
Japanese encephalitis virus (Japan, Southeast Asia, Malaysia).
Venezuelan equine encephalitis virus (Central and South America).
Dengue virus (Southern Asia, Africa, South America).
Rift Valley fever virus (east central Africa).
Murray Valley encephalitis virus (Australia).
Powassan encephalitis virus (Canada).
Nipah virus (Malaysia and Bangladesh).

VISION LOSS, ACUTE, PAINFUL

ICD-10CM #	H53.139	Sudden visual loss, unspecified eye

Acute angle-closure glaucoma.
Corneal ulcer.
Uveitis.
Endophthalmitis.

Factitious.
Somatization syndrome.
Trauma.

VISION LOSS, ACUTE, PAINLESS

ICD-10CM #	H53.139	Sudden visual loss, unspecified eye

Retinal artery occlusion.
Optic neuritis.
Retinal vein occlusion.
Vitreous hemorrhage.
Retinal detachment.
Exudative macular degeneration.
CVA.
Ischemic optic neuropathy.
Factitious.
Somatization syndrome, anxiety reaction.

VISION LOSS, ACUTE, PEDIATRIC AGE[20]

ICD-10CM #	Varies with specific diagnosis

Carotid dissection.[a]
Cortical blindness.
Anoxic encephalopathy.
Benign occipital epilepsy.[a]
Hydrocephalus.[a]
Hypoglycemia.[a]
Hypertension[a] (malignant or accelerated).
Hyperviscosity.
Hypotension.
Migraine.[a]
Occipital metastatic disease.
Posttraumatic transient cerebral blindness.
Systemic lupus erythematosus.
Toxic[a] (e.g., cyclosporine).
Trauma.
Disorders affecting the optic nerves.
Optic neuropathy.[a]
Demyelinating.
Idiopathic optic neuritis.
Multiple sclerosis.
Neuromyelitis optica.
Ischemic.
Toxic.
Traumatic.
Pituitary apoplexy.
Pseudotumor cerebri.[a]
Retinal disease.
Central retinal artery occlusion.
Migraine.
Trauma.

[a]Denotes the most common conditions and the ones with disease-modifying treatments.

VISION LOSS AFTER DIVING[112]

ICD-10CM #	H53.139	Sudden visual loss, unspecified eye

DIFFERENTIAL DIAGNOSIS OF DECREASED VISION AFTER DIVING

Decompression sickness.
Arterial gas embolism.
Bubbles under contact lenses.
Displaced contact lens.
Antifog agent keratopathy.
Contact lens adherence syndrome.
Transdermal scopolamine
Hyperoxic myopia.
Oxymetazoline optic neuropathy.
Diving-induced migraine phenomena.
Eye disorders not related to diving.

VISION LOSS, CHILDREN

ICD-10CM # H53.9 Unspecified visual disturbance

Craniopharyngioma.
Hereditary optic atrophy.
Optic nerve glioma.
Glioma of chiasm.
Albinism.
Optic nerve hypoplasia.

VISION LOSS, CHRONIC, PROGRESSIVE

ICD-10CM # H54.7 Unspecified visual loss

Cataract.
Macular degeneration.
Cerebral neoplasm.
Refractive error.
Open-angle glaucoma.

VISION LOSS, MONOCULAR, TRANSIENT

ICD-10CM # H54.7 Unspecified visual loss

Thromboembolism.
Vasculitis.
Migraine (vasospasm).
Anxiety reaction.
CNS tumor.
Temporal arteritis.
Multiple sclerosis.

VISION LOSS, PROGRESSIVE, PEDIATRIC AGE[20]

ICD-10CM # Varies with specific diagnosis

Compressive optic neuropathies.
   Aneurysm.[a]
   Arteriovenous malformations.[a]
   Craniopharyngioma.[a]
   Hypothalamic and optic tumors.
   Pituitary adenoma.[a]
   Pseudotumor cerebri.[a]

[a]. Denotes the most common conditions and the ones
   with disease-modifying treatments.

Disorders of the lens.
   Cataract.
   Dislocation of the lens.
Hereditary optic atrophy.
   Leber hereditary optic neuropathy.
   Wolfram syndrome.
Intraocular tumors.
Tapetoretinal degenerations.
   Abnormal carbohydrate metabolism.
      Mucopolysaccharidosis.
      Primary hyperoxaluria.
   Abnormal lipid metabolism.
      Abetalipoproteinemia.
      Hypobetalipoproteinemia.
      Multiple sulfatase deficiency.
      Neuronal ceroid lipofuscinosis.
      Niemann-Pick disease.
      Refsum disease.
Other syndromes of unknown etiology.
   Bardet-Biedl syndrome.
   Cockayne syndrome.
   Laurence-Moon syndrome.
   Refsum disease.
   Usher syndrome.

VISUAL HALLUCINATIONS[101]

ICD-10CM # Varies with specific diagnosis

Blindness/sensory deprivation—Charles Bonnet
   syndrome.
Palinopsia.
Dementia-producing diseases.
   Alzheimer disease.
   Dementia with Lewy bodies.[a]
   Parkinson disease.[b]
Intoxications.
   Alcoholic hallucinosis.
   Delirium tremens (DTs).
Hallucinogens.
   Amphetamines.
   Cocaine.
   Lysergic acid diethylamide (LSD).
   Phencyclidine (PCP).
Medicines.
   Atropine, scopolamine.
   Levodopa and dopamine agonists.
   Steroids.
Migraine with aura (classic migraine).
Narcolepsy: hypnopompic (awakening) and hyp-
   nagogic (falling asleep) hallucinations.
Seizures.
Peduncular hallucinations.

[a] Although visual hallucinations are likely to complicate almost
   any form of dementia, they are characteristic of dementia
   with Lewy bodies.
[b] Dopaminergic medications such as levodopa-carbidopa
   (Sinemet) are more likely than Parkinson disease itself to
   produce hallucinations.

VISUAL IMPAIRMENT, ELDERLY PATIENT[101]

ICD-10CM # Varies with specific diagnosis

Cataracts.
Diabetic retinopathy.

Macular degeneration.
Glaucoma.
Presbyopia and other accommodation problems.
Temporal (giant cell) arteritis.
Visual agnosia and cortical blindness from mul-
   tiple strokes or Alzheimer disease.

VITREOUS HEMORRHAGE[98]

ICD-10CM # H43.13 Vitreous hemorrhage,
                     bilateral

CAUSES OF VITREOUS HEMORRHAGE

Acute posterior vitreous detachment associated
   either with a retinal tear or avulsion of a pe-
   ripheral vessel.
Proliferative retinopathies:
   Diabetic.
   Following retinal vein occlusion.
   Sickle cell disease.
   Eales disease.
   Vasculitis.
Miscellaneous retinal disorders:
   Macroaneurysm.
   Telangiectasis.
   Capillary hemangioma.
Trauma:
   Blunt.
   Penetrating.
   Iatrogenic.
Systemic:
   Bleeding disorders.
   Terson syndrome.

VOCAL CORD PARALYSIS

ICD-10CM # J38.00 Paralysis of vocal cords
                     and larynx, unspecified
            J38.01 Paralysis of vocal cords
                     and larynx, unilateral
            J38.02 Paralysis of vocal cords
                     and larynx, bilateral

Neoplasm: primary or metastatic (e.g., lung,
   thyroid, parathyroid, mediastinum).
Neck surgery (parathyroid, thyroid, carotid end-
   arterectomy, cervical spine).
Idiopathic.
Viral, bacterial, or fungal infection.
Trauma (intubation, penetrating neck injury).
Cardiac surgery.
RA.
Multiple sclerosis.
Parkinsonism.
Toxic neuropathy.
CVA.
CNS abnormalities: hydrocephalus, Arnold–Chiari
   malformation, meningomyelocele.

VOLUME DEPLETION[18]

ICD-10CM # E86.9 Volume depletion,
                    unspecified

GI losses:

Upper: bleeding, nasogastric suction, vomiting.

Lower: bleeding, diarrhea, enteric or pancreatic fistula, tube drainage.

Renal losses:

Salt and water: diuretics, osmotic diuresis, postobstructive diuresis, acute tubular necrosis (recovery phase), salt-losing nephropathy, adrenal insufficiency, renal tubular acidosis.

Water loss: diabetes insipidus.

Skin and respiratory losses:

Sweat, burns, insensible losses.

Sequestration without external fluid loss:

Intestinal obstruction, peritonitis, pancreatitis, rhabdomyolysis, internal bleeding.

VOLUME EXCESS[18]

ICD-10CM # Varies with specific diagnosis

Primary Renal Sodium Retention (Increased Effective Circulating Volume)

Renal failure, nephritic syndrome, acute glomerulonephritis.

Primary hyperaldosteronism.

Cushing syndrome.

Liver disease.

Secondary Renal Sodium Retention (Decreased Effective Circulating Volume)

Heart failure.

Liver disease.

Nephrotic syndrome (minimal change disease).

Pregnancy.

VOMITING

ICD-10CM #	R11.10	Vomiting, unspecified
	R11.11	Vomiting without nausea
	R11.12	Projectile vomiting

GI disturbances:

Obstruction: esophageal, pyloric, intestinal.

Infections: viral or bacterial enteritis, viral hepatitis, food poisoning, gastroenteritis.

Pancreatitis.

Appendicitis.

Biliary colic.

Peritonitis.

Perforated bowel.

Diabetic gastroparesis.

Other: gastritis, PUD, IBD, GI tract neoplasms.

Drugs: morphine, digitalis, cytotoxic agents, bromocriptine.

Severe pain: MI, renal colic.

Metabolic disorders: uremia, acidosis/alkalosis, hyperglycemia, DKA, thyrotoxicosis.

Trauma: blows to the testicles, epigastrium.

Vertigo.

Reye syndrome.

Increased intracranial pressure.

CNS disturbances: trauma, hemorrhage, infarction, neoplasm, infection, hypertensive encephalopathy, migraine.

Radiation sickness.

Nausea and vomiting of pregnancy, hyperemesis gravidarum.

Motion sickness.

Bulimia, anorexia nervosa.

Psychogenic: emotional disturbances, offensive sights or smells.

Severe coughing.

Pyelonephritis.

Boerhaave syndrome.

Carbon monoxide poisoning.

VOMITING, NEONATAL[29]

ICD-10CM # R11.10 Vomiting, unspecified

CAUSES OF NEONATAL VOMITING

Anatomic Causes

Esophagus, trachea, great vessels:

Stricture.

Web.

Tracheoesophageal fistula.

Laryngeal cleft.

Double aortic arch.

Stomach and duodenum:

Pyloric stenosis.

Duodenal atresia (usually noted on the first day of life).

Small and large intestine:

Volvulus secondary to malrotation.

Incarcerated hernia.

Hirschsprung disease (secondary to obstipation).

Necrotizing enterocolitis.

Genitourinary:

Testicular torsion.

Nonanatomic Causes

Infection:

Septicemia.

Meningitis.

Urinary tract infection.

Gastroenteritis.

Otitis media.

Increased intracranial pressure:

Cerebral edema.

Subdural hematoma.

Hydrocephalus.

Brain tumor.

Congenital adrenal hyperplasia (salt-losing variety).

Inborn errors of metabolism.

Renal disease.

VULVAR LESIONS[55]

ICD-10CM #	N77.0	Ulceration of vulva in diseases classified elsewhere
	N90.7	Vulvar cyst
	N90.89	Other specified noninflammatory disorders of vulva and perineum

	D07.1	Carcinoma in situ of vulva
	N90.89	Other specified noninflammatory disorders of vulva and perineum
	N90.5	Atrophy of vulva

RED LESION

Infection/Infestation

Fungal infection:

Candida.

Tinea cruris.

Intertrigo.

Pityriasis versicolor.

Sarcoptes scabiei.

Erythrasma: *Corynebacterium minutissimum.*

Granuloma inguinale: *Calymmatobacterium granulomatis.*

Folliculitis: *Staphylococcus aureus.*

Hidradenitis suppurativa.

Behçet syndrome.

Inflammation

Reactive vulvitis.

Chemical irritation:

Detergent.

Dyes.

Perfume.

Spermicide.

Lubricants.

Hygiene sprays.

Podophyllum.

Topical 5-FU.

Saliva.

Gentian violet.

Semen.

Mechanical trauma: scratching.

Vestibular adenitis.

Essential vulvodynia.

Psoriasis.

Seborrheic dermatitis.

Neoplasm

Vulvar intraepithelial neoplasia (VIN):

Mild dysplasia.

Moderate dysplasia.

Severe dysplasia.

Carcinoma-in-situ.

Vulvar dystrophy.

Bowen disease.

Invasive cancer:

Squamous cell carcinoma.

Malignant melanoma.

Sarcoma.

Basal cell carcinoma.

Adenocarcinoma.

Paget disease.

Undifferentiated.

WHITE LESION

Vulvar dystrophy:

Lichen sclerosus.

Vulvar dystrophy.

Vulvar hyperplasia.

Mixed dystrophy.

VIN.
Vitiligo.
Partial albinism.
Intertrigo.
Radiation treatment.

DARK LESION

Lentigo.
Nevi (mole).
Neoplasm (see "Neoplasm, Vulvar," below).
Reactive hyperpigmentation.
Seborrheic keratosis.
Pubic lice.

ULCERATIVE LESION

Infection
Herpes simplex.
Vaccinia.
Treponema pallidum.
Granuloma inguinale.
Pyoderma.
Tuberculosis.
Noninfectious
Behçet disease.
Crohn disease.
Pemphigus.
Pemphigoid.
Hidradenitis suppurativa (see "Neoplasm, Vulvar," below).
Neoplasm
Basal cell carcinoma.
Squamous cell carcinoma.
Vulvar tumor <1 cm:
  Condyloma acuminatum.
  Molluscum contagiosum.
  Epidermal inclusion.
  Vestibular cyst.
  Mesonephric duct.
  VIN.
  Hemangioma.
  Hidradenoma.
  Neurofibroma.
  Syringoma.
  Accessory breast tissue.
  Acrochordon.
  Endometriosis.
  Fox-Fordyce disease.
  Pilonidal sinus.
Vulvar tumor >1 cm:
  Bartholin cyst or abscess.
  Lymphogranuloma venereum.
  Fibroma.
  Lipoma.
  Verrucous carcinoma.
  Squamous cell carcinoma.
  Hernia.
  Edema.
  Hematoma.
  Acrochordon.
  Epidermal cysts.
  Neurofibromatosis.
  Accessory breast tissue.

VULVAR PAIN[99]

ICD-10CM #	N94.81	Vulvodynia
	R10.2	Pelvic and perineal pain

DISEASES ASSOCIATED WITH VULVAR PAIN, NOT QUALIFYING FOR THE DIAGNOSIS OF VULVODYNIA

Podophyllin overdose.
Condylox (podofilox) overdose.
Behçet disease.
Aphthous ulcers.
Herpes (simplex and zoster).
Candidiasis.
Trichomonas.
Chancroid.
Sjögren disease.
Contact dermatitis.
Endometriosis.
Pemphigus.
Pemphigoid.
Atrophy.
Lichen sclerosus.
Lichen planus.
Crohn disease.
Bartholin abscess.
Trauma.
Imperforate hymen.
Prolapsed urethra.
Vulvar intraepithelial neoplasia.
Carcinoma.

VULVITIS, GRANULOMATOUS

ICD-10CM #	N76.2	Acute vulvitis
	N76.3	Subacute and chronic vulvitis

Differential diagnosis of granulomatous vulvitis
Syphilis.
Lymphogranuloma venereum.
Mycobacteria.
Fungus.
Bacillary angiomatosis.
Folliculitis.
Ruptured pilosebaceous unit.
Ruptured cyst.
Crohn disease.
Vulvitis granulomatosa.
Hydradenitis suppurativa.

WEAKNESS, ACUTE, EMERGENT[10]

ICD-10CM #	M62.81	Muscle weakness (generalized)

Demyelinating disorders (Guillain-Barré, chronic inflammatory demyelinating polyneuropathy [CIDP]).
Myasthenia gravis.
Infectious (poliomyelitis, diphtheria).
Toxic (botulism, tick paralysis, paralytic shellfish toxin, puffer fish, newts).

Metabolic (acquired or familial hypokalemia, hypophosphatemia, hypermagnesemia).
Metal poisoning (arsenic, thallium).
Porphyria.

WEAKNESS, GRADUAL ONSET

ICD-10CM #	M62.81	Muscle weakness (generalized)

Depression.
Malingering.
Anemia.
Hypothyroidism.
Medications (e.g., sedatives, antidepressants, narcotics).
CHF.
Renal failure.
Liver failure.
Respiratory insufficiency.
Alcoholism.
Nutritional deficiencies.
Disorders of motor unit.
Basal ganglia disorders.
Upper motor neuron lesions.

WEAKNESS, NONNEUROMUSCULAR CAUSES

ICD-10CM #	G93.3	Postviral fatigue syndrome
	R53.1	Weakness
	R53.81	Other malaise
	R53.83	Other fatigue

Anxiety disorder.
Infectious process.
Anemia.
Renal insufficiency.
Hyperventilation.
Malignancy.
Hypothyroidism.
Hypotension.
Hypercapnia.
Hypoglycemia.
Cardiac arrhythmias.
Hepatic insufficiency.
Electrolyte imbalance.
Malnutrition.
Cerebrovascular insufficiency.

WEIGHT GAIN

ICD-10CM #	R63.5	Abnormal weight gain
	E66.9	Obesity, unspecified

Sedentary lifestyle.
Fluid overload.
Discontinuation of tobacco abuse.
Endocrine disorders (hypothyroidism, hyperinsulinism associated with maturity-onset DM, Cushing syndrome, hypogonadism, insulinoma, hyperprolactinemia, acromegaly).

Medications (nutritional supplements, oral contraceptives, glucocorticoids, etc.).
Anxiety disorders with compulsive eating.
Laurence-Moon-Biedl syndrome, Prader-Willi syndrome, other congenital diseases.
Hypothalamic injury (rare; <100 cases reported in medical literature).

WEIGHT LOSS

ICD-10CM # R63.4 Abnormal weight loss

Malignancy.
Psychiatric disorders (depression, anorexia nervosa).
New-onset DM.
Malabsorption.
COPD.
AIDS.
Uremia, liver disease.
Thyrotoxicosis, pheochromocytoma, carcinoid syndrome.
Addison disease.
Intestinal parasites.
Peptic ulcer disease.
Inflammatory bowel disease.
Food faddism.
Postgastrectomy syndrome.

WHEEZING

ICD-10CM # R06.2 Wheezing

Asthma.
COPD.
Interstitial lung disease.
Infections (pneumonia, bronchitis, bronchiolitis, epiglottitis).
Cardiac asthma.
GERD with aspiration.
Foreign body aspiration.
Pulmonary embolism.
Anaphylaxis.
Obstruction of airway (neoplasm, goiter, edema or hemorrhage from trauma, aneurysm, congenital abnormalities, strictures, spasm).
Carcinoid syndrome.

WHEEZING, PEDIATRIC AGE[45]

ICD-10CM # R06.2 Wheezing

Reactive airways disease.
Atopic asthma.
Infection-associated airway reactivity.
Exercise-induced asthma.
Salicylate-induced asthma and nasal polyposis.
Asthmatic bronchitis.
Other hypersensitivity reactions:
  Hypersensitivity pneumonitis.
  Tropical eosinophilia.
  Visceral larva migrans.

Allergic bronchopulmonary aspergillosis.
Aspiration:
  Foreign body.
  Food, saliva, gastric contents.
  Laryngotracheoesophageal cleft.
  Tracheoesophageal fistula, H-type.
  Pharyngeal incoordination or neuromuscular weakness.
Cystic fibrosis.
Primary ciliary dyskinesia.
Cardiac failure.
Bronchiolitis obliterans.
Extrinsic compression of airways:
  Vascular ring.
  Enlarged lymph node.
  Mediastinal tumor.
  Lung cysts.
Tracheobronchomalacia.
Endobronchial masses.
Gastroesophageal reflux.
Pulmonary hemosiderosis.
Sequelae of bronchopulmonary dysplasia.
"Hysterical" glottic closure.
Cigarette smoke, other environmental insults.

WRIST AND HAND PAIN[35]

ICD-10CM # S69.90XA Unspecified injury of unspecified wrist, hand, and finger(s), initial encounter

Articular

Arthritis of the wrist, MCP, PIP, or DIP as a result of:	Trauma, hypermobility, sprain.
	RA (wrist, MCP, PIP joints).
	Osteoarthritis (first CMC, PIP, and DIP joints).
	Other forms of arthritis: gout, psoriatic arthritis, infection.
	Joint neoplasm.

Periarticular

Subcutaneous.	RA nodules, gouty tophi, painful subcutaneous calcific nodules in scleroderma, glomus tumor of the nail bed.
Palmar fascia.	Dupuytren contracture.
Tendon sheath.	Wrist extensor tenosynovitis, including de Quervain tenosynovitis and extensor carpi radialis tenosynovitis.
	Wrist volar flexor tenosynovitis (including carpal tunnel syndrome).
	Thumb flexor tenosynovitis (trigger or snapping thumb).

	Finger flexor tenosynovitis (trigger finger).
	Pigmented villonodular tenosynovitis (giant cell tumor of the tendon sheath).
Acute calcific periarthritis ganglion.	Wrist, MCP, and rarely the PIP and DIP joints.

Osseous

Bone lesions.	Fractures; neoplasm; infection; osteonecrosis, including Kienböck disease (lunate) and Preiser disease (scaphoid).

Neurologic
Nerve entrapment syndromes

Median nerve.	Carpal tunnel syndrome (at the wrist).
	Pronator teres syndrome (at the pronator teres).
	Anterior interosseous nerve syndrome.
Ulnar nerve.	Cubital tunnel syndrome (at the elbow).
	Guyon canal (at the wrist).
Posterior interosseous nerve syndrome.	Radial nerve palsy (spiral groove syndrome).
Lower brachial plexus.	Thoracic outlet syndrome, Pancoast tumor.
Cervical nerve roots.	Herniated cervical disk, tumors.

Spinal Cord Lesion

Spinal tumors, syringomyelia.

Vascular

Vasoplastic disorders with Raynaud phenomenon.	Scleroderma, occupational vibration syndrome.
Small- or large-vessel vasculitis.	With digital ischemia, ischemic ulcers (e.g., SLE, RA, and Takayasu arthritis).

Referred Pain

Cervical spine disorders.	Shoulder–hand syndrome and causalgia.
Reflex sympathetic dystrophy syndrome.	
Cardiac.	Angina pectoris.

CMC, Carpometacarpal; DIP, distal interphalangeal; MCP, metacarpophalangeal; PIP, proximal interphalangeal; RA, rheumatoid arthritis; SLE, systemic lupus erythematosus.

WRIST AND HAND PAIN, IN DIFFERENT AGE GROUPS[41]

ICD-10CM # S69.80XA Other specified injuries of unspecified wrist, hand and finger(s), initial encounter
S69.90XA Unspecified injury of unspecified wrist, hand and finger(s), initial encounter

COMMON CAUSES OF WRIST AND HAND PAIN IN DIFFERENT AGE GROUPS

Childhood (2 to 10 yr)
Intraarticular
Infection.
Periarticular
Fracture.
Osteomyelitis.
Adolescence (10 to 18 yr)
Intraarticular
Infection.
Periarticular
Trauma.
Osteomyelitis.
Tumors.
Ganglion.
Idiopathic wrist pain.
Early Adulthood (18 to 30 yr)
Intraarticular
Inflammatory arthritis.
Infection.
Osteoarthritis.
Periarticular
Peripheral nerve entrapment.
Tendonitis.
Referred
Cervical.
Adulthood (30 to 50 yr)
Intraarticular
Inflammatory arthritis.
Infection.
Osteoarthritis.
Periarticular
Peripheral nerve entrapment.
Tendonitis.
Referred
Cervical.
Chest.
Cardiac.
Old age (>50 yr)
Intraarticular
Inflammatory arthritis.
Osteoarthritis.
Periarticular
Peripheral nerve entrapment.
Tendonitis.
Referred
Cervical.
Chest.
Cardiac.

WRIST PAIN

ICD-10CM #	S69.80XA	Other specified injuries of unspecified wrist, hand and finger(s), initial encounter
	S69.90XA	Unspecified injury of unspecified wrist, hand and finger(s), initial encounter

MECHANICAL

Osteoarthritis.
Ligament tear.
Fracture.
Ganglion.
De Quervain tenosynovitis.
Avascular necrosis (scaphoid, lunate).
Nonunion of scaphoid or lunate.
Neoplasm.

METABOLIC

Pregnancy.
Diabetes.
Gout.
Pseudogout.
Paget disease.
Acromegaly.
Hypothyroidism.
Hyperparathyroidism.

INFECTIOUS

Osteomyelitis.
Septic arthritis.
Cat-scratch disease.
Tick bite (Lyme disease, babesiosis).
Tuberculosis.

NEUROLOGIC

Peripheral neuropathy.
Nerve injury (median, ulnar, radial nerve).
Thoracic outlet compression syndrome.
Distal posterior interosseous nerve syndrome.

RHEUMATOLOGIC

Psoriasis.
RA.
SLE, mixed connective tissue disorder (MCTD).
Scleroderma.

MISCELLANEOUS

Granulomatous (sarcoidosis).
Amyloidosis.
Multiple myeloma.
Leukemia.

XANTHOMAS[70]

ICD-10CM #	L99	Other disorders of skin and subcutaneous tissue in diseases classified elsewhere

Differential Diagnosis of Xanthomas
Eruptive xanthomas:
  Non-Langerhans cell histiocytosis.
Xanthoma disseminatum.
Papular xanthoma.
Generalized eruptive histiocytomas.
Indeterminate cell histiocytosis.
Rosai-Dorfman disease.
Juvenile xanthogranuloma (micronodular form).
Xanthomatous lesions of Langerhans cell histiocytosis.
Disseminated granuloma annulare.
Tuberous xanthomas:

Erythema elevatum diutinum.
Multicentric reticulohistiocytosis.
Tendinous xanthomas:
  Giant cell tumor of the tendon sheath.
  Rheumatoid nodule.
  Subcutaneous granuloma annulare.
  Erythema elevatum diutinum.
Xanthelasma:
  Syringomas.
  Necrobiotic xanthogranuloma.
  Adult-onset asthma and periocular xanthogranuloma (AAPOX).
  Sebaceous hyperplasia.
  Palpebral sarcoidosis.

XEROPHTHALMIA[25]

ICD-10CM #	H11.149	Conjunctival xerosis, unspecified, unspecified eye

MEDICATIONS

Tricyclic antidepressants: amitriptyline, doxepin.
Antihistamines: diphenhydramine, chlorpheniramine, promethazine, and many cold and decongestant preparations.
Anticholinergic agents: antiemetics such as scopolamine, antispasmodic agents such as oxybutynin chloride.

ABNORMALITIES OF EYELID FUNCTION

Neuromuscular disorders.
Aging.
Thyrotoxicosis.

ABNORMALITIES OF TEAR PRODUCTION

Hypovitaminosis A.
Stevens-Johnson syndrome.
Familial diseases affecting sebaceous secretions.

ABNORMALITIES OF CORNEAL SURFACES

Scarring from past injuries and herpes simplex infection.

XEROSTOMIA[25]

ICD-10CM #	K11.7	Disturbances of salivary secretion
	R68.2	Dry mouth, unspecified

MEDICATIONS

Tricyclic antidepressants: amitriptyline, doxepin.
Antihistamines: diphenhydramine, chlorpheniramine, promethazine, and many cold and decongestant preparations.
Anticholinergic agents: antiemetics such as scopolamine, antispasmodic agents such as oxybutynin chloride.

DEHYDRATION

Debility.
Fever.

POLYURIA

Alcohol intake.
Arrhythmia.
Diabetes.

PREVIOUS HEAD AND NECK IRRADIATION SYSTEMIC DISEASES

Sjögren syndrome.
Sarcoidosis.
Amyloidosis.
HIV infection.
Graft-versus-host disease.

Y – Differential Diagnosis

YELLOW URINE

ICD-10CM # R82 Other abnormal findings in urine

Normal coloration.
Concentrated urine.
Use of multivitamin supplements.
Diet rich in carrots.
Use of Cascara.
Urinary tract infection.

REFERENCES

1. Mandell GL: *Mandell, Douglas, and Bennett's principles and practice of infectious diseases*, ed 6, New York, Churchill Livingstone.
2. Talley NJ, Martin CJ: *Clinical gastroenterology*, ed 2, Sydney, Churchill Livingstone.
3. Feldman M et al: *Sleisenger and Fordtran's gastrointestinal and liver disease*, ed 10, Philadelphia, 2016, Elsevier.
4. Townsend CM: *Sabiston textbook of surgery*, ed 21, Philadelphia, 2022, Elsevier.
5. Cherry JD: *Feigin and Cherry's pediatric infectious diseases*, ed 8, Philadelphia, 2019, Elsevier.
6. Kassirer J: *Practical rheumatology*, London, Mosby.
7. Vincent JL et al: *Textbook of critical care*, ed 6, Philadelphia, Saunders.
8. Firestein GS et al: *Kelly's textbook of rheumatology*, ed 9, Philadelphia, Saunders.
9. Floege J et al: *Comprehensive clinical nephrology*, ed 4, Philadelphia, Saunders.
10. Marx JA: *Rosen's emergency medicine*, ed 8, Philadelphia, 2014, Saunders.
11. Skorecki K: *Brenner & Rector's the kidney*, ed 10, Philadelphia, 2016, Elsevier.
12. Cameron P et al: *Textbook of adult emergency medicine*, ed 5, 2020, Elsevier.
13. Mason RJ: *Murray & Nadel's textbook of respiratory medicine*, ed 5, Philadelphia, Saunders.
14. Parrillo JE, Dellinger RP: *Critical care medicine, principles of diagnosis and management in the adult*, ed 5, Philadelphia, 2019, Elsevier.
15. Rumack CM: *Diagnostic ultrasound*, ed 4, Philadelphia, 2011, Elsevier.
16. Ronco C: *Critical care nephrology*, ed 3, Philadelphia, 2019, Elsevier.
17. Stein JH: *Internal medicine*, ed 5, St Louis, Mosby.
18. Andreoli TE et al: *Cecil essentials of medicine*, ed 5, Philadelphia, Saunders.
19. Kliegman RM et al: *Nelson textbook of pediatrics*, ed 19, Philadelphia, Saunders.
20. Pina-Garza J, James KC: *Fenichel's clinical pediatric neurology*, ed 8, Philadelphia, 2019, Elsevier.
21. Grainger RG, Allison D: *Grainger & Allison's diagnostic radiology, a textbook of medical imaging*, ed 4, London, Churchill Livingstone.
22. Flint PW et al: *Cummings otolaryngology*, ed 7, Philadelphia, 2021, Elsevier.
23. Hoekelman R: *Primary pediatric care*, ed 3, St Louis, Mosby.
24. Goldman L, Ausiello D: *Cecil textbook of medicine*, ed 21, Philadelphia, Saunders.
25. Noble J: *Primary care medicine*, ed 3, St Louis, Mosby.
26. Kassirer J: *Current therapy in adult medicine*, ed 4, St Louis, Mosby.
27. Parrillo JE, Dellinger RP: *Critical care medicine, principles of diagnosis and management in the adult*, ed 4, Philadelphia, 2014, Elsevier.
28. Adkinson NF et al: *Middleton's allergy principles and practice*, ed 8, Philadelphia, 2014, Saunders.
29. Adams JG et al: *Emergency medicine, clinical essentials*, ed 2, Philadelphia, 2013, Elsevier.
30. Melmed S et al: *Williams textbook of endocrinology,* ed 12, Philadelphia, Saunders.
31. Hoffmann R et al: *Hematology: basic principles and practice*, ed 5, Philadelphia, Churchill Livingstone.
32. Gabbe SG: *Obstetrics*, ed 6, Philadelphia, Saunders.
33. Harrington J: *Consultation in internal medicine*, ed 2, St Louis, Mosby.
34. Hoffman R et al: *Hematology: basic principles and practice*, ed 6, Philadelphia, Saunders.
35. Hochberg MC: *Rheumatology*, ed 7, Philadelphia, 2019, Elsevier.
36. Melmed S et al: *Williams textbook of endocrinology*, ed 14, Philadelphia, 2020, Elsevier.
37. Boxt LM, Abbara S: *Cardiac imaging: the requisites*, ed 4, Philadelphia, 2016, Elsevier.
38. Jankovic J et al: *Bradley and Daroff's neurology in clinical practice*, ed 8, Philadelphia, 2022, Elsevier.
39. Goldman L, Braunwald E: *Braunwauld primary cardiology*, Philadelphia, Saunders.
40. Canoso J: *Rheumatology in primary care*, Philadelphia, Saunders.
41. Carr A, Hamilton W: *Orthopedics in primary care*, ed 2, Philadelphia, Saunders.
42. Bennett JE et al: *Mandell, Douglas, and Bennett's principles and practice of infectious diseases*, ed 8, Philadelphia, 2015, Saunders.
43. Barkin RM, Rosen P: *Emergency pediatrics: a guide to ambulatory care*, ed 5, St Louis, Mosby.
44. Bowling B: *Kanski's clinical ophthalmology*, ed 8, Philadelphia, 2016, Elsevier.
45. Behrman RE: *Nelson textbook of pediatrics*, ed 16, Philadelphia, Saunders.
46. Custer JW, Rau RE: *The Harriet Lane handbook*, ed 18, St Louis, Mosby.
47. Souhami RL, Moxham J: *Textbook of medicine*, ed 4, London, Churchill Livingstone.
48. Webb WR et al: *Fundamentals of body CT*, ed 4, Philadelphia, 2015, Saunders.
49. Swaiman KF et al: *Swaiman's pediatric neurology, principles and practice*, ed 6, Philadelphia, 2017, Elsevier.
50. Kryger M et al: *Principles and practice of sleep medicine*, ed 7, Philadelphia, 2023, Elsevier.
51. Kliegman R: *Practical strategies in pediatric diagnosis and therapy*, Philadelphia, Saunders.
52. Pope TL et al: *Musculoskeletal imaging*, ed 2, Philadelphia, 2014, Saunders.
53. Firestein GS et al: *Firestein & Kelley's textbook of rheumatology*, ed 11, Philadelphia, 2021, Elsevier.
54. Specht N: *Practical guide to diagnostic imaging*, St Louis, Mosby.
55. Danakas G: *Practical guide to the care of the gynecologic/obstetric patient*, St Louis, Mosby.
56. Marcdante KJ et al: *Nelson essentials of pediatrics*, ed 9, Philadelphia, 2023, Elsevier.
57. Siedel HM: *Mosby's guide to physical examination*, ed 4, St Louis, Mosby.
58. Zipes DP: *Braunwald's heart disease, a textbook of cardiovascular medicine*, ed 11, Philadelphia, 2019, Elsevier.
59. Goldman L, Schafer AI: *Goldman Cecil medicine*, ed 24, Philadelphia, Saunders.
60. Gorbach SL: *Infectious diseases*, ed 2, Philadelphia, Saunders.
61. Fuhrman BP et al: *Pediatric critical care*, ed 4, Philadelphia, Saunders.
62. Wiederholt WC: *Neurology for non-neurologists*, ed 4, Philadelphia, Saunders.
63. Conn R: *Current diagnosis*, ed 9, Philadelphia, Saunders.
64. Cameron JL, Cameron AM: *Current surgical therapy*, ed 10, Philadelphia, Saunders.
65. Spec A et al: *Comprehensive review of infectious diseases*, 2020, Elsevier.
66. Stern TA: *Massachusetts General Hospital handbook of general hospital psychiatry*, ed 7, Philadelphia, 2018, Elsevier.
67. Rakel RE: *Principles of family practice*, ed 6, Philadelphia, Saunders.
68. Kliegman RM: *Nelson textbook of pediatrics*, ed 21, Philadelphia, 2020, Elsevier.
69. Ryan ET et al: *Hunter's tropical medicine and emerging infectious diseases*, ed 10, 2020, Elsevier.
70. Bolognia JL et al: *Dermatology*, ed 4, 2018, Elsevier.
71. Hoffman R: *Hematology, basic principles and practice*, ed 7, Philadelphia, 2018, Elsevier.
72. Kaufman DM et al: *Kaufman's clinical neurology for psychiatrists*, ed 8, Philadelphia, 2017, Elsevier.
73. Paller AS, Mancini AU: *Hurwitz clinical pediatric dermatology*, ed 5, 2016, Elsevier.
74. Broaddus VC et al: *Murray & Nadel's textbook of respiratory medicine*, ed 7, Philadelphia, 2022, Elsevier.
75. Weinberger SE et al: *Principles of pulmonary medicine*, ed 7, Philadelphia, 2019, Elsevier.
76. Seller RH: *Differential diagnosis of common complaints*, ed 4, Philadelphia, Saunders.
77. Mahanty S, Nutman TB: Eosinophilia and eosinophil-related disorders. In Middleton EJ et al (eds): *Allergy: principles and practice*, ed 4, St Louis, Mosby-Year Book, p. 1077.

Differential Diagnosis

II

78. Sellke FW et al: *Sabiston & Spencer surgery of the chest*, ed 9, Philadelphia, 2016, Elsevier.

79. Eberlein M: A fall in Ghana, *Am J Med* 122:1091, 2009.

80. Moore WT, Eastman RC: *Diagnostic endocrinology*, ed 2, St Louis, Mosby.

81. Schwarz MI: *Interstitial lung disease,* ed 2, St Louis, Mosby.

82. Swain R, Snodgrass JG: Managing groin pain, *Phys Sportsmed* 23(56), 1995.

83. Cameron JL, Cameron AM: *Current surgical therapy*, ed 12, Philadelphia, 2017, Elsevier.

84. Habif TP: *Clinical dermatology*, ed 6, Philadelphia, 2016, Elsevier.

85. Goldberg RJ: *The care of the psychiatric patient*, ed 3, St Louis, Mosby.

86. Mann DL et al: *Braunwald's heart disease*, ed 10, Philadelphia, 2015, Elsevier.

87. Bonow RO et al: *Braunwauld's heart disease*, ed 9, Philadelphia, Elsevier.

88. Park MK: *Park's pediatric cardiology for practitioners*, ed 6, Philadelphia, 2014, Saunders.

89. *Wein AU: Campbell-Walsh urology*, ed 11, Philadelphia, 2016, Elsevier.

90. Hochberg MC et al: *Rheumatology*, ed 5, St Louis, Mosby.

91. Palay D: *Ophthalmology for the primary care physician*, St Louis, Mosby.

92. Callen JP: *Color atlas of dermatology*, ed 2, Philadelphia, WB Saunders.

93. Carlson KJ: *Primary care of women*, ed 2, St Louis, Mosby.

94. Goldman L, Schafer AI: *Goldman-Cecil medicine*, ed 26, Philadelphia, 2020, Elsevier.

95. Bain BJ et al: *Dacie and Lewis practical haematology*, ed 12, Philadelphia, 2017, Elsevier.

96. Talley NJ et al: *Essentials of internal medicine*, ed 4, Chatswood, 2021, Elsevier Australia.

97. Khan MG: *Rapid ECG interpretation*, Philadelphia, Saunders.

98. Kanski JJ, Bowling B: *Clinical ophthalmology, a systematic approach*, ed 7, Philadelphia, Saunders.

99. Crum CP: *Diagnostic gynecologic and obstetric pathology*, ed 3, Philadelphia, 2018, Elsevier.

100. James WD: *Andrews' diseases of the skin*, ed 12, Philadelphia, 2016, Saunders.

101. Kaufman DM et al: *Kaufman's clinical neurology for psychiatrists*, ed 9, Philadelphia, 2023, Elsevier.

102. Gershenson DM et al: *Comprehensive Gynecology*, ed 8, Philadelphia, 2022, Elsevier.

103. Weinberger SE et al: *Principles of pulmonary medicine*, ed 5, Philadelphia, Saunders.

104. Nseyo UO: *Urology for primary care physicians*, Philadelphia, Saunders.

105. Tschudy MM, Arcara KM: *The Harriet Lane handbook*, ed 19, Philadelphia, Mosby.

106. Niederhuber JE et al: *Abeloff's clinical oncology*, ed 6, Philadelphia, 2020, Elsevier.

107. Grant LA, Griffin N: *Grainger & Allison's diagnostic radiology essentials*, ed 2, Philadelphia, 2019, Elsevier.

108. Baude AI: *Infectious diseases and medical microbiology*, ed 2, Philadelphia, Saunders.

109. Henry JB: *Clinical diagnosis and management by laboratory methods*, ed 20, Philadelphia, Saunders.

110. Boyer KM: Nonbacterial pneumonia. In Feigin RD, Cherry JD, editors: *Textbook of pediatric infectious diseases*, ed 4, Philadelphia, 1998, WB Saunders, pp 260-273.

111. Hull KM et al: The expanding spectrum of systemic autoinflammatory disorders and their rheumatic manifestations, *Curr Opin Rheumatol* 15:61-69, 2003.

112. Auerbach P: *Wilderness medicine*, Philadelphia, Saunders.

113. Wilson JD: *Williams textbook of endocrinology*, ed 9, Philadelphia, Saunders.

114. Copeland LJ: *Textbook of gynecology*, ed 2, Philadelphia, Saunders.

115. Lipshultz LI et al: *Urology and the primary care practitioner*, ed 3, Philadelphia, Elsevier.

SECTION III

Clinical Algorithms

PLEASE NOTE: These algorithms are designed to assist clinicians in the evaluation and treatment of patients. They may not apply to all patients with a particular disorder and are not intended to replace the clinician's individual judgment.

Additional algorithms content is available at Elsevier eBooks+ (eBooks.Health.Elsevier.com).

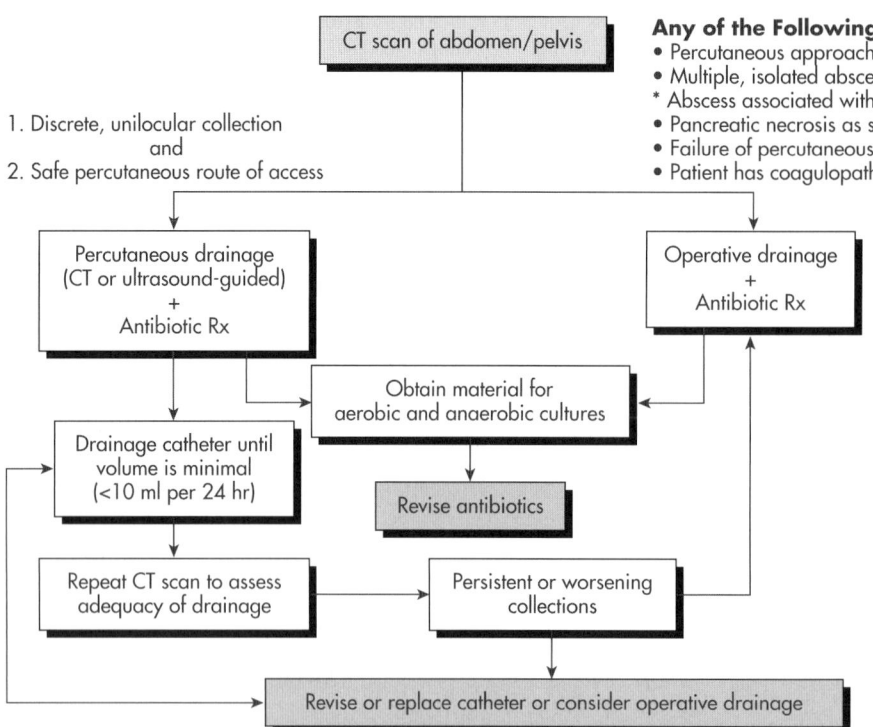

FIG. 1 Approach to management of intraabdominal abscesses including indications for consideration of percutaneous versus operative drainage. *CT,* Computed tomography; *Rx,* treatment. (From Parrillo JE, Dellinger RP: *Critical care medicine, principles of diagnosis and management in the adult,* ed 5, Philadelphia, 2019, Elsevier.)

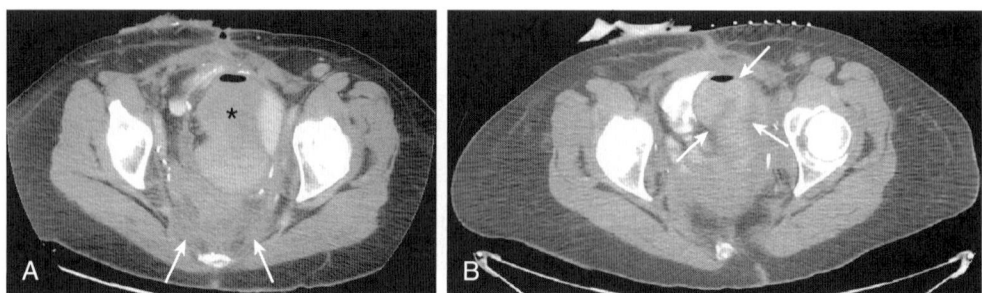

FIG. 2 A, Axial computed tomography (CT) image shows an apparently rim-enhancing structure containing gas *(asterisk)* in the deep pelvis adjacent to tethered bowel loops in a patient with prior pelvic irradiation. The structure could represent an abscess or a dilated loop of small bowel. The presacral inflammation *(arrows)* is related to radiation change. **B,** CT image obtained 2 h later shows ingested oral contrast in this structure *(arrows)* confirming that this is a bowel loop rather than an abscess. (From Feldman M et al: *Sleisenger and Fortran's gastrointestinal and liver disease,* ed 10, Philadelphia, 2016, Elsevier.)

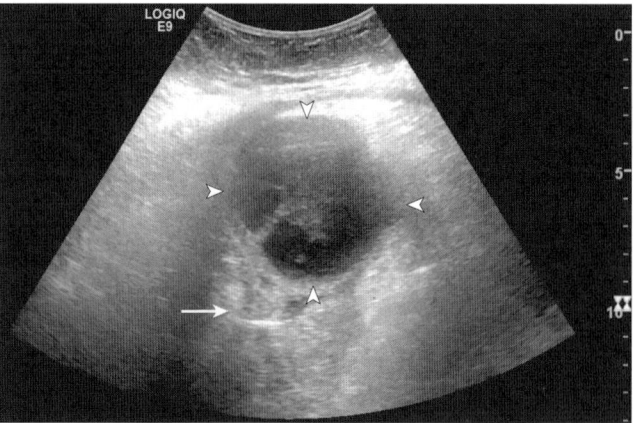

FIG. 3 Abdominal ultrasound of a typical abscess *(arrowheads)* demonstrating central decreased echogenicity, thickened wall, and debris arising anterior to the descending colon *(arrow)* in a patient with diverticulosis compatible with a diverticular abscess. (From Feldman M et al: *Sleisenger and Fortran's gastrointestinal and liver disease,* ed 10, Philadelphia, 2016, Elsevier.)

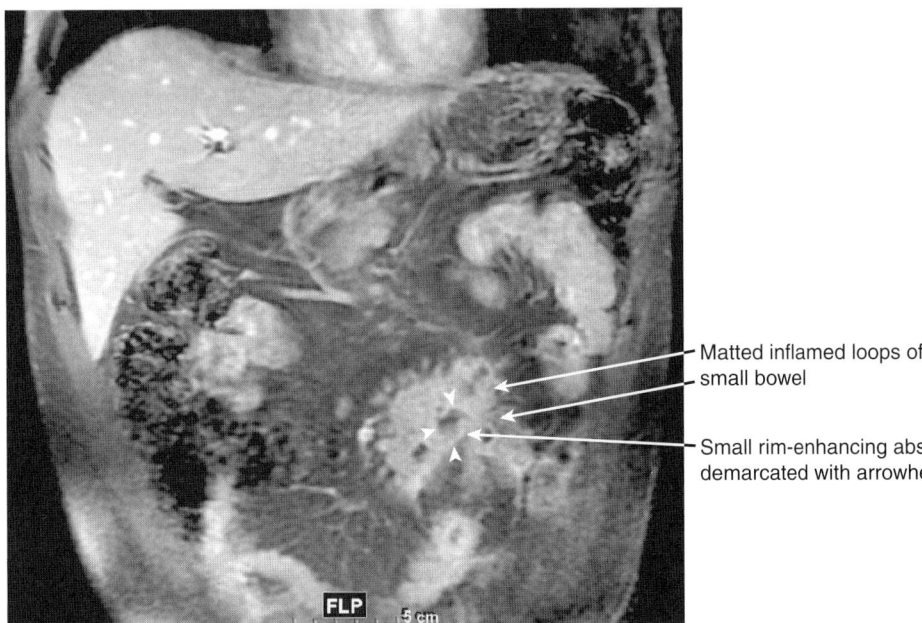

FIG. 4 **Coronal magnetic resonance image with gadolinium contrast of a patient with Crohn disease showing a small rim-enhancing collection *(arrowheads)* interposed between several loops of inflamed bowel *(arrows)* compatible with an interloop abscess.** Interloop abscesses are not amenable to percutaneous drain placement. (From Feldman M et al: *Sleisenger and Fortran's gastrointestinal and liver disease,* ed 10, Philadelphia, 2016, Elsevier.)

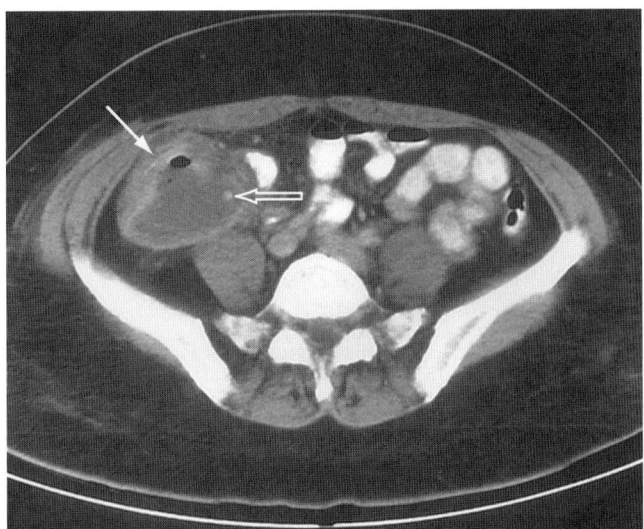

FIG. 5 **Axial computed tomography demonstrating a right lower quadrant abscess *(closed arrow)* with an appendicolith *(open arrow)*.** Such extraluminal appendicoliths may predict clinical failure with percutaneous drainage. (From Feldman M et al: *Sleisenger and Fortran's gastrointestinal and liver disease,* ed 10, Philadelphia, 2016, Elsevier.)

Clinical Algorithms

III

BOX 1 Causes of Intraabdominal Abscesses

Abdominal trauma
Appendicitis
Cholecystectomy and other operations or invasive procedures
Crohn disease
Diverticulitis
Neoplastic disease
Pancreatitis
Perforated hollow viscus (e.g., duodenal or gastric ulcer)

From Feldman M et al: *Sleisenger and Fortran's gastrointestinal and liver disease,* ed 10, Philadelphia, 2016, Elsevier.

BOX 2 Clinical Risk Factors for Intraabdominal Abscess

Chronic glucocorticoid use
Increasing age
Malnutrition
Preexisting organ dysfunction
Transfusion
Underlying malignancy

From Feldman M et al: *Sleisenger and Fortran's gastrointestinal and liver disease,* ed 10, Philadelphia, 2016, Elsevier.

BOX 3 Antibiotic Choices in the Treatment of Intraabdominal Infections

Single-Agent Therapy
Second-Generation Cephalosporins
   Cefoxitin
Carbapenems
   Imipenem-cilastatin
   Meropenem
   Doripenem
   Ertapenem (no *Pseudomonas* coverage)
Extended-Spectrum Penicillin–β-Lactamase Inhibitor Combinations
   Piperacillin sodium-tazobactam
   Ticarcillin disodium-clavulanate
Glycylcyclines
   Tigecycline
Combination Therapy (Antiaerobe[a] + Antianaerobe)
Third- or Fourth-Generation Cephalosporins
   Ceftriaxone + metronidazole
   Cefotaxime + metronidazole
   Ceftazidime (*Pseudomonas* coverage) + metronidazole
   Cefepime (*Pseudomonas* coverage) + metronidazole
Fluoroquinolones
   Ciprofloxacin + metronidazole
   Levofloxacin + metronidazole
   Moxifloxacin[b]

[a]Aminoglycoside therapy as an antiaerobic drug should not be used in routine practice owing to an increase in nephrotoxicity and possible worsened patient outcomes with its use.
[b]Moxifloxacin has adequate anaerobic coverage, making metronidazole unnecessary.
From Feldman M et al: *Sleisenger and Fortran's gastrointestinal and liver disease,* ed 10, Philadelphia, 2016, Elsevier.

TABLE 1   Comparison of Common Causes of Acute Abdominal Pain

Cause	Onset	Location	Character	Descriptor	Radiation	Intensity
Appendicitis	Gradual	Periumbilical area early; RLQ late	Diffuse early; localized later	Aching	None	++
Cholecystitis	Acute	RUQ	Localized	Constricting	Scapula	++
Pancreatitis	Acute	Epigastrium, back	Localized	Boring	Midback	++ to +++
Diverticulitis	Gradual	LLQ	Localized	Aching	None	++ to +++
Perforated peptic ulcer	Sudden	Epigastrium	Localized early, diffuse later	Burning	None	+++
Small bowel obstruction	Gradual	Periumbilical area	Diffuse	Cramping	None	++
Mesenteric ischemia, infarction	Sudden	Periumbilical area	Diffuse	Agonizing	None	+++
Ruptured abdominal aortic aneurysm	Sudden	Abdomen, back, flank	Diffuse	Tearing	None	+++
Gastroenteritis	Gradual	Periumbilical area	Diffuse	Spasmodic	None	+ to ++
Pelvic inflammatory disease	Gradual	Either LQ, pelvis	Localized	Aching	Upper thigh	++
Ruptured ectopic pregnancy	Sudden	Either LQ, pelvis	Localized	Sharp	None	++

+, Mild; ++, moderate; +++, severe; *LLQ*, left lower quadrant; *LQ*, lower quadrant; *RLQ*, right lower quadrant; *RUQ*, right upper quadrant.
From Feldman M et al: *Sleisenger and Fortran's gastrointestinal and liver disease,* ed 10, 2016, Elsevier.

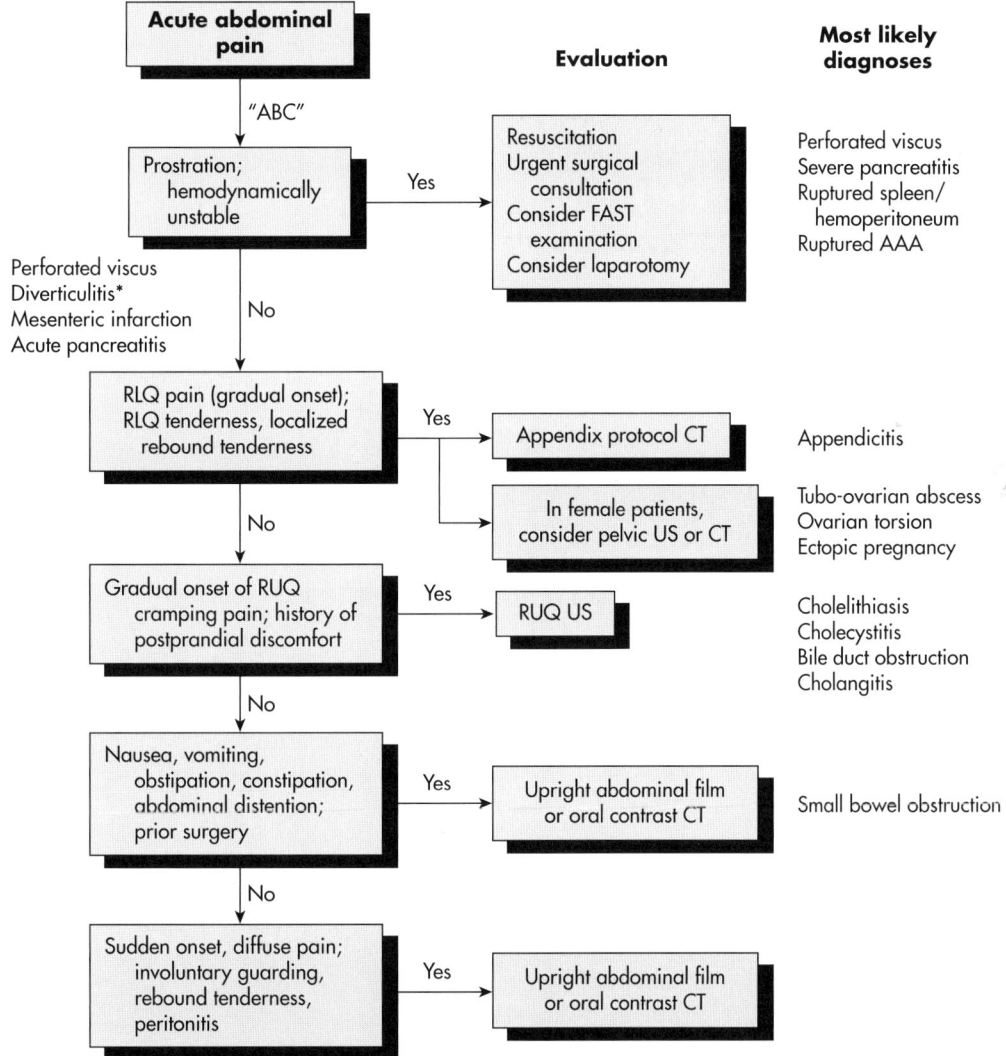

FIG. 6 **An approach to the urgent evaluation of abdominal pain.** Specific complaints and physical examination findings are coupled with appropriate radiologic imaging. *For left lower quadrant pain, the most likely diagnosis is diverticulitis. *AAA,* Abdominal aortic aneurysm; *ABC,* airway, breathing, circulation; *CT,* computed tomography; *FAST,* focused abdominal sonogram for trauma; *RLQ,* right lower quadrant; *RUQ,* right upper quadrant; *US,* ultrasound. (From Feldman M et al: *Sleisenger and Fortran's gastrointestinal and liver disease,* ed 10, Philadelphia, 2016, Elsevier.)

Clinical Algorithms

III

BOX 4 Nonsurgical Causes of the Acute Abdomen

Endocrine and Metabolic Causes
Acute intermittent porphyria
Addisonian crisis
Diabetic crisis

Hereditary Mediterranean fever
Uremia

Hematologic Causes
Acute leukemia
Sickle cell crisis

Toxins and Drugs
Black widow spider poisoning
Lead poisoning
Other heavy metal poisoning
Narcotic withdrawal

From Townsend CM et al: *Sabiston textbook of surgery,* ed 21, St Louis 2022, Elsevier.

BOX 5 Surgical Acute Abdominal Conditions

Hemorrhage
Aortoduodenal fistula after aortic vascular graft
Arteriovenous malformation of the gastrointestinal tract
Bleeding gastrointestinal diverticulum
Hemorrhagic pancreatitis

Intestinal ulceration
Leaking or ruptured arterial aneurysm
Mallory-Weiss syndrome
Ruptured ectopic pregnancy
Solid organ trauma
Spontaneous splenic rupture

Infection
Appendicitis
Cholecystitis
Diverticulitis
Hepatic abscess
Meckel diverticulitis
Psoas abscess

Ischemia
Buerger disease
Ischemic colitis
Mesenteric thrombosis or embolism
Ovarian torsion
Strangulated hernia
Testicular torsion

Obstruction
Cecal volvulus
Gastrointestinal malignancy
Incarcerated hernias
Inflammatory bowel disease
Intussusception
Sigmoid volvulus
Small bowel obstruction

Perforation
Boerhaave syndrome
Perforated diverticulum
Perforated gastrointestinal cancer
Perforated gastrointestinal ulcer

From Townsend CM et al: *Sabiston textbook of surgery,* ed 21, St Louis 2022, Elsevier.

BOX 6 Laboratory Tests for Abdominal Pain

- White blood cell count with differential
- Hemoglobin
- Platelets
- Electrolytes
- Creatinine and blood urea nitrogen
- Amylase and lipase
- Total and fractionated serum bilirubin
- Serum lactate levels
- Viral hepatitis panel
- Urinalysis
- Urine human chorionic gonadotropin
- *Clostridium difficile* culture and toxin assay

From Townsend CM et al: *Sabiston textbook of surgery,* ed 21, St Louis 2022, Elsevier.

TABLE 2 Abdominal Examination Signs

History	Physical Exam	Likely Diagnosis
Danforth sign	Shoulder pain on inspiration	Hemoperitoneum
Inspection		
Cruveilhier sign	Varicose veins at umbilicus	
Cullen sign	Periumbilical bruising	
Grey Turner sign	Local areas of discoloration near umbilicus and flanks	
Ransohoff sign	Yellow discoloration of umbilical region	
Palpation		
Aaron sign	Pain or pressure in epigastrium or anterior chest with persistent firm pressure applied to McBurney point	Acute appendicitis
Bassler sign	Sharp pain created by compressing appendix between abdominal wall and iliacus	Chronic appendicitis
Blumberg sign	Transient abdominal wall rebound tenderness	Peritoneal inflammation
Carnett sign	Loss of abdominal tenderness when abdominal wall muscles contracted	Intraabdominal source of abdominal pain
Chandelier sign	Extreme pelvic pain with movement of the cervix	Pelvic inflammatory disease
Courvoisier sign	Palpable gallbladder when jaundice is present	Periampullary mass
Fothergill sign	Abdominal wall mass that does not cross midline and is palpable when rectus is contracted	Rectus muscle hematoma
Iliopsoas sign	Elevation of extended leg against resistance is painful	Retrocecal acute appendicitis
Murphy sign	Pain caused by inspiration while applying pressure to right upper abdomen	Acute cholecystitis
Obturator sign	Flexion and external rotation of right thigh creates hypogastric pain	Pelvic abscess or inflammatory mass (appendicitis)
Rovsing sign	Pain at McBurney point when palpating the left lower quadrant	Acute appendicitis
Ten Horn sign	Pain caused by gentle traction of right testicle	Acute appendicitis

From Townsend CM et al: *Sabiston textbook of surgery*, ed 21, St Louis 2022, Elsevier.

TABLE 3 Differential Diagnosis of Pain by Location (List Is Not Exhaustive)

Right upper quadrant

Hepatobiliary pathology
Duodenal ulcer, duodenitis
Renal colic, pyelonephritis
Retrocecal appendicitis
Pneumonia, pulmonary embolism

Right lumbar or flank

Renal colic, pyelonephritis
Aortic aneurysm
Psoas abscess
Appendicitis

Right lower quadrant

Appendicitis
Ectopic pregnancy, tuboovarian pathology, endometriosis, pelvic inflammatory disease
Urinary tract infection, ureteric colic
Diverticulitis
Hernia
Aortic aneurysm
Testicular torsion, epididymoorchitis

Pain radiating to the back

Perforated peptic ulcer
Acute pancreatitis
Abdominal aortic aneurysm, aortic dissection

Epigastrium

Gastritis, peptic ulcer
Hepatobiliary pathology
Pancreatitis
Aortic aneurysm
Early appendicitis
Myocardial infarction

Midline or periumbilical

Visceral pain from midgut structures
Early appendicitis
Aortic aneurysm

Suprapubic

Cystitis, bladder pathology
Urinary tract infection
Prostatitis
Ectopic pregnancy, tuboovarian pathology, endometriosis, pelvic inflammatory disease

Left upper quadrant

Gastritis, peptic ulcer
Renal colic, pyelonephritis
Splenic pathology
Pancreatitis
Pneumonia

Left lumbar or flank

Renal colic, pyelonephritis
Aortic aneurysm
Psoas abscess

Left lower quadrant

Similar to causes for right lower quadrant pain except for appendicitis (very rarely left-sided)

Note: Pain from inflammatory bowel disease, diverticulitis, colitis, gastroenteritis, volvulus, intestinal obstruction, adhesions, ischemic colitis, and constipation may localize to any part of the abdomen.
From Cameron P et al: *Textbook of adult emergency medicine*, ed 5, Philadelphia, 2019, Elsevier.

Clinical Algorithms

III

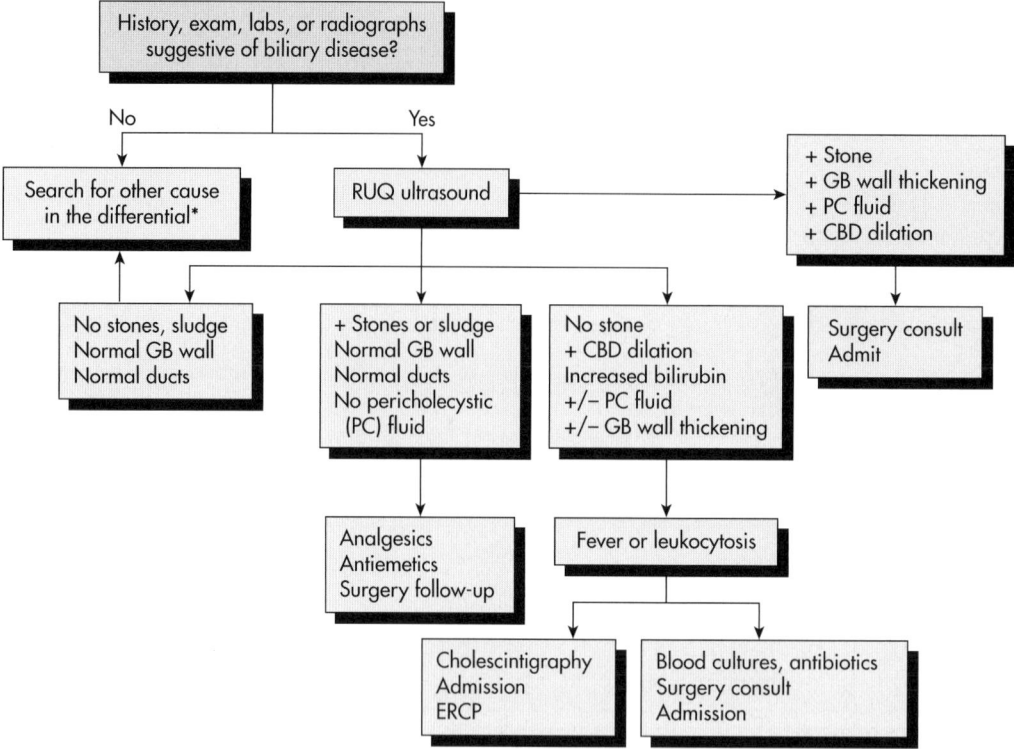

FIG. 7 Treatment algorithm for right upper quadrant *(RUQ)* pain. *Refer to Section II, Differential Diagnosis: Abdominal Pain, Right Upper Quadrant. *CBD,* Common bile duct; *ERCP,* endoscopic retrograde cholangiopancreatography; *GB,* gallbladder; *RUQ,* right upper quadrant; +, with; −, without; ±, with or without. (From Adams JG et al: *Emergency medicine, clinical essentials,* ed 2, Philadelphia, 2013, Elsevier.)

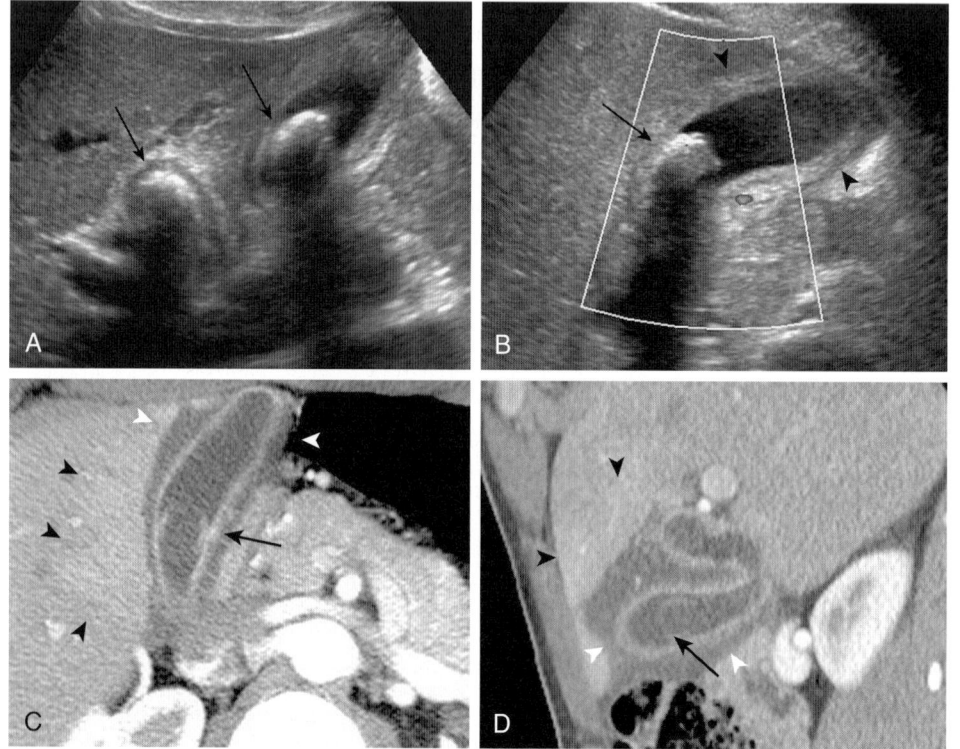

FIG. 8 A 43-yr-old man with acute cholecystitis. Ultrasound images (**A** and **B**) demonstrate echogenic, shadowing gallstones *(arrows)* with gallbladder wall thickening *(arrowheads)* in a patient in whom a sonographic Murphy sign was elicited. Axial (**C**) and sagittal (**D**) portal venous phase computed tomography images reveal a gallstone *(arrows),* as well as a thickened gallbladder wall *(white arrowheads).* Although not acquired in the arterial phase of contrast, hepatic hyperenhancement consistent with secondary inflammation is nevertheless seen *(black arrowheads).* These findings are specific for this life-threatening complication and should be recognized and treated urgently. (From Soto JA, Lucey BC: *Emergency radiology, the requisites,* ed 2, Philadelphia, 2017, Elsevier.)

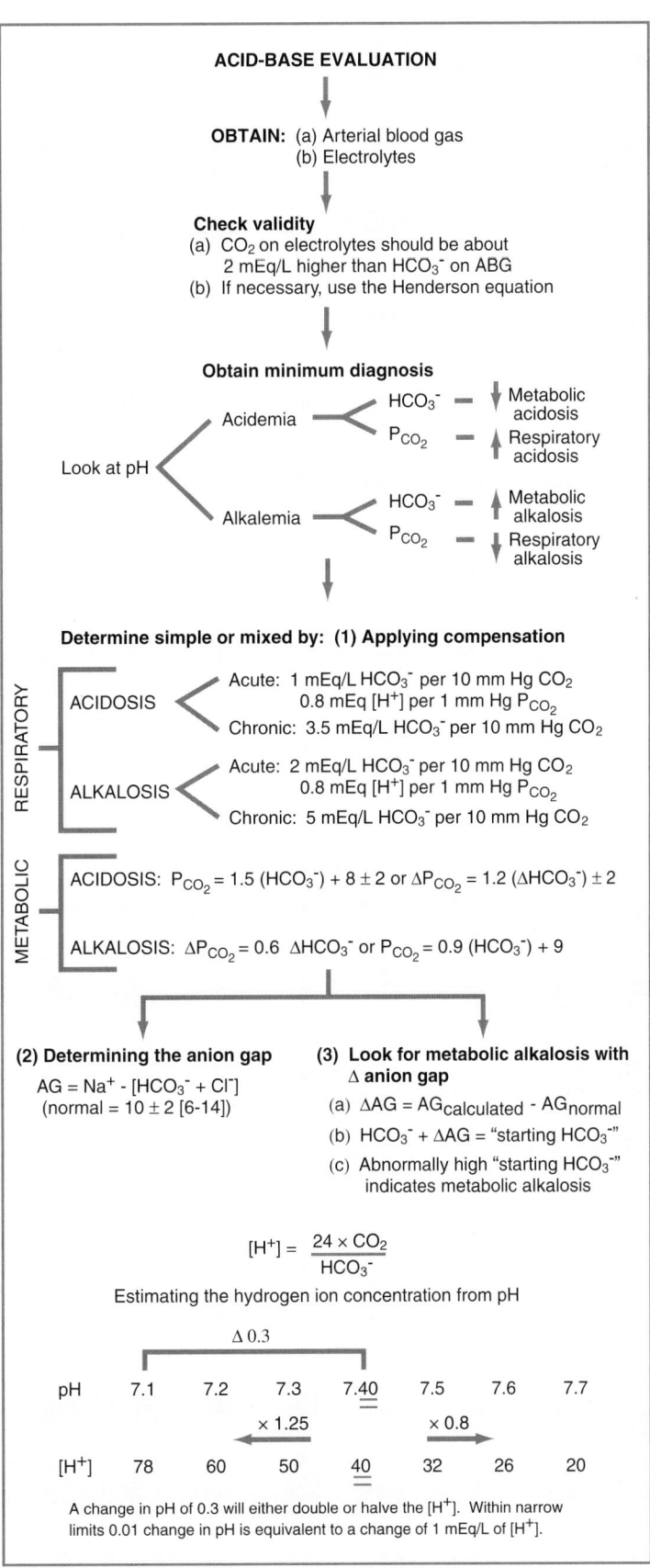

FIG. 9 Scheme for assessing acid-base homeostasis. *ABG,* Arterial blood gases; *AG,* anion gap; *PCO₂,* partial pressure of carbon dioxide. (Modified from Andreoli TE [ed]: *Cecil essentials of medicine,* ed 7, Philadelphia, 2008, Saunders.)

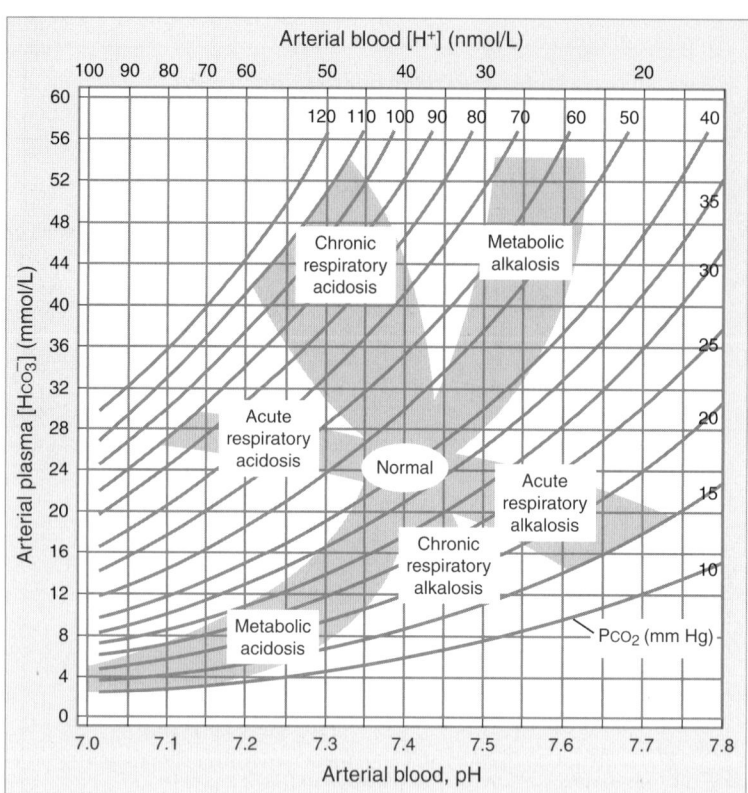

FIG. 10 Acid base normogram. Shaded areas represent 95% confidence limits of normal respiratory and metabolic compensations for primary disturbances. Points outside shaded areas represent a mixed disorder, assuming absence of laboratory error. (From Vincent JL et al: *Textbook of critical care,* ed 6, Philadelphia, 2011, Saunders.)

TABLE 4 Rules of Chronic Compensation

Primary Disorder	Secondary Compensation	EXAMPLES	
		Primary Change	Compensation
↑ P_{CO_2}	↑ HCO_3^-: 4 mEq/L for each 10 mm Hg increase in P_{CO_2} (±3 mEq/L)	P_{CO_2}: 40 → 80	HCO_3^-: 24 → 40 pH: 7.1 → 7.32
↓ P_{CO_2}	↓ HCO_3^-: 2.5 mEq/L for each 10 mm Hg decrease in P_{CO_2} (±3 mEq/L)*	P_{CO_2}: 40 → 20	HCO_3^-: 24 → 19 pH: 7.70 → 7.60
↓ HCO_3^-	↓ P_{CO_2}: 1-1.5 mm Hg for each mEq/L decrease in HCO_3^-	HCO_3^-: 24 → 9	P_{CO_2}: 40 → 25 pH: 7.00 → 7.20
↑ HCO_3^-	↑ P_{CO_2}: 0.5-1.0 mm Hg for each mEq/L increase in HCO_3^-	HCO_3^-: 24 → 34	P_{CO_2}: 40 → 50 pH: 7.56 → 7.46

*HCO_3^- seldom falls below 18 mEq/L in acute and 16 mEq/L in chronic respiratory alkalosis.
From Broaddus VC et al: *Murray & Nadel's textbook of respiratory medicine,* ed 7, Philadelphia 2022, Elsevier.

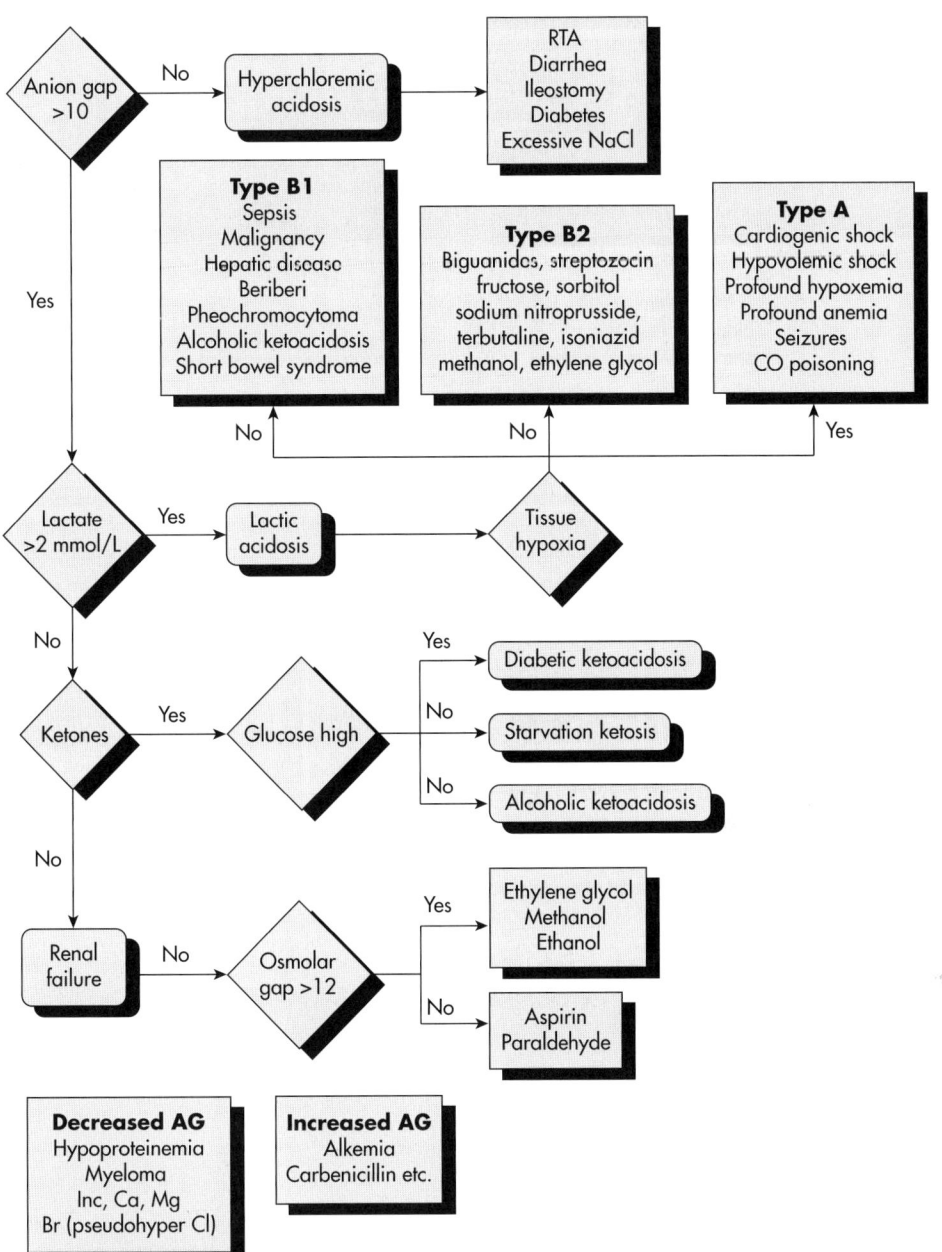

FIG. 11 Diagnostic approach to metabolic acidosis. *AG,* Anion gap; *CO,* carbon monoxide; *RTA,* renal tubular acidosis. (From Vincent JL et al: *Textbook of critical care,* ed 7, Philadelphia, 2017, Elsevier.)

Clinical
Algorithms

III

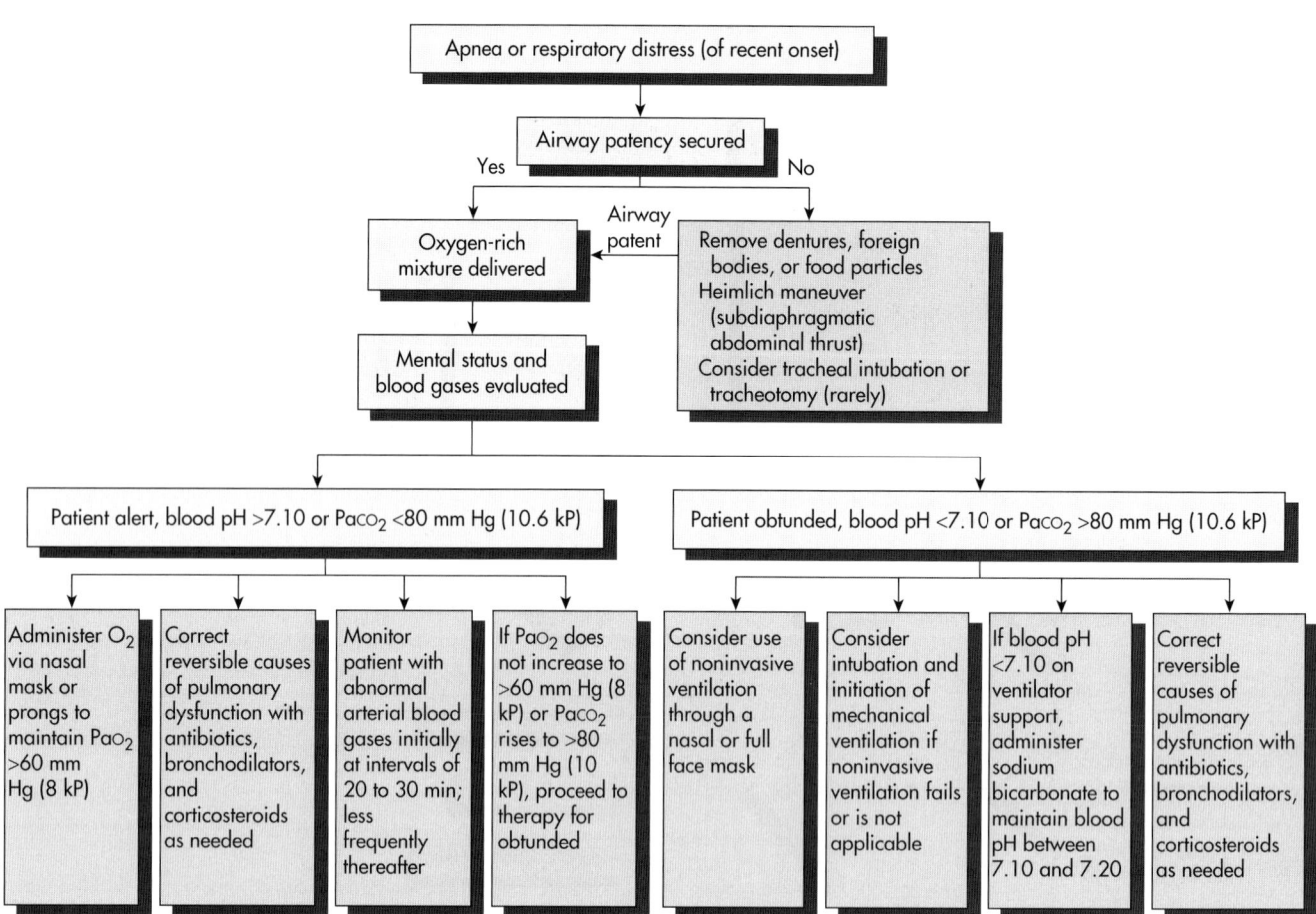

FIG. 12 Algorithm for management of acute respiratory acidosis. *PCO₂*, Partial pressure of carbon dioxide.
(From Johnson R et al: *Comprehensive clinical nephrology*, ed 5, Philadelphia, 2015, Saunders.)

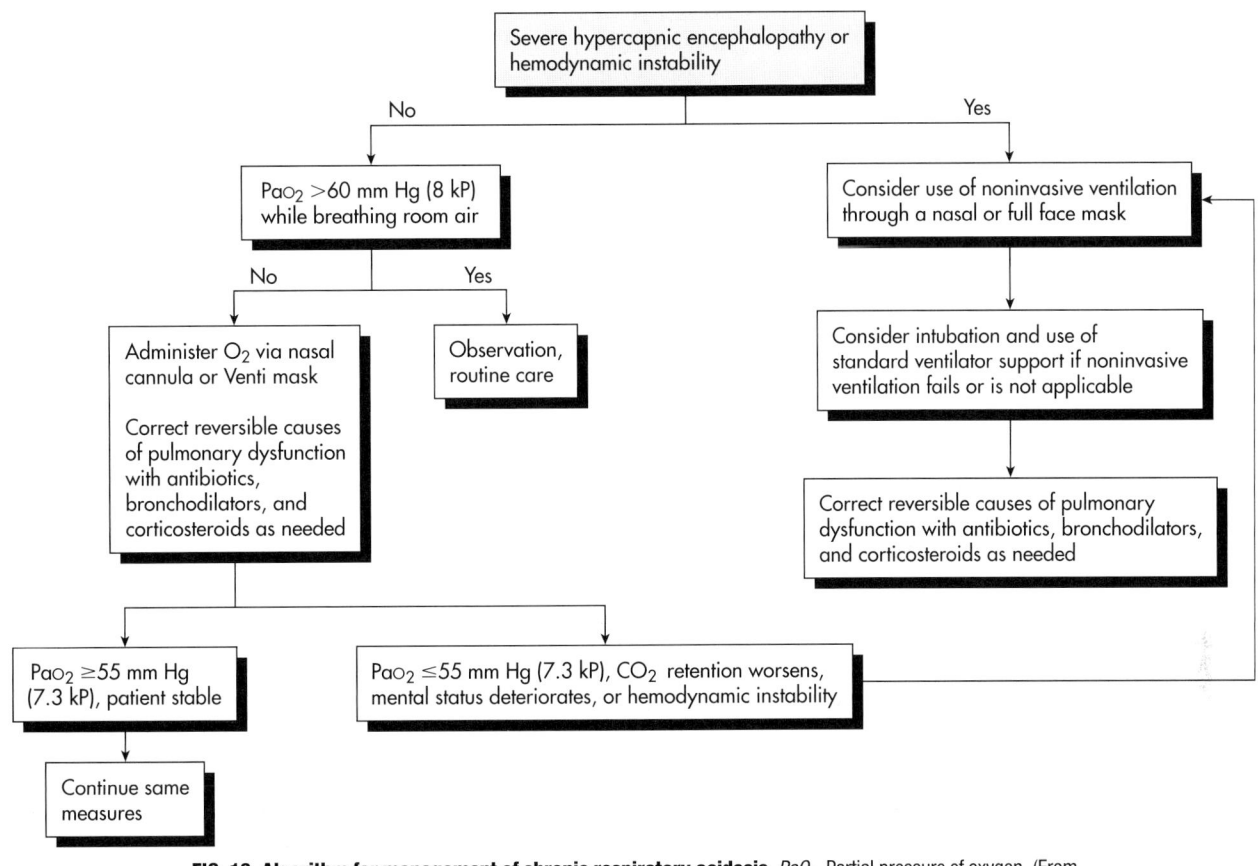

FIG. 13 Algorithm for management of chronic respiratory acidosis. *PaO₂,* Partial pressure of oxygen. (From Johnson R et al: *Comprehensive clinical nephrology,* ed 5, Philadelphia, 2015, Saunders.)

Clinical Algorithms

TABLE 5 Causes of Chronic Alveolar Hypoventilation/Respiratory Acidosis

	Site of Defect	Condition
Defects in respiratory drive	Central and peripheral chemoreceptors	Brainstem lesions Primary alveolar hypoventilation syndrome (Ondine curse), extreme obesity (Pickwickian syndrome) Spinal cord lesions
Neuromuscular defects	Neuromuscular	Motor neuron disease: Critical illness polyneuropathy, multiple sclerosis, amyotrophic lateral sclerosis
	Muscular disease	Myasthenia gravis, critical illness myopathy
Defects in respiratory mechanics and gas exchange	Lung	Increased dead space: Chronic obstructive pulmonary disease, chronic pulmonary embolism Increased lung elastance: Pulmonary fibrosis Increased chest wall elastance: Extreme obesity, fibrothorax, kyphoscoliosis Increased respiratory resistance: Airway stenosis, chronic obstructive pulmonary disease

From Ronco C: *Critical care nephrology,* ed 3, Philadelphia, 2019, Elsevier.

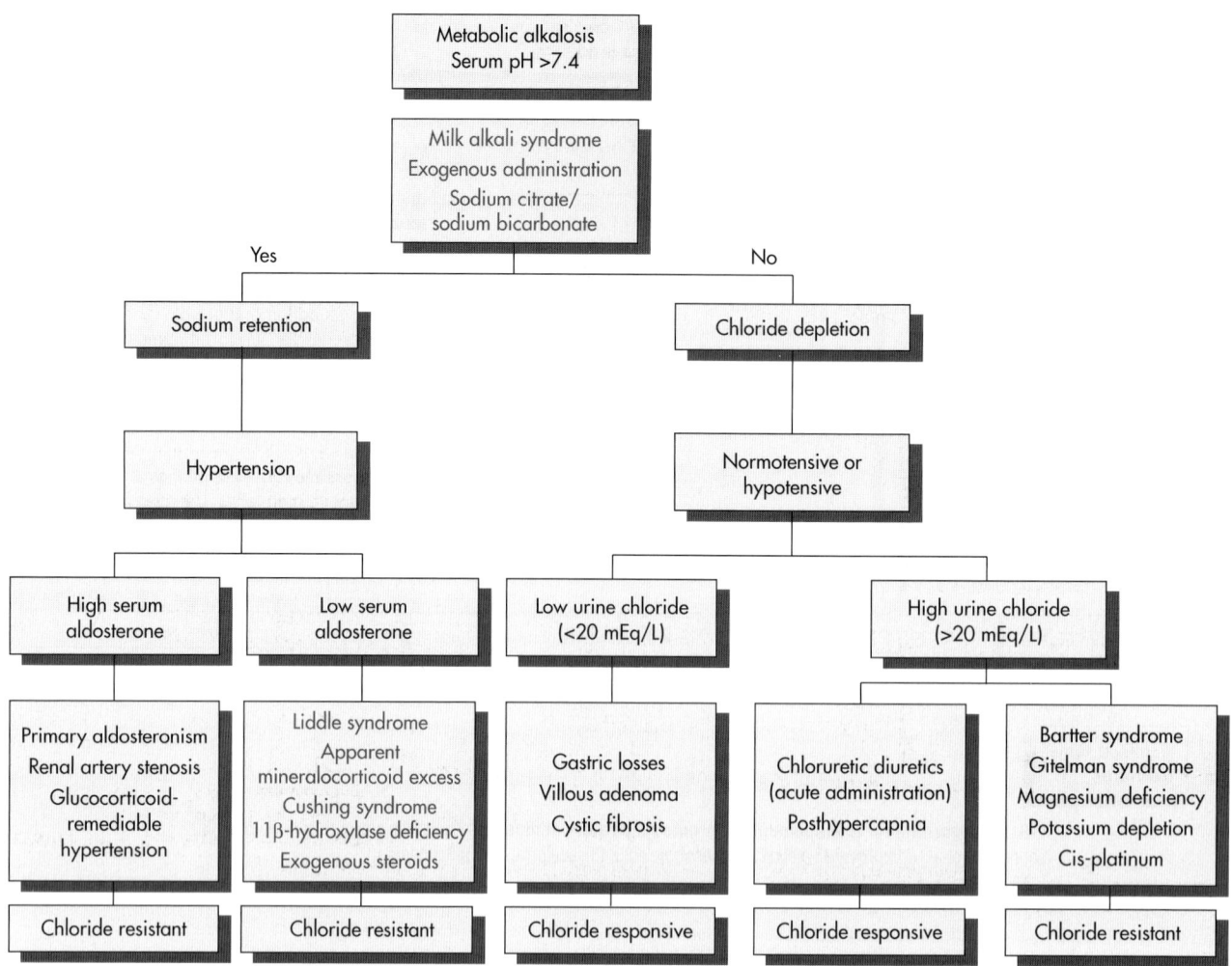

FIG. 16 Differential diagnosis of metabolic alkalosis. (From Ronco C: *Critical care nephrology,* ed 3, Philadelphia, 2019, Elsevier.)

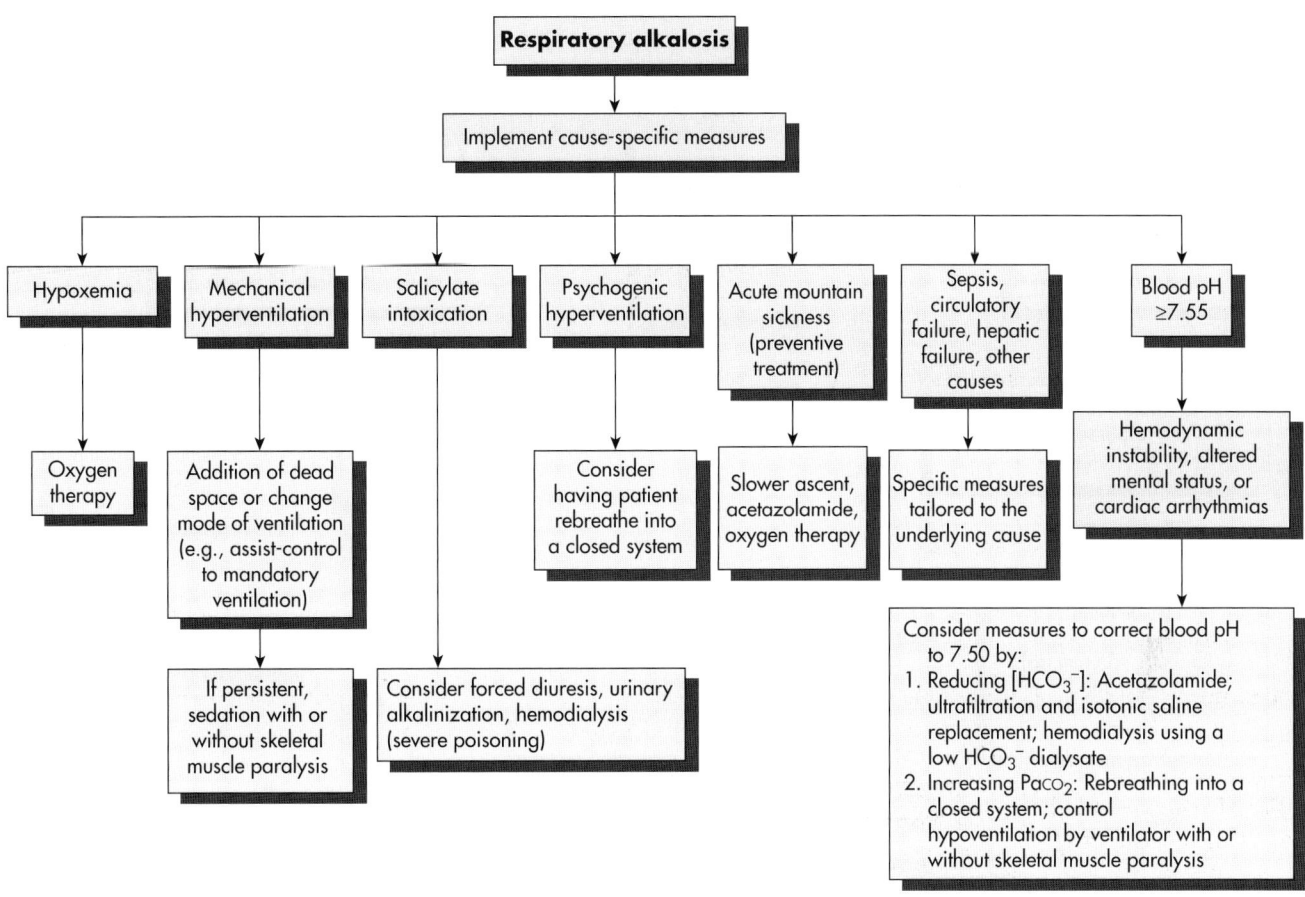

FIG. 17 Recommended treatment of respiratory alkalosis. *PCO₂*, Partial pressure of carbon dioxide. (From Johnson R et al: *Comprehensive clinical nephrology,* ed 5, Philadelphia, 2015, Saunders.)

Clinical Algorithms

III

TABLE 6   Causes of Alveolar Hyperventilation/Respiratory Alkalosis

	Site of Defect	Condition
Defects in respiratory drive	*Central chemoreceptors*	*Voluntary hyperventilation psychogenic:* Pain, panic attack
		Central neurogenic hyperventilation: Brainstem injuries, brain tumors
		Hormonal: Increased progesterone levels in pregnancy and liver cirrhosis
		Infectious: Meningitis, encephalitis
		Thermal hyperpnea: Fever, hyperthermia
		Intoxication: Salicylate, topiramate
		Therapeutic: Doxapram
	Peripheral chemoreceptors	*Increased activity of peripheral chemoreceptors:* Hypoxic pulmonary disease, high altitude
		Increased activity of lung receptors, e.g., pulmonary edema, pneumonia, pulmonary embolism, interstitial fibrosis
Iatrogenic		*Mechanical ventilation:* Excessive mechanical ventilation (accidental, or therapeutic for traumatic brain injury)
		Extracorporeal gas exchange: Excessive extracorporeal CO_2 removal

From Ronco C: *Critical care nephrology,* ed 3, Philadelphia, 2019, Elsevier.

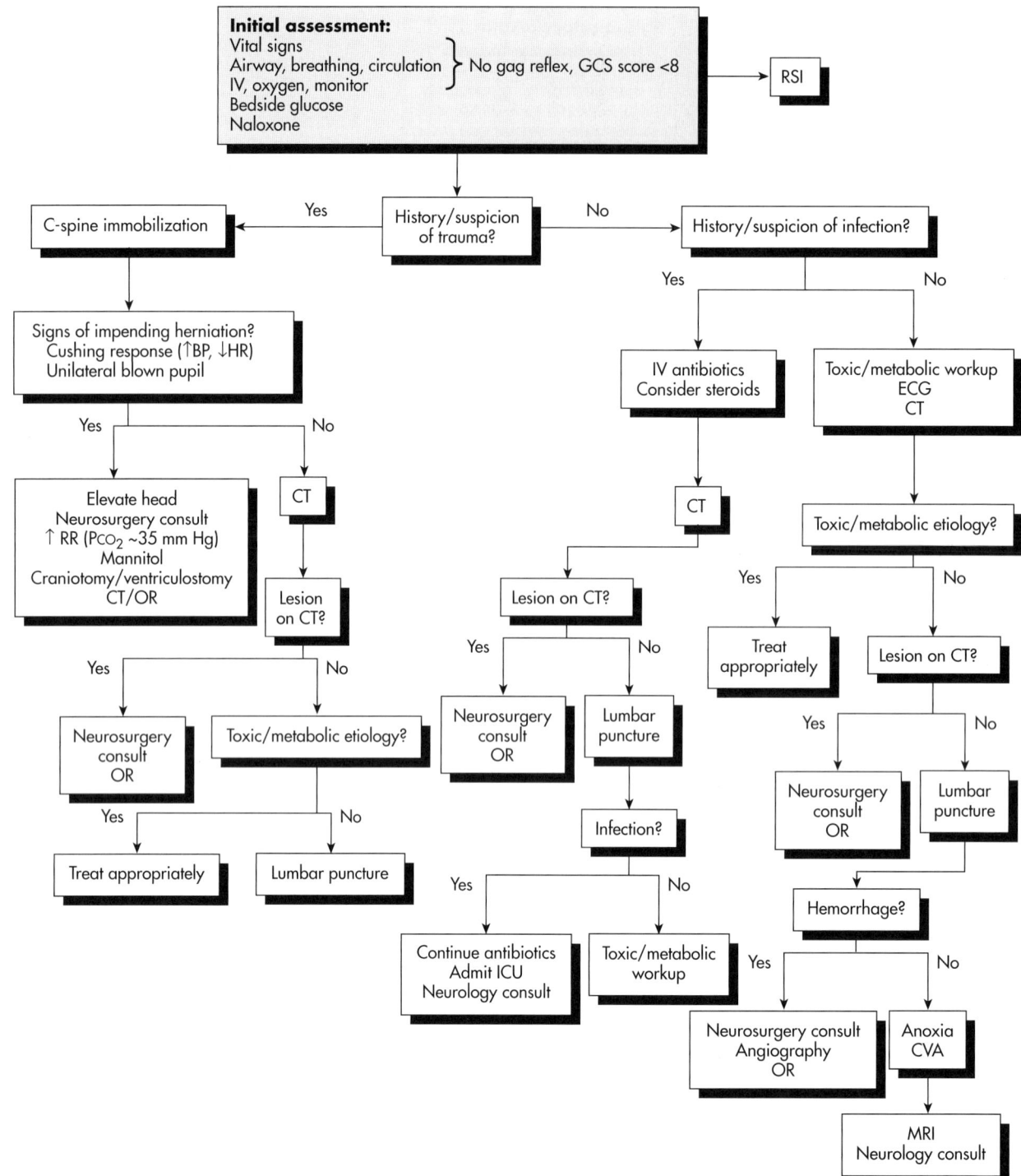

FIG. 19 Diagnostic approach to altered mental status and coma. *BP,* Blood pressure; *C-spine,* cervical spine; *CT,* computed tomography; *CVA,* cerebrovascular accident; *ECG,* electrocardiography; *GCS,* Glasgow Coma Scale; *HR,* heart rate; *ICU,* intensive care unit; *IV,* intravenous; *MRI,* magnetic resonance imaging; *OR,* operating room; *PCO₂,* Partial pressure of carbon dioxide; *RR,* respiratory rate; *RSI,* rapid-sequence intubation. (From Adams JG et al: *Emergency medicine, clinical essentials,* ed 2, Philadelphia, 2013, Elsevier.)

Hb below expected and/or falling over time
- Female: Black Hb <11.5g/dl, white <12.2 g/dl
- Males: Black Hb <12.7g/dl, white <13.2g/dl

Review patient history
- Signs and symptoms and risk factors, attention to iron deficiency (blood thinners or bleeding)

Review prior hematologic laboratories
- Assess available past hemoglobin values

Routine laboratory tests
- Complete blood count, white blood cell differential, RBC indices
- Iron studies: Serum ferritin, serum iron, total iron binding capacity, transferrin saturation
- Vitamin B12
- Serum creatinine for est. GFR
- C-reactive protein
- Reticulocyte count
- Thyroid stimulating hormone
- RBC or serum folate (only when specific risk factors)

Diagnostic considerations of common anemias in older adults　　　　　**Treatment considerations**

Micronutrient deficiency
- Iron deficiency: Serum ferritin <30–50 ng/ml
- Vitamin B12 deficiency: B12 level <200 pg/ml with a methylmalonic acid level >0.4 μmol/L
- Folate deficiency: Serum folate <4.0 ng/ml or RBC folate <316 ng/ml

- IDA: Once daily oral and treat any cause or risk factor for bleeding
- B12: 1000 mcg daily po

Chronic kidney disease
- Estimated GFR <60 ml/min/1.73m^2 body surface area

- Assess for other causes of anemia and treat
- Refer to nephrologist if Hb <10 g/dl
- Consider iron therapy +/− ESA

Anemia of inflammation
- Presence of a subacute or chronic inflammatory condition without evidence of kidney disease and/or vitamin deficiency
- Elevated CRP, low iron saturation and normal/low total iron binding capacity

- Treat underlying inflammatory condition
- Consider iron therapy if functional iron deficiency (e.g., ferritin <100 ng/ml and/or iron saturation <20%)

- **Hematologic malignancy or other**
- Abnormal peripheral smear, thrombocytopenia below 120 x 10^9/L, neutropenia below 1000 10^9/L, unexplained MCV > 100 fL or red cell transfusions

- Refer to hematologist for bone marrow examination

Unexplained anemia
- Typically mild anemia (Hb 10–12 g/dl), normal MCV, without evidence of above etiologies of anemia

- CBC every 6 mo when the Hb level is 2 g/dl below age and race adjusted normal values but the Hb trajectory is stable

Clinical
Algorithms

FIG. 25　Workup of older adult presenting with anemia. (From Warshaw G et al: *Ham's primary care geriatrics,* ed 7, Philadelphia, 2022, Elsevier.)

TABLE 8   Anemia Workup

	Parameters	Interpretation
History	Diet (meat and green vegetables)	Risk of malnutrition if lacking: Suggests susceptibility to iron and folic acid deficiency
	Blood loss	Obvious gastrointestinal bleeding Chronic subclinical blood loss (e.g., NSAIDs, colon polyps, hereditary telangiectasias, menorrhagia)
	Gastrointestinal surgery	Gastrectomy or ileal resection: Vitamin B_{12} deficiency Small bowel resections: Iron, folate deficiency
	Comorbidity	Chronic infections and inflammatory disorders suggest risk of anemia of chronic disease
Examination	Pallor	Severity of anemia
	Icterus	May suggest hemolysis
	Lymphadenopathy, hepatomegaly, splenomegaly, bone tenderness	Coexistence of another primary hematologic disorder
	Evidence of portal hypertension	Hypersplenism and potential for variceal bleed
Red cell size and hemoglobinization	Microcytic hypochromic	Iron deficiency Thalassemia Anemia of chronic disease Sideroblastic anemia
	Normocytic	Acute bleeding Bone marrow infiltration Aplastic anemia Renal failure
	Macrocytic	Vitamin B_{12}/folate deficiencies Myelodysplasia Medication effects Other medical conditions: Hypothyroidism, liver impairment

NSAIDs, Nonsteroidal antiinflammatory drugs.
From Talley NJ et al: *Essentials of internal medicine,* ed 4, Chatswood, NSW, 2021, Elsevier Australia.

TABLE 9   Differentiating Features of Microcytic Anemias*

Test	Iron-Deficiency Anemia	Thalassemia Minor[†]	Anemia of Inflammation[‡]
Serum iron	Low	Normal	Low
Serum iron-binding capacity	High	Normal	Low or normal
Serum ferritin	Low	Normal or high	Normal or high
Marrow iron stores	Low or absent	Normal or high	Normal or high
Marrow sideroblasts	Decreased or absent	Normal or increased	Normal or increased
Free erythrocyte protoporphyrin	High	Normal or slightly increased	High
Hemoglobin A_2 or F	Normal	High beta-thalassemia; normal alpha-thalassemia	Normal
Red blood cell distribution width[§]	High	Normal	Normal/↑

*See Table 11 for definition of microcytosis.
[†]Alpha-thalassemia minor can be diagnosed by the presence of Bart hemoglobin on newborn screening.
[‡]Usually normochromic; 25% of cases are microcytic.
[§]Red blood cell distribution width quantitates the degree of anisocytosis (different sizes) of red blood cells.
From Marcdante KJ et al: *Nelson essentials of pediatrics,* ed 9, Philadelphia, 2023, Elsevier.

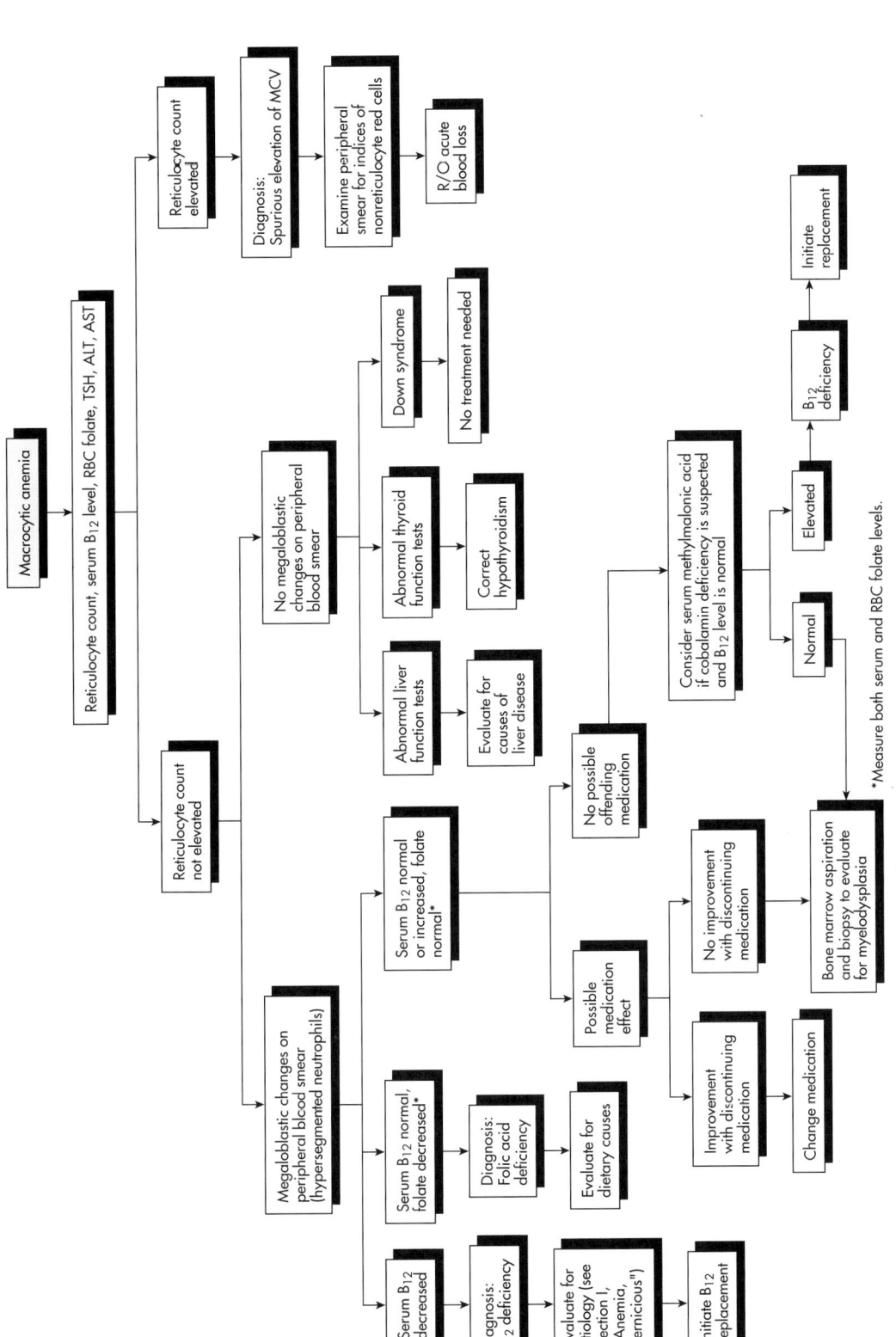

FIG. 26 Differential diagnosis of macrocytic anemia. *ALT,* Alanine transaminase; *AST,* aspartate aminotransferase; *MCV,* mean corpuscular volume; *RBC,* red blood cell; *R/O,* rule out; *TSH,* thyroid-stimulating hormone. (Modified and updated from Rakel RE [ed]: *Principles of family practice,* ed 7, Philadelphia, 2007, Saunders.)

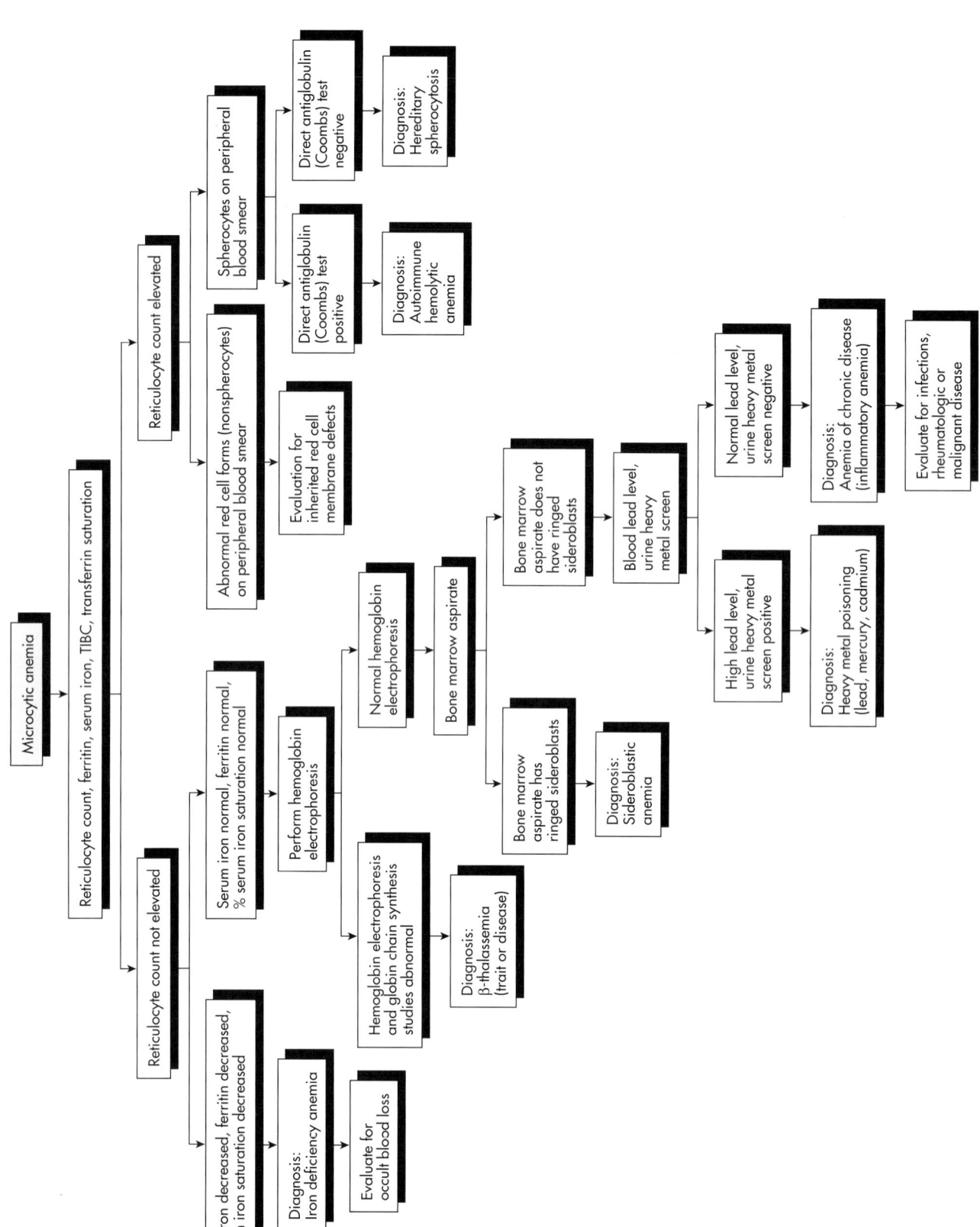

FIG. 27 Differential diagnosis of microcytic anemia. *TIBC,* Total iron binding capacity. (Modified and updated from Rakel RE [ed]: *Principles of family practice,* ed 7, Philadelphia, 2007, Saunders.)

TABLE 10   Differential Diagnosis of Microcytic Hypochromic Anemia

Parameter	Iron-Deficiency Anemia	Anemia of Chronic Disease (Anemia of Inflammation)	Thalassemias	Sideroblastic Anemia
MCV	↓	↓ / N	↓	↓ / N
Serum iron	↓	↓	N	↑
Transferrin saturation	↓	↓ / N	N	↑
TIBC	↓	↓ / N	N	N
Serum transferrin receptor	↑	↓	N	N / ↑
Serum ferritin	↓	↑ / N	N	↑
Serum hepcidin	↓	↑	N / ↓	↓
Bone marrow iron stores	↓	↑ / N	↑ / N	↑ / N Ring sideroblasts

MCV, Mean cell volume; *N,* normal; *TIBC,* total iron-binding capacity.
Talley NJ et al: *Essentials of internal medicine,* ed 4, Chatswood, NSW, 2021, Elsevier Australia.

TABLE 11   Stages in the Development of Iron Deficiency Anemia

Hemoglobin (g/dL)	Peripheral Smear	Serum Iron (μg/dL)	Bone Marrow Iron	Serum Ferritin (ng/ml)
13+ (normal)	nc/nc	50-150	Fe^{2+}	*Male:* 40-340 *Female:* 40-150
10-12	nc/nc	↓	Fe^{2+} absent, erythroid hyperplasia	<12
8-10	hypo/nc	↓	Fe^{2+} absent, erythroid hyperplasia	<12
<8	hypo/micro*	↓	Fe^{2+} absent, erythroid hyperplasia	<12

Hypo/micro, Hypochromic, microcytic; *hypo/nc,* hypochromic, normocytic; *nc/nc,* normochromic, normocytic.
*Microcytosis, determined by a mean corpuscular volume (in fL) <2 standard deviations (SD) below the mean, must be adjusted for age (e.g., −2 SD at 3-6 mo = 74; at 0.5-2 yr = 70; at 2-6 yr = 75; at 6-12 yr = 77; and at 12-18 yr = 78).
From Andreoli TE et al: *Cecil essentials of medicine,* ed 4, Philadelphia, 1997, Saunders.

BOX 9   Causes of Iron Deficiency

Inadequate Intake
- Veganism, dietary choices

Inadequate Absorption
- High gastric pH or antacid therapy
- Excess tannins and phytates in diet
- Bowel resection
- Celiac disease
- Inflammatory bowel disease

Increased Physiologic Requirement
- Pregnancy and breastfeeding
- Infancy, puberty

Increased Loss
- Gastrointestinal blood loss
- Genitourinary blood loss
- Menorrhagia
- Operative blood loss
- Parasitosis
- Trauma
- Excessive phlebotomy

From Talley NJ et al: *Essentials of internal medicine,* ed 4, Chatswood, NSW, 2021, Elsevier Australia.

Clinical Algorithms

III

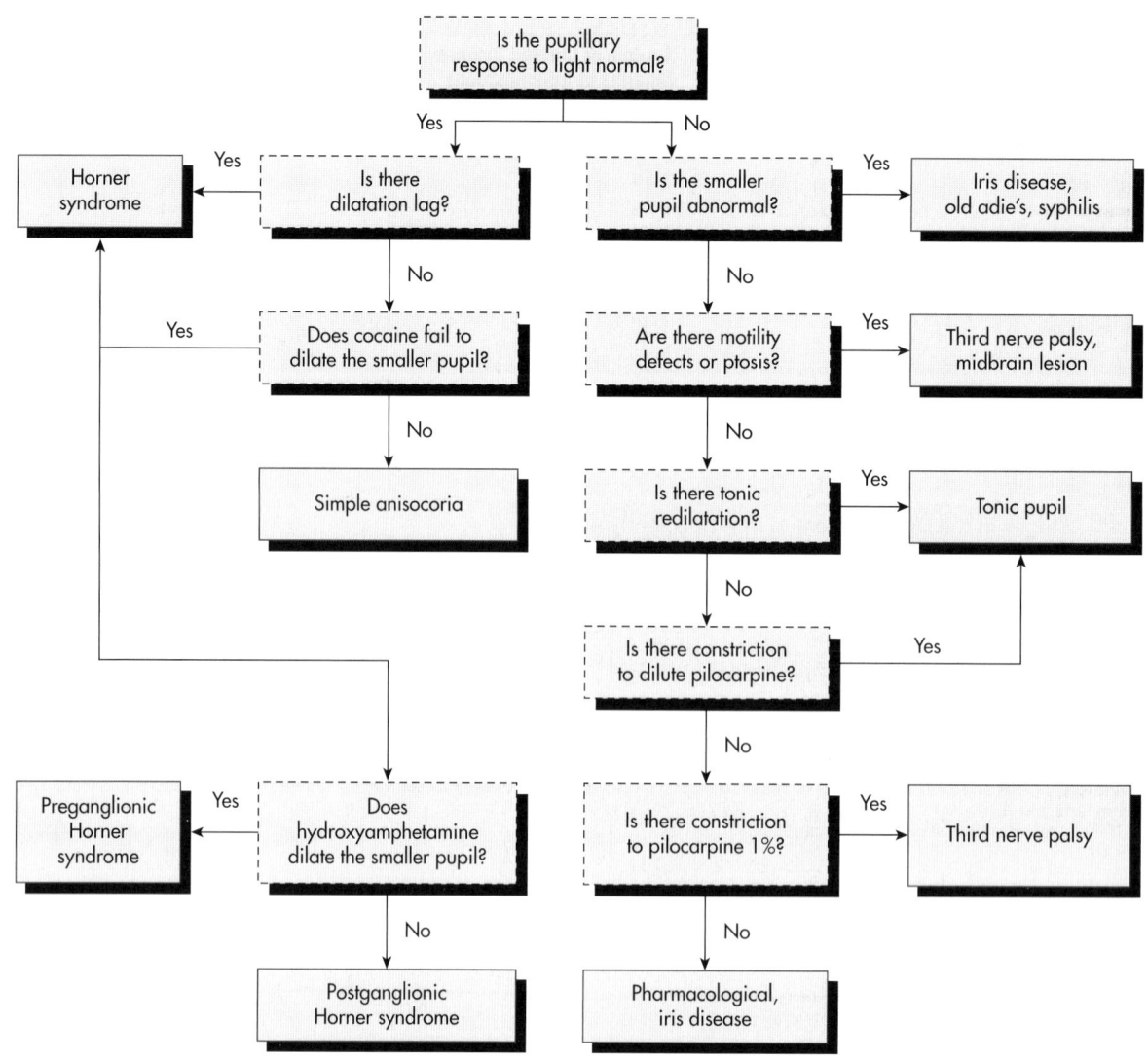

FIG. 28 Flowchart with systematic guidelines for evaluation of anisocoria. (From Jankovic J et al: *Bradley and Daroff s neurology in clinical practice,* ed 8, Philadelphia, 2022, Elsevier.)

TABLE 12 Diagnostic Pupillary Eyedrop Testing

Testing	Mechanism of Action	Diagnostic Utility and Expected Response
Anisocoria Greater in the Light (Abnormal Larger Pupil)		
Dilute pilocarpine (0.0625% or 0.1%)	Parasympathomimetic; direct sphincter stimulation	Tonic pupil will constrict and pupil affected by oculomotor palsy may constrict (denervation supersensitivity)
		Normal pupil and pupil affected by pharmacologic blockade will not respond
Pilocarpine (1%)	Parasympathomimetic; direct sphincter stimulation	Normal pupil and pupil affected by oculomotor palsy will constrict fully
		Pupil affected by pharmacologic blockade will not or only partially respond
Anisocoria Greater in the Dark (Abnormal Smaller Pupil)		
Cocaine (2%-10%)	Inhibits norepinephrine reuptake at the sympathetic terminus	Horner pupil will not dilate
		Normal pupil will dilate
Hydroxyamphetamine (1%)	Induces third-order sympathetic neuron to release any stored norepinephrine	Preganglionic (first- or second-order neuron) Horner pupil will dilate
		Postganglionic (third-order neuron) Horner pupil will not dilate
Apraclonidine (0.5%)	Weak sympathetic agonist	Horner pupil will dilate (denervation supersensitivity)
		Normal pupil will not change or will constrict slightly

From Jankovic J et al: *Bradley and Daroff s neurology in clinical practice,* ed 8, Philadelphia, 2022, Elsevier.

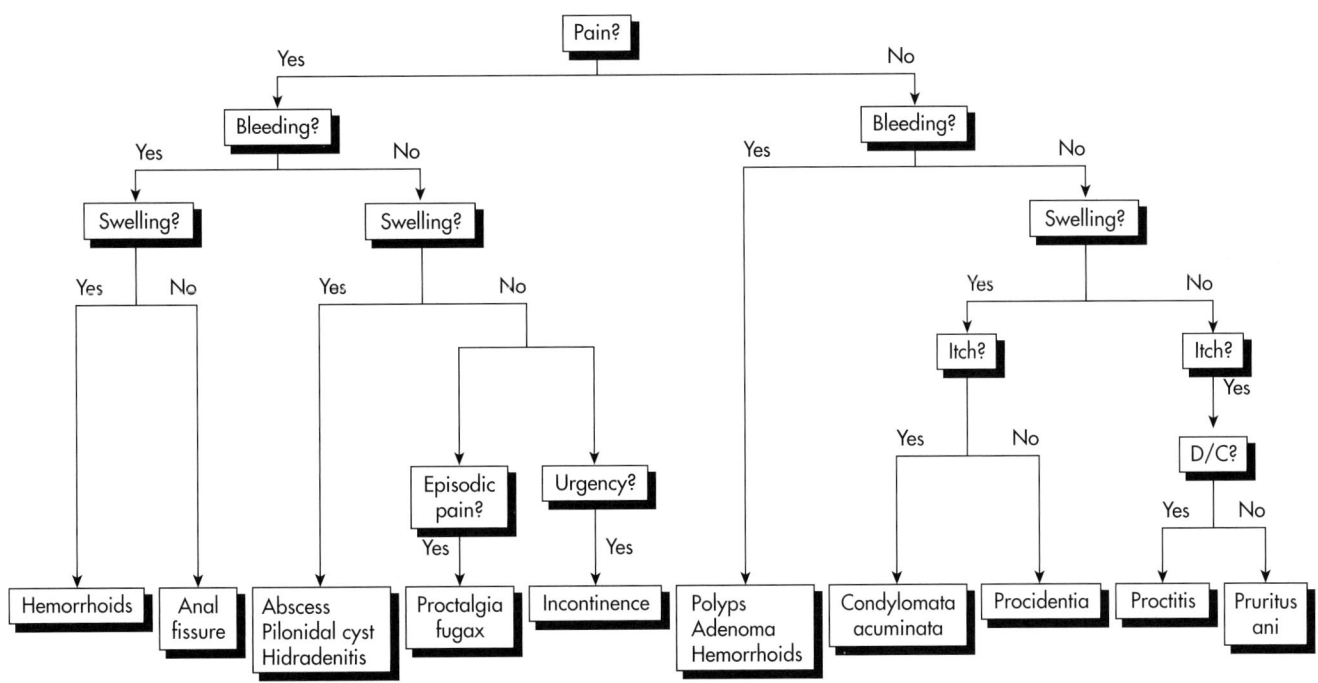

FIG. 30 Algorithm for anorectal complaints. *D/C,* Discharge. (From Marx JA et al: *Rosen's emergency medicine,* ed 8, Philadelphia, 2014, Saunders.)

BOX 10   The WASH Regimen for Management of Hemorrhoids

- *W*arm water
- *A*nalgesic agents
- *S*tool softeners
- *H*igh-fiber diet

From Marx JA et al: *Rosen's emergency medicine,* ed 8, Philadelphia, 2014, Saunders.

BOX 11   Medical History in Diagnosis of Anorectal Disorders

Anorectal History
- Pain
- Bleeding
- Swelling
- Itching
- Discharge
- Urgency

Gastrointestinal History
- Change in bowel habits (straining, flatus, color, consistency, frequency)
- Nausea or vomiting
- Incontinence of stool
- Underlying GI disease (Crohn disease, cancer, polyps)

Systemic Disease History
- Diabetes mellitus
- Coagulopathy
- Cancer
- HIV infection

Sexual History of the Anus
- Penetration
- Known STDs
- Assault

From Marx JA et al: *Rosen's emergency medicine,* ed 8, Philadelphia, 2014, Saunders.

ICD-10CM #		
	M54.5	Low back pain
	L29	Pruritus
	M54.89	Other dorsalgia
	M54.9	Dorsalgia, unspecified
	F45.42	Pain disorder with related psychological factors
	M54.08	Panniculitis affecting regions of neck and back, sacral and sacrococcygeal region
	S23.9XXA	Sprain of unspecified parts of thorax, initial encounter
	M43.27	Fusion of spine, lumbosacral region
	M43.28	Fusion of spine, sacral and sacrococcygeal region
	M53.2X7	Spinal instabilities, lumbosacral region
	M53.3	Sacrococcygeal disorders, not elsewhere classified

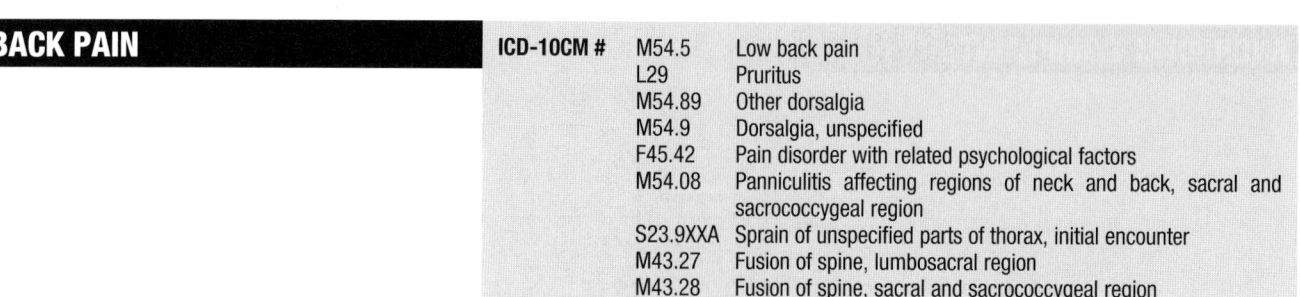

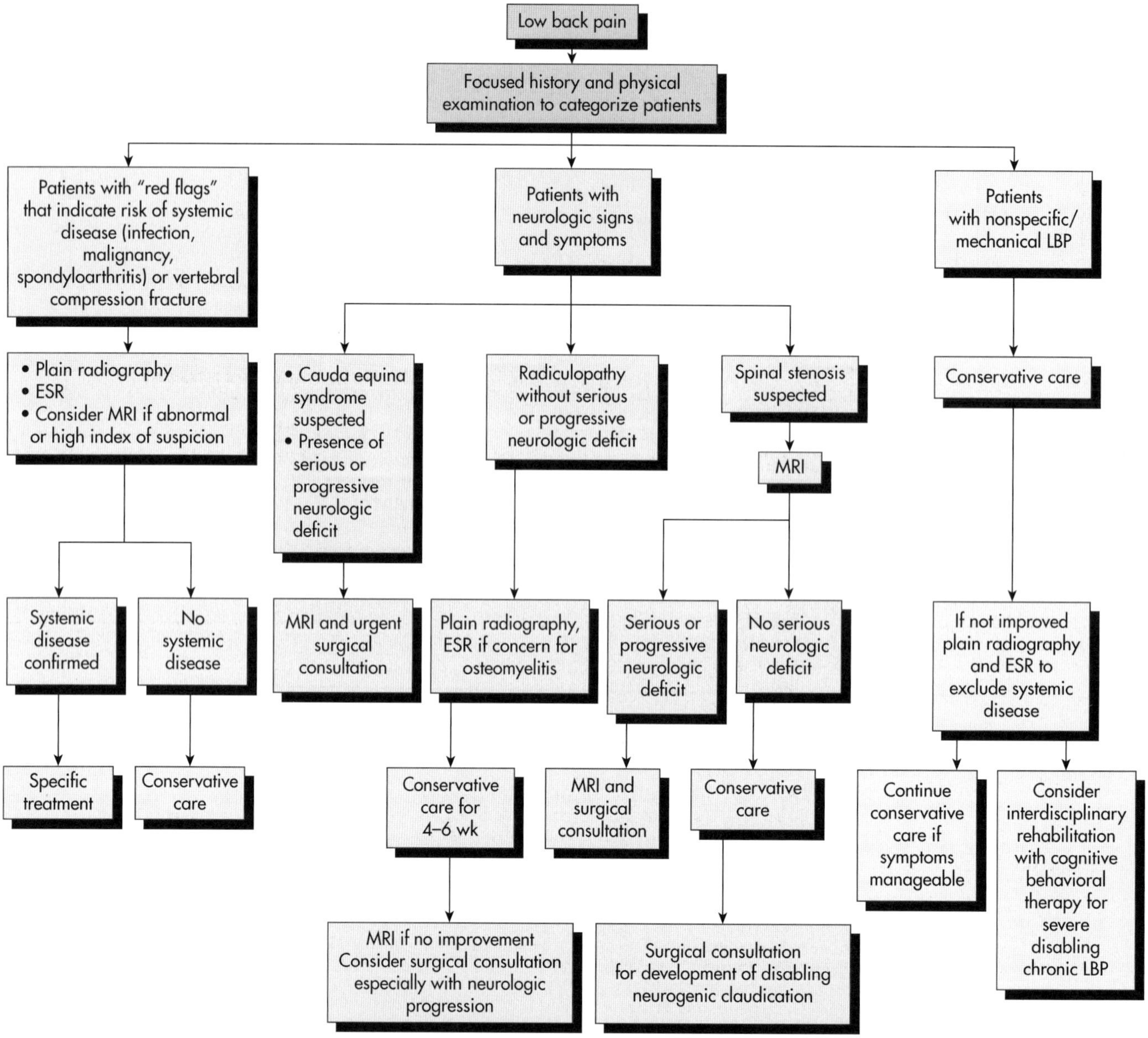

FIG. 33 Algorithm for the differential diagnosis and treatment of low back pain. *ESR,* Erythrocyte sedimentation rate; *LBP,* low back pain. (From Firestein GS et al: *Firestein & Kelley's textbook of rheumatology,* ed 11, Philadelphia, 2021, Elsevier.)

TABLE 13 Red Flags for Potentially Serious Conditions

Possible Fracture	Possible Tumor or Infection	Possible Cauda Equina Syndrome
From Medical History		
Major trauma, such as vehicle accident or fall from height	Age over 50 or under 20 yr	Saddle anesthesia
	History of cancer	Recent onset of bladder dysfunction, such as urinary retention, increased frequency, or overflow incontinence
Minor trauma or even strenuous lifting (in older or potentially osteoporotic patient)	Constitutional symptoms, such as recent fever or chills or unexplained weight loss	
	Risk factors for spinal infection: Recent bacterial infection (e.g., urinary tract infection), intravenous drug abuse, or immune suppression (from steroids, transplant, or human immunodeficiency virus)	Severe or progressive neurologic deficit in the lower extremity
	Pain that worsens when supine; severe nighttime pain	

ICD-10CM #		
	M54.5	Low back pain
	L29	Pruritus
	M54.89	Other dorsalgia
	M54.9	Dorsalgia, unspecified
	F45.42	Pain disorder with related psychological factors
	M54.08	Panniculitis affecting regions of neck and back, sacral and sacrococcygeal region
	S23.9XXA	Sprain of unspecified parts of thorax, initial encounter
	M43.27	Fusion of spine, lumbosacral region
	M43.28	Fusion of spine, sacral and sacrococcygeal region
	M53.2X7	Spinal instabilities, lumbosacral region
	M53.3	Sacrococcygeal disorders, not elsewhere classified

TABLE 14   Motor and Sensory Function of Lumbosacral Nerves

Nerve	Origin	Motor Function	Sensory Function
Femoral	Lumbar plexus, L2-L4	Extension of knee, flexion of thigh	Anterior thigh
Saphenous	Distal sensory branch of femoral nerve	None	Inside aspect of lower leg
Lateral femoral cutaneous	Branch of lumbar plexus, L2-L3	None	Lateral thigh
Obturator	Lumbar plexus, L2-L4	Adduction of thigh	Medial aspect of upper thigh
Sciatic	Combined roots from lumbosacral plexus, partially separated into tibial and peroneal divisions	Foot plantar (tibial division) and dorsiflexion (peroneal division), foot inversion (tibial) and eversion (peroneal)	Lateral, anterior, and posterior aspects of lower leg and foot
Tibial	Lumbosacral plexus, L4-S3	Plantar flexion and inversion of foot	Posterior lower leg and sole of foot
Peroneal	Lumbosacral plexus, L5-S2	Dorsiflexion and eversion of foot	Dorsum of foot and lateral lower leg
Superficial peroneal	Distal sensory branch of peroneal nerve	None	Dorsum of foot
Sural	Cutaneous branches of peroneal and tibial nerves	None	Lateral foot to sole

From Jankovic J et al: *Bradley and Daroff's neurology in clinical practice,* ed 8, Philadelphia, 2022, Elsevier.

TABLE 15   Classification of Lower Back and Lower Limb Pain

Type	Examples
Mechanical pain	Facet pain
	Bony destruction
	Sacroiliac joint inflammation
	Osteomyelitis
	Diskitis
	Lumbar spondylosis
Neuropathic pain	Polyneuropathy
	Radiculopathy from disk disease, zoster, and diabetes
	Mononeuropathy including sciatic, femoral, lateral femoral cutaneous, and peroneal neuropathies
	Plexopathy from cancer, abscess, hematoma, and autoimmune processes
Nonneurologic pain	Urolithiasis
	Retroperitoneal mass
	Ovarian cyst or carcinoma
	Endometriosis

From Jankovic J et al: *Bradley and Daroff's neurology in clinical practice,* ed 8, Philadelphia, 2022, Elsevier.

TABLE 16   Differential Diagnosis of Lower Back and Leg Pain

Disorder	Clinical Features	Diagnostic Findings
Radiculopathy	Back pain radiating into leg in a dermatomal distribution. Sensory loss and motor loss are in a root distribution. Increased pain with coughing or straining.	Suspected when neuropathic pain radiates from back down into leg in a single root distribution. Disk or mass can be seen on MRI or CT. Zoster and diabetes can cause radiculopathy without abnormal studies.
Plexopathy	Back and leg pain with a neuropathic character, dysesthesias, burning, or electric sensation. Back pain can develop when cause is mass lesion in region of plexus.	Suspected when patient has leg pain in more than one peripheral nerve or root distribution. MRI of plexus or CT of abdomen and pelvis can show mass or hematoma.
Spinal stenosis	Pain in lower back, buttocks, and legs, especially with standing, walking, and lumbar spine extension.	MRI or CT shows obliteration of subarachnoid space.

CT, Computed tomography; *MRI,* magnetic resonance imaging.
From Jankovic J et al: *Bradley and Daroff's neurology in clinical practice,* ed 8, Philadelphia, 2022, Elsevier.

ICD-10CM #		
	M54.5	Low back pain
	L29	Pruritus
	M54.89	Other dorsalgia
	M54.9	Dorsalgia, unspecified
	F45.42	Pain disorder with related psychological factors
	M54.08	Panniculitis affecting regions of neck and back, sacral and sacrococcygeal region
	S23.9XXA	Sprain of unspecified parts of thorax, initial encounter
	M43.27	Fusion of spine, lumbosacral region
	M43.28	Fusion of spine, sacral and sacrococcygeal region
	M53.2X7	Spinal instabilities, lumbosacral region
	M53.3	Sacrococcygeal disorders, not elsewhere classified

TABLE 17   Differential Diagnosis of Isolated Lower Back Pain

Disorder	Clinical Features	Diagnostic Findings
Sacroiliac joint inflammation	Pain lateral to spine where sacrum inserts into top of iliac bone. Pain is exacerbated by movement and pressure but does not radiate down leg.	Clinical diagnosis. Radiographs can show degenerative changes in joint. Bone scan shows increased uptake in region.
Facet pain	Unilateral or bilateral paraspinal pain without radiation. Pain is increased by spine motion, especially extension.	Clinical diagnosis. Radiographs can show facet degeneration.
Ovarian cyst or cancer	Pain in hip and lower back, often but not always extending into lower quadrant. Bowel disturbance may develop with advanced disease.	Abdominal and pelvic CT shows mass lesion in ovary.
Endometriosis	Usually pelvic pain but occasionally pain in back and legs. Pain is often timed to menses.	Diagnosis suspected during pelvic examination. Vaginal ultrasound is supportive. Laparoscopy is diagnostic.
Retroperitoneal mass, abdominal aortic aneurysm, abscess, hematoma	Pain in back. May be bilateral to spine. May be associated with superimposed neuropathic pain in cases with plexus or proximal nerve involvement.	CT or MRI shows hematoma, aneurysm, eroding vertebral bodies, or abdominal mass.
Urolithiasis	Pain in upper to mid-back laterally that may radiate to groin. No radiation into leg.	Radiographs may show stones. Intravenous pyelography typically shows obstruction of flow. Contrasted abdominal CT usually shows the stone and obstruction.
Diskitis	Pain in lower back exacerbated by movement. Some patients may have radiation of pain to abdomen, hip, or leg.	MRI shows characteristic changes in disk and surrounding tissues.

CT, Computed tomography; *MRI,* magnetic resonance imaging.
From Jankovic J et al: *Bradley and Daroff's neurology in clinical practice,* ed 8, Philadelphia, 2022, Elsevier.

TABLE 18   Diagnostic Studies for Lower Back and Lower Limb Pain

Diagnostic Test	Advantages	Disadvantages
Magnetic resonance imaging	Sensitive for identification of lumbar disk herniation, spinal stenosis, paravertebral mass in region of plexus, perineural tumors, and diskitis.	May overemphasize structural lesions. May miss vascular lesions of spinal cord. Paravertebral disorders may be overlooked if they are not the focus of interest. Cannot be performed on patients with some implanted metallic and electrical devices.
Noncontrast CT	Shows osteophytes and lateral disk herniations best. Can show bone fractures and extension of fragments into regions that may contain neural elements.	Cannot identify neural elements without intrathecal contrast. Disk herniations without bone involvement may be missed.
Myelography with postmyelographic CT	Many neurosurgeons consider this the definitive test for identification of lumbar disk herniation, osteophytes, and intervertebral foraminal stenosis. Postmyelographic CT should be routinely performed.	May miss far-lateral herniations. Is invasive with a small risk of serious adverse effects.
Nerve conduction studies and EMG	Sensitive for identification of specific nerve root or peripheral neuropathic involvement.	Patients may have clinically significant radiculopathy without EMG evidence of denervation (or vice versa if radiculopathy is old).
Diskogram	Can identify disk anatomy in comparison with bony and neural anatomy. May confirm disk level if it produces pain that reproduces patient's complaints.	Invasive test, but risk of serious complications is low. Seldom performed in routine practice.

CT, Computed tomography; *EMG,* electromyography.
From Jankovic J et al: *Bradley and Daroff's neurology in clinical practice,* ed 8, Philadelphia, 2022, Elsevier.

```
┌─────────────────────────────────────┐
│ Assess reason for referral, previous │
│ diagnosis/investigations, and patient's │
│ concerns about bleeding.             │
└─────────────────────────────────────┘
                    │
                    ▼
┌─────────────────────────────────────────────────┐
│ Evaluate the history for unprovoked, unexpected,  │
│ significant, and recurrent bleeding (current and  │
│ previous). Assess for symptoms of bruising,       │
│ prolonged bleeding with cuts, nosebleeds, gum and │
│ oral bleeding, gastrointestinal bleeding, joint or│
│ muscle bleeds, urinary tract bleeding, and other  │
│ bleeding (e.g., intracranial, umbilical stump).   │
│ Evaluate the drug history and family history of   │
│ bleeding problems. Evaluate other medical         │
│ problems. Determine the nature and timing of any  │
│ abnormal bleeding with challenges (right away,    │
│ within hours or days after) and the severity      │
│ (e.g., required transfusion, longer hospital stay,│
│ developed large hematomas).                       │
└─────────────────────────────────────────────────┘
                    │
                    ▼
┌─────────────────────────────────────────────────┐
│ If symptoms suggest an underlying bleeding        │
│ problem, evaluate whether the cause could be an   │
│ acquired or congenital problem (e.g., symptoms    │
│ from childhood, positive family history).         │
└─────────────────────────────────────────────────┘
                    │
                    ▼
┌─────────────────────────────────────────────────┐
│ If bleeding problems are new, consider potential  │
│ reasons and triggers (e.g., a first major         │
│ hemostatic challenge could be the first           │
│ presentation of a mild bleeding disorder; trigger │
│ could be drugs, development of an immune disorder,│
│ or blood, endocrine, liver, or renal disease).    │
└─────────────────────────────────────────────────┘
                    │
                    ▼
┌─────────────────────────────────────────────────┐
│ Formulate a differential diagnosis for the        │
│ potential inherited and acquired causes that      │
│ should be investigated.                           │
└─────────────────────────────────────────────────┘
```

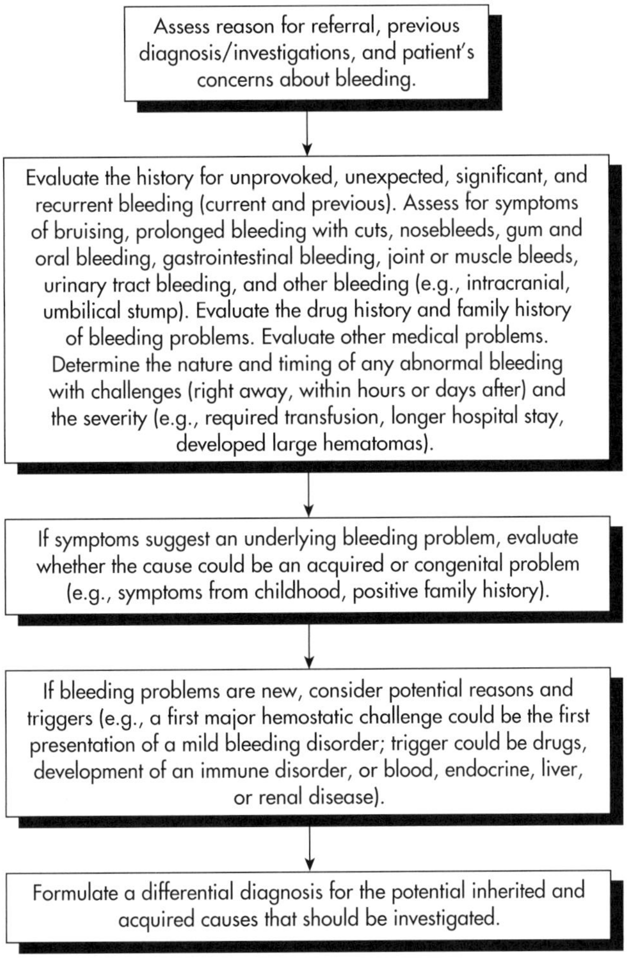

FIG. 34 Steps to evaluate bleeding and bruising problems. (From Hoffman R: *Hematology, basic principles and practice*, ed 7, Philadelphia, 2018, Elsevier.)

Clinical Algorithms

III

TABLE 19 Differential Diagnosis of Bleeding Problems	
Major Categories	**Comments**
No bleeding disorder	Symptoms do not reflect a bleeding disorder and have another explanation (e.g., a surgical bleed, not caused by a bleeding disorder).
Possible bleeding disorder	The laboratory findings are nondiagnostic, and the bleeding history is considered equivocal (e.g., unexplained serious bleed with one surgical procedure; unexplained menorrhagia without other bleeding problems).
Definite bleeding disorder, undefined or indeterminate type	The bleeding history is consistent with a bleeding disorder; however, the laboratory findings are nondiagnostic. Commonly the bleeding history resembles mild to moderate defects in platelet function or von Willebrand factor. The diagnosis should only be made once an adequate evaluation for common bleeding disorders (e.g., for von Willebrand disease and platelet aggregation and release defects) is completed. If testing is not complete, the classification should indicate the types of conditions excluded or not excluded, for example mild mucocutaneous bleeding problem, von Willebrand disease excluded, mild mucocutaneous bleeding problem, platelet release defects not yet excluded.
Definite bleeding disorder with cause	The symptoms and laboratory findings are considered diagnostic of a bleeding disorder. Tables 20 and 21 summarize many of and define the potential inherited and acquired causes.

From Hoffman R: *Hematology, basic principles and practice*, ed 7, Philadelphia, 2018, Elsevier.

TABLE 20 Differential Diagnosis of Congenital Bleeding Disorders

Disorder	Comments
Fibrinogen deficiency or dysfunction	Deficiencies can be mild-moderate hypofibrinogenemia or severe afibrinogenemia. Fibrinogen function is abnormal in dysfibrinogenemias, which can present with bleeding, thrombosis, or both. Fibrinogen levels can be reduced in some dysfibrinogenemias.
X-linked coagulation factor deficiencies—hemophilia	Presentation is influenced by the degree of deficiency. Factor VIII deficiency is more common than factor IX deficiency. If factor VIII is low, von Willebrand disease needs to be excluded as the cause.
Rarer, coagulation factor deficiencies	Deficiencies can affect factors XI, V, II, VII, or X, and the presentation is dependent on the severity of the deficiency. Hereditary deficiencies of multiple coagulation factors are rare (e.g., of factors V and VIII, or multiple vitamin K-dependent coagulation factors for congenital defects impairing γ-carboxylation) and can easily be excluded by measuring multiple factors.
Fibrinolytic defects	Causes include disorders caused by loss of function, such as α2-antiplasmin or PAI-1 deficiency, and by gain-of-function defects, such as Quebec platelet disorder (overexpression of urokinase plasminogen activator in megakaryocytes).
von Willebrand disease	Causes include quantitative (partial type 1 to severe type 3) and qualitative defects (loss of function in type 2M and 2A, gain of function in type 2B and platelet-type). Type 1 von Willebrand disease can be confused with low von Willebrand factor levels (e.g., because of blood group O).
Platelet disorders	These conditions can affect platelet number, function, or both. The most common type of platelet function disorder is a platelet secretion defect, which may or may not also impair aggregation responses. Disorders of platelet function are commonly subclassified by the nature of the defect, such as the following: • Defects of membrane receptors for adhesive proteins (e.g., Glanzmann thrombasthenia and Bernard-Soulier syndrome) or agonists (e.g., $P2Y_{12}$ deficiency) • Defects of signaling or secretion (the largest subcategory) • Cytoskeletal defects (e.g., MYH9-related disorders) • Storage pool disorders (e.g., gray platelet syndrome, dense granule deficiency, $\alpha\gamma$-storage pool deficiency, Quebec platelet disorder) • Defects of procoagulant function (e.g., Scott syndrome)
Vascular disorders	Congenital vascular malformation, including hereditary hemorrhagic telangiectasia, Ehlers-Danlos syndrome

MYH9, Myosin heavy polypeptide 9; *PAI-1*, plasminogen activator inhibitor 1.
From Hoffman R: *Hematology, basic principles and practice*, ed 7, Philadelphia, 2018, Elsevier.

TABLE 21 Differential Diagnosis of Acquired Bleeding Problems

Disorder	Comments
Drug induced	Aspirin, NSAIDs, other platelet function inhibitors (e.g., $P2Y_{12}\alpha_{IIb}\beta_3$ inhibitors), anticoagulants, fibrinolytic drugs, and antidepressants are common causes.
Acquired factor deficiencies	The causes can be immune (e.g., acquired factor VIII deficiency, acquired factor V deficiency) or nonimmune. Reductions in multiple factors can result from vitamin K deficiency, treatment with vitamin K antagonists, liver disease, hemodilution, and rarely snakebites. Severe acquired hypofibrinogenemia is commonly caused by a postpartum coagulopathy or severe liver disease. Prothrombin deficiency occurs with some lupus anticoagulants. Amyloidosis can cause an acquired factor X deficiency, which may be associated with reductions in other coagulation factors synthesized in the liver if the liver is involved.
Disseminated intravascular coagulation	The manifestations can include thrombocytopenia, consumption of coagulation factors, including fibrinogen, and impairment of hemostatic mechanisms from the fibrin/fibrinogen degradation products. Causes are wide ranging and include postpartum consumptive states, prostate and other cancers, and snakebites.
Acquired von Willebrand disease	The cause can be immune (often in association with an IgG paraprotein) or nonimmune (e.g., increased proteolysis of von Willebrand factor with stenotic aortic valvular disease).
Immune thrombocytopenia	Bleeding is usually influenced by the extent of the thrombocytopenia. Some autoantibodies interfere with platelet membrane receptor function, causing bleeding disproportionate to the thrombocytopenia.
Nondrug-induced, acquired platelet function disorders	The cause can be immune (see earlier) or nonimmune, typically from bone marrow disorders, although secretion defects can be secondary to Cushing syndrome or hypothyroidism.
Liver disease	Liver disease can cause thrombocytopenia, deficiencies of coagulation factors, hypofibrinogenemia and dysfibrinogenemia, and increased fibrinolysis. In mild liver disease, factor VII and sometimes factors XI and XII are low. Fibrinogen is often increased in early liver disease, and if low, the finding suggests severe liver disease.
Renal disease	Anemia is an important predictor of uremic bleeding. Uremic bleeding is typically associated with severe renal impairment.
Hypothyroidism	Hypothyroidism can cause an acquired von Willebrand disease and acquired defects in platelet function.
Cushing syndrome	This syndrome should be suspected when there are symptoms and findings suggestive of Cushing syndrome or treatment with systemic or topical glucocorticoids.
Surgical bleeding	This is often a diagnosis of exclusion, although the procedural notes sometimes document that a technical problem was encountered that led to abnormal bleeding.
Vitamin K deficiency	Newborns are at risk, as are individuals with malabsorption and/or receiving broad-spectrum antibiotics that reduce vitamin K production by reducing gut bacteria. Older adults are also at greater risk for developing vitamin K deficiency because of reduced stores from poorer intake of vitamin K. If the patient does not respond to parenteral vitamin K, other causes should be considered.
Vitamin C deficiency (scurvy)	This diagnosis should be considered when there is lethargy with skin and gum bleeding (perifollicular hemorrhages, gum bleeding with swelling). The condition is rare in developed countries. The cause is usually a very poor diet or malabsorption.

IgG, Immunoglobulin G; *NSAID*, nonsteroidal antiinflammatory drug.
From Hoffman R: *Hematology, basic principles and practice*, ed 7, Philadelphia, 2018, Elsevier.

BOX 12   The Laboratory Manifestations of Bleeding Disorders

- The laboratory manifestations of bleeding disorders can include abnormalities from the following:
  - The underlying hemostatic defect
  - Bleeding complications (e.g., anemia, iron deficiency, coagulopathy secondary to hemodilution after resuscitation for a massive bleed, development of red cell antibodies after transfusion)
  - False-positive abnormalities (e.g., prolonged aPTT caused by incidental mild factor XII deficiency, which is found in about 1 of 200 patients, or a lupus anticoagulant, which can be a transient finding in about 5% of hospitalized patients)
  - Extremes of normal variation (e.g., mildly low von Willebrand factor levels in an individual who is blood group O, absent secondary aggregation with epinephrine in adjusted platelet-rich plasma aggregation studies)

From Hoffman R: *Hematology, basic principles and practice,* ed 7, Philadelphia, 2018, Elsevier.

BOX 13   Influences on Presenting Problems

When evaluating a bleeding history, it is important to recognize that the presenting problems are influenced by the following factors:
- The nature and severity of the defect, and the presence of single or multiple risk factors for bleeding
- Whether the bleeding problem is congenital or acquired
- Antecedent exposure to hemostatic challenges (such as surgery, dental extraction, menses, and childbirth) and the risk for bleeding with each of these challenges
- The presence of other medical problems (e.g., renal, hepatic, or thyroid disease), including anemia
- Variability in the bleeding symptoms experienced by individuals without bleeding disorders (e.g., nosebleeds, bruising) and by individuals with known bleeding disorders, even within families with the same defect
- Local factors (e.g., sun-damage to the skin, vascular lesions, diverticular disease, or cancerous lesions in the gastrointestinal tract) and the possibility of nonaccidental trauma
- Treatments that increase the risk for bleeding (e.g., antiplatelet drugs, such as aspirin and nonsteroidal antiinflammatory drugs used for pain control, anticoagulant therapy, etc.)
- Whether treatments were used to prevent or control bleeding
- Whether treatments prescribed for other reasons may have reduced bleeding (e.g., reduced menstrual bleeding while on oral contraceptives to prevent pregnancy)

From Hoffman R: *Hematology, basic principles and practice,* ed 7, Philadelphia, 2018, Elsevier.

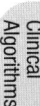

Clinical Algorithms

BOX 14   Case 1: Illustration of a Mild, Inherited Bleeding Problem

A 77-yr-old man who is starting treatment for multiple myeloma was discovered to have a prolonged activated partial thromboplastin time. Review of his records indicated that the abnormality was present on a previous admission for spinal cord compression, which was treated with surgery. He required 4 units of packed red blood cells several days after this surgery because of delayed postoperative bleeding. There was no other bleeding history. He was found to have mild factor IX deficiency, unrelated to the myeloma, and his daughter proved to be a carrier of this defect.

From Hoffman R: *Hematology, basic principles and practice,* ed 7, Philadelphia, 2018, Elsevier.

BOX 15   Case 2: Illustration of the Importance of Assessing Both Personal and Familial Bleeding Problems

A 22-yr-old woman was referred for evaluation of a possible platelet disorder. She had a history of menorrhagia (4 days out of 7 days of menstrual flow were heavy when not on treatment), prolonged nosebleeds in childhood, and hematuria with urinary tract infections. She did not have thrombocytopenia, and she had no exposure to major hemostatic challenges. Her father, uncle, and grandfather had a striking bleeding history, and two of them had thrombocytopenia. The bleeding in her relatives included joint bleeds with trauma and severe, delayed-onset bleeding after trauma and surgery (usually more than a day later), which continued for weeks despite platelet transfusions. One of these relatives reported no bleeding when he had a tooth extracted while receiving fibrinolytic inhibitor therapy. Although menorrhagia is not specific to any one type of bleeding disorder, the delayed bleeding in affected relatives suggests a possible autosomal dominant disorder and either a fibrinolytic defect of a factor defect or deficiency (e.g., affected relatives). Because of the family history of thrombocytopenia, joint bleeds, and delayed bleeding, which did not respond well to platelet transfusions, testing was done for the Quebec platelet disorder. Genetic testing for duplication mutation of the urokinase plasminogen activator gene confirmed this diagnosis in the patient and her relatives. The case illustrates the importance of evaluating both the personal and family bleeding history and highlights the fact that bleeding-symptom severity can vary among affected family members, in part because of their different exposures to challenges and treatments.

From Hoffman R: *Hematology, basic principles and practice,* ed 7, Philadelphia, 2018, Elsevier.

BOX 16 Case 3: Illustration of the Importance of Assessing Bleeding Problems Over Time

A 72-yr-old man was referred for evaluation of a severe bleed after receiving a single dose of low–molecular-weight heparin for unconfirmed deep vein thrombosis. He had a history of a similar bleeding episode several years previously while on warfarin treatment for atrial fibrillation. There was no other bleeding history, and the patient subsequently developed a spontaneous iliopsoas bleed. He had undergone numerous surgeries earlier in life without any bleeding problems, and there was no family history of bleeding. The bleeding history suggested the possibility of an acquired bleeding problem, possibly acquired von Willebrand disease or an acquired factor XIII deficiency. Diagnostic testing indicated that he had acquired factor XIII deficiency. This case illustrates the fact that there may be more than one risk factor for bleeding: In this case, several exposures to anticoagulants triggered bleeding in a patient with an acquired factor deficiency. On initial treatment of his iliopsoas bleed with factor XIII concentrate, there was partial neutralization of the infused factor followed by accelerated clearance, consistent with acquired factor XIII deficiency secondary to an autoantibody.

From Hoffman R: *Hematology, basic principles and practice,* ed 7, Philadelphia, 2018, Elsevier.

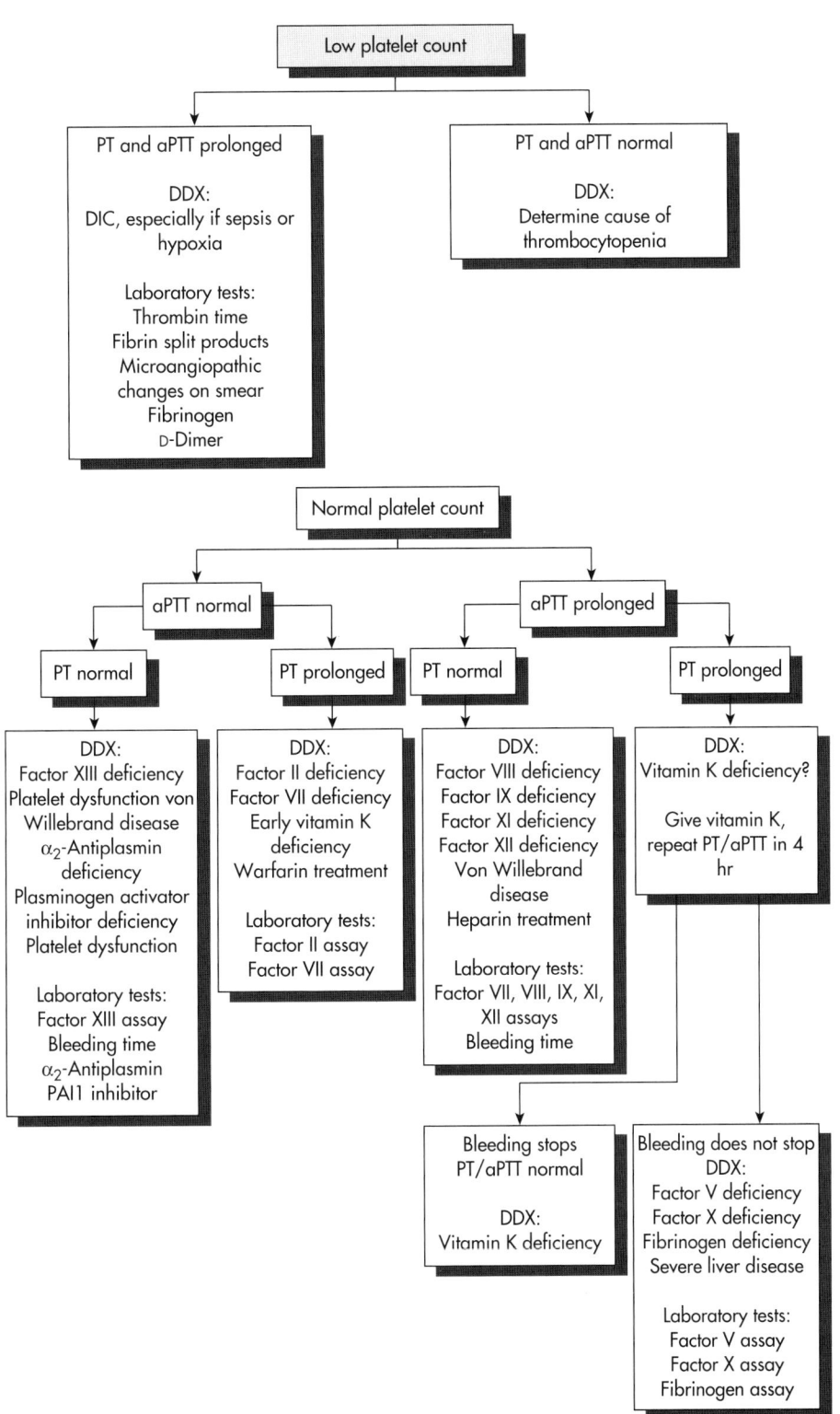

FIG. 35 Differential diagnosis *(DDx)* of bleeding disorders. *aPTT,* Activated partial thromboplastin time; *DIC,* disseminated intravascular coagulation; *PT,* prothrombin time. (From Hughes HK, Kahl LK: *The Harriet Lane handbook,* ed 21, St Louis, 2018, Mosby.)

Clinical
Algorithms

III

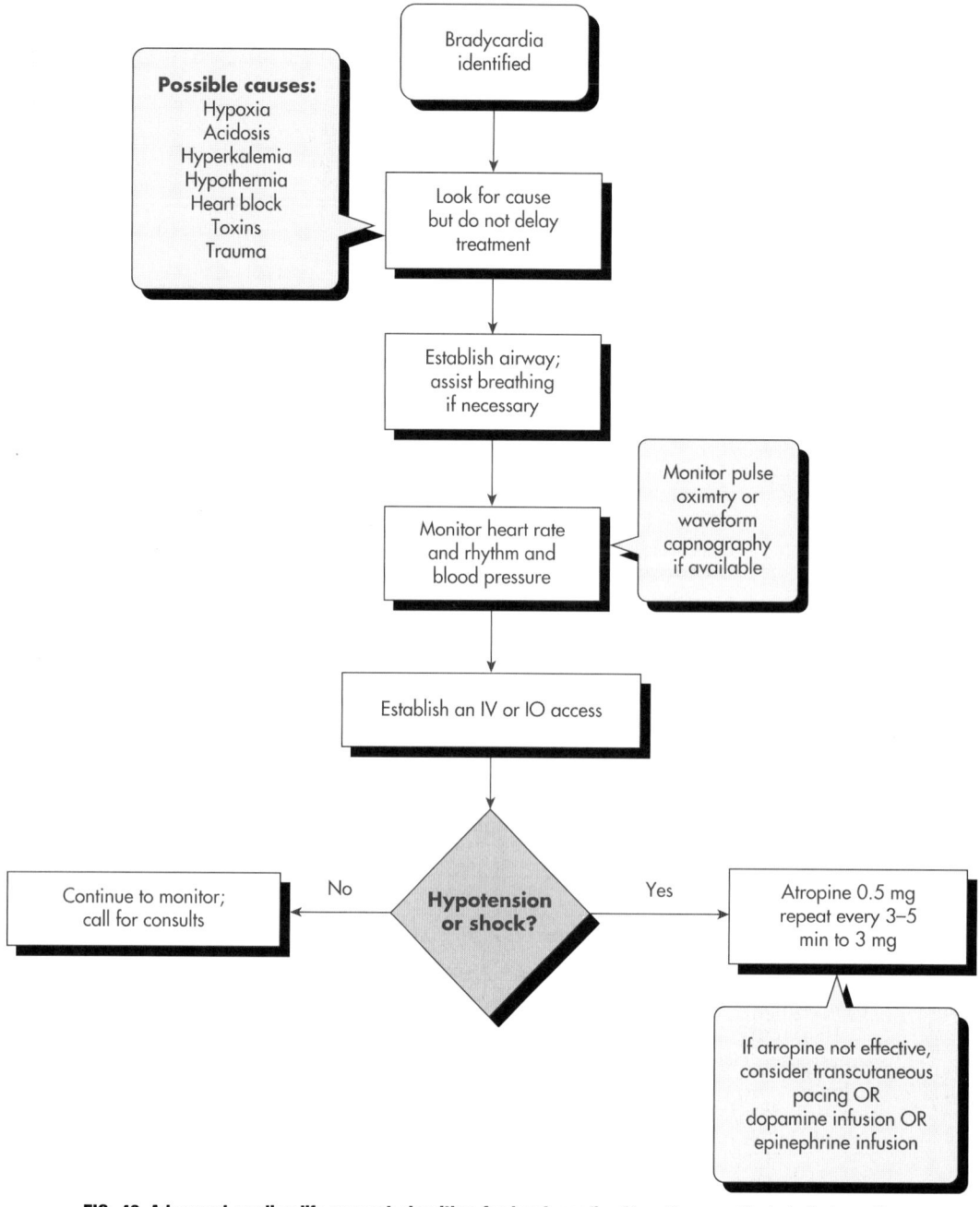

FIG. 40 Advanced cardiac life support algorithm for bradycardia. (From Newman M et al: *Perioperative medicine*, ed 2, Philadelphia, 2022, Elsevier.)

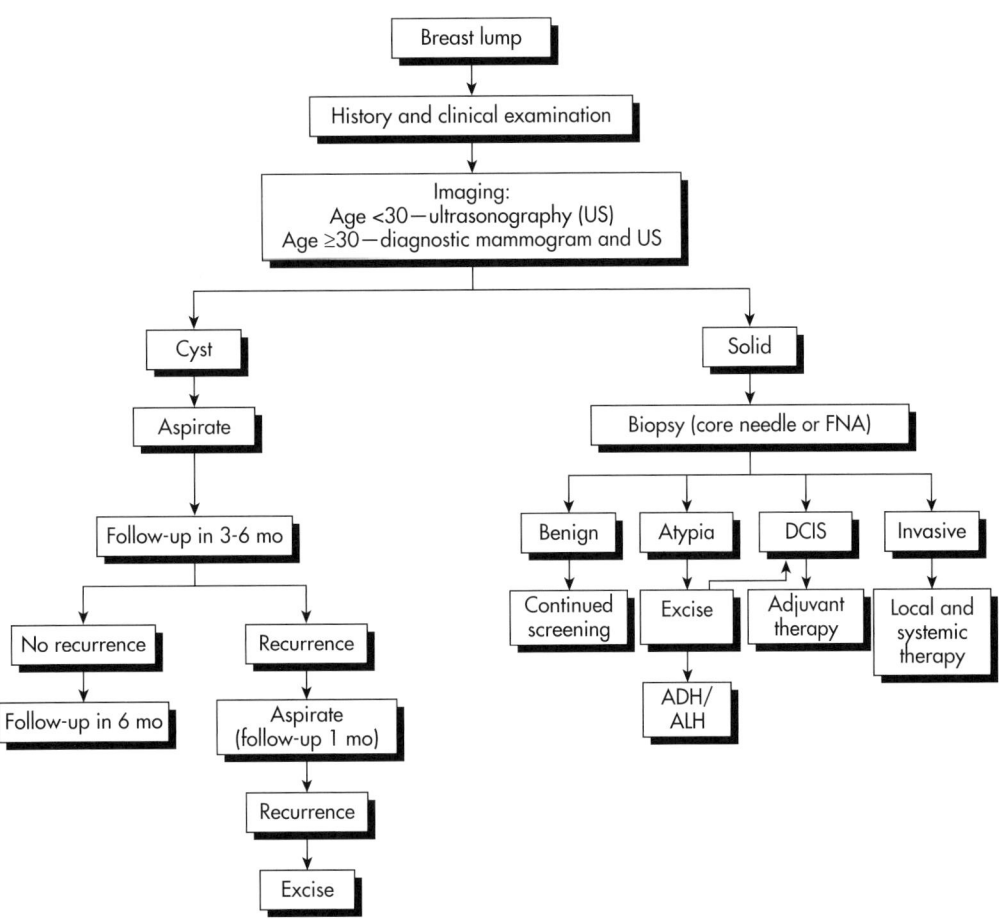

FIG. 41 Algorithm for breast lump management. *ADH,* Atypical ductal hyperplasia; *ALH,* atypical lobular hyperplasia; *DCIS,* ductal carcinoma in situ; *FNA,* fine-needle aspiration. (From Niederhuber JE: *Abeloff's clinical oncology,* ed 6, Philadelphia, 2020, Elsevier.)

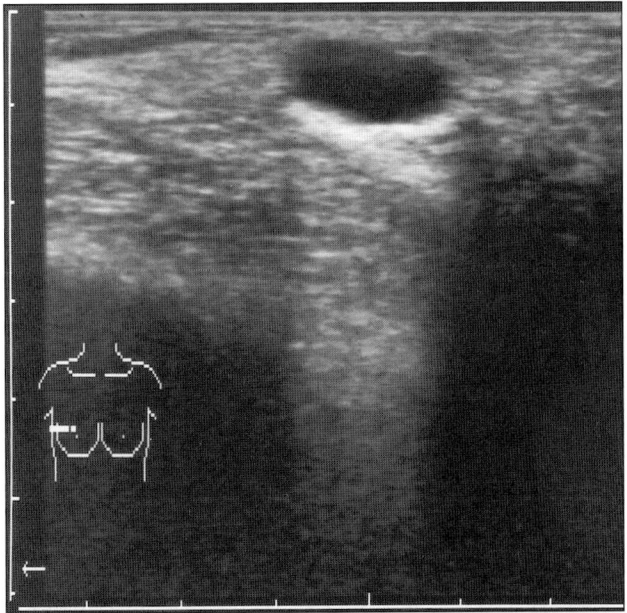

FIG. 42 Ultrasound image of the breast showing the palpable lump to be cystic. Cystic lesions have a characteristic hypoechoic pattern, with prominent acoustic shadowing. (From Niederhuber JE: *Abeloff's clinical oncology,* ed 6, Philadelphia, 2020, Elsevier.)

ICD-10CM #		
	I51.7	Cardiomegaly
	Q24.8	Other specified congenital malformations of heart
	I11.9	Hypertensive heart disease without heart failure
	I11.0	Hypertensive heart disease with heart failure
	Q23.8	Other congenital malformations of aortic and mitral valves

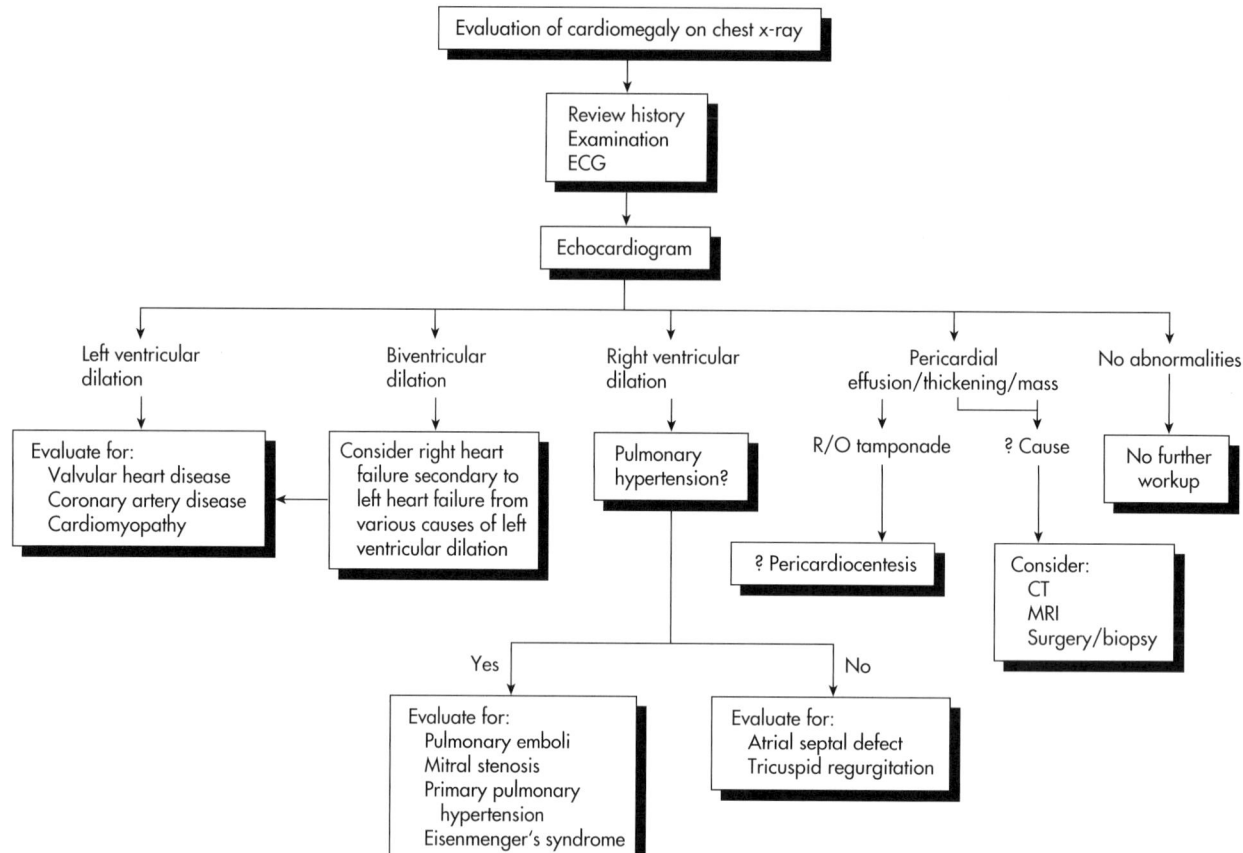

FIG. 47 Approach to the patient with cardiomegaly. When cardiomegaly is found on the chest radiograph, the history and physical examination should be reviewed and an electrocardiogram *(ECG)* performed before obtaining a two-dimensional Doppler echocardiographic study. Cardiomegaly may be explained by left ventricular dilation, biventricular dilation, right ventricular dilation, or pericardial abnormalities, or it may be found to be spurious on the echocardiogram. Rarely, isolated abnormalities of the atrium, particularly the left atrium, may cause abnormalities on the chest radiograph but will not cause true cardiomegaly. Depending on the echocardiographic findings, further tests can help elucidate the cause of echocardiographically confirmed cardiomegaly. *CT*, Computed tomography; *MRI*, magnetic resonance imaging; *R/O*, rule out. (From Goldman L, Braunwald E [eds]: *Primary cardiology,* ed 2, Philadelphia, 2003, Saunders.)

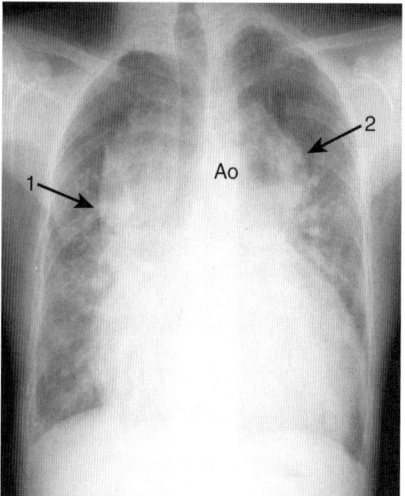

FIG. 48 "Snowman" heart in a 36-yr-old man with increasing shortness of breath. Posteroanterior chest film examination shows cardiomegaly and increased pulmonary blood flow. The superior mediastinum is widened, the result of dilation of the left vertical vein *(arrow 2)* and the right-sided superior vena cava *(arrow 1)*. The trachea is displaced by a normal left-sided aortic arch *(Ao)*. (From Boxt LM, Abbara S: *Cardiac imaging: the requisites,* ed 4, Philadelphia, 2016, Elsevier.)

CARDIOMEGALY ON CHEST X-RAY—cont'd

ICD-10CM #		
	I51.7	Cardiomegaly
	Q24.8	Other specified congenital malformations of heart
	I11.9	Hypertensive heart disease without heart failure
	I11.0	Hypertensive heart disease with heart failure
	Q23.8	Other congenital malformations of aortic and mitral valves

1709

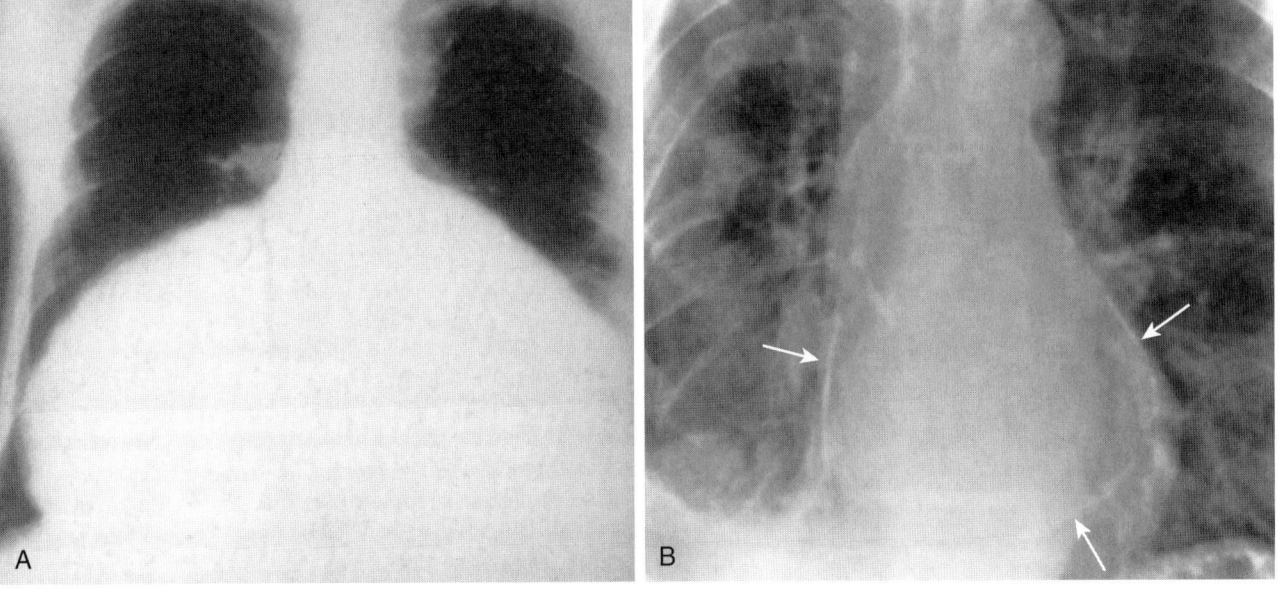

FIG. 49 Chest radiographs in a patient with a very large pericardial effusion. A, "Water bottle" sign. **B,** A patient with constrictive pericarditis and pericardial calcifications *(white arrows).* (From Vincent JL et al: *Textbook of critical care,* ed 7, Philadelphia, 2017, Elsevier.)

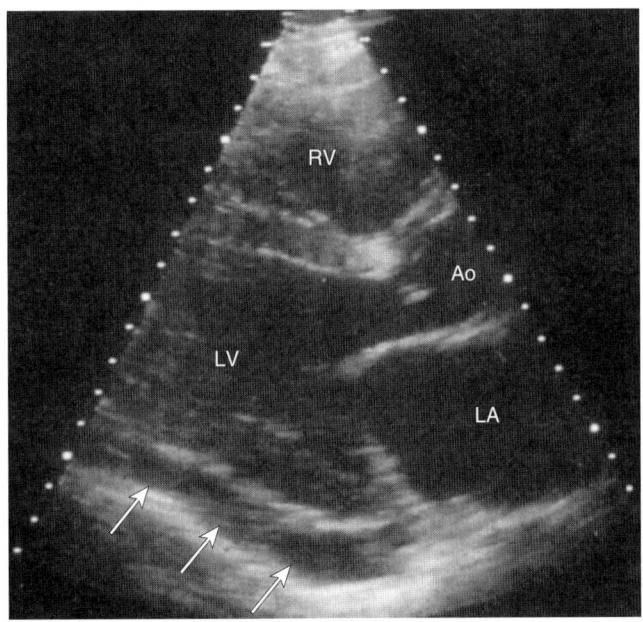

FIG. 50 Echocardiographic findings in a small to moderate pericardial effusion *(white arrows).* *Ao,* Aortic root; *LA,* left atrium; *LV,* left ventricle; *RV,* right ventricle. (From Vincent JL et al: *Textbook of critical care,* ed 7, Philadelphia, 2017, Elsevier.)

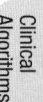

Clinical
Algorithms

III

ICD-10CM #   I51.7   Cardiomegaly
             Q24.8   Other specified congenital malformations of heart
             I11.9   Hypertensive heart disease without heart failure
             I11.0   Hypertensive heart disease with heart failure
             Q23.8   Other congenital malformations of aortic and mitral valves

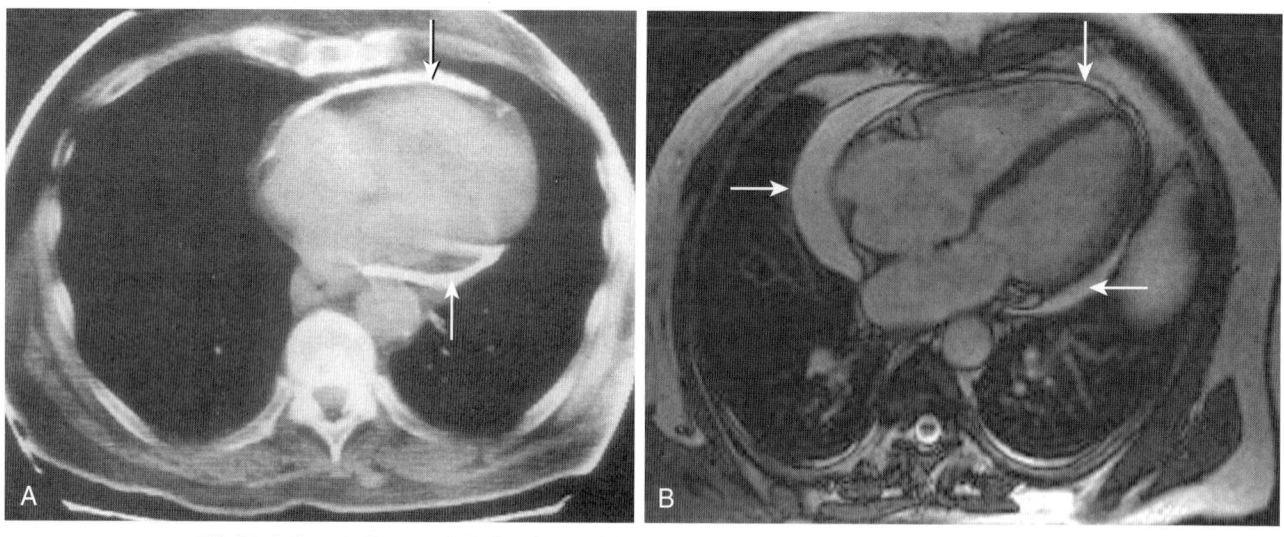

FIG. 51 A, Computed tomography findings in constrictive pericarditis. *White vertical arrows* are depicting thickened pericardium and pericardial calcification. **B,** The magnetic resonance imaging results of a patient with effusive-constrictive pericarditis are shown in the right image. *Horizontal arrows* show a loculated pericardial effusion, and the *vertical arrow* shows thickened pericardium. (From Vincent JL et al: *Textbook of critical care,* ed 7, Philadelphia, 2017, Elsevier.)

CARDIOMEGALY ON CHEST X-RAY—cont'd	ICD-10CM #	I51.7	Cardiomegaly	1711
		Q24.8	Other specified congenital malformations of heart	
		I11.9	Hypertensive heart disease without heart failure	
		I11.0	Hypertensive heart disease with heart failure	
		Q23.8	Other congenital malformations of aortic and mitral valves	

TABLE 24   Diagnosis of Cardiac Tamponade

Clinical presentation	Elevated systemic venous pressure,* hypotension,[†] pulsus paradoxus,[‡] tachycardia,[§] dyspnea, or tachypnea with clear lungs
Precipitating factors	Drugs (cyclosporine, anticoagulants, thrombolytics), recent cardiac surgery, indwelling instrumentation, blunt chest trauma, malignancies, connective tissue disease, renal failure, septicemia[‖]
ECG	Can be normal or nonspecifically changed (ST-T wave), electrical alternans (QRS, rarely T), bradycardia (end stage), electromechanical dissociation (agonal phase)
Chest radiograph	Enlarged cardiac silhouette with clear lungs
M-mode/two-dimensional echocardiogram	Diastolic collapse of the anterior RV free wall,[¶] RA collapse, LA and rarely LV collapse, increased LV diastolic wall thickness "pseudohypertrophy," IVC dilation (no collapse in inspiration), "swinging heart"
Doppler	Tricuspid flow increases and mitral flow decreases during inspiration (reverse in expiration)
	Systolic and diastolic flows are reduced in systemic veins in expiration and reverse flow with atrial contraction is increased
M-mode color Doppler	Large respiratory fluctuations in mitral/tricuspid flows
Cardiac catheterization	Confirmation of the diagnosis and quantification of the hemodynamic compromise
	RA pressure is elevated (preserved systolic × descent and absent or diminished diastolic y descent)
	Intrapericardial pressure is also elevated and virtually identical to RA pressure (both pressures fall in inspiration)
	RV mid-diastolic pressure is elevated and equal to the RA and pericardial pressures (no dip-and-plateau configuration)
	Pulmonary artery diastolic pressure is slightly elevated and may correspond to the RV pressure
	Pulmonary capillary wedge pressure is also elevated and nearly equal to intrapericardial and right atrial pressure
	LV systolic and aortic pressures may be normal or reduced
	Documenting that pericardial aspiration is followed by hemodynamic improvement**
	Detection of coexisting hemodynamic abnormalities (LV failure, constriction, pulmonary hypertension)
	Detection of associated cardiovascular diseases (cardiomyopathy, coronary artery disease)
RV/LV angiography	Atrial collapse and small hyperactive ventricular chambers
Coronary angiography	Coronary compression in diastole

ECG, Electrocardiogram; *IVC,* inferior vena cava; *LA,* left atrium; *LV,* left ventricle; *QRS,* Q wave, R wave, S wave; *RA,* right atrium; *RV,* right ventricle.

*Jugular venous distention is less notable in hypovolemic patients or in "surgical tamponade." An inspiratory increase or lack of fall of pressure in the neck veins (Kussmaul sign), when verified by tamponade or after pericardial drainage, indicates effusive-constrictive disease.

[†]Heart rate is usually greater than 100 beats per min but may be lower in patients with hypothyroidism or uremia.

[‡]Pulsus paradoxus is defined as a drop in systolic blood pressure greater than 10 mm Hg during inspiration, while diastolic blood pressure remains unchanged. It is easily detected by simply feeling the pulse, which diminishes significantly during inspiration. Clinically significant pulsus paradoxus is apparent when the patient is breathing normally. When this sign is present only in deep inspiration, it should be interpreted with caution. The magnitude of pulsus paradoxus is evaluated by sphygmomanometry. If pulsus paradoxus is present, the first Korotkoff sound is not heard equally well throughout the respiratory cycle but only during expiration at a given blood pressure. The blood pressure cuff is therefore inflated above the patient's systolic pressure. Then it is slowly deflated, while the clinician observes the phase of respiration. During deflation, the first Korotkoff sound is intermittent. Correlation with the patient's respiratory cycle identifies a point at which the sound is audible during expiration but disappears when the patient breathes in. As the cuff pressure drops further, another point is reached when the first blood pressure sound is audible throughout the respiratory cycle. The difference in systolic pressure between these two points is the clinical measure of pulsus paradoxus. Pulsus paradoxus is absent in tamponade complicating an atrial septal defect and in patients with significant aortic regurgitation.

[§]Occasional patients are hypertensive, especially if they have preexisting hypertension.

[‖]Febrile tamponade may be misdiagnosed as septic shock.

[¶]Right ventricular collapse can be absent in elevated right ventricular pressure and right ventricular hypertrophy or in right ventricular infarction.

**If after drainage of the pericardial effusion, the intrapericardial pressure does not fall below atrial pressure, effusive-constrictive disease should be considered.

From Vincent JL et al: *Textbook of critical care,* ed 7, Philadelphia, 2017, Elsevier.

Clinical Algorithms

III

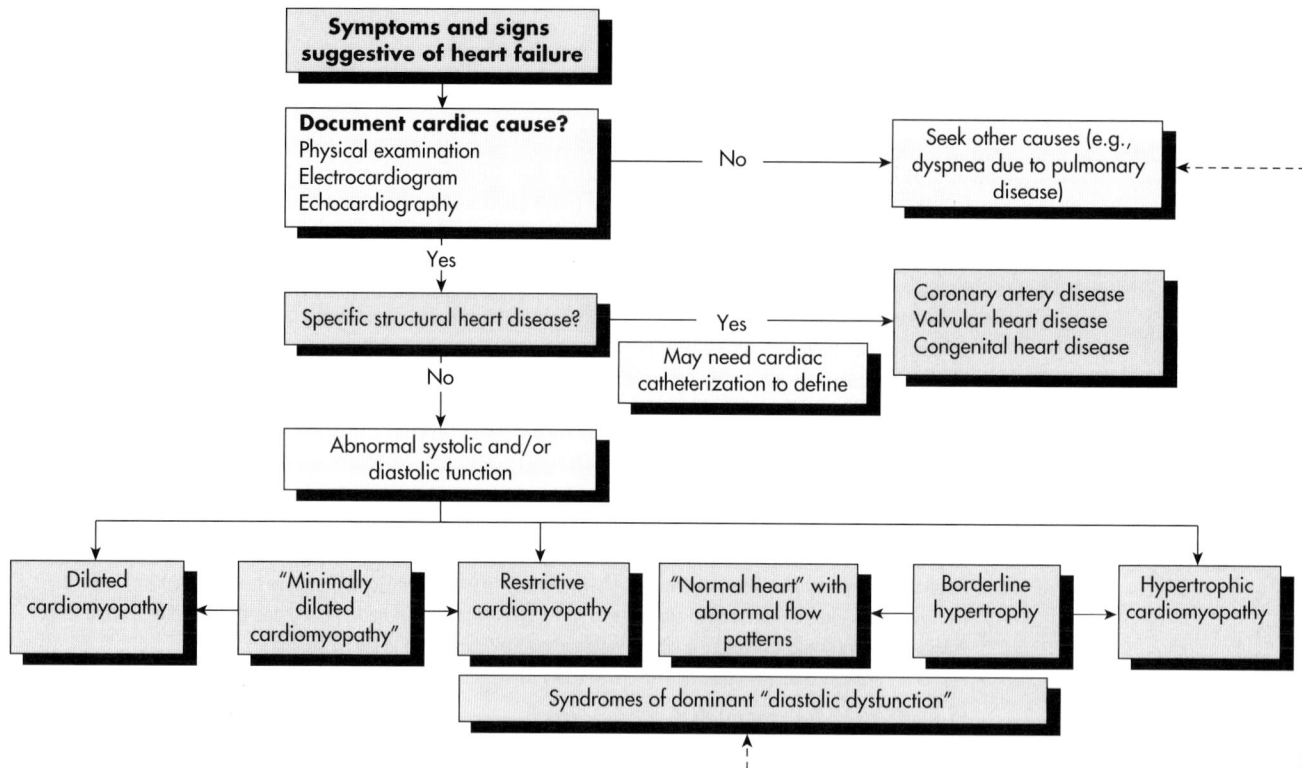

FIG. 52 Initial approach to classification of cardiomyopathy. The evaluation of symptoms or signs consistent with heart failure first includes confirmation that they can be attributed to a cardiac cause. Although this conclusion is often apparent from routine physical examination and electrocardiography, echocardiography serves to confirm cardiac disease and provides clues to the presence of other cardiac diseases, such as focal abnormalities suggesting primary valve disease or congenital heart disease. Having excluded these conditions, cardiomyopathy is generally considered to be dilated, restrictive, or hypertrophic, as shown in the figure. Patients with apparently normal cardiac structure and contraction are occasionally found to demonstrate abnormal intracardiac flow patterns consistent with diastolic dysfunction but should also be evaluated carefully for other causes of their symptoms. Most patients with so-called diastolic dysfunction also demonstrate at least borderline criteria for left ventricular hypertrophy, frequently in the setting of chronic hypertension and diabetes. A moderately decreased ejection fraction without marked dilation or a pattern of restrictive cardiomyopathy is sometimes referred to as minimally dilated cardiomyopathy, which may represent either a distinct entity or a transition between acute and chronic disease. (From Goldman L, Schafer AI: *Goldman Cecil medicine,* ed 25, Philadelphia, 2016, Saunders.)

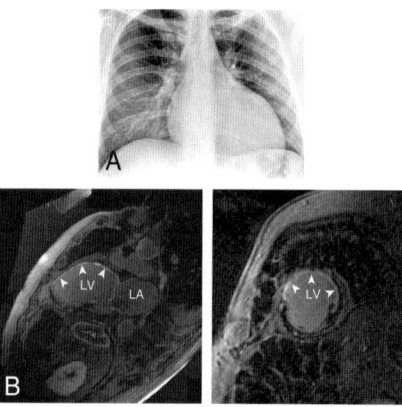

FIG. 53 Dilated cardiomyopathy. A, The heart shows enlargement of all four chambers. The azygos vein and superior vena cava are slightly dilated, reflecting high central venous pressure. **B,** Delayed enhanced magnetic resonance images demonstrate ischemic dilated cardiomyopathy. Extensive subendocardial delayed hyper-enhancement *(arrowheads)* demonstrates features of old myocardial infarction—it follows a vascular territory (the left anterior descending), it is based on the subendocardium, and there is thinning of the affected myocardium. *LA,* Left atrium; *LV,* left ventricle. (Boxt LM, Abbara S: *Cardiac imaging: the requisites,* ed 4, Philadelphia, 2016, Elsevier.)

TABLE 25 Classification of the Cardiomyopathies by Phenome and Genome

	PHENOME			GENOME		
Type	Morphology	Physiology	Pathology	Systemic Conditions or Diseases, Clinically Relevant Features, Classic Risk Factors, Associations	Nonsyndromic, Usually Single Gene	Syndromic
Dilated (DCM)	LV/RV dilation with minimal or no wall thickening	Reduced contractility is the primary defect; variable degree of diastolic dysfunction	Myocyte hypertrophy; scattered fibrosis	Hypertension; alcohol use; thyrotoxicosis, myxedema; persistent tachycardia; toxins, e.g., chemotherapy, especially anthracyclines; radiation; pregnancy	Diverse gene ontology with >30 genes implicated	Diverse array of associated conditions, especially muscular dystrophies (MDs): Emery-Dreifuss MD, limb-girdle MD, Duchenne/Becker MD; Laing distal myopathy; Barth syndrome; Kearns-Sayre; others
Restrictive (RCM)	Usually normal chamber sizes; minimal wall thickening	Contractility normal or near-normal with a marked increase in end-diastolic filling pressure	Specific to type, diagnosis: Amyloid, iron, glycogen storage disease, others	Endomyocardial fibrosis, amyloid, sarcoid, scleroderma, Churg-Strauss syndrome, cystinosis, lymphoma, pseudoxanthoma elasticum, hypereosinophilic syndrome, carcinoid	If not associated with a systemic genetic disease (e.g., hemochromatosis), genetic cause found most commonly to result from sarcomeric gene mutations	Gaucher disease, hemochromatosis, Fabry disease, familial amyloidosis. Mucopolysaccharidoses, Noonan syndrome
Hypertrophic (HCM)	Usually normal or reduced internal chamber dimension; wall thickening pronounced, especially septal hypertrophy	Systolic function increased or normal	Myocyte hypertrophy, classically with disarray	Severe hypertension can confound clinical, morphologic diagnosis	Mutations of genes encoding sarcomeric proteins	Noonan/Leopard, Danon, Fabry, WPW, Friedrich ataxia, MERRF, MELAS
Arrhythmogenic cardiomyopathy (ACM)	Scattered fibrofatty infiltration, classically of the right ventricle but also commonly involving the left ventricle; RV dilation, LV dilation, or both are common although not universal	Ventricular arrhythmias (VT, VF) early or late, reduced contractility with progressive disease; can mimic DCM	Islands of fatty replacement; fibrosis	Palmoplantar keratoderma, wooly hair in Naxos syndrome	Mutations of genes encoding proteins of the desmosome	Naxos syndrome
Left ventricular noncompaction (LVNC)	Ratio of noncompacted to compacted myocardium increased; normal chamber dimensions varying to a DCM phenotype	Normal to reduced systolic function	Myocardium normal and ranging to findings consistent with other coexisting cardiomyopathy	Phenotype has been observed in the setting of other types of cardiomyopathy	Various cardiomyopathy genes associated but uncertain whether genetic cause or developmental defect during organogenesis; see text	
Infiltrative	Usually thickened walls; occasional dilation	Restrictive physiology; systolic function usually mildly reduced	Specific to type, diagnosis: Amyloid, iron, glycogen storage disease, others		See "RCM" above	See "RCM" above
Inflammatory	Normal or dilated without hypertrophy	Reduced systolic function	Inflammatory infiltrates	Hypereosinophilic syndrome (see text), acute myocarditis		
Ischemic	Normal or dilated without hypertrophy	Reduced systolic function	Areas of infarcted myocardium	Hypercholesterolemia, hypertension, diabetes, cigarette smoking, family history	Familial hypercholesterolemia; other heritable lipid disorders	Familial hypercholesterolemia
Infectious	Normal or dilated without hypertrophy	Reduced systolic function		Specific to infection	Viral (especially acute myocarditis); protozoal (e.g., Chagas); bacterial, direct infection (e.g., Lyme disease), or from acute cellular toxicity as a result of systemic toxins (Streptococcus, gram-negatives, etc.)	Genetic predisposition to infection and/or variable response to infective agent

LV, Left ventricle; *MELAS,* mitochondrial encephalopathy, lactic acidosis, and stroke-like symptoms; *MERRF,* myoclonic epilepsy associated with ragged red fibers; *RV,* right ventricle; *VF,* ventricular fibrillation; *VT,* ventricular tachycardia; *WPW,* Wolff-Parkinson-White syndrome.
From Mann DL et al: *Braunwald's heart disease,* ed 10, Philadelphia, 2015, Elsevier.

Clinical Algorithms

III

ICD-10CM #   R07.4   Pain(s) chest
R07.2   Pain(s) heart
R07.3   Pain(s) chest anterior wall

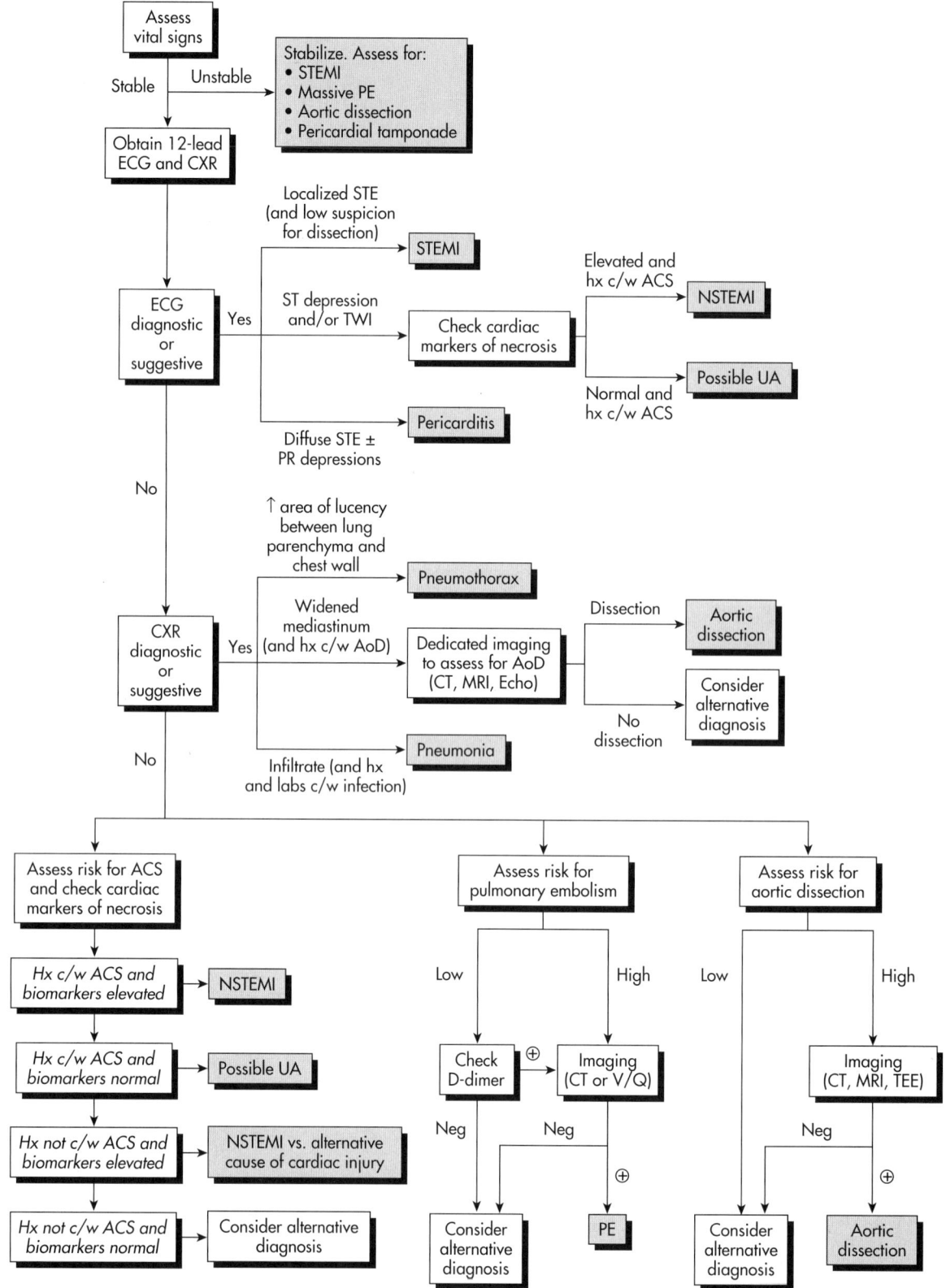

FIG. 55 Algorithm for the initial diagnostic approach to a patient with chest pain. *ACS*, Acute coronary syndrome; *AoD*, aortic dissection; *c/w*, consistent with; *CT*, computed tomography; *CXR*, chest x-ray film; *ECG*, electrocardiogram; *Echo*, echocardiography; *hx*, history; *MRI*, magnetic resonance imaging; *NSTEMI*, non–ST-segment elevation myocardial infarction; *PE*, pulmonary embolism; *STE*, ST-segment elevation; *STEMI*, ST-segment elevation myocardial infarction; *TEE*, transesophageal echocardiography; *UA*, unstable angina; *TWI*, T wave inversion; *V/Q*, ventilation-perfusion scan. (From Zipes DP: *Braunwald's heart disease, a textbook of cardiovascular medicine,* ed 11, Philadelphia, 2019, Elsevier.)

CHEST PAIN—cont'd

ICD-10CM # R07.4 Pain(s) chest
R07.2 Pain(s) heart
R07.3 Pain(s) chest anterior wall

1715

TABLE 26 Differential Diagnosis of Chest Pain in Adults

Diagnosis	Pain	Characteristics	ECG	CXR	Associated Features
Angina pectoris	Substernal, constricting	Transient, effort-related	Local ST depression; occasional elevation	Normal	Relief with NTG
MI	Substernal, crushing	Persistent, severe	Local ST elevation or depression	Possible vascular congestion or cardiomegaly	Relief with opiates; possible hypotension; ↑ troponin
Pulmonary embolism	Pleuritic	Sudden onset with dyspnea	Nonspecific; occasional RV strain	Normal or opacities ± small pleural effusion	Risk factor(s) for venous thrombosis
Pulmonary hypertension	Gradual onset	Associated with dyspnea, fatigue, and edema	Tall right precordial R waves, right axis deviation, RV strain	Prominent pulmonary arteries	Exclude pulmonary thromboembolism and interstitial lung disease
Bacterial pneumonia	Pleuritic	Onset in minutes to hours	Normal	Consolidation	Fever, productive cough
Pneumothorax	Sharp, unilateral	Sudden onset with dyspnea	Normal	Collapsed lung	Asthenic habitus, recurrence
Pericarditis	Pleuritic	Either side; gradual onset; pain referred to trapezius	Generalized ST elevation	Possible enlarged silhouette	Friction rub
Aortic dissection	Substernal, severe	Radiation to the back	Nonspecific; LVH or inferior MI	Widened mediastinum	Prostration, loss of pulse, aortic insufficiency
Esophageal spasm/reflux	Substernal	May mimic angina; burning	Normal or ST-T changes	Normal	Relief with NTG or antacids
Costochondritis	Dull-achy, localized	↑ by cough or deep breath	Normal	Normal	Localized tenderness
Mediastinitis	Interscapular, upper back, can be pleuritic	Severe	Normal	Widened mediastinum, mediastinal emphysema	Associated with fever, odynophagia
Herpes zoster	Sharp, unilateral	Dysesthesia	Normal	Normal	Vesicular rash

CXR, Chest radiograph; *ECG,* electrocardiography; *LVH,* left ventricular hypertrophy; *MI,* myocardial infarction; *NTG,* nitroglycerin; *RV,* right ventricular.
From Broaddus VC et al: *Murray & Nadel's textbook of respiratory medicine,* ed 7, Philadelphia, 2022, Elsevier.

Clinical Algorithms

III

TABLE 27 Differential Diagnosis of Pediatric Chest Pain

COMMON	UNCOMMON/RARE
Musculoskeletal	Cardiac
Costochondritis	Ischemia (coronary artery abnormalities, severe AS or PS, HOCM, cocaine)
Trauma or muscle overuse/strain	Infection/inflammation (myocarditis, pericarditis, Kawasaki disease)
Pulmonary	Dysrhythmia
Asthma (often exercise induced)	Musculoskeletal
Severe cough	Abnormalities of rib cage/thoracic spine
Pneumonia	Tietze syndrome
Gastrointestinal	Slipping rib
Reflux esophagitis	Tumor
Psychogenic	Pulmonary
Anxiety, hyperventilation	Pleurisy
Miscellaneous	Pneumothorax, pneumomediastinum
Precordial catch syndrome (Texidor twinge)	Pleural effusion
Sickle cell vasoocclusive crisis	Pulmonary embolism
Idiopathic	Gastrointestinal
	Esophageal foreign body
	Esophageal spasm
	Psychogenic
	Conversion symptoms
	Somatization disorders
	Depression

AS, Aortic stenosis; *HOCM,* hypertrophic obstructive cardiomyopathy; *PS,* pulmonary stenosis.
From Marcdante KJ et al: *Nelson essentials of pediatrics,* ed 9, Philadelphia, 2023, Elsevier.

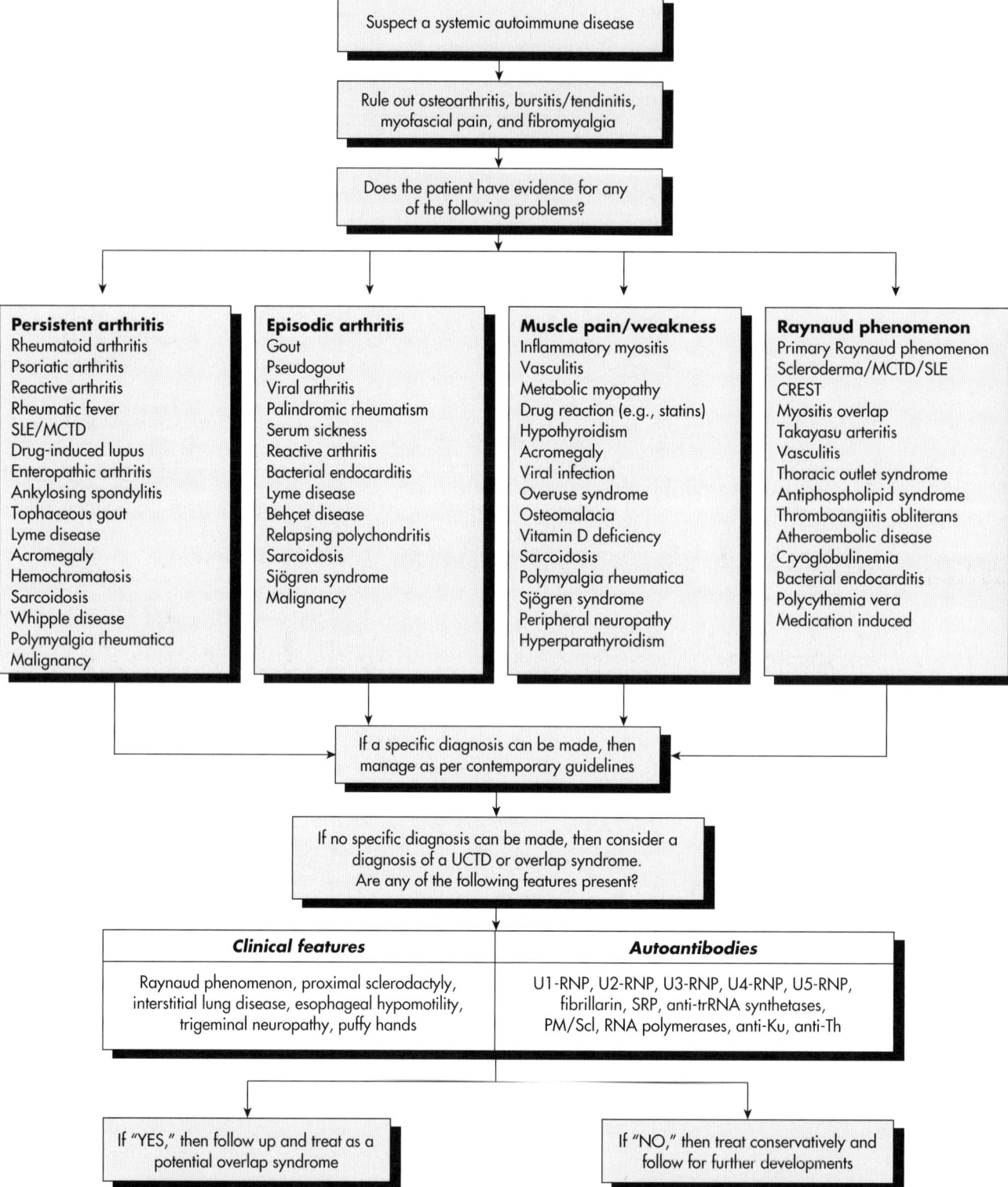

FIG. 56 Algorithm for evaluating patients with undifferentiated connective tissue disease (UCTD). *CREST,* Calcinosis, Raynaud phenomenon, esophageal dysmotility, sclerodactyly, and telangiectasia; *MCTD,* mixed connective tissue disease; *PM/Scl,* polymyositis/scleroderma; *RNA,* ribonucleic acid; *SLE,* systemic lupus erythematosus; *SRP,* signal recognition particle; *trRNA,* transfer ribonucleic acid; *UCTD,* undifferentiated connective tissue disease. (From Firestein GS et al: *Kelley and Firestein's textbook of rheumatology,* ed 10, Philadelphia, 2017, Elsevier.)

CONNECTIVE TISSUE LABORATORY SCREENING TESTS

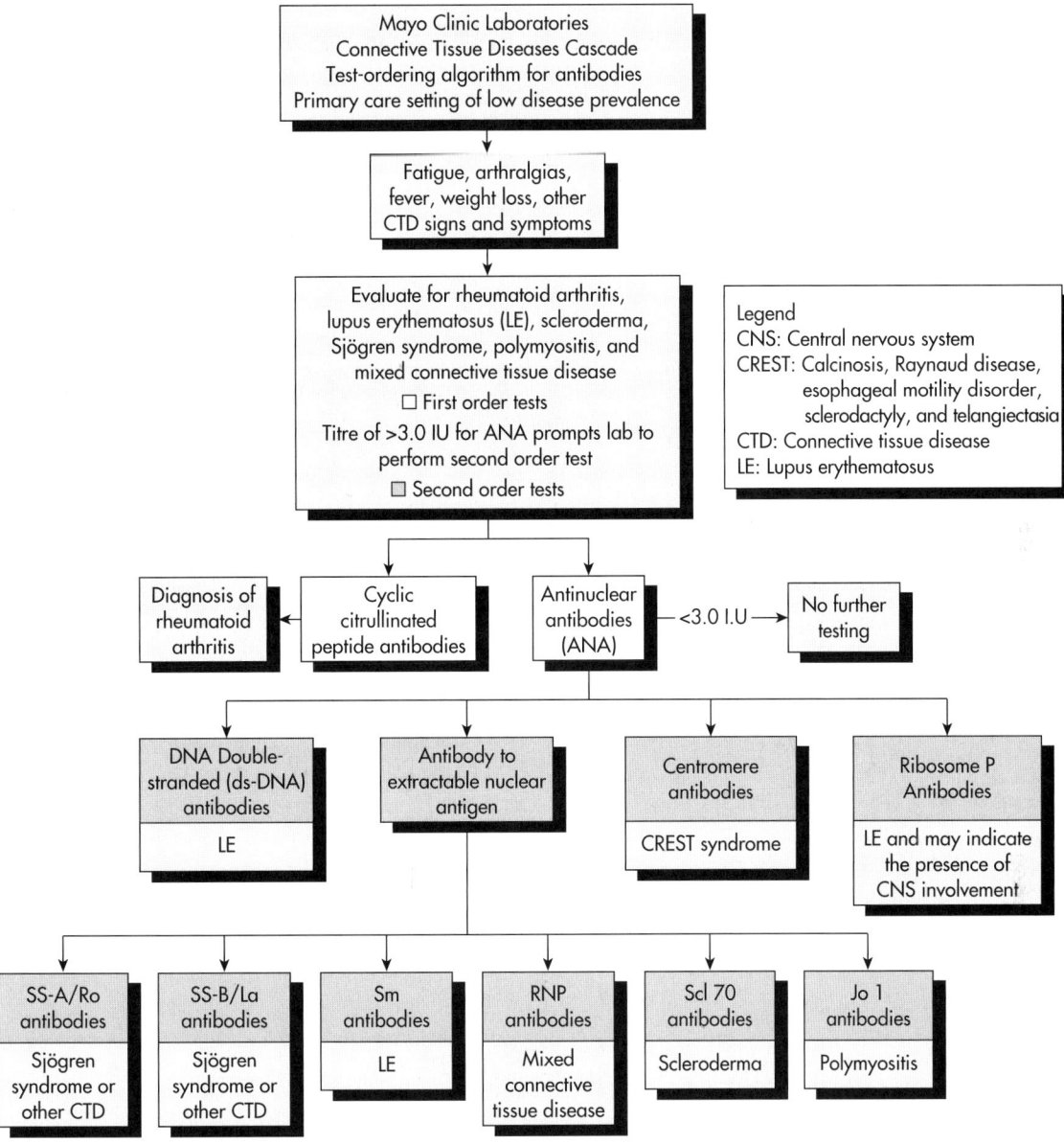

FIG. 57 **Subacute cutaneous lupus erythematosus.** Papulosquamous pattern. Lesions are confined to exposed areas on the upper half of the body. *DNA*, Deoxyribonucleic acid; *RNP*, ribonucleoprotein. (From Habif TP: *Clinical dermatology, a color guide to diagnosis and therapy*, ed 6, Philadelphia, 2016, Elsevier.)

Clinical Algorithms

III

TABLE 28   Autoantibody Tests for Connective Tissue Diseases

Antibody	Clinical Significance
Antinuclear antibodies	Screening for SLE and PSS
Centromere antibodies	Marker for CREST
Histone antibodies	To exclude drug-induced LE
ENA: Sm antibodies	Marker for SLE
RNP antibodies	SLE, MCTD, scleroderma
SS-A (Ro)/SS-B (La) antibodies	SLE, Sjögren syndrome, SCLE, and others
Scl-70 antibodies	Marker for scleroderma
Jo-1 antibodies	Marker for polymyositis
Ku (Ki) antibodies	Polymyositis/scleroderma overlap, SLE
Phospholipid antibodies (lupus anticoagulant)	Marker for SLE subset with thrombosis: Frequent aborters

CREST, Calcinosis, Raynaud phenomenon, esophageal dysmotility, sclerodactyly, and telangiectasia; ENA, extractable nuclear antigen; LE, lupus erythematosus; MCTD, mixed connective tissue disease; PSS, progressive systemic sclerosis; RNP, ribonucleoprotein; SCLE, subacute cutaneous lupus erythematosus; SLE, systemic lupus erythematosus.
From Habif TP: Clinical dermatology, a color guide to diagnosis and therapy, ed 6, Philadelphia, 2016, Elsevier.

TABLE 29   Diagnostic Significance of Immunologic Findings in Serum and Skin Biopsies in Connective Tissue Diseases

Disease	Biopsy Findings: Direct Immunofluorescence	Serum Findings	Relevance
Systemic LE	LE band (granular immune deposits, IgG, and/or IgM) IgA, C3 at DEJ in lesional and/or normal skin (over 90% in sun-exposed skin)	ANA elevated titers (about 95%-99%); nDNA antibodies about 50%-75%; DNP antibodies <50%; Sm antibodies in about 20%; RNP antibodies in about 5%-30%; SS-A antibodies in about 30%-40%; SS-B antibodies in about 1%-15%; phospholipid antibodies in about 30%-50%; PCNA antibodies in about 2%-10%; Ku(Ki) antibodies in about 10%	DIF, ANA, and ENA usually diagnostic; nDNA and Sm antibodies are diagnostic markers
Discoid LE	LE band, mostly IgG and C in lesion ONLY	Essentially negative; ANA titers usually in normal range	LE band highly characteristic
Subacute, cutaneous LE	LE band in lesion	ANA positive in 70%; SS-A (Ro) antibodies positive in more than 60%	DIF and anti–SS-A (Ro) highly characteristic
Neonatal LE	LE band in lesion (about 50%)	ANA positive in 30%; antibodies to SS-A (Ro) in 100%; antibodies to SS-B (La) in about 60%	DIF and anti–SS-A (Ro) highly characteristic
Drug-induced LE	LE band in lesion (rare)	ANA positive in more than 90%; histone positive about 90%; other antibodies to nDNA and ENA negative	DIF and histone antibodies in absence of other nuclear antibodies highly characteristic
Mixed connective tissue disease	Nuclear IgG or LE band in normal and/or lesional epidermis	Speckled ANA antibodies in more than 95% and RNP antibodies in more than 90%	Serology and/or DIF of nuclei diagnostic for MCTD, SLE, or PSS
Sjögren syndrome	Negative	ANA positive in about 55%; antibodies to SS-A (Ro) in 43%-88%; SS-B (La) in 14%-60%; RF positive	Positive serum results support diagnosis
Progressive systemic sclerosis (scleroderma)	Nucleolar IgG in epidermis in few cases; most negative	ANA (about 85%) speckled or nucleolar; centromere antibody in CREST (70%-90%); Scl-70 antibodies in diffuse sclerosis (45%) and in acrosclerosis (15%-20%)	DIF limited value; centromere antibodies are diagnostic marker in CREST; Scl-70 antibodies are diagnostic marker in scleroderma
Polymyositis/dermatomyositis	Negative	ANA usually positive (more than 80%); Jo-1 antibodies in 30% PM, 10% DM; SS-A (Ro) antibodies in 55% PM/scleroderma overlap; Ku (Ki) antibodies in 10% PM/scleroderma overlap	Limited value, but positive serum results support diagnosis
Rheumatoid arthritis	Negative	ANA usually negative or low titer; RF positive in about 90%; RNA positive in about 70%-90% and 95% of RF-negative cases	Positive serum results support diagnosis

ANA, Antinuclear antibodies; CREST, calcinosis, Raynaud phenomenon, esophageal dysmotility, sclerodactyly, and telangiectasia; DEJ, dermal-epidermal junction; DIF, direct immunofluorescence; DM, dermatomyositis; DNP, deoxyribonucleoprotein protein; ENA, extractable nuclear antigen; Ig, immunoglobulin; LE, lupus erythematosus; MCTD, mixed connective tissue disease; nDNA, nuclear deoxyribonucleic acid; PCNA, proliferating cell nuclear antigen; PM, polymyositis; PSS, progressive systemic sclerosis; RF, rheumatoid factor; RNA, antibodies to rheumatoid arthritis-associated nuclear antigen; RNP, ribonucleoprotein; SLE, systemic lupus erythematosus.
From Habif TP: Clinical dermatology, a color guide to diagnosis and therapy, ed 6, Philadelphia, 2016, Elsevier.

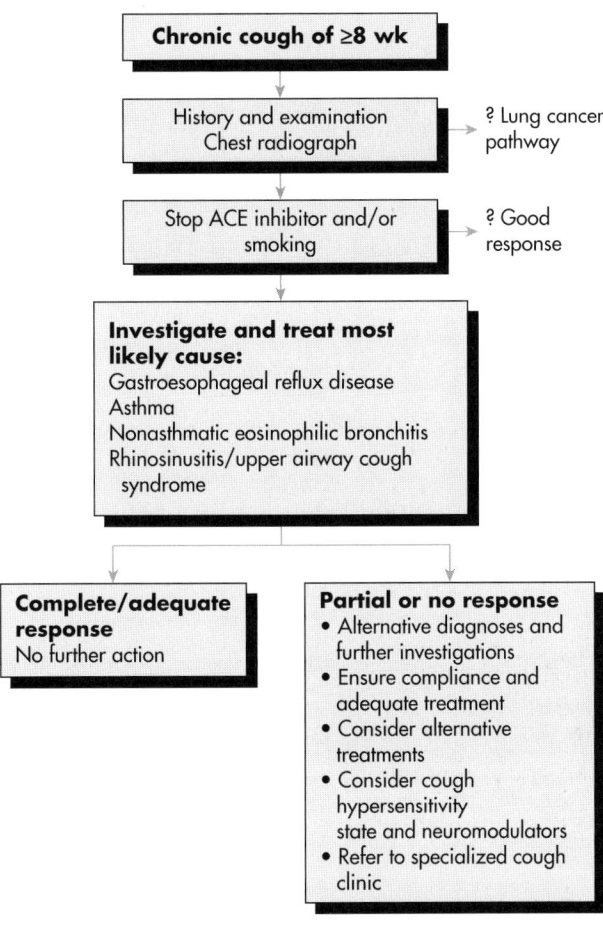

FIG. 59 Algorithm for the management of chronic cough in adult patients. For a chronic cough lasting for >8 wk, the evaluation and management should be methodical. After a thorough history and physical examination and chest imaging to exclude lung cancer or other intrathoracic pathology, and after stopping angiotensin-converting enzyme (ACE) inhibitor and/or smoking, the workup proceeds through the most common likely entities. These are listed as gastroesophageal reflux disease, asthma, nonasthmatic eosinophilic bronchitis and rhinosinusitis, or upper airway cough syndrome. Exclusion can be determined either by investigations or trial of therapy or both. Ultimately, patients with persistent chronic cough can be referred to specialized cough clinics for alternative diagnosis and treatment. (From Broaddus VC et al: *Murray & Nadel's textbook of respiratory medicine*, ed 7, Philadelphia, 2022, Elsevier.)

Clinical Algorithms

III

TABLE 30   Testing Characteristics of Diagnostic Protocol for Evaluation of Chronic Cough

Tests	Diagnosis	Positive Predictive Value (%)	Negative Predictive Value (%)
Sinus radiograph	Sinusitis	57-81	95-100
Methacholine inhalation challenge	Asthma	60-82	100
Modified barium esophagography	GERD, esophageal stricture	38-63	63-93
Esophageal pH*	GERD	89-100	>100
Bronchoscopy	Endobronchial mass/lesion	50-89	100

GERD, Gastroesophageal reflux disease.
*24-hr esophageal pH monitoring.
From Goldman L, Schafer AI (eds): *Goldman's Cecil medicine*, ed 24, Philadelphia, 2012, Saunders.

TABLE 31 Definitions and Common Causes of Cough in Adults and Children

Age Group	Type of Cough	Duration (wk)	Common Causes
Adults	Acute	<3	Common cold Exacerbation of lung disease (e.g., asthma) Acute environmental exposure Acute cardiopulmonary disease
	Subacute	3-8	Postinfectious cough Pertussis infection Exacerbation of underlying lung disease (e.g., asthma, COPD, bronchiectasis)
	Chronic	>8	ACEI therapy Smoking/chronic bronchitis Underlying lung disease UACS Asthma NAEB GERD
Children	Acute	<4	Common cold Exacerbation of underlying lung disease Acute cardiopulmonary disease
	Chronic	>4	Asthma Protracted bacterial bronchitis Tracheobronchomalacia Chronic rhinosinusitis Recurrent aspiration GERD Underlying lung disease (e.g., bronchiectasis) Pulmonary infections (e.g., pertussis)

ACEI, Angiotensin-converting enzyme inhibitor; *COPD,* chronic obstructive pulmonary disease; *GERD,* gastroesophageal reflux disease; *NAEB,* nonasthmatic eosinophilic bronchitis; *UACS,* upper airway cough syndrome.
From Adkinson NF et al: *Middleton's allergy principles and practice,* ed 8, Philadelphia, 2014, Saunders.

TABLE 32 Common Causes of Cough

Acute Infections
Tracheobronchitis
Bronchopneumonia
Viral pneumonia
Acute-on-chronic bronchitis
Pertussis
Chronic infections
Bronchiectasis
Tuberculosis
Cystic fibrosis

Airway Diseases
Asthma
Eosinophilic bronchitis
Cough-variant asthma
Chronic bronchitis
COPD
Chronic postnasal drip
Parenchymal Diseases
Interstitial pulmonary fibrosis
Emphysema
Sarcoidosis

Tumors
Lung cancer
Benign airway tumors
Mediastinal tumors
Aspirated Foreign Bodies
Middle ear pathology
Cardiovascular Diseases
Left ventricular failure
Pulmonary infarction
Aortic aneurysm
Other Diseases
Gastroesophageal reflux disease
Laryngopharyngeal reflux
Recurrent microaspiration
Endobronchial sutures
Obstructive sleep apnea
Laryngeal dysfunction
Drugs
Angiotensin-converting enzyme inhibitors

From Broaddus VC et al: *Murray & Nadel's textbook of respiratory medicine,* ed 7, Philadelphia, 2022, Elsevier.

TABLE 33   Diagnostic Evaluation of Chronic Cough

- History and physical examination.
- Chest radiograph, particularly in smokers.
- Initial evaluation may lead to diagnosis of chronic bronchitis in cigarette smokers and of angiotensin-converting enzyme inhibitor cough. Discontinue cigarette smoking and offending drug.
- Further diagnostic evaluation on basis of initial evaluation:
  1. If suggestive of postnasal drip, order a computed tomography (CT) scan of sinuses, and allergy tests.
  2. If suggestive of asthma, request a record of peak expiratory flow measurements at home for 2 wk and a bronchoprovocation test with histamine or methacholine, and/or a trial of antiasthma treatment.
  3. If suggestive of gastroesophageal reflux disease, request 24-h pH monitoring and, if necessary, an endoscopic examination of the esophagus or a barium swallow series.
  4. If the chest radiograph is abnormal, consider examination of sputum and a fiberoptic bronchoscopy. A high-resolution CT scan of the thorax and further lung function evaluation may be necessary.
- Treat specifically for associated conditions. The cause(s) of cough is (are) determined when specific therapies eliminate or improve the cough. There may be more than one associated cause for the cough.

From Broaddus VC et al: *Murray & Nadel's textbook of respiratory medicine*, ed 7, Philadelphia, 2022, Elsevier.

TABLE 34   Potential Complications From Excessive Cough

Respiratory
Pneumothorax
Subcutaneous emphysema
Pneumomediastinum
Pneumoperitoneum
Laryngeal damage

Cardiovascular
Cardiac dysrhythmias
Loss of consciousness

Central Nervous System
Syncope
Headaches
Cerebral air embolism

Musculoskeletal
Intercostal muscle pain
Rupture of rectus abdominis muscle
Increase in serum creatine phosphokinase
Cervical disc prolapse

Gastrointestinal
Esophageal perforation
Other
Social embarrassment
Depression
Sleep disruption
Urinary incontinence
Disruption of surgical wounds
Subconjunctival hemorrhage
Petechiae
Purpura

From Broaddus VC et al: *Murray & Nadel's textbook of respiratory medicine*, ed 7, Philadelphia 2022, Elsevier.

TABLE 35   Treatments for Chronic Cough

Treating the Specific Underlying Cause(s)

Asthma, cough-variant asthma	Bronchodilators and inhaled corticosteroids
Eosinophilic bronchitis	Inhaled corticosteroids; leukotriene inhibitors
Allergic rhinitis and postnasal drip	Topical nasal steroids and antihistamines
	Topical nasal anticholinergics (with antibiotics, if indicated)
Gastroesophageal reflux	Conservative measures
	Histamine H_2-antagonist or proton pump inhibitor
Angiotensin-converting enzyme inhibitor	Discontinue and replace with alternative drug such as angiotensin II receptor antagonist
Chronic bronchitis/COPD	Smoking cessation
	Treat for COPD
Bronchiectasis	Postural drainage
	Treat infective exacerbation and airflow obstruction
Infective tracheobronchitis	Appropriate antibiotic therapy
	Treat any postnasal drip

Symptomatic Antitussive Treatment: Neuromodulators (Only After Consideration of Cause of Cough)

Chronic cough (all)	Speech and language therapy
Chronic cough affecting quality of life	Amitriptyline
	Gabapentin
Chronic refractory cough	Slow-release morphine

From Broaddus VC et al: *Murray & Nadel's textbook of respiratory medicine*, ed 7, Philadelphia, 2022, Elsevier.

BOX 17 Pitfalls and Errors in the Diagnosis and Management of Chronic Cough in Adults

General Considerations
- Failing to consider that UACS, asthma/NAEB, and/or GERD are likely when the chest radiograph is normal or near-normal in appearance and the patient is a nonsmoker and is not taking an ACEI
- Failing to include UACS, asthma/NAEB, and/or GERD in the differential diagnosis because clinical or radiographic evidence confirms the presence of an "obvious" cause of the patient's cough (e.g., solitary pulmonary nodule, idiopathic pulmonary fibrosis)
- Not recognizing multiple simultaneous causes of cough
- Failing to continue treatment trials long enough to accurately assess their effectiveness
- Prematurely diagnosing "unexplained" cough before a bronchoscopy has been performed to assess for unsuspected airway disease
- Mistakenly diagnosing "unexplained" cough or diagnosing psychogenic cough before a complete evaluation for cough has been performed

Upper Airway Cough Syndrome
- Failing to realize that UACS can manifest as cough productive of phlegm
- Not recognizing that chronic cough can be the sole manifestation of UACS in at least 20% of the cases
- Failing to consider sinusitis as a cause of UACS
- Mistakenly assuming that selective histamine H_1 receptor antagonists are effective in treating nonallergic causes of UACS
- Missing allergic rhinitis because symptoms are perennial
- Missing aspirin-exacerbated disease in a patient with nasal polyps

Asthma/NAEB
- Failing to realize that these conditions can sometimes manifest as cough productive of phlegm
- Not recognizing that chronic cough can sometimes be the sole manifestation of asthma (so-called cough variant asthma)
- Mistakenly assuming that a positive result on bronchial challenge (e.g., methacholine challenge) is diagnostic of asthma when it is merely *consistent* with the diagnosis
- Failing to consider NAEB when the bronchial challenge test yields a negative result
- Not recognizing that inhaled medications can sometimes provoke cough
- Failing to consider occupational and environmental causes of asthma/NAEB

Gastroesophageal Reflux Disease
- Failing to realize that GERD can sometimes manifest as cough productive of phlegm
- Not recognizing that chronic cough can sometimes be the sole manifestation of GERD (so-called silent GERD)
- Mistakenly concluding that cough cannot be due to GERD simply because cough does not resolve with relief of gastrointestinal symptoms
- Not considering nonacid reflux and mistakenly assuming that cough will always respond to acid suppression
- Failing to assess the adequacy of GERD treatment by using 24-h monitoring of esophageal pH and impedance
- Not recognizing coexisting diseases (e.g., sleep apnea) and medications (e.g., nitrates, progesterone) that may impair the effectiveness of GERD treatment
- Failing to recognize that surgery may help when intensive medical therapy has failed

Angiotensin-Converting Enzyme Inhibitor
- Failing to consider ACEI therapy as a cause of chronic cough simply because the cough predated initiation of the ACEI
- Mistakenly concluding that ACEI therapy is not the cause of chronic cough because the cough did not resolve within 1-3 wk of stopping the ACEI

From Adkinson NF et al: *Middleton's allergy principles and practice*, ed 8, Philadelphia, 2014, Saunders.

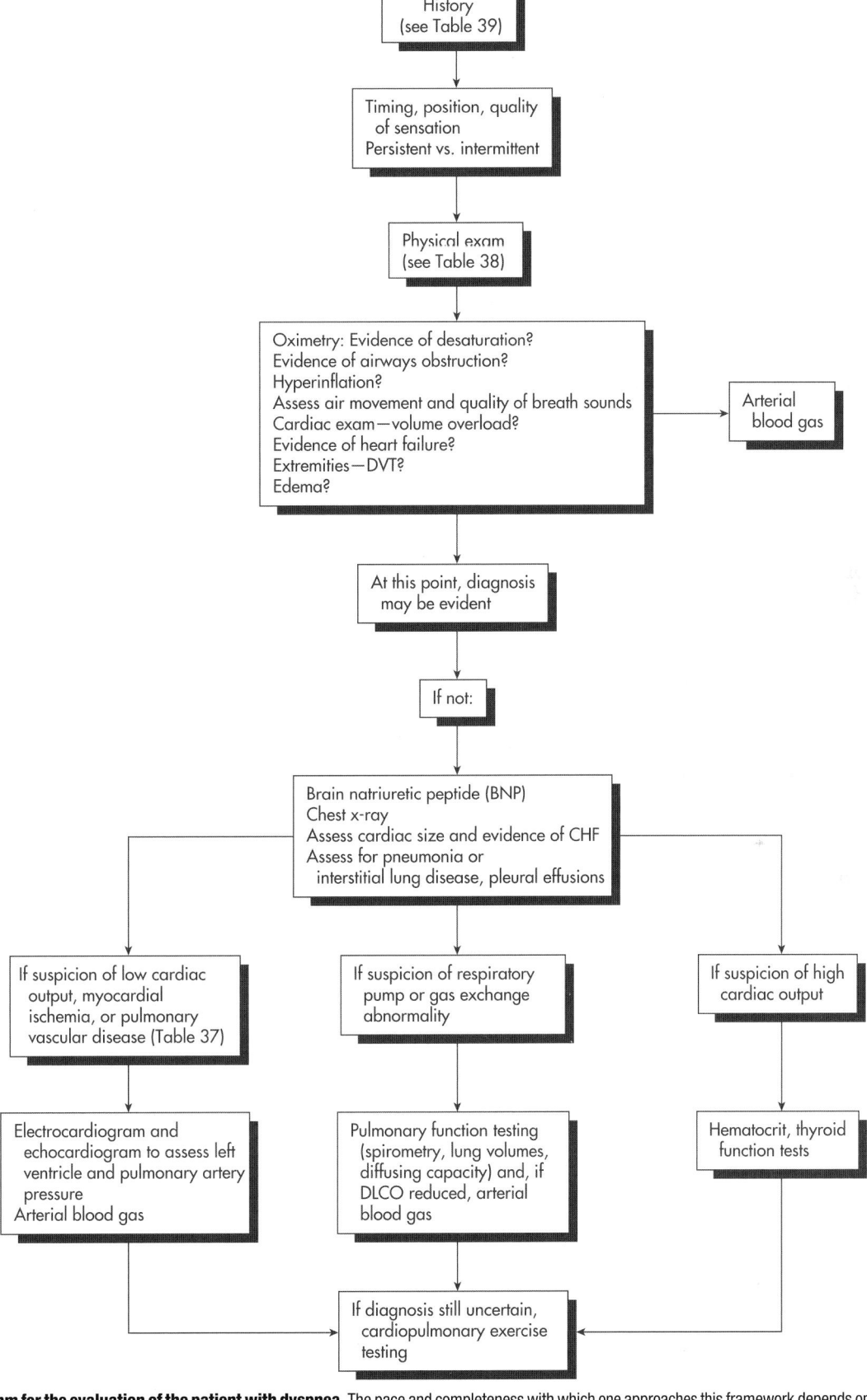

FIG. 66 Algorithm for the evaluation of the patient with dyspnea. The pace and completeness with which one approaches this framework depends on the intensity and acuity of the patient's symptoms. In a patient with severe, acute dyspnea, for example, an arterial blood gas measurement may be one of the first laboratory evaluations, whereas this measurement might not be obtained until much later in the workup in a patient with chronic breathlessness of unclear cause. A therapeutic trial of a medication, for example, a bronchodilator, may be instituted at any point if one is fairly confident of the diagnosis based on the data available at that time. *CHF,* Congestive heart failure; *DLCO,* diffusing capacity of the lung for carbon monoxide; *DVT,* deep venous thrombosis. (Modified from Schwartzstein RM, Feller-Kopman D: Approach to the patient with dyspnea. In Braunwald E, Goldman L [eds]: *Primary cardiology,* ed 2, Philadelphia, 2003, Saunders.)

Clinical Algorithms

TABLE 37 Differential Diagnoses for Acute Dyspnea

Organ System	Critical Diagnoses	Emergent Diagnoses	Nonemergent Diagnoses
Pulmonary	Airway obstruction	Spontaneous pneumothorax	Pleural effusion
	Pulmonary embolus	Asthma	Neoplasm
	Noncardiogenic edema	Cor pulmonale	Pneumonia (CAP score ≤70)
	Anaphylaxis	Aspiration	COPD
	Ventilatory failure	Pneumonia (CAP score >70)	
Cardiac	Pulmonary edema	Pericarditis	Congenital heart disease
	Myocardial infarction		Valvular heart disease
	Cardiac tamponade		Cardiomyopathy
Primarily Associated with Normal or Increased Respiratory Effort			
Abdominal		Mechanical interference	Pregnancy
		Hypotension, sepsis from ruptured viscus, bowel obstruction, inflammatory or infectious process	Ascites obesity
Psychogenic			Hyperventilation syndrome
			Somatization disorder
			Panic attack
Metabolic or endocrine	Toxic ingestion	Renal failure	Fever
	DKA	Electrolyte abnormalities	Thyroid disease
		Metabolic acidosis	
Infectious	Epiglottitis	Pneumonia (CAP score >70)	Pneumonia (CAP score ≤70)
Traumatic	Tension pneumothorax	Simple pneumothorax, hemothorax	Rib fractures
	Cardiac tamponade	Diaphragmatic rupture	
	Flail chest		
Hematologic	Carbon monoxide poisoning	Anemia	
	Acute chest syndrome		
Primarily Associated with Decreased Respiratory Effort			
Neuromuscular	CVA, intracranial insult	Multiple sclerosis	ALS
	Organophosphate poisoning	Guillain-Barré syndrome	Polymyositis
		Tick paralysis	Porphyria

ALS, Amyotrophic lateral sclerosis; *CAP,* community-acquired pneumonia; *COPD,* chronic obstructive pulmonary disease; *CVA,* cerebrovascular accident; *DKA,* diabetic ketoacidosis.
From Marx JA et al: *Rosen's emergency medicine,* ed 8, Philadelphia, 2014, Saunders.

TABLE 38 Pivotal Findings in Physical Examination

Sign	Physical Finding	Diagnoses to Consider
Vital signs	Tachypnea	Pneumonia, pneumothorax
	Hypopnea	Intracranial insult, drug or toxin ingestion
	Tachycardia	PE, traumatic chest injury
	Hypotension	Tension pneumothorax
	Fever	Pneumonia, PE
General appearance	Cachexia, weight loss	Malignancy, acquired immune disorder, mycobacterial infection
	Obesity	Hypoventilation, sleep apnea, PE
	Pregnancy	PE
	Barrel chest	COPD
	"Sniffing" position	Epiglottitis
	"Tripoding" position	COPD or asthma with severe distress
	Traumatic injury	Pneumothorax (simple, tension), rib fractures, flail chest, hemothorax, pulmonary contusion

Table 38   Pivotal Findings in Physical Examination—cont'd

Sign	Physical Finding	Diagnoses to Consider
Skin and nails	Tobacco stains or odor	COPD, malignancy, infection
	Clubbing	Chronic hypoxia, intracardiac shunts, or pulmonary vascular anomalies
	Pallid skin or conjunctivae	Anemia
	Muscle wasting	Neuromuscular disease
	Bruising	Chest wall: Rib fractures, pneumothorax
		Diffuse: Thrombocytopenia, chronic steroid use, anticoagulation
	Subcutaneous emphysema	Rib fractures, pneumothorax, tracheobronchial disruption
	Hives, rash	Allergic reaction, infection, tick-borne illness
Neck	Stridor	Upper airway edema or infection, foreign body, traumatic injury, anaphylaxis
	JVD	Tension pneumothorax, COPD or asthma exacerbation, fluid overload or CHF, PE
Lung examination	Wheezes	CHF, anaphylaxis
		Bronchospasm
	Rales	CHF, pneumonia, PE
	Unilateral decrease	Pneumothorax, pleural effusion, consolidation, rib fractures or contusion, pulmonary contusion
	Hemoptysis	Malignancy, infection, bleeding disorder, CHF
	Sputum production	Infection (viral, bacterial)
	Friction rub	Pleurisy
	Abnormal respiratory pattern (e.g., Cheyne-Stokes)	Intracranial insult
Chest examination	Crepitance or pain on palpation	Rib or sternal fractures
	Subcutaneous emphysema	Pneumothorax, tracheobronchial rupture
	Thoracoabdominal desynchrony	Diaphragmatic injury with herniation; cervical spinal cord trauma
	Flail segment	Flail chest, pulmonary contusion
Cardiac examination	Murmur	PE
	S_3 or S_4 gallop	PE
	S_2 accentuation	PE
	Muffled heart sounds	Cardiac tamponade
Extremities	Calf tenderness, Homans sign	PE
	Edema	CHF
Neurologic examination	Focal deficits (motor, sensory, cognitive)	Stroke, intracranial hemorrhage causing central abnormal respiratory drive; if long-standing, risk of aspiration pneumonia
	Symmetric deficits	Neuromuscular disease
	Diffuse weakness	Metabolic or electrolyte abnormality (hypocalcemia, hypomagnesemia, hypophosphatemia), anemia
	Hyporeflexia	Hypermagnesemia
	Ascending weakness	Guillain-Barré syndrome

CHF, Congestive heart failure; *COPD*, chronic obstructive pulmonary disease; *JVD*, jugular venous distention; *PE*, pulmonary embolism.
From Marx JA et al: *Rosen's emergency medicine*, ed 8, Philadelphia, 2014, Saunders.

Clinical Algorithms

III

TABLE 39   Diagnostic Table: Patterns of Diseases Often Resulting in Dyspnea

Disease	History (Dyspnea)	Associated Symptoms	Signs and Physical Findings	Tests
Pulmonary embolism	HPI: Abrupt onset, pleuritic pain, immobility (travel, recent surgery) PMH: Malignancy, DVT, PE, hypercoagulability, oral contraception, obesity	Diaphoresis, exertional dyspnea	Tachycardia, tachypnea, low-grade fever	• Pulse oximetry, ABG (A-a gradient), D-dimer • ECG (dysrhythmia, right-sided heart strain) • CXR (Westermark sign, Hampton hump), spiral CT, MRV • Pulmonary angiogram • Ultrasound positive for DVT
Pneumonia	Fever, productive cough, chest pain	Anorexia, chills, nausea, vomiting, exertional dyspnea, cough	Fever, tachycardia, tachypnea, rales, or decreased breath sounds	CXR, CBC, sputum and blood cultures
Bacterial	SH: Tobacco use			Pulse oximetry Waveform capnography if altered mental status, ABG if capnography unavailable and acid-base derangement or hypercarbia suspected
Viral	Exposure (e.g., influenza, varicella)			
Opportunistic	Immune disorder, chemotherapy			
Fungal or parasitic	Exposure (e.g., birds), indolent onset	Episodic fever, nonproductive cough		
Pneumothorax	Abrupt onset: Trauma, chest pain, thin males more likely to have spontaneous pneumothorax	Localized chest pain	Decreased breath sounds, subcutaneous emphysema, chest wall wounds or instability	• CXR: Pneumothorax, rib fractures, hemothorax • Ultrasound: Pneumothorax, pleural effusion
Simple				Ultrasound positive for pneumothorax
Tension	Decompensation of simple pneumothorax	Diaphoresis	JVD, tracheal deviation, muffled heart sounds, cardiovascular collapse	Clinical diagnosis: Requires immediate decompression. May verify via bedside ultrasound
COPD or asthma	Tobacco use, medication noncompliance, URI symptoms, sudden weather change	Air hunger, diaphoresis	• Retractions, accessory muscle use, tripoding, cyanosis • "Shark fin" capnograph	• CXR: Rule out infiltrate, pneumothorax, atelectasis (mucus plug) • Ultrasound: Distinguish from heart failure Waveform capnography
	PMH: Environmental allergies FH: Asthma			
Malignancy	Weight loss, tobacco, or other occupational exposure	Dysphagia	Hemoptysis	CXR, chest CT: Mass, hilar adenopathy, focal atelectasis
Fluid overload	• Gradual onset, dietary indiscretion or medication noncompliance, chest pain • PMH: Recent MI, diabetes, CHF	Worsening orthopnea, PND	JVD, peripheral edema, S_3 or S_4 gallop, new cardiac dysrhythmia, hepatojugular reflux	• CXR and/or ultrasound: Pleural effusion, interstitial edema, Kerley B lines, cardiomegaly • ECG: Ischemia, dysrhythmia • NT-proBNP
Anaphylaxis	Abrupt onset, exposure to allergen	Dysphagia	Oral swelling, stridor, wheezing, hives	

A-a, Alveolar-arterial; *ABG,* arterial blood gas; *CBC,* complete blood count; *CHF,* congestive heart failure; *COPD,* chronic obstructive pulmonary disease; *CT,* computed tomography; *CXR,* chest x-ray examination; *DVT,* deep vein thrombosis; *ECG,* electrocardiogram; *FH,* family history; *HPI,* history of present illness; *JVD,* jugular venous distention; *MI,* myocardial infarction; *MRV,* magnetic resonance venography; *NT-proBNP,* amino-terminal pro–B-type natriuretic peptide; *PE,* pulmonary embolism; *PMH,* past medical history; *PND,* paroxysmal nocturnal dyspnea; *SH,* social history; *URI,* upper respiratory infection.
From Marx JA et al: *Rosen's emergency medicine,* ed 8, Philadelphia, 2014, Saunders.

TABLE 40   Relationships among Qualities of Dyspnea, Physiology, and Symptomatic Treatment

Quality of Dyspnea	Physiology	Symptomatic Treatment
Air hunger, urge to breathe, need more air	Stimulation of respiratory controller via chemoreceptors, pulmonary receptors, vascular receptors	Supplemental oxygen; nasal flow of gas; cool air on the face; chest wall vibration; inhaled furosemide; opiates
Chest tightness	Stimulation of airway receptors	Inhaled bronchodilators (beta agonists, anticholinergics, steroids)
Cannot get a deep breath	Stimulation of respiratory controller; dynamic hyperinflation	Breathing retraining (slower breathing); pursed lips breathing
Increased work or effort to breathe	Mechanical load on the respiratory system; neuromuscular weakness	Inspiratory muscle training; noninvasive ventilation/BPAP
Breathing more	Increased ventilation; stimulation of metaboreceptors in muscles	Exercise training
All qualities	Altered perception/processing of information centrally	Desensitization treatment in pulmonary rehabilitation; morphine

BPAP, Bilevel positive airway pressure.
From Broaddus VC et al: *Murray & Nadel's textbook of respiratory medicine,* ed 7, Philadelphia, 2022, Elsevier.

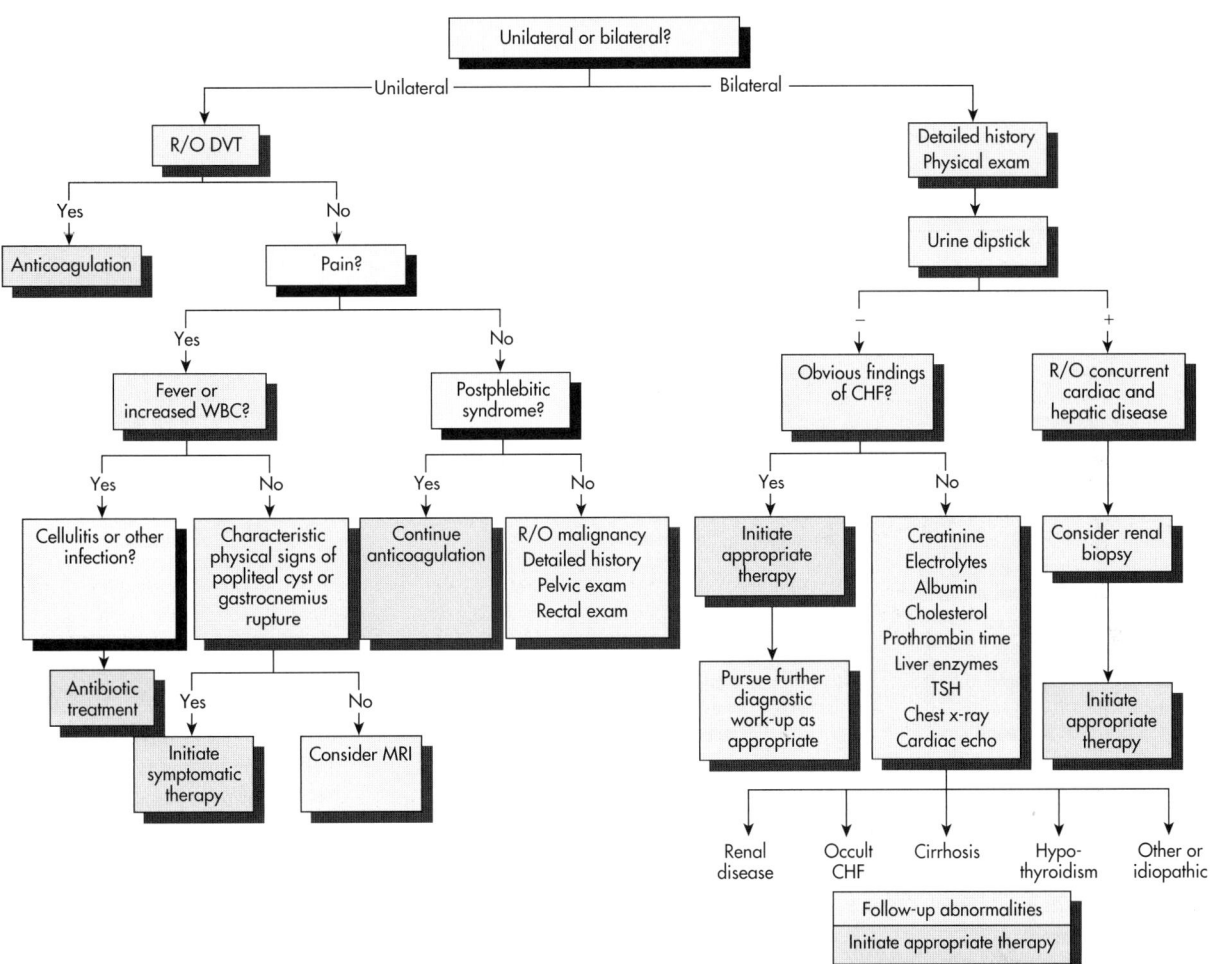

FIG. 68 Diagnostic approach to patients with edema. *CHF,* Congestive heart failure; *DVT,* deep vein thrombosis; *MRI,* magnetic resonance imaging; *R/O,* rule out; *TSH,* thyroid-stimulating hormone; *WBC,* white blood cell count. (From Chertow G: Approach to the patient with edema. In: Braunwald E, Goldman L [eds]: *Primary cardiology,* ed 2, Philadelphia, 2003, Saunders.)

Clinical
Algorithms

ICD-10CM #	D75.0	Familial erythrocytosis
	D75.1	Secondary polycythemia
	D45	Polycythemia vera
	P61.1	Polycythemia neonatorum

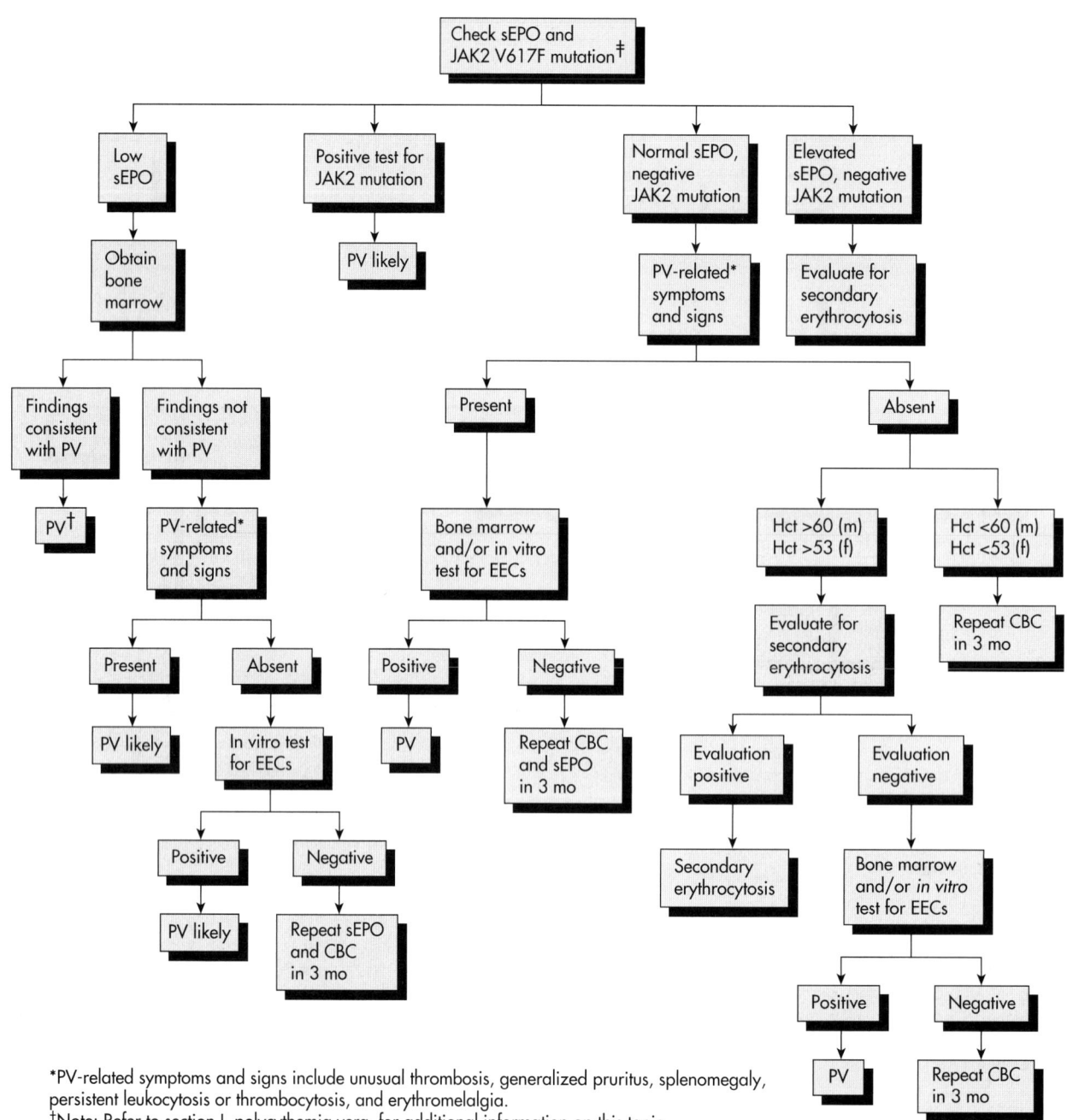

*PV-related symptoms and signs include unusual thrombosis, generalized pruritus, splenomegaly, persistent leukocytosis or thrombocytosis, and erythromelalgia.
†Note: Refer to section I, polycythemia vera, for additional information on this topic.
‡The JAK2 mutation is found in >95% of patients with PV and can be used for diagnostic purposes.

FIG. 71 A diagnostic approach to acquired erythrocytosis. *CBC,* Complete blood cell count; *EEC,* endogenous (spontaneous) erythroid colonies; *f,* female; *Hct,* hematocrit; *m,* male; *PV,* polycythemia vera; *sEPO,* serum erythropoietin level. (Modified from Goldman L, Schafer AL [eds]: *Cecil textbook of medicine,* ed 24, Philadelphia, 2012, Saunders.)

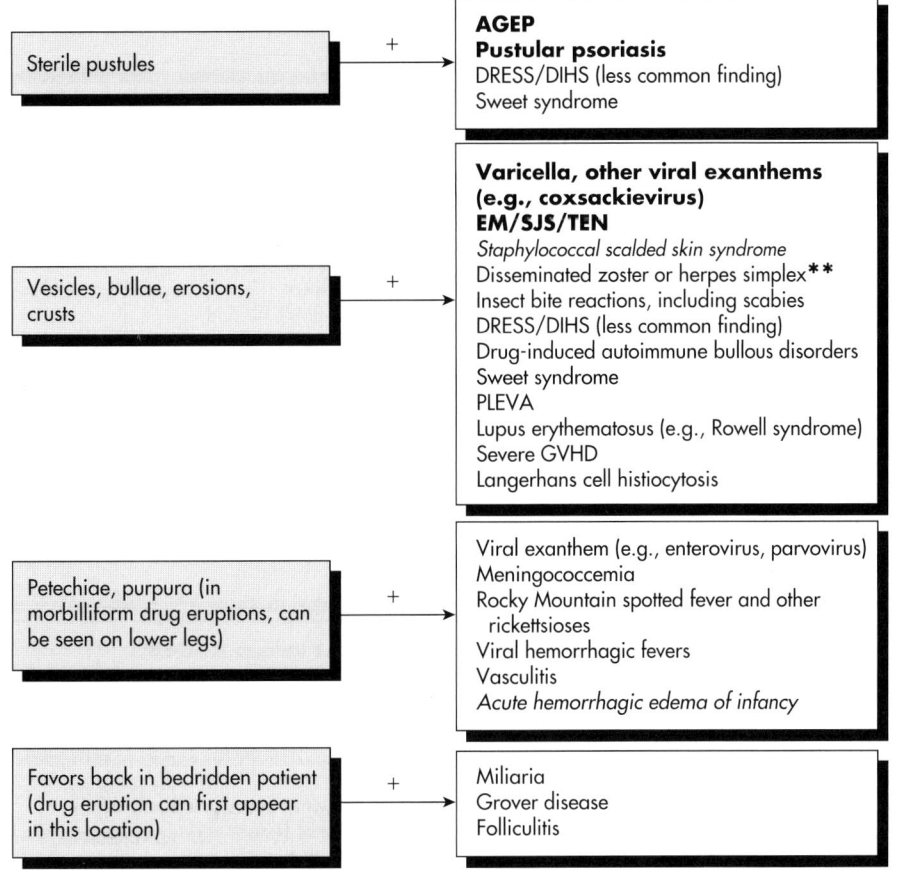

Sterile pustules → +

AGEP
Pustular psoriasis
DRESS/DIHS (less common finding)
Sweet syndrome

Vesicles, bullae, erosions, crusts → +

Varicella, other viral exanthems (e.g., coxsackievirus)
EM/SJS/TEN
Staphylococcal scalded skin syndrome
Disseminated zoster or herpes simplex**
Insect bite reactions, including scabies
DRESS/DIHS (less common finding)
Drug-induced autoimmune bullous disorders
Sweet syndrome
PLEVA
Lupus erythematosus (e.g., Rowell syndrome)
Severe GVHD
Langerhans cell histiocytosis

Petechiae, purpura (in morbilliform drug eruptions, can be seen on lower legs) → +

Viral exanthem (e.g., enterovirus, parvovirus)
Meningococcemia
Rocky Mountain spotted fever and other rickettsioses
Viral hemorrhagic fevers
Vasculitis
Acute hemorrhagic edema of infancy

Favors back in bedridden patient (drug eruption can first appear in this location) → +

Miliaria
Grover disease
Folliculitis

**Immunocompromised host
AGEP = acute generalized exanthematous pustulosis
DIHS = drug-induced hypersensitivity syndrome
DRESS = drug reaction with eosinophilia and systemic symptoms (additional findings include lymphadenopathy, atypical lymphocytosis, hepatitis, myocarditis and renal dysfunction as well as facial swelling > vesicles or sterile pustules)
EM/SJS/TEN = erythema multiforme/Stevens–Johnson syndrome/toxic epidermal necrolysis
GVHD = graft-versus-host disease
PLEVA = pityriasis lichenoides et varioliformis acuta

FIG. 78 Approach to the differential diagnosis of an exanthematous drug reaction. With a few exceptions (e.g., pityriasis rosea, drug-induced autoimmune bullous disorders), patients with these entities may be febrile. Entities in italics occur primarily in children. Toxic shock syndrome can be staphylococcal or streptococcal. Drug-induced autoimmune bullous disorders: Bullous pemphigoid or linear IgA bullous dermatosis > drug-induced pemphigus. *AGEP*, Acute generalized exanthematous pustulosis; *CMV*, cytomegalovirus; *DIHS*, drug-induced hypersensitivity syndrome; *DRESS*, drug reaction with eosinophilia and systemic symptoms; *EBV*, Epstein-Barr virus; *EM*, erythema multiforme; *Ig*, immunoglobulin; *GVHD*, graft versus host disease; *SJS*, Stevens-Johnson syndrome; *TEN*, toxic epidermal necrolysis. (From Bolognia JL: *Dermatology*, ed 4, Philadelphia, 2018, Elsevier.)

Clinical
Algorithms

III

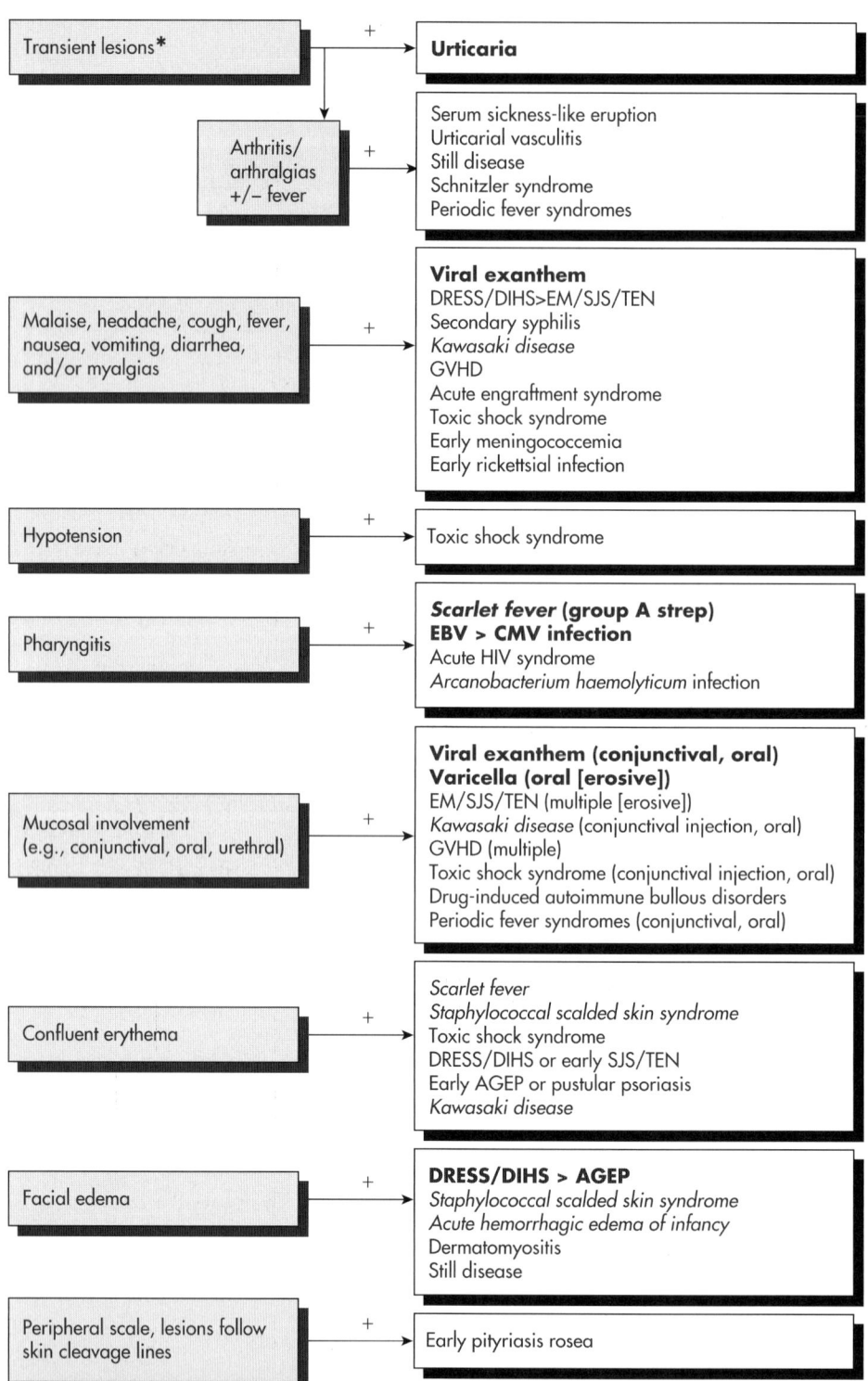

Transient lesions* → **Urticaria**

Arthritis/ arthralgias +/− fever →
Serum sickness-like eruption
Urticarial vasculitis
Still disease
Schnitzler syndrome
Periodic fever syndromes

Malaise, headache, cough, fever, nausea, vomiting, diarrhea, and/or myalgias →
Viral exanthem
DRESS/DIHS>EM/SJS/TEN
Secondary syphilis
Kawasaki disease
GVHD
Acute engraftment syndrome
Toxic shock syndrome
Early meningococcemia
Early rickettsial infection

Hypotension → Toxic shock syndrome

Pharyngitis →
***Scarlet fever* (group A strep)**
EBV > CMV infection
Acute HIV syndrome
Arcanobacterium haemolyticum infection

Mucosal involvement (e.g., conjunctival, oral, urethral) →
Viral exanthem (conjunctival, oral)
Varicella (oral [erosive])
EM/SJS/TEN (multiple [erosive])
Kawasaki disease (conjunctival injection, oral)
GVHD (multiple)
Toxic shock syndrome (conjunctival injection, oral)
Drug-induced autoimmune bullous disorders
Periodic fever syndromes (conjunctival, oral)

Confluent erythema →
Scarlet fever
Staphylococcal scalded skin syndrome
Toxic shock syndrome
DRESS/DIHS or early SJS/TEN
Early AGEP or pustular psoriasis
Kawasaki disease

Facial edema →
DRESS/DIHS > AGEP
Staphylococcal scalded skin syndrome
Acute hemorrhagic edema of infancy
Dermatomyositis
Still disease

Peripheral scale, lesions follow skin cleavage lines → Early pityriasis rosea

*Individual lesions last <24 hr, which can be documented by outlining them with ink; exceptions include urticarial vasculitis and, occasionally, Schnitzler or periodic fever syndromes

FIG. 78, cont'd

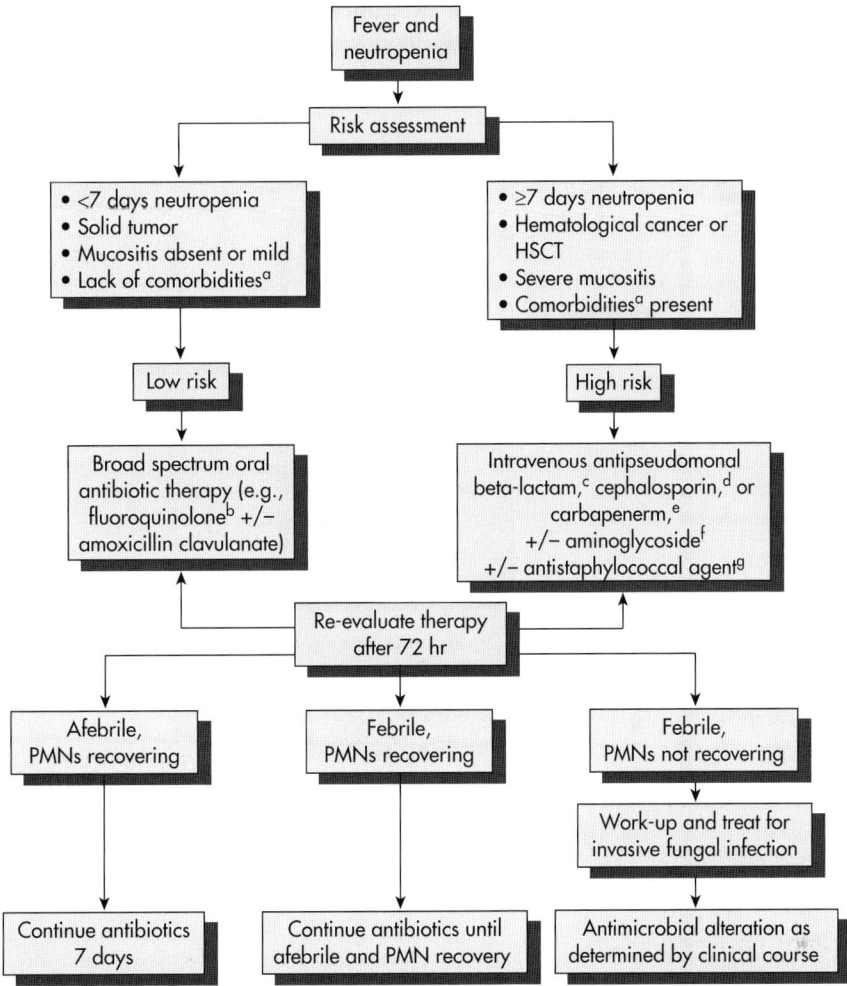

a Hypotension, altered mental status, neurologic changes, respiratory failure, abdominal pain, hemorrhage, cardiac compromise or new arrhythmia, catheter tunnel infection, extensive cellulitis, acute renal or liver failure
b Institution sensitivity dependent, ciprofloxacin, levofloxacin, moxifloxacin
c Drug selection and dosing institution-specific: Piperacillin tazobactam, ticarcillin/clavulanate
d Drug selection and dosing institution-specific: Ceftazidime
e Imipenem, cefepime/cilastatin, meropenem, doripenem
f Gentamicin, tobramycin, or amikacin
g Drug selection and institution-specific: Vancomycin, linezolid, daptomycin, ceftaroline

FIG. 80 Approach to patient with fever and neutropenia. *HSCT,* Hematopoietic stem cell transplant; *PMN,* polymorphonuclear neutrophil. (From Hoffman R: *Hematology: basic principles and practice,* ed 7, Philadelphia, 2018, Elsevier.)

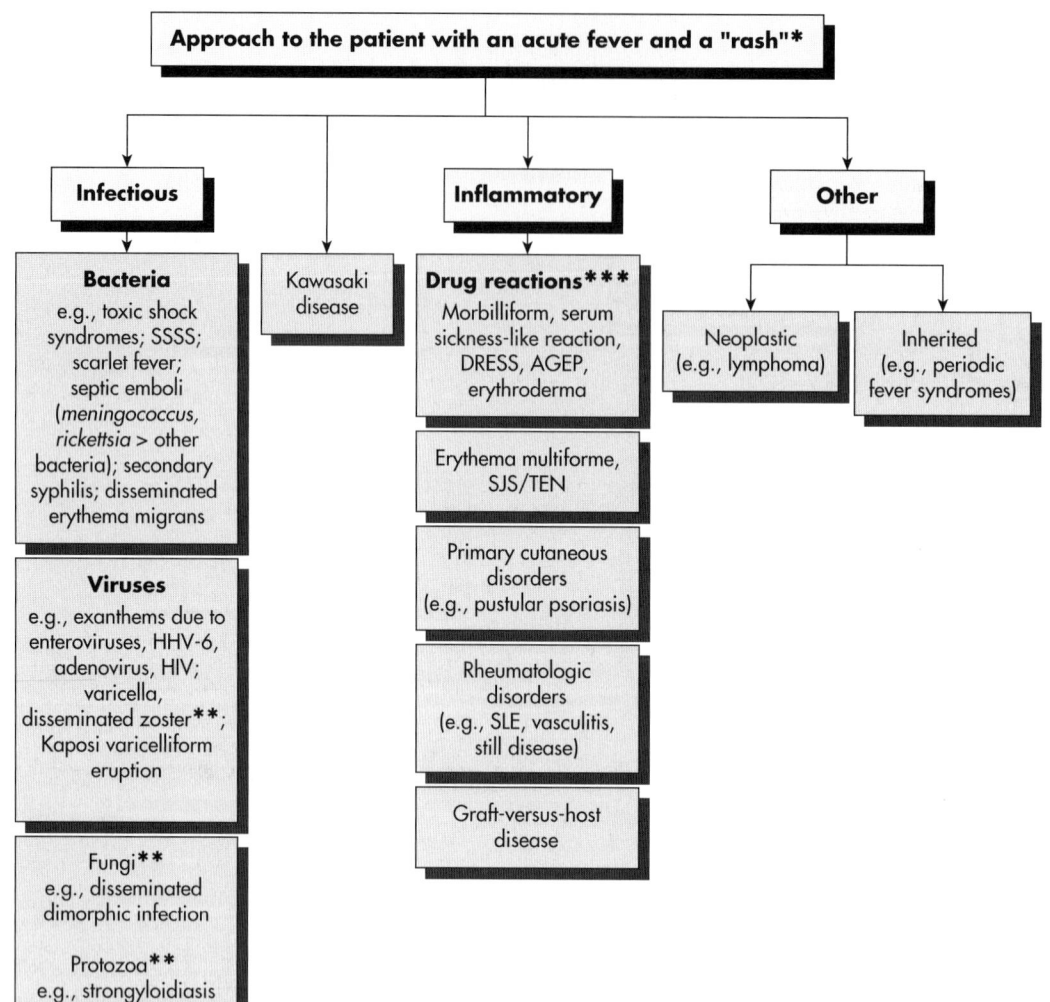

     * Not a single site as in cellulitis, necrotizing fasciitis
     ** More likely in immunocompromised patient
     *** Early on, more serious drug reactions, e.g., DRESS, may resemble a morbilliform eruption

FIG. 82 Approach to the patient with an acute fever and a "rash." *AGEP*, Acute generalized exanthematous pustulosis; *DRESS*, drug reaction with eosinophilia and systemic symptoms (also referred to as drug-induced hypersensitivity syndrome [DIHS]); *HHV*, human herpes virus; *HIV*, human immunodeficiency virus; *SJS*, Stevens-Johnson syndrome; *SLE*, systemic lupus erythematosus; *SSSS*, staphylococcal scalded skin syndrome; *TEN*, toxic epidermal necrolysis. (From Bolognia J: *Dermatology*, ed 4, Philadelphia, 2018, Elsevier.)

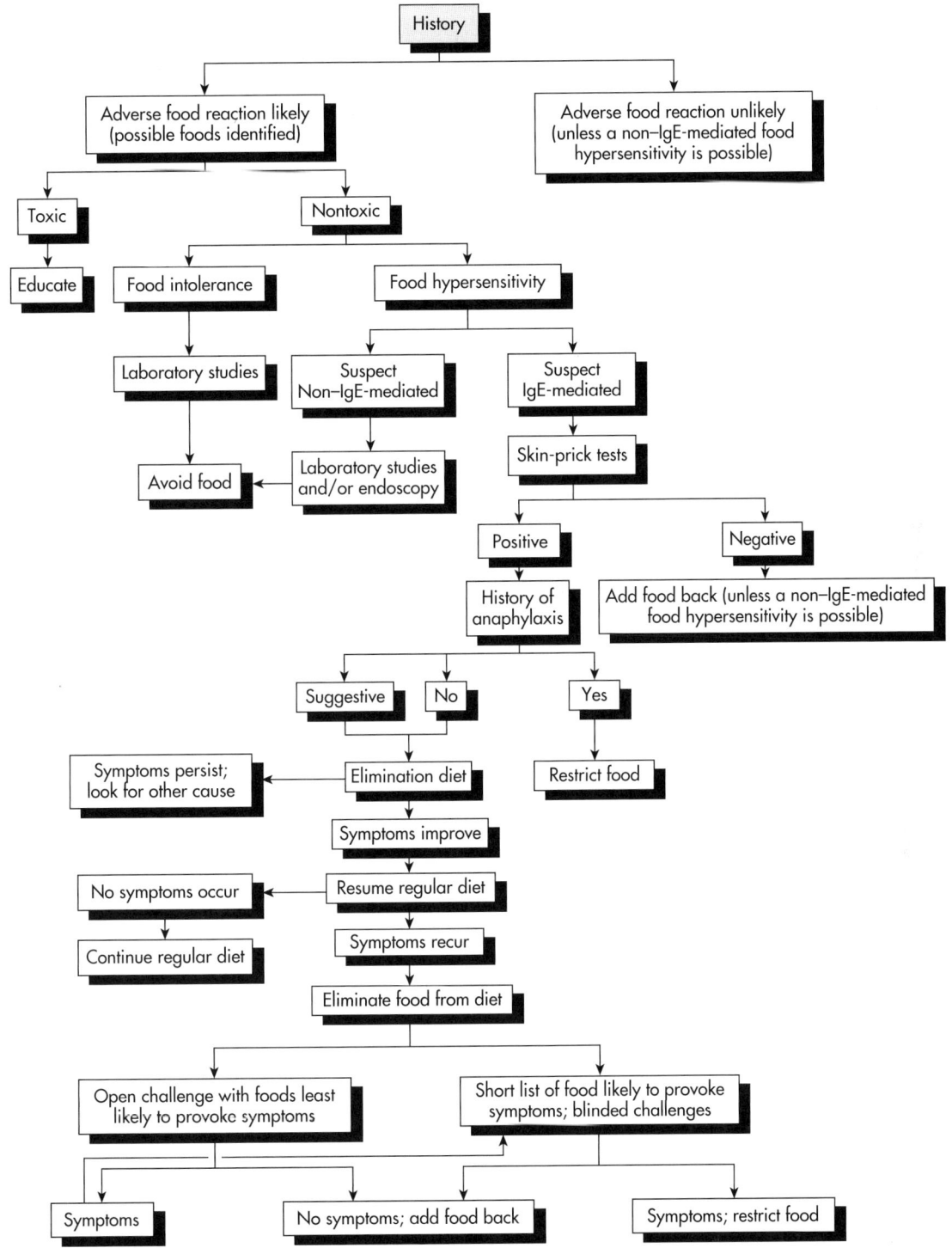

FIG. 83 Algorithm for the evaluation and management of adverse food reactions. *Ig,* Immunoglobulin. (From Feldman M et al: *Sleisenger and Fortran's gastrointestinal and liver disease,* ed 10, Philadelphia, 2016, Elsevier.)

Clinical
Algorithms

III

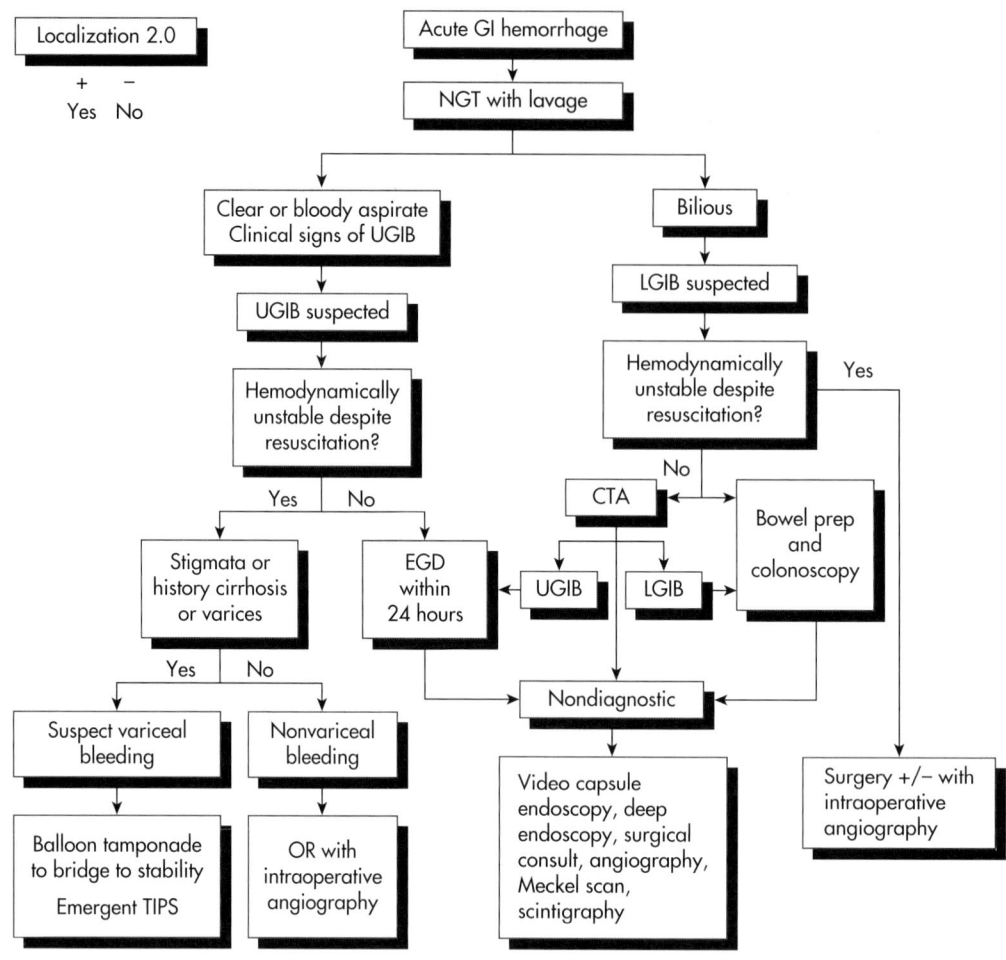

FIG. 84 Algorithm for the diagnosis of acute GI hemorrhage. *CTA,* Computed tomography angiogram; *EGD,* esophagogastroduodenoscopy; *GI,* gastrointestinal; *LGIB,* lower GI bleed; *NGT,* nasogastric tube; *TIPS,* transjugular intrahepatic portosystemic shunt; *UGIB,* upper GI bleed. (From Townsend CM et al: *Sabiston textbook of surgery,* ed 21, St Louis, 2022, Elsevier.)

TABLE 44	Suspected Source of GI Bleeding as Suggested by a Patient's History
Suspected Source of Bleeding	**Patient History**
Nasopharynx	History of nasopharyngeal radiation
	Recurrent epistaxis
	Prior nasopharyngeal malignancy
Lungs	Hemoptysis
Esophageal ulceration	GERD
	Heartburn
	Heavy alcohol use
	Odynophagia
	Pill ingestion
	Traumatic nasogastric tube placement
Esophageal cancer	Dysphagia
	Weight loss
Mallory-Weiss tear	Alcohol binge
	Vomiting
Cameron lesions	Large hiatal hernia
Esophageal or gastric varices or portal hypertensive gastropathy	Chronic liver disease
	Cirrhosis
	Heavy alcohol use

Table 44 Suspected Source of GI Bleeding as Suggested by a Patient's History—cont'd

Suspected Source of Bleeding	Patient History
Gastric angiodysplasia	Chronic kidney disease
Peptic ulcer	Epigastric discomfort
	Frequent aspirin or other NSAID use
	History of PUD
Gastric cancer	Early satiation
	Weight loss
Primary aortoenteric fistula	Prior severe acute unexplained bleeding
Secondary aortoenteric fistula	Prior surgical repair of an abdominal aortic aneurysm with synthetic graft
Ampulla of Vater	Recent endoscopic sphincterotomy
Bile ducts	Recent liver biopsy or cholangiography
Pancreatic ducts	Pancreatitis
	Pseudocyst
	Recent pancreatography
Small intestinal malignancy	Hereditary nonpolyposis colorectal cancer
	History of intraabdominal metastatic cancer
	Intermittent small intestinal obstruction
	Recurrent unexplained GI bleeding
	Weight loss
Meckel diverticulum	Unexplained GI bleeding since childhood
Small intestinal or colonic ulcerations	Use of aspirin or other NSAID
Small intestinal telangiectasias	Frequent nosebleeds
	Hereditary hemorrhagic telangiectasia (Osler-Weber-Rendu disease)
Small intestinal angiodysplasia	Age >60 yr
Colonic diverticulosis	Hematochezia without abdominal pain
	History of diverticulosis
Colonic neoplasia	Change in bowel habits
	Personal or family history colon neoplasia
	Subacute bleeding
	Weight loss
Ischemic colitis	Cardiovascular disease
	Hematochezia with abdominal pain or discomfort
UC	Bloody diarrhea
	Family history of IBD
	History of UC
Crohn disease	Chronic abdominal discomfort
	Family history of IBD
	History of Crohn disease
Anal fissure	Hematochezia with anal pain
Hemorrhoids	Dripping blood with bowel movements
	Hematochezia with normal bowel movements
Postpolypectomy ulcer	Recent colonoscopy with polypectomy
	Use of anticoagulants or antiplatelet drugs
Colonic or small intestinal angioectasias	Age >70 yr
	Cardiovascular disease
	Recurrent bleeding of variable severity
Anastomotic ulceration	Prior intestinal surgical anastomosis
Radiation enteritis or proctitis	History of abdominal radiation therapy

From Feldman M et al: *Sleisenger and Fortran's gastrointestinal and liver disease*, ed 10, Philadelphia, 2016, Elsevier.

Clinical Algorithms

III

TABLE 45   Evaluation of Gastrointestinal Bleeding, Pediatric Patient

Laboratory Investigation

All Patients

CBC and platelet count

Coagulation tests: prothrombin time, partial thromboplastin time

Tests of liver dysfunction: AST, ALT, GGT, bilirubin

Occult blood test of stool or vomitus

Blood type and crossmatch

Evaluation of Bloody Diarrhea

Stool culture or PCR, *Clostridium difficile* toxin

Sigmoidoscopy or colonoscopy

CT or MRI enteroscopy

Evaluation of Rectal Bleeding with Formed Stools

External and digital rectal examination

Sigmoidoscopy or colonoscopy

Meckel scan

Mesenteric arteriogram

Video capsule endoscopy

Initial Radiologic Evaluation

All Patients

Abdominal x-ray series

Evaluation of Hematemesis

Barium upper GI series if endoscopy not available

Evaluation of Bleeding with Pain and Vomiting (Bowel Obstruction)

Abdominal x-ray series

Pneumatic or contrast enema

Upper GI series

ALT, Alanine aminotransferase; *AST,* aspartate aminotransferase; *CBC,* complete blood count; *CT,* computed tomography; *GGT,* γ-glutamyltransferase; *GI,* gastrointestinal.
From Marcdante KJ et al: *Nelson essentials of pediatrics,* ed 9, Philadelphia, 2023, Elsevier.

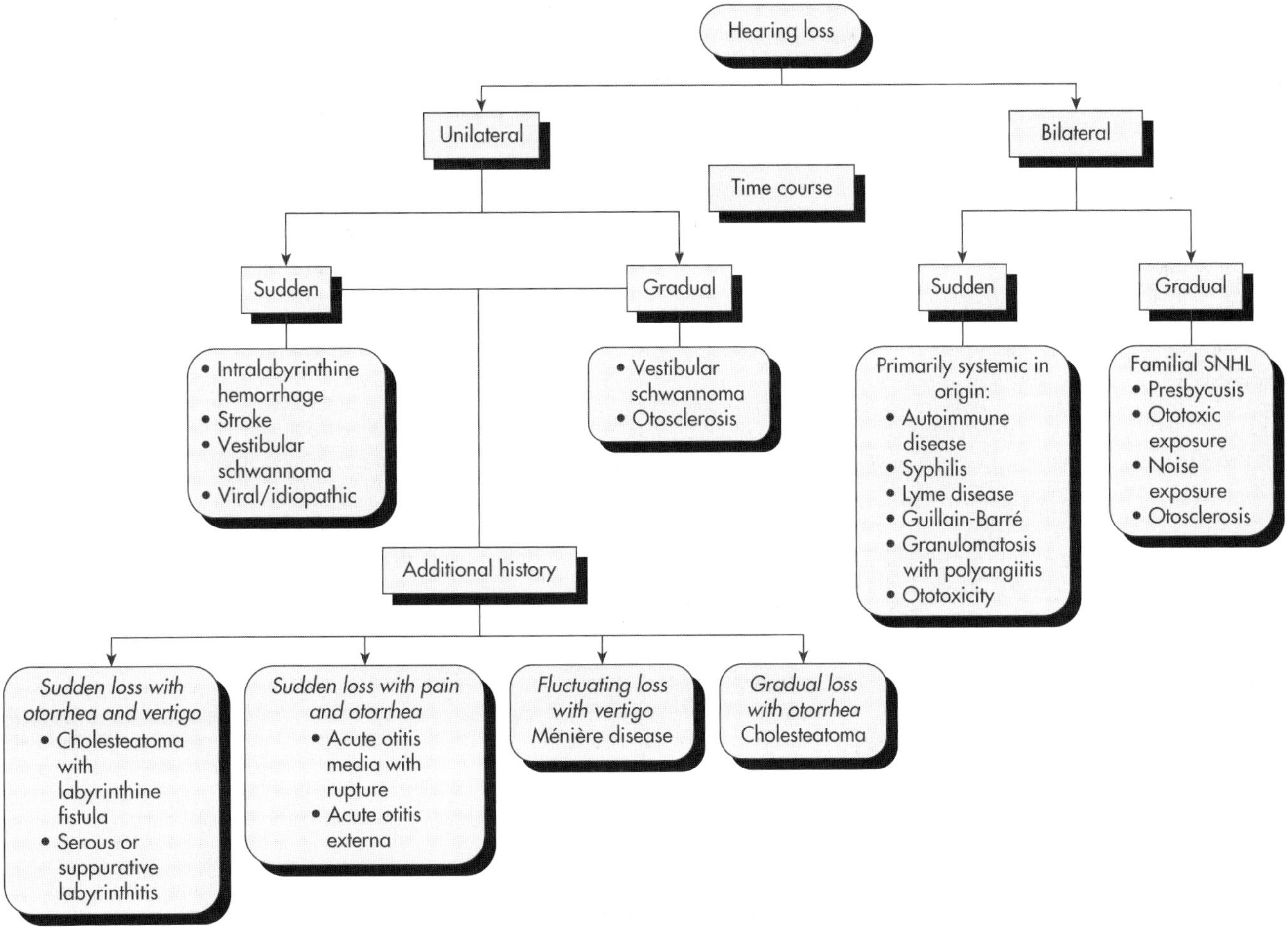

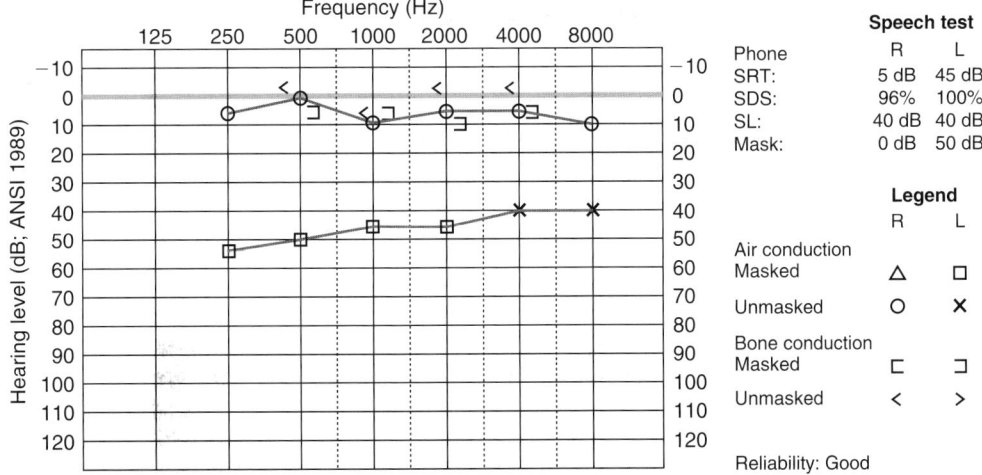

FIG. 88 Establishing a differential diagnosis with a chief complaint of hearing loss. This algorithm encourages the clinician to consider the patient complaint in categorical differential diagnosis families. It is not exhaustive. *SNHL,* Sensorineural hearing loss. (From Flint PW et al: *Cummings otolaryngology, head and neck surgery,* ed 7, Philadelphia, 2021, Elsevier.)

FIG. 89 An audiogram showing a clinically significant left-sided conductive hearing loss. Note the airbone gap, normal speech discrimination, and normal masked bone conduction in the left ear. *SDS,* Speech discrimination score; *SL,* sensory level; *SRT,* speech reception threshold. (From Flint PW et al: *Cummings otolaryngology, head and neck surgery,* ed 7, Philadelphia, 2021, Elsevier.)

Clinical
Algorithms

III

TABLE 47 Lesions That Cause Hearing Loss

	Description of Pathology	Onset/Course	Actions or Treatment	Prognosis
Conductive Lesion				
Foreign body	Mass in external canal blocks sound conduction	Acute onset associated or not with pain, drainage, or odor	Removal. Evaluate for infection. Evaluate for TM perforation	Excellent
Otitis externa	Edema and detritus obstruct external canal	Rapid onset. Pain, edema, swelling. Drainage, odor often present	Aural toilet to remove debris. Topical (±oral) antibiotics. Evaluate for necrotizing otitis	Excellent if treated appropriately
Exostosis	Bony growths obstruct canal. Often seen with prolonged exposure to cold water (divers)	Slow insidious onset. No pain or drainage unless causes complete obstruction	Evaluate for infection. Reassure patient. Refer to ENT	Good
Tympanosclerosis	TM scarring from perforations or infections. Decreased mobility impairs sound conduction	Slow onset following perforations, trauma, or infections	ENT referral. Reassurance	Variable
Perforated TM	Disruption of TM integrity results in impaired transmission of sound to ossicle	Acute onset. May follow direct trauma or sudden barotrauma. May have sudden relief from pain if caused by otitis media	Treat infectious causes. Counsel on importance of keeping water out of ear canal. ENT referral	Good
Sterile effusion (barotrauma)	Fluid in middle ear dampens conduction through ossicles	Often following flight, diving, or URI. Bubbles can cause intermittent pain	Decongestants. Evaluate for infection. Follow-up	Excellent
Acute otitis media	Pus (or fluid) in middle ear dampens conduction through ossicles	Acute to subacute onset, often following URI. Often associated with pain ± fever	Antibiotics (unless viral cause suspected), decongestants, pain control	Excellent if treated appropriately
Cholesteatoma	Trapped stratified squamous epithelial mass in middle ear. Interferes with ossicle conduction	Slow onset. Often history of previous perforations or chronic infections	ENT referral	Variable. May destroy ossicles or erode into surrounding structures
Glomus tumor	Vascular tumor occupies middle ear space. Interferes with ossicle conduction	Slow onset. May be associated with rushing pulsatile sensation	ENT referral	Variable
Cancer	Squamous cell most common. Obstructs external canal	Slow onset. Often noticed first by others. Painless unless occlusion causes otitis externa	ENT referral. Evaluate for secondary infection	Variable
Sensorineural Lesion				
Perilymph fistula (inner ear barotrauma)	Disruption of round or oval window allows leakage of perilymph into middle ear	Sudden onset of hearing loss often with tinnitus and vertigo. Frequently follows straining or abrupt change in pressure. Turning in direction of fistula exacerbates symptoms	Complete bed rest. Elevate head of bed and avoid increases in CSF pressure. Severe symptoms or noncompliance may require hospitalization. ENT consultation for possible oval or round window patch	Variable
Viral cochleitis	Cochlear inflammation. Often following URI	Rapid onset. Often following URI	Steroids often used (no good data)	Variable
Presbycusis	Age-related hearing loss May be related to previous chronic noise exposure	Slow onset. Usually symmetric. High frequencies most affected. Tinnitus may occur	Hearing aid may help with both hearing loss and tinnitus	Variable
Acoustic neuroma	Benign schwannoma of 8th cranial nerve	Slow onset. Usually unilateral. May exhibit tinnitus, vertigo. May exhibit facial hyperesthesias or twitching	May require surgical excision if symptoms debilitating	Variable
Ototoxic agents	Direct toxicity to inner ear structures	Variable onset. High frequency most affected. Exposure to ototoxic drugs. May have associated tinnitus	Stop use of offending agent	Variable. Hearing loss at time of stopping offending agent is usually permanent
Multiple sclerosis	Multiple demyelinating lesions interfere with nerve conduction	Often other associated neurologic findings. May wax and wane	Standard multiple sclerosis treatment (steroids, cytotoxic agents)	Variable
Stroke/CVA	Focal ischemic lesion of auditory nerve or auditory cortex	Sudden onset. Often associated with other neurologic deficits	Treat CVA risk factors (ASA, anticoagulants, glycemic control, BP control)	Variable
Meningitis	Infection enters inner ear through CNS-perilymph connection. Damages organ of Corti	Follows clinical picture of meningitis	Treat infection. Steroids may limit inflammation and damage	Variable

Table 47 Lesions That Cause Hearing Loss—cont'd

	Description of Pathology	Onset/Course	Actions or Treatment	Prognosis
Ménière disease (endolymphatic hydrops)	Abnormal homeostasis of inner ear fluids (clinical diagnosis; definitive diagnosis made histologically)	Episodic spells of vertigo. Associated sensation of fullness, tinnitus, and SNHL or auditory distortion. Low-frequency ranges most affected	Reduce salt, caffeine, nicotine (vasoconstrictors) intake. Consider diuretics, antihistamines, anticholinergics, ENT referral	Variable
Chronic noise exposure	Direct mechanical damage to cochlear structures and hair cells	Slow onset. Usually high frequency most affected	Prevention measures (earplugs). Stop exposure	Usually permanent
Skull trauma	Interruption of cranial nerve VIII, ossicle disruption, or shearing effects on organ of Corti	Sudden onset after trauma	ENT consultation for possible surgical repair	Variable: Ossicle disruption has better prognosis than nerve or organ of Corti damage
Autoimmune causes	Vascular or neuronal inflammatory changes	Bilateral asymmetric SNHL. May be fluctuating or progressive. Often other systemic autoimmune findings	Outpatient autoimmune evaluation. Steroids and cytotoxic agents may slow progression	Variable

ASA, Acetylsalicylic acid; *BP,* blood pressure; *CNS,* central nervous system; *CSF,* cerebrospinal fluid; *CVA,* cerebrovascular accident; *ENT,* ear, nose, and throat; *SNHL,* sensorineural hearing loss; *TM,* tympanic membrane; *URI,* upper respiratory infection.
From Adams JG et al: *Emergency medicine, clinical essentials,* ed 2, Philadelphia, 2013, Elsevier.

TABLE 48 A Summary of Diagnostic Audiology Tests and Applications

Audiologic Test Battery	Hearing acuity	*Air conduction thresholds*	Measures function of the external, middle, and inner ear.
		Bone conduction thresholds	Measures function of the inner ear, bypassing external and middle ear structures.
	Speech testing	*Speech detection threshold (SDT)*	The speech (spondee word) level where an individual can discern the presence of a speech signal 50% of the time.
		Speech reception threshold (SRT)	The intensity level where an individual can correctly repeat spondee words 50% of the time.
		Speech recognition	Measures an individual's ability to recognize speech—typically monosyllabic words presented at supra-threshold levels, under well-controlled conditions. Testing may be open or closed set.
		Subjective report scales	Questionnaires or inventories related to everyday listening situations for adults or that use parental reporting to evaluate a child's listening skills in his or her daily environment.
Evaluating Middle Ear Function	Tympanometry		Measures the acoustic immittance of the tympanic membrane and middle ear ossicular chain as a function of air pressure variations in the ear canal. Estimates intratympanic pressure, eustachian tube function, tympanic membrane integrity and mobility, and continuity of the ossicular chain.
	Stapedial reflexes		Determines the softest level of sound that will elicit stapedial muscle contraction. Typically occurs at 70-100 dB HL for a normal-hearing ear.
	Acoustic reflex decay		Measures the ability of the stapedius muscle to maintain sustained contraction. A response is abnormal if its amplitude decreases to half or less of its original measurement over 5 sec.
Objective Tests for Differential Diagnostic Applications	Otoacoustic emissions	*Transient-evoked otoacoustic emissions*	Audiofrequency signals generated by outer hair cells measured in the ear canal elicited by a transient, brief stimulus such as a click or tone burst. Presence indicates cochlear outer hair cell integrity.
		Distortion-product otoacoustic emissions	Audiofrequency signals generated by outer hair cells measured in the ear canal elicited by a pair of pure tones separated by a specific frequency difference. Presence indicates cochlear outer hair cell integrity.
	ECochG		Measurement of neuroelectric events at the tympanic membrane or promontory generated by cochlear structures and the auditory nerve in response to acoustic stimulation. Response may consist of the cochlear microphonic, summating potential, and/or action potential.
	Sonomotor responses	*C-VEMP and O-VEMP*	

Clinical Algorithms

III

Continued

Table 48 A Summary of Diagnostic Audiology Tests and Applications—cont'd

			Vestibular evoked myogenic potentials elicited from the sternocleidomastoid muscle (inferior vestibular nerve) or inferior rectus/inferior oblique of contralateral eye (superior vestibular nerve) that are useful to evaluate the function of the superior versus inferior vestibular nerve.
	Auditory brainstem response	*Threshold estimation ABR*	Surface-recorded averaged responses to click or tone burst stimuli that represent activity of the distal portion of the auditory pathway. Wave V threshold may be used to estimate behavioral auditory thresholds.
		Neurodiagnostic ABR	Surface-recorded averaged response to click stimuli that represents activity of the distal portion of the auditory pathway. Responses are typically assessed for amplitude, morphology, and absolute and inter-peak latencies of waves I–V.
	Auditory steady-state response		Far-field recording of EEG activity evoked using a continuous sinusoidal acoustic stimulus that is amplitude and frequency modulated at slow rates. Response presence/absence is analyzed automatically using statistical procedures.
	Electrically evoked auditory potentials	*Electrically evoked ABR*	Surface-recorded averaged responses to electrical stimuli delivered to promontory or via a cochlear implant that represents activity of the distal portion of the auditory pathway.
		Electrically evoked compound action potential	Recording of the synchronized discharge of a large number of electrically stimulated auditory nerve fibers. The primary response is a single negative peak (N1) occurring at 0.3-0.5 ms with amplitude up to 2-3 mV.
		Electrically evoked middle-latency response	A series of electrically evoked vertex-positive peaks that occur within a time window of 10-50 ms after stimulation and is thought to be generated by neurons in the auditory midbrain and primary cortex.
		Cortical auditory evoked potentials	Most frequently refers to the long-latency, obligatory P1–N1–P2 complex. Components have latencies between 70 and 300 ms and arise from cortical or precortical levels of the auditory system.
Evaluating Functional HL	PTA/SRT agreement		The average of the air conduction thresholds at 500, 1000, and 2000 Hz should agree with the speech reception threshold within 5 dB.
	Stenger test		A tone is presented to the better ear at 10 dB above its threshold simultaneously with an identical tone to the poorer ear at 10 dB below its voluntary threshold. The individual will respond if the hearing loss is genuine. A nonresponse is a positive Stenger test and indicates pseudohypacusis.

ABR, Auditory brainstem responses; *C-VEMP*, cervical vestibular evoked myogenic potential; *ECochG*, electrocochleography; *HL*, hearing level; *O-VEMP*, ocular vestibular-evoked myogenic potential; *PTA*, pure-tone average; *SDT*, speech detection threshold; *SRT*, speech reception threshold.
From Flint PW et al: *Cummings otolaryngology, head and neck surgery*, ed 7, Philadelphia, 2021, Elsevier.

TABLE 49 History Taking for a Chief Complaint of Hearing Loss

Duration	What difficulty is this causing the individual?
Progression	Prior ear infection/trauma/surgery
Slow versus rapid	Noise exposure
Sudden	Family history of hearing loss
Fluctuating	Ototoxic medication exposure
Symmetric or asymmetric?	Prior amplification experience
Associated ear symptoms	
Tinnitus	
Vertigo	
Otalgia	
Otorrhea	

From Flint PW et al: *Cummings otolaryngology, head and neck surgery*, ed 7, Philadelphia, 2021, Elsevier.

TABLE 50 Red Flags for Hearing Loss History

Unilateral	Otalgia
Sudden onset	Accompanying cranial nerve signs
Fluctuation	Numbness
Rapidly progressive	Diplopia
Vertigo or ataxia	Facial paresis
Otorrhea	Voice/swallowing changes

From Flint PW et al: *Cummings otolaryngology, head and neck surgery*, ed 7, Philadelphia, 2021, Elsevier.

TABLE 51 History Taking for a Chief Complaint of Tinnitus

Duration	Associated ear symptoms
Progression	Vertigo
Slow versus rapid	Hearing loss
Sudden	Otalgia
Fluctuating	Otorrhea
Symmetric or asymmetric?	Prior ear infection/trauma/surgery
Pulsatile or nonpulsatile?	Noise exposure
How does it sound?	Family history of hearing loss
Mitigating factors	Caffeine or other stimulant consumption
Prior therapies	

From Flint PW et al: *Cummings otolaryngology, head and neck surgery*, ed 7, Philadelphia, 2021, Elsevier.

TABLE 52 Interpreting the Weber and Rinne Tuning Fork Tests

	Weber to Left	**Weber to Right**
Rinne + AU	SNHL AD (or mild CHL AS)	SNHL AS (or mild CHL AD)
Rinne − AS	CHL AS	Mixed HL AS[a]
Rinne − AD	Mixed HL AD[a]	CHL AD
Rinne − AU	CHL AS, Mixed HL AD	CHL AD, Mixed HL AS

AD, Right ear; *AS*, left ear; *AU*, bilateral; *CHL*, conductive HL; *HL*, hearing loss; *SNHL*, sensorineural hearing loss.
[a]It is also possible that the Rinne could be heard in the normal-hearing contralateral ear in cases of profound SNHL in the test ear due to inability to mask.
From Flint PW et al: *Cummings otolaryngology, head and neck surgery*, ed 7, Philadelphia, 2021, Elsevier.

TABLE 53 Hearing Loss Classification and Features

Criteria	Classification	Comment
Causality	Genetic	Hereditary
	Environmental	Nonhereditary
	Multifactorial	
Time of onset	Congenital	At birth
	Acquired	Develops any time after birth
Age of onset	Prelingual	Before speech development
	Postlingual	After speech development
Clinical presentation	Nonsyndromic	Hearing loss only symptom
	Syndromic	Hearing loss and other symptoms
Anatomic defect	Conductive	Dysfunction of outer or middle ear
	Sensorineural	Dysfunction of inner ear or auditory nerve
	Mixed	
Severity	Slight	16-25 dB
	Mild	26-40 dB
	Moderate	41-55 dB
	Moderately severe	56-70 dB
	Severe	71-90 dB
	Profound	>90 dB

Clinical Algorithms

III

Continued

Table 53   Hearing Loss Classification and Features—cont'd

Criteria	Classification	Comment
Frequency loss	Low frequency	<500 Hz
	Mid frequency	501-2000 Hz
	High frequency	>2000 Hz
Ears affected	Unilateral	One ear affected
	Bilateral	Both ears affected
	Symmetric	Both ears affected equally
	Asymmetric	Both ears not affected equally
Prognosis	Stable	Severity remains unchanged
	Progressive	Severity increases over time

From Flint PW et al: *Cummings otolaryngology, head and neck surgery*, ed 7, Philadelphia 2021, Elsevier.

TABLE 54   Quantification of Hearing Impairment

Impairment (%)	Pure Tone Average (dB)[a]	Residual Hearing (%)
100	91	0
80	78	20
60	65	40
30	45	70

[a]Pure tone average of 500, 1000, 2000, and 3000 Hz.
From Flint PW et al: *Cummings otolaryngology, head and neck surgery*, ed 7, Philadelphia 2021, Elsevier.

TABLE 55   Differential Diagnosis of Sudden Sensorineural Hearing Loss

Category	Etiology
Infectious	Serous or suppurative labyrinthitis Viral (e.g., mumps, rubella, rubeola, varicella zoster, herpes simplex, HIV/AIDS, mononucleosis, Lassa fever, Zika, West Nile virus) Bacterial (e.g., Streptococcal meningitis, syphilis, Lyme, mycoplasma, cryptococcal meningitis)
Neoplastic	Acoustic neuroma/vestibular schwannoma Meningioma Epidermoid Hemangioma Arachnoid cyst Temporal bone metastasis, meningeal carcinomatosis Lymphoma, leukemia, myeloma
Traumatic	Acoustic trauma Temporal bone fracture, penetrating trauma Inner ear concussion Perilymphatic fistula Barotrauma
Ototoxic	Ototoxic medications (e.g., aminoglycosides, chemotherapeutics) Medication overuse or abuse (e.g., acetaminophen/opiate combinations, heroin, methadone, cocaine)
Immunologic	Autoimmune inner ear disease Autoimmune disease (e.g., Cogan syndrome, systemic lupus erythematosus, granulomatosis with polyangiitis, polyarteritis nodosa, relapsing polychondritis, sarcoidosis) Multiple sclerosis
Vascular	Cerebrovascular accident Vertebrobasilar insufficiency Migraine Sickle cell disease Macroglobulinemia Cardiopulmonary bypass
Developmental	Large vestibular aqueduct
Idiopathic	Idiopathic sudden sensorineural hearing loss Ménière disease Nonorganic hearing loss (factitious, malingering, or conversion disorder)

From Flint PW et al: *Cummings otolaryngology, head and neck surgery*, ed 7, Philadelphia 2021, Elsevier.

TABLE 56 Comparison of Conventional Hearing Aids and Implantable Hearing Devices

Device	Sensor	Actuator	Regulatory Approval	Totally/Partially Implanted	Surgical Placement	Audiologic Indications	MRI	Special Advantages/ Disadvantages	EAC Occlusion
Conventional digital BTE device	External BTE microphone	Acoustic, to TM	Yes	NA	NA	Mild to severe CHL or SNHL	NA	No surgery required; visible; EAC occlusion	Yes, unless open fit
Conventional digital CIC device	External microphone at lateral end of CIC device	Acoustic, to TM	Yes	NA	NA	Mild to moderate CHL or SNHL	NA	No surgery required, low visibility; EAC occlusion	Yes
Esteem (Envoy Medical)	Piezoelectric, coupled to malleus/TM	Piezoelectric, to stapes	FDA CE mark	Total	Transmastoid, mandatory partial incus removal		No	Very high power; requires partial incus removal	No
Carina (Cochlear)	Subcutaneous microphone	Piezoelectric, to incus	CE mark, FDA Phase II clinical trials	Total	Transmastoid	Moderate to severe	No	High-powered output, fully implantable; ossicles remain intact; adjustable for ossicular abnormalities	No
Vibrant Soundbridge (Med-EI)	External BTE microphone	Electromagnetic, clipped to incus	FDA CE mark	Partial	Transmastoid and endaural		No	First FDA approved; largest install base	No
Baha (Cochlear)	External microphone	Electromagnetic vibrator, coupled to titanium screw in skull	FDA CE mark	Partial	Cortical skull bone screw	CHL, inability to tolerate conventional HA, SSD	Yes	Simple placement, nothing in ear or mastoid	No
Ponto (Oticon Medical)	External microphone	Electromagnetic vibrator, coupled to titanium screw in skull	FDA CE mark	Partial	Cortical skull bone screw	CHL, inability to tolerate conventional HA, SSD	Yes	Simple placement, nothing in ear or mastoid	No
Alpha 2 (Sophono)	External microphone	Electromagnetic vibrator, transcutaneously coupled to osseointegrated implant	FDA CE mark	Partial	Cortical skull bone well and screws	CHL unable to tolerate conventional HA, SSD	No	No percutaneous abutment	No
Bonebridge (Med-EI)	External microphone	Electromagnetic vibrator, transcutaneously coupled to osseointegrated implant	CE mark	Partial	Cortical skull bone well and screws	CHL, inability to tolerate conventional HA, SSD	No	No percutaneous abutment	No
SoundBite (Sonitus Medical)	External BTE microphone	Piezoelectric, to maxillary molars	FDA CE mark	NA	NA	CHL inability to tolerate conventional HA, SSD	NA	No surgery required; visible; EAC occlusion	No

BTE, Behind the ear; *CE*, Communauté Européenne; *CHL*, conductive hearing loss; *CIC*, completely in canal; *EAC*, external auditory canal; *FDA*, U.S. Food and Drug Administration; *HA*, hearing aid; *MRI*, magnetic resonance imaging; *NA*, not applicable; *SMHL*, sensorineural hearing loss; *SSD*, single-sided deafness; *TM*, tympanic membrane.
From Flint PW et al: *Cummings otolaryngology, head and neck surgery*, ed 7, Philadelphia 2021, Elsevier.

Clinical Algorithms

III

BOX 18   History and Physical Examination for Hearing Loss

Onset
- Age at onset
- Abrupt versus gradual
- Progressive, intermittent, or continuous
- Antecedent illness
- Duration of symptoms

Associated Symptoms
- Tinnitus
- Dizziness or vertigo
- Aural fullness
- Pain
- Allergy symptoms
- Actions that change intensity of symptoms
- Distorted auditory perception
- Worsening with pregnancy or oral contraceptive use

Further History
- Family history of hearing loss
- Occupational noise exposure
- Recreational noise exposure
- Trauma
- Surgical history
- Previous or current drainage from ear
- Quality of drainage
- Systemic infections and treatments
- Meningitis
- Syphilis
- Previous use of a hearing aid
- Ototoxic medications
- Cancer chemotherapy
- Antibiotics
- Recent air travel
- Recent underwater diving

Examination
- Complete head and neck examination
- Cranial nerve examination
- Otoscopy with microscope as needed
- Otoneurologic examination as indicated
- Tuning fork testing (256 Hz, 512 Hz, 1024 Hz)
- Weber test
- Rinne test

Radiographic and Laboratory Evaluation
- Computed tomography as indicated
- Magnetic resonance imaging as indicated
- Erythrocyte sedimentation rate; fluorescent treponemal antibody, absorbed; Lyme titers; complete blood count; thyroid function tests; electrolytes; urinalysis (additional studies are indicated to work up suspected systemic diseases)

Audiometric Evaluation
- Pure tone audiometry
- Air conduction
- Bone conduction
- Speech testing
- Speech reception threshold
- Speech discrimination testing
- Immittance testing
- Static compliance
- Tympanometry
- Acoustic reflexes

Additional Audiometric Testing
- Auditory brain stem response
- Electrocochleography
- Otoacoustic emissions

From Flint PW et al: *Cummings otolaryngology, head and neck surgery*, ed 7, Philadelphia 2021, Elsevier.

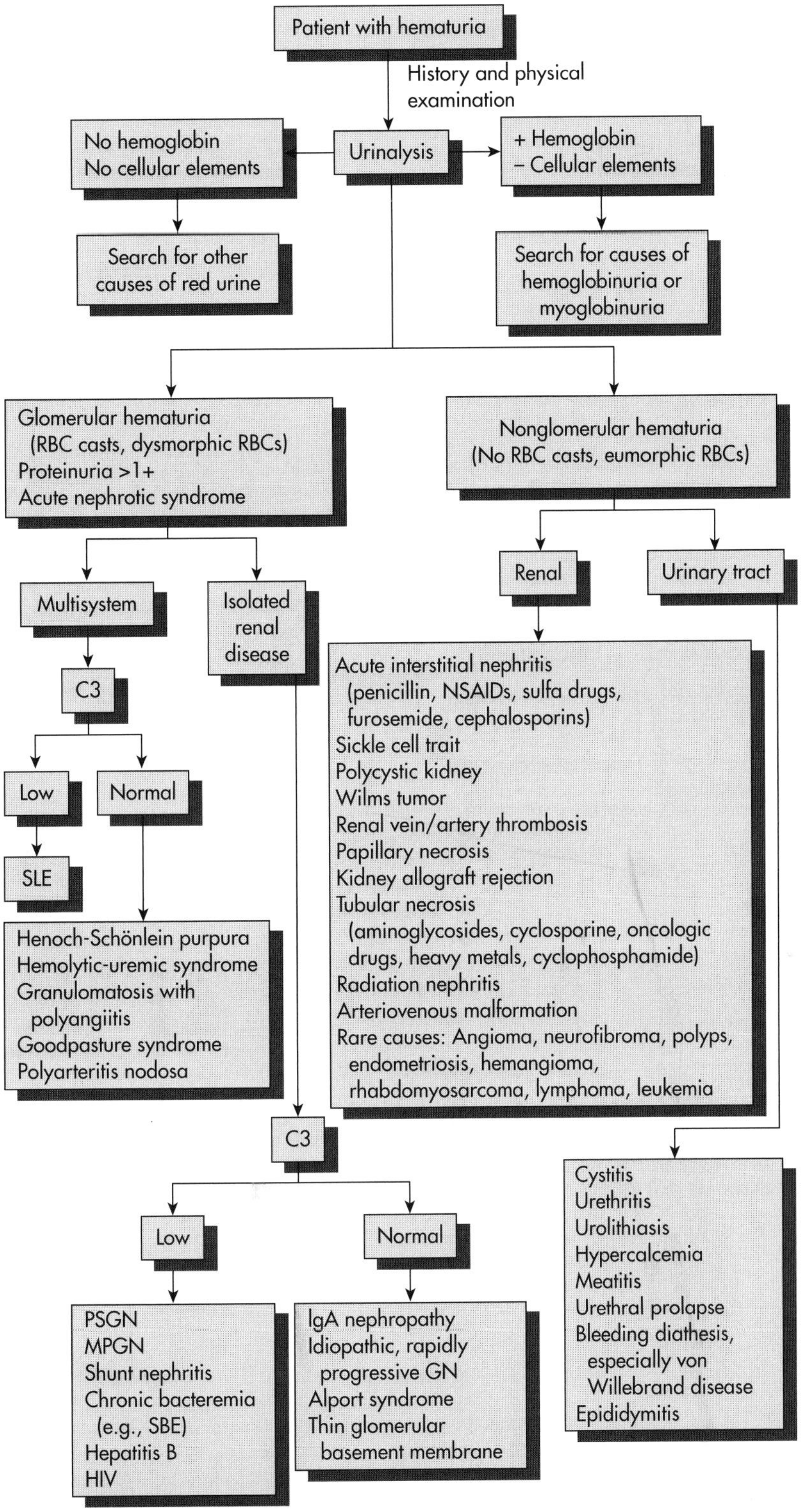

Patient with hematuria

History and physical examination

No hemoglobin
No cellular elements ← Urinalysis → + Hemoglobin
– Cellular elements

Search for other causes of red urine

Search for causes of hemoglobinuria or myoglobinuria

Glomerular hematuria
(RBC casts, dysmorphic RBCs)
Proteinuria >1+
Acute nephrotic syndrome

Nonglomerular hematuria
(No RBC casts, eumorphic RBCs)

Renal   Urinary tract

Multisystem   Isolated renal disease

C3

Low   Normal

SLE

Henoch-Schönlein purpura
Hemolytic-uremic syndrome
Granulomatosis with polyangiitis
Goodpasture syndrome
Polyarteritis nodosa

Acute interstitial nephritis
(penicillin, NSAIDs, sulfa drugs, furosemide, cephalosporins)
Sickle cell trait
Polycystic kidney
Wilms tumor
Renal vein/artery thrombosis
Papillary necrosis
Kidney allograft rejection
Tubular necrosis
(aminoglycosides, cyclosporine, oncologic drugs, heavy metals, cyclophosphamide)
Radiation nephritis
Arteriovenous malformation
Rare causes: Angioma, neurofibroma, polyps, endometriosis, hemangioma, rhabdomyosarcoma, lymphoma, leukemia

C3

Low   Normal

PSGN
MPGN
Shunt nephritis
Chronic bacteremia
(e.g., SBE)
Hepatitis B
HIV

IgA nephropathy
Idiopathic, rapidly progressive GN
Alport syndrome
Thin glomerular basement membrane

Cystitis
Urethritis
Urolithiasis
Hypercalcemia
Meatitis
Urethral prolapse
Bleeding diathesis, especially von Willebrand disease
Epididymitis

Clinical Algorithms

FIG. 91 Diagnostic strategy for hematuria. *GN,* Glomerulonephritis; *HIV,* human immunodeficiency virus; *Ig,* immunoglobulin; *MPGN,* membranoproliferative glomerulonephritis; *NSAIDs,* nonsteroidal antiinflammatory drugs; *PSGN,* poststreptococcal glomerulonephritis; *RBC,* red blood cell; *SBE,* subacute bacterial endocarditis; *SLE,* systemic lupus erythematosus. (From The Johns Hopkins Hospital et al: *The Harriet Lane handbook,* ed 21, St Louis, 2018, Elsevier.)

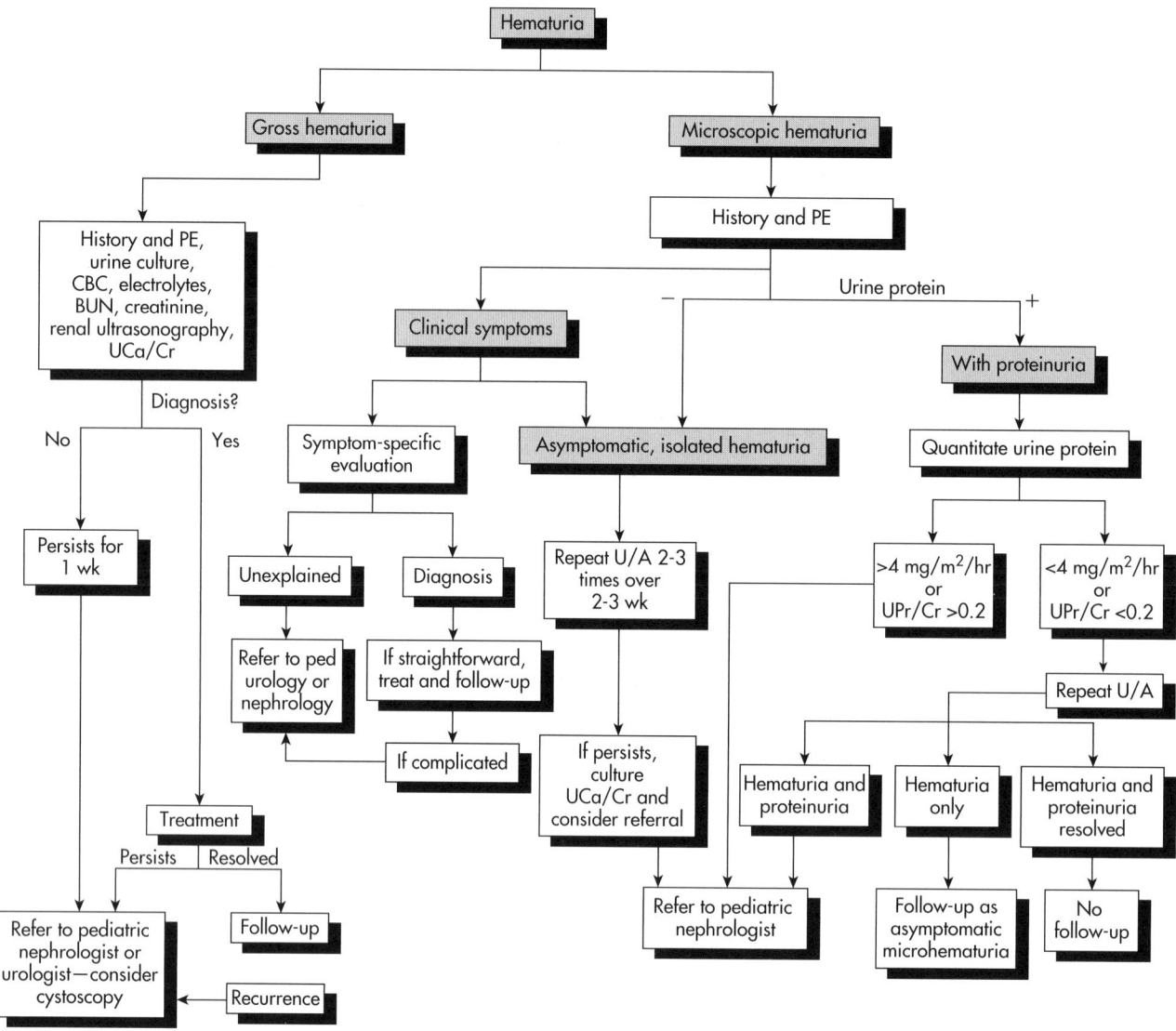

FIG. 92 Algorithm for the treatment of hematuria. *BUN,* Blood urea nitrogen; *CBC,* complete blood cell count; *PE,* physical examination; *U/A,* urinalysis; *UCa/Cr,* urinary calcium/creatinine ratio; *UPr/Cr,* urinary protein/creatinine ratio. (From Wein AJ et al: *Campbell-Walsh urology,* ed 11, Philadelphia, 2016, Elsevier.)

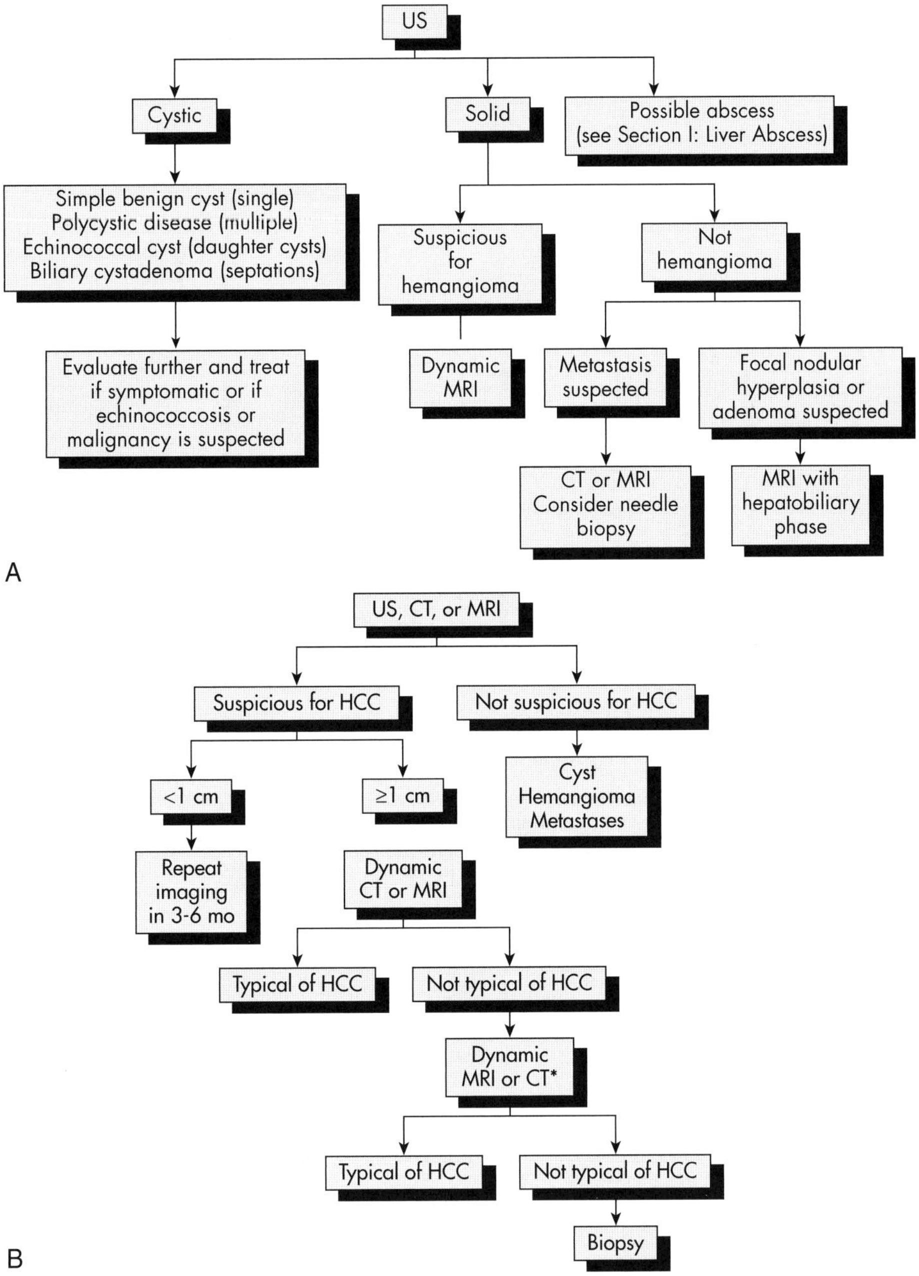

US

Cystic

Solid

Possible abscess
(see Section I: Liver Abscess)

Simple benign cyst (single)
Polycystic disease (multiple)
Echinococcal cyst (daughter cysts)
Biliary cystadenoma (septations)

Suspicious
for
hemangioma

Not
hemangioma

Evaluate further and treat
if symptomatic or if
echinococcosis or
malignancy is suspected

Dynamic
MRI

Metastasis
suspected

Focal nodular
hyperplasia or
adenoma suspected

CT or MRI
Consider needle
biopsy

MRI with
hepatobiliary
phase

A

US, CT, or MRI

Suspicious for HCC

Not suspicious for HCC

<1 cm

≥1 cm

Cyst
Hemangioma
Metastases

Repeat
imaging
in 3-6 mo

Dynamic
CT or MRI

Typical of HCC

Not typical of HCC

Dynamic
MRI or CT*

Typical of HCC

Not typical of HCC

Biopsy

B

FIG. 93 A, Algorithm for the approach to the management of a patient, not known to have cirrhosis, with a hepatic mass (often incidental, possibly symptomatic). B, Algorithm for the approach to the management of a patient with known or suspected cirrhosis and a hepatic mass (found on routine surveillance, because of symptoms, or because of an increasing alpha-fetoprotein level). *Perform imaging modality not previously performed. *CT,* Computed tomography; *HCC,* hepatocellular carcinoma; *MRI,* magnetic resonance imaging; *US,* ultrasound. (From Feldman M et al: *Sleisenger and Fortran's gastrointestinal and liver disease,* ed 10, Philadelphia, 2016, Elsevier.)

Clinical
Algorithms

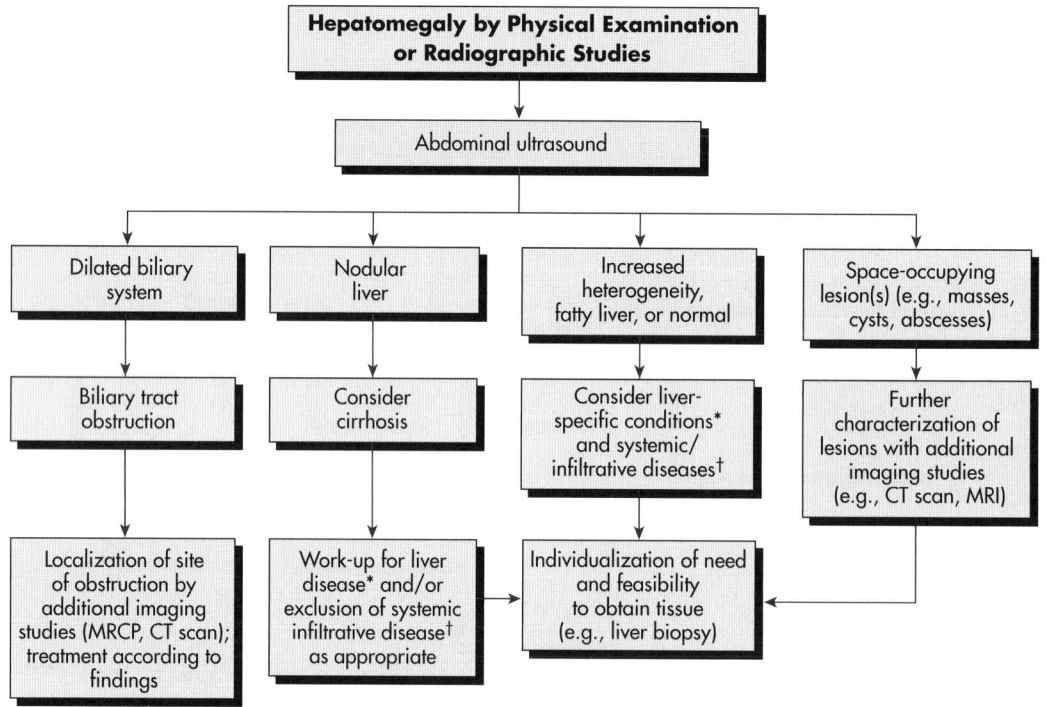

FIG. 94 Diagnostic approach to hepatomegaly. *Conditions to be excluded include viral hepatitis; alcohol- and drug-induced liver disease; steatohepatitis; autoimmune liver diseases; and metabolic disorders, including hemochromatosis, Wilson disease, and α 1-antitrypsin deficiency. †Systemic and infiltrative diseases include amyloidosis, lymphoma, sarcoidosis, and infectious processes such as disseminated tuberculosis and fungemia. *CT*, Computed tomography; *MRCP*, magnetic resonance cholangiopancreatography; *MRI*, magnetic resonance imaging. (From Goldman L, Shafer AI: *Goldman-Cecil medicine*, ed 26, Elsevier, 2020.)

TABLE 57 Approach to Common Hepatic Complaints

Presentation	Common Symptoms	Common Physical Signs	Diagnostic Studies	Common Diagnoses
Ascites	Abdominal distention and pain, ankle edema	Flank dullness Shifting dullness Fluid wave	Ultrasound with Doppler Diagnostic paracentesis Urinalysis	Cirrhosis Budd-Chiari syndrome Heart failure Nephrotic syndrome
Hepatic encephalopathy	Sleep disorientation, confusion, coma	Asterixis Altered mentation Fetor hepaticus	Serum ammonia Blood cultures Stool hemoccult Serum creatinine and electrolytes	Decompensated cirrhosis Acute liver failure Other metabolic encephalopathies (renal, respiratory)
Hepatic mass	None or abdominal pain	Hepatic bruit or rub	α-Fetoprotein Ultrasound CT scan MRI Biopsy	Benign lesions: Hemangioma, adenoma, focal nodular hyperplasia Malignant lesions: Hepatocellular carcinoma, cholangiocarcinoma, metastases
Abdominal pain	Nausea, vomiting, fever	Right upper quadrant tenderness Palpable gallbladder Murphy sign	Ultrasound HIDA scan Paracentesis for ascites if present	Biliary colic Acute cholecystitis Hepatic congestion Hepatic metastases

CT, Computed tomography; *HIDA*, hepatobiliary iminodiacetic acid; *MRI*, magnetic resonance imaging.
From Goldman L, Shafer AI: *Goldman-Cecil medicine*, ed 26, Philadelphia, 2020, Elsevier.

BOX 19   Clinical Clues Suggesting Chronic Liver Disease

Symptoms
- Fatigue, pruritus, bleeding, abdominal pain, nausea, anorexia, myalgia, jaundice, dark urine, pale stools, fever, weight loss; may be no symptoms

Signs
Peripheral signs of chronic liver disease with hepatocellular dysfunction:
- Spider nevi, palmar erythema, white nails, gynecomastia, body hair loss, testicular atrophy, hepatomegaly

Signs of portal hypertension:
- Splenomegaly, ascites, peripheral edema

Signs of poor hepatocellular synthetic function:
- Bruising, peripheral edema (reflecting depleted coagulation factors and albumin levels)

Signs of end-stage liver disease:
- Wasting, progressive severe fatigue, encephalopathy (asterixis, fetor, coma)

From Talley NJ et al: *Essentials of internal medicine*, ed 4, Chatswood, NSW, 2021, Elsevier Australia.

BOX 20   Causes of Hepatomegaly

1. Diffusely enlarged and smooth
Massive
- Metastatic disease
- Alcoholic liver disease with fatty infiltration
- Myeloproliferative diseases (e.g., polycythemia rubra vera, myelofibrosis)

Moderate
- The above causes
- Hematologic disease (e.g., chronic myeloid leukemia, lymphoma)
- Fatty liver (e.g., diabetes mellitus)
- Hemochromatosis

Mild
- The above causes
- Hepatitis (viral, drugs)
- Cirrhosis
- Biliary obstruction
- Granulomatous disorders (e.g., sarcoidosis)
- Infiltrative disorders (e.g., amyloidosis)
- Human immunodeficiency virus infection

2. Diffusely enlarged and irregular
- Metastatic disease
- Cirrhosis
- Hydatid disease
- Polycystic liver disease

3. Localized swelling
- Riedel lobe (a normal variant—the lobe may even be palpable in the right lumbar region)
- Metastasis
- Large simple hepatic cyst
- Hydatid cyst
- Hepatoma
- Liver abscess (e.g., amebic abscess)

4. Hepatosplenomegaly
- Chronic liver disease with portal hypertension
- Hematologic disease (e.g., myeloproliferative disease, lymphoma)
- Infection (e.g., acute viral hepatitis, infectious mononucleosis)
- Infiltration (e.g., amyloidosis, sarcoidosis)
- Connective tissue disease (e.g., systemic lupus erythematosus)

From Talley NJ et al: *Essentials of internal medicine*, ed 4, Chatswood, NSW, 2021, Elsevier Australia.

Clinical
Algorithms

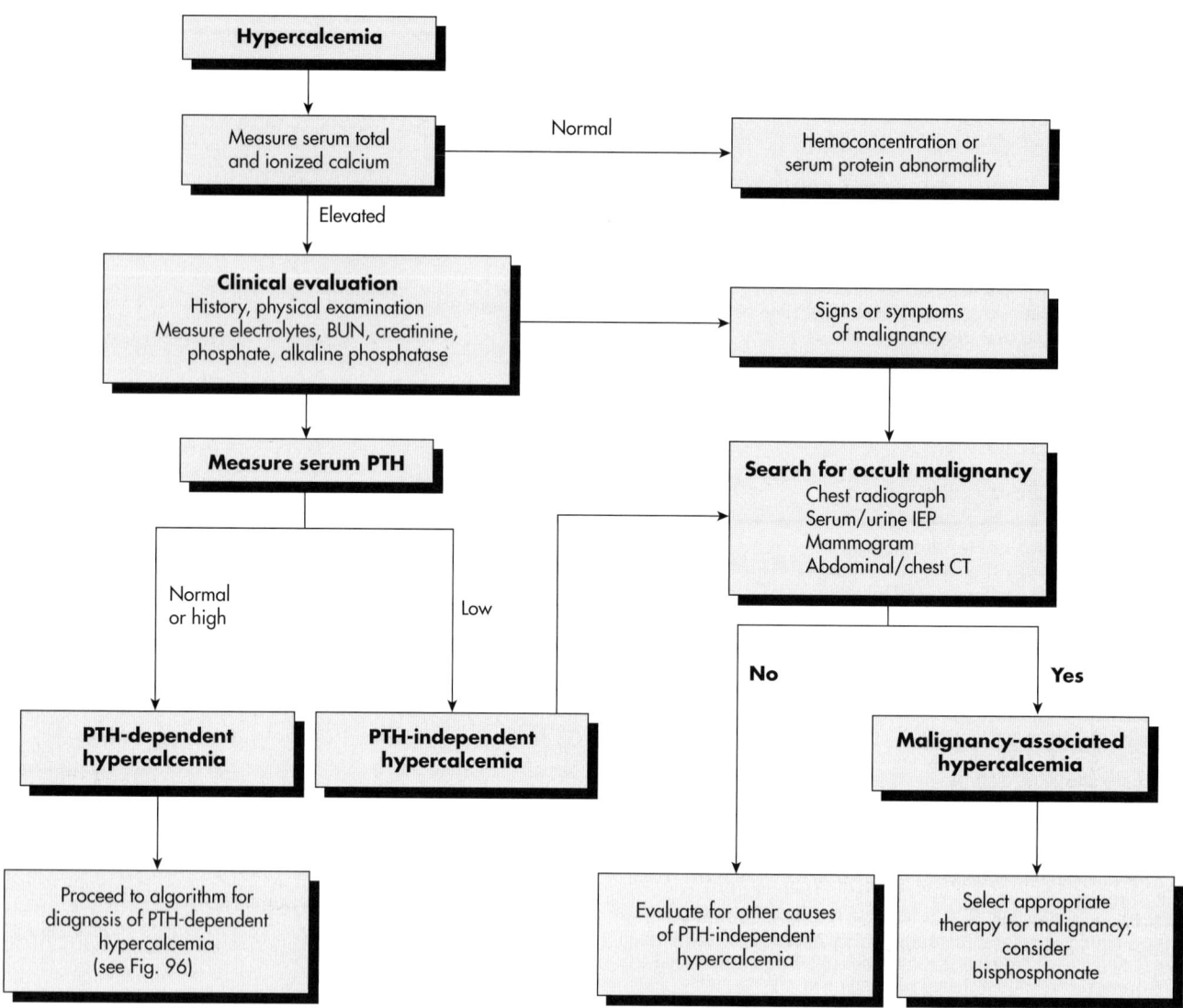

FIG. 95 Approach to the management of the hypercalcemic patient. *BUN,* Blood urea nitrogen; *CT,* computed tomography; *IEP,* immunoelectrophoresis; *PTH,* parathyroid hormone. (From Melmed S et al. *Williams textbook of endocrinology,* ed 14, Philadelphia, 2019, Elsevier.)

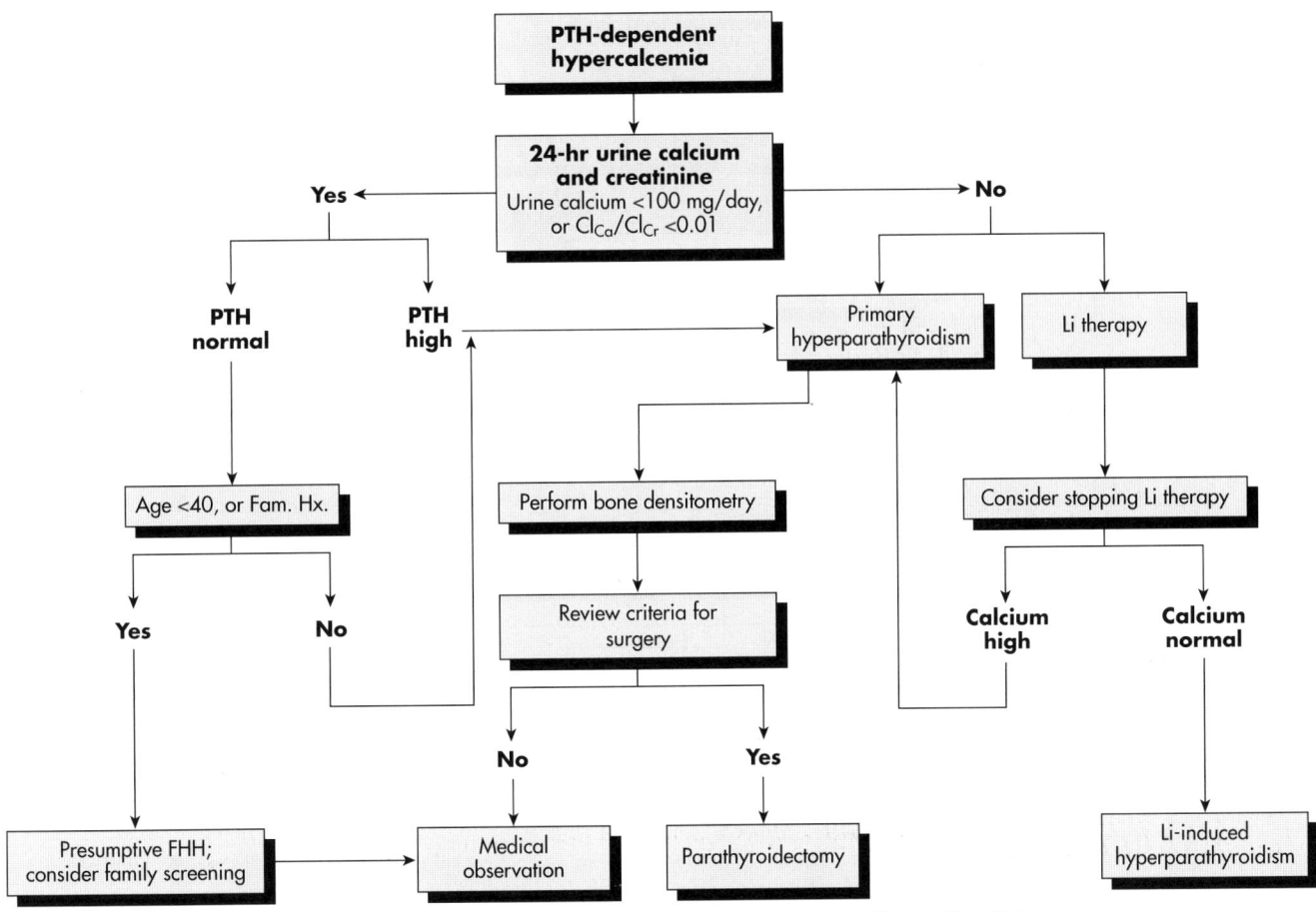

FIG. 96 Approach to the management of the hypercalcemic patient with parathyroid hormone–dependent hypercalcemia. *Cl,* Clearance; *Fam. Hx.,* family history; *FHH,* familial hypocalciuric hypercalcemia; *Li,* lithium; *PTH,* parathyroid hormone. (From Melmed S et al. *Williams textbook of endocrinology*, ed 14, Philadelphia, 2019, Elsevier.)

DIAGNOSTIC IMAGING

- Radiograph of painful bones (r/o bone neoplasm, multiple myeloma)
- Tc-99m parathyroid scan (r/o parathyroid adenoma)
- Ultrasound of parathyroid glands
- Ultrasound of kidneys (r/o renal cell carcinoma)

LAB EVALUATION

- Serum calcium level
- PTH level
- Serum phosphate, magnesium, alkaline phosphatase, albumin
- Electrolytes, BUN, creatinine
- 24-h urine collection for calcium
- Urinary cyclic AMP
- PSA (if prostate carcinoma is suspected)
- Serum and urine protein immunoelectrophoresis (if multiple myeloma suspected)

TABLE 58   Important Physiologic Changes in Bone and Mineral Diseases

CONDITION	CALCIUM	PHOSPHATE	PARATHYROID HORMONE	25(OH)D
Primary hypoparathyroidism	↓	↑	↓	Nl
Pseudohypoparathyroidism	↓	↑	↑	Nl
Vitamin D deficiency	Nl(↓)	↓	↑	↓
Familial hypophosphatemic rickets	Nl	↓	Nl (sl↑)	Nl
Hyperparathyroidism	↑	↓	↑	Nl
Immobilization	↑	↑	↓	Nl

25(OH)D, 25-hydroxyvitamin D; *Nl,* normal; *sl,* slight; ↑, high; ↓, low.
From Marcdante KJ et al: *Nelson essentials of pediatrics*, ed 9, Philadelphia, 2023, Elsevier.

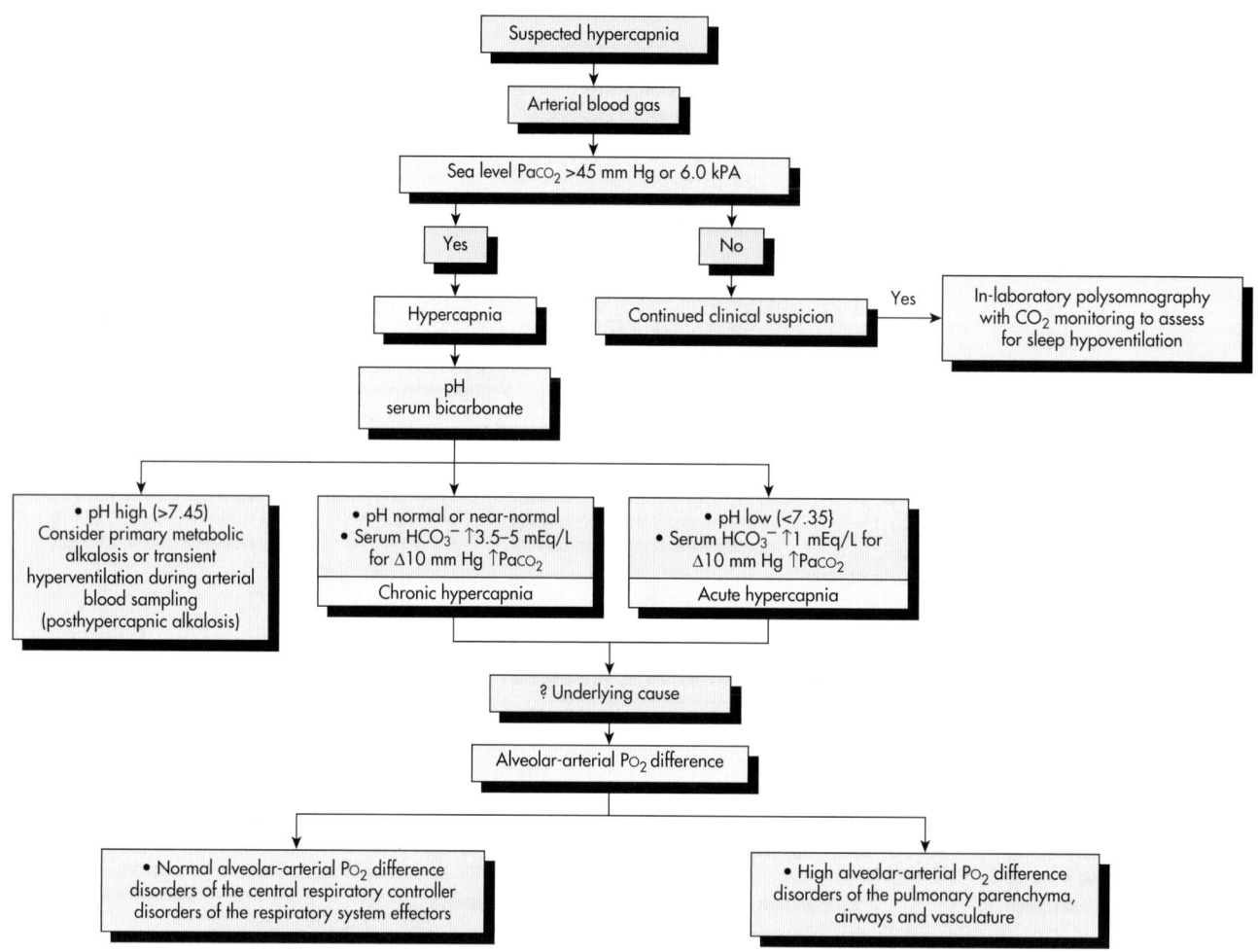

FIG. 97 Algorithm demonstrating a diagnostic approach to a patient with suspected hypercapnia. paO_2, Alveolar pO_2; paO_2, arterial pO_2; $paCO_2$, alveolar pCO_2; $paCO_2$, arterial pCO_2. (From Broaddus VC et al: *Murray & Nadel's textbook of respiratory medicine*, ed 7, Philadelphia, 2022, Elsevier.)

TABLE 59 Classification of Hypercapnic Diseases

	MECHANISM	DIAGNOSIS	TREATMENT
ACQUIRED DISEASE			
Narcotic overdose	Reduced central drive	History, narcotized pupils, toxicology	Supportive care, naloxone
Acute severe asthma	Severe airflow obstruction, high dead space	Typical history, wheezing on examination, low FEV_1/FVC	Bronchodilators, antiinflammatories, mechanical ventilation (usually invasive)
Acute exacerbation of COPD	Airflow obstruction, high dead space	History, cigarette smoking, low FEV_1/FVC, infectious etiology	Bronchodilators, antiinflammatories, noninvasive ventilation
Obesity-hypoventilation syndrome	Low respiratory system compliance, high upper airway resistance, low central drive	High BMI, lack of other diagnoses; blunted carbon dioxide response	Weight loss, nocturnal bilevel positive airway pressure
Neuromuscular disease (e.g., myasthenia gravis, ALS, polymyositis, GBS/AIDP)	Lack of respiratory muscle force	Immediate orthopnea, low VC, low MIPs/MEPs	Underlying cause, nocturnal noninvasive ventilation, supportive care
Severe parenchymal lung disease, e.g., COPD	Lack of alveolar surface area; high pulmonary dead space and work of breathing	Typical history, smoking, low FEV_1 and FEV_1/FVC	Bronchodilator, antiinflammatory therapy, possible nocturnal noninvasive ventilation, smoking cessation
Kyphoscoliosis	Low respiratory system compliance	Physical examination	Supportive care, noninvasive ventilation
CONGENITAL DISEASE			
Central congenital hypoventilation syndrome	*PHOX2B* mutation, lack of central drive	Genetic testing	Supportive care, mechanical ventilation (usually noninvasive)

AIDP, Acute inflammatory demyelinating polyneuropathy; *ALS*, amyotrophic lateral sclerosis; *BMI*, body mass index; *COPD*, chronic obstructive pulmonary disease; *FEV₁*, forced expiratory volume in 1 second; *FVC*, forced vital capacity; *GBS*, Guillain-Barré syndrome; *MEPs*, maximal expiratory pressures; *MIPs*, maximal inspiratory pressures; *VC*, vital capacity.
From Goldman L, Shafer AI: *Goldman-Cecil medicine*, ed 26, Philadelphia, 2019, Elsevier.

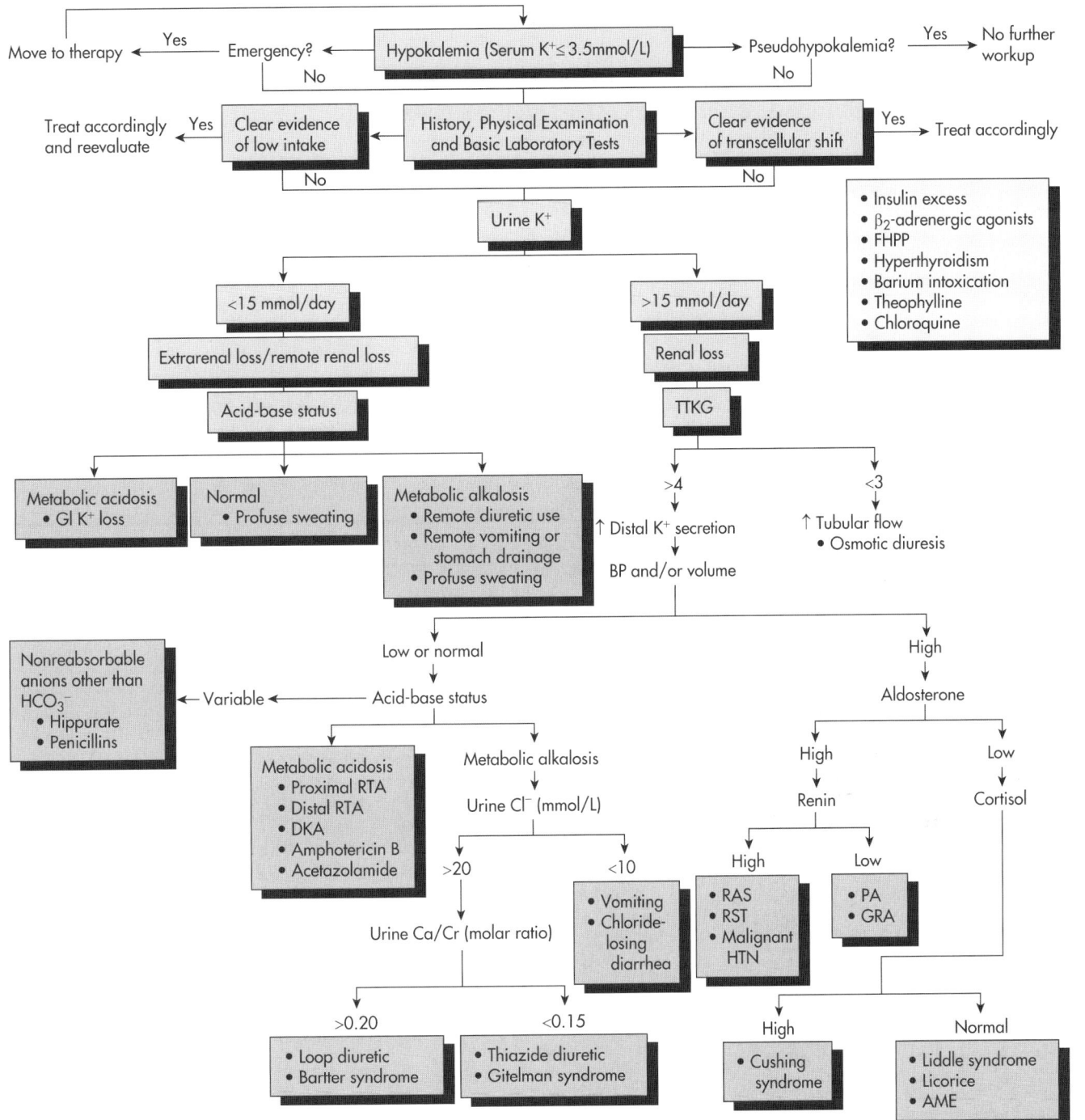

FIG. 101 Clinical approach to hypokalemia. *AME,* Apparent mineralocorticoid excess; *BP,* blood pressure; *CCD,* cortical collecting duct; *DKA,* diabetic ketoacidosis; *FHPP,* familial hypokalemic periodic paralysis; *GI,* gastrointestinal; *GRA,* glucocorticoid-remediable aldosteronism; *HTN,* hypertension; *PA,* primary aldosteronism; *RAS,* renal artery stenosis; *RST,* renin-secreting tumor; *RTA,* renal tubular acidosis; *TTKG,* transtubular potassium gradient. (From Skorecki K et al: *Brenner & Rector's the kidney,* ed 10, Philadelphia, 2016, Elsevier.)

Clinical Algorithms

III

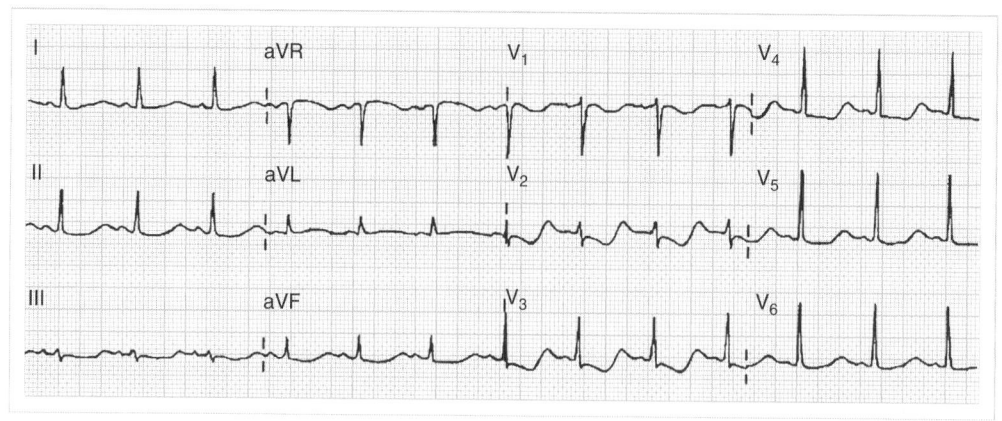

FIG. 102 Hypokalemia. This 12-lead ECG shows the findings of hypokalemia, including ST depression (which can mimic myocardial ischemia), flattening of T waves, prolongation of the QT interval, and increased prominence of the U wave. The merging of the T and U waves makes distinguishing and measuring them more difficult. In this case the potassium level was 1.5 mEq/L. (From Olshansky B et al: *Arrhythmia essentials*, ed 2, Philadelphia, 2017, Elsevier.)

BOX 21   Causes of Acute Hypokalemia

- Treatment of diabetic ketoacidosis
- Refeeding syndrome
- Rapid cell production
  Vitamin B_{12} treatment of pernicious anemia
  GM-CSF treatment of leukopenia
- Pharmacologic agents
  β_2-Adrenoceptor agonists
  Epinephrine
  Soluble barium salts
- Hypokalemic periodic paralysis
  Familial
  Sporadic
  Thyrotoxic
- Pseudohypokalemia

From Parrillo JE, Dellinger RP: *Critical care medicine, principles of diagnosis and management in the adult*, ed 5, Philadelphia, 2019, Elsevier.

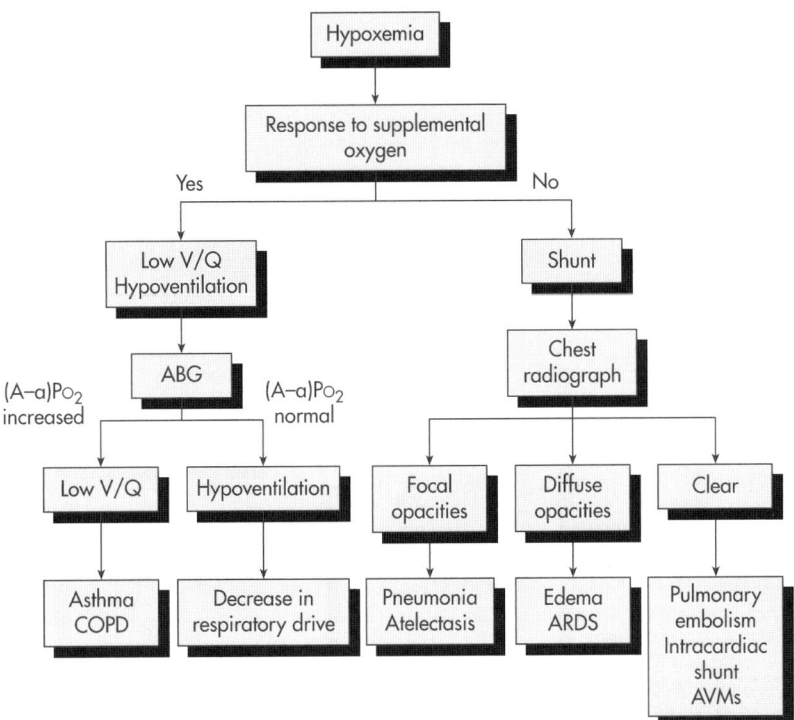

FIG. 105 A simplified algorithm for distinguishing the major clinical causes of hypoxemia. Clinically, the most important first step is in knowing whether the patient responds well to supplemental oxygen. If the response is good, the likely mechanisms are low ventilation-perfusion (V/Q) or hypoventilation; if so, an arterial blood gas (ABG) determination will be the next step. If the response to oxygen is poor, one is likely dealing with a shunt. Imaging with chest radiography will help determine the likely cause and next steps, recognizing that the chest radiograph is not as sensitive as chest computed tomography. *ARDS,* Acute respiratory distress syndrome; *AVMs,* arteriovenous malformations. (From Broaddus VC et al: *Murray & Nadel's textbook of respiratory medicine,* ed 7, Philadelphia, 2022, Elsevier.)

TABLE 62 The Danger of Undetected Hypoventilation When a Patient Is Receiving Supplemental Oxygen*

	paO$_2$	paCO$_2$
Room air	55	50
2 L/min	110	50
2 L/min	97.5	60
2 L/min	85	70
Room air	**30**	70

*In this patient receiving supplemental oxygen, the arterial pCO$_2$ starts to rise. With each 10 mm Hg rise, the arterial pO$_2$ falls 12.5 mm Hg (see text), although the arterial pO$_2$ (and oxygen saturation, not shown) never falls into a range to trigger the pulse oximeter. At the higher arterial pCO$_2$, supplemental oxygen becomes a lifeline. The supplemental oxygen in effect allows the arterial pCO$_2$ to rise without detection of a drop in oxygen saturation by the pulse oximeter. Removing the oxygen when the paCO$_2$ has risen can lead to a precipitous fall in arterial pO$_2$ (the calculated value of 30). *paCO$_2$,* Arterial partial pressure of carbon dioxide; *paO$_2$,* arterial partial pressure of oxygen.
All values in mm Hg.

INFECTIONS OF SOFT TISSUE, JOINTS, AND BONE

ICD-10CM #	T84.3	Infection and inflammatory reaction
	M00.9	Pyogenic arthritis, unspecified
	M86.9	Osteomyelitis unspecified
	M79.9	Soft tissue disorder, unspecified

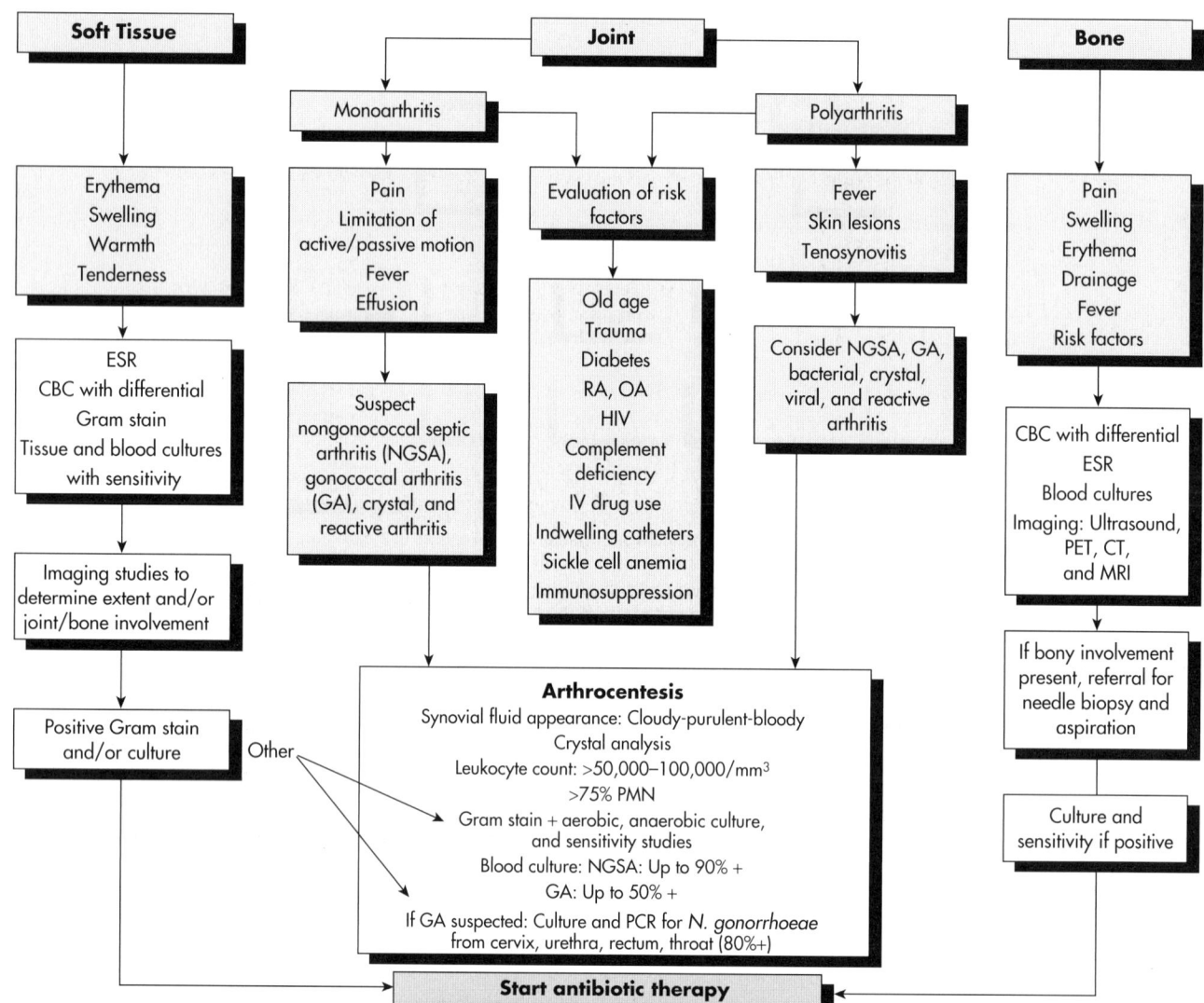

FIG. 107 Clinical evaluation of infections of soft tissues, joints, and bone. *CBC*, Complete blood count; *CT*, computed tomography; *ESR*, erythrocyte sedimentation rate; *HIV*, human immunodeficiency virus; *IV*, intravenous; *MRI*, magnetic resonance imaging; *OA*, osteoarthritis; *PCR*, polymerase chain reaction; *PET*, positron emission tomography; *PMN*, polymorphonuclear leukocyte; *RA*, rheumatoid arthritis. (From Goldman L, Schafer AI: *Goldman Cecil medicine*, ed 25, Philadelphia, 2016, Saunders.)

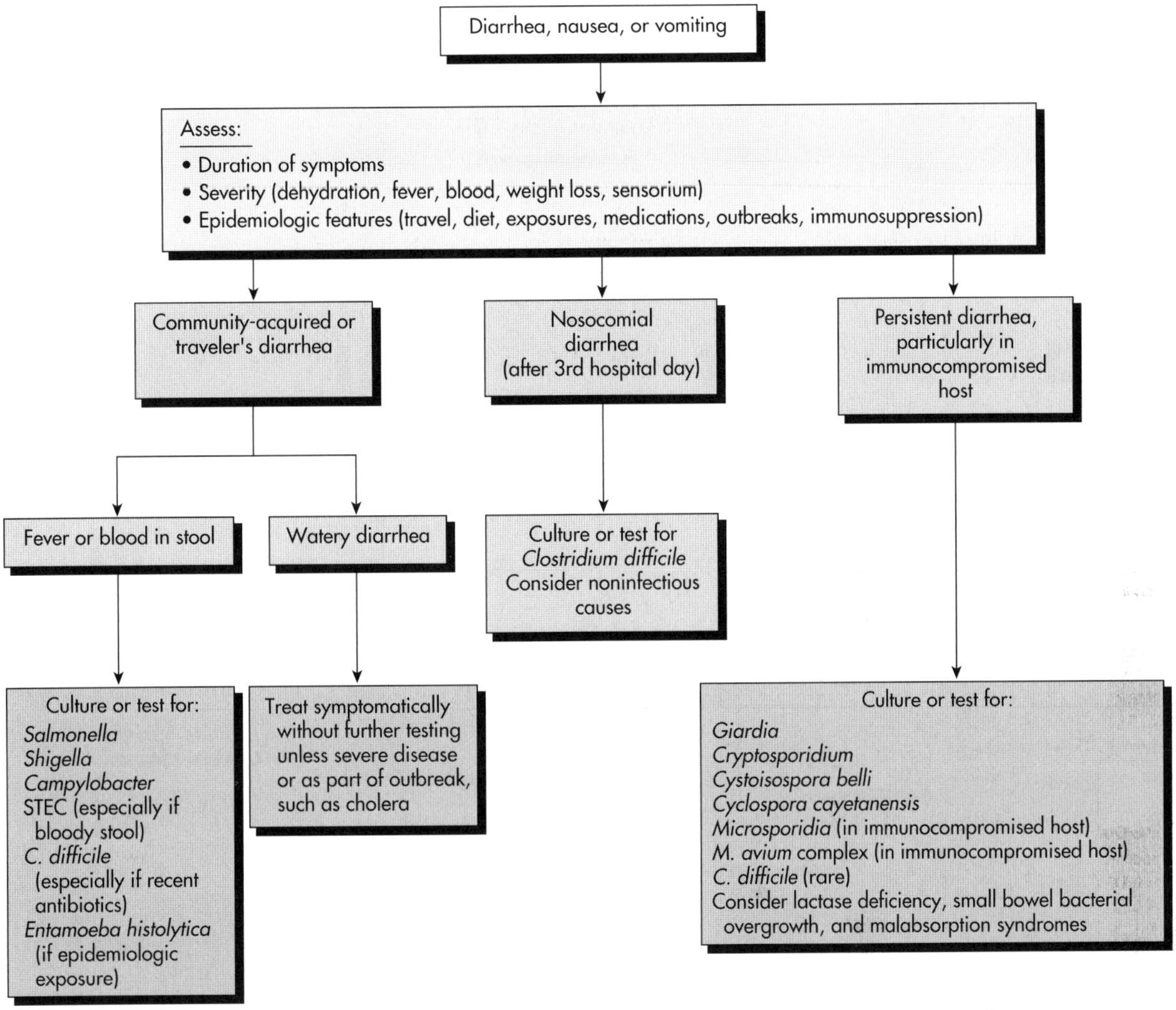

Diarrhea, nausea, or vomiting

Assess:
- Duration of symptoms
- Severity (dehydration, fever, blood, weight loss, sensorium)
- Epidemiologic features (travel, diet, exposures, medications, outbreaks, immunosuppression)

Community-acquired or traveler's diarrhea

Nosocomial diarrhea (after 3rd hospital day)

Persistent diarrhea, particularly in immunocompromised host

Fever or blood in stool

Watery diarrhea

Culture or test for *Clostridium difficile* Consider noninfectious causes

Culture or test for:
Salmonella
Shigella
Campylobacter
STEC (especially if bloody stool)
C. difficile (especially if recent antibiotics)
Entamoeba histolytica (if epidemiologic exposure)

Treat symptomatically without further testing unless severe disease or as part of outbreak, such as cholera

Culture or test for:
Giardia
Cryptosporidium
Cystoisospora belli
Cyclospora cayetanensis
Microsporidia (in immunocompromised host)
M. avium complex (in immunocompromised host)
C. difficile (rare)
Consider lactase deficiency, small bowel bacterial overgrowth, and malabsorption syndromes

FIG. 108 Approach to diagnosis of infectious diarrhea. *STEC,* Shiga toxin-producing *Escherichia coli.* (From Bennett JE et al: *Mandell, Douglas, and Bennett's principles and practice of infectious diseases,* ed 8, Philadelphia, 2015, Saunders.)

Clinical Algorithms

III

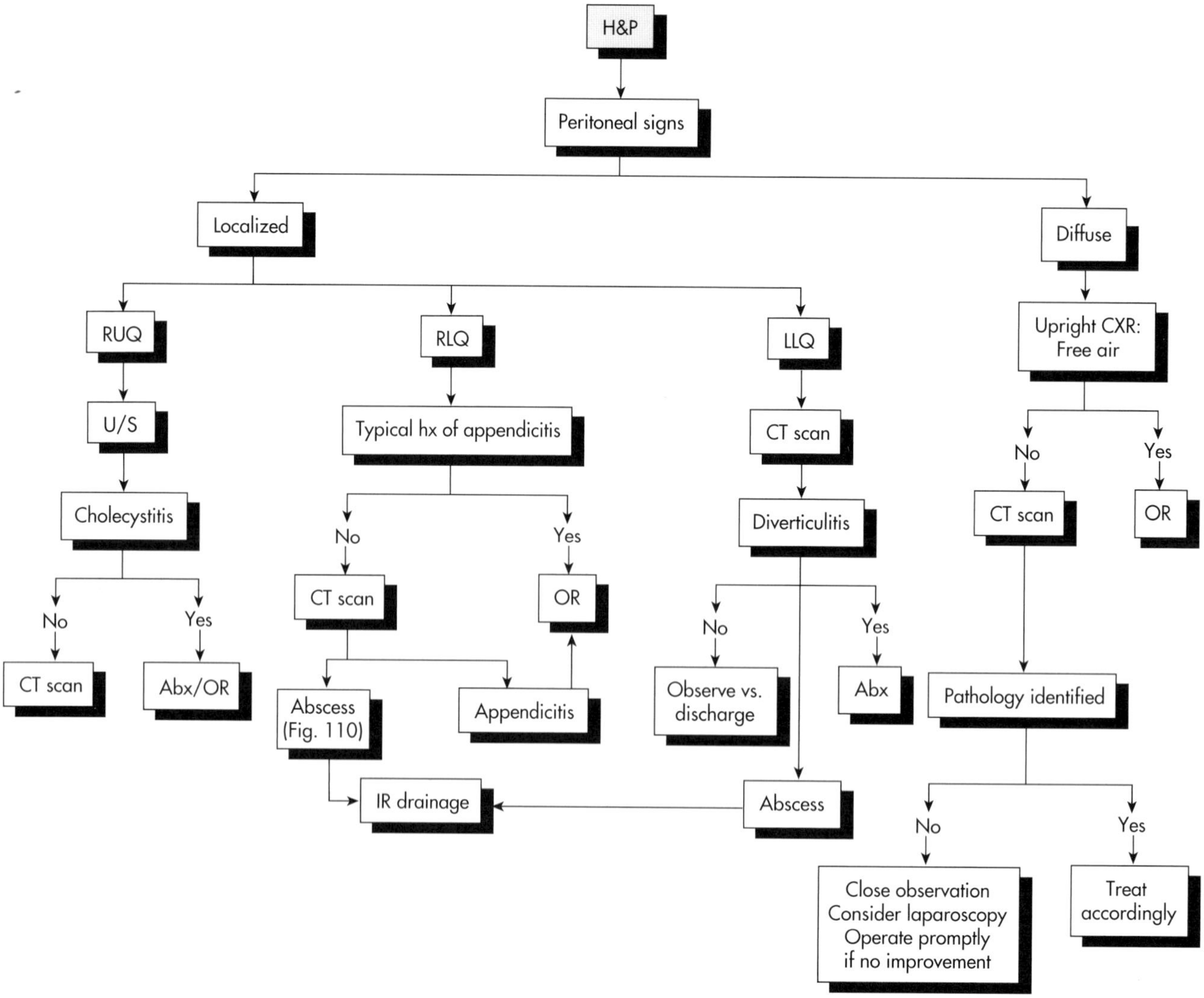

```
                    ┌─────┐
                    │ H&P │
                    └──┬──┘
                       │
              ┌────────────────┐
              │ Peritoneal signs│
              └────────┬────────┘
         ┌─────────────┴──────────────────────────────────┐
    ┌─────────┐                                      ┌─────────┐
    │Localized│                                      │ Diffuse │
    └────┬────┘                                      └────┬────┘
  ┌──────┼──────────────────┬──────────────┐              │
┌─────┐        ┌─────┐    ┌─────┐    ┌──────────────┐
│ RUQ │        │ RLQ │    │ LLQ │    │ Upright CXR: │
└──┬──┘        └──┬──┘    └──┬──┘    │   Free air   │
   │              │          │       └──────┬───────┘
┌─────┐  ┌────────────────┐ ┌─────────┐  No │      Yes
│ U/S │  │Typical hx of   │ │ CT scan │ ┌───────┐  ┌────┐
└──┬──┘  │ appendicitis   │ └────┬────┘ │CT scan│  │ OR │
   │     └────────┬───────┘      │      └───┬───┘  └────┘
┌────────────┐  No       Yes ┌─────────────┐   │
│Cholecystitis│ ┌───────┐ ┌────┐│Diverticulitis│ ┌───────────────────┐
└──────┬──────┘ │CT scan│ │ OR ││              │ │Pathology identified│
   No      Yes  └───┬───┘ └────┘└──────┬───────┘ └─────────┬─────────┘
┌───────┐ ┌──────┐  │      No        Yes      No         Yes
│CT scan│ │Abx/OR│ ┌──────────┐┌────────────┐ ┌──────────────┐┌──────┐
└───────┘ └──────┘ │ Abscess  ││Appendicitis│ │Observe vs.   ││ Abx  │
                   │(Fig. 110)│└────────────┘ │discharge     │└──────┘
                   └────┬─────┘                └──────────────┘
                  ┌───────────┐         ┌─────────┐
                  │IR drainage│◄────────│ Abscess │
                  └───────────┘         └─────────┘
```

Close observation
Consider laparoscopy
Operate promptly
if no improvement

Treat accordingly

FIG. 109 Algorithm for the diagnosis and management of patients with suspected intraabdominal infection. *Abx,* Antibiotics; *CT,* computed tomography; *CXR,* chest radiograph; *H&P,* history and physical exam; *hx,* history; *IR,* interventional radiology; *LLQ,* left lower quadrant; *OR,* operating room; *RLQ,* right lower quadrant; *RUQ,* right upper quadrant; *U/S,* ultrasound. (From Cameron JL, Cameron AM: *Current surgical therapy,* ed 10, Philadelphia, 2011, Saunders.)

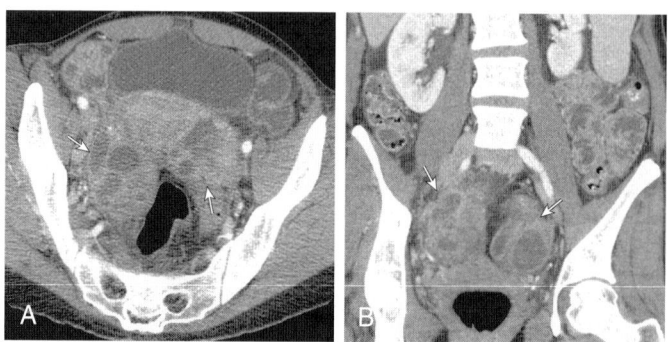

FIG. 110 Axial (A) and coronal (B) postcontrast computed tomographic images showing bilateral tuboovarian abscesses *(arrows).* (From Fielding JR et al: *Gynecologic imaging,* Philadelphia, 2011, Saunders.)

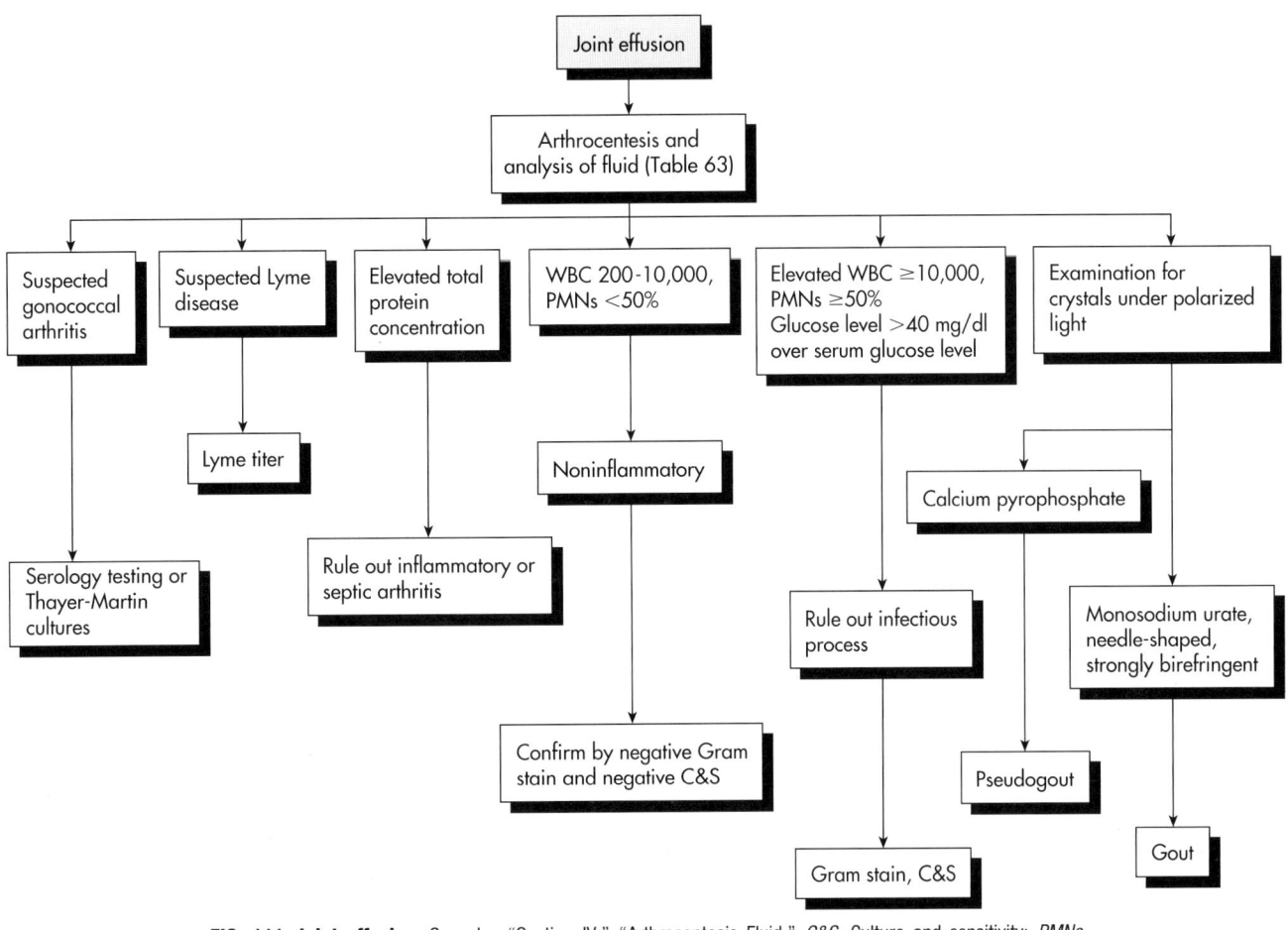

FIG. 111 Joint effusion. See also "Section IV," "Arthrocentesis Fluid." *C&S,* Culture and sensitivity; *PMNs,* polymorphonuclear leukocytes; *WBC,* white blood cell count.

TABLE 63 Indications for Arthrocentesis

Undiagnosed Arthritis with Effusion

Characterize type of arthritis
Noninflammatory (WBC <2000/mm^3)
- Inflammatory (WBC >2000/mm^3)
- Septic (WBC >50,000/mm^3)
- Definitive diagnosis
- Gout (urate crystals)
- Pseudogout (calcium pyrophosphate dihydrate crystals)
- Septic arthritis (Gram stain [rare] or culture)

Undiagnosed Arthritis without Effusion

May be definitive in gout (knee, first metatarsophalangeal joint)

Patient with Known Diagnosis

Septic arthritis (repeated taps for adequate drainage)
Other types of arthritis for symptomatic relief (with or without injection)*

WBC, White blood cells.
*Most studies show improved effect if fluid is aspirated before injection.
From Firestein GS et al: *Kelley's textbook of rheumatology,* ed 9, Philadelphia, 2013, Saunders.

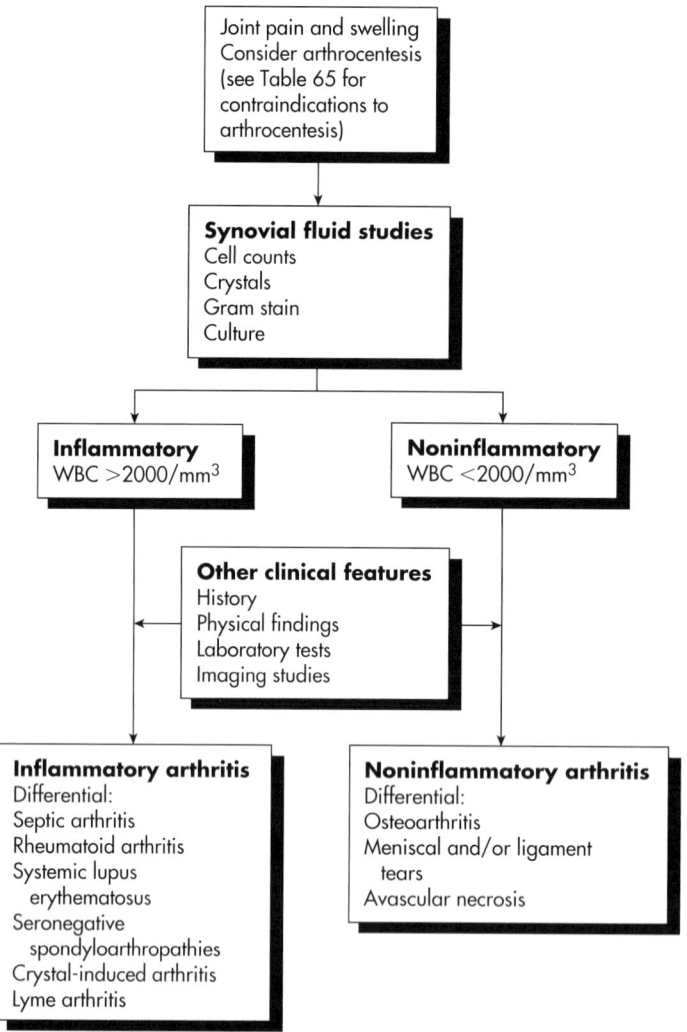

FIG. 112 Diagnostic approach for swollen joints. *WBC,* White blood cell count. (From Goldman L, Schafer AL [eds]: *Cecil textbook of medicine,* ed 24, Philadelphia, 2012, Saunders.)

TABLE 64 Clinical and Radiologic Findings in Joint Disease

Condition	Site of Involvement	Discriminatory Findings
Primary osteoarthritis (F>M •>45 yr)	Hands	PIP and DIP joint involvement (Heberden and Bouchard nodes) • No osteopenia
	Large joints (e.g., hip, knee)	Joint space narrowing • Subchondral sclerosis • Subchondral cysts • Marginal osteophytes
	Spine	Degenerative disc disease • Spondylosis deformans • Apophyseal joint involvement • Spinal stenosis • Foraminal stenosis
Erosive osteoarthritis (affects middle-aged females)	Hands	PIP and DIP joint involvement • Joint ankylosis • 'Gull-wing' deformities (central erosions and marginal osteophytes)

Table 64   Clinical and Radiologic Findings in Joint Disease—cont'd

Condition	Site of Involvement	Discriminatory Findings
Rheumatoid arthritis (F>M • Rh factor positive)	Hand and wrist	Symmetric arthritis • MCP and PIP joint involvement • Periarticular (early) and diffuse (late) osteopenia • Marginal erosions • Subluxation (swan neck and boutonnière deformities) • Periostitis is uncommon
	Large joints	Joint space narrowing • Marginal erosions • Synovial cysts • Protrusio acetabulae
	Spine	Atlantoaxial subluxation
Juvenile idiopathic arthritis (M = F• affects children)	Hands	Joint ankylosis • Florid periosteal reaction • Osteopenia
	Large joints (e.g., knee)	Abnormalities of growth and maturation • Epiphyseal overgrowth and premature closure of the physis • Widened intercondylar notch
	Cervical spine	Apophyseal joint fusion • Atlantoaxial subluxation
Psoriatic arthritis (M>F•nail changes • HLA-B27 +ve)	Upper extremities (e.g., hands)	"Sausage" digit • DIP joint involvement • Terminal tuft erosion • Pencil-in-cup deformity • Joint ankylosis • Arthritis mutilans • Periosteal reaction • No osteopenia
	SI joints	Asymmetric or unilateral sacroiliitis
	Spine	Coarse syndesmophytes
Reites syndrome (affects young male adults)	Lower extremities (e.g., foot)	Hallux involvement • Periosteal reaction • Calcaneal erosions • Osteopenia not prominent
	Spine	Coarse syndesmophytes
	SI joints	Asymmetric or unilateral sacroiliitis
Ankylosing spondylitis (M>F• affects young adults• HLA-B27 +ve in 95%)	SI joints	Bilateral symmetric sacroiliitis • Ankylosis
	Spine	Anterior vertebral body squaring • Syndesmophytes • Paravertebral ossification • Bamboo spine
	Pelvis	"Whiskering" of the iliac crests and ischial tuberosities
Enteropathic arthropathies	SI joints	Symmetric sacroiliitis
Gout (M>F)	Hands and feet (especially the great toe)	MTP joint of the great toe • Juxta-articular erosions • Punched-out lesions with an overhanging margin • No periarticular osteopenia • Tophi
CPPD crystal deposition disease (M = F)	Any peripheral joint • Predilection for the knee	Degenerative changes • Chondrocalcinosis • Paucity of subchondral sclerosis
HA crystal deposition disease (M = F)	Predilection for the shoulder (supraspinatus tendon)	Periarticular calcification
Hemochromatosis (M>F)	Hands	2nd and 3rd MCP joint involvement ("squared" metacarpal heads) • Joint space narrowing • "Hooklike" osteophytes • Numerous subchondral cysts

Clinical Algorithms

III

Continued

Table 64   Clinical and Radiologic Findings in Joint Disease—cont'd

Condition	Site of Involvement	Discriminatory Findings
Alkaptonuria (ochronosis) (M = F)	Intervertebral discs • SI joints • Large joints	Degenerative changes: Disc calcification • Joint space narrowing • Periarticular sclerosis
Systemic lupus erythematosus (F>M • affects young adults)	Hands	Reversible MCP joint subluxation
Scleroderma (F>M • affects adults)	Hands	IP joint arthritis • Acroosteolysis • Soft tissue calcifications
Mixed connective tissue disease (overlap syndrome)	Hands	PIP joint, MCP joint, mid-carpal involvement • Soft tissue swelling, calcifications, or atrophy
Multicentric reticulohistiocytosis (F>M)	Hands and feet	DIP joint and carpal involvement • Soft tissue swelling • Articular erosions • No osteopenia
Polymyositis/dermatomyositis	Proximal extremities	Soft tissue calcification
	Hands	DIP joint erosions
Sarcoidosis	Distal and middle phalanges of the hands and feet	Punched-out cystlike lesions • "Lacelike" appearance
Hemophilic arthropathy (affecting males—but with female carriers)	Predilection for large joints (e.g., knee)	Epiphyseal overgrowth • Juxtaarticular osteopenia • Erosion and cartilage destruction • Widened intercondylar and trochlear notches • Squared patella
Neuropathic arthropathy	Any joint	5 "Ds": Normal bone **D**ensity • Joint **D**istension • Bony **D**ebris • Joint **D**isorganization • **D**islocation
Hypertrophic osteoarthropathy	Tubular bones (radius and ulna > tibia and fibula)	Diaphyseal and metaphyseal painful periostitis

CPPD, Calcium pyrophosphate deposition disease; *DIP*, distal interphalangeal; *F*, female; *HA*, hydroxyapatite; *HLA*, human leukocyte antigen; *IP*, interphalangeal; *M*, male; *MCP*, metacarpophalangeal; *MTP*, metatarsophalangeal; *PIP*, proximal interphalangeal; *Rh*, Rhesus; *SI*, sacroiliac.
From Grant LA, Griffin N: *Grainger & Allison's diagnostic radiology essentials*, ed 2, Philadelphia, 2019, Elsevier.

TABLE 65   Contraindications to Arthrocentesis and Joint Injection

Contraindication	Comment
Established infection in nearby structures (e.g., cellulitis, septic bursitis)	Sometimes gout mimics cellulitis, creating a confusing picture
Septicemia (theoretic risk of introducing organism into joint)	Need to tap suspected septic joints in septic patients
Disrupted skin barrier (e.g., psoriasis)	Do not tap through lesions
Bleeding disorder (not absolute, but use more care)	Risk of bleeding very low, even in patients taking warfarin
Septic joint	Steroid injection contraindicated
Prior lack of response	Relative contraindication
Difficult-to-access joint	Relative contraindication without imaging aid

From Firestein GS et al: *Kelley's textbook of rheumatology*, ed 9, Philadelphia, 2013, Saunders.

TABLE 66 Synovial Fluid Characteristics in Clinical Situations, with Imaging and Investigation Techniques to Identify the Cause

Diagnosis	Cells	Microorganisms	Appearance	Imaging Modality	Comments
Bacterial arthritis	Neutrophils, 10,000->100,000	Gram stain usually positive	Turbid/pus	May need ultrasound to aspirate dryness	Systemic symptoms, Gram stain, blood and synovial fluid culture
Gonococcal arthritis	Neutrophils, 10,000-100,000	Gram stain usually positive	Turbid/pus	May need ultrasound to aspirate dryness	Systemic symptoms, Gram stain, blood and synovial fluid culture
Crystal arthritis	Neutrophils, 10,000->100,000	—	Turbid/pus	Radiographs, CPPD	Presence of appropriate crystals Acute serum urate unreliable
Tuberculous arthritis	Mononuclear 5000-50,000	Acid-fast stain often negative, may need to culture synovial tissue	Turbid/pus		At-risk population; Ziehl-Neelsen stain biopsy may be necessary
Inflammatory monoarthropathies	Neutrophils 5000-50,000	—	Slightly turbid	Ultrasound/MRI for early synovitis and erosions	Serum autoantibodies such as RF, ACPA, ANA
Osteoarthritis	Mononuclear 0-2000	—	Clear	Radiographic changes	Usually noninflammatory CPPD may be present
Internal derangement	Red blood cells	—	Clear/turbid	MRI	Arthroscopy may be necessary
Trauma	Red blood cells	—	Clear/turbid	Radiographs	Tc bone scan may aid diagnosis if radiograph normal
Ischemic necrosis		—		MRI in early disease	XR abnormal only in advanced cases
Uncommon Causes					
Sarcoidosis	Mononuclear, 5000-20,000	—		CXR	
PVNS	Red blood cells	—	Turbid	Ultrasound and MRI	Synovial biopsy essential
Charcot disease	Mononuclear, 0-2000	—		Radiographs	CPPD may be present
Lyme disease	Neutrophils, 0-5000	—	Clear/turbid		SF eosinophilia may be found Serology for *Borrelia*
Amyloid	Mononuclear, 2000-10,000	—	Turbid		Synovial biopsy for Congo red stain

ACPA, Anticitrullinated protein antibody; *ANA,* antinuclear antibody; *CPPD,* calcium pyrophosphate dehydrate deposition; *CXR,* chest radiograph; *PVNS,* pigmented villonodular synovitis; *RF,* rheumatoid factor; *SF,* synovial fluid; *Tc,* technetium; *XR,* radiograph.
From Firestein GS et al: *Firestein & Kelley's textbook of rheumatology,* ed 11, Philadelphia, 2021, Elsevier.

Clinical Algorithms

III

TABLE 67   The Differential Diagnosis of Polyarthritis

Disease Category	Specific Disease	Mono-, Oligo-, or Polyarthritis (Most Common Presentation)
Infections		
Viral	Parvovirus B19	Poly
	Rubella virus	Poly
	Hepatitis A, B, C	Poly
	HIV	Oligo, poly
	Alphaviruses, including Chikungunya infection	Poly
Bacterial	Gram-positive and gram-negative infections	Mono, occasionally oligo/poly
	Initial phase of gonorrhea	Poly
	Later phase of gonorrhea	Mono
	Early phase of Lyme arthritis	Poly
	Later phase of Lyme arthritis	Oligo, mono
Diseases Triggered by Infection but Presumed to Be Autoimmune		
Reactive arthritis	After urogenital infections (*Chlamydia* and *Ureaplasma*); after gastrointestinal infections (*Yersinia*, *Shigella*, *Campylobacter*, and *Salmonella*)	Mono, oligo, poly
Acute rheumatic fever	After infection with group A streptococcus	Oligo
Autoimmune Diseases		
Primary arthritides	Rheumatoid arthritis	Poly
	Psoriatic arthritis	Oligo, poly
	Spondyloarthropathies	Oligo, poly
	Juvenile inflammatory arthritis	Mono, oligo, poly
Transient and recurring polyarthritides	Palindromic rheumatism	Poly
	Recurrent symmetric seronegative synovitis with pitting edema (RS3PE syndrome)	Poly
Systemic autoimmune disease	Systemic lupus erythematosus	Poly
	Mixed connective tissue disease	Poly
	Primary Sjögren syndrome	Poly
	Progressive systemic sclerosis and limited scleroderma	Poly
	Behçet disease	Oligo, poly
	Sarcoidosis	Oligo, poly
	Vasculitis	Poly
Autoinflammatory diseases	Adult-onset Still disease	Oligo, poly
	Familial Mediterranean fever and other cryopyrin-associated fever syndromes	Poly
	Various genetic autoinflammatory conditions usually manifested first in childhood	Poly
Degenerative diseases	Includes erosive inflammatory osteoarthritis	Poly
Osteoarthritis		
Hypertrophic osteoarthropathy		Poly
Osteonecrosis		Mono, oligo
Metabolic Diseases		
Thyroid diseases	Hypothyroidism	Mono, oligo
Hemochromatosis	Hyperthyroidism (Graves disease; early phase of Hashimoto disease)	Oligo, poly
Hemoglobinopathies	Sickle cell anemia	Oligo, poly
Hemochromatosis	Thalassemia	Oligo, poly
Crystal diseases	Gout	Mono (initial), oligo, poly (late stage)
	Pseudogout	Mono, oligo, poly
Deposition diseases	Glycogen storage diseases; amyloid deposition in primary amyloidosis; mucopolysaccharidoses; light- and heavy-chain deposition diseases; others	Oligo, poly
Drug-Induced Diseases		
Vasculitic drug reactions, serum sickness		Poly

From Firestein GS et al: *Firestein & Kelley's textbook of rheumatology*, ed 11, Philadelphia, 2021, Elsevier.

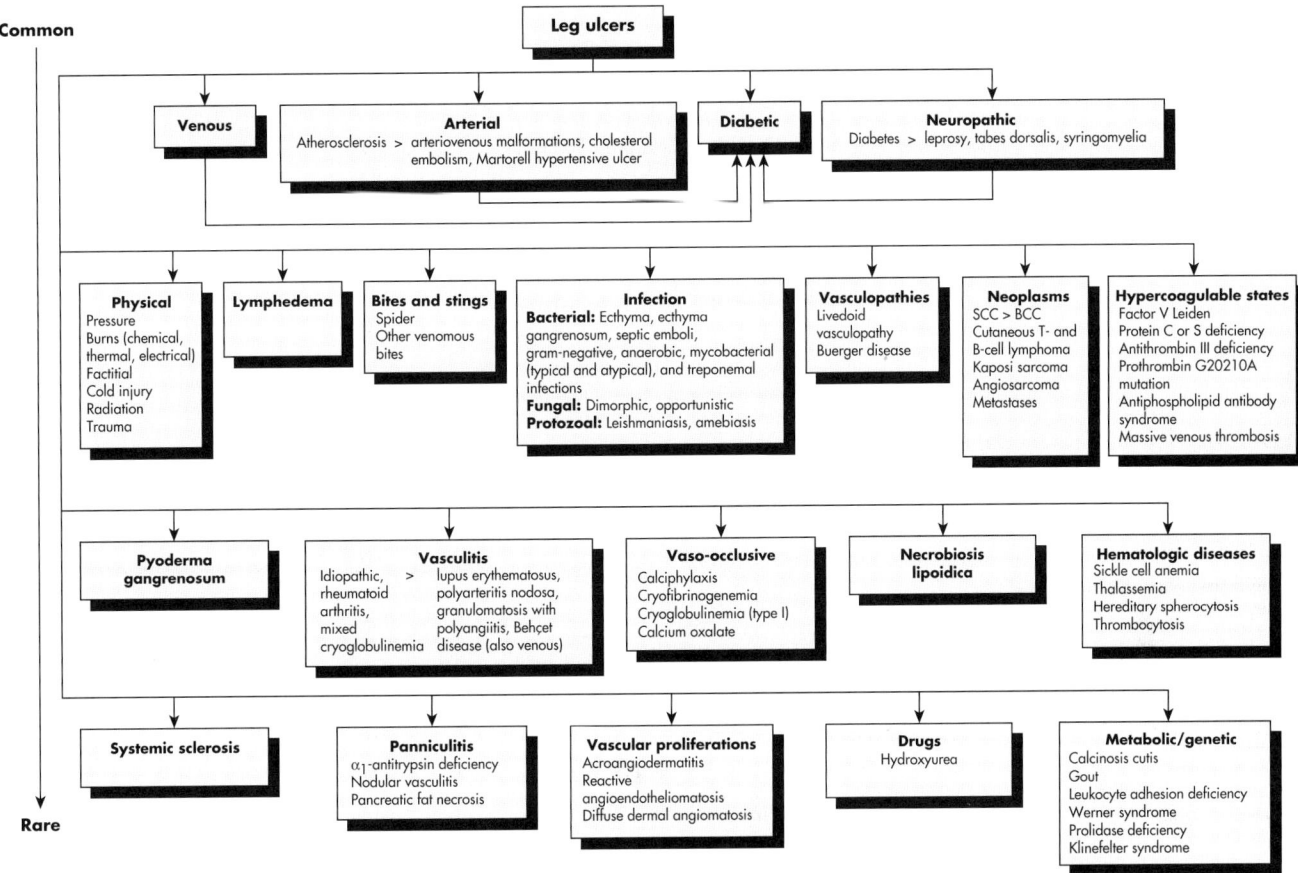

FIG. 113 Causes of leg ulcers. Patients with Behçet disease also develop lower extremity ulcers due to vasculitis and/or venous insufficiency related to deep vein thromboses, and, occasionally, erosive pustular dermatosis is a cause of leg ulcers. Hydroxyurea-induced leg ulcers are often on the malleolus or tibial crest, exceedingly painful, and surrounded by atrophic skin. (From Bolognia J: *Dermatology*, ed 4, Philadelphia, 2018, Elsevier.)

Clinical
Algorithms

III

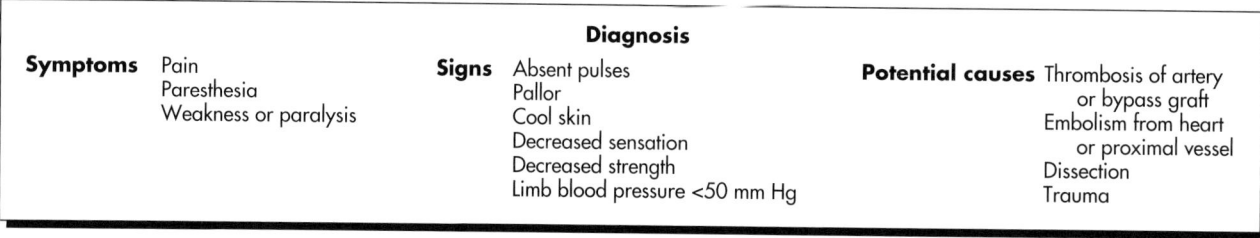

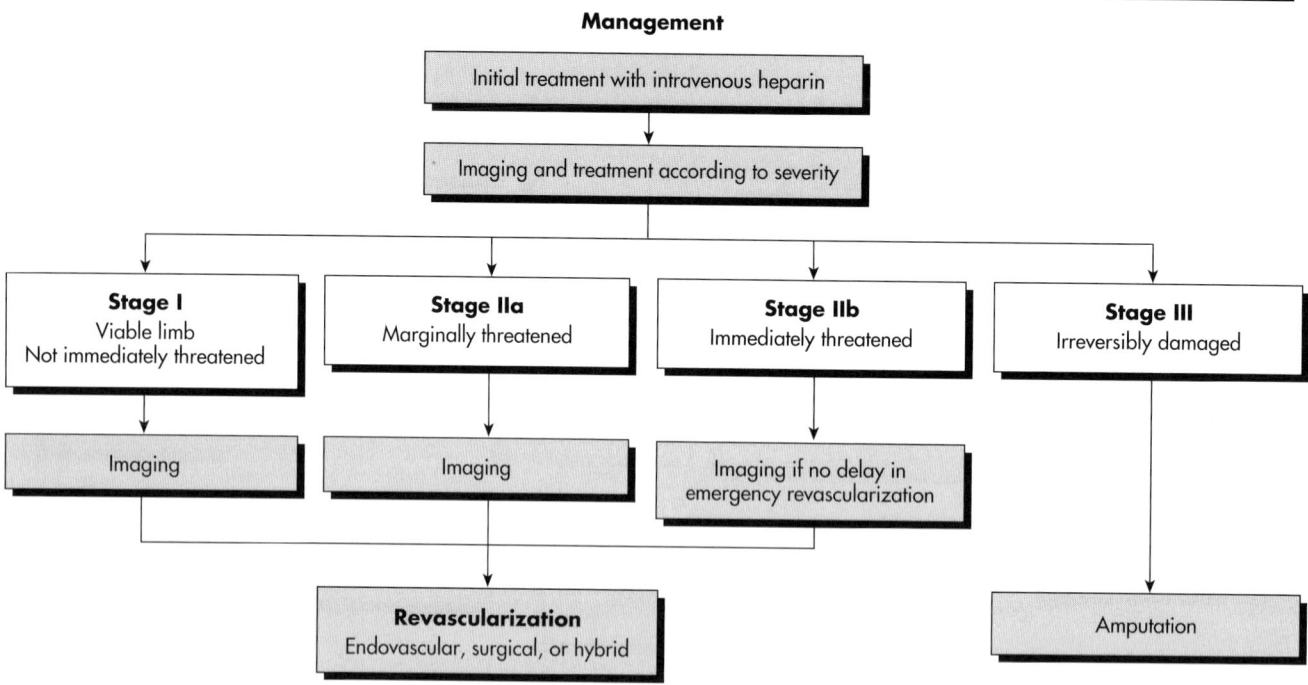

FIG. 114 Diagnostic and treatment approach for patients presenting with acute limb ischemia. (From Zipes DP: *Braunwald's heart disease, a textbook of cardiovascular medicine,* ed 11, Philadelphia, 2019, Elsevier.)

TABLE 68   Rutherford Classification of Acute Limb Ischemia

Category	Description/Prognosis	CLINICAL EXAMINATION		DOPPLER SIGNAL	
		Sensory Loss	**Muscle Weakness**	**Arterial**	**Venous**
I. Viable	Not immediately threatened	None	None	Audible	Audible
II. Threatened					
IIa. Marginally	Salvageable if promptly treated	Minimal (toes) or none	None	(Often) audible	Audible
IIb. Immediately	Salvageable with immediate revascularization	More than toes, associated with rest pain	Mild, moderate	(Usually) audible	Audible
III. Irreversible	Major tissue loss or permanent damage inevitable	Profound, anesthetic	Profound, paralysis (rigor)	Inaudible	Inaudible

From Hoffman R: *Hematology, basic principles and practice,* ed 7, Philadelphia, 2018, Elsevier.

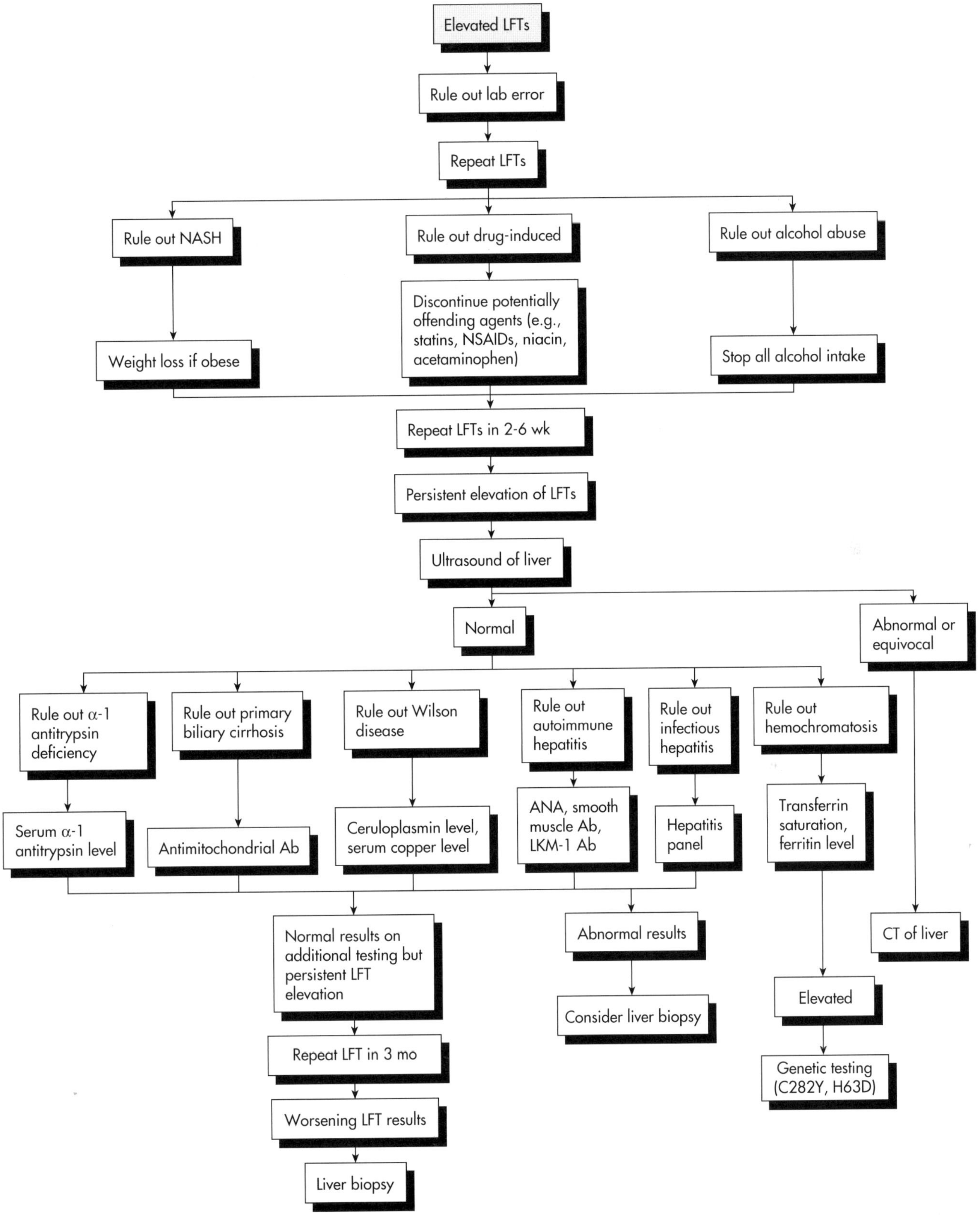

```
                          ┌─────────────────┐
                          │  Elevated LFTs   │
                          └────────┬─────────┘
                                   │
                          ┌────────▼─────────┐
                          │ Rule out lab error│
                          └────────┬─────────┘
                                   │
                          ┌────────▼─────────┐
                          │   Repeat LFTs    │
                          └────────┬─────────┘
```

```
  ┌──────────────┐      ┌──────────────────┐      ┌────────────────────┐
  │ Rule out NASH│      │Rule out drug-induced│    │Rule out alcohol abuse│
  └──────┬───────┘      └─────────┬────────┘      └──────────┬─────────┘
         │                        │                          │
         │              ┌─────────▼────────┐                 │
         │              │ Discontinue potentially            │
         │              │ offending agents (e.g.,│           │
         │              │ statins, NSAIDs, niacin,│          │
         │              │ acetaminophen)   │                 │
  ┌──────▼───────┐      └─────────┬────────┘      ┌──────────▼─────────┐
  │Weight loss if obese│          │                │ Stop all alcohol intake│
  └──────────────┘                │                └────────────────────┘
```

```
                          ┌──────────────────┐
                          │ Repeat LFTs in 2-6 wk│
                          └────────┬─────────┘
                                   │
                          ┌────────▼──────────────┐
                          │ Persistent elevation of LFTs│
                          └────────┬──────────────┘
                                   │
                          ┌────────▼─────────┐
                          │ Ultrasound of liver│
                          └────────┬─────────┘
```

```
                    ┌──────────┐              ┌──────────────────┐
                    │  Normal  │              │ Abnormal or equivocal│
                    └────┬─────┘              └──────────┬───────┘
```

Rule out α-1 antitrypsin deficiency	Rule out primary biliary cirrhosis	Rule out Wilson disease	Rule out autoimmune hepatitis	Rule out infectious hepatitis	Rule out hemochromatosis
Serum α-1 antitrypsin level	Antimitochondrial Ab	Ceruloplasmin level, serum copper level	ANA, smooth muscle Ab, LKM-1 Ab	Hepatitis panel	Transferrin saturation, ferritin level

```
  ┌────────────────────────┐        ┌──────────────────┐      ┌──────────┐
  │ Normal results on        │       │ Abnormal results │      │CT of liver│
  │ additional testing but   │       └────────┬─────────┘      └──────────┘
  │ persistent LFT elevation │                │
  └───────────┬────────────┘       ┌──────────▼─────────┐    ┌──────────┐
              │                      │Consider liver biopsy│    │ Elevated │
  ┌───────────▼────────────┐       └────────────────────┘    └────┬─────┘
  │  Repeat LFT in 3 mo     │                                      │
  └───────────┬────────────┘                              ┌────────▼──────────┐
              │                                            │ Genetic testing    │
  ┌───────────▼────────────┐                               │ (C282Y, H63D)      │
  │  Worsening LFT results  │                               └────────────────────┘
  └───────────┬────────────┘
              │
  ┌───────────▼────────────┐
  │     Liver biopsy        │
  └────────────────────────┘
```

FIG. 115 Liver function test elevations. *Ab,* Antibody; *ANA,* antibody to nuclear antigens; *CT,* computed tomography; *LFTs,* liver function tests; *LKM,* liver-kidney microsome; *NASH,* nonalcoholic steatohepatitis; *NSAIDs,* nonsteroidal antiinflammatory drugs.

Clinical Algorithms

III

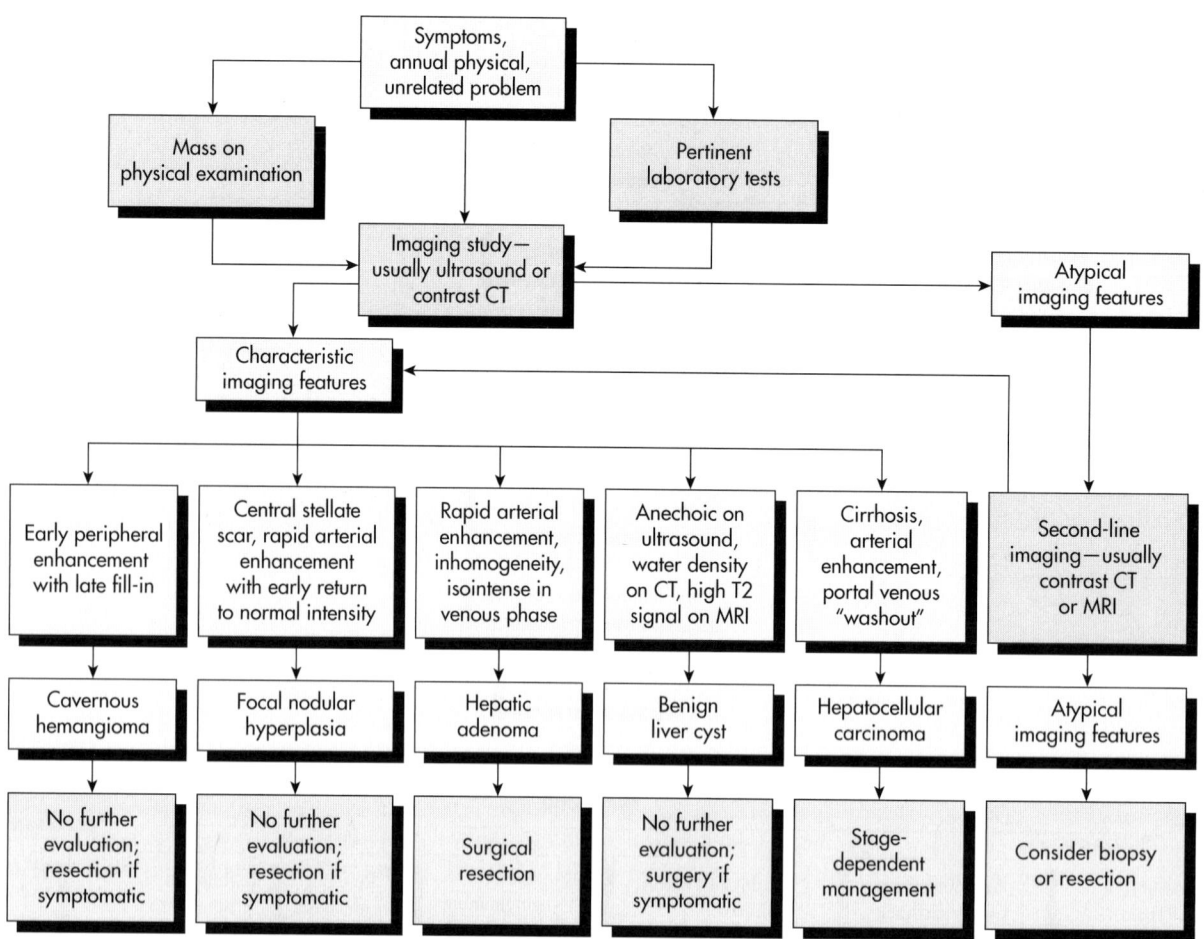

FIG. 116 Approach to evaluating the patient with a mass lesion in the liver. This flow chart shows an algorithm for evaluating and managing common liver mass lesions. *CT,* Computed tomography; *MRI,* magnetic resonance imaging. (From Roberts LR: Liver and biliary tract tumors. In Goldman L, Schafer AI [eds]: *Goldman's Cecil medicine,* ed 24, Philadelphia, 2012, Saunders.)

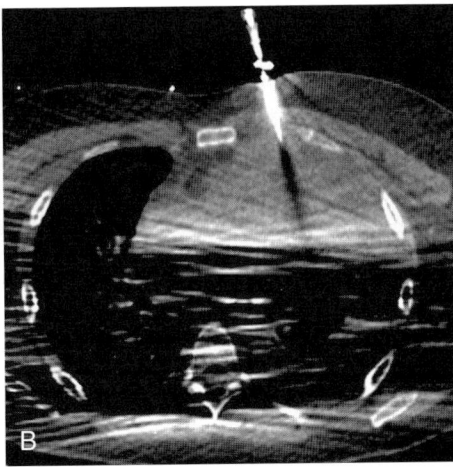

FIG. 117 Bulky anterior mediastinal mass with CT-guided needle aspiration. (A) A 45-yr-old man presenting with hoarseness was found to have a 12 × 10 × 11 cm anterior mediastinal mass. On this noncontrast computed tomography (CT) image, there is central necrosis and mass effect with concurrent left pleural effusion. **(B)** CT-guided needle aspiration of the mass. The needle is lateral to the sternum. The final diagnosis was primary mediastinal B-cell lymphoma. (From Broaddus VC et al: *Murray & Nadel's textbook of respiratory medicine*, ed 7, Philadelphia, 2022, Elsevier.)

Clinical Algorithms

III

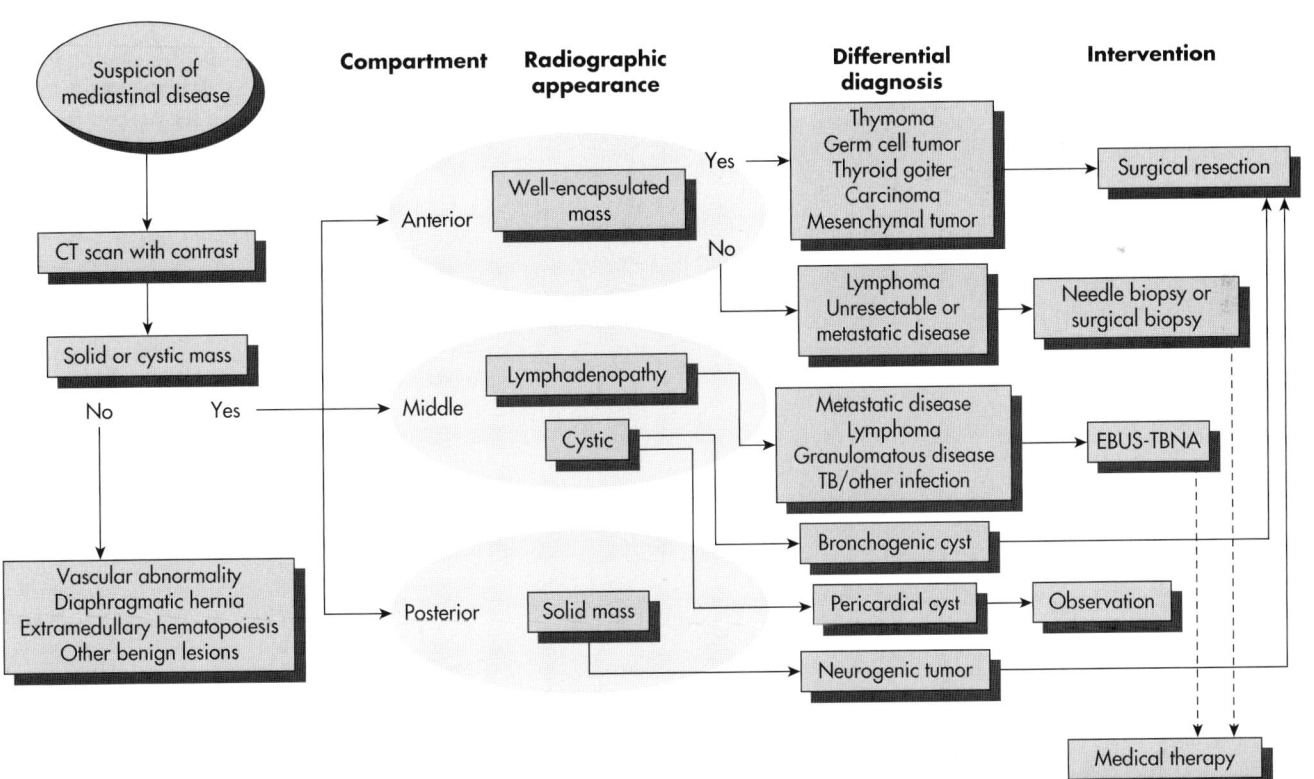

FIG. 118 Suggested algorithm for the diagnostic approach to mediastinal masses. *CT,* Computed tomography; *EBUS-TBNA,* endobronchial ultrasound-guided transbronchial needle aspiration; *TB,* tuberculosis. (From Broaddus VC et al: *Murray & Nadel's textbook of respiratory medicine*, ed 7, Philadelphia, 2022, Elsevier.)

TABLE 69   Disorders Presenting as a Mass in the Mediastinum

Anterior/Prevascular Mediastinum	Middle/Visceral Mediastinum	Posterior/Paravertebral Mediastinum
Thymic neoplasms	Lymphadenopathy	Neurogenic tumors
Germ cell tumors	Reactive and granulomatous inflammation	Meningocele
Teratoma	Metastasis	Diaphragmatic hernia (Bochdalek)
Seminoma	Angiofollicular lymphoid hyperplasia (Castleman disease)	Extramedullary hematopoiesis
Nonseminomatous germ cell tumors	Lymphoma	Lymphadenopathy
Embryonal cell carcinoma	Developmental cysts	Lesions arising from posterior spine
Choriocarcinoma	Pericardial cyst	Metastases
Lymphoma	Foregut duplication cysts	Discitis/osteomyelitis
Hodgkin lymphoma	Bronchogenic cyst	Thoracic duct cyst
Non-Hodgkin lymphoma	Enteric cyst	
Thyroid neoplasms/goiter	Others	
Parathyroid neoplasms	Vascular enlargements (i.e., descending aortic aneurysm)	
Mesenchymal tumors	Diaphragmatic hernia (hiatal)	
Lipoma	Esophageal lesions	
Fibroma	Carcinoma	
Lymphangioma	Diverticula	
Hemangioma	Varices	
Mesothelioma		
Sarcoma		
Diaphragmatic hernia (Morgagni)		
NUT midline carcinoma		
Lymphadenopathy		
Vascular lesions		

NUT, Nuclear protein in testis.
From Broaddus VC et al: *Murray & Nadel's textbook of respiratory medicine*, ed 7, Philadelphia, 2022, Elsevier.

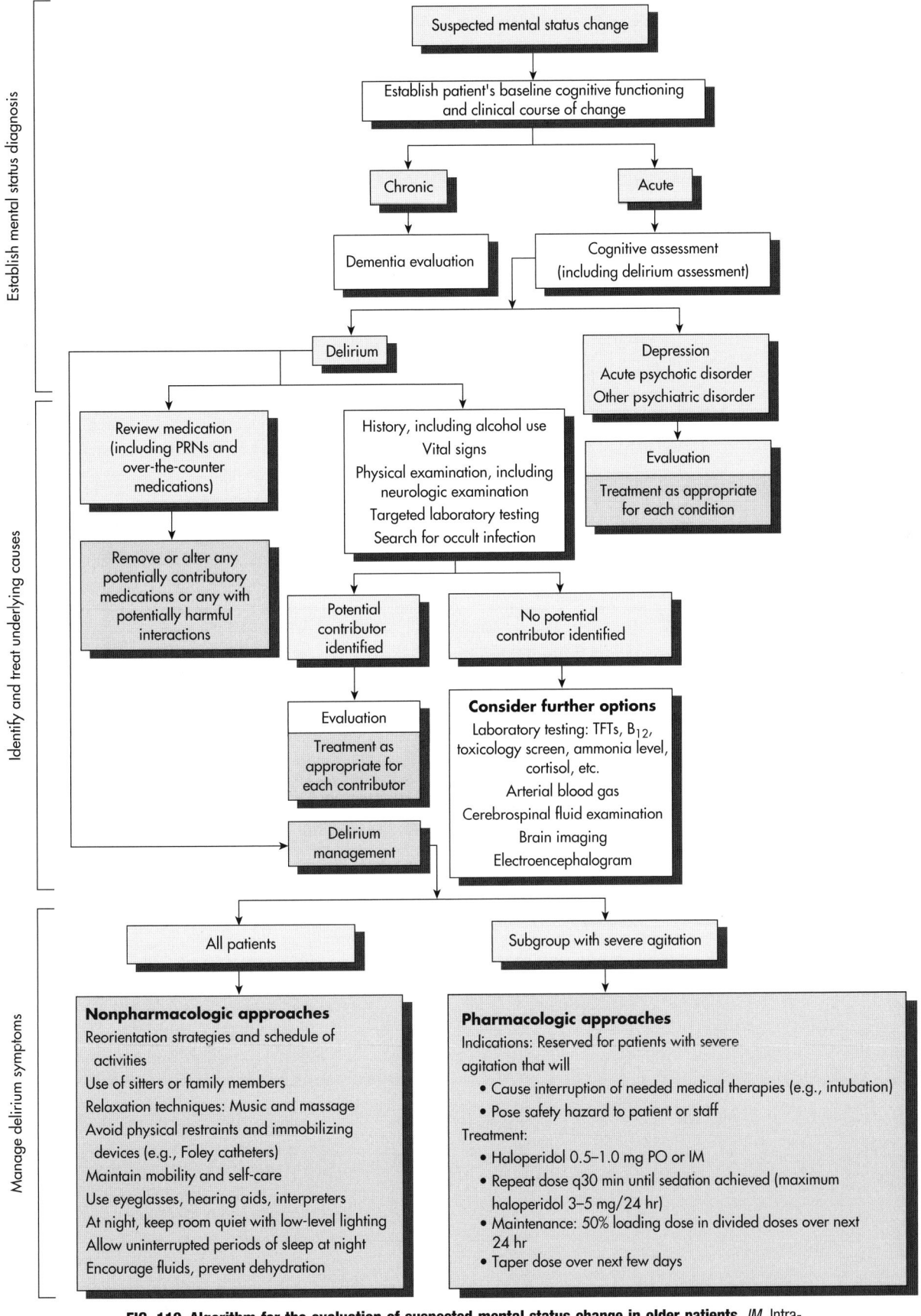

FIG. 119 Algorithm for the evaluation of suspected mental status change in older patients. *IM,* Intramuscular; *PO,* by mouth; *PRN,* as needed; *TFTs,* thyroid function tests. (From Goldman L, Schafer AI: *Goldman Cecil medicine,* ed 25, Philadelphia, 2016, Saunders.)

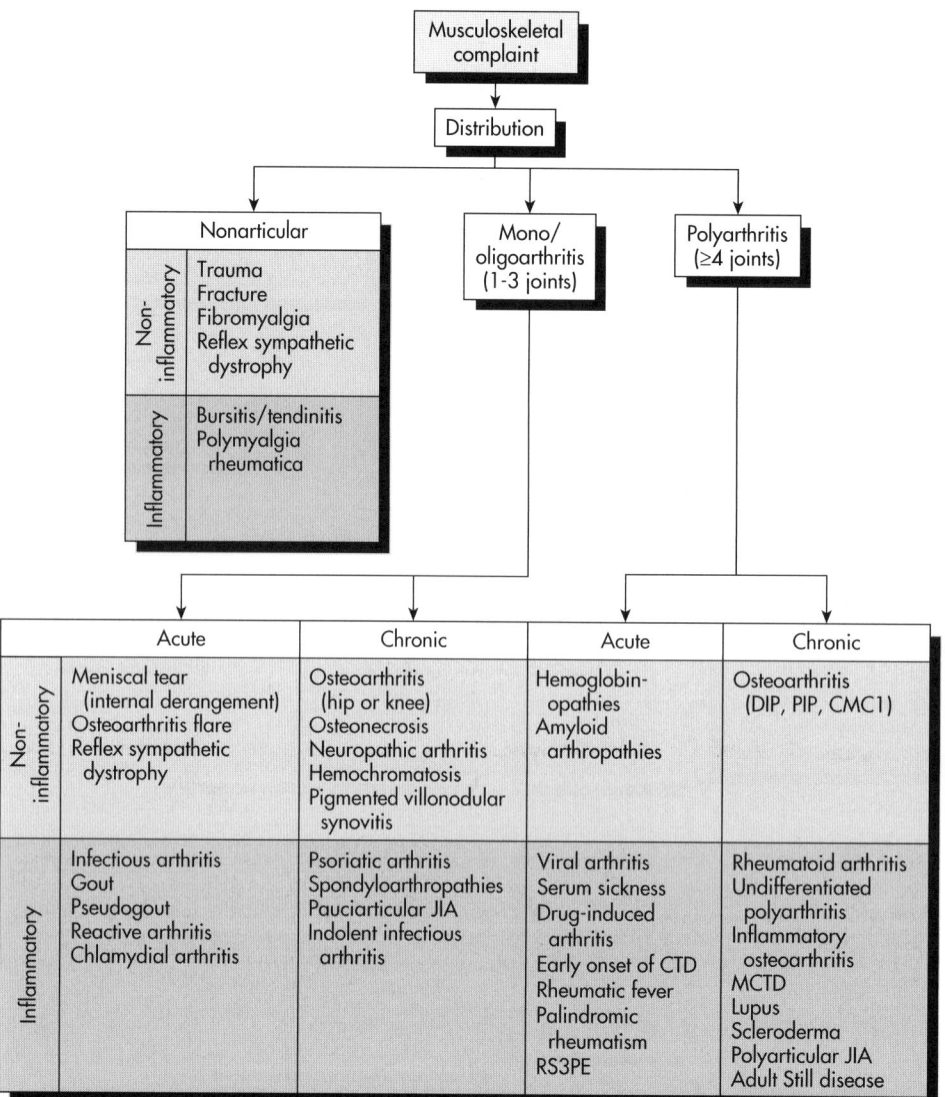

FIG. 120 Algorithm for assessing initial history and examination. *CMC*, Carpometacarpal; *CTD*, connective tissue disease; *DIP*, distal interphalangeal; *JIA*, juvenile idiopathic arthritis; *MCTD*, mixed connective tissue disease; *PIP*, proximal interphalangeal. (From Firestein GS et al: *Kelley's textbook of rheumatology*, ed 9, Philadelphia, 2013, Saunders.)

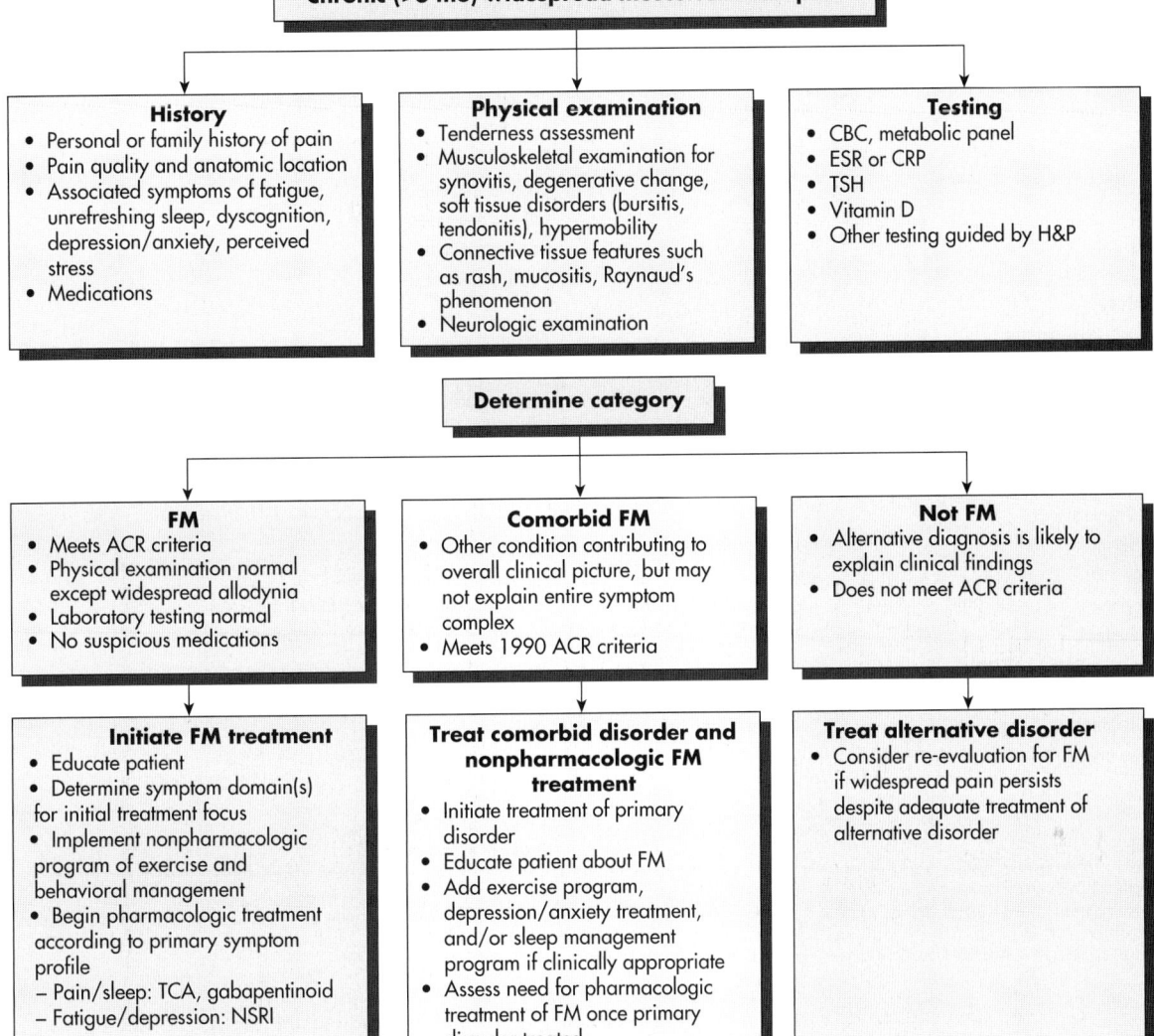

FIG. 121 Strategy for evaluation and initial management of patients with chronic widespread musculoskeletal pain. After initial evaluation, patients may be diagnosed with fibromyalgia (FM), FM comorbid with another diagnosis, or not FM. The figure presents strategies for initial management of each category. *ACR,* American College of Rheumatology; *CBC,* complete blood cell count; *CRP,* C-reactive protein; *ESR,* erythrocyte sedimentation rate; *H&P,* history and physical examination; *NSRI,* norepinephrine serotonin reuptake inhibitor; *TCA,* tricyclic antidepressants; *TSH,* thyroid-stimulating hormone. (From Firestein GS et al: *Firestein & Kelley's textbook of rheumatology,* ed 11, Philadelphia, 2021, Elsevier.)

TABLE 70 Differential Diagnosis of Diffuse Myalgias

Diagnosis	Findings[a]
Inflammatory	
Polymyalgia rheumatica	Elevated ESR and/or CRP
Seronegative spondyloarthropathies	Abnormal imaging
Connective tissue diseases	Positive serologies
Systemic vasculitis	Systemic inflammation, end-organ damage
Infectious	
Hepatitis C	Positive antibodies
HIV	Positive antibodies
Lyme disease	Positive antibodies
Parvovirus B19	Positive antibodies
Epstein-Barr virus	Positive antibodies
Noninflammatory	
Degenerative joint/spine disease	Abnormal imaging
Fibromyalgia	Widespread allodynia/hyperalgesia
Myofascial pain	Localized allodynia/hyperalgesia
Joint hypermobility	Joint hypermobility
Metabolic myopathies	Abnormal muscle biopsy
Endocrine	
Hypo- or hyperthyroidism	Abnormal thyroid function tests
Hyperparathyroidism	Elevated serum calcium
Addison disease	Abnormal serum cortisol
Vitamin D deficiency	Low serum vitamin D
Neurologic Diseases	
Multiple sclerosis	Abnormal neurologic examination and imaging
Neuropathic pain	Reasonable cause or abnormal imaging
Psychiatric Diseases	
Major depressive disorder	Positive depression screening
Drugs	
Statins	History of exposure
Aromatase inhibitors	History of exposure

CRP, C-reactive protein; *ESR*, erythrocyte sedimentation rate.

[a]Recommended routine testing includes ESR or CRP and thyroid-stimulating hormone. Other diagnostic testing should be guided by risk profile and history and physical examination. Repeated diagnostic testing is discouraged.

From Firestein GS et al: *Firestein & Kelley's textbook of rheumatology*, ed 11, Philadelphia, 2021, Elsevier.

TABLE 71 Patterns of Arthritis

	PATTERN				
	Monoarthritis	**Inflammatory Spinal Disease Sacroiliitis**	**Asymmetrical Large Joint Arthritis**	**Symmetrical Small Joint Arthritis (MCP, PIP, MTP)**	**DIP Hands**
Differential diagnosis	Trauma Hemophilia Septic Gout Pseudogout	Ankylosing spondylitis Psoriatic arthritis IBD	Psoriatic arthritis Reactive arthritis IBD	RA SLE Psoriatic arthritis	Inflammatory OA (if involves PIP and first CMC) Psoriatic arthritis
Further investigations	X-ray Aspirate for crystals and culture	Review personal and family history HLA- B27 X- ray lumbar spine and SI joints MRI sacroiliac joints	Review personal and family history Examine scalp and buttocks for psoriasis Examine for conjunctivitis and urethritis Infection screen	Examine for rheumatoid nodules, skin rashes, serositis or mucositis Urinalysis RF, CCP antibodies, ANA X-ray hands and feet	X-ray hands

ANA, Antinuclear antibodies; *CCP*, cyclic citrullinated peptides; *CMC*, carpometacarpophalangeal; *DIP*, distal interphalangeal; *HLA*, human leukocyte antigen; *IBD*, inflammatory bowel disease; *MCP*, metacarpophalangeal; *MTP*, metatarsophalangeal; *OA*, osteoarthritis; *PIP*, proximal interphalangeal; *RA*, rheumatoid arthritis; *RF*, rheumatoid factor; *SI*, sacroiliac; *SLE*, systemic lupus erythematosus.

From Talley NJ et al: *Essentials of internal medicine*, ed 4, Chatswood, 2021, Elsevier Australia.

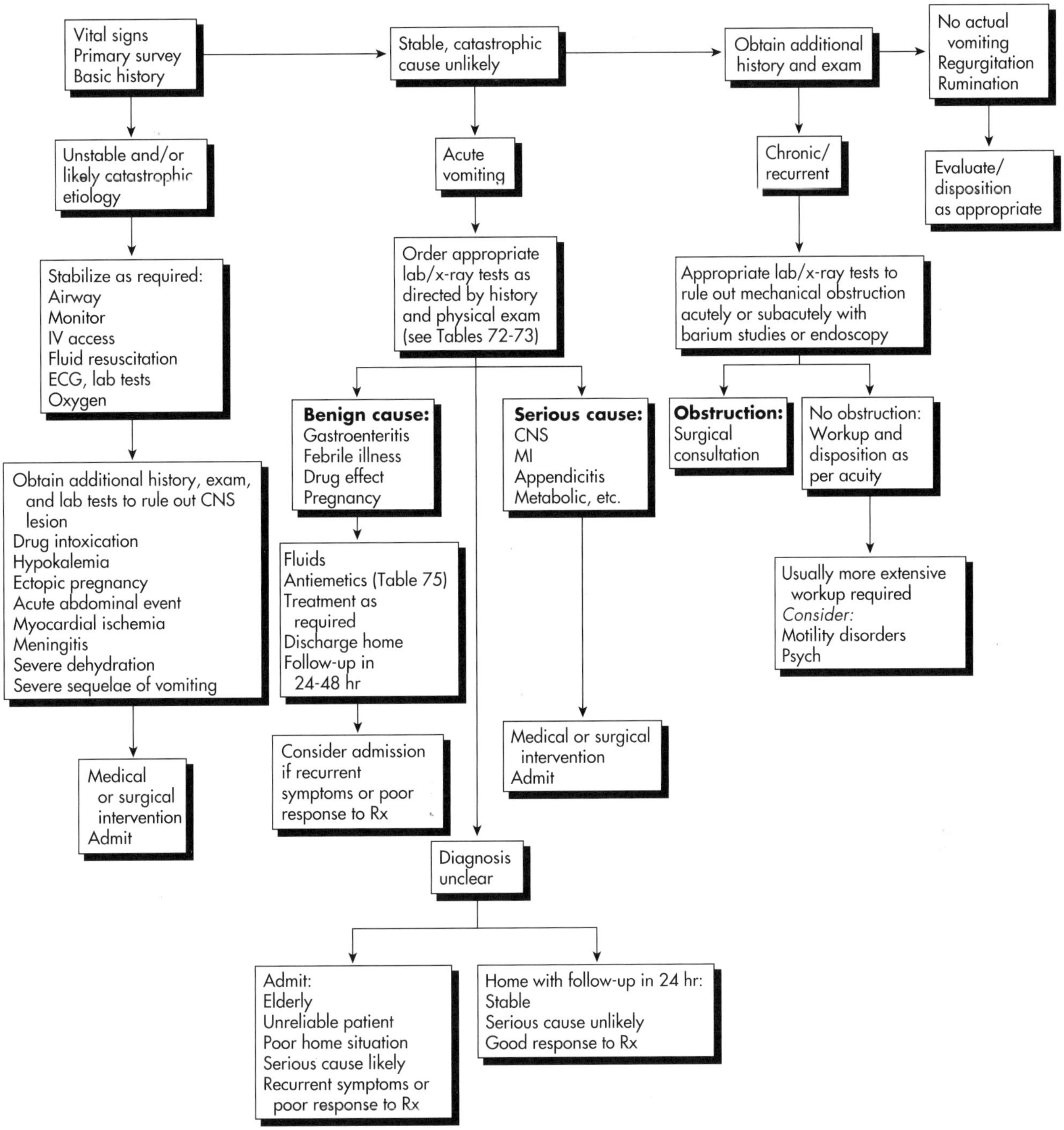

Vital signs
Primary survey
Basic history

Stable, catastrophic
cause unlikely

Obtain additional
history and exam

No actual
vomiting
Regurgitation
Rumination

Unstable and/or
likely catastrophic
etiology

Acute
vomiting

Chronic/
recurrent

Evaluate/
disposition
as appropriate

Stabilize as required:
Airway
Monitor
IV access
Fluid resuscitation
ECG, lab tests
Oxygen

Order appropriate
lab/x-ray tests as
directed by history
and physical exam
(see Tables 72-73)

Appropriate lab/x-ray tests to
rule out mechanical obstruction
acutely or subacutely with
barium studies or endoscopy

Benign cause:
Gastroenteritis
Febrile illness
Drug effect
Pregnancy

Serious cause:
CNS
MI
Appendicitis
Metabolic, etc.

Obstruction:
Surgical
consultation

No obstruction:
Workup and
disposition as
per acuity

Obtain additional history, exam,
and lab tests to rule out CNS
lesion
Drug intoxication
Hypokalemia
Ectopic pregnancy
Acute abdominal event
Myocardial ischemia
Meningitis
Severe dehydration
Severe sequelae of vomiting

Fluids
Antiemetics (Table 75)
Treatment as
required
Discharge home
Follow-up in
24-48 hr

Usually more extensive
workup required
Consider:
Motility disorders
Psych

Medical
or surgical
intervention
Admit

Consider admission
if recurrent
symptoms or poor
response to Rx

Medical or surgical
intervention
Admit

Diagnosis
unclear

Admit:
Elderly
Unreliable patient
Poor home situation
Serious cause likely
Recurrent symptoms or
poor response to Rx

Home with follow-up in 24 hr:
Stable
Serious cause unlikely
Good response to Rx

FIG. 122 Approach to the patient with nausea and vomiting. *CNS,* Central nervous system; *ECG,* electro-cardiogram; *IV,* intravenous; *MI,* myocardial infarction; *Psych,* psychogenic; *Rx,* treatment. (From Marx JA et al: *Rosen's emergency medicine,* ed 8, Philadelphia, 2014, Saunders.)

Clinical Algorithms

TABLE 72 Differential Diagnosis of Nausea and Vomiting

Etiologic Category	Critical Diagnoses	Emergent Diagnoses	Nonemergent Diagnoses
Gastrointestinal (GI)	• Boerhaave syndrome • Ischemic bowel • GI bleeding	• Gastric outlet obstruction • Pancreatitis • Cholecystitis or cholangitis • Bowel obstruction or ileus • Ruptured viscus • Appendicitis • Peritonitis • Spontaneous bacterial peritonitis	• Gastritis • Gastroparesis • Peptic ulcer disease • Inflammatory bowel disease • Biliary colic • Hepatitis • Gastroenteritis
Neurologic	• Intracerebral bleed • Meningitis	• Migraine • CNS tumor • Raised ICP	
Endocrine	• DKA	• Adrenal insufficiency • Uremia	• Thyroid
Pregnancy		• Hyperemesis gravidarum	• Nausea and vomiting of pregnancy
Drug toxicity		• Acetaminophen • Digoxin • Aspirin • Theophylline	
Therapeutic drug use			• Aspirin • Antibiotics • Erythromycin • Ibuprofen • Chemotherapy
Drugs of abuse			• Narcotics • Narcotic withdrawal • Alcohol
Genitourinary		• Gonadal torsion	• Urinary tract infection • Poisoning • Nephrolithiasis
Miscellaneous	• Myocardial infarction • Sepsis	• Carbon monoxide • Electrolyte disorders • Organophosphate poisoning	• Motion sickness • Labyrinthitis

CNS, Central nervous system; *DKA*, diabetic ketoacidosis; *ICP*, intracranial pressure.
From Marx JA et al: *Rosen's emergency medicine*, ed 8, Philadelphia, 2014, Saunders.

TABLE 73 Disorders Commonly Associated with Vomiting

Disorder	History	Prevalence	Physical Examination	Useful Tests	Comments
Nausea and vomiting of pregnancy (NVP)	Vomiting occurs predominantly in the morning. Associated breast tenderness. NVP typically starts in wk 4-7, peaks in wk 10-16, and disappears by wk 20. Vomiting that begins after wk 12 or continues past wk 20 should prompt a search for another cause.	Very common Affects 75% of all pregnancies	Benign abdomen	Urine pregnancy test Serum electrolytes, urine ketones to exclude hyperemesis gravidarum	Consider NVP in all females of childbearing age. Prognosis for mother and infant is excellent. NVP is associated with a decreased risk of miscarriage, fetal growth retardation, and fetal mortality.
Hyperemesis gravidarum	Severe, protracted form of NVP. No universally accepted definition of the disease. Generally accepted hallmarks include 5% weight loss, ketonuria, and electrolyte disturbance. Hyperemesis is associated with multiple gestation, molar pregnancy, and nulliparity.	Uncommon Affects <1% of pregnancies	Signs of dehydration Benign abdomen	β-hCG Urinalysis for ketones Serum electrolytes Ultrasound examination to exclude molar pregnancy or multiple gestation	Most studies have found no adverse outcomes for the fetus. A few studies, however, have shown a correlation with fetal growth retardation.

Table 73   Disorders Commonly Associated with Vomiting—cont'd

Disorder	History	Prevalence	Physical Examination	Useful Tests	Comments
Gastroenteritis	Fever, diarrhea, and crampy abdominal pain. Vomiting and pain occur early, usually followed by diarrhea within 24 h.	Very common	Benign abdomen	Usually not necessary	Early gastroenteritis, when only vomiting and periumbilical pain are present, may be confused with early appendicitis. Diarrhea is usually in the diagnosis of gastroenteritis.
Gastritis	Epigastric pain, belching, bloating, fullness, heartburn, and food intolerance. Use of NSAIDs or ETOH common.	Very common	Mild epigastric tenderness may be present.	Lipase and pregnancy test may be necessary to exclude other diagnoses.	Removal of inciting agent along with antacid therapy will resolve symptoms in most patients.
Peptic ulcer disease (PUD)	Epigastric pain present in 90% of cases. Classically, duodenal ulcer pain is relieved by food whereas gastric ulcer pain is made worse. Presence of severe pain should raise suspicion of perforation.	Very common	Mild epigastric tenderness	Hemoglobin if bleeding is suspected Heme-positive stool Upright abdominal film if perforation is suspected	Three major causes of PUD are NSAIDs, *Helicobacter pylori* infection, and hypersecretory states.
Biliary disease	Abdominal pain may be midepigastric or right upper quadrant (RUQ). Onset frequently after a fatty meal. May have history of similar episodes in the past.	Very common	RUQ tenderness present in most cases. If instructed to breathe deeply during palpation in the RUQ, the patient experiences heightened tenderness and inspiratory arrest (Murphy sign).	WBCs Lipase Serum bilirubin Alkaline phosphatase RUQ ultrasound examination ERCP	Normal temperature, WBCs, and spontaneous resolution of symptoms suggest biliary colic. Fever, Murphy sign, elevated WBCs, and suggestive ultrasound indicate cholecystitis.
Myocardial infarction (MI)	Patients typically have substernal chest pain that may radiate to left arm or jaw. Often associated with dyspnea, diaphoresis, or dizziness.	Common	Patients often are anxious and in distress from pain. No diagnostic examination findings.	ECG (new Q waves, ST segment changes, or T wave inversions) troponin	Not all patients have chest pain. A subset of patients, particularly diabetics and elders, may have only nausea, vomiting, and epigastric discomfort.
Diabetic ketoacidosis (DKA)	Polydipsia and polyuria occur early Without treatment, altered mental status and coma may develop. In patients with long-standing diabetes, DKA may be triggered by infection, trauma, MI, or surgery.	Common	"Fruity" breath odor results from serum acetone. Tachypnea occurs with attempts to "blow off" carbon dioxide to compensate for metabolic acidosis. Signs of dehydration may be present. Severe cases often manifest with altered mental status or coma.	Serum glucose, urine ketones, ABGs	DKA may be the first manifestation of diabetes in some patients. These patients often do not recognize the importance of polydipsia and polyuria. They often report only nausea, vomiting, and epigastric pain.
Pancreatitis	Presenting symptom is epigastric pain, which often radiates to the back. Most cases are caused by gallstones or alcoholism. Other causes include hypercalcemia, hyperlipidemia, drugs (sulfas and thiazides), ERCP.	Common	Epigastric tenderness is present. Associated paralytic ileus may cause abdominal distention and decreased bowel sounds. Frank shock may be present in severe cases.	Lipase WBCs, serum glucose, LDH, AST Hematocrit, BUN, calcium, ABGs	Criteria correlating with higher mortality: *At admission*—age >55 yr, WBCs >16,000/mm^3, glucose >200 dl, base deficit >4, LDH >350 IU/L, AST >250 U/L *Within 48 hr*—Hct drop of 10%, BUN >2 mg/dl, pO$_2$ <60 mm Hg, calcium <8 mg, fluid sequestration >4 L
Appendicitis	Abdominal pain classically begins in periumbilical region and later moves to right lower quadrant. Anorexia is common.	Common	Localized tenderness over right lower quadrant. Low-grade fever may be present.	WBCs Ultrasound Abdominal CT	Early appendicitis can be a difficult diagnosis to make. It is still frequently missed on the first physician encounter.

Clinical Algorithms

III

Continued

Table 73 Disorders Commonly Associated with Vomiting—cont'd

Disorder	History	Prevalence	Physical Examination	Useful Tests	Comments
Bowel obstruction	Classically, abdominal pain consists of intermittent cramps occurring at regular intervals. The frequency of the cramps varies with the level of the obstruction; the higher the level, the more frequent the cramps. The location of the pain also varies with the level of the obstruction; high obstruction causes epigastric pain, midlevel obstruction causes periumbilical pain, colonic obstruction causes hypogastric pain.	Common	Abdominal distention, mild diffuse tenderness, and high-pitched "tinkling" bowel sounds may be present. Thorough search for hernias should be performed.	Supine and upright plain abdominal films Abdominal CT	Adhesions, hernias, and tumors account for 90% of bowel obstructions. Other causes include intussusception, volvulus, foreign bodies, gallstone ileus, inflammatory bowel disease, stricture, cystic fibrosis, and hematoma.
Carbon monoxide (CO) poisoning	Headache is usually present. CO poisoning often occurs during winter months when furnaces are turned on. Family members may have similar symptoms if they also have been exposed.	Uncommon	No reliable signs of early CO poisoning	CO level	Because CO is a tasteless, odorless gas, patients may not realize they have been exposed. It is important to keep a high index of suspicion during the cold months.
Boerhaave syndrome	Patients may have neck, chest, or epigastric pain. Forceful, protracted vomiting usually causes the tear. Most cases follow a bout of heavy eating and drinking. Other reported causes include childbirth, defecation, seizures, and heavy lifting.	Uncommon	Tachypnea, tachycardia, and hypotension may be present. Escaped air from the esophagus may produce subcutaneous emphysema. Air in the mediastinum produces a "crunching" sound as the heart beats (Hamman sign).	CXR may show pleural effusion, widened mediastinum, pneumothorax, or pneumomediastinum. Esophagogram with water-soluble contrast is definitive.	The classic presentation includes forceful vomiting, severe chest pain, subcutaneous emphysema, and multiple CXR findings. There is a growing body of evidence that most cases do not have this "classic" picture. In more subtle presentations, the diagnosis can be difficult to make.

ABGs, Arterial blood gases; *AST,* aspartate aminotransferase; β-*hCG,* β-human chorionic gonadotropin; *BUN,* blood urea nitrogen; *CT,* computed tomography; *CXR,* chest radiography; *ECG,* electrocardiogram; *ERCP,* endoscopic retrograde cholangiopancreatography; *ETOH,* ethyl alcohol; *Hct,* hematocrit; *LDH,* lactate dehydrogenase; *NSAID,* nonsteroidal antiinflammatory drug; pO_2, partial pressure of oxygen; *RUQ,* right upper quadrant; *WBC,* white blood cell.
From Marx JA et al: *Rosen's emergency medicine,* ed 8, Philadelphia, 2014, Saunders.

TABLE 74 Etiology of Nausea and Vomiting in Pediatric Age Groups

Etiologic Category	Newborn	Infant	Child	Adolescent
Infectious	Sepsis, meningitis, UTI, thrush	Pneumonia, otitis media, thrush	Gastroenteritis	Gastroenteritis, URI
Anatomic	Atresia and webs, malrotation, stenosis, meconium ileus, Hirschsprung disease	Pyloric stenosis, intussusception, Hirschsprung disease	Bezoars, chronic granulomatous disease	PUD, superior mesenteric syndrome
Gastrointestinal	Reflux, overfeeding, gastric outlet obstruction, volvulus	Reflux, gastritis, milk intolerance	Appendicitis, pancreatic, hepatitis, other food intolerance	Achalasia, hepatitis
Neurologic	Subdural hematoma, hydrocephalus	Subdural hematoma	Neoplasia, migraine, Reye syndrome, motion sickness, hypertension	Neoplasia, migraine, motion sickness, hypertension
Metabolic	Organic or amino acidemias, urea cycle defects, galactosemia, hypercalcemia, phenylketonuria, kernicterus	Hereditary fructose intolerance, disorders of fatty acid metabolism, uremia, adrenal hyperplasia, kernicterus	Diabetes, vitamin A excess	Diabetes, pregnancy, acute intermittent porphyria
Other	Idiopathic, cardiac failure	Rumination, cardiac failure	Cyclic vomiting syndrome, toxins, food poisoning, Munchausen syndrome by proxy	Psychogenic, anorexia

PUD, Peptic ulcer disease; *URI,* upper respiratory infection; *UTI,* urinary tract infection.
Adapted from Li HK, Sunku BK: Vomiting and nausea. In Wyllie R, Hyams JS (eds): *Pediatric gastrointestinal and liver disease: pathophysiology, diagnosis, management,* Philadelphia, 2005, Saunders, pp. 127-149. From Marx JA et al: *Rosen's emergency medicine,* ed 8, Philadelphia, 2014, Saunders.

TABLE 75   Commonly Used Medications for the Treatment of Nausea and Vomiting

Medication	Dose	Comments
Promethazine (Phenergan)	*Adult:* 12.5-25 mg IV, IM, PO, or by rectum *Pediatric:* 0.25-1 mg/kg/dose q4-6h prn IV, IM, PO, or by rectum; max 25 mg/dose	May be repeated every 4-6 h until cessation of vomiting. May cause dry mouth, dizziness, blurred vision. Boxed warning for use under 2 yr old.
Prochlorperazine (Compazine)	*Adult:* 5-10 mg IM or PO; 2.5-10 mg IV; 25 mg by rectum *Pediatric:* 0.4 mg/kg/24 h tid-qid PO or by rectum; 0.1-0.15 mg/kg/dose tid-qid IM; max 40 mg/24 h	May be repeated every 4 h IV or IM or every 12 h by rectum until cessation of vomiting. May cause lethargy, hypotension, extrapyramidal effects.
Metoclopramide (Reglan)	*Adult:* 10 mg IM or IV, may repeat q6h *Pediatric:* 1-2 mg/kg/dose q2-6h IV q2-3h	May cause dystonic reactions, tardive dyskinesia, neuroleptic malignant syndrome.
Ondansetron (Zofran)	*Adult:* 4 mg IV single dose *Pediatric:* Up to 40 kg: 0.1 mg/kg; >40 kg: 4 mg/dose IV single dose	May cause headache, dizziness, and musculoskeletal pain.

IM, Intramuscularly; *IV,* intravenously; *PO,* orally; *prn,* as needed; *q,* every.
From Marx JA et al: *Rosen's emergency medicine,* ed 8, Philadelphia, 2014, Saunders.

Clinical
Algorithms

III

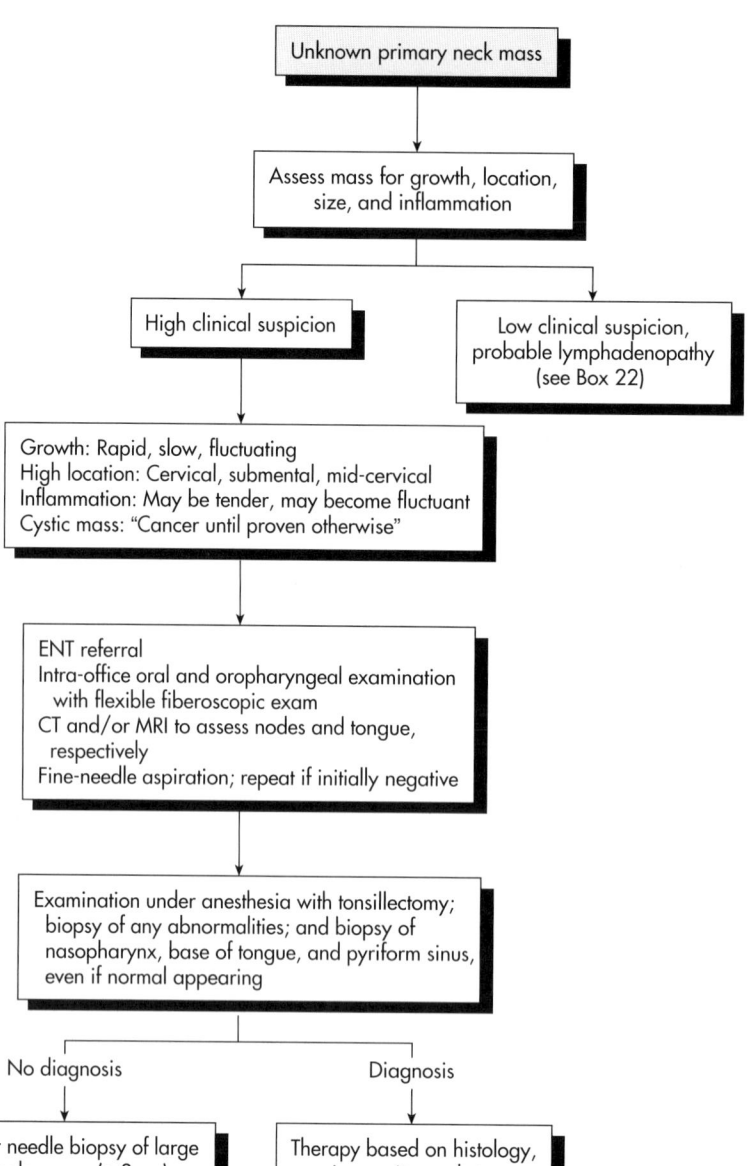

FIG. 123 Evaluation of an unknown primary neck mass. *CT,* Computed tomography; *ENT,* ear, nose, and throat; *MRI,* magnetic resonance imaging. (From Goldman L, Schafer AL [eds]: *Cecil textbook of medicine,* ed 24, Philadelphia, 2012, Saunders.)

BOX 22 An Approach to the Patient with Lymphadenopathy

- Does the patient have a known illness that causes lymphadenopathy? Treat and monitor for resolution.
- Is there an obvious infection to explain the lymphadenopathy (e.g., infectious mononucleosis)? Treat and monitor for resolution.
- Are the nodes very large and/or very firm and thus suggestive of malignancy? Perform a biopsy.
- Is the patient very concerned about malignancy and unable to be reassured that malignancy is unlikely? Perform a biopsy.
- If none of the preceding are true, perform a complete blood cell count, and if it is unrevealing, monitor for a predetermined period (usually 2-6 wk). If the nodes do not regress or if they increase in size, perform a biopsy.

From Goldman L, Ausiello D (eds): *Cecil textbook of medicine,* ed 23, Philadelphia, 2008, Saunders.

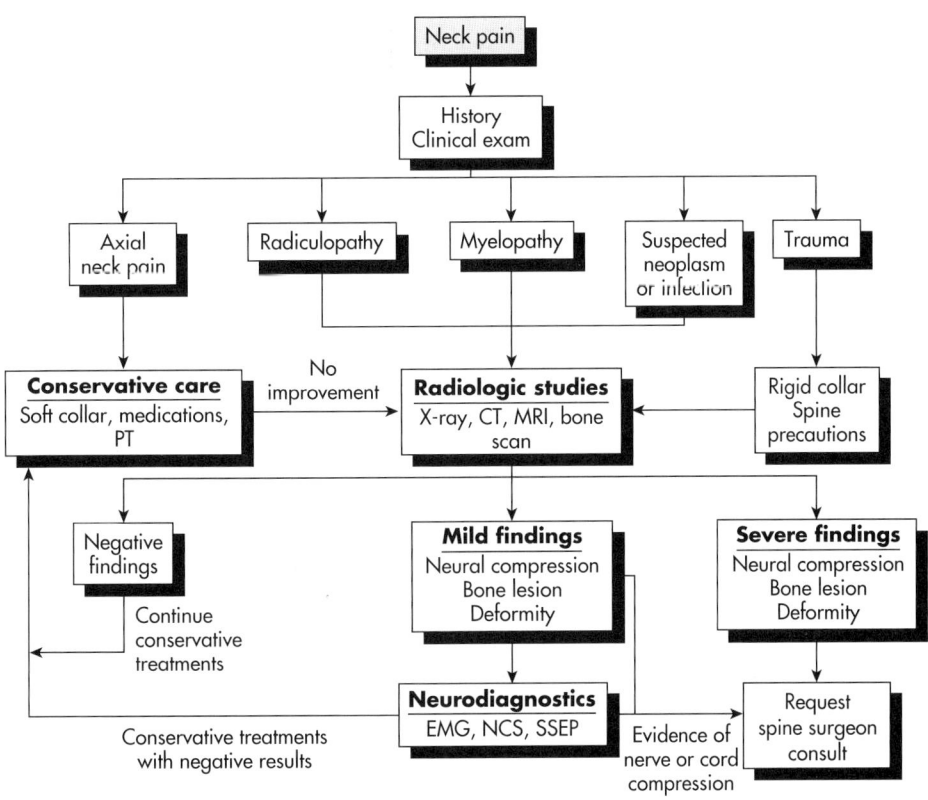

FIG. 124 **Algorithm of neck pain.** *CT,* Computed tomography; *EMG,* electromyogram; *MRI,* magnetic resonance imaging; *NCS,* nerve conduction study; *PT,* physical therapy; *SSEP,* somatosensory evoked potentials. (From Firestein GS et al: *Kelley's textbook of rheumatology,* ed 9, Philadelphia, 2013, Saunders.)

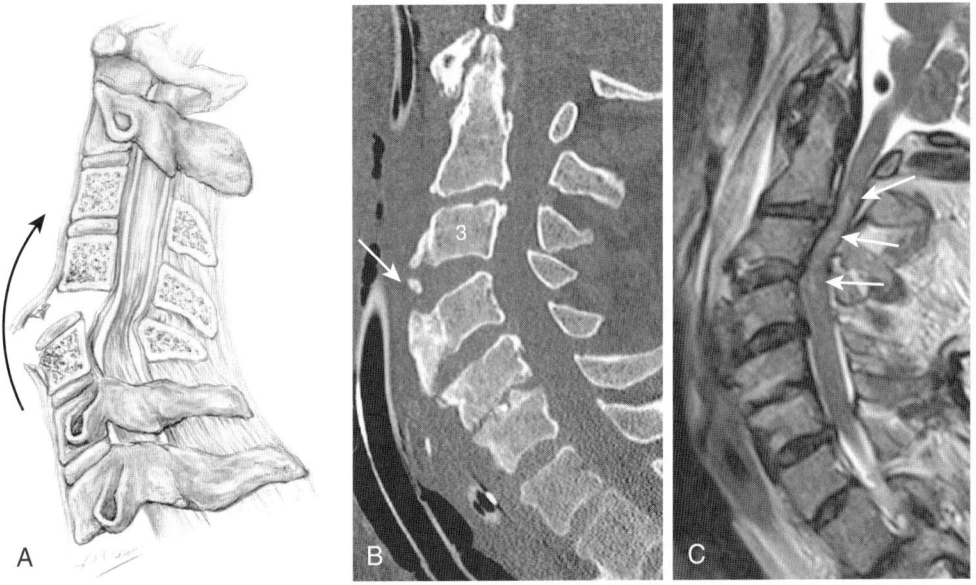

FIG. 125 **Extension injury. A,** Drawing shows mechanism and injury. There is a small avulsion from the anterosuperior margin of the vertebra immediately below the affected level. Note the wide disk space and retrolisthesis, hallmarks of this injury. The spinal cord is frequently injured in this setting. **B,** Sagittal reconstructed computed tomography image shows widening of the C3 disk space with an avulsed fragment of bone *(arrow)* and retrolisthesis. **C,** T2-weighted magnetic resonance image shows cord hemorrhage *(arrows)*. The patient is quadriplegic. (From Pope TL et al: *Musculoskeletal imaging,* ed 2, Philadelphia, 2015, Elsevier.)

TABLE 76   Differential Diagnosis of Common Causes of Axial Neck Pain

Etiology	Cause	Characteristics	Physical Exam	Treatment
Trauma	• Irritation of muscles, facets, intervertebral discs, and ligaments (i.e., "whiplash") • Bony fractures	History of trauma Neck stiffness Pain worsens with movement May have accompanying neurologic deficits	• Guarding of the neck muscles leading to reduced ROM • Severe midline tenderness with fractures • Moderate tenderness with whiplash type injuries • Neurologic deficit	Physical therapy and antiinflammatories may be beneficial in the case of whiplash Bracing may be necessary for minor fractures Surgical intervention may be necessary for instability or neurologic compression
Degenerative Changes (Nonneuropathic)	• Irritation of zygapophyseal (facet) joints • Irritation of cervical discs	Often chronic in nature Pain radiates to shoulders Suboccipital headaches Facet pain improves with injections targeting the joint capsule or block of dorsal primary ramus	• Limited neck range of motion • Facet pain worsened by palpation of paraspinal region • Discogenic pain worsened by midline palpation • Discogenic pain worsened with neck extension and rotation	• Physical therapy, antiinflammatories • Medial branch blocks or radiofrequency ablation for facet pain • Surgical intervention may be considered if instability or deformity is present
Cervical Radiculopathy	• Herniated cervical disc • Spondylosis • Noncompressive pathologies (diabetes, herpes zoster, etc.)	• Sharp, shooting pain • Radiation into the associated dermatome	• Positive Spurling sign • Numbness, tingling, and/or pain in associated dermatomes • Weakness in associated myotomes	1. Physical therapy, antiinflammatories, oral steroids, and epidural steroid injections 2. Surgery for failure of conservative therapy or if weakness is present
Cervical Stenosis	• Spondylosis • Congenitally narrow canal • Postsurgical • Traumatic • Rheumatologic	• Often accompanied by myelopathy (deterioration in fine motor skills, gait and balance disturbances, incontinence, etc.)	• Broad-based, spastic gait • Hyperreflexia • Weakness • Positive Hoffman sign	• Symptomatic treatment may be beneficial in the absence of a neurologic deficit • Surgical intervention warranted in the presence of neurologic deficits or hyperreflexia
Myofascial Pain	• Chronic irritation of neck muscles • May be due to postural or biomechanical imbalance, trauma, emotional stress, and endocrine or hormone abnormalities	• Dull and persistent pain without clear exacerbating or alleviating factors • Sometimes worsened with neck flexion • May be associated with fibromyalgia	• Patient may have trigger points, or palpable muscle bands that refer pain when pressure is applied	• Physical therapy and antiinflammatories • Psychotherapy • Trigger point injections
Rheumatologic Disease • Rheumatoid arthritis (RA) • Ankylosing spondylitis (AS) • Others	• Joint inflammation • Cervical stenosis • Musculoskeletal strain from cervicothoracic kyphotic deformity in AS	• Morning stiffness and rigidity • RA may lead to atlanto-axial instability • AS may lead to cervicothoracic kyphosis	• Additional symptoms related to systemic disorder	• Physical therapy and antiinflammatories may be considered to alleviate symptoms • Surgery may be necessary to address instability or deformity
Infection • Osteomyelitis • Diskitis • Epidural abscess	• Bone destruction • Irritation of periosteal nerves • Instability • Altered biomechanics	• Severe neck pain that is present at rest and worsened with movement • Signs/symptoms of infection • Patients with history of IVDU or immunocompromise	• Severe pain that is worsened with movement • Neurologic deficits may be due to epidural abscess • Stigmata of bacteremia	• IV antibiotics • Surgery may be necessary in the presence of an epidural abscess • Bracing may offer symptomatic relief
Neoplasm • Metastatic tumors • Multiple myeloma/plasmacytoma • Primary bone tumors	• Bone destruction • Irritation of periosteal nerves • Mechanical instability	• Neck pain worsens with movement • Pain awakens patient from sleep • Systemic symptoms such as unexplained weight loss, anorexia, malaise, etc.	• Severe neck tenderness • Neck pain worsens with movement • Neurologic deficits present from epidural tumor	• Symptomatic treatment with antiinflammatories and pain medications • Radiation • Surgical intervention may be warranted for decompression and/or stabilization

Table 76 Differential Diagnosis of Common Causes of Axial Neck Pain—cont'd

Etiology	Cause	Characteristics	Physical Exam	Treatment
Vascular				
• Cervical carotid dissection	• Traumatic or spontaneous tear in the tunica intima • Blood enters the space between the inner and outer wall	• Sudden onset • Tearing sensation • Headache • Facial or eye pain • Pulsatile tinnitus • Ischemic events	• Horner syndrome • Carotid bruit • Expanding hematoma • Neurologic deficit	• Antiplatelet agents, anticoagulants, stenting
Postsurgical				
• Pseudoarthrosis (failed fusion) • Postsurgical iatrogenic instability	• Hardware loosening • Instability due to disruption of disc and joints	• Improvement in neck pain after surgery ("honeymoon period") with worsening neck and interscapular pain	• Painful range of motion in the neck • History of cervical surgery	• Revision surgical procedure

From Firestein GS et al: *Firestein & Kelley's textbook of rheumatology*, ed 11, Philadelphia, 2021, Elsevier.

TABLE 77 Rheumatologic Disorders Causing Neck Pain

- Rheumatoid arthritis
    1. Without disease of the C1-C2 joint
    2. With structural cervical abnormalities
        a. C1-C2 subluxation
        b. C1-C2 facet involvement
- Spondyloarthropathies
    1. Ankylosing spondylitis
    2. Reactive arthritis
    3. Psoriatic arthritis
    4. Enteropathic arthritis
- Polymyalgia rheumatica
- Osteoarthritis
- Fibromyalgia
- Nonspecific musculoskeletal pain
- Miscellaneous spondyloarthropathies
    1. Whipple disease
    2. Behçet disease
    3. Paget disease
    4. Acromegaly
    5. Ossification of the posterior longitudinal ligament
    6. Diffuse idiopathic skeletal hyperostosis

From Firestein GS et al: *Firestein & Kelley's textbook of rheumatology*, ed 11, Philadelphia, 2021, Elsevier.

ICD-10CM #
H92.0	Otalgia
H92.01	Otalgia, right ear
H92.02	Otalgia, left ear
H92.03	Bilateral otalgia
H92 .09	Unspecified otalgia
H92.1	Otorrhea
H92. 13	Bilateral otorrhea
H92.11	Otorrhea, right ear
H92.12	Otorrhea, left ear
H92.10	Otorrhea, unspecified ear

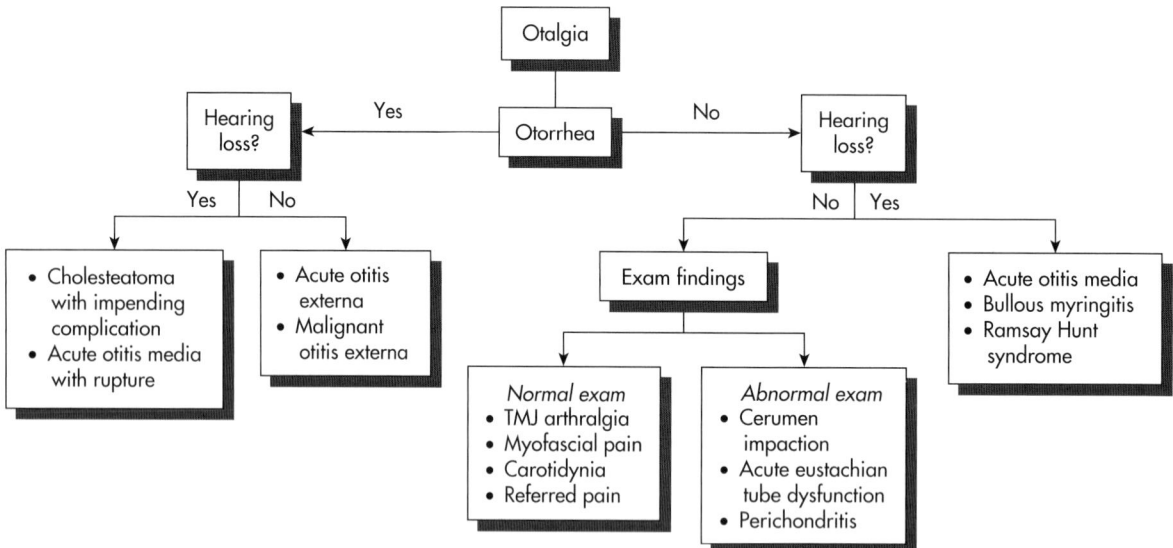

FIG. 127 Establishing a differential diagnosis with a chief complaint of otalgia. This algorithm encourages the clinician to consider the patient complaint in categoric differential diagnosis families. It is not exhaustive. (From Flint PW et al: *Cummings otolaryngology, head and neck surgery*, ed 7, Philadelphia, 2021, Elsevier.)

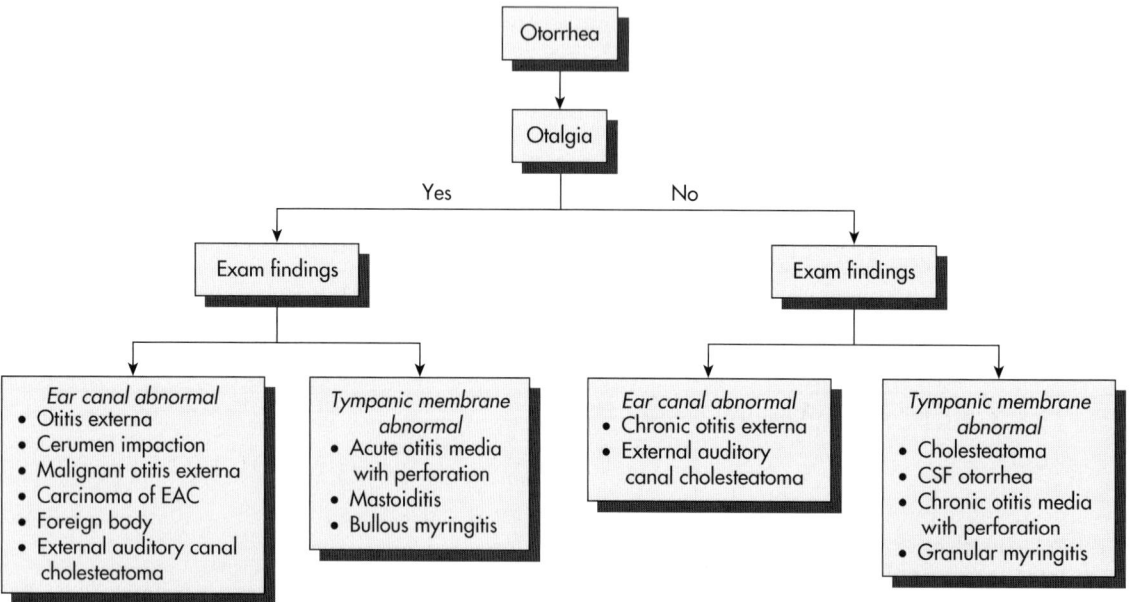

FIG. 128 Establishing a differential diagnosis with a chief complaint of otorrhea. This algorithm encourages the clinician to consider the patient complaint in categoric differential diagnosis families. It is not exhaustive. *CSF,* Cerebrospinal fluid; *EAC,* external auditory canal. (From Flint PW et al: *Cummings otolaryngology, head and neck surgery*, ed 7, Philadelphia, 2021, Elsevier.)

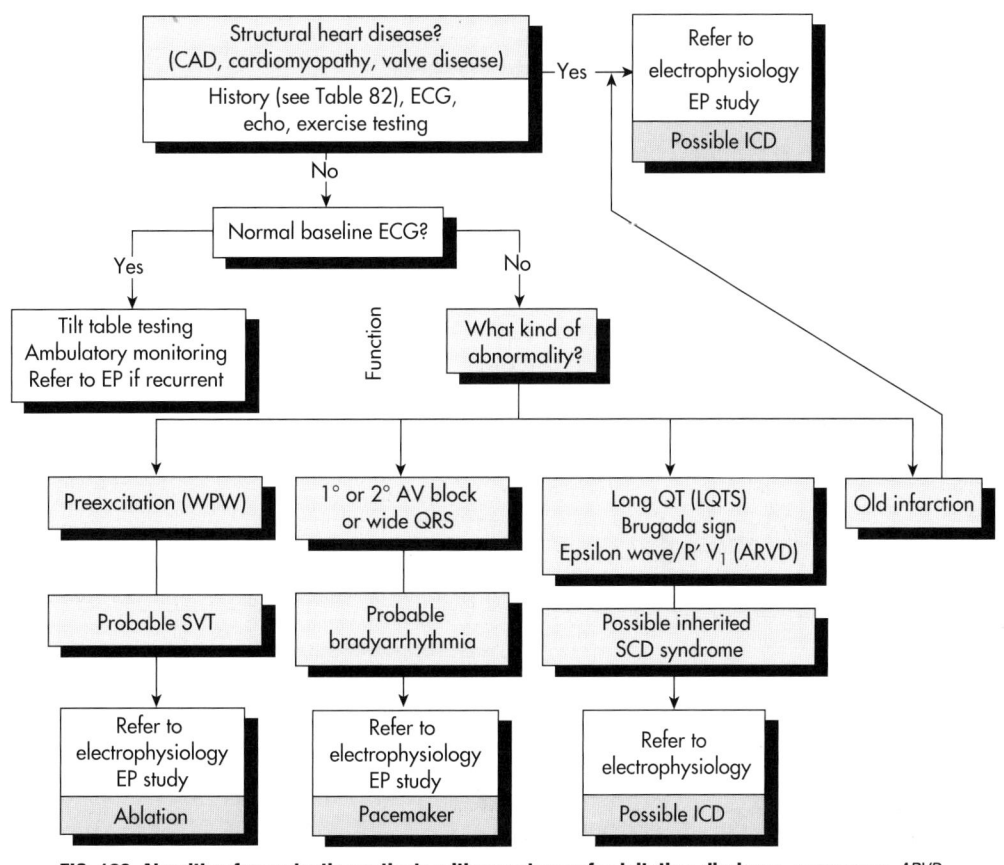

FIG. 129 Algorithm for evaluating patients with symptoms of palpitation, dizziness, or syncope. *ARVD,* Arrhythmogenic right ventricular dysplasia; *AV,* atrioventricular; *CAD,* coronary artery disease; *ECG,* electrocardiogram; *echo,* echocardiogram; *EP,* electrophysiology; *ICD,* implantable cardioverter-defibrillator; *LQTS,* long QT syndrome; *SCD,* sudden cardiac death; *SVT,* supraventricular tachycardia; *WPW,* Wolff-Parkinson-White syndrome. (From Goldman L, Schafer AI: *Goldman Cecil medicine,* ed 25, Philadelphia, 2016, Saunders.)

Clinical Algorithms

III

TABLE 80 Items to Be Covered in History of Patient with Palpitation

Does the Palpitation Occur:	If So, Suspect:
As isolated "jumps" or "skips"?	Extrasystoles
In attacks known to be of abrupt beginning, with a heart rate of 120 beats/min or over, with regular or irregular rhythm?	Paroxysmal rapid heart action
Independent of exercise or excitement adequate to account for the symptom?	Atrial fibrillation, atrial flutter, thyrotoxicosis, anemia, febrile states, hypoglycemia, anxiety state
In attacks developing rapidly, though not absolutely abruptly, unrelated to exertion or excitement?	Hemorrhage, hypoglycemia, tumor of the adrenal medulla
In conjunction with the taking of drugs?	Tobacco, coffee, tea, alcohol, epinephrine, ephedrine, aminophylline, atropine, thyroid extract, monoamine oxidase inhibitors
On standing?	Postural hypotension
In middle-aged women, in conjunction with flushes and sweats?	Menopausal syndrome
When the rate is known to be normal and the rhythm regular?	Anxiety state

From Goldman L, Braunwald E: Chest discomfort and palpitation. In Isselbacher KJ et al (eds): *Harrison's principles of internal medicine,* ed 13, New York, 1994, McGraw-Hill.

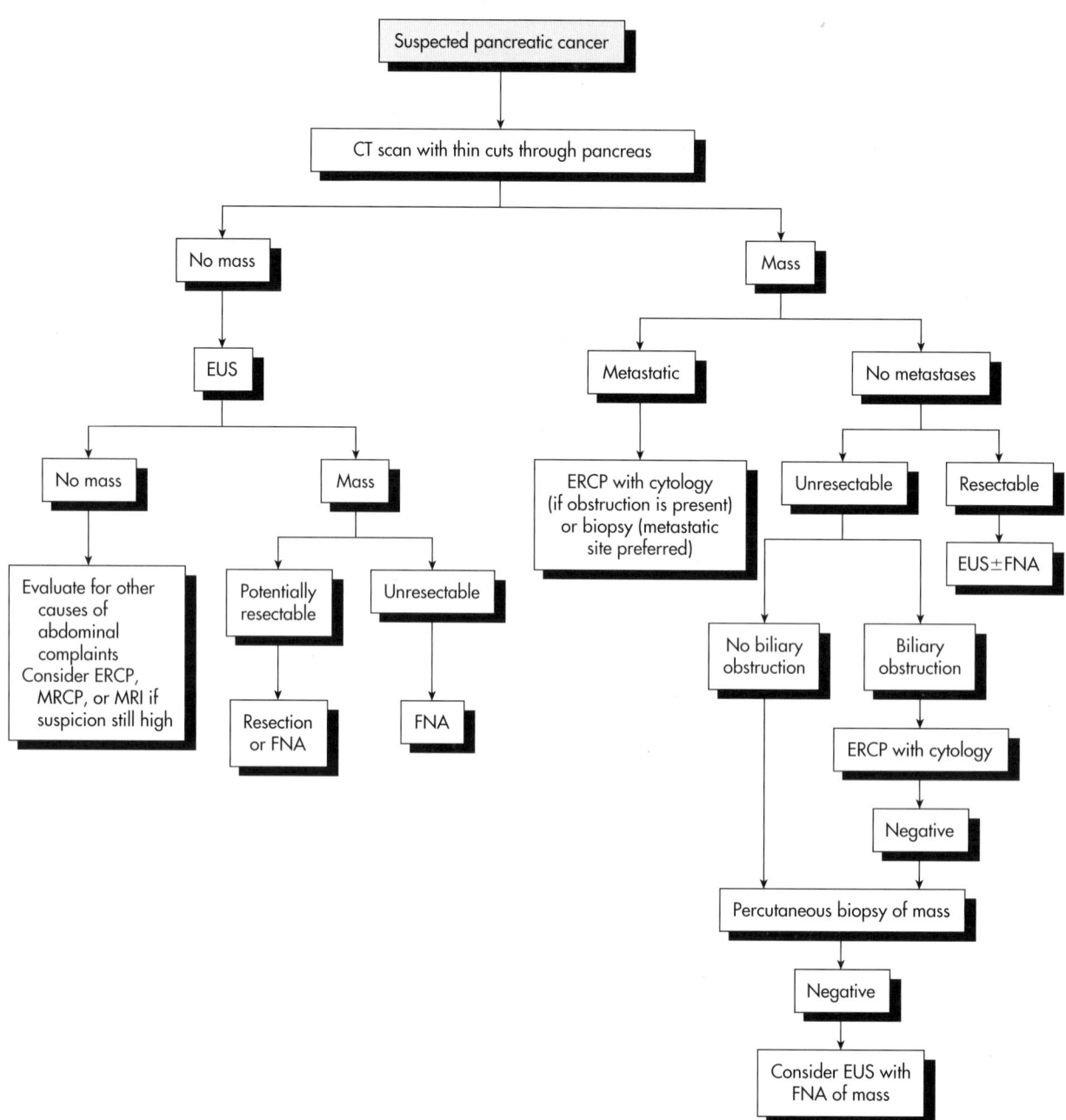

FIG. 132 Diagnostic algorithm for pancreatic cancer. Intraoperative fine-needle aspiration (FNA) if found inoperable during surgery. *CT,* Computed tomography; *ERCP,* endoscopic retrograde cholangiopancreatography; *EUS,* endoscopic ultrasonography; *MRCP,* magnetic resonance cholangiopancreatography; *MRI,* magnetic resonance imaging. (From Goldman L, Schafer AL [eds]: *Cecil textbook of medicine,* ed 24, Philadelphia, 2012, Saunders.)

History and Physical Exam (Table 81)

Most likely gynecologic based on H&P?

— Yes → Pregnant?
— No → Urinary complaints and/or + dipstick?

Pregnant?
— Yes
— No

Urinary complaints and/or + dipstick?
— Yes → UTI / Ureteral stone
— No → Abdominal tenderness or rebound?

Pregnant? Yes:
- 1st trimester → Definite IUP on ultrasound?
- >1st trimester → Placental abruption / Placenta previa / SAB / Round ligament pain / Labor

Pregnant? No:
- Unilateral symptoms/signs?
  - Yes → Torsion / Salpingitis/TOA / Ruptured ovarian cyst / Mittelschmerz
  - No → PID / Endometritis / Dysmenorrhea / Fibroids

Definite IUP on ultrasound?
- Yes → Threatened abortion / Corpus luteum cyst
- No → Ectopic pregnancy (Fig. 137) / Spontaneous abortion / Early pregnancy

Abdominal tenderness or rebound?
- Yes → Appendicitis / Diverticulitis / IBD / IBS / Other
- No → Musculoskeletal / Abuse / Depression / Psychogenic

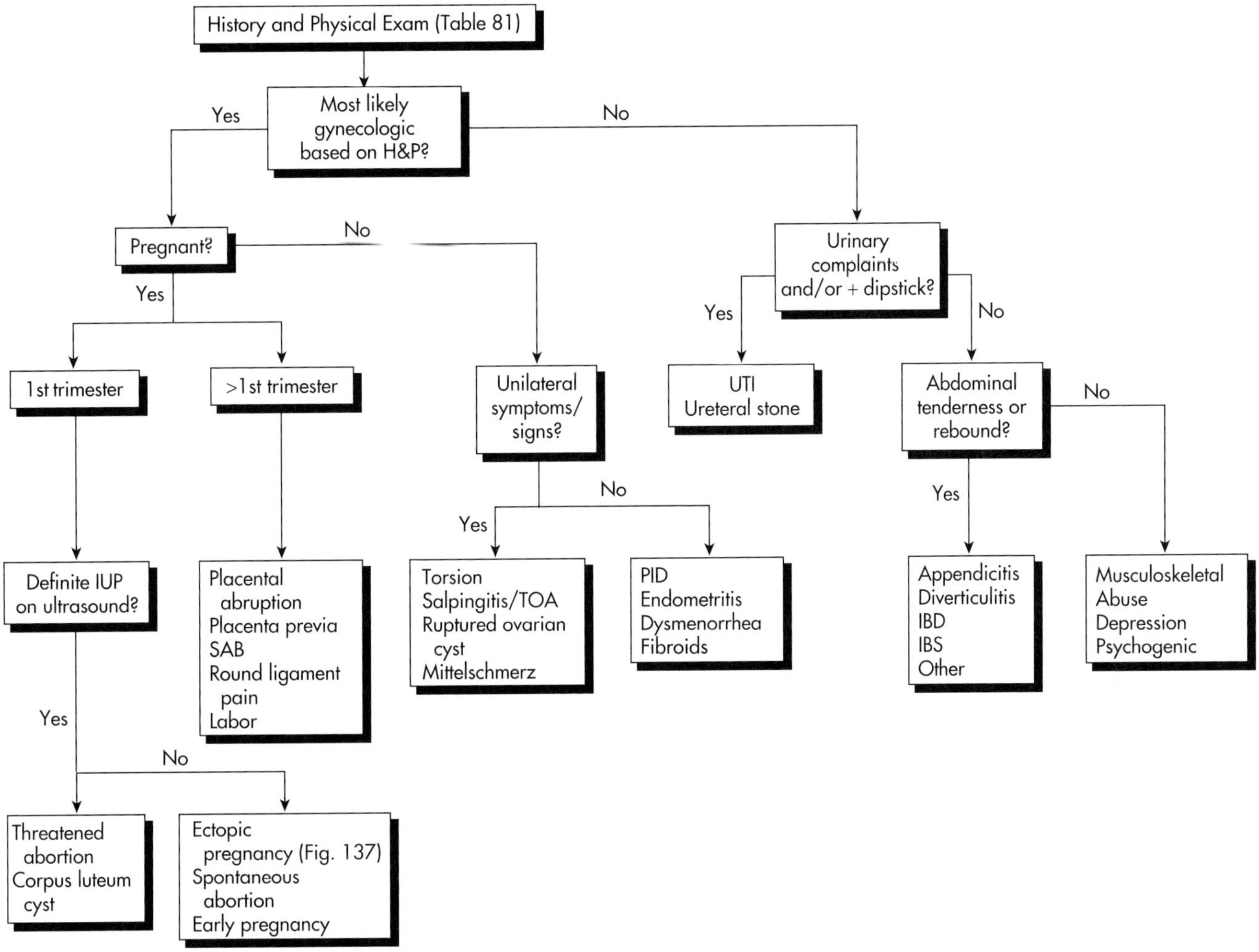

FIG. 133 Diagnostic algorithm for acute pelvic pain. *H&P,* History and physical; *IBD,* inflammatory bowel disease; *IBS,* irritable bowel syndrome; *IUP,* intrauterine pregnancy; *PID,* pelvic inflammatory disease; *SAB,* spontaneous abortion; *TOA,* tuboovarian abscess; *UTI,* urinary tract infection. (From Marx JA et al: *Rosen's emergency medicine,* ed 8, Philadelphia, 2014, Saunders.)

Clinical Algorithms

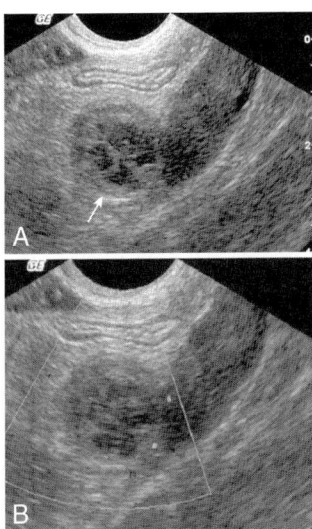

FIG. 134 Ectopic pregnancy seen as mixed-echogenicity mass. A 30-yr-old woman presented with left lower quadrant pain at 7 wk gestation and β-hCG of 500 mIU/ml and falling over a 3-day period. **A,** In the left adnexa, medial to the left ovary, there was a 2-cm mass *(arrow)* with mixed echogenicity, and **B,** only minimal peripheral vascularity. A left ectopic pregnancy was confirmed and, based on a falling β-hCG, was treated expectantly and resolved without complication. (From Rumack CM et al: *Diagnostic ultrasound,* ed 4, Philadelphia, 2011, Elsevier.)

TABLE 81   Differentiation of Common or Potentially Catastrophic Causes of Pelvic Pain

Causative Disorder or Condition	Pain History	Associated Symptoms	Supporting History	Prevalence in ED	Physical Examination	Useful Tests	Atypical or Additional Aspects
Ectopic pregnancy (critical if ruptured)	Classically severe, sharp, lateral pelvic pain, but severity, location, and quality highly variable	Vaginal bleeding (often mild, can be absent)	Missed period; history of previous ectopic pregnancy, infertility, pelvic surgery, PID, or IUD use	Common	Classically unilateral adnexal tenderness, adnexal mass, and CMT	Pelvic US, quantitative β-hCG, T&C, laparoscopy	Cannot reliably exclude diagnosis based on history and physical examination. Severe pain, hypotension, or peritonitis suggests rupture
Ruptured ovarian cyst (emergent—critical with significant hemorrhage; otherwise, urgent)	Abrupt moderate to severe lateral pain	Light-headedness if bleeding is severe; rectal pain arises from fluid in cul-de-sac		Uncommon	Hypotension and tachycardia if blood loss is significant; possible peritonitis	Pelvic US, CBC, T&C	Physical examination findings often do not correlate with volume of blood in pelvis at US
Ovarian torsion (emergent)	Acute onset of moderate to severe lateral pain	Nausea and vomiting	History of ovarian mass or cyst	Uncommon	Adnexal mass and tenderness, possible peritonitis	US with Doppler flow studies, laparoscopy	Torsion can be intermittent
Appendicitis (emergent)	Duration often <48 h, generalized followed by localized RLQ pain	Low-grade fever, nausea, anorexia	Migration of pain to RLQ from center, abdominal pain before vomiting	Common	RLQ tenderness, possible peritonitis	US or CT in unclear cases	Early in course, tenderness may be minimal or poorly localized
PID, TOA (TOA: Emergent; PID: Urgent-emergent)	Without TOA, pain usually bilateral. May manifest acutely within 48 h or subacutely with up to 3 wk of pain	Fever, vaginal discharge	Vaginal discharge, history of PID, history of unprotected intercourse or multiple partners	PID: Common TOA: Uncommon	Pus from cervical os, CMT, adnexal tenderness. Peritonitis suggests severe PID or TOA	CBC, ESR, CRP, pelvic US, laparoscopy, cervical cultures, cervical smear for WBCs	History and physical examination may be inaccurate for diagnosis, particularly in patients with subacute presentation
UTI (urgent)	Pain with urination. Patient may have flank pain from associated pyelonephritis	Urinary urgency and frequency; fever and vomiting if patient has associated pyelonephritis	Recent urologic procedure, prior history of UTI	Common	Suprapubic tenderness, flank tenderness and fever with pyelonephritis	Urinalysis, urine culture (if recurrent or complicated)	WBCs can be present in urine with PID and appendicitis. RBCs present in urine with hemorrhagic cystitis
Ureteral colic (urgent)	Acute onset, manifests within hours. Pain is lateral, usually moderate to severe. Often radiates into the groin or costovertebral angle or flank	Nausea and vomiting	Prior history of stones	Common	Patient often appears uncomfortable, but physical examination can be otherwise unremarkable	Urinalysis: Hematuria present in approximately 80% of cases. Renal ultrasound for hydronephrosis. Abdominal CT	If stone is at ureterovesicular junction, patient can have localized pain that can mimic appendicitis or other acute pelvic pathology
Unruptured ovarian cyst or tumor	Lateral ache, gradual onset	Often minimal	Prior history of similar pain	Common	Lateral pelvic tenderness, with or without a mass	Pelvic US	
Endometriosis	Unilateral or bilateral pelvic pain, often recurrent	Dysmenorrhea, dyspareunia	Prior history of same type of pain in association with menstrual cycle	Common	Unilateral or bilateral adnexal tenderness, occasionally pelvic mass present, peritoneal findings uncommon	Pelvic US, laparoscopy	Symptoms can mimic other types of pelvic pathology; laparoscopy often is needed for confirmation

β-hCG, β-Human chorionic gonadotropin; *CBC,* complete blood count; *CMT,* cervical motion tenderness; *CRP,* C-reactive protein; *CT,* computed tomography; *ED,* emergency department; *ESR,* erythrocyte sedimentation rate; *IUD,* intrauterine device; *PID,* pelvic inflammatory disease; *RBC,* red blood cell; *RLQ,* right lower quadrant; *T&C,* type and crossmatch; *TOA,* tuboovarian abscess; *US,* ultrasonography; *UTI,* urinary tract infection; *WBC,* white blood cell.

From Marx JA et al: *Rosen's emergency medicine,* ed 8, Philadelphia, 2014, Saunders.

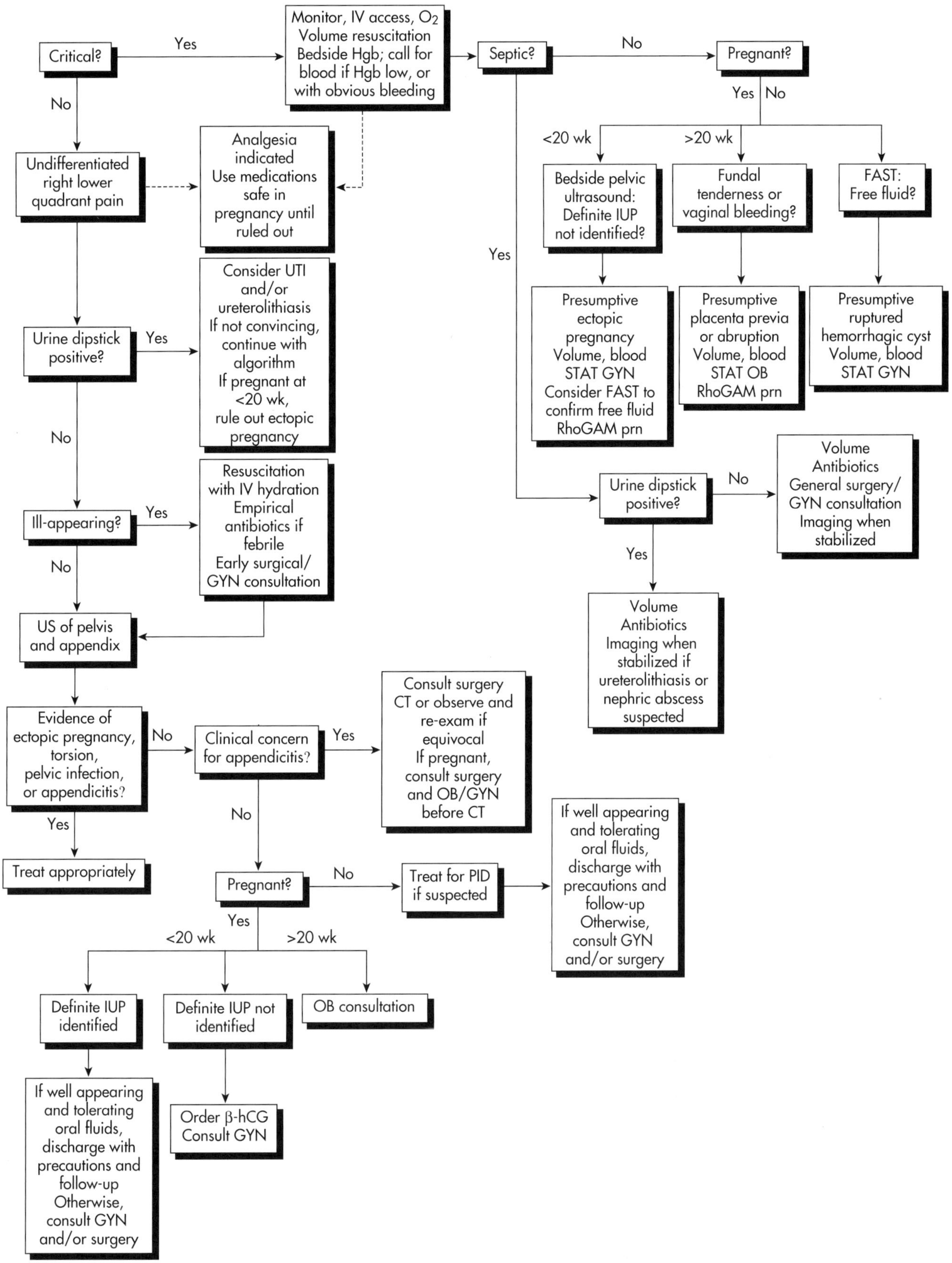

Critical? — Yes → Monitor, IV access, O₂ / Volume resuscitation / Bedside Hgb; call for blood if Hgb low, or with obvious bleeding — Septic?

Critical? — No → Undifferentiated right lower quadrant pain

Monitor box ⤏ (dashed) Analgesia indicated / Use medications safe in pregnancy until ruled out

Undifferentiated right lower quadrant pain ⤏ (dashed) Analgesia indicated / Use medications safe in pregnancy until ruled out

Undifferentiated right lower quadrant pain → Urine dipstick positive?

Urine dipstick positive? — Yes → Consider UTI and/or ureterolithiasis / If not convincing, continue with algorithm / If pregnant at <20 wk, rule out ectopic pregnancy

Urine dipstick positive? — No → Ill-appearing?

Ill-appearing? — Yes → Resuscitation with IV hydration / Empirical antibiotics if febrile / Early surgical/ GYN consultation

Ill-appearing? — No → US of pelvis and appendix

US of pelvis and appendix → Evidence of ectopic pregnancy, torsion, pelvic infection, or appendicitis?

Evidence of ectopic pregnancy, torsion, pelvic infection, or appendicitis? — No → Clinical concern for appendicitis?

Evidence of ectopic pregnancy, torsion, pelvic infection, or appendicitis? — Yes → Treat appropriately

Clinical concern for appendicitis? — Yes → Consult surgery / CT or observe and re-exam if equivocal / If pregnant, consult surgery and OB/GYN before CT

Clinical concern for appendicitis? — No → Pregnant?

Pregnant? — No → Treat for PID if suspected → If well appearing and tolerating oral fluids, discharge with precautions and follow-up / Otherwise, consult GYN and/or surgery

Pregnant? — Yes — <20 wk → Definite IUP identified

Pregnant? — Yes — >20 wk → OB consultation

Definite IUP not identified

Definite IUP identified → If well appearing and tolerating oral fluids, discharge with precautions and follow-up / Otherwise, consult GYN and/or surgery

Definite IUP not identified → Order β-hCG / Consult GYN

Septic? — No → Pregnant?

Septic? — Yes → Urine dipstick positive?

Pregnant? — Yes — <20 wk → Bedside pelvic ultrasound: Definite IUP not identified?

Pregnant? — Yes — >20 wk → Fundal tenderness or vaginal bleeding?

Pregnant? — No → FAST: Free fluid?

Bedside pelvic ultrasound: Definite IUP not identified? → Presumptive ectopic pregnancy / Volume, blood / STAT GYN / Consider FAST to confirm free fluid / RhoGAM prn

Fundal tenderness or vaginal bleeding? → Presumptive placenta previa or abruption / Volume, blood / STAT OB / RhoGAM prn

FAST: Free fluid? → Presumptive ruptured hemorrhagic cyst / Volume, blood / STAT GYN

Urine dipstick positive? — No → Volume / Antibiotics / General surgery/ GYN consultation / Imaging when stabilized

Urine dipstick positive? — Yes → Volume / Antibiotics / Imaging when stabilized if ureterolithiasis or nephric abscess suspected

FIG. 135 Management algorithm for acute pelvic pain: Critical patients and right lower quadrant pain presentations. β-hCG, β-Human chorionic gonadotropin; CT, computed tomography; FAST, focused assessment with sonography for trauma; GYN, gynecology; Hgb, hemoglobin; IUP, intrauterine pregnancy; IV, intravenous; OB, obstetrics; PID, pelvic inflammatory disease; prn, as needed; STAT, immediately; US, ultrasound; UTI, urinary tract infection. (From Marx JA et al: Rosen's emergency medicine, ed 8, Philadelphia, 2014, Saunders.)

Clinical Algorithms

ICD-10CM #	G60.9	Hereditary and idiopathic neuropathy, unspecified
	G57.10	Meralgia paresthetica, unspecified lower limb
	G90.09	Other idiopathic peripheral autonomic neuropathy

APPROACH TO EVALUATION OF PERIPHERAL NEUROPATHIES

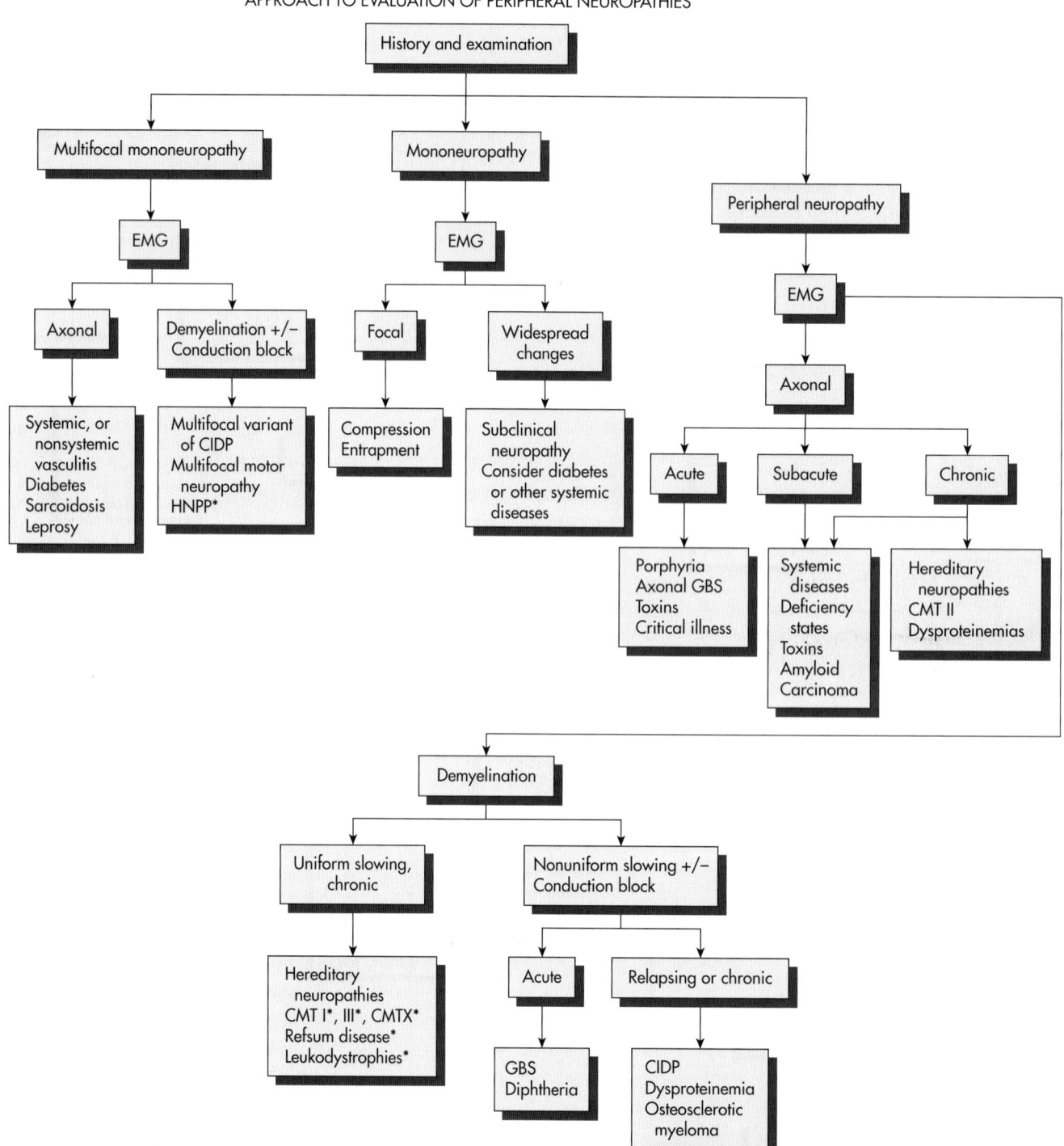

FIG. 136 Diagnostic approach to evaluation of a patient with peripheral neuropathy. Electromyography *(EMG)* denotes electrodiagnostic studies including nerve conduction studies and needle EMG. DNA diagnostic testing or specific biochemical tests are available for conditions marked with asterisks. *CIDP*, Chronic inflammatory demyelinating polyradiculoneuropathy; *CMT*, Charcot-Marie-Tooth disease; *CMTX*, Charcot-Marie-Tooth disease X-linked; *GBS*, Guillain-Barré syndrome; *HNPP*, hereditary liability to pressure palsies. (From Jankovic J et al: *Bradley and Daroff's neurology in clinical practice*, ed 8, Philadelphia, 2022, Elsevier.)

PERIPHERAL NEUROPATHY—cont'd

ICD-10CM #		
	G60.9	Hereditary and idiopathic neuropathy, unspecified
	G57.10	Meralgia paresthetica, unspecified lower limb
	G90.09	Other idiopathic peripheral autonomic neuropathy

1791

TABLE 82 Peripheral Nerve Lesions of the Arm

Lesion	Clinical Findings	Electromyography Findings
Median Neuropathy		
Carpal tunnel syndrome	Weakness and wasting of abductor pollicis brevis if severe; sensory loss on palmar aspect of first through third digits	Slow median motor and sensory NCV through the carpal tunnel; denervation of abductor pollicis brevis if severe
Anterior interosseous syndrome	Weakness of flexor digitorum profundus, pronator quadratus, flexor pollicis longus	Denervation in flexor digitorum profundus, flexor pollicis longus, pronator quadratus
Pronator teres syndrome	Weakness of distal median-innervated muscles; tenderness of pronator teres	Slow median motor NCV through proximal forearm denervation of distal median-innervated muscles
Compression at the ligament of Struthers	Weakness of distal median-innervated muscles	As for pronator teres syndrome, with the addition of denervation of pronator teres
Ulnar Neuropathy		
Palmar branch damage	Weakness of dorsal interossei; no sensory loss	Normal ulnar NCV; denervation of first dorsal interosseus but not abductor digiti minimi
Entrapment at Guyon canal	Weakness of ulnar intrinsic muscles; numbness over fourth and fifth digits	Slow ulnar motor and sensory NCV through wrist
Entrapment at or near the elbow	Weakness of ulnar intrinsic muscles; numbness over fourth and fifth digits	Slow ulnar motor NCV across elbow, denervation in first dorsal interosseus, abductor digiti minimi, and ulnar half of flexor digitorum profundus
Radial Neuropathy		
Posterior interosseus syndrome	Weakness of finger and wrist extensors; no sensory loss	Denervation in wrist and finger extensors; sparing of the supinator and extensor carpi radialis
Compression at the spiral groove	Weakness of finger and wrist extensors; triceps usually spared; sensory loss on dorsal aspects of first digit	Slow radial motor NCV across spiral groove; denervation in distal radial-innervated muscles; triceps may be affected with proximal lesions

NCV, Nerve conduction velocity.
From Jankovic J et al: *Bradley and Daroff's neurology in clinical practice*, ed 8, Philadelphia, 2022, Elsevier.

TABLE 83 Peripheral Nerve Lesions of the Leg

Lesion	Clinical Findings	Electromyography Findings
Sciatic neuropathy	Weakness of tibial- and peroneal-innervated muscles, with sensory loss on posterior leg and foot	Denervation distally in tibial- and peroneal-innervated muscles
Peroneal neuropathy	Weakness of foot extension and eversion and toe extension	Denervation in tibialis anterior; NCV across fibular neck may be slowed
Tibial neuropathy	Weakness of foot plantar flexion	Denervation of gastrocnemius
Femoral neuropathy	Weakness of knee extension; weakness of hip flexion if psoas involved	Denervation in quadriceps, sometimes psoas

NCV, Nerve conduction velocity.
From Jankovic J et al: *Bradley and Daroff's neurology in clinical practice*, ed 8, Philadelphia, 2022, Elsevier.

Clinical Algorithms

III

TABLE 84 Radiculopathies

Level	Motor Deficit	Sensory Deficit
Cervical Radiculopathy		
C5	Deltoid, biceps	Lateral upper arm
C6	Biceps, brachioradialis	Radial forearm and first and second digits
C7	Wrist extensors, triceps	Third and fourth digits
C8	Intrinsic hand muscles	Fifth digit and ulnar forearm
T1	Intrinsic muscles of the hand, especially APB	Axilla
Lumbar Radiculopathy		
L2	Psoas, quadriceps	Lateral and anterior thigh
L3	Psoas, quadriceps	Lower medial thigh
L4	Tibialis anterior, quadriceps	Medial lower leg
L5	Peroneus longus, gluteus medius, tibialis anterior, extensor hallucis longus	Lateral lower leg
S1	Gastrocnemius, gluteus maximus	Lateral foot and fourth and fifth digits

APB, Abductor pollicis brevis.
From Jankovic J et al: *Bradley and Daroff's neurology in clinical practice*, ed 8, Philadelphia, 2022, Elsevier.

ICD-10CM # G60.9   Hereditary and idiopathic neuropathy, unspecified
G57.10 Meralgia paresthetica, unspecified lower limb
G90.09 Other idiopathic peripheral autonomic neuropathy

TABLE 85   Some of the More Common Causes of Peripheral Neuropathy

Disease	Sensory	Motor	Autonomic	Fiber Size	Common Clinical Presentation
Diabetes	+++	±	++	S > L	Burning starting in feet; 'glove and stocking'
Alcohol	+++	±	++	S > L	Burning in feet Often cerebellar, ocular or cognitive features
Critical illness	++	++	++	Mixed	Weakness, difficulty weaning from ventilator
Vitamin B₁₂	+++	−	−	L > S	Sensory ataxia; often dorsal column signs
Uremia	+++	±	+	S > L	Glove and stocking
Malignancy	+++	++	±	Variable	Variable; may have other neurologic features; may have cachexia and muscle weakness
Liver failure	+++	+	±	Often S > L	Glove and stocking
Paraprotein	++	++	−	Both	Slowly progressive glove and stocking
Anti-MAG	++	++	+	S > L	Glove and stocking
MGUS	++	++	+	Both	Progressive sensorimotor involvement with other features of myeloma
POEMS	++	±	+++	S >> L	Painful neuropathy with autonomic dysfunction
Amyloidosis					
Chemotherapy (platinum, taxanes, etc.)	+++	+	±	L > S	Glove and stocking pattern—may be rapidly progressive with repeat exposure
HIV	+++	+	±	Both	Progressive glove and stocking
Hereditary (multiple disorders)	Variable	Variable	Variable	Variable	Typically do not have dysesthesia or pain (may be present late)

HIV, Human immunodeficiency virus; *L*, large; *MAG*, myelin-associated glycoproteins; *MGUS*, monoclonal gammopathy of uncertain significance; *POEMS*, polyneuropathy, organomegaly, endocrinopathy, M-spike, skin changes; *S*, small. *L > S* indicates that large fibers are affected more than small fibers.
From Talley NJ et al: *Essentials of internal medicine*, ed 4, Chatswood, NSW, 2021, Elsevier Australia.

BOX 23   Indications for Nerve Biopsy

Nerve Biopsy Is Diagnostic and Essential for Diagnosis
- Vasculitis*
- Amyloidosis*
- Sarcoidosis*
- Hansen disease (leprosy)
- Giant axonal neuropathy
- Tumor infiltration
- Polyglucosan body disease

Nerve Biopsy Is Suggestive and Only Supportive of Diagnosis
- Charcot-Marie-Tooth disease types 1 and 3
- Chronic inflammatory demyelinating polyradiculoneuropathy
- Paraproteinemic neuropathy (immunoglobulin M monoclonal gammopathy with antimyelin-associated glycoprotein antibody)

*Consider combined distal nerve and muscle biopsies.
From Jankovic J et al: *Bradley and Daroff's neurology in clinical practice*, ed 8, Philadelphia, 2022, Elsevier.

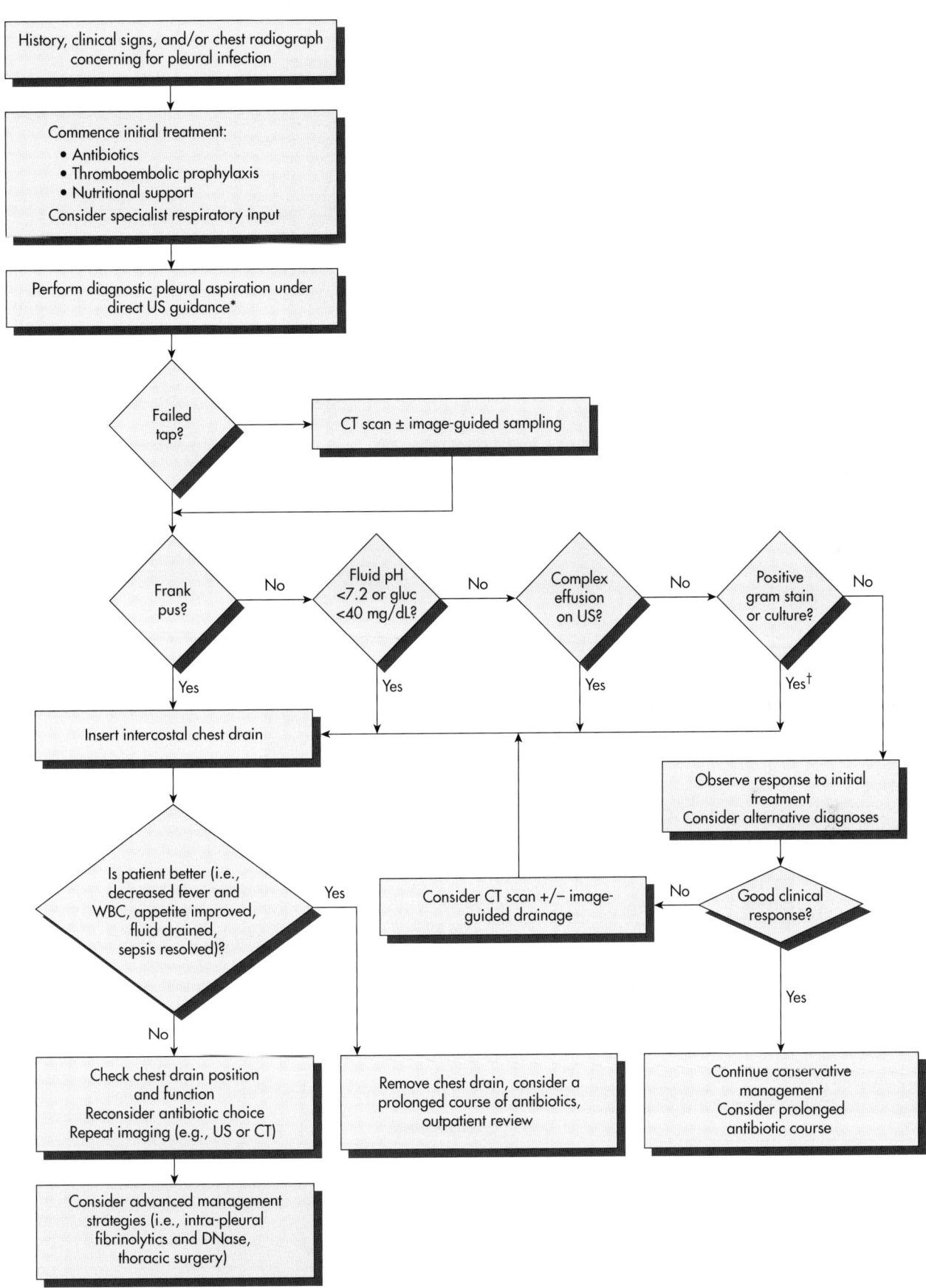

FIG. 138 Algorithm demonstrating the investigation and management of suspected pleural infection.
*Ideally this should be performed before administration of antibiotics; however, treatment should not be delayed if aspiration cannot be performed immediately. †A positive pleural culture or Gram stain result usually means that a chest drain is required; however, the patient's clinical course should be considered when making this decision. *CT,* Computed tomography; *US,* ultrasound; *WBC,* white blood cells. (From Broaddus VC et al: *Murray & Nadel's textbook of respiratory medicine,* ed 7, Philadelphia, 2022, Elsevier.)

Clinical
Algorithms

III

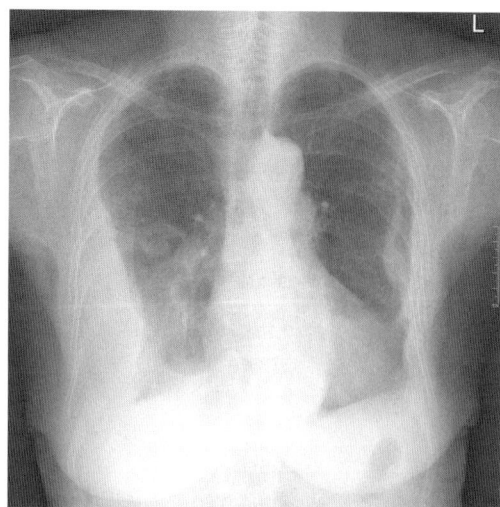

FIG. 139 Pleural empyema seen on a frontal chest radiograph. The D-shaped opacity, suggesting an extraparenchymal process, is commonly seen in cases of pleural infection. (From Broaddus VC et al: *Murray & Nadel's textbook of respiratory medicine*, ed 7, Philadelphia, 2022, Elsevier.)

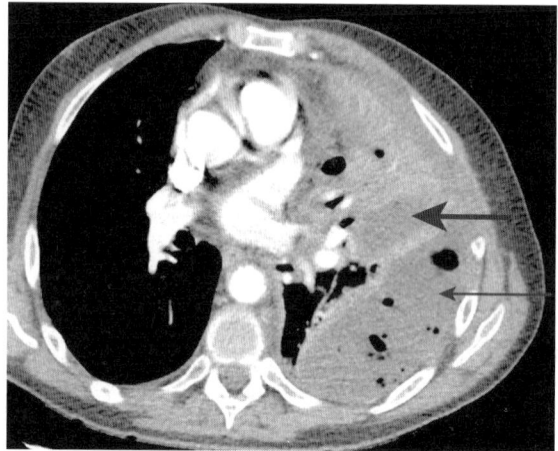

FIG. 140 Contrast-enhanced chest computed tomography showing both pleural empyema and a lung abscess. With contrast-enhanced computed tomography, pleural lesions can be discriminated from parenchymal lesions. The *thin arrow* shows empyema, and the *thick arrow* indicates a lung abscess. Note the lenticular shape of the empyema in contrast to the rounded shape of the abscess. The pleural collection does not have a visible "wall," whereas the abscess wall is thick and irregular. Within the empyema are multiple separate locules of gas, suggesting that the pleural collection is septated. Also see Table 86 for features that differentiate between empyema and lung abscess. (From Broaddus VC et al: *Murray & Nadel's textbook of respiratory medicine*, ed 7, Philadelphia, 2022, Elsevier.)

TABLE 86   Key Differences Between the Radiographic Appearance of Pleural Infection and Lung Abscesses

Empyema	Lung Abscess
Lenticular shape	Rounded
Surrounding lung often compressed	Boundary between lung and fluid indistinct, with necrosis of lung
Margins of collection creating obtuse angles with chest wall	Contact with chest wall made at acute angle
Thick smooth wall	Thick irregular wall
No vessels close by	Vessels seen passing through or near collection

From Broaddus VC etal: *Murray & Nadel's textbook of respiratory medicine*, ed 7, Philadelphia, 2022, Elsevier.

SOLID & PART-SOLID NODULES

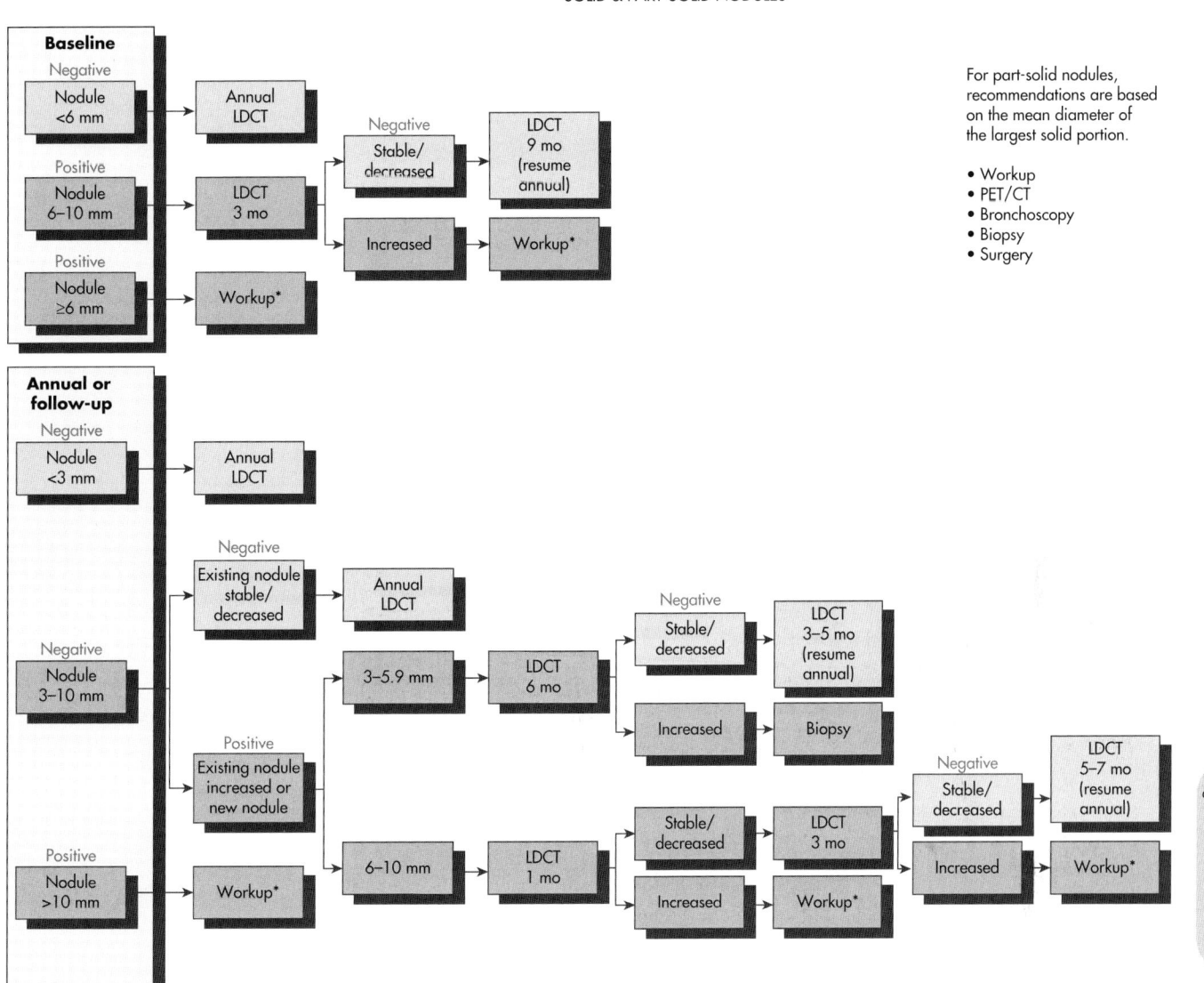

For part-solid nodules, recommendations are based on the mean diameter of the largest solid portion.

- Workup
- PET/CT
- Bronchoscopy
- Biopsy
- Surgery

A

FIG. 146 The diagnostic algorithm for (A) solid or part-solid nodules and (B) nonsolid nodules. This algorithm was created through discussion by a multidisciplinary group composed of thoracic surgeons, radiologists, pulmonologists, oncologists, and pathologists. *Workup is at the discretion of the treating physicians but typically consists of a PET/CT and tissue diagnosis, either by bronchoscopy, CT-guided biopsy, or for highly suspicious nodules, minimally invasive surgery. *CT,* Computed tomography; *LDCT,* low-dose computed tomography; *PET,* positron emission tomography. (From Sellke FW: *Sabiston & Spencer surgery of the chest,* ed 9, Philadelphia, 2016, Elsevier. The Fleischner Society recommendations for computed tomography follow-up of pulmonary nodules are summarized in Tables 87-89.)

Clinical Algorithms

III

NONSOLID NODULES

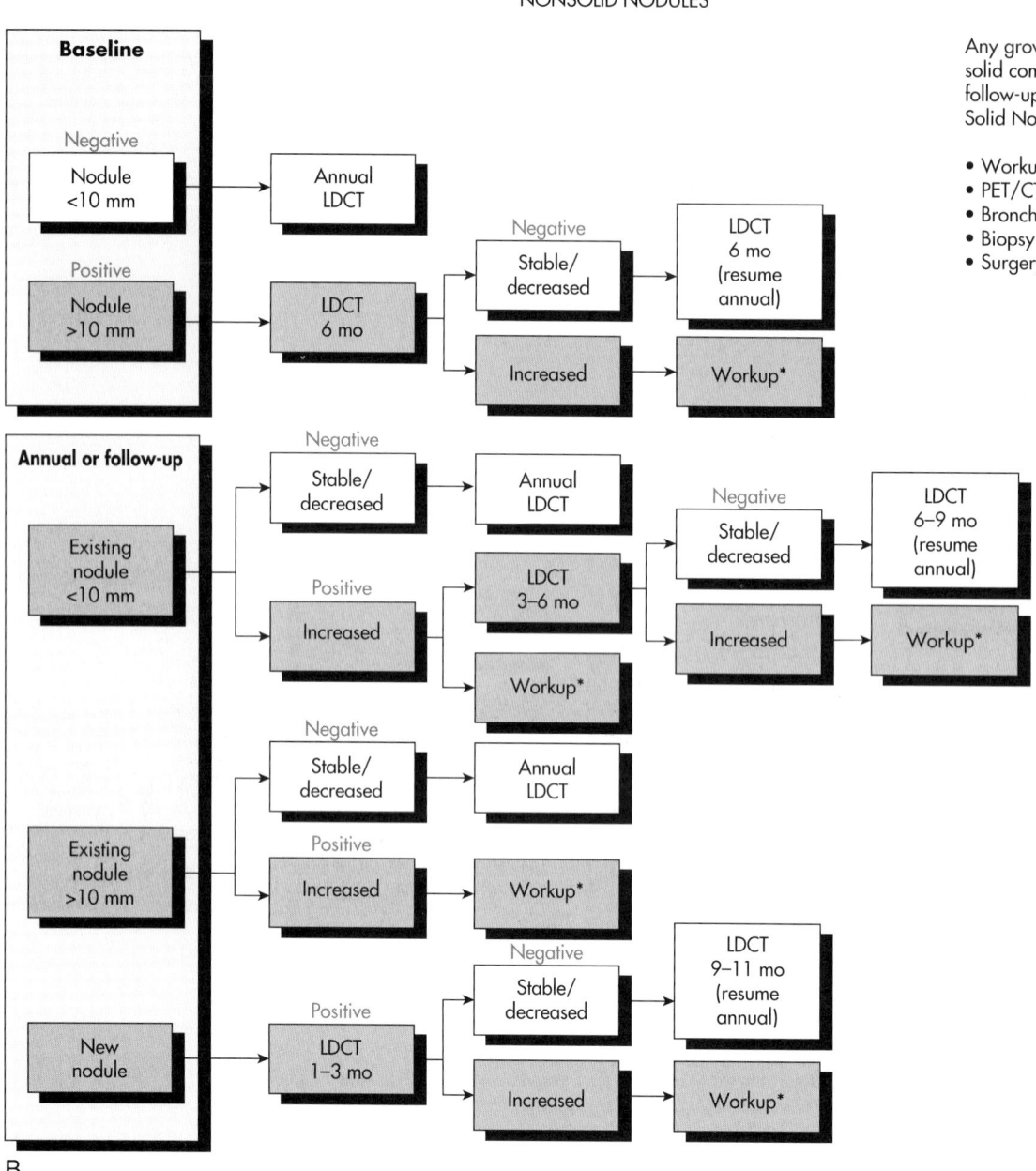

Any growth or development of solid components prompts follow-ups as per Solid & Part-Solid Nodule algorithm.

- Workup
- PET/CT
- Bronchoscopy
- Biopsy
- Surgery

B

FIG. 146 cont'd

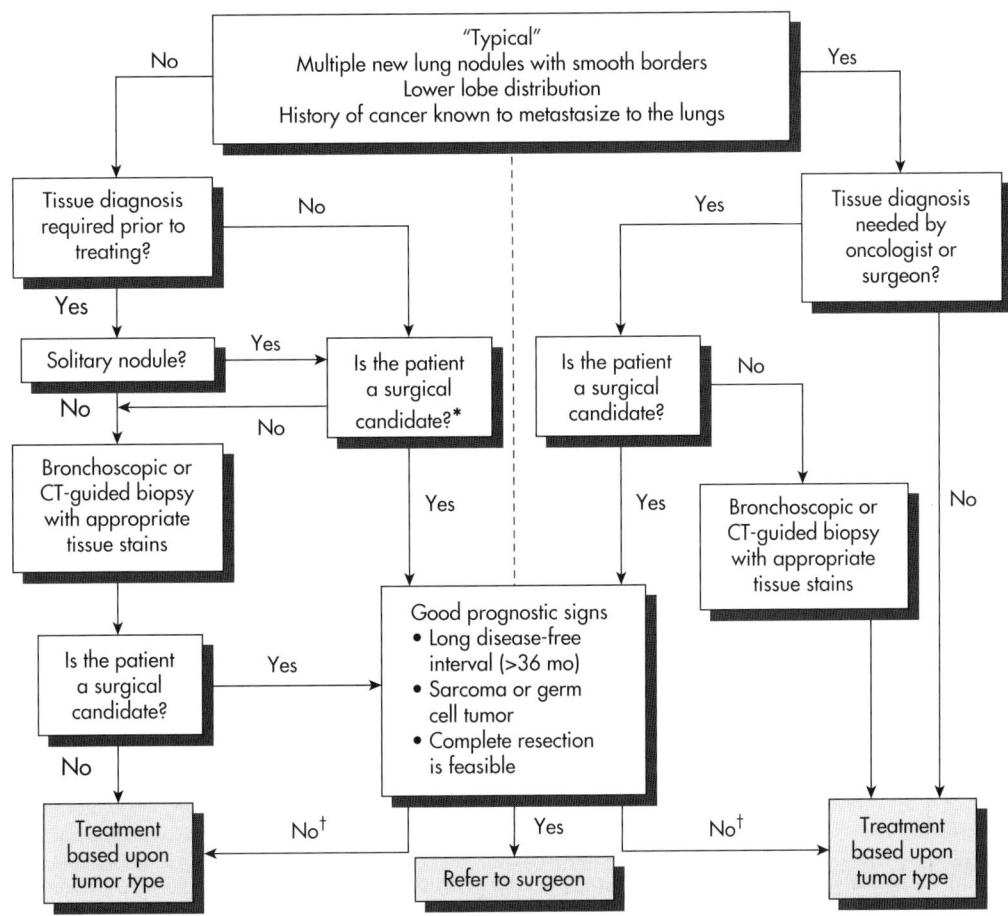

FIG. 147 Suggested management algorithm for patients with known prior cancer and new lung nodule or nodules. Decisions take into account the typical or atypical appearance of a lung nodule in a patient with prior known cancer, the utility of a tissue diagnosis to the treating physicians, the physiologic fitness of the patient for surgery, and the known prognostic indicators for a favorable outcome after metastectomy. Each patient should be managed individually, within the context of the skills and experience of local providers with the varied diagnostic and therapeutic options. *Patients at high risk for primary lung cancer may be considered for diagnostic lobectomy, when appropriate. †These are suggested criteria for surgical resection of lung metastases, and multidisciplinary teams should make this decision. Radiofrequency ablation or stereotactic ablative body radiotherapy may also be an excellent choice for these patients. *CT,* Computed tomography. (From Broaddus VC et al: *Murray & Nadel's textbook of respiratory medicine,* ed 7, Philadelphia, 2022, Elsevier.)

TABLE 87   Fleischner Society Recommendations for Computed Tomography (CT) Follow-Up (FU) of Solid Nodules*

Nodule Size	Low-Risk Patient	High-Risk Patient
≤4 mm	No FU CT needed (FU is optional)	FU CT at 12 mo; if unchanged, no further FU
>4-6 mm	FU CT at 12 mo; if unchanged, no further FU	FU CT at 6-12 mo, then at 18-24 mo if no change
>6-8 mm	FU CT at 6-12 mo, then at 18-24 mo if no change	FU CT at 3-6 mo, then at 9-12 and 24 mo if no change
>8 mm	Options: FU CT at 3, 9, and 24 mo; positron emission tomography; biopsy; video-assisted thoracic surgery	

*Nodule size is average of length and width. Low-risk patient, minimal or absent history of smoking or other known risk factors; high-risk patient, history of smoking or other known risk factors.
From Webb WR et al: *Fundamentals of body CT*, ed 4, Philadelphia, 2015, Saunders.

TABLE 88   Fleischner Society Recommendations for Computed Tomography (CT) Follow-Up (FU) of Solitary Ground-Glass Opacity (GGO) or Part-GGO Nodules

Nodule Type	Recommendation	Additional Remarks
Solitary pure GGO ≤5 mm	No FU CT required	Use 1-mm slices to confirm nodule is pure GGO
Solitary pure GGO >5 mm	FU CT at 3 mo; if persistent, yearly FU for at least 3 yr	Positron emission tomography of limited value and not recommended
Solitary part-solid nodules	FU CT at 3 mo; if persistent and solid component <5 mm, yearly FU for at least 3 yr; if persistent and solid component ≥5 mm, then biopsy or resection	Consider positron emission tomography if nodule >1 cm

From Webb WR et al: *Fundamentals of body CT*, ed 4, Philadelphia, 2015, Saunders.

TABLE 89   Fleischner Society Recommendations for Computed Tomography (CT) Follow-Up (FU) of Multiple Ground-Glass Opacity (GGO) or Part-GGO Nodules

Nodule Type	Recommendation	Additional Remarks
Multiple pure GGO ≤5 mm	FU CT at 2 and 4 yr	Consider alternate cause for GGO nodules
Multiple pure GGO >5 mm; no dominant lesion	FU CT at 3 mo; if persistent, yearly FU for at least 3 yr	Positron emission tomography of limited value and not recommended
Dominant part-solid nodule(s)	FU CT at 3 mo; if persistent, then biopsy or resection, particularly if solid component ≥ 5 mm	Consider lung-sparing surgery in patients with a dominant lesion suspicious for lung cancer

From Webb WR et al: *Fundamentals of body CT*, ed 4, Philadelphia, 2015, Saunders.

PURPURA

ICD-10CM # D69.0   Allergic purpura
D69.2   Other nonthrombocytopenic purpura
D69.49 Other primary thrombocytopenia
M31.1   Thrombotic microangiopathy

1799

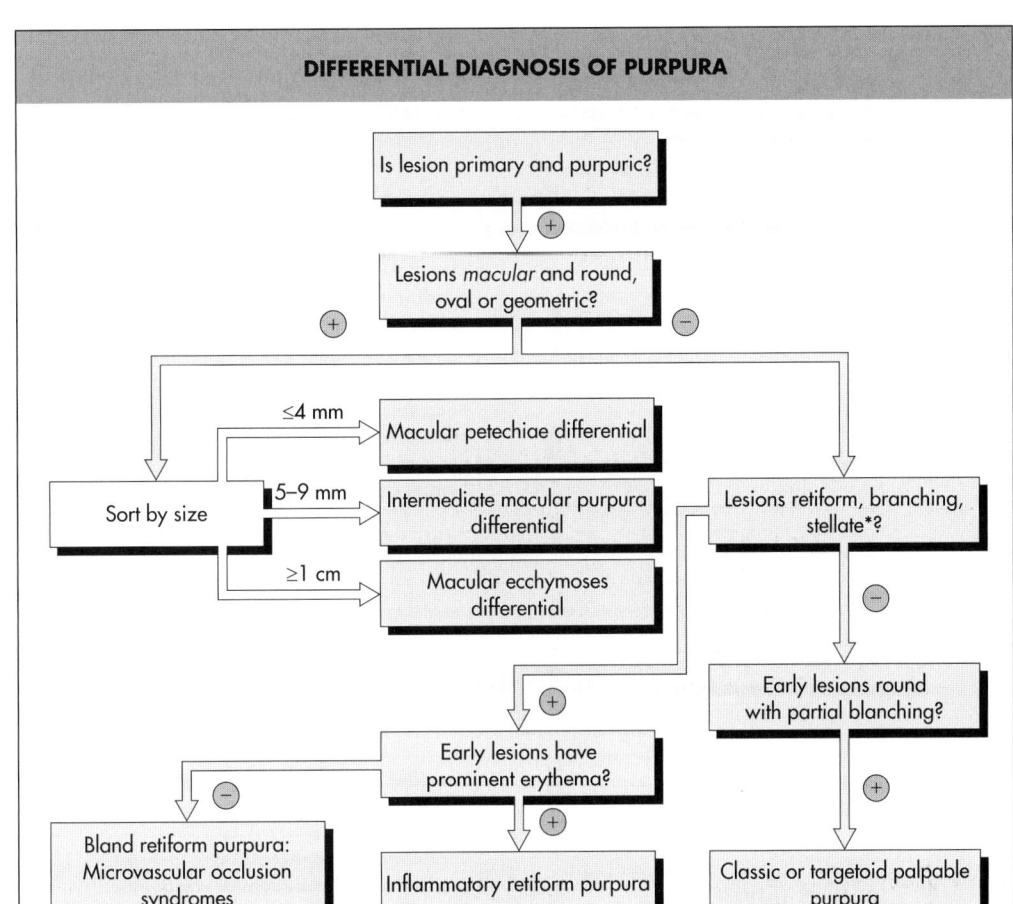

FIG. 148 Differential diagnosis of purpura. *Very few lesions are truly stellate, that is, characterized by a central area of necrosis or hemorrhage with radiating extensions, but some authors continue to use this term to describe these lesions. (From Bolognia J: *Dermatology,* ed 4, Philadelphia, 2018, Elsevier.)

Clinical
Algorithms

III

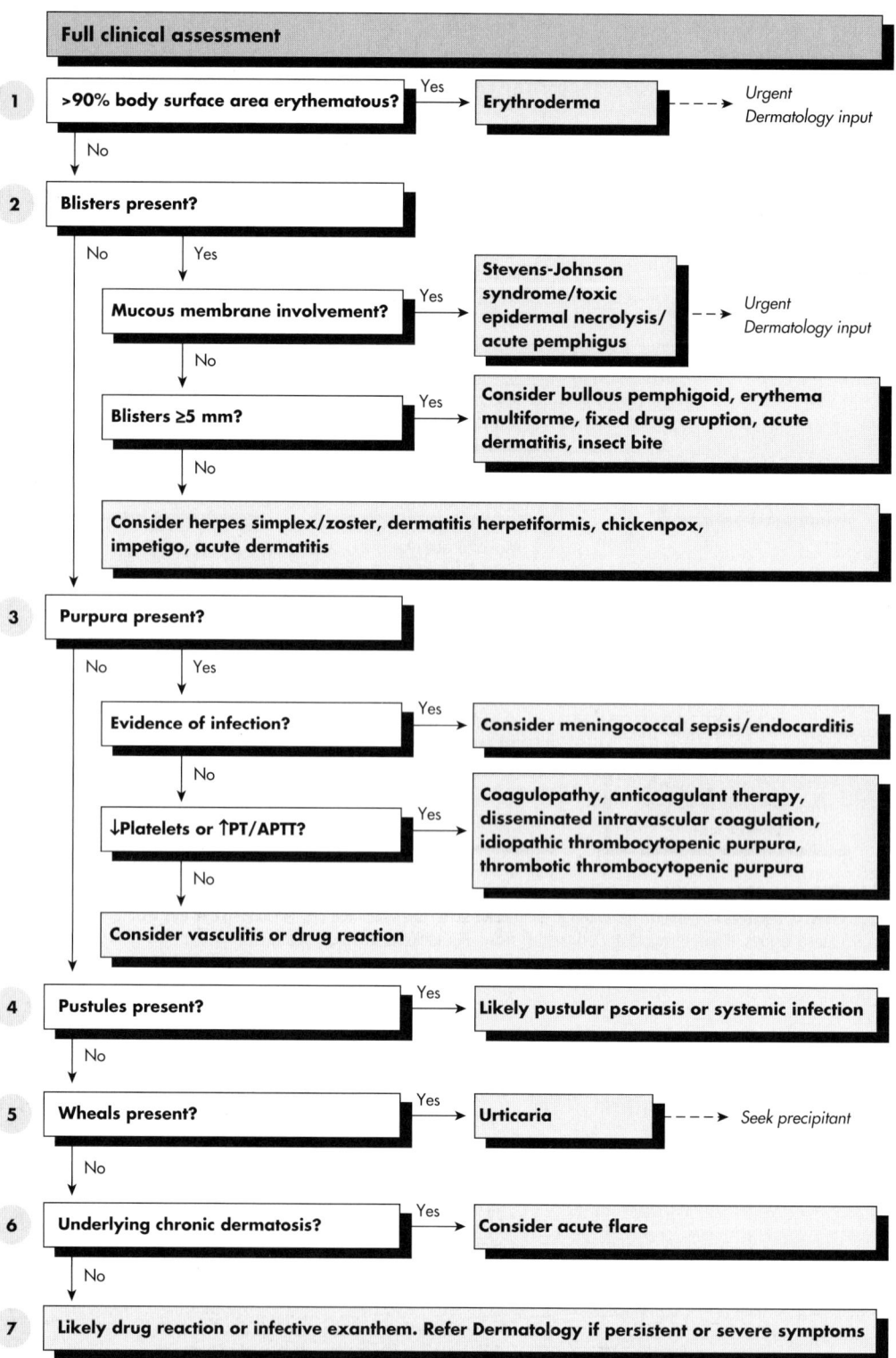

FIG. 149 Rash: Acute generalized skin eruption. *APTT,* Activated partial thromboplastin time; *PT,* prothrombin time. (From Gawkrodger DJ: *Dermatology ICT,* ed 4, Edinburgh, 2008, Churchill Livingstone; Japp AG, Robertson C: *Macleod's clinical diagnosis,* ed 2, Philadelphia, 2018, Elsevier.)

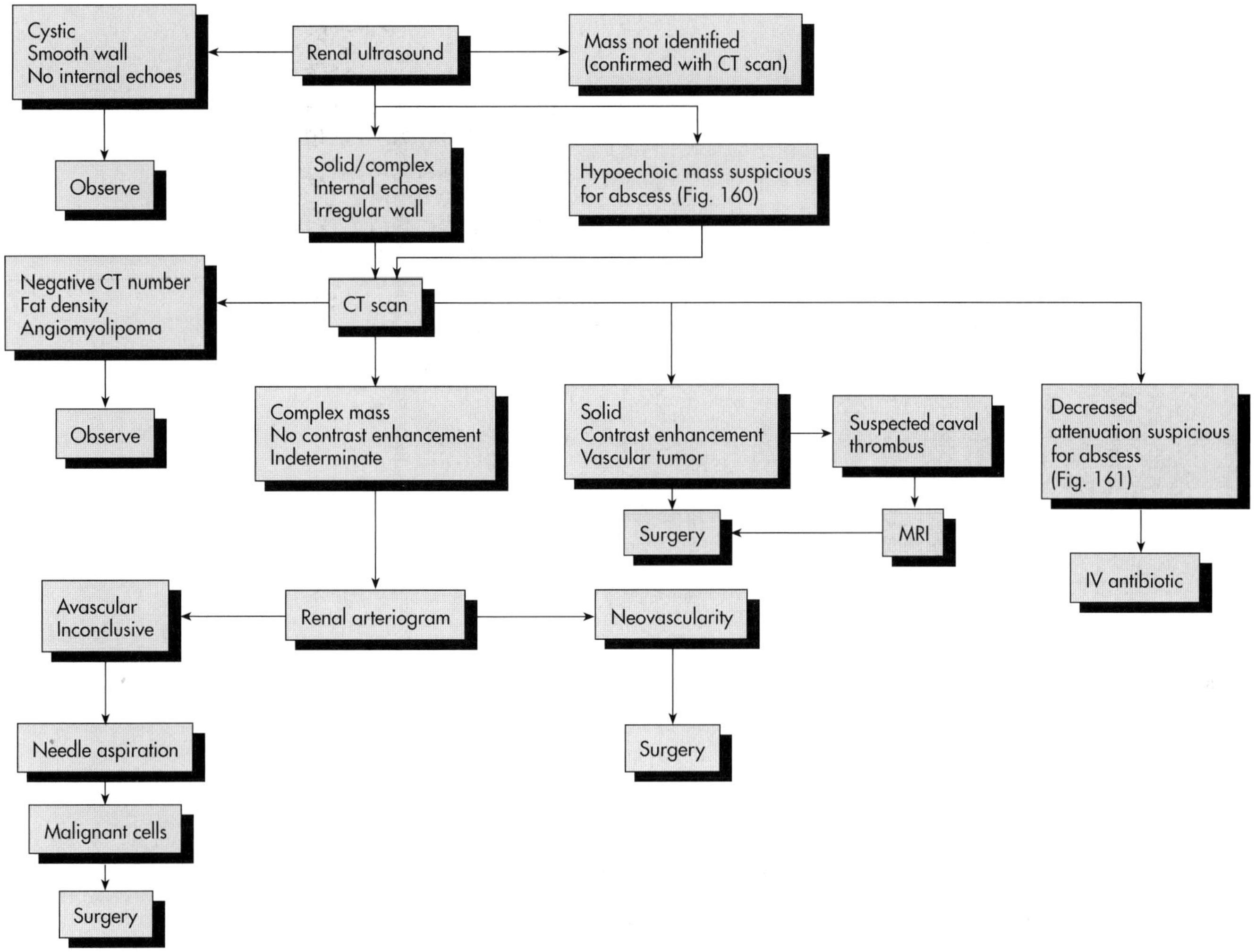

Cystic
Smooth wall
No internal echoes

Renal ultrasound

Mass not identified
(confirmed with CT scan)

Observe

Solid/complex
Internal echoes
Irregular wall

Hypoechoic mass suspicious
for abscess (Fig. 160)

Negative CT number
Fat density
Angiomyolipoma

CT scan

Observe

Complex mass
No contrast enhancement
Indeterminate

Solid
Contrast enhancement
Vascular tumor

Suspected caval
thrombus

Decreased
attenuation suspicious
for abscess
(Fig. 161)

Surgery

MRI

IV antibiotic

Avascular
Inconclusive

Renal arteriogram

Neovascularity

Surgery

Needle aspiration

Malignant cells

Surgery

FIG. 157 Evaluation of a patient with a renal mass on renal ultrasound. *CT,* Computed tomography; *MRI,*
magnetic resonance imaging. (Modified from Williams RD: Tumors of the kidney, ureter, and bladder. In Goldman L,
Schafer AL [eds]: *Cecil textbook of medicine,* ed 23, Philadelphia, 2008, Saunders.)

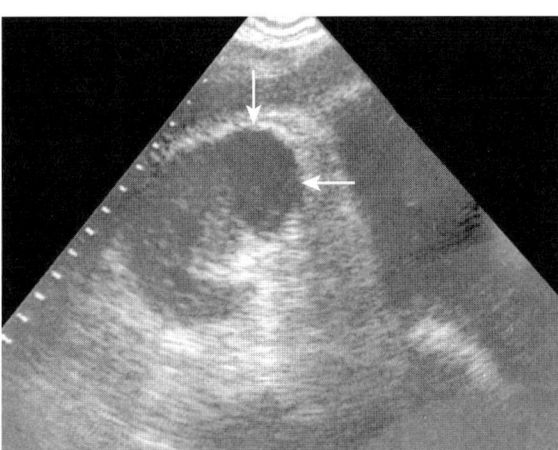

FIG. 158 Acute renal abscess. Transverse ultrasound image of the right kidney demonstrates a poorly marginated
rounded focal hypoechoic mass *(arrows)* in the anterior portion of the kidney. (From Wein AJ et al: *Campbell-Walsh
urology,* ed 11, Philadelphia, 2016, Elsevier.)

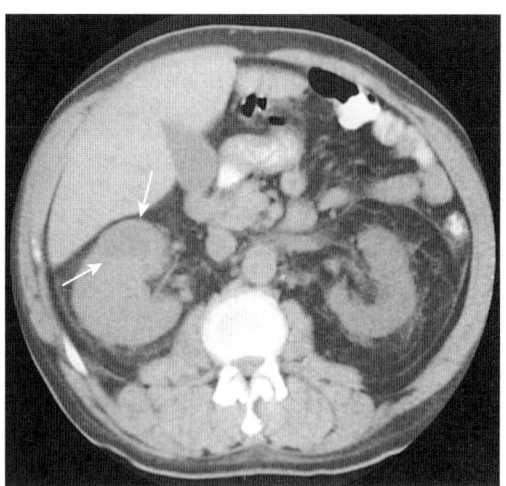

FIG. 159 Acute renal abscess. Nonenhanced computed tomography scan through the mid-pole of the right kidney demonstrates right renal enlargement and an area of decreased attenuation *(arrows)*. After antimicrobial therapy, a follow-up scan showed complete regression of these findings. (From Wein AJ et al: *Campbell-Walsh urology,* ed 11, Philadelphia, 2016, Elsevier.)

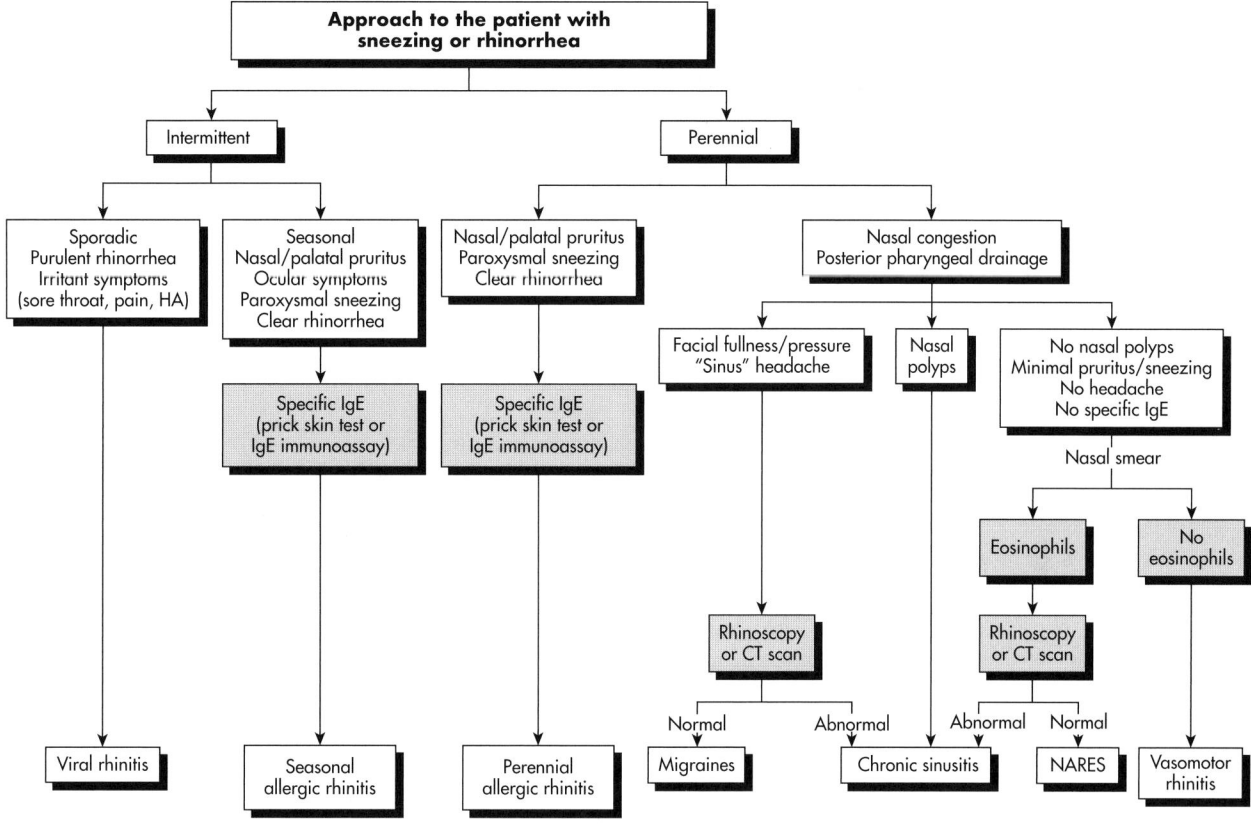

FIG. 161 Approach to the patient with rhinitis symptoms. *CT,* Computed tomography; *HA,* headache; *IgE,* immunoglobulin E; *NARES,* nonallergic rhinitis with eosinophilia syndrome. (From Goldman L, Shafer AI: *Goldman-Cecil medicine,* ed 26, Philadelphia, 2020, Elsevier.)

TABLE 92   Differential Diagnosis of Rhinitis

Allergic

Seasonal allergic rhinitis
Perennial allergic rhinitis

Inflammatory

Infectious rhinitis (viral)
Nonallergic rhinitis with eosinophilia syndrome
Chronic sinusitis with or without nasal polyposis
Laryngopharyngeal reflux

Hormonal

Pregnancy, oral contraceptives, perimenopause
Hypothyroidism
Hyperthyroidism

Rhinitis Medicamentosa

Topical or, less commonly, oral decongestants
Antihypertensives
Antidepressants
Cocaine

Vasomotor

Irritant induced (pollution, cigarette smoke)
Cold air induced
Gustatory (food induced)

Anatomic

Nasal septal deviation
Tumor, neoplasm
Foreign body
Cerebrospinal fluid leak
Atrophic (postsurgical or trauma)

From Goldman L, Shafer AI: *Goldman-Cecil medicine*, ed 26, Philadelphia, 2020, Elsevier.

Clinical
Algorithms

III

ICD-10CM # N44.2 Benign cyst of testis
N44.8 Other noninflammatory disorders of the testis
N50.3 Cyst of epididymis
N50.8 Other specified disorders of male genital organs

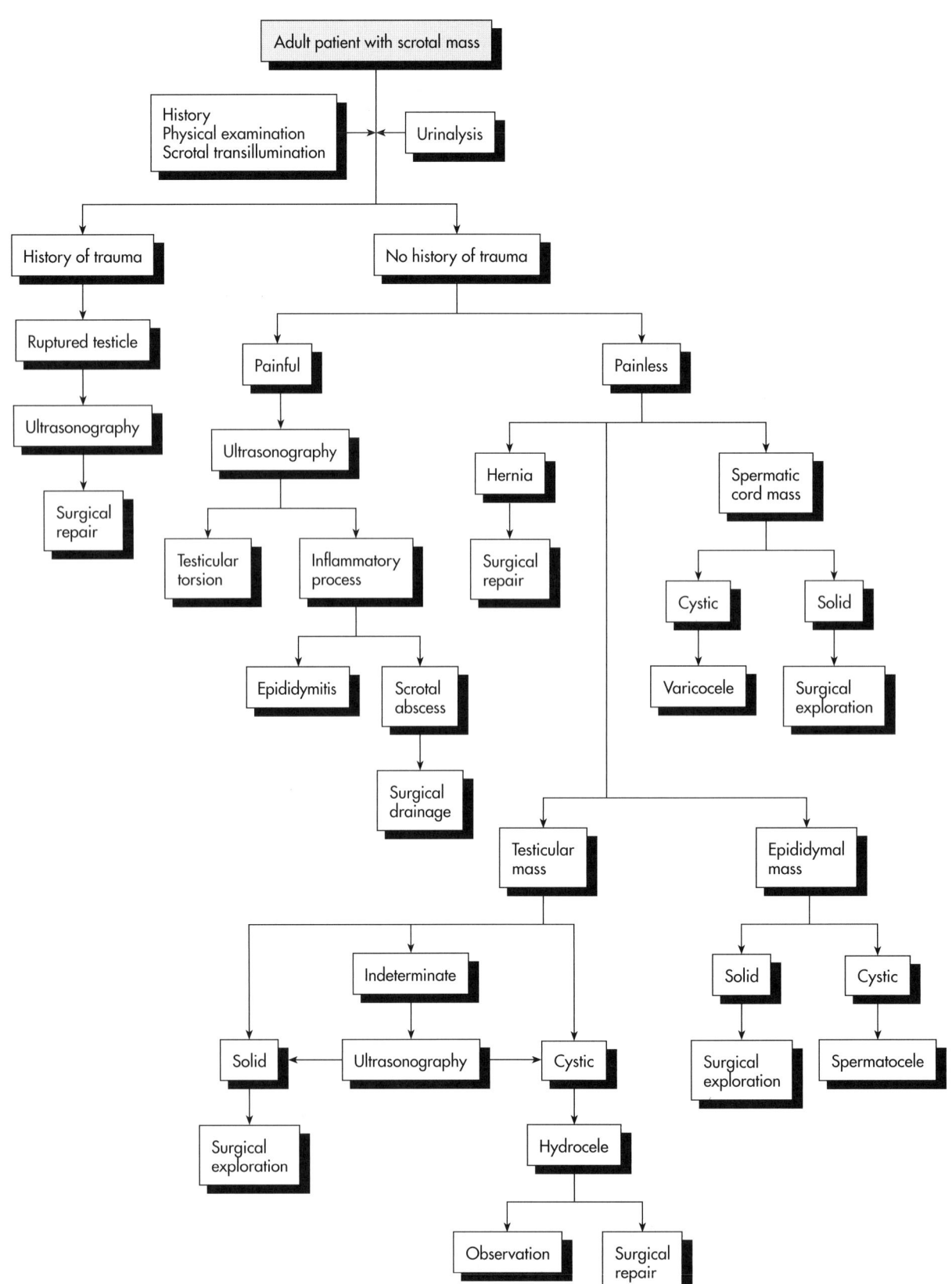

FIG. 162 Evaluation of scrotal mass. (Modified from Greene HL et al [eds]: *Decision making in medicine*, ed 2, St Louis, 1998, Mosby.)

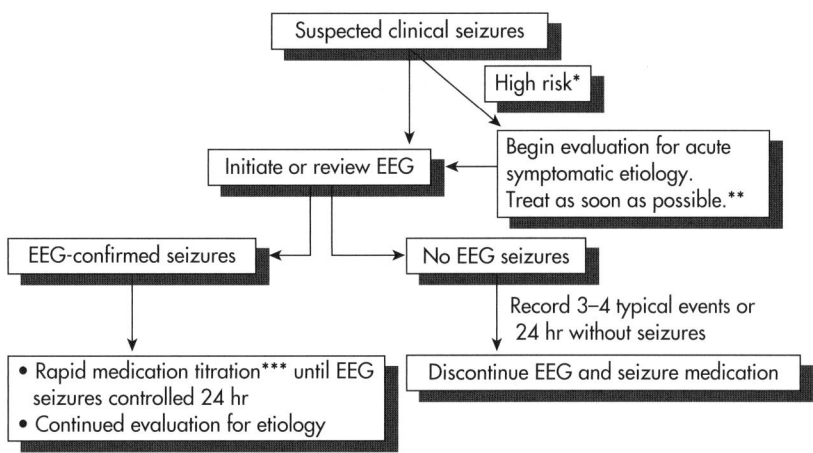

FIG. 163 Assessment algorithm for newborns with suspected seizures. *EEG*, Electroencephalogram. (From Swaiman KF: *Swaiman's pediatric neurology, principles and practice*, ed 6, Philadelphia, 2017, Elsevier.)

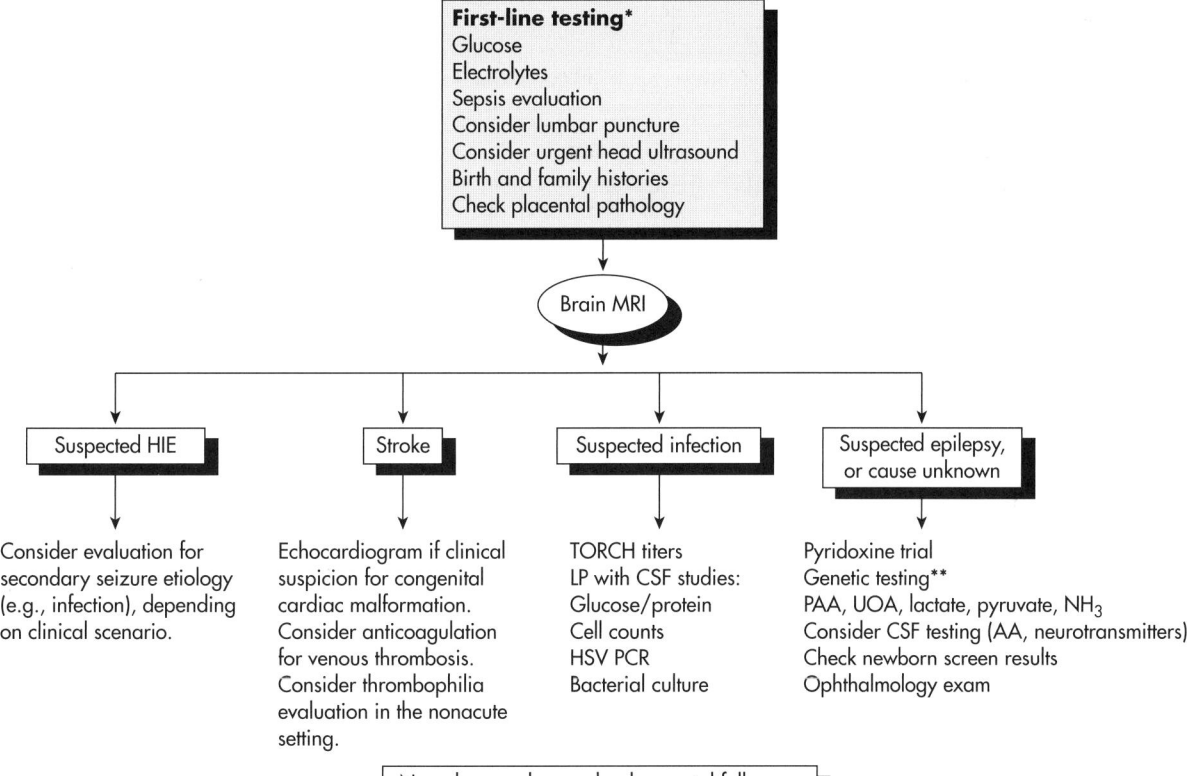

**Genetic testing can include karyotype, chromosomal microarray, epilepsy gene panel, or single gene testing.

FIG. 164 Assessment algorithm for newborns with seizures. *First-line testing should occur simultaneously with initiation of electroencephalography (and empiric seizure treatment in high-risk clinical scenarios). Most infants should receive neuroimaging, and brain magnetic resonance imaging *(MRI)* is the preferred neuroimaging modality. Second-line testing depends on the clinical scenario and MRI findings. Newborns with seizures are at high risk for long-term neurodevelopmental disability and epilepsy, and so they require careful follow-up by appropriate clinicians. *CSF,* Cerebrospinal fluid; *HIE,* hypoxic ischemic encephalopathy; *HSV,* herpes simplex virus; *LP,* lumbar puncture; *PCR,* polymerase chain reaction; *TORCH,* Toxoplasma gondii, other viruses, rubella, cytomegalovirus, and herpes simplex. (From Swaiman KF: *Swaiman's pediatric neurology: principles and practice,* ed 6, Philadelphia, 2017, Elsevier.)

Clinical Algorithms

III

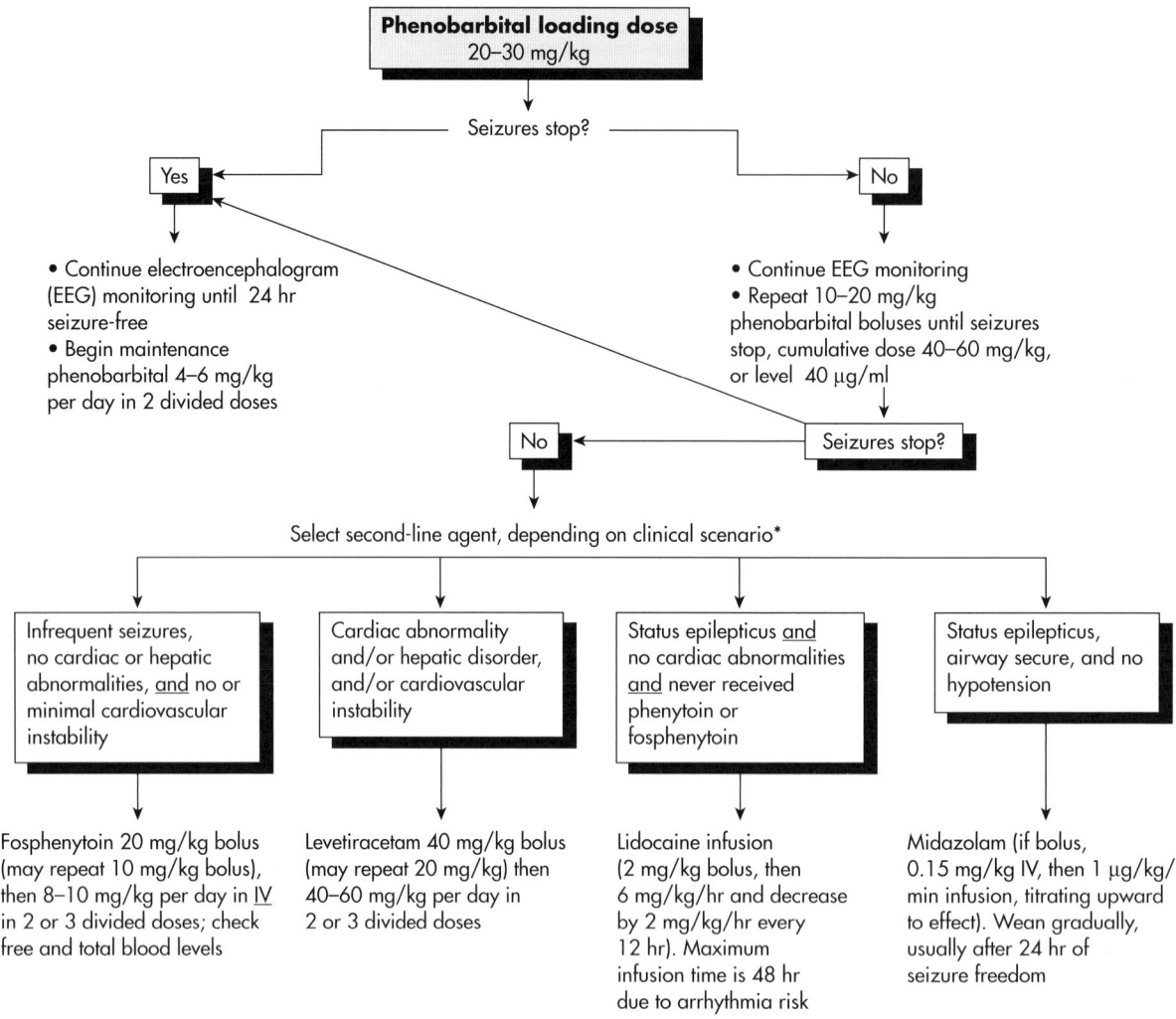

Phenobarbital loading dose
20–30 mg/kg

Seizures stop?

Yes

No

- Continue electroencephalogram (EEG) monitoring until 24 hr seizure-free
- Begin maintenance phenobarbital 4–6 mg/kg per day in 2 divided doses

- Continue EEG monitoring
- Repeat 10–20 mg/kg phenobarbital boluses until seizures stop, cumulative dose 40–60 mg/kg, or level 40 µg/ml

Seizures stop?

No

Select second-line agent, depending on clinical scenario*

Infrequent seizures, no cardiac or hepatic abnormalities, and no or minimal cardiovascular instability

Cardiac abnormality and/or hepatic disorder, and/or cardiovascular instability

Status epilepticus and no cardiac abnormalities and never received phenytoin or fosphenytoin

Status epilepticus, airway secure, and no hypotension

Fosphenytoin 20 mg/kg bolus (may repeat 10 mg/kg bolus), then 8–10 mg/kg per day in IV in 2 or 3 divided doses; check free and total blood levels

Levetiracetam 40 mg/kg bolus (may repeat 20 mg/kg) then 40–60 mg/kg per day in 2 or 3 divided doses

Lidocaine infusion (2 mg/kg bolus, then 6 mg/kg/hr and decrease by 2 mg/kg/hr every 12 hr). Maximum infusion time is 48 hr due to arrhythmia risk

Midazolam (if bolus, 0.15 mg/kg IV, then 1 µg/kg/min infusion, titrating upward to effect). Wean gradually, usually after 24 hr of seizure freedom

*If the infant has acute symptomatic seizures, select from these options, based on comorbidities and seizure severity. If the newborn has epilepsy (e.g., lissencephaly, tuberous sclerosis), consider levetiracetam, topiramate, or oxcarbazepine as second- or third-line treatments.

FIG. 165 Suggested treatment algorithm for neonatal seizures. The rapidity of medication administration will depend on local guidelines and resources. Frequent assessment of treatment response is recommended. *IV*, Intravenous. (From Swaiman KF: *Swaiman's pediatric neurology: principles and practice*, ed 6, Philadelphia, 2017, Elsevier.)

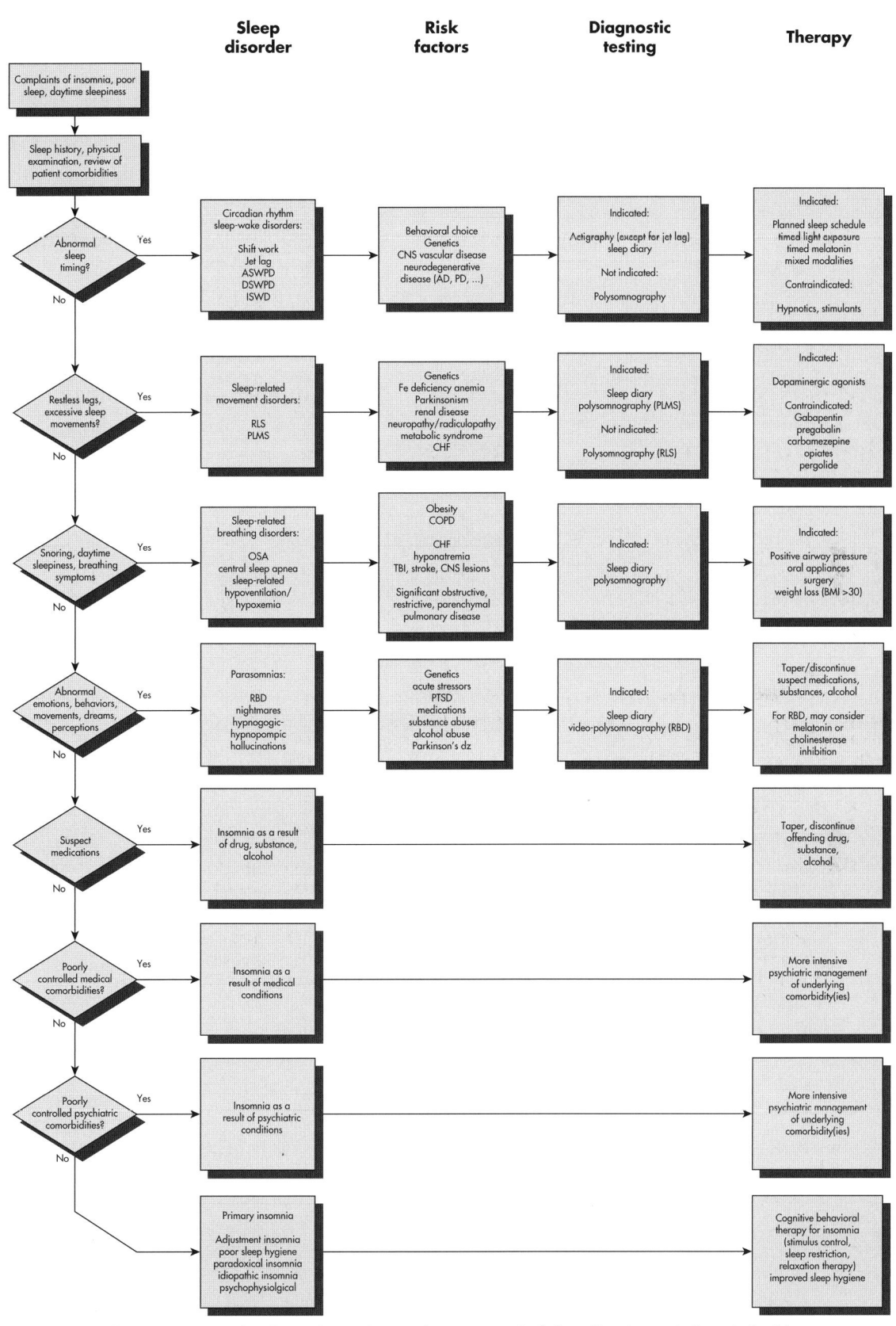

FIG. 173 Flowchart for diagnosis, workup, and management of sleep disorders not characterized by hypersomnia. The first column depicts the flowchart that differentiates among specific sleep disorders, the second column delineates the specific family of sleep disorders associated with the target symptom, the third column notes risk factors associated with the chosen family of sleep disorders, the fourth column notes specific diagnostic modalities that may be required beyond a standard history/physical examination/lab studies, and the fifth column notes specific treatment indications and contraindications. (From Warshaw GA et al: *Ham's Primary Care Geriatrics*, Ed. 7, Philadelphia, 2022, Elsevier.)

Clinical
Algorithms

III

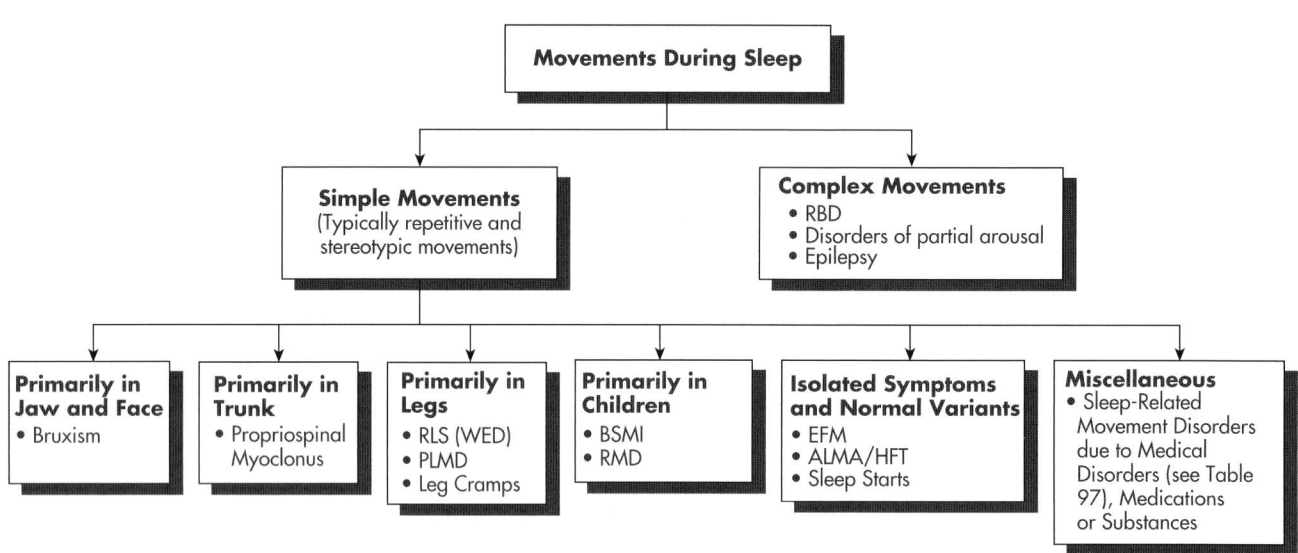

FIG. 174 Flow chart for the approach to the differential diagnosis of sleep-related movement disorders. *WED,* Willis-Ekbom disease; *RMD,* rhythmic movement disorder. *ALMA,* Alternating leg muscle activation; *BSMI,* benign sleep myoclonus of infancy; *EFM,* excessive fragmentary myoclonus; *HFT,* hypnagogic foot tremor; *PLMD,* periodic limb movement disorder; *RBD,* rapid eye movement *(REM)* sleep behavior disorder; *RLS (WED),* restless legs syndrome. (From Kryger M et al: *Principles and practice of sleep medicine,* ed 6, Philadelphia, 2017, Elsevier.)

TABLE 97   Distinguishing Features of Nocturnal Events

Feature	Disorders of Arousal	Sleep-Related Eating Disorder	REM Behavior Disorder	Recurrent Isolated Sleep Paralysis	Exploding Head Syndrome	Psychogenic Events	Nocturnal Seizures
Behavior	Confused; semipurposeful movement with eyes open	Eating typically high-calorie foods; eyes open	Sometimes combative with eyes closed	Episodes of inability to move	Painless sensation of explosion inside the head	Variable	Dependent on the portion of brain involved
Age of onset	Childhood and adolescence	Variable	Older adult	Variable	Adult	Adolescence to adulthood	Variable
Time of occurrence	First third of night	First half of night	During REM	Typically on awakening	Usually near sleep onset but can be variable	Anytime	Anytime
Frequency of events	Less than one per night	Variable	Multiple per night	Variable less than weekly	Rare	Variable	Frontal seizures— multiple per night
Duration	Minutes	Minutes	Seconds to minutes	Seconds to minutes	Seconds	Variable minutes or longer	Usually under 3 min
Memory of event	Usually none	Usually none or limited	Dream recall	Yes	Yes	None	Usually none
Stereotypical movements	No	No	No	No	Similar sensation	No	Yes
Polysomnogram findings	Arousals from slow wave sleep	Arousal from NREM sleep	Excessive electromyogram tone during REM sleep	Arousal from REM sleep	Usually occurs in light sleep	Occur from awake state	Potentially epileptiform activity

REM, Rapid eye movement; *NREM,* nonrapid eye movement.
From Kryger M et al: *Principles and practice of sleep medicine,* ed 6, Philadelphia, 2017, Elsevier.

SORE THROAT

ICD-10CM # J02.9 Acute pharyngitis, unspecified   **1809**
             J31.2 Chronic pharyngitis
             J02.0 Streptococcal pharyngitis

DIAGNOSTIC ALGORITHM

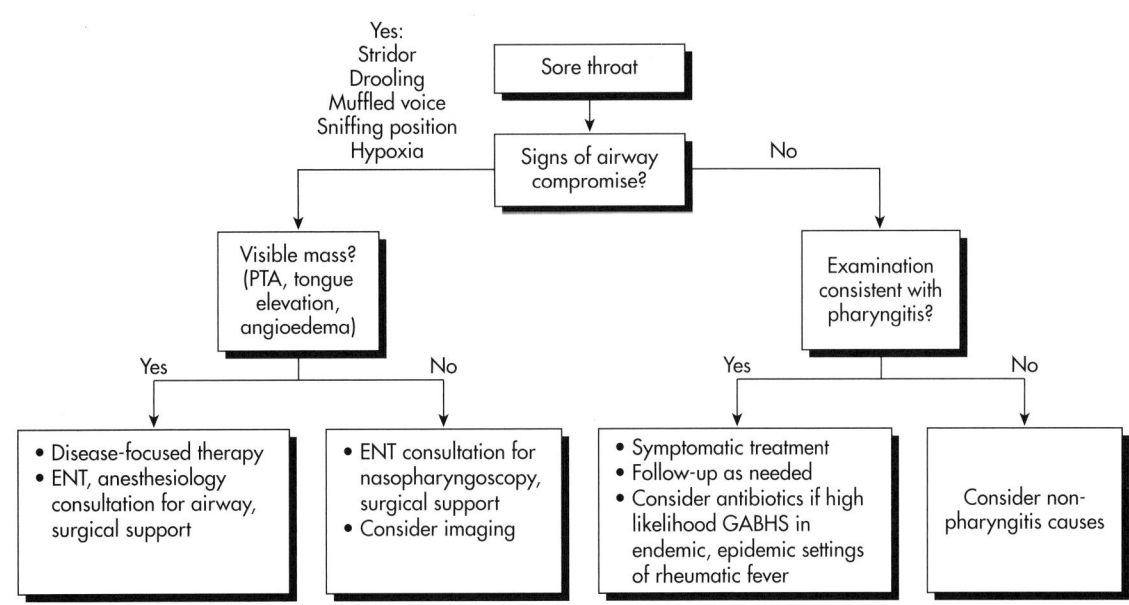

MANAGEMENT ALGORITHM

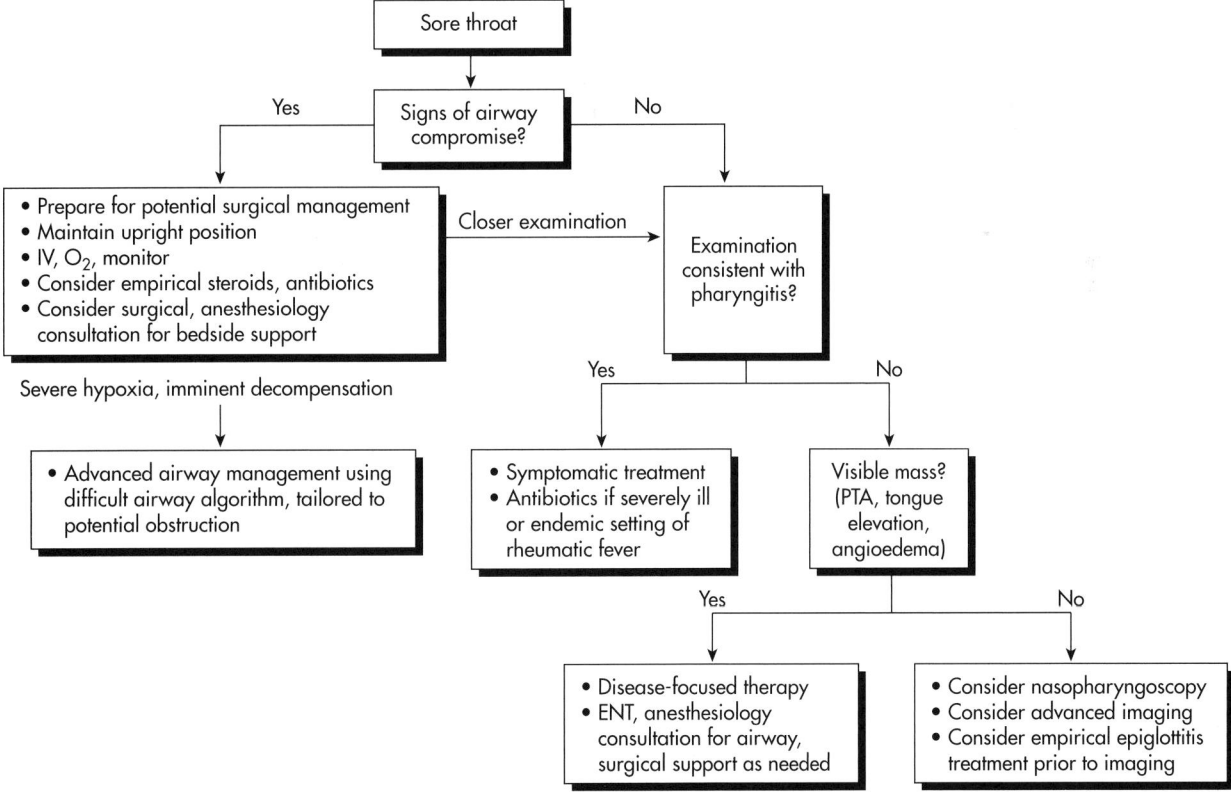

FIG. 175 Clinical approach to the patient with sore throat—diagnosis (A) and management (B). Refer to Section I topics Pharyngitis/Tonsillitis and Epiglottitis for additional information. *ENT,* Ear-nose-throat; *GABHS,* group A beta-hemolytic streptococcus; *IV,* intravenous; *PTA,* peritonsillar abscess. (From Marx JA et al: *Rosen's emergency medicine*, ed 8, Philadelphia, 2014, Saunders.)

Clinical
Algorithms

III

TABLE 98 Differential Diagnosis of Sore Throat

Type of Pharyngitis	Nature of Patient	Nature of Symptoms	Predisposing Factors	Physical Findings	Diagnostic Studies
Without Pharyngeal Ulcers					
Viral	All ages	Pain in throat Rapid onset Systemic symptoms	—	Exudate less likely than with streptococcal infections	—
Infectious mononucleosis	Adolescents and young adults Uncommon in elderly	Gradual onset	—	Low-grade temperature Occasional exudate Posterior cervical adenopathy Hepatosplenomegaly	Monospot test
Streptococcal pharyngitis	Patients younger than 25 yr, especially age 6-12 yr	Pain in throat Rapid onset Few systemic symptoms	Fall and winter Streptococcal infection in family Diabetes	Marked erythema and throat swelling Temperature >101° F Tender anterior cervical nodes Scarlatiniform rash Tonsillar exudate more likely than with viral infection	Culture Rapid streptococcal antigen screening Increased antistreptolysin O titer
Gonococcal pharyngitis	Most common in male homosexuals and people with anogenital gonorrhea	Often no symptoms	Orogenital sex	—	Culture
Sinusitis with postnasal drip	Adults	Mild throat soreness Symptoms often worse with recumbency	—	Evidence of sinusitis Postnasal drip	CT/flexible rhinoscopy (in recalcitrant cases)
Allergic pharyngitis	—	—	Seasonal allergies	No fever Intermittent postnasal drip Swollen pharynx with minimal injection	Allergy testing
With Pharyngeal Ulcers					
Herpangina	More common in children	Painful ulcers on tonsils, pillars, or uvula	Immunosuppression Summer and autumn	Vesicles 1-2-mm ulcers	Serologic tests
Fusospirochetal infection (Vincent angina)	Children and people with poor oral hygiene	Painful ulcers Bleeding gums Foul breath	—	No vesicles Ulcerative gingivitis Gray, necrotic ulcers 2-30-mm ulcers Pseudomembrane	Gram stain: Spirochetes
Candidiasis	Children Immunosuppressed patients Those taking antibiotics	—	Immunosuppression Antibiotics Inhaled steroids	3-11-mm ulcers No vesicles	KOH smear: *Candida* culture
Herpes simplex	Most common in children	Not usually a cause of sore throat	Immunosuppression	1-2-mm painful ulcers Vesicles present on lips, gingivae, buccal mucosa, or tongue	Tzanck smear (not very sensitive) viral culture, PCR, herpes simplex virus antibody assay

CT, Computed tomography; *PCR*, polymerase chain reaction.
Modified from Seller RH, Symons AB: *Differential diagnosis of common complaints*, ed 7, Philadelphia, 2018, Elsevier.

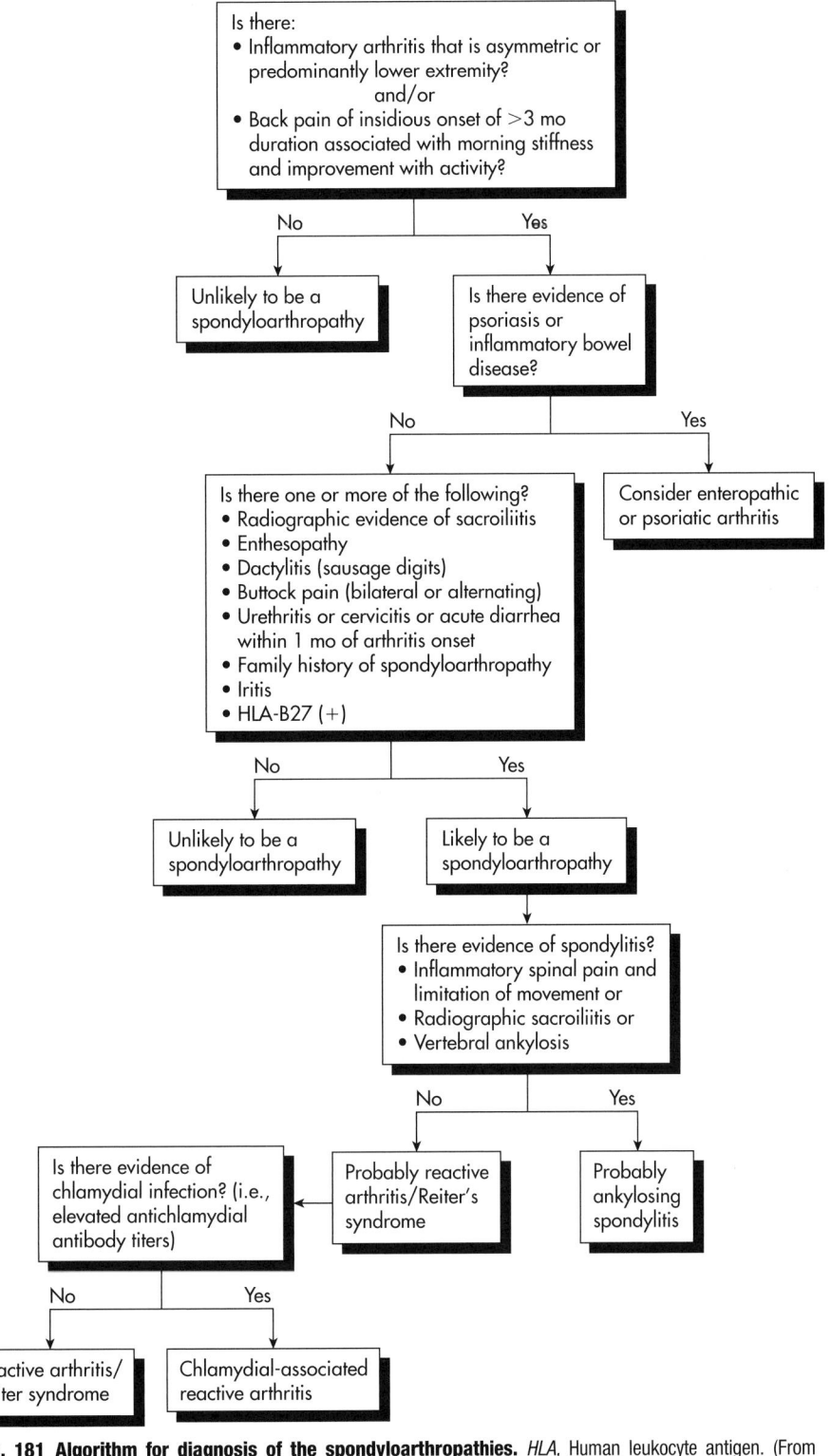

FIG. 181 Algorithm for diagnosis of the spondyloarthropathies. *HLA,* Human leukocyte antigen. (From Goldman L, Schafer AL: *Cecil textbook of medicine,* ed 24, Philadelphia, 2012, Saunders.)

Clinical
Algorithms

III

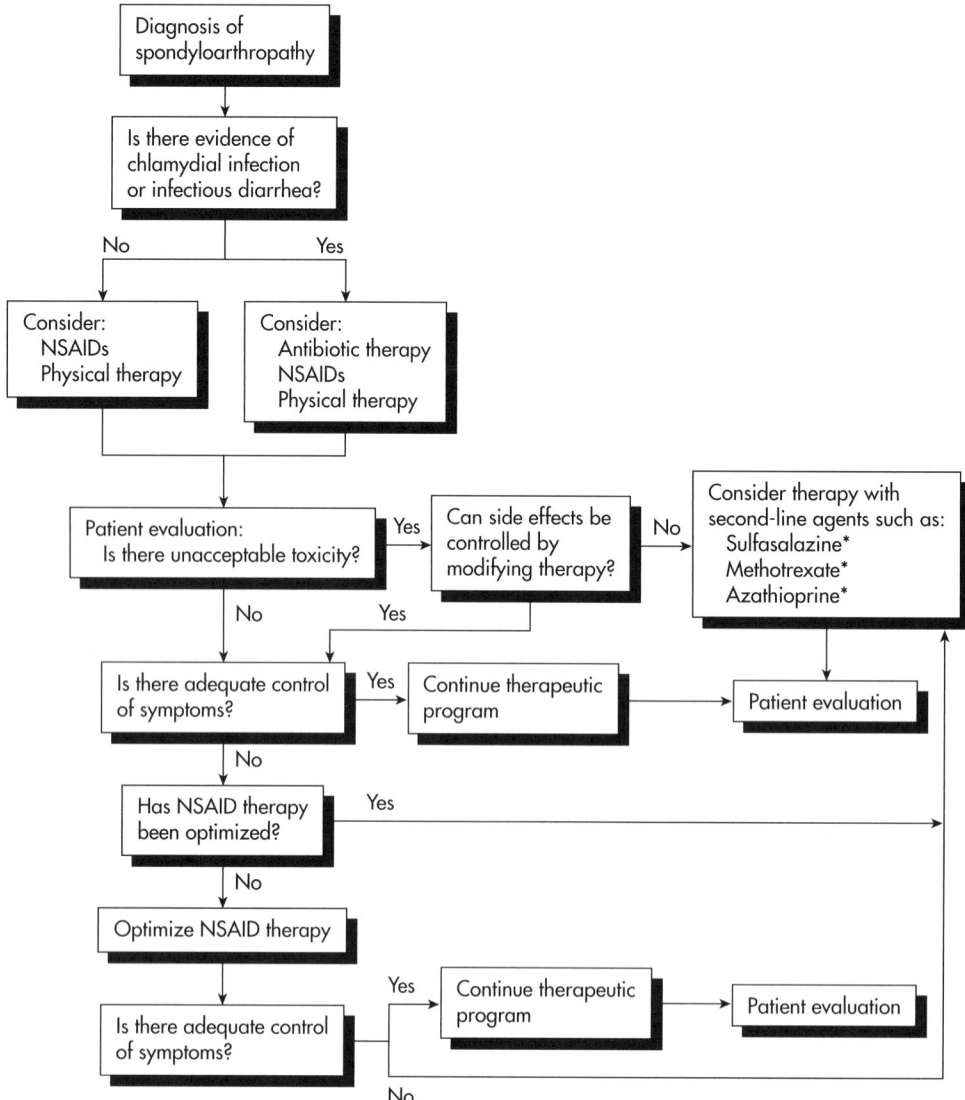

*Not approved by the FDA for treatment of spondyloarthropathies.

FIG. 182 Treatment algorithm for patients with a spondyloarthropathy. *FDA,* Food and Drug Administration; *NSAID,* nonsteroidal antiinflammatory drug. (From Goldman L, Schafer AL: *Cecil textbook of medicine,* ed 24, Philadelphia, 2012, Saunders.)

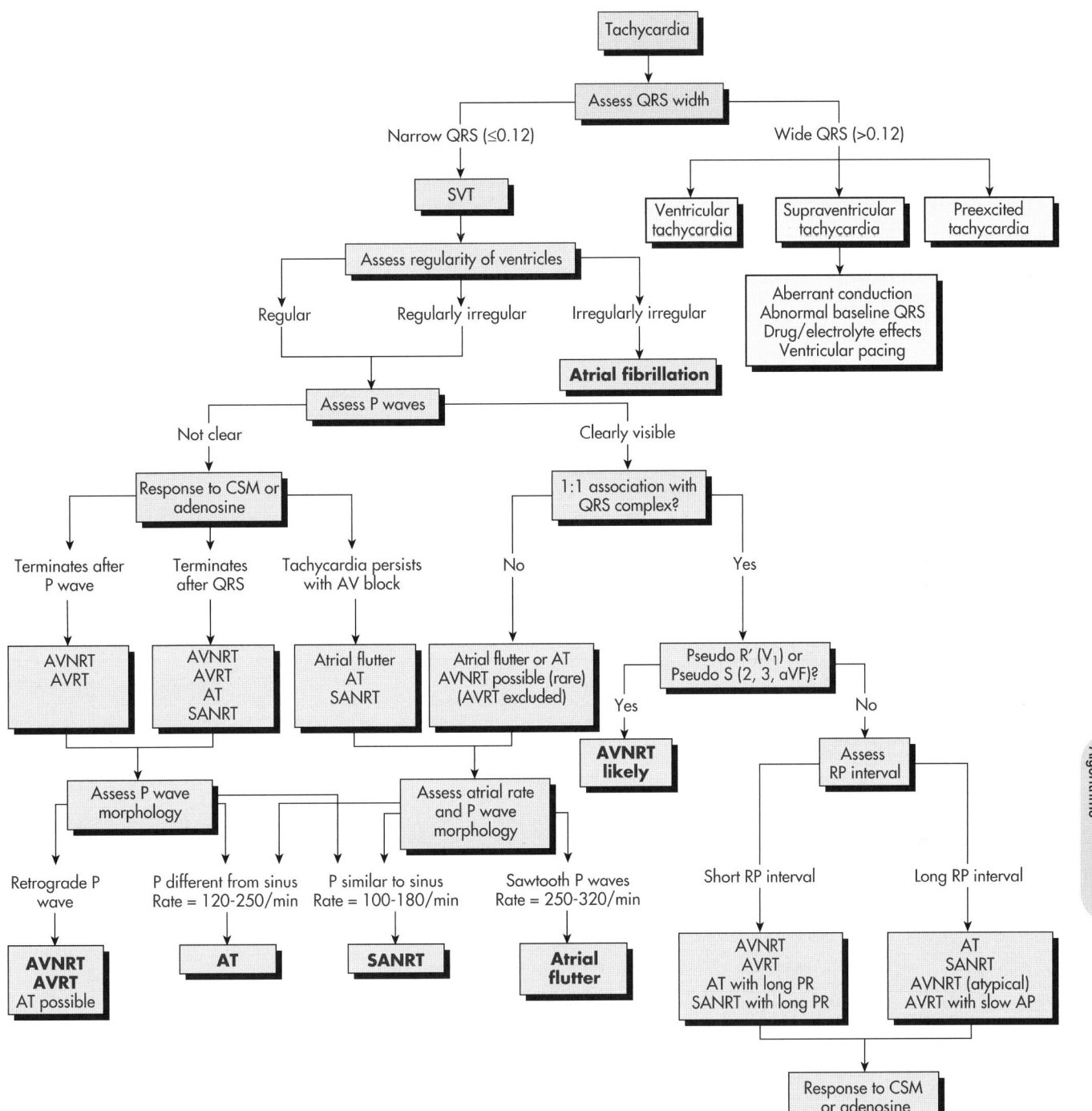

FIG. 183 Stepwise approach to diagnosis of the type of tachycardia based on a 12-lead electrocardiogram during the episode. The initial step is to determine whether the tachycardia has a wide or narrow QRS complex. For wide-complex tachycardia, see Table 100; the remainder of the algorithm is helpful in diagnosis of the type of narrow-complex tachycardia. *AP,* Accessory pathway; *AT,* atrial tachycardia; *AV,* atrioventricular; *AVNRT,* atrioventricular nodal reentrant tachycardia; *AVRT,* atrioventricular reciprocating tachycardia; *CSM,* carotid sinus massage; *SANRT,* sinoatrial nodal reentry tachycardia; *SVT,* supraventricular tachycardia. (From Zipes DP: *Braunwald's heart disease, a textbook of cardiovascular medicine,* ed 11, Philadelphia, 2019, Elsevier.)

Clinical
Algorithms

III

TABLE 100 Electrocardiographic Distinctions for Diagnosis of Wide-QRS Complex Tachycardia

Favor Supraventricular Tachycardia	Favor Ventricular Tachycardia
Initiation with a premature P wave	Initiation with a premature QRS complex
Tachycardia complexes identical to those in resting rhythm	Tachycardia beats identical to PVCs during sinus rhythm
"Long-short" sequence preceding initiation	"Short-long" sequence preceding initiation
Changes in the P-P interval preceding changes in the R-R interval	Changes in the R-R interval preceding changes in the P-P interval
QRS contours consistent with aberrant conduction (V_1, V_6)	QRS contours inconsistent with aberrant conduction (V_1, V_6)
Slowing or termination with vagal maneuvers	AV dissociation or other non-1:1 AV relationship
Onset of the QRS to its peak (positive or negative) <50 msec	Onset of the QRS to its peak (positive or negative) ≥50 msec
	Fusion beats, capture beats
QRS duration ≤0.14 sec	QRS duration >0.14 sec
Normal QRS axis (0 to +90 degrees)	Left axis deviation (especially −90 to 180 degrees)
	Concordant R wave progression pattern
	Contralateral bundle branch block pattern from the resting rhythm
	Initial R, q, or r >40 msec or notched Q in aVR
	Absence of an "rS" complex in any precordial lead

AV, Atrioventricular; *aVR,* augmented vector right; *PVC,* premature ventricular complexes.
From Zipes DP: *Braunwald's heart disease, a textbook of cardiovascular medicine,* ed 11, Philadelphia, 2019, Elsevier.

TACHYCARDIA, NARROW COMPLEX

ICD-10CM # I49.02   Ventricular flutter
         I49.8   Other specified cardiac arrhythmias
         R00.1   Bradycardia, unspecified

1815

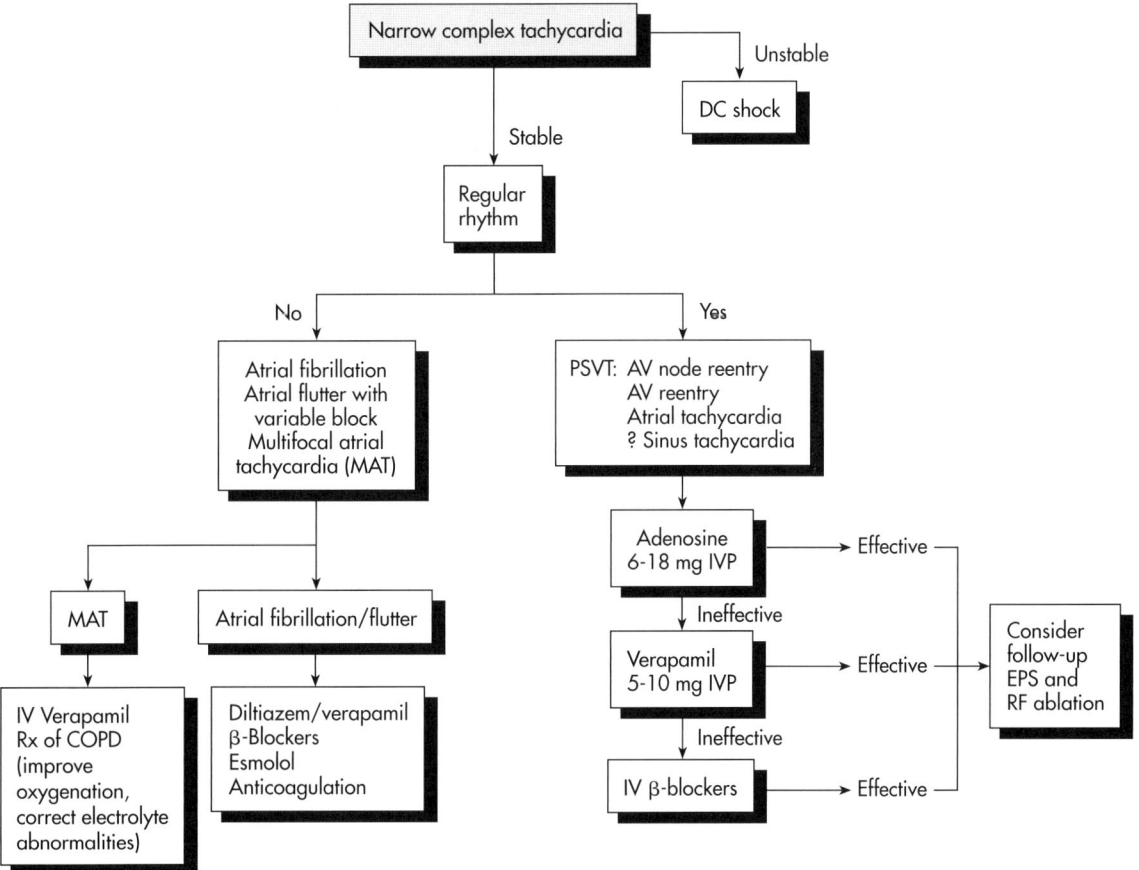

FIG. 184 Evaluation and management of narrow complex tachycardia. *AV,* Atrioventricular; *COPD,* chronic obstructive pulmonary disease; *DC,* direct current; *EPS,* electrophysiologic studies; *IV,* intravenous; *IVP,* intravenous push; *PSVT,* paroxysmal supraventricular tachycardia; *RF,* radiofrequency; *Rx,* treatment.

Clinical
Algorithms

III

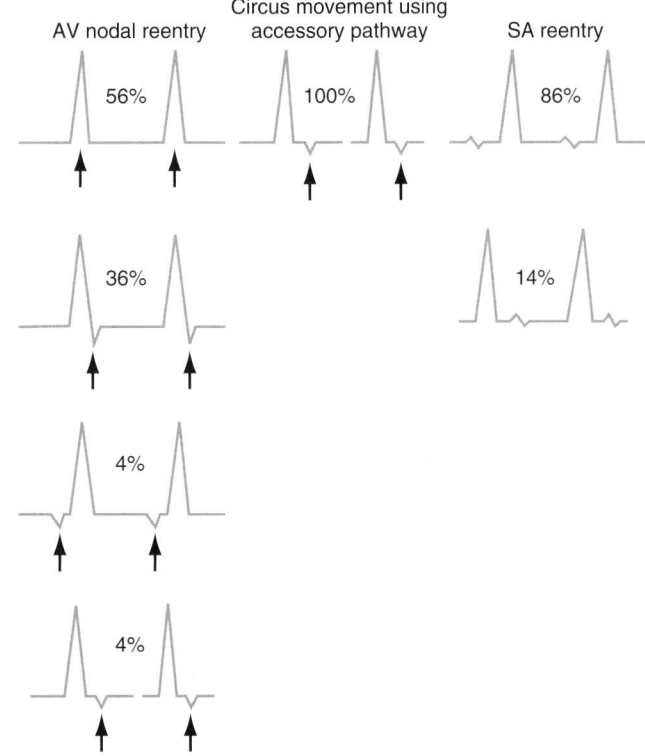

FIG. 185 Location of P waves in common causes of regular narrow-complex tachycardia. *AV,* Atrioventricular; *SA,* sinoatrial. (From Marriott HJL, Conover MB: *Advanced concepts in dysrhythmias,* ed 2, St Louis, 1989, Mosby. In Marx JA et al: *Rosen's emergency medicine,* ed 8, Philadelphia, 2014, Saunders.)

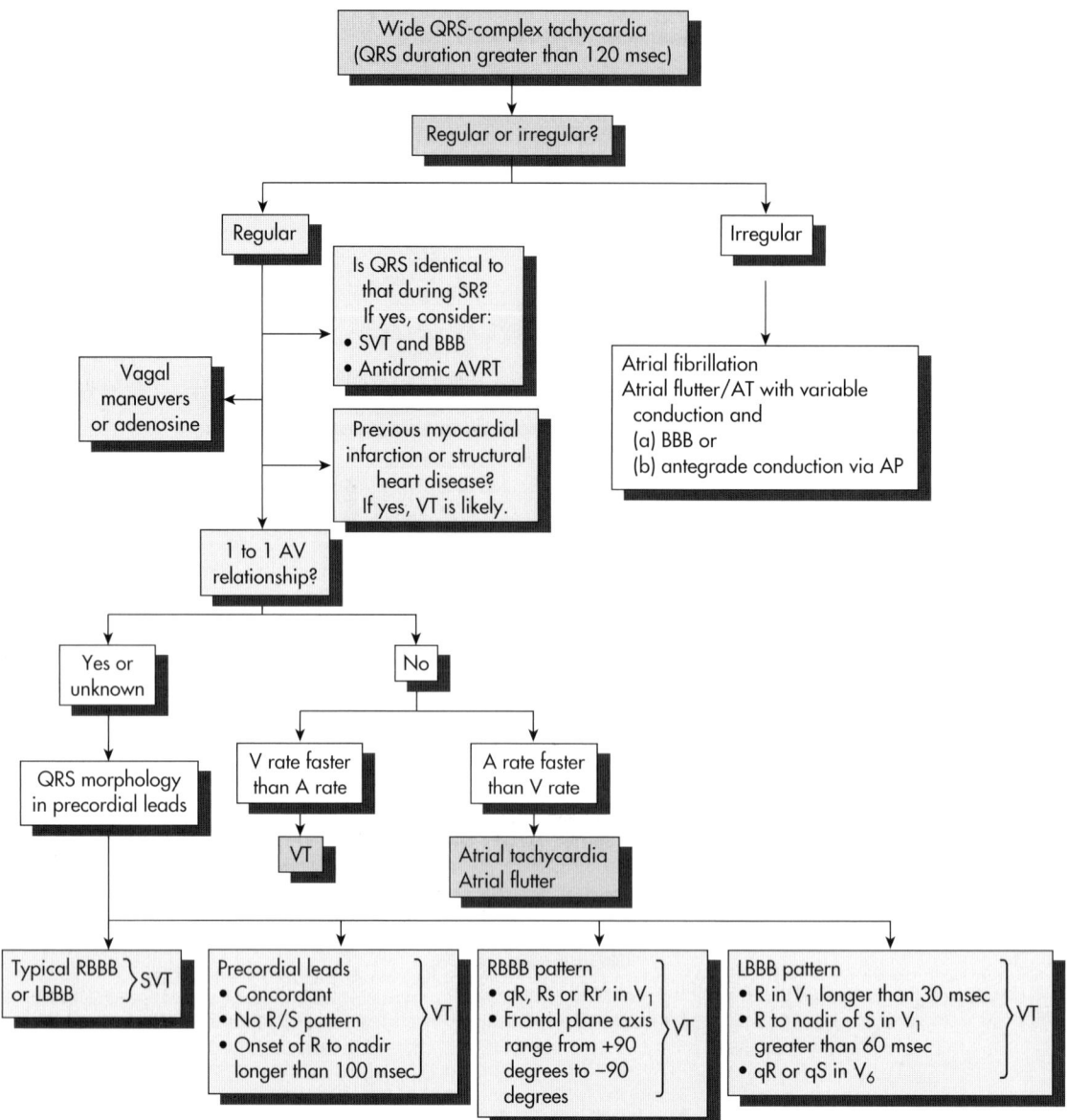

FIG. 187 Algorithm for diagnosis of wide-QRS tachycardia. *AP,* Accessory pathway; *AT,* atrial tachycardia; *AV,* atrioventricular; *AVRT,* AV reentrant tachycardia; *BBB,* bundle branch block; *LBBB,* left bundle branch block; *RBBB,* right bundle branch block; *SVT,* supraventricular tachycardia; *VT,* ventricular tachycardia. (From Bloomstrom-Lundqvist C et al: ACC/AHA/ESC guidelines for the management of patients with supraventricular arrhythmias—executive summary: a report of the American College of Cardiology/American Heart Association Task Force on Practice Guidelines and the European Society of Cardiology Committee for Practice Guidelines [Writing Committee to Develop Guidelines for the Management of Patients with Supraventricular Arrhythmias], *Circulation* 108:1871, 2003; Mann DL et al: *Braunwald's heart disease,* ed 10, Philadelphia, 2015, Elsevier.)

TABLE 101 Stepwise Criteria Favoring Ventricular Tachycardia Patients with Wide-Complex Tachycardias Using Different Algorithms

ACC/AHA/ESC Algorithm*	Kindwall Criteria[†]	Wellens Criteria[‡]	Brugada Criteria[§]	Miller criteria[§]
See Fig. 187	R >30 ms in V_1 or V_2 → VT	AV dissociation → VT	Absence of RS complex in all precordial leads → VT	Initial R wave in aVR → VT
	Any Q in V_6 → VT	QRS width >140 ms → VT	Longest R/S interval >100 ms in any precordial lead → VT	aVR with initial r or q >40 sec in duration → VT
	>60 ms to S wave nadir in V_1 or V_2 → VT	Left axis deviation >−30° → VT	AV dissociation → VT	aVR with a notch on the descending limb of a negative-onset and predominantly negative QRS in aVR → VT
	Notched downstroke S wave in V_1 or V_2 → VT	If RBBB morphology, monophasic or biphasic QRS in V_1 → SVT or R-to-S ratio of <1 in V_6 → VT	If RBBB morphology, monophasic R or qR in V_1 → VT R taller than R′ → VT rS in V_6 → VT	In aVR, mV of initial 40 msec divided by terminal 40 msec ($v/v_t \leq 1$) → VT
		If LBBB morphology, S in V_1-V_2 → VT	If LBBB morphology, initial R >40 ms in duration → VT Slurred or notched S in V_1 or V_2 → VT Beginning Q or QS in V_6 → VT	

ACC, American College of Cardiology; *AHA*, American Heart Association; *AV*, atrioventricular; *aVR*, augmented vector right; *ESC*, European Society of Cardiology; *LBBB*, left bundle branch block; *RBBB*, right bundle branch block; *VT*, ventricular tachycardia.

*Blomström-Lundqvist C et al: ACC/AHA/ESC guidelines for the management of patients with supraventricular arrhythmias—executive summary: a report of the American College of Cardiology/American Heart Association Task Force on Practice Guidelines and the European Society of Cardiology Committee for Practice Guidelines (Writing Committee to Develop Guidelines for the Management of Patients with Supraventricular Arrhythmias). *Circulation* 108:1871, 2003.

[†]Kindwall KE et al: Electrocardiographic criteria for ventricular tachycardia in wide complex left bundle branch block morphology tachycardias. *Am J Cardiol* 61:1279, 1988.

[‡]Wellens HJ et al: The value of the electrocardiogram in the differential diagnosis of a tachycardia with a widened QRS complex. *Am J Med* 64:27, 1978.

[§]Brugada P et al: A new approach to the differential diagnosis of a regular tachycardia with a wide QRS complex. *Circulation* 83:1649, 1991.

‖Vereckei A et al: New algorithm using only lead aVR for differential diagnosis of wide QRS complex tachycardia. *Heart Rhythm* 5:89, 2008.

From Bloomstrom-Lundqvist C et al: ACC/AHA/ESC guidelines for the management of patients with supraventricular arrhythmias—executive summary: a report of the American College of Cardiology/American Heart Association Task Force on Practice Guidelines and the European Society of Cardiology Committee for Practice Guidelines [Writing Committee to Develop Guidelines for the Management of Patients with Supraventricular Arrhythmias], *Circulation* 108:1871, 2003; Mann DL et al: *Braunwald's heart disease*, ed 10, Philadelphia, 2015, Elsevier.

Clinical Algorithms

III

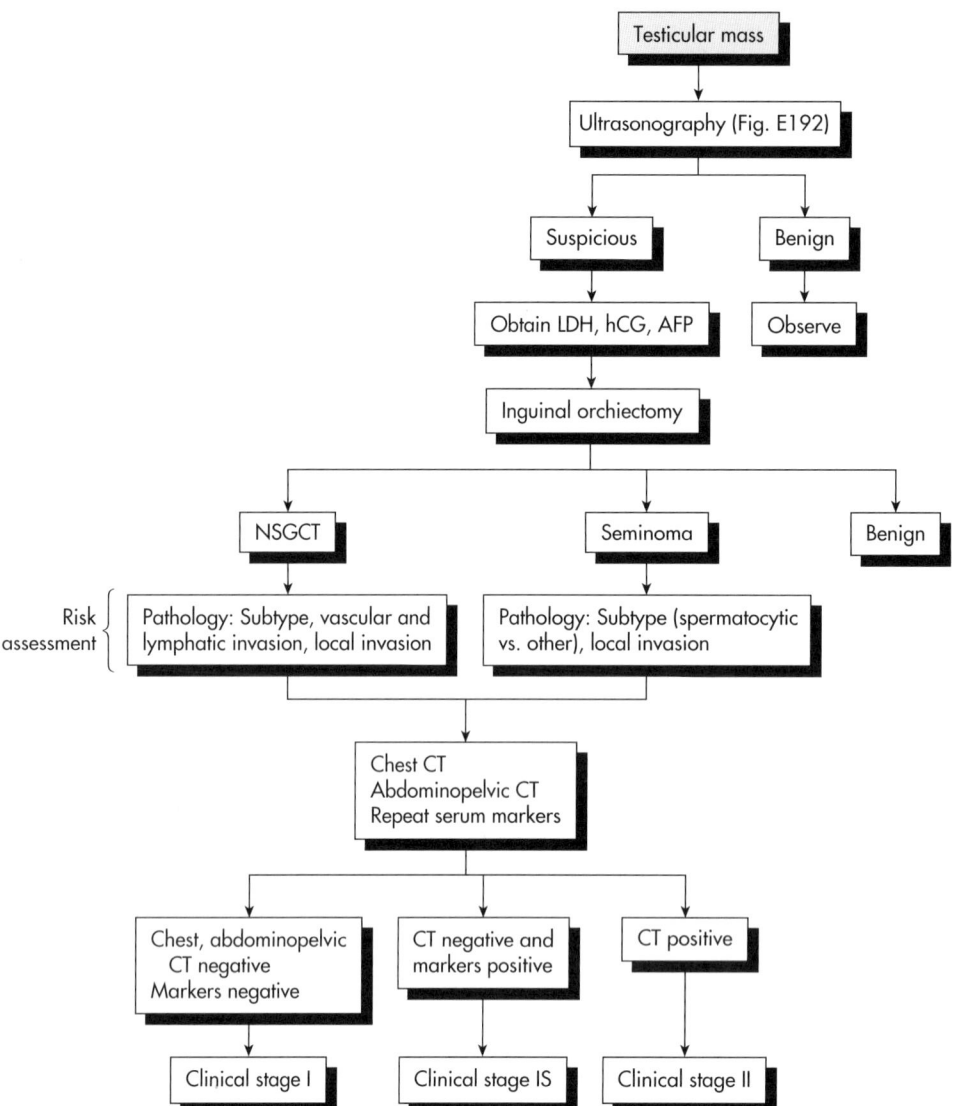

FIG. 188 Diagnosis, staging, and risk assessment of patients with testicular germ cell tumor. See "Section I Topic Testicular Cancer" for additional information. *AFP,* α-Fetoprotein; *CT,* computed tomography; *hCG,* human chorionic gonadotropin; *LDH,* lactic dehydrogenase; *NSGCT,* nonseminoma germ cell tumor. (From Abeloff MD: *Clinical oncology,* ed 4, New York, 2007, Churchill Livingstone.)

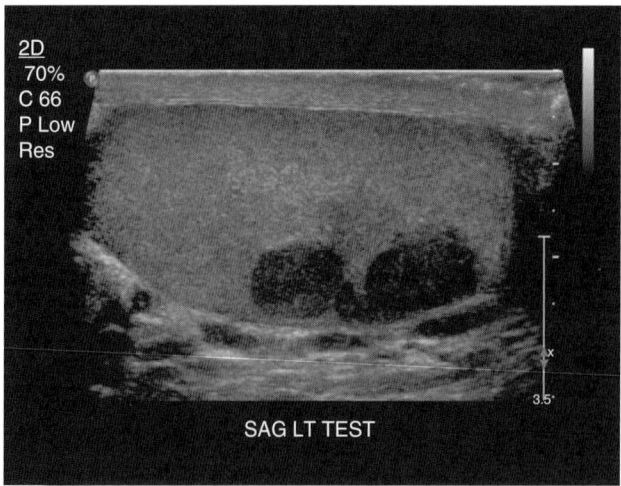

FIG. 189 Sagittal view of ultrasound of left testis showing multinodular hypoechoic intratesticular lesion confirmed to be pure seminoma at orchiectomy. (From Wein AJ et al: *Campbell-Walsh urology,* ed 11, Philadelphia, 2016, Elsevier.)

URETHRAL DISCHARGE OR DYSURIA

ICD-10CM # R36   Urethral discharge
R36.9 Urethral discharge, unspecified
R36.0 Urethral discharge without blood

1819

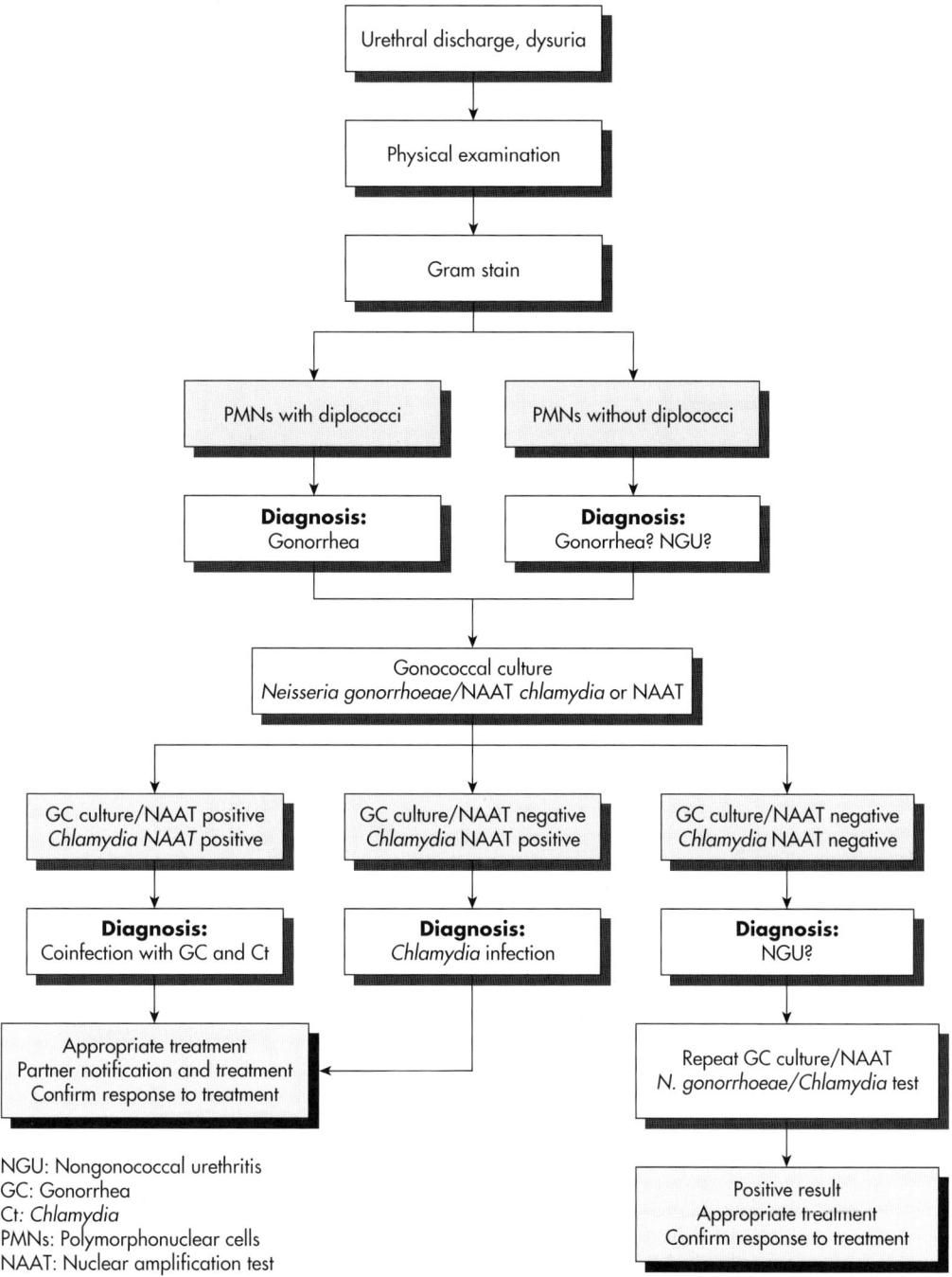

FIG. 193 **Diagnostic algorithm for evaluation of urethral discharge or dysuria.** (From Bolognia J: *Dermatology,* ed 4, Philadelphia, 2018, Elsevier.)

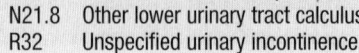

ICD-10CM #
R33.9   Retention of urine, unspecified
N21.8   Other lower urinary tract calculus
R32   Unspecified urinary incontinence

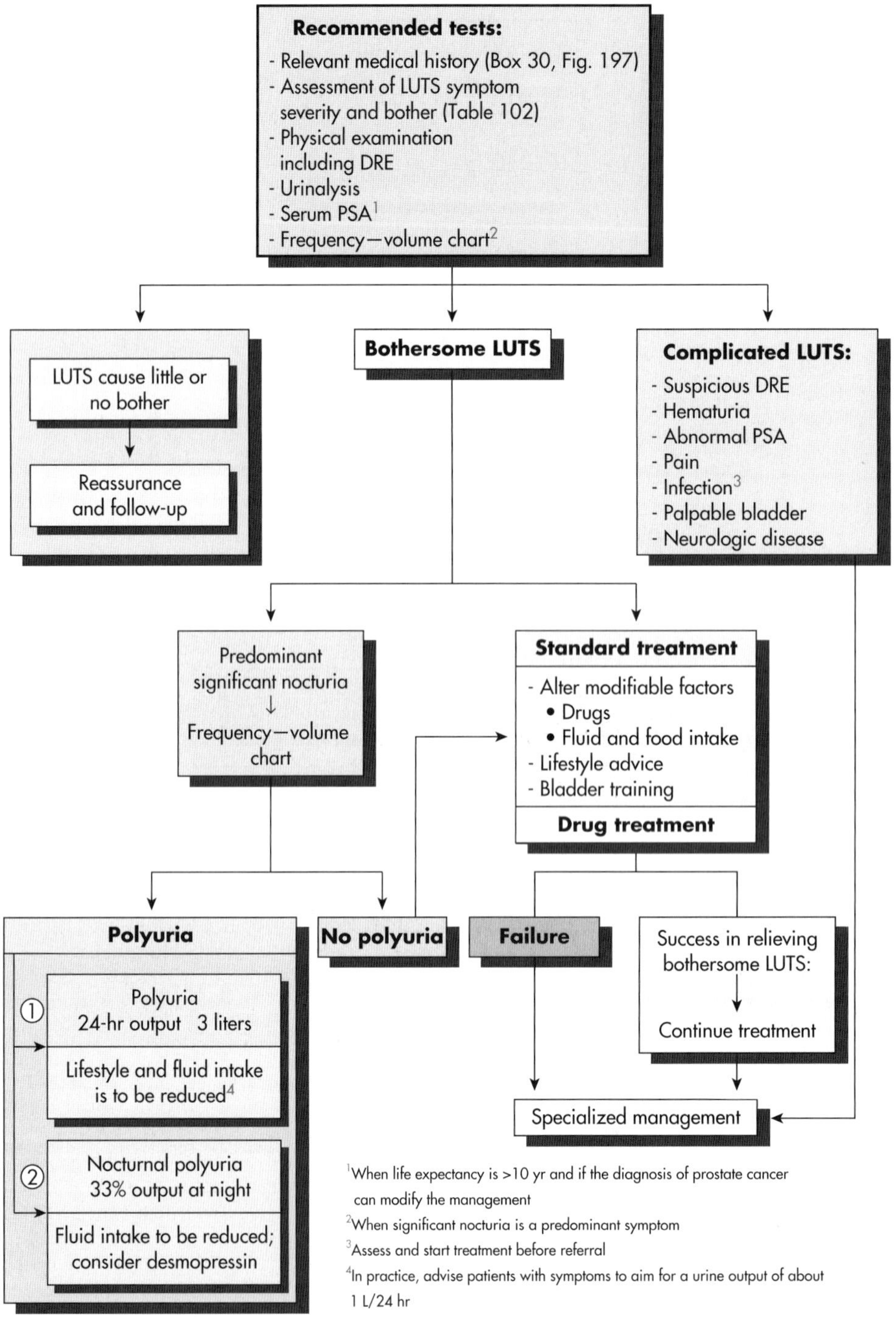

Recommended tests:
- Relevant medical history (Box 30, Fig. 197)
- Assessment of LUTS symptom severity and bother (Table 102)
- Physical examination including DRE
- Urinalysis
- Serum PSA[1]
- Frequency—volume chart[2]

Bothersome LUTS

LUTS cause little or no bother

→ Reassurance and follow-up

Complicated LUTS:
- Suspicious DRE
- Hematuria
- Abnormal PSA
- Pain
- Infection[3]
- Palpable bladder
- Neurologic disease

Predominant significant nocturia
↓
Frequency—volume chart

Standard treatment
- Alter modifiable factors
  • Drugs
  • Fluid and food intake
- Lifestyle advice
- Bladder training

Drug treatment

Polyuria

① Polyuria 24-hr output 3 liters

Lifestyle and fluid intake is to be reduced[4]

② Nocturnal polyuria 33% output at night

Fluid intake to be reduced; consider desmopressin

No polyuria

Failure

Success in relieving bothersome LUTS:

Continue treatment

Specialized management

[1] When life expectancy is >10 yr and if the diagnosis of prostate cancer can modify the management
[2] When significant nocturia is a predominant symptom
[3] Assess and start treatment before referral
[4] In practice, advise patients with symptoms to aim for a urine output of about 1 L/24 hr

FIG. 194 Basic management of lower urinary tract symptoms *(LUTS)* in men. *DRE,* Digital rectal examination; *PSA,* prostate-specific antigen. (From Fillit HM: *Brocklehurst's textbook of geriatric medicine and gerontology,* ed 8, Philadelphia, 2017, Elsevier.)

URINARY SYMPTOMS, LOWER URINARY TRACT—cont'd

ICD-10CM #	R33.9	Retention of urine, unspecified
	N21.8	Other lower urinary tract calculus
	R32	Unspecified urinary incontinence

1821

BOX 30 Causes of Male Lower Urinary Tract Symptoms

Benign prostatic enlargement (secondary to benign prostatic hyperplasia)
Urinary tract infection
Prostatitis
Overactive bladder
Neurogenic bladder dysfunction
Urethral stricture
Bladder neck contracture
Phimosis
Urinary tract stones
Bladder tumor
Advanced prostate cancer
Foreign body in the bladder
Medications, illicit drugs, and dietary factors (including caffeine, alcohol, ketamine, and decongestants)
Diabetes mellitus

From Fillit HM: *Brocklehurst's textbook of geriatric medicine and gerontology*, ed 8, Philadelphia, 2017, Elsevier.

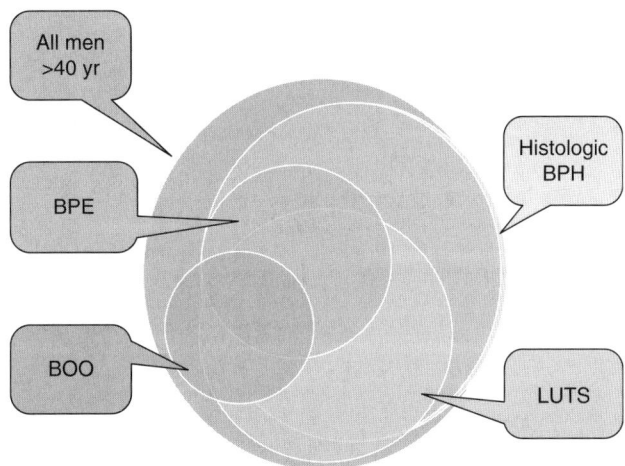

FIG. 195 Occurrence of LUTS with and without BOO, BPE, or BPH. *BOO,* Bladder outflow obstruction; *BPH,* benign prostate hyperplasia; *BPE,* benign prostate enlargement; *LUTS,* lower urinary tract symptoms. (From Fillit HM: *Brocklehurst's textbook of geriatric medicine and gerontology,* ed 8, Philadelphia, 2017, Elsevier.)

TABLE 102 International Continence Society Definitions of Lower Urinary Tract Symptoms

Voiding symptoms	• *Hesitancy* is difficulty in initiating micturition, resulting in a delay in the onset of voiding after being ready to pass urine.
	• *Slow stream* is the perception of reduced urine flow, usually compared to previous performance or in comparison to others.
	• *Splitting or spraying* of the urine stream.
	• *Intermittent stream* (intermittency) is the term used to describe urine flow that stops and starts, on one or more occasions, during micturition.
	• *Straining* to void describes the muscular effort used to initiate, maintain, or improve the urinary stream.
	• *Terminal dribble* is the term used to describe a prolonged final part of micturition, when the flow has slowed to a trickle or dribble.
Storage symptoms	• *Increased daytime frequency* is the complaint by the patient who considers that he voids too often during the day.
	• *Nocturia* is the complaint that the man has to wake at night one or more times to void.
	• *Urgency* is the complaint of a sudden compelling desire to pass urine that is difficult to defer.
	• *Urinary incontinence* is the complaint of any involuntary leakage of urine.
Postmicturition symptoms	• *Feeling of incomplete emptying* is a self-explanatory term for a feeling experienced by the individual after passing urine.
	• *Postmicturition dribble* is the term used to describe the involuntary loss of urine immediately after finishing passing urine, usually after leaving the toilet.

From Fillit HM: *Brocklehurst's textbook of geriatric medicine and gerontology*, ed 8, Philadelphia, 2017, Elsevier.

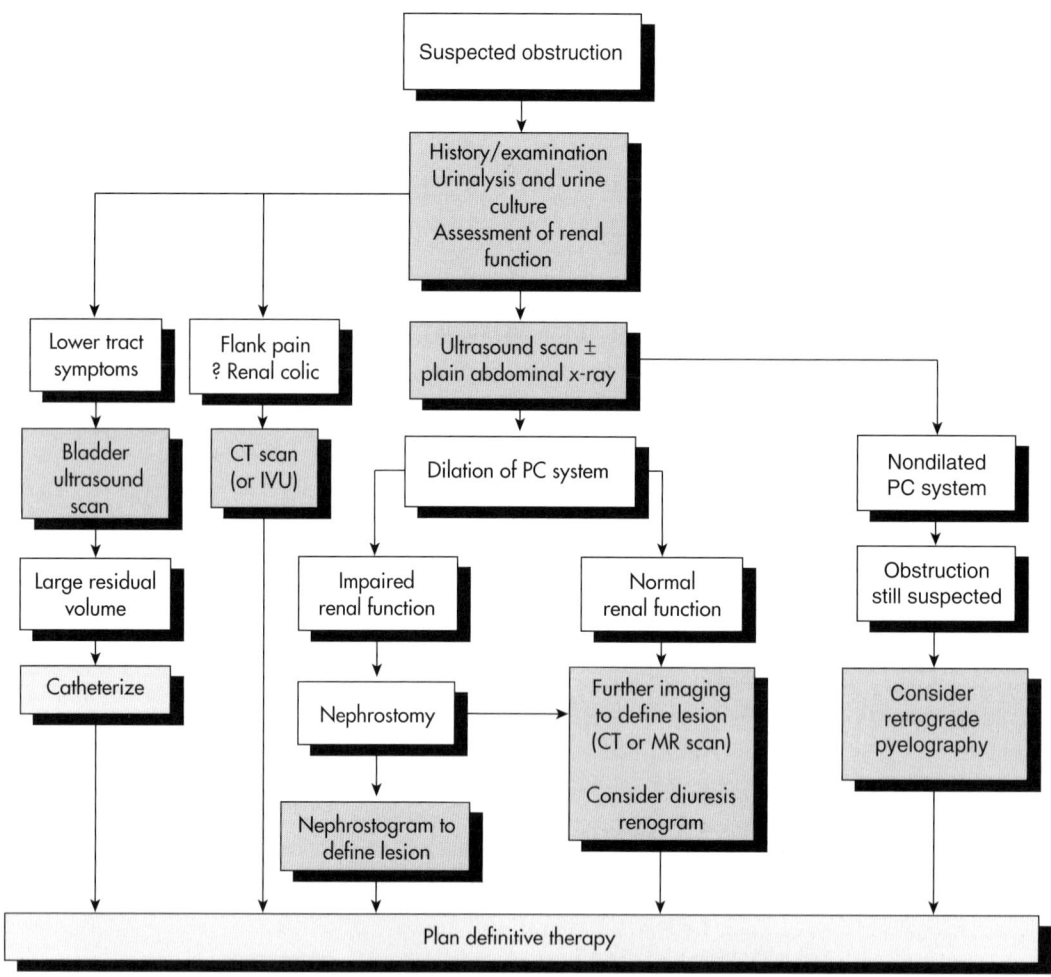

FIG. 196 Investigation and management of suspected urinary tract obstruction. A full history should be taken and a thorough examination performed, together with urinalysis, urine microscopy and culture, and measurement of renal function and serum electrolytes. Ultrasound is a useful first-line investigation for any patient with suspected urinary tract obstruction. Computed tomography *(CT)* is now the preferred imaging technique when renal calculi are suspected. Either CT or magnetic resonance *(MR)* urography can accurately diagnose both the site and cause of obstruction in most cases. If there is renal impairment, a nephrostomy allows the effective relief of the obstruction and time for renal function to recover while definitive therapy is planned. *IVU,* Intravenous urography; *PC,* pelvicalyceal. (From Johnson R et al: *Comprehensive clinical nephrology,* ed 5, Philadelphia, 2015, Saunders.)

BOX 31   Diagnostic Tests Used in Obstructive Uropathy

Upper Urinary Tract Obstruction
- Sonography (ultrasound)
- Plain films of the abdomen (KUB)
- Excretory or intravenous pyelography (very rarely needed)
- Retrograde pyelography
- Isotopic renography
- Computed tomography (helical CT)
- Magnetic resonance imaging
- Pressure flow studies (the Whitaker test)

Lower Urinary Tract Obstruction
- Some of the tests listed at left
- Cystoscopy
- Voiding cystourethrogram
- Retrograde urethrography
- Urodynamic tests
- Debimetry
- Cystometrography
- Electromyography
- Urethral pressure profile

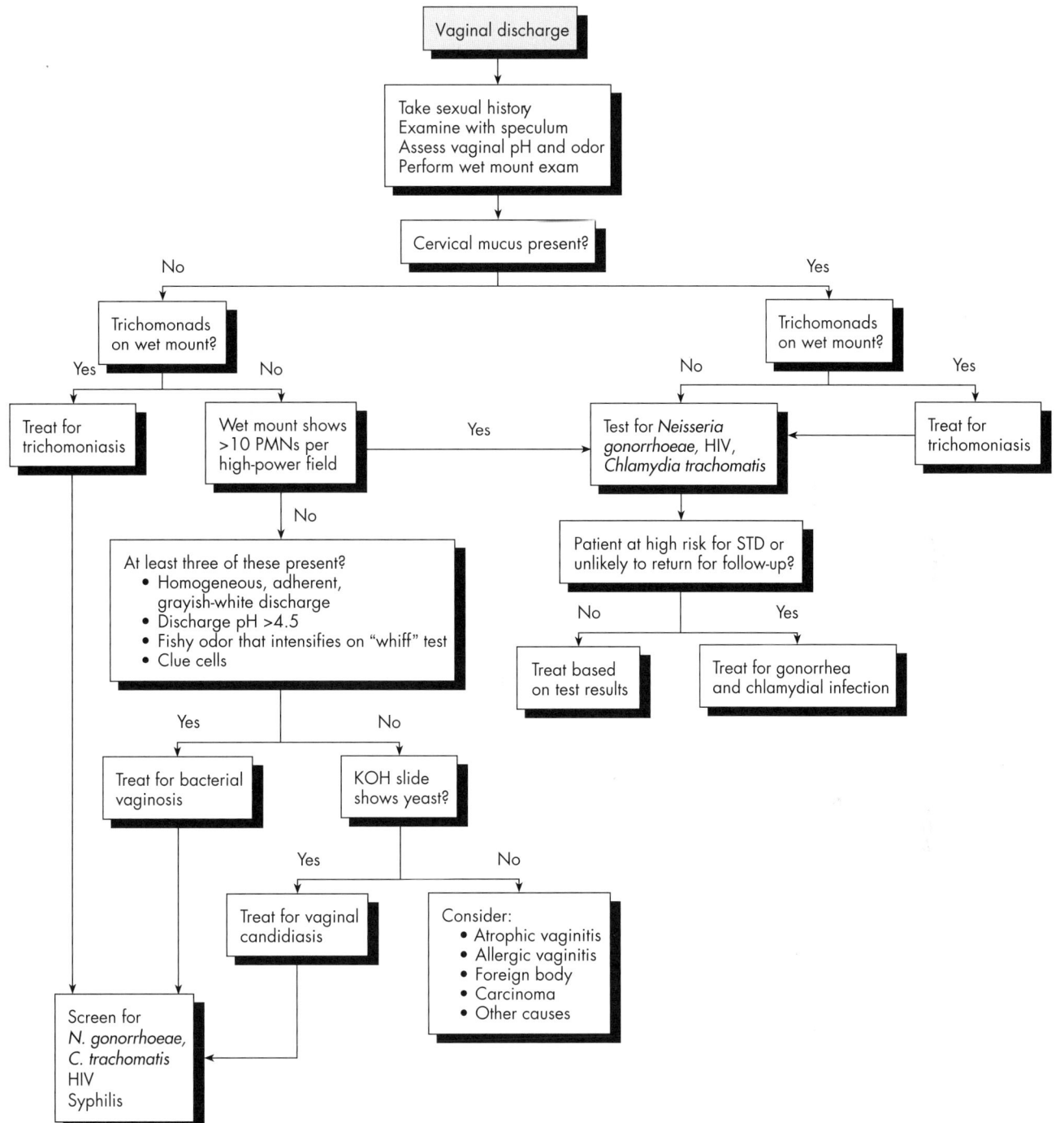

FIG. 197 Evaluation of vaginal discharge. See "Section I" topics "Vaginitis," "Fungal and Vaginitis," "Trichomonas" for additional information. *HIV*, Human immunodeficiency virus; *KOH*, potassium hydroxide; *PMN*, polymorphonuclear leukocyte; *STD*, sexually transmitted disease.

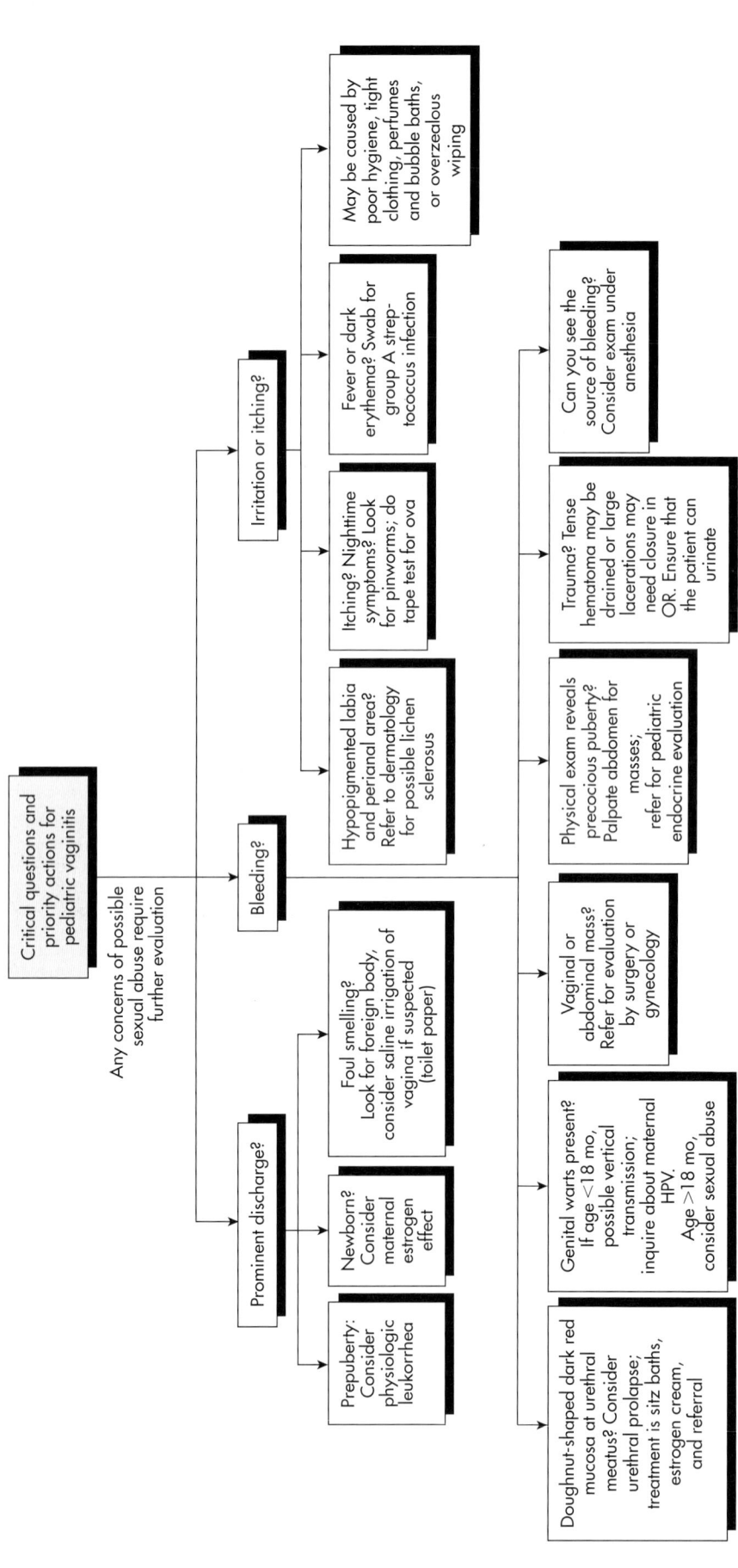

FIG. 198 Algorithm showing critical questions and priority actions for pediatric vaginitis. Additional information available in Section I topic Vaginitis, Prepubescent. *HPV,* Human papillomavirus; *OR,* operating room. (From Adams JG et al: *Emergency medicine: clinical essentials,* ed 2, Philadelphia, 2013, Elsevier.)

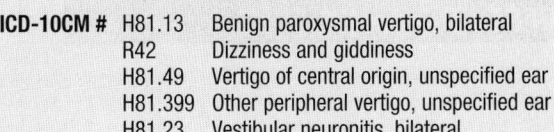

ICD-10CM #		
	H81.13	Benign paroxysmal vertigo, bilateral
	R42	Dizziness and giddiness
	H81.49	Vertigo of central origin, unspecified ear
	H81.399	Other peripheral vertigo, unspecified ear
	H81.23	Vestibular neuronitis, bilateral

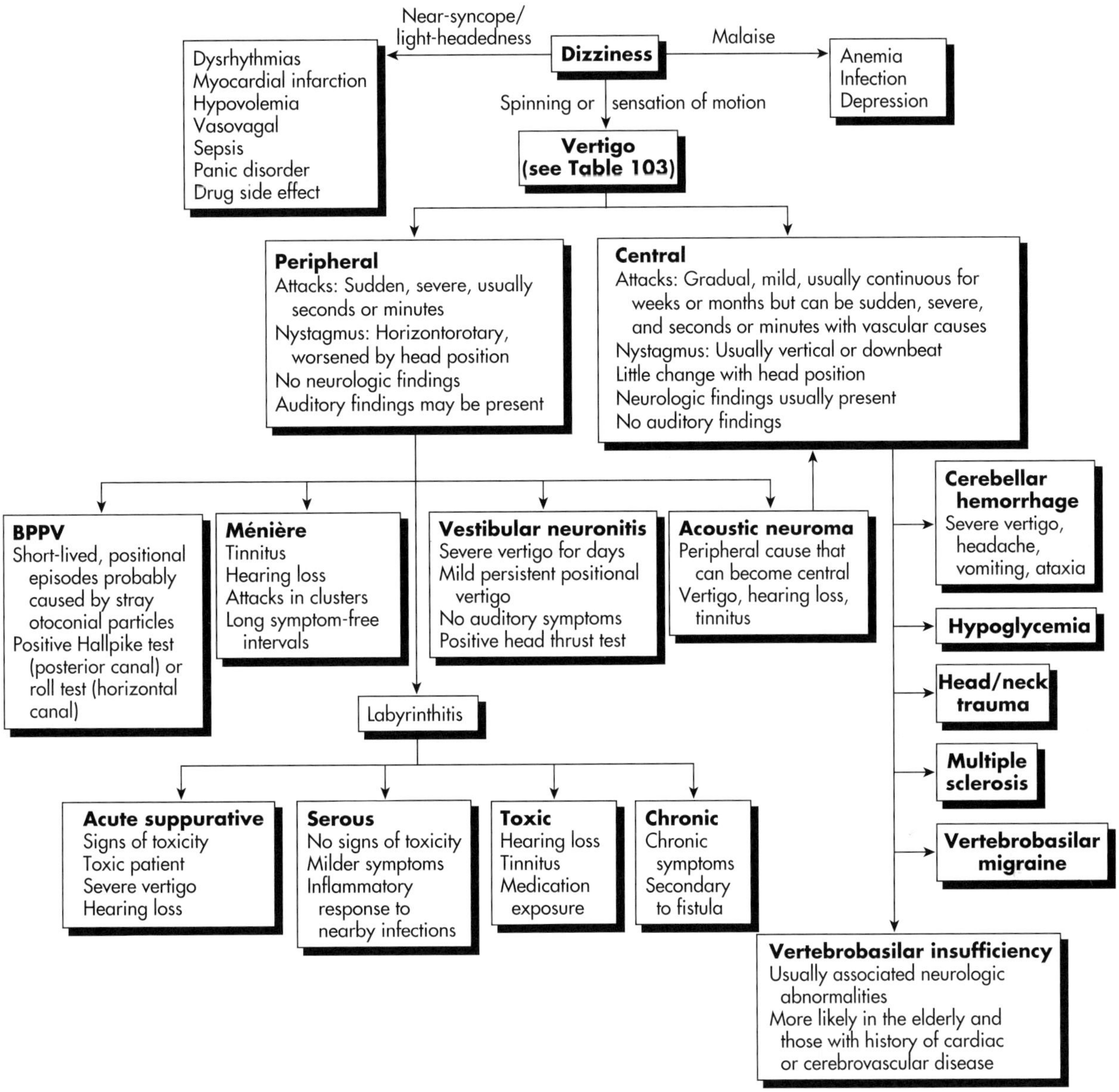

1825

Dizziness

Near-syncope/ light-headedness →
- Dysrhythmias
- Myocardial infarction
- Hypovolemia
- Vasovagal
- Sepsis
- Panic disorder
- Drug side effect

Malaise →
- Anemia
- Infection
- Depression

Spinning or sensation of motion →

Vertigo (see Table 103)

Peripheral
Attacks: Sudden, severe, usually seconds or minutes
Nystagmus: Horizontorotary, worsened by head position
No neurologic findings
Auditory findings may be present

Central
Attacks: Gradual, mild, usually continuous for weeks or months but can be sudden, severe, and seconds or minutes with vascular causes
Nystagmus: Usually vertical or downbeat
Little change with head position
Neurologic findings usually present
No auditory findings

BPPV
Short-lived, positional episodes probably caused by stray otoconial particles
Positive Hallpike test (posterior canal) or roll test (horizontal canal)

Ménière
Tinnitus
Hearing loss
Attacks in clusters
Long symptom-free intervals

Vestibular neuronitis
Severe vertigo for days
Mild persistent positional vertigo
No auditory symptoms
Positive head thrust test

Acoustic neuroma
Peripheral cause that can become central
Vertigo, hearing loss, tinnitus

Cerebellar hemorrhage
Severe vertigo, headache, vomiting, ataxia

Hypoglycemia

Head/neck trauma

Multiple sclerosis

Vertebrobasilar migraine

Labyrinthitis

Acute suppurative
Signs of toxicity
Toxic patient
Severe vertigo
Hearing loss

Serous
No signs of toxicity
Milder symptoms
Inflammatory response to nearby infections

Toxic
Hearing loss
Tinnitus
Medication exposure

Chronic
Chronic symptoms
Secondary to fistula

Vertebrobasilar insufficiency
Usually associated neurologic abnormalities
More likely in the elderly and those with history of cardiac or cerebrovascular disease

FIG. 201 Diagnostic algorithm for dizziness and vertigo. Also see "Section I" topics "Vestibular Neuronitis," "Acoustic Neuroma," "Labyrinthitis," "Ménière Disease," and "Benign Paroxysmal Positional Vertigo." *BPPV,* Benign paroxysmal positional vertigo. (From Marx JA et al: *Rosen's emergency medicine,* ed 8, Philadelphia, 2014, Saunders.)

Clinical Algorithms

III

TABLE 103 Differential Diagnosis of Patients with True Vertigo

Cause	History	Associated Symptoms	Physical
Peripheral			
• Benign paroxysmal positional vertigo	Short-lived, positional, fatigable episodes	Nausea, vomiting	Single position can precipitate vertigo. Positive result on Hallpike test (posterior semicircular canal) or Roll test (horizontal canal).
• Serous	Mild to severe positional symptoms. Usually coexisting or antecedent infection of ear, nose, throat, or meninges.	Mild to severe hearing loss can occur	Usually nontoxic patient with minimal fever elevation.
• Acute suppurative	Coexisting acute exudative infection of the inner ear. Severe symptoms.	Usually severe hearing loss, nausea, vomiting	Febrile patient showing signs of toxicity. Acute otitis media.
• Toxic	Gradually progressive symptoms: Patients on medication causing toxicity.	Hearing loss that may become rapid and severe, nausea and vomiting	Hearing loss. Ataxia common feature in chronic phase.

Continued

ICD-10CM #	H81.13	Benign paroxysmal vertigo, bilateral
	R42	Dizziness and giddiness
	H81.49	Vertigo of central origin, unspecified ear
	H81.399	Other peripheral vertigo, unspecified ear
	H81.23	Vestibular neuronitis, bilateral

Table 103 Differential Diagnosis of Patients with True Vertigo—cont'd

Cause	History	Associated Symptoms	Physical
• Ménière disease	Recurrent episodes of severe rotational vertigo usually lasting hours. Onset usually abrupt. Attacks may occur in clusters. Long symptom-free remissions.	Nausea, vomiting, tinnitus, hearing loss	Positional nystagmus not present.
• Vestibular neuritis	Sudden onset of severe vertigo, increasing in intensity for hours, then gradually subsiding over several days but can last weeks to months. Can be worsened with positional change. Sometimes history of infection or toxic exposure that precedes initial attack. Highest incidence is found in third and fifth decades.	Nausea, vomiting. Auditory symptoms do not occur.	Spontaneous nystagmus toward the involved ear may be present.
• Acoustic neuroma	Gradual onset and increase in symptoms. Neurologic signs in later stages. Most occur in women aged 30-60.	Hearing loss, tinnitus. True ataxia and neurologic signs as tumor enlarges.	Unilateral decreased hearing. True truncal ataxia and other neurologic signs when tumor enlarges. May have diminution or absence of corneal reflex. Eighth cranial nerve deficit may be present.
Central			
• Vertebrobasilar insufficiency	Should be considered in any patient of advanced age with isolated new-onset vertigo without an obvious cause. More likely with history of atherosclerosis. Can occur with neck trauma. Initial episode usually lasts seconds to minutes.	Often headache. Usually neurologic symptoms including dysarthria, ataxia, weakness, numbness, double vision. Tinnitus and deafness uncommon.	Neurologic deficits usually present, but initially neurologic examination can be normal.
• Cerebellar hemorrhage	Sudden onset of severe symptoms.	Headache, vomiting, ataxia	Signs of toxicity. Dysmetria, true ataxia. Ipsilateral sixth cranial nerve palsy may be present.
• Occlusion of posterior inferior cerebellar artery (Wallenberg syndrome)	Vertigo associated with significant neurologic complaints.	Nausea, vomiting, loss of pain and temperature sensation, ataxia, hoarseness	Loss of pain and temperature sensation on the side of the face ipsilateral to the lesion and on the opposite side of the body, paralysis of the palate, pharynx, and larynx. Horner syndrome (ipsilateral ptosis, miosis, and decreased facial sweating).
• Head trauma	Symptoms begin with or shortly after head trauma. Positional symptoms most common type after trauma. Self-limited symptoms that can persist weeks to months.	Usually mild nausea	Occasionally, basilar skull fracture.
• Vertebrobasilar migraine	Vertigo almost always followed by headache. Patient has usually had similar episodes in past. Most patients have a family history of migraine. Syndrome usually begins in adolescence.	Dysarthria, ataxia, visual disturbances, or paresthesias usually precede headache	No residual neurologic or otologic signs are present after attack.
• Multiple sclerosis	Vertigo presenting symptom in 7%-10% and appears in the course of the disease in a third. Onset may be severe and suggest labyrinth disease. Disease onset usually between ages 20 and 40. Often history of other attacks with varying neurologic signs or symptoms.	Nausea and vomiting, which may be severe	May have horizontal, rotary, or vertical nystagmus. Nystagmus may persist after the vertiginous symptoms have subsided. Bilateral internuclear ophthalmoplegia and ataxic eye movements suggest multiple sclerosis.
• Temporal lobe epilepsy	Can be initial or prominent symptom in some patients with the disorder.	Memory impairment, hallucinations, trancelike states, seizures	May have aphasia or convulsions.
• Hypoglycemia	Should be considered in diabetics and any other patient with unexplained symptoms.	Sweating, anxiety	Tachycardia, mental status change may be present.

From Marx JA et al: *Rosen's emergency medicine*, ed 8, Philadelphia, 2014, Saunders.

VERTIGO—cont'd

ICD-10CM #		
	H81.13	Benign paroxysmal vertigo, bilateral
	R42	Dizziness and giddiness
	H81.49	Vertigo of central origin, unspecified ear
	H81.399	Other peripheral vertigo, unspecified ear
	H81.23	Vestibular neuronitis, bilateral

1827

TABLE 104 Distinguishing Among Common Peripheral and Central Vertigo Syndromes

Cause	History of Vertigo	Duration of Vertigo	Associated Symptoms	Physical Examination
Peripheral				
• Vestibular neuritis	Single prolonged episode	Days to weeks	Nausea, imbalance	"Peripheral" nystagmus, positive head-thrust test, imbalance
• BPPV	Positionally triggered episodes	<1 min	Nausea	Characteristic positionally triggered burst of nystagmus
• Ménière disease	May be triggered by salty foods	Hours	Unilateral ear fullness, tinnitus, hearing loss, nausea	Unilateral low-frequency hearing loss
• Vestibular paroxysmia	Abrupt onset; spontaneous or positionally triggered	Seconds	Tinnitus, hearing loss	Usually normal
• Perilymph fistula	Triggered by sound or pressure changes	Seconds	Hearing loss, hyperacusis	Nystagmus triggered by loud sounds or pressure changes
Central				
• Stroke/TIA	Abrupt onset; spontaneous	Stroke, >24 h; TIA, <24 h	Brainstem, cerebellar	Spontaneous "central" nystagmus; gaze-evoked nystagmus; focal neurologic signs; negative head-thrust test; skew deviation
• MS	Subacute onset	Minutes to weeks	Unilateral visual loss, diplopia, incoordination, ataxia	"Central" types or rarely "peripheral" types of spontaneous or positional nystagmus; usually other focal neurologic signs
• Neurodegenerative disorders	May be spontaneous or positionally triggered	Minutes to hours	Ataxia	"Central" types of spontaneous or positional nystagmus; gaze-evoked nystagmus; impaired smooth pursuit; cerebellar, extrapyramidal and frontal signs
• Migraine	Onset usually associated with typical migraine triggers	Seconds to days	Headache, visual aura, photo-/phonophobia	Normal interictal examination; ictal examination may show "peripheral" or "central" types of spontaneous or positional nystagmus
• Familial ataxia syndromes	Acute-subacute onset; usually triggered by stress, exercise, or excitement	Hours	Ataxia	"Central" types of spontaneous or positional nystagmus Ictal, or even interictal, gaze-evoked nystagmus; ataxia; gait disorders

BPPV, Benign paroxysmal positional vertigo; *MS*, multiple sclerosis; *TIA*, transient ischemic attack.
From Jankovic J et al: *Bradley and Daroff's neurology in clinical practice*, ed 8, Philadelphia, 2022, Elsevier.

Clinical Algorithms

III

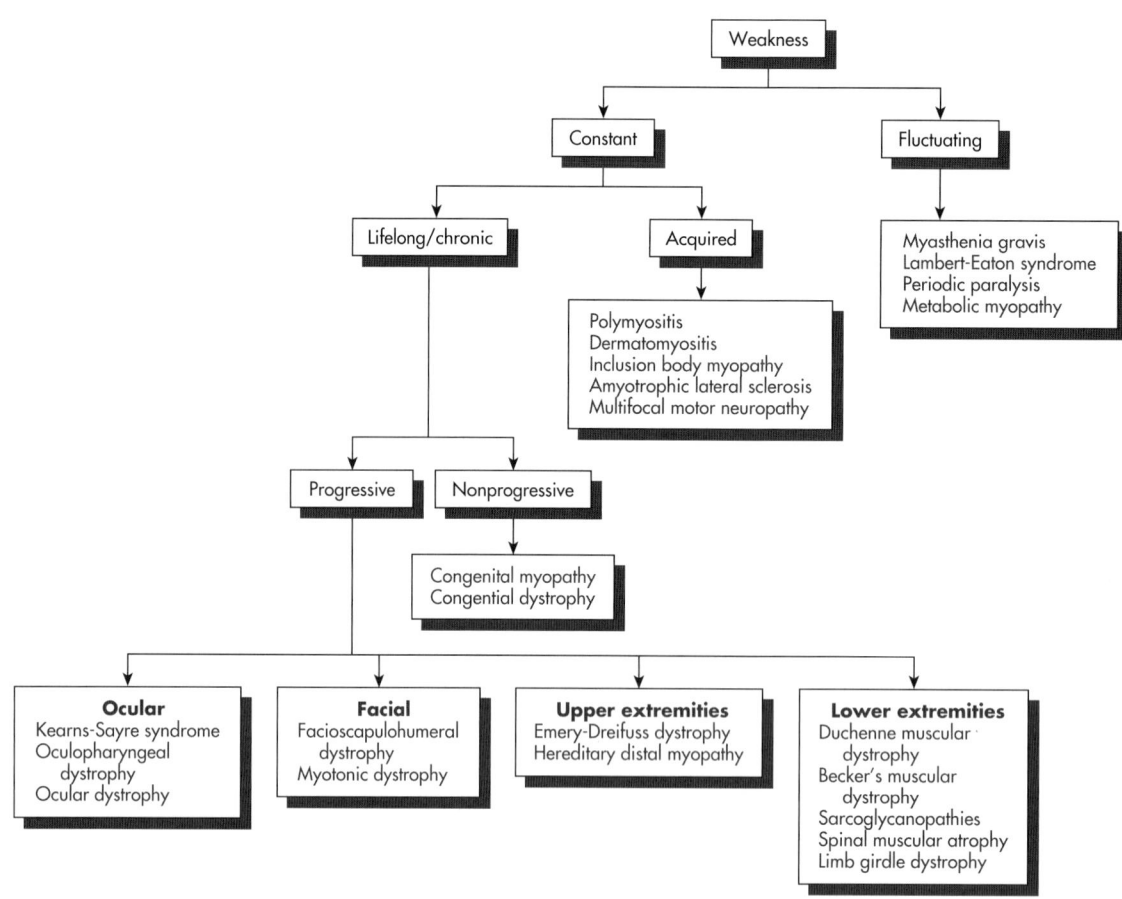

FIG. 204 Algorithm for the diagnostic approach to the patient with weakness. (From Jankovic J et al: *Bradley and Daroff's neurology in clinical practice*, ed 8, Philadelphia, 2022, Elsevier.)

TABLE 106   Critical and Emergent Causes of Neuromuscular Weakness

Critical Diagnoses

Cerebral cortex or subcortical	Ischemic or hemorrhagic cerebrovascular accident (CVA)
Brainstem	Ischemic or hemorrhagic CVA
Spinal cord	Ischemia, compression (disc, abscess, or hematoma)
Peripheral nerve	Acute demyelination (Guillain-Barré syndrome)
Neuromuscular junction	Myasthenic or cholinergic crisis Botulism Tick paralysis Organophosphate poisoning
Muscle	Rhabdomyolysis

Emergent Diagnoses

Cerebral cortex or subcortical	Tumor, abscess, demyelination
Brainstem	Demyelination
Spinal cord	Demyelination (transverse myelitis) Compression (disk, spondylosis)
Peripheral nerve	Compressive plexopathy (hematoma, aneurysm) Paraneoplastic vasculitis uremia
Muscle	Inflammatory myositis

From Marx JA et al: *Rosen's emergency medicine*, ed 8, Philadelphia, 2014, Saunders.

TABLE 107   Clinical Signs That Point to the Origin of Neuromuscular Weakness

Sign	UMNs	LMNs	NMJ	Myopathy
Atrophy	None	Severe	Mild	Mild
Fasciculation	None	Common	None	None
Deep tendon reflexes	Hyperreflexic	Areflexic/hyporeflexic	Normal/hyporeflexic	Normal/hyporeflexic
Distribution of weakness	Pyramidal/regional	Distal/segmental	Variable/fatigable weakness	Proximal > distal
Tone	Spastic	Decreased/flaccid	Decreased/flaccid	Normal/decreased
Plantar response	Upgoing	Downgoing or absent	Downgoing or absent	Downgoing or absent

LMNs, Lower motor neurons; *NMJ,* neuromuscular junction; *UMNs,* upper motor neurons.
From Cameron P et al: *Textbook of adult emergency medicine,* ed 5, Edinburgh, 2019, Elsevier.

Clinical
Algorithms

III

ICD-10CM #   R53.1   Weakness
                M62.81   Muscle weakness (generalized)

TABLE 108   Nonneuromuscular Conditions Associated with Weakness

Condition	Manifestations
Anemia	Breathlessness and fatigue usually worse with acute-onset anemia
Cardiac failure	Fatigue and weakness are common symptoms of heart failure in elderly patients, especially weakness in females over 50 yr
Malignancy	Paraneoplastic syndromes (e.g., generalized wasting)
Psychologic disorders	Depression/anxiety, psychosis, medication side effects, malingering
Malnutrition	Institutionalized patients, impoverished elderly, anorexia nervosa
Chronic fatigue syndrome	Possibly postviral syndrome
Rheumatologic disorders	Rheumatoid arthritis, systemic lupus erythematosus, fibromyalgia
Medications	Many medications have been associated with weakness; the commonly encountered ones include glucocorticoids, statins, antiretrovirals, alcohol, colchicine, and polypharmacy, especially in the elderly
Acute electrolyte derangement (e.g., hypokalemia and hyperkalemia, hypocalcemia)	Acute-onset weakness and/or tetany with hypocalcemia
Sepsis	Acidosis, deranged metabolic state
Dehydration	Lethargy/fatigue
Hypothyroidism	Lethargy, cold intolerance, weight gain, weakness
Chronic disease	Respiratory, renal, hepatic failure

From Cameron P et al: *Textbook of adult emergency medicine*, ed 5, Edinburgh, 2019, Elsevier.

TABLE 109   Key Features of Conditions Associated with the Symptom of Weakness

Disease	Pathophysiology	Assessment	ED Management
Primary Neurologic			
Guillain-Barré syndrome, most common cause of acute symmetric weakness	Immune-mediated polyradiculopathy Postinfective (15%-40%), esp. due to *Campylobacter* or viral infection; >50% are idiopathic	Suggestive history (e.g., diarrhea) Symmetric ascending flaccid weakness; loss of DTRs; early facial palsy common; ± autonomic dysfunction Serial assessment of respiratory function crucial to predict need for intubation/ventilation CSF high protein with normal glucose and cell count	Supportive care; early intubation for respiratory failure Early neurology and ICU consultation Early administration of IVIG ± plasmapheresis beneficial Corticosteroids *not* indicated
Myasthenia gravis, localized variant more common Myasthenic crises/respiratory decompensation (rare) are main ED issues	Immune-mediated Ach receptor dysfunction; may be precipitated by thymic disorders	Fluctuating, fatigable weakness of voluntary muscles, especially ocular muscles or proximal limbs. Cranial nerve involvement with ptosis in >25% cases; ± dysphagia, weakness of masticatory muscles; normal sensation; normal reflexes Improves with rest Serial respiratory assessment if severe Ice-pack test if there is ptosis	Supportive care Avoid potential precipitants including corticosteroids Anticholinesterase treatment as directed by neurologist
Multiple sclerosis, relapsing/remitting course most common	Immune-mediated scattered neuron demyelination; affects motor, sensory, visual, and cerebellar function Classically ≥2 separate episodes of neurologic dysfunction indicating white matter or spinal cord lesions at distinct locations	Acute exacerbations, acute worsening of clinical signs; variable weakness, hypertonicity, spasticity, clonus, altered pain/temp/vibration and proprioceptive senses Lhermitte sign Optic neuritis in up to 30% with acute central vision loss, afferent papillary defect, red desaturation lung puncture, MRI, evoked potentials in consultation with neurologist	Pulse methylprednisolone therapy for exacerbations Supportive care for generalized weakness Neurology consultation Long-term disease modification and lifestyle strategies (e.g., vitamin D)
Cord compression	Spinal stenosis ± malignancy or infection	Thorough neurologic examination Red flags (e.g., fever, malignancy, IVDU warrant MRI)	Neurosurgical consultation Decompression, antibiotics, targeted radiotherapy as indicated
Myopathies			
Congenital Dystrophin disorders, Duchenne muscular dystrophy (DMD); Becker muscular dystrophy (BMB) DMD/BMD, mitochondrial disorders	X-linked dystrophin gene dysfunction Males affected more severely by DMD; life expectancy to early 20s; BMD of later onset less severe	Generalized weakness Usual ED presentation is acute deterioration with respiratory compromise Spirometry/respiratory assessment Mitochondrial disorders—variable episodic weakness and fluctuating consciousness	Supportive care Discussion with patient, advocates, neurologists regarding appropriateness of intensive intervention Consider advance care directives Ventilatory support as appropriate

Table 109   Key Features of Conditions Associated with the Symptom of Weakness—cont'd

Disease	Pathophysiology	Assessment	ED Management
Acquired Metabolic/electrolyte disorders Hypokalemic periodic paralysis Endocrine Cushing disease Addison disease Thyrotoxicosis Toxic Statins, corticosteroids	Variable weakness; may be acute episodic weakness with hypokalemia ± thyrotoxicosis Drug-induced or history of endocrine myopathies suggestive	Periodic paralysis; may be preceded by vomiting/diarrheal illness; may have family history Check electrolytes, especially K^+ ECG if K^+ deranged Endocrine—assess for other stigmata of endocrinopathy (e.g., cushingoid, addisonian)	Electrolyte (K^+) reconstitution Supportive care Correct endocrine abnormalities Discontinue offending medications
Intoxications			
Botulism due to *Clostridium botulinum* toxin	Deranged neurotransmission Ingested botulinum toxin prevents Ach release at NMJ	History of ingestion GI symptoms in 50% Descending flaccid paralysis Postural hypotension, diplopia, blurred vision, ptosis, dysphagia, respiratory compromise, progressing to limb weakness Ileus common	Supportive care ICU admission for ventilatory support as needed Specific antiserum in consultation with toxicology/neurology
Tetanus due to *Clostridium tetani* tetanospasmin toxin Endemic in developing countries	Impaired inhibitory neurotransmission causing skeletal muscle spasm and rigidity Classically infected deep wounds in nonimmunized patients	Suggestive history—recent wound, vulnerable patient (e.g., elderly, nonimmune) Trismus/dysphagia common early; progressive to painful skeletal muscle spasms; exacerbated by minor stimuli (e.g., touch) May be a localized form Clinical diagnosis	Supportive care, ICU for ventilatory support and sedation Tetanus antitoxin Tetanus immunization is protective Antibiotics (penicillin) to treat clostridial infection
Tick paralysis due to tick toxin, ascending flaccid paralysis mimics Guillain-Barré syndrome	Impaired neurotransmission *Ixodes holocyclus* (Australian paralysis tick) Death from respiratory paralysis	Mostly children in tick-endemic area ± tick found on patient; ataxia, weakness ± extraocular palsy/dysphagia May progress after tick removal to generalized/respiratory paralysis	Tick removal/observation sufficient in most cases If severe, ventilatory support Antiserum administration as directed by toxicology/neurology
Marine intoxications Ciguatera Puffer fish Blue-ringed octopus	Ciguatera toxin (from reef fish) Tetrodotoxin (puffer fish, blue-ringed octopus) block sodium channels and impair neurotransmission Tetrodotoxin also acts on CTZ and impairs ventilation	History of tropical fish ingestion; onset of symptoms within a few hours Ciguatera—paresthesias, electrical sensations in response to hot/cold Tetrodotoxin—progressive flaccid weakness with respiratory compromise	Supportive treatment esp. ventilatory support

CSF, Cerebrospinal fluid; *CTZ*, chemoreceptor trigger zone; *DTRs*, deep tendon reflexes; *ECG*, electrocardiogram; *ED*, emergency department; *GI*, gastrointestinal; *ICU*, intensive care unit; *IVDU*, intravenous drug user; *IVIG*, intravenous immunoglobulin; *MRI*, magnetic resonance imaging; *NMJ*, neuromuscular junction.
From Cameron P et al: *Textbook of adult emergency medicine*, ed 5, Edinburgh, 2019, Elsevier.

Clinical Algorithms

III

BOX 32   Progressive Proximal Weakness

- Spinal cord disorders
- Juvenile spinal muscular atrophies
  - Autosomal dominant
  - Autosomal recessive
- GM$_2$ gangliosidosis (hexosaminidase A deficiency)
- Myasthenic syndromes
  - Acquired limb-girdle myasthenia
  - Slow-channel syndrome
- Muscular dystrophies
  - Bethlem myopathy
  - Dystrophinopathies
  - Facioscapulohumeral syndrome
  - Severe childhood autosomal recessive muscular
- Dystrophy
- Inflammatory myopathies
  - Dermatomyositis[a]
  - Polymyositis[a]
- Metabolic myopathies
  - Acid maltase deficiency[a]
  - Carnitine deficiency[a]
  - Debrancher enzyme deficiency[a]
  - Lipid storage myopathies
  - Mitochondrial myopathies
  - Myophosphorylase deficiency
- Endocrine myopathies
  - Adrenal cortex[a]
  - Parathyroid[a]
  - Thyroid[a]

[a]Denotes the most common conditions and the ones with disease-modifying treatments.
From Pina-Garza J, James KC: *Fenichel's clinical pediatric neurology*, ed 8, Philadelphia, 2019, Elsevier.

BOX 33   Progressive Distal Weakness

- Spinal cord disorders
- Motor neuron diseases
  - Juvenile amyotrophic lateral sclerosis
  - Monomelic
  - Spinal muscular atrophies
    - Autosomal dominant forms
    - Autosomal recessive forms
- Neuropathies
- Hereditary motor sensory neuropathies
  - Charcot-Marie-Tooth disease
  - Familial amyloid neuropathy
  - Giant axonal neuropathy (16q24)
  - Other genetic neuropathies
  - Other lipid neuropathies
  - Pyruvate dehydrogenase deficiency
  - Refsum disease
  - Sulfatide lipidosis: metachromatic leukodystrophy
- Neuropathies with systemic diseases
  - Drug-induced[a]
  - Systemic vasculitis[a]
  - Toxins[a]
  - Uremia[a]
- Idiopathic neuropathy
  - Chronic axonal neuropathy[a]
  - Chronic demyelinating neuropathy[a]
- Myopathies
  - Autosomal dominant childhood myopathy
  - Autosomal dominant infantile myopathy
  - Autosomal recessive distal (Miyoshi) myopathy
  - Inclusion body myopathies
  - Myotonic dystrophy
- Scapulo (humeral) peroneal syndrome
  - Emery-Dreifuss muscular dystrophy type 1
  - Emery-Dreifuss muscular dystrophy type 2
  - Scapuloperoneal myopathy
  - Scapuloperoneal neuronopathy

[a]Denotes the most common conditions and the ones with disease-modifying treatments.
From Pina-Garza J, James KC: *Fenichel's clinical pediatric neurology*, ed 8, Philadelphia, 2019, Elsevier.

Clinical
Algorithms

III

ICD-10CM # R53.1   Weakness
M62.81   Muscle weakness (generalized)

BOX 34   Acute Generalized Weakness

Infectious Disorders
- Acute infectious myositis
- Acute inflammatory polyradiculoneuropathy[a] (Guillain-Barre syndrome)
- Acute axonal neuropathies
- Chronic inflammatory polyradiculoneuropathy[a] (CIDP)
- Enterovirus infections

Metabolic Disorders
- Acute intermittent porphyria
- Hereditary tyrosinemia

Neuromuscular Blockade
- Botulism[a]
- Corticosteroid-induced quadriplegia[a]
- Intensive care unit weakness
- Tick paralysis[a]

Periodic Paralysis
- Andersen-Tawil syndrome
- Familial hypokalemic[a] (FPPI)
- Familial hyperkalemic[a] (FPPII)
- Familial normokalemic (FPPIII)

[a]Denotes the most common conditions and the ones with disease-modifying treatments.
From Pina-Garza J, James KC: *Fenichel's clinical pediatric neurology*, ed 8, Philadelphia, 2019, Elsevier.

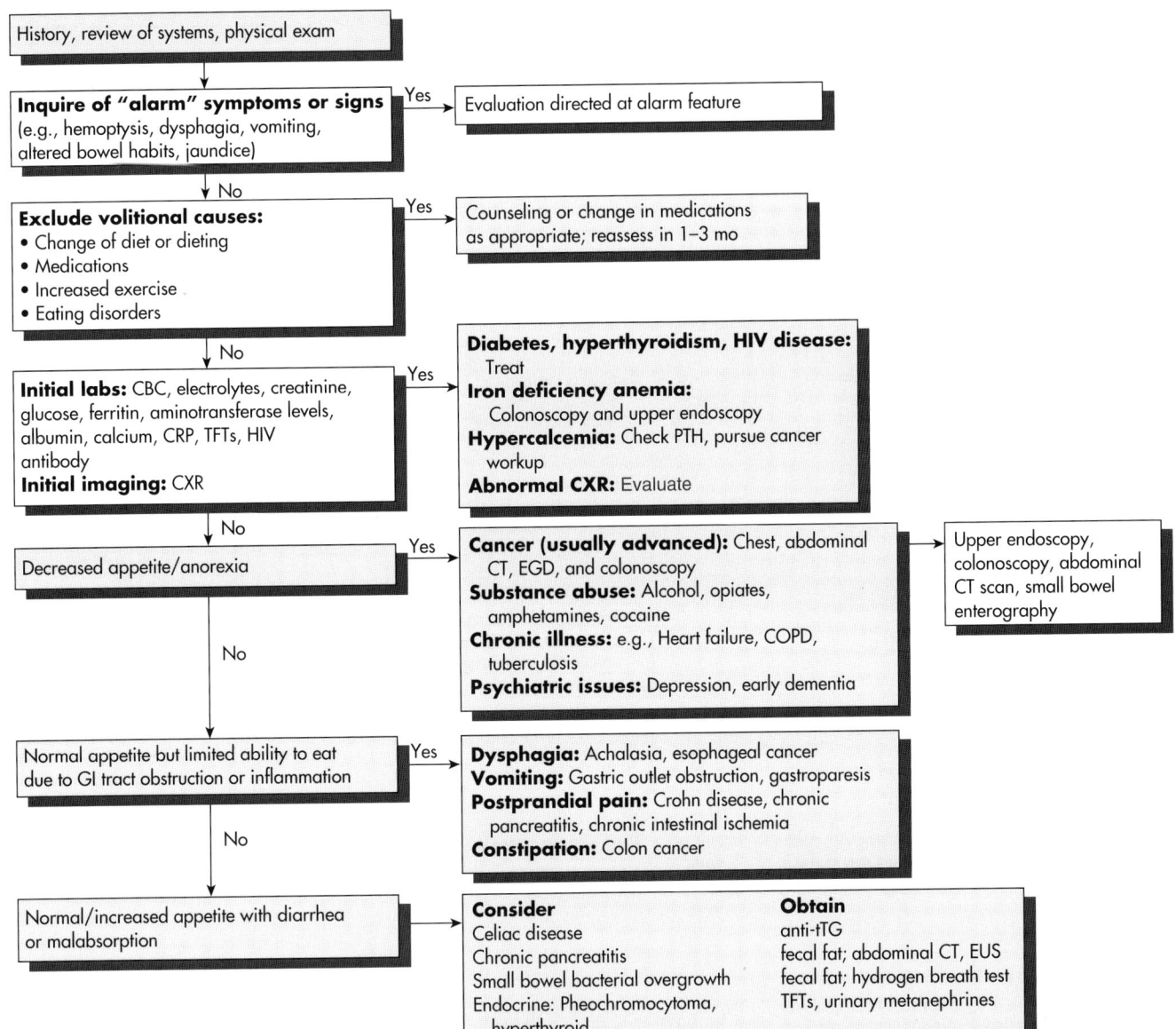

FIG. 206 Approach to the patient with unintentional weight loss of more than 5%. *CBC*, Complete blood count; *COPD*, chronic obstructive pulmonary disease; *CRP*, C-reactive protein; *CT*, computed tomography; *CXR*, chest radiograph; *EGD*, esophagogastroduodenoscopy; *EUS*, endoscopic ultrasound; *GI*, gastrointestinal; *HIV*, human immunodeficiency virus; *PTH*, parathyroid hormone; *TFTs*, thyroid function tests; *tTG*, tissue transglutaminase. (From Goldman L, Schafer AI: *Goldman Cecil medicine*, ed 25, Philadelphia, 2016, Saunders.)

WEIGHT LOSS, UNINTENTIONAL—cont'd

TABLE 110   Causes of Involuntary Weight Loss

Condition	Quality	Duration	Aggravating or Relieving Factors	Associated Symptoms or Signs	Diagnostic Studies
Weight Loss Secondary to Gastrointestinal Causes					
GI, pancreatic, or hepatobiliary malignant disease	Progressive, fast	Months	Better with cancer therapy (e.g., surgery, XRT, chemotherapy)	Dysphagia (esophageal); anorexia, nausea, vomiting (gastric, small or large bowel obstruction); visible or occult blood in stool; altered bowel habits; jaundice or hepatomegaly (biliary obstruction, hepatic tumor, metastatic disease); iron deficiency anemia	CBC, FOBT, ferritin, CEA, CA19-9, AFP, EGD, colonoscopy, abdominal CT, PET
Malabsorption (poor absorption of nutrients due to pancreatic insufficiency, small intestinal mucosal disorders, or bacterial overgrowth)	Progressive, slow	Months to years	Diarrhea or steatorrhea, excessive flatulence; worse with eating and resolves with NPO status	Usually associated with increased appetite; may have anemia (iron, B_{12}, folate), osteoporosis, or osteomalacia (vitamin D, calcium, phosphorus); easy bruising (vitamin K), night blindness (vitamin A)	72-h stool for fecal fat; fecal elastase; vitamins A and D and INR; calcium, ferritin, B_{12}, albumin; celiac disease antibodies (e.g., anti-tTG, antiendomysial antibodies); EGD with small bowel biopsy; breath test for bacterial overgrowth
Inflammatory bowel disease (especially Crohn disease)	Progressive, slow	Months	Eating causes pain, cramps, increased diarrhea and urgency; improved by low-residue diet or NPO status	Bloody stools, abdominal cramps and pain, perianal disease, extraintestinal manifestations (e.g., oral ulcers, uveitis, erythema nodosum, arthralgias)	CBC, albumin, ESR, CRP, colonoscopy with biopsies, CT or MR enterography, wireless capsule study
GI motility disorders	Intermittent, slow	Years	Worse with eating	Nausea, vomiting, distention, diarrhea, or constipation may be present	EGD and colonoscopy, gastric emptying study, CT or MR enterography, surgical full-thickness intestinal biopsies
Cirrhosis	Muscle wasting with edema, so weight may increase	Months to years	Worse with salt or fluid intake	Ascites, peripheral edema	Liver biopsy
Chronic intestinal ischemia	Progressive	Months to years	Worse with eating	Afraid to eat; postprandial abdominal pain, nausea; associated atherosclerotic disease	CT or MR angiography
Weight Loss Secondary to Nongastrointestinal Causes					
Poor or inadequate calorie intake due to social factors	Intermittent or progressive, acute (hospitalized) or chronic	Days to months to years	Common in elderly, teenagers; exacerbated by poor dentition or poorly fitting dentures	Will eat if food is made available	Review dietary log and how food is obtained and prepared
Medications	Intermittent or progressive	Months	Worse with medication; resolves with discontinuation of offending drug	Anorexia, nausea, vomiting	Review drug profile
Non-GI malignant disease	Progressive	Months	Better with cancer therapy (e.g., surgery, XRT, chemotherapy)	Anorexia, nausea, vomiting; pain; metastatic disease	Calcium, cortisol; CT for underlying disease, PET
Endocrine disorders: DM, hyperthyroidism, adrenal insufficiency	DM—appetite increased or decreased, early satiety; hyperthyroidism—increased appetite	Months to years	Worse with disease chronicity	DM: Gastroparesis, neuropathy, retinopathy, nephropathy; Adrenal insufficiency: Nausea, vomiting, diarrhea, abdominal pain	Serum glucose, TFT, cortisol
Chronic infections, including HIV and TB	Progressive, fast	Months	Better with directed therapy, megestrol acetate (Megace)	Nausea, anorexia, other infections	HIV test, PPD, cultures, biopsies if necessary
Systemic inflammatory disorders	Progressive, moderate	Months to years	Better with directed therapy, megestrol acetate (Megace)	Arthritis, rash, vasculitis	ANA, RF, ESR, CRP

Table 110 Causes of Involuntary Weight Loss—cont'd

Condition	Quality	Duration	Aggravating or Relieving Factors	Associated Symptoms or Signs	Diagnostic Studies
Chronic renal failure	Progressive, slow; edema may increase weight	Months to years	Better with dialysis, megestrol acetate (Megace)	Nausea, anorexia, weight gain	BUN, Cr, 24-h creatinine clearance
Advanced COPD or heart failure	Progressive, slow	Months to years	Better with oxygen and specific treatment	Fatigue, dyspnea, edema, wasting	Pulmonary function testing or two-dimensional echocardiography
Psychiatric illness: Depression, manic-depressive illness	Progressive, slow	Months to years	Depression common in elderly; flat affect; manic phase associated with hyperactivity and decreased intake	Psychologic testing	
Psychogenic eating disorders—anorexia nervosa, bulimia	Intermittent or progressive	Months to years	Worse with stressors	Refusal to eat, loss of tooth enamel, calluses and healing ulcerations of hand	Psychiatric testing
Substance abuse (alcohol, opiates, CNS stimulants)	Intermittent or progressive	Months	Resolves with discontinuation	Anorexia, nausea, vomiting	Careful interview; patients may deny or minimize

AFP, α-Fetoprotein; *ANA,* antinuclear antibody; *BUN,* blood urea nitrogen; *CBC,* complete blood count; *CEA,* carcinoembryonic antigen; *CNS,* central nervous system; *COPD,* chronic obstructive pulmonary disease; *Cr,* creatinine; *CRP,* C-reactive protein; *CT,* computed tomography; *DM,* diabetes mellitus; *EGD,* esophagogastroduodenoscopy; *ESR,* erythrocyte sedimentation rate; *FOBT,* fecal occult blood test; *GI,* gastrointestinal; *HIV,* human immunodeficiency virus; *INR,* international normalized ratio; *MR,* magnetic resonance; *NPO,* nothing orally; *PET,* positron emission tomography; *PPD,* purified protein derivative; *RF,* rheumatoid factor; *TB,* tuberculosis; *TFT,* thyroid function test; *tTG,* tissue transglutaminase; *XRT,* x-ray therapy.
From Goldman L, Shafer AI: *Goldman-Cecil medicine,* ed 26, Philadelphia, 2020, Elsevier.

SECTION IV

Laboratory Tests and Interpretation of Results

This section contains over 300 commonly performed laboratory tests. In general, the tests are discussed in the following format:

1. Laboratory test.
2. Normal range in adult patients. Normal values are given using the present (traditional) reference interval, followed by the Système Internationale (SI) reference interval, the conversion factor (CF), and the suggested minimum increment (SMI).
3. Common abnormalities, such as a positive test or increased or decreased value.
4. Causes of abnormal result.
5. The normal ranges may differ slightly, depending on the laboratory. The reader should be aware of the "normal range" of the particular laboratory performing the test. Every attempt has been made to present current laboratory test data, with an emphasis on practical considerations.

ACE LEVEL
See "ANGIOTENSIN-CONVERTING ENZYME"

ACETONE (serum or plasma)
Normal: Negative
Elevated in: Diabetic ketoacidosis (DKA), starvation, isopropanol ingestion

ACETYLCHOLINE RECEPTOR (AChR) ANTIBODY
Normal: <0.03 nmol/L
Elevated in: Myasthenia gravis. Changes in AChR concentration correlate with the clinical severity of myasthenia gravis after therapy and during therapy with prednisone and immunosuppressants. False-positive AChR antibody results may be found in patients with Eaton-Lambert syndrome.

ACID-BASE REFERENCE VALUES
See Tables 1, 2, and 3. Fig. 1 illustrates the relationship between bicarbonate and pCO_2 in a variety of clinical disorders.

ACID PHOSPHATASE (serum)
Normal range: 0 to 5.5 U/L (0 to 90 nkat/L [CF: 16.67; SMI: 2 nkat/L])
Elevated in: Carcinoma of the prostate, other neoplasms (breast, bone), Paget disease, osteogenesis imperfecta, malignant invasion of bone, Gaucher disease, multiple myeloma, myeloproliferative disorders, benign prostatic hypertrophy, prostatic palpation or surgery, hyperparathyroidism, liver disease, chronic renal failure, idiopathic thrombocytopenic purpura, bronchitis

ACID SERUM TEST
See "HAM TEST"

ACTIVATED CLOTTING TIME (ACT)
Normal: This test is used to determine the dose of protamine sulfate to reverse the effect of heparin as an anticoagulant during angioplasty, cardiac surgery, and hemodialysis. The accepted goal during cardiopulmonary bypass surgery is usually 400-500 sec.

ACTIVATED PARTIAL THROMBOPLASTIN TIME (APTT, aPTT)
See "PARTIAL THROMBOPLASTIN TIME"

ADRENOCORTICOTROPIC HORMONE (ACTH)
Normal: 9 to 52 pg/ml. Table E4 describes patterns of serum levels of ACTH and cortisol in different adrenal gland disorders.
Elevated in: Addison disease, ectopic ACTH-producing tumors, congenital adrenal hyperplasia, Nelson syndrome, pituitary-dependent Cushing disease
Decreased in: Secondary adrenocortical insufficiency, hypopituitarism, adrenal adenoma or adrenal carcinoma

ALANINE AMINOPEPTIDASE
Normal:
Male: 1.11 to 1.71 mcg/ml
Female: 0.96 to 1.52 mcg/ml
Elevated in: Liver or pancreatic disease, ethanol use, oral contraceptive use, malignancy, tobacco use, pregnancy
Decreased in: Abortion

ALANINE AMINOTRANSFERASE (ALT, SGPT)
See Fig. E2 for an algorithm for the evaluation of elevated ALT. Table E5 describes patterns of liver function tests in liver disorders.
Normal range: 0 to 35 U/L (0.058 μkat/L [CF: 0.02 μkat/L])
Elevated in: Liver disease (hepatitis, cirrhosis, Reye syndrome), hepatic congestion, infectious mononucleosis, myocardial infarction, myocarditis, severe muscle trauma, dermatomyositis/polymyositis, muscular dystrophy, drugs (antibiotics, narcotics, antihypertensive agents, heparin, labetalol, statins, NSAIDs, amiodarone, chlorpromazine, phenytoin), malignancy, renal and pulmonary infarction, seizures, eclampsia, shock liver

TABLE 1 Commonly Used Acid-Base Reference Values for Arterial and Venous Plasma or Serum (Averaged From Various Sources)

	ARTERIAL		VENOUS	
	Conventional Units	SI Units*	Conventional Units	SI Units*
pH	7.40 (7.35-7.45)	7.40 (7.35-7.45)	7.37 (7.32-7.42)	7.37 (7.32-7.42)
Pco_2	40 mm Hg (35-45)	5.33 kPa (4.67-6.10)	45 mm Hg (45-50)	6.10 kPa (5.33-6.67)
Po_2	80-100 mm Hg	10.66-13.33 kPa	40 mm Hg (37-43)	5.33 kPa (4.93-5.73)
HCO_3- (CO_2 combining power)	24 mEq/L (20-28)	24 mmol/L (20-28)	26 mEq/L (22-30)	26 mmol/L (22-30)
CO_2 content	25 mEq/L (22-28)	25 mmol/L (22-28)	27 mEq/L (24-30)	27 mmol/L (24-30)

*International system.
From Ravel R: *Clinical laboratory medicine*, ed 6, St Louis, 1995, Mosby.

TABLE 2 Summary of Laboratory Findings in Primary Uncomplicated Respiratory and Metabolic Acid-Base Disorders*

Disorder	Pco_2	pH	Base Excess
Acute primary respiratory hypoactivity (respiratory acidosis)	Increase	Decrease	Normal/positive
Acute primary respiratory hyperactivity (respiratory alkalosis)	Decrease	Increase	Normal/negative
Uncompensated metabolic acidosis	Normal	Decrease	Negative
Uncompensated metabolic alkalosis	Normal	Increase	Positive
Partially compensated metabolic acidosis	Decrease	Decrease	Negative
Partially compensated metabolic alkalosis	Increase	Increase	Positive
Chronic primary respiratory hypoactivity (compensated respiratory acidosis)	Increase	Normal	Positive
Fully compensated metabolic alkalosis	Increase	Normal	Positive
Chronic primary respiratory hyperactivity (compensated respiratory alkalosis)	Decrease	Normal	Negative
Fully compensated metabolic acidosis	Decrease	Normal	Negative

*Base excess results refer to negative (−) values more than 22 and positive (+) values more than 12.
From Vincent JL et al: *Textbook of critical care*, ed 7, Philadelphia, 2017, Elsevier. Adapted and updated from Bidani A, Tauzon DM, Heming TA: Regulation of whole body acid-base balance. In DuBose TD, Hamm LL (eds): *Acid base and electrolytes disorders: a companion to Brenner and Rector's the kidney*, Philadelphia, 2002, Saunders, p. 1-21.

TABLE 3 Acid-Base Abnormalities and Appropriate Compensatory Responses for Simple Disorders

Primary Acid-Base Disorders	Primary Defect	Effect on pH	Compensatory Response	Expected Range of Compensation	Limits of Compensation
Respiratory acidosis	Alveolar hypoventilation ($\uparrow$ P_{CO_2})	$\downarrow$	$\uparrow$ Renal HCO_3- reabsorption ($HCO_3-\uparrow$)	Acute: $\Delta[HCO_3-] = +1$ mEq/L for each $\uparrow\Delta P_{CO_2}$ of 10 mm Hg	$[HCO_3-] = 38$ mEq/L
				Chronic: $\Delta[HCO_3-] = +4$ mEq/L for each $\uparrow\Delta P_{CO_2}$ of 10 mm Hg	$[HCO_3-] = 45$ mEq/L
Respiratory alkalosis	Alveolar hyperventilation ($\downarrow$ P_{CO_2})	$\uparrow$	$\downarrow$ Renal HCO_3- reabsorption ($HCO_3-\downarrow$)	Acute: $\Delta[HCO_3-] = -2$ mEq/L for each $\downarrow\Delta P_{CO_2}$ of 10 mm Hg	$[HCO_3-] = 18$ mEq/L
				Chronic: $\Delta[HCO_3-] = -5$ mEq/L for each $\downarrow\Delta P_{CO_2}$ of 10 mm Hg	$[HCO_3-] = 15$ mEq/L
Metabolic acidosis	Loss of HCO_3- or gain of H^+ ($\downarrow$ HCO_3-)	$\downarrow$	Alveolar hyperventilation to $\uparrow$ pulmonary CO_2 excretion ($\downarrow$ P_{CO_2})	$P_{CO_2} = 1.5[HCO_3-] + 8 \pm 2$ $P_{CO_2} =$ last 2 digits of pH $\times$ 100 $P_{CO_2} = 15 + [HCO_3-]$	$P_{CO_2} = 15$ mm Hg
Metabolic alkalosis	Gain of HCO_3- or loss of H^+ ($\uparrow$ HCO_3-)	$\uparrow$	Alveolar hypoventilation to $\downarrow$ pulmonary CO_2 excretion ($\uparrow$ P_{CO_2})	$P_{CO_2} = +0.6$ mm Hg for $\Delta[HCO_3-]$ of 1 mEq/L. $P_{CO_2} = 15 + [HCO_3-]$	$P_{CO_2} = 55$ mm Hg

From Vincent JL et al: *Textbook of critical care,* ed 7, Philadelphia, 2017, Elsevier. Adapted and updated from Bidani A, Tauzon DM, Heming TA: Regulation of whole body acid-base balance. In DuBose TD, Hamm LL (eds): *Acid base and electrolytes disorders: a companion to Brenner and Rector's the kidney,* Philadelphia, 2002, Saunders, p. 1-21.

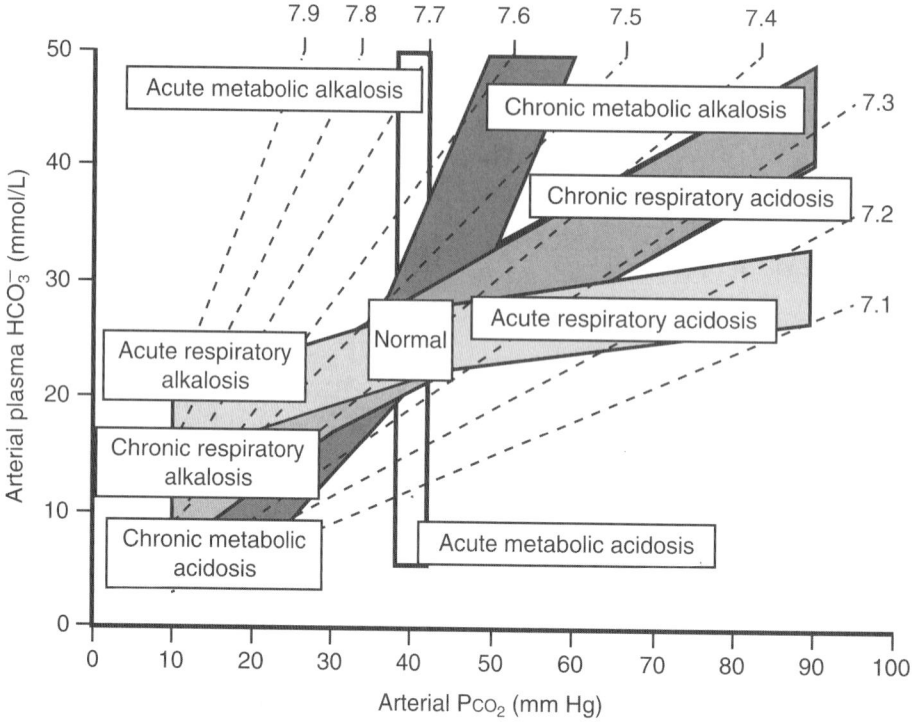

FIG. 1 The relation between bicarbonate ($HCO-^3$) and pCO_2 in a variety of clinical disorders. The 95% confidence levels for acute and chronic respiratory and metabolic abnormalities are denoted by the colored boxes. The vertical transparent bar indicates the absence of any change in arterial pCO_2 with acute changes in $HCO-^3$. However, the respiratory response to the onset of metabolic acidosis and alkalosis is rapid, and the metabolic band rotates clockwise toward the chronic metabolic position within a matter of minutes to hours. Compensatory metabolic responses to respiratory changes in arterial pCO_2 are much slower, making it easier to observe the acute respiratory bands before metabolic compensation. (From Broaddus VC et al: *Murray & Nadel's textbook of respiratory medicine,* ed 7, Philadelphia, 2022, Elsevier.)

ALBUMIN (serum)

Normal range: 4 to 6 g/dl (40 to 60 g/L [CF:10; SMI: 1 g/L])
Elevated in: Dehydration (relative increase)
Decreased in: Liver disease, nephrotic syndrome, poor nutritional status, rapid intravenous (IV) hydration, protein-losing enteropathies (e.g., inflammatory bowel disease), severe burns, neoplasia, chronic inflammatory diseases, pregnancy, oral contraceptives, prolonged immobilization, lymphomas, hypervitaminosis A, chronic glomerulonephritis

ALCOHOL DEHYDROGENASE

Normal: 0 to 7 U/L
Elevated in: Drug-induced hepatocellular damage, obstructive jaundice, malignancy, inflammation, infection

ALDOLASE (serum)

Normal range: 0 to 6 U/L (0 to 100 nkat/L [CF: 16.67; SMI: 20 nkat/L])

Elevated in: Muscular dystrophy, rhabdomyolysis, dermatomyositis/polymyositis, trichinosis, acute hepatitis and other liver diseases, myocardial infarction, prostatic carcinoma, hemorrhagic pancreatitis, gangrene, delirium tremens, burns

Decreased in: Loss of muscle mass, late stages of muscular dystrophy

ALDOSTERONE

Normal range:
Recumbent: 50 to 150 ng/L
Upright: 150 to 300 ng/L
(Highest levels in neonates, decreasing over time to adult levels.) The normal renin-angiotensin-aldosterone axis is illustrated in Fig. E3.

Elevated in: Primary aldosteronism, secondary aldosteronism, pseudoprimary aldosteronism. Table E6 differentiates the various causes of hyperaldosteronism.

Decreased in: Patients with hypertension: Diabetes mellitus; Turner syndrome; acute alcohol intoxication; excess secretion of deoxycorticosterone, corticosterone, and 18-hydroxycorticosterone

Patients without hypertension: Addison disease, hypoaldosteronism resulting from renin deficiency, isolated aldosterone deficiency. Table E7 differentiates the various causes of hypoaldosteronism.

ALKALINE PHOSPHATASE (ALP) (serum)

See Fig. E4 for investigating a raised ALP in general practice.
See Fig. E5 for an approach to elevated ALP.

Normal range: 30 to 120 U/L (0.5 to 2 μkat/L [CF:0.01667; SMI: 0.1 μkat/L])

Elevated in: LIVER AND BILIARY TRACT ORIGIN
Extrahepatic bile duct obstruction
Intrahepatic biliary obstruction
Liver cell acute injury
Liver passive congestion
Drug-induced liver cell dysfunction
Space-occupying lesions
Primary biliary cirrhosis
Sepsis
BONE ORIGIN (OSTEOBLAST HYPERACTIVITY)
Physiologic (rapid) bone growth (childhood and adolescence)
Metastatic tumor with osteoblastic reaction
Fracture healing
Paget disease of bone
CAPILLARY ENDOTHELIAL ORIGIN
Granulation tissue formation (active)
PLACENTAL ORIGIN
Pregnancy
Some parenteral albumin preparations
OTHER
Thyrotoxicosis
Benign transient hyperphosphatasemia
Primary hyperparathyroidism

Decreased in: Hypothyroidism, pernicious anemia, hypophosphatemia, hypervitaminosis D, malnutrition

ALPHA-1-ANTITRYPSIN (serum)

Normal range: 110 to 140 mg/dl
Decreased in: Homozygous or heterozygous deficiency

ALPHA-1-FETOPROTEIN (serum)

See "α-1 FETOPROTEIN"

ALT

See "ALANINE AMINOTRANSFERASE"

ALUMINUM (serum)

Normal range: 0 to 6 ng/ml
Elevated in: Chronic renal failure on dialysis, parenteral nutrition, industrial exposure

AMA

See "ANTIMITOCHONDRIAL ANTIBODY"

AMEBIASIS SEROLOGIC TEST

Test description: Test is used to support the diagnosis of amebiasis caused by *Entamoeba histolytica*. Serum acute and convalescent titers are drawn 1 to 3 wk apart. A fourfold increase in titer is the most indicative result.

AMINOLEVULINIC ACID (δ-ALA) (24-h urine collection)

Normal: 1.5 to 7.5 mg/day
Elevated in: Acute porphyrias, lead poisoning, DKA, pregnancy, anticonvulsant drugs, hereditary tyrosinemia
Decreased in: Alcoholic liver disease

AMMONIA (serum)

See Box E1 for the differential diagnosis of hyperammonemia.
See Fig. E6 for an approach to hyperammonemia in pediatric patients.

Normal range: 10 to 80 μg/dl (5 to 50 μmol/L [CF: 0.5872; SMI: 5 μmol/L])
Elevated in: Hepatic failure, hepatic encephalopathy, Reye syndrome, portacaval shunt, drugs (diuretics, polymyxin B, methicillin)
Decreased in: Drugs (neomycin, lactulose, tetracycline), renal failure

AMYLASE (serum)

Normal range: 0 to 130 U/L (0 to 2.17 μkat/L [CF: 0.01667; SMI: 0.01 μkat/L])
Elevated in: Acute pancreatitis, pancreatic neoplasm, abscess, pseudocyst, ascites, macroamylasemia, perforated peptic ulcer, intestinal obstruction, intestinal infarction, acute cholecystitis, appendicitis, ruptured ectopic pregnancy, salivary gland inflammation, peritonitis, burns, diabetic ketoacidosis, renal insufficiency, drugs (morphine), carcinomatosis (of lung, esophagus, ovary), acute ethanol ingestion, mumps, prostate tumors, postendoscopic retrograde cholangiopancreatography, bulimia, anorexia nervosa (Table E8)
Decreased in: Advanced chronic pancreatitis, hepatic necrosis, cystic fibrosis

AMYLASE, URINE

See "URINE AMYLASE"

AMYLOID A PROTEIN (serum)

Normal: <10 mcg/ml
Elevated in: Inflammatory disorders (acute phase-reacting protein), infections, acute coronary syndrome, malignancies

ANA

See "ANTINUCLEAR ANTIBODY"

ANCA

See "ANTINEUTROPHIL CYTOPLASMIC ANTIBODY"

ANDROSTENEDIONE (serum)

Normal:
Male: 75 to 205 ng/dl
Female: 85 to 275 ng/dl
Elevated in: Congenital adrenal hyperplasia, polycystic ovary syndrome, ectopic ACTH-producing tumor, Cushing syndrome, hirsutism, hyperplasia of ovarian stroma, ovarian neoplasm
Decreased in: Ovarian failure, adrenal failure, sickle cell anemia

ANGIOTENSIN II

Normal: 10 to 60 pg/ml
Elevated in: Hypertension, congestive heart failure (CHF), cirrhosis, renin-secreting renal tumor, volume depletion
Decreased in: ACE inhibitor drugs, angiotensin-converting enzyme inhibitor (ARB) drugs, primary aldosteronism, Cushing syndrome

ANGIOTENSIN-CONVERTING ENZYME (ACE level)

Normal range: <40 nmol/ml/min (<670 nkat/L [CF: 16.67; SMI: 10 nkat/L])
Elevated in: Sarcoidosis, primary biliary cirrhosis, alcoholic liver disease, hyperthyroidism, hyperparathyroidism, diabetes mellitus, amyloidosis, multiple myeloma, lung disease (asbestosis, silicosis, berylliosis, allergic alveolitis, coccidioidomycosis), Gaucher disease, leprosy

ANH

See "ATRIAL NATRIURETIC HORMONE"

ANION GAP (AG)

The AG is the net change difference between the cations Na^+, K^+, and the anions Cl^- and HCO_3^-.
    See Fig. E7 for charge balance in blood plasma.
    See Tables E9, E10, E11.

Normal range: 9 to 14 mEq/L
Elevated in: Lactic acidosis, ketoacidosis (diabetes, alcoholic starvation), uremia (chronic renal failure), ingestion of toxins (paraldehyde, methanol, salicylates, ethylene glycol), hyperosmolar nonketotic coma, antibiotics (carbenicillin)
Decreased in: Hypoalbuminemia, severe hypermagnesemia, IgG myeloma, lithium toxicity, laboratory error (falsely decreased sodium or overestimation of bicarbonate or chloride), hypercalcemia of parathyroid origin, antibiotics (e.g., polymyxin)

ANTICARDIOLIPIN ANTIBODY (ACA)

Normal range: Negative. Test includes detection of IgG, IgM, and IgA antibodies to phospholipid, cardiolipin
Present in: Antiphospholipid antibody syndrome, chronic hepatitis C

ANTICOAGULANT

See "CIRCULATING ANTICOAGULANT"

ANTIDIURETIC HORMONE

Normal range: mOsm/kg 295 to 300 (4 to 12 pg/ml)
Elevated in: SIADH, antipsychotic medications, ectopic ADH from systemic neoplasm, Guillain-Barré syndrome, central nervous system (CNS) infections, brain tumors, nephrogenic diabetes insipidus
Decreased in: Central diabetes insipidus, nephritic syndrome, psychogenic polydipsias, demeclocycline, lithium, phenytoin, alcohol. Table E12 describes the water deprivation test used for diagnosing and classifying diabetes insipidus. Table E13 summarizes tests in the differential diagnosis of water homeostasis. Causes of polyuria due to water diuresis are described in Box E2.

ANTI-DNA

Normal range: Absent
Present in: Systemic lupus erythematosus, chronic active hepatitis, infectious mononucleosis, biliary cirrhosis

ANTI-DS DNA

Normal: <25 U
Elevated in: Systemic lupus erythematosus

ANTIGLOBULIN TEST

See "DIRECT ANTIGLOBULIN (COOMBS DIRECT)"
    See "INDIRECT ANTIGLOBULIN (COOMBS INDIRECT)"

ANTIGLOMERULAR BASEMENT ANTIBODY

See "GLOMERULAR BASEMENT MEMBRANE ANTIBODY"

ANTIHISTONE

Normal: <1 U
Elevated in: Drug-induced lupus erythematosus

ANTIMITOCHONDRIAL ANTIBODY (AMA, Mitochondrial antibody)

Normal range: <1:20 titer
Elevated in: Primary biliary cirrhosis (85% to 95%), chronic active hepatitis (25% to 30%), cryptogenic cirrhosis (25% to 30%)

ANTINEUTROPHIL CYTOPLASMIC ANTIBODY (ANCA)

Positive test: Cytoplasmic pattern (c-ANCA): Positive in granulomatosis with polyangiitis (see Fig. E8 and Table E14 for approach to patient with positive c-ANCA)

Perinuclear pattern (p-ANCA): Positive in inflammatory bowel disease, primary biliary cirrhosis, primary sclerosing cholangitis, autoimmune chronic active hepatitis, crescentic glomerulonephritis (see Table E14 for approach to patient with positive p-ANCA)

ANTINUCLEAR ANTIBODY (ANA)

Fig. E9 describes an algorithm for the use of antinuclear antibodies in the diagnosis of connective tissue disorders. See Fig. E10 for approach to positive ANA pattern. Table E15 shows the frequency of antinuclear antibodies in autoimmune and nonrheumatic diseases.

Normal range: <1:20 titer
Positive test: Systemic lupus erythematosus (more significant if titer >1:160), drugs (phenytoin, ethosuximide, primidone, methyldopa, hydralazine, carbamazepine, penicillin, procainamide, chlorpromazine, griseofulvin, thiazides), chronic active hepatitis, autoimmune thyroid disease (positive ANA is found in up to 45% of patients), idiopathic thrombocytopenic purpura, multiple sclerosis, rheumatoid arthritis, scleroderma, mixed connective tissue disease, necrotizing vasculitis, Sjögren syndrome, tuberculosis, pulmonary interstitial fibrosis. Positive ANA results are nonspecific and can be found in healthy individuals (13.8% of the adult general population). Table E16 describes diseases associated with ANA subtypes. Fig. 11 illustrates various fluorescent ANA test patterns.

ANTI-RNP ANTIBODY

See "EXTRACTABLE NUCLEAR ANTIGEN"

ANTI-SCL-70

Normal: Absent
Elevated in: Scleroderma

ANTI-SM (anti-Smith) **ANTIBODY**

See "EXTRACTABLE NUCLEAR ANTIGEN"

ANTI-SMOOTH MUSCLE ANTIBODY

See "SMOOTH MUSCLE ANTIBODY"

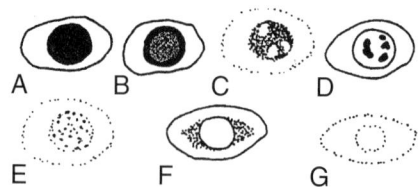

FIG. 11 Fluorescent antinuclear antibody test patterns (HEP-2 cells). A, Solid (homogeneous). **B,** Peripheral (rim). **C,** Speckled. **D,** Nucleolar. **E,** Anticentromere. **F,** Antimitochondrial. **G,** Normal (nonreactive).

ANTISTREPTOLYSIN O TITER (Streptozyme, ASLO titer)

Normal range for adults: <160 Todd units
Elevated in: Streptococcal upper airway infection, acute rheumatic fever, acute glomerulonephritis, increased levels of β-lipoprotein

NOTE: A fourfold increase in titer between acute and convalescent specimens is diagnostic of streptococcal upper airway infection regardless of the initial titer.

ANTITHROMBIN III

See Table E17.

Normal range: 81% to 120% of normal activity; 17 to 30 mg/dl
Decreased in: Hereditary deficiency of antithrombin III, disseminated intravascular coagulation, pulmonary embolism, cirrhosis, thrombolytic therapy, chronic liver failure, postsurgery, third trimester of pregnancy, oral contraceptives, nephrotic syndrome, IV heparin >3 days, sepsis, acute leukemia, carcinoma, thrombophlebitis
Elevated in: Warfarin drugs, postmyocardial infarction

APOLIPOPROTEIN A-1 (Apo A-1)

Normal: Desirable >120 mg/dl
Elevated in: Familial hyperalphalipoproteinemia, statins, niacin, estrogens, weight loss, familial cholesteryl ester transfer protein (CETP) deficiency
Decreased in: Familial hypoalphalipoproteinemia, Tangier disease, diuretics, androgens, cigarette smoking, hepatocellular disorders, chronic renal failure, nephritic syndrome, coronary heart disease, cholestasis

APOLIPOPROTEIN B (Apo B)

Normal: Desirable <100 mg/dl; high risk >120 mg/dl
Elevated in: High saturated fat diet, high-cholesterol diet, hyperapobetalipoproteinemia, familial combined hyperlipidemia, anabolic steroids, diuretics, β-blockers, corticosteroids, progestins, diabetes, hypothyroidism, chronic renal failure, liver disease, Cushing syndrome, coronary heart disease
Decreased in: Statins, niacin, low-cholesterol diet, malnutrition, abetalipoproteinemia, hypobetalipoproteinemia, hyperthyroidism

ARTERIAL BLOOD GASES

Normal range:
P_{O_2}: 75 to 100 mm Hg
P_{CO_2}: 35 to 45 mm Hg
HCO_3^-: 24 to 28 mEq/L
pH: 7.35 to 7.45
Abnormal values: Acid-base disturbances (see the following)
METABOLIC ACIDOSIS
Causes of metabolic acidosis by net acid excretion are summarized in Box E3.
Metabolic acidosis with increased AG (AG acidosis)
Lactic acidosis (see Box E4)
Ketoacidosis (diabetes mellitus, alcoholic ketoacidosis)
Uremia (chronic renal failure)
Ingestion of toxins (paraldehyde, methanol, salicylate, ethylene glycol)
High-fat diet (mild acidosis)

EXTRARENAL ACIDOSIS: INCREASE IN NET ACID EXCRETION

Gastrointestinal loss of bicarbonate
Ingestion of acids or acid precursors: Ammonium chloride, sulfur-containing compounds
Acid precursors or toxins: Salicylate, ethylene glycol, methanol, toluene, acetaminophen, paraldehyde
Organic acidosis:
- L-lactic acidosis
- D-lactic acidosis
- Ketoacidosis
- Pyroglutamic acidosis
Metabolic acidosis with normal AG (hyperchloremic acidosis)
Renal tubular acidosis (including acidosis of aldosterone deficiency)
Intestinal loss of HCO_3^- (diarrhea, pancreatic fistula)

Carbonic anhydrase inhibitors (e.g., acetazolamide)
Dilutional acidosis (as a result of rapid infusion of bicarbonate-free isotonic saline)
Ingestion of exogenous acids (ammonium chloride, methionine, cystine, calcium chloride)
Ileostomy
Ureterosigmoidostomy
Drugs: Amiloride, triamterene, spironolactone, β-blockers
RESPIRATORY ACIDOSIS
Pulmonary disease (chronic obstructive pulmonary disease [COPD], severe pneumonia, pulmonary edema, interstitial fibrosis)
Airway obstruction (foreign body, severe bronchospasm, laryngospasm)
Thoracic cage disorders (pneumothorax, flail chest, kyphoscoliosis)
Defects in muscles of respiration (myasthenia gravis, hypokalemia, muscular dystrophy)
Defects in peripheral nervous system (amyotrophic lateral sclerosis, poliomyelitis, Guillain-Barré syndrome, botulism, tetanus, organophosphate poisoning, spinal cord injury)
Depression of respiratory center (anesthesia, narcotics, sedatives, vertebral artery embolism or thrombosis, increased intracranial pressure)
Failure of mechanical ventilator
METABOLIC ALKALOSIS
Divided into chloride-responsive (urinary chloride <15 mEq/L) and chloride-resistant forms (urinary chloride level >15 mEq/L)
CHLORIDE-RESPONSIVE

Vomiting
Nasogastric (NG) suction
Diuretics
Posthypercapnic alkalosis
Stool losses (laxative abuse, cystic fibrosis, villous adenoma)
Massive blood transfusion
Exogenous alkali administration
CHLORIDE-RESISTANT

Hyperadrenocorticoid states (Cushing syndrome, primary hyperaldosteronism, secondary mineralocorticoidism [licorice, chewing tobacco])
Hypomagnesemia
Hypokalemia
Bartter syndrome
RESPIRATORY ALKALOSIS
Hypoxemia (pneumonia, pulmonary embolism, atelectasis, high-altitude living)
Drugs (salicylates, xanthines, progesterone, epinephrine, thyroxine, nicotine)
CNS disorders (tumor, cerebrovascular accident [CVA], trauma, infections)
Psychogenic hyperventilation (anxiety, hysteria)
Hepatic encephalopathy
Gram-negative sepsis
Hyponatremia
Sudden recovery from metabolic acidosis
Assisted ventilation

ARTHROCENTESIS FLUID

Reference intervals for synovial fluid constituents are described in Table 18. Also see Fig. E12.
Interpretation of results:
1. **Color:** Normally it is clear or pale yellow; cloudiness indicates inflammatory process or presence of crystals, cell debris, fibrin, or triglycerides.
2. **Viscosity:** Normally it has a high viscosity because of hyaluronate; when fluid is placed on a slide, it can be stretched to a string >2 cm in length before separating (low viscosity indicates breakdown of hyaluronate [lysosomal enzymes from leukocytes] or the presence of edema fluid).
3. **Mucin clot:** Add 1 ml of fluid to 5 ml of a 5% acetic acid solution and allow 1 min for the clot to form; a firm clot (does not fragment on shaking) is normal and indicates the presence of large molecules of hyaluronic acid (this test is nonspecific and infrequently done).

TABLE 18 Reference Intervals for Synovial Fluid Constituents

Constituent	Synovial Fluid	Plasma
Total protein	1-3 g/dl	6-8 g/dl
Albumin	55%-70%	50%-65%
α1-Globulin	6%-8%	3%-5%
α2-Globulin	5%-7%	7%-13%
β-Globulin	8%-10%	8%-14%
γ-Globulin	10%-14%	12%-22%
Hyaluronic acid	0.3-0.4 g/dl	
Glucose	70-110 mg/dl	70-110 mg/dl
Uric acid	2-8 mg/dl	2-8 mg/dl
Lactate	9-29 mg/dl	9-29 mg/dl

From McPherson RA, Pincus MR (eds): *Henry's clinical diagnosis and management by laboratory methods,* ed 23, Philadelphia, 2017, Elsevier.

4. **Glucose:** Normally it approximately equals serum glucose level; a difference of more than 40 mg/dl is suggestive of infection.
5. **Protein:** Total protein concentration is <2.5 g/dl in the normal synovial fluid; it is elevated in inflammatory and septic arthritis.
6. Microscopic examination for crystals.
   a. **Gout:** Monosodium urate crystals
   b. **Pseudogout:** Calcium pyrophosphate dihydrate crystals

ASO TITER
See "ANTISTREPTOLYSIN O TITER"

ASPARTATE AMINOTRANSFERASE (AST, SGOT)
Normal range: 0 to 35 U/L (0 to 0.58 μkat/L [CF: 0.01667, SMI: 0.01μkat/L])
Elevated in: *HEART*
Acute myocardial infarction
Pericarditis (active—some cases)
LIVER
Hepatitis virus, Epstein-Barr, or cytomegalovirus infection
Active cirrhosis
Liver passive congestion or hypoxia
Alcohol- or drug-induced liver dysfunction
Space-occupying lesions (active)
Fatty liver (severe)
Extrahepatic biliary obstruction (early)
Drug-induced
SKELETAL MUSCLE
Acute skeletal muscle injury
Muscle inflammation (infectious or noninfectious)
Muscular dystrophy (active)
Recent surgery
Delirium tremens
KIDNEY
Acute injury or damage
Renal infarct
OTHER
Intestinal infarction
Shock
Cholecystitis
Acute pancreatitis
Hypothyroidism
Heparin therapy (60% to 80% of cases)
Fig. E2 describes an approach to the evaluation of AST elevation.
Box E5 describes causes of elevated serum aminotransferase levels.

ATRIAL NATRIURETIC HORMONE (ANH)
Normal: 20 to 77 pg/ml
Elevated in: CHF, volume overload, cardiovascular disease with high filling pressure
Decreased with: Prazosin and other alpha blockers

B-TYPE NATRIURETIC PEPTIDE (BNP)
Normal range: Up to 100 mcg/L. Natriuretic peptides are secreted to regulate fluid volume, blood pressure, and electrolyte balance. They have activity in both the central and peripheral nervous systems. In humans the main source of circulatory BNP is the heart ventricles.
Elevated in: Heart failure. This test is useful to differentiate heart failure patients from those with chronic obstructive pulmonary disease presenting with dyspnea. Levels are also increased in asymptomatic left ventricular dysfunction, arterial and pulmonary hypertension, cardiac hypertrophy, valvular heart disease, arrhythmia, and acute coronary syndrome. See Fig. 13.

BASOPHIL COUNT
Key causes of basophilia are summarized in Box 6.
Normal range:
0.4% to 1% of total white blood cells (WBCs); 40 to 100/mm^3
Elevated in: Leukemia, inflammatory processes, polycythemia vera, Hodgkin lymphoma, hemolytic anemia, after splenectomy, myeloid metaplasia, myxedema
Decreased in: Stress, hypersensitivity reaction, steroids, pregnancy, hyperthyroidism, postirradiation

BICARBONATE
Normal:
Arterial: 21 to 28 mEq/L
Venous: 22 to 29 mEq/L
Elevated in: Metabolic alkalosis, compensated respiratory acidosis, diuretics, corticosteroids, laxative abuse
Decreased in: Metabolic acidosis, compensated respiratory alkalosis, acetazolamide, cyclosporine, cholestyramine, methanol or ethylene glycol poisoning

BILE, URINE
See "URINE BILE"

BILIRUBIN, DIRECT (conjugated bilirubin)
Normal range: 0 to 0.2 mg/dl (0 to 4 μmol/L [CF: 17.10; SMI: 2 μmol/L])
Elevated in: Hepatocellular disease, biliary obstruction, drug-induced cholestasis, hereditary disorders (Dubin-Johnson syndrome, Rotor syndrome)

BILIRUBIN, INDIRECT (unconjugated bilirubin)
Normal range:
0 to 1.0 mg/dl (2 to 18 μmol/L [CF: 17.10; SMI: 2 μmol/L])
Elevated in:
Increased bilirubin production (if normal liver, serum unconjugated bilirubin is usually less than 4 mg/100 ml)
Hemolytic anemia
Acquired
Congenital
Resorption from extravascular sources
Hematomas
Pulmonary infarcts
Excessive ineffective erythropoiesis
Congenital (congenital dyserythropoietic anemias)
Acquired (pernicious anemia, severe lead poisoning; if present, bilirubinemia is usually mild)
Defective hepatic unconjugated bilirubin clearance (defective uptake or conjugation)
Severe liver disease
Gilbert syndrome

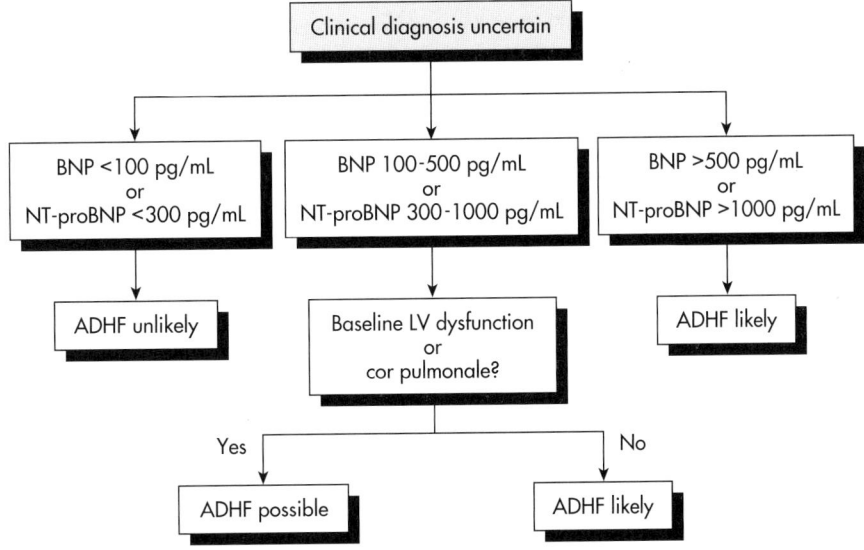

FIG. 13 Interpretation of natriuretic peptide levels. *ADHF,* Acute decompensated heart failure; *BNP,* B-type natriuretic peptide; *LV,* left ventricle; *NT-proBNP,* inactive N-terminal fragment of BNP. (From Adams JG et al: *Emergency medicine, clinical essentials,* ed 2, Philadelphia, 2013, Elsevier.)

BOX 6   Key Causes of Basophilia

Myeloproliferative disease
Allergic—food, drugs, foreign proteins
Infectious—variola, varicella
Chronic hemolytic anemia—especially postsplenectomy
Inflammatory—collagen vascular disease, ulcerative colitis

From McPherson RA, Pincus MR: *Henry's clinical diagnosis and management by laboratory methods,* ed 23, St Louis, 2017, Elsevier.

Crigler-Najjar type I or II
Drug-induced inhibition
Portacaval shunt
Congestive heart failure
Hyperthyroidism (uncommon)

BILIRUBIN, TOTAL

See Fig. E14, Table E19, and Table E20 for evaluation of hyperbilirubinemia and liver disease.

Normal range: 0 to 1.0 mg/dl (2 to 18 μmol/L [CF: 17.10, SMI: 2 μmol/L])

Elevated in: Liver disease (hepatitis, cirrhosis, cholangitis, neoplasm, biliary obstruction, infectious mononucleosis), hereditary disorders (Gilbert disease, Dubin-Johnson syndrome), drugs (steroids, statins, niacin, acetaminophen, diphenylhydantoin, phenothiazines, penicillin, erythromycin, clindamycin, captopril, amphotericin B, sulfonamides, azathioprine, isoniazid, 5-aminosalicylic acid, allopurinol, methyldopa, indomethacin, halothane, oral contraceptives, procainamide, tolbutamide, labetalol), hemolysis, pulmonary embolism or infarct, hepatic congestion secondary to congestive heart failure

BILIRUBIN, URINE

See "URINE BILE"

BLADDER TUMOR ASSOCIATED ANTIGEN

Normal:
≤14 U/ml. Test is used to detect bladder cancer recurrence. Sensitivity 57% to 83% and specificity 68% to 72%.

Elevated in: Bladder cancer, renal stones, nephritis, UTI, hematuria, renal cancer, cystitis, recent bladder or urinary tract trauma

BLEEDING TIME (modified Ivy method)

See Fig. E15 for evaluation of patients with prolonged bleeding time.
Normal range: 2 to 9.5 min
Elevated in: Thrombocytopenia, capillary wall abnormalities, platelet abnormalities (Bernard-Soulier disease, Glanzmann disease), drugs (aspirin, warfarin, antiinflammatory medications, streptokinase, urokinase, dextran, β-lactam antibiotics, moxalactam), disseminated intravascular coagulation, cirrhosis, uremia, myeloproliferative disorders, von Willebrand disease

Bleeding time tests are no longer performed at many hospitals and have been replaced by the platelet function analyzer (PFA-100) assay.

BLOOD TYPE

Blood components must be serologically compatible with the recipient. ABO compatibility is the primary consideration. Transfused red cells must be compatible with recipient antibodies, and transfused plasma must be compatible with recipient red cells. Therefore, whole blood must be of identical ABO type to the recipient. Red blood cells contain a limited amount of plasma and need to be compatible but not necessarily identical to the ABO type of the recipient. Similarly, plasma and platelet concentrates contain few, if any, red cells. ABO-compatible blood component selection is summarized in Table 21. Red blood cells

TABLE 21   ABO Compatibility

Donor Type	RECIPIENT TYPE			
	O	**A**	**B**	**AB**
O	R	R	R	R
	P			
A		R		R
		P		
B			R	R
			P	
AB				R
	P	P	P	P

P, Plasma-containing components (platelets, fresh frozen plasma) are compatible; *R,* red cells are compatible.
From McPherson RA, Pincus MR: *Henry's clinical diagnosis and management by laboratory methods,* ed 23, St Louis, 2017, Elsevier.

Laboratory Tests

IV

must also be negative for clinically significant antigens when transfused to alloimmunized recipients. It is highly desirable to transfuse only Rh-negative red cells to Rh-negative recipients because there is approximately a 30% risk for immunization to Rh(D). This is particularly important for women of childbearing potential because of the risk for hemolytic disease of the newborn in subsequent pregnancies. Special considerations apply to recipients of ABO-incompatible hematopoietic progenitor cell transplants. During the course of transplantation, such individuals will change their blood type. Transfused red cells should be compatible with both donor and recipient isohemagglutinins, and transfused plasma–containing components should be compatible with both donor and recipient red cells. Thus, the optimal choice for such a patient will depend on current and expected future typing results.

BLOOD VOLUME, TOTAL

Normal range: 60 to 80 ml/kg
Elevated in: Polycythemia vera, pulmonary disease, CHF, renal insufficiency, pregnancy, acidosis, thyrotoxicosis
Decreased in: Anemia, hemorrhage, vomiting, diarrhea, dehydration, burns, starvation

BNP

See "B-TYPE NATRIURETIC PEPTIDE"

BORDETELLA PERTUSSIS SEROLOGY

Test description: Polymerase chain reaction (PCR) of nasopharyngeal aspirates or secretions is used to identify *Bordetella pertussis,* the organism responsible for whooping cough.

BRCA ANALYSIS

DESCRIPTION OF ANALYSIS
Comprehensive BRCA analysis:
BRCA1: Full sequence determination in both forward and reverse directions of approximately 5500 base pairs comprising 22 coding exons and one noncoding exon (exon 4) and approximately 800 adjacent base pairs in the noncoding intervening sequence (intron). Exon 1, which is noncoding, is not analyzed. The wild-type *BRCA1* gene encodes a protein comprising 1863 amino acids.
BRCA2: Full sequence determination in both forward and reverse directions of approximately 10,200 base pairs comprising 26 coding exons and approximately 900 adjacent base pairs in the noncoding intervening sequence (intron). Exon 1, which is noncoding, is not analyzed. The wild-type *BRCA2* gene encodes a protein comprising 3418 amino acids.
The noncoding intronic regions of *BRCA1* and *BRCA2* that are analyzed do not extend more than 20 base pairs proximal to the 5' end and 10 base pairs distal to the 3' end of each exon.
Single-site BRCA analysis: DNA sequence analysis for a specified mutation in *BRCA1* and/or *BRCA2.*
Multisite 3 BRCA analysis: DNA sequence analysis of specific portions of *BRCA1* exon 2, *BRCA1* exon 20, and *BRCA2* exon 11 designed to detect only mutations 187delAG and 5385insC in *BRCA1* and 6174delT in *BRCA2.*
Interpretive Criteria:
"Positive for a deleterious mutation": Includes all mutations (nonsense, insertions, deletions) that prematurely terminate ("truncate") the protein product of *BRCA1* at least 10 amino acids from the C-terminus, or the protein product of *BRCA2* at least 110 amino acids from the C-terminus (based on documentation of deleterious mutations in *BRCA1* and *BRCA2*). In addition, specific missense mutations and noncoding intervening sequence (IVS) mutations are recognized as deleterious on the basis of data derived from linkage analysis of high-risk families, functional assays, biochemical evidence, and/or demonstration of abnormal messenger ribonucleic acid (mRNA) transcript processing.
"Genetic variant, suspected deleterious": Includes genetic variants for which the available evidence indicates a likelihood, but not proof, that the mutation is deleterious. The specific evidence supporting such an interpretation will be summarized for individual variants on each such report.
"Genetic variant, favor polymorphism": Includes genetic variants for which available evidence indicates that the variant is highly unlikely to contribute substantially to cancer risk. The specific evidence supporting such an interpretation will be summarized for individual variants on each such report.
"Genetic variant of uncertain significance": Includes missense mutations and mutations that occur in analyzed intronic regions whose clinical significance has not been determined, as well as chain-terminating mutations that truncate *BRCA1* and *BRCA2* distal to amino acid positions 1853 and 3308, respectively.
"No deleterious mutation detected": Includes nontruncating genetic variants observed at an allele frequency of approximately 1% of a suitable control population (providing that no data suggest clinical significance), as well as all genetic variants for which published data demonstrate absence of substantial clinical significance. Also includes mutations in the protein-coding region that neither alter the amino acid sequence nor are predicted to significantly affect exon splicing, and base pair alterations in noncoding portions of the gene that have been demonstrated to have no deleterious effect on the length or stability of the mRNA transcript.
There may be uncommon genetic abnormalities in *BRCA1* and *BRCA2* that will not be detected by *BRCA* analysis. This analysis, however, is believed to rule out the majority of abnormalities in these genes, which are believed responsible for most hereditary susceptibility to breast and ovarian cancer.
"Specific variant/mutation not identified": Specific and designated deleterious mutations or variants of uncertain clinical significance are not present in the individual being tested. If one (or rarely two) specific deleterious mutations have been identified in a family member, a negative analysis for the specific mutation(s) indicates that the tested individual is at the general population risk of developing breast or ovarian cancer.

BREATH HYDROGEN TEST (hydrogen breath test)

Normal: This test is for bacterial overgrowth. H_2 excretion fasting: 4.6 ± 5.1, after lactulose, early increase <12. Lactulose usually results in a colonic response >30 min after ingestion.
Elevated in: A high fasting breath H_2 level and an increase of at least 12 ppm within 30 min after lactulose challenge are indicative of bacterial overgrowth in the small intestine. The increase must precede the colonic response.
False positives in: Accelerated gastric emptying, laxative use
False negatives in: Use of antibiotics and patients who are nonhydrogen producers

BUN

See "UREA NITROGEN, BLOOD"

C282Y AND H63D MUTATION ANALYSIS

PROCEDURE:
Detection of the C282Y and H63D mutations is accomplished by amplification of exons 2 and 4 of the *HFE* gene on chromosome 6 by polymerase chain reaction (PCR) followed by allele-specific hybridization and chemiluminescent detection of hybridized probes. H63D is viewed by some as a polymorphism rather than a mutation because of its prevalence in the population, because 15% of the individuals affected with hereditary hemochromatosis (HH) are compound heterozygotes for C282Y and H63D and about 1% of patients are H63D homozygotes, which suggests that H63D may be causative in the development of the disorder at reduced penetrance.

INTERPRETATION OF RESULTS:
Homozygosity for the C282Y mutation has been associated with an increased risk of being affected with HH compared with the general population. The genotype is observed in 60% to 90% of individuals affected with HH and occurs in less than 1% of the general population. However, approximately 25% of asymptomatic individuals with this genotype do not develop the disorder.

C3
See "COMPLEMENT"

C4
See "COMPLEMENT"

CALCITONIN (serum)
Normal range: <100 pg/ml (<100 ng/L [CF: 1; SMI: 10 ng/L])
Elevated in: Medullary carcinoma of the thyroid (particularly if level >1500 pg/ml), carcinoma of the breast, apudomas, carcinoids, renal failure, thyroiditis

CALCIUM (serum)
Laboratory values in various altered states of calcium metabolism are summarized in Table E22.
See Figs. E16 and E17.

Normal range: 8.8 to 10.3 mg/dl (2.2 to 2.58 μmol/L [CF: 0.2495; SMI: 0.02 μmol/L])

ELEVATED
Relatively common
Neoplasia
Bone primary
Myeloma
Acute leukemia
Nonbone solid tumors
Breast
Lung
Squamous nonpulmonary
Kidney
Neoplasm secretion of parathyroid hormone-related protein (PTHrP, "ectopic PTH")
Primary hyperparathyroidism
Thiazide diuretics
Tertiary (renal) hyperparathyroidism
Idiopathic
Spurious (artifactual) hypercalcemia
Dehydration
Serum protein elevation
Laboratory technical problem (lab error)
Relatively uncommon
Sarcoidosis
Hyperthyroidism
Immobilization (mostly seen in children and adolescents)
Diuretic phase of acute renal tubular necrosis
Vitamin D intoxication
Milk-alkali syndrome
Addison disease
Lithium therapy
Idiopathic hypercalcemia of infancy
Acromegaly
Theophylline toxicity
Table E23 describes the laboratory differential diagnosis of hypercalcemia.
Box E7 describes the differential diagnosis of hypercalcemia in older adults.
DECREASED
Artifactual
Hypoalbuminemia
Hemodilution
Primary hypoparathyroidism
Pseudohypoparathyroidism
Vitamin D related
Vitamin D deficiency
Malabsorption
Renal failure
Magnesium deficiency
Sepsis
Chronic alcoholism

Tumor lysis syndrome
Rhabdomyolysis
Alkalosis (respiratory or metabolic)
Acute pancreatitis
Drug-induced hypocalcemia
Large doses of magnesium sulfate
Anticonvulsants
Mithramycin
Gentamicin
Cimetidine
Table E24 describes the laboratory differential diagnosis of hypocalcemia.

CALCIUM, URINE
See "URINE CALCIUM"

CANCER ANTIGEN 15-3 (CA 15-3)
Normal: <30 U/ml
Elevated in: Approximately 80% of women with metastatic breast cancer. Clinical sensitivity is 0.60, specificity 0.87, positive predictive value 0.91. This test is generally used to predict recurrence of breast cancer and evaluate response to therapy. May also be elevated in liver cancer, pancreatic cancer, ovarian cancer, colorectal cancer. Elevations can also occur with benign breast and liver disease.

CANCER ANTIGEN 27-29 (CA 27-29)
Normal: <38 U/ml
Elevated in: Approximately 75% of women with metastatic breast cancer. Clinical sensitivity is 0.57, specificity 0.97, positive predictive value 0.83, negative predictive value 0.92. This test is generally used to predict recurrence of breast cancer and evaluate response to therapy. May also be elevated in liver cancer, pancreatic cancer, ovarian cancer, colorectal cancer. Elevations can also occur with benign breast and liver disease.

CANCER ANTIGEN 72-4 (CA 72-4)
Normal: <4.0 ng/ml
Elevated in: Gastric cancer (elevated in >50% of patients). Often used in combination with CA 72-4, CA 19-9, and CEA to monitor gastric cancer after treatment.

CANCER ANTIGEN 125 (CA 125)
Normal range: <1.4%
This test uses an antibody against antigen from tissue culture of an ovarian tumor cell line. Various published evaluations report sensitivity of about 75% to 80% in patients with ovarian carcinoma. There is also an appreciable incidence of elevated values in nonovarian malignancies and in certain benign conditions (see "BENIGN" below). Test values may transiently increase during chemotherapy.
MALIGNANT
Epithelial ovarian carcinoma, 75% to 80% (range, 25% to 92%; better in serous than mucinous cystadenocarcinoma)
Endometrial carcinoma, 25% to 48% (2% to 90%)
Pancreatic carcinoma, 59%
Colorectal carcinoma, 20% (15% to 56%)
Endocervical adenocarcinoma, 83%
Squamous cervical or vaginal carcinoma, 7% to 14%
Lung carcinoma, 32%
Breast carcinoma, 12% to 40%
Lymphoma, 35%
BENIGN
Cirrhosis, 40% to 80%
Acute pancreatitis, 38%
Acute peritonitis, 75%
Endometriosis, 88%
Acute pelvic inflammatory disease, 33%
Pregnancy first trimester, 2% to 24%
During menstruation (occasionally)
Renal failure (?frequency)
Normal persons, 0.6% to 1.4%

CAPTOPRIL STIMULATION TEST

Normal: Test performed by giving 25 mg captopril orally after overnight fast. Patient should be seated during test. After captopril, aldosterone <15 ng/dl, renin >2 ng angiotensin L/ml/h.

Interpretation of results: In patients with primary aldosteronism, plasma aldosterone remains high and plasma renin activity remains low after captopril.

CARBAMAZEPINE (Tegretol)

Normal therapeutic range: 4 to 12 mcg/ml

CARBAMAZEPINE LEVEL

Therapeutic range and general information are summarized in Table 25.

CARBOHYDRATE ANTIGEN 19-9

Normal: <37.0 U/ml

Elevated in: GI cancer, most frequently pancreatic cancer. Amount of elevation has no relation to tumor mass. Elevations can also occur with cirrhosis, cholangitis, and chronic or acute pancreatitis.

CARBON DIOXIDE, PARTIAL PRESSURE

Normal:
Male: 35 to 48 mm Hg
Female: 32 to 45 mm Hg
Elevated in: Respiratory acidosis
Decreased in: Respiratory alkalosis

CARBON MONOXIDE

See "CARBOXYHEMOGLOBIN"

CARBOXYHEMOGLOBIN

Normal range: Saturation of hemoglobin <2%; smokers <9%
Elevated in: Smoking, exposure to smoking, exposure to automobile exhaust fumes, malfunctioning gas-burning appliances

CARCINOEMBRYONIC ANTIGEN (CEA)

Normal range:
Nonsmokers: 0 to 2.5 ng/ml (0 to 2.5 µg/L [CF: 1; SMI: 0.1 µg/L])
Smokers: 0 to 5 ng/ml (0 to 5 µg/L [CF: 1; SMI: 0.1 µg/L])
Elevated in:
Colorectal carcinomas*, pancreatic carcinomas, and metastatic disease (usually produce higher elevations: >20 ng/ml)
Carcinomas of the esophagus, stomach, small intestine, liver, breast, ovary, lung, and thyroid (usually produce lesser elevations)
Benign conditions (smoking, inflammatory bowel disease, hypothyroidism, cirrhosis, pancreatitis, infections) (usually produce levels <10 ng/ml)

CAROTENE (serum)

Normal range: 50 to 250 µg/dl (0.9 to 4.6 µmol/L [CF: 0.01863; SMI: 0.1 µmol/L])
Elevated in: Carotenemia, chronic nephritis, diabetes mellitus, hypothyroidism, nephrotic syndrome, hyperlipidemia
Decreased in: Fat malabsorption, steatorrhea, pancreatic insufficiency, lack of carotenoids in diet, high fever, liver disease

CATECHOLAMINES, URINE

See "URINE CATECHOLAMINES"

CBC

See "COMPLETE BLOOD COUNT"

CD40 LIGAND

Normal: <5 mcg/L. CD40 ligand is a soluble protein that is shed from activated leukocytes and platelets and used in risk stratification for acute coronary syndrome.
Elevated in: Acute coronary syndrome. Increased CD40 ligand is associated with higher incidence of death or nonfatal myocardial infarction (MI).

CD4+ T-LYMPHOCYTE COUNT (CD4+ T cells)

Calculated as total WBC × % lymphocytes × % lymphocytes stained with CD4.

This test is used primarily to evaluate immune dysfunction in HIV infection. It is useful as a prognostic indicator and as a criterion for initiating prophylaxis for several opportunistic infections that are sequelae of HIV infection. Progressive depletion of CD4+ T lymphocytes is associated with an increased likelihood of clinical complications (Table E26).

CEA

See "CARCINOEMBRYONIC ANTIGEN"

CEREBROSPINAL FLUID (CSF)

Adult lumbar CSF reference values are summarized in Table 27. CSF proteins in various central nervous system diseases are described in Table E28.

Interpretation of results:
Appearance of the fluid
Clear: Normal.
Yellow color (xanthochromia) in the supernatant of centrifuged CSF within 1 h or less after collection is usually the result of previous bleeding (subarachnoid hemorrhage); it may also be caused by increased CSF protein, melanin from meningeal melanosarcomas, or carotenoids.
Pinkish color is usually the result of a bloody tap; the color generally clears progressively from tubes 1 to 4 (the supernatant is usually crystal clear in traumatic taps).
Turbidity usually indicates the presence of leukocytes (bleeding introduces approximately 1 WBC/500 RBCs into the CSF).

TABLE 25 Carbamazepine (Tegretol)

Purpose	Treatment of Generalized Tonic-Clonic Seizures, Simple Partial Seizures, Complex Partial Seizures, Trigeminal Neuralgia, and Glossopharyngeal Neuralgia
General adult dose	Oral: 0.8-1.2 g/day maintenance for seizure control; 0.2-1.2 g/day for neuralgia
Usual bioavailability	70%
Half-life	Initially approximately 35 hr; approximately 8-20 h after 3-4 wk of administration
General therapeutic range	4-12 mcg/ml
General toxic level	>12 mcg/ml
Transport	60%-70% plasma protein bound
Metabolism	Hepatic: Carbamazepine-10,11-epoxide (active); carbamazepine-10,11-transdihydrodiol (inactive)
Elimination	1%-2% unchanged in urine
Steady state	3-7 days
Mechanism of action	Decreases sodium and calcium ion influx into repeatedly depolarizing CNS neurons; reduces excitatory synaptic transmission in the spinal trigeminal nucleus
Toxic effects	Drowsiness, ataxia, dizziness, nausea, vomiting, involuntary movements, abnormal reflexes, irregular pulse

CNS, Central nervous system.
From McPherson RA, Pincus MR: *Henry's clinical diagnosis and management by laboratory methods,* ed 23, St Louis, 2017, Elsevier.

---

*To detect colorectal cancer, the sensitivity of CEA ranges from 68% for a threshold of 10 mcg/L to 82% for a threshold of 2.5 mcg/L, and the specificity ranges from 97% for a threshold of 10 mcg/L to 80% for a threshold of 2.6 mcg/L.

TABLE 27 Adult Lumbar CSF Reference Values

Analyte	Conventional Units	SI Units
Protein	15-60 mg/dL	0.15-0.60 g/L
Prealbumin	2%-7%	
Albumin	56%-76%	
α_1-Globulin	2%-7%	
α_2-Globulin	4%-12%	
β-Globulin	8%-18%	
γ-Globulin	3%-12%	
Electrolytes		
Osmolality	280-300 mOsm/L	280-300 mmol/L
Sodium	135-150 mEq/L	135-150 mmol/L
Potassium	2.6-3.0 mEq/L	2.6-3.0 mmol/L
Chloride	115-130 mEq/L	115-130 mmol/L
Carbon dioxide	20-25 mEq/L	20-25 mmol/L
Calcium	2.0-2.8 mEq/L	1.0-1.4 mmol/L
Magnesium	2.4-3.0 mEq/L	1.2-1.5 mmol/L
Lactate	10-22 mg/dL	1.1-2.4 mmol/L
pH		
Lumbar fluid	7.28-7.32	
Cisternal fluid	7.32-7.34	
pCO$_2$		
Lumbar fluid	44-50 mm Hg	
Cisternal fluid	40-46 mm Hg	
pO$_2$	40-44 mm Hg	
Other Constituents		
Ammonia	10-35 µg/dL	6-20 µmol/L
Glutamine	5-20 mg/dL	0.3-1.4 mmol/L
Creatinine	0.6-1.2 mg/dL	45-92 µmol/L
Glucose	50-80 mg/dL	2.8-4.4 mmol/L
Iron	1-2 µg/dL	0.2-0.4 µmol/L
Phosphorus	1.2-2.0 mg/dL	0.4-0.7 mmol/L
Total lipid	1-2 mg/dL	0.01-0.02 g/L
Urea	6-16 mg/dL	2.0-5.7 mmol/L
Urate	0.5-3.0 mg/dL	30-180 µmol/L
Zinc	2-6 µg/dL	0.3-0.9 µmol/L

CSF, Cerebrospinal fluid; *pCO$_2$,* partial pressure of carbon dioxide; *pO$_2$,* partial pressure of oxygen.
From McPherson RA, Pincus MR: *Henry's clinical diagnosis and management by laboratory methods,* ed 23, St Louis, 2017, Elsevier.

CSF pressure: Elevated pressure can be seen with meningitis, meningoencephalitis, pseudotumor cerebri, mass lesions, and intracerebral bleeding.

Cell count: In the adult the CSF is normally free of cells (although up to five mononuclear cells/mm^3 is considered normal); the presence of granulocytes is never normal.

Neutrophils: Seen in bacterial meningitis, early viral meningoencephalitis, and early tuberculosis (TB) meningitis. Box 8 summarizes causes of increased CSF neutrophils.

Increased lymphocytes: TB meningitis, viral meningoencephalitis, syphilitic meningoencephalitis, fungal meningitis. Causes of CSF lymphocytosis are summarized in Box 9.

CSF plasmacytosis: Box 10 describes inflammatory and infectious causes of CSF plasmacytosis.

CSF eosinophilia: Causes of CSF eosinophilic pleocytosis are summarized in Box 11.

Protein: Serum proteins are generally too large to cross the normal blood-CSF barrier; however, increased CSF protein is seen with meningeal inflammation, traumatic tap, increased CNS synthesis, tissue degeneration, obstruction to CSF circulation, and Guillain-Barré syndrome. Mean concentrations of plasma and CSF proteins are summarized in Table E29.

BOX 8 Causes of Increased CSF Neutrophils

Meningitis
  Bacterial meningitis
  Early viral meningoencephalitis
  Early tuberculous meningitis
  Early mycotic meningitis
  Amebic encephalomyelitis
Other infections
  Cerebral abscess
  Subdural empyema
  AIDS-related CMV radiculopathy
Following seizures
Following CNS hemorrhage
  Subarachnoid
  Intracerebral
Following CNS infarct
Reaction to repeated lumbar punctures
Injection of foreign material in subarachnoid space (e.g., methotrexate, contrast media)
Metastatic tumor in contact with CSF

AIDS, Acquired immunodeficiency virus; *CMV,* cytomegalovirus; *CNS,* central nervous system; *CSF,* cerebrospinal fluid.
From McPherson RA, Pincus MR: *Henry's clinical diagnosis and management by laboratory methods,* ed 23, St Louis, 2017, Elsevier.

BOX 9 Causes of CSF Lymphocytosis

Meningitis
Viral meningitis
Tuberculous meningitis
Fungal meningitis
Syphilitic meningoencephalitis
Leptospiral meningitis
Bacterial due to uncommon organisms
Early bacterial meningitis where leukocyte counts are relatively low
Parasitic infestations (e.g., cysticercosis, trichinosis, toxoplasmosis)
Aseptic meningitis due to septic focus adjacent to meninges
Degenerative Disorders
Subacute sclerosing panencephalitis
Multiple sclerosis
Drug abuse encephalopathy
Guillain-Barré syndrome
Acute disseminated encephalomyelitis
Other Inflammatory Disorders
HaNDL syndrome (headache with neurologic deficits and CSF lymphocytosis)
Sarcoidosis
Polyneuritis
CNS periarteritis

CNS, Central nervous system; *CSF,* cerebrospinal fluid.
From McPherson RA, Pincus MR: *Henry's clinical diagnosis and management by laboratory methods,* ed 23, St Louis, 2017, Elsevier.

Conditions associated with increased CSF total protein are summarized in Box 12.

Glucose
Decreased glucose is seen with bacterial meningitis, TB meningitis, fungal meningitis, subarachnoid hemorrhage, and some cases of viral meningitis.
A mild increase in CSF glucose can be seen in patients with very elevated serum glucose levels.

BOX 10 Inflammatory and Infectious Causes of CSF Plasmacytosis

Acute viral infections
Guillain-Barré syndrome
Multiple sclerosis
Parasitic CNS infestations
Sarcoidosis
Subacute sclerosing panencephalitis
Syphilitic meningoencephalitis
Tuberculous meningitis

CNS, Central nervous system; *CSF,* cerebrospinal fluid.
From McPherson RA, Pincus MR: *Henry's clinical diagnosis and management by laboratory methods*, ed 23, St Louis, 2017, Elsevier.

BOX 11 Causes of CSF Eosinophilic Pleocytosis

Commonly Associated With
Acute polyneuritis
CNS reaction to foreign material (drugs, shunts)
Fungal infections
Idiopathic eosinophilic meningitis
Idiopathic hypereosinophilic syndrome
Parasitic infections

Infrequently Associated With
Bacterial meningitis
Leukemia/lymphoma
Myeloproliferative disorders
Neurosarcoidosis
Primary brain tumors
Tuberculous meningoencephalitis
Viral meningitis

CNS, Central nervous system; *CSF,* cerebrospinal fluid.
Modified from Kjeldsberg CR, Knight JA: *Body fluids: laboratory examination of amniotic, cerebrospinal, seminal, serous and synovial fluids*, ed 3, Chicago, 1993, American Society for Clinical Pathology, with permission. In McPherson RA, Pincus MR: *Henry's clinical diagnosis and management by laboratory methods*, ed 23, St Louis, 2017, Elsevier.

Table E30 describes CSF findings in infectious and inflammatory diseases of the central nervous system and meninges.

Causes of xanthochromia are summarized in Table E31.

CERULOPLASMIN (serum)

Normal range: 20 to 35 mg/dl (200 to 350 mg/L [CF: 10; SMI: 10 mg/L])
Elevated in: Pregnancy, estrogens, oral contraceptives, neoplastic diseases (leukemias, Hodgkin lymphoma, carcinomas), inflammatory states, systemic lupus erythematosus, primary biliary cirrhosis, rheumatoid arthritis
Decreased in: Wilson disease (values often <10 mg/dl), nephrotic syndrome, advanced liver disease, malabsorption, total parenteral nutrition, Menkes syndrome

CHLAMYDIA GROUP ANTIBODY SEROLOGIC TEST

Test description: Acute and convalescent sera is drawn 2 to 4 wk apart. A fourfold increase in titer between acute and convalescent sera is necessary for confirmation. A single titer ≥1:64 is considered indicative of psittacosis or lymphogranuloma venereum (LGV).

CHLAMYDIA TRACHOMATIS PCR

Test description: Test is performed on endocervical swab, urine, and intraurethral swab (Table E32).
Normal: Negative

CHLORIDE (serum)

Normal range: 95 to 105 mEq/L (95 to 105 mmol/L [CF: 1; SMI: 1 mmol/L])
Elevated in: Dehydration, excessive infusion of normal saline solution, cystic fibrosis (sweat test), hyperparathyroidism, renal tubular disease, metabolic

BOX 12 Conditions Associated With Increased CSF Total Protein

Traumatic Spinal Puncture
Increased blood-CSF permeability
Arachnoiditis (e.g., following methotrexate therapy)
Meningitis (bacterial, viral, fungal, tuberculous)
Hemorrhage (subarachnoid, intracerebral)
Endocrine/metabolic disorders
  Milk-alkali syndrome with hypercalcemia
  Diabetic neuropathy
  Hereditary neuropathies and myelopathies
  Decreased endocrine function (thyroid, parathyroid)
  Other disorders (uremia, dehydration)
Drug Toxicity
Ethanol, phenothiazines, phenytoin
CSF Circulation Defects
Mechanical obstruction (tumor, abscess, herniated disk)
Loculated CSF effusion
Increased Immunoglobulin (Ig)G Synthesis
Multiple sclerosis
Neurosyphilis
Subacute sclerosing panencephalitis
Increased IgG Synthesis and Blood-CSF Permeability
Guillain-Barré syndrome
Collagen vascular diseases (e.g., lupus, periarteritis)
Chronic inflammatory demyelinating polyradiculopathy

CNS, Central nervous system; *CSF,* cerebrospinal fluid.
From McPherson RA, Pincus MR: *Henry's clinical diagnosis and management by laboratory methods*, ed 23, St Louis, 2017, Elsevier.

acidosis, prolonged diarrhea, drugs (ammonium chloride administration, acetazolamide, boric acid, triamterene)
Decreased in: Congestive heart failure, syndrome of inappropriate antidiuretic hormone secretion, Addison disease, vomiting, gastric suction, salt-losing nephritis, continuous infusion of D_5W, thiazide diuretic administration, diaphoresis, diarrhea, burns, diabetic ketoacidosis

CHLORIDE (sweat)

Normal: 0 to 40 mmol/L
Borderline/indeterminate: 41 to 60 mmol/L
Consistent with cystic fibrosis: >60 mmol/L
  False low results can occur with edema, excessive sweating, and hypoproteinemia.

CHLORIDE, URINE

See "URINE CHLORIDE"

CHOLECYSTOKININ-PANCREOZYMIN (CCK, CCK-PZ)

Normal: <80 pg/ml
Elevated in: Pancreatic disease, celiac disease, gastric ulcer, postgastrectomy, irritable bowel syndrome (IBS), fatty food intolerance

CHOLESTEROL, HIGH-DENSITY LIPOPROTEIN

See "HIGH-DENSITY LIPOPROTEIN CHOLESTEROL"

CHOLESTEROL, LOW-DENSITY LIPOPROTEIN

See "LOW-DENSITY LIPOPROTEIN CHOLESTEROL"

CHOLESTEROL, TOTAL

Normal range: Varies with age
  Generally <200 mg/dl (<5.20 mmol/L [CF: 0.02586; SMI: 0.05 mmol/L])
Elevated in: Primary hypercholesterolemia, biliary obstruction, diabetes mellitus, nephrotic syndrome, hypothyroidism, primary biliary cirrhosis, high-cholesterol diet, pregnancy third trimester, myocardial infarction, drugs

(steroids, phenothiazines, oral contraceptives). Classic hyperlipidemia phenotypes are summarized in Table E33.

Decreased in: Medications (statins, niacin), starvation, malabsorption, sideroblastic anemia, thalassemia, abetalipoproteinemia, hyperthyroidism, Cushing syndrome, hepatic failure, multiple myeloma, polycythemia vera, chronic myelocytic leukemia, myeloid metaplasia, Waldenström macroglobulinemia, myelofibrosis

CHORIONIC GONADOTROPINS, HUMAN (serum) (hCG)

Normal range, serum:
Female, premenopausal: <0.8 IU/L; postmenopausal <3.3 IU/L
Male: <0.7 IU/L
Elevated in:
Pregnancy, choriocarcinoma, gestational trophoblastic neoplasia (including molar gestations), placental site trophoblastic tumors; human antimouse antibodies (HAMA) can produce false serum assay for hCG.
The principal use of this test is to diagnose pregnancy. The concentration of hCG increases significantly during the initial 6 wk of pregnancy.
Normal range:
Varies with gestational stage:
1 wk: 5 to 50 mU/ml
1 to 2 wk: 50 to 550 mU/ml
2 to 3 wk: Up to 5000 mU/ml
3 to 4 wk: Up to 10,000 mU/ml
4 to 5 wk: Up to 50,000 mU/ml
2 to 3 mo: 10,000 to 100,000 mU/ml
  Peak values approaching 100,000 IU/L occur 60 to 70 days following implantation.
  hCG levels generally double every 1 to 3 days. In patients with concentration <2000 IU/L, an increase of serum hCG <66% after 2 days is suggestive of spontaneous abortion or ruptured ectopic gestation.

CHYMOTRYPSIN

Normal: <10 mcg/L
Elevated in: Acute pancreatitis, chronic renal failure, oral enzyme preparations, gastric cancer, pancreatic cancer
Decreased in: Chronic pancreatitis, late cystic fibrosis

CIRCULATING ANTICOAGULANT (lupus anticoagulant)

Normal: Negative
Detected in: Systemic lupus erythematosus, drug-induced lupus, long-term phenothiazine therapy, multiple myeloma, ulcerative colitis, rheumatoid arthritis, postpartum, hemophilia, neoplasms, chronic inflammatory states, AIDS, nephrotic syndrome
  NOTE: The name is a misnomer because these patients are prone to hypercoagulability and thrombosis.

CK

See "CREATINE KINASE"

CLONIDINE SUPPRESSION TEST

Interpretation of results: Clonidine inhibits neurogenic catecholamine release and will cause a decrease in plasma norepinephrine into the reference interval in hypertensive subjects without pheochromocytoma. Test is performed by giving 4.3 mcg clonidine/kg orally after overnight fast. Norepinephrine is measured at 3 h. Result should be within established reference range and decrease to <50% of baseline concentration. Lack of decrease in norepinephrine is suggestive of pheochromocytoma.

CLOSTRIDIUM DIFFICILE TOXIN ASSAY (stool)

Normal: Negative
Detected in: Antibiotic-associated diarrhea and pseudomembranous colitis

CO

See "CARBOXYHEMOGLOBIN"

COAGULATION FACTORS

A differential diagnosis of abnormal coagulation screening tests is described in Table 34.
See Table E35 for characteristics of coagulation factors.
See Table E36 for differential diagnosis of low factor VIII.

Factor reference ranges:
V: >10%
VII: >10%
VIII: 50% to 170%
IX: 60% to 136%
X: >10%
XI: 50% to 150%
XII: >30%
Table E37 describes screening laboratory results in coagulation factor deficiencies. Characterization of coagulation factors and their deficiencies is summarized in Table E38.

COBALAMIN, SERUM

See "VITAMIN B12"

COLD AGGLUTININS TITER

Normal range: <1:32
Elevated in
Primary atypical pneumonia (*Mycoplasma* pneumonia), infectious mononucleosis, CMV infection
Others: Hepatic cirrhosis, acquired hemolytic anemia, frostbite, multiple myeloma, lymphoma, malaria

COMPLEMENT

Inherited deficiencies in complement and complement-related proteins are summarized in Table E39.

TABLE 34 Differential Diagnosis of Abnormal Coagulation Screening Tests

IV

Abnormal Activated Partial Thromboplastin Time (APTT) Alone

Associated with bleeding: VIII, IX, and XI defects

Not associated with bleeding: XII, prekallikrein (PK), high molecular weight kininogen, lupus anticoagulants

Abnormal Prothrombin Time (PT) Alone

Factor VII defects

Combined Abnormal APTT and PT

Medical conditions: Anticoagulants, disseminated intravascular coagulation (DIC), liver disease, vitamin K deficiency, massive transfusion

Rarely dysfibrinogenemia; factor X, V, and II defects

From McPherson RA, Pincus MR: *Henry's clinical diagnosis and management by laboratory methods,* ed 23, St Louis, 2017, Elsevier.

BOX 13 Definitions

Classical pathway: C1, C4, C2, C3, and the terminal components.

Alternative pathway: Factor B, factor D, properdin, and the terminal components.

Lectin activation pathway: MBL, MASP1, MASP2, C3, and the terminal components.

Anaphylatoxins: C3a, C4a, C5a. These are mediators of smooth muscle contraction, degranulation of mast cells, enhanced neutrophil aggregation, increased vascular permeability.

Opsonization: Renders a particle more easily phagocytosed

C3 tickover: This term occasionally is used to describe spontaneous C3 hydrolysis.

Membrane attack complex (terminal components): C5, C6, C7, C8, C9

CH50: Used to define the dilution of serum capable of lysing 50% of sensitized sheep red cells. This assay measures the intactness of the classical pathway through the terminal components.

AH50: Used to define the dilution of serum capable of lysing 50% of non-sensitized rabbit red cells. This assay measures the intactness of the alternative pathway through the terminal components.

From Adkinson NF et al: *Middleton's allergy principles and practice*, ed 8, Philadelphia, 2014, Saunders.

Normal range
C3: 70 to 160 mg/dl (0.7 to 1.6 g/L [CF: 0.01; SMI: 0.1 g/L])
C4: 20 to 40 mg/dl (0.2 to 0.4 g/L [CF: 0.01; SMI: 0.1 g/L])
Abnormal values:
Decreased C3: Active SLE, immune complex disease, acute glomerulonephritis, inborn C3 deficiency, membranoproliferative glomerulonephritis, infective endocarditis, serum sickness, autoimmune/chronic active hepatitis
Decreased C4: Immune complex disease, active SLE, infective endocarditis, inborn C4 deficiency, hereditary angioedema, hypergammaglobulinemic states, cryoglobulinemic vasculitis
NOTE: The complement system has daunting nomenclature; accordingly, some basic definitions are given in Box 13.

COMPLETE BLOOD COUNT (CBC)

Common types of anemias and their diagnostic workups are summarized in Table 40.

See Fig. E18, which describes an algorithm for the evaluation of patients with neutropenia.

White blood cells 3200 to 9800/mm^3 (3.2 to 9.8 × 10^9/L [CF: 0.001; SMI: 0.1 × 10^9/L])
Red blood cells
Male: 4.3 to 5.9 × 10^6/mm^3 (4.3 to 5.9 × 10^{12}/L [CF: 0.001; SMI: 0.1 × 10^{12}/L])
Female: 3.5 to 5 × 10^6/mm^3 (3.5 to 5 × 10^{12}/L [CF: 0.001; SMI: 0.1 × 10^{12}/L])
Hemoglobin
Male: 13.6 to 17.7 g/dl (136 to 172 g/L [CF: 10; SMI: 1 g/L])
Female: 12 to 15 g/dl (120 to 150 g/L [CF: 10; SMI: 1 g/L])
Hematocrit
Male: 39% to 49% (0.39 to 0.49 [CF: 0.01; SMI: 0.01])
Female: 33% to 43% (0.33 to 0.43 [CF: 0.01; SMI: 0.01])
Mean corpuscular volume (MCV): 76 to 100 μm^3 (76 to 100 fL [CF: 1; SMI: 1 fL])
Mean corpuscular hemoglobin (MCH): 27 to 33 pg (27 to 33 pg [CF: 1; SMI: 1 pg])
Mean corpuscular hemoglobin concentration (MCHC): 33 to 37 g/dl (330 to 370 g/L [CF: 10; SMI: 10 g/L])
Red blood cell distribution width index (RDW): 11.5% to 14.5%
Platelet count: 130 to 400 × 10^3/mm^3 (130-400 × 10^9/L [CF: 1; SMI: 5 × 10^9/L])
Differential:

TABLE 40 Common Types of Anemias and Their Diagnostic Workups*

Anemia	Cause	Common Analyte Abnormality
Hypoproliferative, microcytic	Iron deficiency	Low ferritin Increased IBC Decreased serum iron Reduced Fe/TIBC ratio Generally increased RDW
Hypoproliferative, microcytic	Anemia of chronic disease	Generally high ferritin Normal IBC Decreased serum iron Normal Fe/TIBC ratio Generally normal RDW
Hyperproliferative, normocytic	Hemolytic anemia	Schistocytosis Increased reticulocytes Low haptoglobin Elevated carboxyhemoglobin Elevated LD and potassium Elevated indirect bilirubin Generally increased RDW
Hypoproliferative, normocytic	Aplastic anemia	Leukopenia Thrombocytopenia Hypocellular bone marrow Generally normal RDW
Hypoproliferative, normocytic	Renal failure	Elevated BUN and creatinine Low erythropoietin Burr cells may be present Generally normal RDW
Hypoproliferative, macrocytic		
Megaloblastic	Vitamin B$_{12}$ and/or folate deficiency	Low vitamin B$_{12}$ and/or folate Hyperlobulated polymorphonuclear leukocytes Macro-ovalocytes Increased RDW
Nonmegaloblastic	Hypothyroidism	Elevated TSH Normal RDW

*Low is equivalent to depressed, and high is equivalent to elevated. Ferritin, haptoglobin, LD, bilirubin, BUN, creatinine, erythropoietin, TSH, and T4 are all expressed as concentrations. All of these analytes are measured in serum.

BUN, Blood urea nitrogen; *Fe*, iron; *IBC*, iron-binding capacity; *LD*, lactate dehydrogenase; *RDW*, red cell distribution width; *TIBC*, total IBC; *TSH*, thyroid-stimulating hormone.

From McPherson RA, Pincus MR: *Henry's clinical diagnosis and management by laboratory methods*, ed 23, St Louis, 2017, Elsevier.

2 to 6 stabs (bands, early mature neutrophils)
60 to 70 segs (mature neutrophils)
1 to 4 eosinophils
0 to 1 basophils
2 to 8 monocytes
25 to 40 lymphocytes

CONJUGATED BILIRUBIN

See "BILIRUBIN, DIRECT"

COPPER (serum)

Normal range: 70 to 140 μg/dl (11 to 22 μmol/L [CF: 0.1574, SMI: 0.2 μmol/L])

Decreased in: Wilson disease, Menkes syndrome, malabsorption, malnutrition, nephrosis, total parenteral nutrition, acute leukemia in remission
Elevated in: Aplastic anemia, biliary cirrhosis, systemic lupus erythematosus, hemochromatosis, hyperthyroidism, hypothyroidism, infection, iron deficiency anemia, leukemia, lymphoma, oral contraceptives, pernicious anemia, rheumatoid arthritis

COPPER, URINE

See "URINE COPPER"

CORTICOTROPIN RELEASING HORMONE (CRH) STIMULATION TEST

Normal: A dose of 0.5 mg of dexamethasone is given every 6 h for 2 days; 2 h after last dose 1 mcg/kg CRH is given IV. Samples are drawn after 15 min. Normally there is a twofold to fourfold increase in mean baseline concentration of ACTH or cortisol. Cortisol >1.4 mcg/L is virtually 100% specific and 100% diagnostic.

Interpretation of results:

Normal or exaggerated response: Pituitary Cushing disease

No response: Ectopic ACTH-secreting tumor

A positive response to CRH or a suppressed response to high-dose dexamethasone has a 97% positive predictive value for Cushing disease. However, a lack of response to either test excludes Cushing disease in only 64% to 78% of patients. When the tests are considered together, negative responses from both have a 100% predictive value for ectopic ACTH secretion.

CORTISOL, PLASMA

Normal range:

Varies with time of collection (circadian variation):

8 A.M.: 4 to 19 μg/dl (110 to 520 nmol/L [CF: 27.59; SMI: 10 nmol/L])

4 P.M.: 2 to 15 μg/dl (50 to 410 nmol/L [CF: 27.59; SMI: 10 nmol/L])

Elevated in: Ectopic adrenocorticotropic hormone production (i.e., oat cell carcinoma of lung), loss of normal diurnal variation, pregnancy, chronic renal failure, iatrogenic, stress, adrenal or pituitary hyperplasia, or adenomas

Decreased in: Primary adrenocortical insufficiency, anterior pituitary hypofunction, secondary adrenocortical insufficiency, adrenogenital syndromes

COOMBS DIRECT

See "DIRECT ANTIGLOBULIN"

COOMBS INDIRECT

See "INDIRECT ANTIGLOBULIN"

COVID-19

Name: Coronavirus

Value: Not detected

Reference range: Not detected

A Not Detected (negative) test result for this test means that SARS-CoV-2 RNA was not present in the specimen above the limit of detection. A negative test does not rule out the possibility of COVID-19 and should not be used as the sole basis for treatment or patient management decisions. If COVID-19 is still suspected, based on exposure history together with other clinical findings, re-testing should be considered in consultation with public health authorities.

Laboratory test results should always be considered in the context of clinical observations and epidemiologic data in making a final diagnosis and patient management decisions.

C-PEPTIDE

Elevated in: Insulinoma, sulfonylurea administration

Decreased in: Insulin-dependent diabetes mellitus, factitious insulin administration

CPK

See "CREATINE KINASE"

C-REACTIVE PROTEIN

Normal range: 6.8 to 820 μg/dl (68 to 8200 μg/L [CF: 10; SMI: 10 μg/L])

Elevated in: Rheumatoid arthritis, rheumatic fever, inflammatory bowel disease, bacterial infections, myocardial infarction, oral contraceptives, third trimester of pregnancy (acute phase reactant), inflammatory and neoplastic diseases. Table 41 shows a comparison of erythrocyte sedimentation rate and C-reactive protein, and Table 42 shows conditions associated with elevated C-reactive protein levels.

TABLE 41 Comparison of Erythrocyte Sedimentation Rate and C-Reactive Protein

	Erythrocyte Sedimentation Rate	C-Reactive Protein
Advantages	Much clinical information in the literature. May reflect overall health status	Rapid response to inflammatory stimuli. Wide range of clinically relevant values are detectable Unaffected by age and gender Reflects value of a single acute phase protein Can be measured on stored sera Quantitation is precise and reproducible
Disadvantages	Affected by age and gender Affected by red blood cell morphology Affected by anemia and polycythemia Reflects levels of many plasma proteins, not all of which are acute phase proteins Responds slowly to inflammatory stimuli Requires fresh sample May be affected by drugs	None

From Firestein GS et al: *Kelley's textbook of rheumatology*, ed 9, Philadelphia, 2013, Saunders.

TABLE 42 Conditions Associated With Elevated C-Reactive Protein Levels

Normal or Minor Elevation (<1 mg/dl)	Moderate Elevation (1-10 mg/dl)	Marked Elevation (>10 mg/dl)
Vigorous exercise	Myocardial infarction	Acute bacterial infection (80%-85%)
Common cold	Malignancies	
Pregnancy	Pancreatitis	Major trauma
Gingivitis	Mucosal infection (bronchitis, cystitis)	Systemic vasculitis
Seizures		
Depression	Most connective tissue diseases	
Insulin resistance and diabetes	Rheumatoid arthritis	
Several genetic polymorphisms		
Obesity		

From Firestein GS et al: *Kelley's textbook of rheumatology*, ed 9, Philadelphia, 2013, Saunders.

C-REACTIVE PROTEIN, HIGH SENSITIVITY (hs-CRP, cardio-CRP)

This is a cardiac risk marker. It is increased in patients with silent atherosclerosis years before a cardiovascular event and is independent of cholesterol level and other lipoproteins. It can be used to help stratify cardiac risk.

Interpretation of Results

Cardio-CRP result (mg/L)	Risk
0.6	Lowest risk
0.7-1.1	Low risk
1.2-1.9	Moderate risk
2.0-3.8	High risk
3.9-4.9	Highest risk
≥5.0	Results may be confounded by acute inflammatory disease. If clinically indicated, a repeat test should be performed in 2 or more wk

Laboratory Tests

IV

CREATINE KINASE (CK, CPK)

Fig. E19 describes a diagnostic approach to creatine kinase elevation.

Normal range: 0 to 130 U/L (0 to 2.16 μkat/L [CF: 0.01667; SMI: 0.01 μkat/L])

Elevated in: Myocardial infarction, myocarditis, rhabdomyolysis, myositis, crush injury/trauma, polymyositis, dermatomyositis, vigorous exercise, muscular dystrophy, myxedema, seizures, malignant hyperthermia syndrome, intramuscular (IM) injections, cerebrovascular accident, pulmonary embolism and infarction, acute dissection of aorta

Decreased in: Corticosteroid use, decreased muscle mass, connective tissue disorders, alcoholic liver disease, metastatic neoplasms

CREATINE KINASE ISOENZYMES

CK-BB

Elevated in: Cerebrovascular accident, subarachnoid hemorrhage, neoplasms (prostate, gastrointestinal tract, brain, ovary, breast, lung), severe shock, bowel infarction, hypothermia, meningitis

CK-MB

Elevated in: Myocardial infarction (MI), myocarditis, pericarditis, muscular dystrophy, cardiac defibrillation, cardiac surgery, extensive rhabdomyolysis, strenuous exercise (marathon runners), mixed connective tissue disease, cardiomyopathy, hypothermia

NOTE: CK-MB exists in the blood in two subforms. MB_2 is released from cardiac cells and converted in the blood to MB_1. Rapid assay of CK-MB subforms can detect MI (CK-$MB_2 \geq 1.0$ U/L, with a ratio of CK-MB_2/CK-$MB_1 \geq 1.5$) within 6 h of onset of symptoms.

Fig. E20 illustrates the time course of CK, AST, troponins, and lactate dehydrogenase (LDH) activity after acute MI.

CK-MM

Elevated in: Crush injury, seizures, malignant hyperthermia syndrome, rhabdomyolysis, myositis, polymyositis, dermatomyositis, vigorous exercise, muscular dystrophy, IM injections, acute dissection of aorta

CREATININE (serum)

Normal range: 0.6 to 1.2 mg/dl (50 to 110 μmol/L [CF: 88.4; SMI: 10 μmol/L]). Fig. E21 illustrates the relationship between creatinine clearance and serum creatinine. Factors that may alter serum creatinine level are described in Box 14.

Elevated in: Renal insufficiency (acute and chronic), decreased renal perfusion (hypotension, dehydration, congestive heart failure), urinary tract infection, rhabdomyolysis, ketonemia

---

BOX 14 Factors That May Alter Serum Creatinine (Cr) Level

Endogenous
Reduced muscle mass: ↓
Hyperbilirubinemia: ↓

Exogenous
Medications inhibiting tubular secretion (trimethoprim, cimetidine): ↑

Medications Interfering with Laboratory Assays*
Flucytosine and cefoxitin: ↑
Catecholamines: ↓

*Varies by assay type used.
From Parrillo JE, Dellinger RP: *Critical care medicine, principles of diagnosis and management in the adult*, ed 4, Philadelphia, 2014, Elsevier.

BOX 15 Cockcroft-Gault Formula to Calculate Creatinine Clearance (C_{cr})

$$C_{cr} = \frac{(140 - \text{age in ear}) \times (\text{lean body weight in kg})}{S_{cr} \text{in mg/dl} - 72}$$

Drugs (antibiotics [aminoglycosides, cephalosporins], hydantoin, diuretics, methyldopa)

The RIFLE criteria for acute kidney injury is summarized in Table E43. A classification of acute kidney injury (AKI) is described in Table E44.

Falsely elevated in: Diabetic ketoacidosis, administration of some cephalosporins (e.g., cefoxitin, cephalothin)

Decreased in: Decreased muscle mass (including amputees and older persons), pregnancy, prolonged debilitation

CREATININE CLEARANCE

Normal range:
75 to 124 ml/min (1.24 to 2.08 ml/sec [CF: 0.01667; SMI: 0.02 ml/sec])
Table E45 shows equations commonly used to estimate renal clearance.

The Cockcroft-Gault formula to calculate creatinine clearance is described in Box 15.

Elevated in:
Pregnancy, exercise

Decreased in:
Renal insufficiency, drugs (cimetidine, procainamide, antibiotics, quinidine)

CREATININE, URINE

See "URINE CREATININE"

CRYOGLOBULINS (serum)

Normal range: Not detectable
Present in: Collagen vascular diseases, chronic lymphocytic leukemia, hemolytic anemias, multiple myeloma, Waldenström macroglobulinemia, chronic active hepatitis, Hodgkin disease

CRYPTOSPORIDIUM ANTIGEN BY EIA (stool)

Normal range: Not detected
Present in: Cryptosporidiosis

CSF

See "CEREBROSPINAL FLUID"

CYSTATIN C

Normal: Cystatin C is a cysteine protease inhibitor that is produced at a constant rate by all nucleated cells. It is freely filtered by the glomerulus and reabsorbed (but not secreted) by the renal tubules with no extrarenal excretion. Its concentration is not affected by diet, muscle mass, or acute inflammation. Normal range when measured by particle-enhanced nephelometric immunoassay (PENIA) is <0.28 mg/L.

Elevated in: Renal disorders. Good predictor of the severity of acute tubular necrosis. Cystatin C increases more rapidly than creatinine in the early stages of GFR impairment. The cystatin C concentration is an independent risk factor for heart failure in older adults and appears to provide a better measure of risk assessment than the serum creatinine concentration.

CYSTIC FIBROSIS PCR

Test description: Test can be performed on whole blood or tissue. Common mutations in the cystic fibrosis transmembrane regulator (CFTR) gene can be used to detect 75% to 80% of mutant alleles.

CYTOMEGALOVIRUS BY PCR

Test description: Test can be performed on whole blood, plasma, or tissue. Qualitative PCR is highly sensitive but may not be able to differentiate between latent and active infection.

D-DIMER

Normal range: <0.5 mcg/ml
Elevated in:
DVT, pulmonary embolism, high levels of rheumatoid factor, activation of coagulation and fibrolytic system from any cause
D-dimer assay by enzyme-linked immunosorbent assay (ELISA) assists in the diagnosis of DVT and pulmonary embolism. This test has significant limitations because it can be elevated whenever the coagulation and fibrinolytic systems are activated and can also be falsely elevated with high rheumatoid factor levels.
A positive D-dimer is suggestive but not diagnostic for pulmonary embolism (PE). Patients with positive D-dimer and clinical suspicion for PE need additional tests such as chest CT to confirm diagnosis.
PE might be ruled out in patients with negative D-dimer and low pretest probability for PE.

DEHYDROEPIANDROSTERONE SULFATE

Normal:

Males:

Ages 19-30:	125-619 mcg/dl
31-50:	59-452 mcg/dl
51-60:	20-413 mcg/dl
61-83:	10-285 mcg/dl

Females:

Ages 19-30:	29-781 mcg/dl
31-50:	12-379 mcg/dl
Postmenopausal:	30-260 mcg/dl

Elevated in: Hirsutism, congenital adrenal hyperplasia, adrenal carcinomas, adrenal adenomas, polycystic ovary syndrome, ectopic ACTH-producing tumors, Cushing disease, spironolactone

DIHYDROTESTOSTERONE (serum, urine)

Normal: Serum: Males: 30 to 85 ng/dl; females: 4 to 22 ng/dl
Urine, 24 h: Males: 20 to 50 mcg/day; females: <8 mcg/day
Elevated in: Hirsutism
Decreased in: 5-α-reductase deficiency, hypogonadism

DEOXYCORTICOSTERONE (11-deoxycorticosterone, DOC) (serum)

Normal: 2 to 19 ng/dl. Normal secretion depends on ACTH and is suppressible by dexamethasone.
Elevated in: Adrenogenital syndromes due to 17- and 11-hydroxylase deficiencies, pregnancy
Decreased in: Preeclampsia

DEXAMETHASONE SUPPRESSION TEST, OVERNIGHT

Normal: Test is performed by giving 1 mg dexamethasone orally at 11 P.M. and measuring serum cortisol at 8 A.M. the following morning. Normal response is cortisol suppression to <3 mcg/dl; if dose of 4 mg dexamethasone is given, cortisol suppression will be to <50% of baseline.

Interpretation of results: Cushing syndrome (<10 mcg/dl), endogenous depression (half of patients suppress test values <5 mcg/dl). Most patients with pituitary Cushing disease demonstrate suppression, whereas patients with adrenal adenoma, carcinoma, and ectopic ACTH-producing tumors do not.

DIGOXIN

Normal therapeutic range: 0.5 to 2 ng/ml
Elevated in: Impaired renal function, excessive dosing, concomitant use of quinidine, amiodarone, verapamil, fluoxetine, nifedipine. Toxicity may occur at a lower blood concentration in the presence of hypokalemia, hypomagnesemia, and hypercalcemia. See Table E46.

DIGOXIN LEVEL

Therapeutic range and general information are summarized in Table 47.

DILANTIN

See "PHENYTOIN"

DIRECT ANTIGLOBULIN (Coombs Direct)

Normal: Negative
Positive: Autoimmune hemolytic anemia, erythroblastosis fetalis, transfusion reactions, drugs (α-methyldopa, penicillins, tetracycline, sulfonamides, levodopa, cephalosporins, quinidine, insulin)
False positive: May be seen with cold agglutinins

DISACCHARIDE ABSORPTION TESTS

Normal: Test is used to diagnose malabsorption due to disaccharide deficiency. It is performed by giving disaccharide orally 1 g/kg body weight to a total of 25 g. Blood is drawn at 0, 30, 60, 90, and 120 min. Normal response is a change in glucose from fasting value >30 mg/dl, inconclusive when increase is 20 to 30 mg/dl, abnormal when increase is >20 mg/dl. Test can also be performed by measuring air at 0, 30, 60, 90, and 120 min. Normal is H_2>20 ppm above baseline level before a colonic response.
Decreased in: Disaccharide deficiency (lactose, fructose, sorbitol), celiac disease, sprue, acute gastroenteritis

DOC

See "DEOXYCORTICOSTERONE"

TABLE 47	Digoxin
Purpose	**Treatment of Congestive Heart Failure and Atrial Fibrillation-Flutter**
General adult dose	Oral: 0.75-1.5 mg for digitalization, 0.125-0.5 mg/day for maintenance
Usual bioavailability	Approximately 60%-85% for tablet or elixir; 90%-100% for liquid-filled capsules
Half-life	Approximately 35-40 hr; however, prolonged in patients with decreased renal function
General therapeutic range	0.5-2 ng/ml
General toxic level	>2 ng/ml, but somewhat variable
Transport	Approximately 20%-25% plasma protein bound
Metabolism	Generally, only small amounts are metabolized (liver, lumen of large intestine)
Elimination	Approximately 50%-75% unchanged in urine
Steady state	Approximately 7 days in undigitalized patients with normal renal function
Mechanism of action	Causes release of calcium ions in T-system of myocardium; slows AV node conduction
Toxic effects	Gastric disturbances, nausea, vomiting, atrial and ventricular arrhythmias, irregular pulse

AV, Atrioventricular.
From McPherson RA, Pincus MR: *Henry's clinical diagnosis and management by laboratory methods,* ed 23, St Louis, 2017, Elsevier.

Laboratory Tests

IV

DONATH-LANDSTEINER (D-L) TEST FOR PAROXYSMAL COLD HEMOGLOBINURIA

Normal: No hemolysis
Interpretation of results: Hemolysis indicates presence of bithermic cold hemolysins or Donath-Landsteiner antibodies (D-L Ab)

DOPAMINE

Normal range: 175 pg/ml
Elevated in: Pheochromocytomas, neuroblastomas, stress, vigorous exercise, certain foods (bananas, chocolate, coffee, tea, vanilla)

D-XYLOSE ABSORPTION

Normal range: 21% to 31% excreted in 5 h
Decreased in: Malabsorption syndrome

D-XYLOSE ABSORPTION TEST

Normal range: URINE: ≥4 g/5 h (5-h urine collection in adults >12 y [25-g dose])
  SERUM: ≥25 mg/dl (adult, 1 h, 25-g dose, normal renal function)
Normal results: In patients with malabsorption, normal results suggest pancreatic disease as an etiology of the malabsorption.
Abnormal results: Celiac disease, Crohn disease, tropical sprue, surgical bowel resection, AIDS. False positives can occur with decreased renal function, dehydration/hypovolemia, surgical blind loops, decreased gastric emptying, vomiting.

ELECTROPHORESIS, HEMOGLOBIN

See "HEMOGLOBIN ELECTROPHORESIS"

ELECTROPHORESIS, PROTEIN

See "PROTEIN ELECTROPHORESIS"

ENA COMPLEX

See "EXTRACTABLE NUCLEAR ANTIGEN"

ENDOMYSIAL ANTIBODIES

Normal: Not detected
Present in: Celiac disease, dermatitis herpetiformis

EOSINOPHIL COUNT

Normal range: 1% to 4% eosinophils (0 to 440/mm^3)
Elevated in: HELMINTHIC PARASITE
Ascaris lumbricoides (invasive larval stage)
Hookworms (invasive larval stage)
Strongyloides stercoralis (initial infection and autoinfection)
Trichinosis
Filariasis
Echinococcus granulosus and *E. multilocularis*
Toxocara species
Animal hookworms
Angiostrongylus cantonensis and *A. costaricensis*
Schistosomiasis
Liver flukes
Fasciolopsis buski
Anisakiasis
Capillaria philippinensis
Paragonimus westermani
"Tropical eosinophilia" (unidentified microfilariae)
NOTE: Table E48 describes an approach to investigation of eosinophilia in returning travelers.

OTHER INFECTIONS/INFESTATIONS
Pulmonary aspergillosis
Severe scabies

ALLERGIES
Asthma
Hay fever
Drug reactions
Atopic dermatitis
AUTOIMMUNE AND RELATED DISORDERS
Polyarteritis nodosa
Necrotizing vasculitis
Eosinophilic fasciitis
Pemphigus
NEOPLASTIC DISEASES
Hodgkin disease
Mycosis fungoides
Chronic myelocytic leukemia
Eosinophilic leukemia
Polycythemia vera
Mucin-secreting adenocarcinomas
IMMUNODEFICIENCY STATES
Hyperimmunoglobulin E with recurrent infection
Wiskott-Aldrich syndrome
OTHER
Addison disease
Inflammatory bowel disease
Dermatitis herpetiformis
Toxic/chemical syndrome
Eosinophilic myalgia syndrome, tryptophan, toxic oil syndrome
Hypereosinophilic syndrome (unknown etiology)
Fig. E22 describes an algorithm for patients with eosinophil disorders.
Table E49 describes hematopoietic neoplasms accompanied by eosinophilia.
Table E50 describes the differential diagnosis of childhood eosinophilia.

EPINEPHRINE, PLASMA

Normal range: 0 to 90 pg/ml
Elevated in: Pheochromocytomas, neuroblastomas, stress, vigorous exercise, certain foods (bananas, chocolate, coffee, tea, vanilla), hypoglycemia (Box E16)

EPSTEIN-BARR VIRUS SEROLOGY

Normal range: IgG antiviral capsid antigen (VCA) <1:10 or negative
Abnormal: IgG anti-VCA >1:10 or positive indicates either current or previous infection.
  IgM anti-VCA >1:10 or positive indicates current or recent infection.
  Anti-Epstein-Barr virus nuclear antigen (EBNA) ≥1.5 or positive indicates previous infection.
  Table E51 and Fig. 23 describe test interpretation.

ERYTHROCYTE SEDIMENTATION RATE (ESR, sed rate, sedimentation rate)

See Table E52 for erythrocyte sedimentation rate ranges in health.

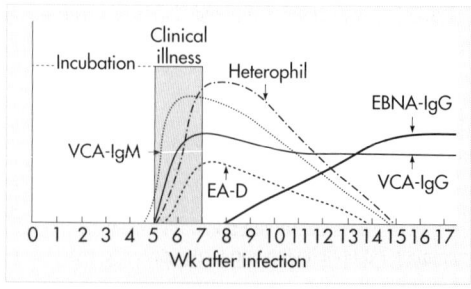

FIG. 23 Tests in Epstein-Barr viral infection. See Table E51 for abbreviations.

Normal range
Male: 0 to 15 mm/h
Female: 0 to 20 mm/h
Elevated in: Collagen vascular diseases, infections, myocardial infarction, neoplasms, inflammatory states (acute phase reactant), hyperthyroidism, hypothyroidism, rouleaux formation
Decreased in: Sickle cell disease, polycythemia, corticosteroids, spherocytosis, anisocytosis, hypofibrinogenemia, increased serum viscosity

ERYTHROPOIETIN (EP)

Normal: 3.7 to 16.0 IU/L by radioimmunoassay
Erythropoietin is a glycoprotein secreted by the kidneys that stimulates RBC production by acting on erythroid-committed stem cells.
Increased in

- **Extremely high:** Generally seen in patients with severe anemia (Hct, <25; Hb<7) such as in cases of aplastic anemia, severe hemolytic anemia, hematologic cancers
- **Very high:** Patients with mild to moderate anemia (Hct, 25 to 35; Hb, 7 to 10)
- **High:** Patients with mild anemia (e.g., AIDS, myelodysplasia)
Erythropoietin can be inappropriately elevated in patients with malignant neoplasms, renal cysts, postrenal transplant, meningioma, hemangioblastoma, and leiomyoma.
Decreased in: Renal failure, polycythemia vera, autonomic neuropathy

ESTRADIOL (serum)

Normal range: Female, premenopausal: 30 to 400 pg/ml, depending on phase of menstrual cycle
Female, postmenopausal: 0 to 30 pg/ml
Male, adult: 10 to 50 pg/ml
Decreased in: Ovarian failure
Elevated in: Tumors of ovary, testis, adrenal, or nonendocrine sites (rare)

ESTROGEN

Normal range (serum):

Males:	20-80 pg/ml
Females:	
Follicular:	60-200 pg/ml
Luteal:	160-400 pg/ml
Postmenopausal:	<130 pg/ml

Normal range (urine):

Males:	4-23 μg/g creatinine
Females:	
Follicular:	7-65 μg/g creatinine
Midcycle:	32-104 μg/g creatinine
Luteal:	8-135 μg/g creatinine

Elevated in: Hyperplasia of adrenal cortex, ovarian tumors producing estrogen, granulosa and thecal cell tumors, testicular tumors
Decreased in: Menopause, hypopituitarism, primary ovarian malfunction, anorexia nervosa, hypofunction of adrenal cortex, ovarian agenesis, psychogenic stress, gonadotropin-releasing hormone deficiency

ETHANOL (blood)

Normal range
Negative (values <10 mg/dl are considered negative)
Ethanol is metabolized at 10 to 25 mg/dl/h. Levels ≥80 mg/dl are considered evidence of impairment for driving. Fatal blood concentration is considered to be >400 mg/dl. Table E53 summarizes the influence of acute ethanol ingestion on ethanol levels and behavior.

EXTRACTABLE NUCLEAR ANTIGEN (ENA complex, anti-RNP antibody, anti-sm, anti-Smith)

Normal: Negative
Present in: Systemic lupus erythematosus, rheumatoid arthritis, Sjögren syndrome, mixed connective tissue disease

FACTOR V LEIDEN

Test Description: PCR test performed on whole blood or tissue. This single mutation, found in 2% to 8% of the general Caucasian population, is the single most common cause of hereditary thrombophilia.

FASTING BLOOD SUGAR

See "GLUCOSE, FASTING"

FBS

See "GLUCOSE, FASTING"

FDP

See "FIBRIN DEGRADATION PRODUCT"

FECAL FAT, QUANTITATIVE (72-h collection)

Normal range: 2 to 6 g/24 h (7 to 21 mmol/dl [CF: 3.515; SMI: 1 mmol/dl])
Elevated in: Malabsorption syndrome

FECAL GLOBIN IMMUNOCHEMICAL TEST

Normal: Negative. This test is performed by immunochromatography on a cellulose strip that has been impregnated with various antibodies. The test uses a small amount of toilet water as the specimen and is placed onto absorbent pads of card similar to traditional occult blood (OB) card. There is no direct handling of stool. This test is specific for the globin portion of the hemoglobin molecule, which confers lower GI bleeding specificity. It specifically detects blood from the lower GI tract; guaiac tests are not lower GI specific. It is more sensitive than typical Hemoccult test (detection limit 50 mcg Hb/g feces versus >500 mcg Hb/g feces for Hemoccult). It has no dietary restrictions and gives no false positives due to plant peroxidases and red meats. It has no medication restrictions. Iron supplements and NSAIDs do not cause false positives. Vitamin C does not cause false negatives.
Positive in: Lower GI bleeding

FERRITIN (serum)

Normal range: 18 to 300 ng/ml (18 to 300 μg/L [CF: 1; SMI: 10 μg/L])
Elevated in: Hyperthyroidism, inflammatory states, liver disease (ferritin elevated from necrotic hepatocytes), neoplasms (neuroblastomas, lymphomas, leukemia, breast carcinoma), iron replacement therapy, hemochromatosis, hemosiderosis. Table E54 summarizes hereditary iron overload disorders.
Decreased in: Iron deficiency anemia

α-1 FETOPROTEIN

Normal range: 0 to 20 ng/ml (0 to 20 μg/L [CF: 1; SMI: 1 μg/L])
Elevated in: Hepatocellular carcinoma (usually values >1000 ng/ml), germinal neoplasms (testis, ovary, mediastinum, retroperitoneum), liver disease (alcoholic cirrhosis, acute hepatitis, chronic active hepatitis), fetal anencephaly, spina bifida, basal cell carcinoma, breast carcinoma, pancreatic carcinoma, gastric carcinoma, retinoblastoma, esophageal atresia

FIBRIN DEGRADATION PRODUCT (FDP)

Normal range: <10 μg/ml
Elevated in: Disseminated intravascular coagulation, primary fibrinolysis, pulmonary embolism, severe liver disease
NOTE: The presence of rheumatoid factor may cause falsely elevated FDP.

FIBRINOGEN

Normal range: 200 to 400 mg/dl (2 to 4 g/L [CF: 0.01; SMI: 0.1 g/L])
Elevated in: Tissue inflammation or damage (acute phase protein reactant), oral contraceptives, pregnancy, acute infection, myocardial infarction

Decreased in: Disseminated intravascular coagulation, hereditary afibrinogenemia, liver disease, primary or secondary fibrinolysis, cachexia

FOLATE (folic acid)

Normal range: Plasma: 2 to 10 ng/ml (4 to 22 nmol/L [CF: 2.266; SMI: 2 nmol/L])

Red blood cells: 140 to 960 ng/ml (550 to 2200 nmol/L [CF: 2.266; SMI: 10 nmol/L])

Decreased in: Folic acid deficiency (inadequate intake, malabsorption), alcoholism, drugs (methotrexate, trimethoprim, phenytoin, oral contraceptives, Azulfidine), vitamin B_{12} deficiency (defective red cell folate absorption), hemolytic anemia. Box E17 summarizes an etiophysiologic classification of folate deficiency.

Elevated in: Folic acid therapy

FOLLICLE-STIMULATING HORMONE (FSH)

Normal range: 5 to 20 mIU/ml

Elevated in: Menopause, primary gonadal failure, alcoholism, castration, Klinefelter syndrome, gonadotropin-secreting pituitary hormones

Decreased in: Pregnancy, polycystic ovary disease, anorexia nervosa, anterior pituitary hypofunction

FREE T_4

See "T_4, FREE"

FREE THYROXINE INDEX

Normal range: 1.1 to 4.3
INCREASED THYROXINE OR FREE THYROXINE VALUES
Laboratory error
Primary hyperthyroidism (T_4/T_3 type)
Severe thyroxine-binding globulin elevation
Excess therapy of hypothyroidism
Excessive dose of levothyroxine
Active thyroiditis (subacute, painless, early active Hashimoto disease)
Familial dysalbuminemic hyperthyroxinemia (some FT_4 kits, especially analog types)
Peripheral resistance to T_4 syndrome
Amiodarone or propranolol
Postpartum transient toxicosis
Factitious hyperthyroidism
Jod-Basedow (iodine-induced) hyperthyroidism
Severe nonthyroid illness
Acute psychosis (especially paranoid schizophrenia)
T_4 sample drawn 2 to 4 h after levothyroxine dose
Struma ovarii
Pituitary thyroid-stimulating hormone-secreting tumor
Certain x-ray contrast media (Telepaque and Oragrafin)
Acute porphyria
Heparin effect (some T_4 and FT_4 kits)
Amphetamine, heroin, methadone, and phencyclidine abuse
Perphenazine or 5-fluorouracil
Antithyroid or anti-IgG heterophil (HAMA) autoantibodies
"T_4" hyperthyroidism
Hyperemesis gravidarum; about 50% of patients
High altitudes
DECREASED THYROXINE OR FREE THYROXINE VALUES
Laboratory error
Primary hypothyroidism
Severe nonthyroid illness
Lithium therapy
Severe thyroxine-binding globulin decrease (congenital, disease, or drug-induced) or severe albumin decrease
Dilantin, Depakene, or high-dose salicylate drugs
Pituitary insufficiency
Large doses of inorganic iodide (e.g., saturated solution of potassium iodide)
Moderate or severe iodine deficiency
Cushing syndrome

High-dose glucocorticoid drugs
Pregnancy, third trimester (low normal or small decrease)
Addison disease; some patients (30%)
Heparin effect (a few FT_4 kits)
Desipramine or amiodarone drugs
Acute psychiatric illness

FTA-ABS (serum)

Normal: Nonreactive
Reactive in: Syphilis, other treponemal diseases (yaws, pinta, bejel), SLE, pregnancy

FUROSEMIDE STIMULATION TEST

Normal: Test is performed by giving 60 mg furosemide orally after overnight fast. Patient should be on a normal diet without medications the wk before the test. Normal results: Renin 1 to 6 ng angiotensin L/ml/h.

Elevated in: Renovascular hypertension, Bartter syndrome, high-renin essential hypertension, pheochromocytoma

No Response in: Primary aldosteronism, low-renin essential hypertension, hyporeninemic hypoaldosteronism

GAMMA-GLUTAMYL TRANSFERASE (GGT)

See "γ-GLUTAMYL TRANSFERASE"

GASTRIN (serum)

Normal range: 0 to 180 pg/ml (0 to 180 ng/L [CF: 1; SMI: 10 ng/L])

Elevated in: Zollinger-Ellison syndrome (gastrinoma), pernicious anemia, hyperparathyroidism, retained gastric antrum, chronic renal failure, gastric ulcer, chronic atrophic gastritis, pyloric obstruction, malignant neoplasms of the stomach, H_2-blockers, omeprazole, calcium therapy, ulcerative colitis, rheumatoid arthritis

GASTRIN STIMULATION TEST

Normal: Gastrin stimulation test after calcium infusion is performed by giving a calcium infusion (15 mg/kg in 500 ml normal saline over 4 h). Serum is drawn in fasting state before infusion and at 1, 2, 3, and 4 h. Normal response is little or no increase over baseline gastrin level.

Elevated in: Gastrinoma (gastrin >400 pg/ml), duodenal ulcer (gastrin level increase <400 ng/L)

Decreased in: Pernicious anemia, atrophic gastritis

GLIADIN ANTIBODIES, IgA AND IgG

Normal: <25 U, equivocal 20 to 25 U, positive >25 U. Test is useful to monitor compliance with gluten-free diet in patients with celiac disease.

Elevated in: Celiac disease with dietary noncompliance

GLOMERULAR BASEMENT MEMBRANE (GBM) ANTIBODY

Normal: Negative
Present in: Goodpasture syndrome

GLOMERULAR FILTRATION RATE

See Box E18 for a summary of common equations for calculating GFR or creatinine clearance. Chronic kidney disease stages based on GFR are summarized in Table 55.
Normal:

Ages 20-29	116 ml/min/1.73 m^2
Ages 30-39	107 ml/min/1.73 m^2
Ages 40-49	99 ml/min/1.73 m^2
Ages 50-59	93 ml/min/1.73 m^2
Ages 60-69	85 ml/min/1.73 m^2
Ages >75	75 ml/min/1.73 m^2

Laboratory Tests and Interpretation of Results

TABLE 55 Chronic Kidney Disease Stages

Stage	eGFR (ml/min/1.73 m²)	Urinalysis Findings
1	≥90	Hematuria, proteinuria, or imaging abnormalities at >3 mo
2	60-89	Hematuria, proteinuria, or imaging abnormalities at >3 mo
3	30-59	↑ or normal
4	15-29	↑ or normal
5	0-14	↑ or normal

eGFR, Estimated glomerular filtration rate.
From Parrillo JE, Dellinger RP: *Critical care medicine, principles of diagnosis and management in the adult*, ed 4, Philadelphia, 2014, Elsevier.

Decreased in: Renal insufficiency, decreased renal blood flow

GLUCAGON

Normal: 20 to 100 pg/ml
Elevated in: Glucagonoma (900 to 7800 pg/ml), chronic renal failure, diabetes mellitus, glucocorticoids, insulin, nifedipine, danazol, sympathomimetic amines
Decreased in: Hyperlipoproteinemia (types III, IV), b-blockers, secretin

GLUCOSE, FASTING (FBS, fasting blood sugar)

Fig. E24 describes the approach to hypoglycemia. An algorithm for evaluation of hypoglycemia in children is described in Fig. E25.
Normal range: 60 to 99 mg/dl (3.8 to 6.0 mmol/L [CF: 0.05551; SMI: 0.1 mmol/L])
Elevated in: Diabetes mellitus, stress, infections, myocardial infarction, cerebrovascular accident, Cushing syndrome, acromegaly, acute pancreatitis, glucagonoma, hemochromatosis, drugs (glucocorticoids, diuretics [thiazides, loop diuretics]), glucose intolerance, impaired fasting glucose
Decreased in: Sulfonylurea therapy, insulin therapy, reactive hypoglycemia (e.g., subtotal gastrectomy), starvation, insulinoma, glycogen storage disorders, severe liver disease or renal disease, ethanol-induced hypoglycemia, mesenchymal tumors that secrete insulin-like hormones

GLUCOSE, POSTPRANDIAL

Normal range: <140 mg/dl (<7.8 mmol/L [CF: 0.05551; SMI: 0.1 mmol/L])
Elevated in: Diabetes mellitus, glucose intolerance
Decreased in: Post gastrointestinal resection, reactive hypoglycemia, hereditary fructose intolerance, galactosemia, leucine sensitivity

GLUCOSE TOLERANCE TEST

Normal values above fasting
30 min: 30 to 60 mg/dl (1.65 to 3.3 mmol/L [CF: 0.05551; SMI: 0.1 mmol/L])
60 min: 20 to 50 mg/dl (1.1 to 2.75 mmol/L [CF: 0.05551; SMI: 0.1 mmol/L])
120 min: 5 to 15 mg/dl (0.28 to 0.83 mmol/L [CF: 0.05551; SMI: 0.1 mmol/L])
180 min: Fasting level or below
Abnormal in: Glucose intolerance, diabetes mellitus, Cushing syndrome, acromegaly, pheochromocytoma, gestational diabetes

GLUCOSE-6-PHOSPHATE DEHYDROGENASE (G6PD) SCREEN (blood)

Normal: G6PD enzyme activity detected
Abnormal: If a deficiency is detected, quantitation of G6PD is necessary; a G6PD screen may be falsely interpreted as "normal" after an episode of hemolysis because most G6PD-deficient cells have been destroyed.

γ-GLUTAMYL TRANSFERASE (GGT)

Normal range: 0 to 30 U/L (0.050 μkat/L [CF: 0.01667; SMI: 0.01 μkat/L])
Elevated in: Chronic alcoholic liver disease, neoplasms (hepatoma, metastatic disease to the liver, carcinoma of the pancreas), systemic lupus

erythematosus, congestive heart failure, trauma, nephrotic syndrome, sepsis, cholestasis, drugs (phenytoin, barbiturates)

GLYCOHEMOGLOBIN (glycated glycosylated hemoglobin), (HbA1c)

Normal range: 4.0% to 5.9%. Glycemic goals in adults are summarized in Table E56.
Elevated in: Uncontrolled diabetes mellitus (glycated hemoglobin levels reflect the level of glucose control over the preceding 120 days), lead toxicity, alcoholism, iron deficiency anemia, hypertriglyceridemia
Decreased in: Hemolytic anemias, decreased red blood cell survival, pregnancy, acute or chronic blood loss, chronic renal failure, insulinoma, congenital spherocytosis, hemoglobin S, C, and D diseases

GROWTH HORMONE

Normal: Male: 1 to 9 ng/ml; female: 1 to 16 ng/ml
Elevated in: Pituitary gigantism, acromegaly, ectopic GH secretion, cirrhosis, renal failure, anorexia nervosa, stress, exercise, prolonged fasting, amphetamines, b-blockers, insulin, levodopa, metoclopramide, clonidine, vasopressin, human growth hormone (HGH) supplementation
Decreased in: Hypopituitarism, pituitary dwarfism, adrenocortical hyperfunction, bromocriptine, corticosteroids, glucose

GROWTH HORMONE RELEASING HORMONE (GHRH)

Normal: <50 pg/ml
Elevated in: Acromegaly caused by GHRH secretion by neoplasms

GROWTH HORMONE SUPPRESSION TEST (after glucose)

Normal: Test is done by giving 1.75 g glucose/kg orally after overnight fast. Blood is drawn at baseline, after 60 min, and after 120 min of glucose load. Normal response is growth hormone suppression to <2 ng/ml or undetectable levels.
Abnormal: There is no or incomplete suppression from the high basal level in gigantism or acromegaly.

HAM TEST (acid serum test)

Normal: Negative
Positive in: Paroxysmal nocturnal hemoglobinuria
False-positive in: Hereditary or acquired spherocytosis, recent transfusion with aged red blood cells, aplastic anemia, myeloproliferative syndromes, leukemia, hereditary dyserythropoietic anemia type II

HAPTOGLOBIN (serum)

Normal range: 50 to 220 mg/dl (0.50 to 2.2 g/L [CF: 0.01; SMI: 0.01 g/L])
Elevated in: Inflammation (acute phase reactant), collagen vascular diseases, infections (acute phase reactant), drugs (androgens), obstructive liver disease
Decreased in: Hemolysis (intravascular more than extravascular), megaloblastic anemia, severe liver disease, large tissue hematomas, infectious mononucleosis, drugs (oral contraceptives)

HBA1c

See "GLYCOHEMOGLOBIN"

HDL

See "HIGH-DENSITY LIPOPROTEIN CHOLESTEROL"

HELICOBACTER PYLORI (serology, stool antigen)

Normal range: Not detected
Detected in: *H. pylori* infection. Positive serology can indicate current or past infection. Positive stool antigen test indicates acute infection (sensitivity and specificity >90%). Stool testing should be delayed at least 4 wk after eradication therapy.

HEMATOCRIT

Normal range:
Male: 39% to 49% (0.39 to 0.49 [CF: 0.01; SMI: 0.01])

Laboratory Tests

IV

Female: 33% to 43% (0.33 to 0.43 [CF: 0.01; SMI: 0.01])
Elevated in: Polycythemia vera, smoking, chronic obstructive pulmonary disease, high altitudes, dehydration, hypovolemia
Decreased in: Blood loss (gastrointestinal, genitourinary) anemia

HEMOGLOBIN

Normal range: Male: 13.6 to 17.7 g/dl (136 to 172 g/L [CF: 10; SMI: 1 g/L])
    Female: 12.0 to 15.0 g/dl (120 to 150 g/L [CF: 10; SMI: 1 g/L])
Elevated in: Hemoconcentration, dehydration, polycythemia vera, chronic obstructive pulmonary disease, high altitudes, false elevations (hyperlipemic plasma, white blood cells >50,000/mm^3), stress
Decreased in: Hemorrhagic (gastrointestinal, genitourinary) anemia

HEMOGLOBIN A$_{1C}$

See "GLYCOHEMOGLOBIN"

HEMOGLOBIN ELECTROPHORESIS

Table E57 describes neonatal hemoglobin electrophoresis patterns, Table 58 summarizes types of hemoglobin, and Table E59 describes classifications of hemoglobinopathies.

TABLE 58   Types of Hemoglobin

	Hemoglobin	Structure	Comment
Normal	A	$\alpha_2\beta_2$	97% of adult hemoglobin
	A$_2$	$\alpha_2\delta_2$	2% of adult Hb; elevated in β-thalassemia
	F	$\alpha_2\gamma_2$	Normal Hb in fetus from 3rd-9th mo; increased in β-thalassemia
Abnormal chain production	H	β_4	Found in α-thalassemia, biologically useless
	Barts	γ_4	Found in α-thalassemia, biologically useless
Abnormal chain structure	S	$\alpha_2\beta_2$	Substitution of valine for glutamic acid in position 6 of β chain
	C	$\alpha_2\beta_2$	Substitution of lysine for glutamic acid in position 6 of β chain

From Ballinger A: *Kumar & Clark's essentials of clinical medicine*, ed 6, Edinburgh, 2012, Saunders.

Normal range: HbA$_1$: 95% to 98%
HbA$_2$: 1.5% to 3.5%
HbF: <2%
HbC: Absent
HbS: Absent

HEMOGLOBIN, GLYCATED

See "GLYCOHEMOGLOBIN"

HEMOGLOBIN, GLYCOSYLATED

See "GLYCOHEMOGLOBIN"

HEMOGLOBIN H

See Table 58.
Normal: Negative
Present in: Hemoglobin H disease, alpha-thalassemia trait, unstable hemoglobin disorders

HEMOGLOBIN, URINE

See "URINE HEMOGLOBIN, FREE"

HEMOSIDERIN, URINE

See "URINE HEMOGLOBIN, FREE"

HEPARIN-INDUCED THROMBOCYTOPENIA ANTIBODIES

Normal: Antigen assay: Negative, <0.45; weak, 0.45-1.0; strong, >1.0
Elevated in: Heparin-induced thrombocytopenia

HEPATITIS A ANTIBODY

Normal: Negative
Present in: Viral hepatitis A; can be IgM or IgG (if IgM, acute hepatitis A; if IgG, previous infection with hepatitis A)
    See Fig. 26 for serologic tests in HAV infection.
    See Table E60 for serologic and virologic tests for hepatitis viruses.

Hepatitis A Viral Infection: Best all-purpose test(s) to diagnose acute HAV infection = HAV-Ab (IgM)
    Best all-purpose test(s) to demonstrate past HAV infection/immunity = HAV-Ab (total)

HEPATITIS A VIRUS-IgM ANTIBODY

Appearance: About the same time as clinical symptoms (3 to 4 wk after exposure; range, 14 to 60 days), or just before beginning of AST/ALT elevation (range, 10 days before to 7 days after)

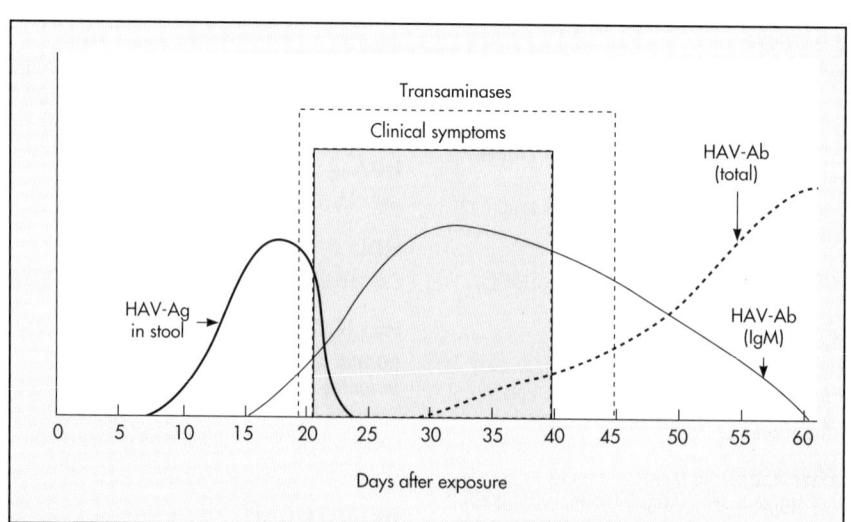

FIG. 26 Serologic tests in hepatitis A viral infection. *HAV,* Hepatitis A virus; *HAV-Ab,* hepatitis A virus antibodies test; *HAV-Ag,* hepatitis A virus antigen test; *Ig,* immunoglobulin.

Peak: About 3 to 4 wk after onset of symptoms (1 to 6 wk)
Becomes nondetectable: 3 to 4 mo after onset of symptoms (1 to 6 mo). In a few cases HAV-IgM antibody can persist as long as 12 to 14 mo.

HEPATITIS A VIRUS TOTAL ANTIBODY

Appearance: About 3 wk after IgM becomes detectable (therefore about the middle of clinical symptom period to early convalescence)
Peak: About 1 to 2 mo after onset
Becomes nondetectable: Remains elevated for life but can somewhat slowly fall

HEPATITIS B SURFACE ANTIGEN (HBsAg)

Normal: Not detected
Detected in: Acute viral hepatitis type B, chronic hepatitis B
Appearance: 2 to 6 wk after exposure (range, 6 days to 6 mo); 5% to 15% of patients are negative at onset of jaundice
Peak: 1 to 2 wk before to 1 to 2 wk after onset of symptoms
Becomes nondetectable: 1 to 3 mo after peak (range, 1 wk to 5 mo)

HEPATITIS B VIRAL INFECTION

See Table 61

Figs. 27, 28, and 29 illustrate antigens and antibodies in hepatitis B infection.

HB$_S$
-Ag
HB$_S$Ag: Shows current active hepatitis B virus (HBV) infection
Persistence over 6 mo indicates carrier/chronic HBV infection
HBV nucleic acid probe: Present before and longer than HB$_S$Ag
More reliable marker for increased infectivity than HB$_S$Ag and/or HB$_e$Ag
-Ab
HB$_S$Ab-total: Shows previous healed HBV infection and evidence of immunity
HB$_C$
-Ab
HB$_C$Ab-IgM: Shows either acute or very recent infection by HBV

In convalescent phase of acute HBV, may be elevated when HB$_S$Ag has disappeared (core window)
Negative HB$_C$Ab-IgM with positive HB$_S$Ag suggests either very early acute HBV or carrier/chronic HBV
HB$_C$Ab-total: Only useful to show past HBV infection if HB$_S$Ag and HB$_C$Ab-IgM are both negative
HB$_E$
-Ag
HB$_e$-AbAg: When present, especially without HB$_e$Ab, suggests increased patient infectivity
HB$_e$Ab-total: When present, suggests less patient infectivity
  HB$_S$Ag positive, HB$_C$Ab negative
  About 5% (range, 0% to 17%) of patients with early-stage HBV acute infection (HB$_C$Ab rises later)
  HB$_S$Ag positive, HB$_C$Ab positive, HB$_S$Ab negative
  Most of the clinical symptom stage
  Chronic HBV carriers without evidence of liver disease ("asymptomatic carriers")
  Chronic HBV hepatitis (chronic persistent type or chronic active type)
  HB$_S$Ag negative, HB$_C$Ab positive, HB$_S$Ab negative
  Late clinical symptom stage or early convalescence stage (core window)
  Chronic HBV infection with HB$_S$Ag below detection levels with current tests
  Old previous HBV infection
  HB$_S$Ag negative, HB$_C$Ab positive, HB$_S$Ab positive
  Late convalescence to complete recovery
  Old infection

HEPATITIS C RNA

Normal: Negative
Elevated in: Hepatitis C. Detection of hepatitis C-RNA is used to confirm current infection and to monitor treatment. Quantitative assays (viral load) are needed before treatment to assess response (<2 log decrease after 12-wk treatment indicates lack of response).

TABLE 61	Serologic Markers of Hepatitis B Infection			
	HBsAg	**anti-HBc**	**anti-HBs**	**IgM anti-HBc**
Susceptible to infection	Negative	Negative	Negative	Negative
Immune due to natural infection	Negative	Positive	Positive	Negative
Immune due to hepatitis B vaccination	Negative	Negative	Positive	Negative
Acutely infected	Positive	Positive	Negative	Positive
Chronically infected	Positive	Positive	Negative	Negative

HBsAg, Hepatitis B surface antigen; *Ig*, immunoglobulin.
From Ballinger A: *Kumar & Clark's essentials of clinical medicine*, ed 6, Edinburgh, 2012, Saunders.

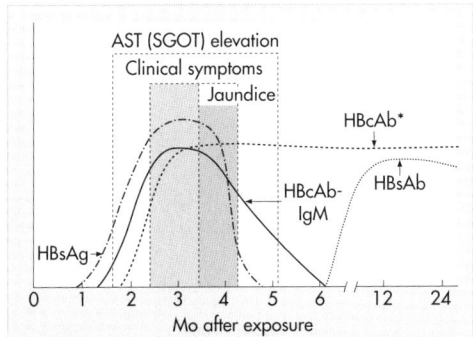

FIG. 27 Hepatitis B virus surface antigen-antibody and core antibodies. Note "core window." *HB$_C$Ab = HB$_C$Ab-IgM + HBCAb-IgG (combined). *AST*, Aspartate aminotransferase; *HBcAb*, hepatitis B core antibody; *HBsAb*, hepatitis B surface antibody; *HBsAg*, hepatitis B surface antigen; *Ig*, immunoglobulin; *SGOT*, serum glutamic-oxaloacetic transaminase.

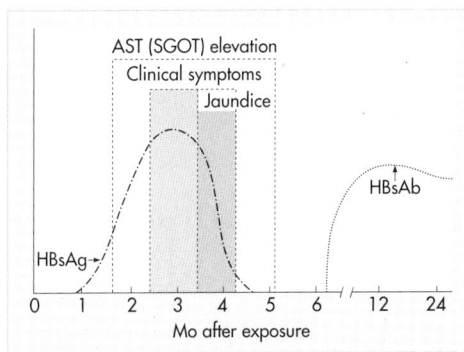

FIG. 28 Hepatitis B virus surface antigen and antibody (HB$_S$Ag and HB$_S$Ab-total). *AST*, Aspartate aminotransferase; *SGOT*, serum glutamic-oxaloacetic transaminase.

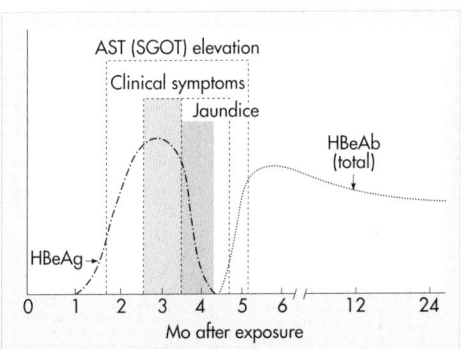

FIG. 29 HBVe antigen and antibody. *AST*, Aspartate aminotransferase; *HBeAb*, hepatitis B e-antibody; *SGOT*, serum glutamic-oxaloacetic transaminase.

HCV

-Ag

HCV nucleic acid probe: Shows current infection by HCV (especially with PCR amplification).

-Ab

HCV-Ab (IgG): Current, convalescent, or old HCV infection.

HAV

-Ag

HAV-Ag by EM Shows presence of virus in stool early in infection.

-Ab

HAV-Ab (IgM): Current or recent HAV infection.
HAV-Ab (total): Convalescent or old HAV infection.

HEPATITIS C VIRAL INFECTION

Fig. 30 illustrates antigens and antibodies in hepatitis C infection. Table 62 summarizes interpretation of patterns of HCV markers.

HEPATITIS D VIRAL INFECTION

Fig. 31 illustrates antigens and antibodies in hepatitis D infection.
Best current all-purpose screening test = HDV-Ab (total)
Best test to differentiate acute from chronic infection = HDV-Ab (IgM)

HEPATITIS DELTA COINFECTION (acute HDV1 acute HBV) OR SUPERINFECTION (acute HDV1 chronic HBV)

HDV

-Ag

HDV-Ag: Shows current infection (acute or chronic) by HDV.
HDV nucleic acid probe: Detects antigen before and longer than HDV-Ag by EIA.

-Ab

HDV-Ab (IgM): High elevation in acute HDV; does not persist
Low or moderate elevation in convalescent HDV; does not persist
Low to high persistent elevation in chronic HDV (depends on degree of cell injury and sensitivity of the assay)
HDV-Ab (total): High elevation in acute HDV; does not persist
High persistent elevation in chronic HDV

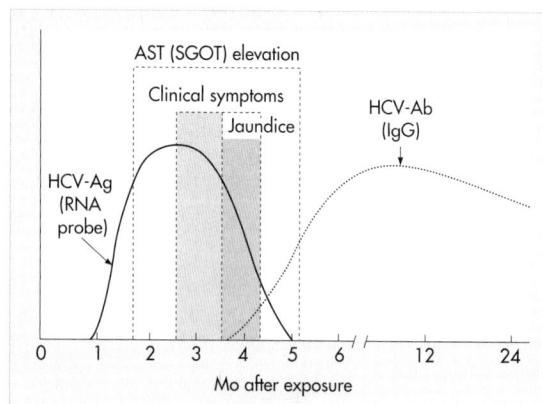

FIG. 30 Hepatitis C virus antigen and antibody. *AST,* Aspartate aminotransferase; *HCV-Ab,* hepatitis C virus antibody; *HCV-Ag,* hepatitis C virus core antigen; *Ig,* immunoglobulin; *RNA,* ribonucleic acid; *SGOT,* serum glutamic-oxaloacetic transaminase.

TABLE 62 Interpretation of Patterns of HCV Markers

Interpretation	Anti-HCV	RIBA	HCV RNA
Acute HCV infection	−	−	+
Active HCV infection	+	+	+
Possible HCV clearance	+	+	−
False-positive HCV test	+	−	−
Requires further study	+	Indeterminate*	−

*Indeterminate result: Only one band positive, or more than one band and nonspecific reactivity.
HCV, Hepatitis C; RIBA, recombinant immunoassay; RNA, ribonucleic acid.
From McPherson RA, Pincus MR: *Henry's clinical diagnosis and management by laboratory methods*, ed 23, St Louis, 2017, Elsevier.

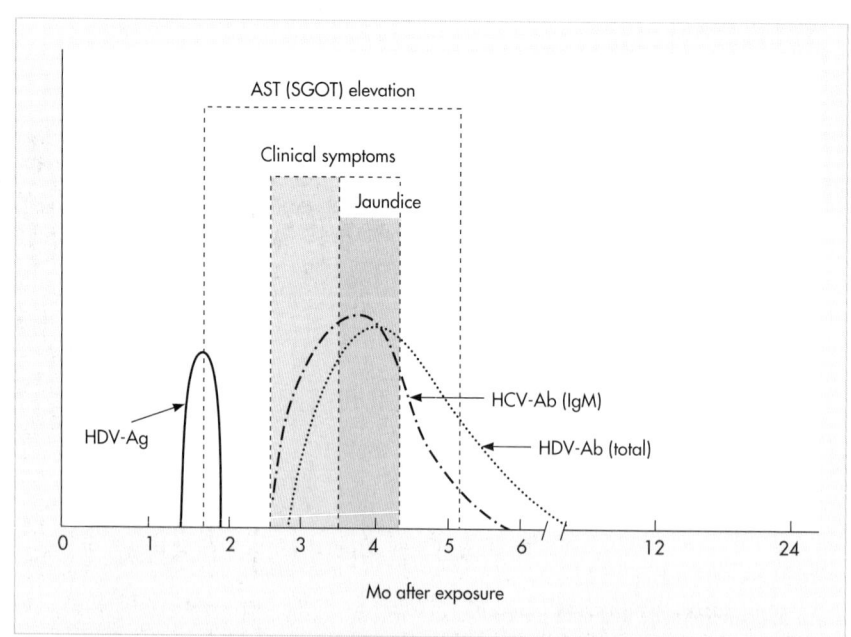

FIG. 31 Hepatitis D virus antigen and antibodies. *AST,* Aspartate aminotransferase; *HCV-Ab,* hepatitis C virus antibody; *HDV-Ab,* hepatitis D virus antibody; *HDV-Ag,* hepatitis D virus antigen; *Ig,* immunoglobulin; *SGOT,* serum glutamic-oxaloacetic transaminase.

HEPATITIS D VIRUS-Ab (IgM)

Appearance: About 10 days after symptoms begin (range, 1 to 28 days)
Peak: About 2 wk after first detection
Becomes nondetectable: About 35 days (range, 10 to 80 days) after first detection (most other IgM antibodies take 3 to 6 mo to become nondetectable)

HEPATITIS D VIRUS-Ag

Detected by DNA probe, less often by immunoassay
Appearance: Prodromal stage (before symptoms); just at or after initial rise in ALT (about a wk after appearance of HB_SAg and about the time HB_CAb-IgM level begins to rise)
Peak: 2 to 3 days after onset
Becomes nondetectable: 1 to 4 days (may persist until shortly after symptoms appear)

HEPATITIS D VIRUS-Ab (total)

Appearance: About 50 days after symptoms begin (range, 14 to 80 days); about 5 wk after HDV-Ag (range, 3 to 11 wk)
Peak: About 2 wk after first detection
Becomes nondetectable: About 7 mo after first detection (range, 4 to 14 mo)

HER-2/*NEU*

Normal: Negative
Present in: 25% to 30% of primary breast cancers. It can also be found in other epithelial tumors, including lung, hepatocellular, pancreatic, colon, stomach, ovarian, cervical, and bladder cancer. Trastuzumab (Herceptin) is a humanized monoclonal antibody against Her-2/*neu*. This test is useful to identify patients with metastatic; recurrent; and/or treatment-refractory, unresectable, locally advanced breast cancer for trastuzumab treatment.

HERPES SIMPLEX VIRUS (HSV)

Test description: The PCR test can be performed on serum biopsy samples, CSF, vitreous humor.

HETEROPHIL ANTIBODY

Normal: Negative
Positive in: Infectious mononucleosis

HFE SCREEN FOR HEREDITARY HEMOCHROMATOSIS

Test description: PCR test can be performed on whole blood or tissue. One mutation (C282Y) and two polymorphisms (H63D, S65C) account for the majority of alleles associated with this disease.

TABLE 64	HLA Antigens Associated With Specific Diseases		
Antigen	**Condition**	**Antigen**	**Condition**
HLA-B27	Ankylosing spondylitis	HLA-B8, Dw3	Celiac disease
	Reiter syndrome	HLA-B8, Dw3	Dermatitis herpetiformis
	Psoriatic arthritis	HLA-B8	Myasthenia gravis
HLA-A10, B18, Dw2	C2 deficiency	HLA-B8	Chronic active hepatitis in children
HLA-A2, B40, Cw3	C4 deficiency	HLA-Drw4	Active chronic hepatitis in adults
HLA-B7, Dw2	Multiple sclerosis	HLA-B13, Bw17	Psoriasis
HLA-A3	Hemochromatosis		

HLA, Human leukocyte antigen.
From Cerra FB: *Manual of critical care,* St Louis, 1987, Mosby.

HIGH-DENSITY LIPOPROTEIN (HDL) CHOLESTEROL

Normal range:
Male: 40 to 70 mg/dl (0.8 to 1.8 mmol/L [CF: 0.02586; SMI: 0.05 mmol/L])
Female: 50 to 90 mg/dl (1.1 to 2.35 mmol/L [CF: 0.02586; SMI: 0.05 mmol/L])
Increased in: Use of gemfibrozil, statins, fenofibrate, nicotinic acid, estrogens, regular aerobic exercise, small (1 oz) daily alcohol intake
Decreased in: Deficiency of apoproteins, liver disease, probucol ingestion, Tangier disease
NOTE: A cholesterol/HDL ratio >4.0 is associated with increased risk of coronary artery disease. Table E63 summarizes significant human apolipoproteins.

HLA ANTIGENS

Associated disorders: See Table 64.

HOMOCYSTEINE (plasma)

Normal range:

0-30 yr:	4.6-8.1 mcmol/L
30-59 yr:	6.3-11.2 mcmol/L (males), 4.5-7.9 mcmol/L (females)
>59 yr:	5.8-11.9 mcmol/L

Increased: Thrombophilic states, B_6, B_{12}, folic acid, riboflavin deficiency, pregnancy, homocystinuria
NOTE: An increased homocysteine level is an independent risk factor for atherosclerosis.

HUMAN CHORIONIC GONADOTROPIN (hCG)

Normal range: Varies with gestational stage:

1 wk:	5-50 mU/ml
1-2 wk:	50-550 mU/ml
2-3 wk:	up to 5000 mU/ml
3-4 wk:	up to 10,000 mU/ml
4-5 wk:	up to 50,000 mU/ml
2-3 mo:	10,000-100,000 mU/ml

Elevated in: Normal pregnancy, hydatidiform mole, choriocarcinoma, germ cell tumors of testicle, some nontrophoblastic neoplasms (e.g., neoplasms of cervix, gastrointestinal tract, ovary, lung, breast)

HUMAN HERPES VIRUS 8 (HHV8)

Test description: PCR test can be performed on whole blood, tissue, bone marrow, and urine. HHV8 is found in all forms of Kaposi sarcoma.

HUMAN IMMUNODEFICIENCY VIRUS ANTIBODY, TYPE 1 (HIV-1)

Normal range: Not detected
Abnormal result: HIV antibodies usually appear in the blood 1 to 4 mo after infection.
Testing sequence: ELISA is the recommended initial screening test. Sensitivity and specificity are >99%. False-positive ELISA may occur with autoimmune disorders, administration of immune globulin manufactured before 1985, within 6 wk of testing, in the presence of rheumatoid factor, in the presence of DLA-DR antibodies in multigravida female, with administration of influenza vaccine within 3 mo of testing, with hemodialysis, with positive plasma reagin test, and with certain medical disorders (hemophilia, hypergammaglobulinemia, alcoholic hepatitis).

Laboratory Tests

IV

A positive ELISA is confirmed with Western blot (Fig. E32). False-positive Western blot may result from connective tissue disorders, human leukocyte antigen antibodies, polyclonal gammopathies, hyperbilirubinemia, presence of antibody to another human retrovirus, or cross-reaction with other non-virus-derived proteins in healthy persons. Undetermined Western blot may occur in AIDS patients with advanced immunodeficiency (caused by loss of antibodies) and in recent HIV infections.

PCR is used to confirm indeterminate Western blot results or negative results in persons with suspected HIV infection.

Fig. 33 describes tests in HIV infection; indications for plasma HIV RNA testing are described in Table E65.

HUMAN IMMUNODEFICIENCY VIRUS TYPE 1 (HIV-1) ANTIGEN (p24), QUALITATIVE (p24 antigen)

Normal range: Negative. This test detects uncomplexed HIV-1 p24 antigen. The core protein p24 is the first detectable protein encoded by the group-specific antigen *(gag)* gene. This protein is a marker for viremia. This test should not be used in place of HIV-1 antibody testing as a screen for HIV-1 infection. HIV-1 p24 may be detectable in the first mo of acute HIV-1 infection and generally falls to undetectable levels during the asymptomatic stage of HIV-1 infection. A negative result does not exclude the possibility of infection or exposure to HIV-1. It is recommended that a negative result be followed with repeat testing at least 8 wk after the original test. This test is used primarily for screening of donated blood and plasma and as an aid for the prognosis of HIV-1 infection.

HUMAN IMMUNODEFICIENCY VIRUS TYPE 1 (HIV-1) VIRAL LOAD

Normal range: HIV-1 RNA, quant. bDNA 3: Less than 50 copies/ml or less than 1.7 log copies/ml

This test should be used only in individuals with documented HIV-1 infection for monitoring the progression of infection, response to antiretroviral therapy, and disease prognosis. It is not indicated for diagnosis of HIV infection.

HUMAN PAPILLOMAVIRUS (HPV)

Test description: PCR test can be performed on cervical smears, biopsies, scrapings, liquid cytology specimen, and anogenital tissues.

HUNTINGTON DISEASE PCR

Test description: PCR can be performed on whole blood. Huntington disease is caused by the expansion of the trinucleotide repeat cytosine-adenine-guanine (CAG) within IT 15 (huntingtin). Pre- and posttest counseling should be performed when ordering this test.

HYDROGEN BREATH TEST

See "BREATH HYDROGEN TEST"

5-HYDROXYINDOLE-ACETIC ACID, URINE

See "URINE 5-HYDROXYINDOLE-ACETIC ACID"

IMMUNE COMPLEX ASSAY

Normal: Negative

Detected in: Collagen vascular disorders, glomerulonephritis, neoplastic diseases, malaria, primary biliary cirrhosis, chronic acute hepatitis, bacterial endocarditis, vasculitis

IMMUNOGLOBULINS

Normal range:

IgA:	50-350 mg/dl (0.5-3.5 g/L [CF: 0.01; SMI: 0.01 g/L])
IgD:	<6 mg/dl (<60 mg/L [CF: 0.01; SMI: 0.01 g/L])
IgE:	<25 μg/dl (<0.00025 g/L [CF: 0.01; SMI: 0.01 g/L])
IgG:	800-1500 mg/dl (8-15 g/L [CF: 0.01; SMI: 0.01 g/L])
IgM:	45-150 mg/dl (0.45-1.5 g/L [CF: 0.01; SMI: 0.01 g/L])

Table E66 summarizes biologic properties of human immunoglobulin isotypes. Box 19 summarizes selected conditions associated with monoclonal immunoglobulins. Disease states associated with polyclonal hyperimmunoglobulinemia are described in Table E67.

Elevated in:

IgA: Lymphoproliferative disorders, Berger nephropathy, chronic infections, autoimmune disorders, liver disease

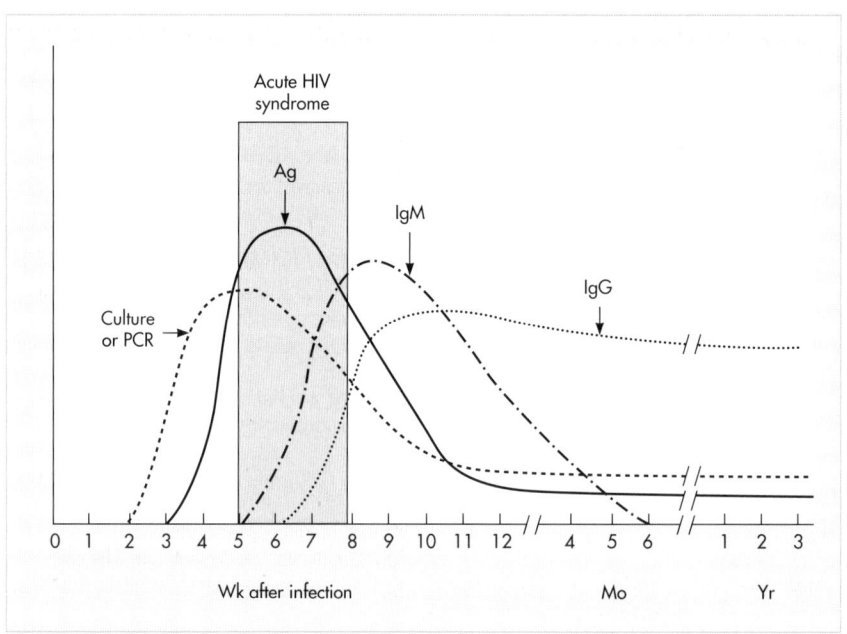

FIG. 33 Tests in human immunodeficiency virus *(HIV)*-1 infection. *Ag,* Antigen; *Ig,* immunoglobulin; *PCR,* polymerase chain reaction. (From Ravel R [ed]: *Clinical laboratory medicine,* ed 6, St Louis, 1995, Mosby.)

BOX 19 Selected Conditions Associated With Monoclonal Immunoglobulins

Multiple myeloma
Macroglobulinemia of Waldenström
Chronic lymphocytic leukemia
Other leukemias
Lymphomas
"Benign" monoclonal gammopathy
Systemic capillary leak syndrome
Amyloidosis
Chronic liver disease such as chronic active hepatitis, primary biliary cirrhosis
Autoimmune disorders, including rheumatoid arthritis, systemic lupus erythematosus, thyroiditis, pernicious anemia, polyarteritis nodosa, Sjögren syndrome
Gaucher disease
Malignancies of various types
Hereditary spherocytosis
HIV infection, including AIDS

From McPherson RA, Pincus MR: *Henry's clinical diagnosis and management by laboratory methods*, ed 23, St Louis, 2017, Elsevier.

IgE: Allergic disorders, parasitic infections, immunologic disorders, IgE myeloma (see Box E20 for summary of nonallergic diseases associated with high levels of IgE. Box 21 summarizes conditions with very high IgE levels)
IgG: Chronic granulomatous infections, infectious diseases, inflammation, myeloma, liver disease
IgM: Primary biliary cirrhosis, infectious diseases (brucellosis, malaria), Waldenström macroglobulinemia, liver disease
Decreased in:
IgA: Nephrotic syndrome, protein-losing enteropathy, congenital deficiency, lymphocytic leukemia, ataxia-telangiectasia, chronic sinopulmonary disease
IgE: Hypogammaglobulinemia, neoplasms (breast, bronchial, cervical), ataxia-telangiectasia, primary biliary cirrhosis (see Box E20)
IgG: Congenital or acquired deficiency, lymphocytic leukemia, phenytoin, methylprednisolone, nephrotic syndrome, protein-losing enteropathy
IgM: Congenital deficiency, lymphocytic leukemia, nephrotic syndrome

---

BOX 21 Conditions Associated With Unusually High Serum Immunoglobulin E Concentrations (≥500 IU/ml)

Allergic bronchopulmonary mycosis
Allergic fungal sinusitis
Atopic dermatitis
Human immunodeficiency virus (HIV) infection
Hyperimmunoglobulin E (hyper-IgE) syndrome
Immunoglobulin E myeloma
Kimura disease
Lymphoma
Netherton syndrome
Systemic helminthic parasitosis
Tuberculosis

From Adkinson NF et al: *Middleton's allergy principles and practice*, ed 8, Philadelphia, 2014, Saunders.

INDIRECT ANTIGLOBULIN (Coombs Indirect)
Normal: Negative
Positive: Acquired hemolytic anemia, incompatible cross-matched blood, anti-Rh antibodies, drugs (methyldopa, mefenamic acid, levodopa)
    Fig. E34 illustrates the mechanism of Coombs test.

INFLUENZA A AND B TESTS
Test description: PCR can be performed on nasopharyngeal swab, wash, or aspirate.
Normal: Negative

INSULIN AUTOANTIBODIES
Normal: Negative
Present in: Exogenous insulin from insulin therapy. The presence of islet cell antibodies indicates ongoing beta cell destruction. This test is useful in the early diagnosis of type 1a diabetes mellitus and in the identification of patients at high risk for type 1a diabetes.

INSULIN, FREE
Normal: <17 mcU/ml
Elevated in: Insulin overdose, insulin resistance syndromes, endogenous hyperinsulinemia
Decreased in: Inadequately treated type 1 diabetes mellitus

INSULIN-LIKE GROWTH FACTOR-1 (IGF-1) (Serum)
Normal range:

Ages 16-24:	182-780 ng/ml
Ages 25-39:	114-492 ng/ml
Ages 40-54:	90-360 ng/ml
Ages >55:	71-290 ng/ml

Elevated in: Adolescence, acromegaly, pregnancy, precocious puberty, obesity
Decreased in: Malnutrition, delayed puberty, diabetes mellitus, hypopituitarism, cirrhosis, old age

INSULIN-LIKE GROWTH FACTOR-II
Normal range: 288 to 736 ng/ml
Elevated in: Hypoglycemia associated with nonislet cell tumors, hepatoma, and Wilms tumor
Decreased in: Growth hormone deficiency

INTERNATIONAL NORMALIZED RATIO (INR)
The INR is a comparative rating of prothrombin time (PT) ratios. The INR represents the observed PT ratio adjusted by the International Reference Thromboplastin. It provides a universal result indicative of what the patient's PT result would have been if measured using the primary World Health Organization International Reference reagent. For proper interpretation of INR values, the patient should be on stable anticoagulant therapy.

RECOMMENDED INR RANGES

Proximal deep vein thrombosis:	2-3
Pulmonary embolism:	2-3
Transient ischemic attacks:	2-3
Atrial fibrillation:	2-3
Mechanical prosthetic valves:	2.5-3.5
Recurrent venous thromboembolic disease:	2.5-3.5

Laboratory Tests

IV

TABLE 68 Serum Iron and Total Iron-Binding Capacity Patterns

SI ↓	TIBC ↓	Chronic diseases; uremia
SI ↓	TIBC ↑	Chronic iron deficiency anemia; pregnancy in third trimester
SI ↑	TIBC ↓	Hemochromatosis iron therapy overload (TIBC may be normal); hemolytic anemia; thalassemia; lead poisoning; megaloblastic anemia; aplastic, pyridoxine deficiency, or other sideroblastic anemias
SI ↑	TIBC ↑	Oral contraceptives; acute hepatitis (some report TIBC is low normal); chronic hepatitis (some patients)
SI ↑	TIBCNL	B_{12} or folate deficiency
SI ↓	TIBCNL	Chronic iron deficiency (some patients); acute infection, surgery, tissue damage
SI NL	TIBC ↑	B_{12}/folate deficiency plus iron deficiency

NL, Normal; *SI*, serum iron; *TIBC*, total iron-binding capacity.

INTRINSIC FACTOR ANTIBODIES

Normal: Negative
Present in: Pernicious anemia (>50% of patients). Cyanocobalamin may give false-positive results.

IRON (Serum)

Normal: Male: 65 to 175 mcg/dl; female: 50 to 1170 mcg/dl
Elevated in: Hemochromatosis, excessive iron therapy, repeated transfusions, lead poisoning, hemolytic anemia, aplastic anemia, pernicious anemia
Decreased in: Iron deficiency anemia, hypothyroidism, chronic infection

IRON-BINDING CAPACITY, TOTAL (TIBC)

Normal range: 250 to 460 μg/dl (45 to 82 μmol/L [CF: 0.1791; SMI: 1 μmol/L])
Elevated in: Iron deficiency anemia, pregnancy, polycythemia, hepatitis, weight loss
Decreased in: Anemia of chronic disease, hemochromatosis, chronic liver disease, hemolytic anemias, malnutrition (protein depletion)
Table 68 describes TIBC and serum iron abnormalities.

IRON SATURATION (% Transferrin Saturation)

Normal:
Male: 20% to 50%
Female: 15% to 50%
Elevated in: Hemochromatosis, excessive iron intake, aplastic anemia, thalassemia, vitamin B_6 deficiency
Decreased in: Hypochromic anemias, GI malignancy

LACTATE (blood)

Normal range: 0.5 to 2.0 mEq/L
Elevated in: Tissue hypoxia (shock, respiratory failure, severe CHF, severe anemia, carbon monoxide or cyanide poisoning), systemic disorders (liver or renal failure, seizures), abnormal intestinal flora (d-lactic acidosis), drugs or toxins (salicylates, ethanol, methanol, ethylene glycol), G6PD deficiency

LACTATE DEHYDROGENASE (LDH)

Normal range: 50 to 150 U/L (0.82 to 2.66 μkat/L [CF: 0.01667; SMI: 0.02 μkat/L])
Elevated in:
Infarction of myocardium, lung, kidney
Diseases of cardiopulmonary system, liver, collagen, central nervous system

Hemolytic anemias, megaloblastic anemias, transfusions, seizures, muscle trauma, muscular dystrophy, acute pancreatitis, hypotension, shock, infectious mononucleosis, inflammation, neoplasia, intestinal obstruction, hypothyroidism

LACTATE DEHYDROGENASE ISOENZYMES

Normal range:
LDH_1: 22%-36% (cardiac, red blood cell) (0.22-0.36 [CF: 0.01, SMI: 0.01])
LDH_2: 35%-46% (cardiac, red blood cell) (0.35-0.46)
LDH_3: 13%-26% (pulmonary) (0.15-0.26)
LDH_4: 3%-10% (striated muscle, liver) (0.03-0.1)
LDH_5: 2%-9% (striated muscle, liver) (0.02-0.09)

Normal ratios:
$LDH_1 < LDH_2$
$LDH_5 < LDH_4$
Abnormal values:
LDH1 > LDH2: Myocardial infarction (can also be seen with hemolytic anemias, pernicious anemia, folate deficiency, renal infarct)
LDH5 > LDH4: Liver disease (cirrhosis, hepatitis, hepatic congestion)

LACTOSE TOLERANCE TEST (serum)

Normal: Test is performed by giving 2 g/kg body weight lactose orally and drawing glucose level at 0, 30, 45, 60, and 90 min. Normal response is change in glucose from fasting value to >30 mg/dl. Inconclusive response is increase of 20 to 30 mg/dl, abnormal response is increase <20 mg/dl. Table E69 summarizes laboratory tests in the differential diagnosis of diarrhea.
Abnormal in: Lactase deficiency

LAP SCORE

See "LEUKOCYTE ALKALINE PHOSPHATASE"

LEAD

Normal: Child, <10 mcg/dl; adult, <25 mcg/dl; acceptable for industrial exposure, <50 mcg/dl
Elevated in: Lead exposure, lead poisoning

LDH

See "LACTATE DEHYDROGENASE"

LDL

See "LOW-DENSITY LIPOPROTEIN CHOLESTEROL"

LEGIONELLA PNEUMOPHILA PCR

Test description: PCR can be performed on lung tissue, water sputum, bronchoalveolar lavage, and other respiratory fluids.

LEGIONELLA TITER

Normal: Negative
Positive in: Legionnaires disease (presumptive: ≥1:256 titer; definitive: fourfold titer increase to ≥1:128)

LEUKOCYTE ALKALINE PHOSPHATASE (LAP)

Normal range: 13 to 100 (33 to 188 U)
Elevated in: Leukemoid reactions, neutrophilia secondary to infections (except in sickle cell crisis—no significant increase in LAP score), Hodgkin disease, polycythemia vera, hairy cell leukemia, aplastic anemia, Down syndrome, myelofibrosis
Decreased in: Acute and chronic granulocytic leukemia, thrombocytopenic purpura, paroxysmal nocturnal hemoglobinuria, hypophosphatemia, collagen disorders

LEUKOCYTE COUNT

See "COMPLETE BLOOD COUNT"

LIPASE

Normal range: 0 to 160 U/L (0 to 2.66 μkat/L [CF: 0.01667; SMI: 0.02 μkat/L])

Elevated in: Acute pancreatitis, perforated peptic ulcer, carcinoma of pancreas (early stage), pancreatic duct obstruction, bowel infarction, intestinal obstruction

LIPOPROTEIN(a)

Normal: Male: 1.35 to 19.6 mg/dl; female: 1.24 to 20.1 mg/dl. Fig. E35 illustrates lipoprotein structure. Table E70 summarizes the major classes of human plasma lipoproteins. The chemical composition of major classes of plasma lipoproteins is described in Table E71.

Elevated in: Coronary artery disease, uncontrolled diabetes, hypothyroidism, chronic renal failure, pregnancy, tobacco use, infections, nephritic syndrome

Decreased in: Niacin, omega-3 fatty acids, estrogens, tamoxifen, statins

LIPOPROTEIN CHOLESTEROL, HIGH-DENSITY

See "HIGH-DENSITY LIPOPROTEIN CHOLESTEROL"

LIPOPROTEIN CHOLESTEROL, LOW-DENSITY

See "LOW-DENSITY LIPOPROTEIN CHOLESTEROL"

LIVER KIDNEY MICROSOME TYPE 1 ANTIBODIES

(LKM1)

Normal: <20 U
Elevated in: Autoimmune hepatitis type 2

LKM1

See "LIVER KIDNEY MICROSOME TYPE 1 ANTIBODIES"

LOW-DENSITY LIPOPROTEIN (LDL) CHOLESTEROL

Normal range: 50 to 130 mg/dl (1.30 to 1.68 mmol/L [CF: 0.02586; SMI: 0.05 mmol/L]). Fig. E36 illustrates the LDL receptor pathway and regulation of cholesterol metabolism.

<70	Optimal in diabetics, prior MI, and patients with cardiac risk factors
100-129	Near or above optimal
130-159	Borderline high
160-189	High
≥190	Very high

LUPUS ANTICOAGULANT

See "CIRCULATING ANTICOAGULANT"

LUTEINIZING HORMONE

Luteinizing hormone (LH) changes during the menstrual cycle are illustrated in Fig. E37. LH changes in different disease states are summarized in Table E72.

Normal range: 5 to 25 mIU/ml

Elevated in: Postmenopause, pituitary adenoma, primary gonadal dysfunction, polycystic ovary syndrome

Decreased in: Severe illness, anorexia nervosa, malnutrition, pituitary or hypothalamic impairment, severe stress

LYME DISEASE ANTIBODY TITER

Normal range: Negative

Positive result: Fig. E38 illustrates the usual serologic response in Lyme disease.

A serologic test is not necessary or helpful for several days after a tick bite because it is only 40% to 50% sensitive in this stage, and a negative test does not rule out the diagnosis.

LYMPHOCYTES

Normal range: 15% to 40%
   Total lymphocyte count = 800 to 2600/mm^3
   Total T lymphocyte = 800 to 2200/mm^3
   CD4 lymphocytes = ≥400/mm^3
   CD8 lymphocytes = 200 to 800/mm^3
   Normal CD4/CD8 ratio is 2.0.

Elevated in: Chronic infections, infectious mononucleosis and other viral infections, chronic lymphocytic leukemia, Hodgkin disease, ulcerative colitis, hypoadrenalism, idiopathic thrombocytopenia

Decreased in: AIDS, bone marrow suppression from chemotherapeutic agents or chemotherapy, aplastic anemia, neoplasms, steroids, adrenocortical hyperfunction, neurologic disorders (multiple sclerosis, myasthenia gravis, Guillain-Barré syndrome)

CD4 lymphocytes are calculated as total white blood cells × % lymphocytes × % lymphocytes stained with CD4. They are decreased in AIDS and other immune dysfunction.

Table E73 describes various lymphocyte abnormalities in peripheral blood. Box E22 summarizes key causes of lymphocytopenia.

MAGNESIUM (serum)

See Figs. E39 and E40.

Normal range: 1.8 to 3.0 mg/dl (0.80 to 1.20 mmol/L [CF: 0.4114; SMI: 0.02 mmol/L])

CAUSES OF HYPERMAGNESEMIA
Decreased renal excretion
Renal failure—glomerular filtration rate less than 30 ml/min
Hyperparathyroidism
Hypothyroidism
Addison disease
Lithium intoxication
Familial hypocalciuric hypercalcemia
Other causes: Usually in association with decrease in glomerular filtration rate
Endogenous loads
Diabetic ketoacidosis
Severe tissue injury: Burns
Exogenous loads
Gastrointestinal
   Magnesium-containing laxatives and antacids
   High-dose vitamin D analogs
Parenteral: Management of toxemia of pregnancy

CAUSES OF HYPOMAGNESEMIA
Alcohol abuse
Diuretic use
Renal losses
Acute and chronic renal failure
Postobstructive diuresis
Acute tubular necrosis
Chronic glomerulonephritis
Chronic pyelonephritis
Interstitial nephropathy
Renal transplantation
Gastrointestinal losses
Chronic diarrhea
Nasogastric suctioning
Short bowel syndrome
Protein-calorie malnutrition
Bowel fistula
Total parenteral nutrition
Acute pancreatitis
Endocrine
Diabetes mellitus
Hyperaldosteronism
Hyperthyroidism
Hyperparathyroidism
Acute intermittent porphyria
Pregnancy

Drugs
Aminoglycosides
Amphotericin
β-agonists
Cisplatin
Cyclosporine
Diuretics
Foscarnet
Pentamidine
Theophylline
Congenital disorders
Familial hypomagnesemia
Maternal diabetes
Maternal hypothyroidism
Maternal hyperparathyroidism

MEAN CORPUSCULAR VOLUME (MCV)

Laboratory features in microcytic hypochromic anemias are summarized in Table E74.
Normal range: 76 to 100 μm^3 (76 to 100 fL [CF: 1; SMI: 1 fL])
Table E75 summarizes clinical conditions not to be confused with megaloblastosis. See Tables E76 and E77 for descriptions of MCV abnormalities. Table E78 describes the usefulness of the MCV and RBC distribution width in the diagnosis of anemia. Table E79 describes peripheral blood film evaluation in a patient with red cell membrane disorder.

METANEPHRINES, URINE

See "URINE METANEPHRINES"

METHYLMALONIC ACID (Serum)

Normal: <0.2 $\mu mol/L$
Elevated in: Vitamin B_{12} deficiency, pregnancy, methylmalonic acidemia

MITOCHONDRIAL ANTIBODY (AMA)

Normal: Negative
Present in: Primary biliary cirrhosis (>90% of patients)

MONOCYTE COUNT

Normal range: 2% to 8%
Elevated in: Viral diseases, parasites, infections, neoplasms, inflammatory bowel disease, monocytic leukemia, lymphomas, myeloma, sarcoidosis
Decreased in: Aplastic anemia, lymphocytic leukemia, glucocorticoid administration
See Table E80 for changes in monocyte number.

MYCOPLASMA PNEUMONIAE PCR

Test description: PCR can be performed on sputum, bronchoalveolar lavage, nasopharyngeal and throat swabs, other respiratory fluids, and lung tissue.

MYELIN BASIC PROTEIN, CEREBROSPINAL FLUID

Normal: <2.5 ng/ml
Elevated in: Multiple sclerosis, CNS trauma, stroke, encephalitis

MYOGLOBIN, URINE

See "URINE MYOGLOBIN"

NEISSERIA GONORRHOEAE PCR

Test description: Test can be performed on endocervical swab, urine, and intraurethral swab
Normal: Negative

NEUTROPHIL COUNT

Normal range: 50% to 70%
Subsets:
Stabs (bands, early mature neutrophils): 2% to 6%
Segs (mature neutrophils): 60% to 70%

Elevated in: Acute bacterial infections, acute myocardial infarction, stress, neoplasms, myelocytic leukemia
Decreased in: Viral infections, aplastic anemias, immunosuppressive drugs, radiation therapy to bone marrow, agranulocytosis, drugs (antibiotics, antithyroidals, clopidogrel), lymphocytic and monocytic leukemias
Box 23 describes various drugs that can cause neutropenia. Table E81 describes miscellaneous inherited neutropenia disorders. Classification of neutropenia is covered in Table E82. Table E83 lists drugs associated with agranulocytosis. Table E84 describes causes of neutrophilia.

NOREPINEPHRINE

Normal range: 0 to 600 pg/ml
Elevated in: Pheochromocytomas, neuroblastomas, stress, vigorous exercise, certain foods (bananas, chocolate, coffee, tea, vanilla)

5'-NUCLEOTIDASE

Normal range: 2 to 16 IU/L (3-27 × 10^8 kat/L [CF: 1.67 × 10^8; SMI: 1 × 10^8 kat/L])
Elevated in: Biliary obstruction, metastatic neoplasms to liver, primary biliary cirrhosis, renal failure, pancreatic carcinoma, chronic active hepatitis

OSMOLALITY (serum)

Normal range: 280 to 300 mOsm/kg (280 to 300 mmol/kg [CF: 1; SMI: 1 mmol/kg])
It can also be estimated by the following formula:

$$2([Na] + [K] + glucose / 18 + BUN / 2.8)$$

The relationship between plasma osmolality and plasma arginine vasopressin is illustrated in Fig. E41.
The relationships between plasma and urine osmolality are illustrated in Fig. E42.
Elevated in: Dehydration, hypernatremia, diabetes insipidus, uremia, hyperglycemia, mannitol therapy, ingestion of toxins (ethylene glycol, methanol, ethanol), hypercalcemia, diuretics
Decreased in: Syndrome of inappropriate diuretic hormone secretion, hyponatremia, overhydration, Addison disease, hypothyroidism

OSMOLALITY, URINE

Normal range: 50 to 1200 mOsm/kg (50 to 1200 mmol/kg [CF: 1; SMI: 1 mmol/kg])
Elevated in: Syndrome of inappropriate antidiuretic hormone secretion, dehydration, glycosuria, adrenal insufficiency, high-protein diet

---

BOX 23 **Drugs That Cause Neutropenia**

Antiarrhythmics: Tocainide, procainamide, propranolol, quinidine
Antibiotics: Chloramphenicol, penicillins, sulfonamides, p-amino-salicylic acid (PAS), rifampin, vancomycin, isoniazid, nitrofurantoin
Antimalarials: Dapsone, quinine, pyrimethamine
Anticonvulsants: Phenytoin, mephenytoin, trimethadione, ethosuximide, carbamazepine
Hypoglycemic agents: Tolbutamide, chlorpropamide
Antihistamines: Cimetidine, brompheniramine, tripelennamine
Antihypertensives: Methyldopa, captopril
Antiinflammatory agents: Aminopyrine, phenylbutazone, gold salts, ibuprofen, indomethacin
Antithyroid agents: Propylthiouracil, methimazole, thiouracil
Diuretics: Acetazolamide, hydrochlorothiazide, chlorthalidone
Phenothiazines: Chlorpromazine, promazine, prochlorperazine
Immunosuppressive agents: Antimetabolites
Cytotoxic agents: Alkylating agents, antimetabolites, anthracyclines, Vinca alkaloids, cisplatin, hydroxyurea, dactinomycin
Other agents: Recombinant interferons, allopurinol, ethanol, levamisole, penicillamine, zidovudine, streptokinase, carbamazepine, clopidogrel, ticlopidine

Decreased in: Diabetes insipidus, excessive water intake, IV hydration with D_5W, acute renal insufficiency, glomerulonephritis

The relationship between plasma urine osmolality and plasma arginine vasopressin in patients with polyuria is illustrated in Fig. E43. Box E24 describes urine osmolality variances in common clinical situations.

OSMOTIC FRAGILITY TEST

Normal: Hemolysis begins at 0.50, w/v [5.0 g/L] and is complete at 0.30, w/v [3.0 g/L] NaCl.

Elevated in: Hereditary spherocytosis, hereditary stomatocytosis, spherocytosis associated with acquired immune hemolytic anemia

Decreased in: Iron deficiency anemia, thalassemias, liver disease, leptocytosis associated with asplenia

PARACENTESIS FLUID

Testing and evaluation of results: Process the fluid as follows:
Tube 1: LDH, glucose, albumin
Tube 2: Protein, specific gravity
Tube 3: Cell count and differential
Tube 4: Save until further notice
Draw serum LDH, protein, albumin.

Gram stain, acid-fast bacilli stain, bacterial and fungal cultures, amylase, and triglycerides should be ordered only when clearly indicated; bedside inoculation of blood-culture bottles with ascitic fluid improves sensitivity in detecting bacterial growth.

If malignant ascites is suspected, consider a carcinoembryonic antigen level on the paracentesis fluid and cytologic evaluation.

In suspected spontaneous bacterial peritonitis (SBP) the incidence of positive cultures can be increased by injecting 10 to 20 ml of ascitic fluid into blood culture bottles.

Peritoneal effusion can be subdivided as exudative or transudative based on its characteristics (see "Section II").

The serum-ascites albumin gradient (serum albumin level-ascitic fluid albumin level [SAAG]) correlates directly with portal pressure and can also be used to classify ascites. Patients with gradients $\geq$1.1 g/dl have portal hypertension, and those with gradients $\leq$1.1 g/dl do not; the accuracy of this method is >95%.

For the differential diagnosis of ascites, refer to Section II.

An ascitic fluid polymorphonuclear leukocyte count >500/µl is suggestive of SBP.

A blood-ascitic fluid albumin gradient. Box E25 summarizes causes of peritoneal effusions. Useful criteria for evaluation of peritoneal lavage is summarized in Box E26. Recommended tests in peritoneal effusions are summarized in Box E27.

PARATHYROID HORMONE (PTH)

Table E85 describes serum PTH and calcium patterns in various disorders.

Normal: Serum, intact molecule 10 to 65 pg/ml
    Plasma 1.0 to 5.0 pmol/L

Elevated in: Hyperparathyroidism (primary or secondary), pseudohypoparathyroidism, anticonvulsants, corticosteroids, lithium, isoniazid (INH), rifampin, phosphates, Zollinger-Ellison syndrome, hereditary vitamin D deficiency

Decreased in: Hypoparathyroidism, sarcoidosis, cimetidine, b-blockers, hyperthyroidism, hypomagnesemia.

PARIETAL CELL ANTIBODIES

Normal: Negative

Present in: Pernicious anemia (>90%), atrophic gastritis (up to 50%), thyroiditis (30%), Addison disease, myasthenia gravis, Sjögren syndrome, type 1 DM

PARTIAL THROMBOPLASTIN TIME (PTT), ACTIVATED PARTIAL THROMBOPLASTIN TIME (APTT)

See Table E86 for interpretation of coagulation protein screening tests.

Normal range: 25 to 41 sec

Elevated in: Heparin therapy, coagulation factor deficiency (I, II, V, VIII, IX, X, XI, XII), liver disease, vitamin K deficiency, disseminated intravascular coagulation, circulating anticoagulant, warfarin therapy, specific factor inhibition (penicillin [PCN] reaction, rheumatoid arthritis), thrombolytic therapy, nephrotic syndrome

NOTE: Useful to evaluate the intrinsic coagulation system.

PEPSINOGEN I

Normal: 124 to 142 ng/ml

Elevated in: Zollinger-Ellison (ZE) syndrome, duodenal ulcer, acute gastritis

Decreased in: Atrophic gastritis, gastric carcinoma, myxedema, pernicious anemia, Addison disease

PH, BLOOD

Normal values: Arterial: 7.35 to 7.45
    Venous: 7.32 to 7.42
    For abnormal values, refer to "ARTERIAL BLOOD GASES."

PH, URINE

See "URINE pH"

PHENOBARBITAL

Therapeutic range and general information are summarized in Table 87.

Normal therapeutic range: 15 to 30 mc g/ml for epilepsy control

PHENYTOIN (Dilantin)

Therapeutic range and general information are summarized in Table 88.

Normal therapeutic range: 10 to 20 mcg/ml

PHOSPHATASE, ACID

See "ACID PHOSPHATASE"

PHOSPHATASE, ALKALINE

See "ALKALINE PHOSPHATASE"

PHOSPHATE (serum)

Phosphate levels in various disorders are summarized in Table E89.

TABLE 87	Phenobarbital
Purpose	**Treatment of Generalized Tonic-Clonic Seizures, Simple Partial Seizures, Anxiety, Insomnia**
General adult dose	Oral: 100-200 mg/day for seizure control; 30-120 mg/day for anxiety; 100-320 mg for sleep induction
Usual bioavailability	Approximately 90%-100%
Half-life	Approximately 5-6 days in adults; approximately 3-4 days in children
General therapeutic range	15-30 mcg/ml for epilepsy control
General toxic level	>40 mcg/ml, although tolerance may develop
Transport	Approximately 40%-60% plasma protein bound
Metabolism	Approximately 75% hepatic:*p*-hydroxyphenobarbital, inactive
Elimination	Approximately 25% unchanged in urine
Steady state	Approximately 14-21 days
Mechanism of action	Stabilizes damaged membranes and raises threshold for neuronal membrane depolarization
Toxic effects	Drowsiness, depression, respiratory depression, coma, sedation, hypotension. Respiratory depression may be caused by rapid intravenous administration

From McPherson RA, Pincus MR: *Henry's clinical diagnosis and management by laboratory methods*, ed 23, St Louis, 2017, Elsevier.

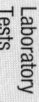

Laboratory Tests

IV

TABLE 88	Phenytoin (Dilantin)
Purpose	**Treatment of Generalized Tonic-Clonic Seizures, Simple Partial Seizures, Complex Partial Seizures**
General adult dose	Oral: 300-400 mg/day maintenance dose
Usual bioavailability	Variable: 30%-95%
Half-life	24 ± 12 hr, and dose dependent
General therapeutic range	10-20 mcg/ml
General toxic level	>20 mcg/ml
Transport	Approximately 90%-95% plasma protein bound
Metabolism	Hepatic: 5-(p-hydroxyphenyl)5-phenylhydantoin, inactive
Elimination	Approximately 5% unchanged in urine
Steady state	Approximately 7-8 days
Mechanism of action	Appears to block sodium and calcium ion influxes into repeatedly depolarizing CNS neurons
Toxic effects	Nystagmus, ataxia, diplopia, drowsiness, coma; rapid intravenous administration may produce cardiovascular collapse and/or CNS depression

CNS, Central nervous system.
From McPherson RA, Pincus MR: *Henry's clinical diagnosis and management by laboratory methods*, ed 23, St Louis, 2017, Elsevier.

Normal range: 2.5 to 5 mg/dl (0.8 to 1.6 mmol/L [CF: 0.3229; SMI: 0.05 mmol/L])
DECREASED
Parenteral hyperalimentation
Diabetic acidosis
Alcohol withdrawal
Severe metabolic or respiratory alkalosis
Antacids that bind phosphorus
Malnutrition with refeeding using low-phosphorus nutrients
Renal tubule failure to reabsorb phosphate (Fanconi syndrome; congenital disorder; vitamin D deficiency)
Glucose administration
Nasogastric suction
Malabsorption
Gram-negative sepsis
Primary hyperthyroidism
Chlorothiazide diuretics
Therapy of acute severe asthma
Acute respiratory failure with mechanical ventilation
INCREASED
Renal failure
Severe muscle injury
Phosphate-containing antacids
Hypoparathyroidism
Tumor lysis syndrome

PLASMA CELLS

Plasma cells are not normally present in circulating blood. They are increased in a variety of chronic infections, in allergic states, in the presence of neoplasms, and in other conditions in which the serum γ-globulin concentration is elevated. Plasma cells have also been recorded in the blood of patients with viral disorders, including rubella, measles, chickenpox, and mumps. They are moderately increased in cutaneous exanthemas, infectious mononucleosis, syphilis, subacute bacterial endocarditis, sarcoidosis, and collagen disease. Rarely, bacterial sepsis may show a peripheral plasmacytosis mimicking plasma cell leukemia. Their increase is usually linked with increases in lymphocytes, monocytes, and eosinophils. Causes and conditions associated with plasmacytosis include those listed in Box E28.

PLASMINOGEN
Normal: Immunoassay (antigen): <20 mg/dl
Elevated in: Infection, trauma, neoplasm, myocardial infarction (acute phase reactant), pregnancy, bilirubinemia
Decreased in: Disseminated intravascular coagulation (DIC), severe liver disease, thrombolytic therapy with streptokinase or urokinase, alteplase

PLATELET AGGREGATION
Normal: Full aggregation (generally >60%) in response to epinephrine, thrombin, ristocetin, adenosine diphosphate (ADP), collagen
Elevated in: Heparin, hemolysis, lipemia, nicotine, hereditary and acquired disorders of platelet adhesion, activation, and aggregation
Decreased in: Aspirin, some penicillins, chloroquine, chlorpromazine, clofibrate, captopril, Glanzmann thrombasthenia, Bernard-Soulier syndrome, Wiskott-Aldrich syndrome, cyclooxygenase deficiency. In von Willebrand disease there is normal aggregation with ADP, collagen, and epinephrine but abnormal agglutination with ristocetin.

PLATELET ANTIBODIES
Normal: Absent
Present in: Idiopathic thrombocytopenic purpura (ITP) (>90% of patients with chronic ITP). Patients with nonimmune thrombocytopenias may have false-positive results.

PLATELET COUNT
A classification of inherited thrombocytopenias by platelet size is described in Table E90.
See Fig. E44 for evaluation of thrombocytosis. Box E29 describes testing for thrombocytopenia. See Table E91 for differential diagnosis. Table E92 describes antibody-mediated thrombocytopenic disorders caused by autoantibodies, alloantibodies, or potentially both. Tables E93 and E94 indicate differential diagnosis of thrombocytopenia in newborns and differential diagnosis of thrombocytopenia in pregnancy, respectively. Table E95 describes laboratory tests used to investigate a patient with thrombocytopenia.
Normal range: 130 to 400 × 10³/mm³ (130 to 400 × 10⁹/L [CF: 1; SMI: 5 × 10⁹/L])
Elevated in:
REACTIVE THROMBOCYTOSIS
Infections or inflammatory states: Vasculitis, allergic reactions, etc.
Surgery and tissue damage: Myocardial infarction, pancreatitis, etc.
Postsplenectomy state
Malignancy: Solid tumors, lymphoma
Iron deficiency anemia, hemolytic anemia, acute blood loss
Uncertain etiology
Rebound effect after chemotherapy or immune thrombocytopenia
Renal disorders: Renal failure, nephrotic syndrome
MYELOPROLIFERATIVE DISORDERS
Chronic myeloid leukemia
Primary thrombocythemia
Polycythemia vera
Idiopathic myelofibrosis
Decreased:
Increased destruction (see Table E96)
Immunologic
Drugs: Quinine, quinidine, digitalis, procainamide, thiazide diuretics, sulfonamides, phenytoin, aspirin, penicillin, heparin, gold, meprobamate, sulfa drugs, phenylbutazone, NSAIDs, methyldopa, cimetidine, furosemide, INH, cephalosporins, chlorpropamide, organic arsenicals, chloroquine
Idiopathic thrombocytopenic purpura
Transfusion reaction: Transfusion of platelets with platelet antigen HPA-1a (PL^A1) in recipients without PL^A1
Fetal/maternal incompatibility
Vasculitis (e.g., systemic lupus erythematosus)
Autoimmune hemolytic anemia
Lymphoreticular disorders (e.g., chronic lymphocytic leukemia)
Nonimmunologic
Prosthetic heart valves
Thrombotic thrombocytopenic purpura

Sepsis
Disseminated intravascular coagulation
Hemolytic-uremic syndrome
Giant cavernous hemangioma
Decreased production
Abnormal marrow
Marrow infiltration (e.g., leukemia, lymphoma, fibrosis)
Marrow suppression (e.g., chemotherapy, alcohol, radiation)
Hereditary disorders (see Table E97)
Wiskott-Aldrich syndrome: X-linked disorder characterized by thrombocytopenia, eczema, and repeated infections
May-Hegglin anomaly: Increased megakaryocytes but ineffective thrombopoiesis
Vitamin deficiencies (e.g., vitamin B_{12}, folic acid)
Splenic sequestration, hypersplenism
Dilutional, secondary to massive transfusion

PLATELET FUNCTION ANALYSIS 100 ASSAY (PFA)

Normal: This test is a two-component assay where blood is aspirated through two capillary tubes, one of which is coated with collagen and ADP (COL/ADP) and the other with collagen and epinephrine (COL/EPI). The test measures the ability of platelets to occlude an aperture in a biologically active membrane treated with COL/ADP and COL/EPI. During the test, the platelets adhere to the surface of the tube and cause blood flow to cease. The closing time refers to the cessation of blood flow and is reported in conjunction with the hematocrit and platelet count. Hematocrit count must be >25% and platelet count >50 K/microliter for the test to be performed.
COL/ADP: 70 to 120 sec
COL/EPI: 75 to 120 sec
Elevated in: Acquired platelet dysfunction, von Willebrand disease, anemia, thrombocytopenia, use of aspirin and NSAIDs

PLEURAL FLUID

Testing and evaluation of results:
Pleural effusion fluid should be differentiated in exudate or transudate.
The initial laboratory studies should be aimed only at distinguishing an exudate from a transudate.
Tube 1: Protein, LDH, albumin.
Tubes 2, 3, 4: Save the fluid until further notice. In selected patients with suspected empyema, a pH level may be useful (generally ≤7.0). See following for proper procedure to obtain a pH level from pleural fluid.
1. A serum/effusion albumin gradient of ≤1.2 g/dl is indicative of exudative effusions, especially in patients with congestive heart failure (CHF) treated with diuretics
2. Note the appearance of the fluid:
   a. A grossly hemorrhagic effusion can be a result of a traumatic tap, neoplasm, or an embolus with infarction.
   b. A milky appearance indicates either of the following:
      (1) Chylous effusion: Caused by trauma or tumor invasion of the thoracic duct; lipoprotein electrophoresis of the effusion reveals chylomicrons and triglyceride levels >115 mg/dl.
      (2) Pseudochylous effusion: Often seen with chronic inflammation of the pleural space (e.g., TB, connective tissue diseases).
3. If transudate, consider CHF, cirrhosis, chronic renal failure, and other hypoproteinemic states and perform subsequent workup accordingly.
4. If exudate, consider ordering these tests on the pleural fluid:
   a. Cytologic examination for malignant cells (for suspected neoplasm).
   b. Gram stain, cultures (aerobic and anaerobic), and sensitivities (for suspected infectious process).
   c. AFB stain and cultures (for suspected TB).
   d. pH: A value <7.0 suggests parapneumonic effusion or empyema; a pleural fluid pH must be drawn anaerobically and iced immediately; the syringe should be prerinsed with 0.2 ml of 1:1000 heparin.
   e. Glucose: A low glucose level suggests parapneumonic effusions and rheumatoid arthritis.
   f. Amylase: A high amylase level suggests pancreatitis or ruptured esophagus.

5. Perplexing pleural effusions are often a result of malignancy (e.g., lymphoma, malignant mesothelioma, ovarian carcinoma), TB, subdiaphragmatic processes, prior asbestos exposure, and postcardiac injury syndrome.
6. Box E30 describes a cellular differential of pleural effusions. Features differentiating exudative from transudative pleural effusion are summarized in Table E98.

POTASSIUM (serum)

Normal range: 3.5 to 5 mEq/L (3.5 to 5 mmol/L [CF: 1; SMI: 0.1 mmol/L])
CAUSES OF HYPERKALEMIA
See Fig. E45 for evaluation and treatment of hyperkalemia, and Fig. E46 for electrocardiographic changes in hyperkalemia.
- Pseudohyperkalemia
  1. Hemolysis of sample
  2. Thrombocytosis
  3. Leukocytosis
  4. Laboratory error
- Increased potassium intake and absorption
  1. Potassium supplements (oral and parenteral)
  2. Dietary: Salt substitutes
  3. Stored blood
  4. Potassium-containing medications
- Impaired renal excretion
  1. Acute renal failure
  2. Chronic renal failure
  3. Tubular defect in potassium secretion
     a. Renal allograft
     b. Analgesic nephropathy
     c. Sickle cell disease
     d. Obstructive uropathy
  4. Hypoaldosteronism
     a. Primary (Addison disease)
     b. Secondary
        (1) Hyporeninemic hypoaldosteronism (type IV renal tubular acidosis [RTA])
        (2) Congenital adrenal hyperplasia
        (3) Drug-induced
        (4) NSAIDs
        (5) ACE inhibitors
        (6) Heparin
        (7) Cyclosporine
  5. Transcellular shifts
     a. Acidosis
     b. Hypertonicity
     c. Insulin deficiency
     d. Drugs
β-blockers
Digitalis toxicity
Succinylcholine
Exercise
Hyperkalemic periodic paralysis
Cellular injury
Rhabdomyolysis
Severe intravascular hemolysis
Acute tumor lysis syndrome
Burns and crush injuries
CAUSES OF HYPOKALEMIA
For the clinical approach to hypokalemia, see Fig. 47.
Decreased intake
Decreased dietary potassium
Impaired absorption of potassium
Clay ingestion
Kayexalate
Increased loss
Renal
Hyperaldosteronism

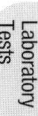

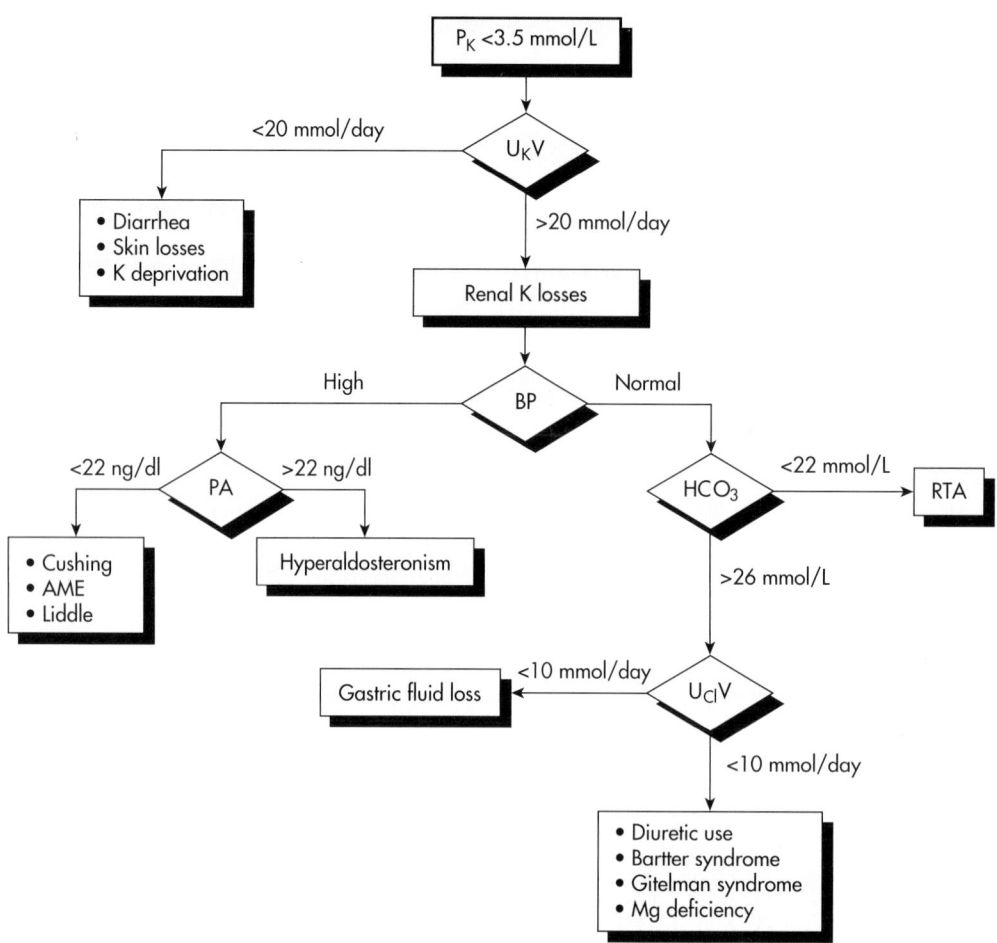

FIG. 47 Diagnostic evaluation of chronic hypokalemia. *AME,* Syndrome of apparent mineralocorticoid excess; *BP,* blood pressure; HCO_3-, bicarbonate; *PA,* stimulated plasma aldosterone (see text); *RTA,* renal tubular acidosis; $U_{Cl}V$, urinary chloride excretion; $U_K V$, urinary potassium excretion. (From Parrillo JE, Dellinger RP: *Critical care medicine, principles of diagnosis and management in the adult,* ed 5, Philadelphia, 2019, Elsevier.)

- Primary
  1. Conn syndrome
  2. Adrenal hyperplasia
- Secondary
  1. Congestive heart failure
  2. Cirrhosis
  3. Nephrotic syndrome
  4. Dehydration
  5. Bartter syndrome

Glycyrrhizic acid (licorice, chewing tobacco)
Excessive adrenal corticosteroids
    Cushing syndrome
    Steroid therapy
    Adrenogenital syndrome
Renal tubular defects
    Renal tubular acidosis
    Obstructive uropathy
    Salt-wasting nephropathy
Drugs
    Diuretics
    Aminoglycosides
    Mannitol
    Amphotericin
    Cisplatin
    Carbenicillin
Gastrointestinal
    Vomiting

Nasogastric suction
Diarrhea
Malabsorption
Ileostomy
Villous adenoma
Laxative abuse
Increased losses from the skin
    Excessive sweating
    Burns
Transcellular shifts
Alkalosis
    Vomiting
    Diuretics
    Hyperventilation
    Bicarbonate therapy
Insulin
    Exogenous
    Endogenous response to glucose
β2-Agonists (albuterol, terbutaline, epinephrine)
Hypokalemia periodic paralysis
    Familial
    Thyrotoxic
Miscellaneous
    Anabolic state
    Intravenous hyperalimentation
    Treatment of megaloblastic anemia
    Acute mountain sickness

POTASSIUM, URINE
See "URINE POTASSIUM"

PROCAINAMIDE
Therapeutic range and general information are summarized in Table 99.
Normal therapeutic range: 4 to 10 mcg/ml

PROGESTERONE (serum)
Normal:
Female: Follicular phase: 15 to 70 ng/dl
Luteal phase: 200 to 2500 ng/dl
Male: 15 to 70 ng/dl
Elevated in: Congenital adrenal hyperplasia, clomiphene, corticosterone, 11-deoxycortisol, dihydroprogesterone, molar pregnancy, lipoid ovarian tumor
Decreased in: Primary or secondary hypogonadism, oral contraceptives, ampicillin, threatened abortion

PROLACTIN
See Fig. E48 for the evaluation of hyperprolactinemia.
Normal range: <20 ng/ml (<20 μg/L [CF: 1; SMI: 1 μg/L])
Elevated in: Prolactinomas (level >200 micrograms/L highly suggestive), drugs (phenothiazines, cimetidine, tricyclic antidepressants, metoclopramide, estrogens, antihypertensives [methyldopa], verapamil, haloperidol), postpartum, stress, hypoglycemia, hypothyroidism, chronic liver disease, end-stage renal disease, brain radiation therapy, polycystic ovary syndrome, seizures, exercise, coitus, lactation. Mild hyperprolactinemia (<100 micrograms/L) can also be caused by large sellar masses, including nonfunctioning pituitary adenoma.

PROSTATE-SPECIFIC ANTIGEN (PSA)
Normal range: 0 to 4 ng/ml
Table E100 describes age-specific reference ranges for PSA.
Elevated in: Benign prostatic hypertrophy, carcinoma of prostate, prostatitis, postrectal examination, prostate trauma
Factors affecting serum PSA are described in Table E101.
NOTE: Measurement of free PSA is useful to assess the probability of prostate cancer in patients with normal digital rectal examination and total PSA between 4 and 10 ng/ml. In these patients, the global risk of prostate cancer is 25%; however, if the free PSA is >25%, the risk of prostate cancer decreases to 8%, whereas if the free PSA is <10%, the risk of cancer increases to 56%. Free PSA is also useful to evaluate the aggressiveness of prostate cancer. A low free PSA percentage generally indicates a high-grade cancer, whereas a high free PSA percentage is generally associated with a slower-growing tumor.
Decreased in: 5-α reductase inhibitors (finasteride, dutasteride), saw palmetto use, antiandrogens

PROSTATIC ACID PHOSPHATASE
Normal: 0 to 0.8 U/L
Elevated in: Prostate cancer (especially in metastatic prostate cancer), BPH, prostatitis, postprostate surgery or manipulation, hemolysis, androgens, clofibrate
Decreased in: Ketoconazole

PROTEIN (serum)
Normal range: 6 to 8 g/dl (60 to 80 g/L [CF: 10; SMI: 1 g/L])
Elevated in: Dehydration, multiple myeloma, Waldenström macroglobulinemia, sarcoidosis, collagen vascular diseases
Decreased in: Malnutrition, low-protein diet, overhydration, malabsorption, pregnancy, severe burns, neoplasms, chronic diseases, cirrhosis, nephrosis

PROTEIN C ASSAY
See Table E102 and Fig. E49.
Normal: 70% to 140%
Elevated in: Oral contraceptives, stanozolol
Decreased in: Congenital protein C deficiency, warfarin therapy, Vitamin K deficiency, renal insufficiency, consumptive coagulopathies

PROTEIN ELECTROPHORESIS (serum)
Normal range:
Albumin: 60% to 75% (0.6 to 0.75 [CF: 0.01; SMI: 0.01])
α-1: 1.7% to 5% (0.02 to 0.05)
α-2: 6.7% to 12.5% (0.07 to 0.13)
β: 8.3% to 16.3% (0.08 to 0.16)
γ: 10.7% to 20% (0.11 to 0.2)
Albumin: 3.6 to 5.2 g/dl (36 to 52 g/L [CF: 0.01; SMI: 1 g/L])
α-1: 0.1 to 0.4 g/dl (1 to 4 g/L)
α-2: 0.4 to 1 g/dl (4 to 10 g/L)
β: 0.5 to 1.2 g/dl (5 to 12 g/L)
γ: 0.6 to 1.6 g/dl (6 to 16 g/L)
Elevated in:
Albumin: Dehydration
α-1: Neoplastic diseases, inflammation
α-2: Neoplasms, inflammation, infection, nephrotic syndrome
β: Hypothyroidism, biliary cirrhosis, diabetes mellitus
γ: See "IMMUNOGLOBULINS"
Decreased in:
Albumin: Malnutrition, chronic liver disease, malabsorption, nephrotic syndrome, burns, systemic lupus erythematosus
α-1: Emphysema (α-1 antitrypsin deficiency), nephrosis
α-2: Hemolytic anemias (decreased haptoglobin), severe hepatocellular damage
β: Hypocholesterolemia, nephrosis
γ: See "IMMUNOGLOBULINS"
Fig. E50 describes serum protein electrophoretic patterns.

PROTEIN S ASSAY
See Table E103.
Normal: 65% to 140%
Elevated in: Presence of lupus anticoagulant
Decreased in: Hereditary deficiency, acute thrombotic events, DIC, surgery, oral contraceptives, pregnancy, hormone replacement therapy, l-asparaginase treatment

PROTHROMBIN TIME (PT)
See Table E104.
Normal range: 10 to 12 sec
Elevated in: Liver disease, oral anticoagulants (warfarin), heparin, factor deficiency (I, II, V, VII, X), disseminated intravascular coagulation, vitamin K

	TABLE 99 Procainamide

Purpose	Treatment of Supraventricular or Ventricular Arrhythmias
General adult dose	Oral: 4 g/day, in divided doses, for maintenance therapy
Usual bioavailability	75%-95%
Half-life	Approximately 3.5 hr in patients with normal renal function
General therapeutic range	4-10 mcg/ml
General toxic level	>12 mcg/ml
Transport	Approximately 15% plasma protein bound
Metabolism	Hepatic: *N*-acetylprocainamide (active), with approximately 7 hr in patients with normal renal function
Elimination	Approximately 50%-60% unchanged in urine
Steady state	Minimum of 12 hr
Mechanism of action	Prolongation of atrial refractory period and decreased myocardial excitability
Toxic effects	Reversible lupus erythematosus–like syndrome, irregular pulse, hypotension, rash, agranulocytosis

From McPherson RA, Pincus MR: *Henry's clinical diagnosis and management by laboratory methods*, ed 23, St Louis, 2017, Elsevier.

IV

Laboratory Tests

deficiency, afibrinogenemia, dysfibrinogenemia, drugs (salicylate, chloral hydrate, diphenylhydantoin, estrogens, antacids, phenylbutazone, quinidine, antibiotics, allopurinol, anabolic steroids). Table E105 describes a differential diagnosis of abnormal coagulation screening tests

Decreased in: Vitamin K supplementation, thrombophlebitis, drugs (glutethimide, estrogens, griseofulvin, diphenhydramine)

PROTOPORPHYRIN (Free erythrocyte)

Normal range: 16 to 36 μg/dl of red blood cells (0.28 to 0.64 μmol/L [CF: 0.0177; SMI: 0.02 μmol/L])

Elevated in: Iron deficiency, lead poisoning, sideroblastic anemias, anemia of chronic disease, hemolytic anemias, erythropoietic protoporphyria

PSA
See "PROSTATE-SPECIFIC ANTIGEN"

PT
See "PROTHROMBIN TIME"

PTH
See "PARATHYROID HORMONE"

PTT
See "PARTIAL THROMBOPLASTIN TIME"

RAPID PLASMA REAGIN (RPR)

Description: Nontreponemal test traditionally used as a screening test for syphilis. It is a quantitative test, and antibody titers can be monitored to assess treatment response.

Normal: Negative

Positive: Syphilis. False-positive results may occur with pregnancy, autoimmune diseases, tuberculosis, and other inflammatory conditions. Positive results should be confirmed with treponemal serologic tests (e.g., T-pallidum enzyme immunoassay [TP-EIA]).

RDW
See "RED BLOOD CELL DISTRIBUTION WIDTH"

RED BLOOD CELL (RBC) COUNT

Normal range: Male: 4.3 to $5.9 \times 10^6/mm^3$ (4.3 to 5.9×10^{12}/L [CF: 1; SMI: 0.1×10^{12}/L])
Female: 3.5 to $5 \times 10^6/mm^3$ (3.5 to 5×10^{12}/L [CF: 1; SMI: 0.1×10^{12}/L])

Elevated in: Polycythemia vera, smokers, high altitude, cardiovascular disease, renal cell carcinoma and other erythropoietin-producing neoplasms, stress, hemoconcentration/dehydration

Decreased in: Anemias, hemolysis, chronic renal failure, hemorrhage, failure of marrow production

RED BLOOD CELL DISTRIBUTION WIDTH (RDW)

Measures variability of red cell size (anisocytosis)
Normal range: 11.5 to 14.5
Normal RDW and elevated mean corpuscular volume (MCV): Aplastic anemia, preleukemia
Normal MCV: Normal, anemia of chronic disease, acute blood loss or hemolysis, chronic lymphocytic leukemia (CLL), chronic myelocytic leukemia, nonanemic enzymopathy or hemoglobinopathy
Decreased MCV: Anemia of chronic disease, heterozygous thalassemia
Elevated RDW and elevated MCV: Vitamin B_{12} deficiency, folate deficiency, immune hemolytic anemia, cold agglutinins, CLL with high count, liver disease
Normal MCV: Early iron deficiency, early vitamin B_{12} deficiency, early folate deficiency, anemic globinopathy
Decreased MCV: Iron deficiency, red blood cell fragmentation, HbH disease, thalassemia intermedia

See Table E106 for combining the reticulocyte count and RBC parameters for diagnosis.

RED BLOOD CELL FOLATE
See "FOLATE"

RED BLOOD CELL MASS (volume)

Normal range: Male: 20 to 36 ml/kg body weight (1.15 to 1.21 L/m^2 body surface area)
Female: 19 to 31 ml/kg body weight (0.95 to 1.00 L/m^2 body surface area)
Elevated in: Polycythemia vera, hypoxia (smokers, high altitude, cardiovascular disease), hemoglobinopathies with high oxygen affinity, erythropoietin-producing tumors (renal cell carcinoma)
Decreased in: Hemorrhage, chronic disease, failure of marrow production, anemias, hemolysis

RED BLOOD CELL MORPHOLOGY

Table E107 describes features of the peripheral blood smear. Table E108 summarizes peripheral blood film evaluation in a patient with red cell membrane disorder. See Fig. E51 for useful peripheral blood and RBC features in the evaluation of anemia.

RENIN (serum)

Blood causes of hypertension associated with high levels of plasma renin are summarized in Box E31. Low levels of renin and hypertension are listed in Box E32.
Elevated in: Drugs (thiazides, estrogen, minoxidil), chronic renal failure, Bartter syndrome, pregnancy (normal), pheochromocytoma, renal hypertension, reduced plasma volume, secondary aldosteronism
Decreased in: Adrenocortical hypertension, increased plasma volume, primary aldosteronism, drugs (propranolol, reserpine, clonidine)
Table 109 describes typical renin-aldosterone patterns in various conditions.

RESPIRATORY SYNCYTIAL VIRUS (RSV) SCREEN

Test description: PCR test can be performed on nasopharyngeal swab, wash, or aspirate

RETICULOCYTE COUNT
See Fig. E52, Fig. E53, and Table E110.

TABLE 109 Typical Renin-Aldosterone Patterns in Various Conditions

	Plasma Renin	Aldosterone
Primary aldosteronism	Low	High
"Low-renin" essential hypertension	Low	Normal
Cushing syndrome	Low	Low-normal
Licorice ingestion syndrome	Low	Low
High-salt diet	Low	Low
Oral contraceptives	High	Normal
Cirrhosis	High	High
Malignant hypertension	High	High
Unilateral renal disease	High	High
"High-renin" essential hypertension	High	High
Pregnancy	High	High
Diuretic overuse	High	High
Juxtaglomerular tumor (Bartter syndrome)	High	High
Low-salt diet	High	High
Addison disease	High	Low
Hypokalemia	High	Low

Normal range: 0.5% to 1.5%

Elevated in: Hemolytic anemia (sickle cell crisis, thalassemia major, autoimmune hemolysis), hemorrhage, postanemia therapy (folic acid, ferrous sulfate, vitamin B_{12}), chronic renal failure

Decreased in: Aplastic anemia, marrow suppression (sepsis, chemotherapeutic agents, radiation), hepatic cirrhosis, blood transfusion, anemias of disordered maturation (iron deficiency anemia, megaloblastic anemia, sideroblastic anemia, anemia of chronic disease)

RHEUMATOID FACTOR

Normal: Negative. Present in titer >1:20

RHEUMATIC DISEASES
Rheumatoid arthritis
Sjögren syndrome
Systemic lupus erythematosus
Polymyositis/dermatomyositis
Mixed connective tissue disease
Scleroderma

INFECTIOUS DISEASES
Subacute bacterial endocarditis
Tuberculosis
Infectious mononucleosis
Hepatitis
Syphilis
Leprosy
Influenza

MALIGNANCIES
Lymphoma
Multiple myeloma
Waldenström macroglobulinemia
Postradiation or postchemotherapy

MISCELLANEOUS
Normal adults, especially the elderly
Sarcoidosis
Chronic pulmonary disease (interstitial fibrosis)
Chronic liver disease (chronic active hepatitis, cirrhosis)
Mixed essential cryoglobulinemia
Hypergammaglobulinemic purpura
RNP
See "EXTRACTABLE NUCLEAR ANTIGEN"

RPR

See "RAPID PLASMA REAGIN"

ROTAVIRUS SEROLOGY

Test description: PCR test is performed on stool specimen
Normal: Negative

SARS-COV-2 ANTIBODIES

Name	Value	Reference Range
SARS-COV-2 ABS Interp.	Negative	Negative
SARS-COV-2 ABS INDEX	0.09	<1.0 (Index)

Index (COI) Value	Interpretation
<1.0	Negative for ANTI-SARS COV 2 antibodies
≥1.0	Positive for ANTI-SARS COV 2 antibodies

The ANTI-SARS-COV-2 assay is intended for the qualitative detection of antibodies to SARS-COV-2 in human serum and as an aid in identifying individuals with an adaptive immune response to SARS-COV-2, indicating recent or prior infection. At the time of this publication, it is unknown for how long antibodies persist following infection and to what degree the presence of antibodies confers protective immunity. This assay should not be used to diagnose acute SARS-COV-2 infection.

Negative results do not preclude acute SARS-COV-2 infection. If acute infection is suspected, direct PCR testing is recommended. False-positive results may occur due to cross-reactivity from preexisting antibodies or other possible causes. This assay has overall sensitivity of 100% and specificity of 99.8% in patients >14 days post-PCR confirmation.

SED RATE

See "ERYTHROCYTE SEDIMENTATION RATE"

SEDIMENTATION RATE

See "ERYTHROCYTE SEDIMENTATION RATE"

SEMEN ANALYSIS

Table 111 describes semen analysis reference ranges.

SGOT

See "ASPARTATE AMINOTRANSFERASE"

SGPT

See "ASPARTATE AMINOTRANSFERASE"

SICKLE CELL TEST

Normal: Negative
Positive in: Sickle cell anemia, sickle cell trait, combination of *Hb S* gene with other disorders such as alpha-thalassemia, beta-thalassemia

SMOOTH MUSCLE ANTIBODY

Normal: Negative
Present in: Chronic acute hepatitis, primary sclerosing cholangitis, primary biliary cirrhosis, autoimmune hepatitis, infectious mononucleosis

SODIUM (serum)

Normal range: 135 to 147 mEq/L (135 to 147 mmol/L [CF: 1; SMI: 1 mmol/L]). Electrolyte concentrations in extracellular and intracellular fluid are summarized in Table E112.
HYPONATREMIA
See Fig. E54.
Common causes of hyponatremia and electrolyte patterns in serum and urine with normal renal function are described in Table E113. Table E114 describes drugs associated with hyponatremia.
Sodium and water depletion (deficit hyponatremia)
Loss of gastrointestinal secretions with replacement of fluid but not electrolytes

TABLE 111 Semen Analysis Reference Ranges

Color	Grayish white
pH	7.3-7.8 (literature range, 7.0-7.8)
Volume	2.0-5.0 ml (literature range, 1.5-6.0 ml)
Sperm count	20-250 million/ml (literature range for upper limit varies from 100-250 million/ml)
Motility	>60% motile <3 h after specimen is obtained (literature range, >40% to >70%)
% Normal sperm	>60% (literature range, >60% to >70%)
Viscosity	Can be poured from a pipet in droplets rather than a thick strand

Vomiting
  Diarrhea
  Tube drainage
Loss from skin with replacement of fluids but not electrolytes
  Excessive sweating
  Extensive burns
Loss from kidney
  Diuretics
  Chronic renal insufficiency (uremia) with acidosis
Metabolic loss
  Starvation with acidosis
  Diabetic acidosis
Endocrine loss
  Addison disease
  Sudden withdrawal of long-term steroid therapy
Iatrogenic loss from serous cavities
  Paracentesis or thoracentesis
Excessive water (dilution hyponatremia)
  Excessive water administration
  Congestive heart failure
  Cirrhosis
  Nephrotic syndrome
  Hypoalbuminemia (severe)
  Acute renal failure with oliguria
Inappropriate antidiuretic hormone (IADH) syndrome
Intracellular loss (reset osmostat syndrome)
False hyponatremia (actually a dilutional effect)
  Marked hypertriglyceridemia
  Marked hyperproteinemia
  Severe hyperglycemia
HYPERNATREMIA
See Fig. E55.
Common causes of hypernatremia and electrolyte patterns in serum and urine with normal renal function are summarized in Table E115
Dehydration is the most frequent overall clinical finding in hypernatremia
Deficient water intake (either orally or intravenously)
Excess kidney water output (diabetes insipidus, osmotic diuresis)
Excess skin water output (excess sweating, loss from burns)
Excess gastrointestinal tract output (severe protracted vomiting or diarrhea without fluid therapy)
Accidental sodium overdose
High-protein tube feedings

STREPTOZYME

See "ANTISTREPTOLYSIN O TITER"

SUCROSE HEMOLYSIS TEST (sugar water test)

Normal: Absence of hemolysis
Positive in:
Paroxysmal nocturnal hemoglobinuria
False positive: Autoimmune hemolytic anemia, megaloblastic anemias
False negative: May occur with use of heparin or EDTA

SUDAN III STAIN (qualitative screening for fecal fat)

Normal: Negative. Test should be preceded by diet containing 100-150 g of dietary fat/day for 1 wk, avoidance of high-fiber diet, and avoidance of suppositories or oily material before specimen collection.
Positive in: Steatorrhea, use of castor oil or mineral oil droplets

SYNOVIAL FLUID ANALYSIS

Table E116 describes the classification and interpretation of synovial fluid analysis. An algorithm for analysis of joint fluid is illustrated in Fig. E56.

T_3 (triiodothyronine)

See Table 117 for T_3 abnormalities.
Normal range: 75 to 220 ng/dl (1.2 to 3.4 nmol/L [CF: 0.01536; SMI: 0.1 nmol/L])

TABLE 117 Findings in Thyroid Function Tests in Various Clinical Conditions

Condition	T_4	FT_4I	T_3	FT_3I	TSH	TSI	TRH Stimulation
Hyperthyroidism							
Graves disease	↑	↑	↑	↑	↓	+	↓
Toxic nodular goiter	↑	↑	↑	↑	↓	−	↓
Pituitary TSH-secreting tumors	↑	↑	↑	↑	↑	−	↓
T_3 thyrotoxicosis	N	N	↑	↑	↓	+,−	↓
T_4 thyrotoxicosis	↑	↑	N	N	↓	+,−	↓
Hypothyroidism							
Primary	↓	↓	↓	↓	↑	+,−	↑
Secondary	↓	↓	↓	↓	↓ N	−	↓
Tertiary	↓	↓	↓	↓	↓, N	−	N
Peripheral unresponsiveness	↑, N	↑, N	↑, N	↑	↑, N	−	N, ↑

↑, Increased; ↓, decreased; +, − variable; *FTI*, free thyroid index; *N*, normal; T_3, triiodothyronine; T_4, thyroxine; *TRH*, thyrotropin-releasing hormone; *TSH*, thyroid-stimulating hormone; *TSI*, thyroid stimulating immunoglobulin.

Abnormal values:
Elevated in hyperthyroidism (usually earlier and to a greater extent than serum T_4)
Useful in diagnosing:
T_3 hyperthyroidism (thyrotoxicosis): Increased T_3, normal free thyroxine index (FTI)
Toxic nodular goiter: Increased T_3, normal or increased T_4
Iodine deficiency: Normal T_3, possibly decreased T_4
Thyroid replacement therapy with liothyronine (Cytomel): Normal T_4, increased T_3 if patient is symptomatically hyperthyroid
Not ordered routinely but indicated when hyperthyroidism is suspected and serum-free T_4 or FTI inconclusive

T_3 RESIN UPTAKE (T_3RU)

Normal range: 25% to 35%
Abnormal values: Increased in hyperthyroidism. T_3 resin uptake (T_3RU or RT_3U) measures the percentage of free T_4 (not bound to protein); it does not measure serum T_3 concentration; T_3RU and other tests that reflect thyroid hormone binding to plasma protein are also known as *thyroid hormone-binding ratios* (THBR).

T_4, FREE (Free thyroxine)

Normal range: 0.8 to 2.8 ng/dl
Elevated in:
Graves disease, toxic multinodular goiter, toxic adenoma, iatrogenic and factitious causes, transient hyperthyroidism.
Serum-free T_4 directly measures unbound thyroxine. Free T_4 can be measured by equilibrium dialysis (gold standard of free T_4 assays) or by immunometric techniques (influenced by serum levels of lipids, proteins, and certain drugs). The FTI can also be easily calculated by multiplying T_4 times T_3RU and dividing the result by 100; the FTI corrects for any abnormal T_4 values secondary to protein binding: FTI = T_4 × T_3RU/100. Normal values equal 1.1 to 4.3.

T_4, SERUM T_4

Normal range: 0.8 to 2.8 ng/dl (10 to 36 pmol/L [CF: 12.87; SMI: 1 pmol/L])
Abnormal values: Serum thyroxine (T_4)
Elevated in:
Graves disease
Toxic multinodular goiter

Toxic adenoma
Iatrogenic and factitious
Transient hyperthyroidism
    Subacute thyroiditis
    Hashimoto thyroiditis
    Silent thyroiditis
Rare causes: Hypersecretion of TSH (e.g., pituitary neoplasms), struma ovarii, ingestion of large amounts of iodine in a patient with preexisting thyroid hyperplasia or adenoma (Jod-Basedow phenomenon), hydatidiform mole, carcinoma of thyroid, amiodarone therapy of arrhythmias

Serum thyroxine test measures both circulating thyroxine bound to protein (represents >99% of circulating T_4) and unbound (free) thyroxine. Values vary with protein binding; changes in the concentration of T_4 secondary to changes in thyroxine-binding globulin (TBG) can be caused by the following:

Increased TBG ($\uparrow T_4$)	Decreased TBG ($\downarrow T_4$)
Pregnancy	Androgens, glucocorticoids
Estrogens	Nephrotic syndrome, cirrhosis
Acute infectious hepatitis	Acromegaly
Oral contraceptives	Hypoproteinemia
Familial	Familial
Fluorouracil, clofibrate	Phenytoin, acetylsalicylic acid (ASA) and other NSAIDs, heroin, methadone, high-dose penicillin, asparaginase, chronic debilitating illness

To eliminate the suspected influence of protein binding on thyroxine values, two additional tests are available: T_3 resin uptake and serum free thyroxine. Table E118 summarizes the effects of pregnancy on thyroid physiology, and Table E119 describes changes in thyroid hormone levels during illness.

TEGRETOL
See "CARBAMAZEPINE"

TESTOSTERONE (total testosterone)
Normal range: Variable with age and sex. Testosterone circulates in plasma mostly bound to plasma proteins and sex hormone-binding globulin (SHBG). Approximately 2% of testosterone circulates in free form (biologically active form). Low testosterone levels in obese patients may be due to reduced levels of SHBG; therefore, it is essential to measure free testosterone when evaluating androgen deficiency in obese patients.

Serum/plasma

Males: 280-1100 ng/dl	Females: 15-70 ng/dl

Urine

Males: 50-135 µg/day	Females: 2-12 µg/day

Elevated in: Testicular tumors, ovarian masculinizing tumors, testosterone replacement therapy
Decreased in: Hypogonadism, obesity, insulin resistance, sleep apnea. Fig. E57 illustrates testosterone level changes with age. The diagnosis of androgen deficiency should be based on at least two morning testosterone measurements (collected on separate days) in a symptomatic patient.

THEOPHYLLINE
Normal therapeutic range: 10 to 20 mcg/ml

THORACENTESIS FLUID
See "PLEURAL FLUID"

THROMBIN TIME (TT), THROMBIN CLOTTING TIME (TCT)
Normal range: 11.3 to 18.5 sec
Elevated in: Thrombolytic and heparin therapy, disseminated intravascular coagulation, hypofibrinogenemia, dysfibrinogenemia
    See Table E120 for synthesizing results of PT, APTT, and TCT. Also see Fig. E58.

THYROGLOBULIN
Normal: 3 to 40 ng/ml. Thyroglobulin is a tumor marker for monitoring the status of patients with papillary or follicular thyroid cancer following resection.
Elevated in: Papillary or follicular thyroid cancer, Hashimoto thyroiditis, Graves disease, subacute thyroiditis

THYROID MICROSOMAL ANTIBODIES
Normal: Undetectable. Low titers may be present in 5% to 10% of normal individuals.
Elevated in: Hashimoto disease, thyroid carcinoma, early hypothyroidism, pernicious anemia

THYROID-STIMULATING HORMONE (TSH)
Changes in TSH levels during illness are summarized in Table E121.
    See Fig. E59 for an algorithmic approach to thyroid testing.
Normal range: 2 to 11 µU/ml (2 to 11 mU/L [CF: 1; SMI: 1 mU/L])
CONDITIONS THAT INCREASE SERUM THYROID-STIMULATING HORMONE VALUES
Laboratory error
Primary hypothyroidism
Synthroid therapy with insufficient dose
Lithium or amiodarone; some patients
Hashimoto thyroiditis in later stage
Large doses of inorganic iodide (e.g., potassium iodide [SSKI])
Severe nonthyroid illness in recovery phase
Iodine deficiency (moderate or severe)
Addison disease
TSH specimen drawn in evening (peak of diurnal variation)
Pituitary TSH-secreting tumor
Therapy of hypothyroidism (3 to 6 wk after beginning therapy [range, 1 to 8 wk]; sometimes longer when pretherapy TSH is over 100 µU/ml)
Acute psychiatric illness
Peripheral resistance to T_4 syndrome
Antibodies (e.g., human antimouse antibody [HAMA]) interfering with monoclonal sandwich method of TSH assay
Telepaque (iopanoic acid) and Oragrafin (ipodate) x-ray contrast media
Amphetamines
High altitudes
CONDITIONS THAT DECREASE SERUM THYROID-STIMULATING HORMONE VALUES
Laboratory error
T_4/T_3 toxicosis (diffuse or nodular etiology)
Excessive therapy for hypothyroidism
Active thyroiditis (subacute, painless, or early active Hashimoto disease)
Multinodular goiter containing areas of autonomy
Severe nonthyroid illness (especially acute trauma, dopamine, or glucocorticoid)
T_3 toxicosis
Pituitary insufficiency
Cushing syndrome (and some patients on high-dose glucocorticoid)

Laboratory
Tests

IV

Jod-Basedow (iodine-induced) hyperthyroidism

Thyroid-stimulating hormone drawn 2 to 4 h after levothyroxine dose

Postpartum transient toxicosis

Factitious hyperthyroidism

Struma ovarii

Radioimmunoassay, surgery, or antithyroid drug therapy for hyperthyroidism 4 to 6 wk (range, 2 wk to 2 yr) after the treatment

Interleukin-2 drugs (3% to 6% of cases) or α-interferon therapy (1% of cases)

Hyperemesis gravidarum

Amiodarone therapy

See Table E119 for changes in thyroid hormone levels during illness.

THYROTROPIN (TSH) RECEPTOR ANTIBODIES

Normal: <130% of basal activity

Elevated in: Values between 1.3 and 2.0 are found in 10% of patients with thyroid disease other than Graves disease. Values >2.8 have been found only in patients with Graves disease.

THYROTROPIN-RELEASING HORMONE (TRH) STIMULATION TEST

Normal: Baseline TSH <11 microU/ml; stimulated TSH: More than double the baseline

In primary hypothyroidism the TSH increase is 2-3× the normal result. In secondary hypothyroidism no TSH response occurs. In tertiary hypothyroidism (hypothalamic failure) there is a delayed rise in the TSH level.

THYROXINE (T$_4$)

Patterns in T$_4$ levels in different thyroid gland conditions are summarized in Table 122.

Normal range: 4 to 11 μg/dl (51 to 142 nmol/L [CF: 12.87; SMI: 1 nmol/L])

Elevated: Hyperthyroidism (see Fig. E59)

TIBC

See "IRON-BINDING CAPACITY, TOTAL"

TISSUE TRANSGLUTAMINASE ANTIBODY

Normal: Negative

Present in: Celiac disease (specificity; 94% to 97%, sensitivity, 90% to 98%), dermatitis herpetiformis

TRANSFERRIN

Normal range: 170 to 370 mg/dl (1.7 to 3.7 g/L [CF: 0.01; SMI: 0.01 g/L])

Elevated in: Iron deficiency anemia, oral contraceptive administration, viral hepatitis, late pregnancy

Decreased in: Nephrotic syndrome, liver disease, hereditary deficiency, protein malnutrition, neoplasms, chronic inflammatory states, chronic illness, thalassemia, hemochromatosis, hemolytic anemia

TRIGLYCERIDES

Normal range: <150 mg/dl (<1.80 mmol/L [CF: 0.01129; SMI: 0.02 mmol/L])

Elevated in: Hyperlipoproteinemias (types I, IIb, III, IV, V), hypothyroidism, pregnancy, estrogens, acute myocardial infarction, pancreatitis, alcohol intake, nephrotic syndrome, diabetes mellitus, glycogen storage disease

Decreased in: Malnutrition, congenital abetalipoproteinemias, drugs (e.g., gemfibrozil, fenofibrate, nicotinic acid, clofibrate)

TRIIODOTHYRONINE

See "T$_3$"

TROPONINS (serum)

Box E33 summarizes the differential diagnosis of elevated troponin other than acute coronary syndrome.

Normal range: 0 to 0.4 ng/ml (negative). If there is clinical suspicion of evolving acute MI or ischemic episode, repeat testing in 5 to 6 h is recommended.

Indeterminate: 0.05 to 0.49 ng/ml. Suggest further tests. In a patient with unstable angina and this troponin I level, there is an increased risk of a cardiac event in the near future.

Strong probability of acute MI: ≥0.05 ng/ml

Cardiac troponin T (cTnT) is a highly sensitive marker for myocardial injury for the first 48 h after MI and for up to 5 to 7 days (see Fig. E21, under "Creatine Kinase Isoenzymes"). It may also be elevated in renal failure, chronic muscle disease, and trauma.

Cardiac troponin I (cTnI) is highly sensitive and specific for myocardial injury (≥CK-MB) in the initial 8 h, peaks within 24 h, and lasts up to 7 days. With progressively higher levels of cTnI, the risk of mortality increases because the amount of necrosis increases.

TSH

See "THYROID-STIMULATING HORMONE"

TT

See "THROMBIN TIME"

TUBERCULIN TEST (PPD)

Abnormal results: See Box 34. Box E35 describes factors associated with false-negative tuberculin tests.

BOX 34 PPD Reaction Size Considered "Positive" (Intracutaneous 5 TU Mantoux Test at 48 h)

5 mm or More

HIV infection or risk factors for HIV

Close recent contact with active TB case

Persons with chest x-ray examination consistent with healed TB

10 mm or More

Foreign-born persons from countries with high TB prevalence in Asia, Africa, and Latin America

IV drug users

Medically underserved low-income population groups (including Native Americans, Hispanics, and Blacks)

Residents of long-term care facilities (nursing homes, mental institutions)

Medical conditions that increase risk for TB (silicosis, gastrectomy, undernourishment, diabetes mellitus, high-dose corticosteroids or immunosuppression Rx, leukemia or lymphoma, other malignancies)

Employees of long-term care facilities, schools, child care facilities, health care facilities

15 mm or More

All others not already listed

TABLE 122 Patterns of Serum Levels of TSH and T$_4$ in Different Thyroid Gland Conditions

Condition	T$_4$ (Most Accurate, Free T$_4$)	TSH	Site of Disease
Euthyroid	Normal	Normal	None
Primary hypothyroidism	Low	High	Thyroid gland
Secondary hypothyroidism	Low	Low to normal	Pituitary
Primary hyperthyroidism	High	Low	Thyroid
Secondary hyperthyroidism	High	High	Pituitary

TSH, Thyroid-stimulating hormone.

From McPherson RA, Pincus MR: *Henry's clinical diagnosis and management by laboratory methods*, ed 23, St Louis, 2017, Elsevier.

HIV, Human immunodeficiency virus; *IV*, intravenous; *PPD*, purified protein derivative; *Rx*, prescription; *TB*, tuberculosis; *TU*, tuberculin units.

UNCONJUGATED BILIRUBIN

See "BILIRUBIN, DIRECT"

UREA NITROGEN, BLOOD (BUN)

Normal range: 8 to 18 mg/dl (3 to 6.5 mmol/L [CF: 0.357; SMI: 0.5 mmol/L])
Box E36 describes factors affecting BUN level independent of renal function.
Elevated in: Dehydration, drugs (aminoglycosides and other antibiotics, diuretics, lithium, corticosteroids), gastrointestinal bleeding, decreased renal blood flow (shock, congestive heart failure, myocardial infarction), renal disease (glomerulonephritis, pyelonephritis, diabetic nephropathy), urinary tract obstruction (prostatic hypertrophy)
Decreased in: Liver disease, malnutrition, third trimester of pregnancy, overhydration, acromegaly, celiac disease

URIC ACID (serum)

Normal range: 2 to 7 mg/dl
Elevated in: Renal failure, gout, excessive cell lysis (chemotherapeutic agents, radiation therapy, leukemia, lymphoma, hemolytic anemia), hereditary enzyme deficiency (hypoxanthine-guanine-phosphoribosyl transferase), acidosis, myeloproliferative disorders, diet high in purines or protein, drugs (diuretics, low doses of ASA, ethambutol, nicotinic acid), lead poisoning, hypothyroidism, Addison disease, nephrogenic diabetes insipidus, active psoriasis, polycystic kidneys
Decreased in: Drugs (allopurinol, febuxostat, high doses of ASA, probenecid, warfarin, corticosteroid), deficiency of xanthine oxidase, syndrome of inappropriate antidiuretic hormone secretion, renal tubular deficits (Fanconi syndrome), alcoholism, liver disease, diet deficient in protein or purines, Wilson disease, hemochromatosis

URINALYSIS

Blood urinalysis abnormalities in various urinary system diseases are summarized in Table E123.
Normal range:
Color: Light straw
  Appearance: Clear
  Ketones: Absent
  pH: 4.5 to 8 (average, 6)
  Protein: Absent
  Glucose: Absent
  Specific gravity: 1.005 to 1.030
  Occult blood absent
  Microscopic examination:
  Red blood cells: 0 to 5 (high-power field)
  White blood cells: 0 to 5 (high-power field)
  Bacteria (spun specimen): Absent
  Casts: 0 to 4 hyaline (low-power field)
  Abnormalities in the microscopic examination of urine are described in Table E124. Causes of abnormal appearance and color of urine are described in Table E125. Urine color changes with commonly used drugs are summarized in Table E126.

URINE AMYLASE

Normal range: 35 to 260 U Somogyi/h (6.5 to 48.1 U/h [CF: 0.185; SMI: 1 U/h])
Elevated in: Pancreatitis, carcinoma of the pancreas

URINE BILE

Normal: Absent
Abnormal: Urine bilirubin: Hepatitis (viral, toxic, drug-induced), biliary obstruction
Urine urobilinogen: Hepatitis (viral, toxic, drug-induced), hemolytic jaundice, liver cell dysfunction (cirrhosis, infection, metastases)

URINE CALCIUM

Normal range: <250 mg/24 h (<6.2 mmol/dl [CF: 0.02495; SMI: 0.1 mmol/dl])
Elevated in: Primary hyperparathyroidism, hypervitaminosis D, bone metastases, multiple myeloma, increased calcium intake, steroids, prolonged immobilization, sarcoidosis, Paget disease, idiopathic hypercalciuria, renal tubular acidosis
Decreased in: Hypoparathyroidism, pseudohypoparathyroidism, vitamin D deficiency, vitamin D-resistant rickets, diet low in calcium, drugs (thiazide diuretics, oral contraceptives), familial hypocalciuric hypercalcemia, renal osteodystrophy, potassium citrate therapy

URINE CAMP

Elevated in: Hypercalciuria, familial hypocalciuric hypercalcemia, primary hyperparathyroidism, pseudohypoparathyroidism, rickets
Decreased in: Vitamin D intoxication, sarcoidosis

URINE CATECHOLAMINES

Normal range: Norepinephrine: <100 μg/24 h (<590 nmol/day [CF: 5.911; SMI: 10 nmol/day])
Epinephrine: <10 μg/24 h (55 nmol/day [CF: 5.458; SMI: 5 nmol/day])
Elevated in: Pheochromocytoma, neuroblastoma, severe stress

URINE CHLORIDE

Normal range: 110 to 250 mEq/day (110 to 250 mmol/day [CF: 1; SMI: 1 mmol/day])
Elevated in: Corticosteroids, Bartter syndrome, diuretics, metabolic acidosis, severe hypokalemia
Decreased in: Chloride depletion (vomiting), colonic villous adenoma, chronic renal failure, renal tubular acidosis

URINE COPPER

Normal range: <40 μg/24 h (<0.6 μmol/day [CF: 0.01574; SMI: 0.2 μmol/day])

URINE CORTISOL, FREE

Normal range: 10 to 110 μg/24 h (30 to 300 nmol/day [CF: 2.759; SMI: 10 nmol/day])
Elevated: See "CORTISOL, PLASMA"

URINE CREATININE (24 h)

Normal range: Male: 0.8 to 1.8 g/day (7 to 16 mmol/day [CF: 8.840; SMI: 0.1 mmol/day])
Female: 0.6 to 1.6 g/day (5.3 to 14 mmol/day)
NOTE: Useful test as an indicator of completeness of 24-h urine collection.

URINE CRYSTALS

Uric acid: Acid urine, hyperuricosuria, uric acid nephropathy
Sulfur: Antibiotics containing sulfa
Calcium oxalate: Ethylene glycol poisoning, acid urine, hyperoxaluria
Calcium phosphate: Alkaline urine
Cystine: Cystinuria

URINE EOSINOPHILS

Normal: Absent
Present in: Interstitial nephritis, acute tubular necrosis, urinary tract infection, kidney transplant rejection, hepatorenal syndrome

URINE GLUCOSE (qualitative)

Normal: Absent
Present in: Diabetes mellitus, renal glycosuria (decreased renal threshold for glucose), glucose intolerance

URINE HEMOGLOBIN, FREE

Normal: Absent
Present in: Hemolysis (with saturation of serum haptoglobin binding capacity and renal threshold for tubular absorption of hemoglobin)

URINE HEMOSIDERIN

Normal: Absent
Present in: Paroxysmal nocturnal hemoglobinuria, chronic hemolytic anemia, hemochromatosis, blood transfusion, thalassemias

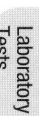

Laboratory Tests

IV

URINE 5-HYDROXYINDOLE-ACETIC ACID (urine 5-HIAA)

Normal range: 2 to 8 mg/24 h (10 to 40 µmol/day [CF: 5.23; SMI: 5 µmol/day])
Elevated in: Carcinoid tumors, after ingestion of certain foods (bananas, plums, tomatoes, avocados, pineapples, eggplant, walnuts), drugs (monoamine oxidase inhibitors, phenacetin, methyldopa, glycerol guaiacolate, acetaminophen, salicylates, phenothiazines, imipramine, methocarbamol, reserpine, methamphetamine). See Table E127.

URINE INDICAN

Normal: Absent
Present in: Malabsorption secondary to intestinal bacterial overgrowth

URINE KETONES (semiquantitative)

Normal: Absent
Present in: Diabetic ketoacidosis, alcoholic ketoacidosis, starvation, isopropanol ingestion

URINE METANEPHRINES

Normal range: 0 to 2.0 mg/24 h (0 to 11.0 µmol/day [CF: 5.458; SMI: 0.5 µmol/day])
Elevated in: Pheochromocytoma, neuroblastoma, drugs (caffeine, phenothiazines, monoamine oxidase inhibitors), stress. Table E128 summarizes medications that may increase metanephrine levels.

URINE MYOGLOBIN

Normal: Absent
Present in: Severe trauma, hyperthermia, polymyositis/dermatomyositis, carbon monoxide poisoning, drugs (narcotic and amphetamine toxicity), hypothyroidism, muscle ischemia
Table 129 differentiates hematuria and hemoglobinuria from myoglobinuria.

URINE NITRITE

Normal: Absent
Present in: Urinary tract infections

URINE OCCULT BLOOD

Normal: Negative
Positive in: Trauma to urinary tract, renal disease (glomerulonephritis, pyelonephritis), renal or ureteral calculi, bladder lesions (carcinoma, cystitis), prostatitis, prostatic carcinoma, menstrual contamination, hematopoietic disorders (hemophilia, thrombocytopenia), anticoagulants, ASA

URINE OSMOLALITY

See "OSMOLALITY, URINE"

URINE PH

Normal range: 4.6 to 8 (average, 6)
Elevated in: Bacteriuria, vegetarian diet, renal failure with inability to form ammonia, drugs (antibiotics, sodium bicarbonate, acetazolamide)
Decreased in: Acidosis (metabolic, respiratory), drugs (ammonium chloride, methenamine mandelate), diabetes mellitus, starvation, diarrhea

URINE PHOSPHATE

Normal range: 0.8 to 2.0 g/24 h
Elevated in: Acute tubular necrosis (diuretic phase), chronic renal disease, uncontrolled diabetes mellitus, hyperparathyroidism, hypomagnesemia, metabolic acidosis, metabolic alkalosis, neurofibromatosis, adult-onset vitamin D-resistant hypophosphatemic osteomalacia
Decreased in: Acromegaly, acute renal failure, decreased dietary intake, hypoparathyroidism, respiratory acidosis

URINE POTASSIUM

Normal range: 25 to 100 mEq/24 h (25 to 100 mmol/day [CF: 1; SMI: 1 mmol/day])
Elevated in: Aldosteronism (primary, secondary), glucocorticoids, alkalosis, renal tubular acidosis, excessive dietary potassium intake
Decreased in: Acute renal failure, potassium-sparing diuretics, diarrhea, hypokalemia
Box E37 describes urine potassium in hypokalemia.

URINE PROTEIN (quantitative)

Normal range: <150 mg/24 h (<0.15 g/day [CF: 0.001; SMI: 0.01 g/day])
Elevated in:
Nephrotic syndrome as a result of primary renal diseases
Malignant hypertension
Malignancies: Multiple myeloma, leukemias, Hodgkin disease
Congestive heart failure
Diabetes mellitus
Systemic lupus erythematosus, rheumatoid arthritis
Sickle cell disease
Goodpasture syndrome
Malaria
Amyloidosis, sarcoidosis
Tubular lesions: Cystinosis
Functional (after heavy exercise)
Pyelonephritis
Pregnancy
Constrictive pericarditis
Renal vein thrombosis
Toxic nephropathies: Heavy metals, drugs
Radiation nephritis
Orthostatic (postural) proteinuria
Benign proteinuria: Fever, heat or cold exposure

URINE SEDIMENT

See Fig. E60 for visual evaluation of common abnormalities. Table E130 summarizes characteristics of amorphous and crystalline urinary sediments.

URINE SODIUM (quantitative)

See Table E131 for use of urine electrolytes in the differential diagnosis of hypokalemia. Table E132 describes urine sodium findings in acute kidney injury (AKI).
Normal range: 40 to 220 mEq/day (40 to 220 mmol/day [CF: 1; SMI: 1 mmol/day])

TABLE 129 Differentiation of Hematuria, Hemoglobinuria, and Myoglobinuria

Condition	Plasma Findings	Urine Findings
Hematuria	Color—normal	Color—normal, smoky, pink, red, brown
		Erythrocytes—many
		Renal—red blood cell casts
		Protein—marked increase
		Lower urinary tract—no casts
		Protein—present or absent
Hemoglobinuria	Color—pink (early)	Color—pink, red, brown
	Haptoglobin—low	Erythrocytes—occasional
		Pigment casts—occasional
		Protein—present or absent
		Hemosiderin—late
Myoglobinuria	Color—normal	Color—red, brown
	Haptoglobin—normal	Erythrocytes—occasional
	Creatine kinase—marked increase	Dense brown casts—occasional
	Aldolase—increased	Protein—present or absent

From McPherson RA, Pincus MR: *Henry's clinical diagnosis and management by laboratory methods,* ed 23, St Louis, 2017, Elsevier.

Elevated in: Diuretic administration, high sodium intake, salt-losing nephritis, acute tubular necrosis, vomiting, Addison disease, syndrome of inappropriate antidiuretic hormone secretion, hypothyroidism, congestive heart failure, hepatic failure, chronic renal failure, Bartter syndrome, glucocorticoid deficiency, interstitial nephritis caused by analgesic abuse, mannitol, dextran, or glycerol therapy, milk-alkali syndrome, decreased renin secretion, postobstructive diuresis

Decreased In: Increased aldosterone, glucocorticoid excess, hyponatremia, prerenal azotemia, decreased salt intake

URINE SPECIFIC GRAVITY

Normal range: 1.005 to 1.030
Elevated in: Dehydration, excessive fluid losses (vomiting, diarrhea, fever), x-ray contrast media, diabetes mellitus, congestive heart failure, syndrome of inappropriate antidiuretic hormone secretion, adrenal insufficiency, decreased fluid intake
Decreased in: Diabetes insipidus, renal disease (glomerulonephritis, pyelonephritis), excessive fluid intake or IV hydration

URINE VANILLYLMANDELIC ACID (VMA)

Normal range: <6.8 mg/24 h (<35 μmol/day [CF: 5.046; SMI: 1 μmol/day])
Elevated in: Pheochromocytoma, neuroblastoma, ganglioblastoma, drugs (isoproterenol, methocarbamol, levodopa, sulfonamides, chlorpromazine), severe stress, after ingestion of bananas, chocolate, vanilla, tea, coffee
Decreased in: Drugs (monoamine oxidase inhibitors, reserpine, guanethidine, methyldopa)

VARICELLA-ZOSTER VIRUS (VZV) SEROLOGY

Test description: Test can be performed on whole blood, tissue, skin lesions, and CSF.

VASOACTIVE INTESTINAL PEPTIDE (VIP)

Normal: <50 pg/ml
Elevated in: Pancreatic VIP-omas, neuroblastoma, pancreatic islet cell hyperplasia, liver disease, multiple endocrine neoplasia (MEN) I, ganglioneuroma, ganglioneuroblastoma

VDRL

Normal range: Negative
Positive test: Syphilis, other treponemal diseases (yaws, pinta, bejel)
   NOTE: A false-positive test may be seen in patients with systemic lupus erythematosus and other autoimmune diseases, infectious mononucleosis, HIV, atypical pneumonia, malaria, leprosy, typhus fever, rat-bite fever, relapsing fever.
   NOTE: See Table E133 for interpretation of serologic tests for syphilis.

VISCOSITY (serum)

Normal range: 1.4 to 1.8 relative to water (1.10 to 1.22 centipoise)
Elevated in: Monoclonal gammopathies (Waldenström macroglobulinemia, multiple myeloma), hyperfibrinogenemia, systemic lupus erythematosus, rheumatoid arthritis, polycythemia, leukemia

VITAMIN B$_{12}$ (cobalamin)

See Box E38 for etiopathophysiologic classification of cobalamin deficiency. Causes of false-positive and false-negative serum cobalamin levels are summarized in Table E134. Table E135 describes causes of megaloblastosis not responding to therapy with cobalamin or folate. Table E136 summarizes indications for prophylaxis with cobalamin or folate.
Normal: 190 to 900 ng/ml
   Causes of vitamin B$_{12}$ deficiency:
a. Pernicious anemia (antibodies against intrinsic factor and gastric parietal cells)
b. Dietary (strict lacto-ovo vegetarians, food faddists)
c. Malabsorption (achlorhydria, gastrectomy, ileal resection, pancreatic insufficiency, drugs [omeprazole, cholestyramine])
   Falsely low levels occur in patients with severe folate deficiency, in patients using high doses of ascorbic acid, and when cobalamin levels are measured after nuclear medicine studies (radioactivity interferes with cobalamin radioimmunoassay).
   Falsely high or normal levels in patients with cobalamin deficiency can occur in severe liver disease and chronic granulocytic leukemia.
   The absence of anemia or macrocytosis does not exclude the diagnosis of cobalamin deficiency.

VITAMIN D, 1,25 DIHYDROXY CALCIFEROL

Normal: 16 to 65 pg/ml
Elevated in: Tumor calcinosis, primary hyperparathyroidism, sarcoidosis, tuberculosis, idiopathic hypercalciuria
Decreased in: Nutritional deficiency, postmenopausal osteoporosis, chronic renal failure, hypoparathyroidism, tumor-induced osteomalacia, rickets, elevated blood lead levels. Table E137 compares vitamin D levels in various disorders. Fig. E61 illustrates vitamin D physiology.

VITAMIN K

Normal: 0.10 to 2.20 ng/ml
Decreased in: Primary biliary cirrhosis, anticoagulants, antibiotics, cholestyramine, GI disease, pancreatic disease, cystic fibrosis, obstructive jaundice, hypoprothrombinemia, hemorrhagic disease of the newborn

VON WILLEBRAND FACTOR

Normal: Levels vary according to blood type; blood type O: 50-150 U/dl; blood type non-O: 90-200 U/dl
Decreased in: von Willebrand disease (however, in type II von Willebrand disease the antigen may be normal but the function is impaired)

SECTION V

Clinical Practice Guidelines

INTRODUCTION

Clinical Practice Guidelines

v

CLINICAL PRACTICE GUIDELINES — IMMUNIZATIONS AND CHEMOPROPHYLAXIS

Childhood and Adolescent Immunizations

TABLE 1   Recommended Child and Adolescent Immunization Schedule for Ages 18 Years or Younger, United States, 2023. (For those who fall behind or start late, see the catch-up schedule [Table 2])

These recommendations must be read with the notes that follow. For those who fall behind or start late, provide catch-up vaccination at the earliest opportunity as indicated by the green bars.
To determine minimum intervals between doses, see the catch-up schedule (Table 2).
From Centers for Disease Control and Prevention.

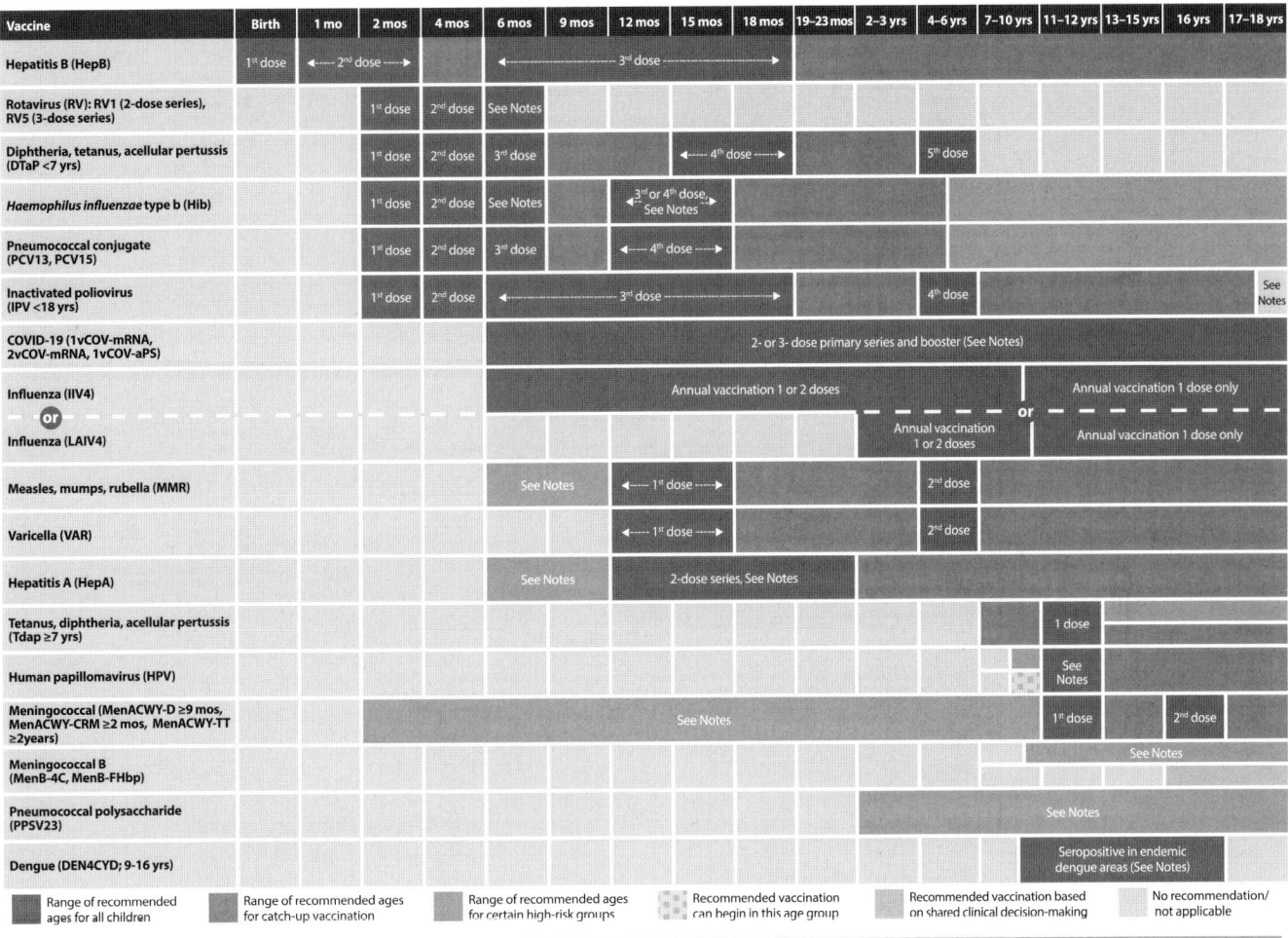

Vaccine	Birth	1 mo	2 mos	4 mos	6 mos	9 mos	12 mos	15 mos	18 mos	19–23 mos	2–3 yrs	4–6 yrs	7–10 yrs	11–12 yrs	13–15 yrs	16 yrs	17–18 yrs
Hepatitis B (HepB)	1st dose	◄---- 2nd dose ----►			◄----------------- 3rd dose ---------------►												
Rotavirus (RV): RV1 (2-dose series), RV5 (3-dose series)			1st dose	2nd dose	See Notes												
Diphtheria, tetanus, acellular pertussis (DTaP <7 yrs)			1st dose	2nd dose	3rd dose		◄---- 4th dose ----►					5th dose					
Haemophilus influenzae **type b (Hib)**			1st dose	2nd dose	See Notes		3rd or 4th dose, See Notes										
Pneumococcal conjugate (PCV13, PCV15)			1st dose	2nd dose	3rd dose		◄---- 4th dose ----►										
Inactivated poliovirus (IPV <18 yrs)			1st dose	2nd dose	◄----------- 3rd dose -----------►							4th dose					See Notes
COVID-19 (1vCOV-mRNA, 2vCOV-mRNA, 1vCOV-aPS)					2- or 3- dose primary series and booster (See Notes)												
Influenza (IIV4)					Annual vaccination 1 or 2 doses							Annual vaccination 1 dose only					
Influenza (LAIV4)											Annual vaccination 1 or 2 doses		Annual vaccination 1 dose only				
Measles, mumps, rubella (MMR)					See Notes		◄---- 1st dose ----►					2nd dose					
Varicella (VAR)							◄---- 1st dose ----►					2nd dose					
Hepatitis A (HepA)					See Notes		2-dose series, See Notes										
Tetanus, diphtheria, acellular pertussis (Tdap ≥7 yrs)														1 dose			
Human papillomavirus (HPV)														See Notes			
Meningococcal (MenACWY-D ≥9 mos, MenACWY-CRM ≥2 mos, MenACWY-TT ≥2years)					See Notes									1st dose		2nd dose	
Meningococcal B (MenB-4C, MenB-FHbp)														See Notes			
Pneumococcal polysaccharide (PPSV23)												See Notes					
Dengue (DEN4CYD; 9-16 yrs)														Seropositive in endemic dengue areas (See Notes)			

■ Range of recommended ages for all children	■ Range of recommended ages for catch-up vaccination	▒ Range of recommended ages for certain high-risk groups	▒ Recommended vaccination can begin in this age group	▒ Recommended vaccination based on shared clinical decision-making	▒ No recommendation/ not applicable

TABLE 2 Recommended Catch-up Immunization Schedule for Children and Adolescents Who Start Late or Who Are More than 1 Month Behind, United States, 2023

The table below provides catch-up schedules and minimum intervals between doses for children whose vaccinations have been delayed. A vaccine series does not need to be restarted, regardless of the time that has elapsed between doses. Use the section appropriate for the child's age. Always use this table in conjunction with Table 1 and the footnotes that follow.
From Centers for Disease Control and Prevention.

		Minimum Interval Between Doses			
Vaccine	**Minimum Age for Dose 1**	**Dose 1 to Dose 2**	**Dose 2 to Dose 3**	**Dose 3 to Dose 4**	**Dose 4 to Dose 5**
	Children age 4 months through 6 years				
Hepatitis B	Birth	**4 weeks**	**8 weeks *and* at least 16 weeks after first dose** minimum age for the final dose is 24 weeks		
Rotavirus	6 weeks Maximum age for first dose is 14 weeks, 6 days.	**4 weeks**	**4 weeks** maximum age for final dose is 8 months, 0 days		
Diphtheria, tetanus, and acellular pertussis	6 weeks	**4 weeks**	**4 weeks**	**6 months**	**6 months**
Haemophilus influenzae type b	6 weeks	**No further doses needed** if first dose was administered at age 15 months or older. **4 weeks** if first dose was administered before the 1st birthday. **8 weeks (as final dose)** if first dose was administered at age 12 through 14 months.	**No further doses needed** if previous dose was administered at age 15 months or older **4 weeks** if current age is younger than 12 months *and* first dose was administered at younger than age 7 months *and* at least 1 previous dose was PRP-T (ActHib®, Pentacel®, Hiberix®), Vaxelis® or unknown **8 weeks *and* age 12 through 59 months (as final dose)** if current age is younger than 12 months *and* first dose was administered at age 7 through 11 months; OR if current age is 12 through 59 months *and* first dose was administered before the 1st birthday *and* second dose was administered at younger than age 15 months; OR if both doses were PedvaxHIB® and were administered before the 1st birthday	**8 weeks (as final dose)** This dose only necessary for children age 12 through 59 months who received 3 doses before the 1st birthday.	
Pneumococcal conjugate	6 weeks	**No further doses needed** for healthy children if first dose was administered at age 24 months or older **4 weeks** if first dose was administered before the 1st birthday **8 weeks (as final dose for healthy children)** if first dose was administered at the 1st birthday or after	**No further doses needed** for healthy children if previous dose was administered at age 24 months or older **4 weeks** if current age is younger than 12 months and previous dose was administered at <7 months old **8 weeks (as final dose for healthy children)** if previous dose was administered between 7–11 months (wait until at least 12 months old); OR if current age is 12 months or older and at least 1 dose was administered before age 12 months	**8 weeks (as final dose)** for children aged 12 through 59 months regardless of risk, or age 60 through 71 months with any risk, who received 3 doses before age 12 months.	
Inactivated poliovirus	6 weeks	**4 weeks**	**4 weeks** if current age is <4 years **6 months (as final dose)** if current age is 4 years or older	**6 months (minimum age 4 years for final dose)**	
Measles, mumps, rubella	12 months	**4 weeks**			
Varicella	12 months	**3 months**			
Hepatitis A	12 months	**6 months**			
Meningococcal ACWY	2 months MenACWY-CRM 9 months MenACWY-D 2 years MenACWY-TT	**8 weeks**	See Notes	See Notes	
	Children and adolescents age 7 through 18 years				
Meningococcal ACWY	Not applicable (N/A)	**8 weeks**			
Tetanus, diphtheria; tetanus, diphtheria, and acellular pertussis	7 years	**4 weeks**	**4 weeks** if first dose of DTaP/DT was administered before the 1st birthday **6 months (as final dose)** if first dose of DTaP/DT or Tdap/Td was administered at or after the 1st birthday	**6 months** if first dose of DTaP/DT was administered before the 1st birthday	
Human papillomavirus	9 years	**Routine dosing intervals are recommended.**			
Hepatitis A	N/A	**6 months**			
Hepatitis B	N/A	**4 weeks**	**8 weeks *and* at least 16 weeks after first dose**		
Inactivated poliovirus	N/A	**4 weeks**	**6 months** A fourth dose is not necessary if the third dose was administered at age 4 years or older and at least 6 months after the previous dose.	A fourth dose of IPV is indicated if all previous doses were administered at <4 years or if the third dose was administered <6 months after the second dose.	
Measles, mumps, rubella	N/A	**4 weeks**			
Varicella	N/A	**3 months** if younger than age 13 years. **4 weeks** if age 13 years or older			
Dengue	9 years	**6 months**	6 months		

TABLE 3 Recommended Child and Adolescent Immunization Schedule by Medical Indication, United States, 2023

Always use this table in conjunction with Table 1 and the notes that follow.
From Centers for Disease Control and Prevention.

VACCINE	Pregnancy	Immunocom-promised status (excluding HIV infection)	HIV infection CD4+ count[a]		Kidney failure, end-stage renal disease, or on hemodialysis	Heart disease or chronic lung disease	CSF leak or cochlear implant	Asplenia or persistent complement component deficiencies	Chronic liver disease	Diabetes
			<15% or total CD4 cell count of <200/mm³	≥15% and total CD4 cell count of ≥200/mm³						
Hepatitis B										
Rotavirus		SCID[b]								
Diphtheria, tetanus, and acellular pertussis (DTaP)										
Haemophilus influenzae type b										
Pneumococcal conjugate										
Inactivated poliovirus										
COVID-19		See Notes		See Notes						
Influenza (IIV4) **or** Influenza (LAIV4)						Asthma, wheezing: 2–4yrs[c]				
Measles, mumps, rubella	*									
Varicella	*									
Hepatitis A										
Tetanus, diphtheria, and acellular pertussis (Tdap)										
Human papillomavirus	*									
Meningococcal ACWY										
Meningococcal B										
Pneumococcal polysaccharide										
Dengue										

Vaccination according to the routine schedule recommended

Recommended for persons with an additional risk factor for which the vaccine would be indicated

Vaccination is recommended, and additional doses may be necessary based on medical condition or vaccine. See Notes.

Precaution–vaccine might be indicated if benefit of protection outweighs risk of adverse reaction

Contraindicated or not recommended–vaccine should not be administered
*Vaccinate after pregnancy

No recommendation/not applicable

a. For additional information regarding HIV laboratory parameters and use of live vaccines, see the *General Best Practice Guidelines for Immunization*, "Altered Immunocompetence," at www.cdc.gov/vaccines/hcp/acip-recs/general-recs/immunocompetence.html and Table 4-1 (footnote J) at www.cdc.gov/vaccines/hcp/acip-recs/general-recs/contraindications.html.
b. Severe Combined Immunodeficiency
c. LAIV4 contraindicated for children 2–4 years of age with asthma or wheezing during the preceding 12 months

Continued

Notes Recommended Child and Adolescent Immunization Schedule for ages 18 years or younger, United States, 2023

For vaccination recommendations for persons ages 19 years or older, see the Recommended Adult Immunization Schedule, 2023.

Additional information

- Consult relevant ACIP statements for detailed recommendations at www.cdc.gov/vaccines/hcp/acip-recs/index.html.
- For calculating intervals between doses, 4 weeks = 28 days. Intervals of ≥4 months are determined by calendar months.
- Within a number range (e.g., 12–18), a dash (–) should be read as "through."
- Vaccine doses administered ≤4 days before the minimum age or interval are considered valid. Doses of any vaccine administered ≥5 days earlier than the minimum age or minimum interval should not be counted as valid and should be repeated as age appropriate. **The repeat dose should be spaced after the invalid dose by the recommended minimum interval.** For further details, see Table 3-2, Recommended and minimum ages and intervals between vaccine doses, in *General Best Practice Guidelines for Immunization* at www.cdc.gov/vaccines/hcp/acip-recs/general-recs/timing.html.
- Information on travel vaccination requirements and recommendations is available at www.cdc.gov/travel/.
- For vaccination of persons with immunodeficiencies, see Table 8-1, Vaccination of persons with primary and secondary immunodeficiencies, in *General Best Practice Guidelines for Immunization* at www.cdc.gov/vaccines/hcp/acip-recs/general-recs/immunocompetence.html, and Immunization in Special Clinical Circumstances (In: Kimberlin DW, Barnett ED, Lynfield Ruth, Sawyer MH, eds. *Red Book: 2021–2024 Report of the Committee on Infectious Diseases*. 32nd ed. Itasca, IL: American Academy of Pediatrics; 2021:72–86).
- For information about vaccination in the setting of a vaccine-preventable disease outbreak, contact your state or local health department.
- The National Vaccine Injury Compensation Program (VICP) is a no-fault alternative to the traditional legal system for resolving vaccine injury claims. All vaccines included in the child and adolescent vaccine schedule are covered by VICP except dengue, PPSV23, and COVID-19 vaccines. COVID-19 vaccines that are authorized or approved by the FDA are covered by the Countermeasures Injury Compensation Program (CICP). For more information, see www.hrsa.gov/vaccinecompensation or www.hrsa.gov/cicp.

COVID-19 vaccination
(minimum age: 6 months [Moderna and Pfizer-BioNTech COVID-19 vaccines], 12 years [Novavax COVID-19 Vaccine])

Routine vaccination

- **Primary series:**
  - **Age 6 months–4 years:** 2-dose series at 0, 4-8 weeks (Moderna) or 3-dose series at 0, 3-8, 11-16 weeks (Pfizer-BioNTech)
  - **Age 5–11 years:** 2-dose series at 0, 4-8 weeks (Moderna) or 2-dose series at 0, 3-8 weeks (Pfizer-BioNTech)
  - **Age 12–18 years:** 2-dose series at 0, 4-8 weeks (Moderna) or 2-dose series at 0, 3-8 weeks (Novavax, Pfizer-BioNTech)
- For **booster dose recommendations** see www.cdc.gov/vaccines/covid-19/clinical-considerations/interim-considerations-us.html

Special situations
Persons who are moderately or severely immunocompromised

- **Primary series**
  - **Age 6 months–4 years:** 3-dose series at 0, 4, 8 weeks (Moderna) or 3-dose series at 0, 3, 11 weeks (Pfizer-BioNTech)
  - **Age 5–11 years:** 3-dose series at 0, 4, 8 weeks (Moderna) or 3-dose series at 0, 3, 7 weeks (Pfizer-BioNTech)
  - **Age 12–18 years:** 3-dose series at 0, 4, 8 weeks (Moderna) or 2-dose series at 0, 3 weeks (Novavax) or 3-dose series at 0, 3, 7 weeks (Pfizer-BioNTech)
- **Booster dose:** see www.cdc.gov/vaccines/covid-19/clinical-considerations/interim-considerations-us.html
- **Pre-exposure prophylaxis** (monoclonal antibodies) may be considered to complement COVID-19 vaccination. See www.cdc.gov/vaccines/covid-19/clinical-considerations/interim-considerations-us.html#immunocompromised

For Janssen COVID-19 Vaccine recipients see COVID-19 schedule at www.cdc.gov/vaccines/covid-19/clinical-considerations/interim-considerations-us.html

Note: Administer an age-appropriate vaccine product for each dose. Current COVID-19 schedule and dosage formulation available at www.cdc.gov/vaccines/covid-19/downloads/COVID-19-immunization-schedule-ages-6months-older.pdf. For more information on Emergency Use Authorization (EUA) indications for COVID-19 vaccines, see www.fda.gov/emergency-preparedness-and-response/coronavirus-disease-2019-covid-19/covid-19-vaccines.

Dengue vaccination
(minimum age: 9 years)

Routine vaccination

- Age 9–16 years living in areas with endemic dengue **AND** have laboratory confirmation of previous dengue infection
  - 3-dose series administered at 0, 6, and 12 months
- Endemic areas include Puerto Rico, American Samoa, US Virgin Islands, Federated States of Micronesia, Republic of Marshall Islands, and the Republic of Palau. For updated guidance on dengue endemic areas and pre-vaccination laboratory testing see www.cdc.gov/mmwr/volumes/70/rr/rr7006a1.htm?s_cid=rr7006a1_w and www.cdc.gov/dengue/vaccine/hcp/index.html
- Dengue vaccine should not be administered to children traveling to or visiting endemic dengue areas.

Diphtheria, tetanus, and pertussis (DTaP) vaccination (minimum age: 6 weeks [4 years for Kinrix® or Quadracel®])

Routine vaccination

- 5-dose series at age 2, 4, 6, 15–18 months, 4–6 years
  - **Prospectively:** Dose 4 may be administered as early as age 12 months if at least 6 months have elapsed since dose 3.
  - **Retrospectively:** A 4th dose that was inadvertently administered as early as age 12 months may be counted if at least 4 months have elapsed since dose 3.

Catch-up vaccination

- Dose 5 is not necessary if dose 4 was administered at age 4 years or older and at least 6 months after dose 3.
- For other catch-up guidance, see Table 2.

Special situations

- **Wound management** in children less than age 7 years with history of 3 or more doses of tetanus-toxoid-containing vaccine: For all wounds except clean and minor wounds, administer DTaP if more than 5 years since last dose of tetanus-toxoid-containing vaccine. For detailed information, see www.cdc.gov/mmwr/volumes/67/rr/rr6702a1.htm.

Recommended Child and Adolescent Immunization Schedule for ages 18 years or younger, United States, 2023

Haemophilus influenzae type b vaccination
(minimum age: 6 weeks)

Routine vaccination

- **ActHIB®, Hiberix®, Pentacel®, or Vaxelis®:** 4-dose series (3-dose primary series at age 2, 4, and 6 months, followed by a booster dose* at age 12–15 months)
  - *Vaxelis® is not recommended for use as a booster dose. A different Hib-containing vaccine should be used for the booster dose.
- **PedvaxHIB®:** 3-dose series (2-dose primary series at age 2 and 4 months, followed by a booster dose at age 12–15 months)

Catch-up vaccination

- **Dose 1 at age 7–11 months:** Administer dose 2 at least 4 weeks later and dose 3 (final dose) at age 12–15 months or 8 weeks after dose 2 (whichever is later).
- **Dose 1 at age 12–14 months:** Administer dose 2 (final dose) at least 8 weeks after dose 1.
- **Dose 1 before age 12 months and dose 2 before age 15 months:** Administer dose 3 (final dose) at least 8 weeks after dose 2.
- **2 doses of PedvaxHIB® before age 12 months:** Administer dose 3 (final dose) at age 12–59 months and at least 8 weeks after dose 2.
- **1 dose administered at age 15 months or older:** No further doses needed
- **Unvaccinated at age 15–59 months:** Administer 1 dose.
- **Previously unvaccinated children age 60 months or older who are not considered high risk:** Do not require catch-up vaccination

For other catch-up guidance, see Table 2. Vaxelis® can be used for catch-up vaccination in children less than age 5 years. Follow the catch-up schedule even if Vaxelis® is used for one or more doses. For detailed information on use of Vaxelis® see www.cdc.gov/mmwr/volumes/69/wr/mm6905a5.htm.

Special situations

- **Chemotherapy or radiation treatment:**
  Age 12–59 months
  - Unvaccinated or only 1 dose before age 12 months: 2 doses, 8 weeks apart
  - 2 or more doses before age 12 months: 1 dose at least 8 weeks after previous dose

  Doses administered within 14 days of starting therapy or during therapy should be repeated at least 3 months after therapy completion.

- **Hematopoietic stem cell transplant (HSCT):**
  - 3-dose series 4 weeks apart starting 6 to 12 months after successful transplant, regardless of Hib vaccination history
- **Anatomic or functional asplenia (including sickle cell disease):**
  Age 12–59 months
  - Unvaccinated or only 1 dose before age 12 months: 2 doses, 8 weeks apart
  - 2 or more doses before age 12 months: 1 dose at least 8 weeks after previous dose
  Unvaccinated persons age 5 years or older
  - 1 dose
- **Elective splenectomy:**
  Unvaccinated persons age 15 months or older
  - 1 dose (preferably at least 14 days before procedure)
- **HIV infection:**
  Age 12–59 months
  - Unvaccinated or only 1 dose before age 12 months: 2 doses, 8 weeks apart
  - 2 or more doses before age 12 months: 1 dose at least 8 weeks after previous dose
  Unvaccinated persons age 5–18 years
  - 1 dose
- **Immunoglobulin deficiency, early component complement deficiency:**
  Age 12–59 months
  - Unvaccinated or only 1 dose before age 12 months: 2 doses, 8 weeks apart
  - 2 or more doses before age 12 months: 1 dose at least 8 weeks after previous dose

*Unvaccinated = Less than routine series (through age 14 months) OR no doses (age 15 months or older)

Hepatitis A vaccination
(minimum age: 12 months for routine vaccination)

Routine vaccination

- 2-dose series (minimum interval: 6 months) at age 12–23 months

Catch-up vaccination

- Unvaccinated persons through age 18 years should complete a 2-dose series (minimum interval: 6 months).
- Persons who previously received 1 dose at age 12 months or older should receive dose 2 at least 6 months after dose 1.

- Adolescents age 18 years or older may receive the combined HepA and HepB vaccine, **Twinrix®**, as a 3-dose series (0, 1, and 6 months) or 4-dose series (3 doses at 0, 7, and 21–30 days, followed by a booster dose at 12 months).

International travel

- Persons traveling to or working in countries with high or intermediate endemic hepatitis A (www.cdc.gov/travel/):
  - **Infants age 6–11 months:** 1 dose before departure; revaccinate with 2 doses (separated by at least 6 months) between age 12–23 months.
  - **Unvaccinated age 12 months or older:** Administer dose 1 as soon as travel is considered.

Hepatitis B vaccination
(minimum age: birth)

Routine vaccination

- 3-dose series at age 0, 1–2, 6–18 months **(use monovalent HepB vaccine for doses administered before age 6 weeks)**
  - Birth weight ≥2,000 grams: 1 dose within 24 hours of birth if medically stable
  - Birth weight <2,000 grams: 1 dose at chronological age 1 month or hospital discharge (whichever is earlier and even if weight is still <2,000 grams).
- Infants who did not receive a birth dose should begin the series as soon as possible (see Table 2 for minimum intervals).
- Administration of 4 doses is permitted when a combination vaccine containing HepB is used after the birth dose.
- **Minimum intervals (see Table 2):** when 4 doses are administered, substitute "dose 4" for "dose 3" in these calculations
- **Final (3rd or 4th) dose:** age 6–18 months (minimum age 24 weeks)
- **Mother is HBsAg-positive**
  - **Birth dose (monovalent HepB vaccine only):** administer **HepB vaccine** and **hepatitis B immune globulin (HBIG)** (in separate limbs) within 12 hours of birth, regardless of birth weight.
  - **Birth weight <2000 grams:** administer 3 additional doses of HepB vaccine beginning at age 1 month (total of 4 doses)
  - **Final (3rd or 4th) dose:** administer at age 6 months (minimum age 24 weeks)
  - Test for HBsAg and anti-HBs at age 9–12 months. If HepB series is delayed, test 1–2 months after final dose. Do not test before age 9 months.

Continued

Notes Recommended Child and Adolescent Immunization Schedule for ages 18 years or younger, United States, 2023

- **Mother is HBsAg-unknown**

If other evidence suggestive of maternal hepatitis B infection exists (e.g., presence of HBV DNA, HBeAg-positive, or mother known to have chronic hepatitis B infection), manage infant as if mother is HBsAg-positive

- **Birth dose (monovalent HepB vaccine only):**
  - Birth weight ≥2,000 grams: administer **HepB vaccine** within 12 hours of birth. Determine mother's HBsAg status as soon as possible. If mother is determined to be HBsAg-positive, administer **HBIG** as soon as possible (in separate limb), but no later than 7 days of age.
  - Birth weight <2,000 grams: administer **HepB vaccine** and **HBIG** (in separate limbs) within 12 hours of birth. Administer 3 additional doses of **HepB vaccine** beginning at age 1 month (total of 4 doses)
- **Final (3rd or 4th) dose:** administer at age 6 months **(minimum age 24 weeks)**
  - If mother is determined to be HBsAg-positive or if status remains unknown, test for HBsAg and anti-HBs at age 9–12 months. If HepB series is delayed, test 1–2 months after final dose. Do not test before age 9 months.

Catch-up vaccination

- Unvaccinated persons should complete a 3-dose series at 0, 1–2, 6 months. See Table 2 for minimum intervals
- Adolescents age 11–15 years may use an alternative 2-dose schedule with at least 4 months between doses (adult formulation **Recombivax HB®** only).
- Adolescents age 18 years or older may receive:
  - **Heplisav-B®:** 2-dose series at least 4 weeks apart
  - **PreHevbrio®:** 3-dose series at 0, 1, and 6 months
  - Combined HepA and HepB vaccine, **Twinrix®:** 3-dose series (0, 1, and 6 months) or 4-dose series (3 doses at 0, 7, and 21–30 days, followed by a booster dose at 12 months).

Special situations

- Revaccination is not generally recommended for persons with a normal immune status who were vaccinated as infants, children, adolescents, or adults.
- **Post-vaccination serology testing and revaccination** (if anti-HBs < 10mIU/mL) is recommended for certain populations, including:
  - Infants born to HBsAg-positive mothers
  - Persons who are predialysis or on maintenance dialysis
  - Other immunocompromised persons
  - For detailed revaccination recommendations, see www.cdc.gov/vaccines/hcp/acip-recs/vacc-specific/hepb.html.

Note: Heplisav-B and PreHevbrio are not recommended in pregnancy due to lack of safety data in pregnant persons

Human papillomavirus vaccination (minimum age: 9 years)

Routine and catch-up vaccination

- HPV vaccination routinely recommended at **age 11–12 years (can start at age 9 years)** and catch-up HPV vaccination recommended for all persons through age 18 years if not adequately vaccinated
- 2- or 3-dose series depending on age at initial vaccination:
  - **Age 9–14 years at initial vaccination:** 2-dose series at 0, 6–12 months (minimum interval: 5 months; repeat dose if administered too soon)
  - **Age 15 years or older at initial vaccination:** 3-dose series at 0, 1–2 months, 6 months (minimum intervals: dose 1 to dose 2: 4 weeks / dose 2 to dose 3: 12 weeks / dose 1 to dose 3: 5 months; repeat dose if administered too soon)
- **Interrupted schedules:** If vaccination schedule is interrupted, the series does not need to be restarted.
- No additional dose recommended when any HPV vaccine series has been completed using the recommended dosing intervals.

Special situations

- **Immunocompromising conditions, including HIV infection:** 3-dose series, even for those who initiate vaccination at age 9 through 14 years.
- **History of sexual abuse or assault:** Start at age 9 years
- **Pregnancy:** Pregnancy testing not needed before vaccination; HPV vaccination not recommended until after pregnancy; no intervention needed if vaccinated while pregnant

Influenza vaccination (minimum age: 6 months [IIV], 2 years [LAIV4], 18 years [recombinant influenza vaccine, RIV4])

Routine vaccination

- Use any influenza vaccine appropriate for age and health status annually:
  - 2 doses, separated by at least 4 weeks, for **children age 6 months–8 years** who have received fewer than 2 influenza vaccine doses before July 1, 2022, or whose influenza vaccination history is unknown (administer dose 2 even if the child turns 9 between receipt of dose 1 and dose 2)
  - 1 dose for **children age 6 months–8 years** who have received at least 2 influenza vaccine doses before July 1, 2022
  - 1 dose for **all persons age 9 years or older**

- For the 2022-2023 season, see www.cdc.gov/mmwr/volumes/71/rr/rr7101a1.htm.
- For the 2023–24 season, see the 2023–24 ACIP influenza vaccine recommendations.

Special situations

- **Egg allergy, hives only:** Any influenza vaccine appropriate for age and health status annually
- **Egg allergy with symptoms other than hives** (e.g., angioedema, respiratory distress) or required epinephrine or another emergency medical intervention: Any influenza vaccine appropriate for age and health status may be administered. If using egg-based IIV4 or LAIV4, administer in medical setting under supervision of health care provider who can recognize and manage severe allergic reactions.
- **Severe allergic reaction (e.g., anaphylaxis) to a vaccine component or a previous dose of any influenza vaccine:** see Appendix listing contraindications and precautions
- **Close contacts (e.g., caregivers, healthcare personnel) of severely immunosuppressed persons who require a protected environment:** these persons should not receive LAIV4. If LAIV4 is given, they should avoid contact with/caring for such immunosuppressed persons for 7 days after vaccination.

Measles, mumps, and rubella vaccination (minimum age: 12 months for routine vaccination)

Routine vaccination

- 2-dose series at age 12–15 months, age 4–6 years
- MMR or MMRV may be administered

Note: For dose 1 in children age 12–47 months, it is recommended to administer MMR and varicella vaccines separately. MMRV may be used if parents or caregivers express a preference.

Catch-up vaccination

- Unvaccinated children and adolescents: 2-dose series at least 4 weeks apart
- The maximum age for use of MMRV is 12 years.
- Minimum interval between *MMRV* doses: 3 months

Recommended Child and Adolescent Immunization Schedule for ages 18 years or younger, United States, 2023

Special situations

• International travel

- **Infants age 6–11 months:** 1 dose before departure; revaccinate with 2-dose series at age 12–15 months (12 months for children in high-risk areas) and dose 2 as early as 4 weeks later.

- **Unvaccinated children age 12 months or older:** 2-dose series at least 4 weeks apart before departure

• In mumps outbreak settings, for information about additional doses of MMR (including 3rd dose of MMR), see www.cdc.gov/mmwr/volumes/67/wr/mm6701a7.htm

Meningococcal serogroup A,C,W,Y vaccination
(minimum age: 2 months [MenACWY-CRM, Menveo], 9 months [MenACWY-D, Menactra], 2 years [MenACWY-TT, MenQuadfi])

Routine vaccination

• 2-dose series at age 11–12 years; 16 years

Catch-up vaccination

• Age 13–15 years: 1 dose now and booster at age 16–18 years (minimum interval: 8 weeks)

• Age 16–18 years: 1 dose

Special situations

Anatomic or functional asplenia (including sickle cell disease), HIV infection, persistent complement component deficiency, complement inhibitor (e.g., eculizumab, ravulizumab) use:

• Menveo**

- Dose 1 at age 2 months: 4-dose series (additional 3 doses at age 4, 6, and 12 months)

- Dose 1 at age 3–6 months: 3- or 4-dose series (dose 2 [and dose 3 if applicable] at least 8 weeks after previous dose until a dose is received at age 7 months or older, followed by an additional dose at least 12 weeks later and after age 12 months)

- Dose 1 at age 7–23 months: 2-dose series (dose 2 at least 12 weeks after dose 1 and after age 12 months)

- Dose 1 at age 24 months or older: 2-dose series at least 8 weeks apart

• Menactra®

- **Persistent complement component deficiency or complement inhibitor use:**

· Age 9–23 months: 2-dose series at least 12 weeks apart

· Age 24 months or older: 2-dose series at least 8 weeks apart

• Anatomic or functional asplenia, sickle cell disease, or HIV infection:

· **Age 9–23 months:** Not recommended

· **Age 24 months or older:** 2-dose series at least 8 weeks apart

· **Menactra®** must be administered at least 4 weeks after completion of PCV series.

• MenQuadfi®

- Dose 1 at age 24 months or older: 2-dose series at least 8 weeks apart

Travel to countries with hyperendemic or epidemic meningococcal disease, including countries in the African meningitis belt or during the Hajj (www.cdc.gov/travel/)**:**

• Children less than age 24 months:

- **Menveo** (age 2–23 months)**

· Dose 1 at age 2 months: 4-dose series (additional 3 doses at age 4, 6, and 12 months)

· Dose 1 at age 3–6 months: 3- or 4-dose series (dose 2 [and dose 3 if applicable] at least 8 weeks after previous dose until a dose is received at age 7 months or older, followed by an additional dose at least 12 weeks later and after age 12 months)

· Dose 1 at age 7–23 months: 2-dose series (dose 2 at least 12 weeks after dose 1 and after age 12 months)

- **Menactra® (age 9–23 months)**

· 2-dose series (dose 2 at least 12 weeks after dose 1; dose 2 may be administered as early as 8 weeks after dose 1 in travelers)

• Children age 2 years or older: 1 dose Menveo**, Menactra®, or MenQuadfi®

First-year college students who live in residential housing (if not previously vaccinated at age 16 years or older) or military recruits:

• 1 dose Menveo**, Menactra®, or MenQuadfi®

Adolescent vaccination of children who received MenACWY prior to age 10 years:

• **Children for whom boosters are recommended** because of an ongoing increased risk of meningococcal disease (e.g., those with complement component deficiency, HIV, or asplenia): Follow the booster schedule for persons at increased risk.

• **Children for whom boosters are not recommended** (e.g., a healthy child who received a single dose for travel to a country where meningococcal disease is endemic): Administer MenACWY according to the recommended adolescent schedule with dose 1 at age 11–12 years and dose 2 at age 16 years.

*Menveo has two formulations: lyophilized and liquid. The liquid formulation should not be used before age 10 years.

Note: Menactra® should be administered either before or at the same time as DTaP. MenACWY may be administered simultaneously with MenB vaccines if indicated, but at a different anatomic site, if feasible.

For MenACWY **booster dose recommendations** for groups listed under "Special situations" and in an outbreak setting and additional meningococcal vaccination information, see www.cdc.gov/mmwr/volumes/69/rr/rr6909a1.htm.

Meningococcal serogroup B vaccination
(minimum age: 10 years [MenB-4C, Bexsero®; MenB-FHbp, Trumenba®])

Shared clinical decision-making

• **Adolescents not at increased risk** age 16–23 years (preferred age 16–18 years) based on shared clinical decision-making:

- **Bexsero®:** 2-dose series at least 1 month apart

- **Trumenba®:** 2-dose series at least 6 months apart (if dose 2 is administered earlier than 6 months, administer a 3rd dose at least 4 months after dose 2)

Special situations

Anatomic or functional asplenia (including sickle cell disease), persistent complement component deficiency, complement inhibitor (e.g., eculizumab, ravulizumab) use:

• **Bexsero®:** 2-dose series at least 1 month apart

• **Trumenba®:** 3-dose series at 0, 1–2, 6 months (if dose 2 was administered at least 6 months after dose 1, dose 3 not needed; if dose 3 is administered earlier than 4 months after dose 2, a 4th dose should be administered at least 4 months after dose 3)

Note: Bexsero® and **Trumenba®** are not interchangeable; the same product should be used for all doses in a series.

For MenB **booster dose recommendations** for groups listed under "Special situations" and in an outbreak setting and additional meningococcal vaccination information, see www.cdc.gov/mmwr/volumes/69/rr/rr6909a1.htm.

Continued

Notes Recommended Child and Adolescent Immunization Schedule for ages 18 years or younger, United States, 2023

Pneumococcal vaccination (minimum age: 6 weeks [PCV13], [PCV15], 2 years [PPSV23])

Routine vaccination with PCV

• 4-dose series at 2, 4, 6, 12–15 months

Catch-up vaccination with PCV

• Healthy children age 24–59 months with any incomplete* PCV series: 1 dose PCV

• For other catch-up guidance, see Table 2.

Note: PCV13 and PCV15 can be used interchangeably for children who are healthy or have underlying conditions. PCV15 is not indicated for children who have received 4 doses of PCV13 or another age appropriate complete PCV13 series.

Special situations

Underlying conditions below: When both PCV and PPSV23 are indicated, administer PCV first. PCV and PPSV23 should not be administered during the same visit.

Chronic heart disease (particularly cyanotic congenital heart disease and cardiac failure); chronic lung disease (including asthma treated with high-dose, oral corticosteroids); diabetes mellitus:

Age 2–5 years

• Any incomplete* series with:
 - 3 PCV doses: 1 dose PCV (at least 8 weeks after any prior PCV dose)
 - Less than 3 PCV doses: 2 doses PCV (8 weeks after the most recent dose and administered 8 weeks apart)

• No history of PPSV23: 1 dose PPSV23 (at least 8 weeks after completing all recommended PCV doses)

Age 6–18 years

• Any incomplete* series with PCV: no further PCV doses needed

• No history of PPSV23: 1 dose PPSV23 (at least 8 weeks after completing all recommended PCV doses)

Cerebrospinal fluid leak, cochlear implant:

Age 2–5 years

• Any incomplete* series with:
 - 3 PCV doses: 1 dose PCV (at least 8 weeks after any prior PCV dose)
 - Less than 3 PCV doses: 2 doses PCV (8 weeks after the most recent dose and administered 8 weeks apart)

• No history of PPSV23: 1 dose PPSV23 (at least 8 weeks after completing all recommended PCV doses)

Age 6–18 years

• No history of either PCV or PPSV23: 1 dose PCV, 1 dose PPSV23 at least 8 weeks later

• Any PCV but no PPSV23: 1 dose PPSV23 at least 8 weeks after the most recent dose of PCV

• PPSV23 but no PCV: 1 dose PCV at least 8 weeks after the most recent dose of PPSV23

Sickle cell disease and other hemoglobinopathies; anatomic or functional asplenia; congenital or acquired immunodeficiency; HIV infection; chronic renal failure; nephrotic syndrome; malignant neoplasms, leukemias, lymphomas, Hodgkin disease, and other diseases associated with treatment with immunosuppressive drugs or radiation therapy; solid organ transplantation; multiple myeloma:

Age 2–5 years

• Any incomplete* series with:
 - 3 PCV doses: 1 dose PCV (at least 8 weeks after any prior PCV dose)
 - Less than 3 PCV doses: 2 doses PCV (8 weeks after the most recent dose and administered 8 weeks apart)

• No history of PPSV23: 1 dose PPSV23 (at least 8 weeks after completing all recommended PCV doses) and a dose 2 of PPSV23 5 years later

Age 6–18 years

• No history of either PCV or PPSV23: 1 dose PCV, 2 doses PPSV23 (dose 1 of PPSV23 administered 8 weeks after PCV and dose 2 of PPSV23 administered at least 5 years after dose 1 of PPSV23)

• Any PCV but no PPSV23: 2 doses PPSV23 (dose 1 of PPSV23 administered 8 weeks after the most recent dose of PCV and dose 2 of PPSV23 administered at least 5 years after dose 1 of PPSV23)

• PPSV23 but no PCV: 1 dose PCV at least 8 weeks after the most recent PPSV23 dose and a dose 2 of PPSV23 administered 5 years after dose 1 of PPSV23 and at least 8 weeks after a dose of PCV

Incomplete series = Not having received all doses in either the recommended series or an age-appropriate catch-up series see Table 2 in ACIP pneumococcal recommendations at www.cdc.gov/mmwr/volumes/71/wr/mm7137a3.htm

For guidance on determining which pneumococcal vaccines a patient needs and when, please refer to the mobile app, which can be downloaded here: www.cdc.gov/vaccines/vpd/pneumo/hcp/pneumoapp.html

Poliovirus vaccination (minimum age: 6 weeks)

Routine vaccination

• 4-dose series at ages 2, 4, 6–18 months, 4–6 years; administer the final dose on or after age 4 years and at least 6 months after the previous dose.

• 4 or more doses of IPV can be administered before age 4 years when a combination vaccine containing IPV is used. However, a dose is still recommended on or after age 4 years and at least 6 months after the previous dose.

Catch-up vaccination

• In the first 6 months of life, use minimum ages and intervals only for travel to a polio-endemic region or during an outbreak.

• IPV is not routinely recommended for U.S. residents age 18 years or older.

Series containing oral polio vaccine (OPV), either mixed OPV-IPV or OPV-only series:

• Total number of doses needed to complete the series is the same as that recommended for the U.S. IPV schedule. See www.cdc.gov/mmwr/volumes/66/wr/mm6601a6.htm?s_%20cid=mm6601a6_w.

• Only trivalent OPV (tOPV) counts toward the U.S. vaccination requirements.
 - Doses of OPV administered before April 1, 2016, should be counted (unless specifically noted as administered during a campaign).
 - Doses of OPV administered on or after April 1, 2016, should not be counted.
 - For guidance to assess doses documented as "OPV," see www.cdc.gov/mmwr/volumes/66/wr/mm6606a7.htm?s_cid=mm6606a7_w.

• For other catch-up guidance, see Table 2.

Special situations

• **Adolescents aged 18 years at increased risk of exposure to poliovirus with:**
 - No evidence of a complete polio vaccination series (i.e., at least 3 doses): administer remaining doses (1, 2, or 3 doses) to complete a 3-dose series
 - Evidence of completed polio vaccination series (i.e., at least 3 doses): may administer one lifetime IPV booster

For detailed information, see: www.cdc.gov/vaccines/vpd/polio/hcp/recommendations.html

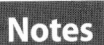 **Notes** Recommended Child and Adolescent Immunization Schedule for ages 18 years or younger, United States, 2023

Rotavirus vaccination
(minimum age: 6 weeks)

Routine vaccination

- **Rotarix®:** 2-dose series at age 2 and 4 months
- **RotaTeq®:** 3-dose series at age 2, 4, and 6 months
- If any dose in the series is either **RotaTeq®** or unknown, default to 3-dose series.

Catch-up vaccination

- Do not start the series on or after age 15 weeks, 0 days.
- The maximum age for the final dose is 8 months, 0 days.
- For other catch-up guidance, see Table 2.

Tetanus, diphtheria, and pertussis (Tdap) vaccination
(minimum age: 11 years for routine vaccination, 7 years for catch-up vaccination)

Routine vaccination

- **Adolescents age 11–12 years:** 1 dose Tdap
- **Pregnancy:** 1 dose Tdap during each pregnancy, preferably in early part of gestational weeks 27–36.
- Tdap may be administered regardless of the interval since the last tetanus- and diphtheria-toxoid-containing vaccine.

Catch-up vaccination

- **Adolescents age 13–18 years who have not received Tdap:** 1 dose Tdap, then Td or Tdap booster every 10 years
- **Persons age 7–18 years not fully vaccinated* with DTaP:** 1 dose Tdap as part of the catch-up series (preferably the first dose); if additional doses are needed, use Td or Tdap.
- **Tdap administered at age 7–10 years:**
  - **Children age 7–9 years** who receive Tdap should receive the routine Tdap dose at age 11–12 years.
  - **Children age 10 years** who receive Tdap do not need the routine Tdap dose at age 11–12 years.
- **DTaP inadvertently administered on or after age 7 years:**
  - **Children age 7–9 years:** DTaP may count as part of catch-up series. Administer routine Tdap dose at age 11–12 years.
  - **Children age 10–18 years:** Count dose of DTaP as the adolescent Tdap booster.
- For other catch-up guidance, see Table 2.

Special situations

- **Wound management** in persons age 7 years or older with history of 3 or more doses of tetanus-toxoid-containing vaccine: For clean and minor wounds, administer Tdap or Td if more than 10 years since last dose of tetanus-toxoid-containing vaccine; for all other wounds, administer Tdap or Td if more than 5 years since last dose of tetanus-toxoid-containing vaccine. Tdap is preferred for persons age 11 years or older who have not previously received Tdap or whose Tdap history is unknown. If a tetanus-toxoid-containing vaccine is indicated for a pregnant adolescent, use Tdap.
- For detailed information, see www.cdc.gov/mmwr/volumes/69/wr/mm6903a5.htm.

Fully vaccinated = 5 valid doses of DTaP OR 4 valid doses of DTaP if dose 4 was administered at age 4 years or older

Varicella vaccination
(minimum age: 12 months)

Routine vaccination

- 2-dose series at age 12–15 months, 4–6 years
- VAR or MMRV may be administered*
- Dose 2 may be administered as early as 3 months after dose 1 (a dose inadvertently administered after at least 4 weeks may be counted as valid)

*Note: For dose 1 in children age 12–47 months, it is recommended to administer MMR and varicella vaccines separately. MMRV may be used if parents or caregivers express a preference.

Catch-up vaccination

- Ensure persons age 7–18 years without evidence of immunity (see *MMWR* at www.cdc.gov/mmwr/pdf/rr/rr5604.pdf) have a 2-dose series:
  - **Age 7–12 years:** Routine interval: 3 months (a dose inadvertently administered after at least 4 weeks may be counted as valid)
  - **Age 13 years and older:** Routine interval: 4–8 weeks (minimum interval: 4 weeks)
  - The maximum age for use of *MMRV* is 12 years.

Continued

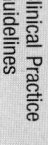

Clinical Practice Guidelines

V

Appendix Recommended Child and Adolescent Immunization Schedule for ages 18 years or younger, United States, 2023

Guide to Contraindications and Precautions to Commonly Used Vaccines

Adapted from Table 4-1 in Advisory Committee on Immunization Practices (ACIP) General Best Practice Guidelines for Immunization: Contraindication and Precautions available at www.cdc.gov/vaccines/hcp/acip-recs/general-recs/contraindications.html *and ACIP's Recommendations for the Prevention and Control of 2022-23 seasonal influenza with Vaccines available at* www.cdc.gov/mmwr/volumes/71/rr/rr7101a1.htm.

> **For COVID-19 vaccine contraindications and precautions see** www.cdc.gov/vaccines/covid-19/clinical-considerations/interim-considerations-us.html#contraindications

Vaccine	Contraindicated or Not Recommended[1]	Precautions[2]
Influenza, egg-based, inactivated injectable (IIV4)	• Severe allergic reaction (e.g., anaphylaxis) after previous dose of any influenza vaccine (i.e., any egg-based IIV, ccIIV, RIV, or LAIV of any valency) • Severe allergic reaction (e.g., anaphylaxis) to any vaccine component[3] (excluding egg)	• Guillain-Barré syndrome (GBS) within 6 weeks after a previous dose of any type of influenza vaccine • Moderate or severe acute illness with or without fever
Influenza, cell culture-based inactivated injectable [(ccIIV4), Flucelvax® Quadrivalent]	• Severe allergic reaction (e.g., anaphylaxis) to any ccIIV of any valency, or to any component[3] of ccIIV4	• Guillain-Barré syndrome (GBS) within 6 weeks after a previous dose of any type of influenza vaccine • Persons with a history of severe allergic reaction (e.g., anaphylaxis) after a previous dose of any egg-based IIV, RIV, or LAIV of any valency. If using ccIIV4, administer in medical setting under supervision of health care provider who can recognize and manage severe allergic reactions. May consult an allergist. • Moderate or severe acute illness with or without fever
Influenza, recombinant injectable [(RIV4), Flublok® Quadrivalent]	• Severe allergic reaction (e.g., anaphylaxis) to any RIV of any valency, or to any component[3] of RIV4	• Guillain-Barré syndrome (GBS) within 6 weeks after a previous dose of any type of influenza vaccine • Persons with a history of severe allergic reaction (e.g., anaphylaxis) after a previous dose of any egg-based IIV, ccIIV, or LAIV of any valency. If using RIV4, administer in medical setting under supervision of health care provider who can recognize and manage severe allergic reactions. May consult an allergist. • Moderate or severe acute illness with or without fever
Influenza, live attenuated [LAIV4, Flumist® Quadrivalent]	• Severe allergic reaction (e.g., anaphylaxis) after previous dose of any influenza vaccine (i.e., any egg-based IIV, ccIIV, RIV, or LAIV of any valency) • Severe allergic reaction (e.g., anaphylaxis) to any vaccine component[3] (excluding egg) • Children age 2–4 years with a history of asthma or wheezing • Anatomic or functional asplenia • Immunocompromised due to any cause including, but not limited to, medications and HIV infection • Close contacts or caregivers of severely immunosuppressed persons who require a protected environment • Pregnancy • Cochlear implant • Active communication between the cerebrospinal fluid (CSF) and the oropharynx, nasopharynx, nose, ear or any other cranial CSF leak • Children and adolescents receiving aspirin or salicylate-containing medications • Received influenza antiviral medications oseltamivir or zanamivir within the previous 48 hours, peramivir within the previous 5 days, or baloxavir within the previous 17 days	• Guillain-Barré syndrome (GBS) within 6 weeks after a previous dose of any type of influenza vaccine • Asthma in persons aged 5 years old or older • Persons with underlying medical conditions (other than those listed under contraindications) that might predispose to complications after wild-type influenza virus infection [e.g., chronic pulmonary, cardiovascular (except isolated hypertension), renal, hepatic, neurologic, hematologic, or metabolic disorders (including diabetes mellitus)] • Moderate or severe acute illness with or without fever

1. When a contraindication is present, a vaccine should NOT be administered. Kroger A, Bahta L, Hunter P. ACIP General Best Practice Guidelines for Immunization. www.cdc.gov/vaccines/hcp/acip-recs/general-recs/contraindications.html
2. When a precaution is present, vaccination should generally be deferred but might be indicated if the benefit of protection from the vaccine outweighs the risk for an adverse reaction. Kroger A, Bahta L, Hunter P. ACIP General Best Practice Guidelines for Immunization. www.cdc.gov/vaccines/hcp/acip-recs/general-recs/contraindications.html
3. Vaccination providers should check FDA-approved prescribing information for the most complete and updated information, including contraindications, warnings, and precautions. Package inserts for U.S.-licensed vaccines are available at www.fda.gov/vaccines-blood-biologics/approved-products/vaccines-licensed-use-united-states

Appendix Recommended Child and Adolescent Immunization Schedule for ages 18 years or younger, United States, 2023

Vaccine	Contraindicated or Not Recommended[1]	Precautions[2]
Dengue (DEN4CYD)	• Severe allergic reaction (e.g., anaphylaxis) after a previous dose or to a vaccine component[3] • Severe immunodeficiency (e.g., hematologic and solid tumors, receipt of chemotherapy, congenital immunodeficiency, long-term immunosuppressive therapy or patients with HIV infection who are severely immunocompromised) • Lack of laboratory confirmation of a previous Dengue infection	• Pregnancy • HIV infection without evidence of severe immunosuppression • Moderate or severe acute illness with or without fever
Diphtheria, tetanus, pertussis (DTaP) Tetanus, diphtheria (DT)	• Severe allergic reaction (e.g., anaphylaxis) after a previous dose or to a vaccine component[3] • For DTaP only: Encephalopathy (e.g., coma, decreased level of consciousness, prolonged seizures) not attributable to another identifiable cause within 7 days of administration of previous dose of DTP or DTaP	• Guillain-Barré syndrome (GBS) within 6 weeks after previous dose of tetanus-toxoid–containing vaccine • History of Arthus-type hypersensitivity reactions after a previous dose of diphtheria-toxoid–containing or tetanus-toxoid–containing vaccine; defer vaccination until at least 10 years have elapsed since the last tetanus-toxoid-containing vaccine • For DTaP only: Progressive neurologic disorder, including infantile spasms, uncontrolled epilepsy, progressive encephalopathy; defer DTaP until neurologic status clarified and stabilized • Moderate or severe acute illness with or without fever
Haemophilus influenzae type b (Hib)	• Severe allergic reaction (e.g., anaphylaxis) after a previous dose or to a vaccine component[3] • For Hiberix, ActHib, and PedvaxHIB only: History of severe allergic reaction to dry natural latex • Less than age 6 weeks	• Moderate or severe acute illness with or without fever
Hepatitis A (HepA)	• Severe allergic reaction (e.g., anaphylaxis) after a previous dose or to a vaccine component[3] including neomycin	• Moderate or severe acute illness with or without fever
Hepatitis B (HepB)	• Severe allergic reaction (e.g., anaphylaxis) after a previous dose or to a vaccine component[3] including yeast • *Pregnancy: Heplisav-B and PreHevbrio are not recommended due to lack of safety data in pregnant persons. Use other hepatitis B vaccines if HepB is indicated[4].*	• Moderate or severe acute illness with or without fever
Hepatitis A–Hepatitis B vaccine [HepA-HepB, (Twinrix®)]	• Severe allergic reaction (e.g., anaphylaxis) after a previous dose or to a vaccine component[3] including neomycin and yeast	• Moderate or severe acute illness with or without fever
Human papillomavirus (HPV)	• Severe allergic reaction (e.g., anaphylaxis) after a previous dose or to a vaccine component[3] • *Pregnancy: HPV vaccination not recommended.*	• Moderate or severe acute illness with or without fever
Measles, mumps, rubella (MMR) Measles, mumps, rubella, and varicella (MMRV)	• Severe allergic reaction (e.g., anaphylaxis) after a previous dose or to a vaccine component[3] • Severe immunodeficiency (e.g., hematologic and solid tumors, receipt of chemotherapy, congenital immunodeficiency, long-term immunosuppressive therapy or patients with HIV infection who are severely immunocompromised) • Pregnancy • Family history of altered immunocompetence, unless verified clinically or by laboratory testing as immunocompetent	• Recent (≤11 months) receipt of antibody-containing blood product (specific interval depends on product) • History of thrombocytopenia or thrombocytopenic purpura • Need for tuberculin skin testing or interferon-gamma release assay (IGRA) testing • Moderate or severe acute illness with or without fever • For MMRV only: Personal or family (i.e., sibling or parent) history of seizures of any etiology
Meningococcal ACWY (MenACWY) [MenACWY-CRM (Menveo®); MenACWY-D (Menactra®); MenACWY-TT (MenQuadfi®)]	• Severe allergic reaction (e.g., anaphylaxis) after a previous dose or to a vaccine component[3] • For MenACWY-D and Men ACWY-CRM only: severe allergic reaction to any diphtheria toxoid– or CRM197–containing vaccine • For MenACWY-TT only: severe allergic reaction to a tetanus toxoid-containing vaccine	• For MenACWY-CRM only: Preterm birth if less than age 9 months • Moderate or severe acute illness with or without fever
Meningococcal B (MenB) [MenB-4C (Bexsero®); MenB-FHbp (Trumenba®)]	• Severe allergic reaction (e.g., anaphylaxis) after a previous dose or to a vaccine component[3]	• Pregnancy • For MenB-4C only: Latex sensitivity • Moderate or severe acute illness with or without fever
Pneumococcal conjugate (PCV)	• Severe allergic reaction (e.g., anaphylaxis) after a previous dose or to a vaccine component[3] • Severe allergic reaction (e.g., anaphylaxis) to any diphtheria-toxoid-containing vaccine or its component[3]	• Moderate or severe acute illness with or without fever
Pneumococcal polysaccharide (PPSV23)	• Severe allergic reaction (e.g., anaphylaxis) after a previous dose or to a vaccine component[3]	• Moderate or severe acute illness with or without fever
Poliovirus vaccine, inactivated (IPV)	• Severe allergic reaction (e.g., anaphylaxis) after a previous dose or to a vaccine component[3]	• Pregnancy • Moderate or severe acute illness with or without fever
Rotavirus (RV) [RV1 (Rotarix®), RV5 (RotaTeq®)]	• Severe allergic reaction (e.g., anaphylaxis) after a previous dose or to a vaccine component[3] • Severe combined immunodeficiency (SCID) • History of intussusception	• Altered immunocompetence other than SCID • Chronic gastrointestinal disease • RV1 only: Spina bifida or bladder exstrophy • Moderate or severe acute illness with or without fever
Tetanus, diphtheria, and acellular pertussis (Tdap) Tetanus, diphtheria (Td)	• Severe allergic reaction (e.g., anaphylaxis) after a previous dose or to a vaccine component[3] • For Tdap only: Encephalopathy (e.g., coma, decreased level of consciousness, prolonged seizures) not attributable to another identifiable cause within 7 days of administration of previous dose of DTP, DTaP, or Tdap	• Guillain-Barré syndrome (GBS) within 6 weeks after a previous dose of tetanus-toxoid–containing vaccine • History of Arthus-type hypersensitivity reactions after a previous dose of diphtheria-toxoid–containing or tetanus-toxoid–containing vaccine; defer vaccination until at least 10 years have elapsed since the last tetanus-toxoid–containing vaccine • For Tdap only: Progressive or unstable neurological disorder, uncontrolled seizures, or progressive encephalopathy until a treatment regimen has been established and the condition has stabilized • Moderate or severe acute illness with or without fever
Varicella (VAR)	• Severe allergic reaction (e.g., anaphylaxis) after a previous dose or to a vaccine component[3] • Severe immunodeficiency (e.g., hematologic and solid tumors, receipt of chemotherapy, congenital immunodeficiency, long-term immunosuppressive therapy or patients with HIV infection who are severely immunocompromised) • Pregnancy • Family history of altered immunocompetence, unless verified clinically or by laboratory testing as immunocompetent	• Recent (≤11 months) receipt of antibody-containing blood product (specific interval depends on product) • Receipt of specific antiviral drugs (acyclovir, famciclovir, or valacyclovir) 24 hours before vaccination (avoid use of these antiviral drugs for 14 days after vaccination) • Use of aspirin or aspirin-containing products • Moderate or severe acute illness with or without fever • If using MMRV, see MMR/MMRV for additional precautions

1. When a contraindication is present, a vaccine should NOT be administered. Kroger A, Bahta L, Hunter P. ACIP General Best Practice Guidelines for Immunization. www.cdc.gov/vaccines/hcp/acip-recs/general-recs/contraindications.html
2. When a precaution is present, vaccination should generally be deferred but might be indicated if the benefit of protection from the vaccine outweighs the risk for an adverse reaction. Kroger A, Bahta L, Hunter P. ACIP General Best Practice Guidelines for Immunization. www.cdc.gov/vaccines/hcp/acip-recs/general-recs/contraindications.html
3. Vaccination providers should check FDA-approved prescribing information for the most complete and updated information, including contraindications, warnings, and precautions. Package inserts for U.S.-licensed vaccines are available at www.fda.gov/vaccines-blood-biologics/approved-products/vaccines-licensed-use-united-states.
4. For information on the pregnancy exposure registries for persons who were inadvertently vaccinated with Heplisav-B or PreHevbrio while pregnant, please visit heplisavbpregnancyregistry.com/ or www.prehevbrio.com/#safety.

VACCINE ADMINISTRATION*

INFECTION CONTROL AND STERILE TECHNIQUE

Persons administering vaccines should follow appropriate precautions to minimize risk for spread of disease. Hands should be cleansed with an alcohol-based, waterless antiseptic hand rub or washed with soap and water between each patient contact. Occupational Safety and Health Administration (OSHA) regulations do not require that gloves be worn when administering vaccinations unless persons administering vaccinations are likely to come into contact with potentially infectious body fluids or have open lesions on their hands. Needles used for injections must be sterile and disposable to minimize the risk for contamination. A separate needle and syringe should be used for each injection. Changing needles between drawing vaccine from a vial and injecting it into a recipient is not necessary. Different vaccines should never be mixed in the same syringe unless specifically licensed for such use, and no attempt should be made to transfer between syringes.

For all intramuscular injections, the needle should be long enough to reach the muscle mass and prevent vaccine from seeping into subcutaneous tissue, but not so long as to involve underlying nerves, blood vessels, or bone. Vaccinators should be familiar with the anatomy of the area where they are injecting vaccine. Intramuscular injections are administered at a 90-degree angle to the skin, preferably into the anterolateral aspect of the thigh or the deltoid muscle of the upper arm depending on the age of the patient.

Decision on needle size and site of injection must be made for each person on the basis of the size of the muscle, the thickness of adipose tissue at the injection site, the volume of the material to be administered, injection technique, and the depth below the muscle surface into which the material is to be injected. Aspiration before injection of vaccines or toxoids (i.e., pulling back on the syringe plunger after needle insertion before injection) is not required because no large blood vessel exists at the recommended injection sites.

INFANTS (AGED <12 MO)

For the majority of infants, the anterolateral aspect of the thigh is the recommended site for injection because it provides a large muscle mass. The muscles of the buttock have not been used for administration of vaccines in infants and children because of concern about potential injury to the sciatic nerve, which is well documented after injection of antimicrobial agents into the buttock. If the gluteal muscle must be used, care should be taken to define the anatomic landmarks. Injection technique is the most important parameter to ensure efficient intramuscular vaccine delivery. If the subcutaneous and muscle tissue are bunched to minimize the chance of striking bone, a 1-inch needle is required to ensure intramuscular administration in infants. For the majority of infants, a 1-inch, 22- to 25-gauge needle is sufficient to penetrate muscle in an infant's thigh. For newborn (first 28 days of life) and premature infants, a 5/8-inch-long needle usually is adequate if the skin is stretched flat between thumb and forefinger and the needle inserted at a 90-degree angle to the skin.

TODDLERS AND OLDER CHILDREN (AGED 12 MO TO 10 YR)

The deltoid muscle should be used if the muscle mass is adequate. The needle size for deltoid site injections can range from 22 to 25 gauge and from 5/8-1 inch on the basis of the size of the muscle and the thickness of adipose tissue at the injection site. A 5/8-inch needle is adequate only for the deltoid muscle and only if the skin is stretched flat between the thumb and forefinger and the needle inserted at a 90-degree angle to the skin. For toddlers, the anterolateral thigh can be used, but the needle should be at least 1 inch in length.

ADOLESCENTS AND ADULTS (AGED >11 YR)

For adults and adolescents, the deltoid muscle is recommended for routine intramuscular vaccinations. The anterolateral thigh also can be used. For men and women weighing <130 lb (<60 kg) a 5/8- to 1-inch needle is sufficient to ensure intramuscular injection. For women weighing 130-200 lb (60-90 kg) and men 130 to 260 lb (60-118 kg), a 1- to $1\frac{1}{2}$-inch needle is needed. For women weighing >200 lb (>90 kg) or men weighing >260 lb (>118 kg), a $1\frac{1}{2}$-inch needle is required.

SUBCUTANEOUS INJECTIONS

Subcutaneous injections are administered at a 45-degree angle, usually into the thigh for infants younger than 12 mo and in the upper-outer triceps area of persons aged 12 mo and older. Subcutaneous injections can be administered into the upper-outer triceps area of an infant if necessary. A 5/8-inch, 23- to 25-gauge needle should be inserted into the subcutaneous tissue.

Immunizations for Adults

RECOMMENDED ADULT IMMUNIZATION SCHEDULE BY AGE GROUP, UNITED STATES, 2023

The *Recommended Adult Immunization Schedule by Age Group, United States* became effective, as recommended by the Advisory Committee on Immunization Practices (ACIP) and approved by the Centers for Disease Control and Prevention (CDC). The adult immunization schedule was also reviewed and approved by the following professional medical organizations:

- American College of Physicians (http://www.acponline.org/)
- American Academy of Family Physicians (http://www.aafp.org/)
- American College of Obstetricians and Gynecologists (http://www.acog.org/)
- American College of Nurse-Midwives (http://www.midwife.org/)

CDC announced the availability of the 2023 adult immunization schedule at https://www.cdc.gov/vaccines/schedules/easy-to-read/adult.html.

The adult immunization schedule describes the age groups and medical conditions and other indications for which licensed vaccines are recommended. The 2023 adult immunization schedule consists of:

- Table 12. Recommended immunization schedule for adults by age group
- Table 13. Recommended immunization schedule for adults by medical condition and other indications
- Footnotes that accompany each vaccine containing important general information and considerations for special populations

Consider the following information when reviewing the adult immunization schedule:

- The tables in the adult immunization schedule should be read with the footnotes that contain important general information and information about vaccination of special populations.
- When indicated, administer recommended vaccines to adults whose vaccination history is incomplete or unknown.
- Increased interval between doses of a multi-dose vaccine does not diminish vaccine effectiveness; therefore, it is not necessary to restart the vaccine series or add doses to the series because of an extended interval between doses.
- Adults with immunocompromising conditions should generally avoid live vaccines, e.g., measles, mumps, and rubella vaccine. Inactivated vaccines, e.g., pneumococcal or inactivated influenza vaccines, are generally acceptable.
- Combination vaccines may be used when any component of the combination is indicated and when the other components of the combination vaccine are not contraindicated.
- The use of trade names in the adult immunization schedule is for identification purposes only and does not imply endorsement by the ACIP or CDC.

Details on vaccines recommended for adults and complete ACIP statements are available at https://www.cdc.gov/vaccines/hcp/acip-recs/index.html. Additional CDC resources include:

- A summary of information on vaccination recommendations, vaccination of persons with immunodeficiencies, preventing and managing adverse reactions, vaccination contraindications and precautions, and other information can be found in *General Recommendations on Immunization* at https://www.cdc.gov/mmwr/preview/mmwrhtml/rr6002a1.htm.

- Vaccine Information Statements that explain benefits and risks of vaccines are available at https://www.cdc.gov/vaccinesafety/Concerns/Index.html.
- Information and resources regarding vaccination of pregnant women are available at http://www.cdc.gov/vaccines/pregnancy/pregnant-women/index.html
- Information on travel vaccine requirements and recommendations is available at https://www.cdc.gov/travel/destinations/list.
- *CDC Vaccine Schedules App* for clinicians and other immunization service providers to download is available at https://www.cdc.gov/vaccines/schedules/.
- *Recommended Immunization Schedule for Children and Adolescents Aged 18 Years or Younger* is available at https://www.cdc.gov/vaccines/schedules/hcp/child-adolescent.html

Report suspected cases of reportable vaccine-preventable diseases to the local or state health department.

Report all clinically significant postvaccination reactions to the Vaccine Adverse Event Reporting System at http://www.vaers.hhs.gov/ or by telephone, 800-822-7967. All vaccines included in the 2022 adult immunization schedule except herpes zoster and 23-valent pneumococcal polysaccharide vaccines are covered by the Vaccine Injury Compensation Program. Information on how to file a vaccine injury claim is available at https://www.hrsa.gov/vaccinecompensation or by telephone, 800-338-2382.

The following acronyms are used for vaccines recommended for adults:

HepA	hepatitis A vaccine
HepA-HepB	hepatitis A and hepatitis B vaccines
HepB	hepatitis B vaccine
Hib	*Haemophilus influenzae* type b conjugate vaccine
HPV vaccine	human papillomavirus vaccine
HZV	herpes zoster vaccine
IIV	inactivated influenza vaccine
LAIV	live attenuated influenza vaccine
MenACWY	serogroups A, C, W, and Y meningococcal conjugate vaccine
MenB	serogroup B meningococcal vaccine
MMR	measles, mumps, and rubella vaccine
MPSV4	serogroups A, C, W, and Y meningococcal polysaccharide vaccine
PCV13	13-valent pneumococcal conjugate vaccine
PPSV23	23-valent pneumococcal polysaccharide vaccine
RIV	recombinant influenza vaccine
Td	tetanus and diphtheria toxoids
Tdap	tetanus toxoid, reduced diphtheria toxoid, and acellular pertussis vaccine
VAR	varicella vaccine

TABLE 12   Recommended Adult Immunization Schedule by Age Group, United States, 2023

These recommendations must be read with the footnotes that follow. From Centers for Disease Control and Prevention.

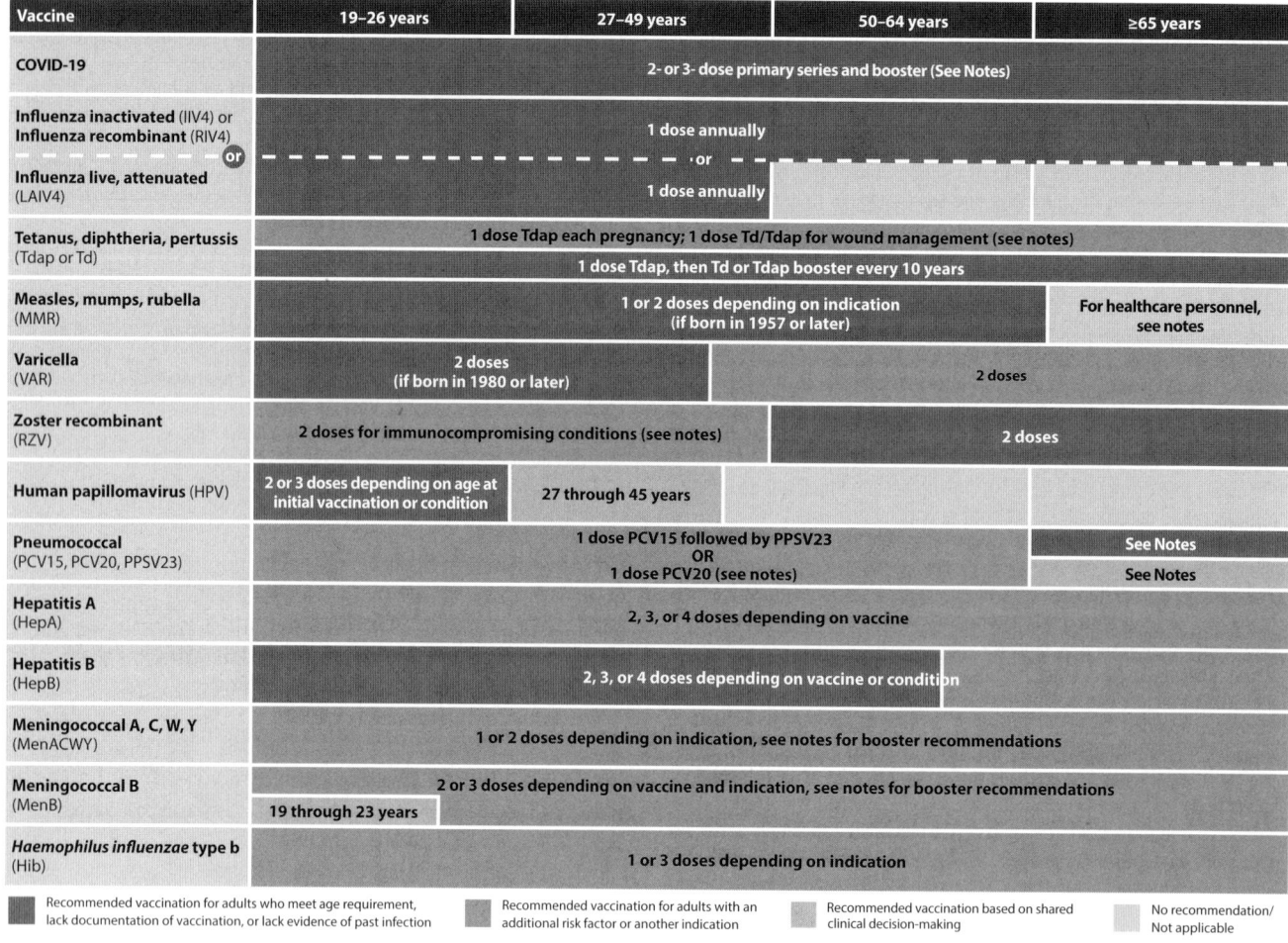

Vaccine	19–26 years	27–49 years	50–64 years	≥65 years
COVID-19	2- or 3- dose primary series and booster (See Notes)			
Influenza inactivated (IIV4) or **Influenza recombinant** (RIV4)	1 dose annually			
Influenza live, attenuated (LAIV4)	1 dose annually			
Tetanus, diphtheria, pertussis (Tdap or Td)	1 dose Tdap each pregnancy; 1 dose Td/Tdap for wound management (see notes)			
	1 dose Tdap, then Td or Tdap booster every 10 years			
Measles, mumps, rubella (MMR)	1 or 2 doses depending on indication (if born in 1957 or later)			For healthcare personnel, see notes
Varicella (VAR)	2 doses (if born in 1980 or later)		2 doses	
Zoster recombinant (RZV)	2 doses for immunocompromising conditions (see notes)		2 doses	
Human papillomavirus (HPV)	2 or 3 doses depending on age at initial vaccination or condition	27 through 45 years		
Pneumococcal (PCV15, PCV20, PPSV23)	1 dose PCV15 followed by PPSV23 OR 1 dose PCV20 (see notes)			See Notes / See Notes
Hepatitis A (HepA)	2, 3, or 4 doses depending on vaccine			
Hepatitis B (HepB)	2, 3, or 4 doses depending on vaccine or condition			
Meningococcal A, C, W, Y (MenACWY)	1 or 2 doses depending on indication, see notes for booster recommendations			
Meningococcal B (MenB)	2 or 3 doses depending on vaccine and indication, see notes for booster recommendations			
	19 through 23 years			
Haemophilus influenzae **type b** (Hib)	1 or 3 doses depending on indication			

Recommended vaccination for adults who meet age requirement, lack documentation of vaccination, or lack evidence of past infection

Recommended vaccination for adults with an additional risk factor or another indication

Recommended vaccination based on shared clinical decision-making

No recommendation/ Not applicable

TABLE 13 Recommended Adult Immunization Schedule by Medical Condition or Other Indication, United States, 2023

These recommendations must be read with the footnotes that follow.
From Centers for Disease Control and Prevention.

Vaccine	Pregnancy	Immuno-compromised (excluding HIV infection)	HIV infection CD4 percentage and count		Asplenia, complement deficiencies	End-stage renal disease, or on hemodialysis	Heart or lung disease; alcoholism[a]	Chronic liver disease	Diabetes	Health care personnel[b]	Men who have sex with men
			<15% or <200 mm³	≥15% and ≥200 mm³							
COVID-19		See Notes									
IIV4 or RIV4 or	1 dose annually										
LAIV4	Contraindicated					Precaution					— or — 1 dose annually
Tdap or Td	1 dose Tdap each pregnancy	1 dose Tdap, then Td or Tdap booster every 10 years									
MMR	Contraindicated*	Contraindicated			1 or 2 doses depending on indication						
VAR	Contraindicated*	Contraindicated			2 doses						
RZV		2 doses at age ≥19 years			2 doses at age ≥50 years						
HPV	Not Recommended*	3 doses through age 26 years			2 or 3 doses through age 26 years depending on age at initial vaccination or condition						
Pneumococcal (PCV15, PCV20, PPSV23)		1 dose PCV15 followed by PPSV23 OR 1 dose PCV20 (see notes)									
HepA					2, 3, or 4 doses depending on vaccine						
HepB	3 doses (see notes)	2, 3, or 4 doses depending on vaccine or condition									
MenACWY		1 or 2 doses depending on indication, see notes for booster recommendations									
MenB	Precaution	2 or 3 doses depending on vaccine and indication, see notes for booster recommendations									
Hib		3 doses HSCT[c] recipients only			1 dose						

■ Recommended vaccination for adults who meet age requirement, lack documentation of vaccination, or lack evidence of past infection

■ Recommended vaccination for adults with an additional risk factor or another indication

■ Recommended vaccination based on shared clinical decision-making

■ Precaution–vaccination might be indicated if benefit of protection outweighs risk of adverse reaction

■ Contraindicated or not recommended–vaccine should not be administered.
*Vaccinate after pregnancy.

■ No recommendation/ Not applicable

a. Precaution for LAIV4 does not apply to alcoholism. **b.** See notes for influenza; hepatitis B; measles, mumps, and rubella; and varicella vaccinations. **c.** Hematopoietic stem cell transplant.

Continued

Notes Recommended Adult Immunization Schedule for ages 19 years or older, United States, 2023

For vaccine recommendations for persons 18 years of age or younger, see the Recommended Child and Adolescent Immunization Schedule.

COVID-19 vaccination

Routine vaccination

- **Primary series:** 2-dose series at 0, 4-8 weeks (Moderna) or 2-dose series at 0, 3-8 weeks (Novavax, Pfizer-BioNTech)

- **Booster dose:** see www.cdc.gov/vaccines/covid-19/clinical-considerations/interim-considerations-us.html

Special situations

Persons who are moderately or severely immunocompromised

- **Primary series**

  - 3-dose series at 0, 4, 8 weeks (Moderna) or 3-dose series at 0, 3, 7 weeks (Pfizer-BioNTech)

  - 2-dose series at 0, 3 weeks (Novavax)

- **Booster dose:** see www.cdc.gov/vaccines/covid-19/clinical-considerations/interim-considerations-us.html

- **Pre-exposure prophylaxis (e.g., monoclonal antibodies)** may be considered to complement COVID-19 vaccination. See www.cdc.gov/vaccines/covid-19/clinical-considerations/interim-considerations-us.html#immunocompromised

For Janssen COVID-19 Vaccine recipients see COVID-19 schedule at www.cdc.gov/vaccines/covid-19/clinical-considerations/interim-considerations-us.html.

Note: Current COVID-19 schedule available at www.cdc.gov/vaccines/covid-19/downloads/COVID-19-immunization-schedule-ages-6months-older.pdf. For more information on Emergency Use Authorization (EUA) indications for COVID-19 vaccines, please visit www.fda.gov/emergency-preparedness-and-response/coronavirus-disease-2019-covid-19/covid-19-vaccines

Haemophilus influenzae type b vaccination

Special situations

- **Anatomical or functional asplenia (including sickle cell disease):** 1 dose if previously did not receive Hib; if elective splenectomy, 1 dose preferably at least 14 days before splenectomy

- **Hematopoietic stem cell transplant (HSCT):** 3-dose series 4 weeks apart starting 6–12 months after successful transplant, regardless of Hib vaccination history

Hepatitis A vaccination

Routine vaccination

- **Not at risk but want protection from hepatitis A** (identification of risk factor not required): 2-dose series HepA (Havrix 6–12 months apart or Vaqta 6–18 months apart [minimum interval: 6 months]) or 3-dose series HepA-HepB (Twinrix at 0, 1, 6 months [minimum intervals: dose 1 to dose 2: 4 weeks / dose 2 to dose 3: 5 months])

Special situations

- **At risk for hepatitis A virus infection:** 2-dose series HepA or 3-dose series HepA-HepB as above

  - **Chronic liver disease** (e.g., persons with hepatitis B, hepatitis C, cirrhosis, fatty liver disease, alcoholic liver disease, autoimmune hepatitis, alanine aminotransferase [ALT] or aspartate aminotransferase [AST] level greater than twice the upper limit of normal)

  - **HIV infection**

  - **Men who have sex with men**

  - **Injection or noninjection drug use**

  - **Persons experiencing homelessness**

  - **Work with hepatitis A virus** in research laboratory or with nonhuman primates with hepatitis A virus infection

  - **Travel in countries with high or intermediate endemic hepatitis A** (HepA-HepB [Twinrix] may be administered on an accelerated schedule of 3 doses at 0, 7, and 21–30 days, followed by a booster dose at 12 months)

  - **Close, personal contact with international adoptee** (e.g., household or regular babysitting) in first 60 days after arrival from country with high or intermediate endemic hepatitis A (administer dose 1 as soon as adoption is planned, at least 2 weeks before adoptee's arrival)

  - **Pregnancy** if at risk for infection or severe outcome from infection during pregnancy

  - **Settings for exposure,** including health care settings targeting services to injection or noninjection drug users or group homes and nonresidential day care facilities for developmentally disabled persons (individual risk factor screening not required)

Hepatitis B vaccination

Routine vaccination

- **Age 19 through 59 years: complete a 2- or 3- or 4-dose series**

  - 2-dose series only applies when 2 doses of Heplisav-B* are used at least 4 weeks apart

  - 3-dose series Engerix-B, PreHevbrio*, or Recombivax HB at 0, 1, 6 months [minimum intervals: dose 1 to dose 2: 4 weeks / dose 2 to dose 3: 8 weeks / dose 1 to dose 3: 16 weeks])

  - 3-dose series HepA-HepB (Twinrix at 0, 1, 6 months [minimum intervals: dose 1 to dose 2: 4 weeks / dose 2 to dose 3: 5 months])

  - 4-dose series HepA-HepB (Twinrix) accelerated schedule of 3 doses at 0, 7, and 21–30 days, followed by a booster dose at 12 months

***Note:** Heplisav-B and PreHevbrio are not recommended in pregnancy due to lack of safety data in pregnant persons.

Notes Recommended Adult Immunization Schedule, United States, 2023

- **Age 60 years or older with** known risk factors for hepatitis B virus infection **should** complete a HepB vaccine series.

- **Age 60 years or older without** known risk factors for hepatitis B virus infection **may** complete a HepB vaccine series.

  - **Risk factors for hepatitis B virus infection include:**

    - **Chronic liver disease** (e.g., persons with hepatitis C, cirrhosis, fatty liver disease, alcoholic liver disease, autoimmune hepatitis, alanine aminotransferase [ALT] or aspartate aminotransferase [AST] level greater than twice upper limit of normal)
    - **HIV infection**
    - **Sexual exposure risk** (e.g., sex partners of hepatitis B surface antigen [HBsAg]-positive persons; sexually active persons not in mutually monogamous relationships; persons seeking evaluation or treatment for a sexually transmitted infection; men who have sex with men)
    - **Current or recent injection drug use**
    - **Percutaneous or mucosal risk for exposure to blood** (e.g., household contacts of HBsAg-positive persons; residents and staff of facilities for developmentally disabled persons; health care and public safety personnel with reasonably anticipated risk for exposure to blood or blood-contaminated body fluids; persons on maintenance dialysis, including in-center or home hemodialysis and peritoneal dialysis, and persons who are predialysis; patients with diabetes)
    - **Incarceration**
    - **Travel in countries with high or intermediate endemic hepatitis B**

Special situations

- **Patients on dialysis:** complete a 3- or 4-dose series

  - 3-dose series Recombivax HB at 0, 1, 6 months (note: use Dialysis Formulation 1 mL = 40 mcg)

  - 4-dose series Engerix-B at 0, 1, 2, and 6 months (note: use 2 mL dose instead of the normal adult dose of 1 mL)

Human papillomavirus vaccination

Routine vaccination

- **HPV vaccination recommended for all persons through age 26 years:** 2- or 3-dose series depending on age at initial vaccination or condition:

  - **Age 15 years or older at initial vaccination:** 3-dose series at 0, 1–2 months, 6 months (minimum intervals: dose 1 to dose 2: 4 weeks / dose 2 to dose 3: 12 weeks / dose 1 to dose 3: 5 months; repeat dose if administered too soon)
  - **Age 9–14 years at initial vaccination and received 1 dose or 2 doses less than 5 months apart:** 1 additional dose
  - **Age 9–14 years at initial vaccination and received 2 doses at least 5 months apart:** HPV vaccination series complete, no additional dose needed

- **Interrupted schedules:** If vaccination schedule is interrupted, the series does not need to be restarted

- **No additional dose recommended when any HPV vaccine series has been completed using the recommended dosing intervals.**

Shared clinical decision-making

- **Some adults age 27–45 years:** Based on shared clinical decision-making, 2- or 3-dose series as above

Special situations

- **Age ranges recommended above for routine and catch-up vaccination or shared clinical decision-making also apply in special situations**

  - **Immunocompromising conditions, including HIV infection**: 3-dose series, even for those who initiate vaccination at age 9 through 14 years.

  - **Pregnancy**: Pregnancy testing is not needed before vaccination; HPV vaccination is not recommended until after pregnancy; no intervention needed if inadvertently vaccinated while pregnant

Influenza vaccination

Routine vaccination

- **Age 19 years or older:** 1 dose any influenza vaccine appropriate for age and health status annually.

  - **Age 65 years or older:** Any one of quadrivalent high-dose inactivated influenza vaccine (HD-IIV4), quadrivalent recombinant influenza vaccine (RIV4), or quadrivalent adjuvanted inactivated influenza vaccine (aIIV4) is preferred. If none of these three vaccines is available, then any other age-appropriate influenza vaccine should be used.

- For the 2022–2023 season, see www.cdc.gov/mmwr/volumes/71/rr/rr7101a1.htm

- For the 2023–2024 season, see the 2023–2024 ACIP influenza vaccine recommendations.

Special situations

- **Egg allergy, hives only:** any influenza vaccine appropriate for age and health status annually

- **Egg allergy–any symptom other than hives** (e.g., angioedema, respiratory distress or required epinephrine or another emergency medical intervention): Any influenza vaccine appropriate for age and health status may be administered. If using egg-based IIV4 or LAIV4, administer in medical setting under supervision of health care provider who can recognize and manage severe allergic reactions.

- **Close contacts (e.g., caregivers, healthcare workers) of severely immunosuppressed persons who require a protected environment:** these persons should not receive LAIV4. If LAIV4 is given, they should avoid contact with/caring for such immunosuppressed persons for 7 days after vaccination.

- **Severe allergic reaction (e.g., anaphylaxis) to a vaccine component or a previous dose of any influenza vaccine:** see Appendix listing contraindications and precautions

Continued

Notes   Recommended Adult Immunization Schedule, United States, 2023

- **History of Guillain-Barré syndrome within 6 weeks after previous dose of influenza vaccine:** Generally, should not be vaccinated unless vaccination benefits outweigh risks for those at higher risk for severe complications from influenza

Measles, mumps, and rubella vaccination

Routine vaccination

- **No evidence of immunity to measles, mumps, or rubella:** 1 dose

  - **Evidence of immunity:** Born before 1957 (health care personnel, see below), documentation of receipt of MMR vaccine, laboratory evidence of immunity or disease (diagnosis of disease without laboratory confirmation is not evidence of immunity)

Special situations

- **Pregnancy with no evidence of immunity to rubella:** MMR contraindicated during pregnancy; after pregnancy (before discharge from health care facility), 1 dose

- **Nonpregnant persons of childbearing age with no evidence of immunity to rubella:** 1 dose

- **HIV infection with CD4 percentages ≥15% and CD4 count ≥200 cells/mm³ for at least 6 months and no evidence of immunity to measles, mumps, or rubella:** 2-dose series at least 4 weeks apart; MMR contraindicated for HIV infection with CD4 percentage <15% or CD4 count <200 cells/mm³

- **Severe immunocompromising conditions:** MMR contraindicated

- **Students in postsecondary educational institutions, international travelers, and household or close, personal contacts of immunocompromised persons with no evidence of immunity to measles, mumps, or rubella:** 2-dose series at least 4 weeks apart if previously did not receive any doses of MMR or 1 dose if previously received 1 dose MMR

- **In mumps outbreak settings,** for information about additional doses of MMR (including 3rd dose of MMR), see www.cdc.gov/mmwr/volumes/67/wr/mm6701a7.htm

- **Health care personnel:**

  - **Born before 1957 with no evidence of immunity to measles, mumps, or rubella:** Consider 2-dose series at least 4 weeks apart for protection against measles or mumps or 1 dose for protection against rubella

  - **Born in 1957 or later with no evidence of immunity to measles, mumps, or rubella:** 2-dose series at least 4 weeks apart for protection against measles or mumps or at least 1 dose for protection against rubella

Meningococcal vaccination

Special situations for MenACWY

- **Anatomical or functional asplenia (including sickle cell disease), HIV infection, persistent complement component deficiency, complement inhibitor (e.g., eculizumab, ravulizumab) use:** 2-dose series MenACWY-D (Menactra, Menveo, or MenQuadfi) at least 8 weeks apart and revaccinate every 5 years if risk remains

- **Travel in countries with hyperendemic or epidemic meningococcal disease, or microbiologists routinely exposed to *Neisseria meningitidis*:** 1 dose MenACWY (Menactra, Menveo, or MenQuadfi) and revaccinate every 5 years if risk remains

- **First-year college students who live in residential housing (if not previously vaccinated at age 16 years or older) or military recruits:** 1 dose MenACWY (Menactra, Menveo, or MenQuadfi)

- For MenACWY **booster dose recommendations** for groups listed under "Special situations" and in an outbreak setting (e.g., in community or organizational settings and among men who have sex with men) and additional meningococcal vaccination information, see www.cdc.gov/mmwr/volumes/69/rr/rr6909a1.htm

Shared clinical decision-making for MenB

- **Adolescents and young adults age 16–23 years (age 16–18 years preferred) not at increased risk for meningococcal disease:** Based on shared clinical decision-making, 2-dose series MenB-4C (Bexsero) at least 1 month apart or 2-dose series MenB-FHbp (Trumenba) at 0, 6 months (if dose 2 was administered less than 6 months after dose 1, administer dose 3 at least 4 months after dose 2); MenB-4C and MenB-FHbp are not interchangeable (use same product for all doses in series)

Special situations for MenB

- **Anatomical or functional asplenia (including sickle cell disease), persistent complement component deficiency, complement inhibitor (e.g., eculizumab, ravulizumab) use, or microbiologists routinely exposed to *Neisseria meningitidis*:** 2-dose primary series MenB-4C (Bexsero) at least 1 month apart or 3-dose primary series MenB-FHbp (Trumenba) at 0, 1–2, 6 months (if dose 2 was administered at least 6 months after dose 1, dose 3 not needed; if dose 3 is administered earlier than 4 months after dose 2, a fourth dose should be administered at least 4 months after dose 3); MenB-4C and MenB-FHbp are not interchangeable (use same product for all doses in series); 1 dose MenB booster 1 year after primary series and revaccinate every 2–3 years if risk remains

- **Pregnancy:** Delay MenB until after pregnancy unless at increased risk and vaccination benefits outweigh potential risks

- For MenB **booster dose recommendations** for groups listed under "Special situations" and in an outbreak setting (e.g., in community or organizational settings and among men who have sex with men) and additional meningococcal vaccination information, see www.cdc.gov/mmwr/volumes/69/rr/rr6909a1.htm

Note: MenB vaccines may be administered simultaneously with MenACWY vaccines if indicated, but at a different anatomic site, if feasible.

Notes Recommended Adult Immunization Schedule, United States, 2023

Pneumococcal vaccination

Routine vaccination

- **Age 65 years or older who have:**

  - **Not previously received a dose of PCV13, PCV15, or PCV20 or whose previous vaccination history is unknown:** 1 dose PCV15 OR 1 dose PCV20. If PCV15 is used, this should be followed by a dose of PPSV23 given at least 1 year after the PCV15 dose. A minimum interval of 8 weeks between PCV15 and PPSV23 can be considered for adults with an immunocompromising condition,* cochlear implant, or cerebrospinal fluid leak to minimize the risk of invasive pneumococcal disease caused by serotypes unique to PPSV23 in these vulnerable groups.

  - **Previously received only PCV7:** follow the recommendation above.

  - **Previously received only PCV13:** 1 dose PCV20 at least 1 year after the PCV13 dose OR complete the recommended PPSV23 series as described here www.cdc.gov/vaccines/vpd/pneumo/downloads/pneumo-vaccine-timing.pdf.

  - **Previously received only PPSV23:** 1 dose PCV15 OR 1 dose PCV20 at least 1 year after the PPSV23 dose. If PCV15 is used, it need not be followed by another dose of PPSV23.

  - **Previously received both PCV13 and PPSV23 but NO PPSV23 was received at age 65 years or older:** 1 dose PCV20 at least 5 years after their last pneumococcal vaccine dose OR complete the recommended PPSV23 series as described here www.cdc.gov/vaccines/vpd/pneumo/downloads/pneumo-vaccine-timing.pdf.

  - **Previously received both PCV13 and PPSV23, AND PPSV23 was received at age 65 years or older:** Based on shared clinical decision-making, 1 dose of PCV20 at least 5 years after the last pneumococcal vaccine dose.

- For guidance on determining which pneumococcal vaccines a patient needs and when, please refer to the mobile app which can be downloaded here: www.cdc.gov/vaccines/vpd/pneumo/hcp/pneumoapp.html

Special situations

- **Age 19–64 years with certain underlying medical conditions or other risk factors** who have

  - **Not previously received a PCV13, PCV15, or PCV20 or whose previous vaccination history is unknown:** 1 dose PCV15 OR 1 dose PCV20. If PCV15 is used, this should be followed by a dose of PPSV23 given at least 1 year after the PCV15 dose. A minimum interval of 8 weeks between PCV15 and PPSV23 can be considered for adults with an immunocompromising condition,* cochlear implant, or cerebrospinal fluid leak

  - **Previously received only PCV7:** follow the recommendation above.

  - **Previously received only PCV13:** 1 dose PCV20 at least 1 year after the PCV13 dose OR complete the recommended PPSV23 series as described here www.cdc.gov/vaccines/vpd/pneumo/downloads/pneumo-vaccine-timing.pdf.

  - **Previously received only PPSV23:** 1 dose PCV15 OR 1 dose PCV20 at least 1 year after the PPSV23 dose. If PCV15 is used, it need not be followed by another dose of PPSV23.

  - **Previously received both PCV13 and PPSV23 but have not completed the recommended series:** 1 dose PCV20 at least 5 years after their last pneumococcal vaccine dose OR complete the recommended PPSV23 series as described here www.cdc.gov/vaccines/vpd/pneumo/downloads/pneumo-vaccine-timing.pdf.

- For guidance on determining which pneumococcal vaccines a patient needs and when, please refer to the mobile app which can be downloaded here: www.cdc.gov/vaccines/vpd/pneumo/hcp/pneumoapp.html

***Note:** Immunocompromising conditions include chronic renal failure, nephrotic syndrome, immunodeficiency, iatrogenic immunosuppression, generalized malignancy, human immunodeficiency virus, Hodgkin disease, leukemia, lymphoma, multiple myeloma, solid organ transplants, congenital or acquired asplenia, sickle cell disease, or other hemoglobinopathies.

****Note:** Underlying medical conditions or other risk factors include alcoholism, chronic heart/liver/lung disease, chronic renal failure, cigarette smoking, cochlear implant, congenital or acquired asplenia, CSF leak, diabetes mellitus, generalized malignancy, HIV, Hodgkin disease, immunodeficiency, iatrogenic immunosuppression, leukemia, lymphoma, multiple myeloma, nephrotic syndrome, solid organ transplants, or sickle cell disease or other hemoglobinopathies.

Polio vaccination

Routine vaccination

Routine poliovirus vaccination of adults residing in the United States is not necessary.

Special situations

- **Adults at increased risk of exposure to poliovirus with:**

  - No evidence of a complete polio vaccination series (i.e., at least 3 doses): administer remaining doses (1, 2, or 3 doses) to complete a 3-dose series

  - Evidence of completed polio vaccination series (i.e., at least 3 doses): may administer one lifetime IPV booster

For detailed information, see: www.cdc.gov/vaccines/vpd/polio/hcp/recommendations.html

Continued

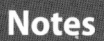 **Notes** Recommended Adult Immunization Schedule, United States, 2023

Tetanus, diphtheria, and pertussis vaccination

Routine vaccination

- **Previously did not receive Tdap at or after age 11 years:** 1 dose Tdap, then Td or Tdap every 10 years

Special situations

- **Previously did not receive primary vaccination series for tetanus, diphtheria, or pertussis:** 1 dose Tdap followed by 1 dose Td or Tdap at least 4 weeks later, and a third dose of Td or Tdap 6–12 months later (Tdap can be substituted for any Td dose, but preferred as first dose), Td or Tdap every 10 years thereafter

- **Pregnancy:** 1 dose Tdap during each pregnancy, preferably in early part of gestational weeks 27–36

- **Wound management:** Persons with 3 or more doses of tetanus-toxoid-containing vaccine: For clean and minor wounds, administer Tdap or Td if more than 10 years since last dose of tetanus-toxoid-containing vaccine; for all other wounds, administer Tdap or Td if more than 5 years since last dose of tetanus-toxoid-containing vaccine. Tdap is preferred for persons who have not previously received Tdap or whose Tdap history is unknown. If a tetanus-toxoid-containing vaccine is indicated for a pregnant woman, use Tdap. For detailed information, see www.cdc.gov/mmwr/volumes/69/wr/mm6903a5.htm

Varicella vaccination

Routine vaccination

- **No evidence of immunity to varicella:** 2-dose series 4–8 weeks apart if previously did not receive varicella-containing vaccine (VAR or MMRV [measles-mumps-rubella-varicella vaccine] for children); if previously received 1 dose varicella-containing vaccine, 1 dose at least 4 weeks after first dose

  - **Evidence of immunity:** U.S.-born before 1980 (except for pregnant persons and health care personnel [see below]), documentation of 2 doses varicella-containing vaccine at least 4 weeks apart, diagnosis or verification of history of varicella or herpes zoster by a health care provider, laboratory evidence of immunity or disease

Special situations

- **Pregnancy with no evidence of immunity to varicella:** VAR contraindicated during pregnancy; after pregnancy (before discharge from health care facility), 1 dose if previously received 1 dose varicella-containing vaccine or dose 1 of 2-dose series (dose 2: 4–8 weeks later) if previously did not receive any varicella-containing vaccine, regardless of whether U.S.-born before 1980

- **Health care personnel with no evidence of immunity to varicella:** 1 dose if previously received 1 dose varicella-containing vaccine; 2-dose series 4–8 weeks apart if previously did not receive any varicella-containing vaccine, regardless of whether U.S.-born before 1980

- **HIV infection with CD4 percentages ≥15% and CD4 count ≥200 cells/mm³ with no evidence of immunity:** Vaccination may be considered (2 doses 3 months apart); VAR contraindicated for HIV infection with CD4 percentage <15% or CD4 count <200 cells/mm³

- **Severe immunocompromising conditions:** VAR contraindicated

Zoster vaccination

Routine vaccination

- **Age 50 years or older*:** 2-dose series recombinant zoster vaccine (RZV, Shingrix) 2–6 months apart (minimum interval: 4 weeks; repeat dose if administered too soon), regardless of previous herpes zoster or history of zoster vaccine live (ZVL, Zostavax) vaccination.

- ***Note:** Serologic evidence of prior varicella is not necessary for zoster vaccination. However, if serologic evidence of varicella susceptibility becomes available, providers should follow ACIP guidelines for varicella vaccination first. RZV is not indicated for the prevention of varicella, and there are limited data on the use of RZV in persons without a history of varicella or varicella vaccination.

Special situations

- **Pregnancy:** There is currently no ACIP recommendation for RZV use in pregnancy. Consider delaying RZV until after pregnancy.

- **Immunocompromising conditions (including persons with HIV regardless of CD4 count)**:** 2-dose series recombinant zoster vaccine (RZV, Shingrix) 2–6 months apart (minimum interval: 4 weeks; repeat dose if administered too soon). For detailed information, see www.cdc.gov/shingles/vaccination/immunocompromised-adults.html

- ****Note:** If there is no documented history of varicella, varicella vaccination, or herpes zoster, providers should refer to the clinical considerations for use of RZV in immunocompromised adults aged ≥19 years and the ACIP varicella vaccine recommendations for further guidance: www.cdc.gov/mmwr/volumes/71/wr/mm7103a2.htm

Appendix Recommended Adult Immunization Schedule, United States, 2023

Guide to Contraindications and Precautions to Commonly Used Vaccines

Adapted from Table 4-1 in Advisory Committee on Immunization Practices (ACIP) General Best Practice Guidelines for Immunization: Contraindication and Precautions available at www.cdc.gov/vaccines/hcp/acip-recs/general-recs/contraindications.html and ACIP's Recommendations for the Prevention and Control of 2022-23 Seasonal Influenza with Vaccines available at www.cdc.gov/mmwr/volumes/71/rr/rr7101a1.htm

---

For COVID-19 vaccine contraindications and precautions see
www.cdc.gov/vaccines/covid-19/clinical-considerations/interim-considerations-us.html#contraindications

---

Vaccine	Contraindicated or Not Recommended[1]	Precautions[2]
Influenza, egg-based, inactivated injectable (IIV4)	• Severe allergic reaction (e.g., anaphylaxis) after previous dose of any influenza vaccine (i.e., any egg-based IIV, ccIIV, RIV, or LAIV of any valency) • Severe allergic reaction (e.g., anaphylaxis) to any vaccine component[3] (excluding egg)	• Guillain-Barré syndrome (GBS) within 6 weeks after a previous dose of any type of influenza vaccine • Moderate or severe acute illness with or without fever
Influenza, cell culture-based inactivated injectable [(ccIIV4), Flucelvax® Quadrivalent]	• Severe allergic reaction (e.g., anaphylaxis) to any ccIIV of any valency, or to any component[3] of ccIIV4	• Guillain-Barré syndrome (GBS) within 6 weeks after a previous dose of any type of influenza vaccine • Persons with a history of severe allergic reaction (e.g., anaphylaxis) after a previous dose of any egg-based IIV, RIV, or LAIV of any valency. If using ccIIV4, administer in medical setting under supervision of health care provider who can recognize and manage severe allergic reactions. May consult an allergist. • Moderate or severe acute illness with or without fever
Influenza, recombinant injectable [(RIV4), Flublok® Quadrivalent]	• Severe allergic reaction (e.g., anaphylaxis) to any RIV of any valency, or to any component[3] of RIV4	• Guillain-Barré syndrome (GBS) within 6 weeks after a previous dose of any type of influenza vaccine • Persons with a history of severe allergic reaction (e.g., anaphylaxis) after a previous dose of any egg-based IIV, ccIIV, or LAIV of any valency. If using RIV4, administer in medical setting under supervision of health care provider who can recognize and manage severe allergic reactions. May consult an allergist. • Moderate or severe acute illness with or without fever
Influenza, live attenuated [LAIV4, Flumist® Quadrivalent]	• Severe allergic reaction (e.g., anaphylaxis) after previous dose of any influenza vaccine (i.e., any egg-based IIV, ccIIV, RIV, or LAIV of any valency) • Severe allergic reaction (e.g., anaphylaxis) to any vaccine component[3] (excluding egg) • Anatomic or functional asplenia • Immunocompromised due to any cause including, but not limited to, medications and HIV infection • Close contacts or caregivers of severely immunosuppressed persons who require a protected environment • Pregnancy • Cochlear implant • Active communication between the cerebrospinal fluid (CSF) and the oropharynx, nasopharynx, nose, ear, or any other cranial CSF leak • Received influenza antiviral medications oseltamivir or zanamivir within the previous 48 hours, peramivir within the previous 5 days, or baloxavir within the previous 17 days.	• Guillain-Barré syndrome (GBS) within 6 weeks after a previous dose of any type of influenza vaccine • Asthma in persons aged 5 years old or older • Persons with underlying medical conditions (other than those listed under contraindications) that might predispose to complications after wild-type influenza virus infection [e.g., chronic pulmonary, cardiovascular (except isolated hypertension), renal, hepatic, neurologic, hematologic, or metabolic disorders (including diabetes mellitus)] • Moderate or severe acute illness with or without fever

---

1. When a contraindication is present, a vaccine should NOT be administered. Kroger A, Bahta L, Hunter P. ACIP General Best Practice Guidelines for Immunization. www.cdc.gov/vaccines/hcp/acip-recs/general-recs/contraindications.html
2. When a precaution is present, vaccination should generally be deferred but might be indicated if the benefit of protection from the vaccine outweighs the risk for an adverse reaction. Kroger A, Bahta L, Hunter P. ACIP General Best Practice Guidelines for Immunization. www.cdc.gov/vaccines/hcp/acip-recs/general-recs/contraindications.html
3. Vaccination providers should check FDA-approved prescribing information for the most complete and updated information, including contraindications, warnings, and precautions. Package inserts for U.S.-licensed vaccines are available at www.fda.gov/vaccines-blood-biologics/approved-products/vaccines-licensed-use-united-states.

Continued

Appendix	Recommended Adult Immunization Schedule, United States, 2023

Vaccine	Contraindicated or Not Recommended[1]	Precautions[2]
Haemophilus influenzae type b (Hib)	• Severe allergic reaction (e.g., anaphylaxis) after a previous dose or to a vaccine component[3] • For Hiberix, ActHib, and PedvaxHIB only: History of severe allergic reaction to dry natural latex	• Moderate or severe acute illness with or without fever
Hepatitis A (HepA)	• Severe allergic reaction (e.g., anaphylaxis) after a previous dose or to a vaccine component[3] including neomycin	• Moderate or severe acute illness with or without fever
Hepatitis B (HepB)	• Severe allergic reaction (e.g., anaphylaxis) after a previous dose or to a vaccine component[3] including yeast • Pregnancy: Heplisav-B and PreHevbrio are not recommended due to lack of safety data in pregnant persons. Use other hepatitis B vaccines if HepB is indicated[4]	• Moderate or severe acute illness with or without fever
Hepatitis A- Hepatitis B vaccine [HepA-HepB, (Twinrix®)]	• Severe allergic reaction (e.g., anaphylaxis) after a previous dose or to a vaccine component[3] including neomycin and yeast	• Moderate or severe acute illness with or without fever
Human papillomavirus (HPV)	• Severe allergic reaction (e.g., anaphylaxis) after a previous dose or to a vaccine component[3] • Pregnancy: HPV vaccination not recommended	• Moderate or severe acute illness with or without fever
Measles, mumps, rubella (MMR)	• Severe allergic reaction (e.g., anaphylaxis) after a previous dose or to a vaccine component[3] • Severe immunodeficiency (e.g., hematologic and solid tumors, receipt of chemotherapy, congenital immunodeficiency, long-term immunosuppressive therapy or patients with HIV infection who are severely immunocompromised) • Pregnancy • Family history of altered immunocompetence, unless verified clinically or by laboratory testing as immunocompetent	• Recent (≤11 months) receipt of antibody-containing blood product (specific interval depends on product) • History of thrombocytopenia or thrombocytopenic purpura • Need for tuberculin skin testing or interferon-gamma release assay (IGRA) testing • Moderate or severe acute illness with or without fever
Meningococcal ACWY (MenACWY) [MenACWY-CRM (Menveo®); MenACWY-D (Menactra®); MenACWY-TT (MenQuadfi®)]	• Severe allergic reaction (e.g., anaphylaxis) after a previous dose or to a vaccine component[3] • For MenACWY-D and MenACWY-CRM only: severe allergic reaction to any diphtheria toxoid–or CRM197–containing vaccine • For MenACWY-TT only: severe allergic reaction to a tetanus toxoid-containing vaccine	• Moderate or severe acute illness with or without fever
Meningococcal B (MenB) [MenB-4C (Bexsero); MenB-FHbp (Trumenba)]	• Severe allergic reaction (e.g., anaphylaxis) after a previous dose or to a vaccine component[3]	• Pregnancy • For MenB-4C only: Latex sensitivity • Moderate or severe acute illness with or without fever
Pneumococcal conjugate (PCV15, PCV20)	• Severe allergic reaction (e.g., anaphylaxis) after a previous dose or to a vaccine component[3] • Severe allergic reaction (e.g., anaphylaxis) to any diphtheria-toxoid–containing vaccine or to its vaccine component[3]	• Moderate or severe acute illness with or without fever
Pneumococcal polysaccharide (PPSV23)	• Severe allergic reaction (e.g., anaphylaxis) after a previous dose or to a vaccine component[3]	• Moderate or severe acute illness with or without fever
Tetanus, diphtheria, and acellular pertussis (Tdap) Tetanus, diphtheria (Td)	• Severe allergic reaction (e.g., anaphylaxis) after a previous dose or to a vaccine component[3] • For Tdap only: Encephalopathy (e.g., coma, decreased level of consciousness, prolonged seizures), not attributable to another identifiable cause, within 7 days of administration of previous dose of DTP, DTaP, or Tdap	• Guillain-Barré syndrome (GBS) within 6 weeks after a previous dose of tetanus-toxoid–containing vaccine • History of Arthus-type hypersensitivity reactions after a previous dose of diphtheria-toxoid–containing or tetanus-toxoid–containing vaccine; defer vaccination until at least 10 years have elapsed since the last tetanus-toxoid–containing vaccine • Moderate or severe acute illness with or without fever • For Tdap only: Progressive or unstable neurological disorder, uncontrolled seizures, or progressive encephalopathy until a treatment regimen has been established and the condition has stabilized
Varicella (VAR)	• Severe allergic reaction (e.g., anaphylaxis) after a previous dose or to a vaccine component[3] • Severe immunodeficiency (e.g., hematologic and solid tumors, receipt of chemotherapy, congenital immunodeficiency, long-term immunosuppressive therapy or patients with HIV infection who are severely immunocompromised) • Pregnancy • Family history of altered immunocompetence, unless verified clinically or by laboratory testing as immunocompetent	• Recent (≤11 months) receipt of antibody-containing blood product (specific interval depends on product) • Receipt of specific antiviral drugs (acyclovir, famciclovir, or valacyclovir) 24 hours before vaccination (avoid use of these antiviral drugs for 14 days after vaccination) • Use of aspirin or aspirin-containing products • Moderate or severe acute illness with or without fever
Zoster recombinant vaccine (RZV)	• Severe allergic reaction (e.g., anaphylaxis) after a previous dose or to a vaccine component[3]	• Moderate or severe acute illness with or without fever • Current herpes zoster infection

1. When a contraindication is present, a vaccine should NOT be administered. Kroger A, Bahta L, Hunter P. ACIP General Best Practice Guidelines for Immunization. www.cdc.gov/vaccines/hcp/acip-recs/general-recs/contraindications.html
2. When a precaution is present, vaccination should generally be deferred but might be indicated if the benefit of protection from the vaccine outweighs the risk for an adverse reaction. Kroger A, Bahta L, Hunter P. ACIP General Best Practice Guidelines for Immunization. www.cdc.gov/vaccines/hcp/acip-recs/general-recs/contraindications.html
3. Vaccination providers should check FDA-approved prescribing information for the most complete and updated information, including contraindications, warnings, and precautions. Package inserts for U.S.-licensed vaccines are available at www.fda.gov/vaccines-blood-biologics/approved-products/vaccines-licensed-use-united-states.
4. For information on the pregnancy exposure registries for persons who were inadvertently vaccinated with Heplisav-B or PreHevbrio while pregnant, please visit heplisavbpregnancyregistry.com/ or www.prehevbrio.com/#safety.

The Advisory Committee on Immunization Practices (ACIP) recommendations and package inserts for vaccines provide information on contraindications and precautions related to vaccines. Contraindications are conditions that increase chances of a serious adverse reaction in vaccine recipients, and the vaccine should not be administered when a contraindication is present. Precautions should be reviewed for potential risks and benefits for vaccine recipient. For a person with a severe allergy to latex, e.g., anaphylaxis, vaccines supplied in vials or syringes that contain natural rubber latex should not be administered unless the benefit of vaccination clearly outweighs the risk for a potential allergic reaction. For latex allergies other than anaphylaxis, vaccines supplied in vials or syringes that contain dry, natural rubber or natural rubber latex may be administered.

TABLE 14 Immunization and Pregnancy

Vaccine	Before Pregnancy	During Pregnancy	After Pregnancy	Type of Vaccine	Route
Hepatitis A	If at high risk for disease	If at high risk for disease	If at high risk for disease	Inactivated	IM
Hepatitis B	Yes, if at risk	Yes, if at risk	Yes, if at risk	Inactivated	IM
Human papillomavirus (HPV)	Yes, if 9-26 yr of age	No, under study	Yes, if 9-26 yr of age	Inactivated	IM
Influenza TIV	Yes	Yes	Yes	Inactivated	IM
Influenza LAIV	Yes, if <50 yr and healthy; avoid conception for 4 wk	No	Yes, if <50 yr and healthy; avoid conception for 4 wk	Live	Nasal spray
MMR	Yes, avoid conception for 4 wk	No	Yes, give immediately postpartum if susceptible to rubella	Live	SC
Meningococcal	If indicated	If indicated	If indicated		
Polysaccharide				Inactivated	SCIM
Conjugate				Inactivated	
Pneumococcal polysaccharide	If indicated	If indicated	If indicated	Inactivated	IM or SC
Tetanus/diphtheria Td	Yes, Tdap preferred	If indicated	Yes, Tdap preferred	Toxoid	IM
Tdap, one dose only	Yes, preferred	If high risk of pertussis; otherwise, Td preferred	Yes, preferred	Toxoid/inactivated	IM
Varicella	Yes, avoid conception for 4 wk	No	Yes, give immediately postpartum if susceptible	Live	SC

IM, Intramuscular; *LAIV,* live, attenuated influenza vaccine; *SC,* subcutaneous; *Tdap,* tetanus and diphtheria toxoids and acellular pertussis; *TIV,* trivalent inactivated influenza vaccine.

TABLE 15 Immunizing Agents and Immunization Schedules for Health Care Workers (HCWs)*

Generic Name	Primary Schedule and Booster(s)	Indications	Major Precautions and Contraindications	Special Considerations
Immunizing Agents Strongly Recommended for Health Care Workers				
Hepatitis B (HB) recombinant vaccine	Two doses IM 4 wk apart; third dose 5 mo after second; booster doses not necessary	**Preexposure:** HCWs at risk for exposure to blood or body fluids	Based on limited data no risk of adverse effects to developing fetuses is apparent. Pregnancy should *not* be considered a contraindication to vaccination of women. Previous anaphylactic reaction to common baker's yeast is a contraindication to vaccination	The vaccine produces neither therapeutic nor adverse effects on HB-infected persons. Prevaccination serologic screening is not indicated for persons being vaccinated because of occupational risk. HCWs who have contact with patients or blood should be tested 1-2 mo after vaccination to determine serologic response
Hepatitis B immune globulin (HBIG)	0.06 ml/kg IM as soon as possible after exposure. A second dose of HBIG should be administered 1 mo later if the HB vaccine series has not been started	**Postexposure prophylaxis:** For persons exposed to blood or body fluids containing HBsAg and who are not immune to HBV infection—0.06 ml/kg IM as soon as possible (but no later than 7 days after exposure)		
Influenza vaccine (inactivated whole-virus and split-virus vaccines)	Annual vaccination with current vaccine Administered IM	HCWs who have contact with patients at high risk for influenza or its complications; HCWs who work in long-term care facilities; HCWs with high-risk medical conditions or who are aged ≥65 yr	History of anaphylactic hypersensitivity to egg ingestion	No evidence exists of risk to mother or fetus when the vaccine is administered to a pregnant woman with an underlying high-risk condition. Influenza vaccination is recommended during second and third trimesters of pregnancy because of increased risk for hospitalization
Measles live-virus vaccine	One dose SC; second dose at least 1 mo later	HCWs[†] born during or after 1957 who do not have documentation of having received two doses of live vaccine on or after the first birthday **or** a history of physician-diagnosed measles or serologic evidence of immunity. Vaccination should be considered for all HCWs who lack proof of immunity, including those born before 1957	Pregnancy; immunocompromised persons,[‡] including HIV-infected persons who have evidence of severe immunosuppression; anaphylaxis after gelatin ingestion or administration of neomycin; recent administration of immune globulin	MMR is the vaccine of choice if recipients are likely to be susceptible to rubella and/or mumps as well as measles. Persons vaccinated between 1963 and 1967 with a killed measles vaccine alone, killed vaccine followed by live vaccine, or with a vaccine of unknown type should be revaccinated with two doses of live measles virus vaccine
Mumps live-virus vaccine	One dose SC; second dose at least 1 mo later	HCWs[†] believed to be susceptible can be vaccinated. Adults born before 1957 can be considered immune	Pregnancy; immunocompromised persons,[‡] history of anaphylactic reaction after gelatin ingestion or administration of neomycin	MMR is the vaccine of choice if recipients are likely to be susceptible to measles and rubella, as well as mumps
Hepatitis A virus (HAV) vaccine	Two doses of vaccine either 6-12 mo apart (HAVRIX), or 6 mo apart (VAQTA)	Not routinely indicated for HCWs in the United States. Persons who work with HAV-infected primates or with HAV in a research laboratory setting should be vaccinated	History of anaphylactic hypersensitivity to alum or, for HAVRIX, the preservative 2-phenoxyethanol. The safety of the vaccine in pregnant women has not been determined; the risk associated with vaccination should be weighed against the risk for hepatitis A in women who may be at high risk for exposure to HAV	

TABLE 15 Immunizing Agents and Immunization Schedules for Health Care Workers (HCWs)*—cont'd

Generic Name	Primary Schedule and Booster(s)	Indications	Major Precautions and Contraindications	Special Considerations
Meningococcal vaccine	One dose in volume and by route specified by manufacturer; single booster for adults 19-21 yr of age if the first dose was given before age 16	Laboratory personnel and others with exposure risk	The safety of the vaccine in pregnant women has not been evaluated; it should not be administered during pregnancy unless the risk for infection is high	
Typhoid vaccine, IM, SC, and oral	IM vaccine: One 0.5-ml/dose, booster 0.5 ml every 2 yr SC vaccine: Two 0.5-ml doses, ≥4 wk apart, booster 0.5 ml SC or 0.1 ID every 3 yr if exposure continues Oral vaccine: Four doses on alternate days. The manufacturer recommends revaccination with the entire 4-dose series every 5 yr	Workers in microbiology laboratories who frequently work with *Salmonella typhi*	Severe local or systemic reaction to a previous dose. Ty21a (oral) vaccine should not be administered to immunocompromised persons[†] or to persons receiving antimicrobial agents	Vaccination should not be considered an alternative to the use of proper procedures when handling specimens and cultures in the laboratory
Vaccinia vaccine (smallpox)	One dose administered with a bifurcated needle; boosters administered every 10 yr	Laboratory workers who directly handle cultures with vaccinia, recombinant vaccinia viruses, or orthopox viruses that infect human beings	The vaccine is contraindicated in pregnancy, in persons with eczema or a history of eczema, and in immunocompromised persons[†] and their household contacts	Vaccination may be considered for HCWs who have direct contact with contaminated dressings or other infectious material from volunteers in clinical studies involving recombinant vaccinia virus
COVID-19	A person is fully vaccinated 2 wk after receiving all recommended doses in the primary series of their COVID-19 vaccination. A person is up to date with their COVID-19 vaccination if they have received all recommended doses in the primary series and boosters when eligible.			
Other Vaccine-Preventable Diseases				
Tetanus and diphtheria and pertussis (Tdap)	Two IM doses 4 wk apart or tetanus and diphtheria toxoid for adults with uncertain or incomplete primary vaccination; third dose 6-12 mo after second dose; booster every 10 yr. Substitute a one-time dose of Tdap for one of the doses of Td, either in the primary series or for the routine booster, whichever comes first	All adults	Except in the first trimester, pregnancy is not a precaution History of a neurologic reaction or immediate hypersensitivity reaction after a previous dose History of severe local (Arthus-type) reaction after a previous dose. Such persons should not receive further routine or emergency doses of Td for 10 yr	Tetanus prophylaxis in wound management[‡]
Pneumococcal polysaccharide vaccine (23 valent)	One dose, 0.5 ml, IM or SC; revaccination recommended for those at highest risk ≥5 yr after the first dose	Adults who are at increased risk of pneumococcal disease and its complications because of underlying health conditions; older adults, especially those age ≥65 who are healthy	The safety of vaccine in pregnant women has not been evaluated; it should not be administered during pregnancy unless the risk for infection is high. Previous recipients of any type of pneumococcal polysaccharide vaccine who are at highest risk for	

Continued

TABLE 15	Immunizing Agents and Immunization Schedules for Health Care Workers (HCWs)*—cont'd			
Generic Name	**Primary Schedule and Booster(s)**	**Indications**	**Major Precautions and Contraindications**	**Special Considerations**
			fatal infection or antibody loss may be revaccinated ≥5 yr after the first dose	
Rubella live-virus vaccine	One dose SC; second dose at least 1 mo later	Indicated for HCWs,[†] both men and women, who do not have documentation of having received live vaccine on or after their first birthday **or** laboratory evidence of immunity. Adults born before 1957, **except women who can become pregnant,** can be considered immune	Pregnancy; immunocompromised persons[†]; history of anaphylactic reaction after administration of neomycin	The risk for rubella vaccine-associated malformations in the offspring of women pregnant when vaccinated or who become pregnant within 3 mo after vaccination is negligible. Such women should be counseled regarding the theoretic basis of concern for the fetus. MMR is the vaccine of choice if recipients are likely to be susceptible to measles or mumps as well as rubella
Varicella-zoster live-virus vaccine	Two 0.5-ml doses SC 4-8 wk apart if ≥13 yr	Indicated for HCWs[†] who do not have either a reliable history of varicella or serologic evidence of immunity	Pregnancy, immunocompromised persons,[‡] history of anaphylactic reaction after receipt of neomycin or gelatin. Avoid salicylate use for 6 wk after vaccination	Vaccine is available from the manufacturer for certain patients with acute lymphocytic leukemia in remission. Because 71%-93% of persons without a history of varicella are immune, serologic testing before vaccination is likely to be cost effective
Varicella-zoster immune globulin (VZIG)	Persons <50 kg: 125 μg/10 kg IM; persons ≥50 kg: 625 μg[§]	Persons known or likely to be susceptible (particularly those at high risk for complications, e.g., pregnant women) who have close and prolonged exposure to a contact case or to an infectious hospital staff worker or patient		Serologic testing may help in assessing whether to administer VZIG. If use of VZIG prevents varicella disease, patient should be vaccinated subsequently

BCG Vaccination

Bacille Calmette-Guérin (BCG) vaccine (TB)	One percutaneous dose of 0.3 ml; no booster dose recommended	Should be considered only for HCWs in areas where multidrug TB is prevalent, a strong likelihood of infection exists, and where comprehensive infection control precautions have failed to prevent TB transmission to HCWs	Should not be administered to immunocompromised persons,[‡] pregnant women	In the United States TB-control efforts are directed toward early identification, treatment of cases, and preventive therapy with isoniazid

Other Immunobiologics That Are or May Be Indicated for HCWs

Immune globulin (hepatitis A)	**Postexposure**—One IM dose of 0.02 ml/kg administered ≤2 wk after exposure	Indicated for HCWs exposed to feces of infectious patients	Contraindicated in persons with IgA deficiency; do not administer within 2 wk after MMR vaccine or 3 wk after varicella vaccine. Delay administration of MMR vaccine for ≥3 mo and varicella vaccine ≥5 mo after administration of immune globulin	Administer in large muscle mass (deltoid, gluteal)

*Persons who provide health care to patients or work in institutions that provide patient care (e.g., physicians, nurses, emergency medical personnel, dental professionals and students, medical and nursing students, laboratory technicians, hospital volunteers, and administrative and support staff in health care institutions).

[†]All HCWs (i.e., medical or nonmedical, paid or volunteer, full time or part time, student or nonstudent, with or without patient-care responsibilities) who work in health care institutions (e.g., inpatient and outpatient, public and private) should be immune to measles, rubella, and varicella.

[‡]Persons immunocompromised because of immune deficiency diseases, HIV infection, leukemia, lymphoma or generalized malignancy, or immunosuppressed as a result of therapy with corticosteroids, alkylating drugs, antimetabolites, or radiation.

[§]Some experts recommend 125 μg/10 kg regardless of total body weight.

HBsAg, Hepatitis B surface antigen; *HBV,* hepatitis B virus; *HIV,* human immunodeficiency virus; *IM,* intramuscular; *MMR,* measles, mumps, rubella vaccine; *SC,* subcutaneous; *TB,* tuberculosis.
Modified from *MMWR* 46(RR-18), 1998.

Recommendations for Providing Sexually Transmitted Diseases Clinical Services

BOX 1 Recommendations for Obtaining a Sexual History and Conducting a Physical Examination as Part of Sexually Transmitted Diseases Care in Primary Care and Sexually Transmitted Diseases Specialty Care Settings*

STD care in primary care settings

- A sexual history and risk assessment **should** be available as part of basic STD care services at the following patient visits:
  1. Initial comprehensive or annual visit
  2. Each visit concerning reproductive, genital, or urologic issues
- A physical examination **should** be available as a basic STD care service for male and female patients with STD-related symptoms, STD-related concerns, or those at high behavioral risk for incident STDs.
- A pelvic examination **should** be available as a basic STD care service.
- A sexual history and risk assessment **could** be available as basic STD care services at each visit unrelated to reproductive, genital, or urologic concerns.
- Anoscopy **could** be available as a basic STD care service.

STD care in STD specialty care settings

- A sexual history and risk assessment **should** be part of specialized STD care services at every visit for patients with STD-related symptoms, STD-related concerns, or concerns about preventing or achieving pregnancy.
- A physical examination **should** be available as a specialized STD care service for male and female patients with STD-related symptoms, STD-related concerns, or high behavioral risk for incident STDs.
- A pelvic examination **should** be available as a specialized STD care service.
- Colposcopy **should** be available as a specialized STD care service for female patients with abnormal Pap smears.
- Anoscopy **should** be available as a specialized STD care service.
- A high-resolution anoscopy **could** be available as a specialized STD care service for patients with abnormal anal Pap smears.

*Primary care setting is defined as a place where patients are evaluated for various health conditions. An STD specialty care setting is defined as a place where the focus is on providing patients with timely, comprehensive, confidential, and culturally sensitive STD care. STD care delivered in STD specialty care settings includes all care delivered in primary care settings.
STD, Sexually transmitted disease.
Barrow RY, Ahmed F, Bolan GA, Workowski KA: Recommendations for providing quality sexually transmitted diseases clinical services, 2020, *MMWR Recomm Rep* 68(No. RR-5):1-20, 2020. https://doi.org/10.15585/mmwr.rr6805a1

BOX 2 Prevention Recommendations for Sexually Transmitted Diseases Care in Primary Care and Sexually Transmitted Diseases Specialty Care Settings*

STD care in primary care settings

- The following prevention services should be available as basic STD care services:
  1. On-site hepatitis B vaccination or referral
  2. On-site HPV vaccination or referral
  3. Brief single STD/HIV prevention counseling session (up to 30 minutes)[†]
  4. PrEP for HIV prevention and nPEP of HIV risk assessment, education, and referral or link to HIV care[†]
  5. Emergency contraceptive pills[§]
  6. Brief contraceptive counseling or referral
  7. Referral or link to HIV care, family planning services, and behavioral health services, if indicated
- The following prevention services could be available as basic STD care services:
  1. On-site condom provision[¶]
  2. On-site hepatitis A vaccination
  3. Provision of PrEP for HIV prevention**
  4. Provision of nPEP of HIV[††]
  5. Moderate-intensity STD behavioral counseling (≥30 minutes)[†]

STD care in STD specialty care settings

- The following prevention services should be available as specialized STD care services:
  1. On-site condom provision
  2. On-site hepatitis A vaccination
  3. On-site hepatitis B vaccination
  4. On-site HPV vaccination
  5. Brief single STD/HIV prevention counseling session (up to 30 minutes)[†]
  6. PrEP for HIV prevention and nPEP of HIV risk assessment, education, counseling, and referral or link to HIV care[†]
  7. Provision of PrEP for HIV prevention[§§]
  8. Provision of nPEP of HIV[¶¶]
  9. Brief contraceptive counseling or referral
  10. Emergency contraceptive pills[§]
  11. Referral or link to HIV care, family planning services, and behavioral health services, if indicated
- The following prevention services could be available as specialized STD care services:
  1. Moderate-intensity STD behavioral counseling (≥30 minutes)[†]
  2. High-intensity STD behavioral counseling (≥2 hr)[†]

*Primary care setting is defined as a place where patients are evaluated for various health conditions. STD specialty care setting is defined as a place where the focus is on providing patients with timely, comprehensive, confidential, and culturally sensitive STD care. STD care delivered in STD specialty care settings includes all care delivered in primary care settings.

[†]Provided by a clinician or other appropriately trained staff.

[§]If emergency contraceptive pills are not available on site or by prescription, patients can be advised that levonorgestrel emergency contraceptive pills are available over the counter and ulipristal acetate emergency contraceptive pills are only available by prescription. Emergency contraceptive pills should be taken as soon as possible within 5 days of unprotected sex.

[¶]Providers can partner with local organizations, such as the local health department and community-based organizations, to procure condoms. In some states, prescriptions can be written for condoms. For certain settings, such as family planning clinics, condoms should be available on site.

**PrEP could be available by starter packs or prescription with on-site follow-up care for basic STD care. If PrEP is not provided, navigator-assisted referral for PrEP should be provided with first appointment made while the patient is on site.

[††]nPEP starter pack (3-7 days of medication) could be available on site, with either on-site follow-up care or referral for basic STD care. nPEP starter pack or complete 28-day course could be available by prescription, with either on-site follow-up care or referral, with first appointment made while the patient is on site. Provision of the complete 28-day nPEP medication supply at the initial visit rather than a starter pack of 3-7 days has been reported to increase likelihood of adherence, especially when patients find returning for multiple follow-up visits difficult. Routinely providing starter packs or the complete 28-day course requires that health care providers stock nPEP drugs in their practice setting or have an established agreement with a pharmacy to stock, package, and urgently dispense nPEP drugs with required administration instructions (https://www.cdc.gov/hiv/pdf/programresources/cdc-hiv-npep-guidelines.pdf).

[§§]PrEP should be available in starter packs or by prescription with on-site follow-up care for specialized STD care. If PrEP is not provided, navigator-assisted referral for PrEP should be provided with first appointment made while the patient is on site.

[¶¶]nPEP starter pack (3-7 days of medication) should be available on site, with either on-site follow-up care or referral to specialized STD care. nPEP complete 28-day course should be available by prescription, with either on-site follow-up care or referral, with first appointment made while the patient is on site. Provision of the complete 28-day nPEP medication supply at the initial visit rather than a starter pack of 3-7 days has been reported to increase likelihood of adherence, especially when patients find returning for multiple follow-up visits difficult.

HIV, Human immunodeficiency virus; *HPV,* human papillomavirus; *nPEP,* nonoccupational postexposure prophylaxis; *PrEP,* preexposure prophylaxis; *STD,* sexually transmitted disease.

Barrow RY, Ahmed F, Bolan GA, Workowski KA: Recommendations for providing quality sexually transmitted diseases clinical services, 2020, *MMWR Recomm Rep* 68(No. RR-5):1-20, 2020. https://doi.org/10.15585/mmwr.rr6805a1

BOX 3 Screening Recommendations for Sexually Transmitted Diseases Care in Primary Care and Sexually Transmitted Diseases Specialty Care Settings*

STD care in primary care settings

- Screening and assessment for the following STDs **should** be available as basic STD care services:
  1. Gonorrhea
  2. Chlamydia
  3. Syphilis
  4. Hepatitis B
  5. Hepatitis C
  6. HIV
  7. Cervical cancer
- Screening and assessment for the following STD **could** be available as a basic STD care service:
  1. Trichomoniasis

STD care in STD specialty care settings

- Screening and assessment for the following STDs **should** be available as specialized STD care services:
  1. Gonorrhea
  2. Chlamydia
  3. Syphilis
  4. Hepatitis B
  5. Hepatitis C
  6. HIV
  7. Cervical cancer
  8. Trichomoniasis
- Screening and assessment for the following STD could be available as a specialized STD care service:
  1. Anal cancer

*Primary care setting is defined as a place where patients are evaluated for various health conditions. STD specialty care setting is defined as a place where the focus is on providing patients with timely, comprehensive, confidential, and culturally sensitive STD care. STD care delivered in STD specialty care settings includes all care delivered in primary care settings.
HIV, Human immunodeficiency virus; *STD,* sexually transmitted disease.
Barrow RY, Ahmed F, Bolan GA, Workowski KA: Recommendations for providing quality sexually transmitted diseases clinical services, 2020, *MMWR Recomm Rep* 68(No. RR-5):1-20, 2020. https://doi.org/10.15585/mmwr.rr6805a1

BOX 4 Partner Services Recommendations for Sexually Transmitted Diseases Care in Primary Care and Sexually Transmitted Diseases Specialty Care Settings*

STD care in primary care settings

- The following partner services **should** be available as basic STD care services:
  1. Guidance regarding notification and care of sex partners
  2. EPT (where legal and where local or state jurisdictions do not prohibit by regulation)[†]
- The following partner services **could** be available as a basic STD care service:
  1. Interactive counseling for partner notification

STD care in STD specialty care settings

- The following partner services **should** be available as specialized STD care services:
  1. Guidance regarding notification and care of sex partners
  2. Interactive counseling for partner notification
  3. EPT (where legal and where local or state jurisdictions do not prohibit by regulation)[†]
  4. Health department DIS elicitation of sex partner information to identify those who might have been exposed and to identify patient follow-up needs[§]

*Primary care setting is defined as a place where patients are evaluated for various health conditions. STD specialty care setting is defined as a place where the focus is on providing patients with timely, comprehensive, confidential, and culturally sensitive STD care. STD care delivered in STD specialty care settings includes all care delivered in primary care settings.
[†]Information on legal status of EPT for each state is available at https://www.cdc.gov/std/ept/legal/default.htm.
[§]Partner services can be provided on site or by referral.
DIS, Disease intervention specialist; *EPT,* Expedited Partner Therapy; *STD,* sexually transmitted disease.
Barrow RY, Ahmed F, Bolan GA, Workowski KA: Recommendations for providing quality sexually transmitted diseases clinical services, 2020, *MMWR Recomm Rep* 68(No. RR-5):1-20, 2020. https://doi.org/10.15585/mmwr.rr6805a1

BOX 5 Evaluation of Sexually Transmitted Disease–Related Conditions Recommendations in Primary Care and Sexually Transmitted Diseases Specialty Care Settings*

STD care in primary care settings

- Evaluation (history and examination) for the following STD-related conditions **should** be available as basic STD care services:
  1. Genital ulcer disease
  2. Male urethritis syndrome
  3. Vaginal discharge
  4. PID
  5. Genital warts
  6. Proctitis[†]
  7. Ectoparasitic infections
  8. Pharyngitis
  9. Epididymitis
  10. Systemic or dermatologic conditions compatible with or suggestive of an STD etiology

STD care in STD specialty care settings

- Evaluation (history and examination) for the following STD-related conditions **should** be available as specialized STD care services:
  1. Genital ulcer disease
  2. Male urethritis syndrome
  3. Vaginal discharge
  4. PID
  5. Genital warts
  6. Proctitis[†]
  7. Ectoparasitic infections
  8. Pharyngitis
  9. Epididymitis
  10. Systemic or dermatologic conditions compatible with or suggestive of an STD etiology

[§]Partner services can be provided on site or by referral.
*Primary care setting is defined as a place where patients are evaluated for various health conditions. STD specialty care setting is defined as a place where the focus is on providing patients with timely, comprehensive, confidential, and culturally sensitive STD care. STD care delivered in STD specialty care settings includes all care delivered in primary care settings.
[†]Evaluation for proctitis might include visual examination of the anus, anorectal examination with a rectal swab, digital anorectal examination, or anoscopy. For specialized STD care, high-resolution anoscopy might be included.
PID, Pelvic inflammatory disease; *STD,* sexually transmitted disease.
Barrow RY, Ahmed F, Bolan GA, Workowski KA: Recommendations for providing quality sexually transmitted diseases clinical services, 2020, *MMWR Recomm Rep* 68(No. RR-5):1-20, 2020. https://doi.org/10.15585/mmwr.rr6805a1

BOX 6 Laboratory Recommendations for Sexually Transmitted Diseases Care in Primary Care and Sexually Transmitted Diseases Specialty Care Settings*

STD care in primary care settings
At the time of the patient visit

- The following general services, equipment, or tests **should** be available as basic STD care services at the time of the patient visit:
    1. Thermometer
    2. pH paper
- The following general services, equipment, or tests **could** be available as basic STD services with test results available during the patient visit:
    1. Phlebotomy
    2. Test for trichomoniasis[†]
    3. Test for bacterial vaginosis[§]
    4. Test for vulvovaginal candidiasis[¶]
    5. Urine dipstick
    6. Urinalysis with microscopy
    7. Test for pregnancy
    8. Test for HIV

Clinical laboratory

- The following tests should be available through clinical laboratory as basic STD care services:
    1. Urogenital NAAT for gonorrhea and chlamydia
    2. Extragenital (pharynx and rectum) NAAT for gonorrhea and chlamydia
    3. Quantitative nontreponemal serologic test for syphilis
    4. Treponemal serologic test for syphilis
    5. HSV viral culture or PCR
    6. HSV serology
    7. Fourth-generation antigen/antibody HIV test
    8. Oncogenic HPV NAATs with Pap smear
    9. nPEP and PrEP
    10. Serologic tests for hepatitis A, B, and C
    11. Test for pregnancy
- The following tests **could** be available through clinical laboratory as basic STD care services:
    1. Gram stain, methylene blue, or gentian violet stain for urethritis
    2. Gonorrhea culture
    3. Gonorrhea antimicrobial susceptibility testing**
    4. NAAT for trichomoniasis

STD care in STD specialty care settings
At the time of the patient visit

- The following general services, equipment, or tests **should** be available as specialized STD care services at the time of the patient visit:
    1. Thermometer
    2. pH paper
    3. Phlebotomy
    4. Test for trichomoniasis[†]
    5. Test for bacterial vaginosis[§]
    6. Test for vulvovaginal candidiasis[¶]
    7. Urine dipstick
    8. Urinalysis with microscopy
    9. Test for pregnancy
    10. Gram stain, methylene blue, or gentian violet stain for urethritis
    11. On-site qualitative nontreponemal serologic test for syphilis
- The following general services, equipment, or tests **could** be available as specialized STD care services with test results available during the patient visit:
    1. Dark-field microscopy for syphilis
    2. Test for HIV

Clinical laboratory

- The following tests **should** be available through a clinical laboratory as specialized STD care services:
    1. Urogenital NAAT for gonorrhea and chlamydia
    2. Extragenital (pharynx and rectum) NAAT for gonorrhea and chlamydia
    3. Quantitative nontreponemal serologic test for syphilis
    4. Treponemal serologic test for syphilis
    5. HSV viral culture or PCR
    6. HSV serology
    7. Fourth-generation antigen/antibody HIV test
    8. Oncogenic HPV NAATs with Pap smear
    9. nPEP and PrEP
    10. Serologic tests for hepatitis A, B, and C
    11. Gonorrhea culture
    12. Gonorrhea antimicrobial susceptibility testing**
    13. NAAT for trichomoniasis

*Primary care setting is defined as a place where patients are evaluated for various health conditions. STD specialty care setting is defined as a place where the focus is on providing patients with timely, comprehensive, confidential, and culturally sensitive STD care. STD care delivered in STD specialty care settings includes all care delivered in primary care settings.

[†]On-site test for trichomoniasis can include wet mount microscopy and OSOM Trichomonas.

[§]On-site test for bacterial vaginosis can include wet mount microscopy, OSOM BVBlue, and Affirm.

[¶]On-site test for vulvovaginal candidiasis can include wet mount microscopy.

**Access needs to be established for transport medium that adequately maintains the viability of *Neisseria gonorrhoeae* until the specimen reaches a laboratory (e.g., transport medium in transport container, transport system, or transport swab). Providers should contact their state or local health department if they have concerns about resistant *N. gonorrhoeae* infection or if assistance is required for culture and antimicrobial susceptibility testing.

HIV, Human immunodeficiency virus; *HSV,* herpes simplex virus; *NAAT,* nucleic-acid amplification test; *nPEP,* nonoccupational postexposure prophylaxis; *PCR,* polymerase chain reaction; *PrEP,* preexposure prophylaxis; *STD,* sexually transmitted disease.

Barrow RY, Ahmed F, Bolan GA, Workowski KA: Recommendations for providing quality sexually transmitted diseases clinical services, 2020, *MMWR Recomm Rep* 68(No. RR-5):1-20, 2020. https://doi.org/10.15585/mmwr.rr6805a1

BOX 7 Persons Recommended to Receive Hepatitis B Vaccination

- All infants
- Unvaccinated children aged <19 yr
- Persons at risk for infection by sexual exposure
  1. Sex partners of hepatitis B surface antigen (HBsAg)-positive persons
  2. Sexually active persons who are not in a long-term, mutually monogamous relationship (e.g., persons with more than one sex partner during the previous 6 mo)
  3. Persons seeking evaluation or treatment for a sexually transmitted infection
  4. Men who have sex with men
- Persons at risk for infection by percutaneous or mucosal exposure to blood
  1. Current or recent injection-drug users
  2. Household contacts of HBsAg-positive persons
  3. Residents and staff of facilities for developmentally disabled persons
  4. Health care and public safety personnel with reasonably anticipated risk for exposure to blood or blood-contaminated body fluids
  5. Hemodialysis patients and predialysis, peritoneal dialysis, and home dialysis patients
  6. Persons with diabetes aged 19-59 yr; persons with diabetes aged ≥60 yr at the discretion of the treating clinician
- Others
  1. International travelers to countries with high or intermediate levels of endemic hepatitis B virus (HBV) infection (HBsAg prevalence of ≥2%)
  2. Persons with hepatitis C virus infection
  3. Persons with chronic liver disease (including persons with cirrhosis, fatty liver disease, alcoholic liver disease, autoimmune hepatitis, and an alanine aminotransferase [ALT] or aspartate aminotransferase [AST] level greater than twice the upper limit of normal)
  4. Persons with human immunodeficiency virus infection
  5. Incarcerated persons
- All other persons seeking protection from HBV infection

From Schillie S et al: Prevention of hepatitis B virus infection in the United States: recommendations of the Advisory Committee on Immunization Practices, *MMWR Recomm Rep* 67(No. RR-1):1-31, 2018.

BOX 8 Testing Anti-Hbs for Health Care Personnel (HCP) Vaccinated in the Past

The issue: An increasing number of HCP have received routine hepatitis B (HepB) vaccination during childhood. No postvaccination serologic testing is recommended after routine infant or adolescent HepB vaccination. Because vaccine-induced antibody to hepatitis B surface antigen (anti-HBs) wanes over time, testing HCP for anti-HBs years after vaccination might not distinguish vaccine nonresponders from responders.

 Guidance for health care institutions: Health care institutions may measure anti-HBs upon hire or matriculation for HCP who have documentation of a complete HepB vaccine series in the past (e.g., as part of routine infant or adolescent vaccination). HCP with anti-HBs <10 mIU/ml should receive one or more additional doses of HepB vaccine and retesting (see Fig. 1). Institutions that decide to not measure anti-HBs upon hire or matriculation for HCP who have documentation of a complete HepB vaccine series in the past should ensure timely assessment and postexposure prophylaxis following an exposure (see Table 25).

 Considerations: The risk for occupational HBV infection for vaccinated HCP might be low enough in certain settings so that assessment of anti-HBs status and appropriate follow-up should be done at the time of exposure to potentially infectious blood or body fluids. This approach relies on HCP recognizing and reporting blood and body fluid exposures and therefore may be applied on the basis of documented low risk, implementation, and cost considerations. Certain HCP occupations have lower risk for occupational blood and body fluid exposures (e.g., occupations involving counseling versus performing procedures), and nontrainees have lower risks for blood and body fluid exposures than trainees. Some settings also will have a lower prevalence of HBV infection in the patient population served than in other settings, which will influence the risk for HCP exposure to HBsAg-positive blood and body fluids.

From Schillie S et al: Prevention of hepatitis B virus infection in the United States: recommendations of the Advisory Committee on Immunization Practices, *MMWR Recomm Rep* 67(No. RR-1):1-31, 2018.

BOX 9 Persons Recommended to Receive Serologic Testing Before Vaccination*

- Human immunodeficiency virus-positive persons[†]
- Persons with elevated alanine aminotransferase/aspartate aminotransferase of unknown etiology[†]
- Hemodialysis patients[†]
- Men who have sex with men[†]
- Past or current persons who inject drugs[†]
- Persons born in countries of high and intermediate hepatitis B virus (HBV) endemicity (HBsAg prevalence ≥2%)
- U.S.-born persons not vaccinated as infants whose parents were born in countries with high HBV endemicity (≥8%)
- Persons needing immunosuppressive therapy, including chemotherapy, immunosuppression related to organ transplantation, and immunosuppression for rheumatologic or gastroenterologic disorders
- Donors of blood, plasma, organs, tissues, or semen

*Serologic testing comprises testing for hepatitis B surface antigen (HBsAg), antibody to HBsAg, and antibody to hepatitis B core antigen.
[†]Denotes persons also recommended for hepatitis B vaccination. Serologic testing should occur before vaccination. Serologic testing should not be a barrier to vaccination of susceptible persons. The first dose of vaccine should typically be administered immediately after collection of the blood for serologic testing.
From Schillie S et al: Prevention of hepatitis B virus infection in the United States: recommendations of the Advisory Committee on Immunization Practices, *MMWR Recomm Rep* 67(No. RR-1):1-31, 2018.

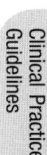

Clinical Practice Guidelines

V

BOX 10   Persons Recommended to Receive Postvaccination Serologic Testing* After a Complete Series of Hepatitis B Vaccination

- Infants born to hepatitis B surface antigen (HBsAg)-positive mothers or mothers whose HBsAg status remains unknown (e.g., when a parent or person with lawful custody safely surrenders an infant confidentially shortly after birth)[†]
- Health care personnel and public safety workers
- Hemodialysis patients and others who might require outpatient hemodialysis (e.g., predialysis, peritoneal dialysis, and home dialysis)
- -infected persons
- Other immunocompromised persons (e.g., hematopoietic stem-cell transplant recipients or persons receiving chemotherapy)
- Sex partners of HBsAg-positive persons

*Postvaccination serologic testing for persons other than infants born to HBsAg-positive (or HBsAg-unknown) mothers consists of anti-HBs.
[†]Postvaccination serologic testing for infants born to HBsAg-positive (or HBsAg-unknown) mothers consists of anti-HBs and HBsAg. Persons with anti-HBs <10 mIU/ml after the primary vaccine series should be revaccinated. Infants born to HBsAg-positive mothers or mothers with an unknown HBsAg status should be revaccinated with a single dose of HepB vaccine and receive postvaccination serologic testing 1-2 mo later. Infants whose anti-HBs remains <10 mIU/ml after single dose revaccination should receive two additional doses of HepB vaccine, followed by postvaccination serologic testing 1-2 mo after the final dose. Based on clinical circumstances or family preference, HBsAg-negative infants with anti-HBs <10 mIU/ml may instead be revaccinated with a mo complete 3-dose series, followed by postvaccination serologic testing performed 1-2 mo after the final dose of vaccine. For others with anti-HBs <10 mIU/ml after the primary series, administration of 3 additional HepB vaccine doses on an appropriate schedule, followed by anti-HBs testing 1-2 mo after the final dose, is usually more practical than serologic testing after ≥1 dose of vaccine.
From Schillie S et al: Prevention of hepatitis B virus infection in the United States: recommendations of the Advisory Committee on Immunization Practices, *MMWR Recomm Rep* 67(No. RR-1):1-31, 2018.

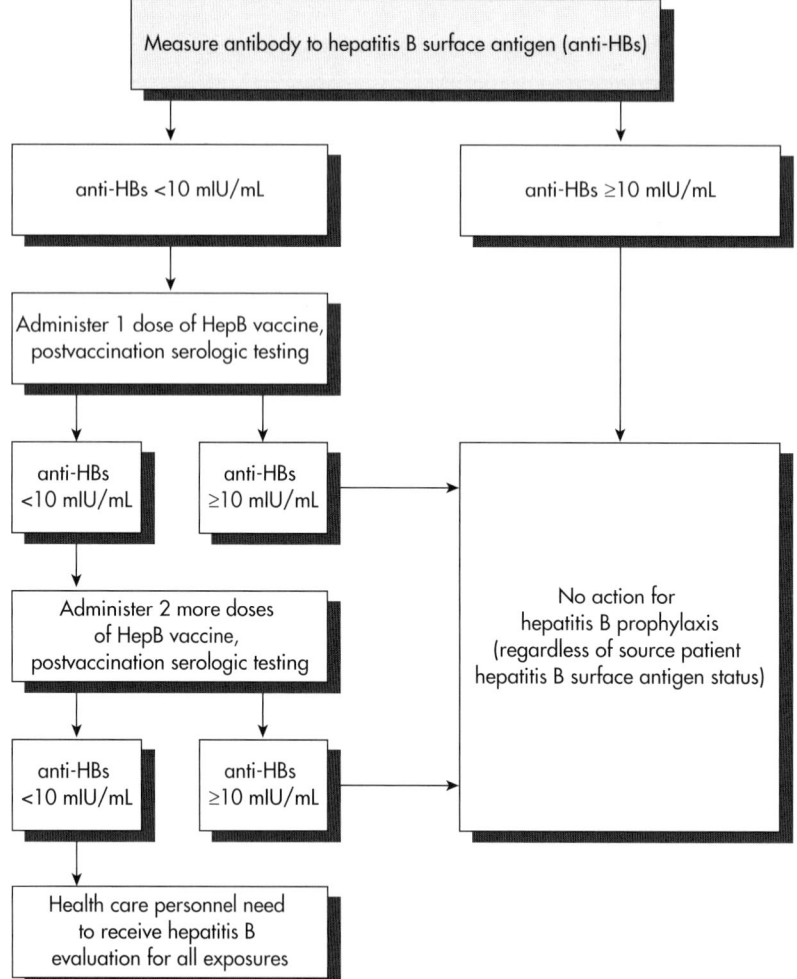

FIG. 1 Preexposure evaluation for health care personnel previously vaccinated with complete ≥3-dose HepB vaccine series who have not had postvaccination serologic testing.*
*Should be performed 1-2 mo after the last dose of vaccine using a quantitative method that allows detection of the protective concentration of anti-HBs (≥10 mIU/ml) (e.g., enzyme-linked immunosorbent assay [ELISA]). (From Schillie S et al: Prevention of hepatitis B virus infection in the United States: recommendations of the Advisory Committee on Immunization Practices, *MMWR Recomm Rep* 67[No. RR-1]:1-31, 2018.) (Source: Adapted from CDC: a comprehensive immunization strategy to eliminate transmission of hepatitis B virus infection in the United States: recommendations of the Advisory Committee on Immunization Practices [ACIP]. Part II: immunization of adults, *MMWR* 55 (No. RR-16), 2006.)

Influenza Treatment and Prophylaxis

BOX 11 Summary of Seasonal Influenza Vaccination Recommendations

Children	Adults
All children aged 6 mo to 18 yr should be vaccinated annually. Children and adolescents at higher risk for influenza complications should continue to be a focus for vaccination efforts as providers and programs transition to routinely vaccinating all children and adolescents, including those who:	Annual vaccination against influenza is recommended for any adult who wants to reduce the risk of becoming ill with influenza or of transmitting it to others. Vaccination is recommended for all adults without contraindications in the following groups, because these persons either are at higher risk for influenza complications, or are close contacts of the persons at higher risk:
<ul><li>Are aged 6 mo to 4 yr (59 mo)</li><li>Have chronic pulmonary (including asthma), cardiovascular (except hypertension), renal, hepatic, cognitive, neurologic/neuromuscular, hematologic, or metabolic disorders (including diabetes mellitus)</li><li>Are immunosuppressed (including immunosuppression caused by medications or by human immunodeficiency virus)</li><li>Are receiving long-term aspirin therapy and therefore might be at risk for experiencing Reye syndrome after influenza virus infection</li><li>Are residents of long-term care facilities</li><li>Will be pregnant during the influenza season</li><li>NOTE: Children aged <6 mo cannot receive influenza vaccination. Household and other close contacts (e.g., day-care providers) of children aged <6 mo, including older children and adolescents, should be vaccinated.</li></ul>	<ul><li>Persons aged ≥50 yr</li><li>Women who will be pregnant during the influenza season</li><li>Persons who have chronic pulmonary (including asthma), cardiovascular (except hypertension), renal, hepatic, cognitive, neurologic/neuromuscular, hematologic, or metabolic disorders (including diabetes mellitus)</li><li>Persons who have immunosuppression (including immunosuppression caused by medications or by human immunodeficiency virus)</li><li>Residents of nursing homes and other long-term care facilities</li><li>Health care personnel</li><li>Household contacts and caregivers of children aged <5 yr and adults aged ≥50 yr, with particular emphasis on vaccinating contacts of children aged <6 mo</li><li>Household contacts and caregivers of persons with medical conditions that put them at higher risk for severe complications from influenza</li></ul>

CDC. Prevention and control of seasonal influenza with vaccines: recommendations of the Advisory Committee on Immunization Practices (ACIP), 2009. *MMWR* 58(No. RR-8), 2009

INDICATIONS FOR USE OF ANTIVIRALS

PERSONS FOR WHOM ANTIVIRAL TREATMENT SHOULD BE CONSIDERED

If possible, antiviral treatment should be started within 48 h of influenza illness onset. The effectiveness of initiating antiviral treatment more than 48 h after illness onset has not been established. Persons for whom antiviral treatment should be considered include:

- Persons hospitalized with laboratory-confirmed influenza (limited data suggest benefit even for persons whose antiviral treatment is initiated more than 48 h after illness onset)
- Persons with laboratory-confirmed influenza pneumonia
- Persons with laboratory-confirmed influenza and bacterial coinfection
- Persons with laboratory-confirmed influenza infection who are at higher risk for influenza complications
- Persons presenting to medical care with laboratory-confirmed influenza within 48 h of influenza illness onset who want to decrease the duration or severity of their symptoms and transmission of influenza to others at higher risk for complications

PERSONS FOR WHOM ANTIVIRAL CHEMOPROPHYLAXIS SHOULD BE CONSIDERED DURING PERIODS OF INCREASED INFLUENZA ACTIVITY IN THE COMMUNITY

- Persons at high risk during the 2 wk after influenza vaccination (after the second dose for children younger than 9 yr who have not previously been vaccinated) if influenza viruses are circulating in the community
- Persons at high risk for whom influenza vaccine is contraindicated
- Family members or health care providers who are unvaccinated and are likely to have ongoing, close exposure to persons at high risk or unvaccinated persons or infants younger than 6 mo
- Persons and their family members and close contacts and health care workers when circulating strains of influenza virus in the community are not matched with vaccine strains
- Persons with immune deficiencies or those who might not respond to vaccination (e.g., persons infected with HIV or other immunosuppressed conditions or who are receiving immunosuppressive medications)
- Unvaccinated staff and persons during response to an outbreak in a closed institutional setting with residents at high risk (e.g., extended-care facilities)

CDC. Prevention and control of influenza: recommendations of the Advisory Committee on Immunization Practices (ACIP), 2008. *MMWR* 57(No.RR-7), 2008.

NOTE: Recommended antiviral medications (neuraminidase inhibitors) are not licensed for chemoprophylaxis of children younger than 1 yr (oseltamivir) or younger than 5 yr (zanamivir). Updates or supplements to these recommendations (e.g., expanded age or risk group indications for licensed vaccines) might be required. Health care providers should be alert to announcements of recommendation updates and should check the Centers for Disease Control and Prevention influenza website periodically for additional information (https://www.cdc.gov/flu).

TESTING AND CLINICAL MANAGEMENT OF HEALTH CARE PERSONNEL POTENTIALLY EXPOSED TO HEPATITIS C VIRUS

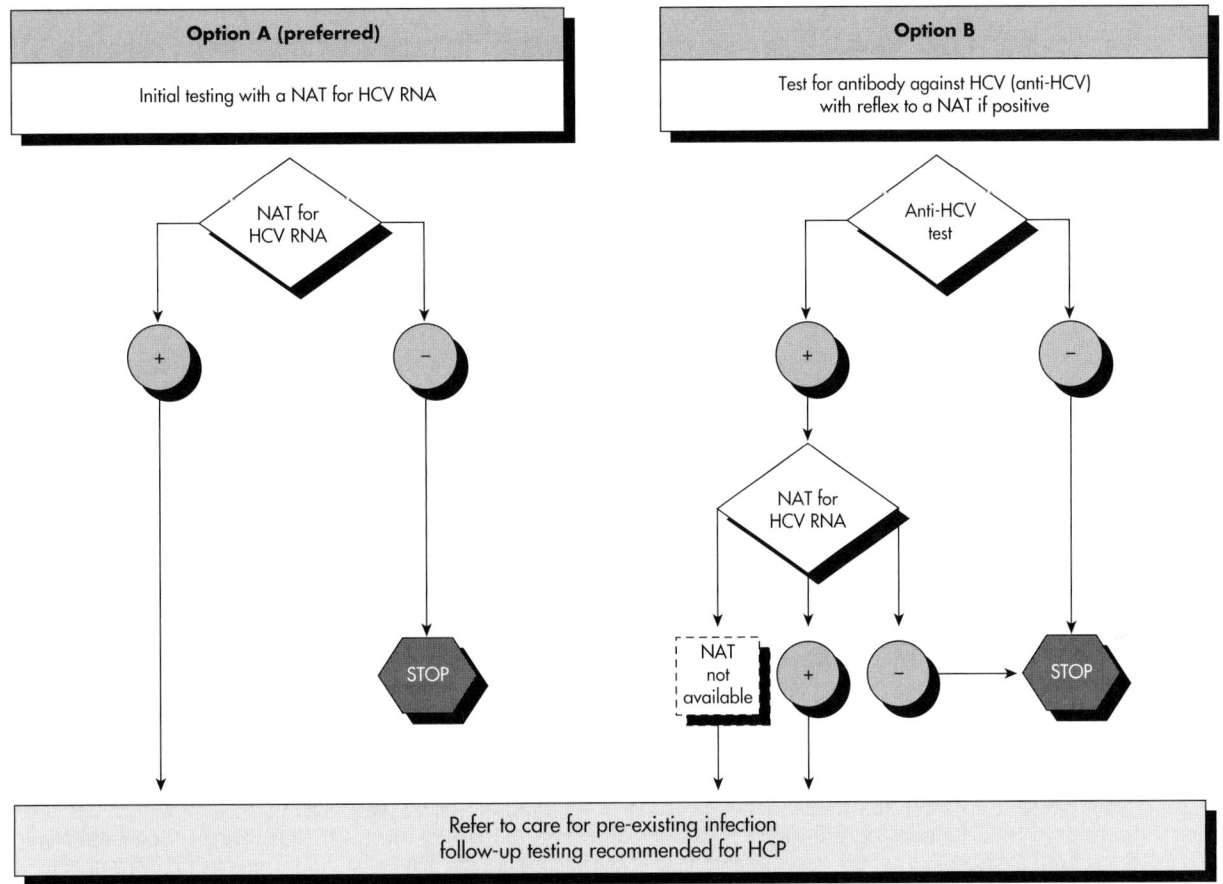

FIG. 2 Testing of source patients after potential exposure of health care personnel to hepatitis C virus—CDC guidance, United States, 2020.* *AASLD-IDSA, American Association for the Study of Liver Diseases and the Infectious Diseases Society of America; HCP, health care personnel; HCV, hepatitis C virus; NAT, nucleic acid test.* *Testing of the source patient should be performed as soon as possible (preferably within 48 h) after exposure. Testing may follow option A (preferred), which is testing with a NAT for HCV RNA, or option B, which is testing for anti-HCV with reflex to a NAT for HCV RNA if positive. If the source patient is known or suspected to have recent behaviors that increase risk for HCV acquisition (e.g., injection drug use within the previous 4 mo) or if risk cannot be reliably assessed, initial testing of the source patient should include an NAT for HCV RNA. A source patient found to be positive for HCV RNA should be referred to care. Follow-up testing of HCP is recommended if the source patient is HCV RNA positive, is anti-HCV positive with HCV RNA status unknown, or cannot be tested. **Persons with detectable HCV RNA at any point** should be referred to care consistent with current AASLD-IDSA guidelines for evaluation and treatment of all persons with acute or chronic HCV infection. Guidance for hepatitis C treatment (https://www.hcvguidelines.org/) is evolving with emerging data on treatment with direct-acting antivirals. (From Moorman AC, de Perio MA, Goldschmidt R et al: Testing and clinical management of health care personnel potentially exposed to hepatitis C virus—CDC Guidance, United States, 2020, *MMWR Recomm Rep* 2020;69(No. RR-6):1-8.)

BOX 12 Testing of Source Patients and Health Care Personnel Potentially Exposed to Hepatitis C Virus—CDC Guidance, United States, 2020

Source-patient testing
- Testing of the source patient may follow option A (preferred), which is testing with a nucleic acid test (NAT) for hepatitis C virus (HCV) RNA, **or** option B, which is testing for anti-HCV with reflex to a NAT if positive.
- If a source patient is known or suspected to have recent behaviors that increase risk for HCV acquisition (e.g., injection drug use within the previous 4 mo) or if risk cannot be reliably assessed, initial testing should include a NAT.
- Follow-up testing of health care personnel (HCP) is recommended if the source patient is HCV RNA positive, is anti-HCV positive with RNA status unknown, or cannot be tested.

HCP testing*
- Baseline testing of HCP for anti-HCV with reflex to a NAT if positive should be conducted as soon as possible (preferably within 48 h) after the exposure and may be simultaneous with source-patient testing.
- If follow-up testing of HCP is recommended based on the source-patient's status, test with an NAT at 3-6 wk postexposure.
- If the HCP is NAT negative at 3-6 wk postexposure, a final test for anti-HCV at 4-6 mo postexposure is recommended.
- A source patient or HCP who is positive for HCV RNA should be referred to care.

*Follow-up testing of HCP is also warranted when concerns exist about specimen integrity, including handling and storage conditions that might have compromised source-patient test results, or if they exhibit any clinical signs of HCV infection.
From Moorman AC, de Perio MA, Goldschmidt R, et al: Testing and clinical management of health care personnel potentially exposed to hepatitis C virus—CDC guidance, United States, 2020, *MMWR Recomm Rep* 69(No. RR-6):1-8, 2020.

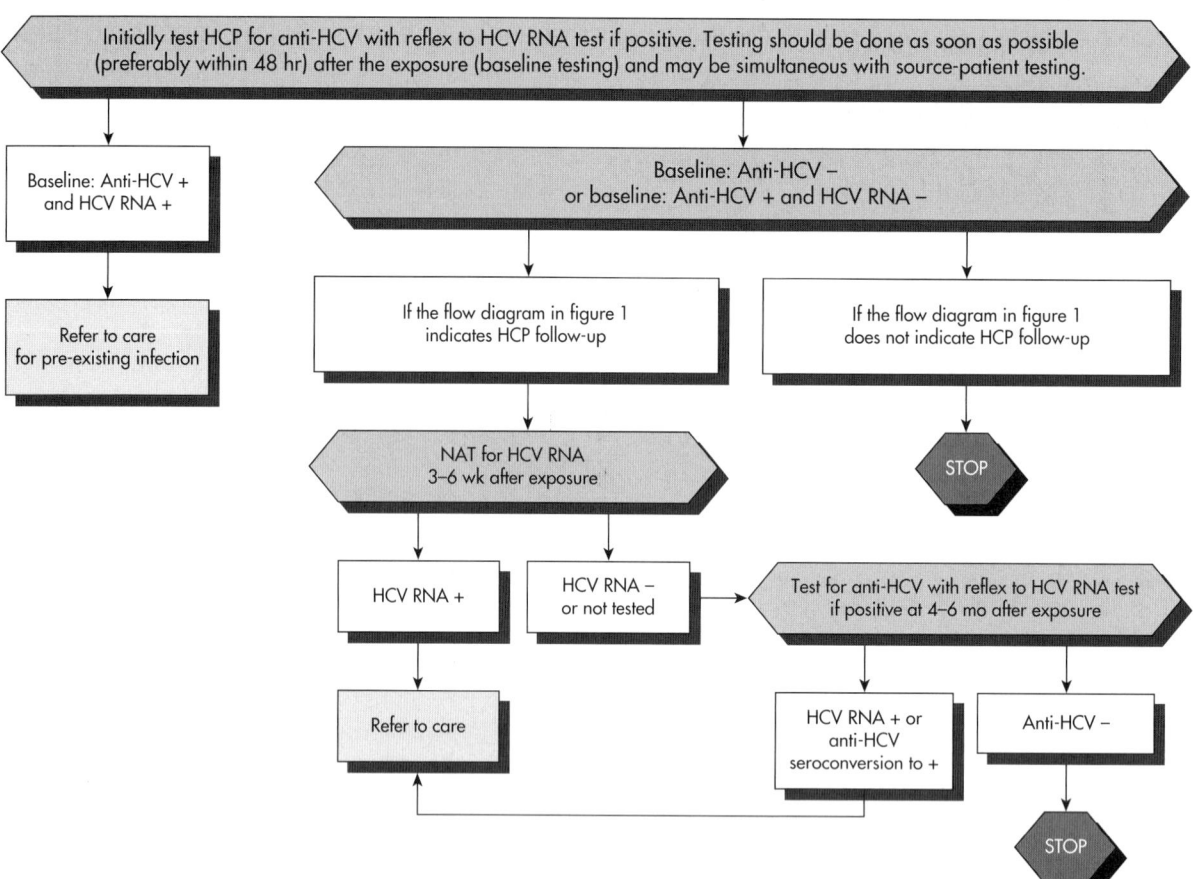

FIG. 3 Testing of health care personnel after potential exposure to hepatitis C virus—CDC guidance, United States, 2020.* *AASLD-IDSA,* American Association for the Study of Liver Diseases and the Infectious Diseases Society of America; *HCP,* health care personnel; *HCV,* hepatitis C virus; *NAT,* nucleic acid test. **Baseline testing of HCP for anti-HCV with reflex to a NAT for HCV RNA if positive should be done as soon as possible** (preferably within 48 h) after the exposure and may be simultaneous with source-patient testing. **If follow-up testing is recommended based on the source-patient's status, test for HCV RNA at 3-6 wk postexposure.** Testing for HCV RNA performed at 6 wk postexposure has the advantage of coinciding with human immunodeficiency virus (HIV) postexposure testing schedules if HIV surveillance is recommended. **If HCV RNA is negative at 3-6 wk postexposure, a final test for anti-HCV at 4-6 mo postexposure is recommended** due to the possibility of intermittent periods of aviremia in acute HCV infection. **If the HCP was anti-HCV positive and HCV RNA negative at baseline, testing at this time should be conducted for HCV RNA detection, as persons successfully treated for HCV infection will remain anti-HCV positive and HCV RNA negative unless reinfected.** Testing performed at 6 mo postexposure has the advantage of coinciding with hepatitis B virus (HBV) postexposure testing schedules if HBV testing is recommended. **HCP with anti-HCV seroconversion and negative HCV RNA should be referred for further evaluation.** False-positive anti-HCV results are known to occur among low-risk populations. Anti-HCV seroconversion occurs on average 8-11 wk after exposure, although cases of delayed seroconversion have been documented among persons with immunosuppression such as in HIV infection. **For persons who had a negative anti-HCV result and are immunocompromised, testing for HCV RNA can be considered.** Also, for persons with a positive anti-HCV and negative HCV RNA result, HCV RNA testing should be repeated if an additional potential HCV exposure occurred within the past 6 mo, clinical evidence of HCV infection is present, or concerns exist about specimen integrity, including handling and storage conditions that might have compromised test results. **Exposed persons who develop viral syndromes suggestive of acute HCV infection at any point** should be retested for HCV RNA. **Persons with detectable HCV RNA at any point** should be referred to care consistent with current AASLD-IDSA guidelines for evaluation and treatment of all persons with acute or chronic HCV infection. Those persons with acute infection should be treated on initial diagnosis without awaiting spontaneous resolution. Guidance for hepatitis C treatment (https://www.hcvguidelines.org/) is evolving with emerging data on treatment with direct-acting antivirals. (From Moorman AC, de Perio MA, Goldschmidt R, et al: Testing and clinical management of health care personnel potentially exposed to hepatitis C virus—CDC guidance, United States, 2020, *MMWR Recomm Rep* 69(No. RR-6):1-8, 2020.)

HIV Testing and Postexposure Prophylaxis

RECOMMENDATIONS FOR HIV TESTING OF ADULTS, ADOLESCENTS, AND PREGNANT WOMEN

RECOMMENDATIONS FOR ADULTS AND ADOLESCENTS

The CDC recommends that diagnostic human immunodeficiency virus (HIV) testing and opt-out HIV screening be a part of routine clinical care in all health care settings while also preserving the patient's option to decline HIV testing and ensuring a provider-patient relationship conducive to optimal clinical and preventive care. The recommendations are intended for providers in all health care settings, including hospital emergency departments, urgent-care clinics, inpatient services, sexually transmitted disease (STD) clinics or other venues offering clinical STD services, tuberculosis (TB) clinics, substance abuse treatment clinics, other public health clinics, community clinics, correctional health care facilities, and primary care settings. The guidelines address HIV testing in health care settings only; they do not modify existing guidelines concerning HIV counseling, testing, and referral for persons at high risk for HIV who seek or receive HIV testing in nonclinical settings (e.g., community-based organizations, outreach settings, or mobile vans).[3]

SCREENING FOR HIV INFECTION

- In all health care settings, screening for HIV infection should be performed routinely for all patients aged 13 to 64 yr. Health care providers should initiate screening unless prevalence of undiagnosed HIV infection in their patients has been documented to be less than 0.1%. In the absence of existing data for HIV prevalence, health care providers should initiate voluntary HIV screening until they establish that the diagnostic yield is less than 1 per 1000 patients screened, at which point such screening is no longer warranted.
- All patients initiating treatment for TB should be screened routinely for HIV infection.
- All patients seeking treatment for STDs, including all patients visiting STD clinics, should be screened routinely for HIV during each visit for a new complaint, regardless of whether the patient is known or suspected to have specific behavior risks for HIV infection.

REPEAT SCREENING

- Health care providers should subsequently test all persons likely to be at high risk for HIV at least annually. Persons likely to be at high risk include users of injection drugs and their sex partners, persons who exchange sex for money or drugs, sex partners of persons who are HIV infected, and men who have sex with men (MSM) or heterosexual persons who themselves or whose sex partners have had more than one sex partner since their most recent HIV test.
- Health care providers should encourage patients and their prospective sex partners to be tested before initiating a new sexual relationship.
- Repeat screening of persons not likely to be at high risk for HIV should be performed on the basis of clinical judgment.
- Unless recent HIV test results are immediately available, any person whose blood or body fluid is the source of an occupational exposure for a health care provider should be informed of the incident and tested for HIV infection at the time the exposure occurs.

CONSENT AND PRETEST INFORMATION

- Screening should be voluntary and undertaken only with the patient's knowledge and understanding that HIV testing is planned.
- Patients should be informed orally or in writing that HIV testing will be performed unless they decline (opt-out screening). Oral or written information should include an explanation of HIV infection and the meanings of positive and negative test results, and the patient should be offered an opportunity

to ask questions and decline testing. With such notification, consent for HIV screening should be incorporated into the patient's general informed consent for medical care on the same basis as are other screening or diagnostic tests; a separate consent form for HIV testing is not recommended.
- Easily understood informational materials should be made available in the languages of the commonly encountered populations within the service area. The competence of interpreters and bilingual staff to provide language assistance to patients with limited English proficiency must be ensured.
- If a patient declines an HIV test, this decision should be documented in the medical record.

DIAGNOSTIC TESTING FOR HIV INFECTION

- All patients with signs or symptoms consistent with HIV infection or an opportunistic illness characteristic of acquired immunodeficiency syndrome (AIDS) should be tested for HIV.
- Clinicians should maintain a high level of suspicion for acute HIV infection in all patients who have a compatible clinical syndrome and who report recent high-risk behavior. When acute retroviral syndrome is a possibility, a plasma RNA test should be used in conjunction with an HIV antibody test to diagnose acute HIV infection.
- Patients or persons responsible for the patient's care should be notified orally that testing is planned, advised of the indication for testing and the implications of positive and negative test results, and offered an opportunity to ask questions and decline testing. With such notification, the patient's general consent for medical care is considered sufficient for diagnostic HIV testing.

HIV SCREENING FOR PREGNANT WOMEN AND THEIR INFANTS

Universal Opt-Out Screening
- All pregnant women in the United States should be screened for HIV infection.
- Screening should occur after a woman is notified that HIV screening is recommended for all pregnant patients and that she will receive an HIV test as part of the routine panel of prenatal tests unless she declines (opt-out screening).
- HIV testing must be voluntary and free from coercion. No woman should be tested without her knowledge.
- Pregnant women should receive oral or written information that includes an explanation of HIV infection, a description of interventions that can reduce HIV transmission from mother to infant, and the meanings of positive and negative test results. They should be offered an opportunity to ask questions and decline testing.
- No additional process or written documentation of informed consent beyond what is required for other routine prenatal tests should be required for HIV testing.
- If a patient declines an HIV test, this decision should be documented in the medical record.

ADDRESSING REASONS FOR DECLINING TESTING

- Providers should discuss and address reasons for declining an HIV test (e.g., lack of perceived risk, fear of the disease, and concerns regarding partner violence or potential stigma or discrimination).
- Women who decline an HIV test because they have had a previous negative test result should be informed of the importance of retesting during each pregnancy.
- Logistical reasons for not testing (e.g., scheduling) should be resolved.
- Certain women who initially decline an HIV test might accept at a later date, especially if their concerns are discussed. Certain women will continue to decline testing, and their decisions should be respected and documented in the medical record.

Timing of HIV Testing
- To promote informed and timely therapeutic decisions, health care providers should test women for HIV as early as possible during each pregnancy. Women who decline the test early in prenatal care should be encouraged to be tested at a subsequent visit.

---

[3]Data from *MMWR* 57(RR-10), 2008.

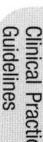

- A second HIV test during the third trimester, preferably less than 36 wk of gestation, is cost effective even in areas of low HIV prevalence and may be considered for all pregnant women. A second HIV test during the third trimester is recommended for women who meet one or more of the following criteria:
- Women who receive health care in jurisdictions with elevated incidence of HIV or AIDS among women aged 15 to 45 yr. In 2004, these jurisdictions included Alabama, Connecticut, Delaware, the District of Columbia, Florida, Georgia, Illinois, Louisiana, Maryland, Massachusetts, Mississippi, Nevada, New Jersey, New York, North Carolina, Pennsylvania, Puerto Rico, Rhode Island, South Carolina, Tennessee, Texas, and Virginia.[4]
- Women who receive health care in facilities in which prenatal screening identifies at least one pregnant woman who is infected with HIV per 1000 women screened.
- Women who are known to be at high risk for acquiring HIV (e.g., users of injection drugs and their sex partners, women who exchange sex for money or drugs, women who are sex partners of persons who are infected with HIV, and women who have had a new or more than one sex partner during this pregnancy).
- Women who have signs or symptoms consistent with acute HIV infection. When acute retroviral syndrome is a possibility, a plasma RNA test should be used in conjunction with an HIV antibody test to diagnose acute HIV infection.

Rapid Testing During Labor
- Any woman with undocumented HIV status at the time of labor should be screened with a rapid HIV test unless she declines (opt-out screening).
- Reasons for declining a rapid test should be explored (see "Addressing Reasons for Declining Testing").

- Immediate initiation of appropriate antiretroviral prophylaxis should be recommended to women on the basis of a reactive rapid test result without waiting for the result of a confirmatory test.

Postpartum/Newborn Testing
- When a woman's HIV status is still unknown at the time of delivery, she should be screened immediately postpartum with a rapid HIV test unless she declines (opt-out screening).
- When the mother's HIV status is unknown postpartum, rapid testing of the newborn as soon as possible after birth is recommended so that antiretroviral prophylaxis can be offered to infants exposed to HIV. Women should be informed that identifying HIV antibodies in the newborn indicates that the mother is infected.
- For infants whose HIV exposure status is unknown and who are in foster care, the person legally authorized to provide consent should be informed that rapid HIV testing is recommended for infants whose biologic mothers have not been tested.
- The benefits of neonatal antiretroviral prophylaxis are best realized when it is initiated within 12 h after birth.

Confirmatory Testing
- Whenever possible, uncertainties regarding laboratory test results indicating HIV infection status should be resolved before final decisions are made regarding reproductive options, antiretroviral therapy, cesarean delivery, or other interventions.
- If the confirmatory test result is not available before delivery, immediate initiation of appropriate antiretroviral prophylaxis should be recommended to any pregnant patient whose HIV screening test result is reactive to reduce the risk for perinatal transmission.

---

[4]A second HIV test in the third trimester is as cost effective as other common health interventions when HIV incidence among women of childbearing age is =17 HIV cases per 100,000 person-yr. In 2004, in jurisdictions with available data on HIV case rates, a rate of 17 new HIV diagnoses per yr per 100,000 women aged 15 to 45 yr was associated with an AIDS case rate of at least nine AIDS diagnoses per yr per 100,000 women aged 15 to 45 yr (CDC, unpublished data, 2005). As of 2004, the jurisdictions listed above exceeded these thresholds. The list of specific jurisdictions where a second test in the third trimester is recommended will be updated periodically based on surveillance data.

BOX 13 Situations for Which Expert Consultation for HIV Postexposure Prophylaxis Is Advised*

- Delayed (i.e., later than 24-36 h) exposure report
  1. The interval after which there is no benefit from postexposure prophylaxis (PEP) is undefined
- Unknown source (e.g., needle in sharps disposal container or laundry)
  1. Decide use of PEP on a case-by-case basis
  2. Consider the severity of the exposure and the epidemiologic likelihood of human immunodeficiency virus (HIV) exposure
  3. Do not test needles or other sharp instruments for HIV
- Known or suspected pregnancy in the exposed person
  1. Does not preclude the use of optimal PEP regimens
  2. Do not deny PEP solely on the basis of pregnancy
- Resistance of the source virus to antiretroviral agents
  1. Influence of drug resistance on transmission risk is unknown
  2. Selection of drugs to which the source person's virus is unlikely to be resistant is recommended if the source person's virus is known or suspected to be resistant to one or more of the drugs considered for the PEP regimen
  3. Resistance testing of the source person's virus at the time of the exposure is not recommended
- Toxicity of the initial PEP regimen
  1. Adverse symptoms such as nausea and diarrhea are common with PEP
  2. Symptoms often can be managed without changing the PEP regimen by prescribing antimotility and/or antiemetic agents
  3. Modification of dose intervals (i.e., administering a lower dose of drug more frequently throughout the day, as recommended by the manufacturer) in other situations might help alleviate symptoms

*Local experts and/or the National Clinicians' Postexposure Prophylaxis Hotline (PEPline [888-448-4911]).

BOX 14 Occupational Exposure Management Resources

National Clinicians' Postexposure Prophylaxis Hotline (PEPline)
Run by University of California—San Francisco/San Francisco General Hospital staff; supported by the Health Resources and Services Administration, Ryan White CARE Act, HIV/AIDS Bureau, AIDS Education and Training Centers, and CDC

Phone: 888-448-4911
Internet: https://nccc.ucsf.edu/clinician-consultation;/pep-post-exposure-prophylaxis/

Hepatitis Hotline

Phone: 888-443-7232
Internet: https://www.cdc.gov/ncidod/diseases/hepatitis/index.htm

Reporting to CDC: Occupationally acquired HIV infections and failures of PEP

Phone: 800-893-0485

HIV Antiretroviral Pregnancy Registry

Phone: 800-258-4263
Fax: 800-800-1052
Address: 1410 Commonwealth Dr., Suite 215, Wilmington, NC 28405
Internet: https://www.apregistry.com/

Food and Drug Administration Report unusual or severe toxicity to antiretroviral agents

Phone: 800-332-1088
Address: MedWatch, HF-2, FDA, 5600 Fishers Lane, Rockville, MD 20857
Internet: https://www.fda.gov/medwatch

HIV/AIDS Treatment Information Service

Internet: http://www.hivatis.org/

BOX 15 Management of Occupational Blood Exposures

Provide Immediate Care to the Exposure Site
- Wash wounds and skin with soap and water
- Flush mucous membranes with water

Determine Risk Associated With Exposure
- Type of fluid (e.g., blood, visibly bloody fluid, other potentially infectious fluid or tissue, and concentrated virus)
- Type of exposure (e.g., percutaneous injury, mucous membrane or nonintact skin exposure, and bites resulting in blood exposure)

Evaluate Exposure Source
- Assess the risk of infection using available information
- Test known sources for HBsAg, anti-HCV, and HIV antibodies (consider using rapid testing)
- For unknown sources, assess risk of exposure to HBV, HCV, or HIV infection
- Do not test discarded needles or syringes for virus contamination

Evaluate the Exposed Person
- Assess immune status for HBV infection (i.e., by history of hepatitis B vaccination and vaccine response)

Give PEP for Exposures Posing Risk of Infection Transmission
- HBV: See Table E5
- HCV: PEP not recommended
- HIV: See Tables E33, E34, and E35
    1. Initiate PEP as soon as possible, preferably within hours of exposure
    2. Offer pregnancy testing to all women of childbearing age not known to be pregnant
    3. Seek expert consultation if viral resistance is suspected
    4. Administer PEP for 4 wk if tolerated

Perform Follow-up Testing and Provide Counseling
- Advise exposed persons to seek medical evaluation for any acute illness occurring during follow-up

HBV Exposures
- Perform follow-up anti-HBs testing in persons who receive hepatitis B vaccine
    1. Test for anti-HBs 1-2 mo after last dose of vaccine
    2. Anti-HBs response to vaccine cannot be ascertained if HBIG was received in the previous 3-4 mo

HCV Exposures
- Perform baseline and follow-up testing for anti-HCV and alanine aminotransferase 4-6 mo after exposure
- Perform HCV RNA at 4-6 wk if earlier diagnosis of HCV infection desired
- Confirm repeatedly reactive anti-HCV enzyme immunoassays with supplemental tests

HIV Exposures
- Perform HIV-antibody testing for at least 6 mo after exposure (e.g., at baseline, 6 wk, 3 mo, and 6 mo)
- Perform HIV-antibody testing if illness compatible with an acute retroviral syndrome occurs
- Advise exposed persons to use precautions to prevent secondary transmission during the follow-up period
- Evaluate exposed persons taking PEP within 72 h after exposure and monitor for drug toxicity for at least 2 wk

HBV, Hepatitis B virus; *HBsAG,* hepatitis B serface antigen; *HCV,* hepatitis C virus; *HIV,* human immunodeficiency virus; *PEP,* postexposure prophylaxis.

Recommendations for Meningococcal Vaccination

BOX 16   Meningococcal Vaccination Recommendations—Advisory Committee on Immunization Practices, United States, 2020

ACIP recommends MenACWY vaccination for the following groups:

- Routine vaccination for adolescents aged 11 or 12 yr, with a booster dose at age 16 yr.
- Routine vaccination of persons aged ≥ 2 mo at increased risk for meningococcal disease (dosing schedule varies by age and indication, and interval for booster dose varies by age at time of previous vaccination):
- Persons with certain medical conditions including anatomic or functional asplenia, complement component deficiencies (e.g., C3, C5-C9, properdin, factor H, or factor D), complement inhibitor (e.g., eculizumab [Soliris] or ravulizumab [Ultomiris]) use, or human immunodeficiency virus infection.
- Microbiologists with routine exposure to *Neisseria meningitidis* isolates.
- Persons at increased risk during an outbreak (e.g., in community or organizational settings, and among men who have sex with men [MSM]).
- Persons who travel to or live in countries in which meningococcal disease is hyperendemic or epidemic.
- Unvaccinated or undervaccinated first-year college students living in residence halls.
- Military recruits.
- Booster doses for previously vaccinated persons who become or remain at increased risk

ACIP recommends MenB vaccination for the following groups:

- Routine vaccination of persons aged ≥ 10 yr at increased risk for meningococcal disease (dosing schedule varies by vaccine brand; boosters should be administered at 1 yr after primary series completion, then every 2-3 yr thereafter):
- Persons with certain medical conditions, such as anatomic or functional asplenia, complement component deficiencies, or complement inhibitor use.
- Microbiologists with routine exposure to *N. meningitidis* isolates.
- Persons at increased risk during an outbreak (e.g., in community or organizational settings, and among MSM).
- Vaccination of adolescents and young adults aged 16-23 yr with a 2-dose MenB series on the basis of shared clinical decision-making. The preferred age for MenB vaccination is 16-18 yr. Booster doses are not recommended unless the person becomes at increased risk for meningococcal disease.
- Booster doses for previously vaccinated persons who become or remain at increased risk.

ACIP, Advisory Committee on Immunization Practices; *MenACWY,* quadrivalent (serogroups A, C, W, Y) meningococcal conjugate vaccine; *MenB,* serogroup B meningococcal vaccine.

From Mbaeyi SA, Bozio CH, Duffy J, et al: Meningococcal vaccination: recommendations of the Advisory Committee on Immunization Practices, United States, 2020, *MMWR Recomm Rep* 69(No. RR-9):1-41, 2020.

Vaccine Websites And Resources

TABLE 45 Vaccine Websites and Resources

Organization	Website
Health Professional Associations	
American Academy of Family Physicians (AAFP)	https://www.familydoctor.org/online/famdocen/home.html
American Academy of Pediatrics (AAP)	https://www.aap.org/
AAP Childhood Immunization Support Program	https://www.aap.org/immunization/
American Association of Occupational Health Nurses (AAOHN)	https://www.aaohn.org/
American College Health Association (ACHA)	https://www.acha.org/
American College of Obstetricians and Gynecologists (ACOG)—Immunization for Women	https://www.immunizationforwomen.org/
American Medical Association (AMA)	https://www.ama-assn.org/
American Nurses Association (ANA)	https://www.nursingworld.org/
American Pharmacists Association (APhA)	https://www.pharmacist.com/
American School Health Association (ASHA)	https://www.ashaweb.org/
American Travel Health Nurses Association (ATHNA)	https://www.athna.org/
Association for Professionals in Infection Control and Epidemiology (APIC)	https://www.apic.org/
Association of State and Territorial Health Officials (ASTHO)	https://www.astho.org/
Association of Teachers of Preventive Medicine (ATPM)	https://www.atpm.org/
National Medical Association (NMA)	https://www.nmanet.org/
Society of Teachers of Family Medicine—Group on Immunization Education	https://www.immunizationed.org/
Nonprofit Groups and Universities	
Albert B. Sabin Vaccine Institute	https://www.sabin.org/
Brighton Collaboration	
Center for Vaccine Awareness and Research—Texas Children's Center	https://www.texaschildrens.org/departments/immunization-project
Children's Vaccine Program	
Every Child by Two (ECBT)	https://www.ecbt.org/
Families Fighting Flu	https://www.familiesfightingflu.org/
GAVI, the Vaccine Alliance	
Health on the Net Foundation (HON)	https://www.hon.ch/
Immunization Action Coalition (IAC)	https://www.immunize.org/
Infectious Diseases Society of America (IDSA)	https://www.idsociety.org/Index.aspx
Institute for Vaccine Safety (IVS), Johns Hopkins Bloomberg School of Public Health	https://www.vaccinesafety.edu/
National Academies: Health and Medicine Division	https://www.nationalacademies.org/hmd/
National Alliance for Hispanic Health	https://www.hispanichealth.org/
National Foundation for Infectious Diseases (NFID)	http://www.nfid.org/
National Foundation for Infectious Diseases (NFID)—Childhood Influenza Immunization Coalition (CIIC)	
National Network for Immunization Information (NNii)	
Parents of Kids with Infectious Diseases (PKIDS)	https://www.pkids.org/
PATH Vaccine Resource Library	
Vaccine Education Center at the Children's Hospital of Philadelphia	https://www.chop.edu/service/vaccine-education-center/home.html
Vaccinate Your Baby	https://www.vaccinateyourbaby.org/
Government Organizations	
Centers for Disease Control and Prevention (CDC)	
Advisory Committee on Immunization Practices (ACIP)	https://www.cdc.gov/vaccines/acip/index.html
ACIP Vaccine Recommendations	https://www.cdc.gov/vaccines/hcp/acip-recs/index.html
Current Vaccine Delays and Shortages	https://www.cdc.gov/vaccines/vac-gen/shortages/
Epidemiology and Prevention of Vaccine-Preventable Diseases (also known as the Pink Book)	https://www.cdc.gov/vaccines/pubs/pinkbook/index.html
Manual for the Surveillance of Vaccine-Preventable Diseases	https://www.cdc.gov/vaccines/pubs/surv-manual/index.html
Public Health Image Library	http://www.phil.cdc.gov/phil/home.asp
Travelers' Health	https://www.cdc.gov/travel/
CDC Health Information for International Travel (also known as the Yellow Book)	https://wwwnc.cdc.gov/travel/yellowbook/2016/table-of-contents
Vaccine Adverse Events Reporting System (VAERS)	
Vaccine Administration: Recommendations and Guidelines	

TABLE 45 Vaccine Websites and Resources—cont'd

Organization	Website
Vaccines and Immunizations	https://www.cdc.gov/vaccines/
Vaccines for Children Program	https://www.cdc.gov/vaccines/programs/vfc/index.html
Vaccines for Children—Vaccine Price List	https://www.cdc.gov/vaccines/programs/vfc/awardees/vaccine-management/price-list/index.html
Vaccine Information Statements	https://www.cdc.gov/vaccines/hcp/vis/index.html
Vaccine Safety	https://www.cdc.gov/vaccinesafety/index.html
Vaccine Storage and Handling	https://www.cdc.gov/vaccines/recs/storage/default.htm
Department of Health and Human Services (HHS)	
National Vaccine Program Office (NVPO)	https://www.hhs.gov/nvpo/
Health Resources and Services Administration	
National Vaccine Injury Compensation Program	https://www.hrsa.gov/vaccinecompensation/
National Institute of Allergy and Infectious Diseases (NIAID)	
Vaccines	https://www.niaid.nih.gov/about/vrc
World Health Organization (WHO)	
Immunization, Vaccines, and Biologicals	https://www.who.int/immunization/en/

From Kliegman RM: *Nelson textbook of pediatrics*, ed 21, Philadelphia, 2020, Elsevier.

Note: Page numbers followed by *f* indicate figures, *b* indicate boxes, *t* indicate tables, and *e* and **bold** indicate online content

1933

Note: Page numbers followed by *f* indicate figures, *b* indicate boxes, *t* indicate tables, and *e* and **bold** indicate online content

Note: Page numbers followed by *f* indicate figures, *b* indicate boxes, *t* indicate tables, and *e* and **bold** indicate online content

Note: Page numbers followed by *f* indicate figures, *b* indicate boxes, *t* indicate tables, and *e* and **bold** indicate online content

---

Note: Page numbers followed by *f* indicate figures, *b* indicate boxes, *t* indicate tables, and *e* and **bold** indicate online content

Note: Page numbers followed by f indicate figures, b indicate boxes, t indicate tables, and e and **bold** indicate online content

Note: Page numbers followed by *f* indicate figures, *b* indicate boxes, *t* indicate tables, and *e* and **bold** indicate online content

---

Note: Page numbers followed by *f* indicate figures, *b* indicate boxes, *t* indicate tables, and *e* and **bold** indicate online content

Gingivitis (Continued)
  necrotizing ulcerative, 605.e7
Gingivostomatitis, herpetic, 1297.e8f
Ginkgo biloba
  for Alzheimer disease, 114
  for claudication, 396
GISTs. See Gastrointestinal stromal tumors
Gitelman syndrome, 245.e5t, 245.e6t, 245.e6
Glandular rosacea, 1222.e2f
Glasdegib, for acute myeloid leukemia, 77
Glasgow Coma Scale, 103, **405.e3t, 494.e7t**, 1132, 1384t
Glatiramer acetate, 923
Glaucoma
  angle-closure, 605.e14–605.e16, 605.e16, 1800.e3f
  narrow-angle, 605.e14
  open-angle, 605.e8–605.e13, 605.e8f, 605.e9f, 605.e10f
  primary angle-closure, 605.e14–605.e16, 605.e14f, 605.e15f
  secondary angle-closure, 605.e16
  in Sturge-Weber syndrome
    manifestations of, 1308.e5–1308.e6
Gleason classification/grading system, for prostate cancer, 1154b, **1154.e1f**, 1154
Glenohumeral dislocation, 605.e17–605.e18
Glenohumeral joint
  instability of, 1223.e7t
  osteoarthrosis of, 1223.e7t
Gliadin, 342
Gliadin antibodies, 1860
Glioblastoma, 193t, **270.e1t**, 272–**273.e1**, 272f, 273f
Glioneuronal tumor, 270
Global aphasia, 151t, 151
Global Initiative for Chronic Obstructive Lung Disease, 105.e10
Global longitudinal strain imaging, for chemical-induced cardiomyopathy, 323.e4
Globose neurofibrillary tangle, 1151.e3f
Glomerular basement membrane antibody, description of, 1860
Glomerular filtration rate, 1860.e1b, 1860–1861
  for cardiorenal syndrome, 333.e4
  for chronic kidney disease, 364
    classification of, 365t
  in contrast-induced acute kidney injury, 415.e5
Glomerulations, 267.e3f
Glomerulonephritis
  acute, 50–**51.e2**, 51t, **51.e1t**
  antigens identified in, 51.e1t
  malignancy associated with, 1538
  poststreptococcal, 51t, **51.e1t**
  rapidly progressive, 51t, **785.e3**, 1538
  renal failure with, 1633
Glomerulopathies
  C3, 50
  with MGUS, 906.e2
  thrombotic, microangiopathic, 1538

Glomerulosclerosis, focal segmental, 1538–1539
Glomus tumor, 1738t–1739t
Glossitis, 605.e19, 605.e19f
Glossodynia, 1539, **1456.e35**
Glossopyrosis, 1456.e35
Glucagon, 1861
Glucagon-like peptide-1 agonists, 463, 474
Glucagonoma, **599.e3t**, 914
Glucocorticoid(s)
  for alcoholic hepatitis, 103
  for ANCA-associated vasculitis, 124
  for Bell palsy, 249
  for blepharitis, 267.e10
  for cirrhosis, 389
  for congenital adrenal hyperplasia, 408.e8
  deficiency of, 1467, 1539
  for electronic cigarette or vaping-associated lung injury, 515.e14
  for hypersensitivity pneumonitis, 740–741
  for IgG4-related disease, 1456.e74
  for lumbar spinal stenosis, 1284.e5
  for myxedema coma, 1456.e93
  for polymyalgia rheumatica, 1126
  for rhabdomyolysis, 1214
  for Still disease, 96.e3–96.e6
  for Takayasu arteritis, 1338.e5–1338.e6
  for vestibular neuritis, 1438.e3
Glucocorticoid-induced transcript 1 gene, 188–192
Glucosamine, for osteoarthritis, 1007.e11
Glucose
  continuous glucose monitoring system, **465.e1f**, 468
  fasting, 1861, **1861.e1f–1861.e2f**
  goals for, 1861.e2t
  mental changes and coma with disorders involving, 1583
  postprandial, 460t, 1861, **1861.e2t**
  preprandial, 460t, **1861.e2t**
  urine, 1881
Glucose tolerance test, 1861
Glucose-6-phosphate dehydrogenase deficiency, 605.e20–605.e21, 605.e20f, 605.e20t, 605.e21t
Glucose-6-phosphate dehydrogenase screen, 1861
Glucuronyl transferase, jaundice and, 1570
Glutaric aciduria type 1, 362.e8t–362.e9t, 502.e4t
Gluten, celiac disease and, 342, **973.e6**
Gluten sensitivity, non-celiac, 973.e6–973.e7, 973.e7t
Gluten-free diet
  for celiac disease, 343
  for dermatitis herpetiformis, 454.e4
Gluten-sensitive enteropathy, 342
Glyburide, 603
Glycemic index, 460
Glyceryl trinitrate, 115.e32
  for heart failure, 639t
Glycogen metabolism, disordered, metabolic myopathies and, 1591
Glycohemoglobin, 1861
Glycolaldehyde, 887.e6

Glycopenia, 756
Glycoprotein IIb/IIIa inhibitors, 44, 944
Glycopyrronium
  for chronic obstructive pulmonary disease, 378t
  for hyperhidrosis, 717.e2
Glycopyrrolate, for hyperhidrosis, 717.e4t
GM1 gangliosidosis, 502.e4t
Gnathostoma spinigerum, **518.e2t–518.e5t**
GnRH. See Gonadotropin-releasing hormone agonists
Goeckerman regimen, 1165
Goiter
  differential diagnosis of, 1539
  evaluation of, 1736.e2f, 1736.e2
  management of, 1736.e2f, 1736.e2
  toxic multinodular, 753
GOLD. See Global Initiative for Chronic Obstructive Lung Disease
GOLD classification system, for chronic obstructive pulmonary disease, 376f
Golfer elbow, 545.e11
Golimumab
  for enteropathic arthritis, 542
  for rheumatoid arthritis, 1220t
  for ulcerative colitis, 1401–1402, 1403t
Golodirsen, 925.e11
Gonadal dysgenesis, 1147
Gonadotropin
  deficiency of, 773–774
  delayed puberty and, 1626
Gonadotropin adenoma, 1090t
Gonadotropin-releasing hormone
  for abnormal uterine bleeding, 8
  for paraphilic disorders, 1042.e5
Gonadotropin-releasing hormone agonists
  for dysmenorrhea, 496t
  for endometriosis, 535–537
  for fertility preservation in women, 570.e4
  for hirsutism, 686.e10
  for premenstrual dysphoric disorder, 1456.e111
  for reversible affirmation in transgender and gender diverse persons, 601.e9
Gonococcal bartholinitis, 606
Gonococcal cervicitis, 606
Gonococcal pharyngitis, 1810t
Gonococcal proctitis, 1401t
Gonococcal urethritis, **606.e1f**, 606, 1405–**1406.e1**
Gonococcal vulvovaginitis, 606
Gonorrhea, 606–**607.e1**, 606.e1f, 1054–**1056.e1**
  purulent urethral discharge, 606.e1f
  skin lesions, 606.e1f
Goodpasture disease, 607.e2–607.e5, 607.e2f, 607.e3t
Goodpasture syndrome, 784t
Goodsall rule, 136.e2
Gorlin sign, 509.e9f, 509.e2
Gorlin syndrome, 270
Gottron sign, 801.e1f
Gout, 608–**610.e2, 608.e1f, 608.e2f, 609.e1f, 610.e1f**, 608t, 610t
  acute, 609b

Gout (Continued)
  chronic, 609b
  classification of, 755.e7t
  hyperuricemia and, 608, **755.e7**
  neutrophils in, 608.e2f
  radiographic findings in, 609.e2f
  treatment of, **610.e1f**, 610t
Gouty arthritis, 308t, **755.e7**
GPC. See Giant papillary conjunctivitis
G6PD deficiency, 605.e20
Graduated compression stockings, for deep vein thrombosis, 441–442
Graft-versus-host disease
  classification of, **610.e5t**
  clinical manifestations of, 610.e3t, 610.e4t
  clinical presentation of, 610.e3, 610.e3t
  definition of, 610.e3
  demographics of, 610.e3
  diagnosis of, 610.e3–610.e4, 610.e3
  epidemiology of, 610.e3
  imaging of, 610.e4
  laboratory tests for, 610.e3
  pathophysiology of, 610.e4f
  physical findings of, 610.e3
  risk factors for, 610.e3
  treatment of, 610.e4–610.e5, 610.e5t
Gram-negative folliculitis, 20
Grand mal seizures, 1243
Granisetron, 355.e21t, 355.e22t, 355.e21
Granular kidney, 809
Granulation tissue–type hemangioma, 1192.e2
Granulocyte-macrophage colony-stimulating factor, for COVID-19 disease, 429
Granuloma
  hepatic, 1548–1549
  noninfectious, 1736.e3f, 1736.e3, 1736.e4t
Granuloma annulare, 610.e7–610.e8, 610.e7f, 610.e8f, 1736.e4t
Granuloma inguinale, 610.e9–610.e10, 610.e10f
Granuloma pyogenicum, 1192.e2
Granulomatosis infantisepticum, 831.e34
Granulomatosis with polyangiitis, **120.e1f, 122.e1f**, 120, **545.e4**, 1429, 1432t
Granulomatous arthritis, 610.e11
Granulomatous dermatitides, 1539
Granulomatous disorders, 1539–1540
Granulomatous hepatitis, drug-induced, 494.e19t
Granulomatous liver disease, 1540
Granulomatous mastitis, 865
Granulomatous mediastinitis, 866.e16
Granulomatous necrotizing scleritis, 1236.e5f
Granulomatous uveitis, 1421.e2
Granulomatous vasculitis, 1663
Granulosa cell tumor, 1136.e12t–1136.e13t
Graves disease, 611–**612.e1**, 611.e1f, 1878t
  Graves ophthalmopathy, 611.e1f

Note: Page numbers followed by *f* indicate figures, *b* indicate boxes, *t* indicate tables, and *e* and **bold** indicate online content

Hyperparathyroidism, 734b, 738b, 733–**738.e1**, 734f, **735.e1f**, 737f, **735.e2f, 735.e3f**, 733t, 735t, 736t, **772.e4**
Hyperphosphatemia
acute, 738.e3
algorithms for, 738.e2f, 738.e3f
in children, 1557
clinical presentation of, 738.e2
definition of, 738.e2
demographics of, 738.e2
diagnosis of, 738.e3f, 738.e2–738.e3, 738.e2, 738.e2–738.e3
differential diagnosis of, 1556–1557
epidemiology of, 738.e2
etiology of, 738.e2
phosphate binders for, 738.e4t
physical findings of, 738.e2
referral for, 738.e3
treatment of, 738.e3, 738.e4t
tumor lysis syndrome and, 1399.e8
workup for, 738.e3f, 738.e2–738.e3
Hyperpigmentation, 1433
algorithm for, 1752.e1f, 1752.e3f
differential diagnosis of, 1557
drugs that cause, 1752.e2t–1752.e3t
of nails, 1752.e3f
Hyperplastic polyposis, 568.e14t
Hyperpotassemia, 718
Hyperprolactinemia, **115.e10, 115.e12,** 774
causing androgen deficiency, 615.e2t
differential diagnosis of, 1557
Hyperreactive airways, 192.e2
Hyperreninemic hypoaldosteronism, 755.e13
Hypersensitivity pneumonitis, 739–**743.e1,** 741f, 742f, **739.e1f,** 739t, 740t, 742t, 784t
Hypersensitivity vasculitis, 1663
Hypersensitivity vesiculobullous diseases, 1665
Hyperserotonemia, 1258
Hypersomnia, of central origin, 950
Hypersplenism, **743.e2–743.e3,** 1558
splenomegaly and, 1646
Hypertension
acute decompensated heart failure-associated, 634
in acute ischemic stroke, 1300–1302
adrenocortical causes of, 1558
antihypertensive drugs for, 748t
aortic coarctation as cause of, **141.e10,** 745t
blood pressure measurement, 744t
characteristics of, 744–**752.e1,** 745t, 746t, 749t
in children, 1558
clinical presentation of, 744
definition of, 744
demographics of, 744
diagnosis of, 744–746
endocrine, 1558
epidemiology of, 744
etiology of, 744, 745t
gestational, 1137
in hemorrhagic stroke, 1305–1307, 1308b

Hypertension (*Continued*)
idiopathic intracranial, 782.e2–782.e3
intraabdominal, 6.e2t
laboratory testing for, 746, 747t
lifestyle modifications for, 746, 747t
malignant, 750, 1876t
physical findings in, 744
portal, 1128–1130, 1128f, **1128.e1f,** 1128t, 1129t, 1130t, 1621–1622
in pregnancy, 749–750, 749t, 1137
pseudohypertension, 750
pulmonary, 1181–**1188.e1,** 1184f, 1185f, **1183.e1f, 1183.e3f,** 1181t, 1182t, 1183t, 1184t, 1185t, **1183.e3t,** 1268
referrals for, 752t
renin-aldosterone pattern in, 1876t
renovascular, 749, 1198
resistant, 750, 1558–1559
secondary, 746b
stroke and, 1308b, 1305–1307, **1308.e3**
treatment of, 746–750, 749t
workup for, 744–746
Hypertensive crisis syndromes, 1559
Hypertensive disorders of pregnancy, 1137
Hypertensive emergencies, 750
Hypertensive encephalopathy, 1559
coma and, 1505
differential diagnosis of, 1521
Hypertensive retinopathy, 1636
Hypertensive urgencies, 750
Hyperthermia, 646
coma and, 1505
malignant, 863b, 864b, 862–**864.e1**
Hyperthyroidism, **612.e1t,** 754b, 753–**755.e1,** 754f, 1878t
Hypertonic hyponatremia, 767
Hypertonicity, 729, **1282.e17**
Hypertrichosis, 1559
congenital, 1559
Hypertriglyceridemia, 725
Hypertriglyceridemic pancreatitis, 1034
Hypertrophic actinic keratosis, 32.e9
Hypertrophic cardiomyopathy, 213t–214t, 327–**330.e2,** 328f, 329f, **327.e1f, 330.e1f,** 330t, **331.e1f,** 1713t
Hypertrophic obstructive cardiomyopathy, 327
Hypertrophic osteoarthropathy, **755.e2–755.e5, 755.e3f, 755.e4f,** 1559–1560, 1760t–1762t
Hypertrophic scars, 1456.e76–1456.e77
Hypertropia, 1297.e9
Hyperuricemia
characteristics of, 755.e6–755.e9, 755.e7f, 755.e8f, 755.e6t
classification of, 755.e7t
gout and, 608
treatment of, 610.e1f
tumor lysis syndrome and, 1399.e8
Hyperventilation
alveolar, 1689t
persistent, 1560
Hypnagogic hallucinations, 950
Hypnopompic hallucinations, 950
Hypoactive delirium, 340.e10

Hypoactive sexual desire disorder, 552t, **755.e10–755.e12, 755.e10f, 1259.e7**
Hypoaldosteronism, 755.e13, 1843.e1t
Hypocalcemia
algorithm for, 1849.e2
differential diagnosis of, 1560, 1851b
laboratory diagnosis of, 1849.e4t
in pediatric patients, 1560
tumor lysis syndrome and, 1399.e8
Hypocapnia, 1560
Hypochondriasis, 755.e14–755.e15, 1282.e12. *See also* **Illness anxiety disorder**
Hypochromic anemia, 1473–1474
Hypocomplementemic urticarial vasculitis, 1456.e71–1456.e72
Hypocomplementemic urticarial vasculitis syndrome, 1456.e71–1456.e72
Hypocretin-1, 950
Hypocretin-2, 950
Hypoestrogenic anovulation, 1606–1607
Hypogammaglobulinemia, 369–370, **1146.e11t**
Hypoglycemia, 757b, 756–**758.e2, 757.e1f,** 758f, 756t, **758.e1t–758.e2t**
in acute ischemic stroke, 1302
coma and, 1505
in diabetes mellitus, **467.e1f,** 467t, 467
differential diagnosis of, 253t–254t, 1560–1561
in infants and children, 1561
Hypoglycemia-associated autonomic failure, 467.e1f
Hypogonadism, 1879.e1f
differential diagnosis of, 1561
male, 759–**765.e1,** 761f, 763t–764t, 765t
primary, 759t
secondary, 760t
Hypogonadotropic hypoestrogenic states, 1606–1607
Hypogonadotropic hypogonadism, **115.e9,** 760, 1561
micropenis with, 1585
Hypokalemia
causes of, 1754b, 1873–1874
diagnosis of, 1753f
differential diagnosis of, 1561–1562
electrocardiographic findings in, 1754f
in pediatric patients, 1562
renin-aldosterone pattern in, 1876t
urine potassium in, 1882.e1b
Hypokalemic alkalosis, with hypercalciuria, 245.e5
Hypokalemic nonperiodic paralysis, 765.e2
Hypokalemic periodic paralysis, **765.e2–765.e3, 765.e3t,** 1615
Hypomagnesemia, 765.e4–765.e7, 765.e4f, 765.e5f, 765.e6t
differential diagnosis of, 1562
in pediatric patients, 1562
Hypomelanotic macules, 1399.e2f, 1399.e4t

Hyponatremia, 766–**769.e1,** 1325, 1326, 1326–1327, 1877–1878, **1877.e2t**–1958t
acute, 767
algorithms for, 768f, **767.e1f, 767.e2f**
brain cell volume changes in, 767.e3f
chronic, 766, 768
clinical presentation of, 766
definition of, 766
demographics of, 766
diagnosis of, 768f, **767.e1f, 767.e2f,** 767
differential diagnosis of, 1562
drugs associated with, 1877.e2t
epidemiology of, 766
etiology of, 766–767, **1877.e2t**–1958t
evaluation of, 1876.e3f
hypertonic, 767
physical findings of, 766
prevention of, 769
recurrence of, 769
referral for, 769
in salt-losing nephropathy, 1227.e3
treatment of, 767–769, **1876.e3f**
Hypo-osmolality, 766
Hypoparathyroidism, 770–**772.e1, 771.e1f,** 770t, 771t
Hypoparathyroidism-deafness-renal dysplasia syndrome, 770
Hypoparathyroidism-retardation-dysmorphism syndrome, 770
Hypopharyngeal cancer, 829.e7b
Hypophosphatemia, 1562–1563
clinical presentation of, 772.e2
definition of, 772.e2
diagnosis of, 772.e4f, 772.e2–772.e4, 772.e2, 772.e2–772.e4
epidemiology of, 772.e2
etiology of, 772.e3f, 772.e2, 772.e2t, 772.e3t
physical findings of, 772.e2
treatment of, 772.e4, 772.e5t
Hypophosphatemic rickets, 1007.e19t
Hypopigmentation, 1563
Hypopituitarism
in acromegaly, 32.e3
characteristics of, 773–776, 776f, **774.e1f,** 773t, 774t, 775t
Hypoplastic anemia, 153.e5
Hypopnea, 989t
Hyporeninemic, hypoaldosteronic renal tubular acidosis, 1203
Hyporeninemic hypoaldosteronism, **755.e13,** 1467
Hypospadias, 776.e2–776.e4, 776.e2f
Hypotension
in acute ischemic stroke, 1302
orthostatic, 1006b, 1006–**1007.e1,** 1007t
in multiple system atrophy, 925.e2, 925.e4t
in parkinsonism, 925.e3, 925.e4t
syncope caused by, 1323–1324
postoperative, 1754.e1f
postural, 1563, 1622
Hypothalamic amenorrhea, 115.e12

Note: Page numbers followed by *f* indicate figures, *b* indicate boxes, *t* indicate tables, and *e* and **bold** indicate online content

---

Note: Page numbers followed by *f* indicate figures, *b* indicate boxes, *t* indicate tables, and *e* and **bold** indicate online content

Note: Page numbers followed by *f* indicate figures, *b* indicate boxes, *t* indicate tables, and *e* and **bold** indicate online content

Note: Page numbers followed by *f* indicate figures, *b* indicate boxes, *t* indicate tables, and *e* and **bold** indicate online content

---

Note: Page numbers followed by *f* indicate figures, *b* indicate boxes, *t* indicate tables, and *e* and **bold** indicate online content

---

Note: Page numbers followed by *f* indicate figures, *b* indicate boxes, *t* indicate tables, and *e* and **bold** indicate online content

Note: Page numbers followed by f indicate figures, b indicate boxes, t indicate tables, and e and **bold** indicate online content

---

Note: Page numbers followed by *f* indicate figures, *b* indicate boxes, *t* indicate tables, and *e* and **bold** indicate online content

---

Note: Page numbers followed by *f* indicate figures, *b* indicate boxes, *t* indicate tables, and *e* and **bold** indicate online content

---

Note: Page numbers followed by *f* indicate figures, *b* indicate boxes, *t* indicate tables, and *e* and **bold** indicate online content

Note: Page numbers followed by *f* indicate figures, *b* indicate boxes, *t* indicate tables, and *e* and **bold** indicate online content

---

Note: Page numbers followed by *f* indicate figures, *b* indicate boxes, *t* indicate tables, and *e* and **bold** indicate online content

---

Note: Page numbers followed by *f* indicate figures, *b* indicate boxes, *t* indicate tables, and *e* and **bold** indicate online content

---

Note: Page numbers followed by *f* indicate figures, *b* indicate boxes, *t* indicate tables, and *e* and **bold** indicate online content

Note: Page numbers followed by f indicate figures, b indicate boxes, t indicate tables, and e and **bold** indicate online content

Note: Page numbers followed by *f* indicate figures, *b* indicate boxes, *t* indicate tables, and *e* and **bold** indicate online content

RCC. *See* Renal cell carcinoma
RCMD-RS. *See* Refractory cytopenia with multilineage dysplasia and ring sideroblasts
RCVS. *See* Reversible cerebral vasoconstriction syndrome
RDW. *See* Red blood cell distribution width
Reactiv. *See* Nitroglycerin ointment
Reactive airway disease, 177, **192.e2**
Reactive arthritis, 135t, **1196.e2–1196.e3**, **1196.e2f**, 1285t
Reactive hemophagocytic lymphohistiocytosis, 96.e6
Reactive lymphohistiocytoses, 686.e13t
Reactive thrombocytosis, 1872
Recanalization, for brainstem ischemic stroke syndromes, 277–278
Recombinant activated factor VII, for hemophilia A, 654.e7
Recombinant tissue plasminogen activator, for acute ischemic stroke, 1303t
Rectal abscess, 1075
Rectal bleeding, 1487
Rectal dysmotility, 409t
Rectal intussusception, 1196.e4
Rectal mass, palpable, 1631
Rectal pain, 1631
Rectal prolapse, 654.e18f, **1196.e4–1196.e5, 1196.e4f**
Rectal ulcer, 1800.e1f
Recti, divarication of, 1462
Rectocele, 1056.e3f
Rectovaginal fistulas, 1421.e16
Rectum, 579t
Recurrent abdominal pain, 813
Recurrent aphthous stomatitis, 153.e2–153.e4, 153.e2f, 153.e2, 153.e4t
Recurrent isolated sleep paralysis, 1808t
Recurrent meningitis, 1582
Recurrent oral aphthae, 153.e2
Recurrent otitis media, 1019t
Recurrent pneumonia, 1618–1619
Recurrent polyserositis, 568.e17
Red blood cell distribution width, 1876
Red blood cells
  abnormal, 1876.e3
  count, 1876
  drugs interfering with, 1473
  mass, 1876
  morphology, 1876
Red cell fragmentation hemolysis, 1631–1632
Red cell sensitization, 1212.e15–1212.e17, 1212.e16f, 1212.e17f
Red degeneration, 1419
Red eye, **408.e11, 408.e13**, 1632, **1800.e2f, 1800.e4f, 1800.e5t**–1860t
  acute, 1632
Red hot joint, 1632
Red pigmentation anomaly, cutaneous, 1504
Red urine, **785.e4**, 1632, 1660
Reed-Sternberg cells, **687.e2f**, 687
Reese-Ellsworth classification system, for retinoblastoma, 1212.e4
Referred hip pain, 1551

Reflex sympathetic dystrophy, 405.e16f, 405.e15
Reflux esophagitis, 600
  pathogenesis of, 600.e1f
  therapy for, 601.e1t
Refractive amblyopia, 115.e2
Refractory anemia, 153.e5
  with ring sideroblasts, 1268.e3
Refractory angina, 125
Refractory ascites, 168t
Refractory cytopenia with multilineage dysplasia and ring sideroblasts, 1268.e3
Refsum disease, 194.e5t
Regional anesthesia, 1024.e16t
Regional enteritis, 432f, 433f, **431.e1f**, 431, 431t
Regional osteoporosis, 1013f
Regorafenib, for colorectal cancer, 404
Regurgitation
  aortic, 142–**145.e1**, 144f, 145f, **143.e1f**, 1662
  tricuspid, **1392.e5–1392.e8, 1392.e5f, 1392.e7f, 1392.e6t, 1392.e8t**, 1662
Rehydration, 599.e10
Reiter disease, 1196.e2
Reiter syndrome, **1196.e2–1196.e3**, 1762t
  characteristics of, **1196.e2f**
  food poisoning and, 588
  HLA antigens associated with, 1865t
Relapsing perichondritis, 1456.e131
Relapsing polychondritis, **131.e131b, 131.e132b**, 1839–1840, **131.e131f, 131.e132f**
Relapsing-remitting multiple sclerosis, 920
Relugolix, for uterine fibroids, 1418
REM behavior disorder, **1208.e1t**, 1808t
REM sleep without atonia, 1208.e1t
Remdesivir, for COVID-19, **424.e8**, 429, 1050
Renal abscess, 1191, 1197–**1197.e1, 1197.e1f**, 1801f, 1802f
Renal acidosis, 1462
Renal allograft dysfunction, 1632
Renal artery occlusion, 1632
Renal artery stenosis, 1198–**1200.e1**, 1198f, 1199f
Renal artery thrombosis, 54t
Renal biopsy
  for acute glomerulonephritis, 51
  for acute kidney injury, 55
  for diabetic kidney disease, 478–479, 479f
  for lupus nephritis, 1334.e1t
Renal carbuncle, 1189
Renal cell carcinoma, 1201–**1202.e1, 1201.e1f**, 1202t
Renal clearance, estimating, 1856.e3
Renal colic, 154t, 1632
Renal cystic disorders, 1632
Renal diseases and disorders
  hydronephrosis, 703–**704.e3, 704.e1f, 704.e2f**
  skin manifestations of, 1632–1633
  tubulointerstitial, 1656–1657
  unilateral, 1876t
Renal failure
  acute, 52, **90.e4**
  chronic, 1633

Renal failure (*Continued*)
  intrinsic or parenchymal causes of, 1633
  pigment-induced acute, 1633
  postrenal causes of, 1633
  prerenal causes of, 1633–1634
Renal infarction, 1634
Renal lupus, 1202.e2–1202.e5, 1202.e4f, 1202.e2t
Renal mass, 1801f
Renal osteodystrophy, 367.e2, 1007.e19
Renal papillary necrosis, 1192
Renal paraneoplastic syndromes, 1611
Renal parenchymal disease, chronic, 1634
Renal pelvis, renal failure caused by, 1633
Renal replacement therapy
  for acute tubular necrosis, 90.e5
  for end-stage renal disease, 538–539
Renal salt wasting, 1227.e2–1227.e3
Renal sclerosis, 809
Renal transplantation, for Bartter syndrome, 245.e6
Renal trauma, 1799f, **1802.e1t**
Renal tubular acidosis, 1203–**1204.e1**, 1204f, 1203t
Renal ultrasound, for diabetic kidney disease, 478
Renal vein thrombosis, 54t, **1204.e2–1204.e3, 1204.e3f**, 1634
Renal-limited lupus, 1202.e2
Renin, serum, 1876
Renin inhibitors, for hypertension, 749
Renin-aldosterone patterns, 1876t
Renin-angiotensin-aldosterone axis, 1841.e2f
Renin-angiotensin-aldosterone system, 333.e3–333.e4
Renin-angiotensin-aldosterone system blockers, for diabetic kidney disease, 479, 483
Renovascular disease, 745t, 1198
Renovascular hypertension, 749, 1198
Repaglinide, 465
Reperfusion
  for acute coronary syndromes, 43t
  for myocardial infarction, 939
Repetitive multifocal paroxysmal atrial tachycardia, 913
RERA. *See* Respiratory event-related arousal
Resin uptake (T3), 1878
Resistant hypertension, 1558–1559
Resisted wrist extension test, for epicondylitis, 545.e11f
Resisted wrist flexion test, 545.e11f
Reslizumab, 184
  for asthma, 185t
Resorption, bone, 1491
Respiratory acidosis
  acute, 1683f, 1686
  algorithm for, 1673, 1714f
  arterial blood gases, 1845
  chronic, 1687, 1687f
  differential diagnosis of, 1463
  laboratory findings in, 1842t–1845t
Respiratory alkalosis
  arterial blood gases, 1845
  differential diagnosis of, 1469

Respiratory alkalosis (*Continued*)
  laboratory findings in, 1842t–1845t
  treatment of, 1689f
Respiratory bronchiolitis-associated interstitial lung disease, 784t, 807t
Respiratory distress
  acute respiratory distress syndrome, 80–**85.e1**, 81f, 82f, 83f, 84f, 80t, 82t
  in newborn, 1205–**1207.e1**, 1206f, 1634–1635
Respiratory dysfunction, 1635
Respiratory event-related arousal, 989t
Respiratory failure, hypoventilatory, 1635
Respiratory infections, in acquired immunodeficiency syndrome, 21
Respiratory insufficiency, 86, 87t
Respiratory muscle weakness, 1635
Respiratory sinus arrhythmia, 1269.e3–1269.e4
Respiratory syncytial virus, 1115–1116
  acute bronchitis caused by, 38t
  croup caused by, 434.e2
  screen, 1876
Respiratory tract candidiasis, 312.e3
Rest pain, with myopathies, 1591
Restless legs syndrome, **1806.e14f**, 1208–**1209.e1**, 1209t, **1208.e1t, 1456.e19**
Rest/resting tremors, 1044f, 1656
Restricting type anorexia nervosa, 136.e8
Restrictive, mechanical orbitopathy, 489.e17
Restrictive cardiomyopathy, 331–**333.e1, 331.e1f**, 1066t, 1713f
  and constrictive pericarditis, **332.e1f**, 332t
Restrictive eye movement, 1297.e9
Retaining urine, 91
Retention, urinary, 91–**92.e1**
Reteplase, 942t
  for myocardial infarction, 939
Reticular dysgenesis, 1146.e12
Reticulocyte count, 1876–1877, **1876.e1t**
  anemia with low, 1474
  differential diagnosis of elevated, 1876.e5
Reticulum cell sarcoma, 1146.e2
Retina
  detachment of, 1209.e2–1209.e3, 1209.e2f, 1209.e3f
  hemorrhage of, 11.e2, 1209.e4–1209.e5, 1209.e4f
  human immunodeficiency virus infection manifestations in, 1554
  tears of, 1209.e2f
Retinal breaks, 1209.e3f
Retinal ischemia, 115
Retinal migraine, amaurosis fugax and, 115
Retinal vein occlusion, 1210–**1212.e1**
  central, 1211.e1f
  clinical presentation of, 1210–1211
  cotton-wool spots, 1211.e1f
  definition of, 1210
  demographics of, 1210
  diagnosis of, 1211

Note: Page numbers followed by *f* indicate figures, *b* indicate boxes, *t* indicate tables, and *e* and **bold** indicate online content

---

Note: Page numbers followed by *f* indicate figures, *b* indicate boxes, *t* indicate tables, and *e* and **bold** indicate online content

Note: Page numbers followed by *f* indicate figures, *b* indicate boxes, *t* indicate tables, and *e* and **bold** indicate online content

---

Note: Page numbers followed by *f* indicate figures, *b* indicate boxes, *t* indicate tables, and *e* and **bold** indicate online content

Note: Page numbers followed by f indicate figures, b indicate boxes, t indicate tables, and e and **bold** indicate online content

---

Note: Page numbers followed by *f* indicate figures, *b* indicate boxes, *t* indicate tables, and *e* and **bold** indicate online content

---

Note: Page numbers followed by *f* indicate figures, *b* indicate boxes, *t* indicate tables, and *e* and **bold** indicate online content

Note: Page numbers followed by *f* indicate figures, *b* indicate boxes, *t* indicate tables, and *e* and **bold** indicate online content

---

Note: Page numbers followed by *f* indicate figures, *b* indicate boxes, *t* indicate tables, and *e* and **bold** indicate online content